Brief Contents

JoAnne Silbert-Flagg, DNP, CPNP, IBCLC, FAAN
Assistant Professor
Clinical Coordinator for the MSN (Entry into Nursing) Program
Coordinator, Pediatric Nurse Practitioner Track
Johns Hopkins University School of Nursing
Baltimore, Maryland

Adele Pillitteri, PhD, RN, PNP
Former Associate Professor
University of Southern California
Los Angeles, California

Maternal & Child Health Nursing

Care of the Childbearing & Childrearing Family

EIGHTH EDITION

Philadelphia • Baltimore • New York • London
Buenos Aires • Hong Kong • Sydney • Tokyo

Acquisitions Editor: Natasha McIntyre
Supervising Development Editor: Heather A. Rybacki
Developmental Editor: Victoria White
Editorial Coordinator: Lauren Pecarich
Marketing Manager: Katie Schlesinger
Production Project Manager: Marian Bellus
Design Coordinator: Holly McLaughlin
Art Director: Jennifer Clements
Manufacturing Coordinator: Karin Duffield
Prepress Vendor: Absolute Service, Inc.

8th edition

Library of Congress Cataloging-in-Publication Data

Names: Silbert-Flagg, JoAnne, author. | Preceded by (work): Pillitteri,
  Adele. Maternal & child health nursing.
Title: Maternal & child health nursing : care of the childbearing &
  childrearing family / JoAnne Silbert-Flagg.
Other titles: Maternal and child health nursing
Description: Eighth edition. | Philadelphia : Wolters Kluwer, [2018] |
  Preceded by Maternal & child health nursing / Adele Pillitteri. 7th
  edition. 2014. | Includes bibliographical references and index.
Identifiers: LCCN 2017035586 | ISBN 9781496348135
Subjects: | MESH: Maternal-Child Nursing | Family Health | Holistic Nursing
Classification: LCC RG951 | NLM WY 157.3 | DDC 618.2/0231--dc23 LC record available at https://lccn.loc.gov/2017035586

LWW.com

CCS1018

I dedicate this book to all the children I have cared for over the years. I hope I have touched your lives as you have touched mine.

— *JoAnne Silbert-Flagg*

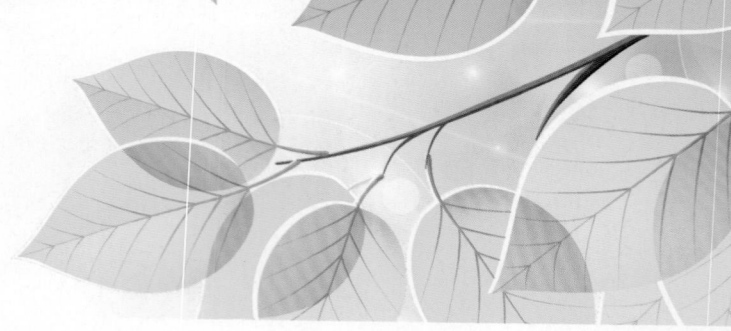

Contributors

Nasreen Bahreman, MSN, RN, PCNS-BC
Nurse at Rales Health Center at KIPP Baltimore
The Ruth and Norman Rales Center for the Integration of
    Health and Education
Johns Hopkins University School of Medicine
Baltimore, Maryland
Chapter 38: Nursing Care of a Family When a Child Needs
    Medication Administration or Intravenous Therapy
Chapter 50: Nursing Care of a Family When a Child Has a
    Vision or Hearing Disorder
Chapter 56: Nursing Care of a Family When a Child Has a
    Long-Term or Terminal Illness

Cheri Barber, DNP, RN, PPCNP-BC, FAANP
Clinical Assistant Professor
Pediatric Nurse Practitioner Programs Coordinator
UMKC School of Nursing and Health Studies
Kansas City, Missouri
Chapter 49: Nursing Care of a Family When a Child Has a
    Neurologic Disorder

Pamela Brandy-Webb, RN, MSN
Assistant Clinical Professor
Prairie View College of Nursing
Prairie View, Texas
Chapter 48: Nursing Care of a Family When a Child Has an
    Endocrine or a Metabolic Disorder

Deborah Busch, DNP, CPNP, IBCLC
Assistant Professor
Johns Hopkins University School of Nursing
Baltimore, Maryland
Chapter 2: Diversity and Maternal Child Nursing
Chapter 17: Nursing Care of a Postpartal Family
Chapter 27: Nursing Care of the Child Born With a
    Physical or Developmental Challenge

Peggy Dorr, DNP, CPNP
Pediatric Nurse Practitioner
Pediatric Sedation Service
University of Maryland Medical Center
Baltimore, Maryland
Chapter 41: Nursing Care of a Family When a Child Has a
    Cardiovascular Disorder

Marlo A. Eldridge, DNP, APRN, CPNP
Director
Pediatric Voiding Improvement Program and International
    Bladder Exstrophy Surgical Preparation Program
Division of Pediatric Urology, Johns Hopkins
    Children's Center
Faculty
The Johns Hopkins University School of Medicine—
    Brady Urological Institute
Baltimore, Maryland
Chapter 46: Nursing Care of a Family When a Child Has a
    Renal or Urinary Tract Disorder

Jennifer Flagg, LCPC, TF-CBT
Therapist
Family and Children's Services of Central Maryland
Baltimore, Maryland
Chapter 54: Nursing Care of a Family When a Child Has an
    Intellectual or Mental Health Disorder

Karen M. Frank, DNP, RNC-NIC, APRN-CNS
Acute and Chronic Care Instructor
Clinical Nurse Specialist Track Coordinator
Johns Hopkins University School of Nursing
Baltimore, Maryland
Chapter 26: Nursing Care of a Family With a
    High-Risk Newborn

Sheila Holdford, MS, RN, APRN-BC, CPNP-PC
Pediatric Primary Mental Health Specialist
Columbus, Ohio
Chapter 54: Nursing Care of a Family When a Child Has an
    Intellectual or Mental Health Disorder

Rita Marie John, EdD, DNP, CPNP, PMHS, FAANP
Pediatric Nurse Practitioner Program Director
Associate Professor of Nursing at CUMC
Columbia University School of Nursing
New York, New York
Chapter 43: Nursing Care of a Family When a Child Has an
    Infectious Disorder

Elizabeth Jordan, DNSc, RNC, FAAN
Associate Dean of Undergraduate Nursing
Associate Professor
University of South Florida College of Nursing
Tampa, Florida
Chapter 9: Nursing Care During Normal Pregnancy and
Care of the Developing Fetus

Colleen Kennedy, DNP, CNM
Certified Nurse Midwife
Johns Hopkins Medical System
Baltimore, Maryland
Chapter 5: The Nursing Role in Reproductive and
Sexual Health
Chapter 6: Nursing Care for the Family in Need of
Reproductive Life Planning
Chapter 7: Nursing Care of the Family Having Difficulty
Conceiving a Child
Chapter 8: The Nursing Role in Genetic Assessment and
Counseling
Chapter 10: Nursing Care Related to Psychological and
Physiologic Changes of Pregnancy
Chapter 12: Nursing Care to Promote Fetal and
Maternal Health
Chapter 13: The Nursing Role in Promoting Nutritional
Health During Pregnancy
Chapter 14: Preparing a Family for Childbirth and Parenting
Chapter 20: Nursing Care of a Family Experiencing
a Pregnancy Complication From a Preexisting or
Newly Acquired Illness
Chapter 21: Nursing Care of a Family Experiencing a
Sudden Pregnancy Complication
Chapter 22: Nursing Care of a Pregnant Family With
Special Needs
Chapter 23: Nursing Care of a Family Experiencing a
Complication of Labor or Birth
Chapter 24: Nursing Care of a Family During a Surgical
Intervention for Birth
Chapter 25: Nursing Care of a Family Experiencing a
Postpartum Complication

Laura Lucas, MS, APRN-CNS, RNC-OB, C-EFM
Clinical Faculty
Johns Hopkins University School of Nursing
Baltimore, Maryland
Chapter 3: The Childbearing and Childrearing Family in the
Community

Rachel Lyons, DNP, CPNP-PC/AC, DCC, CEN
Clinical Associate Professor
Rutgers, The State University of New Jersey
Camden, New Jersey
Chapter 36: Nursing Care of a Family With an Ill Child
Chapter 37: Nursing Care of a Family When a Child Needs
Diagnostic or Therapeutic Modalities
Chapter 51: Nursing Care of a Family When a Child Has a
Musculoskeletal Disorder

Kim Mudd, BSN, MSN
Research Nurse Manager
Division of Pediatric Allergy/Immunology
Johns Hopkins University School of Medicine
Baltimore, Maryland
Chapter 42: Nursing Care of a Family When a Child Has an
Immune Disorder

Shawna Mudd, DNP, CPNP-AC, PNP-BC
Assistant Professor
Johns Hopkins University School of Nursing
Baltimore, Maryland
Chapter 40: Nursing Care of a Family When a Child Has a
Respiratory Disorder

Saribel Garcia Quinones, DNP, PPCNP-BC
Clinical Assistant Professor
New York University Rory Meyers College of Nursing
New York, New York
Chapter 52: Nursing Care of a Family When a Child Has an
Unintentional Injury
Chapter 55: Nursing Care of a Family in Crisis:
Maltreatment and Violence in the Family

Audra N. Rankin, DNP, APRN, CPNP
Instructor
Johns Hopkins University School of Nursing
Baltimore, Maryland
Chapter 40: Nursing Care of a Family When a Child Has a
Respiratory Disorder

Kathryn Kushto Reese, MSRN
Nursing Instructor
Johns Hopkins University School of Nursing
Baltimore, Maryland
Chapter 38: Nursing Care of a Family When a Child Needs
Medication Administration or Intravenous Therapy
Chapter 50: Nursing Care of a Family When a Child Has a
Vision or Hearing Disorder

Kathy Ruble, RN, CPNP, PhD
Assistant Professor
Johns Hopkins University School of Medicine
Director, Survivorship Program
Division of Pediatric Oncology
Johns Hopkins Hospital
Baltimore, Maryland
Chapter 53: Nursing Care of a Family When a Child Has a
Malignancy

JoAnne Silbert-Flagg, DNP, CPNP, IBCLC, FAAN
Assistant Professor
Clinical Coordinator for the MSN (Entry into Nursing)
    Program
Coordinator, Pediatric Nurse Practitioner Track
Johns Hopkins University School of Nursing
Baltimore, Maryland
Chapter 19: Nutritional Needs of a Newborn
Chapter 28: Principles of Growth and Development
Chapter 29: Nursing Care of a Family With an Infant
Chapter 30: Nursing Care of a Family With a Toddler
Chapter 31: Nursing Care of a Family With a Preschool
    Child
Chapter 32: Nursing Care of a Family With a School-Age
    Child

Elizabeth Sloand, PhD, CRNP, FAAN
Associate Professor
Chair, Acute and Chronic Care Department
Johns Hopkins University School of Nursing
Baltimore, Maryland
Chapter 18: Nursing Care of a Family With a Newborn

Tedra S. Smith, DNP, CRNP, CPNP-PC, CNE
Assistant Professor
Nurse Practitioner Track Director
The University of Alabama at Birmingham School of
    Nursing
Birmingham, Alabama
Chapter 44: Nursing Care of a Family When a Child Has a
    Hematologic Disorder
Chapter 47: Nursing Care of a Family When a Child Has a
    Reproductive Disorder

Barbara Stone, MSN, RNC-LRN, IBCLC, RLC
Director of Associate Degree Nursing
Odessa College
Odessa, Texas
Chapter 13: The Nursing Role in Promoting Nutritional
    Health During Pregnancy

Brigit VanGraafeiland, DNP, CRNP
Assistant Professor
Johns Hopkins University School of Nursing
Baltimore, Maryland
Chapter 33: Nursing Care of a Family With an Adolescent

Kelly J. Vasquenza, RN, CPNP
Pediatric Nurse Practitioner
Pediatric Pain Management and Palliative Care Service
Department of Pediatric Anesthesiology and
    Critical Care Medicine
Johns Hopkins Hospital
Charlotte R. Bloomberg Children's Center
Baltimore, Maryland
Chapter 39: Pain Management in Children

Lynne Weissman, DNP, RN, MS, CPNP, FNP-BC
Director
Family Nurse Practitioner and Doctor of
    Nursing Practice Programs
Assistant Professor
Dominican College Prusmack Center
Blauvelt, New York
Chapter 34: Child Health Assessment
Chapter 35: Communication and Teaching With Children
    and Families

Lindsay Wilson, MSN, RN, CPNP
Lead Nurse Practitioner
Pediatric Gastroenterology, Hepatology, and Nutrition
Johns Hopkins Children's Center
Baltimore, Maryland
Chapter 45: Nursing Care of a Family When a Child Has a
    Gastrointestinal Disorder

Erin M. Wright, DNP, CNM, APHN-BC
Instructor
Community Public Health Nursing
Johns Hopkins University School of Nursing
Baltimore, Maryland
Chapter 1: A Framework for Maternal and
    Child Health Nursing
Chapter 4: Home Care and the Childbearing and
    Childrearing Family
Chapter 11: Nursing Care Related to Assessment of
    a Pregnant Family
Chapter 15: Nursing Care of a Family During Labor
    and Birth
Chapter 16: The Nursing Role in Providing Comfort During
    Labor and Birth

M. Elizabeth M. Younger, CRNP, PhD
Assistant Professor
Pediatrics
Johns Hopkins University School of Medicine
Baltimore, Maryland
Chapter 42: Nursing Care of a Family When a Child Has an
    Immune Disorder

Reviewers

Anna Alexander, MS, RNC-OB
Department of Labor and Delivery
Carroll Community College
Westminster, Maryland

Barbara Baldwin
Clinical Nursing Professor
Lehman College
Bronx, New York

Mary Louise Batty, RN, MN
Nurse Clinician III
Faculty of Nursing
University of New Brunswick
Fredericton, New Brunswick, Canada

Kathleen Borge, MS, RNC-MNN, CNE
Faculty
Women and Children's Health
Samaritan Hospital School of Nursing
Troy, New York

Michele Brimeyer, MSN, WHNP-BC
Assistant Professor
University of Florida College of Nursing
Gainesville, Florida

Kim Cooper, RN, MSN
Dean
School of Nursing
Ivy Tech Community College
Terre Haute, Indiana

Nicole de Bosch Kemper, RN, MSN, CCNE
Instructor 1
Team Lead Year 3 POP
University of British Columbia Okanagan
Kelowna, British Columbia, Canada

Debbie Diamond, MSN, ARNP, FNP-BC
Nursing Faculty
Baptist Health South Florida/Nova Southeastern University
Miami, Florida

Kelly Duffy, EdD, MSN, RN
Senior Professor
School of Nursing
Daytona State College
Daytona Beach, Florida

Nancy Fleming, HBScN, MAEd
Professor
Confederation College
Thunder Bay, Ontario, Canada

Larecia Gill, MSN/Ed, RN
Associate Professor of Nursing
Assistant Chair of Nursing
Albany State University
Albany, Georgia

Tamara Hryshchuk, MS, RNC-NIC
Interim Site Director
School of Nursing Faculty
Langston University—Tulsa Campus
Tulsa, Oklahoma

Jessica Huber, RN, MSN, CCRN, CPN
Course Coordinator/Instructor
Undergraduate Nursing Program
Carlow University
Pittsburgh, Pennsylvania

Arlene C. Jones, DNP
Director
Nursing Education
Pearl River Community College
Poplarville, Mississippi

Christine Krause, MSN, CPNP
Associate Director
Adjunct Faculty
Aria Health School of Nursing
Penn State Abington
Trevose, Pennsylvania

Rochelle Kuhn, RN, MS, NP
Nursing Instructor
Aria Health School of Nursing
Trevose, Pennsylvania

Brenda Lennon, MS, RN-BC-C, MNN
Nursing IV Course Chair
Memorial College of Nursing
St. Peter's Health Partners
Albany, New York

Glenn Murphy, MSN, RN, CNE
Assistant Clinical Professor
College of Nursing and Health Professions
Drexel University
Philadelphia, Pennsylvania

Maureen Murt, MSN
Instructor
Department of Professional Studies
Bucks County Community College
Newtown, Pennsylvania

Dave Patterson, BN
Instructor
Faculty of Nursing
University of Calgary
Calgary, Alberta, Canada

Katherine Raker, MSN-Midwifery, CNM
Tenure-Track Faculty Member
Obstetrics/Gynecology and Nursing Department
Geisinger Medical Center and Bloomsburg University
Bloomsburg, Pennsylvania

Cheri Reece, MSN
Assistant Professor of Nursing
Albany State University
Albany, Georgia

Frances Reynolds, MSN
Associate Professor
Howard Community College
Columbia, Maryland

Sheryl Sandahl, DNP, RN, CNP, MPH
Associate Professor and Chair, Department of
    Undergraduate Nursing
The College of St. Scholastica
Duluth, Minnesota

Debbie Treloar, PhD
ADN Faculty
Department of Allied Health
East Mississippi Community College
Scooba, Mississippi

Queen Walters, MSN, DNP, RN
Nursing Faculty
Pearl River Community College
Poplarville, Mississippi

Irene Westlake, MSN
Faculty LVN to RN (ADN)
Texas State Technical College
Sweetwater, Texas

Michele Wolff, MSN, BSN, RN
Professor of Nursing
Saddleback College
Mission Viejo, California

Preface

I am honored that Adele Pillitteri has entrusted me to continue her legacy with the eighth edition of this textbook. As the author of the previous editions, she was committed to a high-quality and student-friendly combined maternal and child health nursing textbook for prelicensure nursing students.

I have provided pediatric health care to a generation of patients as a pediatric nurse practitioner (PNP) at Columbia Medical Practice in Columbia, Maryland. When I joined the faculty of Johns Hopkins University School of Nursing 16 years ago, I was asked to offer hospital clinical instruction to maternal child and pediatric nursing students. In providing maternity instruction, I realized I was not providing adequate breastfeeding support to the mothers in my pediatric practice. I became an International Board Certified Lactation Consultant (IBCLC) to ensure expert breastfeeding support for the parents in my pediatric primary care practice. I have practiced as both a PNP and an IBCLC for over 10 years, and this has been a rewarding part of my practice. These experiences opened my eyes to the importance of understanding the influence of maternal health care on child health nursing, and I am now dedicated to a combined approach to educate nursing students.

Together with the content experts who assisted in the revision of this edition, I have tried to ensure it is accurate and relevant for the prelicensure nursing student. Based on the recommendation of reviewers, many of the features that have evolved over previous editions continue to appear here with some new changes. As an instructor in the classroom of the content in this textbook, I am acutely aware of the pressure on faculty to present relevant and engaging information to their students. The instructor resources that accompany this edition have been expanded and will promote the acquisition of knowledge for the students and promote their critical thinking and lessen the time required for faculty preparation.

Maternal & Child Health Nursing: Care of the Childbearing and Childrearing Family, Eighth Edition, continues to present maternal–child health care not as two separate disciplines but as a continuum of knowledge. Care has been taken to eliminate redundant content. The book is designed for prelicensure nursing students to use either in a combined maternal–child health course or in two separate courses, regardless of the order of the content. It discusses current evidence-based practice related to family-centered maternal child and pediatric care while also promoting a sensitive, holistic outlook on nursing practice. Basic themes include the experience of wellness and illness as family-centered events, the perception of pregnancy and childbirth as periods of wellness, and the importance of knowing normal child development in the planning of nursing care. Themes also reflect changes in healthcare delivery and the importance of meeting the needs of culturally diverse populations.

The Changing Healthcare Scene

As this book is being published, Americans face many unknowns in health care as legislative changes are debated. Preventive health care during pregnancy and throughout childhood is crucial for our nation to survive and prosper. Many diseases and disabilities of adulthood are influenced by the care that pregnant women and their children receive. As health care in the United States continues to evolve and change, nurses will retain an integral role in ensuring preventive needs are addressed.

The 2020 National Health Goals are referenced throughout this book, but it was written with the 2030 National Health Goals in mind. Care has been taken to include content that represents the diversity of the population with regard to race, ethnicity, sexual orientation, and gender identity. National Health Goals for lesbian, gay, bisexual, and transgender (LGBT) persons were added for the first time in 2020. This edition sought to respond by addressing recommendations from The Joint Commission for cultural competency when caring for this population. Nurses are taking an ever-increasing role in the provision of health care for the maternal and child health population. As the population becomes more diverse, it is imperative that nurses understand the cultural beliefs of all individuals. Nursing care requires a greater focus on care planning, communication, evidence-based therapeutic interventions, and critical thinking.

Nursing issues that grow out of the current climate of change include:

- The accentuation of Nursing Care Planning and the Nursing Process: The care planning process provides the structuring framework for coordinating communication that will result in safe and effective care. By structuring the text to reflect this process, students can begin to conceptualize how they will use textbook knowledge in nursing practice to diagnose, plan, deliver, and monitor patients to maximize optimal outcomes. In addition, Nursing Process Overview boxes included at the beginning of each chapter provide a strong theoretical underpinning for nursing process and ways to use the nursing process in clinical practice.
- An emphasis on 2020 National Health Goals: As a way to focus care and research, National Health Goals have gained wider attention at a time when there is a greater need than ever to be wise in the choice of how

dollars are spent. Students can familiarize themselves with how these goals can be applied directly to maternal and child health care by referring to the Nursing Care Planning Based on 2020 National Health Goals displays that appear in each chapter.

- Incorporation of the Centers for Disease Control and Prevention (CDC) Maternity Practices in Infant Nutrition and Care (mPINC) Survey which supports hospital practices that create a supportive environment for breastfeeding prenatally and continue through discharge
- The necessity for nurses to be active participants in redefining quality in health care: A major way nurses can do this is by joining with the Institute of Medicine to help define required competencies for practice. Included in each chapter are multiple-choice questions based on the Quality and Safety Education for Nurses (QSEN) competencies, so students can better envision how these competencies can be applied to practice.
- The importance of basing nursing care on evidence-based practice: The variety of new care settings, as well as the diversity of roles in which nurses practice, is reflected both in the proliferation of community-based nursing facilities and also in the increase in the numbers of nurse-midwives, women's health, pediatric, and neonatal nurse practitioners. This new edition places emphasis on the need for nurses to read and apply research to practice by demonstrating how recent research applies directly to a patient scenario woven throughout each chapter. In addition, boxes on Nursing Care Planning Using Assessment, Nursing Care Planning Based on Responsibility for Pharmacology, and Nursing Care Planning Using Procedures illustrate how medical science is applied to care.
- The need to coordinate care: With a growing ambulatory population, nurses assume the increasingly important role as coordinators for healthcare teams. Interprofessional Care Maps in each chapter demonstrate how the nursing process works for a specific patient throughout the care cycle.
- The responsibility of health teaching with families as a cornerstone of nursing: The teaching role of the nurse has greater significance in the new healthcare milieu as the emphasis on preventive care and short stays in acute care settings create the need for families to be better educated in their own care. Nursing Care Planning Based on Family Teaching displays present detailed health information for the family, emphasizing the importance of a partnership between nurses and patients in the management of health and illness. Nursing Care Planning to Empower a Family boxes provide students with the type of information families need to learn how to participate in and improve both family and individual health.
- The obligation to individualize care according to sociocultural uniqueness: This is a reflection of both greater cultural sensitivity and an increasingly diverse population of caregivers and care recipients. Greater emphasis is being placed on the implications of multiple sociocultural factors in how they affect responses to health and illness. Nursing Care Planning Tips for Effective Communication boxes give examples of ways to improve nurse–patient communication. Nursing Care Planning to Respect Cultural Diversity displays demonstrate solutions in areas of caregiving that differs among patients of various cultures.

Organization of the Text

Maternal & Child Health Nursing follows the family from prepregnancy through pregnancy, labor, birth, and the postpartal period; it then follows the child and the family from birth through adolescence. Coverage includes ambulatory and inpatient care and focuses on primary as well as secondary and tertiary care.

The book is organized in eight units:

Unit 1 provides an introduction to maternal and child health nursing. A framework for practice is presented as well as current trends and the importance of considering childbearing and childrearing within a diverse sociodemographic and family/community context. This focus includes attention to health disparities and the provision of care in the home as well as the hospital setting.

Unit 2 examines the nursing role in preparing families for childbearing and childrearing and discusses reproductive and sexual health, the role of the nurse in genetic counseling, reproductive life planning, and the concerns of the subfertile family.

Unit 3 presents the nursing role in caring for a pregnant family during pregnancy, birth, and the postpartal period and serving as a fetal advocate. A separate chapter details the role of the nurse in providing comfort during labor and birth.

Unit 4 addresses the nursing role when a woman develops a complication of pregnancy, labor or birth, or has a complication during the postpartal period. Separate chapters address the role of the nurse when a woman has a preexisting illness, develops a complication during pregnancy or the postpartal period, has a unique concern, or chooses or needs a cesarean birth. A final chapter details care of the high-risk newborn or a child born with a physical or a developmental challenge.

Unit 5 discusses the nursing role in health promotion during childhood. The chapters in this unit cover principles of growth and development and care of the child from infancy through adolescence, including child health assessment and communication and health teaching with children and families.

Unit 6 presents the nursing role in supporting the health of children and their families. The effects of illness on children and their families, diagnostic and therapeutic procedures, medication administration, and pain management are addressed, with respect to care of the child and family in hospital, home, and ambulatory settings.

Unit 7 examines the nursing role in restoring and maintaining the health of children and families when illness occurs. Disorders are presented according to body systems so that students have a ready orientation for locating content.

Unit 8 discusses the nursing role in restoring and maintaining the mental health of children and families. Separate chapters discuss the role of the nurse when intimate partner violence or child maltreatment or mental, long-term, or fatal illness is present.

Pedagogic Features

Each chapter in the text is organized to provide a complete learning experience for the student. Numerous pedagogic features are included to help a student understand and increase retention. Important elements include:

- **Chapter Objectives:** Learning objectives are included at the beginning of each chapter to identify outcomes expected after the material in the chapter has been mastered.
- **Key Terms:** Terms that would be new to a student are listed at the beginning of each chapter in a ready reference list. Terms are shown in boldface type where they are defined in the text. Definitions also appear online in the Glossary.
- **Chapter-Opening Scenarios:** Short scenarios appear at the beginning of each chapter. These vignettes are designed to help students appreciate that nursing care is always individualized and provide a taste of what is to come in the chapter. Throughout the chapter, open-ended and multiple-choice questions related to the scenario connect learning with patient care.
- **Nursing Process Overview:** Each chapter begins with a review of nursing process in which specific suggestions, such as examples of nursing diagnoses and outcome criteria helpful to modifying care in the area under discussion, are presented. These reviews are designed to improve students' preparation in clinical areas, so they can focus their care planning and apply principles to practice.
- **Nursing Diagnoses and Related Interventions:** A consistent format highlights the nursing diagnoses and related interventions throughout the text. A special heading draws the students' attention to these sections where individual nursing diagnoses and outcome evaluation are detailed for the major conditions and disorders discussed.
- **QSEN Checkpoint Questions:** Throughout the text, NCLEX-style multiple-choice QSEN Checkpoint Questions appear to help students check their progress and reward them for their comprehension. They relate the chapter-opening scenario to the six QSEN competencies: safety, quality improvement, evidence-based practice, team work and collaboration, informatics, and patient-centered care. Students can check their work by reading the answers provided in the Appendix.
- **What If . . . Questions:** These critical thinking questions, formatted to reflect NCLEX style, also appear throughout each chapter in the text. They ask readers to apply the information just acquired in the patient scenario presented in the chapter opening, thus maximizing learning and emphasizing critical thinking. Suggested solutions are supplied on thePoint.
- **Tables and Displays:** Numerous tables and displays summarize important information or provide extra detail on topics so that a student has ready references to this information.
  - **Nursing Care Planning Based on 2020 National Health Goals:** To emphasize the nursing role in accomplishing the healthcare goals of our nation, these displays state specific ways in which maternal and child health nursing can provide better outcomes for families. They help the student to appreciate the importance of national healthcare planning and the influence that nurses can have in creating a healthier nation.
  - **Nursing Care Planning Tips for Effective Communication:** This feature presents tips to apply communication skills in practice and provides case examples of effective communication, illustrating for the student how an awareness of communication can improve the patient's understanding and positively impact outcomes.
  - **Nursing Care Planning Based on Family Teaching:** These boxes present detailed health teaching information for the family, emphasizing the importance of a partnership between nurses and patients in the management of health and illness.
  - **Nursing Care Planning Based on Responsibility for Pharmacology:** These boxes provide quick reference for medications that are commonly used for the health problems described in the text. They give the drug name (brand and generic, if applicable), dosage, pregnancy category, side effects, and nursing implications.
  - **Nursing Care Planning Using Procedures:** Techniques of procedures specific to maternal and child health care are boxed in an easy-to-follow two-column format, often enhanced with color figures.
  - **Nursing Care Planning Using Assessment:** These visual guides provide head-to-toe assessment information for overall health status or specific disorders or conditions.
  - **Nursing Care Planning: Interprofessional Care Maps:** Because nurses rarely work in isolation, but rather as a member of a healthcare team or unit, interprofessional care maps written for specific patients are included in each chapter to demonstrate the use of the nursing process, provide examples of critical thinking, and clarify nursing care for specific patient needs. These Interprofessional Care Maps not only demonstrate nursing process but also accentuate the increasingly important role of the nurse as a coordinator of patient care.
  - **Nursing Care Planning to Respect Cultural Diversity:** These boxes help students appreciate how care delivery should alter to meet the needs of each patient in a country that continually attracts immigrants from throughout the world.
  - **Nursing Care Planning to Empower a Family:** Because patient education is an important nursing responsibility, these boxes provide students with the type of information families need to learn how to participate in improving their health.
- **NEW! Unfolding Patient Stories:** Written by the National League for Nursing, these Unfolding Patient Stories are an engaging way to begin meaningful conversations in the classroom. These vignettes, which appear in relevant chapters, feature patients from Wolters Kluwer's *vSim for Nursing: Maternity and Pediatric* (co-developed with Laerdal Medical) and DocuCare products; however, each Unfolding Patient Story in the book stands alone, not requiring purchase of these products.
- **NEW! Concept Mastery Alerts:** These Concept Mastery Alerts clarify common misconceptions as identified by Lippincott's Adaptive Learning Powered by PrepU.
- **Key Points:** A review of important points is highlighted at the end of each chapter to help students monitor their own comprehension.
- **Critical Thinking Care Studies:** To involve a student in the decision-making realities of the clinical setting, each chapter ends with an additional case scenario, followed by several thought-provoking questions. These could also serve as a basis for conference or class discussion. Suggested answers are supplied on thePoint.

Teaching and Learning Package

RESOURCES FOR INSTRUCTORS

Tools to assist you with teaching your course are available upon adoption of this text at http://thepoint.lww.com/Flagg8e.

- **Pre-Lecture Quizzes:** These exercises ask students to recall information. Based on the main points of the chapter, each of the five true/false statements and five fill-in-the-blank questions will help you determine whether students have read the chapters. Answers are provided.
- **Assignments:** Grouped into Written Assignments, Group Assignments, Clinical Assignments, and Web Assignments, the Assignments package will give you a means to gauge students' understanding of the textbook material. The Assignments give students many chances to test their own knowledge of the chapter concepts as well as their developing critical thinking skills. Suggested Answers are provided.
- **Discussion Topics:** With these topics, you can initiate and foster classroom discussion or assign them for use outside the classroom. Each Discussion Topic is designed to help students make a connection between the textbook and application. Suggested Answers are provided.
- **E-Book:** Online access to the book's full text and images gives you an easy-to-transport format.
- **PowerPoint Presentations With Guided Lecture Notes:** The PowerPoint presentations provide you with visual aids to support your lectures or classroom lessons. The accompanying Guided Lecture Notes offer brief talking points you can use along with the presentations.
- **Test Generator:** The Test Generator lets you put together exclusive new tests from a bank containing hundreds of questions to help you in assessing your students' understanding of the material. Test questions link to chapter learning objectives. This test generator comes with a bank of more than 1,100 questions.
- **Image Bank:** Access to downloadable photographs and illustrations from this textbook offer you the ability to use them in your PowerPoint slides or as you see fit throughout your course.

RESOURCES FOR STUDENTS

Students can access all these learning tools using the code printed in the front of their textbooks by visiting http://thepoint.lww.com/Flagg8e.

- **NCLEX-Style Review Questions:** These *application-level* questions provide students the opportunity to test themselves on their ability to apply specific nursing actions based on what a nurse should know and what a nurse should do in a specific situation related to the chapter content. They also give students experience in answering questions of the type that will appear on the NCLEX.
- **Suggested Readings:** This list of journal articles provides students with the information needed to do more in-depth reading relevant to the topics included in the chapter.
- **Answers and Rationales:** Suggested Answers to the each chapter's What If . . . and Critical Thinking Care Study questions allow students to gauge whether they are on the right track by providing the main points that they are expected to address in answering these questions.
- **Patient Scenarios:** A patient care scenario details a full health history and examination findings pertinent to each chapter's content. Each scenario includes 25 related NCLEX-style questions to help students sharpen their skills and grow more familiar with NCLEX-type questions. Completing these exercises serve as an excellent review of the chapter content.
- **Journal Articles:** Updated for the new edition, online articles offer students the opportunity to read current research related to each chapter's material as available in Lippincott Williams & Wilkins journals.
- **Watch & Learn Video Clips:** These audiovisual aides cover both maternal and child care topics:
  - Developmental Tasks of Pregnancy: 1st Trimester, Accepting the Pregnancy
  - Developmental Tasks of Pregnancy: 2nd Trimester, Accepting the Baby
  - Developmental Tasks of Pregnancy: 3rd Trimester, Preparing for Parenthood
  - Vaginal Birth
  - Scheduled Cesarean Birth
  - Assisting the Patient With Breastfeeding
  - Developmental Considerations in Caring for Children: Infants
  - Developmental Considerations in Caring for Children: Toddlers
  - Developmental Considerations in Caring for Children: Preschoolers
  - Developmental Considerations in Caring for Children: School Agers
  - Developmental Considerations in Caring for Children: Adolescents
  - Care of the Hospitalized Child: Introduction
  - Care of the Hospitalized Child: Medication Administration
  - Care of the Hospitalized Child: Play
  - Care of the Hospitalized Child: Pain Management
  - Care of the Hospitalized Child: Parent and Family Participation
- **Spanish–English Audio Glossary:** This auditory aide provides helpful terms and phrases for communicating with patients who speak Spanish.

A Fully Integrated Course Experience

We are pleased to offer an expanded suite of digital solutions and ancillaries to support instructors and students using *Maternal & Child Health Nursing*, Eighth Edition. To learn more about any solution, please contact your local Wolters Kluwer representative.

LIPPINCOTT COURSEPOINT+

Lippincott CoursePoint+ is an integrated digital learning solution designed for the way students learn. It is the only nursing education solution that integrates:

- **Leading content in context:** Content provided in the context of the student learning path engages students and encourages interaction and learning on a deeper level.
- **Powerful tools to maximize class performance:** Course-specific tools, such as adaptive learning powered by PrepU, provide a personalized learning experience for every student.

- **Real-time data to measure students' progress:** Student performance data provided in an intuitive display lets you quickly spot which students are having difficulty or which concepts the class as a whole is struggling to grasp.
- **Preparation for practice:** Integrated virtual simulation and evidence-based resources improve student competence, confidence, and success in transitioning to practice.
  - *vSim for Nursing*: Codeveloped by Laerdal Medical and Wolters Kluwer, vSim for Nursing simulates real nursing scenarios and allows students to interact with virtual patients in a safe, online environment.

- *Lippincott Advisor for Education*: With over 8,500 entries covering the latest evidence-based content and drug information, Lippincott Advisor for Education provides students with the most up-to-date information possible while giving them valuable experience with the same point-of-care content they will encounter in practice.
- **Training services and personalized support:** To ensure your success, our dedicated educational consultants and training coaches will provide expert guidance every step of the way.

thePoint® is a trademark of Wolters Kluwer.

Acknowledgments

I would like to express my appreciation to the contributors of this edition. All of them have very busy personal and professional lives, yet they took the time and effort to update the content in their area of expertise through many revisions. I especially want to thank one contributor, Colleen Kennedy, who was referred to me by a colleague. When I contacted her about possible chapters, she volunteered for 13 chapters. I was hesitant, as this was much more than any other contributor. She not only completed all of her chapters on time but also volunteered to assist with additional chapters and contributed heavily to the diversity and maternal child nursing chapter.

I want to thank my family for their support and encouragement: my husband Jon, for never complaining about my editing late into the night; my daughter Jennifer, for contributing to the mental health disorder chapter; my son Chris; my daughter-in-law Melissia; and my 1-year-old grandson, Andrew. Sharing the pregnancy and birth of my grandson kept me focused on why maternal child nursing is such a special and personal field of nursing practice. To my stepchildren Sarah, Daniel, Lauren, and Anna, even though I didn't give birth to you and wasn't in your lives in your early years, I have enjoyed watching you grow into responsible young adults these past 5 years. Lastly, I want to thank Victoria White, the Developmental Editor, and Heather A. Rybacki, the Supervising Development Editor, of this edition. I was fortunate to have a professional team who provided expert guidance during every step of this journey.

JoAnne Silbert-Flagg, **DNP, CPNP, IBCLC, FAAN**

Contents

UNIT 6   The Nursing Role in Supporting the Health of Ill Children and Their Families

Case Studies in This Book

Cases That Unfold Within Chapters

Critical Thinking Care Studies

UNIT 1

Maternal and Child Health Nursing Practice

1

A Framework for Maternal and Child Health Nursing

Anna Chung is an early premature neonate who will be transported to a regional center for care about 30 miles from the community where she was born. Her parents, Melissa and Robert, tell you they are worried about their tiny daughter being cared for by strangers so many miles away. They're also concerned how they will be able to pay for or give informed consent for this special level of care. Melissa, 42 years old, feels too exhausted to leave the hospital only 2 days after having a cesarean birth. She wonders how she and her husband will be able to visit the new baby because of her exhaustion and because their first child, Miecko, 6 years old, is on home care for pneumonia. Robert wonders how Miecko will react to having an ill rather than a healthy sister.

This chapter discusses competencies, philosophies, challenges, and new roles for nurses in maternal–child health care and how these challenges and changes mold and affect care.

What are some healthcare issues evident in the previous scenario? What would be your nursing role with Mrs. Chung? With her two children?

KEY TERMS

evidence-based practice

fertility rate

infant mortality rate

maternal and child health nursing

nursing research

patient advocacy

Quality & Safety Education for Nurses (QSEN)

scope of practice

OBJECTIVES

After mastering the contents of this chapter, you should be able to:

1. View the areas of maternal and child health as a continuum with a seamless flow between the two areas.
2. Identify the specific goals and philosophies of maternal and child health nursing and apply these to nursing practice.
3. Identify 2020 National Health Goals as an important guide to understanding the health of the nation and goals that nurses can help the nation achieve.
4. Describe the evolution, scope, competencies, and professional roles of nurses in maternal and child health nursing.
5. Describe family-centered care and ways maternal and child health nursing could be made both more family centered and respectful of diversity.
6. Using the nursing process, plan nursing care that includes the six competencies of Quality & Safety Education for Nurses (QSEN): Patient-Centered Care, Teamwork & Collaboration, Evidence-Based Practice (EBP), Quality Improvement (QI), Safety, and Informatics.
7. Define and use common statistical terms used in the field, such as infant and maternal mortality.
8. Use critical thinking to identify areas of nursing care that could benefit from additional research or application of evidence-based practice.
9. Integrate knowledge of maternal and child health nursing with the interplay of nursing process, the six competencies of QSEN, and Family Nursing to achieve quality maternal and child health nursing care.

Goals and Philosophies of Maternal and Child Health Nursing

The area of childbearing and childrearing families is a major focus of nursing practice in promoting health for the next generation. Comprehensive preconception and prenatal care is essential in ensuring a healthy outcome for mother and child. Although childbearing and childrearing are often viewed as two separate entities, they are interrelated, and a deeper understanding is achieved when they are viewed as a continuum (Fig. 1.1) (Burkhard, 2013).

The primary goal of both **maternal and child health nursing** is the promotion and maintenance of optimal family health. Major philosophical assumptions about combined maternal and child health nursing are listed in Box 1.1. Maternal and child health nursing extends from preconception to menopause with an expansive array of health issues and healthcare providers. Examples of the scope of practice include:

- Preconception health care
- Care of women during three trimesters of pregnancy and the puerperium (the 6 weeks after childbirth, sometimes termed the fourth trimester of pregnancy)

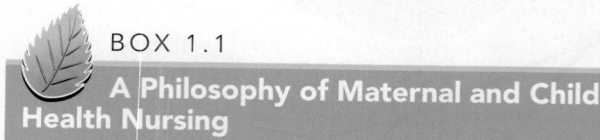

BOX 1.1

A Philosophy of Maternal and Child Health Nursing

Maternal and child health nursing is:

- Family centered; assessment should always include the family as well as an individual.
- Community centered; the health of families is both affected by and influences the health of communities.
- Evidence based; this is the means whereby critical knowledge increases.
- A challenging role for nurses and a major factor in keeping families well and optimally functioning.

A maternal and child health nurse:

- Considers the family as a whole and as a partner in care when planning or implementing or evaluating the effectiveness of care.
- Serves as an advocate to protect the rights of all family members, including the fetus.
- Demonstrates a high degree of independent nursing functions because teaching and counseling are major interventions.
- Promotes health and disease prevention because these protect the health of the next generation.
- Serves as an important resource for families during childbearing and childrearing as these can be extremely stressful times in a life cycle.
- Respects personal, cultural, and spiritual attitudes and beliefs as these so strongly influence the meaning and impact of childbearing and childrearing.
- Encourages developmental stimulation during both health and illness so children can reach their ultimate capacity in adult life.
- Assesses families for strengths as well as specific needs or challenges.
- Encourages family bonding through rooming-in and family visiting in maternal and child healthcare settings.
- Encourages early hospital discharge options to reunite families as soon as possible in order to create a seamless, helpful transition process.
- Encourages families to reach out to their community so the family can develop a wealth of support people they can call on in a time of family crisis.

Figure 1.1 Maternal and child health nursing includes care of the pregnant woman, child, and family. **(A)** During a prenatal visit, a nurse assesses that a pregnant woman's uterus is expanding normally. **(B)** During a health maintenance visit, a nurse assesses a child's growth and development. (© Barbara Proud.)

- Care of infants during the perinatal period (the time span beginning at 20 weeks of pregnancy to 4 weeks [28 days] after birth)
- Care of children from birth through late adolescent
- Care in a variety of hospital and home care settings

Regardless of the setting, a family-centered approach is the preferred focus of nursing care (Papp, 2012). The health of an individual and his or her ability to function as a member of a family can strongly influence and improve overall family functioning.

Family-centered care enables nurses to better understand individuals and their effect on others and, in turn, to provide more holistic care (Hedges, Nichols, & Filoteo, 2012). It includes encouraging rooming-in with the mother by the mother's partner or support person and with the child by

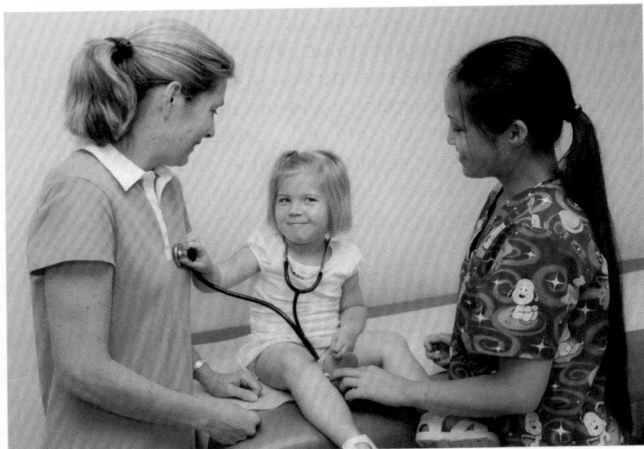

Figure 1.2   A nurse involves the mother in a physical exam to promote family-centered care.

BOX 1.2

Nursing Care Planning Based on Family Teaching

TIPS FOR SELECTING A FAMILY-CENTERED HEALTHCARE SETTING

Q. Melissa Chung asks you, "With so many healthcare settings available, how do we know which one to choose?"

A. When selecting a setting, asking the following questions can help you decide what is best for your family:

- If the setting is for child care, are personnel interested in you as well as your child? If the setting is a maternal care site, do they ask about family concerns as well as individual ones?
- Can the setting be reached easily? (Going for preventive care when well or for continuing care when ill should not be a chore.)
- Will the staff provide continuity of care so you'll always see the same primary care provider if possible?
- Does the physical setup of the facility provide for a sense of privacy, yet a sense that healthcare providers share pertinent information so you do not have to repeat your history at each visit?
- Is the cost of care and the number of referrals to specialists explained clearly?
- Are preventive care and health education stressed? (Keeping well is as important as recovering from illness.)
- Is health education done at your learning level?
- Do healthcare providers respect your opinion and ask for your input on healthcare decisions?
- Will the facility still be accessible if a family member becomes disabled?

their caregiver. Family members are encouraged to provide physical and emotional care based on the individual situation and their comfort level. Nurses provide guidance and monitor the interaction between family members to promote the health and well-being of the family unit. (Fig. 1.2).

Box 1.2 provides guidance on how to assist a family choose a healthcare setting that is family-centered. Family teaching boxes of this kind are found in all chapters as examples of the type of health teaching important in maternal and child health care.

Maternal and Child Health Goals and Standards

Healthcare technology has contributed to a number of important advances in maternal and child health care. Through immunization, childhood diseases such as measles and poliomyelitis almost have been eradicated. New fertility drugs and fertility techniques allow more couples to conceive. The ability to prevent preterm birth and improve the quality of life for both preterm and late preterm infants has increased dramatically. As specific genes responsible for children's health disorders are identified, stem cell therapy may make it possible to replace diseased cells with new growth cells and cure these illnesses. In addition, a growing trend toward healthcare consumerism, or self-care, has made childbearing and childrearing families active participants in their own health monitoring.

Access to health care and social determinants of health impact the role of the nurse and the health of the patient. These factors have expanded the roles of nurses in maternal and child health and, at the same time, have made the delivery of quality maternal and child health nursing care a challenge.

2020 NATIONAL HEALTH GOALS

The importance a society assigns to human life can best be measured by the concern a nation places on its most vulnerable members—its elderly, its disadvantaged, and its youngest citizens. In light of this, in 1979, the U.S. Public Health Service first formulated healthcare objectives for the nation.

Healthcare goals are reviewed every 10 years. In 2010, new goals to be achieved by 2020 were set (U.S. Department of Health and Human Services [DHHS], 2010). The 2030 goals are scheduled for presentation in 2020. Many of these objectives directly involve maternal and child health care because improving the health of these age groups will have long-term effects on the population. The two main overarching national health goals are:

- To increase quality and years of healthy life.
- To eliminate health disparities.

A new objective added in 2010 recommends that 100% of prelicensure programs in nursing include core content on counseling for health promotion and disease prevention, cultural diversity including for lesbian, gay, bisexual, and transgender (LGBT) populations, evaluation of health sciences literature, environmental health, public health systems, and global health, all important areas for maternal and child health and discussed throughout this text (DHHS, 2010).

The 2020 National Health Goals are intended to help citizens more easily understand the importance of health promotion and disease prevention and to encourage wide participation in improving health in the next decade. It's important for maternal and child health nurses to be familiar with these goals because nurses play such a vital role in helping the nation achieve these objectives through both practice and research (see www.healthypeople.gov). The goals also serve as the basis for grant funding and financing of evidence-based practice. Each of the following sections highlights goals as they relate to that specific area of care.

GLOBAL HEALTH GOALS

The United Nations (UN) and the World Health Organization established millennium health goals in 2000 in an effort to improve health worldwide. As with 2020 National Health Goals, these concentrate on improving the health of women and children because increasing the health in these two populations can have such long-ranging effects on general health. These Global Health Goals are:
- To end poverty and hunger.
- To achieve universal primary education.
- To promote gender equality and empower women.
- To reduce child mortality.
- To improve maternal health.
- To combat HIV/AIDS, malaria, and other diseases.
- To ensure environmental sustainability.
- To develop a global partnership for development.

The establishment of global health goals is a major step forward in improving the health of all people, as contagious diseases, poverty, and gender inequality do not respect national boundaries but follow people across the world and into all nations (UN, 2000).

Health Setting Magnet Status

Magnet status is a credential furnished by the American Nurses Credentialing Center (ANCC), an affiliate of the American Nurses Association, to hospitals that meet a rigorous set of criteria designed to improve the strength and quality of nursing care. Hospitals who achieve Magnet status meet criteria in five major categories:
- *Transformational leadership.* This is the ability of nurses in the designated organization to convert their organization's values, beliefs, and behaviors in order to create a high professional level of nursing care.
- *Structural empowerment.* This refers to the ability to provide an innovative environment where strong professional practice can flourish with regard to the hospital's mission, vision, and values.
- *Exemplary professional practice.* The setting demonstrates a comprehensive understanding of the role of nursing; the application of that role with patients, families, communities, and the interdisciplinary team is clear, so new knowledge and evidence can be applied to nursing care.
- *New knowledge, innovation, and improvements.* The organization demonstrates strong nursing leadership, empowered professionals, and exemplary practice while contributing to patient care.
- *Empirical quality results.* The hospital demonstrates solid structure and processes where strong professional practice can flourish and where the mission, vision, and values come to life as the organization achieves the outcomes believed to be important for the organization (ANCC, 2012).

Magnet hospitals typically demonstrate a high level of nursing job satisfaction and a low staff nurse turnover rate and have policies in place that include nurses in data collection and decision making about patient care. These hospitals demonstrate they value staff nurses, involve them in research-based practice, and encourage and reward them for obtaining additional degrees in nursing. All nurse managers and nurse leaders in Magnet-designated hospitals must have either a baccalaureate or master's degree in nursing.

Not all hospitals can qualify for Magnet status; the desirability of being named a Magnet hospital, however, has encouraged all hospitals to examine their nursing environment and bring about changes that improve working conditions, stress evidence-based practice, and improve the education level of their nurses (Hess, Desroches, Donelan, et al., 2011). According to the ANCC, "Magnet hospitals attract and maintain top talent; improve patient care, safety and satisfaction; foster a collaborative culture; advance nursing standards and practice; and grow business and financial success" (ANCC, n.d.).

A Framework for Maternal and Child Health Nursing Care

Maternal and child health nursing can be visualized within a framework in which nurses use nursing process, nursing theory, and Quality & Safety Education for Nurses (QSEN) competencies to care for families during childbearing and childrearing years and through the four phases of health care:
- Health promotion
- Health maintenance
- Health restoration
- Health rehabilitation

Examples of these phases of health care as they relate to maternal and child health are shown in Table 1.1.

NURSING PROCESS

Nursing care, at its best, is designed and implemented in a thorough manner, using an organized series of steps, to ensure quality and consistency of care (Carpenito, 2012). The nursing process, a scientific form of problem solving, serves as the basis for assessing, making a nursing diagnosis, planning, implementing, and evaluating care. It is a process broad enough to serve as the basis for modern nursing care because it is applicable to all healthcare settings, from the home to ambulatory clinics to intensive care units.

Because nurses rarely work in isolation but rather as a member of an interprofessional team, interprofessional care maps and checkpoint questions on teamwork and collaboration are included throughout the text to demonstrate the use of the nursing process as well as to provide examples of critical thinking, clarify nursing care for specific patient needs, and accentuate the increasingly important role of nurses as coordinators of care for a collaborative team.

NURSING THEORY

One of the requirements of a profession (together with other critical determinants, such as members who set their own standards, self-monitor their practice quality, and participate in research) is that a discipline's knowledge flows from a base of established theory.

TABLE 1.1 DEFINITIONS AND EXAMPLES OF PHASES OF HEALTH CARE

Term	Definition	Examples
Health promotion	Educating parents and children to follow sound health practices through teaching and role modeling	Teaching women the importance of rubella immunization before pregnancy; providing preteens with information about safer sex practices well before they are likely to become sexually active
Health maintenance	Intervening to maintain health when risk of illness is present	Encouraging women to be partners in prenatal care; teaching parents the importance of safeguarding their home by childproofing against poisoning
Health restoration	Using conscientious assessment to be certain that symptoms of illness are identified and interventions are begun to return patient to wellness most rapidly	Caring for a woman during a complication of pregnancy such as gestational diabetes or a child during an acute illness such as pneumonia
Health rehabilitation	Helping prevent complications from illness; helping a patient with residual effects achieve an optimal state of wellness and independence; helping a patient to accept inevitable death	Encouraging a woman with gestational trophoblastic disease (abnormal placenta growth) to continue therapy or a child with a renal transplant to continue to take necessary medications

 Concept Mastery Alert

Make note of the differences between health *promotion* and health *maintenance*: Health maintenance involves intervening to maintain health *when risk of disease is present*, for example, teaching a group of sexually active adolescents about contraception and prevention of sexually transmitted infections. Health promotion involves education when no specific risk is present.

Nursing theories are designed to offer helpful ways to view patients so nursing activities can be created to best meet patient needs—for example, Calistra Roy's theory stresses that an important role of the nurse is to help patients adapt to change caused by illness or other stressors (Roy, 2011); Dorothea Orem's theory concentrates on examining patients' ability to perform self-care (Orem & Taylor, 2011); Patricia Benner's theory describes the way nurses move from novice to expert as they become more experienced and prepared to give interprofessional care (Benner, 2011). Using a theoretical basis such as these can help you appreciate the significant effect of a child's illness or the introduction of a new member on the total family.

Other issues most nursing theorists address include how nurses should be viewed or what the goals of nursing care should be. Extensive changes in the scope of maternal and child health nursing have occurred as health promotion (teaching, counseling, supporting, and advocacy, or keeping parents and children well) has become a greater priority in care (Salsman, Grunberg, Beaumont, et al., 2012). As promoting healthy pregnancies and keeping children well protects not only patients at present but also the health of the next generation, maternal–child health nurses fill these expanded roles to a unique and special degree.

QSEN: QUALITY & SAFETY EDUCATION FOR NURSES

In 2007, the Robert Wood Johnson Foundation challenged nursing leaders to improve the quality of nursing care and to build the knowledge, skills, and attitudes necessary to help achieve that level of care into prelicensure and graduate programs (Disch, 2012).

Because of this challenge, the QSEN Learning Collaborative created six competencies deemed necessary for quality care (Cronenwett, Sherwood, & Gelmon, 2009). These competencies included five competencies that originated from a study by the Institute of Medicine: (a) patient-centered care, (b) teamwork and collaboration, (c) quality improvement, (d) informatics, and (e) evidence-based practice. The QSEN Learning Collaborative added safety as the sixth competency.

Throughout all phases of **QSEN**, the overall goal is to address the challenge of preparing future nurses with the abilities necessary to continuously improve the quality and safety of the healthcare systems in which they work. Definitions for each of the six competencies along with examples of the knowledge, skills, and attitudes necessary to achieve quality maternal and child health care are shown in Box 1.3.

EVIDENCE-BASED PRACTICE

Evidence-based practice existed as an important element of nursing practice prior to the development of QSEN; it has since been incorporated into QSEN as one of its competencies. **Evidence-based practice** is the conscientious, explicit, and judicious use of current best evidence to make decisions about the care of patients (Falk, Wongsa, Dang, et al., 2012). Evidence can be a combination of research, clinical expertise, and patient preferences or values.

Use of evidence such as that obtained from randomized controlled trials helps to move healthcare actions from "just tradition" to a more solid and therefore safer, scientific basis. The Cochrane Database (listed in PubMed, Ovid, and MEDLINE) is a good source for discovering evidence-based practices as the organization consistently reviews, evaluates, and reports the strength of health-related research (Dong, Chen, & Yu, 2012).

QSEN Checkpoint Questions: Evidence-Based Practice are included in chapters throughout the text and contain summaries of current maternal and child health research followed by questions to assist you in developing a questioning attitude regarding current nursing practice or in thinking of ways to incorporate research findings into care.

BOX 1.3

QSEN Competencies in Relation to the Chung Family

Competency	Knowledge	Skills	Attitudes
Patient-Centered Care			
The patient or designee is thought of as the source of control and full partner in the provision of compassionate and coordinated care based on respect for the patient's preferences, values, and needs.	Take an admission history detailing the Chung family's composition. Document the roles of family members and who will be the chief childcare provider.	Encourage Anna's family to spend as much time as possible with her while she is hospitalized; assess that she will have family support on transition to home.	Don't think of admitting Anna to the neonatal care nursery as a single patient but rather as admitting her family to the setting.
Teamwork and Collaboration			
Nurses function effectively within nursing and interprofessional teams, fostering open communication, mutual respect, and shared decision making as they achieve quality patient care.	Familiarize yourself with how many other healthcare providers will be interacting with Anna (e.g., neonatologist, nurse practitioner, nutritionist) to help appreciate how frightening having to meet so many people could be to a family.	Discuss with Anna's parents what problems, if any, they will have visiting so other team members can help reassure and support them when they visit.	Consider and respect Anna's parents as integrative members of her healthcare team.
Evidence-Based Practice			
Nurses integrate the best current evidence with clinical expertise and patient/family preferences and values for delivery of optimal health care.	Read journal articles related to new evidence about healthy families or neonatal care to be better prepared to help Anna seamlessly transition from one setting to the next.	Implement evidence-based practice so Anna's family are confident that care is based on credible research.	Value the need for change based on new evidence so you can explain to Anna's family with confidence any need for change in care.
Quality Improvement (QI)			
Nurses use data to monitor the outcomes of care and use improvement methods to design and test changes to continuously improve the quality and safety of healthcare systems.	View QI as an important role for all healthcare professionals beginning with prelicensure students.	Use whatever aids, such as checklists, flow sheets, or patient information forms, necessary in order to provide seamless nursing care from nursery admission to home.	Appreciate that continuous QI is an essential part of successful working with and respecting families.
Safety			
Nurses minimize the risk of harm to patients and providers through both system effectiveness and individual performance.	Learn the requirements for a safe healthcare setting for a vulnerable preterm infant.	Be certain Anna receives developmental stimuli as well as is cared for in an environment that promotes a sense of security and is as free from pain as possible.	Recognize families under stress do not "hear" instructions well and so may need these repeated or provided in a written form as well as orally.
Informatics			
Nurses use information and technology to communicate, manage knowledge, mitigate error, and support decision making.	Keep records and documentation current so various healthcare providers can keep informed in order to provide seamless care shifts and setting shifts in care.	Document care in an electronic health record so it can be available to various healthcare providers.	Recognize that documentation must be complete to be valuable (in audit reviews, what wasn't documented as being done is considered as not done).

NURSING RESEARCH

Nursing research (the systematic investigation of problems that have implications for nursing practice usually carried out by nurses) plays an important role in evidence-based practice as bodies of professional knowledge only grow and expand to the extent people in that profession are able to carry out research (Christian, 2012). Examining nursing care in this way results in improved and cost-effective patient care as it provides evidence for action and justification for implementing activities.

A classic example of how the results of nursing research can influence nursing practice is the application of research carried out by Rubin (1963) concerning mothers' initial approaches to their newborns. Before the publication of this study, nurses assumed a woman who did not immediately hold and cuddle her infant at birth was a "cold" or unfeeling mother. After observing a multitude of new mothers, Rubin concluded attachment is not a spontaneous procedure; rather, it more commonly begins with only fingertip touching, then over the next few days, moves to "motherly" actions such as hugging and kissing. Armed with Rubin's findings, nurses today are better able to differentiate healthy from unhealthy bonding behavior in new mothers. Additional nursing research in this area (see Chapter 17) has provided further substantiation regarding the importance of this original investigation.

Some examples of current questions that warrant nursing investigation in the area of maternal and child health nursing include:

- What is the most effective stimulus to encourage women to come for prenatal care or parents to bring children for health maintenance visits?
- How can nurses be instrumental in fostering diversity and inclusion in care?
- How much self-care should young children be expected (or encouraged) to provide during an illness?
- What is the effect of market-driven health care on the quality of maternal–child nursing care?
- What active measures can nurses take to reduce the incidence of child or intimate partner violence?
- How can nurses best help families cope with the stress of a complication of pregnancy or a child's long-term illness?
- How can nurses help prevent violence such as homicide in communities and modify the effects of violence on families?
- What information do maternal and child health nurses need to know about alternative therapies, such as herbal remedies, so their practices remain current?

QSEN Checkpoint Question 1.1

TEAMWORK & COLLABORATION

A nursing assistant informed the nurse that Mr. Chung asked why the hospital where his baby is being cared for is termed a "Magnet hospital." The nurse would want team members to know which rationale?

  a. Magnet hospitals are those who care for the most acutely ill patients.
  b. The designation is one assigned by the American Medical Association.
  c. The hospital has met high standards for nursing competency.
  d. The term refers to hospitals that only admit a limited number of patients.

Look in Appendix A for the best answer and rationale.

A Changing Discipline

Maternal and child health is an ever-changing area of nursing. This happens because childhood infections, such as pertussis (whooping cough) and measles (Rubeola), can now be prevented so children do not usually require care for these conditions. At the same time, illnesses that could not be treated before, such as cystic fibrosis or hypertension of pregnancy, can now be treated, so the number of settings and critical aspects of care increases.

TRENDS IN THE MATERNAL AND CHILD HEALTH NURSING POPULATION

Not only patterns of illness but also variations in social structure, family lifestyle (a way of living in which families cope with social, physical, psychological, and economic variables in their life), and responsibilities continue to constantly change. Table 1.2 summarizes some of these changes that have directly altered assessment and planning care for maternal and child health nurses.

MEASURING MATERNAL AND CHILD HEALTH

Measuring what constitutes the area of maternal and child health is not as simple as defining whether patients are ill or well because individual patients and healthcare practitioners can maintain different perspectives on illness and wellness. A more objective view of health can be provided by using national or regional health statistics to describe degrees of illness (Box 1.4).

Birth Rate

The birth rate in the United States has continued to gradually decrease in recent years to 13.4 per 1,000 population in 2014 (Fig. 1.3). It has substantially decreased from a high of 30.2 per 1,000 population in 1909 (Hamilton et al., 2015).

Early in the century, births to teenage girls were steadily increasing; however, due to additional counseling and increased availability of contraception, particularly long–acting, reversible contraception such as the intrauterine device, this rate is now steadily declining (presently at 24.2/1,000 from a high of 618/1,000 in 1961) (Finer & Zolna, 2016; Hamilton et al., 2015).

The birth rate for women 20 to 24 years of age (79.0/1,000) is gradually declining as well, as women choose to postpone having children until past college age. In contrast, the number of children born to women older than 40 years of age is steadily increasing (presently at 10.6/1,000 from a low of almost no births in this age group in 1901 (Hamilton et al., 2015).

Fertility Rate

The **fertility rate** tends to be low in countries where there are fewer nutritional resources because poor nutrition makes conceiving difficult, as well as in countries where the proportion of young adult men is low because of war or disease. This rate tends to be high in countries where the average woman has access to good nutrition and feels safe to begin a family. The U.S. fertility rate is currently at 62.9%, a rate typical of a healthy, high-resource country (Hamilton et al., 2015).

TABLE 1.2 TRENDS IN MATERNAL AND CHILD HEALTH CARE AND IMPLICATIONS FOR NURSING

Trend	Implications for Nursing
Families are not as extended as in previous generations, so contain fewer members.	Fewer family members are available as support people in a time of crisis. Nurses are called on to fulfill this role more than ever before.
The number of single-parent families is increasing so rapidly it now equals the number of nuclear families in the United States.	A single parent may have fewer financial resources than dual-employed parents. Nurses need to be aware of alternative care options and available to provide a backup opinion as needed.
Ninety percent of women in the United States work outside their home at least part time; many women are the main wage earner for their family.	Health care must be scheduled at times a working parent can come for care for herself or can bring a child for care. Problems of latchkey (self-care) children and the number and safety of child care centers need to be addressed.
Families are more mobile than previously; there is an increase in the number of homeless women and children.	Good interviewing and health monitoring are necessary with mobile families so a health database can be established and there can be continuity of care.
Both child and intimate partner violence is increasing in incidence.	Screening for child or intimate partner violence should be included in all family assessments. Nurses must be aware of the legal responsibilities for reporting violence.
Families are more health conscious than ever before; the use of websites to monitor their health or ask health questions is rapidly increasing.	Families are ripe for health education; providing evidence-based information can be a major nursing role.
Health care must respect cost containment by creating "healthcare homes" or "medical homes."	Comprehensive care is necessary in primary care settings because referral to specialists may not be an option depending on a family's type or lack of health insurance.
Patient advocacy is necessary as it is easy for families to feel lost in the healthcare system.	**Patient advocacy** is safeguarding and advancing the interests of patients and their families. Familiarity with the healthcare services available in a community, establishing and maintaining a relationship with families, as well as helping them make informed choices about what course of action to take or what services would be best to use are important nursing roles.

BOX 1.4

Common Statistical Terms Used to Report Maternal and Child Health

Birth rate: The number of births per 1,000 population.

Fertility rate: The number of pregnancies per 1,000 women of childbearing age.

Fetal death rate: The number of fetal deaths (over 500 g) per 1,000 live births.

Neonatal death rate: The number of deaths per 1,000 live births occurring at birth or in the first 28 days of life.

Perinatal death rate: The number of deaths during the perinatal time period (beginning when a fetus reaches 500 g, about week 20 of pregnancy, and ending about 4 to 6 weeks after birth); it is the sum of the fetal and neonatal rates.

Maternal mortality rate: The number of maternal deaths per 100,000 live births that occur as a direct result of the reproductive process.

Infant mortality rate: The number of deaths per 1,000 live births occurring at birth or in the first 12 months of life.

Childhood mortality rate: The number of deaths per 1,000 population in children aged 1 to 14 years.

Figure 1.3 Birth rates by age of mother: United States, 1990–2014. (Hamilton, B. E., Martin, J. A., Osterman, M. J., et al. [2015]. Births: Final data for 2014. *National Vital Statistics Report, 64*[12], 6.)

Fetal Death Rate

Fetal deaths before birth but greater than 20 weeks gestation occur because of maternal factors (such as premature cervical dilation and maternal hypertension) and also because of fetal factors (such as chromosomal abnormalities or poor placental attachment). The cause of many fetal deaths cannot be documented or occur for unknown reasons. Fetal death rate is important in evaluating the health of a nation because it reflects the overall quality of maternal health and whether common services such as prenatal care are available. A renewed emphasis on both preconception and prenatal care has helped to reduce the U.S. rate from a number as high as 18% in 1950 to 5.96% in 2013 (Hamilton et al., 2015).

Neonatal Death Rate

This rate reflects not only the quality of care available to women during pregnancy and childbirth but also the quality of care available to infants during the first month of life. According to the Centers for Disease Control and Prevention (CDC's) most recent data, the number of infant deaths per 100,000 live births in 2014 was 582.1. The leading causes of death during this time are prematurity with associated low birth weight or congenital malformations, maternal complications of pregnancy, sudden infant death syndrome (SIDS), and injuries (Hamilton et al., 2015).

The proportion of infants born with low birth weight is about 11.39% of all births. The number of low–birth-weight infants has declined after steadily increasing since 2006 and was 8.02% in 2013. Infants born to women under the age of 20 years and between the ages of 40 and 54 years had the highest rate of neonatal and infant deaths.

Infant Mortality Rate

The **infant mortality rate** of a country is a good index of its general health because it measures the quality of pregnancy care, overall nutrition, and sanitation, as well as infant health and available care. This rate is the traditional standard used to compare the health of a nation with previous years or with other countries.

Thanks to the introduction of prenatal care and other community health measures (such as efforts to encourage breastfeeding, require immunizations, initiate better unintentional injury prevention measures [e.g., requiring car seats], and reduce SIDS or the sudden death of an infant less than 1 year of age that cannot be explained after a thorough investigation of the cause of death), in combination with the many technologic advances available for care, the U.S. infant mortality rate has decreased by 86%, from 47.0 in 1940 to 5.96 per 1,000 live births in 2013 (Heron, Hoyert, Murphy, et al., 2009; Matthews, MacDorman, & Thoma, 2015) (Fig. 1.4).

Unfortunately, infant mortality is not equal among all Americans. For example, the rate is higher among Native Alaskan, Native American, and Black infants than it is for White, Asian or Pacific Islander, or non-Hispanic newborns. These differences are thought to be related to a combination of factors, including an unequal provision of and access to health care in different communities (Hamilton et al., 2015).

The infant mortality rate also varies greatly from state to state within the United States (Table 1.3). For example, in the state of Mississippi, the area with the highest infant mortality (9.25), the rate is over twice that of Massachusetts, the state with the lowest rate (4.21) (Matthews et al., 2015).

Worldwide, one would expect the United States, which has one of the highest gross national products in the world and

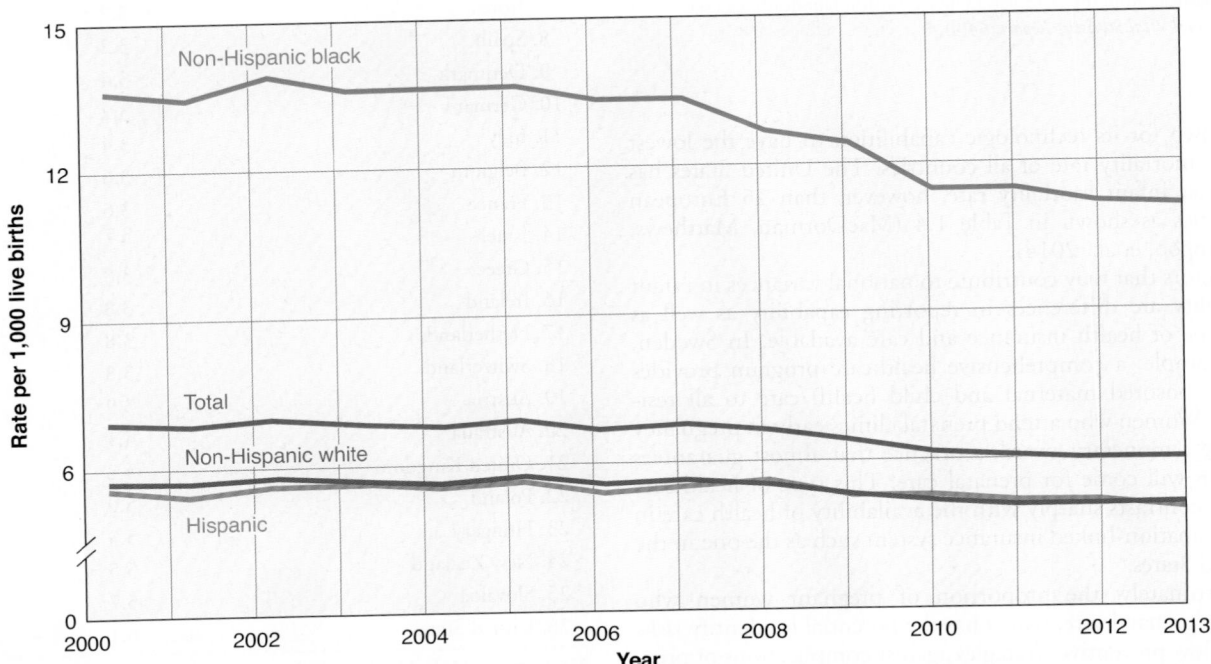

Figure 1.4   Infant mortality rates by race and Hispanic origin of mother: United States, 2005 and 2013. (Matthews, T. J., MacDorman, M. F., & Thoma, M. E. [2015]. Infant mortality statistics from the 2013 period linked birth/infant death data set. *National Vital Statistics Report, 64*[9], 5.)

*Note: Number of pregnancy-related deaths per 100,00 live births per year.

Figure 1.5   Trends in pregnancy-related mortality in the United States 1987–2012. (Centers for Disease Control and Prevention. [2016]. *Pregnancy Mortality Surveillance System.* Atlanta, GA: Author.)

preconception, prenatal, labor and birth, and postnatal care such as:
- Increased participation of women in prenatal care
- Greater detection of disorders such as ectopic pregnancy or placenta previa and prevention of related complications through the use of ultrasound
- Increased control of complications associated with hypertension of pregnancy
- Decreased use of anesthesia with childbirth
- Ability to better prevent or control hemorrhage and infection

This dramatic overall decrease is not a cause for celebration, however. Although the rates of maternal mortality had begun to increase again in 2011 to 17.8% and in some areas to as high as 24 per 100,000 live births, it showed a decline in 2012 to 15.8%. The increasing rate was associated with more cesarean births, more gestational hypertension related to pre-existing hypertensive disorders, and a lack of health insurance for many Americans. Nurses who are alert to the signs and symptoms of hypertension are invaluable guardians of the health of pregnant women and newborns (Clark, 2012). Although some of the causes for maternal mortality remain unclear, known causes include:
- Noncardiovascular disease
- Cardiovascular disease
- Infection or sepsis
- Hemorrhage
- Cardiomyopathy
- Pulmonary embolism
- Hypertensive disorders of pregnancy
- Stroke
- Amniotic fluid embolism
- Anesthesia complications (CDC, 2016b)

QSEN Checkpoint Question 1.2

INFORMATICS

Mrs. Chung's doctor has told her that her baby's most dangerous time will be until the perinatal period ends. When does the perinatal period take place?
- a. From the day of birth until 1 month afterward
- b. During the time the infant will be on ventilator support
- c. From the 20th week of pregnancy to 4 to 6 weeks after birth
- d. Until the infant's body temperature stabilizes following birth

Look in Appendix A for the best answer and rationale.

Child Mortality Rate

Like the infant mortality rate, the child mortality rate in the United States is also declining, although about 25 countries have better rates (UNICEF, 2016). In 1980, for example, the mortality rate was about 6.4% for children aged 1 to 4 years. In 2014, it was 25.5 per 100,000. Children in the prepubescent period (age 5 to 14 years) have the lowest mortality rate of any child age group, at 13 per 100,000. Between 15 and 24 years of age, the rate increases to 64.8 per 100,000 (NCHS, 2016).

The most frequent causes of childhood death are shown in Box 1.5. Notice unintentional injuries are the leading cause of death in children, although many of these accidents are largely preventable through education about the value of car seats and seat belt use, the dangers of drinking/drug abuse and driving, and the importance of pedestrian safety.

BOX 1.5

Major Causes of Death in Childhood

UNDER 1 YEAR

1. Congenital malformations and chromosomal abnormalities
2. Disorders related to short gestation age and low birth weight
3. Maternal complications of pregnancy
4. Sudden infant death syndrome
5. Unintentional injuries (accidents)

1 TO 4 YEARS

1. Unintentional injuries (accidents)
2. Congenital malformations and chromosomal abnormalities
3. Homicide
4. Malignant neoplasms
5. Diseases of the heart

5 TO 9 YEARS

1. Unintentional injuries (accidents)
2. Malignant neoplasms
3. Congenital anomalies
4. Homicide
5. Diseases of the heart

10 TO 14 YEARS

1. Unintentional injuries (accidents)
2. Suicide
3. Malignant neoplasms
4. Congenital anomalies
5. Homicide

15 TO 24 YEARS

1. Unintentional injuries (accidents)
2. Suicide
3. Homicide
4. Malignant neoplasm
5. Diseases of the heart

Center for Disease Control and Prevention. (2016). *10 Leading causes of death by age group United States–2014*. Atlanta, GA: Author.

A particularly disturbing mortality statistic is the high incidence of homicide and suicide in the 10- to 19-year-old age group (more girls than boys attempt suicide, but boys are more successful). Although school-age children and adolescents may not voice feelings of depression or anger during a healthcare visit, such underlying feelings may actually be a primary concern (Bridge, McBee-Strayer, Cannon, et al., 2012; CDC, 2016c). Nurses who are alert to cues of depression or anger can be instrumental in detecting these emotions and lowering the risk of self-injury.

Childhood Morbidity Rate

Health problems commonly occurring in large proportions of children today include respiratory disorders (including asthma and tuberculosis), gastrointestinal disturbances, and

consequences of injuries. Obesity rates for children aged 2 to 19 years now average 17% (CDC, 2016a). Obesity in school-age children can lead to cardiovascular disorders, self-esteem issues, and type 2 diabetes, so counseling children about maintaining a healthy weight is an important nursing responsibility (Junnila, Aromaa, Heinonen, et al., 2012). Morbid obesity in pregnant women can lead to complications during pregnancy, at birth, and following birth (Machado, 2012).

As more immunizations for childhood diseases become available, fewer children in the United States are affected by common childhood communicable diseases. Continued education about the benefits of immunization against rubella (German measles) is still needed because if a woman contracts this form of measles during pregnancy, her infant can be born with severe congenital malformations.

In 2014, vaccination coverage achieved the 90% coverage target for Healthy People 2020 for children aged 19 to 35 months. These targets include vaccination against measles, mumps, rubella, hepatitis B, polio, and varicella. Although the decline in the overall incidence of preventable childhood diseases is encouraging and most regions of the country report strong adherence to recommended vaccination schedules, many children are still not fully immunized. Reasons cited include religious, philosophical, and medical exemptions, as well as limited access to care. A 2015 outbreak of measles in the state of California revealed that 68 of the infected children had not received their MMR vaccination. There is a potential for childhood infectious diseases to increase again if immunization is not maintained as a high national priority (Hill, Elam-Evans, Yankey, et al., 2015).

The advent of the HIV has changed care in all areas of nursing but has particular implications for maternal and child health nursing. Sexually active teenagers are at risk for becoming infected with HIV through sexual contact. Infected women may transmit the virus to a fetus during pregnancy through placental exchange or at birth through body secretions (Owen, 2012).

Nurses play a vital role in helping to prevent the spread of HIV by educating adolescents and late adolescents about safer sexual practices (Nachman, Chernoff, Williams, et al., 2012) (see Chapter 5). Follow standard infectious precautions in all areas of nursing practice to safeguard yourself, other healthcare providers, and patients from the spread of this and other infections.

A number of infectious diseases that are increasing in incidence include syphilis; genital herpes; hepatitis A, B, and C; and tuberculosis. The rise in syphilis, hepatitis C, and genital herpes probably stems from an increase in nonmonogamous sexual relationships and lack of safer sex practices. The increase in hepatitis B is due largely to drug abuse and the use of infected injection equipment. One reason for the increase in hepatitis A is shared diaper-changing facilities in day care centers. Tuberculosis, once considered close to eradication, has experienced such a resurgence that one form occurs as an opportunistic disease in HIV-positive persons and is particularly resistant to usual therapy (Hesseling, Kim, Madhi, et al., 2012). Methicillin-resistant *Staphylococcus aureus* is an infection that often occurs in hospitals, causes skin infections or pneumonia, and is also growing in incidence (Moran, Krishnadasan, Gorwitz, et al., 2012).

The incidence of social concerns, such as intimate partner violence and child maltreatment, remains high. Twelve million adults report experiencing intimate partner violence and 10 million children under the age of 18 years experience maltreatment at the hands of a caregiver ranging from neglect to sexual abuse (Sumner, Mercy, Dahlberg, et al., 2015). Pregnant women are at increased risk for adverse maternal and fetal outcomes as a result of intimate partner violence (James, Brody, & Hamilton, 2013):

- 28.4% of pregnant women report experiencing emotional abuse.
- 13.8% of pregnant women report experiencing physical abuse.
- 8% of pregnant women report experiencing sexual abuse.

Also increasing in incidence is autism spectrum disorder, a range of complex neurodevelopment disorders characterized by social impairment, communication difficulty, and repetitive stereotyped patterns of behavior (Dworzynski, Ronald, Bolton, et al., 2012). The estimated prevalence of ASD based on 2014 data was 2.24%, a significant increase from the estimated annualized prevalence of 1.25% based on 2011–2013 data (Zablotsky, Black, Maenner, et al., 2015).

TRENDS IN THE HEALTHCARE ENVIRONMENT

The settings for health care as well as nursing roles are changing, with the goal of being able to better meet the needs of increasingly well-informed and vocal consumers.

Initiating Cost Containment

Cost containment refers to reducing the cost of health care by closely monitoring the costs of personnel, use and brands of supplies, length of hospital stays, inpatient to outpatient ratios as is clinically appropriate, number of procedures carried out, and number of referrals requested while maintaining quality care (Dolopolous, 2016). Examples of delegation responsibility or teamwork to make care more cost-effective or family centered are highlighted in "Interprofessional Care Maps" throughout this text. Examples of effective communication are shown in "Effective Communication" boxes throughout chapters.

Changes in Health Insurance Coverage

Prior to the Affordable Care Act (ACA) in 2010, the United States was unique among developed countries in that its healthcare system was privately financed or controlled by work sites. This contrasts with other countries where national health insurance has been available to everyone and with no connection to a person's employment. Because of this unique system, the United States spent about 17.5% of its gross national product on health care, whereas other countries, for example, Switzerland, spent less yet had healthier citizens (A. B. Martin, Hartman, Benson, et al., 2016). The increase in expenditure is related to the increase in numbers of individuals who have health insurance and obtain healthcare services as a result of the ACA. In the United States, populations most likely to not have health insurance both prior to and after the ACA include late adolescents, individuals who have moved recently or are unemployed, and those who have low incomes. Nurses have important roles at healthcare agencies to ensure people receive comprehensive care and encourage more children and women to receive preventive care.

Increasing Alternative Settings and Styles for Health Care

The past 100 years have seen several major shifts in settings for maternity and child care. At the turn of the 20th century, for example, most births took place in the home, with only the very poor or ill giving birth in "lying-in" hospitals. By 1940, about 40% of live births occurred in hospitals. By 2014, the figure has risen to 98.5%. Out-of-hospital births account for a total of 1.5% of births, with 68% of those occurring in the home and 30.9% occurring in a freestanding birth center. This is the highest rate of home births since 1989 (Hamilton et al., 2015).

This statistic is predicted to increase in the future because increasing numbers of women are choosing home birth or birthing in freestanding alternative birth centers. Women who give birth in these alternative settings feel they have a greater control of their birth experience and their family can be more involved in the birth. Alternative settings also allow more practice opportunities for nurses in advanced practice roles, such as nurse-midwives (Osborne & Hanson, 2012).

An important outcome of this movement is that hospitals have responded to consumers' demands for more natural childbirth environments by refitting labor and delivery suites as homelike birthing rooms, often called labor-delivery-recovery (LDR) or labor-delivery-recovery-postpartum (LDRP) rooms (Fig. 1.6). Partners, family members, and other support people can stay with the woman in labor as if they were home and so can feel a part of the childbirth. Couplet care—care for both the mother and newborn by a primary nurse—is encouraged after the birth. Whether childbirth takes place at home, in a birthing center, or in a hospital, the goal is to keep it as natural as possible while ensuring the protection experienced healthcare providers offer.

Healthcare settings for children are also changing. Patients' homes, community centers, or school-based or retail setting emergent care clinics are examples of places in which comprehensive health care may be administered. Retail clinics or emergent care clinics located in shopping malls are often staffed by nurse practitioners, so nurses play a vital role in seeing such healthcare settings do not limit continuity of care (Rohrer, Garrison, & Angstman, 2012).

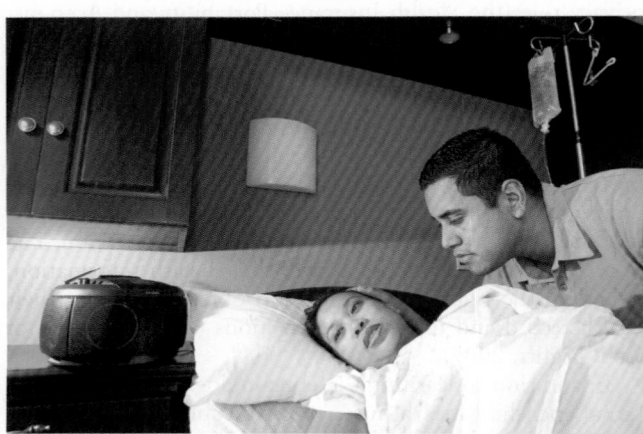

Figure 1.6   A couple, soon to be parents, share a close moment in a birthing room.

In ambulatory settings of this nature, a nurse practitioner may provide immunizations, screenings, health and safety education, counseling, crisis intervention, or parenting classes. This form of community-based care has the potential to provide cost-effective health promotion, disease prevention, and patient care to large numbers of children and families in an environment familiar to them.

More and more, children and women experiencing a pregnancy complication or an acute illness, who might otherwise have been admitted to a hospital, are now being cared for in ambulatory clinics or at home. Separating a child from his or her family during a long hospitalization has been shown to be potentially harmful to the child's development, so any effort to reduce the incidence of separation has a positive effect (see Chapter 36). Avoiding long hospital stays for women during pregnancy is also a preferable method of care because it helps to maintain family integrity.

Ambulatory or non–hospital-based care requires intensive health teaching by the nursing staff and follow-up by home care or community health nurses to ensure a smooth transition to and from this setting. Teaching parents of an ill child or a woman with a complication of pregnancy what danger signs to watch for that will warrant immediate attention includes not only imparting self-care information but also providing support and reassurance that the patient or parents are capable of accomplishing this level of care.

Increasing Use of Technology

The use of technology is increasing in all healthcare settings. The field of assisted reproduction technology such as in vitro fertilization and the possibility of stem cell research are forging new pathways (Palermo, Neri, Monahan, et al., 2012). Charting by computer into electronic health records and monitoring fetal heart rates by Doppler ultrasonography are other examples (Stewart, Letourneau, Masuda, et al., 2011). Using an electronic charting system has the ability to allow different healthcare providers to share information (e.g., an X-ray taken at one site can be reviewed at another, a caregiver can be alerted to all the medicines a pregnant woman has been prescribed). As long as privacy is maintained, the system allows for a coordination of care never before possible.

To protect patient privacy, the DHHS has established a privacy rule (the Health Insurance Portability and Accountability Act, commonly referred to as HIPAA) that creates national standards to protect individuals' medical records and other personal health information and applies to healthcare providers who conduct healthcare transactions electronically. The rule requires appropriate safeguards be put into place to protect the privacy of personal health information and sets limits and conditions on the uses and disclosures that may be made of such information without patient authorization. The rule also gives patients rights over their health information, including the rights to examine and obtain a copy of their health record and to request corrections (DHHS, Office of Civil Rights, 2007).

In addition to learning these technologies and rules, maternal and child health nurses must be able to explain their use and their advantages to patients. Otherwise, patients may find new technologies more frightening than helpful to them.

QSEN Checkpoint Question 1.3

QUALITY IMPROVEMENT

Nurses must always be aware of quality improvement because as society changes with new situations, nursing care must make responding adjustments. Which of the following is a trend that will influence the care that the Chung family's new baby is likely to receive?

a. More and more children are treated in ambulatory, not hospital, settings so nurses will be less significant in the future.

b. Immunizations are available for all childhood infectious diseases so the Chungs' baby will never need treatment for these.

c. The use of multiple technologies can make parents feel overwhelmed unless they receive nursing support.

d. Prematurely born infants, assuming their mother received prenatal care, rarely need long-term or follow-up care.

Look in Appendix A for the best answer and rationale.

Meeting Work Needs of Pregnant and Breastfeeding Women

As many as 90% of women work at least part time outside their home, and many pregnant women want to continue to work during a pregnancy (in many families, women earn more than their spouse or partner, making them the primary wage earner in the family). Following the birth of their child, however, women may want or need a leave from work to care for their newborn.

The Family Medical Leave Act of 1993 is a federal law that requires employers with 50 or more employees to provide a minimum of 12 weeks of unpaid, job-protected leave to employees under four circumstances crucial to family life:

- Birth of the employee's child
- Adoption or foster placement of a child with the employee
- Need for the employee to care for a parent, spouse, or child with a serious health condition
- Inability of the employee to perform his or her functions because of a serious health condition

A serious health condition is defined as "an illness, injury, impairment, or physical or mental condition involving such circumstances as inpatient care or incapacity requiring 3 workdays' absence" (U.S. Department of Labor, 1995). Specifically mentioned in the law is any period of incapacity due to pregnancy or for prenatal care with or without treatment. Illness must be documented by a healthcare provider. Nurse practitioners and nurse-midwives are specifically listed as those who can document a health condition, so they have an equal role with physicians in alerting women to this benefit. Although not as generous a program as many other developed countries, paid leave helps appreciably with the care of an ill child or a woman who is ill during pregnancy.

Whether women should be able to breastfeed at work is a controversial subject for many people (Hojnacki, Bolton, Fulmer, et al., 2012). In 2010, President Obama signed into law the Patient Protection and Affordable Care Act (PPACA), which mandates work settings with more than 50 employees to provide "reasonable break time for a woman to express breast milk for her nursing child for 1 year after the child's birth each time such employee has need to express milk." Employers are also required to provide "a place, other than a bathroom, that is shielded from view and free from intrusion for a setting to express breast milk."

This law has had a major impact on allowing women to continue breastfeeding while working full-time. To support the aim of the law, many employers are now also allowing women to breastfeed at work if doing so does not disrupt their work schedule or work outcome.

Regionalizing Intensive Care

To avoid duplication of care sites, communities are establishing centralized maternal or pediatric health services. Such planning creates one site that is properly staffed and equipped for potential problems rather than a number of lesser equipped sites. When a newborn, older child, or parent is hospitalized in a regional center, the family members who have been left behind need a great deal of support. They may feel they have "lost" their infant, child, or parent unless healthcare personnel can keep them abreast of the ill family member's progress by means of phone calls or snapshots and by encouraging the family to visit as soon as possible.

When regionalization concepts of newborn care were first introduced, transporting the ill or premature newborn to the regional care facility was the method of choice (Fig. 1.7). Today, if it is known in advance that a child may be born with a life-threatening condition, it may be safer to transport the mother to the regional center at the time of birth because the

Figure 1.7 A nurse prepares an infant transport incubator to move a premature infant to a regional hospital. Helping with the safe movement of pregnant women and ill newborns to regional centers is an important nursing responsibility. (© Caroline Brown, RNC, MS, DEd.)

uterus has advantages as a transport incubator that far exceed those of any commercial incubator yet designed.

Important arguments against regionalization for pediatric care include children will feel homesick in strange settings, become overwhelmed by the number of sick children they see, and grow frightened because they are miles from home. An important argument against regionalization of maternal care is that being away from her community and support network places a great deal of stress on the woman and her family and limits her primary care provider's participation in her care. These are important considerations. Because nurses more than any other healthcare group set the tone for hospitals, they are responsible for ensuring patients and families feel as welcome in a regional center as they would have been in a small hospital. Staffing should be adequate to allow sufficient time for nurses to comfort frightened children and prepare them for new experiences or to support a frightened pregnant woman and her family. Documenting the importance of such actions allows them to be incorporated in critical pathways and preserves the importance of the nurse's role (LeFlore, Thomas, Zielke, et al., 2011).

What If . . . 1.1
Melissa Chung has to remain in her local hospital after the birth of her new baby for an extended time while her baby is cared for at a regional center. How could the nurse at the regional center help her keep in touch with her new baby?

Increasing Use of Alternative Treatment Modalities

There is a growing tendency for families to use alternative forms of therapy, such as acupuncture or therapeutic touch, in addition to or instead of traditional healthcare measures. Nurses have an increasing obligation to be aware of complementary or alternative therapies as they have the potential to either enhance or detract from the effectiveness of traditional therapy (D. Adams, Cheng, Jou, et al., 2011). Unfortunately, many nurses (47% to 52%) do not feel comfortable discussing these therapies with their patients (Chang & Chang, 2015).

Healthcare providers who are unaware of the existence of some alternative forms of therapy may lose an important opportunity to capitalize on the positive features of that particular therapy. For instance, it would be important to know that an adolescent who is about to undergo a painful procedure is experienced at meditation because asking the adolescent if she wants to meditate before the procedure could help her relax. Not only could this increase her comfort, but it could also offer her a feeling of control over a difficult situation. People are using an increasing number of herbal remedies, such as drinking herbal teas during pregnancy to relieve morning sickness. Asking about these at a health assessment is important to prevent drug interactions (Dennehy, 2011). Boxes which highlight the importance of both nursing responsibility for pharmacology and respecting cultural diversity are shown in chapters throughout the text to accent these areas of care (Box 1.6).

QSEN Checkpoint Question 1.4

EVIDENCE-BASED PRACTICE

A growing body of knowledge suggests skin-to-skin contact between mother and baby immediately after birth provides numerous benefits, including regulating heartbeat and temperature for the baby and promoting feelings of calm and well-being in both mother and baby. To see if fathers were interested in participating in this form of care (often called kangaroo care), researchers interviewed seven new fathers who had spent time in skin-to-skin interaction with their newborn. Findings showed kangaroo care allowed fathers to feel more in control and also that they were doing something good for their infant (Blomqvist, Rubertsson, Kylberg, et al., 2012).

Based on the previous study, what action would the nurse take?

a. Assess whether Mr. Chung is willing to try skin-to-skin care.

b. Suggest neither parent use skin-to-skin care to prevent infection.

c. Encourage Mr. Chung to praise his wife when she provides skin-to-skin care.

d. Apologize to his wife because men do skin-to-skin care more effectively than women.

Look in Appendix A for the best answer and rationale.

BOX 1.6

Nursing Care Planning to Respect Cultural Diversity

The term *alternative healthcare practices* refers to therapy such as acupuncture, homeopathy, therapeutic touch, herbalism, and chiropractic care, or nontraditional sources of care such as tribal medicine or Hispanic herbalists such as *yerberos* or *curanderos*. Some people seek out these types of therapy or alternative providers before consulting a traditional healthcare provider; others consult with them after they perceive they have received inadequate care by a traditional provider. Still, others rely on these methods as their major form of health care and therapy.

Respect for these forms of care can be instrumental in showing families their sociocultural traditions are important in their plan of care. Assessing what alternative measures are being used is also important because the action of an herb can interfere with prescribed medications. For example, the consumption of traditional ethnic remedies such as *Jin Bu Huan*, a Chinese herbal medicine to relieve pain, can cause adverse effects such as life-threatening bradycardia and respiratory depression. Lead poisoning has resulted from ingestion of *greta*, a traditional Hispanic remedy used as a laxative.

Increasing Reliance on Home Care

Shortened hospital stays have resulted in a transition from hospital to home of many women and children before they are optimally ready to care for themselves. In some instances, ill children and women with complications of pregnancy may choose to remain at home for care rather than be hospitalized. This has created a "second system" of care requiring many additional care providers (Turnbull & Osborn, 2012).

Nurses can be instrumental in assessing women and children at hospital discharge and help them plan the best type of continuing care, devise and modify procedures for home care, and sustain patients' morale so a transition to home is seamless. Home care as a unique and expanding area in maternal and child health nursing is discussed in Chapter 4.

What If . . . 1.2

Melissa Chung demands her 6-year-old, diagnosed with pneumonia, be hospitalized even though it is the clinic's policy to have such children cared for at home by their parents. Would the nurse advocate for hospitalization?

HEALTHCARE CONCERNS AND ATTITUDES

As we progress through the 21st century, there are likely to be even more changes as the United States actively works toward effective health goals and improved health care for all citizens. These steps can create new concerns.

Increasing Concern for Quality of Life

In the past, health care of women and children was focused on maintaining physical health. Today, many patients view quality of life to be as important as physical health, so the scope of health care has expanded to include the assessment of psychosocial facets of life in such areas as self-esteem and independence. Good interviewing skills are necessary to elicit this information at healthcare visits. Nurses can not only help obtain such information but also plan ways to improve quality of life in the areas the patient considers most important.

One way in which quality of life is being improved for children with chronic illness is the national mandate to allow them to attend regular schools, guaranteeing entrance despite severe illness or use of medical equipment such as a ventilator (Public Law 99-452, U.S. 99th Congress, 1986). Under this same law, adolescents who are pregnant cannot be excluded from school. School nurses or nurses asked to be consultants to schools play important roles in honoring these children's rights and making these changes possible.

Increasing Awareness of the Individuality and Diversity of Patients

Maternal and child patients do not fit easily into any set mold. Varying family structures, cultural backgrounds, socioeconomic levels, and individual circumstances lead to unique and diverse patients. Women having children may range in age from 12 or 13 years to women having their first pregnancy after the age of 40 (Johnson & Tough, 2012).

Family structure varies; about 43.9% of babies are born to women outside of marriage. LGBT couples raise families, conceiving children through alternative insemination or adoption. As a result of advances in research and therapy, women who were once unable to have children, such as those with cystic fibrosis, are now able to manage a full-term pregnancy. Individuals with cognitive and physical challenges who once would have been isolated from childbearing are now able to establish families and rear children.

Many families who have emigrated from other countries enter the U.S. healthcare system for the first time during a pregnancy or with a sick child. This requires sensitivity to sociocultural aspects of care on the part of healthcare providers, as people not used to non–government-sponsored health care can easily be lost in the U.S. system. They may have different cultural beliefs about health and illness than their healthcare provider. Some families may live in unsafe neighborhoods and so may not feel safe with home care. All of these concerns require increased nursing attention (see Chapter 2).

What If . . . 1.3
Melissa Chung is concerned because she's already 42 years old and wants to have a third child in a few years. Are many women delaying childbirth until their 40s? Does the nurse anticipate this trend will continue into the future?

Empowerment of Healthcare Consumers

In part because of the influence of market-driven care and a strengthened focus on health promotion and disease prevention, individuals and families have recently begun to take increased responsibility for their own health. For most families, this means learning preventive measures such as following a more nutritious diet and planning regular exercise; for some families, this means adopting an entirely new lifestyle. When a family member is ill, learning more about the illness, participating in the treatment plan, and preventing the illness from returning can offer a sense of empowerment. Parents want to stay with their ill child in the hospital and are eager for information about their child's health and ways they can contribute to the decision-making process. They may question a treatment or care plan if they believe it is not in their child's best interest. If healthcare providers do not provide answers to a patient's questions or are insensitive to needs, many healthcare consumers are willing to take their business to another healthcare setting or rely totally on therapies or information they find from websites (Gallagher, Bell, Waddell, et al., 2012).

Nurses can promote empowerment of parents and children by respecting their views and concerns, regarding parents as important participants in their own or in their child's health, keeping them informed, and helping and supporting them to make decisions about care. Although a nurse may have seen 25 patients already in a particular day, he or she can make each patient feel as important as the first by showing a warm manner and keen interest. Boxes on ways to help empower families at home or at healthcare facilities are shown in following chapters.

QSEN Checkpoint Question 1.5

SAFETY

Mrs. Chung waited until she was 42 years old to have her second baby. She asks the nurse if that is the reason her baby was born prematurely. Which statement would be the most reassuring for her?
  a. "It's hard to say because so few women over 40 years are having babies today."
  b. "No one can say for certain. You did all you could to ensure a healthy pregnancy."
  c. "It's good to see you taking responsibility for your child's prematurity."
  d. "You should ideally have had your children as a teenager as that's the safest time."

Look in Appendix A for the best answer and rationale.

Legal Considerations of Maternal–Child Practice

Legal concerns arise in all areas of health care. Maternal and child health nursing carries some legal concerns above and beyond other areas of nursing because care is often given to patients who are not of legal age for giving consent. Additionally, reproductive healthcare rights and laws are complex and vary from state to state. These issues require specific attention when caring for expectant families. New technologies (e.g., assisted reproduction, surrogate motherhood, umbilical cord sampling, safety of new medicines with children, and end-of-life decisions) can lead to potential legal action, especially if patients are uninformed about the reason or medical necessity for these procedures.

Nurses are legally responsible for protecting the rights of their patients, including confidentiality, and are accountable for the quality of their individual nursing care and that of other healthcare team members. New regulations on patient confidentiality guarantee patients can see their medical record if they choose, but health information must be kept confidential from others (Duffy, 2011). Unfortunately, although nurses recognize the need for patient privacy, it is not practiced at the same rates. Patients are also not aware of the importance for their own medical record privacy (Kim, Han, & Kim, 2016).

Understanding the **scope of practice** (the range of services and care that may be provided by a nurse based on state requirements) and standards of care can help nurses practice within appropriate legal parameters.

Documentation is essential for justifying actions. This concern is long lasting because children who feel they were wronged by healthcare personnel can bring a lawsuit at the time they reach legal age. This means a nursing note written today may need to be defended as many as 21 years into the future. The specific legal ramifications of procedures or care are discussed in later chapters as procedures or treatment modalities are described. Personal liability insurance is strongly recommended for all nurses, so they do not incur great financial losses during a malpractice or professional negligence lawsuit.

Nurses need to be conscientious about obtaining informed consent for invasive procedures in children and determining if pregnant women are aware of any risk to the fetus associated with a procedure or test. A parent can be contacted by phone or e-mail if not present with the child at the time the consent is needed.

In divorced or blended families (those in which two adults with children from previous relationships now live together), it is important to establish who has the right to give consent for health care. Adolescents who support themselves or who are pregnant are frequently termed "emancipated minors" or "mature minors" and have the right to sign for their own health care.

The term "wrongful birth" is the birth of a disabled child whose pregnancy the parents would have chosen to end if they had been informed about the disability during pregnancy. "Wrongful life" is a claim that negligent prenatal testing on the part of a healthcare provider resulted in the birth of a disabled child. "Wrongful conception" denotes that a contraceptive measure failed, allowing an unwanted child to be conceived and born. As many genetic disorders can be identified prenatally, the scope of both "wrongful birth" and "wrongful life" grows yearly (Whitney & Rosenbaum, 2011).

If a nurse knows the care provided by another practitioner was inappropriate or insufficient, he or she is legally responsible for reporting the incident. Failure to do so can lead to a charge of negligence or breach of duty.

QSEN Checkpoint Question 1.6

PATIENT-CENTERED CARE

Melissa Chung is concerned as to how she will give consent for procedures for her newborn baby because the baby is hospitalized so far away. Which statement would be best to reassure her?

a. "Informed consent is not needed for newborn care as newborns are underage."
b. "Newborn care requires parental consent only for procedures that will involve pain."
c. "Healthcare providers can omit informed consent if the parent is not present with the child."
d. "Consent is required: you can be contacted by telephone or e-mail for long distance consultation."

Look in Appendix A for the best answer and rationale.

Ethical Considerations of Practice

Some of the most difficult ethical quandaries in health care today are those that involve children and their families. Examples include:

- Conception issues, especially those related to in vitro fertilization, embryo transfer, ownership of frozen oocytes or sperm, and surrogate motherhood
- Pregnancy termination
- Fetal rights versus rights of the mother
- Stem cell research
- Resuscitation (and length of its continuation)
- Number of procedures or degree of pain a child should be asked to endure to achieve a degree of better health
- Balance between modern technology and quality of life
- Difficulty maintaining confidentiality of records when there are multiple caregivers

Legal and ethical aspects of issues are often intertwined, which makes the decision-making process in this area complex. Because maternal and child health nursing is so strongly family centered, it is common to encounter some situations in which the interests of one family member are in conflict with those of another or the goals of a healthcare provider are different from the family's. Maintaining privacy yet aiding problem solving in these instances can be difficult but is a central nursing role (Kim et al., 2016). Nurses can help patients by providing factual information and supportive listening, and helping the family and healthcare providers clarify their values.

The Pregnant Woman's Bill of Rights and the UN Declaration of Rights of the Child (available at http://thePoint .lww.com/Flagg8e) provide guidelines for determining the rights of women and children with regard to maternal and child health care.

What If . . . 1.4

The nurse is particularly interested in exploring one of the 2020 National Health Goals with respect to maternal and child health (see p. 5). What would be a possible research topic to explore, pertinent to these goals, that would be applicable to the Chung family and could also advance evidence-based practice?

KEY POINTS FOR REVIEW

- Standards of maternal and child health nursing practice have been formulated by the American Nurses Association to serve as guidelines for practice.
- QSEN competencies, combined with the nursing process, provide a sound method of care for expanding areas of practice.
- Nursing research and use of evidence-based practice are methods by which maternal and child health nursing expands and improves.
- The most meaningful and important measure of maternal and child health is the infant mortality rate, which is the number of deaths among infants from birth to 1 year of age per 1,000 live births. This rate is declining steadily, but in the United States, it is still higher than in 25 European countries.
- Trends in maternal and child health nursing include changes in the settings of care, increased concern about healthcare costs, improved preventive care, and family-centered care.
- Practice roles in maternal and child health nursing are expanding rapidly as nurses become more versed in evidence-based practice and technologic skills.
- Maternal and child health care have both legal and ethical considerations and responsibilities over and above those in other areas of practice because of the role of the fetus and child.

CRITICAL THINKING CARE STUDY

Tommy is a 10-year-old who has asthma. He is home schooled after having two serious asthma attacks at school because he is allergic to the cleaning product used in his primary school classroom. His mother is pregnant with a new brother or sister but hasn't come for prenatal care because she noticed the clinic uses the same cleaning solution and doesn't want her new baby to develop an allergy to it. At the same time, she wants a sonogram so she can see if she's having a girl or boy.

1. Nurses work in a wide range of settings in maternal and child health. What actions could you take to help Tommy get back to school and his mother begin to come for prenatal care?

2. Cost containment along with limitations of health insurance make it important for nurses to be aware of the cost of supplies and procedures. Is having a sonogram just to know the sex of a fetus a good use of healthcare funds?

3. Homelessness is becoming an increasing concern in modern society. Suppose Tommy's family became homeless? How do you anticipate this will affect their overall health?

RELATED RESOURCES

Explore these additional resources to enhance learning for this chapter:
- Student resources on thePoint, including answers to the What If . . . and Critical Thinking Care Study questions, http://thepoint.lww.com/Flagg8e
- Adaptive learning powered by PrepU, http://thepoint.lww.com/prepu

REFERENCES

Adams, D., Cheng, F., Jou, H., et al. (2011). The safety of pediatric acupuncture: A systematic review. *Pediatrics, 128*(6), e1575–e1587.

American Nurses Credentialing Center. (2012). *Magnet Recognition Program® model.* Silver Springs, MD: Author.

American Nurses Credentialing Center. (n.d.). *Testimonials & case studies.* Retrieved from http://www.nursecredentialing.org/Magnet/Program Overview/WhyBecomeMagnet/MagnetTestimonials

Benner, P. (2011). Formation in professional education: An examination of the relationship between theories of meaning and theories of the self. *Journal of Medicine and Philosophy, 36*(4), 342–353.

Blomqvist, Y. T., Rubertsson, C., Kylberg, E., et al. (2012). Kangaroo mother care helps fathers of preterm infants gain confidence in the paternal role. *Journal of Advanced Nursing, 68*(9), 1988–1996.

Bridge, J. A., McBee-Strayer, S. M., Cannon, E. A., et al. (2012). Impaired decision making in adolescent suicide attempters. *Journal of the American Academy of Child & Adolescent Psychiatry, 51*(4), 394–403.

Burkhard, A. (2013). A different life: Caring for an adolescent or young adult with severe cerebral palsy. *Journal of Pediatric Nursing, 28*(4), 357–363.

Carpenito, L. J. (2012). *Nursing diagnosis: Application to clinical practice* (14th ed.). Philadelphia, PA: Lippincott Williams & Wilkins.

Centers for Disease Control and Prevention. (2016a). *Overweight and obesity.* Atlanta, GA: Author.

Centers for Disease Control and Prevention. (2016b). *Pregnancy Mortality Surveillance System.* Atlanta, GA: Author.

Centers for Disease Control and Prevention. (2016c). *10 Leading causes of death by age group United States–2014.* Atlanta, GA: Author.

Chang, H. Y., & Chang, H. L. (2015). A review of nurses' knowledge, attitudes, and ability to communicate the risks and benefits of complementary and alternative medicine. *Journal of Clinical Nursing, 24*(11–12), 1466–1478.

Christian, B. J. (2012). Translating research into everyday practice—the essential role of pediatric nurses. *Journal of Pediatric Nursing, 27*(2), 184–185.

Clark, S. (2012). Strategies for reducing maternal mortality. *Seminars in Perinatology, 36*(1), 42–47.

Cronenwett, L., Sherwood, G., & Gelmon, S. B. (2009). Improving quality and safety education: The QSEN Learning Collaborative. *Nursing Outlook, 57*(6), 304–312.

Dennehy, C. (2011). Omega–3 fatty acids and ginger in maternal health: Pharmacology, efficacy, and safety. *Journal of Midwifery & Women's Health, 56*(6), 584–590.

Disch, J. (2012). QSEN? What's QSEN? *Nursing Outlook, 60*(2), 58–59.

Dong, Y., Chen, S. J., & Yu, J. L. (2012). A systematic review and meta-analysis of long-term development of early term infants. *Neonatology, 102*(3), 212–221.

Dopoulos, J. (2016). Hospital cost-containment strategies that earn the respect of rating agencies. *Healthcare Financial Management, 70*(1), 32–35.

Duffy, M. (2011). iNurse: Patient privacy and company policy in online life. *American Journal of Nursing, 111*(9), 65–69.

Dworzynski, K., Ronald, A., Bolton, P., et al. (2012). How different are girls and boys above and below the diagnostic threshold for autism spectrum disorders? *Journal of the American Academy of Child & Adolescent Psychiatry, 51*(8), 788–797.

Falk, J., Wongsa, S., Dang, J., et al. (2012). Using an evidence-based practice process to change child visitation guidelines. *Clinical Journal of Oncology Nursing, 16*(1), 21–23.

Finer, L. B., & Zolna, M. R. (2016). Declines in unintended pregnancy in the United States, 2008–2011. *N Engl J Med, 374*(9), 843–852.

Gallagher, F., Bell, L., Waddell, G., et al. (2012). Requesting cesareans without medical indications: An option being considered by young Canadian women. *Birth, 39*(1), 39–47.

Hedges, C. C., Nichols, A., & Filoteo, L. (2012). Relationship-based nursing practice: Transitioning to a new care delivery model in maternity units. *Journal of Perinatal & Neonatal Nursing, 26*(1), 27–36.

Heron, M. P., Hoyert, D. L., Murphy, S. L., et al. (2009). *Deaths: Final data for 2006* (National Vital Statistics Report Vol. 15, No. 14). Hyattsville, MD: National Center for Health Statistics. Retrieved from http://www.cdc.gov/nchs/data/nvsr/nvsr57/nvsr57_14.pdf

Hess, R., Desroches, C., Donelan, K., et al. (2011). Perceptions of nurses in Magnet® hospitals, non-magnet hospitals, and hospitals pursuing magnet status. *Journal of Nursing Administration, 41*(7–8), 315–323.

Hesseling, A. C., Kim, S., Madhi, S., et al. (2012). High prevalence of drug resistance amongst HIV-exposed and infected children in a tuberculosis prevention trial. *International Journal of Tuberculosis & Lung Disease, 16*(2), 192–195.

Hill, H. A., Elam-Evans, L. D., Yankey, D., et al. (2015). National, state, and selected local area vaccination coverage among children aged 19-35 months—United States, 2014. *Morbidity and Mortality Weekly Report, 64*(33), 889–896.

Hojnacki, S. E., Bolton, T., Fulmer, I. S., et al. (2012). Development and piloting of an instrument that measures company support for breastfeeding. *Journal of Human Lactation, 28*(1), 20–27.

James, L., Brody, D., & Hamilton, Z. (2013). Risk factors for domestic violence during pregnancy: A meta-analytic review. *Violence and Victims, 28*(3), 359–380.

Johnson, J. A., & Tough, S. (2012). Delayed child-bearing. *Journal of Obstetrics & Gynaecology Canada, 34*(1), 80–93.

Junnila, R., Aromaa, M., Heinonen, O. J., et al. (2012). The weighty matter intervention: A family-centered way to tackle an overweight childhood. *Journal of Community Health Nursing, 29*(1), 39–52.

Kim, K., Han, Y., & Kim, J. S. (2016). Nurses' and patients' perceptions of privacy protection behaviours and information provision. *Nursing Ethics.* Advance online publication. doi:10.1177/0969733015622059

LeFlore, J., Thomas, P. E., Zielke, M. A., et al. (2011). Educating neonatal nurse practitioners in the 21st century. *Journal of Perinatal & Neonatal Nursing, 25*(2), 200–205.

MacDorman, M. F., Matthews, T. J., Mohangoo, A. D., et al. (2014). International comparisons of infant mortality and related factors: United States and Europe, 2010. *National Vital Statistics Reports, 63*(5), 1–6.

Machado, L. S. (2012). Cesarean section in morbidly obese parturients: Practical implications and complications. *North American Journal of Medical Sciences, 4*(1), 13–18.

Martin, A. B., Hartman, M., Benson, J., et al. (2016). National health spending in 2014: Faster growth driven by coverage expansion and prescription drug spending. *Health Affairs (Project Hope), 35*(1), 150–160.

Matthews, T. J., MacDorman, M. F., & Thoma, M. E. (2015). Infant mortality statistics from the 2013 period linked birth/infant death data set. *National Vital Statistics Reports, 64*(9), 1–30.

Moon, R.Y. (2016). SIDS and other sleep-related infant deaths: evidence base for 2016 Updated Recommendations for a Safe Infant Sleeping Environment. *Pediatrics, 138*(5).

Moran, G. J., Krishnadasan, A., Gorwitz, R. J., et al. (2012). Prevalence of methicillin-resistant *Staphylococcus aureus* as an etiology of community-acquired pneumonia. *Clinical Infectious Diseases, 54*(8), 1126–1133.

Nachman, S., Chernoff, M., Williams, P., et al. (2012). Human immunodeficiency virus disease severity, psychiatric symptoms, and functional outcomes in perinatally infected youth. *Archives of Pediatric & Adolescent Medicine, 166*(6), 528–535.

National Center for Health Statistics. (2016). *Child health.* Retrieved from https://www.cdc.gov/nchs/fastats/child-health.htm

Orem, D. E., & Taylor, S. G. (2011). Reflections on nursing practice science: The nature, the structure, and the foundation of nursing sciences. *Nursing Science Quarterly, 24*(1), 35–41.

Osborne, K., & Hanson, L. (2012). Directive versus supportive approaches used by midwives when providing care during the second stage of labor. *Journal of Midwifery & Women's Health, 57*(1), 3–11.

Owen, S. M. (2012). Testing for acute HIV infection: Implications for treatment as prevention. *Current Opinion in HIV AIDS, 7*(2), 125–130.

Palermo, G. D., Neri, Q. V., Monahan, D., et al. (2012). Development and current applications of assisted fertilization. *Fertility & Sterility, 97*(2), 248–259.

Papp, L. M. (2012). Longitudinal associations between parental and children's depressive symptoms in the context of interparental relationship functioning. *Journal of Child & Family Studies, 21*(2), 199–207.

Rohrer, J. E., Garrison, G. M., & Angstman, K. B. (2012). Early return visits by pediatric primary care patients with otitis media: A retail nurse practitioner clinic versus standard medical office care. *Quality Management in Health Care, 21*(1), 44–47.

Roy, C. (2011). Research based on the Roy adaptation model: Last 25 years. *Nursing Science Quarterly, 24*(4), 312–320.

Rubin, R. (1963). Maternal touch. *Nursing Outlook, 11*(2), 828–829.

Salsman, J. M., Grunberg, S. M., Beaumont, J. L., et al. (2012). Communicating about chemotherapy-induced nausea and vomiting: A comparison of patient and provider perspectives. *Journal of National Comprehensive Cancer Network, 10*(2), 149–157.

Stewart, M., Letourneau, N., Masuda, J. R., et al. (2011). Online solutions to support needs and preferences of parents of children with asthma and allergies. *Journal of Family Nursing, 17*(8), 357–379.

Sumner, S. A., Mercy, J. A., Dahlberg, L. L., et al. (2015). Violence in the United States: Status, challenges, and opportunities. *JAMA, 314*(5), 478–488.

Turnbull, C., & Osborn, D. A. (2012). Home visits during pregnancy and after birth for women with an alcohol or drug problem. *Cochrane Database of Systematic Reviews*, (1), CD004456.

United Nations. (2000). *Millennium health goals, 2000–2015.* New York, NY: Author.

U.S. 99th Congress. (1986). Public Law 99-452. Congressional Record, 132 (1986): 1.

U.S. Department of Health and Human Services. (2010). *Healthy people 2020.* Washington, DC: Author.

U.S. Department of Health and Human Services, Office of Civil Rights. (2007). *Medical privacy—National standards to protect the privacy of personal health information: The Health Insurance Portability and Accountability Act.* Hyattsville, MD: U.S. Department of Health and Human Services.

U.S. Department of Labor. (1995). The Family and Medical Leave Act of 1993: Final rule. *Federal Register, 60*(4), 2179–2279.

Whitney, D. W., & Rosenbaum, K. N. (2011). Recovery of damages for wrongful birth. *Journal of Legal Medicine, 32*(2), 167–204.

Zablotsky, B., Black, L. I., Maenner, M. J., et al. (2015). *Estimated prevalence of autism and other developmental disabilities following questionnaire changes in the 2014 National Health Interview Survey* (National Health Statistics Report No. 87). Hyattsville, MD: National Center for Health Statistics. Retrieved from https://www.cdc.gov/nchs/data/nhsr/nhsr087.pdf

2

Diversity and Maternal Child Nursing

*M*aria Rodriques is a 12-year-old child who is hospitalized for surgical repair of a broken tibia, which was fractured when she rode her bicycle into a busy street.

In planning care for Maria, you assume, because her culture is Hispanic, her family orientation will be male dominant, her time focus will be on the present, and her nutrition preferences will be Mexican American.

You are surprised on the second day of her hospital stay to hear Maria tell you she feels "second class." Her father has been asked for more input about her care than she has. She hasn't been given any milk to drink so is worried her bone will not heal. She's concerned she won't be able to play soccer by next month, but no one else seems worried about that.

The previous chapters described the standards and philosophy of maternal and child health nursing. This chapter adds information on caring for families from diverse cultures as well as sexual and gender identities. Such information can both enrich care and help improve the health of childbearing and childrearing families.

If you had really planned care in this way, of what would you have been guilty? What would have been a better approach for determining Maria's cultural preferences?

KEY TERMS

acculturation
assimilation
bisexual
cisgender
cultural awareness
cultural competence
cultural humility
cultural values
culture
culture-specific values
culture universal values

discrimination
diversity
ethnicity
ethnocentrism
gay
gender dysphoria
gender expression
gender identity
heterosexual
homosexual
lesbian

minority
mores
norms
prejudice
race
sex assigned at birth
stereotyping
taboos
transcultural nursing
transgender
transition

OBJECTIVES

After mastering the contents of this chapter, you should be able to:

1. Identify common areas or concerns relating to cultural diversity, sexual orientation, and gender identity and apply these to nursing practice.

2. Identify 2020 National Health Goals related to diversity considerations and specific ways nurses can help the nation achieve these goals.

3. Assess a family for aspects of cultural diversity that might influence the way the family responds to childbearing and childrearing.

4. Assess a family for the ways in which sexual orientation or gender identity may affect how a family responds to childbearing and childrearing.

5. Formulate nursing diagnoses related to culturally influenced aspects of nursing care.

6. Develop outcomes to assist families who have specific cultural and sociodemographic needs so they can thrive in their community as well as manage seamless transitions across different healthcare settings.

7. Using the nursing process, plan nursing care that includes the six competencies of Quality & Safety Education for Nurses (QSEN): Patient-Centered Care, Teamwork & Collaboration, Evidence-Based Practice (EBP), Quality Improvement (QI), Safety, and Informatics.

8. Implement nursing care to assist a family adapt to today's changing sociocultural environment.

9. Evaluate expected outcomes for achievement and effectiveness of care to be certain that expected outcomes have been achieved.

10. Integrate aspects of cultural diversity with the interplay of nursing process, the six competencies of QSEN, and Family Nursing to achieve quality maternal and child health nursing care.

Diversity in a population means there is a mixture or variety of sociodemographic groups, experiences, and beliefs in the population. **Culture** is a view of the world and a set of traditions a specific social group uses and transmits to the next generation. The United States is an example of a country with varied ethnic and racial backgrounds, cultural groups, sexual orientations and gender identities, and socioeconomic conditions, so you are likely to see a wide range of behaviors and family structures exhibited in any healthcare setting.

Families have evolved dramatically from a nuclear family with male and female parents with children. Families can be multigenerational or single parent, and they can have same-sex parents or friends of parents as parental figures. Families can be recombined through divorce. Children can be adopted, fostered, or biologically related to the parental figures (Fig. 2.1).

Cultural differences occur across not only different ethnic backgrounds but also different sociodemographic groups (Gagné,

Frohlich, & Abel, 2015). Adolescents, urban youth, those with hearing impairment, and gay, or lesbian, or transgender couples have separate cultures from the mainstream, and respecting these cultures is just as important as respecting ethnic differences. A parent who has been deaf since birth, for example, expects her deaf culture to be respected by having healthcare professionals locate a sign language interpreter for her while she is in labor. A lesbian mother will want to be asked, "Is your partner or wife here?" rather than, "Is your husband here?" at a well-child visit.

Assessing for diverse backgrounds and beliefs of families and patients can reveal why people choose the type of preventive health measures they do or why they seek a particular type of care. Nurses also need to be mindful when doing research to include all cultural and sociodemographic groups in research samples, so more can be learned about cultural preferences in relation to nursing interventions and care. Box 2.1 shows 2020 National Health Goals that reference cultural and sociodemographic influences on health care.

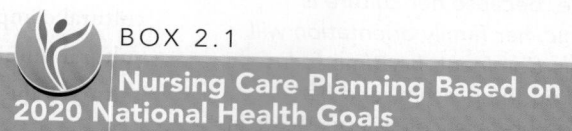

BOX 2.1

Nursing Care Planning Based on 2020 National Health Goals

A number of 2020 National Health Goals are directly concerned with health practices that can be influenced by cultural diversity and lesbian, gay, bisexual, and transgender (LGBT) health:

- Increase the proportion of pregnant women who receive early and adequate prenatal care from a baseline of 70.5% to a target of 77.6%.
- Increase the proportion of mothers who breastfeed their babies in the early postpartum period from a baseline of 43.5% to a target of 60.6%.
- Increase the proportion of healthy full-term infants who are put down to sleep on their backs from a baseline of 69.0% to a target of 75.9%.
- Increase the proportion of young children who receive all vaccines that have been recommended for universal administration from a baseline of 68% to a target of 80%.
- Reduce the rate of suicide from 11.3 per 100,000 to 10.2 per 100,000, a 10 % decrease.
- Reduce the adolescent suicide attempt rate from 1.9 per 100 to 1.7 per 100, a 10% decrease.
- Increase the proportion of homeless people who suffer with mental illness who are able to receive mental health services from 37% to 41% (U.S. Department of Health and Human Services, 2010; see www.healthypeople.gov).

Nurses can help the nation achieve these goals by helping design prenatal and childcare services that take into account cultural diversity and LGBT health and by promoting the nutritional and immunologic advantages of breastfeeding in a culturally competent manner.

Figure 2.1 Various cultural preferences are evident in childrearing. Many extended family members, such as grandparents, are the primary caregivers today.

What If . . . 2.1

When the nurse talks to Mrs. Anna Rodriques, the nurse determines she is pregnant but hasn't gone for prenatal care yet. She states before coming to the clinic she wants to visit a *yerbero* who will both predict her child's sex and guarantee a safe birth. Would recommending she have a sonogram (which also could predict the fetal sex) likely be as satisfying for her?

Nursing Process Overview

FOR CARE THAT RESPECTS CULTURAL DIVERSITY

ASSESSMENT

An assessment of cultural diversity factors is important so care can be planned based not on predetermined assumptions but on the actual preferences of a family. Remember, poverty is a major problem for many minority ethnic groups. Many characteristic responses described as cultural limitations are actually the consequences of poverty (e.g., parents seeking medical care for their children late in the course of an illness or a woman not taking prenatal vitamins during pregnancy). Solving these problems may be a question of locating adequate financial resources and may not be related to cultural differences.

To assess patients for aspects of diversity, assess them as individuals, not as one of a group. Note particularly any cultural characteristic that differs from the usual expectations of your care setting, so potential conflicts can be acknowledged and culturally competent care can be planned. Specific areas to assess, along with suggested questions to help explore these areas, are shown in Table 2.1. Sexual orientation and gender identity content are discussed later in this chapter.

NURSING DIAGNOSIS

Several nursing diagnoses speak to the consequences of ignoring cultural preferences in care, including:

- Powerlessness related to expectations of care not being respected
- Impaired verbal communication related to limited English proficiency
- Imbalanced nutrition, less than daily requirements, related to unmet cultural food preferences
- Anxiety related to a cultural preference for not wanting to bathe while ill
- Fear related to possible ethnic discrimination

OUTCOME IDENTIFICATION AND PLANNING

Planning needs to be very specific for individual families because cultural diversity preferences tend to be very personal. You might want to begin care with an in-service education for team members who are unfamiliar with a particular cultural practice and its importance to a specific family involved. You also might want to ask if your agency could change a policy to accommodate a family's cultural preferences, such as the length of visiting hours, types of food served, or type of hospital clothing provided (e.g., women from the Middle East may only feel comfortable in long-sleeved gowns and with head scarves).

This type of planning can be beneficial not only because it makes health care more acceptable to families but also because it can motivate providers to examine policies, question the rationale behind them, and initiate more diverse care.

ONLINE RESOURCES

Resources for Diversity Education

National Association of Hispanic Nurses	www.nahnnet.org
National Black Nurses Association	www.nbna.org
Transcultural Nursing Society	www.tcns.org
National Coalition of Ethnic Minority Nurse Associations	http://www.ncemna.org /associations.htm
The Joint Commission *Advancing Effective Communication, Cultural Competence, and Patient- and Family-Centered Care for the Lesbian, Gay, Bisexual, and Transgender (LGBT) Community: A Field Guide*	https://www.jointcommission .org/lgbt/
World Professional Association for Transgender Health	http://www.wpath.org/

TABLE 2.1 ASSESSING FOR CULTURAL VALUES

Area of Assessment	Questions to Ask or Observations to Make
Ethnicity	Where were the parents and grandparents born? What ethnicity does the family state is theirs?
Communication	What's the main language used in the home?
Touch	Does the family typically touch or hug each other? Do they mainly use intimate or conversational space?
Time	Is being on time important? Is planning for the future important?
Pain	Do family members express pain or remain stoic in the face of it? What do family members believe best relieves pain?
Family structure	Is the family nuclear? Extended? Single parent? Are the parents same sex? Are family roles clear?
Male and female roles	Is the family male or female dominant? What is the patient's gender identity and what pronouns does he or she use?
Religion	What is the family's religion? Do members actively practice? Will any of their beliefs directly affect your care or their treatment?
Health beliefs	What does the family believe makes one healthy? Causes illness? Makes illness better? Do members use alternative therapies or traditional medical practices?
Nutrition	Does the family mainly eat ethnic foods? Are the foods they enjoy easily available in their community?
Community	Is the predominant culture in the community the same as the family's? Can members name a neighbor they could call on in a crisis?

IMPLEMENTATION

When implementing care, be certain not to force your cultural values on others. Appreciate that such values are ingrained and usually very difficult to change (in yourself as well as in others). An example of implementing care might be to make arrangements for a new Native American mother to take home the placenta after birth of her child if that is important to her, or planning home care for a Chinese American child whose family uses herbal medicine. It might be to establish a network of healthcare agency personnel or personnel from a nearby university or importing firm to serve as interpreters. It might be educating a child, family, or community about the reason for a hospital practice. Don't feel that you or your healthcare agency are always the ones who must adapt; however, a particular situation may call for both sides to adjust (cultural negotiation).

OUTCOME EVALUATION

Assessing whether expected outcomes have been met should reveal that a family's diversity preferences have been considered and respected during care. If this was not achieved, procedures or policies may need to be modified until this can be realized. Examples of expected outcomes that might be established include:

- Parents list three ways they are attempting to preserve cultural traditions in their children.
- Child states she no longer feels socially isolated because of her family's differences.
- Family members state they have learned to substitute easily purchased foods for traditional but unavailable foods to obtain adequate nutrition.
- Child with severe hearing impairment writes that he feels communication with ambulatory care staff has been adequate.
- Adolescent patient states he is ready to tell family about gender identity or sexual orientation.

Methods to Respect Diversity in Maternal and Child Health Nursing

Almost all nations have a set of people who are its dominant or advantaged group. They hold the greater share of wealth in the nation and hold the majority of political offices. Almost all nations also have **minority** or disadvantaged groups, groups not necessarily fewer in number but who hold less power and wealth.

It's important to avoid stereotyping and assumptions rooted in accepting the dominant group as the norm; it can prevent you from planning care that is accurate, individualized, and valued. At the same time, it is important not to ignore cultural characteristics in an attempt to not stereotype, because most people take pride in their cultural heritage.

- **Stereotyping** is expecting a person to act in a characteristic way without regard to his or her individual traits.
- **Prejudice** is a negative attitude toward members of a group or is an intellectual act.
- **Discrimination** is the action of treating people differently based on their physical or cultural traits or is a doing act.

Cultural differences cause behavior to vary widely from one community to another. Given the multicultural mix in large communities, almost any behavior can be considered appropriate for some individuals at some time and place. The way people respond to pain is another example of a trait that is heavily influenced by culture. Some women and children scream with pain; others remain stoic and quiet. Both are "proper" responses, just culturally different.

Stereotyping is generally derogatory in nature such as "Men never diaper babies well" or "Japanese women are never assertive." The phenomenon usually occurs because of lack of exposure to people in a particular group and, consequently, a lack of understanding of the wide range of differences among people. Traditionally, a person whose culture differs most drastically from the dominant culture suffers the greatest amount of rejection or prejudice because they are least able to assimilate (Bergsieker, Leslie, Constantine, et al., 2012). In the previous examples, the first speaker, having seen one man change diapers poorly, assumes he represents the entire male population. The second speaker demonstrates lack of knowledge of a changing culture.

You can acknowledge and celebrate a patient's culture without stereotyping by such actions as respecting a patient's cultural needs when completing a nutrition assessment or ensuring a patient has the opportunity to perform her cultural traditions during labor, such as reciting a Hispanic lullaby to "call her child outside."

It is also important to acknowledge sexual- and gender-based diversity. Assessing for sexual orientation is not appropriate as a routine part of every health assessment. However, it should be included when relevant, such as when discussing adolescent development or before providing reproductive life planning information, during pregnancy, and after childbirth. Gender identity can greatly impact how a person feels during a standard health assessment. Therefore, it is a good idea to assess for these needs as a routine part of providing care.

When scanning a list of characteristics typically seen with people of a specific culture or sociodemographic group, the key is to remember those behaviors may not apply at all to your patient. *Ask* what things are important to the individual.

Understanding Cultural Diversity in Maternal and Child Health Nursing

In the past, the United States was viewed as a giant cultural "melting pot," where all new arrivals gave up their native country's traditions and values and became Americans. Today, many people question the idea that America was ever a melting pot; instead, the preferred concept is of a "salad bowl," in which cultural traditions and values are tossed together but with all their individual crispness and flavor retained.

Maintaining ethnic traditions this way strengthens and enriches family life. It provides security to younger family members as they realize they are one of a continuing line of people who have a past and will have a future (Fig. 2.2 and Box 2.2). Women are often called the "keepers of the culture" or the people most influential in passing on cultural traditions from one generation to another and in honoring the many cultural traditions of childbirth and childrearing (Lauderdale, 2015).

Figure 2.2 Cultural traditions passed from one generation to the next offer a sense of security to children.

CULTURAL COMPETENCY FOR NURSES

Transcultural nursing is care guided by cultural aspects and respects individual differences (Darnell & Hickson, 2015). Nursing care is about improving the health of individuals and populations. Developing cultural competency is an important aspect of complete care for patients. Box 2.3 addresses cultural competency terminology for nurses.

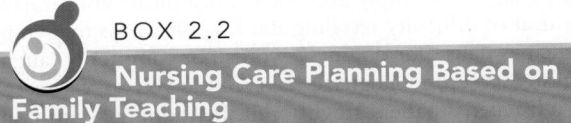

BOX 2.2
Nursing Care Planning Based on Family Teaching

PRESERVING A FAMILY'S CULTURAL HERITAGE

Q. Mrs. Rodriques tells you, "I'm proud of my family's ethnic traditions. What are good ways to help my family preserve these?"

A. Preserving individual heritage traditions while living in another culture calls for creative planning. Some common suggestions for doing this include:

- Plan an "ethnic night" once per week when only ethnic food is served. Encourage children to invite friends for the meal and discuss the traditions behind the various foods.
- Reserve one night per week when family members speak only the native language, if a foreign language is part of your tradition, so children come to value both languages.
- Choose books for children written by authors from your culture or that positively describe your culture. Read them together as a family and discuss the story.
- Monitor television for programs that focus positively on your culture. Watch them with your children and comment on how such traditions enrich family life.
- Speak to your children about your childhood and traditions and values at bedtime or "talk time," so they can appreciate how long these values have been revered by your family.
- Celebrate holidays in your traditional manner. Including cultural influences in holiday celebrations adds a rich ingredient and feeling of security to these occasions.

QSEN Checkpoint Question 2.1

QUALITY IMPROVEMENT

While she is in the hospital, Maria Rodriques, 12 years old, makes the following statements. The nurse determines which statement most clearly suggests she received culturally competent care?

  a. "My doctor is funny; he tells jokes and makes me laugh."
  b. "The nurses keep asking me who makes decisions in my family."
  c. "I'm sure my leg will heal quickly; the nurse said I'm an overall healthy person."
  d. "The nurse asked me what I like to eat and then brought me the taco I wanted."

Look in Appendix A for the best answer and rationale.

The way people react to health care is a cultural value (Chen, Wei, Yeh, et al., 2013). **Cultural values** are preferred ways of acting based on cultural traditions (Giger, 2016). They often arise from environmental conditions (in a country where water is scarce, daily bathing is not valued; in a country where meat is scarce, ethnic recipes use little meat).

BOX 2.3
Cultural Competency Terminology for Nurses

- **Culture-specific values** are norms and patterns of behavior unique to one particular culture.
- **Culture universal values** refers to values, norms, and patterns shared across almost all cultures.
- **Ethnicity** refers to the cultural group into which a person was born, although the term is sometimes used in a narrower context to mean only race.
- **Race**, a social construct, refers to a category of people who share a socially recognized physical characteristic, often skin color or facial features. It can also refer to a group of people who share the same ancestry.
- **Acculturation** refers to the loss of ethnic traditions because of disuse.
  - Cultural **assimilation** means people blend into the general population or adopt the values of the dominant culture.
  - **Ethnocentrism** is the belief one's own culture is superior to all others.
  - **Cultural awareness** is being aware cultural differences exist.
  - **Cultural competence** is respecting cultural differences or diversity.
  - **Cultural humility** is a lifelong process of self-reflection and self-critique that begins, not with an assessment of a patient's beliefs, but rather with an assessment of your own.

Source: Darnell, L. K., & Hickson, S. V. (2015). Cultural competent patient-centered nursing care. *The Nursing Clinics of North America*, 50(1), 99–108; and Gallagher, R. W., & Polanin, J. R. (2015). A meta-analysis of educational interventions designed to enhance cultural competence in professional nurses and nursing students. *Nurse Education Today*, 35(2), 333–340.

They form early in life and strongly influence the manner in which people plan for childbearing and childrearing as well as the way they respond to health and illness (Mireles-Rios & Romo, 2014). Differing cultural values can be a major source of conflict between parents and children because children learn opposing values from friends and school peers. Nurses can be instrumental in helping relieve this type of conflict by always including a cultural assessment at a healthcare visit (Yang, Kuo, Wang, et al., 2014).

The usual values of a group are termed **mores** or **norms**. Expecting women to come for prenatal care and parents to bring children for immunizations are examples of norms in the United States, but these are not beliefs worldwide or even among all Americans (Tangherlini, Roychowdhury, Glenn, et al., 2016).

Actions not acceptable to a culture are called **taboos**. Three universal taboos are murder, incest, and cannibalism. Issues such as abortion, robbery, and lying are controversial taboos because these are taboos only to some people, not everyone. For instance, some cultures do not put emphasis on individual property ownership and therefore would not understand the concept of robbery. Other cultures will put social harmony, appeasing the other person, at a higher priority than the absolute truth.

A great deal of ethnocentrism has existed because of intolerance toward any behavior that was not like white, middle-class Americans, and a belief that the American way (which actually was the Northern European way) was the "best" way. A more modern philosophy is that the world is large enough to accommodate a diversity of ideas and behaviors, and that there is probably no "best" way to accomplish anything.

Numerous levels of cultural intolerance or acceptance persist because people hold different beliefs along a cultural competence continuum (Fig. 2.3). When planning nursing care, try to not only respect these cultural differences but also help people share their cultural beliefs with their entire care team so that their preferences will be considered and respected.

COMMUNICATION PATTERNS

Communication patterns (not only what people say but also how they say it) are influenced strongly by culture.

Language

Communication problems can arise from both translation difficulties and from dialect differences within a country. Something as simple as a New Englander adding an "r" sound to the end of words (saying "idear" instead of "idea") can make an explanation difficult to follow for a non–New Englander. The slow cadence of a person from the South may seem strange to someone who is used to the rapid speech pattern of New York City residents. African American Vernacular English may be used by Black patients who often have a dialect unique to their area. To care for such patients, learn their dialect's cadence and common words but don't attempt to use them yourself, unless that is your dialect. Trying to speak in a dialect not your own could be misinterpreted as mockery.

When caring for patients who speak a different dialect or language than your own, always ask them to repeat your instruction to be certain it was interpreted correctly. Repeat what the patient said so he or she can confirm you understood correctly. Don't be reluctant to ask for an interpreter to help clarify forms, such as informed consent for surgery or wishes regarding right-to-life care, as necessary.

People who ordinarily associate only with members of their own culture, and therefore always speak their native language, can have great difficulty detailing a health history in English when they are or their child is ill because their ability to cope and to express themselves in any language when they are stressed may be at a low point (Meuter, Gallois, Segalowitz, et al., 2015). Some patients prefer to consult a Chinese herbalist or a Hispanic *yerbero* or *curandero* rather than or in connection with other healthcare providers because they can relate health problems with no language barrier.

Children who are embarrassed or bashful about speaking another language may simply not talk at a healthcare visit or have a great deal of difficulty recalling the English words for symptoms such as nausea or dizziness, words not commonly taught in English as a second language class. Unless you appear receptive as a listener, a patient might omit mentioning a symptom rather than try to pantomime it or describe it in a different way.

Listening to English instructions and translating them into another language is another area that can cause confusion. The statement "I need you to wait," for example, is easy to translate as "I need your weight."

Working with an interpreter also can cause miscommunication. General tips for working with interpreters are shown in Box 2.4. It is unacceptable to have a family member serve as an interpreter. There may be cultural limitations that change how the information you are stating is being interpreted for a parent or partner. Additionally, the medical terminology used in the healthcare system is best translated by a trained professional interpreter.

Be certain cultural variations are as respected in written communications as they are in oral communications. In many instances, written communication is even more problematic

CULTURAL DESTRUCTIVENESS	CULTURAL BLINDNESS	CULTURAL AWARENESS	CULTURAL SENSITIVITY	CULTURAL COMPETENCE	CULTURAL HUMILITY
Making everyone fit the same cultural pattern and excluding of those who don't fit—forced assimilation. Emphasis on differences as barriers.	Do not see or believe there are cultural differences among people. Everyone is the same.	Being aware that we all live and function within a culture of our own and that our identity is shaped by it.	Understanding and accepting different cultural values, attitudes, and behaviors.	The capacity to work effectively and with people, integrating elements of their culture—vocabulary, values, attitudes, rules, and norms. Translation of knowledge into action.	The lifelong process of self-reflection and self-critique that begins, not with an assessment of a client's belief but rather an assessment of your own.

Figure 2.3 A cultural competence continuum.

BOX 2.4

Nursing Care Planning to Empower a Family

WHEN A FAMILY HAS LIMITED ENGLISH PROFICIENCY

1. Many people can speak a second language better than they can read it. Assess each patient's reading level as well as speaking level and rewrite information at an easier level if necessary.
2. Ask an interpreter to translate and copy material into the family's primary language as necessary so it can be clearly understood.
3. Be certain rooms in your healthcare agency, such as bathrooms, are labeled with international symbols that do not require reading ability.
4. Learn a few phrases, such as "Good morning" or "This won't hurt," from other languages and use them in interactions with patients to show you're receptive to participating in solving language difficulties.
5. Use hand gestures or draw a figure, if need be, to help ensure productive communication. Imparting health information is what is important for safe care, not worrying how you look.
6. When using an interpreter, do not ignore the person seeking health care in preference to the interpreter. Observe facial expressions for confirmation that a person understands instructions. Use short sentences; avoid slang words that don't interpret accurately.

than oral communication because many people can speak a second language but cannot write or read it. Using short, easy sentences and being certain not to use words with double meanings when writing instructions for patients are important techniques (Box 2.5).

QSEN Checkpoint Question 2.2

TEAMWORK & COLLABORATION

Maria Rodriques is a 12-year-old student. What advice should the nurse provide to an unlicensed care provider about communicating effectively with Maria?
  a. "Speak in a clear and natural tone when you're talking with Maria."
  b. "Maria is Hispanic, so avoid talking about current children's movies."
  c. "Maria's first language is Spanish, so avoid talking about difficult topics."
  d. "If possible, try to speak to Maria in an accent that's similar to hers."

Look in Appendix A for the best answer and rationale.

Nonverbal Communication

Some people gesture wildly to express any topic; others rarely raise their hands. Whether people look at one another when talking is also culturally determined. Chinese Americans, for example, may not make eye contact during a conversation. This social custom shows respect for the position of the

BOX 2.5

Nursing Care Planning Tips for Effective Communication

Anna Rodriques, Maria's mother, brings her 4-year-old son to your pediatric clinic because she thinks he has an ear problem. She speaks minimal English, and a neighbor, who speaks English and Spanish has accompanied her to provide assistance.

Tip: It is not appropriate to use a family member or friend to provide interpretation for a non–English-speaking patient/parent. A medical interpreter is used because a family member or friend may not understand medical words well enough to interpret them correctly. In this scenario, the nurse should call the hospital interpreter line to assist with communication. Effectively using an interpreter adds additional responsibility to history taking.

Nurse: [addressing the neighbor] I appreciate your taking the time to assist Mrs. Rodriques with her visit today. To ensure I get all the information correct and she understands our instructions, I am going to call a medical interpreter who will assist us by phone.

Neighbor: That would be helpful.

Nurse: [addressing the medical interpreter on the phone line] Would you ask Mrs. Rodriques what concerns she has about her son?

Mrs. Rodriques: [through the interpreter] I saw him sticking something in his ear and now it hurts.

Nurse: [through the interpreter] When did this happen?

Mrs. Rodriques: [through the interpreter] Yesterday; there was some blood on his pillow this morning. I hope he didn't damage his ear.

Nurse: [through the interpreter] I will let the nurse practitioner know. Let me take his temperature and get his weight. Are there any other concerns that you have?

Mrs. Rodriques: [through the interpreter] No, he seems fine otherwise. I just want his ear checked.

Neighbor: I am glad you got the interpreter as she told me there was blood on the pillow this morning, but I didn't know he stuck something in his ear. I thought he may have had an ear infection.

healthcare professional and is a compliment, not an avoidance issue.

Touch, such as whether to greet another person with a kiss or a hug, is a form of communication and thus is culturally determined. Some people don't like to be hugged. Some prefer to bow in contrast to shaking hands. Some Asian Americans feel rumpling the hair or palpating fontanelles is an intrusive gesture because they believe the head is the seat of the body's spirit and should not be touched (Andrews, 2015).

Tattoos are becoming more commonplace in the United States and therefore more accepted. Tattoos are often meaningful for the patient. It is important that nursing care reflects respect for individual differences in body modification (Liszewski, Kream, Helland, et al., 2015).

Use of Conversational Space

People of different cultures use the space around them differently:

- *Intimate space* is the space closely surrounding a person. Physical examinations are conducted in this very tight space because palpation and auscultation are parts of the examination.
- Conversational space is usually 18 in. to 4 ft away.
- Beyond 4 ft is *business space*, as this amount of distance allows room for a desk between parties.
- *Public space* is any distance beyond business space such as shouting across a parking lot. Use of the Internet or telephone can vary from private space ("I have a secret to tell you") to public space (conversation in a chat room).

Everyone has had the uncomfortable experience of speaking to someone who moves closer to him or her than expected or invades his or her intimate space while talking. Likewise, everyone has had someone shout something he or she wanted to be kept confidential (violation of public space). Being aware that the use of space can vary from person to person helps you to respect the use of space for patients when giving health instructions.

Respect for modesty is another way to respect a patient's space. Be aware that women from Middle Eastern cultures adhere to a level of modesty exceeding what you may appreciate, so it's a courtesy to add additional modesty sheets for physical examinations.

TIME ORIENTATION

The cultural pattern in the United States is geared toward punctuality regarding appointments. "Time is money" is an often-quoted axiom. In some South Asian cultures, however, the use of time contrasts greatly—being late for appointments is a sign of respect (giving the person you are meeting time to organize and be prepared for your arrival). Other cultures believe time is to be enjoyed. For such a person, there is no such thing as wasted time.

Women who do not have a strict time orientation may have difficulty following a strict medical regimen. If they are told, for example, to give a child a medication at 8 AM, noon, and 6 PM daily and to return for another appointment at 2 PM in a week's time, you may need to stress that the medication should be taken three times a day, not necessarily at the specific times, but returning for a checkup at a set time is important because their primary healthcare provider is only available at that time.

Another way time orientation differs is in whether a culture concentrates on the past, the present, or the future. The dominant U.S. culture is oriented to the present and future. People are expected to not only take care of themselves in the present but also make plans for the future. Other cultures are oriented toward the past: They carefully preserve traditions, allowing only the slightest changes or variations in practices. Still, others are oriented toward the present; saving money for college (a future-oriented action) might seem important to you but would not be a high priority in these cultures.

If a family's orientation is for the present or the past, members may have difficulty accepting a long-term rehabilitation plan. They may need to be motivated by indications of progress (e.g., last week, all their child could do was sit up; today, he was able to walk two or three steps).

People with strong religious convictions may be future oriented (looking forward to a future existence better than their present one on Earth). The Amish and some Native Americans are examples of past-oriented cultures: They adhere to time-honored traditions that do not include technologic advances. People from lower socioeconomic groups tend to be present oriented because the struggle just to get through each day limits them to the present. People with different time orientations tend to make different healthcare decisions based on their outlook (Boyle, 2015).

FAMILY STRUCTURE

The way families structure themselves and the roles family members play are yet a further area that is culturally determined. In most cultures, the nuclear family is most common. In other cultures, extended families and single-parent families may be more desired or common (see Chapter 3 for family structures).

Some cultures stress that family boundaries should be carefully guarded or information about a family should not be given freely at healthcare visits (a way of keeping the family intact and unique and perhaps also as a reflection of mistrust of outside influences). Other families willingly share the same information. When caring for children, be certain to identify a child's primary caregiver before asking what the child likes or giving healthcare instructions because which family member cares for the child can vary by culture.

CONCEPTS OF MALE AND FEMALE ROLES

In many cultures, the man is the dominant figure. In a strongly male-dominant culture, if approval for hospital admission or therapy is needed, the man would prefer to give this approval. A woman might be unable to offer an opinion of her own health or be too embarrassed to submit to a physical examination from a male healthcare provider unless a female nurse was also present. Some women insist on female-only providers for all aspects of care. A woman's pregnancy may have resulted not from a mutual decision but from sexual relations she felt she could not refuse (Martin-de-las-Heras, Velasco, de Dios Luna, et al., 2015). The incidence of intimate partner violence may be higher in male-dominant cultures and may rise even higher with pregnancy (Donovan, Spracklen, Schweizer, et al., 2016). See Chapter 55 for an in-depth discussion of intimate partner violence and how it increases with any type of stress situation.

As a contrast, in some cultures, women are the dominant person in their family. The oldest woman in the home may be the one to give consent for treatment or hospital admission.

Evaluating male and female roles this way can help you understand the impact of illness on a family. If a woman is the family's dominant person and can no longer make her usual decisions because she is ill during pregnancy, for example, the entire family can be thrown into confusion. If the woman is a nondominant member, you may have to act as an advocate for her with a more dominant partner (Darnell & Hickson, 2015).

What If . . . 2.2
Mr. Rodriques says he wants no role in labor when his wife, Anna, has her new baby. Would the nurse encourage him to time contractions (a typical role for fathers) or allow him to sit quietly in a corner of the room as he prefers?

RELIGION AND SPIRITUALITY

There are wide variations in religious and spiritual practices, and many of these are culturally determined. Because religion guides a person's overall life philosophy, it influences how people feel about health and illness, what foods they eat, and their preferences about birth and death rituals (Whitley, 2016). Knowing which religion a family practices can help you locate the correct religious support person if one is needed. It helps in planning care if you know a woman or adolescent wants a time or times set aside daily for private prayer or if they intend to fast, such as during Ramadan. It guides implementation because many practices, such as whether the family eats meat, what and when holidays are celebrated, whether ill newborns should be baptized, and what clothing is proper to wear in public, are all dictated by religious beliefs. It also can have important implications for decision making during a difficult pregnancy or for childhood terminal care.

HEALTH BELIEFS

Even health beliefs are not universal. For example, most people are familiar with the current controversy about whether male circumcision is necessary. More surprising to many people is the belief that, in some cultures, female genital cutting (amputation of the clitoris and perhaps a portion of the vulva) is practiced. Although, as outsiders, this practice seems like a poor health decision, there is often acceptance of it and an expectation that it will be done for all females in the culture (Farage, Miller, Tzeghai, et al., 2015).

The cause of illness is another area strongly culturally influenced. People in developed countries, for example, understand that illness is caused by documented factors such as bacteria, viruses, or trauma. In other cultures, illness may be viewed primarily as a punishment from God, the effect of an evil spirit, or as the work of a person who wishes harm to the sick person.

People who believe their own sins caused an illness may not be highly motivated to take medication or other measures to get well again since they do not believe penicillin can cure them. People with such beliefs may receive more comfort from a spiritualist or counselor than from their primary healthcare provider. Another consequence may be reluctant to ask for pain medication if they believe the pain is necessary to be rid of the illness. Understanding different beliefs of this kind allows you to better work out mutual goals even when opposing beliefs are present. Box 2.6 shows an interprofessional care map illustrating how compromise may be necessary in both nursing and team planning in order to respect cultural diversity.

QSEN Checkpoint Question 2.3

SAFETY

Maria tells the nurse she rates the pain she has from bruising as 5 on a 10-point scale. The nurse offers to bring her a tablet of acetaminophen (Tylenol). Her grandmother produces a packet of herbs from her purse and says, "Good. I'll give her a family remedy along with that." The nurse recognizes

which statement is the most culturally respectful response?

   a. "Wonderful. I'm sure herbs will complement what your doctor prescribed."
   b. "I wouldn't bother with that. Drugs are much more likely to be effective."
   c. "Good. I understand you people often use home cures for many things."
   d. "Let's check first to be certain the herbs won't cause an interaction."

Look in Appendix A for the best answer and rationale.

Pregnancy is an area where illness concepts vary widely, as women's concepts of whether pregnancy is a time of wellness or illness and whether breastfeeding is a desired choice differ a great deal across the world (Jones, Power, Queenan, et al., 2015). Most American women, for example, visit healthcare facilities early in pregnancy, follow prenatal directives, and at birth, allow a healthcare provider to supervise the birth. In other cultures, pregnancy and childbearing are considered such natural processes that a healthcare provider is unnecessary. The woman knows the special rules and taboos she must follow to ensure a safe birth and depends on close friends rather than healthcare providers to guide her safely through labor and birth. She may plan to breastfeed until the next child is born or for as long as 5 years. Unless differences such as these are respected, it is difficult to plan prenatal or newborn care that meets individual women's needs.

The type of therapy people choose to restore health is also dependent on culture. When a parent notices a child has an upper respiratory infection, for example, he or she may immediately call a healthcare provider for a formal prescription. Another parent will depend on an herbal or "natural" self-help method. Be aware when taking health histories that many people today from all cultures rely on complementary or alternative therapies. Knowing about these is a way to be certain a medication that has been prescribed will not counteract or be synergistic with what herbs are being used (Pallivalappila, Stewart, Shetty, et al., 2014).

What If . . . 2.3

The Rodriques family tells the nurse they believe the accident that caused Maria's broken leg was "God's will," not Maria's fault. How would the nurse address patient education about street safety without interfering with the family's cultural beliefs?

QSEN Checkpoint Question 2.4

INFORMATICS

The nurse is including Maria's nursing care plan with her discharge instructions so a visiting community nurse can make her change from reduced activity to full sports participation as seamless as possible.

BOX 2.6

Nursing Care Planning

AN INTERPROFESSIONAL CARE MAP FOR A CHILD NEEDING CULTURAL DIVERSITY CONSIDERATIONS

Maria Rodriques is a 12-year-old child who is hospitalized following surgical repair of a broken tibia, which was fractured when she rode her bicycle into a busy street. She has a cast on her right leg, bruising on her body, and is being evaluated for a concussion. She will be on bed rest for 3 days and then allowed to learn crutch walking.

Family-Centered Assessment: Maria lives with her mother, Anna; her father, Carlos; and a 4-year-old brother, Jose. She attends a local grade school and enjoys playing video games and reading Harry Potter books. Her mother is 4 months pregnant.

Patient-Centered Assessment: Temperature, 99.4°F; pulse, 86 beats/min; respirations, 24 breaths/min. Observed lying on side, gritting teeth as if in pain. Hands clenched and eyes tearing. When asked if she has pain, she stated, "No. I'm okay." Father patted her arm and said to her, "We're proud you're so brave." Cast on right leg dry and intact. Toes warm to touch. Intravenous fluid infusing without difficulty. Oral intake primarily tea and soup. Patient's mother states, "She needs 'hot' foods to get better. Can't she have some mangos?"

Nursing Diagnosis: Pain related to tissue trauma of surgery, with cultural belief to not voice pain

Outcome Criteria: Patient accepts pain medication when offered; nonverbal expressions of pain are minimal to absent. Patient begins to eat and manage self-care.

Team Member Responsible	Assessment	Intervention	Rationale	Expected Outcome
Activities of Daily Living, Including Safety				
Nurse/physical therapist	Assess what self-care activities child feels ready to begin.	Plan a program of self-care possible within constraints of limited ambulation.	Ability to complete self-care can add to self-esteem and supply physiologic benefits.	Patient feeds self, is out of bed in 3 days, and completes hygiene measures at 12-year-old level.
Teamwork and Collaboration				
Nurse/pain management team	Assess pain level on a 1–10 scale. Determine what child feels would relieve pain best.	Consult with pain management team to establish a pain management plan for patient.	Optimal health care is a collaborative practice.	Child states pain management plan is acceptable to her. Rates her pain level as below 2 on a 1–10 scale.
Procedures/Medications for Quality Improvement				
Nurse	Assess for both verbal and nonverbal indicators of pain.	Offer pain medication as prescribed before pain becomes acute.	Offering medication relieves the patient of the responsibility to ask for relief. It also allows her to have some choice and control in her care.	Child's chart documents pain medication was offered every 4 hours during waking hours.
Nutrition				
Nurse/nutritionist	Assess whether the child has food preferences that are not being met by hospital service.	Encourage the family to bring in foods from home that meet child's cultural preferences.	Allowing the family to bring in foods demonstrates respect for their culture and increases the child's sense of security and being cared for.	Patient increases nutrient intake by including foods brought from home.

Patient-Centered Care

Nurse	Assess the child's knowledge of broken bones and bruising and why trauma leads to head concussions.	Explain the physiology of injuries to child so she understands why she has pain.	Explanations help a child of this age minimize fear.	Patient states she understands her injuries and why hospitalization is necessary; states asking for something to relieve pain is expected and acceptable.

Spiritual/Psychosocial/Emotional Needs

Nurse	Assess whether child has unmet needs other than pain relief.	Explain to child you want to help, but she needs to verbally express her needs to enable you to do so.	Children may imagine healthcare providers are all knowing.	Child agrees to participate in expressing the presence of other factors, such as loneliness or fear.

Informatics for Seamless Healthcare Planning

Nurse	Assess with child what modifications she thinks she will need to make to adjust to cast after returning home.	Help parents plan adjustments their child may need in order to return to school (transportation, etc.).	Well-informed parents and children are able to make informed decisions.	Child attends school daily because of modifications she has made in usual lifestyle.

Which aspect of her care planning could be regarded as an act of discrimination?
  a. Documenting the fact that Maria's mother is responsible for making most of the family's decisions.
  b. Cautioning against Maria's participation in the local soccer league because she is unlikely to fit in.
  c. Adding to her electronic health record a list of foods Maria does not eat because of her preference for Mexican American dishes.
  d. Documenting the fact that Maria's priest plays an important role in the family's spiritual life.

Look in Appendix A for the best answer and rationale.

NUTRITION PRACTICES

Foods and their methods of preparation are yet another area strongly related to culture. In many instances, children cannot find any food on a hospital menu that appeals to them because of cultural likes or dislikes. A typical Japanese diet, for example, includes many vegetables such as bean sprouts, broccoli, mushrooms, water chestnuts, and alfalfa. Both children and adults with this preference tire quickly of the macaroni and cheese that is common to a middle-class American menu. Fortunately, in most instances, a family member can provide food that is appealing culturally and is still within prescribed dietary limitations.

When counseling a woman about nutrition during pregnancy, remember that respect for culturally preferred foods is important (Brunst, Wright, DiGioia, et al., 2014). People from other cultures, for example, tend to eat much less meat than those from the United States. Adequate protein is ingested, however, by mixing sources of incomplete protein such as beans and rice. Some women may omit various foods during pregnancy because they believe a particular food will mark a baby (eating strawberries will cause birthmarks, eating raisins will cause brown spots) or they believe it is necessary to eat "hot" or "cold" foods to ensure optimal fetal growth. Pregnancy is usually considered a "hot" condition, so it may be difficult for a woman who is trying to eat only "cold" foods to agree to increase her intake of meat, usually considered a "hot" food. Asian women may believe in a similar pattern of required balances (yin and yang).

Before beginning nutrition counseling, try to learn what the dominant type of food that is stocked in stores in the community of your healthcare agency because women who cannot buy the foods you recommend in their own neighborhood may not eat well because of the inconvenience (and increased cost) involved in shopping elsewhere (Fig. 2.4).

Figure 2.4 Families select different foods and family customs because of cultural diversity preferences.

PAIN RESPONSES

A person's response to pain is both individually and culturally determined (Boissoneault, Bunch, & Robinson, 2015). Although people may all have the same *threshold sensation* (the amount of stimulus that results in pain), their *pain threshold* (the point at which the individual reports a stimulus is painful) and *pain tolerance* (the point at which an individual withdraws from a stimulus) vary greatly.

These differences are so great, one woman in labor might report her contractions as "agonizing" each time she feels one, whereas a woman in the room next to her, experiencing the same degree of sensation, might barely change her facial expression and report her pain as tolerable. It is important to assess each person individually because there are so many possible responses to pain. Strategies to help recognize cultural influences on pain management or degree of pain include:

• Appreciate that the meaning of pain varies among people and cultures.
• Appreciate that people do not all communicate or express their level of pain in the same way.
• Recognize that the communication of pain may not be acceptable within a culture.
• Develop an awareness of your personal values and beliefs as they may affect how you respond to people in pain.
• Use an assessment tool, such as a 1-to-10 scale, to assist in measuring pain so you are certain you are being as objective as possible (Giger, 2016).

Assessing differing responses to pain that occur because of cultural differences is an important nursing role. Further assessment of pain and its meaning to people is discussed in Chapters 16 and 39.

What If . . . 2.4

The nurse is particularly interested in exploring one of the 2020 National Health Goals with respect to cultural diversity (see Box 2.1). What would be a possible research topic to explore, pertinent to this goal that would be applicable to Maria's family and also would advance evidence-based practice?

Understanding Sexual Orientation in Maternal and Child Health Nursing

There are some major barriers for healthcare providers when caring for individuals who are different from them. One of these barriers is the potential for personal bias. This barrier can only be addressed through self-reflection, trying to understand why these differences might bother you, and setting those feelings aside while taking care of patients. The other major barrier is language. Nurses need to know the right words to describe patients and to discuss their differences with them so that they don't feel threatened. These two issues, self-reflection and expanding knowledge and vocabulary, are key parts of becoming a culturally competent nurse.

Understanding sexual orientation is part of providing culturally competent health care. There are three main types of sexual orientation: heterosexual, homosexual, and bisexual. See Box 2.7 for important terminology for nurses.

DEVELOPMENT OF SEXUAL ORIENTATION

It is not yet known how sexual orientation develops, although there is evidence that sexual orientation is genetically determined or develops due to the effect of estrogen or testosterone in utero. Even before puberty, most individuals attracted to the same gender realize they are "different" in that they are not interested in opposite-sex classmates.

It is during adolescence, in seeking a sense of identity, that they realize the reason they feel "different" is because they are lesbian, gay, or bisexual (LGB). This can cause additional stress during adolescent development because revealing their sexual orientation to family and friends or "coming out" may be difficult. There are high rates of homelessness (22% of homeless youth are LGB) and suicide (suicide attempts were present in up to 70% of surveyed LGB individuals) among LGB adolescents (Flentje, Leon, Carrico, et al., 2016; Miranda-Mendizábal, Castellví, Parés-Badell, et al., 2017). Part of the reason these high rates occur may be because LGB teenagers don't know where to turn for help in a heterosexual-dominant culture (Castellanos, 2016; McDermott, 2015). Although attitudes are changing, some people refuse to associate with LGB

BOX 2.7

Sexual Orientation Terminology for Nurses

Heterosexual: A heterosexual person is someone who finds sexual fulfillment with a member of the opposite gender. Straight is often used in place of heterosexual.

Homosexual: A homosexual person is someone who finds sexual fulfillment with a member of his or her own sex. This term is often disparaged in the LGB community. Same-sex partner and gay (for men or women) can be umbrella terms to use instead of homosexual.

Gay: Male-identified individuals who are sexually attracted to male partners. This term is also sometimes used to refer to both men and women who have same-sex partners.

Lesbian: Female-identified individuals who are sexually attracted to female partners.

MSM*: Men who have sex with men.

WSW*: Women who have sex with women.

Bisexual: People are bisexual if they achieve sexual satisfaction from both same-sex and heterosexual relationships.

*Both men who have sex with men (MSM) and women who have sex with women (WSW) include individuals who may not self-identify as gay or homosexual but who may have sex with people of the same gender. They are also terms used in medical or public health publications instead of the terms *homosexual*, *gay*, or *lesbian*.

people to such an extent that the fear-based term *homophobia* exists (Herek, 2015).

HEALTHCARE BARRIERS BASED ON SEXUAL ORIENTATION

Although LGB people often have demonstrated behaviors consistent with an LGB identity from early childhood, late adolescence is the time most persons begin to identify as LGB and when they are ready to reveal this to healthcare providers. LGB patients may be hesitant to reveal their sexual orientation to healthcare providers because they are often the victims of bullying, family rejection, and sexual assault.

In one study, 30% of LGB patients had a negative experience with a healthcare provider because of their sexual orientation (Macapagal, Bhatia, & Greene, 2016). Because of expected or actual discrimination in the healthcare setting, LGB individuals may enter care late and may be at increased risk for adverse health conditions, including sexually transmitted infections (STIs), unwanted pregnancy, and mental health issues (Knight & Jarrett, 2017). They may also need help or suggestions for communicating with friends or family who are having difficulty accepting their sexual orientation. It is important for healthcare providers to be extremely sensitive to these needs.

Men who have sex with men (MSM) may need counseling to help them avoid acquiring HIV and other STIs because issues such as avoiding contact through anal intercourse or vaccination against hepatitis A and human papillomavirus

(HPV) may not be routinely covered in sex education classes (King, Gilson, Beddows, et al., 2015).

There is also a belief that women who have sex with women (WSW) are at much lower risk for contracting STIs. Although there may be a lower incidence of HIV in this population, there is still risk for HPV and herpes simplex virus (HSV) as these are transmitted via skin-to-skin contact. Additionally, WSW may use sex toys that can transmit infection between partners. WSW are inadequately screened for STIs and pap smears because of this inaccurate belief (Agénor, Muzny, Schick, et al., 2017).

Growing a family as an LGB patient is common and is accomplished through multiple routes. Female partners may use sperm donation from a known or unknown partner to achieve pregnancy. They can use intrauterine insemination at home or with a fertility specialist. They may also achieve pregnancy through in vitro fertilization. Sometimes, only one partner carries the fetus; other times each partner has one or more pregnancies to complete their families (Yeshua, Lee, Witkin, et al., 2015). Male partners may use their own sperm and an egg donor. Sometimes, that egg donor carries the pregnancy as well; other times, a third person is involved called a gestational carrier, or surrogate, who shares none of her genetic material with the baby but carries and delivers the baby (Fig. 2.5) (Blake, Carone, Raffanello, et al., 2017). Additionally, adoption is a common course of action couples use to grow their families.

Additional barriers exist for LGB families. Many couples will pursue a second parent adoption. This means an extra cost in the form of legal fees are required to ensure that each parent will have rights to custody and care of the child. Birth certificates vary by state with regard to who is listed as parent to the child. Same-sex couples may face stigma from healthcare professionals, their family, or the public as they try to grow their family, attend prenatal care, and deliver or attend the delivery of their babies. Although rare, there have been instances of doctors refusing to care for the children of same-sex parents (Phillip, 2015). A meta-analysis of Nordic women's experience as same-sex couples seeking prenatal care found that they had anxiety about discussing their sexual orientation for fear of change in the quality of care they would receive from their provider (Wells & Lang, 2016).

Figure 2.5 Some couples seek a surrogate to assist with childbearing. (iStock.com/oscarhdez.)

QSEN Checkpoint Question 2.6

EVIDENCE-BASED PRACTICE

Parenting by same-sex couples and child outcomes has often been questioned. A study looked at 43 female same-sex couples, 52 male same-sex couples, and 95 different-sex couples who were all parents. The couples were matched for demographic qualities. No differences were found in the children's well-being, the parent–child relationships, or use of professional or informal support by the parents (Bos, Kuyper, & Gartrell, 2017). Sofia Garcia, who is a 28-year-old lesbian and Maria's aunt, presents for prenatal care with her mother. Her mother states that the baby will have problems because there is no man in the house.

Based on this study, which statement helps the nurse address Sofia's mother's concerns?
a. "The child will have male influence through his or her grandfathers."
b. "Children raised in same-sex parent houses do just as well as children raised with different sex parents."
c. "Every family faces challenges in raising their children. This will just be another challenge that they will encounter."
d. "Do you feel Sofia will not do a good job raising her child?"

Look in Appendix A for the best answer and rationale.

COMMUNICATION RELATED TO SEXUAL ORIENTATION

Assuming anything about patients is a barrier to good communication. When asking about a patient's needs, ask about the patient's partner or partners. Once information is gathered about the gender of the patient's partner or partners, make sure to tailor education to the patient's specific needs. A nurse can build trust and ensure the individual will return for care as needed by

BOX 2.8

Gender Identity Terminology for Nurses

Cisgender: when an individual feels their gender and their sex match
Transgender: when an individual feels their gender and their sex do not match
MTF: male-to-female transition; usually prefers female pronouns
FTM: female-to-male transition; usually prefers male pronouns
Hormone replacement therapy: use of estrogens and antiandrogens for MTF individuals and testosterone for FTM individuals to gain characteristics of their gender identity
Gender affirmation surgery: surgical procedures to change body characteristics to match an individual's gender identity

using neutral terminology and asking what the patient needs. It is important to address mental and social healthcare needs in this population given the incidence of bullying, victimization, and mental health issues (Knight & Jarrett, 2017).

The Joint Commission has recommendations for changes that can be made across organizations to increase effective communication with LGB patients. Rewriting policy to include LGB populations or incorporating new language into existing policy is an important step. Adopting a nondiscrimination policy and having that policy posted clearly for employees and visitors can help ease the anxiety LGB families may feel. Visiting policies should reflect changing families, and a patient should be able to name his or her support people, independent of his or her support person's legal status as a spouse or adoptive parent. There should also be clear pathways to report any discrimination against LGB families (The Joint Commission, 2011).

Understanding Gender Identity in Maternal and Child Health Nursing

A person has both a sexual orientation and a gender identity. There are multiple terms related to gender identity that are important for nurses to know, see Box 2.8.

Gender identity is the inner sense a person has of being male or female, which may be the same as or different from sex assigned at birth. **Sex assigned at birth** is usually based on a person's chromosomal sex: male (XY) or female (XX). There have been cases of individuals born intersex, with ambiguous genitalia, where sex was assigned based on a provider's assessment of the genitalia alone. **Gender expression** refers to the behavior a person exhibits, which may or may not be the same as the person's gender identity or sex assigned at birth. Sexual orientation and gender identity are separate from each other. Just like a cisgender man could be attracted to women (heterosexual) or men (gay), a transgender man could also be attracted to women (heterosexual) or men (gay).

DEVELOPMENT OF GENDER IDENTITY

A **transgender** person is an individual whose gender identity does not match the sex assigned at birth (Unger, 2015). There is not much information about the development of gender identity. **Gender dysphoria** is the realization one's physical sex and gender are mismatched, which can cause a lot of stress and anxiety.

Young children may start to notice they feel different from others, especially in the cultural context of gendered toys and clothes (Rodgers, 2017). An important way to increase open communication with children who are transitioning is to discuss what gender they identify with and which pronouns they would like the nurse to use when addressing them. They also may choose a new name that feels more in line with their gender. Addressing them by their preferred name and preferred pronouns will build trust.

Parents of transgender children often need support and guidance as they struggle with changes in their family. They may benefit from family therapy and support groups. Children who are transgender may do better with social pressure and bullying if they have a supportive family who affirms their gender. Families can find support through organizations like PFLAG (www.pflag.org) and the Human Rights Campaign (www.hrc.org) (Human Rights Campaign, 2016).

Transgender people will often go through **transition**, where they begin to live as the gender they feel they are. Many will seek a provider who can provide them with hormone replacement therapy to attain the characteristics of their gender.

Some may also choose to have gender affirmation surgery (previously termed *sex change operations*) so they appear cosmetically as the sex they feel they really are. They may have top and bottom surgery or just top surgery. Top surgery refers to having the breasts removed or breast implants placed. Bottom surgery refers to having a vagina or penis created. A person may choose to only have top surgery because bottom surgery can complicate the ability to enjoy sex. Others may choose bottom surgery because having the genitalia of the wrong sex can interfere with their ability to enjoy sex or enjoy life (Gorton & Erickson-Schroth, 2017). Surgical options may also be limited by the cost of care as not all insurance companies will cover these procedures. A female-to-male (FTM) transgender individual who decides not to have bottom surgery will still need regular gynecologic care, such as pap smears, and he may be able to carry a pregnancy.

HEALTHCARE BARRIERS BASED ON GENDER IDENTITY

Just as LGB individuals are the victims of bullying, sexual assault, and societal isolation, transgender individuals are often more marginalized. Transgender women face twice the victimization rates that cisgender women do (Sterzing, Ratliff, Gartner, et al., 2017). Transgender individuals have higher rates of negative experiences in healthcare settings than their LGB or heterosexual counterparts (Macapagal et al., 2016).

FTM transgender individuals may seek pregnancy and find it difficult to obtain an understanding provider, one who they can trust and who can care for their specific needs related to pregnancy, gender dysphoria, and lactation (MacDonald, Noel-Weiss, West, et al., 2016). It is necessary to stop testosterone hormone therapy to successfully carry a pregnancy. The cessation of testosterone and the changes that occur with pregnancy (growing belly, increased mammary tissue if still present) can cause huge shifts in an individual's mental well-being and can lead to increased gender dysphoria (Obedin-Maliver & Makadon, 2016). Although pregnancy progression and delivery are essentially the same for FTM transgender patients as for any other pregnant patient, there are more considerations related to mental health, chest (breast) feeding, and when to reinitiate testosterone therapy after delivery. Listing of gender on birth certificates and legal protections for partners may be additional barriers to consider for transgender patients (Tornello & Bos, 2017).

COMMUNICATION RELATED TO GENDER IDENTITY

With transgender patients, just as with any other patient, it is important not to make assumptions. A patient may be listed as a sex that they don't agree with on their medical chart. It is best to ask which pronouns (he, she, his, her) to use. A partner's gender should not be assumed either. It is crucial for a nurse to ask these questions to show sensitivity to this population's needs and to build trust with the patient.

KEY POINTS FOR REVIEW

- Culture is an organized structure that guides behavior into acceptable ways for a group of people. Usual customs are termed *mores* or *norms*. Actions that are not acceptable to a culture are termed *taboos*.
- *Stereotyping* is expecting a person to act in a characteristic way without regard to his or her individual traits. *Prejudice* is *thinking* people are different in some way. *Discrimination* involves *treating* people differently based on their physical or cultural traits.
- Each culture differs to some degree from every other. Most people are proud of these differences or cultural traits.
- Cultural practices usually arise from environmental conditions and are transmitted by both formal and informal ways from generation to generation.
- Although cultural concepts adapt from time to time, they tend to remain constant among tight-knit populations.
- There is wide variation within a culture concerning values and actions because individuals make up the group and individually express their cultural heritage.
- People bring cultural values and beliefs to nursing interactions, and these affect nursing and health care.
- Cultural aspects that are important to assess are communication patterns; use of conversational space; response to pain; time, work, and family orientation; and social organization including nutrition, family roles, and health beliefs.
- LGB individuals can experience discrimination because of their sexual orientation. They are less likely to receive adequate health care because of perceived or actual bias by the healthcare profession.
- Transgender individuals often face social stressors and healthcare barriers. Transgender individuals will benefit from gender-affirming behaviors from family and healthcare providers.
- Because of social stigma surrounding sexual orientation and gender identity, lesbian, gay, bisexual, and transgender (LGBT) individuals have much higher rates of homelessness, suicide attempts, and victimization.
- Parents of LGBT children will need extra support to adapt to their children's changing needs.
- Considering cultural diversity when caring for a family not only meets QSEN competencies but also best meets the family's total needs.

CRITICAL THINKING CARE STUDY

Rhea Bhaskar is a 32-year-old woman, 20 weeks pregnant, whom you meet at a prenatal clinic. She works as a computer programmer for a wicker import company. She has a 12-year-old daughter from a previous marriage. She has been married to Siddharth, who sells real estate for 6 months. Rhea is concerned because they have just moved to a new community and her daughter (whose father was Black) "hates" their new house and her new school; she also feels as if she "doesn't fit in." She no longer likes to eat at home because Rhea has begun using Indian spices, such as curry, when she cooks to please her new husband. Rhea asks you if cooking more "soul food" the way she used to would make her daughter feel more like part of her family and new community. Rhea is also not pleased with her prenatal clinic; when she said she wanted rhubarb tea as her only fluid to drink during labor, wanted silence during the birth, and to keep her placenta to be turned into capsules for her to take afterward, the charge nurse told her she could not give her the placenta as that would be against infection rules and rhubarb tea wasn't on their list of approved beverages.

1. Rhea is trying to integrate two cultures. Will changing only one thing, such as preparing food differently, make a difference in how her 12-year-old feels about fitting in with their new lifestyle? What are other suggestions you might make to help her daughter adapt to a new family lifestyle?

2. Was the nurse accurate when she said taking a placenta home would be against infection guidelines? Were Rhea's other requests so difficult to carry out that a birth center couldn't adapt to meet them?

3. Rhea's daughter feels she's different than other children at her school. What ideas could you suggest to Rhea to help her daughter better adjust to her new school and community?

RELATED RESOURCES

Explore these additional resources to enhance learning for this chapter:
- Student resources on thePoint, including answers to the What If . . . and Critical Thinking Care Study questions, http://thepoint.lww.com/Flagg8e
- Adaptive learning powered by PrepU, http://thepoint.lww.com/prepu

REFERENCES

Agénor, M., Muzny, C. A., Schick, V., et al. (2017). Sexual orientation and sexual health services utilization among women in the United States. *Preventative Medicine, 95*, 74–81.
Andrews, M. M. (2015). Culturally competent nursing care. In M. M. Andrews & J. S. Boyle (Eds.), *Transcultural concepts in nursing care* (7th ed., pp. 30–54). Philadelphia, PA: Wolters Kluwer.
Bergsieker, H. B., Leslie, L. M., Constantine, V. S., et al. (2012). Stereotyping by omission: Eliminate the negative, accentuate the positive. *Journal of Personality and Social Psychology, 102*(6), 1214–1238.
Blake, L., Carone, N., Raffanello, E., et al. (2017). Gay fathers' motivations for and feelings about surrogacy as a path to parenthood. *Human Reproduction, 32*, 860–867.
Boissoneault, J., Bunch, J. R., & Robinson, M. (2015). The roles of ethnicity, sex, and parental pain modeling in rating of experienced and imagined pain events. *Journal of Behavioral Medicine, 38*(5), 809–816.
Bos, H. M., Kuyper, L., & Gartrell, N. K. (2017). A population-based comparison of female and male same-sex parent and different-sex parent households. *Family Process*. Advance online publication. doi:10.1111/famp.12278
Boyle, J. S. (2015). Culture, family & community. In M. M. Andrews & J. S. Boyle (Eds.), *Transcultural concepts in nursing care* (7th ed., pp. 317–358). Philadelphia, PA: Wolters Kluwer.
Brunst, K. J., Wright, R. O., DiGioia, K., et al. (2014). Racial/ethnic and sociodemographic factors associated with micronutrient intakes and inadequacies among pregnant women in an urban US population. *Public Health Nutrition, 17*(9), 1960–1970.
Castellanos, H. D. (2016). The role of institutional placement, family conflict, and homosexuality in homelessness pathways among Latino LGBT youth in New York City. *Journal of Homosexuality, 63*(5), 601–632.
Chen, Y. C., Wei, S. H., Yeh, K. W., et al. (2013). Learning strengths from cultural differences: A comparative study of maternal health-related behaviors and infant care among Southern Asian immigrants and Taiwanese women. *BMC International Health and Human Rights, 13*(1), 5.
Darnell, L. K., & Hickson, S. V. (2015). Cultural competent patient-centered nursing care. *The Nursing Clinics of North America, 50*(1), 99–108.
Donovan, B. M., Spracklen, C. N., Schweizer, M. L., et al. (2016). Intimate partner violence during pregnancy and the risk for adverse infant outcomes: A systematic review and meta-analysis. *British Journal of Gynaecology, 123*(8), 1289–1299.
Farage, M. A., Miller, K. W., Tzeghai, G. E., et al. (2015). Female genital cutting: Confronting cultural challenges and health complications across the lifespan. *Women's Health, 11*(1), 79–94.
Flentje, A., Leon, A., Carrico, A., et al. (2016). Mental and physical health among homeless sexual and gender minorities in a major urban US city. *Journal of Urban Health, 93*(6), 997–1009.
Gagné, T., Frohlich, K. L., & Abel, T. (2015). Cultural capital and smoking in young adults: Applying new indicators to explore social inequalities in health behaviour. *European Journal of Public Health, 25*(5), 818–823.
Giger, J. N. (2016). *Transcultural nursing: Assessment and intervention* (7th ed.). St. Louis, MO: Elsevier.
Gorton, R. N., & Erickson-Schroth, L. (2017). Hormonal and surgical treatment options for transgender men (female-to-male). *The Psychiatric Clinics of North America, 40*(1), 79–97.
Herek, G. M. (2015). Beyond "homophobia": Thinking more clearly about stigma, prejudice, and sexual orientation. *The American Journal of Orthopsychiatry, 85*(5 Suppl.), S29–S37.
Human Rights Campaign. (2016). *Supporting & caring for transgender children*. Washington, DC: Gabe Murchison.
Jones, K. M., Power, M. L., Queenan, J. T., et al. (2015). Racial and ethnic disparities in breastfeeding. *Breastfeeding Medicine, 10*(4), 186–196.
King, E. M., Gilson, R., Beddows, S., et al. (2015). Human papillomavirus DNA in men who have sex with men: Type-specific prevalence, risk factors and implications for vaccination strategies. *British Journal of Cancer, 112*(9), 1585–1593.
Knight, D. A., & Jarrett, D. (2017). Preventive health care for women who have sex with women. *American Family Physician, 95*(5), 314–321.
Lauderdale, J. (2015). Transcultural perspectives in childbearing. In M. M. Andrews & J. S. Boyle (Eds.), *Transcultural concepts in nursing care* (7th ed., pp. 120–152). Philadelphia, PA: Wolters Kluwer.
Liszewski, W., Kream, E., Helland, S., et al. (2015). The demographics and rates of tattoo complications, regret, and unsafe tattooing practices: A cross-sectional study. *Dermatologic Surgery, 41*(11), 1283–1289.
Macapagal, K., Bhatia, R., & Greene, G. J. (2016). Differences in healthcare access, use, and experiences within a community sample of racially diverse lesbian, gay, bisexual, transgender, and questioning emerging adults. *LGBT Health, 3*(6), 434–442.
MacDonald, T., Noel-Weiss, J., West, D., et al. (2016). Transmasculine individuals' experiences with lactation, chestfeeding, and gender identity: A qualitative study. *BMC Pregnancy and Childbirth, 16*, 106.
Martin-de-las-Heras, S., Velasco, C., de Dios Luna, J., et al. (2015). Unintended pregnancy and intimate partner violence around pregnancy in a population-based study. *Women and Birth, 28*(2), 101–105.
McDermott, E. (2015). Asking for help online: Lesbian, gay, bisexual and trans youth, self-harm and articulating the "failed" self. *Health, 19*(6), 561–577.
Meuter, R. F., Gallois, C., Segalowitz, N. S., et al. (2015). Overcoming language barriers in healthcare: A protocol for investigating safe and effective communication when patients or clinicians use a second language. *BMC Health Services Research, 15*, 371.
Miranda-Mendizábal, A., Castellví, P., Parés-Badell, O., et al. (2017). Sexual orientation and suicidal behaviour in adolescents and young adults: Systematic review and meta-analysis. *The British Journal of Psychiatry*. Advance online publication. doi:10.1192/bjp.bp.116.196345
Mireles-Rios, R., & Romo, L. F. (2014). Latina daughters' childbearing attitudes: The role of maternal expectations and education communication. *Developmental Psychology, 50*(5), 1553–1563.
Obedin-Maliver, J., & Makadon, H. J. (2016). Transgender men and pregnancy. *Obstetric Medicine, 9*(1), 4–8.
Pallivalappila, A. R., Stewart, D., Shetty, A., et al. (2014). Complementary and alternative medicine use during early pregnancy. *European Journal of Obstetrics, Gynecology, and Reproductive Biology, 181*, 251–255.
Phillip, A. (2015, February 19). Pediatrician refuses to treat baby with lesbian parents and there's nothing illegal about it. *The Washington Post*. Retrieved from https://www.washingtonpost.com/news/morning-mix/wp/2015/02/19/pediatrician-refuses-to-treat-baby-with-lesbian-parents-and-theres-nothing-illegal-about-it/?utm_term=.08139d073dd8
Rodgers, S. M. (2017). Transitional age lesbian, gay, bisexual, transgender, and questioning youth: Issues of diversity, integrated identities, and mental health. *Child and Adolescent Psychiatric Clinics of North America, 26*(2), 297–309.

Sterzing, P. R., Ratliff, G. A., Gartner, R. E., et al. (2017). Social ecological correlates of polyvictimization among a national sample of transgender, genderqueer, and cisgender sexual minority adolescents. *Child Abuse & Neglect, 67*, 1–12.

Tangherlini, T. R., Roychowdhury, V., Glenn, B., et al. (2016). "Mommy blogs" and the vaccination exemption narrative: Results from a machine-learning approach for story aggregation on parenting social media sites. *JMIR Public Health and Surveillance, 2*(2), e166.

The Joint Commission. (2011). *Advancing effective communication, cultural competence, and patient- and family-centered care for the lesbian, gay, bisexual, and transgender (LGBT) community: A field guide.* Oak Brook, IL: Author. Retrieved from www.jointcommision.org/assets/1/18/LGBTFieldGuide.pdf

Tornello, S. L., & Bos, H. (2017). Parenting intentions among transgender individuals. *LGBT Health, 4*(2), 115–120.

Unger, C. A. (2015). Care of the transgender patient: A survey of gynecologists' current knowledge and practice. *Journal of Women's Health, 24*(2), 114–118.

U.S. Department of Health and Human Services. (2010). *Healthy people 2020.* Washington, DC: Author.

Wells, M. B., & Lang, S. N. (2016). Supporting same-sex mothers in the Nordic child health field: A systematic literature review and meta-synthesis of the most gender equal countries. *Journal of Clinical Nursing, 25*(23–24), 3469–3483.

Whitley, R. (2016). Ethno-racial variation in recovery from severe mental illness: A qualitative comparison. *Canadian Journal of Psychiatry, 61*(6), 340–347.

Yang, H. J., Kuo, Y. J., Wang, L., et al. (2014). Culture, parenting, and child behavioral problems: A comparative study of cross-cultural immigrant families and native-born families in Taiwan. *Transcultural Psychiatry, 51*(4), 526–544.

Yeshua, A., Lee, J. A., Witkin, G., et al. (2015). Female couples undergoing IVF with partner eggs (Co-IVF): Pathways to parenthood. *LGBT Health, 2*(2), 135–139.

3

The Childbearing and Childrearing Family in the Community

Marlo Hanovan is a 32-year-old woman with a 12-year-old child, Charles, from a first marriage. She is presently married to Stone, 35 years old, who has two children from a first marriage: James, 17 years old, and Brian, 2 years old. James and Brian are both well, but Charles has been sick since birth with cystic fibrosis, a genetic disease that compromises his gastrointestinal and respiratory function. Mrs. Hanovan, a full-time bookkeeper, also attends a community college to study photography. She is 4 months pregnant with a new baby. Because Stone is unemployed, she tells the nurse on many days her income is stretched so far, she's forced to choose between routine health care for her family and groceries.

The previous chapters discussed the philosophy of maternal and child health nursing and how cultural traditions affect families. This chapter adds information about healthy communities and the structure of families and how nurses can help ensure healthy family outcomes.

Are the Hanovans a well or a dysfunctional family? How typical is their structure? What are some concerns they may need help in resolving?

OBJECTIVES

After mastering the contents of this chapter, you should be able to:

1. Describe what constitutes a healthy community.
2. Identify common family structures and functions and the roles within families; use critical thinking to analyze ways families are changing in modern society.
3. Identify 2020 National Health Goals related to the family and specific ways nurses can help the nation achieve these goals.
4. Assess a family for structure and healthy function.
5. Formulate nursing diagnoses related to family health.
6. Develop expected outcomes to help a family achieve optimal health as well as manage seamless transitions across differing healthcare settings.
7. Using the nursing process, plan nursing care that includes the six competencies of Quality & Safety Education for Nurses (QSEN): Patient-Centered Care, Teamwork & Collaboration, Evidence-Based Practice (EBP), Quality Improvement (QI), Safety, and Informatics.
8. Implement nursing care to teach a family more effective wellness behaviors or to help a family modify its lifestyle to adjust to a pregnancy or accommodate an ill child.
9. Evaluate outcome criteria for achievement and effectiveness of care to be certain expected outcomes have been achieved.
10. Integrate knowledge of families with the interplay of nursing process, the six competencies of QSEN, and Family Nursing to promote quality maternal and child health nursing care.

Humans have always tended to live in groups, such as families and communities, but the types of families and communities formed and the goals established have changed as technology has changed and life has become more complicated (Lavoie-Tremblay, Bonin, Bonneville-Roussy, et al., 2012). For example, when families lived on farms, they were extended or had a wealth of relatives and friends or a community close by to provide both physical and psychological support. As more people moved into cities, families became typically nuclear with only two parents and children present. Less support in terms of family members was available.

In 2015, 35% of children younger than 18 years of age live in a single-family household (Kids Count Data Center, 2015). This has important implications when planning nursing care because parents in these types of families may not have even one other adult to offer them support. This causes families to look more and more to healthcare providers, especially nurses, for guidance when a problem with pregnancy or childrearing occurs.

Figure 3.1 Families are a universal among almost all civilizations.

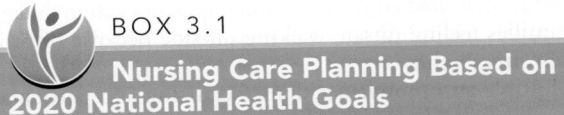

BOX 3.1

Nursing Care Planning Based on 2020 National Health Goals

The 2020 National Health Goals are goals set in place by the U.S. Department of Health and Human Services (DHHS, 2010) to improve the health of the nation for the next millennium and are kept current by updates every 10 years. A number of 2020 National Health Goals focus on ways to improve the quality of families or community life. Representative of these include:

- Increase the percentage of adult smokers aged 18 years and older attempting to stop smoking from 48.3% to 80%.
- Increase the proportion of young children who are screened for an autism spectrum disorder (ASD) and other developmental delays by 24 months of age from a present level of 19.5% to 21.5%.
- Reduce postpartum relapse of smoking among women who quit smoking during pregnancy.
- Increase the proportion of children with special health-care needs who receive their care in family-centered, comprehensive, and coordinated environments from a present level of 20.4% to 22.4%.
- Increase the rate of infants who are breastfed until 6 months from 43.5% to 60.6%.
- Reduce physical violence directed at women by male partners to no more than 27 per 1,000 couples from a current baseline of 30 per 1,000 couples (DHHS, 2010; see www.healthypeople.gov).

Nurses can help the nation meet these goals for healthier family living by assessing families and their environment to identify families at risk, assisting with counseling, and maintaining contact with families to ensure that as a family grows, its changing needs can be recognized and met. Intimate partner violence and child maltreatment are further discussed in Chapter 55.

Families are important to children's growth because no other social group has the potential to provide the depth of support and long-lasting emotional ties as a person's own family. What people learn in their family determines how they relate to people, what moral values they follow, and the molding of their basic perspectives on both the present and the future (Parker, Mandleco, Olsen Roper, et al., 2011).

Maintaining healthy family life is so important to the health and welfare of the nation: Several 2020 National Health Goals speak directly to maintaining healthy family and community life (Box 3.1). Because families have such influence on individuals and individuals on families, nursing care that considers not only a single patient but also his or her family is defined as **family-centered nursing**. It has a strong focus in modern nursing practice.

For a family to adjust to a dramatic change, such as a new family member or an ill child, a family must have structure and roles flexible enough to be able to adjust to the changes pregnancy or a long-term medicine or nutrition regimen for a child bring. The roles individuals assume in the family and their ability to adjust to new roles as their family's structure or situation changes play a major factor in whether a family can adjust to and work through difficult times to achieve a positive family outcome.

Because families do not live in isolation, the family's ability to thrive in and gain strength from a community is equally important. Always consider the strengths, vulnerabilities, and patterns of both a patient's family and the surrounding community to encourage healthy coping mechanisms and to improve overall family health (Fig. 3.1).

Nursing Process Overview

FOR PROMOTION OF FAMILY HEALTH

ASSESSMENT

Assessment of the structure and function, as well as the strengths and challenges, of families provides information on the ability of a family to remain well during either calm or stressful times. It can reveal the meaning of a current health situation for a family as well as the emotional support an individual family member can expect from other family members or the community. This can be vital to understanding what a pregnancy or childhood illness will mean to different family members, especially if not all members appear to be in agreement.

NURSING DIAGNOSIS

Nursing diagnoses formulated for families and the community generally relate to the family's ability to handle stress and to provide a positive environment for the growth and development of the members. Examples include:

- Impaired parenting related to unplanned pregnancy
- Parental role conflict related to prolonged separation from the child during a long hospital stay
- Interrupted family processes related to emergency hospital admission of the oldest child
- Ineffective family coping mechanisms related to an inability to adjust to the mother's illness during pregnancy
- Readiness for enhanced family coping mechanisms related to improved perceptions of the child's capabilities
- Health-seeking behaviors related to the birth of a first child
- Inadequate community support for family related to pregnancy

OUTCOME IDENTIFICATION AND PLANNING

Planning for nursing care is most effective if it includes a design that is both family- and community-centered and also both appropriate and desired by the majority of family members; otherwise, opposing family members can resist following the plan.

It would not be helpful, for example, to suggest a mother quit work to better supervise a child's medication regimen if she is the sole wage earner for her family. Helping all family members assume a portion of the responsibility for safe medicine administration might be a more workable solution. To help parents keep up to date on health insurance issues, family leave, and family rights, an interesting website to recommend is the National Partnership for Women & Families (www.nationalpartnership.org). In addition, the National Safety Council (www.nsc.org) discusses what families can do to help make their home and community safer. The Nurse-Family Partnership (www.nursefamilypartnership.org) offers useful information on helping first-time parents effectively succeed.

IMPLEMENTATION

Implementations to improve family health should flow smoothly if family members have agreed on a plan of action in support of one another. It may be necessary in some instances, however, to encourage family members to agree to a plan or to abide by a chosen plan. Otherwise, they can expend needless energy carrying out activities counterproductive or in direct opposition to their major goal.

OUTCOME EVALUATION

An evaluation should reveal not only that a goal has been achieved but also that the family feels more cohesive after working together toward the goal. If the evaluation does not reveal these two factors, reassess the goal as necessary

to determine whether further interventions are required or whether the goal was inadequate. Examples of expected outcomes that might be established include:

- Family members state they are adapting well to a newborn joining the family.
- The mother states she feels prepared to manage home care for her ill child.
- Parents state they have arranged the family finances to accommodate new healthcare expenses for the family.
- The grandmother states she will omit trans-fatty acids from cooking to better safeguard the health of her family.

Maternal–Child Nursing Care and the Community

Nursing a community refers to nurses' ability and responsibility to help make communities safer by participating in community activities and organizations with the goal of strengthening the community. Nursing activities originate out of the family assessment. Identified community nursing issues can include:

- Families feeling unsafe walking outside because of broken street lights
- Multiple automobile accidents occurring at a particular street corner due to a malfunctioning traffic light
- Need for better signage at a nearby park to indicate a duck pond is over 3 ft deep

It is easy to fall into the mindset that a single telephone call or an e-mail about a problem won't make a difference. But if all nurses took on their neighborhoods as clients, the number of telephone calls or e-mails could become far too many to be ignored by city officials or others in charge of community design and safety. Examples of nursing activities in the community include:

- Participating in fundraising charity events such as a walkathon
- Encouraging a block of homeowners to form a block parent association to ensure safe passage for students to and from school or activities
- Organizing adolescents from a local high school to begin a reading program at a grade school to increase interest in reading and improve the literacy rate in their neighborhood

Knowing the individual aspects of a community also helps you understand why some people reach the illness level they do before they seek health care (e.g., a woman living in a rural area has no transportation to prenatal care until her partner comes home from work, a 5-year-old child develops measles because there are no free immunization services in his community).

THE FAMILY AS PART OF A COMMUNITY

Because the health of individuals and their families are influenced by the health of their community, it is important to become acquainted with the community in which you practice or where a specific patient lives. Families rarely live alone on islands; instead, they are a part of and interact with their surrounding community to buy food, use transportation, and receive wages for work (Jilcott, Vu, Morgan, et al., 2012).

A **community** can be defined in many ways, but it is generally understood to be a group of individuals interacting within a limited geographic area (Allender, 2013). When asked what

Figure 3.2 Community assessment reveals unsafe conditions that can lead to illness, such as mold. (© fotosearch.com.)

community they are from, people may mention an entire city, a school district, a geographic district (e.g., "the East Side"), a street name (e.g., "Pine Street area"), or a natural marking (e.g., "the Lower Creek area"). A community assessment can reveal if there are aspects about the community that contributed to a person's illness (and therefore need to be corrected). It also helps determine whether a person will be able to return to their community without extra help and counseling after recovering from an illness (Fig. 3.2).

Community assessment consists of examining the various systems that are present in almost all communities to see whether they are functioning adequately. For example, it is easier for you to prepare a woman or child for return to a community after childbirth or a hospital stay if you know specific features such as information about the water supply whether the area consists of apartments or homes, or if there is public transportation.

Table 3.1 summarizes common areas to assess in relation to communities. Drawing an **ecomap** or a diagram of a family's relationship to its community can help identify what community resources are being used by a family or the family's "fit" into the community.

Family Structures

How well a family works together when times are good and how well it can organize itself against potential threats depends on both its structure (who its members are) and its function (the activities or roles family members carry out). Recognizing different family structures can help you better focus on family-centered care as well as provide a family-friendly environment for health care.

THE CONCEPT OF FAMILY

A **family** is defined by the U.S. Census Bureau (USCB, 2015) as "a householder and one or more other people living in the same household who are related by birth, marriage, or adoption."

This definition is workable for gathering comparative statistics but has limitations when assessing a family for its

TABLE 3.1 ASSESSING A COMMUNITY

Area of Assessment	Questions to Ask
Age span	Is the community a "young," a "settled-in," or a "retired" one? Is the family within the usual age span of residents in the community and thereby assured of support people?
Education	If the family has school-age children, are there schools nearby? Is there a public library for self-education? Is there easy access to such places if the person becomes physically challenged? If a special program such as diet counseling is needed, does it exist?
Environment	Are environmental risks present, such as air pollution? Busy highways? Train yards? Pools of water where drowning could occur? Could hypothermia be a problem?
Financial status	Is there a high rate of unemployment in the community, which could increase the crime rate? What is the average occupation? Will this family have adequate finances to manage comfortably in this neighborhood? Are supplemental aid programs available?
Health care	Is there a healthcare agency the family can use for comprehensive care? Is it convenient in terms of finances, time, and transportation? Is it accessible for people with disability?
Housing	Are houses mainly privately owned or apartments or condos? Are homes close enough together to afford easy contact? Are they in good repair? Will new construction or deteriorated housing be a safety problem?
Politics	Is the community active politically? Can adults reach a local polling place to vote, or do they know how to apply for absentee ballots?
Recreation	Are recreational activities of interest available? Are they economically feasible? Are there some sites that are apt to create health problems such as ski resorts (broken bones), a lake (drowning), or horse racing tracks (smoke-filled air)?
Spirituality	Is there a facility where the family can worship as they choose? Is there a mixture of worship centers to show the community accepts cultural diversity?
Safety	Is there adequate protection so family members can feel safe to hike or jog? Do they feel safe to remain home alone? Do they know about available hotlines and local police and fire department numbers? Do houses have smoke and carbon monoxide alarms in the bedrooms and near the kitchen?
Culture	What is the dominant culture in the community? Does the family fit into this environment? Are foods that are culturally significant available?
Transportation	Is there public transportation? Will family members have access to it if they become physically challenged?

health concerns or support people available because some families are made up of unrelated couples, and at points in life, not all family members live together.

Allender (2013) defines the family in a much broader context as "two or more people who live in the same household [usually], share a common emotional bond, and perform certain interrelated social tasks." This is a better working definition for healthcare providers because it addresses the broad range of types of families apt to be encountered in healthcare settings.

FAMILY TYPES

What type of family a person belongs to changes over time, as a family is affected by birth, death, possibly divorce, and the growth of family members. For the purposes of assessing families, two basic family types can be described:

- **Family of orientation** (the family one is born into; or oneself, parents, and siblings, if any)
- **Family of procreation** (a family one establishes; or oneself, spouse or significant other, and children, if any)

Almost all families, regardless of their type, share common activities, and those activities influence the health and activities of their members (Chapman, Watkins, Zappia, et al., 2012). Specific descriptions of types vary greatly depending on how many members are present, people's roles, generational issues, means of family support, and sociocultural influences (Box 3.2).

The Childfree or Childless Family

A childfree or childless family is composed of two people living together without children. This category refers to a growing trend of a voluntary choice to not have children and be childfree. With the many opportunities that are offered to women, there may be a delay in marriage and in planning for a family.

BOX 3.2

Nursing Care Planning to Respect Cultural Diversity

Although families are more mobile today than in the past, cultural values and characteristics tend to remain constant. Knowing some of the basic norms and taboos of different cultural groups allows you to understand the differences behind varying practices, a family's value system, and the degree of support family members are able to provide.

Some cultures, for example, respect elderly family members, depend on them for advice, and ensure they receive health care; other families are more oriented to the present and so treat older family members with less respect. Some cultures have extended families; others have a high number of single-parent families. Whether families are headed by men or women is also culturally determined.

Poverty tends to be a problem for nondominant (minority) ethnic groups. Some characteristic responses sometimes described as cultural limitations are actually the consequences of poverty—for example, a mother seeking medical care for her child late in the course of an illness or late in pregnancy is just as apt to be a financial influence as a cultural one. Solving this type of problem may be a question of locating financial resources rather than modifying care to respect cultural patterns.

The increased choice and availability of contraception also assists to prevent pregnancy, allowing a couple to plan for a family. The couple who experiences issues with infertility and is childless may also be included in this type of family (Davidson, London, & Ladewig, 2016).

- **Positive aspects:** companionship, possibly shared resources
- **Potential negative aspects:** feelings of guilt for the couple who decided to delay a family and who then may experience infertility issues

The Cohabitation Family

Cohabitation families are composed of couples, perhaps with children, who live together but remain unmarried. Although such a relationship may be temporary, it may also be as long-lasting as a legal marriage. Couples may choose cohabitation for a variety of personal or financial reasons. Statistically, however, couples who cohabit before marriage have a higher divorce rate than those who do not (Cherlin, 2012).

- Cohabitation provides the same benefits as a legal marriage and included companionship and financial security while the couple is together. It does not always provide for long-term financial security or additional legal benefits if the couple ends the relationship. When children are involved in the relationship, determining custody and financial care may be an issue.

The Nuclear Family

The traditional nuclear family is composed of two parents and children. In the past, it was the most common family structure seen worldwide. Today, however, in the United States, the number of nuclear families has declined to about 46% of families due to the increase in divorce, acceptance of single parenthood, and remarriage (Pew Research Center, 2015). The biggest advantage of a nuclear family is its ability to provide support to family members because, with its small size, people know each other well and can feel genuine affection and support for and from each other. Unfortunately, in a time of crisis, this same characteristic may become a challenge to a family because there are few family members to share the burden or look at a problem objectively. Helping nuclear families locate and reach out to support people in their extended family or community during a crisis can be an important nursing responsibility.

The binuclear family is a family created by divorce when the child is raised in two families. Joint custody allows both the biologic mother and father to spend varying amounts of time with the child(ren) in a joint venture. The children may alternate between two homes with each parent co-parenting (Davidson et al., 2016).

- **Positive aspects:** support for family members; sense of security
- **Possible negative aspects:** may lack support people in a crisis situation

The Extended (Multigenerational) Family

An extended family includes not only a nuclear family but also other family members such as grandmothers, grandfathers, aunts, uncles, cousins, and grandchildren. An advantage of such a family is it contains more people to serve as resources during crises and provides more role models for behavior or values (Keene, Prokos, & Held, 2012). In a typical extended family, however, there is usually only one main income provider, a situation which can strain the family's resources, and to include all family members in shared decisions may be difficult. When assessing such families, remember that, because many members are present, a parent's strongest support person may not be the spouse, and a child's primary caregiver may not be his or her biologic parent. The grandmother, an aunt, or another sibling, for example, may provide the largest amount of support or child care, so may be the person best prepared to talk about a child's health. Helping the family maintain meaningful communication between all members is an important nursing responsibility (Box 3.3).

- **Positive aspects:** many people for child care and member support
- **Possible negative aspects:** Resources may be stretched thin because of few wage earners.

BOX 3.3

Nursing Care Planning to Empower a Family

TIPS TO IMPROVE FAMILY COMMUNICATION

Q. Suppose Mrs. Hanovan says to you, "My family doesn't communicate well. How can I improve this?"

A. Traditionally, families gathered for an evening meal, and this practice allowed a set period of time each day for interaction, problem solving, and conflict resolution while problems were still small. If sit-down-together meals aren't possible because of busy work or school schedules, suggestions for better communication could include:

- Plan a time (even 15 minutes) daily when all family members "touch base" with each other.
- Have all members check in daily by e-mail or a text message.
- Use a telephone answering machine to leave daily messages.
- Set up a bulletin or chalkboard that family members can check each day for messages.
- Plan an earlier wake-up time two or three mornings per week so all family members can sit and have breakfast together.
- Reserve one night a week as "family night," when the family plans a special activity to do together such as play a board game or watch a favorite movie.
- Agree family night is off limits for cell phones, television, computers, iPods, etc., so family members are not distracted by outside sources.
- Limit the amount of time children work on their computers in their own bedrooms or spend in sedentary activities such as television watching; encourage more time in creative activities, discussing the day's events, or participating in an activity where all family members are brought together.
- Plan special activities for holidays or weekends that involve the whole family such as a hike or picnic or visiting a museum or park.
- Participate in each other's activities (e.g., if one member is playing in a ball game, all family members come and watch).

The Single-Parent Family

Single-parent families play a large role in childrearing. Unfortunately, low income is often a problem encountered by single-parent families, especially if a woman is the head of the household. Women's incomes for the same jobs are lower than men's by about 28% (U.S. Bureau of Labor Statistics, 2014). Single parents have difficulty working full-time plus taking total care of young children. Trying to fulfill several central roles (mother and father) is not only time-consuming but also mentally and physically exhausting and, in many instances, not rewarded.

Such a parent may develop low self-esteem if things are not going well, especially if a spouse left them for another or if the other parent refuses to help with child support or shared custody. Single-parent fathers may have difficulty with home management or child care if they had little experience with those roles before the separation. It's important to identify low self-esteem because it has the potential to interfere with decision making and impede daily functioning.

Single-parent families have a special strength, however, as such a family can offer a child a rich parent–child relationship as well as increased opportunities for self-reliance and independence.

If there has been a divorce, one parent may have been given legal custody of the children or both parents may share custody (Carlsund, Eriksson, Löfstedt, et al., 2013). Either way, both parents often participate in decision making. At a time of illness, both may stay with an ill child in the hospital and be eager to receive reports of the child's progress. Identifying who is the custodial parent is especially important when consent forms for care need to be signed, so be certain this is clearly marked in the child's healthcare records.

Another type of single-parent family that has emerged is the single-mother family. The single-mother family is typically designed by choice as a woman desires a family. Her desire for a family then guides her choice to enter motherhood by a variety of methods including adoption or donor insemination (Davidson et al., 2016). Women who choose to be a single parent are often financially secure with their education completed, but they may have no desire to marry or have not met someone they wish to marry or with whom they want to have children.

- **Positive aspects:** ability to offer a unique and strong parent–child bond
- **Possible negative aspects:** Resources may/may not be limited.

QSEN Checkpoint Question 3.1

PATIENT-CENTERED CARE

It's important that care extends to include the concerns of a patient's family. Mrs. Hanovan and Charles were a single-parent family before Mrs. Hanovan remarried. What is the most common challenge among single-parent families that nurses must address when planning care?

 a. Education is frequently compromised.
 b. Finances can be extremely limited.
 c. Communication is often limited.
 d. Emotional engagement is often lacking.

Look in Appendix A for the best answer and rationale.

The Blended Family

In a **blended family** (a remarriage or reconstituted family), a divorced or widowed person with children marries someone who also has children. Although the arrangement is apt to be a positive one because it creates a nuclear family, childrearing problems can arise in this type of family from rivalry among the children for the attention of a parent. In addition, each spouse may encounter difficulties in helping rear the other's children if their philosophy of childrearing differs from the biologic parent's, particularly in terms of discipline. Children may not welcome a stepparent because they have not yet resolved their feelings about the separation of their biologic parents (through either divorce or death); they may believe the stepparent threatens their relationship with their biologic parent. They may become extremely distressed at seeing their other biologic parent move into another home and become a stepparent to other children.

Children also may have heard so many stories about evil stepparents from children's books that they come into the new family already prejudiced against their new parent.

Although blended families usually lessen financial difficulties, finances can be severely limited, especially if one or both parents are obligated to pay child support for children from a previous relationship while supporting the children of the current marriage. If there is economic disparity between what a biologic parent earns and a stepparent earns, conflicts and distorted expectations can occur between parents. Nurses can be instrumental in offering emotional support to members of a blended family until these adjustments for mutual living can be resolved (Box 3.4).

- **Positive aspects:** increased security and resources; exposure to different customs or culture may help children become more adaptable to new situations
- **Possible negative aspects:** rivalry or competition among children; difficulty adjusting to a stepparent

BOX 3.4

Nursing Care Planning Based on Family Teaching

TIPS FOR REDUCING FAMILY STRESS

Q. Suppose Mr. Hanovan tells you he is worried because the tension level in his family is growing so bad he fears his wife will leave him. He asks you, "How can my family better manage stress?"

A. Managing stress calls for interventions specific to each family, but some general suggestions include:

- Try to describe why you and family members feel so stressed. Almost nothing limits the extent of a threat more than being able to describe it accurately (put a fence around it). Detailing a problem is the beginning of problem solving.
- Recognize stress levels differ from person to person. Because one person is not upset by some condition does not mean another person will not be. On the other hand, if a situation does not annoy a person, that person should not feel he or she has to react to it just because someone else does.
- Anticipate life events and plan for them to the extent possible. Anticipatory guidance will not totally prepare you for a coming event but will at least assist you in preparing for the event.
- Try to reduce the number of stressors coming at you by turning off television, dimming the lights, and spending time with just your inner self.
- Ask yourself if you really need to accomplish all the tasks piling up around you. Do you need to volunteer to be a schoolroom helper this month? Does the garage really need to be cleaned this week?
- Face a situation as honestly as possible. As a rule, knowing the exact nature of a threat is less stressful than a "something-is-out-there" feeling. On the other hand, do not feel compelled to face intense threats, such as a serious complication of pregnancy or a fatal illness in a child, until you have had time to mobilize your defenses, or you may feel overwhelmed.
- Learn to change those things you cannot accept and accepting those things you cannot change. Trial and error is often required to determine the difference.
- Consider that a total change may be unnecessary; a simple modification in one thing will create a cascade or be enough to make a difference.
- Reach out for support. When you are under stress, it's easy to become so involved in the problem you don't realize people around you want to help. Sometimes, people closest to you are under the same threat and so are no longer able to offer support. When this happens, you might have to call on second- or third-level support people (extended family or the community) for help.
- Remind family members that unintentional injuries increase when people are under stress. A person worrying about a complication of pregnancy, for example, is more apt to have an automobile accident than a person who is stress free. Children are more apt to poison themselves when the family is under stress as parents are more apt to leave pills on counters during this time.
- Remember that action feels good during stress. Doing something brings a sense of control over feelings of helplessness and disorganization. Action often is so satisfying that people write threatening letters or shout harmful remarks they later regret. Channel your energy into therapeutic action (such as going for a long walk and quietly reflecting) instead.
- Do not rush decisions or make final adaptive outcomes to a stressful situation. As a rule, major decisions should be delayed at least 6 weeks after a stressful event; 6 months is even better.
- Reach out to give support when others are being threatened. Survival is a collaborative effort of social groups; a favor offered now can be called in when you are in need at a later date.

The LGBT Family

Lesbian, gay, bisexual, and transgender (LGBT) couples live together as partners for companionship, financial security, and sexual fulfillment, or form the same structure as a nuclear family. Now that laws in the United States have changed to legally sanction gay marriage, this type of family has increased in number. Such a relationship offers support in times of crisis comparable to that offered by a traditional nuclear or cohabitation family.

Some LGBT families include children from previous heterosexual marriages or through the use of alternative insemination, adoption, or surrogate motherhood. On June 26, 2015, the Supreme Court ruled that states cannot ban same sex marriage. However, lack of understanding by healthcare providers of the strength and richness of these unions can further impede healthcare response (Chapman et al., 2012).

What If . . . 3.1

The Hanovan family identifies their main family problems as a poor financial base, a serious family illness, and limited family communication. Would this change if they were an extended family? A single-parent family? A cohabitation family?

The Foster Family

Children whose parents can no longer care for them may be placed in a foster or substitute home by a child protection agency (Kubiak, Kasiborski, Karim, et al., 2012). Foster parents may have children of their own; they receive remuneration for care of the foster child. Theoretically, foster home placement is temporary until children can be returned to their own parents. Unfortunately, if return does not become possible, children may be raised to adulthood in a series of foster care families. Such children can experience a high level of insecurity, concerned that they will have to soon move again. In addition, they may have some emotional difficulties related to the reason they were removed from their original home (Taussig, Culhane, Garrido, et al., 2012).

Most foster parents are as concerned with health care as biologic parents and can be depended on to follow healthcare instructions conscientiously. When caring for children from foster homes, be certain to determine who has legal responsibility to sign for health care for the child (a foster parent may or may not have this responsibility).

- **Positive aspects:** prevents children from being raised in large orphanage settings
- **Possible negative aspects:** insecurity and inability to establish meaningful relationships because of frequent moves

The Adoptive Family

Families of a great many types (nuclear, extended, cohabitation, blended, single parent, gay, and lesbian) adopt children today. No matter what the family structure is, adopting brings joy and fulfillment to a family. Adoption can also offer a number of challenges for both the adopting parents and the child as well as for any other children in the family (Jones, 2012).

Regardless of whether the adoption was arranged privately or through an adoption agency, new parents should visit a healthcare facility shortly after a child is placed in their home, so a baseline of health information on the child can be established,

potential problems can be discussed, and solutions can be explored (Niemann & Weiss, 2012). If the birth mother of an adopted child ate inadequately or received little prenatal care, for example, the adopted child is at a higher risk for abnormal neurologic development than usual. Children from war-torn or poverty-stricken countries have a greater risk of having illnesses such as hepatitis B, intestinal parasites, and growth restriction. They may lack routine immunizations or have delayed motor development from having been raised in a restricted institutional setting (Roeber, Tober, Bolt, et al., 2012).

When assessing a family with a newly adopted child, be certain to determine the stage of parenting the parents have reached. Nonadopting parents have 9 months to prepare physically and emotionally for a coming child. Adoptive parents may be asked to make the mental steps toward parenthood in as little as 24 hours.

If partners have low self-esteem because they were unable to conceive, they may need reassurance at healthcare visits that they are functioning as well as other parents. With the increase in foreign adoptions, parents often express a conflict between trying to preserve the child's native culture and socializing the child into the community and so appreciate having this problem addressed as well.

Also, be certain to assess siblings' responses to an adopted child. Biologic children (whether born before or after the adoption) may feel inferior to the adopted child because they were "just born," not "chosen." They may, however, feel superior because they are the "real" children of the parents. These feelings can interfere with their relationship with the adopted child as well as their parents if not discussed and resolved.

It is generally accepted that adopted children should be told as early as they can understand they are adopted (at about 2 or 3 years). Knowing this from early childhood is not nearly as stressful as accidentally stumbling onto the information when they are school-age or adolescents. At least by 4 years, children are old enough to fully understand the story of their adoption: They grew inside the body of another woman who, because she could not care for them after they were born, gave them to the adopting parent to raise and love. It's important for parents not to criticize a birth mother as part of the explanation as children need to know for their own self-esteem their birth parents were good people and they were capable of being loved by them. Things just didn't work out that way.

When children are first told they are adopted, they may exhibit "honeymoon behavior" or may try to behave perfectly for fear of being given away again. After this honeymoon period, children may deliberately test their parents to see whether, despite bad behavior such as disobeying a house rule or even shoplifting, the parents will still keep them. It helps parents to put this behavior in perspective if they are aware it may happen. Nonadopted children may also use the same testing strategies on some occasions.

Counseling an adopted child or forming a relationship with one as a healthcare provider carries additional responsibility: making certain the relationship is not ended abruptly or thoughtlessly. When ending a relationship, try to introduce the person who will continue health supervision to the child, so the child doesn't feel abandoned for a second time.

When hospitalized, all preschoolers worry about being abandoned and left in the hospital. Preschoolers who have just been told they were adopted or were chosen by their adoptive parents "from all the babies in the hospital nursery" may be terribly afraid they are now being returned to the hospital to be given back. Parents of an adopted child may need additional help in preparing the child for the hospital experience and also should be encouraged to stay with the child in the hospital as much as possible to reduce this type of postadoption fear.

As adopted children enter puberty and begin to think about having children of their own, they may begin to worry if they will make good parents or fail at parenthood as did their birth mother. Some children of this age feel a lack of a sense of identity because they do not know who their birth parents are. It's common for them to spend time tracing records to try to locate their birth parents. Counsel adopting parents that this is not a criticism of their care but a normal consequence of being adopted. Children seek their birth parents not because they do not love their adoptive parents but because they need information to know where they fit into the eternal scheme of life.

- **Positive aspects:** Children grow up well cared for and experiencing a sense of love; a woman who relinquishes her child for adoption can feel a sense of relief her baby will have a lifestyle better than what she could provide.
- **Possible negative aspects:** Divorce of the adopting parents can be devastating if the child views himself as the cause of the separation or as a child unable to find a secure family for a second time.

Family Functions and Roles

A family is a small community group and, as such, works best if it can designate certain people to complete necessary tasks. Otherwise, it is easy for work in a family to be duplicated or never completed. The roles family members view as appropriate for themselves are usually the ones they saw their own parents fulfilling. As each new generation takes on the values of the previous generation, family traditions and culture pass to the next generation.

Because family roles tend to be more flexible and often not as well defined as in the past, an important part of a family assessment is to identify what roles family members have assumed. Most families, for example, can identify an individual who serves as the *wage earner* or who supplies the bulk of the income for the family. In the past, this was typically the father. Today, it may just as easily be both mother and father. In dual-earner families, the mother contributes as much as 40% of the total family income (Smith, 2015). Also usually identified can be the *financial manager* (the person who determines how money will be spent), the *problem solver*, the *decision maker*, the *nurturer*, the *health manager*, the *environmentalist*, the *culture bearer*, and the *gatekeeper* or the person who allows information into and out of the family (Table 3.2). Identifying what these roles consist of and who fulfills these roles in a family allows you to work with a specific person and for assessment or counseling to be most effective (Fig. 3.3). If a hospitalized child will need continued care after he or she returns home, for example, it would be important to identify and contact the nurturing member of the family because this person is probably the one who will supervise or give the needed care at home so it can continue seamlessly. Be careful not to make assumptions about which family members play which roles based on gender or stereotyping because every family operates differently. Although nurturing has typically been thought of as a female characteristic, many men best fill this role today.

FAMILY TASKS

In addition to family roles, Duvall and Miller (1990) identified eight tasks essential for a family to perform to survive as a healthy unit. These tasks differ in degree from family to family and depend on the growth stage of the family, but they are usually present to some extent in all families. Wellness behaviors such as these may decrease during periods of heightened stress. Therefore, assessing families for these characteristics is helpful to better establish the extent of stress on a family as well as to empower the family to move toward healthier family behaviors.

- *Physical maintenance:* A healthy family provides food, shelter, clothing, and health care for its members. Being certain a family has enough resources to provide for a new or ill member is an important assessment. Box 3.5 shows an example of using effective communication to assess for a family's unique needs.
- *Socialization of family members:* This task includes being certain that children feel part of the family and learning appropriate ways to interact with people outside the family such as teachers, neighbors, or police. It means the family has an open communication system among family members and outward to the community.
- *Allocation of resources:* This involves determining which family needs will be met and their order of priority,

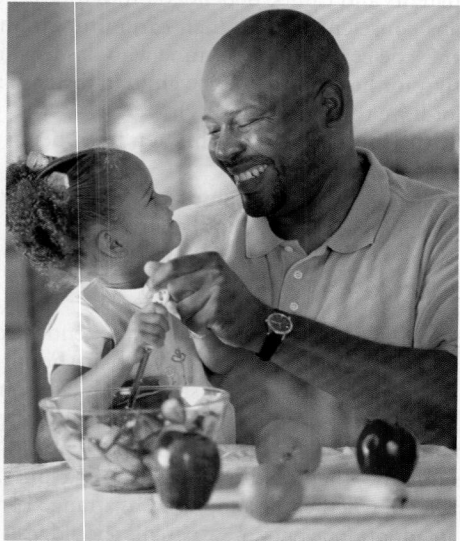

Figure 3.3 A healthy family supports each member and performs roles flexibly. Here, a father and daughter help fix dinner.

TABLE 3.2 PLANNING NURSING CARE BASED ON ASSESSMENT

Area of Assessment	Questions to Ask
Type of family	How many family members live in the home? What are their ages and relationships?
Financial support	Who is responsible for the family's income? Are finances adequate? Is money divided evenly among family members?
Safety	Is the home safe from fire or unintentional injuries? (Are smoke alarms present and police and fire numbers posted?) If there are small children, are poisons put on high shelves or in locked cabinets? Are prescription medicines and alcohol in safe places?
Environment	Is there adequate space? Heat? Hot water? Adequate plumbing?
Health	What is a typical breakfast? Lunch? Dinner? Do members monitor the amount of saturated fat and trans-fatty acids in their diet? Do they receive adequate sleep? Do they have a primary care health provider? Are immunizations current? Is there a balance between work and recreation? Does the family feel it copes with problems adequately?
Emotional support within family	Do members eat together or spend an equal amount of time with each other daily? Do they band together to defend each other from outsiders?
Emotional support outside family	Is the family active in community organizations or activities? Do they visit (or are they visited by) friends and relatives? Can the family name at least one outside person they can always rely on for help in a time of crisis?
Cultural diversity	Are there specific customs or traditions that will affect health care? Can they obtain favorite foods locally? What holidays do they celebrate?
Spirituality	Does the family have a religious affiliation? Do members attend religious services? Are there foods or activities restricted in relation to this that might influence care planning?
Family roles	
Nurturer	Who is the primary caregiver to children or a physically or cognitively challenged member?
Provider	Who brings in the bulk of the family's income?
Decision maker	Who makes decisions, particularly in the area of lifestyle, and how leisure time is spent?
Financial manager	Who supervises the family finances (pays the bills, provides savings for the future)?
Problem solver	Who does the family depend on to provide a solution to problems?
Health manager	Who makes healthcare decisions, ensures family members keep health appointments, immunizations are kept current, and preventive care such as a mammogram for the mother is scheduled?
Culture bearer	Who maintains family and community customs so children can develop a sense of where they belong in history?
Environmentalist	Who is responsible for recycling and not wasting electricity or water?
Gatekeeper	Who determines what information will be released from the family, or what new information can be introduced?

including not only material goods but also affection and space. In healthy families, there is justification, consistency, and fairness in the distribution. In many families, resources are limited, so for example, no one has new shoes. A danger sign would be a family in which one child is barefoot, whereas the others wear $100 sneakers.

- *Maintenance of order:* This task includes establishing family values, establishing rules about expected family responsibilities and roles, and enforcing common regulations for family members such as using "time out" for toddlers. In healthy families, members know the family rules and respect and follow them; in dysfunctional families, you may see a flagrant disregard of rules.
- *Division of labor:* Healthy families not only evenly divide the workload among members but are also flexible enough to interchange workloads as needed.
- *Reproduction, recruitment, and release of family members:* Often, not a great deal of thought is given to who lives in a family; membership often happens more by changing circumstances than by true choice. Having to accept a new infant into an already crowded household may make a pregnancy a less-than-welcome event; allowing a late adolescent to move to a college dorm may be viewed as abandonment by a close-knit family.

- *Placement of members into the larger society:* Healthy families realize they do not have to operate alone but can reach out to other families or their community for help as needed. They are able to select community resources, such as schools, affiliations, a place to worship, a birth setting, a hospital, hospice, or a political group, that correlate with the family's beliefs and values. A family that lives in a community with a culture or values different from its own may find this a difficult task.
- *Maintenance of motivation and morale:* Healthy families are able to maintain a sense of unity and pride in their family. When this is present, it helps members defend the family against threats as well as allows them to support each other during a crisis. It means parents are growing with and through the experience of their children the same as children grow through contact with their parents. Assessing whether a feeling of loyalty to other family members is present tells you a lot about the overall health of a family.

What If . . . 3.2
Charles complains to the nurse he has to do more than his share of the work in his family because he's expected to keep his own room clean and his 2-year-old brother doesn't have to do that. How would the nurse respond to him?

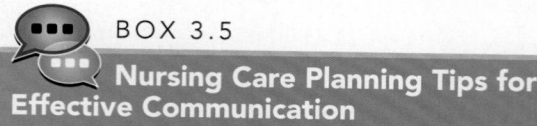

BOX 3.5

Nursing Care Planning Tips for Effective Communication

The Hanovan family consists of Mr. and Mrs. Hanovan and three children: James, 17 years old; Charles, 12 years old; and Brian, 2 years old. You notice Brian has missed many health maintenance visits, and he is underimmunized.

Tip: Assess for the unique needs of a family prior to providing patient education. In our zeal to educate people about good health practices, it is easy to rush in and teach. Unless a family's needs are met, people may agree to comply with a better health regimen but then be unable to do so because their original need was not met.

Nurse: It's good to see you in clinic today, Mrs. Hanovan. I know money is a problem, but you've got to start coming more until Brian gets caught up with his immunizations.

Mrs. Hanovan: It's hard with a 2-year-old.

Nurse: Is there anything I could do to make coming to the clinic easier?

Mrs. Hanovan: I should never come. Brian's outgrown his car seat so it's illegal for me to drive him here.

Nurse: Let me give you the number of an agency you can call to borrow a seat, not only so you can come to the clinic more often but so you can take him out safely at other times as well.

DEVELOPMENTAL STAGES

Families, like individuals, not only have specific tasks to carry out but also pass through predictable developmental stages (Duvall & Miller, 1990). To assess whether a family is using stage-appropriate health promotion activities, it is helpful to first determine what stage the family is experiencing. The age of the oldest child is used to mark the stage. Because families are delaying the age at which they marry and have a first child and parents are living longer, the lengths of stages 7 and 8 are growing longer, whereas stage 1 is growing shorter (Table 3.3).

QSEN Checkpoint Question 3.3

QUALITY IMPROVEMENT

The Hanovan family consists of two parents plus James, 17 years old; Charles, 12 years old; and Brian, 2 years old. Mrs. Hanovan is 4 months pregnant. When examining how to improve the quality of the nurse's health teaching with the Hanovan family, which of Duvall's family life stages would the nurse consider the family currently experiencing?

a. Pregnancy stage
b. Preschool stage
c. Launching stage
d. Adolescent stage

Look in Appendix A for the best answer and rationale.

TABLE 3.3 DEVELOPMENTAL STAGES AND GOALS FOR FAMILIES

Developmental Stages	Goal
Marriage (stage 1)	• Establish a mutually satisfying relationship. • Learn to relate well to their families of orientation. • Engage in reproductive life planning, if applicable.
The early childbearing family (stage 2)	• Integrate the new member into the family. • Make whatever financial and social adjustments are necessary to meet the needs of the new member while continuing to meet the meets of the parents.
The family with a preschool child (stage 3)	• Prevent unintentional injuries (accidents) such as poisoning or falls. • Begin socialization through play dates, child care, or nursery school settings.
The family with a school-age child (stage 4)	• Promote children's health through immunizations, dental care, and routine health assessments. • Promote child safety related to home and automobiles. • Encourage socialization experiences outside the home such as sports participation, music lessons, or hobby activities. • Encourage a meaningful school experience to make learning a lifetime concern, not one of merely 12 years.
The family with an adolescent (oldest child is between 13 and 20 years of age) (stage 5)	• Loosen ties enough to allow an adolescent more freedom while still remaining safe. • Begin to prepare adolescents for life on their own.
The launching stage family: the family with a late adolescent (stage 6)	• Change their role from mother or father to once-removed support persons or guideposts. • Encourage independent thinking and adult-level decision skills in their child.
The family of middle-aged parents (stage 7)	• Adjust to "empty nest" syndrome by reawakening their relationship with their supportive partner. • Prepare for retirement so when they reach that stage they will not be unprepared socially or financially.
The family in retirement or older age (stage 8)	• Maintain heath by preventive care in light of aging. • Participate in social, political, and neighborhood activities to keep active and enjoy this stage of life.

Assessment of Family Structure and Function

Family characteristics can be assessed on a variety of levels and in varying degrees of detail. The type of family data collected and the method of collection should match the way in which the assessment data will be used.

General characteristics of family type and functioning can be assessed using observation and general history questions (see Table 3.2). If more detailed information about family environment and roles is required, using an assessment tool specifically developed for that purpose can be most effective.

THE WELL FAMILY

Assessment of psychosocial family wellness requires a measurement of how the family relates and interacts as a unit, including communication patterns, bonding, roles and role relationships, division of tasks and activities, governance, decision making, problem solving, and leadership within the family unit. Assessment also looks at how the family relates to the outside community.

A **genogram** is a diagram that details family structure and provides information about the family's health history and the roles of various family members across several generations. It can provide a basis for discussion and analysis of family interaction at healthcare visits (Fig. 3.4).

 Concept Mastery Alert

A genogram provides details about family structure and health rather than specifics about an individual patient.

Another aspect of family assessment is to document the "fit" of a family into their community. This is done by means of an ecomap, a diagram of family and community relationships (Fig. 3.5). To construct such a map, first draw a circle in the center to represent the family. Around the outside, draw circles that represent the family's commu-

nity contacts such as church, school, neighbors, or other organizations. Families who "fit" well into their community usually have many outside circles or community contacts. A mark of families who are new to a community is that they have few community contacts because they have not formed these as of yet. This pattern is also the mark of an abusive or dysfunctional family if such a family deliberately keeps outside people separate from them. Constructing such a map helps you assess the emotional support that will be available to a family in a time of crisis. A family whom you assess as having few connecting lines between its members and the community may need increased nursing contact and support to remain a well family. Box 3.6 shows an interprofessional care map illustrating both nursing and team planning for the Hanovan family.

 What If . . . 3.3

The nurse discovers the Hanovan family is "out of sync" with its community (they are the only family on their block who does not work at the local factory, they attend a different church than many, they are having a new baby when many neighbors have college-age children). How could the nurse help them fit into their community better?

CHANGING PATTERNS OF FAMILY LIFE

Family life has changed significantly across the world during the past 50 years due to many complex and interrelated factors, such as an increase in divorce, families in which both parents work outside the home (dual-earner families), the legalization of marriage for LGBT couples, single-parent families, and shared childrearing responsibilities. Many more couples delay marriage and childrearing today until they are completely finished with school and established in their careers. This delay has implications for fertility and the need for assisted reproduction technology.

Understanding the impact these changes have on family structure and family life can help you create care plans that are realistic and better meet the needs of today's families.

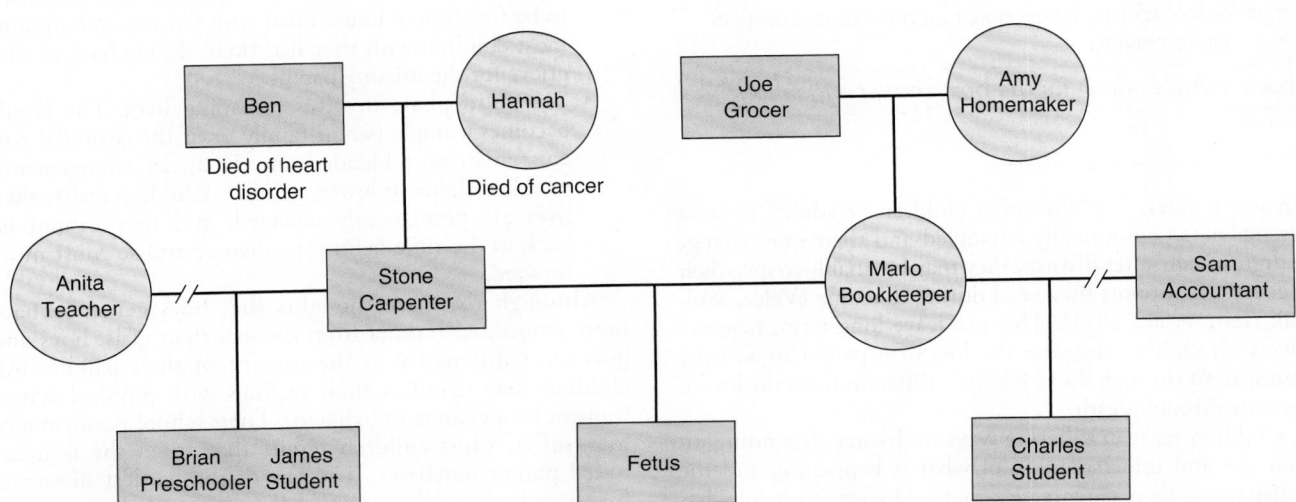

Figure 3.4 A genogram of the Hanovan family showing three generations. Males are shown by squares, females by circles.

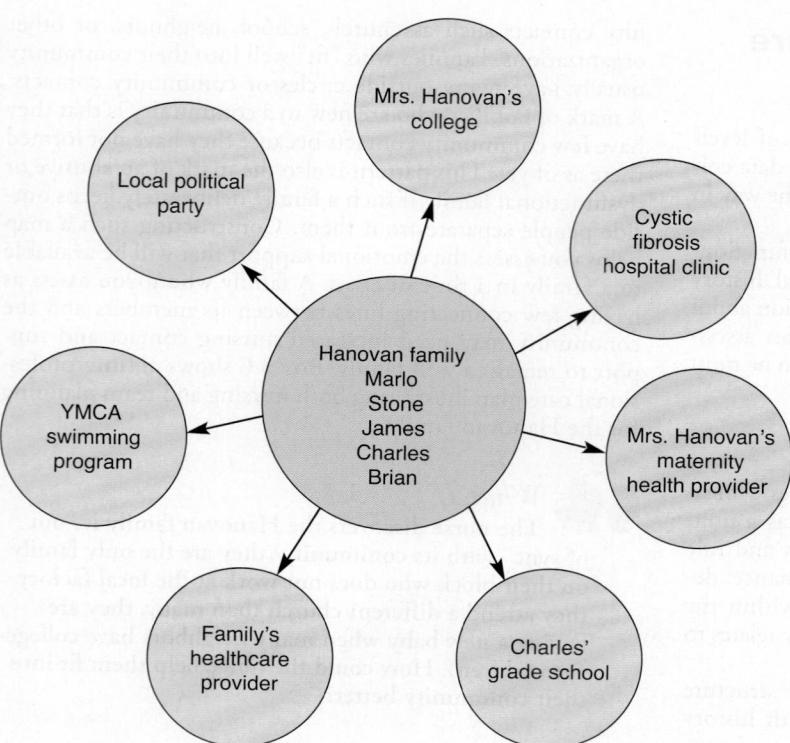

Figure 3.5 An ecomap of the Hanovan family's relationship to its community. The family members are shown in the center circle; the outer circles show community contacts.

QSEN Checkpoint Question 3.4

SAFETY

Because of smaller families, the supervision of children may be delegated to many different caregivers during a day's time. What age group has the most automobile-related unintentional injuries if not supervised conscientiously?

a. Infants, because child car seats are often installed incorrectly
b. Toddlers, because they walk in front of cars in parking lots
c. School-age children, because they ride school buses almost daily
d. Adolescents, because of alcohol or distraction while driving

Look in Appendix A for the best answer and rationale.

Increased Divorce Rate

Divorce is rarely easy for either children or adults. Because parents are so emotionally entangled and their roles change so dramatically after divorce, they may be unable to give their children the support they need during this time (Vélez, Wolchik, Tein, et al., 2011). This can leave long-term, negative effects on children because the loss of a parent or favorite grandparent through divorce is little different from the loss of a parent through death.

Children react in differing ways to divorce depending on their age and understanding of what is happening and the explanations their parents give them. Divorce, as a rule, has

three separate phases in which children follow a course similar to grief.

- The first phase is apt to be an antagonistic time as parents realize they are no longer compatible, marked by quarreling, hurt feelings, and whispered conversations. This phase can be particularly upsetting for children because they usually haven't been told what is happening as yet. They may assume the quarreling is their fault (i.e., if they had behaved better, this wouldn't be happening).
- The second phase is the actual separation stage. Everyone in the family is forced to take on an unfamiliar role, perhaps move to a new home, and probably realize a marked difference in finances. Although it is comforting to be free from a house filled with tension and arguing, most children wish they had their old life back as they grieve for the missing parent.
- The third phase involves reshaping lives. The family becomes a single-parent family or, if the custodial parent remarries, a blended one. Financial arrangements, whether higher or lower, stabilize. Children realize their lives are permanently changed, and they cannot go back to the time before the divorce and so must move forward.

Although there are thoughts that boys generally have more emotional trauma from divorce than girls, boys and girls react differently to the divorce of their parents. All children may manifest their feelings with physical symptoms or by a change in behavior. Their school performance may suffer. Most children report that when the noncustodial parent remarries, it is one of the hardest moments for them because at that point they have no choice but to

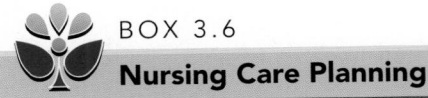

BOX 3.6

Nursing Care Planning

AN INTERPROFESSIONAL CARE MAP FOR A FAMILY WITH AN ILL CHILD

Charles Hanovan is a 12-year-old child with cystic fibrosis whom you care for in the hospital. As you prepare him for discharge, his mother tells you, "He refuses to do his afternoon chores assigned to him and has been 'acting out' in school for the past month. He refuses to speak to family members and argues about what to eat. He's supposed to independently take his medicine and do chest expansion exercises after school but refuses to do them."

Charles states, "I'm tired of being nagged all the time, and of being so different from everyone else. And I want to get out of the house, not stay home alone. Imagine how much worse things will get when the new baby comes."

Family Assessment: Blended middle-class family, which lives in an older three-bedroom home in the central city. Father is disabled from an on-the-job accident 1 year ago; does not participate in any community activities. Mother works as a bookkeeper and also attends a community college; she is 4 months pregnant and active in local political party. Patient is a middle child with two stepbrothers, age 17 years and age 2 years. Mother swims weekly at the local YMCA; the rest of family refuses to go with her. Charles is responsible for homework and cleaning kitchen after school while he is home alone (father is at physical therapy visits). Admits to having few close friends. Two neighbors are available in case of emergency during his alone time.

Patient Assessment: Respiratory rate: 26 breaths/min. Appears thin and pale. Productive cough with tenacious sputum. Lungs with fine bilateral rales.

Nursing Diagnosis: Interrupted family processes related to effect of child's illness and situational stressors limiting communication

Outcome Criteria: Family demonstrates greater participation in family activities, interaction with ill child, and positive methods of communication by 3 months' time.

Charles states he feels more family attachment and increased self-esteem by 3 months' time.

Team Member Responsible	Assessment	Intervention	Rationale	Expected Outcome
Activities of Daily Living, Including Safety				
Nurse	Interview family about family structure and roles.	Complete a family genogram and ecogram. Prioritize needs for each family member.	Family interview, genogram, and ecogram profile will show how family members relate and interact with each other and community and should help prioritize and focus care.	Family supplies interview, genogram, and ecogram information; follow-up visits prioritize the family needs they've identified.
Nurse	Help family select a common activity that can be enjoyed by all members to help decrease sense of loneliness.	Encourage participation in this activity, initially once per month, then twice per month, and then weekly.	Participation in a group activity fosters bonding. Gradually increasing the frequency of the activity promotes integration into the family routine.	Patient maintains a schedule documenting his participation in the selected family activity.
Teamwork and Collaborations				
Nurse/social worker	Assess which community agencies have after-school programs that Charles could attend.	Contact local community organizations with patient and set up a visit. Ask the school nurse or guidance counselor to provide contacts, if needed.	Contacting the organization with the patient offers support and helps reduce any possible anxiety with new situations. School personnel provide additional support and reassurance.	Patient visits at least one local or school agency by next healthcare visit.

Continued on following page

BOX 3.6

Nursing Care Planning (continued)

Team Member Responsible	Assessment	Intervention	Rationale	Expected Outcome
Procedures/Medications for Quality Improvement				
Nurse	Assess and list all of child's required exercises, therapy, and medications.	Demonstrate procedures, if necessary, and ask patient to return demonstrations. Help patient incorporate regimens into usual routine.	Review and redemonstration help to reinforce measures and ensure patient is doing them correctly. Incorporating them into patient's routine helps to promote positive adjustment and decreases feelings of being different.	Patient redemonstrates procedures with 90% accuracy. Incorporate at least one exercise or medication into usual routine. Taking greater responsibility for therapy should enhance patient's sense of "growing up" and decrease need for reminders.
Nurse/physical or respiratory therapist	Help family assess which family member could serve as backup support for child's exercise and medication regimens.	Meet with family and plan a schedule that will allow a backup family member to participate in child's exercise and therapy regimens so he isn't alone.	Family involvement divides the responsibility and minimizes the risk of added stress on the family system.	Family members state they use a checklist to ensure one of them is available to cooperate with and encourage patient to follow treatment regimen. Patient states he is adhering to treatment regimen 90% of time.
Nutrition				
Nurse/ nutritionist	Assess nutrition needs based on medical prescription.	Review special diet needed by patient with patient and father (food preparer). Brainstorm foods patient would like to eat.	Both the food preparer and the patient need to be well informed about a special diet.	Both patient and father state they understand a special diet is necessary and describe breakfast, lunch, and dinner choices that adhere to the diet.
Nurse/ nutritionist	Assess family's eating habits.	Encourage family to eat together as a family unit at least two times per week.	Eating together should help patient comply with nutrition plan and also provide a time for family sharing and communication.	Family reports they eat at least two meals per week together or, if not possible, arrange for an alternate "sharing time."
Patient-Centered Care				
Nurse	Assess patient's and family's present knowledge of his illness.	Review with patient and parents the cause and therapy for illness based on their present knowledge base.	Building on a patient's knowledge base facilitates teaching and learning and minimizes repetition.	Patient and family state they understand the underlying cause of illness and importance of treatments.
Nurse	Assess with patient what a typical school day consists of; how many friends he can identify.	Brainstorm with patient ways he could make a new friend or "fit in" at school better.	A feeling of "being different" can be detrimental to self-esteem.	Patient states he has made at least one new friend by 2 months' time; feels a "better fit" at school.
Psychosocial/Spiritual/Emotional Needs				
Nurse	Help each family member identify his or her greatest stressor.	Help family members reduce stress by teaching better problem-solving techniques such as time or anger management.	Identifying problems is the first step in effective problem solving. Use of therapeutic measures such as time management can reduce stress.	Family members identify the greatest stressors in their family life and techniques they are using to decrease stress by next healthcare visit.

Informatics for Seamless Healthcare Planning

Nurse/case manager	Assess home rules and delegation of responsibilities. Meet with family to identify where support may be needed when child returns home.	Encourage joint cooperation in household tasks so patient doesn't feel so isolated when home alone.	Joint ownership of household tasks encourages a sense of family.	Family members demonstrate they have a family schedule that evens out tasks and involves all members.
Nurse/case manager	Assess what community resources are available to support the Hanovans, such as the Cystic Fibrosis Foundation.	Meet with family to gauge their interest in using identified community organizations as resources.	Community resources can provide additional support in areas of need.	Family members state they have attended at least one Parents of Cystic Fibrosis Children or similar meeting by 3 months' time.

accept the finality of the divorce (Angarne-Lindberg & Wadsby, 2012).

Although all three stages of divorce are stressful for children, following a divorce, a redeeming feature may be that children may actually feel less stress than they experienced living in a home where there was a high level of conflict between parents. To help them adjust to their changing situation, children need an explanation of why the divorce occurred and assurance that it was not their fault. The parent who will now be raising them may need help in avoiding playing the role of the injured party or portraying the former partner as dishonorable, selfish, or unreliable. Although a former spouse was not a good marriage partner, he or she may have been a good parent and may be well loved and missed by the children (Sigal, Wolchik, Tein, et al., 2012).

QSEN Checkpoint Question 3.5

EVIDENCE-BASED PRACTICE

In previous years, few parents asked for shared or joint custody of their children following a divorce. Today, this type of custody is seen in as many as 30% of custody arrangements. To investigate whether joint custody of this type—where a child spends some time in both parents' homes following a divorce—poses behavioral risks such as increased smoking or drug use, researchers interviewed a cohort of 15-year-old Swedish teenagers.

Findings revealed adolescents living in shared physical custody had higher rates of health risk behaviors such as beginning smoking or drinking alcohol compared with adolescents from two-parent families (60% and 50% higher, respectively). At the same time, adolescents in this study had significantly lower rates of these health risk behaviors than their counterparts in single-parent families (Carlsund et al., 2013).

Suppose Mr. and Mrs. Hanovan divorce. Based on this study, what would be an important responsibility when the nurse is discharging James, an adolescent, from a hospital stay to his homecare setting?

a. The nurse should suggest his mother, who will be his primary caregiver, to quit work so he will be able to have a stay-at-home mother for his care.

b. The nurse should assess the parent's custodial pattern to be certain a responsible adult will be available no matter which home James returns to.

c. The nurse should assure his parents that shared custody is a common pattern today and therefore does not pose a risk to teenagers; otherwise, no one would choose it.

d. The nurse should assume the parents are responsible adults and will sensibly solve any problems that arise according to their custodial agreement.

Look in Appendix A for the best answer and rationale.

Decreased Family Size

The U.S. birth rate has declined steadily from 1900 to the present, putting the United States at a rate of almost zero population growth or with fewer births each year than deaths. The average number of children in families has decreased from 4 or 5 at the beginning of the last century to 2.1 children today (National Center for Health Statistics, 2012). Because parents in small families spend less total time providing direct child care, this limits parents' experience in childrearing so the amount of childrearing counseling time by nurses needed per parent increases. As children have fewer older sibling role models than before, they may need more counseling in behaviors such as how to manage stress, how to survive a failing grade at school, or how to deal with a sports team's loss.

Increased Dual-Parent Employment

As many as 60% of women of childbearing age work full-time outside their home, and as many as 90% work at least part-time (Cherlin, 2012). The implication of this trend for healthcare providers is that healthcare facilities need to schedule appointments at times when parents are free to come (parents will willingly miss work if their child is sick but not necessarily for a health maintenance or a routine prenatal visit). Instructions about how to give medication must take into account both the child's and the parents' schedules. For instance, help parents tailor administration of medicine to the times they will be with the child to supervise the administration (perhaps before breakfast, following after-school child care, and at bedtime) rather than suggesting the more traditional 10 AM, 2 PM, and 6 PM schedule.

The amount of time spent watching television and what websites are being visited are important for parents to monitor with self-care school-age children. It is important for children to learn to live in a fast-paced world, but parents need to be certain children understand news of world events are reported over and over. Otherwise, serial repetition of that type can frighten children because it may seem as if 100 airplanes have crashed instead of one airplane crash being reported over and over.

To avoid exposure to excessive violence on television, the American Academy of Pediatrics (AAP) recommends children's television viewing time be limited until they reach 2 years of age (AAP, 2012). Many parents restrict this through school age so children have adequate time to spend with friends and on required homework. Caution parents that they need to monitor time spent on the Internet because of the misinformation posted and the risk from Internet predators.

Dual-parent employment has increased the number of children attending day care centers or after-school programs (Copeland, Sherman, Kendeigh, et al., 2012). This high attendance rate may have an impact on health care as well because children attending day care centers have an increased incidence of infections such as acute diarrhea and upper respiratory infections. They may engage in less gross motor activities than children playing at home. Helping parents choose a quality day care center or after-school program that takes the necessary precautions against infections and includes physical as well as academic activities can be a nursing responsibility (see Chapter 31).

Dual working parents may also require school-age children to spend some time alone after school before their parents return from work. Helping parents prevent loneliness in these "latchkey" or "self-care" children as well as helping children make good use of their time alone can be another important nursing responsibility (see Chapter 32).

QSEN Checkpoint Question 3.6

INFORMATICS

The amount of technology and media that children are exposed to increases yearly. What is the youngest age the nurse would suggest the Hanovan family introduce their new baby to television viewing based on the recommendation of the AAP?

   a. 1 year
   b. 18 months
   c. 2 years
   d. 4 years

Look in Appendix A for the best answer and rationale.

HIGH LEVELS OF VIOLENCE IN FAMILIES

An alarming statistic in today's families is that the incidence and reports of intimate partner violence and child maltreatment remain high (Centers for Disease Control and Prevention, 2016). This is apparently related to high stress levels in families and better reporting of violence and maltreatment. Detecting these behaviors begins with the awareness that they occur. Both intimate partner violence and child maltreatment are discussed in detail in Chapter 55.

What If . . . 3.4

The nurse is particularly interested in exploring one of the 2020 National Health Goals with respect to healthy families (see Box 3.1). What would be a possible research topic to explore pertinent to this goal that would be applicable to the Hanovan family and also would advance evidence-based practice?

KEY POINTS FOR REVIEW

- Families exist within communities; assessment of the community and the family's place in the community yields important information on family functioning and abilities.
- A family is a group of people who share a common emotional bond and perform certain interrelated social tasks.
- Because families work as a unit, the unmet needs of any member can spread to become the unmet needs of all family members.
- Common types of families include nuclear, extended, single-parent, blended, cohabitation, LGBT, foster, and adopted families.
- Common family tasks are physical maintenance, socialization of family members, allocation of resources, maintenance of order, division of labor, reproduction, recruitment and release of members, placement of members into the larger society, and maintenance of motivation and morale.
- Common life stages of families are marriage; early childbearing; families with preschool, school-age, and adolescent children; launching stage; middle-years families; and the family in retirement.
- Changes in patterns of family life that are occurring include dual-parent employment, increased divorce rates, reduced family size, and social problems such as intimate partner violence.
- Considering a family as a unit (a single patient) helps in planning nursing care that not only meets QSEN competencies but also best meets the family's total needs.
- Because families exist within communities, assessment of the community and the family's place in the community yields further information on family functioning and abilities.

CRITICAL THINKING CARE STUDY

The Garcia family consists of Mr. Garcia, 42 years old; Mrs. Garcia, 36 years old; Mrs. Garcia's mother, 62 years old; Jose, 14 years old; Anna, 12 years old; and Carlos, 4 years old. Mr. Garcia works as a city bus driver. All six members live in a crowded apartment in the center of the city. Mrs. Garcia recently solved the problem of someone needing to care for her mother who has Alzheimer disease by quitting her job as a secretary to care for her. She tells the nurse she used to enjoy entertaining her children's friends but now asks them not to visit because her mother needs quiet.

1. What type of family do the Garcia's represent? Who do you think is the family problem solver? The health supervisor? The gatekeeper?

2. What is the stage of the Garcia family? Would their situation be different if the children were other ages?

3. Carlos was adopted because his mother, Mrs. Garcia's sister, died in a car accident. What are special concerns of adopted children you need to consider when giving nursing care?

RELATED RESOURCES

Explore these additional resources to enhance learning for this chapter:
- Student resources on thePoint, including answers to the What If . . . and Critical Thinking Care Study questions, http://thepoint.lww.com/Flagg8e
- Adaptive learning powered by PrepU, http://thepoint.lww.com/prepu

REFERENCES

Allender, J. A. (2013). *Community & public health nursing*. Philadelphia, PA: Lippincott Williams & Wilkins.
American Academy of Pediatrics. (2012). *Where we stand: TV viewing time*. Washington, DC: Author.
Angarne-Lindberg, T., & Wadsby, M. (2012). Psychiatric and somatic health in relation to experience of parental divorce in childhood. *International Journal of Social Psychiatry, 58*(1), 16–25.
Carlsund, A., Eriksson, U., Löfstedt, P., et al. (2013). Risk behaviour in Swedish adolescents: Is shared physical custody after divorce a risk or a protective factor? *European Journal of Public Health, 23*(1), 3–8.
Centers for Disease Control and Prevention. (2016). *Intimate partner violence: Data sources*. Retrieved from http://www.cdc.gov/violenceprevention/intimatepartnerviolence/datasources.html
Chapman, R., Watkins, R., Zappia, T., et al. (2012). Second-level hospital health professionals' attitudes to lesbian, gay, bisexual and transgender parents seeking health for their children. *Journal of Clinical Nursing, 21*(5–6), 880–887.
Cherlin, A. J. (2012). *Public and private families: An introduction* (7th ed.). New York, NY: McGraw-Hill.
Copeland, K. A., Sherman, S. N., Kendeigh, C. A., et al. (2012). Societal values and policies may curtail preschool children's physical activity in child care centers. *Pediatrics, 129*(2), 265–274.

Davidson, M. C., London, M. L., & Ladewig, P. W. (2016). *Olds' maternal-newborn nursing & women's health across the lifespan* (10th ed.). Upper Saddle River, NJ: Pearson Education.
Duvall, E. M., & Miller, B. (1990). *Marriage and family development*. Philadelphia, PA: Lippincott Williams & Wilkins.
Jilcott, S. B., Vu, M. B., Morgan, J., et al. (2012). Promoting use of nutrition and physical activity community resources among women in a family planning clinic setting. *Women & Health, 52*(1), 55–70.
Jones, V. F. (2012). Comprehensive health evaluation of the newly adopted child. *Pediatrics, 129*(1), e214–e223.
Keene, J. R., Prokos, A. H., & Held, B. (2012). Grandfather caregivers: Race and ethnic differences in poverty. *Sociological Inquiry, 82*(1), 49–77.
Kids Count Data Center. (2015). *Children in single-parent families*. Retrieved from http://datacenter.kidscount.org/data/tables/106-children-in-single-parent-families#detailed/1/any/false/573,869,36,868,867/any/429,430
Kubiak, S. P., Kasiborski, N., Karim, N., et al. (2012). Does subsequent criminal justice involvement predict foster care and termination of parental rights for children born to incarcerated women? *Social Work in Public Health, 27*(1–2), 129–147.
Lavoie-Tremblay, M., Bonin, J. P., Bonneville-Roussy, A., et al. (2012). Families' and decision makers' experiences with mental health care reform: The challenge of collaboration. *Archives of Psychiatric Nursing, 26*(4), e41–e50.
National Center for Health Statistics. (2012). Changing demographics. *National Vital Statistics Reports, 58*(1), 2–4.
Niemann, S., & Weiss, S. (2012). Factors affecting attachment in international adoptees at 6 months post adoption. *Children and Youth Services Review, 34*(1), 205–212.
Parker, J. A., Mandleco, B., Olsen Roper, S., et al. (2011). Religiosity, spirituality, and marital relationships of parents raising a typically developing child or a child with a disability. *Journal of Family Nursing, 17*(1), 82–104.
Pew Research Center. (2015). *Parenting in America: Outlook, worries, aspirations are strongly linked to financial situation*. Retrieved from http://www.pewsocialtrends.org/2015/12/17/1-the-american-family-today/
Roeber, B. J., Tober, C. L., Bolt, D. M., et al. (2012). Gross motor development in children adopted from orphanage settings. *Developmental Medicine and Child Neurology, 54*(6), 527–531.
Sigal, A. B., Wolchik, S. A., Tein, J. Y., et al. (2012). Enhancing youth outcomes following parental divorce: A longitudinal study of the effects of the new beginnings program on educational and occupational goals. *Journal of Clinical Child and Adolescent Psychology, 41*(2), 150–165.
Smith, K. (2015). *Women as economic providers: Dual-earner families thrive as women's earnings rise*. Retrieved from http://scholars.unh.edu/cgi/viewcontent.cgi?article=1244&context=carsey
Taussig, H. N., Culhane, S. E., Garrido, E., et al. (2012). RCT of a mentoring and skills group program: Placement and permanency outcomes for foster youth. *Pediatrics, 130*(1), e33–e39.
U.S. Bureau of Labor Statistics. (2014). *Highlight of women's earnings in 2013*. Retrieved from http://www.bls.gov/opub/reports/womens-earnings/archive/highlights-of-womens-earnings-in-2013.pdf
U.S. Census Bureau. (2015). Washington, DC: Author. Retrieved from https://ask.census.gov/faq.php?id=5000&faqId=439
U.S. Department of Health and Human Services. (2010). *Healthy people 2020*. Washington, DC: Author.
Vélez, C. E., Wolchik, S. A., Tein, J. Y., et al. (2011). Protecting children from the consequences of divorce: A longitudinal study of the effects of parenting on children's coping processes. *Child Development, 82*(1), 244–257.

4

Home Care and the Childbearing and Childrearing Family

Lisa Puente, a 16-year-old, is 20 weeks pregnant. She was admitted to the hospital for 3 days at week 14 of her pregnancy. Due to excessive vomiting and weight loss, she was placed on a nutritional supplement regimen that included gastrostomy feedings. Her condition improved over a 6-week time period, but at 20 weeks gestation, her blood pressure increased to 160/90 mmHg and she was diagnosed with gestational hypertension. She was placed on bed rest with fetal and uterine surveillance at home. She reports difficulty resting at home: boredom with school assignments and decreased visits from friends (and boyfriend). You notice she's missed at least three doses of her antihypertensive agent. She requests her care be provided in the hospital instead of at home.

Previous chapters discussed healthy communities, family structure, and how cultural traditions affect families. This chapter adds information about families and their community as they prepare to care for themselves or an ill family member at home.

Is Lisa a good candidate for home care? What additional interventions would she need to make home care more successful?

KEY TERMS

direct care
home care
hospice care

indirect care
skilled home nursing care

OBJECTIVES

After mastering the contents of this chapter, you should be able to:

1. Describe the usual nursing and patient concerns when home care is required during pregnancy or childhood.

2. Identify 2020 National Health Goals related to home care during pregnancy and childhood that nurses can help the nation achieve.

3. Assess a pregnant woman or child and their community for likely success with home care.

4. Formulate nursing diagnoses related to care of a child or pregnant patient at home.

5. Identify expected outcomes for a family requiring home care as well as help manage seamless transitions across differing healthcare settings.

6. Using the nursing process, plan nursing care that includes the six competencies of Quality & Safety Education for Nurses (QSEN): Patient-Centered Care, Teamwork & Collaboration, Evidence-Based Practice (EBP), Quality Improvement (QI), Safety, and Informatics.

7. Implement nursing care to meet the needs of a pregnant woman or child on home care such as teaching techniques of intravenous therapy or suggesting ways to keep in contact with significant others.

8. Evaluate outcome criteria for achievement and effectiveness of nursing care to be certain expected outcomes have been achieved.

9. Integrate knowledge of home care with the interplay of nursing process, the six competencies of QSEN, and Family Nursing to promote quality maternal and child health nursing care.

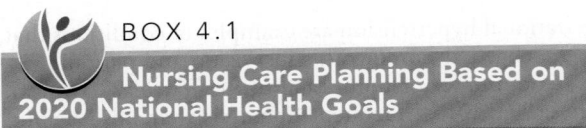

BOX 4.1
Nursing Care Planning Based on 2020 National Health Goals

National Health Goals are concerned with eliminating common infectious diseases of childhood and reducing complications of pregnancy. These measures are important because both eliminating common infections and complications of pregnancy could reduce the hours spent in home care.

- Increase to at least 77% the proportion of all pregnant women who receive early and adequate prenatal care, from a baseline of 70.5%.
- Reduce the rate of preterm births, from a baseline of 12.7% to a target of 11.4%.
- Reduce or eliminate vaccine-preventable diseases such as measles (from 115 to 30 cases per year), pertussis (from 2,777 to 2,500 cases per year), and varicella (chickenpox) (from 482,535 to 100,000 cases per year) and keep poliomyelitis at zero cases per year (U.S. Department of Health and Human Services, 2010; see www.healthypeople.gov).

Nurses can help the nation achieve these goals by helping women better accept and adhere to home care if it is advised during pregnancy. They can remind parents how important it is to have children routinely immunized so children no longer contract "childhood infections."

Home care, as the name suggests, is care of persons in their homes, provided by employees of a certified home healthcare or community healthcare agency. In recent years, hospital stays have decreased, and the need for home care has increased.

Postsurgical children or those recovering from an acute illness are often appropriate patients for home care. Women who receive comprehensive prenatal care during the entire course of their pregnancy have more positive birth and postpartum outcomes (Bernstein & VanBuren, 2013). Home care can be a means of promoting personalized prenatal surveillance and initiating specific health teaching for high-risk pregnancies. Pregnant women who require these additional resources are appropriate for home care (Olander, Atkinson, Edmunds, et al., 2012). Many children in terminal stages of disease are also cared for at home (**hospice care** or palliative care).

Assessing and orienting families to home care, home visiting supervising and coordinating home health personnel, providing health teaching, and evaluating the appropriateness of continuing home care are important nursing responsibilities. Box 4.1 shows 2020 National Health Goals that speak to home care.

Nursing Process Overview

FOR THE PREGNANT WOMAN OR CHILD ON HOME CARE

ASSESSMENT

Being able to assess communities and families is an important role for the nurse in home care. The shorter length of hospital stays has resulted in an increase in the need for expanded home care for pregnant women and ill children. Patients who are candidates for home care are seen and evaluated initially in an ambulatory or acute healthcare setting. After this treatment, they are discharged to a home care program. A family assessment will ensure that care is congruent with the family's usual self-care or childrearing practices.

NURSING DIAGNOSIS

Nursing diagnoses for home care may address the physiologic reason for supervised home care or the effect of the experience on the family, such as:

- Deficient knowledge related to complication of pregnancy and necessary procedures and treatments needed
- Interrupted family processes related to need for home care
- Ineffective role performance related to bed rest at home
- Social isolation related to the need for home care
- Anxiety related to complication of pregnancy, which has required home care

Home care of a child can place a heavy burden on a family as the stress of being responsible for an ill child's daily health status can have a negative impact on a parent's self-esteem or a couple's marriage; it can prevent parents from spending time with their other children or each other. Examples of possible nursing diagnoses that arise out of these factors include:

- Readiness for enhanced family coping related to increased time together because of home care
- Health-seeking behaviors related to skills needed to continue home care
- Risk for delayed growth and development related to lack of usual childhood activities
- Interrupted family processes related to dependence of ill child
- Disabled family coping related to changes in family routine brought about by home care needs of ill child

OUTCOME IDENTIFICATION AND PLANNING

Both outcome identification and planning for home care require close collaboration between the healthcare providers supervising care at home and the family experiencing home care. Reviewing the family's needs and expectations and their congruency with the nursing expectations are an important aspect of nursing care. Local organizations can provide assistance to families on home care. Women, Infants, and Children (WIC) supplies food for qualifying children as well as women during pregnancy, and Literacy Volunteers offers help to increase reading levels so families can better understand healthcare directions or increase their health literacy. Several national and international organizations also have online resources available to families.

ONLINE RESOURCES

Home Healthcare Nurses Association	www.hhna.org
International Association for Hospice & Palliative Care	www.hospicecare.com
National Association for Home Care & Hospice	www.nahc.org

IMPLEMENTATION

Interventions performed for a patient at home range from patient and family teaching and counseling to hands-on nursing care.

The home care nurse assists with the patient and family's psychological well-being and provides patients and families with resources for coping with stress from the caregiving responsibilities. If a child has a terminal illness, parents may require support to express their grief. Nursing care is similar to those performed in an acute care facility. Home care nurses need to have the same background and level of expertise as acute care nurses. They are usually required to have previous acute care experience as they are functioning with more independence and less supervision than nurses in the hospital setting.

OUTCOME EVALUATION

A home setting is less structured than a healthcare facility. Goals may need to be adjusted to reflect this aspect, and goals may need to be adjusted based on individual and/or family circumstances.

The outcome evaluation for the pregnant woman receiving home care includes determining whether the woman and her fetus are stable and progressing as expected in the home environment and whether, with the woman's input, home care is acceptable. For many women, successful home care will mean the difference between a premature birth and a successful term pregnancy.

Examples of outcome criteria for pregnant women could include:
- Patient demonstrates adequate skill at performing home monitoring procedures.
- Patient verbalizes changes in condition she will need to report to her healthcare provider.
- Patient participates as a member of the family within limitations imposed by pregnancy complication.
- Family members state they have adjusted to home care of mother.
- Patient states she is able to maintain contact with friends and family despite complete bed rest at home.

Examples of outcome criteria for an ill child might include:
- Parents state they have been able to make adjustments to accommodate care of an ill child at home.
- Child states he or she enjoys respite care in hospice setting one weekend per month.
- Parents state they are actively trying to supply adequate growth experiences for siblings in light of home care of oldest child.

Understanding Home Care

Home care is possible because parenteral nutrition, fetal monitoring, pharmacy care, mental health care, and laboratory analysis are now available in the home setting. Voluntary agencies may assist with transportation to and from healthcare facilities for specialized testing, such as X-rays. Home care educators may provide individual instruction (Clark, Gates, McKiernan, et al., 2016; Miller-Matero, Dykuis, Albujoq, et al., 2016; Vivian-Taylor, Roberts, Chen, et al., 2012).

Pregnant women with complications such as preterm labor that has been halted, hyperemesis gravidarum (a severe manifestation of nausea and vomiting of pregnancy), and gestational hypertension are examples of conditions that can be managed at home with supervision and periodic visits by a community or home care nurse (Theilla, Ławiński, Cohen, et al., 2015). Frequent home visits are also helpful to monitor the health of newborns who were born at low birth weights or who arrived prematurely. These visits are met with high levels of family satisfaction (Awindaogo, Smith, & Litt, 2015).

Advantages of home care include:
- It prevents extensive disruption of the family. For children who are acutely but not terminally ill, this extra emotional support may not be as immediately important as physical care. For those who are chronically ill or dying, being close to their family and friends may be the most important aspect of their care. For these children, home care is ideal (Ergün, Sülü, & Başbakkal, 2011).
- It is less costly for the healthcare delivery system. It is less costly to care for pregnant women or children at home rather than in a hospital setting largely because the number of healthcare personnel needed is reduced. Home care can also reduce the cost of care when monitoring is the main type of care needed.
- Technologic advances have made it possible for potentially complicated procedures, such as ventilator therapy, to be performed safely at home.
- It presents the opportunity to focus not only on a specific health problem but also on promoting healthy behaviors for the entire family. For example, to prevent a child or woman from being exposed to secondary smoke, family members should agree to establish a "smoke-free" home, allowing a family illness to improve the lifestyle of a whole family (Ashford & Westneat, 2012).
- It can increase a woman's or child's self-confidence and self-efficacy because it allows for more self-care and often more control of circumstances.
- Families can be better assessed in their own environment than in an agency environment because family interactions, values, and priorities are more obvious at home than in a healthcare setting.
- Home visits provide a private, one-on-one opportunity for health teaching.

Disadvantages of home care include:
- Cost containment has to be weighed against the safety and quality of care. Not all home settings are safe for care, and not all families have the commitment necessary, so it is not an alternative for all families. In addition, although home care is cost-effective for healthcare agencies, it may not be cost-effective for the family. Costs that health insurance would have paid for had the patient been hospitalized, such as dressings and medications, may no longer be covered once the person is transferred to home care. This means it can actually increase the cost for an individual family if the family's insurance does not cover the cost of nursing visits or necessary supplies.
- The physical care required (e.g., tracheal suctioning or a complicated medication regimen) can be overwhelming for family caregivers.
- A financial strain can arise if at least one parent or a spouse has to quit work and, therefore, cannot earn an income.
- Bed rest at home can cause social isolation and a disruption of normal family life.

What If . . . 4.1

Lisa's mother is concerned she will become exhausted because of the need for Lisa's around-the-clock care. What suggestions could the nurse offer to make home care more successful?

FEATURES OF HOME CARE

Home care visits vary in frequency depending on a patient's condition and the ability of the patient or family to learn and maintain specific procedures. In some settings, telephone, e-mail, and chat room contacts are set up to link healthcare providers with families so questions can be answered immediately even when the healthcare provider isn't physically present in the home.

Home care is not a level of care adequate for everyone or every situation, so evaluating whether a family is a good candidate for home care is the first assessment needed. Based on this evaluation, the number of home care visits and which provider would be best for home visits can be determined.

Concept Mastery Alert

Home nursing care is deemed "skilled" when a specific provider-prescribed procedure is indicated, such as medication administration, monitoring, or dressing changes.

Care at home may include:

- **Direct care**, in which a nurse remains in continual attendance or visits frequently and actually administers care
- **Indirect care**, in which a nurse plans and supervises care given by others, such as home care assistants

Nursing care is considered **skilled home nursing care** if it includes primary healthcare provider–prescribed procedures such as dressing changes, administration of medication, health teaching, or observation of a woman's or child's progress or status through such activities as monitoring vital signs or fetal heart rate. Whether nursing care is categorized as skilled or not can determine whether it will be paid for by third-party payers.

Frequency of visits varies with individual factors. For example:

- Those patients whose conditions are categorized as low risk probably need only weekly visits; a home healthcare aide may make the majority of visits.
- Those at intermediate risk need one to three visits per week; a nurse is necessary for the level of care needed.
- Those at high risk may need as many as seven visits per week; a nurse combined with other team members such as a nursing assistant, physical therapist, or a respiratory therapist will be needed for this complex level of care.

Assessing a Family for Home Care

The initial assessment includes an interview with the patient and family; a thorough health history and physical examination to document a woman's or child's current status; and

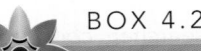

BOX 4.2

Nursing Care Planning Based on Respect for Cultural Diversity

Whether home care is successful is strongly influenced by cultural expectations (Hines, 2012). This may be especially true with regard to male–female roles in a home. In a family in which men and women share responsibilities, care tasks as well as time away from the stress of home care can be distributed equally. In contrast, in cultures in which the male is dominant and child care is strictly delegated to women, a woman can become exhausted from trying to keep her house clean, prepare meals, care for her husband and other children, and also care for a medically fragile child. In male-dominant cultures, the idea of a man giving care to his wife or an ill child contradicts a usual pattern. If a woman is the dominant member of the household, becoming a passive, cared-for partner may be extremely difficult for her.

Because the structure of families is culturally determined, home care may be easier in some cultures than in others. If the family is extended, for example, a mother may be so involved in the care of other family members, such as an older adult, she is unable to rest adequately at home or add enough time to care for an ill child to her other responsibilities. In such a family, however, there may be many people to offer care and support, so home care will be ideal.

Some cultures stress women must be active during pregnancy to help ensure a small baby and therefore an easier birth. That can make bed rest difficult if a woman wants to be active rather than resting. The culture of a particular community might oppose the use of technology, so a family living there might not like having a van to supply needed oxygen or intravenous equipment parked outside. Assessing each family individually helps determine how cultural diversity may affect that particular family and how to individual plans.

an environmental, community, and social assessment. Family motivation and preparation are factors that contribute to successful home care.

THE INTERVIEW

Assessment begins with an interview to determine the current structure and function of the family. Identifying family roles (see Chapter 3), such as who are the wage earner(s), the decision maker(s), the nurturer(s), or the problem solver(s), is an important component of the interview. Incorporating the current structure and function of the family to support the new activities of home care are addressed (Box 4.2).

QSEN Checkpoint Question 4.1

EVIDENCE-BASED PRACTICE

Adolescents may spend hours each day on social media websites or talking with friends. To determine if adolescents on home care experience depression from lack of social interaction, researchers conducted an online survey of 422 adolescents on home care. Findings from the survey revealed adolescents voiced positive aspects to solitude, but they also strongly rejected wanting or liking spending time alone. They expressed feelings such as fear, boredom, and separation anxiety. Those who reported feeling lonely were significantly less likely to enjoy being home alone during the day than those who weren't experiencing loneliness (Ruiz-Casares, 2012).

Lisa Puente is alone all day at home because both of her parents work. Based on the study, the nurse would make which recommendation to help Lisa prevent loneliness?

a. She could arrange to go on brief outings with her friends.
b. She could begin keeping a reflective diary of her thoughts and feelings.
c. She and friends could all download a book to their e-readers and then discuss it by phone or online.
d. She could keep up with her cheerleading squad by cheering along with them on Skype.

Look in Appendix A for the best answer and rationale.

After assessing present family structure and function, the nurse identifies ways family members think the illness and care at home will change their lives. This could include a wide range of changes such as increased expenses, the need for a parent or spouse to take a leave from work, the need for family members to help with frequent ambulatory healthcare visits, and the need to arrange for child care for other children. Because these needs change as the course of an illness changes, assessment must be ongoing.

Other assessments focus on likely adherence to medical, preventive, or medication regimens and whether the family will be able to safely monitor the patient's health at home. Additional assessment regarding other services or resources the family will need, such as the services of a home healthcare assistant or further nursing visits to ensure home care, is optimal. Future visits focus on continuing the assessment and evaluation of patient progress and readiness to help the woman or child move to another level of health care.

The term *resources* refers not only to material objects (such as a hospital bed, oxygen, fetal home monitor) but also whether a family is ready to deal with the chronic stress of home care. For example, pregnant parents may have to quit work to become home care patients. One parent of an ill child usually has to do the same. This automatically reduces a family's income, which can lead to severe financial problems.

HEALTH HISTORY AND PHYSICAL EXAM

A home care plan is developed based on the health history and physical exam. This plan may include teaching the patient or family how to obtain required health parameters. Teaching may also include ensuring the family has received cardiopulmonary resuscitation (CPR) instruction.

Typically, women receiving home care are taught how to self-assess various health parameters such as blood pressure, temperature, pulse, protein in the urine, serum glucose (with the use of a glucometer), fundal height, fetal movement, fetal heart rate, and uterine contractions. Parents or other family members of ill children invariably need to assess vital signs, comfort level, oxygenation (by means of an oximeter), and side effects of medications. When teaching these assessments, be certain to spend enough time with the patient and/or family so they thoroughly understand both the reason for the assessment and the procedure for doing it.

At subsequent home care visits, assess not only the results of the measurements but also whether they are being done correctly and consistently.

ENVIRONMENTAL ASSESSMENT

An assessment of the family's environment ascertains whether the home's physical surroundings will be adequate for home care (Table 4.1). Table 4.2 lists additional important assessments to make depending on the age of a child.

TABLE 4.1 ASSESSING A HOME FOR SAFE HOME CARE

Category of Information	Conditions to Note
Safety	Is there a smoke and carbon monoxide detector in the patient's bedroom? Do caregivers know the emergency call system procedure in their community? Does the primary caregiver know what steps to take if the patient is suddenly worse?
Oxygen therapy	If oxygen will be used, is there a sign to omit smoking in the room? Is the oxygen away from a fireplace, gas space heater, or gas stove? Does the family know not to light candles near oxygen in a power failure or for a birthday?
Space	Is there a bathroom in easy proximity to the patient's bedroom? Is there a working refrigerator if medicine needs to be kept cold? Is there adequate storage space for supplies? Does the family know how to reorder supplies?
Patient support	Is there a family member who will be the consistent caregiver? Does this person understand the importance of this role? Identify the roles of family members such as who are the wage earner(s), the decision maker(s), the nurturer(s), or the problem solver(s).
Electricity	Is the home well lit? Are there adequate three-pronged plugs needed for the care equipment available? Has the power company been notified if an electrical appliance is necessary for life support? What would be the caregiver's actions in a power failure? Do they need to purchase a battery power source?
Environment	Is the home a house or an apartment? Will the bedroom used for care be upstairs or downstairs? Is the home smoke-free? Is there evidence of roaches, rats, mice, or fleas?
Nutrition	Are food preparation areas in the kitchen clean? If a special diet is necessary, does the person who will do the cooking have adequate knowledge of food preparation?

TABLE 4.2 ASSESSING A HOME FOR HOME CARE OF CHILDREN BY AGE GROUP

Age	Points to Assess
Newborn or infant	Is there a suitable sleeping place? Do side rails of a crib lock securely? Are safe sleeping practices being used? Is there a freezer if stored breast milk will be used? Is there protection from mosquitoes? Is the home free of rodents that might attack a small infant? Is the infant kept safe from secondary smoking?
Toddler and preschooler	Is there a safe area for play free from stairs and poisoning possibilities? Are there screens or locks on windows to prevent a child from crawling out onto a ledge? Is there provision for stimulation and learning activities?
School-age child and adolescent	What is the provision for schooling (possibly an intercom with a regular classroom or home tutor)? Is peer interaction possible? If adolescent is self-medicating, will reminder sheets or some other reminder system be necessary?

Beginning Home Care

Discharge planners in acute care settings can be instrumental in helping set the stage for home care by discussing the need for continued health supervision as well as helping patients begin to establish personal goals for home care. A number of steps are then necessary for an actual home visit to be successful. These steps can be divided into previsit, visit, and postvisit phases.

PREPARING FOR A HOME VISIT

Typically, a first home visit is made within 24 hours of discharge or notice from an acute care or ambulatory care facility. A patient's referral form will inform the nurse of the patient's plan of care and treatment, and the nurse can generate a list of supplies needed for the visit. During a home visit, it is crucial to demonstrate respect for the patient's and family's privacy, beliefs, lifestyles, routines, culture, and requests.

As a part of individualizing care, telephone a patient or family in advance to verify the address and arrange a mutually convenient time for a visit. Ethical and legal aspects of nursing care, such as confidentiality, informed consent, Health Insurance Portability and Accountability Act (HIPAA) requirements, decision making, and patient rights commonly associated with acute care nursing, are applicable to home care.

ENSURING PERSONAL SAFETY

Home care visits are often made by an individual nurse. Steps to assure personal safety during the visit are crucial. Safety tips for traveling in an unfamiliar community are shown in Box 4.3.

BOX 4.3

Safety Tips for Home Healthcare Travel and Visits

- Plan your trip in advance using a reliable map of the area, a navigation system, or a computer mapping program so you don't become lost in a strange neighborhood.
- Let an agency member know where you are going and when you expect to return.
- Keep your automobile in good repair and filled with gasoline or electrically charged so you don't run out of gas and can avoid having to make stops at unfamiliar service stations.
- Park your car in a well-lit, busy area. Lock the car door.
- Lock any valuables in the trunk of your car before you leave the healthcare agency, not after you park in front of a home so no one sees you do this.
- Do not leave valuable objects such as expensive electronic equipment in your car or a briefcase on the seat that someone might think contains drugs, so the car is not a target for car thieves.
- Learn the location of public phones in the area or keep a cellular phone with you.
- If you suspect someone is following you in your car, drive to the nearest police or fire station.
- Do not carry a purse or backpack that suggests you are carrying a large sum of money, drugs, or valuables. If you suspect someone is following you while you are walking, walk into a business establishment.
- Carry only minimal supplies so your hands are free to defend yourself. Walk determinedly, as if you have a purpose and are in charge of your environment and situation.
- Avoid shortcuts through alleys or unoccupied areas; drive or walk on main or busy streets.
- Avoid approaching homes by a dark, back alley; use the front door or a busy hallway.
- Use special caution in stairwells and elevators. Leave a stairwell or elevator if a potentially threatening person enters.
- When you first enter a home, assess it for personal safety. Ask who is at home. If there are animals in the house, ask if they are friendly.
- If there are animals, take precautions to avoid getting bitten by fleas (sit on a kitchen chair, not an upholstered one).
- Be cautious about accepting food or drink if you are not certain about the hygiene of the dishes or food. Decline it gracefully with an excuse such as "I'm trying to cut down on the amount of coffee I drink" or "It's against my agency's rules."
- Look under your car when approaching it and in the back seat before entering it to be certain no one is there. Relock your car door immediately once inside.
- Have your car keys in your hand when you leave the house so you can unlock and enter your car quickly.
- If either you or your patient is in personal danger, call 911 for help. Leave a home immediately if you feel threatened or unsafe.

PATIENT-CENTERED CARE

The nurse needs to make a first home visit with Lisa, 16 years old, following a hospital stay. Which action by the nurse is best?

a. Telephoning her home to establish a time both she and a parent will be present.

b. Dropping in unannounced so the nurse can obtain a true picture of Lisa's home conditions.

c. Visiting at a time Lisa will be there by herself so she can better express her feelings.

d. E-mailing Lisa the 10 AM arrival time; the nurse can expect a parent to also be home at that time.

Look in Appendix A for the best answer and rationale.

LOGISTICS OF THE VISIT

Home visits may occur in a variety of settings from a house, an apartment, a mobile home, or a shelter. You need to determine the route to the visit prior to departing for the visit. Upon arrival at the home, knock or ring the bell and wait for someone to physically or verbally invite you to enter (even though you don't want the patient to get out of bed to let you in, walking in without permission could be interpreted as a home invasion). Greet the patient, any other family members present, and pets if they come to greet you. Dogs typically serve a guard function, and you want them to view you as a friendly, not a threatening, visitor. Occasionally, advance arrangements, such as having a neighbor let you in, may be necessary if a woman lives alone and cannot walk down a stairway or a long hallway to answer the door.

As in any healthcare setting, hand washing following universal precautions prior to patient contact and an assessment is required. Most home care nurses carry antibacterial gel or disposable wipes with them for hand washing, as these facilities in a home may not be convenient or available. Consent for care may need to be obtained.

ASSESSING THE PATIENT

At the initial home visit, you are going to conduct a thorough health assessment, including a social history, a current health history, and a focused physical examination.

Provide privacy and confidentiality when obtaining the health history and performing a physical examination. Despite the informality of the setting, appropriate interviewing and physical assessment skills are indicated (Box 4.4) (Polat, Bayrak Kahraman, Kaynak, et al., 2015).

Throughout the assessment, evaluate the patient's needs and provide instructions and reinforcement on any specific areas that are necessary. Assess compliance with the instructions for activity orders. If bed rest is required, ask how this is being achieved to ensure it is congruent with the medical orders. At the conclusion of the visit, ensure the family has a realistic understanding of the medical diagnosis and prescription instructions as well as knowledge of when to seek immediate care for particular signs and symptoms. Prescription instructions include the family's ability to obtain the prescription, and instructions on when to seek immediate care

---

BOX 4.4

Nursing Care Planning Tips for Effective Communication

Lisa is receiving home care because of hyperemesis of pregnancy and elevated blood pressure. She lost 15 lb at the beginning of pregnancy but now, at 20 weeks, has gained back the lost pounds, plus 2 lb extra, since beginning supplemental gastrostomy feedings every day. A home healthcare assistant visits her three times per week to supervise her nutrition. She always seems pleased to be visited by a home care nurse once per week.

Tip: Because home settings are more informal than those of healthcare agencies, it is easy to forget a home is a healthcare setting. Be careful to maintain therapeutic and structured communication during the health interview. Avoid overly relaxed communication with potentially leading questions.

Nurse: Hello, Lisa. How is everything?

Lisa: Great.

Nurse: Are you doing your own gastrostomy feedings?

Lisa: Right.

Nurse: Do you have any concerns about those?

Lisa: They make me throw up once—maybe twice—a day.

Nurse: I need to do a more thorough assessment.

---

include knowing who to contact based on the time and presentation of signs and symptoms.

Plans for a follow-up visit should be provided prior to the end of the visit.

What If . . . 4.2

Lisa's family lives in a trailer park. Their nearest neighbor stops the nurse at every visit to ask how Lisa is doing. How would the nurse answer her?

ASSESSING THE HOME ENVIRONMENT

During the home visit, it is important to assess the home environment to assure basic safety needs are met (Fig. 4.1). This means verifying and answering the following:

- Are the water, electricity, heat, and refrigeration in good working order?
- Are there working smoke alarms?
- Is the structure adequate, including functional windows and doors?
- Is the home free of rodents, insects, and lead-based paint?
- Is the bathroom accessible to the patient?
- Is the telephone within reach of the patient?
- If medical equipment, such as a hospital bed, wheelchair, or oxygen, is required, is the house suitable for the equipment?
- Is the flooring and layout of the room appropriate for a wheelchair?
- Are shelves and cabinets accessible if the person is using a wheelchair?
- Are bathing facilities appropriate and accessible?

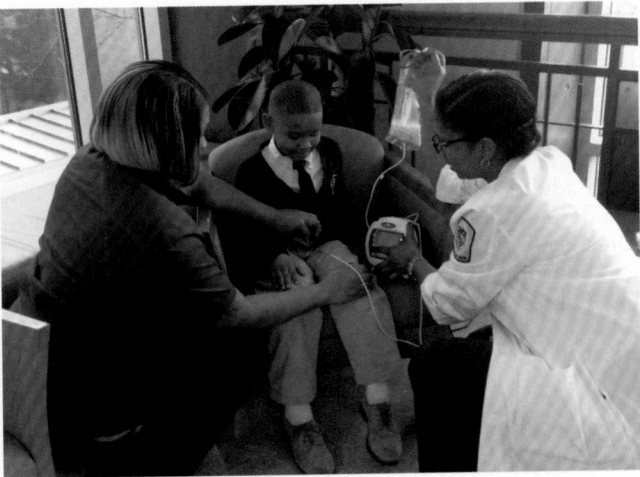

Figure 4.1   Procedures need to be incorporated into the family routine. Here, a young boy gets his gastrostomy tube feeding prior to leaving for school. A nurse assists the family with this new procedure.

QSEN Checkpoint Question 4.3

SAFETY

In the middle of a visit to Lisa's home, her former boyfriend arrives and threatens he will "punch" both Lisa and the nurse if the nurse doesn't leave. What action by the nurse is best?

a. Telling him threatening someone is not mature behavior and he should stop
b. Suggesting Lisa have her parents change their locks so this man can't visit again
c. Leaving the home and notify the agency of the unsafe circumstances for the nurse
d. Telephoning 911 and reporting that both the patient and the nurse are being threatened

Look in Appendix A for the best answer and rationale.

HOME CARE ASSISTANTS

Effective home care requires a team of healthcare providers, including a supervising primary healthcare provider, home care nurses, and other persons such as health equipment suppliers and home care assistants. Home health assistants can supply the bulk of personal care services such as assisting with or providing hygiene, assisting with ambulation, or helping to feed patients. Home care assistants have varied levels of preparation depending on their home health or community healthcare agency policies and the level of care they are being asked to provide.

When working with unlicensed assistive personnel, be certain you are familiar with their level of ability and education, so you assign care that is appropriate to their level of certification.

What If . . . 4.3
   When visiting Lisa, the nurse discovers large mouse holes in the bedroom that will be used by her new baby. What would the nurse do next?

POSTVISIT PLANNING

Postvisit planning consists of completing all required documentation identified in the assessment, care provided, evaluation of care, and planning for future care. Billing information as required by the agency is to be completed. Any changes in health status, needs for prescriptions renewals, or requests for updating and revising the plan of care should be communicated to the primary healthcare provider. Privacy rules (HIPAA regulations) apply the same as in hospital or ambulatory care settings.

FOLLOW-UP VISITS

Subsequent home visits are planned depending on the patient's circumstances. A second visit could be scheduled as often as the next day or as infrequently as once per month depending on the level of supervision required.

QSEN Checkpoint Question 4.4

INFORMATICS

Lisa says one reason she doesn't like home care is because private things about her won't be respected. The nurse could assure her of which of the following?

a. Privacy rules (HIPAA) apply to home care health records the same as hospital records.
b. It is a problem, but the nurse will do try to respect her privacy and gain her confidence as much as possible.
c. The nurse won't keep a record of home care procedures so she doesn't need to worry.
d. Electronic home care records are protected by copyright rules the same as all records.

Look in Appendix A for the best answer and rationale.

 Nursing Diagnoses and Related Interventions

Nursing Diagnosis: The family process is interrupted related to the stress of caring for ill family member at home.

Outcome Evaluation: Family members state they feel able to manage home care; family meets weekly to discuss problems and share accomplishments.

HEALTH PROMOTION

Nursing responsibilities for birthing parents and children receiving home care vary greatly because the reason for home care and the actions needed vary so greatly. Typical interventions carried out in homes are concerned with promoting both a healthy environment and healthy family function.

Identify a Child's Primary Caregiver

Although traditionally the primary caregiver for an ill child is the mother, in today's families, if another parent works more flexible hours, they may be the parent best able to give the bulk of care. In some homes, a grandparent or an older sibling will be the person primarily responsible for care. Arrange to include this person in planning and problem solving because this person knows best what strategy of care will be most effective with the child as well as what strategy will be most appropriate in light of the physical layout of the home and the family's financial ability and lifestyle.

Determine Knowledge (Health Literacy) Level of Family

Before anyone can be cared for at home, teaching will be required so the family understands the illness and principles of care. Include in teaching both the things that must be learned immediately and additional care measures that will need to be taught as the patient's condition changes. Box 4.5 shows an interprofessional care map illustrating both nursing and team planning and education for a family cared for in their community.

Identify Available Resources

Assess where the nearest fire and rescue company are located in relation to the home in case CPR is necessary, whether a backup resource is available to power needed equipment if a blackout should occur, and if the patient can be evacuated easily in case of a fire.

Promote Healthy Family Functioning

A family that is supportive of all family members and provides an environment conducive to each member's continued growth and development is more likely to be able to manage home care than a family with a history of ineffective or destructive coping strategies (e.g., a family in which parents have unrealistic expectations of family members, a family with a history of abusive relationships, or members who do not cope effectively with stressors). A careful assessment is necessary because even a family that appears to be functioning well may become so adversely affected by factors such as the loss of employment income, resentment over missed promotions, or cramped living space all caused by home care that its members' ability to be successful can fail. Remember, every family operates differently and handles stress in different ways. This means events that may seem overwhelming for a visiting healthcare provider may actually be easy for the family to handle. Conversely, problems that seem minor could be disruptive enough to affect the family's ability to continue adequate care at home.

Many women fulfill multiple roles in their family, such as financial manager, peacemaker, problem solver, nurturer, and decision maker. Even when a woman is on bed rest, help her to continue in these roles to ensure the family's usual functioning because support people often have great difficulty assuming these roles in her place. In some families, the ill child may fill one of these roles and so needs to be encouraged to continue in the role as well.

As a general rule, support people can only be supportive if they understand the need for and importance of their role. Arranging for a homemaker service to help care for children or an aging parent or to help with light housework may be necessary to prevent support people from feeling stretched so thin when the usual manager of the home is ill. At home visits, ask a woman how her support people are coping and if there are ways this experience could be made easier for them as well as for her. The ability to be allowed to make decisions about her own care can make a significant difference in whether a woman thinks her home care experience is satisfactory.

HEALTH MAINTENANCE

Health maintenance actions are a step beyond health promotion or are taken when a specific risk of ill health is present.

Maintain Skin Integrity

Both adults and children who are on long-term home care can develop skin ulcers the same as hospital patients if their caretakers don't use preventive measures against this (e.g., good nutrition, position changes, cleaning skin, and promoting mobility) (Kottner, Boronat, Blume-Peytavi, et al., 2015).

Promote Elimination

Constipation occurs at a high rate during pregnancy and can occur in children on bed rest from lack of exercise. Encourage a diet high in fiber and fluid to minimize this problem.

Ensure Bed Rest

One solution to help both adults and children cope with the stress of bed rest is for them to keep busy in some way, such as using their time to learn a new skill. Most women can name activities they would like to do but have never had time before to begin. For example, bed rest could provide an ideal time for an individual to catch up on reading previously neglected for a long time (Fig. 4.2).

Electronic readers make it possible for women and children to download reading material immediately. If a woman has children, she could spend part of her time reading to them. She could also use the time to take a home-study course, learn to knit, write a short story, or study for a certifying examination related to her work. In any event, helping her plan meaningful activities such as these can help her view home care not as wasted time but as time invested in her family or career (Box 4.6).

Children need to involve themselves in schoolwork or play, perhaps by learning a new game or solving sudoku or crossword puzzles. Otherwise, they may spend their time simply watching television or napping.

Although play is a universal activity of children, not all parents realize how important it is to children, so nurses can play an important role in teaching this. When a child is not proficient in English and English is the language of the healthcare provider, games such as stacking blocks or building with Tinkertoys can be played despite communication difficulty. Playing recordings of well-loved children's songs can also be effective because the child doesn't need to be able to understand the words to enjoy the music or clap with the rhythm.

Teach Monitoring of Vital Signs

Monitoring vital signs in the home does not differ from monitoring them in a healthcare agency. Although the mercury thermometer has been banned in many states due to concerns about poisoning, there may be a rare few in the home setting still. The family should be advised to properly dispose of the mercury thermometer and obtain an electronic one.

Blood pressure is best measured on the same arm and when the person is in the same position (lying down or sitting up) each time. Using an automated cuff simplifies taking blood pressure. These can be purchased for a low cost from pharmacies or from home care agencies.

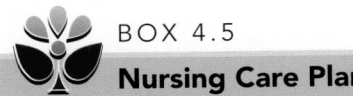

BOX 4.5

Nursing Care Planning

AN INTERPROFESSIONAL CARE MAP FOR A PREGNANT ADOLESCENT AT HOME ON BED REST

Lisa Puente is a 16-year-old who is 20 weeks pregnant. Since the beginning of her pregnancy, she had been vomiting at least four times daily and was losing weight. At 14 weeks, she was admitted to the hospital for 3 days and placed on a program of gastrostomy feedings. She managed well until last week when she was also diagnosed with gestational hypertension and placed on bed rest with fetal and uterine surveillance at home. She tells you it's impossible for her to rest at home: She's bored with school assignments and her friends (and boyfriend) no longer visit. You notice she's missed at least three doses of her antihypertensive agent. She asks to be hospitalized again for care.

Family Assessment: Patient lives with parents in a two-story home. Patient's bedroom is on second floor with bathroom located approximately 20 ft from patient's bed. Patient's mother is primary wage earner in the family; works full-time as a travel agent. Husband drives a delivery van; is home until noon daily.

Patient Assessment: Vital signs: temperature, 98.4°F; pulse, 76 beats/min; respirations, 22 breaths/min; blood pressure (BP), 144/94 mmHg; fetal heart rate (FHR), 148 beats/min. Mild facial edema, +1 protein in urine, 2-lb weight gain in last week.

Nursing Diagnosis: Ineffective coping related to need for bed rest secondary to nausea and gestational hypertension.

Outcome Criteria: Patient identifies methods to continue in school while maintaining bed rest, expresses increased satisfaction with imposed bed rest, and is able to maintain bed rest until fetal maturity. BP remains 140/80 mmHg or less, FHR within acceptable parameters, urine for protein remains +1 or less, weight gain limited to 1 lb/week, edema limited and without increase for the duration of pregnancy.

Team Member Responsible	Assessment	Intervention	Rationale	Expected Outcome
Activities of Daily Living, Including Safety				
Nurse	Assess vital signs, including heart rate, BP, and FHR at every visit.	Instruct patient how to take own vital signs. Review how to do a "count-to-10" assessment daily to assess fetal movement.	Assessment of vital signs and fetal activity provides a baseline for future comparison and evidence of the patient's and fetus's status.	Patient demonstrates she is able to accurately obtain own pulse, BP, and fetal activity. Findings compare with nurse's weekly findings.
Teamwork and Collaboration				
Nurse/primary healthcare provider	Assess what care services are most appropriate for an adolescent patient.	Arrange for home care visits by hospital home care team. Care assistant: daily; registered nurse: once a week.	Home care functions best when it is part of a "seamless" service.	Patient agrees to services of hospital home care team.
Procedures/Medications for Quality Improvement				
Nurse	Assess random urine specimen for protein at each home visit.	Instruct patient to assess urine specimen and weigh herself every day.	Proteinuria +1 suggests potentially limited kidney function or infection.	Patient voices an understanding of need for bed rest and adheres to restriction.
	Assess what patient interprets home bed rest to mean.	Review concept of complete bed rest. Arrange for a bedside commode if necessary.	Weight gain suggests fluid retention. Bed rest will reduce symptoms of gestational hypertension.	Patient demonstrates ability to carry out procedures accurately.
Nutrition				
Nurse/nutritionist	Obtain a 24-hour recall of gastrostomy feeding pattern to determine if nutritional intake is adequate.	Ensure patient is using the prescribed liquid feeding; encourage additional fluid intake.	An adequate nutritional intake is needed for fetal growth.	Patient describes a 24-hour intake of gastrostomy feedings adequate for pregnancy.

Continued on following page

BOX 4.5
Nursing Care Planning (continued)

Team Member Responsible	Assessment	Intervention	Rationale	Expected Outcome
Patient-Centered Care				
Nurse/social worker	Assess what patient feels are her chief needs that could make her more agreeable to remaining on bed rest at home.	Assist patient with planning effective bed rest; discuss possible sources of help from friends and family.	Planning concrete methods to make bed rest more tolerable alleviates stress.	Patient demonstrates ways she has adapted to bed rest restrictions.
	Assess what measures would make her more agreeable to continuing school work.	Urge parents to speak to school for more creative schooling arrangements.	Collaboration with school officials should help teenager to remain in school.	Patient voices plan for creative measures taken so she can remain in contact with school.
Psychosocial/Spiritual/Emotional Needs				
Nurse	Discuss usual activities with patient and how lack of these has led to boredom.	Encourage patient to plan activities such as reading and listening to music that are both enjoyable and compatible with bed rest.	Discussion provides baseline information to identify patient's needs, beliefs, and responsibilities.	Patient lists at least three restful activities she can use to occupy her day so she feels less boredom.
Informatics for Seamless Healthcare Planning				
Nurse	Assess for readiness to continue with home care.	Instruct patient and family to report increased blood pressure or sharp headache to primary care provider.	Knowledge of danger signs allows for early identification and prompt intervention.	Patient lists signs and symptoms she will report to primary care provider if they should occur.

Teach Self-Monitoring of Uterine Height, Contractions, and Fetal Heart Rate

Uterine (fundal) height during pregnancy is measured by using a paper tape measure according to McDonald's rule (see Chapter 9). If a woman is asked to record weekly fundal height measurements, demonstrate the correct technique and have her give a return demonstration, as this measurement varies greatly depending on where the tape measure is placed. Be sure a woman is measuring the height in the same manner each time.

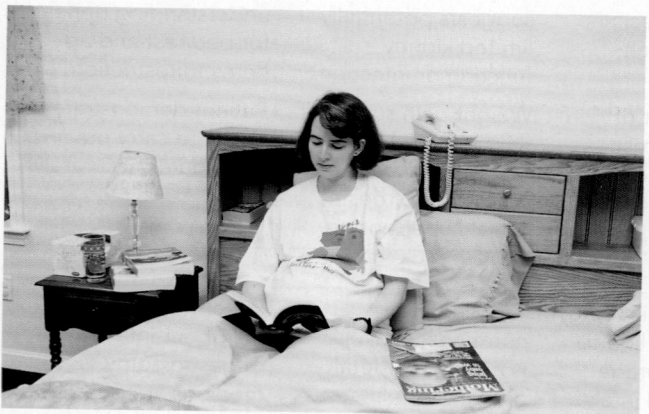

Figure 4.2 Bed rest can be stressful. Helping a woman who is on bed rest identify enjoyable and productive activities to pass the time can help ease stress.

Many women conduct fetal movement counts (also called kick counts) daily (see Chapter 9) to help assess fetal well-being (Hantoushzadeh, Sheikh, Shariat, et al., 2015).

Fetal heart rate (FHR) is usually recorded by the home care nurse at each home visit. In addition, a patient may be taught how to obtain this herself. FHR can be recorded by listening with a Doppler, a fetoscope, or an electronic monitoring device supplied as part of her home care program.

The patient can self-monitor uterine contractions using a uterine monitor, the same as in a healthcare facility, or by palpation (see Chapter 15). A nonstress test can be conducted using a portable monitor no bigger than 3 × 4 in. in size. A birthing parent straps this device to the abdomen for 20 to 30 minutes at a set time every day or at any time they feel contractions or are concerned about the lack of fetal movement (Fig. 4.3). The monitor records both uterine contractions and FHR. At the conclusion of the monitoring period, the tracing is transmitted to a central facility for evaluation.

If you discover a woman is omitting something such as counting fetal movement, spend some time asking why she's omitting it. It may be because she's unsure she's doing it correctly, or it may be because she's afraid it will reveal her fetus is not doing well (the philosophy of what she doesn't know won't hurt her). It's helpful to try to turn her fear into positive action; discovering decreased fetal movement will allow a healthcare provider to initiate an action to save her baby and so is a helpful step, not one to fear.

BOX 4.6

Nursing Care Planning Based on Empowering a Family

Q. Lisa tells you, "I feel like I'm wasting my time being home all the time this way. Tell me what to do to keep busy."

A. Try these suggestions:

- Concentrate on school work; make this a time to really delve into a subject.
- Ask your teacher if there is a special project you could work on from home while on bed rest for extra credit.
- Renew an old hobby or begin a new one such as solving crossword puzzles.
- Ask someone to bring you books on newborn care from the library or download them on an electronic reader (you'll be an expert on newborn care by the time your baby is born).
- Telephone your friends. Rest next to a telephone so friends know they won't be disturbing you when they return calls.
- Catch up on your correspondence. Friends and family will be surprised and delighted to receive a letter as so few people write them anymore.
- Investigate whether there is a local community project (such as telephoning for a political campaign, urging neighbors to write letters of support for a new playground) you could work on while on bed rest.
- E-mail friends or join a social media site (if you have a limited data plan, be conscious of the extra charges that might result). If you have a Skype connection, invite friends to show you what is new with them.
- Learn a second language; many books and websites are available on this.
- Take a mail-order or Internet course on something you want to learn more about (such as creative writing, learning to be a paralegal, how to cook French sauces).
- Ask your home care nurse about preparation-for-childbirth information or download a book on this. By conscientiously practicing breathing exercises while on bed rest, you can become well prepared for labor and birth.

QSEN Checkpoint Question 4.5

TEAMWORK & COLLABORATION

Since Lisa has begun eating oral food after gastrostomy feedings were discontinued, she has begun to develop constipation. What measure would the nurse want the team members to suggest she take to help prevent this?

  a. Drink more milk, as increased calcium prevents constipation.
  b. Walk for at least half an hour daily to stimulate peristalsis.
  c. Drink at least eight full glasses of a fluid, such as water, daily.
  d. Eat more frequent small meals instead of three large ones daily.

Look in Appendix A for the best answer and rationale.

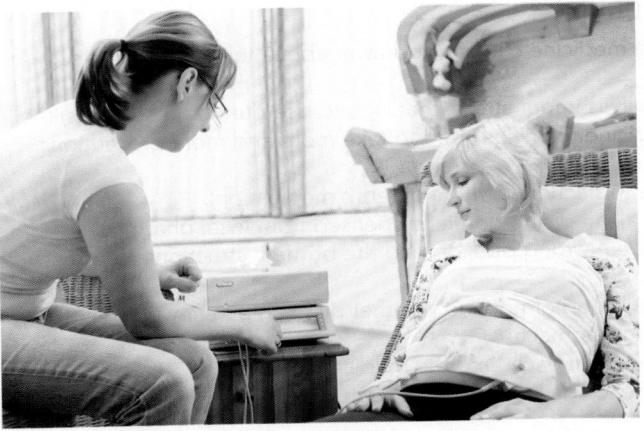

Figure 4.3 Fetal heart rate and uterine contractions can be recorded successfully by women at home. (Kzenon/Shutterstock.com)

HEALTH INTERVENTION

Health intervention begins when illness is present so that symptoms are not allowed to progress to a more serious state.

Explain Advances in Technology

A family may assume one advantage of home care is that their child will no longer be held captive by so much monitoring or oxygen equipment as surrounded the child in a hospital. Because so much of equipment is portable, however, a child on home care can receive the same level of monitoring as in a hospital. Parents may also need to adjust to receiving instructions over the Internet. Webcasting or telemedicine by a healthcare agency can be used to supply them information, treat patient conditions, lend encouragement, and answer questions they have about care (Given, Bunting, O'Kane, et al., 2015).

Caution adolescents there are some downsides to too much Internet use as there is an apparent association between depression and spending excessive amounts of time on social media chat rooms, so much so, a syndrome termed "Facebook depression" has been identified (Blachnio, Przepiórka, & Pantic, 2015).

Parents also need to alert children and adolescents that not all websites are safe to visit because of the possibility that sexual predators also visit such sites, putting them at risk (Khurana, Bleakley, Jordan, et al., 2015).

Provide Health Teaching

Because the home setting is private, a home care visit can provide many more opportunities for one-on-one health teaching than a healthcare agency setting. An important aspect of teaching for a pregnant parent might be providing childbirth education because a woman on bed rest will not be able to attend formal classes. For a child, it could be teaching the whole family about the child's illness and why the current therapy is needed.

Provide for Safe Medicine Administration

Most people receiving home care are prescribed some type of medicine, such as a tocolytic for pregnant women to halt preterm labor or chemotherapy for children because of cancer (Ewen, Combs, Popelas, et al., 2012). Review the rules of safe medication administration with the family to minimize mistakes such as taking the medicine more frequently than prescribed or forgetting to take it (Box 4.7).

Provide for Adequate Nutrition and Hydration

A pregnant parent who is on home care often needs help maintaining adequate nutrition. If ordinarily she is the person who plans menus, shops for food, and cooks for the family, other family members must assume these roles. If other family members are inexperienced at cooking, the entire family, including the pregnant woman, may not eat enough healthy foods.

As ill children don't get as much activity as usual, they may not be as hungry at mealtime as usual. You may need to make suggestions for healthy snacks so a child's total daily intake is adequate even if not a lot of food is eaten at formal meals.

All women during pregnancy should drink six to eight full glasses of fluid a day to obtain adequate fluid for effective kidney function and placental exchange (Harnisch, Harnisch, & Harnisch, 2012). Be certain women on bed rest have a supply of fluid close to their bed, such as a bottle of water, so they can do this easily.

Many pregnant women or children on home care receive intravenous therapy as a route of medication or fluid administration. Women with hyperemesis gravidarum (uncontrolled vomiting during pregnancy) or an isolated incidence oligohydramnios (less than normal amount of amniotic fluid) receive it as a means of hydration (Gizzo, Noventa, Vitagliano, et al., 2015). Women and children with blood dyscrasias may receive blood transfusions in the home (Marouf, 2011).

Because peripheral intravenous lines frequently become dislodged, in the home setting, intravenous fluid is often administered by a central line or a peripherally inserted central catheter (PICC) line threaded to a central blood vessel. Many drugs, especially antibiotics, are given through bagged "piggyback"

infusions kept frozen until the time of administration. Specially pressurized fluid containers allow for fast and easy administration of special solutions. To be certain fluid infuses slowly and accurately, an intravenous infusion pump is strongly recommended. Be certain a woman or a family member knows how to operate a pump, how to monitor intravenous insertion sites for inflammation and infiltration, how to protect the site from becoming infected (e.g., cover it with plastic rather than letting it get wet), when to remind a healthcare provider the site should be changed, and how to monitor the amount and kind of fluid or medication infused.

Home Enteral Nutrition

Chronically ill children and women who have hyperemesis gravidarum may receive nutrition by a gastrostomy or nasogastric tube. The supplies necessary for enteral feedings, such as feeding tubes and enteral pumps, are available for rent or purchase through pharmacies, medical supply houses, or the home care agency. Such tubes are usually changed every 2 to 4 weeks. The home care nurse will most likely be the person responsible for changing the tube, but this depends on the home care agency's policies. In addition to assessing the amount of formula infused by this route, be certain the woman or a family member is familiar with all aspects of care for the tube, equipment, and administration of the feeding. Caution the family to monitor the amount of formula for the feedings they have on hand so they don't run out, especially over weekends or holidays when their supplier may be closed. Patients on enteral feedings probably will need to weigh themselves periodically and record their weight. They may need to test blood serum for glucose with a glucometer. Be certain they use the same scale, wear consistent clothing, and know when to call for advice if they are unsure if their weight is remaining adequate.

Total Parenteral Nutrition

Total parenteral nutrition (TPN) is yet another way to supply complete nutrition and fluid to patients on home care. The home care agency or a separate vendor will furnish and

BOX 4.7

Nursing Care Planning Based on Family Teaching

SAFETY TIPS FOR SAFELY TAKING MEDICINE AT HOME

- Keep drugs in a safe place. In most homes, this is in a locked medicine cabinet or drawer above the height a child could reach.
- Keep alert that most childhood poisonings occur when a family is under stress; that is, because during these times, the family can forget usual procedures such as locking away medicine. Families need to take more and more precautions the higher the stress level rises in the home.
- Never take medicine in front of children (children can imitate this action with the parent's medication).
- Don't pour or prepare medicine in the dark. Because almost all medicine bottles dispensed from local pharmacies look and feel the same, it is easy to pour the wrong liquid, extract the wrong pills, or read the bottle instructions incorrectly without adequate light.
- Read instructions as to whether medicine should be taken with food or not and whether pills can be chewed or not. Try and drink a full glass of water with pills to ensure they reach the stomach.
- Create a reminder sheet and hang it in a prominent place. Cross off each time the medication is taken.
- Purchase a medicine box with an individual compartment for each day of the week. Such boxes help to eliminate confusion over whether medicine was taken or not.

deliver the formula, tubing, clean dressings, and an infusion pump. The formula, which consists of amino acids, hypertonic glucose, vitamins, and minerals in solution, needs to be stored in the patient's refrigerator until 1 to 2 hours before use; it is then removed from the refrigerator and allowed to warm to room temperature. Women and children requiring this type of intravenous nutritional therapy usually have a central venous access device such as a central venous catheter or PICC line inserted. The home care nurse plays a key role in teaching family members about the therapy and also in assessing the woman's or child's response to therapy.

Throughout therapy, be certain the patient or a family member knows how to monitor the infusion of the solution and the patency of the tube, how to change dressings (if that will be their responsibility), how to observe the insertion site for redness or inflammation, and how to assess body temperature for a possible infection. They also must be aware of any restrictions that should be adhered to (such as no baths if the water level will rise above the catheter insertion site) and the interval at which blood should be drawn for monitoring. Because TPN solutions are hypertonic, a woman or a family member needs to obtain blood glucose levels as necessary, test them with a glucometer, and keep a record of these. Be sure the family knows what findings they should report immediately to a healthcare provider.

Teach Self-Monitoring by Serum or Urine Testing

Women who develop gestational diabetes will be required to self-monitor their serum glucose level using a glucometer at least once daily, some three or four times daily (Evensen, 2012). Children with diabetes need to do these actions as well (Garg & Hirsch, 2012). Both women and children need support to be conscientious about continuing to do these actions when home care extends for a long time. A nurse can be instrumental in being the person to supply this support.

Manage Pain

Children who are on home care after surgery or those with a chronic or terminal illness may need efficient pain management for long periods of time. Be certain parents understand the principles of pain management such as to give medication before pain becomes acute. A detailed discussion with other pain management philosophies is discussed in Chapter 39.

QSEN Checkpoint Question 4.6

QUALITY IMPROVEMENT

Lisa has been on home care for a long time. Which of her following statements would worry the nurse most about whether her home is a safe place for home care?
a. "My mother is trying to quit smoking; she usually goes outside to smoke."
b. "If the lights go out, I know the circuit breaker is located in the garage."
c. "A police report says there's never been a robbery in this neighborhood."
d. "My father had the paint in the bathroom tested last year and it is lead-free."

Look in Appendix A for the best answer and rationale.

Health Rehabilitation

Health rehabilitation begins at the point complications have arisen and a patient is learning to adapt to chronic illness or take active steps toward restoring function. It can also mean accepting end-of-life care.

LONG-TERM HOME CARE

Although many families are good candidates for home care in the beginning, they have difficulty maintaining this high level of commitment as home care becomes long term. They may need both advice and support to continue to adapt constructively to the changing phases of an illness. They can develop low self-esteem and depression, feelings which can harm a marital relationship or prevent parents from spending time with other children (Fig. 4.4).

Help families maintain healthy functioning by promoting communication with each other and encouraging family members to identify and share their feelings about the situation at home. Encourage members to voice the frustration they can feel at being constantly confined at home or what they perceive to be a lack of progress in the ill person's condition. If a child has a terminal illness, support parents to express their grief and not grow discouraged because the work they are accomplishing is making the child comfortable. Continued successful coping will require the family to acknowledge and take seriously the impact of home care on each family member and work together to solve identified problems. To do this effectively, they may need to renegotiate roles and responsibilities within the family or seek outside help.

Children on home care need to continue with school if at all possible so they can maintain contact with friends, so they don't fall behind a grade level, and so they can continue the stimulation of learning. This means parents should make some sort of arrangement for schooling either through their local school district (many schools can establish a telecommunication setup for children ill at home) or investigate their ability to home school.

When a family has difficulty functioning well at the beginning of home care or does not adjust readily to continued care, nursing measures to support family functioning become

Figure 4.4   Home care of a child is family care. Here, a brother helps his sister transfer to a wheelchair.

even more important. A family whose coping strategies are maladaptive may not be able to care for a sick family member at home for long without strong nursing and other healthcare professional support.

What If . . . 4.4

The nurse is particularly interested in exploring one of the 2020 National Health Goals with respect to home care (see Box 4.1). What would be a possible research topic to explore pertinent to this goal that would be applicable to Lisa's family and also advance evidence-based practice?

Unfolding Patient Stories: Olivia Jones • Part 1

Olivia Jones, a 23-year-old gravida 1 para 0 at 30 weeks gestation, is being seen for a routine prenatal visit. She presents with mild edema and elevation in blood pressure requiring placement on bed rest at home. She is active in the local Baptist church and lives with her mother, who works during the day. What home care and community resources can the nurse consider to help her with symptom monitoring and maintenance of bed rest at home? (Olivia Jones's story continues in Chapter 13.)

Care for Olivia and other patients in a realistic virtual environment: **vSim** *for Nursing* (thepoint.lww.com /vSimMaternityPed). Practice documenting these patients' care in DocuCare (thepoint.lww.com /DocuCareEHR).

KEY POINTS FOR REVIEW

- Advantages of home care include the ability to provide care to chronically ill children and women with a complication of pregnancy in a cost-effective manner while keeping families intact and encouraging them to provide meaningful comfort and support.

- Disadvantages of home care include possible fatigue for families, possible financial hardship if there is a loss of job for the primary caregiver, and social isolation and disruption of normal home life.

- Home care requires careful planning and a combined effort between healthcare providers and the family to ensure collaboration and continuity of care.

- Not all homes are ideal for home care. Assessing that a primary family care provider is present; that the family is knowledgeable about the care necessary; necessary resources are available; and safety features such as a smoke detector, a safe area for oxygen storage, and a working refrigerator for food or medicine are present are important nursing actions.

- Parents may need respite care to continue to be effective care providers for children just as professionals need time off. Help family members take turns giving care so each has some free time during the week.

- Considering a family as both a single patient and as part of a community helps in planning nursing care that meets not only QSEN competencies but also the family's total needs.

CRITICAL THINKING CARE STUDY

Kimi Toi Hackett is a 23-year-old who just gave birth to a baby boy named Harding. She lives in a high-rise condo that was recently converted into apartments from an unused warehouse in the center of the city. Harding weighs 5.5 lb, has congenital heart disease, and will be cared for at home until he gains 5 more pounds and can have his heart repaired. He's being breastfed; his care instructions include never letting him cry, keeping him away from people with infections, and being certain he gets adequate sleep. Kimi Toi used to be a nanny for two school-age children before she quit work to take care of Harding. Her husband works nights at the post office. Kimi calls you for advice because she doesn't know any of her neighbors and so has no one to help her keep Harding from crying. Harding sleeps instantly if she puts him in his car seat and drives around the block, but she's afraid to go into the underground parking garage at night because there's no night guard. She feels she has moved into a totally wrong community; all of her neighbors are well-to-do businessmen or retired older adults.

1. Kimi Toi feels she and her husband have made a poor choice when they chose to move into a loft. Moving to any new community can be a major adjustment for a family. What are community features this family should have investigated before they bought a loft?

2. Kimi Toi is afraid to walk down to the parking garage at night to get her car. What suggestions could you make to help Harding stop crying in place of driving him around the block?

3. The Hacketts' building was just redone so it's easy to assume their condo has all the qualities needed for home care. To be certain, what questions would you want to ask Kimi Toi about the loft?

RELATED RESOURCES

Explore these additional resources to enhance learning for this chapter:
- Student resources on thePoint, including answers to the What If . . . and Critical Thinking Care Study questions, http://thepoint.lww.com/Flagg8e
- Adaptive learning powered by PrepU, http://thepoint.lww.com /prepu/

REFERENCES

Ashford, K., & Westneat, S. (2012). Prenatal hair nicotine analysis in homes with multiple smokers. *The Nursing Clinics of North America, 47*(1), 13–20.

Awindaogo, F., Smith, V. C., & Litt, J. S. (2015). Predictors of caregiver satisfaction with visiting nurse home visits after NICU discharge. *Journal of Perinatology, 36*(4), 325–328.

Bernstein, H. B., & VanBuren, G. (2013). Normal pregnancy. In A. H. DeCherney, L. Nathan, N. Laufer, et al. (Eds.), *Current diagnosis & treatment: Obstetrics & gynecology* (11th ed., pp. 141–153). New York, NY: McGraw-Hill.

Blachnio, A., Przepiórka, A., & Pantic, I. (2015). Internet use, Facebook intrusion, and depression: Results of a cross-sectional study. *European Psychiatry, 30*(6), 681–684.

Clark, J. A., Gates, B. J., McKeirnan, K. C., et al. (2016). Assessed value of consultant pharmacist services in a home health care agency. *The Consultant Pharmacist, 31*(3), 161–167.

Ergün, S., Sülü, E., & Ba bakkal, Z. (2011). Supporting the need for home care by mothers of children with hemophilia. *Home Healthcare Nurse, 29*(9), 530–538.

Evensen, A. E. (2012). Update on gestational diabetes mellitus. *Primary Care, 39*(1), 83–94.

Ewen, B. M., Combs, R., Popelas, C., et al. (2012). Chemotherapy in home care: One team's performance improvement journey toward reducing medication errors. *Home Healthcare Nurse*, 30(1), 28–37.

Garg, S. K., & Hirsch, I. B. (2012). Self-monitoring of blood glucose. *International Journal of Clinical Practice*, 66(175), 2–7.

Given, J. E., Bunting, B. P., O'Kane, M. J., et al. (2015). Tele-mum: A feasibility study for a randomized controlled trial exploring the potential for telemedicine in the diabetes care of those with gestational diabetes. *Diabetes Technology & Therapeutics*, 17(12), 880–888.

Gizzo, S., Noventa, M., Vitagliano, A., et al. (2015). An update on maternal hydration strategies for amniotic fluid improvement in isolated oligohydramnios and normohydramnios: Evidence from a systematic review of literature and meta-analysis. *PloS One*, 10(12), e0144334.

Hantoushzadeh, S., Sheikh, M., Shariat, M., et al. (2015). Maternal perception of fetal movement type: The effect of gestational age and maternal factors. *The Journal of Maternal-Fetal & Neonatal Medicine*, 28(6), 713–717.

Harnisch, J. M., Harnisch, P. H., & Harnisch, D. R., Sr. (2012). Family medicine obstetrics: Pregnancy and nutrition. *Primary Care*, 39(1), 39–54.

Hines, D. (2012). Cultural competence: Assessment and education resources for home care and hospice clinicians. *Home Healthcare Nurse*, 30(1), 38–45.

Khurana, A., Bleakley, A., Jordan, A. B., et al. (2015). The protective effects of parental monitoring and internet restriction on adolescents' risk of online harassment. *Journal of Youth and Adolescence*, 44(5), 1039–1047.

Kottner, J., Boronat, X., Blume-Peytavi, U., et al. (2015). The epidemiology of skin care provided by nurses at home: A multicentre prevalence study. *Journal of Advanced Nursing*, 71(3), 570–580.

Marouf, R. (2011). Blood transfusion in sickle cell disease. *Hemoglobin*, 35(5–6), 495–502.

Miller-Matero, L. R., Dykuis, K. E., Albujoq, K., et al. Benefits of integrated behavioral health services: The physician perspective. *Families, Systems & Health*, 34(1), 51–55.

Olander, E. K., Atkinson, L., Edmunds, J. K., et al. (2012). Promoting healthy eating in pregnancy: What kind of support services do women say they want? *Primary Health Care Research & Development*, 13(3), 237–243.

Polat, Ü., Bayrak Kahraman, B., Kaynak, I., et al. (2015). Relationship among health-related quality of life, depression and awareness of home care services in elderly patients. *Geriatrics & Gerontology International*, 16(11), 1211–1219.

Ruiz-Casares, M. (2012). "When it's just me at home, it hits me that I'm completely alone": An online survey of adolescents in self-care. *The Journal of Psychology*, 146(1–2), 135–153.

Theilla, M., Ławiński, M., Cohen, J., et al. (2015). Safety of home parenteral nutrition during pregnancy. *Clinical Nutrition*. Advance online publication. doi:10.1016-5614(15)00338-6

U.S. Department of Health and Human Services. (2010). *Healthy people 2020*. Washington, DC: Author.

Vivian-Taylor, J., Roberts, C., Chen, J., et al. (2012). Motor vehicle accidents during pregnancy: A population-based study. *British Journal of Obstetrics and Gynaecology*, 119(4), 499–503.

UNIT 2

The Nursing Role in Preparing Families for Childbearing and Childrearing

5

The Nursing Role in Reproductive and Sexual Health

Suzanne and Kevin Matthews, a young adult couple, planned to have a baby as soon as they married; however, it took Suzanne 1 year before she conceived. Now, 12 weeks pregnant, she comes to your clinic for a prenatal visit. In tears, she states, "My husband isn't interested in me anymore. We haven't had sex since I became pregnant." Kevin states, "I'm afraid I'll hurt the baby."

Previous chapters presented the scope of maternal and child health nursing and how the structure, function, and culture of families can have a significant impact on health. This chapter adds information about how to educate patients and their families about anatomy, physiology, and sexual health to better prepare them for childbearing and childrearing.

How would you counsel Suzanne and Kevin Matthews?

KEY TERMS

adrenarche	cystocele	puberty
andrology	gonad	rectocele
anteflexion	gynecology	retroflexion
anteversion	gynecomastia	retroversion
aspermia	laparoscopy	spermatic cord
bicornuate uterus	menarche	
culdoscopy	oocyte	

OBJECTIVES

After mastering the contents of this chapter, you should be able to:

1. Describe anatomy and physiology pertinent to reproductive and sexual health.
2. Discuss 2020 National Health Goals that nurses can help the nation achieve related to reproductive health.
3. Assess a couple for anatomic and physiologic health and readiness for childbearing.
4. Assess a couple for reproductive planning and sexual health needs related to sexual orientation and gender identity if pertinent.
5. Formulate nursing diagnoses related to reproductive and sexual health.
6. Develop expected outcomes for reproductive and sexual health education to manage seamless transitions across differing healthcare settings.
7. Using the nursing process, plan nursing care that includes the six competencies of Quality & Safety Education for Nurses (QSEN): Patient-Centered Care, Teamwork & Collaboration, Evidence-Based Practice (EBP), Quality Improvement (QI), Safety, and Informatics.
8. Implement nursing care related to reproductive and sexual health, such as educating middle school children about menstruation.
9. Evaluate expected outcomes for achievement and effectiveness of care.
10. Integrate knowledge of preparation for childbearing with the interplay of nursing process, the six competencies of QSEN, and Family Nursing to promote quality maternal and child health nursing care.

Whether or not someone is planning on childbearing, everyone is wiser for being familiar with reproductive anatomy and physiology and his or her own body's reproductive and sexual health. Patients and their partners who are planning on childbearing may become curious about reproductive physiology and the changes they will undergo during pregnancy. Patients who are pregnant are also often interested about physiologic changes, so nurses are frequently asked by both patients and their partners about reproductive and gynecologic health (Callegari, Ma, & Schwarz, 2015).

Although the general public is becoming increasingly sophisticated about their bodies because of courses in school on sexual health, misunderstandings about sexual health, conception (preventing or promoting), and childbearing still abound. When caring for children of school age or adolescence, they may ask you a variety of detailed questions about sexual or reproductive health they heard about in class but didn't really understand. For instance, many adolescents want to know more about what is a "normal" menstrual period; late adolescents may want to know what the "normal" expected frequency is for sexual relations.

A general rule in answering a question about sexual relations is normal sexual behavior includes any act mutually satisfying to both sexual partners. Actual frequency and type of sexual activity vary widely. According to a definition by the Centers for Disease Control and Prevention (CDC, 2014),

sexual health is not just an absence of disease, dysfunction, or infirmity but a condition of physical, emotional, and psychosocial well-being.

Encouraging patients to ask questions about sexual health is one of the most important contributions nurses can make. With this attitude, sexual and reproductive health problems can be openly discussed and made as solvable as other health concern. If this is an area that you were raised to not discuss freely, learning to be comfortable with the topic and your own sexuality can be the first step needed (Johnson & Williams, 2015).

A sample of 2020 National Health Goals that speak directly to improving reproductive or sexual health are shown in Box 5.1.

Nursing Process Overview

FOR PROMOTION OF REPRODUCTIVE AND SEXUAL HEALTH

ASSESSMENT

Problems of sexual or reproductive health may not be evident on first meeting with patients because it may be difficult for people to bring up the topic until they feel more secure with your relationship. This makes good follow-through and planning important because even if people find the courage to discuss a problem once, they may be unable to do so again. If the problem is ignored or forgotten through a change in caregivers, the problem can go unsolved.

Any change in physical appearance (such as occurs with puberty or with pregnancy) can intensify or create a sexual or reproductive concern. The person with a sexually transmitted infection (STI); excessive weight loss or gain; a disfiguring scar from surgery or an unintentional injury; hair loss such as occurs with chemotherapy; surgery, inflammation, or infection of reproductive organs; chronic fatigue or pain; spinal cord injury; or the presence of a retention catheter needs to be assessed for problems regarding sexual role as well as other important areas of reproductive functioning.

NURSING DIAGNOSIS

Common nursing diagnoses used with regard to reproductive health include:
- Health-seeking behaviors related to reproductive functioning
- Anxiety related to inability to conceive after 6 months without contraception
- Pain related to uterine cramping from menstruation
- Disturbance in body image related to early development of secondary sex characteristics
- Risk for infection related to high-risk sexual behaviors

Diagnoses relevant to sexual health may include:
- Sexual dysfunction related to as yet unknown cause
- Altered sexuality patterns related to chronic illness
- Self-esteem disturbance related to recent reproductive tract surgery
- Altered sexuality patterns related to fear of harming a fetus
- Anxiety related to fear of contracting an STI
- Health-seeking behavior related to learning responsible sexual practices

---

BOX 5.1

Nursing Care Planning Based on 2020 National Health Goals

A number of 2020 National Health Goals speak directly to reproductive and sexual health:

- Increase the proportion of adolescents who, by age 15 years, have never engaged in sexual intercourse to 80.2% of girls and 79.2% of boys from baselines 72.9% and 72.0%.
- Increase to at least 91.3% the proportion of sexually active 15- to 19-year-olds at risk for unintended pregnancy who used contraception at last sexual intercourse from a baseline of 83.0%.
- Reduce deaths from cancer of the uterine cervix to no more than 2.2 per 100,000 women, from a baseline rate of 2.4 per 100,000.
- Reduce breast cancer deaths to no more than 20.6 per 100,000 women, from a baseline rate of 22.9 per 100,000.
- Improve the health, safety, and well-being of lesbian, gay, bisexual, and transgender (LGBT) individuals (developmental goal) (U.S. Department of Health and Human Services, 2010; see www.healthypeople.gov).

Nurses help the nation achieve these goals by educating adolescents about abstinence as well as refusal skills, safer sex practices, and the advantage of obtaining a vaccine against human papillomavirus (HPV), the virus associated with cervical cancer. The need to participate in screening activities such as vulvar and testicular self-examination are also important to teach.

OUTCOME IDENTIFICATION AND PLANNING

A major part of nursing care in this area is to empower patients to feel control over their bodies. Plan health teaching to provide patients with knowledge about their reproductive system and specific information about ways to alleviate discomfort or prevent reproductive disease. It is also essential to design care that demonstrates acceptance of all sexual orientations and gender identities equally.

ONLINE RESOURCES

Resources for Reproductive Planning, Contraception, and Sexual Health

Centers for Disease Control and Prevention	www.cdc.gov
It Gets Better Organization: a helpful referral website for LGBT persons	www.itgetsbetter.org/
Not 2 Late: a detailed patient resource for emergency contraception explanations	http://ec.princeton.edu/
Planned Parenthood	www.plannedparenthood.org
Sexuality and U: a Canadian website that provides tips for sexual health and reproductive life planning. See their interactive program *Choosing Wisely*, which helps women select their ideal birth control method.	www.SexualityandU.ca

Resources for Fertility Support and Assistance

American Society for Reproductive Medicine	www.asrm.org
The National Infertility Association: a referral website for support groups and resources for couples with subfertility	www.resolve.org

Resources for Genetic Assessment and Counseling

American Association of Klinefelter Syndrome Information and Support	www.AAKSIS.org
March of Dimes Foundation	www.marchofdimes.com
National Down Syndrome Society	www.ndss.org
National Fragile X Foundation	http://fragileX.org
National Human Genome Research Institute	www.genome.gov
Turner Syndrome Society	www.turnersyndrome.org

IMPLEMENTATION

A primary nursing role concerning reproductive anatomy and physiology is education because both female and male patients may feel more comfortable asking questions of nurses rather than other healthcare providers. For example, nurses may be asked about contraception or fertility needs, STI prevention, or concerns related to congenital health conditions.

It is important to address potential concerns of patients of all sexual orientations and gender identities when providing reproductive and sexual health education. For example, include a discussion about anal or oral–genital sex practices when presenting information on safer sex.

OUTCOME EVALUATION

The evaluation must be ongoing in the area of reproductive health because health education needs to change with circumstances and increased maturity. For example, the needs of a woman at the beginning of a pregnancy may be different from her needs at the end.

How people feel about themselves sexually also changes. Their concept of themselves may have a great deal to do with how quickly they recover from an illness, how quickly they are ready to begin self-care after childbirth, or even how motivated they are as an adolescent to accomplish activities in life phases that depend on being sure of their sexuality or gender.

Examples of expected outcomes include:
- Patient states he is taking precautions to prevent contracting an STI.
- Patient states she is better able to manage symptoms of premenstrual dysphoric syndrome.
- Couple state they have achieved a mutually satisfying sexual relationship.

Assessing and Meeting Reproductive Concerns

An assessment in the area of reproductive health begins with interviewing to determine a patient's knowledge level of the reproductive process, STIs, concerns about his or her reproductive functioning, or safer sex practices (Box 5.2). This area of health interviewing takes practice, and the conviction that exploring sexual health is as important as exploring less emotionally involved areas of health, such as dietary intake or activity level. The 14-year-old girl, who is not yet menstruating, for instance, may be anxious about that fact but may be reluctant to say so unless asked directly.

A statement such as the following invites discussion: "Although many of your friends at school may be menstruating, it's not at all uncommon for some girls not to begin their periods until age 15 or 16 years. How do you feel about not yet having your period?" This combination of providing information and while interviewing may encourage an adolescent to discuss not only her possible concern about delayed **menarche** (the beginning of menstruation) but also other areas that will reveal her knowledge or lack of knowledge about reproductive health. Specific questions to include in a sexual history are shown in Box 5.3.

During a physical examination, it's important to include observation for normal distribution of body hair such as triangle-shaped pubic hair in women and diamond-shaped pubic hair in men, normal genital and breast development, and signs and symptoms of STIs. Many STIs are asymptomatic, so it is important to assess whether the patient is at risk for contracting

BOX 5.2

Nursing Care Planning Tips for Effective Communication

Kevin brings his 16-year-old nephew, Mark, into your healthcare clinic because Mark has had painful urination for 2 days. A culture is taken to determine whether he has contracted a sexually transmitted infection (STI).

Tip: Ask specific, open-ended follow-up questions to ensure a positive exchange of information and effective health teaching. Remain nonjudgmental to encourage the individual to continue to elaborate. Adolescents are often so concerned about protecting their privacy from adults they may initially offer as little information as possible at a healthcare visit, especially in regard to sexual issues.

Nurse: Mark, because you're sexually active, your symptoms suggest you may have contracted a sexually transmitted infection.

Mark: Uh-huh.

Nurse: Do you practice safer sex?

Mark: Uh, yeah.

Nurse: What measures do you take?

Mark: My girlfriend's on the pill, so that's all we need to know, isn't it?

Nurse: Let's talk about the different kinds of protection needed to prevent pregnancy and STIs.

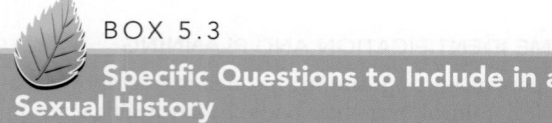

BOX 5.3

Specific Questions to Include in a Sexual History

Are you sexually active?
Is your sexual partner of the same or a different gender?
How many sexual partners have you had in the past 6 months?
Are you satisfied with your sex life? If not, why not?
Do you have any concerns about your sex life? If so, what are they? What would you like to change?
What measures do you take to practice safer sex?
For those at high risk of contracting HIV: Are you using pre-exposure prophylaxis (PrEP) to reduce your chances of HIV infection?
Have you ever contracted a sexually transmitted infection or are you worried you have one now?
Have you ever experienced a problem such as maintaining an erection, erectile dysfunction, failure to achieve orgasm, or pain during intercourse?
If you're sexually active, are you using a method to prevent pregnancy?
Are you satisfied with your current reproductive planning method? Do you have any questions about it?
For adolescents and women under the age of 27 years: Are you vaccinated against human papillomavirus (HPV)?

such an infection (see Chapters 33 and 47 for documentation of stages of sexual development and signs of STIs).

To help patients better understand reproductive functioning and sexual health, specific teaching might include:

- Explaining to a school-age boy that nocturnal emissions are normal
- Teaching an early adolescent about normal anatomy and physiology and the process of reproduction
- Teaching a young adolescent safer sex practices
- Explaining reproductive physiology to a couple who wish to become pregnant

Teaching may be in response to a direct question posed by a parent (Box 5.4). It is often enhanced by the use of illustrations from books or journals, video clips, or models of internal and external reproductive organs. Nursing interventions in this area, however, should include much more than just distributing educational materials. You need to follow up by asking if the education material answered the patient's questions. In addition, offer empathy for a patient's concerns, such as a woman's worry that increased tension before menstruation is a symptom of premenstrual dysphoric syndrome, to help her validate her suspicions. Websites set up by health professionals

BOX 5.4

Nursing Care Planning Based on Family Teaching

COMMUNICATING GENDER AND SEXUALITY TO CHILDREN

Q. Suzanne asks you, "Is it all right to call body parts by nicknames, such as 'peter' for penis, when we talk to children? Or should we use the anatomic name?"

A. Although this decision is strictly up to parents, using anatomic names is usually advised. This prevents children from thinking of one part of their body as so different from others (and perhaps dirty or suspect) it can't be called by its real name. Additionally, using correct names for genitalia can help the child to communicate if he or she has been a victim of sexual assault.

Q. Kevin asks you, "Will it be important to give our child unisex toys?"

A. Gender involves more than the toys children use for play. If parents are concerned about coercing children into particular gender roles through play, they need to begin by monitoring their own perspective. Once they project a feeling, roles are interchangeable, such as both genders participate in sports and both parents cook and do dishes, the general home milieu does more than any one action to teach this principle to children.

can be an ideal method for adolescents to learn more about their bodies and safer sex practices because they can do this in a private, nonjudgmental setting (Guilamo-Ramos, Lee, Kantor, et al., 2015). Again, follow-up is important to be certain the content was understood and the adolescent didn't also visit websites with misleading information.

Discussing the subject of reproduction in a matter-of-fact way, or treating menstruation as a positive sign of growth in a woman rather than as a burden, can help patients assume a positive attitude about these subjects and can serve as a valuable intervention.

Reproductive Development

Reproductive development begins at the moment of conception and continues through life.

INTRAUTERINE DEVELOPMENT

Sex assigned at birth is generally determined at the moment of conception by chromosome information, which is supplied by the sperm that joins with the ovum to create the new life. A **gonad** is a body organ that produces the cells necessary for reproduction (the ovary in females, the testis in males). At approximately week 5 of intrauterine life, mesonephric (wolffian) and paramesonephric (müllerian) ducts, the tissue that will become ovaries and testes, have already formed. By week 7 or 8, in chromosomal males, this early gonadal tissue begins formation of testosterone. Under the influence of testosterone, the mesonephric duct develops into male reproductive organs and the paramesonephric duct regresses. If testosterone is not present by week 10, the paramesonephric duct becomes dominant and develops into female reproductive organs. When ovaries form, all of the **oocytes** (cells that will develop into eggs throughout the woman's mature years) are already present (Edmonds, 2012).

At about week 12 of intrauterine life, the external genitals begin to develop. In males, penile tissue elongates and the ventral surface of the penis closes to form a urethra. In females, with no testosterone present, the uterus, labia minora, and labia majora form. If, for some reason, testosterone secretion is halted in utero, a chromosomal male could be born with female-appearing genitalia (ambiguous genitalia). If a pregnant woman should be prescribed a form of testosterone or, because of a metabolic abnormality, she produces a high level of testosterone, a chromosomal female could be born with male-appearing genitalia (Kumar, 2012).

PUBERTAL DEVELOPMENT

Puberty is the stage of life at which secondary sex changes begin. In most girls, these changes are stimulated when the hypothalamus synthesizes and releases gonadotropin-releasing hormone (GnRH), which then triggers the anterior pituitary to release follicle-stimulating hormone (FSH) and luteinizing hormone (LH). FSH and LH are termed gonadotropin (*gonad* = "ovary"; *tropin* = "growth") hormones not only because they begin the production of androgen and estrogen, which in turn initiate secondary sex characteristics, but also because they continue to cause the production of eggs and

influence menstrual cycles throughout women's lives (Eggers, Ohnesorg, & Sinclair, 2014).

The mechanism that initiates this pubertal change is not well understood, but the hypothalamus apparently serves as a gonadostat or regulation mechanism to "turn on" gonad functioning. Although it is not proven, the general consensus is a girl must reach a critical weight of approximately 95 lb (43 kg) or develop a critical mass of body fat before the hypothalamus is triggered to send initial stimulation to the anterior pituitary gland to begin the formation of FSH and LH. Probably because of the combination of better nutrition and increased obesity, girls are beginning puberty at earlier ages than ever before (8 to 11 years of age) (Maron, 2015). Studies of female athletes and girls with anorexia nervosa demonstrate that delays or halts in menstruation are related to the lack of body fat or energy expenditure (Mountjoy, Sundgot-Borgen, Burke, et al., 2014). The phenomenon of what triggers puberty is even less understood in boys but is probably also related to body weight.

There may be different needs and developmental routes for transgender individuals, whose sex assigned at birth, and gender do not match. Although this section uses gendered pronouns, it is important for nurses to be aware of resources that address transgender patient health and development needs such as The Joint Commission's (2011) *Advancing Effective Communication, Cultural Competence, and Patient- and Family-Centered Care for the Lesbian, Gay, Bisexual, and Transgender (LGBT) Community: A Field Guide.*

The Role of Androgen

Androgenic hormones are the hormones responsible for muscular development, physical growth, and the increase in sebaceous gland secretions that cause typical acne in both boys and girls during adolescence. In males, androgenic hormones are produced by the adrenal cortex and the testes and, in females, by the adrenal cortex and the ovaries.

The level of the primary androgenic hormone, testosterone, is low in males until puberty (between ages 12 and 14 years) when it rises to influence pubertal changes in the testes, scrotum, penis, prostate, and seminal vesicles; the appearance of male pubic, axillary, and facial hair; laryngeal enlargement with its accompanying voice change; maturation of spermatozoa; and closure of growth plates in long bones (termed **adrenarche**). In girls, testosterone influences enlargement of the labia majora and clitoris and the formation of axillary and pubic hair.

The Role of Estrogen

When triggered at puberty by FSH, ovarian follicles in females begin to excrete a high level of the hormone estrogen. This increase influences the development of the uterus, fallopian tubes, and vagina; typical female fat distribution; hair patterns; and breast development. It also closes the epiphyses of long bones in girls the same way testosterone closes the growth plate in boys. The beginning of breast development is termed thelarche, which usually starts 1 to 2 years before menstruation.

Secondary Sex Characteristics

Adolescent sexual development has been categorized into stages (Tanner, 1990). There is wide variation in the time required for adolescents to move through these developmental stages; however, the sequential order is fairly constant. In girls, pubertal changes typically occur as:

- Growth spurt
- Increase in the transverse diameter of the pelvis
- Breast development
- Growth of pubic hair
- Onset of menstruation
- Growth of axillary hair
- Vaginal secretions

The average age at which menarche (the first menstrual period) occurs is 12.4 years of age (Ledger, 2012). It may occur as early as age 9 years or as late as age 17 years, however, and still be within a normal age range. Irregular menstrual periods are the rule rather than the exception for the first year or two. Menstrual periods do not become regular until ovulation occurs consistently, and this does not tend to happen until 1 to 2 years after menarche (see Chapter 33 for a discussion of the use of oral estrogen–based contraceptives to help regulate menstrual periods in girls). Unlike the production of ova in girls, spermatozoa in boys do not begin in intrauterine life and is not produced in a cyclic pattern; rather, they are produced in a continuous process. The production of ova stops at menopause. In contrast, sperm production continues from puberty throughout the male's life.

Secondary sex characteristics of boys usually occur in the order of:

- Increase in weight
- Growth of testes
- Growth of face, axillary, and pubic hair
- Voice changes
- Penile growth
- Increase in height
- Spermatogenesis (production of sperm)

QSEN Checkpoint Question 5.1

PATIENT-CENTERED CARE

Suzanne Matthews tells the nurse she's worried she might be subfertile because both breast development and her first menstrual period occurred later than most of her friends. To increase her self-esteem and meet her learning needs, the nurse could assure her of what fact?

a. Adrenarche, the development of breasts, typically occurs before the first menstrual period.
b. Breast development, termed mamarche, is not fully complete until about age 25 years.
c. The time for development of breasts varies a great deal and is termed thelarche.
d. Menarche, the term for breast development, typically occurs before 12 years of age.

Look in Appendix A for the best answer and rationale.

The Male Reproductive System

Although the structures of the female and male reproductive systems differ greatly in both appearance and function, they are homologues; that is, they arise from the same or matched embryonic origin. **Andrology** is the study of the male reproductive organs. The male reproductive system consists of both external and internal divisions (Fig. 5.1).

MALE EXTERNAL STRUCTURES

External genital organs of the male include the testes (which are encased in the scrotal sac) and the penis.

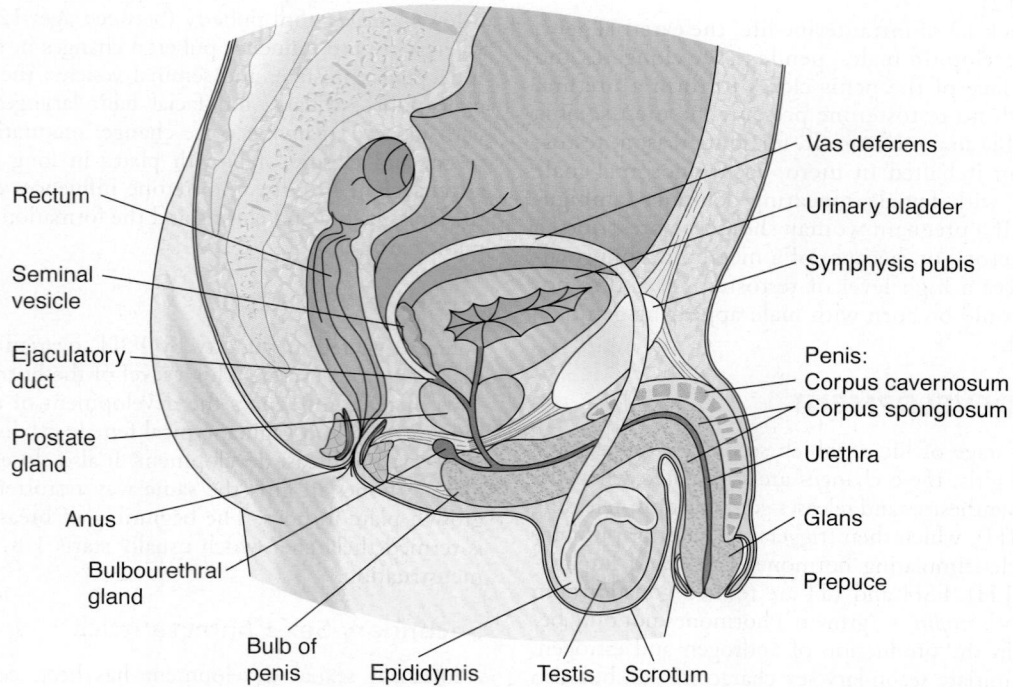

Figure 5.1   The male internal and external reproductive organs.

The Scrotum

The scrotum is a rugated, skin-covered, muscular pouch suspended from the perineum. Its functions are to support the testes and help regulate the temperature of sperm. In very cold weather, the scrotal muscle contracts to bring the testes closer to the body. In very hot weather, or in the presence of fever, the muscle relaxes, allowing the testes to fall away from the body. In this way, the temperature of the testes can remain as even as possible to promote the production and viability of sperm.

The Testes

The testes are two ovoid glands, 2 to 3 cm wide, that rest in the scrotum. Each testis is encased by a protective white fibrous capsule and is composed of a number of lobules. Each lobule contains interstitial cells (Leydig cells) that produce testosterone and a seminiferous tubule that produces spermatozoa.

Testes in a fetus first form in the pelvic cavity and then descend late in intrauterine life (about the 34th to 38th week of pregnancy) into the scrotal sac. Because this descent occurs so late in pregnancy, many male infants born preterm still have undescended testes. These infants need to be monitored closely to be certain their testes do descend at what would have been the 34th to 38th week of gestational age because testicular descent does not occur as readily in extrauterine life as it does in utero. Testes that remain in the pelvic cavity (cryptorchidism) may not produce viable sperm and have a four to seven times increased rate of testicular cancer (Fantasia, Aidlen, Lathrop, et al., 2015).

Although spermatozoa are produced in the testes, they reach maturity through a complex sequence of events. First, the hypothalamus releases GnRH, which in turn influences the anterior pituitary gland to release FSH and LH, the same as in women. FSH in men is responsible for the release of androgen-binding protein (ABP). LH is responsible for the release of testosterone from the testes. ABP and testosterone then combine to promote sperm formation. When the production of testosterone reaches a peak amount, a feedback effect on the hypothalamus and anterior pituitary gland is created, which slows the production of FSH and LH and ultimately decreases or regulates sperm production.

In most males, one testis is slightly larger than the other and is suspended slightly lower in the scrotum than the other (usually the left one). Because of this, testes tend to slide past each other more readily on sitting or muscular activity, and there is less possibility of trauma to them. Most body structures of importance are more protected than the testes (e.g., the heart is surrounded by ribs of hard bone). However, spermatozoa do not survive at a temperature as high as that of the internal body, so the location of the testes outside the body, where the temperature is about 1°F lower than body temperature, provides protection for sperm survival (Huether & McCance, 2012).

Normal testes feel firm and smooth and are egg shaped. Beginning in early adolescence, boys need to learn testicular self-examination so they can detect tenderness or any abnormal growth in testes (see Chapter 34).

The Penis

The penis is composed of three cylindrical masses of erectile tissue in the penis shaft. The urethra passes through these layers of tissue, allowing the penis to serve as both the outlet

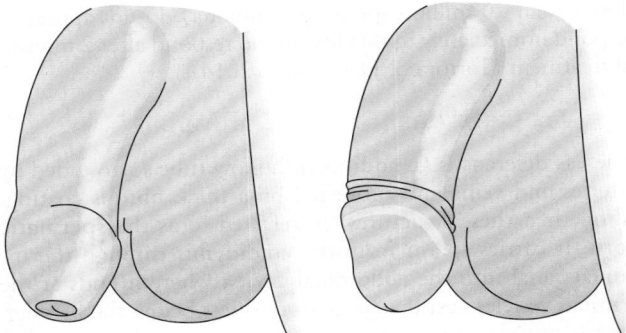

Figure 5.2   An uncircumcised and a circumcised penis.

for the urinary and reproductive tracts in men. With sexual excitement, nitric oxide is released from the endothelium of blood vessels. This causes dilation and an increase in blood flow to the arteries of the penis (engorgement). The ischiocavernosus muscle at the base of the penis, under stimulation of the parasympathetic nervous system, then contracts, trapping both venous and arterial blood in the three sections of erectile tissue. This leads to distention (and erection) of the penis.

At the distal end of the organ is a bulging, sensitive ridge of tissue called the glans. A retractable casing of skin, the prepuce, protects the nerve-sensitive glans at birth. Based on religious or cultural beliefs, many male infants have the prepuce tissue removed surgically (circumcision) shortly after birth (Fig. 5.2). Although controversial to some, the American Academy of Pediatrics (AAP) advises that the health benefits of male circumcision outweigh its medical risks; however, the benefits are not strong enough to recommend every male newborn be circumcised. The AAP advises that circumcision decisions should be made in consultation with parents with consideration of their cultural or religious beliefs. Its advantages allow for lower rates of urinary tract infections, HIV, STIs, and penile cancer. Its disadvantages include surgical complications, such as bleeding and pain, and reduction of sensation with sexual stimulation (AAP, 2012; Bossio, Pukall, & Steele, 2014).

MALE INTERNAL STRUCTURES

The male internal reproductive organs are the epididymis, the vas deferens, the seminal vesicles, the ejaculatory ducts, the prostate gland, the urethra, and the bulbourethral glands (see Fig. 5.1).

The Epididymis

The seminiferous tubule of each testis leads to a tightly coiled tube, the epididymis, which is responsible for conducting sperm from the tubule to the vas deferens, the next step in the passage to the outside. Because each epididymis is so tightly coiled, its length is extremely deceptive: It is actually over 20 ft long. Some sperm are stored in the epididymis, and a part of the alkaline fluid (semen, or seminal fluid that contains a basic sugar and protein) that will surround sperm at maturity is produced by the cells lining the epididymis.

Sperm are immobile and incapable of fertilization as they pass through or are stored at the epididymis level. It takes at least 12 to 20 days for them to travel the length of the tube and a total of 65 to 75 days for them to reach full maturity. This is one reason that **aspermia** (absence of sperm) and oligospermia (fewer than 20 million sperm per milliliter) do not appear to respond immediately to therapy but do respond after 2 months of treatment (Tortora & Derrickson, 2014).

The Vas Deferens (Ductus Deferens)

The vas deferens is an additional hollow tube surrounded by arteries and veins and protected by a thick fibrous coating. Altogether, these structures are referred to as the **spermatic cord**. It carries sperm from the epididymis through the inguinal canal into the abdominal cavity, where it ends at the seminal vesicles and the ejaculatory ducts below the bladder. Sperm complete maturation as they pass through the vas deferens. They are still not mobile at this point, however, probably because of the fairly acidic medium of semen.

The Seminal Vesicles

The seminal vesicles are two convoluted pouches that lie along the lower portion of the bladder and empty into the urethra by ejaculatory ducts. These glands secrete a viscous alkaline liquid with a high sugar, protein, and prostaglandin content. Sperm become increasingly motile because this added fluid surrounds them with a more favorable pH environment.

The Prostate Gland

The prostate is a chestnut-sized gland that lies just below the bladder and allows the urethra to pass through the center of it, like the hole in a doughnut. The gland's purpose is to secrete a thin, alkaline fluid, which, when added to the secretion from the seminal vesicles, further protects sperm by increasing the naturally low pH level of the urethra.

The Bulbourethral Glands

Two bulbourethral, or Cowper's, glands lie beside the prostate gland and empty by short ducts into the urethra. They supply one more source of alkaline fluid to help ensure the safe passage of spermatozoa. Semen, therefore, is derived from the prostate gland (60%), the seminal vesicles (30%), the epididymis (5%), and the bulbourethral glands (5%).

The Urethra

The urethra is a hollow tube leading from the base of the bladder, which, after passing through the prostate gland, continues to the outside through the shaft and glans of the penis. It is about 8 in. (18 to 20 cm) long. Like other urinary tract structures, it is lined with mucous membrane.

QSEN Checkpoint Question 5.2

QUALITY IMPROVEMENT

Suppose Kevin Matthews tells the nurse he is planning on having a vasectomy after the birth of his new child but is worried about having his testes removed this way. The nurse would want the clinic's educational material on vasectomy to clearly state that this procedure involves which of the following structures?

   a. The seminal vesicles
   b. The epididymis
   c. The vas deferens
   d. The ducts of the bulbourethral glands

Look in Appendix A for the best answer and rationale.

The Female Reproductive System

The female reproductive system, like the male, has both external and internal components. The study of the female reproductive organs is **gynecology**.

FEMALE EXTERNAL STRUCTURES

The structures that form the female external genitalia are termed the vulva (from the Latin word for "covering") and are illustrated in Figure 5.3.

The Mons Veneris

The mons veneris is a pad of adipose tissue located over the symphysis pubis, the pubic bone joint. Covered by a triangle of coarse, curly hairs, the purpose of the mons veneris is to protect the junction of the pubic bone from trauma.

The Labia Minora

Immediately posterior to the mons veneris spread two hairless folds of connective tissue, the labia minora. Before menarche, these folds are fairly thin; by childbearing age, they have become firm and full; and after menopause, they atrophy and again become much smaller. Normally, the folds of the labia minora are pink in color; the internal surface is covered with mucous membrane, and the external surface is covered with skin. The area is abundant with sebaceous glands, so localized sebaceous cysts may occur here. Women who perform monthly vulvar examinations are able to detect infection or other abnormalities of the vulva such as sebaceous cysts or herpes lesions.

The Labia Majora

The labia majora are two folds of tissue, fused anteriorly but separated posteriorly, which are positioned lateral to the labia minora and composed of loose connective tissue covered by epithelium and pubic hair. The labia majora serve as protection for the external genitalia; they shield the outlets to the urethra and vagina. Trauma to the area, such as occurs from childbirth or rape, can lead to extensive edema formation because of the looseness of the connective tissue base.

Other External Organs

The *vestibule* is the flattened, smooth surface inside the labia. The openings to the bladder (the urethra) and the uterus (the vagina) both arise from this space. The *clitoris* is a small (approximately 1 to 2 cm), rounded organ of erectile tissue at the forward junction of the labia minora. It's covered by a fold of skin, the prepuce; is sensitive to touch and temperature; and is the center of sexual arousal and orgasm in a woman. Arterial blood supply for the clitoris is plentiful. When the ischiocavernosus muscle surrounding it contracts with sexual arousal, the venous outflow for the clitoris is blocked and this leads to clitoral erection.

In nations which allow it, young girls approaching puberty may be circumcised or have their clitoris removed with the labia minora excised as well. Aside from being a very painful procedure, female circumcision can lead to contractions and scarring of the vulva that make vaginal childbirth difficult because the vagina is unable to expand with birth (Nour, 2015).

Figure 5.3 The female external genitalia.

Two Skene glands (paraurethral glands) are located on each side of the urinary meatus; their ducts open into the urethra. Bartholin glands (vulvovaginal glands) are located on each side of the vaginal opening with ducts that open into the proximal vagina near the labia minora and hymen. Secretions from both of these glands help to lubricate the external genitalia during coitus. The alkaline pH of their secretions also helps to improve sperm survival in the vagina. If the Skene glands or the Bartholin glands (the most common site) become infected, they swell, feel tender, and produce a serous discharge.

The *fourchette* is the ridge of tissue formed by the posterior joining of the labia minora and the labia majora. This is the structure that sometimes tears (laceration) or is cut (episiotomy) during childbirth to enlarge the vaginal opening.

Posterior to the fourchette is the perineal muscle (often called the perineal body). Because this is a muscular area, it stretches during childbirth to allow enlargement of the vagina and passage of the fetal head. Many exercises suggested for pregnancy (such as Kegel exercises, squatting, and tailor sitting) are aimed at making the perineal muscle as flexible as it can be to allow for optimal expansion during birth and to prevent tearing of this tissue.

The *hymen* is a tough but elastic semicircle of tissue that covers the opening to the vagina during childhood. It is often torn during the time of first sexual intercourse. However, because of the use of tampons and active sports participation, many girls who have not had sexual relations can also have torn hymens at the time of their first pelvic examination. Occasionally, a girl has an imperforate hymen, or a hymen so complete that it does not allow for the passage of menstrual blood from the vagina (hematocolpometra) or for sexual relations until it is surgically incised (Fischer & Kwan, 2014).

The Vulvar Blood Supply

The blood supply of female external genitalia is mainly from the pudendal artery and a portion is from the inferior rectus artery. Venous return is through the pudendal vein.

Pressure on this vein by the fetal head during pregnancy can cause extensive back pressure and development of varicosities (distended veins) in the labia majora and in the legs. A disadvantage of this rich blood supply is that trauma to the area, such as occurs from pressure during childbirth or a bicycle seat injury, can cause large hematomas. An advantage is that it contributes to the rapid healing of any tears in the area after childbirth or other injury (Huether & McCance, 2012).

The Vulvar Nerve Supply

The anterior portion of the vulva derives its nerve supply from the ilioinguinal and genitofemoral nerves (L1 level). The posterior portions of the vulva and vagina are supplied by the pudendal nerve (S3 level). Such a rich nerve supply makes the area extremely sensitive to touch, pressure, pain, and temperature. Luckily, at the time of birth, normal stretching of the perineum causes a temporary loss of sensation to the area, limiting the amount of local pain felt during childbirth.

FEMALE INTERNAL STRUCTURES

Female internal reproductive organs (Fig. 5.4) include the ovaries, the fallopian tubes, the uterus, and the vagina.

The Ovaries

The ovaries are approximately 3 cm long by 2 cm in diameter and 1.5 cm thick, or the size and shape of almonds. They are grayish-white and appear pitted, with minute indentations on the surface.

The ovaries are located close to and on both sides of the uterus in the lower abdomen. Normally, they lie so low they cannot be located by abdominal palpation. Only if an abnormality exists, such as an enlarging ovarian cyst, can the resulting tenderness and enlargement be evident on lower left or lower right abdominal palpation.

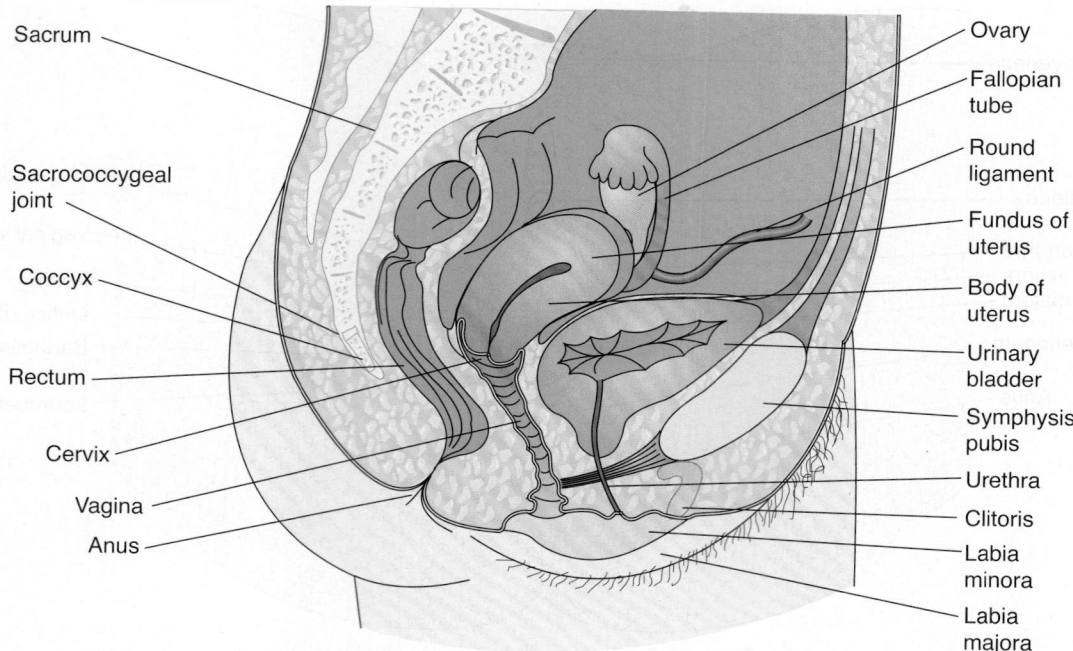

Figure 5.4   The female internal reproductive organs.

The function of the two ovaries is to produce, mature, and discharge ova (the egg cells). In the process of producing ova, the ovaries also produce estrogen and progesterone and initiate and regulate menstrual cycles. If the ovaries are removed before puberty (or are nonfunctional), the resulting absence of estrogen normally produced by the ovaries prevents maturation and maintenance of secondary sex characteristics; in addition, pubic hair distribution will assume a more male than female pattern.

The ovaries are held suspended and in close contact with the ends of the fallopian tubes by three strong ligaments that attach both to the uterus and the pelvic wall. Ovaries are unique among pelvic structures in that they are not covered by a layer of peritoneum. Because they are not covered this way, ova can readily escape from them and enter the uterus by way of the fallopian tubes. Because they are suspended in position rather than being firmly fixed, an abnormal tumor or cyst growing on them can enlarge to a size easily twice that of the organ before pressure on surrounding organs or the ovarian blood supply leads to symptoms of compression. This is the reason ovarian cancer continues to be one of the leading causes of death from cancer in women (the tumor can grow without symptoms for an extended period) (Sundar, Neal, & Kehoe, 2015).

The Division of Reproductive Cells (Gametes)

At birth, each ovary contains approximately 2 million immature ova (oocytes), which were formed during the first 5 months of intrauterine life. Although these cells have the unique ability to produce a new individual, they basically contain the usual components of cells: a cell membrane, an area of clear cytoplasm, and a nucleus that contains chromosomes.

One way they do differ from all other body cells is in the number of chromosomes their nuclei contain. All other human cells have 46 chromosomes: 22 pairs of autosomes (paired matching chromosomes) and 1 pair of sex chromosomes (two X sex chromosomes in the female and an X and a Y sex chromosome pair in the male). In contrast to this, reproductive cells (both ova and spermatozoa) have only half the usual number of chromosomes. This is so that, when sperm and egg combine (fertilization), the new individual formed will not have twice the needed number but, rather, 46 chromosomes. The manner in which reproductive cells divide causes this change in chromosome number.

Other cells in the body undergo cell division by *mitosis*, or daughter cell division; prior to a point of division, all the chromosomes are duplicated, leaving both new daughter cells with the right number of chromosomes.

In intrauterine life, oocytes divide by one typical mitotic division. Division activity then halts until puberty, when a second type of cell division, *meiosis* (cell reduction division), occurs. In the male, this reduction division occurs just before the spermatozoa mature. In the female, it occurs just before ovulation. After this reduction division, a typical ovum will have 22 autosomes and an X sex chromosome; a spermatozoon will have 22 autosomes and either an X or a Y sex chromosome. A new individual formed from the union of an ovum and the X-carrying spermatozoon will be female (an XX chromosome pattern); an individual formed from the union of an ovum and the Y-carrying spermatozoon will be male (an XY chromosome pattern).

The Maturation of Oocytes

Between 5 and 7 million ova form in utero. Most never develop beyond a primitive state and then atrophy, so by birth, only about 2 million are still present. By age 7 years, only about 500,000 are present in each ovary; by 22 years of age, the count is down to 300,000; and by menopause, or the end of the fertile period in females, none are left (all have either matured or atrophied).

The Fallopian Tubes

The fallopian tubes arise from each upper corner of the uterine body and extend outward and backward until each opens at its distal end, next to an ovary. Fallopian tubes are approximately 10 cm long in a mature woman. Their function is to convey the ovum from the ovaries to the uterus and to provide a place for fertilization of the ovum by sperm.

Although a fallopian tube is a smooth, hollow tunnel, it is anatomically divided into four separate parts (Fig. 5.5).

- The most proximal division, the interstitial portion, is the part of the tube that lies within the uterine wall. This portion is only about 1 cm in length; its lumen is only 1 mm in diameter.
- The next distal portion is the isthmus. This is about 2 cm in length and, like the interstitial tube, remains extremely narrow. This is the portion of the tube that is cut or sealed in a tubal ligation, or tubal sterilization procedure.
- The ampulla is the third and also the longest portion of the tube. It is about 5 cm in length and is the portion of the tube where fertilization of an ovum usually occurs.
- The infundibular portion is the most distal segment of the tube. It is about 2 cm long, funnel shaped, and covered by fimbria (small hairs) that help to guide the ovum into the fallopian tube.

The lining of the fallopian tubes is composed of a mucous membrane, which contains both mucus-secreting and ciliated (hair-covered) cells. Beneath this mucous lining are connective tissue and a circular muscle layer. The muscle layer is important because it is able to produce peristaltic motions that help conduct the ovum the length of the tube (probably also aided by the action of the ciliated lining and the mucus, which acts as a lubricant). The mucus produced may also serve as a source of nourishment for the fertilized egg because it contains protein, water, and salts.

Because the fallopian tubes are open at their distal ends, a direct pathway exists from the external genital organs, through the vagina to the uterus and tubes, to the peritoneum. This open pathway is what makes conception possible. It also, however, can lead to infection of the peritoneum (peritonitis) if germs spread from the perineum through the uterus and tubes to the pelvic cavity. For this reason, clean technique must be used during pelvic examinations. During labor and birth, vaginal examinations are done with sterile technique to ensure no organisms can enter by this route.

The Uterus

The uterus is a hollow, muscular, pear-shaped organ located in the lower pelvis, posterior to the bladder and anterior to the rectum. During childhood, it is about the size of an olive; the cervix is the largest portion and the uterine body is the smallest part. When a girl reaches about 8 years of age, an increase in the size of the organ begins. This growth is so slow, however, the young woman is closer to 17 years old before the uterus reaches its adult size and changes its proportions so that the body cavity, not the cervix, is its largest portion. Small uterine size may be a contributing factor to the number of low–birth-weight babies typically born to adolescents younger than this age (March of Dimes Foundation, 2012).

With maturity, a uterus is about 5 to 7 cm long, 5 cm wide, and, in its widest upper part, 2.5 cm deep. In a nonpregnant state, it weighs approximately 60 g. The function of the uterus is to receive the ovum from the fallopian tube; provide a place for implantation and nourishment; furnish protection to a growing fetus; and, at maturity of the fetus,

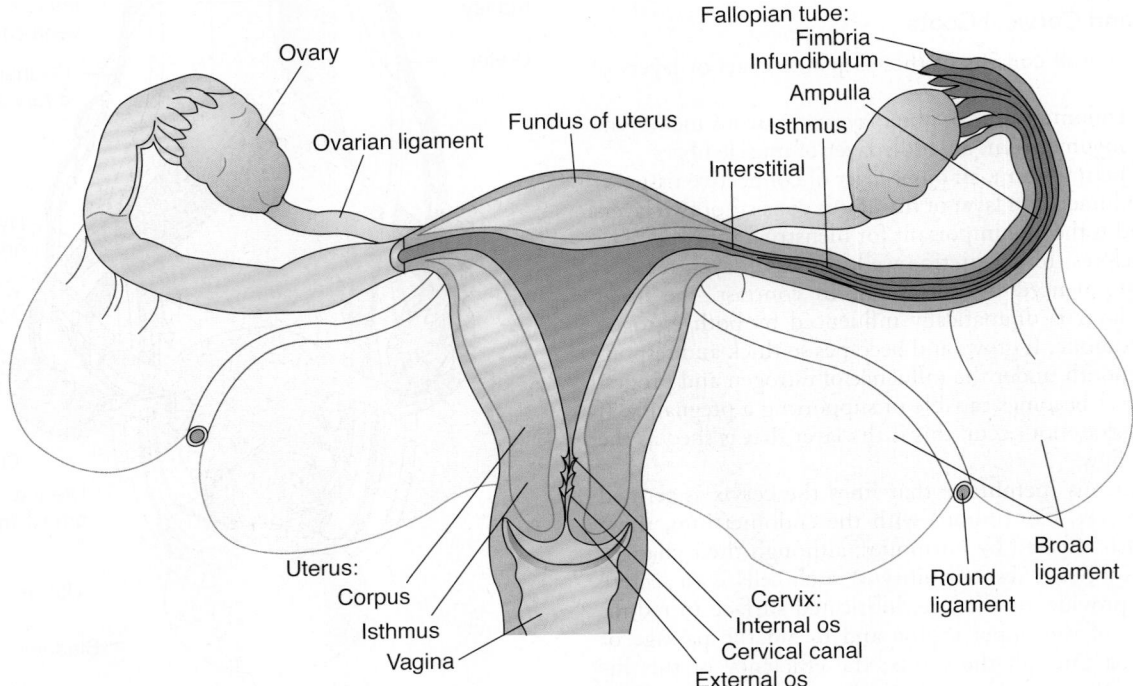

Figure 5.5 An anterior view of female reproductive organs showing the relationship of the fallopian tubes and body of the uterus.

expel it from a woman's body. After a pregnancy, the uterus never returns to exactly its nonpregnant size but remains approximately 9 cm long, 6 cm wide, 3 cm thick, and 80 g in weight.

Anatomically, the uterus consists of three divisions: the body or corpus, the isthmus, and the cervix.

- The body of the uterus is the uppermost part and forms the bulk of the organ. The lining of the cavity is continuous with the fallopian tubes, which enter at its upper aspects (the cornua). The portion of the uterus between the points of attachment of the fallopian tubes is termed the fundus. During pregnancy, the body of the uterus is the portion of the structure that expands to contain the growing fetus. The fundus is the portion that can be palpated abdominally to determine the amount of uterine growth during pregnancy, to measure the force of uterine contractions during labor, and to assess that the uterus is returning to its nonpregnant state after childbirth.
- The isthmus is a short segment between the body and the cervix. In the nonpregnant uterus, it is only 1 to 2 mm in length. During pregnancy, this portion also enlarges greatly to aid in accommodating the growing fetus. It is the portion where the incision most commonly is made when a fetus is born by a cesarean birth.
- The cervix is the lowest portion of the uterus. It represents about one third of the total uterine size and is approximately 2 to 5 cm long. About half of it lies above the vagina and half extends into the vagina. Its central cavity is termed the cervical canal. The opening of the canal at the junction of the cervix and isthmus is the internal cervical os; the distal opening to the vagina is the external cervical os. The level of the external os is at the level of the ischial spines (an important relationship in estimating the level of the fetus in the birth canal at the time of birth).

Uterine and Cervical Coats

The uterine wall consists of three separate coats or layers of tissue:

- The endometrium, an inner layer of mucous membrane
- The myometrium, a middle layer of muscle fibers
- The perimetrium, an outer layer of connective tissue

The endometrium layer of the uterus consists of two layers of cells and is the one important for menstrual function. The cell layer closest to the uterine wall, the basal layer, remains stable, uninfluenced by hormones. In contrast, the inner glandular layer is dramatically influenced by both estrogen and progesterone. It grows and becomes so thick and responsive each month under the influence of estrogen and progesterone that it becomes capable of supporting a pregnancy. If pregnancy does not occur, this is the layer that is shed as the menstrual flow.

The mucous membrane that lines the cervix is termed the endocervix. Continuous with the endometrium, these cells are also affected by hormones, although their changes are more subtle. A responsibility of such cells is to secrete mucus to provide an alkaline, lubricated surface to reduce the acidity of the upper vagina and to aid the passage of spermatozoa through the cervix; the efficiency of this lubrication increases or wanes depending on hormone stimulation. At the point in the menstrual cycle when estrogen

production is at its peak, as many as 700 ml of mucus per day are produced; at the point estrogen is at its lowest level, only a few milliliters are produced. During pregnancy, so much mucus is produced, the endocervix becomes plugged with mucus, forming a seal to keep out ascending infections (the operculum).

Both the lower outer surface of the cervix and the internal cervical canal are lined not with a mucous membrane but with a stratified squamous epithelium, similar to that lining the vagina. Locating the point at which this tissue changes from epithelium to mucous membrane (squamocolumnar junction) is important when obtaining a Papanicolaou smear (a test for cervical cancer) because this tissue interface is most dynamic in cellular growth and is often the origin of cervical cancer (Gueye & Diaz-Montes, 2015).

The myometrium, or muscle layer of the uterus, is composed of three interwoven layers of smooth muscle, the fibers of which are arranged in longitudinal, transverse, and oblique directions. This intertwining network of fibers is what offers extreme strength to the organ so when the uterus contracts at the end of pregnancy to expel the fetus, equal pressure is

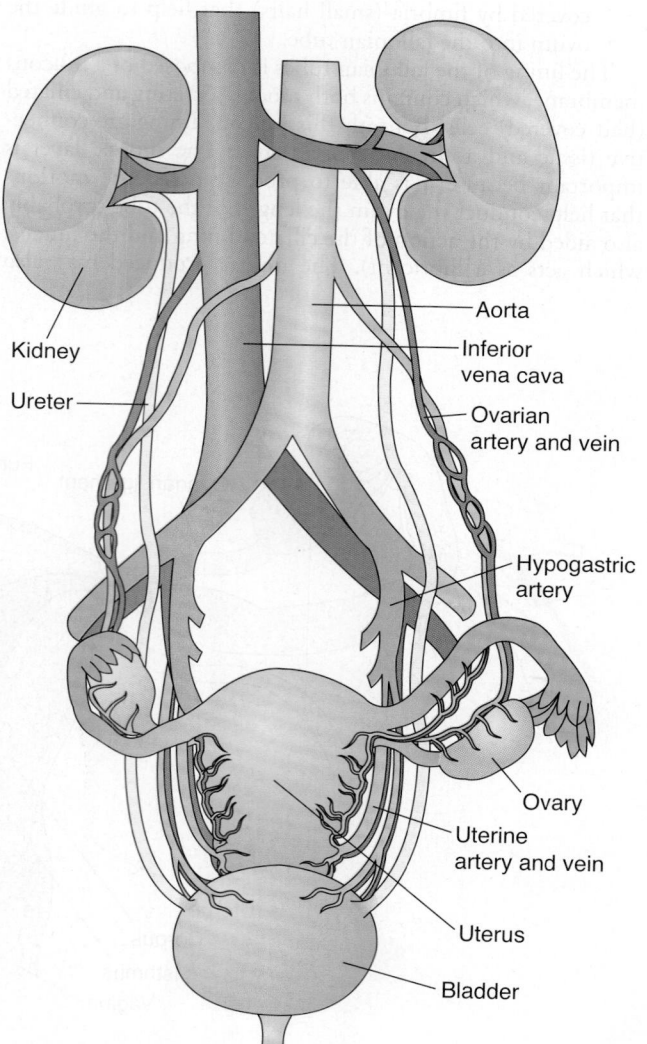

Figure 5.6   Blood supply to the uterus.

exerted at all points throughout the cavity. Another function of the myometrium is to constrict the fallopian tubes at the point they enter the fundus, preventing regurgitation of menstrual blood into the tubes. The myometrium also holds the internal cervical os closed during pregnancy to prevent a preterm birth. After childbirth, the interlacing network of fibers is able to constrict the blood vessels coursing through the layers, thereby limiting the amount of blood loss. Myomas, or benign fibroid (leiomyoma) tumors that can interfere with conception or birth, arise from the myometrium (Huether & McCance, 2012).

The purpose of the perimetrium, the outermost layer of the uterus, is to add further strength and support to the organ.

Uterine Blood Supply

The large descending abdominal aorta divides to form two iliac arteries; these then form the hypogastric arteries and the uterine arteries, which supply the uterus (Fig. 5.6). Because the uterine blood supply is not far removed from the aorta this way, it is guaranteed to be copious and adequate to supply the growing needs of a fetus. As an additional guarantee that enough blood will be available, after supplying the ovaries with blood, the ovarian artery (a direct subdivision of the aorta) joins the uterine artery and adds more blood to the uterus.

The blood vessels that supply the cells and lining of the uterus look tortuous against the sides of the uterine body in nonpregnant women. As a uterus enlarges with pregnancy, the vessels "unwind" and stretch as another guarantee that the uterus will maintain an adequate blood supply as the organ grows larger. The uterine veins follow the same twisting course as the arteries; they empty into the internal iliac veins.

An important organ relationship to be aware of is the close proximity of uterine blood vessels and ureters. Ureters pass from the kidneys on their way to the bladder directly behind the ovarian vessels, near the fallopian tubes (see Fig. 5.5). This close anatomic relationship has implications in procedures such as tubal ligation, cesarean birth, and hysterectomy (removal of the uterus) because a ureter this close to the fallopian tubes can be injured if bleeding during surgery is controlled by clamping of the uterine or ovarian vessels.

This is a reason a first voiding after uterine or tubal surgery is measured and assessed carefully for color or the presence of blood.

Uterine Nerve Supply

The uterus is supplied by both efferent (motor) and afferent (sensory) nerves. The efferent nerves arise from the T5 through T10 spinal ganglia. The afferent nerves join the hypogastric plexus and enter the spinal column at T11 and T12. The fact that sensory innervation from the uterus registers lower in the spinal column than does motor control has implications for controlling pain in labor. An anesthetic solution can be injected to stop the pain of uterine contractions at the T11 and T12 levels without stopping motor control or contractions (which are registered higher, at the T5 to T10 level). This is the principle of both epidural and spinal anesthesia (see Chapter 16).

Uterine Supports

The uterus is suspended in the pelvic cavity by a number of ligaments that also help support the bladder; it is further supported by a combination of fascia and muscle. Because the uterus is suspended this way, it is free to enlarge without discomfort during pregnancy. If its ligaments become overstretched during pregnancy, however, they may not support the bladder well afterward, and the bladder can then herniate into the anterior vagina (a **cystocele**), possibly causing frequent urinary infections from status of urine (Fig. 5.7A). If the rectum pouches into the vaginal wall, a **rectocele** (Fig. 5.7B) develops, possibly leading to constipation (Podzemny, Pescatori, & Pescatori, 2015).

A fold of peritoneum behind the uterus is the posterior ligament. This forms a pouch (Douglas cul-de-sac) between the rectum and uterus. Because this is the lowest point of the pelvis, any fluid (such as blood) released from a condition, such as a ruptured tubal (ectopic) pregnancy, tends to collect in this space. The space can be examined for the presence of fluid or blood to help in diagnosis by inserting a culdoscope through the posterior vaginal wall (**culdoscopy**) or a laparoscope through the abdominal wall (**laparoscopy**) (Sholapurkar, 2015).

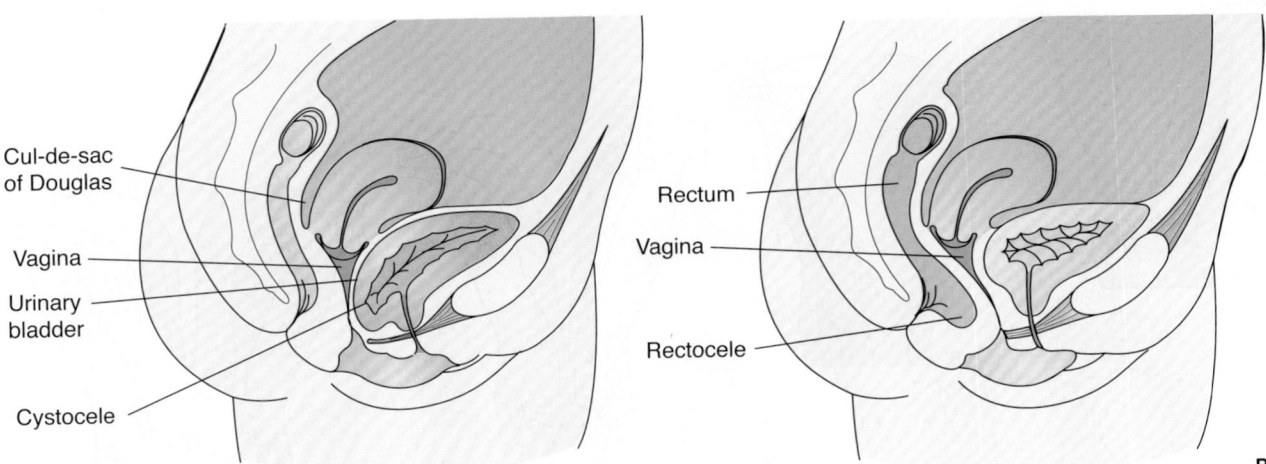

Cul-de-sac of Douglas

Vagina

Urinary bladder

Cystocele

Rectum

Vagina

Rectocele

A   **B**

Figure 5.7   **(A)** A cystocele. The bladder has herniated into the anterior wall of the vagina. **(B)** A rectocele. The posterior of the vagina is herniated.

The *broad ligaments* are two folds of peritoneum that cover the uterus in the front and back and extend to the pelvic sides to help steady the uterus. The *round ligaments* are two fibrous, muscular cords that pass from the body of the uterus through the broad ligaments and down into the inguinal canal, inserting into the fascia of the vulva. The round ligaments act as additional "stays" to further steady the uterus. If a pregnant woman moves quickly, she may pull one of these ligaments, causing a quick, sharp pain of frightening intensity in one of her lower abdominal quadrants. Pain of this type calls for conscientious assessment or it can be mistaken for labor or appendicitis pain.

What If . . . 5.1
Suzanne Matthews decides to have a tubal ligation (clamping of the fallopian tubes) after the birth of her baby. The nurse notices the first time she voids following surgery that her urine looks blood tinged. Would the nurse assume the urine was contaminated by vaginal secretions so its appearance is innocent? Or would the nurse report this as a potentially serious finding (her surgery was on her reproductive, not her urinary, system)?

Uterine Deviations

A number of uterine deviations (i.e., shape and position) can interfere with fertility or pregnancy and so are helpful to recognize. When a uterus first forms in intrauterine life, it is split by a longitudinal septum into two portions. As the fetus matures, this septum dissolves, so, typically at birth, no remnant of the division remains. In some women, half of the septum or even the entire septum never atrophies, so the uterus remains as two separate compartments. Still, other women have oddly shaped "horns" at the junction of the fallopian tubes—a **bicornuate uterus**. Any of these malformations may decrease the ability to conceive or to carry a pregnancy to term (Owens & Green, 2015). Some examples of these types of uterine formation are shown in Figure 5.8. The specific effects of these deviations on fertility and pregnancy are discussed in later chapters.

Ordinarily, the body of the uterus tips slightly forward. Positional deviations of the uterus that are commonly seen include (Fig. 5.9):
- **Anteversion**: The entire uterus tips far forward.
- **Retroversion**: The entire uterus tips far back.
- **Anteflexion**: The body of the uterus is bent sharply forward at the junction with the cervix.
- **Retroflexion**: The body of the uterus is bent sharply back just above the cervix.

Minor variations of these positions do not tend to cause reproductive problems. Extreme abnormal flexion or version positions may interfere with fertility because the sharp bend can block the deposition or migration of sperm.

The Vagina

The vagina is a hollow, musculomembranous canal located posterior to the bladder and anterior to the rectum. It extends from the cervix of the uterus to the external vulva. Its function is to act as the organ of intercourse and to convey sperm to the cervix. With childbirth, it expands to serve as the birth canal.

> **Concept Mastery Alert**
>
> Even though the vagina opens to the outside, it is considered an internal reproductive organ.

When a woman lies on her back, as she does for a pelvic examination, the course of the vagina is inward and downward. Because of this downward slant and the angle of the uterine cervix, the length of the anterior wall of the vagina is about 6 to 7 cm and the length of the posterior wall is 8 to 9 cm. At the cervical end of the structure, there are recesses on all sides, termed the posterior, anterior, and lateral fornices. The posterior fornix serves as a place for the pooling of semen after coitus; this allows for a large number of sperm to remain close to the cervix and encourages sperm migration into the cervix.

Figure 5.8   (A) A normal uterus. **(B)** A bicornuate uterus. **(C)** A septum-dividing uterus. **(D)** A double uterus. Abnormal shapes of uterus allow less placenta implantation space.

Normal position

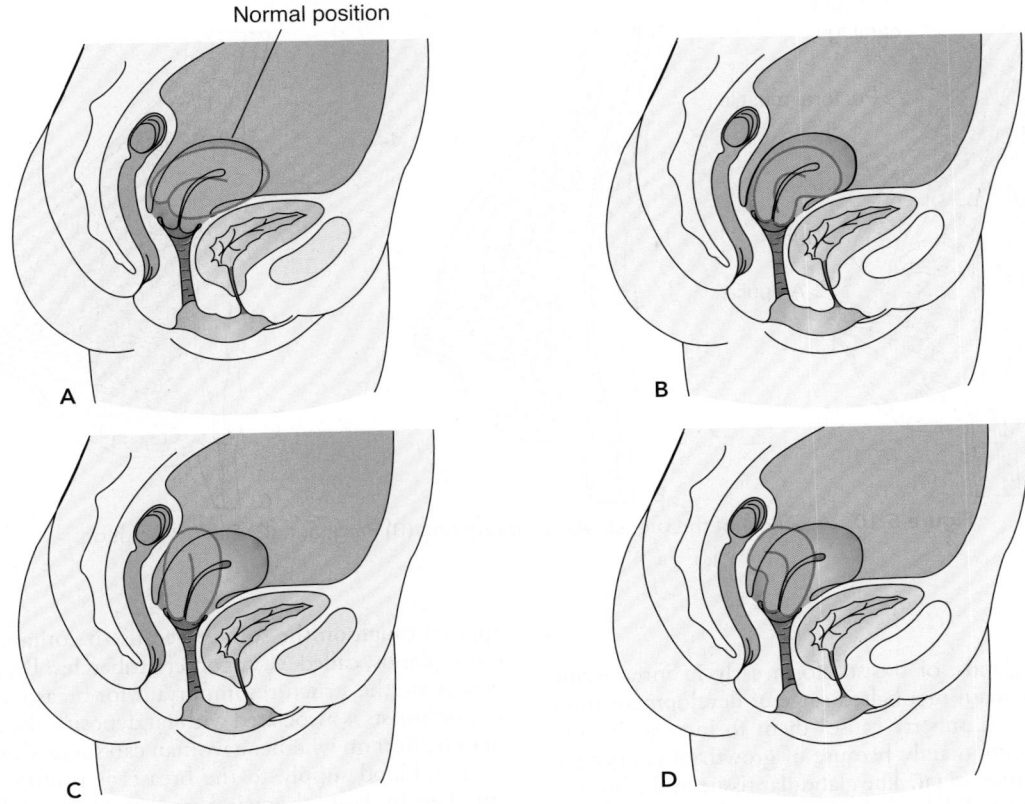

Figure 5.9 Uterine flexion and version. **(A)** Anteversion. **(B)** Anteflexion. **(C)** Retroversion. **(D)** Retroflexion.

The vaginal wall is so thin at the fornices that an examiner can palpate the bladder through the anterior fornix, the ovaries through the lateral fornices, and the rectum through the posterior fornix.

The vagina is lined with stratified squamous epithelium similar to that covering the cervix. Under this, it has a middle connective tissue layer and a strong muscular wall. Normally, the walls contain many folds or rugae that lie in close approximation to each other. These folds make the vagina very elastic and able to expand so much that at the end of pregnancy, a full-term baby can pass through without tearing. A circular muscle at the external opening of the vagina, called the bulbocavernosus muscle, acts as a voluntary sphincter. Relaxing and tensing this external vaginal sphincter muscle a set number of times each day (Kegel exercises) makes it more supple for birth and helps maintain tone after birth.

The blood supply to the vagina is furnished by the vaginal artery, a branch of the internal iliac artery. Vaginal tears at childbirth tend to bleed profusely because of this rich blood supply. The same rich blood supply, however, is also the reason any vaginal trauma at birth heals rapidly.

The vagina has both sympathetic and parasympathetic nerve innervations originating at the S1–S3 levels. Despite this dual nerve supply, the vagina is not an extremely sensitive organ. Sexual excitement, often attributed to a vaginal origin, is actually mainly a clitoral function.

Mucus produced by the vaginal lining has a rich glycogen content. When this glycogen is broken down by the lactose-fermenting bacteria that frequent the vagina (Döderlein bacillus), lactic acid is formed. This causes the usual pH of the vagina to be acidic, a condition detrimental to the growth of pathologic bacteria, so even though the vagina connects directly to the external surface, infection of the vagina does not readily occur. You can advise women not to use vaginal douches or sprays as a daily hygiene measure so they do not clear away this natural acidic medium because this would invite infection (Sheth & Keller, 2015).

QSEN Checkpoint Question 5.3

TEAMWORK & COLLABORATION

On physical examination, Suzanne Matthews is found to have a cystocele. The nurse should confirm that the vocational nurse who is contributing to Suzanne's care knows that a cystocele can cause which of the following?
  a. A fear of developing cancer from the sebaceous vulvar cyst that develops
  b. Nagging pain from protrusion of the lower intestine into the posterior vagina
  c. Bleeding from the prolapse of the uterine body and cervix into the distal vagina
  d. Urinary infection from the pocket caused by pressure against the anterior vaginal wall

Look in Appendix A for the best answer and rationale.

Figure 5.10   Anatomy of the breast. **(A)** Nonpregnant. **(B)** Pregnant. **(C)** During lactation.

The Breasts

The mammary glands, or breasts, form early in intrauterine life. They then remain in a halted stage of development until a rise in estrogen at puberty causes them to increase in size. This increase occurs mainly because of growth of connective tissue plus deposition of fat. The glandular tissue of the breasts, necessary for successful breastfeeding, remains undeveloped until a first pregnancy begins. Boys, especially those who are obese, may notice a temporary increase in breast size at puberty, termed **gynecomastia** (Narula & Carlson, 2014). If boys are not prepared that this is a normal change of puberty, they may be concerned that they are developing abnormally.

Breasts are located anterior to the pectoral muscle (Fig. 5.10), and, in many women, breast tissue extends well into the axilla. When palpating for breast health, always include the axillary region in the examination, or this breast tissue can be missed. It is not uncommon for women or men to have supernumerary breast tissue along mammary lines on the front of their body. The nipple on these auxiliary sites may look like a mole, so adolescents may report this as a "mole changing in color" or be concerned they have skin cancer. You can assure them supernumerary breast tissue or nipples are not uncommon and are innocent findings.

Women should be aware of the usual appearance of their breasts (breast awareness) so they can report any change in contour or density to their healthcare provider.

Milk glands of the breasts are divided by connective tissue partitions into approximately 20 lobes. All of the glands in each lobe produce milk by acinar cells and deliver it to the nipple via a lactiferous duct. The nipple has approximately 20 small openings through which milk is secreted. An ampulla portion of the duct, located just posterior to the nipple, serves as a reservoir for milk before breastfeeding.

The nipple is composed of smooth muscle capable of erection on manual or sucking stimulation. On stimulation, it transmits sensations to the posterior pituitary gland to release oxytocin, which then acts to constrict milk glands and push milk forward into the ducts that lead to the nipple (a let-down reflex). The skin surrounding the nipples is darkly pigmented out to about 4 cm and termed the *areola*. The area

appears rough on the surface because it contains many sebaceous glands, called Montgomery tubercles. Because the milk glands are the structures important for breastfeeding and the size of breasts is associated with fat deposits, the size of breasts has no effect on whether a woman can successfully breastfeed.

The blood supply to the breasts is profuse because it is supplied by large thoracic branches of the axillary, internal mammary, and intercostal arteries. This effective blood supply is necessary so milk glands can be supplied with nutrients and fluid to make possible a plentiful supply of milk for breastfeeding. Unfortunately, this rich blood connection also aids in the metastasis of breast cancer if cancer is not discovered early (Huether & McCance, 2012).

MENSTRUATION

A menstrual cycle (the female reproductive cycle) is episodic uterine bleeding in response to cyclic hormonal changes. The purpose of a menstrual cycle is to bring an ovum to maturity and renew a uterine tissue bed that will be necessary for the ova's growth should it be fertilized. Because menarche may occur as early as 9 years of age, it is good to include health teaching information on menstruation to both school-age children and their parents as early as fourth grade as part of routine care. It is a poor introduction to sexuality and womanhood for a girl to begin menstruation unwarned and unprepared for the important internal function it represents.

The length of menstrual cycles differs from woman to woman, but the average length is 28 days (from the beginning of one menstrual flow to the beginning of the next). It is not unusual for cycles to be as short as 23 days or as long as 35 days. The length of the average menstrual flow (termed menses) is 4 to 6 days, although women may have flows as short as 2 days or as long as 9 days (Ledger, 2012).

Because there is such variation in length, frequency, and amount of menstrual flow and also in the onset of menarche, many women have questions about what is considered normal. Contact with healthcare personnel during a routine health examination or prenatal visit may be their first opportunity to ask questions they have had for some time. Table 5.1 summarizes the normal characteristics of menstruation for quick reference.

TABLE 5.1 CHARACTERISTICS OF NORMAL MENSTRUAL CYCLES

Characteristic	Description
Beginning (menarche)	Average age at onset, 12.4 years; average range, 9–17 years
Interval between cycles	Average, 28 days; cycles of 23–35 days not unusual
Duration of menstrual flow	Average flow, 4–6 days; ranges of 2–9 days not abnormal
Amount of menstrual flow	Difficult to estimate; average 30–80 ml per menstrual period; saturating a pad or tampon in less than 1 hr is heavy bleeding
Color of menstrual flow	Dark red; a combination of blood, mucus, and endometrial cells
Odor	Similar to marigolds

The Physiology of Menstruation

Four body structures are involved in the physiology of the menstrual cycle: the hypothalamus, the pituitary gland, the ovaries, and the uterus. For a menstrual cycle to be complete, all four organs must contribute their part; inactivity of any part results in an incomplete or ineffective cycle (Fig. 5.11).

The Hypothalamus

The release of GnRH (also called luteinizing hormone–releasing hormone [LHRH]) from the hypothalamus initiates the menstrual cycle. GnRH then stimulates the pituitary gland to send the gonadotropic hormone to the ovaries to produce estrogen. When the level of estrogen rises, release of GnRH is repressed and no further menstrual cycles will occur (the principle that

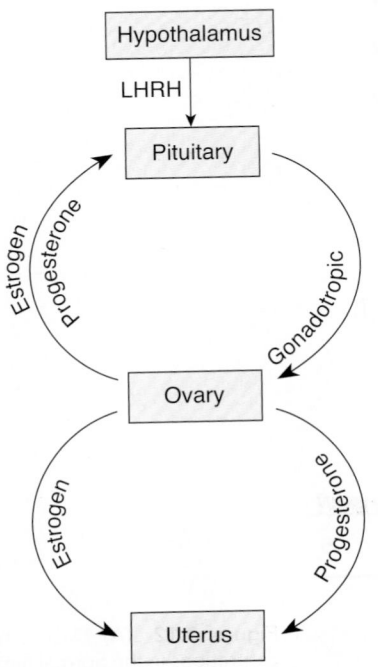

Figure 5.11 The interaction of pituitary–uterine–ovarian functions in a menstrual cycle.

birth control pills use to eliminate menstrual flows). Excessive levels of pituitary hormones can also inhibit release.

During childhood, the hypothalamus is apparently so sensitive to the small amount of estrogen produced by the adrenal glands, release of GnRH is suppressed. Beginning with puberty, the hypothalamus becomes less sensitive to estrogen feedback, so every month in females, the hormone is released in a cyclic pattern.

Diseases of the hypothalamus, which cause deficiency of this releasing factor, can result in delayed puberty. Likewise, a disease that causes early activation of GnRH can lead to abnormally early sexual development or precocious puberty (Neely & Crossen, 2014) (see Chapter 47).

The Pituitary Gland

Under the influence of GnRH, the anterior lobe of the pituitary gland (the adenohypophysis) produces two hormones:
- FSH, a hormone active early in the cycle that is responsible for maturation of the ovum
- LH, a hormone that becomes most active at the midpoint of the cycle and is responsible for ovulation, or release of the mature egg cell from the ovary. It also stimulates growth of the uterine lining during the second half of the menstrual cycle.

The Ovaries

FSH and LH are called gonadotropic hormones because they cause growth (trophy) in the gonads (ovaries). Every month during the fertile period of a woman's life (from menarche to menopause), one of the ovary's oocytes is activated by FSH to begin to grow and mature. As the oocyte grows, its cells produce a clear fluid (follicular fluid) that contains a high degree of estrogen and some progesterone. As the follicle surrounding the oocyte grows, it is propelled toward the surface of the ovary. At full maturity, the follicle is visible on the surface of the ovary as a clear water blister approximately 0.25 to 0.5 in. across. At this stage of maturation, the small ovum (barely visible to the naked eye, about the size of a printed period) with its surrounding follicular membrane and fluid is termed a *graafian follicle*.

By day 14 or the midpoint of a typical 28-day cycle, the ovum has divided by mitotic division into two separate bodies: a primary oocyte, which contains the bulk of the cytoplasm, and a secondary oocyte, which contains so little cytoplasm that it is not functional. The structure also has accomplished its meiotic division, reducing its number of chromosomes to the haploid (having only one member of a pair) number of 23.

After an upsurge of LH from the pituitary at about day 14, prostaglandins are released and the graafian follicle ruptures. The ovum is set free from the surface of the ovary, a process termed *ovulation*. It is swept into the open end of a fallopian tube. It is important to teach women that ovulation does not necessarily occur on the 14th day of their cycle; it occurs 14 days *before the end of their cycle*. If their menstrual cycle is only 20 days long, for example, their day of ovulation would be day 6 (14 days before the end of the cycle). If their cycle is 44 days long, ovulation would occur on day 30, not at the halfway point—day 22.

After the ovum and the follicular fluid have been discharged from the ovary, the cells of the follicle remain in the form of a hollow, empty pit. The FSH has done its work at this point and now decreases in amount. The second pituitary hormone, LH, continues to rise in amount and directs the follicle cells left behind in the ovary to produce lutein, a bright-yellow fluid high in progesterone. With lutein production, the follicle is renamed a *corpus luteum* (yellow body).

The basal body temperature of a woman drops slightly (by 0.5° to 1°F) just before the day of ovulation because of the extremely low level of progesterone that is present at that time. It rises by 1°F on the day after ovulation because of the concentration of progesterone, which is thermogenic. The woman's temperature remains at this elevated level until approximately day 24 of the menstrual cycle, when the progesterone level again decreases (Huether & McCance, 2012). Therefore, taking body temperature daily is one method of assessing if ovulation has occurred.

If conception (fertilization by a spermatozoon) occurs as the ovum proceeds down a fallopian tube and the fertilized ovum implants on the endometrium of the uterus, the corpus luteum remains throughout the major portion of the pregnancy (to about 16 to 20 weeks). If conception does not occur, the

unfertilized ovum atrophies after 4 or 5 days, and the corpus luteum (now called a "false" corpus luteum) remains for only 8 to 10 days. As the corpus luteum regresses, it is gradually replaced by white fibrous tissue, and the resulting structure is termed a corpus albicans (white body). Figure 5.12A summarizes the times when ovarian hormones are secreted at peak levels during a typical 28-day menstrual cycle to cause these changes.

The Uterus

Figure 5.12B also illustrates uterine changes that occur monthly as a result of stimulation from the estrogen and progesterone produced by the ovaries.

The First Phase of the Menstrual Cycle (Proliferative)

Immediately after a menstrual flow (which occurs during the first 4 or 5 days of a cycle), the endometrium, or lining of the uterus, is very thin, approximately one cell layer in depth.

Figure 5.12 (A) Plasma hormone concentrations in the normal female reproductive cycle. **(B)** Ovarian events and uterine changes during the menstrual cycle.

As the ovary begins to produce estrogen (in the follicular fluid, under the direction of the pituitary FSH), the endometrium begins to proliferate so rapidly the thickness of the endometrium increases as much as eightfold from day 5 to day 14. This first half of a menstrual cycle is interchangeably termed the proliferative, estrogenic, follicular, or postmenstrual phase.

The Second Phase of the Menstrual Cycle (Secretory)

After ovulation, the formation of progesterone in the corpus luteum (under the direction of LH) causes the glands of the uterine endometrium to become corkscrew or twisted in appearance and dilated with quantities of glycogen (an elementary sugar) and mucin (a protein). It takes on the appearance of rich, spongy velvet. This second phase of the menstrual cycle is termed the progestational, luteal, premenstrual, or secretory phase.

The Third Phase of the Menstrual Cycle (Ischemic)

If fertilization does not occur, the corpus luteum in the ovary begins to regress after 8 to 10 days, and therefore, the production of progesterone decreases. With the withdrawal of progesterone, the endometrium of the uterus begins to degenerate (at about day 24 or day 25 of the cycle). The capillaries rupture, with minute hemorrhages, and the endometrium sloughs off.

The Fourth Phase of the Menstrual Cycle (Menses)

Menses, or a menstrual flow, is composed of a mixture of blood from the ruptured capillaries; mucin; fragments of endometrial tissue; and the microscopic, atrophied, and unfertilized ovum.

Menses is actually the end of an arbitrarily defined menstrual cycle. Because it is the only external marker of the cycle, however, the first day of menstrual flow is used to mark the beginning day of a new menstrual cycle.

Contrary to common belief, a menstrual flow contains only 30 to 80 ml of blood; if it seems to be more, it is because of the accompanying mucus and endometrial shreds. The iron loss in a typical menstrual flow is approximately 11 mg. This is enough loss that many adolescent women could benefit from a daily iron supplement to prevent iron depletion during their menstruating years (Bitzer, Sultan, Creatsas, et al., 2014).

QSEN Checkpoint Question 5.4

INFORMATICS

The nurse documents the fact that Suzanne Matthews typically has a menstrual cycle of 34 days. If she had coitus on days 8, 10, 15, and 20 of her last cycle, which is the day on which she most likely conceived?
a. The 8th day
b. The 10th day
c. Day 15
d. Day 20

Look in Appendix A for the best answer and rationale.

Cervical Changes

The mucus of the uterine cervix also changes in structure and consistency each month during a menstrual cycle. At the beginning of each cycle, when estrogen secretion from the ovary

is low, cervical mucus is thick and scant. Sperm survival in this type of mucus is poor. At the time of ovulation, when the estrogen level has risen to a high point, cervical mucus becomes thin, stretchy (spinnbarkeit), and copious. Sperm penetration and survival in this thin mucus are both excellent. Because progesterone becomes the major influencing hormone during the second half of the cycle, cervical mucus again thickens and sperm survival is again poor.

Women can analyze cervical mucus changes to help plan coitus so it coincides with ovulation if they want to increase their chance of becoming pregnant or plan to avoid coitus at the time of ovulation to prevent pregnancy (natural family planning; see Chapter 6) by analyzing how thick or thin is cervical mucus. During ovulation, the body of the cervix is softer and the os is slightly open compared with the rest of the cycle when it is firm and the os is closed as another indication of ovulation.

The Fern Test

An interesting property of cervical mucus just before ovulation when estrogen levels are high is the ability to form fernlike patterns on a microscope slide when allowed to dry. This pattern is known as arborization or ferning (Fig. 5.13). When progesterone is the dominant hormone, as it is just after ovulation, this fern pattern is no longer discernible. Cervical mucus, therefore, can be examined at midcycle for ferning

A

B

Figure 5.13 **(A)** A ferning pattern of cervical mucus occurs with high estrogen levels. **(B)** Incomplete ferning during secretory phase of cycle. (From Scott, J. R. [1990]. *Danforth's obstetrics and gynecology* [6th ed.]. Philadelphia, PA: J. B. Lippincott.)

Figure 5.14 Spinnbarkeit is the property of cervical mucus to stretch a distance before breaking.

to detect whether a high estrogen surge is present. Women who do not ovulate usually show a ferning pattern throughout their menstrual cycle (progesterone levels never become dominant), or they never demonstrate it because their estrogen levels never rise.

The Spinnbarkeit Test

At the height of estrogen secretion, yet another property of cervical mucus is the ability to stretch into long strands, a contrast to its thick, viscous state when progesterone is the dominant hormone. That means performing this test, known as *spinnbarkeit*, at the midpoint of a menstrual cycle is another way to demonstrate high levels of estrogen are being produced and, by implication, ovulation is about to occur. A woman can do this herself by stretching a mucus sample between thumb and finger, or it can be tested in an examining room by smearing a cervical mucus specimen on a slide and stretching the mucus between the slide and cover slip (Fig. 5.14).

Sexual Health

Sexuality is a multidimensional phenomenon that includes feelings, attitudes, and actions. It has both biologic and cultural diversity components. It encompasses and gives direction to a person's physical, emotional, social, and intellectual responses throughout life.

Sexuality has always been a part of human life, but only in the past few decades has it been studied scientifically. One common finding of researchers has been that feelings and attitudes about sex vary widely across cultures and individuals. Although the sexual experience is unique to each individual, sexual physiology (how the body responds to sexual arousal) has common features (Resetkova & Rogers, 2015).

THE SEXUAL RESPONSE CYCLE

Two of the earliest researchers of sexual response were Masters and Johnson. In 1966, they published the results

of a major study based on more than 10,000 episodes of sexual activity among more than 600 men and women (Masters, Johnson, & Kolodny, 1998). In this study, they described the human sexual response as a cycle with four discrete stages: excitement, plateau, orgasm, and resolution. Whether stages are felt as separate steps this way or blended into one smooth process of desire, arousal, and orgasm is individualized.

Excitement

Excitement occurs with physical and psychological stimulation (sight, sound, emotion, or thought) that causes parasympathetic nerve stimulation. This leads to arterial dilation and venous constriction in the genital area. The resulting increased blood supply leads to vasocongestion and increasing muscular tension. In women, this vasocongestion causes the clitoris to increase in size and mucoid fluid to appear on vaginal walls for lubrication. The vagina widens in diameter and increases in length. Breast nipples become erect. In men, penile erection occurs as well as scrotal thickening and elevation of the testes. In both sexes, there is an increase in heart and respiratory rate and blood pressure.

Plateau

The plateau stage is reached just before orgasm. In the woman, the clitoris is drawn forward and retracts under the clitoral prepuce, the lower part of the vagina becomes extremely congested (formation of the orgasmic platform), and there is increased breast nipple elevation.

In men, vasocongestion leads to distention of the penis. Heart rate increases to 100 to 175 beats/min and respiratory rate to about 40 breaths/min.

Orgasm

Orgasm occurs when stimulation proceeds through the plateau stage to a point at which a vigorous contraction of muscles in the pelvic area expels or dissipates blood and fluid from the area of congestion. The average number of contractions for the woman is 8 to 15 contractions at intervals of 1 every 0.8 seconds. In men, muscle contractions surrounding the seminal vessels and prostate project semen into the proximal urethra. These contractions are followed immediately by three to seven propulsive ejaculatory contractions, occurring at the same time interval as in the woman, which force semen from the penis (Masters et al., 1998).

As the shortest stage in the sexual response cycle, orgasm is usually experienced as intense pleasure affecting the whole body, not just the pelvic area. It is also a highly personal experience: Descriptions of orgasms vary greatly from person to person.

Resolution

The resolution is a 30-minute period during which the external and internal genital organs return to an unaroused state. For the male, a refractory period occurs during which further orgasm is impossible. Women do not go through this refractory period, so it is possible for women who are interested and properly stimulated to have additional orgasms immediately after the first.

THE INFLUENCE OF THE MENSTRUAL CYCLE ON SEXUAL RESPONSE

During the second half of the menstrual cycle—the luteal phase—there is increased fluid retention and vasocongestion in the woman's lower pelvis. Because some vasocongestion is already present at the beginning of the excitement stage of the sexual response, women appear to reach the plateau stage more quickly and achieve orgasm more readily during this time. Women also may be more interested in initiating sexual relations during this time.

THE INFLUENCE OF PREGNANCY ON SEXUAL RESPONSE

Pregnancy is another time in life when there is vasocongestion of the lower pelvis because of the blood supply needed by a rapidly growing fetus. This causes some women to experience their first orgasm during their first pregnancy. Following a pregnancy, many women continue to experience increased sexual interest because the new growth of blood vessels during pregnancy lasts for some time and continues to facilitate pelvic vasocongestion. These differences in response are why discussing sexual relationships is an important part of health teaching during pregnancy. At a time when a woman may want sexual contact very much, she needs to be free of myths and misconceptions, such as the notion that orgasm will cause a spontaneous miscarriage. Although the level of oxytocin, the hormone that rises with labor, does appear to rise in women after orgasm, this rise is not enough that women should worry that sexual relations will lead to premature labor in the average woman.

For some women, the increased breast engorgement that accompanies pregnancy results in extreme breast sensitivity during coitus. Foreplay that includes sucking or massaging of the breasts may also cause release of oxytocin, but it is not contraindicated unless the woman has a history of premature labor. Box 5.5 shows an interprofessional care map illustrating both nursing and team planning for reproductive and sexual health.

MASTURBATION

Masturbation is self-stimulation for erotic pleasure; it can also be a mutually enjoyable activity for sexual partners. It offers sexual release, which may be interpreted by the person as overall tension or anxiety relief. Masters et al. (1998) reported women may find masturbation to orgasm the most satisfying sexual expression and use it more commonly than men.

SEXUAL HARASSMENT AND VIOLENCE

Sexual gratification can be experienced in a number of ways. What is considered normal varies greatly among cultures, although general components of accepted sexual activity are that it is an activity of adults with privacy, consent, and lack of force included. Sexual violence or violence in general occurs when one partner does not respect these boundaries. This is a particular concern for maternal and child health nurses because intimate partner violence tends to occur at an increased frequency during pregnancy (Van Parys, Deschepper, Michielsen, et al., 2015). Young children and adolescents are also persons targeted for sexual maltreatment. All forms of maltreatment or partner violence are discussed in Chapter 55.

Sexual harassment is unwanted, repeated sexual advances, remarks, or behavior toward another that is offensive to the recipient or interferes with job or school performance. It can involve actions as obvious as a job superior demanding sexual favors from an employee, or it could be a man or woman sending sexist jokes by e-mail to another person in the department. In school, it can refer to bullying (Eom, Restaino, Perkins, et al., 2015).

Two types exist. One is *quid pro quo* (an equal exchange), in which an employer asks for something in return for sexual favors, such as a hiring or promotion preference. The second is a *hostile work environment*, in which an employer creates an environment in which an employee feels uncomfortable and exploited (such as being addressed as "honey" or "babe," asked to wear revealing clothing, or working where walls are decorated with sexist posters).

Sexual harassment rules apply to same-gender as well as opposite-gender harassment. In addition to causing occupational disruption, sexual harassment may be so distressing that it can lead to short- or long-term psychosocial consequences for victims and their families such as emotional distress (e.g., anxiety, depression, posttraumatic stress disorder, substance abuse), interpersonal conflict, and impaired intimacy and sexual functioning (Eom et al., 2015).

Sexual harassment has been illegal in the United States since 1964. Patients who report being subjected to harassment should be advised to report the situation to their personnel supervisor. Nurses should be aware of sexual harassment guidelines in their own work setting and likewise report such behavior to keep their workplace free of this type of strain.

INDIVIDUALS WITH UNIQUE NEEDS OR CONCERNS

A number of individuals have special concerns related to reproductive health.

The Individual With a Disability

Individuals who are physically challenged have sexual desires and needs the same as all others (Chou, Lu, & Pu, 2015). They may, however, have difficulty with sexual identity or sexual fulfillment because of their disability. Males with upper spinal cord injury, for example, may have difficulty with erections and ejaculation because these actions are governed at the spinal level. Manual stimulation of the penis or psychological stimulation can, however, achieve erection in most men with spinal cord lesions, allowing the man a satisfying sexual relationship with his partner. Most women with spinal cord injuries cannot experience orgasm but are able to conceive and have children.

Any person who interprets a procedure such as a colostomy as disfiguring may be reluctant to participate in sexual activities, fearing the sight of an apparatus will diminish their partner's satisfaction. People with chronic pain such as from arthritis may be too uncomfortable to enjoy sexual relations. Individuals with urinary catheters may be concerned about their ability to enjoy coitus with the catheter in place. For women, a retention catheter should not interfere with coitus. Men can be taught how to replace their own catheter, so they can remove it for sexual relations. In all instances in which one sexual partner is disabled in some way, the response of a

BOX 5.5

Nursing Care Planning

AN INTERPROFESSIONAL CARE MAP FOR A COUPLE NEEDING SEXUAL COUNSELING

Suzanne and Kevin Matthews, a young adult couple, 6 months pregnant, come to your antepartal clinic for a routine visit. Suzanne, in tears, states, "My husband isn't interested in me anymore. We haven't had sex since I became pregnant." The couple engaged in coitus two to three times per week prior to this pregnancy. Kevin states, "I'm afraid I'll hurt the baby."

Family Assessment: Couple has been married for 4 years; lives in two-bedroom apartment in the central city. Husband works as a high school teacher; wife works as a baker in a local coffeehouse.

Patient Assessment: A previous pregnancy, 2 years ago, ended at 8 weeks with a spontaneous miscarriage. Blood pressure today is 118/70 mmHg; overall health is "good."

Nursing Diagnosis: Altered sexuality pattern related to pregnancy and fear of harming fetus.

Outcome Criteria: Couple states they recognize coitus is not harmful in normal pregnancy; reports engaging in sexual intercourse as well as pleasurable noncoital sexual activities by next visit if desired.

Team Member Responsible	Assessment	Intervention	Rationale	Expected Outcome
Activities of Daily Living, Including Safety				
Nurse	Assess sexual concerns.	Encourage couple to continue routine prenatal care. Discuss alternative sexual activities, such as cuddling or massage.	As pregnancy progresses, discomfort, fatigue, and increasing abdominal size may interfere with a satisfying sexual relationship.	Couple continues prenatal care; describes other means of sexual expression.
Teamwork and Collaboration				
Nurse/primary care provider	Assess signs and symptoms of pregnancy; note any indication of complications.	Consult with team primary care provider to be certain the patient has no contraindications to remaining sexually active during pregnancy.	Sexual relations may be contraindicated in a few women who have had previous miscarriages or if vaginal bleeding is present.	The couple's primary care provider supplies information on if the couple can remain sexually active throughout pregnancy.
Procedures/Medications for Quality Improvement				
Nurse	Assess whether alternative types of sexual activity would fulfill couple's needs.	Review alternative sexual positions for optimal comfort and pleasure, such as side-lying.	Alternative sexual positions may be necessary to provide comfort late in pregnancy, as the woman's abdomen expands.	Couple describes alternative positions or other ways they relate to each other.
Patient-Centered Care				
Nurse/primary care provider	Assess what couple understands about reproductive anatomy and usual sexual response.	Explain sexual relations are allowed during pregnancy until labor begins. Use charts and illustrations to show how the fetus is protected in utero.	Barring complications, couples can engage in sexual intercourse and activity to the extent it is comfortable and desired. Visual aids enhance learning.	Couple states they understand sexual relations are allowed during a normal pregnancy.

Psychosocial/Spiritual/Emotional Needs

Nurse	Assess whether couple knows hormones can change sexual desire during pregnancy.	Encourage the couple to talk openly about their feelings, concerns, desires, and changes in interest to each other throughout the pregnancy.	Physical and psychological changes occur in both the pregnant woman and her partner throughout pregnancy. Open communication enhances the relationship.	Couple reports they are able to voice their feelings and concerns during the pregnancy.
Nurse	Assess what communication pattern couple uses to share information with each other.	Teach importance of a couple maintaining good communication.	Beginning a sound communication pattern during pregnancy can lay a foundation for a sound future relationship.	Couple reports they appreciate the importance of good communication for their ongoing relationship.

Informatics for Seamless Healthcare Planning

Nurse	Assess whether couple's questions and concerns were answered satisfactorily.	Review concern about sexual relations at each visit as indicated.	Continued interest in a couple's problem allows them to continue to voice concerns.	Patient's electronic health record includes a notation about the questions that were asked and answered at subsequent visits.

loving partner does much to enhance body image and feelings of adequacy of a mate. Encouraging these patients to ask questions and work on specific difficulties is a nursing role.

Sexuality is a facet of rehabilitation that has not always received attention. If a person can accomplish activities of daily living such as eating, elimination, and mobility, then he or she is often considered to be leading a normal or near-normal life. However, establishing a satisfying sexual relationship is an important part of living as well and so should be included in assessments of patients in rehabilitation programs.

The Individual With a Hypoactive Sexual Desire

Lessened interest in sexual relations is normal in some circumstances, such as after the death of a family member, a divorce, or a stressful job change. The support of a caring sexual partner or relief of the tension causing the stress allows a return in sexual interest.

Decreased sexual desire can also be a side effect of many medicines. Chronic diseases, such as peptic ulcers or chronic pulmonary disorders that cause frequent pain or discomfort, may interfere with a man's or a woman's overall well-being and interest in sexual activity. Obese men and women may not feel as much satisfaction from sexual relations as others because they have difficulty achieving deep penetration due to the bulk of their abdomens. An individual with an STI such as genital herpes may choose to forgo sexual relations rather than inform a partner of the disease. Some women experience a decrease in sexual desire during perimenopause. Administration of androgen (testosterone) to women may be helpful at that time because it can improve interest in sexual activity (Wright & O'Connor, 2015).

What If . . . 5.2

The nurse is interested in exploring one of the 2020 National Health Goals related to reproductive or sexual health (see Box 5.1). Most government-sponsored money for nursing research is allotted based on these goals. What research topics would be appropriate to explore these goals and advance evidence-based practice?

KEY POINTS FOR REVIEW

- The reproductive and sexual organs form early in intrauterine life, and full functioning occurs at puberty.
- The female internal organs of reproduction include the ovaries, the fallopian tubes, the uterus, and the vagina.
- The female external organs of reproduction include the mons veneris, the labia minora and majora, the vestibule, the clitoris, the fourchette, the perineal body, the hymen, and the Skene and the Bartholin glands.
- The male external reproductive structures are the penis, scrotum, and testes. Internal organs are the epididymis, the vas deferens, the seminal vesicles, the ejaculatory ducts, the prostate gland, the urethra, and the bulbourethral glands.
- A menstrual cycle is periodic uterine bleeding in response to cyclic hormones. Menarche is the first menstrual period. Menopause is the end of menstruation. Menstrual cycles are possible because of the interplay between the hypothalamus, the pituitary gland, the ovaries, and the uterus.
- Masters et al. (1998) identified a sexual response cycle consisting of excitement, plateau, orgasm, and resolution stages.

- Educating people about reproductive function is an important primary health strategy because it teaches people to better monitor their own health through vulvar or testicular self-examination.

- Considering reproductive and sexual health in a patient assessment helps in planning nursing care that not only meets QSEN competencies but also best meets a family's total needs.

CRITICAL THINKING CARE STUDY

Josephine Rice is 26 years old, works as a nurse on an oncology service, and has been married for 6 years. Her husband, Peter, 28 years of age, is a race car driver. They have been trying to have a child for 4 years. A fertility study revealed that this is probably because Josephine doesn't ovulate every month. A specialist suggested she lose weight (her body mass index is 27.5) and try in vitro fertilization. She confides in you she feels the fault is not ovulation. It's because, unknown to her family, she had a Plan B abortion while in college and this is her "payback."

1. Does Josephine have risk factors because of her work? Are these more apt to be the reason for her subfertility than her former abortion?
2. Does Peter's job also create risk factors?
3. Was Josephine well advised to lose weight?
4. What patient education would you provide regarding Plan B?

RELATED RESOURCES

Explore these additional resources to enhance learning for this chapter:
- Student resources on thePoint, including answers to the What If . . . and Critical Thinking Care Study questions, http://thepoint.lww.com/Flagg8e
- Adaptive learning powered by PrepU, http://thepoint.lww.com/prepu

REFERENCES

American Academy of Pediatrics. (2012). *Where we stand: Circumcision.* Evanston, IL: Author.

Bitzer, J., Sultan, C., Creatsas, G., et al. (2014). Gynecological care in young women: A high-risk period of life. *Gynecological Endocrinology, 30*(8), 542–548.

Bossio, J. A., Pukall, C. F., & Steele, S. (2014). A review of the current state of the male circumcision literature. *The Journal of Sexual Medicine, 11*(12), 2847–2864.

Callegari, L. S., Ma, E. W., & Schwarz, E. B. (2015). Preconception care and reproductive planning in primary care. *The Medical Clinics of North America, 99*(3), 663–682.

Centers for Disease Control and Prevention. (2014). *Sexual health.* Retrieved from http://www.cdc.gov/sexualhealth/default.html#who

Chou, Y. C., Lu, Z. Y., & Pu, C. Y. (2015). Attitudes toward male and female sexuality among men and women with intellectual disabilities. *Women & Health, 55*(6), 663–678.

Edmonds, D. K. (2012). Normal and abnormal development of the genital tract. In D. K. Edmonds (Ed.), *Dewhurst's textbook of obstetrics & gynaecology* (8th ed., pp. 421–434). Chichester, United Kingdom: Wiley-Blackwell.

Eggers, S., Ohnesorg, T., & Sinclair, A. (2014). Genetic regulation of mammalian gonad development. *Nature Reviews. Endocrinology, 10*(11), 673–683.

Eom, E., Restaino, S., Perkins, A. M., et al. (2015). Sexual harassment in middle and high school children and effects on physical and mental health. *Clinical Pediatrics, 54*(5), 430–438.

Fantasia, J., Aidlen, J., Lathrop, W., et al. (2015). Undescended testes: A clinical and surgical review. *Urologic Nursing, 35*(3), 117–126.

Fischer, J. W., & Kwan, C. W. (2014). Emergency point-of-care ultrasound diagnosis of hematocolpometra and imperforate hymen in the pediatric emergency department. *Pediatric Emergency Care, 30*(2), 128–130.

Gueye, A. H., & Diaz-Montes, T. P. (2015). Cervical cancer. In C. T. Johnson, J. L. Hallock, J. L. Bienstock, et al. (Eds.), *The Johns Hopkins manual of gynecology and obstetrics* (5th ed., pp. 592–610). Philadelphia, PA: Wolters Kluwer.

Guilamo-Ramos, V., Lee, J. J., Kantor, L. M., et al. (2015). Potential for using online and mobile education with parents and adolescents to impact sexual and reproductive health. *Prevention Science, 16*(1), 53–60.

Huether, S. E., & McCance, K. L. (2012). *Understanding pathophysiology* (5th ed.). St. Louis, MO: Mosby.

Johnson, S. D., & Williams, S. L. (2015). Solution-focused strategies for effective sexual health communication among African American parents and their adolescents. *Health & Social Work, 40*(4), 267–274.

Kumar, S. (2012). Fetal anomalies. In D. K. Edmonds (Ed.), *Dewhurst's textbook of obstetrics & gynaecology* (8th ed., pp. 219–229). Chichester, United Kingdom: Wiley-Blackwell.

Ledger, W. L. (2012). The menstrual cycle. In D. K. Edmonds (Ed.), *Dewhurst's textbook of obstetrics & gynaecology* (8th ed., pp. 487–494). Chichester, United Kingdom: Wiley-Blackwell.

March of Dimes Foundation. (2012). *Teenage pregnancy.* White Plains, NY: Author.

Maron, D. F. (2015). Why girls are starting puberty early. *Scientific American, 312*(5), 28, 30.

Masters, W. H., Johnson, V. E., & Kolodny, R. C. (1998). *Heterosexuality.* New York, NY: Smithmark.

Mountjoy, M., Sundgot-Borgen, J., Burke, L., et al. (2014). The IOC consensus statement: Beyond the female athlete triad—relative energy deficiency in sport (RED-S). *British Journal of Sports Medicine, 48*(7), 491–497.

Narula, H. S., & Carlson, H. E. (2014). Gynaecomastia—pathophysiology, diagnosis, and treatment. *Nature Reviews. Endocrinology, 10*(11), 684–698.

Neely, E. K., & Crossen, S. S. (2014). Precocious puberty. *Current Opinion in Obstetrics & Gynecology, 26*(5), 332–338.

Nour, N. M. (2015). Female genital cutting: Impact on women's health. *Seminars in Reproductive Medicine, 33*(1), 41–46.

Owens, L., & Green, I. (2015). Anatomy of the female pelvis. In C. T. Johnson, J. L. Hallock, J. L. Bienstock, et al. (Eds.), *The Johns Hopkins manual of gynecology and obstetrics* (5th ed., pp. 326–340). Philadelphia, PA: Wolters Kluwer.

Podzemny, V., Pescatori, L. C., & Pescatori, M. (2015). Management of obstructed defecation. *World Journal of Gastroenterology, 21*(4), 1053–1060.

Resetkova, N., & Rogers, L. (2015). Female sexual response and sexual dysfunction. In C. T. Johnson, J. L. Hallock, J. L. Bienstock, et al. (Eds.), *The Johns Hopkins manual of gynecology and obstetrics* (5th ed., pp. 546–554). Philadelphia, PA: Wolters Kluwer.

Sheth, S., & Keller, J. M. (2015). Infections of the genital tract. In C. T. Johnson, J. L. Hallock, J. L. Bienstock, et al. (Eds.), *The Johns Hopkins manual of gynecology and obstetrics* (5th ed., pp. 356–378). Philadelphia, PA: Wolters Kluwer.

Sholapurkar, S. L. (2015). Diagnostic and management modalities in early tubal ectopic pregnancy with focus on safety. *Human Reproduction Update, 21*(5), 692–693.

Sundar, S., Neal, R. D., & Kehoe, S. (2015). Diagnosis of ovarian cancer. *BMJ, 351*, h4443.

Tanner, J. M. (1990). *Fetus into man: Physical growth from conception to maturity* (2nd ed.). Cambridge, MA: Harvard University Press.

The Joint Commission. (2011). *Advancing effective communication, cultural competence, and patient- and family-centered care for the lesbian, gay, bisexual, and transgender (LGBT) community: A field guide.* Oak Brook, IL: Author. Retrieved from www.jointcommission.org/assets/1/18/LGBTFieldGuide.pdf

Tortora, G. J., & Derrickson, B. H. (2014). The reproductive systems. In G. J. Tortora & B. H. Derrickson (Eds.), *Principles of anatomy and physiology* (14th ed., pp. 974–1021). Hoboken, NJ: Wiley.

U.S. Department of Health and Human Services. (2010). *Healthy people 2020.* Washington, DC: Author.

Van Parys, A. S., Deschepper, E., Michielsen, K., et al. (2015). Intimate partner violence and psychosocial health, a cross-sectional study in a pregnant population. *BMC Pregnancy and Childbirth, 15*, 278.

Wright, J. J., & O'Connor, K. M. (2015). Female sexual dysfunction. *The Medical Clinics of North America, 99*(3), 607–628.

Nursing Care for the Family in Need of Reproductive Life Planning

Seventeen-year-old Dana Crews has come to your community health clinic for a routine gynecologic exam. She tells you she is sexually active and her boyfriend "sometimes" uses a condom. She trusts he will "stop in time" when they aren't using one. She doesn't want to take birth control pills because she can't afford them and also she's afraid her parents will find out she's broken her abstinence pledge if they see the pills.

The previous chapter described the anatomy and physiology of the male and female reproductive systems and the importance of sexual health. This chapter adds information about ways to prevent pregnancy or to plan and space children. Such information builds a base for both care and health teaching of families.

What additional health teaching does Dana need to be well informed about reproductive life planning?

KEY TERMS

abstinence

barrier methods

basal body temperature

cervical cap

coitus

coitus interruptus

contraceptive

diaphragm

elective termination of pregnancy

female condom

fertile days

fertility awareness

intrauterine device

laparoscopy

male condom

natural family planning

reproductive life planning

spermicide

transdermal contraception

tubal ligation

vasectomy

OBJECTIVES

After mastering the contents of this chapter, you should be able to:

1. Describe common methods of reproductive life planning and the advantages, disadvantages, and risk factors associated with each.

2. Identify 2020 National Health Goals related to reproductive life planning that nurses can help the nation achieve.

3. Formulate nursing diagnoses related to reproductive life planning concerns.

4. Using the nursing process, plan nursing care that includes the six competencies of Quality & Safety Education for Nurses (QSEN): Patient-Centered Care, Teamwork & Collaboration, Evidence-Based Practice (EBP), Quality Improvement (QI), Safety, and Informatics.

5. Implement nursing care related to reproductive life planning, such as educating adolescents about the use of condoms as a safer sex practice as well as to prevent unintended pregnancy.

6. Evaluate expected outcomes for achievement and effectiveness of care.

7. Integrate knowledge of reproductive life planning with the interplay of nursing process, the six competencies of QSEN, and Family Nursing to promote quality maternal and child health nursing care.

Reproductive life planning includes all the decisions an individual or couple make about whether and when to have children, how many children to have, and how they are spaced. Some couples you will meet want counseling about how to avoid conception. Others want information on increasing fertility and about their ability to conceive. Others need counseling because a **contraceptive** (a measure to halt conception) has failed (Bond, 2013).

Intentional pregnancies are important for the health of children because when a pregnancy is unintended or mistimed, both short-term and long-term consequences can result. The woman may be less likely or less careful to:

• Seek prenatal care
• Breastfeed
• Protect her fetus from harmful substances

A disproportionate share of women who bear children whose conception was unintended are adolescents; such women are less apt to complete high school or college and more likely to require public assistance and/or live in poverty than their peers who are not mothers. The child of such a pregnancy is at greater risk for low birth weight, dying in the first year of life, being maltreated, and not receiving sufficient resources for healthy development (Centers for Disease Control and Prevention [CDC], 2015).

Planning for reproductive choices is so important that several 2020 National Health Goals speak directly to this area of care (Box 6.1).

BOX 6.1

Nursing Care Planning Based on 2020 National Health Goals

A number of 2020 National Health Goals speak directly to reproductive life planning:

• Increase the proportion of adolescents who receive formal instruction on abstinence before 18 years of age from a baseline of 87.2% to a target of 95.9%.
• Increase the proportion of females less than 15 years of age who have never had sexual intercourse from a baseline of 82.9% to a target of 91.2%; of males, from 82.0% to 90.2%.
• Reduce the proportion of females experiencing pregnancy despite use of a reversible contraceptive method from a baseline of 12.4% to a target of 9.9%.
• Increase the proportion of intended pregnancies from a baseline of 51% to a target of 56%.
• Decrease the proportion of births occurring within 18 months of a previous birth from a baseline of 35.3% to a target of 31.7% (U.S. Department of Health and Human Services, 2010; see www.healthypeople.gov).

Nurses can help the nation achieve these objectives by teaching people, especially adolescents, about contraceptive options while being cautious to avoid indirectly encouraging sexual activity among teens.

Nursing Process Overview

FOR REPRODUCTIVE LIFE PLANNING

ASSESSMENT

As a result of changing social values and lifestyles, many people today are able to talk easily about reproductive life planning. Other people, however, may be uncomfortable with this topic and may not voice their interest in the subject independently. For this reason, at health assessments, ask patients if they want more information or need any help with reproductive life planning as part of obtaining a basic health history.

NURSING DIAGNOSIS

Because reproductive life planning touches so many facets of life, nursing diagnoses can differ greatly depending on the circumstances and individual preferences. Examples might include:

• Readiness for enhanced knowledge regarding contraception options related to a desire to prevent pregnancy
• Deficient knowledge related to use of a diaphragm
• Spiritual distress related to partner's preferences for contraception
• Decisional conflict regarding choice of birth control because of health concerns
• Decisional conflict related to unintended pregnancy
• Powerlessness related to failure of chosen contraceptive
• Altered sexuality pattern related to fear of pregnancy
• Risk for ineffective health maintenance related to lack of knowledge about natural family planning methods

PLANNING AND IMPLEMENTATION

When establishing expected outcomes for care in this area, be certain plans are realistic for each couple. If a woman has a history of poor compliance with medication, for instance, it might not be realistic for her to plan on taking an oral contraceptive every day. If she only desires temporary contraception, tubal ligation or vasectomy for her partner would certainly be inappropriate. Be certain when counseling to be sensitive to a couple's spiritual, cultural, and moral beliefs before suggesting possible methods. It is equally important to explore your own beliefs and values before counseling. This not only helps develop self-awareness of how these beliefs affect nursing care, but it also allows you to become more sensitive to the beliefs of others.

Patients are required to provide informed consent for surgical contraceptive methods or procedures such as vasectomy or tubal ligation. The risks, benefits, alternatives, and proper use of the method and the patient's understanding of his or her rights and responsibilities should be included in the consent form as this helps ensure patients have weighed their options and know the procedure may be irreversible. If you are helping to obtain a consent signature, always do so in the presence of a witness. It is also helpful to refer patients to online resources for further information (see Chapter 5).

OUTCOME EVALUATION

Evaluation is important in reproductive life planning because anything that causes patients to discontinue or misuse a particular method will leave them at risk of pregnancy.

Reassess early (within 1 to 3 weeks) after a couple begins a new method of contraception to prevent such an occurrence. Evaluate not only whether a chosen method is effective but also whether the woman and her partner are satisfied or have further questions. Examples of expected outcomes include:

- Patient voices confidence in chosen contraceptive method by next visit.
- Patient expresses satisfaction with chosen method at follow-up visit.
- Patient consistently uses chosen method without pregnancy for 1 year.

Assessment for Contraception Options and Possible Contraindications

As many as 93% of women of childbearing age in the United States use some form of contraception (CDC, 2015). Major benefits of this increase in contraception include decreases in unintended adolescent pregnancies, the need for "morning after" or postcoital medications, and elective terminations of pregnancy (CDC, 2015).

Important things to consider when helping a couple choose a method that will be right for them include:

- Personal values
- Ability to use a method correctly
- If the method will affect sexual enjoyment
- Financial factors
- If a couple's relationship is short term or long term
- Prior experiences with contraception
- Future plans

For counseling to be successful, it is necessary to understand how various methods of contraception work and how they compare in terms of benefits and disadvantages (Box 6.2). In addition to assessing to determine the best contraceptive option, be certain to emphasize safer sex practices. Although there are many contraceptive options for reliable pregnancy prevention, only condoms (both male and female) provide protection against sexually transmitted infections (STIs) or HIV—an important concern if a relationship is not a monogamous one.

Many postpartum services distribute printed information on contraception packaging to women at discharge. Women are then invited to ask questions as necessary about the material. Read these materials carefully to be certain they are accurate before distributing them and, if suggestions are needed, make them to the correct healthcare committee. Be certain to make it clear you are available to answer questions about contraception; otherwise, women are in such a hurry to take their newborn home, they tend to postpone questions "until later," a time when the question may be too late to be effective or a healthcare provider is no longer available.

Consider each person's lifestyle and overall health, as these influence what type of conception a woman will choose (Box 6.3). Morbidly obese women, for example, may need to choose different types than women with an average body mass index (Mody & Han, 2014). Women in a male-dominant family may have little choice as to what reproductive life planning method they can choose. If their partner does

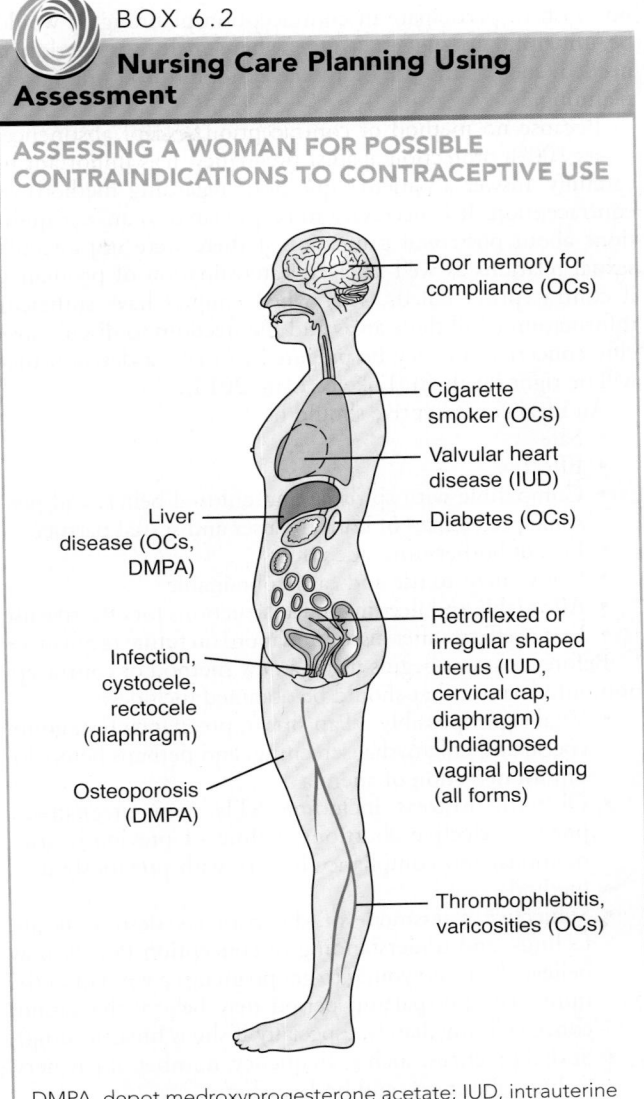

BOX 6.2

Nursing Care Planning Using Assessment

ASSESSING A WOMAN FOR POSSIBLE CONTRAINDICATIONS TO CONTRACEPTIVE USE

- Poor memory for compliance (OCs)
- Cigarette smoker (OCs)
- Valvular heart disease (IUD)
- Diabetes (OCs)
- Liver disease (OCs, DMPA)
- Retroflexed or irregular shaped uterus (IUD, cervical cap, diaphragm) Undiagnosed vaginal bleeding (all forms)
- Infection, cystocele, rectocele (diaphragm)
- Osteoporosis (DMPA)
- Thrombophlebitis, varicosities (OCs)

DMPA, depot medroxyprogesterone acetate; IUD, intrauterine device; OCs, oral contraceptives.

BOX 6.3

Nursing Care Planning to Respect Cultural Diversity

People differ greatly in the way they desire or accept information on reproductive life planning, depending on individual preferences and sociocultural influences. For example, certain religions do not believe a method beyond abstinence or fertility awareness is right to use. People with lower incomes cannot afford surgical procedures or methods such as daily combination pills. Be certain while counseling in this area that you do not impose your own values on people but rather work together to identify a system that your patient will be able to follow consistently.

not wish to participate in contraception planning, it would be unhelpful to suggest a type where male cooperation is needed, such as the use of a male condom or natural family planning.

Because no method of contraception, except abstinence, offers 100% protection against pregnancy, it is important to carefully answer a patient's questions regarding methods of contraception. It is necessary to be prepared to answer questions about postcoital protection if there were unprotected sexual relations as well as elective termination of pregnancy if contraception failed. Only when couples have sufficient information in all these areas and the freedom to discuss specific concerns can they be prepared to make a decision that will be right for them (Loke & Lam, 2014).

An ideal contraceptive should be:
* Safe
* Effective
* Compatible with spiritual and cultural beliefs and personal preferences of both the user and sexual partner
* Free of bothersome side effects
* Convenient to use and easily obtainable
* Affordable and needing few instructions for effective use
* Free of effects (after discontinuation) on future pregnancies

Before a patient begins using a new method of contraception, information that should be obtained includes:
* Vital signs, possibly a Pap smear, pregnancy test, gonococcal and chlamydial screening, and perhaps hemoglobin for detection of anemia
* Obstetric history, including STIs, past pregnancies, previous elective abortions, failure of previously used methods, and compliance history with previously used methods
* Subjective assessment of the patient's desires, needs, feelings, and understanding of conception (a teen may believe she is too young to get pregnant; a woman in the immediate postpartum period may believe she cannot conceive immediately, especially if she is breastfeeding)
* Sexual practices, such as frequency, number of partners, feelings about sex, and body image

How well contraceptive methods meet ideal requirements is discussed with each type. The range of effectiveness of frequently used contraceptive methods is shown in Table 6.1. This table shows the effectiveness of each method by listing the *ideal failure rate* (the number of unintended pregnancies that will occur in 1 year) for couples who use the method consistently and correctly and also the *failure rate* for routine use (less-than-perfect use). A method that shows a large difference between the ideal failure rate and the actual failure rate may not be easy and convenient to use.

Natural Family Planning

Natural family planning methods, also called periodic abstinence methods, are, as the name implies, methods that involve no introduction of chemical or foreign material into the body (Oman & Burke, 2015).

Many people hold spiritual beliefs that rule out the use of birth control pills or devices. Others simply believe a "natural" way of planning pregnancies is best for them, one that will involve no expense, does not introduce a foreign substance into their body, and has no risk to a fetus should they become pregnant. The effectiveness of these methods varies greatly from a 2% ideal failure rate to about a 25% failure rate, depending mainly on the couple's ability to refrain from having sexual relations on **fertile days** or days in which a woman is most likely to become pregnant (Rodriguez, Darney, Elman, et al., 2015).

ABSTINENCE

Abstinence, or refraining from sexual relations, has a theoretical 0% failure rate and is also the most effective way to prevent STIs. Due to the natural human sexual drive, patients may find it difficult to adhere to abstinence because they may deny the possibility of sexual activity and fail to plan for pregnancy and STI prevention. Because it is difficult for many couples to adhere to abstinence, the method has a high failure rate (Schalet, Santelli, Russell, et al., 2014).

Many sex education classes for adolescents advocate abstinence as the only contraceptive measure, so teenagers and young adults who take these courses may know little about other options. When discussing abstinence as a contraceptive method, be certain to provide information not only on the method but also suggestions for ways to comply with this method (Box 6.4). A worry is adolescents who make "abstinence pledges" to not have sexual intercourse until they are married may "tune out" not only additional information on contraception but also on safer sex practices. Then, if they break their pledge (about 50% do), that could leave them more vulnerable to STIs and pregnancy than others (Schalet et al., 2014).

Periodic Abstinence

Periodic abstinence is a method to avoid pregnancy by avoiding sex on the days a woman may conceive. Methods for determining the days when a woman could conceive are under "Fertility Awareness Methods."

LACTATION AMENORRHEA METHOD

When a woman is breastfeeding, there is a natural suppression of both ovulation and menses (Pratts & Lawson, 2015).

Lactation amenorrhea method (LAM) is a safe birth control method (a failure rate of about 1% to 5%) if:
* An infant is:
  * Under 6 months of age
  * Being totally breastfed at least every 4 hours during the day and every 6 hours at night
  * Receives no supplementary feedings, and
* Menses has not returned

After 6 months, or if the infant begins to receive supplemental feedings or isn't sucking well, the use of LAM as an effective birth control method becomes questionable and the woman probably should be advised to choose another method of contraception (Lopez, Grey, Chen, et al., 2014). A woman should also consider a different method of contraception once her baby begins sleeping through the night, even if this occurs before the child reaches 6 months of age.

COITUS INTERRUPTUS

Coitus interruptus (withdrawal) is one of the oldest known methods of contraception. The couple proceeds with coitus until the moment of ejaculation. Then, the man withdraws

TABLE 6.1 CONTRACEPTION FAILURE RATES

Type of Contraceptive	Ideal Failure Rate (%) Perfect Use[a]	Failure Rate (%) Typical Use	Advantages	Disadvantages
Natural Family Planning				
Abstinence	100%	85%	Acceptable to all religious groups No cost	Requires high motivation and periods of abstinence
Lactation, amenorrhea	1%–5% (under 6 months)	95% (after 6 months)	Effective while infant is totally breastfed; approved by all religions and cultures	Temporary measure Not reliable if infant takes supplemental feedings
Calendar	1%–9%	25%	No cost	Requires motivation, cooperation
Standard day method: CycleBeads	5%	12%–13%	Visual aid can improve compliance Available as iPhone app	Initial cost May need to mark on a calendar they have moved a bead rather than rely on memory
Basal body temperature (BBT)	3%	25%	Cost of thermometer	Requires motivation and cooperation by male partner
Ovulation method	3%	25%	No cost	Requires motivation and cooperation by male partner
Symptothermal	0.4%	25%	No cost	Requires motivation and cooperation from male partner
Two-day method	3%–4%	13%–14%	No cost	Requires motivation and cooperation from male partner
Withdrawal	4%	22%	A male-controlled method	Sperm may be present in pre-ejaculatory fluid
Barrier Methods				
Spermicide	18%	28%	Easy to use Sold over the counter	May leave an annoying vaginal discharge
Male condom	2%	18%	Protects against STIs Male responsibility No prescription necessary	Requires interruption of sexual activity
Female condom	5%	21%	Protection against STIs	Insertion may be difficult
Sponge (parous woman)	20%	24%	Easy to insert No prescription	May cause leakage Necessary to take measures to avoid danger of TSS
Sponge (nulliparous woman)	9%	12%	Easy to insert No prescription	May cause leakage Necessary to take measures to avoid TSS
Diaphragm	6%	12%	Easy to insert	Prescription needed Necessary to take measures to avoid TSS
Cervical cap (parous woman)	23%	35%	Can leave in place for several days if desired	May be difficult to insert Can irritate cervix Necessary to take measures to avoid TSS
Cervical cap (nulliparous woman)	9%	18%	Can leave in place for several days if desired	May be difficult to insert Can irritate cervix Necessary to take measures to avoid TSS

Continued on following page

TABLE 6.1 CONTRACEPTION FAILURE RATES (Continued)

Type of Contraceptive	Ideal Failure Rate (%) Perfect Use[a]	Failure Rate (%) Typical Use	Advantages	Disadvantages
Hormonal Methods				
Transdermal patch	0.3%	9%	Easy to apply	Irritation at local site
Vaginal ring	0.3%	9%	Easy to insert	May need reminder to insert
Combination oral contraceptives (COCs)	0.3%	9%	Coitus independent	Continual cost
				Possible side effect of thrombophlebitis
Progestin-only pills (mini-pills)	0.5%	5%–8%	Coitus independent	Continual cost
			No side effects of COCs	
Injectable progesterone (DMPA)	0.2%	6%	Coitus independent	Continual cost
			Dependable for 12 weeks	Continual injections
Intradermal implant (Nexplanon)	0.05%	0.05%	Coitus independent	Initial cost
			Dependable for 5 years	Appearance on arm
IUD (copper T)	0.6%	0.8%	No memory or motivation needed	Cramping, bleeding
				Expulsion possible
Mirena IUD	0.2%	0.2%	No memory or motivation needed	Cramping, bleeding
				Expulsion possible
Surgical Methods				
Female sterilization	0.5%	0.5%	Permanent and highly reliable	Initial cost
				Irreversible
Male sterilization	0.1%	0.15%	Permanent and highly reliable	Initial cost
				Irreversible
Postcoital (Emergency) Methods				
Postcoital pills	1%–2%	25%	Can be purchased over the counter	May cause nausea
Postcoital IUD	0.1%	0.1%–2%	Can be inserted up to 5 days after unprotected coitus	Visit to a healthcare provider is needed within 5 days (120 hr) of unprotected coitus
			Can be left in place as contraceptive measure	

[a]Couples who use the method consistently and correctly during a year's time.
DMPA, depot medroxyprogesterone acetate; IUD, intrauterine device; STI, sexually transmitted infection; TSS, toxic shock syndrome.
Modified from Centers for Disease Control and Prevention. (2014). Appendix D: Contraceptive effectiveness. *Morbidity and Mortality Weekly Report, 63*(4), 47.

 BOX 6.4

Nursing Care Planning to Empower a Family

SUGGESTIONS FOR PROMOTING ABSTINENCE

Q. Dana, 17 years old, asks you, "How can I avoid being pressured into unwanted sex?"

A. A few suggestions are:

- Discuss with your partner in advance which sexual activities you will permit and which you will not.
- Try to avoid high-pressure situations such as a party with known drug use, excessive alcohol consumption; for teenagers: no adult supervision.
- Be certain your partner understands when you say, "No," you mean it.
- Make it clear your partner understands you consider being forced into relations against your wishes the same as rape, not simply irresponsible conduct.
- Do not accept any drug to "help you relax" or "be cool," as such a drug could impair your judgment. The drug could also be the "date rape" drug flunitrazepam (Rohypnol), which causes loss of memory for recent events.

and spermatozoa are emitted outside the vagina. Unfortunately, ejaculation may occur before withdrawal is complete and, despite the caution used, some spermatozoa may be deposited in the vagina. Furthermore, because there may be a few spermatozoa present in pre-ejaculation fluid, fertilization may occur even if withdrawal seems controlled (Killick, Leary, Trussell, et al., 2011). For these reasons, coitus interruptus is only about 82% effective, and the method should be used with caution as it also can lead to STIs (Jones, Lindberg, & Higgins, 2014).

POSTCOITAL DOUCHING

Douching following intercourse, no matter what solution is used, is ineffective as a contraceptive measure as sperm may be present in cervical mucus as quickly as 90 seconds after ejaculation, long before douching could be accomplished.

FERTILITY AWARENESS METHODS

Fertility awareness methods rely on detecting when a woman will be capable of impregnation (fertile) so she can use periods of abstinence during that time. There are a variety of ways to determine a fertile period, such as using a calendar to calculate the period of time based on a set formula, using a visual tool such as "CycleBeads," measuring the woman's body temperature, observing the consistency of cervical mucus, or employing a combination of these methods (Taylor, Aldad, McVeigh, et al., 2012). The methods consider the typical length of sperm survival (anywhere from 3 to more than 5 days) and the length of time an ova is ripe for fertilization (about 1 day). Based on this, a fertile period exists from about 5 days before ovulation to 1 day after.

Calendar (Rhythm) Method

The calendar method requires a couple to abstain from coitus on the days of a menstrual cycle when the woman is most likely to conceive. To plan for this, the woman keeps a diary of about six menstrual cycles. To calculate "safe" days, she subtracts 18 from the shortest cycle she documented. This number predicts her first fertile day. She then subtracts 11 from her longest cycle. This represents her last fertile day. If she had six menstrual cycles ranging from 25 to 29 days, her fertile period would be from the 7th day (25 [the shortest cycle] − 18) to the 18th day (29 [the longest cycle] − 11). To avoid pregnancy, she would avoid coitus during those days (Fig. 6.1A). When used conscientiously, the method has a low failure rate; in typical use, however, this rate rises substantially because of irregular menstrual cycles, miscalculation, or disregard for predicted fertile days.

Basal Body Temperature Method

Just before the day of ovulation, a woman's **basal body temperature** (BBT), or the temperature of her body at rest, falls about 0.5°F. At the time of ovulation, her BBT rises a full Fahrenheit degree (0.2°C) because of the rise in progesterone with ovulation. This pattern serves as the basis for the BBT method of contraception (Taylor et al., 2012).

To use this method, the woman takes her temperature, either orally or with a tympanic thermometer, each morning immediately after waking before she rises from bed or undertakes any activity; this is her BBT. A woman who works nights should take her temperature after awakening from her longest sleep period, no matter what the time of day. As soon as a woman notices a slight dip in temperature followed by an increase, she knows she has ovulated. She refrains from

Figure 6.1 **(A)** A typical month showing predicted fertile days using the calendar method as a natural family planning method. **(B)** A typical month using the cervical mucus method of natural family planning. Unmarked days are those predicted to be unfertile and therefore safe for sexual relations.

having **coitus** (sexual relations) for the next 3 days (the possible life of the discharged ovum).

Because sperm can survive from 3 to 5 days and rarely as many as 7 days in the female reproductive tract, it is usually recommended that the couple combine this method with a calendar method, so they abstain for a few days before ovulation as well. The BBT method has an ideal failure rate as low as 3% but a failure rate of 25% (see Table 6.1). For more information on BBT and how it also can be used to aid conception, see Chapter 7 and Figure 7.2.

A problem with assessing BBT for fertility awareness is that many factors can affect BBT. For example, a temperature rise caused by illness could be mistaken as the signal of ovulation. If this happens, a woman could mistake a fertile day for a safe one. Changes in the woman's daily schedule, such as starting an aerobic program or getting up earlier than usual, could also affect BBT.

Cervical Mucus Method (Billing's Method)

Yet another method to predict ovulation is to use the changes in cervical mucus that occur naturally with ovulation (Fig. 6.1B). Before ovulation each month, the cervical mucus is thick and does not stretch when pulled between the thumb and finger. Just before ovulation, mucus secretion increases. On the day of ovulation (the peak day), it becomes copious, thin, watery, and transparent. It feels slippery (like egg white) and stretches at least 1 inch before the strand breaks, a property known as *spinnbarkeit* (see Chapter 5, Fig. 5.14). In addition, breast tenderness and an anterior tilt to the cervix occur. All the days on which cervical mucus is copious, and for at least 3 to 4 days afterward, are considered to be fertile days, or days on which the woman should abstain from coitus to avoid conception (Oman & Burke, 2015).

A woman using this method must be conscientious about assessing her vaginal secretions every day, or she will miss the change in texture and amount. The feel of vaginal secretions after sexual relations is unreliable because seminal fluid (the fluid containing sperm from the male) has a watery, post-ovulatory consistency and can be confused with ovulatory mucus. Figure 6.1B shows a hypothetical month using this method. This method has a potentially high failure rate because of difficulty in interpreting mucus status (Blackwell, Vigil, Alliende, et al., 2016). Because sperm have a life span from 3 to more than 5 days, a woman needs to abstain for at least 4 days prior to the appearance of estrogen-influenced mucus; therefore, this method should be combined with a calendar method for best results.

Two-Day Method

To use a 2-day method, a woman assesses for vaginal secretions daily. If she feels secretions for 2 days in a row, she avoids coitus that day and the day following as the presence of secretions suggests fertility. The method requires conscientious daily assessment and results in about 12 days per month in which she should avoid coitus, the same as a calendar method (Aksel, Sinai, & Yee, 2012).

Symptothermal Method

The symptothermal method of birth control combines the cervical mucus and BBT methods (Wettstein & Bourgeois, 2014). The woman takes her temperature daily, watching for the rise in temperature that marks ovulation. She also analyzes her cervical mucus every day and observes for other signs of ovulation such as *mittelschmerz* (midcycle abdominal pain) or if her cervix feels softer than usual. The couple then abstains from intercourse until 3 days after the rise in temperature or the fourth day after the peak of mucus change. The symptothermal method, because it assesses more clues to ovulation, is more effective than either the BBT or the cervical mucus method alone (ideal failure rate about 2%).

Standard Days Method: CycleBeads

This method is designed for women who have menstrual cycles between 26 and 32 days (Igras, Sinai, Mukabatsinda, et al., 2014). A woman purchases a circle of beads that helps her predict fertile days (Fig. 6.2). The first bead on the ring is red and marks the first day of her menstrual flow; this is followed by six brown beads which indicate "safe" days. Twelve glow-in-the-dark white beads, which mark fertile days (during which she needs to abstain from coitus), and 13 additional brown "safe" days follow. The woman advances one bead per day during the month. If she reaches a dark brown bead (appears on the 27th day) before she begins her next menses, her cycle is too short for the method to be reliable. If she reaches the end of the string of beads (32 days) before menses, she knows her cycle is too long for the method to be reliable. The system is easy to use, and, if a woman wants a more technology-based system than using a circle of beads, there is an iPhone app available in place of actual beads (iCycleBeads). The system is easy to understand; most women, however, need to use a calendar to check off daily that they have moved a bead or they can lose track of the system.

Ovulation Detection

Still another method to predict ovulation is by the use of an over-the-counter ovulation detection kit. These kits detect the midcycle surge of luteinizing hormone (LH) that can be detected in urine 12 to 24 hours before ovulation. Such kits are 98% to 100% accurate in predicting ovulation. Although they are fairly expensive and not intended to be used as a contraceptive aid, combining a cervical mucus assessment and the ovulation detector to mark the peak fertile day is becoming the method of choice for many families. An ovulation detector can be used in the future to help conception when the couple is ready to have children.

Marquette Model

This method combines the use of ovulation detection with other signs of ovulation (cervical mucus, BBT, cervix position and softness) to avoid pregnancy during a woman's fertile period. It was developed in the late 1990s by nurses and doctors at Marquette University in Wisconsin.

Side Effects and Contraindications for Natural Family Planning

Natural family planning methods do not have side effects. If there is a contraindication to their use, it would be for couples who must prevent conception (perhaps because the woman is taking a drug that would be harmful to a fetus or the couple absolutely does not want the responsibility of children) because the failure rate of all forms is about 25%.

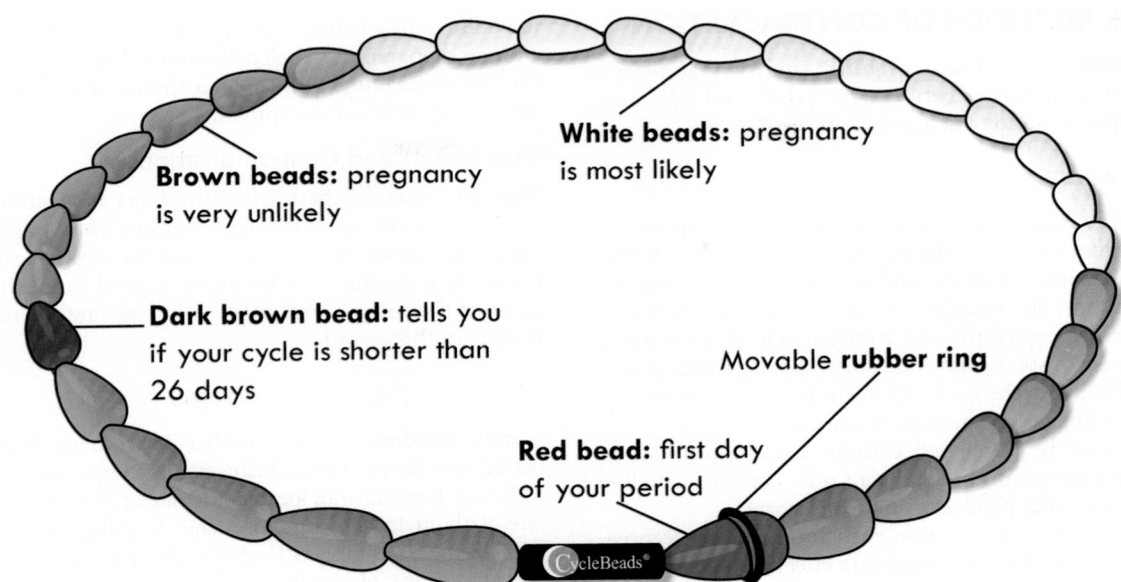

Figure 6.2 With CycleBeads, a woman moves one bead every day to predict her fertile days if her menstrual cycles range from 26 to 32 days. (Courtesy of Cycle Technologies, Inc., Washington, DC.)

Natural Family Planning and Effect on Pregnancy

Natural family planning methods have no effect if a woman should get pregnant while using them as well as no effect on future pregnancies.

Natural Family Planning and Effect on Sexual Enjoyment

Once a couple is certain of a woman's nonfertile days using one of the natural planning methods, more spontaneity in sexual relations is possible than with methods that involve vaginal insertion products. However, the required days of abstinence may make a natural planning method unsatisfactory and unenjoyable for a couple. Coitus interruptus may be unenjoyable because of the need to withdraw before ejaculation.

Natural Family Planning and the Adolescent

Natural methods of family planning (with the exception of abstinence) are usually not the contraceptive method of choice for adolescents as they require a great deal of thought and persistence. Adolescent boys may lack the control or experience to use coitus interruptus effectively. Girls tend to have occasional anovulatory menstrual cycles for several years after menarche and so may not experience definite cervical changes or an elevated body temperature each month. In addition, these methods require adolescents to say "no" to sexual intercourse on fertile days, a task that may be difficult to complete under peer pressure.

Natural Family Planning and the Perimenopausal Woman

Perimenopausal women are good candidates for natural family planning methods because they may not be able to use hormonal methods such as birth control pills because of risk to them if they have a history of high blood pressure, thromboembolic disease, or cigarette smoking. As menopause approaches, however, they may not have as much cervical mucus as previously, causing the contrast between fertile and nonfertile days more difficult to detect. Additionally, their menstrual cycles could become unpredictable, causing issues with detecting fertile days.

Natural Family Planning and the Postpartal Woman

After a successful pregnancy, most women are interested in delaying their next pregnancy until their new baby is older. This makes them good candidates for natural family planning as they can breastfeed with these methods without worrying about hormonal contamination or a decrease in breast milk. However, a postpartal woman often ovulates before her first menstrual cycle and should be warned that she could become pregnant even before her return to menses.

QSEN Checkpoint Question 6.1

PATIENT-CENTERED CARE

Suppose Dana, 17 years old, tells the nurse she wants to use a fertility awareness method of contraception. How should the nurse best meet Dana's learning needs?
  a. The nurse should teach her to record if she feels hot and whether she is perspiring heavily.
  b. The nurse should teach her to assess whether her cervical mucus is thin and watery.
  c. The nurse should teach her to monitor her emotions for sudden anger or crying.
  d. The nurse should teach her to assess whether her breasts feel sensitive to cool air.

Look in Appendix A for the best answer and rationale.

BARRIER METHODS OF CONTRACEPTION

Barrier methods are forms of birth control that place a chemical or latex barrier between the cervix and advancing sperm so sperm cannot reach and fertilize an ovum.

Spermicides

A **spermicide** is an agent that causes the death of spermatozoa before they can enter the cervix. It is a chemical barrier method and is often used in combination with other physical barrier methods. Spermicides not only actively kill sperm but also change the vaginal pH to a strong acid level, a condition not conducive to sperm survival. They do not protect against STIs. In addition to the general benefits for barrier contraceptives, the advantages of spermicides include:

- They may be purchased without a prescription or an appointment with a healthcare provider, so they allow for greater independence and lower costs.
- When used in conjunction with another contraceptive, they increase the other method's effectiveness.
- Various preparations are available, including gels, creams, sponges, films, foams, and vaginal suppositories.

Gels or creams are easily inserted into the vagina before coitus with the provided applicator (Fig. 6.3). The woman should do this no more than 1 hour before coitus. If she chooses to douche to remove the spermicide afterward (no need to do this), she should wait 6 hours after coitus to ensure the agent has completed its spermicidal action.

Another form of spermicidal protection is a film of glycerin impregnated with a spermicidal agent that is folded and inserted vaginally. On contact with vaginal secretions or precoital penile emissions, the film dissolves and a carbon dioxide foam forms to protect the cervix against invading spermatozoa.

Still, other vaginal products are cocoa butter and glycerin-based vaginal suppositories containing a spermicide. Because it takes about 15 minutes for a suppository to dissolve, it must be inserted 15 minutes before coitus.

Foam-impregnated synthetic sponges are moistened to activate the impregnated spermicide and then inserted vaginally to block sperm access. Well liked by most users, they are easy to insert and have an ideal failure rate of 9% and a typical use failure rate of about 16% to 20% (CDC, 2014). Caution women preparations labeled "feminine hygiene" products are for vaginal cleanliness and are not spermicidal; therefore, they are not effective contraceptives.

Side Effects and Contraindications

Vaginally inserted spermicidal products are contraindicated in women with acute cervicitis because they might further irritate the cervix. Some women find the vaginal leakage after use of these products bothersome. Vaginal suppositories, because of the cocoa butter or glycerin base, are the most bothersome in this regard.

Male and Female Condoms

A **male condom** is a latex rubber or synthetic sheath that is placed over the erect penis before coitus to trap sperm (Fig. 6.4). Male condoms have an ideal failure rate of 2% and a true failure rate of about 15% because breakage or spillage occurs in up to 15% of uses (see Table 6.1). A big advantage of male condoms is they are one of the few "male-responsibility" birth control measures available. In addition, no healthcare visit or prescription is needed. They are recommended for partners who do not maintain a monogamous relationship because although latex condoms do not necessarily offer protection against diseases spread by skin-to-skin contact such as human papillomavirus (HPV), syphilis, or genital herpes, they do prevent the spread of STIs such as gonorrhea and chlamydia; their use has become a major part of the fight to prevent infection from HIV.

To be effective, a condom must be applied before any penile–vulvar contact as even pre-ejaculation fluid may contain some sperm. The condom should be positioned so it is loose enough at the penis tip to collect the ejaculate without placing undue pressure on the condom. The penis (with the condom held carefully in place) must be withdrawn before it begins to become flaccid after ejaculation to prevent sperm from leaking from the now loosely fitting sheath into the vagina.

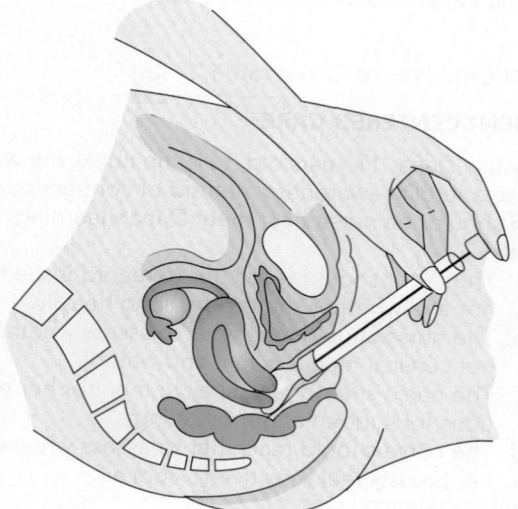

Figure 6.3 Vaginal insertion of a spermicidal agent.

Figure 6.4 Proper application of a male condom. Being certain space is left at the tip helps to ensure the condom will not break with ejaculation.

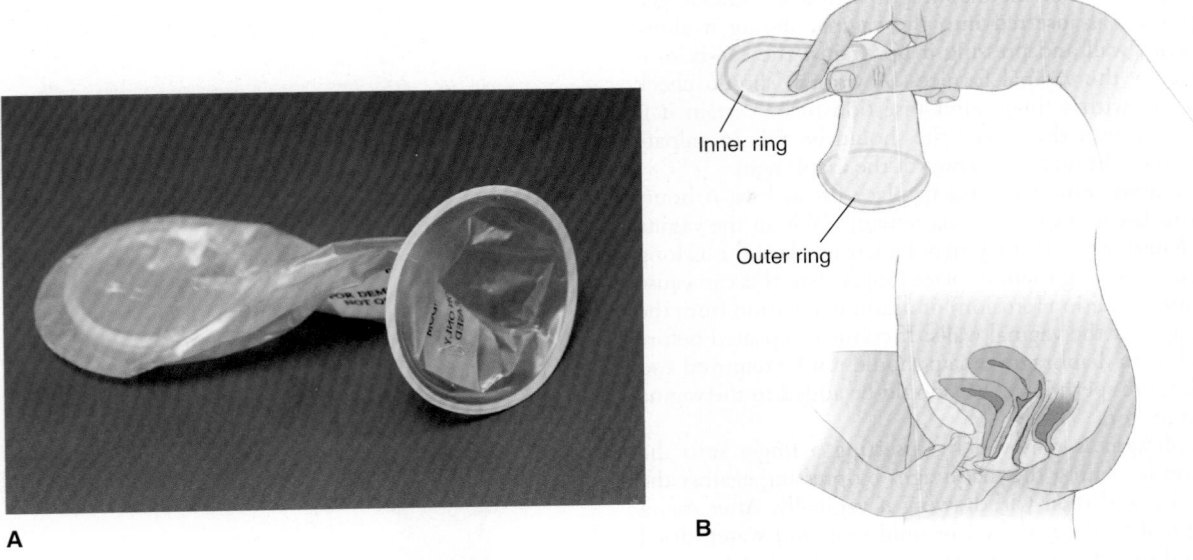

A

B

Figure 6.5 (A) A female condom. Such a device is effective protection against both sexually transmitted infections and pregnancy. **(B)** Insertion technique.

Female condoms are sheaths made of latex or polyurethane, prelubricated with a spermicide so, similarly to male condoms, they offer protection against conception as well as STIs, including HIV. The inner ring (closed end) covers the cervix, and the outer ring (open end) rests against the vaginal opening. The sheath may be inserted any time before sexual activity begins and then removed after ejaculation occurs. Like male condoms, they are intended for one-time use (Fig. 6.5). They can be purchased without a prescription but are more expensive than male condoms. Male and female condoms should not be used together or there is an increased chance of tearing one or the other. The ideal failure and usual failure rate of female condoms equals those of male condoms, 5% and 15% (CDC, 2014). Because they prevent skin-to-skin contact STIs, they are the only woman-controlled safer sex method available (Brawner, Alexander, Fannin, et al., 2015). Despite these features, they have not gained great popularity, probably because of their bulk and difficulty to use.

Side Effects and Contraindications

There are no contraindications to the use of either male or female condoms except for sensitivity or allergy to latex. If either the male or his partner has a sensitivity or allergy to latex, polyurethane or natural membrane types can be used. Couples should be cautioned that these types of condoms do not offer the same level of protection against STIs.

Diaphragms and Cervical Caps

A **diaphragm** is a circular rubber disk that is placed over the cervix before intercourse to mechanically halt the passage of sperm (Fig. 6.6). Although use of a spermicide to coat a diaphragm is not required, using a spermicidal gel with one combines a barrier and a chemical method of contraception so one is usually added. With the use of a spermicide, the failure rate of the diaphragm is as low as 6% (ideal) to 18% (typical use) (see Table 6.1).

A diaphragm is prescribed and fitted initially by a health-care provider to ensure a correct fit. Because the shape of a woman's cervix changes with pregnancy, miscarriage, cervical surgery (dilatation and curettage [D&C]), or elective termination of pregnancy, teach women to return for a second fitting if any of these circumstances occur. A woman should also have the fit of the diaphragm checked if she gains or loses more than 15 lb because this could also change her pelvic and vaginal contours.

A

B

C

D

Figure 6.6 Proper insertion of a diaphragm. **(A)** After spermicidal jelly or cream is applied to the rim, the diaphragm is pinched between the fingers and thumb. **(B)** The folded diaphragm is then inserted into the vagina and pushed backward as far as it will go. **(C)** To check for proper positioning, the woman should feel the cervix to be certain it is completely covered by the soft rubber dome of the diaphragm. **(D)** To remove the diaphragm, a finger is hooked under the forward rim and the diaphragm is pulled down and out.

Before expected coitus, after first coating the inside rim and center portion of the diaphragm with a spermicide gel, the diaphragm is inserted into the vagina, sliding it along the posterior wall and pressing it up against the cervix so it is gripped by the vaginal fornices. A woman should check a diaphragm with a finger after insertion to be certain it is fitted well up over the cervix; she should be able to palpate the cervical os through the center of the diaphragm.

Diaphragms should remain in place for at least 6 hours after coitus because spermatozoa remain viable in the vagina for that length of time; they may be left in place for as long as 24 hours. Leaving them in place longer than this can cause cervical inflammation (erosion) or urethral irritation from the pressure against the vaginal walls. If coitus is repeated before 6 hours, both a diaphragm or cap should not be removed and replaced; more spermicidal gel should be added to the vagina by an applicator.

A diaphragm is removed by inserting a finger into the vagina and loosening the diaphragm by pressing against the anterior rim and then withdrawing it vaginally. After use, a diaphragm should be washed in mild soap and water, dried gently, and stored in its protective case. With this care, a diaphragm will last for 2 years, after which it should be replaced.

Side Effects and Contraindications

Diaphragms may not be effective if a uterus is prolapsed, retroflexed, or anteflexed to such a degree the cervix is also displaced in relation to the vagina. Intrusion on the vagina by a cystocele or rectocele where the walls of the vagina are displaced by bladder or bowel may also make insertion of a diaphragm difficult. Users of diaphragms may experience a higher number of urinary tract infections (UTIs) than nonusers probably because of pressure on the urethra. Diaphragms should not be used in the presence of acute cervicitis, herpes virus infection, or a papillomavirus infection because the close contact of the rubber and the use of a spermicide can cause additional irritation. Other contraindications include:

- History of toxic shock syndrome (TSS; a staphylococcal infection introduced through the vagina)
- Allergy to rubber or spermicides
- History of recurrent UTIs

To prevent TSS (see Chapter 47) while using a diaphragm or cervical cap (discussed in the following), advise women to:

1. Wash their hands thoroughly with soap and water before insertion or removal.
2. Do not use a diaphragm during a menstrual period.
3. Do not leave a diaphragm in place longer than 24 hours.
4. Be aware of the symptoms of TSS, such as elevated temperature, diarrhea, vomiting, muscle aches, and a sunburn-like rash.
5. If symptoms of TSS should occur, immediately remove the diaphragm and telephone a healthcare provider.

Cervical Caps

A **cervical cap** is made of soft rubber shaped like a thimble, which fits snugly over the uterine cervix (Fig. 6.7). The failure rate is estimated to be as high as 23% (ideal) to 35% (typical use) because caps tend to dislodge more readily than diaphragms during coitus (see Table 6.1). The precautions for use are the same as for diaphragm use except caps can be kept in place longer (up to 48 hours) because they do not put pressure on the vaginal walls or urethra.

Figure 6.7 A cervical cap is placed over the cervix and used with a spermicidal jelly the same as a diaphragm.

Many women cannot use cervical caps because their cervix is too short for the cap to fit properly. Like diaphragms, they must be fitted individually by a healthcare provider. They include a small strap, which can be grasped for easy removal. They are contraindicated in any woman who has:

- An abnormally short or long cervix
- A current abnormal Pap smear
- A history of TSS
- An allergy to latex or spermicide
- A history of cervicitis or cervical infection
- A history of cervical cancer
- Undiagnosed vaginal bleeding

They may not be as effective in parous women as they are for those who have never had children because the cervix does not conform as well to a thimble shape after childbirth.

QSEN Checkpoint Question 6.2

QUALITY IMPROVEMENT

Dana, 17 years old, wants to try female condoms as her reproductive planning method. If the nurse was creating a relevant educational handout, it should include which of the following directives?

- a. The hormone that condom use stimulates may cause mild weight gain.
- b. Female condoms should be inserted before any penile penetration.
- c. Women should coat the condom with a spermicide before use.
- d. Female condoms, unlike male condoms, can be reused after being washed.

Look in Appendix A for the best answer and rationale.

Barrier Methods and Effect on Pregnancy

If conception should occur while using a barrier method, there is no reason to think the fetus will be affected. Some women worry a sperm that survived a spermicide must have been weakened by migrating through it and, therefore, will produce a child with problems. They can be assured conception most likely occurred because the product did not completely cover the cervical os, so the sperm that reached the uterus was free of the product and unharmed.

Barrier Methods and Effect on Sexual Enjoyment

Although barrier methods must be inserted fairly close to the time of coitus, most couples find the inconvenience of insertion only a minor problem. If a couple is concerned the method does not offer enough protection, worrying about becoming pregnant may interfere with sexual enjoyment. Some couples find the foam or moisture irritating to vaginal and penile tissue during coitus and, therefore, are unable to use them.

Some men report that condoms dull their enjoyment of coitus; some couples do not like the fact the man must withdraw promptly after ejaculation (not true for female condoms). For some couples, concern that a condom may break or slip may inhibit sexual pleasure.

Use of a vibrator as a part of foreplay, frequent penile insertion, or the woman-superior position during coitus may dislodge a diaphragm or cap; therefore, these may not be the contraceptive of choice for some couples. Some couples may find the precaution that more spermicidal gel should be added to the vagina if coitus is repeated before 6 hours restricting. An advantage of the diaphragm or cap is they allow sexual relations during menses (although see the earlier precaution on TSS). They may also offer some protection against STIs.

What If . . . 6.1
Dana, 17 years old, tells the nurse she and a friend intend to share a diaphragm because they don't have enough money to each buy one. Is this good planning?

Barrier Methods and the Adolescent

Many adolescents use spermicides as their chief method of birth control because no parental permission or extensive expense is involved. Because of the nontraditional settings in which adolescents may engage in coitus (cars or couches), some young women find inserting the product awkward and consequently may not use it, even though they have purchased it and intended to be more cautious.

Adolescents may be fitted for either diaphragms or caps. Because an adolescent girl's vagina will change in size as she matures and begins sexual relations, these devices may not remain as effective as they do with older women and so need refitting more often. Adolescents may need to be reminded that pelvic examinations will be necessary to ensure the diaphragm or cap continues to fit properly. Some adolescents may not know where their cervix is or how to feel for it when checking the placement of a diaphragm. Use an anatomic diagram or model to show them or give them a mirror to use to view their own cervix during a pelvic examination. Caution them not to accidentally tear the diaphragm with long or sharp fingernails.

Male adolescents are showing increased ability to use condoms responsibly. They may need to be cautioned that condoms should never be reused due to concern for infection and wear on the condom itself that could cause STI transmission or pregnancy. Adolescent boys who have infrequent coitus may have condoms they have owned and stored for a long time. The effectiveness of these old condoms, especially if they are carried in a warm pocket, is questionable. For many adolescent couples, use of a dual method, such as a vaginally inserted spermicide by the girl and a condom by her partner, is a preferred method of birth control. These two methods used in conjunction increase effectiveness (Kottke, Whiteman, Kraft, et al., 2015).

Barrier Methods and the Perimenopausal Woman

Women older than 35 years have a higher incidence of cystocele or rectocele than younger women so diaphragms or cervical caps may not be the ideal contraceptive for them. Spermicide foam can help lubricate the vagina to increase sexual enjoyment in women nearing menopause. The use of vaginal film or suppository is not recommended as lessened vaginal secretions might prevent the film or suppository from dissolving completely.

Barrier Methods and the Postpartal Woman

Vaginal spermicides are appealing to postpartal women as they can be purchased over the counter and have no effect on breastfeeding and so can be used in the short time period before a postpartal checkup when a more permanent form of contraception can be discussed and prescribed.

As the cervix changes considerably with childbirth, women must be refitted for diaphragms and cervical caps after childbirth. This is usually done at a 4- or 6-week checkup.

What If . . . 6.2
Dana asks the nurse to help her choose a barrier contraceptive method. What method of reproductive life planning would the nurse recommend? Would the nurse's recommendation be different if she had a guaranteed monogamous relationship?

Hormonal Contraception

Hormonal contraceptives are, as the name implies, hormones that when taken orally, transdermally, intravaginally, or intramuscularly, cause such fluctuations in a normal menstrual cycle that ovulation or sperm transport does not occur.

ORAL CONTRACEPTIVES

Oral contraceptives, commonly known as the pill, OCs (for **o**ral **c**ontraceptive), or COCs (for **c**ombination **o**ral **c**ontraceptives), are composed of varying amounts of natural estrogen (17β-estradiol, estradiol valerate) or synthetic estrogen (ethinyl estradiol) combined with a small amount of synthetic progesterone (progestin). The estrogen acts to suppress follicle-stimulating hormone (FSH) and LH to suppress ovulation. The progesterone action causes a decrease in the permeability of cervical mucus and so limits sperm motility and access to ova. Progesterone also interferes with tubal transport and endometrial proliferation to such an extent the possibility of implantation is significantly decreased.

Combination Oral Contraceptives

Popular COCs prescribed in the United States are:
- *Monophasic* pills, which contain fixed doses of both estrogen and progestin throughout a 21-day cycle
- *Biphasic*, or preparations that deliver a constant amount of estrogen throughout the cycle but varying amounts of progestin
- *Triphasic* and *tetraphasic* preparations, which vary in both estrogen and progestin content throughout the cycle

Typical pills are supplied in 28-pill dispensers (21 active pills and 7 placebo pills) labeled with the day of the cycle they should be taken. Newer forms designed to eliminate menses are supplied in 84-day dispensers (see the following). Caution women to always take pills in the order designated by the dispenser or the progesterone level could be inaccurate and ineffective for that day (Fig. 6.8).

COCs must be prescribed by a healthcare provider after screening for eligibility. If the woman is over the age of 21 years and due for a routine exam, a pelvic exam and Pap smear are usually completed at this visit as well. When used correctly, COCs are 99.9% effective. Because women occasionally forget to take them, however, and because of individual physiologic differences, the typical failure rate is closer to 5% (CDC, 2014).

Oral contraceptives have benefits in addition to preventing pregnancy, such as decreasing incidences of:
- Dysmenorrhea, because of lack of ovulation
- Premenstrual dysphoric syndrome and acne because of the increased progesterone levels
- Iron deficiency anemia because of the reduced amount of menstrual flow
- Acute pelvic inflammatory disease (PID) and resulting tubal scarring
- Endometrial and ovarian cancer, ovarian cysts, and ectopic pregnancies
- Fibrocystic breast disease

- Possibly osteoporosis, endometriosis, uterine myomata (fibroid uterine tumors), and possibly rheumatoid arthritis
- Colon cancer (Bahamondes, Bahamondes, & Shulman, 2015)

Because estrogen interferes with lipid metabolism, it may also lower the concentration of low-density lipoproteins (LDL) and increase the high-density lipoprotein (HDL) level.

Women can set a start date for a cycle of pills in one of four ways:
- Sunday start: Take the first pill on the first Sunday after the beginning of a menstrual flow.
- Quick start: Begin pills as soon as they are prescribed. Beginning pills immediately after a prescription is filled may increase compliance, reducing unintended pregnancies.
- First day start: Begin pills on the first day of menses.
- After childbirth, a woman should start the contraceptive on a day (or Sunday) closest to 2 weeks after birth; after an elective termination of pregnancy, she could begin on a chosen day or the first Sunday after the procedure.

Because COCs are not effective for the first 7 days, advise women to use a second form of contraception during the initial 7 days that they take pills. A woman begins a second dispenser of pills the day after finishing the first dispenser. Menstrual flow will begin during the 7 days on which she is taking the placebo tablets.

If a woman does not want to have menstrual flows, she can eliminate her period by beginning a new cycle of pills immediately after finishing the active pills in a dispenser instead of taking the placebo pills. This can be done routinely or to accommodate special circumstances.

With extended-use pills, pills are taken for 84 days and a woman will have a menstrual flow only every 3 months or 4 times a year. Ethinyl estradiol 20 mcg and levonorgestrel 90 mcg (Lybrel) is a new low-dose combination estrogen and progestin pill that is taken 365 days a year without a placebo or pill-free interval so menstrual periods are completely eliminated for 1 year. Such pills are especially attractive to physically active women or those who have long work schedules such as military deployment (Goyal, Borrero, & Schwarz, 2012). Extensive study documents that suppressing menstrual flows for long periods this way appears to have no long-term effects (Oman & Burke, 2015).

The key to being certain ovulation suppressants are effective is for women to take them consistently and conscientiously. Some women may set an alarm on their phone to alert them it is time to take their pill. Other women may leave them in plain sight on bathroom or kitchen counters so they are reminded to take them. Caution women with young children that this is a potentially dangerous practice. Poisoning with increased blood clotting from the high estrogen content could result if a small child ingested the pills accidentally (urge the woman to use her calendar or some other method to remind her). Women who have difficulty remembering to take a contraceptive in the morning may find it easier to take a daily pill at bedtime or with a meal (the time of day makes no difference; it is the consistency that is important) (Box 6.5). Also, some women find taking pills at bedtime rather than in the morning has the advantage of eliminating any nausea they otherwise may experience.

Figure 6.8 Counseling women on how to follow an oral contraceptive schedule and what to do if they miss a day or more is an important nursing responsibility. (© Caroline Brown, RNC, MS, DEd.)

BOX 6.5

Nursing Care Planning Based on Family Teaching

SUGGESTIONS ON ORAL CONTRACEPTIVE MANAGEMENT

Q. Dana, 17 years old, asks you, "What do I do if I forget to take an oral contraceptive pill?"

A. The answer differs, depending on your situation:

1. If the pill omitted was one of the placebo ones, ignore it and just take the next pill on time the next day.
2. If you forgot to take one of the active pills, take it as soon as you remember. Continue the following day with your usual pill schedule. Doing so might mean taking two pills on one day if you don't remember until the second day, but that's all right. *Missing one pill this way should not initiate ovulation.*
3. If you miss two consecutive active pills, take two pills as soon as you remember. Then, continue the following day with your usual schedule. You may experience some breakthrough bleeding (vaginal spotting) with two forgotten pills. Do not mistake this bleeding for your menstrual flow. *Missing two pills may allow ovulation to occur, so an added contraceptive such as a spermicide should be used for the remainder of the month.*
4. If you miss three or more pills in a row, throw out the rest of the pack and start a new pack of pills. *You might not have a period because of this routine and should use extra protection until 7 days after starting a new pack of pills.*
5. If you think you might be pregnant, stop taking pills and notify your healthcare provider.

QSEN Checkpoint Question 6.3

SAFETY

Suppose Dana, 17 years old, chooses to use a COC as her family planning method. What is a danger sign of COCs the nurse would ask her to report?

   a. A stuffy or runny nose
   b. Arthritis-like symptoms
   c. Weight gain over 5 lb
   d. Severe migraine headache

Look in Appendix A for the best answer and rationale.

Progestin-Only Pills (Mini-Pills)

Oral contraceptives containing only progestins are popularly called mini-pills and, like combination types, must be taken conscientiously every day. Without estrogen content, ovulation may occur, but because the progestins have not allowed the endometrium to develop fully or sperm to freely access the cervix, fertilization and implantation will not take place.

Side Effects and Contraindications of All Oral Contraceptives

The main side effects women may experience with COCs are:

- Nausea
- Weight gain
- Headache
- Breast tenderness
- Breakthrough bleeding (spotting outside the menstrual period)
- Monilial vaginal infections
- Mild hypertension
- Depression

Side effects such as nausea and breakthrough bleeding usually subside after a few months of pill use. They may be lessened by using a different routine or brand of contraceptive.

It is no longer believed the use of COCs leads to an increased risk of myocardial infarction, and the risk of increased clotting or blood pressure elevation is low. Nevertheless, COCs are not routinely prescribed for women with a history of thromboembolic disease or a family history of cerebral or cardiovascular accident, who have migraine with aura, or who smoke because of the increased tendency toward clotting as an effect of the increased estrogen (Karch, 2015).

Advise all women taking COCs to notify their healthcare provider if symptoms of myocardial or thromboembolic complications occur, such as:

- Chest pain (pulmonary embolus or myocardial infarction)
- Shortness of breath (pulmonary embolus)
- Severe headache (cerebrovascular accident)
- Severe leg pain (thrombophlebitis)
- Eye problems, such as blurred vision (hypertension, cerebrovascular accident)

It is also recognized that COCs can interfere with glucose metabolism. For this reason, women with diabetes mellitus or a history of liver disease, including hepatitis, are evaluated individually before COCs are prescribed. The World Health Organization (WHO) recommends women who experience migraines with an aura or those who take certain drugs for seizures avoid the use of oral contraceptives as these women may be at an increased risk for cerebrovascular accident (WHO, 2011). Box 6.6 lists all risk factors and contraindications the WHO has associated with COCs. Oral contraceptives apparently do not increase the risk of breast cancer as was once feared and actually decrease the incidence of ovarian and uterine cancer (Oman & Burke, 2015).

COCs typically increase or strengthen the action of some drugs such as caffeine and corticosteroids. They may also interact with drugs such as acetaminophen, anticoagulants, and some anticonvulsants by reducing their therapeutic effect, so women may be advised to temporarily change their method of birth control while prescribed these drugs. Several drugs, such as barbiturates, griseofulvin, isoniazid, penicillin, and tetracycline, decrease the effectiveness of COCs, so women might want to change their contraceptive method temporarily while taking these drugs (Karch, 2015).

BOX 6.6
Estrogen-Based Oral Contraceptive Use

Contraindications

- Breastfeeding and less than 6 weeks postpartum
- Aged 35 years or older and smoking 15 or more cigarettes per day
- Multiple risk factors for arterial cardiovascular disease, such as older age, smoking, diabetes, moderate or severe hypertension
- Current or history of deep vein thrombosis or pulmonary embolism
- Major surgery that requires prolonged immobilization
- Current or history of ischemic heart disease or cerebrovascular accident
- Complicated valvular heart disease
- Migraine with focal neurologic symptoms (migraine with aura)
- Current breast cancer or diabetes with nephropathy, retinopathy, neuropathy, vascular disease, or diabetes of more than 20 years' duration
- Severe cirrhosis or liver tumors
- Women taking certain seizure drugs such as phenobarbital or phenytoin (Dilantin) and women taking rifabutin for tuberculosis treatment
- Women prescribed certain broad-spectrum antibiotics such as tetracycline

From World Health Organization. (2015). *Medical eligibility criteria for contraceptive use* (5th ed.). Geneva, Switzerland: Author.

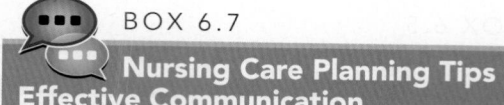

BOX 6.7
Nursing Care Planning Tips for Effective Communication

You notice Dana, 17 years old, is reading a pamphlet on oral contraceptives while she waits to be seen by the nurse practitioner.

Tip: Take the time to help a woman assess how particular measures fit her lifestyle, ask follow-up questions, and avoid advice with a "one size fits all" philosophy. Reproductive life planning measures have to be individualized to fit a person's lifestyle; otherwise, they are quickly discontinued.

Nurse: Is that pamphlet helpful? Tell you everything you need to know?

Dana: Not really. I need a way to remind me to take a pill every day.

Nurse: Will that be a problem?

Dana: Duh. I think so.

Nurse: Your pill dispenser is meant to serve as a daily reminder. If that doesn't work for you, I could help you make out a reminder chart for your mirror. As a long-term solution, though, have you thought about using a method that doesn't require a reminder more than once a month such a vaginal ring? Or not at all such as an IUD? Why don't I discuss different types with you so you can think about some more options?

When discussing COCs, be certain to assess both a woman's ability to pay for them and her ability to follow instructions faithfully (Box 6.7). Women using COCs should return for a yearly follow-up visit (for a pelvic examination, Pap smear, and breast examination), as long as they continue to use this form of birth control. Women without risk factors may continue to take low-dose OCs until they reach menopause.

Progestin-only pills have the disadvantage of causing more breakthrough bleeding than combination pills, but they are just as effective and do not pose a danger of thromboembolism (WHO, 2011). These pills are taken every day, even through the menstrual flow. Because they do not interfere with milk production, they may be taken during breastfeeding.

Oral Contraceptives and Effect on Sexual Enjoyment

For the most part, not having to worry about becoming pregnant because of the reliability of the contraceptive can make sexual relations more enjoyable for a couple. Some women appear to lose interest in coitus after taking COCs for about 18 months, possibly because of the long-term effect of altered hormones in their body. Sexual interest increases again after they change to another form of contraception. Some women experience nausea from COCs and find this interferes with sexual enjoyment as well as with other activities. If they are having side effects with one brand, they might be able to take another brand that has a different strength of estrogen without problems.

ESTROGEN/PROGESTERONE TRANSDERMAL PATCH

Transdermal contraception refers to patches that slowly but continuously release a combination of estrogen and progesterone (Fig. 6.9). Patches are applied each week for 3 weeks. No patch is applied the fourth week. During the week on which the woman is patch free, a menstrual flow will occur. After the patch-free week, a new cycle of 3 weeks on, 1 week off begins again. The efficiency of transdermal patches is

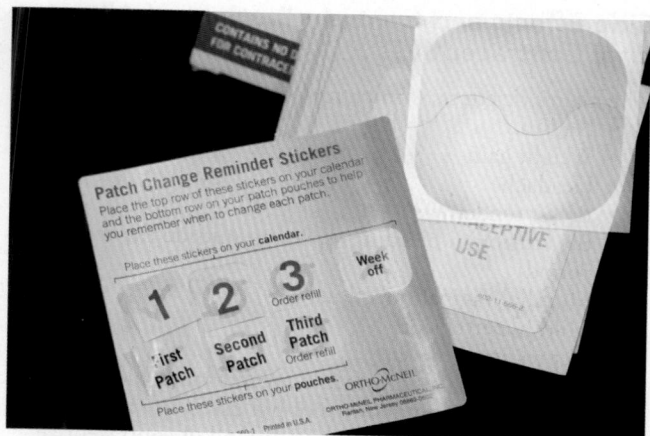

Figure 6.9   Estrogen/progesterone-based patches help adherence because they need attention only once a week. They may be applied on the arms, the trunk, or buttocks.

equal to COCs, although they may be less effective in women who are obese. Because they contain estrogen, they have the same risk for thromboembolic symptoms as COCs.

Patches may be applied to one of four areas: upper outer arm, upper torso (front or back, excluding the breasts), abdomen, or buttocks. They should not be placed on any area where makeup, lotions, or creams will be applied; at the waist where bending might loosen the patch; or anywhere the skin is red, irritated, or has an open lesion.

Patches can be worn in the shower, while bathing, or while swimming. If a patch does come loose, the woman should remove it and immediately replace it with a new patch. No additional contraception is needed if the woman is sure the patch has been loose for less than 24 hours. If the woman is not sure how long the patch has been loose, she should remove it and apply a new patch to start a new 4-week cycle, with a new day 1 and a new week to change the patch. She also should use a backup contraception method, such as a condom or spermicide for the first week of this new cycle.

Although mild breast discomfort as well as irritation at the application site may occur, one reason transdermal patches are so effective is the woman does not need to remember to take a daily pill.

VAGINAL ESTROGEN/PROGESTIN RINGS (NuvaRing)

An etonogestrel/ethinyl estradiol vaginal ring (NuvaRing) is a flexible silicone vaginal ring that, when placed in the vagina, continually releases a combination of estrogen and progesterone (Fig. 6.10). The ring is inserted vaginally by the woman and left in place for 3 weeks and then removed for 1 week with menstrual bleeding occurring during the ring-free week (Bitzer, 2012). The hormones released are absorbed directly by the mucous membrane of the vagina, thereby avoiding a "first pass" through the liver, as happens with COCs; this is an advantage for women with liver disease. Rings do not need

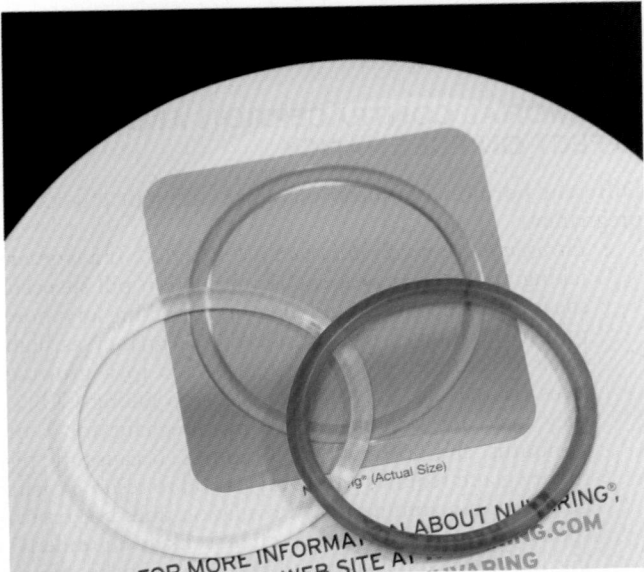

Figure 6.10 A vaginal ring. Progesterone is gradually released to be absorbed by the vaginal walls.

to be removed for intercourse. The effectiveness is equal to COCs. Women may need to mark a conspicuously posted calendar to remind themselves to remove and replace the ring. Some women may need to be encouraged to use vaginal rings, as introducing a ring vaginally may at first seem more complicated than taking a pill every day. Some women may experience vaginal discomfort or infection, both of which would make the ring an undesirable method of contraception. Women should be counseled that if they should take out the ring for more than 4 hours for any purpose, they should replace it with a new ring and use a form of barrier protection for the next 7 days.

SUBDERMAL HORMONE IMPLANTS

A progestin-filled miniature rod no bigger than a matchstick, etonogestrel implant (Nexplanon) can be embedded just under the skin on the inside of the upper arm where it will slowly release progestin over a period of 3 years. Once embedded, the implant is barely noticeable; it appears as an irregular crease on the skin, simulating a small vein. As with oral progestin, the implant is able to effectively suppress ovulation, thicken cervical mucus, and change the endometrium lining, making implantation difficult.

The rod is inserted as an in-office procedure with the use of a local anesthetic during menses or no later than day 7 of a menstrual cycle to be certain a woman is not pregnant at the time of insertion. It can be placed immediately after an elective termination of pregnancy or 6 weeks after the birth of a baby. An implant is so effective, the failure rate is less than 1%, comparable to oral contraception (CDC, 2014).

A major disadvantage of the implant method is its cost, although for most women, the procedure is covered under the regulations of the Affordable Care Act. However, a major advantage of this long-term reversible contraceptive is that compliance issues associated with COCs are eliminated. Rod insertion also offers an effective and reliable alternative to COCs' estrogen-related side effects. Sexual enjoyment is not inhibited, as may happen with condoms, spermicides, diaphragms, and natural family planning methods. An implant can be used during breastfeeding without an effect on milk production. Implants may also be used in adolescents. The rapid return to fertility after removal is an advantage for women when they become ready to begin a family.

Side Effects and Contradictions

Side effects include weight gain, irregular menstrual cycle (heavy bleeding, spotting, breakthrough bleeding, and amenorrhea), depression, scarring at the insertion site, and need for removal.

Contraindications to a subdermal rod are pregnancy, desire to be pregnant within 1 year, and undiagnosed uterine bleeding. A complication that can occur is an infection at the insertion site, although this is very rare. Most people who ask to have them removed do so because of irregular or heavy menstrual flows (Berenson, Tan, & Hirth, 2015).

INTRAMUSCULAR INJECTIONS

A single intramuscular injection of depot medroxyprogesterone acetate or DMPA (Depo-Provera), a progesterone given every 12 weeks, inhibits ovulation, alters the endometrium, and thickens the cervical mucus so sperm progress is difficult (Box 6.8).

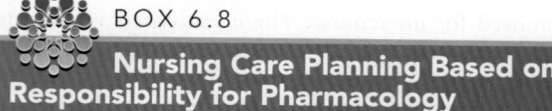

BOX 6.8

Nursing Care Planning Based on Responsibility for Pharmacology

DEPOT MEDROXYPROGESTERONE ACETATE

Classification: Contraceptive

Action: Depot medroxyprogesterone acetate (DMPA) is a progesterone derivative that inhibits the secretion of pituitary gonadotropins, thereby altering the endometrium and preventing follicular maturation and ovulation (Karch, 2015).

Pregnancy Category: X

Dosage: 150 mg intramuscular injection every 3 months

Possible Adverse Effects: Spotting, breakthrough bleeding, amenorrhea, irregular menstrual flow, headaches, weight fluctuations, fluid retention, edema, rash or acne, abdominal discomfort, glucose intolerance, pain at injection site, or osteoporosis (loss of bone density).

Nursing Implications

- Advise patient to have a routine physical examination that includes breast examination, pelvic examination, and Pap smear.
- Caution the patient that potential side effects such as weight gain may occur.
- Advise patient to maintain a high calcium intake to reduce development of osteoporosis.
- Advise the patient to report pain or swelling of the legs, acute chest pain, or shortness of breath; tingling or numbness in the extremities; loss of vision; sudden severe headaches; dizziness; or fainting; these could be signs of potentially serious cardiovascular complications.

The effectiveness rate of this method is almost 100%, making it an increasingly popular contraceptive method (CDC, 2014). The injection is made deep into a major muscle (buttocks, deltoid, or thigh) before the fifth day after the beginning of a menstrual flow. Be sure the woman does not massage the injection site after administration so the drug can absorb slowly from the muscle.

Intramuscular injections have the advantage of long-term reliability without many of the side effects and contraindications associated with COCs. There also is no visible sign a birth control measure is being used as with a subdermal implant, making them attractive to adolescents. However, the thought of weight gain may not be appealing (Modesto, de Nazaré Silva dos Santos, Correia, et al., 2015).

Because DMPA contains only progesterone, it can be used during breastfeeding, although women should wait about 6 weeks after birth for the first injection. Advantageous effects are reductions in ectopic pregnancy, endometrial cancer, endometriosis, and, for unknown reasons, the frequency of sickle cell crises (Taylor et al., 2012).

The woman must return to a healthcare provider for a new injection every 12 weeks for the method to remain reliable. A reminder system, such as a postcard mailed by the prescribing agency, may be necessary to be certain women return on time for their next injection. Alternative methods of administration, such as allowing pharmacists to give the injections or selling them over the counter so women can inject themselves, are being investigated and might increase compliance.

Side Effects and Contraindications

Common side effects include headache, weight gain, depression, irregular or heavy menstrual cycles for 1 year, and no menstrual bleeding after the first year. DMPA may also impair glucose tolerance in women at risk for diabetes so it should be prescribed cautiously for this population. Because there also may be an increase in the risk for osteoporosis from a loss of bone mineral density, women need to include an adequate amount of calcium in their diet (up to 1,200 mg/day) and engage in weight-bearing exercise daily to minimize this risk.

The manufacturer of DMPA has added a "black box" warning for women not to use the method long term (not over 2 years) to protect against bone loss. For this reason, although often prescribed to adolescents, DMPA should be prescribed with caution to this age group, as this is during the time when the bulk of their calcium deposits are being laid down (Modesto, Bahamondes, & Bahamondes, 2015).

QSEN Checkpoint Question 6.4

TEAMWORK AND COLLABORATION

Suppose Dana, 17 years old, chooses intramuscular injections of DMPA as her method of reproductive life planning. What instructions would the nurse want members of the care team to give her with regard to this method?

a. "Encourage Dana to limit cigarette smoking to no more than one pack per day."

b. "Encourage Dana to drink a glass of milk or take a calcium supplement daily."

c. "Teach Dana not to swim for longer than an hour at any one time."

d. "Teach Dana not to expose the injection site to direct sunlight."

Look in Appendix A for the best answer and rationale.

HORMONAL CONTRACEPTION AND EFFECT ON PREGNANCY

Different hormonal applications have different effects on pregnancy.

- *Estrogen/progestin combination pills (COCs).* If a woman taking an estrogen/progestin combination pill suspects she is pregnant, she should discontinue taking any more pills if she intends to continue the pregnancy as high levels of estrogen might be teratogenic to a growing fetus (Karch, 2015). After women stop taking COCs, they may not be able to become pregnant for 1 or 2 months, and possibly 6 to 8 months, because the pituitary gland requires a recovery period to resume cyclic gonadotropin stimulation. If ovulation does not return spontaneously after this time, there is likely an underlying hormonal imbalance and ovulation can be stimulated by administration of FSH, LH, clomiphene citrate (Clomid), or letrozole (Femara) to restore fertility.

- *Progestin-impregnated rings or progestin patches.* If a woman using a progestin ring or patch becomes pregnant, the progestin should have no effect on a developing fetus. After discontinuing both methods, women become fertile again immediately.
- *Subdermal implants.* If a woman becomes pregnant while using a subdermal implant, the rod can be removed; although, because the implant releases only progestin, there should be no effect on the fetus. At the end of 3 years, when the implant is removed (a 5- to 10-minute procedure), the woman will be fertile again almost immediately.
- *DMPA.* DMPA, like other progestin products, should have no effect if a woman becomes pregnant. A worrisome post-use effect for some women, however, is that the return to fertility is often delayed by 6 to 12 months.

HORMONAL CONTRACEPTION AND THE ADOLESCENT

It is usually recommended that adolescent girls have well-established menstrual cycles for at least 2 years before beginning COCs. This reduces the chance the estrogen content will cause permanent suppression of pituitary-regulating activity. Estrogen has the side effect of causing the epiphyses of long bones to close and growth to halt; therefore, waiting at least 2 years also helps ensure the preadolescent growth spurt will not be halted. Because adolescents' compliance with most medications is low, adolescent girls may not take either combined or progestin-only pills reliably enough to make them effective. COCs have side benefits of improving facial acne in some girls because of the increased estrogen/androgen ratio created and also decreasing dysmenorrhea, both of which are appealing to most adolescents and may increase their compliance rate. The pill may be prescribed to some adolescents specifically to decrease dysmenorrhea, especially if endometriosis is present (Evans & Sutton, 2015) (see Chapter 47).

HORMONAL CONTRACEPTION AND THE PERIMENOPAUSAL WOMAN

As women near menopause, they are likely over the age of 35 years and so are less likely to be good candidates for COCs than when they were younger, especially if they smoke. However, most healthy women over the age of 35 years may remain on COCs if they have no other risk factors. If she is not a good candidate, help women in this age group find an alternative method that will meet their personal preferences as well as still be maximally effective for them, such as an intrauterine device, progestin-only patches, or vaginal rings (Brotherston, 2015).

HORMONAL CONTRACEPTION AND THE POSTPARTAL WOMAN

It has been recommended that women who are lactating should not take estrogen-based contraceptives as a small amount of the hormone will not only be excreted in breast milk but will also reduce the amount of breast milk formed. Due to conflict in recent evidence about whether estrogen-based contraceptives affect milk supply, women who want hormonal contraception are, therefore, usually prescribed progestin-only pills, progesterone-activated vaginal rings, etonogestrel implant (Nexplanon), or IUDs until they are no longer breastfeeding (Pieh Holder, 2015).

Intrauterine Devices

An **intrauterine device** (IUD) is a small plastic device that is inserted into the uterus through the vagina. IUDs can be either hormonal or nonhormonal. Although a popular choice worldwide because they are almost 100% effective and need no memory aide, IUDs are used by only a relatively small number of U.S. women. That number is increasing in recent years, however (Conti & Shaw, 2015).

Even though the insertion of foreign objects into the uterus for contraceptive purposes dates back thousands of years (ancient camel drivers used uterine stones for their animals), the mechanism of action for the method is still not fully understood. The method is thought, however, to prevent fertilization as well as to create a local sterile inflammatory reaction that prevents implantation. When copper is added to the device, the possibility sperm will not be able to successfully cross the uterine space and reach the ovum increases as well.

IUDs may be used by women who have never had children as well as those who have. The device must be fitted by a healthcare provider who first performs a pelvic examination and, in women with high risk for STIs, a test for gonorrhea and chlamydia. The device is usually inserted before a woman has had coitus after a menstrual flow, so the healthcare provider can be assured the woman is not pregnant at the time of insertion. The copper IUD can also be used within 5 days of unprotected sex as a form of emergency contraception.

The device is inserted in a collapsed position and then opens to its final shape in the uterus when the inserter is withdrawn. The woman may feel a sharp cramp as the device is passed through the internal cervical os, but she will not feel the IUD after it is in place. Properly fitted, such devices are contained wholly within the uterus, although an attached string protrudes through the cervix into the vagina. Women may continue to use tampons or menstrual cups for menstrual flow with no danger of dislodging an IUD (Wiebe & Trouton, 2012).

Four types are commonly approved for use in the United States, but that number is increasing as companies expand their product line and other companies create generic versions:
- Copper T380 (ParaGard) is a T-shaped plastic device wound with copper. It is effective for 10 years, after which time it should be removed and replaced with a new IUD.
- Levonorgestrel-releasing intrauterine system 52 mg (Mirena or Liletta) IUD, which features a drug reservoir of progesterone in the stem (Fig. 6.11). The progesterone (levonorgestrel) in the drug reservoir gradually diffuses into the uterus through the plastic; it both prevents endometrium proliferation and thickens cervical mucus. Because it reduces endometrium proliferation, it also has the potential to reduce endometrial cancer (Oman & Burke, 2015). It is effective for 5 years (possibly as long as 7 years). Many women using the Mirena will have a cessation of menses or periodic light spotting instead of a normal menses.
- Levonorgestrel-releasing intrauterine system 13.5 mg (Skyla) IUD, which is manufactured by the same company as Mirena, has a lower dose of progesterone in the stem. It works similarly to Mirena and is effective for

Intrauterine device

Uterus

Intrauterine device

Figure 6.11 Intrauterine devices using copper or levonorgestrel. (From Beckmann, C. R. B., Ling, F. W., Herbert, W. N. P., et al. [2014]. *Obstetrics and gynecology* [7th ed.]. Baltimore, MD: Lippincott Williams & Wilkins.)

3 years. Women are more likely to have unscheduled bleeding with Skyla than with Mirena.

• Levonorgestrel-releasing intrauterine system 19.5 mg (Kyleena) IUD, which is manufactured by the same company as Mirena, has a lower dose of progesterone in the stem as compared to Mirena but higher than that of Skyla. It is approved for 5 years and has a bleeding profile similar to Mirena. Women may choose this over Mirena due to the lower dose of progesterone but the benefits of Mirena in terms of duration of use and lower rates of breakthrough bleeding.

All the IUD types have an ideal failure rate as low as 0.1% (see Table 6.1). They have several advantages over other contraceptives in that only one insertion is necessary, so there is no continuing expense. They are appropriate for women who are at risk for complications associated with estrogen-based side effects. With the copper IUD, there is little change in the timing of menstrual flows, although monthly flow may be heavier. Teach women to regularly check after each menstrual flow to make sure the IUD string is in place and to obtain a yearly pelvic examination as usual.

SIDE EFFECTS AND CONTRAINDICATIONS

A woman may notice some spotting or uterine cramping the first 2 or 3 weeks after IUD insertion. Ibuprofen, a prostaglandin inhibitor, is helpful in relieving the pain. Rarely, a woman continues to have cramping and spotting after insertion; in such instances, she may expel the device spontaneously. If this happens, she should use an alternative method of birth control until she can visit her healthcare provider to have a new one inserted (or choose a different type of protection). Nulliparous women may have a higher percentage of spontaneous expulsion than others.

It was once a concern nulliparous women could not be fitted with IUDs and any woman with an IUD in place might have a higher risk for PID than others. Nulliparous women

can be fitted (although they may have a slightly higher rate of expulsion); infection is no longer a concern because the vaginal string no longer conducts fluid (Oman & Burke, 2015). The Mirena IUD may actually help resist infection because of the change created in the cervical mucus.

Use of an IUD may be contraindicated for a woman whose uterus is distorted in shape (the device might perforate the uterine wall). The copper IUD use also is not advised for a woman with severe dysmenorrhea (painful menstruation) or menorrhagia (heavy bleeding) because use may increase the incidence of these conditions. Because use of a copper IUD can cause heavier than usual menstrual flow, a woman with anemia also may not be considered a good candidate for a copper IUD.

EFFECT ON PREGNANCY

If a woman with an IUD in place suspects she is pregnant, she should alert her primary healthcare provider. The woman will receive an early sonogram to document placement of the IUD and rule out ectopic pregnancy. Following confirmation of the IUD's location, it may be left in place during the pregnancy, but it is usually removed vaginally to prevent the possibility of infection or spontaneous miscarriage during the pregnancy.

INTRAUTERINE DEVICES AND THE ADOLESCENT

IUDs and etonogestrel implant (Nexplanon), long-acting reversible contraceptives (LARCs), are now recommended for adolescents by the American Academy of Pediatrics (AAP) due to their efficacy and high rates of continuation (Usinger, et al., 2016).

INTRAUTERINE DEVICES AND THE PERIMENOPAUSAL WOMAN

Women who are premenopausal are, overall, good candidates for IUDs.

INTRAUTERINE DEVICES AND THE POSTPARTAL WOMAN

Although postpartum insertion of an IUD is usually done at a 6-week postpartal checkup, it can be done immediately after childbirth (also immediately after a spontaneous or induced abortion or at the time of a cesarean birth (Goldthwaite & Shaw, 2015). An IUD inserted immediately this way does not affect uterine involution or the uterus's return to its prepregnant uterine size, but it is associated with a higher rate of expulsion (Goldthwaite & Shaw, 2015). Yet another time for the copper IUD insertion is after unprotected sex as postcoital protection (Oman & Burke, 2015).

Surgical Methods of Reproductive Life Planning

Surgical methods of reproductive life planning, often called sterilization, include tubal ligation for women and vasectomy for men. Tubal ligation is chosen by about 16% of all women in the United States of childbearing age as their contraceptive of choice. Vasectomy is the contraceptive method of choice for about 5% of men, making these two procedures a very popular option for couples older than 30 years of age (Daniels, Daugherty, & Jones, 2014). Many people choose these surgical methods because they are some of the most effective methods of contraception besides abstinence, involve no further costs, and should have no effect on sexual enjoyment. Although both sexes should think of these procedures as permanent before they have them, between 6% and 7% of both men and women in the United States who have had these procedures ask to have the procedures reversed (Herrel, Goodman, Goldstein, et al., 2015).

Reversal techniques may be much more complicated and expensive than the sterilization itself, and success rates are only 70% to 80%. For this reason, surgical methods should be chosen with great thought and care. These procedures may not be recommended for individuals whose fertility is important to their self-esteem. Counseling should be especially intensive for men and women younger than 30 years of age because the possibility of divorce, death of a sexual partner, loss of a child, or remarriage could change a person's philosophy toward childbearing.

VASECTOMY

In a **vasectomy**, a small puncture wound (referred to as "no-scalpel technique") is made on the scrotum. The vas deferens on each side are then pulled forward, cut and tied, cauterized, or plugged, blocking the passage of spermatozoa (Cameron & Glasier, 2012) (Fig. 6.12). A vasectomy can be done under local anesthesia in an ambulatory setting, such as in a primary healthcare provider's office or a reproductive life planning clinic. The man may experience a small amount of local pain afterward, which can be managed by taking a mild analgesic and applying ice to the site. Although the procedure is about 99.5% effective, spermatozoa, which were present in the vas deferens at the time of surgery, can remain viable for as long as 6 months.

Therefore, although the man can resume sexual intercourse within 1 week, an additional birth control method should be used until two negative sperm reports at about 6 and 10 weeks have been obtained (proof all sperm in the vas deferens have been eliminated, usually requiring 10 to 20 ejaculations).

Some men resist the concept of vasectomy because they are not sufficiently aware of their anatomy to know exactly what the procedure will involve. They can be assured a vasectomy does not interfere with the production of sperm; the testes continue to produce sperm as always, but the sperm simply do not pass beyond the plugged vas deferens and are absorbed at that point. The man will still have full erection capacity and continue to produce testosterone. Because he also continues to form seminal fluid, he will ejaculate seminal fluid; it will just not contain sperm.

There are very few complications associated with a vasectomy. A hematoma at the surgical site may occur, although this is seen less frequently with "no scalpel" or puncture incisions. The procedure may also be associated with the development of urolithiasis (kidney stones). A few men develop chronic pain after vasectomy (postvasectomy pain syndrome); having the procedure reversed relieves this pain (Horovitz, Tjong, Domes, et al., 2012).

Figure 6.12 A vasectomy. **(A)** The left vas deferens being cut with surgical scissors. **(B)** The cut ends of the vas deferens are cauterized or clamped to completely ensure blockage of the passage of sperm.

Some men develop autoimmunity or form antibodies against sperm following a vasectomy, so even if reconstruction is successful, sperm may not have good mobility or be incapable of fertilization. Men who want their sperm to be available for the future can have it sperm banked before vasectomy.

 Concept Mastery Alert

Vasectomy can be reversed, but the procedure is complicated, expensive, and success rates are low.

TUBAL LIGATION

Sterilization of women could include removal of the uterus or ovaries (hysterectomy), but it usually refers to a minor surgical procedure, such as **tubal ligation**, where the fallopian tubes are occluded by cautery, crushed, clamped, or blocked, thereby preventing passage of both sperm and ova. A fimbriectomy, or removal of the fimbria at the distal end of the tubes, is another possible but little used technique. Tubal ligation has a 99.5% effectiveness rate (CDC, 2014). It also is associated with a decreased incidence of ovarian cancer.

After a menstrual flow and before ovulation, with the woman under general or local anesthesia, an incision as small as 1 cm is made just under the woman's umbilicus by laparoscopy technique. **Laparoscopy** is a surgical procedure where a small incision is made in the abdomen for the purpose of viewing or performing surgery on the organs of the pelvis or abdomen. During a laparoscopic tubal ligation, a lighted laparoscope is inserted through the incision. Carbon dioxide then may be pumped into the incision to lift the abdominal wall upward and out of the line of vision. A surgeon locates the fallopian tubes by viewing the field through a laparoscope. An electrical current to coagulate tissue is then passed through the instrument for 3 to 5 seconds, or the tubes are clamped by plastic, metal, or rubber rings and then cut; they also may be filled with a silicone gel to seal them. All procedures provide immediate contraception.

The woman is discharged from the hospital a few hours after the procedure. She may notice a day or two of abdominal discomfort caused by local necrosis if clips were used, and she may notice abdominal bloating for the first 24 hours, until the carbon dioxide infused at the beginning of the procedure is absorbed. The presence of carbon dioxide can also cause sharp diaphragmatic or shoulder pain if some of the carbon dioxide escapes under the diaphragm and presses on ascending nerves. Possible complications include bowel perforation, hemorrhage, and the risks of general anesthesia if this was used.

A newer system, Essure, consists of a spring-loaded mechanism that, when inserted through the vagina and uterus into a fallopian tube (a hysteroscopy procedure), releases a soft micro-insert into the tube (Fig. 6.13). This procedure is preferred over the traditional surgical tubal ligation for women who are very obese and would therefore be a difficult surgical case. It is also preferred by patients who would like to avoid a surgical procedure through their abdomen. The procedure is done as an in-office or operating room procedure. Women must use a second form of contraception afterward until at 3 months, an infusion sonogram, hysterosalpingogram, or magnetic resonance imaging (MRI) is done to confirm the fallopian tubes

Figure 6.13 An Essure procedure blocks the fallopian tubes by a coiled spring introduced vaginally.

are firmly blocked (la Chapelle, Veersema, Brölmann, et al., 2015). The U.S. Food and Drug Administration (FDA) held a conference on Essure's safety and effectiveness in September of 2015 after receiving complaints from providers and patients. Although Essure has not been pulled off the market, the FDA is seeking more information related to complications of Essure including persistent pelvic pain, allergic reactions, perforation of the fallopian tubes, and spontaneous expulsion of the device through the vagina (FDA, 2016).

Women may return to having coitus as soon as 2 to 3 days after the procedure. Be certain they understand tubal ligation, unlike a hysterectomy, does not affect the menstrual cycle, so they will still have a monthly menstrual flow.

Side Effects and Contraindications

If tubal ligation surgery is done by laparoscopy, an umbilical hernia or ureter or bowel perforation are possible complications. Extensive obesity might require a full laparotomy to allow adequate visualization. A number of women develop vaginal spotting, intermittent vaginal bleeding, and even severe lower abdominal cramping after tubal ligation—symptoms termed *posttubal ligation syndrome*. Removal of the fallopian tubes appears to relieve these symptoms.

Not only is it difficult to reconstruct fallopian tubes after tubal ligation but there is also a possibility that, afterward, the anastomosis site could cause an ectopic (tubal) pregnancy because of its irregular surface. If a silicone gel has been instilled into the tubes as a blocking agent, this can be removed at a later date to reverse the procedure much more easily. As with a vasectomy, however, woman should view tubal ligation as a permanent, irreversible procedure as the length of their tube may be shortened afterward, interfering with fertilization (Messinger, Alford, Csokmay, et al., 2015); otherwise, they can develop postprocedural regret. However, women could turn to in vitro fertilization (IVF) as a method to have future children (see Chapter 7).

Effect on Pregnancy

Because both vasectomy and tubal ligation are nearly 100% effective, pregnancy rarely occurs. If it should, there is no effect on the fetus. If sperm were present in a woman's fallopian tube prior to ligation, an ovum could be fertilized in the blocked tube, causing an ectopic pregnancy.

SURGICAL METHODS AND EFFECT ON SEXUAL ENJOYMENT

Both tubal ligation and vasectomy may lead to increased sexual enjoyment because they largely eliminate the possibility of pregnancy. However, if either partner changes his or her mind about having children, the surgery may become an issue between them that interferes not only with sexual enjoyment but also with their entire relationship.

SURGICAL METHODS AND THE ADOLESCENT

As a rule, counsel adolescents to use more temporary forms of birth control because their future goals may change so drastically that what they think they want at age 16 or 18 years may not be what they desire at age 30 years. Later, if they still feel a vasectomy or tubal ligation is the method of reproductive life planning for them, the option will still be available.

SURGICAL METHODS AND THE PERIMENOPAUSAL WOMAN

When a woman realizes childbearing for her is complete, a vasectomy for her partner or tubal ligation for her are the two most frequently requested forms of contraception as they require no further expense or motivation for success.

SURGICAL METHODS AND THE POSTPARTAL WOMAN

Tubal ligation can be done as soon as 4 to 6 hours after the birth of a baby or after an elective termination of a pregnancy, although it may be more common at 12 to 24 hours after birth. The abdominal distention at this time may make locating the tubes difficult, so a mini-laparotomy may be used. Such procedures can be done in an ambulatory surgery department with the woman under local anesthesia.

QSEN Checkpoint Question 6.5

INFORMATICS

Dana, 17 years old, e-mails the nurse to ask how a tubal ligation prevents pregnancy. To be certain she's fully informed, which would be the nurse's best answer?
  a. Sperm can no longer reach the ova because fallopian tubes are blocked.
  b. Sperm cannot enter the uterus because the cervical entrance is blocked.
  c. Prostaglandins released from the cut fallopian tubes effectively kill sperm.
  d. The ovary no longer releases ova because there is nowhere for them to go.

Look in Appendix A for the best answer and rationale.

EMERGENCY POSTCOITAL CONTRACEPTION

A number of regimens, often referred to as "morning-after pills," are available for emergency postcoital contraception (EC), which is needed after unprotected voluntary coitus or involuntary situations such as rape (American College of Obstetricians and Gynecologists [ACOG], 2015). Two types are most common:
  • High-dose progestin-based pills
  • Insertion of a copper IUD
  It may be important to explain to women postcoital methods such as Plan B One-Step and Next Choice (the most frequently used forms) do not cause abortion; the pills work by inhibiting ovulation and interfering with fertilization by slowing the transport of sperm. An IUD creates changes in the endometrium and cervical mucus to also slow or prevent sperm transport (ACOG, 2015).
  Levonorgestrel 1.5 mg (Plan B One-Step and Next Choice) are available over the counter without a prescription by males or females. Studies show that, despite their age, young adolescents are able to read the pamphlet instructions and take the pills just as independently as adults (McCarthy, 2013). One or two pills, depending on the brand, containing a high dose of levonorgestrel, a progestin, are taken anytime within 72 hours (3 days) of unprotected coitus to interrupt a pregnancy.
  A newer form of pill, ulipristal acetate (known as ella) requires a prescription and may be taken as late as 120 hours (5 days) after unprotected intercourse (ACOG, 2015). The dose is the same (one pill). Most women expect the pills will begin a menstrual flow; caution them this will not happen, although they may notice some spotting from the change of hormones in their body. Their next menstrual flow may begin either earlier or later than usual.
  Overall, the rate of effectiveness for EC if taken within 72 hours is about 75% (ACOG, 2015). Be certain women know the pills do not protect against STIs and they will not continue to protect against pregnancy should coitus recur. A woman needs to begin a protective measure for this or use a postcoital method again.
  An ethical question that was asked when postcoital pills were first approved was whether the availability of EC would encourage risky sexual behavior; this does not seem to be so. It is important women don't think of postcoital contraception as a routine contraceptive method but as a true emergency measure (Raymond & Cleland, 2015). The chief side effect is nausea; if a woman notices this, she can take an over-the-counter antiemetic. Rh-negative women do not need Rho(D) immune globulin (RhoGAM) injections after postcoital pills or IUD insertion because a fetus never formed, thus negating isoimmunization (see Chapter 26 for a full discussion of Rh-negative blood, isoimmunization, and pregnancy).
  Although EC pills have the potential to greatly reduce the number of unintended pregnancies and abortion, fear of side effects, reluctance to have a pelvic examination (not necessary), lack of knowledge about how to use the pills, and reluctance to ask a family pharmacist for the pills limit the number of these products being sold (Upadhya, Santelli, Raine-Bennett, et al., 2017). Internet drug companies can serve as a resource for EC as they provide both privacy protection and competitive prices. Such sites are appreciated by young adults and also can supply education on different reproductive life planning methods for the future (Gawron & Turok, 2015).

A postcoital IUD is inserted by a healthcare provider with the same technique as for routine use. It can then be left in place and continue as the woman's reproductive life planning method so unprotected intercourse will not happen again.

What If . . . 6.3

Dana does not follow the nurse's advice for reproductive life planning and needs a prescription for Plan B One-Step for EC. Her mother asks the nurse to give her something so painful she'll not want to engage in unprotected coitus again. Would the nurse agree to her philosophy of care?

The Couple With Unique Needs

Reproductive life planning can be a greater concern than usual for a couple with a physical or cognitive challenge, as finding a suitable contraceptive may be more difficult for them than for other couples. For example, a man who has unsteady coordination might not have adequate hand coordination to place a condom effectively. A woman with a similar handicap might have difficulty inserting a diaphragm or vaginal ring; a woman who is cognitively challenged might not understand the need to take COCs daily. Morbidly obese patients can also have difficulty with diaphragm insertion and may notice estrogen patches and implants may not supply an adequate dosage of drug to be effective. Women with recurrent convulsions (epilepsy) may be unable to take COCs because of the interaction of estrogen with common seizure medications (Taylor et al., 2012). For these reasons, subdermal implants, IUDs, or surgical intervention may be the ideal contraceptive for many couples with a disability.

Future Trends in Contraception

Although COCs contain much less estrogen today than originally, estrogen remains responsible for most of the side effects associated with COCs. Therefore, studies are being conducted using even lower doses and different forms of estrogen. Biodegradable implants that do not have to be removed or an estrogen-based gel that is rubbed onto the skin may be used in the future. A progesterone-filled vaginal ring that is permanently implanted is yet another possibility. A birth control vaccine consisting of antibodies against human chorionic gonadotropin hormone is a distant possibility. Injections of testosterone for males (which halts sperm production, just as estrogen halts ova production in women) are being tested at major centers. Hormone-related male contraception, however, has inherent problems; because sperm production is continuous, there is not just one event (ovulation) to halt. Administration of FSH and LH to men could stop sperm production through effects on the pituitary and hypothalamus. However, this approach would also decrease production of testosterone, which is necessary for male muscle strength. Until the matter of how to balance the amount of needed testosterone and excessive testosterone (which produces aggression) is solved, hormonal male contraception remains an elusive concept (Zdrojewicz, Konieczny, Papier, et al., 2015).

Until some method is found that satisfies all of the criteria for an ideal contraceptive (completely safe, no side effects, low cost, easy availability, easy reversibility, and user acceptability), both women and men need opportunities to discuss options to find the method right for them. Box 6.9 shows an interprofessional care map illustrating both nursing and team planning for reproductive life planning.

QSEN Checkpoint Question 6.6

EVIDENCE-BASED PRACTICE

Declines in adolescent pregnancy rates have increased from 2007 to 2012; rates dropped 36% in women 15 to 19 years old. Determinants for the decrease in the pregnancy rate in this group could be related to individual, household, community, or other influences. The decrease in pregnancy rate could also be related to how often adolescents are having sex, how often they are using birth control, or how often they are choosing abortion after unexpected pregnancy occurs. The National Survey of Family Growth surveyed high school students and found a modest decline in sexual activity, a large increase in contraceptive use, and that the use of abortion remained the same from 1995 to 2002. A reexamination of data from the same survey from 2007 to 2012 found there was no change in sexual activity, an increase in contraceptive use, and a stable use of abortion (Lindberg, Santelli, & Desai, 2016).

Assuming Dana is a typical 17-year-old adolescent, her likelihood of giving birth in 2012 is mostly related to which of the following factors?

a. Her partner and she decided to choose abstinence.
b. She has access to a provider who provides abortion services.
c. She has access to a provider who prescribes birth control.
d. Her community frowns upon adolescent pregnancy.

Look in Appendix A for the best answer and rationale.

Unfolding Patient Stories: Carla Hernandez • Part 1

Carla Hernandez, a 32-year-old gravida 2 para 1, is accompanied by her husband during a routine prenatal visit. They want to discuss options for preventing a future pregnancy after delivery of their second child. What information can the nurse prepare to help them make an informed decision? What questions asked by the nurse can help guide the discussion toward methods that correspond with their beliefs and values? (Carla Hernandez's story continues in Chapter 15.)

Care for Carla and other patients in a realistic virtual environment: **vSim** *for Nursing* (thepoint.lww.com /vSimMaternityPed). Practice documenting these patients' care in DocuCare (thepoint.lww.com /DocuCareEHR).

BOX 6.9

Nursing Care Planning

AN INTERPROFESSIONAL CARE MAP FOR AN ADOLESCENT SEEKING CONTRACEPTIVE INFORMATION

Seventeen-year-old Dana Crews has come to your community health clinic for a pelvic examination and Pap smear. She is sexually active and tells you her boyfriend "sometimes" uses a condom. She trusts he will "stop in time" when they aren't using one. She doesn't want to take birth control pills because she can't afford it and she's afraid her parents will find out she's broken her abstinence pledge if they see the dispenser.

Family Assessment: Patient lives at home with parents and younger sister, 12 years old. Father works as a Boy Scout administrator. Mother is a stay-at-home mom. Patient states family finances are "good; no problem."

Patient Assessment: Past medical history is negative for major health problems. Menarche at age 12 years. Menstrual cycles range from 28 to 35 days, with a moderately heavy flow lasting 5 to 7 days. She has enough cramping monthly she "has to stay home from school for 1 day." Last menstrual flow was 1 week ago. Denies history of STIs or other reproductive problems. Weight is appropriate for height. Secondary sex characteristics are present. You notice her smoking a cigarette outside in the parking lot. Following her healthcare visit, she is prescribed Ortho-ovum 7/7/7, a 28-day-cycle triphasic oral contraceptive. Decided against DMPA because of cost.

Nursing Diagnosis: Readiness for enhanced knowledge related to knowledge deficit concerning contraception

Outcome Criteria: Patient identifies options available to her; states valid reasons for method chosen; demonstrates correct use of and appropriate follow-up care for chosen method; voices satisfaction with method chosen within 1 month.

Team Member Responsible	Assessment	Intervention	Rationale	Expected Outcome
Activities of Daily Living, Including Safety				
Nurse	Assess patient's lifestyle.	Discuss when she will take pill and where she will store them. Help make out a reminder sheet. Caution against smoking while taking an estrogen-based pill.	Reviewing lifestyle may reveal potential reasons why the method could be ineffective or not continued.	Patient describes lifestyle to healthcare provider and actively participates in devising lifestyle changes that will add to contraceptive's effectiveness.
Teamwork and Collaboration				
Nurse/nurse practitioner	Consult with nurse practitioner to determine whether method patient chooses will be optimal, safe, and effective.	Secure prescription for medication.	Effective health care is a collaborative effort drawing on interdisciplinary expertise.	Consultation reveals the contraceptive method patient has chosen will be optimal, safe, and effective; patient receives prescription.
Procedures/Medications for Quality Improvement				
Nurse/nurse practitioner	Assess what additional information patient needs to use chosen form of contraception effectively. Determine if patient has questions regarding pelvic examination or other procedures scheduled.	Help complete pre-prescription procedures such as a Pap test and pelvic examination. Review method of administration of prescription and steps to take if she forgets to take a pill.	Medication administration invariably requires discussion to help patients comply. Nurses can be invaluable in lending psychological and physical support during procedures.	Procedures necessary for prescription are carried out safely with optimal respect for patient privacy and concern. Patient states she understands the importance of prescription procedures to ensure her safety.

Continued on following page

BOX 6.9

Nursing Care Planning (continued)

Team Member Responsible	Assessment	Intervention	Rationale	Expected Outcome
Nutrition				
Nurse/nutritionist	Determine whether patient commonly eats a dietary source of folic acid such as green vegetables.	Discuss with patient that oral contraceptive use can lead to folic acid deficiency.	Knowledge of side effects is important to create informed consumers.	Patient acknowledges she needs to be conscious of the need for folic acid; names two good sources of folic acid in food.
Patient-Centered Care				
Nurse	Determine whether patient has any further questions regarding chosen contraceptive measure.	Have patient repeat information for return demonstration.	Instruction provides an opportunity for learning to improve compliance.	Patient describes the action of oral contraceptives and the need to take them conscientiously.
Psychosocial/Spiritual/Emotional Needs				
Nurse	Assess if patient has discussed with boyfriend that contraception is different than safer sex practices.	Review and discuss the need for safer sex practices in addition to contraception.	Safer sex practices promote health, empower the patient, and minimize the risk of STIs.	Patient acknowledges need for safer sex practices to prevent STIs and states she will ask her partner to use a condom.
Informatics for Seamless Healthcare Planning				
Nurse	Assess if patient understands she will need continued health supervision while on an oral contraceptive.	Explain the need for routine follow-up in 1 month and yearly pelvic examinations.	Follow-up is essential for evaluating adherence and satisfaction and for reducing the risk of possible complications.	Patient states she will return for a follow-up visit in 1 month and every year thereafter.

STI, sexually transmitted infection.

Elective Termination of Pregnancy

Unsupervised abortions are terminations of pregnancy performed by unskilled people, often under less than sterile conditions at any point in pregnancy. An **elective termination of pregnancy** is a procedure performed by a knowledgeable healthcare provider to end a pregnancy before fetal viability. Such procedures are also referred to as therapeutic, medical, or induced abortions. In 2011, the abortion rate in the United States was 16.9 per 1,000 women aged 15 to 44 years (Jones & Jerman, 2014). Whereas unsupervised abortions carry a high risk for infection or excessive bleeding that can lead to death, the maternal mortality rate for elective terminations is only 0.6 per 100,000 procedures. This rate correlates to elective termination being about 11 times safer for women than childbirth, for which the mortality rate is closer to 6 per 100,000 births (Zane, Creanga, Berg, et al., 2015).

Elective terminations of pregnancy would be needed less often if women were aware of emergency contraception and how to use it within 120 hours of unprotected coitus.

Reasons that elective terminations are most often requested are for a pregnancy that:

- Threatens a woman's life, such as pregnancy in a woman with class IV heart disease
- Involves a fetus found on amniocentesis to have a chromosomal defect
- Is unwanted because it is the result of rape or incest
- Is unwanted because a woman chooses not to have a child at this time in her life for such reasons as being too young, not wanting to be a single parent, wanting no more children, having financial difficulties, or from failed contraception

The majority of pregnancy terminations are done for this last reason.

In the United States, although drugs to induce abortion safely are available, elective termination of pregnancy is still mainly a surgical procedure. Nurses employed in healthcare agencies where induced abortions are performed are asked to assist with such procedures as a part of their duties.

Women should be educated that elective termination is not ideal as a method of reproductive life planning but should be used as remediation for failed contraception. In addition, women should be counseled about other options such as adoption or single parenthood before the procedure (Chervenak & McCullough, 2012).

In 1973, the U.S. Supreme Court ruled elective terminations must be legal in all states as long as the pregnancy is less than 12 weeks. Individual states regulate whether termination of second-trimester pregnancies are allowed and can prohibit termination of third-trimester pregnancies that are not life threatening. They can also mandate additional regulations regarding the procedures, such as requiring a 24-hour waiting period for counseling or requiring parental approval for minors. Whether a particular institution or healthcare provider performs elective termination services depends on the policy and choice of that institution or individual.

MEDICALLY INDUCED TERMINATION

Mifepristone (RU-486 or Mifeprex) is a progesterone antagonist that blocks the effect of progesterone, preventing implantation of the fertilized ovum and therefore causing the pregnancy to be lost. Mifepristone is not solely used for induced terminations and so may also be prescribed to women for regression of uterine leiomyomas or detoxification in cocaine overdose. When used for a medical termination of pregnancy, the compound is taken as a single oral dose any time before 63 days gestational age followed by buccal or vaginal misoprostol (Cytotec) (a prostaglandin), which causes uterine contractions (Chen & Creinin, 2015). Some women may also be prescribed an antibiotic as prophylactic protection against infection.

Another medical regimen is methotrexate (Trexall) and misoprostol (Cytotec). Methotrexate (also used to end ectopic pregnancies or trophoblastic disease; see Chapter 21) interferes with the DNA synthesis of dividing cells and so prevents growth of the zygote. A mifepristone/misoprostol regimen is about 96% effective; methotrexate/misoprostol is slightly lower (Oman & Burke, 2015).

Because the blood type of the conceptus is unknown with either medical or surgical termination, all women with Rh-negative blood should receive Rho(D) immune globulin (RhoGAM or RHIG) at the time the mifepristone is prescribed or within 72 hours after the procedure to prevent the buildup of antibodies in the event the conceptus was Rh positive (Aitken, 2015). (See Chapter 26 for a full discussion of Rh isoimmunization.)

Medically induced termination of pregnancy is contraindicated if a woman has:

- A confirmed or suspected ectopic pregnancy (only methotrexate is used and the woman needs additional follow-up)
- An IUD in place
- A serious medical condition such as chronic adrenal failure
- A history of current long-term systemic corticosteroid therapy
- A history of allergy to mifepristone, misoprostol, or other prostaglandins
- A hemorrhagic disorder or is taking concurrent anticoagulant therapy

Advantages of medically induced over surgical termination include the decreased risk of damage to the uterus through instrument insertion and decreased use of anesthesia necessary for surgically performed procedures. The complications of medically induced termination include nausea and vomiting, diarrhea, severe uterine cramping, incomplete abortion, and the possibility of prolonged bleeding.

A woman can expect to have mild vaginal spotting and perhaps cramping for 2 weeks postprocedure. Caution her to use sanitary pads rather than tampons and not to douche to help avoid infection. She should not take aspirin for discomfort as this can increase bleeding (advise acetaminophen [Tylenol] instead).

She can resume regular activities but avoid heavy lifting or strenuous exercise for about 3 days. Her usual menstrual period will return in 2 to 4 weeks. It's best if she doesn't have sexual relations until a scheduled checkup to avoid infection, but if she does, she should advise her partner to use a condom to avoid a second pregnancy.

It's important that she notify her healthcare provider if she has heavy vaginal bleeding (more than two pads saturated in 1 hour), passing of clots, abdominal pain or tenderness, oral temperature over 102.4°F, or if she notices severe depression or sadness. As a last measure, she should be certain to keep her follow-up appointment in about 2 weeks for postprocedure ultrasonography or a pregnancy test to ensure the pregnancy has ended and obtain contraceptive counseling so she can avoid a repeat procedure.

SURGICAL ELECTIVE TERMINATION PROCEDURES

Elective surgical terminations involve several different techniques, depending on the gestational age at the time the termination is performed.

Menstrual extraction or suction evacuation is performed on an ambulatory basis 5 to 7 weeks after the last menstrual period. A narrow polyethylene catheter is introduced through the vagina into the cervix and uterus; the lining of the uterus that would be shed with a normal menstrual flow is suctioned and removed by the vacuum pressure of a syringe (Fig. 6.14A). The procedure causes only a minimum of discomfort (perhaps slight uterine cramping).

D&C is used when the gestational age of a pregnancy is still less than 13 weeks. This is done in an ambulatory setting using a paracervical anesthetic block that does not eliminate all pain but limits what the woman experiences to cramping and a feeling of pressure. The cervix is dilated and the uterus is scraped clean with a curette, removing the zygote and trophoblast cells with the uterine lining (Fig. 6.14B). D&C has a potential risk of uterine perforation from the instruments used and carries an increased risk of uterine infection compared with menstrual extraction because of the greater cervical dilatation.

Dilatation and vacuum extraction (D&E) is used with terminations between 12 and 16 weeks of gestation. They are done in either an inpatient or ambulatory setting. In some centers, dilatation of the cervix is begun the day before the procedure by administration of buccal misoprostol or insertion of a laminaria tent (seaweed that has been dried and sterilized) into the cervix. In a moist body part such as the cervix, the seaweed absorbs fluid and swells in size. Over a 24-hour period, gradually, painlessly, and without trauma, it dilates the cervix enough for a vacuum extraction tip to be inserted. There is some concern that if a woman needs frequent surgical dilatation of the cervix, as would occur from frequent

Figure 6.14 Techniques of surgical elective termination of pregnancy. **(A)** Menstrual extraction. **(B)** Dilatation and curettage (D&C). **(C)** Dilatation and vacuum extraction (D&E). **(D)** Saline induction.

Prostaglandin or a saline induction is used if a pregnancy is between 16 and 24 weeks (Fig. 6.14D) and is done on an inpatient or same-day surgery basis. Following oral misoprostol or vaginal laminaria to prepare the cervix for dilatation, prostaglandin F2 or E2 is administered followed by a 20% saline injection into the uterus. The saline, because it is hypertonic, causes fluid shifts and sloughing of the placenta and endometrium.

A dilute intravenous solution of oxytocin (Pitocin) to assist the start of contractions may also be used. Pain from the procedure is similar to natural birth but can be controlled by analgesics and breathing exercises.

Oxytocin administration is discussed in Chapter 23. As with the woman receiving oxytocin for term labor, the woman needs to be observed carefully for signs of water intoxication (fluid accumulating in body tissue), such as severe headache and confusion. A serious potential complication of saline administration is hypernatremia from accidental injection of the hypertonic saline solution into a blood vessel within the uterine cavity. This could cause interstitial fluid to shift into the blood vessels in an attempt to equalize osmotic pressure and result in serious hypertension and dehydration of tissue. If an intravascular puncture should occur, the woman immediately experiences an increased pulse rate, a flushed face, and a severe headache. The injection must be stopped immediately and an intravenous solution such as 5% dextrose is begun to dilute the saline solution and restore fluid balance.

After expulsion of the products of conception after about 12 to 36 hours, all the tissue expelled should be examined to determine whether the entire conceptus (fetus and placenta and membranes) have been expelled. If a woman wishes to see the fetus, wrap it as if it were a full-term infant and allow her to do this to begin effective grieving or closure. Assess for vaginal hemorrhage following the procedure, the same as after a term birth. If a procedure is prolonged, a woman may develop disseminated intravascular coagulation (see Chapter 21), making her very susceptible to hemorrhage because her blood clotting mechanism has become compromised.

Hysterotomy, or removal of the fetus by surgical intervention, is similar to a cesarean birth (see Chapter 24) and is performed if the gestational age of the pregnancy is more than about 20 to 24 weeks. Surgery is necessary at this point because the uterus becomes resistant to the effect of oxytocin as it reaches this phase of pregnancy and so may not respond to saline induction, even with the assistance of oxytocin. Furthermore, the chance is great at this gestational age that, because the uterus is so enlarged, it will not contract well afterward, leading to hemorrhage. Because this is so late in pregnancy, fewer than 1% of surgical terminations are done using this technique.

Partial birth abortion was a surgical technique formerly used during the last 3 months of pregnancy if the fetus was discovered to have a congenital anomaly that would be incompatible with life or would result in a severely compromised child. With the advent of so many reproductive life planning methods and early fetal screening measures, this late-in-pregnancy procedure is no longer needed and is believed to be unethical by many (Greasley, 2014). For these reasons, this type of termination is no longer legal in the United States.

abortion procedures, it could lead to a cervix that dilates so easily it would not remain contracted during a subsequent pregnancy. Therefore, laminaria dilatation is often chosen for young women who may have more than one pregnancy termination in their lifetime as the gradual dilation of a cervix by this method helps to safeguard their childbearing potential. Antibiotic prophylaxis may be initiated at the time of the laminaria insertion, and the woman is cautioned not to have sexual relations until the process is complete to protect against infection.

For the actual procedure, a narrow suction tip is introduced into the cervix (Fig. 6.14C). A suction pump or vacuum container gently evacuates the uterine contents over a 15-minute period. The woman will feel pain as the cervical dilatation is performed and some pressure and cramping, similar to menstrual cramps, during suction, but it is not a markedly painful procedure.

PSYCHOLOGICAL ASPECTS OF ELECTIVE TERMINATION OF PREGNANCY

Women of all ages request elective terminations. For such a procedure, the usual profile is a woman who:

- Is young; 18% of women obtaining abortions are teenagers, women in their 20s account for more than 50% of abortions.
- Is unmarried, 45% of all women seeking abortions
- Has had a previous live birth; 61% of abortions are obtained by women who have one or more child.
- Undergoes the procedure to end an unintended pregnancy; 75% of women report economic issues limiting their ability to care for a child.
- Has not taken any or adequate protection against becoming pregnant; however, 51% of women seeking abortion used contraception during the month they got pregnant, either condoms or a hormonal method.
- Abortions are provided to women of all races, 1/3 white women, 1/3 black women, 1/4 Hispanic women, and 9% to women of other races.
- Most women obtaining abortion are low income, 42% below the federal poverty line, and 27% just above the federal poverty line (Guttmacher Institute, 2014).

Only 1.9% of women seeking elective termination of pregnancy do so for reasons associated with rape. However, around 20% of women are raped at some point in their life (Perry, Zimmerman, Al-Saden, et al., 2015). As many as 4% to 8% of women suffer intimate partner violence that not only leads to pregnancy but also increases in the level of violence experienced during the pregnancy (Wilbur & Dennis, 2015) (see Chapter 55).

Be certain to give women undergoing termination procedures the same kind of explanations and support that women in labor receive (women do not share termination experiences with each other the way they share labor experiences, so women usually have little advance education as to what to expect). Remembering that this is not a decision taken lightly helps in planning nursing care aimed at making an elective termination as nontraumatic as possible.

The majority of women report they are relieved with their decision following an elective termination of pregnancy (Andersson, Christensson, & Gemzell-Danielsson, 2014). Those few who express sadness and guilt may need to be referred for professional counseling so they can integrate and accept this event in their lives.

What If . . . 6.4
The nurse is particularly interested in exploring one of the 2020 National Health Goals in respect to reproductive life planning (see Box 6.1). What possible research topic could the nurse explore that is pertinent to this goal, applicable to Dana, and would advance evidence-based practice?

KEY POINTS FOR REVIEW

- Reproductive life planning involves personal decisions based on each individual's background, experiences, and sociocultural beliefs. It involves thorough planning to be certain the method chosen is acceptable and can be used effectively.
- Natural family planning (periodic abstinence and fertility awareness) methods are varied but involve determining the fertile period each month and then avoiding sexual relations during that time.
- Oral contraceptives are combinations of estrogen and progesterone or progesterone-only pills. They provide a reliable form of contraception outside of abstinence. Women who are breastfeeding, are older than 40 years of age, and who smoke are not candidates for COCs because the estrogen can reduce breast milk supply as well as lead to cardiovascular complications such as thromboembolism. Progestin-only oral contraceptives do not contain estrogen, so do not have cardiovascular risk; they can be used during breastfeeding.
- A subdermal implant (renewed every 3 years), intramuscular injections of DMPA (renewed every 3 months), transdermal patches, and vaginal rings are also effective family planning methods.
- IUDs are small plastic devices wound with copper or filled with slow-acting progesterone placed in the uterus to prevent fertilization and implantation and are highly effective forms of birth control.
- Barrier methods of contraception include the diaphragm, cervical cap, sponges, vaginal spermicides, and condoms (male and female). Such methods are low in cost but are not as effective as ovulation suppressant methods. Use of diaphragms may be associated with UTIs.
- Postcoital or "Plan B" protection involves administration of a high dose of progesterone that prevents FSH release, which then prevents ovulation. A copper-wound IUD may also be used for postcoital protection; its insertion creates changes in the endometrium and cervical mucus to slow or prevent sperm transport.
- Surgical methods of contraception are tubal ligation in women and vasectomy in men. Counsel individuals who wish to undergo these procedures that they are largely irreversible and should not be considered lightly.
- An elective termination of pregnancy can be accomplished medically by administration of mifepristone and misoprostol or surgically by menstrual extraction, D&C, D&E, or prostaglandin or saline induction. Counsel women not to think of elective termination of pregnancy as a contraceptive method but as a recourse to be used if preventive measures fail. Women who are Rh negative need to receive Rho(D) immune globulin after these procedures.
- When counseling patients about reproductive life planning, nurses have the second responsibility to teach about safer sex practices. Such thoroughness not only helps in planning care that meets QSEN guidelines but also best meets the family's total needs.

CRITICAL THINKING CARE STUDY

Eve, 27 years old, and Lamar, 33 years, are a young couple who have just gotten married. They both are heavy smokers. Eve had a miscarriage before marriage when they were using a cervical mucus method of natural planning. It's important to her now not to become pregnant again for 2 years so she can finish a master's degree in psychology. Lamar wants a contraceptive that when discontinued will allow fertility to return immediately. He also wants a contraceptive that will prevent sexually transmitted diseases.

1. What contraceptive would you recommend as best for Eve?

2. Lamar has special requests. What contraceptive would best meet his needs?

3. Is it safe to use a contraceptive method for as long as 2 years? What if Eve has another miscarriage, making her over 30 years by the time she's pregnant for the third time?

RELATED RESOURCES

Explore these additional resources to enhance learning for this chapter:

- Student resources on thePoint, including answers to the What If . . . and Critical Thinking Care Study questions, http://thepoint.lww.com/Flagg8e
- Adaptive learning powered by prepU, http://thepoint.lww.com/prepu

REFERENCES

Aitken, S. L. (2015). Rh₀D immune globulin products for prevention of alloimmunization during pregnancy. *American Journal of Health-System Pharmacy, 72*(4), 267–276.

Aksel, S., Sinai, I., & Yee, K. A. (2012). Female genital cutting and other intravaginal practices: Implications for TwoDay Method use. *Journal of Biosocial Science, 44*(5), 631–635.

American College of Obstetricians and Gynecologists, Committee on Health Care for Underserved Women. (2014). ACOG Committee Opinion no. 592: Sexual assault. *Obstetrics and Gynecology, 123*(4), 905–909.

American College of Obstetricians and Gynecologists. (2015). Practice Bulletin No. 152: Emergency contraception. *Obstetrics and Gynecology, 126*(3), e1–e11.

Andersson, I. M., Christensson, K., & Gemzell-Danielsson, K. (2014). Experiences, feelings and thoughts of women undergoing second trimester medical termination of pregnancy. *PLoS One, 9*(12), e115957.

Bahamondes, L., Bahamondes, M. V., & Shulman, L. P. (2015). Non-contraceptive benefits of hormonal and intrauterine reversible contraceptive methods. *Human Reproduction Update, 21*(5), 640–651.

Berenson, A. B., Tan, A., & Hirth, J. M. (2015). Complications and continuation rates associated with 2 types of long-acting contraception. *American Journal of Obstetrics and Gynecology, 212*(6), 761.e1–761.e8.

Bitzer, J. (2012). The vaginal ring (NuvaRing®) for contraception in adolescent women. *Gynecological Endocrinology, 28*(2), 125–129.

Blackwell, L. F., Vigil, P., Alliende, M. E., et al. (2016). Monitoring of ovarian activity by measurement of urinary excretion rates using the ovarian monitor, part IV: The relationship of the pregnanediol glucuronide threshold to basal body temperature and cervical mucus as markers for the beginning of the post-ovulatory infertile period. *Human Reproduction, 31*(2), 445–453.

Bond, S. (2013). No-cost contraception reduces unintended pregnancies and abortion rates at a population level. *Journal of Midwifery & Women's Health, 58*(2), 226–227.

Brawner, B. M., Alexander, K. A., Fannin, E. F., et al. (2015). The role of sexual health professionals in developing a shared concept of risky sexual behavior as it relates to HIV transmission. *Public Health Nursing, 33*(2),139–150.

Brotherston, J. (2015). Contraception meets HRT: Seeking optimal management of the perimenopause. *The British Journal of General Practice, 65*(638), e630–e632.

Cameron, S. T., & Glasier, A. (2012). Contraception and sterilization. In D. K. Edmonds (Ed.), *Dewhurst's textbook of obstetrics & gynaecology* (8th ed., pp. 495–512). Oxford, United Kingdom: Wiley-Blackwell.

Centers for Disease Control and Prevention. (2014). Appendix D: Contraceptive effectiveness. *Morbidity and Mortality Weekly Report, 63*(4), 47.

Centers for Disease Control and Prevention. (2015). *Unintended pregnancy prevention.* Washington, DC: Author.

Chen, M. J., & Creinin, M. D. (2015). Mifepristone with buccal misoprostol for medical abortion: A systematic review. *Obstetrics and Gynecology, 126*(1), 12–21.

Chervenak, F., & McCullough, L. B. (2012). Responsibly counselling women about the clinical management of pregnancies complicated by severe fetal anomalies. *Journal of Medical Ethics, 38*(7), 397–398.

Conti, J., & Shaw, K. (2015). Update on long-acting reversible methods. *Current Opinion in Obstetrics & Gynecology, 27*(6), 471–475.

Daniels, K., Daugherty, J., & Jones, J. (2014). Current contraceptive status among women aged 15–44: United States, 2011–2013. *NCHS Data Brief*, (173), 1–8.

Evans, G., & Sutton, E. L. (2015). Oral contraception. *The Medical Clinics of North America, 99*(3), 479–503.

Gawron, L. M., & Turok, D. K. (2015). Pills on the World Wide Web: Reducing barriers through technology. *American Journal of Obstetrics and Gynecology, 213*(4), 500.e1–500.e4.

Goldthwaite, L. M., & Shaw, K. A. (2015). Immediate postpartum provision of long-acting reversible contraception. *Current Opinion in Obstetrics & Gynecology, 27*(6), 460–464.

Goyal, V., Borrero, S., & Schwarz, E. B. (2012). Unintended pregnancy and contraception among active-duty servicewomen and veterans. *American Journal of Obstetrics and Gynecology, 206*(6), 463–469.

Greasley, K. (2014). The pearl of the 'pro-life' movement? Reflections on the Kermit Gosnell controversy. *Journal of Medical Ethics, 40*(6), 419–423.

Guttmacher Institute. (2014). *Induced abortion in the United States.* New York, NY: Author.

Herrel, L. A., Goodman, M., Goldstein, M., et al. (2015). Outcomes of microsurgical vasovasostomy for vasectomy reversal: A meta-analysis and systematic review. *Urology, 85*(4), 819–825.

Horovitz, D., Tjong, V., Domes, T., et al. (2012). Vasectomy reversal provides long-term pain relief for men with the post-vasectomy pain syndrome. *The Journal of Urology, 187*(2), 613–617.

Igras, S., Sinai, I., Mukabatsinda, M., et al. (2014). Systems approach to monitoring and evaluation guides scale up of the standard days method of family planning in Rwanda. *Global Health, Science and Practice, 2*(2), 234–244.

Jones, R. K., & Jerman, J. (2014). Abortion incidence and service availability in the United States, 2011. *Perspectives on Sexual and Reproductive Health, 46*(1), 3–14.

Jones, R. K., Lindberg, L. D., & Higgins, J. A. (2014). Pull and pray or extra protection? Contraceptive strategies involving withdrawal among US adult women. *Contraception, 90*(4), 416–421.

Karch, A. M. (2015). *Lippincott's nursing drug guide.* Philadelphia, PA: Lippincott Williams & Wilkins.

Killick, S. R., Leary, C., Trussell, J., et al. (2011). Sperm content of pre-ejaculatory fluid. *Human Fertility, 14*(1), 48–52.

Kottke, M., Whiteman, M. K., Kraft, J. M., et al. (2015). Use of dual methods for protection from unintended pregnancy and sexually transmitted diseases in adolescent African American women. *Journal of Pediatric and Adolescent Gynecology, 28*(6), 543–548.

la Chapelle, C. F., Veersema, S., Brölmann, H. A., et al. (2015). Effectiveness and feasibility of hysteroscopic sterilization techniques: A systematic review and meta-analysis. *Fertility and Sterility, 103*(6), 1516–1525.e1–3.

Lindberg, L., Santelli, J., & Desai, S. (2016). Understanding the decline in adolescent fertility in the United States, 2007-2012. *The Journal of Adolescent Health, 59*(5), 577–583.

Loke, A. Y., & Lam, P. L. (2014). Pregnancy resolutions among pregnant teens: Termination, parenting or adoption? *BMC Pregnancy and Childbirth, 14*, 421.

Lopez, L. M., Grey, T. W., Chen, M., et al. (2014). Strategies for improving postpartum contraceptive use: Evidence from non-randomized studies. *Cochrane Database of Systematic Reviews*, (11), CD011298.

McCarthy, M. (2013). US approves "morning after" pill without prescription for women 15 years or older. *BMJ, 346*, f2909.

Messinger, L. B., Alford, C. E., Csokmay, J. M., et al. (2015). Cost and efficacy comparison of in vitro fertilization and tubal anastomosis for women after tubal ligation. *Fertility and Sterility, 104*(1), 32.e4–38.e4.

Modesto, W., Bahamondes, M. V., & Bahamondes, L. (2015). Prevalence of low bone mass and osteoporosis in long-term users of the injectable contraceptive depot medroxyprogesterone acetate. *Journal of Women's Health, 24*(8), 636–640.

Modesto, W., de Nazaré Silva dos Santos, P., Correia, V. M., et al. (2015). Weight variation in users of depot-medroxyprogesterone acetate, the levonorgestrel-releasing intrauterine system and a copper intrauterine device for up to ten years of use. *The European Journal of Contraception & Reproductive Health Care, 20*(1), 57–63.

Mody, S. K., & Han, M. (2014). Obesity and contraception. *Clinical Obstetrics and Gynecology, 57*(3), 501–507.

Oman, S., & Burke, A. E. (2015). Family planning: Contraception, sterilization, and abortion. In C. T. Johnson, J. L. Hallock, J. L. Bienstock, et al. (Eds.), *The Johns Hopkins manual of gynecology and obstetrics* (5th ed., pp. 421–438). Philadelphia, PA: Wolters Kluwer.

Perry, R., Zimmerman, L., Al-Saden, I., et al. (2015). Prevalence of rape-related pregnancy as an indication for abortion at two urban family planning clinics. *Contraception, 91*(5), 393–397.

Pieh Holder, K. L. (2015). Contraception and breastfeeding. *Clinical Obstetrics and Gynecology, 58*(4), 928–935.

Pratts, M. E., & Lawson, S. (2015). Postpartum care and breast-feeding. In C. T. Johnson, J. L. Hallock, J. L. Bienstock, et al. (Eds.), *The Johns Hopkins manual of gynecology and obstetrics* (5th ed., pp. 286–294). Philadelphia, PA: Wolters Kluwer.

Raymond, E. G., & Cleland, K. (2015). Clinical practice. Emergency contraception. *The New England Journal of Medicine, 372*(14), 1342–1348.

Rodriguez, M. I., Darney, B. G., Elman, E., et al. (2015). Examining quality of contraceptive services for adolescents in Oregon's family planning program. *Contraception, 91*(4), 328–335.

Schalet, A. T., Santelli, J. S., Russell, S. T., et al. (2014). Invited commentary: Broadening the evidence for adolescent sexual and reproductive health and education in the United States. *Journal of Youth and Adolescence, 43*(10), 1595–1610.

Taylor, H. S., Aldad, T. S., McVeigh, E., et al. (2012). *Oxford American handbook of reproductive medicine.* New York, NY: Oxford University Press.

Upadhya, K. K., Santelli, J. S., Raine-Bennett, T. R., et al. (2017). Over-the-counter access to oral contraceptives for adolescents. *Journal of Adolescent Health.* Advance online publication. doi:10.1016/j.jadohealth.2016.12.024

Usinger, K. M., Gola, S. B., Weis, M., et al. (2016). Intrauterine contraception continuation in adolescents and young women: A systematic review. *Journal of Pediatric and Adolescent Gynecology, 29*(6), 659–667.

U.S. Department of Health and Human Services. (2010). *Healthy people 2020.* Washington, DC: Author.

U.S. Food and Drug Administration. (2016). *FDA activities: September 2015 advisory committee to discuss Essure safety and effectiveness.* Retrieved from http://www.fda.gov/MedicalDevices/ProductsandMedicalProcedures/ImplantsandProsthetics/EssurePermanentBirthControl/ucm452254.htm

Wettstein, R. H., & Bourgeois, C. (2014). *The complete symptothermal guide: Ecological birth control & pregnancy achievement.* Lully, Switzerland: SymptoTherm.

Wiebe, E. R., & Trouton, K. J. (2012). Does using tampons or menstrual cups increase early IUD expulsion rates? *Contraception, 86*(2), 119–121.

Wilbur, M. B., & Dennis, A. E. (2015). Intimate partner and sexual violence. In C. T. Johnson, J. L. Hallock, J. L. Bienstock, et al. (Eds.), *The Johns Hopkins manual of gynecology and obstetrics* (5th ed., pp. 439–450). Philadelphia, PA: Wolters Kluwer.

World Health Organization. (2011). *Family planning: A global handbook for providers.* Geneva, Switzerland: Author.

Zane, S., Creanga, A. A., Berg, C. J., et al. (2015). Abortion-related mortality in the United States: 1998-2010. *Obstetrics and Gynecology, 126*(2), 258–265.

Zdrojewicz, Z., Konieczny, R., Papier, P., et al. (2015). Brdt bromodomains inhibitors and other modern means of male contraception. *Advances in Clinical and Experimental Medicine, 24*(4), 705–714.

7

Nursing Care of the Family Having Difficulty Conceiving a Child

Cheryl and Bob Carl, married when they were both 25 years old, planned to wait 5 years before beginning their family so they could save money for a house. On the day they moved into their new home, Cheryl stopped taking her birth control pills. At the end of a year, however, she still was not pregnant so she began fertility testing. Three years later, they are now undergoing their second cycle of in vitro fertilization and embryo transfer. The Carls have applied for a second mortgage on their house to finance the fertility testing. At a healthcare visit, Mrs. Carl states, "This is my fault because I'm so rigid. Look how I had to buy the house before I could even consider getting pregnant, and now we'll probably lose it. I've made our whole life revolve around trying to get pregnant instead of enjoying life."

Previous chapters described normal ovulation and conception and ways to prevent pregnancy. This chapter adds information about care of the couple who is unable to conceive.

How could you best help the Carls?

KEY TERMS

alternative insemination

anovulation

cryptorchidism

endometriosis

erectile dysfunction

in vitro fertilization

pelvic inflammatory disease

sperm count

sperm motility

spermatogenesis

sterility

subfertility

varicocele

OBJECTIVES

After mastering the contents of this chapter, you should be able to:

1. Describe common causes of difficulty with conception or subfertility in both men and women.

2. Identify 2020 National Health Goals related to subfertility that nurses can help the nation achieve.

3. Describe common assessments necessary to detect subfertility.

4. Formulate nursing diagnoses related to subfertility.

5. Identify expected outcomes for a subfertile couple to help them manage seamless transitions across differing healthcare settings.

6. Using the nursing process, plan nursing care that includes the six competencies of Quality & Safety Education for Nurses (QSEN): Patient-Centered Care, Teamwork & Collaboration, Evidence-Based Practice (EBP), Quality Improvement (QI), Safety, and Informatics.

7. Implement nursing care designed to improve subfertility and increase ability to conceive a child, such as health teaching about ovulation and conception.

8. Evaluate outcomes for achievement and effectiveness of nursing care to be certain expected outcomes have been achieved.

9. Integrate knowledge of fertility and subfertility with the interplay of nursing process, the six competencies of QSEN, and Family Nursing to promote quality maternal and child health nursing care.

Many marriage customs, such as throwing rice, originate from ancient rituals to promote fertility. The existence of such common rituals is an indication of the importance of having children for most couples and society as a whole.

Infertility is a term used to describe the inability to conceive a child or sustain a pregnancy to birth. A couple is said to be *infertile* if they have not become pregnant after at least 1 year of unprotected sex. Because most couples have the potential to conceive but are just less able to conceive without additional help, the term **subfertility** is more often used today. Subfertility affects as many as 8% to 12% of couples who desire children (Kumar & Singh, 2015).

Couples who feel they need fertility testing consist of a wide range of people: many are married couples; some are planning to marry; some desire to remain single but bear a child; and some are lesbian, gay, bisexual, or transgender (LGBT) and want to have a child through an assisted fertility method. Occasionally, others are looking for assurance they are unable to have children so they can discontinue a contraceptive method (although they'll need to be cautioned to maintain safer sex practices if their relationship isn't monogamous). People who are discontinuing using condoms so a woman can become pregnant need this same safer sex caution.

When a couple first begins fertility counseling, they usually have fears and anxieties not only about their ability to conceive but also about what an identified problem will mean to their future lifestyle and family. Without information about the cause of their subfertility, each may blame the other or carry unexpressed anger toward his or her partner. Some couples may strongly desire a child but feel anxious about impending parenthood, which would bring with it a loss of independence. For all these reasons, subfertility screening and counseling can be both an emotionally difficult and a physically demanding process, often creating a high level of strain on a couple's relationship, especially if they don't maintain open communication (Galhardo, Moura-Ramos, Cunha, et al., 2015). The level of stress a couple is experiencing is important because increased family stress can produce a higher than usual level of intimate partner violence (Hasanpoor-Azghdy, Simbar, & Vedadhir, 2015). Having healthy children when they are wanted is such a priority in health care that a 2020 National Health Goal aimed at reducing subfertility was established (Box 7.1).

BOX 7.1
Nursing Care Planning Based on 2020 National Health Goals

One of the 2020 National Health Goals identified by *Healthy People 2020* directly addresses the problem of subfertility:

- Reduce the proportion of woman aged 18 to 44 years who have impaired fecundity (fertility) from 12% to a target of 10.8% (U.S. Department of Health and Human Services, 2010; see www.healthypeople.gov).

To meet this health objective, nurses need to keep active in health promotion, identify and help prevent problems that could lead to subfertility such as poor nutrition early in life, and play active roles in teaching patients about safer sex practices (see Chapter 5) so the incidence of sexually transmitted infections and pelvic inflammatory disease can be reduced.

Nursing Process Overview

FOR A COUPLE WITH SUBFERTILITY

ASSESSMENT

Subfertility assessment used to require many months and many tests, all of which had the potential to interfere with a couple's self-image, self-esteem, and lifestyle. Today, a subfertility investigation is usually limited to only three assessments: semen analysis, ovulation monitoring, and tubal patency. Even with this more directed approach to evaluation, a nursing assessment often reveals that one or both partners feel inadequate or angry and frustrated by what has happened to them and their need to undergo testing. Questions such as "How do you feel about what has happened?" or "How do you think your partner feels about not being able to conceive?" may be enough to encourage partners to express these concerns.

Talking with both partners together may be advantageous because they may feel more comfortable speaking about their problem together. It is important, however, to spend some time alone with each patient in case there is anything a partner wishes to discuss privately. This might be the only opportunity for one of them to ask that one "silly" question or voice a fear he or she believes is too foolish to ask or bring up in front of his or her partner.

NURSING DIAGNOSIS

Nursing diagnoses related to subfertility are likely to focus on psychosocial issues associated with the inability to conceive and the potentially nerve-wracking process of fertility testing and management. Examples of possible diagnoses include:

- Fear related to possible outcome of subfertility studies
- Situational low self-esteem related to the apparent inability to conceive
- Anxiety related to what the process of fertility testing will entail
- Deficient knowledge related to measures to promote fertility
- Anticipatory grieving related to failure to conceive or sustain a pregnancy
- Powerlessness related to repeated unsuccessful attempts at achieving conception
- Hopelessness related to perception of no viable alternatives to usual conception

If required tests interfere with a couple's relationship (including sexual patterns), "sexual dysfunction related to command performance of subfertility therapy" might be applicable.

EXPECTED OUTCOMES AND PLANNING

In establishing expected outcomes with a couple undergoing fertility testing and counseling, be certain the couple realizes even after the reason for their subfertility is identified, fertility may not be instantaneous. In some instances, a couple may need to change or modify their goals if tests begin to show what they first wanted—to have a child without medical intervention—is impossible. Participation in a support group may allow a couple to work through the stress fertility testing places on their lives. It is helpful to refer patients to online resources for further information and support (see Chapter 5).

IMPLEMENTATION

Fertility testing can be costly for a couple because not all health insurance programs provide reimbursement for these procedures. Because of this, be certain couples are informed beforehand of specific estimates of the cost of testing or therapy so they can budget and plan their resources and the next steps they want taken.

Suggesting a couple combine involvement with fertility testing with ongoing activities or beginning new activities together, such as taking a night school course, planting a garden, or learning a new sport or hobby, is a way of helping them reduce the feeling that their entire existence revolves around the testing procedures. It also may help provide them with time for sharing experiences and increasing intimacy, helping to compensate for any decreased enjoyment that comes from "scheduled" sexual relations.

Throughout testing, couples need thorough education about the various procedures being done. Make sure to review any specific instructions about preprocedural and postprocedural care. Depending on their motivations, a couple's reaction to study results may vary from relief, to stoic acceptance, to grief for children never to be born. Each partner may wonder whether the other will be able to continue the relationship if he or she turns out to be the subfertile one. Couples need the active support of healthcare personnel from the first day they brace themselves to ask "Exactly why are we childless?" until the end, regardless of the results.

OUTCOME EVALUATION

Examples of expected outcomes in this area include:
- The patient rearranges work plans to manage the schedule of fertility testing by 1 month's time.
- The couple verbalizes they understand their individual subfertility problem after preliminary testing.
- The couple demonstrates a high level of self-esteem after fertility studies, even in the face of disappointing study outcomes.

For a couple with the problem of subfertility, an evaluation is best if it is ongoing because, as circumstances around them change, so may their goals and desires. Until they can accept an alternative method of having children—adoption or an assisted reproductive technique such as **alternative insemination** (deposition of sperm into a woman's cervix or uterus) or **in vitro fertilization** (IVF; the union of sperm and ovum under laboratory conditions)—former plans to have children have been crushed.

Continuing or future evaluations are also important because a couple who decides at age 20 years to choose child-free living may change their minds at a later date. In the same way, a couple who chooses an assisted reproductive technique may decide after a number of unsuccessful attempts that they are no longer interested in this method of conception. Keeping the evaluation as an ongoing process allows such plans to be modified as necessary. Because establishing fertility is an ever changing field of study, encourage couples seen for subfertility who couldn't conceive but are still interested in having a child to contact their subfertility setting every 6 to 12 months to inquire about new discoveries in the field and if any of these might apply to their situation.

Subfertility

Subfertility is said to exist when a pregnancy has not occurred after at least 1 year of engaging in unprotected coitus (Hamilton, 2012). In *primary subfertility*, there have been no previous conceptions; in *secondary subfertility*, there has been a previous viable pregnancy but the couple is unable to conceive at present. **Sterility** is the inability to conceive because of a known condition, such as the absence of a uterus.

In about 40% of couples with a subfertility problem, the cause of subfertility is multifactorial; in other words, more than one reason for the loss of full fertility is involved. In about 30% of couples, it is the man who is subfertile; in 70%, it is the woman. Of women seen for a fertility evaluation, 20% to 25% experience ovulatory failure; another 20% experience tubal, vaginal, cervical, or uterine problems. In about 10% of couples, no known cause for the subfertility can be discovered despite all the diagnostic tests currently available. Such couples are categorized as having unexplained subfertility (Oman & Burke, 2015).

Some couples, because they are unaware of the average length of time it takes to achieve a pregnancy, may worry they are subfertile when they are not. On average, if they engage in coitus about four times per week, 65% to 75% of couples will conceive within 6 months; 90% within 12 months. These periods will be longer if sexual relations are less frequent (Ghadir, Ambartsumyan, & Decherny, 2013).

Couples who engage in coitus daily, hoping to cause early impregnation, may actually have more difficulty conceiving than those who space coitus every other day. This is because too-frequent coitus can lower a man's sperm count to a level below optimal fertility. All couples who focus their sexual relations on trying to increase sperm/ovum exposure by scheduling sex may find their lives governed by temperature charts and "good days" and "bad days" to such an extent that their relationship suffers.

Age is related to subfertility. Because of this gradual decline in fertility, women who defer pregnancy into their late 30s are apt to have more difficulty conceiving than their younger counterparts. Women who are using oral, injectable, or implanted hormones for contraception may have difficulty becoming pregnant for several months after discontinuing these medications, although most women return to normal cycles within 1 month. Most couples can benefit from some practical information on how to increase their chances of achieving conception on their own (Box 7.2).

What If . . . 7.1

The nurse hears Cheryl Carl repeat she believes her subfertility problem is her fault because she's too rigid. Does a rigid personality affect fertility? How could the nurse help Cheryl feel more comfortable about what has happened in her life?

Fertility Assessment

The age of a couple and the degree of apprehension they feel about possible subfertility can make a difference in determining when they should be referred for fertility evaluation. Although some healthcare plans or specific settings set limits on the age range in which fertility testing can be scheduled, such as not before age 18 years and not after age 45 years,

BOX 7.2

Nursing Care Planning to Empower a Family

Q. Cheryl Carl asks you, "Is there anything we can do to help increase our chances of conception?"

A. The following are time-honored suggestions to help aid conception:

- Determine the time of ovulation through the use of basal body temperature or analysis of cervical secretions and then plan sexual relations for every other day around the time of ovulation.
- Although frequent intercourse may stimulate sperm production, men need sperm recovery time after ejaculation to maintain an adequate sperm count. This is why coitus every other day, rather than every day, during the fertile period will probably yield faster results.
- The male-superior position is the best position for coitus to achieve conception because it places sperm closest to the cervical opening.
- The male should try for deep penetration so ejaculation places sperm as close as possible to the cervix. Elevating a woman's hips on a small pillow can facilitate sperm being deposited near the opening to the cervix.
- A woman should remain on her back with knees drawn up for at least 20 minutes after ejaculation to help sperm remain near the cervix.
- Don't use douching or lubricants before or after intercourse so vaginal pH is unaltered, which can interfere with sperm mobility.
- Eat a diet high in slowly digested carbohydrates, low in saturated or trans fats, and moderate in protein.
- Maintain a body weight that results in a body mass index between 18.5 and 24.9.
- Exercise about 30 minutes per day to help keep blood glucose and insulin levels stabilized.
- Choose a new activity the two of you can do together, such as learning how to bowl or ballroom dance, so you create an activity separate from planning a baby. This not only helps to pass the time in a positive way but also offers a positive outlook for a month when you don't conceive.

other settings do not establish such limits, allowing couples of any age to benefit from assessment.

As a rule:

- If a woman is younger than 35 years of age, it is usually suggested she have an evaluation after 1 year of subfertility.
- If a woman is older than 35 years, she should be seen after 6 months. Referral is recommended sooner because assisted reproductive strategies such as IVF, as well as common alternatives to natural childbearing such as adoption, are also limited by age. It would be doubly unfortunate if a couple delayed fertility testing so long they not only learned they could not conceive but also were considered to be "too old" to be prospective parents by alternative methods.
- If the couple is extremely apprehensive or knows of a specific problem that could be causing their difficulty in conceiving, studies should never be delayed, regardless of the couple's age (Fritz & Speroff, 2010).

Because most fertility tests are conducted in ambulatory settings, nurses play key roles on fertility teams to help achieve this goal, such as:

- Educating couples about the variety of tests and procedures that may be performed
- Helping patients identify and express their feelings about their desire to have a child
- Helping patients express how far they are willing to go in testing and procedures to achieve a child or how they might feel if, at the end of testing, it is revealed pregnancy will not be possible
- Assuming responsibility for health assessment, patient education, and counseling
- Helping educate couples about advanced techniques of assisted reproduction, many of which are complex and

demand knowledgeable, ongoing involvement from the couple
- Counseling patients about available alternatives when pregnancy cannot be achieved, such as adoption or child-free living

No matter what problem is suspected, basic fertility assessment begins with a health history and physical examination of both sexual partners.

QSEN Checkpoint Question 7.1

PATIENT-CENTERED CARE

Cheryl is unhappy that she waited until she bought a house to plan on having a child. What fact could the nurse cite to Cheryl?

   a. She should have begun trying to conceive by age 25 years, but her outcome should still be positive.

   b. She asked for testing well before the average woman, who asks at age 30 years.

   c. Waiting for 1 year after being unable to conceive is the average time for seeking help.

   d. We all make decisions in life that later on we wish we had not made.

Look in Appendix A for the best answer and rationale.

HEALTH HISTORY

Nurses often assume the responsibility for the initial history taking with a subfertile couple. Because of the wide variety of factors that may be responsible for subfertility, it is critical to

BOX 7.3

Initial History Taking for the Subfertile Couple

History taking for men should include:

- His general health
- A typical 24-hr food intake, including alternative therapies such as herbs and whether he ingests alcohol, uses recreational drugs, or smokes or uses tobacco
- If he had a congenital health problem, such as hypospadias or cryptorchidism (defined later) or a past illness such as mumps orchitis, urinary tract infection, or a sexually transmitted disease that could affect fertility
- If he ever had radiation to his testes because of childhood cancer, X-rays, or an industrial accident
- If he had an operation such as surgical repair of a hernia or torsion of the testes, which could have compromised the blood supply to his testes
- If he has any current illness, particularly an endocrine one or a low-grade infection
- If his job or lifestyle involves sitting all day
- What his sexual practices are, such as frequency of coitus, masturbation, coital positions used, or if he ever experiences failure to achieve ejaculation
- What past contraceptive measures, if any, he has used or if he has children from a previous relationship

History taking for women should include:

- Her general health
- Nutrition, including an adequate source of folic acid and avoidance of trans fats
- Current or past reproductive tract problems, such as infections
- Past history of a childhood cancer treated with radiation that might have reduced ovarian function or any exposure to occupational hazards, such as X-rays or toxic substances
- Abdominal or pelvic operations that could have compromised blood flow to pelvic organs
- Overall health, emphasizing endocrine problems such as galactorrhea (breast nipple secretions) or symptoms of thyroid dysfunction (always tired or hyperactive)
- If she is from a country that allows the practice, ask about female circumcision because this can leave vulvar scars that interfere with penetration and deposition of sperm close to the cervix
- History of contraceptive use
- Past pregnancies, miscarriages, or abortions
- If she can detect ovulation through such symptoms as breast tenderness, midcycle "wetness," or lower abdominal pain (*mittelschmerz*)
- The use of douches or intravaginal medications or sprays that could interfere with vaginal pH
- A menstrual history, including age of menarche; length, regularity, and frequency of menstrual periods; amount of flow; and any difficulties the woman experiences, such as dysmenorrhea or premenstrual dysphoric disorder (PDD) (see Chapter 47)

include a thorough history. Examples of important questions to include for a minimum history for both men and women are addressed in Box 7.3.

Asking about alternative therapies is also important because a couple who wants to have a child could be simultaneously investigating nontraditional methods that they have heard will aid in conception (Read, Carrier, Whitley, et al., 2014). Asking about herbs they may be using can reveal use of an herb that could be causing subfertility or one that would interfere with any procedure or medication prescribed for them after their subfertility investigation is complete.

Most couples assume subfertility is the woman's problem. Many women, even after a careful explanation that the problem is their male partner's and not theirs, continue to show low self-esteem, as if the fault did rest with them. While obtaining health histories, be certain to take time with each partner individually and as a couple to encourage questions and to discuss overall attitudes toward sexual relations, pregnancy, and parenting. A frank discussion centered on resolving the couple's fears and clearing up any long-standing confusion or misinformation will help to set a positive tone for future interactions and, hopefully, establish a feeling of trust and increased self-esteem. Talking with both partners can also help them clarify their feelings about subfertility and why they are seeking help in this area of their life (Box 7.4).

It is not unusual to see a couple move through steps of denial, anger, bargaining, and depression before they reach a level of acceptance that they are different in this one area of life from others but that they are not limited in their ability to achieve in other areas. Acceptance in this way helps them make adjustments in their wants or plans and feel fulfilled again.

PHYSICAL ASSESSMENT

After a thorough history, both men and women need a complete physical examination. For men, important aspects of this include whether secondary sexual characteristics, such as pubic hair, are present as well as no genital abnormalities, such as the absence of a vas deferens or the presence of undescended testes or a **varicocele** (enlargement of a testicular vein), are present. A hydrocele (a collection of fluid in the tunica vaginalis of the scrotum) is rarely associated with subfertility but should be documented if present.

For women, a thorough physical assessment, including a breast and thyroid examination, is necessary to rule out current illness. Of particular importance, again, are secondary sex characteristics, which indicate maturity and suggest good pituitary function (see Chapter 33 for a discussion of Tanner stages). A complete pelvic examination, including a Pap test (see Chapter 11), is needed to rule out anatomic disorders and infection.

Cheryl Carl has been trying to get pregnant for 4 years. She and her husband agreed to in vitro fertilization at a cost of approximately $10,000 per month, even though her religion does not approve of this technique. Every time you see her at the fertility clinic, she seems sadder than the previous time.

Tip: Support patients and help them find ways to continue to feel good about themselves to maintain self-esteem. Be careful not to criticize patients for making choices that were not the same as yours would have been. Patients may not make the same choices about fertility testing or management you might make because such decisions are based on individual circumstances and situations.

Nurse: How is everything going, Mrs. Carl?

Mrs. Carl: Fine. I'm just tired of no results.

Nurse: Considering you have been trying for such a long time, I think you're doing very well.

Mrs. Carl: Being patient is hard.

Nurse: Think of how well learning to be patient the way you're doing now will help you become a good parent.

FERTILITY TESTING

Basic fertility testing is geared toward answering three questions:

1. Is there sperm of good quality and number available?
2. Are ova (eggs) available (i.e., woman is ovulating)?
3. Is it possible for the sperm and egg to meet in a receptive environment?

To answer these questions, only three tests are commonly used: semen analysis in men and ovulation monitoring and tubal patency assessment in women. Nurses play key roles in preparing couples for these tests, helping them schedule the studies appropriately, and supporting them while they wait for results (Allan & Mounce, 2015).

Additional testing for men, if warranted, can include urinalysis; a complete blood count; blood typing, including Rh factor; a serologic test for syphilis; a test for the presence of HIV; erythrocyte sedimentation rate (an increased rate indicates inflammation); protein-bound iodine (a test for thyroid function); cholesterol level (arterial plaques could interfere with pelvic blood flow); and follicle-stimulating hormone (FSH), luteinizing hormone (LH), and testosterone levels (Niederberger, 2016).

Advanced testing for women may include a rubella titer; a serologic test for syphilis; an HIV evaluation; a thyroid uptake determination; and assays for FSH, estrogen, LH, and serial progesterone levels. If a woman has a history of galactorrhea (breast milk secretions), a serum prolactin level will be obtained, as increased prolactin levels reduce the secretion of pituitary hormones. A pelvic sonogram may be performed to rule out ovarian, tubal, or uterine structural disorders.

Factors That Cause Male Subfertility

The factors that most commonly lead to male subfertility include:

- Disturbance in **spermatogenesis** (production of sperm cells)
- Inadequate production of FSH and LH in the pituitary, which stimulates the production of sperm
- Obstruction in the seminiferous tubules, ducts, or vessels, which prevent the movement of spermatozoa
- Qualitative or quantitative changes in the seminal fluid, which prevent **sperm motility** (movement of sperm)
- Development of autoimmunity, which immobilizes sperm
- Problems in ejaculation or deposition, which prevents spermatozoa from being placed close enough to a woman's cervix to allow ready penetration and fertilization
- Chronic or excessive exposure to X-rays or radioactive substances, general ill health, poor diet, and stress, all of which may interfere with sperm production

LIMITED SPERM COUNT

The **sperm count** is the number of sperm in a single ejaculation or in a milliliter of semen. The minimum sperm count considered normal has:

- Thirty-three to 46 million sperm per milliliter of seminal fluid, or 50 million per ejaculation
- Fifty percent of sperm that are motile
- Thirty percent that are normal in shape and form

Spermatozoa must be produced and maintained at a temperature slightly lower than body temperature to be fully motile. This is why the testes, in which sperm are produced and stored, are suspended in the scrotal sac away from body heat. Any condition that significantly increases body temperature, such as a chronic infection from tuberculosis or recurrent sinusitis, has the potential to raise scrotal heat enough to lower a sperm count. Actions that directly increase scrotal heat, such as working at a desk job or driving a great deal every day (e.g., salesmen, motorcyclists) may have lower sperm counts compared with men whose occupations allow them to be ambulatory at least part of each day. Frequent use of hot tubs or saunas may also lower sperm counts. Maintaining an ideal body weight (body mass index [BMI] of 18.5 to 24.9) is a general preventative health measure. Excessive weight may alter testosterone production and sperm production (Calderon, Gomez-Martin, Vega-Pinero, et al., 2016).

Congenital abnormalities are yet another reason sperm count may be lowered. Abnormalities may include **cryptorchidism** (undescended testes) if surgical repair was not completed until after puberty or if the spermatic cord became twisted after the surgery.

A varicocele, or varicosity (enlargement) of the internal spermatic vein, can also increase temperature and congestion within the testes, which may slow and disrupt spermatogenesis. Although more research is needed to determine whether a varicocele does increase temperature, surgical removal of the varicocele (varicocelectomy) may decrease warmth and improve fertility in some men (Agarwal & Esteves, 2016).

Other conditions that may inhibit sperm production include:

- Past trauma to the testes
- Surgery on or near the testicles that has resulted in impaired testicular circulation
- Endocrine imbalances, particularly of the thyroid, pancreas, or pituitary glands
- Drug use or excessive alcohol use
- Environmental factors, such as exposure to X-rays or radioactive substances

Men who are exposed to radioactive substances in their work environment should be provided with adequate protection of the testes. When you are assisting with pelvic X-rays, be certain men and boys are furnished a protective lead shield to guard against radiation to the testes.

Testing for Sperm Number and Availability

A number of common tests, such as semen analysis and sperm motility, help to identify whether adequate sperm are present for conception.

Analysis of Pituitary Hormones

A blood test and analysis can determine whether adequate levels of FSH and LH are present. When a man has typical male features (such as facial hair growth, laryngeal prominence, and a deeper voice), limited sperm count is rarely a problem.

Semen Analysis

On average, ejaculation for a semen analysis should produce a minimum of 1.4 to 1.7 ml of semen and should contain a minimum of 33 to 46 million spermatozoa per milliliter

BOX 7.5

Nursing Care Planning Based on Family Teaching

TIPS FOR ENSURING AN ACCURATE SEMEN ANALYSIS

Q. Bob Carl asks you, "What is the right way to do a semen sample?"

A. Effective guidelines include:

- Abstain from intercourse or masturbation for about 3 days.
- Use a clean, dry plastic or glass container with a secure lid to collect the sample.
- Collect the specimen as close as possible to your usual time of sexual activity.
- Avoid using any lubricants before you collect the specimen.
- After you've collected the specimen in the container, close it securely and write down the time you collected it.
- Take the specimen to the laboratory or healthcare provider's office immediately so it can be analyzed within 1 hour of collection.
- Keep the specimen at body temperature while transporting it. Carrying it next to your chest is one way to do this.

of fluid (World Health Organization, 2010). Semen analysis includes the following steps:

1. The patient is instructed to be sexually abstinent 2 to 4 days prior to the analysis.
2. The patient ejaculates by masturbation into a clean, dry specimen jar or a special condom (one without spermicide).
3. The number of sperm in the specimen are counted and then examined under a microscope within 1 hour of ejaculation (Box 7.5).

The analysis may need to be repeated after 2 or 3 months because spermatogenesis is an ongoing process and 30 to 90 days is needed for new sperm to reach maturity. If patients are reluctant to have their sperm counted at a healthcare facility, they have the option to use various self-test kits to test sperm motility at home. These kits are available online. If the man has a vas deferens obstruction, sperm can be obtained by testes biopsy.

Concept Mastery Alert

Semen specimens should be kept at body temperature during transportation. Patients can be advised to carry the specimen next to the body in an inside pocket to accomplish this goal.

Sperm Penetration Assay and Antisperm Antibody Testing

For impregnation to take place, sperm must be mobile enough to navigate the vagina, uterus, and a fallopian tube to reach the ova. Although sperm penetration studies are rarely necessary, they may be scheduled to determine whether a man's sperm, once they reach an ovum, can penetrate it effectively. With the use of an assisted reproductive technique such as IVF, poorly mobile sperm or those with poor penetration can be injected directly into a woman's ovum under laboratory conditions (intracytoplasmic sperm injection), bypassing the need for sperm to be fully mobile.

What If . . . 7.2
While the Carls are undergoing IVF, Cheryl's mother asks the nurse, "How can I ever love a child created in a 'test tube'?" How would the nurse answer her?

Therapy for Increasing Sperm Count and Motility

If sperm are present but the total count is low, a man may be advised to abstain from coitus for 7 to 10 days at a time to increase the count. Ligation of a varicocele (if present) and changes in lifestyle, such as avoiding recreational marijuana use, wearing looser clothing, avoiding long periods of sitting, and avoiding prolonged hot baths, may also help reduce scrotal heat and increase the sperm count.

OBSTRUCTION OR IMPAIRED SPERM MOTILITY

In some men, adequate sperm are manufactured, but there is obstruction at some point along the pathway spermatozoa must travel to reach the outside: the seminiferous tubules, the epididymis, the vas deferens, the ejaculatory duct, or the urethra (see Chapter 5, Fig. 5.1). Diseases such as *mumps orchitis* (testicular inflammation and scarring due to the mumps virus), epididymitis (inflammation of the epididymis), and infections such as gonorrhea or ascending urethral infection can result in this type of obstruction because adhesions form and occlude sperm transport (Han, Liu, Zhou, et al., 2016). Congenital stricture of a spermatic duct may occasionally be seen. Benign hypertrophy of the prostate gland occurs in most men beginning at about 50 years of age. Pressure from the enlarged gland on the vas deferens can then interfere with sperm transport. Infection of the prostate, through which the sperm and seminal fluid must pass, or infection of the seminal vesicles (spread from a urinary tract infection) can change the composition of the seminal fluid enough to reduce sperm motility.

A few men who have vasectomies develop an autoimmune reaction or form antibodies that immobilize their own sperm after the procedure; they also may experience long-term pain unless the procedure is reversed (Horovitz, Tjong, Domes, et al., 2012). It is conceivable that men with obstruction in the vas deferens from other causes, such as scarring after an infection, could also develop an autoimmune reaction that immobilizes sperm the same way.

Anomalies of the penis, such as hypospadias (urethral opening on the ventral surface of the penis), epispadias (urethral opening on the dorsal surface), or Peyronie disease (a bent penis) can cause sperm to be deposited too far from the sexual partner's cervix to allow optimal cervical penetration. Extreme obesity in a male may also interfere with effective penetration and deposition (Campbell, Lane, Owens, et al., 2015).

Testing for Sperm Transport Disorders

Sperm transport disorders are suspected when FSH and LH hormones, which stimulate the production of sperm, are adequate but the sperm count remains limited.

Therapy for Sperm Transport Disorders

If sperm are not able to pass through the vas deferens because of obstruction, surgery to relieve the obstruction is extensive, costly, and may not have a positive outcome. A better solution can be extracting sperm from a point above the blockage and injecting it into the vagina or uterus of the man's partner by intrauterine insemination (IUI) (Bahadur, Ilahibuccus, Al-Habib, et al., 2015). If the problem appears to be that sperm are immobilized by vaginal secretions due to an immunologic factor, the response can be reduced by abstinence or condom use for about 6 months. However, to avoid this prolonged time interval (which is difficult for a couple who want to have a child immediately), washing of the sperm followed by IUI may be preferred. The administration of corticosteroids to a woman may have some effect in decreasing sperm immobilization because it reduces her immune response and antibody production.

EJACULATION PROBLEMS

Erectile dysfunction or the inability to achieve an erection (formerly called impotence), which may occur from psychological problems; diseases such as a cerebrovascular accident, diabetes, or Parkinson disease; use of certain antihypertensive agents; as well as the discontinuation of finasteride, a drug used for male pattern baldness (Glina, Roehrborn, Esen, et al., 2015), may result in erectile dysfunction. This condition is *primary* if the man has never been able to achieve erection and ejaculation and *secondary* if the man was able to achieve ejaculation in the past but now has difficulty. Erectile dysfunction can be a difficult problem to solve if it is associated with stress because this is not easily relieved.

Premature ejaculation (ejaculation before penetration) is another factor that may interfere with the proper deposition of sperm. It is another problem often attributed to psychological causes. Adolescents may experience it until they become more experienced in sexual techniques.

Testing for Ejaculation Concerns

Ejaculation concerns are identified by a sexual history. It may be difficult for a man to discuss this area of his life, especially if a nurse is female, so skillful patient interviewing technique is required.

Therapy for Ejaculation Concerns

Solutions for erectile dysfunction include psychological or sexual counseling as well as the use of a phosphodiesterase inhibitor, such as sildenafil (Viagra) or tadalafil (Cialis) (see Chapter 5). Dapoxetine, a short-acting selective serotonin reuptake inhibitor, is a drug that has been developed especially for the treatment of premature ejaculation and shows good results when taken about 1 hour before planned coitus (Yue, Dong, Hu, et al., 2015).

QSEN Checkpoint Question 7.2

SAFETY

The Carls introduce themselves to the nurse as an "infertile" couple. As a safety measure, the nurse would want them to understand which of the following?
  a. Couples are not termed infertile until they have been trying to conceive for 2 years.
  b. Infertility can cause depression, so the couple should report any feeling of sadness.
  c. If their relationship is not monogamous, they still need to use safer sex practices.
  d. Infertility is related to antibiotic-resistant infections, so they need to be tested for these.

Look in Appendix A for the best answer and rationale.

Factors That Cause Female Subfertility

The factors that cause subfertility in women are analogous to those causing subfertility in men:
  • Limited production of FHS or LH, which interfere with ova growth
  • Anovulation (faulty or inadequate expulsion of ova)
  • Problems of ova transport through the fallopian tubes to the uterus
  • Uterine factors, such as tumors or poor endometrial development
  • Cervical and vaginal factors, which immobilize spermatozoa
  • Poor nutrition, increased body weight, and lack of exercise, which may compound these problems

ANOVULATION

The steps of ova formation and ovulation are described in Chapter 5. **Anovulation** (absence of ovulation or release of ova from the ovary), the most common cause of subfertility in women, may occur from a genetic abnormality such as Turner syndrome (hypogonadism), in which there is limited ovarian tissue available to produce ova. More often, it results from a hormonal imbalance caused by a condition such as hypothyroidism, which interferes with hypothalamus-pituitary-ovarian interaction. Ovarian tumors or polycystic ovary syndrome may also produce anovulation due to feedback stimulation on the pituitary. Chronic or excessive exposure to X-rays or radioactive substances, general ill health, poor diet, and stress may all contribute to poor ovarian function (Fritz & Speroff, 2010).

Nutrition, body weight, and exercise are all important for adequate ova production because they all influence the blood glucose/insulin balance (Best & Bhattacharya, 2015). When either glucose or insulin levels are too high, they can disrupt the production of FSH and LH, leading to ovulation failure. Vitamin D may also be instrumental in maintaining pituitary hormone levels (Shahrokhi, Ghaffari, & Kazerouni, 2016).

The ideal body weight to maintain is a BMI of 18.5 to 24.9. Eating slowly digested carbohydrate foods (e.g., brown rice, pasta, dark bread, beans) and fiber-rich vegetables (e.g., asparagus, broccoli) rather than easily digested carbohydrate foods (e.g., white bread, cold breakfast cereals) can not only increase fertility by keeping insulin levels balanced but also may prevent gestational diabetes when a woman becomes pregnant (Sanabria-Martínez, García-Hermoso, Poyatos-León, et al., 2015).

Exercising 30 minutes per day by walking or doing mild aerobics also helps to regulate blood glucose levels and increase fertility, complementing healthy eating habits. Stress may play a role in limiting ovulation as this may lower hypothalamic secretion of the gonadotropin-releasing hormone (GnRH), which then lowers the production of LH and FSH, which leads to anovulation.

Decreased body weight or a body fat ratio of less than 10%, as may occur in female athletes such as competitive runners or in women who are excessively lean or anorexic, can reduce pituitary hormones such as FSH and LH and halt ovulation (termed hypogonadotrophic hypogonadism) (Fritz & Speroff, 2010).

The most frequent cause, however, for anovulation is naturally occurring variations in ovulatory patterns or polycystic ovary syndrome, a condition in which the ovaries produce excess testosterone, thus lowering FSH and LH levels, which then causes irregular and unpredictable menstrual cycles (Ecklund & Usadi, 2015).

Polycystic ovary syndrome is associated with metabolic syndrome, which is diagnosed in patients with:

- Waist circumference of 35 in. or more in women
- Fasting blood glucose over 100 mg/dl
- Serum triglycerides over 150 mg/dl
- Blood pressure over 135/85 mmHg
- High-density lipoprotein cholesterol over 50 mg/dl
- Development of hirsutism (unwanted body hair) (Ebrahimi-Mamaghani, Saghafi-Asl, Pirouzpanah, et al., 2015).

Metabolic syndrome is also associated with increased cardiac disease, so efforts to reduce weight and lower triglycerides and cholesterol can improve heart health as well. It is discussed further in Chapter 11.

Testing for Anovulation

Many tests to detect ovulation can be completed independently by women at home, giving them both a sense of control over what is happening and the ability to learn more about the functioning of their bodies.

Ovulation Monitoring

The fastest way to investigate if ovulation is occurring is to measure the woman's serum progesterone level during the luteal phase of her menstrual cycle (about day 21 to day 28 of a typical cycle). If this is elevated, it implies a corpus luteum has formed or ovulation has occurred.

The least costly way to determine a woman's ovulation pattern is to ask her to record her basal body temperature (BBT) for at least 4 months. To determine this, a woman takes her temperature each morning, before getting out of bed or engaging in any activity, eating, or drinking, using a special BBT or tympanic thermometer. She plots this daily temperature on a monthly graph while noting any conditions that might affect her temperature, such as an infection or sleeplessness. At the time of ovulation, the BBT can be seen to dip slightly (about 0.5°F), it then rises to a level about 1 degree higher than her preovulation temperatures and then stays at that level until 3 or 4 days before the next menstrual flow. This increase in BBT marks the time of ovulation because it occurs immediately after ovulation (and at the beginning of the luteal phase of the menstrual cycle, which can occur only if ovulation has occurred). If the temperature rise does not last at least 10 days, it suggests a woman has a luteal phase defect (progesterone is not being produced long enough in a cycle so adequate endometrium for implantation can be laid down). Typical graphs of BBT are shown in Figure 7.1.

What If . . . 7.3

Cheryl Carl tells the nurse she works nights as a cocktail waitress, goes to bed at 4 AM, and then wakes at 6 AM to drive her husband to work. Starting at noon, she sleeps for 4 or 5 hours before getting up to go to work. When during the day should the nurse tell her is the best time to record her BBT?

Ovulation Determination by Test Strip

Various brands of commercial kits are available for assessing the upsurge of LH that occurs just before ovulation and can be used in place of BBT monitoring. A woman dips a test strip into a midmorning urine specimen and then compares it with the kit instructions for a color change. Such kits are purchased over the counter, are easy to use, and have the advantage of marking the point just before ovulation occurs rather than just after ovulation, as is the case with BBT. They are not as economical as simple temperature recording, but they are advantageous for women with irregular work or daily activity, which can make BBT measurements inaccurate.

Several test kits can be found online that contain materials to test both FSH on the third day of a woman's menstrual cycle (an abnormally high level is an indicator her ovaries are not responding well to ovulation) as well as sperm motility for the male. The woman's result is available in 30 minutes; the man's result is available in 10 minutes. The kits are expensive but can be helpful to a couple as a first step in self-fertility

Basal body temperature

A Ovulation without conception

B Ovulation with conception

C Anovulatory cycle

Figure 7.1 Basal body temperature graph. **(A)** A woman's temperature dips slightly at midpoint in the menstrual cycle and then rises sharply, which is an indication of ovulation. Toward the end of the cycle (the 24th day), her temperature begins to decline, indicating progesterone levels are falling and she did not conceive. **(B)** A woman's temperature rises at the midpoint in the cycle and remains at that elevated level past the time of her normal menstrual flow, suggesting pregnancy has occurred. **(C)** There is no preovulatory dip, and no rise of temperature anywhere during the cycle. This is the typical pattern of a woman who does not ovulate.

testing. Be certain the woman realizes this is not a test of her time of ovulation but a test whether she has adequate FSH to stimulate egg growth; therefore, she shouldn't use the test at the midpoint of her menstrual cycle.

Polycystic ovary syndrome can be detected by examining the woman's menstrual history, but even if a woman experiences regular monthly menstruation, it does not necessarily indicate she is also ovulating on a regular basis (Balen, 2012). Fasting-glucose, testosterone, and estrogen levels are analyzed. A pelvic sonogram can be used to confirm cysts are present on the ovaries and may be the cause of subfertility (Hamilton, 2012).

Therapy for Anovulation

If a disturbance in ovulation is identified as the subfertility concern, administration of GnRH is a possibility (this will stimulate the pituitary to secrete more FSH and LH). Therapy with clomiphene citrate (Clomid) or letrozole (Femara), a newer drug, may also be used to stimulate ovulation (Box 7.6). In other women, ovarian follicular growth can be stimulated by the administration of combinations of FSH and LH in conjunction with administration of human chorionic gonadotropin (hCG) to produce ovulation. If increased prolactin levels are identified, bromocriptine (Parlodel) is added to the medication regimen to reduce prolactin levels and allow for the rise of pituitary gonadotropins (Karch, 2015).

Administration of either clomiphene citrate or gonadotropins may overstimulate an ovary, causing multiple ova to come to maturity, and possibly resulting in multiple births. Counsel women who receive these agents that this is a possibility.

TUBAL TRANSPORT PROBLEMS

Difficulty with tubal transport usually occurs because scarring has developed in the fallopian tubes, which is typically caused by chronic salpingitis (chronic pelvic inflammatory disease). This could also result from a ruptured appendix or from abdominal surgery, which involved infection that spread to the fallopian tubes and left adhesion formation in the tubes. Complete tubal obstruction is the chief problem if a woman had a tubal ligation in years past but now wants to become pregnant.

Pelvic inflammatory disease (PID) is infection of the pelvic organs: the uterus, fallopian tubes, ovaries, and their supporting structures. The initial source of the infection is usually a sexually transmitted disease such as chlamydia or gonorrhea. PID occurs at a rate of about 25 per 100 women; in other words, one-fourth of all women will experience this type of infection in a lifetime. About 12% of those who acquire PID will be left subfertile because of tubal scarring (Sheth & Keller, 2015).

PID invasion of fallopian tubes is most apt to occur at the end of a menstrual period because menstrual blood provides such an excellent growth medium for bacteria. There also is a loss of the normal cervical mucus barrier at this time, which increases the risk of initial invasion. When PID is left unrecognized and untreated, it enters a chronic phase, which causes the scarring that can lead to stricture of the fallopian tubes and the resulting fertility problem.

There is a higher incidence of PID among women who have multiple sexual partners (Oman & Burke, 2015). Based on this, it is good advice for women to limit the number of

BOX 7.6

Nursing Care Planning Based on Responsibility for Pharmacology

CLOMIPHENE CITRATE (CLOMID)

Action: Clomiphene citrate (Clomid) is an estrogen agonist commonly used to stimulate the ovary. The drug binds to estrogen receptors, decreasing the number of available estrogen receptors, which falsely signals the hypothalamus to increase follicle-stimulating hormone and luteinizing hormone secretion. This results in ovulation (Karch, 2015).

Pregnancy Category: X

Dosage: Initially, 50 mg/day orally for 5 days (started anytime if no menstrual flow has occurred recently or about the fifth day of the cycle if menstrual flow is occurring). If ovulation does not occur with this initial therapy, the drug can be followed by a prescription of 100 mg/day for 5 days started as early as 30 days after the initial course of therapy. This second course may be repeated one more time.

Possible Adverse Effects: abdominal discomfort, distention, bloating, nausea, vomiting, breast tenderness, vasomotor flushing, ovarian enlargement, ovarian overstimulation, multiple births, and visual disturbances

NURSING IMPLICATIONS

- Ensure women have had a pelvic examination and baseline hormonal studies before therapy.
- Review medication scheduling. Urge women to use a calendar or some other system to mark their treatment schedule and also to determine and plot ovulation.
- Remind patients that timing intercourse with ovulation is important for achieving pregnancy.
- Advise patients 24-hour urine samples may be periodically necessary.
- Caution patients to report any bloating, stomach pain, blurred vision, unusual bleeding, bruising, or visual changes.
- Inform patients that therapy can be repeated for a total of three courses; if no results are obtained, therapy will be discontinued at that point.

Figure 7.2 Insertion of a contrast medium for a sonohysterosalpingogram. The contrast medium outlines the uterus and fallopian tubes on sonogram to demonstrate patency.

their sexual partners or always insist on condom protection to help reduce the incidence of sexually transmitted infections and possibly subfertility.

Testing for Tubal Patency

Ultrasound or X-ray imaging and direct visualization by a hysteroscope of fallopian tubes are all effective methods used to determine the patency of fallopian tubes.

Sonohysterosalpingogram

A sonohysterosalpingogram is a sonographic examination of the fallopian tubes and uterus using an ultrasound contrast agent introduced into the uterus through a narrow catheter inserted into the uterine cervix (Fig. 7.2) followed by intravaginal scanning. If the tubes are patent, they will fill with the contrast medium and be detailed on the ultrasound screen. The procedure is contraindicated if infection of the vagina, cervix, or uterus is present (infectious organisms might be forced through the tubes into the pelvic cavity); it is usually scheduled just following a menstrual flow when a woman could not be pregnant.

Although only a small amount of contrast medium is used, it does slightly distend the uterus and tubes, possibly causing momentary painful uterine cramping. After the study, the small amount of contrast medium used drains out through the vagina. Although it is possible that the procedure could be therapeutic as well as diagnostic as the pressure of the solution could break up adhesions as it passes through the fallopian tubes, this is unlikely because the amount of contrast medium used is so small. Although extremely rare, the procedure carries a small risk of infection (a chlamydia screen before the procedure is usually advised); although unlikely, an allergic reaction to the contrast medium or embolism from the medium entering a uterine blood vessel could also occur.

Hysterosalpingogram

A hysterosalpingogram is similar to a sonohysterosalpingogram except a radiopaque contrast medium is used and the fallopian tubes are revealed by X-ray. This procedure uses more contrast medium than with the sonogram technique so the force of the injected solution may actually break up tubal adhesions, and thus may be therapeutic as well as diagnostic. Because an X-ray is used, which might be harmful to a growing pregnancy, the procedure must be scheduled immediately following a menstrual flow when pregnancy could not be present.

Transvaginal Hydrolaparoscopy

Transvaginal hydrolaparoscopy is begun with the instillation of a paracervical local anesthetic block followed by introduction of a hysteroscope into an incision just behind the cervix through the cul-de-sac of Douglas into the peritoneal cavity. About 200 ml of normal saline is then introduced to move the bowel away from the uterus so the posterior wall of the uterus, the ovaries, and the fallopian tubes can be assessed. Tubal patency can be evaluated if, following the insertion of a small amount of dye into the cervix, it can be viewed exiting the fimbrial end of the tubes. At the end of the procedure, the fluid is drained from the peritoneal cavity; the small incision will heal without stitches (Lo Monte, Capobianco, Piva, et al., 2015).

Therapy for Lack of Tubal Patency

If the subfertility problem is identified as tubal insufficiency from inflammation, the prescription of diathermy or steroid administration may be helpful to reduce adhesions. Hystero-salpingography (instillation of a contrast dye under X-ray monitoring) can be attempted to see if the force of the dye insertion will break adhesions. Canalization of the fallopian tubes and plastic surgical repair (microsurgery) are other possible treatments. If peritoneal adhesions or nodules of endometriosis are holding the tubes fixed and away from the ovaries, these can be removed by laparoscopy or laser surgery (Magos, 2012).

It is possible for fallopian tubes, which have been ligated as a contraception procedure, to be reopened surgically but the success of the operation is not more than 70% to 80%. Also, the irregular incision line left by surgery can result in an ectopic pregnancy (i.e., a tubal pregnancy) if a fertilized ovum is stopped at the irregular point (Malacova, Kemp-Casey, Bremner, et al., 2015). IVF is more commonly used today and more apt to result in a viable pregnancy.

QSEN Checkpoint Question 7.3

TEAMWORK & COLLABORATION

Cheryl Carl is scheduled to have a sonohysterosalpingography. Which of the following instructions would the nurse want the care team members to know so patient teaching can be consistent?

a. She may feel some mild cramping when the contrast medium is inserted.
b. The X-ray of the uterus will reveal any fibroid tumors or adhesions present.
c. She will not be able to conceive for at least 3 months after the procedure.
d. Many women experience mild bleeding for up to 2 hours as an aftereffect.

Look in Appendix A for the best answer and rationale.

UTERINE CONCERNS

Tumors such as fibromas (leiomyomas) may be a rare cause of subfertility if they block the entrance of the fallopian tubes into the uterus or limit the space available on the uterine wall for effective implantation. A congenitally deformed uterine cavity may also limit implantation sites, but this also is rare.

Endometriosis and poor secretion of estrogen or progesterone are more common uterine reasons for subfertility as these result in inadequate endometrial formation (overproduction or underproduction), which then interferes with implantation and embryo growth.

Endometriosis refers to the implantation of uterine endometrium, or nodules, that have spread from the interior of the uterus to locations outside the uterus (Woo & Yates, 2015). The occurrence of endometriosis may indicate the endometrial tissue has different or more friable qualities than usual (perhaps due to a luteal phase defect) and therefore is a type of endometrium that also does not support embryo implantation as well as usual.

Endometriosis symptoms begin in adolescence, with the most common sites of endometrium spread to the fallopian tubes, the cul-de-sac of Douglas, the ovaries, the uterine ligaments, and the outer surface of the uterus and bowel (Fig. 7.3). Some evidence of endometriosis occurs in as many as 50% of women, usually from reflux through the fallopian tubes at the time of menstruation. If viable particles of endometrium, which enter a tube this way, begin to proliferate, they can cause tubal obstruction; growths on the ovaries can displace fallopian tubes away from the ovaries, preventing the entrance of ova into the tubes. Peritoneal macrophages, which are drawn to nodules of endometrium, can destroy sperm.

Testing for Uterine Concerns

Tests to determine if a uterine concern is leading to subfertility include a sonogram or hysteroscopy to view the structure of the uterus, blood work to analyze for hormones, and perhaps an endometrial biopsy.

Hysteroscopy

Hysteroscopy is visual inspection of the uterus through the insertion of a hysteroscope (a thin hollow tube) through the vagina, cervix, and into the uterus. This is helpful to further evaluate uterine adhesions, malformations, or other abnormalities such as fibroid tumors or polyps that were discovered on sonogram imaging. Women are screened for chlamydia before the examination to avoid introduction of bacteria into the uterus.

Uterine Endometrial Biopsy

Uterine endometrial biopsy may be used to reveal an endometrial problem, such as a luteal phase defect. If the endometrium sample removed by biopsy resembles a corkscrew (a typical progesterone-dominated endometrium) seen in the second half of a menstrual cycle, this suggests ovulation has occurred. Although very diagnostic of progesterone-associated concerns, endometrial biopsies are being performed less commonly than they once were, having been replaced with serum progesterone level evaluations that are simpler and also suggest ovulation has occurred.

If an endometrial biopsy is required, it is done 2 or 3 days before an expected menstrual flow (day 25 or 26 of a typical 28-day menstrual cycle). After a paracervical block and a screen for chlamydia, a thin probe and biopsy forceps are introduced through the cervix. A woman may experience mild-to-moderate discomfort from maneuvering the instruments. There may be a moment of sharp pain as the biopsy specimen is taken from the anterior or posterior uterine wall. Possible complications include pain, excessive bleeding, infection, and uterine perforation. This procedure is contraindicated if pregnancy is suspected (although the chance it would interfere

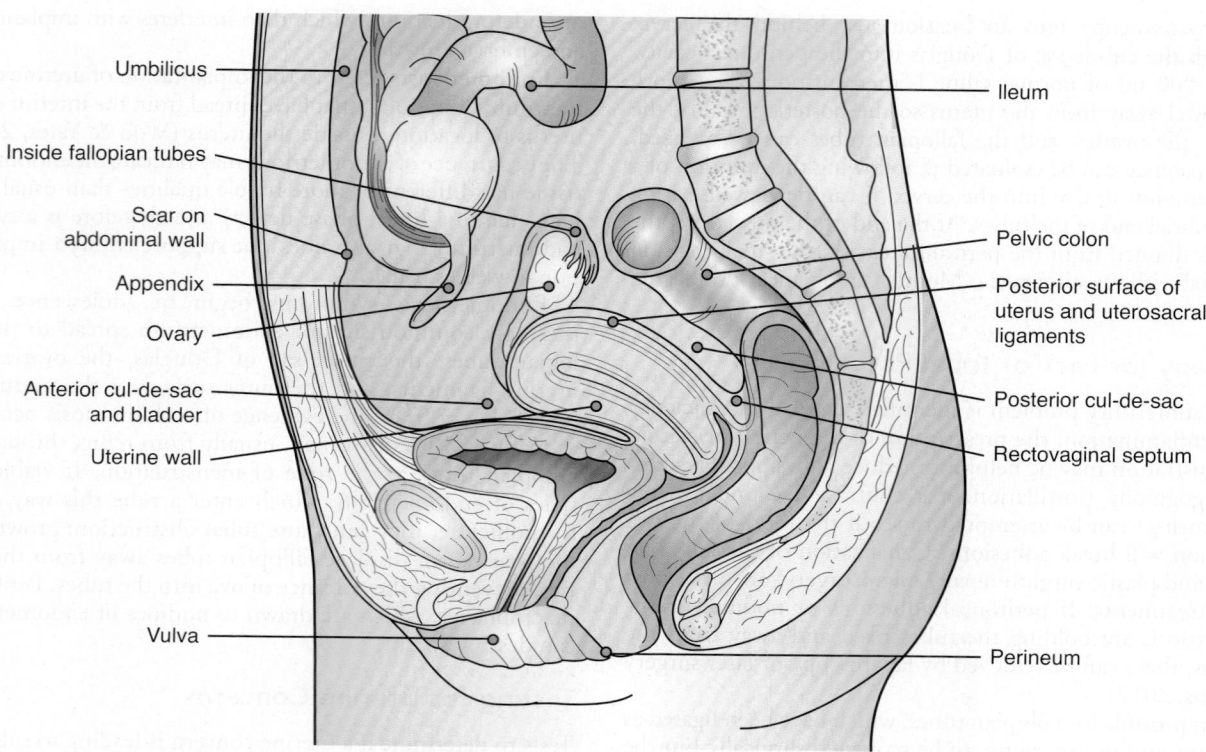

Labels (clockwise from top left):
Umbilicus
Inside fallopian tubes
Scar on abdominal wall
Appendix
Ovary
Anterior cul-de-sac and bladder
Uterine wall
Vulva
Ileum
Pelvic colon
Posterior surface of uterus and uterosacral ligaments
Posterior cul-de-sac
Rectovaginal septum
Perineum

Figure 7.3 Common sites of endometriosis formation.

with a pregnancy is probably less than 10%) or if an infection such as acute PID or cervicitis is present. Caution the woman that she might notice a small amount of vaginal spotting after the procedure. For follow-up, she needs to telephone her primary care provider if she develops a temperature greater than 101°F, has a large amount of bleeding, or passes clots. She needs to telephone the healthcare agency when she has her next menstrual flow because this helps "date" the endometrium and the accuracy of the analysis.

Laparoscopy

Laparoscopy is the introduction of a thin, hollow, lighted tube (a fiber optic telescope or laparoscope) through a small incision in the abdomen, just under the umbilicus, to examine the position and state of the fallopian tubes and ovaries. This allows an examiner to view whether the ovaries are close enough to the fallopian tubes to allow an ovum to enter. It is rarely done unless the results of a uterosalpingography are abnormal because it involves general anesthesia, which is necessary because of the pain caused by extensive maneuvering. It is scheduled during the follicular phase of a menstrual cycle. The woman is positioned in a steep Trendelenburg position (which brings the reproductive organs down out of the pelvis). Carbon dioxide is usually introduced into the abdomen to move the abdominal wall outward and to offer better visualization. Women may feel bloating of the abdomen from the infusion of the carbon dioxide after such a procedure. If some carbon dioxide escapes under the diaphragm, they may feel extremely sharp shoulder pain from the pressure of the gas on the cervical nerves.

During the procedure, a contrast medium can be injected into the uterus through a polyethylene cannula placed in the cervix to assess tubal patency (if tubes are patent, the dye will appear in the abdominal cavity). A scope may be passed directly into a fallopian tube to reveal information about the presence and condition of the fimbria and the tubal lining. If fimbria have been destroyed by PID, the chance for a normal conception is in doubt because ova seem to be unable to enter a tube if fimbrial currents are absent.

Therapy for Uterine Concerns

If the problem of subfertility appears to be a luteal phase defect, this can be corrected by progesterone vaginal suppositories begun on the third day of a woman's temperature rise and continued for the next 6 weeks (if pregnancy occurs) or until a menstrual flow begins.

If a myoma (fibroid tumor) or intrauterine adhesions are found to be interfering with fertility, a myomectomy, or surgical removal of the tumor and adhesions, can be scheduled (Bailey, Jaslow, & Kutteh, 2015). If the growth is small, this can be done by a hysteroscopic ambulatory procedure. During the procedure, an intrauterine device (IUD) may be inserted to prevent the uterine sides from touching and forming new adhesions; the woman may be prescribed estrogen for 3 months as another method to prevent adhesion formation. This treatment can be difficult for a woman to accept because preventing pregnancy (using an IUD) is exactly what she does not want to do. Be certain she has a good explanation of the IUD's purpose and that it can be easily removed in about 1 month's time.

For problems of abnormal uterine formation, such as a septate uterus, surgery is also available. However, these defects are usually related to early pregnancy loss, not initial subfertility. Endometriosis can be treated both medically and surgically; treatment is discussed in Chapter 47 with other causes of dysmenorrhea.

VAGINAL AND CERVICAL CONCERNS

At the time of ovulation, the cervical mucus is thin and watery and can be easily penetrated by spermatozoa for a period of 12 to 72 hours. If coitus is not synchronized with this time, the cervical mucus may be too thick to allow spermatozoa to penetrate the cervix. Infection or inflammation of the cervix (erosion) can also cause cervical mucus to thicken so much that spermatozoa cannot penetrate it easily or survive in it. A stenotic cervical os or obstruction of the os by a polyp may further compromise sperm penetration. This is rarely enough of a problem to be the sole cause of subfertility, however. A woman who has undergone dilatation and curettage (D&C) procedures several times or cervical conization (cervical surgery) should be evaluated in light of the possibility that scar tissue and tightening of the cervical os has occurred.

Infection of the vagina can cause the pH of vaginal secretions to become acidotic, thus limiting or destroying the motility of spermatozoa. Some women appear to have sperm-immobilizing or sperm-agglutinating antibodies in their blood plasma, which act to destroy sperm cells in the vagina or cervix. Either of these immune-based problems can limit the ability of sperm to survive in the vagina and enter the uterus.

Testing and Therapy for Vaginal and Cervical Concerns

If sperm do not appear to survive in vaginal secretions because secretions are too scant or tenacious, a woman may be prescribed low-dose estrogen therapy to increase mucus production during days 5 to 10 of her cycle. Conjugated estrogen (Premarin) is a type of estrogen prescribed for this purpose.

If a vaginal infection is present, the infection will be treated according to the causative organism based on culture reports (see Chapter 47). Vaginal infections such as trichomoniasis and moniliasis tend to recur, requiring close supervision and follow-up. If the woman's sexual partner is the source of infection, and is therefore reinfecting her, the partner needs antibiotic therapy as well. Caution women who are prescribed metronidazole (Flagyl) for a *Trichomonas* infection; although no studies have shown fetal malformations after its use, it may be teratogenic early in pregnancy and therefore should not be continued if the woman suspects she has become pregnant.

Unexplained Subfertility

In a small percentage of couples, no known cause for subfertility can be discovered. It may be that the problem of one partner alone is not significant, but when combined with a small problem in the other partner, together, these become sufficient to create subfertility. It is obviously discouraging for couples to complete a fertility evaluation and be told their inability to conceive cannot be explained. Offer active support to help the couple find alternative solutions at this point, such as continuing to try to conceive, using an assisted reproductive technique, choosing to adopt, or agreeing to a child-free life.

QSEN Checkpoint Question 7.4

INFORMATICS

Cheryl Carl is diagnosed as having endometriosis as a cause of her subfertility. The nurse would want her electronic health record to reflect the fact that this condition interferes with fertility because of which of the following?
- a. The ovaries stop producing estrogen and progesterone.
- b. The uterine cervix becomes very inflamed and swollen.
- c. Pressure on the pituitary leads to decreased FSH levels.
- d. Endometrial implants obstruct both of the fallopian tubes.

Look in Appendix A for the best answer and rationale.

Assisted Reproductive Techniques

If ovulation, sperm production, or sperm mobility problems cannot be corrected, assisted reproductive strategies are the next step for a couple to consider. Before beginning any of these procedures, urge a woman to be in excellent health by discontinuing smoking or recreational drug behaviors, ingesting a diet high in protein, and having a BMI within a normal range of 18.5 to 24.9. She probably also will have, if she has not already had them, tests for HIV and hepatitis C; a hormone profile including levels of FSH, LH, estrogen, and progesterone to test for ovarian reserves (whether ovaries have the capacity to produce multiple oocytes); as well as an intravaginal sonogram to visual usual structures. Whether a woman feels comfortable choosing assisted reproduction is strongly socioculturally related, as people on a limited budget and without health insurance may not be able to afford these therapies, or their religion or cultural beliefs may make these unacceptable procedures. LGBT couples may also feel uncomfortable seeking reproductive advice. In all instances, culturally sensitive care is required by the nurse (Box 7.7).

ALTERNATIVE INSEMINATION

Alternative or IUI is the instillation of sperm from a masturbatory sample into the female reproductive tract by means of a cannula to aid conception at the time of ovulation (Kop, van Wely, Mol, et al., 2015). The sperm can either be instilled into the cervix (intracervical insemination) or directly into the uterus (IUI) at the time of predicted ovulation. BBT charting, mucus analysis, or urinary test kits for LH can be used to detect the day of ovulation (Hamilton, 2012).

Either the male partner's sperm (alternative insemination by male partner) or donor sperm (alternative insemination by donor) can be used. These procedures are used if the male partner has no sperm or an inadequate sperm count, if a woman has a vaginal or cervical factor that interferes with sperm motility, or a woman has hormonal issues

BOX 7.7

Nursing Care Planning to Respect Cultural Diversity

Obtaining a sexual history is often difficult because cultural taboos can make couples feel uncomfortable discussing this part of their life. Simple factors, such as how often couples engage in sexual relations, for example, are influenced by culture and religion. For example, according to Orthodox Jewish law, a couple may not engage in sexual relations for 7 days following menstruation (the *nida* period). This practice can result in fertility problems if a woman ovulates within the 7-day period. Some cultures forbid alternative insemination because preserving male lineage is so important. The Roman Catholic Church does not approve of in vitro fertilization or any form of conception outside the body. Being aware of cultural differences can help you understand the different ways couples react to a diagnosis of subfertility and help you appreciate the full meaning of this diagnosis to an individual couple.

affecting fertility. Donor insemination can be used if the man has a known genetic disorder he does not want to be transmitted to children or if a woman does not have a male partner. It is also a useful procedure for men who underwent a vasectomy but now wish to have children. In the past, men who underwent chemotherapy or radiation for testicular cancer had to accept being child-free afterward because they were no longer able to produce sperm. Today, sperm can be cryopreserved (frozen) in a sperm bank before

radiation or chemotherapy and then used for alternative insemination afterward (Araki, Yao, Asayama, et al., 2015).

One disadvantage of using cryopreserved sperm is that it tends to have slower motility than unfrozen specimens. However, although the rate of conception may be lower from this source, there appears to be no increase in the incidence of congenital anomalies in children conceived by this method, and sperm remain viable even after years of storage.

To prepare for alternative insemination, a woman receives an injection of clomiphene (Clomid) or FSH 1 month prior to the insemination so follicle growth of ova is stimulated and a day of ovulation can be predicted. On the selected day of insemination (confirmed by a serum analysis of progesterone), the sperm sample is instilled next to her cervix using a device similar to a cervical cap or diaphragm, or sperm are injected directly into the uterus using a flexible catheter (Fig. 7.4).

Donors for alternative insemination are volunteers who have no history of disease and no family history of possible inheritable disorders. The blood type, or at least the Rh factor, can be matched with the woman's to prevent incompatibility. Sperm can be selected according to desired physical or mental characteristics if desired. If FSH was used to stimulate follicle growth, caution women that the chance for a multiple birth (twins or triplets) increases so she can be prepared for this (Trew & Lavery, 2012).

Because conception through alternative insemination takes an average of 6 months to achieve, and some couples may have religious or ethical beliefs that prohibit the use of sperm from either the male partner or a donor, it may not be right for every couple. Also, because it can be a discouraging process for a couple to have to wait 6 months (or longer) to see results, couples may need support to continue the technique.

Figure 7.4 Alternative insemination. **(A)** Sperm are deposited next to the cervix, or **(B)** injected directly into the uterine cavity.

Some states have specific laws regarding inheritance, child support, and responsibility concerning children conceived by donor insemination, which may also limit whether a couple finds the technique desirable.

IN VITRO FERTILIZATION

In vitro fertilization (IVF) is most often used for couples who have not been able to conceive because the woman has obstructed or damaged fallopian tubes. It is also used when the man has oligospermia or a very low sperm count. IVF may also be helpful for couples when an absence of cervical mucus prevents sperm from entering the cervix or antisperm antibodies cause immobilization of sperm. In addition, couples with unexplained subfertility of long duration may be helped by IVF.

For the procedure, one or more mature oocytes are removed from a woman's ovary by laparoscopy and fertilized by exposure to sperm in a laboratory. About 40 hours after fertilization, the laboratory-grown fertilized ova (now zygotes) are inserted into a woman's uterus, where, ideally, one or more of them will implant and grow.

A donor ovum, rather than the woman's own ovum, can be used for a woman who does not ovulate or who carries a sex-linked disease she does not want to pass on to her children.

Young women who had extensive ovarian radiation or ovaries removed before surgery for ovarian cancer can have oocytes cryopreserved before surgery and used for IVF (Brezina, Ding, Ke, et al., 2015).

As with alternative insemination, 1 month before the procedure, the woman is given FSH to stimulate oocyte growth. Beginning about the 10th day of the menstrual cycle, the ovaries are examined daily by sonography to assess the number and size of developing ovarian follicles. When a follicle appears to be mature, a woman is given an injection of hCG, which causes ovulation in 38 to 42 hours.

A needle is then introduced intravaginally and guided by ultrasound, and the oocyte is aspirated from its follicle. Because of the drugs given to induce ova maturation, many oocytes may ripen at once, and perhaps as many as 3 to 12 can be removed. The oocytes chosen are incubated for at least 8 hours to ensure viability. In the meantime, the male partner or donor supplies a fresh or frozen semen specimen. The sperm cells and oocytes are mixed and allowed to incubate in a growth medium. Genetic analysis to reveal chromosomal abnormalities or the potential sex can be completed at this point.

In the past, many sperm were necessary even under laboratory conditions to allow sperm to make their way through the resistant zona pellucida surrounding the ovum. A number of techniques, such as creating passages through the resistant cells (i.e., zona drilling), have been discovered to help sperm cross the zona. In some instances, it has been possible to inject sperm directly under the zona pellucida (i.e., intracytoplasmic sperm injection). This is the technique that makes it possible for fertilization to take place with only one sperm. Worry that this technique could lead to an increased number of birth defects is unproven (Thornhill, Fanning, Davis, et al., 2015).

After fertilization of the chosen oocytes occurs, the zygotes formed almost immediately begin to divide and grow. By 40 hours after fertilization, they will have undergone their first cell division. In the past, multiple eggs were chosen and implanted to ensure a pregnancy resulted, but this technique also resulted in many multiple births. Because newborns from multiple births have a much smaller chance of surviving the neonatal period than others, today if a woman is under 35 years of age, only one or two fertilized eggs are chosen and transferred back to her uterine cavity through the cervix by means of a thin catheter. In women age 40 years, up to five embryos may be transferred (Duke & Christianson, 2015) (Fig. 7.5).

Figure 7.5 Steps involved in in vitro fertilization. **(A)** Ovulation. **(B)** Capture of ova (done here intra-abdominally). **(C)** Fertilization of ova and growth in culture medium. **(D)** Insertion of fertilized ova into uterus.

If the couple desires, any eggs that are not used can be cryopreserved for use at a later time. As with sperm cryopreservation, egg cryopreservation presents a range of ethical and religious dilemmas as to who should "own" them if the couple should divorce or disagree about their disposal at a later date.

A lack of progesterone can occur if the corpus luteum was injured by the aspiration of the follicle. Therefore, progesterone or LH may be prescribed to a woman following IVF if it is believed she will not produce enough on her own to support implantation. Proof the zygote has implanted can be demonstrated by a routine serum pregnancy test as early as 11 days after transfer. A few women develop an ovarian hyperstimulation syndrome with IVF. Their ovaries become swollen and painful and they may have accumulating abdominal and lung fluid. Women need to report these symptoms so ovarian stimulation can be halted until their ovaries return to normal; removing a number of oocytes and cryopreserving them can reduce the need for further stimulation with future procedures (Thomsen & Humaidan, 2015).

In some centers, nurse practitioners are the healthcare providers who complete oocyte removal and transfer. In all centers, nurses have a responsibility to supply support and counseling to help sustain a couple through the process. The recovery rate for harvesting ripened eggs is high (about 90%), as is the ability to fertilize eggs by sperm in vitro. However, the overall live birth rate by IVF is as low as 41% to 43% per treatment cycle for women under 35 years; it is as low as 13% to 18% for woman age 40 years (American Pregnancy Association, 2015).

About 25% of pregnancies end in spontaneous miscarriage (the same rate as for natural pregnancies). Once a pregnancy has been successfully established, a woman's prenatal care is the same as for any pregnancy, although the pregnancy may be categorized as high risk because women who have IVF procedures tend to be older than average, may be obese, and may have accompanying uterine concerns (Ensing, Abu-Hanna, Roseboom, et al., 2015). Because the couple was committed to the procedure, the typical couple adjusts to pregnancy and parenthood well. Encourage the woman and offer support for breastfeeding so she can be as successful with this as other women (de Lacey, Peterson, & McMillan, 2015).

If a sonogram reveals that a multiple pregnancy of more than two zygotes has been achieved, selective termination of gestational sacs until only two remain may be recommended to help ensure the pregnancy will come to term. This is done by intra-abdominal injection of potassium chloride into the gestational sacs chosen to be eliminated (Gupta, Fox, Feinberg, et al., 2015). This is obviously a difficult decision for a couple to agree upon, so they may need maximum support at this step.

IVF is expensive (about $12,000 to $17,000 per cycle) and is available only at specialized centers. A complication of maternal infection can occur if bacteria are introduced at any point in the transfer. Waiting to be accepted by a center's program and then waiting for the time to obtain the oocyte, allow for laboratory growth, and then pregnancy success is a major psychological strain. Couples report a feeling of social isolation during this time and weariness answering friends' and family's questions about when they will have a baby. Supply empathic support for them through this difficult time.

Box 7.8 illustrates interprofessional care map for nursing and team planning for a couple who are having difficulty conceiving a child.

GAMETE INTRAFALLOPIAN AND ZYGOTE INTRAFALLOPIAN TRANSFER

In gamete intrafallopian transfer (GIFT) procedures, ova are obtained from ovaries exactly as in IVF. Instead of waiting for fertilization to occur in the laboratory, however, both ova and sperm are instilled, within a matter of hours, using a laparoscopic technique, into the open end of a patent fallopian tube. Fertilization then occurs in the tube, and the zygote moves to the uterus for implantation. It requires at least one patent fallopian tube; it may be a preferred procedure by some couples because conception occurs in the fallopian tube and so is not contradictory to their religious beliefs.

Zygote intrafallopian transfer (ZIFT) is similar to IVF in that the egg is fertilized in the laboratory, but like GIFT, the fertilized egg is transferred by laparoscopic technique into the end of a waiting fallopian tube. Although available, this technique is little used today because of the extensive laparoscopic technique needed.

SURROGATE EMBRYO TRANSFER

Surrogate embryo transfer is an assisted reproductive technique for a woman who does not produce ova. For the process, the oocyte is donated by a friend, relative, or an anonymous donor (Check, Wilson, Levine, et al., 2015). The menstrual cycles of the donor and recipient are synchronized by administration of gonadotropic hormones. At the time of ovulation, the donor's ovum is removed by a transvaginal, ultrasound-guided procedure. The oocyte is then fertilized in the laboratory by the recipient woman's partner's sperm (or donor sperm) and placed in the recipient woman's uterus by embryonic transfer. Once pregnancy occurs, it progresses the same as an unassisted pregnancy.

QSEN Checkpoint Question 7.6

EVIDENCE-BASED PRACTICE

It is generally agreed that breast milk is the natural and best food for babies for the entire first year or at least until 6 months. To see if women who had babies through assisted reproductive techniques such as IVF choose to breastfeed as much as women having babies without an assisted technique, researchers interviewed 183 women who conceived using an assisted technique whether they breastfed their baby or not. Results showed that more women who conceived with the help of an assisted technique began breastfeeding than others (89.3% vs. 83.3%). By 3 months, however, a smaller number of women who had used an assisted technique were exclusively breastfeeding (46% vs. 57%); at 8 months, only 23% were still breastfeeding versus 57% of nonassisted women. Researchers attributed the decline in breastfeeding among women who used an assisted technique to more anxiety late in pregnancy and possibly to receiving suboptimal advice about assisted

BOX 7.8
Nursing Care Planning

AN INTERPROFESSIONAL CARE MAP FOR A COUPLE SEEKING A FERTILITY EVALUATION

Cheryl and Bob Carl married when they were both 25 years old. Three years later, they are now undergoing their second cycle of in vitro fertilization and embryo transfer. They have applied for a second mortgage on their house to finance the fertility testing. Today, at a visit, Mrs. Carl stated, "This is my fault because I'm so rigid. Look how I had to buy the house before I could even consider getting pregnant, and now we'll probably lose it. I've made our whole life revolve around trying to get pregnant instead of enjoying life."

Family Assessment: Couple live in three-bedroom, middle-income home; husband works as a bank manager; wife works as a receptionist in a medical office. Husband reports finances as "not good." Couple both appear discouraged about their apparent inability to have children.

Patient Assessment: Past medical history negative for any major health problems; wife reports a menstrual cycle of 5 days' duration with moderate flow every 30 to 37 days; never any dysmenorrhea. Used a combined estrogen/progestin oral contraceptive for 6 years; discontinued 3 years ago. Baseline laboratory studies and vital signs within normal limits.

Nursing Diagnosis: Situational low self-esteem related to seeming inability to conceive

Outcome Criteria: Couple verbalizes feelings about subfertility and effect on self-esteem; participates actively in care and treatment decisions; states they feel some control over situation and required treatment.

Team Member Responsible	Assessment	Intervention	Rationale	Expected Outcome
Activities of Daily Living, Including Safety				
Nurse	Assess couple's lifestyle to identify areas in which they are successful.	Review and reinforce with patient activities they have achieved successfully.	Identifying positive attributes can provide a foundation for rebuilding self-esteem.	Couple names at least three positive achievements, such as graduating from college or planting a garden.
	Assess if there is a common interest they could draw upon.	Ask couple to propose a new activity that would interest both of them.	Beginning a new activity can eliminate total concentration on fertility management.	Couple names and begins to participate in a new activity by 2 weeks' time.
Teamwork and Collaboration				
Nurse/social worker	Assess the couple's community for available community resources.	Ask couple if they would like a referral to a support group, such as Resolve.	A national organization can help provide effective support during a family crisis.	Couple confirms they have contacted an outside support group and have attended at least one meeting or online chat group.
Procedures/Medications for Quality Improvement				
Nurse/primary healthcare provider	Assess whether couple needs a review of IVF procedure and how their participation is important for success.	Encourage patients to ask questions about procedure; if prescribed an ovulation stimulant, review dosage, and administration schedule.	Fully informed patients are better able to participate in their own care.	Patients state they understand procedure and are interested in being an active part of it by asking questions and demonstrating successful medication adherence.

Continued on following page

BOX 7.8

Nursing Care Planning (continued)

Team Member Responsible	Assessment	Intervention	Rationale	Expected Outcome
Nutrition				
Nurse/ nutritionist	Assess whether couple ingests a healthy diet in light of busy lifestyle.	Remind patient to take prenatal vitamin (because of folic acid content) during fertility studies to be well prepared when pregnancy is achieved.	Folic acid is necessary in early pregnancy to help prevent neural tube anomalies. Overall health may contribute to fertility.	Patient demonstrates she has filled her prenatal vitamin prescription and confirms she takes them daily. Patient lists a healthy diet and states she does not smoke or take recreational drugs.
Patient-Centered Care				
Nurse	Assess whether couple is continuing to have a positive relationship in light of the diagnosis of unexplained subfertility.	Help partners review reasons they married, other than to have children.	Helping a couple find common interests can help them remain a couple and better prepare them for a parenting partnership.	Couple states they are taking steps to remain a close couple in light of the stress and possible negative results of assisted reproduction.
Spiritual/Psychosocial/Emotional Needs				
Nurse	Attempt to identify what it means to have unexplained subfertility for each patient, individually and as a couple.	Clarify any misconceptions patients may have about unexplained subfertility.	Misconceptions can negatively affect self-esteem.	Patients accurately describe situation and manifest adequate self-esteem.
Informatics for Seamless Healthcare Planning				
Nurse	Assess whether couple has any further questions about assisted reproduction and how they are active partners in the procedure. Assess for intimate partner violence.	It is common for assisted reproduction to be extremely stressful. After pregnancy is achieved, waiting for a much-desired pregnancy to come to term can be just as stressful.	Identifying and describing stressful situations can help the couple prepare for them. Unresolved, stress can lead to intimate partner violence.	Couple states they feel well equipped to manage whatever changes assisted reproduction brings to their life.
	Determine who the couple has to turn to for support outside of healthcare providers.	Discuss possible support persons and groups.	Additional support can assist in reinforcing positive attributes, thus enhancing self-esteem.	Patients list at least two persons or groups to use for support.

reproduction and breastfeeding from healthcare providers (Hammarberg, Fisher, Wynter, et al., 2011).

Based on the previous study, assuming Cheryl Carl's IVF is successful and she becomes pregnant, what would the nurse advise her during her pregnancy?

a. "You may be unable to breastfeed because with IVF, you develop immune factors."

b. "You should breastfeed as this will increase your fertility for a second pregnancy."

c. "After your child's birth, you should be able to begin breastfeeding effectively."

d. "Try not to worry; worry causes hormones necessary for vaginal birth to decrease."

Look in Appendix A for the best answer and rationale.

PREIMPLANTATION GENETIC DIAGNOSIS

The individual retrieval of oocytes and their fertilization under laboratory conditions has led to close inspection and recognition of differences in sperm and oocytes. After the oocytes are fertilized in IVF and ZIFT procedures, the DNA of both sperm and oocytes can be examined for specific genetic abnormalities such as Down syndrome or hemophilia (Dahdouh, Balayla, Audibert, et al., 2015).

Couples participating in intrauterine transfer and alternative insemination can also have the sex of their children predetermined using these methods. Such techniques can be useful because popular methods to influence the sex of a child (such as douching with a baking soda mixture before coitus to have a boy or with a vinegar solution to have a girl) have been proven to be more folklore than scientific fact. Allowing couples to choose the sex of children has ethical concerns because it could result in skewed male/female ratios if used by a majority of couples.

Alternatives to Childbirth

For some couples, even treatment for subfertility with procedures such as IVF is not successful. These couples need to consider still other options.

SURROGATE MOTHERS

A surrogate mother is a woman who agrees to carry a pregnancy to term for a subfertile couple or an LGBT couple (Dar, Lazer, Swanson, et al., 2015). The surrogate may provide the ova, which is then impregnated by the man's sperm in the laboratory. In other instances, the ova and sperm both may be donated by the subfertile couple; in a third technique, both donor ova and sperm are used. Surrogate mothers are often friends or family members who assume the role out of friendship or compassion, or they can be referred to the couple through an agency or attorney and receive monetary reimbursement for their expenses. The subfertile couple can enjoy the pregnancy as they watch it progress in the surrogate.

A number of ethical and legal problems arise if the surrogate mother decides at the end of pregnancy that she has formed an attachment to the fetus and wants to keep the baby despite the prepregnancy agreement she signed. Court decisions have been split on whether the surrogate or the subfertile couple has the right to the child. Another potential problem occurs if the child is born imperfect and the subfertile couple then no longer wants the child. Who should have responsibility in this instance? For these reasons, the couple and the surrogate mother must be certain they have given adequate thought to the process and to what will be the outcome should these problems occur before they attempt surrogate mothering.

ADOPTION

Adoption is an alternative for subfertile and LGBT couples, those individuals who have genetic-related health conditions or health conditions that would make pregnancy high risk. There are now fewer children available for adoption in the United States than there were in the past. Couples often consider physically or cognitively challenged children or children born outside the United States for adoption. The process of adoption is discussed in Chapter 3 with different types of families.

CHILD-FREE LIVING

Child-free living is another option available to both fertile and subfertile couples. For many subfertile couples who have been through the rigors and frustrations of subfertility testing and unsuccessful treatment regimens, child-free living may emerge as the option they finally wish to pursue. A couple in the midst of fertility testing may begin to reexamine their motives for pursuing pregnancy and may decide pregnancy and parenting are not worth the emotional or financial cost of future treatments. They may decide the additional stress of going through an adoption is not for them either, or they may simply decide children are not necessary for them to complete their family unit.

Child-free living can be as fulfilling as having children because it allows a couple more time to help other people and contribute to society through personal accomplishments. It has advantages for a couple in that it also allows time for both members to pursue careers. They can travel more or have more time and money to pursue hobbies or continue their education. If a couple still wishes to include children in their lives in some way, many opportunities are available to do this through family connections (most parents welcome offers from siblings or other family members to share in childrearing), through volunteer organizations (such as Big Brother or Big Sister programs), or through local schools and town recreational programs.

Many couples who believe overpopulation is a major concern choose child-free living even if subfertility is not present. Parents who choose child-free living typically rate their marriage as happier than for those with children probably because of the decreased expense involved and the availability of more free time, which allow them greater freedom in life (Avison & Furnham, 2015).

What If . . . 7.4
The nurse is particularly interested in exploring one of the 2020 National Health Goals with respect to subfertility (see Box 7.1). What would be a possible research topic to explore pertinent to this goal that would be applicable to the Carl family and that would also advance evidence-based practice?

KEY POINTS FOR REVIEW

- Subfertility is said to exist when a pregnancy has not occurred after 1 year of unprotected coitus. Sterility refers to the inability to conceive due to a known condition.

- About 14% of couples experience subfertility. The incidence increases with the age of the couple.

- Subfertility testing can be an intense psychological stressor for couples. Help couples to not only persist through the experience but also maintain their relationship as a couple.

- Couples who are told a subfertility problem has been discovered are apt to suffer a loss of self-esteem. Offering support to help them recognize that they are still productive, healthy people in other aspects of their lives helps in planning nursing care that not only meets QSEN competencies but best meets the family's total needs.

- Male factors that contribute to subfertility are inadequate sperm count, obstruction or impaired sperm motility, and problems with ejaculation. Female factors that cause subfertility are problems with ovulation, cervical or tubal transport, or impaired implantation.

- Basic subfertility assessment procedures consist of a health history; a physical examination; laboratory tests to document general health; and specific tests for semen, ovulation, tubal patency, and uterine environment.

- Measures to induce fertility are aimed at improving sperm number and transport, decreasing infections, stimulating ovulation, improving nutrition, and regulating hormones.

- Alternative insemination, donor egg transfer, IVF, adoption, surrogate motherhood, and child-free living are all possible solutions for subfertile and LGBT couples.

CRITICAL THINKING CARE STUDY

Laura, age 40 years, has had three miscarriages in the first trimester, and she and her husband are anxious to have their first child. She is considering a surrogate because she is worried she will have another miscarriage with a subsequent pregnancy.

1. What further information do you want to ask her to assist with her decision making?

2. How would you address her concerns about attempting another pregnancy?

3. Laura's husband prefers they adopt because he is unsure about using a surrogate. How would you address his concerns?

RELATED RESOURCES

Explore these additional resources to enhance learning for this chapter:
- Student resources on thePoint, including answers to the What If . . . and Critical Thinking Care Study questions, http://thepoint.lww.com/Flagg8e
- Adaptive learning powered by PrepU, http://thepoint.lww.com/prepu

REFERENCES

Agarwal, A., & Esteves, S. C. (2016). Varicocele and male infertility: Current concepts and future perspectives. *Asian Journal of Andrology, 18*(2), 161–162.

Allan, H., & Mounce, G. (2015). Managing infertility in primary care. *Practice Nursing, 26*(9), 440–443.

American Pregnancy Association. (2015). *In vitro fertilization.* Irving, TX: Author.

Araki, Y., Yao, T., Asayama, Y., et al. (2015). Single human sperm cryopreservation method using hollow-core agarose capsules. *Fertility and Sterility, 104*(4), 1004–1009.

Avison, M., & Furnham, A. (2015). Personality and voluntary childlessness. *Journal of Population Research, 32*(1), 45–67.

Bahadur, G., Ilahibuccus, A., Al-Habib, A., et al. (2015). Intrauterine insemination practice and the UK NICE guidelines. *Human Reproduction, 30*(5), 1277–1278.

Bailey, A. P., Jaslow, C. R., & Kutteh, W. H. (2015). Minimally invasive surgical options for congenital and acquired uterine factors associated with recurrent pregnancy loss. *Women's Health, 11*(2), 161–167.

Balen, A. (2012). Polycystic ovary syndrome and secondary amenorrhea. In D. K. Edmonds (Ed.), *Dewhurst's textbook of obstetrics & gynaecology* (8th ed., pp. 513–533). Malden, MA: Blackwell Publishing.

Best, D., & Bhattacharya, S. (2015). Obesity and fertility. *Hormone Molecular Biology and Clinical Investigation, 24*(1), 5–10.

Brezina, P. R., Ding, J., Ke, R. W., et al. (2015). Fertility preservation through oocyte cryopreservation in a patient with ovarian dysgerminocarcinoma: A case report. *Journal of Reproductive Medicine, 60*(9–10), 441–444.

Calderon, B., Gomez-Martin, J. M., Vega-Pinero, B., et al. (2016). Prevalence of male secondary hypogonadism in moderate to severe obesity and its relationship with insulin resistance and excess body weight. *Andrology, 4*(1), 62–67.

Campbell, J. M., Lane, M., Owens, J. A., et al. (2015). Paternal obesity negatively affects male fertility and assisted reproduction outcomes: A systematic review and meta-analysis. *Reproductive BioMedicine Online, 31*(5), 593–604.

Check, J. H., Wilson, C., Levine, K., et al. (2015). Improved implantation and live delivered pregnancy rates following transfer of embryos derived from donor oocytes by single injection of leuprolide in mid-luteal phase. *Clinical and Experimental Obstetrics & Gynecology, 42*(4), 429–430.

Dahdouh, E. M., Balayla, J., Audibert, F., et al. (2015). Technical update: Preimplantation genetic diagnosis and screening. *Journal of Obstetrics and Gynaecology Canada, 37*(5), 451–463.

Dar, S., Lazer, T., Swanson, S., et al. (2015). Assisted reproduction involving gestational surrogacy: An analysis of the medical, psychosocial and legal issues: Experience from a large surrogacy program. *Human Reproduction, 30*(2), 345–352.

de Lacey, S. L., Peterson, K., & McMillan, J. (2015). Child interests in assisted reproductive technology: How is the welfare principle applied in practice? *Human Reproduction, 30*(3), 616–624.

Duke, C. M. P., & Christianson, M. S. (2015). Infertility and assisted reproductive technologies. In J. L. Bienstock, H. Fox, E. E. Wallach, et al. (Eds.), *The Johns Hopkins manual of gynecology and obstetrics* (5th ed., pp. 467–484). Philadelphia, PA: Wolters Kluwer.

Ebrahimi-Mamaghani, M., Saghafi-Asl, M., Pirouzpanah, S., et al. (2015). Association of insulin resistance with lipid profile, metabolic syndrome, and hormonal aberrations in overweight or obese women with polycystic ovary syndrome. *Journal of Health, Population and Nutrition, 33*(1), 157–167.

Ecklund, L. C., & Usadi, R. S. (2015). Endocrine and reproductive effects of polycystic ovarian syndrome. *Obstetrics and Gynecology Clinics of North America, 42*(1), 55–65.

Ensing, S., Abu-Hanna, A., Roseboom, T. J., et al. (2015). Risk of poor neonatal outcome at term after medically assisted reproduction: A propensity score-matched study. *Fertility and Sterility, 104*(2), 384–390.

Fritz, M. A., & Speroff, L. (2010). Female infertility. In M. A. Fritz & L. Speroff (Eds.), *Clinical gynecologic endocrinology and infertility* (8th ed., pp. 1137–1191). Philadelphia, PA: Lippincott Williams & Wilkins.

Galhardo, A., Moura-Ramos, M., Cunha, M., et al. (2015). The infertility trap: How defeat and entrapment affect depressive symptoms. *Human Reproduction, 31*(2), 419–426.

Ghadir, S., Ambartsumyan, G., & Decherny, A. H. (2013). Infertility. In A. H. DeCherney, L. Nathan, T. M. Goodwin, et al. (Eds.), *Current diagnosis and treatment: Obstetrics and gynecology* (11th ed., pp. 879–888). Columbus, OH: McGraw-Hill/Lange.

Glina, S., Roehrborn, C. G., Esen, A., et al. (2015). Sexual function in men with lower urinary tract symptoms and prostatic enlargement secondary to benign prostatic hyperplasia: Results of a 6-month, randomized, double-blind, placebo-controlled study of tadalafil coadministered with finasteride. *The Journal of Sexual Medicine, 12*(1), 129–138.

Gupta, S., Fox, N. S., Feinberg, J., et al. (2015). Outcomes in twin pregnancies reduced to singleton pregnancies compared with ongoing twin pregnancies. *American Journal of Obstetrics and Gynecology, 213*(4), 580.e1–580.e5.

Hamilton, M. (2012). Infertility. In D. K. Edmonds (Ed.), *Dewhurst's textbook of obstetrics & gynaecology* (8th ed., pp. 567–579). Oxford, United Kingdom: Wiley.

Hammarberg, K., Fisher, J. R., Wynter, K. H., et al. (2011). Breastfeeding after assisted conception: A prospective cohort study. *Acta Paediatrica, 100*(4), 529–533.

Han, H., Liu, S., Zhou, X. G., et al. (2016). Aetiology of obstructive azoospermia in Chinese infertility patients. *Andrologia, 48*(7), 761–764.

Hasanpoor-Azghdy, S. B., Simbar, M., & Vedadhir, A. (2015). The social consequences of infertility among Iranian women: A qualitative study. *International Journal of Fertility and Sterility, 8*(4), 409–420.

Horovitz, D., Tjong, V., Domes, T., et al. (2012). Vasectomy reversal provides long-term pain relief for men with the post-vasectomy pain syndrome. *Journal of Urology, 187*(2), 613–617.

Karch, A. M. (2015). *Lippincott nursing drug guide.* Philadelphia, PA: Wolters Kluwer.

Kop, P. A., van Wely, M., Mol, B. W., et al. (2015). Intrauterine insemination or intracervical insemination with cryopreserved donor sperm in the natural cycle: A cohort study. *Human Reproduction, 30*(3), 603–607.

Kumar, N., & Singh, A. K. (2015). Trends of male factor infertility, an important cause of infertility: A review of literature. *Journal of Human Reproductive Sciences, 8*(4), 191–196.

Lo Monte, G., Capobianco, G., Piva, I., et al. (2015). Hysterosalpingo contrast sonography (HyCoSy): Let's make the point! *Archives of Gynecology and Obstetrics, 291*(1), 19–30.

Magos, A. (2012). Hysteroscopy and laparoscopy. In D. K. Edmonds (Ed.), *Dewhurst's textbook of obstetrics & gynaecology* (8th ed., pp. 448–470). Oxford, United Kingdom: Wiley.

Malacova, E., Kemp-Casey, A., Bremner, A., et al. (2015). Live delivery outcome after tubal sterilization reversal: A population-based study. *Fertility and Sterility, 104*(4), 921–926.

Niederberger, C. S. (2016). Male infertility. In A. J. Wein, L. R. Kavoussi, A. W. Partin, et al. (Eds.), *Campbell-Walsh urology* (11th ed., pp. 556–579). Philadelphia, PA: Elsevier.

Oman, S., & Burke, A. E. (2015). Family planning: Contraception, sterilization, and abortion. In J. L. Bienstock, H. Fox, E. E. Wallach, et al. (Eds.), *The Johns Hopkins manual of gynecology and obstetrics* (5th ed., pp. 421–438). Philadelphia, PA: Wolters Kluwer.

Read, S. C., Carrier, M., Whitley, R., et al. (2014). Complementary and alternative medicine use in infertility: Cultural and religious influences in a multicultural Canadian setting. *Journal of Alternative and Complementary Medicine, 20*(9), 686–692.

Sanabria-Martínez, G., García-Hermoso, A., Poyatos-León, R., et al. (2015). Effectiveness of physical activity interventions on preventing gestational diabetes mellitus and excessive maternal weight gain: A meta-analysis. *British Journal of Obstetrics and Gynecology, 122*(9), 1167–1174.

Shahrokhi, S. Z., Ghaffari, F., & Kazerouni, F. (2016). Role of vitamin D in female reproduction. *Clinica Chimica Acta, 455,* 33–38.

Sheth, S., & Keller, J. (2015). Infections of the genital tract. In J. L. Bienstock, H. Fox, E. E. Wallach, et al. (Eds.), *The Johns Hopkins manual of gynecology and obstetrics* (5th ed., pp. 356–378). Philadelphia, PA: Wolters Kluwer.

Thomsen, L., & Humaidan, P. (2015). Ovarian hyperstimulation syndrome in the 21st century: The role of gonadotropin-releasing hormone agonist trigger and kisspeptin. *Current Opinion in Obstetrics and Gynecology, 27*(3), 210–214.

Thornhill, J. A., Fanning, D. M., Davis, N. F., et al. (2015). Testicular sperm extraction and intracytoplasmic sperm injection: Outcomes in a specialist fertility centre. *Irish Medical Journal, 108*(9), 263–265.

Trew, G., & Lavery, S. (2012). Assisted reproduction. In D. K. Edmonds (Ed.), *Dewhurst's textbook of obstetrics & gynaecology* (8th ed., pp. 580–596). Oxford, United Kingdom: Wiley.

U.S. Department of Health and Human Services. (2010). *Healthy people 2020.* Washington, DC: Author.

Woo, I., & Yates, M. (2015). Menstrual disorders: Endometriosis, dysmenorrhea & premenstrual dysphoric syndrome. In J. L. Bienstock, H. Fox, E. E. Wallach, et al. (Eds.), *The Johns Hopkins manual of gynecology and obstetrics* (5th ed., pp. 503–512). Philadelphia, PA: Wolters Kluwer.

World Health Organization. (2010). *WHO laboratory manual for the examination & processing of human semen* (5th ed.). Geneva, Switzerland: Author.

Yue, F. G., Dong, L., Hu, T. T., et al. (2015). Efficacy of dapoxetine for the treatment of premature ejaculation: A meta-analysis of randomized clinical trials on intravaginal ejaculatory latency time, patient-reported outcomes, and adverse events. *Urology, 85*(4), 856–861.

8

The Nursing Role in Genetic Assessment and Counseling

*A*my Alvarez, 26 years old, is a woman you meet at a genetic counseling center. She was adopted as a newborn and never felt a need to locate her birth parents because her adoptive parents provided her with a "close-to-perfect" childhood. After college, she married the most eligible bachelor in her hometown. She is now pregnant with her first child. At 15 weeks into her pregnancy, after serum and sonography testing, she has been advised her child may have translocation Down syndrome. She asks you, "How could this happen? There's no disease like that in either of our families. Can you imagine how this will change my life?"

Previous chapters described common family types and how they are affected by sociocultural and community influences. This chapter discusses information about the necessary assessments, care, and guidelines for counseling of families if it is discovered there is a potential for a genetic disorder in the family. Such information can influence the health of a childbearing or childrearing family for generations to come.

How would you answer Amy?

KEY TERMS

alleles	genes	heterozygous
chromosomes	genetics	homozygous
cytogenetics	genome	karyotype
dermatoglyphics	genotype	phenotype

OBJECTIVES

After mastering the contents of this chapter, you should be able to:

1. Identify 2020 National Health Goals related to genetic disorders that nurses can help the nation achieve.
2. Assess a family for adjustment to the probability of inheriting a genetic disorder.
3. Formulate nursing diagnoses related to genetic disorders.
4. Establish expected outcomes that meet the needs of the family undergoing genetic assessment and counseling as well as manage seamless transitions across differing healthcare settings.
5. Using the nursing process, plan nursing care that includes the six competencies of Quality & Safety Education for Nurses (QSEN): Patient-Centered Care, Teamwork & Collaboration, Evidence-Based Practice (EBP), Quality Improvement (QI), Safety, and Informatics.
6. Implement nursing care such as counseling a family with a genetic disorder.
7. Evaluate expected outcomes for achievement and effectiveness of care.
8. Integrate knowledge of genetic disorders with the interplay of nursing process, the six competencies of QSEN, and Family Nursing to promote quality maternal and child health nursing care.

As many as 1 in 20 newborns inherits a genetic disorder. As many as 70% of pediatric hospital admissions may be for genetic-influenced disorders (Simpson, Holzgreve, & Driscoll, 2012). The possibility a child could have a genetic disorder crosses the minds of most pregnant women and their partners at some point during pregnancy, whether or not there is any family history of such disorders. This causes pregnant couples to ask healthcare providers about their chances of having a child with a genetic disorder and about genetic testing (Tasker, McClure, & Acerini, 2013).

Genetics is the study of the way such disorders occur. Because genetics is a constantly changing field of study, it is important for nurses to keep current with new advances so they can appreciate how a new discovery will affect a family and the child's therapy or if it could cure the child (Minear, Alessi, Allyse, et al., 2015). Twenty years ago, for example, most children with cystic fibrosis (a disorder of lung and pancreatic dysfunction) died in early childhood. Today, with good management, such children live into adulthood because the gene mutation that causes the disorder has been identified, giving hope for an eventual cure for this puzzling illness, including a new view of counseling (Prakash, Moore, & Yáñez-Muñoz, 2016).

Due to the Human Genome Project and the determination of the location of specific genes in the human genome, it has become a national priority to improve screening techniques for genetic disorders, and a number of 2020 National Health Goals speak to this area of maternal and child health (Box 8.1).

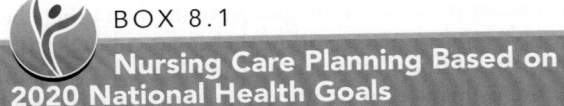

BOX 8.1

Nursing Care Planning Based on 2020 National Health Goals

A number of 2020 National Health Goals speak directly to genetic diseases and screening, including:

- Increase the number of states (and the District of Columbia) that verify through linkage with vital records all newborns are screened shortly after birth for conditions mandated by their state-sponsored screening program from 21% to 45%.
- Reduce the proportion of children diagnosed with a disorder through newborn blood spot screening who experience developmental delay requiring special education services from 15.1% to 13.6%.
- Increase the proportion of screen-positive children who receive follow-up testing within the recommended time period from 98.1% to 100%.
- Increase the proportion of youth with special healthcare needs whose healthcare provider has discussed transition planning from pediatric to adult health care from 41.2% to 45.3%.
- Reduce the number of children and youth with disabilities (aged 21 years and younger) living in congregate care residences from 28,890 to 26,001 (U.S. Department of Health and Human Services, 2010; see www.healthypeople.gov).

Nurses can help the nation achieve these goals by being sensitive to the need for and educating parents about genetic screening in preconception, prenatal, and birth settings.

Nursing Process Overview

FOR GENETIC ASSESSMENT AND COUNSELING

ASSESSMENT

Assessment measures for genetic disorders begin with a detailed family history, preferably of three generations; a physical examination of both the parents and any affected children; and an ever-growing series of laboratory assays of blood, amniotic fluid, and maternal and fetal cells. For example, in the first trimester, women are offered a routine sonogram screening (a nuchal translucency scan) and an analysis of maternal serum levels of α-fetoprotein (MSAFP), pregnancy-associated plasma protein A (PAPP-A), and free beta hCG to evaluate for chromosomal disorders in the fetus. (**Chromosomes** are threadlike structures of nucleic acids and protein found in the nucleus of most living cells, carrying genetic information in the form of genes.) Additionally, women over the age of 35 years may be offered a more accurate noninvasive blood test, circulating cell-free DNA (cfDNA) testing, to screen for chromosomal disorders. Chorionic villi sampling (CVS) and amniocentesis are both techniques that may be offered to women who are older than 35 years of age, or to those whose genetic testing is abnormal, to diagnose chromosomal genetic disorders. The CVS and amniocentesis are diagnostic tests that assess the **karyotype** (a graphic representation of the chromosomes present)—when fetal chromosomes are photographed and displayed, which can provide a definite answer about the presence or absence of chromosomal disorders. Couples who already know of the existence of a genetic disorder in their family or those who have had a previous child born with a congenital anomaly can opt for cfDNA testing, CVS, or amniocentesis, independent of their age, for more accurate screening and diagnosis of chromosomal disorders. Nurses serve as members of genetic assessment and counseling teams to help obtain the initial family history, assist with the physical examination, obtain blood serum for analysis, and assist with procedures such as amniocentesis as part of this process.

The decision to undergo either CVS or amniocentesis is a major one for a couple because, as a rule, they are not making a decision simply for CVS or amniocentesis; if the analysis from these reveals their child has a disorder, they then have to make a second decision about the future of the pregnancy.

Deciding to terminate a pregnancy based on a laboratory finding is rarely easy. If a couple decides to terminate the pregnancy, they need support for their decision to end the pregnancy. If they decide not to terminate the pregnancy, they may need support during the remainder of the pregnancy and in the days following birth. If a couple could not believe what the test showed was true, only when they inspect the baby and see the test was accurate—the child does have a genetic disorder—do they grasp the reality of what has happened. This can result in long-lasting depression, guilt, or grief for the perfect child they had hoped for at the beginning of the pregnancy.

NURSING DIAGNOSIS

Typical nursing diagnoses related to the area of genetic disorders include:

- Decisional conflict related to continuation of genetic-affected pregnancy
- Fear related to outcome of genetic screening tests
- Situational low self-esteem related to identified chromosomal disorder
- Deficient knowledge related to inheritance pattern of the family's inherited disorder
- Readiness for enhanced knowledge related to potential for genetic transmission of disease
- Altered sexuality pattern related to fear of conceiving a child with a genetic disorder

OUTCOME IDENTIFICATION AND PLANNING

Outcome identification and planning for families undergoing a genetic assessment differ according to the types of assessments performed and the results obtained. This may include determining what information the couple needs to know before testing can proceed or helping couples arrange for further assessment measures. When counseling such families, it is helpful to guide them to concentrate on short-term goals and actions or to help them look first at the immediate needs of their family, the fetus, and the newborn and later on at what type of continued follow-up will be necessary. For instance, after the birth, will the baby need to be hospitalized for immediate surgical correction of accompanying congenital anomalies, or will the parents be able to take the baby home? The kind of special schooling the child will need is a decision that can wait until later.

Help identify healthcare personnel with whom the parents will need to maintain contact during the next few months such as a surgeon or an orthopedist. Ensuring the parents have healthcare providers they know they can turn to, especially when they are moving out of the denial stage, helps them move forward to their next step in accepting their child's diagnosis faster.

It is also helpful to identify support people who can assist the parents during their time of disorganization. Support people may include the usual family resources, such as grandparents or other family members. In some families, however, these people are as disturbed by the diagnosis as the parents and therefore cannot offer their usual support. Refer parents to helpful websites and other resources when appropriate.

IMPLEMENTATION

Parental reactions to the knowledge their child has a possible genetic disorder or to the birth of a child with a genetically inherited disorder usually involves a grief reaction, similar to that experienced by parents whose child has died at birth (their "perfect" child is gone). Both parents may pass through stages of shock and denial ("This cannot be true"), anger ("It's not fair this happened to us"), and bargaining ("If only this would go away") before they reach reorganization and acceptance ("It has happened to us and it is all right"). For some couples, a genetic disorder is diagnosed during the pregnancy; for others, it may not be discovered until birth or possibly not even until the child is of school age. For these parents, these reactions will occur at that later point of diagnosis. Support couples in whatever stage they have reached when you care for them and help them work through and adjust to their child's diagnosis.

OUTCOME EVALUATION

Examples of expected outcomes for a family with a known genetic disorder include:

- Couple states they feel capable of coping no matter what the outcome of genetic testing.
- Patient accurately states the chances of a genetic disorder occurring in her next child.
- Couple states they have resolved their feelings of low self-esteem related to birth of a child with a genetic disorder.

A couple's decisions about genetic testing and childbearing do not necessarily remain constant. For example, a decision made at age 25 years not to have children because of a potential genetic disorder may be difficult to maintain at age 30 years because the couple sees many of their friends with growing families. Be certain such couples have the contact information of a genetic counselor. Urge them to call periodically for news of recent advances in genetic screening techniques or disease therapy so they can remain current and well informed for future planning.

Genetic Disorders

Inherited or genetic disorders are disorders that can be passed from one generation to the next because they result from some disorder in the gene or chromosome structure. Genetic disorders occur in some ethnic groups more than others because people tend to marry within their own cultural group (Box 8.2). In addition, concern is increasing that some genetic disorders may occur due to occupational hazards, such as toxic substances in the environment of workplaces (Kiku, Voronin, & Golokvhast, 2015).

Genetic disorders occur at the moment an ovum and sperm fuse or even earlier, in the meiotic division phase of the ovum or sperm when the chromosome count is halved from 46 to 23. Some genetic disorders are so severe that fetal growth cannot continue past that point. This early cell

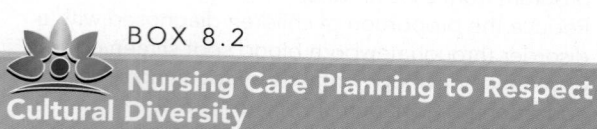

BOX 8.2

Nursing Care Planning to Respect Cultural Diversity

Different ancestry backgrounds cause different genetic disorders to be more common in some ethnic groups than in others. The blood disorder β-thalassemia, for example, occurs most frequently in families of Greek or Mediterranean heritage, whereas α-thalassemia occurs most often in persons from the Philippines or Southeast Asia. Sickle-cell anemia occurs most often in people with an African ancestry. Tay-Sachs disease, a deterioration of muscle and mental facilities, occurs most often in people of eastern Jewish ancestry.

It is important that families who are at high risk for particular genetic disorders such as these be informed of the incidence of these disorders among those of their ethnic heritage and offered genetic screening as appropriate during preconception counseling.

division is so precarious, in fact, that up to 50% of first trimester spontaneous miscarriages may occur as the result of chromosomal disorders (McNair & Altman, 2015). Other genetic disorders do not affect life in utero, so the result of the disorder only becomes apparent at the time of fetal testing or after birth. **Cytogenetics** is the study of chromosomes by light microscopy and the method by which chromosomal aberrations are identified.

Women having in vitro fertilization (IVF) can have both the egg and sperm examined for genetic disorders of single-gene or chromosome concerns before implantation. With ongoing stem cell research, it may be possible not only to identify aberrant genes for disorders this way but also to insert healthy genes in their place using stem cell implantation (Daughtry & Chavez, 2016). Gene replacement therapy is encouraging in the treatment of blood, neural tube, eye, and congenital metabolic disorders as well as for cancers and immunodeficiency syndromes (Kumar, Dunn, & Carcao, 2016; Wang, Liu, Xiang, et al., 2015).

Stem cells can be obtained from bone marrow (adult cells), embryos, or umbilical cord blood (embryonic stem cells). After giving birth, some women today privately bank or donate a sample of cord blood to a public stem cell bank so stem cells can be available for bone marrow or other cell transplantation procedures if someone in their community needs them. A second large source of adult stem cells for replacement therapy is menstrual blood; this also may be a contribution women can make toward stem cell research (Du, Yuan, Qu, et al., 2016).

Neither the American Congress of Obstetricians and Gynecologists (ACOG) nor the American Academy of Pediatrics (AAP) recommends private cord blood banking unless the family has a relative with a disorder known to be treatable by a stem cell transplant because banking is costly and the length of viability of stem cells is unknown, so an infant's own stem cells might not be available if the child should develop a disease in the future (Armitage, 2016).

NATURE OF INHERITANCE

Genes are the basic units of heredity that determine both the physical and cognitive characteristics of people. Composed of segments of DNA, they are woven into strands in the nucleus of all body cells to form chromosomes.

In humans, each cell, with the exception of the sperm and ovum, contains 46 chromosomes (44 autosomes and 2 sex chromosomes). Spermatozoa and ova each carry only half of the chromosome number (23 chromosomes). For each chromosome in a sperm cell, there is a like chromosome of similar size, shape, and function in the ovum. Because genes are always located at fixed positions on chromosomes, there are two like genes (**alleles**) on autosomes for every trait in the ovum and sperm. The one chromosome that does not have a mirror match is the chromosome for determining sex. If in the zygote formed from the union of a sperm and ovum, the sex chromosomes are both type X (large symmetric), the individual is genetically female (Fig. 8.1A). If one sex chromosome is an X and one a Y (a smaller type), the individual is genetically male (Fig. 8.1B).

A person's **phenotype** refers to his or her outward appearance or the expression of genes. A person's **genotype** refers to his or her actual gene composition. It is impossible to predict a person's genotype from the phenotype, or outward appearance.

A person's **genome** is the complete set of genes present (about 50,000 to 100,000). A normal genome is abbreviated

Figure 8.1 Photomicrographs of human chromosomes karyotypes. **(A)** A normal female karyotype. **(B)** A normal male karyotype.

Figure 8.2 Karyotype of trisomy 21. (Courtesy of Dr. Kathleen Rao, Dept. of Ped., UNC.)

as 46XX or 46XY (the designation of the total number of chromosomes plus a graphic description of the sex chromosomes present). If a chromosomal aberration exists, it is listed after the sex chromosome pattern. In such abbreviations, the letter *p* stands for short arm disorders and *q* stands for long arm disorders. For example, the abbreviation 46XX5p— is the abbreviation for a female with 46 total chromosomes but with the short arm of chromosome 5 missing (cri-du-chat syndrome). In Down syndrome, the person has an extra chromosome 21, so this is abbreviated as 47XX21+ or 47XY21+(Fig. 8.2).

MENDELIAN INHERITANCE: DOMINANT AND RECESSIVE PATTERNS

The principles of genetic inheritance of disease are the same as those that govern genetic inheritance of other physical characteristics, such as eye or hair color. These principles were discovered and described by Gregor Mendel, an Austrian naturalist, in the 1800s and are known as Mendelian laws.

A person who has two like genes for a trait—two healthy genes, for example (one from the mother and one from the father)—is said to be **homozygous** for that trait. If the genes differ (a healthy gene from the mother and an unhealthy gene from the father, or vice versa), the person is said to be **heterozygous** for that trait. Many genes are dominant in their action over others. When dominant genes are paired with nondominant (recessive) ones, the dominant genes are always expressed in preference to the recessive genes (a gene for brown eyes, for example, is dominant over one for blue eyes; a child born with a gene for brown eyes and a recessive one for blue eyes will have brown eyes). An individual with two homozygous genes for a dominant trait is said to be *homozygous dominant*; an individual with two genes for a recessive trait is said to be *homozygous recessive*.

Genetic Counseling and Testing

It is advantageous for an individual concerned with the possibility of transmitting a disease to his or her children to ask for genetic counseling at a preconception health visit for advice on the inheritance of disease because counseling can serve to:
- Provide concrete, accurate information about the process of inheritance and inherited disorders
- Reassure people who are concerned their child may inherit a particular disorder that the disorder will not occur
- Allow people who are affected by inherited disorders to make informed choices about future reproduction
- Allow people to pursue potential interventions that may exist such as fetal surgery
- Allow families to begin preparation for a child with special needs

Genetic counseling can result in making individuals feel "well" or free of guilt for the first time in their lives if they discover a disorder they were worried about is not an inherited one but rather occurred by chance.

In other instances, counseling can result in informing individuals they are carriers of a trait responsible for a child's condition. Even when people understand they had no control over this, knowledge about passing a genetic disorder to a child can cause guilt and self-blame. Marriages and relationships can end unless both partners receive adequate support.

It is essential that information revealed in genetic screening be kept confidential because such information could be used to damage a person's reputation or harm a future career or relationship. This necessity to maintain confidentiality prevents healthcare providers from alerting other family members about the inherited characteristic unless the member requesting genetic assessment has given consent for the information to be revealed. In some instances, a genetic history reveals information that a family doesn't want the other members to know, such as that a child has been adopted, is the result of alternative insemination, or that the current husband is not the child's father. The member of the family seeking counseling has the right to decide whether this information may be shared with other family members.

Keeping information secure is assured by the Genetic Information Nondiscrimination Act of 2008, which bars employers from using individuals' genetic information when making hiring, firing, job placement, or promotion decisions (Soo-Jin Lee & Borgelt, 2014). The act also prohibits group health plans and health insurers from denying coverage to a healthy individual or charging that person higher premiums based solely on a genetic predisposition to developing a disease in the future.

The ideal time for discussing whether the possibility of a genetic disorder exists is before a first pregnancy at a preconception health visit (Fletcher & Russo, 2015). Some couples take this step even before committing themselves to marriage, so they can offer not to involve their partner in a marriage if children of the marriage would be subject to a serious inherited disorder. Other couples first become aware of the need for genetic counseling after the birth of a first child with a disorder or fetal genetics testing (like first trimester screening, cfDNA, CVS, or amniocentesis) reveals that a chromosomal disorder may exist.

If a couple did not receive counseling before a first pregnancy, it is best if they receive it before a second pregnancy. A couple may not be ready for this, however, until the initial shock of their first child's condition and the grief reaction that may accompany it have run their course. Only then are they ready for information and decision making (Box 8.3).

BOX 8.3

Nursing Care Planning Based on Family Teaching

GENETIC SCREENING

Q. Amy Alvarez is anxious to have her fetus's health confirmed. She asks you, "Why do I have to wait so late in pregnancy for genetic studies by amniocentesis?"

A. A genetic analysis is done on skin cells obtained from amniotic fluid. The test cannot be scheduled until enough amniotic fluid is present for analysis, which is about the 15th week of pregnancy. Fortunately, it is possible to do an analysis of fetal red cells circulating in maternal blood very early (at about 10 weeks) in pregnancy.

Q. Why do laboratories take so long to return karyotyping results?

A. Karyotyping has traditionally (and by necessity) been done on cells at the metaphase (center phase) of division, so the laboratory had to delay testing until the cells had grown to reach this phase. New techniques now allow an analysis to be done immediately so results are available much sooner.

Q. If there are no inherited diseases in a couple's family, should the couple have a karyotype done "just to be sure" before they have their first baby?

A. A genetic analysis is not routinely recommended unless there is evidence or suspicion of genetic disease in the family. Remember, karyotyping reveals only diseases present on chromosomes. A "perfect" karyotype, therefore, doesn't guarantee a newborn will not be ill in a noninherited way.

Even if a couple decides not to have more children, be certain they know genetic counseling is available for them should their decision change. Also be certain they are aware that as their children reach reproductive age, they too may benefit from genetic counseling. Couples who are most apt to benefit from a referral for genetic testing or counseling include:

- *A couple who has a child with a congenital disorder or an inborn error of metabolism.* Many congenital disorders occur because of teratogenic invasion during pregnancy that has gone unrecognized. Learning the disorder occurred by a chance occurrence rather than inheritance is important because the couple will not have to spend the remainder of their childbearing years concerned another child may be born with the disorder (although a chance circumstance could occur again). If a definite teratogenic agent, such as a drug a woman took during pregnancy, can be identified, the couple can be advised about preventing this occurrence in a future pregnancy.

- *A couple whose close relatives have a child with a genetic disorder such as a chromosomal disorder or an inborn error of metabolism.* It is difficult to predict the expected occurrence of many "familial" or multifactorial disorders because they may involve more than one abnormal gene. In these instances, counseling should include educating the couple about the disorder, treatment available, and the prognosis or outcome of the disorder. Based on this information, the couple can make an informed reproductive choice about children.

- *Any individual who is a known carrier of a chromosomal disorder.* Understanding his or her own chromosome structure and the process by which future children could be affected can help such individuals make an informed choice about reproduction and also alert the person to the importance of fetal karyotyping during any future pregnancy. Box 8.4 shows an interprofessional care map illustrating both nursing and team planning for a woman concerned about genetic disorders.

- *Any individual who has an inborn error of metabolism or chromosomal disorder.* Any person with a disease should know the inheritance pattern of the disease and should be aware if prenatal diagnosis is possible for his or her particular disorder.

- *A consanguineous (closely related) couple.* The more closely related two people are, the more genes they have in common, so the more likely it is that a recessively inherited disease will be expressed. A brother and sister, for example, have about 50% of their genes in common; first cousins have about 12% of their genes in common.

- *Any woman older than 35 years of age and any man older than 55 years of age.* This is directly related to the association between advanced parental age and the occurrence of Down syndrome.

- *Couples of ethnic backgrounds in which specific illnesses are known to occur.* Mediterranean people, for example, have a high incidence of thalassemia, a blood disorder; those with a Chinese ancestry have a high incidence of glucose-6-phosphate dehydrogenase (G6PD) deficiency, a blood disorder where destruction of red cells can occur (Panepinto, Punzalan, & Scott, 2015).

BOX 8.4

Nursing Care Planning

AN INTERPROFESSIONAL CARE MAP FOR A COUPLE CONCERNED ABOUT GENETIC DISORDERS IN FUTURE CHILDREN

Amy Alvarez is a woman you meet at a genetic counseling center. She was adopted as a newborn and never felt a need to locate her birth parents because her adoptive parents provided a "close-to-perfect" childhood for her. After college, she married the most eligible bachelor in her hometown. She is now pregnant with her first child. At 15 weeks into her pregnancy, she has been advised that her child may have translocation Down syndrome. She asks you, "Why is this happening? There's no disease like this in either of our families."

Family Assessment: Patient's family history is unknown because she was adopted. Husband's family has no history of Down syndrome but does have two cousins who are cognitively challenged. Patient is presently attending law school. Husband works as a county public defender. Family lives in condo by lake front. Finances rated as "good."

Patient Assessment: Patient's and husband's past medical histories show no evidence of major health problems. Pregnancy is at 15 weeks. Maternal serum α-fetoprotein showed decreased level.

Nursing Diagnosis: Readiness for enhanced knowledge related to possible genetic disorder inheritance.

Outcome Criteria: Couple accurately states the cause of this genetic disorder and agrees to further genetic testing to confirm fetal diagnosis and describes range of options open to them so any decision they make regarding the pregnancy is an informed one.

Team Member Responsible	Assessment	Intervention	Rationale	Expected Outcome
Activities of Daily Living, Including Safety				
Nurse/nurse practitioner	Obtain a detailed history of the patient and spouse, including information about family members and other relatives.	Perform a physical examination to document current health.	A thorough history and physical examination provide baseline information to direct need for follow-up.	Couple participates fully in health examination, so family history obtained is as complete as possible.
Teamwork and Collaboration				
Nurse/genetic counselor	Assess whether couple would like to speak to an expert in the field of genetics to clarify their understanding.	Refer patient to genetic counselor so they can be aware of exact inheritance pattern and options available.	Couples cannot make informed choices without being aware of extent of problem.	Couple meets with genetic counselor within 1 week.
Procedures/Medications for Quality Improvement				
Nurse/primary healthcare provider	Perform genetic testing. Develop a family genogram for patient and spouse.	Be certain couple receives written documentation of chromosome disorder to take to genetic counselor.	A family genogram may provide additional information about the patient's and spouse's family histories.	Couple receives results of test in a timely and appropriate manner. A family genogram is developed and maintained with electronic health documentation.
Nutrition				
Nurse/dietitian	Assess the couple's nutrition patterns.	Analyze whether couple maintains healthy diet during testing and consultation period.	A healthy diet during pregnancy is important if pregnancy will be continued.	Patient confirms she continues to take prenatal vitamins and adequate protein intake.

Patient-Centered Care

Nurse/nurse practitioner	Ask couple if they have further questions about their particular inheritance pattern.	Review with the couple the mode of transmission and chances for manifesting Down syndrome in children.	Down syndrome may be inherited at a higher incidence in a balanced translocation carrier than in others.	Couple accurately describes the mode of transmission of Down syndrome.

Spiritual/Psychosocial/Emotional Needs

Nurse	Assess whether couple would be interested in contacting the hospital's religious counselor for support or learning activities to reduce stress.	If requested, instruct the couple in positive coping mechanisms. Include activities such as information sharing, relaxation and breathing exercises, and physical activity.	Positive coping mechanisms assist in controlling fear and minimizing its intensity, thus promoting effective problem solving.	Couple demonstrates positive coping mechanisms. Couple states the emotional support they received throughout their period of genetic screening and counseling was adequate.

Informatics for Seamless Healthcare Planning

Nurse/social worker	Assess community for support organizations available.	If the couple chooses to continue the pregnancy, refer them to national support group (e.g., Down Syndrome Foundation) and local parents support group.	Additional counseling and support may be necessary as pregnancy progresses. Community resources can help reduce feelings of isolation and loneliness.	Couple records the names and telephone numbers of support groups as well as the genetic counseling team and states they will keep numbers available if they should need further information.

NURSING RESPONSIBILITIES

Nurses play important roles in assessing for signs and symptoms of genetic disorders, in offering support to individuals who seek genetic counseling, and in helping with reproductive genetic testing procedures.

A great deal of time may need to be spent offering support for a grieving couple confronted with the reality of how tragically the laws of inheritance have affected their lives. Direct counseling is a role for nurses only if they are adequately prepared in the study of genetics, however, because without this background, genetic counseling can be dangerous and destructive (Box 8.5).

Whether one is acting as the nurse member of a genetic counseling team or as a genetic counselor, some common principles apply.

- The individual or couple being counseled needs a clear understanding of the information provided. People may listen to the statistics of their situation ("Your child has a 25% chance of having this disease") and construe a "25% chance" to mean if they have one child with the disease, they can then have three other children without any worry. A 25% chance, however, means *with each pregnancy*, there is a 25% chance the child will have the disease (chance has no "memory" of what has already happened). It is as if the couple had four cards, all aces, with the ace of spades representing the disease. When a card is drawn from the set of

BOX 8.5

Nursing Care Planning Tips for Effective Communication

Amy Alvarez tells you her mother has advised her not to have any more children rather than risk having another child with Down syndrome.

Tip: Reassure the patient while explaining the need for enough time to obtain accurate information. Because we live in an age in which information can be obtained quickly, people tend to believe predictions about the inheritance of disorders can also be supplied quickly. Because Amy is a balanced translocation carrier, more aspects than her age must be considered when predicting her chance for having children with Down syndrome.

Nurse: Hello, Amy. What's the reason you've come to the clinic today?

Amy: I need to know what is the chance all my children will have Down syndrome.

Nurse: That isn't the kind of question I can answer off the top of my head. Let me ask you some questions about your family to get started and then we can talk to a genetic counselor to get your answer.

four, the chance of it being the ace of spades is one in four (25%). When the couple is ready to have a second child, it is as if the card drawn during the first round is returned to the set, so the chance of drawing the ace of spades in the second draw is exactly the same as in the first draw. Similarly, the couple's chance of having a child with the disease remains one in four in each successive pregnancy.

- It is never appropriate for a healthcare provider to impose his or her own values or opinions on others. Individuals with known inherited diseases in their family must face difficult decisions, such as how much genetic testing to undergo or whether to terminate a pregnancy that will result in a child with a specific genetic disease. Be certain couples have been told all the options available to them and then leave them to think about the options and make their decision by themselves. Help them to understand that no one is judging their decision because they are the ones who must live with the decision in the years to come.

QSEN Checkpoint Question 8.2

EVIDENCE-BASED PRACTICE

If it is predicted during a pregnancy that a couple will have a child with Down syndrome, the couple is asked to make a choice whether they want to continue the pregnancy or terminate it at that point. To discover how couples feel about having a child with Down syndrome, researchers surveyed 2,044 parents on the mailing lists of six nonprofit Down syndrome organizations. The majority of parents reported they are happy with their decision to have their child and find their sons and daughters great sources of love and pride. Ninety-nine percent reported they love their affected son or daughter, 97% reported being proud of them, 79% felt their outlook on life was more positive because of them, only 5% felt embarrassed by them, and only 4% regretted having them. In a following study, siblings also reported their relationship with their affected sibling as a positive one. Less than 10% felt embarrassed, and less than 5% expressed a desire to trade their sibling in for another brother or sister (Skotko, Levine, & Goldstein, 2011a, 2011b).

Based on the findings of the previous studies, how would the nurse answer Mrs. Alvarez's question, "Can you imagine how this will change my life?"

a. "You're right. Having a genetically affected child can potentially be a serious burden."
b. "Don't worry so much about what others think; just concentrate on your own life."
c. "Change can create good things in life; I believe as a door closes, a window opens."
d. "Would it help if you talk to a family who has a child with Down syndrome?"

Look in Appendix A for the best answer and rationale.

THE ASSESSMENT FOR GENETIC DISORDERS

A genetic assessment begins with careful study of the pattern of inheritance in a family. A history, physical examination of family members, and laboratory analysis, such as karyotyping or DNA analysis, are performed to define the extent of the problem and the chance of inheritance. Parents can obtain a DNA analysis from a profit-making private laboratory (direct-to-consumer marketing), but this is rarely advised because genetic results usually need to be accompanied by counseling to be certain parents understand the often-complicated result narrative.

History

Taking a health history for a genetic diagnosis can be difficult because the facts detailed may evoke uncomfortable emotions such as sorrow, guilt, or inadequacy in parents. Try, however, to obtain information and document diseases in family members for a minimum of three generations because a history can be a chief tool in discovering transmitted disorders (Edelman, Lin, Doksum, et al., 2014). Remember to include half brothers and sisters or anyone related in any way as family. Document the mother's age because some disorders increase in incidence with age. Document also whether the parents are consanguineous or related to each other.

Documenting the family's ethnic background can reveal risks for certain disorders that occur more commonly in some ethnic groups than others. If the couple seeking counseling is unfamiliar with their family history, ask them to talk to senior family members about other relatives (grandparents, aunts, uncles) before they come for an interview about such instances as spontaneous miscarriage or children in the family who died at birth. In many instances, these children died of unknown chromosomal disorders or were miscarried because of 1 of the 70 or more known chromosomal disorders inconsistent with life.

Many people have only sketchy information about their families, such as "The baby had some kind of nervous disease" or "Her heart didn't work right." Attempt to obtain as much information as you can by asking the couple to describe the appearance or activities of the affected individual ("She had no left side to her heart") or asking for permission to obtain health records.

An extensive prenatal history of any affected person should be obtained to determine whether environmental conditions could account for the condition. Based on the previous information, draw a family genogram (Fig. 8.3). Such a diagram helps to not only identify the possibility of a chromosomal disorder occurring in a particular couple's children but also identify other family members who might benefit from genetic counseling.

When a child is born dead, parents are advised to have a chromosomal analysis and autopsy performed on the infant. If, at some future date, they wish genetic counseling, this would allow their genetic counselor to have additional medical information.

Physical Assessment

Because genetic disorders often occur in varying degrees of expression, a careful physical assessment of any family member with a disorder, that person's siblings, and the couple seeking counseling is necessary because it is possible that

Female with disease

Male with disease

Well male

Figure 8.3 Family genogram: X-linked dominant inheritance.

TABLE 8.1 COMMON PHYSICAL CHARACTERISTICS OF CHILDREN WITH CHROMOSOMAL SYNDROMES

Characteristic	Probable Syndrome
Late closure of fontanelles	Down syndrome
Bossing (prominent forehead)	Fragile X syndrome
Microcephaly (small head)	Trisomy 18, trisomy 13
Low-set ears	Trisomy 18, trisomy 13
Slant of eyes	Down syndrome
Epicanthal fold	Down syndrome
Abnormal iris color	Down syndrome
Large tongue	Down syndrome
Prominent jaw	Fragile X syndrome
Low-set hairline	Turner syndrome
Multiple hair whorls	Trisomy 18, trisomy 13
Webbed neck	Turner syndrome
Wide-set nipples	Trisomy 13
Heart disorders	Many syndromes
Large hands	Fragile X syndrome
Clinodactyly (curved little finger)	Down syndrome
Overriding of fingers	Trisomy 18
Rocker-bottom feet	Trisomy 18
Abnormal dermatoglyphics (fingerprints)	Down syndrome
Simian crease on palm	Down syndrome
Absence of secondary sex characteristics	Klinefelter syndrome, Turner syndrome

another family member has such a minimal expression of the disorder, it has gone previously undiagnosed. During inspection, pay particular attention to certain body areas, such as the space between the eyes; the height, contour, and shape of ears; the number of fingers and toes; and the presence of webbing because these often suggest structural genetic disorders. **Dermatoglyphics** (the study of surface markings of the skin) is also helpful because unusual fingerprints, abnormal palmar creases, hair whorls, or coloring of hair are also present with some disorders.

Careful inspection of newborns is often the first time a child with a potential chromosomal disorder is identified. Infants with multiple congenital anomalies, those born at less than 35 weeks gestation, and those whose parents have had other children with chromosomal disorders need extremely close assessment. Table 8.1 lists the physical characteristics suggestive of some common inherited syndromes in children.

Screening and Diagnostic Testing

Many screening and diagnostic tests are available to provide clues or to diagnose disorders. Before pregnancy, DNA analysis or karyotyping of both parents and an already affected child provides a picture of the family's genetic pattern and can be used for prediction in future children. Once a woman is pregnant, several other tests may be performed to help in the prenatal diagnosis of a genetic disorder. These include first trimester nuchal translucency and hormonal screening, cfDNA testing, quadruple test analysis, CVS, amniocentesis, percutaneous umbilical blood sampling (PUBS), and sonography. All of these tests not only reveal important information but also create ethical and personal concerns for parents because, if an abnormality is discovered, parents are asked to make a decision whether to continue the pregnancy (Hume & Chasen, 2015). Table 8.2 highlights these screening techniques and diagnostic tests.

What If . . . 8.1
Amy tells the nurse, "My family will be so ashamed if a genetic defect happens in our family." What does her statement tell the nurse about her family's knowledge of genetic disorders?

REPRODUCTIVE ALTERNATIVES

Some couples are reluctant to seek genetic counseling because they are afraid they will be told it would be unwise to have children. Helping them to realize viable alternatives for having a family exist can allow them to seek the help they need.

Alternative insemination by donor (AID) is an option for couples if the genetic disorder is one inherited by the male partner or is a recessively inherited disorder carried by both partners. AID is available in all major communities and can permit the couple to experience the satisfaction and enjoyment of a usual pregnancy (Duke & Christianson, 2015).

If the inherited problem is one arising from the female partner, surrogate embryo transfer is an assisted reproductive technique that is a possibility (Check, Wilson, Levine, et al., 2015). For this, an oocyte is donated by a friend or relative or provided by an anonymous donor, which is then fertilized by the male partner's sperm in the laboratory and implanted into a woman's uterus. Like AID, donor embryo transfer offers the couple a chance to experience a usual pregnancy.

Use of a surrogate mother (a woman who agrees to be alternately inseminated, typically by the male partner's sperm, and bear a child for the couple) is yet another possibility (Dar, Lazer, Swanson, et al., 2015). All of these procedures are expensive and, depending on individual circumstances, may have disappointing success rates. Assisted reproductive techniques are discussed in more detail in Chapter 7.

TABLE 8.2 GENETIC DISORDER SCREENING AND DIAGNOSTIC TESTS

Test Type	Timing	Process	Risks	Results
Preimplantation diagnosis	Day 3 or day 5 embryo	Cell sample obtained from day 3 or day 5 embryo prior to implantation in mother during in vitro fertilization process	Invasive to embryo, risk of destruction of embryo	Only 9–11 of chromosomes can be evaluated from sample.
Nuchal translucency	11–14 weeks	Ultrasound to assess thickness at fetus's neck, maternal blood draw	Noninvasive, ultrasound and maternal blood draw	Screening test for Down syndrome, trisomy 18 and 13
cfDNA	11+ weeks, can be done as early as 7 weeks	Maternal blood draw, fetal cell fragments in maternal blood are assessed	Noninvasive, maternal blood draw	Screening test for abnormal amounts of chromosomes and microdeletions in fetal DNA
Chorionic villi sampling	10–12 weeks	Biopsy of placenta (Fig. 8.4)	Invasive, risk of miscarriage	Diagnostic test for karyotype (Fig. 8.1)
Maternal quadruple marker screen	15–20 weeks	Maternal blood draw	Noninvasive, maternal blood draw	Screening test for Down syndrome, trisomy 18 and 13
Amniocentesis	15–18 weeks	Collection of amniotic fluid containing fetal skin cells through maternal abdomen	Invasive, risk of miscarriage	Diagnostic for fetal karyotype; Table 8.3 shows common chromosomal disorders that can be diagnosed through amniocentesis.
Percutaneous umbilical blood sampling	>17 weeks	Fetal umbilical blood sampling through maternal abdomen (Fig. 8.5)	Invasive, risk of miscarriage	Diagnostic for fetal karyotype and fetal blood diseases
Fetal anatomy ultrasound	18–22 weeks, ideal timing	Ultrasound of the fetal anatomy	Noninvasive, ultrasound	Screening test for visual fetal anomalies (cleft lip, etc.)
Fetoscopy	Second and third trimesters	Small camera and instruments passed into the amniotic sac to view and treat anomalies	Invasive, risk of miscarriage	Often used to treat disorders like twin-to-twin transfusion
Newborn screening	Day 2–several weeks after birth	A blood sample via heel prick or blood draw from newborn	Noninvasive, blood draw from newborn	Screening for genetic disorders via serum DNA or other factors

cfDNA, cell-free DNA.

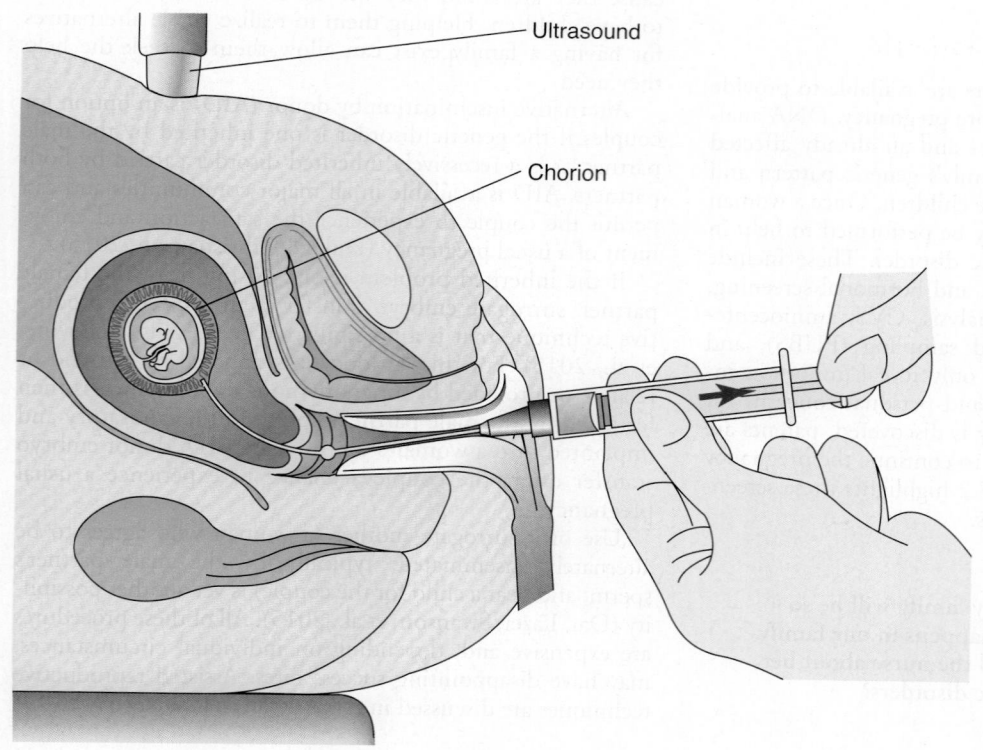

— Ultrasound

— Chorion

Figure 8.4 Chorionic villi sampling. Because the villi arise from trophoblast cells, their chromosome structure is the same as in the fetus.

TABLE 8.3 COMMON GENETIC DISORDERS THAT CAN BE DETECTED BY MATERNAL SERUM, AMNIOCENTESIS, OR CHORIONIC VILLUS SAMPLING

Syndrome	Chromosomal Characteristics	Clinical Signs in Child
Down syndrome	Extra chromosome 21	Cognitively challenged
		Protruding tongue
		Epicanthal folds
		Hypotonia
Translocation Down syndrome	Translocation of a chromosome, perhaps 21/14	Same clinical signs as trisomy 21
Trisomy 18	Extra chromosome 18	Cognitively challenged
		Congenital malformations
Trisomy 13	Extra chromosome 13	Cognitively challenged
		Multiple congenital malformations
		Eye agenesis
Cri-du-chat syndrome	Deletion of short arm of chromosome 5	Cognitively challenged
		Facial structure anomalies
		Peculiar catlike cry
Fragile X syndrome	Distortion of the X chromosome	Cognitively challenged
Philadelphia chromosome	Deletion of one arm of chromosome 21	Chronic granulocytic leukemia
Turner syndrome	Only one X chromosome present (45XO)	Short stature
		Streak ovaries
		Infertility
		Webbed neck
Klinefelter syndrome	An extra X chromosome present (47XXY)	Small testes
		Gynecomastia
		Subfertility

Figure 8.5 Percutaneous umbilical blood sampling. Blood is withdrawn from the umbilical cord using an amniocentesis technique.

Adoption is an alternative many couples can also find rewarding (see Chapter 3). Lastly, choosing to remain child free should not be discounted as a viable option. Many couples who have every reason to think they will have healthy children choose this alternative because they believe their existence is full and rewarding without the presence of children.

Diagnosis of a disorder during pregnancy with prompt treatment at birth to minimize the prognosis and outcome of the disorder is another route to explore. Termination of a pregnancy that reveals a chromosomal or metabolic disorder is also an option.

Help couples decide on a solution that is correct for them, not one they sense you or a counselor feels would be best. They need to consider the ethical philosophy or beliefs of other family members when making their decision, although ultimately, they must do what they believe is best for them as a couple. A useful place to start counseling is with values clarification, to be certain a couple understands what is most important to them.

FUTURE POSSIBILITIES

Stem cell research is looking at the possibility immature cells from a healthy embryo (stem cells) could be implanted into an embryo with a known abnormal genetic makeup, replacing the abnormal cells or righting the affected child's genetic composition (Davidson, Mason, & Pera, 2015). Although presently possible, stem cell research is costly and produces some ethical questions (e.g., Is it ethical to change the life course of a fetus who has no rights? Is it ethical to use embryo cells as a source of stem cells?).

LEGAL AND ETHICAL ASPECTS OF GENETIC SCREENING AND COUNSELING

Nurses can be instrumental in making sure couples who seek genetic counseling receive results in a timely manner and with compassion about what the results may mean to future childbearing. Always keep in mind several legal responsibilities of genetic testing, counseling, and therapy including:

- Participation by couples or individuals in genetic screening must be elective.
- People desiring genetic screening must sign an informed consent for the procedure.
- Results must be interpreted correctly yet provided to the individuals as quickly as possible.
- The results must not be withheld from the individuals and must be given only to those persons directly involved.
- After genetic counseling, persons must not be coerced to undergo procedures such as abortion or sterilization. Any procedure must be a free and individual decision.

Failure to heed these guidelines could result in charges of invasion of privacy, breach of confidentiality, or psychological injury caused by "labeling" someone or imparting unwarranted fear and worry about the significance of a disease or carrier state. If couples are identified as being at risk for having a child with a genetic disorder and are not informed of the risk and offered an appropriate diagnostic procedure such as amniocentesis during a pregnancy, they can bring a "wrongful birth" lawsuit if their child is born with the unrevealed genetic disorder.

 What If . . . 8.2
Amy Alvarez is pregnant with twins. One twin fetus is diagnosed as having Down syndrome and the other is not. How would the nurse counsel her if she wanted to abort the affected child when the procedure also might endanger the child without the disorder?

Unfolding Patient Stories: Amelia Sung • Part 1

 Amelia Sung is 36 years old and 8 weeks pregnant with her second child. She tells the nurse that she is considering an amniocentesis due to her age. What information would the nurse include when providing education on an amniocentesis? (Amelia Sung's story continues in Chapter 20.)
Care for Amelia and other patients in a realistic virtual environment: *vSim for Nursing* (thepoint.lww.com/vSim MaternityPed). Practice documenting these patients' care in DocuCare (thepoint.lww.com/DocuCareEHR).

Common Chromosomal Disorders Resulting in Physical or Cognitive Developmental Disorders

A number of chromosomal disorders are easily detected at birth on physical examination. Many of these disorders leave children cognitively challenged (discussed in Chapter 54).

Figure 8.6 An infant with trisomy 13 syndrome has **(A)** a cleft lip and palate and **(B)** supernumerary digits (polydactyly). (© NMSB/Custom Medical Stock Photograph.)

TRISOMY 13 SYNDROME (47XY13+ OR 47XX13+)

In trisomy 13 syndrome (Patau syndrome), the child has an extra chromosome 13 and is severely cognitively challenged. The incidence of the syndrome is low, approximately 0.45 per 1,000 live births. Midline body disorders such as cleft lip and palate, heart disorders (particularly ventricular septal defects), and abnormal genitalia are present. Other common findings include microcephaly with disorders of the forebrain and forehead, eyes that are smaller than usual (microphthalmos) or absent, and low-set ears (Gezer, Ekin, Gezer, et al., 2015). Most of these children do not survive beyond early childhood (Fig. 8.6).

TRISOMY 18 SYNDROME (47XY18+ OR 47XX18+)

Children with trisomy 18 syndrome (Edwards syndrome) have three copies of chromosome 18. The incidence is approximately 0.23 per 1,000 live births. These children are severely cognitively challenged and tend to be small for gestational age, have markedly low-set ears, a small jaw, congenital heart defects, and usually misshapen fingers and toes (the index finger deviates or crosses over other fingers). Also, the soles of their feet are often rounded instead of flat (rocker-bottom feet). As in trisomy 13 syndrome, most of these children do not survive beyond infancy (Karaman, Aydin, & Göksu, 2015).

CRI-DU-CHAT SYNDROME (46XX5P− OR 46XY5P−)

Cri-du-chat syndrome is the result of a missing portion of chromosome 5. In addition to an abnormal cry, which sounds much more like the sound of a cat than a human infant's cry, children with cri-du-chat syndrome tend to have a small head, wide-set eyes, a downward slant to the palpebral fissure of the eye, and a recessed mandible. They are severely cognitively challenged (Levy & Marion, 2015).

TURNER SYNDROME (45X0)

The child with Turner syndrome (gonadal dysgenesis) has only one functional X chromosome. The child is short in stature and has only streak (small and nonfunctional) ovaries. She is sterile and, with the exception of pubic hair, secondary sex characteristics do not develop at puberty. The hairline at the nape of the neck is low set, and the neck may appear to be webbed and short (Fig. 8.7). A newborn may have appreciable edema of the hands and feet and a number of congenital anomalies, most frequently coarctation (stricture) of the aorta as well as kidney disorders. The incidence of the syndrome is approximately 1 per 10,000 live births. The disorder can be identified on a sonogram during pregnancy (a nuchal translucency scan) because of the extra skin at the sides of the neck (Levy & Marion, 2015).

Although children with Turner syndrome may be severely cognitively challenged, difficulty in this area is more commonly limited to learning disabilities. Socioemotional adjustment problems may accompany the syndrome because of the lack of fertility and if the nuchal folds are prominent.

Human growth hormone administration can help children with Turner syndrome achieve additional height (Ranke, 2015). If treatment with estrogen is begun at approximately 13 years of age, secondary sex characteristics will appear, and osteoporosis from a lack of estrogen during growing years may be prevented. If females continue taking estrogen for 3 out of every 4 weeks, this produces withdrawal bleeding which

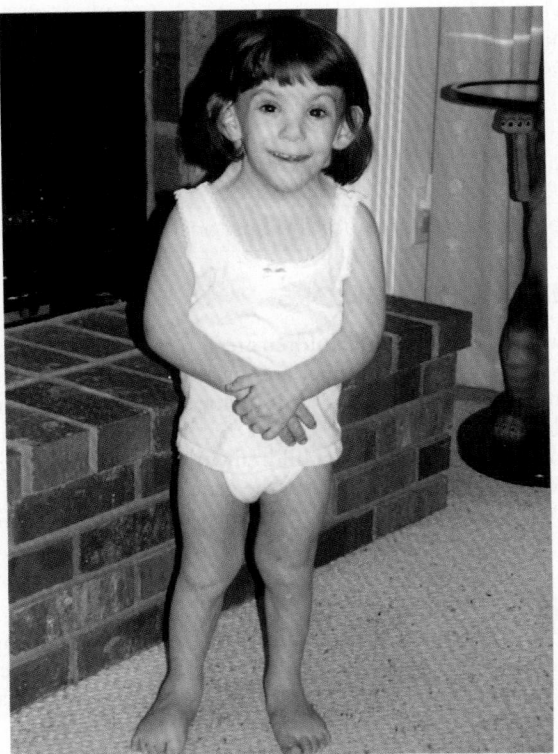

Figure 8.7 A 3-year-old with Turner syndrome. Note the wide neck folds.

results in a menstrual flow. This flow, however, does not correct the basic problem of sterility; ovarian tissue is scant and inadequate for ovulation because of the basic chromosomal aberration. A woman with Turner syndrome could, however, have IVF with surrogate oocyte transfer in order to become pregnant (Levitsky, Luria, Hayes, et al., 2015).

KLINEFELTER SYNDROME (47XXY)

Children with Klinefelter syndrome are males with an extra X chromosome. Characteristics of the syndrome may not be noticeable at birth. At puberty, secondary sex characteristics do not develop; the child's testes remain small and produce ineffective sperm (Palma Sisto & Heneghan, 2015). Affected individuals tend to develop gynecomastia (increased breast size) and have an increased risk of male breast cancer. The incidence of the syndrome is about 1 per 1,000 live births. Karyotyping can be used to reveal the additional X chromosome.

FRAGILE X SYNDROME (46XY23Q−)

Fragile X syndrome is the most common cause of cognitive challenge in males. It is an X-linked disorder in which one long arm of an X chromosome is defective, which results in inadequate protein synaptic responses (Contractor, Klyachko, & Portera-Cailliau, 2015). The incidence of the syndrome is about 1 in 4,000 males.

Before puberty, boys with fragile X syndrome may typically demonstrate maladaptive behaviors such as hyperactivity, aggression, or autism. They may have reduced intellectual functioning, with marked deficits in speech and arithmetic (Vekeman, Gauthier-Loiselle, Faust, et al., 2015). On physical exam, frequent findings identified are a large head, a long face with a high forehead, a prominent lower jaw, large protruding ears, and obesity. Hyperextensive joints and cardiac disorders may also be present. After puberty, enlarged testicles may become evident. Affected individuals are fertile and can reproduce.

Carrier females may show some evidence of the physical and cognitive characteristics. Although intellectual function from the syndrome cannot be improved, a combination of stimulants, α agonists, atypical antipsychotics, and serotonin reuptake inhibitors may improve symptoms of poor concentration and impulsivity (Espinel, Charen, Huddleston, et al., 2015).

DOWN SYNDROME (TRISOMY 21) (47XY21+ OR 47XX21+)

Trisomy 21, the most frequently occurring chromosomal disorder, occurs in about 1 in 800 pregnancies. In women who are older than 35 years of age, the incidence is as high as 1 in 100 live births (Levy & Marion, 2015).

The physical features of children with Down syndrome are so marked that fetal diagnosis is possible by sonography in utero. The nose is broad and flat. The eyelids have an extra fold of tissue at the inner canthus (an epicanthal fold), and the palpebral fissure (opening between the eyelids) tends to slant laterally upward. The iris of the eye may have white specks, called Brushfield spots. The tongue is apt to protrude from the mouth because the oral cavity is smaller than usual. The back of the head is flat, the neck is short, and an extra pad of fat at the base of the head causes the skin to be so loose it can be lifted easily and so thin it can be revealed on a fetal sonogram (Fig. 8.8A).

The ears may be low set. Muscle tone is poor, giving the newborn a rag doll appearance. This muscle tone can be so

Figure 8.8 **(A)** Typical facial features of a child with Down syndrome. **(B)** A simian line, a horizontal crease seen in children with Down syndrome. (© SPL/Custom Medical Stock Photograph.)

lax that the child's toe can be touched against the nose (not possible in the average mature newborn). The fingers of many children with Down syndrome are short and thick, and the little finger is often curved inward. There may be a wide space between the first and second toes and between the first and second fingers. The palm of the hand shows a peculiar crease (a simian line) or a single horizontal crease rather than the usual three creases in the palm (Fig. 8.8B).

Children with Down syndrome are usually cognitively challenged to some degree. The challenge can range from an IQ of 50 to 70 to a child who is profoundly affected (IQ less than 20). The extent of the cognitive challenge is not evident at birth, but the fact the brain is not developing well is usually evidenced by a head size smaller than the 10th or 20th percentile at well-child healthcare visits.

Internally, congenital heart disease, especially an atrioventricular defect, is common. Stenosis or atresia of the duodenum, strabismus, and cataract disorders may also be present. In addition, the child's immune function may be altered because as these children grow, they are prone to upper respiratory tract infections. Probably due to a second gene aberration, they tend to develop acute lymphocytic leukemia about 20 times more frequently than the general population (Izraeli, 2015). Even if children are born without an accompanying disorder such as heart disease or don't develop leukemia, their life span usually is limited to only 50 to 60 years because aging seems to occur faster than usual.

It's important for children with Down syndrome to be enrolled in early educational and play programs so they can develop to their full capacity (see Chapter 54). Because they are prone to infections, sensible precautions such as using a good hand washing technique are important when caring for them. The enlarged tongue may interfere with swallowing and cause choking unless the child is fed slowly. Because their neck may not be fully stable, an X-ray to ensure stability is recommended before they engage in strenuous activities such as competitive sports or Special Olympics. As with all

newborns, these infants need a physical examination at birth to enable the detection of the genetic disorder and the initiation of parental counseling, support, and future planning.

QSEN Checkpoint Question 8.3

TEAMWORK & COLLABORATION

Amy Alvarez's child is born with Down syndrome. What is a common physical feature of newborns with this disorder that the nurse would want all of the team members to recognize?

a. Spastic neck muscles
b. An unusual pattern of palm creases
c. A white lock of forehead hair
d. Wrinkles on the soles of the feet

Look in Appendix A for the best answer and rationale.

CHILDHOOD TUMORS

A number of cancers in children are also associated with chromosomal aberrations. Chief among these are retinoblastoma (chromosome 13), Wilms tumor (chromosome 11), and neuroblastoma (chromosome 1 or 11; Venkatesan, Natarajan, & Hande, 2015). Siblings of children with these cancers need to be tested to reveal if they carry the gene aberration as well and followed closely by a healthcare provider so early diagnosis and therapy can begin.

What If . . . 8.3

The nurse is particularly interested in exploring one of the 2020 National Health Goals with respect to genetic disorders (see Box 8.1). What would be a possible research topic to explore pertinent to this goal that would be applicable to Amy's family and that would also advance evidence-based practice?

KEY POINTS FOR REVIEW

- Genetic disorders are those resulting from a distortion in the structure or number of genes or chromosomes. Genetics, the study of gene variation, includes examining how and why such disorders occur.

- A phenotype is a person's outward appearance. Genotype refers to the actual gene composition. A person's genome is the complete set of genes present. A karyotype is a graphic representation of the chromosomes present.

- A person is homozygous for a trait if he or she has two like genes for the trait. A person is heterozygous if he or she has two unlike genes for the trait.

- Mendelian laws predict the likely incidence of recessive or dominant diseases.

- Genetic counseling can be a role for nurses with advanced preparation and education. An assessment of genetic disorders consists of a health history, physical examination, and screening and diagnostic studies such as first trimester screening, cfDNA testing, CVS, and amniocentesis.

- Some karyotyping tests, such as CVS and amniocentesis, introduce a risk of spontaneous or threatened miscarriage. Be certain women undergoing these tests remain in the healthcare facility for at least 30 minutes after these procedures to be certain vaginal bleeding, uterine cramping, or abnormal fetal heart rate is not present. Women with an Rh-negative blood type need Rh immune globulin administration after these procedures.

- An important aspect of genetic counseling is respecting a couple's right to privacy. Be certain information gained from testing remains confidential and is not given indiscriminately to others, including other family members.

- Common genetic disorders include Down syndrome (trisomy 21), trisomy 13, trisomy 18, Turner syndrome (45XO), and Klinefelter syndrome (47XXY). Most of these syndromes include some degree of cognitive challenge.

- People who are told a genetic disorder does exist in their family may suffer a loss of self-esteem. Offering support to help them deal with the feelings they experience helps in planning nursing care that not only meets QSEN competencies but also best meets the family's total needs.

CRITICAL THINKING CARE STUDY

Gabby Castro, 24 years of age, works as a police officer; her dream is to become a homicide detective. She learned last week her brother, Alex, 26 years of age, has fragile X syndrome. She always knew he was aggressive (and now is serving a jail term for armed robbery), but she thought his aggression was because they moved a lot when they were little and so she thought he never had a chance to achieve in school. Gabby's fiancé, Stanley, 25 years of age, is a manager in his family's hardware store. He asks if the reason she enjoys being a police officer (he views this as mainly a man's occupation) could be because she's missing her X chromosomes. He wants her to have a DNA analysis before they get married to be certain a son won't have fragile X syndrome.

1. Fragile X syndrome is one of the most frequently seen chromosomal abnormalities in boys. Is it true this is associated with aggression? Could the family's frequent moves have contributed to the syndrome?

2. Is it probable that Gabby carries a gene for fragile X syndrome? Is it fair for Stanley to ask her to have a DNA analysis before he agrees to marry her?

3. Stanley asks if the reason Gabby wants to be a detective could be because her X chromosomes are missing. Is this likely? Would you recommend Gabby rethink her relationship with Stanley before agreeing to marriage?

RELATED RESOURCES

Explore these additional resources to enhance learning for this chapter:
- Student resources on thePoint, including answers to the What If . . . and Critical Thinking Care Study questions, http://thepoint.lww.com/Flagg8e
- Adaptive learning powered by PrepU, http://thepoint.lww.com/prepu

REFERENCES

Armitage, S. (2016). Cord blood banking standards: Autologous versus altruistic. *Frontiers in Medicine, 2*, 94.

Check, J. H., Wilson, C., Levine, K., et al. (2015). Improved implantation and live delivered pregnancy rates following transfer of embryos derived from donor oocytes by single injection of leuprolide in mid-luteal phase. *Clinical and Experimental Obstetrics & Gynecology, 42*(4), 429–430.

Contractor, A., Klyachko, V. A., & Portera-Cailliau, C. (2015). Altered neuronal and circuit excitability in fragile X syndrome. *Neuron, 87*(4), 699–715.

Dar, S., Lazer, T., Swanson, S., et al. (2015). Assisted reproduction involving gestational surrogacy: An analysis of the medical, psychosocial and legal issues: Experience from a large surrogacy program. *Human Reproduction, 30*(2), 345–352.

Daughtry, B. L., & Chavez, S. L. (2016). Chromosomal instability in mammalian pre-implantation embryos: Potential causes, detection methods, and clinical consequences. *Cell and Tissue Research, 363*(1), 201–225.

Davidson, K. C., Mason, E. A., & Pera, M. F. (2015). The pluripotent state in mouse and human. *Development, 142*(18), 3090–3099.

Du, X., Yuan, Q., Qu, Y., et al. (2016). Endometrial mesenchymal stem cells isolated from menstrual blood by adherence. *Stem Cells International, 2016*, 3573846.

Duke, C. M. P., & Christianson, M. S. (2015). Infertility and assisted reproductive technologies. In C. T. Johnson, J. L. Hallock, J. L. Bienstock, et al. (Eds.), *The Johns Hopkins manual of gynecology and obstetrics* (5th ed., pp. 467–484). Philadelphia, PA: Wolters Kluwer.

Edelman, E. A., Lin, B. K., Doksum, T., et al. (2014). Implementation of an electronic genomic and family health history tool in primary prenatal care. *American Journal of Medical Genetics. Part C, Seminars in Medical Genetics, 166C*(1), 34–44.

Espinel, W., Charen, K., Huddleston, L., et al. (2015). Improving health education for women who carry an FMR1 premutation. *Journal of Genetic Counseling, 25*(2), 228–238.

Fletcher, W., & Russo, M. (2015). Preconception counseling and prenatal care. In C. T. Johnson, J. L. Hallock, J. L. Bienstock, et al. (Eds.), *The Johns Hopkins manual of gynecology and obstetrics* (5th ed., pp. 58–77). Philadelphia, PA: Wolters Kluwer.

Gezer, C., Ekin, A., Gezer, N. S., et al. (2015). Prenatal karyotype results of fetuses with nuchal edema, cystic hygroma, and non-immune hydrops. *Clinical and Experimental Obstetrics & Gynecology, 42*(5), 586–589.

Hume, H., & Chasen, S. T. (2015). Trends in timing of prenatal diagnosis and abortion for fetal chromosomal abnormalities. *American Journal of Obstetrics and Gynecology, 213*(4), 545.e1–545.e4.

Izraeli, S. (2015). The acute lymphoblastic leukemia of Down syndrome—genetics and pathogenesis. *European Journal of Medical Genetics, 59*(3), 158–161.

Karaman, A., Aydin, H., & Göksu, K. (2015). Concomitant omphalocele, anencephaly and arthrogryposis associated with trisomy 18. *Genetic Counseling, 26*(1), 77–79.

Kiku, P., Voronin, S., & Golokhvast, K. (2015). Congenital anomalies in Primorsky region. *The International Journal of Risk & Safety in Medicine, 27,* S19–S20.

Kumar, R., Dunn, A., & Carcao, M. (2016). Changing paradigm of hemophilia management: Extended half-life factor concentrates and gene therapy. *Seminars in Thrombosis and Hemostasis, 42*(1), 18–29.

Levitsky, L. L., Luria, A. H., Hayes, F. J., et al. (2015). Turner syndrome: Update on biology and management across the life span. *Current Opinion in Endocrinology, Diabetes, and Obesity, 22*(1), 65–72.

Levy, P. A., & Marion, R. W. (2015). Chromosomal disorders. In K. J. Marcdante & R. M. Kliegman (Eds.), *Nelson essentials of pediatrics* (7th ed., pp. 156–160). Philadelphia, PA: Elsevier Saunders.

McNair, T., & Altman, K. (2015). Miscarriage and recurrent pregnancy loss. In C. T. Johnson, J. L. Hallock, J. L. Bienstock, et al. (Eds.), *The Johns Hopkins manual of gynecology and obstetrics* (5th ed., pp. 438–447). Philadelphia, PA: Wolters Kluwer.

Minear, M. A., Alessi, S., Allyse, M., et al. (2015). Noninvasive prenatal genetic testing: Current and emerging ethical, legal, and social issues. *Annual Review of Genomics and Human Genetics, 16,* 369–398.

Palma Sisto, P. A., & Heneghan, M. (2015). Disorders of puberty. In K. J. Marcdante & R. M. Kliegman (Eds.), *Nelson essentials of pediatrics* (7th ed., pp. 589–595). Philadelphia, PA: Elsevier Saunders.

Panepinto, J. A., Punzalan, R. C., & Scott, J. P. (2015). Anemia. In K. J. Marcdante & R. M. Kliegman (Eds.), *Nelson essentials of pediatrics* (7th ed., pp. 509–522). Philadelphia, PA: Elsevier Saunders.

Prakash, V., Moore, M., & Yáñez-Muñoz, R. J. (2016). Current progress in therapeutic gene editing for monogenic diseases. *Molecular Therapy. 24*(3), 465–474.

Ranke, M. B. (2015). Why treat girls with Turner syndrome with growth hormone? Growth and beyond. *Pediatric Endocrinology Reviews, 12*(4), 356–365.

Simpson, J. L., Holzgreve, W., & Driscoll, D. A. (2012). Genetic counseling and genetic screening. In S. G. Gabbe, J. R. Niebyl, J. L. Simpson, et al. (Eds.), *Obstetrics: Normal and problem pregnancies* (6th ed., pp. 193–209). Philadelphia, PA: Elsevier Saunders.

Skotko, B. G., Levine, S. P., & Goldstein, R. (2011a). Having a brother or sister with Down syndrome: Perspectives from siblings. *American Journal of Medical Genetics. Part A, 155A*(10), 2348–2359.

Skotko, B. G., Levine, S. P., & Goldstein, R. (2011b). Having a son or daughter with Down syndrome: Perspectives from mothers and fathers. *American Journal of Medical Genetics. Part A, 155A*(10), 2335–2347.

Soo-Jin Lee, S., & Borgelt, E. (2014). Protecting posted genes: Social networking and the limits of GINA. *The American Journal of Bioethics, 14*(11), 32–44.

Tasker, R. C., McClure, R., & Acerini, C. (2013). Genetics. In R. C. Tasker, R. McClure, & C. Acerini (Eds.), *Oxford handbook of paediatrics* (2nd ed., pp. 925–952). Oxford, United Kingdom: Oxford University Press.

U.S. Department of Health and Human Services. (2010). *Healthy people 2020.* Washington, DC: Author.

Vekeman, F., Gauthier-Loiselle, M., Faust, E., et al. (2015). Patient and caregiver burden associated with fragile X syndrome in the United States. *American Journal on Intellectual and Developmental Disabilities, 120*(5), 444–459.

Venkatesan, S., Natarajan, A. T., & Hande, M. P. (2015). Chromosomal instability—mechanisms and consequences. Mutation research. *Genetic Toxicology and Environmental Mutagenesis, 793,* 176–184.

Wang, W., Liu, F., Xiang, B., et al. (2015). Stem cells as cellular vehicles for gene therapy against glioblastoma. *International Journal of Clinical and Experimental Medicine, 8*(10), 17102–17109.

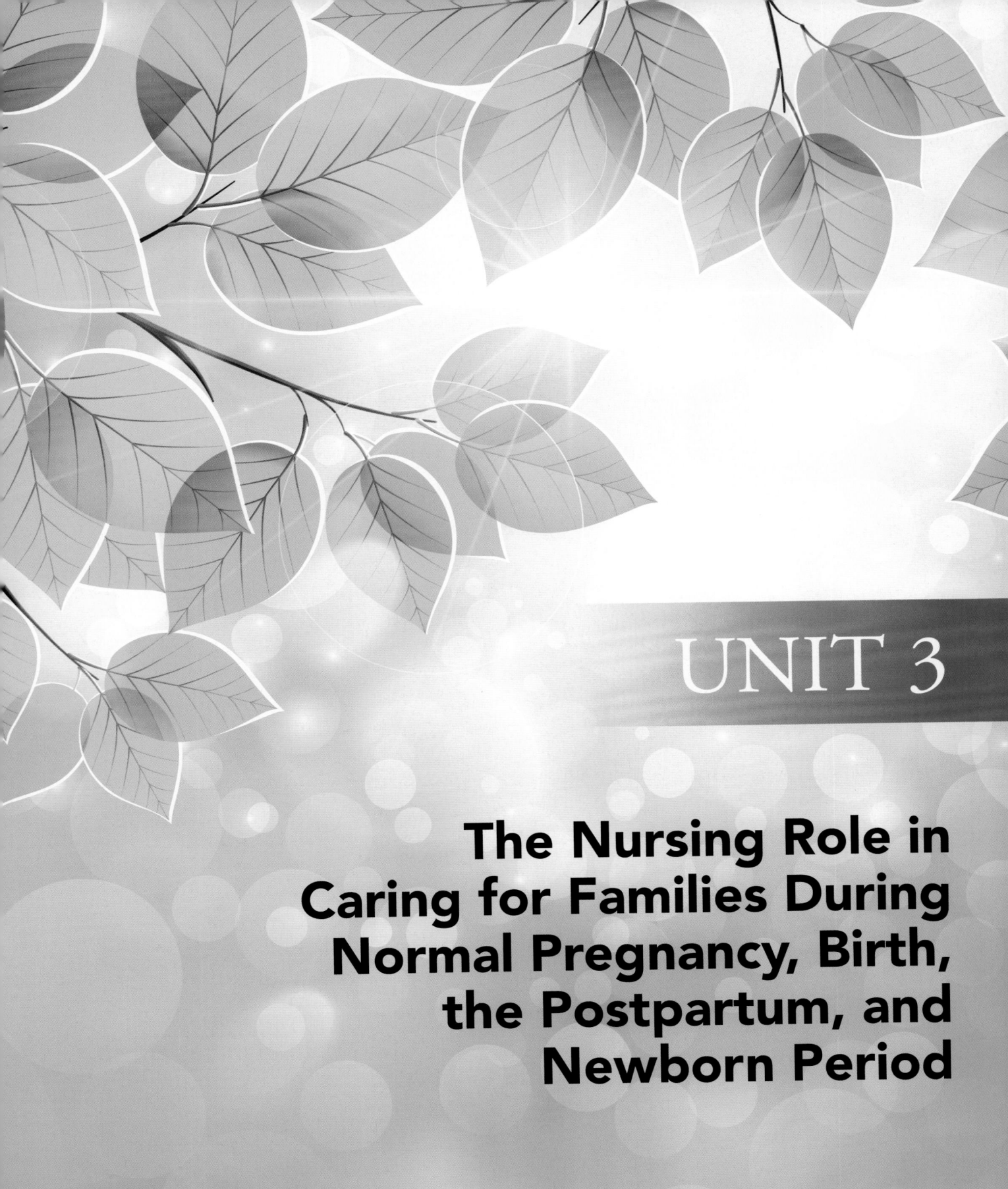

UNIT 3

The Nursing Role in Caring for Families During Normal Pregnancy, Birth, the Postpartum, and Newborn Period

9

Nursing Care During Normal Pregnancy and Care of the Developing Fetus

*L*iz Calhorn, an 18-year-old, is 20 weeks pregnant. Although she says she knows she should have stopped smoking before pregnancy, she has not been able to do this as yet. Twice during the pregnancy (at the 4th and 10th week), she drank beer at summer picnics. Today, at a clinic visit, she tells you she has felt her fetus move. She states, "Feeling the baby move made me realize there's someone inside me, you know what I mean? It made me realize it's time I started being more careful with what I do." Liz works at a fast-food restaurant. Her boyfriend (the father of fetus) is supportive but has no money to give her. Patient states, "I'm not getting married. Just not ready for that big commitment yet."

Feeling a fetus move is often the trigger that makes having a baby "real" for many women. The more women know about fetal development before and after this event, the easier it is for them to begin to think of the pregnancy not as something interesting happening to them but as an act producing a separate life. A previous chapter described reproductive anatomy. This chapter adds information about fetal growth and development and assessment of fetal health.

In light of Liz's revelation, what additional health teaching does she need?

KEY TERMS

- age of viability
- amniotic membrane
- cephalocaudal
- chorionic membrane
- chorionic villi
- decidua
- embryo
- estimated date of birth
- fertilization
- fetoscopy
- fetus
- foramen ovale
- hydramnios
- implantation
- McDonald's rule
- meconium
- nonstress test
- oligohydramnios
- organogenesis
- surfactant
- trophoblast
- umbilical cord
- zygote

OBJECTIVES

After mastering the contents of this chapter, you should be able to:

1. Describe the growth and development of a fetus by gestational age in weeks.
2. Identify 2020 National Health Goals addressing fetal growth and development and address how nurses can help the nation achieve these goals.
3. Assess fetal growth and development through maternal and pregnancy landmarks.
4. Formulate nursing diagnoses related to the needs of a fetus.
5. Establish expected outcomes to meet the perceived needs of a growing fetus as well as manage a seamless transition from fetus to newborn.
6. Using the nursing process, plan nursing care that includes the six competencies of Quality & Safety Education for Nurses (QSEN): Patient-Centered Care, Teamwork & Collaboration, Evidence-Based Practice (EBP), Quality Improvement (QI), Safety, and Informatics.
7. Implement nursing care to help ensure both a safe fetal environment and a safe pregnancy outcome.
8. Evaluate expected outcomes for achievement and effectiveness of care.
9. Integrate knowledge of fetal growth and development with the interplay of nursing process, the six competencies of QSEN, and Family Nursing to promote quality maternal and child health nursing care.

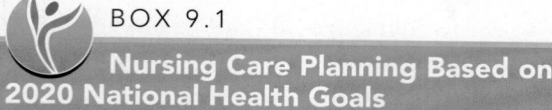

BOX 9.1

Nursing Care Planning Based on 2020 National Health Goals

A number of 2020 National Health Goals address fetal growth.

- Reduce the fetal death rate (death between 20 and 40 weeks of gestation) to no more than 5.6 per 1,000 live births from a baseline of 6.2 per 1,000.
- Reduce low birth weight to an incidence of 7.8% of live births and very low birth weight to 1.4% of live births from baselines of 8.2% and 1.5%.
- Increase the proportion of women of childbearing potential with an intake of at least 400 mg of folic acid from fortified foods or dietary supplements from a baseline of 23.8% to 26.2% (U.S. Department of Health and Human Services, 2010; see www.healthypeople.gov).

Folic acid deficiency in pregnancy can lead to midline closure defects such as neural tube disorders. Nurses can help the nation achieve these goals by urging women to plan their pregnancies so they can enter the pregnancy in good health and with an optimum folic acid level. Educating women about the importance of attending prenatal care is another important role.

It is a unique situation to provide care for the patient who cannot be evaluated directly. The healthy development of the unborn child, referred to as the **fetus**, pregnancy can determine the health of the newborn, and health as a newborn is a positive predictor for health throughout the individual's life span

Unit 3 addresses the nursing role and care you might expect to provide to families during normal pregnancy, birth, and the postpartum and newborn periods. This chapter focuses on the structures of the female reproductive system that must function in harmony to sustain and promote the newborn's growth and development, the various stages of fetal development, and assessment of normal fetal development. Because you cannot have healthy children without healthy intrauterine growth, several 2020 National Health Goals speak to the importance of protecting fetal growth (Box 9.1).

Nursing Process Overview

TO HELP ENSURE FETAL HEALTH

ASSESSMENT

Assessing fetal growth throughout pregnancy, by measuring fundal height and fetal heart rate, is important because these signs of fetal development provide guidelines for determining the well-being of a fetus. For the expectant family, knowledge about fetal growth and development can help a woman understand some of the changes going on in her body as well as allow all family members to begin thinking about and accepting a new member to their family. For this reason, assessing fetal development at prenatal visits and conveying the findings are important, providing the family in as much detail as parents' request.

NURSING DIAGNOSIS

Common nursing diagnoses related to growth and development of the fetus focus on the pregnant woman and the family as well as the fetus. Examples might include:

- Readiness for enhanced knowledge related to usual fetal development
- Anxiety related to lack of fetal movement
- Deficient knowledge related to the need for good prenatal care for healthy fetal well-being

OUTCOME IDENTIFICATION AND PLANNING

Plans for care should include ways to educate potential parents about teratogens (i.e., any substance harmful to a fetus) that have the potential to interfere with fetal health. Outcome criteria established for teaching about fetal growth should be realistic and based on the parents' previous knowledge and desire for information. When additional assessment measures are necessary, such as an amniocentesis or an ultrasound examination, add this information to the teaching plan, explaining why further assessment is necessary and what the parents can expect from the procedure.

Refer women and their families to online resources for further information when appropriate. Helpful resources addressing pregnancy, birth, and postpartal care are available.

ONLINE RESOURCES

Online Resources for Prenatal, Childbirth, and Postpartal Care

American Academy of Pediatrics	http://www2.aap.org/breastfeeding/
Coalition for Improving Maternity Services	www.motherfriendly.org
International Childbirth Education Association (Parent-focused resource for childbirth preparation)	www.icea.org
La Leche League International (Breastfeeding resource with Spanish content)	www.llli.org
LactMed, U.S. National Library of Medicine (Database on drug and chemical exposure for breastfeeding mothers)	http://toxnet.nlm.nih.gov/cgi-bin/sis/htmlgen?LACT
Lamaze International (Parent-focused resource for childbirth preparation)	www.lamaze.org
March of Dimes	www.marchofdimes.com
MedlinePlus, U.S. National Library of Medicine (Resource for medication use during pregnancy)	https://medlineplus.gov/pregnancyandmedicines.html
National Institute of Child Health and Human Development	www.nichd.nih.gov
Office on Women's Health, U.S. Department of Health and Human Services	www.womenshealth.gov

Office on Women's Health,
U.S. Department of Health
and Human Services
(Government-sponsored
breastfeeding resource)

https://www.womenshealth.gov/breastfeeding/

U.S. Department of
Agriculture (USDA)

www.choosemyplate.gov

Women, Infants and
Children (WIC) Special
Supplemental Food
Program
(Resource for financial or
nutritional counseling)

www.fns.usda.gov/wic

IMPLEMENTATION

Most expectant parents are interested in learning about how mature their fetus is at various points in pregnancy as this helps them visualize their expected newborn. This, in turn, helps them to understand the importance of implementing healthy behaviors, such as eating well and avoiding substances that may be dangerous to a fetus such as recreational drugs. Viewing a sonogram and learning the fetal sex is a big step toward helping initiate bonding between the parents and the infant. Remember each woman's pregnancy is unique to her; be certain implementations are individualized for each woman for the best chance of outcome success.

OUTCOME EVALUATION

An outcome evaluation related to fetal growth and development usually focuses on determining whether a woman or family has made any changes in lifestyle necessary to ensure fetal growth and whether a woman voices confidence that her baby is healthy and growing. Examples of expected outcomes include:
- Parents describe smoke-free living by next prenatal visit.
- Patient records number of movements fetus makes during 1 hour daily.
- Couple attends all scheduled prenatal visits.
- Patient states she is looking forward to the birth of her baby.

The Nursing Role and Nursing Care During Normal Pregnancy and Birth

Thanks to the work of modern research and photographers who have been able to capture the process of fertilization and fetal development by ultrasound and high-tech photography, nurses can better understand and assess fetal growth and development.

Attending to the psychological and physiologic changes of pregnancy assures the health of the mother, and a healthy mother is a positive predictor for a healthy baby. A pregnant woman's body systems undergo specific changes during pregnancy to support the growth of the fetus (see Chapter 10). Accurate evaluation of these changes through assessment of the pregnant woman and her family will help you identify those changes that require an intervention (see Chapter 11).

You can foster a healthy outcome by obtaining a complete history and providing a physical examination that focuses on those components that influence fetal development. Vital signs are monitored following a recommended interval during pregnancy. Prenatal visits include standard guidelines, which may be altered if a pregnancy is at risk due to complications. Nursing care for the laboring mother (see Chapters 15 and 16), postpartum care for the mother and newborn (see Chapter 17), and newborn care of the term infant (see Chapter 18) decrease the need for interventions.

Stages of Fetal Development

In just 38 weeks, a fertilized egg (ovum) matures from a single cell to a fully developed fetus ready to be born. Although different cultures or religions debate the point at which life begins, for ease of discussion, all agree fetal growth and development can be divided into three time periods:
- Pre-embryonic (first 2 weeks, beginning with fertilization)
- Embryonic (weeks 3 through 8)
- Fetal (from week 8 through birth)

Table 9.1 lists common terms used to describe the fetus at various stages in this growth.

FERTILIZATION: THE BEGINNING OF PREGNANCY

Fertilization (also referred to as conception and impregnation) is the union of an ovum and a spermatozoon. This usually occurs in the outer third of a fallopian tube, termed the *ampullar portion*.

Usually, only one of a woman's ova reaches maturity each month. Once the mature ovum is released (i.e., ovulation), fertilization must occur fairly quickly because an ovum is capable of fertilization for only about 24 hours (48 hours at the most). After that time, it atrophies and becomes nonfunctional. Because the functional life of a spermatozoon is also about 48 hours, possibly as long as 72 hours, the total critical time span during which sexual relations must occur for fertilization to be successful is about 72 hours (48 hours before ovulation plus 24 hours afterward).

As the ovum is extruded from the graafian follicle of an ovary with ovulation, it is surrounded by a ring of mucopolysaccharide fluid (the zona pellucida) and a circle of cells (the corona radiata). The ovum and these surrounding cells (which increase the bulk of the ovum and serve as protective buffers against injury) are propelled into a nearby fallopian tube by currents initiated by the fimbriae—the fine, hairlike structures that line the openings of the tubes. A combination

TABLE 9.1 TERMS USED TO DESCRIBE FETAL GROWTH

Name	Time Period
Ovum	From ovulation to fertilization
Zygote	From fertilization to implantation
Embryo	From implantation to 5–8 weeks
Fetus	From 5–8 weeks until term
Conceptus	Developing embryo and placental structures throughout pregnancy
Age of viability	The earliest age at which fetuses survive if they are born is generally accepted as 24 weeks or at the point a fetus weighs more than 500–600 g

of peristaltic action of the tube and movements of the tube cilia help propel the ovum along the length of the tube.

Normally, an ejaculation of semen averages 2.5 ml of fluid containing 50 to 200 million spermatozoa per milliliter or an average of 400 million sperm per ejaculation (Welliver, Benson, Frederick, et al., 2016). At the time of ovulation, there is a reduction in the viscosity (thickness) of the woman's cervical mucus, which makes it easy for spermatozoa to penetrate it. Sperm transport is so efficient close to ovulation that spermatozoa deposited in the vagina generally reach the cervix within 90 seconds and the outer end of a fallopian tube within 5 minutes after deposition.

The mechanism whereby spermatozoa are drawn toward an ovum is probably a species-specific reaction, similar to an antibody–antigen reaction. Spermatozoa move through the cervix and the body of the uterus and into the fallopian tube, toward a waiting ovum by the combination of movement by their flagella (tails) and uterine contractions.

All of the spermatozoa that reach the ovum cluster around its protective layer of corona cells. Hyaluronidase (a proteolytic enzyme) is released by the spermatozoa and dissolves the layer of cells protecting the ovum. Under ordinary circumstances, only one spermatozoon is able to penetrate the cell membrane of the ovum. Once it penetrates the cell, the cell membrane changes composition to become impervious to other spermatozoa. An exception to this is the formation of gestational trophoblastic disease in which multiple sperm enter an ovum; this leads to abnormal zygote formation (DiGiulio, Wiedaseck, & Monchek, 2012) (see Chapter 21).

Immediately after penetration of the ovum, the chromosomal material of the ovum and spermatozoon fuse to form a **zygote**. Because the spermatozoon and ovum each carried 23 chromosomes (22 autosomes and 1 sex chromosome), the fertilized ovum has 46 chromosomes. If an X-carrying spermatozoon entered the ovum, the resulting child will have two X chromosomes and will be assigned female at birth (XX). If a Y-carrying spermatozoon fertilized the ovum, the resulting child will have an X and a Y chromosome and will be assigned male at birth (XY).

Fertilization is never a certain occurrence because it depends on at least three separate factors:
- Equal maturation of both sperm and ovum
- Ability of the sperm to reach the ovum
- Ability of the sperm to penetrate the zona pellucida and cell membrane and achieve fertilization

Out of this single-cell fertilized ovum (zygote), the future child and also the accessory structures needed for support during intrauterine life (placenta, fetal membranes, amniotic fluid, and umbilical cord) will form.

IMPLANTATION

Once fertilization is complete, a zygote migrates over the next 3 to 4 days toward the body of the uterus, aided by the currents initiated by the muscular contractions of the fallopian tubes. During this time, mitotic cell division, or cleavage, begins. The first cleavage occurs at about 24 hours; cleavage divisions continue to occur at a rate of about one every 22 hours so by the time the zygote reaches the body of the uterus; it consists of 16 to 50 cells. Over the next 3 or 4 days, large cells tend to collect at the periphery of the ball, leaving a fluid space surrounding an inner cell mass. At this stage, the structure is termed a *blastocyst*. The cells in the outer ring are **trophoblast** cells. They are the part of the structure that will later form the placenta and membranes. The inner cell mass (embryoblast cells) is the portion of the structure that will form the embryo.

Implantation, or contact between the growing structure and the uterine endometrium, occurs approximately 8 to 10 days after fertilization. About 8 days after ovulation, the blastocyst sheds the last residues of the corona and zona pellucida, brushes against the rich uterine endometrium (in the second [secretory] phase of the menstrual cycle), and settles down into its soft folds. The stages to this point are depicted in Figure 9.1.

Figure 9.1 Ovulation, fertilization, and implantation. The blastocyst is differentiated into three germ layers—the ectoderm, mesoderm, and endoderm. Cells at the periphery are trophoblast cells that mature into the placenta.

Implantation usually occurs high in the uterus on the posterior surface. If the point of implantation is low in the uterus, the growing placenta may occlude the cervix and make birth of the child difficult (placenta previa) because the placenta can block the birth canal. Almost immediately, the blastocyst burrows deeply into the endometrium and establishes an effective communication network with the blood system of the endometrium. Once implanted, the zygote is called an **embryo**.

Implantation is an important step in pregnancy because as many as 50% of zygotes never achieve it (Gardosi, 2012). In these instances, the pregnancy ends as early as 8 to 10 days after conception, often before a woman is even aware she was pregnant. Occasionally, a small amount of vaginal spotting appears on the day of implantation because capillaries are ruptured by the implanting trophoblast cells. A woman who normally has a particularly scant menstrual flow could mistake implantation bleeding for her menstrual period. If this happens, the predicted date of birth of her baby (based on the time of her last menstrual period) will be calculated 4 weeks late.

QSEN Checkpoint Question 9.1

TEAMWORK & COLLABORATION

Liz Calhorn, 18 years of age, asks how much longer her nurse practitioner will refer to the baby inside her as an embryo. To ensure team members use terms consistently, the nurse would want them to know the conceptus is classified as an embryo at what time?

   a. At the time of fertilization
   b. When the placenta forms
   c. From implantation until 20 weeks
   d. From implantation until 5 to 8 weeks

Look in Appendix A for the best answer and rationale.

Embryonic and Fetal Structures

The placenta and membranes, which will serve as the fetal lungs, kidneys, and digestive tract in utero as well as help provide protection for the fetus, begin growth in early pregnancy in coordination with embryo growth.

THE DECIDUA OR UTERINE LINING

After fertilization, the corpus luteum in the ovary continues to function rather than atrophying under the influence of human chorionic gonadotropin (hCG) secreted by the trophoblast cells. This hormone also causes the uterine endometrium to continue to grow in thickness and vascularity instead of sloughing off as in a usual menstrual cycle. The endometrium is now typically termed the **decidua** (the Latin word for "falling off") because it will be discarded after birth of the child.

CHORIONIC VILLI

As early as the 11th or 12th day after fertilization, miniature villi, resembling probing fingers and termed **chorionic villi**, reach out from the trophoblast cells into the uterine endometrium to begin formation of the placenta. Chorionic villi have a central core consisting of connective tissue and fetal capillaries surrounded by a double layer of cells, which produce

various placental hormones, such as hCG, somatomammotropin (human placental lactogen [hPL]), estrogen, and progesterone. The middle layer, the *cytotrophoblast* or Langhans' layer, appears to have a second function to protect the growing embryo and fetus from certain infectious organisms such as the spirochete of syphilis early in pregnancy. Because this layer of cells disappears between the 20th and 24th week of pregnancy, this is why syphilis is not considered to have a high potential for fetal damage early in pregnancy, only after the point at which cytotrophoblast cells are no longer present. The layer appears to offer little protection against viral invasion at any point, increasing the vulnerability of the fetus to viruses (Stohl & Satin, 2011).

THE PLACENTA

The placenta (Latin for "pancake," which is descriptive of its size and appearance at term) grows from a few identifiable trophoblastic cells at the beginning of pregnancy to an organ 15 to 20 cm in diameter and 2 to 3 cm in depth, covering about half the surface area of the internal uterus at term (Huppertz & Kingdom, 2012).

Circulation

Placental circulation is shown in Figure 9.2. As early as the 12th day of pregnancy, maternal blood begins to collect in the intervillous spaces of the uterine endometrium surrounding the chorionic villi. By the third week, oxygen and other nutrients such as glucose, amino acids, fatty acids, minerals, vitamins, and water osmose from the maternal blood through the cell layers of the chorionic villi into the villi capillaries. From there, nutrients are transported to the developing embryo.

Placental transfer is dynamic, allowing all but a few substances to cross from the mother into the fetus. Because almost all drugs are able to cross into the fetal circulation, it is important that a woman take no nonessential drugs (including alcohol and nicotine) during pregnancy (Ordean, Kahan, Graves, et al., 2015). For example, alcohol perfuses across the placenta and may cause fetal alcohol spectrum disorder (e.g., unusual facial features, low-set ears, and cognitive challenge). Because it's difficult to tell what quantity is "safe," pregnant women are advised to drink no alcohol during pregnancy to avoid these disorders (Rogers & Worley, 2012).

Theoretically, because the exchange process depends on osmosis, there is no direct exchange of blood cells between the embryo and the mother during pregnancy. Occasionally, however, fetal cells do cross into the maternal bloodstream as well as fetal enzymes such as α-fetoprotein (AFP) produced by the fetal liver (this allows testing of fetal cells for genetic analysis as well as the level of AFP in the maternal blood).

As the number of chorionic villi increases with pregnancy, the villi form an increasingly complex communication network with the maternal bloodstream. Intervillous spaces grow larger and larger, becoming separated by 30 or more partitions or septa. These compartments, known as cotyledons, are what make the maternal side of the placenta look rough and uneven.

To provide enough blood for exchange, the rate of uteroplacental blood flow in pregnancy increases from about 50 ml/min at 10 weeks to 500 to 600 ml/min at term. No additional maternal arteries appear after the first 3 months of pregnancy; instead, to accommodate the increased blood

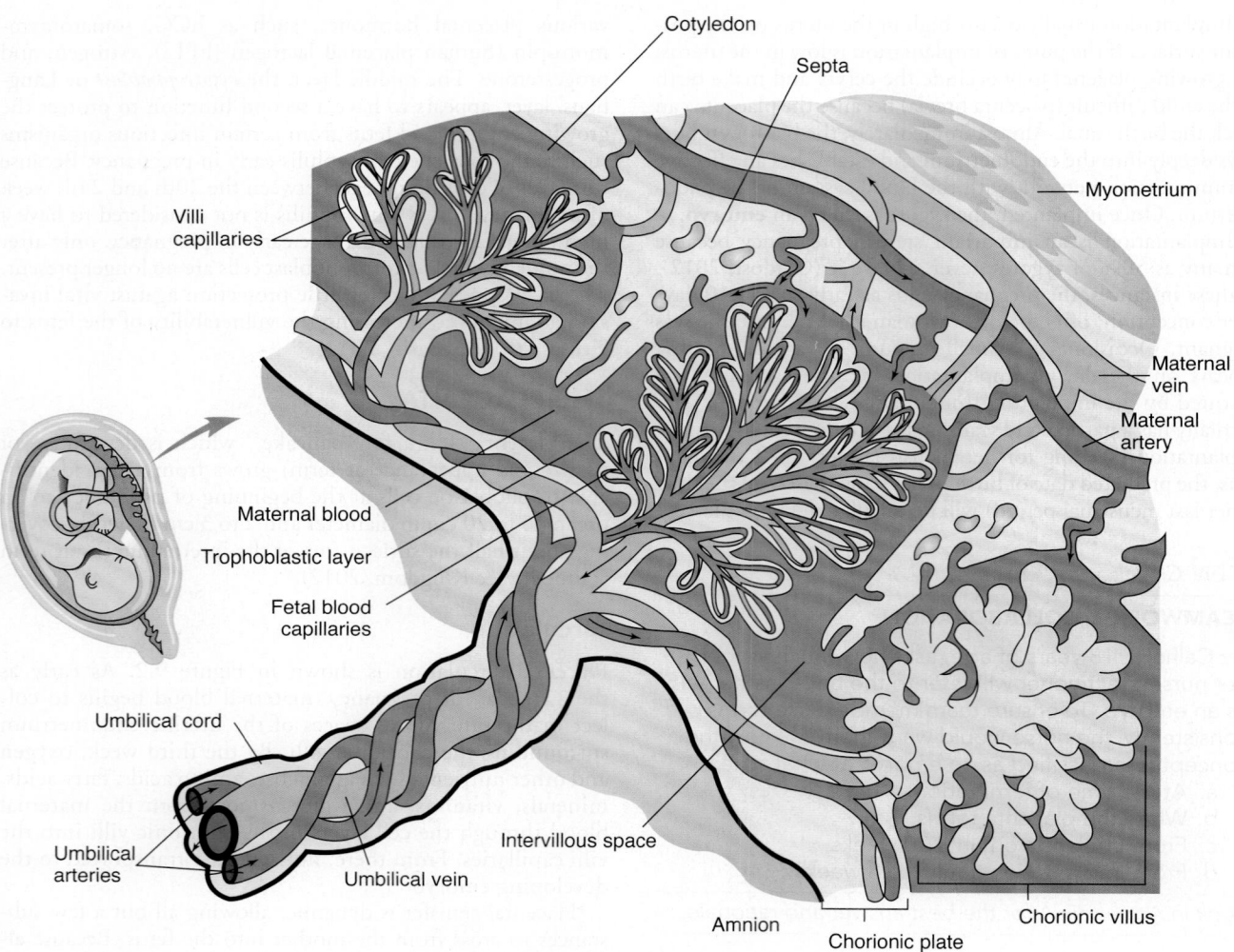

Figure 9.2 Placental circulation.

flow, the arteries increase in size. The woman's heart rate, total cardiac output, and blood volume all increase to supply blood to the placenta (Pipkin, 2012). Braxton Hicks contractions, the barely noticeable uterine contractions present from about the 12th week of pregnancy on, aid in maintaining pressure in the intervillous spaces by closing off the uterine veins momentarily with each contraction.

Uterine perfusion and placental circulation are most efficient when the mother lies on her left side, as this position lifts the uterus away from the inferior vena cava, preventing blood from becoming trapped in the woman's lower extremities. If the woman lies on her back and the weight of the uterus compresses on the vena cava, known as vena cava syndrome, placental circulation can be so sharply reduced that supine hypotension (i.e., very low maternal blood pressure and poor uterine circulation) can occur (Coad & Dunstall, 2011a).

At term, the placental circulatory network has grown so extensively that a placenta weighs 400 to 600 g (1 lb), one-sixth the weight of the newborn. If a placenta is smaller than this, it suggests circulation to the fetus may have been compromised and/or inadequate. A placenta bigger than this also may indicate circulation to the fetus was threatened because it suggests the placenta was forced to spread out in an unusual manner to maintain a sufficient blood supply. The fetus of a woman with diabetes may also develop a larger than usual placenta from excess fluid collected between cells.

Endocrine Function

Besides serving as the source of oxygen and nutrients for the fetus, the syncytial (outer) layer of the chorionic villi develops into a separate and important hormone-producing system.

Human Chorionic Gonadotropin

The first placental hormone produced, hCG, can be found in maternal blood and urine as early as the first missed menstrual period (shortly after implantation has occurred). Levels vary throughout pregnancy. The pregnant woman's blood serum will be completely negative for hCG within 1 to 2 weeks after birth. Finding no serum hCG after birth can be used as proof that placental tissue is no longer present.

hCG's purpose is to act as a fail-safe measure to ensure the corpus luteum of the ovary continues to produce progesterone and estrogen so the endometrium of the uterus is maintained. hCG also may play a role in suppressing the maternal immunologic response so placental tissue is not detected and rejected as a foreign substance. Because the structure of hCG is similar to that of luteinizing hormone of the pituitary gland, if the fetus is male, it exerts an effect on the fetal testes to begin testosterone production and maturation of the male reproductive tract (Huppertz & Kingdom, 2012).

At about the eighth week of pregnancy, the outer layer of cells of the developing placenta begins to produce progesterone, making the corpus luteum, which was producing progesterone, no longer necessary. In coordination with this, the production of hCG, which sustained the corpus luteum, begins to decrease at this point.

Progesterone

Estrogen is often referred to as the "hormone of women," and progesterone as the "hormone that maintains pregnancy." This is because, although estrogen influences a female appearance, progesterone is necessary to maintain the endometrial lining of the uterus during pregnancy. It is present in maternal serum as early as the fourth week of pregnancy as a result of the continuation of the corpus luteum. After placental production begins (at about the 12th week), the level of progesterone rises progressively during the remainder of the pregnancy. This hormone also appears to reduce the contractility of the uterus during pregnancy, thus preventing premature labor.

Estrogen

Estrogen (primarily estriol) is produced as a second product of the syncytial cells of the placenta. Estrogen contributes to the woman's mammary gland development in preparation for lactation and stimulates uterine growth to accommodate the developing fetus.

Human Placental Lactogen (Human Chorionic Somatomammotropin)

hPL is a hormone with both growth-promoting and lactogenic (i.e., milk-producing) properties. It is produced by the placenta beginning as early as the sixth week of pregnancy, increasing to a peak level at term. It promotes mammary gland (breast) growth in preparation for lactation in the mother. It also serves the important role of regulating maternal glucose, protein, and fat levels so adequate amounts of these nutrients are always available to the fetus.

Placental Proteins

In addition to hormones, the placenta also produces a number of plasma proteins. The function of these has not been well documented, but they may contribute to decreasing the immunologic impact of the growing placenta and help prevent hypertension of pregnancy (discussed in Chapter 21) (Song, Li, & An, 2015).

THE AMNIOTIC MEMBRANES

The chorionic villi on the medial surface of the trophoblast (i.e., those that are not involved in implantation because they do not touch the endometrium) gradually thin until they become the **chorionic membrane**, the outermost fetal membrane. The amniotic membrane, or amnion, forms beneath the chorion (Fig. 9.3). The **amniotic membrane** is a dual-walled sac with the chorion as the outmost part and the amnion as the innermost part. The two fuse together as the pregnancy progresses, and by term, they appear to be a single sac. They have no nerve supply, so when they spontaneously rupture at term (a pregnant woman's "water breaks") or are artificially ruptured via a procedure, neither the pregnant woman nor the fetus experiences any pain (Coad & Dunstall, 2011b).

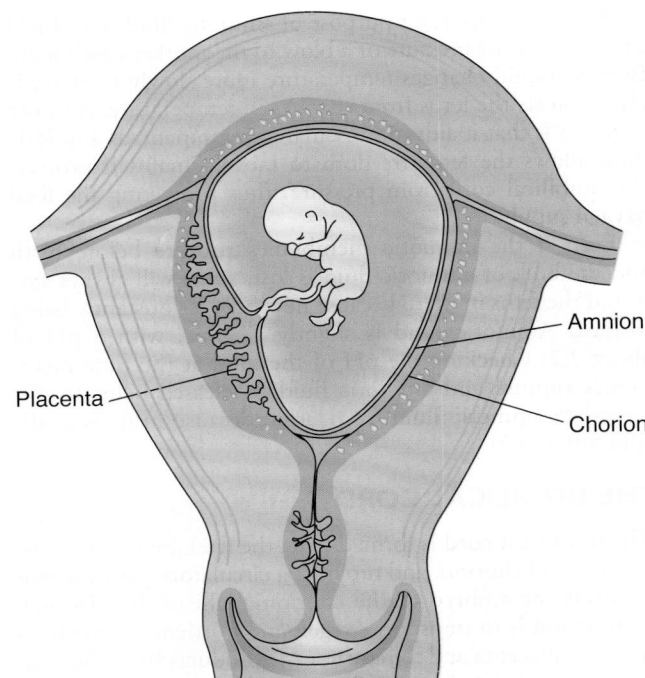

Figure 9.3 Membranes, with embryo lying within amniotic sac.

In contrast to the chorionic membrane, the second membrane (the amniotic membrane) not only offers support to amniotic fluid but also actually produces the fluid. In addition, it produces a phospholipid that initiates the formation of prostaglandins, which may be the trigger that initiates labor.

THE AMNIOTIC FLUID

Amniotic fluid never becomes stagnant because it is constantly being newly formed and absorbed by direct contact with the fetal surface of the placenta. The major method of absorption, however, happens within the fetus. Because the fetus continually swallows the fluid, it is absorbed from the fetal intestine into the fetal bloodstream. From there, it goes to the umbilical arteries and to the placenta and is exchanged across the placenta to the mother's bloodstream.

At term, the amount of amniotic fluid has grown so much it ranges from 800 to 1,200 ml. If for any reason the fetus is unable to swallow (esophageal atresia or anencephaly are the two most common reasons), excessive amniotic fluid or **hydramnios** (more than 2,000 ml in total or pockets of fluid larger than 8 cm on ultrasound) will result (Ghionzoli, James, David, et al., 2012). Hydramnios may also occur in women with diabetes because hyperglycemia causes excessive fluid shifts into the amniotic space (Perović, Garalejić, Gojnić, et al., 2012).

Early in fetal life, as soon as the fetal kidneys become active, fetal urine adds to the quantity of the amniotic fluid. A disturbance of kidney function, therefore, may cause **oligohydramnios** or a reduction in the amount of amniotic fluid. Oligohydramnios can be detected by ultrasound. The amniotic fluid index is measured, and it should be at least 5 cm. The vertical pocket of amniotic fluid should be greater than 2 cm (American Congress of Obstetricians and Gynecologists [ACOG], 2014). The appropriate amount of amniotic fluid ensures adequate kidney function.

The most important purpose of amniotic fluid is to shield the fetus against pressure or a blow to the mother's abdomen. Because liquid changes temperature more slowly than air, it also protects the fetus from changes in temperature. Another function is that it aids in muscular development, as amniotic fluid allows the fetus freedom to move. Finally, it protects the umbilical cord from pressure, thus protecting the fetal oxygen supply.

Even if the amniotic membranes rupture before birth and the bulk of amniotic fluid is lost, some will always surround the fetus in utero because new fluid is constantly being formed. Amniotic fluid is slightly alkaline, with a pH of about 7.2. Checking the pH of the fluid at the time membranes rupture and amniotic fluid is released helps to differentiate amniotic fluid from urine because urine is acidic (pH 5.0 to 5.5).

THE UMBILICAL CORD

The **umbilical cord** is formed from the fetal membranes, the amnion and chorion, and provides a circulatory pathway that connects the embryo to the chorionic villi of the placenta. Its function is to transport oxygen and nutrients to the fetus from the placenta and to return waste products from the fetus to the placenta. It is about 53 cm (21 in.) in length at term and about 2 cm (0.75 in.) thick. The bulk of the cord is a gelatinous mucopolysaccharide called Wharton jelly, which gives the cord body and prevents pressure on the vein and arteries that pass through it.

An umbilical cord contains only one vein (carrying blood from the placental villi to the fetus) and two arteries (carrying blood from the fetus back to the placental villi). The number of veins and arteries in the cord is always assessed and recorded at birth because about 1% to 5% of infants are born with a cord that contains only a single vein and artery. Of these infants, 15% to 20% are found to have accompanying chromosomal disorders or congenital anomalies, particularly of the kidney and heart (Schneider, 2011).

The rate of blood flow through an umbilical cord is rapid (350 ml/min at term). The adequacy of blood flow (blood velocity) through the cord, as well as both systolic and diastolic cord pressure, can be determined by ultrasound examination. Counting the number of coils in the cord may be used as a prediction of healthy fetal growth, as hypocoiling is associated with maternal hypertension and hypercoiling is associated with respiratory distress in the newborn (Chitra, Sushanth, & Raghavan, 2012).

Because the rate of blood flow through the cord is so rapid, it is unlikely a knot or twist in the cord will interfere with the fetal oxygen supply. In about 20% of all births, a loose loop of cord is found around the fetal neck (nuchal cord) at birth (Hoh, Sung, & Park, 2012). If this loop of cord is removed before the newborn's shoulders are born (not usually hard to do) so there is no traction on it, the oxygen supply to the fetus remains unimpaired.

The walls of the umbilical cord arteries are lined with smooth muscle. When these muscles contract after birth, the cord arteries and vein are compressed to prevent hemorrhage of the newborn through the cord. Because the umbilical cord contains no nerve supply, it can be clamped and cut at birth without discomfort to either the child or mother.

QSEN Checkpoint Question 9.2

SAFETY

Liz Calhorn tells the nurse she is worried her baby will be born with a congenital heart disease. What assessment of the umbilical cord at birth would be most important to help detect congenital heart defects?
  a. Assessing whether the pH of the Wharton jelly is higher than 7.2
  b. Assessing whether the umbilical cord has two arteries and one vein
  c. Measuring the length of the cord to be certain it is longer than 3 ft
  d. Determining that the umbilical cord is neither green nor yellow stained

Look in Appendix A for the best answer and rationale.

Origin and Development of Organ Systems

Following the moment of fertilization, the zygote, which later becomes an embryo and then a fetus, begins to grow at an active pace.

STEM CELLS

During the first 4 days of life, zygote cells are termed *totipotent stem cells*, or cells so undifferentiated they have the potential to grow into any cell in the human body. In another 4 days, as the structure implants and becomes an embryo, cells begin to show differentiation or lose their ability to become any body cell. Instead, they are slated to become specific body cells, such as nerve, brain, or skin cells, and are *termed pluripotent stem cells*. In yet another few days, the cells grow so specific they are termed *multipotent*, or are so specific they cannot be deterred from growing into a particular body organ such as spleen or liver or brain (Chen, Sun, Li, et al., 2016).

ZYGOTE GROWTH

As soon as conception has taken place, development proceeds in a **cephalocaudal** (head-to-tail) direction; that is, head development occurs first and is followed by development of the middle and, finally, the lower body parts. This pattern of development continues after birth as shown by the way infants are able to lift up their heads approximately 1 year before they are able to walk.

PRIMARY GERM LAYERS

As a fetus grows, body organ systems develop from specific tissue layers called germ layers. At the time of implantation, the blastocyst already has differentiated to a point at which three separate layers of these cells are present: the *ectoderm*, the *endoderm*, and the *mesoderm* (see Fig. 9.1). Each of these germ layers develops into specific body systems (Table 9.2). Knowing which structures arise from each germ layer is helpful to know because coexisting congenital disorders found in newborns usually arise from the same germ layer. For example, a fistula between the trachea and the esophagus (both of which arise from the endoderm layer) is a common birth anomaly.

TABLE 9.2 ORIGIN OF BODY TISSUE

Germ Layer	Body Portions Formed
Ectoderm	Central nervous system (brain and spinal cord)
	Peripheral nervous system
	Skin, hair, nails, and tooth enamel
	Sense organs
	Mucous membranes of the anus, mouth, and nose
	Mammary glands
Mesoderm	Supporting structures of the body (connective tissue, bones, cartilage, muscle, ligaments, and tendons)
	Upper portion of the urinary system (kidneys and ureters)
	Reproductive system
	Heart, lymph, and circulatory systems and blood cells
Endoderm	Lining of pericardial, pleura, and peritoneal cavities
	Lining of the gastrointestinal tract, respiratory tract, tonsils, parathyroid, thyroid, and thymus glands
	Lower urinary system (bladder and urethra)

In contrast, it is rare to see a newborn with a malformation of the heart (which arises from the mesoderm) and also a malformation of the lower urinary tract (which arises from the endoderm). One reason rubella infection is so serious in pregnancy is because this virus is capable of infecting all three germ layers so can cause congenital anomalies in a myriad of body systems (White, Boldt, Holditch, et al., 2012).

All organ systems are complete, at least in a rudimentary form, at 8 weeks gestation (the end of the embryonic period). During this early time of **organogenesis** (organ formation), the growing structure is most vulnerable to invasion by teratogens (i.e., any factor that affects the fertilized ovum, embryo, or fetus adversely, such as a teratogenic medicine; an infection such as toxoplasmosis; cigarette smoking; or alcohol ingestion) (Box 9.2). Figure 9.4 illustrates critical periods of fetal growth when it is most important for women to minimize their exposure to teratogens. The effect of individual teratogens and how to avoid them is discussed in Chapter 12.

CARDIOVASCULAR SYSTEM

The cardiovascular system is one of the first systems to become functional in intrauterine life. Simple blood cells joined to the walls of the yolk sac progress to become a network of blood vessels and a single heart tube, which forms as early as the 16th day of life and beats as early as the 24th day. The septum that divides the heart into chambers develops during the sixth or seventh week; heart valves develop in the seventh week. The heartbeat may be heard with a Doppler instrument as early as the 10th to 12th week of pregnancy. An electrocardiogram (ECG) may be recorded on a fetus as early as the 11th week, although early ECGs are not accurate until conduction is more regulated at about the 20th week of pregnancy.

The heart rate of a fetus is affected by oxygen level, activity, and circulating blood volume, just as in adulthood. After the 28th week of pregnancy, when the sympathetic nervous system matures, the heart rate stabilizes, and a consistent heart rate of 110 to 160 beats/min is assessed.

Fetal Circulation

Fetal circulation (Fig. 9.5) differs from extrauterine circulation because the fetus derives oxygen and excretes carbon dioxide not from gas exchange in the lungs but from exchange in the placenta.

Blood arriving at the fetus from the placenta is highly oxygenated. This blood enters the fetus through the umbilical vein (which is still called a vein even though it carries oxygenated blood because the direction of the blood is toward the fetal heart). Specialized structures present in the fetus then shunt blood flow to first supply the most important organs of the body: the liver, heart, kidneys, and brain. Blood flows from the umbilical vein to the ductus venosus, an accessory vessel that discharges oxygenated blood into the fetal liver, and then connects to the fetal inferior vena cava so oxygenated blood is directed to the right side of the heart. Because there is no need for the bulk of blood to pass through the lungs, the bulk of this blood is shunted as it enters the right atrium into the left atrium through an opening in the atrial

BOX 9.2

Nursing Care Planning Based on Family Teaching

Q. Liz Calhorn tells you, "I have to work. How can I guard against fetal teratogens at work?"

A. Here are a number of helpful tips:

- Ask your employer for a statement on hazardous substances at your work site; discuss your need to avoid these substances during pregnancy.
- Ask your employer to maintain a smoke-free site if that is not already a rule.
- Avoid any room, such as a coffee room, where smokers gather.
- Refrain from drinking alcohol, a frequent accompaniment to work lunches or social functions; ask for nonalcoholic drinks to be available at such events.
- Locate a fellow coworker who will "buddy" with you to help you avoid alcohol or tobacco at work activities.
- If quitting smoking is difficult, try a supportive telephone or Internet quitline. Ask your primary healthcare provider before using a nicotine patch, nicotine gum, or bupropion (Zyban), a drug to assist smokers to quit. Both nicotine and Zyban are category C drugs; Zyban is particularly contraindicated in women with symptoms of gestational hypertension as it can cause seizures in high doses.

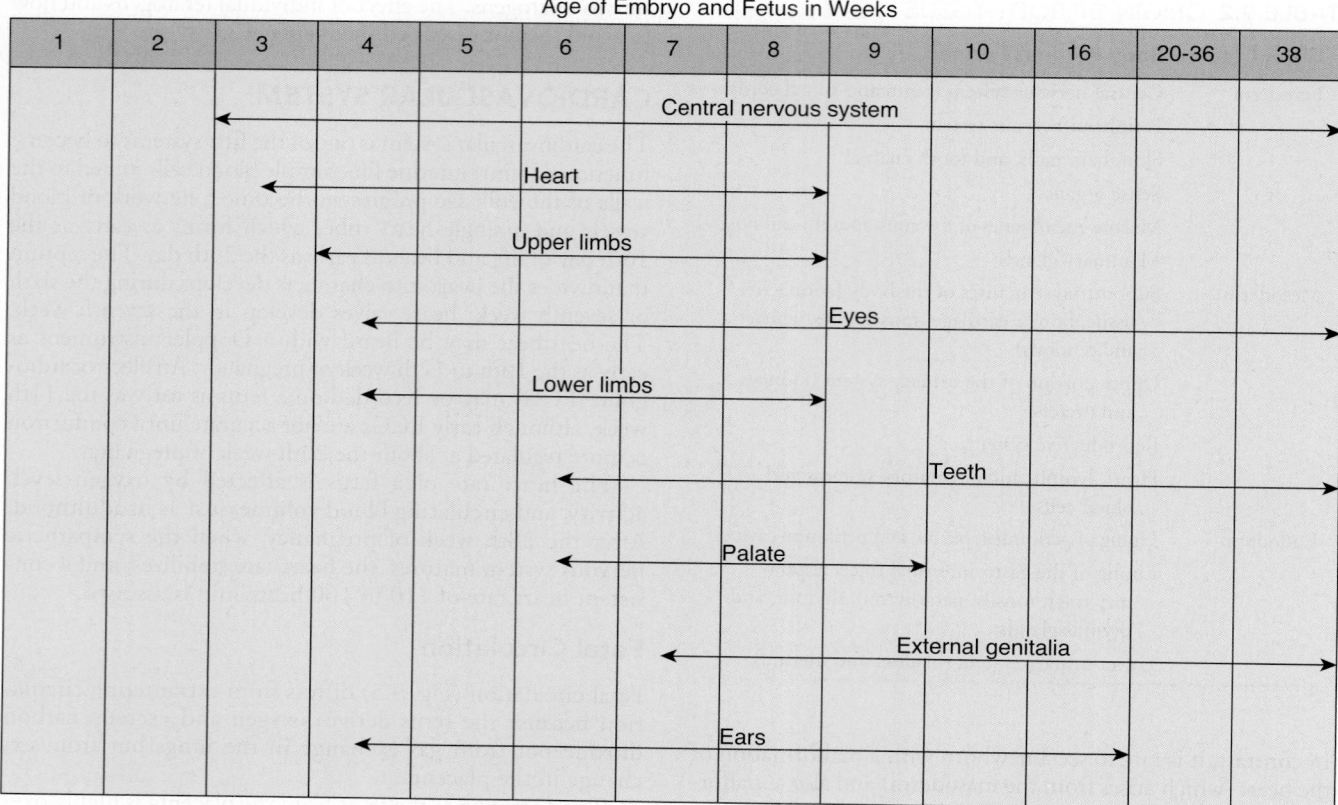

Figure 9.4   Critical periods of fetal growth.

septum called the **foramen ovale**. From the left atrium, it follows the course of adult circulation into the left ventricle, then into the aorta, and out to body parts.

A small amount of blood that returns to the heart via the vena cava does leave the right atrium by the adult circulatory route; that is, through the tricuspid valve into the right ventricle and then into the pulmonary artery and lungs to service the lung tissue. However, the larger portion of even this blood is shunted away from the lungs through an additional structure, the *ductus arteriosus*, directly into the descending aorta.

As the majority of blood cells in the aorta become deoxygenated, blood is transported from the descending aorta through the umbilical arteries (which are called arteries because they carry blood away from the fetal heart) back through the umbilical cord to the placental villi, where new oxygen exchange takes place.

At birth, an infant's oxygen saturation level is 95% to 100% and pulse rate is 80 to 140 beats/min. Because there is a great deal of mixing of blood in the fetus, the oxygen saturation level of fetal blood reaches only about 80%. A normal fetal heart rate is 110 to 160 beats/min, supplying needed oxygen to cells. Even with this low blood oxygen saturation level, however, carbon dioxide does not accumulate in the fetal system because it rapidly diffuses into maternal blood across a favorable placental pressure gradient.

Fetal Hemoglobin

Fetal hemoglobin differs from adult hemoglobin in several ways. It has a different composition (two α and two γ chains compared with two α and two β chains of adult hemoglobin). It is also more concentrated and has greater oxygen affinity,

two features that increase its efficiency. Because hemoglobin is more concentrated, a newborn's hemoglobin level is about 17.1 g/100 ml compared with a normal adult level of 11 g/100 ml; a newborn's hematocrit is about 53% compared with a normal adult level of 45%.

The change from fetal to adult hemoglobin levels begins before birth (γ cells are exchanged for β cells), but the process is still not complete at birth. Major blood dyscrasias, such as sickle cell anemia, tend to be defects of the β-hemoglobin chain, which is why clinical symptoms of these disorders do not become apparent until the bulk of fetal hemoglobin has matured to adult hemoglobin, at about 6 months of age (Panepinto & Scott, 2011).

RESPIRATORY SYSTEM

At the third week of intrauterine life, the respiratory and digestive tracts exist as a single tube. Like all body tubes, initially, this forms as a solid structure, which then canalizes (i.e., hollows out). By the end of the fourth week, a septum begins to divide the esophagus from the trachea. At the same time, lung buds appear on the trachea.

Until the seventh week of life, the diaphragm does not completely divide the thoracic cavity from the abdomen. This causes lung buds to extend down into the abdomen, reentering the chest only as the chest's longitudinal dimension increases and the diaphragm becomes complete (at the end of the seventh week). If the diaphragm fails to close completely, the stomach, spleen, liver, or intestines may be pulled up into the thoracic cavity. This causes the child to be born with intestine present in the chest (i.e., diaphragmatic hernia), compromising the lungs and perhaps displacing the heart (Gowen, 2011).

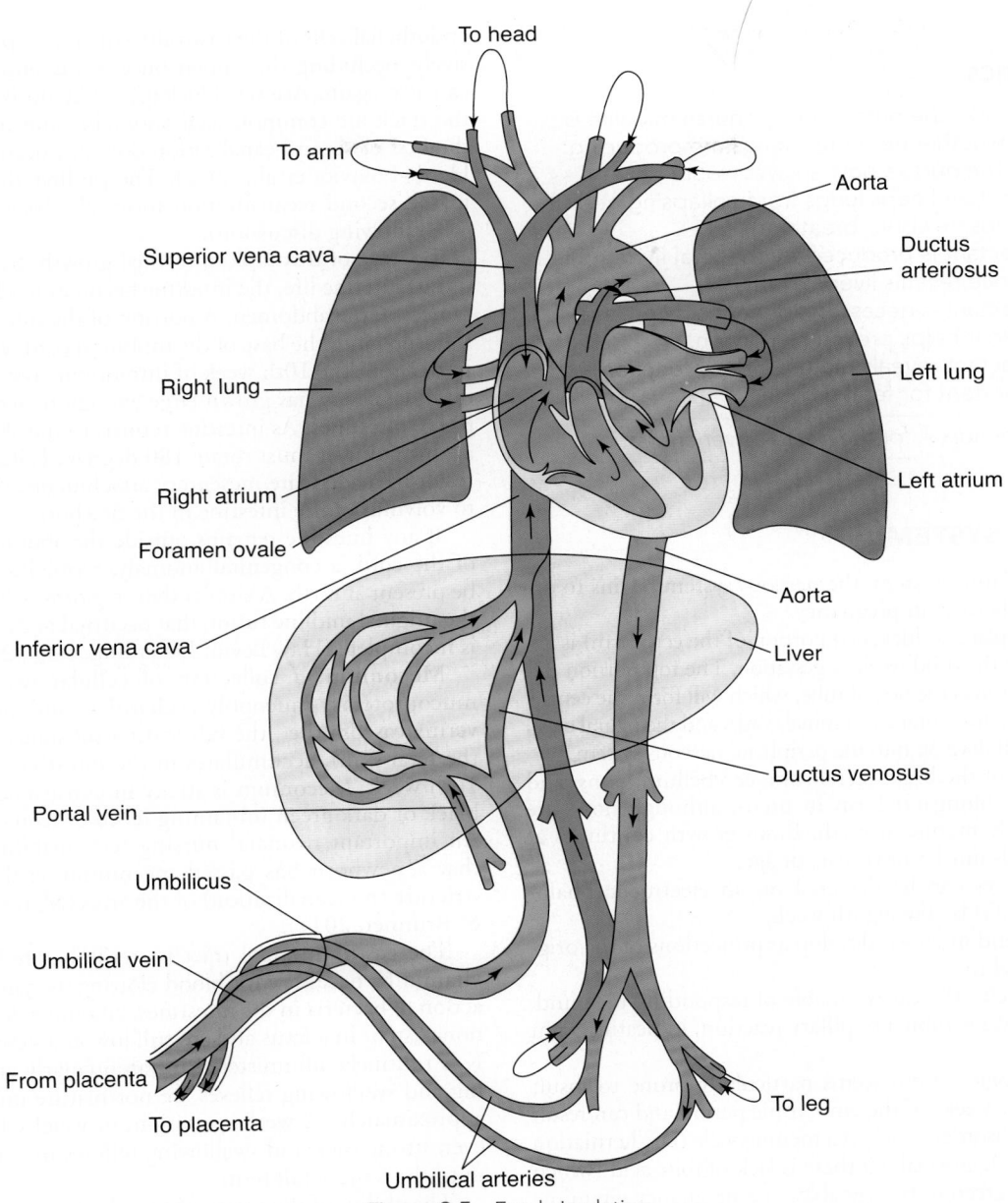

Figure 9.5   Fetal circulation.

Other important respiratory developmental milestones include:

- Spontaneous respiratory practice movements begin as early as 3 months gestation and continue throughout pregnancy.
- Specific lung fluid with a low surface tension and low viscosity forms in alveoli to aid in expansion of the alveoli at birth; it is rapidly absorbed shortly after birth.
- **Surfactant**, a phospholipid substance, is formed and excreted by the alveolar cells of the lungs beginning at approximately the 24th week of pregnancy. This decreases alveolar surface tension on expiration, preventing alveolar collapse and improving the infant's ability to maintain respirations in the outside environment at birth (Rojas-Reyes, Morley, & Soll, 2012).

Surfactant has two components: lecithin and sphingomyelin. Early in the formation of surfactant, sphingomyelin is the chief component. At approximately 35 weeks, there is a surge in the production of lecithin, which then becomes the chief component by a ratio of 2:1. As a fetus practices breathing movements, surfactant mixes with amniotic fluid. Using an amniocentesis technique, an analysis of the lecithin/sphingomyelin (L/S) ratio in surfactant (whether lecithin or sphingomyelin is the dominant component) is a primary test of fetal maturity. Respiratory distress syndrome, a severe breathing disorder, can develop if there is a lack of surfactant or it has not changed to its mature form at birth (see Chapter 26).

Any interference with the blood supply to the fetus, such as placental insufficiency or maternal hypertension, may raise steroid levels in the fetus and enhance surfactant development. Synthetically increasing steroid levels in the fetus (e.g., the administration of betamethasone to the mother late in pregnancy) can also hurry alveolar maturation and surfactant production without interfering with permanent lung function prior to a preterm birth (Smith, 2016).

NERVOUS SYSTEM

Like the circulatory system, the nervous system begins to develop extremely early in pregnancy.

• A neural plate (a thickened portion of the ectoderm) is apparent by the third week of gestation. The top portion differentiates into the neural tube, which will form the central nervous system (brain and spinal cord), and the neural crest, which will develop into the peripheral nervous system.
• All parts of the brain (cerebrum, cerebellum, pons, and medulla oblongata) form in utero, although none are completely mature at birth. Brain growth continues at high levels until 5 or 6 years of age.
• Brain waves can be detected on an electroencephalogram (EEG) by the eighth week.
• The eye and inner ear develop as projections of the original neural tube.
• By 24 weeks, the ear is capable of responding to sound, and the eyes exhibit a pupillary reaction, indicating sight is present.

The neurologic system seems particularly prone to insult during the early weeks of the embryonic period and can result in neural tube disorders, such as a meningocele (i.e., herniation of the meninges), especially if there is lack of folic acid (which is contained in green leafy vegetables and pregnancy vitamins) (Cohen & Uddin, 2011). All during pregnancy and at birth, the system is vulnerable to damage if anoxia should occur.

ENDOCRINE SYSTEM

The function of endocrine organs begins along with neuro-system development.

• The fetal pancreas produces insulin needed by the fetus (insulin is one of the few substances that does not cross the placenta from the mother to the fetus).
• The thyroid and parathyroid glands play vital roles in fetal metabolic function and calcium balance.
• The fetal adrenal glands supply a precursor necessary for estrogen synthesis by the placenta.

DIGESTIVE SYSTEM

The digestive tract separates from the respiratory tract at about the fourth week of intrauterine life and, after that, begins to grow extremely rapidly. Initially solid, the tract canalizes (hollows out) to become patent. Later in the pregnancy, the endothelial cells of the gastrointestinal tract proliferate extensively, occluding the lumen once more, and the tract must canalize again. Atresia (blockage) or stenosis (narrowing) of the track are common fetal anomalies and develop if either the first or second canalization does not occur (Lin, Munsie, Herdt-Losavio, et al., 2012). The proliferation of cells shed in the second recanalization forms the basis for meconium (see following discussion).

Because of this rapid intestinal growth, by the sixth week of intrauterine life, the intestine becomes too large to be contained by the abdomen. A portion of the intestine, therefore, is pushed into the base of the umbilical cord, where it remains until about the 10th week of intrauterine life or until the abdominal cavity has grown large enough to accommodate the bulky intestines. As intestine returns to the abdominal cavity at this point, it must rotate 180 degrees. Failure to do so can result in inadequate mesentery attachments, possibly leading to volvulus of the intestine in the newborn.

If any intestine remains outside the abdomen in the base of the cord, a congenital anomaly, termed *omphalocele*, will be present at birth. A similar defect, *gastroschisis*, occurs when the original midline fusion that occurred at the early cell stage is incomplete (Hay, Levin, Deterding, et al., 2016).

Meconium, a collection of cellular wastes, bile, fats, mucoproteins, mucopolysaccharides, and portions of the vernix caseosa (i.e., the lubricating substance that forms on the fetal skin), accumulates in the intestines as early as the 16th week. Meconium is sticky in consistency and appears black or dark green (obtaining its color from bile pigment). An important neonatal nursing responsibility is recording that a newborn has passed meconium as this rules out a stricture (noncanalization) of the anus (Marcelis, de Blaauw, & Brunner, 2011).

The gastrointestinal tract is sterile before birth. Because vitamin K, necessary for blood clotting, is synthesized by the action of bacteria in the intestines, vitamin K levels are almost nonexistent in a fetus and are still low in a newborn (vitamin K is routinely administered intramuscularly at birth). Sucking and swallowing reflexes are not mature until the fetus is approximately 32 weeks gestation, or weighs 1,500 g. However, strong suck and swallowing reflexes may not be present until the fetus is full term.

The ability of the gastrointestinal tract to secrete enzymes essential for carbohydrate and protein digestion is mature at 36 weeks. However, amylase, an enzyme found in saliva and necessary for digestion of complex starches, does not mature until 3 months after birth. Many newborns have also not yet developed lipase, an enzyme needed for fat digestion (a reason breast milk is the best food for newborns because its digestion does not depend on these enzymes).

The liver is active throughout intrauterine life, functioning as a filter between the incoming blood and the fetal circulation and as a deposit site for fetal stores such as iron and glycogen. Unfortunately, during intrauterine life, the fetal liver is unable to prevent recreational drugs or alcohol ingested by the mother from entering the fetal circulation and possibly causing birth anomalies (Singer, Moore, Fulton, et al., 2012). Newborns need careful assessment at birth for hypoglycemia (low blood sugar) and hyperbilirubinemia (excessive breakdown products from destroyed red blood cells), two serious problems that can occur in the first 24 hours after birth because, although active, liver function is still immature.

MUSCULOSKELETAL SYSTEM

During the first 2 weeks of fetal life, cartilage prototypes provide position and support to the fetus. Ossification of this cartilage into bone begins at about the 12th week and continues all through fetal life and into adulthood. Carpals, tarsals, and sternal bones generally do not ossify until birth is imminent. A fetus can be seen to move on ultrasonography as early as the 11th week, although the mother usually does not feel this movement (*quickening*) until 16 to 20 weeks of gestation. It is usually felt earlier in multigravida women.

> ### What If . . . 9.1
> Liz Calhorn repeats that not only have her feelings toward her baby changed since she felt the baby move but she's also more interested in how to keep him safe now. How would the nurse modify the health teaching with her because of this?

REPRODUCTIVE SYSTEM

A child's sex is determined at the moment of conception by a spermatozoon carrying an X or a Y chromosome and can be ascertained as early as 8 weeks by chromosomal analysis or analysis of fetal cells in the mother's bloodstream. At about the sixth week after implantation, the gonads (i.e., ovaries or testes) form. If testes form, testosterone is secreted, apparently influencing the sexually neutral genital duct to form other male organs (i.e., maturity of the wolffian, or mesonephric, duct). In the absence of testosterone secretion, female organs will form (i.e., maturation of the müllerian, or paramesonephric, duct). This is an important phenomenon because if a woman should unintentionally take an androgen or an androgen-like substance during this stage of pregnancy, a child who is chromosomally female could appear more male than female at birth. If deficient testosterone is secreted by the testes, both the müllerian (female) duct and the wolffian (male) duct could develop (i.e., pseudohermaphroditism, or intersex) (Kutney, Konczal, Kaminski, et al., 2016).

The testes first form in the abdominal cavity and do not descend into the scrotal sac until the 34th to 38th week of intrauterine life. Because of this, many male preterm infants are born with undescended testes. These boys need a follow-up to be certain their testes do descend when they reach what would have been the 34th to 38th week of gestational age because testicular descent does not always occur as readily in extrauterine life as it would have in utero. Testes that do not descend (cryptorchidism) require surgery as they are associated with poor sperm production and possibly testicular cancer later in life (Kelsey, Barker, Bartz, et al., 2016).

URINARY SYSTEM

Although rudimentary kidneys are present as early as the end of the fourth week of intrauterine life, the presence of kidneys does not appear to be essential for life before birth because the placenta clears the fetus of waste products. Urine, however, is formed by the 12th week and is excreted into the amniotic fluid by the 16th week of gestation. At term, fetal urine is being excreted at a rate of up to 500 ml/day. An amount of amniotic fluid less than usual (oligohydramnios) suggests fetal kidneys are not secreting adequate urine and that there is a kidney, ureter, or bladder disorder (Kumar, 2012).

The complex structure of the kidneys gradually develops during intrauterine life and continues to mature for months afterward. The loop of Henle, for example, is not fully differentiated until the fetus is born. Glomerular filtration and concentration of urine in the newborn are still not efficient because the ability to concentrate urine is still not mature at birth. Early in the embryonic stage of urinary system development, the bladder extends as high as the umbilical region, and there is an open lumen between the urinary bladder and the umbilicus. If this fails to close, (termed a *patent urachus*), this is revealed at birth by the persistent drainage of a clear, acid–pH fluid (urine) from the umbilicus (Samra, McGrath, & Wehbe, 2011).

INTEGUMENTARY SYSTEM

The skin of a fetus appears thin and almost translucent until subcutaneous fat begins to be deposited underneath it at about 36 weeks. Skin is covered by soft downy hairs (lanugo) that serve as insulation to preserve warmth in utero as well as a cream cheese–like substance, vernix caseosa, which is important for lubrication and for keeping the skin from macerating in utero. Both lanugo and vernix are still present at birth.

IMMUNE SYSTEM

Immunoglobulin (Ig) G maternal antibodies cross the placenta into the fetus as early as the 20th week and certainly by the 24th week of intrauterine life to give a fetus temporary passive immunity against diseases for which the mother has antibodies. These often include poliomyelitis, rubella (German measles), rubeola (regular measles), diphtheria, tetanus, infectious parotitis (mumps), hepatitis B, and pertussis (whooping cough). Infants born before this antibody transfer has taken place have no natural immunity and so need more than the usual protection against infectious disease in the newborn period.

A fetus only becomes capable of active antibody production late in pregnancy. Generally, it is not necessary for a fetus to produce antibodies because they need to be manufactured only to counteract an invading antigen, and antigens rarely invade the intrauterine space. Because IgA and IgM antibodies (the types which develop to actively counteract infection) cannot cross the placenta, their presence in a newborn is proof that the fetus has been exposed to an infection.

MILESTONES OF FETAL GROWTH AND DEVELOPMENT

When fetal milestones occur can be confusing because the life of the fetus is typically measured from the time of ovulation or fertilization (ovulation age), but the length of a pregnancy is more commonly measured from the first day of the last menstrual period (gestational age). Because ovulation and fertilization take place about 2 weeks after the last menstrual period, the ovulation age of the fetus is always 2 weeks less than the length of the pregnancy or the gestational age.

Both ovulation and gestational age are typically reported in lunar months (4-week periods) or in trimesters (3-month periods) rather than in weeks. In lunar months, a total pregnancy is 10 months (40 weeks or 280 days) long; a fetus grows in utero for 9.5 lunar months or three full trimesters (38 weeks or 266 days).

Figure 9.6 Human embryos at different stages of life. **(A)** Implantation in uterus 7 to 8 days after conception. **(B)** The embryo at 32 days. **(C)** At 37 days. **(D)** At 41 days. **(E)** Between 12 and 15 weeks. (Petit Format/Nestle/Science Source/Photo Researchers.)

The following discussion of fetal developmental milestones is based on gestational weeks because it is helpful when talking to expectant parents to correlate fetal development with the way they measure pregnancy—from the first day of the last menstrual period. Figure 9.6 illustrates the comparative size and appearance of human embryos and fetuses at different stages of development.

End of Fourth Gestational Week

- The length of the embryo is about 0.75 cm; weight is about 400 mg.
- The spinal cord is formed and fused at the midpoint.
- The head is large in proportion and represents about one third of the entire structure.
- The rudimentary heart appears as a prominent bulge on the anterior surface.
- Arms and legs are bud-like structures; rudimentary eyes, ears, and nose are discernible.

End of Eighth Gestational Week

- The length of the fetus is about 2.5 cm (1 in.); weight is about 20 g.
- Organogenesis is complete.
- The heart, with a septum and valves, beats rhythmically.
- Facial features are definitely discernible; arms and legs have developed.
- External genitalia are forming, but sex is not yet distinguishable by simple observation.
- The abdomen bulges forward because the fetal intestine is growing so rapidly.
- A sonogram shows a gestational sac, which is diagnostic of pregnancy (Fig. 9.7).

End of 12th Gestational Week (First Trimester)

- The length of the fetus is 7 to 8 cm; weight is about 45 g.
- Nail beds are forming on fingers and toes.
- Spontaneous movements are possible, although they are usually too faint to be felt by the mother.
- Some reflexes, such as the Babinski reflex, are present.
- Bone ossification centers begin to form.
- Tooth buds are present.
- Sex is distinguishable on outward appearance.

Figure 9.7 Sonogram showing the characteristic circle diagnostic of pregnancy (the gestational sac). (From Stephenson, S. R. [2012]. *Diagnostic medical sonography: Obstetrics and gynecology* [3rd ed.]. Baltimore, MD: Lippincott Williams & Wilkins.)

- Urine secretion begins but may not yet be evident in amniotic fluid.
- The heartbeat is audible through Doppler technology.

End of 16th Gestational Week

- The length of the fetus is 10 to 17 cm; weight is 55 to 120 g.
- Fetal heart sounds are audible by an ordinary stethoscope.
- Lanugo is well formed.
- Both the liver and pancreas are functioning.
- The fetus actively swallows amniotic fluid, demonstrating an intact but uncoordinated swallowing reflex; urine is present in amniotic fluid.
- Sex can be determined by ultrasonography.

End of 20th Gestational Week

- The length of the fetus is 25 cm; weight is 223 g.
- Spontaneous fetal movements can be sensed by the mother.
- Antibody production is possible.
- Hair, including eyebrows, forms on the head; vernix caseosa begins to cover the skin.
- Meconium is present in the upper intestine.
- Brown fat, a special fat that aids in temperature regulation, begins to form behind the kidneys, sternum, and posterior neck.
- Passive antibody transfer from mother to fetus begins.
- Definite sleeping and activity patterns are distinguishable as the fetus develops biorhythms that will guide sleep/wake patterns throughout life.

End of 24th Gestational Week
(Second Trimester)

- The length of the fetus is 28 to 36 cm; weight is 550 g.
- Meconium is present as far as the rectum.
- Active production of lung surfactant begins.
- Eyelids, previously fused since the 12th week, now open; pupils react to light.
- Hearing can be demonstrated by response to sudden sound.
- When fetuses reach 24 weeks, or 500 to 600 g, they have achieved a practical low-end age of viability if they are cared for after birth in a modern intensive care nursery.

End of 28th Gestational Week

- The length of the fetus is 35 to 38 cm; weight is 1,200 g.
- Lung alveoli are almost mature; surfactant can be demonstrated in amniotic fluid.
- Testes begin to descend into the scrotal sac from the lower abdominal cavity.
- The blood vessels of the retina are formed but thin and extremely susceptible to damage from high oxygen concentrations (an important consideration when caring for preterm infants who need oxygen).

End of 32nd Gestational Week

- The length of the fetus is 38 to 43 cm; weight is 1,600 g.
- Subcutaneous fat begins to be deposited (the former stringy, "little old man" appearance is lost).
- Fetus responds by movement to sounds outside the mother's body.

- An active Moro reflex is present.
- Iron stores, which provide iron for the time during which the neonate will ingest only breast milk after birth, are beginning to be built.
- Fingernails reach the end of fingertips.

End of 36th Gestational Week

- The length of the fetus is 42 to 48 cm; weight is 1,800 to 2,700 g (5 to 6 lb).
- Body stores of glycogen, iron, carbohydrate, and calcium are deposited.
- Additional amounts of subcutaneous fat are deposited.
- Sole of the foot has only one or two crisscross creases compared with a full crisscross pattern evident at term.
- Amount of lanugo begins to diminish.
- Most fetuses turn into a vertex (head down) presentation during this month.

End of 40th Gestational Week
(Third Trimester)

- The length of the fetus is 48 to 52 cm (crown to rump, 35 to 37 cm); weight is 3,000 g (7 to 7.5 lb).
- Fetus kicks actively, sometimes hard enough to cause the mother considerable discomfort.
- Fetal hemoglobin begins its conversion to adult hemoglobin.
- Vernix caseosa starts to decrease after the infant reaches 37 weeks gestation and may be more apparent in the creases than the covering of the body as the infant approaches 40 weeks or more gestational age.
- Fingernails extend over the fingertips.
- Creases on the soles of the feet cover at least two thirds of the surface.

In primiparas (i.e., women having their first baby), the fetus often sinks into the birth canal during the last 2 weeks of pregnancy, giving the mother a feeling the load she is carrying is less. This event, termed *lightening*, is a fetal announcement that the fetus is in a ready position and birth is nearing.

DETERMINATION OF ESTIMATED BIRTH DATE

It is impossible to predict with a high degree of accuracy the exact day an infant will be born because fewer than 5% of pregnancies end exactly 280 days from the last menstrual period; fewer than half end within 1 week of the 280th day.

Traditionally, this date was referred to as the estimated date of confinement (EDC). Because women are no longer "confined" after childbirth, the acronym EDB (**estimated date of birth**) is more commonly used today.

If fertilization occurred early in a menstrual cycle, the pregnancy will probably end "early"; if ovulation and fertilization occurred later than the midpoint of the cycle, the pregnancy will end "late." Because of these normal variations, a pregnancy ending 2 weeks before or 2 weeks after the calculated EDB is considered well within the normal limit (38 to 42 weeks). Gestational age wheels and birth date calculators, which can be used to predict a birth date are available, but calculation by Naegele's rule is the standard method used to predict the length of a pregnancy (Box 9.3).

BOX 9.3

Naegele's Rule

To calculate the date of birth by this rule, count backward 3 calendar months from the first day of a woman's last menstrual period and add 7 days. For example, if the last menstrual period began May 15, you would count back 3 months (April 15, March 15, February 15) and add 7 days, to arrive at the predicted date of birth as February 22.

What If . . . 9.2

Liz Calhorn first came to the prenatal clinic on August 5 and told the nurse she had her last menstrual period from March 13 to March 18. What would be her child's EDB?

Assessment of Fetal Growth and Development

Tests for fetal growth and development are commonly done for a variety of reasons, including to:

- Predict the outcome of the pregnancy
- Manage the remaining weeks of the pregnancy
- Plan for possible complications at birth
- Plan for problems that may occur in the newborn infant
- Decide whether to continue the pregnancy
- Find conditions that may affect future pregnancies

Both fetal growth and development can be compromised if a fetus has a metabolic or chromosomal disorder that interferes with normal growth, if the supporting structures such as the placenta or cord do not form normally, or if environmental influences such as the nicotine in cigarettes causes fetal growth restriction (including testes growth in a male fetus) (Virtanen, Sadov, & Toppari, 2012).

Nursing responsibilities for these assessment procedures include verifying that a signed consent form has been obtained as needed (which is necessary if the procedure poses any risk to the mother or fetus that would not otherwise be present), being certain the woman and her support person are aware of what the procedure will entail and any potential risks, preparing the woman physically and psychologically, providing support during the procedure, assessing both fetal and maternal responses during and after the procedure, providing any necessary follow-up care, and managing equipment and specimens. Box 9.4 shows an interprofessional care map illustrating both nursing and team planning for fetal care, including assessment procedures.

Providing follow-up care may include being certain a couple understands the results of a test and how to interpret it. When a result is positive, parents feel assured their infant is growing well. When results are not encouraging, a couple may experience a mixture of emotions. They may express being committed to the pregnancy but express concerns regarding a desire to protect their child, themselves, and their family from the burden of having a child with a severe disability. In some instances, they will be asked to make a life and death decision depending on the results. Quiet listening so a couple has time to thoroughly think through what option will be right for them may be difficult to do but is usually the soundest action for healthcare providers (Reed & Berrier, 2016).

HEALTH HISTORY

Like all assessments, a fetal assessment begins with a health history. Ask the mother specifically about any prepregnancy illnesses such as gestational diabetes or heart disease because these both can interfere with fetal growth. Ask about any drugs a woman takes; for instance, common drugs taken for recurrent seizures can be teratogenic and therefore pose a risk in pregnancy (Mawhinney, Campbell, Craig, et al., 2012). Inquire about nutritional intake because if a woman is not eating a well-balanced diet, she may not be taking in enough nutrients for fetal growth (Whitney & Rolfes, 2012). Be certain to also ask about personal habits such as cigarette smoking, both prescription and recreational drug use, alcohol consumption, and exercise because all of these may influence glucose/insulin balance and fetal growth. Most women are aware alcohol ingestion can harm a fetus (e.g., fetal alcohol spectrum disorder) but many are not yet aware of fetal tobacco syndrome (Wong, Ordean, & Kahan, 2011). This syndrome applies to the fetus of a woman who smokes more than five cigarettes a day and who is born growth restricted (i.e., birth weight under 2,500 g at term). Smoking may also be a cause of ectopic (tubal) pregnancy as fallopian tubes may become irritated (Shao, Zou, Wang, et al., 2012).

Most women instinctively protect a fetus growing inside them so pregnancy may be the push they need to improve their lifestyle (Box 9.5). Asking if a woman has had any exposure to teratogens can reveal exposure to such substances as chemicals, paint fumes, cleaning products, poor air quality, or a loud noise level (Krueger, Horesh, & Crossland, 2012). Asking about unintentional injuries or intimate partner violence can help reveal whether the pregnant woman and fetus could have suffered any trauma from these sources (e.g., intimate partner violence tends to increase during pregnancy because of the stress a pregnancy can create) (Dalton, 2012).

PHYSICAL EXAMINATION

A physical examination of the mother is the second step in evaluating fetal health. Assess maternal weight and general appearance because both obesity and underweight are clues that the mother's nutrition may not be adequate for sound fetal growth (Warren, Rance, & Hunter, 2012). Bruises may indicate intimate partner violence that could have bruised the fetus as well. An elevated blood pressure may be the beginning of hypertension of pregnancy, which can restrict fetal growth (Vest & Cho, 2012).

QSEN Checkpoint Question 9.4

EVIDENCE-BASED PRACTICE

To investigate whether there are any psychosocial predictors of women who smoke during pregnancy, a cross-sectional analysis of a birth cohort was reviewed. In this prospective study, the answers to questionnaires completed by 514 mothers shortly after the birth of their full-term infants found that 14.8% of the participants smoked. Of those women responded that they smoked during pregnancy,

BOX 9.4

Nursing Care Planning

AN INTERPROFESSIONAL CARE MAP FOR A WOMAN UNDERGOING FETAL STUDIES

Liz Calhorn, an 18-year-old, is about 20 weeks pregnant (can't remember date of last menstrual period). Although she says she knows she should have stopped smoking before pregnancy, she has not been able to do this as yet. Twice during the pregnancy (at the 4th and 10th week), she drank beer at summer picnics. Today, at a clinic visit, she tells you she has felt her fetus move. She states, "Feeling the baby move made me realize there's someone inside me, you know what I mean? It made me realize it's time I started being more careful with what I do." Liz works at a fast food restaurant. Boyfriend (father of fetus) is supportive but has no money to offer her for support. Patient states, "I'm not getting married. Just not ready for that level of commitment yet."

Family Assessment: Patient lives in one-bedroom apartment; supports self by working at a fast food restaurant. States, "My parents would help out if I begged them, but I'm not going to do that."

Patient Assessment: Patient smokes a pack of cigarettes a day. Takes aspirin, 10 g, for almost daily sinus headaches. No recreational drug use.
Nutrition: Breakfast: None, to help control her weight.
             Lunch: A hotdog and salad. One diet cola.
             Dinner: Macaroni and cheese; applesauce. One cup coffee.
             Snack: Half bag of potato chips and cream-cheese dip.
Physical examination: Fundal height is 16 cm. Fetal heart tones by Doppler at 160 beats/min. Has been advised to have an ultrasound done to assess for fetal growth and to date pregnancy.

Nursing Diagnosis: Risk for altered fetal growth related to inadequate nutrition and alcohol and nicotine consumption

Outcome Criteria: Patient consents to sonogram for fetal growth assessment; reports lessened alcohol and cigarette use at the next visit.

Team Member Responsible	Assessment	Intervention	Rationale	Expected Outcome
Activities of Daily Living, Including Safety				
Nurse	Ask patient to describe a "typical day" to reveal any actions possibly detrimental to fetal growth.	Discuss common actions unsafe during pregnancy, such as smoking and drinking alcohol.	Knowing what constitutes unsafe practices during pregnancy is a woman's best safeguard against fetal harm.	Patient states she will stop drinking alcohol; is using a supportive Internet quitline to help reduce smoking.
Teamwork and Collaboration				
Primary healthcare provider/nurse	Determine whether sonogram department has appointments free in coming week.	Schedule sonogram 1 week in advance with sonogram department.	Patient believes she might be 20 weeks pregnant. Fundal height, recent fetal movements correspond more closely to 16 weeks.	Patient reports for scheduled ultrasound in 1 week.
Procedures/Medications for Quality Improvement				
Nurse	Assess what prescription or over-the-counter or alternative therapies patient is using.	Discuss with patient inadvisability of taking aspirin during pregnancy; suggest she take acetaminophen (Tylenol) instead.	Acetylsalicylic acid (aspirin) can lead to bleeding or prolonged pregnancy.	Patient reports at next prenatal visit she takes acetaminophen for any pain.

Continued on following page

BOX 9.4

Nursing Care Planning (continued)

Team Member Responsible	Assessment	Intervention	Rationale	Expected Outcome
Nutrition				
Nurse/nutritionist	Ask patient for a 24-hour recall nutrition history.	Discuss the advisability of eating breakfast while pregnant to help avoid hypoglycemia in fetus.	Knowing what constitutes a healthy diet helps ensure a fetus will receive adequate nutrients.	Patient reports at prenatal visits she eats breakfast before leaving for work in the morning; includes more protein in intake.
Patient-Centered Care				
Nurse	Determine whether patient understands ultrasound is not an X-ray, so it is not harmful to the fetus.	Instruct patient about preparation for sonogram (drink fluid; avoid emptying bladder).	A well-prepared patient is more apt to result in an effective procedure and a satisfied patient.	Patient will describe accurate preparations for procedure; receives printed instructions for ambulatory ultrasound.
Spiritual/Psychosocial/Emotional Needs				
Primary healthcare provider/nurse	Assess the extent of factors, such as alcohol and cigarette use, that could have led to intrauterine growth restriction.	Review the possibility with patient that her pregnancy dating may be wrong because fundal height is below usual. Alternate cause could be fetal growth restriction.	Understanding contributors to fetal health is necessary for women to make informed choices during pregnancy.	Patient states she understands the discrepancy in fundal height and weeks gestation following explanation.
Informatics for Seamless Healthcare Planning				
Nurse/primary healthcare provider	Perform complete assessment to help ensure continuity of care with other services.	Mark chart as high-risk patient for intrauterine growth restriction (fundal height below average for weeks gestation).	Documenting risk factors helps to safeguard the fetus.	The patient chart documents high-risk status.

BOX 9.5

Nursing Care Planning to Respect Cultural Diversity

Different cultures have different ideas as to what foods to eat, how much exercise is good during pregnancy, and whether fetal tests for well-being are ethical. Cultural beliefs also affect everyday things, such as believing it is wrong to have a photograph taken during pregnancy because that will alert unknown spirits that the woman is pregnant (the origin of lullabies were songs to keep away Lilith, an avenging creature in Jewish folklore who was thought to bring harm to babies). Believing photographs are harmful may make a woman reluctant to have a sonogram taken during pregnancy; unlike most women, she may not like a photograph of the ultrasound for a baby keepsake.

Some religions also do not support a full range of contraception options; in these instances, the nurse can assist by recommending other natural family planning options that align with the woman's preferences.

they were also more likely to have the following characteristics: lower education, maternal age less than 20 years, unmarried, history of elective abortion, history of unplanned pregnancy, lack of emotional acceptance of the pregnancy by the mother and father, emotional distress, and alcohol consumption (Širvinskienė, Žemaitienė, Jusienė, et al., 2016).

Based on the previous study, which statement by Liz Calhorn would make the nurse most worried she might have difficulty quitting smoking during the remainder of her pregnancy?
   a. "I sometimes do have a few beers on the weekend with my boyfriend."
   b. "When I feel tense, I like to shop. It really takes away that bad feeling."
   c. "I'm trying to stop smoking so I won't have to smoke around my baby."
   d. "My mother had five children with no trouble; why am I so different?"

Look in Appendix A for the best answer and rationale.

ESTIMATING FETAL HEALTH

A number of procedures, both noninvasive and invasive, are used to evaluate fetal health. Because there are many procedures, helping a woman with a high-risk pregnancy maintain a sense of control or empowerment as she is scheduled for them is an important nursing responsibility (Box 9.6).

Fetal Growth

As a fetus grows, the uterus expands to accommodate its size. Although not evidence grounded, typical fundal (top of the uterus) measurements are:

- Over the symphysis pubis at 12 weeks
- At the umbilicus at 20 weeks
- At the xiphoid process at 36 weeks

McDonald's rule, another symphysis–fundal height measurement (although, again, not documented to be thoroughly reliable), is an easy method of determining midpregnancy growth. Typically, tape measurement from the notch of the symphysis pubis to over the top of the uterine fundus as a woman lies supine is equal to the week of gestation in centimeters between the 20th and 31st weeks of pregnancy (e.g., in a pregnancy of 24 weeks, the fundal height should be 24 cm) (Fig. 9.8).

Figure 9.8 Measuring fundal height from the superior aspect of the pubis to the fundal crest. The tape is pressed flat against the abdomen for the measurement.

A fundal height much greater than this standard suggests a multiple pregnancy, a miscalculated due date, a large-for-gestational-age (LGA) infant, hydramnios (increased amniotic fluid volume), or possibly even gestational trophoblastic disease (see Chapter 21). A fundal measurement much less than this suggests the fetus is failing to thrive (e.g., intrauterine growth restriction), the pregnancy length was miscalculated, or an anomaly interfering with growth has developed. McDonald's rule becomes inaccurate during the third trimester of pregnancy because the fetus is growing more in weight than in height during this time.

ASSESSING FETAL WELL-BEING

A number of actions or procedures are helpful in detecting and documenting the fetus is not only growing but also apparently healthy.

Fetal Heart Rate

Fetal heart sounds can be heard and counted as early as the 10th to 11th week of pregnancy by the use of an ultrasound Doppler technique (Fig. 9.9). This is done routinely at every prenatal visit past 10 weeks.

BOX 9.6

Nursing Care Planning to Empower a Family

Women may find the names of tests like maternal serum α-fetoprotein (MSAFP) and substances being tested for (acetylcholinesterase) so confusing that they feel as if their life is being taken over by scheduled tests or exams. To help a woman maintain control:

- Encourage her to ask questions until her primary healthcare provider simplifies instructions or test results enough that she thoroughly understands them.
- Encourage her to set the time and date of appointments if possible so she can fit fetal testing in with her schedule rather than be expected to appear "on command."
- Encourage her to bring her significant other with her for fetal testing so he or she hears the same explanation she does and so that person can also ask questions rather than hearing the information second hand.
- Don't refer to a fetus as "it" during testing because that is such an impersonal term. If the woman has chosen a name, use that while referring to her fetus; otherwise, use "he or she."
- Respect modesty during exams where the woman's abdomen will be exposed. Movie stars are often pictured today with their pregnant abdomen on view, but not every woman wants her body exposed unnecessarily that way.
- Remember that late in pregnancy, women's movements can be painful and may feel awkward, so respect that asking a woman to step up and lie on an examining table is not asking her to complete an easy task. Offer help as necessary but also remember feeling independent is an empowering feeling.

Figure 9.9 Measuring fetal heart rate with a Doppler transducer, which detects and broadcasts the fetal heart rate to the parents-to-be as well as you.

Daily Fetal Movement Count (Kick Counts)

Fetal movement that can be felt by the mother (quickening) occurs at approximately 18 to 20 weeks of pregnancy and peaks in intensity at 28 to 38 weeks. After that time, a healthy fetus moves with a degree of consistency at about 10 times per hour. In contrast, a fetus who is not receiving enough nutrients because of poor maternal nutrition or placental insufficiency has greatly decreased movements. The technique for "kick counts" varies from institution to institution, but a typical method used is to ask women with high-risk pregnancies to:

- Lie in a left recumbent position after a meal.
- Observe and record the number of fetal movements (kicks) their fetus makes until they have counted 10 movements.
- Record the time (typically, this is under an hour).
- If an hour passes without 10 movements, they should walk around a little and try a count again.
- If 10 movements (kicks) cannot be felt in a second 1-hour period, they should telephone their primary healthcare provider. The fetus could be healthy but sleeping during this time, so lack of typical movements may not be serious, but it is an indication for further assessment.

Kick counts are particularly useful in growth-restricted or postterm pregnancies to reveal if a fetus is still receiving adequate nutrition (Caughey, 2012). Make certain the woman knows fetal movements do vary, especially in relation to sleep cycles, her activity, and the time since she last ate. Otherwise, she can become unduly worried her fetus is in jeopardy when the fetus is asleep or just having an inactive time.

What If . . . 9.3

The nurse gives instructions to Liz Calhorn to count fetal movements (count kicks) daily after lunch, and she tells the nurse she can't do that because she snacks all day long rather than eats at regular times. Which would be more important: that she should count kicks after meals or that she do it every day?

Rhythm Strip Testing

The term "rhythm strip testing" refers to an assessment of fetal well-being and assesses the fetal heart rate for a normal baseline rate. For this, help the woman into a semi-Fowler's position (either in a comfortable lounge chair or on an examining table or bed with an elevated backrest) to prevent her uterus from compressing the vena cava and causing supine hypotension syndrome during the test. Attach an external fetal heart rate monitor abdominally (Fig. 9.10A). Record the fetal heart rate for 20 minutes.

The baseline reading refers to the average rate of the fetal heartbeat. Variability denotes the small changes in rate that occur from second to second if the fetal parasympathetic nervous system is receiving adequate oxygen and nutrients. In the rhythm strip in Figure 9.10B, for example, the baseline (average) of the fetal heartbeat is 130 beats/min. Variability is present.

Long-term variability reflects the state of the fetal sympathetic nervous system. On a rhythm strip, it is the differences in heart rate that occur over the 20-minute time period. Note in Figure 9.10B how the heart rate varies from 150 to 130 beats/min. Because the average fetus moves about twice every 10 minutes, and movement causes the heart rate to increase, there will typically be two or more instances of fetal heart rate acceleration in a 20-minute rhythm strip.

Variability is rated as:

- Absent: No peak-to-trough range is detectable.
- Minimal: An amplitude range is detectable but the rate is 5 beats/min or fewer.
- Moderate or normal: An amplitude range is detectable; rate is 6 to 25 beats/min.
- Marked: An amplitude range is detectable; rate is greater than 25 beats/min (ACOG, 2009).

Rhythm strip testing requires a woman to remain in a fairly fixed position for 20 minutes. Keep her well informed of the importance and purpose of the test and be certain she understand the meaning of the results after the test. Electronic fetal heart rate recording is further discussed in Chapter 15 as it can also be used to assess fetal well-being at the beginning of labor.

Nonstress Testing

A **nonstress test** measures the response of the fetal heart rate to fetal movement. Position the woman and attach both a fetal heart rate and a uterine contraction monitor. Instruct the woman to push the button attached to the monitor (similar to a call bell) whenever she feels the fetus move. This will create a dark mark on the paper tracing at these times.

When the fetus moves, the fetal heart rate should increase approximately 15 beats/min and remain elevated for 15 seconds. It should decrease to its average rate again as the fetus quiets (Fig. 9.10C). If no increase in beats per minute is noticeable on fetal movement, further testing may be necessary to rule out poor oxygen perfusion of the fetus.

A nonstress test usually is done for 20 minutes. The test is said to be reactive (healthy) if two accelerations of fetal heart rate (by 15 beats or more) lasting for 15 seconds occur after movement within the time period. The test is nonreactive (fetal health may be affected) if no accelerations occur with the fetal movements. The results also can be interpreted as nonreactive if no fetal movement occurs or if there is low short-term fetal heart rate variability (less than 6 beats/min) throughout the testing period (Bienstock, Fox, Wallach, et al., 2015).

If a 20-minute period passes without any fetal movement, it may only mean that the fetus is sleeping, although other reasons for lessened variability are maternal smoking, drug use, or hypoglycemia. Although not evidence based, if you give the woman an oral carbohydrate snack, such as orange juice, it can cause her blood glucose level to increase enough to cause fetal movement. The fetus also may be stimulated by a loud sound (discussed later) to cause movement.

Because both rhythm strip and nonstress testing are noninvasive procedures and cause no risk to either the pregnant woman or fetus, they can be used as screening procedures in all pregnancies. They can be conducted at home daily as part of a home monitoring program for the woman who is having a complication of pregnancy. If a nonstress test is nonreactive, an additional fetal assessment, such as a biophysical profile test, will be scheduled.

Vibroacoustic Stimulation

For acoustic (sound) stimulation, a specially designed acoustic stimulator is applied to the mother's abdomen to produce a sharp sound of approximately 80 dB at a frequency of 80 Hz, thus startling and waking the fetus (Bienstock et al., 2015).

During a standard nonstress test, if a spontaneous acceleration has not occurred within 5 minutes, apply a single 1- to

Figure 9.10 Rhythm strip and nonstress testing of fetal heart rate. **(A)** The woman sits in a comfortable chair to avoid supine hypotension. Both a uterine contraction monitor and fetal heart rate monitor are in place on her abdomen. (Photograph by Melissa Olson, with permission of Chestnut Hill Hospital, Philadelphia, PA.) **(B)** A rhythm strip. The upper strip signifies heart rate; the lower strip indicates uterine activity. *Arrows* signal fetal movement. **(C)** Baseline fetal heart rate on this strip is 130 to 132 beats/min. This strip shows fetal heart rate acceleration in response to fetal movement, shown by arrows. (Photograph by Melissa Olson, with permission of Chestnut Hill Hospital, Philadelphia, PA.)

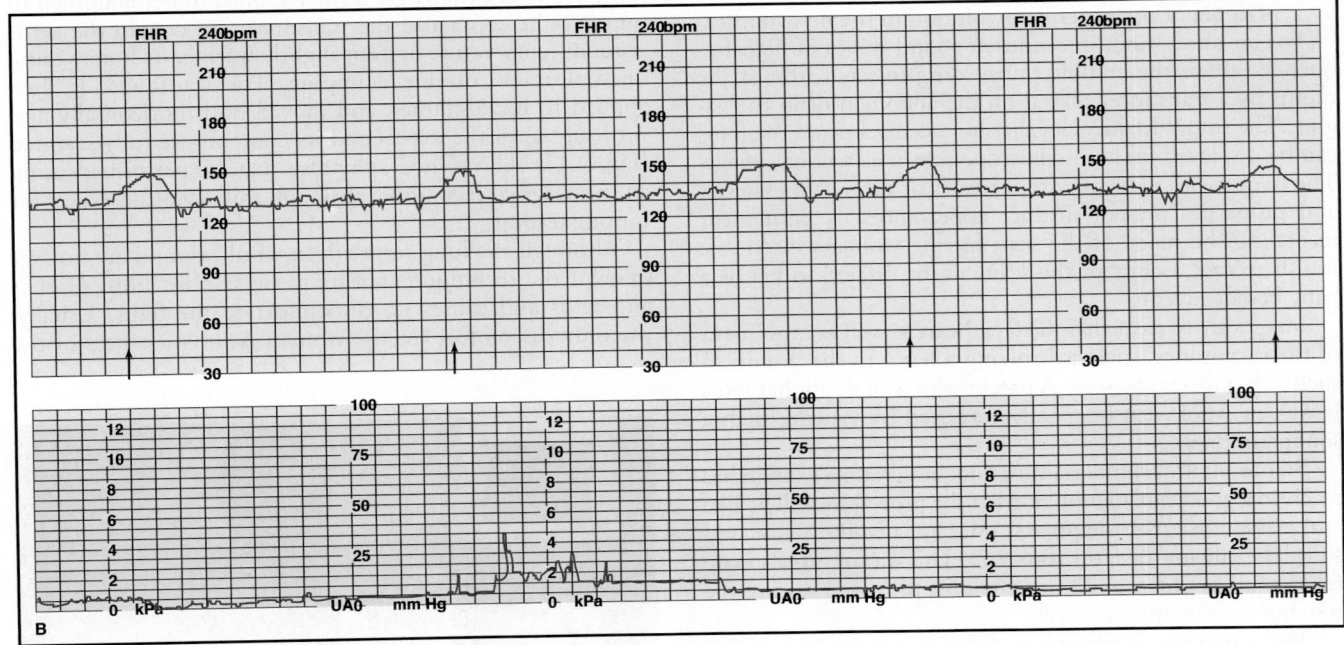

2-second sound stimulation to the lower abdomen. This can be repeated again at the end of 10 minutes if no further spontaneous movement occurs, so two movements within the 20-minute window can be evaluated.

Ultrasonography

Ultrasonography, which measures the response of sound waves against solid objects, is a much-used tool for fetal health assessments. It can be used to:

- Diagnose pregnancy as early as 6 weeks gestation.
- Confirm the presence, size, and location of the placenta and amniotic fluid.
- Establish a fetus is growing and has no gross anomalies such as hydrocephalus; anencephaly; or spinal cord, heart, kidney, and bladder concerns.
- Establish the sex if a penis is revealed.
- Establish the presentation and position of the fetus.
- Predict gestational age by measurement of the biparietal diameter of the head or crown-to-rump measurement.
- Discover complications of pregnancy, such as the presence of an intrauterine device, hydramnios (excessive amniotic fluid) or oligohydramnios (lessened amniotic fluid), ectopic pregnancy, missed miscarriage, abdominal pregnancy, placenta previa (a low-implanted placenta), premature separation of the placenta, coexisting uterine tumors, or multiple pregnancy. Genetic disorders such as Down syndrome and fetal anomalies such as neural tube disorders, diaphragmatic hernia, or urethral stenosis also can be diagnosed. Fetal death can be revealed by a lack of heartbeat and respiratory movement.
- After birth, a sonogram may be used to detect a retained placenta or poor uterine involution in the new mother.

For an ultrasound, intermittent sound waves of high frequency (above the audible range) are projected toward the uterus by a transducer placed on the abdomen or in the vagina. The sound frequencies that bounce back from the fetus can be displayed on an oscilloscope screen as a visual image. The frequencies returning from tissues of various thicknesses and properties present distinct appearances. A permanent record can be made of the scan for the woman's electronic health record; a copy of the scan can be offered to her as a baby book souvenir.

Images are so clear that the fetal heart as well as movement of the extremities, such as bringing a hand to the mouth to suck a thumb, can be seen. A parent who is in doubt her fetus is well or whole can be greatly reassured by viewing such a sonogram image.

Before an ultrasound examination, be certain a woman has received a good explanation of what the procedure will be like and reassurance that the process does not involve X-rays and so will be safe for the fetus (Box 9.7). This means it is also safe for the father of the child to remain in the room during the test and see the images as well.

The sound waves reflect best if the uterus can be held stable so it is helpful if the woman has a full bladder at the time of the procedure. To ensure this, ask her to drink a full glass of water every 15 minutes beginning 90 minutes before the procedure and to not void until after the procedure.

Help the woman up to an examining table and drape her for modesty, but with her abdomen exposed. To prevent supine hypotension syndrome, place a towel under her right buttock to tip her body slightly so the uterus will roll away

💬 Nursing Care Planning Tips for Effective Communication

Liz Calhorn is scheduled for an ultrasound. She is 20 weeks pregnant with her first child. She has been coming to her prenatal visits by herself. She has not missed any scheduled appointments. Liz is healthy and has had no complications thus far with her pregnancy.

Tip: Avoid becoming so engrossed in sharing personal feelings that you forget to listen to what the patient is actually saying. Consider what the patient wants and carefully listen for any underlying fears.

Nurse: Do you have any questions about what will happen, Liz?

Liz: I guess. I can't decide if I want to know my baby's sex or not.

Nurse: That's an individual decision. What things are you thinking about?

Liz: I think I'd rather be surprised. I know I don't want a boy.

Nurse: You don't want a boy?

Liz: A guy got me into this trouble. The last thing I need is another one around the house.

Nurse: Let's talk about what it will mean if you should have a boy.

from the vena cava. A gel is then applied to her abdomen to improve the contact of the transducer. Be certain the gel is at room temperature or even slightly warmer or it may cause uncomfortable uterine cramping. The transducer is then applied to her abdomen and moved both horizontally and vertically until the uterus and its contents are fully scanned (Fig. 9.11). Ultrasonography also may be performed using an intravaginal technique, although this is not necessary for routine testing.

Although the long-term effects of ultrasound are not yet known, the technique appears to be safe for both mother and fetus and causes no discomfort to the fetus. Usually, the only discomfort for the woman is the messiness of the

Figure 9.11 A sonogram being recorded. Notice the mother's interest in being able to see her baby's first photograph.

Figure 9.12 A sonogram at 26 weeks gestation showing measurement of the biparietal diameter. (From Cosby, K. S., & Kendall, J. L. [2014]. *Practical guide to emergency ultrasound* [2nd ed.]. Philadelphia, PA: Wolters Kluwer.)

contact lubrication and a strong desire to void before the scan is completed. Taking home a photograph of the sonographic image can enhance bonding because it is proof the pregnancy exists and the fetus appears well. As desirable as it is, however, caution women against having ultrasound images done just for the purpose of having "keepsake" photographs. Commercial firms offering these services are not well regulated, and their equipment may be outdated and unsafe.

In medical practice, a number of specific features are studied by sonogram.

Biparietal Diameter

Ultrasonography may be used to predict fetal maturity by measuring the biparietal diameter (side-to-side measurement) of the fetal head. In 80% of pregnancies in which the biparietal diameter of the fetal head is 8.5 cm or greater, it can be predicted the infant will weigh more than 2,500 g (5.5 lb) at birth or is at a fetal age of 40 weeks.

Figure 9.12 is a sonogram showing the biparietal diameter of a fetus at 26 weeks. Figure 9.13 shows a fetus close to term.

Doppler Umbilical Velocimetry

Doppler ultrasonography measures the velocity at which red blood cells in the uterine and fetal vessels travel. Assessment of the blood flow through uterine blood vessels is helpful to determine the vascular resistance present in women with gestational diabetes or hypertension and whether resultant placental insufficiency is occurring. Decreased velocity is an important predictor that uterine growth restriction will occur because it reveals that only a limited number of nutrients are able to reach the fetus (Kaponis, Harada, Makrydimas, et al., 2011).

Placental Grading for Maturity

Placentas can be graded by ultrasound based on the particular amount of calcium deposits present in the base. Placentas are graded as:
- 0: between 12 and 24 weeks
- 1: 30 to 32 weeks
- 2: 36 weeks
- 3: 38 weeks (Because fetal lungs are apt to be mature by 38 weeks, a grade 3 placenta suggests the fetus is mature.)

Amniotic Fluid Volume

The amount of amniotic fluid present is yet another way to estimate fetal health because a portion of the fluid is formed by fetal kidney output. If a fetus is becoming so stressed in utero that circulatory and kidney function is failing, urine output and, consequently, the volume of amniotic fluid will decrease. A decrease in amniotic fluid volume puts the fetus at risk for compression of the umbilical cord with interference of nutrition as well as lack of room to exercise and maintain muscle tone. Between 28 and 40 weeks, the total pockets of amniotic fluid revealed by sonogram average 12 to 15 cm. An amount greater than 20 to 24 cm indicates hydramnios (i.e., excessive fluid, perhaps caused by inability of the fetus to swallow). An amount less than 5 to 6 cm indicates oligohydramnios (i.e., decreased amniotic fluid, perhaps caused by poor perfusion and kidney failure).

Nuchal Translucency

Children with a number of chromosome anomalies have unusual pockets of fat or fluid present in their posterior neck, which show on sonograms as nuchal translucency. Chromosomal anomalies associated with this are discussed in Chapter 7.

QSEN Checkpoint Question 9.5

PATIENT-CENTERED CARE

Liz Calhorn is scheduled to have an ultrasound examination and the nurse wants to ensure that she understands and is prepared for this procedure to mitigate her anxiety. What instruction would the nurse give her before her examination?
- a. "Use the restroom immediately before the procedure to reduce your bladder size."
- b. "The intravenous fluid used to dilate your uterus does not hurt the fetus."
- c. "You will need to drink at least three glasses of water before the procedure."
- d. "You can have medicine for the pain of any contractions caused by the test."

Look in Appendix A for the best answer and rationale.

Figure 9.13 A sonogram showing a fetus close to term.

TABLE 9.3 BIOPHYSICAL PROFILE SCORING

Assessment	Instrument	Criteria for a Score of 2
Fetal breathing	Sonogram	At least one episode of 30 s of sustained fetal breathing movements within 30 min of observation
Fetal movement	Sonogram	At least three separate episodes of fetal limb or trunk movement within a 30-min observation
Fetal tone	Sonogram	The fetus must extend and then flex the extremities or spine at least once in 30 min.
Amniotic fluid volume	Sonogram	A pocket of amniotic fluid measuring more than 2 cm in vertical diameter must be present
Fetal heart reactivity	Nonstress test	Two or more accelerations of fetal heart rate of 15 beats/min lasting 15 s or more following fetal movements in a 20-min period

Biophysical Profile

A biophysical profile combines five parameters (i.e., fetal reactivity, fetal breathing movements, fetal body movement, fetal tone, and amniotic fluid volume) into one assessment. The fetal heart and breathing record measures short-term central nervous system function; the amniotic fluid volume helps measure long-term adequacy of placental function. The scoring for a complete profile is shown in Table 9.3. By this system, each item has the potential for scoring a 2, so 10 would be the highest score possible. A biophysical profile is more accurate in predicting fetal well-being than any single assessment (Oyelese & Vintzileos, 2011). Because the scoring system is similar to an Apgar score determined at birth on infants, it is often referred to as a fetal Apgar score.

Biophysical profiles may be done as often as daily during a high-risk pregnancy. The fetal scores are as follows:

- A score of 8 to 10 means the fetus is considered to be doing well.
- A score of 6 is considered suspicious.
- A score of 4 denotes a fetus potentially in jeopardy.

For simplicity, some centers use only two assessments (amniotic fluid index [AFI] and a nonstress test) for the analysis. Referred to as a modified biophysical profile, this predicts short-term viability by the nonstress test and long-term viability by the AFI. A healthy fetus should show a reactive nonstress test and an AFI range between 5 and 25 cm (Bienstock et al., 2015). Nurses play a large role in obtaining the information for both a modified and a full biophysical profile by obtaining either the nonstress test or the sonogram reading.

Magnetic Resonance Imaging

Magnetic resonance imaging (MRI) is yet another way to assess a growing fetus. Because the technique apparently causes no harmful effects to the fetus or woman, MRI has the potential to replace or complement ultrasonography as a fetal assessment technique because it can identify structural anomalies or soft tissue disorders (O'Connor, Rooks, & Smith, 2012). An MRI may be most helpful in diagnosing complications such as ectopic pregnancy or trophoblastic disease (see Chapter 21) because later in a pregnancy, fetal movement (unless the fetus is sedated) can obscure the findings.

Maternal Serum

Because a number of trophoblast cells pass into the maternal bloodstream beginning at about the seventh week of pregnancy, maternal serum analysis can reveal information about the pregnant woman as well as the fetus.

Maternal Serum α-Fetoprotein

AFP is a substance produced by the fetal liver that can be found in both amniotic fluid and maternal serum (maternal serum α-fetoprotein [MSAFP]). The level is abnormally high if the fetus has an open spinal or abdominal wall defect because the open defect allows more AFP to enter the mother's circulation than usual. Although the reason is unclear, the level is low if the fetus has a chromosomal defect such as Down syndrome. MSAFP levels begin to rise at 11 weeks gestation and then steadily increase until term. Traditionally assessed at the 15th week of pregnancy, between 85% and 90% of neural tube anomalies and 80% of babies with Down syndrome can be detected by this method (Rogers & Worley, 2012).

Maternal Serum for Pregnancy-Associated Plasma Protein A

Pregnancy-associated plasma protein A (PAPP-A) is a protein secreted by the placenta; low levels in maternal blood are associated with fetal chromosomal anomalies, including trisomies 13, 18, and 21 or small-for-gestational-age (SGA) babies. A high PAPP-A level may predict an LGA baby.

Quadruple Screening

Quadruple screening analyzes four indicators of fetal health: AFP, unconjugated estriol (UE; an enzyme produced by the placenta that estimates general well-being), hCG (also produced by the placenta), and inhibin A (a protein produced by the placenta and corpus luteum associated with Down syndrome).

As with the measurement of MSAFP, quadruple testing requires only a simple venipuncture of the mother. Because it measures four separate values, it is the most common of the maternal serum tests used today (Manipalviratn, Trivax, & Huang, 2013).

Fetal Gender

Although fetal gender is usually determined by an ultrasound screen at about 4 months, it can be determined as early as 7 weeks by analysis of maternal serum. This early diagnosis could be helpful to a woman who has an X-carrying genetic disorder so she could discover if she has a male fetus who could inherit the disease or a female fetus who will be disease-free (Mortarino, Garagiola, Lotta, et al., 2011). Screening of this type has some ethical connotations because if the fetus is determined to be the "wrong" gender, there could be serious consequences for the now unwanted child.

Invasive Fetal Testing

If a genetic or growth concern is identified by noninvasive measures, a number of invasive measures allow for more refined investigation. Examples include chorionic villi sampling and amniocentesis (see Chapter 8).

If the woman has Rh-negative blood, Rho(D) immune globulin (RhIG; RhoGAM) is administered after the procedure to prevent fetal isoimmunization or help ensure maternal antibodies will not form against any placental red blood cells that might have accidentally been released into the maternal bloodstream during the procedure.

Amniotic fluid (obtained through amniocentesis, Fig. 9.14) can be analyzed for:

- AFP
- Acetylcholinesterase, another compound that rises to high levels if a neural tube anomaly is present
- Bilirubin determination. The presence of bilirubin may be analyzed if a blood incompatibility is suspected. If bilirubin is going to be analyzed, the specimen must be free of blood or a false-positive reading will occur.
- Chromosome analysis. A few fetal skin cells are always present in amniotic fluid so these cells may be cultured and stained for karyotyping for genetic analysis. Examples of genetic diseases that can be detected by prenatal amniocentesis and their significance to health are discussed in Chapter 7.
- Color. Normal amniotic fluid is the color of water; late in pregnancy, it may have a slightly yellow tinge. A strong yellow color suggests a blood incompatibility (the yellow results from the presence of bilirubin released from the breakdown of red blood cells). A green color suggests meconium staining, a phenomenon associated with fetal distress.
- Fibronectin. Fibronectin is a glycoprotein that plays a part in helping the placenta attach to the uterine decidua. Early in pregnancy, it can be assessed in the woman's cervical mucus, but the amount then fades until, after 20 weeks of pregnancy, it is no longer present in cervical mucus. As labor approaches and cervical dilation begins, it can be found again in cervical or vaginal fluid. Damage to fetal membranes from cervical dilatation releases a great deal of the substance, so detection of fibronectin in either the amniotic fluid or in the mother's vagina late in pregnancy can serve as an announcement that preterm labor may be beginning.
- Inborn errors of metabolism. A number of inherited diseases that are caused by inborn errors of metabolism can be detected by amniocentesis. For a condition to be identified, an errant enzyme must be present in the amniotic fluid as early as the time of the procedure. Examples of illnesses that can be detected in this way are sickle cell disease, cystic fibrosis, muscular dystrophy, Tay-Sachs disease, and maple syrup urine disease (an amino acid disorder).
- L/S ratio. Lecithin and sphingomyelin are the protein components of the lung enzyme surfactant that the alveoli begin to form at the 22nd to 24th weeks of pregnancy. Following an amniocentesis, the L/S ratio may be determined quickly by a shake test (if bubbles appear in the amniotic fluid after shaking, the ratio is mature), but the specimen is then sent for laboratory analysis for a definite analysis. An L/S ratio of 2:1 is traditionally accepted as lung maturity. Infants of mothers with severe diabetes may have false-mature readings of lecithin because stress to the infant in utero tends to mature lecithin pathways early. This means fetal values must be considered in light of the presence of maternal diabetes or the infants may be born with mature lung function but be immature overall (a fragile giant), causing them to not do well in postnatal life (Hay et al., 2016). Some

Figure 9.14 Amniocentesis. A pocket of amniotic fluid is located by sonogram. A small amount of fluid is removed by needle aspiration.

laboratories interpret a ratio of 2.5:1 or 3:1 as a mature indicator in infants of women with diabetes.

- Phosphatidylglycerol and desaturated phosphatidylcholine. These are additional compounds, in addition to lecithin and sphingomyelin, found in surfactant. Pathways for these compounds mature at 35 to 36 weeks. Because they are present only with mature lung function, if they are present in the sample of amniotic fluid, it can be predicted with even greater confidence that respiratory distress syndrome is not likely to occur.

QSEN Checkpoint Question 9.6

QUALITY IMPROVEMENT

Liz Calhorn is scheduled to have an amniocentesis to test for fetal maturity. To help make sure the procedure is successful, what instruction would be best to give her before this procedure?

a. "Void (pee) immediately before the procedure to reduce the size of your bladder."
b. "The X-ray used to reveal your fetus's position will have no long-term fetal effects."
c. "The IV fluid used to dilate your uterus is isotonic saline so will not hurt the fetus."
d. "Your fetus will have less amniotic fluid for the rest of pregnancy, but that's all right."

Look in Appendix A for the best answer and rationale.

Percutaneous Umbilical Blood Sampling

Percutaneous umbilical blood sampling (PUBS; also called cordocentesis or funicentesis) is the aspiration of blood from the umbilical vein for analysis. After the umbilical cord is located by sonography, a thin needle is inserted by amniocentesis technique into the uterus and is then guided by ultrasound until it pierces the umbilical vein. A sample of blood is then removed for blood studies, such as a complete blood count, direct Coombs test, blood gases, and karyotyping. To ensure the blood obtained is fetal blood, it is submitted to a Kleihauer–Betke test, which measures the difference between adult and fetal hemoglobin. If a PUBS test reveals that the fetus is anemic, blood may be transfused into the cord using this same technique. Because the umbilical vein continues to ooze for a moment after the procedure, there is a high chance fetal blood could enter the maternal circulation after the procedure, so RhIG is given to Rh-negative women to prevent sensitization. Fetal heart rate and uterine contractions need to be monitored before and after the procedure to be certain uterine contractions are not beginning and also by ultrasound to be certain no bleeding is evident. This procedure carries little additional risk to the fetus or woman over amniocentesis and can yield information not available by any other means, especially about blood dyscrasias.

Fetoscopy

The use of a **fetoscopy**, in which the fetus is visualized by inspection through a fetoscope (an extremely narrow, hollow tube inserted by amniocentesis technique), can be yet another way to assess fetal well-being. This method allows direct visualization of both the amniotic fluid and the fetus (Richter, Wergeland, DeKoninck, et al., 2012). If a photograph is taken through the fetoscope, it can document a problem or reassure parents that their infant is perfectly formed. The main reasons the procedure is used are to:

- Confirm the intactness of the spinal column.
- Obtain biopsy samples of fetal tissue and fetal blood samples.
- Determine meconium staining is not present.
- Perform elemental surgery, such as inserting a polyethylene shunt into the fetal ventricles to relieve hydrocephalus or anteriorly into the fetal bladder to relieve a stenosed urethra. It may be possible to repair a neural tube defect such as meningocele or improve the outcome of myelomeningocele by fetoscopy (Danzer, Johnson, & Adzick, 2012).

The earliest time in pregnancy a fetoscopy can be performed is approximately the 16th or 17th week. For the procedure, the mother is draped as for amniocentesis. A local anesthetic is injected into the abdominal skin. The fetoscope is then inserted through a minor abdominal incision. If the fetus is very active, meperidine (Demerol) may be administered to the woman to help sedate the fetus to avoid fetal injury by the scope and allow for better observation.

A fetoscopy carries a small risk of premature labor or amnionitis (infection of the amniotic fluid). To avoid infection, the woman may be prescribed antibiotic therapy after the procedure. The number of procedures performed by a fetoscopy is limited because of the manipulation involved and the ethical quandary of the mother's autonomy being compromised by fetal needs if further procedures are necessary such as asking the pregnant woman to undergo general anesthesia so the fetus can have surgery.

Women With Unique Needs or Concerns

Fetal assessment can be more difficult in some women than others. For example, it is more difficult to hear fetal heart sounds in a morbidly obese woman. If the straps for fetal heart rate monitors are not long enough to circle a woman's abdomen, they may need to be held in place manually. If a woman is not easily mobile, she can have difficulty obtaining a clean catch urine for protein and glucose testing. Be ready to assist in these circumstances as needed.

Women who are wheelchair challenged can remain in their wheelchair for fetal heart rate monitoring. All individuals who use wheelchairs need to periodically press on the armrests with their hands and raise their buttocks off the seat of the wheelchair to help prevent pressure ulcers as the danger of ulcers increases with pregnancy because of the added weight. During a lengthy test, a woman may need to take a break to stretch; mark the break on a rhythm strip so a sudden corresponding fetal movement on the strip is not misinterpreted.

Remember that women who are hearing challenged will not be able to hear their baby's heartbeat by Doppler assessment. Observing a rhythm strip is a better method to prove to them their fetus appears healthy. In contrast, a woman who is visually impaired would be most assured by listening to the beeping of a Doppler rather than the blurry outlines (for her) of a rhythm strip. Women with special needs are further discussed in Chapter 22. Assess each woman individually to be certain each has obtained and understands the results of fetal assessments accurately and doesn't have continuing questions about her baby's health.

What If . . . 9.4

The nurse is particularly interested in exploring one of the 2020 National Health Goals in respect to fetal health (see Box 9.1). What would be a possible research topic to explore pertinent to this goal that would be applicable to Liz and her family and also advance evidence-based practice?

Unfolding Patient Stories: Brenda Patton • Part 1

Brenda Patton is 18 years old at 24 weeks gestation with her first child. During the prenatal visit, what questions would the nurse ask to evaluate fetal well-being? What factors can interfere with normal growth and development of the fetus? Describe the assessments the nurse performs to monitor fetal growth and development. (Brenda Patton's story continues in Chapter 22.)

Care for Brenda and other patients in a realistic virtual environment: *vSim for Nursing* (thepoint.lww.com/vSimMaternityPed). Practice documenting these patients' care in DocuCare (thepoint.lww.com/DocuCareEHR).

KEY POINTS FOR REVIEW

- Being aware of healthy fetal growth helps in planning nursing care that not only meets Quality & Safety Education for Nurses (QSEN) competencies but also best meets a family's need for health teaching.

- The union of a single sperm and egg (fertilization) signals the beginning of pregnancy.

- The fertilized ovum (zygote) travels by way of a fallopian tube to the uterus, where implantation takes place in about 8 days.

- From implantation to 5 to 8 weeks, the growing structure is called an embryo. The period after 8 weeks until birth is the fetal period.

- Growth of the umbilical cord, amniotic fluid, and amniotic membranes proceeds in concert with fetal growth. The placenta produces a number of important hormones: estrogen, progesterone, hPL, and hCG.

- Various methods to assess fetal growth and development include fundal height, fetal movement, fetal heart tones, ultrasonography, MRI, MSAFP, amniocentesis, PUBS, quadruple screening, and fetoscopy.

- A biophysical profile is a combination of fetal assessments that predicts fetal well-being better than measuring single parameters.

CRITICAL THINKING CARE STUDY

Maeve is a 35-year-old woman who is about 3 months pregnant. She recently broke her fibula in a touch football game and so has her leg encased in a midcalf level cast. It's not a walking cast, so she will be using a wheelchair for the next 6 weeks. She's worried she'll gain too much weight because she's no longer active. Because she's not sure of the date of her last menstrual period, she'd like a sonogram done to date her pregnancy. She asks if that can be done with her in a wheelchair.

1. How would you answer Maeve's question about using her wheelchair for a sonogram?

2. What other special considerations does Maeve need with regard to fetal health because she uses a wheelchair?

3. Maeve asks you if her baby has hair yet. That's important to her because if her baby is a boy she doesn't want him to be as bald as her husband, who at 36, has already lost most of his hair.

RELATED RESOURCES

Explore these additional resources to enhance learning for this chapter:

- Student resources on thePoint, including answers to the What If . . . and Critical Thinking Care Study questions, http://thepoint.lww.com/Flagg8e
- Adaptive learning powered by PrepU, http://thepoint.lww.com/prepu

REFERENCES

American College of Obstetricians and Gynecologists. (2009). ACOG Practice Bulletin No. 106: Intrapartum fetal heart rate monitoring: Nomenclature, interpretation and general management principles. *Obstetrics and Gynecology, 114*(1), 192–202.

American College of Obstetricians and Gynecologists. (2014). ACOG Practice Bulletin No. 145: Antepartum fetal surveillance. *Obstetrics & Gynecology, 124,* 182–192.

Bienstock, J. L., Fox, H. E., Wallach, E. E., et al. (2015). *The Johns Hopkins manual of gynecology and obstetrics* (5th ed.). Philadelphia, PA: Wolters Kluwer.

Caughey, A. G. (2012). Post-term pregnancy. In D. K. Edmonds (Ed.), *Dewhurst's textbook of obstetrics & gynaecology* (8th ed., pp. 269–286). Oxford, United Kingdom: Wiley-Blackwell.

Chen, S., Sun, R., Li, X., et al. (2016). Recent perspectives of stem cells use in cardiac disorders. *Hellenic Journal of Cardiology*. Advance online publication. doi:10.1016/j.hjc.2016.11.031

Chitra, T., Sushanth, Y. S., & Raghavan, S. (2012). Umbilical coiling index as a marker of perinatal outcome: An analytical study. *Obstetrics and Gynecology International, 2012,* 213689.

Coad, J., & Dunstall, M. (2011a). Physiological adaptation to pregnancy. In J. Coad & M. Dunstall (Eds.), *Anatomy and physiology for midwives* (3rd ed., pp. 257–288). London, United Kingdom: Elsevier/Churchill Livingstone.

Coad, J., & Dunstall, M. (2011b). The placenta. In J. Coad & M. Dunstall (Eds.), *Anatomy and physiology for midwives* (3rd ed., pp. 173–198). London, United Kingdom: Elsevier/Churchill Livingstone.

Cohen, S., & Uddin, S. (2011). Primary and preventive care. In K. J. Hurt, M. W. Guile, J. L. Bienstock, et al. (Eds.), *The Johns Hopkins manual of gynecology and obstetrics* (4th ed., pp. 1–14). Philadelphia, PA: Lippincott Williams & Wilkins.

Dalton, M. (2012). Domestic violence and sexual assault. In D. K. Edmonds (Ed.), *Dewhurst's textbook of obstetrics & gynaecology* (8th ed., pp. 798–804). Oxford, United Kingdom: Wiley-Blackwell.

Danzer, E., Johnson, M. P., & Adzick, N. S. (2012). Fetal surgery for myelomeningocele: Progress and perspectives. *Developmental Medicine & Child Neurology, 54*(1), 8–14.

DiGiulio, M., Wiedaseck, S., & Monchek, R. (2012). Understanding hydatidiform mole. *The American Journal of Maternal/Child Nursing, 37*(1), 30–34.

Gardosi, J. (2012). Normal fetal growth. In D. K. Edmonds (Ed.), *Dewhurst's textbook of obstetrics & gynaecology* (8th ed., pp. 26–34). Oxford, United Kingdom: Wiley-Blackwell.

Ghionzoli, M., James, C. P., David, A. L., et al. (2012). Gastroschisis with intestinal atresia—predictive value of antenatal diagnosis and outcome of postnatal treatment. *Journal of Pediatric Surgery, 47*(2), 322–328.

Gowen, C. W., Jr. (2011). Respiratory diseases of the newborn. In K. J. Marcdante, R. M. Kliegman, H. B. Jenson, et al. (Eds.), *Nelson essentials of pediatrics* (6th ed., pp. 237–244). Philadelphia, PA: Saunders/Elsevier.

Hay, W. W., Jr., Levin, M. J., Deterding, R. R., et al. (Eds.). (2016). *Current diagnosis and treatment: Pediatrics* (23rd ed.). Columbus, OH: McGraw-Hill/Lange.

Hoh, J. K., Sung, Y. M., & Park, M. I. (2012). Fetal heart rate parameters and perinatal outcomes in fetuses with nuchal cords. *The Journal of Obstetrics and Gynaecology Research, 38*(2), 358–363.

Huppertz, B., & Kingdom, J. C. P. (2012). The placenta and fetal membranes. In D. K. Edmonds (Ed.), *Dewhurst's textbook of obstetrics & gynaecology* (8th ed., pp. 16–25). Oxford, United Kingdom: Wiley-Blackwell.

Kaponis, A., Harada, T., Makrydimas, G., et al. (2011). The importance of venous Doppler velocimetry for evaluation of intrauterine growth restriction. *Journal of Ultrasound Medicine, 30*(4), 529–545.

Kelsey, M., Barker, J., Bartz, S., et al. (2016). Endocrine disorders. In W. W. Hay Jr., M. J. Levin, R. R. Deterding, et al. (Eds.), *Current diagnosis & treatment: Pediatrics* (23rd ed., pp. 1007–1044). New York, NY: McGraw-Hill/Lange.

Krueger, C., Horesh, E., & Crosland, B. A. (2012). Safe sound exposure in the fetus and preterm infant. *Journal of Obstetric, Gynecologic, & Neonatal Nursing, 41*(2), 166–170.

Kumar, S. (2012). Fetal anomalies. In D. K. Edmonds (Ed.), *Dewhurst's textbook of obstetrics & gynaecology* (8th ed., pp. 219–229). Oxford, United Kingdom: Wiley-Blackwell.

Kutney, K., Konczal, L., Kaminski, B., et al. (2016). Challenges in the diagnosis and management of disorders of sex development. *Birth Defects Research, 108*(4), 293–308.

Lin, S., Munsie, J. P., Herdt-Losavio, M. L., et al. (2012). Maternal asthma medication use and the risk of selected birth defects. *Pediatrics, 129*(2), e317–e324.

Manipalviratn, S., Trivax, B., & Huang, A. (2013). Genetic disorders & sex chromosome disorders. In A. H. DeCherney, L. Nathan, T. M. Goodwin, et al. (Eds.), *Current diagnosis & treatment: Obstetrics & gynecology* (11th ed., pp. 67–96). Columbus, OH: McGraw-Hill/Lange.

Marcelis, C., de Blaauw, I., & Brunner, H. (2011). Chromosomal anomalies in the etiology of anorectal malformations: A review. *American Journal of Medical Genetics, 155A*(11), 2692–2704.

Mawhinney, E., Campbell, J., Craig, J., et al. (2012). Valproate and the risk for congenital malformations: Is formulation and dosage regime important? *Seizure, 21*(3), 215–218.

Mortarino, M., Garagiola, I., Lotta, L. A., et al. (2011). Non-invasive tool for foetal sex determination in early gestational age. *Haemophilia, 17*(6), 952–956.

O'Connor, S. C., Rooks, V. J., & Smith, A. B. (2012). Magnetic resonance imaging of the fetal central nervous system, head, neck, and chest. *Seminars in Ultrasound, CT, and MR, 33*(1), 86–101.

Ordean, A., Kahan, M., Graves, L., et al. (2015). Obstetrical and neonatal outcomes of methadone-maintained pregnant women: A Canadian multisite cohort study. *Journal of Obstetrics and Gynaecology Canada, 37*(3), 252–257.

Oyelese, Y., & Vintzileos, A. M. (2011). The uses and limitations of the fetal biophysical profile. *Clinics in Perinatology, 38*(1), 47–64.

Panepinto, J. A., & Scott, J. P. (2011). Hematology. In K. J. Marcdante, R. M. Kliegman, H. B. Jenson, et al. (Eds.), *Nelson essentials of pediatrics* (6th ed., pp. 555–584). Philadelphia, PA: Saunders/Elsevier.

Perović, M., Garalejić, E., Gojnić, M., et al. (2012). Sensitivity and specificity of ultrasonography as a screening tool for gestational diabetes mellitus. *The Journal of Maternal-Fetal & Neonatal Medicine, 25*(8), 1348–1353.

Pipkin, F. B. (2012). Maternal physiology. In D. K. Edmonds (Ed.), *Dewhurst's textbook of obstetrics & gynaecology* (8th ed., pp. 5–15). Oxford, United Kingdom: Wiley-Blackwell.

Reed, A. R., & Berrier, K. L. (2016). A qualitative study of factors influencing decision-making after prenatal diagnosis of down syndrome. *Journal Genetic Counseling.* Advance online publication. doi:10.1007/s10897-016-0061-8

Richter, J., Wergeland, H., DeKoninck, P., et al. (2012). Fetoscopic release of an amniotic band with risk of amputation: Case report and review of the literature. *Fetal Diagnosis and Therapy, 31*(2), 134–137.

Rogers, V. L., & Worley, K. C. (2012). Obstetrics & obstetric disorders. In S. J. McPhee, M. A. Papadakis, & M. W. Rabow (Eds.), *Current medical diagnosis & treatment* (51st ed., pp. 760–786). Columbus, OH: McGraw-Hill/Lange.

Rojas-Reyes, M. X., Morley, C. J., & Soll, R. (2012). Prophylactic versus selective use of surfactant in preventing morbidity and mortality in preterm infants. *Cochrane Database of Systematic Reviews*, (3), CD000510.

Samra, H. A., McGrath, J. M., & Wehbe, M. (2011). An integrated review of developmental outcomes and late-preterm birth. *Journal of Obstetric, Gynecological & Neonatal Nursing, 40*(4), 399–411.

Schneider, D. S. (2011). The cardiovascular system. In K. J. Marcdante, R. M. Kliegman, H. B. Jenson, et al. (Eds.), *Nelson essentials of pediatrics* (6th ed., pp. 525–555). Philadelphia, PA: Saunders/Elsevier.

Shao, R., Zou, S., Wang, X., et al. (2012). Revealing the hidden mechanisms of smoke-induced fallopian tubal implantation. *Biology of Reproduction, 86*(4), 131.

Singer, L. T., Moore, D. G., Fulton, S., et al. (2012). Neurobehavioral outcomes of infants exposed to MDMA (Ecstasy) and other recreational drugs during pregnancy. *Neurotoxicology and Teratology, 34*(3), 303–310.

Širvinskienė, G., Žemaitienė, N., Jusienė, R., et al. (2016). Smoking during pregnancy in association with maternal emotional well-being. *Medicina, 52*(2), 132–138.

Smith, G. C. (2016). Antenatal betamethasone for women at risk for late preterm delivery. *The New England Journal of Medicine, 375*(5), 486.

Song, J., Li, Y., & An, R. F. (2015). Identification of early-onset preeclampsia-related genes and microRNAs by bioinformatics approaches. *Reproductive Sciences, 22*(8), 954–963.

Stohl, H., & Satin, A. J. (2011). Perinatal infections. In K. J. Hurt, M. W. Guile, J. L. Bienstock, et al. (Eds.), *The Johns Hopkins manual of gynecology and obstetrics* (4th ed., pp. 137–153). Philadelphia, PA: Lippincott Williams & Wilkins.

U.S. Department of Health and Human Services. (2010). *Healthy people 2020.* Washington, DC: Author.

Vest, A. R., & Cho, L. S. (2012). Hypertension in pregnancy. *Cardiology Clinics, 30*(3), 407–423.

Virtanen, H. E., Sadov, S., & Toppari, J. (2012). Prenatal exposure to smoking and male reproductive health. *Current Opinion in Endocrinology, Diabetes & Obesity, 19*(3), 228–232.

Warren, L., Rance, J., & Hunter, B. (2012). Feasibility and acceptability of a midwife-led intervention programme called 'Eat Well Keep Active' to encourage a healthy lifestyle in pregnancy. *BMC Pregnancy and Childbirth, 12*(1), 27.

Welliver, C., Benson, A. D., Frederick, L., et al. (2016). Analysis of semen parameters during 2 weeks of daily ejaculation: A first in humans study. *Translational Andrology and Urology, 5*(5), 749–755.

White, S. J., Boldt, K. L., Holditch, S. J., et al. (2012). Measles, mumps, and rubella. *Clinical Obstetrics and Genecology, 55*(2), 550–559.

Whitney, E. N., & Rolfes, S. R. (2012). Life cycle nutrition: Pregnancy and lactation. In E. N. Whitney & S. R. Rolfes (Eds.), *Understanding nutrition* (pp. 468–496). Belmont, CA: Wadsworth Publishing.

Wong, S., Ordean, A., & Kahan, M. (2011). SOGC clinical practice guidelines: Substance use in pregnancy: No. 256, April 2011. *International Journal Gynaecology & Obstetrics, 114*(2), 190–202.

Nursing Care Related to Psychological and Physiologic Changes of Pregnancy

KEY TERMS

Lauren Maxwell is a part-time model who has come to your clinic for her first prenatal visit. She has a 3-year-old at home. She tells you she missed her period 4 weeks ago and immediately took a home pregnancy test. She's happy it was positive but also sad because she had to turn down a modeling assignment in Paris for the summer. "I want to have a second child," she explains, "Just not so soon." You suspect she's also anxious because she says, "I know there's no turning back but what will a second child do to my career?" She adds her husband, John, doesn't seem a bit worried. "Is that a good thing or not?" she asks. She also seems concerned about being a good parent as she says, "I'd die if I turn into the same kind of parent as my mother."

In addition to the positive home pregnancy test, Lauren presents with amenorrhea, breast tenderness, fatigue, and morning sickness. She's interested in learning when she will begin to look pregnant and what she can do for the morning sickness.

Previous chapters discussed reproductive anatomy and physiology. This chapter adds information about the physiologic and psychological changes that occur in both a woman and her partner during pregnancy. Knowing such information can help you protect the health of a family and a fetus for the next 9 months.

What psychological development tasks of pregnancy does Lauren need to complete? Should you assure her that her worry about being a good parent is unfounded?

- ballottement
- Braxton Hicks contractions
- Chadwick's sign
- couvade syndrome
- diastasis
- Goodell's sign
- Hegar's sign
- lightening
- linea nigra
- melasma
- Montgomery's tubercles
- multipara
- operculum
- polyuria
- primigravida
- quickening
- striae gravidarum

OBJECTIVES

After mastering the contents of this chapter, you should be able to:

1. Describe common psychological and physiologic changes that occur with pregnancy and the relationship of the changes to pregnancy diagnosis.
2. Identify 2020 National Health Goals related to preconception counseling and prenatal care that nurses can help the nation achieve.
3. Assess a woman and her support team for psychological adjustment to the physiologic changes that occur with pregnancy.
4. Formulate nursing diagnoses related to adjustments necessary because of psychological and physiologic changes of pregnancy.
5. Identify expected outcomes in relation to a family's psychological and physical adaptation to pregnancy to help them manage seamless transitions across differing healthcare settings.
6. Using the nursing process, plan nursing care that includes the six competencies of Quality & Safety Education for Nurses (QSEN): Patient-Centered Care, Teamwork & Collaboration, Evidence-Based Practice (EBP), Quality Improvement (QI), Safety, and Informatics.
7. Implement nursing care, such as health teaching related to the expected changes of pregnancy.
8. Evaluate outcomes for achievement and effectiveness of goals to be certain expected outcomes have been achieved.
9. Integrate knowledge of psychological and physiologic changes of pregnancy with the interplay of nursing process, the six competencies of QSEN, and Family Nursing to promote quality maternal and child health nursing care.

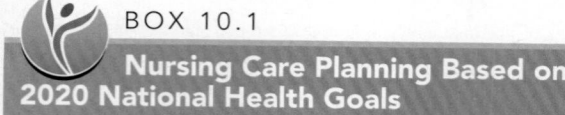

BOX 10.1

Nursing Care Planning Based on 2020 National Health Goals

A number of 2020 National Health Goals speak to the care necessary because of physiologic and psychological changes of pregnancy:

- Increase abstinence from alcohol, cigarettes, and illicit drugs among pregnant women from baselines of 89.4%, 89.6%, and 94.9% to target levels of 98.4%, 98.6%, and 100%.
- Reduce maternal deaths from a baseline of 12.7/100,000 live births to a target of 11.4/100,000.
- Increase the proportion of pregnant women who receive early and adequate prenatal care from a baseline of 70.5% to a target level of 77.6% (U.S. Department of Health and Human Services, 2010; see www.healthypeople.gov).

Nurses can help the nation achieve these objectives by being certain women receive counseling in nutrition, safer sex practices, and low uses of alcohol and tobacco before pregnancy so they can enter intended pregnancies in the best health possible.

Patients are often interested in learning more about the physical or psychological changes that pregnancy brings because these changes both verify the reality and mark the progress of pregnancy.

Physiologic changes of pregnancy occur gradually but eventually affect all of a woman's organ systems. They are necessary changes because they allow a woman's body to be able to provide oxygen and nutrients for her growing fetus as well as extra nutrients for her own increased metabolism. They also ready her body for labor and birth and for lactation (breastfeeding) once her baby is born (Bernstein & VanBuren, 2013). Despite the magnitude of these changes, such as a woman's blood volume doubling in amount, they are all extensions of normal physiology. At the end of pregnancy, her body will virtually return to its prepregnant state.

Psychological changes of pregnancy occur in response not only to the physiologic alterations happening but also to the increased responsibility associated with welcoming a new and completely dependent person to a family.

Because pregnancy changes are extensions of normal psychological and physiologic baselines, pregnancy represents a time of wellness, not of illness. A major responsibility for nurses caring for pregnant women and their families is to help the family maintain a feeling of wellness throughout the pregnancy and into early parenthood (Rogers & Worley, 2016). Box 10.1 shows 2020 National Health Goals relevant to these changes that come with pregnancy.

Nursing Process Overview

FOR HEALTHY ADAPTATION TO PREGNANCY

ASSESSMENT

Ideally, assessment for pregnancy begins before the pregnancy with preconception counseling. During a preconception assessment, evaluate a woman's overall health status, nutritional intake (ask specifically about sufficient intake of folic acid and protein), and lifestyle (especially drinking, smoking, and recreational drug habits); identify any potential problems (such as a risk for ectopic pregnancy because of tubal scarring); and identify a woman's understanding and expectations of conception, pregnancy, and parenthood.

In early pregnancy, be certain you establish a trusting relationship with a woman so she will see you as a person who is capable of counseling her and helping her solve problems and in whom she will be able to confide about any worries she has. Continue to assess a woman's health and nutritional status as well as the well-being of her fetus at all prenatal visits. Physical changes can be learned through health history, physical assessment, and laboratory tests. An assessment in psychological areas is obtained primarily through interviewing and should include societal, cultural, family, and personal influences as a woman adapts to pregnancy.

NURSING DIAGNOSIS

Examples of nursing diagnoses involving the changes that occur with pregnancy include:

- Altered breathing patterns related to respiratory system changes of pregnancy
- Disturbed body image related to weight gain from pregnancy
- Deficient knowledge related to normal changes of pregnancy
- Imbalanced nutrition, less than body requirements, related to early morning nausea
- Powerlessness related to unintended pregnancy
- Possible impaired health and prenatal care behaviors associated with cultural beliefs

OUTCOME IDENTIFICATION AND PLANNING

Planning nursing care in connection with the physiologic and psychological changes of pregnancy should involve a plan to review the common concerns women have about being pregnant before changes occur, so there are no surprises. Refer patients to helpful websites and other resources when appropriate (see Chapter 9).

IMPLEMENTATION

Most women of childbearing age have a mental picture of themselves or a good idea of how they will look in a dress before they try it on. They participate in sports or other activities that conform to that self-image. Then, in a span of 9 months, they gain 25 to 30 lb and their figure changes so drastically that their prepregnancy clothes may no longer fit. At the beginning of a pregnancy, a woman may feel constantly nauseated; toward the end, the extra weight and the strain of waiting may make her feel tired and short of breath. Endocrine changes can make her feel moody and quick to cry.

Help women at prenatal visits to voice their concerns about the changes happening to them so any worry brought on by these changes does not lead to a stressful 9 months for them or prevent solid bonding with their baby.

OUTCOME EVALUATION

Evaluation should determine whether a woman has really "heard" your teaching. Remember that people under stress do not always comprehend well, so it is not unusual for a woman who is worried about her pregnancy to pocket away information, thinking, "I'll concentrate on that when it happens to me, not now." Then, when a particular change does happen, she realizes she has forgotten what you said. Examples of outcome criteria you might strive for include:

- Patient states she is able to continue her usual lifestyle throughout pregnancy.
- Family members describe ways they have adjusted their lifestyles to accommodate the mother's fatigue.
- Couple states they appreciate the physiologic changes of pregnancy and even though they are causing discomfort, they know these are healthy changes.

Psychological Changes of Pregnancy

Pregnancy is such a huge change in a woman's life; it brings about more psychological changes than any other life event besides puberty (Fletcher & Russo, 2015). How a woman adjusts to a pregnancy depends a great deal on psychological aspects, such as the environment in which she was raised, the messages about pregnancy her family communicated to her as a child, the society and culture in which she lives as an adult, and whether the pregnancy has come at a good time in her life (Silveira, Ertel, Dole, et al., 2015).

For many women, a prenatal visit is the first time they have seen a healthcare provider since childhood. Guidance given during this time can be instrumental in not only guiding a woman safely through a pregnancy but also connecting her back with ongoing health care.

SOCIAL INFLUENCES

From the first part of the 20th century until about the 1960s, there was such heavy emphasis on medical management for women during pregnancy that it conveyed the idea that pregnancy was a 9-month-long illness. The pregnant woman went alone to a physician's office for care; at the time of birth, she was separated from her family, hospitalized in seclusion from visitors, and even from the new baby for 1 week afterward so the newborn could be fed by nurses.

Today, pregnancy is viewed as a healthy span of time best shared with a supportive partner and/or family. Women bring their families for prenatal care visits as well as to watch the birth. Women choose what level of pain management they want to use for labor and birth; many women choose to breastfeed their newborn.

How well a pregnant woman and her partner feel during pregnancy and are prepared to meet the challenges this new responsibility brings is related to their cultural background, their personal beliefs, the experiences reported by friends and relatives, as well as by the current plethora of information available on the Internet. Nurses play an important role in teaching women about their healthcare options as well as continuing to work with other healthcare providers to "demedicalize" or humanize childbirth (Heatley, Watson, Gallois, et al., 2015).

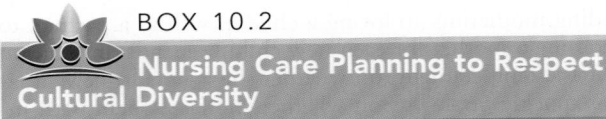

BOX 10.2

Nursing Care Planning to Respect Cultural Diversity

Women react differently on realizing they are pregnant based on their individual circumstances and their cultural expectations.

Women eat different foods during pregnancy based on what they perceive will be "good" or "bad" for their infant. Assess women's intake carefully to be certain a particular woman is not eating nonfood substances such as ice cubes or raw flour, for instance (called pica), during pregnancy. These habits result from a woman entering pregnancy with low iron stores so iron-deficient anemia results. Cravings such as ice cubes are harmless to a fetus, but asking about pica can reveal women eating substances such as paint chips or sniffing gasoline, which could be harmful to fetal growth.

CULTURAL INFLUENCES

A woman's cultural background may strongly influence how active a role she wants to take in her pregnancy because certain beliefs and taboos can place restrictions on her behavior and activities (Guelfi, Wang, Dimmock, et al., 2015). To learn about the beliefs of a particular woman and her partner, ask at prenatal visits if there is anything the couple believes should or should not be done to make the pregnancy successful and keep the fetus healthy. Supporting these beliefs shows respect for the individuality of a woman and her knowledge of good health (Box 10.2).

Before evidence-based practice was available to scientifically support why pregnancy brought about changes in a woman's body, different societies devised differing explanations about why changes occurred. These myths became so well engrained in cultures that some persist to the present. For example, a belief that lifting your arms over your head during pregnancy will cause the cord to twist or that watching a lunar eclipse will cause a birth deformity are still believed by women in some cultures (Lauderdale, 2016). Find a compromise that will assure a woman that these are not really harmful to a fetus but that still respects these beliefs.

FAMILY INFLUENCES

The family in which a woman was raised can be influential to her beliefs about pregnancy because it is part of her cultural environment. If she and her siblings were loved and their births were seen as a pleasant outcome of their family, she is more likely to have a positive attitude toward learning she is pregnant than if she and her siblings were blamed for the breakup of a marriage or a relationship, for example. A woman who views mothering as a positive activity is more likely to be pleased when she becomes pregnant than one who does not value mothering.

INDIVIDUAL DIFFERENCES

A woman's ability to cope with or adapt to stress plays a major role in how she can resolve any conflict she feels at becoming a mother. This ability to adapt (e.g., to being a mother without needing mothering, to loving a child as well as a partner, to becoming a mother for each new child) depends, in part, on her basic temperament, on whether she adapts to new situations quickly or slowly, on whether she faces them with intensity or maintains a low-key approach, and on whether she has had experience coping with change and stress (Guedes & Canavarro, 2014).

The extent to which a woman feels secure in her relationship with the people around her, especially the father of her child or her chief support person, is usually also important to her acceptance of a pregnancy. Anxiety as to whether her partner may soon disappear, leaving her alone to raise a child, may make her reexamine whether her pregnancy is a wise life step.

Yet another influence on how women perceive pregnancy as a positive or negative experience is past experiences (Muzik, McGinnis, Bocknek, et al., 2016). A woman who thinks of brides as young but mothers as old may believe pregnancy will rob her of her youth. If she's concerned about her appearance, she may worry pregnancy will permanently stretch her abdomen and breasts. She may also worry pregnancy will rob her financially and ruin her chances of job promotion (referred to as a "mommy track") (Misri & Swift, 2015).

These are real feelings and must be taken seriously when assessing or counseling pregnant women. Women who do not have a supportive partner may look to healthcare providers during pregnancy to fill the role of an attentive listener (Adeniran, Aboyeji, Fawole, et al., 2015).

Partner's Adaptation

The more emotionally attached a partner is to a pregnant woman, the closer the partner's attachment is apt to be to the child (Fuertes, Faria, Beeghly, et al., 2016). Whether partners are able to form a close relationship with each other, as well as accept a pregnancy and a coming child, depends on the same factors that affect the pregnant woman's decision making: cultural background, past experience, and relationships with family members (Fortinash & Holoday Worret, 2012).

Although partners may be inarticulate about such emotional factors, they may be able to convey such feelings by a touch or a caress, which is one reason a partner's presence is always desirable at a prenatal visit and certainly in a birthing room.

The Psychological Tasks of Pregnancy

During the 9 months of pregnancy, a woman and her partner run a gamut of emotions, ranging from surprise at finding out about the pregnancy (or wishing she were not), to pleasure and acceptance as they begin to identify with the coming child at the middle of pregnancy, to worry for themselves and the child, to acute impatience near the end of pregnancy (Table 10.1). Once the child is born, a woman and her partner may feel surprised again that the pregnancy is over and they really do have a child.

From a physiologic standpoint, it is fortunate that a pregnancy is 9 months long because this gives the fetus time to mature and be prepared for life outside the protective uterine environment. From a psychological standpoint, the 9-month period is also fortunate because it gives a family time to prepare emotionally as well. These psychological changes are frequently termed "guaranteeing safe passage" for the fetus (Box 10.3).

TABLE 10.1 COMMON PSYCHOLOGICAL CHANGES THAT OCCUR WITH PREGNANCY

Psychological Change	Description
First trimester task: Accepting the pregnancy	The woman and her partner both spend time recovering from the surprise of learning they are pregnant and concentrate on what it feels like to be pregnant. A common reaction is ambivalence, or feeling both pleased and not pleased about the pregnancy.
Second trimester task: Accepting the fetus	The woman and her partner move through emotions such as narcissism and introversion as they concentrate on what it will feel like to be a parent. Role-playing and increased dreaming are common.
Third trimester task: Preparing for the baby and end of pregnancy	The woman and her partner prepare clothing and sleeping arrangements for the baby but also grow impatient as they ready themselves for birth.

Although the average woman is happy to be pregnant, don't underestimate the effect the emotional and physical upheavals brought about by the hormonal changes of pregnancy can cause. These can be so tremendous that they can influence whether a pregnancy is carried to term, which may not only lead to poor acceptance of the child but also to postpartum depression or, in rare instances, psychosis (Biaggi, Conroy, Pawlby, et al., 2016; Lilliecreutz, Larén, Sydsjö, et al., 2016).

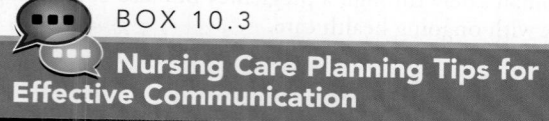

BOX 10.3

Nursing Care Planning Tips for Effective Communication

You have seen Lauren Maxwell in your prenatal clinic every month for the last 3 months. At visits, she answers questions but rarely volunteers any information. You'd like her to talk more about how she feels about her pregnancy and her plans for the new baby.

Tip: Focus on the patient's concerns, allowing her to express them fully. Avoid cutting off the conversation by talking too much about your own needs and expectations. Some people are naturally shy and are not interested in casual conversations at healthcare visits. Others are not talkative because they are not aware healthcare providers are interested in them as individuals.

Nurse: Good morning. Lauren. How are you today?

Lauren: Tired.

Nurse: Tell me about that.

Lauren: I am so tired by noon every day I can't get any work done. I should never have gotten pregnant.

Nurse: You're so tired you can barely get your work done?

Lauren: No one in our financial situation should be having a baby.

FIRST TRIMESTER: ACCEPTING THE PREGNANCY

The Woman

The task of women during the first trimester of pregnancy is to accept the reality of the pregnancy; later will come the task of accepting the baby. Most cultures structure celebrations around important life events such as coming of age, marriages, birthdays, and deaths, all of which have rituals to help individuals face and accept the coming change in their lives. A diagnosis of pregnancy is a similar rite of passage, but an unusual one among passages, because the suspicion of pregnancy is made initially not on something happening but the absence of something: a missed menstrual flow.

With the availability and common use of reproductive planning measures today, it would seem few pregnancies would still be a surprise. In reality, as many as 49% of pregnancies are still unintended, unwanted, or mistimed (Centers for Disease Control and Prevention [CDC], 2015). Because no woman can be absolutely confident in advance that she will be able to conceive until it happens, even planned pregnancies are a surprise to some extent because a woman can be amazed it either happened so quickly or took so long.

QSEN Checkpoint Question 10.1

EVIDENCE-BASED PRACTICE

How women feel about being pregnant has a great deal to do with how anxious they are about becoming pregnant. To investigate whether women look forward to a second birth or whether anxiety about their first birth makes them reluctant to have a second child, researchers interviewed 908 women who had given birth to at least one child, asking them to "please describe your feelings when you think about giving birth in the future."

Results showed that two thirds of women who responded had mostly positive feelings; one third of women stated they were frightened of future childbirth. The qualitative analysis resulted in an overall theme of women feeling a mixture of both dread and delight at the thought of a second pregnancy (Rilby, Jansson, Lindblom, et al., 2012).

Based on the previous study, which statement by Lauren would make the nurse believe she's having a typical reaction to her second pregnancy?

   a. "I'm feeling good about having a second baby, but a bit worried at the same time."

   b. "I think having a second child is going to be totally wonderful. I'm sure it will be so much easier."

   c. "I'm really looking forward to watching my two children play together in the future."

   d. "I'd rather my husband had this one; knowing what it all involves makes it even harder."

Look in Appendix A for the best answer and rationale.

Following their initial surprise, women often experience feelings less than pleasure and closer to anxiety or a feeling of *ambivalence*. Ambivalence doesn't mean positive feelings counteract negative feelings and a woman is left feeling nothing. Instead, it refers to the interwoven feelings of wanting and not wanting, feelings which can be confusing to an ordinarily organized woman.

Fortunately, most women who were not happy about being pregnant at the beginning are able to change their attitude toward their pregnancy by the time they feel the child move inside them. Some healthcare plans provide for a routine sonogram at about this time in pregnancy, between 18 and 22 weeks, to date the pregnancy and to assess for growth anomalies. This can be a major step in promoting acceptance because women can see a beating heart or a fetal outline or can learn the sex of their fetus (Lindberg, Maddow-Zimet, Kost, et al., 2015).

Although most women self-diagnose their pregnancy by using a urine pregnancy test strip, hearing their pregnancy officially diagnosed at a first prenatal visit is another step toward accepting a pregnancy. Because this happens, woman often comment after such a visit they feel "more pregnant" or it makes a first visit more than an ordinary one. Early diagnosis is important because the earlier a woman realizes she is pregnant or comes for a first prenatal visit, the sooner she can begin to safeguard fetal health by measures such as discontinuing all drugs not specifically prescribed or approved by her primary healthcare provider (Chakraborty, Anstice, Jacobs, et al., 2015).

The Partner

In the past, partners were forgotten persons in the childbearing process. Unwed fathers were dismissed as not interested in either the pregnancy or the woman's health. A female partner was completely ignored. In actuality, all partners are important and should be encouraged to play a continuing emotional and supportive role in a pregnancy.

Accepting the pregnancy for a partner means not only accepting the certainty of the pregnancy and the reality of the child to come but also accepting the woman in her changed state. Like women, partners may also experience a feeling of ambivalence. A partner may feel proud and happy at the beginning of pregnancy, for example. Soon, however, it's easy to begin to feel both overwhelmed with what the loss of a salary will mean to the family if the woman has to quit work, and a feeling close to jealousy of the growing baby who, although not yet physically apparent, seems to be taking up a great deal of the woman's time and thought (Da Costa, Zelkowitz, Dasgupta, et al., 2015). Remember, once partners feel an attachment to a coming child, they can then feel as deep a sense of loss as the woman if the pregnancy should end before term or the baby is born with a unique concern. In addition, they may not have anyone to turn to for support because no one recognizes how involved they were in the pregnancy. To help both male and female partners resolve these feelings, be certain to make partners feel welcome at prenatal visits or during fetal testing, provide an outlet for them to discuss concerns, and offer parenting information as necessary.

QSEN Checkpoint Question 10.2

QUALITY IMPROVEMENT

Lauren wasn't totally happy about learning that she was pregnant. What psychological task is important

for the woman to complete during the first trimester of her pregnancy?
   a. Accepting morning sickness nausea
   b. Accepting the fact that she is pregnant
   c. Appreciating the responsibility of having a baby
   d. Choosing a name for her baby

Look in Appendix A for the best answer and rationale.

SECOND TRIMESTER: ACCEPTING THE BABY

As soon as fetal movements can be felt, psychological responses of both partners usually begin to change.

The Woman

During the second trimester, the psychological task of a woman is to accept she is having a baby, a step up from accepting the pregnancy. This change usually happens at **quickening**, or the first moment a woman feels fetal movement. Until a woman experiences for herself this proof of the child's existence and although she ate to meet nutritional needs and took special vitamins to help the fetus grow, it seemed more like just another part of her body. With quickening, the fetus becomes a separate identity. She then may imagine herself as a mother, teaching her child the alphabet or how to ride a bicycle. This anticipatory role-playing is an important activity for midpregnancy as it leads her to a greater concept of her condition and helps her realize she is more than just pregnant—there is a separate human being inside her.

Women often use the term "it" to refer to their fetus before quickening but begin to use *he* or *she* afterward. Some women continue to use *it*, however, so doing so is not a sign of poor attachment but an individual preference as some women believe referring to the child as "she" or "he" will bring bad luck or disappointment if the sonogram report was wrong.

Most women can pinpoint a moment during each pregnancy when they knew definitely they wanted their child. The firmer this attachment, the less postpartum depression they are apt to experience (Brummelte & Galea, 2015).

For a woman who carefully planned the pregnancy, this moment of awareness may occur as soon as she recovers from the surprise of learning she has actually conceived. For others, it may come when she announces the news to her parents and hears them express their excitement or when she sees a look of pride on her partner's face. For example, shopping for baby clothes for the first time, setting up the crib, or seeing a blurry outline on a sonogram screen may suddenly make the coming baby seem real and desired (Fig. 10.1).

Accepting the baby as a welcome addition to the family might not come, however, until labor has begun or a woman first hears her baby's cry or feeds her newborn. If a woman has a complication of pregnancy, it could take several weeks after the baby is born for her to accept that the birth was real and to come to terms with motherhood.

A good way to measure the level of a woman's acceptance of her coming baby is to measure how well she follows prenatal instructions. Until a woman views the growing life inside her as something desired, it may be difficult for her to

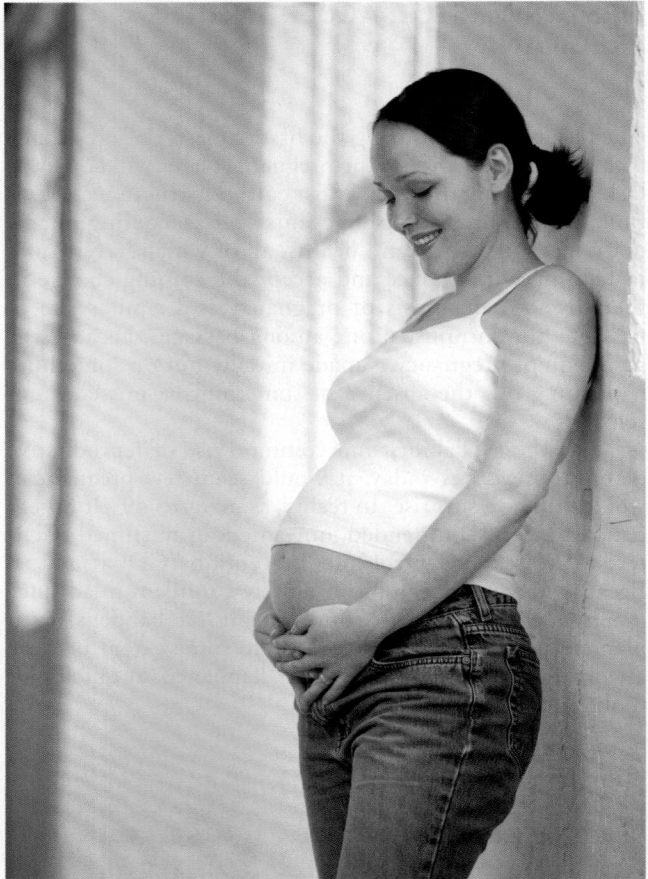

Figure 10.1 A growing abdomen and fluttering fetal movements help to make a pregnancy a reality.

substitute a high-protein food for her favorite high-calorie coffee drink, for instance. After all, until her abdomen begins to enlarge, watching herself gain weight may be the most certain proof she has that she is pregnant.

The Partner

As a woman begins to actively prepare for the coming baby, a partner increasingly may feel as if he or she is left standing in the wings, waiting to be asked to take part in the event. To compensate for this feeling, a partner may become overly absorbed in work, striving to produce something concrete on the job as if to show the woman is not the only one capable of creating something. This preoccupation with work may limit the amount of time a partner spends with family or is available for prenatal visits, just when the pregnant woman most needs emotional support.

Some men may have difficulty enjoying the pregnancy because they have been misinformed about sexuality, pregnancy, and women's health. A man might believe, for example, that breastfeeding will make his wife's breasts no longer attractive or that after birth, sexual relations will no longer be enjoyable. Such a man needs education to correct misinformation. Read the pamphlets supplied by your prenatal healthcare setting and ask: Do they contain mainly information about childbirth and pregnancy from a woman's perspective? Would they be relevant to a supportive partner?

THIRD TRIMESTER: PREPARING FOR PARENTHOOD

During the third trimester, couples usually begin "nest-building" activities, such as planning the infant's sleeping arrangements, choosing a name for the infant, and "ensuring safe passage" by learning about birth. These preparations are evidence the couple is completing the third trimester task of pregnancy or preparing for parenthood.

Couples at this point are usually interested in attending prenatal classes and/or classes on preparing for childbirth. It's helpful to ask a couple what specifically they are doing to get ready for birth to see if they are interested in taking such a class and to document how well prepared they will be for the baby's arrival. Attending a childbirth education class or one on preparing for parenthood can not only help a couple accept the fact they are about to become parents but also expose them to other parents as role models who can provide practical information about pregnancy and child care (Jones, Feinberg, & Hostetler, 2014). Chapter 14 discusses the usual curriculum of childbirth and parenthood education classes.

Although pregnancy is a happy time for most women, certain external life contingencies such as an unwanted pregnancy, financial difficulties, lack of emotional support, or high levels of stress can slow the psychological work of pregnancy or attachment to the child (Biaggi et al., 2016) (Box 10.4). During prenatal visits, ask such questions as "Is pregnancy what you thought it would be?" or "Has anything changed in your home life since you last came to clinic?" to reveal if any situation that could potentially interfere with bonding has occurred. It is unrealistic to believe any one healthcare professional has all the solutions to the problems couples reveal when asked these questions. An interprofessional approach (referral to a nutritionist, a primary healthcare provider, or social services) is often necessary to help solve some of these multifaceted problems.

ADDITIONAL PREPARATION WORK TO COMPLETE IN PREGNANCY

In addition to the three main tasks of pregnancy, more subtle emotions also surface or need to be worked through.

Reworking Developmental Tasks

An important task to complete during pregnancy is working through previous life experiences or Erikson's developmental tasks of autonomy, industry, and identity (Erikson, 1993). Needs and wishes that have been repressed for years may surface to be studied and reworked, often to an extreme extent along these lines.

Fear of being separated from family or fear of dying are common preschool fears that can be revived during pregnancy. A clue that might signal a woman's distress over this could be "Am I ever going to make it through this?" Such an expression might simply mean she is tired of her backache, but it also might be a plea for reassurance she will survive this event in her life.

Part of gaining a sense of identity is establishing a working relationship with parents, which may still be an awkward one since adolescence. For the first time in her life, a woman during pregnancy can begin to empathize with the way her mother used to worry because she's already begun to worry about her child when she feels no movement for a few hours. This can make her own mother become more important to her and a new, more equal relationship may develop.

Teenagers who are pregnant need to resolve the double conflict of still establishing a sense of identity (teenagers are still children developmentally) at the same time they are planning to be a mother. Unless these feelings are examined and resolved, teenagers can have a difficult time thinking about enjoying their pregnancy or becoming a mother.

A partner needs to do the same reworking of old values and forgotten developmental tasks. A man has to rethink his relationship with his father, for example, to understand better what kind of father he will be. Some men may have had emotionally distant fathers and wish to be more emotionally available to their own children. Support from healthcare providers and exposure to caring role models can be instrumental in helping a man achieve this goal.

Role-Playing and Fantasizing

Another step in preparing for parenthood is role-playing, or fantasizing about what it will be like to be a parent. Just as a child learns what to do by following a mother as she sets a table or balances her checkbook, a pregnant woman may begin to spend time with other pregnant women or mothers of young children to learn how to be a mother. As a part of this role-playing process, women's dreams tend to focus on the pregnancy and concerns about keeping themselves and their coming child safe.

BOX 10.4

Assessing Events That Could Contribute to Difficulty Accepting a Pregnancy

- Pregnancy is unintended.
- Learning the pregnancy is a multiple, not a single one.
- Learning the fetus has a developmental abnormality.
- Pregnancy is less than 1 year after a previous one.
- Family has to relocate during pregnancy (involves a need to find new support people).
- The woman has a role reversal (a previously supporting person becomes dependent or vice versa).
- The main family support person suffers a job loss.
- The woman's relationship ends because of partner infidelity.
- There is a major illness in self, partner, or a relative.
- There is loss of a significant other.
- Complications of pregnancy occur, such as severe hypertension.
- The woman has a series of devaluing experiences such as failure in school or work.

There is concern that a young adolescent will have inadequate role models for motherhood; they are either other teens her age, who typically are not interested in a commitment to mothering, or possibly her own mother, who may have struggled with poverty or her own lack of support. Try to locate good role models (e.g., in classes for mothers, at the healthcare agency, or in a social agency) for adolescents so they can find a good maternal role model to copy and modify their own behavior.

A woman's partner also has the same role-playing to do during pregnancy, to imagine himself or herself as the parent of a boy or a girl. A partner who is becoming a parent for the first time may have to change a view of being a carefree individual to being a significant member of a family unit. If the partner already is a parent from a former relationship, he or she has to cast aside the parent-of-one identity to accept a parent-of-two image, and so forth.

Other support persons who will have an active role in raising the child, such as grandparents, close friends, or an ex-spouse, also have to work out their roles with regard to the pregnancy and impending parenthood. This may be particularly difficult because the roles for these support persons may not be clearly defined, and no role model may be apparent (Hayslip, Blumenthal, & Garner, 2015).

EMOTIONAL RESPONSES THAT CAN CAUSE CONCERN IN PREGNANCY

Because of all the tasks that need to be worked through during a pregnancy, emotional responses can vary greatly, but common reactions include grief, narcissism, introversion or extroversion, body image and boundary concerns, couvade syndrome, stress, mood swings, and changes in sexual desire. These are all normal, so it is helpful to caution a pregnant woman and her partner that these common changes may occur so they're not alarmed if they appear. Otherwise, a partner can misinterpret the woman's mood swings, decreased sexual interest, introversion, or narcissism not as changes from pregnancy but as a loss of interest in their relationship.

Grief

The thought that grief can be associated with such a positive process as having a child seems at first incongruent. But before a woman can take on a mothering role, she has to give up or alter her present role as she will never be the woman she has been in exactly the same way again. She will never be able to be as irresponsible and carefree again, or perhaps sleep soundly for the next few years. All of this takes mental preparation, which may manifest as a form of grief, as she incorporates her new role as a mother into her other roles as daughter, wife, business professional, or friend. Partners must also incorporate a new role as a parent into their other roles in life.

Narcissism

Self-centeredness (narcissism) may be an early reaction to pregnancy. A woman who previously perhaps was barely conscious of her body, who dressed in the morning with little thought about what to wear, suddenly begins to concentrate on these aspects of her life. She dresses so her pregnancy will or will not show. She may lose interest in her job or community events because the work seems alien to the more important event taking place inside her.

Narcissism may also be revealed by changes in activity. A woman may stop playing tennis, for example, even though her primary healthcare provider has assured her it will do no harm in moderation. She may criticize her partner's driving, although it never bothered her before. She does these things to unconsciously protect her body and her baby. Her partner may demonstrate the same behavior by reducing risky activities, such as mountain biking, trying to ensure he or she will be present to raise their child.

This need of a woman to protect her body has implications for nursing care. It means a woman may regard unnecessary nudity as a threat to her body (e.g., be sure to drape properly for pelvic and abdominal examinations). She may resent casual remarks such as "Oh my, you've gained weight" (i.e., a threat to her appearance) or "You don't like milk?" (i.e., a threat to her judgment).

There is a tendency to organize health instructions during pregnancy around the baby: "Be sure to keep this appointment. You want to have a healthy baby." "You really ought to eat more protein for the baby's sake." This approach may be particularly inappropriate early in pregnancy, before the fetus stirs and before a woman is convinced not only that she is pregnant but also that there is a baby inside her. At early stages, a woman may be much more interested in doing things for herself because it is her body, her tiredness, and her well-being that will be directly affected (e.g., "Eat protein because it keeps your fingernails from breaking" or "Protein will give you long-term energy").

Introversion Versus Extroversion

Introversion, or turning inward to concentrate on oneself and one's body, is a common finding during pregnancy. Some women, however, react in an entirely opposite fashion and become more extroverted. They are more active, appear healthier than ever before, and are more outgoing. This tends to occur in women who are finding unexpected fulfillment in pregnancy, perhaps who had seriously doubted they would be lucky enough or fertile enough to conceive. Such a woman regards her expanding abdomen as public proof of her ability to fulfill the maternal role. Although these changes may make a woman become more varied in her interests during pregnancy, she may be puzzling to those around her who liked her for her quiet and self-contained manner.

Body Image and Boundary

Body image (i.e., the way your body appears to yourself) and body boundary (i.e., a zone of separation you perceive between yourself and objects or other people) both change during pregnancy as a woman begins to envision herself as a mother or becoming "bigger" in many different ways. Changes in concept of body boundaries are so startling that a pregnant woman may walk far away from an object such as a table to avoid bumping against it. At the same time, she may perceive herself as needing body boundaries as if her body were delicate and easily harmed.

Stress

Because pregnancy brings with it such a major role change, it can cause extreme stress in a woman who was not planning to be pregnant or if she finds her lifestyle changing dramatically after she becomes pregnant. Stress in pregnancy, like stress at any time, can make it difficult for a woman to make decisions, be as aware of her surroundings as usual, or maintain time management with her usual degree of skill. This may cause people who were dependent on her before pregnancy to feel neglected because now that she is pregnant, she seems to have strength only for herself. If a woman was in a violent relationship before the pregnancy, the increased stress of pregnancy is apt to cause even more violence. Privately asking whether intimate partner violence has ever occurred in the past to help predict if it could occur during pregnancy is an important part of prenatal interviewing (Van Parys, Deschepper, Michielsen, et al., 2015).

To help families keep their perspective for the full length of a pregnancy, remind them that any decrease in the ability to function that happens to a pregnant woman is a reaction to the stress of pregnancy. A woman may need to remind an employer that any lack of decision-making ability is no different than in people who are feeling stress because of marital discord or a loved one's illness. Pregnancy may actually be less stressful and less of a concern than those situations because of its predictable 9-month duration.

Depression

Depression—a feeling of sadness marked by loss of interest in usual things, feelings of guilt or low self-worth, disturbed sleep, low energy, and poor concentration—is a common finding in late adolescents. Depression causes as many as 15% of women to enter pregnancy feeling depressed; others grow depressed during pregnancy, especially if they lack a meaningful support person (Chojenta, Lucke, Forder, et al., 2016). Screening for women who have a history of depression is important at a preconception visit as common drugs prescribed for depression can be teratogenic to a fetus as well as cause hypertension in the woman (Zoega, Kieler, Nørgaard, et al., 2015). It is also important to investigate if the woman has a meaningful support person or the stress and anxiety that can come with pregnancy can increase depression substantially and lead to postpartum depression (see Chapter 25).

A woman with few support people around her almost automatically has more difficulty adjusting to and accepting a pregnancy and a new child than women with more support. A woman who begins a pregnancy with a strong support person and then loses that person through trauma, illness, separation, or divorce needs special attention with regard to loneliness and depression. Evaluate her carefully as to how she is managing and give her extra support as needed because her feeling of loss is likely to be extremely acute. Knowing she has supportive healthcare providers she can call on when needed is the one thing that may make her pregnancy acceptable to her.

QSEN Checkpoint Question 10.3 ✓

TEAMWORK & COLLABORATION

Lauren Maxwell is aware she's been showing some narcissism since becoming pregnant. How would the nurse describe this phenomenon to an unlicensed care provider?

a. She feels pulled in multiple directions.
b. She feels a need to sleep more than usual.
c. Her thoughts tend to be mainly about herself.
d. She often feels emotionally "numb."

Look in Appendix A for the best answer and rationale.

Couvade Syndrome

Many partners experience physical symptoms such as nausea, vomiting, and backache to the same degree or even more intensely than their partners during a pregnancy; some begin to gain weight along with their partner. As a woman's abdomen begins to grow, partners may perceive themselves as growing larger too, as if they were the ones who were experiencing changing boundaries the same as the pregnant woman. These symptoms apparently result from stress, anxiety, and empathy for the pregnant woman. The phenomenon is common enough that it has been given a name: **couvade syndrome** (from the French word "to hatch"). The more a partner is involved in or attuned to the changes of the pregnancy, the more symptoms a partner may experience. A close marital relationship, which this reflects, can increase the strength of the partner–infant attachment (Fuertes et al., 2016). Such symptoms are only worrisome and require psychological attention if they become so extreme that they create intolerable emotional stress.

What If . . . 10.2

John finds himself calling in sick at least 3 days a week because of "nausea." Because his wife, Lauren, is 5 months pregnant, would the nurse assume his symptoms are because of couvade syndrome?

Emotional Lability

Mood changes occur frequently in a pregnant woman, partly as a symptom of narcissism (i.e., her feelings are easily hurt by remarks that would have been laughed off before) and partly because of hormonal changes, particularly the sustained increase in estrogen and progesterone. Mood swings may be so common that they can make a woman's reaction to her family and to healthcare routines unpredictable. She may cry over her children's bad table manners at one meal, for example, and find the situation amusing or even charming at the next. Caution families that such mood swings occur beginning with early pregnancy so they can accept them as part of a normal pregnancy (Box 10.5).

Changes in Sexual Desire

Most women report their sexual desire changes, at least to some degree, during pregnancy. Women who formerly were worried about becoming pregnant might truly enjoy sexual relations for the first time during pregnancy. Others might feel a loss of desire because of their increase in estrogen, or they might unconsciously view sexual relations as a threat to the fetus they must protect. Some may worry coitus could bring on early labor.

During the first trimester, most women report a decrease in libido because of the nausea, fatigue, and breast tenderness that accompany early pregnancy. During the second trimester, as blood flow to the pelvic area increases to supply the placenta, libido and sexual enjoyment can rise markedly. During the third trimester, sexual desire may remain high, or it may decrease because of difficulty finding a comfortable position and increasing abdominal size. When a couple knows early in pregnancy such changes may occur, it's easier for them to interpret these in the correct light or as a normal change, not as loss of interest in a sexual partner or as a diminishment of the strength of the total relationship (Yıldız, 2015). Suggestions for helping women and their partners adjust to these circumstances are discussed in Chapter 12.

Changes in the Expectant Family

Most parents are aware that their older children need preparation when a new baby is on the way; however, knowing preparation is needed and being prepared to explain where babies come from are two different things. For this reason, many couples appreciate suggestions from healthcare providers as to how this task can be accomplished.

Both preschool and school-age children may need to be assured periodically during pregnancy a new baby will be an addition to the family and will not replace them or change their parents' affection for them. Preparing a child for the birth of a sibling is discussed in Chapters 14 and 31 with other growth and development concerns.

The Confirmation of Pregnancy

A medical diagnosis of pregnancy serves to date when the birth will occur and also helps predict the existence of a high-risk status. Most women who come to a healthcare facility for a diagnosis of pregnancy have already guessed they are pregnant based on a multitude of subjective symptoms as well as having completed a home pregnancy test, so a healthcare visit is more a confirmation of pregnancy than a diagnosis. If a pregnancy was planned, this official confirmation of pregnancy produces a feeling of intense fulfillment and achievement. If the pregnancy was not planned (remember almost half of pregnancies are unintended), it can result in an equally extreme crisis state.

From the day a pregnancy is officially confirmed, most women try to eat a more nutritious diet, give up cigarette smoking and alcohol ingestion, and stop taking nonessential medications. Because a woman may not take these measures before confirmation of her pregnancy, this makes early confirmation of pregnancy important. If a woman does not wish to continue the pregnancy, early confirmation is also imperative; therapeutic termination of pregnancy should be carried out at the earliest stage possible for the safest outcome (Gerdts, Dobkin, Foster, et al., 2016).

Before there were sonograms and maternal serum pregnancy tests, pregnancy was diagnosed on symptoms reported by the woman and the signs elicited by a healthcare provider. These signs and symptoms, still important today, are traditionally divided into three classifications: presumptive (subjective symptoms), probable (objective signs), and positive (documented signs) (Table 10.2).

PRESUMPTIVE (SUBJECTIVE) SYMPTOMS

Presumptive symptoms are those which, when taken as single entities, could easily indicate other conditions (Fletcher & Russo, 2015). These findings, discussed in connection with the body system in which they occur, are experienced by the woman but cannot be documented by an examiner (Box 10.6).

PROBABLE SIGNS

In contrast to presumptive symptoms, probable signs of pregnancy are objective and so can be verified by an examiner. Although they are more reliable than presumptive symptoms, they still do not positively diagnose a pregnancy (Box 10.7).

Laboratory Tests

The commonly used laboratory tests for pregnancy are based on the use of a venipuncture or a urine specimen to detect the presence of human chorionic gonadotropin (hCG), a hormone created by the chorionic villi of the placenta, in the urine or blood serum of the pregnant woman. Because these tests are only accurate 95% to 98% of the time, positive results from these tests are considered probable rather than positive signs.

In the nonpregnant woman, no units of hCG will be detectable because there are no trophoblast cells producing hCG. In the pregnant woman, trace amounts of hCG appear in her serum as early as 24 to 48 hours after implantation and reach a measurable level (about 50 milli-International Unit/ml 7 to 9 days after conception. Levels peak at about 100 milli-International Unit/ml between the 60th and 80th day of gestation. After that point, the concentration of hCG declines again so, at term, it is again barely detectable in serum or urine.

Home Pregnancy Tests

A number of brands for pregnancy testing are available over the counter, take only 2 to 3 minutes to complete, and have a high degree of accuracy (97% to 99%) if the instructions are followed exactly because they can detect as little as 35 milli-International

TABLE 10.2 PRESUMPTIVE, PROBABLE, AND POSITIVE INDICATIONS OF PREGNANCY

Time From Implantation (Weeks)	Presumptive Finding	Probable Finding	Positive Finding	Description
1		Maternal serum test		A venipuncture of blood serum reveals the presence of human chorionic gonadotropin hormone
2	Breast changes			Feelings of tenderness, fullness, tingling; enlargement and darkening of areola
2	Nausea, vomiting			Nausea or vomiting on arising or when fatigued
2	Amenorrhea			Absence of menstruation
3	Frequent urination			Sense of having to void more often than usual
6		Chadwick's sign		Color change of the vagina from pink to violet
6		Goodell's sign		Softening of the cervix
6		Hegar's sign		Softening of the lower uterine segment
6		Sonographic evidence of gestational sac		Characteristic ring is evident
8			Sonographic evidence of fetal outline	Fetal outline can be seen and measured by sonogram
10–12			Fetal heart audible	Doppler ultrasound reveals heartbeat
12	Fatigue			General feeling of tiredness
12	Uterine enlargement			Uterus can be palpated over symphysis pubis
16		Ballottement		When lower uterine segment is tapped on a bimanual examination, the fetus can be felt to rise against the abdominal wall
18	Quickening			Fetal movement felt by woman
20			Fetal movement felt by examiner	Fetal movement can be palpated through abdomen
20		Braxton Hicks contractions		Periodic uterine tightening occurs
20		Fetal outline felt by examiner		Fetal outline can be palpated through abdomen
24	Linea nigra			Line of dark pigment forms on the abdomen
24	Melasma			Dark pigment forms on face
24	Striae gravidarum			Stretch marks form on abdomen

Unit/ml of hCG. For the test, a woman dips a reagent strip into her stream of urine. A color change or the appearance of two bars on the strip denotes pregnancy.

Tips to give the woman for successful testing include:
- Check the expiration date on the package to be certain the kit has not expired; an outdated kit can give false-positive results.
- Read the instruction pamphlet provided with the test, noting especially the time period you should wait before reading the result, and follow this instruction carefully.
- A concentrated urine sample such as a first urine in the morning tests best. Don't drink a large quantity of water beforehand because this can dilute a urine sample.
- Read the test results at the exact time the instructions dictate. Reading the strip after the designated time can cause inaccurate results (e.g., denoting that you are pregnant when you are not).
- Some prescription medicines, like methadone or chlordiazepoxide, may cause false-positive results. Contact your healthcare provider if you get an unexpected positive result

and ask if any medication you are taking could cause that result.
- Early prenatal care is the best safeguard to ensure a successful pregnancy. If your test result is positive, your next step should be to make a healthcare appointment as early as possible to begin care.

Most manufacturers suggest a woman wait until at least the day of the missed menstrual period to test. If a woman thinks she is pregnant but gets a negative result, she could repeat the test 1 week later if she still has not had a menstrual flow. If symptoms of pregnancy persist after two tests, she needs to see her healthcare provider as she might have another condition causing the amenorrhea; she would need appropriate diagnosis and therapy for this.

A worry about the common use of home test kits is that because women do not have to come to a healthcare setting for confirmation of pregnancy, they may not seek prenatal care until something seems to be going wrong with their pregnancy or until they feel they need to arrange added healthcare provider coverage for the birth. After a positive pregnancy

BOX 10.6

Nursing Care Planning Using Assessment

ASSESSING A WOMAN FOR PRESUMPTIVE SYMPTOMS OF PREGNANCY

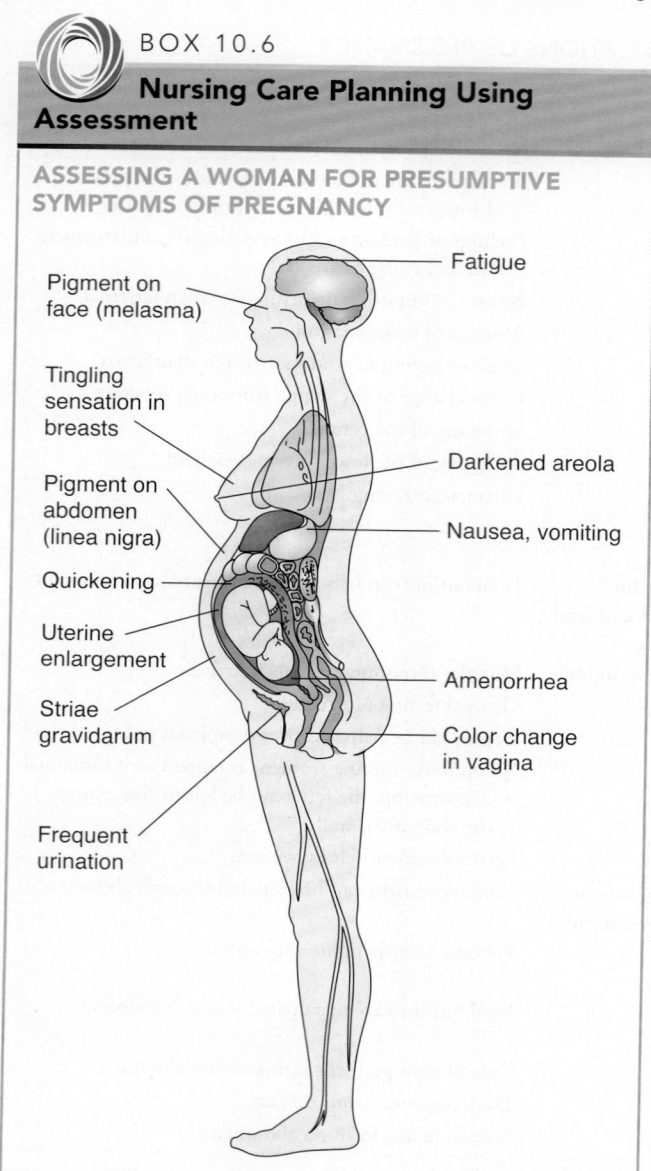

Pigment on face (melasma)
Fatigue
Tingling sensation in breasts
Darkened areola
Pigment on abdomen (linea nigra)
Nausea, vomiting
Quickening
Uterine enlargement
Striae gravidarum
Amenorrhea
Color change in vagina
Frequent urination

BOX 10.7

Nursing Care Planning Using Assessment

ASSESSING A WOMAN FOR PROBABLE SIGNS OF PREGNANCY

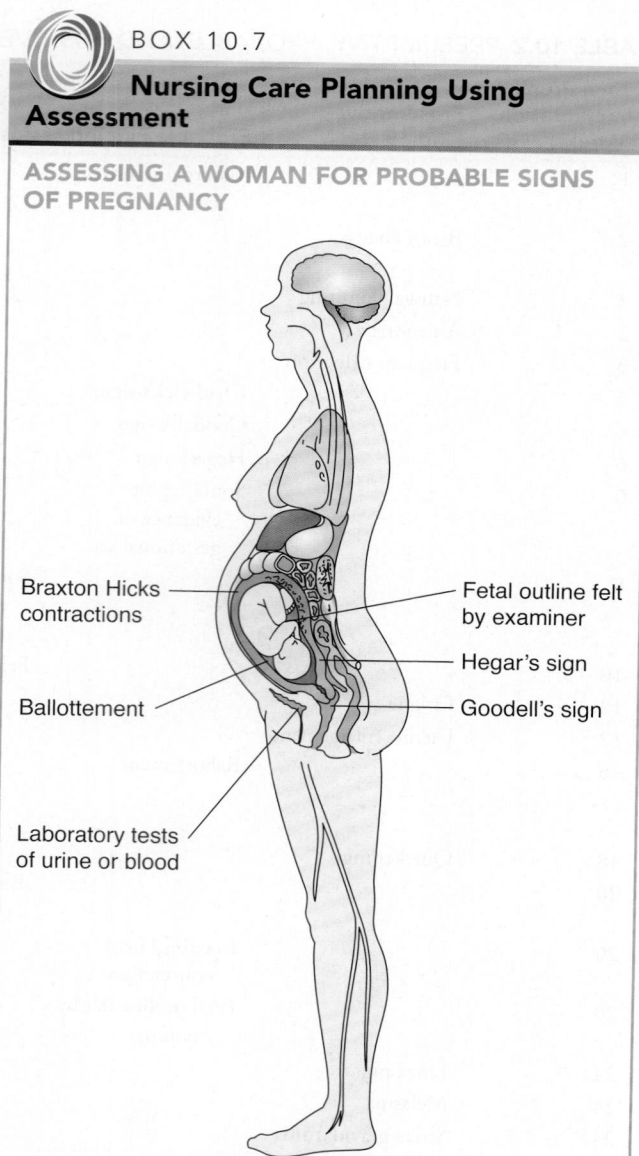

Braxton Hicks contractions
Fetal outline felt by examiner
Hegar's sign
Ballottement
Goodell's sign
Laboratory tests of urine or blood

test, the first step should therefore be to arrange for prenatal care (Attilakos & Overton, 2012).

POSITIVE SIGNS OF PREGNANCY

There are only three documented or positive signs of pregnancy:

1. Demonstration of a fetal heart separate from the mother's
2. Fetal movements felt by an examiner
3. Visualization of the fetus by ultrasound

Demonstration of a Fetal Heart Separate From the Mother's

Although a fetal heart beat cannot be heard through an ordinary stethoscope until 18 to 20 weeks of pregnancy, an echocardiography can demonstrate a heartbeat as early as 5 weeks. An ultrasound can reveal a beating fetal heart as early as the sixth to seventh week of pregnancy. Doppler instrumentation that converts ultrasonic frequencies to audible frequencies is able to detect fetal heart sounds as early as the 10th to 12th week of gestation.

The fetal heart rate ranges between 120 and 160 beats/min. Sounds are more difficult to hear if a woman's abdomen has a great deal of subcutaneous fat or if there is a larger-than-normal amount of amniotic fluid present (polyhydramnios). They are heard best when the position of the fetus is determined by palpation and the stethoscope is placed over the area of the fetal back.

Fetal Movements Felt by an Examiner

Fetal movements may be felt by a woman as early as 16 to 20 weeks of pregnancy. An objective examiner can discern fetal movements at about the 20th to 24th week of pregnancy unless the woman is extremely obese. This outside evaluation is considered the more reliable assessment because a woman could mistake the movement of gas through her intestines for fetal movement.

Visualization of the Fetus by Ultrasound

Ultrasound is the most common method for confirmation of pregnancy today. If a woman is pregnant, a characteristic ring, indicating the gestational sac, will be revealed on an oscilloscope screen as early as the fourth to sixth week of pregnancy. This method also gives information about the site of implantation and whether a multiple pregnancy exists. By the eighth week, a fetal outline can be seen so clearly that the crown-to-rump length can be measured to establish the gestational age of the pregnancy. Seeing the fetal outline on a sonogram is also clear proof for a couple that they are pregnant if they had any doubt up to that point (Zheng, 2012b).

 Concept Mastery Alert

Although *probable signs* of pregnancy (such as laboratory tests, ballottement, and softening of the cervix) are objective and can be verified by an examiner, they are not reliable enough to positively diagnosis a pregnancy. The only three *positive signs* of pregnancy are demonstration of a fetal heartbeat separate from the mother's, fetal movement felt by an examiner, and visualization of the fetus by ultrasound.

QSEN Checkpoint Question 10.4

INFORMATICS

Lauren Maxwell did a urine pregnancy test but was surprised to learn a positive result is not a sure sign of pregnancy. As the nurse is recording her result in the electronic health record, she asks what a positive sign would be. The nurse should cite what finding?

a. She has noticed consistent abdominal and uterine growth.
b. She can feel her fetus move more than once per hour.
c. A serum tests reveals hCG.
d. A fetal heartbeat can be seen during an ultrasound exam.

Look in Appendix A for the best answer and rationale.

Physiologic Changes of Pregnancy

Physiologic changes that occur during pregnancy are the basis for the signs and symptoms used to confirm a pregnancy. They can be categorized as local (i.e., confined to the reproductive organs) or systemic (i.e., affecting the entire body). For easy reference, Table 10.3 summarizes the changes that occur during a typical 40-week pregnancy.

REPRODUCTIVE SYSTEM CHANGES

Reproductive tract changes are those involving the uterus, ovaries, vagina, and breasts.

Uterine Changes

The most obvious alteration in a woman's body during pregnancy is the increase in size of the uterus to accommodate the growing fetus. Over the 10 lunar months of pregnancy, the uterus increases in length, depth, width, weight, wall thickness, and volume.

- Length grows from approximately 6.5 cm to 32 cm.
- Depth increases from 2.5 cm to 22 cm.
- Width expands from 4 cm to 24 cm.
- Weight increases from 50 g to 1,000 g.
- Early in pregnancy, the uterine wall thickens from about 1 cm to about 2 cm; toward the end of pregnancy, the wall thins to become supple and only about 0.5-cm thick.
- The volume of the uterus increases from about 2 ml to more than 1,000 ml. This makes it possible for a uterus to hold a 7-lb (3,175-g) fetus plus 1,000 ml of amniotic fluid for a total of about 4,000 g.

This great uterine growth is due partly to formation of a few new muscle fibers in the uterine myometrium but principally to the stretching of existing muscle fibers (by the end of pregnancy, muscle fibers in the uterus because of fibroblastic

TABLE 10.3 TIMETABLE FOR PHYSIOLOGIC CHANGES OF PREGNANCY

Location of Change	First Trimester	Second Trimester	Third Trimester
Cardiovascular	Blood volume increasing Pseudoanemia may occur Clotting factors increasing	Blood pressure slightly decreased	Blood pressure returns to prepregnancy levels
Ovarian	Corpus luteum active	Corpus luteum fading	
Uterine	Steady increased growth	Placenta producing estrogen and progesterone, steady increased growth	Steady increased growth
Cervix	Softening begins	Softening increases	"Ripe"
Vaginal	White discharge present		Increasing in amount
Musculoskeletal		Progressive cartilage softening Lordosis increasing	Possible back or pelvic girdle pain
Pigmentation		Progressively increasing	
Kidney	Maternal glomerular filtration rate increasing Glycosuria begins and increases Aldosterone increased, aiding retention of sodium and fluid		
Gastrointestinal		Slowed peristalsis	
Thyroid	Increased metabolic rate		

tissue that forms between them, are two to seven times longer than they were before pregnancy). Because uterine fibers simply stretch during pregnancy and are not newly built, the uterus is able to return to its prepregnant state at the end of the pregnancy with little difficulty and almost no destruction of tissue (Edmonds, 2012).

By the end of the 12th week of pregnancy, the uterus is large enough that it can be palpated as a firm globe under the abdominal wall, just above the symphysis pubis. An important factor to assess regarding uterine growth at healthcare visits is its constant, steady, and predictable increase in size (Fig. 10.2).

- By the 20th or 22nd week of pregnancy, it typically reaches the level of the umbilicus.
- By the 36th week, it usually touches the xiphoid process and can make breathing difficult.
- About 2 weeks before term (the 38th week) for a **primigravida**, a woman in her first pregnancy, the fetal head settles into the pelvis and the uterus returns to the height it was at 36 weeks.

This settling of the fetus into the midpelvis is termed **lightening** because a woman's breathing is so much easier that she feels as if her load is lightened. The point at which lightening will occur is not predictable in a **multipara** (a woman who has had one or more children). In such women, it may not occur until labor begins.

Uterine height is measured from the top of the symphysis pubis to over the top of the uterine fundus (Zheng, 2012a). Although growth of a uterus implies a pregnancy is causing the increase in size because a uterine tumor could also cause uterine growth, uterine growth is only a presumptive symptom of pregnancy.

The exact shape of the expanding uterus can be influenced by the position of the fetus. As the uterus grows larger, it pushes the intestines to the sides of the abdomen, elevates the diaphragm and liver, compresses the stomach, and puts pressure on the bladder. It usually remains in the midline during pregnancy, although it may be pushed slightly to the right side because of the larger bulk of the sigmoid colon on the left. A woman may worry there will not be enough room inside her abdomen for this much increase in size. You can assure her the abdominal contents will readily shift to accommodate uterine enlargement (Fig. 10.3).

Uterine blood flow increases during pregnancy as the placenta requires more and more blood for perfusion. Doppler ultrasonography has shown that, before pregnancy, uterine blood flow is 15 to 20 ml/min. By the end of pregnancy, it expands to as much as 500 to 750 ml/min, with 75% of that volume going to the placenta. Measuring an increase in placenta blood volume and velocity is an important gauge of fetal health (Khong, Kane, Brennecke, et al., 2015).

Circulation to the uterus increases so much that toward the end of pregnancy, one sixth of a woman's blood supply is circulating through the uterus at any given time; this means uterine bleeding in pregnancy has to always be regarded as serious because it could result in sudden and major blood loss. Caution women to contact their healthcare provider if any vaginal bleeding occurs during pregnancy.

A bimanual examination (two fingers of an examiner are placed in the vagina, the other hand on the abdomen) can demonstrate, during a pregnancy, that the uterus feels more anteflexed, larger, and softer to the touch than usual. At about the sixth week of pregnancy (at the time of the second missed menstrual flow), the lower uterine segment just above the cervix becomes so soft when it is compressed between examining fingers on bimanual examination that the wall feels as thin as tissue

Figure 10.2 Fundus height at various weeks of pregnancy.

36 weeks
40 weeks
32 weeks
28 weeks
24 weeks
20–22 weeks
16 weeks
12 weeks

Figure 10.3 Crowding of abdominal contents late in pregnancy.

Liver pushed up
Stomach compressed
Bladder largely in pelvis, therefore frequent urination

Figure 10.4 Examining for Hegar's sign. If the sign is present, the wall of the uterus is softer than usual.

paper (Fletcher & Russo, 2015). This extreme softening of the lower uterine segment is known as **Hegar's sign** (Fig. 10.4).

During the 16th to 20th week of pregnancy, when the fetus is still small in relation to the amount of amniotic fluid present, if the lower uterine segment is tapped sharply during a pelvic exam, the fetus can be felt to bounce or rise in the amniotic fluid up against a hand placed on the abdomen. This phenomenon, termed **ballottement** (from the French word *ballotter*, meaning "to quake"), may, however, also be simulated by a loosely attached uterine tumor and, therefore, is no more than a probable sign of pregnancy.

Between the 20th and 24th week of pregnancy, the uterine wall becomes thinned to such a degree a fetal outline within the uterus may be palpated by a skilled examiner. Because a tumor with calcium deposits could simulate a fetal outline, palpation of what seems to be a fetus, like other uterine assessments, does not constitute a sure confirmation of pregnancy.

Uterine contractions begin early in pregnancy, at least by the 12th week, and are present throughout the rest of pregnancy, becoming stronger and harder as the pregnancy advances. A woman experiences them as waves of hardness or tightening across her abdomen. If a hand is placed on her abdomen, an examiner may be able to feel these contractions as well; an electronic monitor can easily measure both the frequency and length of such contractions.

These "practice" contractions, termed **Braxton Hicks contractions**, serve as warm-up exercises for labor and also play a role in ensuring the placenta receives adequate blood. They may become so strong in the last month of pregnancy that a woman mistakes them for labor contractions (i.e., false labor). One way they can be differentiated from true contractions is that true contractions cause cervical dilation, and Braxton Hicks contractions do not (Attilakos & Overton, 2012). Although these contractions are always present with pregnancy, they also could accompany any growing uterine mass; so, like ballottement, they are no more than a probable sign of pregnancy.

Amenorrhea

Amenorrhea (i.e., an absence of a menstrual flow) occurs with pregnancy because of the suppression of follicle-stimulating hormone (FSH) by rising estrogen levels. In a healthy woman who has menstruated previously, the absence of a menstrual flow strongly suggests impregnation has occurred. Amenorrhea, however, also heralds the onset of menopause or could result from unrelated reasons such as uterine infection, anxiety (perhaps over becoming pregnant), a chronic illness such as severe anemia, hormonal imbalance, or undue stress. It also is seen in athletes who train strenuously, especially in long-distance runners and ballet dancers if their body fat percentage drops below a critical point (Mountjoy, Sundgot-Borgen, Burke, et al., 2014). Amenorrhea is, therefore, only a presumptive symptom of pregnancy.

Cervical Changes

In response to the increased level of circulating estrogen produced by the placenta during pregnancy, the cervix of the uterus becomes more vascular and edematous than usual. A mucus plug, called the **operculum**, forms to seal out bacteria and help prevent infection in the fetus and membranes. Increased fluid between cells causes it to soften in consistency, and increased vascularity causes it to darken from a pale pink to a violet hue (**Goodell's sign**).

The consistency of a nonpregnant cervix can be compared with that of the nose; the consistency of a pregnant cervix more closely resembles an earlobe. Just before labor, the cervix becomes so soft it takes on the consistency of butter or is said to be "ripe" for birth (Wu & Chou, 2015).

Vaginal Changes

Under the influence of estrogen, the vaginal epithelium and underlying tissues increase in size as they become enriched with glycogen. Muscle fibers loosen from their connective tissue base in preparation for great distention at birth. This increase in the activity of the epithelial cells results in a slight white vaginal discharge throughout pregnancy (but this is only a presumptive symptom as vaginal infections also produce discharges).

An increase in the vascularity of the vagina parallels the vascular changes in the uterus. The resulting increase in circulation changes the color of the vaginal walls from their normal light pink to a deep violet (**Chadwick's sign**).

Vaginal secretions before pregnancy have a pH value greater than 7 (an alkaline pH). During pregnancy, the pH level falls to 4 or 5 (an acid pH), which helps make the vagina resistant to bacterial invasion for the length of the pregnancy. This occurs because of the action of *Lactobacillus acidophilus*, a bacteria that grows freely in the increased glycogen environment, which increases the lactic acid content of secretions.

Ovarian Changes

Ovulation stops with pregnancy because of the active feedback mechanism of estrogen and progesterone produced early in pregnancy by the corpus luteum and late in pregnancy by the placenta. This feedback causes the pituitary gland to halt production of FSH and luteinizing hormone (LH); without stimulation from FSH and LH, ovulation does not occur.

The corpus luteum that was created after ovulation continues to increase in size on the surface of the ovary until about the 16th week of pregnancy, by which time the placenta takes over as the chief provider of progesterone and estrogen. The corpus luteum, no longer essential for the continuation of the pregnancy, regresses in size and appears white and fibrous on the surface of the ovary (a corpus albicans).

QSEN Checkpoint Question 10.5

PATIENT-CENTERED CARE

Lauren Maxwell's doctor told her she had a positive Chadwick's sign. When she asks the nurse what this means, the best answer would be which of the following?

a. "Your abdomen feels soft and tender, a normal finding."

b. "Your uterus has tipped forward, a potential complication."

c. "Your cervical mucus feels sticky, just as it should feel."

d. "Your vagina looks dark in color, a typical pregnancy sign."

Look in Appendix A for the best answer and rationale.

CHANGES IN THE BREASTS

Subtle changes in the breasts may be one of the first physiologic changes of pregnancy a woman notices (at about 6 weeks) (Fig. 10.5). Typical changes are a feeling of fullness, tingling, or tenderness that occurs because of the increased stimulation of breast tissue by the high estrogen level in her body. As the pregnancy progresses, breast size increases because of growth in the mammary alveoli and in fat deposits. The areola of the nipple darkens, and its diameter increases from about 3.5 cm (1.5 in.) to 5 cm or 7.5 cm (2 or 3 in.). There is additional darkening of the skin surrounding the areola in some women, forming a secondary areola.

Early in pregnancy, the breasts begin readying themselves for the secretion of milk. By the 16th week, colostrum—the thin, watery, high-protein fluid that is the precursor of breast milk—can be expelled from the nipples. As vascularity of the breasts increases, blue veins may become prominent over the surface of the breasts. The sebaceous glands of the areola (**Montgomery's tubercles**), which keep the nipple supple and help to prevent nipples from cracking and drying during lactation, enlarge and become protuberant.

Talking to women during pregnancy about breast changes and how these changes are devised to aid breastfeeding can be the trigger that alerts women to the importance of breastfeeding for their baby (Pratts & Lawson, 2015).

SYSTEMIC CHANGES

Although the physiologic changes first noticed by a woman are apt to be those of the reproductive system, changes also occur in almost all body systems.

Endocrine System

Almost all aspects of the endocrine system increase during pregnancy in order to support fetal growth (Table 10.4) (Burton & Jauniaux, 2015).

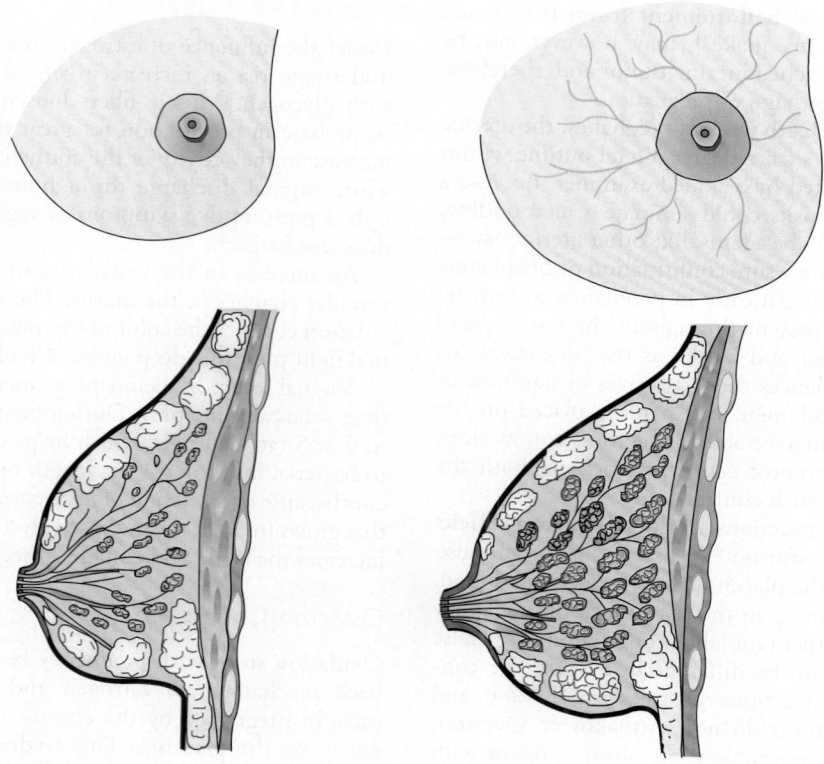

Nonpregnant   Pregnant

Figure 10.5   Comparison of nonpregnant and pregnant breasts.

Immune System

Immunologic competency during pregnancy decreases, probably to prevent a woman's body from rejecting the fetus as if it were a transplanted organ. Immunoglobulin G (IgG) production is particularly decreased, which can make a woman more prone to infection during pregnancy. A simultaneous increase in the white blood cell count may help to counteract this decrease in the IgG response.

TABLE 10.4 ENDOCRINE SYSTEM CHANGES IN PREGNANCY

Placenta*	Produces estrogen and progesterone (which help maintain the pregnancy), hCG (which allows detection of early pregnancy), and other hormones during pregnancy that impact growth of the baby and uterus and timing and onset of labor
Pituitary gland*	Late in pregnancy produces increased levels of prolactin (milk production); produces oxytocin which is necessary for labor contractions
Thyroid[†]	Increases levels of hormones that increase the basal metabolic rate by 20% and can lead to increased emotional lability, perspiration, tachycardia, and palpitations[†]
Adrenal glands*	Increases levels of corticosteroids and aldosterone inhibit immune response, thereby preventing rejection of fetus
Pancreas*	Increases insulin production but insulin is less effective due to estrogen, progesterone, and other hormones that are antagonists to insulin. This allows for more glucose to be circulating in the maternal blood stream to be available to the fetus.

hCG, human chorionic gonadotropin.

*Cunningham, F., Leveno, K., Bloom, S., et al. (2014). Maternal physiology. In F. Cunningham, K. Leveno, S. Bloom, et al. (Eds.), *William's obstetrics* (24th ed., pp. 46–79). New York, NY: McGraw-Hill.

[†]Medici, M., Korevaar, T. I., Visser, W. E., et al. (2015). Thyroid function in pregnancy: What is normal? *Clinical Chemistry, 61*(5), 704–713.

Integumentary System

As the uterus increases in size, the abdominal wall must stretch to accommodate it. This stretching (plus possibly increased adrenal cortex activity) can cause rupture and atrophy of small segments of the connective layer of the skin, leading to streaks (**striae gravidarum**) on the sides of the abdominal wall and sometimes on the thighs (Fig. 10.6). During the months after birth, striae gravidarum lighten to a silvery color (striae albicantes or atrophicae), and, although permanent, they become barely noticeable.

Often, the abdominal wall has difficulty stretching enough to accommodate the growing fetus, causing the rectus muscles underneath the skin to actually separate, a condition known as **diastasis**. If this happens, after pregnancy, the separation can be assessed through physical exam, and physical therapy can be offered for persistent diastasis.

The umbilicus is stretched by pregnancy to such an extent that by the 28th week, its depression becomes obliterated and it is pushed so far outward in some women, it appears as if it has turned inside out, protruding as a round bump at the center of the abdominal wall.

Extra pigmentation generally appears on the abdominal wall because of melanocyte-stimulating hormone from the pituitary. A narrow, brown line (**linea nigra**) may form, running from the umbilicus to the symphysis pubis and separating the abdomen into right and left halves (see Fig. 10.6). Darkened or reddened areas may appear on the face as well, particularly on the cheeks and across the nose. This is known as **melasma** (chloasma) or the "mask of pregnancy." With the decrease in the level of melanocyte-stimulating hormone after pregnancy, these areas lighten but do not always disappear.

Vascular spiders or telangiectasias (small, fiery-red branching spots) sometimes develop on the skin, particularly on the thighs. Palmar erythema, as mentioned earlier, may occur on the hands. Both of these symptoms result from the increased level of estrogen in the body; telangiectasias may fade but not completely disappear after pregnancy. The activity of sweat glands increases throughout the body beginning early in pregnancy, leading to increased perspiration. Fewer hairs

Figure 10.6 Skin changes in pregnancy: striae gravidarum and linea nigra. (sokolenok/Shutterstock.com)

on the head enter a resting phase because of overall increased metabolism, so scalp hair growth is increased.

Respiratory System

A local change that often occurs in the respiratory system is marked congestion, or "stuffiness," of the nasopharynx, a response, again, to increased estrogen levels. Women may worry this stuffiness indicates an allergy or a cold. Not realizing it is a symptom of pregnancy, some women take over-the-counter cold medications or antihistamines in an effort to relieve the congestion. Ask women at prenatal visits if they are taking any kind of medicine for this to detect this possibility and to be certain the medication they are taking is safe during pregnancy.

Because the uterus enlarges so much during pregnancy, the diaphragm, and ultimately, the lungs, receive an increasing amount of pressure. Toward the end of pregnancy, this can actually displace the diaphragm by as much as 4 cm upward. Even with all this crowding, however, a woman's vital capacity (the maximum volume exhaled after a maximum inspiration) does not decrease during pregnancy because, although the lungs are crowded in the vertical dimension, they can still expand horizontally. Two major changes do occur with pregnancy: a more rapid than usual breathing rate (18 to 20 breaths/min) and a chronic feeling of shortness of breath (Pipkin, 2012).

The physiologic reasons for those changes include:

- Residual volume (the amount of air remaining in the lungs after expiration) is decreased up to 20% because of the pressure of the diaphragm.
- Tidal volume (the volume of air inspired) is increased up to 40% as a woman draws in deeper breaths trying to increase the effectiveness of her air exchange.
- Total oxygen consumption increases by as much as 20%.
- The increased level of progesterone appears to set a new level in the hypothalamus for acceptable serum carbon dioxide levels (PCO_2) because, during pregnancy, a woman's body tends to maintain a PCO_2 at closer to 32 mmHg than the usual 40 mmHg. This low PCO_2 level is helpful as it causes a favorable CO_2 gradient at the placenta (i.e., because the fetal CO_2 level is higher than that in the mother, CO_2 crosses readily from the fetus to the mother).
- To keep the mother's pH level from becoming acidic because of the load of CO_2 being shifted to her from the fetus, increased expiration (mild hyperventilation) to blow off excess CO_2 begins early in pregnancy.
- At full term, a woman's total ventilation capacity may have risen by as much as 40%. This increased ventilation may become so extreme toward the end of pregnancy that a woman develops a respiratory alkalosis or exhales more than the usual amount of CO_2. To compensate, kidneys excrete plasma bicarbonate in urine to lower this pH. This results in increased urination or **polyuria**, a sign of pregnancy.
- The slight increase in pH in serum because of the changed expiratory effort is advantageous because it slightly increases the binding capacity of maternal hemoglobin and thereby raises the oxygen content of maternal blood (PO_2), from a usual level of about 92 mmHg to about 106 mmHg. This can be advantageous to fetal

TABLE 10.5 RESPIRATORY CHANGES DURING PREGNANCY

Variable	Change
Vital capacity	No change
Tidal volume	Increased by 30%–40%
Respiratory rate	Increased by 1 or 2 breaths/min
Residual volume	Decreased by 20%
Plasma PCO_2	Decreased to about 27–32 mmHg
Plasma pH	Increased to 7.40–7.45
Plasma PO_2	Increased to 104–108 mmHg
Respiratory minute volume	Increased by 40%
Expiratory reserve	Decreased by 20%

growth because it helps ensure good oxygenation of the fetus.

- The total respiratory changes and the compensating mechanisms that occur in the respiratory system can be described as a chronic respiratory alkalosis fully compensated by a chronic metabolic acidosis (Cunningham, Leveno, Bloom, et al., 2014).

Changes in respiratory function during pregnancy are summarized in Table 10.5.

Temperature

Early in pregnancy, body temperature increases slightly because of the secretion of progesterone from the corpus luteum (the temperature, which increased at ovulation, remains elevated). As the placenta takes over the function of the corpus luteum at about 16 weeks, the temperature usually decreases to normal.

Cardiovascular System

Changes in the circulatory system are extremely significant to the health of a fetus because they determine whether there will be adequate placental and fetal circulation for oxygenation and nutrition. Table 10.6 summarizes these changes.

What If . . . 10.3
Lauren's husband is worried because his wife sometimes has heart palpitations and often seems short of breath. He tells the nurse, "She eats almost nothing to stay 'model-slim.' Should she even have tried to have another child?" How would the nurse answer him?

Gastrointestinal System

At least 50% of women experience some nausea and vomiting early on in pregnancy. For many women, this is the first sensation a woman experiences with pregnancy (it can be noticed even before the first missed menstrual period). It is most apparent early in the morning, on rising, or if a woman becomes fatigued during the day.

Known as morning sickness, nausea and vomiting begins to be noticed at the same time levels of hCG and progesterone begin to rise, so these may contribute to its cause.

TABLE 10.6 CHANGES IN THE CARDIOVASCULAR SYSTEM AND CARDIOVASCULAR NEEDS DURING PREGNANCY

Assessment Factor	Prepregnancy	Pregnancy	Reason
Cardiac output		25%–50% increase	Increased blood volume
Heart rate (beats/min)	70–80	80–90	Increased blood volume
Blood volume (ml)	4,000	5250	Compensate for blood loss at birth, ensure transport of nutrients to fetus[*]
Red blood cell mass (mm^3)	4.2 million	4.65 million	Increased blood volume requires increased RBCs
Leukocytes (mm^3)	7,000	25,000–30,0000	To accommodate increased blood volume
Fibrinogen (mg/dl)	300	450	To accommodate increased blood volume
Blood pressure (BP)		Decreases in second trimester, rises to prepregnancy level in third trimester (Fig. 10.7)	Increased heart rate and cardiac output usually cause no change in BP.
Iron		Need 800 μg more daily	Fetal growth, increase in maternal red blood cells[†]
Folic acid		Need 400 μg daily	Low folic acid leads to large nonfunctioning red blood cells and increase risk for fetal neural tube and abdominal wall defects
Peripheral blood flow		Impaired blood return from lower extremities through the pelvis (due to weight of the baby)	Leads to edema and varicosities in vulva, rectum, and legs[‡]
Supine hypotension syndrome		Lying supine compresses the vena cava, blood return to the heart decreases (Fig. 10.8)	Decreased cardiac output and hypotension leading to faintness and palpitations and possibly fetal hypoxia[**]
Blood constitution		Increased clotting factors, platelets, white blood cells, lipids. Decreased protein level	Increased clotting factors and platelets help with bleeding during delivery, white blood cells increase to protect against infection and as a result of blood volume increases, blood lipids increase to provide energy to the fetus. Protein decreases as a result of the proteins being used by the fetus and can lead to edema.[††]

RBCs, red blood cells.

[*]Bernstein, H. B., & VanBuren, G. (2013). Normal pregnancy. In A. H. DeCherney, L. Nathan, T. M. Goodwin, et al. (Eds.), *Current diagnosis and treatment: Obstetrics and gynecology* (11th ed., pp. 141–153). Columbus, OH: McGraw-Hill/Lange.

[†]Whitney, E. N., & Rolfes, S. R. (2016). Life cycle nutrition: Pregnancy & lactation. In E. N. Whitney & S. R. Rolfes (Eds.), *Understanding nutrition* (14th ed., pp. 473–508). Belmont, CA: Wadsworth Publishing.

[‡]Pipkin, F. B. (2012). Maternal physiology. In D. K. Edmonds (Ed.), *Dewhurst's textbook of obstetrics & gynaecology* (6th ed., pp. 5–15). Oxford, United Kingdom: Wiley.

[**]Wu, E. S., & Hueppchen, N. A. (2015). Surgical disease and trauma in pregnancy. In J. L. Bienstock, H. Fox, E. E. Wallach, et al. (Eds.), *The Johns Hopkins manual of gynecology and obstetrics* (5th ed., pp. 277–285). Philadelphia, PA: Lippincott Williams & Wilkins.

[††]Attilakos, G., & Overton, T. G. (2012). Antenatal care. In D. K. Edmonds (Ed.), *Dewhurst's textbook of obstetrics & gynaecology* (6th ed., pp. 42–52). Oxford, United Kingdom: Wiley.

Figure 10.7 Blood pressure determination is an important assessment during pregnancy. Normally, this does not elevate during pregnancy. (iofoto/Shutterstock.com)

Figure 10.8 Supine hypotension can occur if a pregnant woman lies on her back. **(A)** The weight of the uterus compresses the vena cava, trapping blood in the lower extremities. **(B)** If a woman turns on her side, pressure is lifted off of the vena cava.

Another reason may be a systemic reaction to increased estrogen levels or decreased glucose levels because glucose is being used in such great quantities by the growing fetus. Nausea usually subsides after the first 3 months, after which time a woman may have a voracious appetite (Festin, 2015). Many alternate or complementary methods to help reduce nausea are available, such as acupuncture or wrist bands (discussed in Chapter 13). Box 10.8 is an interprofessional care map illustrating both nursing and team planning for a woman with nausea of pregnancy.

In addition to nausea, other gastrointestinal tract changes occur:

- Although the acidity of stomach secretions decreases during pregnancy, heartburn can readily result from reflux of stomach contents into the esophagus, caused by both the upward displacement of the stomach by the uterus, and a relaxed cardioesophageal sphincter, caused by the action of relaxin produced by the ovary. Interventions for heartburn are discussed in Chapter 13.
- As the uterus increases in size, it pushes the stomach and intestines toward the back and sides of the abdomen. At about the midpoint of pregnancy, this pressure may be sufficient to slow intestinal peristalsis and the emptying time of the stomach, leading to renewed heartburn, constipation, and flatulence.
- Pressure from the uterus on veins returning from the lower extremities can lead to hemorrhoids.
- The entire gastrointestinal tract may become less active from the combined actions of relaxin and progesterone. This natural slowing of the stomach and intestine can be helpful because the blood supply is reduced in the gastrointestinal tract as more blood is drawn to the uterus.
- Women with chronic gastric reflux usually find their condition either improved because the acidity of the stomach is decreased or worsened because of upward uterine pressure.
- Because of the gradual slowing of the gastrointestinal tract, decreased emptying of bile from the gallbladder may result. This can lead to reabsorption of bilirubin into the maternal bloodstream, giving rise to a symptom of generalized itching (subclinical jaundice). A woman who has had gallstones may have an increased tendency for stone formation during pregnancy as a result of the increased plasma cholesterol level and additional cholesterol incorporated in bile.
- Some pregnant women notice hypertrophy at their gum lines and bleeding of gingival tissue when they brush their teeth. There also may be increased saliva formation (hyperptyalism), probably as a local response to increased levels of estrogen. This is an annoying but not a serious problem.
- A lower-than-normal pH of saliva may lead to increased tooth decay if tooth brushing is not done conscientiously. This can be a problem for homeless women or any women who do not have frequent access to a place to brush their teeth.

Urinary System

Like other systems, the urinary system undergoes specific physiologic changes during pregnancy, including alterations in fluid retention and renal, ureter, and bladder function. These changes, summarized in Table 10.7, result from:

- Effects of high estrogen and progesterone levels
- Compression of the bladder and ureters by the growing uterus
- Increased blood volume that increases kidney production of more urine
- Postural influences

Musculoskeletal System

Calcium and phosphorus needs are increased during pregnancy because an entire fetal skeleton must be built. As pregnancy advances, a gradual softening of a woman's pelvic ligaments and joints occurs to create pliability and to facilitate passage of the baby through the pelvis at birth. This softening is probably caused by the influence of both the ovarian hormone relaxin and placental progesterone. This excessive mobility of joints can cause discomfort late in pregnancy, especially if there is a separation of the symphysis pubis. Separation this way causes acute pain and makes walking difficult and painful.

BOX 10.8

Nursing Care Planning

AN INTERPROFESSIONAL CARE MAP FOR A WOMAN EXPERIENCING HER SECOND PREGNANCY

Lauren Maxwell is a part-time model who explains to you, "I was planning on getting pregnant. Just not so soon." You suspect she's anxious about the pregnancy because she also says, "I know there's no turning back, but what will this do to my career?"

Family Assessment: The Maxwells have been married for 3.5 years and live in a two-bedroom apartment. Husband, John, works as a chef in a nearby Italian restaurant. Patient, Lauren, works part-time as a model while she attends cooking school. Finances are listed as "tight" but "okay."

Patient Assessment: Lauren presents with amenorrhea, breast tenderness, fatigue, and morning sickness. She is interested in when she will begin to look pregnant and what she can do for the morning sickness (she has eaten almost nothing for 2 days).

Nursing Diagnoses: Altered nutrition pattern related to nausea of early pregnancy.
   Anxiety related to pregnancy and becoming a parent.

Outcome Criteria: Patient states she is able to eat at least one full meal a day despite nausea; names two complementary therapies she is using to decrease nausea; states she is managing anxiety through self-help measures with support from significant others.

Team Member Responsible	Assessment	Intervention	Rationale	Expected Outcome
Activities of Daily Living, Including Safety				
Nurse	Determine whether patient is able to carry out usual activities (attending work and/or school, keeping house) by obtaining a health history.	Work with patient to see if modifications (going to work later, giving more home responsibility to husband) could help alleviate symptoms.	Documenting whether patient can complete normal activities helps to verify extent of concerns.	Patient reports she is able to attend school and work part-time as long into pregnancy as she desires.
Teamwork and Collaboration				
Nurse/nutritionist	Assess if patient would like additional suggestions for dealing with nausea from team expert.	Consult with nutritionist if nausea interferes with eating in 1 week.	Nausea can become extreme if not recognized as potentially serious in early pregnancy.	Patient meets with nutritionist if she still describes incapacitating nausea at 1-week telephone follow-up.
Procedures/Medications for Quality Improvement				
Nurse/primary healthcare provider	Assess whether patient would like to try a complementary therapy, such as a motion sickness band or eating dry crackers before meals.	Review pros and cons of any alternative therapy chosen with patient.	Many alternative therapies are effective at reducing symptoms of nausea during pregnancy.	Patient states she has tried at least one alternative therapy by 1-week follow-up telephone call.
Nutrition				
Nurse/nutritionist	Ask patient to list 24-hour recall nutrition history. Ask if pregnancy weight gain causes her anxiety because of her modeling career.	Examine 24-hour recall history and analyze for nutrition deficits. Make suggestions for better intake.	Documenting the problem best identifies its extent. Anxiety can compound nausea.	Patient gives 24-hour recall history and helps determine any nutritional deficits and possible solutions.

Continued on following page

BOX 10.8

Nursing Care Planning (continued)

Team Member Responsible	Assessment	Intervention	Rationale	Expected Outcome
Patient-Centered Care				
Nurse	Determine whether patient had the same degree of nausea with her first pregnancy and, if so, how she managed symptoms.	Provide clinic pamphlet to patient; discuss with patient how nausea, although uncomfortable, is a usual symptom of early pregnancy.	Recognizing that a symptom is normal can help a patient accept discomfort. Nausea of pregnancy responds to many self-help measures.	Patient reports at 1-week follow-up phone call she recognizes nausea as a normal part of early pregnancy and is taking active steps to relieve it.
Psychosocial/Spiritual/Emotional Needs				
Nurse	Assess if patient is concerned about the differences in her feelings and her husband's feelings toward pregnancy will interfere with their relationship.	Urge patient to discuss pregnancy fears with husband.	Differences in reactions to pregnancy can potentially interfere with degree of support from significant other.	Patient says she has discussed her fears with her husband and will continue to do so as pregnancy progresses.
Informatics for Seamless Healthcare Planning				
Nurse	Assess if patient has any further questions before she leaves the clinic.	"Brainstorm" with patient as needed to help her determine a solution to any concerns identified.	Unanswered questions can lead to increased anxiety over coming weeks.	Patient confirms her questions have been answered; has telephone number for clinic if further concerns arise.

TABLE 10.7 URINARY TRACT CHANGES DURING PREGNANCY

Variable	Change
Renal function	Changes to excrete waste from maternal and fetal blood supplies
Glomerular filtration rate	Increased by 50%
Blood urea nitrogen	Decreased by 25%, BUN of 15 mg/100 ml or higher is abnormal
Creatinine	Decreased in pregnancy, creatinine clearance should be 90–180 ml/min in 24-hour urine sample, serum creatinine greater than 1 mg/100 ml is abnormal
Renal threshold for sugar	Decreased to allow slight spillage
Ureter and bladder function	Increase in urinary output but also physiologic increase in urinary stasis (bladder infections and pyelonephritis are more likely)
Bladder capacity	Increased by 1,000 ml
Diameter of ureters	Increased by 25%
Frequency of urination	Increased slightly in first trimester, last 2 weeks of pregnancy increases to 10–12 times per day
Fluid retention	Increased aldosterone production causes increased sodium reabsorption and fluid retention

Solomon, J. S., & Altaus, J. E. (2015). Preterm labor & premature rupture of membranes. In J. L. Bienstock, H., Fox, E. E. Wallach, et al. (Eds.), *The Johns Hopkins manual of gynecology and obstetrics* (5th ed., pp. 128–138). Philadelphia, PA: Wolters Kluwer.

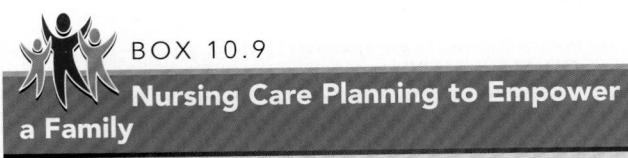

BOX 10.9
Nursing Care Planning to Empower a Family

Q. You notice Lauren Maxwell rubbing her back at a prenatal visit. She asks how she can keep her backache from becoming worse.

A. Backache is a common symptom of pregnancy because of the strain the extra uterine weight puts on lower vertebrae. Common measures to relieve backache in pregnancy include:

- Limit the use of high heels because they add to the natural lordosis of pregnancy.
- Try to rest daily with feet elevated.
- Walk with head high and pelvis straight.
- Pelvic rocking (see Chapter 14) at the end of the day may relieve pain for the night.

Backache should be reported if:

- It is experienced as waves of pain (i.e., could be preterm labor).
- There are accompanying urinary symptoms, such as frequency and pain on urination (i.e., could be a urinary tract infection).
- The back is tender at the point of backache (i.e., could be pyelonephritis or a kidney infection or a ruptured vertebrae).
- Rest doesn't relieve it (i.e., could be a muscle strain).

To change her center of gravity and make ambulation easier, a pregnant woman tends to stand straighter and taller than usual. This stance is sometimes referred to as the "pride of pregnancy." Standing this way, with the shoulders back and the abdomen forward, however, creates a lordosis (forward curve of the lumbar spine), which may lead to chronic backache, particularly in older women (Cakmak, Ribeiro, & Inanir, 2016) (Box 10.9).

Patients With Unique Concerns in Pregnancy

TRANSGENDER PATIENTS

Transgender men (men whose sex assigned at birth was female) may seek pregnancy. Discontinuation of testosterone hormone therapy and the physiologic changes of pregnancy will often bring up self-identity issues. Being a transgender or gender variant individual can feel isolating, and this isolation can deepen during pregnancy. Many transgender male patients will need extra support during the preconception time period as well as during the pregnancy itself (Ellis, Wojnar, & Pettinato, 2014).

Transgender women (women whose sex assigned at birth was male) may really want to carry a pregnancy and, with new medical research on uterus transplants, may be able to do so. Uterus transplants are still in the early stages and have not yet been attempted for transgender women (Murphy, 2015).

PATIENTS WITH DISABILITIES

Women with disabilities may also have specific concerns about how to care for themselves during pregnancy and for their child when he or she is born, and they need a careful assessment of their feelings about having a baby and any special adjustments they may need to make during pregnancy (Horner-Johnson, Darney, Kulkarni-Rajasekhara, et al., 2016). Assess if they are concerned their child may be born with their disability. Research or ask a knowledgeable team member to be certain your advice will be accurate before assuring them this is not apt to happen.

RESTLESS LEG SYNDROME AND CARPAL TUNNEL SYNDROME

Two other concerns that arise more frequently in pregnant women than others are restless leg syndrome and carpal tunnel syndrome.

Carpal tunnel syndrome is named for the Greek word *karpos* meaning "wrist" and the narrow space where the median nerve passes between the bones of the wrist. Repetitive movements, such as typing or swinging a tennis racket, can irritate the nerve resulting in sensations of pain, tingling, and numbness. Probably because of the effect of the hormone relaxin secreted by the placenta, pregnant women seem to be more susceptible to this condition than others (Meems, Truijens, Spek, et al., 2015). Actions women can take to avoid the syndrome and usual therapy is discussed in Chapter 49.

Restless leg syndrome is the uncontrollable urge to move the legs, often accompanied by itching, tingling, or aching to such an extent a person has difficulty falling or staying asleep (Oyieng'o, Kirwa, Tong, et al., 2016). It tends to occur more often in pregnant women and people with iron deficiency than others. Therapy for the condition is discussed in Chapter 51.

What If . . . 10.4

The nurse is particularly interested in exploring one of the 2020 National Health Goals with regard to psychological or physiologic changes in pregnancy (see Box 10.1)? What would be a possible research topic to explore pertinent to this goal that would be applicable to Lauren or her family and that would also advance evidence-based practice?

KEY POINTS FOR REVIEW

- The ability of a woman to accept and enjoy a pregnancy depends on social, cultural, family, and individual influences.
- The psychological tasks of pregnancy are centered on ensuring safe passage for the fetus. They consist of, in the first trimester, accepting the pregnancy; in the second trimester, accepting the baby; and in the third trimester, preparing for parenthood.
- Common emotional responses that occur with pregnancy can include grief, narcissism, introversion or extroversion, stress, couvade syndrome, body image and boundary confusion, emotional lability, and changes in sexual desire.
- Physiologic changes that occur with pregnancy are both local, such as uterine, ovarian, and vaginal changes as well as systemic changes such as those that occur in the endocrine, respiratory, cardiovascular, urinary, and immune systems.

- Women may have read about the expected psychological and physiologic changes of pregnancy but once they are experiencing them may find them more intense than anticipated.
- The confirmation of pregnancy may be assisted by three levels of findings: presumptive (subjective), probable (objective), and positive (documented).
- The positive signs of pregnancy are demonstration of a fetal heartbeat separate from the mother's, fetal movement felt by an examiner, and visualization of a fetus by ultrasound.
- Although a woman may be in a prenatal healthcare setting for only an hour, if her pregnancy is confirmed at that visit, she invariably feels "more pregnant" when she leaves. Early diagnosis or confirmation is important so a woman can begin to change unhealthy habits or have adequate time to carry out a therapeutic termination of pregnancy.
- Teaching women common psychological and physiologic changes that occur with pregnancy helps to plan nursing care that not only meets QSEN competencies but also best meets a family's total needs.

CRITICAL THINKING CARE STUDY

Joella Sanchez is a 22-year-old woman who just realized she is pregnant. She is delighted with the news, and so she was surprised to hear her 4-year-old daughter, Michelle, scream that she didn't want a brother or sister. Joella and Michelle both live with Joella's mother in a two-bedroom house. Her mother's reaction to learning about the pregnancy was to ask, "How will I fit another crib in here?" Joella works nights as a nurse's assistant at a local nursing home. Her supervisor's reaction was to frown and say, "Don't ask me to change your work schedule because you're tired all the time."

1. Is Michelle's reaction to learning a new sibling is on the way unusual? What could Joella do to win her over about the new baby?
2. Both Joella's mother and her work supervisor don't sound happy about the new baby either. What could Joella do to win them over?
3. Joella is happy about her pregnancy but surrounded by a circle of negative reactions. Could this affect her acceptance of the pregnancy? What patient education can you provide to assist her in responding to these reactions?

RELATED RESOURCES

Explore these additional resources to enhance learning for this chapter:
- Student resources on thePoint, including answers to the What If . . . and Critical Thinking Care Study questions, http://thepoint.lww.com/Flagg8e
- Adaptive learning powered by PrepU, http://thepoint.lww.com/prepu

REFERENCES

Adeniran, A. S., Aboyeji, A. P., Fawole, A. A., et al. (2015). Male partner's role during pregnancy, labour and delivery: Expectations of pregnant women in Nigeria. *International Journal of Health Sciences, 9*(3), 305–313.
Attilakos, G., & Overton, T. G. (2012). Antenatal care. In D. K. Edmonds (Ed.), *Dewhurst's textbook of obstetrics & gynaecology* (6th ed., pp. 42–52). Oxford, United Kingdom: Wiley.
Bernstein, H. B., & VanBuren, G. (2013). Normal pregnancy. In A. H. DeCherney, L. Nathan, T. M. Goodwin, et al. (Eds.), *Current diagnosis and treatment: Obstetrics and gynecology* (11th ed., pp. 141–153). Columbus, OH: McGraw-Hill/Lange.
Biaggi, A., Conroy, S., Pawlby, S., et al. (2016). Identifying the women at risk of antenatal anxiety and depression: A systematic review. *Journal of Affective Disorders, 191*, 62–77.
Brummelte, S., & Galea, L. A. (2015). Postpartum depression: Etiology, treatment and consequences for maternal care. *Hormones and Behavior, 77*, 153–166.
Burton, G. J., & Jauniaux, E. (2015). What is the placenta? *American Journal of Obstetrics and Gynecology, 213*(4), S6.e1–S6.e4.
Cakmak, B., Ribeiro, A. P., & Inanir, A. (2016). Postural balance and the risk of falling during pregnancy. *The Journal of Maternal-Fetal & Neonatal Medicine, 29*(10), 1623–1625.
Centers for Disease Control and Prevention. (2015). *Unintended pregnancy prevention*. Hyattsville, MD: Author.
Chakraborty, A., Anstice, N. S., Jacobs, R. J., et al. (2015). Prenatal exposure to recreational drugs affects global motion perception in preschool children. *Scientific Reports, 5*, 16921.
Chojenta, C. L., Lucke, J. C., Forder, P. M., et al. (2016). Maternal health factors as risks for postnatal depression: A prospective longitudinal study. *PLoS One, 11*(1), e014724.
Cunningham, F., Leveno, K., Bloom, S., et al. (2014). Maternal physiology. In F. Cunningham, K. Leveno, S. Bloom, et al. (Eds.), *William's obstetrics* (24th ed., pp. 46–79). New York, NY: McGraw-Hill.
Da Costa, D., Zelkowitz, P., Dasgupta, K., et al. (2015). Dads get sad too: Depressive symptoms and associated factors in expectant first-time fathers. *American Journal of Men's Health*. Advance online publication. doi:10.1177/1557988315606963
Edmonds, D. K. (2012). Puerperium and lactation. In D. K. Edmonds (Ed.), *Dewhurst's textbook of obstetrics & gynaecology* (6th ed., pp. 365–376). Oxford, United Kingdom: Wiley.
Ellis, S. A., Wojnar, D. M., & Pettinato, M. (2014). Conception, pregnancy, and birth experiences of male and gender variant gestational parents: It's how we could have a family. *Journal of Midwifery and Women's Health, 60*(1), 62–69.
Erikson, E. (1993). *Childhood and society* (3rd ed.). New York, NY: Norton.
Festin, M. (2015). Nausea and vomiting in early pregnancy. *American Family Physician, 92*(6), 516–517.
Fletcher, W., & Russo, M. L. (2015). Preconception counseling and prenatal care. In J. L. Bienstock, H. Fox, E. E. Wallach, et al. (Eds.), *The Johns Hopkins manual of gynecology and obstetrics* (5th ed., pp. 58–77). Philadelphia, PA: Wolters Kluwer.
Fortinash, K. M., & Holoday Worret, P. A. (2012). Therapeutic communication: Interviews and interventions. In K. M. Fortinash & P. A. Holoday Worret (Eds.), *Psychiatric mental health nursing* (5th ed., pp. 59–86). St. Louis, MO: Elsevier/Mosby.
Fuertes, M., Faria, A., Beeghly, M., et al. (2016). The effects of parental sensitivity and involvement in caregiving on mother-infant and father-infant attachment in a Portuguese sample. *Journal of Family Psychology, 30*(1), 147–156.
Gerdts, C., Dobkin, L., Foster, D. G., et al. (2016). Side effects, physical health consequences, and mortality associated with abortion and birth after an unwanted pregnancy. *Women's Health Issues, 26*(1), 55–59.
Guedes, M., & Canavarro, M. C. (2014). Psychosocial adjustment of couples to first-time parenthood at advanced maternal age: An exploratory longitudinal study. *Journal of Reproductive & Infant Psychology, 32*(5), 425–440.
Guelfi, K. J., Wang, C., Dimmock, J. A., et al. (2015). A comparison of beliefs about exercise during pregnancy between Chinese and Australian pregnant women. *BMC Pregnancy & Childbirth, 15*(1), 1–8.
Hayslip, B., Jr., Blumenthal, H., & Garner, A. (2015). Social support and grandparent caregiver health: One-year longitudinal findings for grandparents raising their grandchildren. *Journals of Gerontology: Social Sciences, 70*(5), 804–812.
Heatley, M. L., Watson, B., Gallois, C., et al. (2015). Women's perceptions of communication in pregnancy and childbirth: Influences on participation and satisfaction with care. *Journal of Health Communication, 20*(7), 827–834.
Horner-Johnson, W., Darney, B. G., Kulkarni-Rajasekhara, S., et al. (2016). Pregnancy among US women: Differences by presence, type, and complexity of disability. *American Journal of Obstetrics and Gynecology, 214*(4), 529.e1–529.e9.
Jones, D. E., Feinberg, M. E., & Hostetler, M. L. (2014). Costs to implement an effective transition-to-parenthood program for couples: Analysis of the Family Foundations program. *Evaluation and Program Planning, 44*, 59–67.

Khong, S. L., Kane, S. C., Brennecke, S. P., et al. (2015). First-trimester uterine artery Doppler analysis in the prediction of later pregnancy complications. *Disease Markers, 2015*, 679730.

Lauderdale, J. (2016). Transcultural perspectives in childbearing. In M. M. Andrews & J. S. Boyle (Eds.), *Transcultural concepts in nursing care* (7th ed., pp. 120–152). Philadelphia, PA: Wolters Kluwer.

Lilliecreutz, C., Larén, J., Sydsjö, G., et al. (2016). Effect of maternal stress during pregnancy on the risk for preterm birth. *BMC Pregnancy and Childbirth, 16*(1), 1–8.

Lindberg, L., Maddow-Zimet, I., Kost, K., et al. (2015). Pregnancy intentions and maternal and child health: An analysis of longitudinal data in Oklahoma. *Maternal & Child Health Journal, 19*(5), 1087–1096.

Medici, M., Korevaar, T. I., Visser, W. E., et al. (2015). Thyroid function in pregnancy: What is normal? *Clinical Chemistry, 61*(5), 704–713.

Meems, M., Truijens, S., Spek, V., et al. (2015). Prevalence, course and determinants of carpal tunnel syndrome symptoms during pregnancy: A prospective study. *BJOG, 122*(8), 1112–1118.

Misri, S., & Swift, E. (2015). Generalized anxiety disorder and major depressive disorder in pregnant and postpartum women: Maternal quality of life and treatment outcomes. *Journal of Obstetrics and Gynaecology Canada, 37*(9), 798–803.

Mountjoy, M., Sundgot-Borgen, J., Burke, L., et al. (2014). The IOC consensus statement: Beyond the female athlete triad—relative energy deficiency in sport (RED-S). *British Journal of Sports Medicine, 48*(7), 491–497.

Murphy, T. F. (2015). Assisted gestation and transgender women. *Bioethics, 29*(6), 389–397.

Muzik, M., McGinnis, E. W., Bocknek, E., et al. (2016). PTSD symptoms across pregnancy and early postpartum among women with lifetime PTSD diagnosis. *Depression and Anxiety, 33*(7), 584–591.

Oyieng'o, D. O., Kirwa, K., Tong, I., et al. (2016). Restless legs symptoms and pregnancy and neonatal outcomes. *Clinical Therapeutics, 38*(2), 256–264.

Pipkin, F. B. (2012). Maternal physiology. In D. K. Edmonds (Ed.), *Dewhurst's textbook of obstetrics & gynaecology* (6th ed., pp. 5–15). Oxford, United Kingdom: Wiley.

Pratts, M. E., & Lawson, S. (2015). Postpartum care & breast-feeding. In J. L. Bienstock, H., Fox, E. E. Wallach, et al. (Eds.), *The Johns Hopkins manual of gynecology and obstetrics* (5th ed., pp. 286–294). Philadelphia, PA: Wolters Kluwer.

Rilby, L., Jansson, S., Lindblom, B., et al. (2012). A qualitative study of women's feelings about future childbirth: Dread and delight. *Journal of Midwifery & Women's Health, 57*(2), 120–125.

Rogers, V. L., & Worley, K. C. (2016). Obstetrics and obstetric disorders. In M. Papadakis, S. McPhee, & M. W. Rabow (Eds.), *Current medical diagnosis & treatment* (55th ed., pp. 783-811). New York, NY: McGraw-Hill/Lange.

Silveira, M. L., Ertel, K. A., Dole, N., et al. (2015). The role of body image in prenatal and postpartum depression: A critical review of the literature. *Archives of Women's Mental Health, 18*(3), 409–421.

U.S. Department of Health and Human Services. (2010). *Healthy people 2020*. Washington, DC: Author.

Van Parys, A. S., Deschepper, E., Michielsen, K., et al. (2015). Intimate partner violence and psychosocial health, a cross-sectional study in a pregnant population. *BMC Pregnancy and Childbirth, 15*(278), 1–8.

Wu, J. L., & Chou, B. (2015). Normal labor and delivery, operative delivery and malpresentations. In C. T. Johnson, J. L. Hallock, J. L. Bienstock, et al. (Eds.), *The Johns Hopkins manual of gynecology and obstetrics* (5th ed., pp. 78–94). Philadelphia, PA: Wolters Kluwer.

Yıldız, H. (2015). The relation between prepregnancy sexuality and sexual function during pregnancy and the postpartum period: A prospective study. *Journal of Sex & Marital Therapy, 41*(1), 49–59.

Zheng, T. (2012a). Prenatal diagnosis. In T. Zheng (Ed.), *Comprehensive handbook of obstetrics & gynecology* (2nd ed., pp. 80–81). Paradise Valley, AZ: Phoenix Medical Press.

Zheng, T. (2012b). Ultrasound in pregnancy. In T. Zheng (Ed.), *Comprehensive handbook of obstetrics & gynecology* (2nd ed., pp. 85–91). Paradise Valley, AZ: Phoenix Medical Press.

Zoega, H., Kieler, H., Nørgaard, M., et al. (2015). Use of SSRI and SNRI antidepressants during pregnancy: A population-based study from Denmark, Iceland, Norway and Sweden. *PLoS One, 10*(12), e0144474.

11

Nursing Care Related to Assessment of a Pregnant Family

Sandra Czerinski is a 29-year-old woman, 12 weeks pregnant, who comes for a first prenatal visit. She is concerned because she did not realize she was pregnant until a week ago. As a result, she has been actively dieting (two diet drinks plus one meal of mainly vegetables daily) and lifting weights at a health club. She has not had a pelvic examination since she was in high school, when she had a vaginal infection. She remembers that examination as being very painful. She is worried she has a urinary tract infection now because she has to "go all the time." She does not want any blood work done because she does not have health insurance.

Previous chapters described normal reproductive anatomy and physiology and the psychological and physiologic changes that occur during pregnancy. This chapter adds information about care needed during pregnancy to help ensure a healthy outcome for both the woman and her child.

What type of health teaching does Sandra need? Is Sandra a high-risk or a low-risk patient?

KEY TERMS

diagonal conjugate

erosion

grand multipara

gravida

ischial tuberosity

lithotomy position

multigravida

multipara

nulligravida

para

primigravida

primipara

speculum

OBJECTIVES

After mastering the contents of this chapter, you should be able to:

1. Describe the areas of health assessment commonly included in prenatal visits.
2. Identify 2020 National Health Goals related to prenatal care that nurses can help the nation achieve.
3. Assess the readiness for parenthood and the health status of a pregnant woman and her family.
4. Formulate nursing diagnoses related to a woman's health status during pregnancy.
5. Identify expected outcomes to help ensure a safe pregnancy as well as manage seamless transitions across healthcare settings.
6. Using the nursing process, plan nursing care that includes the six competencies of Quality & Safety Education for Nurses (QSEN): Patient-Centered Care, Teamwork & Collaboration, Evidence-Based Practice (EBP), Quality Improvement (QI), Safety, and Informatics.
7. Implement nursing care such as establishing a risk score for a patient during pregnancy.
8. Evaluate expected outcomes for the childbearing family to establish achievement and effectiveness of goals.
9. Integrate knowledge of pregnancy health assessment with the interplay of nursing process, the six competencies of QSEN, and Family Nursing to promote quality maternal and child health nursing care.

Prenatal care, essential for ensuring the overall health of newborns and their mothers, is a major strategy for helping to reduce complications of pregnancy such as the number of preterm or low–birth-weight babies born each year (Mehta & Sokol, 2013). Prenatal care is so important that several 2020 National Health Goals directly address it (Box 11.1).

Ideally, preparation for a healthy pregnancy begins during a woman's childhood as good preparation includes a lifetime of an adequate intake of calcium and vitamin D to prevent rickets (which can distort pelvic size), adequate immunizations against contagious diseases so a woman has protection against viral diseases such as rubella and varicella during pregnancy, and maintenance of an overall healthy lifestyle to ensure the best state of health possible for a woman and her partner when entering pregnancy. Preconception care and risk assessment should be provided at every healthcare visit throughout the childbearing years for both men and women.

Other phases of an overall healthy lifestyle are a positive attitude about sexuality, womanhood, and childbearing. Once a woman becomes sexually active, preparation for a successful pregnancy includes practicing safer sex, regular pelvic examinations, and prompt treatment of any sexually transmitted infection to prevent complications that could lead to subfertility (Price, Ades, Soldan, et al., 2016). It also includes not smoking, drinking alcohol, or using recreational drugs. Acquisition and use of reproductive life planning information can help ensure each pregnancy is intended and wanted.

The initial prenatal visit is the first time many women have been to a healthcare facility since their routine health maintenance visits of childhood and adolescence. It also may be the first time they have had an appointment that focuses more on health promotion than on the diagnosis of disease. A woman usually comes with a specific goal in mind for the visit, such as confirming her pregnancy. However, a prenatal visit is much more than this; it is also a time for health promotion, pregnancy education, and encouraging a pattern of healthy behaviors for the family to use in the future. Individualized teaching varies depending on the lifestyle, age, and parity of a woman and her degree of family support (Hussein, Kai, & Qureshi, 2016).

Urging her to continue prenatal care is important because lack of prenatal care is associated with pregnancy complications such as preterm birth (Demont-Heinrich, Hawkes, Ghosh, et al., 2014).

Nursing Process Overview

FOR PRENATAL CARE

ASSESSMENT

The first prenatal visit is a time to establish baseline data relevant to a woman's health and identify health-promotion strategies that will be important at every prenatal visit. This begins by obtaining a detailed health and sexual history including screening for the risk of teratogen (any factor that may adversely affect the fetus) exposure as well as any concerns a woman has about her pregnancy. Explaining why specific assessment data are important has the potential to lead to health teaching. For instance, while you are weighing a woman, discuss the importance of a healthy body mass index (BMI) and how her expected weight gain over the coming months will be calculated based on her prepregnancy value. Relating assessment information and health-promotion activities this way helps keep a woman and her family both well informed and eager to comply with further healthcare recommendations.

NURSING DIAGNOSIS

Although most women probably have used a home pregnancy kit to find out if they are pregnant, the first prenatal visit officially confirms this, so nursing diagnoses usually focus on the response of a woman and her family to that information. Examples include:

- Decisional conflict related to desire to be pregnant
- Risk for ineffective coping related to confirmation of unintended pregnancy

Nursing diagnoses appropriate to prenatal care include:

- Health-seeking behaviors related to guidelines for nutrition and activity during pregnancy
- Deficient knowledge regarding exposure to teratogens during pregnancy
- Health-seeking behaviors related to strong cultural desire to have a healthy child
- Risk for injury to fetus related to lifestyle choices

OUTCOME IDENTIFICATION AND PLANNING

Be certain to reserve sufficient time at prenatal visits so care can be thorough and there is enough time to set realistic goals and expected outcomes with both a birthing parent and her partner, if needed. Establishing a pattern of regular appointments is crucial to the provision of effective, individualized prenatal care, so be certain a patient schedules an appointment for a

---

BOX 11.1

Nursing Care Planning Based on 2020 National Health Goals

A number of 2020 National Health Goals speak directly to the importance of prenatal care:

- Increase the proportion of pregnant women who receive early and adequate prenatal care from a baseline of 70.5% to a target of 77.6%.
- Increase the proportion of pregnant women who attend a series of prepared childbirth classes (developmental).
- Increase the proportion of women delivering a live birth who received preconception care services and practiced key recommended preconception health behaviors (developmental).
- Increase the proportion of women of childbearing potential who have an intake of at least 400 mg of folic acid from fortified foods or dietary supplements before pregnancy from a baseline of 23.8% to a target level of 26.2%.
- Increase the proportion of mothers who achieve a recommended weight gain during their pregnancies (developmental) (U.S. Department of Health and Human Services. 2010; see www.healthypeople.gov).

Nurses can help the nation achieve these goals by educating women and their families about the importance of both preconception and prenatal care as well as making sites for prenatal care "family friendly" or maximally receptive to women and families.

following visit. Ask if she has transportation to the healthcare facility because lack of transportation can be a major reason women don't consistently attend prenatal care.

It will be important to emphasize the need to visit reliable websites as not all websites about pregnancy are evidence based or monitored by a healthcare provider of any type. Refer patients and their families to helpful websites and other resources when appropriate (see Chapter 9).

IMPLEMENTATION

An important nursing intervention at prenatal visits is teaching women and their families about a safe pregnancy lifestyle. Women often discount prepared lists, believing their pregnancy is too personal to be a condition for which there are routine lists of advice. Advice, therefore, needs to be individualized for each woman. For visual learners, it can be helpful to offer a woman and her partner pamphlets that cover the same topics discussed verbally. Be certain all printed materials you give to families are consistent with what you say and with the views of the patient's obstetric healthcare provider. In addition, reinforce to the woman that she should feel free to call or e-mail the healthcare setting between visits with any problems or questions. Some women may feel reluctant to "bother" a healthcare provider outside of scheduled visits unless you give them this permission.

OUTCOME EVALUATION

Evaluation during prenatal visits should concentrate on a woman's initial understanding of the goals for care during pregnancy and assessing outcomes established for specific concerns. Examples of expected outcomes include:

- Couple state they have reached a mutual decision to both stop smoking.
- Patient states she feels well informed about the common body changes of pregnancy and actions to take to relieve any discomfort these cause.
- Patient lists ways to avoid exposure to teratogens at her work site during pregnancy.

Health Promotion and Assessment Before and During Pregnancy

The overall purposes of prenatal care are to:
- Establish a baseline of present health
- Determine the gestational age of the fetus
- Monitor fetal development and maternal well-being
- Identify women at risk for complications
- Minimize the risk of possible complications by anticipating and preventing problems before they occur
- Provide education about pregnancy, lactation, and newborn care

THE PRECONCEPTION VISIT

Preconception care is best if it is not provided at a single visit but included at every healthcare visit for all women of childbearing age. Before planning a pregnancy, a woman should schedule a specific appointment with her primary care provider to obtain accurate reproductive life planning information,

receive reassurance about fertility (based on a thorough health history and physical examination), and identify any problems that may need correction to help ensure fertility (Bienstock, Fox, & Wallach, 2015). At this visit, her hemoglobin level and blood type (including Rh factor) may be determined and, if appropriate, a Papanicolaou (Pap) smear taken (a cervical swab obtained to rule out cervical cancer) (American Congress of Obstetricians and Gynecologists [ACOG], 2015). If a vaginal infection such as chlamydia is found to be present, this can be treated to help ensure fertility. Yeast infections do not tend to interfere with fertility, although, if present, they should be treated as well. Be certain to counsel women on the importance of a diet with adequate protein, folic acid, iron, and vitamins. A prenatal vitamin may be prescribed to ensure folic acid intake will be adequate for pregnancy. Stress the importance of early prenatal care for when pregnancy occurs. If vaccinations are not current, women can be immunized against influenza at a preconception visit (Marshall, McMillan, Andrews, et al., 2016).

CHOOSING A HEALTHCARE PROVIDER FOR PREGNANCY AND CHILDBIRTH

Once a woman becomes pregnant, her next step is to choose a primary healthcare provider to care for her throughout the pregnancy and birth. Nurses contribute to the success of prenatal care through individualized assessment, counseling, and educating. Many clinics and group practices provide an initial educational seminar for women in the early stages of their pregnancy, often led by a nurse, nurse-midwife or nurse practitioner. Some practices form cohorts of women to meet monthly (cluster prenatal care) and discuss their concerns to be certain they will have support from others during pregnancy (Barger, Faucher, & Murphy, 2015; Ickovics, Earnshaw, Lewis, et al., 2016; Trotman, Chhatre, Darolia, et al., 2015). Box 11.2 summarizes ways prenatal care can be individualized so all women feel comfortable in prenatal settings and return for continuing care.

QSEN Checkpoint Question 11.1

EVIDENCE-BASED PRACTICE

One of the first things a woman who suspects she is pregnant must do is choose a primary healthcare provider to guide her through her pregnancy. Many women ask, "What type of care provider should I choose?"

To investigate whether pregnancy care and outcomes differed when women chose a nurse-midwife rather than a physician as their primary care provider, researchers examined 15 different trials involving 17,674 women researchers interviewed a sample of 6,421 Canadian women, all 15 years of age or older, all who had given birth to a singleton baby, and all who were living with their infant. Results of the study showed women whose primary prenatal care provider was a nurse-midwife were more likely to be satisfied with their maternity care experience and information provided on pregnancy and birth topics and have improved outcomes for both the birthing parent and the infant. They were prescribed fewer ultrasounds and were more likely to attend prenatal classes.

They were almost half as likely to have labor induced and 7.33 times more likely to experience a medication-free birth, experienced fewer inductions, forceps or vacuum deliveries, amniotomies, episiotomies, preterm births, and fewer overall fetal or neonatal deaths before 24 weeks gestation. Women who chose midwifery led continuity care had higher rates of unmedicated childbirth (Sandall, Soltanni, Gates, et al., 2016). Postpartally, they were more likely to initiate and maintain breastfeeding at 3 and 6 months (O'Brien, Chalmers, Fell, et al., 2011).

Based on the previous study, if Sandra asks the nurse if she should choose a nurse-midwife as her primary care provider, how would the nurse best answer her question?

  a. "Of course. Nurses are always more 'patient friendly' than physicians."
  b. "Who you choose is such a personal choice; I shouldn't give you any advice."
  c. "Nurse-midwives tend to use less medication with birth. Is that important to you?"
  d. "Nurse-midwives don't talk to women as much as doctors. Would you like that?"

Look in Appendix A for the best answer and rationale.

HEALTH ASSESSMENT DURING THE FIRST PRENATAL VISIT

Women should schedule a first prenatal visit as soon as they suspect they are pregnant. Although evidence-based practice is investigating whether the number of prenatal visits traditionally scheduled is still needed during a usual pregnancy, after the first prenatal visit, return appointments are usually scheduled every 4 weeks through the 28th week of pregnancy, every 2 weeks through the 36th week, and then every week until birth. Women categorized as high risk are followed more frequently.

An important focus of all prenatal visits, in addition to education about pregnancy and helping a woman achieve a healthy pregnancy lifestyle, is to assure women that their pregnancy is progressing well. Another important action is to screen for danger signs that might reveal a complication is beginning. The major causes of serious illness or death during pregnancy for women today are hypertension, hemorrhage, embolism, infection, morbid obesity, and anesthesia-related complications such as intrapartum cardiac arrest (Centers for Disease Control and Prevention [CDC], 2016d).

Screening at a first prenatal visit to detect subtle signs of any of these conditions includes an extensive health history, a complete physical examination (including a pelvic examination), and obtaining blood and urine specimens for laboratory analysis. Ultrasonography has decreased the need to manually measure pelvic diameters for this purpose.

QSEN Checkpoint Question 11.2

PATIENT-CENTERED CARE

Sandra Czerinski feels healthy, so she asks the nurse why she needs to bother coming for prenatal care. What benefit should the nurse cite when responding to Sandra's statement?

  a. Discovering any allergies can reduce the risk of preterm labor.
  b. It allows for the collection of accurate epidemiologic and demographic data.
  c. It provides time for education about pregnancy and birth.
  d. It provides important time to interact with a prenatal group.

Look in Appendix A for the best answer and rationale.

BOX 11.2

Suggestions to Individualize Prenatal Care

- Schedule appointments for women within 1 week after they first call the healthcare setting so they see the healthcare site as one interested in meeting their particular needs.
- Try to schedule further appointments at times convenient for a birthing parent and her support person and with the obstetric care provider of choice depending on the type of practice. Some patients choose to see one provider exclusively, whereas some choose to meet as many people in a group practice as possible during the course of their pregnancy.
- Ask whether there are outside pressures, such as having to report for work or older children coming home from school, that make a certain time of day for appointments best.
- Try to schedule appointments so there won't be a long wait time because later in pregnancy, a woman may feel uncomfortable sitting for a long stretch of time. Almost every woman is too busy to spend unnecessary time waiting at healthcare facilities.
- Make waiting time at the site educational by providing materials such as pamphlets or videos on pregnancy in the waiting room.

- Provide privacy for assessments such as blood pressure and weight.
- Be certain that pregnant women meet healthcare providers while fully clothed and upright, not naked and in a lithotomy position on an examining table.
- Encourage women to feel responsible for their health record. If a woman's first language is not English, contact an interpreter if necessary to be certain she understands prenatal instructions and will feel free to ask questions.
- Educate pregnant women about care options and encourage them to participate in making decisions about their care.
- Encourage family members and friends to accompany the patient for prenatal care. Allow them to enter the examination room and participate in all aspects of care to the extent they and the woman desire.
- Be certain women have a specific person's name and that person's phone number or e-mail contact in case they have any pregnancy-related questions before their next visit.

The Initial Interview

Because obtaining an initial health history can be time-consuming, a woman may be asked to complete some necessary forms before arrival. Appropriate interviewing techniques, however, are important to obtain a thorough and meaningful health history and the rapport established by face-to-face interviewing with healthcare personnel may be as much a reason a woman returns for follow-up care as her desire to be assured her pregnancy is progressing normally (Box 11.3). Some women are extremely frightened at the thought of birth and thus need education and assurance about this as well (Rouhe, Salmela-Aro, Toivanen, et al., 2015).

Remember that pregnancy symptoms are subtle, so a woman may not regard certain information as important, causing her to provide vague answers instead of specific information in these areas. She may be unaware, for example, that she is the only person who knows the answer to a question such as "How do you feel about being pregnant?" or "Have you been taking anything for your nausea in the morning?" For best success, remember the following:

- Interviewing is best accomplished in a private, quiet setting. Pregnancy is too private an affair to be discussed in a crowded hallway or a full waiting room.
- Caution a woman that a first visit may be lengthy because of all the things that need to be accomplished. This prevents a woman from trying to fit the visit in between other errands or from having to terminate the interview because of another appointment.
- Be certain to ask how a patient wants you to address her taking into account gender identification. Make certain she also knows your name and understands your role. If she views you as someone only gathering preliminary data, she may be willing to discuss superficial facts (name, address, phone number, and the like) but will resist discussing more intimate things (her feelings toward this pregnancy, the difficulty she has reworking old fears, or how scared she is about birth).

SUPPORT PERSON'S ROLE

Both partners and young children accompany women for prenatal care (Fig. 11.1). Some women bring a female friend or a relative as their best support person. If family members are present, should they be included in an initial interview? As a whole, interviewing is most effective if it is a one-to-one interaction because a woman may be unwilling to mention certain concerns when her family is present for fear of worrying them.

If childbearing is to be a family affair, however, it is important to determine a partner's degree of acceptance of the pregnancy and how well prepared he or she is of assuming a new parenting role. Including the fetus's siblings in a prenatal visit also provides them an opportunity to be involved.

Interviewing a woman alone and then inviting the support person and family to join her while you talk about pregnancy symptoms with them as a family can be an effective compromise. In addition, providing some private interview time with a partner allows the partner to express any of his or her concerns or worries.

If a woman wishes, a partner can accompany her during the physical examination. After confirmation of pregnancy, include the partner in healthcare information or suggestions.

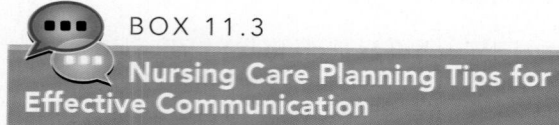

BOX 11.3
Nursing Care Planning Tips for Effective Communication

Sandra has come to her obstetrician's office for a first prenatal visit.

Tip: Ask additional questions to prompt patients to elaborate. Such questions often reveal poor nutrition, poor exercise, or risky pregnancy patterns such as alcohol intake. Most people are not aware how much information can be revealed by a typical day history, so they give only a scant description of their day.

Nurse: The first thing I'd like you to do is describe what a typical day is like for you.

Ms. Czerinski: I don't have typical ones. Or very interesting ones.

Nurse: What about yesterday? Could you describe that to me?

Ms. Czerinski: Up at 7:00, at work by 9:00. A friend picked me up after work and we celebrated his birthday. Back home and in bed by 10:00. That's it.

Nurse: What did you have for breakfast?

Ms. Czerinski: Nothing. I was far too rushed to eat.

Nurse: Dinner?

Ms. Czerinski: We went to a bar. Cheese blintzes, I think. And beer. A lot of beer.

COMPONENTS OF THE HEALTH HISTORY

An initial interview includes both present and past history. General principles of interviewing are discussed in Chapter 34. Included in Table 11.1 is a review of elements pertinent to a pregnancy history.

Demographic Data

Demographic data usually obtained include name, age (additional testing such as genetic screening may be necessary if she is over age 35 years), address, telephone number, e-mail address, religion, ethnicity, type and place of employment, and health insurance information.

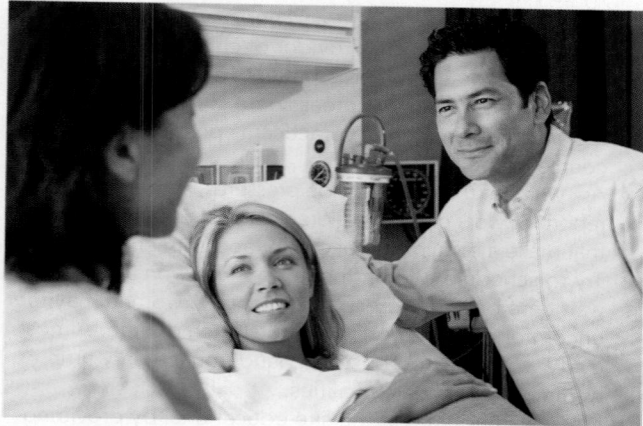

Figure 11.1 Including a support person in the labor room who also was involved in the prenatal preparation is helpful to the mother. (Monkey Business Images/Shutterstock.com)

TABLE 11.1 PATIENT PROFILE: TYPICAL DAY AND SOCIAL HISTORY FOR A PREGNANT PATIENT

	Recommended Questions	Findings That Require Further Action	Patient Education
Nutrition	Can you provide a 24-hour recall of food you've eaten today? Do you ever vomit excess food you've eaten after meals? (see Chapter 54 for discussion of eating disorders) Are you happy with your weight? Are you on a diet now?	An affirmative answer may indicate an eating disorder (see Chapter 54) Dieting is not advised during pregnancy to be certain a fetus receives adequate nutrients for growth	Women need to take a prenatal vitamin that contains folic acid (minimum 400 mg/day) all during pregnancy. Although the vitamin is found in vegetable and fruit sources, women are unable to eat enough of these natural sources to achieve an adequate amount. Prenatal vitamins also supply higher amounts of iron (30 mg on average).
Exercise	What type of exercise do you enjoy each week? How much and how frequently do you exercise each week?	Although good for her, if a woman hikes or camps, it can put her at risk for exposure to Lyme disease, an infection carried by deer ticks. Ask if she knows about precautions to prevent this disease (see Chapter 43).	Asking about the type, amount, and frequency of exercise helps determine her routine pattern and whether that will be consistent with a recommended level for pregnancy (ACOG, 2016b; Haakstad, Torset, & Bø, 2016). Daily exercise is healthy for women all through life and has been demonstrated to reduce common pregnancy discomforts. Suggestions for exercise that should be safe during pregnancy are provided in Chapter 12.
Hobbies	What hobbies do you enjoy?	Working with lead-based glazes and ceramics can cause exposure to lead, a known teratogen (Ford, 2015).	Most hobbies are harmless, but certain ones need to be discontinued or carefully managed during pregnancy.
Tobacco, alcohol, and drug consumption	Do you smoke cigarettes? If so, how often? Do you drink alcohol? If so, how often? Do you use any drugs, such as marijuana or cocaine, recreationally? Do you use any drugs intravenously? (Although this type of information under usual circumstances may not be readily revealed, most women will answer these questions honestly during pregnancy because they are concerned about protecting the health of their fetus.)	If a woman answers vaguely about how much she smokes or drinks ("I drink socially" or "I only smoke occasionally"), ask her to clarify exactly what she means by "socially" or "occasionally" so you can more accurately evaluate the frequency of these events.	Drugs and alcohol are associated with preterm or low–birth-weight infants (Roozen, Peters, Kok, et al., 2016). Intravenous drugs increase the risk of exposure to HIV and hepatitis B through the use of contaminated needles.
Medication and herbal therapy	Do you take any medications, prescribed or over-the-counter? Do you take any herbal preparations?	Tetracycline, an antibiotic commonly prescribed for facial acne, causes long bone defects in the fetus and will need to be discontinued during pregnancy (Karch, 2013). Many women take herbal supplements to relieve the nausea of early pregnancy. Even seemingly innocent alternative therapies could be detrimental if they stimulate uterine contractions or in any other way interfere with fetal health.	The effect on a growing fetus by all medications, both prescribed and over-the-counter, will have to be evaluated.

Continued on following page

TABLE 11.1 PATIENT PROFILE: TYPICAL DAY AND SOCIAL HISTORY FOR A PREGNANT PATIENT (Continued)

	Recommended Questions	Findings That Require Further Action	Patient Education
Intimate partner violence	Beginning with a normalizing statement can open the door to communication: All couples argue, but have you ever been in a situation where you were fighting and felt unsafe?" Other types of question you could ask include: Have you ever been hurt by anyone? Are you afraid of anyone? Have you ever been forced to have sex when you didn't want to?	Women and adolescents who are trapped in a violent intimate partner relationship need to be identified because both the amount and severity of violence are apt to increase with pregnancy (L. James, Brody, & Hamilton, 2013).	

Chief Concern

The chief concern is the reason the woman has come to the healthcare setting—in this instance, the fact that she is or thinks she is pregnant.

- Document the date of her last menstrual period, whether it was normal for her and whether she has used a home test pregnancy kit.
- Elicit information about the usual signs that occur with early pregnancy, such as nausea, vomiting, breast changes, or fatigue.
- Ask if she is feeling any discomfort with her pregnancy, such as constipation, backache, or frequent urination.
- Ask also about any danger signs of pregnancy, such as bleeding, abdominal pain, continuous headache, visual disturbances, or swelling of the hands and face.
- Document whether the pregnancy was intended. If you feel uncomfortable asking about this directly, use a statement such as "All pregnancies are a bit of a surprise. Is that how it was with this one?" Another way to word such a question might be "Some couples plan on having children right away; some plan on waiting. How was it with you?" If a woman says the pregnancy was not intended, explore with her if she has reached a decision about whether to continue with the pregnancy. A question such as "Some women change their mind about wanting a baby once they realize they are pregnant; some don't. How has it been for you?" is an effective way to obtain this type of information because it indicates that either answer is possible and acceptable. You just want her to tell you which is happening.

Family Profile

Obtaining information about the woman's family structure and function early in an interview helps you get to know her, identify her important support persons, shape the nature and kind of questions you want to ask, and evaluate the possible impact of the woman's culture on care. It also lays a foundation for health teaching. Areas important to ask about include:

- Marital status and support people available, and if a partner will be accompanying her for visits. As a rule, both married and unmarried women want you to know their married status because they want to alert you if they do not have a firm support person available. Box 11.4 offers suggestions to help make a partner feel like an important part of prenatal visits.
- Educational level of her and her partner (helps you estimate the level of teaching you will need to plan).
- If she works outside the home, exactly what her job consists of; for example, does it involve heavy lifting, long hours of standing in one position, or handling a toxic substance (all actions that may need to be modified during pregnancy)?
- Size and structure of the apartment or house. You'll need this information so you can talk with her in the coming months about space for a baby. If she is restricted from climbing stairs more than once or twice a day during the last part of pregnancy or after birth, knowing whether essential rooms are located on the ground floor is helpful.

BOX 11.4

Nursing Care Planning Based on Family Teaching

Q. Sandra asks you, "What can I do to make sure my boyfriend feels involved with my prenatal care?"

A. Have you tried these ideas?

- Ask for appointments to be scheduled at a time that is convenient for both of you.
- A prenatal visit can be lengthy. Be certain your partner reserves enough time so the visit doesn't become more of an inconvenience than an enjoyable event.
- Ask your partner to accompany you into the examining room at visits so you both can share your pregnancy progress or decisions.
- Be certain your partner listens to the fetal heart at visits as soon as it can be heard.
- If a sonogram is scheduled, ask your partner to view it with you (it's an exciting moment for both of you to see your fetus moving).

- Family composition. It is important to assess not only the structure of the home but also who the patient lives with and what the relationships are. This is helpful for identifying support persons in addition to identifying any potential issues that may exist in the living situation.
- Lifestyle. Are finances a problem? Does the woman take usual safety precautions such as use of a seat belt when in her car? Does she smoke, drink alcohol, or use recreational drugs? Does she have smoke and carbon monoxide monitors in her home?
- Document whether a woman has recently experienced any lifestyle changes such as a change in status from independence to dependence, a chronic illness, the death or loss of a significant person, a geographic move, financial hardship, or lack of support people. These are all examples of stressful situations that could hinder a woman's ability to accept her pregnancy and child.

History of Past Illnesses

Questions about a woman's past medical history are important because a past condition can become active during or immediately following pregnancy. Representative diseases that pose potential difficulty during pregnancy include kidney disease, heart disease (coarctation of the aorta and heart valve problems cause concern most often), hypertension, sexually transmitted infections (including hepatitis B and C, herpes, and HIV), diabetes, thyroid disease, recurrent seizures, gallbladder disease, urinary tract infections, varicosities, phenylketonuria, tuberculosis, and asthma.

It is also important to ask whether a woman had childhood diseases such as chickenpox (varicella), mumps (epidemic parotitis), measles (rubeola), German measles (rubella), and poliomyelitis or if she has had immunizations against these illnesses. Confirm whether a woman has had a human papillomavirus (HPV) vaccine; many women are not yet aware that the vaccine has the potential not only to prevent HPV infections but also to prevent cervical cancer. It is now routinely prescribed for both male and female adolescents (CDC, 2016b).

From the information obtained about common infectious diseases and immunizations, you can estimate the degree of antibody protection a woman has against these diseases if she is exposed to them during her pregnancy. Pregnant women appear to develop more complications from influenza (the flu), for example, than others, so a woman who will be pregnant during the flu season (October through May) should receive an influenza vaccine (Marshall et al., 2016).

She cannot be immunized with the oral Sabin poliomyelitis vaccine or with the vaccine against measles, mumps, or rubella because the vaccines for these contain live viruses that could be harmful to the fetus if the virus crossed the placenta (McLean, Fiebelkorn, Temte, et al., 2013). Because many women don't know if they have ever had rubella, almost all women have blood drawn for an antibody titer against rubella at a first prenatal visit. After birth, a woman who shows a high titer could then be immunized against the disease to provide fetal protection for a following pregnancy.

Be certain to ask also about any allergies, including any drug sensitivities. This information will not only be important for prenatal treatment of any potential infections or conditions that may occur during pregnancy but also will alert the birth team if someone has an allergy and is unable to communicate that for any reason.

Any past surgical procedures are also important to document because adhesions resulting from past abdominal surgery such as a ruptured appendix could interfere with uterine growth. If a birthing parent has had a prior cesarean birth, the details will be important to know for planning route of delivery and to evaluate placental location.

History of Family Illnesses

Identifying any illnesses that occur frequently in a woman's relatives can help identify potential problems a woman or her infant could experience during pregnancy or after birth. Ask specifically about cardiovascular and renal disease, diabetes, cognitive impairment, blood disorders, and any known genetically inherited diseases or congenital anomalies.

Day History/Social Profile

Information about a woman's current nutrition, elimination, sleep, recreation, and interpersonal interactions can be elicited best by asking a woman to describe what her typical day is like. If any of this information is not reported spontaneously as she describes her day, ask for additional details. An overview is provided in Table 11.2.

GYNECOLOGIC HISTORY

In the past, most women had children early in their childbearing years, so they experienced few reproductive tract or women's health disorders, such as breast disease, before pregnancy. Today, with women delaying conception of their first child past 30 years of age, it is not unusual to discover a woman who has had a reproductive tract or breast disorder. Table 11.3 lists common gynecologic illnesses that occur and their possible significance in pregnancy.

Menstrual History

A woman's past experience with her reproductive system may have some influence on how well she accepts a pregnancy as well as whether she'll develop a complication. Information to obtain includes her age of menarche (first menstrual period) and how well she was prepared for it. Ask about her usual cycle, including the interval, duration, amount of menstrual flow, and any discomfort she feels. If she has discomfort with periods, document when the discomfort occurs, how long it lasts, and what she does to relieve it.

This is important because some women with severe dysmenorrhea can be looking forward to pregnancy because it will mean 9 months without discomfort. However, if she describes menstrual cramps as "horrible" and wonders "how I live through them some months," you can anticipate that she might need additional counseling to help her prepare for the pain of labor. Anticipate the need for counseling in the postpartum period about active ways to relieve menstrual discomfort when menstrual periods resume (see Chapter 47).

Perineal and Breast Self-Examination

Perineal self-examination is inspecting the external genitalia monthly for signs of infection or lesions (see Chapter 34 for the technique). Immigrants from other countries may have had female genital cutting (clitoris removed) in childhood;

this needs to be documented because scarring and strictures may limit the size of the vaginal opening (Box 11.5).

Breast self-examination is no longer thought to yield enough reliable information to be continued as a monthly self-care routine, but women should be alerted to normal breast changes during pregnancy and about the responsibility to begin having mammograms when they reach 40 to 45 years of age depending on risk status (American Cancer Society [ACS], 2015). Clinical breast examination in women of average risk has not been shown to be effective in average risk women at any age. However, it may be helpful in identifying any anatomical issues with breastfeeding that may occur (King, Brucker, Kriebs, et al., 2015).

Past Surgery

Any type of past surgery on the reproductive tract is important to document because it can influence a woman's ability to conceive and give birth. For example, if a woman had tubal surgery following an ectopic pregnancy, her statistical risk of another tubal pregnancy is greater than usual because of possible tubal scarring. If she had uterine surgery, a cesarean birth may be necessary because her uterus may not be able to contract as efficiently as usual because of a surgical scar or she may be at risk for uterine rupture. If she has undergone frequent dilatation and curettage of the uterus or cervical biopsies, her cervix may be weakened or unable to remain closed for 9 months, leading

to preterm birth unless she has a surgical procedure (cerclage) to prevent premature dilation (see Chapter 21).

Concept Mastery Alert

Tubal surgery following an ectopic pregnancy may cause tubal scarring, which increases the patient's risk of a subsequent ectopic pregnancy.

Reproductive Planning

Ask also about what reproductive planning method, if any, a woman has been using. Occasionally, a woman may become pregnant with an intrauterine device (IUD) in place. If this occurs, its location needs to be evaluated prior to making the decision to proceed with removal. Another woman, not certain she is pregnant, may be continuing to take an oral contraceptive. If a pregnancy is confirmed, you can assure her taking the pill while pregnant will not cause fetal harm but she should discontinue taking it for the remainder of pregnancy (Charlton, Mølgaard-Nielsen, Svanström, et al., 2016).

Sexual History

Be certain to obtain a sexual history, including the number of sexual partners and the use of safer sex practices, to establish a woman's risk for contracting a sexually transmitted infection

TABLE 11.2 TYPICAL ASSESSMENTS FOR A FIRST PREGNANCY VISIT

Health History	
Demographic data	Name, address, age, ethnicity, telephone number, health insurance
Chief concern (her reason for coming for prenatal care)	Was this pregnancy intended? When was the woman's last normal menstrual period (LNMP)? Any exposure to infectious diseases or ingestion of drugs other than those prescribed since a woman thinks she has been pregnant?
Family and social profile	What is the birthing parent's family composition? Do they have a support person? What is their occupation? Source of income? Level of exercise? Hobbies? Substance use? Living conditions? Nutrition? Sleep pattern? Tobacco and alcohol use?
Past medical history	Any past history of abdominal surgery, kidney disease, heart disease, hypertension, sexually transmitted infections, diabetes, or allergies? Are all immunizations up to date?
Gynecologic history	When was menarche? What is length of menstrual cycle? Duration of menstrual flow? History of dysmenorrhea? Any gynecologic surgeries?
Obstetric history	Any previous pregnancies? When? Type and outcome of birth? Any history of previous miscarriages or therapeutic abortions?
Review of systems	Brief review of all body systems
Physical Examination	
Baseline data	Height, weight, prepregnancy body mass index, vital signs, fundal height measurement (after 12 weeks), fetal heart sounds
System assessment	Full physical examination to confirm general health
Pelvic examination	General assessment; Pap smear (if age appropriate) and human papillomavirus (HPV) culture; additional cultures for chlamydia, gonorrhea; pelvic measurements may be taken
Laboratory Assessment	
Blood	Complete blood count, serologic test for syphilis, blood type and Rh, maternal serum α-fetoprotein (MSAFP), pregnancy-associated plasma protein A (PAPP-A), antibody titer against Rh, hepatitis B and possibly C, rubella, varicella and HIV
Urinalysis	Clean catch for glucose, protein, and culture
Tuberculosis	Purified protein derivative (PPD; Mantoux) test or serum test
Ultrasound	To date pregnancy or confirm fetal health (if date of last menstrual period is unknown)

TABLE 11.3 COMMON GYNECOLOGIC DISORDERS SEEN IN PREGNANCY

Disorder	Possible Symptoms	Significance and Suggested Therapy
Disorders of the Vulva		
Cysts or infection of Skene or Bartholin glands	Cysts appear as asymptomatic swelling at the sides of the urinary meatus or vestibule; if infected, glands appear swollen and reddened and can be painful	Such cysts are surgically incised to prevent blockage of the gland duct. Infections are treated with antibiotics.
Condylomata acuminata	Painless cauliflower-like lesion on vulva	Tends to occur in women with chronic vaginitis. Caused by the same virus that causes common warts. Removed by cryocautery or knife excision, or treated with medication.
Lichen sclerosis	Whitish papules on the vulva; asymptomatic	No need for removal; the area is biopsied, however, because leukoplakia, a potentially cancerous condition, has an almost identical appearance.
Leukoplakia	Thick, gray, patchy epithelium that cracks; possibly a premalignant state that infects easily, accompanied by itching and pain	Therapy involves hydrocortisone and frequent return visits to healthcare personnel (every 6 months) for observation to detect any changes suggestive of carcinoma.
Carcinoma of the vulva	A shallow vulvar ulcer that does not heal	Vulvar cancer occurs most often in postmenopausal women; represents only 3%–4% of all reproductive tract cancers in women. Therapy is vulvectomy—vagina is left intact, and sexual relations and pregnancy, with cesarean birth to prevent tearing of fibrotic vulvar tissue, may be possible afterward.
Female genital cutting	Surgical removal of the clitoris; possibly vagina is sewed closed	Illegal in United States; done as a cultural ritual in young girls from African and Middle Eastern countries. Vaginal stricture may need to be excised to allow for menstrual flow and childbirth.
Disorders of the Vagina and Cervix		
Cervical polyp	Red, vascular, protruding pedunculated tissue that bleeds readily with trauma	May be discovered because of vaginal spotting on coitus, tampon insertion, or vaginal examination. Removed vaginally by excision. Often associated with chronic cervical inflammation.
Cervicitis (erosion)	Reddened cervical tissue with a whitish exudate	Douching with a vinegar solution aids healing. May be treated with cryosurgery if extensive.
Nabothian cyst	Clear shining circles on cervix from blocked gland ducts	No therapy necessary.
Cervical carcinoma	Postcoital spotting, unexplained vaginal discharge, or spotting between menstrual periods	The most frequent type of reproductive tract malignancy seen; risk factors include coitus with multiple partners or uncircumcised males, herpes type 2 or human papillomavirus (HPV) infections. Diagnosed by Pap test or colposcopy. Therapy is conization, radiation, or surgical excision. Pregnancy is possible following cervical carcinoma; cesarean birth may be necessary because of fibrotic cervical tissue. HPV vaccine can reduce the incidence.
Disorders of the Ovaries		
Endometrial cyst	Chocolate-brown cyst on tender enlarged ovary; may cause acute pain if rupture occurs	Endometriosis is the cause; occurs in women age 20–40 years. Therapy is surgical excision; ovary may or may not be removed depending on extent of cyst.
Follicular cyst	Amenorrhea and possibly dyspareunia; ovary tender and enlarged	Cysts typically regress after 1 or 2 months; low-dose oral contraceptive may be prescribed for 6–12 weeks to suppress ovarian activity; estrogen may be continued for 6 months.
Polycystic ovary syndrome	A syndrome of chronic follicular cysts, anovulation, insulin resistance, and excess testosterone production leading to perimenopausal onset of hirsutism, obesity, subfertility, and elevated triglycerides	Excess testosterone secretion by ovaries leads to inhibition of follicle-stimulating hormone and anovulation, causing subfertility. Weight loss, reduction in triglycerides and cholesterol levels, clomiphene citrate therapy to induce ovulation, and a combination of spironolactone (Aldactone) with estrogen-progestin oral contraceptives to reduce hirsutism are all used as therapy.
Corpus luteum cyst	Delayed menstrual flow followed by prolonged bleeding; ovary enlarged and tender	A corpus luteum persists rather than atrophies. Most regress in about 2 months; a low-dose oral contraceptive may be prescribed for 6 weeks to suppress ovarian activity.
Dermoid cyst	Asymptomatic; ovary enlarged on examination	Cyst originates from embryonic tissue; may contain hair, cartilage, and fat. Most common ovarian tumor of childhood; also occurs at age 30–50 years. Therapy is surgical resection.

Continued on following page

TABLE 11.3 COMMON GYNECOLOGIC DISORDERS SEEN IN PREGNANCY (Continued)

Disorder	Possible Symptoms	Significance and Suggested Therapy
Serous cystadenoma	Bilateral; asymptomatic except for signs of pelvic pressure	The most common type of ovarian cyst; high malignancy rate of 20%–30%. Therapy is surgical resection.
Carcinoma	Asymptomatic; intermenstrual bleeding	Ovarian cancer originates in epithelial tissue most often in women over 50 years of age. Tendency may be inherited; environmental contamination such as use of talcum powder may play a role in development. Therapy is hysterectomy and salpingo-oophorectomy.
Disorders of the Uterus		
Endometrial polyp	Intermenstrual bleeding	Polyp is removed by dilatation and curettage.
Leiomyomas (fibroids)	Asymptomatic or with increased menstrual flow; uterus may be enlarged	Muscle and fibrous connective tissue form in response to estrogen stimulation. May increase in size during pregnancy; may cause interference with cervical dilatation and result in postpartal hemorrhage. Stress to the myometrium by uterine contractions may be the original cause of formation. Therapy is embolization (blocking the blood supply), oral contraceptives or gonadotropin-releasing hormone agonists to lower estrogen level, surgical resection (myomectomy), or hysterectomy if childbearing is complete.
Endometrial carcinoma	Vaginal bleeding between menstrual periods	Diagnosis is by endometrial washing, not Pap test. Initial therapy is hysterectomy.
Uterine prolapse	Vaginal pressure and low back pain	The uterus has descended into the vagina due to overstretching of uterine supports and trauma to the levator ani muscle. Occurs most often in women who had insufficient prenatal care, birth of a large infant, a prolonged second stage of labor, bearing-down efforts or extraction of a baby before full dilatation, instrument birth, and poor healing of perineal tissue postpartally. Therapy is surgery to repair uterine supports or placement of a pessary, a plastic uterine support. Women with pessaries in place need to return for a pelvic examination every 3 months to have the pessary removed, cleaned, and replaced and the vagina inspected; otherwise, vaginal infection or erosion of the vaginal walls can result. Surgical replacement is also possible.

BOX 11.5

Nursing Care Planning to Respect Cultural Diversity

Female genital cutting is the removal of a portion or all of the female genitalia done in early adolescence as a way of attempting to controlling sexual activity in girls before marriage. The practice arises from religious or cultural customs.

Both the clitoris and the labia minora may be removed; the labia majora may be stitched closed. If keloid formation or scarring occur, the vaginal opening may be so obstructed that neither menstrual flow nor childbirth may be possible; coitus can be difficult and painful. Female genital cutting is seen most in women from African and Middle Eastern nations. The practice is illegal in the United States and opposed by the World Health Organization because it violates a woman's right to well health and physical integrity. It is an important assessment to make when obtaining a health history at preconception or first prenatal visits because it influences not just sexual health but the ability to conceive and whether vaginal childbirth will be possible.

such as herpes (a viral infection spread by direct contact) or hepatitis C (a viral infection spread by contact with blood or by intercourse with a partner who is infected). Include history taking regarding patients' sexual orientation and gender identity as there are increasing numbers of patients who grow more comfortable discussing their lesbian, gay, bisexual, and transgender healthcare requirements with their providers. It is the responsibility of the healthcare team to be aware of recent evidence-based practices to best serve these patients (Makadon & Goldhammer, 2015).

Stress Incontinence

As part of any woman's gynecologic history, assess for the possibility of stress incontinence (incontinence of urine on laughing, coughing, deep inspiration, jogging, or running). Urinary incontinence occurs with these actions because they cause the diaphragm to descend, which then increases overall abdominal pressure and bladder tension; increased tension leads to sudden emptying if the woman lacks strength in her perineal muscles or bladder supports. Commonly, this weakness occurs from past difficult births, the birth of large infants, grand multiparity, or instrument births. During pregnancy, stress incontinence can become intensified from the increasing abdominal pressure of the growing uterus. Some women, however, accept this incontinence as a normal consequence of childbearing and may not report it unless asked.

Women can relieve stress incontinence to some degree by strengthening perineal muscles with the use of Kegel exercises (periodic tightening of the perineal muscles; see Chapter 12). Surgical correction to increase support to the bladder neck could be performed following the pregnancy.

QSEN Checkpoint Question 11.3

INFORMATICS

The nurse is reviewing Sandra's electronic health record. While doing so, the nurse asks Sandra to clarify and confirm her surgical history. Why is it important to ask Sandra about past surgery during a pregnancy health history?

a. Previous use of general anesthetics is a risk factor for preterm labor.

b. Adhesions from surgery could potentially limit uterine growth.

c. Previous experience with surgery means that she will likely be comfortable in a hospital setting.

d. Abdominal incisions are associated with potential uterine rupture.

Look in Appendix A for the best answer and rationale.

OBSTETRIC HISTORY

Do not assume the current pregnancy is a woman's first pregnancy simply because she is very young or says she has only recently been married. She may have had an adolescent pregnancy or this could be a second marriage. For each previous pregnancy, document the newborn's sex and the place and date of birth. Review the pregnancy briefly by asking:

- Was the pregnancy intended?
- How did the pregnancy go, overall? Did she have any complications, such as vaginal spotting, swelling of her hands or feet, falls, or surgery?
- Did she take any medication? If so, what and why?
- Did she receive prenatal care? If so, when did she start?
- What was the duration of the pregnancy?
- What was the duration of labor? Was it what she expected? Worse? Better?
- What was the type of birth? Vaginal or cesarean? Vertex or breech? In a healthcare facility or at home? What type of anesthesia, if any, was used?
- Did she have stitches following birth?
- Did she have any complications following birth, such as excessive bleeding or infection?
- What was the infant's birth weight and sex? Did the infant cry right away? What was the infant's Apgar score?
- Was any special care needed for the baby, such as suctioning, oxygen, or an incubator?
- Was the baby discharged from the healthcare setting with her?
- What is the child's present state of health?

Ask also about any previous miscarriages or therapeutic abortions and whether she had any complications during or following those. If a woman's blood type is Rh negative, ask

TABLE 11.4 TERMS RELATED TO PREGNANCY STATUS

Key Terms	Definition
Para	The number of pregnancies that have reached viability, regardless of whether the infants were born alive
Gravida	A woman who is or has been pregnant
Primigravida	A woman who is pregnant for the first time
Primipara	A woman who has given birth to one child past age of viability
Multigravida	A woman who has been pregnant previously
Grand multipara	A woman who has carried five or more pregnancies to viability
Multipara	A woman who has carried two or more pregnancies to viability
Nulligravida	A woman who has never been and is not currently pregnant

if she received Rh immune globulin (RhIG [RhoGAM]) after miscarriages, abortions, or previous births, so you will know whether Rh sensitization could have occurred. In conjunction, ask if she has ever had a blood transfusion to establish possible risk of hepatitis B or HIV exposure or Rh sensitization from a blood transfusion.

After this history of previous pregnancies is obtained, rate the woman's status with respect to the number of times she has been pregnant, including the present pregnancy (her gravida status) and the number of children over the age of viability (20 weeks gestation) she has previously delivered (her para status). Table 11.4 explains these terms. For example, a woman who had two previous pregnancies that ended in miscarriages at 12 weeks (under the age of viability) and is now pregnant is a gravida 3, para 0. If she had given birth from the two previous pregnancies and is now pregnant, she would be gravida 3, para 2.

A more comprehensive system for classifying pregnancy status (GTPAL or GTPALM) provides greater detail on a woman's pregnancy history. By this system, the gravida classification remains the same, but para is broken down as follows:

T: the number of full-term infants born (infants born at 37 weeks or after)

P: the number of preterm infants born (infants born before 37 weeks)

A: the number of spontaneous miscarriages or therapeutic abortions

L: the number of living children

Using this system, a woman in the first example who is pregnant and has two children at home would be gravida 3, para 2002 (GTPAL) or gravida 3, para 2002 (GTPAL). A multigestation pregnancy is considered as one para. For example, a woman who had term twins, then one preterm infant, and is now pregnant again would be a gravida 3, para 2103 (GTPAL).

What If . . . 11.1

A pregnant woman has the following past history: a boy born at 39 weeks gestation, alive and well; a girl born at 40 weeks gestation, alive and well; and a girl born at 33 weeks gestation, alive and well. How would the nurse summarize her gravida and para status?

REVIEW OF SYSTEMS

A review of systems completes the subjective information of a health history. Use a systematic approach, such as head to toe, and explain what you will be doing by an explanation such as "I'm going to start at the top of your head and go through to your toes, asking about body parts or systems and any diseases you may have had." A review of systems helps women recall concerns they forgot to mention earlier, such as a urinary tract infection, a condition that can influence the outcome of pregnancy and thus would be important to your history taking.

The following body systems and questions about conditions constitute the minimum information to be addressed in a review of systems for a first prenatal visit:

- *Head*: Headache? Head injury? Seizures? Dizziness? Fainting?
- *Eyes*: Vision? Glasses or contacts needed? Diplopia or double vision? Infection? Glaucoma? Cataract? Pain? Recent changes? Last vision examination and outcome?
- *Ears*: Infection? Discharge? Earache? Hearing loss? Tinnitus? Vertigo?
- *Nose*: Epistaxis (nose bleeds)? Discharge? How many colds a year? Allergies? Postnasal drainage? Sinus pain?
- *Mouth and pharynx*: Dentures? Condition of teeth? Toothaches? Any bleeding of gums? Hoarseness? Difficulty in swallowing? Tonsillectomy? Last dental examination and outcome?
- *Neck*: Stiffness? Masses?
- *Breasts*: Lumps? Secretion? Pain? Tenderness?
- *Respiratory system*: Cough? Wheezing? Asthma? Shortness of breath? Pain? Serious chest illness, such as tuberculosis or pneumonia?
- *Cardiovascular system*: History of heart murmur? History of heart disease such as rheumatic fever or Kawasaki disease? Hypertension? Any pain? Palpitations? Anemia? Does she know her blood pressure? Has she ever had a blood transfusion?
- *Gastrointestinal system*: What was her prepregnancy weight? Vomiting? Diarrhea? Constipation? Change in bowel habits? Rectal pruritus? Hemorrhoids? Pain? Ulcer? Gallbladder disease? Hepatitis? Appendicitis?
- *Genitourinary system*: Urinary tract infection? Hematuria? Frequent urination? Sexually transmitted infection? Pelvic inflammatory disease? Hepatitis B? HIV? Did she have a problem getting pregnant? Is subfertility a concern?
- *Extremities*: Varicose veins? Pain or stiffness of joints? Any fractures or dislocations? Carpal tunnel syndrome? Restless leg syndrome?
- *Skin*: Any rashes? Acne? Psoriasis?

INTERVIEW CONCLUSION

End an interview by asking if there is anything you have not covered that the woman wants to discuss; this gives her one more chance to ask any questions she has about this new life experience. Explore any further concerns she mentions because these can be equally as important as her first concern mentioned.

Physical Examination

The next step in health assessment is physical examination. Ask a woman to void for a clean-catch urine specimen before the examination because this will provide a urine specimen for either immediate dipstick or laboratory testing of bacteria, protein, glucose, and ketone determinations. In addition, an empty bladder makes the pelvic examination more comfortable and, by reducing bladder size, allows for easier identification of pelvic organs. If you are not already familiar with obtaining a clean-catch urine specimen, Box 11.6 provides instructions.

A physical examination at a first prenatal visit typically includes inspection of major body systems, with emphasis on the changes that occur with pregnancy or that could signal a developing complication. General techniques of physical examination are discussed in Chapter 34.

BASELINE HEIGHT/WEIGHT AND VITAL SIGN MEASUREMENT

A woman's weight and height are measured at a first prenatal visit to establish a pregnancy BMI to serve as a baseline for future comparison. Record this assessment with her prepregnancy BMI, if available, to determine how much weight she has already gained or lost (Fig. 11.2). When obtaining women's weight, be certain to convey an air of "weight gain is healthy" so a woman feels comfortable gaining 30 to 40 lb during pregnancy (many patients, especially younger ones, with a lower BMI need to gain 40 lb to help ensure a healthy fetus).

Measure vital signs, including blood pressure, respiratory rate, and pulse rate, again, for baseline levels. A sudden increase in blood pressure and a sudden weight gain are both danger signs that gestational hypertension may be occurring. A sudden increase in pulse or respirations could suggest undetected bleeding. If close monitoring of blood pressure will be necessary during pregnancy, teach a support person or the woman herself how to do this so the woman can continue assessing blood pressure at home.

ASSESSMENT OF BODY SYSTEMS

Physical examination always begins with an inspection of general appearance to form an overall impression of a woman's health and well-being. General appearance is important because the manner in which people dress, the way they speak, and the body posture they assume all suggest how they feel about themselves. Remember that not all women are thoroughly happy about being pregnant. After the general assessment, examine the patient head-to-toe by beginning with the head and scalp and ending with the extremities and the skin (Table 11.5).

What If . . . 11.2

Sandra's job at a commercial laundry ironing sheets keeps her on her feet for long periods. Is she likely to be exposed to toxic substances doing this work? Is there a greater opportunity than usual for her to develop upper respiratory infections? What effect might her job have on her hips and posture?

MEASUREMENT OF FUNDAL HEIGHT AND FETAL HEART SOUNDS

At about 12 to 14 weeks of pregnancy, the uterus becomes palpable as a firm globular sphere showing over the symphysis pubis. It grows to reach the umbilicus at 20 to 22 weeks and the xiphoid process of the sternum at 36 weeks. In primiparas, it then often returns to about 4 cm below the xiphoid process because of "lightening" for the rest of pregnancy. If

BOX 11.6

Nursing Care Planning Using Procedures

OBTAINING A CLEAN-CATCH URINE SPECIMEN

Purpose: Helping a woman obtain a clean-catch urine specimen

Procedure	Principle
1. Ask the woman to wash her hands.	1. Handwashing helps prevent spread of microorganisms.
2. She then needs to open the commercial clean-catch urine specimen kit and moisten the cotton balls with the antiseptic solution or open the prepared antiseptic wipes.	2. Preparation enhances efficiency and decreases the possibility of contamination during the procedure.

3. a. Ask the woman to sit on the commode and separate her labia with her nondominant hand.	3. Cleansing helps prevent microorganisms from entering the urine specimen.

b. She should then cleanse her perineum, washing from front to back, using a cotton ball or wipe for only one stroke and then discarding it.	Cleansing from front to back prevents bringing rectal contamination forward.

4. Caution her to avoid touching the inside of the container or cap.	4. Careful handling of equipment prevents contamination.

Continued on following page

BOX 11.6

Nursing Care Planning Using Procedures (continued)

Procedure	Principle
5. The woman should begin urinating, allowing the first urine to flow into the toilet. Next, she should hold the container under the urine stream until approximately 10–20 ml has been obtained. Once the specimen is obtained, she can remove the container, release her hand from her labia, and finish voiding into the toilet.	5. The first flow of urine washes microorganisms and debris from the urinary meatus and thus shouldn't be collected. Collecting the specimen midstream helps ensures that a sterile specimen is obtained.

Procedure	Principle
6. To finish, she should cap the specimen container, wash her hands, and bring the specimen to you. Encourage her to report whether she felt any pain on urination.	6. Capping the container prevents inadvertent spilling and possible contamination of the specimen. Pain on urination is a symptom of urinary tract infection.

Figure 11.2 A woman weighs in at a prenatal visit. Pregnant women may need reassurance that gaining weight aids fetal growth. (© Barbara Proud.)

a woman is past 12 weeks of a pregnancy, assess whether the fundus of the uterus is palpable, measure the fundal height (from the top notch of the symphysis pubis to the superior aspect of the fundus), and plot the height on a graph such as the one shown in Figure 11.3; plotting uterine growth at each visit this way can help detect any unusual variation in uterine or fetal growth. If an abnormality is detected, further investigation with ultrasound can be scheduled to determine the cause of the unusual increase or lack of growth.

Auscultate for fetal heart sounds (a rate of 110 to 160 beats/min is normal) by Doppler if the pregnancy is past 10 weeks (the lower limit at which they can usually be heard). Palpate for fetal outline and position after the 28th week as a further estimation of fetal size and growth.

QSEN Checkpoint Question 11.4

QUALITY IMPROVEMENT

Sandra reports that the palms of her hands are always itchy, and the nurse notices scratches on them when you perform a physical examination. The nurse's plan of care should specify that this problem is most likely due to what factor in women who are pregnant?

a. Anxiety or fear about the pregnancy
b. A potential Rh incompatibility
c. Peripheral edema related to changes in fluid and electrolyte levels
d. A common reaction to increasing estrogen levels

Look in Appendix A for the best answer and rationale.

TABLE 11.5 HEAD-TO-TOE ASSESSMENT FOR PREGNANT PATIENT

System	Signs and Symptoms That Require Further Action	Considerations and Actions
General appearance and mental status	Poor hygiene	Assess for IPV.
	Soiled or inappropriate clothing	Consider social and mental health components.
	Inappropriate affect	
	Multiple bruises or lacerations	
Head and scalp	Dry or sparse hair	Provide nutritional counseling.
	Lack of hygiene	Consider social and mental health components.
	Headache	Assess BP.
Eyes	Eyelid edema	Asses BP: concern for hypertensive disorder.
	Swollen optic disk	Assess diabetic status.
	Visual changes	
Nose and sinuses	Nasal congestion	Patient education about this normal discomfort of pregnancy; avoid the use of any medicated nasal spray as it can lead to or exacerbate hypertension.
	Tender sinuses	Consider infection.
Ears	Feeling of fullness	Patient education about normal discomfort of pregnancy
	Pain or discharge	Concern for infection
Mouth, teeth, throat	Poor dentition/oral hygiene	Refer to dentist. Provide documentation of pregnancy.
	Gingival hypertrophy	Patient education about normal discomfort of pregnancy
Neck	Enlarged thyroid or nodule on thyroid	Consider thyroid disorder or nutritional deficiency.
Lymph nodes	Palpable	Assess for symptoms and signs of infection or illness.
Breasts	Normal changes:	Patient education about these normal discomforts and changes in pregnancy
	• Darker areola	
	• Prominent Montgomery's tubercles	Concern for breast cancer
	• Increase in size	
	• Breast tenderness	
	• Prominent vascularization	
	• Colostrum from nipples	
	• Enlarged supernumerary nipples	
	Abnormal changes:	
	• Masses, lesions, peau d'orange, nipple retraction	
Heart	Murmur	May be a normal change in pregnancy but requires evaluation
	Supine hypotension and/or heart palpitations	Patient education about normal changes and proper positioning in pregnancy
Lungs	Dyspnea in third trimester	Patient education about normal discomforts and changes in pregnancy
	Increased respiratory rate	
Back	Backache	Discuss posture and normal discomforts of pregnancy.
	Scoliosis	Consider anesthesia consult for planned epidural.
Rectum	Hemorrhoids	Patient education about normal discomforts and changes in pregnancy
		Recommend over the counter hemorrhoid remedies.
Extremities and skin	Relaxed or loose joints	Patient education about normal discomforts and changes in pregnancy
	Itching palms and soles of feet	Requires medical evaluation for liver condition
	Edema	Assess for temporal relationship. This could be dependent edema and normal, or it may be a symptom of a serious condition related to hypertension. Obtain BP.

IPV, intimate partner violence; BP, blood pressure.

Figure 11.3 Plotting uterine height on a uterine height graph at prenatal visits (recorded typically after 12 weeks gestation) helps to monitor whether fundal height is increasing.

PELVIC EXAMINATION

A pelvic examination reveals information on the health of both a woman's internal and external reproductive organs. The following equipment is required:

- A **speculum** (a metal or plastic instrument with movable flat blades; Fig. 11.4)
- A spatula and/or broom for cervical sampling
- Clean examining gloves
- Lubricant
- A glass slide or liquid collection device for a Pap smear
- A culture tube
- Two or three sterile cotton-tipped applicators or cytobrushes for obtaining cervical cultures
- A good examining light
- A movable stool at correct sitting height

Pelvic examinations have the reputation of being painful and causing a loss of modesty. If this is a first pregnancy and the patient is under the age of 21 years, it may be the first time a woman has ever had this type of examination. Having heard stories about how painful these examinations can be may cause a woman to tense just thinking about it. When pelvic muscles are tense, however, not only can the examination become painful but also an examiner has difficulty assessing the status of pelvic organs. This examination may be particularly difficult if a patient has a history of sexual abuse or assault.

Allow a woman the opportunity to talk with the person performing the examination while sitting up, before being placed in a lithotomy position, because this can enhance her sense of self-esteem and control. Many women want their support person to remain with them at the head of the table during the examination. In addition, it is customary, especially on an initial visit, for a nurse or nursing assistant to be in the room with a woman for a pelvic examination to offer additional support. This is true whether the examiner is male or female.

After the woman empties her bladder, have her lie in a **lithotomy position** (on her back with her thighs flexed and her feet resting in the examining table stirrups; Fig. 11.5). If a woman is uncomfortable in a lithotomy position, the exam can be done with her lying flat on a bed or table with her knees raised. Make sure her buttocks extend slightly beyond

A   B   C

Figure 11.4 Insertion of a vaginal speculum. **(A)** Blades held obliquely on entering the vagina. **(B)** Blades rotated to horizontal position as they pass the introitus. **(C)** Blades separated by depressing thumbpiece and elevating handle. The position of the blades is maintained by adjusting a thumbscrew.

Figure 11.5 A lithotomy position used for a pelvic examination. Help position a woman with her buttocks just over the edge of the table. Drape appropriately for modesty.

the end of the examining table if possible. Place a pillow under her head or slightly elevate the head of the examination table to help her relax her abdominal muscles. Properly drape her with a draw sheet over her abdomen that extends over her legs for modesty.

When serving as a support person, remember to remain at the head of the table so you can hold a woman's hand or put a hand on her shoulder if she needs the support of physical contact. Give explanations of what is happening, what she might be feeling (such as pressure), and what the examiner is doing as needed. Conversation with the examiner over her head is not helpful. Suggesting a woman breathe in and out (not hold her breath as she is likely to do) is a good technique to help her relax (holding her breath pushes the diaphragm down and makes the pelvic organs tense and unyielding).

External Genitalia

A pelvic examination begins with inspection of the external genitalia. Any signs of inflammation, infection, ulcerations, lesions, vaginal discharge, or circumcision are noted.

A herpes simplex 2 viral infection appears as clustered, pinpoint vesicles on an erythematous (reddened) base on the vulva that feel painful when touched or irritated. It is important that these are detected during pregnancy because the presence of herpes lesions on the vulva or vagina at the time of birth may necessitate cesarean birth to prevent exposing the fetus to the virus during passage through the birth canal. Note the presence of a herpes infection in the woman's record so she can receive prophylactic treatment at the end of her pregnancy to prevent neonatal transmission during birth which could result in a life-threatening neonatal infection (S. H. James & Kimberlin, 2015).

Next, the Skene glands that empty into the urethra and Bartholin glands that enter into the posterior vagina are checked for size and consistency. If they are swollen or emit a discharge, the discharge is cultured because an infection here could be caused by something as simple as streptococci; it may also be a more serious infection such as gonorrhea or chlamydia that could cause subfertility in the woman and conjunctivitis in her newborn.

Problems with vaginal muscle wall support, such as a rectocele (a forward pouching of the rectum into the posterior vaginal wall) or a cystocele (a pouching of the bladder into the anterior vaginal wall), are usually evaluated next. To reveal these, while the labia are gently separated to allow a view of the vaginal walls, a woman is asked to bear down as if she were moving her bowels, an action that will reveal irregular pouching on the vaginal walls.

Internal Genitalia

To view the cervix, the vagina must be opened and held open with a speculum. When fully inserted and rotated to this horizontal position, the blades are opened and the cervix becomes visible. They are secured in the open position by a thumb screw (metal speculum) or sliding latch (plastic speculum) at the side (see Fig. 11.4C).

With the speculum in place, the cervix is inspected for position. Normally, the uterine cervix is centered in the vagina; the cervix of a retroverted uterus will be positioned anteriorly, and the cervix of an anteverted uterus is positioned posteriorly. The cervix color (a nonpregnant cervix is light pink; in pregnancy, it changes to almost purple) and any lesions, ulcerations, discharge, or otherwise abnormal appearance are documented.

In a nulligravida (a woman who is not now or never has been pregnant), the cervical os appears round and small (Fig. 11.6A1). In a woman who has had a previous vaginal birth, the cervical os has much more of a slitlike appearance (see Fig. 11.6A2). If a woman had a cervical tear during a previous birth, the cervical os may appear as a transverse crease the width of the cervix or a typical star-like (stellate) formation (see Fig. 11.6A3).

If a cervical infection is present, cervical lesions (herpes simplex 2; see Fig. 11.6B1), chancre (syphilis; see Fig. 11.6B2), or a mucus discharge may be present. With infection, the epithelium of the cervical canal often enlarges and spreads onto the area surrounding the os, giving the cervix a reddened appearance that bleeds easily (**erosion**; see Fig. 11.6B3).

Typical infections that might be found are trichomoniasis, candidal (yeast) infection, gonorrhea, and chlamydia. Trichomoniasis, a protozoal infection, if present, causes petechial spots on the vaginal walls, cervical redness, and a profuse, whitish, bubbly discharge. It is important that trichomoniasis and bacterial vaginosis be treated in pregnancy as there is a link between these infections and preterm birth (Meites, Gaydos, Hobbs, et al., 2015). A candidal infection causes an itching and burning sensation in addition to producing a clumpy

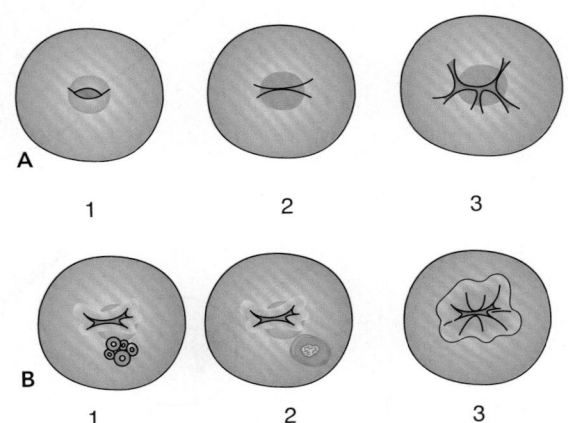

Figure 11.6 (A) Appearances of the cervix. *(1)* Nulligravida cervix. *(2)* Cervix after childbirth. *(3)* "Stellate" cervix seen after mild cervical tearing. **(B)** Possible cervical lesions. *(1)* Herpes simplex 2. *(2)* Chancre of syphilis. *(3)* Erosion or infection.

cheese-like discharge that may cause bleeding if scraped away from the vaginal walls. A gonorrhea infection presents with a thick, greenish-yellow discharge and extreme inflammation. Chlamydia is called a "silent" or "invisible" infection because it shows almost no external symptoms but internally may cause a mucopurulent cervical discharge and slight cervical redness (Price et al., 2016). Cultures for gonorrhea and chlamydia should be collected during the initial pelvic exam and between 35 and 37 weeks for patients aged 25 years and under.

A nonpregnant woman needs medication to relieve discomfort from these infections. A pregnant woman needs medication to not only relieve discomfort but also prevent preterm birth or transmission of the infection to the newborn as the newborn passes through the birth canal at term (S. H. James & Kimberlin, 2015; Meites et al., 2015). A candidal infection in the newborn, for example, causes thrush or *oral candidiasis*. A chlamydia infection can cause pneumonia or conjunctivitis in a newborn. Gonorrhea causes such a severe conjunctivitis that it can lead to blindness (Workowski & Bolan, 2015). Specific therapies for these infections are discussed in Chapter 47.

Carcinoma of the cervix appears as an irregular, granular growth. Cervical polyps (red, soft, pedunculated benign protrusions) are also occasionally seen at the os to the cervix. Women should have a first Pap smear to detect cervical cancer when they reach 21 years of age and then every 3 years thereafter (ACOG, 2016a).

Papanicolaou Smear

A Pap smear is taken from the endocervix at a first prenatal visit to be certain a precancerous or cancerous condition of the uterine cervix, vulva, or vagina is not present (Fig. 11.7).

In addition, a photograph of the cervix may be taken to document the appearance of a suspicious lesion on the cervix or confirm that a previous lesion from an infection has healed.

The most commonly used classification system used to interpret Pap smears is the Bethesda system shown in Table 11.6. Be certain when discussing results of Pap exams with woman that they are not overinterpreting results (Nayar & Wilbur, 2015). As shown in Table 11.6, the first three levels describing squamous cells reveal some abnormal cells are present, but only the last category indicates that cancer is present.

Women who engage in anal intercourse may have an anal swab taken as well as vaginal swabs to detect anal squamous neoplasms. The technique for obtaining an anal Pap smear is the same as that for vaginal specimens (a cytobrush is used). Caution the patient that she may have slight rectal bleeding following this procedure so she isn't unnecessarily concerned.

What If . . . 11.3

The foot of an examining table in a clinic faces the room door, leaving women to feel exposed if someone should walk in unexpectedly. This saves an examiner steps, but is this the best position for the table?

Vaginal Inspection

Before the vaginal speculum is removed, a culture for trichomoniasis (microscope slide wet mount sample) or group B *Streptococcus* (done at 35 to 37 weeks gestation) may be taken. Some Pap test specimen can be analyzed for gonorrhea,

1 Endocervical collection

2 Cervical collection

3 Vaginal pool collection

Figure 11.7 Obtaining a Papanicolaou smear from the cervix.

TABLE 11.6 INTERPRETATION OF PAP SMEARS BY THE BETHESDA SYSTEM

Finding	Interpretation
Negative	No precancerous or cancerous cells are found.
Squamous Cells	
Atypical squamous cells (ASC)	Some cells appear different than normal but cannot be classified as precancerous.
Low-grade squamous intraepithelial lesion (LSIL)	Mild precancerous changes may have been found in some cells.
High-grade squamous intraepithelial lesion (HSIL)	Moderate to severe precancerous changes may have been found in some cells.
Squamous cell carcinoma	Cancerous cells are present.
Glandular Cells	
Atypical glandular cells	There is an increased risk of precancer or cancerous cells.
Adenocarcinoma	Cancerous cells are present.

From Mackay, H. T. (2012). Gynecologic disorders. In S. J. McPhee, M. Papadekis, & M. W. Radow (Eds.), *Current medical diagnosis and treatment*, (pp. 727–759). Columbus, OH: McGraw-Hill.

chlamydia, and HPV, so a separate swab for these infections is not required. Treatment to eliminate all of these infections during early pregnancy helps guard maternal, fetal, and newborn health (Meites et al., 2015).

In a nonpregnant woman, vaginal walls are light pink; pregnancy may turn them dark blue to purple. Any areas of inflammation, ulceration, lesions, or discharge should be noted.

Examination of Pelvic Organs

Following the speculum examination, a bimanual (two-handed) examination is performed to assess the position, contour, consistency, and tenderness of pelvic organs (Fig. 11.8).

Abnormalities that can be noted by bimanual examination include ovarian cysts, enlarged fallopian tubes (perhaps from pelvic inflammatory disease), and an enlarged uterus. An early sign of pregnancy (Hegar's sign) is elicited on bimanual examination as well (see Chapter 10, Fig. 10.4).

Rectovaginal Examination

After a bimanual pelvic examination, the hand is withdrawn from the vagina. The index finger is reinserted into the vagina and the middle finger into the rectum. By palpating the tissue between the examining fingers in this way, it is possible to assess the strength and irregularity of the posterior vaginal wall. This maneuver may be slightly uncomfortable for a woman because of rectal pressure.

After completing the examination, any excess lubricant is wiped away from the vaginal and rectal openings. Be certain to wipe front to back to prevent bringing rectal contamination forward from the rectum to the vagina. Box 11.7 shows an interprofessional care map illustrating both nursing and team planning for a first prenatal visit including support during a pelvic examination.

Figure 11.8 A bimanual examination to determine uterine size.

QSEN Checkpoint Question 11.5

TEAMWORK & COLLABORATION

Sandra has not had a pelvic examination since she was in high school. Consequently, the nurse-midwife has asked the nurse to help make her more at ease during her first prenatal pelvic examination. What action should the nurse take?

a. Have her take a deep breath and hold it as long as she can during the examination.

b. Tell her to bear down slightly as the speculum is inserted.

c. Encourage her to moan in a low-pitched tone because this will push down the diaphragm.

d. Teach her to breathe slowly and evenly while being examined.

Look in Appendix A for the best answer and rationale.

The Pelvis: Establishing Adequacy for Childbirth

The pelvis is a bony ring formed by four united bones: the two innominate (flaring hip) bones, which form the anterior and lateral portion of the ring, and the coccyx and sacrum, which form the posterior aspect (Fig. 11.9). The pelvis serves both to support and protect pelvic organs.

- Each innominate bone is divided into three parts: *ilium, ischium,* and *pubis.*
- The ilium forms the upper and lateral portion. The flaring superior border forms the prominence of the hip (the crest of the ilium).

BOX 11.7

Nursing Care Planning

AN INTERPROFESSIONAL CARE MAP FOR A WOMAN'S FIRST PRENATAL VISIT

Sandra Czerinski is a 29-year-old woman, 12 weeks pregnant, who comes for a first prenatal visit. She's concerned because she didn't realize she was pregnant until a week ago. As a result, she has been actively dieting plus lifting weights at a health club. She hasn't had a pelvic examination since she was in high school, when she had a vaginal infection. She remembers that exam as being very painful. She is worried she has a urinary tract infection now because she has to "go all the time." She does not want any blood work done because she is not sure if her health insurance will cover the entire fee.

Family Assessment: Single woman; lives by herself in one-bedroom apartment. Works at a laundry. Boyfriend is a roofing salesman; out of town 4 days a week

Patient Assessment: Gravida 1, para 0. Last menstrual period 3 months ago. Had nausea last month but thought it was the "flu."

Menarche at age 11 years; menstrual cycle every 29 days, 6 days duration with moderate flow and mild cramps. Past history positive for sinusitis; appendectomy at age 12 years. Smokes about 1/2 pack per day, "more when I'm stressed at work"; denies alcohol use. "I drink club soda with lime or mineral water."

ROS: Height, 5 ft 5 in.; prepregnancy weight, 160 lb (BMI: 27.5 or overweight). Slight gingival hyperplasia; breasts full and slightly tender

Pelvic examination by nurse-midwife: cervical os round, clean, and slightly soft; uterus enlarged and soft; + Chadwick's sign, + Hegar's sign, + Goodell's sign. Uterine height palpable at one finger over symphysis pubis. Fetal heart rate via Doppler at 152 beats/min.

Remainder of physical examination within normal limits. Weight today: 177 lb.

Nursing Diagnosis: Health-seeking behaviors related to guidelines for healthy pregnancy

Outcome Criteria: Patient states importance of stopping smoking, identifies measures she will take to reduce number of cigarettes smoked per day, and states she will no longer try to lose weight. Makes appointment for follow-up visits.

Team Member Responsible	Assessment	Intervention	Rationale	Expected Outcome
Activities of Daily Living, Including Safety				
Nurse/ nurse-midwife	Assess patient's expectations about the pregnancy, including if she expects to continue to work and continue present lifestyle.	Discuss the effect of pregnancy on her partner and any religious or cultural beliefs that would interfere with her ability to adapt to pregnancy changes.	Assessing expectations is important to assist a woman in identifying areas of need and adaptation necessary for pregnancy.	Patient describes the likely effect of the pregnancy on herself and partner; identifies areas where she anticipates life changes.
Teamwork and Collaboration				
Nurse/ nurse-midwife	Fully assess symptoms of urinary frequency to rule out urinary tract infection; collect clean-catch urine specimen.	Discuss with patient the need for a few laboratory tests to ensure a safe pregnancy.	Urinary tract infections are associated with preterm birth. Patient is concerned regarding her coverage of health insurance.	Nurse-midwife documents urinary tract infection and prescribes or give samples of appropriate antibiotic if indicated.
Procedures/Medications for Quality Improvement				
Nurse/ nurse-midwife	Establish baseline findings of present health.	Obtain initial health history and physical exam.	Initial assessment provides a baseline for future comparison and identification of factors that may place a patient at risk.	Patient receives a thorough initial assessment, to lay a psychological and physiologic foundation of healthcare information for prenatal care.
Nurse	Obtain additional measures of wellness during pregnancy.	Obtain weight, vital signs, and urine and blood specimens.	A baseline weight and vital signs are necessary for future comparison.	Patient's weight and vital signs are monitored and compared with previous values at each prenatal visit.

Nutrition

Nurse/nutritionist	Obtain a 24-hour nutrition recall.	Discuss with patient her increased nutritional needs during pregnancy. Provide information about a high-protein diet with prenatal vitamin supplementation.	A well-balanced diet with adequate fluid intake and use of prenatal vitamins helps to ensure an optimal environment for fetal growth and development.	Patient voices an understanding of the increased food she needs during pregnancy. Patient voices she will discontinue dieting.

Patient-Centered Care

Nurse	Assess if patient is interested in decreasing smoking during pregnancy.	Instruct patient in the effects of smoking on the fetus. Assist patient with methods to reduce and stop smoking, if possible.	Nicotine in cigarettes has been shown to be teratogenic to a fetus.	Based on the fetal effects of nicotine, patient describes a plan to stop smoking at least until after the birth and, ideally, long term.
Nurse	Assess if patient is aware of the danger signs of pregnancy she will need to report immediately should they occur.	Instruct patient about possible danger signs. Emphasize that although these signs are important, they do not necessarily mean something is wrong.	Knowledge of possible danger signs allows for early detection and prompt intervention should it be necessary.	Patient and partner list danger signs of pregnancy to report immediately.

Psychosocial/Spiritual/Emotional Needs

Nurse	Assess if patient has questions or concerns about success of pregnancy.	Assure patient that concern during pregnancy is a normal response. Include information about physiologic and psychological changes of pregnancy.	Anxiety can interfere with ability to adjust to pregnancy. Reviewing information reinforces understanding.	Patient describes any concerns about pregnancy and receives appropriate information or assurance.

Informatics for Seamless Healthcare Planning

Nurse	Assess whether patient will have any difficulty continuing with prenatal care.	Assist patient with setting up appointments for future visits keeping in mind that she is concerned about her health insurance coverage.	Assisting with setting appointments helps to ensure adherence.	Patient states plan for expected antepartal care visits and affirms her willingness to adhere to the plan.

- The ischium is the inferior portion.
- At the lowest portion of the ischium are two projections: the ischial tuberosities, or the part of the bone on which a person sits. These projections are important markers used to determine lower pelvic width.
- The ischial spines are small projections that extend from the lateral aspects of the pelvis into the pelvic cavity. They mark the midpoint of the pelvis. Their location is used to assess the level to which a fetus has descended into the birth canal just before or during labor.
- Where the two anterior portions of the innominate bone meet is the symphysis pubis.
- The sacrum is the upper posterior portion of the pelvic ring. There is a marked anterior projection of this bone at the point where it touches the lower lumbar vertebrae (the sacral prominence), which is used as a landmark when securing pelvic measurements.
- The coccyx, just below the sacrum, is composed of five very small bones fused together. Although the bone itself is stiff, there is a degree of movement possible in the joint between the sacrum and the coccyx (the sacrococcygeal joint). This movement is important during labor because it permits the coccyx to be pressed backward, allowing more room for the fetal head to pass through the bony pelvic ring at birth.

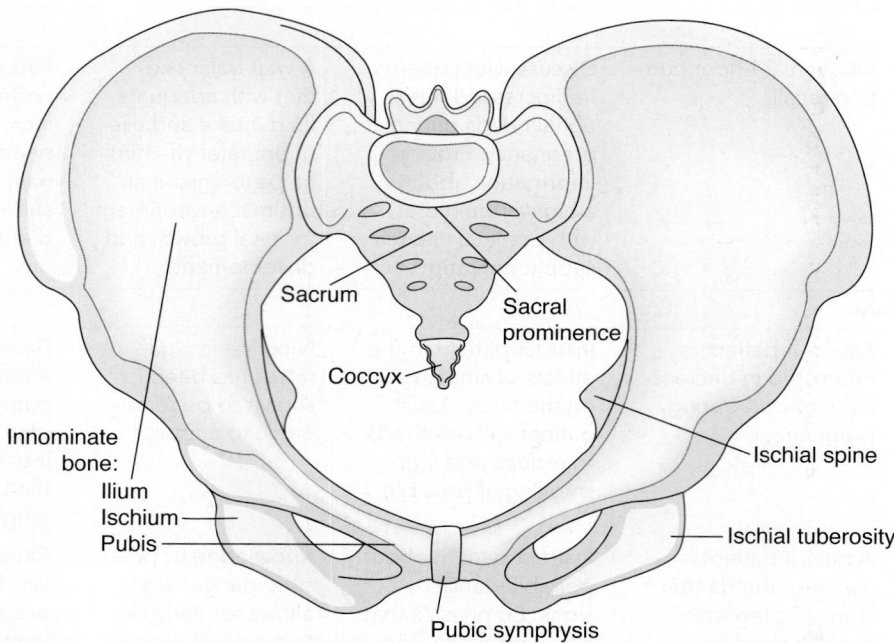

Figure 11.9 Structure of the pelvis.

For obstetric purposes, the pelvis is further divided into the false pelvis (the superior half) and the true pelvis (the inferior half) (Fig. 11.10). The false pelvis supports the uterus during the late months of pregnancy and aids in directing the fetus into the true pelvis for birth. The false pelvis is divided from the true pelvis only by an imaginary line, the linea terminalis. This imaginary line is drawn from the sacral prominence at the back of the pelvis to the superior aspect of the symphysis pubis at the front.

Other important terms in relation to the pelvis are the inlet, the outlet, and the pelvic cavity.

- The *inlet* is the entrance to the true pelvis, or the upper ring of bone through which the fetus must pass to be born vaginally. It is at the level of the linea terminalis or is marked by the sacral prominence in the back, the ilium on the sides, and the superior aspect of the symphysis pubis in the front. If you looked down at the pelvic inlet, the passageway would appear heart-shaped because of the jutting sacral prominence. It is wider transversely (sideways) than in the anteroposterior dimension.
- The *outlet* is the inferior portion of the pelvis, or that portion bounded in the back by the coccyx, on the sides by the ischial tuberosities, and in the front by the inferior aspect of the symphysis pubis. In contrast to the inlet of the pelvis, the greatest diameter of the outlet is its anteroposterior diameter.
- The *pelvic cavity* is the space between the inlet and the outlet. This space is not a straight but a curved passage; the purpose of its curve is to slow and control the speed of birth. The snugness of the cavity also serves to compress the chest of the fetus as he or she passes through. This helps to expel lung fluid and mucus and thereby better prepare lungs for good aeration at birth.

For a baby to be born vaginally, he or she must be able to pass through the inlet, the cavity, and the outlet of the pelvic

bone. This is not a problem for the average fetus; it may, however, be a problem if the mother is a young adolescent who has not yet achieved full pelvic growth (girls younger than age 14 years are most prone to this difficulty) or a woman who has had a pelvic injury from something such as an automobile accident.

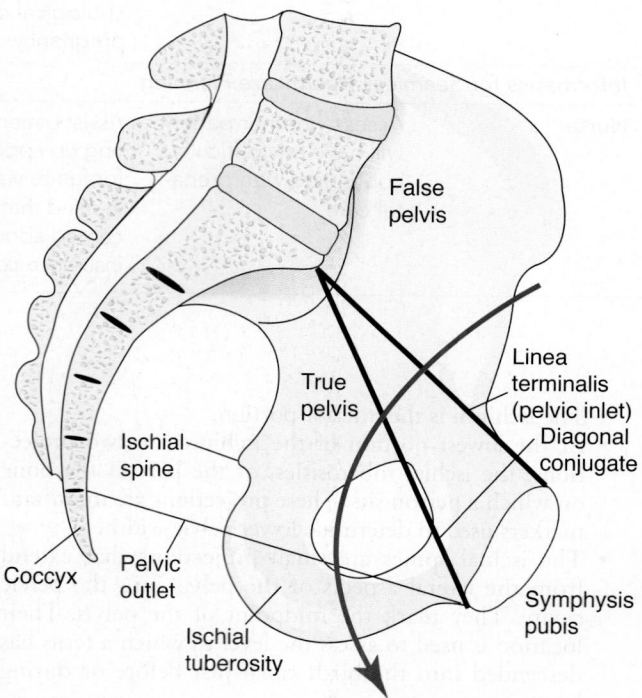

Figure 11.10 True and false pelvis. Portion above linea terminalis is false pelvis; portion below is true pelvis. *Arrow* shows "stovepipe" curve the fetus must follow to be born.

Estimating Pelvic Size

It is impossible to predict from the outward appearance of a woman whether her pelvic ring will be adequate for a fetus to pass through its center without difficulty.

Differences in pelvic contour occur mainly because of hereditary factors, but disease such as rickets, now rarely seen in the United States but still a concern in undeveloped countries, may cause contraction of the pelvis and severely narrow the pelvic outlet (Okeke, Enwereji, Onwuka, et al., 2015).

Once a woman has given birth vaginally, her pelvis has been proven adequate for vaginal birth, so it is unnecessary for pelvic measurements to be repeated unless she had an intervening history or trauma to the pelvis between pregnancies.

Types of pelvises found in women can be categorized into four groups (Fig. 11.11): android, anthropoid, gynecoid, and platypelloid.

- A *gynecoid*, or "female," pelvis has an inlet that is well rounded forward and backward and has a wide pubic arch. This pelvic type is ideal for childbirth.
- In an *android*, or "male," pelvis, the pubic arch forms an acute angle, making the lower dimensions of the pelvis extremely narrow. A fetus may have difficulty exiting from this type of pelvis.
- In an *anthropoid*, or "ape-like," pelvis, the transverse diameter is narrow; the anteroposterior diameter of the inlet is larger than usual. Even though the inlet is large, the shape of the pelvis does not accommodate a fetal head as well as a gynecoid pelvis.

- A *platypelloid*, or "flattened," pelvis has a smoothly curved oval inlet, but the anteroposterior diameter is shallow. A fetal head might not be able to rotate to match the curves of the pelvic cavity.

Internal pelvic measurements reveal the diameters of the inlet and outlet and can be obtained by pelvimetry at the time of a routine sonogram examination done to date a pregnancy. The following measurements are most commonly determined:

- The **diagonal conjugate** is the measurement between the anterior surface of the sacral prominence and the posterior surface of the symphysis pubis. The average measurement is 10.5 to 11 cm.
- The **ischial tuberosity** diameter is the distance between the ischial tuberosities, or the transverse diameter of the outlet (the narrowest diameter at that level, or the one most apt to cause a misfit). It is made at the medial and lowermost aspect of the ischial tuberosities at the level of the anus. A diameter of 11 cm is considered adequate because it will allow the widest diameter of the fetal head, or 9 cm, to pass freely through the outlet.

Laboratory Assessment

A number of laboratory studies are included as part of assessment at a first prenatal visit to confirm general health and rule out sexually transmitted infection that could injure a growing fetus. Normal levels for these studies are available at http://thePoint.lww.com/Flagg8e.

Figure 11.11 Types of pelves. **(A)** *Android*, or "male," pelvis. **(B)** *Anthropoid*, or "ape-like," pelvis. **(C)** *Gynecoid*, or "female," pelvis. **(D)** *Platypelloid*, or "flattened," pelvis.

URINALYSIS

Urine is tested for proteinuria (protein in urine), glycosuria (glucose in urine), nitrites (bacteria in urine), and pyuria (white blood cells in urine suggesting an infection). All four of these can be assessed by point of care tests, or the urine can be sent for microscopic examination in a laboratory.

BLOOD SERUM STUDIES

The following serum studies are usually obtained at a first prenatal visit:

1. A complete blood count, including hemoglobin or hematocrit and red cell index to determine the presence of anemia, a white blood cell count to determine infection, and a platelet count to estimate clotting ability.
2. A genetic screen for common ethnically inherited diseases. African American women, for example, may have a blood sample taken to screen for sickle-cell trait or disease and glucose-6-phosphate dehydrogenase (G6PD). Asian and Mediterranean women may have this done for β-thalassemia, those with Jewish ancestry may have this done for Tay-Sachs disease, and Caucasian women may be tested to see if they are a carrier for cystic fibrosis.
3. A serologic test for syphilis (venereal disease research laboratory [VDRL] or rapid plasma reagin test). If syphilis is present, it must be treated early in pregnancy before fetal damage occurs.
4. Blood typing (including Rh factor). Blood type is documented because blood may have to be made available if a woman has bleeding during pregnancy and to detect the possibility of ABO and Rh isoimmunization.
5. Cultures for chlamydia and gonorrhea should be collected for each patient at the initial pelvic examination. By identifying these often asymptomatic infections, the patient can be appropriately treated with antibiotics and the risk of neonatal morbidity reduced. A test of cure should be done for these conditions as well as a repeat culture between 35 and 37 weeks. All patients aged 25 years and under should have a repeat gonorrhea and chlamydia test at 35 to 37 weeks regardless of prior infection status.
6. Maternal serum α-fetoprotein (MSAFP) and pregnancy-associated plasma protein A. Both of these levels will be elevated if a neural tube or abdominal defect is present in the fetus; they may be decreased if a chromosomal anomaly is present. These tests are not routinely done at a first prenatal visit because they are most accurate if scheduled between 16 and 18 weeks of pregnancy. If levels are elevated or decreased, a sonogram or amniocentesis will be prescribed to clarify fetal health (Choi, Van Riper, & Thoyre, 2012).
7. An indirect Coombs test (determination of whether Rh antibodies are present in an Rh-negative woman). This test is generally repeated at 28 weeks of pregnancy. If an Rh-negative woman's titer is not elevated, she will be offered RhIG (RhoGAM) at 28 weeks of pregnancy, after any procedure that might cause placental bleeding (amniocentesis or external version), and within 72 hours after delivery.
8. Serum antibody titers for rubella, hepatitis B (HBsAg), hepatitis C, varicella (chickenpox) may be assessed. These tests determine whether a woman is protected against these diseases if exposure should occur during pregnancy. Vaccines against these diseases can then be offered in the postpartum period. HBsAg testing may be repeated at about 36 weeks.
9. HIV screening. The CDC recommends that all women be tested in early pregnancy for HIV, and those at high risk should be retested in the third trimester (CDC, 2016a). High-risk criteria include women who have used or are using intravenous drugs; have engaged in sex with multiple partners; have had sexual partners who are infected or are at risk because they are bisexual, intravenous drug users, or hemophiliac; or received a blood transfusion between 1977 and 1985. Screening for HIV is done by an enzyme-linked immunosorbent assay (ELISA) on a blood sample. If this is positive, the finding is confirmed by a second test (a Western blot). Testing for HIV early in pregnancy allows a woman who is found to be HIV antibody positive the opportunity to begin therapy with a combination of anti-retrovirals which can decrease the risk of her infant acquiring the virus. It also allows a woman the option of choosing to terminate a pregnancy if she chooses. Because there is still no cure for HIV infection, some women may choose not to have a blood titer taken because they would rather not know they have the illness. Screening is increased in states who use the opt out method for HIV testing. This means that the patient will have HIV testing done along with their other serum testing unless they specifically ask not to be tested for this virus. Because HIV testing is controversial, be certain the information given about test results is relayed accurately and with tact and compassion (a high blood antibody titer means the woman has been exposed to the virus, not that she is necessarily infected). The result of HIV testing, like all patient information, is confidential; be certain not to report this information to anyone other than the woman.
10. If a woman has a history of previously unexplained fetal loss, has a family history of diabetes, has had babies who were large for gestational age (9 lb or more at term), has a BMI over 30, or has glycosuria, she will need to be scheduled for a 50-g oral 1-hour glucose loading or tolerance test (sometimes called a glucose challenge test) toward the end of the first trimester (12 weeks) to rule out gestational diabetes The addition of a serum (HgA1C) has the best predictive value for identifying diabetes (Hughes, Moore, Gullam, et al., 2015).

If she is not high risk, she will have this test prescribed routinely at the 24th to 28th week of pregnancy. A glucose challenge test analyzes how well a woman's body is able to process sugar or whether the insulin-antagonistic effects of placental hormones are counteracting pancreatic insulin and causing an elevated blood glucose (a sign of gestational diabetes, which as many as 2% to 5% of woman develop during pregnancy). Normally, a woman's plasma glucose level should not exceed 130 to 140 mg/dl at 1 hour after glucose ingestion (see Chapter 20 for a discussion of further testing and nursing responsibilities for women with diabetes in pregnancy).

TUBERCULOSIS SCREENING (MANTOUX TEST)

The incidence of tuberculosis is on the rise as more people with lowered immune system function, such as a woman with HIV infection, contract tuberculosis and then spread it to others through coughing. Consequently, a woman's primary care provider may prescribe a purified protein derivative (PPD) tuberculin test for a woman as a test for tuberculosis.

For this test, a small amount (0.1 ml) of tuberculin units are injected by a needle and syringe intradermally (just under the top layer of skin). In 48 to 72 hours, the area is inspected. If the woman has tuberculosis, has been exposed to tuberculosis, or has received the bacille Calmette–Guérin (BCG) vaccine for tuberculosis, a reddened, raised, hardened area (called induration) will appear at the injection site. If the induration area is at least 10 cm in diameter, the test is considered positive (a person has been either exposed to tuberculosis or has tuberculosis); in a person with a lowered immune response, 5 cm can be considered a positive result.

If a woman has a positive result, a chest X-ray will be prescribed to assess her current disease status. Women are often reluctant to have X-rays done during pregnancy because they know radiation is harmful to a growing fetus. You can assure her that her fetus will be protected as long as she is given a lead apron to cover her abdomen.

Tuberculosis screening may also be done by a blood serum test called an interferon-gamma release assay (IGRA). IGRA testing is the preferred method because:

- In a woman who has a history of tuberculosis or who has received the BCG vaccine, a PPD test can cause an extreme reaction. BCG vaccine is not administered to people in the United States, but women from other countries may have received it.
- It can offer results for a woman who states it will be difficult for her to return for a follow-up appointment for a PPD test to be read and interpreted.

Screening for tuberculosis early in pregnancy is important because it is a chronic and debilitating disease that increases the risk of miscarriage. Further, the change in the shape of the maternal lung tissue as the growing uterus presses on the lungs may reactivate already healed lesions, thus worsening the disease (LaCourse, Greene, Dawson-Hahn, et al., 2016).

ULTRASONOGRAPHY

If the date of the last menstrual period is unknown, a woman will be scheduled for a sonogram to confirm the pregnancy length and document healthy fetal growth at 7 to 11 weeks of pregnancy. An ultrasound may also be done, ideally between 11 and 13 weeks of pregnancy, as a part of a first trimester screening to assess for increased risk of Down syndrome. A sonogram can be scheduled between 16 and 20 weeks gestation to verify healthy fetal structures and gender. Be certain women know that a sonogram done under 8 weeks will show only the presence of a gestation sac, not a moving, kicking fetus, so their expectations of what they will see are not disappointing (Gonçalves, 2016).

Risk Assessment

Following information gathering at a first prenatal visit, findings are analyzed to determine whether a pregnancy is apt to continue with a good outcome or there is likely to be some risk that it will end before term or with an unfavorable fetal or maternal outcome (a high-risk pregnancy).

Table 11.7 lists a minimum of factors that would identify a pregnancy as high risk. A woman identified as high risk will need close observation during prenatal visits to be certain the

pregnancy is progressing well; the infant born of a woman identified this way needs close observation in the neonatal period until it is confirmed the newborn is responding well to postuterine life.

Risk assessment should be updated at each prenatal visit because events can cause a pregnancy first rated as low risk to change to high risk. Chapters 20 through 22 discuss specific conditions that cause high-risk pregnancy and nursing for these responsibilities.

Signs Indicating Possible Complications of Pregnancy

Although most signs that suggest a complication may be occurring appear toward the end of pregnancy, women need to be aware of what these are from the beginning. To introduce the topic of danger signs, assure a woman you have every reason to believe she is going to have a normal, uncomplicated pregnancy (assuming that is true) but, if any danger signs do occur, you want her to be informed as to what they are so she can inform her healthcare provider by telephone or e-mail immediately. Be certain you give her an alternate contact number to call if the healthcare facility is closed. Assure her as well that if one of these danger signs should occur, it serves merely as a signal of the possibility that something may be happening, not that something serious has already happened. It is important for her to report a danger sign immediately, though, so it can be dealt with before something harmful does occur. A pregnant woman should report the following signs or symptoms immediately:

- Vaginal bleeding. A woman should report vaginal bleeding, no matter how slight, because some of the serious bleeding complications of pregnancy begin with only slight spotting. If a woman reports bleeding, ask her how she discovered the blood. If she found it on toilet paper following a bowel movement, she's probably reporting spotting from hemorrhoids. Until the bleeding is found to be innocent this way, however, all women with spotting need further evaluation.
- Persistent vomiting. Once- or twice-daily vomiting is not uncommon during the first trimester of pregnancy. Persistent, frequent vomiting is not normal nor is vomiting that continues past the 12th week of pregnancy. Persistent or extended vomiting depletes the nutritional supply available to a fetus and thus is a danger to the pregnancy. (See Chapter 13 for an in-depth discussion of persistent vomiting [hyperemesis gravidarum].)
- Chills and fever or pain on urination. Chills and fever may be symptoms of a relatively benign gastroenteritis, but they also may indicate an intrauterine infection, a potentially serious complication for both a woman and a fetus. Pain on urination is a symptom of a urinary infection, which is potentially serious because these infections are associated with preterm birth. Because a woman cannot make a definite determination about the cause of a fever herself, further evaluation by a healthcare provider is necessary.
- Sudden escape of clear fluid from the vagina. When a gush of clear fluid is discharged suddenly from the vagina, it means the membranes have ruptured and mother and fetus are now both threatened because the uterine cavity

TABLE 11.7 ASSESSMENTS THAT MIGHT CATEGORIZE A PREGNANCY AS AT RISK

Assessment	Risk Factors
Obstetric history	Existing uterine or cervical anomaly
	History of subfertility, recurrent miscarriages, or grand multiparity
	Last pregnancy less than 1 year previous
	History of abnormal Pap smear
	Previous premature cervical dilatation, preterm labor, preterm birth, low–birth-weight infant, or cesarean birth
	Previous macrosomic infant or multiple gestation
	Previous abnormal gestational trophoblastic disease
	Previous ectopic pregnancy or stillborn/neonatal death
	Previous infant with neurologic deficit, birth injury, or congenital anomaly
Past illness history	A chronic disease such as diabetes mellitus, heart disease, renal disease, or chronic hypertension
	Emotional disorder or cognitive challenge
	Family history of severe inherited disorders
	Fibroid tumors or previous surgeries on reproductive organs
	Maternal reproductive tract anomalies or malignancy
	Seizure disorders
	Sexually transmitted infections
	Surgery required during pregnancy
Current obstetric status	Abnormal fetal surveillance tests
	Abnormal presentation; fetal version necessary
	Premature separation of the placenta or placenta previa
	Cervical cerclage
	Limited prenatal care
	Maternal weight loss or weight gain less than 10 lb by midpregnancy
	Multiple gestation or hydramnios (excessive amniotic fluid)
	Gestational hypertension or preeclampsia
	Premature rupture of membranes or preterm labor
	Rh sensitization
	Sexually transmitted infection
Psychosocial factors	Attempt or ideation of self-injury
	Dangerous occupation
	Lack of support people
	Inadequate finances; inadequate nutrition or poor housing
	Lack of acceptance of pregnancy
Demographic factors	Maternal age under 16 years or over 40 years
Lifestyle	Alcohol use during pregnancy
	Smoking greater than 10 cigarettes a day or living with a person who smokes this much
	Heavy lifting or long periods of standing
	Recreational drug use
	Unusual stress

is no longer sealed against infection. If a fetus is small so the head does not fit snugly into the cervix, the umbilical cord may prolapse. If the fetal head then presses on the misplaced cord, oxygenation can be compromised and the fetus will be in immediate and grave danger. Alerting a healthcare provider to any sudden escape of fluid is crucial so a safe and controlled birth can be planned.

Occasionally, a woman confuses stress incontinence (involuntary loss of urine on coughing or sneezing or lifting a heavy object) for membranes breaking. In this situation, vaginal examination typically reveals that the membranes are still intact

and the pregnancy is not in danger. Urine can be identified by Nitrazine paper as urine is acidotic (the test strip turns yellow), whereas amniotic fluid is alkaline (the strip turns blue).

- Abdominal or chest pain. Abdominal or chest pain at any time is a signal something is abnormal, so a woman should also report these immediately. Some women may think abdominal pain is normal because the growing uterus is deflecting other organs from their usual alignment, but a pregnant uterus normally expands painlessly. Abdominal pain is therefore a sign of some other problem, such as a tubal (ectopic) pregnancy, separation of the placenta, preterm labor, or something unrelated to the pregnancy but perhaps equally serious, such as appendicitis, ulcer, or pancreatitis. Chest pain and shortness of breath may indicate a pulmonary embolus, a complication that can follow thrombophlebitis.

- Gestational hypertension. Gestational hypertension refers to a potentially severe and even fatal elevation of blood pressure that occurs during pregnancy usually after 20 weeks of pregnancy. A number of symptoms signal that gestational hypertension is developing:
  - Rapid weight gain (over 2 lb/week in the second trimester, over 1 lb/week in the third trimester)
  - Swelling of the face or fingers
  - Flashes of light or dots before the eyes
  - Dimness or blurring of vision
  - Severe, continuous headache
  - Decreased urine output
  - Right upper quadrant pain unrelated to fetal position
  - Blood pressure increased above 140/90 mmHg

One by one, these are vague symptoms, so a woman may need some help appreciating they are important enough to report during pregnancy. Some edema of the ankles during pregnancy is normal, for example, particularly if it occurs after a woman has been on her feet all day. Swelling of the hands (ask if she has noticed if her rings are tight) or face (difficulty opening eyes in the morning because of edema of the eyelids), however, indicates edema that is more extensive than usual. Visual disturbances or a continuous headache may signal cerebral edema or acute hypertension.

Be certain a woman is not reporting symptoms such as visual difficulties and headaches she had before she became pregnant. If she had the same symptoms before pregnancy as she is reporting now, she may need to see an ophthalmologist rather than her obstetrician for help with the problem. (See Chapter 21 for an in-depth discussion of gestational hypertension.)

- Increase or decrease in fetal movement. Because a fetus normally moves more or less the same amount every day, an unusual increase or decrease in movement suggests a fetus responding to a need for more oxygen. Be certain to ask a woman about typical fetal movements and whether she has noticed any increase or decrease in this rate. If there has been a change, she is a candidate for further testing such as a fetal "kick count" or a nonstress test. Common tests of fetal movement and health of this type are discussed in Chapter 9.
- Uterine contractions before 37 weeks of pregnancy. Women do have faint and irregular Braxton Hicks contractions prior to this point, but regular rhythmic contractions before 37 weeks suggest preterm birth is beginning. A woman needs to lie down, drink a glass of water to ensure she is well hydrated, and telephone her obstetric care provider. Such contractions may be innocent, but it is better to report them than to ignore them and allow a preterm birth to continue.

QSEN Checkpoint Question 11.6

SAFETY

The nurse is reviewing danger signs of pregnancy with Sandra. In the interests of safety, which of the following would the nurse tell her to report if it should occur?

   a. Her uterus becomes palpable over the symphysis pubis before 12 weeks.
   b. Blue veins appear and can be readily observed on both of her breasts.
   c. She gains more than 3 lb a week beginning at 20 weeks.
   d. She tends to lose her balance when she wears high-heeled shoes.

Look in Appendix A for the best answer and rationale.

Be certain that after a first prenatal visit, a woman understands she needs to continue with spaced prenatal care. No one likes surprises, so reviewing with a woman what she can expect at future visits can help her understand the importance of keeping them. Box 11.8 lists components of assessments and care important for these continuing prenatal visits.

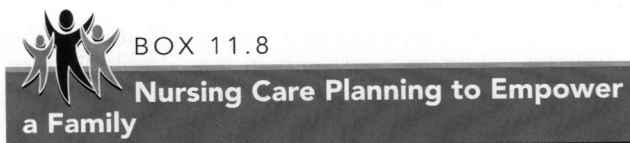

BOX 11.8

Nursing Care Planning to Empower a Family

ASSESSMENTS AND INTERVENTIONS A WOMAN CAN EXPECT AT CONTINUING PRENATAL VISITS

Health Interview

Interim history or new personal or family developments since last visit (every visit)
Review of danger signs of pregnancy (every visit)
Review of symptoms of beginning labor (every visit)
Any new concerns with pregnancy or family since last visit (every visit)

Physical Examination

Blood pressure (every visit)
Clean-catch urine for glucose, protein, and leukocytes (every visit)
Blood serum level for maternal serum α-fetoprotein (MSAFP) and pregnancy-associated plasma protein A (PAPP-A) (at 16 weeks)
VDRL test for syphilis if possibility of new exposure
Glucose screen (24–28 weeks)
Glucose challenge (24–28 weeks), if warranted
Anti-Rh titer (28 weeks)
Group B *Streptococcus* (GBS) screen (35–37 weeks)

Fetal Health

Fetal heart rate counted (every visit)
Fundal height measured (every visit)
Questions about quickening (first fetal movement, which occurs at 16–20 weeks) or continuing fetal movement (every visit)
Ultrasound dating of pregnancy (if necessary)
Ultrasound evaluation for fetal health (about 20 weeks)

What If . . . 11.4

The nurse is interested in exploring one of the 2020 National Health Goals related to prenatal care (see Box 11.1). Most government-sponsored money for nursing research is allotted based on these goals. What would be a possible research topic to explore pertinent to these goals that would be applicable to Sandra or her family and also advance evidence-based practice?

KEY POINTS FOR REVIEW

- The purpose of prenatal care is to establish a baseline of present health, determine the gestational age of the fetus, monitor fetal development, identify women at risk for complications, and minimize the risk of possible complications of pregnancy by anticipating and preventing problems before they occur as well as providing time for education about pregnancy and possible dangers. Planning nursing care that includes these things and not only meets QSEN competencies but also best meets the family's total needs.

- Prenatal care has the potential to reduce the incidence of preterm birth and the infant mortality rate.

- A first prenatal visit confirms a pregnancy, but it is also a time for important assessments such as a health history, physical examination, and laboratory tests. The physical examination includes measurement of fundal height and assessment of fetal heart sounds if the pregnancy is beyond 12 weeks, a pelvic examination (including a Pap smear and HPV test), and possibly an estimation of pelvic size.

- A first prenatal visit sets the tone for visits to follow. Maintaining a supportive manner is helpful to establish rapport and allow a woman to feel comfortable returning for future care.

- Common pelvic types include gynecoid (well-rounded with a wide pubic arch), anthropoid (narrow), platypelloid (flattened), and android (male or with a sharp pubic arch). A gynecoid pelvis is ideal for childbearing; however, vaginal birth is often achieved with other pelvis shapes.

- For a pelvic examination, pregnant women should remain in a lithotomy or supine position for as short a time as possible to help prevent thromboembolism and supine hypotension syndrome.

- Danger signs for women to report during pregnancy are vaginal bleeding, persistent vomiting, chills and fever, escape of fluid from the vagina, abdominal or chest pain, swelling of the face and fingers, shortness of breath not related to activity, vision changes or continuous headache, rhythmic cramping, burning with urination, and a pronounced decrease in fetal movement.

- Remember that a family, not a woman alone, is having a baby, and include family members in procedures and health teaching as desired.

CRITICAL THINKING CARE STUDY

Macie is a 40-year-old, G5 T3 P0 A1 L2 woman pregnant with her fifth child. She had a miscarriage with her second pregnancy, and her last child died at 3 months from sudden infant death syndrome (SIDS). Her other two children are healthy, ages 5 and 3 years. She has heard that using pacifiers and putting babies to sleep on their backs decreases the chance of SIDS and is worried she caused her baby girl's death.

1. Pregnancy creates a vulnerable period for Macie because she may be dealing with both losses from her previous pregnancies. What actions can you take to ensure that Macie will discuss openly her fears and concerns about this pregnancy?

2. Macie works as a cheerleading coach. Her husband works at adding insulation to homes. What special questions would you want to ask her about her job to see if it poses some concerns during pregnancy? About her husband's job?

3. How could grieving for the loss of her children affect Macie's adaptation to this pregnancy?

RELATED RESOURCES

Explore these additional resources to enhance learning for this chapter:
- Student resources on thePoint, including answers to the What If . . . and Critical Thinking Care Study questions, http://thepoint.lww.com/Flagg8e
- Adaptive learning powered by PrepU, http://thepoint.lww.com/prepu

REFERENCES

American Cancer Society. (2015). Breast cancer screening for women at average risk: 2015 Guideline update from the American cancer society. *JAMA, 314*(15), 1599–1614.

American Congress of Obstetricians and Gynecologists. (2015). *The Pap test: Committee opinion*. Washington, DC.

American Congress of Obstetricians and Gynecologists. (2016a). *Abnormal cervical cancer screening test results*. Washington DC: Author.

American Congress of Obstetricians and Gynecologists. (2016b). *Exercise and fitness*. Washington, DC: Author.

Barger, M., Faucher, M. A., & Murphy, P. A. (2015). Part II: The centering pregnancy model of group prenatal care. *Journal of Midwifery & Women's Health, 60*(2), 211–213.

Bienstock, J. L., Fox, H. E., & Wallach, E. E. (2015). *The Johns Hopkins manual of gynecology and obstetrics* (5th ed.). Philadelphia, PA: Lippincott Williams & Wilkins.

Centers for Disease Control and Prevention. (2016a). *HIV among pregnant women, infants and children*. Atlanta, GA: Author.

Centers for Disease Control and Prevention. (2016b). Human papillomavirus-associated cancers: United States, 2008–20012. *MMWR: Morbidity & Mortality Weekly Report, 65*(26), 661–666.

Centers for Disease Control and Prevention. (2016d). *Pregnancy mortality surveillance system*. Atlanta, GA: Author.

Charlton, B. M., Mølgaard-Nielsen, D., Svanström, H., et al. (2016). Maternal use of oral contraceptives and risk of birth defects in Denmark: Prospective, nationwide cohort study. *BMJ, 352*, h6712.

Choi, H., Van Riper, M., & Thoyre, S. (2012). Decision making following a prenatal diagnosis of Down syndrome: An integrative review. *Journal of Midwifery & Women's Health, 57*(2), 156–164.

Demont-Heinrich, C. M., Hawkes, A. P., Ghosh, T., et al. (2014). Risk of very low birth weight based on perinatal periods of risk. *Public Health Nursing, 31*(3), 234–242.

Ford, J. H. (2015). Data from the PALS (Pregnancy and Lifestyle Study), a community-based study of lifestyle on fertility and reproductive outcome. *Open Health Data, 3*(1), e2.

Gonçalves, L. F. (2016). Three-dimensional ultrasound: A role in early pregnancy? In J. S. Abramowics (Ed.), *First-trimester ultrasound* (pp. 213–221). New York, NY: Springer.

Haakstad, L. A., Torset, B., & Bø, K. (2016). What is the effect of regular group exercise on maternal psychological outcomes and common pregnancy complaints? An assessor blinded RCT. *Midwifery, 32,* 81–86.

Hughes, R. C., Moore, M. P., Gullam, J. E., et al. (2015). An early pregnancy HbA1c ≤5.9%(41 mmol/mol) is optimal for detecting diabetes and identifies women at increased risk of adverse pregnancy outcomes. *Obstetrical & Gynecological Survey, 70*(3), 151–153.

Hussein, N., Kai, J., & Qureshi, N. (2016). The effects of preconception interventions on improving reproductive health and pregnancy outcomes in primary care: A systematic review. *The European Journal of General Practice, 22*(1), 42–52.

Ickovics, J. R., Earnshaw, V., Lewis, J. B., et al. (2016). Cluster randomized controlled trial of group prenatal care: Perinatal outcomes among adolescents in New York City health centers. *American Journal of Public Health, 106*(2), 359–365.

James, L., Brody, D., & Hamilton, Z. (2013). Risk factors for domestic violence during pregnancy: A meta-analytic review. *Violence and Victims, 28*(3), 359–380.

James, S. H., & Kimberlin, D. W. (2015). Neonatal herpes simplex virus infection: Epidemiology and treatment. *Clinics in Perinatology, 42*(1), 47–59, viii.

Karch, A. M. (2013). *2013 Lippincott's nursing drug guide.* Philadelphia, PA: Lippincott Williams & Wilkins.

King, T. L., Brucker, M. C., Kriebs, J. M., et al. (2015). *Varney's midwifery.* Jones & Bartlett.

LaCourse, S. M., Greene, S. A., Dawson-Hahn, E. E., et al. (2016). Risk of adverse infant outcomes associated with maternal tuberculosis in a low burden setting: A population-based retrospective cohort study. *Infectious Diseases in Obstetrics and Gynecology, 2016,* 6413713.

Makadon, H. J., & Goldhammer, H. (2015). Taking a sexual history and creating affirming environments for lesbian, gay, bisexual, and transgender people. *Journal of the Mississippi State Medical Association, 56*(12), 358–362.

Marshall, H., McMillan, M., Andrews, R. M., et al. (2016). Vaccines in pregnancy: The dual benefit for pregnant women and infants. *Human Vaccines & Immunotherapeutics, 12*(4), 848–856.

McLean, H. Q., Fiebelkorn, A. P., Temte, J. L., et al. (2013). Prevention of measles, rubella, congenital rubella syndrome, and mumps, 2013: Summary recommendations of the advisory committee on immunization practices (ACIP). *Morbidity and Mortality Weekly Report, 62*(RR-04), 1–34.

Mehta, S. H., & Sokol, R. J. (2013). Assessment of at-risk pregnancy. In A. H. DeCherney, L. Nathan, N. Laufer, et al. (Eds.), *Current diagnosis and treatment: Obstetrics and gynecology* (11th ed., pp. 223–233). Columbus, OH: McGraw-Hill/Lange.

Meites, E., Gaydos, C. A., Hobbs, M. M., et al. (2015). A review of evidence-based care of symptomatic trichomoniasis and asymptomatic trichomonas vaginalis infections. *Clinical Infectious Diseases, 61*(Suppl. 8), S837–S848.

Nayar, R., & Wilbur, D. C. (2015). The Pap Test and Bethesda 2014. "The reports of my demise have been greatly exaggerated." (after a quotation from Mark Twain). *Acta Cytologica, 59,* 121–132.

O'Brien, B., Chalmers, B., Fell, D., et al. (2011). The experience of pregnancy and birth with midwives: Results from the Canadian maternity experiences survey. *Birth, 38*(3), 207–215.

Okeke, T. C., Enwereji, J. O., Onwuka, C. I., et al. (2015). A single institution study of attitudes of primigravidae to routine clinical pelvimetry. *British Journal of Medicine and Medical Research, 8*(11), 931–936.

Price, M. J., Ades, A. E., Soldan, K., et al. (2016). The natural history of Chlamydia trachomatis infection in women: A multi-parameter evidence synthesis. *Health Technology Assessment, 20*(22), 1–250.

Roozen, S., Peters, G. J., Kok, G., et al. (2016). Worldwide prevalence of fetal alcohol spectrum disorders: A systematic literature review including meta-analysis. *Alcoholism, Clinical and Experimental Research, 40*(1), 18–32.

Rouhe, H., Salmela-Aro, K., Toivanen, R., et al. (2015). Group psychoeducation with relaxation for severe fear of childbirth improves maternal adjustment and childbirth experience—a randomised controlled trial. *Journal of Psychosomatic Obstetrics and Gynaecology, 36*(1), 1–9.

Sandall, J., Soltani, H., Gates, S., et al. (2016). Midwife-led continuity models versus other models of care for childbearing women. *Cochrane Database of Systematic Reviews,* (4), CD004667.

Trotman, G., Chhatre, G., Darolia, R., et al. (2015). The effect of centering pregnancy versus traditional prenatal care models on improved adolescent health behaviors in the perinatal period. *Journal of Pediatric and Adolescent Gynecology, 28*(5), 395–401.

U.S. Department of Health and Human Services. (2010). *Healthy people 2020.* Washington, DC: Author.

Workowski, K. A., & Bolan, G. A. (2015). Sexually transmitted diseases treatment guidelines, 2015. *Morbidity and Mortality Weekly Report Recommendations and Reports, 64*(RR-03), 1–137.

12

Nursing Care to Promote Fetal and Maternal Health

*J*ulberry Adams, a single, 30-year-old woman, is 4 months pregnant when you first see her in a prenatal clinic. She works as a curator for an art gallery but has missed work this past week because of nausea. She is worried she will not be able to work past 6 months of her pregnancy because her job involves a great deal of walking. She has already stopped her volunteer work teaching children's swimming at the YMCA. She wants to travel to see her sister in St. Louis because her sister is very ill but has heard pregnant women should not drive more than 100 miles at a time. She asks you if marijuana would help reduce her early pregnancy nausea.

Previous chapters discussed normal reproductive anatomy and physiology and the changes that occur with pregnancy. This chapter adds information about the usual health teaching women need during pregnancy to ensure a healthy outcome for themselves and their child.

What additional health teaching does Ms. Adams need?

KEY TERMS

cytomegalovirus

fetal alcohol spectrum

herpes simplex virus (HSV)

leukorrhea

Sims position

teratogen

toxoplasmosis

OBJECTIVES

After mastering the contents of this chapter, you should be able to:

1. Describe common lifestyle behaviors important for a healthy pregnancy outcome.
2. Identify 2020 National Health Goals related to a healthy pregnancy lifestyle that nurses can help the nation achieve.
3. Assess a woman for minor discomforts of pregnancy and corresponding measures to counteract such discomforts as well as healthy lifestyle practices and concerns during pregnancy.
4. Formulate nursing diagnoses concerned with a healthy pregnancy.
5. Identify expected outcomes to promote a healthy pregnancy, such as limiting exposure to teratogens, as well as manage seamless transitions across differing healthcare settings.
6. Using the nursing process, plan nursing care that includes the six competencies of Quality & Safety Education for Nurses (QSEN): Patient-Centered Care, Teamwork & Collaboration, Evidence-Based Practice (EBP), Quality Improvement (QI), Safety, and Informatics.
7. Implement nursing care to promote healthy practices during pregnancy.
8. Evaluate outcomes for achievement and effectiveness of care.
9. Incorporate knowledge of a healthy lifestyle with the interplay of the nursing process, the six competencies of QSEN, and Family Nursing to promote quality maternal and child health nursing care.

The health of a fetus and the health of a mother are inextricably linked. Generally, a woman who eats well and takes care of her own health during pregnancy provides a healthy environment for fetal growth and development. However, a woman may need instructions on exactly what constitutes a healthy lifestyle during pregnancy. Most women have questions regarding how much extra rest they need, what type of exercise they can continue, and whether all the changes going on in their bodies, some of which bring them at least slight daily discomfort, are normal. Because of this, a major role in promoting maternal and fetal health is education about these subjects. Providing empathetic advice about ways to prevent or alleviate minor discomforts of pregnancy and keeping abreast of the latest evidence-based practice studies on maternal exposure to **teratogens** (factors detrimental to fetal health) are all part of this role. Because the health of women is so important to a nation, the United Nations (UN) lists "improve maternal health" and "reduce child mortality" as Millennium Global Health Goals (UN, 2015). Because effective prenatal care is such an important means to improve women's health, the 2020 National Health Goals speak to the importance of all pregnant women receiving counseling and prenatal care (Box 12.1).

BOX 12.1

Nursing Care Planning Based on 2020 National Health Goals

A number of 2020 National Health goals speak to the importance of women maintaining a healthy lifestyle during pregnancy:

- Increase the proportion of pregnant women who receive early and adequate prenatal care from a baseline of 70.5% to a target of 77.6%.
- Increase to 100% from a baseline of 94.9% the proportion of pregnant women who abstain from illicit drugs during pregnancy.
- Increase to 98.5% from a baseline of 89.6% the proportion of pregnant women who abstain from cigarette smoking during pregnancy.
- Increase to 95% from a baseline of 90% the proportion of pregnant women who abstain from alcohol during pregnancy.
- Increase to 100% from a baseline of 95% the proportion of pregnant women who abstain from binge drinking (i.e., drinking a large amount of alcohol over a short time with the primary intention of becoming intoxicated) during pregnancy (U.S. Department of Health and Human Services, 2010; see www.healthypeople.gov).

Because nurses are important members of prenatal healthcare teams, they play an important role in ensuring women are aware that preconception and early pregnancy care are important. Evidence-based practice and nursing research to answer such questions as to which aspects of preconception care are most important in reducing pregnancy complications and which are effective incentives to make women come in early for prenatal care would be important to help the nation meet these goals.

Nursing Process Overview

FOR HEALTH PROMOTION OF A FETUS AND MOTHER

ASSESSMENT

A thorough health history, physical evaluation, and initial laboratory data are obtained at a first prenatal visit. A continuing assessment concentrates on screening for any abnormalities in physical or emotional health that might be occurring and for the possibility of teratogens in the pregnant woman's environment. Encourage the woman to discuss whatever concerns she is having during all visits. Although some of these concerns may represent minor common body changes associated with a normal pregnancy, others may be early indicators of potential problems such as gestational hypertension or gestational diabetes. Knowing what is happening as soon as possible allows you to provide information and guidance on ways to alleviate any discomforts of pregnancy and also allows you to alert a woman's obstetric provider (nurse-midwife or obstetrician) of your findings as soon as they appear.

NURSING DIAGNOSIS

Examples of nursing diagnoses related to health promotion of the pregnant woman and fetus include:

- Health-seeking behaviors related to interest in maintaining optimal health during pregnancy
- Anxiety related to body changes of pregnancy
- Risk of deficient fluid volume related to gestational nausea and vomiting
- Disturbed body image related to changes in appearance with pregnancy
- Risk of altered sexual patterns related to fear of harming fetus during pregnancy
- Disturbed sleep pattern related to frequent need to empty bladder during night
- Risk for fetal injury related to intimate partner violence

OUTCOME IDENTIFICATION AND PLANNING

When establishing goals and outcomes, be certain that plans are individualized and realistic for a woman's situation and lifestyle. Try to turn long-term goals into more manageable, short-term ones if possible. For example, a goal of reducing smoking during pregnancy may be more realistic than a goal of stopping smoking forever. Eliminating the pressure of making a major permanent lifestyle change this way can help a woman concentrate her efforts on herself and her fetus over the next several months. Continued reinforcement of her progress could then help her to continue reducing the number of cigarettes smoked or to quit smoking altogether after the baby is born so she can provide a smoke-free environment for her child. Similarly, you cannot set a goal for a woman to be free of the nausea of early pregnancy. The best you can expect to accomplish is to be certain she maintains good nutrition and adequate weight gain in the face of it.

Often, helping a woman plan to avoid teratogens is difficult because a total change in lifestyle and environment, such as not smoking, not drinking alcohol, or changing a work environment, may be impossible. Fortunately, most women are highly motivated to complete a pregnancy satisfactorily. With this level of motivation, planning becomes the task of determining the best route to achieve a goal rather than educating about the need for goal achievement.

Be certain women do not consult online pregnancy forums where lay people are the main contributors as these may contain anecdotal information that is often misleading or incorrect. Refer women to helpful websites and other resources when appropriate (see Chapter 9).

IMPLEMENTATION

The major intervention associated with health promotion during pregnancy is education. Although the average woman is aware minor body changes will occur with pregnancy, these changes may seem extreme when they are happening to *her*. Often, adolescent girls are uninformed about common minor body changes during pregnancy because they lack a set of peers with pregnancy experience and so are surprised by them. Even an adolescent who knows it is normal for breast tenderness to occur during pregnancy may not be sure the amount she is feeling is normal. A woman who had a mental image of herself as someone who would not gain much weight during pregnancy may be very concerned because she is, in fact, gaining a great deal of weight. Education about minor body changes can switch this type of worry situation into a pleasant reminder that the pregnancy is progressing as expected.

OUTCOME EVALUATION

An evaluation is an ongoing process at prenatal healthcare visits. Expected outcomes developed with a woman at one prenatal visit need to be assessed at the next. Examples of expected outcomes include:

- Patient states measures she will use to manage increased discomfort from hemorrhoids formed during pregnancy.
- Patient reports she is resting for half an hour twice a day.
- Patient verbalizes positive statements about her appearance.
- Patient and her partner both state they have stopped smoking.
- Patient expresses positive feelings about the manner in which her prenatal care providers accommodated her cultural needs.
- Patient documents by use of a pedometer that she walks the length of a city block daily.

Health Promotion During Pregnancy

Women in prenatal care settings create an ideal teaching audience because the average woman is eager to learn more about her pregnancy and the steps she can take to maintain health during pregnancy. In addition to general health teaching, good role modeling, such as not smoking in prenatal settings and exhibiting a healthy lifestyle including sound nutrition and exercise, is important (Power, Wilson, Hogan, et al., 2013).

When planning teaching strategies, a woman's receptiveness to instruction is key. Regardless of how excited and pleased a woman is about being pregnant, she can assimilate only so much information at one time. It is important, therefore, to be selective about the health information you

BOX 12.2
Nursing Care Planning to Respect Cultural Diversity

What people do to keep well is culturally influenced. Some women, for example, may rely on herbs and folk remedies for minor discomforts of pregnancy; others feel a need to rely on only medical management.

Implementing prenatal care to meet the needs of all of the different cultures represented in the United States includes careful assessment to identify individual needs. It then may include providing special classes in prenatal health, exploring how health-promotion regimens fit with women's cultural belief systems, and maintaining an attitude of advocacy to help women adjust to a more formal healthcare system than they are used to.

provide and include those points most relevant to the individual woman. For example, you would want to discuss varicosity prevention more for a woman with a history of varicosities in a former pregnancy than for one who is pregnant for the first time and is athletic. Keep in mind that health measures taught must be maintained for an extended time—40 weeks. To help a woman follow changes for this long, choose individualized priorities, so health advice is specific and meaningful (Box 12.2).

Also remember the basic tenet of teaching and learning: Learning is enhanced when the information has direct and immediate application to that person. This principle means devising a plan that spaces out health-promotion and health-maintenance information into two sections. The first should include teaching those measures that are immediately applicable; the second should come later and include those measures that have relevance only toward the end of pregnancy.

Remind the woman at every visit to bring problems to her healthcare provider's attention as soon as she becomes worried; otherwise, a provider has no opportunity to take the necessary measures to prevent long-term discomfort or symptoms. For example, common minor body changes associated with early pregnancy are shown in Box 12.3. Many women, however, do not mention these discomforts or body changes unless specifically asked because they may not be aware of their significance to a pregnancy or because they are reluctant to take up a busy healthcare provider's time for little things. To illustrate, a woman experiencing constipation may not mention it early enough to take preventive measures against the occurrence of hemorrhoids, which can become a long-term problem not only throughout the pregnancy but afterward as well.

 Concept Mastery Alert

The technique of *anticipatory guidance* (i.e., psychologically preparing a person for an unfamiliar event) can be helpful in promoting fetal and maternal health. Knowing what to expect can help a patient prepare for what is ahead and lead to more effective coping and better health.

BOX 12.3

Nursing Care Planning Using Assessment

ASSESSING A WOMAN FOR MINOR BODY CHANGES OF PREGNANCY

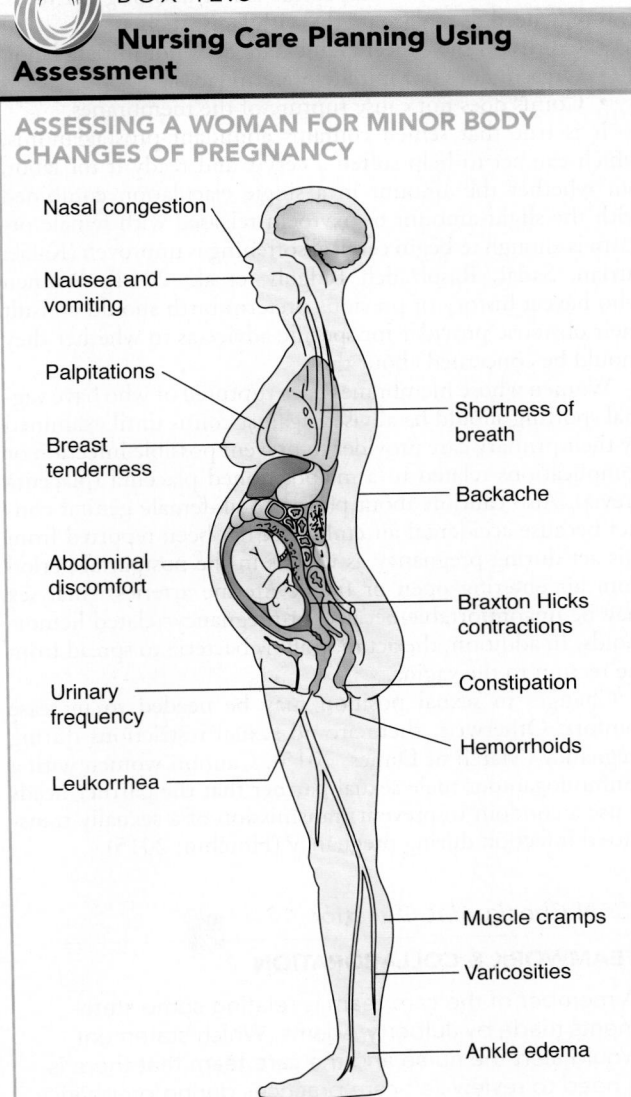

- Nasal congestion
- Nausea and vomiting
- Palpitations
- Breast tenderness
- Abdominal discomfort
- Urinary frequency
- Leukorrhea
- Shortness of breath
- Backache
- Braxton Hicks contractions
- Constipation
- Hemorrhoids
- Muscle cramps
- Varicosities
- Ankle edema

SELF-CARE NEEDS

Because pregnancy is a state of wellness, few special care measures or advice other than common sense measures about self-care are needed. Many women, however, have heard different warnings about what they should or should not do during pregnancy, which may mean that they need some help separating fact from fiction. Doing so may enable the woman to enjoy her pregnancy unhampered by unnecessary restrictions. In no other area of nursing, except possibly infant feeding, does there seem to be as many misconceptions or inappropriate information available to women.

Bathing

During pregnancy, sweating tends to increase because a woman excretes waste products for both herself and the fetus. She also has an increase in vaginal discharge. For these reasons, daily tub baths or showers are recommended. Women should

not soak for long periods in extremely hot water or in hot tubs, however, as heat exposure for a lengthy time could lead to hyperthermia in the fetus and birth defects, specifically esophageal atresia, omphalocele, and gastroschisis (Wilde, Petersen, & Niswander, 2014).

As pregnancy advances, a woman may have difficulty maintaining her balance when getting in and out of a bathtub. If so, she should change to showering or sponge bathing for her own safety. If membranes rupture or vaginal bleeding is present, tub baths become contraindicated because there might be a danger of developing a uterine infection.

Breast Care

Women need to make few changes related to breast care during pregnancy. A general rule is: as her breast size increases, a woman should be certain to wear a firm, supportive bra with wide straps to spread breast weight across the shoulders. Interestingly, evidence shows that a woman's breasts enlarge more if the fetus she carries is male than if the fetus is female (Żelaźniewicz & Pawłowski, 2015). Regardless of fetal sex, women may need to buy a larger bra size halfway through pregnancy to accommodate breast changes. Assuming a woman plans on breastfeeding, recommend she choose bras suitable for this (open in the front), so she can continue to use them after the baby's birth.

At about the 16th week of pregnancy, colostrum secretion begins in the breasts. The sensation of a fluid discharge from the breasts can be frightening unless a woman has been cautioned of this possibility. Teach her to wash her breasts with clear tap water (no soap, because that could be drying and cause her nipples to crack) daily to remove the colostrum and reduce the risk of infection. After washing, she should dry her nipples well by patting them with a soft towel.

If colostrum secretion is profuse, a woman may need to place gauze squares or breast pads inside her bra, changing them frequently to maintain dryness. Otherwise, constant moisture next to the breast nipples can cause nipple excoriation, pain, and fissuring. Asking about colostrum at prenatal visits provides a good time to also discuss the benefits of breastfeeding for both a woman and her child (see Chapter 19).

Dental Care

There is a strong correlation between poor oral health and preterm birth, so maintaining good oral health during pregnancy is important (Gupta, Jain, Mohan, et al., 2015). Without adequate brushing, gingival tissue tends to hypertrophy and, unless a pregnant woman brushes her teeth well, pockets of plaque form readily between the swollen gum line and teeth, possibly leading to periodontal diseases (Papapanou, 2015).

When bacteria in the mouth interact with sugar, this lowers the pH of the mouth, creating an acid medium that can lead to etching or destruction of the enamel of teeth (i.e., tooth decay). Because 9 months is a fairly long time to be without preventive dental care, in addition to stressing brushing on arising, after meals, and at bedtime, encourage pregnant women to see their dentists regularly for routine examination and cleaning. Encourage women to snack on nutritious foods, such as fresh fruits and vegetables rather than sugar-rich snacks to reduce the amount of sugar in contact with their teeth. If a woman has trouble avoiding sweet snacks such as candy, suggest eating snacks that dissolve easily (like a chocolate bar) rather than one that remains in the mouth a long time (like chewy caramel). This helps to minimize the level of sugar in the mouth and its long-term contact with teeth.

Women should question the need for X-rays during pregnancy; however, if these are necessary for dental health, they can be done safely as long as a woman's abdomen is shielded with a lead apron.

Perineal Hygiene

Women have increased vaginal discharge during pregnancy and so need to maintain good perineal hygiene. Caution them to always wipe front to back after voiding to prevent bringing contamination forward from the rectum. Even if the vaginal discharge seems excessive, douching is contraindicated because the force of the irrigating fluid could cause the solution to enter the cervix, leading to a uterine infection. In addition, douching alters the pH of the vagina, leading to an increased risk of vaginal bacterial growth (Sheth & Keller, 2015).

Clothing

Maternity clothing should be comfortable. Women should be cautioned to avoid garters, extremely firm girdles with panty legs, and knee-high stockings during pregnancy because these may impede lower extremity circulation. Suggest wearing shoes with a moderate-to-low heel to minimize pelvic tilt and possible backache as well as to reduce the risk of falling.

SEXUAL ACTIVITY

Sexual changes occur during pregnancy. Many of these changes were reviewed in Chapter 5.

Asking a woman at a prenatal visit if she has any questions about sexual activity allows her to voice concerns about coitus (Box 12.4). This conversation allows a woman to feel more

comfortable and secure that coitus is not harming her fetus. You may need to replace myths with facts, such as:
- Coitus on the expected due date does not initiate labor.
- Orgasm does not initiate preterm labor.
- Coitus does not cause rupture of the membranes.

It is true that semen contains abundant prostaglandins, which can act to help soften a cervix and ready it for labor, but whether the amount in a single ejaculation combined with the slight amount of oxytocin released with female orgasm is enough to begin cervical softening is unproven (Kafaei Atrian, Sadat, Rasolzadeh Bidgoly, et al., 2014). Women who have a history of previous preterm birth should consult their obstetric provider for specific advice as to whether they should be concerned about this.

Women whose membranes have ruptured or who have vaginal spotting should be advised against coitus until examined by their primary care provider to prevent possible infection or complications related to a malpositioned placenta (placenta previa). Also caution about partner oral–female genital contact because accidental air embolism has been reported from this act during pregnancy as well as in the postpartal period from air entering open or fragile uterine arteries. Anal sex may be uncomfortable because of pregnancy-related hemorrhoids. In addition, the act may allow bacteria to spread from the rectum to the vagina.

Changes in sexual position may be needed to increase comfort. Otherwise, there are no sexual restrictions during pregnancy (March of Dimes, 2015). Caution women with a nonmonogamous male sexual partner that the partner needs to use a condom to prevent transmission of a sexually transmitted infection during pregnancy (Hotchin, 2015).

QSEN Checkpoint Question 12.1

TEAMWORK & COLLABORATION

A member of the care team is relating some statements made by Julberry Adams. Which statement would alert the nurse and the care team that there is a need to review self-care practices during pregnancy with the patient?
- a. "I take either a shower or tub bath because I know both are safe."
- b. "I wash my breasts with clear water, not with soap, every day."
- c. "I know if my partner uses a condom it can tear fetal membranes."
- d. "I'm wearing low-heeled shoes to try to avoid backache."

Look in Appendix A for the best answer and rationale.

EXERCISE

Extreme exercise in women has been associated with difficulty conceiving but after pregnancy occurs, moderate exercise is healthy (Wahlqvist, Krawetz, Rizzo, et al., 2015). During pregnancy, exercise can offer a general sense of well-being. It also helps prevent circulatory stasis in the lower extremities. For some women, teaching about exercise focuses on both helping them realize the need for exercise and urging them to get enough. Others may need to be cautioned to restrict

---

> 💬 BOX 12.4
> ### Nursing Care Planning Tips for Effective Communication
>
> Julberry Adams is 4 months pregnant and no longer lives with the father of her baby.
>
> *Tip:* Health teaching is an art separate from teaching morality. Avoid cutting off communication by making a judgment about the information a patient might need. Actively listen to your patient, focus on the patient's needs and concerns, and supply the information the patient has requested.
>
> **Nurse:** Do you have any questions, Ms. Adams?
>
> **Julberry:** How long into pregnancy can I have sex?
>
> **Nurse:** Basically, as long as you're comfortable and you don't have any complications.
>
> **Julberry:** Good. My new boyfriend made me promise to ask today.
>
> **Nurse:** Since you mentioned a new partner, let's review STI testing and condom use during pregnancy. Do you have any other questions about sex during pregnancy that you or your partner were wondering about?

exercise, such as for those who participate in contact sports like touch football or unrefereed soccer.

As a rule, average, well-nourished women should exercise during pregnancy about three times weekly for 30 consecutive minutes (Fletcher & Russo, 2015). Their exercise program should consist of 5 minutes of warm-up exercises, an active "stimulus" phase of 20 minutes, and then 5 minutes of cool-down exercises. Movements that exercise large muscle groups rhythmically, such as walking, are best but the type of activity chosen should depend on their interests. Advise women to eat a protein and a complex carbohydrate such as peanut butter and whole wheat bread at least 15 minutes before exercise to keep blood sugar from falling during exercise and to drink water before and after to prevent dehydration.

As a rule, a woman can continue any sport she participated in before pregnancy unless it was one that involved body contact, such as soccer. If a woman is a competent horsewoman, for example, there is little reason for her to discontinue riding until it becomes uncomfortable. Pregnancy is not the time to learn to ride, however, because a beginning rider is at greater risk for being thrown than an experienced one. The same principle applies to skiing and bicycling. An accomplished skier or bicyclist may continue the activity in moderation until balance becomes a problem. Pregnancy is not the time to learn to ski or ride a bicycle, however, because the lack of skill could result in many falls.

The intensity of the exercise program depends on cardiopulmonary fitness. Both pregnant and nonpregnant women should exercise at 70% to 85% of their maximum heart rate. The easiest way to calculate this is for women to subtract their age from 220 and then calculate 70% or 85% of that number. For example, after exercise, a 23-year-old woman should have a pulse range of 137 to 167 beats/min ($220 - 23$ [$= 197$] $\times$ 70% [$= 137.90$] or 85% [$= 167.4$]). For a woman of 35 years, this target range would be 129 to 157 beats/min. An additional way for women to assess if they are exercising too strenuously is to evaluate their ability to continue talking while exercising. If a woman is too short of breath to do this, she is exercising beyond her target heart rate.

Because walking is the best exercise during pregnancy, women should be encouraged to take a walk daily unless inclement weather, many levels of stairs, or an unsafe neighborhood are contraindications. Yoga is also a good exercise as long as positions are limited to those in which pregnant women are able to maintain balance (Polis, Gussman, & Kuo, 2015). Jogging, in contrast, is questioned because of the strain the extra weight of pregnancy places on the knees. Late in pregnancy, jogging can also cause pelvic pain from relaxed symphysis pubis movement.

Swimming is a good activity for pregnant women and, like bathing, is not contraindicated as long as membranes are intact. It not only increases muscle tone but may help relieve backache. Diving, long-distance swimming, or any other activity carried out to a point of extreme fatigue should be avoided. A moderate-impact aerobics program such as dancing is well tolerated during pregnancy, but a high-impact aerobics program is usually contraindicated because it can be strenuous on both pelvic and knee joints (Erdener & Budgett, 2016).

An epidemiologic study suggests an elevation of maternal body temperature by 2°C for at least 24 hours can cause a range of fetal defects, but there is little information on thresholds for shorter exposures such as occur with exercise. Use of hot tubs and saunas after workouts, similar to a hot bath, should be limited to no longer than 15 minutes, again on the chance these can lead to hyperthermia in the fetus and birth defects, specifically esophageal atresia, omphalocele, and gastroschisis (Agopian, Tinker, Lupo, et al., 2014).

General guidelines for exercise during pregnancy are highlighted in Box 12.5. Beginning an exercise program during pregnancy not only offers the advantage of being healthy during pregnancy but also provides long-term benefits such as:
- Lowering cholesterol levels
- Reducing the risk of osteoporosis
- Increasing energy levels
- Maintaining a healthy body weight
- Decreasing the risk of heart disease
- Increasing self-esteem and well-being

Women who know they have an incompetent cervix or have had cerclage to correct this and women who develop any complication of pregnancy such as bleeding, gestational hypertension, preterm rupture of membranes, preterm labor, or whose fetus is growth restricted should consult with their obstetric provider before beginning or continuing an exercise program.

SLEEP

The optimal condition for body growth occurs when growth hormone secretion is at its highest level—that is, during sleep. This, plus the overall increased metabolic demand of pregnancy, appears to be the physiologic reason pregnant women require an increased amount of sleep or at least need rest to build new body cells during pregnancy.

Pregnant women rarely have difficulty falling asleep at night because of this increased physiologic need for sleep. If a woman does have trouble falling asleep, drinking a glass of warm milk may help. Relaxation exercises (e.g., lying quietly, systematically relaxing neck muscles, shoulder muscles, arm muscles) also may be effective.

A good resting or sleeping position is a left-sided **Sims position**, with the top leg forward (Fig. 12.1). This position puts the weight of the fetus on the bed, not on the woman, and allows good circulation in lower extremities.

Be certain a woman knows to avoid resting flat on her back because supine hypotension syndrome (i.e., faintness, diaphoresis, and hypotension from the pressure of the expanding uterus on the inferior vena cava) can develop in this position. If needed, placing a rolled pillow behind her can act as a reminder not to turn onto her back. Also, be certain women know not to rest with their knees sharply bent either when sitting or lying down because of the increased risk of venous stasis that this causes below the knee.

Sleep deprivation during pregnancy is associated not only with fatigue in the woman but also with the possibility of growth restriction in her fetus (Tsai, Lin, Wu, et al., 2016). To obtain enough sleep and rest during pregnancy, pregnant women may need to begin sleep earlier in the evening as well as schedule a rest period during the afternoon (Maness & Khan, 2015).

Late in pregnancy, a woman often finds herself awakened from sleep at short, frequent intervals by the activity of her fetus. Pregnant women also have a higher incidence

BOX 12.5

Nursing Care Planning Based on Family Teaching

GUIDELINES FOR EXERCISE IN PREGNANCY

Q. Julberry Adams asks you, "How much should I be exercising now that I'm pregnant?"

A. New and intense exercise should never be started for the first time during pregnancy. Use the following recommendations as guidelines for safe exercise:

1. Perform scheduled exercise periods (about three times per week for 30 minutes) rather than engaging in intermittent activity.
2. Do not perform vigorous exercise in hot, humid weather or if you have a fever to avoid overexerting yourself or developing hyperthermia.
3. Avoid activities that require jumping, jarring motions, or rapid changes in direction such as jogging because your joints may be unstable late in pregnancy.
4. Exercise on a wooden floor or a tightly carpeted surface to reduce shock to the abdomen or knees and to provide a sure footing.
5. To avoid muscle cramping, avoid exercises and motions that involve deep flexion or joint extension, such as stretching with the toes extended.
6. Always start your exercise program by warming up for approximately 5 minutes with activities such as slow walking or stationary cycling with low resistance.
7. End your exercise program with a period of gradually declining activity that includes gentle, stationary stretching. Because of the increased risk of joint injury, do not stretch to the point of maximum resistance.
8. Measure your heart rate at times of peak activity. Talk with your obstetric provider about target heart rate and limits and don't exceed them.
9. When getting up from lying on the floor, do so gradually to prevent dramatic blood pressure changes or stretching of the round ligament, which can lead to sharp abdominal pain.
10. Drink liquids liberally before and after exercise to prevent dehydration. If necessary, interrupt your activity to replenish fluids.
11. Eat a protein and complex carbohydrate snack before exercise to help maintain serum glucose levels.
12. If you were sedentary before pregnancy, begin your exercise program with physical activity of very low intensity and advance your activity level gradually.
13. Stop any activity and contact your obstetric provider if any unusual symptoms appear such as dizziness or vaginal bleeding.
14. Perform strenuous activities for no longer than 20 minutes.
15. To prevent supine hypotension syndrome do not exercise in the supine position (lying flat on your back) after the fourth month of pregnancy.
16. Avoid exercises that employ a Valsalva maneuver (holding your breath while bearing down) because this action increases blood pressure and decreases blood supply to the fetus.
17. Make sure your caloric intake is adequate to meet not only the extra energy needs of pregnancy but also those of the exercise performed.

---

of "restless leg syndrome" (waking at night because of spontaneous leg movement) than nonpregnant women. Pramipexole dihydrochloride (Mirapex), a class C drug frequently recommended for restless leg syndrome, should not be taken during pregnancy (Schneider, Krafft, Manconi, et al., 2015).

Frequent waking such as this can lead to loss of rapid eye movement (REM) sleep. Loss of REM sleep causes a

woman to feel anxious and not well rested, even though she has slept her usual number of hours. Pyrosis (heartburn), dyspnea (shortness of breath), snoring, or sleep apnea (particularly in obese women) also can cause a woman to wake up, especially if she has been lying flat. Recommend sleeping with two or three pillows or on a couch with an armrest in these instances.

EMPLOYMENT

Changes in public assistance laws that encourage women to seek employment have led to more women working during pregnancy than ever before. Unless a woman's job involves exposure to toxic substances, lifting heavy objects, other kinds of excessive physical strain, long periods of standing or sitting, or having to maintain body balance, there are few reasons a woman cannot continue to work throughout pregnancy. Women may, however, experience some discrimination from fellow workers (Lee, Symanski, Lupo, et al., 2016).

Figure 12.1 A modified Sims position is a good rest position during pregnancy. Notice the weight of the fetus rests on the bed.

Women who are unable to continue working are protected from loss of employment benefits during pregnancy by federal law (Public Law 95-555) unless they work for a company with fewer than 15 employees.

According to federal law, an employer cannot:

- Deprive women of seniority rights, in pay or promotion, because they take a maternity leave
- Treat women returning from maternity leave as new hires, starting over on the eligibility period for pension and other benefits
- Force pregnant women to leave their job if they are able to and want to continue working
- Refuse to hire women just because they are pregnant or fire them for the same reason
- Refuse to cover employees' normal pregnancy and birth expenses in the company health plan or pay less for pregnancy than for other medical conditions
- Refuse to pay sick leave or disability benefits to women whose difficult pregnancies keep them off the job

Passed in 1993, the Family and Medical Leave Act is another federal law that guarantees women the right to 12 weeks of unpaid, job-protected leave on the birth of a child; the adoption or foster placement of a child; when a woman is needed to care for a parent, spouse, or child with a serious health condition; or because of a serious health condition from which she suffers (29 C.F.R. 825.11). Specifically mentioned in this law is any period of incapacity because of pregnancy or for prenatal care. Families need to be educated about this important law because many women are still not aware they can take time off from work during pregnancy or spend time with a new baby. In addition, women may be able to qualify for provisions under the Americans with Disabilities Act (ADA) if their reason for quitting work is because of a physical or mental impairment that substantially limits one or more major life activities (ADA Amendments Act, 2008).

Some occupations are hazardous during pregnancy and should be discontinued because they bring women into contact with harmful substances. For example, nurses working with anesthetic gases in operating rooms or dental offices are reported to have a higher incidence of spontaneous miscarriage and, possibly, congenital anomalies in children than nurses working in other locales, probably because of exposure to nitrous oxide (National Institute for Occupational Safety and Health [NIOSH], 2010). Nurses working with chemotherapy agents may also be at risk and so should wear gloves to protect themselves from exposure to these drugs. Ribavirin (Virazole), an antiviral formerly used to treat respiratory syncytial virus (RSV) infections, is also apparently teratogenic. It is administered by inhalation to individuals with RSV in hematopoietic cell or heart and lung transplant recipients or orally to chronic hepatitis C patients. Both male and females trying to conceive and women who are pregnant should avoid inhaling the drug (Karch, 2015).

Other problems that can occur with employment include interference with adequate rest and nutrition. Urge a woman who works outside her home to put her feet up and rest when performing tasks that can be done in that position. Review what she eats at fast-food restaurants or packs for herself to be certain she plans ways to make lunch as nutritious as if she were eating at home.

Most women work to augment or supply family income, not for fun. Even those who could afford to leave their jobs may not be willing to sacrifice the collegial relationships and sense of fulfillment derived from work, or the lifestyle their income allows them to enjoy. Counseling them to reserve periods during the day for rest and to eat a healthy diet is more effective than suggesting they resign from their jobs during pregnancy to get more rest (Box 12.6).

 BOX 12.6

Nursing Care Planning to Empower a Family

GUIDELINES FOR PREGNANT WOMEN WORKING OUTSIDE THEIR HOME

Q. Julberry Adams asks you, "Now that I'm pregnant, can I continue to work at the art gallery?"

A. Use the following suggestions as guidelines for safe work practices during pregnancy:

- Plan rest periods during your break periods rather than running errands, etc.
- Try to use at least part of your lunch hour to rest. Lie on your left side in a break room if possible. If this is not possible, then rest sitting with your legs elevated.
- If your job involves long periods of standing, think of times you could sit and elevate your legs (working in a low file drawer, reading time in a classroom, etc.).
- Walk around periodically to avoid prolonged standing or sitting in one position if possible; stretch your back periodically to avoid backache.
- Wear support hose to improve venous return to your lower extremities.
- Avoid excessive overtime or working longer than 8-hour shifts.
- Empty your bladder every 2 hours to help prevent urinary tract infection.
- Get extra rest on weekends or days off.
- Take great caution when working around equipment that requires good balance. Avoid ladders late in pregnancy, when balance can be a problem.
- Learn your target heart rate for exercise. If your job involves strenuous exercise, stop and rest at the point your target heart rate is exceeded.
- Be certain you are not relying on fast foods for lunch. Take time to pack or purchase nutritious foods.

QSEN Checkpoint Question 12.2

QUALITY IMPROVEMENT

The nurse is reviewing an educational pamphlet that has been frequently provided to pregnant women. What statement from the pamphlet suggests that revision is necessary?

a. "You may want to jog rather than walk to get an increased amount of exercise."

b. "Be certain to rest or sleep on your side, not flat on your back."

c. "Plan to pack a lunch every day so that you won't eat junk food."

d. "Try to walk around your desk every hour to help leg circulation."

Look in Appendix A for the best answer and rationale.

TRAVEL

Because we live in such a mobile society, many women have questions about travel during pregnancy. Early in a normal pregnancy, there are no restrictions unless the woman needs to travel to a malaria-prone, Zika virus, or other at-risk region (where she would need vaccine protection). If a woman is susceptible to motion sickness, advise her not to take any medication for this unless it is specifically prescribed or approved by her primary care provider. Suggest she use a "sea-sick" wrist or acupuncture band for this instead. Late in pregnancy, travel plans should take into consideration the possibility of early labor, requiring birth at a strange setting where a woman's obstetric history will be unknown.

Regardless of the month of her pregnancy, if a woman plans to spend time at a remote location, such as could happen to a migrant worker, or a woman taking a family vacation at a campsite, be certain she has investigated the location of a nearby healthcare facility should an unexpected complication occur (van den Akker & van Roosmalen, 2016). Caution her not to eat unwashed fruits or vegetables or raw meats and not to drink unpurified water. If she is going to be away from home for an extended time, she should make arrangements to visit a healthcare provider in that area so she can keep the schedule of her regular prenatal visits. Encourage her to make these plans far enough in advance so her records can be copied and carried by her or, with her consent, an electronic record can be forwarded to the interim healthcare provider. Also, make certain she has enough of her prescribed vitamin supplement plus adequate prescriptions for refills as necessary.

Advise a woman who is taking a long trip by automobile to plan for frequent rest or stretch periods. Preferably every hour, but at least every 2 hours, she should get out of the car and walk a short distance. This break relieves stiffness and muscle aches and improves lower extremity circulation, helping prevent varicosities, hemorrhoids, and thrombophlebitis.

Pregnant women may drive automobiles as long as they fit comfortably behind the steering wheel. They should use seat belts like everyone else. Occasionally, uterine rupture has been reported from seat belt use, but overall evidence confirms seat belts reduce mortality among pregnant women in car accidents, as they do for everyone (Fletcher & Russo, 2015). Both shoulder harnesses and lap belts should be used. The lap belt should be worn as snugly as comfortable so that it fits under the abdominal bulge and across the pelvic bones.

Figure 12.2 Encourage women to wear seat belts during pregnancy. The bottom strap should cross beneath the abdomen.

The shoulder harness should be snug but comfortable, worn across the shoulder, chest, and upper abdomen. A pad may be placed under the shoulder harness at the neck to avoid chafing (Fig. 12.2).

Pregnancy is also a time for the family to think about transportation safety for the newborn. Purchasing a car seat is an investment that not only is legally required for transporting infants but also helps guarantee their safety. Families who cannot afford to purchase an infant car seat may want to ask friends or relatives about the possibility of borrowing one they may no longer need. Many hospitals and local Red Cross chapters provide infant seats on a rental or loan basis for families who may find it difficult to obtain one in other ways. An easy way to determine if a used car seat is up-to-date is to check the website http://www.safercar.gov/parents/CarSeats/Car-Seat-Safety.htm.

Traveling by plane for women is not contraindicated during pregnancy as long as the plane has a well-pressurized cabin (which is true of commercial airlines but not of all small private planes), the woman is offered an extension seat belt as needed, and the woman is not required to sit in one position for a long time (Tucker, 2014).

Some airlines do not permit women who are more than 7 months pregnant to board; others require written permission from her provider. Advise a woman to investigate these restrictions by calling the airline or a travel agency before making such travel plans.

With businesses becoming global, more women than ever before are asked to travel internationally. Women who travel abroad may need additional safety measures such as a vaccine for protection against cholera or antibiotic prophylaxis for malaria before they can safely enter certain countries (Tucker, 2014). The influenza vaccine is recommended if it is flu season (October through May) for all pregnant women (Sukumaran, McCarthy, Kharbanda, et al., 2015).

Before accepting or allowing any immunization, however, a woman should ask her provider to verify it will be safe. All live virus vaccines (e.g., measles, mumps, rubella, and yellow fever) are contraindicated during pregnancy and should not be administered unless the risk of the disease outweighs the risk to the pregnancy because live virus vaccines can cross the placenta and infect the fetus. Pregnancy does not alter indications for rabies vaccine because without the vaccine, a fatal disease could occur. Tetanus is also treated the same in pregnant women as in others.

What If . . . 12.1

Julberry Adams tells the nurse she usually drives to her parents' home for vacation but can't this year because she no longer fits behind the wheel of her compact car. She asks the nurse if it would be better for her to take the train or fly. How would the nurse best respond?

MINOR BODY CHANGES OF PREGNANCY: THE FIRST TRIMESTER

Although most women are pleased to discover they are pregnant, for some women, the symptoms of early pregnancy cause much discomfort. Providing empathetic and sound advice about ways to relieve discomfort helps promote overall health and well-being. Although these early symptoms are classified as minor, they may not seem minor to a woman who wakes each morning feeling so nauseated she wonders if she will ever feel like herself again. Each of these symptoms has the potential to lead to secondary problems that could be serious, so signs and symptoms need to be identified as they occur.

Nursing Diagnoses and Related Interventions

Nursing Diagnosis: Health-seeking behaviors related to learning more about minor body changes of early pregnancy, such as morning nausea

Outcome Evaluation: Patient states she is familiar with early body changes of pregnancy and will take measures to relieve them.

Because each woman's experience is unique, nursing diagnoses and care must be developed according to each woman's individual needs. Additional nursing diagnoses that might be developed for women experiencing the minor body changes of early pregnancy include:

- Health-seeking behaviors related to interest in using herbal remedies to relieve discomfort early in pregnancy
- Constipation related to reduced peristalsis in pregnancy
- Fatigue related to increased physiologic need for sleep and rest during pregnancy
- Acute pain related to frequent muscle cramps secondary to physiologic changes of pregnancy
- Disturbed sleep pattern related to frequent movement of fetus during night

Breast Tenderness

Breast tenderness is often one of the first symptoms noticed in early pregnancy and may be most noticeable on exposure to cold air. For most women, the tenderness is minimal and transient, something they are aware of but not something that overly concerns them. If the tenderness is enough to cause discomfort, encourage a woman to wear a bra with a wide shoulder strap for support and to dress warmly to avoid cold drafts if cold increases symptoms. If actual pain exists, the presence of conditions such as nipple fissures or other explanations for the pain, such as breast abscess, need to be ruled out.

Palmar Erythema

Palmar erythema, or palmar pruritus, occurs in early pregnancy and is probably caused by increased estrogen levels. Constant redness or itching of the palms can make a woman believe she has developed an allergy. Explain that this type of itching in early pregnancy is normal to prevent a woman from spending time and effort trying different soaps or detergents or attempting to implicate certain foods she has eaten as the cause of her discomfort. She may find calamine lotion to be soothing. As soon as a woman's body adjusts to the increased level of estrogen, the erythema and pruritus disappear (Coad & Dunstall, 2011).

Nausea, Vomiting, Constipation, and Pyrosis

At least half of pregnant women experience gastrointestinal symptoms such as nausea, vomiting, constipation, and pyrosis. Because these symptoms are related to nutrition, they are discussed in Chapter 13.

Fatigue

Fatigue is extremely common in early pregnancy, probably because of increased metabolic requirements (Haakstad, Torset, & Bø, 2016). Much of it can be relieved by increasing the amount of rest and sleep. Some women, however, are reluctant to take time out of their day to do this. They know pregnancy is not an illness and so they proceed as if nothing is happening to them. Rarely is there justification during a normal pregnancy for women to take extra days off from work because of their condition, but it is also unrealistic to proceed as if nothing is happening. Fatigue can increase the amount of morning nausea a woman experiences. If she becomes too tired, she may not eat properly and nutrition can suffer. If she remains on her feet without at least one break during a day, the risk for varicosities and the danger of thromboembolic complications increase.

For all these reasons, ask women at prenatal visits whether they manage to have at least one short rest period every day. A woman who works outside her home at a job that requires her to be on her feet most of the day might use part of her lunch hour to sit with her feet elevated (Fig. 12.3). After she returns home from work in the evening, she may need to modify her customary routine from typical activities such as cooking dinner or watching a child's soccer game to resting, then cooking dinner or going to the soccer game, or resting while her partner cooks dinner.

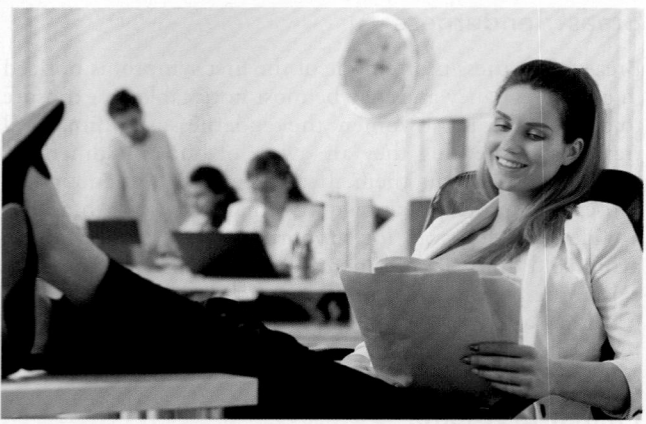

Figure 12.3 A "feet-up" break during a workday helps prevent ankle edema. (Photographee.eu/Shutterstock.com)

Figure 12.4 Relieving a leg cramp in pregnancy. Pressing down on the knee and pressing the toes backward (dorsiflexion) relieves most cramps. Here, a woman's partner helps.

QSEN Checkpoint Question 12.3 ✓

EVIDENCE-BASED PRACTICE

Almost all women experience a number of minor discomforts during pregnancy. To investigate whether these symptoms are serious enough to lead to depression, researchers scored 1,507 Australian women during their first pregnancy on a depression inventory questionnaire. The women were also asked what minor body changes they were experiencing. The most frequent body changes reported were exhaustion (86.9%), morning nausea (64.3%), back pain (45.6%), constipation (43.5%), and severe headache or migraine (29.5%). Women who reported five or more physical health problems were 3 times more likely to also report depressive symptoms (Perlen, Woolhouse, Gartland, et al., 2013).

Based on the previous study, which statement by Julberry would give the nurse the most concern that she should be assessed at her next prenatal visit as to whether she could be depressed?

a. "I wake up every morning with backache. Do I need a new mattress?"
b. "I like the job I do, although I come home exhausted almost every day."
c. "Between the headache, the backache, and the nausea, pregnancy isn't fun."
d. "The amount of constipation I have is a surprise; I don't usually get that."

Look in Appendix A for the best answer and rationale.

Muscle Cramps

Decreased serum calcium levels, increased serum phosphorus levels, and, possibly, interference with circulation commonly cause muscle cramps of the lower extremities during pregnancy. This problem is best relieved if a woman lies on her back momentarily and extends the involved leg while keeping her knee straight and dorsiflexing the foot until the pain disappears (Fig. 12.4).

Taking a calcium supplement, which would lower the phosphorus level, may be helpful. If a woman is experiencing frequent leg cramps, she may be advised to take magne-

sium lactate or citrate once in the morning and again in the evening as these bind phosphorus in the intestinal tract and thereby lower its circulating level; however, there is a lack of strong evidence that this decreases the frequency or intensity of leg cramps (Zhou, West, Zhang, et al., 2015). Elevating lower extremities frequently during the day to improve circulation and avoiding full leg extension, such as stretching with the toes pointed, may also be helpful. Typically, muscle cramps are a minor symptom of pregnancy, but the pain is extreme and the intensity of the contraction can be frightening. Always ask at prenatal visits if this is a problem. Otherwise, women may not realize cramping is pregnancy related and so fail to report it.

Hypotension

Supine hypotension is a symptom that occurs when a woman lies on her back and the uterus presses on the inferior vena cava, impairing blood return to her heart (Wang, Xu, Zhou, et al., 2015). A woman experiences an irregular heart rate and a feeling of apprehension. Relieving the problem is simple: If a woman turns or is turned onto her side, pressure is removed from the inferior vena cava, blood flow is restored, and the symptoms quickly fade. To prevent the syndrome, advise pregnant women to always rest or sleep on their side, not their back. If they can only fall asleep on their back, they should insert a small firm pillow under their right hip to cause the weight of their uterus to shift off their inferior vena cava.

If a woman rises suddenly from a lying or sitting position or stands for an extended time in a warm or crowded area, she may faint from the same phenomenon (blood pooling in the pelvic area or lower extremities). Rising slowly and avoiding extended periods of standing prevents this problem. If a woman should feel faint, sitting with her head lowered—the same action as for any person who feels faint—alleviates the problem.

Varicosities

Varicosities, or the development of tortuous leg veins, commonly form in pregnancy because the weight of the distended uterus puts pressure on the veins returning blood from the lower extremities (Attilakos & Overton, 2012). This causes blood pooling and vessel distention. The veins

Figure 12.5 Position to relieve varicosities. The mother keeps a pad under her right hip to prevent supine hypotensive syndrome.

become enlarged, inflamed, and painful. Although usually confined to the lower extremities, varicosities can extend up to and including the vulva. They occur most frequently in women with a family history of varicose veins, those who are obese, and those who have a large fetus or a multiple pregnancy. Urge such women to take active measures to prevent varicosities beginning in early pregnancy; if left until late in pregnancy, the best they will be able to accomplish is relief of pain from already formed varicosities.

Resting in a Sims position or on the back with the legs raised against the wall (with a small firm pillow under their right hip) or elevated on a footstool for 15 to 20 minutes twice a day is a good precaution (Fig. 12.5). Caution women not to sit with their legs crossed or their knees bent and to avoid constrictive knee-high hose or garters.

Some women who developed varicosities during a previous pregnancy may need elastic support stockings for relief of varicosities in a second pregnancy. If a woman needs to wear these, urge her to put them on before she arises in the morning because once she is on her feet, blood pooling begins, and the stockings will be less effective. When applied properly, the stockings should reach an area above the point of distention.

Be certain a woman understands the stockings she buys should be labeled "medical support hose." Otherwise, as many pantyhose manufacturers advertise their stockings as giving "firm support," she may assume erroneously this is sufficient for her.

Because it stimulates venous return, exercise is as effective as rest periods for alleviating varicosities. Most women assume they do not need set exercise periods during pregnancy because they work hard at other activities. If they analyze the type of work they do, however, they may realize a great deal of their work leads to venous stasis of their lower extremities. Women stand in one position to wash dishes, run a copying machine, defend a patient in court, process a part on an assembly line, or teach a class. Sitting at a desk for prolonged periods of time with legs bent at the knee also encourages venous stasis.

To increase circulation, advise women to break up these long periods of sitting or standing with a "walk break" at least twice a day. As a rule, their families or fellow workers will

benefit by accompanying them on such walks as partners may discover that when they analyze their day, they, too, sit more than walk during their workday.

Vitamins C, A, and B complex are all important for circulatory health. Vitamin C appears to be most important as it is necessary for the formation of blood vessel collagen and endothelium. Ask at prenatal visits if women are taking a daily prenatal vitamin as well as including fresh fruit or juice in their diet every day as yet another measure to help prevent varicosities.

What If . . . 12.2
Julberry knows taking a prenatal vitamin every day is important but is having trouble remembering to take one. What are some suggestions the nurse could make to help her remember to take this daily?

Hemorrhoids

Hemorrhoids (i.e., varicosities of the rectal veins) occur commonly in pregnancy because of pressure on these veins from the bulk of the growing uterus (Zielinski, Searing, & Deibel, 2015). Daily bowel evacuation to prevent constipation, drinking adequate fluid, eating adequate fiber, and resting in a modified Sims position are all helpful measures to both prevent these and relieve pain. At day's end, assuming a knee–chest position (Fig. 12.6) for 10 to 15 minutes is an excellent way to reduce the pressure on rectal veins. A knee–chest position may initially make a woman feel light-headed. If this happens, advise her to remain in this position for only a few minutes at first and then gradually increase the time until she can maintain the position comfortably for about 15 minutes.

In addition to the previous measures, a stool softener such as docusate sodium (Colace) may be recommended if a woman already has hemorrhoids when she enters pregnancy. Replacing external hemorrhoids with gentle finger pressure and applying witch hazel, a cold compress, or over-the-counter hemorrhoid cream are other helpful measures to relieve pain. Hydrocortisone-pramoxine (Proctofoam-HC) is a prescription medication that is also helpful and is safe for the fetus (Lohsiriwat, 2015). As with varicosities, think prevention, not just providing help for already established hemorrhoids.

Figure 12.6 Knee–chest position. Because the weight of the uterus is shifted forward, this position promotes free flow of urine from the kidneys (preventing urinary tract stasis and infection) and better circulation in the rectal area (preventing hemorrhoids).

PATIENT-CENTERED CARE

Julberry Adams tells the nurse she has developed painful hemorrhoids. She admits that she is embarrassed to discuss this problem but acknowledges that it needs to be addressed. The best advice to give her would be which of the following?

    a. "Take a tablespoon of mineral oil with each of your meals."

    b. "Omit most of the fiber from your diet. This will prevent constipation."

    c. "Lie on your stomach daily to drain blood from rectal veins."

    d. "Witch hazel pads feel cool against swollen hemorrhoids."

Look in Appendix A for the best answer and rationale.

Heart Palpitations

On sudden movement, such as turning over in bed, a pregnant woman may experience a bounding palpitation of the heart (Nelson-Piercy, 2012). This is probably because of circulatory adjustments necessary to accommodate her increased blood supply. Although only momentary, the sensation can be frightening because the heart seems to stop for an instant or skip a beat. It is reassuring for women to learn heart palpitations are normal and are to be expected on occasion. Only if they occur very frequently or continuously or are accompanied by pain should they be a concern. Gradual, slow movements will help prevent this from happening.

Frequent Urination

Frequent urination occurs in early pregnancy because the growing uterus presses on the anterior bladder. This sensation lasts about 3 months, beginning as early as the first or second missed menstrual period, disappears in midpregnancy as the uterus rises above the bladder, and then returns again in late pregnancy as the fetal head presses against the bladder (Fig. 12.7).

Caution women not to wait but to void as often as necessary, as urine stasis can lead to infection. When a woman reports frequency of urination, be certain this is the only urinary symptom she is experiencing. Ask her about any burning or pain on urination or whether she has noticed any blood in her urine, which are signs of a urinary tract infection.

Women should not restrict their fluid intake to diminish frequency of urination, as fluids are necessary to allow their blood volume to double. Decreasing daily caffeine intake due to the risks caffeine poses for low birth weight may have the added benefit of reducing urinary frequency. Most importantly, a woman needs to understand voiding more frequently is a normal pregnancy finding. The sensation of frequency will probably return after lightening (the settling of the fetal head into the inlet of the pelvis at pregnancy's end). Unless she is cautioned, she may worry at that time that she has a urinary tract infection. Again, unless other symptoms are present, she can be assured this is a normal finding.

Occasionally, a woman notices stress incontinence (involuntary loss of urine on coughing or sneezing) during pregnancy. Although this is largely unpreventable, doing Kegel exercises (alternately contracting and relaxing perineal muscles; Box 12.7) not only helps strengthen urinary control but also directly strengthens perineal muscles for birth (Sangsawang & Sangsawang, 2015).

Abdominal Discomfort

Some women experience uncomfortable feelings of abdominal pressure early in pregnancy. Women with a multiple pregnancy may notice this throughout pregnancy. Many pregnant women typically stand with their arms crossed in front of them because the weight of their arms resting on their abdomen relieves this discomfort.

When a woman stands up quickly, she may experience a pulling pain, sometimes sharp and frightening, in her right or left lower abdomen from tension on a round ligament. She can prevent this from happening by always rising slowly from a lying to a sitting or from a sitting to a standing position.

A   B   C

Figure 12.7 Bladder changes during pregnancy. **(A)** Early pregnancy: The uterus presses against the bladder, causing frequent urination. **(B)** Middle pregnancy: Urinary frequency is relieved. **(C)** Late pregnancy: The uterus is again pressing on the bladder, leading to the recurrence of urinary frequency.

BOX 12.7
Kegel Exercises

Kegel exercises are exercises designed to strengthen the pubococcygeal muscles. Each is a separate exercise and should be done about three times per day.

1. Squeeze the muscles surrounding the vagina as if stopping the flow of urine. Hold for 3 seconds. Relax. Repeat this sequence 10 times.
2. Contract and relax the muscles surrounding the vagina as rapidly as possible 10 to 25 times.
3. Imagine you are sitting in a bathtub of water and squeeze muscles as if sucking water into the vagina. Hold for 3 seconds. Relax. Repeat this action 10 times.
4. Caution: Don't regularly start and stop the flow of urine during urination to try and strengthen muscles as this can lead to incomplete emptying of the bladder.

It may take as long as 6 weeks of exercise before pubococcygeal muscles are strengthened. In addition to strengthening urinary control and preventing stress incontinence, Kegel exercises can lead to increased sexual enjoyment because of tightened vaginal muscles and can help avoid tearing of the perineum with childbirth.

Because round ligament pain may simulate the abrupt pain that occurs with ruptured ectopic pregnancy, a woman's description of the pain needs to be evaluated carefully. If ectopic pregnancy is suggested, she should be referred to her obstetric provider (Fletcher & Russo, 2015).

Leukorrhea

Leukorrhea, a whitish, viscous vaginal discharge or an increase in the amount of normal vaginal secretions, occurs in response to the high estrogen level and the increased blood supply to the vaginal epithelium and cervix in pregnancy. A daily bath or shower to wash away accumulated secretions and prevent vulvar excoriation usually controls this problem. Wearing cotton underpants and sleeping at night without underwear can be helpful to reduce moisture and possible vulvar excoriation. Some women may need to wear a perineal pad to absorb the discharge. Caution women not to use tampons because this could lead to stasis of secretions and subsequent infection. Advise women to contact their obstetric provider if there is a change in the color, odor, or character of this discharge as these suggest infection. Caution women not to douche; douching is contraindicated generally and especially throughout pregnancy because fluid could be forced into the uterine cervix (Sheth & Keller, 2015).

A woman with vulvar itching (pruritus) accompanying a vaginal discharge needs additional evaluation because this strongly indicates infection. Be certain that when describing pruritus, the woman is not describing burning on urination, which is a sign of an early bladder infection (which also needs therapy, but of a different type). Therapy for common vaginal infections, such as candidiasis, that present with pruritus are discussed in Chapter 47.

Avoiding tight underpants and pantyhose may help prevent vulvar and vaginal infections, particularly yeast infections.

Although over-the-counter medications for yeast infections are available, caution women to contact their healthcare provider rather than self-treat vaginal infections during pregnancy so their healthcare provider knows that infections are occurring.

A woman who is uncomfortable about discussing this part of her body or who associates vaginal infections with poor hygiene or sexually transmitted infections may be reluctant to mention an irritating vaginal discharge at a healthcare visit. At each prenatal visit, therefore, be sure to ask women specifically whether they are experiencing this problem.

What If . . . 12.3
Julberry Adams tells the nurse she has urinary frequency. She also reports a white vaginal discharge. What questions would the nurse need to ask to evaluate whether she is experiencing a normal finding of pregnancy or a possible urinary tract infection?

MINOR BODY CHANGES OF PREGNANCY: SECOND AND THIRD TRIMESTERS

At about the midpoint of pregnancy (the 20th to 24th weeks), a woman is usually ready for further health teaching that relates to the new symptoms that occur in the latter half of pregnancy. As she starts to view the child within her as a separate person, she becomes interested in discussing and making plans for the signs and symptoms of beginning labor, birth, and the infant's care. The midpoint of a pregnancy is also a good time to review precautionary measures to prevent constipation, varicosities, and hemorrhoids, as these increase in intensity as the pregnancy progresses.

Nursing Diagnoses and Related Interventions

Nursing Diagnosis: Health-seeking behaviors related to learning more about the minor body changes of late pregnancy such as Braxton Hicks contractions

Outcome Evaluation: Patient states she feels confident in self-managing the minor body changes of late pregnancy.

Examples of other possible nursing diagnoses associated with the minor body changes of middle-to-late pregnancy are:

- Pain related to almost constant backache
- Acute abdominal pain related to sudden postural change in pregnancy
- Anxiety related to shortness of breath, resulting from expanding uterine pressure on the diaphragm
- Deficient knowledge related to beginning signs of labor

Muscular/Skeletal Discomfort

As pregnancy advances, a lumbar lordosis develops and postural changes necessary to maintain balance lead to backache (see Box 12.3). Wearing shoes with low-to-moderate heels reduces the amount of spinal curvature necessary to maintain an upright posture. Encouraging a woman to walk with her pelvis tilted forward (i.e., putting pelvic support under the weight of the fetus) is also helpful. In addition, applying local heat from a heating pad may aid in relieving backache (Liddle & Pennick, 2015).

To avoid back strain and worsen the condition, advise women to squat rather than bend over to pick up objects. Also encourage women to always lift objects by holding them close to the body. For some women, a firmer mattress during this time may be required. Sliding a board under the mattress is a cost-effective alternative for achieving a firmer sleeping surface rather than buying a new mattress. Pelvic rocking or tilting, an exercise described in Chapter 14, also helps to prevent and relieve backache.

Obtaining a detailed account of a woman's back symptoms is crucial because back pain can be an initial sign of a bladder or kidney infection. Too often, women are observed at a prenatal visit only lying in a lithotomy position on an examining table. Always assess the manner in which a woman walks and what type of shoes she wears as she moves from a waiting room to an examining room to evaluate whether her posture or shoes could be a cause of backache.

Generally, acetaminophen (Tylenol) is considered to be safe and effective for relieving this type of pain during pregnancy. Acupuncture can also be effective (Carr, 2015). Caution women not to take herbal remedies, muscle relaxants, or other analgesics (or any other medication) for back pain without first consulting their obstetric provider.

A second skeletal problem that occurs at a greater incidence during pregnancy than at any other time is carpel tunnel syndrome or pain at the wrist from compression of the median nerve. Therapy for this is discussed in Chapter 49.

Headache

Many women experience headaches during pregnancy, apparently from their expanding blood volume, which puts pressure on cerebral arteries. Trying to reduce any possible causative situations, such as eye strain or tension, may lessen the number of headaches they experience. Resting with an ice pack on the forehead and taking a usual adult dose of acetaminophen usually furnishes adequate relief (Spierings & Sabin, 2016). Compounds with ibuprofen (Motrin, Advil) (class C drugs) are not usually recommended because they cause premature closure of the ductus arteriosus in the fetus. Additionally, they have been found to contribute to fetal renal damage, low amniotic fluid, and fetal intracranial hemorrhage. Although a few women who have migraine headaches find these worsen during pregnancy, most women notice considerable improvement with this type of headache because of increased estrogen levels (see Chapter 49). Caution women that if a headache seems unusually intense or continuous, they should report it to their primary care provider as a continuous sharp headache may be a sign of high blood pressure, a danger sign of pregnancy.

Dyspnea

As the expanding uterus places pressure on the diaphragm, lung compression and shortness of breath result. A woman will notice this primarily at night if she lies flat. She will definitely notice it on exertion. To relieve nighttime dyspnea, advise her to sleep with her head and chest elevated so the weight of the uterus falls away from her diaphragm. As pregnancy progresses, she may require two or more pillows to sleep at night and she may need to limit her activities during the day to prevent exertional dyspnea. Always question women about this important symptom at prenatal visits to be certain the sensation is not continuous, which could describe a respiratory disorder (Goland, Perelman, Asalih, et al., 2015).

Ankle Edema

Most women experience some swelling of their ankles and feet during late pregnancy, most noticeably at the end of the day. Women are often first conscious of this when they kick off their shoes to rest and then cannot put them on again comfortably.

As long as proteinuria and hypertension are absent, ankle edema of this nature is a normal occurrence of pregnancy. It is probably caused by general fluid retention and reduced blood circulation in the lower extremities because of uterine pressure. This simple edema can be relieved best by resting in a left side-lying position because this increases the kidney's glomerular filtration rate and also allows for good venous return. Sitting for half an hour in the afternoon and again in the evening with the legs elevated is also helpful. Caution women to avoid wearing constricting clothing such as panty girdles or knee-high stockings because these impede lower extremity circulation and venous return.

Although ankle edema is common, it is important not to dismiss a report of lower extremity edema as insignificant until you are certain a woman does not exhibit any signs such as proteinuria, edema of other, nondependent body parts, or has had a sudden increase in weight as these, in conjunction with ankle edema, are beginning signs of gestational hypertension (Ohno, Terauchi, Tamakoshi, et al., 2016).

Braxton Hicks Contractions

Beginning as early as the 8th to 12th week of pregnancy, the uterus periodically contracts and then relaxes again (Coad & Dunstall, 2011). Early in pregnancy, these sensations, termed Braxton Hicks contractions, are not apt to be noticeable. By middle or late pregnancy, the contractions become so strong a woman who tenses at the sensation may experience pain, similar to a forceful menstrual cramp. Although these contractions are not a sign of beginning labor, women should telephone or e-mail their primary care provider to report them so they can be evaluated. A rhythmic pattern of even very light but persistent contractions could be a beginning sign of preterm labor.

QSEN Checkpoint Question 12.5

INFORMATICS

Julberry Adams has done some online research about the ankle edema that she typically experiences by the end of each day. Which statement by her would reveal that she has read accurate information about the cause of this?

a. "I know this is a beginning complication; I'll call my doctor tonight."
b. "I understand this is from eating too much salt; I'll restrict that more."
c. "I'll rest with my feet up to take pressure off my leg veins."
d. "I know this is from gaining too much weight; I'll start to diet tomorrow."

Look in Appendix A for the best answer and rationale.

Preventing Fetal Exposure to Teratogens

A teratogen is any factor, chemical or physical, that adversely affects the fertilized ovum, embryo, or fetus. A fetus is extremely vulnerable to environmental injury, specifically at the beginning or early weeks of pregnancy. Although the causes of many anomalies occurring in utero are still unknown, many specific teratogenic factors have been isolated.

EFFECTS OF TERATOGENS ON A FETUS

Several factors influence the amount of damage a teratogen can cause. The strength of the teratogen is the first one. For example, radiation is a known teratogen. In small amounts (everyone is exposed to some radiation every day, such as from the rays of the sun), it causes no damage. However, in large doses (e.g., a woman received radiation to treat cancer of the cervix during pregnancy), serious fetal defects or death could occur (Basta, Bak, & Roszkowski, 2015).

The timing of the teratogenic insult is a second factor that makes a significant difference. If a teratogen is introduced before implantation, for example, either the zygote is destroyed or it appears unaffected. If the insult occurs when the main body systems are being formed (in the second to eighth weeks of embryonic life), a fetus is very vulnerable to injury. During the last trimester, the potential for harm again decreases because all the organs of a fetus are formed and are merely maturing. The times when different anatomic areas of a fetus are most likely to be affected by teratogens are shown in Chapter 9, Figure 9.4.

Two exceptions to the rule that deformities usually occur in early embryonic life are the effects caused by the organisms of syphilis and **toxoplasmosis**. These two infections can cause abnormalities in organs that were originally formed normally. Intimate partner violence is another teratogen that can be responsible for injury to a fetus at any stage of pregnancy (Demelash, Nigatu, & Gashaw, 2015).

A third factor determining the effects of a teratogen is the teratogen's affinity for specific body tissues. Lead and mercury, for example, attack and disable nervous tissue (Dórea, 2015). Thalidomide (Immunoprin), originally used to treat nausea in pregnancy, is now prescribed for cancer therapy, and it may cause limb defects (Coombes, 2016). Tetracycline (Apo-Tetra), a common antibiotic, causes tooth enamel deficiencies, and possibly, long bone deformities. The rubella virus affects many organs, with the eyes, ears, heart, and brain the four most commonly attacked (Karch, 2015).

Nursing Diagnoses and Related Interventions

Nursing Diagnosis: Health-seeking behaviors related to learning more about avoiding teratogens that can affect fetal growth

Outcome Evaluation: Patient states she feels confident in monitoring her environment for the presence of possible teratogens.

Much of the health history information obtained at prenatal visits is taken to help determine if there is a possibility a woman is unknowingly being exposed to teratogens during her pregnancy. Examples of nursing diagnoses associated with maternal exposure to teratogens include:

- Health-seeking behavior related to mother's interest in avoiding exposure to harmful substances she could contact at work
- Risk for fetal injury related to lack of knowledge about teratogenicity of alcohol, drugs, and tobacco
- Risk for fetal infection related to transmission from mother to fetus of genital herpes

TERATOGENIC MATERNAL INFECTIONS

Teratogenic maternal infections involve viral, bacterial, or protozoan organisms, which cross the placenta from mother to fetus. Most infections that may detract from a healthy pregnancy outcome cause relatively mild, flu-like symptoms in the woman but can have much more serious effects on a fetus or newborn. Preventing and predicting fetal injury from an infection is complicated because when a disease is subclinical (without any symptoms in the mother), it is difficult to analyze any effect on the fetus.

When newborns are tested to see if antibodies against the common infectious teratogenic diseases are present, the test is described collectively under the umbrella term TORCH, an acronym for toxoplasmosis, rubella, cytomegalovirus, and herpes simplex virus (Neu, Duchon, & Zachariah, 2015.). Some laboratories spell the test as TORSCH to show they also screen for syphilis. Still, other laboratories identify the O with "other infections," which could include hepatitis B virus (HBV) or chlamydia (discussed in Chapter 47). In addition to TORCH screening, ask women if it is all right to screen them for human immunodeficiency virus (HIV); you must obtain separate permission for this test (Camacho-Gonzalez, Kingbo, Boylan, et al., 2015).

Malaria

Malaria in humans is caused by intraerythrocytic protozoa of the genus *Plasmodium* transmitted to humans by the bite of an infected female *Anopheles* mosquito. Healthcare providers can contact it from infected blood products. During pregnancy, women can transmit malaria to a fetus. Most malaria infections in the United States occur among people who have traveled to areas where malaria is epidemic, such as Africa or South America.

A number of drugs, such as chloroquine (Aralen) in the first trimester and mefloquine (Lariam) in the second or third trimesters, are helpful. Women who will be visiting an area known to be epidemic for malaria can begin treatment as prophylaxis up to 2 weeks before travel (Tinto, Sevene, Dellicour, et al., 2015).

Toxoplasmosis

Toxoplasmosis, a protozoan infection, is spread most commonly through contact with uncooked meat, although it may also be contracted through handling cat stool in soil or cat litter (Hampton, 2015).

As many as 1 in 900 pregnancies may be affected by toxoplasmosis. Prepregnancy serum analysis can be done to identify women who have never had the disease and so are susceptible (about 50% of women). Removing a cat from the home during pregnancy as a means of prevention is not necessary as long as the cat is healthy. However, taking in a new cat, which could be infected, is unwise. Instruct pregnant women to avoid undercooked meat and also not to change a cat litter box or garden in soil in an area where cats may defecate to avoid exposure to the disease. Also, reinforce proper hand washing after handling uncooked meat.

Rubella (German Measles)

The rubella virus usually causes only a mild rash and mild systemic illness in a woman, but the teratogenic effects on a fetus can be devastating, such as hearing impairment, cognitive and motor challenges, cataracts, cardiac defects (most commonly patent ductus arteriosus and pulmonary stenosis), restricted intrauterine growth (i.e., small for gestational age), thrombocytopenic purpura, and dental and facial clefts, such as cleft lip and palate (Grant, Reef, Dabbagh, et al., 2015).

Typically, a rubella titer from a pregnant woman to estimate whether a woman is susceptible to rubella is obtained on the first prenatal visit. A titer greater than 1:8 suggests immunity to the disease. A titer of less than 1:8 suggests a woman is susceptible to viral invasion. A titer that is greatly increased over a previous reading or is initially extremely high suggests a recent infection has occurred.

A woman who is not immunized before pregnancy cannot be immunized during pregnancy because the vaccine contains a live virus that would have effects similar to those occurring with a subclinical case of rubella. After rubella immunization, a woman is advised not to become pregnant for about 3 months, until the rubella virus is no longer active. Immediately after a pregnancy, assess whether a woman who has a low rubella titer would like to be immunized to provide protection against rubella in future pregnancies.

An increasing concern is women who demonstrate antibodies against rubella yet still become reinfected during pregnancy. Because of this, all pregnant women should avoid contact with children with rashes. Infants who are born to mothers who had rubella during pregnancy may be capable of transmitting the disease for a time after birth. Because of this, such an infant is isolated from other newborns during the newborn period. Be certain a woman is aware her infant might infect others, including pregnant women. Nurses who care for pregnant women or newborns should receive immunization against rubella to ensure they neither spread nor contract the disease (CDC, 2016).

Herpes Simplex Virus (Genital Herpes Infection)

Genital **herpes simplex virus (HSV)** is a sexually transmitted infection spread by intimate contact. The first time a woman contracts an HSV infection, systemic involvement occurs. The virus spreads into the bloodstream (viremia) and, if a woman is pregnant, can cross the placenta to a fetus, thus posing substantial fetal risk (Lopez-Medina, Cantey, & Sánchez, 2015). Typically, HSV-2 is the cause of genital outbreaks and is caused by genital-to-genital contact. Increasingly, HSV-1 can cause genital outbreaks and is often transmitted during oral sex. The management of genital herpes is the same whether HSV-1 or HSV-2 is the cause.

If the infection takes place in the first trimester, severe congenital anomalies or spontaneous miscarriage can occur.

If the infection invades during the second or third trimester, there is a high incidence of premature birth, intrauterine growth restriction, neurologic disease, and continuing infection of the newborn at birth. Mortality may be as high as 60% (Martin & Satin, 2015).

If a woman has had oral HSV, typically HSV-1, infections (popularly called cold sores) before contracting genital herpes, or if the genital outbreak is a recurrence, antibodies to the virus in her system help reduce the severity of the outbreak and help prevent spread of the virus to the fetus across the placenta.

If genital lesions are present at the time of birth, however, a fetus may contract the virus from direct exposure during birth. For this reason, if a woman has existing genital lesions at the time of birth, cesarean birth is usually advised to reduce the risk of this route of infection. This awareness of the placental spread of HSV has increased the importance of obtaining information about exposure to HSV or any painful perineal or vaginal lesions that might indicate this infection at prenatal visits through conscientious history taking.

Acyclovir (Zovirax) or valacyclovir (Valtrex) can both be safely administered to women who develop lesions during pregnancy as well as to their newborns at birth (Groves, 2016). Either drug is recommended daily as prophylaxis at 36 weeks of pregnancy to prevent a lesion at the time of birth. The primary mechanism for protecting a fetus, however, is disease prevention. Urging women to practice safer sex is important to lessen their exposure to this and other sexually transmitted infections.

Cytomegalovirus

Cytomegalovirus (CMV), a member of the HSV family, is another teratogen that can cause extensive damage to a fetus while causing few symptoms in a woman (Martin & Satin, 2015). It is not sexually transmitted but spreads from person to person by droplet infection such as occurs with sneezing. If a woman acquires a primary CMV infection during pregnancy and the virus crosses the placenta, the infant may be born with severe neurologic challenges (e.g., hydrocephalus, microcephaly, or spasticity) or with eye damage (e.g., optic atrophy or chorioretinitis), hearing impairment, or chronic liver disease. The newborn's skin may be covered with large petechiae (i.e., "blueberry-muffin" lesions). Because a woman has almost no symptoms, she may not even be aware she contracted an infection. Diagnosis in the mother or infant can be established by the isolation of CMV antibodies in blood serum. Unfortunately, there is no treatment for the infection even if it presents in the mother with enough symptoms to allow detection. Because there is no treatment or vaccine for the disease, routine screening for CMV during pregnancy is not recommended. Advise women to wash hands thoroughly before eating and to avoid crowds of young children at daycare or nursery school settings to help prevent exposure (Drew, Stapleton, Abu, et al., 2015).

Like HSV, a primary CMV infection may become latent, reactivating periodically. These recurrences are not thought to have a teratogenic effect on a fetus, but they can cause infection of a newborn during birth from genital secretions or postpartum from exposure to CMV-infected breast milk. CMV infection contracted at or shortly after birth is not associated with serious adverse effects except in babies of very low birth weight.

Syphilis

Syphilis, a sexually transmitted infection, is of great concern for the maternal–fetal population. Despite the availability of accurate screening tests and proven medical treatment, it is growing in incidence; it places a fetus at risk for intrauterine or congenital syphilis (Su, Brooks, Davis, et al., 2016). Early in pregnancy, when the cytotrophoblast layer of the chorionic villi is still intact, the causative spirochete of syphilis, *Treponema pallidum*, apparently cannot cross the placenta and damage the fetus. When this layer atrophies at about the 16th to 18th week of pregnancy, however, the spirochete can cross and cause extensive fetal damage. If syphilis is detected in the mother and treated with an antibiotic such as intramuscular benzathine penicillin (Bicillin L-A) in the first trimester, a fetus is rarely affected. If left untreated beyond the 18th week of gestation, hearing impairment, cognitive challenge, osteochondritis, and fetal death are possible.

For these reasons, serologic screening (either by a venereal disease research laboratory [VDRL] or a rapid plasma reagin [RPR] test) is done at a first prenatal visit; the test may then be repeated again close to term (the eighth month) if recent exposure is a concern. Even when a woman has been treated with antibiotics, the serum titer remains high up to 200 days; an increasing titer, however, suggests reinfection has occurred. In an infant born to a woman with syphilis, the serologic test for syphilis may remain positive for up to 3 months even though the disease was treated during pregnancy.

The newborn with congenital syphilis may have congenital anomalies, extreme rhinitis (sniffles), and a characteristic syphilitic rash, all of which identify the baby as high risk at birth (Akahira-Azuma, Kubota, Hosokawa, et al., 2015). When the baby's primary teeth come in, they are often oddly shaped (i.e., Hutchinson teeth). As the infant requires long-term follow-up, medical and nursing care of the newborn with congenital syphilis is discussed in Chapter 47. As with all sexually transmitted infections, prevention through safer sex practices is key.

Other Viral Diseases

It is difficult to detect other viral teratogens, but rubeola (measles), coxsackievirus, infectious parotitis (mumps), varicella (chickenpox), poliomyelitis, influenza, and viral hepatitis all may be teratogenic. Women are advised to be vaccinated against influenza before pregnancy. If contracted during pregnancy, parvovirus B19, the causative agent of erythema infectiosum (also called fifth disease) and a common viral disease in school-age children, can cross the placenta and attack the red blood cells of the fetus. Infection with the virus during early pregnancy is associated with fetal death. If the infection occurs late in pregnancy, the infant may be born with severe anemia and congenital heart disease (American College of Obstetricians and Gynecologists, 2015).

TERATOGENIC MATERNAL EXPOSURES

Potentially Teratogenic Vaccines

Live virus vaccines, such as measles, human papillomavirus (HPV), mumps, rubella, and poliomyelitis (Sabin type), are contraindicated during pregnancy because they may transmit a viral infection to a fetus (Fletcher & Russo, 2015). Care must be taken in routine immunization programs at high

Figure 12.8 A woman needs to think twice before taking an over-the-counter medicine during pregnancy to be certain it will be safe for both herself and her fetus.

schools to be certain adolescents about to be vaccinated are not pregnant. Women who work in biologic laboratories where vaccines are manufactured are well advised to use protective gear or not to work with live virus products during pregnancy.

Teratogenic Drugs

Many women assume the rule of being cautious with drugs during pregnancy applies only to prescription drugs and continue to take over-the-counter drugs or herbal supplements freely during pregnancy. Although not all drugs cross the placenta (heparin, for example, does not because of its large molecular size), most do (Fig. 12.8).

To help ensure the safety of drugs during pregnancy, the U.S. Food and Drug Administration (FDA, n.d.) rates drugs according to five categories in relation to pregnancy (Table 12.1). Always look for a drug's listed category before administering it to a pregnant woman to be certain it will be safe to administer. In addition, two principles always govern drug intake during pregnancy:

- Any drug or herbal supplement, under certain circumstances, may be detrimental to fetal welfare. Therefore, during pregnancy, women should not take any drug or supplement not specifically prescribed or approved by their obstetric provider.
- A woman of childbearing age should not take any drug other than one prescribed by a obstetric provider to avoid exposure to a drug should she become pregnant.

The classic example of a drug that can cause harm in pregnancy is thalidomide (Immunoprin), which was once liberally prescribed for morning nausea in Europe. Never approved for use in the United States, thalidomide caused amelia or phocomelia (i.e., total or partial absence of extremities) in 100% of instances when taken between the 34th and 45th day of pregnancy. Thalidomide is again available as it is effective as an anticancer drug, specifically for patients with multiple myeloma or hepatic cancer, so women still need to be cautioned about its detrimental fetal effects (Sherbet, 2015).

Finasteride (Propecia), a drug taken by both men and women to restore hair growth, is an example of a drug that may be readily available in a modern home but which is

TABLE 12.1 FDA PREGNANCY RISK CATEGORIES OF DRUGS

Category	Description	Example
A	No risk to fetus. Studies have not shown risk of fetal harm.	Thyroid hormone (Synthroid)
B	No risk in animal studies. Well-controlled studies in pregnant women are not available. It is assumed there is little to no risk in pregnant women.	Insulin aspart (NovoLog)
C	Animal studies indicate risk to the fetus. Controlled studies on pregnant women are not available. Risk versus benefit of the drug must be determined.	Docusate sodium (Colace)
D	Risk to the human fetus has been proven. Risk versus benefit of the drug must be determined. Could be used in lifesaving situations.	Lithium citrate (Lithobid)
X	Risk to the human fetus has been proven. Risk outweighs the benefit so the drug should be avoided during pregnancy.	Thalidomide (Immunoprin)

From U.S. Food and Drug Administration. (n.d.). *FDA pregnancy categories.* Washington, DC: Author.

documented to cause fetal deformities (Varothai & Bergfeld, 2014). Other examples of drugs capable of being teratogenic are shown in Box 12.8.

Almost all recreational drugs put a fetus at risk in two ways: The drug may have a direct teratogenic effect and, if taken intravenously, the drug increases the mother's risk of exposure to diseases such as HIV and hepatitis B and C (Kamarulzaman & Altice, 2015).

Narcotics such as meperidine (Demerol) and heroin have long been implicated as having serious impacts on intrauterine growth. The use of marijuana alone apparently does not, although the accompanying lifestyle may lead to fetal growth restriction and preterm birth (Roth, Satran, & Smith, 2015).

Cocaine, particularly in crack form, is potentially harmful to a fetus because it causes severe vasoconstriction in the mother, thus compromising placental blood flow and perhaps dislodging the placenta. Its use is associated with spontaneous miscarriage, preterm labor, meconium staining, and intrauterine growth restriction (Fletcher & Russo, 2015). Whether cocaine causes long-term effects in the infant remains controversial (Forray & Foster, 2015). See Chapter 22 for more information on the potential hazards of cocaine or heroin use during pregnancy.

An area of recreational drug use rising in incidence is that of inhalant abuse ("huffing"). Substances frequently used as inhalants include gasoline, butane lighter fluid, Freon, glue, and nitrous oxide (NIOSH, 2010). Although the teratogenic properties of these inhalants are not well studied, they all carry the possibility of a respiratory distress effect on the mother, which could limit the oxygen supply to a fetus. They are used most often by adolescents as they are easy to obtain on a limited budget.

Herbs

Herbs are not regulated by the FDA in the same way as medications; therefore, they are not rated with regard to their safety in pregnancy. Even though most are safe, American ginseng, used to improve general well-being, has been associated with birth defects; and St. John's wort, an herb taken as a mood enhancer, can interfere with the action of seizure-control drugs, such as phenytoin (Dilantin) and phenobarbital (Phenobarb), and so should be avoided by women prescribed such drugs (National Center for Complementary and Alternative Medicine [NCCAM], 2010).

Green tea, a common breakfast drink, was thought to interfere with the absorption of folic acid, but this has not been confirmed in further studies. As folic acid is needed in pregnancy to help prevent birth defects, women could avoid it in pregnancy or when hoping to soon become pregnant (Gormack, Peek, Derraik, 2015). As with medicine, women should not take herbs in pregnancy until they discuss the herbs' safety with their obstetric provider.

Teratogenicity of Alcohol

Evidence confirms that when women consume a large quantity of alcohol during pregnancy, their babies demonstrate a high incidence of characteristic congenital craniofacial deformities including short palpebral fissures, a thin upper lip, an upturned nose, as well as cognitive impairment **fetal alcohol spectrum** (Charness, Riley, & Sowell, 2016). Fetuses cannot remove the breakdown products of alcohol from their body. The large buildup of these leads to vitamin B deficiency and accompanying neurologic damage.

Because of individual variations in metabolism, it is impossible to define a safe level of alcohol consumption. Women, therefore, should be screened for alcohol use at a first prenatal visit and are best advised to abstain from alcohol completely for the remainder of their pregnancy. Be certain to ask about binge drinking (e.g., consuming more than four alcoholic drinks in an evening with the intention of becoming intoxicated) because women may refer to this as only "occasional drinking." If necessary, refer women with alcohol addiction to an alcohol treatment program as early in pregnancy as possible to help them reduce their alcohol intake.

Teratogenicity of Tobacco

Cigarette smoking is associated with infertility in women. If used by a pregnant woman, it has been shown to cause fetal growth restriction. In addition, a fetus may be at greater risk for being stillborn and, after birth, may be at a greater risk than others for sudden infant death syndrome (Mohlman & Levy, 2016).

Low birth weights in infants of smoking mothers result from vasoconstriction of the uterine vessels, an effect of nicotine. This limits the blood supply to a fetus. Another contributory effect may be related to inhaled carbon monoxide. Secondary smoke, or inhaling the smoke of another person's cigarettes, may be as harmful as actually smoking because of inhaled carbon monoxide. All prenatal healthcare settings should be smoke-free environments for this reason.

BOX 12.8

Nursing Care Planning Based on Responsibility for Pharmacology

SOME POTENTIALLY OR POSITIVELY TERATOGENIC DRUGS

Category	Example	Drug Use	Teratogenic Effect
Alcohol (ethanol)	Wine, beer, whiskey	Social use	Fetal alcohol spectrum disorder
Analgesics	Acetylsalicylic acid (aspirin)	Minor pain relief	Prolonged pregnancy; maternal bleeding
	Nonsteroidal anti-inflammatory drugs (NSAIDs)		Patent ductus arteriosus
Antineoplastics	Methotrexate (Trexall)	Chemotherapy	Multiple anomalies
	Cyclophosphamide (Cytoxan)	Chemotherapy	Multiple anomalies
Androgens	Danazol (Cyclomen)	Endometriosis	Masculinization of female fetus
Anticonvulsants	Phenytoin (Dilantin)	Seizures	Fetal hydantoin syndrome
	Valproic acid (Depakote)		Neural tube defects
	Carbamazepine (Tegretol)		Neural tube defects
	Lamotrigine (Lamictal)		Possibly fetal anomalies
Anticoagulants	Warfarin (Coumadin)	Anticoagulation	Fetal bleeding or anomalies
Antidepressants	Imipramine (Tofranil)	Elevate mood	Cardiovascular anomalies
Antidiabetic agents	Chlorpropamide (Apo-Chlorpropamide)	Lower blood glucose	Neonatal hypoglycemia
Antischizophrenic	Lithium (Lithobid)	Schizophrenia	Polyhydramnios
Antithyroid	Methimazole (Tapazole)	Hypothyroidism	Hypothyroidism in fetus
Antibiotics	Sulfonamides	Infection	Hyperbilirubinemia in newborn
	Tetracycline (Apo-Tetra)	Infection	Teeth and bone deformities
Antihelmintics	Lindane (Gammallin)	Eradication of lice	Manufacturer recommends limiting exposure to two dosages
Antivirals	Ribavirin (Rebetol)	Respiratory infection, chronic hepatitis C	Multiple anomalies
Angiotensin-converting enzyme inhibitors	Enalapril (Vasotec); captopril (Capoten)	Reduce hypertension	Oligohydramnios (reduced amount of amniotic fluid)
Caffeine	Coffee, soft drinks, chocolate	Social use	Low birth weight
Hypoglycemics	Tolbutamide (Orinase)	Type 2 diabetes	Profound hypoglycemia in newborn
Nicotine	Tobacco	Relaxation	Growth restriction
Radiopharmaceuticals	Iodide-131 (Hicon)	Diagnostic studies	May destroy thyroid of fetus
Narcotics	Cocaine	Social pleasure	Dysmorphic and central nervous system (CNS) anomalies
	Heroin		Growth restriction; narcotic abstinence in newborn
Tranquilizers	Diazepam (Valium)	Reduce anxiety	Growth restriction; CNS dysfunction, hypotonia, respiratory depression
Vaccines (live)	Rubella (ProQuad)	Provide immunity	Possible infection in fetus
Vitamin A derivatives	Acitretin (Soriatane)	Psoriasis	Craniofacial, cardiac, CNS anomalies

Source: Briggs, G. G., Freeman, R. K., Towers, C. V., et al. (2017). *Drugs in pregnancy and lactation* (11th ed.). Philadelphia, PA: Wolters Kluwer.

If a woman cannot stop smoking during pregnancy (and, realistically, many women cannot), reducing the number of cigarettes smoked per day should help diminish adverse effects on a fetus as well as also protect a woman's own health from long-term illnesses, such as chronic respiratory diseases, in the future.

The best way to urge women to discontinue smoking is to educate them about the risks to themselves and their fetus at the first prenatal visit and then offer a support program to help them throughout the pregnancy. It may be effective to encourage women to sign a contract with their healthcare provider to try to stop or to join a smoking-cessation program. Be certain pregnant women know it would be best if they didn't enter a stop-smoking program that uses drug therapy such as nicotine patches until it is clear if such patches are not harmful to a fetus (Coleman, Chamberlain, Davey, et al., 2015). Box 12.9 shows an interprofessional care map illustrating both nursing and team planning to address decreasing alcohol and tobacco use during pregnancy.

BOX 12.9

Nursing Care Planning

AN INTERPROFESSIONAL CARE MAP FOR A PREGNANT WOMAN WITH THREATS TO FETAL HEALTH

Julberry Adams, a single, 30-year-old woman, is 4 months pregnant when you first see her in a prenatal clinic. She works as a curator for an art gallery but has missed work this past week because of nausea. She's worried she will not be able to work past 6 months of her pregnancy because her job involves a great deal of walking. She has already stopped her volunteer work teaching children's swimming at the YMCA. She wants to travel to see her sister in St. Louis because her sister is very ill but has heard pregnant women should not drive more than 100 miles. She asks you if marijuana would help reduce her early pregnancy nausea.

Family Assessment: Patient lives by herself in one-bedroom apartment. Rates finances as "Good, unless I have to quit work because of pregnancy." She asks you, "Will I have to have an ultrasound? I'm worried about that."

Patient Assessment: Gravida 1, para 0. Unsure of date of last menstrual period, but it was about 11 weeks ago. Uterine height barely above symphysis. Fetal heart rate at 148 beats/min by Doppler. History of frequent sinus headaches. "I use Sudafed (pseudoephedrine) at least three to four times a week; sometimes other things." Smokes one-half pack of cigarettes "some days." Drinks two to three glasses of wine per week at art gallery functions. Denies history of marijuana or other recreational drug use.

Nursing Diagnosis: Risk for fetal injury related to knowledge deficit concerning possible fetal exposure to teratogens

Outcome Criteria: Patient reports a decrease in smoking to less than 10 cigarettes per day and no alcohol consumption by next prenatal visit; verbalizes no use of recreational drugs, including marijuana.

Patient states she has contacted healthcare provider about whether she should continue to use sinus medications.

Team Member Responsible	Assessment	Intervention	Rationale	Expected Outcome
Activities of Daily Living, Including Safety				
Nurse	Assess what activities patient wants to participate in during pregnancy.	Discuss with the patient her desired activities and any modification necessary for pregnancy.	Finding a match between desired activities and necessary modifications will help with adherence.	Patient discusses what activities she intends to continue during pregnancy and ways to modify them as necessary.
Nurse/obstetric provider	Assess patient's work and travel plans.	Assure patient she can continue to work and can travel to visit her sister.	Reassurance helps patient maintain usual lifestyle.	Patient states she will continue work and maintain contact with sister.
Teamwork and Collaboration				
Nurse/obstetric provider	Assess what medications patient is currently taking.	Consult with healthcare provider about safety of over-the-counter (OTC) sinus medications.	Not all OTC medications are safe during pregnancy.	Patient states she will follow recommendations of obstetric provider regarding medications.
Procedures/Medications for Quality Improvement				
Nurse/obstetric provider	Anticipate the need for follow-up ultrasound examination to date pregnancy.	Explain the need for ultrasound exam to assess dating and possible fetal growth restriction because of alcohol and cigarette smoking habits.	Teratogen exposure may have slowed fetal growth, which will be revealed by ultrasound exam. Date of last menstrual period is unknown.	Patient states she understands the purpose of the ultrasound exam and will allow exam to be scheduled.
Nutrition				
Nurse/nutritionist	Assess patient's lifestyle to identify beverages she could substitute for alcohol, measures she could use for nausea.	Suggest patient replace alcohol consumption with caffeine-free beverages. Suggest measures to combat nausea and vomiting, such as dry crackers or acupuncture band.	Alcohol consumption during pregnancy is associated with fetal alcohol spectrum disorder. Decreasing nausea to increase food intake aids fetal growth and development.	Patient voices intent to replace alcohol consumption with caffeine-free beverages. Patient suggests measures that appeal to her to reduce nausea and vomiting.

Patient-Centered Care

Nurse/obstetric provider	Assess whether patient has tried any nonmedicinal measures to relieve sinus headaches.	Discuss with patient possible nonmedicinal measures to assist with sinus headache relief, such as saline nasal sprays, humidification, and warm compresses to nasal area.	Complementary comfort measures may provide symptomatic relief without danger to the fetus.	Patient describes two complementary therapies she will try to relieve sinus congestion.

Psychosocial/Spiritual/Emotional Needs

Nurse/social worker	Discuss with patient whether her current support system is adequate.	Help patient locate at least one person she can depend on if a pregnancy emergency should arise.	Pregnancy can be a very stressful time for a woman who lacks a secure support system.	Patient telephones or e-mails the healthcare facility with questions rather than relying on nonexperienced friends for information; names one reliable support person.

Informatics for Seamless Healthcare Planning

Nurse	Assess extent of cigarette smoking.	Encourage the patient to decrease smoking and quit if possible. Offer suggestions to accomplish this goal, including use of sugar-free gums or candies, distraction, and activity. Refer to a smoking-cessation group if appropriate.	Cigarette use during pregnancy can lead to fetal growth restriction. Support and suggestions provide concrete measures to assist patient with cutting down and quitting.	Patient voices intention to decrease smoking and, if possible, quit smoking during pregnancy.

Environmental Teratogens

Teratogens such as impure air or water can be as damaging to a fetus as those that are directly or deliberately ingested. Women are exposed to these through contact at home or at work sites. Breathing air filled with pollutants, for example, has been shown to lead to fetal growth restriction (Forde, Dewailly, Robertson, et al., 2014).

Metal and Chemical Hazards

Pesticides and carbon monoxide, such as from automobile exhaust, should be avoided as these are examples of chemical teratogens. Arsenic, a byproduct of copper and lead smelting, used in pesticides, paints, and leather processing; formaldehyde, used in paper manufacturing; and mercury, used in the manufacture of electrical apparatuses and found in high proportions in swordfish and tuna, are all teratogens that can be found at work sites.

Lead poisoning generally is considered a problem of young children who eat lead-based paint chips, but it can be a fetal hazard as well. Women may ingest lead by drinking water that travels through old pipes that are leaking lead, by "sniffing" lead-based gasoline, or eating paint chips (paint tastes sweet and may be eaten as a symptom of pica).

Lead ingestion during pregnancy may lead to a newborn who is both cognitively and neurologically challenged (Dórea, 2015).

Radiation

Rapidly growing cells are extremely vulnerable to destruction by radiation. This makes radiation a potent teratogen to unborn children because they have such a high proportion of rapidly growing cells. Radiation produces a range of malformations depending on the stage of development of the embryo or fetus and the strength and length of exposure. If the exposure occurs before implantation, for example, the growing zygote apparently is killed. If the zygote is not killed, it survives apparently unharmed. The most damaging time for exposure and subsequent damage is from implantation to 6 weeks after conception (a time when many women are not yet aware they are pregnant). The nervous system, brain, and the retinal innervation are growing rapidly at this time and so are most affected (CDC, 2014).

Even with this danger of radiation, X-rays to maternal parts other than the pelvis, including computerized tomography (CT) can be performed safely during pregnancy as long as a lead pelvic shield is provided (Nelson-Piercy, 2012). If a woman of childbearing age requires a pelvic

X-ray for any reason, this should be scheduled during the first 10 days of a menstrual cycle (when pregnancy is unlikely because ovulation has not yet occurred); during pregnancy, X-rays of the pelvis should be avoided except in emergency situations. Even fluoroscopy, which uses lower radiation doses than regular X-ray photography, should also be avoided during pregnancy—again, except in an emergency. A serum pregnancy test to rule out pregnancy can be completed on women who have reason to believe they might be pregnant before diagnostic tests involving X-rays are scheduled.

X-rays should be taken at term only if the data obtained are vitally important for birth and cannot be obtained by any other means. Sonography and magnetic resonance imaging can be used for confirmation of situations such as a multiple pregnancy because these do not appear to be teratogenic (Siauve, Chalouhi, Deloison, et al., 2015). Although still being investigated, long-term use of slight radiation sources, such as a computer, microwave oven, or cellular phone, also do not appear to be teratogenic (Shah & Farrow, 2014).

In addition to immediate fetal damage, evidence demonstrates that radiation can have long-lasting effects on the health of a child. There appears to be an increased risk of cancer in children who are exposed to radiation in utero. Exposure of the fetal gonads could lead to a genetic mutation that will not be evident until the next generation (Brent, 2015).

Hyperthermia and Hypothermia

Hyperthermia to a fetus can be detrimental to growth because it interferes with cell metabolism. This can occur from the use of saunas, hot tubs, or tanning beds; from a work environment next to a furnace, such as in welding or steel making; or from a high maternal fever early in pregnancy (4 to 6 weeks). For this reason, advise pregnant women not to use hot tubs, saunas, or tanning beds during pregnancy.

The effect of hypothermia on pregnancy is not well known. Because the uterus is an internal organ, a woman's body temperature would have to be lowered significantly before a great deal of fetal temperature change would result.

Teratogenic Maternal Stress

There is some evidence that a pregnancy filled with anxiety and worry beyond the usual amount could produce physiologic changes through their effects on the sympathetic division of the autonomic nervous system. The primary change this would cause includes constriction of the peripheral blood vessels (i.e., a fight-or-flight syndrome). If the anxiety is prolonged, the constriction of uterine vessels (the uterus is a peripheral organ) could substantially interfere with the blood and nutrient supply to a fetus (Latendresse, Wong, Dyer, et al., 2015).

It is important to remember these phenomena are characteristic only of long-term, extreme stress, not the normal anxiety of pregnancy. Personal tragedies such as a house fire, illness or death of one's partner, difficulty with relatives, marital discord, living in a war zone, and illness or death of another child are examples of stressful situations that might provoke this excessive level of anxiety.

It's not easy to help a woman resolve complex problems of this type during pregnancy because they are complicated. To prevent maternal stress from becoming severe, advise

counseling for women with low stress levels at prenatal care visits before the levels become extreme.

Infections That Cause Illness at Birth

A number of infections are not teratogenic to a fetus during pregnancy but are harmful if they are present at the time of birth. Gonorrhea, candidiasis, chlamydia, streptococcus B, and hepatitis B infections are examples of these. Chapters 45 and 47 discuss the effects of these infections on maternal, fetal, and neonatal health.

QSEN Checkpoint Question 12.6

SAFETY

Julberry Adams makes the following statements. Which one would the nurse rate as the safest practice?
 a. "My brother takes medicine for heartburn; if I think of it, I'll borrow his."
 b. "I'm going to get a measles shot; I don't want measles while I'm pregnant."
 c. "There are so many medicines for headache; I'll ask my doctor what to take."
 d. "I know all over-the-counter medicine is safe; that's why it's over the counter."

Look in Appendix A for the best answer and rationale.

Preparation for Labor

At about the midpoint of pregnancy, along with cautioning women about new minor body changes and possible teratogenic threats, it is a good time to review the signs or symptoms that signal the beginning of labor so women will not be surprised by these happenings or dismiss them as something other than the important events that they are. These are discussed in the following sections and summarized in Table 12.2.

TABLE 12.2 BEGINNING SIGNS AND SYMPTOMS OF LABOR

Sign or Symptom	Cause
Lightening	Sinking of the fetal head into the true pelvis
Slight loss of weight	As progesterone level falls, more fluid is excreted, slightly lowering body weight
Excess energy	Burst of adrenaline to provide energy for labor
Backache	Beginning but unrecognized uterine contractions
Ripening of the cervix	Prostaglandins soften the cervix to allow for shortening and dilatation
Rupture of membranes	Membranes have ruptured with release of amniotic fluid
Show	Internal cervical mucus plug has been released
Uterine contractions	True beginning of labor

PRELIMINARY SIGNS OF LABOR

In the days or hours before labor begins, a woman often experiences subtle signs or symptoms that signal labor is imminent. Because these signs and symptoms are subtle, they are easily missed if a woman is not informed of them in advance.

Lightening

In primiparas, *lightening*, or descent of the fetal presenting part (usually the fetal head) into the pelvis, occurs approximately 10 to 14 days before labor begins. This fetal descent changes a woman's abdominal contour because it positions the uterus lower and more anterior in the abdomen. Lightening gives a woman relief from the diaphragmatic pressure and shortness of breath she has been experiencing and in this way "lightens" her load. Lightening probably occurs early in primiparas this way because of tight abdominal muscles. In multiparas, it is not as dramatic and usually occurs on the day of labor or even after labor has begun. As the fetus sinks lower into the pelvis, a woman may experience shooting leg pains from the increased pressure on a sciatic nerve, increased amounts of vaginal discharge, and urinary frequency from pressure on her bladder.

Increase in Energy

A woman may awaken on the morning of labor full of energy, in contrast to the feeling of chronic fatigue that she has been feeling for the previous month. This increase in activity is related to a boost in epinephrine release, which is initiated by a decrease in progesterone production by the placenta. This additional epinephrine prepares a woman's body for the work of labor ahead. It's important that the woman recognizes this sensation for what it is or she may use this burst of energy to clean her house or finish paperwork at the office and exhaust herself before labor begins. If she can recognize this symptom as an initial sign of labor, she can conserve her energy in preparation for labor.

Slight Loss of Weight

As progesterone level falls, body fluid is more easily excreted from the body. This increase in urine production can lead to a weight loss between 1 and 3 lb.

Backache

Because labor contractions begin in the back, an intermittent backache stronger than usual may be the first symptom a woman notices.

Braxton Hicks Contractions

In the last week or days before labor begins, a woman usually notices extremely strong Braxton Hicks contractions. A woman having her first child may have such difficulty distinguishing between these and true contractions that she may come to the labor unit of a hospital or birthing center believing she is in labor. It is discouraging for a woman when this happens (strong Braxton Hicks contractions cause true discomfort) to be told she is not in true labor and should return home. When this happens, you can assure the woman that misinterpreting labor signals is common. Remind her that if contractions have become strong enough to be mistaken for true labor, true labor is not far away.

Ripening of the Cervix

Ripening of the cervix is an internal sign seen only on pelvic examination. Throughout pregnancy, the cervix feels softer than usual to palpation, similar to the consistency of an earlobe (Goodell's sign). At term, the cervix becomes still softer (described as "butter soft"), and it tips forward. Cervical ripening this way is an internal announcement that labor is very close at hand.

SIGNS OF TRUE LABOR

Signs of true labor involve both uterine and cervical changes. The contrast between true and false labor is summarized in Chapter 15, Table 15.3.

Uterine Contractions

True labor contractions usually begin in the back and sweep forward across the abdomen similar to the tightening of a rubber band. They gradually increase in frequency and intensity over a period of hours. Because contractions are involuntary and come without warning, their intensity can be frightening in early labor. Helping a woman appreciate that she can predict when her next one will occur and therefore can control the degree of discomfort she feels by using breathing exercises offers her a sense of control.

Advise a woman to telephone her primary care provider when contractions begin to alert healthcare personnel that she is in labor. Her healthcare provider will advise her as to what point in labor she should come to the healthcare facility she has chosen or when to begin preparations for home birth if that is her choice. The typical time for this is when contractions are 5 minutes apart, but this will vary depending on a woman's past and present pregnancy history. In all instances, if a woman should become exceptionally anxious, be home alone, or have a long drive, she should be given options as to when it would be best for her to leave home.

Show

As the cervix softens and ripens, the mucus plug that filled the cervical canal during pregnancy is expelled. The exposed cervical capillaries seep blood as a result of pressure exerted by the fetus. This blood, mixed with mucus, takes on a pink tinge and is referred to as "show" or "bloody show." Women need to be aware of this event so they do not think they are bleeding abnormally.

Rupture of the Membranes

Labor may begin with rupture of the membranes, experienced either as a sudden gush or as a scanty, slow seeping of clear fluid from the vagina. Some women may worry if their labor begins with a rupture of the membranes because they have heard labor will then be "dry," and this will cause it to be difficult and long. Actually, amniotic fluid continues to be produced until delivery of the membranes after the birth of their child, so no labor is ever "dry." Early rupture of the membranes can actually be advantageous as it can cause the fetal head to settle snugly into the pelvis, aiding cervical dilation and shortening labor.

A woman should telephone her obstetric provider immediately when her membranes rupture as two risks are associated with ruptured membranes: intrauterine infection and prolapse of the umbilical cord (which could cut off the oxygen supply to the fetus) (Maher & Heavey, 2015). In most instances, the fetal head is already snugly fitting the cervix, so prolapse is not a concern. If labor does not spontaneously begin by 24 hours after membrane rupture and the pregnancy is at term, labor will likely be induced to help reduce the risk of infection.

What If . . . 12.4

The nurse is particularly interested in exploring one of the 2020 National Health Goals with respect to fetal and maternal health (see Box 12.1). What would be a possible research topic to explore pertinent to this goal that would be applicable to Julberry or her family and that would also advance evidence-based practice?

KEY POINTS FOR REVIEW

- Prenatal education is an important part of prenatal care. The more women know about measures they should take during pregnancy to safeguard their health, the more likely they will be to avoid substances or activities harmful to fetal growth.

- Urge women to find the best way for them to modify their individual lifestyle for pregnancy as this helps in planning nursing care that not only meets QSEN competencies but also best meets the family's total needs. Remember, pregnancy is 9 months long, so modifications must be agreeable to the woman or she will not maintain them over such a long time.

- Women need to make provisions for rest periods during their day and to be aware of any potential teratogens at a work site, such as exposure to radiation or heavy metals.

- Women who travel should plan for break periods to avoid congestion in their lower extremities. Seat belts should be used when traveling by car. On an airplane, a woman may need to ask for an extension seat belt.

- Common minor body changes of early pregnancy include breast tenderness, constipation, palmar erythema, nausea and vomiting, fatigue, muscle cramps, pain from varicosities or hemorrhoids, heart palpitations, frequency of urination, and leukorrhea. If women know these symptoms may occur, they will not interpret them as complications but usual events.

- Minor body changes of middle or late pregnancy include backache, dyspnea, ankle edema, Braxton Hicks contractions, sleep disturbance, restless leg syndrome, and carpal tunnel syndrome. Caution women that contractions could be a sign of labor.

- Women should take active measures to avoid exposure to infectious diseases such as rubella, HIV, hepatitis B and C, cytomegalovirus, HSV, syphilis, and toxoplasmosis during pregnancy.

- Counsel pregnant women about the necessity to avoid the use of any drug or herbal supplement not specifically approved by their obstetric provider as well as alcohol and tobacco.

- It is almost impossible for a woman to modify a behavior, such as smoking, if her support person does not agree to change also. Including a woman's family in care is an important way to help support persons understand the need for the modification and increasing cooperation.

- Beginning signs of labor for which a pregnant woman should be alert include lightening, show, excess energy, rupture of membranes, and uterine contractions.

CRITICAL THINKING CARE STUDY

Emma Hennigan is a 34-year-old woman who is 3 months pregnant with her second pregnancy. She has a 2-year-old son at home. She tells you this pregnancy has not "been fun" because it is so different from her first pregnancy. She has had nausea, fatigue, and frequent urination 24/7 for the last 3 months. She wants to quit her job as a short-order cook so she can feel better, but her boyfriend won't let her "even consider this" as they need the money. The only thing she does all week to feel "like her old self" or to make the pregnancy "bearable" is to jog around a neighborhood park two times a day.

1. Emma wants to quit work so she feels better. Would you recommend she do this?

2. Emma needs to use a restroom often at work because she has the symptom of frequent urination. This is difficult, however, because this involves a long walk and time away from cooking. She asks if drinking less fluid will help relieve this symptom. How would you advise her?

3. Emma has two breaks during the day during which she jogs—the only activity that is making her pregnancy "bearable." Would you encourage her to continue doing this for the remainder of her pregnancy?

RELATED RESOURCES

Explore these additional resources to enhance learning for this chapter:

- Student resources on thePoint, including answers to the What If . . . and Critical Thinking Care Study questions, http://thepoint.lww.com/Flagg8e
- Adaptive learning powered by PrepU, http://thepoint.lww.com/prepu

REFERENCES

ADA Amendments Act of 2008, Pub. L. 110-325, 122, Stat 3555 (2008).

Agopian, A. J., Tinker, S. C., Lupo, P. J., et al. (2014). Proportion of neural tube defects attributable to known risk factors. *Birth Defects Research Part A: Clinical and Molecular Teratology, 97*(1), 42–46.

Akahira-Azuma, M., Kubota, M., Hosokawa, S., et al. (2015). Republication: Two premature neonates of congenital syphilis with severe clinical manifestations. *Tropical Medicine and Health, 43*(3), 165–170.

American College of Obstetricians and Gynecologists. (2015). Practice Bulletin No. 151: Cytomegalovirus, parvovirus B19, varicella zoster, and toxoplasmosis in pregnancy. *Obstetrics and Gynecology, 125*(6),1510–1525.

Attilakos, G., & Overton, T. G. (2012). Antenatal care. In D. K. Edmonds (Ed.), *Dewhurst's textbook of obstetrics & gynaecology* (6th ed., pp. 42–52). Oxford, United Kingdom: Wiley.

Basta, P., Bak, A., & Roszkowski, K. (2015). Cancer treatment in pregnant women. *Contemporary Oncology, 19*(5), 354–360.

Brent, R. L. (2015). Protection of the gametes embryo/fetus from prenatal radiation exposure. *Health Physics, 108*(2), 242–274.

Camacho-Gonzalez, A. F., Kingbo, M. H., Boylan, A., et al. (2015). Missed opportunities for prevention of mother-to-child transmission in the United States. *AIDS, 29*(12), 1511–1515.

Carr, D. J. (2015). The safety of obstetric acupuncture: Forbidden points revisited. *Acupuncture in Medicine, 33*(5), 413–419.

Centers for Disease Control and Prevention. (2014). *Radiation and pregnancy: A fact sheet for clinicians.* Washington, DC: Author.

Centers for Disease Control and Prevention. (2016). *Pregnancy and rubella.* Retrieved from https://www.cdc.gov/rubella/pregnancy.html

Charness, M. E., Riley, E. P., & Sowell, E. R. (2016). Drinking during pregnancy and the developing brain: Is any amount safe? *Trends in Cognitive Science, 20*(2), 80–82.

Coad, J., & Dunstall, M. (2011). Physiological adaptation to pregnancy. In J. Coad & M. Dunstall (Eds.), *Anatomy & physiology for midwives* (pp. 257–288). London, United Kingdom: Elsevier/Churchill Livingstone.

Coleman, T., Chamberlain, C., Davey, M. A., et al. (2015). Pharmacological interventions for promoting smoking cessation during pregnancy. *Cochrane Database of Systematic Reviews,* (12), CD010078.

Coombes, R. (2016). Attacking the devil: The thalidomide story. *BMJ, 352,* i353.

Demelash, H., Nigatu, D., & Gashaw, K. (2015). A case-control study on intimate partner violence during pregnancy and low birth weight, southeast Ethiopia. *Obstetrics and Gynecology International.* Advance online publication. doi:10.1155/2015/394875

Dórea, J. G. (2015). Maternal risk factors associated with lead, mercury and cadmium. *The Journal of Maternal-Fetal & Neonatal Medicine.* Advance online publication. doi:10.3109/14767058.2015.1118042

Drew, R. J., Stapleton, P., Abu, H., et al. (2015). Pregnancy outcomes of mothers with detectable CMV-specific IgM antibodies: A three-year review in a large Irish tertiary referral maternity hospital. *Infectious Diseases in Obstetrics and Gynecology, 2015,* 218080.

Erdener, U., & Budgett, R. (2016). Exercise and pregnancy: Focus on advice for the competitive and elite athlete. *British Journal of Sports Medicine, 50*(10), 567.

Family and Medical Leave Act of 1993, Pub. L. No. 103-3, 107 Stat. 6 (1993).

Fletcher, W., & Russo, M. L. (2015). Preconception counseling and prenatal care. In J. L. Bienstock, H. Fox, E. E. Wallach, et al. (Eds.), *The Johns Hopkins manual of gynecology and obstetrics* (5th ed., pp. 58–77). Philadelphia, PA: Wolters Kluwer.

Forde, M. S., Dewailly, E., Robertson, L., et al. (2014). Prenatal exposure to persistent organic pollutants and polybrominated diphenyl ethers in 10 Caribbean countries. *Environmental Research, 133,* 211–219.

Forray, A., & Foster, D. (2015). Substance use in the perinatal period. *Current Psychiatry Reports, 17*(11), 1–11.

Goland, S., Perelman, S., Asalih, N., et al. (2015). Shortness of breath during pregnancy: Could a cardiac factor be involved? *Clinical Cardiology, 38*(10), 598–603.

Gormack, A. A., Peek, J. C., Derraik, J. G., et al. (2015). Many women undergoing fertility treatment make poor lifestyle choices that may affect treatment outcome. *Human Reproduction, 30*(7), 1617–1624.

Grant, G. B., Reef, S. E., Dabbagh, A., et al. (2015). Global progress toward rubella and congenital rubella syndrome control and elimination—2000-2014. *Morbidity and Mortality Weekly Report, 64*(37), 1052–1055.

Groves, M. J. (2016). Genital herpes: A review. *American Family Physician, 93*(11), 928–934.

Gupta, S., Jain, A., Mohan, S., et al. (2015). Comparative evaluation of oral health knowledge, practices and attitude of pregnant and non-pregnant women, and their awareness regarding adverse pregnancy outcomes. *Journal of Clinical and Diagnostic Research, 9*(11), ZC26–ZC32.

Haakstad, L. A., Torset, B., & Bø, K. (2016). What is the effect of regular group exercise on maternal psychological outcomes and common pregnancy complaints? An assessor blinded RCT. *Midwifery, 32,* 81–86.

Hampton, M. M. (2015). Congenital toxoplasmosis: A review. *Neonatal Network, 34*(5), 274–278.

Hotchin, R. (2015). The forgotten link between sexual health and pregnancy. *The Practising Midwife, 18*(5), 32–34.

Kafaei Atrian, M., Sadat, Z., Rasolzadeh Bidgoly, M., et al. (2014). The association of sexual intercourse during pregnancy with labor onset. *Iranian Red Crescent Medical Journal, 17*(1), e16465.

Kamarulzaman, A., & Altice, F. L. (2015). Challenges in managing HIV in people who use drugs. *Current Opinion in Infectious Diseases, 28*(1), 10–16.

Karch, A. M. (2015). *Lippincott's nursing drug guide.* Philadelphia, PA: Lippincott Williams & Wilkins.

Latendresse, G., Wong, B., Dyer, J., et al. (2015). Duration of maternal stress and depression: Predictors of newborn admission to neonatal intensive care unit and postpartum depression. *Nursing Research, 64*(5), 331–341.

Lee, L. J., Symanski, E., Lupo, P. J., et al. (2016). Data linkage between the National Birth Defects Prevention Study and the Occupational Information Network (O*NET) to assess workplace physical activity, sedentary behaviors, and emotional stressors during pregnancy. *American Journal of Industrial Medicine, 59*(2), 137–149.

Liddle, S. D., & Pennick, V. (2015). Interventions for preventing and treating low-back and pelvic pain during pregnancy. *Cochrane Database of Systematic Reviews,* (9), CD001139.

Lohsiriwat, V. (2015). Treatment of hemorrhoids: A coloproctologist's view. *World Journal of Gastroenterology, 21*(31), 9245–9252.

Lopez-Medina, E., Cantey, J. B., & Sánchez, P. J. (2015). The mortality of neonatal herpes simplex virus infection. *The Journal of Pediatrics, 166*(6), 1529.e1–1532.e1.

Maher, M. D., & Heavey, E. (2015). When the cord comes first: Umbilical cord prolapse. *Nursing, 45*(7), 53–56.

Maness, D. L., & Khan, M. (2015). Nonpharmacologic management of chronic insomnia. *American Family Physician, 92*(12), 1058–1064

March of Dimes. (2015). *Sex during pregnancy.* White Plains, NY: Author.

Martin, S., & Satin, A. J. (2015). Perinatal infections. In J. L. Bienstock, H. Fox, E. E. Wallach, et al. (Eds.), *The Johns Hopkins manual of gynecology and obstetrics* (5th ed., pp. 146–163). Philadelphia, PA: Wolters Kluwer.

Mohlman, M. K., & Levy, D. T. (2016). Disparities in maternal child and health outcomes attributable to prenatal tobacco use. *Maternal and Child Health Journal, 20*(3), 701–709.

National Center for Complementary and Alternative Medicine. (2010). *Herbs at a glance.* Washington, DC: Author.

National Institute for Occupational Safety and Health. (2010). *Pocket guide to chemical hazards.* Washington, DC: Author.

Nelson-Piercy, C. (2012). Heart disease in pregnancy. In D. K. Edmonds (Ed.), *Dewhurst's textbook of obstetrics & gynaecology* (6th ed., pp. 111–120). Oxford, United Kingdom: Wiley.

Neu, N., Duchon, J., & Zachariah, P. (2015). TORCH infections. *Clinics in Perinatology, 42*(1), 77–103.

Ohno, Y., Terauchi, M., Tamakoshi, K., et al. (2016). The risk factors for labor onset hypertension. *Hypertension Research, 39*(4), 260–265.

Papapanou, P. N. (2015). Systemic effects of periodontitis: Lessons learned from research on atherosclerotic vascular disease and adverse pregnancy outcomes. *International Dental Journal, 65*(6), 283–291.

Perlen, S., Woolhouse, H., Gartland, D., et al. (2013). Maternal depression and physical health problems in early pregnancy: Findings of an Australian nulliparous pregnancy cohort study. *Midwifery, 29*(3), 233–239.

Polis, R. L., Gussman, D., & Kuo, Y. H. (2015). Yoga in pregnancy: An examination of maternal and fetal responses to 26 yoga postures. *Obstetrics and Gynecology, 126*(6), 1237–1241.

Power, M. L., Wilson, E. K., Hogan, S. O., et al. (2013). Patterns of preconception, prenatal and postnatal care for diabetic women by obstetrician-gynecologists. *Journal of Reproductive Medicine, 58*(1–2), 7–14.

Roth, C. K., Satran, L. A., & Smith, S. M. (2015). Marijuana use in pregnancy. *Nursing for Women's Health, 19*(5), 431–437.

Sangsawang, B., & Sangsawang, N. (2015). Is a 6-week supervised pelvic floor muscle exercise program effective in preventing stress urinary incontinence in late pregnancy in primigravid women? A randomized controlled trial. *European Journal of Obstetrics & Gynecology and Reproductive Biology, 197,* 103–110.

Schneider, J., Krafft, A., Manconi, M., et al. (2015). Open-label study of the efficacy and safety of intravenous ferric carboxymaltose in pregnant women with restless legs syndrome. *Sleep Medicine, 16*(11), 1342–1347.

Shah, S. G., & Farrow, A. (2014). Systematic literature review of adverse reproductive outcomes associated with physiotherapists' occupational exposures to non-ionising radiation. *Journal of Occupational Health, 56*(5), 323–331.

Sherbet, G. V. (2015). Therapeutic potential of thalidomide and its analogues in the treatment of cancer. *Anticancer Research, 35*(11), 5767–5772.

Sheth, S., & Keller, J. (2015). Infections of the genital tract. In J. L. Bienstock, H. Fox, E. E. Wallach, et al. (Eds.), *The Johns Hopkins manual of gynecology and obstetrics* (5th ed., pp. 322–348). Philadelphia, PA: Wolters Kluwer.

Siauve, N., Chalouhi, G. E., Deloison, B., et al. (2015). Functional imaging of the human placenta with magnetic resonance. *American Journal of Obstetrics and Gynecology, 213*(4 Suppl.), S103–S114.

Spierings, E. L., & Sabin, T. D. (2016). De novo headache during pregnancy and puerperium. *The Neurologist, 21*(1), 1–7.

Su, J. R., Brooks, L. C., Davis, D. W., et al. (2016). Congenital syphilis: Trends in mortality and morbidity in the United States, 1999 through 2013. *American Journal of Obstetrics and Gynecology, 214*(3), 381.e1–381.e9.

Sukumaran, L., McCarthy, N. L., Kharbanda, E. O., et al. (2015). Safety of tetanus toxoid, reduced diphtheria toxoid, and acellular pertussis and influenza vaccinations in pregnancy. *Obstetrics and Gynecology, 126*(5), 1069–1074.

Tinto, H., Sevene, E., Dellicour, S., et al. (2015). Assessment of the safety of antimalarial drug use during early pregnancy (ASAP): Protocol for a multicenter prospective cohort study in Burkina Faso, Kenya and Mozambique. *Reproductive Health, 12*(1), 1–9.

Tsai, S. Y., Lin, J. W., Wu, W. W., et al. (2016). Sleep disturbances and symptoms of depression and daytime sleepiness in pregnant women. *Birth, 43*(2), 176–183.

Tucker, R. (2014). Advising pregnant women on miminising travel risks. *Nursing Times, 110*(14), 19–21.

United Nations. (2015). *The millennium development goals report 2015, summary.* New York, NY: Author.

U.S. Department of Health and Human Services. (2010). *Healthy people 2020.* Washington, DC: Author.

U.S. Food and Drug Administration. (n.d.). *FDA pregnancy categories.* Washington, DC: Author.

van den Akker, T., & van Roosmalen, J. (2016). Maternal mortality and severe morbidity in a migration perspective. Best Practice & Research. *Clinical Obstetrics & Gynaecology, 32*, 26–38.

Varothai, S., & Bergfeld, W. (2014). Androgenetic alopecia: An evidence-based treatment update. *American Journal of Clinical Dermatology, 15*(3), 217–230.

Wahlqvist, M. L., Krawetz, S. A., Rizzo, N. S., et al. (2015). Early-life influences on obesity: From preconception to adolescence. *Annals of the New York Academy of Sciences, 1347*, 1–28.

Wang, X., Xu, J. M., Zhou, F., et al. (2015). Maternal position and development of hypotension in patients undergoing cesarean section under combined spinal-epidural anesthesia of intrathecal hyperbaric ropivacaine. *Medical Science Monitor, 21*, 52–58.

Wilde, J. J., Petersen, J. R., & Niswander, L. (2014). Genetic, epigenetic, and environmental contributions to neural tube closure. *Annual Review of Genetics, 48*, 583–611.

Żelaźniewicz, A., & Pawłowski, B. (2015). Breast size and asymmetry during pregnancy in dependence of a fetus's sex. *American Journal of Human Biology, 27*(5), 690–696.

Zhou, K., West, H. M., Zhang, J., et al. (2015). Interventions for leg cramps in pregnancy. *Cochrane Database of Systematic Reviews,* (8), CD010655.

Zielinski, R., Searing, K., & Deibel, M. (2015). Gastrointestinal distress in pregnancy: Prevalence, assessment, and treatment of 5 common minor discomforts. *The Journal of Perinatal & Neonatal Nursing, 29*(1), 23–31.

13

The Nursing Role in Promoting Nutritional Health During Pregnancy

KEY TERMS

bariatric surgery

body mass index

complete protein

Hawthorne effect

hypercholesterolemia

hyperplasia

hypertrophy

incomplete protein

lactase

obese

overweight

pica

pyrosis

underweight

Tori Alarino, 19 years old, is 4 months pregnant. She works at a fast-food restaurant and eats breakfast and lunch at the restaurant. Her partner, Alessa, works four evenings a week, so Tori cooks for herself on those evenings. She dislikes milk, so she drinks milkshakes as a source of calcium. She is concerned because she has already gained 23 lb. She craves oranges, eating six to eight of them a day. She tells you, "I thought pregnant women always craved pickles and ice cream. What's wrong with me?"

Previous chapters described reproductive normal anatomy and physiology, the changes associated with pregnancy, and common discomforts and danger signs of pregnancy. This chapter adds information about prenatal nutrition, an important aspect to help ensure a healthy outcome for both a woman and her child.

What nutritional counseling does Tori need?

OBJECTIVES

After mastering the contents of this chapter, you should be able to:

1. Discuss recommendations for healthy nutrition during pregnancy.
2. Identify 2020 National Health Goals related to pregnancy nutrition that nurses can help the nation achieve.
3. Assess a woman for nutritional adequacy during pregnancy.
4. Formulate nursing diagnoses related to nutritional concerns during pregnancy.
5. Develop expected outcomes to assist a pregnant woman to achieve optimal nutrition during pregnancy as well as manage seamless transitions across differing healthcare settings.
6. Using the nursing process, plan nursing care that includes the six competencies of Quality & Safety Education for Nurses (QSEN): Patient-Centered Care, Teamwork & Collaboration, Evidence-Based Practice (EBP), Quality Improvement (QI), Safety, and Informatics.
7. Implement nursing care that encourages healthy nutritional practices during pregnancy.
8. Evaluate outcomes for achievement and effectiveness of nursing care to be certain expected outcomes have been achieved.
9. Integrate knowledge of nutrition and pregnancy with the interplay of nursing process, the six competencies of QSEN, and Family Nursing to promote quality maternal and child health nursing care.

Figure 13.1 The Choose MyPlate guide to healthy eating. Note that the word protein is substituted for meat; vegetables occupy the largest portion on the plate. (From U.S. Department of Agriculture. [2012]. *Choose my plate: A guide to daily food choices.* Washington, DC: Author.)

Although adequate nutrition during pregnancy cannot guarantee a good pregnancy outcome, it does make an important contribution because both the nutritional state a woman brings into pregnancy and her nutrition during pregnancy have a direct bearing on her health and on fetal growth and development. A poor diet, such as one deficient in folic acid before and during pregnancy, for example, is associated with fetal growth restriction or birth anomalies such as neural tube defects (Atta, Fiest, Frolkis, et al., 2016).

Good nutrition during pregnancy is recognized as so important that the subject is addressed in 2020 National Health Goals (Box 13.1).

Nursing Process Overview

FOR PROMOTING NUTRITIONAL HEALTH DURING PREGNANCY

ASSESSMENT

An assessment begins with a woman's preconception nutrition patterns. From this assessment, determine whether a patient is eating healthy food sources and healthy proportions of food (Fig. 13.1). Also, evaluate any cultural, environmental, or social lifestyles that could affect eating habits. A 24-hour recall history followed by a physical examination to document weight and vitality are the best ways to secure necessary information, confirm well-balanced nutrition, and identify areas for teaching and learning.

NURSING DIAGNOSIS

Nursing diagnoses related to the nutritional status of a pregnant woman consider the desired health and growth of both the fetus and the woman. A woman who is eating large amounts of

nutritionally inferior food and a woman who has difficulty eating because of fatigue or nausea may both be at risk for the same problem: fetal growth restriction. Being sensitive to a woman's concern about maintaining her own appearance can help her keep a healthy perspective about "eating for two" and the need to gain sufficient weight. Examples of nursing diagnoses include:

- Imbalanced nutrition, less than body requirements, related to increased physiologic needs
- Imbalanced nutrition, less than body requirements, related to nausea every morning
- Health-seeking behaviors related to determining best food choices in pregnancy
- Imbalanced nutrition, more than body requirements, related to overeating or poor food choices
- Deficient knowledge related to need for increased intake of nutrients and calories during pregnancy

OUTCOME IDENTIFICATION AND PLANNING

In large health centers, nutritionists are available to meet with women prenatally and help them plan nutrition during pregnancy. In other settings, a nutritionist may be available only for women with special needs, so the responsibility for nutrition advice falls directly on nurses. When helping a woman set expected outcomes for improving her nutrition, be certain to consider all the cultural and lifestyle factors that give different meanings to food. Because food is an expensive commodity, consider financial resources as well. Teaching about long-term outcomes such as building iron stores or bone mass is as important as short-term goals, such as to eat better for a week. Eating more nutritious foods for a week will probably not lead to a radical change. However, continuing a healthy eating pattern throughout the pregnancy (and maintaining it throughout life) will bring about important changes and help prepare a woman for feeding her family nutritionally for the years to come. Refer to helpful websites and other resources when appropriate (see Chapter 9).

IMPLEMENTATION

As anyone who has ever tried to change a nutritional pattern knows, this can be a lonely and seemingly unrewarding endeavor as results occur slowly. Begin by emphasizing the physiologic basis for nutritional needs in pregnancy (a woman is building a whole new person). Based on this, explain what nutritional deficits you have identified and then show the woman how to change her nutritional pattern to improve this situation.

Pregnant women are usually highly motivated to adopt healthy behaviors for the sake of their baby's health; although they still need support and encouragement because this can involve a major life change, such as eating a different lunch than everyone around them is eating, getting up 15 minutes earlier to prepare breakfast rather than just dashing to work with only coffee, or resisting having a soft drink with dinner and drinking a calcium-fortified drink, like almond milk, instead.

Asking women to list what foods they eat daily and to bring in a chart to show you at a prenatal visit is an effective motivating technique. In research studies, this is called a **Hawthorne effect**, or a positive change in behavior that occurs because of the attention received. Because of this effect, the average woman will eat better than she usually does so her list of food looks better when she presents it. As soon as she realizes these better eating patterns are making her feel better, she will hopefully continue them indefinitely.

OUTCOME EVALUATION

When evaluating whether a woman's nutritional pattern has been improved, rely on the most important assessments: weight, energy level, general appearance, bowel function, hydration status, and, when available, hemoglobin and urinalysis findings. Urge women to be honest about whether they are actually following a nutrition plan. If they are not, it probably means the plan did not fit their lifestyle or degree of motivation. Examples of outcomes that would demonstrate improved nutrition include:

- Patient demonstrates weekly menus that include three main meals and two snacks per day.
- By next prenatal visit, patient demonstrates knowledge of meat and nonmeat sources of protein by providing menus of meals eaten in the last week that include fish, eggs, beans, or peanut butter.
- Patient verbalizes correct information about calcium needs during pregnancy.
- Patient states she is able to make up later in the day meals missed because of nausea.
- Patient's food lists for 1 week include three sources of calcium per day.
- Patient describes pattern she is using to drink at least eight glasses of fluid daily.

Relationship of Maternal Nutrition and Fetal Health

During pregnancy, a woman must eat adequately to not only support her own nutrition but also to supply enough nutrients so the fetus can grow. Adequate protein and calcium intake is vital because so much of these are needed by the fetus to build a strong body framework. Adequate protein may also help prevent complications of pregnancy such as gestational hypertension or preterm birth. Either deficiencies or overuse of vitamins may contribute to poor intrauterine growth (Johnston, Sharma, & Abe, 2016). Therefore, a pregnant woman should be counseled to consult her primary care provider prior to taking any new vitamin or herbal supplement aside from her prescribed prenatal vitamin.

Early in pregnancy, fetal growth occurs largely by an increase in the number of cells formed (**hyperplasia**); late in pregnancy, it occurs mainly by enlargement of existing cells (**hypertrophy**). This means a fetus deprived of adequate nutrition early in pregnancy could be small for gestational age because of an inadequate number of cells formed in the body. Later on, although the number of cells may be normal, restricted growth can occur because cells cannot grow to their full potential. To ensure early pregnancy deficiencies do not occur, encourage women of childbearing age to follow a healthy nutrition plan before pregnancy (preconception care) that specifically supplies adequate folic acid (400 µg/day) (Fletcher & Russo, 2015). Otherwise, in the time before a woman recognizes she is pregnant (about 6 weeks), her poor diet and lack of important nutrient stores could already have seriously impaired fetal growth (Atta et al., 2016).

Pregnancy provides opportune nutrition "teaching moments" as a woman finds herself suddenly more interested in her weight and well-being than usual (C. L. Martin, Siega-Riz, Sotres-Alvarez, et al., 2016). Always comment on the things a woman is doing correctly rather than what she is doing wrong. Positive reinforcement, a basic rule of teaching, enhances learning, self-esteem, and compliance more than criticism. Remember, women will have some degree of nutritional "backsliding" on holidays and special events. To help prevent this, a woman needs to make definite, concrete plans for what foods to avoid as well as how to substitute healthy foods for them.

Be careful when nutrition counseling not to make general statements such as "Eat high-protein foods." Food in the supermarket, after all, is not labeled "high protein"; it's labeled meat, cheese, and so forth. Based on this, provide advice whenever possible in more specific terms such as "Eat three servings of some type of protein, like meat, eggs, fish, beans or nuts, every day." An effective counseling session should also include teaching the patient how to read a food label and adequately measure serving size.

The word "diet" has come to mean a form of unpleasant food denial for most women. Rather than talk about a "pregnancy diet," therefore, talk about "foods that are best for you during pregnancy" or "pregnancy nutrition." These terms not only sound more positive but also refer more closely to what you are encouraging a woman to do: Eat healthy meals.

Giving a woman a clearly written list of suggested foods may be a help to some women. Be certain a list of that type is short, clear, and specific. Complicated lists of foods or a list of don'ts tend to be overwhelming and, therefore, ignored.

RECOMMENDED WEIGHT GAIN DURING PREGNANCY

One of the things women begin to wonder about when they first realize they are pregnant is how much weight they will gain during pregnancy. As a rule, the average woman should gain 11.3 to 15.8 kg (25 to 35 lb) during pregnancy. To predict individual weight gain, first calculate a woman's

BOX 13.2
Nursing Care Planning Using Assessment

ASSESSING MATERNAL WEIGHT GAIN

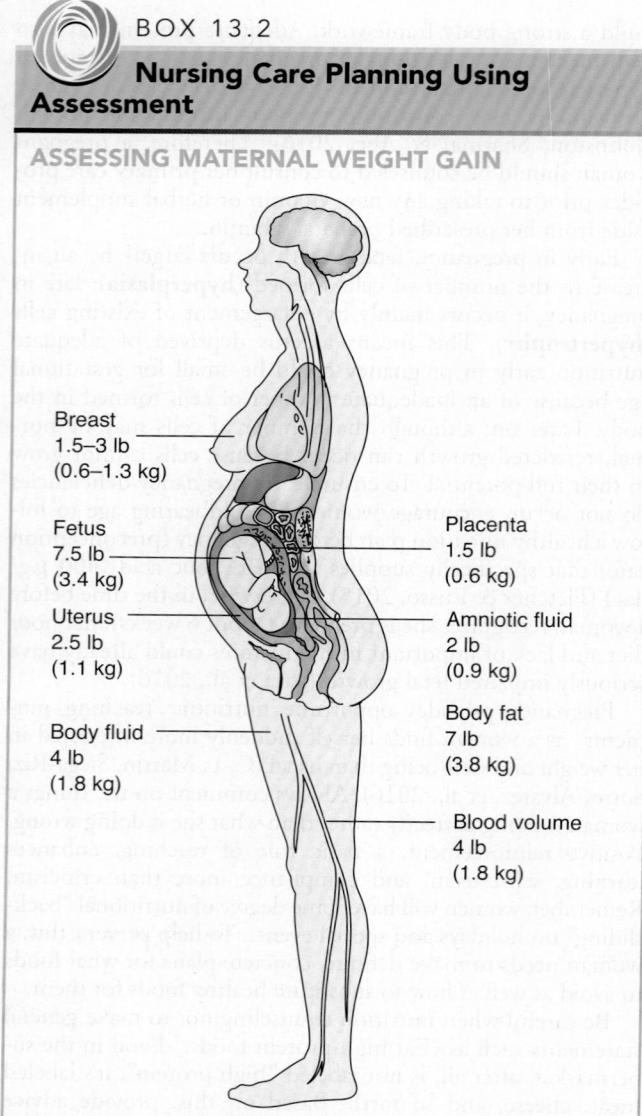

Breast
1.5–3 lb
(0.6–1.3 kg)

Fetus
7.5 lb
(3.4 kg)

Uterus
2.5 lb
(1.1 kg)

Body fluid
4 lb
(1.8 kg)

Placenta
1.5 lb
(0.6 kg)

Amniotic fluid
2 lb
(0.9 kg)

Body fat
7 lb
(3.8 kg)

Blood volume
4 lb
(1.8 kg)

body mass index (BMI) or the ratio of body fat to weight and height. This can be done most easily by visiting a web-sites such as the one run by the National Heart, Lung and Blood Institute (www.nhlbi.nih.gov/health/educational/lose _wt/BMI/bmicalc.htm). A BMI calculator for children and teenagers can be found at www.apps.nccd.cdc.gov/dnpabmi /calculator.aspx.

Women whose weight falls into the normal BMI category (18.5 to 24.9) should aim to gain 25 to 35 lb; **underweight** women or those whose BMI is less than 18.5 should gain 28 to 40 lb; **overweight** women (a BMI over 25 to 29.9) should gain 15 to 25 lb; and **obese** women (a BMI over 30) should gain 11 to 20 lb (Institute of Medicine [IOM] & National Research Council, 2009).

Weight gain in pregnancy occurs from both fetal growth and an accumulation of maternal stores (Box 13.2) and in-creases by approximately 0.8 kg (1.5 lb) per month during the first trimester and then 0.4 kg (1 lb) per week during the last two trimesters (a trimester minimum weight gain of 4.5 lb, 12 lb, and 12 lb, respectively). Although this may seem to be a lot of weight gain, women can be assured most of the weight gained with pregnancy is easily lost afterward.

- To ensure adequate fetal nutrition, advise women not to diet to lose weight during pregnancy.
- A woman who reaches the midpoint of pregnancy and has gained less than 10 lb needs to have her daily nutri-tion intake reevaluated as low weight gain is associated with fetal growth restriction.
- Even obese women need to gain a minimum of 0.5 lb per week or 11 to 15 lb total to help ensure adequate fetal growth.
- Weight gain will be higher for a multiple pregnancy than for a single pregnancy (Table 13.1). You can encourage women who are pregnant with multiple fetuses to gain at least 1 lb per week for a total of 37 to 54 lb.
- Sudden increases in weight suggest fluid retention or polyhydramnios (excessive amniotic fluid); a loss of weight suggests illness and should also be carefully eval-uated at prenatal visits.

The Woman Who Is Underweight

A woman who enters a pregnancy underweight needs nu-tritional counseling just as much as an overweight woman. Underweight is defined as a state in which a woman's weight is 10% to 15% less than the ideal weight for her height, or a BMI of less than 18.5. Most women who are underweight tire easily because they have an accompanying iron-deficiency anemia. Even when underweight women gain more weight than usual during a pregnancy, they still tend to have a higher than usual incidence of low–birth-weight infants and preterm birth (Akahoshi, Arima, Miura, et al., 2016). This is one reason why preconception healthcare visits and assessments are so important.

TABLE 13.1 TOTAL WEIGHT GAIN DURING PREGNANCY, BY PREPREGNANCY BODY MASS INDEX (BMI)

Prepregnancy BMI	BMI+ (kg/m²) (WHO)	Total Weight Gain Range (lb) Single Fetus	Total Weight Gain Range (lb) Multiple Fetuses[a]
Underweight	<18.5	28–40	
Normal weight	18.5–24.9	25–35	37–54
Overweight	25.0–29.9	15–25	31–50
Obese (includes all classes)	≥30.0	11–20	25–42

WHO, World Health Organization.
[a]Weight gain recommendations for multiple fetuses are provisional.
Institute of Medicine & National Research Council. (2009). *Weight gain during pregnancy: Reexamining the guidelines.* Washington, DC: The National Academies Press.

Women may be underweight for a variety of reasons, including:

- Dieting for weight loss
- Inability to buy adequate food while impoverished (however, many low-income women are obese rather than underweight because starchy foods are less expensive than those with a higher protein content, such as meat and eggs)
- Excessive worry or stress, which can lead to a loss of appetite
- Depression, which can cause a chronic loss of appetite
- An eating disorder, such as anorexia nervosa or bulimia, in which a woman has developed an unhealthy relationship with food (Kimmel, Ferguson, Zerwas, et al., 2016) (see Chapter 54)

The primary reason women are underweight, however, is insufficient intake of food because of chronic, poor nutritional habits.

Convincing women who are underweight to eat more may be difficult because you are asking women to change lifelong eating habits. Counseling also can be challenging because you are asking her to take in additional food during the first trimester of pregnancy when fetal need is greatest and a woman has nausea and vomiting.

Begin counseling by asking a woman for a 24-hour nutrition recall. Total daily caloric intake for the underweight woman may need to be as high as 3,200 calories (500 to 1,000 calories more than the usual specified daily amount). Work with women to develop menus based on well-planned meals rather than on quick take-out foods. Suggest additional calories in the form of a concentrated formula such as an instant liquid breakfast drink. Be certain a woman understands that this should not be a high-protein drink used for high-protein dieting regimens. High-protein diets of this nature are not recommended for long-term use by anyone, but they should be completely avoided by women during pregnancy.

A 500-calorie increase over normal requirements should result in a weight gain of an additional pound per week. Be certain to plan for this additional gain when the total weight gain during pregnancy is calculated at each office visit. Otherwise, the total weight gain of a woman may seem excessive when it is actually healthy.

If a lack of nutritional stores makes a woman feel tired, urge her to schedule adequate rest periods daily so she can feel sufficiently energetic to prepare nutritious meals. Be certain she is taking her prescribed vitamin and iron supplements. Additional nutritional counseling during the postpartum period may be necessary so she can maintain better nutrition throughout her life and enter a subsequent pregnancy (if she desires one) in a state of nutritional health.

The Woman Who Is Overweight

A woman is considered overweight if she is 20% above ideal weight or has a BMI over 25. She is considered obese if she is 50% above ideal body weight for height, or her BMI is above 30. As many as 60% of women in the United States are overweight; 35% are obese (Centers for Disease Control and Prevention [CDC], 2016). Less-educated women and those living in poverty tend to be more overweight than others. Obesity during pregnancy is serious because it is associated with an increased incidence of gestational diabetes and gestational hypertension (Simhan, 2016).

Although obesity may occur from hypothyroidism, it most often occurs as a result of excessive caloric intake and decreased energy expenditure. It becomes a problem during pregnancy because:

- Pregnancy causes circulatory volume to increase by 20% to 50% and metabolism to increase to meet the demands of the pregnancy, placing additional stress on a possibly already overworked body.
- It is often difficult to hear fetal heart tones in an obese woman; palpating for position and size of a fetus at birth is also difficult.
- Obese women are at increased risk for giving birth to infants with macrosomia (excessive fetal growth); this increases the incidence of cesarean births in this population (Declercq, MacDorman, Osterman, et al., 2015).
- Performing a cesarean birth, if necessary, may be difficult because of the excessive adipose tissue that must be incised to reach the uterus.
- The pregnancies of obese women are more apt to be prolonged, leading to postmature infants.
- Ambulating during pregnancy and immediately afterward is more difficult because of the increased energy expenditure necessary, increasing the risk of complications such as thrombophlebitis and pneumonia.
- Many overweight women are hypertensive when they enter pregnancy and develop severe gestational hypertension (Stang & Huffman, 2016).

Most obesity is caused by overeating, but the habit of overeating has many causes. For some women, overeating is a habit learned in childhood when they were told to "clean their plate"; for others, it is a coping mechanism for stress. Because pregnancy can be stressful, it may be a particularly difficult time for a woman to change her food intake pattern. If a woman has been serving her family, as well as herself, an excessive amount of calories, then the entire family may have to change their eating pattern to bring about a change in a woman's intake. The children of obese women also tend to be obese probably because of excessive food served to them combined with the lack of physical exercise (Saltzman, Pineros-Leano, Liechty, et al., 2016).

Dieting to reduce weight is not recommended during pregnancy. If carbohydrates are reduced too much, the body will use protein and fat for energy, thus depriving the fetus of protein for growth (Bodnar, Siminerio, Himes, 2016), which can also lead to ketoacidosis. Although the long-term effects of mild ketoacidosis on a fetus are not well studied, it can be avoided if the daily caloric intake, even in the most obese woman, does not go below 1,500 to 1,800 per day.

Overweight women tend to exercise less than women of normal weight. Try to encourage all pregnant women, including overweight or obese women, to engage in an exercise program, such as walking, in conjunction with dietary changes.

Helping a woman look at her nutrition in terms of empty calorie versus nutritious foods may help her to eat less fatty and more protein-rich foods. Early in pregnancy, when she is eager to appear pregnant, may be the most difficult time to limit intake. Stress that a fetus grows best on nutritious foods, not necessarily those with the most calories. Provide additional nutritional counseling in the postpartum period so she can prepare more nutritious meals in the future for herself and her growing family. If successful, she will not enter another pregnancy severely overweight.

The Woman Who Is Morbidly Obese

When a woman weighs over 300 lb or has a BMI over 40, she is classified as morbidly obese. During a pregnancy, she presents with a series of special care problems because she is even more prone to complications of pregnancy, such as:

- Gestational or type 2 diabetes
- Hypertension
- Back pain
- Thrombophlebitis or thromboembolism (she may be prescribed support hose to aid lower leg circulation)
- Difficulty sleeping or sleep apnea (which may make her feel tired over and above normal pregnancy fatigue)
- Difficulty hearing fetal heart sounds and palpating for fetal position
- Difficulty exercising
- Prolonged pregnancy with a high rate of cesarean birth (Renes, Barka, Gyurkovits, et al., 2017)

Children born of an obese mother may develop obesity, diabetes, and cardiovascular diseases later in life at a higher proportion than average weight women (Barbour, 2014).

At a prenatal visit, morbidly obese women may need special care equipment furnished for them such as a wider examining table, a larger examining gown, a wider wheelchair, and longer straps for fetal monitoring equipment than usual. Be discreet when arranging for this type of equipment for a woman as she may be sensitive to her appearance and weight.

Although women with morbid obesity generally eat larger amounts of food, take a nutrition history to be assured their larger intake includes protein-rich, not empty-calorie, foods.

COMPONENTS OF HEALTHY NUTRITION FOR THE PREGNANT WOMAN

The old saying that a pregnant woman must "eat for two" is not as much a myth as it is a truism. It does not mean, however, a woman should eat enough for two adults, just enough to provide nutrients for herself and a growing fetus. To do this, many women will not have to increase by much the quantity of food they eat, but they will have to increase the quality.

A good way to feel assured a woman is eating the right kinds of foods during pregnancy is to compare the foods she eats to the U.S. Department of Agriculture (USDA, 2012) food guidelines (see Fig. 13.1).

Common suggestions for a healthy intake are shown in Box 13.3. When discussing nutrition and portion size using a representative plate, remember to refer to servings of food rather than milligrams or percentages because this is how a woman will measure the amount she plans to eat.

Energy (Calorie) Needs

The average recommended daily allowance (RDA) of calories for women of childbearing age is 2,200. An additional 300 calories, or a total caloric intake of 2,500 calories, is recommended to meet the increased needs of pregnancy (Whitney & Rolfes, 2016). In addition to supplying energy for a fetus, this increase provides calories to sustain an elevated metabolic rate in the mother because of increased thyroid function and her increased workload from the extra weight she carries. If a woman should begin restricting her carbohydrate intake so her calorie intake is below this in order to avoid gaining weight, her body will begin to break down protein to supply energy, depriving a fetus of essential protein, and possibly resulting in ketoacidosis,

BOX 13.3

Nursing Care Planning to Empower a Family

Healthy Eating Begins With Building a Healthy Plate of Food

- Fill half of your plate with fruits and vegetables.
- Switch to skim or 1% milk.
- Make at least half of your grains whole grains.
- Vary your protein food choices so you include lean sources.

Cut Back on Foods High in Solid Fats, Added Sugars, and Salt

- Read food labels and eliminate foods high in sodium.
- Try to eliminate foods high in solid (saturated) fat.

Eat the Right Amount of Calories for You

- Enjoy your food but eat less.
- Cook more often at home, where you are in control of what's in your food.
- When eating out, choose lower calorie menu options.

Model Good Nutrition

- Provide healthy snacks as well as healthy meals.
- Remember that you are your children's most important role model.
- Don't just tell children to eat their vegetables—show them that you eat and enjoy vegetables every day.

a possible cause of fetal growth restriction and newborn neurologic disorders.

Advise women to obtain their carbohydrate calories from complex carbohydrates (cereals and grains) rather than simple carbohydrates (sugar and sweets) because complex carbohydrates are more slowly digested. Doing so will help regulate glucose and insulin levels more consistently. Do not recommend sugar substitutes for women during pregnancy because a pregnant woman needs sugar to maintain glucose levels. Even obese women should never consume fewer than 1,500 calories per day (Whitney & Rolfes, 2016).

When helping a woman plan an increased caloric intake, consider her lifestyle. For example, many women commonly skip meals, have erratic eating patterns, or rely on fast and convenience foods. During pregnancy, in addition to carbohydrate calories, a woman needs protein calories furnished by eating foods rich not only in protein but also in fat, iron, and other essential nutrients. Suggest preparing snacks such as carrot sticks or cheese and crackers early in the day, when fatigue is usually less, and keeping them readily available in the refrigerator. Otherwise, later in the day when she is tired, a woman may snack on empty-calorie foods such as pretzels and doughnuts simply because they require no preparation.

Measuring fundal height at prenatal visits is an indirect way to assess if a woman's nutrition intake is adequate. The easiest method for determining if a woman's caloric intake is adequate is assessing if she is gaining weight. Keep in mind a woman's weight gain pattern is as important as the total weight gain. Even if a woman has surpassed her target weight before the end of the third trimester, encourage her not to restrict her caloric intake. She should continue to gain weight because a fetus grows rapidly during these final weeks.

Protein Needs

The RDA for protein in women is 34 to 46 g. During pregnancy, the need for protein increases to 71 g daily. If protein needs are met, overall nutritional needs are likely to be met as well (with the possible exceptions of vitamins A, C, and D) because of the high incorporation of other nutrients with protein foods. If protein intake is inadequate, iron, B vitamins, calcium, and phosphorus also will probably be inadequate. Vitamin B_{12} is found almost exclusively in animal protein, so if animal protein is excluded from the diet, vitamin B_{12} deficiency can occur unless this is supplemented. This is why it is important to ascertain whether your patient follows a vegetarian or vegan diet during your initial assessment. Such a diet may lead to serious vitamin deficiencies that can affect both the mother and fetus unless supplements are added.

Meat, poultry, fish, yogurt, eggs, and milk best supply extra protein because the protein in these forms contains all nine essential amino acids required (**complete proteins**). The protein in nonanimal sources does not contain all essential amino acids (and so is an **incomplete protein** source). It is possible to provide all amino acids by combining nonanimal or incomplete proteins. Proteins that when cooked together provide all essential amino acids are termed *complementary proteins*. Examples are beans and rice, legumes and rice, or beans and wheat.

A woman with a family history of high cholesterol levels (**hypercholesterolemia**) probably should not eat more than two or three eggs per week. She also should monitor her intake of red meat because of the high cholesterol content. Encourage such women to eat lean meat, to cook with olive oil instead of lard or butter, and to remove the skin from poultry to reduce its fat content. She also should not eat lunch meats such as bologna or salami as food staples because their protein content may not be high, their fat content is invariably exceptionally high, and they may be a source of *Listeria*, a bacteria harmful to fetal growth (Pfaff & Tillett, 2016).

Milk is another rich source of protein. Unfortunately, some women resist drinking it because it can be high in calories and fat. Others cannot drink it because of lactose intolerance. Women who are lactose intolerant can add a lactase supplement to milk (which predigests milk and makes it possible for them to drink it without discomfort) or substitute soy milk (Sethi, Tyagi, & Anurag, 2016). Nonfat milk supplies the same amount of protein as regular milk with half the calories of regular milk and so can be recommended. Buttermilk, although it contains a large amount of sodium, can also be substituted for milk; chocolate or another flavoring can be added to make milk palatable. Yogurt, cheese, cream soup, custards, and eggnogs are yet other good substitutes for milk.

QSEN Checkpoint Question 13.1

TEAMWORK & COLLABORATION

Tori Alarino has a BMI of 25 and is considered to be slightly overweight. The interprofessional team should recommend what range of weight gain during her pregnancy?
 a. 10 to 12 lb
 b. 15 to 25 lb
 c. 30 to 35 lb
 d. 40 to 60 lb

Look in Appendix A for the best answer and rationale.

Fat Needs

Omega-3 fatty acids, particularly linoleic acid, are fats that are essential for new cell growth but that cannot be manufactured by the body. Vegetable oils such as safflower, corn, olive, peanut, and cottonseed; fatty fish; omega-3–infused eggs; and omega-3–infused spreads are all good sources (Lauritzen, Brambilla, Mazzocchi, et al., 2016). Pregnant women should ingest 200 and 300 mg of omega-3 fatty acids daily. An added advantage of using vegetable oils rather than animal-based oils (butter) is that they have low cholesterol contents. For this reason, they are recommended for all adults as a means of preventing hypercholesterolemia and coronary heart disease. Because some fish may be contaminated by mercury, alert women that the American Pregnancy Association (APA) recommends that marlin, orange roughy, tilefish, swordfish, shark, king mackerel, and bigeye and yellowfin tuna should be avoided during pregnancy. For information regarding other types of fish, the Natural Resources Defense Council has a list of fish and their mercury levels all women can assess to be informed on what they are consuming (APA, 2016).

Vitamin Needs

The intake of vitamins as a daily dietary supplement has become common place. Many women will already be taking a woman's multivitamin, or, if they were intending pregnancy, a prenatal vitamin (Box 13.4). Although the requirements for both fat- and water-soluble vitamins increase during pregnancy to support the growth of new fetal cells, there is new evidence that supplementation with a multivitamin does not improve maternal or fetal outcomes. The best way for a woman to help ensure she and her baby have necessary nutrients is by consuming a well-balanced diet. Folic acid is the only vitamin recommended for daily supplementation as the evidence is clear that adequate folic acid helps prevent neural tube defects (World Health Organization [WHO], 2016). Vitamin requirements are discussed in greater detail in Table 13.2.

Mineral Needs

Minerals are necessary for building new cells in a fetus. Because they are found in so many foods and because mineral absorption appears to improve during pregnancy, mineral deficiency, with the exception of iron, is rare. Mineral requirements are discussed in Table 13.3.

What If . . . 13.1

Tori Alarino insists drinking milkshakes is a good source of calcium. How would the nurse advise her?

Fiber Needs

Constipation can occur during pregnancy because bowel peristalsis slows due to the effect of progesterone and pressure of the uterus on the intestine. Eating fiber-rich foods (i.e., foods consisting of parts of the plant cell wall resistant to normal digestive enzymes such as fruit, broccoli, and asparagus) is a natural way to prevent constipation because the bulk of the fiber left in the intestine aids evacuation. Fiber also has the advantage of lowering cholesterol levels and may remove carcinogenic contaminants from the intestine. Eating fiber-rich foods this way is a better choice for preventing constipation

BOX 13.4

Nursing Care Planning Based on Responsibility for Pharmacology

PRENATAL VITAMINS (MATERNA)

Action: A vitamin and mineral combination used to treat or prevent a lack of vitamins or minerals before, during, and after pregnancy and during breastfeeding. The folic acid content helps prevent megaloblastic anemia in the mother and neural tube defects in the fetus.

Ingredients: Selected ingredients are vitamin A (1,000 International Units), vitamin D (400 Units), vitamin E (30 International Units), vitamin C (85 mg), vitamin B_1 (1.4 mg), vitamin B_2 (1.4 mg), vitamin B_6 (1.9 mg), vitamin B_{12} (2.6 mcg), niacin (18 mg), folic acid (1 mg), pantothenic acid (6 mg), calcium (250 mg), iron (27 mg), copper (1 mg), zinc (7.5 mg), and magnesium (50 mg) (Wyeth Ayerst Pharmaceuticals, 2012).

Dosage: One tablet daily prior to conception, during pregnancy, and when breastfeeding

Possible Side Effects: Nausea, bloating

Possible Adverse Effects: Folic acid may mask the signs of pernicious anemia.

Nursing Implications

- A woman should start taking a prenatal multivitamin at least 10 weeks prior to conception (when she is trying to conceive or planning a pregnancy). She should continue to take this until she stops breastfeeding.
- Tablets are best taken with a meal to help the tablet disintegrate and to maximize nutrient absorption as well as to minimize the potential for gastrointestinal upset among women sensitive to iron.
- If a woman has difficulty swallowing a tablet, she can crush it and mix the crushed tablet in a liquid such as milk or fruit juice.
- Materna can be purchased without a prescription so women can begin taking the medication preconception or before they have made a prenatal healthcare visit.
- Encourage women to take the medication exactly as prescribed; caution women not to exceed the recommended dosage.
- Assist with ways to remind women to take the medication, such as a note on the refrigerator.
- Advise women to keep prenatal vitamins, like all medications, out of the reach of small children to prevent accidental poisoning from the high folate level.

TABLE 13.2 VITAMIN NEEDS FOR THE PREGNANT WOMAN

Vitamin	Essential Functions	Signs of Deficiency	Relevant Foods and Supplementation	Recommended Amounts	Evidence-Based Evaluation
Vitamin D	Aids calcium absorption, formation of bones/teeth, and immune function	Low birth weight, increased rates of preeclampsia	Fortified milk, eggs, salmon	No standard, suggested 600 IU daily	Not recommended to improve maternal or perinatal outcomes by WHO; concern for adverse effects—fat-soluble vitamin
Vitamin A	New cell growth, healthy skin, oral health, vision	Tender gums or tongues, cracks in skin around mouth, poor night vision	Dark green and yellow vegetables and fruits, liver, milk, butter, cheese, eggs	In areas where vitamin A deficiency is a severe public health problem: 10,000 IU daily or 25,000 IU weekly	Not recommended to improve maternal or perinatal outcomes by WHO; only to improve night vision during pregnancy; concern for overdose—fat-soluble vitamin
Vitamin C	Antioxidant, collagen formation	Scurvy, easy bruising, swollen and bleeding gums	Fresh vegetables and fruit	Suggested 85 mg daily	No benefit seen with standard supplementation with vitamin C; not recommended to improve maternal or perinatal outcomes by WHO
Folic acid	Red blood cell formation, prevents neural tube defects	Megaloblastic anemia, fetal neural tube defects	Fresh vegetables and fruit	400 μg daily	Clear evidence of benefit, WHO recommends daily supplementation

IU, International Units; WHO, World Health Organization.

De-Regil, L. M., Palacios, C., Lombardo, L. K., et al. (2016). Vitamin D supplementation for women during pregnancy. *Cochrane Database of Systematic Reviews*, (1), CD008873; Devakumar, D., Fall, C. H., Sachdev, H. S., et al. (2016). Maternal antenatal multiple micronutrient supplementation for long-term health benefits in children: A systematic review and meta-analysis. *BMC Medicine*, 14, 90; World Health Organization. (2016). *WHO recommendations on antenatal care for a positive pregnancy experience*. Geneva, Switzerland: Author; Haider, B. A., & Bhutta, Z. A. (2015). Multiple-micronutrient supplementation for women during pregnancy. *Cochrane Database of Systematic Reviews*, (11), CD004905; McCauley, M. E., van den Broek, N., Dou, L., et al. (2015). Vitamin A supplementation during pregnancy for maternal and newborn outcomes. *Cochrane Database of Systematic Reviews*, (10), CD008666; Rumbold, A., Ota, E., Nagata, C., et al. (2015). Vitamin C supplementation in pregnancy. *Cochrane Database of Systematic Reviews*, (9), CD004072.

TABLE 13.3 MINERAL NEEDS FOR THE PREGNANT WOMAN

Mineral	Essential Functions	Relevant Foods and Supplementation	Recommended Amounts	Evidence-Based Evaluation
Calcium	Calcification of fetal bones (as early as 8 weeks)	Milk, cheese, yogurt, leafy greens, almonds	Adolescents—1,300 mg, Adults—1,000 mg	In populations with low dietary intake, supplementation is recommended; reduces risk of preeclampsia
Iodine	Thyroid gland function	Iodized salt, seafood, cranberries	Suggested 250 µg daily where iodized salt use is less than 20%	Strong evidence that populations without iodized salt need supplementation
Iron	Fetal cell development, physiologic anemia of pregnancy	Organ meats, eggs, leafy greens, whole grains, enriched breads, dried fruit	30–60 mg elemental iron daily	Strong evidence supplementation reduces maternal anemia, puerperal sepsis, low birth weight, and preterm birth
Fluoride	Tooth development	Fluoridated water	Supplements only warranted in areas without fluorinated water	Lack of evidence suggesting routine supplementation
Zinc	Immune health	Oysters, red meat, poultry, beans, nuts, whole grains, dairy products	Supplementation only in context of research	Not standard recommended by WHO given lack of evidence

Gernard, A. D., Schulze, K. J., Stewart, C. P., et al. (2016). Micronutrient deficiencies in pregnancy worldwide: Health effects and prevention. *Nature Reviews Endocrinology, 12,* 274–289; World Health Organization. (2016). *WHO recommendations on antenatal care for a positive pregnancy experience.* Geneva, Switzerland: Author.

than taking a fiber laxative as it allows a woman to receive nutrients from the food as well as prevents constipation (Kee, Hayes, & McCuistion, 2015).

Fluid Needs

Extra amounts of water are needed during pregnancy to promote kidney function because a woman must excrete waste products for two. Eight glasses of fluid daily (e.g., two glasses of fluid over and above a daily quart of milk) is a common recommendation.

QSEN Checkpoint Question 13.2

INFORMATICS

The nurse helps Tori evaluate some claims on a website aimed at pregnant women. The nurse identifies which statement from the website as most accurate?
a. "It's best to take your iron pills with milk."
b. "If you prefer, you can crush your iron pills to disguise the taste."
c. "Iron pills are most effective if taken with a carbonated beverage."
d. "Orange juice is an acceptable beverage to take with your iron pills."

Look in Appendix A for the best answer and rationale.

FOODS TO AVOID OR LIMIT IN PREGNANCY

Foods to avoid during pregnancy include those that are known to be teratogenic and, because a woman's immunologic resistance is lowered, those that may spread bacteria, such as:
- Raw eggs and undercooked chicken (danger of salmonella)
- Soft unpasteurized cheese (can harbor *Listeria* bacteria)
- Raw milk
- Raw seafood and sushi (can harbor hepatitis A virus)

- Cold cuts (deli meats should be heated until steaming to kill any bacteria)
- Alcoholic beverages (known to cause fetal alcohol spectrum disorder)
- Saccharin (has a long half-life and so can reach toxic levels in a fetus)
- Fish with high mercury content such as mackerel and swordfish
- Weight loss diets or supplements (women need additional nutrients, not less in pregnancy)
- Caffeine (excessive amounts may be a cause of miscarriage, although research is still ongoing)

Foods With Caffeine

Caffeine is thought of by many women as an incidental ingredient in beverages. However, it is a central nervous system stimulant capable of increasing heart rate, urine production in the kidneys, and secretion of acid in the stomach.

A daily intake of over three cups of coffee per day may interfere with fertility (Sharma, Biedenharn, Fedor, et al., 2013). Caffeine has also been associated with an increased risk of miscarriage (Sharma et al., 2013).

Women who want to limit their caffeine intake need to limit not only the amount of coffee they drink but also other sources of caffeine such as chocolate, soft drinks, energy drinks, and tea. If a woman has difficulty omitting these common foods from her diet, she can still reduce the amount of caffeine she ingests by modifying food preparation. For example, instant coffee has less caffeine than brewed coffee. Decaffeinated coffee, as the name implies, contains almost no caffeine.

Tea, like coffee, varies in caffeine content depending on the type and time of brewing, as the longer tea brews, the greater the caffeine content. Both herbal teas that do not contain caffeine and decaffeinated teas are readily available.

Soft drinks do not naturally contain caffeine, an addictive substance; it is added to soft drinks by their manufacturer to increase product sales. To limit the amount of caffeine consumed, encourage pregnant women to choose from the many caffeine-free types available or, better, to drink water, which will help them stay hydrated without extra empty calories or caffeine.

What If . . . 13.2

Tori Alarino states, "I love coffee. There's always a pot brewing where I work, and everyone drinks it on morning breaks." What suggestions could the nurse make to help Tori reduce her caffeine intake?

Artificial Sweeteners

Artificial sweeteners are used to improve the taste and to limit the caloric content of foods. It is probably safest for pregnant women to reduce their intake of these because they need the glucose of regular sugar to help supply daily energy. Many nonnutritive sweeteners are approved by the U.S. Food and Drug Administration (FDA) as safe for pregnancy, including sucralose (Splenda), aspartame (NutraSweet), acesulfame-K (Ace K), neotame, stevia, and advantame, but large amounts of these sweeteners should probably be avoided until safety in pregnancy is thoroughly confirmed. The use of saccharin is not recommended during pregnancy because it is eliminated so slowly from the fetal bloodstream that it could rise to toxic amounts (Araújo, Martel, & Keating, 2014).

Weight Loss Diets

As a rule, measures to protect against excessive weight gain during pregnancy are wise because excessive weight gain is difficult for women to lose after pregnancy and is part of the reason for the present obesity epidemic (Luke, Kirby, & Wright, 2016). In contrast, weight reduction is not wise. Liquid diets and/or diets that are combined with weight-reducing drugs are particularly contraindicated because they may lead to fetal ketoacidosis and poor growth. If women have been following such diets before becoming pregnant, they may enter pregnancy with so few nutritional stores that additional vitamin and mineral supplementation may be necessary.

QSEN Checkpoint Question 13.3 ✓

EVIDENCE-BASED PRACTICE

Gaining too much weight in pregnancy can lead to complications in the mother such as gestational diabetes; in addition, the fetus can gain excess weight with possible long-term weight problems. To see how much weight gain women perceived they needed in pregnancy, nurse researchers surveyed 54 women who were less than 20 weeks pregnant. Results of the questionnaire showed 39% of the women were overweight or obese before pregnancy. Daily caloric intake ranged from 599 to 5,856 calories. Women in all racial/ethnic groups were taking in less than recommended amounts of protein, carbohydrates, calcium, iron, folate, and fiber. Central American Hispanic women were the group who perceived they needed to gain the most weight for a healthy pregnancy; Caribbean black women, as a group, perceived they needed to gain the least weight (Brooten, Youngblut, Golembeski, et al., 2012).

This study demonstrated the average woman was taking in less nutrients than required during pregnancy. How should the nurse best advise Tori about what foods she should eat during pregnancy?
a. "Protein makes you gain weight too rapidly so keep all your meat portions small."
b. "Eat as much as you like all during pregnancy; you can always diet close to term."
c. "Make sure that you work plenty of leafy green vegetables into your diet."
d. "Iron causes constipation so limit your intake of iron-rich foods any way you can."

Look in Appendix A for the best answer and rationale.

Assessing Nutritional Health

Women who follow good nutrition practices before pregnancy come into pregnancy in better health and are best prepared to avoid pregnancy complications (Cheikh Ismail, Bishop, Pang, et al., 2016). The best method for assessing a woman's nutritional intake before pregnancy or during pregnancy is to ask a woman to describe a "typical day," or a 24-hour nutrition recall, to isolate usual patterns and possible nutritional risk factors (Table 13.4). First, ask if yesterday was a typical day. If it was, ask a woman to list all the food she ate within the past

TABLE 13.4 COMMON NUTRITIONAL RISK FACTORS DURING PREGNANCY

Risk	Rationale
Adolescent (less than 18 years old)	Adolescents require nutrition for both their own growth and fetal growth.
Short intervals between pregnancies	A woman's body has not had time to replace nutritional stores depleted during a previous pregnancy.
Low income	Family may not have resources to purchase iron-rich foods to meet pregnancy nutritional needs.
Food fads or dieting	Foods eaten may not be those adequate for pregnancy.
Drug use (including cigarettes and alcohol)	Drugs may be ingested in preference to healthy foods as well as cause teratogenic effects.
Existence of a chronic illness requiring a special diet	Intake may be low in an essential substance such as carbohydrates or protein.
Underweight or overweight	Underweight and overweight status may indicate chronic inadequate nutrition.
Multiple pregnancy	A woman must supply enough nutrition for multiple fetal development.
Anemic at conception	A woman has no iron stores for fetal growth.
Lactose intolerance	A woman may not be ingesting adequate calcium for fetal skeletal growth.
Post–bariatric surgery	A woman may not be able to eat large enough portions to meet pregnancy nutritional needs.

24 hours, starting with when she awakened until she went to sleep. Be certain she includes all snack foods as well as sit-down meals. This method of history taking yields much more accurate information than asking a woman how often she eats specific foods.

In addition to actual food intake, ask if a woman thinks she has any problem with nutrition (such as cravings). Also, assess the circumstances of eating, such as cultural preferences, who prepares food in the family, and how many meals are eaten outside the home weekly, as these are important to form a total nutrition picture (Table 13.5). To strengthen history findings, assess a woman's prepregnancy weight and calculate her BMI. People with poor nutrition are typically overweight or underweight and show typical physical signs. Table 13.6 lists important physical examination assessments that suggest a good nutritional intake or evidence of poor nutrition. After obtaining a full nutritional pattern, compare the types and amounts of food the woman eats with those shown in Figure 13.1 to see if all food groups and adequate amounts are included. Comparing foods from the person's 24-hour recall with a food guide is helpful because it shows patients that what they thought was a "perfect" intake is imperfect, or what they thought was a "little" problem actually involves the loss of an entire food group. Once a woman sees such a deficit exists, she may be more motivated to improve her nutrition. Such a picture also offers an instant reward for a woman who is including all food groups every day.

TABLE 13.5 AREAS TO ASSESS FOR A TOTAL NUTRITION HISTORY

Area of Assessment	Pertinent Questions
Food preparation	Who does the cooking at your house?
	Do you cook for people besides yourself?
	How do you usually prepare food (fried or baked)?
	What spices or condiments do you commonly use?
	What type of oil do you use for frying (saturated or unsaturated)?
Food pattern	How many meals do you eat on a typical day?
	Which is your biggest meal?
	How many snacks do you eat a day? What are they?
	How many meals do you eat outside your home?
	Where do you eat them? Cafeteria? Fast-food store? Restaurant? Bagged lunch?
	Are there any foods you cannot or will not eat? Why?
Financial concerns	Does your family have enough money for food?
	Who does the food shopping?
	Would you eat differently if more money were available?
	Do you use any supplementary financial programs such as the SNAP or WIC programs?
Activity level	Are you normally active or sedentary? (An active lifestyle increases calorie need.)
Lifestyle	Were you dieting before you became pregnant?
	Were you taking oral contraceptives before pregnancy?
	Do you take supplemental vitamins? What type? How many?
	Do you drink alcohol? What type? How much?
	Do you smoke cigarettes? How many?
Health	Do you have any allergies to food?
	Do you have any trouble with chewing or digestion?
	What is your bowel movement frequency?
	What is your stress level? Does stress affect your appetite?
	Are you ill in any way, such as with heart disease or inflammatory bowel disease?
	If you have a secondary illness? Are there foods you cannot eat?
Personal food preferences	Are you always hungry for a particular food?
	Do you ever eat things that are not food such as ice chips or laundry starch?
	Are there any foods you particularly enjoy or dislike?
	Are there any foods you feel are harmful or particularly beneficial during pregnancy?
	Do you have any cultural or religious preferences that influence what you eat?
Family dietary patterns	Is anyone in your family on a special diet?
	Is anyone obviously overweight or underweight?
	Does your family eat meals together?
	Is mealtime a social time?

TABLE 13.6 PHYSICAL SIGNS AND SYMPTOMS OF ADEQUATE PREGNANCY NUTRITION

Assessment Area	Signs of Good Nutrition	Signs of Poor Nutrition
Hair	Shiny; strong, with good body	Hair dull and lifeless (possible protein deficit)
Eyes	Good eyesight, particularly at night; conjunctiva moist and not pale	Pale and dry conjunctiva (iron and fluid deficit); difficulty with night vision (vitamin A deficit)
Mouth	No cavities in teeth; no swollen or inflamed gum line; no cracks or fissures at corners of mouth; mucous membrane moist and pink; tongue smooth and nontender	Fissures at corners of mouth; tongue rough and tender (vitamin A deficit); mucous membrane pale (iron deficit)
Neck	Normal contour of thyroid gland	Thyroid gland enlarged (iodine deficit)
Skin	Smooth, with normal color and turgor; no ecchymotic or petechial areas present	Rough texture; poor turgor (fluid deficit) Vitamin K deficiency leads to petechia
Extremities	Normal muscle mass and circumference; normal strength and mobility; edema limited to slight ankle involvement; normal reflexes	Poor muscle tone; diminished reflexes (protein deficit)
Fingernails and toenails	Smooth; pink; normal contour	Pale; break easily; little growth (protein deficit)
Weight	Within normal limits of ideal weight before pregnancy; following normal pattern of pregnancy weight gain	Overweight or underweight; unusually slow or rapid weight gain (inadequate or excessive carbohydrate)
Blood pressure	Within normal limits for length of pregnancy	Decreased from anemia (iron deficit); increased from hypertension

Promoting Nutritional Health During Pregnancy

Be certain plans made for improving nutritional patterns take into account a woman's lifestyle, family preferences, financial resources, customs, and cultural desires because she and her family must follow them for 9 months for them to be successful (Fig. 13.2).

FAMILY CONSIDERATIONS

Meal planning is best if it involves the entire family because even if a woman is receptive to changing her eating habits, she may have difficulty carrying out recommendations if her family resists the change. In families where a member has a special nutritional need, such as restricted sodium, change

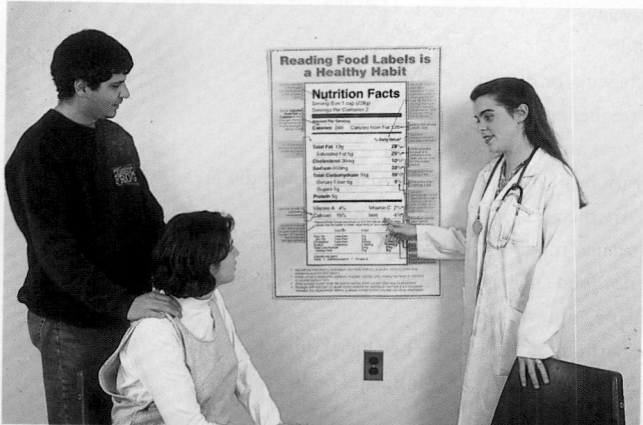

Figure 13.2 Encourage pregnant women and their partners to eat a varied diet with a high iron and protein content. This may be difficult for a woman early in pregnancy because of nausea and late in pregnancy because of fatigue. (© Barbara Proud.)

may be even more difficult. You may need to speak with the person who prepares meals for a pregnant adolescent as well as the adolescent to be certain recommended changes will be carried out.

FINANCIAL CONSIDERATIONS

Food is costly, so to provide the extra servings required during pregnancy, a woman must spend more on food for herself per week than she was spending previously. Women generally view this increased expense as an investment in their child's health and do not regard it as a burden. A woman on a marginal income, however, although she understands the importance of this, may have difficulty actually doing it. If this occurs, review what foods the woman is eating to be certain she is not filling her plate with less expensive starchy foods, such as pasta, in preference to higher protein foods such as meat. Help her secure available financial assistance such as from the Supplemental Nutrition Assistance Program (SNAP) or the Women, Infants and Children (WIC) Special Supplemental Food Program if needed.

Since 1939, under the SNAP program, a family with a low income can be issued an Electronic Benefit Transfer (EBT) or debit card that can be used to buy food items. SNAP cards cannot be used to buy hot and prepared food, cigarettes, alcohol, personal care items, paper commodities, pet food, household supplies, or medication. The amount of the debit card varies depending on the needs of the family. In general, a family of four whose monthly income is under $2,000 can increase their monthly food buying power by as much as $650 per month (USDA, 2016).

The advantage of this type of supplemental program is to help provide money for food but that places almost no restrictions on what foods, except for those mentioned previously. For a low-income family, it can make the difference between a healthy intake and a low-nutrient one.

WIC is a federal program that provides nutritional support for low-income women and children not only to reduce the risk of low birth weight but also to aid with the cost of new-born nutrition. Established in 1972, WIC is funded by the Food and Nutrition Service of the USDA. The program supplies supplemental foods and nutrition education for:

- Pregnant women
- Postpartum women up to 6 months
- Nursing mothers up to 1 year
- Children from birth to age 5 years

Each state defines the income eligibility level for its cit-izens, but the eligibility for all programs is based on three criteria: income level, geographic area, and nutritional risk. To receive food, patients must live in an area that has been designated as a funding area. The nurse or nutritionist in the healthcare facility determines possible risk and nutritional need and helps enroll a family in the program. Factors consid-ered that put pregnant women at nutritional risk include age (an adolescent or woman over age 40 years), poor obstetric history such as previous spontaneous miscarriage, a short pe-riod between pregnancies, having given birth to a previous low–birth-weight infant, gestational diabetes, anemia, poor weight gain, or inadequate consumption of food by nutrition history.

For the pregnant woman, foods typically offered by the program include those with high-quality protein, iron, cal-cium, and vitamins A and C, such as fresh fruits and veg-etables, eggs, milk, legumes, whole grain cereals and breads, and canned fish. Vegetarian families or those with allergies can receive tofu and soy-based beverages or foods. At pre-determined intervals, WIC patients are reevaluated to see if the program supplements are helpful or still necessary. WIC has been successful at improving nutrition during pregnancy because it not only supplies additional food to recipients but also provides periodic evaluations for nutritional counseling (Andreyeva & Leudicke, 2015).

The school lunch program is yet another federal program that can furnish some pregnant adolescents with nutritional help. Millions of schoolchildren qualify for free or reduced-price school breakfasts or lunches designed to provide one third of requirements for protein, vitamin A, vitamin C, iron, calcium, and calories. Communities are working hard to re-place burgers, fries, and burritos with salads, fresh fruits, sim-ply prepared meats, and whole grain breads in schools. Soft drinks are being replaced with fat-free milk or water.

For many adolescents, this improved menu may repre-sent the most nutritious meal they eat all day. Because there is a selection of food choices that can be made, a pregnant adolescent or one with other special needs may need some individual counseling to allow her to choose foods best for her, not those her friends are eating (Adams, Bruening, Ohri-Vachaspati, et al., 2016).

CULTURAL CONSIDERATIONS

When helping plan nutrition during pregnancy, try to sug-gest foods that are individually or culturally favored, as these are the foods women tend to enjoy most and so will eat most consistently. Common cultural differences to be aware of during nutritional counseling are shown in Box 13.5. Remember when counseling using such a table, not to ste-reotype women into cultural boxes. "Americanized" women may prepare few foods from their ethnic background because their spouse or significant other is of a contrasting culture with differing preferences.

MANAGING COMMON PROBLEMS AFFECTING NUTRITIONAL HEALTH

Specific nutrition problems may result from a number of factors or circumstances during pregnancy.

Nausea and Vomiting

As many as three fourths of pregnant women report nausea and vomiting in early pregnancy (Rogers & Worley, 2016). No definite cause has been established for this symptom of early pregnancy, but it may be related to:

- Sensitivity to the high level of chorionic gonadotropin hormone produced by the trophoblast cells
- High estrogen or progesterone levels
- Lowered maternal blood sugar caused by the needs of the developing embryo
- Lack of pyridoxine (vitamin B_6)
- Diminished gastric motility

Nausea is aggravated by fatigue and possibly by emotional disturbances. Most women notice the sensation as early as the first missed menstrual period and experience it through the first 3 months of pregnancy. The sensation is usually most intense on rising but may occur from smelling certain foods or while a woman is preparing meals. Vomiting at least once daily is com-mon. Women who work nights and sleep days often experience "evening sickness" because that is the time when they arise.

The traditional solution for preventing nausea is for women to keep dry crackers, such as saltines, by their bedside and eat a few before rising because increasing carbohydrate intake seems to relieve nausea better than any other nutrition remedy. Sucking on sour candies may serve the same purpose. A woman may then eat a light breakfast or delay breakfast until 10 AM or 11 AM, or past the time her nausea seems to persist. To be certain she maintains good food intake during pregnancy even in the face of nausea, urge her to be certain to compensate for any missed meals later in the day. If preparing food for others makes her feel queasy, she might try to give this responsibility to another family member, at least through the worst phase of this symptom. Preparing and freezing meals ahead of time, perhaps at night when the nausea is less bothersome, may also help.

Other therapy such as acupressure, anti–motion sickness wrist bands, and avoiding fluid with meals are other measures

BOX 13.5

Nursing Care Planning to Respect Cultural Diversity

CHARACTERISTICS OF CERTAIN ETHNIC DIETS

Group and Place of Origin	Staple Foods	Common Customs
Hispanic Americans from Puerto Rico	Steamed white rice; many varieties of beans; starchy vegetables, such as cassavas or yams; salted fish or pork; sugared fruit juices; cafe con leche (coffee and hot milk)	Milk is rarely consumed as a beverage. Most foods are cooked for long periods of time or fried. Malt beer is believed to be nutritious and may be given to children and breastfeeding mothers.
Hispanic Americans from Mexico, Central America	Many varieties of beans; steamed rice; corn products such as tortillas; chili peppers, fresh fruit, potatoes; meat; fish; poultry; eggs; milk cheeses; milk custards and bread puddings	Most vegetables are cooked for a long time so they lose most of their nutritional value. Diet is high in fiber and starch. Animal fat is frequently added during food preparation. Diet may be inadequate in calcium, iron, vitamin A, and vitamin C.
Hispanic Americans from Cuba	Stews and casseroles; soup is served daily; fried foods, especially fish, poultry, and eggs; rice; many varieties of beans	Fruits and vegetables are not eaten on a regular basis. Main meal is usually served at lunch.
Southern African Americans from West Africa	Hominy grits; biscuits; corn bread; rice; legumes; sweet potatoes; okra; green leafy vegetables cooked in salt pork; pork, poultry, and fish; thick stews; bread puddings; pies and sweets	African American food patterns are similar to Caucasians in same region. Northern African Americans may be unfamiliar with "soul food." Frying is common; diet tends to be high in fat and salt, low in calcium.
Chinese Americans (diets vary sometimes with region)	Rice; wheat noodles; many seasonal cooked vegetables and fruits; various shoots; soybean products such as tofu, soy sauces, and soy milk; small portions of meat, fish, poultry, and seafood	Yin (feminine)–yang (masculine) concept of balancing intake; moderation is valued. Diet is high in fiber and many nutrients, is low in fat, and may be low in protein.
Japanese Americans	Rice; vegetables; tofu, bean paste, and soy sauce; fruits; salads; fish, green tea; milk is rarely used by adults	Foods are broiled, steamed, boiled, and stir fried. Meat portions are small. Diet is low in fat, rich in nutrients, high in sodium.
Vietnamese Americans	Rice, rice noodles; curries of asparagus and potatoes; salads; tropical fruits and vegetables; small portions of poultry; eggs; fish; nuoc mam (a strong, fermented fish sauce)	Rice may be eaten at every meal. Lactose intolerance is common. Little fat is used in preparation. Diet may be low in iron and calcium.
Native Americans	Southeast: corn; cornmeal; coontie (flour from a palmlike plant); fried breads; vegetables; alligator, snake, wild hog, duck, fish, and shellfish; Northeast: many berries, beans; corn; pumpkins; fish, lobster, and wild game; Midwest: bison; beans; corn; fruits and vegetables; Southwest: corn, beans, squash, pumpkins, chili peppers, melons, cactus; Northwest: salmon, other fish, bear, elk, wild fruits, nuts, wild greens.	Food has great religious and social significance. Corn is a status food for most tribes. Milk is seldom used; calcium intake may be low.

Source: Dudek, S. (2010). *Nutrition essentials for nursing practice* (6th ed.). Philadelphia, PA: Lippincott Williams & Wilkins.

effective for many women. It is a good rule for women not to go longer than 3 to 4 hours between meals during pregnancy to prevent hypoglycemia. To prevent this from happening, women may need to eat a snack before bedtime to compensate for a late breakfast. Some women are able to tolerate fruit and raw vegetables during the morning before other food. Urge a woman to experiment with soups or vegetable drinks

she may not usually think of as breakfast foods but that can give her early-morning calories.

Common measures to take to relieve nausea are summarized in Box 13.6. Caution women against self-medicating for nausea by using a scopolamine patch, a drug used for motion sickness. Although it has not been proven unsafe for pregnancy, it is not intended for long-term use. Also caution

BOX 13.6

Nursing Care Planning Based on Family Teaching

MEASURES TO REDUCE AND EVALUATE NAUSEA DURING PREGNANCY

Q. Tori Alarino tells you, "I've been nauseated ever since I became pregnant. What can I do to make this better?"

A. Common nonpharmacologic measures you can take to *prevent* nausea include:

- Be aware between 50% and 90% of women experience nausea during pregnancy, so what you are experiencing is absolutely normal.
- Eat a few dry crackers, toast, or a sour ball before you get out of bed in the morning to increase your carbohydrate intake.
- Eat small but frequent meals rather than large infrequent ones.
- Avoid greasy or highly seasoned food.
- Delay breakfast until nausea passes (or dinner if it is evening nausea).
- Make up missed meals at some other time of the day to maintain nutrition.
- Avoid sudden movements and fatigue because these may increase or cause nausea.
- Eat a snack before bedtime so delaying breakfast won't cause you to go a long time between meals.
- Purchase a wrist acupressure band (purchased in travel stores for motion sickness) or schedule an acupuncture visit.

If nausea is present:

- Try sipping a carbonated beverage.
- Try a walk outside in the fresh air or take deep breaths through an open window.

Notify your healthcare provider if:

- You vomit more than once daily.
- You are losing weight rather than gaining it.
- You have not gained the projected amount of weight for your week of pregnancy.
- You are unable to make up for lost meals some other time of the day.
- You have signs of dehydration such as little urine output.
- Nausea has lasted past 12 weeks of pregnancy.
- The amount of nausea you are feeling is interfering with what you want to do in a day's time.

---

against taking excessive amounts of antacids containing sodium bicarbonate as their sodium content could cause fluid retention.

About 10% of women have nausea and vomiting that are so acute they need additional measures to feel comfortable and to prevent fluid and nutrient shortages. Pyridoxine HCl (vitamin B_6) or a combination of pyridoxine HCl plus doxylamine succinate (Unisom) can be prescribed. Dimenhydrinate (Dramamine) is an H_1 receptor antagonist that also can be helpful (O'Donnell, McParlin, Robson, et al., 2016). Fortunately, nausea usually disappears spontaneously as women enter their fourth month of pregnancy. If it persists beyond this month or is so extreme in early pregnancy that it interferes with nutrition, it may indicate the development of hyperemesis gravidarum, a serious complication of pregnancy and a complication for which the woman needs additional therapy (O'Donnell et al., 2016).

Cravings

Cravings for food or aversions to certain foods during pregnancy are so common they are considered a normal part of adaptation to pregnancy.

When taking a nutrition history, ask if a woman notices any particular cravings. As long as this is a healthy type of food, help her plan an intake that includes the food, at least in moderation, to help her enjoy her pregnancy without feeling guilty.

Some women report a craving for foods such as oranges or chocolate. Others, however, crave a nonfood substance (termed **pica**, from the Latin for magpie, a bird that is an indiscriminate eater). The most common form of pica in the past was a craving for laundry starch. Today, women are more apt to report cravings for clay, dirt, cornstarch, or ice cubes (Miao, Young, & Golden, 2015).

Although some of these items do no harm in themselves, the ingestion of large quantities of nonfood substances can leave a woman deficient in nutrients essential for a healthy pregnancy outcome (Box 13.7).

Always ask women at prenatal visits if they crave any nonfood items, as most women do not supply this information unless asked directly. They worry you will find their behavior odd, or they may not realize their habit is pregnancy related as much as being a nervous habit.

Stopping the woman from eating the nonfood substance may be difficult because the habit may be deeply ingrained. Because pica is a symptom that often accompanies iron-deficiency anemia, suggest that her primary care provider assess her serum iron levels as correcting this underlying problem with an iron supplement may correct the pica. At subsequent visits, be certain to assess if a woman's hemoglobin is increasing and ask if she has noticed any difference in her cravings.

Diminished Gastric Mobility

As peristalsis slows from the effect of progesterone and the weight of a growing uterus presses against her bowel, constipation occurs in nearly 50% of pregnant women (Rungsiprakam,

BOX 13.7

Nursing Care Planning Tips for Effective Communication

Tori comes to your prenatal clinic, and you want to obtain her nutrition history.

Tip: Ask specific questions about the patient's individual nutrition intake. Most people believe they eat well and so respond that their nutrition is adequate if asked only general questions. Only when they are asked to describe what they ate during one day is the truth revealed. For example, eating ice cubes may reflect iron-deficiency anemia.

Nurse: Hi, Tori. Are you eating a nutritious diet?

Tori: I eat everything in sight. No problem.

Nurse: Tell me what you ate yesterday.

Tori: A muffin and coffee for breakfast, a milkshake for lunch, a hamburger and fries for supper. A soft drink before bed. And ice cubes. I suck on them all day like candy.

Nurse: Let's talk about ways you might get some fruit and vegetables into your day.

Laopaiboon, Sangkomkamhang, et al., 2015). Discuss preventive measures with women early in pregnancy to help them avoid this problem. Encourage them to evacuate their bowels regularly (many women neglect this first simple rule); increase the amount of roughage in their diet by eating raw fruits, bran, and vegetables; and drink at least eight 8-oz glasses of water daily.

Some women find that prescribed oral iron supplements contribute to constipation. Because this supplement is necessary to build fetal iron stores, help a woman find a method to relieve or prevent constipation other than omitting taking the supplement.

Women should not use mineral oil to relieve constipation as it can prevent absorption of fat-soluble vitamins A, D, E, and K, vitamins necessary for both good fetal and maternal health. Enemas also should be avoided because their action might initiate labor. Over-the-counter laxatives are also contraindicated, as are all nonessential drugs during pregnancy, unless specifically prescribed or sanctioned by a woman's primary healthcare provider. If dietary measures and attempts at regular bowel evacuation fail, a stool softener such as docusate sodium (Colace) or evacuation suppositories such as glycerin may be helpful.

Some women have extensive flatulence accompanying constipation. Recommend avoiding gas-forming foods, such as cabbage or beans, to help control this problem.

Pyrosis

Pyrosis (heartburn) is a burning sensation along the esophagus caused by regurgitation of gastric contents into the lower esophagus (Phupong & Hanprasertpong, 2015). In pregnancy, it may accompany early nausea; it may also persist beyond the resolution of nausea and even increase in severity as pregnancy advances.

Pyrosis is probably caused by decreased gastric motility (an effect of progesterone, which slows gastric emptying) as well as the effect of pressure from the expanding uterus pushing up against the stomach. Common suggestions to help prevent reflux into the esophagus and relieve pain are:

- Eat small meals frequently rather than large meals.
- Sleep on the left side with two pillows to elevate the upper torso.
- Do not lie down immediately after eating; try to wait at least 2 hours.
- Avoid fatty and fried foods, coffee, carbonated beverages, tomato products, and citrus juices.

Aluminum hydroxide (Amphojel, pregnancy class N or not classified) or a combination of aluminum and magnesium hydroxide (Maalox, class B) may be prescribed for relief. If these do not relieve the discomfort, an H_2 receptor antagonist such as cimetidine (Tagamet, class B) or ranitidine (Zantac, class B) may be prescribed (Attilakos & Overton, 2012). Be certain a woman understands this "chest" pain is from her gastrointestinal tract and, although it is called heartburn, it has nothing to do with her heart.

Hypercholesterolemia

Women with a family history of hypercholesterolemia may enter pregnancy with already elevated cholesterol levels. During pregnancy, increasing progesterone levels cause a further elevation. Combined with intrahepatic cholestasis, this can lead to an increased risk for gallstone formation (cholelithiasis) and cardiovascular disease during pregnancy. Preventing cholelithiasis is important because gallstones can cause extremely sharp pain. Fortunately, surgery to remove gallstones during pregnancy is possible with new ambulatory laparotomy techniques.

A woman who has had difficulty with hypercholesterolemia before pregnancy may need to continue to eat only moderate amounts of fat during pregnancy to prevent any increase in cholesterol. Helpful ways to reduce cholesterol include:

- Exercising daily
- Eating oat cereal
- Broiling, grilling, or baking meat rather than frying it
- Using a minimum of salad oils
- Substituting new omega-3 products in place of butter
- Eating fish high in omega-3 oil, such as salmon or trout

Although tuna is also high in omega-3 oil, current recommendations are for pregnant women to limit their intake of tuna, swordfish, and mackerel because of their potentially high mercury content (APA, 2016). Eating raw fish is also not advised because of the danger of parasitic contamination.

Urge women to check with their healthcare provider about the wisdom of continuing to take cholesterol-lowering drugs (statins such as Lipitor, class X) during pregnancy because these drugs are proven to be teratogenic (Bateman, Hernandez-Diaz, Fischer, et al., 2015). A low-cholesterol diet will automatically be lower in calories than the average diet because oils and fats add many calories. Therefore, be certain women watching their fat intake are taking in enough calories for adequate weight gain during pregnancy. Also make certain a woman includes some oil daily (perhaps as olive oil on a salad) so she has included a source of omega-3 oil in her daily intake.

PATIENT-CENTERED CARE

The nurse identifies which statement by Tori as suggesting she has developed pica?
   a. "I eat the erasers off pencils. It helps relieve my heartburn."
   b. "I can't eat a thing before 11 o'clock every morning."
   c. "I notice I've been hungry for lemon cookies lately."
   d. "I crave oranges; can't get enough of them every day."

Look in Appendix A for the best answer and rationale.

Women With Unique Needs

A number of lifestyles make it difficult for women to enter pregnancy with sound nutrition stores or to make the healthiest nutrition choices during pregnancy. Such women need careful assessments and counseling during pregnancy to help them modify their lifestyle enough so they can meet nutritional needs.

THE ADOLESCENT

A pregnant adolescent needs a higher caloric intake (2,400 calories per day) than a mature woman to supply energy because of the dual demand of consuming enough food to provide for fetal growth and for her own continuing growth. The nutrients most often lacking from a typical adolescent diet tend to be calcium, iron, folic acid, and total calories. Look for sources of these when analyzing a teenager's pregnancy intake.

An adolescent who is trying to hide an unintended pregnancy may eat very little to keep her abdomen from growing or eat a lot hoping the overall weight she gains will hide the size of her abdomen. She may have been on a diet before pregnancy and want to continue this to "not get fat." Because she's not meeting nutritional needs with any of these eating patterns, she runs a high risk of developing anemia, which can lead to fetal growth restriction and possibly preterm birth (Menon, Ferguson, Thomson, et al., 2016).

In their search for identity, adolescents may avoid foods their parents see as important, such as milk, warm cereal, vegetables, or fruit, and indulge instead in foods such as soft drinks, potato chips, and French fries. If they eat lunch or breakfast at a school cafeteria, finding healthy food choices may be difficult.

To help an adolescent plan nutritional intake for pregnancy, respect her right to reject traditional foods as long as what she does eat includes sufficient nutrients. A cheese and sausage pizza, a glass of milk, and an apple compose a lunch that provides all basic food groups (meat: sausage; bread: pizza crust; vegetable: tomato sauce; dairy: cheese and milk; fruit: apple). A fish or hamburger taco (fish or hamburger, salsa, sour cream, and taco shell) plus a mango or tangerine provides the same.

Most adolescents snack frequently during the day. Toward the end of pregnancy, when preparing nutritious snacks becomes more difficult because of fatigue, you may notice they list more and more "junk food" when detailing what they eat. Advising them to prepare nutritious snacks such as carrot sticks or cheese bites early each day when they have more energy might be helpful. This way, if they are tired later in the day, eating a nutritious snack will not involve so much effort.

Because adolescents often do not prepare the foods they eat, you may need to speak to a parent or a support person (with permission) who does prepare foods to alter the adolescent's nutrition pattern. Encourage the food preparer to suggest a number of foods that would fill a deficit and let the adolescent choose from them to provide a sense of control.

Adolescents with eating disorders (bulimia or anorexia nervosa) enter pregnancy with major nutrient deficiencies. It is important to identify these teens at the first pregnancy visit so they can receive close supervision and supplementation of specific nutrients as needed (Kimmel et al., 2016).

THE WOMAN OLDER THAN 40 YEARS OF AGE

Today, many women are older than 40 years by the time they have their first child, and many more are older than 40 years when they have their second or third child (J. A. Martin, Hamilton, Osterman, et al., 2015). The nutritional needs of women in this age group are not well studied, but it is obvious women in this age group should maintain the same careful pregnancy nutrition as younger women. Because women in this age group may have slightly decreased kidney function, they should be certain to maintain a high fluid intake to remove waste products for themselves and for their fetus. They need adequate calcium to prevent bone density loss. Many women at this point in life may also be caring for elderly parents and/or have delayed childbearing to establish a career; this means they may eat whatever they are preparing for elderly parents or depend on packed or fast-food lunches for at least part of their nutrition. Focus your nutrition counseling on maintaining adequate nutrition during pregnancy, based on these changing lifestyles.

THE WOMAN WITH A STRESSFUL LIFESTYLE

A stressful lifestyle can interfere with pregnancy nutrition as such women may simply have too many other stresses in their lives to concentrate on eating healthy meals. Examples of women who have this problem might be a busy executive trying to meet project time lines; one taking care of an ill child, partner, or aging parents; or one who is homeless or lacking enough money to purchase adequate food. Women who live in a situation with intimate partner violence may not have enough freedom to select what foods they prepare or serve to include all food groups every day. A conscientious assessment of women at first prenatal visits (hopefully at preconception visits) can help identify women in this group and provide the additional support they need to achieve adequate nutrition and a safe pregnancy outcome.

THE WOMAN WITH NUTRITIONAL DEFICIENCIES

The Woman With Decreased Nutritional Stores

A woman with high parity or a short interval between pregnancies or one who has been dieting rigorously to lose weight before pregnancy may enter pregnancy with such depleted nutritional reserves she has little to draw on during the first part of pregnancy. If her folic acid intake has been inadequate, her fetus is susceptible to neural tube defects (Temel, Erdem, Voorham, et al., 2015). This shortage of nutrients may become critical during the time she is unable to eat well because of the usual nausea and vomiting of pregnancy. Be alert for:

- Women from low-income families, who may enter pregnancy with anemia because they haven't been able to purchase iron-rich foods
- Women who used diuretics for a dieting program, who may be deficient in potassium as this can be removed in urine by some diuretics
- Women who have been taking oral contraceptives, who may have decreased folate stores
- Women who were using intrauterine devices or who have menorrhagia (heavy menstrual flow), who may be deficient in iron from excessive blood loss with menstrual flows
- Women who drink alcohol excessively, who may be deficient in thiamine

Women with these decreased nutritional stores need to be identified early in pregnancy through history taking so they can be referred to a nutritionist for specific nutritional counseling. They may need additional supplements during pregnancy to help restore a particular nutrient.

The Woman Who Has Been Dieting or Following a Food Fad

Women who have been dieting and those who have been following a food fad such as eating nothing but cabbage soup are another group who may enter pregnancy with nutrient deficiencies. Be certain to ask if a woman has been dieting at a first prenatal visit.

The Woman Who Eats Many Fast-Food Meals

As many as 70% of women with children work at least part-time outside their homes (Bureau of Labor Statistics, 2013). This means nutritional counseling for pregnancy must include helping women who rely on packed lunches or fast-food meals to ingest adequate pregnancy nutrition. One big difficulty with fast-food restaurants is the limited choice of food available. This can cause a woman to grow tired of the same thing and either eat little or have little choice but to eat foods with more empty calories than nutritionally effective ones. Unless there is a salad bar, the menu is apt to be particularly limited in fruits and vegetables. It is helpful to advise her to carry an apple or other fruit to eat along with what she selects from the menu to achieve a better food balance.

Caution women that fast-food restaurants have been associated with outbreaks of infection due to undercooked hamburger (*Escherichia coli*) or contaminated salad bars (*Salmonella*). Caution women to inspect a salad bar for cleanliness and order hamburgers well done to prevent gastrointestinal upsets of severe vomiting and diarrhea, which could lead to a serious fluid and electrolyte imbalance (Torso, Voorhees, Forest, et al., 2015).

A packed lunch poses few problems in pregnancy as long as a woman uses creativity in preparation so she does not grow so tired of packed lunches that she reduces her noontime intake or substitutes fast food in their place. Packing her lunch at bedtime rather than in the morning, when she may feel nauseated (and therefore packs little because nothing looks good), is a good recommendation early in pregnancy. Late in pregnancy, a woman may feel too tired at bedtime to do this and so could change back to preparing it in the morning when she may have more energy.

Including a thermos with a cream soup is a good way to add milk and calcium to her diet. Packing sliced oranges or cucumbers, tomatoes, or apples helps to make a lunch nutritious and also makes food available for a midmorning or midafternoon snack. Having these snacks available prevents her from having long stretches of time without eating or eating empty-calorie foods from vending machines. Box 13.8 is an interprofessional care map illustrating both nursing and team planning for sound nutrition for a woman who works outside her home during pregnancy.

The Woman Who Cannot Obtain Culturally Preferred Foods

Because the United States is such a blend of different cultures and people move rapidly from place to place for various reasons, a pregnant woman may find herself living in a community where grocery stores do not stock the foods she is most comfortable eating. If she lives in an apartment, she also has no opportunity to grow any favorites. This situation presents a good opportunity to discuss what she can find as substitutes. Fortunately, most major stores carry a wide range of ethnic foods. Support a woman's efforts to speak to her grocery store manager to stock an item she prefers as practice for motherhood when she will need to learn to serve as a strong supporter or advocate for her child.

THE WOMAN WHO HAS HAD BARIATRIC SURGERY

Bariatric surgery is a weight-control method to reduce overeating by surgically reducing stomach size from about 30 to 40 oz to 3 to 4 oz. For gastric bypass surgery, the smaller, upper part of the stomach is stapled to separate it from the rest of the stomach, thereby reducing the amount of food a woman can eat. Next, the small intestine is rerouted and connected to the smaller stomach pouch, lessening the amount of nutrient absorption possible. In Lap-Band surgery, a silicone rubber band is placed around the top of the stomach, creating a small stomach pouch and reducing the amount of food a woman can eat at any one time. A sleeve gastrectomy is a laparoscopic procedure where the greater curve of the stomach is removed, again, reducing the size of the stomach and the amount that can be eaten at any one meal. A sleeve gastrectomy has the advantage of being a laparoscopy procedure and so requires only a small incision, and like Lab-Band surgery, the pyloric value to the small intestine is left intact.

Gastric bypass surgery results in an average of 60% to 80% loss in presurgery weight; banding and sleeve gastrectomy result in a 45% to 50% weight loss (Monson & Jackson, 2016). Although once limited to mature women, the number of adolescents who are having these types of surgeries is increasing, so ask about bariatric surgery in teenagers as well as mature women (Inge, Courcoulas, Jenkins, et al., 2016).

Both women and adolescents are advised not to become pregnant for about 18 months after a gastric bypass and for 6 months after banding or sleeve gastrectomy. This is the period of greatest weight loss, during which it would be difficult to supply enough nutrients for sound fetal growth.

BOX 13.8

Nursing Care Planning

AN INTERPROFESSIONAL CARE MAP FOR A PREGNANT WOMAN WITH AN INADEQUATE NUTRITIONAL PATTERN

Tori Alarino, 19 years of age, is 4 months pregnant. She works at a fast-food restaurant and eats breakfast and lunch at the restaurant. Her partner, Alessa, works four evenings a week, so Tori cooks for herself on those evenings. She dislikes milk, so she drinks milkshakes as a source of calcium. She is concerned because she has already gained 23 lb. She craves oranges, eating six to eight of them a day. She tells you, "I thought pregnant women always craved pickles and ice cream. What's wrong with me?"

Family Assessment: Patient lives with her partner in a four-bedroom home; partner works as an electrician. Patient's father (aged 58 years) lives with them since recent divorce.

Patient Assessment: Primigravida; last menstrual period (LMP) 16 weeks ago. Height: 5 ft 6 in. Prepregnancy weight: 110 lb (10 lb under desirable weight for height); BMI 17.8 (underweight). Weight today: 116 lb (minimum weight gain for first trimester). History of weight problem during adolescence; usually controls weight by eating only one main meal per day. Reports feeling tired and "rundown." 24-hour dietary recall: Breakfast: 1 cup coffee with muffin; lunch: 1 milkshake; dinner: 1 hamburger with French fries and 1 milkshake; snacks: 8-oz soft drink.

Nursing Diagnosis: Imbalanced nutrition: less than body requirements related to desire to control weight

Outcome Criteria: Patient reports increased intake of foods adequate in calories, high in iron, calcium, and protein by next prenatal visit.
    Demonstrates weight gain appropriate for stage of pregnancy and prepregnancy weight.

Team Member Responsible	Assessment	Intervention	Rationale	Expected Outcome
Activities of Daily Living, Including Safety				
Nurse	Assess if the patient's fatigue is interfering with adequate food preparation.	If fatigue is a problem, recommend preparing food early in day when less fatigued.	Fatigue can increase nausea/vomiting in early pregnancy and can interfere with food preparation throughout pregnancy.	Patient states she is willing to cook and realizes eating fast food at all meals may not meet her nutrition needs during pregnancy.
Teamwork and Collaboration				
Nurse/primary healthcare provider/nutritionist	Assess nutrition requirements based on patient's BMI and individual preferences.	Consult with nutritionist about recommended caloric and mineral requirements.	Caloric recommendations may need to be increased in light of patient's BMI and prepregnancy and current weight.	An ideal nutrition plan is created with patient's input.
Procedures/Medications for Quality Improvement				
Nurse	Assess if patient has experience with keeping a journal.	Ask if patient will record all food and fluid intake for 1 week; review with patient at next visit.	Keeping a journal provides concrete evidence of patient's adherence to nutritional plan.	Patient brings log to next prenatal visit and reviews it with prenatal staff.
Nutrition				
Nurse/nutritionist	Assess if patient could eat more food prepared at home.	Suggest foods that patient's father or partner could prepare. Provide written information as needed.	Involving other family members could improve nutrition for entire family. Printed information enhances learning.	Patient and nutritionist prepare a schedule in which all family members participate in food preparation.

Continued on following page

BOX 13.8

Nursing Care Planning (continued)

Team Member Responsible	Assessment	Intervention	Rationale	Expected Outcome
Patient-Centered Care				
Nurse/nutritionist	Assess if there are nutritious food choices for the patient at the fast-food restaurant.	Discuss other possible food choices with patient.	Knowledgeable patients can best follow a nutritious meal plan.	Patient lists foods she will include for healthy pregnancy nutrition; if none available, pack own lunch.
Psychosocial/Spiritual/Emotional Needs				
Nurse	Question patient about food likes and dislikes. Investigate any cultural influences on food choices.	Ask patient to list foods in each food group that she enjoys cooking or eating.	Ascertaining food preferences and cultural influences provides a baseline for future food selections and suggestions.	Patient lists foods she prefers and knows she can eat consistently.
Informatics for Seamless Healthcare Planning				
Nurse	Assess best times for patient to return for prenatal appointments based on work/family obligations.	Schedule a follow-up nurse appointment in 1 week if possible.	Changing nutritional habits and behaviors can be difficult. Scheduling close follow-up provides an opportunity for evaluation and instruction.	Patient states she will return for follow-up nutritional counseling.

After surgery, all women are required to maintain a conscientious diet of small but healthy portions as well as to take daily a chewable or liquid multivitamin supplement that includes iron, folate, vitamin B_{12}, vitamin A, vitamin B_1 (thiamine), and zinc. Ask if women have been taking their supplement to establish whether they are entering pregnancy with vitamin deficits. Urge them to eat their protein source first in a meal, so they are certain to ingest enough protein.

If a woman does neglect eating a small meal and eats a large one or one extremely rich in calories (e.g., birthday cake with butter cream frosting, ham with buttered sweet potatoes), this can cause a "dumping syndrome" or sudden symptoms of nausea, bloating, and diarrhea. Be certain to mark the chart of a woman who has had bariatric surgery, so her primary healthcare provider can decide if a 50-g glucose tolerance test will be safe or stimulate acute dumping symptoms. Because a woman who has undergone bariatric surgery will have an overall small intake during pregnancy, her weight gain will be less than others; she is prone to develop iron, protein, folic acid, and vitamin B_{12} deficiencies. Women who have had a gastric bypass are also prone to fat-soluble vitamin (vitamins A, D, E, and K) deficiencies because fat is no longer well absorbed.

Women may ask if bariatric surgery was a wise choice for them. You can assure them that following their surgery and subsequent weight loss, they are better candidates for pregnancy than they were when they were morbidly obese. They also have a lesser chance of developing gestational hypertension and gestational diabetes, both serious complications of pregnancy (Monson & Jackson, 2016).

THE WOMAN WHO IS VEGETARIAN

Some women are vegetarians because of religious guidelines or moral conviction. Others turn to vegetarianism to both maintain healthy nutrition and avoid excess fat and food contaminants. Vegetarian diets are have been shown to be protective in pregnancy (Pistollato, Sumalla Cano, Elio, et al., 2015).

Most women vegetarians are closer to their ideal weight and have lower serum cholesterol and blood pressure levels than women who eat a more typical American diet. Nurses may find many pregnant women, therefore, who want to exclude meat from their intake (Pistollato et al., 2015). Vegetarians vary as to what they can eat:

- Lacto-ovo vegetarians eat no animal flesh or fish, but dairy products and eggs are allowed.
- Lacto-vegetarians eat no meat, fish, or eggs, but dairy products are allowed.
- Vegans eat nothing derived from an animal, including butter and eggs.
- Semi-vegetarians usually restrict meat, fish, and poultry.
- Macrobiotics eat whole grains such as brown rice and vegetables; they avoid meat, eggs, milk, and cheese.

To replace meat, fish, and poultry at meals, women need to eat three or more servings a day of both fruits and vegetables, six or more servings per day of grains, and two or more servings per day of legumes such as kidney, black, or lima beans. Most vegetarians are knowledgeable about nutrients needed and can discuss what foods are high in various nutrients and how they incorporate such foods into their daily intake.

Special concerns during pregnancy are that vegetarians may lack vitamin B_{12} (meat is the chief source of this), an adequate intake of calcium because milk is a prime source of this (recommend dark green vegetables or soy milk to supplement this), and vitamin D (fortified soy milk and sunlight are good sources of this). Urge women who are vegetarians to remember to take their daily prenatal supplement, like all women, to ensure adequate iron and folic acid. Vegetarian nutrition for their new infant is discussed in Chapter 29.

THE WOMAN WITH A MULTIPLE PREGNANCY

Twinning occurs naturally at about 4 in every 1,000 births, but the increased use of intrauterine fertilization has caused the number of multiple births to increase to as high as 15 per 1,000 births (Kilby & Oepkes, 2012). A woman with a multiple pregnancy tends to gain more weight overall and at a faster pace than a woman carrying a single child because of the increased fetal weight.

- A woman with a normal BMI should gain 37 to 54 lb.
- A woman with an overweight BMI, 31 to 50 lb.
- A woman with an obese BMI, 25 to 42 lb (IOM & National Research Council, 2009).

To sustain her own nutrition stores, a woman with a multiple pregnancy must ingest high levels of protein and carbohydrate as well as iron and folic acid. For this reason, a multiple pregnancy needs to be recognized early so nutritional supplements as well as overall close supervision can be added as needed (Kilby & Oepkes, 2012) (see Chapter 21).

> *What If . . . 13.3*
>
> **Tori Alarino is pregnant with a multiple pregnancy and tells the nurse she is "eating for three." The nurse notices on her list of foods that she lists three desserts every day for lunch. Will this hurt her or just add a few extra pounds?**

THE WOMAN WHO SMOKES OR USES DRUGS OR ALCOHOL

The specific effects of alcohol, cigarette smoking, and substance use on fetal growth are discussed in Chapter 22. In addition to specific teratogenic fetal effects, these substances can lead to general nutrition problems because a woman is ingesting these substances rather than eating nutritious foods.

THE WOMAN WITH A CONCURRENT HEALTH PROBLEM

Any health concern that requires rigid salt, protein, or carbohydrate restriction poses a potential threat to fetal nutrition. That means women who have medical problems such as kidney disease, diabetes, tuberculosis, bulimia, inflammatory bowel disease, celiac disease, or anorexia nervosa should consult their primary care provider before pregnancy because of the specific metabolic disorders involved with these illnesses. Women who develop gestational diabetes need the same type of nutrition counseling. Nursing interventions and nutrition concerns for women with major health problems such as these are discussed in Chapter 20.

The Woman With Lactose Intolerance

The sugar in milk is called lactose. In the intestines, lactose is broken down into glucose and galactose by the enzyme **lactase**. Most of the world's population has sufficient lactase as an infant to make this conversion, but the amount of lactase available fades by school age. After this point, people can have difficulty digesting lactose or become lactose intolerant. African Americans, Native Americans, and Asians tend to have the highest percentage of lactose intolerance (approximately 70% of African American adults cannot drink milk). Those most able to tolerate milk are Northern Europeans and their descendants (Silanikove, Leitner, & Merin, 2015).

When people who are lactose intolerant drink milk, they experience nausea, diarrhea, cramps, gas, and a general feeling of bloating. For these women, fortified soy milk is a good substitute; it is rich in protein, calcium, and vitamin D and is easily digestible. Women who don't like the taste of soy milk may be able to eat cheese because the processing of cheese changes its lactose content; yogurt may also be tolerated. Lactase tablets to be chewed before ingesting milk products can be prescribed to supplement absent lactase, although the woman needs to consult with her primary healthcare provider before taking these as they are a class N drug (not assigned a pregnancy category of safety). Even if a woman does take lactase tablets, a calcium supplement (1,200 mg daily) and a vitamin D supplement (400 International Units) may also be prescribed. This is because the amount of cheese or yogurt needed to replace the calcium of milk is too large to be practical. Because milk is also a good source of protein, be sure to assess whether, without milk, a woman's intake of protein is adequate.

Because many baby magazines, television advertisements, and government pamphlets on pregnancy repeatedly mention that it is important to drink milk during pregnancy, you may need to explain to a woman with lactose intolerance as long as she ingests the same nutrients from other foods, the actual drinking of milk is not important.

QSEN Checkpoint Question 13.6

SAFETY

Tori describes the foods she eats daily. Which nutritional risk does the nurse identify as most likely if Tori is a vegetarian?
  a. Lack of iron
  b. Lack of vitamin C
  c. Lack of folic acid
  d. Lack of vitamin B$_{12}$

Look in Appendix A for the best answer and rationale.

The Woman With Phenylketonuria

Phenylketonuria (PKU) is an inherited disorder in which a person cannot convert phenylalanine, an essential amino acid, into tyrosine. Without conversion, phenylalanine accumulates in the person's blood serum, eventually leaving the bloodstream to invade body cells. When brain cells are invaded, severe cognitive impairment and accompanying neurologic damage, such as recurrent seizures, develop (see Chapter 48). A fetus of a woman with uncontrolled PKU can develop a cognitive impairment, microcephaly, intrauterine growth restriction, and neurologic damage from exposure to excessive phenylalanine levels (Marcdante & Kliegman, 2015).

Women with the disorder need to avoid foods high in phenylalanine, which are those high in protein such as meat and legumes; examples of foods low in phenylalanine are fruits and vegetables such as orange juice, bananas, squash, spinach, and peas. Children with PKU follow a diet with restricted phenylalanine intake until at least past adolescence. A woman with PKU should consult her healthcare provider when she is planning to become pregnant and, if she is not following a restricted intake, should return to a low-phenylalanine diet for at least 3 months before she becomes pregnant. She then follows this low-phenylalanine diet during the pregnancy and as long as she is breastfeeding. A woman needs to discuss with her primary healthcare provider if she should continue to take sapropterin dihydrochloride (Kuvan), a drug to lower phenylalanine serum levels, during pregnancy as it is a class C category drug (its safety during pregnancy is unproven) (Karch, 2015).

Because a PKU diet is restrictive, a woman needs support during pregnancy to adhere to such restricted intake. It is particularly disappointing to have to follow the diet if a woman does not become pregnant immediately because each month she is "prepregnant" extends the period she has to follow the restrictions. Women with PKU are usually well informed about their particular nutritional needs. Although they may wish they could eat more liberally, they are aware phenylalanine is destructive to developing brain cells. Not following a restricted plan could leave their future child severely cognitively challenged (Murphy, 2015).

The Woman With Hyperemesis Gravidarum

Hyperemesis gravidarum (sometimes called pernicious or persistent vomiting) is nausea and vomiting of pregnancy prolonged past week 16 of pregnancy or that is so severe that dehydration, ketonuria, and significant weight loss occur within the first 12 weeks of pregnancy (O'Donnell et al., 2016). It occurs at an incidence of 2% in pregnant women. The cause is unknown, but women with the disorder may have increased thyroid function because of the thyroid-stimulating properties of human chorionic gonadotropin. Some studies reveal it is associated with *Helicobacter pylori*, the same bacteria that cause peptic ulcers (Cardaropoli, Rolfo, & Todros, 2014).

With hyperemesis gravidarum, weight loss can be severe because, with so much nausea and vomiting, a woman cannot maintain her usual nutrition. Urine may test positive for ketones, evidence the woman's body is breaking down stored fat and protein for cell growth. An elevated hematocrit concentration may be detected at a monthly prenatal visit because the inability to retain fluid has resulted in hemoconcentration (which is dangerous because it can lead to thromboembolism). In contrast, concentrations of sodium, potassium, and chloride may be reduced because of a woman's low intake; hypokalemic alkalosis may develop from loss of hydrochloric acid from the stomach. In some women, ataxia and confusion, caused by deficiency of vitamin B_1 (thiamine), develops. If left untreated, a woman with hyperemesis may become so dehydrated she can no longer provide a fetus with essential nutrients for growth, and intrauterine growth restriction or preterm birth can result (McCarthy, 2012).

Assessment

Always try to determine exactly how much nausea and vomiting women are having during pregnancy. Ask the patient to describe the events of the day before:

- How late into the day did the nausea last?
- How many times did she vomit and how much?
- What was the total amount of food she was able to eat?

Therapeutic Management

Women with hyperemesis gravidarum may need to be hospitalized for about 24 hours to document and monitor their intake, output, and blood chemistries and to restore hydration.

All oral food and fluids are usually withheld for the first 24 hours. Intravenous fluid (e.g., 3,000 ml Ringer's lactate with added vitamin B_1) may be administered to increase hydration. An antiemetic, such as metoclopramide (Reglan, pregnancy class B), may be prescribed to control vomiting. Throughout this period, carefully measure intake and output, including the amount of vomitus, so the degree of hydration can best be evaluated.

If there is no vomiting after the first 24 hours of oral restriction, small amounts of clear fluid can be started and the woman discharged home, usually with a referral for home care. If she can continue to take clear fluid without vomiting, small quantities of dry toast, crackers, or cereal can be added every 2 or 3 hours, after which the woman may be gradually advanced to a soft diet and then to a regular diet. If vomiting returns at any point, enteral or total parenteral nutrition may be prescribed to ensure she receives adequate nutrition (O'Donnell et al., 2016).

 Nursing Diagnoses and Related Interventions

The main challenge in the beginning of excessive vomiting is fluid deficiency. As hyperemesis of pregnancy continues, lack of total nutrition becomes a concern. A woman with hyperemesis gravidarum needs the opportunity to express how she feels about this strange phenomenon that is happening to her and how it feels to live with ever present nausea. Some women are under such psychosocial stress from this they appreciate counseling to help them decide whether to terminate a pregnancy or allow it to go to completion.

Nursing Diagnosis: Imbalanced nutrition, less than body requirements, related to prolonged vomiting

Outcome Evaluation: Patient ingests 2,200 calories daily or receives supplemental nutrition intravenously or enterally.

Like the typical nausea and vomiting of pregnancy, the vomiting of hyperemesis gravidarum may be precipitated by fatigue and the smell of cooking. Encourage a woman to serve herself small portions so the amount on her plate does not appear overwhelming. If she is hospitalized, try to limit her exposure to food odors. Be certain hot foods are served hot, and cold foods are served cold. Check to be certain food carts smelling of food such as fish, bacon, or coffee are not parked outside her room door.

An emesis basin is an important piece of equipment for a woman who is vomiting. Put it out of sight, though, and not on a bedside table, so a woman is not constantly reminded of vomiting. Do not urge a woman who is already struggling to eat to "Eat just a little more. You don't want to hurt your baby." Urging women to eat in this way may cause them to feel guilty on top of feeling so nauseated.

If a woman is receiving total parenteral nutrition, she needs her blood tested for glucose about twice daily. If her blood glucose is elevated, it suggests the infusion solution contains more glucose than her body's metabolism can process. In contrast, if ketones are present in her urine, it means her body is not receiving enough nutrients and is breaking down protein. If either of these findings is positive, she needs a nutrition reassessment to see if she needs a change in her prescription for the enteral or total parenteral therapy.

Fortunately, despite its extreme symptoms, if hyperemesis is identified early in pregnancy and managed, it will not lead to pregnancy loss or low birth weight but rather to a healthy pregnancy.

KEY POINTS FOR REVIEW

- Assessment of nutritional health should include a health history (24-hour recall) and physical examination.
- Aiding women to include about 300 additional calories daily to provide energy, spare protein, and provide for fetal growth requirements not only helps meet QSEN competencies but also best meets a woman's pregnancy needs.
- Important minerals necessary for pregnancy include iron, iodine, calcium, fluoride, sodium, and zinc. Most women need to take an iron supplement to prevent iron-deficiency anemia and may need additional calcium and vitamin D supplementation as well.
- Women should monitor their intake of caffeine and artificial sweeteners during pregnancy and should restrict alcohol and tobacco to the lowest amounts possible.
- Remind women to use prescribed prenatal vitamins rather than over-the-counter ones during pregnancy because prescribed vitamins contain additional folic acid, calcium, and iron supplements. Be certain women regard pregnancy vitamins as medication and follow the medication rule: Take nothing other than medications specifically recommended by their primary care providers, or else toxicity could result.
- Advise pregnant women not to go longer than 3 to 4 hours between meals to avoid hypoglycemia.
- Common nutrition concerns associated with pregnancy include nausea and vomiting, constipation, cravings (including pica), and pyrosis.
- Women who are at high risk for inadequate nutrition include those who are adolescent or over age 40 years; those who have decreased nutrition stores; and women with a multiple pregnancy or who are lactose intolerant, underweight, or overweight. Others at high risk are those with a secondary health concern; who are on a special diet; who use recreational drugs, including alcohol or cigarettes; and those who experience hyperemesis gravidarum (extreme nausea and vomiting).
- Hyperemesis gravidarum is nausea and vomiting of pregnancy that extends past 16 weeks of pregnancy or that is too extreme to allow for adequate nutrition. Women with this condition may need antiemetic medication or nutrition supplemented by total parenteral nutrition or enteral feedings.

CRITICAL THINKING CARE STUDY

Annette Milano is 26 years old and is 5 months pregnant. She has a PhD in psychology and lives alone in an apartment near the university where she teaches. She tells you she "didn't mean" to get pregnant and also that she is afraid to go outside at night because gangs "own" her neighborhood. She began feeling nauseated early in pregnancy and has continued to feel this way into her fifth month. She vomits three or four times a day.

24-hour nutrition recall:
Breakfast: none
Lunch: 1 cup of tea, a few dry crackers
Dinner: 1 slice pizza, 1 glass chocolate milk
Snack: 1 apple

Annette knows she is eating very little but tells you, "I have a PhD, so I'm not stupid. You can trust me when I say this is the amount I've always eaten, so it is all right for me."

1. Is Annette's food intake adequate for pregnancy? How would you respond to her admonition she is not stupid?
2. Suppose Annette is hospitalized so she can receive total parental nutrition. What common steps would you want to take to try to decrease her feeling of nausea?
3. You want to assess Annette daily for dehydration. What would be important factors to assess to see if she is well hydrated?

Unfolding Patient Stories: Olivia Jones • Part 2

Think back to Chapter 4, where you met Olivia Jones, a 23-year-old, gravida 1, para 0 at 30 weeks gestation, who presents with signs and symptoms of preeclampsia requiring bedrest at home. She is obese and informs the nurse that she is eating less due to nausea and unemployment. What are important nursing assessments for nutrition evaluation and nutritional requirements during pregnancy? Outline a nursing plan of care that promotes nutritional health for Olivia, addressing her identified problems and educational needs.

Care for Olivia and other patients in a realistic virtual environment: **vSim** for Nursing (thepoint.lww.com /vSimMaternityPed). Practice documenting these patients' care in DocuCare (thepoint.lww.com /DocuCareEHR).

RELATED RESOURCES

Explore these additional resources to enhance learning for this chapter:
- Student resources on thePoint, including answers to the What If . . . and Critical Thinking Care Study questions, http://thepoint.lww.com/Flagg8e
- Adaptive learning powered by PrepU, http://thepoint.lww.com /prepu

REFERENCES

Adams, M. A., Bruening, M., Ohri-Vachaspati, P., et al. (2016). Location of school lunch salad bars and fruit and vegetable consumption in middle schools: A cross-sectional plate waste study. *Journal of the Academy of Nutrition and Dietetics, 116*(3), 407–416.

Akahoshi, E., Arima, K., Miura, K., et al. (2016). Association of maternal pre-pregnancy weight, weight gain during pregnancy, and smoking with small-for-gestational-age infants in Japan. *Early Human Development, 92,* 33–36.

American Pregnancy Association. (2016). *Mercury levels in fish.* Irving, TX: Author.

Andreyeva, T., & Luedicke, J. (2015). Incentivizing fruit and vegetable purchases among participants in the Special Supplemental Nutrition Program for Women, Infants, and Children. *Public Health Nutrition, 18*(1), 33–41.

Araújo, J. R., Martel, F., & Keating, E. (2014). Exposure to non-nutritive sweeteners during pregnancy and lactation: Impact in programming of metabolic diseases in the progeny later in life. *Reproductive Toxicology, 49,* 196–201.

Atta, C., Fiest, K. M., Frolkis, A. D., et al. (2016). Global birth prevalence of spina bifida by folic acid fortification status: A systematic review and meta-analysis. *American Journal of Public Health, 106*(1), e24–e34.

Attilakos, G., & Overton, T. G. (2012). Antenatal care. In D. K. Edmonds (Ed.), *Dewhurst's textbook of obstetrics & gynaecology* (6th ed., pp. 42–52). Oxford, United Kingdom: Wiley.

Barbour, L. A. (2014). Changing perspectives in pre-existing diabetes and obesity in pregnancy: Maternal and infant short- and long-term outcomes. *Current Opinion in Endocrinology, Diabetes, and Obesity, 21*(4), 257–263.

Bateman, B. T., Hernandez-Diaz, S., Fischer, M. A., et al. (2015). Statins and congenital malformations: Cohort study. *BMJ, 350,* h1035.

Bodnar, L. M., Siminerio, L. L., Himes, K. P., et al. (2016). Maternal obesity and gestational weight gain are risk factors for infant death. *Obesity, 24*(2), 490–498.

Brooten, D., Youngblut, J. M., Golembeski, S., et al. (2012). Perceived weight gain, risk, and nutrition in pregnancy in five racial groups. *Journal of the American Academy of Nurse Practitioners, 24*(1), 32–42.

Bureau of Labor Statistics. (2013). *Economic news release: Table 5. Employment status of the population by sex, marital status, and presence of own children under 18, 2014-2015 annual averages.* Retrieved from http://www.bls.gov/news.release/famee.t05.htm

Cardaropoli, S., Rolfo, A., & Todros, T. (2014). Helicobacter pylori and pregnancy-related disorders. *World Journal of Gastroenterology, 20*(3), 654–664.

Centers for Disease Control and Prevention. (2016). *Defining adult overweight and obesity.* Washington, DC: Author.

Cheikh Ismail, L., Bishop, D. C., Pang, R., et al. (2016). Gestational weight gain standards based on women enrolled in the Fetal Growth Longitudinal Study of the INTERGROWTH-21st Project: A prospective longitudinal cohort study. *BMJ, 352,* i555.

Declercq, E., MacDorman, M., Osterman, M., et al. (2015). Prepregnancy obesity and primary cesareans among otherwise low-risk mothers in 38 U.S. states in 2012. *Birth, 42*(4), 309–318.

Fletcher, W., & Russo, M. L. (2015). Preconception counseling and prenatal care. In J. L. Bienstock, H. E. Fox, E. E. Wallach, et al. (Eds.), *The Johns Hopkins manual of gynecology and obstetrics* (5th ed., pp. 58–78). Philadelphia, PA: Lippincott Williams & Wilkins.

Inge, T. H., Courcoulas, A. P., Jenkins, T. M., et al. (2016). Weight loss and health status 3 years after bariatric surgery in adolescents. *New England Journal of Medicine, 374*(2), 113–123.

Institute of Medicine & National Research Council. (2009). *Weight gain during pregnancy: Reexamining the guidelines.* Washington, DC: The National Academies Press.

Johnston, E. O., Sharma, A. J., & Abe, K. (2016). Association between maternal multivitamin use and preterm birth in 24 states, pregnancy risk assessment monitoring system, 2009–2010. *Maternal and Child Health Journal, 20*(9), 1825–1834.

Karch, A. M. (2015). *Lippincott's nursing drug guide.* Philadelphia, PA: Lippincott Williams & Wilkins.

Kee, J. L., Hayes, E. R., & McCuistion, L. E. (2015). Drugs for gastrointestinal tract disorders. In J. L. Kee, E. R. Hayes, & L. E. McCuistion (Eds.), *Pharmacology: A nursing process approach* (pp. 676–692). St. Louis, MO: Elsevier/Saunders.

Kilby, M. D., & Oepkes, P. (2012). Multiple pregnancy. In D. K. Edmonds (Ed.), *Dewhurst's textbook of obstetrics & gynaecology* (6th ed., pp. 230–246). Oxford, United Kingdom: Wiley.

Kimmel, M. C., Ferguson, E. H., Zerwas, S., et al. (2016). Obstetric and gynecologic problems associated with eating disorders. *The International Journal of Eating Disorders, 49*(3), 260–275.

Lauritzen, L., Brambilla, P., Mazzocchi, A., et al. (2016). DHA effects in brain development and function. *Nutrients, 8*(1), 1–17.

Luke, S., Kirby, R. S., & Wright, L. (2016). Postpartum weight retention and subsequent pregnancy outcomes. *The Journal of Perinatal & Neonatal Nursing, 34*(4), 292–301.

Marcdante, K. J., & Kliegman, R. M. (2015). Amino acid disorders. In K. J. Marcdante & R. M. Kliegman (Eds.), *Nelson essentials of pediatrics* (7th ed., pp. 174–176). Philadelphia, PA: Saunders/Elsevier.

Martin, C. L., Siega-Riz, A. M., Sotres-Alvarez, D., et al. (2016). Maternal dietary patterns during pregnancy are associated with child growth in the first 3 years of life. *The Journal of Nutrition, 146*(11), 2281–2288.

Martin, J. A., Hamilton, B. E., Osterman, M. J. K., et al. (2015). Births: Final data for 2013. *National Vital Statistics Reports, 64*(1), 1–65.

McCarthy, A. (2012). Miscellaneous medical disorders. In D. K. Edmonds (Ed.), *Dewhurst's textbook of obstetrics & gynaecology* (6th ed., pp. 173–184). Oxford, United Kingdom: Wiley.

Menon, K. C., Ferguson, E. L., Thomson, C. D., et al. (2016). Effects of anemia at different stages of gestation on infant outcomes. *Nutrition, 32*(1), 61–65.

Miao, D., Young, S. L., & Golden, C. D. (2015). A meta-analysis of pica and micronutrient status. *American Journal of Human Biology, 27*(1), 84–93.

Monson, M., & Jackson, M. (2016). Pregnancy after bariatric surgery. *Clinical Obstetrics and Gynecology, 59*(1), 158–171.

Murphy, E. (2015). Medical problems in obstetrics: Inherited metabolic disease. *Best Practice & Research. Clinical Obstetrics & Gynaecology, 29*(5), 707–720.

O'Donnell, A., McParlin, C., Robson, S. C., et al. (2016). Treatments for hyperemesis gravidarum and nausea and vomiting in pregnancy: A systematic review and economic assessment. *Health Technology Assessment, 20*(74), 1–268.

Pfaff, N. F., & Tillett, J. (2016). Listeriosis and toxoplasmosis in pregnancy: Essentials for healthcare providers. *The Journal of Perinatal & Neonatal Nursing, 30*(2), 131–138.

Phupong, V., & Hanprasertpong, T. (2015). Interventions for heartburn in pregnancy. *Cochrane Database of Systematic Reviews,* (9), CD011379.

Pistollato, F., Sumalla Cano, S., Elio, I., et al. (2015). Plant-based and plant-rich diet patterns during gestation: Beneficial effects and possible shortcomings. *Advances in Nutrition, 6*(5), 581–591.

Rénes, L., Barka, N., Gyurkovits, Z., et al. (2017). Predictors of caesarean section—a cross-sectional study in Hungary. *Journal of Maternal-Fetal & Neonatal Medicine.* Advance online publication. doi:10.1080/14767058.2017.1285888

Rogers, V. L., & Worley, K. C. (2016). Obstetrics and obstetric disorders. In M. A. Papadakis, S. J. McPhee, & M. W. Rabow (Eds.), *Current medical diagnosis & treatment* (55th ed., pp. 783–811). Columbus, OH: McGraw-Hill.

Rungsiprakarn, P., Laopaiboon, M., Sangkomkamhang, U. S., et al. (2015). Interventions for treating constipation in pregnancy. *Cochrane Database of Systematic Reviews,* (9), CD011448.

Saltzman, J. A., Pineros-Leano, M., Liechty, J. M., et al. (2016). Eating, feeding, and feeling: Emotional responsiveness mediates longitudinal associations between maternal binge eating, feeding practices, and child weight. *International Journal of Behavioral Nutrition and Physical Activity, 13,* 89.

Sethi, S., Tyagi, S. K., & Anurag, R. K. (2016). Plant-based milk alternatives an emerging segment of functional beverages: A review. *Journal of Food Science and Technology, 53*(9), 3408–3423.

Sharma, R., Biedenharn, K. R., Fedor, J. M., et al. (2013). Lifestyle factors and reproductive health: Taking control of your fertility. *Reproductive Biology and Endocrinology, 11,* 66.

Silanikove, N., Leitner, G., & Merin, U. (2015). The interrelationships between lactose intolerance and the modern dairy industry: Global perspectives in evolutionary and historical backgrounds. *Nutrients, 7*(9), 7312–7331.

Simhan, H. N. (2016). Antepartum care of the obese patient. *Clinical Obstetrics and Gynecology, 59*(1), 148–157.

Stang, J., & Huffman, L. G. (2016). Position of the academy of nutrition and dietetics: Obesity, reproduction, and pregnancy outcomes. *Journal of the Academy of Nutrition and Dietetics, 116*(4), 677–691.

Temel, S., Erdem, O., Voorham, T. A., et al. (2015). Knowledge on preconceptional folic acid supplementation and intention to seek for preconception care among men and women in an urban city: A population-based cross-sectional study. *BMC Pregnancy and Childbirth, 15,* 340.

Torso, L. M., Voorhees, R. E., Forest, S. A., et al. (2015). Escherichia coli O157:H7 outbreak associated with restaurant beef grinding. *Journal of Food Protection, 78*(7), 1272–1279.

U.S. Department of Agriculture. (2012). *Choose my plate: A guide to daily food choices.* Washington, DC: Author.

U.S. Department of Agriculture. (2016). *Supplemental nutrition assistance program (SNAP).* Washington, DC: Author.

U.S. Department of Health and Human Services. (2010). *Healthy people 2020.* Washington, DC: Author.

Whitney, E. N., & Rolfes, S. R. (2016). Life cycle nutrition: Pregnancy & lactation. In E. N. Whitney & S. R. Rolfes (Eds.), *Understanding nutrition* (pp. 473–508). Stamford, CT: Cengage Learning.

World Health Organization. (2016). *WHO recommendations on antenatal care for a positive pregnancy experience.* Geneva, Switzerland: Author.

Wyeth Ayerst Pharmaceuticals. (2012). *Product information.* Philadelphia, PA: Author.

14

Preparing a Family for Childbirth and Parenting

*E*lena Garza is a 30-year-old woman who is pregnant with her second child. During her first pregnancy, she did not attend any childbirth classes and received an epidural for the birth. During a prenatal visit for her current pregnancy, Elena tells you she would now like to have a more natural birth in a birthing center. She asks you for information on childbirth education classes. Her partner, Joe, a Navy Seal, wants Elena to go to the hospital and have an epidural like the last time. He says, "The doctors know what they're doing. Just let them do their job." After further speaking with Joe, you discover he doesn't want Elena to go through the pain of natural childbirth because he fears he may be out of town when she's in labor.

Previous chapters discussed normal reproductive anatomy and physiology and nursing care necessary during pregnancy. This chapter adds information about ways couples can make labor and birth a more satisfying experience. The information helps protect the mental as well as the physical health of both women and children throughout the continuum of pregnancy, birth, and childrearing.

How can you help alleviate some of Joe's concerns and best advise the Garzas on preparations for childbirth?

KEY TERMS

alternative birthing centers (ABCs)

birthing bed

birthing chair

birthing room

cleansing breath

conditioned reflexes

conscious relaxation

consciously controlled breathing

distraction

doula

effleurage

gating control theory of pain perception

labor-birth-recovery-postpartum room (LBRP)

Leboyer method

psychoprophylactic

vaginal birth after cesarean (VBAC)

OBJECTIVES

After mastering the contents of this chapter, you should be able to:

1. Describe common preparations for childbirth and parenting, including common settings for birth.

2. Identify 2020 National Health Goals related to preparation for parenthood and how nurses can help the nation achieve these goals.

3. Assess the readiness of a couple for childbirth with regard to choice of birth attendant, preparation for labor, and birth setting.

4. Formulate nursing diagnoses related to preparation for childbirth and parenting.

5. Identify expected outcomes for a couple preparing for childbirth and parenting while helping them manage seamless transitions across differing healthcare settings.

6. Using the nursing process, plan nursing care that includes the six competencies of Quality & Safety Education for Nurses (QSEN): Patient-Centered Care, Teamwork & Collaboration, Evidence-Based Practice (EBP), Quality Improvement (QI), Safety, and Informatics.

7. Implement nursing care to assist a couple in selecting and preparing for an alternative birth setting such as a freestanding clinic or their home as well as support a woman during labor by controlled breathing.

8. Evaluate outcome criteria for achievement and effectiveness of care.

9. Integrate knowledge of prepared childbirth with the interplay of nursing process, the six competencies of QSEN, and Family Nursing to promote quality maternal and child health nursing care.

> BOX 14.1
>
> ### Nursing Care Planning Based on 2020 National Health Goals
>
> Preparation-for-childbirth classes supply information not only on how to prepare for childbirth but also on how to parent. A number of 2020 National Health Goals that speak directly to such classes or counseling include:
>
> - Increase the proportion of pregnant women who attend a series of prepared childbirth classes (Developmental).
> - Increase the proportion of pregnant women who receive early and adequate prenatal care from a baseline of 70.5% to a target of 77.6%.
> - Increase the proportion of women delivering a live birth who received preconception care services and practiced key recommended preconception health behaviors (Developmental) (U.S. Department of Health and Human Services, 2010; see www.healthypeople.gov).
>
> Nurses have a direct role in helping the nation achieve these objectives by participating as instructors in preparation for childbirth and parenting classes as well as teaching and supervising prenatal care.

As active consumers of health care, expectant families can find themselves faced with a wide array of choices for a childbirth experience and preparation for parenting. Three important decisions families need to make before labor include:

- Choice of birth attendant
- Choice of setting
- How much and what type of analgesic they want to use in labor

For example, a woman may elect to have her family doctor, an obstetrician, or a nurse-midwife as her birth attendant. She may choose to be supported by her intimate partner, other family members, friends, or a **doula** (a woman experienced in childbirth who provides continuous emotional and physical support). She may choose to give birth in a birthing center or a hospital with specially equipped birthing rooms (MacDorman, Mathews, & Declercq, 2014).

No matter what setting the woman or couple choose, expectant parents are well advised to be as prepared as possible for the physical and emotional aspects of childbirth (Black, Entwistle, Bhattacharya, et al., 2016). Box 14.1 shows 2020 National Health Goals related to preparation for childbirth and parenting.

Nursing Process Overview

FOR CHILDBIRTH AND PARENTING EDUCATION

ASSESSMENT

Assessing each woman's or couple's readiness for decision making about childbirth as well as providing foundation information early in the process can help a woman or couple make plans for childbirth. Some couples have a clear idea of where and how they wish their child's birth to occur from the moment they realize they are pregnant. Others cannot even consider the actual birth until they have adjusted to the idea of pregnancy.

Childbirth education is not just for primiparas because if a woman expecting her second or third child has waited several years between children, she usually appreciates refresher information as much as a primipara hungers for new information. Whether a woman is a primipara or multipara, ask whether either she or her support person wants to attend childbirth or parenting courses. Provide appropriate information on what classes are available and how and when they should enroll.

NURSING DIAGNOSIS

Nursing diagnoses tend to cluster around whether the woman or couple is sure of their decision about the birth setting and childbirth preparation. Examples include:

- Health-seeking behaviors related to learning more about childbirth and newborn care
- If there is a lack of a support person, the following diagnoses might apply:
  - Ineffective coping related to lack of a support person
  - Anxiety related to absence of significant other
- For a couple unable to make a decision about a childbirth setting, an appropriate diagnosis might be decisional conflict related to lack of information about advantages and disadvantages of various childbirth settings.
- If there are older children in the family, a nursing diagnosis might be anxiety related to sibling role in pending birth event and sibling ability to welcome a new family member.

OUTCOME IDENTIFICATION AND PLANNING

When planning with couples for labor and birth, goals that are set should seem both realistic and flexible. For example, the goal of preparation is to help couples make informed choices rather than to follow a rigid plan.

Not all women want to go through labor without analgesia, so setting a goal to do so would be unrealistic for such a woman. The majority of women, however, want to participate as fully as possible in their labor and birth experience, so setting a goal for them to do that would be very realistic. Some women may be reluctant to attend a childbirth preparation course because of fear attending will mean they are committing themselves to a medication-free birth. You can assure them that learning about medications or other methods to reduce the pain of childbirth does not mean they have to use one or the other of these methods. In the same way, women who are certain they want medication before having taken a class will not be held to this afterward.

Refer couples to helpful websites and other resources when appropriate (see Chapter 9).

IMPLEMENTATION

Be certain to provide a woman and her partner with information on the benefits and drawbacks of birthing options without influencing them in a particular direction. To remain objective, examine your own attitudes, cultural influences, and values related to childbirth and explore how these beliefs might differ from those of your patients (Box 14.2). Referring couples to a childbirth preparation course can provide many answers for them in a sympathetic group setting, where feelings and anxieties can be shared. Be familiar with the content of courses available in your community so you can be certain the courses you suggest are appropriate for individual couples and present adequate and accurate information.

Review the arrangements a woman needs to make for labor and birth at the midpoint of pregnancy. No matter how calm a woman seems when discussing these details, many women experience some fear at the last minute and will forget what they need to do when labor begins. Be certain a woman has thought through arrangements for transportation to the hospital or birthing center and for child care if she has other children at home. Be certain a woman who anticipates a home birth has organized her home and purchased supplies for birth well in advance of her expected due date.

OUTCOME EVALUATION

Evaluate whether expected outcomes for childbirth education have been achieved during the last few prenatal visits. By this time, a woman or couple should know where the baby will be born and should have worked out transportation and child care details. Encourage women who will be coached through childbirth by their partners or another support person to continue practicing breathing and relaxation techniques together up to the time of birth so they do not lose these skills. A final evaluation as to whether the couple was satisfied with their birth setting or preparation choices takes place after the birth. Examples of expected outcomes that would demonstrate the success of interventions include:

- The couple states they feel prepared for childbirth.
- The patient states she feels confident she can use breathing exercises for contractions as long as 70 seconds.
- The patient has made preparations for a doula to support her during labor.
- The sibling states she is ready to welcome a new brother or sister into the family.
- The couple states they were well prepared for birth and that it was both a satisfying and a growth experience for them.

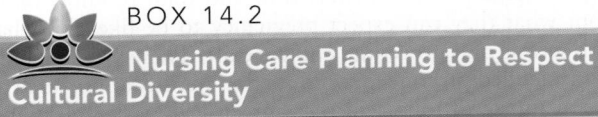

BOX 14.2
Nursing Care Planning to Respect Cultural Diversity

Whether women want or are able to take a childbirth and parenting preparation course depends a great deal on cultural and socioeconomic factors and individual choices. In some cultures, for example, the advice of a friend or family member carries more weight than the advice of a professional healthcare practitioner. A very old cross-cultural belief is a knife placed under the mattress will "cut the pain" better than a Lamaze program, so you may need to advocate to allow this type of pain relief. Asking each woman separately whether she is interested in a course and being certain women are fully informed about the options available are two ways to be certain all women receive as much advice and knowledge as they wish about childbirth.

Who women choose as a support person or coach in labor also differs depending on one's cultural background. Some women would not think of choosing anyone but their male partner; whereas others' first choice would be a female relative or friend. Assess each couple individually to be certain cultural preferences such as these are respected.

Childbirth Education

Although parenting is unarguably an important occupation, it is one of the few occupations that requires no formal education, no examination to test a person's ability to take on such a role, and no refresher course to ensure a parent is following healthy standards of childrearing. Assessing whether couples need preparation for childbirth or parenting classes or encouraging them to take one can therefore be extremely important to make childbirth a satisfying experience, to help a family bond with its new member, and to help couples become effective parents (Box 14.3).

Preparation for childbirth courses that teach this material should be individualized to meet the parents' needs. Classes should be personalized and structured for women with special needs such as adolescents, career women, women who are physically challenged, or those experiencing a high-risk pregnancy. There also are classes available to help prepare siblings or grandparents learn more about their role. Women having a **vaginal birth after cesarean (VBAC)** or women who are having a scheduled cesarean birth can attend classes specially designed for them (Horey, Kealy, Davey, et al., 2013).

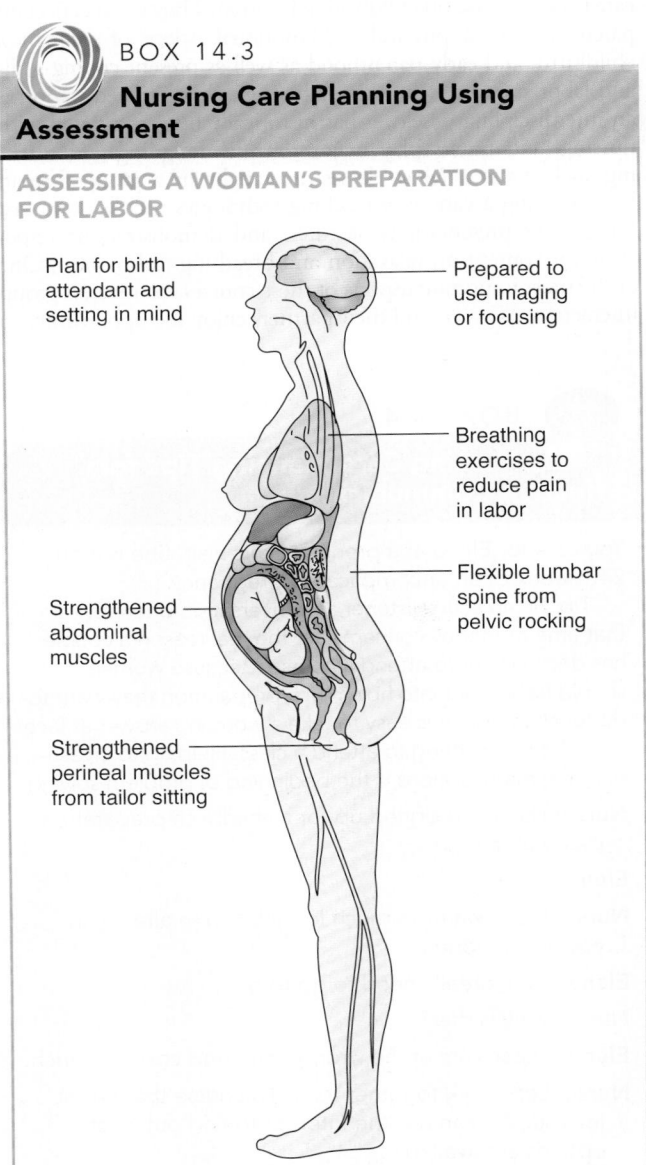

BOX 14.3
Nursing Care Planning Using Assessment

ASSESSING A WOMAN'S PREPARATION FOR LABOR

- Plan for birth attendant and setting in mind
- Prepared to use imaging or focusing
- Breathing exercises to reduce pain in labor
- Flexible lumbar spine from pelvic rocking
- Strengthened abdominal muscles
- Strengthened perineal muscles from tailor sitting

Preparation for childbirth courses initially began in the early 1900s to encourage women to come for prenatal care (Godin, Alton, Gangodawilage, et al., 2015). Classes continue today because, with all the birth choices available, they fulfill an important need for education about labor and childbirth. As many as 15% of women express fear or anxiety about what will happen in labor, so counseling can be very important to alleviate this fear (Ternström, Hildingsson, Haines, et al., 2016).

The overall goals of childbirth education are to prepare expectant parents emotionally and physically for childbirth while promoting wellness behaviors that can be used by parents and families for life. Women usually enjoy such classes because they offer them a sense of "family" if their intimate partner also attends as well as create a sense of empowerment or confidence that they will be knowledgeable enough to participate fully in their birth experience.

CHILDBIRTH EDUCATORS AND METHODS OF TEACHING

Childbirth educators are usually healthcare providers who have a professional degree in the helping professions as well as a certificate from a course on childbirth education. They teach expectant parents about the physical and emotional aspects of pregnancy, childbirth, and early parenthood as well as present coping skills and labor support techniques. Although childbirth education is an interdisciplinary field, it has historically been associated with nursing, and nurses play major roles in designing and teaching such courses. Most classes are taught in a group format, incorporating a variety of teaching techniques such as DVD or PowerPoint presentations, lectures, and demonstrations (especially for content on relaxation and breathing techniques). One of the most important aspects of these courses, however, is group interaction. Women and their partners enjoy the opportunity to share their fears and hopes about their pregnancy and upcoming birth with others as they learn together (Box 14.4).

The Childbirth Plan

Most classes for expectant parents urge couples to make a written childbirth plan to include information such as their choice of setting, birth attendant, special needs such as the extent of family participation they wish during labor, birthing positions, medication options, plans for the immediate postpartum period, baby care, and family visitation—all measures to give them a better sense of control (Hidalgo-Lopezosa, Rodríguez-Borrego, & Muñoz-Villanueva, 2013).

Urge couples to make these decisions at least 1 month before the expected day of birth. This way, if an expectant couple has a strong desire in a certain area, this gives them time to communicate their wish so it can be accommodated if possible. If plans are left to the last minute, the couple may find decisions determined by agency policy or the circumstances at the moment rather than by their input.

When talking to couples about their birth plan, be certain it includes flexibility as well as is centered on the ultimate goal of childbirth: a healthy baby and healthy parents rather than concentration on a limited goal, such as not having fetal monitoring or using a particular birthing position. This is because in the event of a complication that requires an emergency cesarean birth, their preference to have the baby without anesthesia will need to be modified. Making a birth plan in a group setting has the advantage of allowing a couple to sort out their questions and feelings about what they want to consider in their plan as they share information with others. Box 14.5 is a sample birth plan.

Preconception Visits

Preconception visits are specific visits for couples who plan to get pregnant within a short time and want to know more about what they can expect pregnancy to be like and what birth setting and procedure choices exist. These visits include recommended preconception nutrition modifications such as a good intake of folic acid (e.g., green leafy vegetables) and protein (e.g., meat, tofu, beans) and perhaps a prenatal vitamin during the time waiting to get pregnant to ensure a healthy fetus (Shannon, Alberg, Nacul, et al., 2014). Box 14.6 lists questions a couple might want to discuss about birth.

BOX 14.4

Nursing Care Planning Tips for Effective Communication

You care for Elena at a prenatal clinic visit. She is in the 24th week of an uncomplicated pregnancy.

Tip: Be an active listener as conversation often reveal that time or money concerns are the real reason a couple has decided not to attend a course. Because women should have input into how much preparation they want to do for childbirth, it is easy to take a woman's answer at face value for not wanting to attend a class. Helping to investigate the many options is the beginning of problem solving.

Nurse: Have you signed up for a childbirth preparation class yet, Elena?

Elena: No.

Nurse: Don't wait too much longer. You're already in your sixth month.

Elena: I don't really need to go to one.

Nurse: Why is that?

Elena: Classes are at the wrong time. And cost too much.

Nurse: Let's work together to find a course that's right for you. We can use the Internet to find out what options are available.

QSEN Checkpoint Question 14.1

PATIENT-CENTERED CARE

Elena, 30 years of age, shows the nurse the birth plan that she has drafted. Which statement by her would help assure the nurse that she has a workable plan?
   a. "I've written down everything I have to have to make labor a success."
   b. "I didn't include anything my boyfriend wanted; I'm the one having the baby."
   c. "My mother strongly suggested I ask for morphine like she did, so I'm going to add that."
   d. "I've tried to keep it flexible because I know circumstances can change."

Look in Appendix A for the best answer and rationale.

BOX 14.5
Birth Plan: Elena Garza

BIRTH ATTENDANTS

Alexander Coppin, MD, and nurse-midwife Kaitlin Brandywine, or whoever is on call for the big day.

BIRTH SETTING

Room Number 1 at Huntington Alternative Birth Center

SUPPORT PERSONS

My boyfriend Joe and my sister Adrienne. Adrienne will serve as my doula.

ACTIVITIES DURING LABOR

I want to walk around or rock in the rocking chair or play Monopoly.
I want to use breathing exercises with contractions.
I want to wear my own nightgown and listen to Lady Antebellum's CD *Own the Night*
I want to wear my glasses, not my contact lenses.
I want to eat "anything chocolate" during labor.
I want to drink raspberry-flavored water to stay hydrated (partner will supply).
I want a walking epidural for pain as soon as I'm far enough dilated to have it.

BIRTH

Position for birth: on my side (no stirrups, please).
No episiotomy please.
Joe wants to cut the cord.
I want my older son to watch if he wants to (my mother will babysit).
I want to cord bank a sample of my baby's blood.
I'm okay with circumcision.
I want the first voice my baby hears to be my voice so no talking please while he's born.

POSTPARTUM

I want to breastfeed immediately and exclusively (will probably need some help).
I want to use skin-to-skin care to keep the baby warm.
I want to room-in constantly.
Joe wants to sleep over on bedside cot.

BOX 14.6
Nursing Care Planning Based on Family Teaching

CHOOSING A BIRTH SETTING

Q. Elena and her partner Joe ask you, "There are so many options available for a birth setting. How do we decide which one to choose?"

A. Choosing a birth setting is a personal decision. Some questions you might want to ask to help with the decision include:

- What type of healthcare provider do I want to supervise my prenatal care and labor and birth? Nurse-midwife? Family doctor? Obstetrician?
- What settings does a particular childbirth provider let me choose from? A birthing room? An alternative birthing center? My home?
- Will the same person be present at prenatal visits as for the birth? Does the setting offer preparation for childbirth or childrearing classes?
- Will I be allowed to choose a birth position? Will I have input into the amount of anesthesia used? Can a doula be with me in labor? Can administration of ophthalmic ointment for the baby's eyes be delayed so it doesn't interrupt bonding? Can I begin breastfeeding immediately? Will nurses who are supportive and informed about breastfeeding be available if I have a problem?
- Will the setting allow my support person to participate? Will he or she be allowed to stay with me throughout labor and birth? Could he or she cut the cord or help with the birth? Can older children participate? Can I record the birth on video or by photographs?
- Is early discharge available? Will a follow-up home visit be included in care?
- If I should have a complication during labor or birth, is there adequate equipment and personnel available for emergency care? If our baby should have a complication, is there provision for immediate emergency care or transport to a high-risk facility? Will my partner be able to go with the baby?

Expectant Parenting Classes

Expectant parenting classes are designed for couples to attend early in pregnancy. They focus on the woman's health during a pregnancy by covering such topics as the psychological and physical changes of pregnancy, pregnancy nutrition, routine health care such as dental checkups, and newborn care. A typical course plan for 8 weeks is shown in Box 14.7.

Both the woman and her support person are invited to classes; the curriculum is individualized for the group members and their needs such as women in the military, sibling preparation, refresher classes for grandparents, classes for expectant adoptive parents, pregnant adolescents, or women with physical disabilities. If all the women in the group already have children, for example, they may not need a tour of a maternity unit as part of the program; instead, they may want to learn what is new in baby food or child care. If all the women in the class work at least part-time, discussion of "brown bag nutrition" and how to include rest periods during work hours might be most useful. If all the women are teenagers, they may be most interested in what is going to happen to their bodies during pregnancy, or what sports are safe to continue. They may also need extended information on how to care for a newborn. They probably will also want a tour of the maternity unit (Fig. 14.1).

BREASTFEEDING CLASSES

Breastfeeding classes are designed to help women learn more about breastfeeding so they not only choose breastfeeding over bottle feeding but also continue with breastfeeding for at least 6 months following their child's birth. Such classes cover the physiology of breastfeeding as well as

BOX 14.7

Sample Outline for Weekly Expectant Parents Classes

Lesson 1: Review of Physiologic Changes of Pregnancy and Fetal Growth

Lesson 2: Personal Care During Pregnancy
  Nutrition, hygiene such as bathing, dental care, exercise, and rest

Lesson 3: Emotional Changes During Pregnancy

Lesson 4: Labor and Birth
  The process of birth, exercises, and breathing techniques, and medication in labor

Lesson 5: Plans for Birth
  Birth settings available, supplies to take to birth settings, tour or film of a typical birth

Lesson 6: The Postpartum Period

Lesson 7: Infant Care
  Nutrition and hygiene

Lesson 8: Reproductive Life Planning

the psychological aspects. Classes are often taught by a certified La Leche League instructor who is an expert on what problems new mothers are apt to encounter (see Chapter 19 for breastfeeding techniques) (Minert, 2014).

What If . . . 14.1

Elena tells the nurse her partner won't be coming to childbirth classes with her because, as a Navy Seal, he may be out of town when she's in labor. She asks the nurse if it is really important to have someone with her. How would the nurse best advise her?

PREPARATION FOR CHILDBIRTH CLASSES

Preparation for childbirth classes focus mainly on explaining the psychological and physiologic changes that occur with childbirth and ways to prevent or reduce the pain of childbirth.

Figure 14.1 An enjoyable part of a preparation-for-parenthood class is touring a maternity service. Here, parents plan for their visit to the hospital through a hospital tour.

Common areas taught include:
- Preparing the expectant woman and her support person for the childbirth experience
- Helping women become more informed about the options available for childbirth
- Explaining the role of both pharmacologic and nonpharmacologic methods of pain control that are useful for labor
- Helping increase the couple's overall enjoyment of and satisfaction with the childbirth experience

In addition to teaching about normal labor and pain relief, classes also include a number of exercises to ready the body for labor.

EXERCISE DURING PREGNANCY

Encourage women to maintain an active exercise program during pregnancy overall because such a program will both increase blood circulation to the fetus and help prevent excessive weight gain in the mother (Wahlqvist, Krawetz, Rizzo, et al., 2015).

Women should not, however, enroll or participate in a formal exercise program without their obstetric provider's approval. They should also not attempt to exercise if any of the danger signs of pregnancy are present and should never exercise to a point of fatigue (Box 14.8).

Prenatal Yoga

Prenatal yoga classes are aimed at helping a woman relax and manage stress better for all times in her life, not just pregnancy.

BOX 14.8

Nursing Care Planning to Empower a Family

EXERCISE GUIDELINES FOR LABOR PREPARATION

Q. Elena asks you, "How can I be sure the exercises I'm doing to be ready for birth won't hurt me or my baby?"

A. Good rules to follow include:

- Always rise from the floor slowly to prevent feeling dizzy from orthostatic hypotension.
- To rise from the floor, roll over to the side first and then push up to avoid strain on the abdominal muscles or round ligaments because this can cause intense pain.
- To prevent leg cramps when doing leg exercises, never point the toes (extend the heel instead).
- To prevent back pain, do not attempt exercises that hyperextend the lower back.
- Do not hold your breath while exercising, because this increases intra-abdominal and intrauterine pressure.
- Do not continue with exercises if any danger signal of pregnancy occurs.
- Never exercise to a point of fatigue.
- Never practice second-stage pushing. Pushing increases intrauterine pressure and could rupture membranes.

Yoga exercises help a woman stay overall fit by their focus on gentle stretching and deep breathing. They can also help a woman experience high self-esteem as she masters difficult levels or positions. Yoga breathing techniques are also useful in labor to help both relaxation and pain management (Polis, Gussman, & Kuo, 2015).

Caution women that as pregnancy progresses, it will become difficult to maintain yoga positions that involve balancing. Urge women to use a chair or a wall for stabilization and to avoid twisting exercises late in pregnancy because when joints soften in preparation for labor, muscle or joint strain could occur.

Perineal and Abdominal Exercises

Women can practice specific exercises to strengthen pelvic and abdominal muscles to make these muscles stronger and more supple for labor. If perineal muscles are supple, this allows for stretching during birth, reduces discomfort, and helps perineal muscles function more efficiently after childbirth, which helps reduce the possibility of urinary incontinence (Mørkved & Bø, 2014).

A woman may begin exercises as early in pregnancy as she likes. Many exercises can be incorporated into daily activities so they take little time from a busy day. It is best, however, for a woman to set aside a specific time each day for practicing exercises; otherwise, her participation may be sporadic. Initially, women should do each exercise only a few times and gradually increase the number with each session.

Tailor Sitting

Although many women may be familiar with tailor sitting, they may have to be retaught the position, so it is done in a way that stretches perineal muscles without occluding blood supply to the lower legs. A woman should put one leg in front of the other, not put one ankle on top of the other to avoid interfering with leg circulation (Fig. 14.2). As she sits in this position,

Figure 14.3 Squatting helps to stretch the muscles of the pelvic floor. Notice the feet are flat on the floor for optimal perineal stretching.

she should then gently push on her knees toward the floor until she feels her perineum stretch. This is a good position to use to watch television, read, talk to friends on the phone, or file papers in a lower cabinet at work. If a woman sits in this position for at least 15 minutes every day, by the end of pregnancy, her perineum should be so supple when she tailor sits, her knees will almost touch the floor if pushed.

Squatting

Squatting (Fig. 14.3) also stretches the perineal muscles and can be a useful position for second-stage labor as well and, like tailor sitting, should be practiced for about 15 minutes a day. For pelvic muscles to stretch, a woman should keep her feet flat on the floor and not raise on her tiptoes. Incorporating squatting into daily activities such as picking up toys from the floor reduces the amount of time a woman must devote to daily exercises.

Pelvic Floor Contractions (Kegel Exercises)

Pelvic floor contractions can be done easily during daily activities. While sitting at her desk or working around the house, a woman can tighten the muscles of her perineum by doing Kegel exercises (see Chapter 12, Box 12.7). Such perineal muscle-strengthening exercises are helpful in the postpartum period to reduce pain and promote perineal healing. They also have long-term effects of increasing sexual responsiveness and helping prevent stress incontinence (Mørkved & Bø, 2014).

Abdominal Muscle Contractions

Abdominal muscle contractions may help strengthen abdominal muscles during pregnancy, help prevent constipation, and help restore abdominal tone after pregnancy. Strong abdominal muscles can also contribute to effective second-stage pushing during labor. Abdominal contractions can be done in a standing or lying position. A woman merely tightens her abdominal muscles and then relaxes them. She can repeat the exercise as often as she wishes during the day.

Figure 14.2 Tailor sitting stretches perineal muscles to make them more supple. Notice that the legs are parallel so one does not compress the other. A woman could use this position for television watching, telephone conversations, or playing with an older child.

Figure 14.4 Pelvic rocking is helpful for relieving backache during pregnancy and labor. To do this, the woman first hollows her back and then arches it.

Pelvic Rocking

Pelvic rocking (Fig. 14.4) helps relieve backache during pregnancy and early labor by making the lumbar spine more flexible. It can be done in a variety of positions: on hands and knees, lying down, sitting, or standing. A woman arches her back, trying to lengthen or stretch her spine. She holds the position for 1 minute and then hollows her back. If a woman does this at the end of the day about five times, it not only increases her flexibility but also helps relieve back pain and make her more comfortable during the night.

QSEN Checkpoint Question 14.2 ✔

SAFETY

Elena asks the nurse which type of exercise is best to strengthen her perineal muscles in anticipation of birth. Which of the following recommendations is safest and most effective?

  a. Walk or jog 20 minutes daily at a fairly rapid pace.
  b. Squat or tailor sit for 15 minutes out of every day.
  c. Periodically bear down as hard as possible while holding her breath.
  d. Lift both of her legs into the air while she lies on her back.

Look in Appendix A for the best answer and rationale.

Birthing Aids

During early labor, a woman needs to discover what activities she could use for **distraction** that would be unique for her such as playing cards or listening to specific music; further into labor, she should plan what she could use as a greater distraction for even stronger contractions such as singing out loud, having her partner massage her back, or center intently on breathing exercises. Caution her partner that by mid-labor, women become so intent on the process of birthing that they no longer want to talk or joke.

In order to help fetal descent and help relieve pain, women can use an exercise ball, a Jacuzzi tub, or change of position such as squatting, swaying with a partner, or rocking in a chair. These alternative pain and descent methods are discussed in Chapter 16 with other measures that are useful in labor but don't involve practice during pregnancy.

Methods to Manage Pain in Childbirth

Beginning in the late 1950s, many specific methods for non-pharmacologic pain reduction during labor were developed. These included the Lamaze, Dick-Read, Kitzinger, and Bradley methods, all named after the professionals who developed them. More recently, childbirth education has moved away from a strict method approach like these to more eclectic ones. Many educators teach a variety of approaches, including the use of complementary or herbal therapies.

Most approaches to reducing discomfort in labor are based on the following three principles:

1. A woman needs to come into labor informed about what causes labor pain and prepared with breathing exercises to use to minimize pain during contractions.
2. A woman experiences less pain if her abdomen is relaxed and the uterus is allowed to rise freely against the abdominal wall with contractions.
3. Using the **gating control theory of pain perception**, distraction techniques can be employed to alter how pain is received (Box 14.9).

 What If . . . 14.2
Elena tells the nurse she does not intend to take a preparation for labor class because she wants to have epidural anesthesia as soon as she is admitted to the hospital in labor. Would the nurse advise her to attend a class?

BRADLEY (PARTNER-COACHED) METHOD

The Bradley method of childbirth, originated by Robert Bradley, is based on the premise that pregnancy and childbirth are joyful, natural processes and that a woman's partner should play an active role during pregnancy, labor, and the early newborn period. During pregnancy, a woman performs muscle-toning exercises and limits or omits foods that contain preservatives, animal fat, or a high salt content. She reduces pain in labor by abdominal breathing. In addition, she is encouraged to walk during labor and to use an internal focal point as a disassociation technique. The method is used at specific centers in the United States and is used widely in Europe, so it may be a favorite method of an immigrant woman. It is taught by certified Bradley instructors (Bradley, Hathaway, Hathaway, et al., 2008).

THE PSYCHOSEXUAL METHOD

The psychosexual method of childbirth was developed by Sheila Kitzinger in England during the 1950s. The method stresses pregnancy, labor and birth, and the early newborn period are some of the most important points in a woman's life. It includes a program of conscious relaxation and levels of progressive breathing that encourage a woman to "flow with" rather than struggle against contractions (Kitzinger, 2011).

THE DICK-READ METHOD

The Dick-Read method is based on an approach proposed by Grantly Dick-Read, an English physician. The premise is

BOX 14.9

Gating Control Mechanisms to Reduce Pain

PAIN FLOWS THROUGH PATHWAYS BECAUSE:

1. The endings of small peripheral nerve fibers detect a stimulus.
2. Small nerve fibers transmit the sensation of pain to cells in the dorsal horn of the spinal cord.
3. Impulses pass through a dense, interfacing network of cells in the spinal cord (the substantia gelatinosa).
4. Immediately, a synapse occurs in a motor nerve that initiates a response at the peripheral site. For example, a woman touches a hot stove, the impulse travels to the spinal cord, immediately returns to her fingers, and the woman jerks her hand away from the stove burner.
5. After this short-circuit synapse, the impulse then continues in the spinal cord to reach the hypothalamus and cortex of the brain.
6. The impulse is interpreted (e.g., the burner is hot) and is perceived as pain.

GATING THEORY OF PAIN CONTROL

The gating theory of pain perception refers to gate control mechanisms in the substantia gelatinosa that are capable of halting an impulse at the level of the spinal cord so the impulse is never perceived at the brain level as pain—a process similar to closing a gate. Techniques that can assist gating mechanisms include:

- *Cutaneous stimulation.* If large peripheral nerves next to an injury site are stimulated, the ability of the small nerve fibers at the injury site to transmit pain impulses appears to decrease. Therefore, rubbing an injured part or applying transcutaneous electrical nerve stimulation (TENS) or heat or cold to the site (cutaneous stimulation) are effective maneuvers to suppress pain. Effleurage, or light massage used in the Lamaze method, also accomplishes this.
- *Distraction.* If the cells in the brain cortex that will register an impulse as pain are preoccupied with other stimuli, a pain impulse cannot register. Different childbirth classes use different breathing, vocalization, or focusing techniques such as imaging to accomplish this. Breathing techniques not only furnish distraction but can increase oxygenation to the mother and fetus.
- *Reduction of anxiety.* Pain impulses are perceived more quickly if a woman is anxious. The third technique of gating, therefore, is to reduce patient anxiety as much as possible. Teaching a woman what to expect during labor is a means of achieving this.

THE LAMAZE PHILOSOPHY

The Lamaze method of prepared childbirth, a philosophy based on the gating control theory of pain relief, is the one most often taught in the United States today (Amis, 2010). The method is based on the theory that through stimulus-response conditioning, women can learn to use controlled breathing to reduce pain during labor. It was originally termed the **psychoprophylactic** method because it focuses on preventing pain in labor (prophylaxis) by use of the mind (psyche). The method was developed in Russia based on Pavlov's conditioning studies but was popularized by a French physician, Ferdinand Lamaze. Formal classes are organized by Lamaze International and the International Childbirth Education Association.

Lamaze preparation is not so much a method to help a woman cope with labor as it is a total philosophy of how to enjoy a safe and satisfying childbirth experience. Information to guide a woman and her coach through pregnancy such as prenatal nutrition, exercises, and common discomforts of pregnancy are discussed in classes along with information to prepare couples for unexpected circumstances of birth, such as malpresentation, cesarean birth, or the need for analgesia or anesthesia.

Throughout the program, the following six major concepts are stressed:

1. Labor should begin on its own, not be induced.
2. Women should walk, move around, and change positions throughout labor.
3. Women should bring a loved one, friend, or doula for continuous support.
4. Interventions that are not medically necessary should be avoided.
5. Women should be allowed to give birth in other positions than on their back and should follow their body's urges to push.
6. Mother and baby should be kept together after birth; it is best for the mother, for the baby, and for breastfeeding (Amis, 2010).

In addition, the following three main principles are taught in the prenatal period related to the gating control method of pain relief:

1. If a couple understands the process of labor and birth, they can enter labor with decreased tension.
2. Concentrating on breathing patterns or imagery or focusing can block incoming pain sensations.
3. **Conditioned reflexes**, or reflexes that automatically occur in response to a stimulus, can also be used to displace pain during labor. For example, a woman is conditioned to relax automatically on hearing a command ("contraction beginning") or at the feel of a contraction beginning. The responses to contractions must be recently conditioned to be effective (because conditioned responses fade if not reinforced). This is the reason it is generally recommended that women attend Lamaze classes in the last trimester of pregnancy. A disadvantage of enrolling so late is that it limits the total amount of time directed to perineal exercises. If labor begins early, a woman may have had little or no practice with this type of exercise.

Lamaze classes are kept small, so there is time for individual instruction and attention to each couple (Fig. 14.5). Advise a woman to bring the support person who will serve as her coach in labor to class with her to practice breathing exercises.

that fear leads to tension, which leads to pain. If a woman can prevent fear from occurring or can break the chain between fear and tension or tension and pain, then she can reduce the pain of labor contractions. A woman achieves lack of fear through education about childbirth, and she achieves reduced pain by focusing on abdominal breathing during contractions (Dick-Read & Gaskin, 2013).

Figure 14.5 Every woman needs to be well prepared for birth. Here, a partner practices a position for pushing. Caution women not to actually push to avoid rupturing membranes.

happen with rapid breathing patterns and can interfere with an adequate fetal oxygen supply. If women do become light-headed during labor from hyperventilation (i.e., develop respiratory alkalosis), breathing into a paper bag can help because it causes rebreathing of exhaled carbon dioxide. The cleansing breath also signals to the woman's partner a contraction is about to begin or has ended.

QSEN Checkpoint Question 14.3

EVIDENCE-BASED PRACTICE

One of the most controversial aspects of childbirth addresses the question of the best birth position for women to use. To evaluate the impact of birth position on maternal risk for obstetric anal sphincter injuries (OASIs), a study was conducted on data from the Stockholm-Gotland Obstetric Database, which included 113,279 singleton spontaneous vaginal births.

The results showed that the lowest risk for OASIS was in the standing position. The highest rates of OASIS were in the lithotomy position. Squatting and birth seat position did increase the risk for OASIS in women who had previously given birth (Elvander, Ahlberg, Thies-Langergren, et al., 2015).

Based on the previous study, what would the nurse like to see included in Elena's birth plan?
  a. "I don't want any medical interventions in labor, like an IV."
  b. "I want to labor the same way that you see women do it on TV and in movies."
  c. "I'm willing to try anything safe that will decrease my risk for tearing."
  d. "I'm afraid I'll get dizzy if I try to sit up or stand during labor."

Look in Appendix A for the best answer and rationale.

Exercises taught vary from teacher to teacher, especially in terms of complexity, but have common features, which are discussed as follows.

Conscious Relaxation

This is learning to relax body parts so, unknowingly, a woman does not remain tense and cause unnecessary muscle strain and fatigue during labor. She practices **conscious relaxation** by deliberately relaxing one set of muscles, then another, and another until her body is completely relaxed. Her support person concentrates on noticing symptoms of tension such as a wrinkled brow, clenched fists, or a stiffly held arm. By either placing a comforting hand on the tense body area or telling a woman to relax that area, the support person can help her to achieve complete relaxation.

The Cleansing Breath

To begin all breathing exercises, a woman breathes in deeply and then exhales deeply (**cleansing breath**). To end each exercise, she repeats this step. It is an important step to take because it limits the possibility of either hyperventilation (blowing off too much carbon dioxide) or hypoventilation (not exhaling enough carbon dioxide), both of which could

Consciously Controlled Breathing

Using **consciously controlled breathing**, or set breathing patterns at specific rates, provides distraction as well as prevents the diaphragm from descending fully and putting pressure on the expanding uterus. To practice, after a cleansing breath, a woman inhales comfortably but fully, and then exhales, with her exhalation a little stronger than her inhalation (to help prevent hypoventilation). She practices breathing in this manner at a controlled pace, depending on the intensity of contractions through the following various levels of breathing:

• *Level 1.* Slow deep chest breathing of comfortable but full respirations at a rate of 6 to 12 breaths/min. This level is used for early contractions in labor when the cervical dilation is between 0 and 3 cm.
• *Level 2.* Lighter and more rapid breathing than level 1. The rib cage should expand but be so light that the diaphragm barely moves. The rate of respirations is up to 40 breaths/min. This is a good level of breathing for contractions when cervical dilation is between 4 and 6 cm.
• *Level 3.* Even more shallow and more rapid breathing. The rate is 50 to 70 breaths/min. As the respirations become faster, the exhalation must be a little stronger than the inhalation to allow good air exchange and to prevent hypoventilation. If a woman practices saying

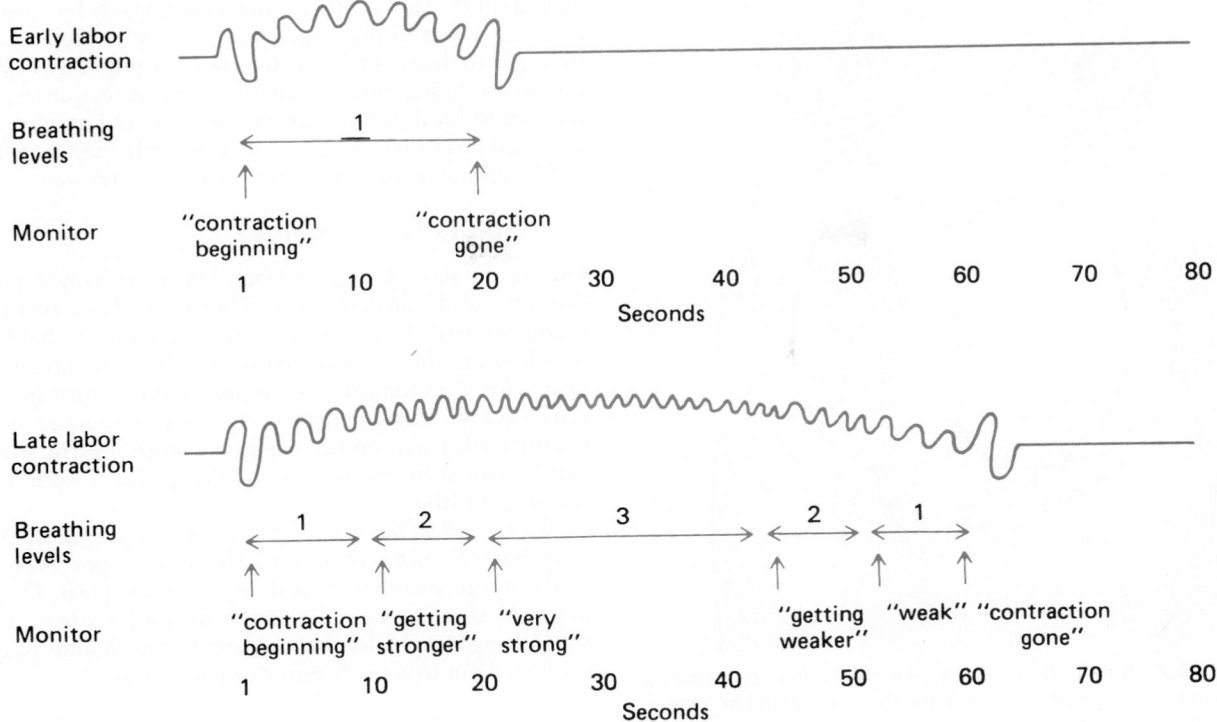

Figure 14.6   An example of differing breathing patterns during a single contraction. 1, 2, and 3 are levels of breathing. A cleansing breath is taken at the beginning and end of the contraction.

"out" with each exhalation, she almost inevitably will make exhalation stronger than inhalation. A woman uses this level for transition contractions when cervical dilation is between 7 and 10 cm. Keeping the tip of her tongue against the roof of her mouth helps prevent her oral mucosa from drying out during such rapid breathing.

- *Level 4.* Another pattern effective for transition contractions is a "pant-blow" pattern, or taking three or four quick breaths (in and out), then a forceful exhalation. Because this type of breathing sounds like a train (breath-breath-breath-huff), it is sometimes referred to as "choo-choo" or "hee-hee-hee-hoo" breathing.
- *Level 5.* Quiet, continuous, very shallow panting at about 60 breaths/min. This can be used during strong contractions or during the second stage of labor to prevent a woman from pushing before full dilatation.

Some courses stop teaching at the point a woman has mastered these levels of breathing; others have her learn to shift from one level to the other on command or at the point she feels a need for more pain relief.

Figure 14.6 illustrates the use of levels of breathing. At the beginning of a mild, early labor contraction, a woman's coach says, "contraction beginning." A woman takes a cleansing breath and then breathes at level 1; she feels no bite from the contraction and so does not need to change to a more involved breathing pattern. Later in labor, contractions are stronger and longer. Now, at the sound of "contraction beginning," a woman takes a cleansing breath and then begins level 1 breathing (three breaths), shifts to level 2 (four to six breaths), and then shifts to level 3 (10 breaths). The contraction is lessening. She shifts down to

level 2 (four to six breaths), then to level 1 (three or four breaths). The contraction is gone. She takes a final cleansing breath.

During actual labor, her coach can tell the strength of contractions by resting a hand on her abdomen or observing a uterine contraction monitor. A coach can tell a woman when to shift breathing levels depending on the coach's estimation of the strength of the contraction with words such as "contraction beginning, getting stronger, now getting weaker, gone." In the time before transition to the second stage of labor, when contractions are longest and strongest, a woman may need to use her level 4 breathing or continuous light panting as well. A woman who can perform all five levels of breathing and maintain relaxation can be assured she is prepared to handle all labor contractions up to the second stage of labor (Lothian, 2014).

Effleurage

One additional technique to encourage relaxation and displace pain in the Lamaze method is **effleurage**, which is French for "light abdominal massage"; it is done with just enough pressure to avoid tickling. To do this, a woman traces a pattern on her abdomen with her fingertips (Fig. 14.7). The rate of effleurage should remain constant even though breathing rates change. Effleurage serves as a distraction technique and decreases sensory stimuli transmission from the abdominal wall, helping limit local discomfort. If an external electronic monitor is in place on the abdomen, effleurage can be done superior or inferior to it or even on the thighs. Effleurage can also be done by the support person.

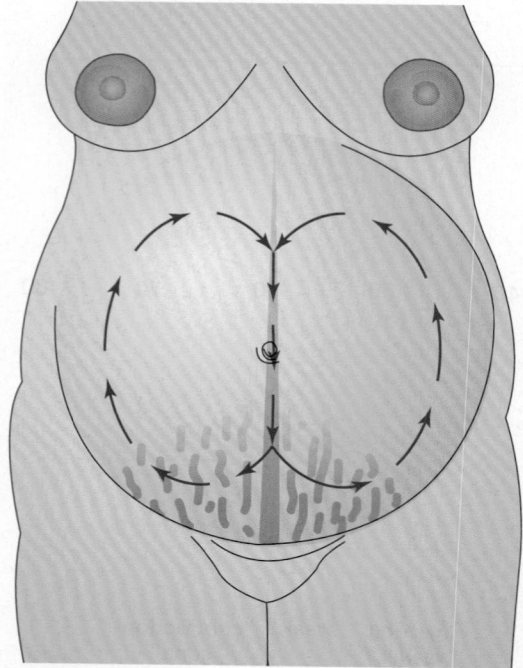

Figure 14.7 Effleurage patterns. During uterine contractions, a woman traces a pattern on her bare abdomen with her fingers.

Focusing or Imagery

Focusing intently on an object (sometimes called "sensate focus") is another method of keeping sensory input from reaching the cortex of the brain (Chuang, Liu, Chen, et al., 2015). For example, a woman brings into labor a photograph of her partner or children, a graphic design, or just something that appeals to her like an ocean scene she can concentrate on

Figure 14.8 A woman chooses what she wishes to focus on during labor. Here, a woman creates a playlist with music that she will focus on during contractions.

during contractions. Other women use imagery by imagining they are in a calm place such as on a beach watching waves rolling in to them or relaxing on a porch swing (Fig. 14.8). Be careful not to step into a woman's line of vision during a contraction to break her concentration on an object; also, don't ask questions or try to talk to women while they are focused and breathing or you will break their concentration.

Second-Stage Breathing

During the second stage of labor, when the baby is pushed down the birth canal, the type of breathing that is best to use is controversial. In the past, women were told to hold their breath while they pushed. Now, it is believed holding the breath for a prolonged time impairs blood return from the vena cava (a Valsalva maneuver), so this practice is now discouraged. Based on this, suggest women breathe any way that is natural for them, except holding their breath during this stage of labor.

Women should not practice pushing during pregnancy or if in labor before the end of the first stage because the possibility they could rupture membranes by doing this is too great. They can practice assuming a good position for pushing (e.g., squatting, sitting upright, leaning on partner) but should always be cautioned not to actually bear down and push.

QSEN Checkpoint Question 14.4

INFORMATICS

Elena's sister-in-law has referred her to a website that outlines the Lamaze method for labor and birth. What is the guiding principle of Lamaze childbirth?
  a. Pain can be interrupted before it registers in the brain as pain.
  b. Labor contractions are rooted in psychology, not physiology.
  c. "Brown pain" like labor contractions is unlike other forms of pain.
  d. Labor contractions can be eliminated by learned mind control techniques.

Look in Appendix A for the best answer and rationale.

PREPARATION FOR CESAREAN BIRTH

Some women choose to have a cesarean birth to help prevent uterine prolapse or urinary incontinence in later years (Black et al., 2016). To ensure a safe birth, a cesarean birth may become necessary during labor. The specific preparations needed for a cesarean birth as well as a VBAC is discussed in Chapter 24.

The Birth Setting

Besides how to best prepare for labor, choosing a birth setting is another important decision that a couple needs to make during pregnancy (Alliman & Phillippi, 2016). This decision depends on a woman's health and that of her fetus, the couple's preferences, and how much and what kind of supervision they want for the birth. Although hospitals are the usual site for birth today in the United States, that has not always been true. Up until the late 1800s, childbirth was conducted in the home setting with little pain relief. Analgesia or anesthesia for childbirth first became popular when Queen Victoria birthed Prince Leopold under chloroform in 1853. Although chloroform relieved pain, it also complicated birth because not only were women asleep for one of the most memorable moments of their life but it also caused them to not be able to push effectively during the second stage of labor, thus making it necessary to use a lithotomy position, an episiotomy, and forceps for birth.

Part of the reason for giving so much anesthesia during birth can be attributed to healthcare providers misinterpreting the moment of birth as the time that produces the greatest degree of discomfort. As a result, women were allowed to labor without pain medication and then were given anesthesia or analgesia right before the baby was born. Although the pain felt at birth is intense, it is over quickly, unlike the hours of labor that precede it, making women not as uncomfortable during the actual birth as they are during labor. Birth is also such an exhilarating time that the excitement of the moment and natural perineal anesthesia can mask pain.

Fortunately, based on women's descriptions of the pain of childbirth, birthing practices have changed to better meet women's needs (Keirns, 2015). Nurses are in a strong position to advocate for making childbirth as "natural" a process as possible and conducted in the least restrictive setting possible. At the same time, nurses have a strong responsibility to encourage parents to respect any restriction that will allow the birth to remain safe.

CHOOSING A BIRTH ATTENDANT AND SUPPORT PERSON

In the United States, most births are supervised by an obstetrician, a physician specializing in labor and birth; a family practitioner; or a nurse-midwife (Hamilton, Martin, Osterman, et al., 2015). In addition to selecting who will medically supervise her baby's birth, many women choose a doula, or a person specially prepared to assist with birth. Doulas can be especially helpful as support people because having such a person present frees the father to enjoy the birth rather than feel occupied with coaching instructions. Although research in the subject is not extensive, there are suggestions that rates of oxytocin augmentation, epidural anesthesia, and cesarean birth can all be reduced by doula support (Kozhimannil, Hardeman, Alarid-Escudero, et al., 2016). With specific education, many nurses are participating as either a doula or special support nurse to women in labor.

CHOOSING A BIRTH SETTING

Women who are low risk for complications may choose hospitals, birthing centers, or their homes as settings for birth. Women who might have a complication are advised to give birth at birthing centers or hospitals. Women with high-risk pregnancies are advised to give birth in hospitals where more immediate emergency care is available.

The Hospital Birth

The maternity services of hospitals have changed a great deal in recent years, having been influenced by the Coalition for Improving Maternity Services (CIMS). This organization rates hospitals as to whether they are mother-friendly or not based on if a woman has the opportunity for any of the following:

- Experience a healthy and joyous birth experience, regardless of her age or circumstances
- Give birth as she wishes in an environment in which she feels nurtured and secure
- Have access to the full range of options for pregnancy, birth, and nurturing her baby
- Receive accurate and up-to-date information about the benefits and risks of all procedures, drugs, and tests suggested for use during pregnancy, birth, and the postpartum period, with the right to informed consent and informed refusal
- Receive support for making informed choices about what is best for her and her baby based on her individual values and beliefs (CIMS, 2015).

To qualify as a mother-friendly hospital, a hospital should not have routine policies that include practices for such things as perineal shaving, admission enemas, withholding food or fluid during labor, rupturing membranes to hurry labor, or the use of continuous intravenous lines or constant fetal monitoring. It also should have low rates of episiotomies, induction for labor, and cesarean births. In contrast, it should also have a high VBAC rate (60% or more [CIMS, 2015]). Urge women to ask their primary care provider if the hospital they recommend is rated as mother-friendly because this should influence both a couple's choice of a hospital and their birth attendant.

The major advantage of a hospital birth is that equipment and expert personnel are readily available if the mother, fetus, or newborn should have a complication. When hospital birth is compared to births at alternative settings as to how many complications occur, women who give birth in hospitals invariably have more complications. Remember, though, that women at high risk for complications choose to give birth at hospitals so, of course, more complications will occur there.

A woman usually comes to the hospital when her contractions are approximately 5 minutes apart and regular in pattern. If she has preregistered at the hospital, she is admitted to a **birthing room** without any separation time from her support person. Birthing rooms are also called labor-birth-recovery rooms (LBRs) or **labor-birth-recovery-postpartum rooms (LBRPs)**. Such rooms are decorated in a homelike way, and couples can bring favorite music or reading materials with them to use during labor (Fig. 14.9).

Women are expected to use a prepared method of childbirth with a minimum of analgesia and anesthesia (although an advantage of a hospital birth is that anesthesia such as an epidural is readily available if needed). The woman's partner or other family members can stay with her throughout labor and birth, allowing a couple and their families to feel they have control over and can share in the birth experience. The bed is used as a labor bed until birth, when it is then converted into a **birthing bed**. Women can choose a birthing position: squatting, supine with head raised, or side-lying. Woman can choose to use a supine recumbent position (on her back with knees flexed) rather than a lithotomy position (legs elevated into stirrups) because such a position reduces tension on the perineum and is not only more comfortable but also may result in fewer perineal tears than with a lithotomy position.

Figure 14.9 A birthing (labor-birth-recovery) room designed to maintain a homelike atmosphere in a hospital setting.

Following birth, additional cabinets in the room are opened and converted into a space for baby care. A support person can cut the umbilical cord if desired. The mother is encouraged to breastfeed immediately. Some hospitals screen women in early labor with an external monitor to evaluate both fetal heart rate and uterine contractions. If the fetal heart rate is good, monitors are then removed and a simple Doppler monitor is used if any periodic screening is needed as labor progresses.

A **birthing chair**, a comfortable reclining chair with a slide-away seat that allows a woman to assume a comfortable position during labor and also furnishes perineal exposure so a birth attendant can assist with the birth, could also be used (Fig. 14.10). The chair has the advantage of maintaining a woman in a semi-Fowler's position, a position that acts with gravity and so may speed the second stage of labor.

Postpartum Care

Women giving birth in LBRPs remain in the room with their families for the rest of their hospital stay. Women giving birth in birthing rooms may be transferred to a postpartum unit after birth where they remain for the length of their hospital stay. Both LBRPs and postpartum units serve as "rooming-in" units in which the infant remains in the mother's room either constantly or for most of the day, whichever is her choice. Urge a couple to keep their newborn with them as much as possible so they have ample time to become acquainted and learn their baby's cues for hunger. Mothers can then breastfeed when the infant is hungry, not according to any schedule. There should be no restrictions on visiting for the primary support person; in many institutions, a rollaway bed can be provided so that the partner can remain constantly. Siblings and friends of the newborn should be allowed to visit as much as the mother chooses. Mother and infant remain in the hospital up to 48 hours and are then discharged home.

QSEN Checkpoint Question 14.5

TEAMWORK & COLLABORATION

Elena wants to use controlled breathing for early labor and the nurse is reviewing with her doula the actions that Elena will take. What should the nurse review with Elena's doula about controlled breathing early in labor?

a. She should try to breathe exclusively through her nose.
b. She should breathe as rapidly as possible to distract from early contractions.
c. If hypoventilation occurs, she should begin to sip on ice water.
d. She should breathe at a rate of 6 to 12 breaths/min for mild contractions.

Look in Appendix A for the best answer and rationale.

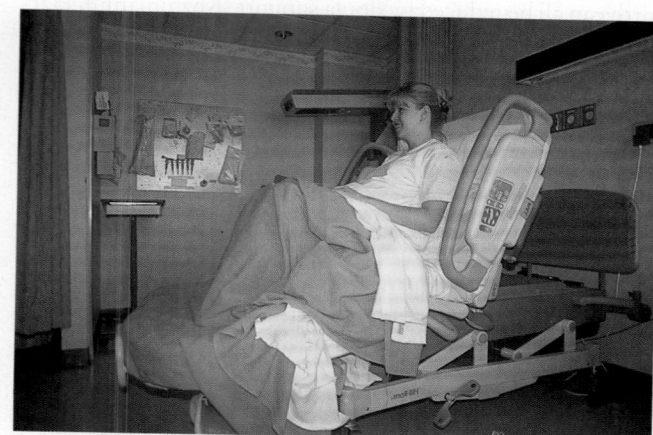

Figure 14.10 **(A)** A birthing chair allows a woman to maintain a semi-Fowler's position. **(B)** A birthing chair used during labor. (© Caroline Brown, RNC, MS, DEd.)

Alternative Birthing Centers

Alternative birthing centers (ABCs) are wellness-oriented childbirth facilities designed to remove childbirth from the acute care hospital setting while still providing medical resources for emergency care should a complication of labor or birth arise. These settings are established inside, next door, or at least within an easy distance to a hospital. The primary birth attendants tend to be nurse-midwives. Because the facility is located outside an acute care setting, where infections abound, the risk of hospital-acquired infection to a woman is thought to be reduced. Women who deliver in ABCs are screened for potential complications before being rated as eligible for admittance. Because of this, the mortality rate of mothers and infants is no higher and may be lower in these out-of-hospital settings than in hospital settings.

Like hospitals, ABCs have LBRPs where a woman and her support person can invite friends and siblings to participate in the birth. In some centers, a central play area for siblings and cooking facilities are also available. ABCs encourage a woman to express her own needs and wishes during the labor process. A minimum of analgesia and anesthesia is provided, and she can choose a birth position. She can bring her own music or distraction objects, and the partner can perform such tasks as cutting the umbilical cord if he or she chooses.

Women remain in an ABC from 4 to 24 hours after birth. Because minimum analgesia or anesthesia is used, a woman recovers quickly after birth and is ready to be discharged early. Box 14.10 shows an interprofessional care map illustrating both nursing and team planning for a birthing center experience.

QSEN Checkpoint Question 14.6

QUALITY IMPROVEMENT

Suppose Elena follows her boyfriend's wishes and decides on a hospital birth. What would be an advantage of hospital birth that can be cited to women considering this birth setting?
   a. She can give birth in a sterile environment.
   b. Both labor and childbirth can generally be pain-free.
   c. Extended high-risk newborn care is available.
   d. Hospital care costs are lower than other settings.

Look in Appendix A for the best answer and rationale.

Home Birth

Home birth is the usual mode of birth in developing countries and is also a popular choice for birth in Europe; however, only about 1% of women in the United States choose this method (MacDorman et al., 2014). Home birth may be supervised by a physician, but nurse-midwives are the more likely choice as a birth attendant in this setting. The Frontier Nursing Service of Kentucky is an example of an organization in the United States that maintains an active and well-accepted program of home birth.

Most women who choose home birth are well educated and from middle-income families. They choose home birth so they are not separated from their family for even a short time; they can have their baby close by after birth to help integrate the child into the family; they can have more control over their childbirth experience; and they can give birth in familiar, low-cost surroundings.

Home birth can have a disadvantage in that it puts responsibility on a woman to prepare her home for the birth and to give full care to the infant after birth. Some women, however willing, may be unable to take on these roles because, passing through their first postpartum or "taking-in" phase, they may feel more comfortable maintaining a dependent-passive role than immediately taking responsibility for the infant's care. They also may feel exhausted from their last weeks of pregnancy or they don't know the best recourse in a crisis situation.

To be a candidate for a home birth, a woman:
- Should be in good overall health
- Must be able to adjust to changing circumstances
- Must have adequate support people to sustain her during labor and to assist her for the first few days after birth

Women with any complication of pregnancy are not good candidates for home birth. Be certain women planning home birth know the following:
- Adequate equipment other than first-line emergency equipment will not be available.
- An abrupt change of goals may be necessary if a complication occurs.
- Both she and her support person may become exhausted because of the responsibility placed on them during labor or the postpartum period.
- She must be prepared to independently monitor her postpartal status.
- Interference with the "taking-in phase" may occur postpartally because she must "take hold" rather than allow herself a rest phase.

 Concept Mastery Alert

The best candidates for home birth are healthy women who can adjust to changing circumstances and who have adequate support systems. A woman who chooses home birth should be interested in learning all she can to prepare for the birth.

CHILDREN ATTENDING BIRTH

Most birthing centers and some hospitals allow children to view the birth of a sibling. It is good advice to suggest that parents and siblings attend a class designed to prepare children to witness a birth beforehand to keep the event from becoming overwhelming. If children will be present, a person separate from the main support person needs to be designated to provide entertainment, explanations, food, and a place for them to nap. This prevents the likelihood that a child who is without supervision during this time will remember the experience as one of rejection rather than an exciting, happy experience. The mother should not be expected to provide such supervision during labor because she will want to concentrate on distraction or breathing techniques.

Help couples to consider whether the birth experience will be a positive and enjoyable one for the family based on the sibling's developmental level and stage. Allowing a child to witness the birth of kittens or puppies might be an alternative way to expose the child to birth.

BOX 14.10

Nursing Care Planning

AN INTERPROFESSIONAL CARE MAP FOR A FAMILY WHO DESIRES BIRTH AT AN ALTERNATIVE BIRTH CENTER

Elena Garza is pregnant with her second child. During her first pregnancy, she did not attend any childbirth classes and received an epidural for the birth. During a prenatal visit for this pregnancy, Elena tells you she would now like to have a more natural birth in a birthing center. She asks you for information on childbirth education classes. Her partner, Joe, a Navy Seal, wants Elena to go to the hospital and have an epidural like she did with her last pregnancy. After further speaking with Joe, you discover he doesn't want Elena to go through the pain of natural childbirth because he fears he may be out of town when she is in labor.

Family Assessment: Elena and Joe live with 4-year-old Josh in an apartment in central downtown. Elena is a stay-at-home mom. Depends on Joe for financial help.

Patient Assessment: Pregnancy progressing without evidence of problems or complications. Gravida 2, para 1, 24 weeks gestation. Patient states she wants to use alternative birth center (ABC) but has not contacted one yet; reports concern over previous hospital birth of son. Wants son Josh, now 4 years old, to be a part of new baby's birth. Her sister has volunteered to serve as a doula. Wants to walk during labor and have a ready supply of "anything chocolate" to eat. No childbirth education classes attended with previous pregnancy; not presently enrolled in any with this pregnancy.

Nursing Diagnosis: Decisional conflict related to choice of birth setting and birth process

Outcome Criteria: Patient and partner state advantages and disadvantages of birth setting options and make final plans for birth and birth setting by 3 weeks' time.
   Patient and partner verbalize goal of healthy mother and baby as motivation for choice of birth setting.

Team Member Responsible	Assessment	Intervention	Rationale	Expected Outcome
Activities of Daily Living, Including Safety				
Nurse	Investigate the type of birth facilities available in local area.	Review the requirements, advantages, and disadvantages for birth setting choices available.	Reviewing options allows the couple to make an informed decision appropriate for their needs.	Patient and partner state they have reviewed and understand options available to them.
Nurse	Ask couple if they have plans for child care of Josh during labor.	Suggest that couple ask a family member to be caretaker for son during the birth.	A caretaker can enhance the experience for the older child by promoting a positive, family-centered event.	Couple states Elena's mother will serve as caretaker for Josh.
Teamwork and Collaboration				
Nurse/nurse-midwife	Assess what family expects of a doula for labor.	Review responsibilities of a doula with Elena's sister.	Doulas can offer strong support in labor; prearrangements help assure everyone has the same labor and birth goals.	Couple confirms they are pleased with sister serving as a doula.
Procedures/Medications for Quality Improvement				
Nurse/obstetric care provider	Determine if there are any contraindications to active positioning such as walking or swaying during labor.	Educate patient about the few situations, such as placenta previa, that would contradict walking in labor.	Using active positions during labor such as walking has the potential to decrease the time of labor unless contraindicated.	Patient states she will be flexible with regard to wishes in labor based on her own and fetal safety but wants a site that welcomes active movement.
Nutrition				
Nurse	Assess whether patient's chosen food option during labor is approved by ABC chosen.	Help patient modify her goals for nutrition during labor as appropriate based on facility requirements.	Because many choices for food exist, coordinating plans with the facility should result in less stress during labor.	Patient confirms eating chocolate is agreeable with chosen agency.

Family-Centered Care

Nurse	Obtain information about local childbirth education classes available.	Assist couple as necessary with selecting class that fits their resources.	Education can enhance the chances of a positive childbirth experience.	Patient attends the chosen childbirth preparation class before the 38th week of pregnancy.
Nurse	Assess if any classes for sibling preparation for birth are available in community.	Help couple plan for mother and son to attend class on sibling preparation for birth or meet with nurse for instruction.	Adequate preparation for all involved improves the chances of a positive experience.	Couple states they will either attend a class for sibling preparation or meet with nurse for information.

Psychosocial/Spiritual/Emotional Needs

Nurse/nurse-midwife	Explore with patient and partner past experiences with childbirth and current expectations and beliefs.	"Debriefing" or encouraging couple to verbalize feelings about unsatisfactory experience helps to alleviate distress.	Verbalization of feelings permits a safe outlet for emotions.	Couple states their overall goal for childbirth is a safe one for mother and new child and so will be flexible if a complication arises.

Informatics for Seamless Healthcare Planning

Nurse	Assess if couple has any further questions about birth centers.	Ascertain couple has phone number for and directions to chosen birthing center.	Advance planning can help avoid increased stress at time of birth.	Couple states they are happy with birth setting decision and prepared to follow through on plans.

Alternative Methods of Birth

In addition to varied settings, several methods of childbirth are popular. These include alternative birth methods such as the Leboyer method of birth, birth under water, and unassisted birthing.

THE LEBOYER METHOD

Frederick Leboyer was a French obstetrician who postulated moving from a warm, fluid-filled intrauterine environment to a noisy, air-filled, brightly lit birth room creates a major shock for a newborn (Leboyer, 2009). With the **Leboyer method**, the birthing room is darkened so there is no sudden contrast in light; the environment is kept pleasantly warm, not chilled; soft music is played, or at least harsh noises are kept to a minimum; the infant is handled gently; the cord is cut late; and the infant is placed immediately after birth into warm bath water.

Some neonatologists question the wisdom of a warm bath because it could reduce spontaneous respirations and allow a high level of acidosis to occur. Late cutting of the cord supplies extra white blood cells to a baby so the newborn can increase resistance to disease but it also could lead to excess blood viscosity. Certainly, soft music, gentle handling, and a welcoming atmosphere are important ingredients for all birth attendants to incorporate into birth. Providing dim lights (or at least not bright, glaring ones) and providing a warm temperature could be given more consideration in most institutions.

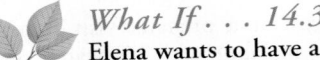

What If . . . 14.3
Elena wants to have a Leboyer birth. How would the nurse prepare her birthing room?

HYDROTHERAPY AND THE WATER BIRTH

Reclining or sitting in warm water during labor can be soothing; the feeling of weightlessness that occurs under water as well as the relaxation from the warm water both can contribute to reducing discomfort in labor. Using this principle, many birthing settings encourage women to not only labor in warm showers or tubs but also to give birth in spa tubs of warm water (Davies, Davis, Pearce, et al., 2015). Women need to ask if this will be an option at their birth setting if they are interested. One disadvantage is that because most women expel feces from pushing in the second stage of labor, the water bath may become contaminated. Most women who choose underwater birth, however, enjoy the experience and are pleased that they chose this method (Koyyalamudi, Sidhu, Cornett, et al., 2016).

UNASSISTED BIRTHING

Unassisted birthing, freebirthing, or couples birth refers to women giving birth without healthcare provider supervision (Snowden, Tilden, Snyder, et al., 2015). It differs from home birth because, using this technique, a woman learns pregnancy care from reading books or articles found on the Internet and then arranges to have her child birth at home, perhaps accompanied by her family or friends, but without healthcare supervision.

Some women choose this method of birth because they believe birth is such a natural process that no medical supervision is necessary. Others choose it because they have no health insurance and so can't afford either a hospital or alternative birth setting (Snowden et al., 2015). Unassisted birthing is potentially dangerous because, if a complication should occur, the woman may not recognize that what is happening is serious until damage to her child or herself results. Even if she recognizes that a problem is occurring, there is a gap of time before emergency help can arrive to assist her, which puts her at risk for harm. Unassisted birthing is particularly dangerous if a woman avoids prenatal care or depends solely on online information because she may be at high risk for a complication but not know it. Educating women that not all online information is reliable and that supervised birth does not mean they have no choice in their care decisions, such as whether they want pain relief or to use a special position for birth, is an effective way to help women make safer choices about birth.

Women With Unique Needs

There are a number of women who have special needs related to preparations for childbirth.

THE WOMAN WITH A DISABILITY

Care of women with disabilities during pregnancy is discussed in Chapter 22. Women with these special circumstances may need additional help to prepare for labor and birth based on their unique concern. It may not be realistic, for example, for a woman who has chronic back pain to practice pelvic rocking; a woman with poor balance may not be able to practice squatting safely. A woman who is immobile or in a wheelchair may have difficulty attending a preparation class if the classroom is not located in a handicapped-accessible building. Women with vision or hearing disabilities can have difficulty following classroom content. A highly stressed woman may not have the patience to concentrate on learning controlled breathing.

Encourage women with special needs to think through any circumstance that will require special adaptation and be certain they include this requirement in their birth plan.

THE WOMAN WITH CULTURAL CONCERNS

Because the United States has such a diverse mixture of cultures, a preparation for labor and birth class can include women from a diverse mix of cultures. Urging women to share cultural traditions enriches discussions at such classes. Be certain to encourage women who are worried that their cultural preferences will not be respected when they are in labor to discuss their concerns with their primary care provider at their next visit. A woman who believes in circumcision as a religious necessity, for example, does not want to listen to a discussion on the pros and cons of circumcision. A woman who wants to be fully clothed during labor may need to plan on bringing her own nonrevealing gown to a birthing center, and she may not want to be offered showering or tub bathing as pain management because these will not respect modesty. Be certain women include these special needs in their written birth plan so they are not overlooked by busy labor service personnel.

THE WOMAN WHO IS OBESE

Women with a body mass index over 30 may have difficulty practicing exercises such as squatting or tailor sitting because not only do these positions require balance but they also may tire easily. Overweight women should, however, have no difficulty preparing for labor by practicing controlled breathing or doing abdominal and perineal strengthening by doing exercises

such as Kegel or abdominal contractions. Urge women to think through what pain management measures they think may cause a problem for them in labor such as leaning forward against a birthing bar or a birthing ball or bathing in warm water (the bar or ball or a plastic tub might not support their weight). For modesty, they may also need to bring their own gown to their birthing center. Encourage women to add what will be important for them to do or not to do on their birthing plan so they remain active participants in the experience.

What If . . . 14.4
The nurse is particularly interested in exploring one of the 2020 National Health Goals with respect to preparation for labor (see Box 14.1). What would be a possible research topic to explore pertinent to this goal that would be applicable to Joe and Elena and that would also advance evidence-based practice?

KEY POINTS FOR REVIEW

- Couples should be encouraged to make a flexible childbirth plan early in pregnancy, which includes a birth attendant, setting, desired method of pain management, and any special wishes.
- Common exercises taught in pregnancy to strengthen perineal muscles are tailor sitting, squatting, and Kegel exercises. Abdominal muscle contraction and pelvic rocking exercises both strengthen the abdominal muscles and help relieve backache.
- Types of childbirth preparations include the Bradley (partner coached), Kitzinger (psychosexual), Dick-Read, and Lamaze methods. Lamaze is the most common method used in the United States.
- Commonly used nonpharmacologic techniques for pain relief in labor are conscious relaxation, consciously controlled breathing, effleurage, focusing, imagery, and hydrotherapy.
- Classes for expectant parents provide information on pregnancy, birth, and child care.
- Common sites for childbirth include hospitals, ABCs, and home settings.
- Couples should determine if their preferred birth setting is rated as mother-friendly before choosing a birth site.
- Considering childbirth as one of the biggest events in a woman's life should help in planning nursing care that not only meets QSEN competencies but also best meets the family's total needs.

CRITICAL THINKING CARE STUDY

Brooke is a 28-year-old woman having her first baby. She has worked as a nurse on a labor and delivery service for the past 3 years. She didn't take a preparation for childbirth class because she felt no material would be presented she didn't already know. She doesn't feel she needs a doula because she has had so much experience with women in labor. Her husband will be with her during labor.

1. Brooke's husband asks you at a prenatal visit if he should time contractions in labor with his watch or by the wall clock. Also, he asks if it will be all right if

Brooke drinks coffee during labor. Why do you think he's asking so many basic questions?

2. Brooke's mother tells you she knows she can't be with Brooke in labor but she wants special permission to hold her new grandson before he's taken away to a nursery. She also wants to make it clear she needs to do that before her ex-husband or his "fluffy" girlfriend have a chance to hold the baby. Does Brooke's mother understand the options available to her in a mother-friendly hospital?

3. Brooke doesn't seem to have shared much information about labor with her family. Can you assume this is because she's so independent she wants to manage her labor by herself, or would you worry she doesn't have a strong support system?

RELATED RESOURCES

Explore these additional resources to enhance learning for this chapter:
• Student resources on thePoint, including answers to the What If . . . and Critical Thinking Care Study questions, http://thepoint.lww.com/Flagg8e
• Adaptive learning powered by PrepU, http://thepoint.lww.com/prepu

REFERENCES

Alliman, J., & Phillippi, J. C. (2016). Maternal outcomes in birth centers: An integrative review of the literature. *Journal of Midwifery & Women's Health*, *61*(1), 21–51.

Amis, D. (2010). *Prepared childbirth: The family way*. New York, NY: Lamaze International.

Black, M., Entwistle, V. A., Bhattacharya, S., et al. (2016). Vaginal birth after caesarean section: Why is uptake so low? Insights from a meta-ethnographic synthesis of women's accounts of their birth choices. *BMJ Open*, *6*(1), e008881.

Bradley, R., Hathaway, M., Hathaway, J., et al. (2008). *Husband-coached childbirth* (5th ed.). New York, NY: Bantam Books.

Chuang, L. L., Liu, S. C., Chen, Y. H., et al. (2015). Predictors of adherence to relaxation guided imagery during pregnancy in women with preterm labor. *The Journal of Alternative and Complementary Medicine*, *21*(9), 563–568.

Coalition for Improving Maternity Services. (2015). *The mother-friendly childbirth initiative*. Retrieved from http://www.motherfriendly.org/MFCI

Davies, R., Davis, D., Pearce, M., et al. (2015). The effect of waterbirth on neonatal mortality and morbidity: A systematic review and meta-analysis. *JBI Database of Systematic Reviews and Implementation Reports*, *13*(10), 180–231.

Dick-Read, G., & Gaskin, I. M. (2013). *Childbirth without fear: The principles and practice of natural childbirth*. London, United Kingdom: Pinter & Martin.

Elvander, C., Ahlberg, M., Thies-Langergren, L., et al. (2015). Birth position and obstetric anal sphincter injury: A population-based study of 113 000 spontaneous births. *BMC Pregnancy and Childbirth*, *15*, 252.

Godin, K. M., Alton, G. D., Gangodawilage, H. P., et al. (2015). Knowledge change associated with participation in prenatal education programs in Ontario: A cohort study. *Canadian Journal of Public Health*, *106*(6), e401–e407.

Hamilton, B. E., Martin, J. A., Osterman, M. J., et al. (2015). Births: Final data for 2014. *National Vital Statistics Reports*, *64*(12), 1–64.

Hidalgo-Lopezosa, P., Rodríguez-Borrego, M. A., & Muñoz-Villanueva, M. C. (2013). Are birth plans associated with improved maternal or neonatal outcomes? *MCN: The American Journal of Maternal Child Nursing*, *38*(3), 150–156.

Horey, D., Kealy, M., Davey, M., et al. (2013). Interventions for supporting pregnant women's decision-making about mode of birth after a caesarean. *Cochrane Database of Systematic Reviews*, (7), CD010041.

Keirns, C. (2015). Watching the clock: A mother's hope for a natural birth in a cesarean culture. *Health Affairs*, *34*(1), 178–182.

Kitzinger, S. (2011). *The new pregnancy & childbirth*. London, United Kingdom: Penguin Books/Dorling Kindersley.

Koyyalamudi, V., Sidhu, G., Cornett, E. M., et al. (2016). New labor pain treatment options. *Current Pain and Headache Reports*, *20*(2), 1–9.

Kozhimannil, K. B., Hardeman, R. R., Alarid-Escudero, F., et al. (2016). Modeling the cost-effectiveness of doula care associated with reductions in preterm birth and cesarean delivery. *Birth*, *43*(1), 20–27.

Leboyer, F. (2009). *Birth without violence*. Rochester, VT: Healing Arts Press.

Lothian, J. A. (2014). Promoting optimal care in childbirth. *The Journal of Perinatal Education*, *23*(4), 174–177.

MacDorman, M. F., Mathews, T. J., & Declercq, E. (2014). Trends in out-of-hospital births in the United States, 1990–2012. *NCHS Data Brief*, *144*, 1–8.

Minert, G. L. (2014). Your key to improving breastfeeding outcomes. *Journal of Obstetric, Gynecologic & Neonatal Nursing*, *43*(Suppl. 1), S55–S55.

Mørkved, S., & Bø, K. (2014). Effect of pelvic floor muscle training during pregnancy and after childbirth on prevention and treatment of urinary incontinence: A systematic review. *British Journal of Sports Medicine*, *48*(4), 299–310.

Polis, R. L., Gussman, D., & Kuo, Y. H. (2015). Yoga in pregnancy: An examination of maternal and fetal responses to 26 yoga postures. *Obstetrics & Gynecology*, *126*(6), 1237–1241.

Shannon, G., Alberg, C., Nacul, L., et al. (2014). Preconception healthcare and congenital disorders: Systematic review of the effectiveness of preconception care programs in the prevention of congenital disorders. *Maternal and Child Health Journal*, *18*(6), 1354–1379.

Snowden, J. M., Tilden, E. L., Snyder, J., et al. (2015). Planned out-of-hospital birth and birth outcomes. *New England Journal of Medicine*, *373*(27), 2642–2653.

Ternström, E., Hildingsson, I., Haines, H., et al. (2016). Pregnant women's thoughts when assessing fear of birth on the Fear of Birth Scale. *Women and Birth*, *29*(3), e44–e49.

U.S. Department of Health and Human Services. (2010). *Healthy people 2020*. Washington, DC: Author.

Wahlqvist, M. L., Krawetz, S. A., Rizzo, N. S., et al. (2015). Early-life influences on obesity: From preconception to adolescence. *Annals of the New York Academy of Sciences*, *1347*, 1–28.

15

Nursing Care of a Family During Labor and Birth

*C*eleste Bailey is a 26-year-old woman having her first baby whom you admit to a birthing room. She has been having labor contractions for 6 hours; her contractions are now 45 seconds long and 3 minutes apart. She tells you she wants to have her baby "naturally" without any analgesia or anesthesia. Her husband, a long distance truck driver, is on his way home but has not arrived yet. Her teenage sister who is with her states she has no idea how to coach her, except to pray. As you finish assessing contractions, Celeste grips her abdomen, screams, and shouts, "I'm breathing just like I'm supposed to do! Why does this hurt so bad?"

Previous chapters discussed the anatomic and physiologic changes that occur in pregnancy as well as effective steps women can take to prepare for labor. This chapter adds information about the process of labor and how to offer effective support and education to a woman in labor. Without this type of support, labor can be a frightening rather than an enjoyable event.

What additional teaching and support does Celeste need so her labor and birth are memorable experiences for her?

KEY TERMS

attitude

breech presentation

cardinal movements of labor

cephalic presentation

crowning

dilatation

doula

effacement

engagement

fetal descent

fetal position

Leopold maneuvers

lie

molding

ripening

station

transition

OBJECTIVES

After mastering the contents of this chapter, you should be able to:

1. Describe common theories explaining the onset of labor and the role of passenger, passage, powers, and psyche in labor.

2. Identify 2020 National Health Goals related to safe labor and birth that nurses can help the nation achieve.

3. Assess a family in labor and birth and identify the woman's readiness, stage, and progression.

4. Formulate nursing diagnoses related to the physiologic and psychological aspects of labor and birth.

5. Develop expected outcomes to meet the needs of a family throughout the labor process as well as manage seamless transitions across differing healthcare settings.

6. Using the nursing process, plan nursing care that includes the six competencies of Quality & Safety Education for Nurses (QSEN): Patient-Centered Care, Teamwork & Collaboration, Evidence-Based Practice (EBP), Quality Improvement (QI), Safety, and Informatics.

7. Implement nursing care for a family during labor such as teaching about the stages of labor.

8. Evaluate expected outcomes for achievement and effectiveness of care.

9. Integrate knowledge of labor and birth with the interplay of nursing process, the six competencies of QSEN, and Family Nursing to promote quality maternal and child health nursing care.

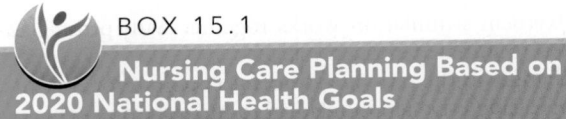

BOX 15.1

Nursing Care Planning Based on 2020 National Health Goals

Because labor and birth are potentially high-risk times for both a fetus and a mother, a number of 2020 National Health Goals speak directly to these:

- Reduce the rate of maternal deaths to no more than 11.4 out of 100,000 live births from a baseline of 12.7 out of 100,000 live births.
- Reduce maternal illness due to pregnancy complications developed during hospitalized labor and delivery from a baseline of 31.1% to a target level of 28.0%.
- Reduce cesarean births among low-risk (full-term, singleton, vertex presentation) women from a baseline of 26.5% to a target of 23.9%.
- Reduce the rate of fetal deaths at 20 or more weeks gestation to no more than 5.6 out of 1,000 live births from a baseline of 6.2 out of 1,000.
- Reduce the rate of fetal and infant deaths during the perinatal period (28 weeks gestation to 7 days after birth) to no more than 5.9 out of 1,000 live births from a baseline of 6.6 out of 1,000 live births (U.S. Department of Health and Human Services, 2010; see www.healthypeople.gov).

Nurses can help the nation achieve these goals by closely monitoring women during labor and birth and by teaching women as much as possible about labor so they are able to use as little analgesia and anesthesia as possible. The less anesthesia and analgesia used, the fewer complications that occur, resulting in reduced fetal or maternal death.

Labor is the series of events by which uterine contractions and abdominal pressure expel a fetus and placenta from the uterus. Regular contractions cause progressive dilatation of the cervix and create sufficient muscular uterine force to allow a baby to be pushed out into the extrauterine world. Labor represents a time of change as it is both an ending and a beginning for the woman, her fetus, and her family (Archie & Roman, 2013).

Labor and birth are unique events, requiring a woman to employ all the psychological and physical coping methods she has available. Regardless of the amount of childbirth preparation or the number of times a woman has been through the birth experience, family-centered nursing care is the approach that best supports the woman as she focuses on the beginning of her new family. This goal for nursing is further emphasized by 2020 National Health Goals (Box 15.1).

Nursing Process Overview

FOR THE WOMAN IN LABOR

ASSESSMENT

A woman in labor is keenly aware of both nonverbal and verbal expressions around her (i.e., not only words spoken but gestures such as eye rolling or sighing). Because of this sensitivity, an assessment must be done quickly yet thoroughly and gently because she may have difficulty being patient, for example, while admission information is obtained or relaxing for a vaginal examination.

Remember that pain is a subjective symptom. Only the woman can evaluate how much she is experiencing or how much she wants to endure. Assess how much discomfort she is experiencing and how she feels about her labor not only by what she scores on a pain scale but also by subtle signs of pain such as facial tenseness, flushing or paleness of the face, hands clenched in a fist, rapid breathing, or rapid pulse rate. Appreciate that the fetus as well as the mother is under stress from the process of labor, so both need vital sign assessments.

NURSING DIAGNOSIS

Nursing diagnoses in labor generally relate to a woman's reaction to labor. Common nursing diagnoses include:

- Pain related to labor contractions
- Anxiety related to process of labor and birth
- Health-seeking behaviors related to management of discomfort of labor
- Situational low self-esteem related to inability to use planned childbirth method

Although the discomfort of labor contractions is commonly referred to as "contractions" rather than "pain," do not omit the word "pain" from a nursing diagnosis because the term strengthens an understanding of the problem as well as alerts a woman she should feel free to ask for something for pain at the point she feels she needs additional help.

OUTCOME IDENTIFICATION AND PLANNING

When establishing expected outcomes for a woman in labor and her partner, be certain they are realistic and that they can be met. Although labor usually takes place over a relatively short time frame (average, 12 hours), it is important not to project a definite time limit for labor to be completed because the length of labor can vary greatly from woman to woman and still be within normal limits. It is necessary also to appreciate the magnitude of labor. It is unlikely all the fear or anxiety experienced during a woman's labor can be completely alleviated. Often, because it is such an unusual and significant experience, the average couple may need guidance in order to be able to employ additional coping measures.

Be certain to incorporate a support person as well as the woman in planning so the experience is a shared one. Although a couple may have learned about the stages of labor and what to expect at each stage during pregnancy, the reality of labor may seem very different from what they imagined. Be certain also that planning is flexible and individualized, allowing the woman to experience the full significance of the event.

IMPLEMENTATION

As much as possible, interventions during labor should always be carried out between contractions so the woman can use a prepared childbirth technique to limit the discomfort of contractions. This calls for good coordination of care among healthcare providers and the woman and her support person. The person a woman chooses to stay with her during childbirth is often culturally determined and varies from being a husband, a significant other or partner, the father of the child, a sister, a parent, or a close friend.

OUTCOME EVALUATION

An evaluation during labor should be ongoing to preserve the safety of the woman and her newborn. After birth, an evaluation helps to determine the woman's opinion of her experience with labor and birth. Ideally, the experience should not only be one she was able to endure but also one that allowed her self-esteem to grow and the family bond to intensify through a shared experience. It is advantageous to talk to women following birth about their labor experience because doing so serves as a means of evaluating nursing care during labor. It also provides a woman the chance to "work through" the experience and incorporate it into her self-image. Possible outcome criteria include:

- Patient states pain during labor was tolerable because of her advance preparation.
- Patient verbalizes that her need for nonpharmacologic comfort measures was met.
- Patient and family members state the labor and birth experience was a positive growth experience for them, both individually and as a family.

Theories of Why Labor Begins

Labor normally begins between 37 and 42 weeks of pregnancy, when a fetus is sufficiently mature to adapt to extrauterine life, yet not too large to cause mechanical difficulty with birth. In some instances, labor begins before a fetus is mature (preterm birth). In others, labor is delayed until the fetus and the placenta have both passed beyond the optimal point for birth (postterm birth).

A number of factors are known to be responsible for the initiation of spontaneous labor, although much is still unknown. Factors such as withdrawal of progesterone, an increase of prostaglandins, and other complex biochemical markers have shown to be at work (Irani & Foster, 2015).

A number of theories, including a combination of factors originating from both the woman and fetus, have been proposed to explain why progesterone withdrawal begins. Some of the theories include:

- The uterine muscle stretches from the increasing size of the fetus, which results in release of prostaglandins.
- The fetus presses on the cervix, which stimulates the release of oxytocin from the posterior pituitary.

- Oxytocin stimulation works together with prostaglandins to initiate contractions.
- Changes in the ratio of estrogen to progesterone occurs, increasing estrogen in relation to progesterone, which is interpreted as progesterone withdrawal.
- The placenta reaches a set age, which triggers contractions.
- Rising fetal cortisol levels reduce progesterone formation and increase prostaglandin formation.
- The fetal membrane begins to produce prostaglandins, which stimulate contractions (Bienstock, Fox, & Wallach, 2015).

The role of prostaglandins answers the often asked question: Does coitus help induce labor? Semen does contain prostaglandins, which can be helpful in softening, also known as "**ripening**," of the cervix; if a cervix is ready to ripen, semen prostaglandins could possibly stimulate the beginning of contractions. Rhythmical contractions brought on by a woman's orgasm can conceivably help as well, although, again, not until a uterus is prepared and ready for labor.

The Components of Labor

A successful labor depends on four integrated concepts, often referred to as the four *P*s:

1. The *passage* (a woman's pelvis) is of adequate size and contour.
2. The *passenger* (the fetus) is of appropriate size and in an advantageous position and presentation.
3. The *powers* of labor (uterine factors) are adequate.
4. The *psyche*, or a woman's psychological state which may either encourage or inhibit labor. This can be based on her past life experiences as well as her present psychological state.

THE PASSAGE

The passage refers to the route a fetus must travel from the uterus through the cervix and vagina to the external perineum (Fig. 15.1).

In most instances, if a disproportion between fetus and pelvis occurs, the pelvis is the structure at fault. If the fetus is the cause of the disproportion, it is often not because the fetal

Figure 15.1   Views of the pelvic inlet and outlet: **(A)** the pelvic inlet, **(B)** the pelvic outlet.

head is too large but because it is presenting to the birth canal at less than its narrowest diameter. Keep this in mind when discussing with parents why an infant may not be able to be born vaginally. It can be upsetting for parents to learn that a child cannot be born vaginally because the mother's pelvis is too small. It can be much more upsetting to think their infant's head is too large because it implies something may be seriously wrong with their baby (and that is rarely true). Avoiding this type of negative thought helps promote good parent–child bonding.

THE PASSENGER

The passenger is the fetus. The body part of the fetus that has the widest diameter is the head, so this is the part least likely to be able to pass through the pelvic ring. Whether a fetal skull can pass depends on both its structure (bones, fontanelles, and suture lines) and its alignment with the pelvis.

Structure of the Fetal Skull

The cranium, the uppermost portion of the skull, is composed of eight bones. The four superior bones—the

frontal (actually two fused bones), the two parietal, and the occipital—are the bones important in childbirth. The other four bones of the skull (sphenoid, ethmoid, and two temporal bones) lie at the base of the cranium and so are of little significance in childbirth because they are never presenting parts (Fig. 15.2).

Fontanelle spaces compress during birth to aid in molding of the fetal head. Their presence can be assessed manually through the cervix after the cervix has dilated during labor. Palpating for fontanelle spaces during a pelvic examination helps to establish the position of the fetal head and whether it is in a favorable position for birth.

Diameters of the Fetal Skull

The shape of a fetal skull causes it to be wider in its anteroposterior diameter than in its transverse diameter. To fit through the inlet of the birth canal best, a fetus must present the smaller diameter (the transverse diameter) of the head to the smaller diameter of the maternal pelvis (the diagonal conjugate); otherwise, progress can be halted and vaginal birth may not be possible. The diameters of the fetal

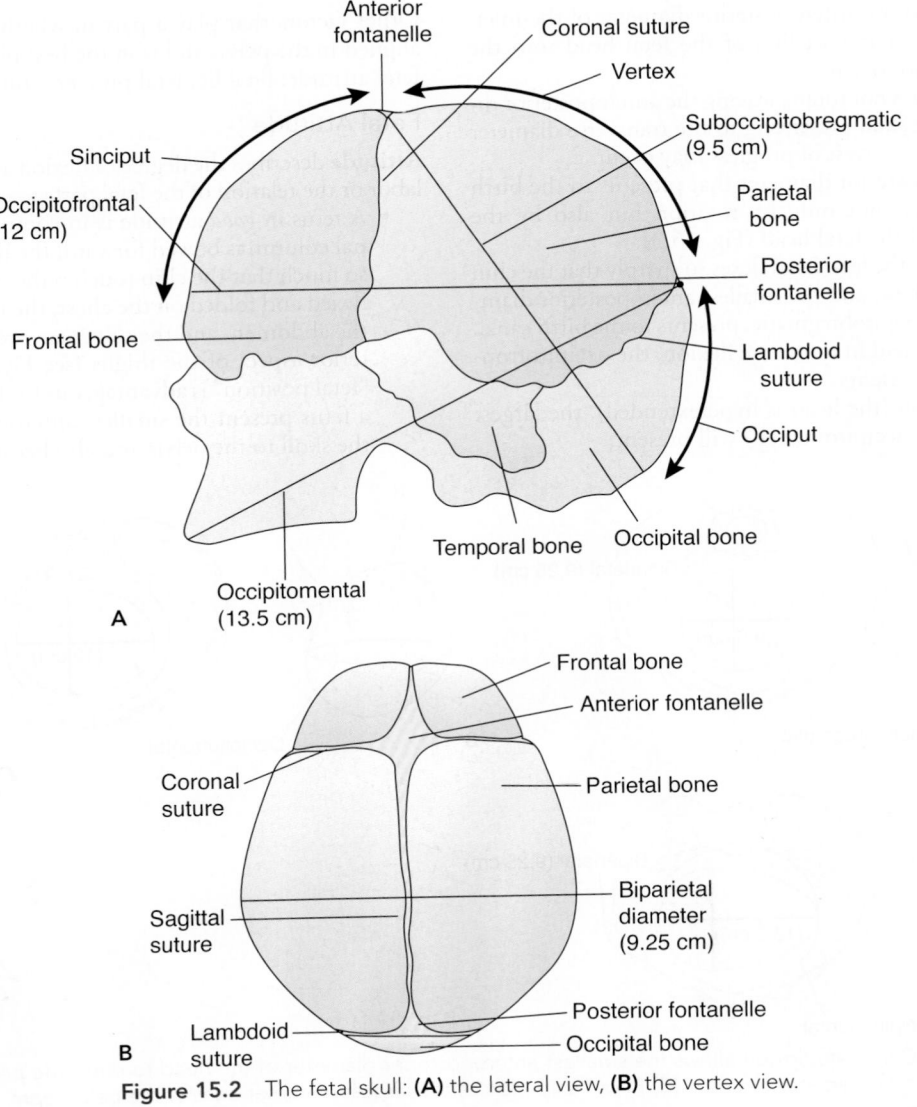

Figure 15.2   The fetal skull: **(A)** the lateral view, **(B)** the vertex view.

skull vary depending on where the measurement is taken (Fig. 15.2A).

- The smallest diameter of the fetal skull is the biparietal diameter or the transverse diameter, which measures about 9.25 cm.
- The smallest anteroposterior diameter is the suboccipitobregmatic measurement (approximately 9.5 cm) and is measured from the inferior aspect of the occiput to the center of the anterior fontanelle.
- The occipitofrontal diameter, measured from the occipital prominence to the bridge of the nose, is approximately 12 cm.
- The occipitomental diameter, which is the widest anteroposterior diameter (approximately 13.5 cm), is measured from the posterior fontanelle to the chin.

The anteroposterior diameter of the pelvis, a space approximately 11 cm wide, is the narrowest diameter at the pelvic inlet, and so the best presentation for birth is when the fetus presents a biparietal diameter (the narrowest fetal head diameter) to this (see Fig. 15.2B). At the outlet, the fetus must rotate to present this narrowest fetal head diameter (the biparietal diameter) to the maternal transverse diameter, a space, again, approximately 11 cm wide.

- If a fetus presents one of the anteroposterior diameters of the skull to the anteroposterior diameter of the inlet, engagement, or the settling of the fetal head into the pelvis, may not occur.
- If the fetus does not rotate, leaving the anteroposterior diameter of the skull presenting to the transverse diameter of the outlet, an arrest of progress may occur.

Which anteroposterior diameter that presents to the birth canal is determined not only by rotation but also by the degree of flexion of the fetal head (Fig. 15.3).

- In full flexion, the fetal head flexes so sharply that the chin rests on the chest, and the smallest anteroposterior diameter, the suboccipitobregmatic, presents to the birth canal.
- If the head is held in moderate flexion, the occipitofrontal diameter presents.
- In poor flexion (the head is hyperextended), the largest diameter (the occipitomental) will present.

It follows that full head flexion is an important aspect of labor because a fetal head presenting a diameter of 9.5 cm will fit through a pelvis much more readily than if the diameter is 12.0 or 13.5 cm.

Molding

Molding is overlapping of skull bones along the suture lines, which causes a change in the shape of the fetal skull to one long and narrow, a shape that facilitates passage through the rigid pelvis. Molding is caused by the force of uterine contractions as the vertex of the head is pressed against the not yet dilated cervix. The overlapping that occurs in the sagittal suture line and, generally, the coronal suture line can be easily palpated on the newborn skull. Parents can be reassured that molding only lasts a day or two and will not be a permanent condition. There is little molding when the brow is the presenting part (described later) because frontal bones are fused. No skull molding occurs when a fetus is breech because the buttocks, not the head, present first. Babies born by cesarean birth when there is no preprocedure labor also typically have no molding.

Fetal Presentation and Position

Other factors that play a part in whether a fetus is properly aligned in the pelvis and is in the best position to be born are fetal attitude, fetal lie, fetal presentation, and fetal position.

Fetal Attitude

Attitude describes the degree of flexion a fetus assumes during labor or the relation of the fetal parts to each other (Fig. 15.4).

- A fetus in *good* attitude is in complete flexion: The spinal column is bowed forward, the head is flexed forward so much that the chin touches the sternum, the arms are flexed and folded on the chest, the thighs are flexed onto the abdomen, and the calves are pressed against the posterior aspect of the thighs (see Fig. 15.4A). This usual "fetal position" is advantageous for birth because it helps a fetus present the smallest anteroposterior diameter of the skull to the pelvis and also because it puts the whole

Figure 15.3 **(A)** Complete flexion allows the smallest anteroposterior diameter of the head to enter the pelvis. **(B)** Moderate flexion causes a larger diameter to enter. **(C)** Poor flexion forces the largest diameter against the pelvic brim so the head is too large to enter the pelvis.

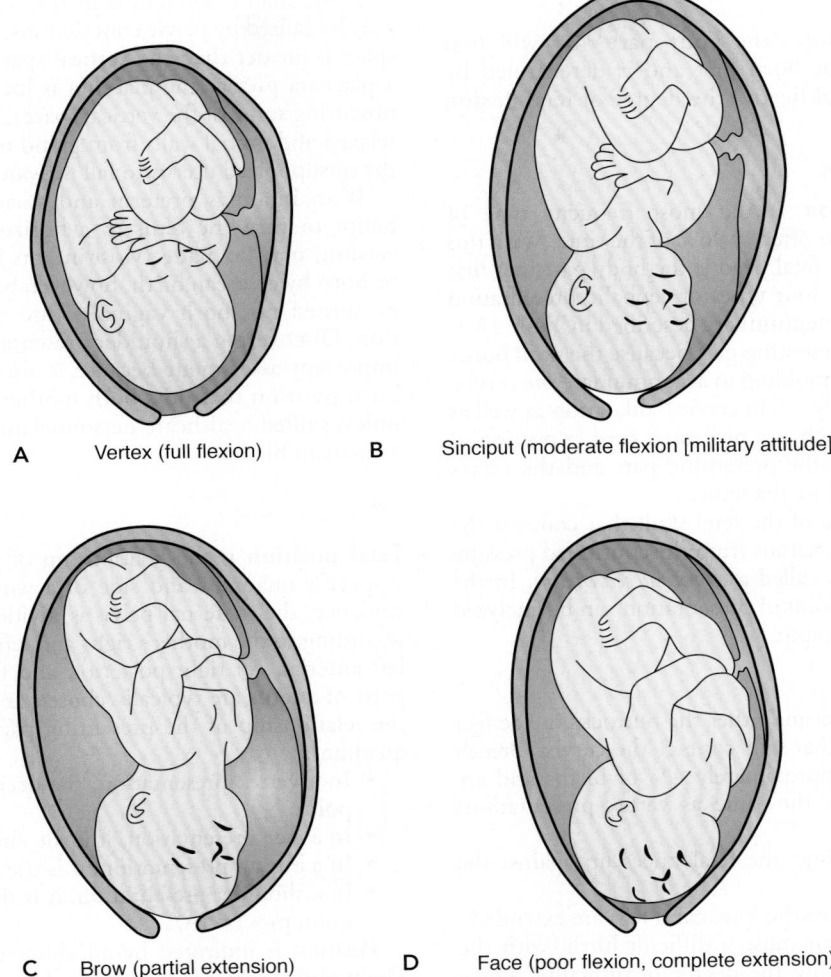

A   Vertex (full flexion)   B   Sinciput (moderate flexion [military attitude])

C   Brow (partial extension)   D   Face (poor flexion, complete extension)

Figure 15.4 Fetal attitude. **(A)** The fetus in full flexion presents the smallest anteroposterior diameter (suboccipitobregmatic) of the skull to the inlet in this good attitude (vertex presentation). **(B)** The fetus is not as well flexed (military attitude) and presents the occipitofrontal diameter to the inlet (sinciput presentation). **(C)** The fetus in partial extension (brow presentation). **(D)** The fetus in complete extension presents a wide (occipitomental) diameter (face presentation).

body into an ovoid shape, occupying the smallest space possible.

- A fetus is in *moderate* flexion if the chin is not touching the chest but is in an alert or "military position" (see Fig. 15.4B). This position causes the next widest anteroposterior diameter, the occipitofrontal diameter, to present to the birth canal. A fair number of fetuses assume a military position early in labor. This does not usually interfere with labor, however, because later mechanisms of labor (descent and flexion) force the fetal head to fully flex.
- A fetus in partial extension presents the "brow" of the head to the birth canal (see Fig. 15.4C).
- If a fetus is in complete extension, the back is arched and the neck is extended, presenting the occipitomental diameter of the head to the birth canal (a face presentation; see Fig. 15.4D). This unusual position usually presents too wide a skull diameter to the birth canal for vaginal birth. Such a position

may occur in an otherwise healthy fetus or may be an indication there is less than the usual amount of amniotic fluid present (oligohydramnios), which is not allowing the fetus adequate movement space. It also may reflect a neurologic abnormality in the fetus causing spasticity.

Fetal Lie

Lie is the relationship between the long (cephalocaudal) axis of the fetal body and the long (cephalocaudal) axis of a woman's body—in other words, whether the fetus is lying in a horizontal (transverse) or a vertical (longitudinal) position. Approximately 96% of fetuses assume a longitudinal lie (with their long axis parallel to the long axis of the woman) (Ferreira, Borowski, Czuba, et al., 2015).

Longitudinal lies are further classified as cephalic, which means the fetal head will be the first part to contact the cervix, or breech, with a foot or the buttocks as the first portion to contact the cervix.

Fetal Presentation

Fetal presentation denotes the body part that will first contact the cervix or be born first and is determined by the combination of fetal lie and the degree of fetal flexion (attitude).

Cephalic Presentation

A **cephalic presentation** is the most frequent type of presentation, occurring as often as 96% of the time. With this type of presentation, the fetal head is the body part that first contacts the cervix. The four types of cephalic presentation (vertex, brow, face, and mentum) are described in Table 15.1. The vertex is the ideal presenting part because the skull bones are capable of effectively molding to accommodate the cervix. This exact fit may actually aid in cervical dilatation as well as prevent complications such as a prolapsed cord (a portion of the cord passes between the presenting part and the cervix and enters the vagina before the fetus).

During labor, the area of the fetal skull that contacts the cervix often becomes edematous from the continued pressure against it. This edema is called a *caput succedaneum*. In the newborn, what was the point of presentation can be analyzed from the location of the caput.

Breech Presentation

A **breech presentation** means either the buttocks or the feet are the first body parts that will contact the cervix. Breech presentations occur in approximately 4% of births and are affected by fetal attitude the same as vertex presentations (Ferreira et al., 2015).

- A good attitude brings the fetal knees up against the fetal abdomen.
- A poor attitude means the knees and legs are extended.

Breech presentation can cause a difficult birth, with the presenting point influencing the degree of difficulty. Three types of breech presentation (complete, frank, and footling) are possible and described in Table 15.2.

Shoulder Presentation

In a transverse lie, a fetus lies horizontally in the pelvis so the longest fetal axis is perpendicular to that of the mother. The presenting part is usually one of the shoulders (acromion process), an iliac crest, a hand, or an elbow (Fig. 15.5). The usual contour of the mother's abdomen at term may appear fuller side to side rather than top to bottom.

Fewer than 1% of fetuses lie transversely. This presentation may be caused by pelvic contractions, in which the horizontal space is greater than the vertical space or by the presence of a placenta previa (the placenta is located low in the uterus, obscuring some of the vertical space). It also can be caused by relaxed abdominal walls from grand multiparity, which allow the unsupported uterus to fall forward (Ferreira et al., 2015).

If an infant is preterm and smaller than usual, an attempt to turn the fetus to a horizontal lie (external fetal version) may be made. Most infants in a transverse lie must be born by cesarean birth, however, because they can neither be turned nor born vaginally due to this "wedged" position. Discovering a shoulder presentation during labor is an important assessment because it almost always identifies a birth position that puts both mother and child in jeopardy unless skilled healthcare personnel are available to complete a cesarean birth.

Fetal Position

Fetal position is the relationship of the presenting part to a specific quadrant and side of a woman's pelvis. For convenience, the maternal pelvis is divided into four quadrants according to the mother's right and left: (a) right anterior, (b) left anterior, (c) right posterior, and (d) left posterior. Four parts of a fetus are typically chosen as landmarks to describe the relationship of the presenting part to one of the pelvic quadrants.

- In a vertex presentation, the occiput (O) is the chosen point.
- In a face presentation, it is the chin (mentum [M]).
- In a breech presentation, it is the sacrum (Sa).
- In a shoulder presentation, it is the scapula or the acromion process (A).

Position is indicated by an abbreviation of three letters. The middle letter denotes the fetal landmark (O for occiput, M for mentum, Sa for sacrum, and A for acromion process). The first letter defines whether the landmark is pointing to the mother's right (R) or left (L). The last letter defines whether the landmark points anteriorly (A), posteriorly (P), or transversely (T).

If the occiput of a fetus points to the left anterior quadrant in a vertex position, for example, this is a left occipitoanterior (LOA) position. If the occiput points to the right posterior quadrant, the position is right occipitoposterior (ROP). LOA is the most common fetal position, and right occipitoanterior

TABLE 15.1 TYPES OF CEPHALIC PRESENTATIONS

Type	Lie	Attitude	Description
Vertex	Longitudinal	Good (full flexion)	The head is sharply flexed, making the parietal bones or the space between the fontanelles (the vertex) the presenting part. This is the most common presentation and allows the suboccipitobregmatic diameter to present to the cervix.
Brow	Longitudinal	Moderate (military)	Because the head is only moderately flexed, the brow or sinciput becomes the presenting part.
Face	Longitudinal	Poor	The fetus has extended the head to make the face the presenting part. From this position, extreme edema and distortion of the face may occur.
Mentum	Longitudinal	Very poor	The fetus has completely hyperextended the head to present the chin, causing the presenting diameter (the occipitomental) to be so wide that vaginal birth may not be possible.

TABLE 15.2 TYPES OF BREECH PRESENTATIONS

Type	Lie	Attitude	Description
Complete	Longitudinal	Good (full flexion)	The fetus has the thighs tightly flexed on the abdomen; both the buttocks and the tightly flexed feet present to the cervix.
Frank	Longitudinal	Moderate	Attitude is moderate because the hips are flexed, but the knees are extended to rest on the chest. The buttocks alone present to the cervix.
Footling	Longitudinal	Poor	Neither the thighs nor lower legs are flexed. If one foot presents, it is a single-footling breech; if both present, it is a double-footling breech.

Figure 15.5   A transverse or shoulder presentation.

(ROA) is the second most frequent. Box 15.2 summarizes possible positions. Six common positions in cephalic presentations are illustrated in Figure 15.6.

Position is important because it can influence both the process and efficiency of labor. Typically, a fetus is born fastest from an ROA or LOA position. Labor can be considerably extended if the position is posterior (ROP or LOP) and may be more painful for a woman because the rotation of the fetal head puts pressure on sacral nerves. Encouraging a woman to rest in a Sims position on the same side as the fetal spine or use a hands and knees position may encourage rotation from an occipitoposterior to an occipitoanterior position prior to and during labor (Simkin, 2010).

Engagement

Engagement refers to the settling of the presenting part of a fetus far enough into the pelvis that it rests at the level of the ischial spines, the midpoint of the pelvis. Descent to this point means the widest part of the fetus (the presenting skull diameter in a cephalic presentation, or the intertrochanteric diameter in a breech presentation) has passed through the pelvis or the pelvic inlet has been proven adequate for birth. In a primipara, nonengagement of the head at the beginning of labor suggests that a possible complication such as an abnormal presentation or position, abnormality of the fetal head, or cephalopelvic disproportion exists. In multiparas, engagement may or may not be present at the beginning of labor. The degree of engagement is established by a vaginal and cervical examination.

- A presenting part that is not engaged is said to be "floating."
- One that is descending but has not yet reached the ischial spines may be referred to as "dipping."

Station

Station refers to the relationship of the presenting part of the fetus to the level of the ischial spines (Fig. 15.7).

- When the presenting fetal part is at the level of the ischial spines, it is at a 0 station (synonymous with engagement).
- If the presenting part is above the spines, the distance is measured and described as minus stations, which range from −1 to −4 cm.

LOP   LOT   LOA

ROP   ROT   ROA

Figure 15.6   The fetal position. All are vertex presentations. A, anterior; L, left; O, occiput; P, posterior; R, right; T, transverse.

BOX 15.2

Examples of Possible Fetal Positions

Vertex Presentation (Occiput)	Breech Presentation (Sacrum)	Shoulder Presentation (Acromion Process)
LOA, left occipitoanterior	LSaA, left sacroanterior	LAA, left scapuloanterior
LOP, left occipitoposterior	LSaP, left sacroposterior	LAP, left scapuloposterior
LOT, left occipitotransverse	LSaT, left sacrotransverse	RAA, right scapuloanterior
ROA, right occipitoanterior	RSaA, right sacroanterior	RAP, right scapuloposterior
ROP, right occipitoposterior	RSaP, right sacroposterior	
ROT, right occipitotransverse	RSaT, right sacrotransverse	

- If the presenting part is below the ischial spines, the distance is stated as plus stations (+1 to +4 cm).
- At a +3 or +4 station, the presenting part is at the perineum and can be seen if the vulva is separated (i.e., it is crowning).

QSEN Checkpoint Question 15.1

TEAMWORK & COLLABORATION

The nurse is collaborating with Celeste Bailey's obstetrician and is planning possible interventions in light of fetal position. Which of the following fetal positions is considered ideal and is most conducive to a birth that requires few interventions by the obstetrician?

   a. Right occipitoanterior with full flexion
   b. Left transverse anterior in moderate flexion
   c. Right occipitoposterior with no flexion
   d. Left sacroanterior with full flexion

Look in Appendix A for the best answer and rationale.

Mechanisms (Cardinal Movements) of Labor

Effective passage of a fetus through the birth canal involves not only position and presentation but also a number of different position changes in order to keep the smallest diameter of the fetal head (in cephalic presentations) always presenting to the smallest diameter of the pelvis. These position changes are

Figure 15.7 The station (anteroposterior view). The station, or degree of engagement, of the fetal head is designated by centimeters above or below the ischial spines. At −4 station, the head is "floating." At 0 station, the head is "engaged." At +4 station, the head is "at outlet."

termed the **cardinal movements of labor**: descent, flexion, internal rotation, extension, external rotation, and expulsion (Fig. 15.8).

Descent

Descent is the downward movement of the biparietal diameter of the fetal head within the pelvic inlet. Full descent occurs when the fetal head protrudes beyond the dilated cervix and touches the posterior vaginal floor. Descent occurs because of pressure on the fetus by the uterine fundus. As the pressure of the fetal head presses on the sacral nerves at the pelvic floor, the mother will experience the typical "pushing sensation," which occurs with labor. As a woman contracts her abdominal muscles with pushing, this aids descent.

Flexion

As descent is completed and the fetal head touches the pelvic floor, the head bends forward onto the chest, causing the smallest anteroposterior diameter (the suboccipitobregmatic diameter) to present to the birth canal. Flexion is also aided by abdominal muscle contraction during pushing.

Internal Rotation

During descent, the biparietal diameter of the fetal skull was aligned to fit through the anteroposterior diameter of the mother's pelvis. As the head flexes at the end of descent, the occiput rotates so the head is brought into the best relationship to the outlet of the pelvis, or the anteroposterior diameter is now in the anteroposterior plane of the pelvis. This movement brings the shoulders, coming next, into the optimal position to enter the inlet, or puts the widest diameter of the shoulders (a transverse one) in line with the wide transverse diameter of the inlet.

Extension

As the occiput of the fetal head is born, the back of the neck stops beneath the pubic arch and acts as a pivot for the rest of the head. The head extends, and the foremost parts of the head, the face and chin, are born.

External Rotation

In external rotation, almost immediately after the head of the infant is born, the head rotates a final time (from the anteroposterior position it assumed to enter the outlet) back to the diagonal or transverse position of the early part of labor. This brings the after coming shoulders into an anteroposterior position, which is best for entering the outlet. The anterior shoulder is born first, assisted perhaps by downward flexion of the infant's head.

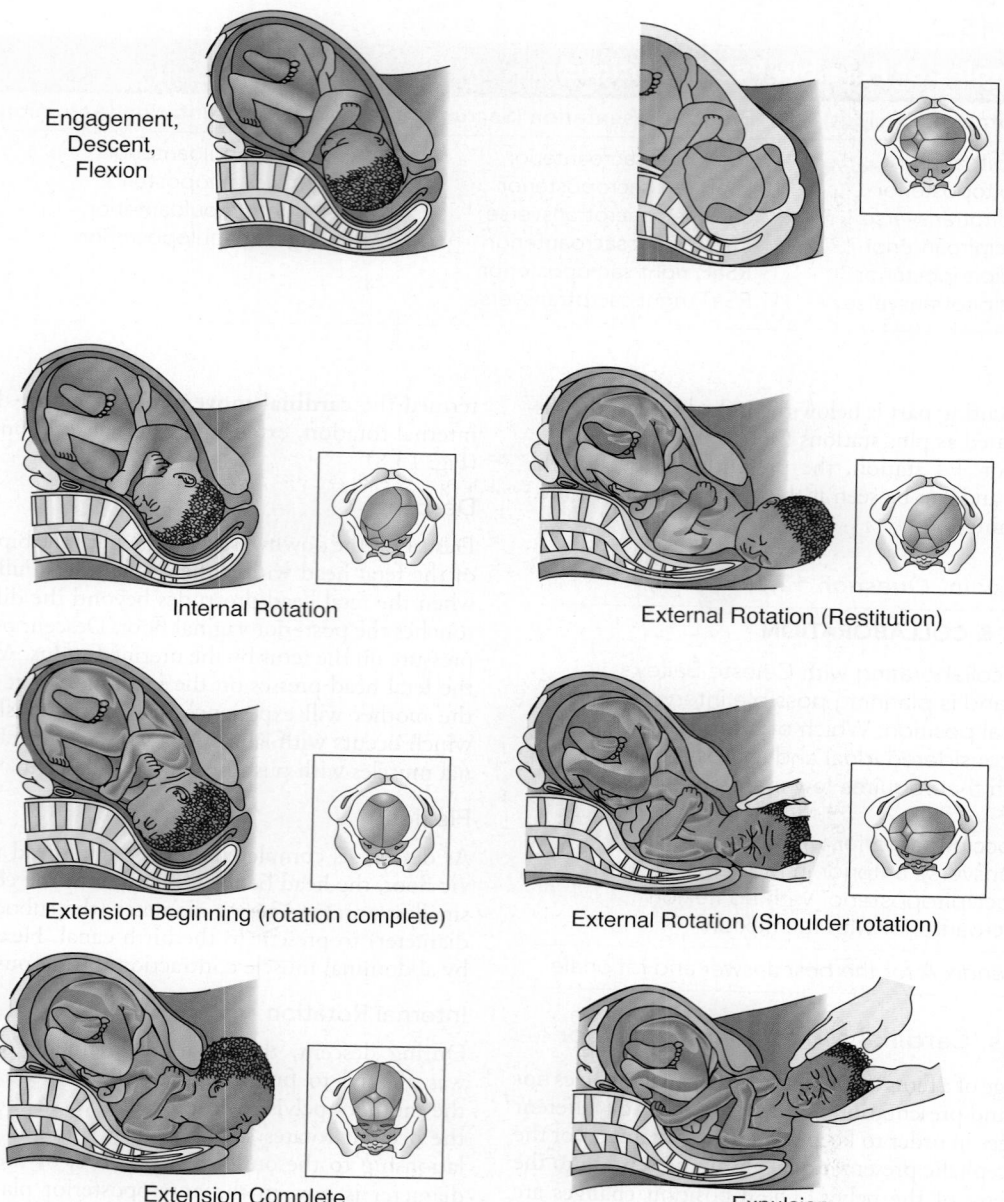

Engagement, Descent, Flexion

Internal Rotation

External Rotation (Restitution)

Extension Beginning (rotation complete)

External Rotation (Shoulder rotation)

Extension Complete

Expulsion

Figure 15.8 The mechanism of normal labor and cardinal positions of the fetus from a left occipitoanterior position.

Expulsion

Once the shoulders are born, the rest of the baby is born easily and smoothly because of its smaller size. This movement, called expulsion, is the end of the pelvic division of labor. For a view of the complete birth sequence, see Figure 15.9.

THE POWERS OF LABOR

The third important requirement for a successful labor is effective powers of labor. This is the force supplied by the fundus of the uterus and implemented by uterine contractions, which causes cervical dilatation and then expulsion of the fetus from the uterus. After full dilatation of the cervix, the primary power is supplemented by use of a secondary power source, the abdominal muscles. It is important for women to understand that they should not bear down with their abdominal muscles to push until the cervix is fully dilated. Doing so impedes the primary force and could cause fetal and cervical damage.

Uterine Contractions

During pregnancy, the uterus begins to contract and relax periodically as if it is rehearsing for labor (Braxton Hicks contractions, or false labor). These contractions are usually mild but can be so strong that a woman mistakes them for true labor. As a rule, even if a woman thinks what she is feeling cannot be true labor, she needs to phone or e-mail her primary care provider to have the contractions further evaluated in case she is mistaking preterm labor for practice contractions. The mark of Braxton Hicks contractions is that they are usually irregular and are painful but do not cause cervical dilation.

6:00 AM: Early in labor, a mother-to-be is supported by her husband and her sister.

9:00 AM: The nurse checks the fetal monitor and documents fetal and maternal status.

10:00 AM: The doctor makes a final check of cervical dilatation and says it's time to push.

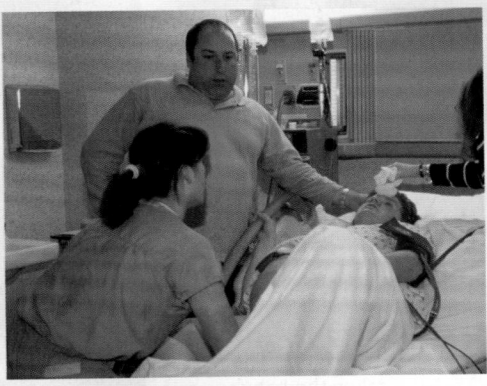

11:15 AM: She pushes from an alternative position, using a support bar.

10:30 AM: The mother pushes in the dorsal recumbent position with her coach.

Figure 15.9 A day in the life of a new family.

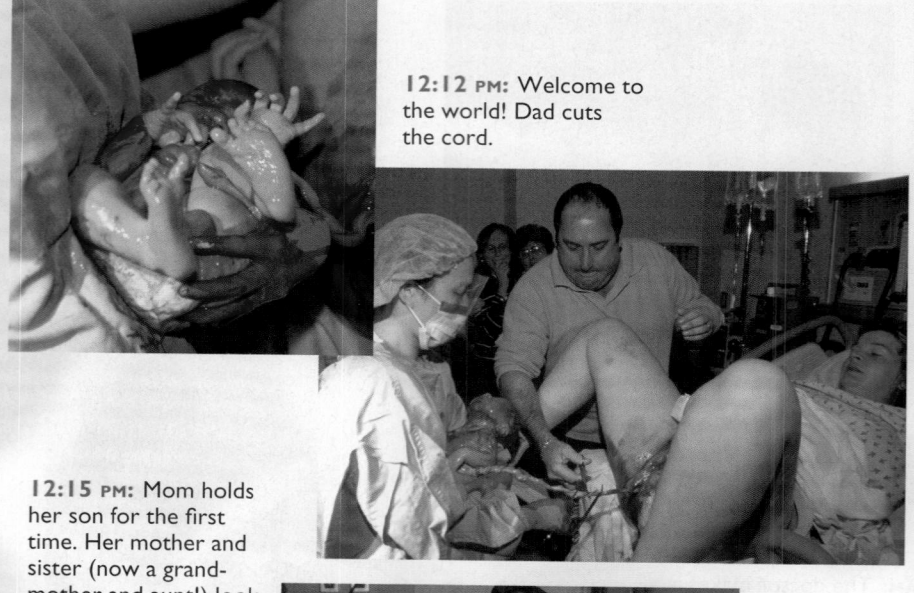

12:12 PM: Welcome to the world! Dad cuts the cord.

12:15 PM: Mom holds her son for the first time. Her mother and sister (now a grand-mother and aunt!) look on.

12:30 PM: The nurse takes the baby's footprints.

1:15 PM: Cleaned and swaddled, the newborn gets a kiss from Mom.

3:00 PM: The new mom gives Stephen his first feeding, with support from the nurse.

5:00 PM: New parents bond with the new member of their family.

Figure 15.9   (continued)

TABLE 15.3 DIFFERENTIATING BETWEEN TRUE AND FALSE LABOR CONTRACTIONS

False Contractions	True Contractions
Begin and remain irregular	Begin irregularly but become regular and predictable
Felt first abdominally and remain confined to the abdomen and groin	Felt first in lower back and sweep around to the abdomen in a wave
Often disappear with ambulation or sleep	Continue no matter what the woman's level of activity
Do not increase in duration, frequency, or intensity	Increase in duration, frequency, and intensity
Do not achieve cervical dilatation	Achieve cervical dilatation

In contrast, effective uterine contractions have rhythmicity, a progressive increase in length and intensity, and accompany dilatation of the cervix. These differences between false and true labor are summarized in Table 15.3. Contractions are assessed according to frequency, duration, and strength.

Origins

Like cardiac contractions, labor contractions begin at a "pacemaker" point located in the uterine myometrium near one of the uterotubal junctions. Each contraction begins at that point and then sweeps down over the uterus as a wave. After a short rest period, another contraction is initiated and the downward sweep begins again.

In early labor, the uterotubal pacemaker may not operate in a synchronous manner. This makes contractions sometimes strong, sometimes weak, and somewhat irregular. This mild incoordination of early labor improves after a few hours as the pacemaker becomes more attuned to calcium concentrations in the myometrium and begins to function effectively.

In some women, contractions appear to originate in the lower uterine segment rather than in the fundus. These are reversed and ineffective and may actually cause tightening rather than dilatation of the cervix. It is difficult to tell from palpation that contractions are being initiated in a reverse pattern. It can be suspected, however, if the woman tells you she feels pain in her lower abdomen before the contraction is readily palpated at the fundus. It is truly revealed only when apparently strong uterine contractions do not cause cervical dilatation.

Some women seem to have additional pacemaker sites in other portions of the uterus. If this is so, contractions can be uncoordinated. Uncoordinated contractions may slow labor and can lead to failure to progress and fetal distress because they may not allow for adequate placental filling. All of these possibilities make evaluating the rate, intensity, and pattern of uterine contractions an important nursing responsibility.

Phases

A contraction consists of three phases: the increment, when the intensity of the contraction increases; the acme, when the contraction is at its strongest; and the decrement, when the intensity decreases (Fig. 15.10). Between contractions, the uterus relaxes. As labor progresses, the relaxation intervals decrease from 10 minutes early in labor to only 2 to 3 minutes. The duration of contractions also changes, increasing from 20 to 30 seconds at the beginning to a range of 60 to 70 seconds by the end of the first stage (López Bernal & Norwitz, 2012).

Contour Changes

As labor contractions progress and become regular and strong, the uterus gradually differentiates itself into two distinct functioning areas: an upper portion, which thickens, and a lower segment, which becomes thin-walled, supple, and passive so the fetus can be pushed out of the uterus easily. The contour of the overall uterus also changes from a round, ovoid structure to an elongated one with a vertical diameter markedly greater than the horizontal diameter. This lengthening straightens the body of the fetus, bringing it into better alignment with the cervix and pelvis. The elongation of the uterus can cause pressure against the diaphragm and causes the often expressed sensation that a uterus is "taking control" of a woman's body.

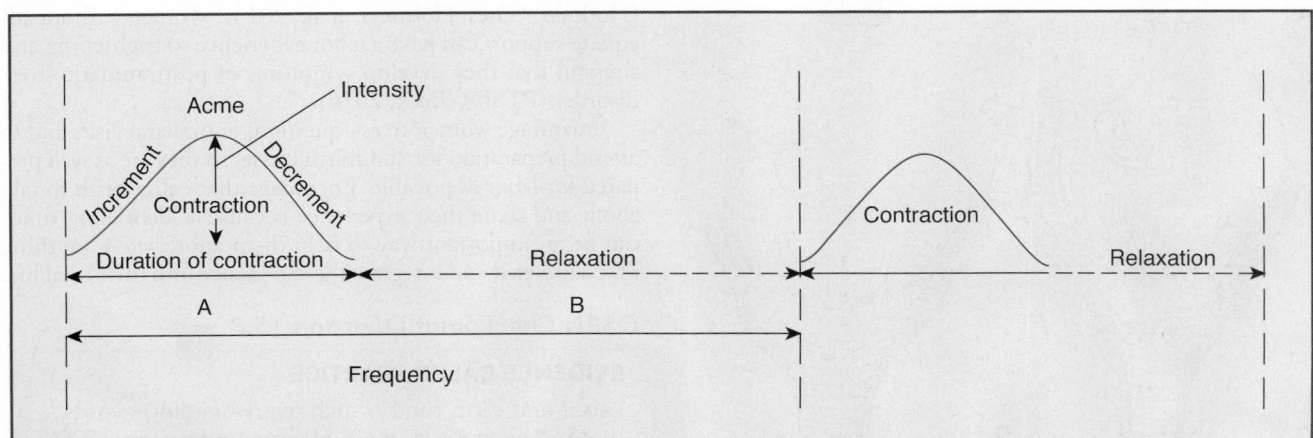

Figure 15.10 The interval and duration of uterine contractions. The frequency of contractions is the time from the beginning of one contraction to the beginning of the next. It consists of two parts: **(A)** the duration of the contraction and **(B)** the period of relaxation. The broken line indicates an indeterminate period because the relaxation time **(B)** is usually of longer duration than the actual contraction **(A)**.

Cervical Changes

Even more marked than the changes in the body of the uterus are two changes that occur in the cervix: effacement and dilatation.

Effacement

Effacement is shortening and thinning of the cervical canal. All during pregnancy, the canal is approximately 1 to 2 cm long. During labor, the longitudinal traction from the contracting uterus shortens the cervix so much that the cervix virtually disappears (Fig. 15.11).

In primiparas, effacement is accomplished before dilatation begins. Be sure to inform women of both effacement and dilation following a pelvic examination. If a woman is told at noon, for example, she is 3 cm dilated and then at 4 PM, she is told she is still 3 cm dilated, it is a discouraging report because it seems as if absolutely nothing has happened in 4 hours. Effacement, however, will have been occurring; telling her about this can be the encouragement she needs to continue breathing or working with contractions.

In multiparas, dilatation may proceed before effacement is complete. Effacement must occur by the end of dilatation, however, before the fetus can be safely pushed through the cervical canal; otherwise, cervical tearing can result.

Figure 15.11 Effacement and dilation of the cervix. **(A)** The beginning of labor. **(B)** Effacement is beginning; dilation is not apparent yet. **(C)** Effacement is almost complete. **(D)** After complete effacement, dilation proceeds rapidly.

Dilatation

Dilatation refers to the enlargement or widening of the cervical canal from an opening a few millimeters wide to one large enough (approximately 10 cm) to permit passage of a fetus (see Fig. 15.11).

Dilatation occurs first because uterine contractions gradually increase the diameter of the cervical canal lumen by pulling the cervix up over the presenting part of the fetus. Secondly, the fluid-filled membranes push ahead of the fetus and serve as an opening wedge. If they are ruptured, the presenting part will serve this same function, although maybe not as effectively.

As dilatation begins, there is an increase in the amount of vaginal secretions (show) because minute capillaries in the cervix rupture and the last of the mucus plug that has sealed the cervix since early pregnancy is released.

QSEN Checkpoint Question 15.2

QUALITY IMPROVEMENT

Celeste Bailey didn't recognize for over an hour that she was in labor. During her prenatal education, Celeste should have been taught to recognize which sign of true labor?
   a. Sudden loss of energy from epinephrine release
   b. "Nagging" but constant pain in the lower back
   c. Urinary urgency from increased bladder pressure
   d. "Show" or release of the cervical mucus plug

Look in Appendix A for the best answer and rationale.

THE PSYCHE

The fourth "P," or a woman's psychological outlook, refers to the psychological state or feelings a woman brings into labor. For many women, this is a feeling of apprehension or fright. For almost everyone, it includes a sense of excitement or awe.

Women who manage best in labor typically are those who have a strong sense of self-esteem and a meaningful support person with them. These factors allow women to feel in control of sensations and circumstances they have never experienced before and which may not be what they pictured (Hodnett, Gates, Hofmeyr, et al., 2013). Women without adequate support can have a labor experience so frightening and stressful that they develop symptoms of posttraumatic stress disorder (PTSD) (Beck, 2016).

Encourage women to ask questions at prenatal visits and to attend preparation for childbirth classes so they are as well prepared for labor as possible. Encourage them after birth to talk about and share their experience because a "debriefing time" can be an important way to help them appreciate everything that happened and integrate the experience into their total life.

QSEN Checkpoint Question 15.3

EVIDENCE-BASED PRACTICE

Labor and birth can be such overwhelming events that between 1% and 6% of women develop PTSD after childbirth. "Hotspots" are moments of extreme distress that strongly influence the development of PTSD. To find what are the hotspots in labor, researchers asked 675 women who experienced a difficult or traumatic birth to complete a questionnaire describing their labor and birth experience. Of the women, 67% reported at least one hotspot during birth and 52.9% had reexperiencing anxiety of these hotspots. Women were more likely to have PTSD if hotspots involved fear and lack of control or if the hotspots concerned interpersonal difficulties or maternal complications compared to complications with the baby (Greenfield, Jomeen, & Glover, 2016).

Based on the previous study, which statement by Celeste would cause the most concern for the nurse that labor could be becoming traumatic for Celeste?
  a. "I'm feeling as if I'm losing a grasp on things."
  b. "I wish my husband was able to be here."
  c. "Pushing is harder to do than I thought it would be."
  d. "I wish this didn't hurt so much."

Look in Appendix A for the best answer and rationale.

The Stages of Labor

Labor is traditionally divided into three stages:
- The first stage of dilatation, which begins with the initiation of true labor contractions and ends when the cervix is fully dilated
- The second stage, extending from the time of full dilatation until the infant is born
- The third or placental stage, lasting from the time the infant is born until after the delivery of the placenta
- The first 1 to 4 hours after birth of the placenta is sometimes termed the "fourth stage" to emphasize the importance of close maternal observation needed at this time.

THE FIRST STAGE

The first stage, which takes about 12 hours to complete, is divided into three segments: a latent, an active, and a transition phase. Traditionally the Freidman's curve, an algorithm for determining normal labor progress, has been utilized in labor settings everywhere. However, new research is discovering that a normal labor can actually take a great deal longer than previously thought (Zhang, Landy, Branch, et al., 2010).

The Latent Phase

The latent or early phase begins at the onset of regularly perceived uterine contractions and ends when rapid cervical dilatation begins. Contractions during this phase are mild and short, lasting 20 to 40 seconds. Cervical effacement occurs, and the cervix dilates minimally. A birthing parent who is multiparous usually progresses more quickly than a nullipara. A woman who enters labor with a "nonripe" cervix will probably have a longer than average latent phase. If a woman wants analgesia at this point, she shouldn't be denied of it, but analgesia given too early in labor is a factor that tends to prolong this phase.

In a woman who is psychologically prepared for labor and who does not tense at each tightening sensation in her abdomen, latent phase contractions cause only minimal discomfort and can be managed by controlled breathing.

During this phase, encourage women to continue to walk about and make preparations for birth, such as doing last-minute packing for her stay at the hospital or birthing center, preparing older children for her departure and the upcoming birth, or giving instructions to the person who will take care of them while she is away. If desired, she could begin alternative methods of pain relief such as aromatherapy, distraction, or acupressure (Steel, Adams, & Sibbritt, et al., 2014). If the woman should come to a birthing setting this early, encourage her to continue to be active and to use any nonpharmacotherapeutic measures she finds effective.

The Active Phase

During the active phase of labor, cervical dilatation occurs more rapidly. Contractions grow stronger, lasting 40 to 60 seconds, and occur approximately every 3 to 5 minutes. Show (increased vaginal secretions) and perhaps spontaneous rupture of the membranes may occur during this time. Encourage women to be active participants in labor by keeping active and assuming whatever position is most comfortable for them during this time, except flat on their back (Iravani, Janghorbani, Zarean, et al., 2015).

This phase can be difficult for a woman because contractions grow so much stronger and last so much longer than they did in the latent phase that she begins to experience true discomfort. It is also both an exciting and a frightening time because it is obvious something dramatic is definitely happening. In a few hours, a woman will have a new baby. Her life will never be the same again.

The Transition Phase

During the **transition** phase, contractions reach their peak of intensity, occurring every 2 to 3 minutes with a duration of 60 to 70 seconds, and a maximum cervical dilatation of 8 to 10 cm occurs. If it has not previously occurred, show will occur as the last of the mucus plug from the cervix is released. If the membranes have not previously ruptured, they will usually rupture at full dilatation (10 cm). By the end of this phase, both full dilatation (10 cm) and complete cervical effacement (obliteration of the cervix) have occurred.

During this phase, a woman may experience intense discomfort that is so strong, it might be accompanied by nausea and vomiting. She may also experience a feeling of loss of control, anxiety, panic, and/or irritability. Because of the intensity and duration of the contractions, it may seem as though labor has taken charge of her. A few minutes before, she may have enjoyed having her forehead wiped with a cool cloth or her back rubbed. Now, she may knock a partner's hand away from her. Her focus turns entirely inward to the task of birthing her baby. As a woman reaches the end of this stage at 10 cm of dilatation, unless she has been administered epidural anesthesia, a new sensation, the irresistible urge to push, usually begins.

What If . . . 15.1
Celeste tells the nurse she is certain her labor is going wrong because it has lasted over 6 hours. Is this an unusually long time for a first stage of labor for a woman having her first child? Would she be comforted by learning the usual length?

THE SECOND STAGE

The second stage of labor is the time span from full dilatation and cervical effacement to birth of the infant. A woman typically feels contractions change from the characteristic crescendo–decrescendo pattern to an uncontrollable urge to push or bear down with each contraction as if to move her bowels. She may experience momentary nausea or vomiting because pressure is no longer exerted on her stomach as the fetus descends into the pelvis. She pushes with such force that she perspires and the blood vessels in her neck become distended.

The fetus begins descent and, as the fetal head touches the internal perineum to begin internal rotation, her perineum begins to bulge and appear tense. The anus may become everted, and stool may be expelled. As the fetal head pushes against the vaginal introitus, this opens and the fetal scalp appears at the opening to the vagina and enlarges from the size of a dime, to a quarter, then a half-dollar. This is termed **crowning**.

It takes a few contractions of this new type for a woman to realize everything is all right, just different, and to appreciate it feels better and less frightening, to push with contractions. As she concentrates on pushing, she may become unaware of the conversation in the room. Pain may disappear as all of her energy and thoughts are directed toward giving birth. As the fetal head is pushed out of the birth canal, it extends and then rotates to bring the shoulders into the best line with the pelvis. The body of the baby is then born.

THE THIRD STAGE

The third stage of labor, the placental stage, begins with the birth of the infant and ends with the delivery of the placenta. Two separate phases are involved: *placental separation* and *placental expulsion*.

After the birth of the infant, the uterus can be palpated as a firm, round mass just below the level of the umbilicus. After a few minutes of rest, uterine contractions begin again, and the organ assumes a discoid shape. It retains this new shape until the placenta has separated, approximately 5 minutes after the birth of the infant.

Placental Separation

As the uterus contracts down on an almost empty interior, there is such a disproportion between the placenta and the contracting wall of the uterus that folding and separation of the placenta occur. Active bleeding on the maternal surface of the placenta begins with separation, which helps to separate the placenta still further by pushing it away from its attachment site. As separation is completed, the placenta sinks to the lower uterine segment or the upper vagina.

The placenta has loosened and is ready to deliver when:
- There is lengthening of the umbilical cord.
- A sudden gush of vaginal blood occurs.
- The placenta is visible at the vaginal opening.
- The uterus contracts and feels firm again.

If the placenta separates first at its center and lastly at its edges, it tends to fold on itself like an umbrella and presents at the vaginal opening with the fetal surface evident. Approximately 80% of placentas separate and present in this way. Appearing shiny and glistening from the fetal membranes, this is called a *Schultze* presentation. If, however, the placenta separates

first at its edges, it slides along the uterine surface and presents at the vagina with the maternal surface evident. It looks raw, red, and irregular, with the ridges or cotyledons that separate blood collection spaces evident; this is called a *Duncan* presentation. Although there is no difference in the outcome, record which way the placenta presented. A simple trick of remembering the presentations is remembering that, if the placenta appears shiny, it is a Schultze presentation. If it looks "dirty" (the irregular maternal surface shows), it is a Duncan presentation (Fig. 15.12).

This stage can take anywhere from 1 to 30 minutes and still be considered normal. Because bleeding occurs as the placenta separates, before the uterus contracts sufficiently to seal maternal capillaries, there is a blood loss of about 300 to 500 ml, not a great amount in relation to the extra blood volume that was formed during pregnancy.

Placental Expulsion

Once separation has occurred, the placenta delivers either by the natural bearing-down effort of the mother or by gentle pressure on the contracted uterine fundus by the primary healthcare provider (a Credé maneuver). Pressure should never be applied to a uterus in a noncontracted state because doing so could cause the uterus to evert (turn inside out), accompanied by massive hemorrhage (Bienstock et al., 2015).

A

B

Figure 15.12 The fetal **(A)** and maternal **(B)** surfaces of the placenta. (Photos by Joe Mitchell.)

BOX 15.3
Nursing Care Planning to Respect Cultural Diversity

It is important for women to understand what is happening to them during labor so they can make informed decisions as to their care. If a woman is not proficient in English, make arrangements to locate an interpreter. If she is hearing challenged, it is the healthcare facility's responsibility to provide an interpreter for her so she can receive adequate explanations of her progress. Remember, whether a woman enjoys being touched or not is in part culturally determined. Assess early in a woman's labor whether she might benefit from such caring measures as having her hand held or her back rubbed or if she wants this only from her support person.

For most healthcare providers in the United States, a placenta has little importance or meaning after its work of fetal oxygenation is done. Worldwide, however, the placenta has continuing importance. Based on this, ask women if they want to take it home with them. In a number of Asian and Native American cultures, it is important to bury the placenta to ensure the child will continue to be healthy. In some parts of China, the placenta is cooked then ground into a powder and eaten to ensure the continued health of the mother (M. F. Moore, 2016). Be certain when supplying placentas to women to take home that you respect standard infection precautions and hospital policy.

If the placenta does not deliver spontaneously, it can be removed manually. It needs to be inspected after delivery to be certain it is intact and part of it was not retained (which could prevent the uterus from fully contracting and lead to postpartal hemorrhage). In recognition of cultural preferences, be certain to ask if a woman wants to take home the placenta because this can be a strong cultural tradition you don't want to break (Box 15.3).

Some women choose to have a cord blood sample withdrawn from the cord to be banked for stem cell transplantation in the future. In some major health centers, women may be asked to donate a placental blood sample for a community stem cell banking program (Sun, Yue, He, et al., 2016).

QSEN Checkpoint Question 15.4

PATIENT-CENTERED CARE

Celeste is anxious for her placenta to deliver so she can move to a rocking chair and help relieve her back pain. To best facilitate Celeste's wishes, which action is best?

   a. Tug gently on the umbilical cord until the placenta comes loose.
   b. Ask Celeste to continue hard pushing as she did to birth her baby.
   c. Push on the lax fundus of her uterus to cause the placenta to loosen.
   d. Assure her that a placenta loosens quickly so the waiting time will not be long.

Look in Appendix A for the best answer and rationale.

Maternal and Fetal Responses to Labor

Labor is a local process that involves the abdomen and reproductive organs, but because it is such an intense process, it has systemic physiologic effects on both a woman and her fetus. Its intensity is so great that almost all body systems are affected by it.

THE MATERNAL PHYSIOLOGIC EFFECTS AND PSYCHOLOGICAL RESPONSES

Pregnancy has effects on many systems of the birthing parent. During labor, there are yet further effects which may require the nurse to deliver specific care to their patient. Knowing and recognizing what is normal and what is not normal can help to ensure safe provision of care (Table 15.4).

The Response to Pain

Cultural factors can strongly influence a woman's experience and satisfaction with labor. In the past, American women were accustomed to expecting hospital procedures and a medical model of care; based on this, they followed instructions with few questions. Today, women are encouraged to help plan their care. In addition, every woman responds to cultural cues in some way. This makes her response to pain, her choice of nourishment, her preferred birthing position, the proximity and involvement of a support person, and customs related to the immediate postpartal period highly individualized.

To make labor a positive experience, be prepared to adapt care to the woman's specific needs. If a woman has traditions that run counter to hospital protocols, address these differences and make arrangements to accommodate her desires, beliefs, or customs, if possible, such as advocating for special foods to eat, ballroom dancing in order to remain upright, or saving the placenta for the mother to take home.

The Response to Fatigue

By the time the date of birth approaches, a woman is generally tired from the normal discomforts of pregnancy and has not slept well for the past month (Nazik & Eryilmaz, 2014). For example, a side-lying position caused backache; when she turned onto her back, her fetus kicked and wakened her; when she turned back to her side, her back ached again. Sleep hunger from this type of discomfort can make it difficult for a woman to perceive situations clearly or to adjust rapidly to new situations. It can make a small deficiency such as a wrinkled sheet appear as a major threatening discrepancy in her care. It can make the process of labor loom as an overwhelming, unendurable experience unless she has competent people with her to offer support, reassurance, and comfort.

The Response to Fear

Women appreciate a review of the labor process early in labor as a reminder that childbirth is not a strange, bewildering event but a predictable and well-documented one. Being taken by surprise—labor moving faster or slower than the woman thought it would or contractions harder and longer than she remembers from last time—can lead a woman to feel out of control and increase the level of pain she experiences. This sense of lack of control combined with pain may cause her to begin to

TABLE 15.4 PHYSIOLOGICAL EFFECTS OF LABOR

System	Response	Recommended Nursing Action
Cardiovascular system	• Cardiac output increases 40%–50% from prelabor levels. • Blood loss at birth is 300–500 ml on average. • Blood pressure may rise with pain response and, due to work of the system during contractions, by an average systolic rise of 15 mmHg per contraction. Epidural anesthesia may cause hypotension.	• Monitor closely for hemorrhage. • Monitor for signs of pathology with hypertensive episodes. Ensure that patients are well hydrated prior to epidural administration. This usually involves an IV fluid bolus (see Chapter 16).
Hematopoietic system	• During labor, WBCs increase to a level of 25,000–30,000 cells/mm^3 compared to 5,000–10,000 cell/mm^3.	• Continue to monitor for any signs of infection.
Respiratory system	• Increased respiratory rate to respond to increased cardiovascular parameters • Total oxygen needs increase 100% during the second stage of labor.	• Monitor for any signs of hyperventilation. If hyperventilation occurs, rebreathing into a paper bag can be helpful. • If needed, use appropriately patterned breathing to regulate respiratory rate.
Temperature regulation	• Temperature may increase up to (1°F). • Diaphoresis occurs with accompanying evaporation to cool and limit excessive warming.	• Monitor for any signs of infection. • Offer cool washcloths for the patient's forehead for comfort if needed.
Fluid balance	• Insensible water loss increases during labor due to diaphoresis and the increase in rate and depth of respirations.	• Encourage women to sip fluid during labor the same as they would if they were exercising to keep hydrated. • If a woman is nauseated by labor, encourage sips of fluid, ice chips, or hard candy to supply some extra fluid.
Urinary system	• Pressure of the fetal head as it descends in the birth canal against the anterior bladder reduces bladder tone or the ability of the bladder to sense filling.	• Ask the birthing parent to void approximately every 2 hours during labor to avoid overfilling because overfilling can decrease postpartal bladder tone.
Musculoskeletal system	• During pregnancy, *relaxin* is secreted from the ovaries causing the cartilage between joints to be more flexible. This allows the joints of the pelvis to be able to open as much as 2 cm in labor to allow for fetal passage.	• Monitor for appropriate mobility and be mindful of fall risks.
Gastrointestinal (GI) system	• Blood shunts to life-sustaining organs causing the GI system to become fairly inactive during labor. • Digestive and emptying time of the stomach becomes lengthened. • Some women experience a loose bowel movement as contractions grow strong.	• Although many hospital protocols dictate that women who present in labor should not partake of oral nutrition, there is little evidence to support this restrictive practice.
Neurologic and sensory response	• Increased pain • Increased respiratory rate	• Where pain registers is important in appreciating why epidural anesthesia is effective. For early labor, the anesthetic block needs to suppress the lower thoracic synapses; for birth, it needs to block sacral nerves. • Discuss nonpharmacologic pain techniques if the patient does not desire medication.
Psychological responses	• Labor can lead to emotional distress because it is not only painful and fatiguing but it also represents the beginning of a major life change for a woman and her partner.	• Offer expeditious care to the patient. • Continue to encourage her process of labor. • Prior to birth, a woman can investigate the services of a doula. • A **doula** is an individual with specialized training who provides physical, emotional, and psychological support to laboring parents. A doula does not perform clinical tasks. However, the simple gift of presence has been shown to reduce the need for analgesia and anesthesia requests, shorten labor times, and increase satisfaction with the birth experience.

worry for her infant and may make her afraid she will not meet her own behavioral expectations. Explain and repeat as necessary that labor is predictable but also variable. Contractions last a certain length and reach a certain intensity but always have a rest period in between so she can have a break from pain. Fear of labor this way releases adrenaline, and adrenaline interferes with oxytocin release and so can limit the effectiveness of uterine contractions (Rouhe, Samelo-Aro, & Toivanen, 2015).

FETAL RESPONSES TO LABOR

The pressure and circulatory changes that occur with contractions not only affect the mother but also can cause detectable physiologic changes in the fetus as well.

The Neurologic System

Uterine contractions exert pressure on the fetal head, so the same response that is involved with any instance of increased intracranial pressure occurs. The fetal heart rate (FHR) decreases by as much as 5 beats/min during a contraction, as soon as contraction strength reaches 40 mmHg; although not measurable, fetal blood pressure also rises. The decrease in FHR appears on a fetal heart monitor as a normal or early deceleration pattern.

The Cardiovascular System

A sufficiently mature fetus is unaffected by the continual variations of heart rate that occur with labor contractions. During a contraction, as the arteries of the uterus become sharply constricted, and the filling of cotyledons almost completely halts, the amount of nutrients, including oxygen, exchanged during this time is greatly reduced, causing a slight but inconsequential fetal hypoxia. The increase in blood pressure caused by increased intracranial pressure raises blood pressure and keeps circulation from falling below normal for the duration of a contraction.

The Integumentary System

The pressure involved in the birth process is often reflected in minimal petechiae or ecchymotic areas on a fetus (particularly the presenting part). There may also be edema of the presenting part (caput succedaneum) from this pressure.

The Musculoskeletal System

The force of uterine contractions tends to push a fetus into a position of full flexion or with the head bent forward, which is the most advantageous position for birth.

The Respiratory System

The process of labor appears to aid in the maturation of surfactant production by alveoli in the fetal lung. Both the pressure applied to the chest from contractions and passage through the birth canal help to clear the respiratory tract of lung fluid. For this reason, an infant born vaginally is usually able to establish respirations more easily than a fetus born by cesarean birth.

Measuring Progress in Labor

A woman's progress in labor is recorded on a labor record (a Partogram) devised by the World Health Organization, or a like form on which vital signs, FHR, cervical dilation, descent of the fetal head, urine tests, and any drugs administered can be recorded.

Remember, when using such forms, how much and what type of analgesia a woman receives in labor can influence the length of labor. Because "norms" on such a record refer to averages, an individual woman's labor can vary greatly from the ideal projected course of labor and still be normal for that woman.

After each cervical examination, cervical dilatation and **fetal descent** (which may be referred to as "moulding") are plotted on the graph. The pattern of cervical dilatation usually plots as a rising S-shaped curve. You may need to remind women that assessments of cervical dilation are subjective, so one examiner may report a different finding from another (Archie & Roman, 2013). At the end of the latent phase of the first stage of labor, cervical dilatation is 3 to 4 cm. As a woman enters the active phase of the first stage, cervical dilation proceeds at a minimum of 1 cm/hr, or about 7 additional hours to reach full dilation (10 cm). The form shows an "alert" line, which marks when 4 hours has passed. Four hours beyond that, an "action" line advises a primary care provider that cervical dilation is taking longer than usual and that an intervention may be necessary to make the labor safe and effective. Maintaining an ongoing record and alerting the care provider that the alert line or action line is approaching are important nursing responsibilities.

MATERNAL DANGER SIGNS OF LABOR

Wide variation exists among individuals in their response to labor and their pattern of labor contractions. Certain signs, however, indicate that the course of events is deviating from usual. These signs, both fetal and maternal, are described in Box 15.4. Nursing care of a woman who is experiencing these signs and so may be developing a complication during labor or birth is addressed in Chapter 23. In addition to problems of cervical dilation or contractions, other symptoms suggest augmentation or intervention of labor are necessary.

High or Low Blood Pressure

Normally, a woman's blood pressure rises slightly in the second (pelvic) stage of labor because of her pushing effort. A systolic pressure greater than 140 mmHg and a diastolic pressure greater than 90 mmHg, or an increase in the systolic pressure of more than 30 mmHg or in the diastolic pressure of more than 15 mmHg (the basic criteria for gestational hypertension), should be reported. Just as important to report is a falling blood pressure because it may be the first sign of intrauterine hemorrhage, although a falling blood pressure from hemorrhage is often associated with other clinical signs of hypovolemic shock, such as apprehension, increased pulse rate, and pallor.

Abnormal Pulse

Most women during pregnancy have a pulse rate of 70 to 80 beats/min. This rate normally increases slightly during the second stage of labor because of the exertion involved. A maternal pulse rate greater than 100 beats/min during labor is unusual and should be reported because it may be another indication of hemorrhage.

BOX 15.4

Nursing Care Planning Using Assessment

ASSESSING FOR DANGER SIGNS OF LABOR

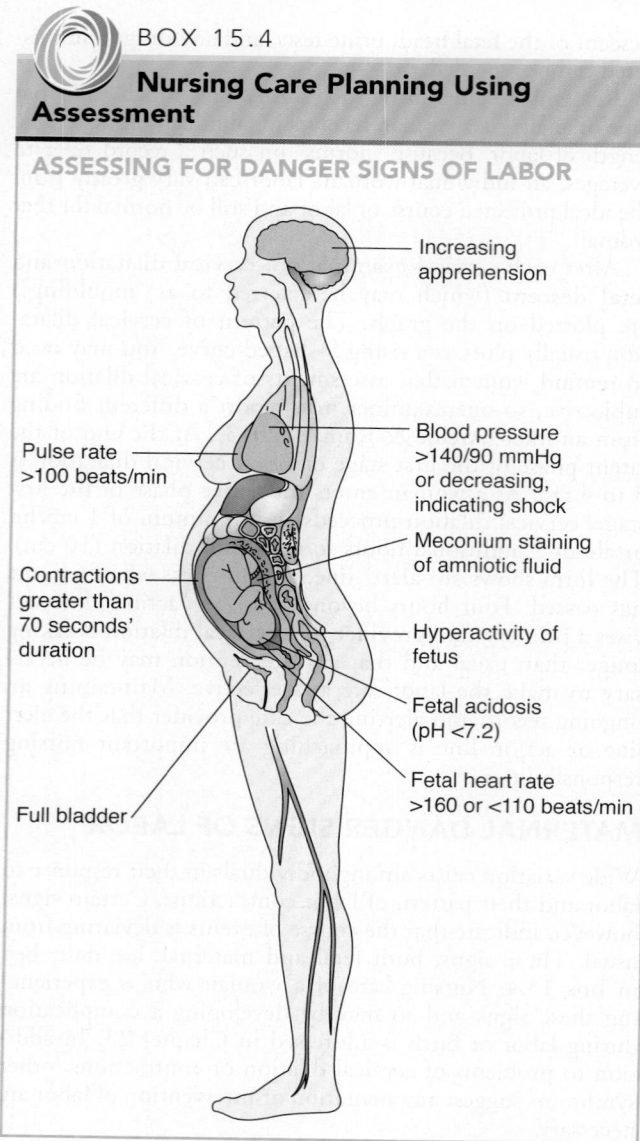

Increasing apprehension

Pulse rate >100 beats/min

Blood pressure >140/90 mmHg or decreasing, indicating shock

Meconium staining of amniotic fluid

Contractions greater than 70 seconds' duration

Hyperactivity of fetus

Fetal acidosis (pH <7.2)

Fetal heart rate >160 or <110 beats/min

Full bladder

Inadequate or Prolonged Contractions

Uterine contractions normally become more frequent, intense, and longer as labor progresses. If they become less frequent, less intense, or shorter in duration, this may indicate uterine exhaustion (inertia). This problem may be correctable but needs augmentation or other interventions to accomplish this.

Observe also if there is a period of relaxation between contractions so the intervillous spaces of the uterus can fill and maintain an adequate supply of oxygen and nutrients for the fetus. As a rule, uterine contractions lasting longer than 70 seconds are becoming long enough to compromise fetal well-being because this interferes with adequate uterine artery filling.

Abnormal Lower Abdominal Contour

If a woman has a full bladder during labor, a round bulge appears on her lower anterior abdomen. This is a danger signal for two reasons: First, the bladder may be injured by the

pressure of the fetal head pressing against it; and second, the pressure of the full bladder may not allow the fetal head to descend. To avoid a full bladder, ask women to try to void about every 2 hours during labor.

Increasing Apprehension

Warnings of psychological danger during labor are as important to consider in assessing maternal well-being as are physical signs. As she approaches the second stage of labor, a woman who is becoming increasingly apprehensive despite clear explanations of unfolding events may not be "hearing" because she has a concern that has not been met. Using an approach such as "You seem more and more concerned. Could you tell me what is worrying you?" may be helpful. Increasing apprehension also needs to be investigated for physical reasons because it can be a sign of oxygen deprivation or internal hemorrhage.

FETAL DANGER SIGNS OF LABOR

As well as observing for a woman's danger signs of pregnancy, observing fetal danger signs is equally important. These fetal danger signs include the following.

High or Low Fetal Heart Rate

As a rule, an FHR of more than 160 beats/min (fetal tachycardia) or less than 110 beats/min (fetal bradycardia) is a sign of possible fetal distress. An equally important sign is a late or variable deceleration pattern revealed on a fetal monitor (described later in this chapter). Frequent monitoring by a fetoscope, Doppler, or a monitor is necessary to detect these changes as they first occur.

Meconium Staining

This is not always a sign of fetal distress but is highly correlated with its occurrence. Meconium staining, a green color in the amniotic fluid, reveals the fetus has had a loss of rectal sphincter control, allowing meconium to pass into the amniotic fluid. It may indicate a fetus has or is experiencing hypoxia, which stimulates the vagal reflex and leads to increased bowel motility. Although meconium staining may be usual in a breech presentation because pressure on the buttocks causes meconium loss, it should always be reported immediately even with breech presentations so its cause can be investigated.

Hyperactivity

Ordinarily, a fetus remains quiet and barely moves during labor. Fetal hyperactivity may be a subtle sign that hypoxia is occurring because frantic motion is a common reaction to the need for oxygen.

Low Oxygen Saturation

Oxygen saturation in a fetus is normally 40% to 70%. A fetus can be assessed for this by a catheter inserted next to the cheek (under 40% oxygenation needs further assessment). If fetal blood is obtained by scalp puncture, the finding of acidosis (blood pH lower than 7.2) suggests fetal well-being is becoming compromised and that further investigation is also necessary.

Maternal and Fetal Assessments During Labor

Women are invariably nervous when they arrive at a hospital or birth center. Nursing assessment is important to detect how they are managing physically and emotionally to this intense event in their life.

THE IMMEDIATE ASSESSMENT OF A WOMAN IN FIRST STAGE OF LABOR

A number of immediate assessment measures are necessary to safeguard maternal and fetal health when a woman first arrives at a birthing facility. After she and her support person are oriented to the area, focus on obtaining this vital assessment data.

The Initial Interview and Physical Examination

Information about the woman's pregnancy can be gained from her prenatal record electronically on admission or if a paper copy has been forwarded to the birth setting beforehand. Additional important data that needs to be obtained includes a description of her labor thus far, her general physical condition, and her preparedness and plans for labor and birth. This amount of information is scant but helps to establish whether the woman is in active labor and needs immediate preparation for birth or whether she has arrived at the birthing setting at an early stage of labor and therefore will benefit most from paced interventions.

Ask about the following:
- Her baby's expected date of birth (EDB)
- When her contractions began
- Amount and character of any show
- Whether rupture of membranes has occurred
- Any known drug allergies
- If she uses any recreational or prescription drugs (women addicted to opioids need special precautions before analgesia is administered for pain management; their newborn may need special care to prevent neonatal abstinence syndrome from opioid withdrawal)
- Past pregnancy and present pregnancy history if her prenatal record is not available. It is important to note the route of delivery with any prior births as well as any complications which may have occurred.
- Her birth plan or what individualized measures she thinks will create a memorable experience for her such as whether she wants analgesia or who she would like to cut the umbilical cord

Assess the following:
- Vital signs: temperature, pulse, respirations, and blood pressure (assess between contractions for comfort and accuracy)
- Nature of her contractions (frequency, duration, and intensity)
- Her rating of pain on a 10-point scale
- What she has done to be prepared for labor such as learning breathing exercises
- Urine specimen for protein and glucose
- Position and presentation of her fetus

It is important to document fetal presentation and position at the beginning of labor because these help predict if the presentation of a body part other than the vertex could be putting a fetus at risk or leading to the possibility labor will be longer than usual because fetal descent will be less effective, causing ineffective dilatation of the cervix. A different presentation could also lead to early rupture of membranes, increasing the possibility of infection, fetal anoxia from cord prolapse, and meconium staining, all of which can lead to cesarean birth or respiratory distress at birth (Barber, Lundsberg, Belanger, et al., 2011).

THE DETAILED ASSESSMENT DURING THE FIRST STAGE OF LABOR

If the woman is in active labor, the history taken on arrival may be the only history obtained until after her baby is born. If birth is not imminent, both a more extensive history and a physical examination can be obtained.

The History

Performing a detailed interview of a woman in labor can be difficult because of the constant interruptions labor contractions cause. Be patient until a contraction ends so you don't interrupt any form of controlled breathing a woman is using. Remember, the longest contraction is rarely more than 60 seconds. If a woman concentrates so intently on a breathing exercise, she completely forgets a question asked just before a contraction, repeat the question as the contraction subsides, as if it had not been asked before, or as if it is no trouble to ask it again.

Current Pregnancy History

Important information needed for a complete history includes documentation of gravida and parity status, a description of this pregnancy (e.g., intended or not, place and pattern of prenatal care, adequacy of nutrition, whether any complications such as spotting, falls, hypertension of pregnancy, infection, alcohol or drug ingestion occurred during pregnancy), plans for labor (e.g., Does she want to have the baby naturally? Will she use breathing exercises? Will her support person be able to remain with her continuously?), and plans for child care (e.g., Will she breastfeed? Has she chosen a primary healthcare provider for the baby? If she's having a boy, does she want him circumcised?).

Past Pregnancy History

Document prior pregnancies, abortions, or miscarriages, including number, dates, types of birth, any complications, and outcomes, including health, sex, and birth weights of previous children.

Past Health History

Document any previous surgeries (abdominal surgical adhesions might interfere with fetal passage), heart disease or diabetes (special precautions will be required during labor and birth), anemia (blood loss at birth may be more important than usual), tuberculosis (she'll need testing after birth to be certain healed lung lesions weren't reactivated by birth), kidney disease or hypertension (blood pressure must be monitored even more carefully than usual), or if she has ever had a sexually transmitted infection such as herpes (the infant may be exposed to the disease by vaginal contact if the disease is active). Determine also whether a woman's lifestyle places her at high risk for prescription or nonprescription drug abuse or HIV exposure.

Family Medical History

Ask if any family member has a condition that could be inherited such as a cognitive challenge, heart disease, blood dyscrasia, diabetes, kidney disease, allergies, seizures, hearing loss, or malignant hyperthermia (a dominantly inherited disorder that causes a dangerous increase in temperature in response to certain anesthetics). If any of these are present, adequate preparation can then be made for a child who might have special needs at birth.

The Physical Examination

After history taking, a woman needs a physical examination, including a pelvic examination, to confirm her general health, the presentation and position of the fetus, and the stage of cervical dilatation. In order to have an HIV test, a woman must sign additional informed consent over and above her usual health facility consent.

The physical assessment during labor begins, as does all physical assessments, with the woman's overall appearance: Does she appear tired? Pale? Ill? Frightened? Are there signs of edema or dehydration? Does she have open lesions anywhere? Be prepared to adapt further examination techniques with regard to a woman's stage of labor, frequency of contractions, and labor progression.

Be certain to palpate for enlargement of neck lymph nodes to detect the possibility of a respiratory infection. Inspect the mucous membrane of her mouth and the conjunctiva of her eyes for color to see if paleness suggests anemia. Examine her teeth for caries or abscesses because an oral infection might account for a postpartal fever. Examine the outer and inner surfaces of her lips carefully to detect herpes lesions (pinpoint vesicles on an erythematous base). Report to her primary care provider if herpetic lesions are present anywhere because, although oral lesions are invariably a type 1 herpes virus (common cold sores), type 2 (genital) herpes virus needs to be identified because this can be lethal to newborns; a woman's obstetric healthcare provider may suggest that the woman with oral herpes lesions take isolation precautions such as not kissing her newborn until the lesions crust.

Auscultate the woman's lungs to be certain they are clear of rales. Listen for normal heart sounds and rhythms as well. Many pregnant women at term have a grade 2 to 3 systolic ejection murmur because of the extra volume of blood that must cross their heart valves. Document if this is noticeable. Next, inspect and palpate her breasts. Are they free of cysts and lumps? Mark the chart of a woman who has a palpable mass in her breasts for reexamination after labor and birth. This is probably an enlarged milk gland but needs further evaluation to be certain it is not something more serious such as a breast malignancy.

Abdominal and Lower Leg Assessment

Assessing a woman's abdomen is important to estimate fetal size by fundal height (which should be at the level of the xiphoid process at term). Palpate and percuss the bladder area (over the symphysis pubis) to detect a full bladder. Assess for abdominal scars to reveal previous abdominal or pelvic surgery that could have left adhesions.

Finally, inspect lower extremities for skin turgor to assess hydration and also for edema and varicose veins. Women with large varicosities are more prone to thrombophlebitis after birth than other women. Severe edema suggests hypertension of pregnancy. A blood pressure 140/90 mmHg or higher can confirm this.

Determining Fetal Position, Presentation, and Lie

Four methods can be used to determine if the fetus is in an optimal position for birth:

- Determining the place on the woman's abdomen where fetal heart tones are heard strongest
- Abdominal inspection and palpation, called Leopold maneuvers
- Vaginal examination
- Sonography

Leopold Maneuvers

Leopold maneuvers are a systematic method of observation and palpation to determine fetal presentation and position and are done as part of a physical examination. Steps for this are described in Box 15.5.

The Vaginal Examination

A vaginal examination is necessary to determine the extent of cervical softening, effacement, and dilatation and to confirm the fetal presentation, position, and degree of descent. These are traditionally done by the primary care provider but, if not available, can be done by a nurse skilled in the technique. Responsibilities for helping with a vaginal examination during labor are shown in Box 15.6.

Vaginal examinations are best done between contractions. Although more of the fetal skull can be palpated during a contraction because the cervix retracts more at that time, an examination during a contraction is more uncomfortable and rarely is justified by the additional amount of information gained. A palpation of membranes during a contraction, when they are under pressure, also can cause them to rupture.

Women are anxious to have frequent reports during labor to reassure them that everything is progressing well, but vaginal exams should be kept to a minimum to prevent infection.

BOX 15.5

Nursing Care Planning Using Procedures

LEOPOLD MANEUVERS

Purpose: Systematically observe and palpate the abdomen to determine fetal presentation and position.

Procedure	Principle
1. Explain the procedure and instruct the woman to void to empty her bladder.	1. Explanation reduces anxiety and enhances cooperation. An empty bladder promotes comfort and allows for more productive palpation because fetal contour will not be obscured by a distended bladder.
2. Wash your hands using warm water. Provide privacy.	2. Hand washing prevents the spread of possible infection. Using warm water aids in patient comfort and prevents tightening of abdominal muscles during palpation.
3. Position the woman supine with knees slightly flexed. Place a small pillow or rolled towel under her left side.	3. Flexing the knees relaxes the abdominal muscles. Using a pillow or towel tilts the uterus off the vena cava, preventing supine hypotension syndrome.
4. Observe the woman's abdomen as to which is the longest diameter and where fetal movement is apparent.	4. The longest diameter (axis) is the length of the fetus. The location of activity most likely reflects the position of the feet.
5. First maneuver: Stand at the foot of the woman, facing her, and place both hands flat on her abdomen. Palpate the superior surface of the fundus. Determine consistency, shape, and mobility.	5. This maneuver determines whether the fetal head or breech is in the fundus. A head feels more firm than a breech, is round and hard, and moves independently of the body (the breech feels softer and moves only in conjunction with the body).

6. Second maneuver: Face the woman, hold the left hand stationary on the left side of the uterus while you palpate with the right hand on the opposite side of the uterus from top to bottom. Repeat palpation using the opposite side.	6. This maneuver locates the back of the fetus. The fetal back feels like a smooth, hard, and resistant surface; the knees and elbows of the fetus on the opposite side feel more like a number of angular bumps or nodules.

Continued on following page

BOX 15.5

Nursing Care Planning Using Procedures (continued)

Procedure	Principle
7. Third maneuver: Gently grasp the lower portion of the abdomen just above the symphysis pubis between the thumb and fingers and try to press the thumb and finger together. Determine any movement and whether the part feels firm or soft.	7. This maneuver determines which part of the fetus is at the inlet and its mobility. If the presenting part moves upward so your fingers and thumb can be pressed together, the presenting part is not engaged (not firmly settled into the pelvis). If the part is firm, it is the head; if soft, then it is the breech.

Procedure	Principle
8. Fourth maneuver: Place fingers on both sides of the uterus approximately 2 in. above the inguinal ligaments, pressing downward and inward in the direction of the birth canal. Allow fingers to be carried downward.	8. This maneuver is only done if the fetus is in a cephalic presentation because it determines fetal attitude and degree of fetal extension into the pelvis. The fingers of one hand will slide along the uterine contour and meet no obstruction, indicating the back of the fetal neck. The other hand will meet an obstruction an inch or so above the ligament—this is the fetal brow. The position of the fetal brow should correspond to the side of the uterus that contained the elbows and knees of the fetus. If the fetus is in a poor attitude, the examining fingers will meet an obstruction on the same side as the fetal back; that is, the fingers will touch the hyperextended head. If the brow is very easily palpated (as if it lies just under the skin), the fetus is probably in a posterior position (the occiput is pointing toward the woman's back).

The woman's primary care provider will tell a woman immediately after an examination about her progress. If giving a progress report, remember that most women are aware of the word dilatation but not effacement. Just saying, "No further dilatation," therefore, is a depressing report. "You're not dilated a lot more, but a lot of thinning is happening and that's just as important" is the same report given in a positive manner. After a vaginal examination, plot the new degree of dilatation and descent of the presenting part on a labor progress graph, as described earlier.

Vaginal examinations should not be done in the presence of fresh bleeding because fresh bleeding may indicate that a placenta previa (implantation of the placenta so low in the uterus that it is encroaching on the cervical os) is present. Performing a vaginal examination in this instance might tear the placenta and cause hemorrhage, resulting in danger to both the mother and fetus. Make certain a primary care provider knows about the fresh bleeding before attempting a vaginal examination.

Women from cultures where female circumcision is allowed may have tightened or obstructed vaginal openings from scarring, which can make a vaginal exam painful. Note this because it also indicates a woman may need a cesarean birth to prevent perineal tearing if her vagina cannot dilate adequately.

Sonography

Although not routine, sonography may be used to determine the diameters of the fetal skull and to determine presentation, position, flexion, and degree of descent of a fetus at the beginning of labor. This is usually done by a portable unit, but if it's necessary for a woman to be transported to another department to have this done, be certain someone accompanies her, so, if labor should become more active, she can be returned quickly to the labor or birth service for needed care.

Assessing Rupture of Membranes

One out of every four labors begins with spontaneous rupture of the fetal membranes. When this occurs, a woman feels a sudden gush or a slow trickle of amniotic fluid from her vagina. This is a startling sensation for most women because it feels as if she has lost bladder control. She may feel embarrassed before she realizes the warm fluid on her perineum and legs is not urine but an unexpected announcement that labor is beginning. If the fluid expelled was only a small amount, there may be a question as to whether the membranes have ruptured.

A sterile vaginal examination using a sterile speculum usually reveals whether amniotic fluid is present in the vagina. After vaginal secretions are obtained with a sterile,

BOX 15.6

Nursing Care Planning Using Procedures

ASSISTING WITH A VAGINAL EXAMINATION

Purpose: Determine cervical readiness for labor and fetal position and presentation.

Procedure	Principle
1. Wash your hands and explain the procedure to the patient. Provide privacy.	1. Hand washing helps prevent the spread of microorganisms. Explanations ensure patient cooperation and compliance. Privacy enhances self-esteem.
2. Assemble equipment, including sterile examining gloves, sterile lubricant, and gauze squares. Ask the woman to turn onto her back with knees flexed (a dorsal recumbent position).	2. Organization and planning improve efficiency. Positioning in this manner allows for good visualization of the perineum. Use of a sterile glove prevents contamination of the birth canal.
3. Discard one drop of clean lubricating solution and drop an ample supply on tips of gloved fingers of examiner.	3. Discarding the first drop of lubricant ensures quantity used will not be contaminated.
4. The examiner places a hand on the outer edges of the woman's vulva and spread her labia while inspecting for lesions. Help look for red, irritated mucous membranes; open, ulcerated sores; and clustered, pinpoint vesicles.	4. Presence of any lesions may indicate an infection and may possibly preclude vaginal birth.
5. Note any fluid escaping from the vagina that could be amniotic fluid, in addition to the presence of the umbilical cord or bleeding.	5. Amniotic fluid implies membranes have ruptured and the umbilical cord may have prolapsed. Bleeding may be a sign of placenta previa. *Vaginal examinations should not be continued if a possible placenta previa exists.*
6. If there is no bleeding or cord visible, the examiner stabilizes the uterus by placing a hand on the woman's abdomen and then introducing the index and middle fingers of the other hand into the vagina, directing them toward the posterior vaginal wall.	6. The posterior vaginal wall is less sensitive than the anterior wall.

7. The examiner touches the cervix with gloved fingers to assess:
  a. Cervical consistency, position, and rate if *firm* or *soft.*
  b. Extent of dilatation and whether an anterior rim or lip of cervix is present.
	7. a. The cervix feels like a circular rim of tissue around a center depression. If firm, it feels similar to the tip of a nose; if soft, it is as pliable as an earlobe.
	  b. An index finger averages about 1 cm; a middle finger about 1.5 cm. If they can both enter the cervix, the cervix is dilated 2.5–3 cm. If there would be room for double the width of two fingers, the dilatation is about 5–6 cm. When the space is four times the width of two fingertips, dilatation is complete at 10 cm.
	  c. Effacement is estimated in a percentage depending on thickness. A cervix before labor is 2–2.5 cm thick. If it is only 1 cm thick, it is 50% effaced. If it is tissue paper thin, it is 100% effaced. With a 100% effaced cervix, dilatation is difficult to feel because the edges of the cervix are so thin.
	  d. The membranes (with a slight amount of amniotic fluid in front of the presenting part) assume the shape of a watch crystal. With a contraction, they bulge forward, become prominent, and can be felt much more readily.

  c. Estimate the degree of effacement.
  d. Estimate whether membranes are intact.

Continued on following page

BOX 15.6

Nursing Care Planning Using Procedures (continued)

Procedure	Principle
8. Next, the examiner locates the ischial spines, identifies the presenting part, and rates the station of the fetus.	8. Ischial spines are palpated as notches at the 4 and 8 o'clock positions of the pelvic outlet. Station is the number of centimeters above or below the spines the presenting fetal part has reached. Identifying the presenting part confirms findings obtained with Leopold maneuvers. The vertex has a hard, smooth feel. Fetal hair may be palpable but massed together and wet, and it may be difficult to appreciate through gloves. Palpating the two fontanelles, one diamond-shaped and one triangular, helps identification. Buttocks feel softer and give under fingertip pressure. Identifying the anus may be possible because the sphincter action will "trap" an examining finger.
9. Next is establishment of the fetal position.	9. The fontanelle palpated is invariably the posterior one because the fetus maintains a flexed position, presenting the posterior not the anterior fontanelle. If it points toward an anterior quadrant, the position is ROA or LOA. In a breech presentation, the anus can serve as a marker for position.
10. Upon withdrawal of the examining hand, help wipe the perineum front to back to remove secretions or examining lubricant. Help patient return to side or sit up.	10. Wiping front to back prevents moving rectal contamination forward to the vagina. Side lying or sitting helps prevent supine hypotension syndrome.
11. Document procedure, assessment findings, and how patient tolerated procedure.	11. Documentation provides a means for communication and evaluation of care and patient outcomes.

cotton-tipped applicator, test them with a strip of Nitrazine paper. Vaginal secretions are usually acid; amniotic fluid, in contrast, is alkaline. If amniotic fluid has passed through the vagina recently, the pH of the vaginal fluid will probably be alkaline (greater than 6.5) when tested by Nitrazine paper (appears blue-green or gray to deep blue). A false blue reading may occur in a woman with intact membranes who has a heavy, bloody show because blood is also alkaline. An additional test that can be done is a fern test (examination of vaginal secretions under a microscope). Because of its high estrogen content, amniotic fluid will show a fern pattern (see Chapter 5, Fig. 5.13A) when dried and examined in this way; urine will not.

If the woman's membranes ruptured at home, ask her to describe the color of the amniotic fluid, the amount, the odor, and the approximate time of rupture. Amniotic fluid should be clear as water. Yellow-stained fluid suggests a blood incompatibility between the mother and fetus (the amniotic fluid is bilirubin stained from the breakdown of red blood cells). Green fluid suggests meconium staining. Although meconium staining is normal in breech births because of compression of the buttocks, in a vertex presentation, it may indicate fetal anoxia. Either way, a fetus with meconium staining needs immediate assessment. After birth, the infant continues to need close assessment at birth to rule out possible meconium aspiration (Lee, Romero, Lee, et al., 2016). If the fluid is malodorous, there could be an infection. If membranes rupture during labor, assess FHR immediately to be certain the umbilical cord hasn't prolapsed and is now being compressed against the cervix by the fetal head. The time of

rupture is important because the potential time clock for an infection begins with ruptured membranes. It's preferable if the baby is born within 24 hours of rupture to reduce the risk of infection.

Assessment of Pelvic Adequacy

Evaluating pelvic adequacy using internal conjugate and ischial tuberosity diameters is generally done during pregnancy either manually or by sonogram, so, by weeks 32 to 36 of pregnancy, a primary care provider can be alerted that cephalopelvic disproportion could occur. Because the diameters obtained during pregnancy have not changed, they are not retaken if already obtained.

Vital Signs

Vital signs are taken at the beginning and then periodically during labor, as summarized in Table 15.5.

Temperature

Temperature is usually obtained every 4 hours during labor. Report a temperature greater than 99°F (37.2°C) because it may indicate the development of infection. Unless there are accompanying symptoms, however, temperature elevation in a woman who has taken little fluid by mouth usually reflects dehydration (urge her to drink at least sips of water to maintain hydration). After rupture of the membranes, temperature should be taken every 2 hours because the possibility for infection markedly increases after that time.

TABLE 15.5 TYPICAL TIME INTERVALS FOR NURSING INTERVENTIONS DURING THE FIRST STAGE OF LABOR

Intervention	Assessment on Admission	Latent Phase (0–3 cm)	Active Phase (4–7 cm)	Transition Phase (8–10 cm)
Assess and Record				
Temperature	X	q4h (unless membranes are ruptured, then q2h)	q4h (unless membranes are ruptured, then q2h)	q4h (unless membranes are ruptured, then q2h)
Pulse	X	q30–60 min	q30–60 min	q15–30 min
Respirations	X	q30–60 min	q30–60 min	q15–30 min
Blood pressure	X	q30–60 min	q30–60 min	q15–30 min
Voiding	X	q2h	q2h	q2h
Fetal heart rate	X	q30–60 min	q15–30 min	q15–30 min
Contractions	X	q30–60 min	q15–30 min	q10–15 min
Perineum	X	q30–60 min	q30 min	q15 min
Provide				
Ambulation and change of position	X	Continuously; question if membranes rupture	Continuously; question if membranes rupture	Continuously
Support	X	Continuously	Continuously	Continuously

Pulse and Respiration

The pulse and respiration rate should be measured and recorded at the same time intervals as temperature. A woman's pulse may be rapid on admission because she is nervous and anxious. After she has become better acquainted with her surroundings and has been assured everything is going well, her pulse usually falls in a range between 70 and 80 beats/min. A persistent pulse rate of more than 100 beats/min could be tachycardia from dehydration or hemorrhage and so needs investigation. Respiratory rate during labor is usually 18 to 20 breaths/min. Do not count respirations during contractions because women tend to breathe rapidly from pain. Conversely, if a woman is using controlled breathing to decrease pain in labor, her respiration rate during contractions can be abnormally slow.

Observe for hyperventilation (rapid, deep respirations) because prolonged hyperventilation can cause a "blowing off" of carbon dioxide and accompanying symptoms of dizziness and tingling of hands and feet. Rebreathing into a paper bag and reassurance the feeling is normal help to reverse this process.

Blood Pressure

Blood pressure is usually measured and recorded every 4 hours as well. As with pulse and respirations, measure blood pressure between contractions, both for a woman's comfort and for accuracy, because maternal blood pressure tends to rise 5 to 15 mmHg during a contraction. An increase in blood pressure at other times is potentially dangerous because it may indicate the development of hypertension of pregnancy. A decrease in blood pressure or a decrease in the pulse pressure (the difference between the systolic and diastolic pressures) may indicate hemorrhage. If a woman received an analgesic agent (such as meperidine), which tends to cause hypotension, check her blood pressure approximately 15 minutes after administration to be certain extreme hypotension did not occur.

Laboratory Analysis

Most women have some preliminary laboratory studies done in early labor.

Blood

Blood is drawn for hemoglobin and hematocrit, a serologic test for syphilis (Venereal Disease Research Laboratory [VDRL] test), hepatitis B antibodies, and blood typing to determine whether a blood incompatibility is likely to exist in the newborn and what type of blood will need to be supplied if the woman should have an acute blood loss. If a woman gives permission for HIV testing, blood for this will be drawn as well.

Urine

Obtain a clean-catch urine specimen and test it at the point of care for protein and glucose, then send it to the laboratory for a complete urinalysis. If a woman reports any symptoms that suggest a urinary tract infection such as burning on urination, blood in urine, extreme frequency, or flank pain, obtain a clean-catch specimen for culture. A woman in labor is able to void most easily if she is allowed to use a bathroom. However, if a woman has ruptured membranes, check whether she should ambulate to a bathroom until it is confirmed the fetal head is well engaged so gravity does not cause a prolapsed cord. Use a bedpan or receptacle placed on a commode to collect any material passed from the vagina so this can be assessed as well.

The Assessment of Uterine Contractions

Depending on the hospital or birthing center policy, most women are monitored by an external contraction monitor for about 20 minutes in early labor. The monitor is then removed, and contractions are assessed intermittently by Doppler because extensive electronic monitoring has not shown to lower fetal mortality with low-risk women, can limit mobility, and can lead to an increase in cesarean birth (Cox & King, 2015). The use of internal fetal monitoring is reserved for high-risk pregnancies and is described in Chapter 24.

Length of Contractions

To determine the length of a contraction with a monitor in place, simply observe the rhythm strip and, using the time line, count the number of seconds the contraction lasted. To determine the beginning of a contraction without a moni-

Figure 15.13 Contractions can be assessed by very gently placing a hand over the fundus of the uterus.

tor, rest a hand on a woman's abdomen at the fundus of the uterus very gently until you sense the gradual tensing and upward rising of the fundus that accompanies a contraction (Fig. 15.13). Time the duration of the contraction from the moment the uterus first tenses until it has relaxed again. It is possible to palpate this tensing approximately 5 seconds before the woman is able to feel the contraction because contractions become palpable when the intrauterine pressure reaches approximately 20 mmHg. However, the pain of a contraction is not usually felt until pressure reaches approximately 25 mmHg.

Intensity of Contractions

The intensity of a contraction refers to its strength. On a monitor, this is the height of the waveform. If you are assessing manually, rate a contraction according to:

- Mild, if the uterus does not feel more than minimally tense
- Moderate, if the uterus feels firm
- Strong, if the uterus feels as hard as a wooden board or you are unable to indent the uterus with your fingertips at the peak of the contraction

After estimating either the intensity or duration of a contraction, recheck the fundus at the conclusion of the contraction to be certain it does relax and becomes soft to the touch again. This demonstrates that the uterus is not in continuous contraction but is providing a relaxation time, during which placental blood vessels can fill to supply the fetus with adequate oxygen.

Frequency of Contractions

Lastly, time the frequency of contractions or how often they are occurring. Frequency is timed from the beginning of one contraction to the beginning of the next (see Fig. 15.10).

Use as light a touch as possible on a woman's abdomen while evaluating contractions or estimating their strength manually.

Otherwise, the uterine fundus can become tender if it has to push against the extra weight of a hand with each contraction, creating unnecessary discomfort for a woman in labor.

What If . . . 15.2

Celeste Bailey refuses to have any electronic fetal monitoring. Would this worry the nurse? Would the nurse try to convince her she needs this?

THE INITIAL FETAL ASSESSMENT

Although fairly passive in labor, a fetus is subjected to extreme pressure by uterine contractions and passage through the birth canal, so it is important to ascertain that the FHR remains within normal limits despite these pressures.

Auscultation of Fetal Heart Sounds

Fetal heart sounds are transmitted best through the convex portion of a fetus because that is the part that lies in closest contact with the uterine wall.

- In a vertex or breech presentation, fetal heart sounds are usually best heard through the fetal back.
- In a face presentation, the back becomes concave so the sounds are best heard through the more convex thorax.
- In breech presentations, fetal heart sounds are heard most clearly high in the uterus, at a woman's umbilicus or above.
- In cephalic presentations, they are heard loudest low in a woman's abdomen.
- In an ROA position, sounds are heard best in the right lower quadrant.
- In an LOA position, sounds are heard best in the left lower quadrant.
- In posterior positions (LOP or ROP), heart sounds may be loudest at a woman's side.

Figure 15.14 illustrates where fetal heart sounds radiate best from various fetal positions.

Hearing fetal heart sounds in these positions not only confirms that the fetus is responding well to labor but also provides confirmatory information about fetal position. Conversely, recognizing fetal position aids in locating fetal heart sounds.

As a rule, determine the FHR every 30 minutes during beginning latent labor, every 15 minutes during active first stage labor, and every 5 minutes during the second stage of labor. This can be done by inspecting an FHR monitoring strip or by periodic auscultation by a fetoscope (a modified stethoscope attached to a headpiece), a Pinard stethoscope (a hollow tube that directs sound into the ear), or a Doppler unit (which uses ultrasound waves that bounce off the fetal heart to produce echoes or clicking noises, which reflect the fetal heartbeat [Fig. 15.15]) as labor progresses.

ELECTRONIC MONITORING

The use of fetal monitors in labor has provoked one of the biggest controversies in modern obstetric health care as their use moved from routine use in the mid-1970s for all women in labor to today when they are used judiciously to prevent intrusion on the childbirth experience and to prevent needless discomfort and distraction to the mother. Monitors are set with automatic alarms that trigger if an

Figure 15.14 Locating fetal heart sounds by fetal position: **(A)** Left occipitoanterior (LOA), **(B)** right occipitoanterior (ROA), **(C)** left occipitoposterior (LOP), **(D)** right occipitoposterior, and **(E)** left sacroanterior (LSaA).

FHR goes below 110 beats/min or above about 170 beats/min and so may ring many times if a woman is active in labor. This causes their use to result in unnecessary cesarean births as well as frightened parents (which could adversely affect early parent–infant bonding).

Monitoring does offer advantages from a healthcare provider's standpoint because observing the FHR on a monitor is quicker than listening with a Doppler and yields information on not only the rate but also on how the FHR responds to a forceful contraction. Use of monitors for a short-term initial assessment followed by intermittent manual monitoring is a compromise solution.

Be certain to inform parents that the FHR can vary greatly during labor so they're not surprised when they see this and also that a monitor is only an aid and should not be the focus of their attention. Otherwise, a couple can become so focused on a monitor screen or paper strip that they lose the ability to concentrate on previously learned relaxation and breathing techniques. When giving care, be sure not to focus solely on the equipment, continue to communicate to the couple, not the machine, and offer support to the woman and her partner as needed.

Initial Electronic Monitoring

Electronic monitoring is noninvasive, easily applied, and does not require cervical dilatation or fetal descent before it can be used, so it can be introduced at any time during labor. The presence and duration of uterine contractions is gained by means of a pressure transducer or tocodynamometer (*toko* is Greek for "contraction") strapped to the woman's abdomen or held in place by stockinette (Fig. 15.16).

Figure 15.15 **(A)** Auscultation of the fetal heartbeat using a fetoscope. (Beth Van Trees/Shutterstock.com) **(B)** A Doppler ultrasound device can be used to monitor fetal heart rate intermittently in low-risk labor. (COLLATERAL/Shutterstock.com) **(C)** A nurse-midwife using a Pinard stethoscope. (Capifrutta/Shutterstock.com)

Place the transducer snugly over the uterine fundus or the area where contractions are most easily felt. The transducer works to convert the pressure originated by the contraction into an electronic signal that is then recorded on graph paper.

The FHR is monitored with the use of an ultrasonic sensor or monitor (see Fig. 15.16) also strapped against a woman's abdomen at the level of the fetal chest. The small Doppler unit converts fetal heart movements into audible beeping sounds and also records them on graph paper.

Figure 15.16 External electronic monitoring in place. Two devices (a transducer for the uterus and an ultrasound sensor for the fetus) are strapped to the woman's abdomen. (busayamol/Shutterstock.com)

A woman who is worried something will happen to her child during labor can find it reassuring to listen to the regular beeping sound of an undistressed fetal heartbeat from a fetal heart transducer. Many women ask for and can have a short graph tracing to save for their baby book.

A disadvantage is the woman may feel discomfort from the straps holding the monitors in place, and the snugness of the sensor head may limit her ability to breathe deeply. If a woman changes her position (and she should change position often during labor), the sensor often needs to be repositioned. Remind a woman that the fetal heart signal may stop when she changes position so she does not think by the silence that her baby's heart has stopped beating.

Urge women not to lie on their backs for monitoring but to rest on their side, sit in a chair, or bend forward over the foot of the bed or a birthing ball or rail so the likelihood of supine hypotension syndrome is not increased.

FETAL HEART RATE AND UTERINE CONTRACTION RECORDS

Labor monitors trace both the FHR and the duration and interval of uterine contractions onto an oscilloscope screen and produce a permanent record on paper rolls (Fig. 15.17). Uterine contraction information is recorded on the bottom half of the paper, whereas FHR is recorded on the top half. Time can be calculated by counting the number of bold vertical lines on the paper (the space between two bold lines represents 60 seconds).

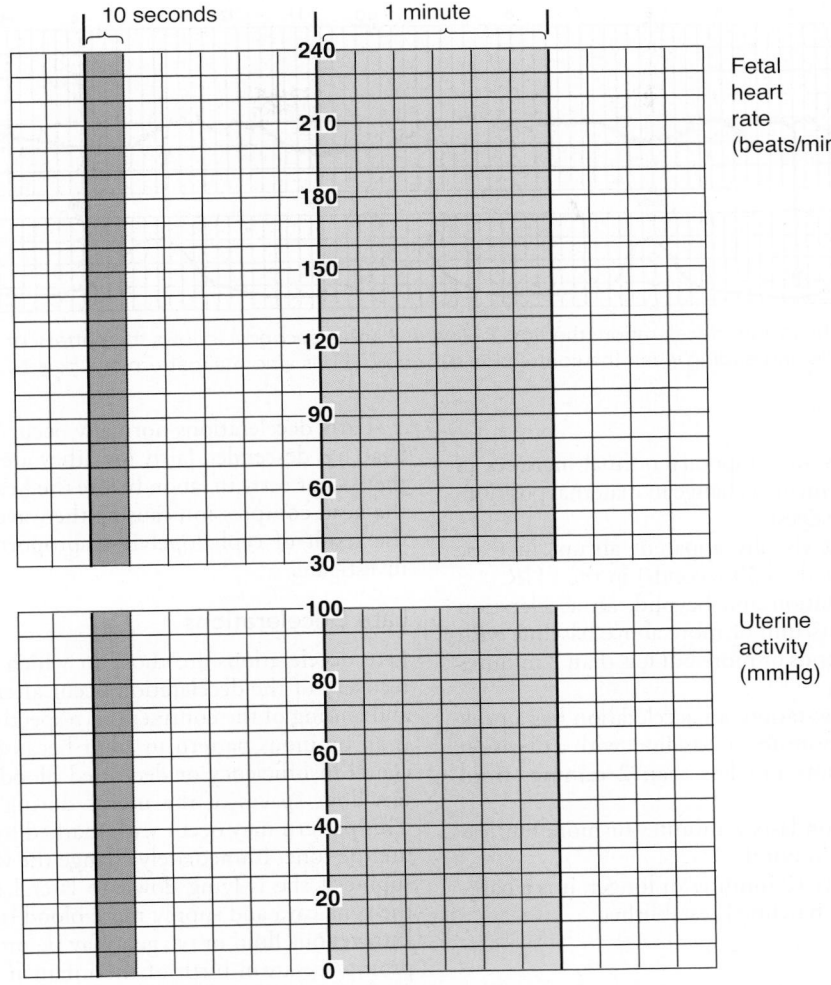

Figure 15.17   A paper strip for recording electronic fetal monitoring data.

FETAL HEART RATE PARAMETERS

Assessing and interpreting FHR patterns involves evaluating three parameters: the baseline rate, variabilities in the baseline rate, and periodic changes in the rate (acceleration and deceleration) (American Congress of Obstetricians and Gynecologists [ACOG], 2009).

The Baseline Fetal Heart Rate

A baseline FHR is determined by analyzing the pace of fetal heartbeats recorded in a minimum of 2 minutes obtained between contractions. A normal rate is 110 to 160 beats/min.

Variability

FHR variability or the difference between the highest and lowest heart rates shown on a strip is one of the most reliable indicators of fetal well-being. Variability is reflected on an FHR tracing as a slight irregularity or "jitter" to the wave. The degree of baseline variability increases (5 to 15 beats/min) when a fetus moves; it slows if a fetus sleeps. If no variability is present, it indicates the natural pacemaker activity of the fetal heart (effects of the sympathetic and parasympathetic nervous systems) may be affected. This may occur

as a response to narcotics or barbiturates administered to a woman in labor, but the possibility of fetal hypoxia and acidosis must also be considered and investigated. Very immature fetuses show diminished baseline variability because of a reduced nervous system response to stimulation and immature cardiac node function.

Variability should be recorded as:
- Absent: No amplitude range is detectable.
- Minimal: Amplitude range is detectable but is 5 beats/min or fewer.
- Moderate (normal): Amplitude range is 6 to 25 beats/min.
- Marked: Amplitude range is greater than 25 beats/min.

Other patterns in the baseline rate that can be detected include fetal bradycardia (FHR is lower than 110 beats/min for 10 minutes) and fetal tachycardia (FHR is faster than 160 beats/min for a 10-minute period).

Periodic Changes

Periodic changes or fluctuations in FHR occur in response to contractions and fetal movement and are described in terms of *accelerations* or *decelerations*. Periodic changes are short-term changes in rate other than baseline; they last from a few seconds to 1 or 2 minutes.

Figure 15.18 Early fetal heart rate deceleration (the time between 2 and 4 seconds) follows the pattern of the contraction starting when the contraction begins and ending when the contraction subsides. This is a normal pattern of a healthy fetus.

Accelerations

Nonperiodic accelerations are temporary normal increases in FHR caused by fetal movement, a change in maternal position, or administration of an analgesic.

- An acceleration is a visually apparent abrupt increase (onset to peak in less than 30 seconds) in the FHR.
- At 32 weeks of gestation and beyond, an acceleration has a peak of 15 beats/min or more above baseline with a duration of 15 seconds or more but less than 2 minutes from onset to return.
- Before 32 weeks of gestation, an acceleration has a peak of 10 beats/min or more above baseline, with a duration of 10 seconds or more but less than 2 minutes from onset to return.
- Prolonged acceleration lasts 2 minutes or more but less than 10 minutes in duration.
- If an acceleration lasts 10 minutes or longer, it is a baseline change or a new baseline is established.

Decelerations

Decelerations are visually apparent, usually symmetrical, periodic decreases in FHR resulting from pressure on the fetal head during contractions as parasympathetic stimulation in response to vagal nerve compression brings about a slowing of FHR. Early deceleration follows the pattern of the contraction, beginning when the contraction begins and ending when the contraction ends. However, the waveform of the FHR change is the inverse of the contraction waveform, or the lowest point of the deceleration occurs with the peak of the contraction (a mirror image of the contraction). The rate rarely falls below 100 beats/min, and it returns quickly to between 110 and 160 beats/min at the end of the contraction (Fig. 15.18).

Early decelerations normally occur late in labor, when the head has descended fairly low; they are viewed as innocent. If they occur early in labor, before the head has fully descended, the head compression causing the waveform change could be the result of cephalopelvic disproportion and is a cause to investigate.

Late Decelerations

Late decelerations are those in which the onset, nadir, and recovery of the deceleration occur after the beginning, peak, and ending of the contraction, respectively (Fig. 15.19). This is an ominous pattern in labor because it suggests uteroplacental insufficiency or decreased blood flow through the intervillous spaces of the uterus during uterine contractions. This pattern may occur with marked hypertonia or increased uterine tone. Immediately change the woman's position from supine if she is lying down to lateral to relieve pressure on the vena cava and supply more blood to the uterus and fetus. Intravenous fluid or oxygen may be prescribed. Prepare for a prompt cesarean birth of the infant if the late decelerations persist or if FHR variability becomes abnormal (absent or decreased).

Prolonged Decelerations

Prolonged decelerations are decelerations that are a decrease from the FHR baseline of 15 beats/min or more and last longer than 2 to 3 minutes but less than 10 minutes. They generally reflect an isolated occurrence, but they may signify a significant event, such as cord compression or maternal hypotension. For this reason, they must be reported and documented. If a deceleration lasts longer than 10 minutes, it is considered a baseline change.

Figure 15.19 Late deceleration (the time between 20 and 22 seconds) occurs after the peak of a contraction and continues beyond the end of the contraction. This is an ominous pattern in labor because it suggests the fetus is growing short of oxygen. The prolonged deceleration (between 26 and 31 seconds) is also ominous.

Figure 15.20 A fetal heart rate (FHR) showing variable and prolonged decelerations. Note the abrupt drop in FHR in both types of decelerations. The variable decelerations return to baseline more quickly than the prolonged deceleration at 26 to 31 minutes, however.

Variable Decelerations

The pattern of variable decelerations refers to decelerations that occur at unpredictable times in relation to contractions. They may indicate compression of the cord, which can be an ominous development in terms of fetal well-being (Fig. 15.20). Cord compression may be occurring because of a prolapsed cord, but it most often occurs because the fetus is simply lying on the cord. It tends to occur more frequently after rupture of the membranes than when membranes are intact, or with oligohydramnios (the presence of less than a normal amount of amniotic fluid), such as occurs in postterm pregnancy or with intrauterine growth restriction. As a first step, change the woman's position from supine to lateral if she is not already lying on her side. If a prolapsed cord is diagnosed as the cause of the variable decelerations, oxygen will be prescribed as well as changing her position to a knee-to-chest one to help relieve pressure on the cord. Because a prolapsed cord is a potential serious complication of labor, nursing care and outcomes are further discussed in Chapter 23.

The Sinusoidal Pattern

In a fetus who is severely anemic or hypoxic, central nervous system control of heart pacing may be so impaired that the FHR pattern resembles a smooth, frequently undulating wave with a cycle frequency of 3 to 5 per minute and persisting 20 minutes or more. Although the cause of this pattern is poorly understood, it is recognized to be as ominous as a late deceleration or variable deceleration pattern and so needs to be reported. For unknown reasons, on occasion,

especially after administration of a narcotic to the mother, a *pseudo*sinusoidal or false sinusoidal pattern may appear. These are usually transient, resolve spontaneously without intervention, and are associated with a good fetal outcome. The pattern may show some variability and perhaps an FHR acceleration. Identifying these is equally important so they can be differentiated from a true sinusoidal pattern.

FHR baseline, variability, and patterns are categorized from 1 to 3 to help establish if a deviation is serious. Knowing these helps you to understand why interventions are initiated at certain points (Table 15.6).

QSEN Checkpoint Question 15.6

INFORMATICS

The nurse assesses Celeste Bailey's uterine contractions and the FHR. Which of the following would the nurse document as a late deceleration?
  a. The FHR began increasing 45 seconds after the contraction was over.
  b. The FHR decreased in rate 30 seconds after the start of a contraction.
  c. The FHR decreased in strength after the 10th consecutive contraction.
  d. A decrease in FHR occurs but is totally unrelated to timing of contractions.

Look in Appendix A for the best answer and rationale.

TABLE 15.6 THE AMERICAN CONGRESS OF OBSTETRICIANS AND GYNECOLOGISTS CATEGORIES OF FETAL HEART RATE MONITORING

Category	Importance	Recommended Action
Category I	FHR factors (baseline and variability) are normal.	Continue routine monitoring; no specific action needed.
Category II	FHR factors are indeterminate.	Continue surveillance and reevaluation.
Category III	FHR tracings are abnormal.	Prompt evaluation is required. Expedite action to determine the cause and resolve the situation is required. This may include but is not limited to provision of maternal oxygen, change in maternal position, discontinuation of labor stimulation, treatment of maternal hypotension, and treatment of tachysystole with FHR changes. If category III tracing does not resolve with these measures, birth should be undertaken.

FHR, fetal heart rate.
From American Congress of Obstetricians and Gynecologists. (2009). ACOG Practice Bulletin No. 106: Intrapartum fetal heart rate monitoring: Nomenclature, interpretation, and general management principle. *Obstetrics & Gynecology, 114*(1), 193–200.

The Care of a Woman During the First Stage of Labor

Labor and birth are natural processes, so the average woman should be able to complete labor and birth without assistance from medical interventions. Nurses can be instrumental in keeping labor as free of unnecessary interventions as possible so it remains not only safe but also a joyful and memorable experience (Association of Women's Health, Obstetric and Neonatal Nurses [AWHONN], 2011). Six major concepts that make labor and birth as natural as possible include the following:

- Labor should begin on its own, not be artificially induced.
- Women should be able to move about freely throughout labor, not be confined to bed.
- Women should receive continuous support from a caring support person during labor.
- No interventions such as intravenous fluid should be used routinely.
- Women should be allowed to assume a nonsupine position such as upright and side lying for birth.
- Mother and baby should be housed together after the birth, with unlimited opportunity for breastfeeding

Because the first stage of labor begins with the start of uterine contractions and takes hours to complete, most women have been having labor contractions for hours before they arrive at a birthing center or hospital. This means, most likely, that they have been experiencing pain and relying on their own or their partner's judgment that everything is going well for a long time. One of their chief needs when they arrive at a birthing setting, therefore, is reassurance their judgment has been correct—everything is going well and the exhaustion and increasing pain they feel is part of usual labor.

BOX 15.7

Nursing Care Planning Tips for Effective Communication

Celeste Bailey is having a great deal of back pain as well as strong uterine contractions.

Tip: Be prepared to repeat instructions as necessary to prevent a woman from becoming confused. Women in labor may be enduring so much pain and are under so much stress that they don't hear or process instructions well. Gently repeat the instructions without reminding them they were previously given the information. A reminder is not therapeutic because it can lower self-esteem and a sense of self-control.

Nurse: You don't look very comfortable, Mrs. Bailey. Would you feel better if you sat in the rocking chair rather than stay in bed?

Celeste: Can I do that?

Nurse: You can use any position comfortable for you.

Celeste: Can I walk over to the window?

Nurse: Whatever is most comfortable.

Celeste: Thank you. You're very understanding.

Nursing Diagnoses and Related Interventions

Nursing Diagnosis: Powerlessness related to duration of labor

Outcome Evaluation: Patient voices she feels in control of happenings, expresses preferences for positions and techniques to control pain, asks questions about her progress, and states feelings about what is happening.

After admission, care during the first stage of labor centers on helping a woman feel confident in her ability to control pain and maintain physiologic stability in the face of it. At first, it is exciting for a woman to feel labor contractions. They are little more than menstrual cramps and project a "this-is-really-happening" sensation. Soon, however, if a woman is not concentrating on controlled breathing, the contractions become biting in their intensity. Despite the fact she is becoming more and more uncomfortable, however, nothing seems to be happening. This can cause a couple to begin to worry something is going wrong—to think because the 9 months are over, that victory should be near, yet it is eluding them. Give couples frequent progress reports during labor, so they do not become discouraged or fearful this way at this seeming lack of progress (Box 15.7).

Help Empower Women. Most women want to feel in control of what is happening to them during labor in order to be able to face this big an event in their life. They accomplish this by stating their preferences, breathing with contractions, and changing their position to the one that makes them most comfortable. In contrast, some women handle the stress of labor by becoming extremely passive and quiet. Still others feel a need to show their emotions by shouting or crying. Help each woman express her feelings in her own way or in the way that works best for her.

Part of the way women react to labor is culturally influenced. Don't stereotype women, however, by studying a list of how a typical Hispanic, Middle Eastern, or Asian woman is most apt to react in labor. Instead, ask each woman what will make her feel most comfortable and able to feel in control. A list of expected behaviors may not apply to some women at all.

Respect Contraction Time. Do not interrupt a woman who is in the middle of breathing exercises during labor to perform a procedure or ask questions because, once her concentration is disrupted, she will feel the pain of the contraction and, if she has been successfully using breathing exercises to reduce pain, suddenly feeling the full force of a contraction can be extremely frightening. She tenses and the pain becomes worse, causing her to doubt her ability to breathe constructively in the face of the next contraction. Instead of interrupting, allow her to finish breathing with her contraction, then ask questions or announce what procedure needs to be done next. (See Chapter 16 for a discussion of pain management techniques during labor.)

Promote Change of Positions. Because the bed is the main piece of furniture in a birthing room, many women assume they are expected to lie quietly in bed during labor. In early labor, however, a woman should be out of bed walking or sitting in a chair, kneeling, squatting, on all fours, or in whatever position she prefers because active movement can shorten the beginning stage of labor (Jones, 2015) (Fig. 15.21). Ballroom dancing or swaying with her partner to music they have brought with them can be a helpful activity. Soaking in a tub of warm water (98.6°F [37°C]) or taking a warm shower with the water directed on the abdomen both feel relaxing and so may also help. Water tubs give a woman buoyancy and so make it easier for her to change position. Remember, they also can make a woman feel drowsy, so never leave a woman alone in a tub. Be certain the tub is kept clean of feces so a vaginal examination can be done with the woman in the tub without worry of vaginal contamination.

The exception to being active in labor is a woman whose membranes have ruptured in early labor. She should lie on her side until it is established the FHR is stable or she has had a vaginal examination by her primary care provider.

If a woman receives medication for pain such as a narcotic, she may need to remain in bed for about 15 minutes afterward to avoid a fall if she should become dizzy from the medication. While she is in bed, encourage her to lie on her left side so the heavy uterus tips forward, away from the vena cava, allowing free blood return from the lower extremities and adequate placental filling and circulation. Most women are comfortable in this position and adjust to it readily. Position the chair for the support person facing her so she doesn't keep turning onto her back to talk. Many institutions have protocols which do not allow women to be ambulatory after the administration of narcotics.

Some women have practiced breathing exercises in a supine position while at home and may need additional coaching to do them in a sitting or dancing position. If a woman feels she must lie on her back during a contraction to make her breathing exercises effective, place a folded towel under her left hip to tilt her uterus to the side. Remind her to return to her side or sit up between contractions.

Help With Fetal Alignment. A baby's birth is easiest from an ROA or LOA position because a fetus that presents in an LOP or ROP position needs to rotate into an anterior position to be born. Either squatting or an "all fours" position may help the fetus turn and shorten labor. A birthing sling, or rebozo, is a long piece of fabric that can be slipped under a woman's back as she lies supine or over the abdomen if she is in a hands-and-knees position (Cohen & Thomas, 2015). A support person uses the sling to gently rock the mother's abdomen, a technique which is advocated as also helping a fetus move into good alignment with the pelvis. It is difficult to find evidence-based practice that birthing slings accomplish this, so they should be used with caution until their worth is more firmly established. There is little need for them with the fetus who is already in good alignment.

Promote Voiding and Provide Bladder Care. A full bladder or bowel can impede fetal descent, so encourage a woman to void, if possible, at least every 2 to 4 hours during labor. The way a full bladder can impede descent of a fetus is illustrated in Figure 15.22. The reason you need to remind a woman to void during labor is because she may mistakenly interpret the discomfort of a full bladder as part of the sensations of labor. You can assess for a full bladder by percussion (an empty bladder sounds dull; a full one sounds resonant). If a woman cannot void and the bladder becomes distended, she may need to be catheterized. Catheterizing a woman in labor is uncomfortable for her and difficult for you: The vulva is edematous from the pressure of the fetal presenting part, stretching the urethral canal downward and making the urethra difficult to locate. For best results, use a small catheter (No. 12 to 14F) and insert it between contractions. Use extremely careful aseptic technique to avoid introducing any microorganisms that might result in a urinary tract infection.

Nursing Diagnosis: Risk for ineffective breathing pattern related to breathing exercises

Outcome Evaluation: Patient's respiratory rate returns to normal limits after a contraction; skin is her usual color, cool, and dry. No reports of light-headedness or tingling/numbness in extremities.

Figure 15.21 Finding a comfortable position during early labor is important. Here, a nurse assists a woman with walking during labor.

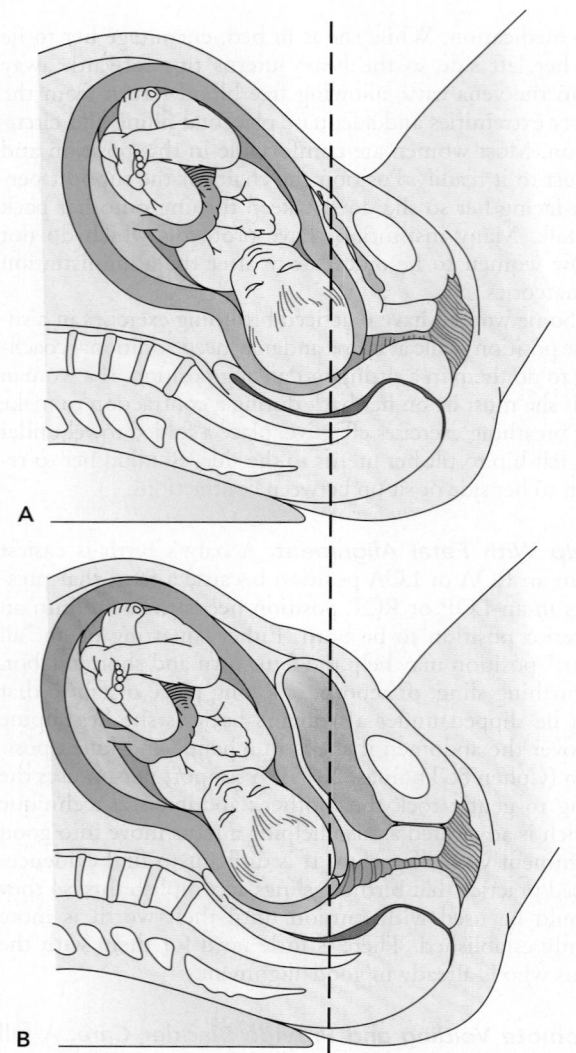

Figure 15.22 The effect of a full bladder on fetal descent. **(A)** The bladder is empty. **(B)** A full bladder impedes fetal progress.

Hyperventilation (an accelerated rate of respiration) occurs when a woman exhales more deeply than she inhales. As a result, extra carbon dioxide is blown off and respiratory alkalosis results. This can occur when a woman is practicing breathing exercises in preparation for labor, but it is most apt to occur during actual labor. The woman feels lightheaded and may have tingling or numbness in her toes and fingertips. If allowed to progress, hyperventilation can lead to loss of consciousness.

The best way to manage hyperventilation is to prevent it. Be certain that when a woman is breathing rapidly, she ends all breathing sessions with a long cleansing breath to help restore carbon dioxide balance. If hyperventilation begins, ask her to breathe in and out into a paper bag, so she rebreathes the carbon dioxide she has exhaled. If a paper bag is unavailable, a woman can use her cupped hands or those of her partner.

Nursing Diagnosis: Anxiety related to stress of labor

Outcome Evaluation: Patient states she feels in control of her situation; she and her support person express confidence in their ability to weather this extraordinary event in their life.

Labor is such an intense process it creates a high level of emotional stress for both the woman and her support person. Ability to tolerate stress (to cope adequately) depends on a person's perception of the event, the support people available, and past experience in using coping mechanisms. Ways to reduce stress in labor, therefore, center on helping a woman to perceive labor clearly, providing opportunities for her partner to provide support, and helping her gain confidence that she can manage this event.

Offer Support. Support needs to come from healthcare personnel as well as a woman's individual support person. There is no substitute for personal touch and contact as a way to provide support during labor (unless she's a person who doesn't like to be touched). Patting an arm while telling a woman she is progressing in labor, brushing away a wisp of hair from her forehead, and wiping her forehead with a cool cloth are indispensable methods of conveying support and produce several benefits.

Effective support can make the difference in helping a woman feel able to continue with labor. In addition, a woman who is touched, who experiences the warmth and friendliness of human contact during labor—a time when she is physically dependent—may handle her newborn (who is also physically dependent and undergoing an adjustment not unlike the one she has just gone through) more warmly and affectionately.

Respect and Promote the Support Person. Be certain to admit a woman's support person to the birthing area along with the woman and encourage him or her to remain with the woman throughout the birth because having someone familiar with her during labor helps to counteract the sensation everything is new and unexpected. Acquaint the support person with the physical layout of the birthing room and point out where supplies such as towels, washcloths, and ice chips are stored, so he or she can get them as necessary. Be certain that all healthcare personnel are aware of whom the support person is and the importance of making him or her feel welcome.

If the support person will be acting as a labor coach, ask whether he or she has attended a prepared childbirth class and exactly how the support person wants to help the woman manage the pain of contractions. If a support person is hesitant to give coaching instructions, it's better to review techniques than to take over. Offer praise not only for the woman but also for the support person as well because watching a birth is often as totally a new experience for this person as for the woman. Relieve the support person as necessary, so he or she can take a break and get something to eat or visit with older children (Fig. 15.23). If older children will view the birth, be certain they are oriented and have a child care provider to entertain them during the long hours of labor.

In addition to having a support person, many women choose a doula or an expert support person to be with them in labor. Having such a person present frees the woman's partner to enjoy the birth rather than feel occupied with coaching instructions. Extensive research on the subject of doula care has demonstrated that rates of oxytocin augmentation, the need for epidural anesthesia,

Figure 15.23 Encouraging a support person so he can continue to give support is an important nursing role. (© Barbara Proud.)

and cesarean birth rates can be reduced through doula support. Additionally, mothers tend to be more satisfied with the birth experience regardless of outcomes (Hodnett et al., 2013).

Support a Woman's Pain Management Needs. Many women plan on using nonpharmacologic pain relief measures such as hydrotherapy (soaking in a tub of warm water or taking a warm shower), position changes, or acupuncture during labor; ask if the woman has planned any of these and what you could do to help her make these effective (Chaillet, Belaid, Crochetière, et al., 2014). Other women want pharmacologic help in labor. Support whichever decision a woman has made coming into labor as well as any change she decides on as labor progresses (see Chapter 16 for a discussion of common nonpharmacologic as well as pharmacologic measures for labor).

Some healthcare providers are reluctant to suggest to a woman that pharmacologic pain relief is available as this might influence her to accept an analgesic rather than continue to use nonpharmacologic methods. Part of being in control, however, is knowing your options and feeling free to elect the one most appropriate at that time. Because pain is subjective, only the woman knows how much pain she can endure and whether she needs some supplemental help to make childbirth the experience she planned.

What If . . . 15.3
Celeste's doula and Celeste's teenage sister disagree on whether Celeste needs medication for pain during labor. Whose suggestion would the nurse pay the most attention to? How could the nurse resolve the issue?

Nursing Diagnosis: Risk for fluid volume deficit related to prolonged lack of oral intake and diaphoresis from the effort of labor

Outcome Evaluation: Patient drinks at least one glass of selected beverage every hour, states she does not feel thirsty; voids at least 30 ml/hr every 2 to 4 hours.

Women need to remain well hydrated during labor, so urge them to drink at least a glass of fluid every hour. Sucking

on ice chips, popsicles, or lollipops can help supply additional fluid. Some women need isotonic sports drinks to prevent secondary uterine inertia (a cessation of labor contractions) as well as to combat generalized dehydration and exhaustion. Even with an adequate fluid intake, a woman's mouth and lips can become uncomfortably dry because of mouth breathing. Applying lip balm to prevent or relieve this discomfort can be helpful.

The Care of a Woman During the Second Stage of Labor

The second stage of labor is the time from full cervical dilatation to birth of the newborn. Even women who have taken childbirth education classes and who believe they are well prepared for any length or type of contractions are surprised at the intensity of the pushing sensation they feel in this stage of labor. Because the feeling to push becomes so strong, some women react to this by growing argumentative and angry, or by crying and screaming. Other women react by tensing their abdominal muscles and trying to resist pushing, thus making the sensation even more painful and frightening. If the woman has not received an epidural for pain management, she should push with contractions and rest in between. In the past, women were told to hold their breath while they did this. Holding the breath for a prolonged time, however, impairs blood return from the vena cava (a Valsalva maneuver), so this should be discouraged. Instead, encourage women to assume any position that is comfortable for them and breathe any way that is natural for them, except by holding their breath while they push (Vaziri, Arzhe, Asadi, et al., 2016) (Box 15.8).

A support person plays a vital role during this time because all of the preparations done up to this point may still not be enough to sustain a woman during these final contractions unless she feels well supported. This participation also creates an important sharing time later after the birth and can give a couple a sense of family for the first time.

Women also need to have an experienced healthcare person with them as they enter this stage of labor to reassure them that the change in contractions is normal and to give knowledgeable support everything is all right. Box 15.9 shows an interprofessional care map illustrating both nursing and team planning for labor.

BOX 15.8
Nursing Care Planning to Empower a Family

Q. Celeste asks you, "How will I know when I should begin to push with labor?"

A. After full cervical dilatation, the baby's head descends in the pelvis to the level of the pelvic floor. When this happens, you'll realize a strong feeling you have to push as if you need to move your bowels. Don't push before that; wait for the natural signal. Pushing is a great moment in labor because as you push (remember not to hold your breath), you no longer feel pain, just a wonderful awareness your baby is about to be born.

BOX 15.9

Nursing Care Planning

AN INTERPROFESSIONAL CARE MAP FOR A WOMAN DURING LABOR AND BIRTH

Celeste Bailey is a 26-year-old woman you admit to a birthing room. She tells you she wants to have her baby "naturally," without any analgesia or anesthesia. Her husband, a long distance truck driver, is on his way home but hasn't arrived as of yet. Her teenage sister is with her. She states she has no idea how to coach her except to pray. As you finish assessing contractions, Celeste grips her abdomen, screams, and shouts, "I'm breathing just like I'm supposed to do! Why does this hurt so bad?"

Family Assessment: Patient lives with husband in fixed rent housing project. Finances rated as "horrible." She says, "If you want to be rich, don't marry a truck driver." Her sister and parents live nearby.

Patient Assessment: Gravida 1, para 0. Contractions of moderate intensity, 45 seconds in duration, 3 minutes apart. Cervix dilated 3 cm, 60% effaced. Membranes intact. Fetal heart rate (FHR), 148 beats/min; fetus in right occipitoanterior (ROA) position. Attended childbirth education classes but appears to be using breathing exercises ineffectively without her coach. Brought a red rose to use as a focusing object. Has not voided for past 4 hours.

Nursing Diagnosis: Pain related to uterine contractions and pressure on pelvic structures from labor

Outcome Criteria: Patient manages her discomfort in labor with nonpharmacologic methods, identifies additional pain relief measures if needed, responds to questions and instructions; states labor and birth were a positive experience for her.

Team Member Responsible	Assessment	Intervention	Rationale	Expected Outcome
Activities of Daily Living, Including Safety				
Nurse	Inspect the patient's suprapubic area and palpate for bladder distention because she has not voided for 4 hours.	Encourage patient to void every 2 hours.	A full bladder contributes to the patient's discomfort and impedes fetal descent, possibly prolonging labor.	Patient has no signs of bladder distention and voids every 2 hours during labor.
Nurse	Assess level of pain from uterine contractions and pelvic pressure by both verbal and nonverbal indicators; use 1–10 pain score.	Review and observe breathing patterns with patient and teenage sister to be certain she is obtaining maximum relief.	Pain is a subjective symptom, so only the patient can determine her degree of pain or what is most helpful to relieve it.	Patient rates her level of pain from labor contractions as good to tolerable. Teenage sister offers effective support.
Teamwork and Collaboration				
Nurse/primary care provider	Ask sister if she will serve as labor coach until husband arrives. Determine if a nurse anesthetist is available in case the patient changes mind about analgesia because husband is not with her.	Demonstrate to sister how to serve as coach. Consult with nurse anesthetist about patient's wish to not receive any pharmacologic pain relief.	Respecting patient's wishes is a prime mode of encouraging self-efficacy. A support person can play a major role in making labor a tolerable experience.	Sister serves as effective labor coach. Pain management team supports patient's wish for no pharmacologic interventions but will be prepared to administer pain relief if patient's wishes change or an emergency should change the patient's goal.
Procedures/Medications for Quality Improvement				
Nurse	Assess what particular care measures, if any, patient desires during labor such as walking or using a water tub.	Establish a birth plan with patient so all staff members can be aware of her individual preferences.	Respecting a patient's choice helps to maintain self-esteem and a feeling of control.	Patient expresses her preferences during labor.

Nutrition

Nurse	Assess when patient last ate. Ask about preferences for fluid during labor.	Provide patient with ice chips, hard candy, or other fluid as desired.	Ice chips or hard candy can relieve mouth dryness from breathing exercises, and fluid is important to prevent dehydration.	Patient states she has no mouth discomfort and does not feel hungry; drinks at least a glass of fluid every hour.

Patient-Centered Care

Nurse	Assess what patient knows about the usual process and time intervals of labor.	Provide information to supplement patient's knowledge of labor; update patient frequently on labor progress.	Frequent updates about patient's progress help to alleviate anxiety.	Patient states she understands the process of usual labor and indicates progress reports are helpful.

Psychosocial/Spiritual/Emotional Needs

Nurse	Assess if physical environment seems conducive to labor.	Provide a comfortable environment. Encourage patient to assume different positions and to change them regularly. Respect the need for focusing during contractions.	A comfortable environment aids in relaxation and minimizes distractions. Position changes promote fetal descent. Interrupting focusing can lessen effectiveness of the technique.	Patient reports environment is comfortable and she feels secure. She assumes a variety of positions during labor as desired. She expresses she is able to use a rose for focus during contractions unimpaired by healthcare providers.

Informatics for Seamless Healthcare Planning

Nurse	Assess how patient evaluates her labor experience.	Help patient voice her satisfaction or dissatisfaction with her labor experience.	Reviewing a possibly traumatic experience helps put it into perspective among life events.	Patient states labor and birth were, at worst, a tolerable experience and, at best, a highlight of her life.

A general timetable for second-stage care is shown in Table 15.7. Be certain to assess fetal heart sounds at the beginning of the second stage to be certain the start of the baby's passage into the birth canal is not occluding the cord and interfering with fetal circulation. Assisting a woman into whatever position she feels will be most effective for pushing (e.g., squatting, sitting upright, leaning forward against her partner) is important to help align the fetal presenting part with the cervix, increase the pelvic diameters, and use the fetal weight to help descent so that a prolonged second stage does not occur. A danger of a prolonged second stage is chorioamnionitis (membrane infection), an increased rate of cesarean birth, and future urinary incontinence (Stephansson, Sandström, Petersson, et al., 2016).

PREPARING THE PLACE OF BIRTH

For a multipara, convert a birthing room into a birth room by opening the sterile packs of supplies on waiting tables when the cervix has dilated. Be certain drapes and materials used for birth are sterile so no microorganisms can be accidentally introduced into the uterus. A table arranged with equipment such as sponges, drapes, scissors, basins, clamps, vaginal packing, and sterile gowns, gloves, and towels can be left, if covered, for up to 8 hours.

A birthing bed is "broken" or the foot folded down to allow the primary care provider ready access to support a crowning newborn head. Be certain that once a bed is broken, someone remains continuously at the foot of the bed so if the fetus is born suddenly, the head and body can be supported and born safely. Some providers do not choose to "break the bed" and instead will accommodate the woman in the birthing position of her choice, whether this be side-lying, hands and knees, standing or on a birthing stool.

To provide for baby care, open the partition at the end of the room to reveal the "baby island," or newborn care area. Such areas include a radiant heat warmer, equipment for suction and resuscitation, and supplies for eye care and identification of the newborn. Turn on the radiant heat warmer in advance, so the bottom mattress is pleasantly warm to the touch at the time of birth. Place sterile towels and a blanket

TABLE 15.7 TIME INTERVALS FOR NURSING INTERVENTIONS DURING THE SECOND STAGE OF LABOR

Intervention	Beginning of Second Stage	Continued Frequency	After Birth of Infant	After Delivery of Placenta
Assess and Record				
Temperature	X	q2h	X	q1h
Pulse	X	q1h	X	q15 min
Respirations	X	q5–30 min	X	q15 min
Blood pressure	X	q5–30 min	X	X
Fetal heart rate	X	q5 min		
Contractions	X	q5 min		
Perineum	X	q15 min	X	q15 min
Provide				
Support	X	Continuously	Continuously	Continuously

on the warmer so they will also be warm when used to dry and cover the infant to help prevent hypothermia.

POSITIONING FOR BIRTH

Women can choose a variety of positions for birth. In the past, a lithotomy position was the preferred position for birth because it offers a clear view of the perineum, but it is no longer a position of choice as a woman lying flat on her back may slow, not help, fetal descent, and lying longer than 1 hour in a lithotomy position can lead to intense pelvic congestion and possibly thrombophlebitis. More effective birth positions include the lateral or Sims position, a dorsal recumbent position (on the back with knees flexed), semi-sitting, or squatting. Using these positions plus warm compresses to the perineum place less tension on the perineum and result in fewer perineal tears (Vaziri, Farahmand, Samsami, et al., 2014).

The Water Birth

Women may not only use a warm water tub for labor comfort and relaxation but also to give birth under water. The increased buoyancy they feel from the water helps them change positions easily; a sitting posture helps with fetal descent (Impey & Child, 2012).

As women begin to push with contractions, they also often move their bowels so the water can become contaminated with feces. Keep the bath water as free as possible by lifting any feces out with a plastic scoop so, if the infant is born in the tub, he or she will be born into as clean an environment as possible.

The baby is born underwater and then immediately brought to the surface for a first breath. A potential difficulty is contamination of the bath water with feces, which could lead to uterine infection or aspiration of contaminated bath water by a newborn, which could lead to pneumonia. Newborns, however, have a dive reflex, which alerts them not to breathe while under water, so this is not usually a problem. A dive reflex may not be operative if the baby's head is brought to the surface before the entire baby is born so the timing of this is important. Maternal chilling when a woman leaves the water is another factor to consider and prevent. Yet another concern is that a short umbilical cord could tear as the baby is brought to the surface. To help prevent this, limit the amount of water in the tub to about 12 in.

Be certain tubs are cleaned with the agency-designated solution at the finish of labor so it will be clean for the next couple.

PROMOTING EFFECTIVE SECOND-STAGE PUSHING

For the most effective pushing during the second stage of labor, a woman should wait to feel the urge to push even though a pelvic exam has revealed she is fully dilated (Lemos, Amorim, Dornelas de Andrade, et al., 2015). Pushing is usually best done from a semi-Fowler's position with legs raised against the abdomen, squatting, or on all fours rather than lying flat to allow gravity to aid the effort (Fig. 15.24). Make sure the woman pushes with contractions and rests between them. She can use short pushes or long, sustained ones, whichever feels more comfortable. Holding the breath during a contraction could cause a Valsalva maneuver or temporarily impede blood return to her heart because of increased intrathoracic pressure, which could then also interfere with blood supply to the uterus. To prevent her from holding her breath during pushing, urge her to grunt or breathe out during a pushing effort (as tennis players do).

If there is a reason such as a nuchal cord (cord located around the baby's neck), which must be removed before the infant is fully born, it may be necessary to prevent a woman from pushing immediately after delivery of the fetal head. To help her do this, ask her to pant with contractions. Because it is difficult to push effectively when she is using her diaphragm for panting, this limits pushing. Remember, however, that pushing is involuntary. Regardless of how much a woman wants to cooperate, stopping this overwhelming urge to push is almost beyond her power. Demonstrating panting with her may be most effective. Be sure she is inhaling adequately with panting. Otherwise, she might hyperventilate and become light-headed. Have her take deep cleansing breaths between contractions to prevent this.

PERINEAL CLEANING AND MASSAGE

Massaging the perineum as the fetal head enlarges the vaginal opening helps to keep it supple and prevent tearing. To remove vaginal or rectal secretions and prepare the cleanest environment for the birth of the baby, the care provider may clean the perineum with a warmed antiseptic such as Ioda-

Figure 15.24 Positions for pushing during second stage labor: **(A)** squatting with support person, **(B)** on all fours, and **(C)** on all fours with chest support. (© Barbara Proud.)

phor (cold solution causes cramping) and then rinse the area with sterile water. If assisting with this, always clean from the vagina outward (so microorganisms are moved away from the vagina, not toward it), using a clean compress for each stroke. Be certain to include a wide area (vulva, upper inner thighs, pubis, and anus). Figure 15.25 shows a typical pattern for cleaning.

THE BIRTH

As soon as the head of a fetus is prominent (approximately 8 cm across) at the vaginal opening, one technique to help the fetus achieve extension and allow the smallest head diameter to present is for the care provider to place a sterile towel over the rectum and press forward on the fetal chin while the other hand presses downward on the occiput (a Ritgen maneuver) (Fig. 15.26). This maneuver, however, is often unnecessary as babies tend to be born easily without this assistance. Pressure should never be applied to the fundus of the uterus to effect birth because uterine rupture could occur.

The woman is asked to continue pushing until the occiput of the fetal head is firmly at the pubic arch. The head is then gently born between contractions if possible. This helps to prevent the head from being expelled too rapidly, creating a major pressure change in the skull, which might then rupture cerebral blood vessels. It also reduces the possibility of a perineal tear. A woman who has not had anesthesia experiences the birth of the head as a flash of pain or a burning sensation, as if someone had momentarily poured hot water on her perineum.

Immediately after birth of the baby's head, the primary care provider passes his or her fingers around the newborn's neck to determine whether a loop of umbilical cord is encircling the neck. It is not uncommon for a single loop of cord to be positioned this way (termed a nuchal cord). If such a

Figure 15.25 The pattern for cleaning the perineum before birth. Cleaning from the birth canal outward moves bacteria away from, not into, the vagina. Numbers refer to the steps of the procedure.

Figure 15.26   The Ritgen maneuver. The *arrow* shows direction of pressure.

Figure 15.27   A child is considered born when the whole body is born. (© Barbara Proud.)

loop is felt, it is gently loosened and drawn down over the fetal head. If it is too tightly coiled to allow this, it is clamped and cut before the shoulders are born. Otherwise, it could tear and interfere with the fetal oxygen supply.

After expulsion of the fetal head, external rotation occurs (a woman can feel this happening by gently touching the head if she wants to). Gentle pressure is then exerted downward on the side of the infant's head by the primary care provider so the anterior shoulder is born. Slight upward pressure on the side of the head allows the anterior shoulder to nestle against the symphysis pubis and the posterior shoulder to be born. The remainder of the body then slides free without any further difficulty.

A child is considered born when the whole body is born. This is the time that should be noted and recorded as the time of birth, which is a nursing responsibility (most primary care providers regard it as their responsibility or pleasure to announce the sex of the infant). The newborn is immediately laid on the mother's naked abdomen and covered with a warmed blanket and cap to conserve heat and encourage mother–infant bonding (E. R. Moore, Anderson, Bergman, et al., 2012). With this, the second stage of labor is complete (Fig. 15.27).

CUTTING AND CLAMPING THE CORD

Cutting the cord is part of the stimulus that initiates a first breath or marks the newborn's most important transition into the outside world, the establishment of independent respirations. The timing of cord clamping, however, varies depending on the parent's preference and the maturity of the infant.

The umbilical cord continues to pulsate for a few minutes after birth and then the pulsation ceases. Delaying cutting (also called physiologic clamping) until pulsation ceases and maintaining the infant at a uterine level allows as much as 100 ml more of blood to pass from the placenta into the fetus than if the infant were held in a superior position or the cord was immediately cut. Delaying cutting, therefore, helps

ensure an adequate red blood cell and white cell count in the newborn (Popat, Robledo, Sebastian, et al., 2016). The timing of cord clamping, however, is individualized because late clamping of the cord this way could cause overinfusion with placental blood and the possibility of polycythemia and hyperbilirubinemia in a susceptible newborn, a particular concern if the infant is preterm.

Before cutting, the cord is clamped with two hemostats placed 8 to 10 in. from the infant's umbilicus. The woman's partner or support person may then have the privilege of cutting the cord between the hemostats. A cord blood sample is often obtained to provide a ready source of infant blood if blood typing or other emergency measures, such as establishing whether fetal acidosis was present, needs to be done. Blood may also be taken for cord blood banking so the family has stem cells available if needed in the future.

The vessels in the cord are then counted to be certain three are present and an umbilical clamp is applied to replace the forceps (Fig. 15.28). Some umbilical clamps in hospitals have an alarm attached that will ring if the infant is taken further than set hospital boundaries, a precaution against newborn abduction.

INTRODUCING THE INFANT

After the cord is cut, it is time for the new parents to spend quality time with their newborn. The infant can remain on the mother's abdomen for skin-to-skin contact. If the woman's partner or support person wants to hold the infant, dry the infant well with a warmed towel, wrap him or her in a sterile blanket, and cover the head with a wrapped towel or cap. Be certain to handle newborns gently but firmly as they are slippery from amniotic fluid and vernix.

Most newborns receive prophylactic eye ointment against the possibility of a chlamydia infection. Don't administer this until after the parents have had this chance to see their infant for the first time (and the infant has had a chance to see them) (see Chapter 18 for continuing infant care such as weighing and measuring). This initial contact is also the optimal time for a mother to begin breastfeeding because an infant seems to be hungry at birth and sucking at the breasts stimulates the release of endogenous oxytocin, encouraging uterine contraction and involution, or the return of the uterus to its prepregnant state (World Health Organization, 2014).

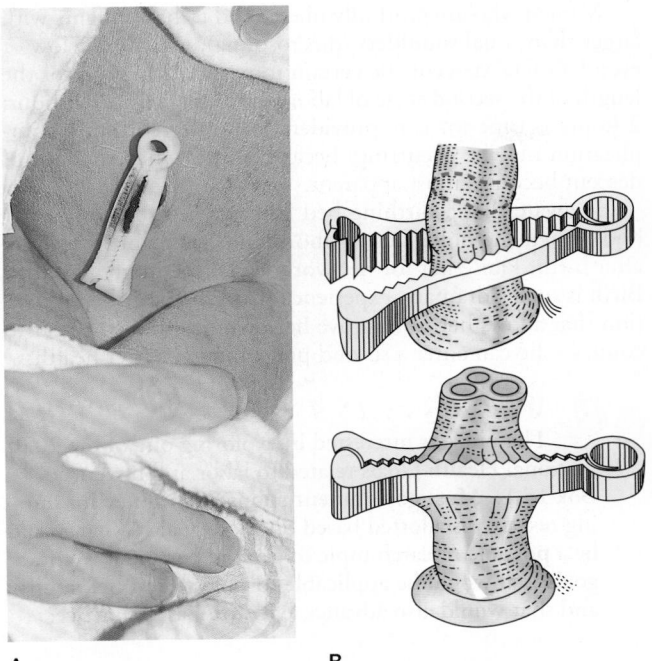

A   **B**

Figure 15.28 **(A)** An umbilical clamp applied to the cord. (© Caroline Brown, RNC, MS, DEd.) **(B)** Placing clamp and locking the clamp.

The Care of a Woman During the Third and Fourth Stages of Labor

The third stage of labor is the time from the birth of the baby until the placenta is delivered. For most women, this is a time of great excitement because the infant has been born, but this can also be a time of feeling anticlimactic because the infant has finally arrived after being anticipated for so long a time.

THE DELIVERY OF THE PLACENTA

The placenta will deliver spontaneously following most births (Begley, Gyte, Devane, et al., 2015). Although this is true in most cases, up to 30 minutes is considered normal. After delivery, the placenta is inspected to be certain it is intact without gross abnormalities and that no cotyledons remain in the uterus. Normally, a placenta is one sixth the weight of the infant. If it is unusually large or small, you may be asked to weigh it.

After the placenta inspection, if the mother's uterus has not contracted firmly on its own, the primary care provider will massage the fundus to urge it to contract. Oxytocin (Pitocin 10 units) may be prescribed to be administered intramuscularly (IM) or per 1,000 ml fluid intravenously (IV) to also help contraction (Karch, 2013). If excessive bleeding with poor uterine contraction remains, an injection of carboprost tromethamine (Hemabate) or methylergonovine maleate (Methergine) is yet another solution to increase uterine contraction and to guard against hemorrhage. It is important to know prior to the second stage whether a woman has a contraindication to either of these drugs such as asthma or hypertension.

The administration of these drugs is a nursing responsibility in most healthcare facilities. Because Pitocin causes hypertension by vasoconstriction, be certain to obtain a baseline blood pressure measurement before administration.

Question the use of such a drug if the woman had an elevated blood pressure during pregnancy that is still present.

The fourth stage of labor includes the first few hours after birth (discussed in Chapter 17). It signals the beginning of dramatic changes because it marks the beginning of both a new life and a new family.

THE PERINEAL INSPECTION

To be certain a woman's perineum did not tear from the pressure of the fetal head, the perineum is carefully inspected after birth. About 3% of women do have a small tear extending backward from the vagina. Perineal tears are rated grade 1 to grade 4, grade 1 being minimal and grade 4 extending to and including the rectum (see Chapter 25 for grading definitions and care).

Most are small enough that no suturing is needed (Dudley, Kettle, & Ismail, 2013). If a tear is large enough to require suturing, a woman usually has enough natural perineal anesthesia from pressure of the fetal head or enough effect from epidural anesthesia, she will not feel pain from the suturing. If she does have pain, a local anesthetic can be given to make the process pain-free.

THE IMMEDIATE POSTPARTUM ASSESSMENT AND NURSING CARE

This is the beginning of the postpartal period or the fourth stage of labor. Because the uterus may be so exhausted from labor that it cannot maintain contraction, there is a high risk for hemorrhage during this time (it is the most dangerous time of birth for the mother). Obtain vital signs (pulse, respirations, and blood pressure) every 15 minutes for the first hour and then according to agency policy or the woman's condition. Pulse and respirations may be fairly rapid immediately after birth (80 to 90 beats/min and 20 to 24 breaths/min), and blood pressure may be slightly elevated due to exertion and excitement of the moment or recent oxytocin administration. Wash the perineum with the agency-designated solution and apply a perineal pad. Palpate a woman's fundus for size, consistency, and position and observe the amount and characteristics of lochia each time you record vital signs.

Return the birthing bed to its original position. Offer a clean gown and a warmed blanket because a woman often experiences chills and a shaking sensation 10 to 15 minutes after birth. This may be due to the low temperature of a birthing room but may also be a result of the sudden release of pressure on pelvic nerves or of excess epinephrine production during labor. In any event, it is a normal phenomenon but can be frightening to the mother if she associates the chills with fever or infection and worry she will be ill at a time when she most wants to be well to care for her new child. You can reassure her this is a transitory sensation, is very common, and passes quickly. Continuing assessments are discussed in Chapter 17 with care of a postpartal family.

The Woman With Unique Concerns in Labor

THE WOMAN WITHOUT A SUPPORT PERSON

Some women choose to labor without their partner—the usual support person—during labor. Other times, a partner is not available due to work or other commitments. Such women then ask a family member or close friend to act as their support person. A woman who brings no support person with her needs a supportive nurse to remain with her continuously during labor.

A woman whose acceptance of her pregnancy was slow to develop due to lack of adequate support people may not have completed the psychological tasks of pregnancy by the time she is in labor. This could make her more apprehensive about being alone and being asked to begin a new life role. Increased assessment of parent–child bonding may be necessary in the immediate postpartal period to be certain her loneliness does not affect her relationship with her child.

THE WOMAN WHO WILL BE PLACING HER BABY FOR ADOPTION

Even if a woman has decided to place her baby for adoption during pregnancy, she needs to be an active participant in her labor and the baby's birth and be allowed to hold her child afterward unless she chooses otherwise. Each state has a set number of days in which a mother must decide whether she wants to keep her baby or decide on adoption. Although this decision may have seemed easier to make during pregnancy, once a woman holds the baby in her arms, the prospect of giving up the child may be more painful than she realized. Offer support no matter what decision she eventually makes; also offer support as to whether she wants to hold the child or begin breastfeeding. Be certain you do not offer influencing advice because the woman is the only person who knows whether keeping this child will be right for her or for the child in the future.

THE WOMAN WITH CULTURAL CONCERNS

A number of women from countries where female genital cutting is part of her culture may have difficulty with a successful second stage of labor because their perineum has so much scar tissue that their vagina cannot dilate adequately for a fetal head to pass. They may need an episiotomy or defibulation (discussed in Chapter 24) to avoid extensive perineal tearing.

THE WOMAN WHO IS MORBIDLY OBESE

The incidence of women who are morbidly obese seen in birth settings is growing yearly (Perlow, Jones, & Ozimek, 2015). Care of women with a high body mass index (BMI) requires a number of special interventions in labor and birth.

On admission, a woman may be unusually fatigued from her efforts to keep active in early labor. Because many overweight women have elevated blood pressure, be certain to assess this on admission (but then repeat it about 15 minutes later when she is more rested to be certain an elevated pressure was not from anxiety). Assess her ankles carefully for edema because this is common from overworked circulation in her lower extremities. Fetal heart sounds may be difficult to auscultate in women who are obese. Electronic monitors may not have straps long enough to hold the sensors snugly in place, so they may have to be handheld or attached by wrapped gauze or stockinette.

It's important for all women to remain active in labor. Be certain to respect modesty of all sized women while helping her change from a soiled gown to a clean one or that she is adequately covered if she plans to walk in the birthing center or hospital hallway.

Women who are morbidly obese tend to have infants with larger than usual shoulders (macrosomia), which can slow or even halt fetal descent. Be certain to particularly monitor the length of the second stage of labor (the average time is 1 hour; 2 hours is time for care providers to be alerted that a complication may be occurring) because this is when the lack of descent becomes most apparent.

Be aware that a birthing bed is narrow in relation to her body when she holds her newborn and begins breastfeeding after birth. Praise her for her work well done in giving birth. Birth is such a dramatic experience that it may be the motivation that allows her to improve her own health in the year to come so she can enter a second pregnancy in better health.

What If . . . 15.4

The nurse is interested in exploring one of the 2020 National Health Goals related to labor and birth (see Box 15.1). Most government-sponsored money for nursing research is allotted based on these goals. What would be a possible research topic to explore pertinent to these goals that would be applicable to Celeste and her family and that would also advance evidence-based practice?

Unfolding Patient Stories: Carla Hernandez • Part 2

Remember Carla Hernandez, a 32-year-old gravida 2, para 1, who you met in Chapter 6. She is at 39 5/7 weeks gestation when her husband brings her to the hospital. How does the nurse determine that she is in active labor? If she is in labor, how will the nurse monitor the progress of labor? What nursing assessments are done to identify the signs of potential complications during labor? What questions would the nurse ask Carla to identify symptoms of potential complications of labor? What nursing interventions can assist the couple's ability to cope with pain and stress experienced during labor?

Care for Carla and other patients in a realistic virtual environment: *vSim for Nursing* (thepoint.lww.com /vSimMaternityPed). Practice documenting these patients' care in DocuCare (thepoint.lww.com /DocuCareEHR).

KEY POINTS FOR REVIEW

- Labor is the series of events by which uterine contractions expel a fetus and placenta from a woman's body.

- The exact reason why labor begins is unknown. It most likely occurs because of an interplay between fetal and uterine factors that registers as progesterone withdrawal.

- Effective labor depends on interactions between the passage, the passenger, the power of contractions, and a woman's psychological readiness.

- Labor is an almost overwhelming experience because it involves intense sensations and emotions never felt before. Urge women to bring a support person with them to help cope with the experience. Orient and explain what is happening to this person as well as the woman in labor.

- The fetal presentation (the fetal body part that will initially contact the cervix), the position (the relationship of the fetal presenting part to a specific quadrant of the woman's pelvis), and the lie (whether the fetus is presenting the head or breech to the birth canal) are important determinants of the success of labor.

- The first stage of labor lasts from the onset of cervical dilatation until dilatation is complete (10 cm). The second stage extends from the time of full dilatation until the infant is born. A third or placental stage lasts from the time the infant is born until after delivery of the placenta. A fourth stage comprises the first few hours after birth.

- Danger signs of labor include an abnormal FHR, meconium staining of amniotic fluid, abnormal maternal pulse or blood pressure, inadequate or prolonged contractions, development of an abnormal lower abdomen contour, or increasing apprehension.

- Monitoring of uterine contractions and FHR is an important nursing responsibility. Fetal bradycardia, tachycardia, and FHR variability are important observations to make.

- Interventions such as keeping a woman active during labor and promoting voiding help to strengthen contractions and make labor more effective.

- Offering psychological support is crucial to maternal well-being and helps in planning nursing care that not only meets QSEN competencies but also best meets the family's total needs.

- Pushing during the second stage of labor should be guided by the woman's need to push. Urge her to breathe out while pushing, if possible.

- The placental stage follows birth and consists of both placental separation and expulsion. Observe for excessive bleeding during this time. Do not pull on the cord to hasten separation because this can lead to uterine inversion.

- A fetus is in potential danger when the membranes rupture because of the possibility of cord prolapse. Always assess FHR at this point to safeguard the fetus.

- A woman is at potential risk for hemorrhage throughout labor because of the possibility that the placenta could dislodge. Following birth, hemorrhage remains a possibility. Assess for vaginal bleeding and vital signs during both times to be certain this is not occurring.

CRITICAL THINKING CARE STUDY

Gail Taylor is an obese-appearing 16-year-old whom you meet as she is admitted to your labor service. Her cervix is fully effaced, 10 cm dilated, and she is pushing. Her mother tells you she didn't know Gail was pregnant because she's been living at her boyfriend's apartment for 8 months. She didn't realize she was in labor until an hour ago when she dropped by the apartment and found the living room set up for a home birth. She pulled Gail into her car and drove her to the hospital, which took over an hour because of early morning freeway traffic. Gail's mother tells you the boyfriend (a 20-year-old college student) is waiting downstairs in the parking lot; she threatened she'd charge him with rape if he came any further inside than the front door of the hospital. Gail received no prenatal care or preparation for labor; when you ask her if she's happy she's having a baby, her mother interrupts and says, "I don't want her to even see it. We'll give it away for adoption."

1. This is a family with a multitude of problems. Did the mother make a good decision when she brought Gail to the hospital in her car rather than dial for emergency help if she was worried about her? Which would have been the best place for Gail to give birth: at an apartment arranged for home birth or in a car on a busy freeway?

2. Gail is automatically a high-risk patient because of her age. What other factors make her high risk?

3. Gail's mother seems to be making decisions for everyone here. Does she have any right to make an adoption decision for Gail?

RELATED RESOURCES

Explore these additional resources to enhance learning for this chapter:
- Student resources on thePoint, including answers to the What If . . . and Critical Thinking Care Study questions, http://thepoint.lww.com/Flagg8e
- Adaptive learning powered by PrepU, http://thepoint.lww.com/prepu

REFERENCES

American Congress of Obstetricians and Gynecologists. (2009). ACOG Practice Bulletin No. 106: Intrapartum fetal heart rate monitoring: Nomenclature, interpretation, and general management principles. *Obstetrics & Gynecology, 114*(1), 193–200.

Archie, C., & Roman, A. S. (2013). Normal & abnormal labor & delivery. In A. H. DeCherney, L. Nathan, T. M. Goodwin, et al. (Eds.), *Current diagnosis and treatment: Obstetrics and gynecology* (11th ed., pp. 154–162). Columbus, OH: McGraw-Hill/Lange.

Association of Women's Health, Obstetric and Neonatal Nurses. (2011). Nursing support of laboring women. *Journal of Obstetric, Gynecologic & Neonatal Nursing, 40*(5), 665–666.

Barber, E. L., Lundsberg, L., Belanger, K., et al. (2011). Contributing indications to the rising cesarean delivery rate. *Obstetrics and Gynecology, 118*(1), 29–38.

Beck, C. T. (2016). Posttraumatic stress disorder after birth: A metaphor analysis. *MCN: The American Journal of Maternal Child Nursing, 41*(2), 76–83.

Begley, C. M., Gyte, G. M. L., Devane, D., et al. (2015). Active versus expectant management for women in the third stage of labour. *Cochrane Database of Systematic Reviews,* (3), CD007412.

Bienstock, J. L., Fox, H. E., & Wallach, E. E. (2015). *The Johns Hopkins manual of gynecology and obstetrics* (5th ed.). Philadelphia, PA: Wolters Kluwer.

Chaillet, N., Belaid, L., Crochetière, C., et al. (2014). Nonpharmacologic approaches for pain management during labor compared with usual care: A meta-analysis. *Birth, 41*(2), 122–137.

Cohen, S. R., & Thomas, C. R. (2015). Rebozo technique for fetal malposition in labor. *Journal of Midwifery & Women's Health, 60*(4), 445–451.

Cox, K. J., & King, T. L. (2015). Preventing primary cesarean births: Midwifery care. *Clinical Obstetrics and Gynecology, 58*(2), 282–293.

Dudley, L., Kettle, C., & Ismail, K. (2013). Secondary suturing compared to non-suturing for broken down perineal wounds following childbirth. *Cochrane Database of Systematic Reviews,* (9), CD008977.

Ferreira, J. C., Borowski, D., Czuba, B., et al. (2015). The evolution of fetal presentation during pregnancy: A retrospective, descriptive cross-sectional study. *Acta Obstetricia et Gynecologica Scandinavica, 94*(6), 660–663.

Greenfield, M., Jomeen, J., & Glover, L. (2016). What is traumatic birth? A concept analysis and literature review. *British Journal of Midwifery, 24*(4), 254–267.

Hodnett, E., Gates, S., Hofmeyr, G., et al. (2013). Continuous support for women during childbirth. *Cochrane Database of Systematic Reviews,* (3), CD003766.

Impey, L., & Child, T. (2012). Labour 1: Mechanism: Anatomy and physiology. In L. Impey & T. Child (Eds.), *Obstetrics & gynaecology* (4th ed., pp. 239–245). West Sussex, United Kingdom: Wiley.

Irani, R. A., & Foster, S. (2015). Overview of the mechanisms of induction of labor. *Seminars in Perinatology, 39*(6), 426–429.

Iravani, M., Janghorbani, M., Zarean, E., et al. (2015). An overview of systematic reviews of normal labor and delivery management. *Iranian Journal of Nursing and Midwifery Research, 20*(3), 293–303.

Jones, L. V. (2015). Non-pharmacological approaches for pain relief during labour can improve maternal satisfaction with childbirth and reduce obstetric interventions. *Evidence Based Nursing, 18*(3), 70.

Karch, A. M. (2013). *2013 Lippincott's nursing drug guide.* Philadelphia, PA: Lippincott Williams & Wilkins.

Lee, J., Romero, R., Lee, K. A., et al. (2016). Meconium aspiration syndrome: A role for fetal systemic inflammation. *American Journal of Obstetrics and Gynecology, 214*(3), 366.e1–366.e9.

Lemos, A., Amorim, M. M. R., Dornelas de Andrade, A., et al. (2015). Pushing/bearing down methods for the second stage of labour. *Cochrane Database of Systematic Reviews,* (10), CD009124.

López Bernal, A., & Norwitz, E. R. (2012).The normal mechanisms of labour. In K. Edmonds (Ed.), *Dewhurst's textbook of obstetrics & gynaecology* (8th ed., pp. 245–268). Oxford, United Kingdom: Wiley.

Moore, E. R., Anderson, G. C., Bergman, N., et al. (2012). Early skin-to-skin contact for mothers and their healthy newborn infants. *Cochrane Database of Systematic Reviews,* (5), CD003519.

Moore, M. F. (2016). Multicultural differences in women's expectations of birth. *ABNF Journal, 27*(2), 39–43.

Nazik, E., & Eryilmaz, G. (2014). Incidence of pregnancy-related discomforts and management approaches to relieve them among pregnant women. *Journal of Clinical Nursing, 23*(11–12), 1736–1750.

Perlow, J. H., Jones, M., & Ozimek, J. (2015). Labor and delivery management of the obese gravida. In G. A. Macones (Ed.), *Management of labor and delivery* (2nd ed., 362–375). London, United Kingdom: Wiley.

Popat, H., Robledo, K. P., Sebastian, L., et al. (2016). Effect of delayed cord clamping on systemic blood flow: A randomized controlled trial. *The Journal of Pediatrics, 178*, 81.e2–86.e2.

Rouhe, H., Salmela-Aro, K., Toivanen, R., et al. (2015). Group psychoeducation with relaxation for severe fear of childbirth improves maternal adjustment and childbirth experience—a randomised controlled trial. *Journal of Psychosomatic Obstetrics & Gynecology, 36*(1), 1–9.

Simkin, P. (2010). The fetal occiput posterior position: State of the science and a new perspective. *Birth, 37*(1), 61–71.

Steel, A., Adams, J., Sibbritt, D., et al. (2014). The influence of complementary and alternative medicine use in pregnancy on labor pain management choices: Results from a nationally representative sample of 1,835 women. *Journal of Alternative & Complementary Medicine, 20*(2), 87–97.

Stephansson, O., Sandström, A., Petersson, G., et al. (2016). Prolonged second stage of labour, maternal infectious disease, urinary retention and other complications in the early postpartum period. *British Journal of Obstetrics and Gynaecology, 123*(4), 608–616.

Sun, C., Yue, J., He, N., et al. (2016). Fundamental principles of stem cell banking. *Advances in Experimental Medicine and Biology, 951*, 31–45.

U.S. Department of Health and Human Services. (2010). *Healthy people 2020.* Washington, DC: Author.

Vaziri, F., Arzhe, A., Asadi, N., et al. (2016). Spontaneous pushing in lateral position versus Valsalva maneuver during second stage of labor on maternal and fetal outcomes: A randomized clinical trial. *Iranian Red Crescent Medical Journal, 18*(10), e29279.

Vaziri, F., Farahmand, M., Samsami, A., et al. (2014). The effects of warm perineum compress during the second phase of labor on first-birth outcomes. *Modern Care Journal, 11*(1), 28–37.

World Health Organization. (2014). *The World Health Organization's infant feeding recommendation.* Retrieved from http://who.int/nutrition/topics/infantfeeding_recommendations/en/

Zhang, J., Landy, H., Branch, D., et al. (2010). Contemporary patterns of spontaneous labor with normal neonatal outcomes. *Obstetrics & Gynecology, 116*(6), 1281–1287.

16

The Nursing Role in Providing Comfort During Labor and Birth

*J*onny Baranca is a primipara in early labor whom you admit to a birthing unit. Her cervix is 3 cm dilated. She tells you her sister had epidural anesthesia that completely obliterated her pain in labor for the birth of her baby 3 months ago. Based on her sister's experience, Jonny expected to be given epidural anesthesia as soon as she arrived at the hospital as she "is in early labor." Her physician, however, asked her to wait until she is 4 cm dilated. When you enter her room, you find her lying on her back in a birthing bed, crying. Her husband shouts his "wife deserves better care than this."

The previous chapter discussed the process of labor and birth and nursing care responsibilities. This chapter adds information to your knowledge base about how to promote comfort during labor. Effective pain management in labor can change labor from an experience so negative it can result in a posttraumatic stress syndrome to a positive, forward-moving experience.

Was the information Jonny received from her sister realistic? What are some immediate interventions you could do to help Jonny better cope with her pain?

KEY TERMS

analgesia
anesthesia
doula
endorphins
epidural anesthesia

pain
pressure anesthesia
pudendal nerve block
reflexology

OBJECTIVES

After mastering the contents of this chapter, you should be able to:

1. Describe the physiologic basis of contractions during labor and how nonpharmacologic therapies, as well as analgesia and anesthesia, can be used to promote a woman's comfort during labor and birth.

2. Identify 2020 National Health Goals related to comfort and drug-free pain management measures effective in childbirth that nurses can help the nation achieve.

3. Assess the degree and type of discomfort a woman is experiencing during labor and birth, including her ability to cope with pain effectively and the maternal and fetal impact of pain management, including side effects and safety.

4. Formulate nursing diagnoses related to the effect of pain or pain management during labor and birth.

5. Establish expected outcomes to meet the needs of a woman experiencing discomfort during labor and birth and manage seamless transitions across differing healthcare settings.

6. Using the nursing process, plan nursing care that includes the six competencies of Quality & Safety Education for Nurses (QSEN): Patient-Centered Care, Teamwork & Collaboration, Evidence-Based Practice (EBP), Quality Improvement (QI), Safety, and Informatics.

7. Implement common complementary and pharmacologic measures for pain management during labor and birth.

8. Evaluate expected outcomes for effectiveness and achievement of care.

9. Integrate knowledge of pain management during labor and birth with the interplay of nursing process, the six competencies of QSEN, and Family Nursing to promote quality maternal and child health nursing care.

Concerns about the discomfort and pain that accompany labor and birth can dominate a pregnant woman's or couple's thoughts during pregnancy; these can become particularly strong as the baby's due date approaches. As discussed in Chapter 14, prepared childbirth classes provide couples with an opportunity to learn and practice a variety of pain management techniques, such as breathing patterns, to help reduce pain in labor.

Often, however, the labor experience is so intense it becomes overwhelming, so administration of an analgesic or a regional anesthetic may be necessary to reduce discomfort sufficiently to allow a woman to regain control over herself and use breathing patterns. If the use of regional anesthesia makes labor a satisfying, positive experience, the intervention can ultimately promote the entire family's health. Some women, however, may feel they have let down themselves, a partner, or childbirth educator by asking for anesthesia; if this happens, asking for pain medication can make labor a negative experience.

Much has been written in nursing literature about using the neutral term *contraction* or other alternative reference instead of *labor pain* to keep from reminding a woman contractions are painful. The theory is a sound one, not only because a woman is experiencing a *contracting* sensation but also because calling it *pain* could magnify fear and tension; tension, in turn, magnifies pain. Remember, however, renaming it will not change its basic nature. Discomfort accompanies labor regardless of what term is used for it. Fortunately, many nursing interventions can help reduce pain, so labor is as fulfilling and rewarding an experience as a woman hoped it would be.

Making labor and birth a memorable experience for families is so important that 2020 National Health Goals have been established to address this topic. These are shown in Box 16.1.

BOX 16.1
Nursing Care Planning Based on 2020 National Health Goals

Because administration of either analgesia or anesthesia during labor can prolong labor and can possibly increase the number of instruments used or risk for cesarean birth, several 2020 National Health Goals are related to the types of pain relief used in labor. Examples include:

- Reduce the maternal mortality rate to no more than 11.4 deaths per 100,000 live births from a baseline of 12.7 per 100,000.
- Reduce the fetal/newborn death rate during the perinatal period (28 weeks of gestation to 7 days after birth) to no more than 5.9 per 1,000 live births from a baseline of 6.6 per 1,000 live births (U.S. Department of Health and Human Services, 2010; see www.healthypeople.gov).

Nurses can help the nation achieve these goals by educating women about the advantages of preparing for childbirth, helping them to use breathing patterns or other complementary and alternative therapies and techniques during labor so they need a minimum of analgesia and anesthesia, and conscientiously monitoring women who receive analgesics and anesthesia.

Nursing Process Overview

FOR PAIN RELIEF DURING LABOR AND CHILDBIRTH

ASSESSMENT

Pain, the sensation of discomfort, is a subjective, personal symptom; it is what the experiencing person says it is and present when the experiencing person says it is present (McCaffery, 1972). It is unique to each individual, so a woman is the only person who can describe or know the extent of her pain. To assess the amount of discomfort a woman is having in labor, listen carefully to not only what she says but also how she rates her discomfort level on a pain assessment scale. Also look for subtle signs such as facial tenseness, flushing or paleness, hands clenched in fists, rapid breathing, or rapid pulse rate.

NURSING DIAGNOSIS

Although pain related to labor contractions is the most obvious nursing diagnosis applicable to labor, it is not the only relevant one because pain can create other problems for the laboring woman that can negatively affect the childbirth experience. If not resolved, these problems can intensify pain. Some women, for example, may become more concerned with their reaction to the pain than to the pain itself. Because of this, applicable nursing diagnoses might include:

- Pain related to labor contractions
- Powerlessness related to the duration and intensity of labor
- Anxiety related to lack of knowledge about "normal" labor process
- Risk for situational low self-esteem related to ineffectiveness of prepared childbirth breathing exercises
- Decisional conflict related to use of analgesia or anesthesia during labor

OUTCOME IDENTIFICATION AND PLANNING

When developing realistic outcomes and planning interventions to manage discomfort during labor, consider the woman's perceptions about childbirth, her past childbirth experiences (if any), and the amount and type of childbirth preparation she and her partner have made. For example, if a woman is using breathing exercises well, expecting she will need medication late in labor is probably not realistic. However, if a woman has not made any preparation as to how she will manage labor contractions, expecting that no medication will be used might be inappropriate.

Be aware that pharmacologic agents used during labor and birth may pose risks for both the woman, such as hypotension, as well as the fetus or neonate, such as bradycardia or respiratory issues at birth. Therefore, when considering use of pharmacologic intervention, the benefit to the woman and the fetus must outweigh the risks of medication use. In addition, a decision to use analgesia or anesthesia may also affect family functioning if the method chosen limits the partner's participation in the birth. Contrarily, the use of a pharmacologic agent may be what a woman could most benefit from, particularly if she has a history of sexual trauma (Nerum, Halvorsen, Straume, et al., 2013).

IMPLEMENTATION

Keeping a woman and her support person informed about their options and how they differ as labor progresses is important. For instance, simply knowing that birth is getting closer can make the next few contractions easier to withstand. Supporting and encouraging a woman to use methods of complementary and alternative therapies for pain management, such as a birthing ball, ambulation, relaxation, and breathing techniques, also are helpful. Offering analgesia or assisting with anesthesia administration during labor or birth requires nursing judgment and a caring presence to help one woman accept analgesia when she needs it and to encourage another to experience childbirth without pharmacologic intervention when that is what she desires.

OUTCOME EVALUATION

Evaluations are ongoing and typically must occur within a short time frame. Examples of short-term expected outcomes that would indicate successful achievement during labor are:

- Patient states pain during labor is within a tolerable level for her.
- Couple reports they feel control throughout the labor process.
- Patient and fetus remain physiologically stable with use of pharmacologic interventions.
- Patient verbalizes satisfaction with current pain control measures.

A long-term evaluation should reveal a woman found labor and birth to be an experience not only endurable but also that it allowed her to grow in self-esteem and the family to grow through a shared experience. Asking a woman to describe her labor experience afterward in relation to pain not only aids an evaluation of whether pain management was adequate but also helps her work through this emotional period of life and integrate it into her previous experiences as well.

Experience of Pain During Childbirth

Pain accompanies labor contractions for several different reasons and manifests itself in different ways for each woman (Box 16.2).

ETIOLOGY OF PAIN DURING LABOR AND BIRTH

Normally, contractions of involuntary muscles, such as the heart, stomach, and intestine, do not cause pain. This concept makes uterine contractions unique because they do cause pain. Several explanations exist for why this happens. During contractions, blood vessels constrict, reducing the blood supply to uterine and cervical cells, resulting in anoxia to muscle fibers. This anoxia can cause pain in the same way blockage of the cardiac arteries causes the pain of a heart attack. As labor progresses and contractions become longer and more intense, the ischemia to cells increases, the anoxia increases, and the pain intensifies.

Pain also probably results from stretching of the cervix and perineum. This phenomenon is the same as the intestinal pain that results when accumulating gas stretches the

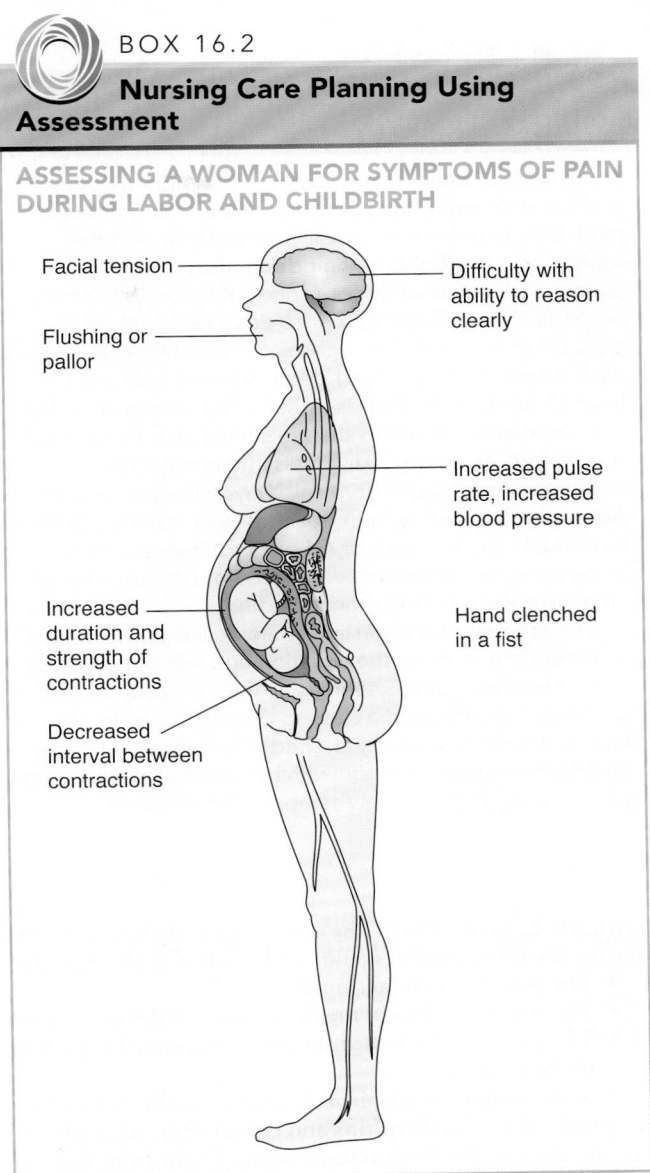

BOX 16.2

Nursing Care Planning Using Assessment

ASSESSING A WOMAN FOR SYMPTOMS OF PAIN DURING LABOR AND CHILDBIRTH

- Facial tension
- Flushing or pallor
- Increased duration and strength of contractions
- Decreased interval between contractions
- Difficulty with ability to reason clearly
- Increased pulse rate, increased blood pressure
- Hand clenched in a fist

intestines. At the end of the transitional phase in labor, when stretching of the cervix is complete and the woman feels she has to push, pain from the contractions often disappears as long as the woman is pushing, until the fetal presenting part causes a final stretching of the perineum.

Additional discomfort in labor may stem from the pressure of the fetal presenting part on tissues, including pressure on surrounding organs, such as the bladder, the urethra, and the lower colon. In addition to these factors, cultural expectations effect how pain is perceived (Box 16.3). All these factors make nursing support, in addition to a doula or a partner, important as it can have a positive influence on pain relief in all situations of labor.

PHYSIOLOGY OF PAIN

Pain is a basic protective mechanism that alerts a person that something threatening is happening somewhere in the body. The Melzack–Wall gate control theory of pain

Nursing Care Planning to Respect Cultural Diversity

Some women believe their expected role during labor is to be stoic and nonverbal even in the face of intense pain. Others believe expressing their discomfort by screaming or verbalizing their discomfort is what is expected. If a woman is not proficient in English, it may be particularly difficult for her to describe her level of discomfort and that she needs some assistance. Assess each woman individually to determine not only what level of comfort she feels is right for her during labor but also the manner in which she feels most able to express discomfort. Assessing individuals in this way rather than relying on a list of "typical" ways Hispanic women, Asian women, and so forth, react to pain achieves better individual care. Because of Americanization, a woman's surname or her appearance may be not be indicative at all of how she wants to manage pain.

The amount of analgesia women desire or will accept is dependent both on the situation and her culture. In a culture in which birth is seen as a "natural" process or if a woman has attended a class to prepare for birth, the less analgesia is generally desired. Any woman who has an effective support person with her generally needs less pharmacologic pain relief than one who does not.

pain relief. Some interventions relieve pain for both the first and second stages of labor, whereas others work for one stage but not both.

PERCEPTION OF PAIN

The amount of discomfort a woman experiences during contractions differs according to her expectations of and preparation for labor; the length of her labor; the position of her fetus; the presence of fear, anxiety, worry, body image, and self-efficacy; and the availability of meaningful people around her to offer support (Fig. 16.1). As a rule, women who believe they can control their situation (have self-efficacy) are more apt to report a satisfactory birth experience than those who do not feel in control (Howarth, Swain, & Treharne, 2011).

Fetal position is a physical variable that influences the degree of pain a woman experiences. If the fetus is in an occiput posterior position, the woman often reports intense or nagging back pain, even between contractions, much more than if a fetus is in an occipitoanterior position (Impey & Child, 2012).

Pain is perceived differently by different individuals because of psychosocial, physiologic, and cultural responses. The body's ability to produce and maintain endorphins may influence a person's overall pain threshold and the amount of pain a person perceives at any given time. Women who come into the labor experience believing the pain will be horrible are usually surprised afterward to realize the agony they expected never materialized. However, women who thought

(Melzack & Wall, 1965), the most widely accepted theory of pain response, proposes pain can be halted at three points:

- The peripheral end terminals
- The synapse points in the dorsal horn of the spinal cord
- The point at which the impulse is interpreted as pain in the brain cortex

Pain in peripheral terminals is automatically reduced by the production of **endorphins** and encephalins, naturally occurring opiates that limit transmission of pain from the end terminals. Pain can be reduced further at these end points by mechanically irritating nerve fibers through an action such as rubbing the skin, which blocks nerve transmission.

A major way to block spinal cord neurotransmitters (i.e., never allowing the pain impulse to cross to a spinal nerve) is by the administration of pain medications. In addition, the brain cortex can be distracted from sensing impulses as pain by such techniques as imagery, thought stopping, and perhaps aromatherapy or yoga.

Sensory impulses of pain from the uterus and cervix synapse at the spinal column at the level of T10 through L1, whereas motor impulses register higher in the cord at T5 through T10. Anesthetic pain relief measures for the first stage of labor, therefore, are designed to stop pain by blocking the lower sensory sites, but not the upper motor sites, so strong contractions can continue.

Sensory impulses from the perineum, which is involved in the second stage of labor, are carried by the pudendal nerve to join the spinal column at S2, S3, and S4. When the perineum is initiating the pain, anesthetic pain relief must block these lower receptor sites. This is an important point to remember when talking to a woman in labor about

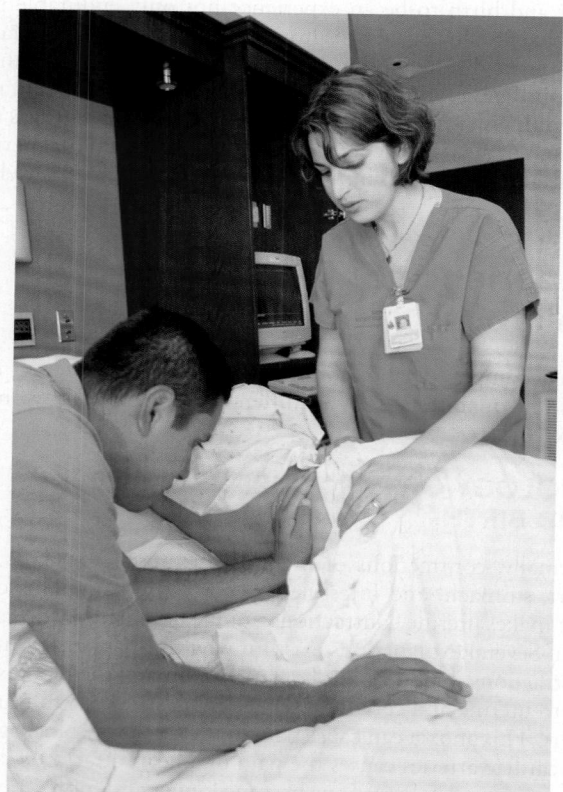

Figure 16.1 The discomfort a woman experiences during childbirth is related to the amount of support she receives from her family and healthcare providers. Here, the woman's support person uses the palm of his hand to apply counter pressure to her lower back, helping to ease back pain.

pain would be minimal can be overwhelmed by its intensity. Unrealistic expectations of labor pain can make a woman so tense during labor her pain feels worse than it would have if she had been relaxed. A woman cannot relax simply because she is instructed to do so by another person, however. Some additional interventions must be used.

Comfort and Nonpharmacologic Pain Relief Measures

The pattern of interventions to promote comfort and manage pain in labor has swung from a philosophy of no intervention (none given because pain in labor was expected), to a philosophy that drug intervention was always required (excessive amounts were given), to the modern approach of empowering women and their partners with information so they can choose how to best relieve pain during labor within the limits of medical safety.

Nurses play a key role in educating women and their support persons about the numerous comfort and pain relief strategies available and making sure certain couples understand the choices available to them along with the benefits and risks (L. Jones, Othman, Dowswell, et al., 2012). Throughout their decision-making process, couples need support for their choices so they can feel confident in the method they choose.

SUPPORT FROM A DOULA OR COACH

Although, historically, women have always attended other women in childbirth, in the past 45 years or so, the father or partner of a woman's child has traditionally served as her chief support person in labor. Some partners or fathers, however, find it difficult to serve as effective coaches because they are so emotionally involved in the birth. Some women prefer to ask a sister, mother, or friend to serve as a coach.

A **doula** is a woman who is experienced in childbirth and postpartum support. These support persons (who may hold certificates as birth or postpartum doulas) provide physical, emotional, and informational support prenatally, during labor and birth, and even at home in the postnatal period. Having an effective doula can increase a woman's self-esteem, speed the labor process, and improve breastfeeding success as well as decrease rates of oxytocin augmentation, epidural anesthesia, cesarean birth, and postpartum complications (Hodnett, Gates, Hormeyr, et al., 2013).

QSEN Checkpoint Question 16.1

PATIENT-CENTERED CARE

Jonny Baranca is having a painful labor. She asks the nurse if she should have hired a doula. The nurse identifies which answer as best?
   a. "Definitely. Doulas time contractions and perform many tasks, taking the burden off you."
   b. "Maybe. Doulas are good at telling you if you are doing everything correctly."
   c. "That's an individual choice, but a doula can serve as an important support person."
   d. "No. A second person giving advice is apt to cause conflict."

Look in Appendix A for the best answer and rationale.

COMPLEMENTARY AND ALTERNATIVE THERAPIES

Complementary and alternative therapies for pain relief involve nonpharmacologic measures that may be used either as a woman's total pain management program or to complement pharmacologic interventions. Most of these interventions are based on the gate control theory concept that distraction can be effective at preventing the brain from processing pain sensations coming into the cortex. Many of the same techniques may help the descent of a fetus. These may include the use of acupressure, position changes, imagery, and other relaxation techniques.

Relaxation

The technique of relaxation, as discussed in Chapter 14, is taught in most preparation for childbirth classes but can be taught in early labor as well. Relaxation keeps the abdominal wall from becoming tense, allowing the uterus to rise with contractions without pressing against the hard abdominal wall. It also serves as a distraction technique because, while concentrating on relaxing, a woman cannot concentrate on pain. Asking a woman to bring favorite music or aromatherapy with her to enjoy in the birthing room, although not evidence based, can help with relaxation. Remember, no aromatic candles should be used because of nearby oxygen outlets.

Focusing and Imagery

Concentrating intently on an object is another method of distraction, or another method of keeping sensory input from reaching the cortex of the brain (Smith, Levett, Collins, et al., 2011). For this technique, a woman uses a photograph of someone important to her or some setting she finds appealing such as a beautiful sunset. She concentrates on the photo during contractions (focusing). A woman can also concentrate on a mental image, such as waves rolling onto a beach (imagery), or chant a word or phrase such as the new baby's name during contractions, all of which help prevent her from concentrating on the pain of contractions. If a woman has never used these techniques before, she may question how effective they are. Urge her to try one of them at least for a few contractions before she dismisses them entirely, as evidence supports their efficacy (Hodnett et al., 2013). Do not ask questions or talk while a woman is using focusing, imagery, or chanting because that is apt to break her concentration and let the sensation of pain break through.

QSEN Checkpoint Question 16.2

EVIDENCE-BASED PRACTICE

To investigate if listening to music can help women feel less pain and anxiety in labor, researchers assigned 30 primiparas expected to have normal spontaneous births to either an experimental group that received routine labor care or a control group that received routine care plus music therapy. Both women and their nurses assessed the degree of pain experienced during labor. Results of the study revealed women who listened to music had significantly lower pain during the latent phase of labor (Simavli, Gumus, Kaygusuz, et al., 2014).

Based on this study, which statement by Jonny represents the best way to use music therapy in labor?
a. "I've brought techno music to play during the second stage so I can push to a rhythm."
b. "I'll need distraction most just before I have to push. I'll save my music until then."
c. "I know music probably won't make a difference but I'll enjoy listening to it anyway."
d. "I brought some romantic music to play during early labor to help me relax."

Look in Appendix A for the best answer and rationale.

Spirituality

For many women, prayer may be the first measure they use to relieve a stress they are facing (Abbaspoor, Moghaddam-Banaem, Ahmadi, et al., 2014). Provide uninterrupted time as needed. Women may bring helpful worship objects such as a Bible or Qur'an into their birthing setting to use during prayer. Remember, these are sacred objects; be careful when changing sheets that you do not accidentally throw such important objects away or let them fall to the floor.

Breathing Techniques

Breathing patterns are taught in most preparation for childbirth classes and are well documented to decrease pain in labor (Dick-Read & Gaskin, 2013). They are largely distraction techniques because a woman concentrating on slow-paced breathing cannot concentrate on pain. Breathing strategies can be taught to a woman in labor if she is not familiar with their advantages before labor (see Chapter 14). Stay with her until she appreciates how useful slow-paced breathing can be and feels comfortable using this technique independently.

Herbal Preparations

Several herbal preparations have traditionally been used to reduce pain with dysmenorrhea or labor, although there is little evidence-based support for their effectiveness. Examples include chamomile tea for its relaxing properties; raspberry leaf tea (women freeze it into ice cubes to suck on), which is thought to strengthen uterine contractions; skullcap; and catnip, which are thought to help with pain. Black cohosh (squawroot), an herb that induces uterine contractions, is not recommended because of the risk of acute toxic effects such as cerebrovascular accident to the mother or fetus (Ulbricht & Windsor, 2015).

Aromatherapy and Essential Oils

Aromatherapy is the use of aromatic oils to complement emotional and physical well-being. Their use is based on the principle that the sense of smell plays a significant role in overall health. When an essential oil is inhaled, its molecules are transported via the olfactory system to the limbic system in the brain. The brain then responds to particular aromas with emotional responses such as relaxation. These oils should not be applied directly to the skin to avoid irritation but are used in a mister so they are inhaled and then carried throughout the body. The oils may be able to penetrate cell walls and transport nutrients or oxygen to the inside of cells. The effects of aromatherapy can range from reducing postcesarean incisional pain to reducing anxiety in the first stage of labor (Fakari, Tabatabaeichehr, Kamali, et al., 2015; Metawie, Amasha, Abdraboo, et al., 2015; Roozbahani, Attarha, Akbari Torkestani, et al., 2015). The evidence regarding the efficacy of aromatherapy continues to be studied with mixed results.

QSEN Checkpoint Question 16.3

INFORMATICS

The nurse offers to teach Jonny controlled breathing to help with pain management until she can receive her epidural. Which instruction by the nurse would be best?
a. "Lie on your back and breathe in slowly while repeating, 'I can do this.'"
b. "Hold your breath as long as you possibly can before exhaling."
c. "Breathe in as slowly as you can and then breathe out just as slowly."
d. "Pant rapidly as this best lifts your abdominal wall off your expanding uterus."

Look in Appendix A for the best answer and rationale.

Heat or Cold Application

The application of heat and cold has always been used for pain relief after injuries such as minor burns or strained muscles. It is only lately that their use has been investigated as effective ways to help relieve the pain of labor. Women who are having back pain may find the application of heat to the lower back by a heating pad, instant hot pack, or warm moist compress extremely comforting. Heat applied to the perineum is proven to provide the dual benefits of soothing and softening the perineum and decreasing the risk of perineal tears (Aasheim, Nilsen, Lukasse, et al., 2011). Caution women if they are going to heat pads in a microwave to test the temperature of the pad on the forearm before applying it to their perineum. **Pressure anesthesia** (pressure to an area of the body that interferes with pain receptors) can dull sensation and, with an overheated pack, patients could sustain a perineal burn without realizing it.

Women who become warm from the exertion of labor find a cool washcloth to the forehead, chest, or back of the neck comforting. Sucking on ice chips to relieve mouth dryness is also refreshing. Immediately following birth, an ice pack applied to the perineum feels soothing, and it helps reduce edema and swelling. Cultural differences exist with preference to heat and cold. This may be evident in dietary choices or compress application (Goyal, 2016). It is imperative that nurses to provide care that is culturally competent and respectful of the practices of their patients.

Bathing or Hydrotherapy

Standing under a warm shower or soaking in a tub of warm water, jet hydrotherapy tub, or whirlpool is another way to apply heat to help reduce the pain of labor (Fig. 16.2) (Harper, 2014). The temperature of water used should be 37°C to prevent hyperthermia of the woman and also the newborn at birth.

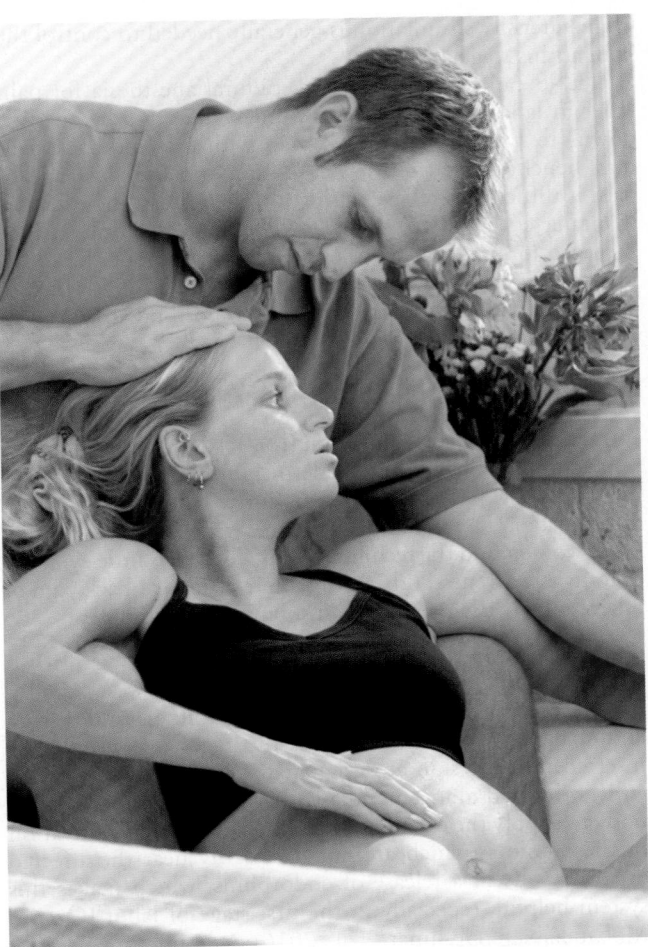

Figure 16.2 A woman in labor enjoys the soothing effects of a warm water bath.

Remind women that plastic or porcelain tubs are slippery, so they should ask for help stepping into and out of them. Do not leave women unsupervised in a tub as they could slip and have difficulty getting their head above water. A support person can join the woman in a tub or shower if she wishes and can continue with back massage or other measures she finds soothing. Timing of contractions, auscultation of fetal heart rate, and vaginal examinations can all be done without the woman needing to leave the water. The birth environment, including the use of hydrotherapy in labor, can help support physiologic birth (Stark, Remynse, & Zwelling, 2016).

Therapeutic Touch and Massage

In a classic work, Krieger (1990) defined therapeutic touch as the laying on of hands to redirect energy fields that lead to pain. It is based on the concept that everyone's body contains energy fields that, when plentiful, lead to health or, when in low supply, result in illness.

Effleurage, the technique of gentle abdominal massage often taught with Lamaze in preparation for childbirth classes is a classic example of therapeutic touch (see Chapter 14, Fig. 14.8). *Reiki* can also promote healing. The term Reiki consists of two Japanese words: *rei*, which means "God's wisdom or the higher power," and *ki*, which means "life force energy." So Reiki is actually "spiritually guided life force energy."

The technique includes "laying on of hands" and is based on the theory that an unseen "life force energy" flows through us and is what causes us to be alive (Rakestraw, 2010). If one's life force energy is low, then a person is more likely to get sick or feel stress. If it is high, a person is more capable of being happy and healthy.

Although the effectiveness of therapeutic touch is not well documented, both touch and massage probably work to relieve pain by increasing the release of endorphins. Both techniques may also work because they serve as forms of distraction. Many women find massage, especially of the lower back or feet, helpful in the first and second stages of labor (L. Jones et al., 2012; Smith et al., 2012).

QSEN Checkpoint Question 16.4

SAFETY

Jonny asks the nurse if she could safely use warm water tub bathing during labor. Which answer by the nurse would be best?

   a. "No. The chilling that sometimes results can lead to hypothermia."

   b. "Yes, as long as your membranes are not ruptured."

   c. "No. This technique will separate you from your partner."

   d. "Yes, as long as you know warm water has no significant effect."

Look in Appendix A for the best answer and rationale.

Yoga and Meditation

Yoga, a term derived from the Sanskrit word for "union," describes a series of exercises that were originally designed to bring people closer to a divine power. It offers a significant variety of proven health benefits, including increasing the efficiency of the heart, slowing the respiratory rate, improving fitness, lowering blood pressure, promoting relaxation, reducing stress, and allaying anxiety. Exercises consist of deep breathing exercises, body postures to stretch and strengthen muscles, and meditation to focus the mind and relax the body. It may be helpful in reducing the pain of labor through its ability to relax the body and possibly through the release of endorphins. Mothers who engage in yoga prenatally have been shown to have a greater sense of self-efficacy and may experience fewer episodes of antenatal depression (Battle, Uebelacker, Magee, et al., 2015; Schwartz, Toohill, Creedy, et al., 2015).

Meditation is a self-directed practice for relaxing the body and calming the mind. Mindfulness-based stress reduction (MBSR), an 8-week intervention program developed by Dr. John Kabat Zinn for patients dealing with issues of chronic pain, is based on the cultivation of intentional awareness of experiences in the present moment. Transcendental meditation (TM) is a simple, natural, and effortless activity done while resting comfortably with the eyes closed. Using one of these techniques, an individual experiences a state of deep rest that can change physical and emotional responses to stress (Chan, 2016). Women can meditate in any position. Do not interrupt a woman using meditation as a pain relief technique if at all possible in order to not break her concentration.

Reflexology

Reflexology is the practice of stimulating the hands, feet, and ears as a form of therapy (Smith, Levett, Collins, et al., 2012). Professional reflexologists apply pressure to specific areas of the hands, feet, and ears to alleviate common ailments such as headache, back pain, sinus colds, and stress. The theory behind reflexology holds that the body is divided into 10 zones that run in longitudinal lines from the top of the head to the tips of the toes. Each of the body's organs and glands is linked to corresponding areas of the hands and feet. Application of pressure to a specific area aims to restore energy to the body and improve the overall condition. The point that corresponds to the uterus is located on the inside ankle about halfway between the ankle bone (malleolus) and the heel. Massaging this area is believed to begin labor or hurry labor, thus creating less pain.

Hypnosis

Hypnosis is yet another method that can be used for pain relief in labor. A woman who wants to use this modality needs to meet with her hypnotherapist during pregnancy. At these visits, she is evaluated for and conditioned for susceptibility to hypnotic suggestion. Close to her last weeks of pregnancy, she is given a posthypnotic suggestion that she will experience a reduction in or absence of pain during labor. Fully awake and able to participate in labor, the woman who is susceptible to hypnotic suggestion may find this may provide a very satisfactory and drug-free method of pain relief (Streibert, Reinhard, Yuan, et al., 2015). A woman who wants to use this system but began labor before the posthypnotic suggestion was given may be very disappointed to find herself in labor without the help she envisioned. Some hypnotists may visit during labor or supply the suggestion over the telephone so a woman can still use the method. Further research is needed to determine the effectiveness of the effects of hypnosis on pain relief in labor (Madden, Middleton, Cyna, et al., 2016).

Biofeedback

Biofeedback is based on the belief that people have control and can regulate internal events such as heart rate and pain responses. Women who are interested in using biofeedback for pain relief in labor must attend several sessions during pregnancy to condition themselves to regulate their pain response. During these sessions, a biofeedback apparatus is used to measure muscle tone or the woman's ability to relax. Evidence is continuing to emerge that shows biofeedback is an effective method for reducing the pain of labor (Janula & Mahipal, 2015).

Transcutaneous Electrical Nerve Stimulation

Transcutaneous electrical nerve stimulation (TENS) works to relieve pain by applying counterirritation to nociceptors (Santana, Gallo, Ferreira, et al., 2016). When two pairs of electrodes are attached to a woman's back to coincide with the T10 through L1 nerve pathways, low-intensity electrical stimulation is given continuously or is applied by the woman herself as a contraction begins. This stimulation blocks the afferent fibers, preventing pain from traveling to the spinal cord synapses from the uterus. As labor and descent progress, the electrodes are moved to stimulate the S2 through S4 level.

High-intensity stimulation is generally needed to control the pain at this stage.

TENS can be as effective as epidural anesthesia for pain relief in labor, although some women object to being "tied down" to the equipment. Women with extreme back pain may benefit most from a TENS unit because this type of pain is difficult to relieve with controlled breathing exercises (Santana et al., 2016). This method may not only reduce the need for epidural anesthesia but also postpone the use of pharmacologic agents (Santana et al., 2016). TENS is further discussed in Chapter 24 as it applies to postoperative pain of a cesarean birth.

Intracutaneous Nerve Stimulation

Intracutaneous nerve stimulation (INS) is a technique of counterirritation involving the intradermal injection of sterile water or saline along the borders of the sacrum to relieve low back pain during labor (Derry, Straube, Moore, et al., 2012). Although some women find the technique helpful, there is little evidence as to its effectiveness; other women prefer to bear back pain or relieve it by massage rather than submit to injections.

Acupuncture and Acupressure

Acupuncture is based on the concept that illness results from an imbalance of energy. To correct the imbalance, needles are inserted into the skin at designated susceptible body points (*tsubos*) located along meridians that course throughout the body to supply the organs of the body with energy. Activation of these points (which are not necessarily near the affected organ) results in a release of endorphins, which makes this system helpful, especially in the first stage of labor (Ozgoli, Mobarakabadi, Heshmat, et al., 2016). Acupuncture may also decrease the duration of labor (Asadi, Maharlouei, Khalili, et al., 2015).

Acupressure is the application of pressure or massage at these same points. It seems to be most effective for low back pain. A common point used for women in labor is Co4 (*Hoku* or *Hegu* point), which is located between the first finger and thumb on the back of the hand. Women may report their contractions feel lighter when a support person holds and squeezes their hand because the support person is accidentally triggering this point. Acupressure can reduce maternal anxiety as well as the length of labor when specific pressure points are used (Akbarzadeh, Masoudi, Zare, et al., 2015).

> *What If . . . 16.1*
>
> The nurse had met Jonny during pregnancy and discovered she did not attend any preparation for childbirth classes because she planned to rely totally on epidural anesthesia for pain relief. Would the nurse have supported her plan? Now that she is in early labor, what are some complementary and alternative therapies the nurse could teach her to use while she waits for anesthesia?

PHARMACOLOGIC MEASURES FOR PAIN RELIEF DURING LABOR

The discovery of ether and chloroform in the 1800s led to the determination that childbirth could be managed relatively pain free. Unfortunately, this goal was achieved by means of complete anesthesia or unconsciousness for the woman during labor and birth. Women, afterward, had difficulty believing the birth was over and that the infant was their child.

This led to an era (late 1960s to the 1980s) in which women refused pharmacologic pain relief in labor and depended entirely on prepared childbirth measures such as breathing patterns. Since the advent of epidural anesthesia, women now have more options regarding how much or what kind of pain relief they want in labor (Anim-Somuah, Smyth, & Jones, 2011).

Pharmacologic management of pain during labor and birth includes **analgesia**, which reduces or decreases awareness of pain, and **anesthesia**, which causes partial or complete loss of pain sensation. For the best results, be certain women are included in the selection of these methods and understand any fetal effects or maternal side effects that might occur.

Virtually all medications given during labor cross the placenta and have some effect on the fetus, which makes it important to do regular assessments of maternal and fetal responses to the administration of systemic medication. However, labor should not test a woman to the limit of her endurance because both analgesia and anesthesia are available. Be sure to caution women not to take acetylsalicylic acid (aspirin) for pain in labor as aspirin interferes with blood coagulation, increasing the risk for bleeding in the newborn or herself. In addition, the manufacturers of pain relief patches such as Salonpas, Absorbine Jr., and Icy Hot caution women not to use these in labor because of the potentially teratogenic effect of the menthol ingredient.

The best approach to pain management for women in labor is to always aid any pharmacologic intervention with a complementary or alternative therapy measure. For example, an intramuscular analgesic can be linked with breathing exercises to make both more effective.

Goals of Pharmacologic Pain Management During Labor

The ideal or goal of medications used during labor is to relax a woman and relieve her discomfort and yet have minimal systemic effects on uterine contractions, her pushing effort, or the fetus (Box 16.4). Whether a drug affects a fetus depends on its ability to cross the placenta and that depends on its molecular weight. Drugs with a molecular weight of less than 600 Da cross very readily; drugs with a molecular weight of

more than 1,000 Da cross poorly. Drugs with highly charged molecules or molecules strongly bound to protein also tend to cross more slowly than others. Fat-soluble drugs cross the easiest.

If a drug causes a systemic response, such as hypotension in a woman, it can result in a decreased oxygen (PO_2) gradient across the placenta, causing the indirect result of fetal hypoxia. If a drug causes confusion or disorientation, a woman may be unable to work effectively with contractions, thus prolonging labor and increasing discomfort for her. A preterm fetus, which has an immature liver and is unable to metabolize or inactivate drugs, is generally more affected by drugs than a term fetus. If a medication causes changes in a fetus, such as a decreased heart rate or central nervous system (CNS) depression, it may be difficult for the newborn infant to initiate respirations at birth, severely compromising the infant in the important first minutes of life. In addition, if a drug reduces or eliminates the bearing down reflex, a woman may have difficulty pushing effectively, which may prolong the second stage and increase the risk for a cesarean birth.

Lastly, because pain is a subjective sensation, some women are most aware of pain early in labor, whereas some report the second stage of labor as the most difficult. The point at which pain medication is needed, therefore, differs from one individual to another and should be given at whatever point an individual woman feels she needs it. When labor is in the active phase of the first stage, medication to relieve discomfort tends to speed labor progress because, with the pain gone, a woman can relax and work with, not against, her contractions. In contrast, at the second stage, epidural anesthesia or a drug that disorients a woman can slow progress and may result in more instrumentation or cesarean births. For all these reasons, no perfect analgesic agent exists for labor or birth that has no effect on labor, the mother, or the fetus.

Preparation for Medication Administration

The type of medication used during labor varies among different healthcare providers and also changes based on new research as the effectiveness and safety of new drugs for use during labor are tested. To be safe, follow The Joint Commission's *2016 National Patient Safety Goals* (The Joint Commission, 2016) and remember the criteria a drug must fulfill to be used in pregnancy at any point. Never give a drug to a pregnant woman unless you know the benefit outweighs

BOX 16.4
Nursing Care Planning Based on Family Teaching

Q. Jonny asks you, "Can I choose what medicine I want to use in labor for pain or do I have to do whatever my doctor says?"

A. A number of helpful rules about pain in labor are:

- You have the right to choose how much pharmacologic pain relief you want to use.
- It's best if analgesia and anesthesia are begun after labor is well established, although this should be balanced against the need for pain relief.
- Any drug used should provide maximum relief for you and have minimal effect on your fetus.
- Constant fetal and maternal monitoring should be available, although periodic monitoring is acceptable.
- Any medicine given should not interfere with the ability of your uterus to contract during labor or interfere with contraction after labor to prevent uterine hemorrhage.

the risk for both of your patients: the mother and the fetus. Be certain to ask about allergies to all medications before administering them during labor as women in distress from pain can be too distracted to mention this unless directly asked.

Prepare a woman for the type of agent prescribed, how it will be administered with an explanation such as "You'll need to lie on your side" as well as what she can expect to happen after administration ("I'll be taking your blood pressure frequently"). Women in labor are under a lot of stress. That can make experiencing surprising body sensations from a drug without preparation about the effects that may occur so frightening it can defeat their individual coping ability and any relaxation potential associated with it.

Opioid (Narcotic) Analgesics

Narcotics may be given during labor because of their potent effect, but all drugs in this category cause maternal respiratory depression as well as fetal CNS depression to some extent and so should be used cautiously (Brimdyr, Cadwell, Widström, et al., 2015).

Timing the administration of narcotics during labor is especially important as, if given too early (before 3 cm cervical dilatation), they tend to slow labor. If given close to birth, because the fetal liver takes 2 to 3 hours to activate a drug, the effect will not be registered in the fetus for 2 to 3 hours after birth. For this reason, narcotics are preferably given when the mother is more than 3 hours away from birth. This allows the peak action of the drug in the fetus to have passed by the time of birth so the newborn breathes easily.

It can be puzzling to see a sleepy baby born to a woman who was given butorphanol tartrate 2 hours before birth, for example, and an alert baby delivered to a woman who had the same drug within 1 hour of birth. In the second instance, the peak action or peak effect has not yet occurred in the infant. This newborn needs careful assessment for the next 4 hours until the drug does reach its peak.

Common opioid analgesics used in labor traditionally include butorphanol tartrate (Stadol), morphine sulfate, nalbuphine (Nubain), meperidine (Demerol), and fentanyl (Sublimaze). None of these drugs completely eliminate the pain of contractions, but they do reduce pain sensation to a level where other nonpharmacologic methods of pain relief can begin to be effective. They all begin to work 15 to 30 minutes after intramuscular administration or about 5 minutes after intravenous (IV) administration. A drawback to all these opioids is they may cause nausea and vomiting in some women. These effects appear to be dose-related (Armstrong & Fernando, 2016). They also produce a feeling of euphoria, so women often report they feel as if they are "floating"; because of this sensation, they may feel they have lost control or are unable to breathe effectively with contractions. Routes of administration and common side effects are shown in Table 16.1.

Because of the fetal effects, whenever a narcotic is given during labor, a narcotic antagonist such as naloxone hydrochloride (Narcan) should be available for administration to the infant at birth if needed (Box 16.5). Carefully observe any infant who received naloxone hydrochloride in the immediate postpartum period because the infant's respirations may become severely depressed again when the drug's effect wears off (Karch, 2013). If severe infant respiratory depression is anticipated, naloxone hydrochloride can be given to a woman

just before birth. It readily crosses the placenta and, because it interferes with or competes for narcotic binding sites, may increase the chance for spontaneous respiratory activity in the newborn.

What If . . . 16.2

Jonny receives no narcotics during labor, yet her newborn is born very sleepy. Would the nurse administer naloxone hydrochloride? Would asking Jonny if she uses recreational drugs be warranted in order to discover the cause of newborn respiratory depression?

Additional Drugs

Additional drugs, such as tranquilizers, may be administered during labor to reduce anxiety or potentiate the action of a narcotic. An example of such a drug is hydroxyzine hydrochloride (Vistaril). These drugs do not relieve pain, so the woman in labor needs pain management measures in addition to these drugs.

Nitrous Oxide

Nitrous oxide inhalation has been widely used in Europe for effective pain relief in labor. In the United States, it is beginning to be used more prevalently. In the past, this method had resulted in adverse neonatal outcomes such as brain cell apoptosis leading to developmental impairment. There was also concern about caregiver and maternal exposure. Over the past decade, nitrous oxide has made a comeback in the United States. Research by Rooks (2011) has shown that in appropriate doses (≤50% blend with oxygen) and with a proper and now standard delivery system, nitrous oxide can be safe for mother, fetus, neonate, and caregivers. It does not affect the pattern or intensity of contractions and does not interfere with normal labor. Apgar scores in neonates whose mothers used nitrous oxide do not significantly differ from those who used other forms of pharmacologic pain relief, or no analgesia (Likis, Andrews, Collins, et al., 2014).

Regional (Local) Anesthesia

Regional anesthesia is the injection of a local anesthetic such as chloroprocaine (Nesacaine) or bupivacaine (Marcaine) to block specific nerve pathways (Anim-Somuah et al., 2011). This achieves pain relief by blocking sodium and potassium transport in the nerve membrane, thereby stabilizing the nerve in a polarized resting state so the nerve is unable to conduct sensations.

Various regional anesthetic injection sites are shown in Figure 16.3. Any woman with a bleeding defect, such as those that may occur with preeclampsia, need to be assessed carefully before regional anesthesia is administered to prevent bleeding at the injection site.

Regional anesthetics have the potential to result in fetal bradycardia. This is not due to the transmission of the drug from maternal to fetal circulation but rather secondary to the effects of maternal hypotension following administration of the medication. This may resolve spontaneously, with position change or with the administration of additional medication (Mohta, Aggarwal, Sethi, et al., 2016). The effects of epidurals on breastfeeding show mixed and contradictory results in the literature (French, Cong, & Chung, 2016).

TABLE 16.1 ANALGESICS AND ANESTHETICS COMMONLY USED IN LABOR AND BIRTH

Type	Drug	Method of Administration	Effect on Mother	Effect on Labor Progress	Effect on Fetus or Newborn
Narcotic analgesic	Butorphanol tartrate (Stadol)	Intramuscular or intravenous	Effective analgesic; withdrawal symptoms if woman is opiate dependent	Possible slowing of labor if given early	Results in some respiratory depression
	Nalbuphine (Nubain)	Intramuscular or intravenous	Effective analgesic; slowing of respiratory rate	Mild maternal sedation	Results in some respiratory depression
	Morphine sulfate	Intrathecal prior to epidural anesthesia	Pruritus; effective analgesia	Possible slowing of labor contractions	Some respiratory depression
	Fentanyl (Sublimaze)	Intravenous	Hypotension; respiratory depression	Slowing of labor if given early	May result in respiratory depression
Lumbar epidural block	Local anesthetic Bupivacaine (Marcaine) Ropivacaine (Naropin)	Injected by anesthesiologist or nurse anesthetist at L3–L4 for first stage of labor; with continuous block, anesthesia will last through birth; fentanyl or morphine possibly added to cerebral spinal fluid first	Rapid onset in minutes lasting 60–90 min; loss of pain perception for labor contractions and birth; possible maternal hypotension	Slowing of labor if given too early; pushing feeling is obliterated, resulting in possible prolonged second stage	May be some differences in response in first few days of life
Pudendal block	Local anesthetic Lidocaine (Xylocaine)	Administered just before birth for perineal anesthesia; injected through vagina	Rapid anesthesia of perineum	None apparent	None apparent
Local infiltration of perineum	Local anesthetic Lidocaine (Xylocaine)	Injected just before episiotomy incision	Anesthesia of perineum almost immediately	None apparent	None apparent
General anesthetic	Thiopental sodium	Intravenous by anesthesiologist or nurse-anesthetist	Rapid anesthesia; also rapid recovery	Forceps required because abdominal pushing is no longer possible	Results in infant being born with central nervous system depression

Source: Karch, A. M. (2013). *2013 Lippincott's nursing drug guide*. Philadelphia, PA: Lippincott Williams & Wilkins.

BOX 16.5

Nursing Care Planning Based on Responsibility for Pharmacology

NALOXONE HYDROCHLORIDE (NARCAN)

Action: Naloxone hydrochloride is a narcotic antagonist that counteracts the effect of narcotic analgesics (Karch, 2013). It is used to counteract respiratory depression in newborns when a woman has received a narcotic analgesic during labor.

Pregnancy Risk Category: B

Dosage: 0.01 mg/kg, administered either intravenously via umbilical vein, subcutaneously, or intramuscularly; repeated at 2- to 3-minute intervals until a response is obtained

Possible Adverse Effects: Hypotension, hypertension, tachycardia, diaphoresis, tremulousness

Nursing Implications

- Anticipate the need for newborn resuscitative measures including the use of naloxone hydrochloride; have resuscitative equipment and emergency drugs readily available.
- If no intravenous access is available, prepare for possible administration via endotracheal tube.
- If no response is seen after two or three doses, question whether the respiratory depression is caused by maternal narcotic administration.
- Continuously monitor all vital signs for changes.
- Remember that the pain-relieving effect of a narcotic will be reversed as the narcotic is cleared from the baby's system; assess for pain in the neonate if a narcotic was given for pain relief.

Local
infiltration
of perineum

Pudendal
block

Pia mater
Arachnoid
Dura mater

Spinal cord
Ligamentum flavum

Subarachnoid space
Epidural space

Lumbar epidural block
Low spinal block
Saddle block

Figure 16.3   Anatomy of the spinal canal and sites of injection for regional anesthesia.

Most importantly, regional anesthesia is able to completely eliminate pain yet allow a woman to be completely awake and aware of what is happening during birth. It can make pushing with second stage labor more difficult, but it does not depress uterine tone, so the uterus remains capable of optimal contraction after birth, thereby helping to prevent postpartal hemorrhage.

In the rare event an infant is born with symptoms of toxicity from a regional anesthetic, an exchange transfusion at birth will remove the anesthetic from the infant's bloodstream. Gastric lavage also will remove a great deal of anesthetic because anesthetics have a strong affinity for acid media, such as stomach acid.

Epidural Anesthesia

The nerves in the spinal cord are protected by several tissue layers.

- The *pia mater* is the membrane adhering to the nerve fibers.
- Surrounding this is the *cerebrospinal fluid* (CSF).
- Next comes the arachnoid membrane and, outside that, the *dura mater*.
- Outside the dura mater is a vacant space (the *epidural space*).
- Beyond it is the *ligamentum flavum*, yet another protective shield for the vulnerable spinal cord (see Fig. 16.3).

An anesthetic agent introduced into the CSF in the subarachnoid space is *spinal injection* or *spinal anesthesia*. An anesthetic agent placed just inside the ligamentum flavum in the epidural space is called **epidural anesthesia**. Anesthetic agents placed in the epidural space at the L4–L5, L3–L4, or L2–L3 interspace block not only spinal nerve roots in the space but also the sympathetic nerve fibers that travel with them. Therefore, these blocks can provide pain relief during both labor and birth. Because a woman no longer experiences

pain, the release of catecholamines (epinephrine) with a β-blocking effect from a pain response is decreased, making this a very effective pain relief measure for labor (Impey & Child, 2012).

Epidural blocks are suitable for almost all women. They are advantageous for women with heart disease, pulmonary disease, diabetes, and sometimes severe gestational hypertension because they make labor virtually pain free and thereby reduce stress from the discomfort of labor. Because the woman does not feel contractions, her physical energy is preserved. Epidural blocks are acceptable for use in preterm labor because the drug has scant effect on a fetus and allows for a controlled and gentle birth with lessened trauma to an immature fetal skull. Because the woman receives no systemic medication, the infant responds more quickly after birth than if systemic narcotic analgesics were used.

The chief concern with epidural anesthesia is its tendency to cause hypotension because of its blocking effect on the sympathetic nerve fibers in the epidural space. This blocking leads to decreased peripheral resistance in the woman's circulatory system. Decreased peripheral resistance causes blood to flow freely into peripheral vessels, and a pseudohypovolemia develops, which registers as hypotension. This risk can be reduced by being certain a woman is well hydrated with 500 to 1,000 ml of IV fluid, such as Ringer's lactate, before the anesthetic is administered. Ringer's lactate is preferable to a glucose solution because too much maternal glucose can cause hyperglycemia with rebound hypoglycemia in the newborn. Be certain a woman does not lie supine after an epidural block but remains on her side to help prevent supine hypotension syndrome.

If hypotension should occur, raising the woman's legs and administering oxygen and additional IV fluid along with an antihypotensive agent such as ephedrine to elevate blood pressure may be necessary to stabilize cardiovascular status. This is an emergency because if the woman is severely hypotensive, blood is shunted away from the uterus and leads to poor perfusion of the placenta, eventually causing fetal distress.

A disadvantage of epidural anesthesia is that the bearing down reflex may be reduced or absent, making it difficult for a woman to push effectively. This may delay fetal descent, thus prolonging the second stage of labor and leading to an increased number of instrument-assisted births (Schrock & Harraway-Smith, 2012). A second stage delay this way occurs primarily when the fetus is in an occipitoposterior position. Changing the woman's position (e.g., to all fours) to help fetal rotation can be helpful to aid descent. For both of these situations, allowing an epidural to wear off by the second stage of labor so that a woman can push with contractions is another option. If this is unsuccessful, an oxytocin IV to help strengthen contractions can be administered. Many women are understandably overwhelmed and disappointed if the epidural is allowed to wear off; the excellent pain control they had may make the return of contraction pain seem extreme. Encouragement and use of nonpharmacologic methods will be critical nursing interventions at this time.

In rare instances, the anesthetic enters the woman's blood circulation instead of settling into the epidural space. Drowsiness, a metallic taste on the tongue, slurred speech, blurred vision, unconsciousness, and seizure, which may lead to cardiac arrest, are alerts this has happened and, again, is an emergency situation. The woman needs oxygen and an anticonvulsant, such as diazepam (Valium) or thiopental sodium (Pentothal) IV, followed by the prompt birth of the fetus to protect the health of the woman and the fetus.

Technique for Administration

Epidural blocks are usually delayed until a woman's cervix is dilated 3 to 5 cm as earlier administration may slow the first stage of labor. Be certain an infusion of Ringer's lactate solution is begun preprocedure and that equipment for blood pressure monitoring is in place and functioning. Help position the woman on her side on her birthing bed. If she curves her back outward, this increases the intravertebral spaces and allows easier access to the injection site.

An epidural block may consist of only an anesthetic injection into the epidural space or a combined method where a low-dose anesthetic is injected into the epidural space and a small dose of an analgesic such as fentanyl is also injected into the CSF space. This combination of drugs and technique is advantageous because it results in a "walking" or "mobile" block, which produces anesthesia up to the level of the umbilicus in 10 to 15 minutes that will last for approximately 40 minutes to 2 hours (Schrock & Harraway-Smith, 2012). Its second advantage is that it allows a woman to move about and walk while anesthesia is in effect. A catheter is left in place attached to a syringe to allow for repeated injections without further injection pain (Fig. 16.4).

Assess a woman's pulse and blood pressure following the injection. Observe for toxic symptoms of hypotension, slurred speech, and rapid pulse, which would occur if the anesthetic was accidentally placed into a blood vessel and not the hollow epidural space. Be certain to review agency policy regarding catheter care before caring for a person with a catheter in place to prevent infection at the site. Proper gowning is encouraged prior to administration for colonization reduction (Siddiqui, Davies, McGeer, et al., 2014).

An epidural block provides anesthesia for uterine contractions but not perineal relaxation. Close to birth, if the woman sits up and an additional dose of anesthesia is added to the catheter, perineal anesthesia will result as well. Leaving the lower anesthesia for late in labor this way is thought to allow for better internal rotation of the fetal head because the perineal muscle is not lax, creating a lessened need for forceps for rotation.

Aftercare for the Woman With an Epidural Anesthesia

Following anesthetic administration, be certain a woman lies on her side, or if on her back, she should place a firm towel under her left hip to avoid hypotension from poor blood

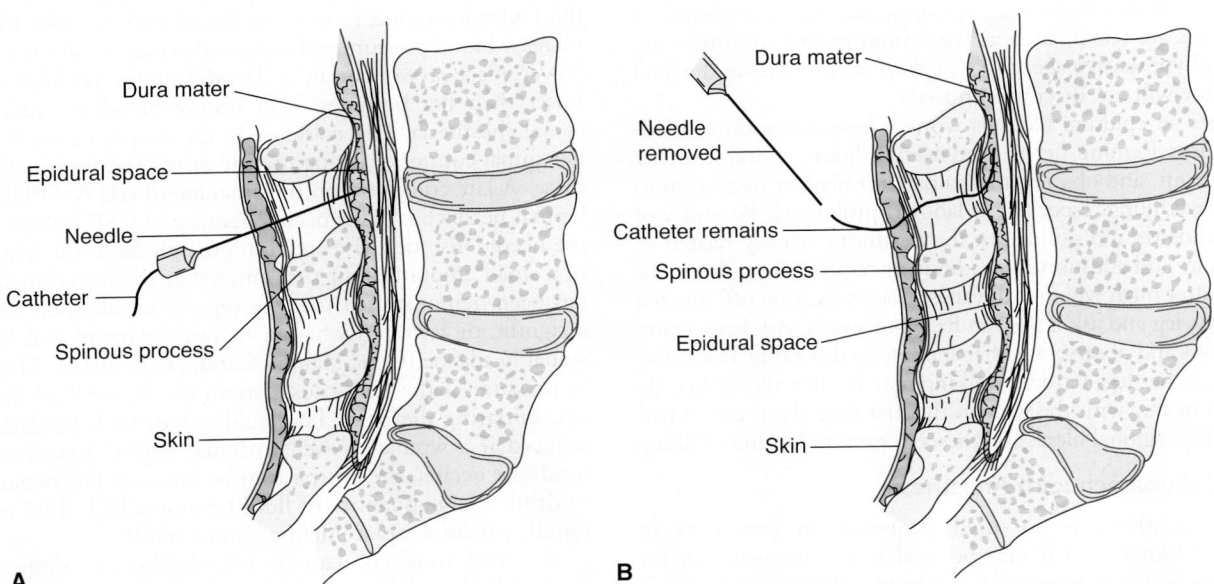

A   **B**

Figure 16.4 Epidural anesthesia. **(A)** A needle is inserted into the epidural space. **(B)** A catheter is threaded into the space; the needle is then removed. The catheter allows medication to be administered intermittently or continuously to relieve pain during labor and childbirth.

return to the heart. To keep her free from discomfort during the duration of labor, anesthetic can be continually infused by an infusion pump, or other doses of anesthetic, termed "top-ups," can be added at intervals. Both techniques are equal in their effect on length of labor, although continuous administration may result in more cesarean births because of difficulty pushing and fetal descent (Siddiqui et al., 2014).

Each time, before an additional top-up dose is administered, ask the woman to say out loud a phrase such as "I can do it" three times. If she is unable to do this, question the dose; lack of fine motor coordination and slurred speech can indicate a slowly occurring toxic reaction.

Yet another technique used to maintain epidural anesthesia is self-administration or patient-controlled epidural analgesia (PCEA). With this technique, following a lockout period when no more anesthetic can be administered to avoid overdosing, an analgesic mixture is delivered whenever the patient presses a button on a PCEA pump (Jokinen, Weibel, Afshari, et al., 2015). This method of administration is advantageous because less anesthetic is required compared with continuous epidural infusion (CEI) and can give the woman a feeling of empowerment as she controls her own pain management.

A nurse should be in continuous attendance as long as epidural anesthesia is being used. When recording vital signs, be aware epidural anesthesia can cause a temporary elevation in temperature, which is not serious unless it rises above 101°F (Sultan, David, Fernando, et al., 2016).

Possible complications that can occur from epidural blocks include hypotension, pruritus (especially if morphine was used), urinary retention, nausea and vomiting, and, rarely, a postpartal dural puncture headache (PDPH) (because the subarachnoid space was entered for the analgesic injection).

To detect if hypotension is occurring, continuously monitor blood pressure for the first 20 minutes after each new injection of anesthetic. Continue to periodically monitor blood pressure throughout the time the anesthetic is in effect to be certain the woman's systolic pressure does not fall to less than 100 mmHg or decrease by 20 mmHg or more in a hypertensive woman. A drop greater than this could be life-threatening to a fetus unless prompt and effective corrective measures are taken, such as repositioning and administering an antihypotensive agent (e.g., ephedrine) to ensure the fetal outcome will not be compromised.

After an epidural block, a woman loses sensation of bladder filling. Remind her to void every 2 hours, monitor intake and output, and observe and palpate for bladder distention to avoid overfilling, especially if labor is prolonged. Be aware of the standards and policies of the healthcare agency related to who may add additional anesthesia or remove the catheter. To assess after birth whether the anesthesia is wearing off, touch a woman's leg and ask if she can feel your touch. Ask her to raise her knees and observe whether she can do this easily. Even after feeling in her legs returns, walking may be difficult for her. Be certain to stay with the woman the first time she is out of bed following regional block anesthesia to prevent her from falling.

Spinal (Subarachnoid) Anesthesia

Spinal anesthesia is not used frequently in preference to epidural blocks, but it may be used in an emergency or for a cesarean birth because the administration technique is simpler than that of an epidural and can be accomplished more rapidly.

Before spinal anesthesia, as a guard against hypotension, an IV fluid such as Ringer's lactate solution is usually begun to ensure good hydration. Be certain the fluid is infusing well before the anesthesia is administered.

For spinal anesthesia, a local anesthetic agent such as bupivacaine (Marcaine) is injected using lumbar puncture technique into the subarachnoid space (into the CSF) at the L3 and L4 interspace. A narcotic agonist such as morphine or fentanyl may be added for additional pain relief. For administration, the woman is usually asked to sit on the side of the bed with legs dangling and head bent. Ask her to bend her head forward so her back curves and the intravertebral spaces open. Be sure either you or her support person steadies her in this sitting position because she is very "front heavy" as a result of her pregnancy and could easily fall forward if not well supported.

After injection, the anesthetic normally rises to the level of T10. Anesthesia up to the umbilicus and including both legs will be achieved. Spinal anesthetic agents may be "loaded" or "weighted" with glucose to make them heavier than CSF. This helps prevent them from rising too high in the spinal canal and interfering with the motor control of the uterus or with respiratory muscles (Drasner & Larson, 2011).

Following the anesthetic injection, if the woman was sitting, the anesthesiologist will ask the woman to lie down. It's important a woman lies down at this time because if she continues to sit upright, the anesthetic will not rise high enough in the canal to achieve pain relief. She must not lie down before this time, however, or the anesthetic could rise too high in the canal. Lying with a pillow under the head is another method to help ensure the anesthesia will be confined to the lower spinal canal.

As mentioned, hypotension from sympathetic blockage in the lower extremities may occur immediately after spinal anesthetic administration. This leads to vasodilation and a decrease in central blood pressure. If hypotension occurs, placental blood perfusion can be compromised. Turn the woman to her left side to reduce vena cava compression. Expect the anesthesiologist to quickly increase the rate of IV fluid administration to increase blood volume; ephedrine to increase blood pressure and oxygen also may be administered. Never place a woman in a Trendelenburg position (head lower than her body) to help restore blood pressure after spinal anesthesia. This could make the anesthetic rise high in her spinal column, causing uterine or respiratory function to cease. A late complication of spinal anesthesia is a PDPH or "spinal headache." This occurs because of CSF leakage from the needle insertion site and also possibly from the irritation of a small amount of air that entered at the injection site. It has been demonstrated that the type of needle used may be a significant factor in whether or not a woman will have a spinal headache (Genç, Sahin, Maral, et al., 2016). The shift in pressure of the CSF causes strain on the cerebral meninges, initiating the pain. The incidence of such headaches is reduced if a woman is well hydrated before injection. If a headache occurs, the postpartum woman can be encouraged to drink a large quantity of fluid because a high fluid intake rapidly provides replacement of spinal fluid.

A spinal headache can be relieved by the administration of hydrocortisone to reduce inflammation (Hanling, Lagrew, Colmenar, et al., 2016). Having the woman lie flat and administering an analgesic also helps. Some women find a cold cloth applied to their forehead helpful. If a headache is incapacitating, it can be treated with a blood patch technique. For this, 10 to 20 ml of blood is withdrawn from an accessible vein and then immediately injected into the epidural space over the spinal injection site. The injected blood clots and seals off any further leakage of CSF (Hanling et al., 2016).

QSEN Checkpoint Question 16.5

TEAMWORK & COLLABORATION

Jonny has chosen to have epidural anesthesia, and the nurse has consequently informed the anesthesiologist. What are two risks that are potentially associated with this form of anesthesia?

- a. Hypotension and a prolonged second stage of labor can occur.
- b. Severe headache and peripheral cyanosis can occur.
- c. Women have increased back pain and abrupt transitions between stages of labor.
- d. Maternal hypertension and a reduced red blood cell count can occur.

Look in Appendix A for the best answer and rationale.

MEDICATION FOR PAIN RELIEF DURING BIRTH

Stretching of the perineum causes pain that occurs during the birth. The simplest form of relief for this type of pain is the natural pressure anesthesia that results from the fetal head pressing against the stretched perineum. This natural anesthesia is often adequate to allow the fetal head to be born with only momentary pain, which, although intense and hot, occurs suddenly and is over quickly. Often, after the hours of hard contractions a woman has come through, this flash of pain seems insignificant. For some women, however, additional medication is needed to reduce the pain of birth.

Local Anesthetics

Local anesthesia reduces the ability of local nerve fibers to conduct pain.

Local Infiltration

Local infiltration is the injection of an anesthetic such as lidocaine (Xylocaine) into the superficial nerves of the perineum along the vulva. The effect lasts for approximately 1 hour, allowing for a less painful birth and suturing of an episiotomy (a cut to enlarge the vagina opening; discussed in Chapter 24).

Pudendal Nerve Block

A **pudendal nerve block** is the injection of a local anesthetic such as bupivacaine (Marcaine) through the vagina to anesthetize the pudendal nerve. It is used for a woman who has not had an epidural to provide a pain-free birth and, if the woman should have an episiotomy, painless surgical suturing and repair. Although a pudendal nerve block is local, assess the fetal heart rate and the mother's blood pressure immediately after the injection to be certain maternal hypotension does not occur.

General Anesthesia

General anesthesia is never preferred for childbirth because it carries the dangers of hypoxia and possible inhalation of vomitus during administration. Because it is used so rarely, you probably will not see this used; if it is used, there are special precautions you need to be aware of. Pregnant women are particularly prone to gastric reflux and aspiration because of increased stomach pressure from the weight of the full uterus beneath it. The gastroesophageal valve at the top of the stomach also may be displaced and possibly functioning improperly. Despite these risks, general anesthesia may be necessary in emergency situations, such as if the placenta loosens before the fetus is born (placental abruption), spinal anesthesia is contraindicated, or an immediate cesarean birth is required.

For complete and rapid anesthesia during childbirth, thiopental sodium (Pentothal), a short-acting barbiturate, is usually the drug of choice. It causes rapid induction of anesthesia and, because it has a short half-life, allows for good uterine contraction afterward and so prevents postpartal hemorrhage. All women who receive a general anesthetic, however, must be observed closely in the postpartal period for uterine relaxation and the risk of uterine atony and postpartal hemorrhage.

For the procedure, after induction with thiopental sodium, the woman is intubated, and anesthesia is then maintained by administration of nitrous oxide and oxygen. Thiopental sodium crosses the placenta rapidly, so an infant born to a woman anesthetized by this method may be slow to respond at birth and may need resuscitation.

Some women comment that their throat feels raw or sore after general anesthesia administration; this is from the insertion and maintenance of an endotracheal tube. Using an anesthetic throat spray or gargle, sipping cold liquids, or sucking on ice chips (as soon as this is safe after general anesthesia) can help to relieve the discomfort.

Preparation for the Safe Administration of General Anesthesia

To ensure safe general anesthesia administration, an anesthesiologist or nurse anesthetist needs a minimum of six drugs readily available:

- Ephedrine to use in the event blood pressure falls
- Atropine sulfate to dry oral and respiratory secretions to prevent aspiration
- Thiopental sodium (Pentothal) for rapid induction
- Succinylcholine (Anectine) to achieve laryngeal relaxation for intubation
- Diazepam (Valium) to control seizures, a possible reaction to anesthetics
- Isoproterenol (Isuprel) to reduce bronchospasm, should aspiration occur

In addition to these medications, an adult laryngoscope, an endotracheal tube, a breathing bag with a source of 100% oxygen, and a suction catheter and suction source should be at hand.

Aspiration of Vomitus

There is a danger of vomiting with a general anesthetic; this can be fatal if a woman's airway becomes occluded by foreign matter. In addition, stomach contents have an acid pH that can cause chemical pneumonitis and secondary infection of the respiratory tract.

Some anesthesiologists may prescribe IV ranitidine (Zantac) or an oral antacid such as sodium citrate to be given before general anesthesia is administered to reduce the level of acid in stomach contents should aspiration occur. Metoclopramide (Reglan) increases gastric emptying and may also be prescribed.

For general anesthesia administration, the woman is asked to lie on her back with a wedge under her left hip to displace the uterus from the vena cava. To reduce the occurrence of hypotension and to establish a line for emergency medications, IV fluid administration is begun. The woman is then given a rapid-induction IV agent, followed by intubation with a cuffed endotracheal tube.

The moments of induction of general anesthesia before the endotracheal tube is safely in place are critical ones for the anesthesiologist. Respect his or her need to concentrate by not talking until the task is achieved.

If aspiration of vomitus should occur following administration, prompt attention is essential. The anesthesiologist suctions the woman's trachea to remove as much foreign material as possible. The woman is intubated, if she was not previously, and given 100% oxygen. IV isoproterenol to reduce bronchospasm and a corticosteroid to reduce inflammation may be given. Positive-pressure ventilation may be initiated. Blood gas analysis and a chest X-ray usually are obtained to determine how much aeration the woman is still capable of achieving.

The woman may receive mechanical ventilation until her overall clinical condition improves, as shown by X-ray films and blood gas concentrations. She may be critically ill at the time of aspiration and, after the cesarean birth, often will be transferred to an intensive care unit for the special care she needs to survive this emergency.

QSEN Checkpoint Question 16.6

QUALITY IMPROVEMENT

There is no reason to think Jonny will need a general anesthetic. But if she did, what type of drug would the nurse want to ensure is readily available on a birthing unit to help minimize the risk of aspiration of vomitus?

a. An anticonvulsant such as diazepam (Valium)
b. A nerve relaxant such as phenobarbital
c. Metoclopramide (Reglan) to speed gastric emptying
d. Oxytocin to increase the effectiveness of labor

Look in Appendix A for the best answer and rationale.

 ## Nursing Diagnoses and Related Interventions

Nursing Diagnosis: Anxiety related to more pain than expected from labor contractions

Outcome Evaluation: Patient identifies beginning and end of contractions, expresses confidence rather than confusion about ongoing process, states she feels less anxious, and is able to concentrate on controlled breathing.

In addition to causing local discomfort, pain can evoke a general stress response (fight-or-flight syndrome). This releases epinephrine, which causes peripheral and uterine vasoconstriction. This can increase the degree of pain experienced because of the resulting increase in tissue anoxia. Reducing anxiety through relaxation techniques such as spaced breathing exercises or through administration of medication to reduce anxiety can reduce vasoconstriction and help reduce pain.

Reduce Anxiety With Explanations of the Labor Process. Planning with women their options for pain relief during labor should begin prenatally (Box 16.6).

During labor, use a standard method of pain assessment, such as asking a woman to rate her pain level on a scale of 1 to 10 or show her a paper with a line marked 1 to 10 if she's more visually oriented, so she can rate her pain. Based on her response, evaluate whether pain relief is adequate and effective.

Introduce natural methods based on the gate control theory of pain relief such as massage or imagery. Be sure to offer careful explanations of what is happening or what will happen during labor because this can help alleviate anxiety and thereby reduce some discomfort.

Be certain to explain the characteristics of contractions (e.g., labor contractions are rhythmic and come and go repeatedly) and reinstruct as necessary. Do not assume a woman is aware of this simply because she is experiencing the contractions. Her pain may be so intense and the intensity so unexpected that she is unaware of any relief between contractions (Box 16.7).

This on/off effect of labor contractions differentiates the pain from that of a toothache or headache, which is continuous. Sometimes, just knowing this can help a woman tolerate the pain even as it increases in intensity.

Do not assume a woman knows such things like when membranes rupture it is painless, that a pink-stained show is normal, or that contractions change in character during labor. A woman having her first child may not know these things. A woman having her second child may not remember what her labor was like the last time, or she may find this time so different (even if it is well within usual limits) she is frightened by it. Be certain to give explanations to a woman's partner or support person as well because it's hard to support someone when you need support yourself. Unless the support person's anxiety and fear are relieved, he or she may start to convey anxiety back to the woman in labor rather than help her relax.

Nursing Diagnosis: Ineffective coping related to combination of uterine contractions and anxiety

Outcome Evaluation: Patient demonstrates effective coping by expressing confidence in her ability to maintain active participation during labor, using continued breathing techniques, expressing the need to change position, and verbalizing confidence in healthcare providers.

Help the Woman Identify Coping Strategies. Because pain is not a new phenomenon for a woman of childbearing age, it can be helpful to ask her to recall methods she usually uses to combat pain or anxiety,

BOX 16.6

Nursing Care Planning to Empower a Family

PAIN RELIEF DURING LABOR

Q. Jonny tells you, "I know my friends have told me pain during labor would be horrible, but what can I do so I won't hurt so much?"

A. Here are some common suggestions to help with pain relief:

- Ask your primary healthcare provider early in pregnancy about pain management options for labor. The options your care provider suggests may actually influence your decision as to whether this is the optimal care provider for you.
- Attend childbirth preparation classes during pregnancy and conscientiously practice breathing or other relaxation exercises. These measures can be adequate all by themselves; if not, they may complement pharmacologic methods of pain relief.
- Make a birth plan detailing what position you choose for labor and other options you want to use. This helps give you a greater sense of control in the face of pain.
- Be certain a support person will be with you during labor. Name a second person or investigate using a doula if you are uncertain whether your usual support person will be available or can fill this role.
- Late in pregnancy, if you are still concerned, let your primary healthcare provider know. In addition to medication for pain relief during labor, medication to reduce anxiety is also available.
- On admission to the hospital, let the medical and nursing staff know you are concerned so they can work with you to find satisfactory pain management.
- The most commonly used options today are oral, intramuscular, or intravenous administration of narcotics or injection of regional anesthesia by epidural block. Ask questions about any method suggested if necessary so you're aware of action and side effects.
- Be aware the choice of receiving analgesia or anesthesia is yours. However, if a complication occurs, be ready to compromise in the interest of safety for yourself and your child.

BOX 16.7

Nursing Care Planning Tips for Effective Communication

Jonny stated early in labor that she didn't want to use any medication for pain relief. As soon as her contractions became 30 seconds in length, however, she requested some analgesia. Her physician prescribed intramuscular butorphanol tartrate (Stadol). Her contractions are now 40 seconds in duration and only moderately strong. She looks increasingly uncomfortable with each contraction.

Tip: Ask the patient to rate her pain on a scale of 1 to 10 rather than just asking how she feels. Assess whether she has a clear understanding of the nature of labor contractions to make it easier for her to manage them. Because women in labor are under stress, they may not hear instructions when they are given.

Nurse: How are you feeling, Jonny? Is there anything I can do for you?

Jonny: I need something stronger for pain.

Nurse: On a scale of 1 to 10, with 1 being little pain and 10 being the worst pain ever, how would you rate the pain you're having?

Jonny: Two, but I know it'll be 10 in another half hour when my contractions get so strong that they're constant.

Nurse: I can assist you with relaxation techniques to lessen your discomfort. Contractions aren't constant and resting in-between contractions is helpful.

such as meditation or applying a cool cloth. Associating labor pain with usual circumstances can go a long way toward helping her collect her resources and decide on a workable pain relief strategy. Box 16.8 shows an interprofessional care map illustrating both nursing and team planning for helping reduce anxiety to manage discomfort during labor.

Provide Comfort Measures. Usually, anyone can tolerate a little discomfort from a backache, being thirsty, having dry lips, or having a leg cramp. However, few people can tolerate having all of these discomforts simultaneously or feeling even one of them while experiencing a labor contraction.

Assist the woman's support person to provide the usual comfort measures that are helpful for anyone with pain, such as reassurance, massage, or a change in position. For dry lips, ice chips to suck on, moistening the lips with a wet cloth, or using a moisturizing jelly or balm can be helpful. A cool cloth to wipe perspiration from the forehead, neck, and chest can keep a woman from feeling overheated.

A woman's sheets and clothing may wrinkle rapidly and stick to her skin if she is perspiring. The waterproof pad under her buttocks will become soiled with vaginal secretions and will begin to feel hot and sticky. Never apply sanitary pads in labor because, although they absorb vaginal secretions well, they also tend to slip out of place, possibly carrying pathogens from the rectal area forward to the vaginal opening. Instead, change waterproof pads frequently. At least halfway through the first stage of labor,

BOX 16.8

Nursing Care Planning

AN INTERPROFESSIONAL CARE MAP FOR A WOMAN REQUIRING COMFORT MEASURES DURING LABOR AND BIRTH

Jonny Baranca is a primipara in early labor whom you admit to a birthing unit. Her contractions are 7 minutes apart, and her cervix is 3 cm dilated. She tells you her sister had epidural anesthesia that completely obliterated her pain in labor for the birth of her baby 3 months ago. Based on her sister's experience, Jonny expected to be given epidural anesthesia as soon as she arrived at the hospital. As she is in early labor, her physician asked her to wait until she is 4 cm dilated. When you enter her room, you find her lying on her back in a birthing bed, crying from pain. Her husband shouts at you that his "wife deserves better care than this."

Family Assessment: Gravida 1, para 0; accompanied by husband who will act as support person and coach. Patient works as clerk in clothing store; husband is physical education major at local university.

Patient Assessment: Contractions are of moderate intensity, every 6 to 7 minutes, with a duration of 35 seconds. Cervix dilated 3 cm, 80% effaced, −1 station. Membranes intact. Fetal heart rate (FHR), 148 beats/min; fetus in right occiput anterior (ROA) position. Attended childbirth education classes but did not practice breathing exercises. Last meal: 3 hours ago; last voided, 2 hours ago.

Nursing Diagnosis: Pain related to effects of uterine contractions and pressure on pelvic structures

Outcome Criteria: Patient confirms discomfort is controlled (pain is a 3 or less on a 1 to 10 pain scale) with either non-pharmacologic or pharmacologic methods; responds to questions and instructions; identifies need for additional pain relief measures if required.

Team Member Responsible	Assessment	Intervention	Rationale	Expected Outcome
Activities of Daily Living, Including Safety				
Nurse	Assess what birth plan the woman wants to follow. Inspect her suprapubic area and palpate for bladder distention.	Remind patient she does not need to remain in bed. Encourage her to void every 2 hours.	Ambulation can increase comfort and progress. A full bladder contributes to discomfort and may impede fetal descent, possibly prolonging labor.	Patient ambulates in early labor. Has no signs of bladder distention; voids every 2 hours during labor.
Teamwork and Collaboration				
Nurse/primary healthcare provider	Locate the on-call healthcare provider to provide anesthetic pain relief when patient reaches 4 cm dilation.	Notify nurse-anesthetist concerning patient's wish to receive an epidural block as soon as possible.	Respecting patient's wishes is a prime method of encouraging self-efficacy.	Pain management team supports patient's wish for pharmacologic intervention; encourages nonpharmacologic measures until epidural anesthetic is appropriate.
Procedures/Medications for Quality Improvement				
Nurse	Assess how patient's husband views his role in labor. Assess if patient will try controlled breathing exercises learned in preparation for labor class.	Refresh controlled breathing and imagery with support of husband. Allow husband occasional breaks. Stay with the patient during this time to provide support.	A support person increases satisfaction with labor; controlled breathing and imagery can be learned during labor.	Support person helps patient with imagery and controlled breathing. Patient allows healthcare providers to substitute for husband so husband can take occasional breaks.

Nutrition

Nurse	Determine what patient would like to eat or drink while in labor.	Provide patient with a beverage at least every hour; food as desired.	Fluid maintains hydration; ice chips or hard candy can relieve mouth dryness from breathing exercises.	Patient states she has no mouth discomfort from breathing; drinks fluid every hour.

Patient-Centered Care

Nurse/nurse anesthetist	Assess if patient still desires epidural anesthesia for pain management.	Provide information on epidural anesthesia as needed; update the couple on labor progress.	Frequent updates on progress help alleviate anxiety and fears that may exacerbate pain.	Couple confirms they are certain epidural anesthesia is their method of choice; receive frequent updates on labor progress.

Psychosocial/Spiritual/Emotional Needs

Nurse	Assess level of patient's pain by verbal, pain scale, and nonverbal indicators. Use 1 to 10 scale and evaluate response to techniques used.	Support patient in her ability to manage pain until her epidural can be given.	Praise can instill a sense of control and motivation to continue to use alternative methods of pain control.	Patient rates her level of pain from labor contractions not above 3 on a 1 to 10 scale.
Nurse	Assess what nonpharmacologic measures (such as music, touch, environmental calm) patient thinks would help complement epidural block and aid comfort.	Provide a comfortable environment: clean sheets, cool washcloth to forehead, closed room door. Refrain from intervening with patient during a contraction.	A comfortable environment aids in relaxation, promoting effective coping. Interrupting the patient's breathing can make the technique ineffective as a pain relief measure.	Patient reports she feels environment is comfortable and complements other pain relief measures.

Informatics for Seamless Healthcare Planning

Nurse	Ask patient and husband to evaluate their labor experience.	Review with patient pain relief measures used and determine which were most effective.	Reviewing a possibly traumatic experience helps to put it into perspective among life events.	Patient and support person state labor and birth were, at worst, a tolerable experience and, at best, a highlight of their lives.

or more frequently as indicated by the woman's condition, change her sheets, offer her a clean gown, and ask if she'd like to bathe or take a shower. These measures can help her feel clean and refreshed, with a ready-to-go-again feeling.

Think of comfort measures for the woman's support person as well. Is the chair by the side of the bed comfortable? Does he or she need to stretch or take a beverage or bathroom break? Could you serve as the coach while the support person makes some phone calls? Breaks such as these allow a partner to come back rested and ready to give support again.

Nursing Diagnosis: Pain related to labor contractions

Outcome Evaluation: Patient states pain is reduced to a tolerable level with techniques used so she is able to handle

or "work with" contractions and demonstrates ability to listen and respond to questions and instructions.

Assist the Woman With Prepared Childbirth Method. Depending on the type of childbirth preparation a woman and her support person have had, the method used may include breathing exercises, distraction by focusing on an external object, acupressure, therapeutic touch, music therapy, guided imagery, self-hypnosis, or a combination of these methods. The use of biofeedback is not well documented in labor but may also be effective.

Even though a woman conscientiously practiced breathing or focusing in a relaxed, fun setting of an antepartal class, the discomfort and stress of labor may make it easy for her to forget what she learned. As necessary, review previously learned breathing techniques with her. Urge her to begin using these early in labor, before contractions become strong, so she gains confidence that they can be effective at diminishing pain. If a woman has had no prior training in breathing exercises, sit with her and teach her a simple breathing pattern, so she can begin to utilize this to relieve some of her pain.

Massage is another pain relief method that can be taught to a woman and her support person during labor. This may be especially useful if a woman is experiencing back pain because rubbing or massaging the sacral area often alleviates that. Firm massage on her shoulders can provide a relaxing distraction from the sensation of internal pressure and pain.

Encourage Comfortable Positioning. An upright position, sitting, walking, or swaying with a partner may be most comfortable for a woman in early labor and aids contractions and descent through gravity (see Chapter 15). If a woman wants to walk and has no support person, walk with her as she may need support during a contraction. Leaning forward against a birthing ball or pelvic rocking between contractions may relieve tense back muscles. If a woman must remain in bed because of a situation such as her membranes have ruptured and the fetal head is not engaged, urge her to keep active within the limits of bed rest and especially not to lie on her back to avoid supine hypotension syndrome. Move bedclothes or monitor leads, if any are attached, as needed to allow her to be able to turn and remain active.

Position changes during the second stage of labor help fetal descent and may shorten labor. Urge a woman to sit, stand, kneel on hands and knees, lie in a lateral recumbent position, squat, or use whatever position she prefers (see Chapter 15). Keep in mind that maintaining these positions often requires assistance from one or two support people to keep an unbalanced woman from falling.

Provide Pharmacologic Pain Relief. Helping a woman decide if and when medication for pain relief should be used requires an in-depth understanding of the available drugs, their effects on the mother and the fetus, and their mechanism and duration of action. It also requires sympathetic listening and counseling skills. Many women come into labor wishing to avoid drugs entirely. Once in labor, they may change their minds but hesitate to say so, especially if their partners also believe a birth without the use of drugs is ideal. Other women come into labor asking to receive something immediately to avoid experiencing any pain. In both instances, provide information about the use of drugs and their ultimate effects. Maintain a supportive presence to help a woman make the best decision for herself and her baby. Some women require analgesia or anesthesia because of a complication. Helping these women and their support persons understand why the medication is necessary calls for equal care and skill. As a rule, record a baseline fetal heart rate and maternal blood pressure and pulse before administering medication; reassess 15 minutes later for fetal and maternal safety.

What If . . . 16.3

Jonny, who is still in early labor, tells the nurse if she can't have an epidural immediately, she wants a general anesthesia. If she can't have that, she will leave the hospital. Her physician has said she cannot justify a general anesthesia for uncomplicated labor. The nurse finds Jonny crying because her doctor won't give her anything for pain. How would the nurse handle this situation?

The Woman With Unique Needs

THE MORBIDLY OBESE WOMAN

Morbidly obese women may have more difficulty using some nonpharmacologic measures for pain relief than other women. For example, be certain a portable birthing tub (looks like a child's plastic pool) will be sturdy enough to support her weight as she leans against the side. Check to be certain the labor room shower is wide enough if she wishes to use warm water sprays for pain management. Remember, birthing beds are not very wide; be cautious when you ask her to turn that she has adequate space to do that. Straddling a chair and leaning against the back may be unsafe if the chair is not strong enough to support her weight.

Analgesic administration may also pose a problem as a usual dose may not be as effective in extremely obese women. Question doses for women who might need a larger amount so they can achieve pain relief. Anesthetic administration may also cause concern as it may be more difficult for an anesthetist to identify the L3–L4 intravertebral space for injection. Although women who are classified as obese do have higher risk of labor complications, they are also at greater risk for procedures such as induction of labor, resulting in cesarean birth (Kerrigan, Kingdon, & Cheyne, 2015).

THE WOMAN WITH CULTURAL CONCERNS

Because of cultural traditions, some women are very opposed to the use of analgesia or anesthesia in labor. Be certain to respect this concern by aiding women in any way possible to use the methods they have chosen for pain control and to not interrupt distraction techniques such as controlled breathing, meditation, or chanting. Mark a nursing care plan as to the woman's preference so other team members don't suggest analgesia. Caution other team members as well to remain quiet while the baby is born if there is a special prayer a partner or the woman wants to say at this time (Goyal, 2016).

In many cultures, childbearing is a woman's field of expertise so male partners may have large gaps of knowledge about what is expected of them during birth. Be certain to explain the purpose of procedures and assist the partner to help with breathing exercises, warming hot pads, making tea, or other comfort measures if the partner wants to help in other ways.

If analgesia or anesthesia becomes necessary because of an unanticipated emergency, talk to the woman and her partner afterward to be certain they understand why the additional pain management method was necessary. Stress that the overriding aim of labor is a healthy mother and healthy baby; using analgesia or anesthesia or using none at all is only different means to achieve that end.

THE WOMAN WITH SUBSTANCE USE DISORDER

The incidence of women who suffer from substance use disorder, and particularly opioid use is rising, so the number of women seen in labor with these concerns is also increasing. Include a question on the use of recreational and prescription drugs when history taking at a woman's admittance to a birthing center. Concern about their baby's health, the possibility of overdosing from an analgesic administered to them during labor, or their newborn acquiring neonatal abstinence syndrome from opioid withdrawal all encourage women to answer a question about illicit drug use honestly. Women addicted to prescription drugs may not realize they are using more of a drug than is healthy for them or their fetus and so may not mention this unless asked directly.

If a woman states she uses illicit drugs, ask what drug she uses and when was the last time she used to prevent administering an analgesic overdose. Be certain the anesthetist who will administer a regional block has this same information. Marijuana is a drug frequently smoked at the beginning of labor by users because it offers such a relaxed feeling. There is little evidence that marijuana has immediate effects on a newborn, but it is important to be cautious because a marijuana user may also be a polysubstance user. A woman needs to alert her primary healthcare provider she used it as an alternative pain measure. Cocaine is also a frequent choice for women beginning labor because, again, it has such a euphoric effect. Cocaine use during pregnancy is associated with loosening of the placenta (placenta abruption) so a woman who has taken this drug needs to be observed closely for signs of poor fetal circulation, such as a decreasing heart rate (Oliveira, Bersusa, dos Santos, et al., 2016).

Women who consistently use opioids may not receive the same pain relief from an analgesic such as butorphanol tartrate (Stadol) as nonusers, so be prepared to suggest alternative measures of pain relief as well. Their newborn may need special care at birth as many newborns of consistent users are small for gestational age and need observation for opioid withdrawal or neonatal abstinence signs (H. E. Jones, Deppen, Hudak, et al., 2015).

Many women who are addicted to opioids are identified during pregnancy and prescribed methadone or buprenorphine to substitute for their drug of addiction. Methadone has the same effect on a newborn as all opioids, so it is equally important that these women identify themselves in labor so their newborn can be closely monitored. Although buprenorphine has similar effects on neonates as methadone, some studies show that there are fewer instances of neonatal abstinence syndrome (Noormohammadi, Forinash, Yancey, et al., 2016).

A typical prescription drug abused by women is hydrocodone-acetaminophen as this is frequently prescribed for chronic pain such as carpal tunnel syndrome or back pain. The half-life of this drug is about 2 hours in addicted women (Kokki, Franco, Raatikainen, et al., 2012). It appears to have little effect on newborns; however, because the compound contains an adult dosage of acetaminophen, the newborn needs to be observed for both withdrawal and liver effects.

THE WOMAN WHO USES TOBACCO

Women who smoke cigarettes typically turn to them when they are stressed, so it may be very difficult for a tobacco user to go without a cigarette if her labor lasts more than 4 hours (and labor typically does). A woman needs to ask her primary healthcare provider if she could use nicotine gum or a patch during labor; nicotine is a pregnancy category C drug, so she needs to alert the team that she is a tobacco user as her infant may have a low birth weight and may need special care (Mei-Dan, Walfisch, Weisz, et al., 2015). Women who use tobacco in pregnancy are at risk for having a neonate with low birth weight, very low birthweight, small for gestational age, preterm, and stillbirth (Inamdar, Croucher, Chokhandre, et al., 2015).

What If . . . 16.4

The nurse is particularly interested in exploring one of the 2020 National Health Goals with respect to analgesia in labor (see Box 16.1). What would be a possible research topic to explore pertinent to this goal that would be applicable to Jonny Baranca's family and that would also advance evidence-based practice?

KEY POINTS FOR REVIEW

- Pain in labor occurs because of anoxia to uterine cells, stretching of the cervix and perineum, and pressure of the presenting part of the fetus on maternal tissues.

- Each person perceives pain differently. Only a woman herself can describe the type or extent of her pain.

- Usually, the better prepared a woman is for childbirth and the more effective her support person is, the less there is a need for analgesia and anesthesia.

- Encourage complementary and alternative therapies such as reducing anxiety, providing changes in position, increasing knowledge, supporting prepared childbirth exercises, and prescribed analgesics or anesthesia as these help in planning/implementing nursing care that not only meets QSEN competencies but also best meets a family's total needs.

- Be certain to ask about allergies to medications before administering them. Women under stress from pain may be too concerned to mention this unless directly asked.

- Women may lose their ability to use controlled breathing after systemic opioid administration because of a light-headed feeling. They may need additional support during this time to be able to continue with a breathing technique until this feeling passes and the analgesic agent begins to have an effect.

- Regional anesthesia, such as epidural anesthesia, is extremely effective at relieving labor pain. Be certain the woman is well hydrated with IV fluid and her blood pressure is within normal limits before assisting with administration of the anesthetic agent.

- Remind all women to lie on their side or place a firm towel under their right hip while in labor to help avoid supine hypotension. During general anesthesia administration, if a woman must lie supine, position a wedge under her right buttock to help prevent hypotension. If hypotension should occur after epidural anesthesia administration, elevating a woman's legs and administering an antihypotensive agent such as ephedrine are emergency measures to help relieve hypotension.

- If an opioid analgesic is used, naloxone hydrochloride (Narcan) must be available to use for possible newborn resuscitation.

- General anesthesia is not administered for an uncomplicated labor because it has risks for both the mother and the infant, but it may still be used in an emergency.

CRITICAL THINKING CARE STUDY

Bailey is a 32-year-old gravida 1, para 0 woman in active labor. She is 6 cm dilated, 40% effaced, and having moderate- to strong-intensity contractions. She has brought some rock-and-roll music with her to play during labor. Her support person is her apartment roommate Cheryl rather than her boyfriend because he "hates hospitals."

1. What is the chance an apartment roommate will make as good a support person in labor for Bailey as the father of her baby? Should she have insisted he come to be with her?

2. Bailey has brought music that is not at all relaxing. It is loud and boisterous. Should you suggest she play music you supply with sounds of the ocean to help her relax?

3. Bailey is using controlled breathing and you hear her roommate say "push" with each contraction as well. What additional information do you need to know if her support person is giving her good advice in labor?

RELATED RESOURCES

Explore these additional resources to enhance learning for this chapter:

- Student resources on thePoint, including answers to the What If . . . and Critical Thinking Care Study questions, http://thepoint .lww.com/Flagg8e

- Adaptive learning powered by PrepU, http://thepoint.lww.com /prepu:

REFERENCES

Aasheim, V., Nilsen, A. B., Lukasse, M., et al. (2011). Perineal techniques during the second stage of labour for reducing perineal trauma. *Cochrane Database of Systematic Reviews*, (12), CD006672.

Abbaspoor, Z., Moghaddam-Banaem, L., Ahmadi, F., et al. (2014). Iranian mothers' selection of a birth method in the context of perceived norms: A content analysis study. *Midwifery*, 30(7), 804–809.

Akbarzadeh, M., Masoudi, Z., Zare, N., et al. (2015). Comparison of the effects of doula supportive care and acupressure at the BL32 point on the mother's anxiety level and delivery outcome. *Iranian Journal of Nursing and Midwifery Research*, 20(2), 239–246.

Anim-Somuah, M., Smyth, R. M., & Jones, L. (2011). Epidural versus non-epidural or no analgesia in labour. *Cochrane Database of Systematic Reviews*, (12), CD000331.

Armstrong, S., & Fernando, R. (2016). Side effects and efficacy of neuraxial opioids in pregnant patients at delivery: A comprehensive review. *Drug Safety*, 39(5), 381–399.

Asadi, N., Maharlouei, N., Khalili, A., et al. (2015). Effects of LI-4 and SP-6 acupuncture on labor pain, cortisol level and duration of labor. *Journal of Acupuncture and Meridian Studies*, 8(5), 249–254.

Battle, C. L., Uebelacker, L. A., Magee, S. R., et al. (2015). Potential for prenatal yoga to serve as an intervention to treat depression during pregnancy. *Women's Health Issues*, 25(2), 134–141.

Brimdyr, K., Cadwell, K., Widström, A. M., et al. (2015). The association between common labor drugs and suckling when skin-to-skin during the first hour after birth. *Birth*, 42(4), 319–328.

Chan, K. P. (2016). Perceptions and experiences of pregnant Chinese women in Hong Kong on prenatal meditation: A qualitative study. *Journal of Nursing Education and Practice*, 6(3), 135.

Derry, S., Straube, S., Moore, R. A., et al. (2012). Intracutaneous or subcutaneous sterile water injection compared with blinded controls for pain management in labour. *Cochrane Database of Systematic Reviews*, (1), CD009107.

Dick-Read, G., & Gaskin, I. M. (2013). *Childbirth without fear: The principles and practice of natural childbirth*. London, United Kingdom: Pinter & Martin.

Drasner, K., & Larson, M. D. (2011). 17 Spinal and epidural anesthesia. In R. D. Miller & M. Pardo (Eds.), *Basics of anesthesia* (pp. 252–283). Philadelphia, PA: Elsevier Saunders.

Fakari, F. R., Tabatabaeichehr, M., Kamali, H., et al. (2015). Effect of inhalation of aroma of geranium essence on anxiety and physiological parameters during first stage of labor in nulliparous women: A randomized clinical trial. *Journal of Caring Sciences*, 4(2), 135–141.

French, C. A., Cong, X., & Chung, K. S. (2016). Labor epidural analgesia and breastfeeding: A systematic review. *Journal of Human Lactation*, 32(3), 507–520.

Genç, M., Sahin, N., Maral, J., et al. (2015). Caesarean section with spinal anesthesia and postspinal headache. *American Journal of Obstetric & Gynecologic Research*, 1(1), 1–7.

Goyal, D. (2016). Perinatal practices & traditions among Asian Indian women. *MCN: The American Journal of Maternal Child Nursing*, 41(2), 90–97.

Hanling, S. R., Lagrew, J. E., Colmenar, D. H., et al. (2016). Intravenous cosyntropin versus epidural blood patch for treatment of postdural puncture headache. *Pain Medicine*. Advance online publication. doi:10.1093 /pm/pnw014

Harper, B. (2014). Birth, bath, and beyond: The science and safety of water immersion during labor and birth. *The Journal of Perinatal Education*, 23(3), 124–134.

Hodnett, E. D., Gates, S., Hofmeyr, G. J., et al. (2013). Continuous support for women during childbirth. *Cochrane Database of Systematic Reviews*, (7), CD003766.

Howarth, A. M., Swain, N., & Treharne, G. J. (2011). Taking personal responsibility for well-being increases birth satisfaction of first time mothers. *Journal of Health Psychology*, 16(8), 1221–1230.

Impey, L., & Child, T. (2012). Labour 2: Management. In L. Impey & T. Child (Eds.), *Obstetrics & gynaecology* (4th ed., pp. 246–265). West Sussex, United Kingdom: Wiley.

Inamdar, A. S., Croucher, R. E., Chokhandre, M. K., et al. (2015). Maternal smokeless tobacco use in pregnancy and adverse health outcomes in newborns: A systematic review. *Nicotine & Tobacco Research*, 17(9), 1058–1066.

Janula, R., & Mahipal, S. (2015). Effectiveness of aromatherapy and biofeedback in promotion of labour outcome during childbirth among primigravidas. *Health Science Journal*, 9(1), 1–5.

Jokinen, J., Weibel, S., Afshari, A., et al. (2015). Patient-controlled analgesia with remifentanil versus alternative parenteral methods for pain management in labour. *Cochrane Database of Systematic Reviews*, (12), CD011989.

Jones, H. E., Deppen, K., Hudak, M. L., et al. (2015). Clinical care for opioid-using pregnant and postpartum women: The role of obstetric providers. *Obstetric Anesthesia Digest*, 35(2), 58–59.

Jones, L., Othman, M., Dowswell, T., et al. (2012). Pain management for women in labour: An overview of systematic reviews. *Cochrane Database of Systematic Reviews*, (3), CD009234.

Karch, A. M. (2013). *2013 Lippincott's nursing drug guide*. Philadelphia, PA: Lippincott Williams & Wilkins.

Kerrigan, A., Kingdon, C., & Cheyne, H. (2015). Obesity and normal birth: A qualitative study of clinician's management of obese pregnant women during labour. *BMC Pregnancy and Childbirth*, 15(1), 1.

Kokki, M., Franco, M. G., Raatikainen, K., et al. (2012). Intravenous oxycodone for pain relief in the first stage of labour—maternal pharmacokinetics and neonatal exposure. *Basic Clinical Pharmacology & Toxicology*, 110(3), 1742–1744.

Krieger, D. (1990). Therapeutic touch: Two decades of research, teaching, and clinical practice. *Imprint*, 37(3), 83–89.

Likis, F. E., Andrews, J. C., Collins, M. R., et al. (2014). Nitrous oxide for the management of labor pain: A systematic review. *Anesthesia & Analgesia*, 118(1), 153–167.

Madden, K., Middleton, P., Cyna, A. M., et al. (2016). Hypnosis for pain management during labour and childbirth. *Cochrane Database of Systematic Reviews*, (5), CD009356.

McCaffery, M. (1972). *Nursing management of the patient with pain*. Philadelphia, PA: Lippincott Williams & Wilkins.

Mei-Dan, E., Walfisch, A., Weisz, B., et al. (2015). The unborn smoker: Association between smoking during pregnancy and adverse perinatal outcomes. *Journal of Perinatal Medicine, 43*(5), 553–558.

Melzack, R., & Wall, P. (1965). Pain mechanisms: A new theory. *Science, 150*(2), 971–982.

Metawie, M. A. H., Amasha, H. A. R., Abdraboo, R. A., et al. (2015). Effectiveness of aromatherapy with lavender oil in relieving post caesarean incision pain. *Journal of Surgery, 3*(2–1), 8–13.

Mohta, M., Aggarwal, M., Sethi, A. K., et al. (2016). Randomized double-blind comparison of ephedrine and phenylephrine for management of post-spinal hypotension in potential fetal compromise. *International Journal of Obstetric Anesthesia, 27*, 32–40.

Nerum, H., Halvorsen, L., Straume, B., et al. (2013). Different labour outcomes in primiparous women that have been subjected to childhood sexual abuse or rape in adulthood: A case-control study in a clinical cohort. *BJOG: An International Journal of Obstetrics & Gynaecology, 120*(4), 487–495.

Noormohammadi, A., Forinash, A., Yancey, A., et al. (2016). Buprenorphine versus methadone for opioid dependence in pregnancy. *Annals of Pharmacotherapy, 50*(8), 666–672.

Oliveira, T. A., Bersusa, A. A. S., dos Santos, T. F., et al. (2016). Perinatal outcomes in pregnant women users of illegal drugs. *Revista Brasileira de Ginecologia e Obstetrícia/RBGO Gynecology and Obstetrics, 38*(4), 183–188.

Ozgoli, G., Mobarakabadi, S. S., Heshmat, R., et al. (2016). Effect of LI4 and BL32 acupressure on labor pain and delivery outcome in the first stage of labor in primiparous women: A randomized controlled trial. *Complementary Therapies in Medicine, 29*, 175–180.

Rakestraw, T. (2010). Reiki: The energy doula. *Midwifery Today With International Midwife, 92*(1), 16–17.

Rooks, J. P. (2011). Safety and risks of nitrous oxide labor analgesia: A review. *Journal of Midwifery & Women's Health, 56*(6), 557–565.

Roozbahani, N., Attarha, M., Akbari Torkestani, N., et al. (2015). The effect of rose water aromatherapy on reducing labor pain in primiparous women. *Complementary Medicine Journal of Faculty of Nursing & Midwifery, 5*(1), 1042–1053.

Santana, L. S., Gallo, R. B. S., Ferreira, C. H. J., et al. (2016). Transcutaneous electrical nerve stimulation (TENS) reduces pain and postpones the need for pharmacological analgesia during labour: A randomised trial. *Journal of Physiotherapy, 62*(1), 29–34.

Schrock, S. D., & Harraway-Smith, C. (2012). Labor analgesia. *American Family Physician, 85*(5), 447–454.

Schwartz, L., Toohill, J., Creedy, D. K., et al. (2015). Factors associated with childbirth self-efficacy in Australian childbearing women. *BMC Pregnancy and Childbirth, 15*(1), 29.

Siddiqui, N. T., Davies, S., McGeer, A., et al. (2014). The effect of gowning on labor epidural catheter colonization rate: A randomized controlled trial. *Regional Anesthesia and Pain Medicine, 39*(6), 520–524.

Simavli, S., Gumus, I., Kaygusuz, I., et al. (2014). Effect of music on labor pain relief, anxiety level and postpartum analgesic requirement: A randomized controlled clinical trial. *Gynecologic and Obstetric Investigation, 78*(4), 244–250.

Smith, C. A., Levett, K. M., Collins, C. T., et al. (2011). Relaxation techniques for pain management in labour. *Cochrane Database of Systematic Reviews*, (12), CD000111.

Smith, C. A., Levett, K. M., Collins, C. T., et al. (2012). Massage, reflexology and other manual methods for pain management in labour. *Cochrane Database of Systematic Reviews*, (2), CD009290.

Stark, M. A., Remynse, M., & Zwelling, E. (2016). Importance of the birth environment to support physiologic birth. *Journal of Obstetric, Gynecologic & Neonatal Nursing, 45*(2), 285–294.

Streibert, L. A., Reinhard, J., Yuan, J., et al. (2015). Clinical study: Change in outlook towards birth after a midwife led antenatal education programme versus hypnoreflexogenous self-hypnosis training for childbirth. *Geburtshilfe und Frauenheilkunde, 75*(11), 1161–1166.

Sultan, P., David, A. L., Fernando, R., et al. (2016). Inflammation and epidural-related maternal fever: Proposed mechanisms. *Anesthesia & Analgesia, 122*(5), 1546–1553.

The Joint Commission. (2016). *2016 National patient safety goals*. Oakbrook Terrace, IL: Author.

Ulbricht, C., & Windsor, R. C. (2015). An evidence-based systematic review of black cohosh (Cimicifuga racemosa, Actaea racemosa) by the Natural Standard Research Collaboration. *Journal of Dietary Supplements, 12*(3), 265–358.

U.S. Department of Health and Human Services. (2010). *Healthy people 2020*. Washington, DC: Author.

17

Nursing Care of a Postpartal Family

*A*s the nurse working on a postpartum unit, you care for Leana Cooper, who gave birth to a healthy 8-lb 2-oz baby girl 6 hours ago. She is on maternity leave from her job as a court reporter. Her husband, Mike, plans to take a week off from work to help take care of the baby.

Leana has not voided since she gave birth. Although her baby latches well, Leana is worried she's not getting enough breast milk. She tells you, "I haven't smoked in 9 months. Can't wait to go home so I can light up." Mike pulls you aside and says, "Sometimes, I see my wife crying for no reason. Why does she get so upset over little things? Isn't she as happy as I am?"

Previous chapters discussed caring for the pregnant woman and her family during the antepartal and intrapartal periods. This chapter adds information about caring for a postpartal woman and family. Nurses are able to play major roles in assessment, promotion of comfort, and education during this period as they help a new family adjust to the many physiologic and psychological changes that occur during this period.

What additional postpartal healthcare teaching does the Cooper family need?

KEY TERMS

afterpains	engorgement	lochia
attachment	engrossment	relaxin
bonding	Homans sign	rooming-in
chloasma	Kegel exercises	striae gravidarum
colostrum	lactogenesis	taking-hold phase
diastasis recti	letting-go phase	taking-in phase
en face position	linea nigra	uterine atony

OBJECTIVES

After mastering the contents of this chapter, you should be able to:

1. Describe the psychological and physiologic changes that occur in a postpartal woman and her family.

2. Identify 2020 National Health Goals related to the postpartal period that nurses can help the nation achieve.

3. Assess the physiologic and psychological changes of the postpartal woman and her family.

4. Formulate nursing diagnoses related to physiologic and psychological transitions of the postpartal period.

5. Develop expected outcomes for a postpartal woman and family related to the changes during this period as well as manage seamless transitions across differing healthcare settings.

6. Using the nursing process, plan nursing care that includes the six competencies of Quality & Safety Education for Nurses (QSEN): Patient-Centered Care, Teamwork & Collaboration, Evidence-Based Practice (EBP), Quality Improvement (QI), Safety, and Informatics.

7. Implement nursing care to aid the progression of physiologic and psychological transitions occurring in a postpartal woman and family.

8. Evaluate outcome criteria for achievement and effectiveness of care.

9. Integrate knowledge of postpartal women and families with the interplay of nursing process, the six competencies of QSEN, and Family Nursing to promote quality maternal and child health nursing care.

The postpartal period, or *puerperium* (from the Latin *puer*, for "child," and *parere*, for "to bring forth"), refers to the 6-week period after childbirth. It is a time of maternal changes that are both retrogressive (involution of the uterus and vagina) and progressive (production of milk for lactation, restoration of the normal menstrual cycle, and beginning of a parenting role). Protecting a woman's health as these changes occur is important for preserving her future childbearing function and for ensuring she is physically well enough to incorporate her new child into her family (Souza, Gülmezoglu, Vogel, et al., 2013). The period is often termed the *fourth trimester of pregnancy*.

The physical care a woman receives during the postpartal period can influence her future health. The physical care of the postpartum mother involves providing comfort and relief from any discomfort from delivery, such as the use of sitz baths and cool compresses to soothe the perineal area. Mothers may often experience temporary difficulty in passing stool in the early postpartum period. This can be addressed with the use of stool softeners and encouraging fluid intake and a high-fiber diet. The emotional support she receives can influence the emotional health of her child and family so much that it can be felt into the next generation (Newton, 2012). Box 17.1 shows 2020 National Health Goals related to the postpartal period that nurses can help the nation achieve.

BOX 17.1

Nursing Care Planning Based on 2020 National Health Goals

The postpartal period is an extremely important one because of the possibility of uterine hemorrhage and because it is the optimal period for parent–child bonding. The 2020 National Health Goals that involve this time period include:

- Reduce the maternal mortality rate to no more than 11.4/100,000 live births from a baseline of 12.7/100,000.
- Increase to at least 82% the proportion of mothers who breastfeed their babies in the early postpartum period from a baseline of 74% and increase the proportion of mothers who still breastfeed at 6 months to 60.6% from a baseline of 43.5%.
- Increase the proportion of worksite lactation support programs to 38% from a baseline of 25%.
- Reduce the proportion of breastfed newborns who receive supplemental formula in the first 2 days from 24% to 14%.
- Increase the proportion of live births that occur in facilities that provide care for lactating mothers and their babies from 2.9% to 8.1%.
- Reduce postpartum relapse of smoking among women who quit smoking during pregnancy (developmental).
- Increase the proportion of women who used contraception to plan their pregnancy (developmental) (U.S. Department of Health and Human Services, 2010; see www.healthypeople.gov).

Nurses can help the nation achieve these goals by maintaining close observation in the immediate postpartal period to detect maternal hemorrhage, encouraging and supporting women as they begin breastfeeding, and ensuring women receive reproductive life planning information if desired.

Nursing Process Overview

FOR A POSTPARTAL WOMAN AND FAMILY

ASSESSMENT

During the puerperium, assessment of a woman is accomplished by health interview; awareness of her prenatal, natal, and medical history; physical examination; and analysis of laboratory data. It is important to ensure that physical changes, such as uterine involution, are occurring by evaluating uterine size and consistency and the amount of lochia flow.

Assessment of a woman's psychological adjustment begins with her reaction to her baby at birth (Was she disappointed or happy with the appearance of her baby? Is she glad to be through with the pregnancy or still longing to be back in it?) and continues with every contact made with the family during and after a hospital stay. Assess the extent and quality of the woman's interaction with her child (Does she hold and talk to the infant?), her overall mood (Do you observe her crying? Does she have long periods of staring into space or not talking?), and her ability to begin infant care and self-care. A woman who feels good about herself, even though she is exhausted from childbirth, usually will try to maintain her appearance. If she is depressed, however, she probably has little energy to do things such as comb her hair or worry about her appearance and may not want to interact with her newborn.

NURSING DIAGNOSIS

Nursing diagnoses during the postpartal period are often "risk for" diagnoses and concerned with a family's ability to accept and bond with a new child or with physiologic considerations. Examples include:

- Health-seeking behaviors related to care of newborn
- Fear related to lack of preparation for child care
- Risk for deficient fluid volume related to postpartal hemorrhage
- Risk for altered family coping related to an additional family member
- Risk for complications in human lactation/breastfeeding
- Uncertainty regarding the infant's well-being if there are congenital anomalies

OUTCOME IDENTIFICATION AND PLANNING

Be certain that outcomes established during this time are realistic in light of a woman's changed life pattern, support from family, and cultural preferences. Most postpartal families remain in the hospital for a relatively short time, only 48 to 72 hours. The postpartum stay in an alternative birth center can be as short as 4 hours. That means outcomes must be devised that can be accomplished and evaluated during this short period of patient contact. If an outcome cannot be evaluated within this short time frame, follow-up home care, ambulatory visits, or phone calls may be necessary.

When planning care in the postpartal period, try to arrange procedures to allow optimal time for family–infant interaction and yet provide adequate time for a woman to rest to prevent exhaustion because this can improve her coping ability and plans for self-care. Nurses can become active in promoting and incorporating the Ten Steps for a Baby-Friendly Initiative strategies (Box 17.2) postpartum to

BOX 17.2

U.S. Baby Friendly Hospital Initiative
Baby-Friendly Ten Steps

1. Have a written breastfeeding policy that is routinely communicated to all health care staff.
2. Train all health care staff in the skills necessary to implement this policy.
3. Inform all pregnant women about the benefits and management of breastfeeding.
4. Help mothers initiate breastfeeding within one hour of birth.
5. Show mothers how to breastfeed and how to maintain lactation, even if they are separated from their infants.
6. Give newborn infants no food or drink other than breast-milk, unless medically indicated.
7. Practice "rooming in"—allow mothers and infants to remain together 24 hours a day.
8. Encourage breastfeeding on demand.
9. Give no pacifiers or artificial nipples to breastfeeding infants.
10. Foster the establishment of breastfeeding support groups and refer mothers to them on discharge from the hospital or birth center.

Reprinted with permission from Baby-Friendly USA. (n.d.). *Ten steps to successful breastfeeding.* Retrieved from http://www.babyfriendlyusa.org/about-us/baby-friendly-hospital-initiative/the-ten-steps

promote breastfeeding and infant-maternal bonding, such as immediate skin-to-skin contact after birth and rooming-in of mom and baby (Baby-Friendly USA, n.d.).

After adequate instruction and assurance that mom and baby are healthy, a woman should be prepared to monitor her own health after she returns home.

Planning should also include ample time for health teaching such as care of the newborn and the need for flexibility in care because the parents do not yet know what their new life will be like or how tired they will become after being awakened frequently during the night. Brainstorming with the parents—practicing to produce at least three different methods of reaching a particular goal—is excellent practice for parenting because giving advice only solves an immediate problem; helping parents learn good problem-solving techniques improves their ability to handle the many challenges that will arise with childrearing. Refer patients and their partners to helpful websites and other resources when appropriate (see Chapter 9).

IMPLEMENTATION

All interventions in the postpartal period should be family-centered, to enhance family functioning and bonding, and geared toward increasing a woman's self-esteem, allowing her to view herself as a new mother and helping her view her new infant as part of her family.

OUTCOME EVALUATION

If a woman fails to make an adequate adjustment to her new life changes, she may have difficulty integrating an infant into the family. This could affect a child's physical and mental health, self-esteem, and ability to form a sense of trust.

Evaluation in the postpartal period, then, involves not only being certain a woman and her baby are safe but also that the woman knows how to maintain her own and her infant's health. Such follow-up evaluation can be done by telephone, during home visits, or during postpartal and well-child assessments. Examples of expected outcomes include:

- The parents spontaneously verbalize at least one positive comment about their child's characteristics before hospital discharge.
- The patient states she believes she will be able to manage newborn care with the support of her significant other.
- The patient's lochial flow is no more than one saturated perineal pad (50 ml) every 3 hours.
- The patient states she is tired but feels able to manage her newborn and family care.
- Physical interaction and holding of the infant appears appropriate and responsive to the infant's needs.

Psychological Changes of the Postpartal Period

The postpartum period is a time of transition, during which a couple gives up concepts such as "childless" or "parents of one" and moves to not only trying out their new role but also determining whether they "fit" their new role. Nurses can help couples acknowledge the extent of the change so that they can gain closure on their previous lifestyle. Opening channels for communication, anticipating new needs, and highlighting potential gains that will occur because of the change are important actions.

BEHAVIORAL ADJUSTMENT: PHASES OF THE PUERPERIUM

In her classic work on maternal behavior, Reva Rubin, a nurse, divided the puerperium into three separate phases (Rubin, 1984). The first of these is the **taking-in phase**, or the time when the new parents review their pregnancy and the labor and birth. The subsequent phases, called the taking-hold and letting-go phases, are times of renewed action and forward movement. At the time these phases of the puerperium were identified, women were hospitalized for 5 to 7 days after childbirth and moved in a paced manner from one step to the next. Today, with a stay in a healthcare facility as short as a few hours, women appear to move through these phases much more quickly and may even experience two different phases at once.

Taking-In Phase

The taking-in phase is largely a time of reflection. During this 1- to 3-day period, a woman is largely passive. She prefers having a nurse attend to her needs and make decisions for her rather than do these things herself. This dependence results partly from her physical discomfort because of afterpains or hemorrhoids, partly from her uncertainty in caring for her newborn, and partly from the exhaustion that follows childbirth.

As part of thinking and pondering about her new role, the woman usually wants to talk about her pregnancy, especially about her labor and birth. She holds her new child with a sense of wonder and asks: Is birth really over? Could this child really have been inside me? She wants to rest to regain her physical strength and experience a calm atmosphere around her to

BOX 17.3
Nursing Care Planning Tips for Effective Communication

Leana Cooper gave birth to a boy 6 hours ago. You want to assess her for postpartal pain, so you enter her hospital room. She is wearing a hospital gown and sitting in the chair by her bed.

Tip: Use therapeutic communication that encourages women to elaborate on their story and avoid any communication that discourages storytelling. Most women are interested in discussing their labor and birth experience in the days immediately after birth as a part of a "taking-in" phase. Repeating the story of how worried they were when labor started, how much pain they had, or how scared they were when their membranes broke helps them put these sensations into perspective and integrate them into their life experiences. Once you have talked about what concerns them most, they'll then be more able to discuss and assess their pain.

Nurse: How are you feeling, Mrs. Cooper?

Mrs. Cooper: Like I'm still rushing around. I called my husband as soon as my water broke. He hit a truck on the way home, though, and afterward, his car wouldn't start. I tried to call—

Nurse: Do you have any pain?

Mrs. Cooper: Just some afterpain. Next, I tried to call my mother, but she couldn't come over because she didn't have a car. My neighbor—

Nurse: Go on.

Mrs. Cooper: He said he'd drive me but then discovered his wife had his car keys.

Nurse: Keep going. It sounds as if you have a lot to get off your mind. Can I do anything to assist or help?

Mrs. Cooper: The whole thing was terrifying. I can't believe I didn't have my baby in the middle of the freeway!

quiet and contain her swirling thoughts. Encouraging her to talk about the birth is an important way to help her integrate the experience into her total life experiences (Box 17.3).

If the birth experience did not go as planned, such as a surprise cesarean delivery or the infant needing specialized care in the neonatal intensive care unit (NICU), encourage the mother to express her feelings regarding the difference from the anticipated birth plan. Being able to acknowledge and articulate her feelings that her preconceived birth plan did not occur as intended is a healthy way to release any negative emotions. Discuss with the mother the possible medical reasons why the birth was different than expected. The birth plan often changes to ensure the safety of the newborn and mother. This will help the mother absorb the new reality and be able to understand the importance of the need to make the necessary changes at birth for her own health and the health of her newborn.

Taking-Hold Phase

After a time of passive dependence, a woman begins to initiate action (the **taking-hold phase**). She prefers to get her

own washcloth or to make her own decisions. Women who give birth without any anesthesia may reach this second phase in a matter of hours after birth.

Concept Mastery Alert

Taking-hold is a time of initiation of action and greater independence as evidenced by performing self-care.

During the taking-in period, a woman may have been too tired to care for her child. Now, she begins to take a stronger interest in her infant and begins maternal role behaviors. As a rule, it is usually best to give a woman a brief demonstration of baby care and then allow her to care for her child herself—with watchful guidance—as she enters this phase.

Although a woman's actions suggest greater independence during this time, she often still feels insecure about her ability to care for her new child. She needs praise for the things she does well, such as supporting the baby's head or beginning breastfeeding, to give her confidence. This positive reinforcement begins in the healthcare facility and continues after discharge, at home and at postpartum and well-baby visits.

Do not rush a woman through the phase of taking-in or prevent her from taking hold when she reaches this point. For many young mothers, learning to make decisions about their child's welfare is one of the most difficult phases of motherhood. It helps if a woman has practice in making such decisions in a sheltered setting, such as a hospital, rather than first taking on that level of responsibility after she is home alone. First-time mothers may need additional guidance and time during this phase compared to multigravida moms, but not always, as in the case of a multigravida mom who is learning to care for twins.

Letting-Go Phase

In this third phase (the **letting-go phase**), a woman finally redefines her new role. She gives up the fantasized image of her child and accepts the real one; she gives up her old role of being childless or the mother of only one or two (or however many children she had before this birth). This process requires some grief work and readjustment of relationships, similar to what occurred during pregnancy. It is extended and continues during the child's growing years. A woman who has reached this phase is well into her new role (Box 17.4).

BOX 17.4
Nursing Care Planning to Respect Cultural Diversity

In the United States, the postpartal period is generally regarded as a time of wellness; early ambulation and eating a varied diet are encouraged. In other cultures, the period after childbirth is regarded primarily as a time of rest. Cultural differences include restricting certain foods, reducing activity levels, or both; taboos and rituals to guard the health of the baby are not uncommon. Assessing women in the postpartal period for cultural variations of these types is important because such variation can explain why a woman might be reluctant to ambulate or why she leaves a lunch uneaten although she said she was hungry.

PATIENT-CENTERED CARE

Leana Cooper has expressed that she is excited to "get to know" her new baby. The nurse determines which of the following actions will support Leana's transition into a postpartal taking-hold phase?

a. Tell her that she did well in labor and that it was "all worth it."
b. Encourage her to take as much time as she needs to recover from her labor.
c. Help her to give her new baby a bath.
d. Encourage her and her husband to choose their baby's name as soon as possible.

Look in Appendix A for the best answer and rationale.

DEVELOPMENT OF PARENTAL ATTACHMENT, BONDING, AND POSITIVE FAMILY RELATIONSHIPS

During pregnancy, almost every woman worries about her ability to be a "good" mother, and this concern does not evaporate as soon as the baby is born. Some women are able to recognize a newborn's needs immediately and to give care with confident understanding right from the start. More often, however, a woman enters into a relationship with her newborn tentatively and with qualms and conflicts that must be addressed before the relationship can be meaningful. Another factor is the infant's inherent personality. Some infants are calm and others are easily excitable. Learning the infant's cues and personality takes time and patience. This is because parental love is only partly instinctive. A major portion develops gradually, in stages such as planning the pregnancy, hearing the pregnancy confirmed, feeling the child move in utero, birthing, touching the baby, and, finally, giving total care to the child.

When a woman has successfully linked with her newborn, it is termed **attachment** or **bonding**. Although a woman carried the child inside her for 9 months, she often approaches her newborn not as someone she loves but more as she would approach a stranger. The first time she holds the infant, she may touch only the blanket. If she unfolds the blanket to examine the baby or count the fingers or toes, she may use only her fingertips for touch (Fig. 17.1). Skin-to-skin contact soon after birth facilitates the early attachment and binding phase. This should ideally occur within the first hour of any birth, even cesarean deliveries, as soon as the mother and baby are stable and last until completion of the first breastfeeding (Moore, Bergman, Anderson, et al., 2016).

Gradually, as a woman holds her child more, she begins to express more warmth, touching the child with the palm of her hand rather than with her fingertips. She smoothes the baby's hair, brushes a cheek, plays with toes, and lets the baby's fingers clasp hers. Soon, she feels comfortable enough to press her cheek against the baby's or kiss the infant's nose; she has successfully bonded or become a mother tending to her child. Looking directly at her newborn's face, with direct eye contact (termed an **en face position**), is a sign a woman is beginning effective attachment. Many fathers can be observed staring at a newborn for long intervals in this same way.

Figure 17.1 A mom and dad begin interaction with their newborn immediately after birth: a very special moment in their life. (© Kathy Sloane.)

Often termed **engrossment**, this action alerts caregivers to how actively the father, as well as the mother, is beginning bonding (Fig. 17.2). The length of time parents take to bond with a child depends on the circumstances of the pregnancy and birth, the wellness and ability of the child to meet the parents' expectations, reciprocal actions by the newborn, and the opportunities the parents have to interact with the child. When pregnancy or newborn complications lead to separation of the mother from her newborn, it places the woman at greater risk for developing posttraumatic stress disorder and interferes with the usual process of bonding (Dale-Hewitt, Slade, Wright, et al., 2012). Guided, supportive interactions, such as pointing out positive parental behaviors and infant responses, enhance positive parent–infant interaction. Helping parents sort out their feelings about being a mother or father and about their new responsibilities through anticipatory guidance also strengthens parent–infant bonding. Facilitating early skin-to-skin bonding between infant and mother has shown to improve breastfeeding durations and outcomes and the emotional stability of both infant and mother (Moore et al., 2016).

Figure 17.2 A nurse encourages a father as he interacts and bonds with his newborn. Note the fingertip touching. (© Caroline Brown, RNC, MS, DEd.)

QUALITY IMPROVEMENT

The nurse observes Leana Cooper holding her newborn. Which position would best reassure the nurse that interventions aimed at promoting bonding have been successful?

   a. She looks directly at her infant's face and talks to him.
   b. She holds the infant over her shoulder and gently burps him.
   c. She sits in a rocking chair and slowly rocks her new infant.
   d. She lies in bed and places the infant on her stomach.

Look in Appendix A for the best answer and rationale.

Figure 17.3 Sibling visiting is important to bring a family together.

Rooming-In

The more time a woman has to spend with her baby, the sooner she can become better acquainted with her child, feel more confident in her ability to care for her baby, and more likely form a sound mother–child relationship (Elliott-Carter & Harper, 2012). In order to qualify as "baby friendly," a hospital must provide "**rooming-in**," or space to keep the infant with the parents (Smith, Moorem, & Peters, 2012).

Rooming-in occurs when the infant remains in the woman's room and the mother and child are together 23 out of 24 hours a day. With both complete and partial rooming-in (infant spends time in newborn nursery), the father and siblings can hold the infant when they visit. In many settings, the father can stay overnight in the mother's room.

Sibling Visitation

Separation from children is often as painful for a mother as it is for her children. Waiting at home, separated from their mother and listening only to telephone reports of what a new brother or sister looks like, can be very difficult for older children. They may picture the new baby as much older than he or she actually is. "He is eating well" may produce an image of a child sitting at a table using a fork and spoon. "He weighs 8 pounds" can be meaningless information. A chance to visit the hospital and see the new baby and their mother reduces feelings that their mother cares more about the new baby than about them. The visit can help to relieve some of the impact of separation and also help to make the baby a part of the family (Fig. 17.3). Assess to be certain siblings are free of contagious diseases such as upper respiratory tract illnesses or recent exposure to chickenpox before they visit. Then, have them wash their hands and, if they choose, hold or touch the newborn with parental assistance.

Encourage the success of a family visit by evaluating if the mother would like to take her pain medication before the visit. If she had a cesarean delivery, protecting her abdomen with padding can decrease anxiety of the siblings about the condition of their mother.

You may need to caution a woman that the opinions of a new brother or sister expressed by her older children may not be complimentary; for example, this baby with little hair may not be their idea of a "pretty baby." If they thought the new baby would be big enough to play with, they may not agree that he is a "big baby."

MATERNAL CONCERNS AND FEELINGS IN THE POSTPARTAL PERIOD

Traditionally, it is assumed the bulk of a woman's concerns in the postpartal period center on the care of her new infant. As a result, classes in the postpartal period have traditionally focused on teaching how to breastfeed and bathe infants. Many women, however, are not as concerned about infant care as they are about their adjustment to a new role change.

Typical issues identified by postpartal women that they would like to hear discussed are breast soreness; regaining their figure; regulating the demands of a job, housework, their partner, and their children; coping with emotional tension and sibling jealousy; and how to combat fatigue.

Abandonment

Many mothers, if given the opportunity, admit to feeling abandoned and less important after giving birth than they did during pregnancy or labor. Only hours before, after all, they were the center of attention, with everyone asking about their health and well-being. Now, suddenly, the baby is everyone's chief interest. Relatives ask about the baby's health; the gifts are all for the baby. Even a woman's primary healthcare provider, who has made her feel so important for the last 9 months, may ask during a visit, "How's that healthy 8-pound boy?" Comments such as this can make a woman experience a sensation very close to jealousy. And how can a good mother be jealous of her own baby?

You can help a woman move past these feelings by verbalizing the problem: "How things have changed! Everyone's asking about the baby today and not about you, aren't they?" These are reassuring words for a woman and help her realize that, although uncomfortable, the feeling she is experiencing is normal.

When a newborn comes home, a father or partner may express much the same feelings as he or she feels resentful of the time the mother spends with the infant. Examination of these competitive feelings can help a couple realize that parenthood involves some compromise in favor of the baby's interests. Making infant care a shared responsibility can help alleviate these feelings and make both partners feel equally involved in the baby's care. You can help parents or partners move past this competitive stage by pointing out positive parenting behaviors, positive self-care behaviors, and the warm infant response to their behaviors.

Disappointment

Another common feeling parents or partners may experience is disappointment in the baby. All during pregnancy, they pictured a chubby-cheeked, curly-haired, smiling girl or boy. They may have instead a thinner baby, without any hair, who seems to cry constantly, or may have a congenital condition. This can make it difficult to feel positive immediately toward a child who does not meet their expectations. It can cause parents to remember their adolescence, when they felt gangly and unattractive, or to experience feelings of inadequacy all over again.

You can never change the sex, size, or look of a child, but in the short time you care for a postpartal family, it is possible for a key person such as a nurse to tip a scale toward acceptance or at least help a person involved to take a clearer look at his or her situation and begin to cope with the new circumstances. As an example, handle the child warmly, to show you find the infant satisfactory or even special. Comment on the child's good points, such as long fingers, lovely eyes, and healthy appetite. Be aware, however, that, culturally, some groups are fearful for the baby if these types of comments are made because they could draw evil influences toward the child.

Postpartal Blues

During the postpartal period, as many as 50% of women experience some feelings of overwhelming sadness or "baby blues" (Baselice & Lawson, 2012). They may burst into tears easily or feel let down and irritable. This phenomenon may be caused by hormonal changes, particularly the decrease in estrogen and progesterone that occurred with delivery of the placenta. Breastfeeding has been shown to help elevate baby blues and counteract the effects of the hormonal drop that occurs after childbirth. For some women, it may be a response to dependence and low self-esteem caused by exhaustion, being away from home, physical discomfort, and the tension engendered by assuming a new role, especially if a woman is not receiving support from her partner. In addition to crying, the syndrome is evidenced by feelings of inadequacy, mood lability, anorexia, and sleep disturbance.

Anticipatory guidance and individualized support from healthcare personnel are important to help the parents understand that this unexpected response is normal. Be certain support persons also receive assurance of this type, or they can think the woman is unhappy with them or the new baby or is keeping some terrible news about the baby secret.

Give the woman a chance to verbalize her feelings and make as many decisions as she wants to help her gain a sense of control and move past this strange postpartal emotion.

Remember, however, not all postpartal women you see crying are doing so because they have baby blues. Perhaps problems at home have become overwhelming. A partner may have been laid off from a job just at this time when they most need money. One of her parents may be ill, or her house may have been damaged by a disaster such as a flood. Encouraging women to talk about their postpartal feelings helps to differentiate between problems that can be handled best with discussion and concerned understanding and those that should be referred to a social service department or a community health agency for additional support.

Women are at greater risk (19% to 48%) for moderate to severe depression after childbirth requiring formal counseling, especially if they are economically stressed or have a comorbid condition such as diabetes (Farr, Dietz, Williams, et al., 2011). Severe psychosis also can occur in women during this time (Heron, Gilbert, Dolman, et al., 2012). Because these are deeper level concerns, postpartal depression beyond the scope of "baby blues" and psychosis are discussed in Chapter 25. If a mother appears to have a level of depression that is beyond baby blues and/or has a history of previous postpartal depression (PPD), closer observation and referral is indicated immediately.

Physiologic Changes of the Postpartal Period

Retrogressive physiologic changes that occur during the postpartal period include those related specifically to the reproductive system as well as other systemic changes (Box 17.5).

REPRODUCTIVE SYSTEM CHANGES

Involution is the process whereby the reproductive organs return to their nonpregnant state. A woman is in danger of hemorrhage from the denuded surface of the uterus until involution is complete (Katz, 2012).

The Uterus

Involution of the uterus involves two processes. First, the area where the placenta was implanted is sealed off to prevent bleeding. Second, the organ is reduced to its approximate pregestational size.

The sealing of the placenta site is accomplished by rapid contraction of the uterus immediately after delivery of the placenta. This contraction pinches the blood vessels entering the 7-cm-wide area left denuded by the placenta and halts bleeding. With time, thrombi form within the uterine sinuses and permanently seal the area. Eventually, endometrial tissue undermines the site and obliterates the organized thrombi, covering and healing the area so completely the process leaves no scar tissue within the uterus so does not compromise future implantation sites.

The same contraction process reduces the bulk of the uterus. Devoid of the placenta and the membranes, the walls of the uterus thicken and contract, gradually reducing the uterus from a container large enough to hold a full-term fetus to one the size of a grapefruit, a phenomenon that can be compared with a rubber band that has been stretched for many months and now is regaining its normal contour. None of the rubber band is destroyed; the shape is simply altered.

ASSESSING THE POSTPARTAL WOMAN

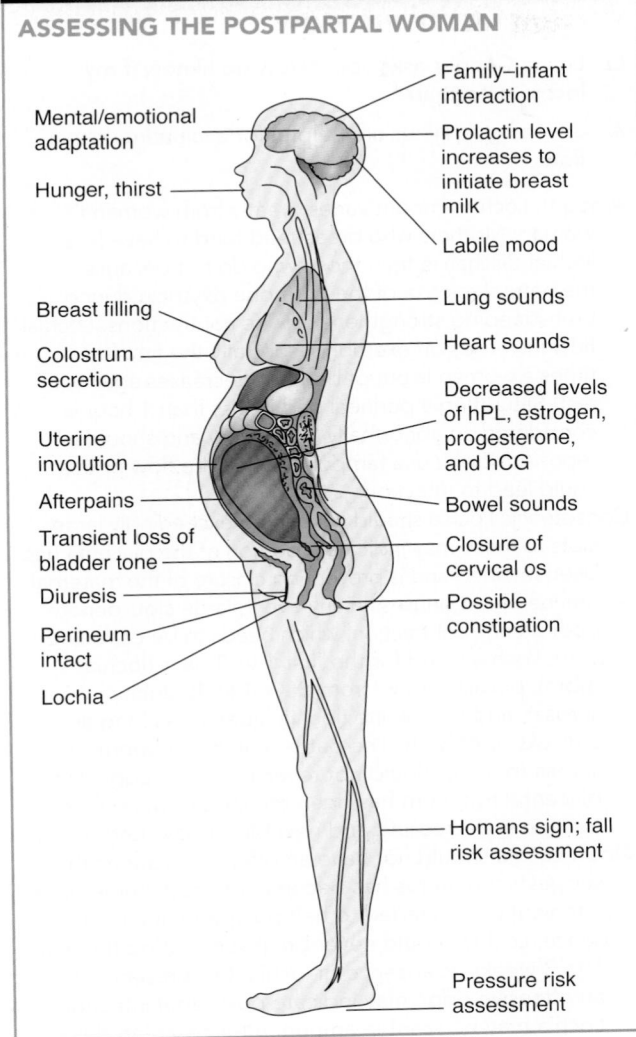

- Mental/emotional adaptation
- Hunger, thirst
- Breast filling
- Colostrum secretion
- Uterine involution
- Afterpains
- Transient loss of bladder tone
- Diuresis
- Perineum intact
- Lochia
- Family–infant interaction
- Prolactin level increases to initiate breast milk
- Labile mood
- Lung sounds
- Heart sounds
- Decreased levels of hPL, estrogen, progesterone, and hCG
- Bowel sounds
- Closure of cervical os
- Possible constipation
- Homans sign; fall risk assessment
- Pressure risk assessment

For this reason, the postpartal period, like pregnancy, is not a period of illness, of necrosing cells being evacuated, but primarily a period of healthy change (Edmonds, 2012).

Immediately after birth, the uterus weighs about 1,000 g. At the end of the first week, it weighs 500 g. By the time involution is complete (6 weeks), it weighs approximately 50 g, similar to its prepregnancy weight. Because uterine contraction begins immediately after placental delivery, the fundus of the uterus is palpable through the abdominal wall, halfway between the umbilicus and the symphysis pubis, within a few minutes after birth. One hour later, it will rise to the level of the umbilicus, where it remains for approximately the next 24 hours. From then on, it decreases by one fingerbreadth, or 1 cm, per day; for example, on the first postpartal day, it will be palpable 1 cm below the umbilicus. In the average woman, by the ninth or tenth day, the uterus will have contracted so much that it is withdrawn into the pelvis and can no longer be detected by abdominal palpation (Fig. 17.4).

The uterus of a breastfeeding mother may contract even more quickly because oxytocin, which is released with breastfeeding, stimulates uterine contractions. Breastfeeding alone, however, is not sufficient to protect against postpartum hemorrhage.

The fundus is normally located in the midline of the abdomen. Occasionally, it can be felt slightly to the right because the bulk of the sigmoid colon forced it to that side during pregnancy and it tends to remain in that position. Assess fundal height shortly after a woman has emptied her bladder for most accurate results because a full bladder can keep the uterus from contracting, pushing it upward and increasing the risk of excess bleeding and blood clot formation in the uterus.

Involution will occur most dependably in a woman who is well nourished and who ambulates early after birth as gravity may play a role. Involution may be delayed by a condition such as the birth of multiple fetuses, hydramnios, exhaustion from prolonged labor, grand multiparity, or physiologic effects of excessive analgesia. Contraction may be ineffective if there is retained placenta or membranes (Samanta, Roy, Mistri, et al., 2013).

An estimation of the consistency of the postpartal uterus is as important as measurement of its height. A well-contracted fundus feels so firm it can be compared with a grapefruit in both size and tenseness. Whenever the fundus feels boggy (soft or flabby), it is not as contracted as it should be, despite its position in the abdomen.

The first hour after birth is potentially the most dangerous time for a woman. If her uterus should become relaxed during this time (**uterine atony**), she will lose blood very rapidly because no permanent thrombi have yet formed at the placental site.

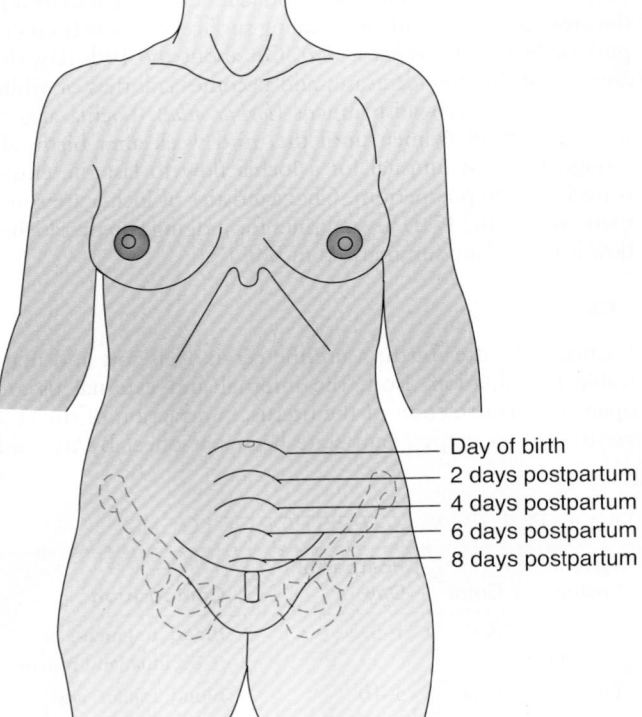

- Day of birth
- 2 days postpartum
- 4 days postpartum
- 6 days postpartum
- 8 days postpartum

Figure 17.4 Uterine involution. The uterus decreases in size at a predictable rate during the postpartal period. After 10 days, it recedes under the pubic bone and is no longer palpable.

In some women, contraction of the uterus after birth causes intermittent cramping termed **afterpains**, similar to that accompanying a menstrual period. Afterpains tend to be noticed most by multiparas than by primiparas and by women who have given birth to large babies or multiple births. In these situations, the uterus must contract more forcefully to regain its prepregnancy size. These sensations are noticed most intensely with breastfeeding, when the infant's sucking causes a release of oxytocin from the posterior pituitary, increasing the strength of the contractions.

Lochia

The separation of the placenta and membranes occurs in the spongy layer or outer portion of the decidua basalis of the uterus. By the second day after birth, the layer of decidua remaining under the placental site (an area 7 cm wide) and throughout the uterus differentiates into two distinct layers. The inner layer attached to the muscular wall of the uterus remains, serving as the foundation from which a new layer of endometrium will be formed. The layer adjacent to the uterine cavity becomes necrotic and is cast off as a vaginal discharge similar to a menstrual flow. This flow, consisting of blood, fragments of decidua, white blood cells, mucus, and some bacteria, is termed **lochia** (Chi, Bapir, Lee, et al., 2010).

The portion of the uterus where the placenta was not attached is so fully cleansed by this sloughing process it will be in a reproductive state in about 3 weeks' time; it takes approximately 6 weeks (the entire postpartal period) for the placental implantation site to be healed.

For the first 3 days after birth, a lochia discharge consists almost entirely of blood, with only small particles of decidua and mucus. Because of its mainly red color, it is termed *lochia rubra*. As the amount of blood involved in the cast-off tissue decreases (about the fourth day) and leukocytes begin to invade the area, as they do with any healing surface, the flow becomes pink or brownish (*lochia serosa*). On about the 10th day, the amount of the flow decreases and becomes colorless or white with streaks of brownish mucus (*lochia alba*). Lochia alba is present in most women until the third week after birth, although it is not unusual for a lochia flow to last the entire 6 weeks of the puerperium. Characteristics of lochia are summarized in Table 17.1. Several rules for judging whether lochia flow is normal are summarized in Box 17.6.

The Cervix

Immediately after birth, a uterine cervix feels soft and malleable to palpation. Both the internal and external os are open. Like contraction of the uterus, contraction of the cervix toward its prepregnant state begins at once. By the end

BOX 17.6

Nursing Care Planning Based on Family Teaching

EVALUATING LOCHIA FLOW

Q. Leana Cooper asks you, "How do I know if my lochia is normal?"

A. Several guidelines are helpful for evaluating lochia flow:

Amount: Lochia amount varies greatly from woman to woman. Mothers who breastfeed tend to have less lochial discharge than those who do not because the natural release of the hormone oxytocin during breastfeeding strengthens uterine contractions. Lochial flow increases on exertion, especially the first few times a woman is out of bed but decreases again with rest. Saturating a perineal pad in less than 1 hour is considered an abnormally heavy flow and should be reported. Don't use tampons to halt the flow or this could lead to infection.

Consistency: Lochia should contain no exceedingly large clots as these may indicate a portion of the placenta has been retained and is preventing closure of the maternal uterine blood sinuses. In any event, large clots denote poor uterine contraction, which needs to be corrected.

Pattern: Lochia is red for the first 1 to 3 days (lochia rubra), pinkish-brown from days 4 to 10 (lochia serosa), and then white (lochia alba) for as long as 6 weeks after birth. The pattern of lochia (rubra to serosa to alba) should not reverse as this suggests a placental fragment has been retained or uterine contraction is decreasing and new bleeding is beginning.

Odor: Lochia should not have an offensive odor as this suggests the uterus has become infected. Immediate intervention is needed to halt postpartal infection.

Absence: Lochia should never be absent during the first 1 to 3 weeks as absence of lochia, like presence of an offensive odor, may indicate postpartal infection. Lochia may be scant in amount after cesarean delivery, but it is never altogether absent.

of 7 days, the external os has narrowed to the size of a pencil opening; the cervix feels firm and nongravid again.

In contrast to the process of uterine involution, in which the changes consist primarily of old cells being returned to their former position by contraction, the process in the cervix does involve the formation of new muscle cells. Because of this, the cervix does not return exactly to its prepregnancy state. The internal os closes as before, but after a vaginal birth, the external os usually remains slightly open and appears slit-like or stellate (star shaped), whereas previously, it was round. Finding this pattern on pelvic examination suggests that childbearing has taken place.

The Vagina

After a vaginal birth, the vagina feels soft, with few rugae, and its diameter is considerably greater than normal. The hymen is permanently torn and heals with small, separate tags of tissue.

TABLE 17.1 CHARACTERISTICS OF LOCHIA

Type of Lochia	Color	Postpartal Day	Composition
Lochia rubra	Red	1–3	Blood, fragments of decidua, and mucus
Lochia serosa	Pink	3–10	Blood, mucus, and invading leukocytes
Lochia alba	White	10–14 (may last 6 weeks)	Largely mucus; leukocyte count high

It takes the entire postpartal period for the vagina to involute (by contraction, as with the uterus) until it gradually returns to its approximate prepregnancy state. Thickening of the walls appears to depend on renewed estrogen stimulation from the ovaries. Because a woman who is breastfeeding may have delayed ovulation, she may continue to have thin-walled or fragile vaginal cells that cause slight vaginal bleeding during sexual intercourse until about 6 weeks' time. If a woman practices Kegel exercises, the strength and tone of the vagina will increase more rapidly (see Chapter 12). This may be important for the sexual enjoyment of both a woman and her partner.

QSEN Checkpoint Question 17.3

SAFETY

The nurse wants to prepare Leana to assess her own health after discharge. Which statement by her would make the nurse worry that she needs added information?

a. "I know about lochia; I'll use tampons just like I do for my periods."
b. "I admit I don't like having lochia, but I understand its purpose."
c. "I know to wash my hands after I change perineal pads and before handling the baby."
d. "I'll look for the color of my lochia to change from red to pink."

Look in Appendix A for the best answer and rationale.

The Perineum

Because of the great amount of pressure experienced during birth, the perineum is edematous and tender immediately after birth. Ecchymosis patches from ruptured capillaries may show on the surface. The labia majora and labia minora typically remain atrophic and softened after birth, never returning to their prepregnancy state. Mothers may experience various levels of tenderness in the perineum area. Suggesting nonpharmacologic comfort measures such as ice or warm packs or a gentle pillow or doughnut pad to sit on will be much appreciated by the mother. Nurses should discuss with the mother's provider available pharmacologic pain relievers, such as acetaminophen or ibuprofen, and administer according to the prescription orders when deemed necessary or by maternal request.

SYSTEMIC CHANGES

The same body systems that were involved in pregnancy are also involved in postpartal changes as the body returns to its prepregnancy state.

The Hormonal System

Pregnancy hormones begin to decrease as soon as the placenta is no longer present. Levels of human chorionic gonadotropin (hCG) and human placental lactogen (hPL) are almost negligible by 24 hours. By week 1, progestin, estrogen, and estradiol are all at prepregnancy levels (estriol may take an additional week before it reaches prepregnancy levels). Follicle-stimulating hormone (FSH) remains low for about 12 days and then begins to rise as a new menstrual cycle is initiated.

The Urinary System

During pregnancy, as much as 2,000 to 3,000 ml of excess fluid accumulates in the body so extensive diaphoresis (excessive sweating) and diuresis (excess urine production) begin almost immediately after birth to rid the body of this fluid. This easily increases the daily urine output of a postpartal woman from a normal level of 1,500 ml to as much as 3,000 ml/day during the second to fifth day after birth. This marked increase in urine production causes the bladder to fill rapidly. Reassure the mother that this is normal and she still needs to continue drinking a healthy amount of fluids daily, especially if she is breastfeeding.

Because during a vaginal birth, the fetal head exerts a great deal of pressure on the bladder and urethra as it passes on the bladder's underside, this may leave the bladder with a transient loss of tone that, together with the edema surrounding the urethra, decreases a woman's ability to sense when she has to void. A woman who has had epidural anesthesia can feel no sensation in the bladder area until the anesthetic has worn off.

To prevent permanent damage to the bladder from overdistention, assess a woman's abdomen frequently in the immediate postpartal period. On palpation, a full bladder is felt as a hard or firm area just above the symphysis pubis. On percussion (placing one finger flat on the woman's abdomen over the bladder and tapping it with the middle finger of the other hand), a full bladder sounds resonant, in contrast to the dull, thudding sound of non–fluid-filled tissue. Pressure on this area may make a woman feel as if she has to void, but she is then unable to do so. As the bladder fills, it displaces the uterus; uterine position and lack of contraction are therefore a second good gauge of whether a bladder is full or empty (Mulder, Schoffelmeer, Hakvoort, et al., 2012).

The hydronephrosis or increased size of ureters that occurred during pregnancy remains present for about 4 weeks after birth. The increased size of these structures, in conjunction with reduced bladder sensitivity, increases the possibility of urinary stasis and urinary tract infection in the postpartal period.

The Circulatory System

The diuresis that is evident between the second and fifth days after birth, as well as the blood loss at birth, acts to reduce the added blood volume a woman accumulated during pregnancy. This reduction occurs so rapidly, in fact, that the blood volume returns to its normal prepregnancy level by the first or second week after birth.

The usual blood loss with a vaginal birth is 300 to 500 ml. With a cesarean delivery, it is 500 to 1,000 ml. A 4-point decrease in hematocrit (proportion of red blood cells to circulating plasma) and a 1-g decrease in hemoglobin value occur with each 250 ml of blood lost. For example, if an average woman enters labor with a hematocrit of 37%, it will be about 33% on the first postpartal day, and hemoglobin will fall from 11 to 10 g/dl. If the woman was anemic during pregnancy, she can expect to continue to be anemic afterward. As excess fluid is excreted, the hematocrit gradually rises (because of hemoconcentration), reaching prepregnancy levels by 6 weeks after birth.

Women usually continue to have the same high level of plasma fibrinogen during the first postpartal weeks as they did during pregnancy. This is a protective measure against hemorrhage. However, this high level also increases the risk of thrombus formation. There is also an increase in the number of leukocytes in the blood. The white blood cell count may be as high as 30,000 cells/mm^3 (mainly granulocytes) compared to a normal level of 5,000 to 10,000 cells/mm^3, particularly if labor was long or difficult. This, too, is part of the body's defense system, a defense against infection and an aid to healing.

Any varicosities that are present from pregnancy will recede, but they rarely return to a completely prepregnant appearance. Although vascular blemishes, such as spider angiomas, fade slightly, they may not disappear completely either. Bilateral ankle edema is not uncommon but should not progress above the knees. This decreases over time as fluid shifts and returns to the circulatory system.

The Gastrointestinal System

Digestion and absorption begin to be active again soon after birth unless a woman has had a cesarean delivery. Almost immediately, the woman feels hungry and thirsty, and she can eat without difficulty from nausea or vomiting during this time.

Hemorrhoids (distended rectal veins) that have been pushed out of the rectum because of the effort of pelvic-stage pushing often are present. Bowel sounds are active, but passage of stool through the bowel may be slow because of the still-present effect of **relaxin** (a hormone which softens and lengthens the cervix and pubic symphysis for preparation of the infant's birth during pregnancy) on the bowel. Bowel evacuation may be difficult because of pain if a woman has episiotomy sutures or from hemorrhoids. Encouraging the mother to eat produce and soluble fiber foods, especially fruits, will help keep her stools naturally soft and ease in her bowel movements.

The Integumentary System

After birth, the stretch marks on a woman's abdomen (**striae gravidarum**) still appear reddened and may be even more prominent than during pregnancy, when they were tightly stretched. Typically, in a White woman, these will fade to a pale white over the next 3 to 6 months; in a Black woman, they may remain as areas of slightly darker pigment. Excessive pigment on the face and neck (**chloasma**) and on the abdomen (**linea nigra**) will become barely detectable by 6 weeks' time. If **diastasis recti** (overstretching and separation of the abdominal musculature) occurred, the area will appear as a slightly indented bluish streak in the abdominal midline. Modified sit-ups help to strengthen abdominal muscles and return abdominal support to its prepregnant level. Diastasis recti, however, may require surgery to correct (Hickey, Finch, & Khanna, 2011).

RETROGRESSIVE CHANGES OF THE PUERPERIUM

The overall effects of postpartal retrogressive changes are exhaustion and weight loss.

Exhaustion

As soon as birth is completed, a woman experiences total exhaustion. For the last several months of pregnancy, she probably experienced some difficulty sleeping. All during labor, she worked hard with little or no sleep. Now, she has "sleep hunger," which may make it difficult for her to cope with new experiences and stressful situations until she has enjoyed a sustained period of sleep.

Weight Loss

The rapid diuresis and diaphoresis during the second to fifth days after birth usually result in a weight loss of 5 lb (2 to 4 kg), in addition to the approximately 12 lb (5.8 kg) lost at birth. Lochia flow causes an additional 2- to 3-lb (1-kg) loss, for a total weight loss of about 19 lb. Additional weight loss is dependent on the amount of pregnancy weight gain and on whether a woman continues active measures to lose weight (Cahill, Freeland-Graves, Shah, et al., 2012). It is also influenced by nutrition, exercise, and breastfeeding. The weight a woman reaches at 6 weeks after birth becomes her baseline postpartal weight unless she continues active measures to lose the weight. In many women, this baseline is higher than their prepregnancy weight and one of the reasons that obesity has become a national health concern (Lipsky, Strawderman, & Olson, 2012). Balancing a newborn, eating healthy foods, and finding the time to exercise becomes a challenge to many mothers. Discussing strategies with her will help to organize her efforts to find balance, such as helpful babysitters, family members, and/or her partner to come and give her needed breaks.

Vital Sign Changes

Vital sign changes in the postpartum period reflect the internal adjustments that occur as a woman's body returns to its prepregnant state.

Temperature

Temperature is always taken orally or tympanically (never rectally) during the puerperium because of the danger of vaginal contamination and the discomfort involved in rectal intrusion.

A woman may show a slight increase in temperature during the first 24 hours after birth because of dehydration that occurred during labor. If she takes in adequate fluid during the first 24 hours, this temperature elevation will return to normal. Most women are thirsty immediately after birth and are eager to take in fluid, so drinking a large quantity of fluid is not a problem unless the woman is nauseated from a birth analgesic.

Any woman whose oral temperature rises above 100.4°F (38°C), excluding the first 24-hour period, is considered by criteria of the Joint Commission on Maternal Welfare to be febrile, and such a high temperature may indicate that a postpartal infection is present (Johnson, Thakar, & Sultan, 2012). Occasionally, when a woman's breasts fill with milk on the third or fourth postpartum day during lactogenesis II, her temperature will rise for a period of hours because of the increased vascular activity involved; this process is termed **engorgement**. If the elevation in temperature lasts longer than a few hours, however, infection may be the reason. An infection of the breast during lactation is termed *mastitis*. Mothers may or may not feel breast pain or experience redness of the breast, but they will often have a high temperature and feel flu-like symptoms such as malaise and fatigue. Mastitis can interfere with lactation, and sometimes, an infant will refuse to nurse on the affected side. The women's medical provider must be notified to initiate antibiotic treatment (congruent with breastfeeding). Mothers should be instructed to continue breastfeeding if the infant will breastfeed from the affected side. If the infant refuses, instruct the mother to pump her breasts to maintain flow (and to avoid clogged ducts) and then offer the affected breast after 12 to 24 hours. Once the mastitis is treated, infants often will resume breastfeeding after 12 to 24 hours. Unless specifically directed otherwise, infants are safe to continue to breastfeed while a mother is being treated for mastitis; there is no reason to provide alternative feeding methods or to wean because of maternal mastitis. Because infection is a major cause of postpartal mortality and morbidity, nurses have the important role of being the healthcare providers who may first detect the problem.

Pulse

A woman's pulse rate during the postpartal period is usually slightly slower than usual. During pregnancy, the distended uterus obstructed the amount of venous blood returning to the heart; after birth, to accommodate the increased blood volume returning to the heart, stroke volume increases. This increased stroke volume reduces the pulse rate to between 60 and 70 beats/min. As diuresis diminishes the blood volume and causes blood pressure to fall, the pulse rate increases accordingly. By the end of the first week, the pulse rate will have returned to normal.

Evaluate pulse rate conscientiously in the postpartal period because a rapid and thready pulse during this time could be a sign of hemorrhage.

Blood Pressure

Blood pressure should also be monitored carefully during the postpartal period because a decrease in this can also indicate bleeding. In contrast, an elevation above 140 mmHg systolic or 90 mmHg diastolic may indicate the development of postpartal hypertension of pregnancy, an unusual but serious complication of the puerperium (Chhabra, Tyagi, Bhavani, et al., 2012) (see Chapter 21).

To evaluate blood pressure, compare a woman's pressure with her prepregnancy level if possible rather than with standard blood pressure ranges; otherwise, if her blood pressure rose during pregnancy, a significant postpartal decrease in pressure could be missed.

Oxytocics, drugs frequently administered during the postpartal period to achieve uterine contraction, cause contraction of all smooth muscle, including blood vessels (Karch, 2013). Consequently, these drugs can increase blood pressure. Always measure blood pressure before administering one of these agents; if blood pressure is greater than 140/90 mmHg, withhold the agent and notify the woman's primary care provider to prevent hypertension and, possibly, a cerebrovascular accident.

A major complication in women who have lost an appreciable amount of blood with birth is orthostatic hypotension, or dizziness that occurs on standing because of the lack of adequate blood volume to maintain nourishment of brain cells. To test whether a woman will be susceptible to this, assess her blood pressure and pulse while she is lying supine. Next, raise the head of the bed fully upright, wait 2 or 3 minutes, and reassess these values. If the pulse rate is increased by more than 20 beats/min and blood pressure is 15 to 20 mmHg lower than formerly, the woman might

be susceptible to dizziness and fainting when she ambulates. Inform the woman's primary care provider of these findings. Advise her to always sit up slowly and "dangle" on the side of her bed before attempting to walk. If she notices obvious dizziness on sitting upright, support her during ambulation to avoid the possibility of a fall. Caution her not to attempt to walk carrying her newborn until her cardiovascular status adjusts to her blood loss.

 What If . . . 17.1
Leana Cooper, now 12 hours postpartum, has an oral temperature of 99°F (37.2°C) and is uncomfortable from profuse diaphoresis and extreme fatigue. What actions would the nurse take?

PROGRESSIVE CHANGES OF THE PUERPERIUM

Two physiologic changes that occur during the puerperium involve progressive changes, or the building of new tissue. Because this requires good nutrition, caution women against strict dieting that would limit cell-building ability during the first 6 weeks after childbirth (Whitney & Rolfes, 2012).

Lactation

The early lactation process, which is driven by hormones from the hypothalamus to the pituitary gland in order to secrete the lactation hormones, is identified by four phases of **lactogenesis** (human milk production). Prolactin hormone is responsible for milk production, and oxytocin is responsible for the let-down reflex arch. A retrained placenta can inhibit this process by causing continual circulation of progesterone, which inhibits prolactin and thus milk production. The lactogenesis I (milk synthesis) process begins around 16 weeks gestation as the glandular luminal cells in the breast begin secreting **colostrum**, a thin, watery prelactation secretion (Wambach & Riordan, 2016). Lactogenesis II is triggered at birth by the delivery of the placenta, when the progesterone hormone (prolactin is no longer inhibited) and other circulating pregnancy hormones suddenly decrease and oxytocin sharply increases as a result of the infant suckling. Oxytocin helps the uterus to shrink to its prepregnancy size; some mothers will feel uterine cramps initially when breastfeeding until the uterus fully involutes. Lactogenesis II is often when mothers feel that their "milk has come in" (engorgement) and occurs from birth to 5 to 10 days postpartum; this is often termed "transitional milk." Lactogenesis III can occur from day 10 until weaning postpartum, when the "mature milk" supply is now driven by the circulating lactation hormones oxytocin and progesterone. Lactogenesis IV occurs after complete weaning and the breasts involute to their prelactation state. Other hormones are associated with breastfeeding, such as endorphins and oxytocin, and may help to mitigate and reduce the risk of developing postpartum depression (Ahn & Corwin, 2015).

The formation of breast milk (lactation) begins in a postpartal woman whether or not she plans to breastfeed (Stuebe, 2012). Early in pregnancy, the increased estrogen level produced by the placenta stimulated the growth of milk glands; breasts increased in size because of these larger glands, accumulated fluid, and some extra adipose tissue. For the first 2 days after birth, an average woman notices little change in her breasts from the way they were during pregnancy because, since mid-way through pregnancy, she has been secreting colostrum. On the third day after birth, her breasts become full and feel tense or tender as milk forms within breast ducts and replaces colostrum. If a mother reports she experienced little or no changes in her breasts during pregnancy, alert her provider and call for a lactation consultation. This may indicate a complication in her breast anatomy and her ability to secrete enough milk. Generally, breastfeeding complications are rare and typically initially stem from a painful latch, a problem that can be addressed quickly. Most American women are able to successfully breastfeed their newborn and even twins or triplets.

Breast milk forms in response to the decrease in estrogen and progesterone levels that follows delivery of the placenta (which stimulates prolactin production and, consequently, milk production) and an increase in prolactin and oxytocin. A woman's breasts become fuller, larger, and firmer as blood and lymph enter the area to contribute fluid to the formation of milk. In many women, breast distention/engorgement is accompanied by a feeling of heat or tenderness. During the engorgement phase, the breast tissue may appear reddened as if an acute inflammatory or infectious process were present and some moms experience increased tenderness or throbbing. This feeling of tension in the breasts on the third or fourth day after birth is termed *primary engorgement*. It fades as the infant begins effective latching and begins transferring colostrum initially followed by milk from the breasts. Whether milk production (lactogenesis) continues will depend on an infant's successful latch, ability to suck, and transfer milk effectively, as this releases oxytocin and prolactin which promotes the lactogenesis process. Mothers who are primigravida tend to have a longer initial lactogenesis phase and may not have an abundance of milk until the fourth to sixth day postpartum. This is normal and does not indicate that a mother cannot breastfeed. Multigravida mothers' breast milk often "arrives" quickly within the first few days and their milk volume tends to be fuller earlier. First-time mothers may need additional breastfeeding support and lots of encouragement and assurance to continue efforts to breastfeed. Whether women continue to breastfeed after hospital discharge is influenced by such factors as lactation support, latch, milk supply, employment, personal habits, and how important they view breastfeeding to be for themselves and their newborn (Busch, Nassar, & Silbert-Flagg, 2015; Gage, Williams, Von Rosen-Von Hoewel, et al., 2012; McCarter-Spaulding, Lucas, & Gore, 2011). The tri-core lactation model is an evidenced-based practice model that can help guide nurses in providing early postpartum lactation promotion (Fig. 17.5); incorporating breastfeeding support, education, and maternal self-efficacy (confidence) strategies to improve a mother's chances of a successful breastfeeding relationship with her infant (Busch, Logan, & Wilkinson, 2014; Busch et al., 2015). Primary care offices that also incorporate the American Academy of Pediatrics (2014) *Ten Steps for Supporting Parents' Choice to Breastfeed Their Baby* have shown to improve the long-term rates and durations of breastfeeding beyond the initial early postpartum period (Box 17.7).

While breastfeeding, women must be certain to drink adequate fluid daily, eat a varied nutritious diet, and check with their healthcare provider before ingesting medicine or alternative therapies such as herbs because most of these can be found in breast milk and their use may not be evidence-based

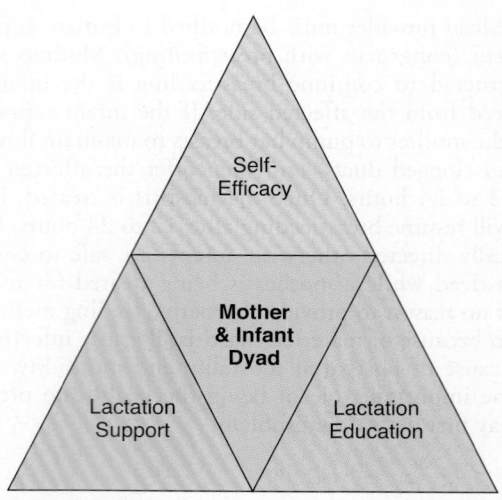

Figure 17.5 The tri-core breastfeeding model. (Reprinted with permission from Busch, D. W., Logan, K., & Wilkinson, A. [2014]. Clinical practice breastfeeding recommendations for primary care: Applying a tri-core breastfeeding conceptual model. *Journal of Pediatric Health Care, 28*[6], 486–496.)

(Schaffir & Czapla, 2012). Breastfeeding techniques are discussed in Chapter 19.

RETURN OF MENSTRUAL FLOW

With the delivery of the placenta, the production of placental estrogen and progesterone ends. The resulting decrease in hormone concentrations causes a rise in production of FSH

BOX 17.7

American Academy of Pediatrics Ten Steps to Support Parents' Choice to Breastfeed

1. Make a commitment to the importance of breastfeeding.
2. Train all staff in skills necessary to support breastfeeding.
3. Inform women and families about the benefits and management of breastfeeding.
4. Assess infants during early follow-up visits.
5. Encourage mothers to breastfeed on demand.
6. Show mothers how to breastfeed and how to maintain lactation when they will be away from their babies.
7. Use appropriate anticipatory guidance that supports exclusive breastfeeding until infants are about 6 months old.
8. Support breastfeeding by providing accurate information about maternal issues.
9. Communicate support for breastfeeding in the office environment.
10. Expand the network of support for breastfeeding.

Reprinted with permission from American Academy of Pediatrics. (2014). *Ten steps to support parents' choice to breastfeed their baby.* Elk Grove Village, IL: Author.

by the pituitary, which leads, with only a slight delay, to the return of ovulation. This initiates the return of normal menstrual cycles.

A woman who is not breastfeeding can expect her menstrual flow to return in 6 to 10 weeks after birth. If she is breastfeeding, a menstrual flow may not return for 3 or 4 months (*lactational amenorrhea*) or, in some women, for the entire lactation period. However, the absence of a menstrual flow does not guarantee that a woman will not conceive during this time because she may ovulate well before menstruation returns (Kramer & Kakuma, 2012).

Nursing Care of a Woman and Family During the First 24 Hours After Birth

A woman remains in a birthing room for at least the first hour after birth so she has time to become acquainted with her newborn and to provide for careful healthcare team observation. Skin-to-skin cuddling with the newborn should be encouraged as well as offering the newborn the breast to try to suckle. She then remains in the room as a postpartal patient or is transferred to a separate postpartal room. With this, the most dangerous hour in childbearing—the first hour after birth—has passed.

Hemorrhage is still a possibility for the first 2 or 3 days after birth, until the myometrial vessels have sclerosed. One of the worries for a woman giving birth at home is that she will not appreciate how dangerous a time this is. With attention focused more on the newborn than on her, postpartal hemorrhage could occur. In the hospital, various healthcare personnel may be involved in caring for a woman: Be certain all members of your healthcare team are knowledgeable about this danger.

Women may have cultural preferences such as the temperature of the room and the fluids they drink. A warm room and drink may be preferred over a cooler room and ice water. Some women may choose not to shower or bathe their newborn immediately for fear that the cool water will cause illness.

ASSESSMENT

Assessment of a postpartal woman includes history, physical examination, and analysis of laboratory findings.

Health History

The technical aspects of a woman's pregnancy, labor, and birth can be learned from her electronic record. Most of this information is best obtained from a woman herself, however, because this supplies not only information on the events of her pregnancy and labor but also her emotions and impressions about them.

Family Profile

Information for a family profile includes age, partner and/or newborn's father, support persons, other children, type of housing and community setting, occupation, education and socioeconomic level, or that information necessary to evaluate the impact a new child will have on the woman and her family. This information also lays a foundation for teaching

self-care and child care specific to the woman's knowledge level and needs.

Pregnancy History

Information for a pregnancy history includes para and gravida status (and the reason for any discrepancy), expected date of birth, whether the pregnancy was intended, and any problems or complications such as spotting or gestational hypertension that occurred during pregnancy. This information helps you gauge a woman's potential for bonding because an unplanned pregnancy or complications arising during pregnancy can interfere greatly with bonding.

Labor and Birth History

It's important to gather information on the length of labor, position of the fetus, type of birth, any analgesia or anesthesia used, problems during labor such as fetal distress, supine hypotension syndrome, and the presence of perineal sutures because this information helps in planning necessary procedures. In addition, explore the mother's thoughts and feelings about labor and birth and whether this was a positive experience for her.

Infant Data

The sex and weight of the infant, Apgar scores, any difficulty at birth such as the need for resuscitation, plans to breastfeed or formula feed, and any congenital anomalies present are the major facts to obtain because, again, this information helps in planning care for the infant and promoting bonding with the parents.

Postpartal Course

To assess a woman's postpartal course and plan anticipatory guidance needed, ask about her general health; her activity level since the birth; a description of lochia; the presence of perineal, abdominal, or breast pain; difficulty with elimination; success with infant feeding; and response of her support person to parenting.

Laboratory Data

Women who had a cesarean delivery, prenatal anemia, or an excessive blood loss will routinely have their hemoglobin and hematocrit levels measured 12 to 24 hours after birth to determine whether blood loss at birth has left them anemic. If the hemoglobin finding is lower than 10.5 g/100 ml, supplemental iron is usually prescribed. It's important that postpartal anemia be detected because the responsibilities of being a new mother, coupled with the additional burden of an undetected low hemoglobin level, can severely tax a woman's energy levels and increase her risk for postpartum depression (East, 2012).

Physical Assessment

During early labor, a woman is given a fairly complete physical examination. During the immediate postpartal period, therefore, repetition of a complete examination is not usually necessary. However, crucial assessments examining particular aspects of health, such as an estimation of nutrition and fluid state, energy level, presence or absence of pain, breast health, fundal height and consistency, lochia amount and character, perineal integrity, and circulatory adequacy, are required.

General Appearance

A woman's general appearance in the postpartal period reveals a great deal about her energy level, her self-esteem, and whether she is moving into a taking-hold phase. Before beginning assessment, ask a woman to void so she has an empty bladder. Observe how much energy she uses when reaching for her robe or walking to the bathroom—does she struggle or move listlessly, or does she accomplish this task quickly? Observe for a cringing expression or hand pressure against her abdomen that suggests pain on movement. Observe whether she has combed her hair and put on her own clothing. Many women choose to sleep in an agency gown to prevent lochia stains on their own clothing, but a woman who is pleased with herself, her pregnancy, and her birth experience is usually anxious to wear her own clothing and "fuss" with her appearance within an hour after birth. The mother may be chatty and enjoy talking with the nurse and inquire about the baby's disposition. In contrast, a woman who is extremely exhausted or depressed probably will not bother with her appearance this way. An overspent mother will often not have the energy to chat and may want to avoid extra conversations. Keep in mind, however, a woman whose labor progressed so rapidly she came to a healthcare agency as an emergency admission may not have had time to pack a comb and brush or her own clothing. Cultural variations also affect appearance and actions.

Hair

Palpate the woman's hair to determine its firmness and strength; whenever a diet is full of nutrients, hair is firm and crisp, whereas if a woman's intake during pregnancy was deficient in nutrients, her hair feels listless and "stringy." Many women begin to lose a quantity of hair in the postpartal period because, during pregnancy, their increased metabolism caused hair to grow rapidly and many hairs to reach maturity at the same time. As the woman's body returns to a normal metabolism level following birth, this rapid-growth hair will be lost, especially around 6 to 12 weeks postpartum. You may need to reassure a woman that hair loss is not a sign of illness but just another aspect of return to her prepregnant state.

Face

Assess the woman's face for evidence of edema such as puffy eyelids or a prominent fold of tissue inferior to the lower eyelid. Normally, this should be negligible. However, in a woman who had gestational hypertension and thus accumulated excessive fluid, it will be evident. It also will become evident in a woman who is developing postpartal hypertension (although this condition is rare). Facial edema is most apparent early in the morning because the woman has been lying flat with her head level during the night.

Eyes

Inspect the color and texture of the inner conjunctiva. If a woman is dehydrated, the area appears dry. The conjunctiva of a woman who is anemic from poor pregnancy nutrition or excessive blood loss is pale. Be alert to possible variations because of skin color, however, as dark-skinned women may have a ruddy conjunctiva appearance even with anemia. Check the electronic record of any woman with paler than usual conjunctivae to determine whether anemia (revealed by a low hemoglobin level) is present.

Breasts

Breast tissue increases in size as breast milk forms. To assess breasts, ask a woman to remove her bra and cover her breasts with a towel or folded sheet to protect modesty. Ask her to raise her hands and tuck them under her head because this stretches and thins breast tissue. Inspect and then palpate for breast size, shape, and color.

Breast tissue should feel soft on palpation on the first and second postpartal day. On the third day, it should begin to feel firm and warm (described as *filling*). On the third or fourth day, breasts appear large and reddened, with taut, shiny skin (engorgement) and, on palpation, feel hard and tense and painful. Because, normally, engorgement causes the entire breast to feel warm or appear reddened, if only one portion of a breast appears this way, inflammation or, possibly, infection of glands or milk ducts (mastitis) is suggested (Katz, 2012). It is also normal for the breast to swell into the axillary area due to lymph node swelling and/or breast tissue engorgement. This is called the tail of Spence area; reassure the mother that this finding is normal.

Occasionally, a firm nodule is detected on palpation. Usually, this is only a temporarily blocked milk duct preventing milk from flowing forward to the nipple. Often, hand massages and warm compresses will help to soften the nodule area. One of the best interventions for engorgement is an effective latch and to have the newborn breastfeed often from both sides initially while the milk is coming in (lactogenesis I and II). If the nodule remains troublesome, note the location of the nodule and report its presence to the woman's primary care provider so that it can be thoroughly reassessed to ascertain whether a fibrocystic or malignant growth unrelated to the pregnancy is present.

Note also whether the breast nipples are normally erect and not inverted. Assess for any cracks, fissures, or the presence of caked milk. Avoid squeezing the nipples because this can be painful. Unnecessary nipple manipulation also may increase the risk of mastitis by providing a portal for infection. If the mother is experiencing a painful latch or the newborn is having difficulty latching and transferring milk, a call to the hospital lactation consultant is warranted immediately.

Uterus

For uterine assessment, position the woman supine so the height of the uterus is not influenced by an elevated position. Observe her abdomen for contour, to detect distention, and for the appearance of striae or a diastasis. If a diastasis is present (a slightly indented, possibly bluish-tinged groove in the midline of the abdomen), measure the width and length by fingerbreadths.

Palpate the fundus of the uterus by placing one hand on the base of the uterus, just above the symphysis pubis, and the other at the umbilicus. Press in and downward with the hand at the umbilicus until you "bump" against a firm globular mass in the abdomen: the uterine fundus (Fig. 17.6). Assess consistency (firm, soft, or boggy), location (midline), and height. For the first hour after birth, the height of the fundus is at the umbilicus or even slightly above it; it then decreases one fingerbreadth in size daily. Measure the distance under the umbilicus in fingerbreadths, such as "2 F↓" or 2 cm beneath the umbilicus. Although this measurement seems less scientific than a measurement of the height of the uterus from the pubis, it is a more certain measurement and demonstrates the gradual decline in size of the uterus.

Figure 17.6 To palpate a uterus, be certain to place one hand at the base of the uterus. This fundus measures about two fingerbreadths below the umbilicus.

Never palpate a uterus without supporting the lower segment because the uterus potentially could invert (turn inside out) if not stabilized, resulting in a massive hemorrhage.

Palpation of a fundus should not cause pain as long as the action is done gently. If the uterus is not firm on palpation, massage it gently with the examining hand; this usually causes the fundus to contract and immediately become firm. Use a gentle rotating motion, never a hard or forceful touch, so that you do not cause pain or cause the uterus to expend excess energy in contracting. If the uterine fundus does not grow firm with massage, extreme atony, possibly retained placenta fragments, or an excess amount of blood loss may be occurring. Notify the woman's primary care provider. Administer oxytocin as prescribed. In addition, placing the woman's infant at her breast will cause endogenous release of oxytocin and achieve the same effect as oxytocin administration.

If massage appears ineffective, the cause of this may be a clot present in the cavity of the uterus. This may be expressed from the uterus by gentle pressure on the fundus but only after the uterus has been massaged and is fairly firm. As mentioned earlier, if fundal pressure is applied with the uterus totally relaxed, fundal pressure could cause inversion of the uterus, an extremely serious complication that leads to rapid hemorrhage. Another reason the uterus may not be well contracted is that a rapidly filling bladder is preventing contraction. If contraction remains inadequate, a lower abdominal ultrasound may be prescribed to help detect an abnormality.

A woman who received no oxytocin after birth to help her uterus contract is at greater risk for poor uterine contraction than is a woman who did receive oxytocin and thus needs frequent uterine assessment (about every 10 to 15 minutes for the first hour).

Once this first hour has passed, height and consistency can be assessed less frequently, depending on institutional policy. By the 9th or 10th day after delivery, the uterus will have become so small that it is no longer palpable above the symphysis pubis.

QSEN Checkpoint Question 17.4

TEAMWORK & COLLABORATION

The nurse is performing massage of Leana's fundus 2 days postpartum. What assessment finding should prompt the nurse to contact Leana's primary care provider immediately?

   a. Leana's fundal height is two fingerbreadths below her umbilicus.
   b. Leana's uterus does not become firm when massaged.
   c. Firm massage of Leana's fundus results in pain.
   d. The fundus is located midline on Leana's abdomen.

Look in Appendix A for the best answer and rationale.

Lochia

A woman can expect to have lochia for 2 to 6 weeks. Characteristics of normal lochia and the change in pattern from red to pink to white were described in Table 17.1.

During the first hour after birth, when the fundus is checked every 15 minutes, also remove the mother's perineal pad and evaluate lochia character, amount, color (rubra, serosa, or alba), odor, and the presence of any clots. If the woman has perineal stitches, be certain the pad is not adhering to those before removing it.

Ask the woman to turn, so you can inspect under her buttocks to be certain blood is not pooling beneath her. If you observe a constant trickle of vaginal flow or a woman is soaking through a pad every 60 minutes, she is losing more than the average amount of blood. It is concerning if the women appears disoriented and/or her vital signs are abnormal. She needs to be examined by her primary care provider to be certain there is no cervical or vaginal tear or that poor uterine contraction is not causing excessive bleeding.

While a woman is at the healthcare facility, inspect her lochia discharge once every 15 minutes for the first hour and then according to the institution's policy (usually hourly for the next 4 hours and then every 8 hours after that). Make certain a woman understands that she should wash her hands after handling pads and must use only her own personal care equipment so that she does not contract or spread infection. Demonstrate good role modeling for hand washing and non-sharing of equipment. Encourage a woman to change perineal pads frequently as she begins self-care because lochia is an excellent medium for bacterial growth that could spread through the vagina to the uterus. The presence of constantly wet pads against an episiotomy suture line also slows healing. Be certain she knows not to use tampons until after she returns for her postpartal checkup to diminish the risk of infection and possibly toxic shock syndrome (see Chapter 47) and to contact her provider if she develops a fever upon returning home. Ensure women are familiar with the criteria for judging the amount and type of normal lochia (see Box 17.6), so they can do this accurately when they return home.

Perineum

While asking a woman to turn on her side to evaluate whether lochia is pooling, also inspect her perineum. If a woman has no episiotomy or a midline one, which side she turns to does not matter. If she has a mediolateral incision, ask her to turn so the incision is on the bottom buttock because this tends to cause less pain and offers better visibility. Gently lift the upper buttock and inspect for ecchymosis, a hematoma, erythema, edema, intactness, and presence of drainage or bleeding from any episiotomy stitches.

Episiotomies are rarely done today because they may increase the risk of extended perineal lacerations. If stitches are present, the suture line is 1 or 2 in. long. If a laceration extends beyond the episiotomy incision, stitches may extend from the vagina back to the rectum or go into the muscle and tissues surrounding the perineal area. The incision line is usually fused (edges sealed) by 24 hours after birth; if it is a midline incision, it may be almost invisible to see because the perineal fold obscures it. If there is clotted lochia along the incision line, review postpartal perineal care so that this does not continue to occur. Before discharge, teach a woman who has stitches how to lie on her back and view her perineum with a handheld mirror, so that, once a day while at home, she can inspect her perineum for redness, sloughing of sutures, pus formation, drainage at the suture line, or development of a hematoma. A hematoma is a collection of blood in the subcutaneous space from bleeding from the episiotomy incision that can become so extensive it causes intense pain and disrupts the suture line (see Chapter 25).

Following perineal assessment, assess the rectal area for the presence of hemorrhoids. If any are present, document their number, appearance, and size in centimeters. Because postpartum women are not on bed rest unless they have a serious complication, assess risk of skin breakdown as per facility protocol using an assessment scale such as the Braden Assessment Scale (Tescher, Branda, Byrne, et al., 2012).

What If . . . 17.2

Leana Cooper, at 18 hours postpartum, tells the nurse she has had to change her perineal pads twice in the last 30 minutes because they were saturated. In addition, the nurse noticed two large clots on her last pad. To guard her safety, what should be the nurse's first action?

Nursing Diagnoses and Related Interventions

Nursing Diagnosis: Risk for fluid volume deficit related to uterine atony

Outcome Evaluation: Patient maintains vital signs within normal range; fundus is firm to palpation; lochia discharge is small to moderate with a minimum of clot formation.

In order to assess if uterine atony is present, frequently assess vital signs, lochia amount, and fundal height. Teach patient the usual involution process and how to check her fundus and evaluate lochia so she can do this after she returns home.

Nursing Diagnosis: Pain related to perineal discomfort, uterine cramping (afterpains), or muscular aches

Outcome Evaluation: Patient states that degree of pain is tolerable; patient demonstrates knowledge of measures for adequate pain relief.

Women experience pain postpartally as a result of uterine contraction as well as from the aftereffects of pushing during labor.

Provide Pain Relief for Afterpains. Pain from uterine contractions is similar to pain from menstrual cramps and can be intense. It's usually helpful to assure a woman that this type of discomfort, although painful, is normal and rarely lasts longer than 3 days. If necessary, either ibuprofen (such as Motrin), which has anti-inflammatory and antiprostaglandin properties, or a common analgesic such as acetaminophen (such as Tylenol) is effective for pain relief. As with any abdominal pain, heat to the abdomen should be avoided because it could cause relaxation of the uterus and subsequent uterine bleeding. Remind the woman that the total 24-hour dose for acetaminophen is 3,000 mg so she does not take an excessive amount after returning home (Karch, 2013).

Relieve Muscular Aches. Many women feel so sore and achy after labor and birth that they describe feeling as if they have "run for miles." A backrub is usually effective for relieving an aching back or shoulders, but some woman may appreciate a mild analgesic such as acetaminophen for the pain. Carefully assess a woman who states she has intense warmth or pain in the calf of her leg on standing because pain in the calf on standing (a position that dorsiflexes the foot) is **Homans sign** and could indicate that thrombophlebitis is present (see later discussion).

Administer Cold and Hot Therapy. Applying an ice or cold pack to the perineum during the first 24 hours reduces perineal edema and the possibility of hematoma formation and also reduces pain and promotes healing and comfort. Be certain not to place ice or plastic directly on the woman's perineum. Use a commercial cold pack, or wrap an ice bag first in a towel or disposable pad, to decrease the chance of a thermal burn (risk of injury increases because the perineum has decreased sensation from edema after birth).

Ice to the perineum after the first 24 hours is no longer therapeutic because, after this time, healing increases best if circulation to the area is encouraged by the use of heat. Dry heat in the form of a perineal hot pack or moist heat with a sitz bath are both effective ways to increase circulation to the perineum, provide comfort, reduce edema, and promote healing.

Commercial hot packs grow warm after they are "cracked" and the chemicals in them combine. Caution women to use a washcloth or gauze square between the pack and their skin to prevent a possible burn.

Promote Perineal Exercises. Some women find that carrying out perineal exercises three or four times a day can greatly relieve perineal edema. The most effective exercise consists of contracting and relaxing the muscles of the perineum 5 to 10 times in succession, as if trying to stop voiding (**Kegel exercises**). This aids comfort by improving circulation to the area and decreasing edema. When repeated frequently, Kegel exercises can also help a woman regain her prepregnant muscle tone and help prevent urinary incontinence (Boyle, Hay-Smith, Cody, et al., 2012).

Give Suture Line Care for Women With an Episiotomy. Although relatively small in size, episiotomy sutures can cause considerable discomfort because the perineum is an extremely sensitive area and the muscles of the perineum are involved in so many activities such as sitting, walking, stooping, squatting, bending, urinating, and defecating.

Because the perineal area heals rapidly, you can assure a woman that discomfort is normal and does not usually last longer than 5 or 6 days. Most primary care providers prescribe a soothing anesthetic cream or spray to be applied to the suture line to reduce discomfort. A cortisone-based cream or warm sitz bath helps to decrease inflammation and relieve tension in the area. Because of their cooling effect, witch hazel–impregnated pads (Tucks) are a mainstay for relief of both perineal and hemorrhoidal discomfort.

In addition to local perineum creams or sprays, a woman may require an oral analgesic such as hydrocodone for the first 24 hours and then a milder one such as acetaminophen for the remainder of the first week. Caution a woman not to use aspirin for pain relief during the postpartal period because it interferes with blood clotting and may increase her risk for hemorrhage from the denuded placental site (Karch, 2013). If a woman is worried she will experience additional discomfort when her episiotomy sutures are removed, you can assure her these sutures will dissolve within 10 days and thus do not need to be removed.

Nursing Diagnosis: Risk for infection (uterine) related to presence of lochia and denuded uterine surface

Outcome Evaluation: Patient's temperature remains below 100.4°F; lochia is present and without foul odor.

Measures to decrease the risk of infection are concerned with not allowing organisms to spread from the perineum into the uterus.

Provide Perineal Care. Postpartal women are particularly prone to a uterine infection because lochia, if allowed to dry and harden on the vulva and perineum, furnishes a rich bed for bacterial growth, which then can spread to the uterus. Because the vagina lies in close proximity to the rectum, there is also always the danger bacteria will spread from the rectum to the vagina. Interruption in skin integrity from an episiotomy also increases a woman's risk for infection.

To reduce these risks, teach a woman to include perineal care as part of her daily bath or shower and after every voiding or bowel movement. For the woman on bed rest during the first hour after birth, you will need to provide this care for her.

Before beginning perineal care, be certain to wash your hands well and pull on clean gloves. This nursing action requires universal precautions. Place a plastic-covered pad under the woman's buttocks to protect the bed from lochia or water. With the woman lying supine, remove her perineal pad from front to back (the direction is important to prevent the portion of the pad that was over her rectal area from sliding forward to contaminate the vaginal opening).

Agencies differ as to the type of cleansing that is done and the articles and solutions used to wash away accumulating lochia. If actual washing is to be done, use a clean gauze square or a clean portion of a washcloth with the designated solution for each stroke, always washing from front to back or from the pubis toward the rectum. Rinse the area in the same manner and pat it dry.

A second common method of cleaning is to spray the perineum with clear tap water from a spray bottle. When doing this, direct the spray toward the front of the perineum and allow it to flow from front to back, from the vaginal to the rectal area to reduce cross-bacterial transmission into the vagina. The labia have a tendency to close and cover the vaginal opening. Do not separate the labia; instead, allow them to perform this protective function. Spray gently to avoid splashing any blood-tinged solution on yourself.

Promote Perineal Self-Care. As soon as a woman is allowed to be out of bed and use a bathroom (if she gave birth without an anesthetic, this is within the first hour after birth), teach her how to carry out her own perineal care.

A postpartum bathroom should have an area close to the toilet where she can place the equipment she needs for care: a spray bottle, sponges to dry, clean pads, and so forth. Remind her of the importance of applying any cream or medication that has been prescribed. Caution her not to flush the toilet until she is standing upright so the flushing water doesn't spray her perineum and increase the risk of infection.

If women are given a clear explanation as to why perineal care is important, they perform it well. Self-care does not eliminate a nurse's responsibility, however, for checking a woman's perineum to assess its condition and the amount and type of lochia flow present. By continuing with these assessments, you remain a woman's first line of defense against both infection and hemorrhage.

Nursing Diagnosis: Disturbed sleep pattern related to exhaustion from and excitement of childbirth

Outcome Evaluation: Patient states she is able to sleep and feels rested during postpartal period.

After birth, a woman is a paradox. She wants to hold and be with the new person in her life. She wants to talk to her support person about the experience, their child, and their future. At the same time, she is so exhausted she falls asleep easily.

Promote Rest in the Early Postpartal Period. Few women are prepared for the degree of fatigue they experience after childbirth. When giving care, try to consolidate procedures to allow as much time for sleep as possible. If a woman has discomfort from hemorrhoids, perineal stitches, or afterpains, be certain to supply adequate pain relief so she can rest comfortably or sleep. Caution her to return her infant to a bassinette if she grows sleepy while feeding or holding the infant as a newborn in a narrow bed could easily fall and be injured.

Some women experience shaking chills immediately or within a half hour after birth. This is caused in part by the pressure changes in the abdomen that occur with reduction in the bulk of the uterus and temperature readjustment in response to the diaphoresis of labor. It also may result from the exhilaration the woman is feeling, combined with exhaustion. In any event, you can assure a woman that shaking chills at this point are very common, so she will not attribute them to developing a cold or other infection. Covering her with a warm blanket and offering a warm drink are usually enough to cause the chill to be transient and allow the woman to fall into a sound, much-needed sleep of about an hour. Although a woman may choose any position to sleep, she may enjoy being able to sleep on her stomach, something she was not able to do during the latter part of pregnancy.

Promote Rest Throughout the Puerperium. You cannot stress too much to women the importance of rest throughout the entire puerperium. Offer suggestions for getting adequate rest after a woman returns home such as sleeping while her baby naps or asking for respite time from baby care so she can nap.

A woman without this type of support can have difficulty balancing the many demands of her new role—being a mother instead of a daughter; a mother as well as a wife; or a mother of three, not two. Overcome by sleep hunger, her judgment and sense of balance can blur. Although it is not the only contributing factor, extreme fatigue is also associated with the development of postpartal depression (Meadows-Oliver, 2012). Learning to breastfeed her infant can also be an overwhelming experience; provide reassurance to the women that this is a normal feeling and suggest that her partner or support person relieve her so she may nap after she breastfeeds.

Nursing Diagnosis: Risk for bathing/hygiene self-care deficit related to exhaustion from childbirth

Outcome Evaluation: Patient takes full daily responsibility for own hygiene.

After childbirth, women often report that their hospital or birthing center room feels too warm; to prove it, they point out how heavily they are perspiring. Postpartal rooms often are kept warm so newborns will be comfortable, but the profuse perspiration a woman is experiencing most likely comes from her body's attempt to regulate fluid, not from the heat of the environment.

You can assure a woman that sweating is a normal postpartal event that is helping to bring her body back to its prepregnant state. If she has profuse diaphoresis, particularly at night, suggest she wear a hospital gown rather than one of her own. She may need frequent gown changes during the day to be comfortable and not become chilled.

Before a woman walks to a shower room on her first postpartal day, perform a fall-risk assessment as identified by your facility protocol. Accompany her in the hallway because she may be more fatigued than she realizes. Encourage her to not make the shower excessively warm and to keep the call light in reach because standing under warm water may make her feel so dizzy that she may need help to walk safely back to bed.

Formerly, women were not allowed to take tub baths after birth, for fear bacteria from the bath water would enter the vagina and cause infection. There appears to be little evidence this is a real danger, however, so if a woman wants to bathe instead of shower after she returns home, she may do so.

Nursing Diagnosis: Imbalanced nutrition, less than body requirements, related to lack of knowledge about postpartal needs

Outcome Evaluation: Patient ingests a 2,200- to 2,700-kcal diet and drinks six to eight glasses of fluid daily.

Postpartal menu planning should include a diet of between 2,200 and 2,300 calories daily including foods high in protein and the vitamins and minerals needed for good tissue repair. An adequate supply of roughage is also important to help restore peristaltic action of the bowel. Women who are breastfeeding need an additional 500 calories (a 2,700-kcal diet) and an additional 500 ml of fluid (these may be from the same source) each day to encourage the production of high-quality breast milk. Most mothers are hungry during the immediate postpartal period and consume an adequate diet without urging.

After hospital discharge, a woman needs to continue to eat a nutritious diet. It's important to stress this because women can become so fatigued during their first weeks at home they are unable to prepare anything but fast-food meals. Neglecting to eat properly leads to more fatigue and, ultimately, to an even less nutritious diet. Encourage the mother to eat and drink frequently, such as every 2 to 3 hours while awake; these can be simple snacks such as an apple and peanut butter (if no allergy) or yogurt and granola.

If a woman has any prenatal vitamins or supplementary iron preparations left over from pregnancy, she should, as a rule, continue to take them until her supply is used. Breastfeeding patients are strongly encouraged to continue taking their prenatal vitamins until they stop nursing their infant. If a woman needs further supplements, her primary care provider will prescribe them for her either on discharge from her birth setting or when she returns for her postpartum checkup (Milman, 2012).

Promote Adequate Fluid Intake. The rapid diuresis and diaphoresis that occur during the second to fifth postpartal days ordinarily result in a weight loss of 5 lb in addition to the approximately 12 lb lost at childbirth.

Women often feel thirsty during this period of rapid fluid loss because they also may have had a limited liquid intake during labor, and so they readily drink a large amount of fluid. You may need to encourage an individual woman to drink more fluid because she is restricting fluid in the hope of preventing her breasts from becoming engorged or is beginning to diet in the hope of bringing her body more quickly back to its nonpregnant slim state. Fluid restriction, however, does little to affect engorgement or weight loss and thus should be discouraged. Instead, encourage a woman to drink at least three to four 8-oz glasses of fluid each day (six to eight glasses if breastfeeding).

Nursing Diagnosis: Risk for impaired urinary elimination or constipation related to loss of bladder and bowel sensation after childbirth

Outcome Evaluation: Patient voids more than 30 ml/hr without urinary retention, beginning 1 hour after birth and has a bowel movement by postpartum day 4. No urinary incontinence is noted.

Because the fetal head pressed on the posterior surface of the bladder during birth, a woman's bladder may have so much edema that the sensation of a full bladder is hard to sense. Bowel peristalsis may also be reduced because a woman's abdominal wall is so lax.

Promote Urinary Elimination. Because the diuresis of the postpartal period begins almost immediately after birth, a woman's bladder begins filling almost immediately. This is potentially serious because a full bladder puts pressure on the uterus and so can interfere with uterine contraction. An overdistended bladder may also damage bladder function. Women who have had epidural anesthesia are particularly prone to inability to sense a full bladder and so can develop urinary retention (Mulder et al., 2012).

Encourage a woman to walk to the bathroom and void at the end of the first hour after birth to help prevent bladder distention; however, some women have too much perineal edema to be able to void this early. A woman with an episiotomy may be reluctant to void because she knows acid urine against her sutures will sting. Most women who have had epidural anesthesia have enough residual effect, however, that even with perineal stitches, voiding at this time is painless. Assist by providing privacy (but remain in close proximity in case a woman feels faint), running water at the sink, or offering the woman a drink of water. Pouring warm tap water over the vulva, if consistent with the agency's policy for perineal care, also may help.

If the woman still has not been able to void by 4 to 8 hours after birth, and bladder distention is present, she will need to be catheterized to relieve bladder pressure. It can be difficult to locate the urethra in a woman after birth because the perineum is edematous. Be certain that, during catheterization, you do not invade the vagina by mistake and thereby carry contamination to the denuded uterus. Occasionally, because of poor tone, the bladder appears to be emptying but actually is retaining large amounts of residual urine that harbors bacteria and can lead to bladder infection.

To detect whether urinary retention is occurring, be certain to measure a first voiding after birth. Whether the bladder is emptying also may be judged by measuring whether the fundal height is decreasing or by palpating or percussing bladder prominence in the lower abdomen. If a woman is voiding less than 100 ml at a time or has a displaced uterus or a palpable bladder, her primary care provider may prescribe catheterization for residual urine after a voiding. As a rule, if the residual urine removed is more than 100 to 150 ml, the catheter is left in place for 12 to 24 hours to give the bladder time to regain its normal tone and to begin to function efficiently.

Fortunately for most women who must be catheterized, the procedure needs to be done only once after birth.

After another 6 to 8 hours have passed and the bladder has filled again, some of the perineal edema has subsided, the bladder has achieved better tone, and the woman is able to void by herself if helped to the bathroom.

Because catheterization can lead to urinary infection, it should not be used indiscriminately. However, it should be done before the woman's bladder is injured or the uterus is displaced and uncontracted, resulting in bleeding.

Some women experience urinary incontinence during the postpartal period, probably resulting from poor perineal tone and sensation. Suggest Kegel exercises to strengthen perineal muscles and eliminate incontinence in the future.

Prevent Constipation. Many women have difficulty moving their bowels during the first week of the puerperium, a condition that can be both worrisome and uncomfortable. Constipation occurs because of relaxation of the abdominal wall and the intestine, now that they are no longer compressed by the bulky uterus. Also, if hemorrhoids or perineal stitches are present, a woman may decline to try to move her bowels for fear of pain.

To prevent constipation, early ambulation, a diet with adequate roughage, and an adequate fluid intake are all helpful measures. Many women are prescribed a stool softener such as docusate sodium (Colace) beginning with the first day after birth (Box 17.8). If a woman has not moved her bowels by the third postpartum day, a mild laxative or cathartic may be prescribed. There is danger in giving cathartics before the third day because the resulting increase in intestinal activity could cause uterine irritation and lead to insufficient contraction.

Prevent Development of Hemorrhoids. The pressure of the fetal head on the rectal veins during birth tends to aggravate or produce hemorrhoids (swollen rectal veins) to

 BOX 17.8

Nursing Care Planning Based on Responsibility for Pharmacology

DOCUSATE SODIUM (COLACE, SURFAK)

Classification: Docusate sodium is a stool softener.

Action: Used in the postpartal period to prevent constipation. It works by lowering the surface tension of feces, allowing water and lipids to penetrate the stool and soften it (Karch, 2013).

Pregnancy Risk Category: C

Dosage: 50–100 mg PO daily.

Possible Adverse Effects: occasional abdominal pain and diarrhea

Nursing Implications

- Encourage a woman to swallow the medication with a full glass of water or juice.
- Instruct a woman to consume high-fiber foods to encourage elimination.
- Encourage activity to promote intestinal motility.

such an extent that some women find hemorrhoidal discomfort to be their chief discomfort in the first few days after birth (Avsar & Keskin, 2010). This discomfort can be relieved by sitz baths, anesthetic sprays, witch hazel or astringent preparations, or preparations such as hydrocortisone acetate (Proctofoam). Gentle manual replacement of hemorrhoidal tissue may also give relief. Assuming a Sims position several times a day aids in good venous return to the rectal area and also reduces discomfort. Increased fluid and the administration of a stool softener can prevent the development of hardened stool, which can irritate hemorrhoids.

Nursing Diagnosis: Risk for ineffective peripheral tissue perfusion related to immobility and increased estrogen level

Outcome Evaluation: Patient demonstrates negative Homans sign and absence of erythema or pain in calves of legs.

Because estrogen, which aids blood clotting, is still elevated following birth, women are at high risk for thrombophlebitis of the leg unless they ambulate quickly after birth.

Assess Peripheral Circulation. As a rule, women who ambulate quickly feel stronger and healthier by the end of their first week and have fewer bowel, bladder, and circulatory complications than those who do not (Fig. 17.7). To determine if peripheral circulation is adequate, assess a woman's thigh for skin turgor. Assess for edema at the ankle and over the tibia on the lower leg. Although this technique is not totally reliable, assess for thrombophlebitis by dorsiflexing a woman's ankle and asking her if she notices pain in her calf on that motion (Homans sign). Assess also for redness in the calf area because thrombophlebitis can be present even with a negative Homans sign. Continue to assess for adequate peripheral circulation once every 8 hours during the woman's stay in a healthcare facility. If you suspect thrombophlebitis, do not massage the area—doing so could cause the thrombophlebitis to become an embolus.

Nursing Diagnosis: Pain related to primary breast engorgement

Outcome Evaluation: Patient states pain from breast engorgement is at a tolerable level.

Figure 17.7 Ambulating postpartum is not always easy but helps to prevent complications.

Prevent/Alleviate Breast Engorgement. If a woman is breastfeeding, encouraging her newborn to attempt to latch at the breast is the main treatment for relief of the tenderness and soreness of primary breast engorgement (breastfeeding techniques are discussed in Chapter 19).

Many women find the application of warm compresses or standing under a warm shower beneficial to relieve the discomfort of engorgement. Instructing a mother how to perform manual expression helps to relieve milk engorgement as well. Good support from a bra also offers relief because it prevents unnecessary strain on the supporting muscles of the breasts and positions the breasts in good alignment. Assess the woman for any intense nipple discomfort or pain. If nipple pain is occurring within the first few days postpartum it is often due to an infant's ineffective latch. Nipple damage from a mislatch can result in a bacterial or yeast infection of the nipple. Nipple pain must be assessed by a lactation consultant and the women's provider prior to discharge and preferably as soon as possible.

A woman who is not breastfeeding may experience strong discomfort for the first few days. When little or no milk is removed from the breasts, however, the accumulation of milk inhibits further milk formation, and engorgement subsides by the third day. An oral analgesic, wearing a snug-fitting bra, avoiding nipple stimulation, or applying cold compresses three or four times a day can all provide relief. Restricting fluid and pumping milk from the breasts are not effective.

Promote Breast Hygiene. Breast care during the postpartal period includes cleanliness and support and is the same whether or not a woman is breastfeeding.

Teach a woman to wash her breasts daily with clear water and gentle soap at the time of her bath or shower and then dry them with a soft towel. It is not necessary for women to wash their breasts more often than daily or use a vast amount of soap because excessive washing means unnecessary skin manipulation.

A woman who has a considerable discharge of colostrum or milk from her breasts (whether breastfeeding or not) should insert clean gauze squares or commercial nursing pads into her bra to absorb the moisture, changing them as often as necessary to keep the nipples dry because if the nipples remain wet for any length of time, fissures may form and lead to infection.

Nursing Diagnosis: Health-seeking behaviors related to future breast health

Outcome Evaluation: Patient states the importance of once-yearly breast examination by a healthcare provider and a yearly to biyearly mammography, if appropriate for her age and risk factors, and her intention to schedule this examination yearly (Oelffinger, Fontham, Etzioni, et al., 2015).

Because breast cancer is a major type of neoplasm in women, all women of childbearing age should know the importance of yearly breast assessment (Granek & Fergus, 2012; Oelffinger et al., 2015). Many women are not interested in hearing about cancer prevention measures during pregnancy because the possibility of developing cancer seems too far removed from what they are doing—creating life. In the postpartal period, they become conscious of the need to remain well to raise this new child to maturity. This makes them more receptive to a review of the importance of a yearly breast exam at healthcare visits.

A breastfeeding woman may occasionally discover a distended milk gland that feels very much like a cyst or tumor, especially in the axillary area (tail of Spence). You can assure her she need not report such distended glands unless they persist beyond two breastfeedings.

Nursing Diagnosis: Health-seeking behaviors related to patient's desire to return to prepregnant weight and appearance

Outcome Evaluation: Patient states realistic goals for return to former appearance; patient is able to demonstrate appropriate exercises.

After childbirth, the abdominal wall and the uterine ligaments remain stretched. The abdomen tends to pouch forward. Wearing a girdle may help a woman feel more comfortable during the first few weeks after birth, but it does not aid, and may actually hinder, strengthening the tone of the abdominal wall. She can best help her abdominal wall return to good tone by using proper body mechanics and posture, getting adequate rest, and performing prescribed exercises such as those described in Table 17.2.

Teach Methods to Promote Uterine Involution. All during the postpartal period, lying on the abdomen gives support to abdominal muscles and may aid involution because it tips the uterus into its natural forward position. If this puts too much pressure on sore breasts, placement of a small pillow under the abdomen usually solves the problem.

It may be dangerous for a woman to assume a knee–chest position until at least the third week after birth because, in a knee–chest position, the vagina tends to open. Because the cervical os is open to some extent until the third week, there is a danger air could enter the vagina and the open cervix, penetrate the open blood sinuses inside the uterus, enter the circulatory system, and cause an air embolism.

Although this would be a rare occurrence, it is good practice for a woman to avoid this position until she returns for a postpartal examination and is assured her cervix has closed. Women who have used a knee–chest position during pregnancy to relieve the pressure of hemorrhoids need to be cautioned that a modified Sims position, such as they used for a rest position during pregnancy, is better for them now.

Nursing Diagnosis: Risk for ineffective sexuality patterns related to physiologic changes of postpartal period

Outcome Evaluation: Patient states she has a satisfactory sexual relationship with her partner; patient demonstrates understanding of both coital and noncoital methods of sexual expression.

At one time, women were cautioned not to resume sexual relations after the birth of a baby until after their medical checkup at 6 weeks. However, there is no apparent physiologic reason to delay sexual relations this long. For most couples, gentle coitus may be resumed as soon as lochia serosa has stopped—about 1 to 2 weeks after birth.

Caution women, however, that sex may be somewhat uncomfortable if it is begun this early because vaginal epithelium is still thin and tender. A woman who is breastfeeding may also notice that breast milk is released from her nipples with sexual arousal. Use of a lubricant will help any mucosal dryness. A female-superior position may be most comfortable because it allows the woman to control the depth of penile penetration. Be sure women receive adequate reproductive planning information, if desired, before they resume sexual relations to prevent another

TABLE 17.2 MUSCLE-STRENGTHENING EXERCISES

Exercise	Description
Abdominal breathing	Abdominal breathing may be started on the first day after birth because it is a relatively easy exercise. Lying flat on her back or sitting, a woman should breathe slowly and deeply in and out five times, using her abdominal muscles. Check by watching her abdominal wall rise that she is actually using these muscles.
Chin-to-chest	The chin-to-chest exercise is excellent for the second day. Lying on her back with no pillow, a woman raises her head and bends her chin forward on her chest without moving any other part of her body while exhaling. She should start this gradually, repeating it no more than 5 times the first time and then increasing it to 10–15 times in succession. The exercise can be done 3 or 4 times a day. She will feel her abdominal muscles pull and tighten if she is doing it correctly.
Perineal contraction	If a woman is not already using this exercise as a means of alleviating perineal discomfort, it is a good one to add on the third day. She should tighten and relax her perineal muscles 10–25 times in succession as if she were trying to stop voiding (Kegel exercises). She will feel her perineal muscles working if she is doing it correctly.
Arm raising	Arm raising helps both the breasts and the abdomen return to good tone and is a good exercise to add on the fourth day. Lying on her back, arms at her sides, a woman moves her arms out from her sides until they are perpendicular to her body. She then raises them over her body until her hands touch and lowers them slowly to her sides. She should rest a moment and then repeat the exercise five times.
Abdominal crunches	It is advisable to wait until the 10th or 12th day after birth before attempting abdominal crunches. Lying flat on her back with knees bent, a woman folds her arms across her chest and raises herself to a sitting position. This exercise expends a great deal of effort and tires a postpartal woman easily. Caution her to begin very gradually and work up slowly to doing it 10 times in a row.

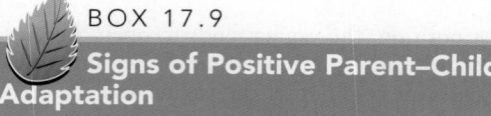

BOX 17.9

Signs of Positive Parent–Child Adaptation

Good parent–child adaptation is demonstrated when a parent:

- Speaks of infant as desirable and attractive
- Is not upset by vomiting, drooling, and the like
- Holds the baby warmly
- Makes eye contact with the infant
- Plays with and soothes the infant
- Talks or sings to the baby
- Expresses confidence that the infant is well
- Finds physical or psychological attributes to admire about the baby
- Is able to discriminate between the baby's signs of hunger or need for sleep

pregnancy so soon (see Chapter 6). If a women experiences intense pain during intercourse, instruct her to consult her gynecologist for further evaluation.

Nursing Diagnosis: Risk for impaired parenting related to inadequate bonding behavior after childbirth

Outcome Evaluation: Parents hold and comfort their infant appropriately and voice positive characteristics of child.

To assess whether bonding is occurring, listen to what parents say about their newborn in the immediate postpartal period. Do they make positive statements, such as "I'm glad he's a boy" or "She's cute," or negative ones, such as "I really hoped it would be a girl" or "She looks like a circus clown with no hair"? First impressions may not be lasting ones; however, negative comments need to be identified, so that extra discussion about issues such as what it feels like to have four boys or not to have the prettiest child in the nursery can take place. Although brief hospital stays are advantageous in many ways, if limited time prevents such discussions from occurring, a family may be discharged from the healthcare agency with not only physical but also educational and emotional needs unmet (Gross, Resnik, Nanda, et al., 2011). Typical signs of good parent–child adaptation are shown in Box 17.9.

QSEN Checkpoint Question 17.5

EVIDENCE-BASED PRACTICE

Many new mothers are not prepared for how much time newborns spend crying (as many as 16 of 24 hours); trying to quiet a newborn can lead to extreme fatigue in a postpartal parent. To investigate the effect of newborn crying on new mothers' ability to rest, researchers conducted a systematic review of studies concerned with newborn crying. Results of the literature review revealed that infant crying during the first 3 months postpartum is responsible for disrupting new mothers' circadian rhythms, reducing opportunities

to rest, and exacerbating tiredness. Incremental exhaustion from infant crying diminishes a parent's ability to concentrate, raises the fear of harming the children, triggers depressive symptoms, and burdens parent–child interaction (Nugent, 2013).

The Neonatal Behavioral Assessment Scale (NBAS) focuses on the dynamic relationship of a newborn with its parents, rather than a passive state, and that newborns are extremely sensitive to their new surroundings and parents (Nugent, 2013). The NBAS uniquely identifies and assess a newborn's 18 reflex behavioral and social competencies and helps to provide a window into the infant's temperament to aid the parents in their parenting techniques.

Based on current research, which comment by Leana would make the nurse worry that she may have a difficult time getting enough sleep after she returns home and understanding her newborn's behavior?

- a. "I didn't think I'd like breastfeeding, but in reality, it's very enjoyable."
- b. "I walk my dog daily; I'm looking forward to walking the baby as well."
- c. "My husband knows nothing about newborns, but he is usually a fast learner."
- d. "I know that the baby will sleep just fine because I've read everything I can about the subject."

Look in Appendix A for the best answer and rationale.

 What If . . . 17.3

Leana Cooper does not have an episiotomy incision; therefore, the nurse expects her to have little perineal discomfort. Instead, she states her perineal pain is excruciating. Would the nurse bring her something for pain or assume she's exaggerating her pain level?

Nursing Care of a Woman and Family in Preparation for Health Agency Discharge

The greatest need of a postpartal woman before discharge from a healthcare agency is education to prepare her to care for herself and her newborn at home. Box 17.10 shows an interprofessional care map illustrating both nursing and team planning for a postpartal woman.

How to bathe and breastfeed the baby, how to care for the infant's cord and circumcision if the infant has one, a review of how much infants sleep during 24 hours, and how to fit a newborn into the family's pattern of living are topics parents like to discuss before discharge. A great deal of teaching can be done by a comment such as "Notice how large all newborns' heads seem" while you are showing the parents how to bathe the baby, or "Babies like to be bundled firmly" while you are helping dress the child, or "Notice how uneven newborn respirations are." This kind of informal instruction saves parents many anxious moments when they are at home. Common instructions for a woman for her first week at home are summarized in Table 17.3.

BOX 17.10

Nursing Care Planning

AN INTERPROFESSIONAL CARE MAP FOR A POSTPARTAL WOMAN

Leana Cooper is 6 hours postpartum after birth of an 8-lb 2-oz baby girl. She states, "I haven't urinated since before the birth. What kind of mother am I going to be if I can't even manage my own care?" Her husband Mike pulls you aside and says, "Sometimes, I see my wife crying for no reason. Why is she so upset over little things? Isn't she as happy as I am?"

Family Assessment: Couple has been married for 3 years. Husband works as a pharmacist. Will be taking a week off to help care for new baby. Leana is on maternity leave from her job as a court reporter.

Patient Assessment: Labor and birth were without incident. Abdomen soft. Uterus 1/2 fingerbreadth above umbilicus, soft, and displaced to the right. Moderate lochia rubra. Bladder firm on palpation above symphysis pubis. Resonant on percussion. Vital signs within acceptable parameters.

Nursing Diagnosis: Altered urinary elimination related to perineal edema and decreased bladder tone from fetal head pressure during labor and birth.

Outcome Criteria: Patient attempts common measures to initiate voiding; voids more than 100 ml within 2 hours' time. Voices she understands crying is a common reaction after birth.

Team Member Responsible	Assessment	Intervention	Rationale	Expected Outcome
Activities of Daily Living, Including Safety				
Nurse	Assess amount of urine voided during labor and reassess fundal height and position.	Discuss importance of drinking fluid to help initiate bladder reflex.	Retention of urine can predispose to infection and uterine atony.	Patient voids 100 ml by 2 hours' time; fundal height is 1 cm below umbilicus after voiding.
Teamwork and Collaboration				
Nurse/primary healthcare provider	Determine which member of patient's primary care team is on call.	If patient has not voided by 8 hours after birth, notify team member.	Bladder distention can interfere with uterine involution; possible loss of bladder tone.	Primary healthcare provider is notified of patient's inability to void.
Procedures/Medications for Quality Improvement				
Nurse	Assess what measures patient thinks would help her to void.	Instigate measures patient suggests, such as ambulating to bathroom and increased privacy.	Respecting patient's preferences helps her to maintain sense of control.	Patient ambulates to bathroom to void with assistance from nurse.
Nutrition				
Nurse	Assess whether intake, both intravenous and oral, has been adequate since birth.	Stress importance of drinking extra water during the postpartum period.	Ample fluid is needed to counteract diuresis and ensure good urine output.	Patient confirms she has been drinking 1 glass of fluid an hour. Knows to drink 6 to 8 glasses of fluid daily.
Patient-Centered Care				
Nurse	Assess patient's knowledge of postpartal care measures.	Teach normal physiologic changes that occur after birth and importance of preventing complications.	The more informed patients are, the more they can participate in self-care.	Patient states she understands the importance of a good fluid output to help prevent urinary tract infection.

Continued on following page

BOX 17.10

Nursing Care Planning (continued)

Team Member Responsible	Assessment	Intervention	Rationale	Expected Outcome
Psychosocial/Spiritual/Emotional Needs				
Nurse	Assess how often episodes of crying occur.	Emphasize "baby blues" are common during the postpartal period.	The change to being a parent is a major role change.	Patient states she views inability to void as a temporary setback, nothing to interfere with her success as a parent.
Informatics for Seamless Healthcare Planning				
Nurse/primary healthcare provider	Assess patient to see whether she understands the importance of monitoring voiding at home.	Once voiding pattern is reestablished, instruct patient in Kegel exercises.	Kegel exercises help strengthen perineal muscles.	Patient describes Kegel exercises she will continue to use to strengthen perineal muscles.

Make certain a woman is aware that she must return to her primary care provider for an examination 4 to 6 weeks after birth for a postpartum exam for herself and that she should make an appointment to take her baby to a primary care provider for an examination within the first 3 to 5 days postpartum. A follow-up consultation with a community lactation consultant and lactation support group is highly recommended, especially with mothers who experience initial difficulties or who are breastfeeding for the first time (Busch et al., 2014; Holmes, McLeod, & Bunik, 2013).

MATERNAL IMMUNIZATIONS

Recent maternal natal immunization guidelines, supported by the Centers for Disease Control and Prevention (CDC, 2017a, 2017b) and the American Congress of

TABLE 17.3 POSTPARTAL DISCHARGE INSTRUCTIONS

Area	Instructions
Work	All women should avoid heavy work (lifting or straining) for at least the first 3 weeks after birth. Women differ in their concept of heavy work, so it is a good idea to explore what a woman considers heavy work. If she plans to do too much, you can perhaps help her to modify her plans. It is usually advised that a woman not return to an outside job for at least 3 weeks (or better, 6 weeks), not only for her own health but also for enjoyment of the early weeks with her newborn.
Rest	A woman should plan at least one rest period each day while her baby sleeps and try to get a good night's sleep. If she has other family members dependent on her, explore the possibility of having a neighbor, another family member, or a person from a community health agency relieve her so she can rest.
Exercise	A woman should limit the number of stairs she climbs to one flight/day for the first week at home. This limitation may involve some planning on her part, especially if her washing machine is in the basement or if she must go up and down stairs to check on her baby. Help her plan for a place for the baby to sleep downstairs to alleviate the second concern. She should continue with muscle-strengthening exercises, such as abdominal crunches.
Hygiene	A woman may take either tub baths or showers. She should continue to apply any perineal cream or ointment. Remind her to cleanse her perineum from front to back after voiding to prevent fecal contamination. Any perineal stitches will be absorbed within 10 days.
Coitus	Coitus is safe as soon as a woman's lochia has turned to alba and, if present, an episiotomy is healed (usually the first week after birth). Vaginal cells may not be as thick as formerly because prepregnancy hormone balance has not yet completely returned to supply lubrication. Use of a contraceptive foam or lubricating jelly will aid comfort. Be certain she knows safer sex precautions.
Contraception	If desired, a woman should begin a contraception measure with the initiation of coitus. If she wants an intrauterine device, this may be fitted immediately after birth or at her first postpartal checkup. Combination oral contraceptives are begun about 2–3 weeks after birth due to clotting factor risks and interference with milk production for women who are breastfeeding (progestin-only oral contraceptives can be started earlier). A diaphragm must be refitted at a 6-week checkup. Until she returns for this checkup, an over-the-counter spermicidal jelly and condoms can provide protection.
Follow-up	A woman should notify her primary care provider if she notices an increase, not a decrease, in lochial discharge, or if lochia serosa or lochia alba becomes lochia rubra; if lochia has a foul odor; if she has a temperature greater than 101°F; or if symptoms of sadness last longer than 2 weeks. A woman should schedule a 4- to 6-week checkup so she can be assured involution is complete and immunization if not previously immunized against the virus associated with cervical cancer (human papillomavirus) can be administered and so reproductive life planning (if desired) can be discussed.

Obstetricians and Gynecologists (ACOG, 2015), recommend that each pregnant woman receive a Tdap and seasonal influenza vaccine with each pregnancy. Determine if this was provided prenatally to the women, and if not, inform her primary provider of the need to administer the Tdap and seasonal influenza (if applicable) vaccines prior to discharge. Other close caregivers of the newborn (partners and grandparents) are also recommended to be up-to-date on their Tdap and influenza vaccines (ACOG, 2015). If a woman does not have an adequate rubella antibody titer and anticipates further pregnancies, she should also be asked if she wants a rubella immunization before discharge and her provider made aware of this need. Women who are Rh negative and who have had an Rh-positive infant will receive Rh$_o$(D) immunoglobulin (RhIG) or Rh antibodies to prevent isoimmunization concerns in a future pregnancy (Kline, 2012).

Be certain that home care instructions for the family are given both verbally and in writing. Getting ready to go home, dressing the baby, seeing him or her in new clothes for the first time, and experiencing the thrill of realizing the baby is really theirs to take home is so exciting that it is easy for oral instructions to go unheard.

Many healthcare agencies have a community liaison person, ideally a nurse, who calls or makes a home visit to women after discharge. This person helps the new mother assess her own health and that of her baby and answers questions from families who lose their instructions or are unable to interpret them after they have returned home.

Making a telephone call to or visiting a family 24 hours after discharge is another way to evaluate whether the family is able to continue self-evaluation and infant care and is able to integrate the new infant into the family. Such calls or visits also have the potential to reduce the number of acute care visits and rehospitalizations for newborns.

POSTPARTAL EXAMINATION

Every woman should have a checkup by her primary care provider at 4 to 6 weeks after birth (the end of the postpartal period) to assure herself and her healthcare provider that she is in good health and has no residual problems from her pregnancy or signs of postpartum depression.

During this examination, the woman's abdominal wall is inspected for tone and to determine that her uterus involution is so complete that the uterus is no longer palpable abdominally. Her breasts are inspected to see whether they have returned to their nonpregnant state if she is not breastfeeding. If she is breastfeeding, assess that she is free of nipple pain or damage and has an established milk supply; discuss any concerns regarding returning to work or school to ensure her goals of breastfeeding are successful. Most important, a thorough internal examination is performed to be certain involution is complete, the ligaments and the pelvic muscle supports have returned to functional alignment, and any lacerations sustained during birth have healed (Table 17.4).

TABLE 17.4 SIX-WEEK PHYSICAL ASSESSMENT

Area of Assessment	Data Collection
History	Assess chief concern, family profile (support system, bonding, self-esteem, family integrity), interval history, and review of systems (urinary system for pain, frequency, or stress incontinence along with gastrointestinal tract and reproductive tract in particular). Assess maternal intake because some new mothers are too fatigued to eat well.
Physical Examination	Expected Findings
General appearance	Alert; positive mood. If not, woman is probably still extremely fatigued.
Weight	Achievement of prepregnant weight; if not, this will be her baseline postpregnant weight.
Hair	Healthy, firm hair; excess loss of hair from early postpartal period has halted.
Eyes	Pink and moist conjunctiva; if pallor persists, diet may be inadequate in iron.
Breasts	
Breastfeeding woman	Full and firm to palpation; blue veins prominent under skin. Areola darkens and nipple elongates. No palpable nodules or lumps. If erythematous or extremely tender, mastitis or nipple fissure may be present. An occasional filled milk gland may present as a lump; reexamine after breastfeeding.
Nonbreastfeeding woman	Return to prepregnant size; no palpable nodules or lumps.
Abdomen	Striae less prominent; linea nigra fading, muscle tone improving. No distended bowel from constipation. No distended bladder from retention. No history of pain, frequency, or blood on urination. Urinary symptoms probably reflect urinary infection that needs specific treatment.
Perineum and uterus	Lochia no longer present; cervix closed; uterus has returned to prepregnant size. Pap test is normal. Ask woman to bear down during pelvic examination to observe for uterine prolapse, rectocele, or cystocele. If involution is not complete, reason for subinvolution must be investigated.
Lower extremities	Varicosities barely noticeable
Rectum	Hemorrhoids receded to prepregnant size or are no longer observable.
Mental	Positive interaction with infant, appropriate personal hygiene (clean hair, etc.). No indication of postpartal depression or psychosis is present.
Laboratory Reports	
Laboratory values	Hct: 37%; Hgb: 11–12 g/100 ml. If these are low, reassess diet; possibly iron supplement may be needed. Rubella antibody titer: 1:8; if low, additional immunization is recommended before a second pregnancy.
Immunization status	Assess need for human papillomavirus (HPV) [Gardasil] or rubella vaccine.

Hct, hematocrit; Hgb, hemoglobin.

If a woman has hemorrhoids or varicosities as a result of the pregnancy, her primary care provider will discuss with her whether further management of these conditions are necessary. Always ask about the possibility of intimate partner violence because this can increase during the postpartal period because of the added stress of adding a new family member (Malta, McDonald, Hegadoren, et al., 2012). Review the necessity of having a breast examination, Papanicolaou (Pap) smear, and pelvic examination every year as a means of screening for breast, cervical, and uterine cancer. If a woman is older than 40 years, include a discussion about the need for mammogram examinations. Encourage women who have stopped smoking during pregnancy to continue to be smoke free as yet another good health measure for both themselves and their new child, especially if she is breastfeeding.

If reproductive life planning was not discussed immediately after birth, this visit is the opportune time for such a discussion. If a woman desires to use a diaphragm or a cervical cap, these can be fitted during this examination. Injectable progesterone (depot medroxyprogesterone acetate) also can be begun at this time or an intrauterine device (IUD) can be placed. Women who are breastfeeding can begin on progesterone-only birth control pills, implant, or an IUD (Academy of Breastfeeding Medicine [ABM], 2015; Costa, Cecatti, Krupa, et al., 2012).

QSEN Checkpoint Question 17.6

INFORMATICS

The nurse cares for Leana Cooper at a 6-week postpartum visit. The nurse reads in Leana's electronic health record that her fundal height has been progressing in a healthy and predicted manner. What should her fundal height be during this current visit?

   a. At least six fingerbreadths below the umbilicus
   b. No longer palpable over the symphysis pubis
   c. Four centimeters below the top of the iliac crest
   d. Still palpable above her pubic hair line

Look in Appendix A for the best answer and rationale.

Nursing Care of a Postpartal Woman and Family With Unique Needs

A WOMAN WHO CHOOSES NOT TO KEEP HER CHILD

Although the availability of birth control information and the availability of postcoital pregnancy protection have reduced the number of unwanted or unintended pregnancies, some women still may complete a pregnancy and then give up their child for adoption immediately after birth. There are numerous reasons for a decision such as this: The pregnancy may have been unplanned, a woman may be unmarried, she may not be ready or want to assume the responsibilities of parenthood, or her marriage may be failing and she does not want to raise a child alone. She may feel that her family is already complete. She may want to finish school before having a child, or she may want to pursue a career.

During pregnancy, most women decide whether they will keep their child. During labor, they express confidence in their decision, but with the actual birth of their child, they may find their resolve wavers. A woman who was certain she was going to surrender her child for adoption may realize she wants to keep the child. A woman who was certain she was going to keep her child could become aware for the first time of the responsibility involved and decide that the best course for the child is adoption. In either event, a woman's feelings can become confused.

For a woman who chooses not to keep her child, the wait in the birthing room for preparations to transfer the baby to a nursery may seem unusually long. She may also be alone, with no partner or support person with her during this time. Every woman has a right to see, hold, and feed her child if she wishes. A woman who is not going to keep her child may feel proud that she has produced a healthy baby. The realization that the baby is well can provide a foundation on which to build a sounder future so she does not have to make this choice again.

Do not attempt to change a woman's mind about keeping her child or placing the child for adoption during the postpartal period because she is extremely vulnerable to suggestion at this time, and such decisions are too long range and too important to be made at such an emotional time. Her earlier conclusion may be the sound one. Instead, offer nonjudgmental support. Be especially aware of your own feelings about this issue to avoid influencing a woman's decision making unnecessarily.

During the taking-in phase of the puerperium, be especially careful that you do not "lead" the woman's thinking. Women enjoy having decisions made for them during this time and may ask what you think is best. An answer such as "You're the one who has to make this decision. What are your thoughts about it?" can help her begin to think through the problem.

It is not uncommon for women who surrender their infants for adoption to experience grief reactions, the same as those of women whose children have died. If a woman decides to surrender her child for adoption, refer her to an official adoption agency, if she has not contacted one already, because an official agency gives a woman the best assurance the parents chosen for her child will be appropriate. This assurance can help relieve any misgivings or guilt she may feel in future years about surrendering the child, such as wondering whether the child is well cared for and is getting everything the mother could have given her.

Some women do not openly voice a wish to give up their child, but their actions demonstrate they feel little attachment to their newborn. A woman who wants to keep her baby has a tentative but eager approach to her newborn, whereas a woman who has doubts is slow to make contact, barely touching the baby even by the time of discharge, and asking few questions about newborn care. When this happens, the hospital social service department can be of assistance in helping the woman plan the child's future.

It is a fallacy to assume that everything will work out once the woman and infant arrive home. The number of children who experience intrafamily maltreatment seen in hospital emergency departments is proof of the harm that can follow when assessment to detect poor parent–child bonding is inadequate in the first few days of life (Louwers, Korfage, Affourtit, et al., 2012).

A WOMAN WHO IS DISCHARGED BUT WHOSE CHILD REMAINS HOSPITALIZED

Newborns who are ill at birth often are transported to a regional center or to a neonatal intensive care nursery for care, a move that automatically separates them from their parents. Encourage parents to take photographs of the baby on their phone or using a camera before transport and to be certain they have the nursery telephone number and the name of a nurse to contact for questions or information. Most transport teams call the parents after they arrive at the transfer hospital to assure them their infant managed the stress of transport well.

Maintaining communication with the nursery is important so parents can begin to bond with their child despite the imposed separation. Urge them to call the nursery at least once daily to ask about their infant. If the infant is hospitalized in the same hospital, help transport the mother to the nursery, so that she can see and, ideally, hold her child daily. Without this assistance, some women will be so overwhelmed by the technology in the nursery, they are reluctant to call or visit. Assure a mother her telephone calls and visits are expected and valued. A new movement is forming to allow the mother to room-in with the baby in "family style" hospital rooms. This allows the mother (and partner/father) to be close and with their baby, especially for breastfeeding and bonding promotion. Visiting in an intensive care nursery is further discussed in Chapter 26.

It is easy for a woman who is separated from her newborn to feel despondent. Be certain to evaluate whether a woman seems depressed or needs additional support to overcome this unexpected outcome to her pregnancy.

A FAMILY WHO IS ADOPTING A CHILD

A family who is adopting an infant may come into the hospital or birthing center to meet their new infant for the first time. Such a couple needs the same introduction to newborn care as biologic parents. Additional needs of adopting parents are discussed in Chapter 3.

What If . . . 17.4

The nurse is interested in exploring one of the 2020 National Health Goals related to postpartal care (see Box 17.1). Most government-sponsored money for nursing research is allotted based on these goals. What would be a possible research topic to explore pertinent to these goals that would be applicable to the Cooper family and also advance evidence-based practice?

KEY POINTS FOR REVIEW

- The postpartal period (puerperium) is the 6-week period after childbirth. Women move through an initial "taking-in" phase, in which they are dependent; a "taking-hold" phase, in which they manifest independence; and a "letting-go" phase, in which the mother role is finally defined.
- Rooming-in is the preferred healthcare agency arrangement for postpartal families because it allows a new family the best chance for quality interaction and promote breastfeeding (Baby-Friendly USA, n.d.; Holmes et al., 2013). The more time new parents spend with a newborn, the more likely it is that effective bonding will occur. Help parents to feel comfortable with their newborn by offering anticipatory guidance and role modeling infant care as this not only helps in planning nursing care that meets QSEN competencies but also best meets the family's total needs.
- "Postpartal blues" are a normal accompaniment to childbirth. You can assure a woman that such feelings are normal and offer supportive care until the emotion passes.

- Uterine involution is the process whereby the uterus returns to its prepregnant state. A uterus decreases in size one fingerbreadth (1 cm) a day until it disappears under the pubic bone at about day 10. Lochia is the name of the vaginal flow after childbirth: The flow is lochia rubra (red) for the first 1 to 3 days, lochia serosa (pink to brown) on days 4 through 10, and lochia alba (white) until 2 to 6 weeks after the birth.
- A woman is at great risk for hemorrhage in the postpartal period, so assessments done to reveal this are some of the most critical assessments made in nursing. Do not discount the importance of these assessments because the overall content of the postpartal period is so focused on wellness.
- Lactation is the production of breast milk. Colostrum is present immediately after birth; milk forms on the third to fourth postpartal day. A feeling of fullness and firmness on this day is termed *filling*; if warmth and discomfort occur, it is termed *engorgement*. Assessing the mother's milk production, infant's latch, painful nipples, and ability to transfer milk is crucial in the early postpartum period.
- Women may need various comfort measures to alleviate pain from uterine pain (afterpains) and breast tenderness. Application of cold or heat and administration of analgesics are important nursing interventions.
- Women need to learn about self-care before healthcare agency discharge, so they can maintain self-care at home. A follow-up telephone call or home visit can be helpful to answer questions. All women should conscientiously return for a health assessment visit at 6 weeks after childbirth to be certain their reproductive organs have returned to their nonpregnant state. Menstrual flow should return within 6 to 10 weeks in the nonbreastfeeding mother or after 3 to 4 months in the breastfeeding mother.

CRITICAL THINKING CARE STUDY

Katie is a 30-year-old primigravida. She is being discharged with her healthy daughter Sarah this evening. Katie delivered vaginally 50 hours ago without complications and is breastfeeding without difficulty. You chart evidence of positive bonding behaviors. Her postdelivery hemoglobin is 9.5 mg/dl. She has a history of depression during high school. Her mother is planning to help for the next few weeks until Katie and Sarah get settled at home.

1. While preparing for Katie's discharge, you would anticipate teaching about which factors that are most concerning to you?
2. Katie's mother is a support person for her, so how can you include her family in the education?
3. What parenting behaviors would indicate positive bonding between Katie and Sarah?

RELATED RESOURCES

Explore these additional resources to enhance learning for this chapter:
- Student resources on thePoint, including answers to the What If . . . and Critical Thinking Care Study questions, http://thepoint.lww.com/Flagg8e
- Adaptive learning powered by PrepU, http://thepoint.lww.com/prepu

REFERENCES

Academy of Breastfeeding Medicine. (2015). ABM Clinical Protocol #13: Contraception during breastfeeding, revised 2015. *Breastfeeding Medicine, 10*(1), 3–12.

Ahn, S., & Corwin, E. (2015). The association between breastfeeding, the stress response, inflammation, and postpartum depression during the postpartum period: Prospective cohort study. *International Journal of Nursing Studies, 52*(10), 1582–1590.

American Academy of Pediatrics. (2014). *Ten steps to support parents' choice to breastfeed their baby.* Elk Grove Village, IL: Author.

American Congress of Obstetricians and Gynecologists. (2015). ACOG Committee Opinion No. 566: Update on immunization and pregnancy: Tetanus, diphtheria, and pertussis vaccination. *Obstetrics and Gynecology, 121*(6), 1411–1414.

Avsar, A. F., & Keskin, H. L. (2010). Haemorrhoids during pregnancy. *Journal of Obstetrics and Gynaecology, 30*(3), 231–237.

Baby-Friendly USA. (n.d.). *Ten steps to successful breastfeeding.* Retrieved from http://www.babyfriendlyusa.org/about-us/baby-friendly-hospital-initiative/the-ten-steps

Baselice, J., & Lawson, S. (2011). Postpartal care and breast-feeding. In K. J. Hurt, M. W. Guile, J. L. Bienstock, et al. (Eds.), *The Johns Hopkins manual of gynecology and obstetrics* (4th ed., pp. 257–264). Philadelphia, PA: Lippincott, Williams & Wilkins.

Boyle, R., Hay-Smith, E. J., Cody, J. D., et al. (2012). Pelvic floor muscle training for prevention and treatment of urinary and faecal incontinence in antenatal and postnatal women. *Cochrane Database of Systematic Reviews,* (10), CD007471.

Busch, D. W., Logan, K., & Wilkinson, A. (2014). Clinical practice breastfeeding recommendations for primary care: Applying a tri-core breastfeeding conceptual model. *Journal of Pediatric Health Care, 28*(6), 486–496.

Busch, D. W., Nassar, L., & Silbert-Flagg, J. (2015). The necessity of breastfeeding—promoting breastfeeding in the primary care setting: A community pilot project applying the tri-core breastfeeding model: Beyond the basics. *Journal of Pregnancy and Child Health, 2*(2), 1–7.

Cahill, J. M., Freeland-Graves, J. H., Shah, B. S., et al. (2012). Determinants of weight loss after an intervention in low-income women in early postpartum. *Journal of the American College of Nutrition, 31*(2), 133–143.

Chhabra, S., Tyagi, S., Bhavani, M., et al. (2012). Late postpartum eclampsia. *Journal of Obstetrics & Gynaecology, 32*(3), 264–266.

Centers for Disease Control and Prevention. (2017a). *Maternal vaccines: Part of a healthy pregnancy.* Retrieved from https://www.cdc.gov/vaccines/pregnancy/pregnant-women/index.html

Centers for Disease Control and Prevention. (2017b). *Recommended immunization schedule for adults aged 19 years or older, United States, 2017.* Retrieved from https://www.cdc.gov/vaccines/schedules/downloads/adult/adult-combined-schedule.pdf

Chi, C., Bapir, M., Lee, C. A., et al. (2010). Puerperal loss (lochia) in women with or without inherited bleeding disorders. *American Journal of Obstetrics and Gynecology, 203*(1), 56.e1–56.e5.

Costa, M. L., Cecatti, J. G., Krupa, F. G., et al. (2012). Progestin-only contraception prevents bone loss in postpartum breastfeeding women. *Contraception, 85*(4), 374–380.

Dale-Hewitt, V., Slade, P., Wright, I., et al. (2012). Patterns of attention and experiences of post-traumatic stress symptoms following childbirth: An experimental study. *Archives of Women's Mental Health, 15*(4), 289–296.

East, M. (2012). Postpartum anaemia. Are we vigilant enough? *Practicing Midwife, 15*(6), 37–39.

Edmonds, D. K. (2012). Puerperium and lactation. In D. K. Edmonds (Ed.), *Dewhurst's textbook of obstetrics & gynaecology* (8th ed., pp. 365–376). Oxford, United Kingdom: Wiley.

Elliott-Carter, N., & Harper, J. (2012). Keeping mothers and newborns together after cesarean: How one hospital made the change. *Nursing for Women's Health, 16*(4), 290–295.

Farr, S. L., Dietz, P. M., Williams, J. R., et al. (2011). Depression screening and treatment among nonpregnant women of reproductive age in the United States, 1990–2010. *Preventing Chronic Disease, 8*(6), A122.

Gage, H., Williams, P., Von Rosen-Von Hoewel, J., et al. (2012). Influences on infant feeding decisions of first-time mothers in five European countries. *European Journal of Clinical Nutrition, 66*(8), 914–919.

Granek, L., & Fergus, K. (2012). Resistance, agency, and liminality in women's accounts of symptom appraisal and help-seeking upon discovery of a breast irregularity. *Social Science & Medicine, 75*(10), 1753–1761.

Gross, S. M., Resnik, A. K., Nanda, J. P., et al. (2011). Early postpartum: A critical period in setting the path for breastfeeding success. *Breastfeeding Medicine, 6*(6), 407–412.

Heron, J., Gilbert, N., Dolman, C., et al. (2012). Information and support needs during recovery from postpartum psychosis. *Archives of Women's Mental Health, 15*(3), 155–165.

Hickey, F., Finch, J. G., & Khanna, A. (2011). A systematic review on the outcomes of correction of diastasis of the recti. *Hernia, 15*(6), 607–614.

Holmes, A. V., McLeod, A. Y., & Bunik, M. (2013). ABM Clinical Protocol #5: Peripartum breastfeeding management for the healthy mother and infant at term, revision 2013. *Breastfeeding Medicine, 8*(6), 469–473.

Johnson, A., Thakar, R., & Sultan, A. H. (2012). Obstetric perineal wound infection: Is there underreporting? *British Journal of Nursing, 21*(5), S28, S30, S32–S35.

Karch, A. M. (2013). *2013 Lippincott's nursing drug guide.* Philadelphia, PA: Lippincott Williams & Wilkins.

Katz, V. L. (2012). Postpartum care. In S. G. Gabbe, J. R. Niebyl, J. L. Simpson, et al. (Eds.), *Obstetrics: Normal and problem pregnancies* (6th ed., pp. 517–532). Philadelphia, PA: Elsevier/Saunders.

Kline, N. E. (2012). Alterations of hematologic function in children. In S. E. Huether & K. L. McCance (Eds.), *Understanding pathophysiology* (5th ed., pp. 535–551). New York, NY: Elsevier Health Sciences.

Kramer, M. S., & Kakuma, R. (2012). Optimal duration of exclusive breastfeeding. *Cochrane Database of Systematic Reviews,* (8), CD003517.

Lipsky, L. M., Strawderman, M. S., & Olson, C. M. (2012). Maternal weight change between 1 and 2 years postpartum: The importance of 1 year weight retention. *Obesity, 20*(7), 1496–1502.

Louwers, E. C., Korfage, I. J., Affourtit, M. J., et al. (2012). Effects of systematic screening and detection of child abuse in emergency departments. *Pediatrics, 130*(3), 457–464.

Malta, L. A., McDonald, S. W., Hegadoren, K. M., et al. (2012). Influence of interpersonal violence on maternal anxiety, depression, stress and parenting morale in the early postpartum: A community based pregnancy cohort study. *BMC Pregnancy & Childbirth, 12*, 153.

McCarter-Spaulding, D., Lucas, J., & Gore, R. (2011). Employment and breastfeeding outcomes in a sample of black women in the United States. *Journal of the National Black Nurses Association, 22*(2), 38–45.

Meadows-Oliver, M. (2012). Screening for postpartum depression at pediatric visits. *Journal of Psychosocial Nursing & Mental Health Services, 50*(9), 4–5.

Milman, N. (2012). Postpartum anemia II: Prevention and treatment. *Annals of Hematology, 91*(2), 143–154.

Moore, E., Bergman, N., Anderson, G., et al. (2016). Early skin-to-skin contact for mothers and their healthy newborn infants. *Cochrane Database of Systematic Reviews,* (11), CD003519.

Mulder, F. E., Schoffelmeer, M. A., Hakvoort, R. A., et al. (2012). Risk factors for postpartum urinary retention: A systematic review and meta-analysis. *British Journal of Obstetrics and Gynaecology, 119*(12), 1440–1446.

Newton, E. R. (2012). Lactation & breastfeeding. In S. G. Gabbe, J. R. Niebyl, J. L. Simpson, et al. (Eds.), *Obstetrics: Normal and problem pregnancies* (6th ed., pp. 533–564). Philadelphia, PA: Elsevier/Saunders.

Nugent, J. K. (2013). The competent newborn and the Neonatal Behavioral Assessment Scale: T. Berry Brazelton's legacy. *Journal of Child and Adolescent Psychiatric Nursing, 26*, 173–179.

Oelffinger, K. C., Fontham, E. T., Etzioni, R., et al. (2015). Breast cancer screening for women at average risk: 2015 guideline update from the American Cancer Society. *JAMA, 314*(15), 1599–1614.

Rubin, R. (1984). *Maternal identity and the maternal experience.* New York, NY; Springer Publishing.

Samanta, A., Roy, S. G., Mistri, P. K., et al. (2013). Efficacy of intra-umbilical oxytocin in the management of retained placenta: A randomized controlled trial. *Journal of Obstetrics & Gynaecology Research, 39*(1), 75–82.

Schaffir, J., & Czapla, C. (2012). Survey of lactation instructors on folk traditions in breastfeeding. *Breastfeeding Medicine, 7*(8), 230–233.

Smith, P. B., Moorem, K., & Peters, L. (2012). Implementing baby-friendly practices: Strategies for success. *MCN: American Journal of Maternal Child Nursing, 37*(4), 228–233.

Souza, J. P., Gülmezoglu, A. M., Vogel, J., et al. (2013). Moving beyond essential interventions for reduction of maternal mortality: A cross-sectional study. *Lancet, 381*(9879), 1747–1755.

Stuebe, A. M. (2012). Postpartum care. In V. Berghella (Ed.), *Obstetric evidence-based guidelines* (2nd ed., pp. 242–249). New York, NY: Informa Healthcare.

Tescher, A. N., Branda, M. E., Byrne, T. J., et al. (2012). All at-risk patients are not created equal: Analysis of Braden pressure ulcer risk scores to identify specific risks. *Journal of Wound, Ostomy & Continence Nursing, 39*(3), 282–291.

U.S. Department of Health and Human Services. (2010). *Healthy people 2020.* Washington, DC: Author.

Wambach, K., & Riordan, J. (Eds.). (2016). *Breastfeeding and human lactation* (5th ed.). Burlington, MA: Jones & Bartlett.

Whitney, E., & Rolfes, S. R. (2012). Life cycle nutrition: Pregnancy and lactation. In E. Whitney & S. R. Rolfes (Eds.), *Understanding nutrition* (pp. 508–545). Belmont, CA: Wadsworth.

Nursing Care of a Family With a Newborn

*C*arlotta Ruiz, a 29-year-old woman, has just given birth to her second child, a 39 weeks and 2 days, 6-lb, 5-oz baby girl named Beth. Apgar scores at 1 and 5 minutes were 6 and 8, respectively. Vital signs are temperature (axillary), 98.2°F (36.8°C); heart rate, 136 beats/min; and respirations, 74 breaths/min. Beth is 18.5 in. long, with a head circumference of 34 cm and a chest circumference of 32 cm. She has a small port-wine birthmark on her right thigh.

While Jose, Carlotta's husband, is in the room, Carlotta tells you she is a "veteran" at baby care. Jose adds, "Little Joe [their 3-year-old] will be so excited to see his new sister. That's all he's been talking about."

When Carlotta is alone, you notice she seems apprehensive about caring for her new daughter. She tells you, "She's so much smaller than Joe was. And why does it sound like she has a cold? Or have this rash all over her? Isn't it bad enough she has a birthmark?"

Previous chapters described the care of a pregnant woman and family during the antepartal, intrapartal, and postpartal periods. This chapter adds information about caring for the family with a newborn. The newborn period is a critical one for a family because it lays the foundation for the rest of the family's childrearing years.

Does Carlotta know as much about newborns as she thought? What additional teaching does this family need?

KEY TERMS

acrocyanosis
acute bilirubin encephalopathy
caput succedaneum
cavernous hemangioma
central cyanosis
cephalohematoma
conduction
convection
erythema toxicum

evaporation
hemangioma
jaundice
lanugo
meconium
milia
mongolian spot
natal teeth
neonatal period
nevus flammeus

newborns
physiologic jaundice
pseudomenstruation
radiation
strawberry hemangioma
subconjunctival hemorrhage
thrush
transitional stool
vernix caseosa

OBJECTIVES

After mastering the contents of this chapter, you should be able to:

1. Describe the normal characteristics of a term newborn.
2. Identify 2020 National Health Goals related to newborn care that nurses could help the nation achieve.
3. Assess a newborn for normal growth and development.
4. Formulate nursing diagnoses related to a newborn or the family of a newborn.
5. Identify expected outcomes for a newborn and family during the first 4 weeks of life to help them manage seamless transitions across different healthcare settings.
6. Using the nursing process, plan nursing care that includes the six competencies of Quality & Safety Education for Nurses (QSEN): Patient-Centered Care, Teamwork & Collaboration, Evidence-Based Practice (EBP), Quality Improvement (QI), Safety, and Informatics.
7. Implement nursing care for a normal newborn, such as instructing parents on the care of their newborn.
8. Evaluate outcome criteria for the achievement and effectiveness of care.
9. Integrate knowledge of newborn growth and development with the interplay of nursing process, the six competencies of QSEN, and Family Nursing to promote quality maternal and child health nursing care.

Newborns undergo profound physiologic changes at the moment of birth (and, probably, psychological changes as well) as they are released from a warm, snug, dark, liquid-filled environment that has met all of their basic needs into a chilly, unbounded, brightly lit, gravity-based, outside world. Within minutes after being plunged into this strange environment, a newborn has to initiate respirations and adapt a circulatory system to extrauterine oxygenation. Within 24 hours, neurologic, renal, endocrine, gastrointestinal, and metabolic functions must be operating competently for life to be sustained.

How well a newborn makes these major adjustments depends on his or her genetic composition, the competency of the recent intrauterine environment, gestational duration, presence of fetal anomalies, the care received during labor and birth, and the care received during the newborn or **neonatal period** (the time from birth through the first 28 days of life) (Swanson & Sinkin, 2015). One half of all deaths that occur during the first year of life occur in the neonatal period and more than one million babies die every year in the first 24 hours after birth—an indication of how hazardous a time this is for an infant (Save the Children, 2014).

Newborn health is so important to families that the 2020 National Health Goals related to newborn health have been revised (Box 18.1). Nurses play a major role in achieving these goals because nurses are uniquely suited to give care to newborns and newborn instructions to parents.

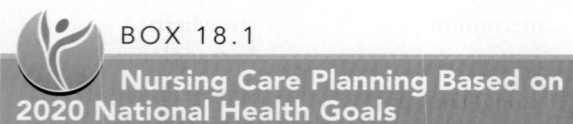

BOX 18.1

Nursing Care Planning Based on 2020 National Health Goals

A number of 2020 National Health Goals speak directly to the newborn period:

- Increase the proportion of mothers who breastfeed their babies in the early postpartal period from a baseline of 74% to 81.9%.
- Increase the proportion of mothers who continue exclusive breastfeeding until their babies are 3 months old from a baseline of 33.6% to 46.2%.
- Increase the percentage of healthy full-term infants who are put to sleep on their backs from a baseline of 69% to 75.9%.
- Reduce the proportion of young children aged 3 to 5 years with dental caries in their primary teeth (which could originate from nighttime bottle feeding) from a baseline of 33.3% to 30%.
- Reduce the perinatal mortality rate to no more than 5.9 per 1,000 live births from a baseline of 6.6 per 1,000 live births (U.S. Department of Health and Human Services, 2010; see www.healthypeople.gov).

Nurses can help the nation achieve these goals by encouraging women to not only begin breastfeeding but to also continue breastfeeding through the first 6 months of life, by advising parents of the importance of placing infants in their own beds and on their backs to sleep, and advising parents of the danger of tooth decay from allowing a baby to drink from a bottle of milk or juice while falling asleep. By discussing early signs and symptoms of illness in a newborn, parents can learn to better evaluate their newborn's health and ask for their primary care provider's opinion before their infant becomes seriously ill.

Nursing Process Overview

FOR HEALTH PROMOTION OF THE TERM NEWBORN

ASSESSMENT

The assessment of a newborn includes a review of the mother's pregnancy history; a physical examination of the infant; an analysis of laboratory reports such as hematocrit, bilirubin, and blood type; and an assessment of parent–child interactions to be certain bonding is beginning. This assessment begins immediately after birth and is continued at every contact during a newborn's birthing center stay, at early home visits, and at well-baby and sick baby visits. Teaching new mothers and their partners to make assessments concerning their infant's temperature, respiratory rate, and overall health is crucial so they can continue to monitor their infant's health at home.

NURSING DIAGNOSIS

Nursing diagnoses associated with newborns center on the difficulty of establishing respirations, beginning nutrition, and assisting with parent–newborn bonding. Examples include:

- Ineffective airway clearance related to mucus in the airway
- Ineffective thermoregulation related to heat loss from exposure in the birthing room
- Imbalanced nutrition, less than body requirements, related to poor sucking reflex
- Readiness for enhanced family coping related to birth of infant
- Health-seeking behaviors related to newborn needs

If a minor deviation from the normal is present, such as a birthmark, a diagnosis such as "Parental fear related to hemangioma on left thigh of newborn" might be relevant.

OUTCOME IDENTIFICATION AND PLANNING

Nursing care planning should take into account the newborn's needs during this transition period, a mother's need for adequate rest during the postpartum period, and the parents' need to become acquainted with their new child. Try to adapt teaching time to the schedules of the mother, her partner, and the newborn. Although the woman must learn as much as possible about newborn care, she also must go home from the healthcare setting with enough energy to practice what she has learned. Important planning measures for newborns include helping them regulate their temperature and helping them grow accustomed to feeding. Refer parents to helpful websites and other resources when appropriate.

IMPLEMENTATION

Role modeling by the nurse during the newborn period is an effective way to help new parents grow confident with their newborn. Parents will be observing you closely. Conserving newborn warmth and energy, to help prevent hypoglycemia and respiratory distress, should be an important consideration during all interventions.

OUTCOME EVALUATION

An evaluation of expected outcomes should reveal that a baby's primary caregiver is able to give beginning newborn care with confidence. Be certain a woman and her partner make arrangements for continued health supervision for their newborn, so the infant's long-term health needs are met.

Examples indicating achievement of outcomes concerning newborns include:

- Infant establishes respirations of 30 to 60 breaths/min.
- Infant maintains temperature at 97.8° to 98.6°F (36.5° to 37°C).
- Mother demonstrates competence in caring for newborn.
- Infant breastfeeds well with a strong sucking reflex.

The Profile of a Newborn

It is not unusual to hear the comment "all newborns look alike" from people viewing a nursery full of babies. In actuality, every child is born with individual physical and personality characteristics that make him or her unique right from the start (Fig. 18.1).

Some newborns are born stocky and short, some are large and bony, and some are thin and rangy. Some have a temperament that causes them to feed greedily, protest procedures loudly, and respond to their parent's inexperienced handling with restlessness and spitting up. Other newborns are sleepy, make no protest over procedures or diaper changes, and seem passive in their new life circumstances. With experience in working with newborns, it becomes easier to differentiate newborns who are merely demonstrating these extremes of normal behavior from those whose behavior or appearance indicates a need for more skilled care because their adjustment to independent life is not progressing smoothly (Box 18.2).

VITAL STATISTICS

Vital statistics measured for a newborn usually consist of the baby's weight, length, and head and chest circumferences. The technique for obtaining these is shown in Chapter 34, along with other aspects of health assessment. Be certain all healthcare providers who care for newborns are aware of safety issues specific to newborn care when taking these measurements, such as not leaving a newborn unattended on a bed or scale and protecting against hypothermia.

BOX 18.2

Nursing Care Planning Using Assessment

ASSESSING THE AVERAGE NEWBORN

Head circumference: 34 to 35 cm

Temperature: 97.6 to 98.6°F axillary

Chest circumference: 32 to 33 cm

Heart rate: 120 to 140 beats/min

Respirations: 30 to 60 breaths/min

Length: 46 to 54 cm

Weight: 2.5 to 3.4 kg

WEIGHT

As long as newborns are breathing well, they are weighed nude and without a blanket soon after birth in the birthing room (Fig. 18.2). Measurements such as body length and head, chest, and abdominal circumferences are also done but can be obtained later because performing these measurements while an infant is still damp exposes the newborn unnecessarily to chilling.

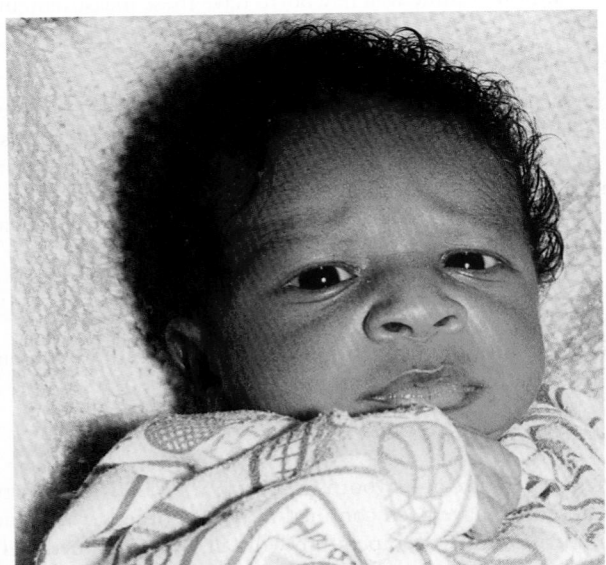

Figure 18.1 Personality is apparent in a newborn from the start. Note the alert, searching interest.

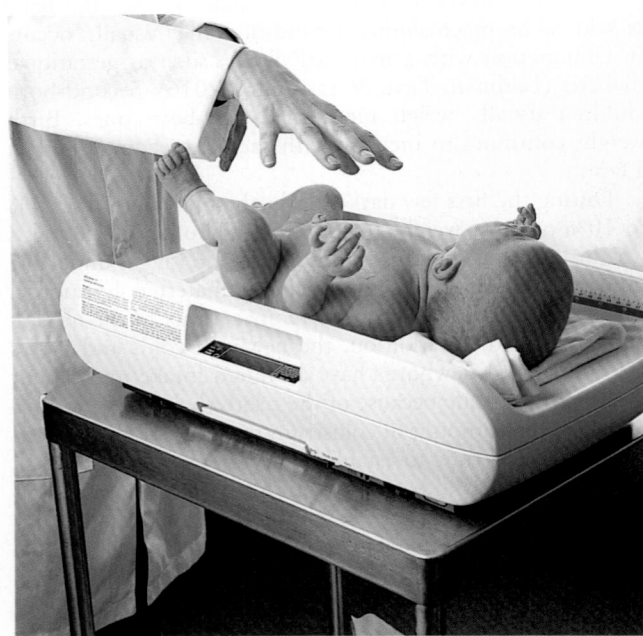

Figure 18.2 Weighing a newborn. Notice the protective hand held over the infant.

A newborn's weight is important because it helps to determine maturity as well as establish a baseline against which all other weights can be compared. Following this initial weight, an infant is weighed nude once a day, at approximately the same time every day, during a hospital or birthing center stay.

The birth weight of newborns varies depending on the racial, nutritional, intrauterine, and genetic factors that were present during conception and pregnancy. The weight in relation to the gestational age should be plotted on a standard neonatal graph, such as those available at the Centers for Disease Control and Prevention (CDC) website based on World Health Organization (WHO) growth standards at http://www.cdc.gov/growthcharts/who_charts.htm#TheWHOGrowthCharts. Plotting weight this way helps identify newborns who are at risk because they are less than usual weight. This information also separates those who are small for their gestational age (newborns who have suffered intrauterine growth restriction) from preterm infants (infants who are healthy but small in weight only because they were born early).

Plotting weight in conjunction with height and head circumference is also helpful because it highlights disproportionate measurements. All three of these measurements should fall near the same percentile in an individual child. For example, a newborn who falls within the 50th percentile for height and weight but whose head circumference is in the 90th percentile may have abnormal head growth. A newborn who is in the 50th percentile for weight and head circumference but in the 3rd percentile for height may have a growth problem. Such discrepancies must be monitored over time to determine trends and any needed interventions.

According to CDC (2010) Growth Chart data, the average birth weight (50th percentile) for a mature female newborn is 3.4 kg (7.5 lb) and for a mature male newborn is 3.5 kg (7.7 lb). Newborn weights vary according to ethnicity and background. The arbitrary lower limit of expected birth weight for all newborns is 2.5 kg (5.5 lb). Birth weight exceeding 4.7 kg (10 lb) is unusual, but weights as high as 7.7 kg (17 lb) have been documented (CDC, 2010).

If a term newborn weighs more than 4.7 kg, the baby is said to be macrosomic, a condition that usually occurs in conjunction with a maternal illness, such as gestational diabetes (Feldman, Tieu, & Yasumura, 2016). Second-born children usually weigh more than first-born ones. Birth weight continues to increase with each succeeding child in a family.

During the first few days after birth, a newborn loses 5% to 10% of birth weight (6 to 10 oz) (Thulier, 2016). This weight loss occurs because a newborn is no longer under the influence of salt- and fluid-retaining maternal hormones. This causes diuresis to begin to remove a part of the infant's high fluid load. In addition, the newborn voids and passes stool. Breastfed newborns have a limited intake until about the third day of life because of the relatively low caloric content and small amount of colostrum they ingest; formula-fed newborns need time to establish effective sucking. This lack of intake also plays a part in weight loss.

After this initial loss of weight, a newborn has about 1 day of stable weight and then begins to gain weight. The breastfed newborn recaptures birth weight within 10 days; a formula-fed infant accomplishes this gain within 7 days. After this, all infants begin to gain about 2 lb per month (6 to 8 oz per week) for the first 6 months of life.

While the newborn is still in the birthing center, compare the weight obtained each day with that of the preceding day to be certain an infant is not losing more than 10% of birth weight because abnormal loss of weight may be the first indication that a newborn has an inborn error of metabolism, such as adrenocortical insufficiency (salt-dumping type) or is becoming dehydrated.

What If . . . 18.1

Mrs. Ruiz tells the nurse she wants to weigh Beth on an infant scale after each feeding to be certain Beth's getting enough breast milk. Would the nurse agree that is a good idea? What would the nurse want Mrs. Ruiz to know before she does this?

Length

A newborn's length at birth in relation to weight is a second important determinant used to confirm that a newborn is healthy.

- The average birth length (50th percentile) of a mature female newborn is 49 cm (19.2 in.).
- For mature males, the average birth length is 50 cm (19.6 in.).
- The lower limit of expected birth length is arbitrarily set at 46 cm (18 in.).
- Although rare, babies with lengths as great as 57.5 cm (24 in.) have been reported.

Head Circumference

Head circumference is measured with a tape measure drawn across the center of the forehead and then around the most prominent portion of the posterior head (the occiput) (see Chapter 34, Fig. 34.5).

- In a mature newborn, the head circumference is usually 34 to 35 cm (13.5 to 14 in.).
- A mature newborn with a head circumference greater than 37 cm (14.8 in.) or less than 33 cm (13.2 in.) should be carefully assessed for neurologic involvement, although some well newborns have these measurements.

Chest Circumference

Chest circumference is measured at the level of the nipples. If a large amount of breast tissue or edema of the breasts is present, this measurement will not be accurate until the edema has subsided. The chest circumference in a term newborn is about 2 cm (0.75 to 1 in.) less than head circumference.

VITAL SIGNS

Vital sign measurements begin to change from those present in intrauterine life at the moment of birth.

Temperature

The temperature of newborns is about 99°F (37.2°C) at birth because they have been confined in their mother's warm and supportive uterus. Temperature will fall almost immediately to below normal because of heat loss, the temperature of birthing rooms (approximately 68° to 72°F [21° to 22°C]), and the infant's immature temperature-regulating mechanisms if the baby is not protected from heat loss at birth and in the moments afterward.

The majority of heat loss occurs because of four separate mechanisms: convection, radiation, conduction, and evaporation (Fig. 18.3).

- **Convection** is the flow of heat from the newborn's body surface to cooler surrounding air. Eliminating drafts, such as from air conditioners, is an important way to reduce convection heat loss.
- **Radiation** is the transfer of body heat to a cooler solid object not in contact with the baby, such as a cold window or air conditioner. Moving an infant as far from the cold surface as possible helps reduce this type of heat loss.
- **Conduction** is the transfer of body heat to a cooler solid object in contact with a baby. For example, a baby placed on the cold base of a warming unit quickly loses heat to the colder metal surface. Covering surfaces with a warmed blanket or towel is necessary to help minimize conduction heat loss.
- **Evaporation** is loss of heat through conversion of a liquid to a vapor. Newborns are wet when born, so they can lose a great deal of heat as the amniotic fluid on their skin evaporates. To prevent this type of heat loss, lay a newborn on the mother's abdomen immediately after birth and cover with a warm blanket for skin-to-skin contact

(Moore, Anderson, Bergman, et al., 2012). In addition, drying the infant—especially the face and hair—also effectively reduces evaporation because the head, which is a large surface area in a newborn, can be responsible for a great amount of heat loss. Covering the hair with a cap after drying further reduces the possibility of evaporation cooling.

A newborn not only loses heat easily by the means just described but also has difficulty conserving heat under any circumstance. Insulation, an efficient means of conserving heat in adults, is not as effective in newborns because they have little subcutaneous fat to provide insulation. Shivering, a means of increasing metabolism and thereby providing heat in adults, is also rarely seen in newborns.

Newborns can conserve heat by constricting blood vessels and moving blood away from the skin. *Brown fat*, a special tissue found in mature newborns, apparently helps to conserve or produce body heat by increasing metabolism as well as regulating body temperature similar to that of a hibernating animal. The greatest amounts of brown fat are found in the intrascapular region, the thorax, and behind the kidneys.

Other ways newborns are able to increase their metabolic rate and produce more heat include kicking and crying. This reaction, however, also forces them to increase their respiratory rate to allow them to take in more oxygen. All newborns can easily become fatigued from this extra exertion, thus

Figure 18.3 Heat loss in the newborn. **(A)** Convection. **(B)** Radiation. **(C)** Conduction. **(D)** Evaporation.

placing additional strain on an already stressed cardiovascular system. An immature newborn with poor lung development may have extreme difficulty making such an adjustment and may fail to deliver sufficient oxygen to body systems.

In addition, as muscles become overstressed, they release lactic acid. Every newborn is born slightly acidotic. Any new buildup of acid created by cold exposure may lead to further acidosis that could be life-threatening.

Drying and placing newborns on their mother's abdomen (covered by a warm blanket), drying and wrapping them and placing them in warmed cribs, or drying and placing them under a radiant heat source is an excellent mechanical measure to help conserve heat or prevent heat loss. Perform all early newborn care speedily and expose the newborn to cool air as little as possible. Be certain that any procedure during which a newborn must be uncovered such as resuscitation or circumcision is done under a radiant heat source.

If chilling is prevented by these methods, a newborn's temperature stabilizes at 98.6°F (37°C) within 4 hours after birth. In contrast to an adult who typically runs an increased temperature with an infection, a newborn may run a subnormal temperature. Therefore, if a newborn's temperature does not stabilize shortly after birth, the cause needs to be investigated to rule out an infection (Ramachandrappa & Jain, 2015).

Pulse

The heart rate of a fetus in utero averages 110 to 160 beats/min. Immediately after birth, as the newborn struggles to initiate respirations, the heart rate may be as rapid as 180 beats/min. Within 1 hour after birth, as the newborn settles down to sleep, the heart rate stabilizes to an average of 120 to 140 beats/min.

The heart rate of a newborn often remains slightly irregular because of immaturity of the cardiac regulatory center in the medulla, and transient murmurs may result from the incomplete closure of fetal circulation shunts. During crying, the rate may rise again to 180 beats/min. In addition, heart rate can decrease during sleep, ranging from 90 to 110 beats/min.

You should be able to palpate femoral pulses in a newborn. Radial and temporal pulses are more difficult to palpate accurately. Therefore, a newborn's heart rate is best determined by listening for an apical heartbeat for a full minute rather than assessing a pulse in an extremity or over the carotid artery. Always palpate for femoral pulses and document that they are present because their absence suggests possible coarctation (narrowing) of the aorta, which is a cardiovascular abnormality (Lissauer, 2015).

Respiration

The respiratory rate of a newborn in the first few minutes of life may be as high as 90 breaths/min. As respiratory activity is established and maintained over the next hour, this rate will settle to an average of 30 to 60 breaths/min. Respiratory depth, rate, and rhythm are likely to be irregular, and short periods of apnea (without cyanosis), sometimes called *periodic respirations*, are also common and normal during this time. Respiratory rate can be observed most easily by watching the movement of a newborn's abdomen because breathing primarily involves the use of the diaphragm and abdominal muscles.

Coughing and sneezing reflexes are present at birth and help clear the airway. Newborns are obligate nose breathers and show signs of distress if their nostrils become obstructed. Short periods of crying, which increase the depth of respirations and aid in aerating deep portions of the lungs, may be beneficial to a newborn. Long periods of crying, however, exhaust the cardiovascular system, become fatiguing, and serve no purpose.

Blood Pressure

The blood pressure of a newborn is approximately 80/46 mmHg at birth. By the 10th day, it rises to about 100/50 mmHg and remains at that level for the infant year. Because measurement of blood pressure in newborns is somewhat inaccurate due to the small size of their arms, it is not routinely measured unless a cardiac anomaly is suspected. For an accurate reading, the cuff width used must be no more than two thirds the length of the upper arm or thigh.

Blood pressure tends to increase with crying (and a newborn cries when disturbed and manipulated by such procedures such as taking blood pressure), so a Doppler method may achieve better results (see Chapters 34 and 36). Hemodynamic monitoring is used when continuous assessment is required.

QSEN Checkpoint Question 18.1

PATIENT-CENTERED CARE

Beth Ruiz, like all newborns, is in danger of losing body heat by conduction. The nurse is taking action to ensure that Beth's body temperature is maintained to protect her health and comfort. Under which condition is heat loss by conduction most likely to occur?

a. A fan is operating in the room.
b. Beth is wet from amniotic fluid at birth.
c. She pulls off the cap the nurse put on her head.
d. The nurse place her on a scale that has not been prewarmed.

Look in Appendix A for the best answer and rationale.

PHYSIOLOGIC FUNCTIONS

Just as changes occur in vital signs after birth, so do changes in all major body systems.

Cardiovascular System

Changes in the cardiovascular system are necessary after birth because now, the lungs are responsible for oxygenating blood that was formerly oxygenated by the placenta. As soon as the umbilical cord is clamped, which stimulates a neonate to take in oxygen through the lungs, fetal cardiovascular shunts begin to close.

With the first breath, blood pressure decreases in the pulmonary artery (the artery leading from the heart to the lungs). As this pressure decreases, the ductus arteriosus, the fetal shunt between the pulmonary artery and aorta, begins to close. At the same time, increased blood flow to the left side of the heart causes the foramen ovale (the opening between the right and left atria) to close because of the pressure against the lip of the structure (permanent closure does not occur for weeks). With the remaining fetal circulatory structures (umbilical vein, two umbilical arteries, and ductus venosus) no longer receiving blood from the placenta, the blood within them clots and closes them, and the vessels atrophy over the next few weeks.

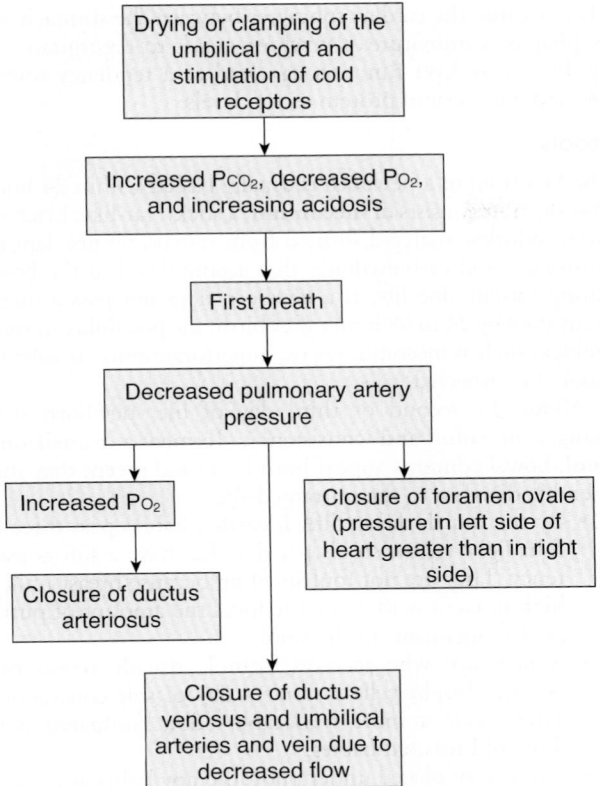

Figure 18.4 Circulatory events at birth.

Figure 18.4 summarizes these respiratory and cardiovascular changes that occur at birth. The peripheral circulation of a newborn remains sluggish for at least the first 24 hours, which can cause cyanosis in the infant's feet and hands (**acrocyanosis**) and for a newborn's feet to feel cold to the touch.

Blood Values

A newborn's blood volume is 80 to 110 ml/kg of body weight or about 300 ml total. Because a newborn has more red blood cells than the average adult, the hemoglobin level averages 17 to 18 g/100 ml of blood (the average for an adult is 11 to 12 g/ml). A newborn's hematocrit is between 45% and 50% (for an adult, 36% to 45%). A newborn's red blood cell count is about 6 million cells/mm³ (for an adult, 3.5 to 5.5 million cells/mm³).

Capillary heel sticks may reveal a falsely high hematocrit or hemoglobin value because of sluggish peripheral circulation. Before obtaining a blood specimen from a heel, warm the foot by wrapping it in a warm cloth to increase circulation and improve the accuracy of this value.

Once proper lung oxygenation has been established, the need for the high red cell count diminishes so, within a matter of days, red cells begin to be destroyed. As these cells are broken down, bilirubin is released and the serum indirect bilirubin level rises. At birth, the indirect bilirubin level is between 1 and 4 mg/100 ml. Any increase over this amount reflects that excessive red blood cells have begun their breakdown (Maheshwari & Carlo, 2016).

A newborn has a corresponding high white blood cell count, about 15,000 to 30,000 cells/mm³ at birth (40,000 cells/mm³ if the birth was stressful). Seeing the count increased, therefore, is not evidence of infection but reflects how stressful an event birth is for a fetus. However, although the high white blood

cell count makes infection difficult to prove in a newborn, infection must not be dismissed as a possibility if other signs of infection such as pallor, respiratory difficulty, or cyanosis are present. Usual blood values in a newborn are available at http://thePoint.lww.com/Flagg8e.

Blood Coagulation

Vitamin K, synthesized through the action of intestinal flora, is responsible for the formation of factor II (prothrombin), factor VII (proconvertin), factor IX (plasma thromboplastin component), and factor X (Stuart-Power factor) in the clotting sequence. Because a newborn's intestine is sterile at birth unless membranes were ruptured more than 24 hours, it will take about 24 hours for flora to accumulate and for ongoing vitamin K to be synthesized. This causes most newborns to be born with a lower than usual level of vitamin K, leading to a prolonged coagulation or prothrombin time.

Because almost all newborns can be predicted to have this diminished blood coagulation ability, vitamin K (Aqua-MEPHYTON) is usually administered intramuscularly into the lateral anterior thigh, the preferred site for all injections in newborns, immediately after birth (Box 18.3). If parents object to an injection, vitamin K can be administered orally,

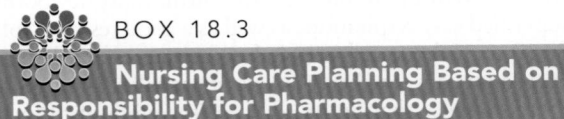

BOX 18.3

Nursing Care Planning Based on Responsibility for Pharmacology

VITAMIN K (PHYTONADIONE, AQUAMEPHYTON)

Action: Vitamin K is used to prevent and treat hemorrhagic disease in newborns. It is a necessary component for the production of certain coagulation factors (II, VII, IX, and X) and is produced by microorganisms in the intestinal tract (Karch, 2013).

Pregnancy Risk Category: C

Dosage: Prophylaxis: 0.5 to 1.0 mg intramuscularly (IM) one time in the first hour after birth; treatment of hemorrhagic disease: 1 to 2 mg IM or subcutaneously (SC) daily

Possible Adverse Reactions: Local irritation, such as pain and swelling at the site of injection.

Nursing Implications

- Anticipate the need for injection within an hour after birth.
- Administer IM injection into a large muscle, such as the anterolateral muscle of a newborn's thigh.
- Be certain to administer the injection at a time it doesn't interrupt parent–child bonding or beginning breastfeeding.
- If giving vitamin K for treatment, obtain prothrombin time before administration (the single best indicator of vitamin K–dependent clotting factors).
- Assess for signs of bleeding in the infant, such as black, tarry stools (different from meconium stools, which have a greenish shade), hematuria (blood in urine), decreased hemoglobin and hematocrit levels, and bleeding from any open wound or at the base of the cord. (These signs would indicate more vitamin K is necessary because bleeding control has not been achieved.)

although it is not as effective (Karch, 2013). Whether giving this orally or by injection, be certain the administration doesn't interfere with parent bonding or beginning breastfeeding as these are also vitally important in the first hours after birth.

The Respiratory System

A first breath is a major undertaking because it requires a tremendous amount of pressure (about 40 to 70 cm H_2O) for a newborn to be able to inflate alveoli for the first time. The reflex to breathe is initiated by a combination of cold receptors; a lowered partial pressure of oxygen (PO_2), which falls from 80 mmHg to as low as 15 mmHg before a first breath; and an increased partial carbon dioxide pressure (PCO_2), which rises as high as 70 mmHg before a first breath.

Some fluid present in the lungs from intrauterine life makes a newborn's first breath possible because fluid eases surface tension on alveolar walls and allows alveoli to inflate more easily than if the lung walls were dry. About one third of this fluid is forced out of the lungs by the pressure of vaginal birth. The rest of the fluid is quickly absorbed by lung blood vessels and lymphatics after the first breath.

Once the alveoli have been inflated this first time, breathing becomes much easier for a baby, requiring only about 6 to 8 cm H_2O pressure. Within 10 minutes after birth, most newborns have established easy respirations as well as a good residual volume. By 10 to 12 hours of age, vital capacity is established at newborn proportions (the heart in a newborn takes up proportionately more space than in an adult, so the amount of lung expansion space available for a large vital capacity is limited).

A baby born by cesarean birth does not have as much lung fluid expelled at birth as one born vaginally and so typically has more difficulty establishing respiration because excessive fluid blocks air exchange space. Preterm newborn alveoli may collapse each time they exhale (because of the lack of pulmonary surfactant). As a result, they also have difficulty establishing effective residual capacity and respirations. In these infants, because alveoli do not open well, the foramen ovale and ductus arteriosus also may not close as usual. This happens because their closure depends on free blood flow through the pulmonary artery and good oxygenation of blood.

Because of the association between ineffective respirations and heart disease, any newborn who had difficulty establishing respirations at birth needs to be examined closely in the postpartal period for a cardiac murmur or any other indication that he or she still has the patent cardiac structures from fetal life, especially a patent ductus arteriosus (Benitz, 2015).

The Gastrointestinal System

Although the gastrointestinal tract is usually sterile at birth, bacteria may be cultured from the tract in most babies within 5 hours after birth and from all babies at 24 hours of life. Most of these bacteria enter the tract through the newborn's mouth from airborne sources. Others may come from vaginal secretions at birth, from hospital bedding, and from contact at the breast. The accumulation of bacteria is helpful because bacteria in the gastrointestinal tract are necessary for digestion through probiotics and for the synthesis of vitamin K.

Although a newborn stomach holds about 60 to 90 ml, a newborn has limited ability to digest everything taken in, especially fat and starch because the pancreatic enzymes, lipase and amylase, remain deficient for the first few months of life.

Also, because the cardiac sphincter between the stomach and esophagus is immature, a newborn tends to regurgitate easily. Immature liver function can lead to a tendency toward lowered glucose and protein serum levels.

Stools

The first stool of a newborn is usually passed within 24 hours after birth. It consists of **meconium**, a sticky, tar-like, blackish-green, odorless material formed from mucus, vernix, lanugo, hormones, and carbohydrates that accumulated in the bowel during intrauterine life. If a newborn does not pass a meconium stool by 24 to 48 hours after birth, the possibility of some problem such as meconium ileus, imperforate anus, or volvulus should be suspected.

About the second or third day of life, newborn stool changes in color and consistency. Termed a **transitional stool**, bowel contents appear both loose and green; they may resemble diarrhea to the untrained eye.

- By the fourth day of life, breastfed babies pass three or four light yellow stools per day that have a soft consistency. They are not foul smelling because breast milk is high in lactic acid, which reduces the amount of putrefactive organisms in the stool.
- A newborn who receives formula usually passes two or three bright yellow stools a day of soft consistency. These have a more noticeable odor, compared with those of breastfed babies.
- A newborn placed under phototherapy lights as therapy for jaundice will have bright green stools because of increased bilirubin excretion.
- Newborns with bile duct obstruction have clay-colored (gray) stools because bile pigments cannot enter the intestinal tract.
- Blood-flecked stools usually indicate an anal fissure.
- Occasionally, a newborn has swallowed some maternal blood during birth and either vomits fresh blood immediately after birth or passes a black tarry stool after two or more days. Whether bleeding is caused by ingestion of maternal blood at birth or newborn bleeding may be differentiated by a dipstick Apt-Downey test. If stools remain black or tarry, this suggests newborn intestinal bleeding rather than swallowed blood.
- If mucus is mixed with stool or the stool is watery and loose, a milk allergy, lactose intolerance, or some other condition interfering with digestion or absorption is suspected.

The Urinary System

The average newborn voids within 24 hours after birth. A newborn who does not take in much fluid for the first 24 hours may void later than this, but the 24-hour point is a general rule. Newborns who do not void within this time need to be assessed for the possibility of urethral stenosis or absent kidneys or ureters.

The kidneys of newborns do not concentrate urine well, making newborn urine usually light colored and odorless. The infant is about 6 weeks of age before much control over reabsorption of fluid in tubules and concentration of urine becomes evident.

A single voiding in a newborn is only about 15 ml and may be easily missed in an absorbent diaper. Specific gravity ranges from 1.008 to 1.010. The daily urinary output for the first 1 or 2 days is about 30 to 60 ml total. By week 1, total daily volume rises to about 300 ml. The first voiding may be pink or dusky because of uric acid crystals that were formed in the bladder in utero; this looks a lot like blood in urine but is an innocent finding. If tested for protein, a small amount may be normally present in voidings for the first few days of life until the kidney glomeruli are more mature. Diapers can be weighed to determine the amount and timing of voiding, which is done when there is a concern.

The possibility of obstruction in the urinary tract can also be assessed by observing the force of the urinary stream in both male and female infants. Males should void with enough force to produce a small projected arc; females should produce a steady stream, not just continuous dribbling. Projecting urine farther than normal may signal urethral obstruction because it indicates urine is being forced through a narrow channel.

The Immune System

Newborns have limited immunologic protection at birth because they are not able to produce antibodies until about 2 months (the reason most immunizations are not administered until 2 months of age). Newborns are, however, born with passive antibodies (immunoglobulin G) passed to them from their mother that crossed the placenta. In most instances, these include antibodies against poliomyelitis, measles, diphtheria, pertussis, chickenpox, rubella, and tetanus. Newborns are routinely administered a hepatitis B vaccine before they leave their birth setting to promote antibody formation against this disease (CDC, 2016). Because the newborn has little natural immunity against herpes simplex, healthcare personnel with herpes simplex eruptions (cold sores) should not care for newborns until the lesions have crusted. Without antibody protection, herpes simplex type 2 infections can become systemic or create a rapidly fatal form of the disease in a newborn (James & Kimberlin, 2015).

The Neuromuscular System

Term newborns demonstrate neuromuscular function by moving their extremities, attempting to control head movement, exhibiting a strong cry, and demonstrating newborn reflexes. Limpness or total absence of a muscular response to manipulation is not normal and suggests narcosis, shock, or cerebral injury. A newborn occasionally makes twitching or flailing movements of the extremities in the absence of a stimulus because of the immaturity of the nervous system; these are common and normal. Newborn reflexes can be tested with consistency by using a number of simple maneuvers.

The Blink Reflex

A blink reflex in a newborn serves the same purpose as it does in an adult—to protect the eye from any object coming near it by rapid eyelid closure. It may be elicited by shining a strong light such as a flashlight into an eye. A sudden movement toward the eye sometimes can elicit the blink reflex, but this is not as reliable.

The Rooting Reflex

If a newborn's cheek is brushed or stroked near the corner of the mouth, the infant will turn the head in that direction. This reflex serves to help a newborn find food; when a mother holds the child and allows her breast to brush the newborn's cheek, the reflex causes the baby to turn toward the breast. The reflex disappears at about the sixth week of life, not coincidentally at the same time a newborn's eyes focus steadily so a food source can be seen.

The Sucking Reflex

When a newborn's lips are touched, the baby makes a sucking motion. Like the rooting reflex, this reflex also helps a newborn find food. The sucking reflex begins to diminish at about 6 months of age. It disappears immediately if it is never stimulated such as in a newborn with a tracheoesophageal fistula who cannot take in oral fluids. It can be maintained in such an infant by offering the child a nonnutritive sucking object such as a pacifier.

The Swallowing Reflex

The swallowing reflex in a newborn is the same as in the adult. Food that reaches the posterior portion of the tongue is automatically swallowed. Gag, cough, and sneeze reflexes also are present in newborns to maintain a clear airway.

The Extrusion Reflex

In order to prevent the swallowing of inedible substances, a newborn extrudes any substance that is placed on the anterior portion of the tongue. If newborns are offered solid food before this reflex fades at 4 months, it will look as if they are rejecting the food. Be certain parents are aware of this reflex so they don't offer solid food this early.

The Palmar Grasp Reflex

Newborns grasp an object placed in their palm by quickly closing their fingers on it (Fig. 18.5). Mature newborns grasp so strongly they can be raised from a supine position and suspended momentarily from an examiner's fingers. This reflex disappears at about 6 weeks to 3 months of age; after it fades, a baby begins to grasp meaningfully.

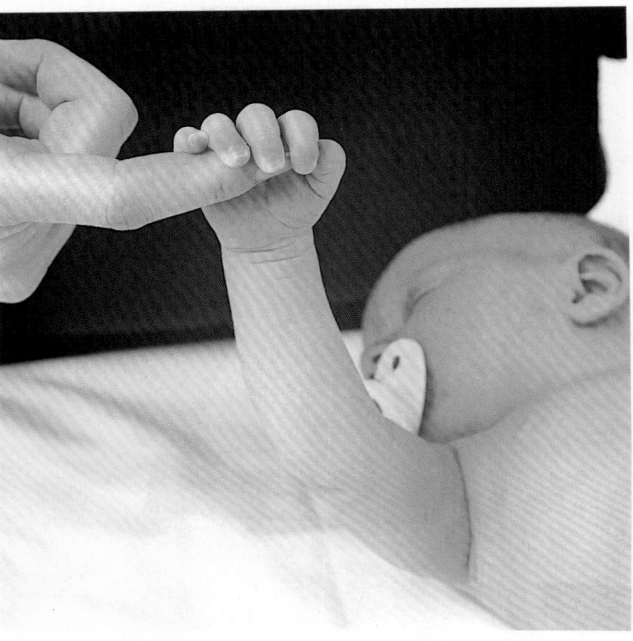

Figure 18.5 The palmar grasp reflex.

The Step (Walk)-in-Place Reflex

Newborns who are held in a vertical position with their feet touching a hard surface will take a few quick, alternating steps (Fig. 18.6). This reflex disappears by 3 months of age.

The Placing Reflex

The placing reflex is elicited by touching the anterior lower leg against a surface such as the edge of a table. The newborn makes a few quick lifting leg motions, as if to step onto the table.

The Plantar Grasp Reflex

When an object touches the sole of a newborn's foot at the base of the toes, the toes grasp in the same manner as the fingers. This reflex disappears at about 8 to 9 months of age in preparation for walking.

The Tonic Neck Reflex

When the arm and leg on the side toward which the head is turned extend, and the opposite arm and leg contract (Fig. 18.7). This posture is most evident in the arms but should not be totally absent in the legs. If you turn a newborn's head to the opposite side, he or she may change the extension and contraction of legs and arms accordingly. It is also called a "boxer" or "fencing reflex." Unlike other reflexes, the purpose or function of this reflex is not known. The reflex typically disappears between the second and third months of life.

The Moro Reflex

A Moro (startle) reflex (Fig. 18.8) can be elicited with a loud noise or by jarring the bassinet. The most accurate method of eliciting the reflex is to hold a newborn in a supine position and then allow the head to drop backward about 1 in. In response to this sudden backward head movement, the newborn first extends arms and legs, then swings the arms into an embrace position and pulls up the legs against the abdomen (Lehman & Schor, 2016). The reflex simulates the

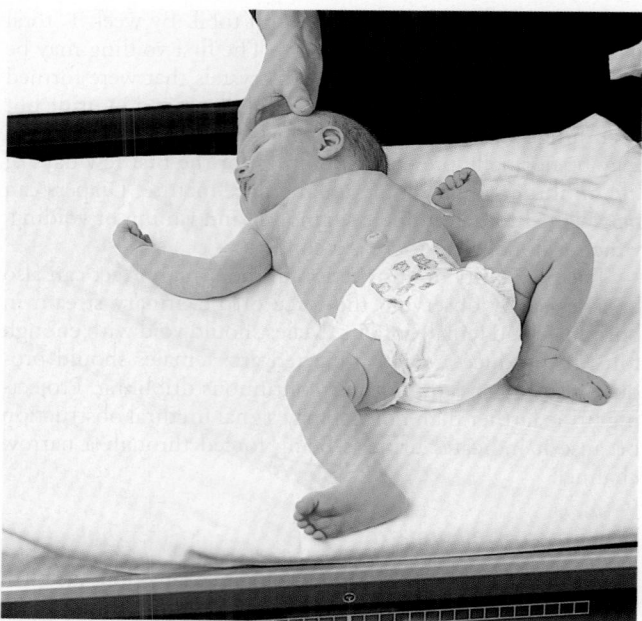

Figure 18.7 The tonic neck reflex.

action of someone trying to ward off an attacker and then covering up to protect the body. It is strong for the first 8 weeks of life and then fades by the end of the fourth or fifth month.

The Babinski Reflex

When the sole of a newborn's foot is stroked in an inverted "J" curve from the heel upward, a newborn fans the toes (positive Babinski sign) (Fig. 18.9). This is in contrast to the adult, who flexes the toes if the foot is stroked this way. The reflex remains positive (toes fan) until at least 3 months of age, when it is supplanted by the down-turning response.

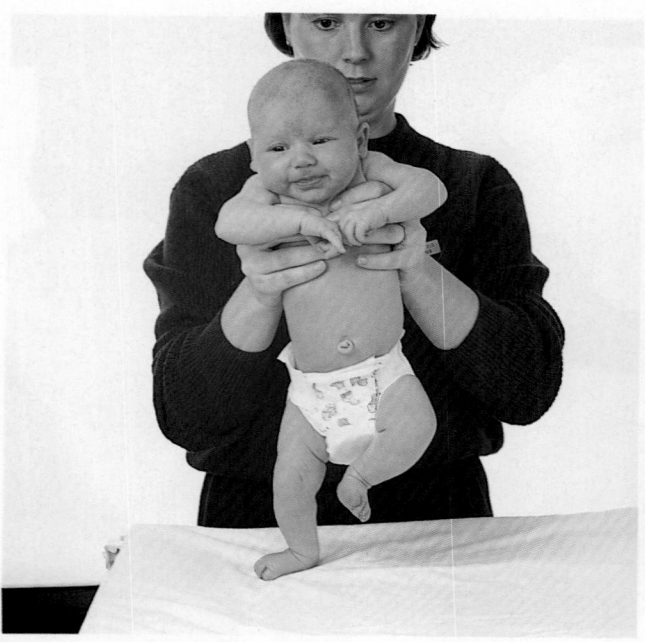

Figure 18.6 The step-in-place reflex.

Figure 18.8 The Moro reflex.

Figure 18.9 The Babinski reflex. When the examiner moves her finger upward, the newborn's toes will fan outward.

The Magnet Reflex

If pressure is applied to the soles of the feet of a newborn lying in a supine position, he or she pushes back against the pressure. This and the two following reflexes are tests of spinal cord integrity.

The Crossed Extension Reflex

When a newborn is lying supine, if one leg is extended and the sole of that foot is irritated by being rubbed with a sharp object, such as a thumbnail, the infant raises the other leg and extends it as if trying to push away the hand irritating the first leg.

The Trunk Incurvation Reflex

When a newborn lies in a prone position and is touched along the paravertebral area on the back by a probing finger, the newborn flexes the trunk and swings the pelvis toward the touch (Fig. 18.10).

Figure 18.10 The trunk incurvation reflex. When the paravertebral area is stroked, the newborn flexes his or her trunk toward the direction of the stimulation.

The Landau Reflex

When a newborn is supported in a prone position by a hand, the newborn should demonstrate some muscle tone. A newborn may not be able to lift the head or arch the back in this position but neither should the infant sag into an inverted "U" position. The latter response indicates extremely poor muscle tone, which needs to be investigated.

The Deep Tendon Reflexes

Both a patellar and a biceps reflex are intact in a newborn (see Chapter 34 for the technique to elicit these).

QSEN Checkpoint Question 18.2

QUALITY IMPROVEMENT

A Moro reflex is the single best assessment of neurologic ability in a newborn. Unit protocols should specify what action for eliciting a Moro reflex in Beth?

    a. Turn her onto her abdomen and see if she can turn her head.
    b. Make a sharp noise, such as clapping your hands.
    c. Lift her head while she is supine and allow it to fall back 1 in.
    d. Gently shake Beth's bassinette until she responds by flailing out her arms.

Look in Appendix A for the best answer and rationale.

The Senses

The senses in newborns, probably because they are so important for survival, are already fully developed at birth.

Hearing

Newborns appear to recognize their mother's voice almost immediately and calm to the sound since they have heard it in utero. In fact, by 25 to 27 weeks gestation, hearing is functional and the fetus can hear the mother's heartbeat and voice. Hearing continues to develop so that the fetus hears a broader range of frequencies throughout gestation and shortly after birth (Clark-Gambelunghe & Clark, 2015). As soon as amniotic fluid drains or is absorbed from the middle ear by way of the eustachian tube within hours after birth, hearing becomes acute. Newborns respond with generalized activity to a sound such as a bell. They appear to have difficulty locating where a sound is coming from.

Vision

A pupillary reflex or ability to contract the pupil is present from birth. The fetus has a blink or squint reflex in response to a bright light in utero by 26 weeks gestation; newborns demonstrate they can see by blinking at a strong light (blink reflex) or by following a bright light or toy a short distance with their eyes as soon as they are born (Clark-Gambelunghe & Clark, 2015). Be certain parents know their newborn cannot follow an object past the midline or appears to lose track of objects easily. Teach also that newborns focus best on black and white objects at a distance of 9 to 12 in.

TABLE 18.1 PERIODS OF REACTIVITY: NORMAL ADJUSTMENT TO EXTRAUTERINE LIFE

Assessment	First Period (First 15–30 min)	Resting Period (30–120 min)	Second Period (2–6 hr)
Color	Acrocyanosis is present.	Color begins to stabilize.	Quick color changes occur with movement or crying.
Temperature	Temperature begins to fall from intrauterine temperature of about 100.6°F (38.1°C).	Temperature stabilizes at about 99°F (37.2°C).	Temperature increases to 99.8°F (37.6°C).
Heart rate	Heart rate is rapid, as much as 180 beats/min while crying.	Heart rate slows to 120–140 beats/min.	Wide swings in rate occur with activity but stabilize at 120–140 beats/min.
Respirations	Breathing is irregular; 30–90 breaths/min while crying; some nasal flaring and occasional retraction may be present.	Breathing slows to 30–50 breaths/min; barreling of chest may occur.	Breathing rate becomes irregular with activity but stabilizes at 30–60 breaths/min.
Activity	Alert; watching	Sleeping	Awakening
Ability to respond to stimulation	Vigorous reaction	Difficult to arouse	Becoming responsive again
Mucus	Visible in mouth	Small amount present while sleeping	Mouth full of mucus, possibly causing gagging
Bowel sounds	Can be heard after first 15 minutes	Present	Often passage of first meconium stool

From Desmond, M. M., Franklin, R. R., Vallvona, C., et al. (1963). The clinical behavior of the newly born: The term infant. *Journal of Pediatrics, 62*(3), 307–325.

Touch

The sense of touch is also well developed at birth. Newborns quiet down at a soothing touch, cry at painful stimuli, and show sucking and rooting reflexes that are elicited by touch.

Taste

A newborn has the ability to discriminate taste because taste buds are developed and functioning even before birth. A fetus in utero, for example, will swallow amniotic fluid more rapidly than usual if glucose is added to sweeten its taste. The swallowing decreases if a bitter flavor is added. After birth, a baby continues to show a preference for sweet over bitter tastes.

Smell

The sense of smell is present in newborns as soon as the nose is clear of lung and amniotic fluid. Newborns probably turn toward their mothers' breasts partly out of recognition of the smell of breast milk and partly as a manifestation of the rooting reflex.

The Physiologic Adjustment to Extrauterine Life

All newborns appear to move through periods of irregular adjustment in the first 6 hours of life, until their body systems stabilize. These periods were first described by Desmond in 1963 and are termed three periods of reactivity (Desmond, Franklin, Vallvona, et al., 1963) (Table 18.1). Newborns who are ill or who had difficulty in utero or at birth may not pass through these typical stages. For example, they may never have periods of alertness or periods of quiet, their vital signs may not fall and rise again but remain rapid, or their temperature may remain subnormal. Demonstration of these typical reactivity patterns indicates a newborn's neurologic system is intact and healthy and the newborn is adjusting well to extrauterine life. Explain these periods to new mothers because the alert periods are ideal periods for mother–infant bonding to begin.

Assessments for Well-Being

A number of traditional standardized assessments as well as a history and physical examination are done at birth to evaluate a newborn for maturity and general well-being.

APGAR SCORING

At 1 minute and 5 minutes after birth, newborns are observed and rated according to an Apgar score, an assessment scale used as a standard for newborn evaluation since 1958 (Apgar, Holaday, James, et al., 1958). As shown in Table 18.2, heart rate, respiratory effort, muscle tone, reflex irritability, and color of the infant are each rated 0, 1, or 2. There is a high correlation between low 5-minute Apgar scores and neurologic illness (American Academy of Pediatrics [AAP], 2015b). The following points are considered in obtaining the rating:

Heart Rate

Auscultating a newborn heart with a stethoscope is the best way to determine heart rate; however, heart rate also may be obtained by observing and counting the pulsations of the umbilical cord at the abdomen if the cord is still uncut.

Respiratory Effort

Respirations are counted by observing chest movements. A mature newborn usually cries and aerates the lungs spontaneously at about 30 seconds after birth. By 1 minute, he or she is maintaining regular, although rapid, respirations. Difficulty with breathing might be anticipated in a newborn whose mother received large amounts of analgesia or general anesthetic during labor or birth.

TABLE 18.2 APGAR SCORING

Apgar scoring is done at one and five minutes after birth. The newborn is considered to be "vigorous" if the initial scores are 7 and above. If the five-minute score is less than 7, scoring is done every five minutes thereafter until the score reaches 7. The numbers in the left-hand column represent the number of points that are assigned to each parameter when the criteria in the corresponding column are met.

	Heart Rate	Respiratory Effort	Muscle Tone	Reflex Irritability	Color
2	Heart rate >100 beats per minute (bpm)	Strong, vigorous cry	Maintains a position of flexion with brisk movements	Cries or sneezes when stimulated[a]	Body and extremities pink
1	Heart rate present, but <100 bpm	Weak cry, slow or difficult respirations	Minimal flexion of extremities	Grimaces when stimulated	Body pink, extremities blue
0	No heart rate	No respiratory effort	Limp and flaccid	No response to stimulation	Body and extremities blue (cyanosis) or completely pale (pallor)

[a]Stimulation is provided by suctioning the infant or by gently flicking the sole of the foot.
Reprinted with permission from Hatfield, N. T., & Kincheloe, C. (2017). *Introductory maternity and pediatric nursing* (4th ed.). Philadelphia, PA: Wolters Kluwer.

Muscle Tone

Term newborns hold their extremities tightly flexed, simulating their intrauterine position. Muscle tone is tested by observing their resistance to any effort to extend their extremities.

Reflex Irritability

One of two possible cues is used to evaluate reflex irritability: response to a suction catheter in the nostrils or response to having the soles of the feet slapped. A baby whose mother was heavily sedated for birth will probably demonstrate a low score in this category.

Color

All infants appear cyanotic at the moment of birth. They grow pink with or shortly after the first breath, which makes the color of newborns correspond to how well they are breathing. Acrocyanosis (cyanosis of the hands and feet) is so common in newborns that a score of 1 in this category can be thought of as normal.

The Respiratory Evaluation

Good respiratory function has the highest priority in newborn care, so the assessment for it is ongoing at every newborn contact. The Silverman-Andersen index, originally devised in 1956 (Silverman & Andersen, 1956), is a standard method, which can be used to estimate degrees of respiratory distress in newborns. For this assessment, a newborn is observed and then scored on each of five criteria (Fig. 18.11).

Concept Mastery Alert

As with any patient, the nurse assesses for pain with vital signs and any procedure.

QSEN Checkpoint Question 18.3

INFORMATICS

Beth Ruiz had Apgar scores of 6 at 1 minute and 8 at 5 minutes after birth. Which of the following are the five areas assessed with Apgar scoring?

  a. Heart rate, respiratory effort, muscle tone, reflex irritability, and color
  b. Respiratory rate, abdominal tone, reflexes, color, and head circumference
  c. Color, breathing rate, cry, amount of brown fat, and response to loud noise
  d. Abdominal tone, persistence, reflexes, blood pressure, and response to pain

Look in Appendix A for the best answer and rationale.

THE ASSESSMENT OF GESTATIONAL AGE

Newborns are said to be term if they are born between 37 and 42 weeks of gestation or within 2 weeks of their due date. Gestational age for an infant born 5 days after the due date would be recorded as 40 + 5; an infant born 3 days before the due date would be recorded as 40 − 3. Specific findings from physical assessment also provide clues to a newborn's gestational age. As early as 1966, Usher and colleagues (Usher, McLean, & Scott, 1966) proposed five criteria to evaluate gestational maturity (Table 18.3). These quick criteria can be used for an assessment of all newborns in a birthing room.

Maturity Rating

Many healthcare facilities do not routinely do maturity testing. They rely on the ultrasound, done at 20 weeks gestation, to assess maturity in most cases. The Ballard or Dubowitz test may be performed if the mother did not have prenatal care or if there is another question regarding maturity of the newborn. Gestational rating scales such as the Ballard or

SCORE

Feature observed	0	1	2
Chest movement	Synchronized respirations	Lag on inspiration	Seesaw respirations
Intercostal retraction	None	Just visible	Marked
Xiphoid retraction	None	Just visible	Marked
Nares dilatation	None	Minimal	Marked
Expiratory grunt	None	Audible by stethoscope	Audible by unaided ear

Total score: 0 indicates no respiratory distress; 1-3 indicate mild distress; 4-6 indicate moderate distress; 7-10 indicate severe distress

Figure 18.11 Grading of neonatal respiratory distress based on the Silverman-Andersen index. (Silverman, W. A., & Andersen, D. H. [1956]. A controlled clinical trial of effects of water mist on obstructive respiratory signs, death rate and necroscopy findings among premature infants. *Pediatrics, 17*[4], 1–9.)

Dubowitz use extensive criteria to assess gestational age. The process of rating the infant, completed shortly after birth, includes physical maturity and neuromuscular maturity (Fig. 18.12). The newborn's skin, lanugo, foot creases, breast maturity, eyes and ears, and genitalia are observed and given a score of −1 to +5, as described in Figure 18.12A. See Chapter 26 for illustrations of mature and immature body features for the scale. For the second half of the examination,

observe or position a newborn as shown in Figure 18.12B. Again, score the child's response numerically from −1 to +5. Then, the total score obtained (on both sections) is compared with the rating scale in Figure 18.12C. Using this standard method to rate maturity helps detect infants who were thought to be term but instead are actually preterm because of a miscalculated due date and who need additional observation and perhaps high-risk care.

TABLE 18.3 CLINICAL CRITERIA FOR GESTATIONAL ASSESSMENT

	Gestation Age (In Weeks)		
Finding	*0–36*	*37–38*	*39 and Over*
Sole creases	Anterior transverse crease only	Occasional creases in anterior two thirds	Sole covered with creases
Breast nodule diameter (mm)	2	4	7
Scalp hair	Fine and fuzzy	Fine and fuzzy	Coarse and silky
Ear lobe	Pliable; no cartilage	Some cartilage	Stiffened by thick cartilage
Testes and scrotum	Testes in lower canal; scrotum small; few rugae	Intermediate	Testes pendulous, scrotum full; extensive rugae

Usher, R., McLean, F., & Scott, K. E. (1966). Judgment of fetal age. *Pediatric Clinics of North America, 13*(4), 835–840.

The Brazelton Neonatal Behavioral Assessment Scale

Term newborns are physically active and emotionally prepared to interact with the people around them. They are people oriented from the beginning, and how much so can be demonstrated by the way they immediately attune to human voices or concentrate on their mother's face (Fig. 18.13).

The *Brazelton Neonatal Behavioral Assessment Scale* is a rating scale of six different categories of behavior: habituation, orientation, motor maturity, variation, self-quieting ability,

SIGN	SCORE						
	−1	0	1	2	3	4	5
Skin	Sticky, friable, transparent	Gelatinous, red, translucent	Smooth pink, visible veins	Superficial peeling and/or rash, few veins	Cracking, pale areas, rare veins	Parchment, deep cracking, no vessels	Leathery, cracked, wrinkled
Lanugo	None	Sparse	Abundant	Thinning	Bald areas	Mostly bald	
Plantar Surface	Heel-toe 40–50mm: −1 <40 mm: −2	>50 mm, no crease	Faint red marks	Anterior transverse crease only	Creases ant. 2/3	Creases over entire sole	
Breast	Imperceptible	Barely perceptible	Flat areola, no bud	Stippled areola, 1–2 mm bud	Raised areola, 3–4 mm bud	Full areola, 5–10 mm bud	
Eye / Ear	Lids fused loosely: −1 tightly: −2	Lids open; pinna flat stays folded	Sl. curved pinna; soft; slow recoil	Well-curved pinna; soft but ready recoil	Formed and firm instant recoil	Thick cartilage; ear stiff	
Genitals (Male)	Scrotum flat, smooth	Scrotum empty; faint rugae	Testes in upper canal; rare rugae	Testes descending; few rugae	Testes down; good rugae	Testes pendulous; deep rugae	
Genitals (Female)	Clitoris prominent and labia flat	Prominent clitoris and small labia minora	Prominent clitoris and enlarging minora	Majora and minora equally prominent	Majora large, minora small	Majora cover clitoris and minora	

SIGN	SCORE						
	−1	0	1	2	3	4	5
Posture							
Square Window	>90°	90°	60°	45°	30°	0°	
Arm Recoil		180°	140°–180°	110°–140°	90°–110°	<90°	
Popliteal Angle	180°	160°	140°	120°	100°	90°	<90°
Scarf Sign							
Heel to Ear							

TOTAL SCORE (NEUROMUSCULAR + PHYSICAL)	Weeks
−10	20
−5	22
0	24
5	26
10	28
15	30
20	32
25	34
30	36
35	38
40	40
45	42
50	44

Figure 18.12 Ballard assessment of gestational age criteria. **(A)** Physical maturity assessment criteria. **(B)** Neuromuscular maturity assessment criteria. *Posture*: With infant supine and quiet, score as follows: arms and legs extended = 0; slight or moderate flexion of hips and knees = 2; legs flexed and abducted, arms slightly flexed = 3; full flexion of arms and legs = 4. *Square window*: Flex hand at the wrist. Exert pressure sufficient to get as much flexion as possible. The angle between hypothenar eminence and anterior aspect of forearm is measured and scored. Do not rotate wrist. *Arm recoil*: With infant supine, fully flex forearm for 5 seconds and then fully extend by pulling the hands and release. Score as follows: remain extended or random movements = 0; incomplete or partial flexion = 2; brisk return to full flexion = 4. *Popliteal angle*: With infant supine and pelvis flat on examining surface, flex leg on thigh and fully flex thigh with one hand. With the other hand, extend leg and score the angle according to the chart. *Scarf sign*: With infant supine, draw infant's hand across the neck and as far across the opposite shoulder as possible. Assistance to elbow is permissible by lifting it across the body. Score according to location of the elbow: elbow reaches opposite anterior axillary line = 0; elbow between opposite anterior axillary line and midline of the thorax = 1; elbow at midline of thorax = 2; elbow does not reach midline of thorax = 3; elbow at proximal axillary line = 4. *Heel to ear*: With infant supine, hold infant's foot with one hand and move it as near to the head as possible without forcing it. Keep pelvis flat on examining surface. **(C)** Scoring for the Ballard assessment scale. The point total from assessment is compared to the left column. The matching number in the right column reveals the infant's age in gestation weeks. (From Ballard, J. L., Khoury, J. C., Wedig, K., et al. [1991]. New Ballard score, expanded to include extremely premature infants. *Journal of Pediatrics, 119*[3], 417–424.)

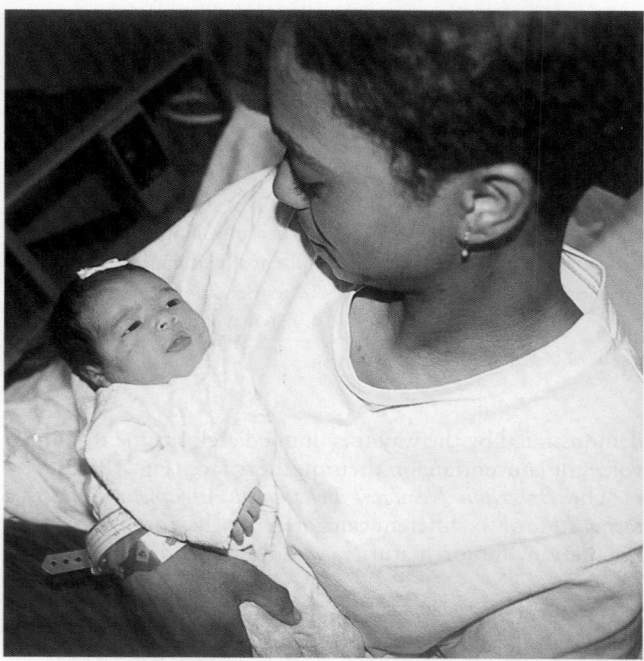

Figure 18.13 A newborn alerts at the sight of her parent's face and sound of her voice.

and social behavior and was devised by Brazelton in the early 1970s (Brazelton, 1973) to evaluate a newborn's behavioral capacity or ability to respond to set stimuli.

A total evaluation takes 20 to 30 minutes to complete. To perform an assessment using the scale requires training to ensure it is used consistently. Unlike many assessment scales, the infant is scored on best performance rather than on average performance. Although not used routinely, many of the items tested on the scale, such as how infants alert to a voice (e.g., eyes widen, head held as if listening) or how they naturally cuddle when held next to their parent, are excellent examples of newborn behavior to point out to parents to help them interact with their newborn.

The Health History

The history of a newborn is obtained from examination of the mother's pregnancy record if this is available, her labor and birth record, and an interview with the mother. Important information to gather includes:

- Any complications of pregnancy such as gestational diabetes, hypertension, premature rupture of membranes, serious falls, or other injuries
- Length of pregnancy and length of labor
- Type of birth (vaginal or cesarean) and whether the infant breathed spontaneously or needed assistance at birth

The Physical Examination

A newborn is given a preliminary physical examination as soon as parents have had an initial time to spend with their new child in addition to height and weight determinations, to establish gestational age and to detect any observable condition such as difficulty breathing, a congenital heart anomaly, or any birthmarks (Table 18.4). This assessment may be the responsibility of the primary care provider or a nurse depending on the facility and circumstances of birth. Always complete such assessments quickly to prevent exposing a newborn to chilling, yet not so swiftly that important findings are overlooked (Gooding & McClead, 2015).

THE APPEARANCE OF A NEWBORN

Although all newborns have similar physical findings, each is unique and has individual differences from all others.

The Skin

General inspection of a newborn's skin includes color, any birthmarks, and general appearance.

The Color

Most term newborns have a ruddier complexion for their first month than they will have later in life because of the increased concentration of red blood cells in their blood vessels and a decrease in the amount of subcutaneous fat, which makes

TABLE 18.4 CONGENITAL ANOMALY APPRAISAL

Procedure	Abnormalities Considered
Inquire for hydramnios or oligohydramnios	Presence of hydramnios (excessive amount of amniotic fluid) suggests congenital gastrointestinal obstruction. Oligohydramnios (lessened amount of amniotic fluid) suggests genitourinary obstruction or extreme prematurity.
Appearance of abdomen	Distended abdomen suggests ascites or tumor.
	Empty abdomen suggests diaphragmatic hernia.
Passage of nasogastric tube (#8 feeding catheter) through nares into stomach	Failure to pass nasogastric tube through nares on either side establishes choanal atresia. Failure to pass it into the stomach confirms presence of esophageal atresia.
Aspiration of stomach contents from feeding tube with recording of color and amount of fluid obtained	With excess of 20 ml of fluid or yellow fluid, duodenal or ileal atresia is suspected.
Insertion of feeding tube into rectum	Failure to pass or obtain meconium on tip suggests imperforate anus or higher obstruction.
Counting of umbilical arteries	The presence of one artery suggests possible congenital urinary or cardiac anomalies or chromosomal trisomy (if other portions of examination are consistent).

Van Leeuwen, G., & Glenn, L. (1968). Screening for hidden congenital anomalies. *Pediatrics, 41*(6), 147–152. Copyright 1968, American Academy of Pediatrics.

blood vessels more visible. Infants with poor central nervous system control or respiratory difficulty may appear pale and cyanotic. In darker skinned newborns, cyanosis may appear as dusky grey or whitish around the child's mouth.

Cyanosis

Generalized mottling of the skin is a common finding in newborns. The lips, hands, and feet are likely to appear blue from immature peripheral circulation (termed *acrocyanosis*). This can be so prominent in some newborns that the infant's hands appear as if a stricture at the wrist must be cutting off circulation because there is usual skin color on one side and blue on the other. Acrocyanosis is a normal finding at birth through the first 24 to 48 hours after birth.

In contrast, **central cyanosis**, or cyanosis of the trunk, is always a cause for concern. Central cyanosis indicates decreased oxygenation that could be occurring as the result of a temporary respiratory obstruction and also could reflect a serious underlying respiratory or cardiac disease. Mucus obstructing a newborn's respiratory tract causes sudden cyanosis and apnea, but this can be relieved by suctioning the mucus from the mouth and nose. In newborns, always suction the mouth before the nose because suctioning the nose first may trigger a reflex gasp, possibly leading to aspiration if there is mucus in the posterior throat. Follow mouth suctioning with suction to the nose because the nose is the chief conduit for air in newborns.

Hyperbilirubinemia

Hyperbilirubinemia is caused by the accumulation of excess bilirubin in blood serum. In the average newborn, the skin and sclera of the eyes begin to appear noticeably yellow on the second or third day of life as a result of a breakdown of fetal red blood cells (called **physiologic jaundice**). This occurs because, as the high red blood cell count built up in utero is being reduced, heme and globin are released.

- Heme is further broken down into iron (which is reused and not involved in the jaundice) and protoporphyrin.
- Protoporphyrin is then broken down into indirect bilirubin, a compound which is fat-soluble and therefore cannot be excreted by the kidneys. In order to be removed from the body, it must be converted by the liver enzyme glucuronyl transferase into direct bilirubin, which is water-soluble, and is then incorporated into the stool and excreted as feces.

Newborns can have difficulty with this process because their immature liver function prevents indirect bilirubin from being converted to direct bilirubin. As long as the buildup of indirect bilirubin that occurs remains in the circulatory system, the red coloring of the blood cells covers the yellow tint of the bilirubin. After the level of this indirect bilirubin rises to more than 7 mg/100 ml, however, bilirubin permeates through the blood vessels to tissue outside the circulatory system and the infant begins to appear jaundiced (Squires & Balistreri, 2016).

Carefully observe infants who are prone to extensive bruising (large, breech, or preterm babies) for **jaundice** because bruising leads to hemorrhage of blood into the subcutaneous tissue or skin; this blood then has to be broken down so can add to the amount of indirect bilirubin accumulating. A **cephalohematoma** is a collection of blood under the periosteum of the skull bone caused by pressure at birth. As the red blood cells in this type of lesion are hemolyzed, additional indirect bilirubin is also released and so can be yet another cause of jaundice (Rozance & Rosenberg, 2017)

Another reason indirect bilirubin levels can increase is if a newborn has an intestinal obstruction because, in this case, stool cannot be evacuated. Intestinal flora in the bowel then breaks down bile into its basic components, one of which is indirect bilirubin. Early feeding of newborns promotes intestinal movement and excretion of meconium and helps prevent indirect bilirubin buildup from this source.

Above normal indirect bilirubin levels are potentially dangerous because, if enough indirect bilirubin (about 20 mg/100 ml) leaves the bloodstream, it can interfere with the chemical synthesis of brain cells, resulting in permanent cell damage, a condition termed **acute bilirubin encephalopathy** or *kernicterus*. If this occurs, permanent neurologic damage, including cognitive, vision, and hearing problems, may result.

The level of jaundice developing in newborns can be grossly judged by estimating the extent to which it has progressed on the surface of the infant's body because it is noticed first in the head and then spreads downward onto the body and legs.

Various commercial devices (transcutaneous bilirubinometry devices) are available to measure skin tone and help in estimating the level of bilirubin present. Although use of these devices rarely replaces serum measurements, they can be used to identify infants who need serum bilirubin determinations.

Treatment for physiologic jaundice or the routine rise in indirect bilirubin in newborns is rarely necessary, except for preventive measures such as early feeding to speed the passage of meconium.

There is no set level at which indirect serum bilirubin requires treatment because other factors, such as age, maturity, and breastfeeding status, affect this determination. If the level rises to more than 10 to 12 mg/100 ml, treatment is usually considered. Phototherapy (exposure of the infant to light to initiate maturation of liver enzymes) is common therapy (see Chapter 26). If this is necessary, the incubator and light source can be moved to the mother's room so the mother is not separated from her baby. Some infants need continued therapy after discharge and receive phototherapy at home either by a light-emitting diode (LED) or fluorescent lights over their crib or a phototherapy blanket (Muchowski, 2014).

Compared with formula-fed babies, a small proportion of breastfed babies may have more difficulty converting indirect bilirubin to direct bilirubin because breast milk contains pregnanediol (a metabolite of progesterone), which depresses the action of glucuronyl transferase. However, breastfeeding alone rarely causes enough jaundice to warrant therapy and in most cases, healthcare providers should promote breastfeeding in infants with jaundice (Muchowski, 2014). A decision to stop breastfeeding in the first 2 weeks of life due to jaundice must be taken very seriously because of the high risk that the interruption will interfere with establishing breastfeeding for the mother–infant dyad.

Pallor

Pallor in newborns is potentially serious because it usually occurs as the result of anemia, which may be caused by a number of circumstances such as:

- Low iron stores caused by poor maternal nutrition during pregnancy.
- Blood incompatibility in which a large number of red blood cells were hemolyzed in utero.
- Fetal–maternal transfusion.

- Inadequate flow of blood from the cord into the infant before the cord was cut.
- Excessive blood loss when the cord was cut.
- Internal bleeding. To detect this, a baby who appears pale should be watched closely for signs of blood in the stool or vomitus.

Newborns identified as having anemia need therapy such as supplemental iron or a packed red cell transfusion to restore their blood volume.

The Harlequin Sign

Occasionally, because of immature blood circulation, a newborn who has been lying on his or her side appears red on the dependent side of the body and pale on the upper side, as if a line had been drawn down the center of the body. This is a transient phenomenon and, although startling, is of no clinical significance. The odd coloring fades immediately if the infant's position is changed or the baby kicks or cries.

Birthmarks

Several common types of birthmarks occur in newborns. It is important to be able to differentiate the various types of hemangiomas that occur because some are more serious than others, and you do not want to give family members false reassurance nor worry them unnecessarily about these lesions.

Hemangiomas

Hemangiomas are vascular tumors of the skin and occur in three distinct types (Table 18.5).

Mongolian Spots

Mongolian spots are collections of pigment cells (melanocytes) that appear as slate-gray patches across the sacrum or buttocks and possibly on the arms and legs of newborns. They tend to occur most often in children of Asian, Southern European, or African ethnicity and disappear by school age without treatment (Smith & Grover, 2016). Be sure to educate parents that these are not bruises.

What If . . . 18.2
Beth's father tells the nurse he's not worried about the port-wine stain on his baby's thigh because he knows all birthmarks fade by school age. How would the nurse respond to him?

Vernix Caseosa

Vernix caseosa is the white, cream cheese–like substance that serves as a skin lubricant in utero. It is typically noticeable on a term newborn's skin, at least in the skin folds, at birth. Document the color of any vernix present because it takes on the color of the amniotic fluid (yellow

TABLE 18.5 VASCULAR DISORDERS OF THE NEWBORN

Type	Description	Location	Treatment

Nevus flammeus	• Two types:
	  ◦ Benign macular purple or dark-red lesion (also called a *port-wine stain*) (see Fig. 18.14A)
	  ◦ Light-pink patches: *stork bites* or *telangiectasia* (see Fig. 18.14B).
	• Present at birth
		Port wine: face, thighs
		Stork bites: nape of neck
			• Port wine:
			  ◦ May spontaneously fade
			  ◦ Cosmetically cover
			  ◦ Laser later in life
			• Stork bites: do not fade; no treatment because usually covered by hair

Infantile hemangiomas (also called *strawberry hemangiomas*)	• Elevated areas formed by immature capillaries and endothelial cells (see Fig. 18.14C) • Appear at birth or within 2 weeks after birth • Size may enlarge up to 1 year of age. • After 1 year of age, hemangiomas tend to be absorbed and shrink in size. By the time the child is 7 years old, 70% have involuted to a reasonable level; most involution completed by 10 years	Can occur anywhere on the infant; most common on scalp, face, neck	• Educate parent about expected increase in size for up to one year and that they are likely to resolve with time. • Propranolol (Inderal) and corticosteroids can be used to reduce size. • Surgical excision is rarely done due to risk for complications.
Cavernous hemangioma	• Caused by dilated vascular spaces • Raised and irregular shape; resemble a strawberry hemangioma (see Fig. 18.14D) • Do not disappear with time • Some may have additional lesions on internal organs such as the spleen or liver.	Most commonly appear on the face, behind the ears, and the neck	• Surgical removal if they interfere with sight or breathing • Steroids, interferon alfa-2a, vincristine, or radiation may reduce size of lesions; risk vs. benefit must be considered • Hematocrit levels to assess for blood loss if child has internal cavernous lesions

Paller, A. S., & Mancini, A. J. (2016). Vascular disorders of infancy and childhood. In A. S. Paller & A. J. Mancini (Eds.), *Hurwitz clinical pediatric dermatology* (5th ed., pp. 279–316). New York, NY: Elsevier; Chinnadurai, S., Fonnesbeck, C., Snyder, K. M., et al. (2016). Pharmacologic interventions for infantile hemangioma: A meta-analysis. *Pediatrics, 137*(2), e20153896.

Figure 18.14   Types of hemangiomas found on a newborn. **(A) Nevus flammeus** (port-wine stain) formed of a plexus of newly formed capillaries in the papillary layer of the corium. It is deep red to purple, does not blanch on pressure, and does not fade with age. **(B)** A telangiectasia or stork beak mark, commonly occurring on nape of neck. It blanches on pressure; although it does not fade, it is not noticeable as it becomes covered by hair. **(C) Strawberry hemangiomas** consist of dilated capillaries in entire dermal and subdermal layers. They continue to enlarge after birth but usually disappear by age 10 years. **(D) Cavernous hemangiomas** consist of a communicating network of venules in subcutaneous tissue and do not fade with age.

vernix implies the amniotic fluid was stained from excessive bilirubin or a blood dyscrasia may be present; green vernix suggests meconium was present in the amniotic fluid).

Handle newborns with gloves to protect yourself from exposure to vernix. Remove only the vernix that is contaminated by meconium or blood (Lovejoy-Bleum, 2014). Never rub it away harshly because newborn skin is tender and breaks in the skin caused by too vigorous attempts at removal could open portals of entry for bacteria.

Lanugo

Lanugo is the fine, downy hair that covers a term newborn's shoulders, back, upper arms, and possibly also the forehead and ears. Postterm infants (born after more than 42 weeks of gestation) rarely have lanugo. Babies born at 37 to 39 weeks, in contrast, have a generous supply of lanugo. Following birth, lanugo is rubbed away by the friction of bedding and clothes against the newborn's skin. By 2 weeks of age, it has usually totally disappeared.

Desquamation

Within 24 hours after birth, the skin of most newborns begins to dry. The dryness is particularly evident on the palms of the hands and soles of the feet and results in areas of peeling similar to those caused by sunburn. This is a reaction to suddenly living in an air-filled rather than a liquid-filled environment. No treatment is needed. Parents may apply mild lotion to prevent excessive dryness if they wish.

Newborns who are postterm and have suffered intrauterine malnutrition may have such extremely dry skin that it has a leathery appearance and there are actual cracks in the skin folds. This should be differentiated from normal desquamation because it helps to diagnose the newborn as postterm.

Milia

Sebaceous glands in a newborn are immature, so at least one pinpoint white papule (a plugged or unopened sebaceous gland) is usually found on a cheek or across the bridge of the nose of every newborn. Such lesions, termed **milia** (Fig. 18.15), disappear by 3 to 4 weeks of age as the sebaceous glands mature and

Figure 18.15 Milia are unopened sebaceous glands frequently found on the nose, chin, or cheeks of a newborn.

Figure 18.17 Forceps marks are commonly found in newborns born by forceps. Such marks are transient and disappear in a day or two.

the plugged ones drain. Advise parents to wait for the milia to resolve spontaneously; recommend that they avoid scratching or squeezing the papule, which could lead to secondary infection.

Erythema Toxicum

Erythema toxicum commonly presents on the skin of most term newborns (Fig. 18.16). The rash usually appears in the first to fourth day of life but may appear as late as 2 weeks of age. It begins with small papules, increases in severity to become erythematous by the second day and then disappears by the third day. It is sometimes called a *flea-bite rash* because the lesions are so minuscule. One of the chief characteristics of the rash is its lack of pattern. It occurs sporadically and unpredictably and may last hours or days. It is probably caused by the newborn's eosinophils reacting to the rough environment of sheets and clothing rather than a smooth liquid against the skin. It requires no treatment. It is important it be differentiated from

lesions of herpes simplex (clustered vesicles) because herpes simplex is a serious finding in a newborn (Paller & Mancini, 2016).

Forceps Marks

Forceps are rarely used for birth today, but if they are used (see Chapter 23), they may leave a circular or linear contusion matching the rim of the forceps blade on the infant's cheek (Fig. 18.17). The mark occurs with normal forceps use and does not denote unskilled or overly vigorous application of forceps. The mark disappears in 1 to 2 days, along with the edema that accompanies it. Closely assess the face of a newborn with a forceps mark especially during a crying episode to be certain the infant's mouth is symmetrical, to detect any potential facial nerve injury requiring further evaluation.

Skin Turgor

Like adult skin, newborn skin should feel resilient if the underlying tissue is well hydrated. Grasp a fold of the skin between your thumb and fingers and evaluate if it feels elastic. When released, the skin should fall back to form a smooth surface. If severe dehydration is present, the skin will not smooth out again but will remain as an elevated ridge. Poor turgor is seen in newborns who suffered malnutrition in utero, who have difficulty sucking at birth, or who have certain metabolic disorders such as adrenocortical insufficiency. Poor turgor always needs to be reported as it suggests poor hydration.

Figure 18.16 Erythema toxicum is found on almost all newborns. The reddish rash consists of sporadic pinpoint papules on an erythematous base. It fades spontaneously in a few days.

QSEN Checkpoint Question 18.4

SAFETY

Beth Ruiz has milia on her nose. What teaching point would constitute a quality and safety risk?
  a. "These will disappear on their own, so you don't need to take any action."
  b. "Wash Beth the same way that the nurse first taught you."
  c. "Try to gently scratch off these spots in a few days."
  d. "Make sure that you keep Beth bundled warmly."

Look in Appendix A for the best answer and rationale.

THE HEAD

A newborn's head usually appears disproportionately large because it is about one fourth of the total body length compared with an adult, whose head is one eighth of total height. Other features include:

- The forehead appears large and prominent.
- The chin appears to be receding, and it quivers easily if the infant is startled or cries.
- If a newborn has hair, the hair should look full bodied; both poorly nourished and preterm infants have thin, lifeless hair.
- If internal fetal monitoring was used during labor (see Chapter 24), a newborn may have a pinpoint ulcer at the point where the monitor was attached.

Fontanelles

The fontanelles are the spaces or openings where the skull bones join. The anterior fontanelle is located at the junction of the two parietal bones and the two fused frontal bones. It is diamond-shaped and measures 2 to 3 cm (0.8 to 1.2 in.) in width and 3 to 4 cm (1.2 to 1.6 in.) in length. The posterior fontanelle is located at the junction of the parietal bones and the occipital bone. It is triangular and measures about 1 to 2 cm (0.4 to 0.7 in.) in length.

The anterior fontanelle can be felt as a soft spot. It should not appear indented (a sign of dehydration) or bulging (a sign of increased intracranial pressure) when the infant is held upright. The fontanelle may bulge if the newborn strains to pass a stool, cries vigorously, or is lying supine. The anterior fontanelle normally closes at 12 to 18 months of age. In some newborns, the posterior fontanelle is so small that it cannot be palpated readily. It closes by the end of the second month.

Sutures

The skull *sutures*, the separating lines of the skull, may override at birth because of the extreme pressure exerted on the head during passage through the birth canal. If the sagittal suture between the parietal bones overrides, the fontanelles are less perceptible than usual. The overriding subsides in 24 to 48 hours.

Suture lines should never appear widely separated in newborns. Wide separation suggests increased intracranial pressure because of abnormal brain formation, abnormal accumulation of cerebrospinal fluid in the cranium (hydrocephalus), or an accumulation of blood from a birth injury such as subdural hemorrhage. Fused suture lines also are abnormal; they require X-ray confirmation and further evaluation because this will prevent the head from expanding with brain growth.

Molding

The part of the infant's head that engaged the cervix (usually the vertex) molds to fit the cervix contours during labor. After birth, this area appears prominent and asymmetric (Fig. 18.18). You can assure parents the head will evolve to a more rounded shape within a few days after birth.

Caput Succedaneum

Caput succedaneum (Fig. 18.19A) is edema of the scalp that forms on the presenting part of the head. It occurs in cephalic births and can either involve wide areas of the head or be so confined that it's the size of a large egg. The edema, which crosses the suture lines, is gradually absorbed and disappears within several days. No treatment is needed (Gooding & McCLead, 2015).

Cephalohematoma

A *cephalohematoma*, a collection of blood between the periosteum of a skull bone and the bone itself, is caused by rupture of a periosteal capillary because of the pressure of birth (see Fig. 18.19B). Although the blood loss is negligible, edema, which appears by 24 hours after birth, appears severe and is well outlined as an egg shape. It may be discolored (black and blue) because of the presence of coagulated blood underneath the periosteum. Unlike a caput, a cephalohematoma is confined to an individual bone, so the associated swelling stops at the bone's suture line.

Cephalohematomas will subside without treatment. It may take weeks for the blood under the periosteum to be absorbed. As the blood breaks down, the infant needs to be observed for jaundice that can occur from the large amount of indirect bilirubin that may be released (Muchowski, 2014).

Craniotabes

Craniotabes is a localized softening of the cranial bones probably caused by pressure of the fetal skull against the mother's pelvic bone in utero. It is more common in first-born infants than in infants born later because of the lower position of the fetal head in the pelvis during the last 2 weeks of pregnancy in primiparous women. With craniotabes, the skull is so soft that the pressure of an examining finger can indent it. The bone then returns to its normal contour after the pressure is removed. The condition corrects itself without treatment after a few months as the infant ingests calcium from milk (Gomella, Cunningham, Eyal, et al., 2013).

Craniotabes is an example of a condition that is normal if seen in a newborn but would be pathologic in an older child or adult (because then it probably would be the result of faulty calcium metabolism or kidney dysfunction).

THE EYES

To inspect the eyes of a newborn, lay the infant in a supine position and lift the head; this maneuver usually causes the baby to open his or her eyes. It's rare to see tears in a newborn because their lacrimal ducts do not fully mature until about 3 months of age. Almost without exception, the irises of the eyes look gray or blue; the surrounding sclera may appear light blue due to its thinness. The iris will assume its permanent color between 3 and 12 months of age.

The eyes should appear clear, without redness or purulent discharge. Occasionally, the administration of an antibiotic ointment such as erythromycin at birth, to protect against chlamydia, has caused the eyes to appear reddened with a slight discharge; if this has occurred, it lasts for about 24 hours of life then clears.

Pressure during birth sometimes ruptures a conjunctival capillary of the eye, resulting in a small **subconjunctival hemorrhage** on the sclera. This appears as a red spot, usually on the inner aspect of the eye, or as a red ring around the cornea. The bleeding is slight, requires no treatment, and is completely absorbed within 2 or 3 weeks. While it may appear as if the baby is bleeding from within the eye and that

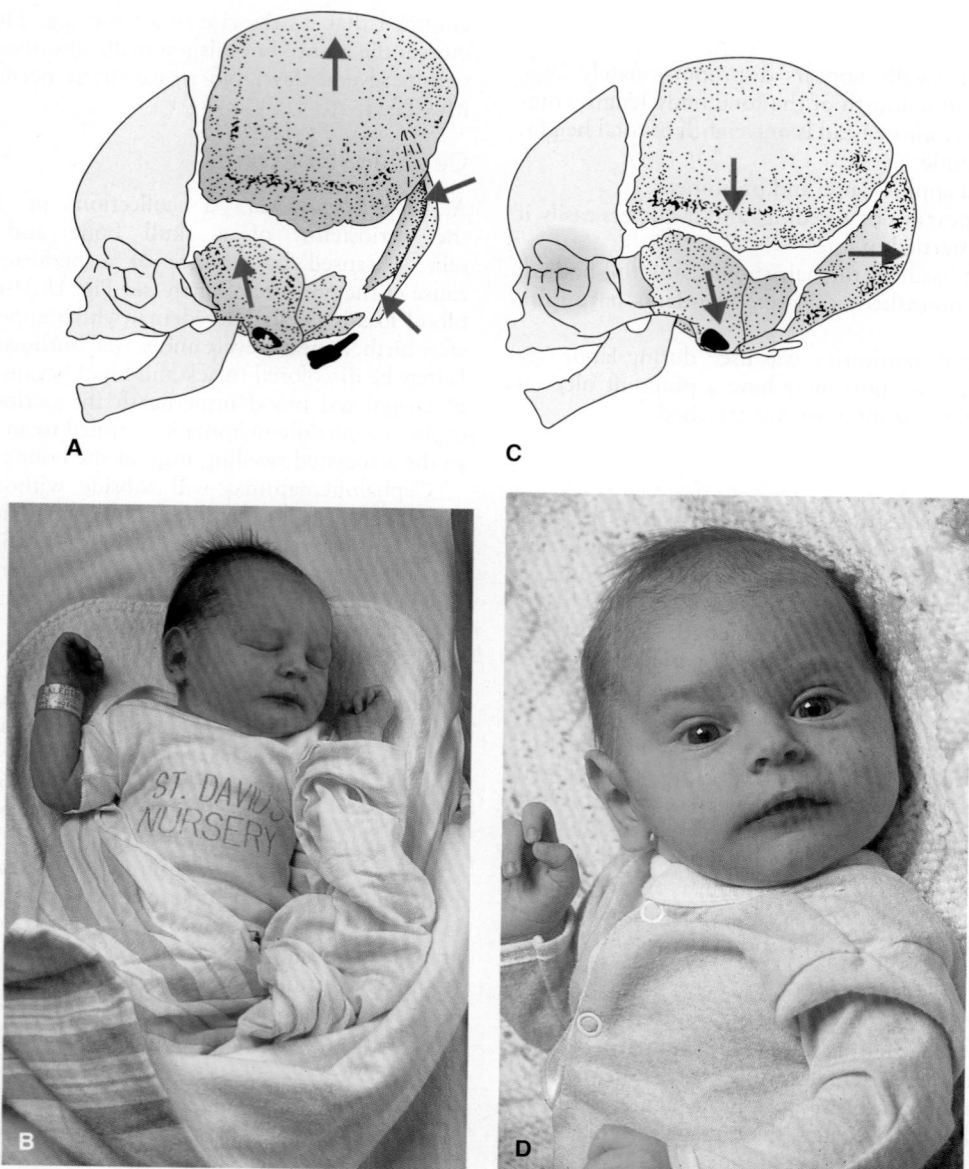

Figure 18.18   Molding. **(A,B)** The infant head molds to fit the birth canal more easily. On palpation, the skull sutures will be felt to be overriding. **(C,D)** The head shape returns to normal within 1 week.

his or her vision might be impaired, you can assure a mother and her partner that these hemorrhages occur often and will soon resolve.

Slight edema is often present around the orbit or on the eyelids and remains for the first 2 or 3 days until the newborn's kidneys are capable of evacuating fluid more efficiently.

Be certain the cornea of each eye appears round and proportionate in size to an adult eye because a cornea that appears larger than usual may be the result of congenital glaucoma. An irregularly shaped pupil or discolored iris may denote a congenital formation such as a coloboma (see Chapter 50). The pupil, as in adults, should appear dark. A white pupil suggests the presence of a congenital cataract, glaucoma, retinoblastoma, or other eye disorder and should be reported (Gomella et al., 2013).

THE EARS

A newborn's external ear is not as completely formed as it will be eventually, so the pinna tends to bend forward easily. In a term newborn, however, the pinna should be strong enough to recoil after bending.

The level of the top part of the external ear should be even to a line drawn from the inner canthus to the outer canthus of the eye and back across the side of the head (see Chapter 34). Ears that are set lower than this are found in infants with certain chromosomal abnormalities, particularly trisomy 18 and 13, syndromes in which there are other physical variations coupled with varying degrees of cognitive impairment (Saenz, Meeks, Tsai, et al., 2016).

A small tag of skin is sometimes found just in front of an ear. Although these tags may be associated with chromosomal

Figure 18.19 **(A)** Caput succedaneum. From pressure of the birth canal, an edematous area is present beneath the scalp. Note how it crosses the midline of the skull. **(B)** Cephalohematoma. A small capillary beneath the periosteum of the skull bone has ruptured, and blood has collected under the periosteum of the bone. Note how the swelling now stops at the midline. Because the blood is contained under the periosteum, it is necessarily stopped by a suture line.

abnormalities or kidney disease, they usually are isolated findings of no consequence. They can be removed by ligation immediately or within the first week of life. Always inspect closely in front of newborns' ears for pinpoint-size openings that may lead down to a hollow sinus because an open track under the skin lined with squamous epithelium may also be present at these sites. The sinus itself is usually small and inconsequential, but advise parents that the closed space can become infected. If this occurs, the site will appear red and swollen and the infant will need an antibiotic ointment. The parents can have the tract removed surgically to prevent further infection.

Amniotic fluid and flecks of vernix usually still fill the ear canal, obliterating the tympanic membrane and its accompanying landmarks; therefore, visualization of the membrane is usually not attempted.

The AAP recommends all newborns be screened for hearing before discharge from their birth setting (AAP, 2013). Hearing screening is done with a reliable standardized method such as the optoacoustic emissions test or automated auditory brainstem response test. While waiting for a hearing examiner, infants can be tested by ringing a small bell held about 6 in. from each ear. A hearing infant will blink, attend to the bell's sound, and possibly startle.

THE NOSE

A newborn's nose usually has milia present and tends to appear large for the face. Always test for choanal atresia (blockage at the rear of the nose) when examining a newborn by closing the infant's mouth while compressing one naris at a time with your fingers. Note any distress with breathing while one side of the nose is blocked this way.

THE MOUTH

A newborn's mouth should open evenly when he or she cries. If one side of the mouth curves more than the other, facial nerve injury may have occurred. The tongue may appear short or "tongue tied" because the frenulum membrane is attached close to the tip. At one time, it was almost routine to snip a newborn's frenulum membrane to lengthen it. Now, this procedure is regarded as unnecessary unless the infant has difficulty sucking or latching because snipping leaves a portal of entry for infection, risks hemorrhage because of the low level of vitamin K in most newborns, and could cause feeding difficulties by making the tongue sore and irritated. As the tongue grows, the frenulum recedes to its adult placement.

Inspect the palate of a newborn to be certain it is intact. Occasionally, one or two small round, glistening, well-circumscribed cysts (Epstein pearls) can be seen on the palate from extra calcium that was deposited in utero. Be sure to inform parents that these pearl-like cysts are insignificant, require no treatment, and will disappear spontaneously within a week. Epstein pearls must be distinguished from **thrush**, a *Candida* infection, which appears on the tongue and sides of the cheeks as white or gray patches and requires treatment with an antifungal drug such as nystatin (Martin, Baumhart, D'Alesio, et al., 2012).

Small, white epithelial pearls (benign inclusion cysts) may be noticed on the gum margins. Like Epstein pearls, no therapy is necessary for these. It is highly unusual for a newborn to have teeth, but sometimes one or two (called **natal teeth**) will have erupted. Any teeth that are present must be evaluated for stability. If loose, they are usually extracted (they remove easily) to prevent possible aspiration during feeding (Martin et al., 2012).

Most newborns have some mucus in the mouth. Newborns born by cesarean birth usually have more mucus than those born by vaginal birth. If a newborn is placed on the side, the mucus drains from the mouth and results in no distress. If the mouth is filled with so much mucus that the neonate seems to be blowing bubbles, suspect a tracheoesophageal fistula. It is important that this be confirmed or ruled out before the newborn is fed; otherwise, formula could be aspirated into the lungs from the inadequately formed esophagus (see Chapter 45 for a discussion of such fistulas).

THE NECK

The neck of a newborn appears short with creased skin folds. The head should rotate or turn freely on it. If the neck is rigid, congenital torticollis, caused by injury to the sternocleidomastoid muscle during birth, might be present (see Chapter 27). In newborns whose membranes were ruptured more than 24 hours before birth, nuchal rigidity may be an early sign of meningitis.

The neck of a newborn is not strong enough to support the total weight of the head but in a sitting position, a newborn should make a momentary effort at head control. When lying prone, newborns can raise the head slightly, usually enough to lift the nose out of mucus or spit-up milk. If they are pulled into a sitting position from a supine position, the head will lag.

The trachea usually appears prominent on the front of the neck. The thymus gland also appears enlarged because of the rapid growth of glandular tissue early in life. Even though the thymus appears to be enlarged and bulging, it is rarely a cause of respiratory difficulty; it plays a critical role in providing immunity so is not removed (Benjamin, Mezu-Ndubuisi, & Maheshwari, 2015).

THE CHEST

The chest in most newborns looks small because the head is so large in proportion to it (an important finding at birth so the largest diameter of the baby is born first). The chest averages 2 cm (0.75 to 1 in.) smaller in circumference than the head and is as wide in the anteroposterior diameter as it is across. Both right and left sides should appear symmetric. At around 2 years of age, the chest measurement typically exceeds that of the head.

The clavicles should appear straight and feel smooth. A *crepitus* (crackling) or an actual separation of one or both clavicles suggests a fracture occurred during birth (can happen with large infants).

A supernumerary nipple (usually found below and in line with the normal nipples) may be present. In both female and male infants, the breasts may be engorged because of the influence of maternal hormones during pregnancy. Occasionally, the breasts may secrete a thin, watery fluid popularly termed *witch's milk*. As soon as the hormones are cleared from the infant's system (about 1 week), the engorgement and fluid will subside. Fluid should never be expressed from infants' breasts because the manipulation could introduce bacteria and lead to *mastitis* (infection of the breast).

Respirations are normally rapid (30 to 60 breaths/min) but not distressed. *Retraction* (drawing in of the chest wall with inspiration) should not be present. An infant who is breathing with retractions (Fig. 18.20) is using such a strong

Figure 18.20 Sternal retractions are a sign of respiratory distress requiring immediate intervention, such as mechanical ventilation or increased oxygen.

force to pull air into the respiratory tract that he or she is pulling in the anterior chest muscle as well. This breathing is not sustainable for a long period of time, and immediate help such as oxygen, is needed.

Because a newborn's lung alveoli open slowly over the first 24 to 48 hours and the baby invariably has mucus in the back of the throat, listening to lung sounds often reveals rhonchi—the sound of air passing over mucus. An abnormal sound, such as grunting, suggests *respiratory distress syndrome*, and a high, crowing sound on inspiration suggests stridor or immature tracheal development, both conditions that need immediate consultation (see Chapter 40).

THE ABDOMEN

The contour of a newborn abdomen looks slightly protuberant. A scaphoid or sunken appearance suggests missing abdominal contents or a diaphragmatic hernia (bowel or other abdominal organs positioned in the chest instead of the abdomen). Bowel sounds show the bowel is beginning peristalsis and should be present within 1 hour after birth. On the right side, the edge of the liver is usually palpable 1 to 2 cm below the costal margin. On the left side, the edge of the spleen may be palpable 1 to 2 cm below the left costal margin.

For the first hour after birth, the stump of the umbilical cord appears as a white, gelatinous structure marked with the blue and red streaks of the one umbilical vein and the two arteries. Any child with a single umbilical artery needs close needs and assessment for anomalies that are frequently associated with the lack of an umbilical artery (Gutvirtz, Walfisch, Beharier, et al., 2016).

Always inspect the cord clamp to be certain it is secure. After the first hour of life, the cord will begin to dry, shrink, and turn brown as if it were the dead end of a vine. By the second or third day, it will have turned black. On day 6 to 10, it breaks free, leaving a granulating area a few centimeters wide that will heal during the following week.

There should be no bleeding at the base of the cord and it should not appear wet. A moist or odorous cord suggests infection, requiring immediate antibiotic therapy to prevent the infectious organisms from entering the newborn's bloodstream and causing septicemia. Moistness at the base of the cord also may indicate a patent urachus (a narrow opening that connects the bladder and the umbilicus), which requires surgical repair (Gleason, Bowlin, Bagli, et al., 2015).

Inspect the base of the cord to be certain no abdominal wall defect such as an umbilical hernia is present. If there is an abdominal wall defect smaller than 2 cm in diameter, it will usually close on its own by school age; a larger defect may require surgical correction. Taping or putting buttons or coins on the cord are home remedies that may be seen. There is no evidence for these actions. To the contrary, heavy taping may worsen the condition by preventing the development of abdominal wall muscle and may also may keep the cord moist, increasing the risk for infection.

When a newborn voids, it demonstrates that there is at least one kidney functioning (but not necessarily two). Attempt to verify the presence of kidneys by deep palpation of the right and left abdomen within the first few hours after birth before the intestines fill with air, making palpation more difficult (see Chapter 34). A small kidney suggests decreased function; an enlarged kidney suggests a polycystic kidney or pooling of urine from a urethral obstruction.

To finish an abdominal assessment, elicit an abdominal reflex. Stroking each quadrant of the abdomen with a finger should cause the umbilicus to move or "wink" in that direction. This superficial abdominal reflex, a test of spinal nerves T8 through T10, is usually present at birth, but may not be observable until it is stronger at about the 10th day of life.

QSEN Checkpoint Question 18.5

TEAMWORK & COLLABORATION

Mrs. Ruiz is preparing to take her new daughter home and has asked an unlicensed care provider when Beth's dried umbilical cord will fall off. The nurse should confirm that the care provider has stated what time?

   a. Day 1
   b. Days 2 to 3
   c. Days 6 to 10
   d. Day 30

Look in Appendix A for the best answer and rationale.

THE ANOGENITAL AREA

Examine the anus to ascertain its presence and patency. Test for anal patency and that the anus is not covered by a membrane (imperforate anus) by gently inserting the tip of your gloved and lubricated little finger. Note the time after birth when the infant first passes meconium. If a newborn does not do so in the first 24 hours, there may be an anatomical or physiologic problem that needs to be assessed.

The Male Genitalia

The scrotum in most male newborns is edematous and has rough rugae on the surface. It may be deeply pigmented in dark-skinned newborns. Both testes should be palpable in the scrotum. If one or both testicles are not present (cryptorchidism), referral is needed to further investigate the problem. This condition could be caused by agenesis (absence of the testes), ectopic testes (the testes are present in the abdomen but

Figure 18.21 Press the nondominant hand against the inguinal ring when palpating the testes.

cannot enter the scrotum because the opening to the scrotal sac is closed), or undescended testes (the vas deferens or artery is too short to allow the testes to descend). Make a practice of pressing your nondominant hand against the inguinal ring before palpating for testes, so they do not slip upward and out of the scrotal sac as you palpate (Fig. 18.21). Newborns with agenesis of the testes are usually referred for investigation of kidney anomalies because the testes arise from the same germ tissue as the kidneys (Hutson & Thorup, 2015)

Always elicit a cremasteric reflex by stroking the internal side of the thigh while inspecting testes (as the skin on the thigh is stroked, the testis on that side moves perceptibly upward). The response is indication that spinal nerves T8 through T10 are intact, although it may be absent before 10 days of age when nerve stabilization is complete.

The penis of newborns appears small, approximately 2 cm long. Shorter length requires referral to an endocrinologist to investigate any other anomalies. Inspect the tip of the penis to be certain the urethral opening is at the tip of the glans, not on the dorsal surface (epispadias) or on the ventral surface (hypospadias). In most newborns, the prepuce (foreskin) slides back very little from the meatal opening, so don't try to retract it.

The Female Genitalia

The vulva in female newborns may appear swollen because of the effect of maternal hormones during intrauterine life. Some female newborns also have a mucus vaginal secretion, sometimes blood tinged (**pseudomenstruation**), which is also caused by maternal hormones. The discharge does not indicate an infection or trauma and disappears in 1 or 2 days.

THE BACK

A newborn normally assumes the position maintained in utero for days after birth, with the back rounded and arms and legs flexed across the abdomen and chest. A child who was born in a frank breech position tends to straighten the legs at the knee and bring them up next to the face. The position of a baby with a face presentation sometimes simulates opisthotonos (backward arching of the spine) for the first week because the curve of the back is concave.

The spine of a newborn typically appears flat in the lumbar and sacral areas; these curves appear after a child is able to sit and walk. Inspect the base of a newborn's spine carefully to be certain there is no pinpoint opening, dimpling, or sinus tract in the skin, which suggest a dermal sinus or spina bifida occulta (see Chapter 27) (Lewis, 2014).

THE EXTREMITIES

The arms and legs of a newborn appear short in proportion to the trunk. The hands seem plump and are typically clenched. Newborn fingernails feel soft and smooth and extend over the fingertips. Test the upper extremities for muscle tone by unflexing the arms for approximately 5 seconds then letting them return to their flexed position (which typically occurs immediately if muscle tone is good). Next, hold the arms down by the sides and note their length. The fingertips on both sides should reach as far as the mid-thigh. Unusually short arms may signify achondroplasia (dwarfism) and would require further evaluation.

Observe for curvature of the little finger, and inspect the palm for a simian crease (a single palmar crease). Although curved fingers and simian creases can occur normally, they are commonly seen in children with Down syndrome (Nussbaum, McInnes, & Willard, 2016).

When a newborn moves, the arms and legs should move symmetrically (unless the infant is demonstrating a tonic neck reflex). Asymmetry suggests birth injury, such as injury to a clavicle or to the brachial or cervical plexus or fracture of a long bone. Assess for webbing (syndactyly) between fingers as well as missing or extra fingers (polydactyly). Test to see whether the fingernails fill immediately after blanching from pressure to test for adequate blood circulation.

Newborn legs appear bowed and short. The sole of the foot is flat because of an extra pad of fat in the longitudinal arch. The foot of a term newborn has many crisscrossed lines on the sole, covering approximately two thirds of the foot. If these creases cover less than two thirds of the foot or are absent, it suggests the infant is preterm.

Move the ankle through a range of motion to evaluate that the heel cord is not unusually tight. Check for ankle clonus by supporting the lower leg in one hand and dorsiflexing the foot sharply two or three times by pressure on the sole of the foot with the other hand. After the dorsiflexion, one or two continued movements are normal. Rapid alternating contraction and relaxation (clonus) is not normal and suggests neurologic or calcium insufficiency. The feet may turn in (varus deviation) because of their former intrauterine position. This is benign if the feet can be brought to the midline position by easy manipulation. When the infant begins to bear weight, the feet will align themselves without treatment.

If a foot does not align readily or will not turn to a definite midline position, a talipes deformity (clubfoot) may be present and warrants specialty referral.

To test if the femur is situated comfortably in the hip socket, with a newborn in a supine position, flex both hips and abduct the legs as far as they will go (typically 180 degrees or the knees touch or nearly touch the surface of the bed) (Fig. 18.22). If the hip joint seems to lock short of this distance (160 to 170 degrees), it suggests hip subluxation (Sankar, Horn, Wells, et al., 2016). Confirm subluxation by holding the infant's legs with the fingers on the greater and lesser trochanters and then abduct the hips; if subluxation is present, a "clunk" of the femur head striking the shallow acetabulum can be heard (Ortolani sign). If the femur can be felt to actually slip in and out of the socket, this is a Barlow sign.

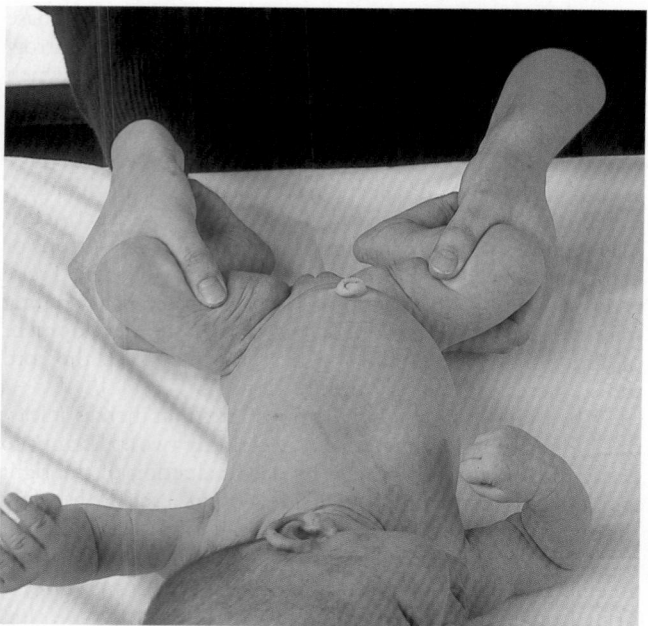

Figure 18.22 Hip abduction in a newborn. Both hips should abduct so completely that they lie almost flat against the mattress (180 degrees).

A subluxated hip may be bilateral or unilateral. Like talipes disorders, it is important that a hip subluxation be identified early because correction is most successful if initiated early.

Lastly, inspect the feet for missing or extra toes or unusual spacing of toes, particularly between the big toe and the others; although this finding can be a normal finding in some families, it is also present in certain chromosomal disorders. When placed on their abdomen, newborns should be capable of bringing their arms and legs underneath them and raising their stomach slightly off the bed. The preterm newborn is not able to do this.

LABORATORY STUDIES

After the first hour of undisturbed rest, depending on health agency policy, newborns may have a heel-stick test for hematocrit, hemoglobin, and hypoglycemia determinations. Hemoglobin is assessed to detect newborn anemia that could have been caused by hypovolemia because of bleeding from placenta previa or abruptio placentae or by a cesarean birth that involved incision into the placenta. Another condition as dangerous as anemia is the presence of excess red blood cells (polycythemia), probably caused by excessive flow of blood into an infant from the umbilical cord. A heel-stick hematocrit reveals both hypovolemia and hypervolemia if they are present. A normal hematocrit at 1 hour of life is about 50% to 55%.

Hypoglycemia, like anemia, produces few symptoms in newborns, so glucose is also tested with the heel capillary blood sample. A serum glucose reading that is less than 40 mg/100 ml of blood (30 mg/100 ml in the first 3 days of life) indicates hypoglycemia. To correct this condition, the infant is prescribed oral glucose or is breastfed immediately because either will elevate the infant's blood sugar to a safe level. It is important to treat hypoglycemia quickly because if brain cells become completely depleted of glucose, brain damage can result. Newborn symptoms of hypoglycemia include jitteriness, lethargy, seizures, and intravenous glucose may be prescribed. A continuous intravenous infusion of glucose may be necessary if the newborn is unable to maintain glucose levels higher than 40 mg/100 ml.

Heel sticks require a minimum of blood and are minimally traumatic.

The Care of a Newborn at Birth

Birthing rooms provide an island for newborn care separate from the supplies needed for the mother's care. Necessary equipment includes a radiant heat table or warmed bassinet; a warm, soft blanket; and equipment for oxygen administration, resuscitation, suction, eye care, identification, and weighing of a newborn.

Newborns should be handled gently at birth. The image of an obstetrician holding a newborn up by the heels and spanking to stimulate breathing exists only in movies because such treatment is probably painful after the months spent in a flexed position in utero. In addition, gentle stimulation, such as rubbing the back, will stimulate breathing.

NEWBORN IDENTIFICATION AND REGISTRATION

Newborn identification is an important nursing responsibility. Nurses must be certain the infant has an identification band in place, so medicine administration or performing procedures can be done safely.

Identification Banding

One traditional form of identification used with newborns is a plastic bracelet with a permanent lock that requires cutting to be removed. A number that corresponds to the mother's hospital number; the mother's name; and the sex, date, and time of the infant's birth are printed on the band. If an identification band is attached to a newborn's arm or leg, two bands should be used because bands can slide off easily. A newer form of identification band has a built-in sensor unit that sounds an alarm—similar to those attached to clothing in department stores to stop shoplifting—if a baby is transported beyond set hospital boundaries (Fig. 18.23).

After identification bands are attached, an infant's footprints may be taken (Fig. 18.24A) and thereafter kept with

Figure 18.23 This newborn is wearing a security band, which sets off an alarm and locks exits if an infant is taken off the unit.

Figure 18.24 **(A)** Footprinting a newborn for identification. **(B)** Newborn footprints.

the baby's electronic record for permanent identification (see Fig. 18.24B). Babies who are born elsewhere and then admitted to the hospital should have bands applied and their footprints taken on admission.

Infant Abduction

Infant identification is important because a newborn may be handed to the wrong mother or be switched or abducted from a healthcare facility. The profile of someone who might abduct a newborn is a woman who has recently lost a pregnancy or had an infant stillborn. She often is someone familiar with hospitals and may pretend to be a volunteer or a healthcare worker and say she needs to take a baby out the mother's room for a procedure. Although rare, all healthcare personnel need to be vigilant, take measures to prevent infant abduction, and alert parents to the danger so they can also be vigilant (Box 18.4) (National Center for Missing & Exploited Children, 2016).

Birth Registration

The primary care provider who supervised a newborn's birth has the responsibility to be certain a birth registration is filed with the Bureau of Vital Statistics for the state in which the infant was born. The infant's name, the mother's name, the father's name (if the mother chooses to reveal this), and the birth date and place are recorded. This official birth information is important for eligibility for school, voting, passports, and Social Security benefits.

BOX 18.4

Nursing Care Planning Based on Family Teaching

MEASURES TO HELP PREVENT ABDUCTION FROM A BIRTH SETTING UNIT

Q. Beth's mother tells you, "I've read babies are being kidnapped from hospitals. How can we make sure that doesn't happen to us?"

A. Although abduction is rare, it can happen. To minimize the risk, use the following guidelines:

- Review the hospital's newborn identification procedure with a nurse so you are familiar with it and can feel comfortable with the safeguards being taken.
- Check that identification bands are in place on your infant as you care for her because these can slide off easily over small hands or feet. If a band or necklace is missing, ask a nurse to replace it immediately.
- Do not allow any person without proper hospital identification to remove your baby from your room. Be certain they describe why they are taking your baby.
- Do not leave your baby unattended in your room. Either return the baby to the nursery or take your baby with you if you are leaving your room, for example, to walk in the hallway.
- Report the presence of any suspicious person you observe in the unit.
- Some hospitals use a microchip system embedded in identification bands, similar to the tag used to thwart shoplifting in department stores, which sounds an alarm if a baby is removed from the unit. If this type of band is used, be certain it is removed before hospital discharge, or it will set off an alarm as you leave.

Birth Record Documentation

The infant's chart is also a vital piece of documentation because it serves as a baseline for the infant's health. It should contain the following:

- Time of birth
- Time the infant breastfed
- Whether respirations were spontaneous or aided
- Apgar score at 1 minute and at 5 minutes of life
- Whether eye prophylaxis was given
- Whether vitamin K was administered
- General condition of the infant
- Number of vessels in the umbilical cord (Fig. 18.25)
- Whether cultures were taken
- Whether the infant voided and whether he or she passed a stool

Figure 18.25 A chart abbreviation for a three-vessel cord.

BOX 18.5

Nursing Care Planning to Respect Cultural Diversity

What new parents believe is usual newborn care is not consistent across cultures and actually varies a great deal. Although it is enjoyable to point out the positive aspects of their new child to parents in order to aid parent–child bonding, in some areas of the world, such as Cambodia and Laos, newborns are not given compliments this way because it is believed compliments could leave them vulnerable to invading spirits. In other cultures, it is vitally important for a newborn to have an amulet (good-luck charm) tied around the neck or wrist to ward off danger. Respect these as important items and leave them in place when caring for the infant.

In the traditional Haitian culture and some Native American cultures, infants are not named immediately but only after a set period of time (to be certain the name will truly reflect the child's personality). Oiling the infant's body and placing a belly band over the umbilical cord (thought to reduce the incidence of umbilical hernias) also are common care practices. Being aware of cultural variations in newborn care such as these helps you plan care specific and meaningful to individual parents and can aid parent–child bonding as well as parent–nurse relationships.

Nursing Diagnoses and Related Interventions

Nursing Diagnosis: Risk for ineffective thermoregulation related to newborn's transition to extrauterine environment

Outcome Evaluation: Newborn establishes axillary temperature of 98.6°F (37°C) by 1 hour after birth.

Following birth, a newborn is placed on the mother's abdomen for a period of skin-to-skin contact to help retain heat. Allow the mother to begin breastfeeding if she wishes and to allow time for parents to enjoy and get acquainted with their newborn. It's important not to interrupt this time because newborns are alert (first period of activity) and respond well to the parents' first tentative touches or interactions with them during this time (Box 18.5). After about 30 minutes, begin routine care such as footprinting and administering eye drops if the parents want eye drops administered. Be certain to adhere to standard infection precautions, such as wearing gloves, when caring for newborns. Grasp a newborn securely when lifting off the mother's abdomen. Newborn skin is slippery, and infants can slip through your hands easily.

All of the measures mentioned previously such as skin-to-skin contact, gently rubbing a newborn dry, swaddling the infant with a blanket, and placing a cap on the infant's head (Fig. 18.26) help to prevent heat loss and also mimic the tight confines of the uterus, which can offer a sense of security and comfort (Pillai Riddell, Racine, Gennis, et al., 2015).

Figure 18.26   A newborn wrapped and capped to conserve body heat.

Although the temperature of newborns who are dried, wrapped, and then held by their parents immediately after birth apparently falls slightly lower than that of infants placed in heated cribs, their core temperature does not fall below safe limits.

At the end of the first hour of life, a newborn can be bathed quickly to remove excess vernix caseosa and blood, then dressed in a shirt and diaper, swaddled in a blanket, and placed in a bassinet or returned to the parents.

During the first day of life, a newborn's temperature is usually taken and recorded every 4 to 8 hours. After that, it is done daily in the healthcare facility unless indicated. If an infant has difficulty maintaining temperature, place him or her in a warmed incubator or on a radiant heat warmer and notify the primary care provider because the infant may be more immature than was estimated or is ill in some way.

Nursing Diagnosis: Risk for ineffective airway clearance related to presence of mucus in mouth and nose at birth

Outcome Evaluation: Neonate maintains a respiratory rate of 30 to 60 breaths/min without evidence of retraction or grunting by 5 minutes after birth.

A number of measures help ensure a newborn is breathing effectively.

Record the First Cry. A crying infant is a breathing infant because the sound of crying is made by a current of air passing over the larynx. The more lusty the cry, the greater the assurance the newborn is breathing deeply and forcefully. Vigorous crying may also help blow off the extra carbon dioxide that makes all newborns slightly acidotic. Although gentleness is necessary to make an infant's transition from intrauterine life to extrauterine life as nontraumatic as possible, there is no need to completely halt the initial crying of a newborn.

A newborn who does not breathe spontaneously at birth or who takes a few quick, gasping breaths but then is unable to maintain respirations needs resuscitation as an emergency measure. An infant with grunting respirations needs careful observation for respiratory distress syndrome (see Chapter 26).

Promote Adequate Breathing Pattern and Prevent Aspiration. Although not done routinely, if a newborn appears to have a great deal of mucus in the mouth following birth, the primary care provider can suction mucus from the infant's mouth with a bulb syringe. If needed, this is done before the infant is laid on the mother's abdomen in order to prevent aspiration of the secretions. If the infant continues to have an accumulation of mucus in the mouth or nose after these first steps, you may need to suction further after the baby is placed under a warmer. Use a bulb syringe or a soft, small (#10 or 12) catheter. Always suction gently to prevent mucous membrane irritation that could leave a portal of entry for infection. Brisk suctioning also has been associated with bradycardia in newborns because of vagal nerve stimulation. With a bulb syringe, decompress the bulb before inserting it into the infant's mouth or nose; otherwise, the force of decompression of the bulb could push secretions back into the pharynx or bronchi. Although the use of the procedure is not standardized, when an infant is born with meconium-stained amniotic fluid, intubation may be performed so deep tracheal suction can be accomplished before the first breath to help prevent meconium aspiration into the lungs. The use of surfactant and inhaled nitric oxide may also be helpful to assist breathing if meconium aspiration has occurred (discussed in Chapter 26) (Carlo & Ambalavanan, 2016).

Nursing Diagnosis: Risk for infection related to newly clamped umbilical cord and exposure of eyes to vaginal secretions

Outcome Evaluation: Area around cord is dry and free of erythema. Eyes are free of inflammation and drainage. Axillary temperature is maintained between 97.6°F and 98.6°F (36.5°C and 37°C).

Inspect and Care for the Umbilical Cord. The umbilical cord pulsates for a moment after an infant is born as a last flow of blood passes from the placenta into the infant. Two clamps are then applied to the cord about 8 in. from the infant's abdomen, and the cord is cut between the clamps. The woman's partner may choose to cut the cord. The infant cord is then reclamped by a permanent cord clamp, such as a Hazeltine or a Kane clamp (see Chapter 15, Fig. 15.28).

Every time you handle a newborn, inspect the cord to be certain it is clamped securely because if it loosens before thrombosis obliterates the umbilical vessels, hemorrhage could result. As previously mentioned, the number of cord vessels should be counted immediately after the cord is cut because they are most visible before drying begins. Until the cord falls off, at about 7 to 10 days of life, be certain diapers are folded below the level of the umbilical cord to help keep the cord dry. Advise parents to keep the cord dry until it falls off. Discourage the use of creams, lotions, and oils near the cord because these tend to slow drying and may invite infection. Remind them to use sponge baths until the cord falls off. Some healthcare agencies recommend that parents apply rubbing alcohol to the cord site once or twice a day to hasten drying. Most agencies recommend using no products because any manipulation of the cord could invite infection (Gooding & McClead, 2015). After the cord falls off, a small, pink, granulating area about a quarter of an inch in diameter may remain. This should also be left clean and dry until it has healed (about 24 to 48 more hours). If the ulcerous area is still present after a week, it may require cautery with silver nitrate (a quick office procedure) to speed healing.

Administer Eye Care. Although the practice may eventually become obsolete, as it is in some countries, most birth settings in the United States and Canada still administer prophylactic eye treatment (erythromycin ointment) to help prevent gonorrheal and chlamydia conjunctivitis. Such infections are usually acquired from the mother as the infant passes through the birth canal; therefore, if a mother is certain she does not have either of these diseases, she can request eye drops not be given. Eye prophylaxis is typically applied immediately after birth and should be given within the first 24 hours for maximal effectiveness (U.S. Preventive Services Task Force, 2011). If it is given, allow parents to interact with their infant before the procedure so their newborn can focus on them without blurry vision caused by the ointment.

If applying eye ointment, always use a single-use tube or package of ointment to avoid transmitting an infection from one newborn to another. First dry the newborn's face with a soft gauze square. Open the newborn's eyes by shading them from the light and then press on both the lower and upper lids one eye at a time with a finger and your thumb. Squeeze a line of ointment along the lower eyelid from the inner canthus outward. Let the eye close to allow the ointment to spread across the conjunctiva.

If it is the healthcare policy to instill eye ointment, babies born at home or other settings such as a car or taxi should have the prophylactic treatment administered on admission to the hospital unless the parents are certain they are both free of gonorrheal and chlamydial infections and they refuse the treatment.

General Infection Precautions. Each newborn's private bassinet should have compartments that hold a supply of diapers, shirts, gowns, and individual equipment for bathing and temperature taking. Avoid sharing of these items to prevent the spread of infection.

Healthcare workers caring for newborns should thoroughly wash their hands and arms to the elbows with an antiseptic soap before handling infants. Although not proven to reduce infections, agency personnel are usually required to wear cover gowns or nursery uniforms when directly caring for infants (Webster & Pritchard, 2011).

Staff members with infections (particularly sore throats, upper respiratory tract infections, or herpes lesions) should be excluded from caring for mothers or infants until the condition has completely cleared. If a mother might have a contagious illness, her newborn should be excluded from her room until there is no longer a possibility of contagion. Daily photographs and videos can help the mother follow the baby's progress. The mother should manually express breast milk during this time to help maintain her milk supply. The mother can resume breastfeeding as soon as it is safe for her infant.

Any baby born outside a hospital or under circumstances conducive to infection, such as rupture of membranes more than 24 hours before birth, should be kept in the mother's room until negative cultures show the newborn is free of infection. Likewise, any newborn in whom symptoms of infection develop should be housed in the mother's room or an isolation nursery to prevent the spread of infection to other babies in a common nursery. Encourage parents to visit the baby to help decrease any worries due to the isolation. When visiting isolation nurseries, parents are required to use the same infection control techniques staff members use such as masks or gowns.

Nursing Care of a Newborn and Family in the Postpartal Period

Newborns are cared for in either a birthing room or a transitional nursery for optimal safety in the first few hours of life. Box 18.6 shows an interprofessional care map illustrating both nursing and team planning for newborn care during a healthcare agency stay.

THE INITIAL FEEDING

The Baby-Friendly Hospital Initiative (BFHI) is a global program sponsored by the WHO and the United Nations Children's Fund (UNICEF) to encourage and recognize hospitals and birthing centers that offer an optimal level of care for infants that promotes breastfeeding.

To qualify as a Baby-Friendly–designated facility, a setting must:

1. Maintain a written breastfeeding policy that is routinely communicated to all healthcare staff.
2. Educate all healthcare staff in skills necessary to implement the written policy.
3. Inform all pregnant women about the benefits and management of breastfeeding.
4. Help mothers initiate breastfeeding within 1 hour of birth.
5. Show mothers how to breastfeed and how to maintain their milk supply, even if they are separated from their infants.
6. Offer breastfed newborns no food or drink other than breast milk unless medically indicated.
7. Practice "rooming in" or allow mothers and infants to remain together 24 hours a day.
8. Encourage unrestricted or "on-demand" breastfeeding.
9. Give breastfeeding infants no pacifiers or artificial nipples.
10. Foster the establishment of breastfeeding support groups and refer mothers to them on discharge from the birth setting (UNICEF, 2016).

After a first feeding in the birthing room, both formula-fed and breastfed infants do best with an "on-demand" schedule (i.e., are fed when they are hungry). Many need to be fed as often as every 1.5 to 2 hours in the first few days and weeks of life. Chapter 19 discusses techniques of both breastfeeding and formula feeding. Nurses can play an important role in helping new mothers establish breastfeeding during the infant's first weeks of life.

BATHING

The Association of Women's Health, Obstetric and Neonatal Nurses recommends that most newborns receive a complete

BOX 18.6

Nursing Care Planning

AN INTERPROFESSIONAL CARE MAP FOR A TERM NEWBORN

Carlotta Ruiz has just given birth to her second child, a 39 weeks and 2 days, 6-lb, 5-oz baby girl. While Jose, Carlotta's husband, is in the room, Carlotta tells you she is a "veteran" at baby care. When Carlotta is alone, however, you notice she seems apprehensive about caring for her new daughter.

Family Assessment: Family is composed of two parents, a 3-year-old sibling, and newborn. They live in a three-bedroom flat over a dry cleaning store. Father clerks in a grocery store; mother works as a school bus driver. Finances rated as "hanging in there."

Patient Assessment: Birth from left occipitoanterior (LOA) position. Apgar score: 6 at 1 minute; 8 at 5 minutes after administration of blow-by oxygen. Respirations are 74 breaths/min. She has a 2 × 3 cm red pigmented area on outer right thigh. Mother attempted breastfeeding in birthing room, but newborn had difficulty sucking because of rapid respirations. Remainder of physical examination within acceptable parameters.

Nursing Diagnosis: Risk for ineffective parenting related to infant's smaller than expected size and birthmark

Outcome Criteria: Respiratory rate is decreased to 30 to 50 breaths/min, infant sucks well at breast every 2 to 3 hours, and mother voices she is pleased with infant's appearance and progress.

Team Member Responsible	Assessment	Intervention	Rationale	Expected Outcome
Activities of Daily Living, Including Safety				
Nurse	Assess respiratory rate every 15 minutes for 1 hour.	Report increase in rate, retractions, or development of nasal flaring or grunting.	Increases in respiratory rate, retractions, nasal flaring, and grunting are signs of respiratory distress.	Infant gradually decreases respiratory rate to 30–50 breaths/min by 24 hours; grunting, retractions, or nasal flaring is not present.
Teamwork and Collaboration				
Nurse/primary care provider	Assess whether parents would like a dermatology consultation for child's birthmark.	Refer parents to dermatology consultant if desired.	A second opinion can help assure parents birthmark is a benign nevus flammeus birthmark.	Parents visit with consultant if desired; state they understand the prognosis for port-wine lesions.
Procedures/Medications for Quality Improvement				
Nurse	Assess if mother is rested enough from birth to give infant first bath.	Assist mother as needed with bath or other newborn care.	Active interaction with a newborn makes the birth more "real" and aids parent–child bonding.	Mother states she would appreciate review of newborn care but feels capable of giving care.
Nutrition				
Nurse	Assess mother's knowledge of breastfeeding.	Assist mother with breastfeeding as needed; remind her that rapid respirations make sucking difficult.	Breast milk is the preferred milk for human newborns; a mother may need assistance if an infant sucks poorly.	Infant and mother establish mutually enjoyable breastfeeding by hospital discharge.
Patient-Centered Care				
Nurse/primary care provider	Review with parents their expectations of new child coming into the hospital (e.g., bigger? prettier? more relaxed?).	Inform parents that rapid respirations are not unusual because of unabsorbed lung fluid. Help them mold expectations with reality.	Providing information and having a frank discussion helps to allay parents' anxieties and fears.	Parents state they were initially surprised by baby's appearance, but are adjusting to think of her as a healthy newborn.

Continued on following page

BOX 18.6
Nursing Care Planning (continued)

Team Member Responsible	Assessment	Intervention	Rationale	Expected Outcome
Psychosocial/Spiritual/Emotional Needs				
Nurse	Assess infant for general physical condition and any additional concerns parents have about infant.	Point out positive attributes of newborn, such as pretty eyes and alert expression.	Pointing out positive areas helps parents focus attention on the unique qualities of their child.	Parents state they appreciate learning more about their newborn from healthcare professionals.
Informatics for Seamless Healthcare Planning				
Nurse	Assess whether parents have made plans for hospital discharge.	Remind parents about importance of car seat, avoiding falls, and aspiration.	Safety awareness plays a big role in preventing unintentional, early age injuries.	Parents state they feel ready to begin parenting their new infant.

sponge bath in 2 to 4 hours after birth when their temperature and vital signs are stable. There is no need to use antibiotic cleansers and no need to remove all vernix (Association of Women's Health, Obstetric and Neonatal Nurses, 2013). Babies of mothers with HIV infection should have a thorough bath immediately to decrease the possibility of HIV transmission. Thereafter, all babies are sponge bathed once a day, although the procedure may be limited to washing only the baby's face, diaper area, and skin folds. Wear gloves when handling newborns until the first bath to avoid exposing your hands to body secretions such as the vernix caseosa.

Plan to help a mother give a first bath before (not after) a feeding to prevent spitting up or vomiting and possible aspiration. Check to be certain the mother's room is warm (about 75°F [24°C]) to prevent chilling. Supply bath water at 98° to 100°F (37° to 38°C), a temperature that feels pleasantly warm to the elbow or wrist, plus a washcloth, towel, comb, and clean diaper and shirt.

As a rule, bathing should proceed from the cleanest parts of the body to the most soiled areas—that is, from the eyes and face to the trunk and extremities and, last, to the diaper area. Wipe a newborn's eyes with clear water from the inner canthus outward, using a clean portion of the washcloth for each eye to prevent spread of infection to the other eye. Remind the mother to wash around the cord with care so she doesn't soak the cord and to give particular care to the creases of skin where milk tends to collect if the child spits up after feedings. If the mother wants to use a mild neutral soap for sponging, be sure she rinses well so no soap is left on the skin (soap is drying and newborns are susceptible to desquamation) and also to dry well. It's good for parents to wash the infant's hair daily during the bath. The easiest way to do this is to first soap the hair with the baby lying in the bassinet. Then, hold the infant in one arm over a basin of water as you would a football (Fig. 18.27). Pour water from the basin over the hair to rinse. Dry the hair well to prevent chilling. Inform the parents that lathering and gently massaging all parts of the head including the soft spots will help prevent buildup of scales.

In male infants, the foreskin of the uncircumcised penis should not be forced back while washing the penis, or

Figure 18.27 A football hold. Such a position supports the infant's head and back and leaves the nurse's or mother's other hand free for assembling or using equipment.

constriction of the penis may result. Wash the vulva of a female infant, wiping from front to back to prevent contamination of the vagina or urethra by rectal bacteria.

Most healthcare agencies do not apply powder or lotion to newborns because some infants are allergic to these products and breathing in powder can cause respiratory distress (adult talcum powders contain zinc stearate, which is irritating to the respiratory tract). If a newborn's skin seems extremely dry and portals for infection are becoming apparent because of cracking in the skin, a lubricant such as Nivea oil, added to the bath water or applied directly to the baby's skin, should relieve the condition.

SLEEPING POSITION

Sudden infant death syndrome (SIDS) is the sudden, unexplained death of an infant younger than 1 year of age. Although the specific cause of SIDS cannot be explained, these interventions have been shown to decrease the incidence of the syndrome: place infant on the back to sleep; use a firm sleep surface; breastfeeding; room sharing without bed sharing; routine immunizations;

consideration of using a pacifier; avoidance of soft bedding, overheating; and exposure to tobacco smoke, alcohol, and illicit drugs (National Institutes of Health [NIH], 2015).

DIAPER AREA CARE

Preventing diaper dermatitis, or diaper rash, is a practice parents need to start from the very beginning with their newborns (Visscher, Adam, Brink, et al., 2014). Advise parents to change diapers frequently and, with each diaper change, wash the area with clear water and dry well. For yourself, wear gloves for diaper care as part of standard precautions.

METABOLIC SCREENING TESTS

Newborns born in a hospital or birthing center are routinely screened for more than 30 metabolic or inherited disorders by a screening technique that requires a small blood sample obtained by a heel stick and then dropped onto special filter paper (Tluczek & De Luca, 2013). Ideally, a baby should have received formula or breast milk for 24 hours before the blood is obtained for best results.

If, for some reason, blood testing is not done before discharge, alert parents that they need to schedule screening tests at an ambulatory visit in 2 to 3 days' time. Always assess at a newborn's first health supervision visit that screening was done.

HEPATITIS B VACCINATION

All newborns born in a hospital or a birthing center receive a first vaccination against hepatitis B within 12 hours after birth; a second dose will then be administered at 1 month and a third one at 6 months. Infants whose mothers are positive for the hepatitis B surface antigen (HBsAg) also receive hepatitis B immune globulin (HBIG) at birth (AAP, 2015a).

VITAMIN K ADMINISTRATION

Newborns are at risk for bleeding disorders during the first week of life because their gastrointestinal tract is sterile at birth and therefore unable to produce vitamin K, a vitamin necessary for blood coagulation. A single dose of 0.5 to 1.0 mg of vitamin K administered intramuscularly within the first hour of life helps prevent such problems (Phillippi, Holley, Morad, et al., 2016).

CIRCUMCISION

Circumcision is the surgical removal of the foreskin of the penis. Except for a baby who has constriction (phimosis) of the foreskin that obstructs the urinary meatal opening (rare), there are few medical indications to circumcise a male newborn. Some parents elect not to have their male infant circumcised because the operation is painful and increases the risk of cold exposure and infection. Scientific evidence shows that circumcision reduces the risk of HIV, human papillomavirus (HPV), and cancer in the male as well as cervical cancer in a female sexual partner, suggesting that the preventive health benefits of male infant circumcision may outweigh the risks. At this point, the AAP has declined to recommend routine circumcision for boys. Therefore, parents are free to evaluate risks and benefits and then make this health decision for their child (AAP, 2012). Circumcision is performed as a religious rite among some groups such as Jewish and Muslim communities. Contraindications for circumcision include a

history of a bleeding tendency in the family or hypospadias or epispadias because the prepuce skin may be needed when a plastic surgeon repairs these defects.

The procedure is best performed during the first or second day of life, after the baby has synthesized enough vitamin K to reduce the chance of faulty blood coagulation rather than immediately after birth when the level of vitamin K is at a low point.

For the procedure, an infant is placed in a supine position and restrained either manually or with a commercial swaddling board. Application of EMLA cream (a *e*utectic *mi*xture of *l*ocal *a*nesthetics) or a similar compound is a popular choice for local anesthesia. Regional block anesthesia may also be used if an anesthetist is involved.

For the actual procedure, a specially designed plastic bell (Plastibell) is fitted over the end of the penis. A suture is then tied around the rim of the bell and a circle of the prepuce is cut away, allowing the remaining foreskin to be

Figure 18.28 The technique for performing circumcision using a Plastibell. **(A)** An incision is made at the top of the foreskin. **(B)** The Plastibell is placed over the head of the penis, and the foreskin is pulled over the Plastibell. **(C)** A suture is tied around the foreskin over the tying groove in the Plastibell. Excess skin beyond the suture is trimmed away. The Plastibell falls off in 3 to 7 days. (Courtesy of Hollister Inc., Libertyville, IL.)

easily retracted and the glans to be fully exposed (Fig. 18.28). The rim of the bell will remain in place for about 1 week and then fall off by itself. While in place, the bell helps protect against infection and bleeding because it prevents the healing penis from sticking to a diaper. Petrolatum ointment may be applied to further decrease the possibility of penile secretions adhering to the diaper and causing pain at a diaper change.

Complications that can occur from circumcision include hemorrhage, infection, and urethral fistula formation. To keep the risk of these complications to a minimum, check the infant for bleeding every 15 minutes for the first hour and observe closely for about 2 more hours. Document that the infant is voiding after the procedure to be certain the urethra is not occluded.

The circumcision site appears red but should not have a strong odor or discharge. A film of light yellow mucus often covers the glans (similar to a scab) by the second day after surgery and should not be washed away because it serves a protective function.

Teach parents to keep the area clean from feces and covered with petrolatum (if used) for about 3 days or until healing is complete. If they notice any redness or tenderness, or if the baby cries as if in constant pain, they should report it to their primary care provider because this suggests an infection.

The Assessment of a Family's Readiness to Care for a Newborn at Home

It is important to assess how prepared each family is to care for their newborn at home to be certain the newborn will remain safe and develop a sense of security. Parents may need to plan changes in their routine, such as shifting their usual dinner time. Their sleep schedules are certain to be disrupted because infants wake during the night for one or more feedings for about the first 4 months of life.

The physical environment of the home to which a newborn will be discharged is important to explore with parents. Pertinent questions and areas to consider include:

- How many other people live in the home? (Infections spread more rapidly in crowded homes.)
- Are there any pets in the home? Will a large dog, for example, be a safe pet around the baby?
- Is there a bed for the baby? (A separate baby bed helps prevent SIDS.)
- Who will be the primary caregiver? (This is the person who needs to be given discharge instructions.)
- Does the mother have anyone to turn to if she has questions about the baby? (This is especially important at night when a primary health provider's office will be closed.)
- Is there a refrigerator in the home? (Formula or breast milk will need to be stored.)
- Is there adequate heat? (An infant needs a temperature of 70° to 75°F during the day and 60° to 65°F at night.)
- Are the windows draft free and screened to keep out insects such as mosquitoes?
- If housing is in poor condition, is there a danger that rodents might attack the baby?
- Is there a danger of lead poisoning? (An older home may have lead-based paint on the walls, which chips and can be eaten by infants.)

- Does the family have a source of income? (If not, what sort of referral is needed to care for the child?)
- Does the mother have a concrete plan for continuing health care for the infant?

These are not prying questions but a means of determining whether the home will be adequate and safe for a newborn. A home assessment will also help the nurse determine when additional resources are needed by the family. In some cases, the home environment may be unsafe and a referral to social services may be necessary before the newborn is discharged.

 Nursing Diagnoses and Related Interventions

Nursing Diagnosis: Health-seeking behaviors related to the needs of a newborn after discharge from the healthcare facility

Outcome Evaluation: Parents state ways in which they have already altered their home and lifestyle to accommodate their newborn and indicate they are prepared for other changes; mother voices relative confidence in her ability to care for a newborn and states names of individuals within her family or community who can serve as resources when needed.

Remind a woman and her partner before discharge to consider how they will care for their child at home. Many couples mull over these concerns during pregnancy, whereas others wait until the child is born to address these important issues.

Mothers who are young, without family support, or those who did not receive regular prenatal care may be particularly unprepared for the hours and effort involved in newborn care. To assist them, try to anticipate problems most relevant to them. If there are other children or pets at home, for example, discuss that sibling or pet jealousy may naturally occur. Check the child's identification band against the mother's band a final time before discharge.

Daily Home Care. Newborns thrive on a gentle rhythm of care and a sense of being able to anticipate what is to come next. At the same time, however, there is no set time at which an infant must be bathed or put to sleep. If the house is cold, a newborn does not need a bath every day. If a parent works evenings, it may be important to have the baby awake later in the evening so that parent has time to spend with the child.

Your aim in helping parents plan their schedule of care is to arrive at one that:

- Offers some consistency (a mother cannot expect an infant to stay awake until midnight five nights a week, then go to sleep at 7 PM on the sixth night)
- Appears to both satisfy the infant and offer the mother and her partner a sense of well-being and contentment with the child

Sleep Patterns. A newborn sleeps an average of 16 hours out of every 24 during the first week home, sleeping about 4 hours at a time. It is exhausting for a parent who is already tired from labor and birth to have to awaken during the night to feed a newborn.

Advise couples that their newborn needs fluid and nutrition, so it is not recommended to eliminate night feedings in the early weeks of life. Teach them not to put formula-fed infants to sleep with a bottle of formula, glucose water, or fruit juice because, after their teeth erupt, having a carbohydrate-rich beverage near their teeth all night can lead to early childhood caries (cavities), a syndrome popularly known as "baby-bottle caries" (Moyer, 2014). Knowing their baby is not sick when she or he wakes up at night, that you are concerned and willing to listen to questions, and that every other parent of a newborn is also up at night does not solve the problem of sleep-deprived parents and caretakers, but it is a help.

Crying. **Newborns** typically cry an average of 2 hours of every 24 during the first 7 weeks of life. The frequency seems to peak at age 6 or 7 weeks and then tapers off.

Almost all infants have a period during the day when they are wide awake and invariably fussy. Help new parents to recognize this as common for most newborns so they don't worry it means their child is ill. Parents might use this fussy time for bathing or playing with the infant. Unfortunately, the most typical time for wakefulness is between 6 and 11 PM, when parents may be tired and least able to tolerate crying. Helping them recognize when they need a break from care during this time can be very helpful. Other family members or close friends who can assist with the baby can be crucial. Taking a break from care can be the difference between a parent shaking a baby (can lead to shaken baby syndrome, which can be lethal) and being rested and able to effectively meet the infant's and family's needs (Allen, 2014).

Whether to use pacifiers to reduce crying is a question parents must decide for themselves, depending on how they feel about them and their infant's needs. It is rare for an infant to have such a need for sucking that the baby must have a pacifier in the mouth constantly. An infant who completes a feeding and still seems restless and discontented, who actively searches for something to put into the mouth, and who sucks on hands and clothes may need the increased sucking activity a pacifier provides. One drawback of pacifiers is the problem of cleanliness: They tend to fall and are then put back into the infant's mouth. Clipping the pacifier onto the infant's shirt helps prevent this problem. If parents use pacifiers, be certain they are of one-piece construction, so loose parts cannot be aspirated. Mothers who are breastfeeding should use pacifiers sparingly until breastfeeding is well established because sucking on a pacifier takes less effort than sucking at a breast (Nyquist, Haggkvist, Hansen, et al., 2013).

QSEN Checkpoint Question 18.6

EVIDENCE-BASED PRACTICE

Shaken baby syndrome, or abusive head trauma caused by a parent or caregiver shaking an infant in anger or frustration, creates a potentially lethal situation because forceful shaking can lead to subdural bleeding. To investigate whether a nurse-initiated program could reduce the incidence of abusive head trauma by shaking, nurse researchers offered an educational program including a leaflet explaining abusive head trauma, helpful ways to cope safely with an infant's crying, and an 8-minute video on the subject given to all new mothers at their hospital. Results of the study showed a decrease from 2.8 injuries per year (14 cases in 5 years prior to the intervention) to 0.7 injuries per year (2 cases in 3 years) or a 75% reduction in injuries following the intervention (Altman, Canter, Patrick, et al., 2011).

The nurse notices Mrs. Ruiz grows irritated with Beth when Beth doesn't suck readily when she begins to breastfeed. Based on the previous study, what is the best action for the nurse to take?
a. Evaluate whether Beth can hear because this may be the underlying problem.
b. List the dangers of shaken baby syndrome for Mrs. Ruiz.
c. Discuss the fact that breastfeeding is a new skill, so infants take time to learn this.
d. Suggest that Mrs. Ruiz ask the physician for a sedative so she can better tolerate newborn crying.

Look in Appendix A for the best answer and rationale.

Car Safety. Automobile accidents are a safety problem all during childhood, beginning with the newborn period. For protection while in automobiles, newborns should always be transported in rear facing car seats placed in the back seat (AAP, 2016) (Fig. 18.29). Without this protection, if a car should stop suddenly, an infant could be seriously injured or die. At a speed of only 30 mph, an infant may hit the dashboard with a force equal to a fall from a three-story building. If an adult holding the infant is not wearing a seat belt, the adult can be thrown against the infant, causing even more damage.

When purchasing a car seat, advise parents to ascertain that the seat meets current federal guidelines. Guidance for parents regarding car seats can be found at an AAP-sponsored website at https://www.healthychildren.org/English/safety-prevention/on-the-go/pages/Car-Safety-Seats-Information-for-Families.aspx. Some hospitals and

Figure 18.29 To be safe, newborns need to ride in an appropriately sized backward facing car set while in an automobile. Be sure every family leaving the healthcare facility is properly equipped.

Red Cross chapters loan infant car seats for temporary use, such as when visiting out of state with grandparents or when first coming home from the hospital. New cars are mandated to be equipped with lower anchors and tethers for safe use of car seats. A mirror can be positioned in the back seat so a parent can observe the infant from the front seat while driving.

The ideal model has a five-point harness with broad straps, which helps spread the force of a collision over the chest and hips, and a shield, which cushions the head. Advise parents not to use a sack sleeper or papoose bunting nor should they wrap the baby in a bulky blanket which could prevent a secure fit of the infant in the seat. To provide extra warmth, a blanket can be draped over the child and straps as needed. To support the baby's head, parents can use a rolled-up receiving blanket or towel on each side of the head or purchase commercial head supports.

Caution parents that plastic car seats grow extremely hot in the summer, so they should test the temperature of the surface before placing their infant into the seat. Stress also that it is as dangerous to not use a car seat as it is to use one improperly, such as not fastening the harness securely or not attaching the seat to the car correctly.

What If . . . 18.3

The nurse notices the Ruiz family does not have a car seat to transport Beth home. Would the discharge nurse insist they will have to stay in the hospital until they purchase a car seat?

Continued Health Maintenance for a Newborn.
Parents do not need to continue to weigh a newborn or take an infant's temperature at home because these practices can cause worry, as weight fluctuates day by day, and infant activity and clothing can influence temperature. Instead, teach parents to judge their infant's state of health by the child's overall appearance, eagerness to eat, general activity, and disposition as well as weight gain assessed at healthcare visits.

Make certain parents make and keep their healthcare appointment for a first newborn assessment according to their primary care provider's schedule (2 to 6 weeks). Just as conscientious healthcare throughout pregnancy promotes the birth of a healthy child, obtaining routine health care promotes optimum health for the newborn from birth through adolescence. Parents must now begin a healthcare program to keep the child well.

What If . . . 18.4

The nurse is particularly interested in exploring one of the 2020 National Health Goals with respect to newborn care (see Box 18.1). What would be a possible research topic to explore pertinent to this goal that would be applicable to both Beth and her family and that would also advance evidence-based practice?

KEY POINTS FOR REVIEW

- A newborn history and physical examination yields important information on the infant's appearance, gestational age, and any factors that suggest additional care is needed.
- Using a standardized method of assessment, such as an Apgar score, is important to assess and document that an infant is adjusting well to extrauterine life.
- Converting from fetal to newborn respiratory function is a major step in extrauterine adaptation. Newborns need particularly close observation during the first few hours of life to determine if this adaptation occurs.
- Maintaining body heat is a second major challenge for newborns. When a procedure requires undressing an infant for an extended period of time, the procedure should be done under a radiant heat source to guard against chilling and hypothermia.
- Newborns may suffer hypoglycemia in the first few hours of life because they use so much energy to establish respirations and maintain heat. Signs of jitteriness and a blood glucose level of less than 40 mg/100 ml by heel stick help to identify hypoglycemia.
- A great deal of nurses' responsibility for newborns is being certain a mother and her partner spend some time with their newborn in the birth setting and give some of the care, so they feel confident in giving care at home. Be certain they are well informed about controversial topics such as circumcision and prophylactic antibiotic eye drops because this helps in planning nursing care that not only meets QSEN competencies and also meets a family's comprehensive needs.
- Assess that identification bands are securely attached while a newborn is hospitalized; match mother's to baby's one last time before discharge. To help prevent the possibility of infant abduction, be certain of the identification of anyone to whom you give a newborn.
- Be certain that caregivers have a car seat to use at discharge for their infant, that they know how to use it properly, and that they know to schedule a well-child visit at 2 to 6 weeks of age.

CRITICAL THINKING CARE STUDY

U2 is a 7-lb, 5-oz neonate born in the "dirty backseat" of a taxi because her 16-year-old mother, Debbie Tillerman, didn't realize she was in labor. The baby's grandparents are angry with Debbie because, although grounded for breaking a house rule, she took the bus to visit her boyfriend out of town and was there when her labor started. Apgar scores were not recorded. The grandparents want the baby moved to the neonatal intensive care unit because, although the baby's weight is that of a term newborn, they are concerned the baby is preterm. "Don't trust anything Debbie tells you about her due date," they tell you. "She lies all of the time."

1. What standardized assessment would you want to do on U2 to assess if she is a preterm or not? Who would you ask to obtain a pregnancy history: Debbie or the grandparents?

2. Debbie is going to call her baby U2 rather than a typical name. Would you be concerned about this? Would

you talk to her about changing it before the birth certificate is filed?

3. What special care will U2 need because she was born in the "dirty backseat" of a taxi cab? Are there any special instructions Debbie will need to know to care for her?

RELATED RESOURCES

Explore these additional resources to enhance learning for this chapter:

- Student resources on thePoint, including answers to the What If . . . and Critical Thinking Care Study questions, http://thepoint.lww.com/Flagg8e
- Adaptive learning powered by PrepU, http://thepoint.lww.com/prepu

REFERENCES

Allen, K. A. (2014). The neonatal nurse's role in preventing abusive head trauma. *Advanced Neonatal Care*, 14(5), 336–342.

Altman, R. L., Canter, J., Patrick, P. A., et al. (2011). Parent education by maternity nurses and prevention of abusive head trauma. *Pediatrics*, 128(5), 164–172.

American Academy of Pediatrics. (2012). Circumcision policy statement. *Pediatrics*, 130(3), 686.

American Academy of Pediatrics. (2013). Supplement to the JCIH 2007 position statement: Principle and guidelines for early intervention after confirmation that a child is deaf or hard of hearing. *Pediatrics*, 131(4), e1324–e1349.

American Academy of Pediatrics. (2015a). *Red Book: 2015 Report of the Committee on Infectious Diseases.* Elk Grove Village, IL: Author.

American Academy of Pediatrics. (2015b). The Apgar score. *Pediatrics*, 136(4), 819–822.

American Academy of Pediatrics. (2016). *State advocacy focus: Child passenger safety.* Retrieved from https://www.aap.org/en-us/advocacy-and-policy/state-advocacy/Documents/CPS.pdf

Apgar, V., Holaday, D. A., James, L. S., et al. (1958). Evaluation of a newborn infant: Second report. *JAMA*, 168(15), 1985–1988.

Association of Women's Health, Obstetric and Neonatal Nurses. (2013). *Neonatal skin care: Evidence-based clinical practice guideline* (3rd ed.). Washington, DC: Author.

Benitz, W. E. (2015). Patent ductus arteriosus. In R. J. Martin, A. A. Fanaroff, & M. C. Walsh (Eds.), *Fanaroff and Martin's neonatal-perinatal medicine* (10th ed., pp. 1223–1229). Philadelphia, PA: Elsevier Saunders.

Benjamin, J., Mezu-Ndubuisi, O. J., & Maheshwari, A. (2015). Developmental immunology. In R. J. Martin, A. A. Fanaroff, & M. C. Walsh (Eds.), *Fanaroff and Martin's neonatal-perinatal medicine* (10th ed., pp. 696–733). Philadelphia, PA: Elsevier Saunders.

Brazelton, T. B. (1973). Neonatal behavior assessment scale. *Clinics in Developmental Medicine*, 50(5), 1–15.

Carlo, W. A., & Ambalavanan, N. (2016). Respiratory tract disorders. In R. M. Kliegman, B. F. Stanton, J. St. Geme, et al. (Eds.), *Nelson textbook of pediatrics* (20th ed., pp. 848–867). Philadelphia, PA: Elsevier.

Centers for Disease Control and Prevention. (2010). *Growth charts.* Atlanta, GA: Author.

Centers for Disease Control and Prevention. (2016). *Immunization schedules.* Retrieved from http://www.cdc.gov/vaccines/schedules/hcp/imz/child-adolescent.html

Clark-Gambelunghe, M. B., & Clark, D. A. (2015). Sensory development. *Pediatric Clinics*, 62(2), 367–384.

Desmond, M. M., Franklin, R. R., Vallvona, C., et al. (1963). The clinical behavior of the newly born: The term infant. *Journal of Pediatrics*, 62(3), 307–325.

Feldman, R. K., Tieu, R. S., & Yasumura, L. (2016). Gestational diabetes screening: The International Association of Diabetes and Pregnancy Study Groups compared with Carpenter-Coustan screening. *Obstetrics & Gynecology*, 127(1), 10–17.

Gleason, J. M., Bowlin, P., Bagli, J., et al. (2015). A comprehensive review of pediatric urachal anomalies and predictive analysis for adult urachal adenocarcinoma. *Journal of Urology*, 193(2), 632–636.

Gomella, T., Cunningham, M., & Eyal, F. G. (2013). Newborn physical examination. In T. Gomella, M. Cunningham, & F. G. Eyal (Eds.), *Neonatology: Management, procedures, on-call problems, diseases, and drugs* (7th ed., pp. 43–64). New York, NY: McGraw-Hill.

Gooding, J. R., & McClead, R. E., Jr. (2015). Initial assessment and management of the newborn. *Pediatric Clinics of North America*, 62(2), 345–365.

Gutvirtz, G., Walfisch, A., Beharier, O., et al. (2016). Isolated single umbilical artery is an independent risk factor for perinatal mortality and adverse outcomes in term neonates. *Archives of Gynecology and Obstetrics*, 294(5), 931–935.

Hutson, J. M., & Thorup, J. (2015). Evaluation and management of the infant with cryptorchidism. *Current Opinions in Pediatrics*, 27(4), 520–524.

James, S. H., & Kimberlin, D. W. (2015). Neonatal herpes simplex virus infection: Epidemiology and treatment. *Clinical Perinatology*, 42(1), 47–59.

Karch, A. M. (2013). *2013 Lippincott's nursing drug guide.* Philadelphia, PA: Lippincott Williams & Wilkins.

Lehman, R. K., & Schor, N. F. (2016). Neurologic evaluation. In R. M. Kliegman, B. F. Stanton, J. St. Geme, et al. (Eds.), *Nelson textbook of pediatrics* (20th ed., pp. 2791–2802). Philadelphia, PA: Elsevier.

Lewis, M. (2014). A comprehensive newborn examination: Part II. Skin, trunk, extremities, neurologic. *American Family Physician*, 90(5), 297–302.

Lissauer, T. (2015). Physical examination of the newborn. In R. J. Martin, A. A. Fanaroff, & M. C. Walsh (Eds.), *Fanaroff and Martin's neonatal-perinatal medicine* (10th ed., pp. 391–406). Philadelphia, PA: Elsevier Saunders.

Lovejoy-Bluem, A. (2014). Newborn skin care guidelines (3rd ed.). *Neonatal Network*, 33(4), 232.

Maheshwari, A., & Carlo, W. A. (2016). Blood disorders. In R. M. Kliegman, B. F. Stanton, J. St. Geme, et al. (Eds.), *Nelson textbook of pediatrics* (20th ed., pp. 880–889). Philadelphia, PA: Elsevier.

Martin, B., Baumhardt, H., D'Alesio, A., et al. (2012). Oral disorders. In B. J. Zitelli, S. C. McIntire, & A. J. Nowalk (Eds.), *Atlas of pediatric physical diagnosis* (6th ed., pp. 775–802). Philadelphia, PA: Elsevier.

Moore, E. R., Anderson, G. C., Bergman, N., et al. (2012). Early skin-to-skin contact for mothers and their healthy newborn infants. *Cochrane Database Systematic Reviews*, (5), CD003519.

Moyer, V. A. (2014). Prevention of dental caries in children from birth through age 5 years: US Preventive Services Task Force recommendation statement. *Pediatrics*, 133(6), 1102–1111.

Muchowski, K. (2014). Evaluation and treatment of neonatal hyperbilirubinemia. *American Family Physician*, 89(11), 873–878.

National Center for Missing & Exploited Children. (2016). *Infant abductions.* Retrieved from http://www.missingkids.org/InfantAbduction

National Institutes of Health. (2015). *About SIDS and safe infant sleep.* Retrieved from https://www.nichd.nih.gov/sts/about/Pages/default.aspx

Nussbaum, R., McInnes, R. R., & Willard, H. F. (2016). The chromosomal and gnomic basis of disease. In R. L. Nussbaum (Ed.), *Thompson & Thompson genetics in medicine* (8th ed. pp. 75–105). Philadelphia, PA: Elsevier.

Nyquist, K., Haggkvist, A., Hansen, M., et al. (2013). Expansion of the Baby-Friendly Hospital Initiative ten steps to successful breastfeeding into neonatal intensive care. *Journal of Human Lactation*, 29(3), 300–309.

Paller, A. S., & Mancini, A. J. (2016). Vascular disorders of infancy and childhood. In A. S. Paller & A. J. Mancini (Eds.), *Hurwitz clinical pediatric dermatology* (5th ed., pp. 279–316). New York, NY: Elsevier.

Phillippi, J. C., Holley, S. L., Morad, A., et al. (2016). Prevention of Vitamin K deficiency bleeding. *Journal of Midwifery Women's Health.* Advance online publication. http://dx.doi.org/10.1111/jmwh.12470

Pillai Riddell, R. R., Racine, N. M., Gennis, H. G., et al. (2015). Non-pharmacological management of infant and young child procedural pain. *Cochrane Database Systematic Reviews*, (12), CD006275.

Ramachandrappa, A., & Jain, L. (2015). The late preterm infant. In R. Martin, A. A. Fanaroff, & M. C. Walsh (Eds.), *Fanaroff and Martin's neonatal-perinatal medicine* (10th ed., pp. 577–591). Philadelphia, PA: Elsevier Saunders.

Rozance, P., & Rosenberg, A. (2017). The neonate. In S. Gabbe, J. Niebyl, J. Simpson, et al. (Eds.), *Obstetrics: Normal and problem pregnancies* (7th ed., pp. 468–498). Philadelphia, PA: Elsevier.

Saenz, M. S., Meeks, N., Tsai, A. C., et al. (2016). Genetics & dysmorphology. In W. W. Hay, J. M. Levin, R. R. Deterding, et al. (Eds.), *Current diagnosis and treatment: Pediatrics* (23rd ed., pp. 1080–1113). Columbus, OH: McGraw-Hill.

Sankar, W. N., Horn, B. D., Wells, L., et al. (2016). The hip. In R. M. Kliegman, B. F. Stanton, J. St. Geme, et al. (Eds.), *Nelson textbook of pediatrics* (20th ed., pp. 3274–3283). Philadelphia, PA: Elsevier.

Save the Children. (2014). *Ending newborn deaths: Ensuring every baby survives.* Retrieved from http://www.savethechildren.org/site/c.8rKLIXMGIpI4E/b.8989373/k.E376/Ending_Newborn_Deaths_Ensuring_Every_Baby_Survives.htm

Silverman, W. A., & Andersen, H. (1956). A controlled clinical trial of effects of water mist on obstructive respiratory signs, death rate and necroscopy findings among premature infants. *Pediatrics, 17*(4), 1–9.

Smith, D., & Grover, T. R. (2016). The newborn infant. In W. W. Hay, M. J. Levin, R. R. Deterding, et al. (Eds.), *Current diagnosis and treatment: Pediatrics* (23rd ed., pp. 10–70). Columbus, OH: McGraw-Hill.

Squires, J. E., & Balistreri, W. F. (2016). Manifestations of liver disease. In R. M. Kliegman, B. F. Stanton, J. St. Geme, et al. (Eds.), *Nelson textbook of pediatrics* (20th ed., pp. 1922–2928.). Philadelphia, PA: Elsevier.

Swanson, J. R., & Sinkin, R. A. (2015). Transition from fetus to newborn. *Pediatric Clinics of North America, 62*(2), 329–343.

Thulier, D. (2016). Weighing the facts: A systematic review of expected patterns of weight loss in full-term, breastfed infants. *Journal of Human Lactation, 32*(1), 28–34.

Tluczek, A., & De Luca, J. M. (2013). Newborn screening policy and practice issues for nurses. *Journal of Obstetric Gynecologic and Neonatal Nursing, 42*(6), 718–729.

Usher, R., McLean, F., & Scott, K. E. (1966). Judgment of fetal age. *Pediatric Clinics of North America, 13*(4), 835–840.

United Nations Children's Fund. (2016). *The Baby-Friendly Hospital Initiative.* Retrieved from https://www.unicef.org/programme/breastfeeding/baby.htm

U.S. Department of Health and Human Services. (2010). *Healthy people 2020.* Washington, DC: Author.

U.S. Preventive Services Task Force. (2011). *Ocular prophylaxis for gonococcal ophthalmia neonatorum: Preventive medication.* Retrieved from http://www.uspreventiveservicestaskforce.org/Page/Document/UpdateSummaryFinal/ocular-prophylaxis-for-gonococcal-ophthalmia-neonatorum-preventive-medication

Visscher, M., Adam, R., Brink, S., et al. (2014). Newborn infant skin: Physiology, development, and care. *Clinics in Dermatology, 33*(3), 271–281.

Webster, J., & Pritchard, M. A. (2011). Gowning by attendants and visitors in newborn nurseries for prevention of neonatal morbidity and mortality. *Cochrane Database of Systematic Reviews*, (3), CD003670.

Nutritional Needs of a Newborn

Linda Satir is a mother of a 7-lb full-term female newborn. During the pregnancy, she and her husband, Paul, both agreed Linda would breastfeed. Linda will be returning to work as an executive assistant after her 6-week maternity leave. She attempted to breastfeed her newborn in the birthing room with minimal success. While you are assisting her with breastfeeding, she says, "Did I make the right choice? Maybe I should formula feed her. Paul could help that way and I won't have to worry about what to do when I'm back at work."

Previous chapters described the care of a woman and family during the antepartal, intrapartal, postpartal, and newborn periods. This chapter addresses the challenges parents face when feeding their newborn.

How would you answer Linda?

KEY TERMS

colostrum

engorgement

interferon

lactoferrin

let-down reflex

lysozyme

prolactin

OBJECTIVES

After mastering the contents of this chapter, you should be able to:

1. Describe nutritional requirements for a term newborn.
2. Identify 2020 National Health Goals related to newborn nutrition.
3. Assess the nutritional intake and feeding method of a newborn to determine if the infant has an adequate nutritional status.
4. Formulate nursing diagnoses related to newborn nutrition.
5. Assist parents with newborn nutrition while they are adapting to their new role.
6. Using the nursing process, plan nursing care that includes the six competencies of Quality & Safety Education for Nurses (QSEN): Patient-Centered Care, Teamwork & Collaboration, Evidence-Based Practice (EBP), Quality Improvement (QI), Safety, and Informatics.
7. Implement nursing care, such as supporting a mother to initiate breastfeeding.
8. Evaluate expected outcomes for achievement and effectiveness of care.
9. Integrate knowledge of newborn nutrition with the interplay of nursing process, the six competencies of QSEN, and Family Nursing to promote quality maternal and child health nursing care.

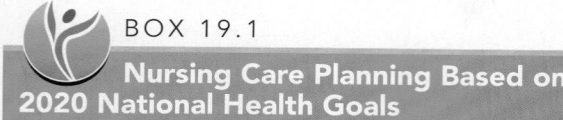

BOX 19.1

Nursing Care Planning Based on 2020 National Health Goals

The 2020 National Health Goals address increasing the proportion of infants who are breastfed. Goals include increasing:

- Ever breastfed to more than 81.9%.
- Exclusive breastfeeding at 3 months to more than 46.2%.
- Exclusive breastfeeding at 6 months to more than 25.5%.
- Breastfeeding at 6 months to more than 60.6%.
- Breastfeeding at a year to more than 34.1%.
- Increasing proportion of employers that have worksite lactation support programs from 25% to 38%.
- Increasing proportion of live births that occur in facilities that provide recommended care for lactating mothers and their babies from 2.9% to 8.1%.

The goals also address reducing:

- Proportion of breastfed newborns who receive supplemental formula within first 2 days from 24.2% to 14.2% (U.S. Department of Health and Human Services, 2010; see www.healthypeople.gov).

Nurses can help the nation achieve these goals by educating women while they are pregnant about the importance of breastfeeding as well as by supporting a family during the subsequent year while a woman is breastfeeding. Home visits with families and well-child health assessments provide opportunities to advocate for continued and exclusive breastfeeding.

Proper nutrition is essential for optimal growth and development, especially in the first few months of life because brain growth proceeds at such a rapid rate during this time. Feeding for a newborn extends beyond the physiologic need of adequate nutrition, however; it also fulfills important psychological needs. During feeding, a parent is close to the infant, and a baby is apt to be particularly sensitive to the parent's demonstration of affection or lack of warmth. The feeding experience, therefore, enables an emotional bond between infant and caregiver and helps provide an environment that enhances the psychosocial development of the infant as well as aids physical growth (Lutter & Morrow, 2013). Box 19.1 shows 2020 National Health Goals related to newborn nutrition.

Nursing Process Overview

FOR PROMOTING NUTRITIONAL HEALTH IN A NEWBORN

ASSESSMENT

An assessment of newborn nutrition begins during pregnancy with an assessment of the mother's and her partner's attitudes and choices about infant feeding. Breastfeeding is widely accepted as the preferred method of human newborn nutrition and should be recommended. However, if a mother chooses not to breastfeed as a personal preference, it is important she not be made to feel guilty for her choice. Most importantly, parents need to feel comfortable with and confident about the feeding method they choose.

Part of a feeding assessment includes recognizing signs of hunger in the newborn. Ask parents if they can identify restlessness, tense body posture, and mouth movements as signs of hunger in their infant. Otherwise, they may wait for their infant to cry, and this is actually a late sign of newborn hunger. Assess adequate intake by monitoring voiding and stooling patterns for the expected quantity and ensuring the newborn wakes for feedings at least every 3 hours after the first 24 hours of life (Box 19.2). Newborns are often sleepy the first 24 hours after birth, and they may not wake for feedings every 3 hours during that time period. If they have no risk factors for hypoglycemia, they may wait longer than 3 hours during the first 24 hours of life. Breastfed newborns may lose up to 3% of birthweight on day 1, 5% of birth weight on day 2, and 7% of birthweight on day 3. A formula-fed newborn's weight loss is not as much as a breastfed newborn. A formula-fed newborn regains birth weight at about 10 days; a breastfed infant does so at about 14 days.

NURSING DIAGNOSIS

Nursing diagnoses in relation to nutrition usually center on a woman's choice regarding the method of feeding or a newborn's nutritional intake and feeding patterns. Examples of nursing diagnoses include:

- Effective breastfeeding related to a well-prepared mother and a healthy newborn who is able to latch properly and transfer milk effectively
- Risk for ineffective breastfeeding related to a poor latch, or ineffective transfer of milk

BOX 19.2

Nursing Care Planning Using Assessment

ASSESSING THE NEWBORN FOR ADEQUATE NUTRITION

Sleeps between feedings

Loses no more than 10% of birth weight

Good skin turgor

Voids six to eight times/day; two to three bowel movements

- Imbalanced nutrition, less than body requirements, related to poor newborn response, poor latch, or ineffective transfer of milk
- Risk for impaired parenting related to inability to exclusively breastfeed the newborn if the mother's desire was to exclusively breastfeed

OUTCOME IDENTIFICATION AND PLANNING

Human milk is the ideal food for newborns. Patient education regarding infant feeding begins during the prenatal period. The discussion should provide the expectant couple with information to make an informed choice about feeding their infant and address their questions and concerns regarding breastfeeding. Maternal and infant risk factors that may interfere with successful breastfeeding should be identified as they arise. Possible risk factors are listed in Table 19.1. There may be medical contraindications to breastfeeding. After birth, a teaching plan addressing the nutritional needs of both the mother and her newborn should be developed. Refer patients and their families to helpful websites and other resources on infant feeding when appropriate (see Chapter 9).

Expectant parents cannot make an informed choice if they are not aware of the nutritional and health benefits of breast milk (Table 19.2). Parents who choose formula feeding can practice behaviors, such as skin-to-skin contact, to promote bonding. They require instructions on formula preparation, safe feeding techniques, and appropriate volumes for newborn and infant feeding. Mothers should consult their pediatric care provider regarding the type and preparation of formula to provide to their newborn.

IMPLEMENTATION

An intervention related to newborn nutrition is supporting a mother's choice of a feeding method and helping her feel confident in her ability to feed her infant. In addition to providing classes on breastfeeding prior to delivery, it is important to provide mothers with information on breastfeeding support groups at the time of discharge. Mothers may need to see a lactation consultant in the following situations:

- LATCH score less than 7 for two consecutive feeds
- Nipple trauma, absence of prenatal breast changes
- Pain throughout feed
- Infant weight loss is 8% of birth weight (less than 2% to 3% per day)
- Inadequate output
- No or limited swallowing after 24 hours of age
- History of unsuccessful breastfeeding
- History of breast surgery

TABLE 19.1 RISK FACTORS THAT MAY INTERFERE WITH SUCCESSFUL BREASTFEEDING

History/Related Maternal Risk Factors	Physical Exam/Related Maternal Risk Factors	History/Related Infant Risk Factors (Including Birth History)	Physical Exam/Related Infant Risk Factors
• Lack of experience breastfeeding	• Abnormal breast tissue distribution, tubular breast	• Anesthesia during labor	• Oral facial abnormalities
• Parity	• Breast surgeries (reduction/augmentation, mastectomy)	• Length of labor, pushing 2 hours or longer	• Palate abnormalities
• Advanced maternal age		• Delivery related (vaginal delivery vs. cesarean section)	• Tongue tie
• History of breast surgery (reduction/augmentation)	• Cracked nipples (nipple infection)	• Use of vacuum, forceps	• Uncoordinated suck
• No breast enlargement during pregnancy	• Type of nipple (inverted nipples, flat, small, large, nipple piercing)	• Type of suctioning at birth, meconium aspiration	• Sleepiness
• Social (no one breastfed in family), cultural beliefs		• Apgar (fetal distress)	• Drug dependent
• Interpersonal violence or other home stressors	• Breast engorgement	• Skin-to-skin postbirth	• Sepsis
• Infertility, using oral contraceptive pills/hormonal birth control	• Edema	• Prematurity (preterm, late preterm)	• Hypoglycemia
• Late or inconsistent prenatal care	• Vasospasm of nipple	• NICU admission (separation from mother)	• Gestational age (preterm, late preterm, full term)
• Depression, hypertension, obesity	• Mastitis, milk duct obstruction, bleb	• Multiples	• LGA or SGA
• Malnutrition, anemia	• Maternal pain level	• Risk for hypoglycemia (SGA, LGA, <37 wk, diabetic mother)	• Jaundice
• Endocrine (thyroid, diabetes, hypertension, obesity)	• Maternal obesity	• Pacifier use first 3 wk	• Caput/cephalohematoma
• Delivery related (vaginal delivery vs. caesarean section), blood loss during delivery, retained placenta fragments	• Poor positioning	• Supplemental formula feeding	• Congenital anomaly
• Pain management, epidural medications	• Poor latch	• History of jaundice or at risk for jaundice	
• Tobacco use, intravenous drug use/substance use, toxicology screen		• Voiding and stools quantity less than expected	
• Early return to work		• Circumcision	
		• Weight loss 10% or greater from birth weight	

NICU, neonatal intensive care unit; SGA, small for gestational age; LGA, large for gestational age.
Flagg, J. (2015). Breastfeeding problems associated with maternal and/or infant risk factors. *Journal of Pregnancy and Child Health, 2*(2), e119.

TABLE 19.2 NUTRITIONAL AND HEALTH BENEFITS OF BREASTFEEDING

Condition	% of Lowered Risk
Lower respiratory tract infections	72
Gastrointestinal infections	64
Otitis media (exclusive vs. formula fed)	50
Atopic dermatitis	42
Diabetes types 1 and 2	19–27/39
Obesity	7–27
Sudden infant death syndrome	36
Childhood leukemias	15–19
Maternal breast cancer	28
Ovarian cancer	21

Source: Ip, S., Chung, M. Raman, G., et al. (2007). *Breastfeeding and maternal and infant health outcomes in developed countries* (AHRQ Publication No. 07-E007). Rockville, MD: Agency for Healthcare Research and Quality.

- Abnormal infant oral anatomy
- Mother of neonatal intensive care unit (NICU) infant/separation from infant
- Late preterm (34 to 36 6/7), small for gestational age (SGA), large for gestational age (LGA)
- Infant jaundice
- Multiple births
- Birth interventions
- Unrelieved fullness or engorgement (Wambach & Riordan, 2016)

Hospitals seeking to improve lactation support or seeking the Baby-Friendly Hospital certification may provide mother's breastfeeding support groups. Components of the United States Baby-Friendly Hospital Initiative* include:

- Have a written breastfeeding policy that is routinely communicated to all healthcare staff.
- Train all healthcare staff in skills necessary to implement policy.
- Inform all pregnant women about the benefits and management of breastfeeding.
- Help mothers initiate breastfeeding within 1 hour of birth.
- Show mothers how to breastfeed and how to maintain lactation, even if they are separated from their infants.
- Give newborn infants no food or drink other than breast milk, unless medically indicated.
- Practice "rooming-in" by allowing mothers and infants to remain together 24 hours a day.
- Encourage breastfeeding on demand.
- Give no pacifiers or artificial nipples to breastfeeding infants.
- Ensure continuity of care, foster the establishment of breastfeeding support groups, and refer mothers to them on discharge from the hospital or clinic.

*Reprinted from Baby-Friendly USA. (2012). *The ten steps to successful breastfeeding*. Retrieved from https://www.babyfriendlyusa.org/about-us/baby-friendly-hospital-initiative/the-ten-steps.

OUTCOME EVALUATION

The evaluation is an important final step to ensure a newborn receives adequate nutrition because unforeseen circumstances, such as jaundice, infant tongue-tie, or late preterm delivery may require the mother to provide expressed breast milk until the problem is resolved. Mothers may need to pump to provide breast milk to their newborns in the following circumstances:

- Infants in NICU
- Infants with weight loss greater or equal to 8%, LATCH scores less or equal to 7 × 2 and in need of supplementation
- Infants close to 24 hours old and who have not nursed
- Mothers using breast shield
- Mothers with a history of breast surgery
- Mothers with medical conditions (i.e., hemorrhage or shock)(Wambach & Riordan, 2016)

There are alternative methods to provide expressed breast milk until successful breastfeeding is established. These include cup feeding, finger feeding, spoon feeding, and bottle feeding. It is possible the introduction of a bottle prior to 3 weeks of age could cause nipple confusion. If a nipple is used, a slow-flow nipple is recommended to encourage the newborn to initiate and control the flow. Full-term healthy newborns may be sleepy the first 24 hours after birth. Unless they are at risk for hypoglycemia, they may be fed at all feeding cues. Risk factors for hypoglycemia in newborns include:

- Preterm (less than 37 weeks gestation)
- Intrauterine growth restriction
- Low birth weight (less than 2.5 kg)
- SGA (less than 10%)
- Maternal diabetes
- LGA (greater than 90%)
- Hypothermia
- Infection/other illness in the newborn
- Severe intrapartum asphyxia
- Maternal use of β-blockers, such as labetalol (Trandate) (Wambach & Riordan, 2016)

Examples suggesting successful expected outcomes related to newborn feeding include:

- Newborn wakes for feedings every 2 to 3 hours after the first 24 hours of life.
- Newborn feeds 10 to 30 ml of formula with iron every 3 to 4 hours after the first 24 hours of life.
- Mother expresses satisfaction with her chosen method of newborn feeding.
- Newborn voids and defecates once within the first 24 hours, twice within the second 24 hours, three times within the third 24 hours, and four times within the fourth 24 hours. From day 5 on, the newborn voids five to six times daily as a measure of adequate hydration. Stools are meconium at birth, brown by day 2, green by day 3 or 4, and then seedy yellow. The newborn usually has one or more stools daily by day 5.

Nutritional Allowances for a Newborn

Nutritional allowances for a newborn need to take into account total calories, protein, vitamins, minerals, and fluid.

CALORIES

Growth in the neonatal period and early infancy is more rapid than in any other period of life (U.S. Department of Agriculture, 2016); therefore, the caloric requirements exceed those at any other age. For example, an infant up to 2 months of age requires 100 to 120 calories per kilogram of body weight (50 to 55 kcal/lb) every 24 hours to provide an adequate amount for maintenance and growth. After 2 months of age, this amount gradually declines until the requirement at 1 year is 100 kcal/kg (45 kcal/lb) per day. In contrast, the adult caloric requirement is 42 kcal/kg (20 kcal/lb) per day (U.S. Department of Agriculture, 2016). During growth spurts, more calories are needed to supply additional energy.

Commercial infant formulas are designed to provide approximately the same number of calories as breast milk, 20 calories per ounce. They contain about 9% to 12% of their calories as protein and 45% to 55% of calories as lactose carbohydrate. The balance (34% to 46%) is fat, of which linoleic acid accounts for about 4%.

PROTEIN

The newborn has a high requirement of protein, which is necessary for the formation of new cells, during this period to provide for a rapid growth of new cells as well as maintenance of existing cells. The nutritional allowance of protein for the first 2 months of life is 2.2 g per kilogram of body weight. Both human milk and commercial formulas provide all the essential amino acids necessary to form protein. Histidine, an amino acid that appears to be essential for infant growth but is not necessary for adult growth, is found in both milk forms.

Unaltered cow's milk is not recommended for newborns because it contains about 16% of its calories as protein, whereas human milk contains about 8%. This means cow's milk can create such a rich solute load (i.e., the amount of urea and electrolytes that must be excreted in the urine) that a newborn's kidneys could be overwhelmed. In addition, cow's milk can cause microscopic bleeding of the gastrointestinal tract, leading to blood loss and anemia. These problems occur because the protein in cow's milk, *casein*, differs from that in human milk, *lactalbumin*, both in composition and in amount. This is important because the amount of casein present in milk determines its curd tension. Because of the increased amount of casein in cow's milk, the curd is large, tough, and difficult to digest, whereas in human milk, the curd is softer and digests easily. This is the rationale behind recommending formula-fed infants be given a commercial formula containing albumin rather than cow's milk. Cow's milk products, such as yogurt and cottage cheese, should not be introduced until 9 to 12 months of age because of this same reason.

FAT

Linoleic acid, an essential fatty acid, is necessary for brain growth and skin integrity in infants. When the amount of linoleic acid is sufficient, the infant can then manufacture docosahexaenoic acid (DHA), an omega-3 fatty acid, and arachidonic acid (ARA), an omega-6 fatty acid, both of which are important for brain growth. Breast milk contains a generous supply of all three of these fatty acids. Commercial formulas contain varying amounts depending on the brand and type of fats included in the formula.

Because fat is so important for brain and nerve growth, use of fat-free milk for long periods in newborns and infants (when other sources of food are not being offered) can result in linoleic acid deficiency. Therefore, parents should not feed fat-free milk as a means of preventing obesity in newborns or young infants. In addition, fat-free milk does not contain sufficient calories for a newborn; it only has about half as many calories as commercial formulas or breast milk.

CARBOHYDRATE

Lactose, the disaccharide found in human milk and added to commercial formulas, appears to be the most easily digested of the carbohydrates. Lactose also improves calcium absorption and aids in nitrogen retention. It produces stools consisting predominantly of gram-positive rather than gram-negative bacteria and therefore decreases the possibility of gastrointestinal illness (which usually results from gram-negative organisms). Adequate lactose also allows protein to be used for building new cells rather than for calories, encouraging normal water balance and preventing abnormal metabolism of fat. Lactose intolerance, which can occur in older children, is rarely present in newborns; they typically use the calories provided by lactose well.

FLUID

It is important to maintain a sufficient fluid intake in newborns because their metabolic rate is so high (and metabolism requires water). In addition, a newborn's body surface area is large in relation to body mass. This means a baby loses water by evaporation much more readily than does an adult, and, because the kidneys of a newborn are not yet capable of fully concentrating urine, a newborn cannot conserve body water by this mechanism to prevent dehydration.

Another difference between newborns and adults is that body water is distributed differently. In a newborn, 30% to 35% of body weight is extracellular fluid; in an adult, this proportion is only 20%. Consequently, if a newborn's extracellular fluid store is depleted through loss of fluid or inadequate fluid intake, as much as 35% of a newborn's fluid component may be lost.

Because of all these factors, a newborn needs 150 to 200 ml/kg (2.5 to 3.0 oz/lb) of water intake every 24 hours (adults require 2,400 ml per day or less than 1 oz/lb). This requirement can be supplied completely by breastfeeding or formula feeding. Fruit juice is not recommended for infants younger than 6 months because it supplies no protein and, if not pasteurized, can carry infectious organisms (American Academy of Pediatrics [AAP], 2012c).

QSEN Checkpoint Question 19.1

PATIENT-CENTERED CARE

A nursing assessment of Linda Satir's plan for her infant's nutrition should begin with which of the following?
  a. An assessment of Linda's beliefs and attitudes about breastfeeding
  b. An assessment of the infant's body mass index and glucose levels
  c. An assessment of Linda's education level and reading ability
  d. An assessment of the infant's ability to suck and swallow

Look in Appendix A for the best answer and rationale.

MINERALS

A number of minerals are particularly important to early growth.

Calcium

Calcium is important to the newborn because a newborn's skeleton grows so rapidly. Because milk is high in calcium, tetany resulting from a low calcium level seldom occurs in infants who suck well, regardless of whether they are fed human milk or commercial formula (U.S. Department of Agriculture, 2016).

Iron

A newborn (37 or more weeks gestation age) whose mother had adequate iron intake during pregnancy will be born with iron stores that, theoretically, will last for the first 3 months of life, until the newborn begins to produce adult hemoglobin. Because not all mothers eat an iron-rich diet during pregnancy (and socioeconomic level is not a good criterion for judging the quality of a diet), the AAP recommends infants who are formula fed ingest an iron-enriched formula for the entire first year of life) (U.S. Department of Agriculture, 2016). Some women who breastfeed are also advised to supplement iron to ensure their infant does not develop iron-deficiency anemia (U.S. Department of Agriculture, 2016).

Fluoride

Fluoride is essential for building sound teeth and for preventing tooth decay. Because teeth are already set in their primary form during pregnancy, it is important for women to drink fluoridated water during pregnancy. A lactating mother should continue drinking fluoridated water (although only a small amount of fluoride passes into breast milk), and formulas should be prepared with fluoridated water. This is an essential point to remember because a mother may think she is helping her child by using bottled, "natural" water in formula rather than chlorinated (and fluoridated) water from a tap.

If a mother is breastfeeding and a source of fluoridated water is not available (the family drinks well, spring, or bottled water or the tap water is not fluoridated), a fluoride supplement, 0.25 mg daily, may be given to the infant beginning at 6 months of age.

VITAMINS

Although both breast milk and commercial formulas contain sufficient vitamins for growth, the AAP now recommends that breastfed newborns be given a supplement of 400 international units per day of vitamin D, beginning in the first few days of life. Newborns who are fully or partially formula fed also benefit from a daily 400 international units vitamin D supplement (U.S. Department of Agriculture, 2016).

Breastfeeding

It is universally agreed that human milk is the preferred food for newborns because it provides numerous health benefits to both a mother and an infant; it remains the ideal nutritional source for infants through the first year of life

(U.S. Department of Agriculture, 2016). Nurses are prime healthcare professionals to teach women about the benefits of breastfeeding and provide anticipatory guidance for problems that may occur. You can also help create an atmosphere conducive to breastfeeding success in healthcare facilities by implementing steps, such as:

- Educating all pregnant women about the benefits and management of breastfeeding
- Helping women initiate breastfeeding within half an hour after birth
- Assisting mothers to breastfeed and maintain lactation even if they should be separated from their infant
- Not giving newborns food or drink other than breast milk unless medically indicated, so they are hungry to breastfeed. Advise women they need not introduce solid food until at least 4 months.
- Not giving newborns pacifiers to quiet them as this can reduce the sucking initiative
- Supporting rooming-in (such as allowing mothers and infants to remain together) 24 hours a day
- Encouraging breastfeeding on demand
- Fostering the establishment of breastfeeding support groups and referring mothers to them on discharge from the birthing center or hospital (Baby-Friendly USA, 2012)

PHYSIOLOGY OF BREAST MILK PRODUCTION

Breast milk is formed in the acinar or alveolar cells of the mammary glands (Fig. 19.1). With the delivery of the placenta following birth, the level of progesterone in a woman's body falls dramatically, stimulating the production of **prolactin**, an anterior pituitary hormone. Prolactin acts on the acinar cells of the mammary glands to stimulate the production of milk. In addition, when an infant sucks at a breast, nerve impulses travel from the nipple to the hypothalamus to stimulate the production of prolactin-releasing factor.

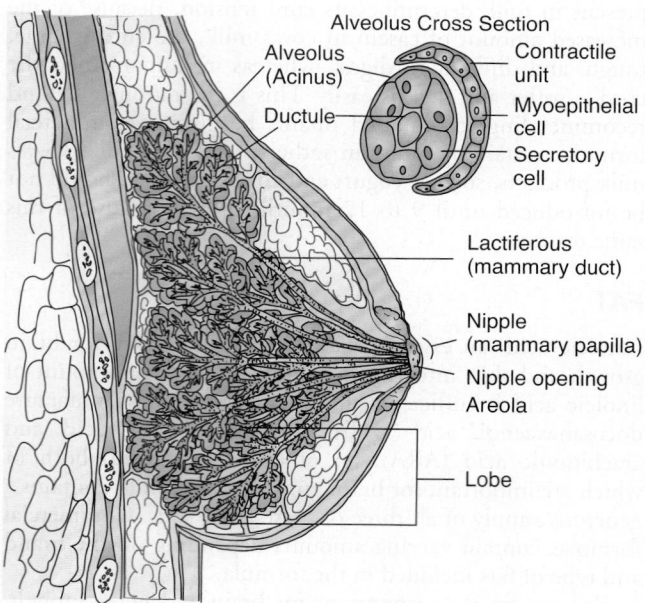

Figure 19.1 Anatomy of the breast.

This factor stimulates further active production of prolactin. Other anterior pituitary hormones, such as adrenocorticotropic hormone, thyroid-stimulating hormone, and growth hormone, probably also play a role in growth of the mammary glands and their ability to secrete milk. Regardless of the gestational age of the infant, the mother should be able to produce a sufficient quantity of breast milk for the infant, providing she empties the breasts through breastfeeding or expressing milk (manually or by using a breast pump). A hospital-grade breast pump is recommended to establish and maintain lactation if the infant is unable to latch and transfer breast milk through breastfeeding (U.S. Department of Agriculture, 2016).

Colostrum, a thin, watery, yellow fluid composed of protein, sugar, fat, water, minerals, vitamins, and maternal antibodies, is secreted by the acinar breast cells starting in the fourth month of pregnancy. For the first 3 or 4 days after birth, colostrum production continues. Because it is high in protein and fairly low in sugar and fat, colostrum is easy to digest and capable of providing adequate nutrition for a newborn until it is replaced by transitional breast milk on the second to fourth day. True or mature breast milk is produced by the 10th day.

Milk flows from the alveolar cells, where it is produced, through small tubules to reservoirs for milk, the lactiferous sinuses, located behind the nipple. This constantly forming milk is called fore milk. Its availability depends very little on the infant's sucking at the breast. As the infant sucks at the breast, oxytocin, released from the posterior pituitary, causes the collecting sinuses of the mammary glands to contract, forcing milk forward through the nipples, making it available for the baby. This action is called a **let-down reflex**. A let-down reflex may also be triggered by the sound of a baby crying or by thinking about the baby. New milk, called hind milk, is formed after the let-down reflex. Hind milk, which is higher in fat than fore milk, is the milk that makes a breastfed infant grow most rapidly. The release of oxytocin has a second advantage in that, by causing smooth muscle contraction, it helps contract the uterus. As a result, a woman may feel a small tugging or cramping in her lower pelvis during the first few days of breastfeeding (i.e., afterpains) (U.S. Department of Agriculture, 2016).

ADVANTAGES OF BREASTFEEDING

Little controversy exists that breastfeeding is the ideal nutrition for human infants. It is contraindicated in only a few circumstances, such as:
- An infant with galactosemia (such infants cannot digest the lactose in milk)
- Herpes lesions on a mother's nipples
- Maternal exposure to radioactive compounds (such as occurs with thyroid testing)
- Mothers receiving antimetabolites or chemotherapeutic agents
- Mothers receiving prescribed medications that would be harmful to an infant, such as lithium or methotrexate
- Women with maternal active, untreated tuberculosis, who need to be evaluated individually depending on the stage of their disease
- Women who are positive for HIV, who are advised not to breastfeed in the United States until further

studies confirm the risk of not breastfeeding outweighs the risk of breast milk transmission of the virus (Academy of Breastfeeding Medicine Protocol Committee, 2010a). In developing countries, women who are HIV positive may be advised to breastfeed because commercial formula is not available.
- Women whose toxicology screens for substance abuse are positive, who need to be evaluated on an individual basis regarding recommendations to breastfeed

Cigarette smoking is not a contraindication to breastfeeding, but women should be aware some nicotine is carried in breast milk. Nicotine has the potential to decrease a mother's milk supply (Reece-Stremtan & Marinelli, 2015). If the infant is exposed to secondhand smoke, it could lead to an increase in respiratory illnesses. The nurse needs to be aware of a number of other situations that call for individual planning in consultation with a lactation consultant.

Advantages of Breastfeeding for Women

A woman gains several physiologic benefits from breastfeeding:
- The release of oxytocin from the posterior pituitary gland aids in uterine involution.
- Breastfeeding may serve a protective function in preventing breast cancer and possibly ovarian cancer.
- A woman may return to her prepregnant weight sooner, and if menstruation is delayed, this may serve as a temporary family planning method.
- Successful breastfeeding can have an empowering effect because it is a skill only a woman can master.
- Breastfeeding reduces the cost of feeding and preparation time for infant feeding.
- A long-term effect may include a decreased risk of hip fractures and osteoporosis in the postmenopausal period for the woman (U.S. Department of Agriculture, 2016).
- Breastfeeding provides an excellent opportunity to enhance a true symbiotic bond between mother and child. Although this does readily occur with breastfeeding, a woman who holds her baby to formula feed can form this bond as well.

Common reasons women give for not exclusively breastfeeding or discontinuing breastfeeding include (a) insufficient milk supply, (b) feeling very tired, (c) having trouble with the infant latching to breast, and (d) wanting to allow their partner to feed the infant (U.S. Department of Agriculture, 2016). According to the Agency for Healthcare Research & Quality, reasons for discontinuing breastfeeding during the first week of life include latching difficulty (47%), soreness/cracked nipples (35%), perceived low milk supply (27%), prefers others to feed baby (8%), and work/school-related issues (6%). Reasons during the first 1 to 3 months of life include perceived low milk supply (37%), work/school related issues (35%), latching difficulty (15%), soreness/cracked nipples (12%), prefer others to feed baby (12%), and partner preference (2%) (Ip, Chung, Raman, 2007). Some women are reluctant to breastfeed because they fear having to be available to feed their baby every 3 or 4 hours will tie them down. Like mothers who formula feed, however, they can leave a bottle with expressed breast milk with a caregiver if they need to be away from their baby at the time of a feeding.

QSEN Checkpoint Question 19.2

EVIDENCE-BASED PRACTICE

The AAP (Hagan, Shaw, & Duncan, 2017) recommends infants be exclusively breastfed for 6 months. To discover the characteristics of women who were exclusively breastfeeding at the time of hospital discharge, researchers studied all term hospital births in the province of Ontario, Canada, for a year. From this pool of over 90,000 infants, 56,865 were identified as still being exclusively breastfed at discharge. Characteristics of women who were exclusively breastfeeding were older age, nonsmoking, higher income, and no pregnancy complications or reproductive assistance. They also had a single rather than twin infants and had attended prenatal classes. Patients of obstetricians were less likely to exclusively breastfeed than those cared for by midwives or family physicians. Women who had a planned cesarean birth were more apt to breastfeed than those who had an unplanned cesarean birth.

Based on the previous findings, which statement by Linda would be the best indicator that she will be successful at exclusive breastfeeding?
  a. "I enjoyed going for prenatal visits."
  b. "I wish my husband earned more money."
  c. "I can't wait until discharge when I can have a cigarette."
  d. "I like having my first baby at 23; I'm young enough to adjust."

Look in Appendix A for the best answer and rationale.

Advantages for Infants

Breastfeeding has major physiologic advantages for infants as well as it does for women. Breast milk contains secretory immunoglobulin A (IgA), which binds large molecules of foreign proteins, including viruses and bacteria, thus keeping them from being absorbed from the gastrointestinal tract.

Lactoferrin is an iron-binding protein in breast milk that interferes with the growth of pathogenic bacteria. The enzyme **lysozyme** in breast milk apparently actively destroys bacteria by lysing (dissolving) their cell membranes, possibly increasing the effectiveness of antibodies. Leukocytes in breast milk provide protection against common respiratory infectious invaders. Macrophages, responsible for producing **interferon** (a protein that protects against viruses), help interfere with virus growth. The bifidus factor is a specific growth-promoting factor for the beneficial bacteria *Lactobacillus bifidus*. The presence of *L. bifidus* in breast milk interferes with the colonization of pathogenic bacteria in the gastrointestinal tract, thus reducing the incidence of diarrhea (U.S. Department of Agriculture, 2016).

In addition to these anti-infective properties, breast milk contains the ideal electrolyte and mineral composition for human infant growth. It is high in lactose, an easily digested sugar that provides ready glucose for rapid brain growth. The protein in breast milk is easily digested, and the ratio of cysteine to methionine (two amino acids) in breast milk favors rapid brain growth in the early months. It contains nitrogen in compounds other than protein, so an infant can receive cell-building materials from sources other than just protein.

Breast milk contains more linoleic acid, an essential fatty acid for skin integrity, and less sodium, potassium, calcium, and phosphorus than do many formulas. Breast milk also has a better balance of trace elements, such as zinc. These levels of nutrients are enough to supply the infant's needs, yet they spare the infant's kidneys from having to process a high renal solute load of unused nutrients. Exclusively breastfeeding for at least 3 to 4 months or longer was found to reduce the incidence of certain allergies in 42% of infants where there was a family history of allergies (U.S. Department of Agriculture, 2016).

Yet, another advantage of breastfeeding is that breastfed newborns appear to be able to regulate their calcium/phosphorus levels better than infants who are formula fed. Decreased calcium levels in a newborn can lead to tetany (muscle spasm). The increased concentration of fatty acid in commercial formulas may bind calcium in the gastrointestinal tract, also increasing the danger of tetany. Breastfeeding may also help prevent excessive weight gain in infants. It has been shown that exclusive breastfeeding into the infant's fourth month of life can decrease obesity as late as adolescence (Wallby, Lagerberg, & Magnusson, 2017).

In addition, a great deal of discussion about the benefits of breastfeeding has centered on the effects of breastfeeding on the formation of the dental arch because babies suck differently from a breast than from a bottle (Fig. 19.2). Babies pull their tongue backward as they suck from a breast. They thrust their tongue forward to suck from a rubber nipple. That may make breastfeeding the best preparation for forming common speech sounds (U.S. Department of Agriculture, 2016).

QSEN Checkpoint Question 19.3

INFORMATICS

Linda asks the nurse why breastfeeding is so beneficial for her newborn. The nurse would want her to know breast milk has which of the following characteristics?
  a. It is more nutritious than formula because it never needs to be warmed.
  b. It will provide immunity as well as nutrients for her newborn.
  c. It will protect her child from gastrointestinal cancer.
  d. It will ensure her baby will never be obese as an adult.

Look in Appendix A for the best answer and rationale.

TECHNIQUES OF BREASTFEEDING

Ask all women during pregnancy whether they plan to breastfeed their newborns because thinking about feeding in advance allows a woman and her partner to make an informed choice. If a partner expresses jealousy at the thought of breastfeeding, early discussion can help address this common sensation, with the eventual realization that parenting will involve many other opportunities for interaction with their child.

No preparation of the nipples is needed during pregnancy. In addition, oxytocin, which is released with nipple stimulation, could lead to preterm labor. Less than 1% of

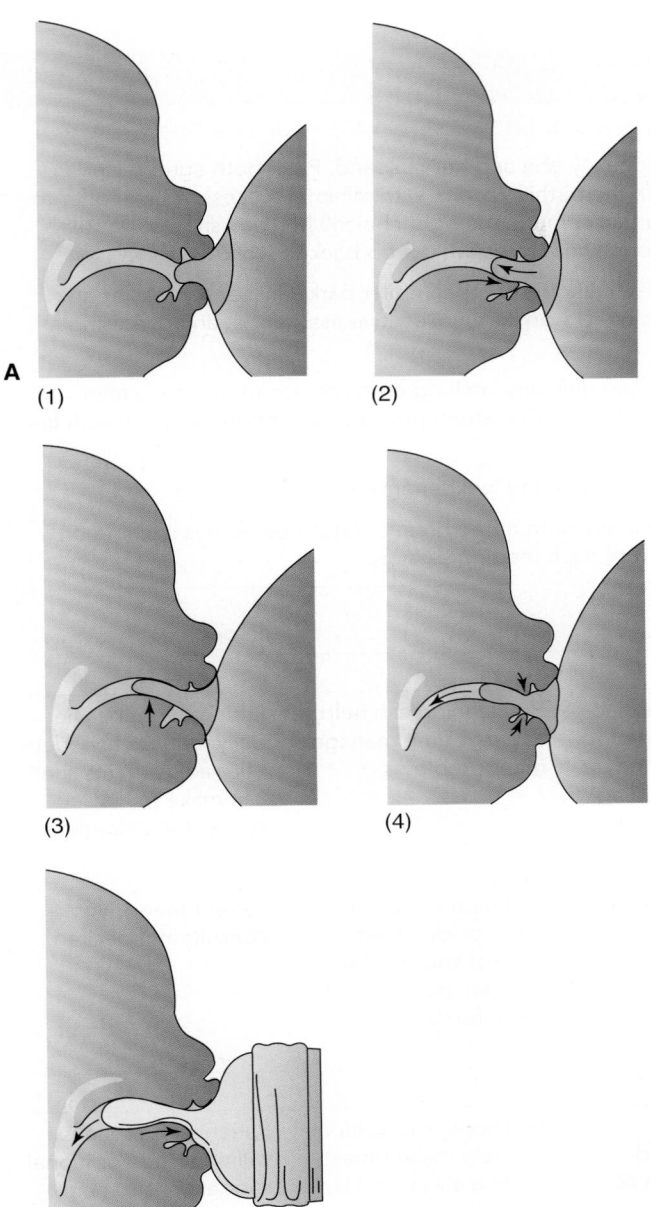

Figure 19.2 Differences in the sucking mechanism. **(A)** Breast-feeding. *(1)* Lips of the infant clamp in a C shape. The cheek muscles contract. *(2)* The tongue thrusts forward to grasp the nipple and areola. *(3)* The nipple is brought against the hard palate as the tongue pulls backward, bringing the areola into the mouth. *(4)* The gums compress the areola, squeezing milk into the back of the throat. **(B)** Formula feeding. The large rubber nipple of a bottle strikes the soft palate and interferes with the action of the tongue. The tongue moves forward against the gums to control the overflow of milk into the esophagus.

woman have inverted nipples. A nipple shield (a plastic shell) may be suggested to help her nipples become more everted (U.S. Department of Agriculture, 2016).

Beginning Breastfeeding

Skin-to-skin contact should be initiated within the first hour of delivery, while the infant is in the first reactivity period (U.S. Department of Agriculture, 2016).

Skin-to-skin contact is defined as placing the undressed infant on the mother's chest against her skin. When placed in this position, the infant will root toward the nipple and initiate a latch. This may be more successful in an unmedicated birth of a full-term infant. A mother breastfeeding for the first time may require additional support (Box 19.3). Pumping with a hospital grade pump or manual expression is an alternative method to provide breast milk to a newborn who is unable to latch or if mother and baby are separated.

Manual expression of breast milk consists of supporting the breast firmly, then placing the thumb and forefinger on the opposite sides of the breast just behind the areolar margin, and first pushing backward toward the chest wall and then downward until secretions begins to flow (Box 19.4). Women should avoid soap on the nipples as it may lead to dryness and skin breakdown. The release of oxytocin by breastfeeding, pumping, or manual expression initiates let-down of milk and also stimulates uterine contraction. The average quantity a mother may produce and guidelines for breast milk storage include 37 ml (7 to 123 ml) within the first 24 hours, 500 ml by day 5, 750 ml/day by month 3, and 800 ml/day by month 6. For mothers of twins, it can vary at approximately 2,100 ml/day.

What If . . . 19.1
Linda told the nurse she doesn't really want to breastfeed but her husband is insisting she do so? What would the nurse do?

Prolonged Jaundice in Breastfed Infants

Jaundice occurs in as many as 15% of breastfed infants because pregnanediol (a breakdown product of progesterone) in breast milk depresses the action of glucuronyl transferase, the enzyme that converts indirect bilirubin (which cannot be excreted) to the direct form, which is then readily excreted in bile (Academy of Breastfeeding Medicine Protocol Committee, 2010b). To prevent this excess buildup of bilirubin (i.e., hyperbilirubinemia) in their newborn, women should feed frequently in the immediate postpartum period because colostrum is a natural laxative and helps promote passage of both meconium and bile. Newborns who are discharged early from their birth setting or born at home need to be observed carefully for jaundice. Breastfeeding rarely results in a serum bilirubin level high enough to warrant therapy or to require discontinuation of breastfeeding, however, because pregnanediol remains in breast milk for only 24 to 48 hours (Academy of Breastfeeding Medicine Protocol Committee, 2010b).

Nursing Diagnoses and Related Interventions for Newborn Nutrition

Nursing Diagnosis: Health-seeking behaviors related to lack of knowledge about lactation and breastfeeding techniques

Outcome Evaluation: Woman states correct information as to how lactation begins and is maintaining an adequate supply; demonstrates effective positioning for baby and herself by 24 hours.

BOX 19.3

Nursing Care Planning

AN INTERPROFESSIONAL CARE MAP FOR A WOMAN WHO IS BREASTFEEDING FOR THE FIRST TIME

Linda Satir is a new mother of a term baby girl. During the pregnancy, she and her husband, Paul, both agreed Linda would breastfeed. She attempted to breastfeed her newborn in the birthing room, with minimal success. As you offer to help her feed her baby for the second time, she says, "Do you think I made the right choice? Maybe I should formula feed her. Paul could help that way and I won't have to worry about what to do when I go back to work."

Family Assessment: Patient lives with husband in two-bedroom trailer in suburban trailer park. Husband works as an interpreter for local chamber of commerce. Linda will be returning to work as an executive assistant at an advertising agency after her 6-week maternity leave.

Patient Assessment: Mother is 2 hours postpartum. Newborn had difficulty latching onto breasts immediately after birth. Nipples without signs of redness or irritation. Breasts slightly firm. Colostrum present. Patient discouraged with first breastfeeding attempt.

Nursing Diagnosis: Risk for ineffective breastfeeding related to anxiety and inexperience

Outcome Criteria: Patient describes ways to properly position a newborn at the breast; states newborn is latching on and sucking; verbalizes increasing satisfaction and confidence with each feeding session.

Team Member Responsible	Assessment	Intervention	Rationale	Expected Outcome
Activities of Daily Living, Including Safety				
Nurse	Assess patient's usual daily activity pattern.	Review with patient activities she may need to adjust to accommodate time for breastfeeding.	Preplanning can help to avoid time management problems.	Patient describes her daily routines and identifies adjustments she can make to aid successful breastfeeding.
Teamwork and Collaboration				
Nurse/lactation consultant	Investigate whether patient would like to speak to a lactation consultant; determine which lactation consultant is available.	If patient agrees, initiate a referral to a lactation consultant.	Lactation consultants can provide an additional source of support, encouragement, and information.	Patient meets with consultant if desired.
Procedures/Medications for Quality Improvement				
Nurse	Observe patient breastfeeding to determine technique she uses.	Make suggestions as necessary regarding technique such as how to break suction, remove newborn from breast, or begin next feeding on breast newborn used most recently.	Additional suggestions can help make breastfeeding successful by encouraging patient to relax during feedings.	Patient states she is willing to try additional suggestions to help improve breastfeeding success.
Nutrition				
Nurse	Assess patient's present daily fluid intake.	Urge patient to drink at least four to six 8-oz glasses of fluid per day.	Adequate fluid intake is essential to maintain an adequate milk supply.	Patient confirms she drinks suggested fluid every day and will continue to do this at home.
Patient-Centered Care				
Nurse/lactation consultant	Assess patient's knowledge about breastfeeding. Allow time for questions.	Educate patient regarding any gaps in knowledge.	The better informed women are about breastfeeding, the more apt they are to feel comfortable with the process.	Patient asks questions regarding areas of breastfeeding of which she is unsure.

Psychosocial/Spiritual/Emotional Needs

Nurse/lactation consultant	Assess what patient thought breastfeeding would be like.	Acknowledge breastfeeding involves newly learned skills and may not be as easy as it looks.	Assurance can increase self-esteem when a person is learning a new skill.	Patient states she is willing to try for a longer time than a few feedings to see if she can be successful at breastfeeding.

Informatics for Seamless Healthcare Planning

Nurse	Assess steps patient intends to take to ensure breastfeeding success after returning home or to work.	Provide feedback and suggestions, reinforcing accomplishments and assisting with any difficulties.	Feedback and positive reinforcement promote self-confidence and learning, enhancing the success and effectiveness of teaching and breastfeeding.	Patient describes well-thought-out plans for continuing breastfeeding and integrating it into her lifestyle.
Nurse	Assess if local support organization is available for referral.	Suggest patient keep telephone numbers of support group and lactation consultant available if she needs additional help while at home or work.	Support can go a long way toward preventing a patient from becoming discouraged once she returns home.	Patient states she will contact support people as necessary if she has questions after discharge.

In cultures where breastfeeding is practiced by almost all mothers, the technique is learned early in life by observation. In the United States, a woman may have had few, if any, opportunities to observe breastfeeding and so may need some advice (Box 19.5). Many hospitals employ International Board Certified Lactation Consultants (IBCLC) who provide lactation support for breastfeeding mothers. IBCLC also provide education and training to hospital staff who provide maternal child care.

Support, adequate instruction, and reassurance from healthcare personnel are important for helping a woman feel secure enough to successfully breastfeed (Barnes, Cox, Doyle, et al., 2010). Rooming-in is ideal for breastfeeding because the infant can be fed with feeding cues. Nurses should discuss safe sleep with new mothers and counsel mothers to place newborns on a firm mattress and on their back with no blankets or covers. The room should be a comfortable temperature, and the newborn should not be exposed to environmental tobacco smoke. Caretakers should avoid excessive alcohol causing intoxication and medications or drugs that alter mental status. Pacifiers may be introduced at 3 weeks of age if breastfeeding is well established and there are no latch concerns (Centers for Disease Control and Prevention, 2016).

Provide Information Regarding Lactation and Proper Positioning Techniques. Mature breast milk may appear thin and blue-tinged in appearance. Some women may need assurance that this color and consistency are normal; otherwise, they may think their milk is not nutritious enough.

Before breastfeeding, recommend a woman wash her hands to be certain they are free of pathogens picked up from handling perineal pads or other sources. Washing her breasts is not necessary unless she notices caked colostrum

on the nipples. There are several positions a mother may use when breastfeeding. The side-lying position (Fig. 19.3) may permit the mother to rest while feeding. This may be difficult as the initial feeding position as it requires the newborn to latch more independently. Figure 19.4A shows a sitting position with a pillow under the newborn. Using a football hold with the newborn supported on a pillow also may be helpful, especially if a mother had a cesarean birth (Fig. 19.4B). This position is also helpful if the baby is having difficulty latching due to large breasts that obstruct the mother's view or less prominent nipples that provide little palate stimulation.

Brushing the infant's cheek with a breast nipple stimulates a newborn's rooting reflex. The newborn will then turn toward the breast. Do not try to initiate a rooting reflex by pressing a baby's face against the mother's breast as this will cause the child to turn away from the mother and toward your hand. An assessment tool such as the LATCH assessment (Table 19.3) can be helpful. This charting system, similar to an Apgar score, provides a systematic method for gathering information about breastfeeding progress. The system assigns a numerical score of 0, 1, or 2 to five key components of breastfeeding; 10 is a perfect score, meaning the woman is ready to independently breastfeed. The LATCH score is a useful tool to identify mother–infant pairs who might benefit from additional skilled support to encourage them to continue exclusive breastfeeding.

During the first few days of life, because they are receiving only colostrum and need the nutrients and fluid obtained by frequent sucking, newborns should be fed with all feeding cues (mouth opening, eyes open, bringing hands to mouth). Frequent feeding also is advantageous to establish a milk supply.

BOX 19.4

Nursing Care Planning Using Procedures

MANUAL BREAST MILK EXPRESSION

Purpose: To assist a woman to manually express milk so she can strengthen her milk supply or supply milk for her newborn should she be separated from the newborn

Procedure	Principle
1. Explain the procedure to the patient.	1. Explanations help decrease anxiety and enhance learning; they also provide information for the patient to carry out the procedure on her own.
2. Assemble equipment, including a clean towel and collection container.	2. Assembling equipment aids in organization and efficiency.
3. Wash your hands and put on clean gloves; have patient wash her hands.	3. Hand washing prevents the transmission of infection; use of gloves protects self and patient from possible infection.
4. Provide privacy and help the woman assume a comfortable sitting position.	4. The let-down reflex may not occur readily if the woman is tense or nervous.
5. Help the woman place her right hand on her right breast, with her right thumb on the top of the breast at the outer limit of the areola and her right fingers underneath the breast. Tell the woman to press inward toward the chest wall (Fig. A).	5. Milk is expressed by pressure on the collecting ducts, not the nipple.

A

Procedure	Principle
6. Help the woman hold the collecting jar just under her nipple.	6. Collecting bottles should be made of plastic marked "safe for infants" as this best preserves antibodies found in milk; having the container close by prevents waste of any breast milk that is expressed.
7. Have the woman slide her hand forward in a milking motion, causing the milk to be expressed from the nipple into the container (Fig. B).	7. Pressure on the lactiferous sinuses pushes milk forward.

B

Procedure	Principle
8. Encourage the woman to move her thumb and fingers around her breast, repeating the technique.	8. Repeating the technique ensures all milk sinuses are emptied.
9. Caution the woman not to use excess force at any point when using the technique.	9. Excess force could damage sensitive breast tissue.
10. After collection, refrigerate milk if it will be used within 24 hours; freeze if this time is longer.	10. Breast milk spoils in the same manner as cow's milk if not protected.
11. Reinforce the woman's success with this maneuver, regardless of the amount of breast milk expressed.	11. Manual breast milk expression is an easy technique to carry out once it is learned, but it can be difficult to grasp at first. Positive reinforcement enhances progress and self-esteem.

BOX 19.5

Nursing Care Planning to Respect Cultural Diversity

Women are recognized as the "keepers of the culture," or the main people who transmit customs to the next generation. Chief among these customs is the preferred method for feeding newborns. The rate of breastfeeding varies in communities from almost 84.6% to a low of 30% as this is both sociodemographically and culturally influenced (AAP, 2012a). If a woman comes from a family where no one has ever breastfed, she may be very interested in being a "pioneer" in her family. Or, she may be more interested in following her family's tradition of formula feeding.

How soon women want to begin breastfeeding after birth is also culturally determined. Although it is recommended women begin this immediately after birth, some cultures believe colostrum is not appropriate for newborns and so have a cultural preference not to begin breastfeeding until milk is present, at about 3 days of age. Be certain to assess each family individually to recognize cultural preferences.

A mother should be taught how to properly take her newborn off the breast while he or she is sucking. This may be necessary if the latch is painful. Teach a woman to insert a clean finger with a short fingernail in the corner of the infant's mouth or pull down the infant's chin to release suction. Otherwise, the baby may pull too hard on the nipple, causing nipple cracking or soreness.

Promote Adequate Sucking. Often, a newborn being breastfed becomes sleepy at the breast, especially in the first 24 hours of life. Jaundice and hypoglycemia are also causes of sleepiness at the breast. To both stimulate milk production effectively and ensure adequate breast milk intake, a woman may need to keep the infant awake and urge him or her to suck. Placing the newborn skin to skin will often provide the proper environment to arouse the newborn to feed.

If an infant is not latching properly, a hospital-grade pump or hand expression may be used to provide express breast milk to the newborn.

Provide Immediate Support if Problems Arise. Successfully breastfeeding their newborn in the hospital increases the likelihood mothers will be successful breastfeeding after discharge (Perry, Ip, Chau, et al., 2013).

The nurse should provide an individual feeding plan to the mother upon discharge, ideally in consultation with an IBCLC. Early follow-up and referral to breastfeeding support groups will promote successful breastfeeding during the newborn period. The first 4 weeks postpartum are usually the most challenging for a new breastfeeding mother. After 4 weeks, breastfeeding, if successfully accomplished, is easier than formula feeding.

Provide Information Regarding Techniques for Burping the Breastfed Baby. Some infants seem to swallow little air when they breastfeed, whereas others swallow a great deal. As a rule, it is helpful to burp newborns after

A

B

Figure 19.4 **(A)** A sitting position for breastfeeding with a nursing pillow. **(B)** A football hold for breastfeeding. (Courtesy of Lourdes Forster, MD, FAAP. From Chung, E. K. [2010]. *Visual diagnosis and treatment in pediatrics.* Philadelphia, PA: Lippincott Williams & Wilkins.)

Figure 19.3 A side-lying position for breastfeeding.

TABLE 19.3 LATCH BREASTFEEDING CHARTING SYSTEM

	0	1	2
L: Latch	Too sleepy or reluctant; no latch achieved	Repeated attempts; necessary to hold nipple in mouth; stimulate to suck	Grasps breast; tongue down; lips flanged; rhythmic sucking
A: Audible swallowing	None	A few swallows with stimulation	Spontaneous and intermittent under 24 hr old; spontaneous and frequent over 24 hr old
T: Type of nipple	Inverted	Flat	Everted (after stimulation)
C: Comfort (breast/nipple)	Engorged; cracked, bleeding, large blisters, or bruises; severe discomfort	Filling; reddened/small blisters or bruises; mild/moderate discomfort	Soft, nontender
H: Hold (positioning)	Full assist (staff holds infant at breast)	Minimal assist (staff places pillows for support, elevates head of bed); teach one side, mother does other; mother takes over feeding	No assist from staff; mother able to position/hold baby by herself

Add up total score. A perfect score is 10, meaning a woman is ready to independently breastfeed.
From Jensen, D., Wallace, S., & Kelsay, P. (1994). LATCH: A breastfeeding charting system and documentation tool. *Journal of Obstetric, Gynecologic, and Neonatal Nursing, 23*(1), 27–32.

they have emptied the first breast and again after the total feeding to help evacuate air from their stomachs.

Placing the baby over one shoulder and gently patting or stroking the back is a time-honored position. However, this position is not always satisfactory for a newborn who has poor head control because a parent may have difficulty supporting the baby and patting the back at the same time.

Holding the baby in a sitting position on the lap and then leaning the child forward against one hand, with the index finger and thumb supporting the head, is often the best position to use. This position provides head support and leaves the other hand free to pat the baby's back (Fig. 19.5). Parents usually need to be shown this method because it does not seem as natural as placing a baby against the shoulder. Laying the baby prone across the lap is yet another alternative position.

Support for a Mother Who Is Breastfeeding Multiple Infants.
Because of in vitro fertilization, an increasing number of women are giving birth to multiple newborns. Reassure women they can provide breast milk to more than one newborn. Nurses can recommend pillow supports designed to allow twins to feed simultaneously. These pillows are similar to the pillows used to support one baby but are wider on the sides to support two babies for simultaneous feedings (Fig. 19.6).

Nursing Diagnosis: Pain related to breast engorgement or sore nipples

Outcome Evaluation: Patient states she is experiencing little or no discomfort; breastfeeds without undue discomfort; infant grasps nipple firmly. Nipples are intact with bruising or blisters. Nipple trauma may be evaluated using the following scale:

- Stage 1: superficial intact
- Stage 2: superficial with tissue breakdown
- Stage 3: partial erosion
- Stage 4: full thickness erosion (Mohrbacher, 2017)

On the third or fourth day after birth, when breast milk volume increases, women often notice breast distention, accompanied by hardness, and tenderness, and the skin may appear red, tense, and shiny. This is physiologic **engorgement**, caused by vascular and lymphatic congestion arising from an increase in the blood and lymph supply to the breasts. Newborns have difficulty latching when breasts are engorged because the areola can be too hard to grasp (Fig. 19.7). A woman also may have difficulty breastfeeding her newborn because her breasts are uncomfortable (Strong, 2011).

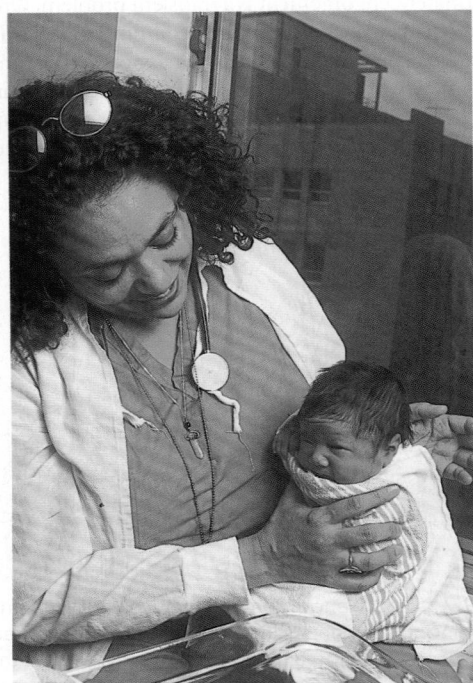

Figure 19.5 A nurse burps a newborn using a sitting position. Notice how the infant's head is supported by the nurse's hand.

Figure 19.6 Breastfeeding multiples. **(A)** Breastfeeding positions for mothers of multiples. (Copyright 2006 by Marvelous Multiples, Inc. Used with permission.) **(B)** The mother of twins may find a wider, firmer pillow easier to use when breastfeeding. (Photo of My Brest Friend Twin Nursing Pillow used with permission from My Brest Friend, https://www.mybrestfriend.com.)

Prevent or Relieve Engorgement. There are few evidence-based methods for relieving engorgement; a common suggestion is to empty the breasts of milk by having the infant feed more often. Unfortunately, a woman's breasts are sometimes so painful it is difficult for her to continue to breastfeed unless she is given something such as a mild analgesic for pain relief. Good breast support from a firm-fitting bra also helps prevent a pulling, heavy feeling.

If an infant cannot grasp a nipple to latch properly because of engorgement, moist heat applied to both breasts or standing under a warm shower for a few minutes before feeding, combined with massage to begin milk flow, often promotes breast softness so a newborn can suck. Manual expression or the use of a breast pump to completely empty the breasts after the baby has breastfed can help maintain or promote a good milk supply during a period of engorgement (Fig. 19.8).

Fortunately, engorgement is a transient problem. Unfortunately, it occurs just as women are beginning to feel skilled at breastfeeding. Because their breasts are swollen, hot, and tender, they may worry an infection has developed or their baby is not getting enough milk. Assure a mother that symptoms of engorgement are actually a normal finding. Assure her that engorgement is only temporary and should begin to subside 24 hours after it first became apparent. If engorgement persists after 24 hours or beyond the first week postpartum, the mother may be experiencing pathologic engorgement and should consult with an IBCLC. Excessive engorgement is a risk factor for mastitis, a breast infection.

Promote Healing of Sore Nipples. Painful nipples may result from:

- Improper positioning of the newborn. The newborn's body should face the mother with the head and body in alignment. The newborn's head should be at a level position or in the sniffing position. When the newborn's chin is on the chest, it cannot open its mouth wide enough to achieve a good latch.
- Improperly removing a newborn from the breast
- Prolonged breastfeeding for comfort after the newborn's nutritional needs are met
- Abnormalities of the palate and/or tongue. A palate that is high arched or flat may affect proper latching. An abnormal frenulum of the lip or tongue may prevent a proper latch. The infant can be provided expressed breast milk through pumping until evaluation by a lactation consultant.

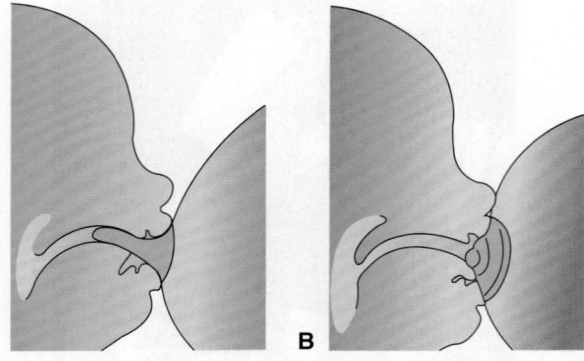

Figure 19.7 Breast engorgement may cause problems when breastfeeding. **(A)** When sucking at a nonengorged breast, the infant's lips compress the areola and fit neatly against the sides of the nipple. The infant also has adequate room to breathe. **(B)** When a breast is engorged, the infant has difficulty grasping the nipple. Breathing ability may also be compromised.

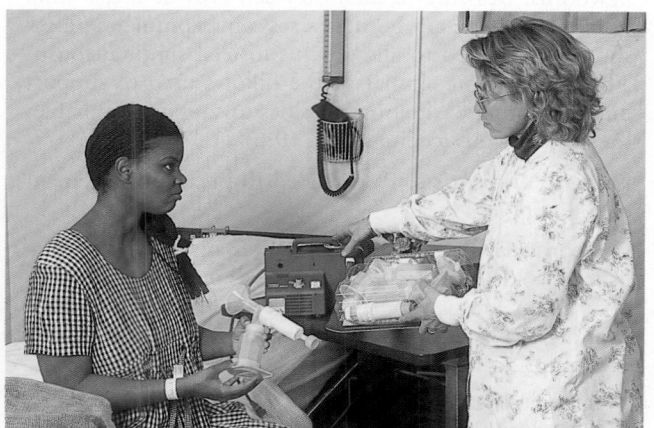

Figure 19.8 A nurse and mother discuss the advantages and disadvantages of an electric breast pump (shown on the table) and a manual pump (shown in the mother's hands).

• Improper use of the breast pump may cause sore nipples. Setting the vacuum at too high a pressure or pumping for an excessive period of time can damage the nipple. Fifteen minutes is usually sufficient to empty the breast. The breast flange comes in a several sizes to accommodate different size nipples. A flange that is an improper size can damage the nipple. Websites such as www.medela.com and www.ameda.com offer guidance on the proper sizing of the breast flange. Hospital pumps have a frequency setting in addition to a vacuum or pressure setting. The frequency should be set high (frequent cycles per minute) to mimic the sucking that a newborn provides at the breast until the milk begins to flow and the frequency can be decreased.

Appropriate nipple care is important to prevent skin breakdown of the nipples. The nurse can also recommend applying a few drops of breast milk to the nipples after feeding and gently massaging it into the areola. The components of breast milk have healing properties.

Sore nipples are not a contraindication to breastfeeding as long as a proper latch is obtained. If the latch is too painful, the mother can pump to provide expressed breast milk to her newborn and ensure her milk supply is protected. A nipple shield, worn while breastfeeding, can protect the nipple while the reasons for poor latch are determined (Figure 19.9A). A nipple shell is worn over the nipple in between feedings to promote healing and protect the nipple from irritation (Figure 19.9B).

Nursing Diagnosis: Anxiety related to inability to measure amount of milk taken by the baby

Outcome Evaluation: Mother states her newborn seems satisfied after feeding and voices confidence her baby is obtaining enough milk; baby voids six to eight times per day after the first week, stools are yellow and frequent, and the newborn is waking for 8 to 12 feedings in a 24-hour period.

Breastfeeding mothers may fear their newborns are not getting adequate amounts of breast milk at each feeding. This may be especially true when the newborn cries for reasons other than hunger. Mothers cannot measure the amount of breast milk the newborn ingests each feeding. Nurses can reassure mothers by instructing them to look for signs the newborn is voiding and defecating within the acceptable range and waking for feedings 8 to 12 times in 24 hours. The newborn can be weighed prior to and after a feeding to determine intake in instances where there are concerns. The scale must be calibrated and have the ability to detect weight gain as little as 2 g. If there are any concerns regarding the newborn's ability to transfer milk or the mother's milk supply, an early discharge appointment with their pediatric care provider is indicated.

What If . . . 19.2

Linda tells the nurse she is unsure her baby is getting enough milk when she breastfeeds. How would the nurse assure Linda that her baby is receiving adequate nutrition?

Nursing Diagnosis: Deficient knowledge related to potential harm to baby from drugs taken by breastfeeding mother

Outcome Evaluation: Mother states she is aware almost all drugs taken may be excreted in breast milk; voices importance of consulting her newborn's primary healthcare provider before taking any medication.

Medication and drugs ingested by the mother are present in human milk in varying degrees. Many factors affect the quantity of the substance in human milk. Substances may transfer to human milk if they obtain high concentrations in maternal plasma, are low in molecular weight (below 500), are low in protein binding, and are high in lipid solubility. The most important determinant is plasma level. As the mother's plasma level rises, the level in human milk rises. As soon as the mother's plasma level falls, an equilibrium forces the substance out of the human milk into the maternal plasma for elimination. This factor is important when considering the timing of substance ingestion by the mother and the timing of the newborn's feeding. Substances that are in human milk may not enter the newborn's circulation

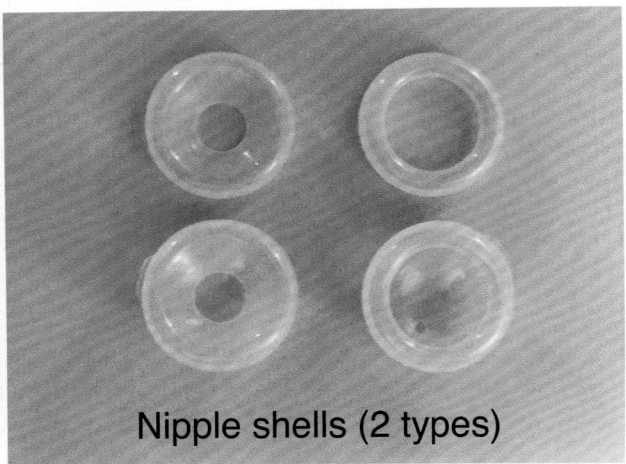

A   **B**

Figure 19.9 **(A)** Nipple shields. **(B)** Nipple shells.

due to several factors. The substance may be destroyed or fail to be absorbed by the newborn's gut. Premature infants (less than 34 weeks) may be more affected by substances than late preterm infants (34 to 36 6/7 weeks or full-term infants (37 or more weeks). During early lactation (days 1 to 3), the volume of milk the newborn ingests is small, so medication the mother is taking postdelivery is not a concern. If the relative infant dose is less than 10%, it is considered safe. Most medications are less than 1%. In most cases, the benefits of breastfeeding outweigh the risks of medication use by the mother. Encourage the mother to consult her pediatric care provider for guidance. A list of drugs breastfeeding mothers should avoid because of their documented harmful effects on infants is available at http://www.thePoint.com/Flagg8e (Hale & Rowe, 2017).

Nursing Diagnosis: Effective breastfeeding related to mother's desire to provide the best nutrition for her child

Outcome Evaluation: Mother states she intends to continue exclusive breastfeeding the first 6 months and add complementary foods at 6 months and continue breastfeeding through the first year and beyond if she desires.

Anticipate Potential Problems and Suggest Methods for Resolving Them. Common problems and solutions that can arise with breastfeeding once a mother returns home are summarized in Table 19.4.

Fatigue can be another problem on returning home if a woman does not take adequate measures to conserve her energy. Sitting relaxed in a comfortable chair with her feet elevated, feeding her baby, and enjoying this time are excellent ways to rest as well as to promote effective feeding.

Remind women a good fluid intake is necessary to maintain an adequate milk supply. Recommend they drink at least four 8-oz glasses of fluid a day; many may need to drink six glasses. They also need to increase their calorie intake by about 500 calories per day.

There are no dietary restrictions when breastfeeding other than eating uncooked or undercooked food, which could present a risk for bacterial infection. Alcohol and caffeine can affect the newborn and should be avoided by the breastfeeding mother.

Positive support by healthcare providers, family, friends and the work environment is important as a protective factor for continuation of breastfeeding.

QSEN Checkpoint Question 19.4

TEAMWORK & COLLABORATION

The discharge coordinator is discussing some of the statements made by Linda. Which of the following would indicate she needs further teaching about breastfeeding from the nurse?

  a. "I know breastfeeding is recommended for the first year of my baby's life."
  b. "To prevent nipple pain, I may need to vary the position I use to feed."
  c. "While breastfeeding, I need to drink at least 12 glasses of fluid a day."
  d. "I recognize that breastfeeding may help me lose some pregnancy weight."

Look in Appendix A for the best answer and rationale.

TABLE 19.4 COMMON CONCERNS OF BREASTFEEDING PARENTS

Concern	Cause	Nursing Interventions
Mother worries about amount of milk being taken.	Mother cannot see the amount taken.	Assure mother the best way to judge amount taken is to note whether infant appears content between feedings and is wetting diapers.
Infant does not suck well.	Possible effect of analgesia from labor.	Adjust feeding pattern to infant's needs; assure mother effect of analgesia is temporary.
	Mother is trying to feed when infant is not hungry.	
	Infant exhausted by crying from hunger.	Encourage rooming-in. Encourage feeding on hunger cues, not on a set schedule.
Mother reports infant's stools are loose and thin.	Stools should be looser and lighter in color than in formula-fed babies.	Examine stools; explain normal stool pattern and transitions.
Father feels shut out of parent–child relationship.	Father does not participate in infant feeding.	Show father other ways of interacting with infant than through feeding.
Mother reports sore nipples.	Infant is not gripping entire areola.	Help infant to grasp nipple correctly; expose nipple to air between feedings; aloe vera or lanolin applied to nipples helps heal tissue.
	The nipple is kept wet.	
Mother reports engorgement.	Lymphatic filling as milk production begins.	Encourage infant to suck (engorgement subsides best if infant can be encouraged to suck); apply warm packs to breasts or have mother take a warm shower before feeding to help soften breast tissue.
Mother is concerned about breastfeeding in public.	A woman may feel uncomfortable breastfeeding at work or other public places.	Encourage a woman to use discretion to avoid confrontation (unless she wants to make a point that breastfeeding is a natural action) and to speak to a work site administrator about comfortable arrangements.

Provide Information on Supplemental Feedings.
Mothers may ask about breast milk collection and storage in preparation for their return to work. Once the infant is sleeping a 4- or 5-hour stretch, the mother could pump after feeding the infant and collect that breast milk for future feedings (U.S. Department of Agriculture, 2016).

Bottles and nipples should be washed using normal dishwashing practice. An easy way to recall breast milk storage is 4 hours at room temperature, 4 days in the refrigerator, and 4 months in the freezer. The bottle used should be plastic and marked "safe for infant feeding"; otherwise, it may contain substances that can leech into stored milk and which may be associated with chromosomal aberrations (Rasmussen & Geraghty, 2011). Commercially prepared formula may be used if expressed breast milk is not available.

Provide Information for a Mother Who Works Outside the Home. Some women return to work while continuing to breastfeed by bringing their infants with them to their workplace. Others express breast milk for a caregiver to give by bottle while they work. As there are many considerations to think about, women should review with their employer the best way for them to continue successful breastfeeding at their work site (Payne & Nicholls, 2010). Federal law has provisions that entitle a mother to the time and a suitable place to pump while at work up through the first year of her child's life (Centers for Disease Control and Prevention, 2016) (Box 19.6).

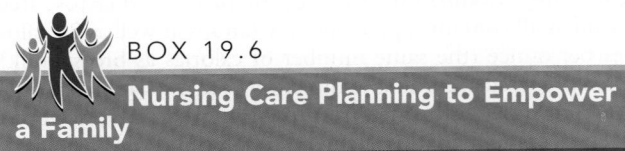

BOX 19.6

Nursing Care Planning to Empower a Family

SUGGESTIONS FOR RETURNING TO WORK WHILE BREASTFEEDING

Q. Linda Satir asks you, "How can I continue to breastfeed after I return to work in 6 weeks?"

A. Common suggestions include:

- Some women are able to arrange for child care near or at their work site so they can breastfeed at lunch or during a morning or afternoon break. Discuss with your employer or your immediate work supervisor whether this would be a possibility for you.
- Breastfeeding can be done in a public place, such as a lounge area, without undue exposure if you wear a smock-type or buttoned blouse that you lift or unfasten only as far as is necessary; covering any bared breast with a shawl or towel ensures modesty.
- If you are not able to breastfeed during work hours, you will need to express milk manually at least once during the day to maintain a milk supply. You might want to rent an electric pump to keep at work. Expressed breast milk can be safely stored in a refrigerator or in an iced container for 24 to 48 hours and used by your caregiver to feed the infant the next day.
- Plastic that does not contain bisphenol A is the best type of storage container for breast milk because antibodies apparently cling to glass and may therefore be lost to the milk.
- Any reminder of a baby may cause leaking of milk from breasts. Wear gauze pads inside your bra to prevent stains on your clothing and keep an extra change of clothing at work. Pressing against your breasts with the heel of your hands may be helpful in halting leakage.
- Drink four to six 8-oz glasses of fluid during the day to ensure a high fluid intake.
- Try to arrive early at your day care center or sitter so you can breastfeed just before leaving the baby.
- Fatigue can interfere with breastfeeding. Relax and enjoy your baby during the time you are home.

What If . . . 19.3
Linda tells the nurse she doesn't know how she will manage breastfeeding when she returns to work. How would the nurse advise her?

Provide Information on Weaning. The AAP (2016) recommends infants be exclusively breastfed for the first 6 months and breastfed with complementary foods for the first year of life; the World Health Organization recommends exclusive breastfeeding for 6 months and continuation for 2 years (U.S. Department of Agriculture, 2016) (Fig. 19.10).

Figure 19.10 Some women choose to breastfeed their child beyond 1 year of age. Accepting various preferences of this kind is important to care planning.

QSEN Checkpoint Question 19.5

SAFETY

When teaching Linda about newborn feeding, the nurse would include which statement(s) to reflect safety and evidence-based practice? Select all that apply.

a. Breastfeeding exclusively for 6 months can reduce the risk of obesity later in life.
b. Maternal benefits of breastfeeding include a decreased risk of breast and ovarian cancer.
c. Benefits to the infant from formula feeding include increased calcium density in the spine.
d. Once breastfeeding is established, pacifier use may help to decrease the risk of sudden infant death syndrome.

Look in Appendix A for the best answer and rationale.

Formula Feeding

Human milk is recognized as the ideal food for the newborn. There are many reasons why mothers do not breastfeed for the first year of life (Box 19.7). These may include partner unsupportive, prefer someone else feed the infant possibly due to maternal fatigue, nipple soreness, newborn fussy or difficult and question whether they are receiving adequate nutrition, returning to work or school, and real or perceived inadequate milk supply.

PREPARING FOR FORMULA FEEDING

Women should use commercial formulas for formula feeding if they choose not to breastfeed because they contain the recommended nutritional requirements.

Commercial Formulas

The contents of commercial formulas are supervised by the U.S. Food and Drug Administration (FDA). Formulas are

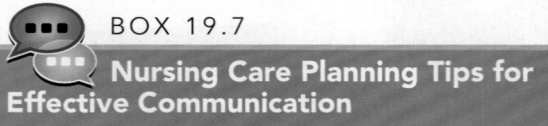

BOX 19.7

Nursing Care Planning Tips for Effective Communication

Mrs. Morgan, Linda's roommate in the hospital, is a new mother who has chosen to formula feed her newborn. You notice on the second day after birth she is studying her baby closely.

Tip: Avoid imposing your opinion on someone because it is not therapeutic. Allowing a woman to explain her individual situation helps you to understand the woman's decision and to offer her support.

Nurse: Is everything all right? You look worried.

Mrs. Morgan: I feel guilty I'm not breastfeeding.

Nurse: What made you decide not to breastfeed?

Mrs. Morgan: I work as an electrician at a construction site. I can't breastfeed or pump milk on a scaffold a hundred feet in the air in freezing weather.

Nurse: Let's talk about how formula feeding seems to be the best option for you.

available in three types: modified milk based, soy based, and elemental (fat, protein, and carbohydrate content is modified, such as in lactose-free formula). Modified milk-based formulas are used for the majority of newborns; lactose-free formulas are used for newborns with lactose intolerance or galactosemia (inability to use sugar). Soy formulas were devised for infants who are allergic to cow's milk protein, although such infants may be given casein hydrolysate formulas, which have protein particles too small to be recognized by the immune system. Elemental formulas are used for infants with protein allergies or fat malnutrition.

If the mother is not breastfeeding, then the newborn should be formula fed and continue on formula for the first year of life. Modified milk-based, soy-based, and lactose-free formulas all contain supplemental vitamins as well as 20 calories per ounce (the same number of calories as breast milk) when prepared according to directions. Advise parents to purchase formula with added iron to ensure that their newborn receives enough of this element to prevent iron-deficiency anemia (Szymlek-Gay, Lönnerdal, Abrams, et al., 2012). Participation in a supplemental food program, such as the Special Supplemental Nutrition Program for Women, Infants and Children (WIC), are available to help low-income parents afford formula (www.fns.usda.gov/wic).

Commercial formulas are supplied in four separate forms:
- Powder that is prepared by adding water as directed
- Condensed liquid that is diluted with an equal amount of water
- Ready-to-feed, which requires no dilution
- Individually prepackaged and prepared bottles of formula

The powder is the least expensive. A single bottle is easy to prepare by vigorous shaking. The prepackaged type does not need refrigeration or preparation (simply remove the bottle cap and it is ready), but it is the most expensive type. Cost should not be the only basis for a parent's choice, however. Tolerance of the formula by the infant and convenience for the parents are also factors.

Calculating a Formula's Adequacy

To calculate the adequacy of a formula, the following may be used:
1. The total fluid ingested for 24 hours must be sufficient to meet the infant's fluid needs: 75 to 90 ml (2.5 to 3 oz) of fluid per pound of body weight (150 to 200 ml/kg) per day.
2. The number of calories required per day is 50 to 55 per pound of body weight (100 to 120 kcal/kg).

For example, a 7-lb infant needs 17.5 to 21 oz (7 lb × 2.5 to 3 oz) of fluid per day. As commercial formula contains 20 calories per ounce, this amount will also supply the infant's calorie needs (350 to 420 calories per day). The total volume can be divided into six feedings of 3 to 3.5 oz each. A 9-lb infant would need 22.5 to 27 oz of fluid per day, supplying 450 to 540 calories per day.

A quick rule of thumb to estimate how much an infant will drink at a feeding is to add two or three to the infant's age in months. After initially taking 0.5 to 1 oz for the first 2 days, a newborn (0 age) will take 2 to 3 oz each feeding; a 3-month-old child, 5 to 6 oz; and a 6-month-old child, 8 oz. As infants change from six to five feedings a day (at about 4 months of age, when they begin to sleep through the night), they begin to take more at each feeding, keeping their total intake the same. Knowing the minimum requirements for fluid and calories per day, being able to calculate whether formula is adequate, and assessing if an infant appears content and is gaining weight allows for evaluating the adequacy of a formula-fed infant's intake.

 ## Nursing Diagnoses and Related Interventions

Nursing Diagnosis: Health-seeking behaviors related to techniques of formula feeding

Outcome Identification: Patient verbalizes knowledge of techniques of formula feeding by hospital discharge.

Provide Information Regarding Supplies Needed. Most parents today do not prepare a full day's supply of formula at once but rather prepare it bottle by bottle, as needed. Caution parents to keep opened cans of liquid formula covered and refrigerated, discarding any unused formula within 24 hours. They should use glass or plastic bottles that are noted to not contain polycarbonate (bisphenol A), as these are the only types safe for infant feeding (Centers of Disease Control and Prevention, 2016).

Nipples for bottles should be firm enough so an infant sucks vigorously. A soft, flabby nipple allows a baby to suck in milk so rapidly the need for sucking may not be satisfied. A way to judge a nipple's adequacy is to hold a bottle of milk with nipple attached upside down. The milk should drip from it at a rate of about one drop per second. Bottle caps to cover nipples are helpful to keep nipples clean when outdoors or during transport.

Provide Information Regarding Formula Preparation. Infant formula of any type must be prepared with careful attention to cleanliness to prevent pathogenic microorganisms from growing in it.

When using presterilized formula, the parent need only do the following to prepare a bottle of formula:

- Wash off the top of the can with warm, soapy water and rinse.
- Open the can and pour the desired amount of formula and water into a previously cleaned bottle.
- Put on the nipple, taking care not to handle the nipple projection.
- Place the bottle cap over the nipple and refrigerate or use to feed immediately.

If using powdered formula, the parent simply combines tap water and the measured amount of powder into a previously cleaned bottle, caps the bottle, and shakes it to mix the ingredients.

Provide Information Regarding Feeding Techniques. Whether to warm formula or not is a parental decision because infants who are fed cooled formula directly from the refrigerator seem to thrive as well as those who are fed warmed formula. The best method to warm formula is to stand the bottle in a bowl of warm water or hold it under a faucet of running hot water for a few minutes. Caution parents not to use a pan on the stove to warm formula because if the pan boils dry, the bottle of milk will burst.

It also is not recommended to warm bottles in a microwave oven because the milk in the center of the bottle can become hotter than that near the sides. Finally, with all warming methods, parents should test the temperature of the formula by allowing a drop or two to fall onto the inside of a wrist to make certain it is not overheated enough to burn the baby's mouth.

With any type of bottle, any contents remaining after a feeding should be discarded, not stored and reused. When sucking, an infant exchanges a small amount of saliva for milk. Because milk is a good growth medium for bacteria and everyone's mouth harbors many bacteria, the bacterial content in reused formula is likely to be high.

Like breastfeeding, formula feeding an infant is a skill that needs some practice. A parent needs a comfortable chair and adequate time (at least half an hour) to enjoy the process and not rush the baby (Fig. 19.11). Holding the baby with the head slightly elevated reduces the danger of aspiration and retention of air bubbles. Caution parents to be certain the nipple is kept filled so the baby sucks milk, not air. Babies in the early weeks should be burped to raise air from their stomach after every ounce of milk taken. The technique is the same as that used for breastfed infants.

Remind parents not to prop up bottles because babies are in danger of aspiration if a bottle is propped. In addition, an increased incidence of otitis media (middle ear infection) has been associated with bottle propping because the infant's head is not upright and formula may enter the eustachian tubes. Propping also can limit the amount of parent–child interaction. Another precaution is not to put a baby to bed with a bottle of formula. This practice can lead to "baby-bottle caries," or tooth decay of the lower teeth (Bishop, 2011) (see Chapter 29), because the formula remains in contact with the teeth for an extended time. Some common problems and solutions that can arise with formula feeding are summarized in Table 19.5.

Figure 19.11 A newborn receives a bottle feeding from her father. Notice the *en face* position: The father and baby are both looking directly at each other.

TABLE 19.5 COMMON CONCERNS OF FORMULA-FEEDING PARENTS

Concern	Possible Causes	Nursing Interventions
Infant sucks for a few minutes and then stops and cries.	Either nipple is blocked and infant is unable to get milk, or flow is too fast and baby has choking sensation.	Show parent how to test flow of milk from the nipple (hold bottle upside down); milk should flow from nipple at rate of about 1 drop per second.
Infant does not burp well after feeding.	Some infants swallow little air with feeding and so don't need extensive burping. Parent may be handling infant too tentatively or not burping effectively.	Observe baby feeding and parent's technique of handling; rubbing newborn's back may be more effective than patting it.
Parent reports constipation in infant.	Bowel movements from formula-fed infants are not as loose as those from breastfed infants, so parents may be concerned.	Examine stools; assure parent and explain normal stool pattern and that straining to pass stool is normal.

QSEN Checkpoint Question 19.6

QUALITY IMPROVEMENT

Linda's husband, Paul, plans to offer their baby bottled breast milk once daily when Linda returns to work. Educational literature available on the unit should include which guideline?

 a. He should stop feeding bottled milk if he notices the baby has loose yellow stools.
 b. He should microwave the milk for a full minute to be certain it is absolutely sterile.
 c. He should prop the bottle so the baby continues to enjoy breastfeeding best.
 d. After the baby drinks from a bottle, he should discard any milk still in the bottle.

Look in Appendix A for the best answer and rationale.

Discharge Planning for Newborn Nutrition

Mothers only remain in a hospital or birthing center for a short time, so teaching parents about either breastfeeding or formula feeding is crucial. Be certain to review a mother's plans for feeding her baby before discharge so there is time to answer any remaining questions. Connect the mother to local breastfeeding support groups in the area.

Review with the mother the criteria to use to assess if her infant is receiving adequate intake based on the recommended voiding and stooling pattern previously described.

Ensure the newborn has a follow-up appointment with a pediatric primary care provider. Nurses can increase a mother's self-confidence by empowering women to learn to make decisions regarding feeding and to not be reluctant to ask for help when they need it.

What If . . . 19.4

The nurse is interested in exploring one of the 2020 National Health Goals related to newborn nutrition (see Box 19.1). Most government-sponsored money for nursing research is allotted based on these goals. What would be a possible research topic to explore pertinent to these goals that would be applicable to the Satir family and that would also advance evidence-based practice?

KEY POINTS FOR REVIEW

- Human milk is the ideal food and the preferred feeding method for newborns because it provides antibodies as well as nutrients. Encourage all mothers to breastfeed by providing them with the knowledge, skill, and support to be successful. This helps in planning nursing care that not only meets QSEN competencies but best meets the family's total needs.

- Linoleic acid is an essential fatty acid that is necessary for growth and skin integrity and cannot be manufactured by the body. It is supplied by both infant formula and human milk but not by fat-free milk.

- Both breast milk and commercial formulas contain 20 kcal/oz. A term newborn requires 120 kcal/kg per day and 150 to 200 ml/kg of fluid per day.

- Encourage mothers who are breastfeeding to drink fluoridated water; formula-feeding mothers should prepare formula using fluoridated water to help build strong teeth in the infant.

- Both breastfed and partially breastfed newborns need supplemental vitamin D (400 IU). Newborns who are formula fed should be fed iron-fortified formula to avoid iron-deficiency anemia; breastfed babies may require an iron supplement for the same reason.

- Drugs pass into breast milk and their effects vary depending on their availability to accumulate in breast milk and the infant's ability to absorb the drug. A breastfeeding mother should consult with her child's pediatric care provider before discontinuing breastfeeding due to concerns with her medication usage. In most cases, the benefits of breastfeeding outweigh the risk of discontinuing breastfeeding due to the mother's medication use.

- If a baby will be formula fed, be certain the parents understand how to prepare the formula.

- Caution parents not to prop bottles because it increases the risk for aspiration and otitis media. It also deprives infants of the pleasure of being held for feedings.

- To avoid baby-bottle caries (decay of the lower teeth), advise parents not to put the newborn to bed with a bottle.

CRITICAL THINKING CARE STUDY

Shannon, 30 years old, and her husband, Jason, have three boys, with the youngest being 17 months old. Shannon has just given birth to her fourth child. Shannon is a smoker and wants to breastfeed her baby girl just like she did with all of her boys. Throughout the pregnancy, multiple ultrasounds were performed to check the baby's growth, which measured the infant 1 week under estimated gestational age. When the baby was born, she weighed 5 lb and 13 oz. In the birthing room, the infant did not latch.

1. Because of the infant's inability to latch on to the breast, what nursing interventions would you include in your plan of care for this infant?

2. On day 2, the newborn weighs 4 lb and 14 oz. Should you be concerned with the amount of weight loss? What should you do?

3. According to the AAP, what should you advise Shannon concerning her smoking habit and breastfeeding? Is her infant at an increased risk for sudden infant death syndrome?

RELATED RESOURCES

Explore these additional resources to enhance learning for this chapter:

• Student resources on thePoint, including answers to the What If . . . and Critical Thinking Care Study questions, http://thepoint.lww.com/Flagg8e

• Adaptive learning powered by PrepU, http://thepoint.lww.com/prepu

REFERENCES

Academy of Breastfeeding Medicine Protocol Committee. (2010a). ABM Clinical Protocol #7: Model breastfeeding policy (revision 2010). *Breastfeeding Medicine, 5*(4), 173–177.

Academy of Breastfeeding Medicine Protocol Committee. (2010b). ABM Clinical Protocol #22: Guidelines for management of jaundice in the breastfeeding infant equal to or greater than 35 weeks' gestation. *Breastfeeding Medicine, 5*(2), 87–93.

American Academy of Pediatrics. (2012a). *Fluoride supplements.* Elk Grove, IL: Author.

American Academy of Pediatrics. (2012c). *Where we stand: Fruit juice.* Elk Grove, IL: Author.

Baby-Friendly USA. (2012). *The ten steps to successful breastfeeding.* Retrieved from https://www.babyfriendlyusa.org/about-us/baby-friendly-hospital-initiative/the-ten-steps

Barnes, M., Cox, J., Doyle, B., et al. (2010). Evaluation of a practice-development initiative to improve breastfeeding rates. *The Journal of Perinatal Education, 19*(4), 17–23.

Bishop, W. P. (2011). Oral cavity. In K. J. Marcdante, R. M. Kliegman, R. E. Behrman, et al. (Eds.), *Nelson essentials of pediatrics* (6th ed., pp. 475–476). Philadelphia, PA: Saunders/Elsevier.

Centers of Disease Control and Prevention. (2016). *Parents and caregivers.* Retrieved from http://www.cdc.gov/sids/Parents-Caregivers.htm

Hale, T. W., & Rowe, H. E. (2017). *Medications & mothers' milk* (17th ed.). New York, NY: Springer Publishing.

Ip, S., Chung, M., Raman, G., et al. (2007). *Breastfeeding and maternal and infant health outcomes in developed countries* (AHRQ Publication No. 07-E007). Rockville, MD: Agency for Healthcare Research and Quality.

Lutter, C. K., & Morrow, A. L. (2013). Protection, promotion, and support and global trends in breastfeeding. *Advances in Nutrition, 4*(2), 213–219.

Mohrbacher, N. (2017). *Nipple pain & trauma: Causes & treatments.* Retrieved from http://lactspeak.com/nancymohrbacher/presentation/nipple-pain-trauma-causes-treatments/

Payne, D., & Nicholls, D. A. (2010). Managing breastfeeding at work: A Foucauldian secondary analysis. *Journal of Advanced Nursing, 66*(8), 1810–1818.

Perry, J. E., Ip, D. K., Chau, P. Y., et al. (2013). Predictors and consequences of in-hospital formula supplementation for healthy breastfeeding newborns. *Journal of Human Lactation, 29*(4), 527–536.

Rasmussen, K. M., & Geraghty, S. R. (2011). The quiet revolution: Breastfeeding transformed with the use of breast pumps. *American Journal of Public Health, 101*(8), 1356–1359.

Strong, G. D. (2011). Provider management and support for breastfeeding pain. *Journal of Obstetric, Gynecologic & Neonatal Nursing, 40*(6), 753–764.

Szymlek-Gay, E. A., Lönnerdal, B., Abrams, S. A., et al. (2012). α-Lactalbumin and casein-glycomacropeptide do not affect iron absorption from formula in healthy term infants. *The Journal of Nutrition, 142*(7), 1226–1231.

U.S. Department of Agriculture. (2016). *Infant feeding guide.* Retrieved from https://wicworks.fns.usda.gov/infants/infant-feeding-guide

U.S. Department of Health and Human Services. (2010). *Healthy people 2020.* Washington, DC: Author.

Wallby, T., Lagerberg, D., & Magnusson, M. (2017). Relationship between breastfeeding and early childhood obesity: Results of a prospective longitudinal study from birth to 4 years. *Breastfeeding Medicine, 12*, 48–53.

Wambach, K., & Riordan, J. (Eds.). (2016). *Breastfeeding and human lactation* (5th ed.). Burlington, MA: Jones & Bartlett.

UNIT 4

The Nursing Role in Caring for a Family During Complications of Pregnancy, Birth, or the Postpartal Period

Nursing Care of a Family Experiencing a Pregnancy Complication From a Preexisting or Newly Acquired Illness

*A*ngelina Gomez, 22 years old, is a gravida 1, para 0 woman, 34 weeks pregnant, whom you meet in the emergency room. Her electronic record shows you she had rheumatic fever with mitral valve stenosis as a child. During this pregnancy, she developed gestational diabetes. At 34 weeks, she has already been hospitalized twice for hyperglycemia. This afternoon, she fainted while participating in her weekly hour-long aerobics class. Her serum glucose at the moment is 207 mg/dl. Blood pressure is 90/40 mmHg; pulse rate is 130 beats/min; the fetal heart rate is 180 beats/min. A uterine monitor shows she is having moderate-strength contractions 7 minutes apart. Angelina asks you, "If exercise is supposed to be good for you, why did this happen?"

Previous chapters discussed normal pregnancy and the minor discomforts that may occur. This chapter adds information about illnesses and other events that can complicate pregnancy when they occur prior to or during pregnancy. As more women wait until they are older than age 30 years to have their first child, more and more women enter pregnancy with a preexisting disorder, such as cardiac or respiratory illness, that can complicate pregnancy.

How would you answer Angelina? Do you think she realizes pregnancy often becomes high risk not because of any one factor but an accumulation of them?

KEY TERMS

deep vein thrombosis (DVT)

glucose challenge test

glycosuria

glycosylated hemoglobin (HbA1c)

high-risk pregnancy

hyperglycemia

hypoglycemia

megaloblastic anemia

orthopnea

paroxysmal nocturnal dyspnea

peripartal cardiomyopathy

OBJECTIVES

After mastering the contents of this chapter, you should be able to:

1. Define *high-risk pregnancy*, including preexisting factors that contribute to its development such as diabetes mellitus or cardiovascular disease.
2. Identify 2020 National Health Goals related to complications of pregnancy that nurses can help the nation achieve.
3. Assess a woman with an illness during pregnancy for changes occurring in the illness because of the pregnancy or in the pregnancy because of the illness.
4. Formulate nursing diagnoses related to the effect of a preexisting or newly acquired illness on pregnancy.
5. Identify expected outcomes that will contribute to a safe pregnancy outcome when illness occurs with pregnancy as well as help families manage seamless transitions across differing healthcare settings.
6. Using the nursing process, plan nursing care that includes the six competencies of Quality & Safety Education for Nurses (QSEN): Patient-Centered Care, Teamwork & Collaboration, Evidence-Based Practice (EBP), Quality Improvement (QI), Safety, and Informatics.
7. Implement nursing care for a woman when illness complicates pregnancy, such as teaching her how to measure blood glucose.
8. Evaluate expected outcomes for achievement and effectiveness of care.
9. Integrate knowledge of high-risk pregnancy and the interplay of nursing process, the six competencies of QSEN, and Family Nursing to promote quality maternal and child health nursing care.

Although pregnancy can be a stressful time, generally, women experience overall good health during pregnancy, perhaps in part because of their extra care and concern in keeping healthy for two. This extra motivation also encourages a woman with a high-risk pregnancy to carefully follow a therapeutic regimen established for her to keep herself and her fetus safe.

Unit 4 addresses the nursing role and care you might provide to families with pregnancy complications, which are common. This chapter focuses on women who enter pregnancy with a chronic condition, such as cardiovascular or kidney disease, and those who experience unintentional injury or develop a chronic illness during pregnancy. Both the woman and the fetus can be at risk for complications. Either the pregnancy can complicate the disease or the disease can complicate the pregnancy, affecting the fetus or leaving the woman less equipped to function in the future or undergo a future pregnancy. Nursing care needs to include close observation of both maternal health and fetal well-being, education for the woman and her family about special danger signs to watch for during pregnancy, and actions to minimize complications whenever possible, including:

- Preventing disorders from affecting the health of the fetus
- Helping a woman regain her health as quickly as possible so she can continue a healthy pregnancy and prepare herself psychologically and physically for labor, birth, and the arrival of her newborn
- Helping a woman learn more about her illness so she can continue to safeguard her health during her childrearing years

Conditions that cause severe symptoms such as a marked change in fluid and electrolyte balance, altered cardiovascular or respiratory function, or severe blood loss are especially dangerous to a fetus (Gregory, Korst, Lu, et al., 2013). Because of this danger, 2020 National Health Goals related to complications of pregnancy have been established (Box 20.1).

BOX 20.1

Nursing Care Planning Based on 2020 National Health Goals

Several National Health Goals are aimed at reducing complications of pregnancy that arise from existing or newly acquired disorders.

- Reduce the rate of fetal deaths to 5.6 per 1,000 live births from a baseline of 6.2 per 1,000 live births.
- Reduce the rate of maternal deaths to 11.4 per 100,000 live births from a baseline of 12.7 per 100,000 live births.
- Reduce the rate of maternal illness and complications during pregnancy to 28 per 100 births from a baseline of 31.1 per 100 births (U.S. Department of Health and Human Services, 2010; see www.healthypeople.gov).

Nurses can help the nation reach these goals by educating women about the importance of entering pregnancy in the best state of health possible. Helping women who have diabetes mellitus understand the importance of pre-pregnancy care so they enter pregnancy without hyperglycemia is an important step toward reducing congenital anomalies in newborns. Supporting women with kidney, heart, or respiratory disease during pregnancy to continue to follow their medical regimen is yet another way.

Nursing Process Overview

FOR CARE OF A WOMAN WITH A PREEXISTING OR NEWLY ACQUIRED ILLNESS

ASSESSMENT

An accurate prenatal assessment of a woman with a preexisting or newly acquired illness requires a thorough understanding of the signs and symptoms of the illness in addition to an understanding of the course of a normal pregnancy (Fig. 20.1). Assessment techniques include objective measures such as establishing baseline vital signs as well as subjective factors such as the extent of edema or level of exhaustion a woman is experiencing. Such assessment is best made by healthcare personnel who care for a woman consistently throughout the pregnancy so that subtle changes can be recognized. It's also important to teach a woman how to assess her own health in relation to objective parameters. She could report exhaustion, for example, in relation to daily activity such as "Two weeks ago I could walk a block without being short of breath. Today I could walk only half a block" or "The last time I was in for a checkup, edema didn't occur until bedtime. Now I notice it every afternoon by the time my son comes home from school."

NURSING DIAGNOSIS

Nursing diagnoses developed for a woman with a high-risk pregnancy address her specific, disease-related condition as well as any therapeutic restrictions her condition might require. Examples of possible nursing diagnoses include:

- Ineffective tissue perfusion (cardiopulmonary) related to poor heart function secondary to mitral valve prolapse during pregnancy
- Pain related to pyelonephritis secondary to uterine pressure on ureters
- Social isolation related to prescribed bed rest during pregnancy secondary to concurrent illness
- Ineffective role performance related to increasing level of daily restrictions secondary to chronic illness and pregnancy

Figure 20.1   It is important to establish baseline vital signs to later identify a complication related to a preexisting condition. (Monkey Business Images/Shutterstock.com)

- Knowledge deficit related to normal changes of pregnancy versus illness complications
- Fear regarding pregnancy outcome related to chronic illness
- Health-seeking behaviors related to the effects of illness on pregnancy
- Situational low self-esteem related to illness during pregnancy

OUTCOME IDENTIFICATION AND PLANNING

Be certain that expected outcomes are realistic in light of a woman's pregnancy and the restrictions placed on her by her health. Remember that one family member with illness affects all family members; therefore, outcomes should relate to the entire family's health.

When making plans with a woman who has a preexisting medical condition, base them on the pattern of her life before the pregnancy. For example, to ensure a pregnant woman receives enough rest during pregnancy, planning for an afternoon rest period each day is usually adequate. However, for a woman with cardiac disease who took two rest periods a day before pregnancy, this would be ineffective because now she probably needs four rest periods. A primary goal for a woman with a severe chronic condition might be to maintain her health during pregnancy so she can remain at home as long as possible, thereby minimizing hospitalization and family disruptions.

Planning for a new illness may be difficult for a woman because of the shock of the diagnosis. Be careful, however, not to make plans for her such as "Your best plan would be to begin strict bed rest." Instead, give a woman the available alternatives such as "There are two possible therapies. Let me review with you the advantages and disadvantages of each one." Allowing a woman to choose among alternatives in this way helps her to participate in her own care and also maintain self-esteem as well as helps her move a step toward parenthood and assuming care for her family.

Refer women and their families to online resources for further information when appropriate. Helpful resources addressing complications of pregnancy and childbirth and support programs are available.

ONLINE RESOURCES

Complications of Pregnancy and Childbirth

American Diabetes Association	www.diabetes.org
American Heart Association	www.americanheart.org
American Pregnancy Association	www.americanpregnancy.org
American Sudden Infant Death Syndrome (SIDS) Institute: a nonprofit dedicated to research, education, and family support promoting infant health	www.sids.org
Centers for Disease Control and Prevention	www.cdc.gov
International Cesarean Awareness Network	www.ican-online.org
March of Dimes Association: a nonprofit that provides patient education on cesarean birth, high-risk newborns, and children born with physical or developmental challenges	www.marchofdimes.com
National Kidney Foundation	www.kidney.org
Sickle Cell Disease Association of America	www.sicklecelldisease.org

Support Programs for Families

Alcoholics Anonymous	www.aa.org
Cleft Palate Foundation	www.cleftline.org
Easterseals Disability Services	www.easterseals.com
Girlshealth.gov: a government program that works to reduce teenage pregnancy	www.girlshealth.gov
Narcotics Anonymous	www.na.org
Newborn Individualized Developmental Care and Assistance Program (NIDCAP) Federation International	www.nidcap.org
Postpartal Support International: a support network for women who are depressed after childbirth	www.postpartum.net
Spina Bifida Association: support network for children and families with spina bifida	www.spinabifidaassociation.org
Substance Abuse and Mental Health Services Administration	www.samhsa.gov

IMPLEMENTATION

Nursing interventions for a pregnant woman with a chronic illness may focus on teaching her new or additional measures to maintain health during the pregnancy. Imaginative solutions to problems may need to be created because, otherwise, a woman may be unable to adjust to the extent of changes she must make.

OUTCOME EVALUATION

If an evaluation of outcomes at healthcare visits reveals that an expected outcome is not being met, a new assessment, analysis, and planning need to be done. In some instances, an outcome is not met because a woman did not understand the need for an additional pregnancy measure. At other times, a woman may need better psychological support to continue to follow a healthcare routine consistently because 9 months is a long time to adhere to restrictions. Make evaluation ongoing to ensure that you know throughout the pregnancy whether interventions are successful. Some examples of outcomes that might be established include:

- Patient states she rests for 2 hours morning and afternoon; dependent edema remains at 1+ or less at next prenatal visit.
- Family members state they are all participating in an exercise program since mother developed gestational diabetes.
- Patient reports no burning on urination or flank pain at next prenatal visit.
- Patient states she understands the importance of taking daily thyroid medicine for total length of pregnancy.

The Nursing Role and Nursing Care During Pregnancy Complications

All types of women desire pregnancy, including those with an underlying disease process, such as diabetes or heart disease, which can worsen with pregnancy. Some complications lead to early pregnancy loss or preterm delivery (see Chapter 21). Other complications arise due to specific characteristics of the mother, such as her age or her use of substances (see Chapter 22). Still, other complications happen during labor itself, related to contractions, to the mother's pelvis, or to the baby (see Chapter 23). At times, complications in pregnancy or during labor lead to cesarean delivery, and nurses need to be prepared to care for the family experiencing this type of delivery (see Chapter 24). Infections or bleeding can also occur in the postpartum period, which can complicate a mother's recovery (see Chapter 25).

IDENTIFYING A HIGH-RISK PREGNANCY

A **high-risk pregnancy** is one in which a concurrent disorder, pregnancy-related complication, or external factor jeopardizes the health of the woman, the fetus, or both.

It's important that women with such pregnancies be identified because illness during pregnancy can complicate not only the pregnancy but also a woman's entire lifestyle and that of her family. In most instances, more than one factor contributes to the classification of a pregnancy as high risk. The pregnancy of a woman with diabetes, for example, is automatically considered as having a greater-than-normal risk because it forces a fetus to grow in an environment in which **hyperglycemia** (increased serum glucose levels) becomes the rule. During such a pregnancy, a woman, worrying that something will happen to her baby, may fail to begin the "pregnancy work" that she must do so bonding can take place. At birth, her child is in double jeopardy: Not only is the baby born with altered glucose metabolism but he or she also is at high risk for poor maternal–child or parent–child attachment.

Remembering that the term "high risk" rarely refers to just one causative factor but includes psychological and social as well as physical aspects helps in the planning of holistic, and ultimately effective, nursing care. Preexisting or newly acquired maternal illnesses that can make a pregnancy high risk are discussed in this chapter. Chapter 21 discusses conditions directly related to pregnancy that can make a pregnancy high risk. Chapter 22 covers populations that are at high risk because of age (younger than 18 years or older than 40 years), the presence of a disability or trauma, or drug abuse.

Cardiovascular Disorders and Pregnancy

The number of women of childbearing age who have heart disease is diminishing as more and more congenital heart anomalies (discussed in Chapter 41) are corrected in early infancy. Also, rheumatic fever is being more actively prevented and treated so that cardiac damage from this disorder is also reduced. For these reasons, cardiovascular disease (even with hypertension included), which was once a major threat to pregnancy, now complicates only approximately 1% of all pregnancies. Cardiovascular disease is still a concern in pregnancy, however, because it can lead to such serious complications. It is responsible for 5% of maternal deaths during pregnancy (Cunningham, Leveno, Bloom, et al., 2014).

The cardiovascular disorders that most commonly cause difficulty during pregnancy are valve damage concerns caused by rheumatic fever or Kawasaki disease and congenital anomalies such as atrial septal defect or uncorrected coarctation of the aorta (Gordon, Jimenez-Fernandez, Daniels, et al., 2014). Aortic dilatation may occur from Marfan syndrome and is also a concern (Easterling & Stout, 2012). As the number of women delaying their first pregnancy until later in life increases, there is a corresponding increase in the incidence of coronary artery disease and varicosities during pregnancy. In contrast, heart disease that occurs specifically with pregnancy (peripartum heart disease) still only rarely occurs as it is apparently unrelated to age. With improved management of women with cardiac disorders, women who might never have risked pregnancy in the past are able to complete pregnancies successfully today.

A woman with cardiovascular disease needs an interprofessional team approach to care during pregnancy. Ideally, she should visit her pregnancy care provider for preconception care so her state of health and baseline data when she is not pregnant can be established. She should begin prenatal care as soon as she suspects she is pregnant (1 week after the first missed menstrual period or as soon as she has a positive home pregnancy test), so her general condition and circulatory system can be monitored from the beginning of pregnancy.

Pregnancy taxes the circulatory system of every woman, even those without cardiac disease, because both the blood volume and cardiac output increases approximately 30% (and up to as much as 50%) during pregnancy. Half of this increase occurs by 8 weeks; it is maximized by midpregnancy (Ayad, Hassanein, Mohamed, et al., 2016).

Because of the increased blood flow past valves, functional (innocent) or transient murmurs can be heard in many women without heart disease during pregnancy. Heart palpitations on sudden exertion are also usual.

The danger of pregnancy in a woman with cardiac disease occurs primarily because of this increase in circulatory volume. The most dangerous time for her is in weeks 28 to 32, just after the blood volume peaks. However, if heart disease is severe, symptoms can occur at the very beginning of pregnancy. Toward the end of pregnancy, her heart may become so overwhelmed by the increase in blood volume that her cardiac output falls to the point vital organs (including the placenta) can no longer be perfused adequately. When this happens, the oxygen and nutritional requirements of her cells and those of the fetus are not met.

The estimation of whether a woman with cardiovascular disease can complete a pregnancy successfully depends on the type and extent of her disease. As a rule, a woman with an artificial but well-functioning heart valve, a woman with a pacemaker implant, and even a woman who has had a heart transplant can expect to have successful pregnancies as long as they have effective prenatal and postnatal care (Abdalla & Mancini, 2014).

To predict a pregnancy outcome, heart disease is divided into four categories based on criteria established by the New York Heart Association (Table 20.1). A woman with

TABLE 20.1 CLASSIFICATION OF HEART DISEASE

Class	Description
I	Uncompromised. Ordinary physical activity causes no discomfort. No symptoms of cardiac insufficiency and no anginal pain.
II	Slightly compromised. Ordinary physical activity causes excessive fatigue, palpitation, and dyspnea or anginal pain.
III	Markedly compromised. During less than ordinary activity, woman experiences excessive fatigue, palpitations, dyspnea, or anginal pain.
IV	Severely compromised. Woman is unable to carry out any physical activity without experiencing discomfort. Even at rest, symptoms of cardiac insufficiency or anginal pain are present.

From Criteria Committee of the New York Heart Association. (1994). *Nomenclature and criteria for diagnosis of diseases of the heart and great vessels* (9th ed.). Boston, MA: Little, Brown & Co.

class I or II heart disease can expect to experience a normal pregnancy and birth. Women with class III can complete a pregnancy by maintaining special interventions such as bed rest. Women with class IV heart disease are usually advised to avoid pregnancy because they are in cardiac failure even at rest and when they are not pregnant.

A WOMAN WITH CARDIAC DISEASE

Cardiac disease can affect pregnancy in different ways depending on whether it involves the left or the right side of the heart.

A Woman With Left-Sided Heart Failure

Left-sided heart failure occurs in conditions such as mitral stenosis, mitral insufficiency, and aortic coarctation. In these instances, the left ventricle cannot move the large volume of blood forward that it has received by the left atrium from the pulmonary circulation. This causes back pressure—the left side of the heart becomes distended, systemic blood pressure decreases in the face of lowered cardiac output, and pulmonary hypertension occurs. When pressure in the pulmonary vein reaches a point of about 25 mmHg, fluid begins to pass from the pulmonary capillary membranes into the interstitial spaces surrounding the lung alveoli and then into the alveoli themselves (pulmonary edema). Pulmonary edema produces profound shortness of breath as it interferes with oxygen–carbon dioxide exchange (Brashers & Huether, 2017). If pulmonary capillaries rupture under the pressure, small amounts of blood leak into the alveoli and the woman develops a productive cough with blood-speckled sputum. Because of the limited oxygen exchange, a woman with left-sided heart failure is at an extremely high risk for spontaneous miscarriage, preterm labor, or even maternal death. As pulmonary edema becomes severe, a woman cannot sleep in any position except with her chest and head elevated (**orthopnea**), as elevating her chest this way allows fluid to settle to the bottom of her lungs and frees space for gas exchange. She may also notice **paroxysmal nocturnal dyspnea**—suddenly waking at night with shortness of breath. This occurs because heart action is

more effective when she is at rest. With the more effective heart action, interstitial fluid returns to the circulation. This overburdens her circulation, causing increased left-side failure and increased pulmonary edema.

If mitral stenosis is present, it is so difficult for blood to leave the left atrium that a secondary problem of thrombus formation can occur from noncirculating blood. If coarctation of the aorta is causing the difficulty, dissection of the aorta from high blood pressure from trying to push blood past the constriction can occur. To prevent thrombus formation, a woman may be prescribed an anticoagulant. If an anticoagulant is required, low–molecular-weight heparin is the drug of choice for early pregnancy because it does not cross the placenta and so does not have teratogenic effects. To decrease the strain on the aorta, antihypertensives may be prescribed to control blood pressure, diuretics to reduce blood volume, and β-blockers to improve ventricular filling. A woman will be scheduled for serial ultrasound and nonstress tests after weeks 30 to 32 of pregnancy to monitor fetal health and to rule out poor placental perfusion (Dennis, 2016).

A Woman With Right-Sided Heart Failure

Right-sided heart failure occurs when the right ventricle is overwhelmed by the amount of blood received by the right atrium from the vena cava. It can be caused by an unrepaired congenital heart defect such as pulmonary valve stenosis, but the anomaly most apt to cause right-sided heart failure in women of reproductive age is Eisenmenger syndrome, a right-to-left atrial or ventricular septal defect with an accompanying pulmonary valve stenosis (Bhatt & DeFaria Yeh, 2015).

With this, congestion of the systemic venous circulation and decreased cardiac output to the lungs occurs. Blood pressure decreases in the aorta because less blood is able to reach it; in contrast, pressure is high in the vena cava from back pressure of blood. Both jugular venous distention and increased portal circulation are evident. The liver and spleen both become distended. Extreme liver enlargement can cause dyspnea and pain in a pregnant woman because the enlarged liver, as it is pressed upward by the enlarged uterus, puts extreme pressure on the diaphragm. Distention of abdominal and lower extremity vessels can lead to exudate of fluid from the vessels into the peritoneal cavity (i.e., ascites) or peripheral edema.

Women who have an uncorrected anomaly of this type may be advised not to become pregnant. If they do plan a pregnancy, because they need oxygen administration and frequent arterial blood gas assessments to ensure fetal growth, they can expect to be hospitalized for at least some days during the last part of pregnancy. During labor, they may need a pulmonary artery catheter inserted to monitor pulmonary pressure. Women with this condition also need extremely close monitoring after epidural anesthesia to minimize the risk of hypotension.

A WOMAN WITH PERIPARTUM HEART DISEASE

An extremely rare condition, **peripartal cardiomyopathy**, can originate in pregnancy in women with no previous history of heart disease (Desplantie, Tremblay-Gravel, Avram, et al., 2015). Although the cause is unknown, this apparently occurs because of the stress of the pregnancy on the circulatory system. The mortality rate can be as high as 50%.

It occurs most often in Black multiparas in conjunction with gestational hypertension. A woman develops signs of myocardial failure such as shortness of breath, chest pain, and nondependent edema. Her heart increases in size (i.e., cardiomegaly). For therapy, she must sharply reduce her physical activity; many women also need a diuretic, an arrhythmia agent, and digitalis therapy to maintain heart function. Low–molecular-weight heparin may be administered to decrease the risk of thromboembolism. Immunosuppressive therapy is yet another possibility to improve symptoms.

If the cardiomegaly persists past the postpartum period, it is generally suggested a woman not to attempt any further pregnancies because the condition tends to recur or worsen in additional pregnancies. At the same time, oral contraceptives are contraindicated because of the danger of thromboembolism that these can create. Some women's disease progresses so much that following pregnancy, a woman may need a heart transplant (Dalzell, Cannon, Simpson, et al., 2015).

ASSESSMENT OF A WOMAN WITH CARDIAC DISEASE

Nurses play a major role in the care of pregnant women with cardiovascular disease because continuous assessment of women's health status, health education, and health-promotion activities are so essential. Assessment begins with a thorough health history to document prepregnancy cardiac status (Box 20.2). Document a woman's level of exercise performance (i.e., what level she can do before growing short of breath and what physical symptoms she experiences, such as cyanosis of the lips or nail beds). Ask if she normally has a cough or edema (it's important that women with cardiac disease always report coughing during pregnancy because pulmonary edema from heart failure may first manifest itself as a simple cough).

Documenting edema is also important because the usual innocent edema of pregnancy must be distinguished from the beginning of edema from heart failure (serious). An important difference is the usual edema of pregnancy involves only the feet and ankles but becomes systemic with heart failure. It can begin as early as the first trimester, and other symptoms such as irregular pulse, rapid or difficult respirations, and perhaps chest pain on exertion will probably also be present. Be certain to record a baseline blood pressure, pulse rate, and respiratory rate in either a sitting or lying position at the first prenatal visit; at future health visits, always obtain these in the same position for the most accurate comparison. Making comparison assessments for nail bed filling (should be <5 seconds) and jugular venous distention can also be helpful throughout pregnancy.

If a woman's heart disease involves right-sided heart failure, assess liver size at prenatal visits. Keep in mind that liver assessments can become difficult and probably inaccurate late in pregnancy because the enlarged uterus presses the liver upward under the ribs and makes it difficult to palpate.

For an additional cardiac status assessment, an electrocardiogram (ECG) or an echocardiogram may be done at periodic points in pregnancy. Assure the woman that an ECG merely measures cardiac electrical discharge and so cannot harm her fetus in any way. Echocardiography uses ultrasound and, likewise, will not harm her fetus.

FETAL ASSESSMENT

At the point that maternal blood pressure becomes insufficient to provide an adequate supply of blood and nutrients

BOX 20.2

Nursing Care Planning Using Assessment

ASSESSING A PREGNANT WOMAN WITH CARDIAC DISEASE

Fatigue

Cough

Increased respiratory rate

Tachycardia

Poor fetal heart tone (FHT) variability from poor tissue perfusion

Decreased amniotic fluid from intrauterine growth restriction

Edema from poor venous return

to the placenta, fetal health can be compromised. For this reason, the infants of women with severe heart disease tend to have low birth weights or be small for gestational age because of acidosis, which develops due to poor oxygen/carbon dioxide exchange or not being furnished with enough nutrients. This can result in preterm labor, which exposes the newborn to the hazards of immaturity as well as low birth weight. If the placenta is not filling well, a fetus may not respond well to labor (evidenced by late deceleration patterns on a fetal heart monitor), and a cesarean birth may be necessary (an increased risk for both the mother and fetus).

Nursing Diagnoses and Related Interventions

Nursing Diagnosis: Deficient knowledge regarding steps to take to reduce the effects of maternal cardiovascular disease on the pregnancy and fetus

Outcome Evaluation: Patient identifies danger signs such as angina pain and steps to take when they occur; maternal blood pressure is maintained above 100/60 mmHg and fetal heart rate at 110 to 160 beats/min.

Be certain that goals and outcomes established with a woman with heart disease are realistic. Not all women with heart disease, for example, will be able to complete a pregnancy successfully; some infants of women with severe involvement will be born with the effects of placental insufficiency, such as neurologic involvement or cognitive challenge. However, there are positive actions a woman with heart disease can take to reduce or eliminate complications during pregnancy, such as increasing periods of rest to strengthen heart action.

Promote Rest. As a rule, women with cardiac disease need two rest periods a day (fully resting, not getting up frequently) and a full night's sleep (not tossing and turning) to obtain adequate rest. Rest should be in the left lateral recumbent position to prevent supine hypotension syndrome and increased heart effort.

Women should plan activities so they stop exercising before the point when cardiac output becomes insufficient to meet systemic body demands causing peripheral and uterine/placental constriction. Be certain they know exactly how much they should limit their exercise. Some women, for example, may need to discontinue employment early in pregnancy rather than work until the end. A prescription to allow "normally heavy" housework may mean nothing more strenuous than dusting to some women. To others, it may mean washing windows, turning mattresses, and shoveling snow. Ask enough questions, therefore, to make certain a woman's definition of "heavy work" is the same as yours and her primary care provider's.

Promote Healthy Nutrition. A woman with cardiac disease may need closer supervision of nutrition during pregnancy than the average woman because she must gain enough weight to ensure a healthy pregnancy and a healthy baby, but she must not gain so much weight that her heart and circulatory system become overburdened.

Be certain she is remembering to take her prenatal vitamins. These contain an iron supplement to help prevent anemia. Anemia is important to prevent because it places an extra burden on the heart because her circulatory system must circulate blood more vigorously than usual to distribute oxygen to all body cells. If a woman was following a sodium-restricted diet before pregnancy, this may be continued during pregnancy; although typically, a woman's sodium intake is only limited, not severely restricted, during pregnancy because it's important to obtain enough sodium to maintain fluid volume and balance as well as furnish an adequate supply of blood to the fetus.

Educate Regarding Medication. Women taking cardiac medication, such as digoxin, before pregnancy may need to increase their maintenance dose because of their expanded blood volume during pregnancy. A woman who was not digoxin dependent before pregnancy may need such therapy prescribed as pregnancy advances and her cardiac output has to be increased or strengthened.

To aid a woman in continuing to think of herself as basically a well person, help her to understand this does not mean her heart function is weakening, but rather, it is only temporarily being stressed by the increased circulatory load of pregnancy. Digoxin also has a unique use during pregnancy as it can be administered to the woman to slow the fetal heart if fetal tachycardia is present. Antihypertensive and arrhythmia agents such as adenosine, β-blockers, and calcium channel blockers to reduce hypertension are safe to use during pregnancy and are also frequently prescribed. Nitroglycerin, a compound often prescribed for angina, although not well studied during pregnancy (a category C drug), is also considered safe (Karch, 2015).

A woman who was taking penicillin prophylactically because she had rheumatic fever as a child (which is often taken for 10 years after the occurrence of rheumatic fever, or at least until age 18 years) should continue to take this drug during pregnancy because penicillin is not known to be a teratogen (a category B drug). Close to the anticipated day of birth, some primary care providers prescribe an additional course of ampicillin, amoxicillin (Amoxil), or clindamycin (Cleocin) to prevent streptococci bacteria from invading the denuded placental site on the uterus and creating a subacute bacterial endocarditis.

It is often difficult to keep healthy women from taking over-the-counter medicines during pregnancy; conversely, it can be just as difficult to encourage women to take medicine prescribed during pregnancy. Help women with heart disease to understand there are valid exceptions to the rule of "no medicine during pregnancy" so they make out reminders to adhere to their prescribed regimen.

What If . . . 20.1

Angelina is diagnosed as having class II heart disease. Because of her work as a fundraiser, she is on her feet all day. What suggestions could the nurse make to help her incorporate more rest into each day?

Educate Regarding Avoidance of Infection. A systemic infection almost automatically increases body temperature, forcing a woman to expend more energy and increase her cardiac output as her metabolism increases, an effect that could be too extreme for a woman with heart disease to withstand. Caution women with heart disease, therefore, to avoid visiting or being visited by people with infections and to alert healthcare personnel at the first indication of an upper respiratory tract infection or urinary tract infection (UTI) so that, if warranted, antibiotic therapy can begin early in the course of the infection. Monthly screening for bacteriuria with a clean-catch urine test at prenatal visits should help detect UTIs.

Be Prepared for Emergency Actions. If women with heart disease overexert during a prenatal visit, they may need supplemental oxygen or cardiac resuscitation. The rules for cardiac resuscitation for women who are pregnant do not differ from the usual technique (Box 20.3).

BOX 20.3

Nursing Care Planning Using Procedures

CARDIOPULMONARY RESUSCITATION DURING PREGNANCY

Purpose: To restore cardiac and respiratory function

Plan	Principle
1. Determine the woman is unconscious and not breathing by shaking and shouting her name.	1. Shaking the shoulders and shouting are effective actions to determine unconsciousness and rouse a woman who may have fainted or is asleep.
2. Call for emergency help and have them bring a cardiac defibrillator.	2. The woman may need more than simple resuscitation.
3. Begin chest compressions. Place both hands on the lower sternum just above the xiphoid process and compress the chest a distance of 2 in. at a rate of 100 times a minute.	3. External chest compressions stimulate the action of the heart to maintain tissue perfusion. Allow chest recoil after each compression.
4. A second rescuer can deliver respiratory ventilations at a rate of 1 breath every 6 to 8 seconds (8 to 10 breaths/min).	4. Ventilation improves oxygenation.
5. If an automated external defibrillator (AED) is necessary, remove any fetal or uterine monitors if these are in place. Follow standard application and procedure according to agency protocol.	5. AED is effective at stimulating heart action and is not detrimental to pregnancy or a fetus.
6. When the emergency rescue team has arrived and relieved you as a first responder, place a rolled or folded towel under the woman's right hip.	6. A towel placed under one hip helps to prevent uterine compression on the vena cava and helps prevent supine hypotension syndrome.

What If . . . 20.2

Angelina tells the nurse she has abruptly discontinued taking the daily penicillin she has been prescribed for her heart disease since childhood. As it has been a long time since she had rheumatic fever, would the nurse recommend she could omit taking this during pregnancy?

Nursing Interventions During Labor and Birth

Frequently assess a woman's blood pressure, pulse, and respirations and monitor fetal heart rate and uterine contractions during labor for women with heart disease to be certain their circulatory system is not failing and the placenta is filling adequately. A rapidly increasing pulse rate (.100 beats/min) is an indication a heart is pumping ineffectively and so has increased its rate in an effort to compensate. Normally, it's good to advise a woman to assume a side-lying position during labor to reduce the possibility of supine hypotension syndrome. If a woman has some pulmonary edema, however, it may be necessary for her to elevate her head and chest (a semi-Fowler's position) to ease the work of breathing. If this is necessary, be certain to place a towel under her right hip to shift the uterus off the vena cava, the same as would happen with a side-lying position. Remember, fatigue is a symptom of heart decompensation. Evaluate women carefully, therefore, to determine whether the fatigue a woman reports is heart or labor related.

Women with extreme heart disease may need oxygen administered during labor because of the need for extra oxygen due to the exertion of labor; continuous hemodynamic monitoring such as by a Swan-Ganz catheter to monitor heart function may be prescribed. Many women with heart disease should not push with contractions, as pushing requires more effort than they should expend. That makes epidural anesthesia the anesthetic of choice for women with heart disease because this decreases the sensation of pushing and can make both labor and birth less taxing. Because of the lack of pushing, low forceps or a vacuum extractor may be used for birth. A woman may be disappointed during labor to learn her labor is not going to be "natural." Stress that these measures may not be what she anticipated, but they can help her achieve her ultimate goal, a healthy newborn and a mother able to care for her new baby.

Postpartum Nursing Interventions

The period immediately after birth is a critical time for a woman with heart disease because, with delivery of the placenta, the blood that supplied the placenta is released into her general circulation, increasing her blood volume by 20% to 40%. During pregnancy, the increase in blood volume that occurred did so over a 6-month period, so her heart had time to gradually adjust to this change. After birth, the increase in pressure takes place within 5 minutes, so the heart must make a rapid and major adjustment (Easterling & Stout, 2012).

To compensate for these circulatory changes, a woman may need a program of decreased activity and possibly anticoagulant and digoxin therapy until her circulation stabilizes. Antiembolic stockings or intermittent pneumatic compression (IPC) boots may be prescribed to increase venous return from the legs. If prophylactic antibiotics had not been started prior to birth, they should be started immediately after birth to discourage subacute bacterial endocarditis caused by the introduction of microorganisms through the placental site.

A woman with heart disease is often interested in close inspection of her baby immediately after birth because she wants to know if her infant has a heart defect or was harmed by any medication she took during pregnancy. Be certain to point out that acrocyanosis is normal in newborns, so she does not interpret her baby's peripheral cyanosis as cardiac inadequacy.

In the postpartum period, a stool softener can be prescribed to prevent straining with bowel movements. Agents to encourage uterine involution, such as oxytocin (Pitocin), should be used with caution because they tend to increase blood pressure, which necessitates increased heart action. As a rule, women with heart disease can breastfeed without difficulty. Kegel exercises are acceptable for perineal strengthening immediately, but the woman should not begin postpartum exercises to improve abdominal tone until her primary care provider approves them. Before discharge, be certain a woman has thought through if she will need help at home, so she can continue getting periods of rest. Also ensure that she schedules a return appointment for a postpartum checkup for both her gynecologic health and her cardiac status.

A WOMAN WITH AN ARTIFICIAL VALVE PROSTHESIS

In the past, women with heart valve prostheses were advised not to become pregnant for fear the increased blood volume gained during pregnancy would overwhelm the artificial valve. Today, evidence shows women with a valve prosthesis can complete a pregnancy safely (Yarrington, Valente, & Economy, 2015). One potential problem involves the use of oral anticoagulants women take to prevent the formation of blood clots at the valve site. Because the usual maintenance drug for this, sodium warfarin (Coumadin), increases the risk of congenital anomalies in infants (pregnancy risk category D), women are usually placed on low–molecular-weight heparin therapy (category C) before becoming pregnant and during pregnancy. Subclinical bleeding from continuous anticoagulant therapy has the potential to cause placental dislodgement. Therefore, observe a woman who is taking an anticoagulant for signs of petechiae and premature separation of the placenta during both pregnancy and labor.

A WOMAN WITH CHRONIC HYPERTENSIVE VASCULAR DISEASE

Women with chronic hypertensive disease enter pregnancy with an elevated blood pressure (140/90 mmHg or above). Hypertension of this kind is usually associated with arteriosclerosis or renal disease, making it a problem for the older pregnant woman. Chronic hypertension can be serious be-

cause it places both the woman and fetus at high risk because of poor heart, kidney, and/or placental perfusion during the pregnancy (Almasi, Pariente, Kessous, et al., 2016). Management includes a prescription of β-blockers and calcium channel blockers to reduce blood pressure by peripheral dilation to a safe level but not to reduce it below the threshold that allows for good placenta circulation. Labetalol (Trandate) and nifedipine (Procardia) are typical drugs that may be prescribed.

A WOMAN WITH VENOUS THROMBOEMBOLIC DISEASE

The incidence of venous thromboembolic disease increases during pregnancy because of a combination of stasis of blood in the lower extremities from uterine pressure and hypercoagulability (the effect of elevated estrogen; Box 20.4). When the pressure of the fetal head at birth puts additional pressure on lower extremity veins, damage can occur to the walls of the

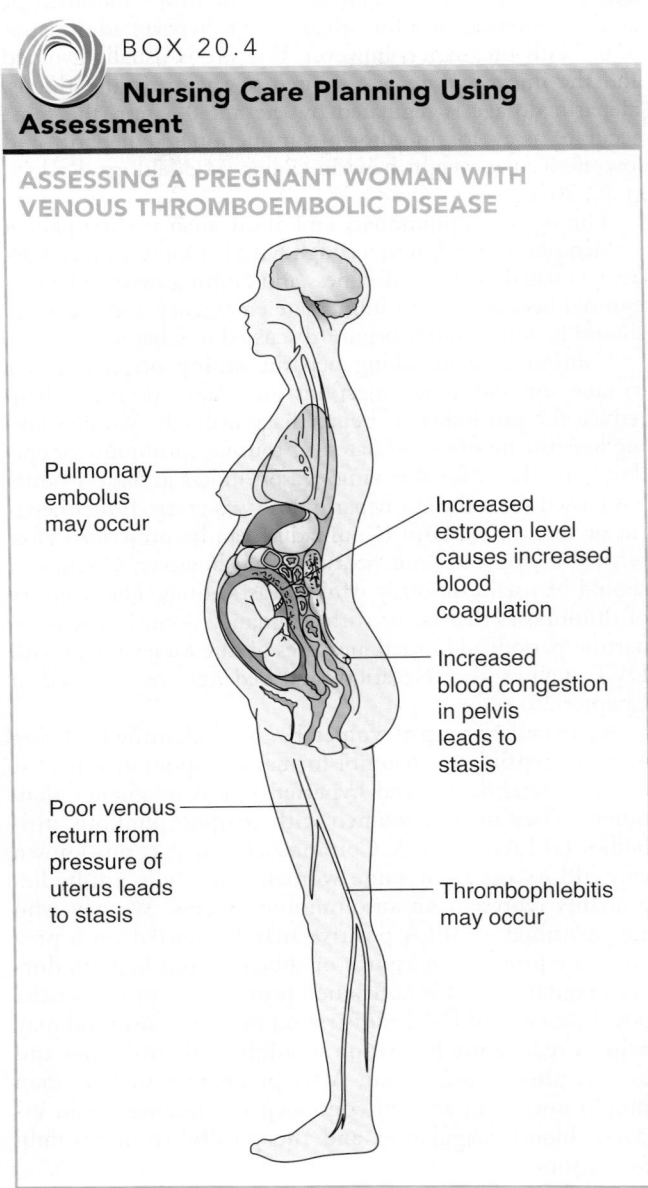

BOX 20.4

Nursing Care Planning Using Assessment

ASSESSING A PREGNANT WOMAN WITH VENOUS THROMBOEMBOLIC DISEASE

Pulmonary embolus may occur

Increased estrogen level causes increased blood coagulation

Increased blood congestion in pelvis leads to stasis

Poor venous return from pressure of uterus leads to stasis

Thrombophlebitis may occur

veins. With this triad of effects in place (stasis, vessel damage, and hypercoagulation), the stage is set for thrombus formation in the lower extremities. The likelihood of **deep vein thrombosis (DVT)**, formation of a blood clot in the veins of the lower extremities, leading to pulmonary emboli is highest in women 30 years of age or older because increased age is yet another risk factor for thrombosis formation (Goodacre & Hunt, 2016).

The risk of thrombus formation can be reduced through common-sense measures such as avoiding the use of constrictive knee-high stockings, not sitting with legs crossed at the knee, and avoiding standing in one position for a long period. If a thrombus does occur during pregnancy, a woman may notice pain and redness usually in the calf of a leg. It is diagnosed by a woman's history and Doppler ultrasonography. In order to keep the thrombus from moving and becoming a pulmonary embolus, a woman will be treated with bed rest and intravenous heparin for 24 to 48 hours. After this, she may be prescribed subcutaneous heparin she can self-inject every 12 or 24 hours for the duration of the pregnancy. It is generally recommended the lower abdomen be used for rotating sites for subcutaneous heparin administration. With pregnancy, however, this site is usually avoided and the injection sites are limited to the arms and thighs. Heparin dosage is regulated by the anti-Xa test, the most accurate assay for monitoring unfractionated heparin and low–molecular-weight heparin (Bates, Middeldorp, Rodger, et al., 2016).

The signs of a pulmonary embolism, such as chest pain, a sudden onset of dyspnea, a cough with hemoptysis, tachycardia or missed beats, or dizziness and fainting need to be recognized because it is an immediate emergency and measures should be immediately begun (discussed in Chapter 25).

Caution women taking heparin during pregnancy not to take any additional injections once labor begins to help reduce the possibility of hemorrhage at birth. Women taking heparin are not candidates for routine episiotomy or epidural anesthesia for this same reason unless at least 4 hours has passed since the last heparin dose was given. Either heparin or sodium warfarin (Coumadin) can be prescribed after birth if a woman is not breastfeeding; however, Coumadin should be used cautiously while breastfeeding. The majority of thromboses that occur with pregnancy occur in the postpartum period; additional measures of care for a woman with DVT, such as heat, elevation, and bed rest are discussed in Chapter 25.

A particular group of women has been identified as being more susceptible to thrombi formation, spontaneous miscarriage, fetal death, and hypertension of pregnancy than others. They include women with antiphospholipid antibodies (aPLAs) (Leaf & Connors, 2017). It is not known why aPLAs occur in some women, but these antibodies probably represent an autoimmune process. Women who are identified as aPLA positive may be started on a prophylactic program of aspirin or subcutaneous heparin during pregnancy that is continued postpartum to reduce the possibility of DVT. Administration of a corticosteroid may help to reduce the formation of additional antibodies and so may also be prescribed. After pregnancy, such women should not begin an oral contraceptive because it can increase blood coagulation and the possibility of thrombi formation.

> ## QSEN Checkpoint Question 20.1
>
> ### PATIENT-CENTERED CARE
>
> Angelina develops a DVT while in the hospital on bed rest and is prescribed low–molecular-weight heparin. The nurse identifies which action as important when planning care for her?
>
> a. Showing her how to self-administer the drug as a rectal suppository
> b. Cautioning her that her hemoglobin level will be closely monitored during therapy
> c. Allowing her to choose a subcutaneous site for the injection
> d. Monitoring her white blood cell count daily for decreased coagulation
>
> *Look in Appendix A for the best answer and rationale.*

Hematologic Disorders and Pregnancy

Hematologic disorders during pregnancy involve either blood formation or coagulation disorders.

ANEMIA AND PREGNANCY

Because the blood volume expands during pregnancy slightly ahead of the red cell count, most women have a pseudoanemia in early pregnancy. This condition is normal and should not be confused with true types of anemia that occur as complications of pregnancy. True anemia is typically considered to be present when a woman's hemoglobin concentration is less than 11 g/dl (hematocrit <33%) in the first or third trimester of pregnancy or when the hemoglobin concentration is less than 10.5 g/dl (hematocrit <32%) in the second trimester (Samuels, 2012).

A Woman With Iron-Deficiency Anemia

Iron-deficiency anemia is the most common anemia of pregnancy, complicating as many as 15% to 25% of all pregnancies (Chmielewska, Dziechciarz, Gieruszczak-Białek, et al., 2016). Many women enter pregnancy with a deficiency of iron stores resulting from a combination of a diet low in iron, heavy menstrual periods, or unwise weight-reducing programs. Iron stores are also apt to be low in women who were pregnant less than 2 years before the current pregnancy or those from low socioeconomic levels who have not had iron-rich diets. Iron-deficiency anemia is confirmed by a corresponding low serum iron level (under 30 μg/dl) and an increased iron-binding capacity (over 400 μg/dl).

Iron is made available to the body by absorption from the duodenum into the bloodstream after it has been ingested. In the bloodstream, it is bound to transferrin for transport to the liver, spleen, and bone marrow. At these sites, it is incorporated into hemoglobin or stored as ferritin.

The type of anemia is characteristically a microcytic (i.e., small red blood cell) and hypochromic (i.e., less hemoglobin than the average red cell) anemia, which occurs when such an inadequate supply of iron is ingested that iron is not available for incorporation into red blood cells.

A woman experiences extreme fatigue and poor exercise tolerance because she cannot transport oxygen effectively. The condition is mildly associated with low birth weight and preterm birth. Because the body recognizes that it needs increased nutrients, some women with this condition develop pica, or the craving and eating of substances such as ice or starch (Rabel, Leitman, & Miller, 2016). It is also associated with restless leg syndrome (Singh, Chaudhary, Sonker, et al., 2016).

To prevent this common anemia, women should take prenatal vitamins containing 27 mg of iron as prophylactic therapy during pregnancy. In addition, they need to eat a diet high in iron and vitamins (e.g., green leafy vegetables, meat, and legumes) so the supplement is truly a supplement. Women who develop iron-deficiency anemia will be prescribed therapeutic levels of medication (120 to 200 mg elemental iron per day), usually in the form of ferrous sulfate or ferrous gluconate.

Iron is absorbed best in an acid medium. Advise women, therefore, to take iron supplements with orange juice or a vitamin C supplement, which supplies ascorbic acid. If they are not already enrolled in the Special Supplemental Nutrition Program for Women, Infants, and Children (WIC) but are eligible (www.fns.usda.gov/wic), making a referral could help ensure a better diet. When women begin to take a prescribed iron supplement, new red blood cells should begin to increase almost immediately, or their reticulocyte count should rise from a range of between 0.5% and 1.5% to 3% and 4% by 2 weeks. Some women report constipation or gastric irritation when taking oral iron supplements. Increasing roughage in the diet and always taking the pills with food can help reduce these symptoms. Ferrous sulfate turns stools black, so caution women about this to prevent them from worrying that they are bleeding internally. If iron-deficiency anemia is severe and a woman has difficulty with oral iron therapy, intravenous iron can be prescribed.

A Woman With Folic Acid–Deficiency Anemia

Folic acid, or folate or folacin, one of the B vitamins, is necessary for the normal formation of red blood cells in the woman as well as being associated with preventing neural tube and abdominal wall defects in the fetus. Folic acid–deficiency anemia occurs most often in multiple pregnancies because of the increased fetal demand; in women with a secondary hemolytic illness in which there is rapid destruction and production of new red blood cells; in women who are taking hydantoin, an anticonvulsant agent that interferes with folate absorption; and in women who have poor gastric absorption, such as in those who have had a gastric bypass for morbid obesity (Pentieva, Selhub, Paul, et al., 2016).

The anemia that develops is a **megaloblastic anemia** (enlarged red blood cells). Because of the size of the cells, the mean corpuscular volume will be elevated in contrast to the lowered level seen with iron-deficiency anemia. Slow to progress, the deficiency may take several weeks to develop or may not be apparent until the second trimester of pregnancy. Full blown, it may be a contributory factor in early miscarriage or premature separation of the placenta.

All women expecting to become pregnant are advised to begin a supplement of 400 μg folic acid daily in addition to eating folate-rich foods (e.g., green leafy vegetables, oranges, dried beans). Over-the-counter women's multivitamin preparations generally do contain adequate folic acid for pregnancy so be certain women are specifically taking a prenatal or women's multivitamin. Women who develop folic acid–deficiency anemia are prescribed even higher or therapeutic levels of folic acid (Clark, Thomson, & Greer, 2012).

A WOMAN WITH SICKLE-CELL ANEMIA

Sickle-cell anemia is a recessively inherited hemolytic anemia caused by an abnormal amino acid in the beta chain of hemoglobin. If the abnormal amino acid replaces the amino acid valine, sickling hemoglobin (HbS) results; if it is substituted for the amino acid lysine, nonsickling hemoglobin (HbC) results. An individual who is heterozygous (i.e., has only one gene in which the abnormal substitution has occurred) has the sickle-cell trait (HbAS). If the person is homozygous (i.e., has two genes in which the substitution has occurred), sickle-cell disease (HbSS) results (Rote & McCance, 2017).

With the disease, the majority of red blood cells are irregular or sickle shaped, so they cannot carry as much hemoglobin as normally shaped red blood cells can. When oxygen tension becomes reduced, as occurs at high altitudes, or blood becomes more viscid than usual, such as occurs with dehydration, the cells clump together because of their irregular shape, resulting in vessel blockage with reduced blood flow to organs. The cells then will hemolyze (i.e., be destroyed), thus reducing the number available and causing a severe anemia.

Approximately 1 in every 10 Blacks has the sickle-cell trait or carries a recessive gene for S hemoglobin but is asymptomatic; theoretically, 1 in every 400 Blacks has the disease, although with interracial marriages increasing, the disease is no longer confined to one ethnic group (Boga & Ozdogu, 2016).

Although the sickle-cell trait does not appear to directly influence the course of pregnancy, preterm birth, growth restriction, miscarriage, or perinatal mortality, rates tend to be higher for women with the homozygous disease. At any time in life, sickle-cell anemia is a threat to life if vital blood vessels such as those to the liver, kidneys, heart, lungs, or brain become blocked. In pregnancy, blockage to the placental circulation can directly compromise the fetus, causing low birth weight and possibly fetal death.

Assessment

All Black women who have not been previously tested should be screened for sickle-cell anemia at a first prenatal visit. Hemoglobin levels for all women with sickle-cell disease should then be obtained throughout pregnancy. A woman with sickle-cell disease may normally have a hemoglobin level of 6 to 8 mg/100 ml. Unless she receives active interventions to raise this level, she will maintain it during pregnancy, potentially reducing oxygen to the fetus. If a hemolytic sickle-cell crisis occurs, a woman's hemoglobin level can fall to 5 or 6 mg/100 ml in a few hours, causing an accompanying rise in indirect bilirubin because the woman cannot conjugate the bilirubin released from so many destroyed red blood cells.

Because a pregnant woman with sickle-cell anemia has vascular stasis, they are more susceptible to bacteriuria than other women; periodically collect a clean-catch urine sample during pregnancy to detect developing bacteriuria while a woman is still asymptomatic.

Throughout pregnancy, monitor a woman's nutritional intake to be certain she is consuming sufficient amounts of folic acid and possibly an additional folic acid supplement, which is necessary for replacing red blood cells that have been destroyed. Women should *not* take a routine iron supplement as sickled cells cannot incorporate iron in the same manner as non-sickled cells. Ensure the woman is drinking at least eight glasses of fluid daily to be certain she is guarding against dehydration. Early in pregnancy, when she may be nauseated, it is easy for her fluid intake to decrease, causing dehydration and a subsequent sickle-cell crisis.

Assess a woman's lower extremities at prenatal visits for varicosities or pooling of blood in leg veins, which can lead to red cell destruction. Standing for long periods during the day increases this pressure, whereas sitting on a chair with the legs elevated or lying on the side in a modified Sims position encourages venous return from the lower extremities. Help a woman plan her day so she has limited long periods of standing and adequate rest periods.

Fetal health is usually monitored during pregnancy by an ultrasound examination at 16 to 24 weeks to assess for intrauterine growth restriction and by weekly nonstress or ultrasound examinations beginning at about 30 weeks. Blood flow through the uterus and placenta may be measured by blood flow velocity. If blood flow velocity is reduced, the chance of intrauterine growth restriction increases.

Therapeutic Management

Interventions to prevent a sickle-cell crisis can include periodic exchange or blood transfusions throughout pregnancy to replace sickled cells with non-sickled cells. An exchange transfusion serves a secondary purpose of removing a quantity of the increased bilirubin resulting from the breakdown of red blood cells as well as restoring the hemoglobin level (Benites, Benevides, Valente, et al., 2016). If a crisis occurs, controlling pain, administering oxygen as needed, and increasing the fluid volume of the circulatory system to lower viscosity are important interventions (see Chapter 44 for a further discussion of therapy for sickle-cell anemia).

If a woman develops an infection that raises her temperature and causes her to perspire more than usual (which creates dehydration) or contracts a respiratory infection that compromises air exchange so that her PO_2 is lowered, hospitalization for observation may be necessary to rule out the development of a sickle-cell crisis and subsequent hemolysis of crowded cells (Oteng-Ntim, Meeks, Seed, et al., 2015).

When the fetus is mature, the time and method of birth are individualized. Be certain to keep a woman in labor well hydrated and help her resist strenuous exertion. If an operative birth is necessary, epidural anesthesia is the method of choice because general anesthesia poses a possible risk of hypoxia. In the postpartal period, early ambulation and wearing pressure stockings or IPC boots can help reduce the risk of thromboembolism from stasis in lower extremities.

Women are generally interested in determining at birth whether their child has inherited the disease. Because the disorder is recessively inherited, if one of the parents has the disease and the other is free of the disease and trait, the chance the child will inherit the disease is zero. If a woman has the disease and her partner has the trait, the chance the child will be born with the disease is 50%. If both parents have the disease, all their children will also have the disease (see Chapter 8).

Electrophoresis of red blood cells obtained from maternal serum or by amniocentesis during pregnancy can reveal the presence of the disease on the few β-hemoglobin chains already present in fetal life. If not assessed during pregnancy, although the symptoms of sickle-cell disease do not become clinically apparent until 3 to 6 months of age, a routine newborn serum screening at birth will also reveal the disease.

QSEN Checkpoint Question 20.2

SAFETY

Angelina is friends with a woman in the clinic who has sickle-cell anemia, and they often talk together about their care. Which statement would alert the nurse that her friend may need further instruction on prenatal care?

a. "I understand why folic acid is important for red cell formation."
b. "I'm careful to drink at least eight glasses of fluid every day."
c. "I take an iron pill every day to help grow new red blood cells."
d. "I've temporarily stopped jogging so I don't risk becoming dehydrated."

Look in Appendix A for the best answer and rationale.

The Woman With Thalassemia

The thalassemias are a group of autosomal recessively inherited blood disorders that lead to poor hemoglobin formation and severe anemia. They occur most frequently in Mediterranean, African, and Asian populations (Charoenboon, Jatavan, Traisrisilp, et al., 2016). Symptoms first appear in childhood. Treatment focuses on combating anemia through such measures as folic acid supplementation and perhaps blood transfusion to infuse hemoglobin-rich red blood cells. Women with thalassemia do not usually take an iron supplement during pregnancy because they could receive an iron overload because iron is infused with blood transfusions. Care of a child with both forms of thalassemia, alpha and beta, is discussed in Chapter 44.

The Woman With Malaria

Malaria is a protozoan infection that is transmitted to people by *Anopheles* mosquitoes (Andrews, Lynch, Eckert, et al., 2015). The infection causes red blood cells to stick to the surface of capillaries causing obstruction of these vessels and resulting in end-organ anoxia and blood not reaching organs effectively.

Although the disorder does not have a high incidence in the United States, newly immigrated women may be infected with it. It's important to consider during pregnancy as it can not only make women high risk for blood clotting during pregnancy but also, if untreated, can be transmitted to a fetus by mother-to-fetus transmission.

The incubation period for the most frequently occurring type is 12 to 14 days. The most noticeable symptoms are elevated liver function tests accompanying fever, malaise, and headache. Because of the altered blood cells, thrombocytopenia (i.e., low platelet count), anemia, and renal failure can develop.

Malaria can be prevented by wearing clothing that covers most of the body as well as using an insect repellent when in an area infested with mosquitoes, sleeping at night with a mosquito net, or keeping windows closed to prevent mosquitoes from entering. As further prevention, urge women to delay travel to endemic areas until after pregnancy if possible.

Treatment is with a combination of antimalarial drugs, which will both stop the course of the disease and help reduce the incidence of low birth weight and preterm birth. Sulfadoxine/pyrimethamine is safe to administer during the last trimester of pregnancy. Chloroquine is safe to administer all during pregnancy and so is the drug of choice (Adeola & Okwilagwe, 2015). Quinine, atovaquone and proguanil (Malarone), or tetracyclines, although effective against the disease, should not be used at any point in pregnancy or with women who are breastfeeding as they are teratogenic.

COAGULATION DISORDERS AND PREGNANCY

Most coagulation disorders are sex linked or occur only in males and so have little effect on pregnancies. However, one of them, von Willebrand disease, is a coagulation disorder inherited as an autosomal dominant trait and so does occur in women (Neff & Sidonio, 2014). Women will have normal platelet counts, but bleeding time is prolonged. Levels of factor VIII–related antigen (VIII-R) and factor VIII coagulation activity (VIII-C) are both reduced. From the time she was a child, a woman with the disorder might have noticed menorrhagia or frequent episodes of epistaxis. If these symptoms were not severe, however, the condition can go undiagnosed until pregnancy when a woman experiences a spontaneous miscarriage or postpartum hemorrhage. Replacement of the missing coagulation factors by infusion of cryoprecipitate or fresh frozen plasma may be necessary before labor to prevent excessive bleeding with birth.

Hemophilia B (Christmas disease, factor IX deficiency) is a sex-linked disorder, so the actual disease occurs only in males. However, female carriers may have such a reduced level of factor IX (only 33% of normal) that hemorrhage with labor or a spontaneous miscarriage can be a serious complication. As with von Willebrand disease, carriers of the disorder need to be identified before pregnancy. Restoration of factor IX levels can be quickly restored by infusion of factor IX concentrate or fresh frozen plasma.

Maternal serum analysis can be used to detect whether a fetus has a coagulation disorder during pregnancy. If there is a family history of a coagulation disorder, before an internal fetal heart rate monitor is attached or fetal scalp blood sampling is done, it should be determined if the fetus has a coagulation defect. If one is present, these procedures are contraindicated because they could result in extensive fetal blood loss.

Idiopathic thrombocytopenic purpura (ITP), which is a decreased number of platelets, is not inherited, can occur at any time in life, and so occasionally occurs during pregnancy. The cause of the condition is unknown, but because symptoms usually occur shortly after a viral invasion such as an upper respiratory tract infection, it is assumed to be an autoimmune reaction (an antiplatelet antibody that destroys platelets is apparently released) (Hisano, Tsukada, Sago, et al., 2015).

Laboratory studies reveal a marked thrombocytopenia (platelet count may be as low as 20,000/mm^3 from a usual count of 150,000/mm^3). Without an adequate level of platelets, the woman is prone to frequent nosebleeds and minute petechiae or large ecchymoses appear on her body.

The illness typically runs a 1- to 3-month limited course, but because a low platelet count also appears with hypertension of pregnancy with HELLP (**h**emolysis, **e**levated **l**iver enzymes, **l**ow **p**latelet count) syndrome, a serious complication of pregnancy (see Chapter 21), the condition is frightening until it is differentiated as ITP. Oral prednisone or a platelet transfusion or plasmapheresis may be administered to temporarily increase the platelet count to prevent increased bleeding at birth. The antiplatelet factor can cross the placenta and cause accompanying platelet destruction in the newborn or allow a newborn to be born with the illness, so a careful assessment of the baby is necessary at birth (see Chapter 44 for care of the child with ITP).

Renal and Urinary Disorders and Pregnancy

Adequate kidney function is important for a successful pregnancy outcome because a woman is excreting waste products not only for herself but also for the fetus. This dual function makes any condition that interferes with kidney or urinary function always potentially serious.

A WOMAN WITH A URINARY TRACT INFECTION

As many as 4% to 10% of nonpregnant women have asymptomatic bacteriuria (i.e., organisms are present in the urine without symptoms of infection). In a pregnant woman, because the ureters dilate from the effect of progesterone, stasis of urine can occur. The minimal presence of abnormal amounts of glucose (**glycosuria**) that also occurs with pregnancy provides an ideal medium for growth for any organisms present. Combined, these factors cause asymptomatic UTIs in as many as 10% to 15% of pregnant women (Widmer, Lopez, Gülmezoglu, et al., 2015). Asymptomatic infections are potentially dangerous because they can progress to pyelonephritis (i.e., infection of the pelvis of the kidney) and are associated with preterm labor and premature rupture of membranes. Women with known vesicoureteral reflux (i.e., backflow of urine into the ureters) tend to develop UTIs or pyelonephritis more often than others. The organism most commonly responsible for UTI is *Escherichia coli* from an ascending infection. A UTI can also occur as a descending infection or can begin in the kidneys from the filtration of organisms present from other body infections. If the infectious organism is determined to be *Streptococcus* B, vaginal cultures should be obtained because streptococcal B infection of the genital tract is associated with pneumonia in newborns.

Assessment

A UTI typically manifests as frequency and pain on urination. With pyelonephritis, a woman develops pain in the lumbar region (usually on the right side) that radiates downward. The area feels tender to palpation. She may have accompanying nausea and vomiting, malaise, pain, and frequency of urination. Her temperature may be elevated only slightly or may be as high as 103° to 104°F (39° to 40°C). The infection usually occurs on the right side because there is greater compression and urinary stasis on the right ureter from the uterus being pushed that way by the large bulk of the intestine on the left side. A urine culture will reveal over 100,000 organisms per milliliter of urine, a level diagnostic of infection.

Therapeutic Management

Obtain a clean-catch urine sample for culture and sensitivity to assess for asymptomatic bacteriuria or symptoms of UTI (see Chapter 11). A sensitivity test will then determine which antibiotic will best combat the infection. Amoxicillin, ampicillin, and cephalosporins are effective against most organisms causing UTIs and are safe antibiotics during pregnancy. The sulfonamides can be used early in pregnancy but not near term because they can interfere with protein binding of bilirubin, which then leads to hyperbilirubinemia in the newborn. Tetracyclines are contraindicated during pregnancy as they cause retardation of bone growth and staining of the deciduous teeth (Karch, 2015).

Nursing Diagnoses and Related Interventions

Nursing Diagnosis: Risk for infection related to stasis of urine with pregnancy

Outcome Evaluation: Oral temperature is below 100.4°F (38°C), and a clean-catch urine specimen has a bacteria count below 100,000 colonies per milliliter.

As part of prenatal education, remind all women during pregnancy of common measures to prevent UTIs, such as:

- Voiding frequently (at least every 2 hours)
- Developing a habit of urinating as soon as the need is felt and emptying the bladder completely when urinating
- Wiping front to back after voiding and bowel movements
- Wearing cotton, not synthetic fiber, underwear
- Voiding immediately after sexual intercourse
- Drinking a glass of cranberry juice daily

The pregnant woman with a UTI needs to take the additional measure of drinking an increased amount of fluid to flush out the infection from the urinary tract. To be most effective, do not simply tell her to "push fluids" or "drink lots of water." Give her a specific amount to drink every day (up to 3 to 4 L per 24 hours) to make certain she increases her fluid intake sufficiently.

A woman can promote urine drainage by assuming a knee–chest position for 15 minutes morning and evening. In this position, the weight of the uterus is shifted forward, releasing the pressure on the ureters and allowing urine to drain more freely.

If a woman has one UTI during pregnancy, the chances are high she will develop another late in pregnancy, when urinary stasis tends to grow even greater. She may, therefore, be kept on prophylactic antibiotics throughout the remainder of the pregnancy. Ask at prenatal visits whether she is continuing to take this type of prophylactic medicine. When women have pain and symptoms of urinary frequency, they usually take medication consistently. When they no longer have any clinical evidence they are ill, their compliance rate may begin to fall dramatically. Urge a woman to post a chart on her refrigerator door or in her bathroom as a reminder to take the medication. Encourage her not to leave the medication on the counter as a reminder because she needs to begin to childproof her home.

Pyelonephritis occurs as an extension of a UTI or infection that originated in or spread to the kidney (Suskind, Saigal, Hanley, et al., 2016). If this develops, a woman may be hospitalized for 24 to 48 hours while she is treated with intravenous antibiotics. After this acute episode, she will be maintained on a drug such as oral nitrofurantoin (Macrodantin) for the remainder of the pregnancy. Acidifying urine by the use of ascorbic acid (vitamin C), which is often recommended in nonpregnant women, is not usually recommended during pregnancy because a newborn can develop scurvy in the immediate neonatal period from vitamin C withdrawal.

After birth, a woman who developed more than one UTI may have an ultrasound scheduled to detect any urinary tract abnormality that might be present, such as vesicoureteral reflux, to help prevent future infections.

QSEN Checkpoint Question 20.3

QUALITY IMPROVEMENT

While reviewing antenatal electronic records, the charge nurse of a prenatal clinic notes that a high number of pregnant women seen in the clinic, including Angelina Gomez, have developed UTIs during their pregnancies. The nurse should emphasize the need for staff nurses to do which of the following?

  a. Ensure that the housekeeping department is adequately cleaning the toilets.
  b. Suggest all women be prescribed a prophylactic antibiotic during their first trimester.
  c. Educate women on the need for sound perineal care during pregnancy.
  d. Urge women to restrict fluid to keep their urine acidic and concentrated.

Look in Appendix A for the best answer and rationale.

A WOMAN WITH A HYPERACTIVE BLADDER

A hyperactive bladder refers to a bladder that contracts more frequently than usual, causing symptoms of frequency, urgency, and incontinence. During pregnancy, these symptoms can increase greatly because of the additional pressure from the uterus on the bladder. Fesoterodine (Toviaz; pregnancy category C), an antispasmodic drug frequently prescribed for the disorder should be used during pregnancy and breastfeeding only if the risk outweighs the benefit until it is proven not to be teratogenic (Kahyaoglu Sut & Balkanli Kaplan, 2016).

A WOMAN WITH CHRONIC RENAL DISEASE

In the past, females with chronic renal disease did not reach childbearing age or were advised not to have children because of their automatic high-risk status during pregnancy. Today, with conscientious prenatal care, women with chronic renal disease and even women who have had renal transplants, can expect to have healthy pregnancies and healthy children (Zhang, Ma, Hao, et al., 2015).

Women with chronic renal disease need to be monitored carefully during pregnancy because their diseased kidneys may not produce erythropoietin, a glycoprotein necessary for red cell formation and so they may develop a severe anemia (Box 20.5). Fortunately, synthetic erythropoietin is now available and is safe to take during pregnancy (Sienas, Wong, Collins, et al., 2013).

Because the glomerular filtration rate normally increases during pregnancy, a woman's serum creatinine level (a measure of kidney function that elevates when kidneys are under stress) may be actually slightly below normal during pregnancy or may fall from a usual level of 0.7 mg/100 ml to about 0.5 mg/100 ml. Women with kidney disease who normally have a serum creatinine level greater than 2.0 mg/dl may be advised not to undertake a pregnancy in case the increased strain on already damaged kidneys leads to kidney failure.

Many women with renal disease routinely take a corticosteroid such as oral prednisone at a maintenance level.

This drug therapy typically is continued throughout pregnancy. Although animal studies have shown an increased incidence of cleft palate from corticosteroid use during pregnancy, this does not appear to be true in humans. The infant may be hyperglycemic at birth, however, because of the suppression of insulin activity by the corticosteroid.

Women with severe renal disease may require dialysis to aid kidney function during pregnancy (Piccoli, Minelli, Versino, et al., 2016). With dialysis, there is a risk of preterm labor, perhaps because progesterone is removed with the dialysis. To prevent this complication, progesterone may be administered intramuscularly before the procedure. If hemodialysis is used, it should be scheduled frequently and for short durations to avoid acute fluid shifts. The heparin administered in connection with hemodialysis is safe during pregnancy because it does not cross the placenta. Even in light of the expanding uterine size, peritoneal dialysis is actually preferred over hemodialysis because it normally causes less drastic fluid shifts. This can be accomplished on an ambulatory basis (continuous ambulatory peritoneal dialysis) throughout pregnancy.

If women are on a low-potassium diet to avoid a buildup of potassium that accumulates because their diseased kidneys do not evacuate it well, they may need a nutrition consultation to be certain they can continue to avoid potassium yet also eat a healthy pregnancy diet. They also may need a great deal of emotional support during pregnancy because they are aware of the stress of pregnancy on damaged kidneys. By being pregnant, they are risking not only the life of the child growing inside them but also their own life. They may also need extra time with their infant at birth for bonding because they may have been too concerned during pregnancy to begin this process.

Although successful pregnancies in women with kidney transplants are to be expected, women should be considered individually to determine whether they will be able to carry a pregnancy to term before a pregnancy is initiated (Kovács, Szabó, Jenei, et al., 2015). Criteria to be evaluated include:

- A woman's general health and the time since the transplant (preferably >2 years)
- A woman's serum creatinine level
- The presence of proteinuria or hypertension or signs of graft rejection
- Medications the woman is taking to reduce graft rejection

It is helpful if the drugs a woman is taking are limited to prednisone to ensure fetal safety during pregnancy.

Respiratory Disorders and Pregnancy

Respiratory diseases have a wide range from mild (e.g., the common cold), to severe (e.g., pneumonia), to chronic (e.g., tuberculosis or chronic obstructive pulmonary disease [COPD]). Any respiratory condition can worsen in pregnancy because the rising uterus compresses the diaphragm, thus reducing the size of the thoracic cavity and available lung space. Any respiratory disorder can also pose serious hazards to the fetus if allowed to progress to the point where the mother's oxygen–carbon dioxide exchange is altered or the mother or fetus cannot receive enough oxygen.

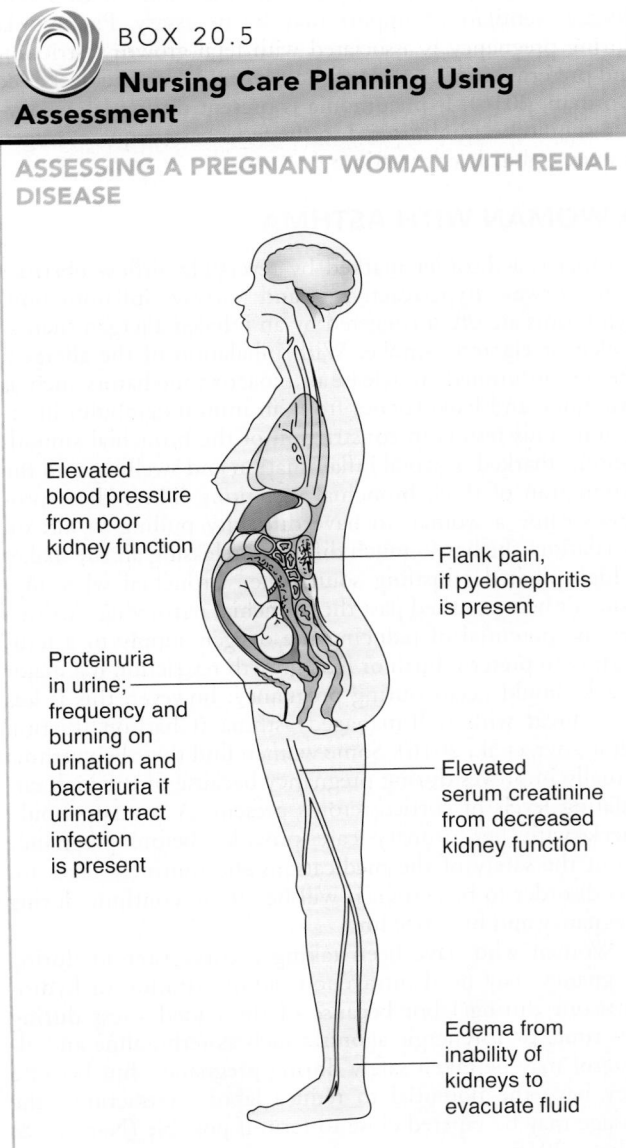

BOX 20.5

Nursing Care Planning Using Assessment

ASSESSING A PREGNANT WOMAN WITH RENAL DISEASE

Elevated blood pressure from poor kidney function

Proteinuria in urine; frequency and burning on urination and bacteriuria if urinary tract infection is present

Flank pain, if pyelonephritis is present

Elevated serum creatinine from decreased kidney function

Edema from inability of kidneys to evacuate fluid

Nursing Diagnoses and Related Interventions

Nursing Diagnosis: Risk for ineffective breathing pattern related to respiratory changes during pregnancy

Outcome Evaluation: Respiratory rate is 16 to 20 breaths/min, PO_2 is above 80 mmHg, PCO_2 is below 40 mmHg, and fetal heart rate is 110 to 160 beats/min with good variability.

Respiratory illnesses in women who are pregnant can become extremely serious and may require therapy such as oxygen and medication to help increase oxygenation in both the woman and her fetus.

A WOMAN WITH ACUTE NASOPHARYNGITIS

Acute nasopharyngitis (i.e., the common cold) tends to be more severe during pregnancy than at other times because, during pregnancy, estrogen stimulation normally causes some degree of nasal congestion. This means that even with a minor cold, a woman can find it difficult to breathe. Women should not take high-dose aspirin as a remedy for a headache, which commonly accompanies an upper respiratory infection. It can interfere with blood clotting in both the mother and fetus as well as cause fetal constricted ductus arteriosus (Karch, 2015). Because common colds are invariably caused by a virus, antibiotic therapy is unnecessary except to prevent a secondary infection. And although most simple cough syrups don't contain ingredients that would make them unsafe for use during pregnancy, women should check with their healthcare provider before taking any over-the-counter medication other than honey and lemon lozenges. Urge women to use simple measures to combat a cold, such as:

- Be sure to get extra rest and sleep and eat a diet high in vitamin C (e.g., orange juice and fruit) to help boost the immune system.
- Take acetaminophen (Tylenol) every 4 hours for aches and pains (up to 3,000 mg/day). Do not take acetylsalicylic acid (Aspirin) during pregnancy because it can interfere with blood clotting.
- Use a room humidifier or apply a medicated vapor rub to the chest, especially at night, to moisten nasal secretions and help mucus drain.
- Use cool or warm compresses to relieve sinus headaches.

A WOMAN WITH INFLUENZA

Influenza is caused by a virus, identified as type A, B, or C. The disease spreads in epidemic form and is accompanied by high fever, extreme prostration, aching pains in the back and extremities, and generally, a sore, raw throat. Contrary to early reports, influenza infection has not been clearly correlated with congenital anomalies in newborns, although it can be a cause of preterm labor. For unknown reasons, some studies have shown a link between influenza during pregnancy and schizophrenia in children born of that pregnancy (Cai, Wan, He, et al., 2015). Treatment includes an antipyretic such as acetaminophen (Tylenol) to control fever. The risk for the woman of not taking oseltamivir (Tamiflu), an oral antiviral drug that is pregnancy category C, is greater than if it is taken, so it should be prescribed and begun immediately during pregnancy (Ghulmiyyah, Alame, Mirza, et al., 2016). Because influenza vaccines are made from inert viruses, women may also be immunized safely against influenza during pregnancy (Polyzos, Konstantelias, Pitsa, et al., 2015).

A WOMAN WITH PNEUMONIA

Pneumonia is the bacterial or viral invasion of lung tissue by pathogens such as *Streptococcus pneumoniae*, *Haemophilus influenzae*, and *Mycoplasma pneumoniae*. After the invasion, an acute inflammatory response occurs in the lung alveoli, causing an exudate of red blood cells, fibrin, and polymorphonuclear leukocytes to flood into the alveoli. This process has the helpful effect of confining the bacteria or virus within segments of the lobes of the lungs, but it also has a less helpful effect of filling alveoli with fluid, blocking off breathing space. If the collection of fluid becomes extreme, it can limit the oxygen available not only to the woman but also to the fetus. Therapy involves the use of an appropriate antibiotic and perhaps oxygen administration. With severe disease, ventilation support may be necessary. Pneumonia during pregnancy is associated with fetal growth restriction and preterm birth because of the oxygen deficit (Leidecker & Dorman, 2016). If pneumonia is present during labor, oxygen should be administered so the fetus has adequate oxygen resources during contractions.

A WOMAN WITH ASTHMA

Asthma is a disorder marked by reversible airflow obstruction, airway hyperreactivity, and airway inflammation. Symptoms are often triggered by an inhaled allergen such as pollen or cigarette smoke. With inhalation of the allergen, there is an immediate release of bioactive mediators such as histamine and leukotrienes from an immunoglobulin interaction. This results in constriction of the bronchial smooth muscle, marked mucosal inflammation and swelling, and the production of thick bronchial secretions. These three processes cause a woman to have difficulty pulling in air; on exhalation, she has so much difficulty releasing air she makes a high-pitched whistling sound (i.e., bronchial wheezing) from air being pushed past the bronchial narrowing. Asthma has the potential of reducing the oxygen supply to a fetus leading to preterm birth or fetal growth restriction if a major attack should occur during pregnancy; however, this is less of a threat with well-managed asthma (Charlton, Pierini, Klungsøyr, et al., 2016). Some women find that their asthma actually improves during pregnancy because of the high circulating levels of corticosteroids present. A woman should check with her primary care provider before pregnancy about the safety of the medications she routinely takes for this disorder to be certain it will be safe to continue during pregnancy and breastfeeding.

Women who have been taking a corticosteroid during pregnancy may need intravenous administration of hydrocortisone during labor because of the added stress during this time. β-Adrenergic agonists such as terbutaline and albuterol may be taken safely during pregnancy, but because they have the potential to reduce labor contractions, the dosage may be tapered close to term if possible (Namazy & Schatz, 2015).

A WOMAN WITH TUBERCULOSIS

Tuberculosis is a disease that should have been eradicated because of the effective treatment available. However, in highly populated areas, the incidence has actually increased and in some areas is at epidemic proportions. Worldwide, it is still one of the leading causes of death.

With tuberculosis, lung tissue is invaded by *Mycobacterium tuberculosis*, an acid-fast bacillus. Macrophages and T lymphocytes surround the invading bacillus, but rather than actually killing it, they merely surround and confine it. Fibrosis, calcification, and a final ring of collagenous scar tissue develop, effectively sealing off the organisms from the body and any further invasion or spread. The antibodies produced will thereafter cause a woman to have a positive response to a Mantoux test (purified protein derivative [PPD]) test.

Assessment

Symptoms of tuberculosis, in addition to a chronic cough, are substantial weight loss, hemoptysis (coughing blood), a low-grade fever, extreme fatigue, and waking at night with night sweats. In high-risk areas, women should undergo skin testing (a PPD test) at their first prenatal visit. Women need to be cautioned that a positive reaction does not necessarily mean they have the disease; it can only mean they have at some time been exposed to tuberculosis and so have antibodies in their system. If a woman has a positive reaction, a chest X-ray (which is safe during pregnancy as long as her abdomen is lead shielded) or a sputum culture for acid-fast bacillus to confirm the diagnosis will be scheduled.

Therapeutic Management

Women with active tuberculosis need treatment during pregnancy (Leidecker & Dorman, 2016). Isoniazid (INH), rifampin (RIF), and ethambutol hydrochloride (Myambutol)—the drugs of choice for tuberculosis—may be given without apparent teratogenic effects. INH, however, may result in a peripheral neuritis if a woman does not also take supplemental pyridoxine (vitamin B_6). Ethambutol has the side effect of causing optic atrophy and loss of green color recognition in the woman. To detect this, test the woman's ability to recognize green at prenatal visits using the color section of a Snellen (eye test) chart. If symptoms develop, inform her health provider about possibly discontinuing the drug.

A woman who had tuberculosis earlier in life must be especially careful to maintain an adequate level of calcium during pregnancy to ensure the calcium tuberculosis pockets in her lungs are not broken down and the disease is not reactivated. A woman is usually advised to wait 1 to 2 years after the infection becomes inactive before attempting to conceive as pressure on the diaphragm from the enlarging uterus changes the shape of the lung and can break open recently calcified pockets more readily than well-calcified lesions. Pockets may also break open during labor from the increased intrapulmonary pressure of pushing. Recent inactive tuberculosis may also become active during the postpartum period as the lung returns to its more vertical prepregnant position following birth.

Although tuberculosis can be spread by the placenta to the fetus, if it is active, it usually is spread to the infant after birth by the mother's coughing. Obtaining a negative sputum culture after birth rules out active tuberculosis. Urge the woman to continue taking her tuberculosis medications as prescribed during breastfeeding as only small amounts of these are secreted in breast milk and so are safe for her infant.

A WOMAN WITH CHRONIC OBSTRUCTIVE PULMONARY DISEASE

COPD is constriction of the airway associated most often with long-term cigarette smoking. When women had their children between 20 and 30 years of age, COPD was rarely associated with pregnancy. Now that more and more women are waiting until age 35 to 40 years to have children, it is now possible to see the condition with pregnancy. Constrictive air disease limits the amount of oxygen that can reach the lungs, so the condition is associated with fetal growth restriction and preterm birth. Women may need additional rest during pregnancy because of fatigue and may need continuous supplemental oxygen during the day. If they experience sleep apnea, they may be prescribed continuous positive airway pressure (CPAP) at night (Karaduman, Sarı, Aydoğan, et al., 2016). During labor, a woman might grow so short of breath from the exertion needed for pushing that she may be advised to have a cesarean birth.

Pregnancy may be the time a woman with COPD realizes she needs to stop smoking not only to preserve her own health but also to be able to supply a smoke-free environment for her baby. Offer support at prenatal visits for her attempt to do this, but caution her it is difficult to stop smoking unless her entire family takes this same step toward wellness.

A WOMAN WITH CYSTIC FIBROSIS

Cystic fibrosis is a recessively inherited disease in which there is generalized dysfunction of the exocrine glands (Leidecker & Dorman, 2016). This dysfunction leads to mucus secretions, particularly in the pancreas and lungs, which become so viscid that normal lung and pancreatic functions become compromised.

Many men with cystic fibrosis are subfertile because their semen is so thick that sperm cannot be motile. Fertility may be lessened in women with the disorder because sperm cannot migrate through viscid cervical mucus. This can make reproductive technologies such as alternative insemination or in vitro fertilization necessary for conception.

Persons with the disease typically show symptoms of chronic respiratory infection and overinflation of their lungs from the thickened mucus present; they have difficulty digesting fat and protein because the pancreas cannot release amylase. During a pregnancy, poor pulmonary function can result in inadequate oxygen supply to the fetus, resulting in an increased risk of growth restriction, preterm labor, and perinatal death. Identifying whether the fetus also has the disease can be done by chorionic villi sampling, amniocentesis, or identification of the abnormal gene on chromosome 7 in fetal cells obtained from the woman's blood serum. Screening for the disorder is included in routine neonatal screening programs after birth (Brennan & Schrijver, 2016).

Therapy for the illness consists of administration of pancrelipase (Pancrease) to supplement pancreatic enzymes. Although pancrelipase is a pregnancy risk category C drug (i.e., teratogenic effects are unknown), it does not appear to affect the fetus, so caution women to continue to take this even with nausea of early pregnancy. Women are often also prescribed a bronchodilator or antibiotic to reduce pulmonary symptoms. They should schedule a preconception meeting with their healthcare provider to discuss whether all of these will be safe during pregnancy. In addition to pharmacologic measures, women with cystic fibrosis must perform chest physiotherapy daily to reduce the buildup of lung secretions; this should continue during pregnancy. As women with the disorder excrete a higher level of sodium in perspiration than others, monitor them carefully during labor to be certain they do not become dehydrated.

Modifications for Pregnancy

Because pancrelipase may interfere with iron absorption, a woman is at greater risk for iron-deficiency anemia during pregnancy than others. Therefore, an iron supplement usually is prescribed. They also have a higher than usual incidence of developing diabetes mellitus because of pancreas involvement; therefore, women also need close monitoring of serum glucose levels at prenatal visits to detect the development of gestational diabetes.

Chest physiotherapy can become difficult late in pregnancy because the process is exhausting, moving to new positions is difficult, and lying prone, a position used frequently in postural drainage, is contraindicated in late pregnancy. To continue this effectively, therefore, a woman may need to plan more frequent and shorter sessions in modified positions (other than prone) during pregnancy (Fig. 20.2). Fetal health will be monitored by ultrasound and nonstress tests to identify intrauterine growth restriction.

Modifications for the Postpartum Period

Help a woman plan how to conserve her energy for infant care in the immediate postpartum period so she does not become exhausted and can enjoy her newborn. The milk of a nursing mother with cystic fibrosis is high in sodium, and potentially places the infant at risk for hypernatremia, so women with cystic fibrosis are usually advised not to breastfeed (Brennan & Schrijver, 2016). Although not their first choice for infant care, you can assure mothers that their infant will do well on formula.

QSEN Checkpoint Question 20.4

TEAMWORK & COLLABORATION

Angelina had tuberculosis as a teenager, and her primary care provider orders a chest X-ray during pregnancy. The nurse would want care team members to know that this is necessary because of which danger of tuberculosis during pregnancy?

a. Calcium deposits that wall off old tuberculosis lesions can break down.
b. Latent tuberculosis can turn to pneumonia if a woman has a folic acid deficit.
c. PPD tests are always negative during pregnancy so tuberculosis often goes undetected.
d. The disease can result in neural tube defects in the fetus.

Look in Appendix A for the best answer and rationale.

Figure 20.2 Modified positions for chest physiotherapy during pregnancy: **(A)** chest physiotherapy for the upper lobes and **(B)** chest physiotherapy for the lower lobes.

Rheumatic Disorders and Pregnancy

Several rheumatic disorders that occur in young adult women can be seen during pregnancy. Because most of these illnesses result in discomfort, the most common primary nursing diagnosis for these is pain. Women may not be able to achieve a pain-free outcome during pregnancy because of the nature of these illnesses, but outcomes should center on a woman stating her pain level is tolerable and that she's finding enjoyment in being pregnant.

A WOMAN WITH RHEUMATOID ARTHRITIS

Juvenile rheumatoid arthritis (JRA; sometimes referred to as chronic rheumatoid arthritis) is a disease of connective tissue marked by joint inflammation and contractures. Most likely the result of an autoimmune response, the disease pathology involves synovial membrane destruction, inflammation with effusion, swelling, erythema, and painful motion of the joints (Ngian, Briggs, Ackerman, et al., 2016). Untreated, formation of granulation tissue fills the joint space, resulting in permanent disfigurement and loss of joint motion.

Women with JRA frequently take corticosteroids, hydroxychloroquine, and nonsteroidal anti-inflammatory drugs (NSAIDs) to prevent joint pain and loss of mobility. Some women may be taking oral aspirin therapy. Although they should continue to take these medications during pregnancy to prevent joint damage, large amounts of salicylates have the potential to lead to increased bleeding at birth or possibly prolonged pregnancy (salicylate interferes with prostaglandin synthesis, so labor contractions are not initiated) (Karch, 2015). The infant may be born with a bleeding defect and may also experience premature closure of the ductus arteriosus because of the drug's effects. For this reason, the woman is asked to decrease her intake of salicylates approximately 2 weeks before term. A number of women also take low-dose methotrexate, a carcinogen (pregnancy risk category X). As a rule, they should stop taking this prepregnancy because of the danger of head and neck defects in the fetus.

Joint symptoms of the disease may improve during pregnancy because of the naturally increased circulating level of corticosteroids in the maternal bloodstream during pregnancy. During the postpartum period, when a woman's corticosteroid levels fall to prepregnancy levels, arthritis symptoms will probably recur (Ngian et al., 2016).

In the postpartum period, the determination as to the safety of breastfeeding must be individualized based on the medication each woman is taking. Those taking NSAIDS, such as ibuprofen, can breastfeed. Those taking methotrexate or large doses of aspirin may be advised not to breastfeed because of the danger to the infant.

A WOMAN WITH SYSTEMIC LUPUS ERYTHEMATOSUS

Systemic lupus erythematosus (SLE) is a multisystem chronic disease of connective tissue that occurs most frequently in woman 20 to 40 years of age (Schreiber, 2016). Widespread degeneration of connective tissue (especially of the heart, kidneys, blood vessels, spleen, skin, and retroperitoneal tissue) occurs with onset of the illness. A marked skin change is a characteristic erythematous butterfly-shaped rash on the face. In the kidneys, fibrin deposits develop, plugging and blocking the glomeruli and leading to necrosis and scarring. The thickening of collagen tissue in the blood vessels can cause vessel obstruction. This obstruction can be life-threatening to a woman if blood flow to vital organs becomes compromised and life-threatening to a fetus if blood flow to the placenta is obstructed. Many women with SLE have aPLAs, which increase the tendency for thrombi to form (Schreiber, 2016). In contrast, marked thrombocytopenia (i.e., decreased platelet count) may be present, so clotting may be deficient. Prior to pregnancy, a woman may be taking a combination of NSAIDS, low–molecular-weight heparin, salicylates, hydroxychloroquine, low-dose prednisone, or azathioprine (an immunosuppressant) to reduce disease symptoms. She can continue these during pregnancy if used with caution but may be asked to reduce the dose of salicylates 2 weeks prior to labor to prevent bleeding in the newborn and premature closure of the ductus arteriosus.

The naturally increased circulation of corticosteroids during pregnancy may lessen symptoms in some women. In others, the chief complication of the disorder—acute nephritis with glomerular destruction—may occur for the first time during pregnancy. With associated nephritis, a woman's blood pressure will rise sharply and she will develop hematuria, proteinuria with decreased urine output, and edema. It is difficult to differentiate these symptoms from the symptoms of gestational hypertension, except that with gestational hypertension, there is no hematuria. Frequent monitoring of serum creatinine levels will be necessary to assess if kidney function is adequate. If this value is over 1.5 mg/dl and proteinuria and a decreased creatinine clearance value are also present, the fetus is seriously threatened with growth restriction and the pregnancy is also threatened to be preterm. Dialysis to remove excess creatinine or plasmapheresis to replace platelets may be necessary to guard against hemorrhage in the woman at birth.

During labor, intravenous hydrocortisone may be administered to help a woman adjust to stress at this time. During the postpartum period, there may be an acute exacerbation of symptoms as corticosteroid levels again fall to normal. Infants of women with SLE may be born with a lupus-like rash, anemia, thrombocytopenia (low platelet count), and neonatal heart block. Such newborn symptoms last about 6 months and then fade. If congenital heart block occurs, a newborn pacemaker may be necessary. Screening for the exact type of autoantibodies present may be helpful in predicting which newborns will be susceptible to this.

Gastrointestinal Disorders and Pregnancy

Although minor gastrointestinal discomforts (such as nausea, heartburn, and constipation) are common during pregnancy, acute abdominal pain and protracted vomiting are causes for concern because complications such as premature separation of the placenta or ectopic pregnancy often manifest with acute abdominal pain and protracted vomiting can lead to dehydration. In some women, sudden abdominal pain is caused by a condition completely unrelated to the pregnancy, such as ulcerative colitis, hepatitis, hiatal hernia, or cholecystitis, conditions that may be known to a woman before she becomes pregnant or that may develop or be discovered during her pregnancy. In either event, they need a clear assessment and therapy to maintain the woman's overall health. Women who have colostomies may ask if they can complete a pregnancy without difficulty; the answer is yes. Even a previous liver transplant is not a contraindication to pregnancy (Margioula-Siarkou, Kalogiannidis, Petousis, et al., 2016).

 Nursing Diagnoses and Related Interventions

Nursing Diagnosis: Imbalanced nutrition, less than body requirements, related to a gastrointestinal disorder during pregnancy

Outcome Evaluation: Patient's weight gain amounts to 25 to 30 lb during pregnancy, hemoglobin is above 11 mg/dl, and specific gravity of urine is below 1.030.

Because most gastrointestinal disorders interfere with nutrition or fluid/electrolyte balance, a major intervention with all of these disorders is to ensure women are taking in adequate food and fluid for their well-being and that of their fetus, and to assess that their disease process is resolving.

A WOMAN WITH APPENDICITIS

The incidence of appendicitis, or inflammation of the appendix, is high in late adolescents and occurs as frequently as 1 in 1,500 to 2,000 pregnancies (Debnath, Sharma, & Maurya, 2016).

Assessment

History taking is important. Appendicitis usually begins with a few hours of nausea and then an hour or two of generalized abdominal discomfort. Then, comes the typical sharp, peristaltic, lower right quadrant pain of acute appendicitis.

Pain from an overstretched round ligament or a ruptured ectopic pregnancy may both cause sharp lower quadrant pain, so the pain from these needs to be differentiated from that of appendicitis. The major difference is that the pain of an over-stretched round ligament fades almost instantly; appendicitis pain not only continues but grows more intense. With an ectopic pregnancy, a woman may experience morning sickness, and the pain she feels is either diffuse or sharp. With appendicitis, the nausea and vomiting is much more intense and the pain is sharp and localized at McBurney point (a point halfway between the umbilicus and the iliac crest on the lower right abdomen). In the pregnant woman, this can shift higher in the abdomen because the appendix is often displaced so far up in the abdomen by the uterus that the pain may resemble the pain of gallbladder disease (Fig. 20.3).

The woman's temperature is usually elevated, a urine sample reveals ketones, and a complete blood count reveals leukocytosis. Because pregnant women typically have an elevated white blood cell (WBC) count, however, an elevated WBC is not as diagnostic in pregnancy as it might be otherwise. An ultrasound or magnetic resonance imaging (MRI) scan will confirm the inflamed appendix.

Advise a woman in an emergency room that while she is waiting to be evaluated for possible appendicitis not to eat any food, drink any liquid, or consume any laxatives because increasing peristalsis could cause an inflamed appendix to rupture.

Therapeutic Management

If a woman is near term (past 37 weeks) and the fetus is believed to be mature, a cesarean birth may be performed along with removal of the inflamed appendix at the same time. If appendicitis occurs early in pregnancy, the inflamed appendix is usually removed by laparoscopy. As long as the

anesthesiologist is aware the woman is pregnant and carefully controls oxygen levels during anesthesia administration, the outcome of both the surgery and the pregnancy will be good.

If the appendix ruptures before surgery, the risk to both mother and fetus increases dramatically. This occurs because, with rupture, infected fecal material escapes into the peritoneum and could spread by the fallopian tubes to the fetus. Also, generalized peritonitis is such an overwhelming infection that it would be difficult for a woman's body to combat it effectively and also maintain the pregnancy. As a third concern, peritoneal adhesions may develop after an appendix ruptures, resulting in future subfertility because of changes in the placement of fallopian tubes (Wu & Hueppchen, 2015).

A WOMAN WITH GASTROESOPHAGEAL REFLUX DISEASE OR HIATAL HERNIA

Gastroesophageal reflux disease (GERD) refers to the reflux of acid stomach secretions into the esophagus (Zielinski, Searing, & Deibel, 2015). Hiatal hernia is a condition in which a portion of the stomach extends and protrudes up through the diaphragm into the esophagus, trapping stomach acid and causing it to reflux into the esophagus. Although these conditions can be present constantly, symptoms most often occur only sporadically after increased peristaltic action. Both conditions may generate symptoms for the first time during pregnancy as the uterus pushes the stomach up against the esophageal valve and increases the reflux of acid or the extent of the hernia. Symptoms include:

- Heartburn, which is particularly extreme when lying supine after a full meal
- Gastric regurgitation
- Dysphagia (difficulty swallowing)

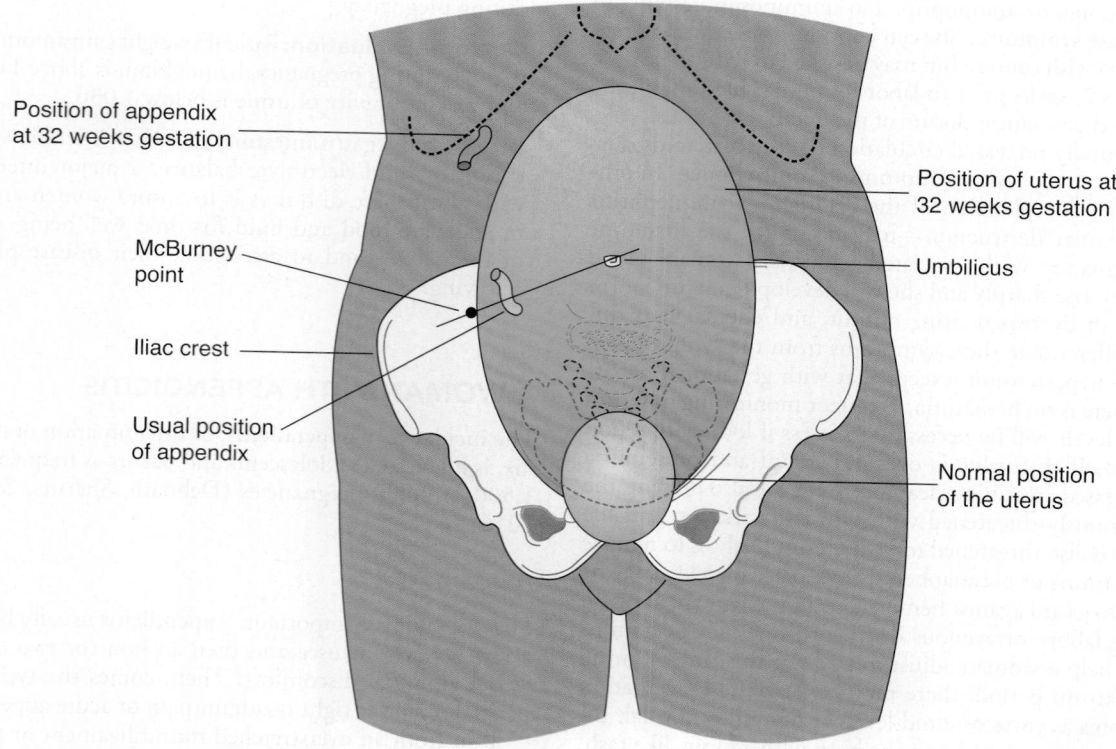

Figure 20.3 The change in position of appendix during pregnancy.

- Possible weight loss because of the stomach pain
- Hematemesis (i.e., vomiting of blood) if extreme esophageal irritation occurs

During pregnancy, these conditions are usually diagnosed by ultrasound, although direct endoscopy could be used. In most women, an over-the-counter antacid or a prescription for a proton pump inhibitor such as esomeprazole magnesium (Nexium; pregnancy category B) will effectively dilute or inhibit gastric acid production and so relieve symptoms. As additional measures, advise a woman to wear clothing that is loose around her waist and to sleep with her head elevated on two or more pillows to help confine stomach secretions. Esomeprazole magnesium has not been studied as to its safety during breastfeeding, but as the uterine pressure is eliminated following birth, the symptoms generally become less noticeable or disappear and the woman no longer needs the drug. Some women may continue to have pain after birth and so need to take an acid inhibitor for several months until their irritated esophagus is completely healed.

A WOMAN WITH CHOLECYSTITIS AND CHOLELITHIASIS

Cholecystitis (i.e., gallbladder inflammation) and cholelithiasis (i.e., gallstone formation) are most frequently associated with women older than 40 years of age, who are obese, are multiparas, and ingest a high-fat diet. Because gallstones form from cholesterol, the hypercholesterolemia that naturally occurs during pregnancy may be the reason an increased incidence of gallstone formation occurs during pregnancy in women prone to these. Symptoms they cause are constant aching and pressure in the right epigastrium, perhaps accompanied by jaundice.

Medical therapy to prevent both conditions is to lower fat intake; however, during pregnancy, women should not eliminate it entirely because of the importance of linoleic acid for fetal brain growth. If symptoms of acute cholecystitis occur during pregnancy, the condition can be diagnosed by ultrasound. It can generally be managed by temporarily halting oral intake to rest the gastrointestinal tract and administering intravenous fluids to provide fluid and nutrients as well as analgesics for pain. Surgery for gallbladder removal by laparoscopic technique may be done during pregnancy if a woman's symptoms cannot be controlled by conservative management (Jorge, Keswani, Veerappan, et al., 2015).

A WOMAN WITH PANCREATITIS

Pancreatitis (i.e., inflammation of the pancreas) is a rare disorder that tends to occur in late adolescents and so may occur during pregnancy (Hacker, Whalen, Lee, et al., 2015). The woman experiences severe epigastric pain, nausea, vomiting, anorexia, and fever. Diagnosis may be difficult as serum amylase, which rises with pancreatitis, is also normally elevated during pregnancy. If serum amylase levels are greater than two times above normal, however, pancreatitis should be suspected. The disorder is treated the same during pregnancy as in nonpregnant women: nasogastric suction, bowel rest, analgesia (because pancreatic pain is sharp), and intravenous hydration through parenteral nutritional supplementation (Xu, Wang, & Zhang, 2015). The inflammation usually subsides within a week. Pregnancy loss, however, can occur from acidosis, hypovolemia, and fetal hypoxia (Abdullah, Kathiresan Pillai, Cheen, et al., 2015).

A WOMAN WITH HEPATITIS

Hepatitis is a liver disease that occurs from invasion of the hepatitis A, B, C, D, or E virus. Hepatitis A is spread mainly by fecal–oral contact (children in day-care settings have a high incidence) or by ingestion of fecally contaminated water or shellfish. It has an incubation period of 2 to 6 weeks. Pregnant women exposed to hepatitis A may be given prophylactic γ-globulin to try to prevent the disease after exposure. This form follows a rather benign course and is not thought to be transmitted to the fetus (Rac & Sheffield, 2014).

Hepatitis B and C are spread by exposure to contaminated blood or blood products or by contact with contaminated semen or vaginal secretions (and so are considered sexually transmitted infections [STIs]). These can be transmitted to the fetus across the placenta. Hepatitis D and E are apparently spread by the same methods as hepatitis B and C but are rarely seen in pregnant women.

Hepatitis C demonstrates few symptoms, and these may not be present for 12 months after exposure. It is, however, the most common cause of chronic liver disease and liver transplantation in the United States (Rac & Sheffield, 2014).

Hepatitis B occurs about 1 in every 2,000 pregnancies (Rac & Sheffield, 2014). It has an incubation period of 6 weeks to 6 months. It occurs in both an acute and chronic form, leading to liver cell necrosis with scarring and an inability to convert indirect to direct bilirubin or to excrete direct bilirubin. Women exposed to the virus receive immune globulin for prophylaxis; a hepatitis B vaccine can be administered to those who are at high risk, such as women who handle blood products, to prevent the illness.

Assessment

With all forms of hepatitis, a woman experiences nausea and vomiting. Her liver area may feel tender to palpation. Urine will turn dark yellow from excretion of bilirubin; stools will be light-colored from lack of bilirubin. Jaundice occurs as a late symptom. On physical examination, hepatomegaly (i.e., enlargement of the liver) is noted. The serum bilirubin level is elevated. Levels of liver enzymes, such as transaminase, are increased. Specific antibodies against the virus can be detected in the blood serum, so women at high risk may be routinely screened for this during pregnancy. If a liver biopsy is necessary for diagnosis, this can be performed safely during pregnancy as this is done under local anesthesia.

Therapeutic Management

A woman is usually prescribed bed rest and encouraged to eat a high-calorie diet because her liver has difficulty converting stored glycogen into glucose in its diseased state and so hypoglycemia can result. A cesarean birth may be planned at term to reduce the possibility of blood exchange between mother and fetus. Follow standard infection precautions when you give care to avoid contact with body fluids.

Hepatitis during pregnancy may lead to spontaneous miscarriage or preterm labor. Unlike most other diseases that cause maximum fetal threat in the first trimester, the later in pregnancy a woman contracts hepatitis B infection, the greater the risk the infant will be affected or develop hepatitis B. If this should occur, it is a serious consequence because a proportion of hepatitis B Ag-positive infants will develop liver cirrhosis or carcinoma later in life (Rac & Sheffield, 2014).

Use precautions during birth to avoid exposure to maternal body fluids. After birth, a woman may breastfeed as the infection is apparently not transmitted by breast milk. The infant should be washed well to remove any maternal blood; hepatitis B immune globulin (HBIG) and the first dose of hepatitis B should be administered (see Chapter 34 for the full immunization series). The infant then needs to be observed carefully for symptoms of infection during the first few months of life and for chronic liver disease as he or she grows older.

A WOMAN WITH INFLAMMATORY BOWEL DISEASE

Crohn disease (i.e., inflammation of the terminal ileus) and ulcerative colitis (i.e., inflammation of the distal colon) occur most often in late adolescents between ages 12 and 30 years. The cause of these diseases is unknown, but an autoimmune process is thought to be responsible. They are also associated with passive and active smoking (Dutta & Chacko, 2016). In both diseases, the bowel develops shallow ulcers. A woman experiences chronic diarrhea, weight loss, occult blood in stool, and nausea and vomiting. If extreme, obstruction and fistula formation with peritonitis can occur. With Crohn disease, malabsorption, particularly of vitamin B (the absorption of which occurs almost entirely in the ileum), can occur. Because of the potential difficulty with absorbing nutrients in both disorders, women with these disorders need careful monitoring for weight gain during pregnancy. There is a potential for fetal growth restriction if extreme malabsorption occurs. Therapy for the disorders is rest for the gastrointestinal tract by administration of total parenteral nutrition. Sulfasalazine (Azulfidine), an anti-inflammatory and a mainstay of therapy, may be continued during pregnancy without fetal injury. Close to birth, the dosage of sulfasalazine, because of its sulfa base, is reduced because it may interfere with bilirubin binding sites and cause neonatal jaundice (Karch, 2015). Infliximab (IFX) and adalimumab (ADA) are other attractive treatment options, but there is still limited data on the benefit/risk profile during pregnancy (Shihab, Yeomans, & De Cruz, 2016).

Neurologic Disorders and Pregnancy

Neurologic illness, as a whole, does not occur at a high incidence in women of childbearing age. However, any neurologic disease with symptoms of seizures must be carefully managed during pregnancy because the anoxia that could be caused by severe seizures could deprive a fetus of oxygen.

A WOMAN WITH A SEIZURE DISORDER

Recurrent seizures have several causes, such as head trauma or meningitis. However, the causes of most recurrent seizures, such as epilepsy, are unknown (i.e., are idiopathic). Recurrent seizures are seen in about 3 to 5 women per 1,000 births.

Therapeutic Management

The goal of care is to establish the best seizure control with the fewest possible number of antiseizure drugs prior to pregnancy. During pregnancy, because almost all antiseizure drugs

are at least mildly teratogenic, dosages may have to be decreased even further to protect the fetus, which unfortunately then increases the risk of seizures (Videman, Tokariev, Stjerna, et al., 2016). Be certain women understand the rule "Do not take medication during pregnancy" does not apply to antiseizure medications so that they continue to conscientiously take them despite the nausea or vomiting of early pregnancy. It is important the levels of antiseizure drugs be monitored and the doses adjusted routinely during pregnancy and again after birth. As blood volume increases with pregnancy, some women may need their dosage increased or their serum level will be diluted. Common drugs prescribed to control seizures are trimethadione (Tridione; pregnancy risk category D); valproic acid (sodium valproate and divalproex sodium; pregnancy risk category D); carbamazepine (Tegretol; pregnancy risk category C); ethosuximide (Zarontin; pregnancy risk category C), a drug often used to control absence seizures; and phenytoin sodium (Dilantin; pregnancy risk category D).

Women who have been taking phenytoin (Dilantin) for some time may have developed chronic hypertension, so a baseline blood pressure should be established early in pregnancy so any changes that occur with pregnancy can be interpreted correctly. Phenytoin (Dilantin) is recognized as the cause of a fetal syndrome, including cognitive impairment, vitamin K deficiency, and a peculiar facial proportion not unlike that of fetal alcohol sequence. To counteract the vitamin K deficiency and prevent hemorrhage in the newborn, women may be prescribed vitamin K during labor or the last 4 weeks of gestation.

 Concept Mastery Alert

Adverse effects of phenytoin sodium (Dilantin) include vitamin K deficiency and possible bleeding. This can be counteracted by administration of vitamin K supplementation in the last 4 weeks of gestation.

 Nursing Diagnoses and Related Interventions

Nursing Diagnosis: Risk for ineffective tissue (placental) perfusion related to hypoxia resulting from maternal seizure

Outcome Evaluation: Patient informs healthcare personnel about history of seizures; states importance of immediate care and oxygen therapy should she begin a seizure. Apgar score of infant is 7 to 10, with no apparent birth anomalies.

Absence seizures (often just a rapid fluttering of the eyelids or a moment's staring into space) should have no effect on a woman or fetus. Tonic–clonic seizures (sustained, full-body involvement) could affect a fetus because spasm of the woman's chest muscles could lead to hypoxia. If a seizure should occur during pregnancy, a woman must be evaluated to be certain the cause of the seizure was the underlying seizure disorder, not a sign of eclampsia (see Chapter 21). Nonpregnant women experiencing tonic–clonic seizures do not need oxygen administered during a seizure, but in pregnancy, administering oxygen by mask is a good prophylaxis to ensure adequate fetal oxygenation.

Woman who have recurrent seizures may worry their children will develop seizures as they grow older. If a woman's seizures were the result of an acquired disorder such as meningitis or head trauma, you can assure her that her child's risk for seizures is no greater than that for any other child. If the etiology of her seizures is unknown, the chance her child also will develop them is slightly higher than in the rest of the population. This prediction is only theoretical, however, and cannot be made without a thorough review of the onset and nature of the woman's disorder. Be certain a woman spends enough time with her newborn so she can become acquainted with the sudden jerking motions that occur in newborns such as when a newborn is startled (Moro reflex) or the jaw quivers after prolonged crying so she doesn't interpret these normal movements as seizure activity.

A WOMAN WITH MYASTHENIA GRAVIS

Myasthenia gravis is an autoimmune disorder characterized by the presence of an IgG antibody against acetylcholine receptors in striated muscle. The presence of the antibody causes failure of the striated muscles to contract, particularly those of the oropharyngeal, facial, and extraocular groups. The disorder usually occurs in 20- to 30-year-olds, although it also is seen in young children. Women with the disorder need to be carefully monitored during pregnancy as pregnancy can cause major exacerbations of the disease (Roth, Dent, & McDevitt, 2015).

The disorder is treated with anticholinesterase drugs such as pyridostigmine (Mestinon) or neostigmine (Prostigmin) and possibly a corticosteroid such as prednisone. These medications may be continued during pregnancy, as the fetus will experience no effects from them. Be certain a woman understands atropine is the lifesaving antidote for neostigmine if an overdose should occur. Plasmapheresis (i.e., removal of and replacement of plasma) to remove immune complexes from the bloodstream may be prescribed to reduce symptoms. It must be carried out gradually during pregnancy, however, to reduce the risk of fluid overload or hypotension. Because smooth muscle is not affected by the disease, labor should occur without complications. Magnesium sulfate (administered to halt preterm labor or treat hypertension of pregnancy) should be avoided at any point in pregnancy because it can diminish the acetylcholine effect and therefore increase disease symptoms.

An infant born to a woman with myasthenia gravis may demonstrate disease symptoms at birth because of the transfer of antibodies (see Chapter 51).

A WOMAN WITH MULTIPLE SCLEROSIS

Multiple sclerosis (MS) occurs predominantly in women of childbearing age, usually between 20 and 40 years of age (Pozzilli & Pugliatti, 2015). With MS, nerve fibers become demyelinated and therefore lose function. Women develop symptoms of fatigue, numbness, blurred vision, and loss of coordination. ACTH (adrenocorticotropic hormone) or a corticosteroid is commonly given to strengthen nerve conduction and both can be administered safely during pregnancy. In contrast, immunosuppressants such as cyclosporine

(Sandimmune), azathioprine (Imuran), and cyclophosphamide (Cytoxan), which are also frequently prescribed, should be used cautiously during pregnancy. Women may continue with plasmapheresis (i.e., withdrawal and replacement of plasma), another treatment regimen, during pregnancy as long as the volume of exchange is well controlled to prevent hypotension. Although women with the disorder may grow increasingly fatigued as pregnancy progresses, pregnancy does not affect the long-term course of MS. In some women, symptoms may actually improve during pregnancy because of the increased circulating corticosteroid levels. Monitor for UTIs at prenatal visits as these tend to occur as a poorly defined consequence of the illness.

Musculoskeletal Disorders and Pregnancy

Falls or other unintentional injuries that may lead to bone fractures or muscle sprains in women of childbearing age are discussed in Chapter 22. A chronic musculoskeletal disorder that is first identified during adolescence and so may play a role in childbearing is scoliosis.

A WOMAN WITH SCOLIOSIS

Scoliosis (i.e., lateral curvature of the spine) begins to be noticed first in girls between 12 and 14 years of age. If it is uncorrected at this time, the curvature progresses until it can interfere with respiration and heart action because of chest compression. Pelvic distortion can interfere with childbirth, especially at the pelvic inlet. If a woman's spine is extremely curved, epidural anesthesia may be difficult to administer for pain management in labor.

Girls with scoliosis may wear a body brace during their adolescent years to maintain an erect posture. Although these braces are not as bulky as they once were, unless they are modified, they cannot be worn during the last half of pregnancy. For surgical correction, girls have stainless steel rods surgically implanted on both sides of their vertebrae to strengthen and straighten their spine. Such rod implantations do not interfere with pregnancy; a woman may notice more than usual back pain, however, from increased tension on back muscles. If a woman's pelvis is distorted, a cesarean birth may be scheduled to ensure a safe birth. Vaginal birth, if permitted, requires the same management as for any woman. With the improved management of scoliosis, the high maternal and perinatal risks associated with the disorder reported in earlier literature no longer exist (Falick-Michaeli, Schroeder, Barzilay, et al., 2015). Plot the course of labor on a labor graph so an unusually long first stage, suggesting cephalopelvic disproportion, can be recognized. Chapter 51 discusses in detail the nursing care of adolescents following surgery to have rods inserted.

Endocrine Disorders and Pregnancy

Endocrine disorders have the potential to be serious complications of pregnancy because enzymes and hormones control so many specific body functions (Krassas, Karras, & Pontikides, 2015).

A WOMAN WITH A THYROID DYSFUNCTION

As a normal effect of pregnancy, the thyroid gland enlarges (i.e., hypertrophies) slightly because of increased vascularity and blood flow. A woman with a preexisting thyroid illness may have difficulty making this pregnancy transition.

 Nursing Diagnoses and Related Interventions

Nursing Diagnosis: Risk for maternal and fetal injury related to preexisting thyroid disorder during pregnancy

Outcome Evaluation: No congenital anomalies are present in infant at birth; Apgar score is 7 to 10. Mother continues prepregnancy level of activities.

Thyroid function is necessary for the regulation of almost all body functions. Problems that affect pregnancy are either those of too little thyroid response (i.e., hypothyroidism) or too great a response (i.e., hyperthyroidism).

A Woman With Hypothyroidism

Hypothyroidism, or underproduction of the thyroid hormone, is a rare condition in late adolescents and especially rare in pregnancy because women with symptoms of untreated hypothyroidism are often anovulatory and unable to conceive. A woman who does conceive can then face another obstacle in that she can have difficulty increasing thyroid functioning to a necessary pregnancy level, which can then lead to early spontaneous miscarriage. Women with hypothyroidism fatigue easily, tend to be obese, their skin is dry (myxedema), and they have little tolerance for cold. It may be associated with an increased incidence of extreme nausea and vomiting (i.e., hyperemesis gravidarum).

Most women with hypothyroidism take levothyroxine (Synthroid) to supplement their lack of thyroid hormone. A woman who is taking levothyroxine needs to consult with her primary care provider when she is planning on becoming pregnant to be certain her dose of this will be high enough to sustain a pregnancy. She needs to come for an early diagnosis and close follow-up as soon as she suspects she is pregnant (1 week past her missed menstrual period). As a rule, her dose of levothyroxine will need to be increased as much as 20% to 30% for the duration of the pregnancy to simulate the increase that would normally occur in pregnancy (Kraut & Farahani, 2015). Be certain a woman realizes the importance of taking this increased dose. Also, caution women that they should take levothyroxine at a different time from any medication containing iron, calcium, or any soy product by about 4 hours to be certain there is no problem with the absorption of the drug (Karch, 2015).

After the pregnancy, the dose of levothyroxine prescribed for pregnancy must be gradually tapered back to the prepregnancy level for both her health and so she can breastfeed safely. Be certain a woman does not continue to take her pregnancy dose (e.g., in trying to be economical and use up her higher dose pills), or she could pass beyond normal thyroid function and develop hyperthyroidism.

A Woman With Hyperthyroidism

Hyperthyroidism, or overproduction of thyroid hormone, causes symptoms such as a rapid heart rate, exophthalmos (i.e., protruding eyeballs), heat intolerance, heart palpitations, and weight loss. Sometimes called Graves disease, it is more apt to be seen in pregnancy than is hypothyroidism. If undiagnosed, a woman may develop heart failure because her heart, already stressed, cannot manage the increasing blood volume that occurs with pregnancy. She is also more prone than the average woman to symptoms of gestational hypertension, fetal growth restriction, and preterm labor.

Hyperthyroidism is normally diagnosed by a nuclear medicine imaging study involving the radioactive uptake of ^{131}I subtype. This diagnostic procedure should not be used during pregnancy because the fetal thyroid would also incorporate this drug, possibly resulting in destruction of the fetal thyroid. Treatment for hyperthyroidism is with thioamides (methimazole [Tapazole] or propylthiouracil [PTU]), which reduce thyroid activity. These drugs, unfortunately, cross the placenta and can lead to congenital hypothyroidism and, consequently, an enlarged thyroid gland (i.e., a goiter) in the fetus. Women should be regulated on the lowest possible dose of the drug and cautioned to keep a careful record of doses taken so they do not forget or unintentionally duplicate a dose, because if a goiter in the fetus enlarges enough, it can obstruct the airway and make resuscitation difficult at birth. Methimazole is the preferred drug for pregnant women as it appears to cross the placenta less easily (Andersen, Olsen, & Laurberg, 2016).

If hyperthyroidism is not regulated during pregnancy, an infant may be born with symptoms of hyperthyroidism because of the excess stimulation he or she receives in utero. The newborn may appear jittery with tachypnea and tachycardia. An assay of fetal cord blood will reveal the level of thyroxine (T_4) and thyroid-stimulating hormone and the need for therapy in the infant. Women receiving smaller or minimal doses of antithyroid drugs may breastfeed, although women receiving large doses of these drugs may be advised not to breastfeed because they are excreted in breast milk (Prunty, Heise, & Chaffin, 2016).

Surgical treatment to reduce the functioning of the maternal thyroid gland can be accomplished, but this is generally not the treatment of choice during pregnancy because of the need for general anesthesia. After a pregnancy, if a woman desires other children, the procedure might be suggested as an interpregnancy procedure so she does not enter a second pregnancy with hyperthyroidism.

A WOMAN WITH DIABETES MELLITUS

Diabetes mellitus is an endocrine disorder in which the pancreas cannot produce adequate insulin to regulate body glucose levels. The disorder affects 3% to 5% of all pregnancies and is the most frequently seen medical condition in pregnancy (Bradley, Duprey, & Castorino, 2016). It is increasing in incidence as more and more obese adolescents develop type 2 diabetes (Klingensmith, Pyle, Nadeau, et al., 2016).

Before insulin was produced synthetically in 1921, women with type 1 diabetes (i.e., diabetes acquired in childhood) died before reaching childbearing age, were subfertile, or had spontaneous miscarriages early in pregnancy. Now that both type 1 and type 2 diabetes can be well managed, three new challenges have developed:

- How to manage both type 1 and type 2 diabetes during pregnancy to achieve a healthy glucose/insulin balance during pregnancy
- How to protect an infant in utero from the adverse effects of increased glucose levels
- How to care for the infant in the first 24 hours after birth until the infant's insulin–glucose regulatory mechanism stabilizes

Reproductive planning may be a fourth concern, as women with diabetes may not be good candidates for oral contraceptives because progesterone interferes with insulin activity and therefore increases blood glucose levels.

Pathophysiology and Clinical Manifestations

The possible etiology and pathology of diabetes mellitus are discussed in detail in Chapter 48. The primary concern for any woman with this disorder is controlling the balance between insulin and blood glucose levels to prevent hyperglycemia or hypoglycemia. Both of these conditions are dangerous during pregnancy not only because of long-term effects on the woman's health but also because of the threat to normal fetal growth. Infants of women with unregulated diabetes are five times more apt to be born large for gestational age or with birth anomalies (Ornoy, Reece, Pavlinkova, et al., 2015).

If a woman's insulin production is insufficient, glucose cannot be used by body cells. The cells register the need for glucose, and the liver quickly converts stored glycogen to glucose to increase the serum glucose level. Because insulin is still not available, however, the body cells still cannot use the glucose, so the serum glucose levels rise (i.e., hyperglycemia). When the level of blood glucose reaches 150 mg/100 ml (normal level is 80 to 120 mg/dl), the kidneys begin to excrete quantities of glucose in the urine (i.e., glycosuria) in an attempt to lower the level. This causes large quantities of fluid to be excreted with urine (i.e., polyuria).

As dehydration begins to occur, the blood serum becomes concentrated and the total blood volume decreases. With the reduced blood flow, cells do not receive adequate oxygen, and anaerobic metabolic reactions cause large stores of lactic acid to pour out of muscles into the bloodstream. To replace needed glucose, fat is mobilized from fat stores and metabolized for energy, pouring large amounts of acidic ketone bodies into the bloodstream.

As the process continues, protein stores are tapped in a final attempt to find a source of energy. Utilizing protein for energy this way reduces the supply of protein to body cells. As cells die, they release potassium and sodium, which is lost from the body in the extensive polyuria. These factors combined create an immediate severe metabolic acidosis. Long-term effects are vascular narrowing that leads to kidney, heart, and retinal dysfunction.

Diabetes During Pregnancy

In type 1 diabetes, which, although unproven, is probably an autoimmune disorder because marker antibodies are present, the pancreas fails to produce adequate insulin for body requirements (Gururaj Setty, Crasto, Jarvis, et al., 2016). In type 2 diabetes, there is a gradual loss of insulin production, but some ability to produce insulin will still be present.

Women with either type 1 or type 2 diabetes who have successful regulation of glucose and insulin metabolism before pregnancy are apt to develop less-than-optimal control during pregnancy because all women experience several changes in the glucose–insulin regulatory system as pregnancy progresses. In all pregnancies, the glomerular filtration of glucose is increased (the glomerular excretion threshold is lowered), causing slight glycosuria. The rate of insulin secretion is increased, and the fasting blood sugar level is lowered. All women appear to develop an insulin resistance as pregnancy progresses or insulin does not seem as effective during pregnancy, a phenomenon that is probably caused by the presence of the hormone human placental lactogen (i.e., chorionic somatomammotropin) and high levels of cortisol, estrogen, progesterone, and catecholamines. This resistance to or destruction of insulin is helpful in a healthy pregnancy because it prevents the maternal blood glucose from falling to dangerous limits. It causes difficulty for a pregnant woman with diabetes because she must then increase her insulin dosage beginning at about week 24 of pregnancy to prevent hyperglycemia.

At the same time, she must guard against **hypoglycemia** (i.e., lowered serum glucose levels) and ketoacidosis caused by the constant use of glucose by the fetus. If a woman has preexisting kidney disease (revealed by proteinuria, decreased creatinine clearance, and hypertension), the risk of hypertension of pregnancy rises markedly (Au, Raynes-Greenow, Turner, et al., 2016).

Infants of women with poorly controlled diabetes tend to be large (>10 lb) because the increased insulin the fetus must produce to counteract the overload of glucose he or she receives acts as a growth stimulant. Hydramnios may develop because a high glucose concentration causes extra fluid to shift and enlarge the amount of amniotic fluid. A macrosomic infant may create birth problems at the end of the pregnancy because of cephalopelvic disproportion. This, combined with an increased risk for shoulder dystocia, may make it necessary for infants of women with diabetes to be born by cesarean birth.

There is also a high incidence of congenital anomaly, especially caudal regression syndrome (failure of the lower extremities to develop), spontaneous miscarriage, and stillbirth in women with uncontrolled diabetes. At birth, neonates are more prone to hypoglycemia, respiratory distress syndrome, hypocalcemia, and hyperbilirubinemia. The first trimester of pregnancy is the most important time for fetal development; if a woman can be kept from becoming hyperglycemic during this time, the chances of a congenital anomaly are greatly lessened (Box 20.6) (Ornoy et al., 2015).

Classification of Diabetes Mellitus

Diabetes is divided into various categories that can be used to predict a pregnancy outcome (Table 20.2). Approximately 2% to 3% of all women who do not begin a pregnancy with diabetes develop the condition during pregnancy, usually at the midpoint of pregnancy when insulin resistance becomes most noticeable. This is termed *gestational diabetes mellitus* (Landon, Catalano, & Gabbe, 2012). The symptoms fade again at the completion of pregnancy, but the risk of developing type 2 diabetes later in life may be as high as 50% to 60%. It is unknown whether gestational diabetes results from inadequate insulin response to carbohydrate, from excessive

BOX 20.6

Nursing Care Planning Using Assessment

ASSESSING A PREGNANT WOMAN WITH DIABETES MELLITUS

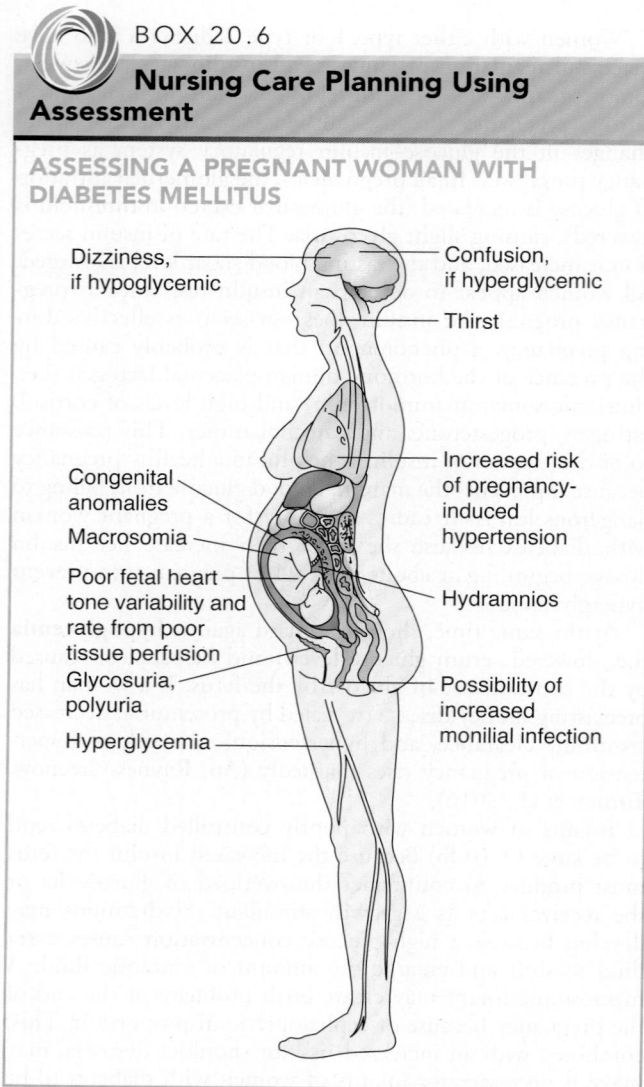

- Dizziness, if hypoglycemic
- Confusion, if hyperglycemic
- Thirst
- Congenital anomalies
- Macrosomia
- Increased risk of pregnancy-induced hypertension
- Poor fetal heart tone variability and rate from poor tissue perfusion
- Hydramnios
- Glycosuria, polyuria
- Possibility of increased monilial infection
- Hyperglycemia

TABLE 20.2 CLASSIFICATION OF DIABETES MELLITUS

Class	Description
Type 1	A state characterized by the destruction of the beta cells in the pancreas that usually leads to absolute insulin deficiency.
	a. Immune-mediated diabetes mellitus results from autoimmune destruction of the beta cells.
	b. Idiopathic type 1 refers to forms that have no known cause.
Type 2	A state that usually arises because of insulin resistance combined with a relative deficiency in the production of insulin.
Gestational diabetes	A condition of abnormal glucose metabolism that arises during pregnancy.
	Possible signal of an increased risk for type 2 diabetes later in life.
Impaired glucose homeostasis	A state between "normal" and "diabetes" in which the body is no longer using and/or secreting insulin properly.
	a. Impaired fasting glucose: a state when fasting plasma glucose is at least 110 but under 126 mg/dl
	b. Impaired glucose tolerance: a state when results of the oral glucose tolerance test are at least 140 but under 200 mg/dl in the 1-hour sample

From American Diabetes Association. (2011). Summary of revisions to the 2011 clinical practice recommendations. *Diabetes Care, 34*(Suppl. 1), S3.

recommended that all pregnant women receive a 50-g **glucose challenge test** between 24 and 28 weeks gestation to determine if they are at risk for gestational diabetes. If the result of that test is 140 mg/dl (some providers use 130 mg/dl as the cutoff), then the woman will need to do a three hour glucose tolerance test.

For this, after a fasting glucose sample is obtained, the woman drinks an oral 100-g glucose solution; a venous blood sample is then taken for glucose determination at 1, 2, and 3 hours later. If two of the four blood samples collected for this test are abnormal or the fasting value is above 95 mg/dl, a diagnosis of diabetes is made. The values that confirm diabetes are reviewed in Table 20.3.

resistance to insulin, or from a combination of both. Risk factors for developing gestational diabetes include:

- Obesity
- Age over 25 years
- History of large babies (10 lb or more)
- History of unexplained fetal or perinatal loss
- History of congenital anomalies in previous pregnancies
- History of polycystic ovary syndrome
- Family history of diabetes (one close relative or two distant ones)
- Member of a population with a high risk for diabetes (Native American, Hispanic, Asian)

Assessment

Because diabetes is such a serious complication in pregnancy, all women should be screened during pregnancy for gestational diabetes. A fasting plasma glucose greater than or equal to 126 mg/dl or a nonfasting plasma glucose greater than or equal to 200 mg/dl meets the threshold for the diagnosis of diabetes and does not need confirmation. It is

TABLE 20.3 ORAL GLUCOSE CHALLENGE TEST VALUES (FASTING PLASMA GLUCOSE VALUES) FOR PREGNANCY FOLLOWING A 100-g GLUCOSE SOLUTION

Test Type	Pregnant Glucose Level (mg/dl)
Fasting	95
1 hr	180
2 hr	155
3 hr	140

Monitoring a Woman With Diabetes

A woman with diabetes (type 1 or type 2) before pregnancy should meet with her primary healthcare provider prior to becoming pregnant; during this period, her condition can be well regulated so that hyperglycemia does not develop during the early weeks of pregnancy, when the tendency for congenital anomalies in the fetus is highest. A woman should use a home test kit to determine she is pregnant so she knows this at the earliest possible time. The best insulin control program for her during pregnancy can then be determined. The measurement of **glycosylated hemoglobin (HbA1c)**, a measure of the amount of glucose attached to hemoglobin, is used to detect the degree of hyperglycemia present. Measuring HbA1c is advantageous not just because it offers a present value of glucose, but because it reflects the average blood glucose level over the past 4 to 6 weeks (i.e., the time the hemoglobin in red blood cells were picking up the glucose). The upper normal level of HbA1c is 6% of total hemoglobin.

A urine culture may be done each trimester to detect asymptomatic UTIs as the increased glucose concentration in urine may lead to increased infection. An ophthalmic examination should be done once during the pregnancy for a woman with gestational diabetes and at each trimester for women with known diabetes because common background retinal changes that are common in diabetes, such as increased exudate (Fig. 20.4), dot hemorrhage, and macular edema, can progress or originate during pregnancy. Laser therapy to halt these changes can be done during pregnancy without risk to the fetus.

Nursing Diagnoses and Related Interventions

Because diabetes is such a complex disorder, associated nursing diagnoses are many and varied. Examples include:

- Risk for ineffective tissue perfusion related to reduced vascular flow
- Imbalanced nutrition, less than body requirements, related to inability to use glucose
- Risk for ineffective coping related to required change in lifestyle

Figure 20.4 Increased exudate in the retina can occur with progressing diabetes during pregnancy. It appears as a "cloud-like" finding obscuring a retinal vessel.

- Risk for infection related to impaired healing accompanying condition
- Deficient fluid volume related to polyuria accompanying the disorder
- Deficient knowledge related to complex health problem
- Health-seeking behaviors related to voiced need to learn home glucose monitoring

The following nursing diagnosis and related interventions illustrate one of the most important facets of the nurse's role in caring for the pregnant woman with diabetes: health teaching. Important topics include nutrition, exercise, insulin administration, blood glucose monitoring, and explanations of the various fetal assessment tests that will be done. Box 20.7 shows an interprofessional care map illustrating both nursing and team planning for a woman with diabetes.

Nursing Diagnosis: Deficient knowledge related to a therapeutic regimen necessary during pregnancy

Outcome Evaluation: Patient states importance of careful attention to nutrition, exercise, and home monitoring of glucose levels during pregnancy; describes nutrition and exercise program; states intention to keep nutrition and exercise constant.

Education Regarding Nutrition During Pregnancy. Women with diabetes need to be aware of how much carbohydrate they eat daily by estimating the total carbohydrate each anticipated meal will contain and then administer a number of units of insulin prior to that based on a predetermined insulin-to-carbohydrate ratio. As children also need to adjust insulin amounts to carbohydrate ratios, carbohydrate counting is discussed in Chapter 48.

Dietary control, or maintaining an adequate glucose intake so hypoglycemia does not occur, may be extremely difficult early in pregnancy because of nausea and vomiting. A 1,800- to 2,400-calorie diet (or one calculated at 30 kcal/kg of ideal weight), divided into three meals and three snacks to try and keep carbohydrate evenly distributed during the day so the glucose level remains constant, is a typical nutrition regimen during pregnancy. Ideally, 20% of dietary calories should be from protein, 40% to 50% from carbohydrate, and up to 30% from fat (Dornhorst & Williamson, 2012).

In addition, a woman's diet should be certain to include a reduced amount of saturated fats and cholesterol and an increased amount of dietary fiber. Increasing fiber decreases postprandial hyperglycemia and so lowers insulin requirements. Women are extremely vulnerable to hypoglycemia at night during pregnancy because of the continuous fetal use of glucose during the time they sleep. Urge a woman to make her final snack of the day one of protein and a complex carbohydrate (e.g., an egg and whole grain toast, hummus and whole grain crackers) to allow slow digestion during the night. If a woman cannot eat because of vomiting or nausea early in pregnancy or heartburn in later pregnancy, she should immediately notify her healthcare provider as she may need temporary intravenous fluid and glucose supplementation. Later in

BOX 20.7

Nursing Care Planning

AN INTERPROFESSIONAL CARE MAP FOR A WOMAN WITH MULTIPLE THREATS TO PREGNANCY

Angelina Gomez, 22 years old, is pregnant with her first child. She fainted this afternoon while participating in an aerobics class.

Family Assessment: Patient lives with the 30-year-old father of her child, Josh. She works as a fundraiser for a movie producer. Josh works as an animation artist. Finances are rated as "workable." She fainted this afternoon while participating in her weekly hour-long aerobics class.

Patient Assessment: Patient had rheumatic fever with mitral stenosis as a child. She developed gestational diabetes early in this pregnancy. Her serum glucose level is 207 mg/dl; her blood pressure (BP) is 100/60 mmHg. A uterine monitor shows moderate-strength uterine contractions 7 minutes apart; fetal heart rate (FHR) is 167 beats/min. She asks you, "If exercise is supposed to be good for you, why did this happen?"

Nursing Diagnosis: Risk for ineffective tissue perfusion (peripheral) related to lowered blood pressure secondary to mitral stenosis and gestational diabetes

Outcome Criteria: BP returns to 120/70 mmHg; pulse rate at 70 to 90 beats/min; fetal heart rate at 110 to 160 beats/min. Serum glucose is less than 126 mg/dl; labor is halted.

Team Member Responsible	Assessment	Intervention	Rationale	Expected Outcome
Activities of Daily Living, Including Safety				
Nurse/primary care provider	Assess whether patient understands it is healthy for her to exercise regularly.	Review with patient the need for consistent diet and exercise to regulate glucose during pregnancy.	Strenuous exercise increases cardiac output, placing additional workload on the heart.	Patient describes a more consistent exercise program to use during pregnancy rather than a once-per-week aerobics class.
Teamwork and Collaboration				
Nurse/emergency room medical care provider	Telephone pregnancy and cardiac care providers and alert them to patient's admission.	Coordinate care with pregnancy and cardiac healthcare providers who know patient best.	Collaboration with pregnancy and cardiac healthcare providers helps ensure a healthy outcome for the woman and fetus.	Both pregnancy and cardiac care providers contact emergency staff to coordinate care.
Procedures/Medications for Quality Improvement				
Nurse/emergency room medical care provider	Monitor patient's BP, pulse rate, FHR, and uterine contractions by continuous monitoring.	Determine patient progress by monitor and physical exam. Inform patient of signs of beginning labor.	Increased FHR (tachycardia) is a sign of possible fetal distress. Uterine contractions could mark the beginning of preterm labor.	Patient voices an understanding labor may be beginning; has confidence in emergency room (ER) staff to manage her condition until her primary care provider arrives.
Nurse/cardiac ultrasound technician/consulting medical care provider	Explain process of echocardiogram to document mitral valve function.	Assure patient echocardiogram is safe during pregnancy. Assist as necessary.	Mitral valve stenosis can lower blood pressure by not allowing adequate blood flow to aorta.	Echocardiogram is recorded in an expedient manner.
Nutrition				
Nurse	Assess serum glucose every 15 minutes by finger stick.	Document pattern of blood glucose. Administer intravenous (IV) fluid, insulin additive as prescribed.	Correcting blood glucose is vital to both maternal and fetal well-being.	Patient's serum glucose is maintained within normal level within 45 minutes.

Patient-Centered Care

Nurse	Assess patient's understanding that her complex situation (both cardiac and diabetes disorders) could be compromising her pregnancy.	Educate patient about need for rest in lateral recumbent position until condition is stabilized.	Activity restriction can help prevent uteroplacental insufficiency and supine hypotension syndrome.	Patient voices she understands need for continuous monitoring and rest. Complies with position for rest.

Psychosocial/Spiritual/Emotional Needs

Nurse	Assess the patient's main support person and ask if she would like him or her notified.	Locate support person and invite him or her to join patient in emergency department.	Anxiety and stressors can increase the workload of the heart. Support person can be instrumental in reducing stress.	Support person arrives and works with staff to alleviate anxiety.

Informatics for Seamless Healthcare Planning

Nurse/primary care provider	Assess if patient is aware of need for admittance to hospital to continue monitoring.	Assist patient in transfer to hospital unit.	Continuous monitoring is necessary to detect if uterine contractions and preterm birth were halted.	Patient is satisfactorily transferred to hospital unit for further monitoring and care.

pregnancy, she must be extremely nutrition conscious to maintain good control of glucose levels and to keep her weight gain to a suitable amount (approximately 25 to 30 lb) in the hope of limiting the size of her infant and making a vaginal birth possible. Urge women, however, not to reduce their intake to below 1,800 calories during pregnancy as an intake this low in carbohydrates can lead to fat breakdown and acidosis.

What If . . . 20.3

Angelina develops gestational diabetes. She's resistant to learn much about her condition, though, because she knows her symptoms are only temporary and will fade at the end of pregnancy. What type of teaching plan would the nurse devise to help her learn in the face of this attitude?

Education Regarding Exercise During Pregnancy. Exercise is another mechanism that lowers serum glucose levels and, therefore, the need for insulin. If a woman begins an exercise program for the first time during pregnancy, she may notice excessive glucose fluctuations at first. Therefore, it's best if she begins her exercise program before pregnancy, when glucose fluctuation can be evaluated and food and snacks adjusted accordingly before a fetus is involved.

With exercise, blood glucose levels decrease because the muscles increase their need for glucose, an effect which lasts for at least 12 hours after exercise. If the arm in which a woman injected insulin is actively exercised, the insulin is released so quickly that it can cause hypoglycemia. To avoid this phenomenon, a woman should eat a snack consisting of a protein or complex carbohydrate before exercise and should maintain a consistent exercise program—she should not do aerobic exercises one day and then none the next, but rather, do 30 minutes of walking every day. In a woman with poor blood glucose control, extreme exercise will cause hyperglycemia and ketoacidosis as the liver both releases glucose and breaks down fatty acids in an attempt to supply enough energy for the exercise, yet the body cannot use them because of inadequate insulin.

Unfolding Patient Stories: Amelia Sung • Part 2

Think back to Amelia Sung, who, as you learned in Chapter 8, is 36 years old and gravida 2 para 1. She is diagnosed with gestational diabetes mellitus at 26 weeks. Explain the areas of education the nurse should provide on diabetes management. How does the nurse evaluate Amelia's understanding of the information provided and her ability to manage diabetes and maintain normal glucose levels?

Care for Amelia and other patients in a realistic virtual environment: **vSim** for Nursing (thepoint.lww .com/vSimMaternityPed). Practice documenting these patients' care in DocuCare (thepoint.lww.com /DocuCareEHR).

TABLE 20.4 THERAPEUTIC MANAGEMENT OF DIABETES DURING PREGNANCY

	Description	Methods	Precautions
Insulin therapy	Needed by pregestational and gestational diabetics who are uncontrolled with diet or oral therapy. Necessary for the cells to take glucose from the bloodstream	Short-acting insulin may be used alone or with an intermediate type. Two thirds of daily insulin needs are given before breakfast and one third before dinner. Insulin should be given subcutaneously and at a 90-degree angle to the skin. The injection site should generally be the same each injection (arms OR legs OR abdomen).	Early in pregnancy, insulin needs may be less. Later in pregnancy, increased insulin may be needed. Women should eat immediately after injecting insulin to avoid hypoglycemia. Different body areas take up insulin at different rates. Rotate within the same type of injection site.
Blood glucose monitoring	Completed four times a day by the patient. The patient pricks her finger and uses a glucometer to determine her blood glucose. She should track these numbers with a chart and bring it to her OB visits. Her provider will determine if any adjustments in her insulin or oral diabetic regimen are needed.	The patient should obtain fasting and 1-hour postprandial values. Her goals include fasting numbers that are 90 and below and postprandial values that are less than 140.	If the patient is hypoglycemic, she should have some carbohydrate rich food, like crackers, and a protein, like milk. Simple sugars can create hyperglycemia and rebound hypoglycemia.
Insulin pump therapy (Fig. 20.5)	An insulin pump is an automatic pump with thin tubing, which is placed subcutaneously, most often on the woman's abdomen. Insulin is given through this tube and injection of insulin is therefore eliminated.	A continuous rate (basal) of insulin is given to the patient through the pump, and the patient can program the pump to give extra doses as boluses prior to meals or correctional doses related to her blood glucose values after meals.	The patient should clean the site daily and cover it with a dressing to keep it clean. The site also needs to be changed every 24–48 hr to ensure optimal absorption and decrease infection.

Therapeutic Management

Because blood glucose levels near normal help minimize the risk of maternal and fetal complications, both women with gestational diabetes and those with overt diabetes need more frequent prenatal visits than usual to ensure close monitoring of their condition and that of the fetus (Table 20.4).

Tests for Placental Function and Fetal Well-Being

Monitoring of fetal well-being will be individualized depending on the woman's overall health. Because women with diabetes tend to have infants with a higher than normal incidence of birth anomalies, a woman will have a serum α-fetoprotein level obtained at 15 to 17 weeks to assess for a neural tube defect and an ultrasound examination performed at approximately 18 to 20 weeks to detect gross abnormalities. A creatinine clearance test may be ordered each trimester. A normal creatinine clearance rate suggests a woman's vascular system is intact because kidney function is normal. By default, this also implies uterine perfusion is also adequate. Placental functioning may also be assessed by a weekly nonstress test or biophysical profile during the last trimester of pregnancy (see Chapter 9) if a woman is in good control, or a daily nonstress test if her regulation is poor.

In addition, a woman may be asked to self-monitor fetal well-being by recording how many movements occur an hour

Figure 20.5 Using an insulin pump during pregnancy is the best assurance that insulin levels will remain constant.

(usually about 10 fetal kicks) (see Chapter 9). Be certain she understands that fetal activity varies depending on her activity and meal patterns to prevent her from becoming frightened by normal variations. An ultrasound examination may be taken at week 28 and then again at weeks 36 to 38 to determine fetal growth, amniotic fluid volume, placental location, and biparietal diameter. Oligohydramnios (i.e., a small amount of amniotic fluid) may indicate fetal growth restriction or a fetal renal abnormality, whereas polyhydramnios (i.e., an excessive amount of amniotic fluid) may indicate gastrointestinal malformation or poorly controlled disease. A lecithin/sphingomyelin ratio by amniocentesis is usually performed by week 36 of pregnancy to assess fetal maturity. In pregnancies complicated by diabetes, this ratio tends not to show maturity as early as in other pregnancies probably because the synthesis of phosphatidylglycerol, the compound that stabilizes surfactant, is delayed if hyperglycemia is present.

Because lung surfactant does not appear to form as early in these fetuses as in others, the presence of phosphatidylglycerol, an ingredient of surfactant, at amniocentesis is used to indicate lung maturity for these infants. Although it is known that administering corticosteroids to the mother during the last week of pregnancy can hasten lung maturity, corticosteroids may also impair fetal insulin release and perhaps fetal pancreatic islet development. Therefore, with a fetus who already has a risk at birth from poor glucose control, corticosteroid use to improve lung maturity is not usually recommended.

Fetal surveillance can be both difficult and time-consuming for a woman. Having to wait during each weekly test to hear how her fetus is doing is emotionally draining, especially for a woman who believes it is somehow her fault all the tests are necessary (it is, after all, her diabetes). She needs support people with her to minimize the feeling she is alone and without support in this crisis.

Timing for Birth

Among the most hazardous times for a fetus during a diabetes-involved pregnancy are weeks 36 to 40 of pregnancy, when the fetus is drawing large stores of maternal nutrients because of his or her large size. In the past, many infants were birthed early by routine cesarean birth at 37 weeks gestation to prevent fetal loss from placental insufficiency during these final weeks; unfortunately, if the fetus was still immature, this relieved one concern but created another, such as respiratory distress syndrome in the infant (infants of women with diabetes may be more prone to this than usual because surfactant is not as mature).

Cesarean birth was chosen because it is difficult to induce labor this early in pregnancy because the cervix is not yet ripe or responsive to labor contractions; babies of women with diabetes are large, making vaginal birth difficult; and a fetus suffering placental dysfunction or insufficiency did not do well in labor.

Today, when an accurate assessment of fetal age is available by amniocentesis and the pregnancy can be maintained within safe limits by the use of nonstress testing for a longer period, the last weeks of pregnancy are not as hazardous as before, and the timing and type of birth is much more individualized.

If at all possible, vaginal birth is preferred. Labor may be induced by rupture of the membranes or an oxytocin infusion after measures to induce cervical ripening (see Chapter 23). Both labor contractions and fetal heart sounds need to be conscientiously monitored during labor to ensure early detection of placental dysfunction. A woman's glucose level is regulated during labor by an intravenous infusion of short-acting or regular insulin with frequent blood glucose assays to prevent hypoglycemia in the mother or rebound hypoglycemia in the newborn (see Chapter 26 for care of the infant of a woman with diabetes at birth).

If a woman will be given an epidural anesthetic, use of an intravenous glucose solution as a plasma volume expander should be avoided to prevent hyperglycemia from developing; Ringer's lactate or 0.9% saline is infused instead.

Postpartum Adjustment

During the postpartum period, a woman who came into pregnancy with diabetes must undergo yet another readjustment to insulin regulation. With insulin resistance gone, often she needs no insulin during the immediate postpartum period; in another few days, however, she will return to her prepregnant insulin requirements. One- or 2-hour postprandial blood glucose determinations help to regulate how much insulin she needs during this adjustment period. A woman with gestational diabetes usually demonstrates normal glucose values by 24 hours after birth and then will need no further diet or insulin therapy. She requires careful observation, however, during the immediate postpartum period because if polyhydramnios was present during pregnancy, she is at risk of hemorrhage from poor uterine contraction. Women with diabetes may breastfeed because insulin is one of the few substances that does not pass into breast milk from the bloodstream (Gururaj Setty et al., 2016).

Because a woman who has had gestational diabetes is at risk for developing type 2 diabetes later in life, she should have glucose testing done during health maintenance visits throughout life. Be certain that women receive contraceptive information as appropriate. Remind women with ongoing diabetes before they plan a second pregnancy that they will need to be certain their disease is stabilized and in good control.

QSEN Checkpoint Question 20.5

INFORMATICS

Angelina is prescribed an insulin pump to administer insulin for her gestational diabetes. What patient education would the nurse want to provide to explain why nighttime is a particularly hazardous time for her fetus during pump therapy?

a. The fetus can develop hyperglycemia from excessive insulin administration.

b. Continuous insulin administration with no food intake can lead to hypoglycemia.

c. Her lack of exercise at night tends to lead to hypercalcemia from muscle disuse.

d. Her lack of fluid intake during the night causes a relative increase in serum insulin levels.

Look in Appendix A for the best answer and rationale.

Mental Illness and Pregnancy

Mental illness may precede or occur with pregnancy the same as it can at any point in life. Schizophrenia tends to have its highest incidence in adolescents and late adolescents and so may occur in young pregnant women. Depression occurs almost four times more commonly in women than in men and often in late adolescents, making it the most common mental illness seen in pregnant women.

Even normal levels of stress make it difficult to use effective coping mechanisms, so pregnancy or childbirth may be the additional stress that reveals mental illness for the first time. Because of this, a woman with a psychiatric disorder is best cared for by a team approach, including both a psychiatric care team and a prenatal care group, to ensure the stress of pregnancy is not exacerbating the mental illness and that distorted perceptions or depression do not complicate the pregnancy. Any psychotropic medication taken by a pregnant woman should be evaluated before pregnancy for possible fetal harm (Urato, 2015). For example, lithium, a mainstay of therapy for mood disorders such as bipolar disorder, and serotonin-reuptake inhibitors used to counteract depression, are potentially teratogenic (Karch, 2015).

As the care of a newborn requires such a major life change, mental illness may also occur in the postpartum period (postpartum depression or psychosis are discussed in Chapter 25).

QSEN Checkpoint Question 20.6

EVIDENCE-BASED PRACTICE

Women who have had a complication of pregnancy have the potential to develop depression in the postpartal period because their pregnancy did not go the way they wanted or imagined. To see what factors tend to be associated with depression in women who develop gestational diabetes, researchers administered a questionnaire to 71 women at 4 to 15 weeks postpartum. Results of the study showed that 34% of the women who developed gestational diabetes showed depressive symptoms; factors most associated with depression were cesarean birth and more weight gain than expected during pregnancy (Nicklas, Miller, Zera, et al., 2013).

Based on the previous study, which statement by Angelina would worry the nurse most that she might develop postpartum depression?
a. "I want to shed some pounds so I'll fit into the new dress I bought for New Year's Eve."
b. "I hated giving insulin to myself; I'm relieved to not be doing that anymore."
c. "My baby is bigger than I expected, but his eyes are beautiful and he's cute."
d. "I think my husband adjusted better to my having diabetes than I did."

Look in Appendix A for the best answer and rationale.

Cancer and Pregnancy

The malignancies most commonly seen with pregnancy are those that occur most frequently in women during childbearing years such as ovarian cancer, uterine cancer, cervical cancer, breast cancer, thyroid cancer, leukemia, melanoma, and Hodgkin lymphoma (Basta, Bak, & Roszkowski, 2015). Although immunologic mechanisms are altered during pregnancy, there is no evidence that pregnant women are more prone to cancer or that pregnancy changes the course of an existing disease.

If a woman is in the first trimester of pregnancy when a malignancy is diagnosed, she and her partner are asked to make a difficult decision: to delay treatment to avoid teratogenic risks to a fetus from treatment (possibly increasing a woman's risk), to end the pregnancy to allow chemotherapy or radiation treatment to be initiated, or to choose chemotherapy or radiation treatment with the knowledge they may cause birth anomalies in the fetus (Karunaratne, Premaratne, Hapuachchige, et al., 2016).

As a rule, women can receive chemotherapy in the second and third trimesters without adverse fetal effects. In contrast, radiation therapy, another modality that is a mainstay of cancer therapy, puts the fetus at risk throughout pregnancy if the fetus is directly exposed.

A biopsy to confirm the diagnosis or surgery to remove a tumor can be completed during pregnancy with the understanding the fetus is at some risk for anoxia if a general anesthesia is used. Cervical conization for cervical cancer has a particularly high fetal risk because the surgery may directly disrupt the pregnancy. With a vaccine against human papillomavirus (HPV) now available, cervical cancer incidence should be seen much less in the future (Luckett & Feldman, 2016). Following surgery of any kind, a woman is at a higher risk of thrombus formation because of the increased coagulation process accompanying pregnancy.

Cancer in a woman does not appear to metastasize to the fetus. This is because the placenta serves as a barrier against this spread and also because the fetus may be capable of resisting the invasion of the foreign cells. Melanoma is the exception to this, as this does seem capable of spreading to the fetus (Jeremić, Jeremić, Stefanović, et al., 2015).

What If . . . 20.4

The nurse is interested in exploring one of the 2020 National Health Goals related to acquired health disorders and pregnancy (see Box 20.1). Most government-sponsored money for nursing research is allotted based on these goals. What would be a possible research topic to explore pertinent to these goals that would be applicable to Angelina's family and that would also advance evidence-based practice?

KEY POINTS FOR REVIEW

- When women with a preexisting disease become pregnant, it is crucial to obtain a thorough history and physical examination at the first prenatal visit to establish a baseline of information on the condition. Documentation by a medication reconciliation form of any medication being taken is important to protect against adverse drug interactions and the possibility of teratogenic effects on the fetus.
- Teaching is an important nursing intervention because a woman with a preexisting illness must modify her usual therapy to adjust to pregnancy. Health teaching and how it affects women's overall health helps in planning nursing

care that not only meets QSEN competencies but also best meets the family's total needs.

- Because blood volume increases by as much as 50% during pregnancy, cardiac function may become inadequate if cardiovascular disease is present. Cardiac illnesses that cause difficulty can be either acquired disorders such as Kawasaki disease and rheumatic fever or congenital disorders such as mitral valve stenosis and coarctation of the aorta.
- Iron-deficiency anemia, sickle-cell anemia, and folic acid–deficiency anemia are examples of various forms of anemia that can also cause complications of pregnancy. Such anemias can result in fetal distress because of inadequate oxygen transport.
- Urinary tract disorders can lead to pregnancy complications because pregnancy increases the workload of the kidneys. UTIs and chronic renal disease are two disorders that may lead to early pregnancy loss.
- Acute nasopharyngitis, asthma, pneumonia, influenza, and tuberculosis are common respiratory disorders seen in pregnancy. The incidence of tuberculosis is on the increase and special assessments and care are needed for these women.
- Juvenile rheumatoid arthritis and systemic lupus erythematosus are examples of rheumatic disorders seen in pregnancy. These disorders generally require large doses of NSAIDs for therapy. Women taking salicylates are advised to decrease use 2 weeks before birth to avoid bleeding disorders in the newborn and premature closure of the ductus arteriosus.
- Some gastrointestinal illnesses that occur with pregnancy are hiatal hernia, cholecystitis, viral hepatitis, inflammatory bowel disease, and appendicitis. If surgery is necessary for conditions such as cholecystitis or appendicitis, it can be performed by laparoscopic technique during pregnancy, but this may result in preterm labor.
- Recurrent seizures are the most frequently seen neurologic condition during pregnancy. Many drugs used to control seizures are teratogenic. Women need to have their medical regimen evaluated before pregnancy to be certain they are regulated on the fewest medications and the lowest dosages possible.
- The major endocrine disorder seen during pregnancy is diabetes mellitus. Gestational diabetes is diabetes that occurs only during pregnancy.

CRITICAL THINKING CARE STUDY

Tawnlee Pawlinsky is a 37-year-old G40030, 30-week pregnant woman who comes to your high-risk prenatal clinic for care. She has chronic hypertension and mitral valve insufficiency, which cause her to be short of breath if she hurries up a ladder at her job as a roofer or runs to catch a bus after work. When you talk about pregnancy nutrition with her, she makes a point that she is a vegan. Her hemoglobin is 9 g/ml; her red blood cells are microcytic and microchromic.

1. Tawnlee is diagnosed as having iron-deficiency anemia. Because she is a vegan, in addition to taking the iron supplement prescribed for her, what foods would you suggest she include daily in meals? Would you suggest

she change her eating philosophy for the remainder of pregnancy to include meat?

2. Suppose Tawnlee ran from the bus stop into the clinic to avoid being late for her appointment. As soon as she reached the reception desk, she fell to the floor. You realize she needs cardiopulmonary resuscitation (CPR). What rate of respiratory/cardiac ratio would you use because she is 30 weeks pregnant?

3. Tawnlee is concerned because she was prescribed enalapril for hypertension before pregnancy but was changed to methyldopa at her prepregnancy consultation. She doesn't feel confident methyldopa will work as well, and she fears she will grow dizzy working on a roof and fall. Would you assure her the medication change was a good one, or urge her to ask her primary care provider to change the prescription back to enalapril so she feels more secure at work?

RELATED RESOURCES

Explore these additional resources to enhance learning for this chapter:
- Student resources on thePoint, including answers to the What If . . . and Critical Thinking Care Study questions, http://thepoint.lww.com/Flagg8e
- Adaptive learning powered by PrepU, http://thepoint.lww.com/prepu

REFERENCES

Abdalla, M., & Mancini, D. M. (2014). Management of pregnancy in the post-cardiac transplant patient. *Seminars in Perinatology, 38*(5), 318–325.
Abdullah, B., Kathiresan Pillai, T., Cheen, L. H., et al. (2015). Severe acute pancreatitis in pregnancy. *Case Reports in Obstetrics and Gynecology, 2015,* 239068.
Adeola, A. A., & Okwilagwe, E. A. (2015). Acceptance and utilisation of sulphadoxine-pyrimethamine and insecticide-treated nets among pregnant women in Oyo state, Nigeria. *Malaria Research and Treatment, 2015,* 1–9.
Almasi, O., Pariente, G., Kessous, R., et al. (2016). Association between delivery of small-for-gestational-age neonate and long-term maternal chronic kidney disease. *The Journal of Maternal-Fetal & Neonatal Medicine, 29*(17), 2861–2864.
Andersen, S. L., Olsen, J., & Laurberg, P. (2016). Antithyroid drug side effects in the population and in pregnancy. *The Journal of Clinical Endocrinology & Metabolism, 101*(4), 1606–1614.
Andrews, K. G., Lynch, M., Eckert, E., et al. (2015). Missed opportunities to deliver intermittent preventive treatment for malaria to pregnant women 2003–2013: A systematic analysis of 58 household surveys in sub-Saharan Africa. *Malaria Journal, 14*(1), 1–10.
Au, C. P., Raynes-Greenow, C. H., Turner, R. M., et al. (2016). Antenatal management of gestational diabetes mellitus can improve neonatal outcomes. *Midwifery, 34,* 66–71.
Ayad, S. W., Hassanein, M. M., Mohamed, E. A., et al. (2016). Maternal and fetal outcomes in pregnant women with a prosthetic mechanical heart valve. *Clinical Medicine Insights: Cardiology, 10,* 11–17.
Basta, P., Bak, A., & Roszkowski, K. (2015). Cancer treatment in pregnant women. *Contemporary Oncology, 19*(5), 354–360.
Bates, S. M., Middeldorp, S., Rodger, M., et al. (2016). Guidance for the treatment and prevention of obstetric-associated venous thromboembolism. *Journal of Thrombosis and Thrombolysis, 41*(1), 92–128.
Benites, B. D., Benevides, T. C., Valente, I. S., et al. (2016). The effects of exchange transfusion for prevention of complications during pregnancy of sickle hemoglobin C disease patients. *Transfusion, 56*(1), 119–124.
Bhatt, A. B., & DeFaria Yeh, D. (2015). Pregnancy and adult congenital heart disease. *Cardiology Clinics, 33*(4), 611–623.
Boga, C., & Ozdogu, H. (2016). Pregnancy and sickle cell disease: A review of the current literature. *Critical Reviews in Oncology/Hematology, 98,* 364–74.

Bradley, P. K., Duprey, M., & Castorino, K. (2016). Identifying key intervention opportunities during a pregnancy complicated by diabetes: A review of acute complications of diabetes during pregnancy. *Current Diabetes Reports, 16*(2), 17.

Brashers, V. L., & Huether, S. E. (2017). Alterations of pulmonary function. In S. E. Huether & K. L. McCance (Eds.), *Understanding pathophysiology* (6th ed., pp. 687–714). St. Louis, MO: Elsevier.

Brennan, M. L., & Schrijver, I. (2016). Cystic fibrosis: A review of associated phenotypes, use of molecular diagnostic approaches, genetic characteristics, progress, and dilemmas. *The Journal of Molecular Diagnostics, 18*(1), 3–14.

Cai, L., Wan, C. L., He, L., et al. (2015). Gestational influenza increases the risk of psychosis in adults. *Medicinal Chemistry, 11*(7), 676–682.

Charlton, R. A., Pierini, A., Klungsøyr, K., et al. (2016). Asthma medication prescribing before, during and after pregnancy: A study in seven European regions. *BMJ Open, 6*(1), e009237.

Charoenboon, C., Jatavan, P., Traisrisilp, K., et al. (2016). Pregnancy outcomes among women with beta-thalassemia trait. *Archives of Gynecology and Obstetrics, 293*, 771–774.

Chmielewska, A., Dziechciarz, P., Gieruszczak-Białek, D., et al. (2016). Effects of prenatal and/or postnatal supplementation with iron, PUFA or folic acid on neurodevelopment: Update. *The British Journal of Nutrition.* Advance online publication. doi:10.1017/S0007114514004243

Clark, P., Thomson, A. J., & Greer, I. A. (2012). Haematological problems in pregnancy. In D. K. Edmonds (Ed.), *Dewhurst's textbook of obstetrics & gynaecology* (8th ed., pp. 151–172). Oxford, United Kingdom: Wiley.

Cunningham, F. G., Leveno, K., Bloom, S. L., et al. (2014). Cardiovascular disease. In F. G. Cunninghan, K. Leveno, S. L. Bloom, et al. (Eds.), *Williams obstetrics* (24th ed., pp. 973–999). New York, NY: McGraw-Hill Education.

Dalzell, J. R., Cannon, J. A., Simpson, J., et al. (2015). Improving outcomes in peripartum cardiomyopathy. *Expert Review of Cardiovascular Therapies, 13*(6), 665–671.

Debnath, J., Sharma, P., & Maurya, V. (2016). Diagnosing appendicitis during pregnancy: Which study when? *American Journal of Obstetrics and Gynecology, 214*(1), 135–136.

Dennis, A. (2016). Valvular heart disease in pregnancy. *International Journal of Obstetric Anesthesia, 25*, 4–8.

Desplantie, O., Tremblay-Gravel, M., Avram, R., et al. (2015). The medical treatment of new-onset peripartum cardiomyopathy: A systematic review of prospective studies. *The Canadian Journal of Cardiology, 31*(12), 1421–1426.

Dornhorst, A., & Williamson, C. (2012). Diabetes & endocrine disease in pregnancy. In D. K. Edmonds (Ed.), *Dewhurst's textbook of obstetrics & gynaecology* (6th ed., pp. 121–136). Oxford, United Kingdom: Wiley.

Dutta, A. K., & Chacko, A. (2016). Influence of environmental factors on the onset and course of inflammatory bowel disease. *World Journal of Gastroenterology, 22*(3), 1088–1100.

Easterling, T. R., & Stout, K. (2012). Heart disease. In S. G. Gabbe, J. R. Niebyl, J. L. Simpson, et al. (Eds.), *Obstetrics: Normal and problem pregnancies* (6th ed., pp. 825–850). Philadelphia, PA: Elsevier/Saunders.

Falick-Michaeli, T., Schroeder, J. E., Barzilay, Y., et al. (2015). Adolescent idiopathic scoliosis and pregnancy: An unsolved paradigm. *Global Spine Journal, 5*(3), 179–184.

Ghulmiyyah, L. M., Alame, M. M., Mirza, F. G., et al. (2016). Influenza and its treatment during pregnancy: A review. *Journal of Neonatal-Perinatal Medicine, 8*(4), 297–306.

Goodacre, S., & Hunt, B. (2016). The problem of pulmonary embolism diagnosis in pregnancy. *British Journal of Haematology, 175*(5), 971–972.

Gordon, C. T., Jimenez-Fernandez, S., Daniels, L. B., et al. (2014). Pregnancy in women with a history of Kawasaki disease: Management and outcomes. *British Journal of Obstetrics and Gynaecology, 121*(11), 1431–1438.

Gregory, K. D., Korst, L. M., Lu, M. C., et al. (2013). AHRQ patient safety indicators: Time to include hemorrhage and infection during childbirth. *Joint Commission Journal of Quality Patient Safety, 39*(3), 114–122.

Gururaj Setty, S., Crasto, W., Jarvis, J., et al. (2016). New insulins and newer insulin regimens: A review of their role in improving glycaemic control in patients with diabetes. *Postgraduate Medical Journal, 92*(1085), 152–164.

Hacker, F. M., Whalen, P. S., Lee, V. R., et al. (2015). Maternal and fetal outcomes of pancreatitis in pregnancy. *American Journal of Obstetrics and Gynecology, 213*(4), 568.e1–568.e5.

Hisano, M., Tsukada, N., Sago, H., et al. (2015). Successful prevention of exacerbation of thrombocytopenia in a pregnant patient with idiopathic thrombocytopenic purpura by anticoagulation treatment. *BMC Pregnancy and Childbirth, 15*, 1–4.

Jeremić, J., Jeremić, K., Stefanović, A., et al. (2015). Pregnancy associated with melanoma and fetal anomalies: A case report and review of literature. *Clinical and Experimental Obstetrics & Gynecology, 42*(3), 386–387.

Jorge, A. M., Keswani, R. N., Veerappan, A., et al. (2015). Non-operative management of symptomatic cholelithiasis in pregnancy is associated with frequent hospitalizations. *Journal of Gastrointestinal Surgery, 19*(4), 598–603.

Kahyaoglu Sut, H., & Balkanli Kaplan, P. (2016). Effect of pelvic floor muscle exercise on pelvic floor muscle activity and voiding functions during pregnancy and the postpartum period. *Neurourology and Urodynamics, 35*(3), 417–422.

Karadaman, M., Sarı, O., Aydoğan, U., et al. (2016). Evaluation of obstructive sleep apnea symptoms in pregnant women with chronic disease. *The Journal of Maternal-Fetal & Neonatal Medicine, 29*(20), 3379–3385.

Karch, A. M. (2015). *Lippincott's nursing drug guide.* Philadelphia, PA: Lippincott Williams & Wilkins.

Karunaratne, K., Premaratne, S., Hapuachchige, C., et al. (2016). Counselling pregnant women with cancer. *Best Practice & Research Clinical Obstetrics & Gynaecology, 33*, 117–123.

Klingensmith, G. J., Pyle, L., Nadeau, K. J., et al. (2016). Pregnancy outcomes in youth with type 2 diabetes: The TODAY study experience. *Diabetes Care, 39*(1), 122–129.

Kovács, D. Á., Szabó, L., Jenei, K., et al. (2015). Pregnancy management of women with kidney transplantation. *Interventional Medicine & Applied Science, 7*(4), 161–165.

Krassas, G., Karras, S. N., & Pontikides, N. (2015). Thyroid diseases during pregnancy: A number of important issues. *Hormones, 14*(1), 59–69.

Kraut, E., & Farahani, P. (2015). A systematic review of clinical practice guidelines' recommendations on levothyroxine therapy alone versus combination therapy (LT4 plus LT3) for hypothyroidism. *Clinical and Investigative Medicine, 38*(6), E305–E313.

Landon, M. B., Catalano, P. M., & Gabbe, S. G. (2012). Diabetes mellitus complicating pregnancy. In S. G. Gabbe, J. R. Niebyl, J. L. Simpson, et al. (Eds.), *Obstetrics: Normal and problem pregnancies* (6th ed., pp. 887–921). Philadelphia, PA: Elsevier/Saunders.

Leaf, R. K., & Connors, J. M. (2017). The role of anticoagulants in the prevention of pregnancy complications. *Clinical and Applied Thrombosis/Hemostasis, 23*(2), 116–123.

Leidecker, K., & Dorman, K. (2016). Pulmonary disorders complicating pregnancy: An overview. *The Journal of Perinatal & Neonatal Nursing, 30*(1), 45–53.

Luckett, R., & Feldman, S. (2016). Impact of 2-, 4- and 9-valent HPV vaccines on morbidity and mortality from cervical cancer. *Human Vaccines & Immunotherapeutics, 12*(6), 1332–1342.

Margioula-Siarkou, C., Kalogiannidis, I., Petousis, S., et al. (2016). Pregnancy after liver transplantation. How safe? A retrospective case-series study in a large tertiary hospital. *The Journal of Maternal-Fetal & Neonatal Medicine, 29*(13), 2120–2124.

Namazy, J. A., & Schatz, M. (2015). Pharmacotherapy options to treat asthma during pregnancy. *Expert Opinion on Pharmacotherapy, 16*(12), 1783–1791.

Neff, A. T., & Sidonio, R. F., Jr. (2014). Management of VWD. *American Society of Hematology, 2014*(1), 536–541.

Ngian, G. S., Briggs, A. M., Ackerman, I. N., et al. (2016). Management of pregnancy in women with rheumatoid arthritis. *The Medical Journal of Australia, 204*(2), 62–63.

Nicklas, J. M., Miller, L. J., Zera, C. A., et al. (2013). Factors associated with depressive symptoms in the early postpartum period among women with recent gestational diabetes mellitus. *Maternal Child Health Journal, 17*(9), 1665–1672.

Ornoy, A., Reece, E. A., Pavlinkova, G., et al. (2015). Effect of maternal diabetes on the embryo, fetus, and children: Congenital anomalies, genetic and epigenetic changes and developmental outcomes. *Birth Defects Research Part C: Embryo Today: Reviews, 105*(1), 53–72.

Oteng-Ntim, E., Meeks, D., Seed, P. T., et al. (2015). Adverse maternal and perinatal outcomes in pregnant women with sickle cell disease: Systematic review and meta-analysis. *Blood, 125*(21), 3316–3325.

Pentieva, K., Selhub, J., Paul, L., et al. (2016). Evidence from a randomized trial that exposure to supplemental folic acid at recommended levels during pregnancy does not lead to increased unmetabolized folic acid concentrations in maternal or cord blood. *The Journal of Nutrition, 146*(3), 494–500.

Piccoli, G. B., Minelli, F., Versino, E., et al. (2016). Pregnancy in dialysis patients in the new millennium: A systematic review and meta-regression analysis correlating dialysis schedules and pregnancy outcomes. *Nephrology Dialysis Transplantation, 31*(11), 1915–1934.

Polyzos, K. A., Konstantelias, A. A., Pitsa, C. E., et al. (2015). Maternal influenza vaccination and risk for congenital malformations: A systematic review and meta-analysis. *Obstetrics & Gynecology, 126*(5), 1075–1084.

Pozzilli, C., & Pugliatti, M. (2015). An overview of pregnancy-related issues in patients with multiple sclerosis. *European Journal of Neurology*, 22(Suppl. 2), 34–39.

Prunty, J. J., Heise, C. D., & Chaffin, D. G. (2016). Graves' disease pharmacotherapy in women of reproductive age. *Pharmacotherapy*, 36(1), 64–83.

Rabel, A., Leitman, S. F., & Miller, J. L. (2016). Ask about ice, then consider iron. *Journal of the American Association of Nurse Practitioners*, 28(2), 116–120.

Rac, M. W., & Sheffield, J. S. (2014). Prevention and management of viral hepatitis in pregnancy. *Obstetrics and Gynecology Clinics of North America*, 41(4), 573–592.

Rote, N. S., & McCance, K. L. (2017). Structure and function of the hematologic system. In S. E. Huether & K. L. McCance (Eds.), *Understanding pathophysiology* (6th ed., pp. 490–512). St. Louis, MO: Mosby.

Roth, C. K., Dent, S., & McDevitt, K. (2015). Myasthenia gravis in pregnancy. *Nursing for Women's Health*, 19(3), 248–252.

Samuels, P. (2012). Hematologic complications of pregnancy. In S. G. Gabbe, J. R. Niebyl, J. L. Simpson, et al. (Eds.), *Obstetrics: Normal and problem pregnancies* (6th ed., pp. 962–979). Philadelphia, PA: Elsevier/Saunders.

Schreiber, K. (2016). Pregnancies in women with systemic lupus erythematosus and antiphospholipid antibodies. *Lupus*, 25(4), 343–345.

Shihab, Z., Yeomans, N. D., & De Cruz, P. (2016). Anti-tumour necrosis factor α therapies and inflammatory bowel disease pregnancy outcomes: A meta-analysis. *Journal of Crohn's & Colitis*, 10(8), 979–988.

Sienas, L., Wong, T., Collins, R., et al. (2013). Contemporary uses of erythropoietin in pregnancy: A literature review. *Obstetrical & Gynecological Survey*, 68(8), 594–602.

Singh, A., Chaudhary, R., Sonker, A., et al. (2016). Importance of donor history of restless leg syndrome and pica to asses iron deficiency. *Transfusion and Apheresis Science*, 54(2), 259–261.

Suskind, A. M., Saigal, C. S., Hanley, J. M., et al. (2016). Incidence and management of uncomplicated recurrent urinary tract infections in a national sample of women in the United States. *Urology*, 90, 50–55.

Urato, A. C. (2015). Are the SSRI antidepressants safe in pregnancy? Understanding the debate. *International Journal of Risk & Safety in Medicine*, 27(2), 93–99.

U.S. Department of Health and Human Services. (2010). *Healthy people 2020*. Washington, DC: Author.

Videman, M., Tokariev, A., Stjerna, S., et al. (2016). Effects of prenatal antiepileptic drug exposure on newborn brain activity. *Epilepsia*, 57(2), 252–262.

Widmer, M., Lopez, I., Gülmezoglu, A. M., et al. (2015). Duration of treatment for asymptomatic bacteriuria during pregnancy. *Cochrane Database of Systematic Reviews*, (11), CD000491.

Wu, E. S., & Hueppchen, N. A. (2015). Surgical disease & trauma in pregnancy. In J. L. Bienstock, H. Fox, E. E. Wallach, et al. (Eds.), *The Johns Hopkins manual of gynecology and obstetrics* (5th ed., pp. 277–285). Philadelphia, PA: Lippincott Williams & Wilkins.

Xu, Q., Wang, S., & Zhang, Z. (2015). A 23-year, single-center, retrospective analysis of 36 cases of acute pancreatitis in pregnancy. *International Journal of Gynecology & Obstetrics*, 130(2), 123–126.

Yarrington, C. D., Valente, A. M., & Economy, K. E. (2015). Cardiovascular management in pregnancy: Antithrombotic agents and antiplatelet agents. *Circulation*, 132(14), 1354–1364.

Zhang, J. J., Ma, X. X., Hao, L., et al. (2015). A systematic review and meta-analysis of outcomes of pregnancy in CKD and CKD outcomes in pregnancy. *Clinical Journal of the American Society of Nephrology*, 10(11), 1964–1978.

Zielinski, R., Searing, K., & Deibel, M. (2015). Gastrointestinal distress in pregnancy: Prevalence, assessment, and treatment of 5 common minor discomforts. *The Journal of Perinatal & Neonatal Nursing*, 29(1), 23–31.

21

Nursing Care of a Family Experiencing a Sudden Pregnancy Complication

Beverly Muzuki, a 20-year-old gravida 2, para 0, 30-week pregnant woman, noticed some mild lower abdominal pain but thought it was irritation from a bladder infection and waited to get help until she went to her scheduled appointment at the hospital. During the night, she woke up twice because of a nagging lower backache. This morning, she has intermittent sharp uterine contractions. "Why am I starting labor so early?" she asks you. "Is it because I'm Rh negative?"

Previous chapters described normal pregnancies and preexisting and newly acquired conditions that can complicate pregnancies. This chapter adds knowledge about complications directly related to the pregnancy.

Were Beverly's actions as informed as they could have been? What additional health teaching might have helped her recognize the signs of preterm labor earlier?

KEY TERMS

abortion

ankle clonus

cervical cerclage

chorioamnionitis

Couvelaire uterus

early pregnancy failure

eclampsia

ectopic pregnancy

erythroblastosis fetalis

gestational trophoblastic disease

HELLP syndrome

hemolytic disease of the newborn

polyhydramnios

isoimmunization

miscarriage

oligohydramnios

placenta previa

postterm pregnancy

preeclampsia

premature cervical dilatation

premature separation of the placenta

preterm labor

preterm rupture of membranes

recurrent pregnancy loss

Rh incompatibility

tocolytic agent

OBJECTIVES

After mastering the contents of this chapter, you should be able to:

1. Describe sudden complications of pregnancy that place a pregnant woman and her fetus at high risk.

2. Identify 2020 National Health Goals related to complications of pregnancy that nurses can help the nation achieve.

3. Assess a woman who is experiencing a complication of pregnancy.

4. Formulate nursing diagnoses that address the needs of a woman and her family experiencing a complication of pregnancy.

5. Identify expected outcomes to minimize the risks to a pregnant woman and her fetus when a sudden complication of pregnancy occurs as well as manage seamless transitions across differing healthcare settings.

6. Using the nursing process, plan nursing care that includes the six competencies of Quality & Safety Education for Nurses (QSEN): Patient-Centered Care, Teamwork & Collaboration, Evidence-Based Practice (EBP), Quality Improvement (QI), Safety, and Informatics.

7. Implement nursing care specific to a woman who has developed a sudden complication of pregnancy, such as teaching her how to recognize the symptoms of preterm labor.
8. Evaluate expected outcomes for effectiveness and achievement of care.
9. Integrate knowledge of complications of pregnancy with the interplay of nursing process, the six competencies of QSEN, and Family Nursing to promote quality maternal and child health nursing care.

Most women who enter pregnancy in good health expect to complete a pregnancy and birth without complications. In a few women, however, unexpected deviations or complications from the course of normal pregnancy occur, which place a severe burden on a woman and her family and her healthcare providers. All families benefit from the support and skill of a professional nurse who helps them work through the stages of pregnancy and prepares them to become new parents. For a family who must take special care to ensure the continuation of pregnancy, the support and skills of a professional nurse are essential to help them carry the baby to term. Hospitalization may be necessary. Once stabilized, a woman has to be monitored carefully until the pregnancy reaches term. As this is done on an ambulatory basis, nurses continue to be instrumental in care (DiMiceli-Zsigmond, Williams, & Richardson, 2015).

The leading complications related directly to pregnancy are thromboembolism, hemorrhage, infection, hypertension of pregnancy, and ectopic pregnancy (Mehta & Sokol, 2013). All of these have the potential to threaten both the life of the mother and the fetus. National Health Goals established to help reduce poor outcomes of complications of pregnancy such as these are shown in Box 21.1.

BOX 21.1

Nursing Care Planning Based on 2020 National Health Goals

Preventing complications of pregnancy is viewed as so important this issue is included in the 2020 National Health Goals.

- Reduce the rate of maternal deaths to 11.4 maternal deaths per 100,000 live births from a baseline of 12.7 per 100,000 live births.
- Reduce the rate of maternal illness and complications because of pregnancy to 28 per 100 births from a baseline of 31.1 per 100 births.
- Reduce the proportion of total preterm births to 11.4% from a baseline of 12.7%.
- Reduce the incidence of low birth weight to 7.1% of live births from a baseline of 8.2% of live births (U.S. Department of Health and Human Services, 2010; see www.healthypeople.gov).

Encouraging all women to come for prenatal care is the best preventive measure for eliminating complications of pregnancy. Nurses working in prenatal settings can help to ensure women are well informed about the normal course of pregnancy so they can actively participate in risk assessment at prenatal visits and also recognize and alert healthcare providers if a complication begins.

Nursing Process Overview

FOR A WOMAN WHO DEVELOPS A COMPLICATION OF PREGNANCY

ASSESSMENT

Nurses often are the first healthcare providers to discover a complication of pregnancy. Always ask women at prenatal visits about any symptoms that might indicate a complication such as pain or vaginal symptoms (e.g., leaking of fluid or bleeding). Provide enough time for a thorough health history so more subtle problems such as headache, blurred vision, or back pains can be discovered and investigated thoroughly. In addition, review the danger signs of pregnancy with women and, if appropriate, significant family members or other support people so potential problems can be recognized early and a healthcare provider can be contacted. Assure women they are free to call whenever they are concerned. Otherwise, they may wait until symptoms become acute rather than call when a symptom is first noticed.

NURSING DIAGNOSIS

Nursing diagnoses pertaining to a woman with a pregnancy complication should reflect both the physical problem and the woman's or family's concern. Some examples include:

- Anxiety related to guarded pregnancy outcome
- Fear of preterm labor ending the pregnancy
- Anticipatory grieving related to uncertain pregnancy outcome
- Deficient knowledge related to signs and symptoms of possible complications
- Risk for infection related to incomplete miscarriage
- Deficient fluid volume related to third-trimester bleeding
- Risk for ineffective tissue perfusion related to gestational hypertension

OUTCOME IDENTIFICATION AND PLANNING

Complications of pregnancy produce emergency situations. Be sure outcomes address both fetal and maternal welfare and often total family welfare. Treatment protocols should be regularly updated and maintained so they are current. Be certain they reflect a current nursing management level, so nurses can act swiftly and independently as needed with lifesaving measures. Once a woman's condition stabilizes, outcome identification can then focus on long-term objectives.

Many women who develop a pregnancy complication may spend a few days in the hospital for therapy and monitoring followed by discharge to their homes. Waiting for a pregnancy that has been threatened this way to come to term can be difficult and fraught with anxiety. Readmission to the healthcare facility, especially when a new complication occurs, compounds these feelings. Be certain planning considers the many feelings this experience can cause. Offer referrals for counseling and/or community support groups for both the woman and her family as needed. Refer patients and their families to helpful websites and other resources when appropriate (see Chapter 20).

IMPLEMENTATION

Interventions for a woman experiencing a complication of pregnancy require an interprofessional approach that speaks to several different areas:

- Continued both healthy maternal and fetal physical growth
- A woman's and family's psychological health
- Continuation of the pregnancy for as long as possible

Maintaining an optimistic attitude of fetal progress is important so a woman does not begin anticipatory grieving for her fetus, which could halt the growth of bonding. If the complication can be contained and the pregnancy continues uninterrupted, this can help protect the mental health of the whole family. If the pregnancy cannot be continued, be available to offer support as the family grieves for the loss of an unborn child and, in rare instances, the loss of future childbearing potential or the woman herself.

OUTCOME EVALUATION

After a pregnancy with complications, a woman has reason to be especially worried about her infant's health at the time of birth. Even though the woman may still be ill herself, help her spend enough time with her child to see that, although perhaps born before term, her infant is well and healthy. Pointing out the infant's ability to follow a light and respond to a voice can help her begin to view the baby as the healthy one she anticipated having. And even though the success or failure of some nursing interventions cannot be fully evaluated until a child is born or into the postnatal period, outcomes should be evaluated throughout the pregnancy if possible. Be aware that after a complication of early pregnancy, a woman cannot help but worry for the remainder of the pregnancy the complication will recur or the original insult to the fetus was severe enough to cause long-term effects. Evaluate the woman and her family's attitude and the woman's physical status at each healthcare visit to be certain she and her family are coping with the situation and adjusting psychosocially.

Unfortunately, even with sustained care, not all fetal outcomes will be optimal. Evaluation will then include the ability of the family to care for an ill infant or grieve if a newborn dies. Examples of expected outcomes include:

- Patient's blood pressure is maintained within acceptable parameters for remainder of pregnancy.
- Couple states they feel able to cope with anxiety associated with the pregnancy complication.
- Patient's signs and symptoms of hypertension of pregnancy do not progress to eclampsia.
- Patient accurately verbalizes crucial signs and symptoms she should immediately report to her primary healthcare provider.
- Couple expresses feelings of sadness over pregnancy loss.
- Patient is able to adhere to the medical treatment regimen and experiences no adverse effects from the treatment.

Bleeding During Pregnancy

Vaginal bleeding during pregnancy is always a deviation from the normal, is always potentially serious, may occur at any point during pregnancy, and is always frightening. It must always be carefully investigated because it can impair both the outcome of the pregnancy and the woman's health or life. The primary causes of bleeding during pregnancy are summarized in Table 21.1.

Although vaginal bleeding may be innocent, any degree of this during pregnancy is a potential emergency because it may mean the placenta has loosened and cut off nourishment to the fetus. Also, the amount of blood visualized may be only a fraction of the blood actually being lost because an undilated cervix and intact membranes contain blood within the uterus. A woman with any degree of bleeding, therefore, needs to be evaluated for the possibility she is experiencing a significant blood loss or is developing hypovolemic shock.

The process of shock due to blood loss is shown in Figure 21.1. Because the uterus is a nonessential body organ, danger to the fetal blood supply occurs when a woman's body begins to decrease blood flow to peripheral organs (although the increased blood volume of pregnancy allows more than normal blood loss before hypovolemic shock processes begin). Signs of hypovolemic shock (Table 21.2) occur when 10% of blood volume, or approximately 2 units of blood, have been lost; fetal distress occurs when 25% of blood volume is lost (Box 21.2). Because "normal" blood pressure varies from woman to woman, it is important to know the baseline blood pressure for a pregnant woman when evaluating for hypovolemic shock.

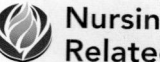 **Nursing Diagnoses and Related Interventions**

Nursing Diagnosis: Risk for deficient fluid volume related to bleeding during pregnancy

Outcome Evaluation: Patient's blood pressure is maintained at above 100/60 mmHg; pulse rate is below 100 beats/min; only minimal bleeding is apparent; fetal heart rate (FHR) is maintained at 120 to 160 beats/min with adequate short- and long-term variability; maternal urine output is greater than 30 ml/hr.

Therapy for hypovolemic shock is aimed at restoring blood volume and halting the source of hemorrhage as quickly as possible (Table 21.3). Monitoring urine output is a good gauge of blood loss because kidneys need sufficient arterial blood flow and pressure to function. If they are not producing urine, it suggests the kidneys are not obtaining adequate blood. If the blood deficit continues so blood cannot reach other major organs, multiorgan failure can result. Obtaining hemoglobin and hematocrit levels and securing a blood sample for typing or cross-matching are essential not only to help predict the extent of blood loss but also to prepare for blood replacement. A woman suspected of having serious bleeding will need intravenous fluid replacement, such as Ringer's lactate, as an early intervention. Use a large-gauge Angiocath (16 or 18) for rapid fluid expansion as this will also allow a blood transfusion to be administered through the same site as soon as blood is available. If respirations are rapid, administer

TABLE 21.1 SUMMARY OF PRIMARY CAUSES OF BLEEDING DURING PREGNANCY

Time	Type	Cause	Assessment	Cautions
First and second trimester	Threatened spontaneous miscarriage (early: under 16 weeks; late: 16 to 24 weeks)	Unknown; possibly chromosomal or uterine abnormalities	Vaginal spotting, perhaps slight cramping	Caution women not to use tampons to halt bleeding as this can lead to infection.
	Imminent (inevitable) miscarriage	Unknown reasons but possibly poor placental attachment	Vaginal spotting, cramping, cervical dilatation	
	Missed miscarriage	Unknown	Vaginal spotting, perhaps slight cramping; no apparent loss of pregnancy	Disseminated intravascular coagulation is associated with missed miscarriage.
	Incomplete spontaneous miscarriage	Unknown; possibly chromosomal or uterine abnormalities	Vaginal spotting, cramping, cervical dilatation, but incomplete expulsion of uterine contents	High risk for uterine infection and hemorrhage
	Complete spontaneous miscarriage	Unknown but possibly chromosomal or uterine abnormalities	Vaginal spotting, cramping, cervical dilatation, and complete expulsion of uterine contents	
	Ectopic (tubal) pregnancy	Implantation of zygote at site other than in uterus, associated with tubal constrictures	Sudden unilateral lower abdominal quadrant pain; minimal vaginal bleeding, possible signs of hypovolemic shock or hemorrhage	May have repeat ectopic pregnancy in future if tubal scarring is bilateral
Second trimester	Gestational trophoblastic disease (hydatidiform mole)	Abnormal proliferation of trophoblast cells; fertilization or division defect	Overgrowth of uterus; highly positive human chorionic gonadotropin (hCG) test; no fetus present on ultrasound; bleeding from vagina of old or fresh blood accompanied by cyst formation	Retained trophoblast tissue may become malignant (choriocarcinoma); follow for 6 months to 1 year with hCG testing
	Premature cervical dilatation	Cervix begins to dilate and pregnancy is lost at about 20 weeks; unknown cause but cervical trauma from dilatation and curettage (D&C) may be associated.	Painless bleeding leading to expulsion of fetus	Can have cervical sutures placed to ensure a second pregnancy
Third trimester	Placenta previa	Low implantation of placenta possibly because of uterine abnormality	Painless bleeding at beginning of cervical dilatation	Don't allow a vaginal examination to minimize placental trauma.
	Premature separation of the placenta (abruptio placentae)	Unknown cause; associated with hypertension; placenta separates from uterus before birth of fetus	Sharp abdominal pain followed by uterine tenderness; vaginal bleeding; signs of maternal hypovolemic shock, fetal distress	Disseminated intravascular coagulation is associated with condition.
	Preterm labor	Many possible etiologic factors such as trauma, substance abuse, hypertension of pregnancy, or cervicitis; increased chance in multiple gestation, maternal illness	Show (pink-stained vaginal discharge) accompanied by uterine contractions becoming regular and effective	Preterm labor may be halted if the cervix is less than 4 cm dilated and the membranes are intact. Corticosteroids are administered to aid fetal lung maturity.

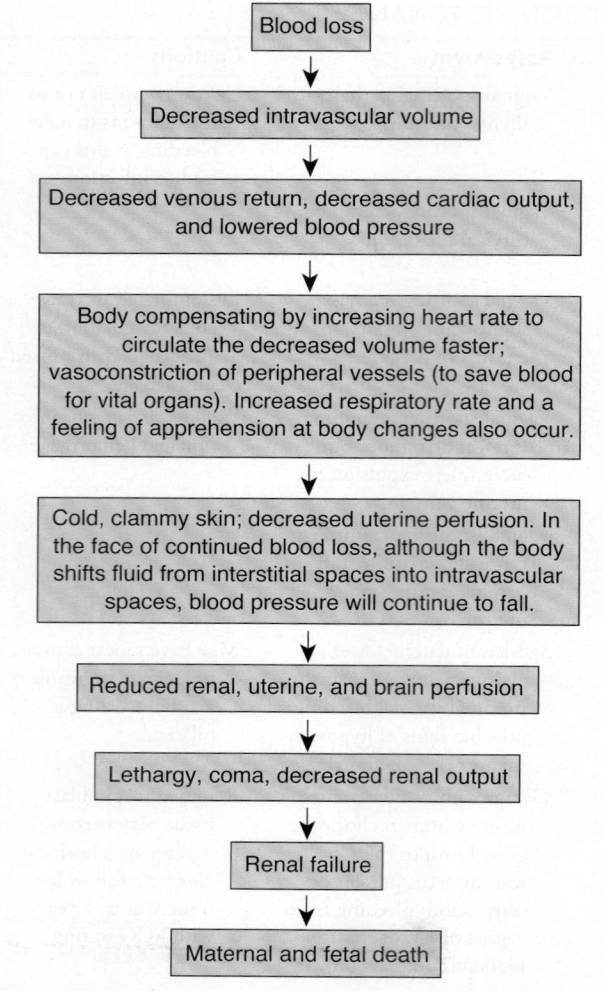

Figure 21.1 The process of shock because of blood loss (hypovolemia).

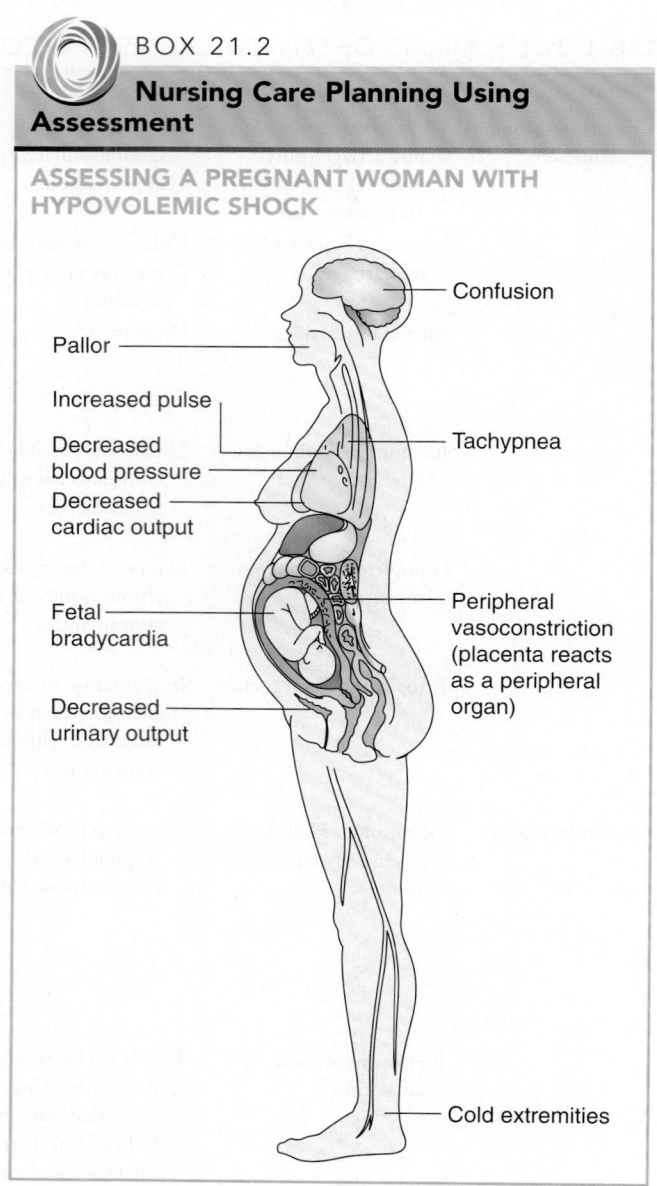

BOX 21.2

Nursing Care Planning Using Assessment

ASSESSING A PREGNANT WOMAN WITH HYPOVOLEMIC SHOCK

TABLE 21.2 SIGNS AND SYMPTOMS OF HYPOVOLEMIC SHOCK

Assessment	Significance
Increased pulse rate	Heart attempts to circulate decreased blood volume.
Decreased blood pressure	Less peripheral resistance is present because of decreased blood volume.
Increased respiratory rate	Respiratory system attempts to increase gas exchange to better oxygenate decreased red blood cell volume.
Cold, clammy skin	Vasoconstriction occurs to maintain blood volume in central body core.
Decreased urine output	Inadequate blood is entering kidneys because of decreased blood volume.
Dizziness or decreased level of consciousness	Inadequate blood is reaching cerebrum because of decreased blood volume.
Decreased central venous pressure	Decreased blood is returning to heart because of reduced blood volume.

TABLE 21.3 EMERGENCY INTERVENTIONS FOR BLEEDING IN PREGNANCY

Intervention	Rationale
Alert healthcare team of emergency situation.	Provides maximum coordination of care
Place woman flat in bed on her side.	Maintains optimal placental and renal function
Begin intravenous fluid such as Ringer's lactate with a 16- or 18-gauge Angiocath.	Replaces intravascular fluid volume; intravenous line is established if blood replacement will be needed
Administer oxygen as necessary at 6–10 L/min by face mask.	Provides adequate fetal oxygenation despite lowered maternal circulating blood volume
Monitor uterine contractions and fetal heart rate by external monitor.	Assesses whether labor is present and fetal status; external system avoids cervical trauma
Omit vaginal examination.	Prevents tearing of placenta if placenta previa is cause of bleeding
Withhold oral fluid.	Anticipates need for emergency surgery
Order type and cross-match of 2 units of whole blood.	Allows for restoring circulating maternal blood volume if needed
Measure intake and output.	Enables assessment of renal function (will decrease to under 30 ml/hr with massive circulating volume loss)
Assess vital signs (pulse, respirations, and blood pressure every 15 min; apply pulse oximeter and automatic blood pressure cuff as necessary).	Provides baseline data on maternal response to blood loss
Assist with placement of central venous pressure or pulmonary artery catheter and blood determinations.	Provides more accurate data on maternal hemodynamic state
Measure maternal blood loss by weighing perineal pads; save any tissue passed.	Provides objective evidence of amount of bleeding; saturating a sanitary pad in less than 1 hr is heavy blood loss; tissue may be abnormal trophoblast tissue
Assist with ultrasound examination.	Supplies information on placental and fetal well-being
Maintain a positive attitude about fetal outcome.	Supports mother–child bonding
Support woman's self-esteem; provide emotional support to woman and her support person.	Assists problem solving, which is lessened by poor self-esteem.

oxygen by mask and monitor oxygen saturation levels by pulse oximetry. A woman needs frequent assessments of vital signs and continuous fetal monitoring; therefore, an external monitoring device should be started.

Urge the woman to rest in a side-lying position (left lateral is preferred) to help prevent vena cava compression. If this is not possible, position her on her back, with a wedge under one hip to minimize uterine pressure on the vena cava and prevent blood from being trapped in the lower extremities (supine hypotension syndrome). Continue to provide information about care and emotional support to her and her family members.

A woman may have a central venous pressure catheter (measures the right atrial pressure or the pressure of blood within the vena cava) or a pulmonary capillary wedge catheter (measures the pressure in the left atrium or the filling pressure in the left ventricle) inserted after bleeding is halted (see Chapter 41). During pregnancy, usual values of these measures differ from the average, so they need to be evaluated in light of the pregnancy. Central venous pressure during pregnancy is 1 to 6 mmHg and pulmonary capillary wedge pressure during pregnancy is 6 to 12 mmHg (Watson & Wilkinson, 2012).

SPONTANEOUS MISCARRIAGE

Abortion is a medical term for any interruption of a pregnancy before a fetus is viable (i.e., able to survive outside the uterus if born at that time), but it is better to speak of these early pregnancy losses as spontaneous miscarriages to avoid confusion with intentional terminations of pregnancies. A viable fetus is usually defined as a fetus of more than 20 to 24 weeks of gestation or one that weighs at least 500 g. A fetus born before this point is considered a **miscarriage** or is termed a premature or immature birth (Sneider, Langhoff-Roos, Sundtoft, et al., 2015).

Spontaneous miscarriage occurs in 15% to 30% of all pregnancies and arises from natural causes (Seifert & Altman, 2015). A miscarriage is an early miscarriage if it occurs before week 16 of pregnancy and a late miscarriage if it occurs between weeks 16 and 20. For the first 6 weeks of pregnancy, the developing placenta is tentatively attached to the decidua of the uterus; during weeks 6 to 12, it is moderately attached. After week 12, the attachment is penetrating and deep. Because of these degrees of attachment achieved at different weeks of pregnancy, it is important to attempt to establish the week of the pregnancy at which bleeding has become apparent. Bleeding before week 6 is rarely severe; bleeding after week 12 can be profuse because the placenta is implanted so deeply. Fortunately, at this time, with such deep placental implantation, the fetus tends to be expelled as in natural childbirth before the placenta separates. Uterine contractions, however, then help to control placental bleeding as they do postpartally. For some women, then, the stage of attachment between weeks 6 and 12 can lead to the most severe, even life-threatening bleeding.

Common Causes

The most frequent cause of miscarriage in the first trimester of pregnancy is abnormal fetal development, due either to a teratogenic factor or to a chromosomal aberration. In other

COPING WITH A SPONTANEOUS MISCARRIAGE

Q. Beverly Muzuki had a spontaneous miscarriage when she was younger. She asks you, "What did I do wrong that time?"

A. Early miscarriage is largely not preventable because it is caused by such things as abnormal chromosome formation or poor uterine implantation—things over which you have no control. Eating a nutritious diet, so you enter a pregnancy in good health and avoiding cigarette smoking or drinking alcohol are sensible recommendations to reduce your risk of miscarriage. If you had extensive blood loss with your miscarriage, be certain to eat iron-rich foods (such as meat and green vegetables) to help restore red blood cells for a second pregnancy.

miscarriages, immunologic factors may be present or rejection of the embryo through an immune response may occur (Surette & Dunham, 2013). Another common cause of early miscarriage involves implantation abnormalities, as up to 50% of zygotes probably never implant securely because of inadequate endometrial formation or from an inappropriate site of implantation. With inadequate implantation, the placental circulation does not develop adequately enough to support the pregnancy. Miscarriage may also occur if the corpus luteum on the ovary fails to produce enough progesterone to maintain the decidua basalis. Progesterone therapy may be attempted to prevent this if this cause is documented (Aytac, Bulgan Kilicdag, Haydardedeoglu, et al., 2016).

Ingestion of alcohol at the time of conception or during early pregnancy can contribute to pregnancy loss because of abnormal fetal growth (Bingham, 2015). Urinary tract infections may be a cause but are more strongly associated with preterm birth. Systemic infections such as rubella, syphilis, poliomyelitis, cytomegalovirus, and toxoplasmosis readily cross the placenta and so may also be responsible. With an infection, if the fetus fails to grow, estrogen and progesterone production by the placenta falls and leads to endometrial sloughing. With the sloughing, prostaglandins are released; uterine contractions and cervical dilatation along with expulsion of the products of the pregnancy begin.

Because miscarriage can occur from so many causes and because the cause is often difficult to determine, couples may have difficulty understanding why it happened to them (Box 21.3).

Assessment

The presenting symptom of spontaneous miscarriage is almost always vaginal spotting. At the first indication of this, a woman should contact her healthcare provider and describe how much spotting she is having and its appearance (e.g., dark or fresh blood). Because a nurse often takes this initial call, guidelines to help assess vaginal bleeding quickly are shown in Table 21.4.

The history of the episode is important to help diagnose the cause. Knowledge of a woman's actions is important to ensure she did not attempt an illegal abortion. Asking what she has done, if anything, to halt the bleeding may reveal she inserted a tampon, for example. If she did, although reporting only slight spotting, she actually has an unknown amount of blood loss and might be bleeding much more heavily than she first reported.

Therapeutic Management

Depending on the symptoms and the description of the bleeding, a woman's primary healthcare provider will decide whether she needs to be seen and, if so, whether she should be seen in an ambulatory setting or the hospital.

Diagnosis

Threatened Miscarriage

Symptoms of a threatened miscarriage begin as vaginal bleeding, initially only scant and usually bright red. A woman may

TABLE 21.4 IMMEDIATE ASSESSMENT OF VAGINAL BLEEDING DURING PREGNANCY

Assessment Factor	Specific Questions to Ask
Confirmation of pregnancy	Does the woman know for certain she is pregnant (positive pregnancy test or healthcare provider confirmation)? A woman who has been pregnant before and states she is certain she is pregnant is probably right, even if she has not yet had her pregnancy confirmed.
Pregnancy length	What is the length of the pregnancy in weeks?
Duration	How long did the bleeding episode last? Is it continuing?
Intensity	How much bleeding occurred? (Ask the woman to compare it to a common measure such as a tablespoon or a cup.)
Description	Was blood mixed with amniotic fluid or mucus? Was it bright red (fresh blood) or dark (old blood)? Was it accompanied by tissue fragments? Was it odorous?
Frequency	Steady spotting? A single episode?
Associated symptoms	Cramping? Sharp pain? Dull pain? Has she ever had cervical surgery (to alert healthcare providers the woman may have cervical sutures in place?)
Action	What was happening at the time the bleeding started? What has she done (if anything) to control bleeding? (Caution her not to insert a tampon so the true extent of the bleeding shows.)
Blood type	Does she know this? (Rh-negative women will need Rh immune globulin to prevent Rh isoimmunization.)

notice slight cramping, but no cervical dilatation is present on vaginal examination. A woman with an apparent threatened miscarriage may be asked to come to the clinic or office to have fetal heart sounds assessed or an ultrasound performed to evaluate the viability of the fetus. Blood may be drawn to test for human chorionic gonadotropin (hCG) hormone at the start of bleeding and again in 48 hours (if the placenta is still intact, the level in the bloodstream should double in this time). If it does not double, poor placental function is suspected and the pregnancy probably will be lost. Avoidance of strenuous activity for 24 to 48 hours is the key intervention, assuming the threatened miscarriage involves a live fetus and presumed placental bleeding. Complete bed rest is usually not necessary as this may appear to stop the vaginal bleeding but only because blood pools vaginally. When a woman does ambulate again, the vaginal blood collection will drain and bleeding will reappear.

Women are apt to be extremely worried at the sight of bleeding. They need to talk with a sympathetic, supportive person about how distressed they are feeling. Women with threatened miscarriages often look for reasons why this could have happened, such as running up a flight of stairs, forgetting to take an iron pill, or getting angry with an older child. Being assured that none of these events causes miscarriage can help to minimize the guilt a woman may feel.

If the spotting with a threatened miscarriage is going to stop, it usually does so within 24 to 48 hours after a woman reduces her activity. Once bleeding stops, she can gradually resume normal activities. Coitus may be restricted for 2 weeks, however, to prevent infection and to avoid inducing further bleeding. As many as 50% of women with a threatened miscarriage continue the pregnancy; for the other 50%, unfortunately, the threatened miscarriage changes to imminent, or inevitable, miscarriage and the pregnancy ends (Ku, Allen, Malhotra, et al., 2015).

Imminent (Inevitable) Miscarriage

A threatened miscarriage becomes an imminent (i.e., inevitable) miscarriage if uterine contractions and cervical dilation occur as, with cervical dilation, the loss of the products of conception cannot be halted. A woman who reports cramping or uterine contractions is usually asked to come to the hospital or office, where she is examined. She should save any tissue fragments she has passed and bring them with her so they can be analyzed for an abnormality such as gestational trophoblastic disease (hydatidiform mole; see later). If no fetal heart sounds are detected and an ultrasound reveals an empty gestational sac or nonviable fetus, her primary healthcare provider may offer medication to help the pregnancy pass or perform a dilatation and curettage (D&C) or a dilation and evacuation (D&E) to ensure all the products of conception are removed (Sajan, Pulikkathodi, Vahab, et al., 2015). Be certain the woman has been told the pregnancy was already lost and that all procedures, such as suction curettage, are to clean the uterus and prevent further complications such as infection and not to end the pregnancy. Save any tissue fragments passed in the labor room, along with any brought from home, so it can be established that all the products of conception have been removed from the uterus. After a woman is discharged, the woman should assess the amount of vaginal bleeding she is having by recording the number of pads she uses; saturating more than one pad per hour is abnormally heavy bleeding.

Complete Miscarriage

In a complete miscarriage, the entire products of conception (fetus, membranes, and placenta) are expelled spontaneously without any assistance. The bleeding usually slows within 2 hours and then ceases within a few days after passage of the products of conception. Because the process is complete, no therapy other than advising the woman to report heavy bleeding is needed.

Incomplete Miscarriage

In an incomplete miscarriage, part of the conceptus (usually the fetus) is expelled, but the membranes or placenta are retained in the uterus. The term "incomplete" can be confusing for women as they may interpret it to mean that because the miscarriage was incomplete, it means the pregnancy will continue. With an incomplete miscarriage, there is a danger of maternal hemorrhage as long as part of the conceptus is retained in the uterus because the uterus cannot contract effectively under this condition. The woman will usually have a D&C or suction curettage to evacuate the remainder of the pregnancy. Again, be certain the woman knows the pregnancy is already lost and that these procedures are being done to protect her from hemorrhage and infection, not to end the pregnancy.

Missed Miscarriage

In a missed miscarriage, also commonly referred to as **early pregnancy failure**, the fetus dies in utero but is not expelled. Women can also find this term misleading because it suggests that if a miscarriage was "missed," then the pregnancy can continue. A missed miscarriage is usually discovered at a prenatal examination when the fundal height is measured and no increase in size can be demonstrated or when previously heard fetal heart sounds can no longer be heard. A woman may have had symptoms of a threatened miscarriage (e.g., painless vaginal bleeding) or she may have had no prior clinical symptoms.

After an ultrasound establishes the fetus has no heart rate, a D&C or D&E may be done to evacuate the pregnancy. If the pregnancy is over 14 weeks in length and, therefore, these procedures are no longer possible, labor can be induced by a prostaglandin suppository or misoprostol (Cytotec) introduced into the posterior fornix of the vagina to cause dilatation, followed by oxytocin stimulation or administration of mifepristone techniques used for elective termination of pregnancy, which cause contractions and birth (Oman & Burke, 2015). If the pregnancy is not actively terminated this way, miscarriage usually occurs spontaneously within 2 weeks. There is a danger of allowing this normal course to happen, however, because disseminated intravascular coagulation (DIC), a coagulation defect, may develop if the nonviable (and possibly toxic) fetus remains too long in utero (Zheng, 2012b).

Most women hope, until the moment the ultrasound shows their fetus no longer has a heart rate, that their baby is alive. They may need support in accepting the reality of the situation (Box 21.4) and need counseling to begin a future pregnancy because of fears they may never be able to carry a baby to full term.

Recurrent Pregnancy Loss

In the past, women who had three spontaneous miscarriages that occurred at the same gestational age were called "habitual aborters." They were advised they were apparently too "nervous" or that something was so wrong with their hormones

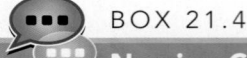

BOX 21.4

Nursing Care Planning Tips for Effective Communication

Beverly's neighbor noticed some vaginal spotting at 10 weeks into her pregnancy. The bleeding stopped spontaneously, but her healthcare provider was unable to hear fetal heart tones. An ultrasound revealed a missed miscarriage. You talk to her neighbor after she has received this news.

Tip: Because many women want so badly to be pregnant, it can be easy for them to "miss" bad news about a pregnancy. Actively listen to ensure there are no misunderstandings. It is also difficult for a shocked patient to absorb all the information after being informed about a miscarriage. Repeat information as necessary or ask for the patient to verbalize the plan.

Nurse: Hello, Vivian. How are you feeling?

Vivian: Fine. I guess this was a small thing.

Nurse: I'm sorry it happened. It must be upsetting.

Vivian: The bleeding was scary. Made me really nervous something was going wrong with the baby.

Nurse: With the baby?

Vivian: Yes. I'm really lucky I missed having a miscarriage.

Nurse: Let me ask your doctor to reexplain what she meant by a missed miscarriage. That's a term that can be confusing.

that childbearing was not for them. Today, the term **recurrent pregnancy loss** is used to describe this miscarriage pattern, and a thorough investigation is done to discover the cause of the loss and to help ensure the outcome of a future pregnancy. Recurrent pregnancy loss occurs in about 1% of women who want to be pregnant. Although many of these losses occur for unknown reasons, possible causes include:

- Defective spermatozoa or ova
- Endocrine factors such as lowered levels of protein-bound iodine (PBI), butanol-extractable iodine (BEI), and globulin-bound iodine (GBI); poor thyroid function; or a luteal phase defect
- Deviations of the uterus, such as septate or bicornuate uterus
- Resistance to uterine artery blood flow
- Chorioamnionitis or uterine infection
- Autoimmune disorders such as those involving lupus anticoagulant and antiphospholipid antibodies (Besharat, Tabandeh, Keshtkar, et al., 2015)

Complications of Miscarriage

As with full-term childbirth, hemorrhage and infection are two of the most likely complications after miscarriage. The risk for Rh isoimmunization and a woman's psychological state also need to be considered.

Hemorrhage

With a complete spontaneous miscarriage, serious or fatal hemorrhage is rare. With an incomplete miscarriage or in a woman who develops an accompanying coagulation defect (usually DIC), major hemorrhage becomes a possibility. Monitor vital signs for any changes to detect possible hypovolemic shock. If excessive vaginal bleeding occurs, immediately position a woman flat and massage the uterine fundus to try to aid contraction, although this may be impossible with an early pregnancy because the small uterus is not palpable above the symphysis pubis (see Chapter 17). Applying pneumatic antishock garments can help maintain blood pressure (FIGO Safe Motherhood and Newborn Health Committee, 2015).

If bleeding doesn't halt, a woman may need a D&C or suction curettage to empty the uterus of the material that is preventing it from contracting and achieving hemostasis. A transfusion may be necessary to replace blood loss. Direct replacement of fibrinogen or another clotting factor may be used to increase coagulation ability.

After a self-limiting complete miscarriage, a woman needs clear instructions on how much bleeding is abnormal (more than one sanitary pad per hour is excessive) and what color changes she should expect in bleeding (gradually changing to a dark color and then to the color of serous fluid as it does with the postpartum woman). Be certain she is aware any unusual odor or passing of large clots is also abnormal. If her primary healthcare provider has prescribed an oral medication such as methylergonovine maleate (Methergine) to aid uterine contraction, review with her why it is being prescribed and the importance of taking it. Some women repress their feelings following a miscarriage, anxious to forget the experience as quickly as possible. Short-term repression this way can be helpful if it helps them with their anger or grief at the loss of the pregnancy. Be careful, however, in repressing the experience a woman does not also repress the memory of her medication and leave herself open to hemorrhage.

QSEN Checkpoint Question 21.1

PATIENT-CENTERED CARE

Beverly Muzuki had a miscarriage when she was younger. After addressing her immediate psychosocial needs, the nurse identifies which advice as best for a woman who says she is miscarrying?

  a. Lie down and remain on bed rest for 24 hours to stop the bleeding.

  b. Continue light activity as usual because most spotting during pregnancy is harmless.

  c. Save any clots or material passed for your healthcare provider to examine.

  d. Use a tampon to put pressure on your cervix and stop the bleeding.

Look in Appendix A for the best answer and rationale.

Infection

The possibility of infection is minimal when pregnancy loss occurs over a short time, bleeding is self-limiting, and instrumentation is limited. However, there is always a possibility it may occur. It tends to develop most often in women who have lost an appreciable amount of blood. Infection is often a reason for excessive blood loss. Observe such women closely to rule out this second and possibly fatal complication. Be certain the woman is familiar with common danger signs of infection, such as fever higher than 100.4°F (38.0°C), abdominal pain or tenderness, and a foul-smelling vaginal discharge. Usually, fever is the most important sign of infection, but it can also be a transient reaction to the period of decreased fluid intake that preceded or shortly followed the miscarriage. Don't dismiss any degree of elevated temperature, however, to avoid overlooking the possibility infection is developing.

The organisms responsible for infection after miscarriage are usually *Escherichia coli* (spread from the rectum forward into the vagina) or group A streptococcus (Eschenbach, 2015). Caution women to always wipe their perineal area from front to back after voiding and particularly after defecation to prevent the spread of bacteria from the rectal area and to decrease the possibility of this source of infection. Be certain to advise the woman not to use tampons (stasis of any body fluid increases the risk of infection).

Infection usually involves the inner lining of the uterus (endometritis), but it may be more extensive and lead to parametritis, peritonitis, thrombophlebitis, or septicemia. The management of these infections is the same as if they were occurring after the safe birth of a child and so are discussed in Chapter 25.

Septic Abortion

A septic abortion is an abortion complicated by infection (Eschenbach, 2015). Infection can occur after a spontaneous miscarriage, but more frequently, it occurs in women who have tried to self-abort or whose pregnancy was aborted illegally using a nonsterile instrument such as a knitting needle. Septic abortion is not common in the United States due to the legal status of abortion, but it is much more common in areas where abortion is illegal or medical care is not readily available. Because the uterus is a warm, moist, dark cavity, once infectious organisms are introduced, they grow rapidly in this environment, particularly if products of conception such as necrotic membranes are still present.

The woman will have symptoms of fever and crampy abdominal pain; her uterus will feel tender to palpation. Left untreated, such an infection can lead to toxic shock syndrome, septicemia, kidney failure, and death (Eschenbach, 2015).

Women with a septic abortion need immediate, intensive assessment and therapy. Typically, complete blood count; serum electrolytes; serum creatinine; blood type and crossmatch; and cervical, vaginal, and urine cultures are obtained. An indwelling urinary (Foley) catheter may be inserted to monitor urine output hourly to assess kidney function. Intravenous fluid to restore fluid volume and to provide a route for high-dose, broad-spectrum antibiotic therapy is begun. A combination of penicillin (gram-positive coverage), gentamicin (gram-negative aerobic coverage), and clindamycin (gram-negative anaerobic coverage) is commonly prescribed to combat the infection.

A central venous pressure or pulmonary artery catheter may be inserted to monitor left atrial filling pressure and hemodynamic status. The removal of all infected or necrotic tissue from the uterus is important, so a D&C or D&E will be performed. A tetanus toxoid given subcutaneously or a tetanus immune globulin given intramuscularly will be prescribed for prophylaxis against tetanus.

Infection following a septic abortion can be so severe that a woman needs to be admitted to an intensive care setting for continuing care. Dopamine and digitalis may be necessary to maintain sufficient cardiac output. Oxygen and perhaps ventilatory support may be necessary to maintain respiratory function.

Assuming a woman recovers from such an intense episode, a final result may be infertility because of uterine scarring or fibrotic scarring of the fallopian tubes. If the infection was caused by a woman trying to self-abort, she needs follow-up social work counseling to assess her home life and aid in identifying resources that could help her avoid having to make that decision in the future.

Isoimmunization

Whenever a placenta is dislodged at any point in pregnancy, either by spontaneous birth or by a D&C/D&E, some blood from the placental villi (the fetal blood) is apt to enter the maternal circulation. If the fetus was Rh positive and the woman is Rh negative, enough Rh-positive fetal blood may enter the maternal circulation to cause **isoimmunization**, or the production of antibodies against Rh-positive blood. If the woman's next child should have Rh-positive blood, these antibodies would attempt to destroy the red blood cells of this infant during the months that infant is in utero (Aitken & Tichy, 2015). Therefore, after a miscarriage, because the blood type of the conceptus is unknown, all women with Rh-negative blood should receive Rh (D antigen) immune globulin (RhIG) to prevent the buildup of antibodies in the event the conceptus was Rh positive.

Powerlessness or Anxiety

As with pregnancy loss for any reason, assess a woman's adjustment to a spontaneous miscarriage. Sadness and grief over the loss or the feeling that a woman has lost control of her life is to be expected. Do not forget to assess a partner's or the extended family's feelings as well, or the potential impact of their grief and possible lack of support for the woman over the pregnancy loss can be missed. Spontaneous miscarriage can be particularly heartbreaking for an older woman because she realizes her window of childbearing is limited.

QSEN Checkpoint Question 21.2

QUALITY IMPROVEMENT

Beverly Muzuki has an Rh-negative blood type. Her electronic record shows she had a previous miscarriage at 16 weeks into her last pregnancy. What medication should the nurse check she received following the miscarriage to minimize isoimmunization?

a. Misoprostol (Cytotec)
b. RhIG (RhoGAM)
c. Ferrous sulfate
d. Packed red blood cell transfusion

Look in Appendix A for the best answer and rationale.

ECTOPIC PREGNANCY

An **ectopic pregnancy** is one in which implantation occurred outside the uterine cavity. The most common site (in approximately 95% of such pregnancies) is in the fallopian tube (Fig. 21.2). Of these fallopian tube sites, approximately 80% occur in the ampullar portion, 12% occur in the isthmus, and 8% are interstitial or fimbrial (Jurkovic, 2012).

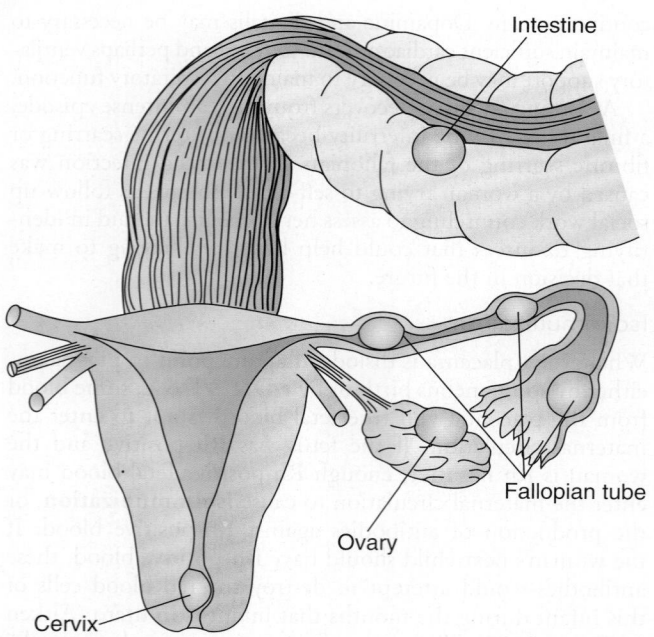

Figure 21.2 The sites at which an ectopic pregnancy may occur.

With most ectopic pregnancy, fertilization occurs as usual in the fallopian tube. Unfortunately, because an obstruction is present, such as an adhesion of the fallopian tube from a previous infection (chronic salpingitis or pelvic inflammatory disease), congenital malformations, scars from tubal surgery, or a uterine tumor pressing on the proximal end of the tube, the zygote cannot travel the length of the tube. It lodges at a strictured site along the tube and implants there instead of in the uterus.

Approximately 2% of pregnancies are ectopic, and because at least minimal bleeding occurs, it is the second most frequent cause of bleeding early in pregnancy. The incidence of ectopic pregnancy appears to be increasing, possibly because of the increasing rate of pelvic inflammatory disease, which can lead to tubal scarring. The incidence is also increased following in vitro fertilization (a woman might be having the in vitro fertilization because she has tubal scarring) and also in women who smoke.

Women who have one ectopic pregnancy have a higher chance of having a subsequent ectopic pregnancy. This is because salpingitis generally leaves scarring, which is bilateral. Congenital anomalies such as webbing (fibrous bands) that block a fallopian tube may also occur in both tubes. For unknown reasons, oral contraceptives used before pregnancy reduce the incidence of ectopic pregnancy (Li, Zhao, Zhu, et al., 2015).

Assessment

With an ectopic pregnancy, there are no unusual symptoms at the time of implantation. The corpus luteum of the ovary continues to function as if the implantation were in the uterus, so, often, no menstrual flow occurs. A woman may begin to experience the usual nausea and vomiting of early pregnancy and a pregnancy test for hCG will be positive. Many ectopic pregnancies are diagnosed because a woman has an early pregnancy ultrasound to date the pregnancy. Magnetic resonance imaging (MRI) is also effective to use for this. If not revealed by an ultrasound, at weeks 6 to 12 of pregnancy (2 to 8 weeks after a missed menstrual period), the zygote grows large enough that

it ruptures the slender fallopian tube. Tearing and destruction of blood vessels and bleeding result. If implantation was in the interstitial portion of the tube (where the tube joins the uterus), rupture can cause severe intraperitoneal bleeding because of the large blood vessels in that part of the tube. Fortunately, the incidence of tubal pregnancies is highest in the ampullar area (the distal third), where the blood vessels are smaller and profuse hemorrhage is less likely. Constant, continued bleeding from this area, however, may result in a large amount of blood loss over time. Therefore, a ruptured ectopic pregnancy is serious regardless of the site of implantation.

A woman usually experiences a sharp, stabbing pain in one of her lower abdominal quadrants at the time of rupture, followed by scant vaginal spotting. The amount of bleeding evident with a ruptured ectopic pregnancy usually does not reveal the actual amount present, however, because the products of conception from the ruptured tube and the accompanying blood may be expelled into the pelvic cavity rather than into the uterus. Blood does not reach the vagina to become evident. At the point the placenta dislodges, progesterone secretion will stop and the uterine decidua will begin to slough, causing additional vaginal bleeding. As soon as the woman becomes hypotensive from blood loss, she will experience light-headedness and a rapid pulse, signs of hypovolemic shock.

Because of these symptoms, any woman with sharp abdominal pain and vaginal spotting needs to be evaluated by her healthcare provider to rule out the possibility of ectopic pregnancy. When helping determine whether an ectopic pregnancy is present, ask a woman what she was doing when she felt the pain, if she had pain but no vaginal bleeding. Occasionally, a woman will move suddenly and pull one of her round ligaments, the anterior uterine supports, which causes a sharp but momentary lower quadrant pain, so this must be ruled out. Vaginal spotting or bleeding does rule out round ligament pain as it would be rare for this phenomenon to be reported in connection with vaginal spotting.

By the time a woman arrives at the hospital or primary healthcare provider's office, she may already be in severe shock, as evidenced by a rapid, thready pulse; rapid respirations; and falling blood pressure. Leukocytosis may be present, not from infection but from the trauma. Temperature is usually normal. A transvaginal ultrasound will demonstrate the ruptured tube and blood collecting in the peritoneum. Either a falling hCG or serum progesterone level suggests the pregnancy has ended. If the diagnosis of ectopic pregnancy is in doubt, a primary healthcare provider may insert a needle through the posterior vaginal fornix into the cul-de-sac under sterile conditions to see whether blood can be aspirated. A laparoscopy or culdoscopy can also be used to visualize the fallopian tube if the symptoms alone do not reveal a clear picture of what has happened. However, ultrasonography alone usually reveals a clear-cut diagnostic picture (Rodgers, Chang, DeBardeleben, et al., 2015).

If a woman waits for a time before seeking help, her abdomen gradually becomes rigid from peritoneal irritation. Her umbilicus may develop a bluish-tinged hue (Cullen sign). She may have continuing extensive or dull vaginal and abdominal pain; movement of the cervix on pelvic examination can cause excruciating pain. She may feel pain in her shoulders as well from blood in the peritoneal cavity causing irritation to the phrenic nerve. A tender mass is usually palpable in Douglas cul-de-sac on vaginal examination.

Therapeutic Management

Some ectopic pregnancies spontaneously end before they rupture and are reabsorbed over the next few days, requiring no treatment. It is difficult to predict when or if this will happen, however, so when an ectopic pregnancy is revealed by an early ultrasound, the woman is shown the sonogram, and after her agreement that therapy could be lifesaving, she is usually medically treated by the intramuscular or less often, oral, administration of methotrexate (Song, Kim, Kim, et al., 2016) (see Chapter 53 for a general discussion of chemotherapy agents of this type). The advantage of this therapy is that the tube is left intact, with no surgical scarring that could cause a second ectopic implantation. Women are treated until a negative hCG titer is achieved. A hysterosalpingogram or ultrasound is usually performed after this to assess that the pregnancy is no longer present and also whether the tube appears fully patent. If an ectopic pregnancy is not discovered early, but rather, only when it ruptures, it creates an emergency situation (Abraham & Seethappan, 2015).

Keep in mind the amount of blood evident with a ruptured ectopic pregnancy is a poor estimate of the actual blood loss. A blood sample needs to be drawn immediately for hemoglobin level, typing and cross-matching, and possibly the hCG level for immediate pregnancy testing, if pregnancy has not yet been confirmed. Intravenous fluid using a large-gauge catheter to restore intravascular volume will be prescribed. Blood then can be administered through this same line as soon as it is matched.

The therapy for ruptured ectopic pregnancy is laparoscopy to ligate the bleeding vessels and to remove or repair the damaged fallopian tube. A rough suture line on a fallopian tube may lead to another tubal pregnancy, so either the tube will be removed or suturing on the tube will be done with microsurgical technique. If a tube is removed, a woman may lose about 5% of her fertility. When she ovulates from either ovary, the egg can be moved into the remaining open tube with the peristaltic motion of that fallopian tube (Talarczyk-Desole, Wróbel, Niepsuj-Biniaś, et al., 2016). As with miscarriage, women with Rh-negative blood should receive RhIG/RhoGAM after an ectopic pregnancy for isoimmunization protection in future childbearing.

Nursing Diagnoses and Related Interventions

Nursing Diagnosis: Powerlessness related to early loss of pregnancy secondary to ectopic pregnancy

Outcome Evaluation: Patient states she feels sad at pregnancy loss but is able to deal with situation; has returned to previous level of activities and has forward-thinking plans.

A woman who has had an ectopic pregnancy not only has grief stages to work through (she has lost a child) but also may have problems of diminished self-image and a sense of powerlessness if surgery included removal of a fallopian tube. Encourage her to verbalize her concerns about this and her possibly reduced potential for future childbearing. This process of working through grief and role image may take weeks to months, but should begin in the hospital, where a woman has professional people to help her through the first days and to determine whether she will need further counseling.

ABDOMINAL PREGNANCY

Very rarely after an ectopic pregnancy ruptures—so rarely the instances are difficult to document—the products of conception are expelled into the pelvic cavity with a minimum of bleeding. The placenta continues to grow in the fallopian tube, spreading perhaps into the uterus for a better blood supply; or it may escape into the pelvic cavity and implant on an organ such as an intestine. The fetus will grow in the pelvic cavity (an abdominal pregnancy). This can also occur if a uterus ruptures because an old uterine scar ruptures during pregnancy (Nassali, Benti, Bandani-Ntsabele, et al., 2016).

In an abdominal pregnancy, the fetal outline is usually easily palpable through the abdomen because it is directly below the abdominal wall, not inside the uterus. A woman may either not be as aware of movements as she would be normally or she may experience painful fetal movements and abdominal cramping with fetal movements. She may report she noticed sudden lower quadrant pain earlier in the pregnancy but, because there was no external bleeding, didn't report it. An ultrasound or MRI will reveal the fetus outside the uterus.

The danger of abdominal pregnancy is that the placenta could infiltrate and erode a major blood vessel in the abdomen, leading to hemorrhage. If implanted on the intestine, it may erode so deeply it causes bowel perforation, leaking of intestinal contents, and peritonitis. The fetus is also at high risk (only about 60% come to term) because without a good uterine blood supply, nutrients may not reach the fetus in adequate amounts leading to the threat of fetal deformity or growth restriction.

At term, the infant must be born through laparotomy. The placenta is often difficult to remove after birth if it has implanted onto an abdominal organ such as the intestine. It may, therefore, be left in place and allowed to absorb spontaneously in 2 or 3 months. A follow-up ultrasound can be used to detect whether this has occurred. If not, a woman can be treated with methotrexate to help the placenta absorb, although this therapy may not be effective because the remaining trophoblasts are no longer fast growing (Nassali et al., 2016).

GESTATIONAL TROPHOBLASTIC DISEASE (HYDATIDIFORM MOLE)

Gestational trophoblastic disease is abnormal proliferation and then degeneration of the trophoblastic villi (Jean-Jacques, 2016). As the cells degenerate, they become filled with fluid and appear as clear fluid-filled, grape-sized vesicles. The embryo fails to develop beyond a primitive start. Abnormal trophoblast cells must be identified because they are associated with choriocarcinoma, a rapidly metastasizing malignancy (Fig. 21.3).

The incidence of gestational trophoblastic disease is approximately 1 in every 1,500 pregnancies. The condition tends to occur most often in women who have a low-protein intake, in women older than 35 years of age, in women of Asian heritage, and in blood group A women who marry blood group O men (Maestá, Berkowitz, Goldstein, et al., 2015).

Two types of molar growth can be identified by chromosome analysis. With a complete mole, all trophoblastic villi swell and become cystic. If an embryo forms, it dies early at only 1 to 2 mm in size, with no fetal blood present in the villi. On chromosomal analysis, although the karyotype is a normal 46XX or 46XY, this chromosome component was contributed only by the father or an "empty ovum" was fertilized and the chromosome material was duplicated (Fig. 21.4A).

Figure 21.3 Gestational trophoblastic disease (hydatidiform mole). (From Rubin, E., & Farber, J. L. [1994]. *Pathology* [2nd ed.]. Philadelphia, PA: JB Lippincott.)

With a partial mole, some of the villi form normally. The syncytiotrophoblastic layer of villi, however, appears swollen and misshapen. The embryo may grow for about 9 weeks but then macerates; some fetal blood may be present in the villi. A partial mole has 69 chromosomes (69XX or 69XY) (a triploid formation in which there are three chromosomes instead of two for every pair: one set supplied by an ovum that apparently was fertilized by two sperm or an ovum fertilized by one sperm in which meiosis or reduction division did not occur). This could also occur if one set of 23 chromosomes was supplied by one sperm and an ovum that did not undergo reduction division supplied 46 (see Fig. 21.4B).

In contrast to complete moles, partial moles rarely lead to choriocarcinoma. Although still above average, hCG titers are

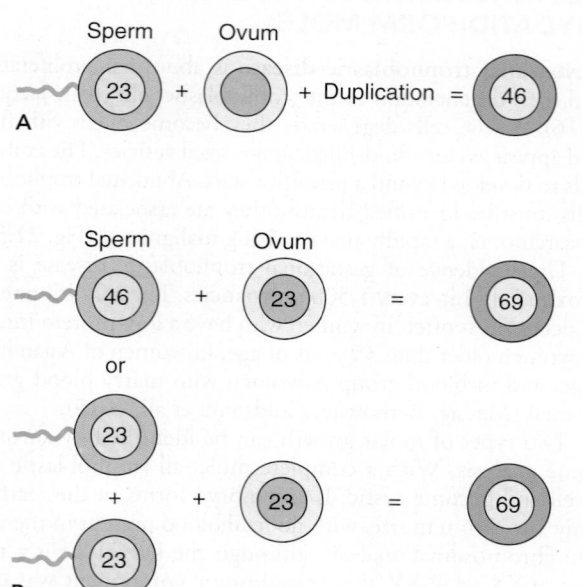

Figure 21.4 Formation of gestational trophoblastic disease (hydatidiform mole). **(A)** A complete mole. **(B)** A partial mole.

lower in partial than in complete moles; titers also return to normal faster after gestational trophoblast evacuation (Savage & Seckl, 2012).

Assessment

Because proliferation of the abnormal trophoblast cells grow so rapidly, the uterus tends to expand faster than usual or the uterus reaches its landmarks (just over the symphysis brim at 12 weeks, at the umbilicus at 20 to 24 weeks) before the usual time. This rapid development is also diagnostic of multiple pregnancy or a miscalculated due date, however, so this finding must be evaluated carefully. Because hCG is produced by the trophoblast cells that are overgrowing, a serum or urine test of hCG for pregnancy will be strongly positive (1 to 2 million International Units compared with a normal pregnancy level of 400,000 International Units).

Results continue to be strongly positive after day 100 of pregnancy, when the level of hCG normally begins to decline. This fact must be evaluated carefully also, however, because highly positive test results can be characteristic of multiple pregnancies with more than one placenta or a miscalculated due date. The nausea and vomiting of early pregnancy is usually marked, probably because of the high hCG level present. Symptoms of gestational hypertension, such as increased blood pressure, edema, and proteinuria, are ordinarily not present before week 20 of pregnancy. With gestational trophoblastic disease, they may appear before this time. An ultrasound will show dense growth (typically a snowflake pattern) but no fetal growth in the uterus. No fetal heart sounds can be heard because there is no viable fetus.

At approximately week 16 of pregnancy, if the structure was not identified earlier by ultrasound, it will identify itself with vaginal bleeding. This may begin as spotting of dark-brown blood resembling prune juice or as a profuse fresh flow. As the bleeding progresses, it is accompanied by discharge of the clear fluid-filled vesicles. This is why it is important for any woman who begins to miscarry at home to bring any clots or tissue passed to the hospital with her. The presence of clear fluid-filled cysts changes the diagnosis from a simple miscarriage to gestational trophoblastic disease.

Therapeutic Management

Therapy for gestational trophoblastic disease is suction curettage to evacuate the abnormal trophoblast cells. Following extraction, women should have a baseline pelvic examination and a serum test for the beta subunit of hCG. The hCG is then analyzed every 2 weeks until levels are again normal. The serum hCG level is then assessed every 4 weeks for the next 6 to 12 months to see if it is declining (half of women will still have a positive reading at 3 weeks; one fourth still have a positive test result at 40 days).

If the level plateaus or increases, it suggests a malignant transformation (i.e., choriocarcinoma) is occurring. During the waiting time for the hCG level to decline, a woman should use a reliable contraceptive such as oral estrogen/progesterone so that a positive pregnancy test (the presence of hCG) resulting from a new pregnancy will not be confused with the increasing level that occurs with a developing malignancy. After 6 months, if hCG levels are still negative, a woman is theoretically free of the risk of a malignancy. By 12 months, she could begin to plan a second pregnancy. Although the development of gestational trophoblastic disease means a pregnancy never materialized and a fetus never formed, a woman may experience the same feeling of loss after evacuation that she would have experienced after the loss of a true pregnancy—she did, after all, believe she was pregnant. In addition, she is faced with the possibility a malignancy may develop as well as also delay her childbearing plans for a year. If she had already put off having a child for some time, this may seem to be an unbearably long time.

Some primary healthcare providers give women who have had gestational trophoblastic disease a prophylactic course of methotrexate. However, because the drug interferes with white blood cell formation (i.e., leukopenia), prophylactic use must be weighed carefully (Stevens, Katzorke, Tempfer, et al., 2015). If malignancy should occur, it can be treated effectively in most instances with methotrexate at that time (Stevens et al., 2015). A second agent such as dactinomycin can be added to the regimen if metastasis occurs.

Women need the opportunity to express their anger and sense of unfairness at this type of event. They may feel inadequate because something went wrong with the pregnancy. They may wonder whether it will happen again in a future pregnancy or whether they will ever be able to have children. Unfortunately, women who have one incidence of gestational trophoblastic disease do have an increased risk of a second molar pregnancy (Maestá et al., 2015). They need early screening with ultrasound during a second pregnancy to be certain this irregular trophoblastic growth is not happening again.

What If . . . 21.1
After having had a gestational trophoblastic disorder, Beverly Muzuki told the nurse she did not believe in birth control because of religious convictions. She did not intend to take the oral contraceptives prescribed following her mole evacuation. How would the nurse best advise her?

CERVICAL INSUFFICIENCY (PREMATURE CERVICAL DILATATION)

Premature cervical dilatation, previously termed an incompetent cervix, refers to a cervix that dilates prematurely and therefore cannot retain a fetus until term (Roman, 2013). It occurs in about 1% of women. The dilatation usually occurs painlessly, so often the first symptom is show (a pink-stained vaginal discharge) or increased pelvic pressure, which then is followed by rupture of the membranes and discharge of the amniotic fluid. Uterine contractions begin and, after a short labor, the fetus is born. Unfortunately, this commonly occurs at approximately week 20 of pregnancy, when the fetus is still too immature to survive.

It is often difficult to explain in a particular instance what caused premature dilatation, although it is associated with increased maternal age, congenital structural defects, and trauma to the cervix, such as might have occurred with a cone biopsy or repeated D&Cs. Although it may be diagnosed by an early ultrasound before symptoms occur, it is usually diagnosed only after the pregnancy is lost.

After the loss of one child because of premature cervical dilatation, a surgical operation termed **cervical cerclage** can be performed to prevent this from happening in a second pregnancy (Gilner & Biggio, 2016).

Figure 21.5   Shirodkar suture for cervical cerclage.

As soon as an ultrasound confirms that the fetus of a second pregnancy is healthy at approximately weeks 12 to 14, purse-string sutures are placed in the cervix by the vaginal route under regional anesthesia. This procedure is called a McDonald or a Shirodkar procedure after the surgeons who perfected the technique. The sutures serve to strengthen the cervix and prevent it from dilating until the end of pregnancy (Fig. 21.5). Still newer techniques allow purse-string sutures to be set before a woman becomes pregnant, providing added assurance she will not begin miscarrying before week 14 of pregnancy. In a McDonald procedure, nylon sutures are placed horizontally and vertically across the cervix and pulled tight to reduce the cervical canal to a few millimeters in diameter. With a Shirodkar technique, sterile tape is threaded in a purse-string manner under the submucous layer of the cervix and sutured in place to achieve a closed cervix. Although routinely accomplished by a vaginal route, sutures may be placed by a transabdominal route.

After cerclage surgery, women remain on bed rest (perhaps in a slight or modified Trendelenburg position) for a few days to decrease pressure on the new sutures. Usual activity and sexual relations can be resumed in most instances after this rest period.

With these procedures, the sutures are removed at weeks 37 to 38 of pregnancy so the fetus can be born vaginally. When a transabdominal approach is used, the sutures must be left in place and a cesarean birth performed.

Women who are discovered to have cervical dilatation but with membranes still intact at a prenatal visit may have emergent cerclage sutures placed in the cervix even at that point as prophylaxis against preterm birth. The success of this procedure is limited, however, compared to preventive suturing (Ragab & Mesbah, 2015).

Be certain to ask women who are reporting painless bleeding (also the symptoms of spontaneous miscarriage) whether they have had past cervical operations to remind them they may have sutures in place. Currently, the prognosis for a successful pregnancy after surgical correction for premature cervical dilatation is very favorable. The success rate with both types of cerclage techniques averages 80% to 90% (Seifert & Altman, 2015).

PLACENTA PREVIA

Placenta previa, a condition of pregnancy in which the placenta is implanted abnormally in the lower part of the uterus, is the most common cause of painless bleeding in the third

Figure 21.6   Degrees of placenta previa: **(A)** low implantation, **(B)** partial placenta previa, and **(C)** total placenta previa.

trimester of pregnancy (Mastrolia, Baumfeld, Loverro, et al., 2016) (Fig. 21.6). It occurs in four degrees: implantation in the lower rather than in the upper portion of the uterus (low-lying placenta), marginal implantation (the placenta edge approaches that of the cervical os), implantation that occludes a portion of the cervical os (partial placenta previa), and implantation that totally obstructs the cervical os (total placenta previa). The degree to which the placenta covers the internal cervical os is generally estimated in percentages: 100%, 75%, 30%, and so forth.

Increased parity, advanced maternal age, past cesarean births, past uterine curettage, multiple gestation, and perhaps a male fetus are all associated with placenta previa. The incidence is approximately 5 per 1,000 pregnancies; it is thought to occur whenever the placenta is forced to spread to find an adequate exchange surface. There is a possibility an increase in congenital fetal anomalies or fetal restricted growth could occur if the low implantation does not allow optimal fetal nutrition or oxygenation, but in actual practice, this rarely happens (Ahmed, Aitallah, Abdelghafar, et al., 2015).

Assessment

Placenta previa is often detected during pregnancy through a routine sonogram done to date the pregnancy. Although many low-lying placentas detected on early ultrasounds migrate upward to a noncervical position, the condition is explained to the woman and she is cautioned to call her healthcare provider at any sign of vaginal bleeding. The bleeding with placenta previa doesn't usually begin, however, until the lower uterine segment starts to differentiate from the upper segment late in pregnancy (approximately week 30) and the cervix begins to dilate. At that point, because the placenta is unable to stretch to accommodate the differing shape of the lower uterine segment or the cervix, a small portion loosens and damaged blood vessels begin to bleed. The bleeding is usually abrupt, painless, bright red, and sudden enough to frighten a woman. It is not associated with increased activity or participation in sports and may stop as abruptly as it began, so that by the time a woman is seen at the healthcare setting, she is no longer bleeding. In other women, it may slow after the initial hemorrhage but linger as continuous spotting.

Therapeutic Management

The bleeding of placenta previa, like that of ectopic pregnancy, creates an emergency situation as the open vessels of the uterine decidua (maternal blood) place the mother at risk for hemorrhage. Because the placenta is loosened, the fetal oxygen and nutrient supply may also be compromised, placing the fetus at risk as well. With the placental loosening, preterm labor (labor that occurs before the end of week 37 of gestation) may begin, posing the additional threat of preterm birth to the fetus.

Immediate Care Measures

To ensure an adequate blood supply to a woman and fetus, place the woman immediately on bed rest in a side-lying position. Be certain to assess:

- Duration of the pregnancy
- Time the bleeding began
- Woman's estimation of the amount of blood—ask her to estimate in terms of cups or tablespoons (a cup is 240 ml; a tablespoon is 15 ml)
- Whether there was accompanying pain
- Color of the blood (red blood indicates bleeding is fresh or is continuing)
- What she has done, if anything, for the bleeding (if she inserted a tampon to halt the bleeding, there may be hidden bleeding)
- Whether there were prior episodes of bleeding during the pregnancy
- Whether she had prior cervical surgery for premature cervical dilatation

Inspect the perineum for bleeding and estimate the present rate of blood loss. Weighing perineal pads before and after use and calculating the difference by subtraction is a good method to determine vaginal blood loss. An Apt or Kleihauer–Betke test (test strip procedures) can be used to detect whether the blood is of fetal or maternal origin. Obtain baseline vital signs to determine whether symptoms of hypovolemic shock are present. Continue to assess blood pressure every 5 to 15 minutes or continuously with an electronic cuff. Never attempt a pelvic or rectal examination with painless bleeding late in pregnancy because any agitation of the cervix when there is a placenta previa might tear the placenta further and initiate massive hemorrhage, possibly fatal to both mother and child.

Attach external monitoring equipment to record fetal heart sounds and uterine contractions (an internal monitor for either fetal or uterine assessment is contraindicated). Hemoglobin, hematocrit, prothrombin time, partial thromboplastin time, fibrinogen, platelet count, type and cross-match, and antibody screen will be assessed to establish baselines, detect a possible clotting disorder, and ready blood for replacement if necessary. Monitor urine output frequently, as often as every hour, as an indicator her blood volume is remaining adequate to perfuse her kidneys. Administer intravenous fluid as prescribed, preferably with a large-gauge catheter to allow for blood replacement through the same line.

A vaginal birth is always safest for an infant. It is essential, therefore, to determine the placenta's location as accurately as possible in the hope that its position will make vaginal birth feasible. If the previa is under 30% by abdominal or intravaginal ultrasound, it may be possible for the fetus to be born past it. If over 30%, and the fetus is mature, the safest birth method for both mother and baby is often a cesarean birth (Kim, Joung, Lee, et al., 2015).

If only a minimum previa is detected by sonogram, the primary healthcare provider may attempt a careful speculum examination of the vagina and cervix to establish the degree of fetal engagement and to rule out another cause for bleeding, such as ruptured varices or cervical trauma. This should be done in an operating room or a fully equipped birthing room so that if hemorrhage does occur with cervical manipulation, an immediate cesarean birth can be carried out to remove the child and the bleeding placenta and contract the uterus. Have oxygen equipment available in case the fetal heart sounds indicate fetal distress, such as bradycardia or tachycardia, late deceleration, or variable decelerations during the exam.

Continuing Care Measures

The point at which a diagnosis of placenta previa is made and the age of the gestation dictate the final management. If labor has begun, bleeding is continuing, or the fetus is being compromised (measured by the response of the FHR to contractions), birth must be accomplished regardless of gestational age. If the bleeding has stopped, the fetal heart sounds are of good quality, maternal vital signs are good, and the fetus is not yet 36 weeks of age, a woman is usually managed by expectant watching. Typically, a woman remains in the hospital on bed rest for close observation for 24 to 48 hours. If the bleeding stops, she can be sent home with a referral for bed rest and home care. Assessments of fetal heart sounds and laboratory tests, such as hemoglobin or hematocrit, are obtained frequently. Betamethasone, a steroid that hastens fetal lung maturity, may be prescribed for the mother to encourage the maturity of fetal lungs if the fetus is less than 34 weeks gestation (Box 21.5).

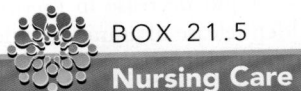

BOX 21.5

Nursing Care Planning Based on Responsibility for Pharmacology

BETAMETHASONE (CELESTONE)

Action: Betamethasone is a corticosteroid that acts as an anti-inflammatory and immunosuppressive agent. It is given to pregnant women 12 to 24 hours before birth to hasten fetal lung maturity if a fetus is less than 34 weeks gestation and help prevent respiratory distress syndrome in the newborn (Karch, 2015).

Pregnancy Risk Category: C

Dosage: 12 to 12.5 mg intramuscularly (IM) initially; may be repeated in 24 hours and again in 1 to 2 weeks

Possible Adverse Effects: Burning, itching, and irritation at the injection site; swelling, tachycardia, headache, dizziness, weight gain, sodium, and fluid retention; and increased risk of infection if used long term.

Nursing Implications

- Explain the purpose of the drug to the patient.
- Administer the initial dose IM. Anticipate the need for repeat dosing within 24 hours and again in 1 to 2 weeks.
- Assist with measures to halt preterm labor if indicated.
- Continue to monitor patient's vital signs and fetal heart rate for changes.
- If patient is also receiving a tocolytic agent, be alert for possible cardiac decompensation as a result of a drug–drug interaction. Observe for signs such as increased pulse, decreased blood pressure, and presence of edema.
- Assess for signs and symptoms of possible infection with long-term use.
- Instruct patient about the possibility that a repeat dose may be necessary.

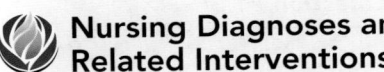

Nursing Diagnoses and Related Interventions

Because the diagnosis of placenta previa with bleeding is an emergency, all goals should reflect the short time frame of the emergency condition.

Nursing Diagnosis: Fear related to outcome of pregnancy after episode of placenta previa bleeding

Outcome Evaluation: Patient discusses concerns with nurse and other healthcare providers; states hearing fetal heartbeat helps to reassure her about baby's health.

Often, it is difficult for a woman who has experienced bleeding late in a pregnancy to wait for the baby to come to term because she wonders whether her infant will be all right. Regardless of her outward appearance, most likely, she is experiencing severe emotional stress. She cannot help but wonder if the next bleeding she experiences will kill her, the infant, or both. Listening to fetal heart sounds and being reassured they are in a healthy range is helpful, as is having a listening ear she can talk to about her fears for both the pregnancy and herself.

Birth

If the pregnancy was past 37 weeks at the time of the initial bleeding, and an amniocentesis analysis for lung maturity shows a positive result (a favorable lecithin/sphingomyelin ratio), a birth decision will generally be made immediately as it is important birth be in a controlled setting in case more than the usual blood loss occurs with birth. If the fetus is not mature, the pregnancy will be allowed to continue to the point bleeding occurs again, labor begins, the fetus shows symptoms of distress, or the fetus is mature. Offer firm support if the birth will be an emergency situation.

If the placenta previa is found to be total, birth through the cervix which is covered by the placenta is impossible and the baby must be born by cesarean birth. If the placenta previa is partial, the amount of the blood loss, the condition of the fetus, and a woman's parity will influence the birth decision. For cesarean birth, if an ultrasound clearly reveals the placental location, a transverse uterine incision may still be possible, although the uterine cut must be made high, possibly vertically above the low implantation site of the placenta.

After birth, most women inspect their child carefully. They may be worried that because of the problem with placental implantation, there might be something wrong with the baby. During the postpartum period, be sure a woman has adequate time with her child to be certain she feels comfortable giving care before she leaves the healthcare facility.

Any woman who has had a placenta previa is more prone than normal to postpartum hemorrhage because the placental site is in the lower uterine segment, which does not contract as efficiently as the upper segment. Also, because the uterine blood supply is less in the lower segment, the placenta tends to grow larger than it would normally, leaving a larger denuded surface area when it is removed. As a second complication, a woman is more likely to develop endometritis because the placental site is close to the cervix, the portal of entry for pathogens.

QSEN Checkpoint Question 21.3

SAFETY

Suppose a sonogram shows Beverly, who is beginning preterm labor, has a placenta previa. The nurse identifies which measure as the priority to ensure her safety?

a. Keep her physically active to avoid a deep vein thrombosis.

b. Perform a daily vaginal exam to assess the extent of the previa.

c. Assess for vaginal bleeding and clear fluid leakage every shift.

d. Keep her nothing by mouth (NPO) as she will need an emergency cesarean birth.

Look in Appendix A for the best answer and rationale.

PREMATURE SEPARATION OF THE PLACENTA (ABRUPTIO PLACENTAE)

Unlike placenta previa, in **premature separation of the placenta** (also called abruptio placentae; Fig. 21.7), the placenta appears to have been implanted correctly. Suddenly, however, it begins to separate and bleeding results. This occurs in about 10 out of 1,000 pregnancies and, because it can lead to extensive bleeding, is the most frequent cause of perinatal death (Ananth, Lavery, Vintzileos, et al., 2016). The separation generally occurs late in pregnancy; even as late as during the first or second stage of labor. Because premature separation of the placenta may occur during an otherwise normal labor, it is important to always be alert to both the amount and kind of pain and vaginal bleeding a woman is having in labor.

The primary cause of premature separation is unknown, but certain predisposing factors are high parity, advanced maternal age, a short umbilical cord, chronic hypertensive disease, hypertension of pregnancy, direct trauma (as from an automobile accident or intimate partner violence), vasoconstriction from cocaine or cigarette use, and thrombophilic conditions that lead to thrombosis formation (Boisramé, Sananès, Fritz, et al., 2014). It also may be caused by **chorioamnionitis** or infection of the fetal membranes and fluid (Hackney, Kuo, Petersen, et al., 2016).

Yet another possible cause is a rapid decrease in uterine volume, such as occurs with sudden release of amniotic fluid as can happen with polyhydramnios. Usually, the fetal head is low enough in the pelvis that when membranes rupture, this prevents loss of the total volume of the amniotic fluid at one time, so normally a rapid reduction in amniotic fluid does not occur.

Assessment

A woman experiences a sharp, stabbing pain high in the uterine fundus as the initial separation occurs. If labor begins with the separation, each contraction will be accompanied by pain over and above the pain of the contraction. Tenderness can be felt on uterine palpation.

Heavy bleeding usually accompanies premature separation of the placenta, although it may not be readily apparent. External bleeding will only be evident if the placenta separates first at the edges, so blood escapes freely into the uterus and then the cervix. In contrast, if the center of the placenta

Partial Separation
(Concealed Hemorrhage)

Partial Separation
(Apparent Hemorrhage)

Complete Separation
(Concealed Hemorrhage)

Figure 21.7 Premature separation of the placenta.

separates first, blood can pool under the placenta, and although bleeding is just as intense, it will be hidden from view. Whether blood is evident or not, signs of hypovolemic shock usually follow quickly. The uterus becomes tense and feels rigid to the touch. If blood infiltrates the uterine musculature, **Couvelaire uterus** or uteroplacental apoplexy, forming a hard, boardlike uterus occurs. As bleeding progresses, a woman's reserve of blood fibrinogen becomes diminished as her body attempts to accomplish effective clot formation, and DIC syndrome can occur (see later).

If a woman is being admitted to the hospital after experiencing symptoms at home, assess when the time the bleeding began, whether pain accompanied it, the amount and kind of bleeding, and her actions to detect if trauma could have led to the placental separation. Initial blood work should include hemoglobin level, typing and cross-matching, and a fibrinogen level and fibrin breakdown products to detect DIC.

Therapeutic Management

Because of the threat to both the woman and the fetus, separation of the placenta is immediately an emergency situation (Heavey & Dahl Maher, 2015). A woman needs a large-gauge intravenous catheter inserted for fluid replacement and oxygen by mask to limit fetal anoxia. Monitor fetal heart sounds externally and record maternal vital signs every 5 to 15 minutes to establish baselines and observe progress. The baseline fibrinogen determination will be followed by additional determinations up to the time of birth. Keep a woman in a lateral, not supine, position to prevent pressure on the vena cava and additional interference with fetal circulation. It is important not to disturb the injured placenta any further. Therefore, do not perform any abdominal, vaginal, or pelvic examination on a woman with a diagnosed or suspected placental separation.

For better prediction of fetal and maternal outcomes, the degrees of placental separation can be graded (Table 21.5). Unless the separation is minimal (grades 0 and 1), the pregnancy must be ended because the fetus cannot obtain adequate oxygen and nutrients. If vaginal birth does not seem imminent, cesarean birth is the birth method of choice. If DIC has developed, cesarean birth may pose a grave risk because of the possibility of hemorrhage during the surgery and later from the surgical incision. Intravenous administration of

TABLE 21.5 PREMATURE SEPARATION OF THE PLACENTA: DEGREES OF SEPARATION

Grade	Criteria
0	No symptoms of separation are apparent from maternal or fetal signs; the diagnosis is made after birth, when the placenta is examined and a segment of the placenta shows a recent adherent clot on the maternal surface.
1	Minimal separation, but enough to cause vaginal bleeding and changes in the maternal vital signs; no fetal distress or hemorrhagic shock occurs, however.
2	Moderate separation; there is evidence of fetal distress; the uterus is tense and painful on palpation.
3	Extreme separation; without immediate interventions, maternal hypovolemic shock and fetal death will result.

fibrinogen or cryoprecipitate (which contains fibrinogen) can be used to elevate a woman's fibrinogen level prior to and concurrently with surgery. With the worst outcome, a hysterectomy might be necessary to prevent exsanguination.

Fetal prognosis depends on the extent of the placental separation and the degree of fetal hypoxia. Maternal prognosis depends on how promptly treatment can be instituted. Death can occur from massive hemorrhage leading to shock and circulatory collapse or renal failure from circulatory collapse.

Any woman who has had bleeding before birth is more prone to infection after birth than the average woman. A woman with a history of premature separation of the placenta, therefore, needs to be observed closely for the development of infection in the postpartum period.

DISSEMINATED INTRAVASCULAR COAGULATION

DIC is an acquired disorder of blood clotting in which the fibrinogen level falls to below effective limits (Cunningham & Nelson, 2015). Early symptoms include easy bruising or bleeding from an intravenous site. Conditions such as premature separation of the placenta, hypertension of pregnancy, amniotic fluid embolism, placental retention, septic abortion, and retention of a dead fetus are all associated with its development (Cunningham & Nelson, 2015). Normally, platelets quickly form a seal over a point of bleeding to prevent further loss of blood. Intrinsic and extrinsic clotting pathways then activate and strengthen this plug with fibrin threads to produce a firm, fixed structure. To prevent too much clotting from occurring, at the same time the clot is being formed, thrombin activates fibrinolysin, a proteolytic enzyme, which begins digestion of excess fibrin threads (anticoagulation). This lysis results in the release of fibrin degradation products.

DIC occurs when there is such extreme bleeding and so many platelets and fibrin from the general circulation rush to the site that there is not enough left in the rest of the body. This results in a paradox: At one point in the circulatory system, the person has increased coagulation, but throughout the rest of the system, a bleeding defect exists. DIC is an emergency because it can result in extreme blood loss. Goals for care should reflect the presence of the emergency.

Blood needs to be drawn for a platelet count (will be decreased to $\leq 100,000/\mu l$), prothrombin (will be low because it depends on the conversion of fibrinogen to fibrin), thrombin time (will be elevated because it measures the time necessary for conversion of fibrinogen to fibrin), fibrinogen (will be decreased to <150 mg/dl because fibrinogen is not available), and fibrin split products (will be >40 mcg/ml reflecting the destruction of fibrinogen or fibrin). A D-dimer analysis is specific for fibrin (not fibrinogen) degradation products and will be abnormal in 90% of patients with DIC (Cunningham & Nelson, 2015).

To stop the process of DIC, the underlying insult that began the phenomenon must be halted. When the insult was a complication of pregnancy, such as premature separation of the placenta, ending the pregnancy by birthing the fetus and delivering the placenta is part of the solution. Next, the marked coagulation must be stopped so that coagulation factors can be freed and normal clotting function can be restored. This is accomplished by the administration of heparin to halt the clotting cascade, first intravenously, then by subcutaneous (SQ) injection. Heparin must be cautiously given close to birth, however, or postpartum hemorrhage could occur from poor clotting after delivery of the placenta. A blood or platelet transfusion may be necessary to replace blood or platelet loss, but this is usually delayed until after heparin therapy so the new blood factors are also not consumed by the coagulation process. Antithrombin III factor, fibrinogen, or cryoprecipitate (which contains fibrinogen) can all be used in place of whole blood for transfusion. If these are not available, fresh frozen plasma or platelets can also aid in restoring clotting function.

It can be confusing for a woman with a disorder such as premature separation of the placenta to have her primary healthcare provider tell her 1-minute bleeding is what he or she is worried about but then hear the next minute an anticoagulant such as heparin has been prescribed. If a woman understands the action of heparin—to discourage blood coagulation—it seems as if this would be exactly the wrong medication. Be certain a woman and her support person have a full explanation of what is happening (i.e., she has an increased risk of hemorrhage because part of her system has tied up coagulation factors; by releasing them, coagulation can be restored throughout the rest of her body) so she can maintain confidence in her caregivers.

Evaluation focuses on determining whether a woman's blood coagulation studies are returning to normal and if any maternal anoxia has occurred, particularly in renal or brain cells from occluded coagulated capillaries. A fetal and newborn assessment is equally important to evaluate the efficiency of the placental circulation in light of the increased clotting (heparin does not cross the placenta so a newborn will not be born with decreased clotting ability).

Preterm Labor

Preterm labor is labor that occurs before the end of week 37 of gestation. It occurs in approximately 9% to 11% of all pregnancies. It is always potentially serious because if it results in the infant's birth, the infant will be immature. Because of this, it is responsible for almost two thirds of all infant deaths in the neonatal period (American College of Obstetricians and Gynecologists [ACOG], 2016a). Any woman having persistent uterine contractions, even if they are mild and widely spaced, should be considered to be in labor. A woman is documented as being in actual labor rather than having false labor contractions if contractions have caused cervical effacement over 80% or dilation over 1 cm.

Maintaining general health during pregnancy is the best preventive measure to avoid preterm birth. Other measures can help prevent an occurrence of preterm birth (Box 21.6). Knowing the signs of labor can help women identify if preterm birth is beginning because some women wait before they seek help for preterm labor because they diagnose back pain or contractions as nothing more than extremely hard Braxton Hicks contractions. Currently, when there is treatment available to delay labor for at least a few days or until a fetus reaches a level of maturity that will allow the newborn to survive in the outside environment, evaluation and the institution of therapy before membranes rupture become vital, as ruptured membranes make it that much more difficult to halt labor.

Why labor begins before a fetus is mature is usually unclear. It is associated, however, with dehydration, urinary tract infection, periodontal disease, chorioamnionitis, and perhaps large fetal size. African American women, adolescents, and those who receive inadequate prenatal care are most susceptible (Parets, Knight, & Smith, 2015). Women who continue to work at strenuous jobs during pregnancy or perform shift work that leads to extreme fatigue may have a higher incidence than others (van Beukering, van Melick, Mol, et al., 2014). Intimate partner violence and the trauma this causes may be yet another cause (Alhusen, Ray, Sharps, et al., 2015).

Common symptoms of early preterm labor women need to identify include a persistent, dull, and low backache; vaginal spotting; a feeling of pelvic pressure or abdominal tightening; menstrual-like cramping; increased vaginal discharge; uterine

BOX 21.6

Nursing Care Planning Based on Family Teaching

MEASURES TO HELP PREVENT A RECURRENCE OF PRETERM LABOR FOR WOMEN ON BED REST

Q. Beverly Muzuki has started preterm labor and so is prescribed bed rest on home care. She asks you, "What else can I do to help prevent having this baby early?"

A. Although there are no guarantees, several actions can be helpful to prevent a recurrence of preterm labor:

- Remain on bed rest (a lounge or couch) except to use the bathroom.
- Drink 8 to 10 glasses of fluids daily (keep a pitcher by your bed so you do not have to get up).
- Keep mentally active by reading or working on a project to prevent boredom.
- Avoid activities that could stimulate labor, such as nipple stimulation.
- Consult your primary care provider regarding whether sexual relations should be restricted.
- Immediately report signs of ruptured membranes (sudden gush of vaginal fluid) or vaginal bleeding.
- Report signs of urinary tract or vaginal infection (e.g., burning or frequency of urination, vaginal itching or pain).
- Keep appointments for prenatal care.

   If uterine contractions recur:

- Empty your bladder to relieve pressure on the uterus.
- Lie down on your left or right side to encourage blood return to the uterus.
- Drink two or three glasses of fluid to increase hydration.
- Contact your healthcare provider to report the incident and ask for further care measures.

contractions; and intestinal cramping. Listen carefully to any woman who has these symptoms or believes she is in preterm labor because beginning symptoms of labor are subtle and best recognized by the woman herself.

It is possible to predict which pregnancies will end early by analyzing changes in the length of the cervix by ultrasound exam and analysis of vaginal mucus for the presence of fetal fibronectin, a protein produced by trophoblast cells (Jung, Park, Ryu, et al., 2016). If this is present in vaginal mucus, it predicts that preterm contractions are ready to occur; absence of the protein predicts that labor will not occur for at least 14 days.

THERAPEUTIC MANAGEMENT

Medical attempts can be made to stop labor if the fetal membranes have not ruptured, fetal distress is absent, there is no evidence that bleeding is occurring, the cervix is not dilated more than 4 to 5 cm, and effacement is not more than 50%.

A woman who is in preterm labor is usually first admitted to the hospital and placed on bed rest to relieve the pressure of the fetus on the cervix. External fetal and uterine contraction monitors are attached to monitor FHR and the intensity of contractions. Intravenous fluid therapy to keep her well hydrated is begun because although not well documented, hydration may help stop contractions. This is thought to be effective because if a woman is dehydrated, the pituitary gland will be activated to secrete antidiuretic hormone, which might cause the pituitary gland to release oxytocin as well, strengthening uterine contractions.

Vaginal and cervical cultures and a clean-catch urine sample are prescribed to rule out infection. If a urinary tract infection is present, the woman will be prescribed an antibiotic that is especially effective for group B streptococcus as this infection can be fatal in a newborn.

DRUG ADMINISTRATION

Terbutaline is a drug approved to prevent and treat bronchospasm (i.e., narrowing of airways) but may be used, off-label, as a **tocolytic agent** (i.e., an agent to halt labor). Terbutaline carries a "black box" warning, however, that it should not be used for over 48 to 72 hours of therapy because of a potential for serious maternal heart problems and death. It should not be used in an outpatient or home setting because its administration requires constant professional assessment (Roman, 2013).

Magnesium sulfate, given intravenously, is used primarily to treat preeclampsia and prevent eclamptic seizures. It was traditionally given to prevent preterm labor as well. However, recent research does not support the use of magnesium as a tocolytic. There are no differences seen between those women receiving magnesium and those receiving no treatment in preterm birth outcomes (Navathe & Berghella, 2016). Magnesium sulfate for fetal neuroprotection is used prior to 32 weeks to help prevent cerebral palsy in premature infants (Nijman, van Vliet, Koullali, et al., 2016).

For reasons not clearly understood, if, in the time between when preterm contractions begin and preterm birth occurs, a woman is administered a corticosteroid such as betamethasone the formation of lung surfactant appears to accelerate, thus reducing the possibility of respiratory distress syndrome or bronchopulmonary dysplasia (Msan, Usta, Mirza, et al.,

2015). During the time labor is being chemically halted, therefore, if the pregnancy is under 34 weeks, a woman may be given two doses of 12 mg betamethasone intramuscularly 24 hours apart or four doses of 6 mg dexamethasone intramuscularly 12 hours apart.

Although the effect of betamethasone lasts for about 7 days, it takes about 24 hours for the drug to begin its effect, so it is important labor be halted for at least 24 hours. If the fetus is not born within the 7-day time span, the dose of betamethasone may be repeated, but this is controversial because any corticosteroid can interfere with glucose regulation in the woman and potentially in the fetus.

> *What If . . . 21.2*
> **The nurse overhears Beverly tell her mother not to come to the hospital to be with her because her baby is so small that her labor should be quick and easy. Would the nurse investigate further or assume Beverly knows what will be best for herself?**

FETAL ASSESSMENT

In addition to supervising tocolytic therapy, be certain to assess overall fetal welfare in the woman who is trying to delay or prevent preterm labor by assessing the FHR and activity (Box 21.7, an interprofessional care map for a woman in preterm labor).

Following this initial therapy and if contractions have ceased and there is evidence of fetal well-being, women with arrested preterm labor can be safely cared for at home as long as they can dependably drink enough fluid to remain well hydrated and, although there is little evidence that strict bed rest prevents preterm labor, a woman limits strenuous activities (Sosa, Althabe, Belizán, et al., 2015). It is also important for women to maintain adequate nutrition and to not smoke cigarettes as both poor nutrition and smoking are risks for preterm birth (Moore, Blatt, Chen, et al., 2016). To help with fetal assessment, a woman may be asked to record a daily fetal "kick" count or "count to 10" test (see Chapter 9 for this technique and Chapter 4 for a discussion of home care).

LABOR THAT CANNOT BE HALTED

In some women, preterm labor is too far advanced (e.g., membranes have ruptured or the cervix is more than 50% effaced and more than 3 to 4 cm dilated) when they are first seen in a healthcare facility for it to be halted. The rupture of membranes, especially, can be thought of as a "point of no return" in stopping or delaying labor because of the increased risk of infection that begins at that point.

If the fetus is very immature at the time labor cannot be halted, a cesarean birth may be planned to reduce pressure on the fetal head and reduce the possibility of subdural or intraventricular hemorrhage from a vaginal birth, although this is controversial because infants born by cesarean birth have a higher incidence of respiratory difficulty, which is already a high risk for a very preterm infant.

Most women assume that if a fetus is preterm, labor for a vaginal birth will be shorter than normal because the infant is still so small. This is not necessarily true, however, because the first stage of labor, the longest stage, proceeds exactly as it would with a term pregnancy. The second stage of labor may be shorter

BOX 21.7

Nursing Care Planning

AN INTERPROFESSIONAL CARE MAP FOR A WOMAN IN PRETERM LABOR

Beverly Muzuki is a 20-year-old gravida 2, para 0, 30-week pregnant woman, whom you see in a prenatal clinic. She has had symptoms of a urinary tract infection for the past few days but didn't call the clinic because she knew she would be in today for her appointment. Yesterday, she noticed some mild lower abdominal pain but thought it was irritation from the bladder infection. During the night, she woke twice because of a nagging lower backache. This morning, she has intermittent sharp uterine contractions. "Why am I starting labor so early?" she asks you. "Is it because I'm Rh negative?"

Family Assessment: Patient, 20 years old, lives in a two-bedroom, third-floor apartment and works as a secretary for local construction firm; husband, 26 years old, is a payroll supervisor at the same firm. Finances rated as, "Who couldn't use more money?"

Patient Assessment: Gravida 2, para 0, 30-week pregnancy. Heart rate, 88 beats/min; respirations, 22 breaths/min; blood pressure, 130/78 mmHg. Fetal heart rate (FHR), 142 beats/min; reports positive fetal movements. Uterine contractions every 7 minutes lasting 40 seconds. Cervical effacement 30%; dilation: 2–3 cm. Intravenous (IV) therapy with magnesium sulfate and IM corticosteroid prescribed.

Nursing Diagnosis: Risk for injury (maternal and fetal) related to preterm labor and tocolytic therapy

Outcome Criteria: Contractions halt after treatment with tocolytic; FHR remains within acceptable parameters; patient remains free of signs and symptoms of adverse effects of tocolytic therapy. Patient verbalizes concerns and fears; participates in decision making and relaxation measures.

Team Member Responsible	Assessment	Intervention	Rationale	Expected Outcome
Activities of Daily Living, Including Safety				
Nurse/primary healthcare provider	Attach contraction and FHR monitors for continuous evaluation of contractions and fetal response.	Institute bed rest with patient in side-lying position.	Bed rest relieves pressure of the fetus on the cervix. Side-lying position enhances uterine perfusion. Uterine and fetal monitoring provides evidence of fetal well-being.	Patient will remain on bed rest until labor contractions halt or further action becomes necessary.
Teamwork and Collaboration				
Nurse/primary healthcare provider	Contact ultrasound personnel.	Obtain patient consent for ultrasound. Arrange for ultrasound to establish fetal health and cervical length.	An ultrasound can document fetal health and cervical dilation.	Patient agrees to procedure; completes preprocedure readiness actions.
Procedures/Medications for Quality Improvement				
Nurse	Assess vital signs of patient. Obtain history of events leading up to beginning of labor.	Obtain laboratory studies, including complete blood count, hemoglobin and hematocrit, and serum electrolytes. Obtain clean-catch urine for culture, vaginal and cervical cultures, and fetal fibronectin as ordered.	Assessment provides a baseline for future comparisons. Urine, vaginal, and cervical cultures help to rule out infection as a causative factor for preterm labor. Fetal fibronectin can help predict whether labor is likely to continue.	Specimens are collected and sent to lab promptly to ensure rapid assessment.

Procedures/Medications for Quality Improvement

Nurse/primary healthcare provider	Assess for contraindications to betamethasone administration. Obtain reports of urine and cervical cultures and fetal fibronectin.	Administer betamethasone to aid fetal lung maturity and an antibiotic for urinary tract infection as prescribed.	Betamethasone, a steroid, helps to decrease the risk of respiratory distress syndrome in the event of premature birth. An antibiotic decreases urinary tract infection.	Patient agrees to betamethasone and antibiotic administration.
Nurse	Establish strength, duration, and frequency of baseline uterine contractions.	Administer magnesium sulfate as prescribed as an IV piggyback with infusion pump for fetal neuroprotection. Continue infusion for 12–24 hours.	Magnesium sulfate helps protect preterm babies from cerebral palsy.	Premature infant, if born, does not suffer from cerebral palsy.
Nurse	Continue maternal and fetal vital sign assessment.	Monitor patient's vital signs and neurologic status closely. Respirations should be at least 12 breaths/min before each magnesium sulfate dose; FHR, 120–160 beats/min; maternal reflexes, 1+ to 2+.	Decreasing urine output, neurologic changes, or decreased respiration or pulse rate are major indicators of magnesium sulfate toxicity. Decreasing FHR can indicate fetal distress.	Patient's and fetal vital signs, neurologic status, intake and output (renal status), and laboratory values remain within normal parameters during infusion.
Nurse	Assess if calcium gluconate is available.	Keep calcium gluconate available at the bedside.	Calcium gluconate is the antidote for magnesium sulfate toxicity.	Calcium gluconate is prepared by the pharmacy and is readily available.

Nutrition

Nurse	Obtain hematocrit and serum electrolyte levels every 4 hours or as ordered.	Assist with or insert an IV line. Begin IV fluid therapy as prescribed.	Hematocrit, electrolyte levels, and IV intake measures the patient's fluid volume status.	IV fluid improves hydration, which may help to minimize contractions.

Patient-Centered Care

Nurse	Assess patient's knowledge of preterm labor.	Instruct patient about preterm labor and about steps to be taken to counteract the process.	A well-informed patient can participate more fully in her own care.	Patient states the cause of preterm labor cannot always be identified; describes the part she can play in halting process.

Psychosocial/Spiritual/Emotional Needs

Nurse	Assess patient's anxiety level over preterm labor. Assess for possible feelings of guilt related to cause of preterm labor.	Help patient to use using relaxation techniques, such as muscle relaxation, breathing, and music. Provide frequent updates about progress. Allow patient to verbalize feelings and concerns.	Relaxation techniques help to decrease anxiety and fear, enhancing feelings of control. Frequent updates about progress help to minimize fear due to the unknown.	Patient verbalizes her feelings about this crisis in her life; demonstrates anxiety but at a level that allows her to cooperate with caregivers.
Nurse	Determine whether patient wants a support person to be with her.	Contact support person as necessary.	The presence of a support person can offer additional comfort to a patient.	Patient names a support person she wants notified about hospital admission.

Continued on following page

BOX 21.7

Nursing Care Planning (continued)

Team Member Responsible	Assessment	Intervention	Rationale	Expected Outcome
Informatics for Seamless Healthcare Planning				
Nurse	Assess patient's home surroundings to determine whether they are appropriate for bed rest and continuing monitoring at home.	Contact home care nurse service to provide monitoring at home.	Monitoring to see if contractions return can safely be done at home with a conscientious and well-informed patient.	Patient states she feels her home and support system will be adequate for home care with self-monitoring; agrees on appointment for first home visit with home care nurse service.

because a small infant can be pushed through the dilated cervix and the birth canal more easily. Because the second stage takes, at most, 1 hour, this means the difference will not be more than 30 minutes to 1 hour. Unless a woman is given this explanation, she may worry not only that her labor is preterm but also that something is going wrong because it is lasting so long. Because of the increased risk for prolapse of the cord around a small head, artificial rupture of the membranes is not done as a rule in preterm labor until the fetal head is firmly engaged.

Analgesic agents are administered with caution because an immature infant will have enough difficulty breathing at birth without the additional burden of being sedated from a drug such as meperidine (Demerol). If a woman wants pharmaceutical pain management for labor, an epidural is preferable.

A woman may feel reassured by having an external fetal monitor during labor because the monitor screen shows evidence that, although her infant is going to be small, heart tones seem to be of good quality and the infant is reacting well to labor. Be certain that if a monitor is attached, the woman rests on her side to help prevent supine hypotension syndrome or an interference with uterine circulation.

Although an episiotomy is not routinely used because the head of a preterm infant is more fragile than that of a mature infant, one may be done to relieve excessive pressure on the head and hopefully reduce the possibility of a subdural or intraventricular hemorrhage. Following birth, the cord of the preterm infant is usually not clamped immediately because this extra amount of blood can help reduce the possibility of preterm anemia and the need for postbirth transfusion (Brocato, Holliday, Whitehurst, et al., 2016).

 Nursing Diagnoses and Related Interventions

Nursing diagnoses for the woman in preterm labor whose labor cannot be halted center around fear for the uncertain outcome of the pregnancy and risk for fetal or newborn injury related to the preterm birth. Be certain these diagnoses and outcomes for care are realistic in light of the threat to fetal and newborn health. Although many measures are available to help the preterm baby adjust to the outside world, a baby born preterm will be at risk for a variety of health problems, especially difficulty with respirations (see Chapter 26).

Nursing Diagnosis: Situational low self-esteem related to feelings of responsibility for preterm labor

Outcome Evaluation: Patient expresses feelings and worries to nurse; states she knows she is not responsible for her labor beginning prematurely.

A woman in preterm labor is undergoing an extreme crisis situation. She cannot help asking herself, "What did I do to cause this?" Time spent taking the initial history or timing contractions presents an opportunity to not only bring that concern out in the open but any others she may have as well. She needs a strong support person with her during labor because if she has not yet taken a preparation for labor class, she may be more concerned than the average woman. Offer frequent assurance during labor that she is breathing well with contractions or just is "doing well." During the postpartum period, she may need continued reassurance as she is being asked to care for a very small and vulnerable-appearing infant. Helping rebuild self-esteem this way, therefore, not only prepares her better for the stress of labor but also prepares her to be a parent to her preterm infant.

QSEN Checkpoint Question 21.4

TEAMWORK & COLLABORATION

Beverly's husband drove her to the emergency room because she was having symptoms of preterm labor. The admitting nurse in the emergency department identifies which action as the priority?
   a. Encourage her to carefully walk so the fetal head maintains pressure on her cervix.
   b. Position her in a side-lying position and assess fetal heart rate and contractions.
   c. Obtain blood for an hCG hormone assessment.
   d. Ensure no one initiates intravenous fluid infusion because hypervolemia exacerbates preterm labor.

Look in Appendix A for the best answer and rationale.

Preterm Rupture of Membranes

Preterm rupture of membranes is rupture of fetal membranes with loss of amniotic fluid before 37 weeks of pregnancy (ACOG, 2016b). This occurs in 5% to 10% of pregnancies. The cause of preterm rupture is unknown, but it is strongly associated with infection of the membranes (i.e., chorioamnionitis). If rupture occurs early in pregnancy this way, it poses a major threat to the fetus as, after a rupture, the seal to the fetus is lost and uterine and fetal infections may occur. A second complication that can result is increased pressure on the umbilical cord from the loss of amniotic fluid (thus, inhibiting the fetal nutrient supply) or cord prolapse (extension of the cord out of the uterine cavity into the vagina past the small fetus), a condition that could also interfere with fetal circulation. Yet another risk to the fetus of remaining in a non–fluid-filled environment is the development of a Potter-like syndrome (i.e., distorted facial features and pulmonary hypoplasia from uterine pressure). In many instances, preterm labor follows rupture of the membranes and ends the pregnancy. If neither labor nor an infection begins, the greater the amount of amniotic fluid that remains (revealed by a sonogram), the better will be the pregnancy outcome (Ekin, Gezer, Taner, et al., 2015).

ASSESSMENT

Rupture of the membranes is suggested by the history. A woman usually describes a sudden gush of clear fluid from her vagina, with continued minimal leakage. Occasionally, a woman mistakes urinary incontinence caused by exertion for rupture of membranes. Amniotic fluid cannot be differentiated from urine by appearance, so a sterile vaginal speculum examination is done to observe for vaginal pooling of fluid. If the fluid is tested with Nitrazine paper, amniotic fluid causes an alkaline reaction on the paper (appears blue) and urine causes an acidic reaction (remains yellow). The fluid can also be tested for ferning, or the typical appearance of a high-estrogen fluid on microscopic examination (amniotic fluid shows this; urine does not). If there is still a question regarding whether the membranes have ruptured, an ultrasound can be used to assess the amniotic fluid index. Because preterm rupture of membranes is associated with vaginal infection, cultures for *Neisseria gonorrhoeae*, group B streptococcus, and chlamydia are usually obtained. Blood is drawn for white blood cell count and C-reactive protein, both of which increase with membrane rupture. Avoid doing routine vaginal examinations because the risk of infection rises significantly when digital examinations are performed after preterm rupture of membranes.

THERAPEUTIC MANAGEMENT

A future hope is that by stem cell engineering, ruptured membranes can be repaired. Currently, however, if labor does not begin within 24 hours and the fetus is estimated to be mature enough by amniocentesis to survive in an extrauterine environment, labor contractions may be induced by intravenous administration of oxytocin so the infant can be born before infection can occur.

If the fetus is not at a point of viability, a woman is offered immediate delivery to end the pregnancy or, if she declines delivery, she is placed on bed rest either in the hospital or at home. If she reaches viability, a corticosteroid is administered to hasten fetal lung maturity. Prophylactic administration of broad-spectrum antibiotics effective against group B streptococcus during this period may both delay the onset of labor and reduce the risk of infection in the newborn sufficiently to allow the corticosteroid to have its effect.

A woman with no signs of infection may be administered a tocolytic agent if labor contractions begin. Although its effectiveness is not well documented, a woman might be given an amnioinfusion (see Chapter 23) to reduce pressure on the fetus or cord and to allow a safer term birth (Hofmeyr, Eke, Lawrie, et al., 2014).

 Nursing Diagnoses and Related Interventions

Nursing Diagnosis: Risk for infection related to preterm rupture of membranes without accompanying labor

Outcome Evaluation: Maternal white blood cell count remains below 20,000/mm^3; maternal temperature is less than 100.4°F (38.0°C) while awaiting fetal maturity.

An infection can be dangerous for both the mother and fetus; so, if at home, a woman is asked to take her temperature about twice a day and to report a fever (a temperature greater than 100.4°F [38.0°C]), uterine tenderness, or odorous vaginal discharge. She should refrain from tub bathing, douching, and coitus because of the danger of introducing infection. The white blood cell count will need to be assessed frequently. A count of more than 18,000 to 20,000/mm^3 suggests infection, especially if the count is increasing over serial blood draws.

Before a woman is discharged to home care, be certain to ask if she has a thermometer and provide her with specific instructions regarding what degree of temperature she should report and if she understands the level of bed rest expected of her. Help her understand the signs and symptoms of infection so her white blood cell count can be assessed as necessary.

Many misconceptions about the difficulty of labor after preterm rupture of the membranes (i.e., "dry labor") exist. You can assure a woman that there is no such thing as a dry labor because amniotic fluid is always being formed by the fetus voiding and through production of fluid by the amnion layer of the fetal membranes.

What If . . . 21.3

Beverly is prescribed bed rest for 24 hours because of preterm contractions, but she tells the nurse she's too busy to "waste time" on bed rest. How can the nurse empower the patient to ask for help from family and friends so she can achieve bed rest? Are there any other suggestions the nurse could provide to help her maintain bed rest?

Hypertensive Disorders in Pregnancy

Gestational hypertension is a condition in which vasospasm occurs in both small and large arteries during pregnancy, causing increased blood pressure. **Preeclampsia** is a pregnancy-related disease process evidenced by increased blood pressure and proteinuria. An older term for preeclampsia was toxemia of pregnancy because researchers pictured the symptoms as being caused by women producing a toxin of some kind in response to the foreign protein of the growing fetus. The condition occurs in 5% to 7% of pregnancies. The cause of the disorder is unknown, although women with antiphospholipid syndrome (APS) or the presence of antiphospholipid antibodies in maternal blood are much more likely to develop preeclampsia (van Hoorn, Hague, van Pampus, et al., 2016). The condition tends to occur most frequently in women of color; those with a multiple pregnancy; primiparas younger than 20 years or older than 40 years of age; women from low socioeconomic backgrounds (perhaps because of poor nutrition); those who have had five or more pregnancies; those who have polyhydramnios (i.e., overproduction of amniotic fluid; refer to later discussion); or those who have an underlying disease such as heart disease, diabetes with vessel or renal involvement, and essential hypertension (Miller, 2012).

PATHOPHYSIOLOGIC EVENTS

The symptoms of preeclampsia affect almost all organs. The vascular spasm that occurs may be caused by the increased cardiac output required by pregnancy, which injures the endothelial cells of the arteries and reduces the action of prostacyclin—a prostaglandin vasodilator—and excess production of thromboxane—a prostaglandin vasoconstrictor and stimulant of platelet aggregation. Usually during pregnancy, blood vessels are resistant to the effects of pressor substances such as angiotensin and norepinephrine, so even with the increased blood supply, blood pressure remains normal during pregnancy. With gestational hypertension, this reduced responsiveness to blood pressure changes appears to be lost because of the prostaglandin release. Vasoconstriction occurs, and blood pressure increases dramatically.

Beginning about the 20th week of pregnancy, almost all body systems begin to be affected. The cardiac system, for example, can easily become overwhelmed because the heart is forced to pump against rising peripheral resistance. This causes a reduced blood supply to organs, most markedly the kidney, pancreas, liver, brain, and placenta. Poor placental perfusion reduces the fetal nutrient and oxygen supply.

Ischemia in the pancreas can result in epigastric pain and an elevated amylase–creatinine ratio. If spasm occurs in the arteries of the retina, vision changes can occur. If this results in retinal hemorrhage, blindness can result.

Vasospasm in the kidney increases blood flow resistance. Degenerative changes then develop in the kidney glomeruli because of back pressure. This leads to increased permeability of the glomerular membrane, allowing the serum proteins albumin and globulin to escape into the urine (i.e., proteinuria). The degenerative changes also result in decreased glomerular filtration, so there is lowered urine output and clearance of creatinine. If increased kidney tubular reabsorption occurs, retention of sodium begins. As sodium retains fluid, edema results. Edema is further increased because, as more protein is lost, the osmotic pressure of the circulating blood falls and fluid diffuses from the circulatory system into the denser interstitial spaces to equalize the pressure (Fig. 21.8). Extreme edema can lead to maternal cerebral and pulmonary edema and seizures (eclampsia).

Yet another effect of the condition is that arterial spasm causes the bulk of the blood volume in the maternal circulation to be pooled in the venous circulation, so on assessment, a woman has a deceptively low arterial intravascular volume. In addition, thrombocytopenia or a lowered platelet count occurs as platelets cluster at the sites of endothelial damage. Measuring hematocrit levels helps to assess the extent of plasma loss to the interstitial space or the extent of the edema (the higher the hematocrit, the more is being lost). A hematocrit level above 40% suggests significant fluid loss into interstitial spaces.

ASSESSMENT

Although women may have additional symptoms such as vision changes, typically hypertension, proteinuria, and edema are considered the classic signs of preeclampsia. Of the three, hypertension and proteinuria are the most significant because extensive edema occurs only after the other two are present (Box 21.8).

Preeclampsia is classified as preeclampsia without severe features, preeclampsia with severe features, and eclampsia,

Figure 21.8 Physiologic changes with gestational hypertension.

BOX 21.8

Nursing Care Planning Using Assessment

ASSESSING THE WOMAN WITH GESTATIONAL HYPERTENSION

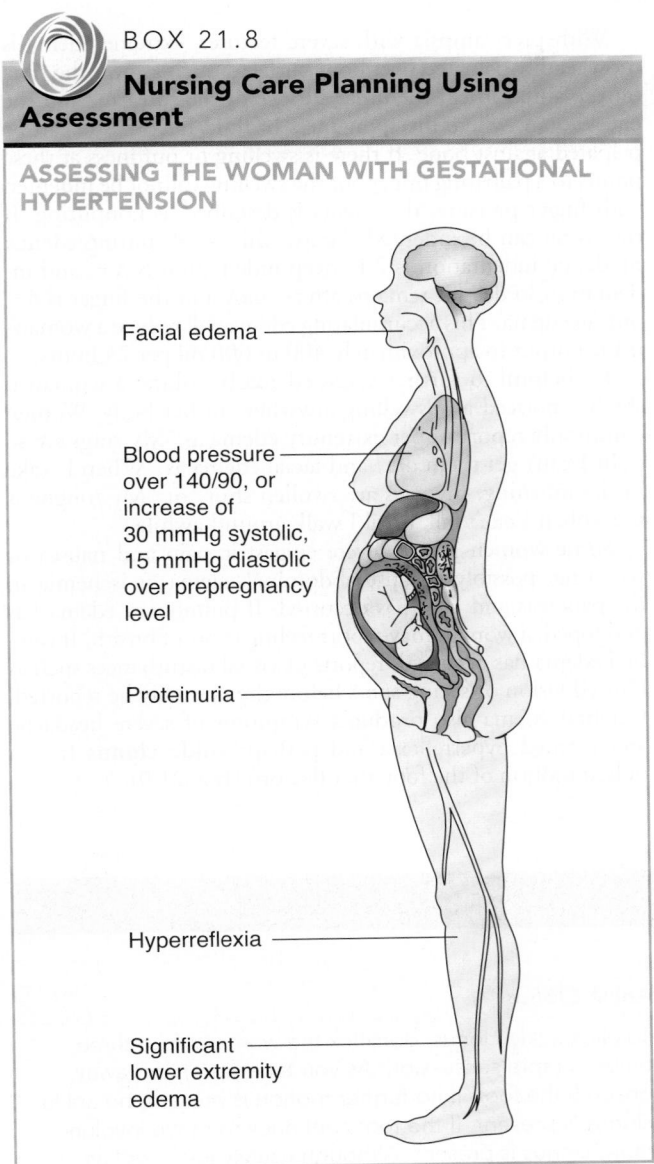

- Facial edema
- Blood pressure over 140/90, or increase of 30 mmHg systolic, 15 mmHg diastolic over prepregnancy level
- Proteinuria
- Hyperreflexia
- Significant lower extremity edema

TABLE 21.6 SYMPTOMS OF GESTATIONAL HYPERTENSION

Hypertension Type	Symptoms
Gestational hypertension	Blood pressure is 140/90 mmHg or systolic pressure elevated 30 mmHg or diastolic pressure elevated 15 mmHg above prepregnancy level; no proteinuria or edema; blood pressure returns to normal after birth
Preeclampsia without severe features	Blood pressure is 140/90 mmHg or systolic pressure elevated 30 mmHg or diastolic pressure elevated 15 mmHg above prepregnancy level; proteinuria of 1+ to 2+ on a random sample; weight gain over 2 lb/week in second trimester and 1 lb/week in third trimester; mild edema in upper extremities or face
Preeclampsia with severe features	Blood pressure is 160/110 mmHg; proteinuria 3+ to 4+ on a random sample and 5 g on a 24-hour sample; oliguria (500 ml or less in 24 hours or altered renal function tests; elevated serum creatinine more than 1.2 mg/dl); cerebral or visual disturbances (headache, blurred vision); pulmonary or cardiac involvement; extensive peripheral edema; hepatic dysfunction; thrombocytopenia; epigastric pain
Eclampsia	Either seizure or coma accompanied by signs and symptoms of preeclampsia are present.

depending on how far development of the syndrome has advanced (Table 21.6). Any woman with a high risk of preeclampsia should be observed carefully for symptoms at prenatal visits. She needs instructions about what symptoms to watch for so she can alert her healthcare provider if symptoms begin to occur between visits.

GESTATIONAL HYPERTENSION

A woman is said to have gestational hypertension when she develops an elevated blood pressure (140/90 mmHg) but has no proteinuria or edema. Perinatal mortality is not increased with simple gestational hypertension, so careful observation but no drug therapy is necessary.

PREECLAMPSIA WITHOUT SEVERE FEATURES

If a seizure from preeclampsia occurs, a woman now has eclampsia, but any status above gestational hypertension and below a point of seizures is preeclampsia. A woman is said to be

preeclamptic without severe features when she has proteinuria (1+ on a urine dip or 300 mg in a 24-hour urine protein collection or 0.3 or higher on a urine protein–creatinine ratio) and a blood pressure rise to 140/90 mmHg, taken on two occasions at least 6 hours apart. The diastolic value of blood pressure is extremely important to document because it is this pressure that best indicates the degree of peripheral arterial spasm present.

A second criterion for evaluating blood pressure is a systolic blood pressure greater than 30 mmHg and a diastolic pressure greater than 15 mmHg above prepregnancy values. This rule is helpful for a woman with preexisting hypertension, but the value of 140/90 mmHg is a more useful cutoff point when there are no baseline data available, such as when a woman seeks prenatal care late in pregnancy.

Average blood pressures in American women are available at http://thePoint.lww.com/Flagg8e. According to these averages, a woman younger than 20 years could have a blood pressure of 98/61 mmHg and still be within normal limits. If her blood pressure was elevated 30 mmHg systolic and 15 mmHg diastolic, it would be only 128/76 mmHg. This is well beneath the traditional warning point of 140/90 mmHg but would represent hypertension for her.

Many women show a trace of protein during pregnancy. Actual proteinuria is said to exist when it registers as 1+ or more (this represents a loss of 1 g/L). A woman with preeclampsia will begin to show proteinuria of 1+ or 2+ on a reagent test strip on a random sample.

Occasionally, women have orthostatic proteinuria (i.e., on long periods of standing, they excrete protein; on bed rest, they do not). If proteinuria is present without other signs of gestational hypertension (no hypertension and no edema), check to see when the specimen was obtained. Ask her to bring in a first morning urine sample next time as that may reveal that orthostatic proteinuria, not preeclampsia, is the cause of protein in her urine.

Edema develops, as mentioned, because of the protein loss, sodium retention, and lowered glomerular filtration rate. The edema can be separated from the typical ankle edema of pregnancy because it begins to accumulate in the upper part of the body as well. A weight gain of more than 2 lb/week in the second trimester or 1 lb/week in the third trimester usually indicates abnormal tissue fluid retention is occurring. No noticeable edema may be present when this sudden increase in weight first occurs or it will be the first symptom a woman notices.

PREECLAMPSIA WITH SEVERE FEATURES

A woman has passed to preeclampsia with severe features when her blood pressure rises to 160 mmHg systolic and 110 mmHg diastolic or above on at least two occasions 6 hours apart at bed rest (the position in which blood pressure is lowest) or her diastolic pressure is 30 mmHg above her prepregnancy level. Marked proteinuria, 3+ or 4+ on a random urine sample or more than 5 g in a 24-hour sample (Olson-Chen & Seligman, 2016).

With preeclampsia with severe features, extreme edema is most readily palpated over bony surfaces, such as over the tibia on the anterior leg, the ulnar surface of the forearm, and the cheekbones, where the sponginess of fluid-filled tissue can be palpated against bone. If there is swelling or puffiness at these points to a palpating finger but the swelling cannot be indented with finger pressure, the edema is described as nonpitting. If the tissue can be indented slightly, this is 1+ pitting edema; moderate indentation is 2+; deep indentation is 3+; and indentation so deep it remains after removal of the finger is 4+ pitting edema. This accumulating edema will reduce a woman's urine output to approximately 400 to 600 ml per 24 hours.

It's helpful to further assess edema by asking a woman if she has noticed any swelling anywhere in her body. Women commonly report upper extremity edema as "My rings are so tight I can't get them off" and facial edema as "When I wake in the morning, my eyes are swollen shut" or "My tongue is so swollen I can't talk until I walk around awhile."

Some women report severe epigastric pain and nausea or vomiting, possibly because abdominal edema or ischemia to the pancreas and liver has occurred. If pulmonary edema has developed, a woman may report feeling short of breath. If cerebral edema has occurred, reports of visual disturbances such as blurred vision or seeing spots before the eyes may be reported. Cerebral edema also produces symptoms of severe headache and marked hyperreflexia and perhaps **ankle clonus** (i.e., a pulsed motion of the foot after flexion) (Box 21.9).

BOX 21.9

Nursing Care Planning Using Procedures

ELICITING A PATELLAR REFLEX AND ANKLE CLONUS

Patellar Reflex	Ankle Clonus
With the woman in a supine position, ask her to bend her knee slightly. Place your hand under her knee to support the leg. Locate the patellar tendon in the midline of the anterior leg just below the kneecap. Strike it firmly and quickly with a reflex hammer or the side of your hand. If the leg and foot move, a patellar reflex is present. The reflex is scored as: 0 = No response; hypoactive; abnormal 1+ = Somewhat diminished response but not abnormal 2+ = Average response 3+ = Brisker than average but not abnormal 4+ = Hyperactive; very brisk; abnormal	To elicit ankle clonus, dorsiflex the woman's foot three times in rapid succession. As you take your hand away, observe the foot. If no further motion is present, no ankle clonus is present. If the foot continues to move involuntarily, clonus is present. Although usually just rated as present or absent, it can be rated as:

Mild = 2 movements
Moderate = 3–5 movements
Severe = Over 6 movements

ECLAMPSIA

Eclampsia is the most severe classification of pregnancy-related hypertensive disorders. A woman has passed into this stage when cerebral edema is so acute a grand mal (tonic–clonic) seizure or coma has occurred. With eclampsia, the maternal mortality can be as high as 20% from causes such as cerebral hemorrhage, circulatory collapse, or renal failure (Gongora & Wenger, 2015).

The fetal prognosis with eclampsia is also poor because of hypoxia, possibly caused by the seizure, with consequent fetal acidosis. If premature separation of the placenta from extreme vasospasm occurs, the fetal prognosis becomes even graver. If a fetus must be born before term, all the risks of immaturity will be faced.

QSEN Checkpoint Question 21.5

INFORMATICS

The nurse routinely assesses all pregnant women for signs of hypertension while interviewing them at the prenatal clinic and then documents the findings in the electronic health record. Which statement by Beverly would the nurse document as possible evidence that she might be developing gestational hypertension?

  a. "My feet are so swollen at night I can't put on my bedroom slippers."
  b. "I never guessed I would feel as tired as I do just from being pregnant."
  c. "My abdomen feels firm, as if I had a blown-up balloon inside me."
  d. "I can live with my puffy feet, but now it's also my hands and wrists."

Look in Appendix A for the best answer and rationale.

 ### Nursing Diagnoses and Related Interventions

The nursing diagnoses used with gestational hypertensive disorders are numerous because the disease process has such wide-ranging effects. Some possible nursing diagnoses include:

- Ineffective tissue perfusion related to vasoconstriction of blood vessels
- Deficient fluid volume related to fluid loss to SQ tissue
- Risk for fetal injury related to reduced placental perfusion secondary to vasospasm
- Social isolation related to prescribed bed rest

NURSING INTERVENTIONS FOR A WOMAN WITH PREECLAMPSIA WITHOUT SEVERE FEATURES

Patients with preeclampsia without severe features prior to full term can be managed at home with frequent follow-up care and fetal testing.

Monitor Antiplatelet Therapy

Because of the increased tendency for platelets to cluster along arterial walls, a mild antiplatelet agent, such as low-dose as-pirin, may prevent or delay the development of preeclampsia (Leaf & Connors, 2015). Because aspirin is such a common over-the-counter drug, be certain women appreciate that this is not something to be taken lightly but a serious drug prescription for them. Be certain they purchase low-dose aspirin (81 mg, sold as baby aspirin) as excessive salicylic levels can cause maternal bleeding at the time of birth.

Promote Bed Rest

When the body is in a recumbent position, sodium tends to be excreted at a faster rate than during activity. Bed rest, therefore, is the best method of aiding increased evacuation of sodium and encouraging diuresis of edema fluid. Be certain women know to rest in a lateral recumbent position to avoid uterine pressure on the vena cava and prevent supine hypotension syndrome.

Promote Good Nutrition

A woman needs to continue her usual pregnancy nutrition while on bed rest. At one time, stringent restriction of salt was advised in order to reduce edema. This is no longer true because stringent sodium restriction may activate the renin–angiotensin–aldosterone system and actually result in increased blood pressure, thus compounding the problem.

Assess if a woman has someone to help her prepare food, or either bed rest or nutrition may be compromised.

Provide Emotional Support

It is difficult for a woman with preeclampsia to appreciate the potential seriousness of symptoms because they are so vague; neither high blood pressure nor protein in urine is something she can see or feel. She is aware edema is present, but it seems unrelated to the pregnancy; after all, it is in her hands and face, not a body area near her growing child.

Women are also used to having severe disorders treated with some form of medication. If no other medicine than low-dose aspirin is prescribed, this can make a woman underestimate the severity of her situation, causing her to take instructions such as getting rest lightly. Almost 90% of women of childbearing age work outside their home at least part time today. In addition, most working women make major financial contributions to the running of their households. If a woman is unmarried, her income is probably her sole support. This makes it seem difficult to leave work on the basis of a few vague symptoms—a little swelling or a little headache—unless the woman receives clear information that, if these early symptoms are ignored, they could worsen to the point that they interfere with both her health and that of her fetus.

Healthcare providers cannot solve financial problems, but be certain to ask enough questions at healthcare visits so financial need, if present, can be determined. Questions such as "What will it mean to your family if you have to be on bed rest?" and "How long a maternity leave does your work allow?" will bring concerns to the surface.

Ask if a woman with small children will need to make child care arrangements so she can get sufficient rest. The woman who spends considerable time chauffeuring school-age children to activities may need to investigate carpooling as an alternative. Ask, "What will it mean to your other children or your husband if you have to rest?" to allow her to begin to examine these problems. Remember, having a wife or mother on bed rest is a stress on the total family, so other family members may need support as well.

Women with beginning signs of preeclampsia will be seen approximately weekly or more frequently for the remainder of pregnancy. Be certain a woman understands that if symptoms worsen before her next healthcare visit, she should report them immediately.

NURSING INTERVENTIONS FOR A WOMAN WITH PREECLAMPSIA WITH SEVERE FEATURES

If a woman's preeclampsia is severe (systolic blood pressure of more than 160 mmHg, diastolic blood pressure of more than 110 mmHg after a woman has been on bed rest; extensive edema; marked proteinuria [3+ to 4+]; cerebral or visual disturbances; marked hyperreflexia; or oliguria [500 ml per 24 hours or less]), a woman may be admitted to a healthcare facility for care. If the pregnancy is greater than 37 weeks, labor can be induced or a cesarean birth performed to end the pregnancy at that point. If the pregnancy is less than 37 weeks, interventions will be instituted to attempt to alleviate the severe symptoms and allow the fetus to come to term. However, if the symptoms persist or worsen, or if the fetal testing shows a compromised fetus, vaginal or cesarean delivery will be necessary even if the pregnancy is preterm.

Support Bed Rest

With preeclampsia with severe features, most women are hospitalized so that bed rest can be enforced and a woman can be observed more closely than she can be on home care. Getting up to use the bathroom is not contraindicated in women with preeclampsia. Visitors are usually restricted to support people such as a partner, father of the child, mother, or older children. Because a loud noise such as a crying baby or a dropped tray of equipment can be sufficient to trigger a seizure that initiates eclampsia, a woman with preeclampsia with severe features is admitted to a private room so she can rest as undisturbed as possible. Raise side rails to help prevent injury if a seizure should occur.

 Concept Mastery Alert

Sudden noises can trigger a seizure in a woman with preeclampsia with severe features.

Darken the room if possible because a bright light can also trigger seizures. However, the room should not be so dark that caregivers need to use a flashlight to make assessments. Shining a flashlight beam into a woman's eyes is the kind of sudden stimulation to be avoided.

Stress is another stimulus capable of increasing blood pressure and evoking seizures in a woman with severe preeclampsia. Be certain, therefore, the woman receives clear explanations of what is happening and what is planned, especially about the need for visitor restrictions and not to "cheat" on bed rest. Allow her opportunities to express her feelings about what is happening or how bewildered she is because the few simple symptoms she noticed 2 weeks ago (e.g., increase in weight, increasing edema) have now developed into a syndrome that may be lethal to her baby and possibly to herself.

Monitor Maternal Well-Being

Take blood pressure frequently (at least every 4 hours) or with a continuous monitoring device to detect any increase, which is a warning that a woman's condition is worsening. Obtain blood studies such as a complete blood count, platelet count, liver function, blood urea nitrogen, and creatine and fibrin degradation products as ordered by the obstetric team to assess renal and liver function and the development of DIC, which often accompanies severe vasospasm, as well as plasma estriol levels (a test of placenta function), and electrolyte levels. Because a woman is at high risk for premature separation of the placenta and resulting hemorrhage, a blood sample for type and cross-match is usually also obtained.

Daily hematocrit levels are used to monitor blood concentration (this level will rise if increased fluid is leaving the bloodstream for interstitial tissue [edema]).

Obtain daily weights at the same time each day as another evaluation of fluid retention. Ensure a woman is wearing the same amount of clothing at each weighing so any change in weight is not influenced by a change in the weight of her clothing.

An indwelling urinary catheter may be inserted to allow accurate recording of output and comparison with intake. Urinary output should be more than 30 ml/hr; an output lower than this suggests oliguria. Urinary proteins and specific gravity are measured and recorded with voiding or hourly if an indwelling catheter is present. A 24-hour urine sample, or a urine protein–creatinine ratio, may be collected for protein and creatinine clearance determinations to evaluate kidney function. A woman with mild preeclampsia spills between 0.5 and 1 g of protein every 24 hours (1+ on a random sample); a woman with severe preeclampsia spills approximately 5 g per 24 hours (3+ to 4+ on an individual specimen). A urine protein–creatinine ratio is above 0.3 with preeclampsia with mild features.

Monitor Fetal Well-Being

Generally, single Doppler auscultation at approximately 4-hour intervals is sufficient at this stage of management. A woman may have a nonstress test or biophysical profile done daily to assess uteroplacental sufficiency (see Chapter 9). If fetal bradycardia occurs, oxygen administration to the mother may be necessary to maintain adequate fetal oxygenation.

Support a Nutritious Intake

A woman needs a diet moderate to high in protein and moderate in sodium to compensate for the protein she is losing in urine. An intravenous fluid line is usually initiated and maintained to serve as an emergency route for drug administration as well as to administer fluid to reduce hemoconcentration and hypovolemia.

Administer Medications to Prevent Eclampsia

A hypotensive drug such as hydralazine (Apresoline), labetalol (Normodyne), or nifedipine may be prescribed to reduce hypertension. These drugs act to lower blood pressure by peripheral dilatation and thus do not interfere with placental circulation. They can, however, cause maternal tachycardia, so assess pulse and blood pressure before and after administration. Diastolic pressure should not be lowered below 80 to 90 mmHg or inadequate placental perfusion could occur. Even with these new drugs, magnesium sulfate (Table 21.7) still remains the drug of choice to prevent eclampsia (ACOG, 2016c). This drug, classified as a cathartic, reduces edema by causing a shift in fluid from the extracellular spaces into the intestine. It also has a central nervous system depressant action (it blocks peripheral neuromuscular transmissions), which lessens the possibility of seizures (Karch, 2015). To achieve an immediate reduction of blood pressure, magnesium sulfate may first be given intravenously in a loading or bolus dose. The drug begins to act almost immediately; unfortunately, the effect lasts only 30 to 60 minutes, so administration must be continuous.

The importance of different serum levels of magnesium sulfate is shown in Box 21.10. For the drug to act as an anticonvulsant, blood serum levels must be maintained at 5 to 8 mg per 100 ml. If the blood serum level rises above this, respiratory depression, cardiac arrhythmias, and cardiac arrest can occur.

The most evident symptoms of overdose from magnesium sulfate administration include decreased urine output, depressed respirations, reduced consciousness, and decreased deep tendon reflexes. Because magnesium is excreted from the body almost entirely through the urine, urine output must be monitored closely to ensure adequate elimination. If severe oliguria should occur (less than 100 ml in 4 hours), excessively high serum levels of magnesium can result. Before you administer further magnesium sulfate, therefore, ensure that urine output is at least 30 ml/hr, with a specific gravity of 1.010 or lower. Respirations should be above 12 breaths/min, a woman should be able to answer questions asked of her such as her name or address, ankle clonus should be minimal, and deep tendon reflexes should be present. Make these assessments every hour if a continuous intravenous infusion is being used.

The easiest deep tendon reflex to assess is the patellar reflex (i.e., knee jerk). Instructions for initiating this reflex and ankle clonus are shown in Box 21.9. If an epidural block has been given for labor anesthesia, assess the biceps or triceps reflex (see Chapter 34).

In addition to making the previous assessments when magnesium sulfate is being given, a solution of 10 ml of a 10% calcium gluconate solution (1 g) should be kept ready nearby for immediate intravenous administration should a woman develop signs and symptoms of magnesium toxicity, as calcium is the specific antidote for magnesium toxicity.

An FHR monitor during pregnancy may show loss of variability of the heartbeat immediately after magnesium therapy; an ultrasound may reveal reduced fetal breathing movements. Observe carefully for other signs of fetal effects, such as late deceleration with labor contractions. Magnesium sulfate is continued for 12 to 24 hours after birth to prevent eclampsia during this period. The dose is then tapered and discontinued. Breastfeeding does not need to be delayed until the medication is discontinued. A long-term effect of magnesium sulfate therapy is osteoporosis. A woman may be started on a course of calcium postpartally to decrease this problem. On the planned day of birth, the baby's primary care provider should be alerted that the woman has been receiving magnesium sulfate. This is because if magnesium sulfate, which crosses the placenta, is given intravenously within 2 hours of a baby's birth, the baby may be born with severe respiratory depression.

NURSING INTERVENTIONS FOR A WOMAN WITH ECLAMPSIA

Degeneration of a woman's condition from preeclampsia with severe features to eclampsia occurs when cerebral irritation from increasing cerebral edema becomes so acute that a seizure occurs. This usually happens late in pregnancy but

TABLE 21.7 DRUGS USED IN PREECLAMPSIA

Drug	Indication	Dosage	Comments
Magnesium sulfate (pregnancy risk category B)	Muscle relaxant; prevents seizures	Loading dose 4–6 g Maintenance dose 1–2 g/hr IV	Infuse loading dose slowly over 15–30 minutes. Always administer as a piggyback infusion. Assess respiratory rate, urine output, deep tendon reflexes, and clonus every hour. Urine output should be over 30 ml/hr and respiratory rate over 12 breaths/min. Serum magnesium level should remain below 7.5 mEq/l. Observe for central nervous system (CNS) depression and hypotonia in infant at birth and calcium deficit in the mother.
Hydralazine (Apresoline) (pregnancy risk category C)	Antihypertensive (peripheral vasodilator); used to decrease hypertension	5–10 mg IV	Administer slowly to avoid sudden fall in blood pressure. Maintain diastolic pressure over 90 mmHg to ensure adequate placental filling.
Diazepam (Valium) (pregnancy risk category D)	Halt seizures	5–10 mg IV	Administer slowly. Dose may be repeated q 5–10 minutes (up to 30 mg/hr). Observe for respiratory depression or hypotension in mother and respiratory depression and hypotonia in infant at birth.
Calcium gluconate (pregnancy risk category C)	Antidote for magnesium intoxication	1 g IV (10 ml of a 10% solution)	Have prepared at bedside as the antidote when administering magnesium sulfate. Administer at 5 ml/min.

Source: Karch, A. M. (2015). *Lippincott's nursing drug guide.* Philadelphia, PA: Lippincott Williams & Wilkins.

BOX 21.10

Nursing Care Planning Based on Responsibility for Pharmacology

MAGNESIUM SULFATE

Action: Magnesium sulfate is a central nervous system depressant that acts to block neuromuscular transmission of acetylcholine to halt convulsions (Karch, 2015).

Pregnancy Risk Category: A

Dosage: Initially, 2–6 g IV administered in a 250-ml solution over a 20-minute period, followed by individually calculated IV infusion at a rate to maintain designated serum levels
- Therapeutic range: 5–8 mg/100 ml
- Patellar reflex disappears: 8–10 mg/100 ml
- Respiratory depression occurs: 15–20 mg/100 ml
- Cardiac conduction defects occur: more than 20 mg/100 ml

Possible Adverse Effects: Flushing, thirst; with toxicity, absence of deep tendon reflexes, respiratory depression, cardiac arrhythmias, cardiac arrest, and decreased urine output

Nursing Implications
- Administer continuous infusion piggybacked into a main IV line so it can be discontinued immediately without interfering with fluid administration.
- Always use an infusion control device to maintain a regular flow rate.

- Assess maternal blood pressure and fetal heart rate continuously with bolus IV administration.
- Assess deep tendon reflexes every 1–4 hours during continuous infusion. Use the patellar reflex. If patient has received epidural anesthesia, use the biceps reflex.
- Monitor intake and output every hour during continuous infusion. Urine output should be 30 ml/hr or greater.
- Assess patient's level of consciousness, including ability to respond to questions, every hour.
- Obtain serum magnesium levels as indicated, usually every 6–8 hours.
- Keep calcium gluconate, the antidote for toxicity, readily available at the bedside.
- Maintain serum blood levels (for anticonvulsant use) at 5–8 mg/100 ml. If blood serum levels rise above this, respiratory depression, cardiac arrhythmias, and cardiac arrest can occur.
- Do not administer additional doses and stop infusion if deep tendon reflexes are absent or if respiratory rate is less than 12–14 breaths/min or urine output is less than 30 ml/hr.
- This drug may cause respiratory depression in the newborn if administered close to birth. Alert neonatal care personnel about this possibility.
- Magnesium sulfate may cause osteoporosis in the mother if given over a long time.

can happen up to 48 hours after childbirth. Immediately before a seizure, a woman's blood pressure rises suddenly from additional vasospasm. The increased cerebral pressure causes her temperature to rise sharply to 103° to 104°F (39.4° to 40°C). She notices blurring of vision or severe headache (from the increased cerebral edema), and her reflexes become hyperactive. She may experience a premonition or aura that "something is happening." Vascular congestion of the liver or pancreas can lead to severe epigastric pain and nausea or vomiting. Urinary output may decrease abruptly to less than 30 ml/hr. However, eclampsia has actually occurred, by definition, only when a woman experiences a seizure.

Tonic–Clonic Seizures

An eclamptic seizure is a tonic–clonic type that occurs in stages. After the preliminary signal or aura that something is happening, all the muscles of the woman's body contract. Her back arches, her arms and legs stiffen, and her jaw closes so abruptly she may bite her tongue. Respirations halt because her thoracic muscles are held in contraction. This phase of the seizure, called the tonic phase, lasts approximately 20 seconds. It may seem longer because a woman may grow slightly cyanotic from the cessation of respirations.

During the second (clonic) stage, the woman's bladder and bowel muscles contract and relax; incontinence of urine and feces may occur. Although a woman begins to breathe during this stage, the breathing is not entirely effective so she may remain cyanotic. The clonic stage of a seizure lasts up to

1 minute. Following this, she will enter an hour long postictal stage, during which she is unconscious.

The priority care for a woman with a tonic–clonic seizure is to maintain a patent airway. To prevent aspiration, turn her onto her side to allow secretions to drain from her mouth. Magnesium sulfate or diazepam (Valium) may be administered intravenously as emergency measures. Assess oxygen saturation via a pulse oximeter. Administer oxygen by face mask as needed to protect fetal oxygenation. Apply an external fetal heart monitor if one is not already in place to assess the FHR. The seizure may announce the beginning of labor, so assess as well for uterine contractions. Check for vaginal bleeding to detect placental separation, although evidence placental separation has occurred will probably appear first on the fetal heart record; vaginal bleeding will strengthen the presumption.

During the postictal stage, a woman cannot be roused except by painful stimuli for 1 to 4 hours. Extremely close observation is therefore as important during this third stage as it was during the first two stages. Be certain to assess for uterine contractions during this stage because if labor begins during this period, the woman will be unable to report the sensation of contractions. Also, the painful stimulus of contractions may initiate another seizure. Be certain to keep the woman on her side so secretions can drain from her mouth. Give her nothing to eat or drink. Remember that with coma, hearing is not necessarily lost, so be certain conversation is limited to those things you would say if she were awake. Continue to check for vaginal bleeding every 15 minutes.

Birth

If the fetus has reached a point of viability, a decision about birth will be made as soon as a woman's condition stabilizes, usually 12 to 24 hours after the seizure. Probably because of the increased stress that has occurred, fetal lung maturity appears to advance rapidly with preeclampsia, so even though the fetus is younger than 37 weeks, the lecithin/sphingomyelin ratio may indicate fetal lung maturity.

Cesarean birth is always more hazardous for the fetus than vaginal birth because of the association of retained lung fluid (see Chapter 26). Furthermore, a woman with severe high blood pressure is not a good candidate for surgery. An additional problem arises: Because her vascular system is low in volume, she may become hypotensive with regional anesthesia, such as an epidural block. The preferred method for birth, therefore, is vaginal with a minimum of anesthesia. If labor does not begin spontaneously, rupture of the membranes or induction of labor with intravenous oxytocin may be instituted. If this is ineffective and the fetus appears to be in imminent danger, cesarean birth becomes the birth method of choice.

NURSING INTERVENTIONS DURING THE POSTPARTUM PERIOD

Postpartum preeclampsia may occur up to 10 to 14 days after birth, although it usually occurs within 48 hours after birth. Therefore, monitoring blood pressure in the postpartum period and at healthcare visits and being alert for preeclampsia, which can occur as late as 2 weeks postbirth, are essential to detect this residual hypertension (Takaoka, Ishii, Taguchi, et al., 2016).

QSEN Checkpoint Question 21.6

EVIDENCE-BASED PRACTICE

Because so many women of childbearing age work at physically demanding occupations, researchers assessed the work lifting requirements of 66,693 pregnant woman when they were at 16 weeks gestational age by phone interview and then analyzed if there was an association between their work lifting characteristics and the development of small-for-gestational-age babies. Results of the study showed no consistent association between the work-related lifting and the incidence of small-for-gestational-age babies (Juhl, Larsen, Anderson, et al., 2014).

Based on the previous study, which statement by Beverly about her job as a secretary at a construction site would give the nurse the most concern regarding fetal health?

a. "I think I likely walk at least a mile every work day."

b. "I rarely have time to eat when I'm at work because I get so busy."

c. "Sometimes, I have to move boxes of files around the office."

d. "I usually help my colleague bring boxes of paper up to the office for the photocopier."

Look in Appendix A for the best answer and rationale.

HELLP Syndrome

HELLP syndrome is a variation of the gestational hypertensive process named for the common symptoms that occur:

- **H**emolysis leads to anemia
- **E**levated **l**iver enzymes lead to epigastric pain
- **L**ow **p**latelets lead to abnormal bleeding/clotting (Pourrat, Coudroy, & Pierre, 2015)

The syndrome occurs in 4% to 12% of patients who have elevated blood pressure during pregnancy. It is a serious syndrome because it results in a maternal mortality rate as high as 24% and an infant mortality rate as high as 35%.

Why some women with elevated blood pressure also develop the HELLP syndrome is unknown. It occurs in both primigravidas and multigravidas and is associated with APS or the presence of antiphospholipid antibodies (Tufano, Coppola, Maruotti, et al., 2015).

In addition to proteinuria, edema, and increased blood pressure, additional symptoms of nausea, epigastric pain, general malaise, and right upper quadrant tenderness from liver inflammation occur. Laboratory studies reveal hemolysis of red blood cells (they appear fragmented on a peripheral blood smear), thrombocytopenia (a platelet count $<100,000/mm^3$), and elevated liver enzyme levels (alanine aminotransferase [ALT] and serum aspartate aminotransferase [AST]), which are all effects of hemorrhage and necrosis of the liver. Because of the low platelet count, women with the HELLP syndrome need extremely close observation for bleeding, in addition to the observations necessary for preeclampsia. Complications associated with the syndrome are subcapsular liver hematoma, hyponatremia, renal failure, and hypoglycemia from poor liver function. Mothers are also at risk for cerebral hemorrhages, aspiration pneumonia, and hypoxic encephalopathy. Fetal complications can include growth restriction and preterm birth (Barnhart, 2015).

Therapy for the condition is transfusion of fresh frozen plasma or platelets in order to improve the platelet count. If hypoglycemia is present, this is corrected by an intravenous glucose infusion. The infant is born as soon as feasible by either vaginal or cesarean birth. Be alert that maternal hemorrhage may occur at birth because of poor clotting ability. Epidural anesthesia may not be possible because of the low platelet count and the high possibility of bleeding at the epidural site. Laboratory results return to normal after birth, the same as preeclamptic symptoms, but the experience of developing the HELLP syndrome is frightening. Women need assurance afterward that symptoms were pregnancy related and so will not return.

Multiple Pregnancy

Multiple gestation is considered a complication of pregnancy because a woman's body must adjust to the effects of more than one fetus. The incidence of multiple births has increased dramatically because of the use of in vitro fertilization, but still only occurs in 2% to 3% of all births (Bush & Pernoll, 2012).

Identical (i.e., monozygotic) twins begin with a single ovum and spermatozoon. In the process of fusion, or in one of the first cell divisions, the zygote divides into two identical individuals. Single-ovum twins usually have one placenta, one

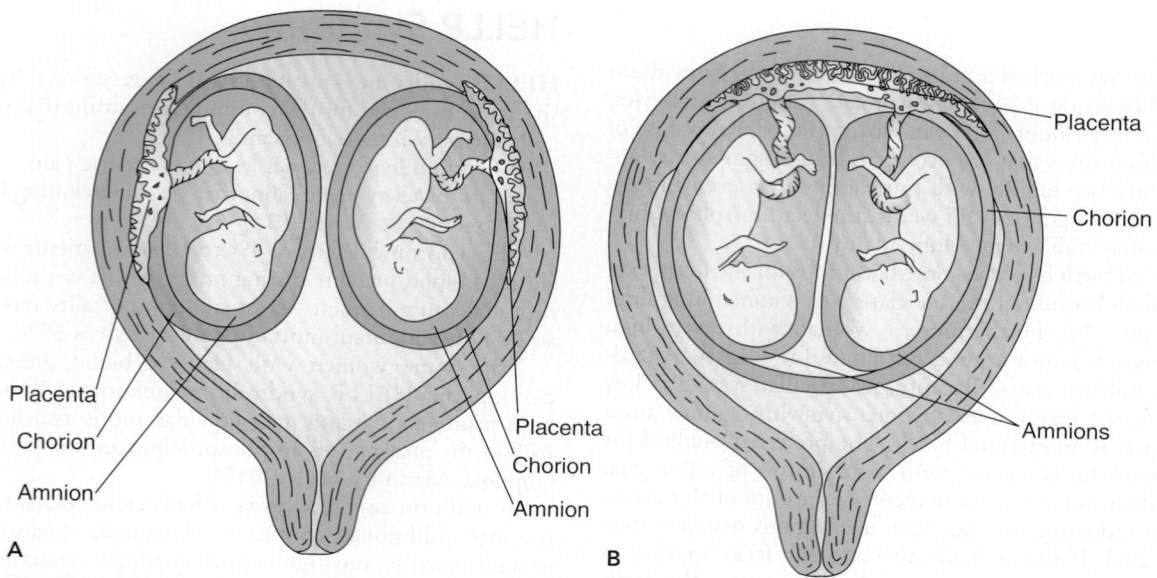

Figure 21.9 Multiple gestations. **(A)** Dizygotic twins showing two placentas, two chorions, and two amnions. **(B)** Monozygotic twins with one placenta, one chorion, and two amnions.

chorion, two amnions, and two umbilical cords. The twins are always of the same sex; they account for one third of twin births. The other two thirds of twins are fraternal (i.e., dizygotic, nonidentical), the result of the fertilization of two separate ova by two separate spermatozoa (possibly not from the same sexual partner). Double-ova twins have two placentas, two chorions, two amnions, and two umbilical cords. The twins may be of the same or a different sex (Fig. 21.9). It is sometimes difficult to determine by ultrasound or at birth whether twins are identical or fraternal because the two fraternal placentas may fuse and appear as one large placenta.

Multiple pregnancies of two to eight children may be single-ovum conceptions, multiple-ova conceptions, or a combination of the two types. Most multiple pregnancies today occur from multiple ova being implanted as an in vitro fertility process. Naturally occurring multiple pregnancies are more frequent in Blacks and Hispanics than Whites. The higher a woman's parity and age, the more likely she is to have a multiple gestation. Inheritance appears to play a role in natural dizygotic twinning; this has a familial maternal pattern of occurrence.

ASSESSMENT

Multiple gestation is suspected early in pregnancy when the uterus begins to increase in size at a rate faster than usual. AFP levels will also be elevated. At the time of quickening, a woman may report flurries of action at different portions of her abdomen rather than at one consistent spot (e.g., where the feet are located). On auscultation of the abdomen, multiple sets of fetal heart sounds can be heard; although if one or more fetus has his or her back positioned toward a woman's back, only one fetal heart sound may be heard.

An ultrasound can reveal multiple gestation sacs early in pregnancy. In some instances, early ultrasound examinations reveal multiple amniotic sacs but then later in pregnancy, in as many as 30% of women, only one fetus remains (i.e., vanishing twin syndrome) (Evron, Sheiner, Friger, et al., 2015). Women who were told they were having twins but

then later in pregnancy find out they are having only one child may grieve for a vanished twin as much as if the baby had died at birth. This emotional response is important in an assessment because it could disrupt pregnancy bonding work.

THERAPEUTIC MANAGEMENT

Women with a multiple gestation are more susceptible to complications of pregnancy such as gestational hypertension, polyhydramnios, placenta previa, preterm labor, and anemia than are women carrying one fetus. Following birth, they are more prone to postpartum bleeding because of the additional uterine stretching that occurred. Because a multiple pregnancy usually ends before term, 25% of low–birth-weight babies are from multiple pregnancies. If monozygotic twins share a common vascular communication, it can lead to overgrowth of one fetus and undergrowth of the second (a twin-to-twin transfusion), resulting in discordant infants (Beauquier-Maccotta, Chalouhi, Picquet, et al., 2016) (see Chapter 26). If a single amnion is present, there can be knotting and twisting of umbilical cords, causing fetal distress or difficulty with birth. Because of the possibility of these complications, a woman with a twin pregnancy needs closer prenatal supervision than a woman with a single gestation to detect these problems as early as possible. A woman carrying more than two fetuses is at greatest risk.

 Nursing Diagnoses and Related Interventions

Nursing Diagnosis: Fatigue related to increased stress on body functioning secondary to multiple gestation

Outcome Evaluation: Patient states she is tired but identifies steps she has taken to minimize fatigue.

Although there is little evidence that strict bed rest helps prolong multiple pregnancies (Fuchs & Senat, 2016), spend time at healthcare visits reviewing with a woman with a multiple pregnancy her need for extra rest, especially in a side-lying position during the day, to increase placental perfusion.

Because the woman is carrying double weight during pregnancy, she may notice extreme fatigue and backaches late in the day. She may have more difficulty resting or sleeping than the average woman because of this greater discomfort and increased fetal activity. As the growing uterus compresses her stomach, she may find her appetite decreasing and her intake falling. To compensate and maintain nutrition, a woman may need to eat six small meals a day rather than three large ones. She must also be sure to take her iron, folic acid, and vitamin supplements.

Toward the end of pregnancy, a woman may have extreme difficulty ambulating because of her excess weight. Her abdomen may become so stretched she feels as if she is going to burst.

Beginning with week 28 of pregnancy, a woman may be asked to come to a healthcare facility for monthly ultrasound examinations or weekly nonstress tests to document normal fetal growth, although this may not be necessary if the pregnancy is going well and the fetuses are growing consistently. If these tests are necessary, be certain that appointments are scheduled to conserve her energy as much as possible.

Nursing Diagnosis: Parental role conflict related to recent discovery of multiple (as opposed to single) pregnancy

Outcome Evaluation: Patient states she is looking forward to caring for multiple infants (or may express concern about her ability to manage their arrival); patient identifies changes she is making in preparation now that more than one baby is expected.

A woman with a multiple pregnancy has to work through an additional role change during pregnancy. First, she must accept that she is pregnant and then accept that she is having a baby. Then suddenly, at a routine office visit, two or more gestational sacs are seen on ultrasound or two or more sets of heart sounds are heard on auscultation. She is told she is going to have more than one child. Now, she has to work through a second role change—for example, becoming a mother of two, not just of one (or more if she has additional children). This role change takes time and so may be difficult to complete, especially if the pregnancy ends early. A woman may need extra help after birth to form a close mother–child relationship with her newborns.

Nursing Diagnosis: Fear concerning her own and the babies' health related to risks of a multiple pregnancy

Outcome Evaluation: Patient accurately states risks of a multiple pregnancy; expresses confidence in healthcare team's ability to care for her and her babies through pregnancy and birth.

In addition to having to work through a role change, a woman with a multiple pregnancy has more reason to fear for her life and the life of her babies than does the average woman. Every woman has heard stories about twins being conjoined or born so prematurely they did not survive. If she has not already heard these stories, someone will be sure to mention them to her before her due date. Unfortunately, all these risks cannot simply be filed away under the heading of untrue stories: Both prematurity and high risk status are real hazards in multiple gestation. Help a woman deal with her fears as positively as possible. It can be helpful to tell her there is no indication so far that her babies are in any danger, so right now it is best to continue doing the things that have to be done; if any problems arise, the healthcare team and the woman's family will be there to support her.

Sometimes a woman is so fearful that her infants will be born too small to survive that she makes no preparations for them. She so lacks confidence in herself she cannot imagine she will be lucky enough or "good" enough to be able to carry a multiple pregnancy to term. Give her assurance during prenatal visits she is managing well, so her self-esteem is maintained at as high a level as possible. When her babies are born and all are healthy, the proof she needs she "deserved" this or was capable of it will be present in her arms. Nursing care at the birth of multiple infants is discussed in Chapter 23.

Polyhydramnios

Usually, the amniotic fluid volume at term is 500 to 1,000 ml. **Polyhydramnios** occurs when there is excess fluid of more than 2,000 ml or an amniotic fluid index above 24 cm (Wiegand, Beamon, Chescheir, et al., 2016).

Polyhydramnios can cause fetal malpresentation because the additional uterine space can allow the fetus to turn to a transverse lie. It also can lead to premature rupture of the membranes from the increased pressure, which then leads to the additional risks of infection, prolapsed cord, and preterm birth.

ASSESSMENT

Amniotic fluid is formed by a combination of the cells of the amniotic membrane and from fetal urine. It is evacuated by being swallowed by the fetus, absorbed across the intestinal membrane into the fetal bloodstream, and transferred across the placenta. Although polyhydramnios can occur separate from fetal involvement, accumulation of amniotic fluid suggests difficulty with the fetus's ability to swallow or absorb, or excessive urine production. Inability to swallow occurs in infants who are anencephalic, who have tracheoesophageal fistula with stenosis, or who have intestinal obstruction (Bishop & Ebach, 2015). Excessive urine output occurs in the fetuses of diabetic women (hyperglycemia in the fetus causes increased urine production).

The first sign of polyhydramnios may be unusually rapid enlargement of the uterus. The small parts of the fetus become difficult to palpate because the uterus is unusually tense. Auscultating the FHR can be difficult because of the depth of the increased amount of fluid surrounding the fetus. A woman may begin to notice extreme shortness of breath as the overly distended uterus pushes up against her diaphragm. She may develop lower extremity varicosities and hemorrhoids because good venous return from the lower extremities is blocked by extensive uterine pressure. The increased amount of fluid will cause increased weight gain. Generally, an ultrasound is done to document the presence of polyhydramnios and to discover a reason for the excessive amount of fluid.

THERAPEUTIC MANAGEMENT

Women with severe polyhydramnios may be admitted to a hospital for bed rest and further evaluation or may be cared for at home. Regardless of the setting, maintaining bed rest helps to increase uteroplacental circulation and reduces pressure on the cervix, which may help prevent preterm labor. Teach a woman that it is vitally important to report any sign of ruptured membranes or uterine contractions. Although not common, there is a possibility that straining to defecate could increase uterine pressure and cause a rupture of membranes. Help her, therefore, avoid constipation by encouraging her to eat a high-fiber diet. Suggest a stool softener if diet alone is ineffective.

Assess vital signs as well as lower extremity edema frequently (the extremely tense uterus puts unusual pressure on both the diaphragm and the vessels of the pelvis). Amniocentesis can be performed to remove some of the extra fluid. Because amniotic fluid is replaced rapidly, however, this has to be repeated almost daily to be effective. Polyhydramnios can also lead to placental separation or rupture of membranes (Zheng, 2012a). If contractions begin, tocolysis may be necessary to prevent or halt preterm labor.

Even with these precautions, in many instances of polyhydramnios, there will be preterm rupture of the membranes because of excessive pressure, followed by preterm birth. To prevent the sudden loss of fluid and the accompanying danger of a prolapsed cord during labor, membranes can be "needled" (a thin needle is inserted vaginally to pierce them) to allow a slow, controlled release of fluid. After birth, the infant must be assessed carefully for factors that may have interfered with the ability to swallow in utero, such as a gastrointestinal blockage.

Oligohydramnios

Oligohydramnios refers to a pregnancy with less than the average amount of amniotic fluid (Kumar, 2012). Because part of the volume of amniotic fluid is formed by the addition of fetal urine, this reduced amount of fluid is usually caused by a bladder or renal disorder in the fetus that is interfering with voiding. It also can occur from severe growth restriction (because of the small size, a fetus is not voiding as much as usual). Because the fetus is so cramped for space, muscles are left weak at birth, lungs can fail to develop (hypoplastic lungs), possibly leading to severe difficulty breathing after birth, and distorted features of the face occur (termed Potter syndrome).

Oligohydramnios is suspected during pregnancy when the uterus fails to meet its expected growth rate. It is confirmed by ultrasound when the pockets of amniotic fluid are less than average. Infants need careful inspection at birth to rule out kidney disease and compromised lung development.

Postterm Pregnancy

A term pregnancy is 38 to 42 weeks long. A pregnancy that exceeds these limits is prolonged (i.e., postterm pregnancy, postmature, or postdate). The infant of such a pregnancy is considered postmature, or dysmature, if there is evidence that placental insufficiency has occurred and interfered with fetal growth. **Postterm pregnancy** occurs in 3% to 12% of all pregnancies (Kortekaas, Kazemier, Ravelli, et al., 2015).

Included in this group are some pregnancies that appear to extend beyond the due date set for them because of a faulty due date. Women who have long menstrual cycles (e.g., 40 to 45 days) do not ovulate on day 14 as in a typical menstrual cycle. Because they ovulate 14 days from the end of their cycle, or on day 26 or 31, their children will be considered "late" by 12 to 17 days.

In other instances, the pregnancy is truly overdue. For some reason, the trigger that initiates labor did not turn on. Such pregnancies can occur in women receiving a high dose of salicylates (for severe sinus headaches or rheumatoid arthritis) that interferes with the synthesis of prostaglandins, which may be responsible for the initiation of labor. It is also associated with myometrial quiescence, or a uterus that (for unknown reasons) does not respond to normal labor stimulation.

Remaining in utero for longer than 2 weeks beyond term creates a danger to a fetus for several reasons. Meconium aspiration is more apt to occur as fetal intestinal contents are more likely to reach the rectum. If the fetus continues to grow, macrosomia could create a birth problem. However, the usual effect of being postterm is lack of growth because a placenta seems to have adequate functioning ability for only 40 to 42 weeks. After that time, it acquires calcium deposits. This exposes a fetus to decreased blood perfusion and a lack of oxygen, fluid, and nutrients (Mission, Marshall, & Caughey, 2015). If oligohydramnios occurs, it can lead to variable decelerations in the FHR from cord compression.

If labor has not begun by 41 weeks, a nonstress test, and/or a biophysical profile may be done to document the state of placental perfusion and the amount of amniotic fluid present. If these are normal, it suggests the due date was miscalculated. If the test results are abnormal or the physical examination or biparietal diameter measured on ultrasound suggests the fetus is term size, labor will be induced. Prostaglandin gel or misoprostol (Cytotec) applied to the vagina to initiate cervical ripening followed by an oxytocin infusion are common methods used to begin labor. If oxytocin is ineffective, cesarean birth may be necessary. Monitor the FHR closely during labor to be certain placental insufficiency is not occurring from aging of the placenta. Nursing care for the postterm infant at birth is discussed in Chapter 26.

Isoimmunization (Rh Incompatibility)

Approximately 15% of Whites and 10% of African Americans in the United States are missing the Rh (D) factor in their blood or have an Rh-negative blood type. **Rh incompatibility** occurs when an Rh-negative mother (one negative for a D antigen or one with a dd genotype) carries a fetus with an Rh-positive blood type (DD or Dd genotype). For such a situation to occur, the father of the child must either be homozygous (DD) or heterozygous (Dd) Rh positive. If the father of the child is homozygous (DD) for the factor, 100% of the couple's children will be Rh positive (Dd). If the father is heterozygous for the trait, 50% of their children can be expected to be Rh positive (Dd). Although blood incompatibility is basically a problem that affects the fetus, it can cause such concern and apprehension in a woman during pregnancy that it becomes a maternal problem as well.

Figure 21.10 Maternal antibody formation against the Rh antigen.

Because people who have Rh-positive blood have a protein factor (the D antigen) that Rh-negative people do not, when an Rh-positive fetus begins to grow inside an Rh-negative mother who is sensitized, her body reacts in the same manner it would if the invading factor were a substance such as a virus—she forms antibodies against the invading substance. The Rh factor exists as a portion of the red blood cell, so these maternal antibodies cross the placenta and cause destruction (i.e., hemolysis) of fetal red blood cells (Fig. 21.10). A fetus can become so deficient in red blood cells from this that a sufficient oxygen transport to body cells cannot be maintained. This condition is termed **hemolytic disease of the newborn or erythroblastosis fetalis**. Management of the infant born with this condition is discussed in Chapter 26.

Theoretically, there is no connection between fetal blood and maternal blood during pregnancy, so the mother should not be exposed to fetal blood. In reality, a small amount of fetal blood does enter maternal circulation (McBain, Crowther, & Middleton, 2015). Procedures such as amniocentesis or percutaneous umbilical blood sampling can allow this to occur. During a first pregnancy, this effect is small. As the placenta separates after birth of the first child, however, there is an active exchange of fetal and maternal blood from damaged villi. This causes most of the maternal antibodies formed against the Rh-positive blood to be formed in the first 72 hours after birth. These become a threat in a second pregnancy.

ASSESSMENT

All women with Rh-negative blood should have an anti-D antibody titer done at a first pregnancy visit. If the results are normal or the titer is minimal (normal is 0; a ratio below 1:8 is minimal), the test is repeated at week 28 of pregnancy. If this is also normal, no therapy is needed.

If a woman's anti-D antibody titer is elevated at a first assessment (1:16 or greater), showing Rh sensitization, the well-being of the fetus in this potentially toxic environment will be monitored every 2 weeks (or more often) by Doppler velocity of the fetal middle cerebral artery, a technique that can predict when anemia is present or fetal red cells are being destroyed (Kamei, Yamaguchi, Sato, et al., 2014).

If the artery velocity remains high, a fetus is not developing anemia and most likely is an Rh-negative fetus. If the reading is low, it means a fetus is in danger, and immediate birth will be carried out providing the fetus is near term. If the fetus is not near term, efforts to reduce the number of antibodies in the woman or replace damaged red cells in the fetus are begun.

THERAPEUTIC MANAGEMENT

To reduce the number of maternal Rh (D) antibodies being formed, RhIG, a commercial preparation of passive Rh (D) antibodies against the Rh factor, is administered to women who are Rh negative at 28 weeks of pregnancy. These cannot cross the placenta and destroy fetal red blood cells because the antibodies are not the IgG class, the only type that crosses the placenta. RhIG (RhoGAM) is given again by injection to the mother in the first 72 hours after birth of an Rh-positive child to further prevent the woman from forming natural antibodies. Because RhIG is passive antibody protection, it is transient, and in 2 weeks to 2 months, the passive antibodies are destroyed. Only those few antibodies that were formed during pregnancy are left. For this reason, every pregnancy is like a first pregnancy in terms of the number of antibodies present, ensuring a safe intrauterine environment for any future pregnancies.

After birth, the infant's blood type will be determined from a sample of the cord blood. If it is Rh positive, the mother will receive the RhIG injection. If the newborn's blood type is Rh negative, no antibodies have been formed in the mother's circulation during pregnancy and none will form, so passive antibody injection (RhIG) is unnecessary.

Although in future years, the problem of Rh sensitization will be greatly reduced, it currently remains a complication of pregnancy, particularly in women who gave birth to a first child in an undeveloped nation where they did not receive passive anti-D antibodies. Other women become sensitized because they did not receive an RhIG injection after an induced abortion, miscarriage, ectopic pregnancy, or amniocentesis.

INTRAUTERINE TRANSFUSION

To restore fetal red blood cells, blood transfusion can be performed on the fetus in utero. This is done by injecting red blood cells by amniocentesis technique directly into a vessel in the fetal cord or depositing them in the fetal abdomen where they migrate into the fetal circulation.

Blood used for transfusion in utero is either the fetus's own type (determined by percutaneous blood sampling) or group O negative if the fetal blood type is unknown. From 75 to 150 ml of washed red cells are used, depending on the age of the fetus. After deposition of the blood in the cord or abdomen, the cannula is withdrawn and a woman is urged to rest for approximately 30 minutes while fetal heart sounds and uterine activity are monitored.

Intrauterine transfusion is not without risk. A cord blood vessel could be lacerated by the needle or the uterus could be so irritated by the invasive procedure that labor contractions begin. For the fetus who is severely affected by isoimmunization, however, such a risk is no greater than that of being left untreated in a destructive intrauterine environment. The mother receives an RhIG injection after the transfusion to help reduce increased sensitization from any blood that might have been exchanged. Transfusion is sometimes done only once during pregnancy, or it may be repeated as often as every 2 weeks. As soon as fetal maturity is reached, as shown by a mature lecithin/sphingomyelin ratio, birth will be induced.

After birth, the infant may require therapy with phototherapy lights to reduce the level of bilirubin released from destroyed red blood cells or an exchange transfusion to remove hemolyzed red blood cells and replace them with healthy blood cells (see Chapter 26). A woman needs to discuss her plans for further childbearing with her healthcare provider and should be provided with contraceptive information if she does not want to undergo the strain of another pregnancy because the constant feeling of wishing that everything was all right but never being certain it was, is more than she may want to endure again.

Fetal Death

Obviously, one of the most severe complications of pregnancy is fetal death. The most likely causes of this include chromosomal abnormalities, congenital malformations, infections such as hepatitis B, immunologic causes, and complications of maternal disease. If fetal death occurs before the time of quickening, a woman will not be aware the fetus has died because she is not able to feel fetal movements. This type of fetal death may be discovered at a routine prenatal visit when no fetal heartbeat can be heard. An ultrasound will reveal that no fetal heartbeat is present.

That a fetus has died early in intrauterine life may also be revealed first by the miscarriage that occurs. With this, a woman begins painless spotting, gradually accompanied by uterine contractions with cervical effacement and dilatation. The fetus is born lifeless and emaciated. Carefully observe all women who give birth to a fetus who has died for excess bleeding because if the fetus has been dead in utero for any length of time, the risk for the development of DIC increases.

If a fetus dies in utero past the point of quickening, a woman will be very aware that fetal movements are suddenly absent. She may lie down or sit in a position that she knows

usually causes fetal movement. Unable to believe something could have happened, she may attribute the lack of movement to "sleeping" or "saving enough strength to be born." Because she is denying what is happening, it may be a full 24 hours before she calls her healthcare facility to report the apparent lack of fetal movement. On assessment, no fetal heartbeat can be heard. An ultrasound will confirm the absence of a fetal heartbeat.

If labor does not begin spontaneously once the fetal death is confirmed, it will be induced through a combination of prostaglandin gel or misoprostol (Cytotec) applied to the vagina to effect cervical ripening and oxytocin administration to begin uterine contractions (Abediasl, Sheikh, Pooransari, et al., 2016). Blood for coagulation studies to detect DIC must be obtained to rule out the possibility of this developing.

 ### Nursing Diagnoses and Related Interventions

Nursing Diagnosis: Powerlessness related to fetal death

Outcome Evaluation: Patient and support person express meaning of pregnancy loss; identify support people/family with whom they can share grief.

Going through labor knowing a fetus is dead is difficult. A woman grieves for both her dead child and her inability to carry a pregnancy to term. She may wonder what she had done to cause this, such as forgetting to take an iron supplement, or may worry she is not as good a woman as others. Give her opportunities to express how she feels about this loss. "This must be a very difficult day for you" is the kind of statement that opens up the topic for discussion. If there are older children, it might be a help to explore how a woman plans to explain the fetal death to them.

Ask a couple about their desire for clergy or religious rites, such as baptism. Encourage a support person to remain with a woman during labor but remember that the support person is grieving too. Although this is a difficult time, encouraging them to express their grief can help to make the fact the pregnancy has ended and allows the couple to begin rebuilding their life.

Labor involving a dead fetus is the same as for a live fetus because every fetus is basically a passive participant during labor. It may be difficult for a woman to use controlled breathing exercises, although encouraging her to use them is helpful in making the experience one of controllable pain. If a woman wishes a high level of analgesia, there is no contraindication to this because there is no living fetus to protect from narcotic effects. An epidural is also an option, as this will guard against poor uterine involution in the postpartum period from heavy analgesic sedation.

Ask if the parents wish to see the child after birth. If they do, wash away obvious blood, swaddle the baby as if he or she were a well newborn, and bring the baby to them. Point out particularly endearing features of the child as these can provide a focus for memories. Some parents may want to keep a lock of the child's hair. Others may want to keep the hospital identification bracelet or take a photograph. Parents may want to name the child. All of these measures are usual responses to grief and help to make the death real to parents, thus letting them begin the healthy process of grieving (Lisy, Peters, Riitano, et al., 2016).

If the child has a congenital anomaly that led to the death, prepare them for this before bringing the child to them and explain how the anomaly affected the child. Explain hospital procedures such as when the body will be released or what additional permission for autopsy is needed. Different communities have different laws concerning whether burial for an immature fetus is necessary. Consult local health department regulations so you can serve as a resource person for parents about this.

A woman needs to remain for only a few hours in the hospital, assuming no complications with labor developed. Many couples ask how soon it will be safe for them to have another child. They will need to consult with their primary care provider with regard to this, because it depends on why the fetal death occurred and whether the birth was cesarean. For some couples, beginning a second pregnancy immediately is a good recommendation. For others, waiting for an interval of time (perhaps 6 months) is better as this gives them more time to work through their grief before starting a new pregnancy. This helps prevent the new baby from becoming a "replacement baby" or someone to take the place of the dead infant rather than a unique individual in his or her own right. This is important in years to come because replacement children are rarely able to live up to the image of what the deceased baby would have been if only that baby had lived.

Prepare the couple for the possibility that they may feel sad on the day the infant would have been born if the pregnancy had been carried to term, or if they visit a friend's child of the age their child would have been. Be certain before a woman is discharged from the healthcare facility that she has a support person she can rely on during the following week or month, when the full impact of the fetal loss registers with her. Be certain she has a return appointment for a postpartal checkup so her physiologic and psychological health can be evaluated at that time.

What If . . . 21.4

The nurse is interested in exploring one of the 2020 National Health Goals related to complications of pregnancy (see Box 21.1). Most government-sponsored money for nursing research is allotted based on these goals. What would be a possible research topic to explore pertinent to these goals that would be applicable to the Muzuki family and that would also advance evidence-based practice?

KEY POINTS FOR REVIEW

- Vaginal bleeding during pregnancy is always serious until ruled otherwise because it has the potential to diminish the blood supply to both the mother and fetus.

- The amount of bleeding that is evident may not be truly indicative of the amount of bleeding occurring because hidden, internal bleeding may also be happening. As a rule, position women with bleeding during pregnancy on their side to improve placental circulation and prevent supine hypotension syndrome.

- Spontaneous miscarriage is the loss of a pregnancy before viability of the fetus (20 to 24 weeks). The majority of these early pregnancy losses are attributed to chromosomal abnormalities. They are classified as threatened, imminent, complete, incomplete, missed, or recurrent pregnancy loss. Women who have a spontaneous miscarriage at home should bring any tissue passed to the hospital for an analysis for gestational trophoblastic disease. APS is an autoimmune disease that may contribute to recurrent miscarriages; therapy is SQ heparin and low-dose aspirin.

- Ectopic pregnancy is implantation outside the uterus, usually in a fallopian tube. If discovered before the tube ruptures, methotrexate can be administered to cause the conceptus to be reabsorbed. If not discovered early, sharp lower quadrant pain occurs at about 6 to 12 weeks as the tube ruptures. A laparoscopy is necessary to remove the conceptus and repair the tube to halt bleeding.

- Gestational trophoblastic disease is abnormal overgrowth of trophoblast cells. If not discovered by an ultrasound early in pregnancy, bleeding and expulsion of the abnormal growth occur at about the 16th week of pregnancy. Women need close follow-up after this because it can lead to choriocarcinoma, a malignancy.

- Premature cervical dilatation occurs when the cervix dilates early in pregnancy before viability of the fetus. Sutures (cervical cerclage) can be placed to prevent the cervix from dilating prematurely this way again in a second pregnancy.

- Placenta previa is low implantation of the placenta so that it crosses the cervical os. If this is not discovered before labor, cervical dilatation may cause the placenta to tear, causing severe blood loss. Women who have symptoms of placenta previa (i.e., painless vaginal bleeding in the third trimester) should not have vaginal examinations done to prevent disruption of the low-implanted placenta.

- Premature separation of the placenta (i.e., abruptio placentae) or placental separation from the uterus before the fetus is born usually occurs late in pregnancy and cuts off blood supply to the fetus. Women with increased parity, those with previous uterine surgery, and those who are cocaine dependent are at highest risk for this. Often, it is manifested by sudden, sharp fundal pain and then a continuing dull pain and vaginal bleeding.

- DIC is a blood disorder that may occur with any trauma, so it can accompany such conditions as premature separation of the placenta and hypertension of pregnancy. Blood coagulation is so extreme at one point in the circulatory system that clotting factors become diminished, resulting in their absence in the remainder of the system. Beginning symptoms of this include easy bruising, petechiae, and oozing from intravenous sites. Heparin is used to stop the local coagulation and free up clotting factors for systemic use.

- Preterm labor is labor that occurs after 20 weeks and before the end of the 37th week of pregnancy. A woman is said to be in preterm labor when she has had uterine contractions every 10 minutes for 1 hour and cervical dilatation begins. Magnesium sulfate, parentally administered, is the drug of choice to halt preterm labor.

- A corticosteroid is also used in preterm labor management because it appears to accelerate the formation of lung surfactant in the fetus.

- Preterm rupture of the membranes is tearing of the fetal membranes with loss of amniotic fluid before the pregnancy is at term. After rupture, there is a high risk of fetal and uterine infection (i.e., chorioamnionitis) and preterm birth.

- Preeclampsia is a unique disorder that occurs with three classic symptoms: hypertension, edema, and proteinuria. It is categorized as preeclampsia or eclampsia. If mild (blood pressure not over 140/90 mmHg), treatment is bed rest and perhaps low-dose aspirin. If severe (blood pressure over 160/110 mmHg), bed rest plus administration of magnesium sulfate will be prescribed. If a seizure occurs, the condition becomes eclampsia. Helping prevent the disease from progressing to this stage not only meets QSEN competencies but also can best meet the family's total needs.

- The HELLP syndrome is a unique form of gestational hypertension marked by hemolysis of red blood cells, elevated liver enzymes, and a low platelet count.

- Multiple gestation puts an additional strain on a woman's physical resources and may lead to preterm birth with immaturity of her infants. Helping a woman plan adequate nutrition and rest during pregnancy are nursing responsibilities.

- Postterm pregnancy is pregnancy that extends beyond 42 weeks. Because the placenta deteriorates at this time, it can cause a fetus to receive decreased nutrients.

- Polyhydramnios is overproduction of amniotic fluid (above 2,000 ml) and is a condition that can lead to ruptured membranes and premature birth because of increased intrauterine pressure. Oligohydramnios is characterized by too little amniotic fluid and suggests a renal disorder may exist in the fetus.

- Isoimmunization (Rh incompatibility) is a possibility when a woman who is Rh negative is sensitized and carries a fetus who is Rh positive. Maternal antibodies form and destroy fetal red blood cells, leading to anemia, edema, and jaundice in the newborn. Being certain that women are screened for blood type and antibody titer early in pregnancy is a nursing responsibility.

CRITICAL THINKING CARE STUDY

Maria Maya is a 37-year-old woman who works part-time in the personnel office at your school. She felt nauseated after receiving the flu vaccine in the health center. Last night, she experienced right-sided lower abdominal pain with scant vaginal spotting. Today, she appears pale. She is diagnosed as having a ruptured ectopic pregnancy. She is scheduled for an emergency laparotomy.

1. Maria questions her diagnosis because she had no idea she was pregnant. How would you respond if she asks you, "Why didn't I have any pregnancy symptoms if I'm really pregnant?"

2. Maria's blood pressure is 90/60 mmHg and she appears very pale. She is refusing, however, to have surgery to end the pregnancy in case there is any chance her baby is still alive. Would you support her decision?

3. Maria's left fallopian tube was so damaged that it was removed in surgery. A week later, she quits her job, sets fire to her apartment, and swallows drain cleaner in a self-injury attempt because "I'm never going to be able to have children, now, am I?" Did Maria receive sound information about what her surgery consisted of?

RELATED RESOURCES

Explore these additional resources to enhance learning for this chapter:
- Student resources on thePoint, including answers to the What If . . . and Critical Thinking Care Study questions, http://thepoint.lww.com/Flagg8e
- Adaptive learning powered by PrepU, http://thepoint.lww.com/prepu

REFERENCES

Abediasl, Z., Sheikh, M., Pooransari, P., et al. (2016). Vaginal misoprostol versus intravenous oxytocin for the management of second-trimester pregnancies with intrauterine fetal death: A randomized clinical trial. *Journal of Obstetrics and Gynaecology Research, 42*(3), 246–251.

Abraham, C., & Seethappan, V. (2015). Spontaneous live recurrent ectopic pregnancy after ipsilateral partial salpingectomy leading to tubal rupture. *International Journal of Surgery Case Reports, 7*, 75–78.

Ahmed, S. R., Aitallah, A., Abdelghafar, H. M., et al. (2015). Major placenta previa: Rate, maternal and neonatal outcomes experience at a Tertiary Maternity Hospital, Sohag, Egypt: A prospective study. *Journal of Clinical and Diagnostic Research, 9*(11), QC17–QC19.

Aitken, S. L., & Tichy, E. M. (2015). Rh(O)D immune globulin products for prevention of alloimmunization during pregnancy. *American Journal of Health-System Pharmacy, 72*(4), 267–276.

Alhusen, J. L., Ray, E., Sharps, P., et al. (2015). Intimate partner violence during pregnancy: Maternal and neonatal outcomes. *Journal of Women's Health, 24*(1), 100–106.

American College of Obstetricians and Gynecologists. (2016a). Practice Bulletin No. 159: Management of preterm labor. *Obstetrics and Gynecology, 127*(1), e29–e38.

American College of Obstetricians and Gynecologists. (2016b). Practice Bulletin No. 160: Premature rupture of membranes. *Obstetrics and Gynecology, 127*(1), e39–e51.

American College of Obstetricians and Gynecologists. (2016c). Practice Bulletin No. 652: Magnesium sulfate use in obstetrics. *Obstetrics and Gynecology, 127*(1), e52–e53.

Ananth, C. V., Lavery, J. A., Vintzileos, A. M., et al. (2016). Severe placental abruption: Clinical definition and associations with maternal complications. *American Journal of Obstetrics and Gynecology, 214*(2), 272.e1–272.e9.

Aytac, P. C., Bulgan Kilicdag, E., Haydardedeoglu, B., et al. (2016). Luteal phase support after mild ovulation induction with intrauterine insemination: An on-going debate. *Gynecological Endocrinology, 32*(7), 543–547.

Barnhart, L. (2015). HELLP syndrome and the effects on the neonate. *Neonatal Network, 34*(5), 269–273.

Beauquier-Maccotta, B., Chalouhi, G. E., Picquet, A. L., et al., (2016). Impact of monochorionicity and twin to twin transfusion syndrome on prenatal attachment, post traumatic stress disorder, anxiety and depressive symptoms. *PloS One, 11*(1), e0145649.

Besharat, M., Tabandeh, A., Keshtkar A., et al. (2015). Evaluation of some plasma coagulation factors in women with spontaneous miscarriage. *International Journal of Fertility and Sterility, 9*(3), 309–312.

Bingham, R. J. (2015). Latest evidence on alcohol and pregnancy. *Nursing for Women's Health, 19*(4), 338–344.

Bishop, W. P., & Ebach, D. R. (2015). The digestive system. In K. J. Marcdante & R. M. Kliegman (Eds.), *Nelson essentials of pediatrics* (7th ed., pp. 417–454). Philadelphia, PA: Saunders/Elsevier.

Boisramé, T., Sananès, N., Fritz, G., et al. (2014). Placental abruption: Risk factors, management and maternal-fetal prognosis. Cohort study over 10 years. *European Journal of Obstetrics & Gynecology and Reproductive Biology, 179*, 100–104.

Brocato, B., Holliday, N., Whitehurst, R. M., Jr., et al. (2016). Delayed cord clamping in preterm neonates: A review of benefits and risks. *Obstetrical & Gynecological Survey, 71*(1), 39–42.

Bush, M. C., & Pernoll, M. L. (2012). Multiple gestation. In D. K. Edmonds (Ed.), *Dewhurst's textbook of obstetrics & gynaecology* (8th ed., pp. 301–309). Oxford, United Kingdom: Wiley.

Cunningham, F. G., & Nelson, D. B. (2015). Disseminated intravascular coagulation syndromes in obstetrics. *Obstetrics and Gynecology, 126*(5), 999–1011.

DiMiceli-Zsigmond, M., Williams, A. K., & Richardson, M. G. (2015). Expecting the unexpected: Perspectives on stillbirth and late termination of pregnancy for fetal anomalies. *Anesthesia & Analgesia, 121*(2), 457–464.

Ekin, A., Gezer, C., Taner, C. E., et al. (2015). Perinatal outcomes in pregnancies with oligohydramnios after preterm premature rupture of membranes. *The Journal of Maternal-Fetal & Neonatal Medicine, 28*(16), 1918–1922.

Eschenbach, D. A. (2015). Treating spontaneous and induced septic abortions. *Obstetrics and Gynecology, 125*(5), 1042–1048.

Evron, E., Sheiner, E., Friger, M., et al. (2015). Vanishing twin syndrome: Is it associated with adverse perinatal outcome? *Fertility and Sterility, 103*(5), 1209–1214.

FIGO Safe Motherhood and Newborn Health Committee. (2015). Non-pneumatic anti-shock garment to stabilize women with hypovolemic shock secondary to obstetric hemorrhage. *International Journal of Gynecology & Obstetrics, 128*(3), 194–195.

Fuchs, F., & Senat, M. V. (2016). Multiple gestations and preterm birth. *Seminars in Fetal and Neonatal Medicine, 21*(2), 113–120.

Gilner, J., & Biggio, J. (2016). Management of short cervix during pregnancy: A review. *American Journal of Perinatology, 33*(3), 245–252.

Gongora, M. C., & Wenger, N. K. (2015). Cardiovascular complications of pregnancy. *International Journal of Molecular Sciences, 16*(10), 23905–23928.

Hackney, D. N., Kuo, K., Petersen, R. J., et al. (2016). Determinants of the competing outcomes of intrauterine infection, abruption, or spontaneous preterm birth after preterm premature rupture of membranes. *The Journal of Maternal-Fetal & Neonatal Medicine, 29*(2), 258–263.

Heavey, E., & Dahl Maher, M. (2015). Placental abruption: Are we going to lose them both? *Nursing, 45*(5), 54–59.

Hofmeyr, G. J., Eke, A. C., Lawrie, T. A., et al. (2014). Amnioinfusion for third trimester preterm premature rupture of membranes. *Cochrane Database of Systematic Reviews*, (3), CD000942.

Jean-Jacques, C. (2016). The hydatidiform mole. *Cell Adhesion & Migration, 10*(1–2), 226–235.

Juhl, M., Larsen, P. S., Anderson, P. K., et al. (2014). Occupational lifting during pregnancy and child's birth size in a large cohort study. *Scandinavian Journal of Work, Environment & Health, 40*(4), 411–419.

Jung, E. Y., Park, J. W., Ryu, A., et al. (2016). Prediction of impending preterm delivery based on sonographic cervical length and different cytokine levels in cervicovaginal fluid in preterm labor. *Journal of Obstetrics and Gynaecology Research, 42*(2), 158–165.

Jurkovic, D. (2012). Ectopic pregnancy. In D. K. Edmonds (Ed.), *Dewhurst's textbook of obstetrics & gynaecology* (8th ed., pp. 77–87). Oxford, United Kingdom: Wiley.

Kamei, K., Yamaguchi, K., Sato, M., et al. (2014). Successful treatment of severe rhesus D-incompatible pregnancy with repeated double-filtration plasmapheresis. *Journal of Clinical Apheresis, 30*(5), 305–307.

Karch, A. M. (2015). *Lippincott's nursing drug guide*. Philadelphia, PA: Lippincott Williams & Wilkins.

Kim, J. H., Joung, E. J., Lee, S. J., et al. (2015). Intraoperative bleeding control during cesarean delivery of complete placenta previa with transient occlusion of uterine arteries. *Obstetrics & Gynecology Science, 58*(6), 522–524.

Kortekaas, J. C., Kazemier, B. M., Ravelli, A. C., et al. (2015). Recurrence rate and outcome of postterm pregnancy, a national cohort study. *European Journal of Obstetrics & Gynecology and Reproductive Biology, 193*, 70–74.

Ku, C. W., Allen, J. C., Jr., Malhotra, R., et al. (2015). How can we better predict the risk of spontaneous miscarriage among women experiencing threatened miscarriage? *Gynecological Endocrinology, 31*(8), 647–651.

Kumar, S. (2012). Fetal anomalies. In D. K. Edmonds (Ed.), *Dewhurst's textbook of obstetrics & gynaecology* (8th ed., pp. 219–229). Oxford, United Kingdom: Wiley.

Leaf, R. K., & Connors, J. M. (2015). The role of anticoagulants in the prevention of pregnancy complications. *Clinical and Applied Thrombosis/Hemostasis, 23*(2), 116–123.

Li, C., Zhao, W. H., Zhu, Q., et al. (2015). Risk factors for ectopic pregnancy: A multi-center case-control study. *BMC Pregnancy and Childbirth, 15*, 1–9.

Lisy, K., Peters, M. D., Riitano, D., et al. (2016). Provision of meaningful care at diagnosis, birth, and after stillbirth: A qualitative synthesis of parents' experiences. *Birth, 43*(1), 6–19.

Maestá, I., Berkowitz, R. S., Goldstein, D. P., et al. (2015). Relationship between race and clinical characteristics, extent of disease, and response to chemotherapy in patients with low-risk gestational trophoblastic neoplasia. *Gynecologic Oncology, 138*(1), 50–54.

Mastrolia, S. A., Baumfeld, Y., Loverro, G., et al. (2016). Placenta previa associated with severe bleeding leading to hospitalization and delivery:

A retrospective population-based cohort study. *The Journal of Maternal-Fetal & Neonatal Medicine, 29*(21), 3467–3471.

McBain, R. D., Crowther, C. A., & Middleton, P. (2015). Anti-D administration in pregnancy for preventing rhesus alloimmunisation. *Cochrane Database of Systematic Reviews*, (9), CD00002.

Mehta, S. H., & Sokol, R. J. (2013). Assessment of high-risk pregnancy. In A. H. DeCherney, L. Nathan, T. M. Goodwin, et al. (Eds.), *Current diagnosis and treatment: Obstetrics and gynecology* (11th ed., pp. 223–233). Columbus, OH: McGraw-Hill/Lange.

Miller, D. A. (2012). Hypertension in pregnancy. In D. K. Edmonds (Ed.), *Dewhurst's textbook of obstetrics & gynaecology* (8th ed., pp. 454–464). Oxford, United Kingdom: Wiley.

Mission, J. F., Marshall, N. E., & Caughey, A. B. (2015). Pregnancy risks associated with obesity. *Obstetrics and Gynecology Clinics of North America, 42*(2), 335–353.

Moore, E., Blatt, K., Chen, A., et al. (2016). Relationship of trimester-specific smoking patterns and risk of preterm birth. *American Journal of Obstetrics and Gynecology, 215*(1), 109.e1–109.e6.

Msan, A. K., Usta, I. M., Mirza, F. G., et al. (2015). Use of antenatal corticosteroids in the management of preterm delivery. *American Journal of Perinatology, 32*(5), 417–426.

Nassali, M. N., Benti, T. M., Bandani-Ntsabele, M., et al. (2016). A case report of an asymptomatic late term abdominal pregnancy with a live birth at 41 weeks of gestation. *BMC Research Notes, 9*(1), 1–5.

Navathe, R., & Berghella, V. (2016). Tocolysis for acute preterm labor: Where have we been, where are we now, and where are we going? *American Journal of Perinatology, 33*(3), 229–235.

Nijman, T. A., van Vliet, E. O., Koullali, B., et al. (2016). Antepartum and intrapartum interventions to prevent preterm birth and its sequelae. *Seminars in Fetal & Neonatal Medicine, 21*(2), 121–128.

Olson-Chen, C., & Seligman, N. S. (2016). Hypertensive emergencies in pregnancy. *Critical Care Clinics, 32*(1), 29–41.

Oman, S., & Burke, A. E. (2015). Family planning: Contraception, sterilization & abortion. In J. L. Bienstock, H. Fox, E. E. Wallach, et al. (Eds.), *The Johns Hopkins manual of gynecology and obstetrics* (5th ed., pp. 421–438). Philadelphia, PA: Lippincott Williams & Wilkins.

Parets, S. E., Knight, A. K., & Smith, A. K. (2015). Insights into genetic susceptibility in the etiology of spontaneous preterm birth. *The Application of Clinical Genetics, 8*, 283–290.

Pourrat, O., Coudroy, R., & Pierre, F. (2015). Differentiation between severe HELLP syndrome and thrombotic microangiopathy, thrombotic thrombocytopenic purpura and other imitators. *European Journal of Obstetrics & Gynecology and Reproductive Biology, 189*, 68–72.

Ragab, A., & Mesbah, Y. (2015). To do or not to do emergency cervical cerclage (a rescue stitch) at 24–28 weeks gestation in addition to progesterone for patients coming early in labor? A prospective randomized trial for efficacy and safety. *Archives of Gynecology and Obstetrics, 292*(6), 1255–1260.

Rodgers, S. K., Chang, C., DeBardeleben, J. T., et al. (2015). Normal and abnormal us findings in early first-trimester pregnancy: Review of the society of radiologists in ultrasound 2012 consensus panel recommendations. *Radiographics, 35*(7), 2135–2148.

Roman, A. S. (2013). Late pregnancy complications. In A. H. DeCherney, L. Nathan, T. M. Goodwin, et al. (Eds.), *Current diagnosis and treatment: Obstetrics and gynecology* (11th ed., pp. 250–266). Columbus, OH: McGraw-Hill/Lange.

Sajan, R., Pulikkathodi, M., Vahab, A., et al. (2015). Expectant versus surgical management of early pregnancy miscarriages—a prospective study. *Journal of Clinical and Diagnostic Research, 9*(10), QC06–QC09.

Savage, P., & Seckl, M. (2012). Gestational trophoblast tumours. In D. K. Edmonds (Ed.), *Dewhurst's textbook of obstetrics & gynaecology* (8th ed., pp. 88–100). Oxford, United Kingdom: Wiley.

Seifert, S., & Altman, K. (2015). Miscarriage and recurrent pregnancy loss. In J. L. Bienstock, H. Fox, E. E. Wallach, et al. (Eds.), *The Johns Hopkins manual of gynecology and obstetrics* (5th ed., pp. 485–495). Philadelphia, PA: Lippincott Williams & Wilkins.

Sneider, K., Langhoff-Roos, J., Sundtoft, I. B., et al. (2015). Validation of second trimester miscarriages and spontaneous deliveries. *Clinical Epidemiology, 7*, 517–527.

Song, T., Kim, M. K., Kim, M. L., et al. (2016). Single-dose versus two-dose administration of methotrexate for the treatment of ectopic pregnancy: A randomized controlled trial. *Human Reproduction, 31*(2), 332–338.

Sosa, C. G., Althabe, F., Belizán, J. M. et al. (2015). Bed rest in singleton pregnancies for preventing preterm birth. *Cochrane Database of Systematic Reviews*, (3), CD003581.

Stevens, F. T., Katzorke, N., Tempfer, C., et al. (2015). Gestational trophoblastic disorders: An update in 2015. *Geburtshilfe Frauenheilkd*, *75*(10), 1043–1050.

Surette, A., & Dunham, S. M. (2013). Early pregnancy risks. In A. H. DeCherney, L. Nathan, T. M. Goodwin, et al. (Eds.), *Current diagnosis and treatment: Obstetrics and gynecology* (11th ed., pp. 234–249). Columbus, OH: McGraw-Hill/Lange.

Takaoka, S., Ishii, K., Taguchi, T., et al. (2016). Clinical features and antenatal risk factors for postpartum-onset hypertensive disorders. *Hypertension in Pregnancy*, *35*(1), 22–31.

Talarczyk-Desole, J., Wróbel, M., Niepsuj-Biniaś, J., et al. (2016). Ectopic pregnancy: Which treatment method least affects fertility? *European Journal of Obstetrics & Gynecology and Reproductive Biology*, *198*, 161–162.

Tufano, A., Coppola, A., Maruotti, G. M., et al. (2015). HELLP syndrome and its relation with the antiphospholipid syndrome. *Blood Transfusion*, *12*(1), 114–118.

U.S. Department of Health and Human Services. (2010). *Healthy people 2020*. Washington, DC: Author.

van Beukering, M. D., van Melick, M. J., Mol, B. W., et al. (2014). Physically demanding work and preterm delivery: A systematic review and meta-analysis. *International Archives of Occupational and Environmental Health*, *87*(8), 809–834.

van Hoorn, M. E., Hague, W. M., van Pampus, M. G., et al. (2016). Low-molecular-weight heparin and aspirin in the prevention of recurrent early-onset pre-eclampsia in women with antiphospholipid antibodies: The FRUIT-RCT. *European Journal of Obstetrics & Gynecology and Reproductive Biology*, *197*, 168–173.

Watson, C. A., & Wilkinson, M. (2012). Monitoring central venous pressure, arterial pressure and pulmonary wedge pressure. *Anaesthesia & Intensive Care Medicine*, *13*(3), 116–120.

Wiegand, S. L., Beamon, C. J., Chescheir, N. C., et al. (2016). Idiopathic polyhydramnios: Severity and perinatal morbidity. *American Journal of Perinatology*, *33*(7), 658–664.

Zheng, T. (2012a). Antepartum testing. In T. Zheng (Ed.), *Comprehensive handbook of obstetrics & gynecology* (2nd ed., pp. 92–95). Paradise Valley, AZ: Phoenix Medical Press.

Zheng, T. (2012b). Spontaneous abortion. In T. Zheng (Ed.), *Comprehensive handbook of obstetrics & gynecology* (2nd ed., pp. 230–233). Paradise Valley, AZ: Phoenix Medical Press.

Nursing Care of a Pregnant Family With Special Needs

*M*indy Carson, 16 years old and 15 weeks pregnant, received a 4-in. laceration on her leg when she was in an automobile accident on her way into prenatal clinic this morning. The father of Mindy's baby, Carlos, does not want Mindy to keep her baby after the birth because he does not want to get married until he finishes graduate school. Mindy insists she is old enough to be a parent and wants to keep her baby. Mindy's mother has accused Carlos of sharing methamphetamine with Mindy. She's worried Mindy has been working as a prostitute to support a substance abuse habit. Mindy turns to you and asks you what you would recommend she do.

Previous chapters discussed high-risk pregnancies for women who are ill when they become pregnant and for those who develop an illness while pregnant. This chapter presents information about women who do not fit the description of the average pregnant woman—a well adult who maintains a healthy lifestyle. Representative of such women who do not fit the description of average pregnant women are very young adolescents, women who have waited until midlife to have their first child, those who are physically or cognitively challenged, those who are unintentionally injured, and those who are substance dependent.

What type of immediate assessment does Mindy need? What qualities would you look for to decide if she is ready to be a parent?

KEY TERMS

adolescence	generativity
advanced maternal age	paracentesis
autonomic dysreflexia	peritoneal lavage
culdocentesis	substance abuse
emancipated minor	substance dependent

OBJECTIVES

After mastering the contents of this chapter, you should be able to:

1. Identify the characteristics and the risks of pregnancy for a pregnant woman who has special needs, such as one who has been injured, an adolescent, a woman over age 40 years, one who is physically or cognitively challenged, or a woman who is substance dependent.

2. Identify 2020 National Health Goals related to women with special needs that nurses can help the nation achieve.

3. Assess a woman with special needs during pregnancy.

4. Formulate nursing diagnoses related to pregnancy for a woman with special needs.

5. Identify expected outcomes for a pregnant woman with special needs to help her manage seamless transitions across differing healthcare settings.

6. Using the nursing process, plan nursing care that includes the six competencies of Quality & Safety Education for Nurses (QSEN): Patient-Centered Care, Teamwork & Collaboration, Evidence-Based Practice (EBP), Quality Improvement (QI), Safety, and Informatics.

7. Implement nursing care for a woman with special needs, such as encouraging her to remain ambulatory during pregnancy.

8. Evaluate outcomes for effectiveness and achievement of care.

9. Integrate knowledge of the risks of pregnancy for women with special needs with the interplay of nursing process, the six competencies of QSEN, and Family Nursing to promote quality maternal and child health nursing care.

The National Center for Health Statistics (NCHS) reported in 2014 that the live birth rate, the number of births per 1,000 women aged 15 to 44 years, was 62.9. This was a slight increase from a previous downward trend in birth rates since 2007. The rate of first births to women under 20 years old has declined by 42% between the years 2000 and 2014. In addition, teen birth rates declined for all races, including Hispanics, hitting a historic low live birth rate of 24.2 (Matthews & Hamilton, 2016). Although reasons for the declines are not clear, younger teens appear to be less sexually active and more of those who are sexually active may be using contraception than in previous years. In contrast, more women have delayed beginning a family until their 30s. As a result, birth rates continue to rise for women aged 40 to 44 years (Martin, Hamilton, & Osterman, 2015; Matthews & Hamilton, 2016).

Adolescents require special consideration during pregnancy because they are physically and psychosocially immature. Women over age 40 years may need special consideration also because they can have difficulty adjusting psychosocially to a first pregnancy and the physical changes that are required (Ben-David, Glasser, Schiff, et al., 2016).

The pregnancy rate is increasing among women who are physically or cognitively challenged as well, including conditions that might have precluded pregnancy a few years ago such as cerebral palsy. Physical and cognitive conditions present a challenge to childbearing and childrearing but do not necessarily prevent women from establishing their own families. Supportive nursing care that considers the limitations imposed by a particular disability while focusing on the normal aspects of childbearing and childrearing combined with a woman's strengths helps to make these pregnancies successful (H. K. Brown, Lunsky, Wilton, et al., 2016).

Women who are substance dependent or who are injured are other high-risk women who require a great deal of nursing support and care. Ideally, a woman should give up substance abuse for the health of a fetus, but that may not be possible. When substance abuse continues, every effort must be made to provide enough prenatal care and attention to protect the fetus in other ways. Women who are injured in automobile accidents or from intimate partner violence can have substantial blood loss that threatens the health of the fetus. They need rapid emergency department assessment and care to be certain fetal health is protected.

Women with special needs have become such a large population of pregnant women that several 2020 National Health Goals have been established in relation to them (Box 22.1).

Nursing Process Overview

FOR CARE OF A PREGNANT WOMAN WITH SPECIAL NEEDS

ASSESSMENT

Assessing the strengths and weaknesses of individual women is always crucial to establish accurate nursing diagnoses and realistic outcomes as well as planning effective nursing care. When a woman has a special need, assessment becomes even more important. Establishing as thorough a database as possible early in pregnancy helps to predict the risks a woman may be exposed to when pregnancy is affected by age extremes, physical or cognitive challenges, an unintentional injury, or an unhealthy lifestyle.

The capacity of a woman with special needs to adapt to pregnancy depends both on her physical capabilities and on her ability to persevere against odds to overcome obstacles. When caring for a woman who is physically challenged, keep in mind physical disabilities occur in degrees; therefore, first establish the impact of the disability on a woman's lifestyle before beginning to offer guidance for care measures during pregnancy. Be certain to assess physical strengths as well as limitations and psychosocial strengths as well as challenges. A woman with a spinal cord injury, for example, is likely to have developed ways of coping in daily life that may never occur to someone who has not experienced that disability.

For some women who are substance dependent, pregnancy may be the impetus they need to stop their substance abuse. Others may only be able to reduce their substance use. In both instances, encourage a woman to keep coming for prenatal care. As long as she feels comfortable with you during regular visits, you may be able to establish a trusting relationship that will eventually provide her with the confidence to try a more healthful pattern of living.

NURSING DIAGNOSIS

Nursing diagnoses established for pregnant women with special needs differ in degree, but not in substance, from the nursing diagnoses established for all pregnant women. For example, if a pregnant adolescent is still growing, sound nutrition is an extremely important issue for both her and her fetus. Examples of nursing diagnoses for women with special needs include:

- Risk for imbalanced nutrition related to combined needs of adolescent and pregnancy
- Risk for fetal injury related to drug and alcohol use
- Impaired physical mobility related to physical disability
- Risk for injury related to unstable balance

BOX 22.1

Nursing Care Planning Based on 2020 National Health Goals

Several National Health Goals have been formulated to improve the health of women with special needs during pregnancy. These include:

- Reduce the pregnancy rate among adolescent females to no more than 105.9 per 1,000 adolescents from a baseline of 117.7 per 1,000 adolescents.
- Increase abstinence from alcohol, cigarettes, and illicit substances among pregnant women to 98.3% from a baselines of 89.4% (alcohol), 100% from a baseline of 95% (binge drinking), 100% from a baseline of 94.9% (illicit drugs), and 98.6% from a baseline of 89.6% (cigarette smoking) (U.S. Department of Health and Human Services, 2010; see www.healthypeople.gov).

Nurses can help the nation achieve these goals by teaching unintentional injury prevention, the dangers and complications of substance dependency, and both the psychological and physical concerns of teenage pregnancy.

- Risk of injury related to potential for unintentional injuries
- Impaired verbal communication related to spastic muscle functioning
- Impaired home maintenance related to a sensory challenge
- Risk for social isolation related to bed rest at home
- Risk for disruption of social interactions related to unclear speech
- Disruption in family dynamics related to serious illness of family's main provider
- Readiness for enhanced family coping related to commitment to have a child in the face of a disabling condition

OUTCOME IDENTIFICATION AND PLANNING

Be especially careful to establish realistic outcomes given a woman's particular condition or situation. An adolescent, for instance, cannot achieve independent decision making if she is not mature enough to do this. A woman who is visually challenged may not be able to read a digital display on a glucometer or use a wall clock to time contractions no matter how much she would like to do these things.

Often, a pregnant woman with a special need already has significant stressors to deal with in her life. **Adolescence**, for example, is a period of growth and change that can be stressful for both the teenager and her family. The woman who is physically challenged constantly copes with a condition that must be considered in all activities, even if she has adjusted completely to the limitations the disability imposes. The substance-dependent woman is confined by a life-threatening habit. A woman who has an unintentional injury may have to temporarily restructure her life to accommodate a hospital admission. Pregnancy brings with it a whole new set of stressors that can be overwhelming if a woman has no outside support. Planning for a pregnant woman with special needs, therefore, often involves identifying support people to help with this added stress. This support can come from family, friends, a professional organization, or healthcare providers. If a woman is not totally independent in her care, some planning may be required with her support person, who may be the person who actually carries out the proposed action. At the same time, be certain to not ignore a woman and plan around her. Only if she approves of the plan can pregnancy be the enjoyable experience it should be. This principle applies to any woman but especially to one with special needs.

Plans should also include ways to strengthen confidence and self-esteem, crucial attributes for a new mother. These also are areas in which a woman with a special need, especially one who perceives herself as too young or too old or who has experienced a physical dysfunction, may not have developed fully. Substance dependence may also be related to feelings of lowered self-worth, which may have been intensified if the substance-dependent woman has tried unsuccessfully to limit her substance intake in the past.

Being certain that plans are established in a wide range of areas helps to ensure planning is comprehensive. Remember to include safe care of the newborn in plans as well because once an infant is born, it may be too late to make these plans in a comprehensive manner. The U.S. Department of Health and Human Services (DHHS) has initiated a special girls' health program through the Office on Women's Health to help reduce teenage pregnancy, which is helpful to use for referral, along with the Substance Abuse & Mental Health Services. Narcotics Anonymous can be helpful to women who are substance dependent. Alcoholics Anonymous is the standby for women with alcohol dependence. Women who feel they will be injured by an intimate partner can locate a shelter by calling their local police department. Refer patients and their families to helpful websites and other resources when appropriate (see Chapter 20).

IMPLEMENTATION

Interventions for the high-risk pregnant woman include promoting a healthy pregnancy and preventing pregnancy complications. Care focuses on teaching and encouraging a woman with any special needs to determine how best to manage her pregnancy according to her particular situation.

A high proportion of adolescents do not seek prenatal care early in pregnancy because they deny they are pregnant. Others may not feel comfortable in a healthcare facility that sees mainly adults. The same may be true of a woman with substance dependency, who fears discrimination from healthcare providers regarding her substance use. A nonjudgmental, welcoming attitude that focuses on the pregnancy and the baby, while avoiding recriminations about a woman's youth or circumstances, is essential to attracting such women to prenatal care and keeping them coming for regular visits. If they hear from a friend that the staff members at the clinic are helpful and not judgmental, they then take the first step into the facility.

OUTCOME EVALUATION

An evaluation of nursing interventions for the care of a pregnant woman with special needs often focuses on a woman's physical and emotional readiness for childbearing, maintenance of fetal health, and a woman's ability to provide a safe and healthy environment for her newborn. Some examples include:

- Patient states she will use walker to maintain balance during pregnancy.
- Adolescent lists a weekly intake of adequate calories, even with frequent meals at fast-food restaurants.
- Family members state they have been able to adjust to changing demands of pregnancy in a mother who is physically challenged.
- Patient reports to methadone maintenance clinic daily and reports no other substance use.
- Patient states she is able to manage a daily rest period even in light of a busy work and travel schedule.
- Patient states she is able to carry out usual lifestyle activities in spite of cast on injured arm.

The Pregnant Adolescent

Adolescent pregnancy is not a new phenomenon. Historically, it was common for women to marry as early as age 12 or 13 years and have their first baby at age 15 years. In today's society, however, marriage and childbearing are life situations thought of as belonging to later years. Reasons for the high number of teenage pregnancies that still continue include:

- Earlier age of menarche in girls (the average age is 12.4 years; many girls begin menstruating at age 9 years and so are ovulating and able to conceive by age 11 years)
- Rates of sexual activity among teenagers
- Lack of knowledge about (or failure to use) contraceptives or abstinence
- Desire by young girls to have a baby

Having an equally young sexual partner can contribute to pregnancy incidence because, in this situation, neither partner may be well versed in contraceptive options (Centers for Disease Control and Prevention [CDC], 2014). In addition, some adolescents become pregnant as the result of rape or incest (Wilson, Casanueva, Smith, et al., 2014).

Failure of adolescents to obtain adequate knowledge of contraceptive measures or abstinence is an issue that can be addressed by healthcare providers. As protective measures are easy to use, the average adolescent should not have difficulty following instructions. Adolescents are also capable of using emergency contraceptive measures correctly and safely. Access to emergency contraception is not associated with increased rates of unprotected intercourse or with higher rates of pregnancy or sexually transmitted infections (STIs) (Potter & Santelli, 2015; Society for Adolescent Health and Medicine, 2016). Unfortunately, providing this type of information does not always resolve the problem because adolescents may lack money to purchase protection such as birth control pills or a diaphragm. In addition, the egocentric phenomenon of adolescence makes a sexually active teenager believe she will not become pregnant (i.e., "It won't happen to me"). Some adolescent girls actually plan pregnancy because they believe being pregnant will free them from an intolerable school or home situation or give them someone to love who will also love them back. It puts a tremendous responsibility on a newborn to furnish love and change a girl's life; child maltreatment can occur when the newborn cannot meet such expectations (Seay, Jahromi, Umaña-Taylor, et al., 2016).

As recently as the 1960s, unmarried pregnant girls were sent to a "secret" home or shelter where they would stay throughout their pregnancy, give birth, place the child for adoption, and then return home as if nothing had happened to them. Today, pregnant teenagers typically remain at home, attend prenatal care, and are seen in maternity care facilities the same as older women do. They give birth in birthing rooms at hospitals, and as many as 90% keep their babies (Martin et al., 2015). Few give birth in alternative birth centers because the risk of cephalopelvic disproportion makes adolescent pregnancies high risk. Home birth is not recommended for the same reason. Offering increased guidance during pregnancy and for child care during the following years for adolescents can be an important nursing role.

DEVELOPMENTAL TASKS

Adolescence is a vulnerable time for pregnancy because the developmental tasks of pregnancy are superimposed on those of adolescence. The developmental tasks of the average adolescent are fourfold: to establish a sense of self-worth or a value system, to emancipate from parents, to adjust to a new body image, and to choose a vocation (Erikson, 1963). A girl in the process of separating from her parents may be devastated by the reality that a baby will soon be dependent on her. She may need her parents' financial help to obtain prenatal care or buy clothing for her new baby. If she must depend on her parents' health insurance, she may feel virtually trapped into dependence. Helping adolescents to make their own healthcare decisions at healthcare visits helps to foster a sense of independence in the middle of this forced dependency. Consider, for example, the decision the adolescent must make about where to place a medication reminder chart: If it hangs in the kitchen, her mother may monitor

it; in her bedroom or in her school locker, she alone will monitor it. An adolescent may not be able to choose when she comes for care (her mother has the car to drive her only on Tuesday afternoons), but during a visit, she can do many things to feel independent, such as weigh herself, hold a mirror to view her pelvic examination, or be interviewed apart from her parents.

Parents may have difficulty allowing a daughter to make her own healthcare decisions. Soon, however, she will be caring for an infant, so she needs this practice in independence and responsibility. You may need to remind parents that a pregnant adolescent is regarded as an **emancipated minor** or a *mature minor*—a person capable of making healthcare decisions—and so may sign permission for her own care. In some states, emancipated minors can qualify and are eligible for special health insurance coverage, so issues with privacy, parental permission, and parental notification are avoided. In August 2002, a new federal rule that is based on requirements contained in the Health Insurance Portability and Accountability Act of 1996 (HIPAA) embodies important protections for minors, along with a significant degree of deference to other laws (both state and federal) and to the judgment of healthcare providers. These provisions represent a compromise between competing viewpoints about the importance of parental access to minors' health information and the availability of confidential adolescent healthcare services (Bayer, Santelli, & Klitzman, 2015). The protection of confidentiality for adolescents is based on recognition that some minors would not seek needed health care for such concerns as sexual activity, pregnancy, HIV, STIs, substance abuse, or mental health if they could not receive it confidentially. Forgoing care because of this would have negative health implications for them as well as society. Maintaining privacy for adolescents needs to be especially respected with the introduction of electronic health records (Bayer et al., 2015).

Pregnancy may interfere with the development of a healthy sexual relationship and cause difficulty in establishing future intimate relationships if a girl realizes her current relationship has led to a situation detrimental to her. To prevent this, it is useful to help her view the pregnancy as a growth-producing experience. Most people can point to a day in their life when they "grew up" (perhaps a day a parent became ill or the day they left home for college). This pregnancy can be that "growing up" revelation for a pregnant adolescent.

Establishing a value system or sense of identity can be difficult if healthcare personnel treat a pregnant adolescent as though she is irresponsible. Encouraging her to continue school is crucial to her self-esteem and to her future as well as to the financial future of her unborn child. Many schools have special programs for pregnant adolescents that include aspects of prenatal care to help ensure pregnant adolescents can stay in school.

PRENATAL ASSESSMENT

Adolescents are considered high-risk patients because they have a high incidence of iron-deficiency anemia and premature labor (Box 22.2). They also have a higher incidence of low–birth-weight infants, a disproportion between fetal and pelvic size, and a high rate of intimate partner violence (Kirbas, Gulerman, & Daglar, 2016; Willie, Powell, & Kershaw, 2016). Early and consistent prenatal care is essential to their health and the health of their baby.

BOX 22.2

Nursing Care Planning Using Assessment

ASSESSING THE PREGNANT ADOLESCENT FOR COMPLICATION RISK

Conflicting development crises

High risk for cephalopelvic disproportion

High risk for premature labor

High risk for hemorrhoids

High risk for iron-deficiency anemia

Unfortunately, many adolescents do not seek prenatal care until late in their pregnancies because they may view not seeking prenatal care as a way of protecting the pregnancy—if they don't tell anyone, no one can suggest they terminate the pregnancy. After the sixth month, abortion is no longer a possibility, so a girl can feel free to come for care without being subjected to this pressure.

Other factors contributing to the lack of prenatal care include:

- Denial she is pregnant
- Lack of knowledge of the importance of prenatal care
- Dependence on others for transportation
- Feeling awkward in a prenatal setting (an adult setting)
- Fear of a first pelvic examination
- Difficulty relating to authority figures

A primary nursing or case management approach that minimizes the number of healthcare providers a teenager is exposed to may be the most effective method for providing care during the prenatal period. Some adolescents do well in group prenatal care because it allows them to interact with peers the same as they do at school.

Health History

Take a detailed health history of an adolescent at the first prenatal visit to establish individual risks. This is best done without a parent present. The girl needs practice in being responsible for her own health, and having to account for her health practices can help her do this. It also helps prevent her from fabricating an answer to please a parent.

Some adolescents come to a facility with concerns such as "weight gain" or "feeling tired all the time" rather than saying they are pregnant, hoping healthcare providers will think of pregnancy as a possible reason for their symptoms. This is part denial and part pregnancy protection. Always be alert to the possibility of pregnancy when an adolescent describes symptoms that are vague and hard to define. If the importance of what she is saying when she mentions feeling "tired" or "nauseated" is dismissed, she may ask if someone will feel her stomach. If told this is not necessary for any of the symptoms she has mentioned, she may describe bigger symptoms, such as "terrible stomach pain." Think of possible pregnancy when you hear such a "growing" history.

Many adolescents want to keep their world totally separate from the adult world, and to do so, they do not voluntarily share information with adults. When interviewing adolescents, be certain to press for the responses needed to allow you to assess them safely. Do not accept statements such as "I eat okay" as a nutrition history or "I'm a very active person" as a history of rest and activity. Ask for details.

If an adolescent delayed seeking health care, ask for the reason for this at her first prenatal visit. Acknowledge that "protecting" the pregnancy is a desirable motive, but continuing with prenatal care will be much more beneficial.

If a parent accompanies a girl, ask the parent separately what, if any, concerns he or she wishes to discuss. A young adolescent is still a daughter, and a parent may be very concerned about her health during this pregnancy, as the parent was at health visits when the girl was being seen for a cold or a sports injury. If the baby's father attends prenatal care, help him to feel welcome. Because he is not married, he does not have a legal right to participate in decisions concerning the pregnancy, abortion, or adoption, but because he is at the visit, he likely is invested in his partner or the baby (Garfield, Duncan, Rutsohn, et al., 2014). If he is an adolescent, he may feel sorrow that because of his age, he cannot provide adequately. If a complication occurs, he may feel genuine grief things are not going well. Allowing him to offer support in the current pregnancy can help him learn more about himself as well as better define his role. In addition, be sure he receives compassionate education on preventing further pregnancies until he is more mature.

Often, adolescent girls have not talked to other pregnant women, so they may need extra teaching about common pregnancy symptoms such as urinary frequency, fatigue, and breast tenderness. Asking what symptoms an adolescent is having and reassuring her they are part of a normal pregnancy can help prevent her from attempting to treat them with potentially teratogenic over-the-counter medications.

As pregnancy progresses, listen for signs of "nest-building" behavior. An adolescent girl may not have the financial resources to buy clothing or a crib, but she may reveal nest-building feelings by asking an increasing number of questions about newborns or saving money to buy a simple baby article such as a pair of booties. This may seem like small involvement, but for a young girl without financial means, a dollar a week is actually large involvement.

Some adolescents have difficulty telling their parents about the pregnancy. Role-playing or simulation may be an effective technique to help them prepare to do this. Some girls report on a second visit their parents were not nearly as angry as they had anticipated. Instead, their parents reacted as if they had been waiting to hear this news, having accepted it as inevitable months before.

Family Profile

Adolescents may leave home if their family disapproves of their pregnancy, thus joining the ranks of homeless or adolescent runaways. Others do not leave home, but separate themselves emotionally from their family. Trying to manage by themselves leaves adolescents with a tremendous financial strain and a devastating sense of loneliness. Be sure to ask a girl at prenatal visits where she is living, what the source of her income is, and whom she would call if she suddenly became ill.

Asking about home life may reveal a dysfunctional family or an incest relationship as the cause of the pregnancy. If the girl is under legal age, incest is considered child maltreatment. Know your local and state laws on this topic and make the necessary report.

Because of family relationship problems, a girl may need help in making arrangements for the next few months of her pregnancy and for child care afterward. If she can no longer live at home, is there a relative she may live with? What kind of financial support does she need? Family and social supports for pregnant adolescents have been shown to be important influences on the maintenance of a healthy pregnancy lifestyle and to help prevent low birth weight in their children (Cheng, Rifas-Shiman, Perkins, et al., 2016; Zeiders, Umaña-Taylor, Jahromi, et al., 2015).

Be certain to ask if the girl is planning to continue with school because pregnancy is an egocentric time when outside interests do not always seem important. Help her to see that the months of pregnancy will go by faster if she keeps busy and remaining in school will be a way of doing this. It also is important in preparing for her future because a high school education will be necessary to obtain enough marketable skills to support herself and her baby. Once she has given birth, returning to school may be difficult because she may have child care problems and because she may feel more mature than her classmates (or her classmates may make her feel this way). Any school that obtains federal money cannot discriminate against students because they are physically challenged. Many states interpret pregnancy as physically challenging, so in those states, a girl cannot be forced to leave school (or even asked to go to an alternate school) because of pregnancy. For some girls, you may need to advocate with a school committee for a proper school placement. Box 22.3 shows an interprofessional care map illustrating both nursing and team planning for a pregnant adolescent.

Day History

Adolescents may be unwilling to provide a detailed day history unless its purpose is well explained. Assure a pregnant teenager the purpose of the history is to learn more about her as a whole person, not to discover if she is doing things during the day she should not be doing. Adolescents are private people so to allow you to walk through their adolescent world for a day is a breach of adolescent philosophy. Ask in particular about nutritional practices, sleep, daily activities, use of drugs or alcohol, and whether she has friends who can support her throughout this experience.

Be certain to include questions about her medication history. Ask if she is taking anything over the counter such as cold remedies or herbal supplements. Impress on a girl the importance of not taking any medication—even nonprescription medication—without prior approval from her healthcare provider. It's possible for pregnancy to become an important growth experience if it provides the motivation some adolescents need to withdraw from recreational substance use.

Physical Examination

Physical examination procedures with pertinent adolescent findings are discussed in Chapter 34. Be certain to explain procedures as you do an examination. A statement such as "Oh, you're starting to have colostrum," a positive finding of pregnancy, may be frightening to an adolescent who does not know what colostrum is. A better way to phrase such a finding might be, "Your breasts are not only healthy but already beginning to produce early breast milk. Later on, we'll talk about the importance of that for newborns." This kind of feedback makes a health examination both a learning experience and relieves anxiety for adolescents, who tend to be very concerned about body appearance.

Adolescents may be at an increased risk for gestational hypertension, probably because of immature blood vessels or an immune response to the foreign protein of their fetus (Waugh & Smith, 2012). Few adolescents know what their blood pressure was prior to pregnancy, so they do not know their nonpregnant pressure. Obtain a baseline pressure at the first prenatal visit and make a point of informing the girl of her reading to encourage active healthcare participation in the future. Adolescents are often active in a waiting room (e.g., walking to get a magazine, returning it, or looking out the window); be certain the girl has 15 minutes of rest before you take a blood pressure or the recording may be falsely high.

Use a Doppler technique to obtain fetal heart tones, if possible, because hearing the fetal heart helps an adolescent acknowledge the reality of her pregnancy. For the same reason, make a point of assessing fundal height from visit to visit to show the baby is growing.

Adolescents with a substance dependency may be reluctant to supply a urine specimen for testing because they are worried you are secretly looking for evidence of substance use. In these instances, you may receive a cupful of water in place of a urine specimen. If in doubt regarding the substance you are testing, check the specific gravity. The specific gravity of water is 1.000, whereas urine specific gravity ranges from 1.003 to 1.030. Most adolescents like to weigh themselves at prenatal visits because weight gain in early pregnancy is proof they are pregnant. It is good practice to make a note of the clothing a girl is wearing the first time she is weighed, such as jeans and a T-shirt, so later weight determinations can be compared accurately. Be certain teenagers know a healthy weight gain is important for fetal growth and that this weight can be lost afterward.

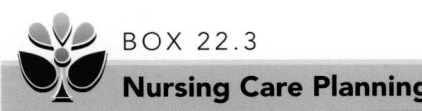

BOX 22.3

Nursing Care Planning

AN INTERPROFESSIONAL CARE MAP FOR A PREGNANT ADOLESCENT

Mindy Carson, 16 years old and 15 weeks pregnant, received a 4-in. laceration on her leg when she was in an automobile accident on her way to the prenatal clinic this morning. The father of Mindy's baby, Carlos, is a college student who does not want Mindy to keep her baby after the birth because he does not want to get married until he finishes graduate school. Mindy insists she is old enough to be a parent and wants to keep her baby. Mindy's mother has accused Carlos of sharing methamphetamine with Mindy. She's also worried Mindy has been working as a prostitute to support a substance habit.

Family Assessment: Lives with family in second-floor apartment above convenience store, which parents own and operate. Is a junior in high school but is "ready to drop out." Cares for 5-year-old sister after school while parents work downstairs.

Patient Assessment: Pale, tired-appearing adolescent female. Failed to come for two previous appointments. Admits to methamphetamine use since becoming pregnant. Hinted she might be using prostitution as income source. Parents want her to end pregnancy; patient wants to continue pregnancy because "Now I can eat anything I want since I'm eating for two." Unhappy with arguing between parents and boyfriend. States, "I'm coming apart at the seams."

Nursing Diagnosis: Altered family processes related to the stress of adolescent pregnancy

Outcome Criteria: Patient and family members demonstrate positive coping mechanisms by communicating effectively; patient identifies plans for self and infant; clarifies relationship desired with father of child. Baby's father (Carlos) participates in pregnancy activities as desired; patient halts risky, unhealthy practices.

Team Member Responsible	Assessment	Intervention	Rationale	Expected Outcome
Activities of Daily Living, Including Safety				
Nurse	Assess the reason patient states she is ready to drop out of school.	Discuss with patient advantages of staying in school during pregnancy.	It is difficult for young women to support themselves and an infant without at least a high school education.	Patient contracts to stay in school through graduation if academically possible.
Teamwork and Collaboration				
Nurse/social worker	Investigate patient's options for schooling if she no longer feels comfortable in her local public school.	Contact the patient's school (with her permission) to explore options for her continued school attendance.	Discussion promotes active problem solving and positive adaptation.	Patient and school personnel agree on a course of action that will optimally benefit the patient.
Nurse/social worker	Assess what community resources are available for withdrawal from methamphetamine.	Discuss the advantages of a withdrawal program during pregnancy.	Almost all substances cross the placenta and reach the fetus.	Patient attends sessions for withdrawal from methamphetamine.
Procedures/Medications for Quality Improvement				
Nurse	Assess what patient expects from prenatal care and if she understands the importance of regular attendance.	Discuss that prenatal care is especially important for adolescents as they are prone to complications because of immature body development.	Prenatal care is the best safeguard against complications of pregnancy and can help ensure early, effective intervention if a complication occurs.	Patient attends all future prenatal care appointments; participates in discussions at these times.
Nutrition				
Nurse/nutritionist	Assess 24-hour dietary recall with patient.	Examine food intake to see if it contains all essential nutrients for pregnancy.	"Eating for two" does not mean eating more; it means eating more nutritious foods.	Patient's 24-hour recall history at next visit shows improvement in nutrients needed during pregnancy.

Continued on following page

BOX 22.3

Nursing Care Planning (continued)

Team Member Responsible	Assessment	Intervention	Rationale	Expected Outcome
Patient-Centered Care				
Nurse	Assess what patient means by "I'm coming apart at the seams" in reference to her lack of support.	Meet with family members (with patient's permission) to see if they could offer more emotional support.	Additional emotional help may be required to cope with the added demands of a teenage pregnancy.	Patient states she is receiving adequate support from a combination of her family, her boyfriend, or healthcare providers.
Psychosocial/Spiritual/Emotional Needs				
Nurse	Assess if patient's disagreement with family over continuing pregnancy is a major stressor.	Assist patient with ways to adapt to changes of pregnancy and responsibility for fetal safety. Support patient's decision to continue pregnancy.	Adolescence is a highly stressful time, especially without parental support, so change can be difficult if not anticipated.	Patient states she is open to changes she knows will occur with pregnancy; will ask healthcare providers for additional suggestions to handle stress as needed.
Informatics for Seamless Healthcare Planning				
Nurse	Assess the best days for patient and boyfriend to attend prenatal care.	Set up follow-up visits with patient and support person; plan teaching strategies and discussion of all parties' needs and concerns as appropriate.	Prenatal care can help detect and prevent complications of pregnancy.	Patient attends prenatal care regularly during remainder of pregnancy.

QSEN Checkpoint Question 22.1

EVIDENCE-BASED PRACTICE

To broaden understanding of the reproductive health education needs of adolescent girls, researchers conducted in-depth interviews with 31 adolescent mothers. These interviews included 15 who experienced a second pregnancy within one year of their first birth and 16 who had not had another pregnancy within 1 year. The group who had not had another pregnancy within a year expressed more independent control of their contraceptive choices than those that had a repeat pregnancy within 1 year. Adolescent mothers should be able to independently make decisions about their contraceptive choices (Conroy, Engelhart, Martins, et al., 2015).

Based on the previous study, if Mindy comes to clinic and tells the nurse her mother will not allow her to make independent decisions about her care, what action would be best?

a. Avoid interfering because the mother is providing helpful input.
b. Tactfully ask the mother to leave the room and then interview Mindy privately.
c. Support Mindy in her attempts to take responsibility for her own care.
d. Supplant Mindy's mother's advice with the nurse's own suggestions that are in Mindy's best interests.

Look in Appendix A for the best answer and rationale.

Nursing Diagnoses and Related Interventions

Nursing Diagnosis: Health-seeking behaviors related to special care necessary for healthy adolescent pregnancy

Outcome Evaluation: Patient states she feels confident in her ability to follow healthy prenatal guidelines to avoid pregnancy complications; asks questions as needed about her pregnancy.

Pregnancy Education

Adolescents usually need a great deal of health teaching during pregnancy because they do not know many of the common measures of care older women have learned from experience. They are also often unwilling to follow healthcare advice that makes them feel different in any way from their peers. However, as adolescents often do not have well-established health practices, they may be extremely adaptable and ready to change health habits for a pregnancy.

Adolescent girls may respond to health teaching that is directed to their own health more than to that of a fetus. A statement such as "Eat a high-protein diet because protein makes your hair shiny [or prevents split fingernails]" often leads to better adherence than a reminder that protein is good for the baby. "Taking the iron supplement should make you feel less tired" might be better than, "It will help build the baby's blood supply," for the same reason. These are truthful statements, and they appeal to an adolescent's preoccupation with self. In addition, this type of health teaching is the only form to which an adolescent who is denying her pregnancy can respond.

Adolescents also need instructions about possible discomforts and changes associated with pregnancy and measures to relieve them (see Chapter 12 for a complete discussion). Many pregnant adolescents, for example, develop hemorrhoids because the disproportion of their body size to a fetus puts extra pressure on pelvic vessels, causing blood to pool in rectal veins. You can assure girls this is a pregnancy-related phenomenon that will resolve when the pregnancy is over.

Adolescents may also develop many striae across the sides of their abdomens because so much stretching of the abdominal skin occurs. Assure them, because of skin elasticity, these marks will probably fade after pregnancy. Chloasma, excess pigment deposition on the face and neck, appears at the same rate in adolescents as in older women. Adolescents, however, may be more conscious of this pigment because, overall, they are more conscious and concerned about their facial appearance. Suggesting a cover makeup and offering reassurance the pigmentation will fade after pregnancy may help.

Nutrition

Good nutrition can be a major problem during an adolescent pregnancy because many girls enter pregnancy with poor nutritional stores from years of eating a less-than-optimal diet. This lack of nutritional stores is serious because, especially in very young adolescents, it can result in preterm births and low–birth-weight newborns. To prevent these complications, a girl should have an intake that both allows for growth of the fetus and also provides for the needs of her own growing body. Otherwise, protein; iron; folic acid; and vitamins A, C, and D deficiencies may become acute. In order to compensate, she may need to gain more weight than a mature woman to supply adequate pregnancy nutrients.

As more and more teenagers are obese today than ever before because of overeating and lack of exercise, many adolescents enter pregnancy overweight or obese. This can lead to macrosomia or overgrowth in a fetus, a situation that leads to an increase in the number of cesarean births (Houde, Dahdouh, Mongrain, et al., 2015). Such adolescents should not actively restrict nutrients during pregnancy; although they are obese, their body may be deficient in protein and vitamins.

Many adolescent girls do not eat well during pregnancy because they simply do not know what constitutes good nutrition. Some girls have little choice in what foods are prepared at home. To change a dietary pattern for these girls, you may have to talk to the person who does the cooking in the family. Besides eating the right amount of food, a pregnant adolescent may need to abandon a food fad she has been following, such as drinking soda, for a glass of orange juice (difficult to do if no one she knows drinks orange juice). The best you may be able to accomplish in this situation is to secure her agreement to switch to noncaffeinated soft drinks.

Remember, if a girl is attending school, she probably eats at least one meal away from home each day, so be certain nutrition education includes how to "brown bag" or buy a nutritious cafeteria lunch (type A school lunches are discussed in Chapter 32). If she travels by school bus, she may leave home by 6:00 AM or 7:00 AM, so she needs suggestions on how to construct a quick but healthy breakfast. Leaving so early creates a second problem of having to wait a long space of time until lunchtime. Suggest midmorning snacks, such as fruit, that also supply vitamins, not just empty calories.

Adolescents traditionally do not take medicine conscientiously, so they may need frequent reminders to take their vitamin or iron supplement. Stress that these are intended to complement nutrition during pregnancy so must not only be purchased but also must be swallowed. For a reminder system, girls may need to post a medication reminder chart at home or in her school locker or to set a reminder on her phone in order to increase adherence.

What If . . . 22.1

Mindy tells the nurse her daily nutrition consists of a liquid diet beverage for breakfast, a salad for lunch, and then cheese pizza for dinner. Will this typical teenage diet be adequate for her during pregnancy?

Activity and Rest

Adolescents vary greatly in their levels of activity. Assess a girl's participation in sports and determine which ones (if any), such as diving, gymnastics, or touch football, may need to be discontinued during pregnancy. Many girls practice sports for the feeling of belonging to a group or for companionship. To prevent her from feeling "shut out" by her friends, you may need to suggest alternative activities such as joining the drama or language club or perhaps inviting friends over once a week to watch a movie so she does not suffer from the loss of companionship.

Planning enough rest time during pregnancy can be yet another area of concern, especially if a girl is acting as if nothing different than usual is happening to her (Box 22.4). If this is so, it may help to explore a typical day and suggest ways to rest without compromising social relationships (e.g., sitting and talking after school rather than walking through the mall).

BOX 22.4

Nursing Care Planning Tips for Effective Communication

You talk to Mindy at a prenatal clinic. She is 16 years old and 15 weeks pregnant, and there is concern that she is using methamphetamines.

Tip: Be careful not to be so intent on giving advice that you forget the first step of effective problem solving: identifying the exact problem that needs solving.

Nurse: Hello, Mindy. How are you feeling?

Mindy: Good, but always tired. You know.

Nurse: Are you getting enough sleep? How about your diet—are you getting enough iron-rich foods?

Mindy: How can I? I work every day after school. I don't always have money for food.

Nurse: Is there anyone who could help you out more? Your boyfriend? A friend?

Mindy: I'm pretty much alone since I got pregnant.

Nurse: As long as you're coming to this clinic, you're not alone. Tell me about a typical day and let's investigate together ways you could get more rest. We can discuss resources to help you get quality food as well.

Physiologic Changes

A young girl may have little knowledge about body functions, so as a rule, all adolescent girls need substantial education on the physiologic changes that will occur during pregnancy. Despite all the health information given to children in school, it is not uncommon to find an adolescent who thinks her baby is growing in her stomach and so is unable to eat large meals for fear of suffocating or drowning her fetus. In addition, specific information about labor and delivery is essential to counteract all the "scare stories" girls may be hearing from their peers. Gaining this type of knowledge is another way pregnancy can be a growth experience. At the end of the pregnancy, this adolescent will know a great deal more about her body and her ability to monitor her health than her average classmate.

Childbirth Preparation

Peer companionship is a strong need for most adolescents. When girls become pregnant, because they are suddenly so different, they may find themselves cut off from fellow classmates. This can make them more inclined, therefore, to join a class of other adolescents in preparation for childbirth. Because being a student is so age appropriate for them, they usually are excellent students in a class. In addition, they have enough childish magical belief operating that they are not skeptical about whether prepared childbirth will work for them. In fact, believing prepared childbirth will work is an important component in a successful prepared childbirth experience, so this becomes a self-fulfilling prophecy.

Birth Decisions

Pelvic measurements should be taken early and carefully in adolescent girls because cephalopelvic disproportion is a real possibility because of the girl's incomplete pelvic growth (Timofeev, Reddy, Huang, et al., 2013). Most girls who are told their baby will have to be born by cesarean birth respond well to the news, and some are actually relieved, because surgery seems controlled and simple compared with the agonies of labor they may imagine. Be certain the information a cesarean birth must be scheduled is shared with the girl and her parents as soon as possible as adolescents want to know the truth. They can regard the withholding of information not as protection but as an indication they are being treated as children.

Plans for the Baby

Adolescents may need additional time at prenatal visits to talk to a good listener about how they feel about being pregnant and becoming a mother. Scared? Bewildered? Numb? Happy? Be certain they know all the options available to them when their baby is born (e.g., keeping the baby, placing the baby in a temporary foster home, adoption). Adolescents, like all women, should be encouraged to breastfeed (Olaiya, Dee, Sharma, et al., 2016). Breast tissue matures with pregnancy, so even very young adolescents are physically capable of breastfeeding.

COMPLICATIONS OF PREGNANCY

As mentioned earlier, adolescent pregnancy carries the increased incidence of iron-deficiency anemia, preterm labor, and cephalopelvic disproportion (see Box 22.2). Fortunately, with conscientious prenatal care, these complications can be minimized.

Iron-Deficiency Anemia

Many adolescent girls are deficient in iron because their low intake cannot balance the amount of iron lost with menstrual flows. Deficiency is revealed by chronic fatigue, pale mucous membranes, and a hemoglobin level less than 11 g/dl. Iron-deficiency anemia is associated with pica, or the ingestion of inedible substances such as blackboard chalk (Lumish, Young, Lee, et al., 2014).

A pregnancy compounds iron-deficiency anemia because a girl must now supply enough iron for fetal growth and her increasing blood volume. All pregnant women should take an iron and folic acid supplement (folic acid is important for red blood cell growth and prevention of neural tube defects), but these are especially important for the adolescent (Menon, Ferguson, Thomson, et al., 2016). Like any other medication prescribed for pregnancy, help an adolescent plan a time each day to take her iron supplement. Review with her how many iron-rich foods she needs to eat daily in addition to this. An iron supplement is not a supplement until her dietary intake is already strong in iron-rich foods.

As soon as her body recognizes it has additional iron, she will begin rapidly forming immature red blood cells. To measure whether the supplemental iron is causing this effect, a reticulocyte count may be scheduled after 2 weeks; if the reticulocyte count is not elevated at this time, it implies a secondary problem exists or, more likely, the girl has not been taking the supplement. Taking a stool swab and assessing it for the black tinge of an iron supplement or reassessing her serum iron level are other methods of assessing for adherence.

Preterm Labor

Adolescents are at high risk for preterm labor, probably because their uteruses are not fully grown (Kirbas et al., 2016). For this reason, review the signs of labor with them by the third month of pregnancy. Stress labor contractions usually begin as only a sweeping contraction no more intense than menstrual cramps. Any vaginal bleeding is suspicious of labor and needs to be reported. Adolescent girls have gained much of their knowledge of labor from television (where a woman suddenly announces she is in labor and within 15 minutes gives birth). Therefore, they may dismiss light contractions as simple discomfort, not realizing they might be the start of labor. If they can recognize labor contractions early, it is more likely premature labor can be halted.

COMPLICATIONS OF LABOR, BIRTH, AND THE POSTPARTUM PERIOD

Cephalopelvic Disproportion

Adolescent labor does not differ from labor in the older woman if cephalopelvic disproportion is absent. The presence of cephalopelvic disproportion is suggested by a lack of engagement at the beginning of labor, a prolonged first stage of labor, and poor fetal descent. Graphing labor progress is an effective way to detect labor that is becoming abnormal or prolonged. Be certain an adolescent has a support person with her in labor so she can relax and breathe effectively with contractions. If this person is also an adolescent, you may need to serve as the true support person, or at least spend considerable time coaching so this person can effectively support the girl in labor.

Postpartum Hemorrhage

Young adolescents are more prone to postpartum hemorrhage than the average woman because, if a girl's uterus is not yet fully developed, it becomes overdistended by pregnancy. An overdistended uterus is more likely not to contract as readily as a normally distended uterus in the postpartum period, thus allowing bleeding to occur (Kawakita, Wilson, Grantz, et al., 2016). Adolescents also may have more frequent or deeper perineal and cervical lacerations than older women because of the size of the infant in relation to their body. Young adolescents, however, are generally healthy and have supple body tissue that allows for adequate perineal stretching. If a laceration does occur, it usually heals readily without complication.

Inability to Adapt Postpartally

Giving birth is such a stress and a major crisis that almost all women have difficulty integrating it into their life. This can make the immediate postpartum period almost an unreal time for an adolescent. A girl may "block out" the hours of labor as if they did not happen. If she was particularly frightened or she received a narcotic for pain, her memory of the labor hours may not be clear. Urge her to talk about labor and birth to make the happening real to her; otherwise, postpartum depression is more apt to occur (Jeha, Usta, Ghulmiyyah, et al., 2015).

Lack of Knowledge About Infant Care

Adolescents show the same positive bonding behavior with their infants as their more mature counterparts (Fig. 22.1). Although they may consider themselves to be knowledgeable in child care because they have babysat for a neighbor's child or a younger sibling, they may lack knowledge of newborn care. They can be overwhelmed in the postpartum period when realizing the baby is their own and child care is not as simple as it seemed. When the child cries, they cannot hand it to someone else; at the end of 4 hours, when they are tired of caring for the baby, they cannot leave and walk away. Although these things were most likely discussed with an

adolescent during pregnancy, these feelings may not become prominent until the child is actually born. Spend time with a girl, observing how she handles her infant. Demonstrate bathing and changing the baby as appropriate. Model good parenting behaviors whenever possible by being aware of how you hold and care for the child.

Unfortunately, most adolescent mothers choose not to breastfeed. This is probably related to a lack of understanding about the importance of breastfeeding, their perception of breastfeeding as something that will "tie them down," and anticipating that this will create a time management conflict when returning to school (Olaiya et al., 2016). Education about the importance of breastfeeding and tips for how to incorporate it into a busy lifestyle can increase the number of adolescents who breastfeed (see Chapter 19). Help young mothers who do not choose to breastfeed to select a feeding method that is satisfying to them and safe for the infant as part of the process of becoming a young, but effective, new mother.

QSEN Checkpoint Question 22.2

INFORMATICS

Mindy was placed on an iron supplement because her hemoglobin level was below normal. What would be the best way to determine if Mindy is taking her iron supplement?
   a. Perform a physical assessment noting if her nail beds have deepened in color.
   b. Ask her to describe in her own words why she has been prescribed an iron supplement.
   c. Look up her laboratory results to see if her reticulocyte count has increased since her last visit.
   d. Analyze her urine for color that would reveal the presence of iron deposits.

Look in Appendix A for the best answer and rationale.

Unfolding Patient Stories: Brenda Patton • Part 2

Recall **Brenda Patton** from Chapter 9, an 18-year-old who is pregnant with her first child. She lives at home with her mother, stepfather, and three siblings (ages 13, 7, and 5 years). She is in a relationship with a boyfriend who is not living in the household. The boyfriend is supportive but uncertain of paternity status. What are the unique family dynamics for a pregnant adolescent and her boyfriend when considering the risks associated with an adolescent pregnancy and the health of the mother and fetus? What assessments and interventions can be incorporated into the nursing plan of care to promote effective prenatal care for an adolescent? What areas of education should the nurse address during prenatal visits?

Care for Brenda and other patients in a realistic virtual environment: *vSim for Nursing* (thepoint.lww.com /vSimMaternityPed). Practice documenting these patients' care in DocuCare (thepoint.lww.com /DocuCareEHR).

Figure 22.1   A new adolescent mother begins to bond with her infant. (Barbara Sauder/Shutterstock.com)

The Pregnant Woman Over Age 40 Years

The incidence of women delaying their first pregnancy until their late 30s or early 40s is increasing so much that 12% of births in the United States today are to women age 35 to 39 years and 3% are to women over age 40 years (Hamilton, Martin, & Osterman, 2015). **Advanced maternal age** is the label for pregnant women 35 years and older at delivery. In the past, it was assumed a woman over 40 years old was past the optimal age for childbearing and so was at risk for many complications. Today, with the exception of a greater incidence of chromosomal abnormality, there is little evidence of serious complications in women older than age 40 years as long as prenatal care is begun early in the pregnancy.

A woman over age 40 years is more likely than a younger woman to enter pregnancy with a previously diagnosed condition, such as hypertension, varicosities, or hemorrhoids. In addition, by age 40 years, a woman usually has a major role change she must undertake during pregnancy, especially if she is well established in a career or has an accustomed routine at home or in her community. During pregnancy, she will need to think through how the pregnancy and childrearing are going to fit into and change her life. Although she may feel rich in the number of support people she perceives around her, she may discover she actually has few "pregnancy support" people because she does not have many friends her age who are also having babies, some even may be close to becoming grandparents. Many of the things these friends remember of pregnancy and labor were their particular highs and lows; the care they received may not reflect current practice. This can leave a woman without access to the daily "shop talk" of other pregnant women or someone to turn to with questions such as whether the backache she is experiencing or frequent need to urinate is normal. On the other hand, because many women delay childbearing today, she may be one of a sizable group of women in her community experiencing pregnancy at this stage of life. For this reason, be certain to assess each woman individually (Box 22.5).

BOX 22.5

Nursing Care Planning to Respect Cultural Diversity

What is perceived as the best time in life to have children is strongly culturally influenced. In developing countries, for example, many people believe having children while young allows parents to grow with children. In other cultures, such as the United States, many believe delaying childbirth until a family is financially secure is best. Because of these various beliefs, what you believe about the perfect time to have a baby may not be the belief of a family for whom you provide care. What may seem like a catastrophe in timing to you may seem like a blessing to someone else (and vice versa). Assess couples by history and observation to determine if childbearing appears to be timed correctly for them. If not, they may need extra time to accept a pregnancy and adapt to becoming parents.

DEVELOPMENTAL TASKS AND PREGNANCY

The developmental challenge of the over-40-years-old age group is to expand their awareness or develop **generativity**— that is, a sense of moving away from themselves and becoming involved with the world or community (Erikson, 1963). Some people assume that once they reach adulthood, the way they are is the way they will always be. They are amazed to find not only do their bodies change (men may lose their hair; women and men both gain weight) but so do their interests. They may now find themselves joining committees and clubs, coaching Little League teams, or organizing fundraising or community events—activities they shunned when younger.

This can cause a woman in this age group who is pregnant to begin to feel ambivalent during the pregnancy because she may want to continue with community activities yet also want to concentrate on the baby growing inside her. Encouraging her to discuss how this conflict feels can help her balance her life and manage two life phases this way.

Women who are having a child after age 40 years tend to fall into one of two groups: those who are having their final child and those who have delayed childbearing because of education or a career and are having their first child. Many adults over the age of 40 years care for aging parents and so may also be dealing with the issues of older adults. These additional responsibilities and obligations can make it difficult for a woman to complete the psychological work of pregnancy. It also may create extra strain on her finances and time and it creates a "sandwich generation," or one pressured by responsibilities by both older and younger family members. Important worries include having enough energy, arranging for child care, and financial and space strains.

PRENATAL ASSESSMENT

A woman over age 40 years, like all women, should begin prenatal care early in pregnancy. A few mistakenly believe their lack of menstruation is the result of early menopause and so do not seek an early healthcare consultation. Fortunately, most women of this age group recognize what is happening, are well informed about the advisability of early prenatal care, and also have adequate health insurance, so they do seek an early appointment.

Health History

Ask women in this age group to document their symptoms of pregnancy, how they feel about the pregnancy, and how it fits into their lifestyle. If a woman did not realize she was pregnant, she may have self-medicated. Ask if she has been taking any medication or herbal remedies to relieve symptoms such as nausea or fatigue. Because a woman is functioning well in a business world does not mean she follows a healthy pregnancy lifestyle. Do not accept answers such as "I drink socially" or "I take the usual drugs" without exploring what those phrases specifically mean.

Family Profile

Some women over age 40 years who are pregnant for the first time have recently changed their life pattern (e.g., become married or became involved in a long-term sexual relationship) or have decided to have a child, perhaps through in vitro fertilization, without a spouse before they are no longer able to conceive. Whereas a younger woman often waits a while after marrying or beginning a relationship with a new partner to become pregnant, a woman over age 40 often plans to become pregnant immediately because she senses her reproductive time clock ticking. Because of this, she may find herself making many adjustments at once (not only to a new life partner, house or apartment, and perhaps community, but also to a pregnancy).

Be certain to identify a woman's source of income. If she has a well-paying job, stopping work because of a pregnancy complication could greatly reduce her family's income. Also evaluate how many people are financially or emotionally dependent on her, such as children from a former marriage, elderly parents, an elderly neighbor, or fellow workers who count on her. During pregnancy, when a woman often needs extra emotional support, feeling responsible for so many people can complicate the pregnancy.

Day History

Ask specifically about a woman's type of work or home responsibilities and estimate the amount of walking or back strain those entail. Ask about recent diet or exercise programs. If a woman belongs to a health club, remind her the use of saunas and hot tubs for longer than 10 minutes at a time is contraindicated during pregnancy because of possible hyperthermia and teratogenic effects of extreme heat on a developing fetus (Agopian, Tinker, Lupo, et al., 2013). Identify personal habits, such as cigarette smoking and alcohol consumption, which could be detrimental to a fetus to determine if counseling to halt or decrease these habits is needed.

Physical Examination

A woman over age 40 years needs a thorough physical examination at her first prenatal visit to establish her general health and to identify any problems, particularly circulatory disturbances, she may have. Inspect her lower extremities thoroughly for varicosities because these are more common in women over age 40 years (Box 22.6). Obtain a urine specimen and test it for specific gravity, glucose, and protein to evaluate overall renal function and the possibility of gestational or type 2 diabetes because older women are more prone than younger women to develop these conditions.

Assess a woman's breasts for any abnormalities, as women over age 40 years are in a higher risk group for breast cancer than are younger women. In addition, as gestational trophoblastic disease (hydatidiform mole) is also more common in women over age 40 years (see Chapter 21), assess carefully for fundal height and fetal movement at prenatal visits.

Chromosomal Assessment

Because the risk for Down syndrome is higher in older women than in younger women, an incidence of about 1 in 100 compared to 1 in 350 women over 35 years, genetic screening is offered to detect if an open spinal cord or chromosomal defect could be present in the fetus. These tests include an ultrasound to examine for nuchal translucency (seen in chromosomal abnormalities) and an analysis of maternal serum levels of α-fetoprotein (MSAFP), pregnancy-associated plasma protein A (PAPP-A), and free beta human chorionic gonadotropin (hCG) to evaluate for chromosomal disorders in the fetus. These tests are done at 11 to 13 weeks.

Women over the age of 35 years may be offered a more accurate noninvasive blood test, circulating free DNA (cfDNA) testing, to screen for chromosomal disorders as early as 10 weeks of gestation. Additionally, chorionic villi sampling (CVS) and amniocentesis are both techniques that may be offered to women who are older than 35 years of age to diagnose chromosomal genetic disorders. The CVS and amniocentesis are diagnostic tests (rather than screening tests); they assess the actual karyotype of the fetus to give a definite answer about the presence or absence of chromosomal disorders. Between 15 and 20 weeks gestation, the MSAFP test is repeated to identify if the fetus is at risk for open neural tube defects (Fletcher & Russo, 2015) (see Chapter 8).

Be certain a woman is prepared for these studies and receives support during them. Alert her that false-positive results can occur; to limit these, positive reports will be confirmed through a chromosomal analysis obtained by CVS or amniocentesis. Some women of this age group do not begin nest building until these tests are completed and they've been assured their child will be healthy.

BOX 22.6

Nursing Care Planning Based on Family Teaching

TIPS ON PREVENTING VARICOSE VEINS

Q. Mindy says to you, "My mother was older when she had me so developed terrible varicose veins. How can I stop that from happening to me?"

A. Although the following activities are not foolproof, incorporating them into your day helps prevent the development of varicose veins.

- Find opportunities, such as a class or lunch break, to elevate your legs on a foot stool.
- Be certain your diet includes vitamin C every day because this is important to strengthen vein walls.
- Rest in a side-lying position with your body tipped slightly forward (Sims position) as this allows leg veins to drain and empty.
- Avoid long periods of standing in one place; take "walk breaks" as active muscle contraction help venous return.
- Avoid sitting with your legs crossed.
- Do not wear anything constricting on your lower legs, such as knee-high stockings.
- If you're prescribed support hose, put them on before you get out of bed in the morning, before veins become swollen, for best results. Don't be fooled into thinking panty hose marked "strong support" are the same as medically prescribed support stockings.

Nursing Diagnoses and Related Interventions

Nursing Diagnosis: Health-seeking behaviors related to special care necessary for healthy pregnancy

Outcome Evaluation: Patient states she feels confident in self-care and her ability to decrease possible complications of pregnancy.

Be certain to adapt prenatal teaching to fit an older woman's lifestyle. If she had not planned on ever being pregnant, she may have isolated herself through the years from "mothering" activities and so, despite her years, may know little about pregnancy and newborn care. Others may have read so extensively that they may know more theoretical information than a woman who has already given birth. Be certain to review information about possible discomforts of pregnancy (see Chapter 12). A pregnant woman over age 40 years, for example, is prone to hemorrhoids because she may have some rectal varicosities present at the beginning of pregnancy. Pain from rectal distention may, in fact, be one of the primary symptoms she reports at a first visit. Review measures to increase comfort from these (see Chapter 12).

Varicosities, like hemorrhoids, develop readily in a woman over age 40 years because she may have had some tendency toward these even before the pregnancy. As with hemorrhoids, her best approach during pregnancy is to prevent formation of these. At the time of birth, be certain to document any degree of varicosity formation so nurses caring for her during the postpartum period can take special precautions to prevent thrombophlebitis because, as with venous stasis present after birth, a woman with varicosities is prone to develop this complication immediately postpartum.

PREGNANCY EDUCATION

Nutrition

Assess the number of meals a woman eats outside her home each week, including those she packs for lunch or eats in restaurants. If she enjoys many of these, she may need tips on how to obtain the same nutrition whether she prepares meals at home or eats them at an office or community function. Urge her to substitute a caffeine-free soft drink in place of an alcoholic beverage at social events. In the same way, substitute milk or juice or decaffeinated coffee for regular coffee. Some women this age normally drink little milk. Rather than getting used to milk again, a woman might appreciate suggestions on other ways to ingest calcium, such as puddings or yogurt or ask her healthcare provider for a calcium supplement.

Prenatal Classes

Because a pregnant woman over age 40 years may be unique in her circle of friends, she may be very interested in joining a childbirth preparation or prenatal exercise class where she is "one of the group" (Fig. 22.2).

Such classes for this age group often center on how to avoid complications such as varicosities, how to integrate pregnancy

Figure 22.2 Exercise classes during pregnancy can provide women with an opportunity to interact with others like themselves while benefiting from a carefully monitored workout. (wavebreakmedia/Shutterstock.com)

with a full-time work position, and supplying discussion time on how women are reacting to this dramatic life change. Be certain a woman or couple plan to set aside a specific time every day to do breathing exercises to be prepared for labor. Otherwise, a busy woman may never find time to get to them and will find herself unprepared in labor.

COMPLICATIONS OF PREGNANCY

The complications of pregnancy most likely to occur in a woman over age 40 years—gestational hypertension, preterm or postterm birth, and cesarean birth—are related to the fact that the woman's circulatory system may not be as competent as when she was younger or her body tissues may not be as elastic as they were once (Box 22.7).

Gestational Hypertension

A woman over age 40 years has a higher risk for gestational hypertension than a younger woman because of blood vessel inelasticity, because hypertension tends to occur more frequently in nulliparas than in multiparas, and because some degree of hypertension may already exist before pregnancy (Ben-David et al., 2016). At any age, the best way to reduce the symptoms of gestational hypertension is for women to take in an adequate supply of protein and obtain adequate rest each day. If a woman works full-time, stopping work to obtain more rest may be difficult not only because she believes she may miss out on a promotion or risk losing her job but also because her income is important to her family; she also is used to being productive, not merely resting all day. To allow her to rest effectively, you may need to help her plan activities she can accomplish on bed rest, such as reworking a school course outline or restructuring her office filing system.

COMPLICATIONS OF LABOR, BIRTH, AND THE POSTPARTUM PERIOD

Complications that occur with a woman over age 40 years related to birth or the immediate period after birth also may be due to the body, which may not be as elastic as it once was.

BOX 22.7

Nursing Care Planning Using Assessment

ASSESSING THE PREGNANT WOMAN OVER 40 YEARS OF AGE FOR COMPLICATIONS

- Gestational hypertension
- Cesarean birth
  Postterm birth
  Preterm birth
- Hemorrhoids
- Varicose veins, thrombophlebitis

Failure to Progress in Labor

Labor in an older primipara may be prolonged because cervical dilatation does not seem to occur as spontaneously as it does in younger women. Graphing labor progress is a good method to use to determine when labor is becoming prolonged. Many women this age may need a cesarean birth if labor becomes so overly prolonged it begins to place a fetus at risk. Encourage a woman to verbalize how she is feeling about her progress throughout labor to allow for reassurance and prompt intervention should problems arise.

Difficulty Accepting the Event

Women over age 40 years may begin to have second thoughts about childbearing this late in life as the reality of a new baby registers with them during the intrapartal and postpartum periods. Although they may have read a great deal about babies during pregnancy, they may state they wish they had read more or felt as confident with this phase of their life as they are about other areas such as their home, office, or classroom.

Review plans for child care and postpartum rest, with an emphasis on helping women learn to balance their lives, especially if they are planning on returning to work soon after the birth. They might appreciate help making child care arrangements. You can assure them well-organized day care programs for preschool children have positive socialization and perhaps nutrition and exercise results (Santos, Daniel, Fernandes, et al., 2015).

Postpartum Hemorrhage

Just as the cervix may not dilate as readily during labor due to inelasticity, the uterus may not contract as readily in the postpartum period. The result of this puts women over 40 years of age at higher risk for postpartum hemorrhage (Debost-Legrand, Rivière, Dossou, et al., 2015). She also may be more prone to perineal–anal tears because her perineum is less supple (Richards, Flanagan, Littman, et al., 2016). Because a woman over age 40 years may be an independent woman who is interested in self-care, she may ask for little help. Respect her need for independence, but at the same time, don't neglect assessing the amount of lochial flow or potential perineal bleeding to be certain these complications are detected.

QSEN Checkpoint Question 22.3

QUALITY IMPROVEMENT

Women over the age of 40 years are at increased risk for developing gestational hypertension. As a result, routine screenings for this health problem have been emphasized on the maternal unit for older mothers. What is the rationale for this change in nursing practice?
  a. Many women over 40 years are underweight before they begin pregnancy.
  b. Older women tend to have a higher fluid intake than do younger women.
  c. Many older women are prone to edema due to their lower activity levels.
  d. The blood vessels of older women may not be as elastic as those of younger women.

Look in Appendix A for the best answer and rationale.

The Pregnant Woman Who Is Physically or Cognitively Challenged

In the past, women with conditions such as vision, hearing, cognitive, neurologic, or orthopedic challenges were sheltered by their families to such an extent women with even moderately physically challenging conditions could not meet potential sexual or marriage partners and so didn't become pregnant. In addition, many people believed this was right or that these individuals should not become pregnant. Today, women with varying degrees of disability attend public school, work in offices, join community organizations, establish sexual relationships, and plan pregnancies just like everyone else.

It is important to urge women with physical or cognitive disabilities to begin with preconception care so medicines they are taking can be evaluated, and careful planning for safe pregnancy care can be started early (H. K. Brown et al., 2016). Because these women (and in some instances, also their support persons) face special problems related to their conditions, nursing care during pregnancy must be designed with these special concerns in mind so the woman's and her family's challenges and needs can be addressed and met (H. K. Brown et al., 2016).

Table 22.1 lists general areas of care that are important in planning for the pregnant woman who is physically or cognitively challenged.

RIGHTS OF THE PHYSICALLY OR COGNITIVELY CHALLENGED PERSON

There are ethical and legal considerations related to women with disabilities. By federal law, persons who are physically disabled must have freedom of access to public buildings by means of ramps or handrails (U.S. Equal Employment Opportunity Commission [USEEOC], 1990). All public healthcare facilities must be in compliance with these laws both in terms of physical facilities and in the true spirit of the law; that is, people should be made to feel psychologically welcome as well as physically able to access the inside of the building. Under the same law, a hospital cannot deny care to a person with a disability even though the disabling condition complicates treatment considerably, possibly requiring extra personnel and time. A woman with a disability has full rights to her child, so the baby cannot be taken from her at birth without her full consent. Likewise, she cannot be forced to terminate a pregnancy or undergo sterilization unless that is her informed decision.

MODIFICATIONS FOR PREGNANCY

Explore with women with a disability at a first prenatal visit the exact nature of their disability and their general self-image to identify what modifications they may need you to plan for care during pregnancy. Some women who are physically or cognitively challenged maintain high self-esteem despite severe limitations and are able to modify and grow with a pregnancy, whereas others have a poor sense of self-esteem that could make change particularly difficult for them. However, for most women, pregnancy will become a special event, a 9-month announcement to everyone that despite their seeming limitations, they are equal to other women and so are capable of participating in one of life's miracles. If a woman is housebound, be certain she is prescribed a prenatal vitamin containing vitamin D and can obtain refills because she is probably not receiving as much sun exposure as those who spend some time outside (Eggemoen, Falk, Knutsen, 2016).

Safety Measures to Explore

Safety is a key area of concern for a pregnant woman who is physically or cognitively challenged. Be certain to assess areas such as if she has emergency contact persons, suppliers of transportation, and individual considerations such as mobility, elimination, and possible autonomic responses. Be certain a woman reviews any medicine she is taking for her primary condition with her pregnancy care provider to be certain this will continue to be safe during pregnancy. Women with recurrent seizures, for example, may need to have their dose of antiseizure medicine reduced during pregnancy because some of these are teratogenic (Laganà, Triolo, D'Amico, et al., 2015).

Emergency Contacts

Evaluate the patient's ability to contact someone in case of a pregnancy-related emergency. Does she have a telephone she can reach readily? Does she know how to activate the emergency medical system (911) in her community? If a woman's speech is not clear, evaluate whether she will be understood while using a telephone to call for help in an emergency. Some women with limited mobility, such as those with a spinal cord injury or cerebral palsy, have a specially designed telephone contact system in their home that connects to a paramedic or hospital emergency service through a beeper system. Check that they intend to maintain this throughout pregnancy. Some women who are hearing challenged use a specially equipped telephone (a telecommunications device for the deaf [TDD]) that prints out messages for them.

TABLE 22.1 AREAS OF PLANNING WITH WOMEN WHO ARE PHYSICALLY OR COGNITIVELY CHALLENGED DURING PREGNANCY

Area	Assessment and Planning Guidelines
Transportation	Ask if a woman has access to transportation for prenatal care and for emergencies.
Pregnancy counseling	Assess the special modifications of care that will need to be made depending on a woman's special challenge. Use additional visual or auditory aids to make your teaching points clear.
Support person	Determine the woman's main support person. In some instances, a woman's condition requires so much assistance during pregnancy you may need to contact community agencies to lend additional support (with her permission).
Health	Do not lose track of a woman's primary health problem. For example, a woman with cerebral palsy may need to continue an active muscle exercise program during pregnancy; a woman with multiple sclerosis may need to change her medication to avoid teratogenic effects.
Work	Assess whether a woman works outside her home and, if work is discontinued during pregnancy, what she could substitute for social contacts.
Recreation	Assess whether a woman's level of activity is adequate, and make concrete suggestions within her limitations if it needs to be increased.
Self-esteem	Assess a woman's level of self-esteem. If it is low, give praise at prenatal visits and help her make pregnancy a growth experience.

Transportation

Assess a patient's ability to come for prenatal care. If a woman depends on a support person for transportation to a healthcare facility, you may have to arrange appointments according to that person's schedule to prevent missed appointments. Ask the woman, in an emergency, if that person is not available, how could she come for care? Women with cognitive or vision challenges, for example, may not qualify for a driver's license and so may need someone, such as a family member or friend, to drive. Women with a mobility challenge may have difficulty transferring into the specially equipped, hand-controlled car they usually drive as pregnancy progresses.

Mobility

All women who use wheelchairs are taught to press with their hands against the armrests and lift their buttocks up off the wheelchair seat for 5 seconds every hour to prevent the formation of pressure ulcers on the buttocks and posterior thighs. Encourage pregnant women to continue to perform this maneuver during pregnancy as the increased weight of a fetus increases her risk for pressure ulcer formation from

Figure 22.3 During pregnancy, a woman who is physically challenged may need to use a wheelchair to help safeguard herself against injury. Assure her that she may still enjoy her independence and daily activities, such as caring for an older child. (Lorena Fernandez/Shutterstock.com)

additional compression. In addition, severe hip flexion from sitting in a wheelchair limits venous return from the lower extremities. For at least 1 hour every morning and afternoon, encourage women who ambulate by wheelchair to decrease the sharp bend at their knees and hips that results from sitting in the chair, to promote venous return and help prevent varicosities and thrombi formation. Resting on a couch for a time or adjusting the footrests of the wheelchair so her legs are not as sharply bent accomplishes this.

If maintaining balance is a problem, a woman may need reevaluation at the midpoint of pregnancy because as the weight of her abdomen increases, she becomes less stable. She may need to use crutches if she did not use them before, or use a wheelchair if she was ambulatory with crutches or a walker before pregnancy. Keep in mind a woman who is physically challenged achieved the degree of ambulation with which she first presents usually only after years of physical therapy and strengthening of leg and arm muscles. Help her see that reducing her degree of independence during pregnancy is not a step backward for her but a step forward, allowing her to have a safe pregnancy without the danger of falling (Fig. 22.3).

Elimination

When mobility is an effort, a woman may not drink as much as usual or use a bathroom as frequently as she would if those actions were effortless. Encourage a high fluid intake and frequent voiding, however, to prevent urinary tract infections. Women who use an indwelling catheter are at especially high risk for contracting urinary tract infections at any time and especially during pregnancy. Women who perform self-catheterization or change their own indwelling catheter may be unable to continue to do this late in pregnancy because the increasing size of their abdomen interferes with their ability to see or reach their perineum comfortably. If this happens, it may be necessary for a woman to arrange for a support person, a home care nurse, or a home health aide to do this for her.

Autonomic Responses

In a woman who has a high spinal cord injury (cervical or high thoracic), observe for **autonomic dysreflexia** during pregnancy, labor, and the immediate postpartum period. This is an exaggerated autonomic response to stimuli. Any irritating condition, such as a distended bladder, increasing uterine size, labor contractions, or breastfeeding, may initiate the response (Castro, Lourenço, & Carrilho, 2014). Without upper motor neuron control to reverse the phenomenon, extreme symptoms such as severe hypertension (300/160 mmHg), throbbing headache, flushing of the skin and profuse diaphoresis above the level of the spinal lesion, nausea, and bradycardia may occur. Immediate action is necessary to protect against a cerebrovascular accident or intraocular damage. Elevate a woman's head to reduce cerebral pressure and locate the irritating stimulus (usually a distended bladder or bowel). If bladder distention is the cause, the woman needs bladder pressure relieved by catheterization if an indwelling catheter is not in place. If a catheter is in place, check to see why it is not draining, then encourage it to drain by unkinking or flushing to allow urine to flow freely again. Anticipate the need for an antihypertensive agent to alleviate the extreme hypertension, although as soon as the source of irritation is removed, symptoms typically fade quickly.

Prenatal Care Modifications to Meet Specific Needs

Physical examination may need to be modified depending on individual circumstances for women with disabilities (H. K. Brown et al., 2016). Although women with disabilities have been followed by healthcare providers most of their lives, they may never have had a pelvic examination before and so need clear instructions about why it is needed and what it will consist of. Many obstetric examining tables are built for the comfort of the examiner and are too high for a woman to transfer to from a wheelchair by simply sliding onto the table. You may need to secure a ramp from the physical therapy department so the wheelchair can be elevated to the level of the table. Woman with a spinal cord injury or cerebral palsy may be unable to maintain their legs in a lithotomy position because of either hip flexion contracture or laxness of leg support. This means a dorsal recumbent position, rather than a lithotomy position, may be required for a pelvic examination.

Women who are cognitively challenged may not be aware of how they became pregnant. If a woman became pregnant because she was taken advantage of sexually, she may need some time to talk and work through this experience before she can agree to a pelvic examination.

If a woman who is visually challenged brings a guide dog with her to a healthcare visit, remember that although the dog's chief function is to offer direction, its instinct causes it to become a woman's protector. Resist petting guide dogs as this may be interpreted by the dog as a threat because it creates a distraction from safeguarding its owner.

When interviewing or teaching visually challenged women, be certain not to use your hands to illustrate points ("I'll need a urine sample of at least this much urine [measured with your fingers]"). Do not use colors as descriptions of objects ("Put on the blue gown"). Use demonstration aids that allow a woman to feel or touch instead. When helping with or performing a physical assessment, let a woman know you are closing the door or drawing a curtain to ensure privacy. Always alert a woman when you are going to touch her, so as not to startle her. Otherwise, you may find yourself facing a growling guide dog that rises to protect her.

If a woman is hearing impaired, she may not be able to see the examiner's face during a pelvic examination. This means any question asked of her during this time will not be understood because she cannot see the examiner's lips to lip read (H. L. Brown, Hughes-Bell, & McDuffie, 2015). Stand by the head of the table and repeat instructions or questions as necessary.

Pregnancy Education

Try to modify health teaching to meet each woman's specific needs. For a woman who is cognitively challenged, for example, instructions about pregnancy may need to be given to her care provider. Those specifically for her might be limited to those few items crucial for safety, such as "Do not drink alcohol or take any medicines except your vitamin pill."

If a woman and her support person are both visually challenged, pamphlets about pregnancy care will not be useful. If the support person can see, offer the pamphlets to him or her, suggesting the support person read them to the pregnant woman as a shared activity. This will not only be helpful to her but will also make the partner a more informed support person. Many visually challenged women have assistive technology

devises such as special audio apps that record and play audio files. Nurses can contact the local branch of the national nonprofit organization Learning Ally (formerly Recording for the Blind and Dyslexic; http://www.learningally.org/) and ask if they have any material already recorded on pregnancy or breastfeeding they can supply. If not, you may be able make an audio file on the assistive technology device, including any information you particularly want a woman to remember or that she seems concerned about. Supply the healthcare facility telephone number at the beginning of the recording as an easy reminder for an emergency and perhaps the date of her next visit as well.

Nutritional education is another area that should be designed based on each patient's specific challenges and usual routine. For example, a woman may only be able to prepare meals that do not require a stove unless her support person is with her. Nutrition counseling, therefore, needs to center on foods that can be prepared without cooking or only microwave warmed.

Activity and exercise, important for any pregnant woman, are just as crucial for a woman who is physically challenged. If exercise is likely to be very reduced in bad weather because she cannot walk safely on slippery snowy sidewalks, be certain a woman understands walking around her home or apartment can provide the same level of exercise as if she were walking around the block or exercising at a health club. Although labor and her child's birth may be modified somewhat because of a physical condition, gaining general knowledge about labor and birth and participating in a shared experience with her partner in a childbirth preparation class are still valuable. If a woman does not have many outside contacts, she may be the person in the class who has the most time to practice breathing exercises and is able to be the most adept at using such a method to control pain in labor.

The woman who is severely hearing challenged usually has heard the many television announcements on not smoking or drinking alcohol during pregnancy because she uses closed captioning. Be certain, however, that she is as aware of this as others. Likewise, if the woman depends on lip reading, be certain she is deciphering new words such as amniotic, gestation, or edema. It often helps to show her the printed words so she can see what your lip motion represents when presenting new pregnancy terms. If a woman speaks with sign language and brings an interpreter with her to translate, be certain to talk to her, not the interpreter, when interviewing.

MODIFICATIONS FOR LABOR AND BIRTH

Women who are physically or cognitively challenged usually need a few adaptations in preparation for labor and birth. Helpful suggestions include:

- A woman with a spinal cord injury may not be able to feel uterine contractions. Late in pregnancy, she will need to palpate her abdomen periodically for tightening or the presence of contractions so she is aware of beginning labor.
- Women with muscle spasticity or spinal cord injury may not be able to push effectively for the second stage of labor and so may need a cesarean or forceps birth.
- Birth from a Sims or dorsal recumbent position is usually best as this avoids a lithotomy position (true for all women).

- Braille watches used by persons who are visually challenged may not have second hands. This means they may need to time the length of contractions by counting their length rather than timing them by a watch.
- During labor, the woman who is hearing challenged cannot hear information on how she is progressing if you are not directly facing her. If she needs to communicate with her support person in sign language, act as an advocate to keep her hands unencumbered by equipment such as an intravenous line. Remember she cannot hear her infant cry at birth. Hand the infant to her as soon as possible after birth so she can see and feel the baby is crying and breathing well.
- Be certain to identify the usual sounds of birthing rooms (the beeping of a monitor, the swish of a central supply routing system, and so forth) for the visually challenged woman as hearing sounds and not being able to identify them can be frightening.

MODIFICATIONS FOR POSTPARTUM CARE

After birth, be certain to assess and teach:
- Whether a woman needs additional support to be successful at breastfeeding.
- Whether she has a return appointment for both herself and her infant for follow-up care; also that the arrangements are within her capabilities, transportation, and understanding.
- Whether she desires contraceptive information and what would be best for her individual circumstances.

Women with disabilities generally feel a need to space pregnancies, but their choices of contraceptive methods can vary widely (Fouquier & Camune, 2015). A woman with poor hand control, for example, might not be able to effectively insert a diaphragm; a woman who is cognitively challenged might not understand the importance of taking an oral contraceptive every day.

Modifications for Planning Child Care

Allow ample time during the first days after birth for mother–child interaction. For example, after birth, a woman who is cognitively challenged may need extra time to understand the transition from "being pregnant" to "having a baby." She may have difficulty learning to judge when her infant is hungry. She may need extra supervision to be certain she does not leave the baby unprotected on a bed. A woman with a spinal cord disability may be particularly interested in inspecting her baby's back. A visually challenged woman will probably want to reassure herself her baby can see. Provide generous time during which she can touch her baby and feel for intact body parts. In contrast, a couple who are hearing challenged may not be pleased to learn their baby can hear as they want the child to be as comfortable as they are in their nonhearing world (Paradis & Koester, 2015). Point out other features such as pretty eyes or long hair to help with bonding.

Breastfeeding has special advantages for women who are physically or cognitively challenged because it is the method of feeding that is not only best for the baby but also requires the least preparation effort on a mother's part. For a woman who is visually challenged and unable to read printed instructions, breastfeeding eliminates formula errors. For a woman who is mobility challenged, it eliminates trips to the refrigerator. Breastfeeding may not be possible for a woman with muscle spasticity, however, because the let-down reflex, which depends on muscle relaxation, may not occur. Be certain women who are cognitively challenged understand they need to feed until the infant is satisfied, not until they are tired of feeding.

Some women will need a referral for home care follow-up and possibly the use of a home health aide to ensure safe child care. Encourage them to think through what baby care equipment will be best for them. Some crib rails lower by pressure on a foot pedal, for example. Others are activated by a waist-high lever. A woman who ambulates by wheelchair usually finds the waist-high lever most convenient because she can reach this most easily. A woman who is hearing impaired needs a flashing rather than a buzzing baby care monitor.

If a woman has difficulty with mobility, ask how she anticipates carrying her infant. Using an anterior baby sling usually works well for the mother who uses a wheelchair. Women who are mobile by crutches or a walker can place the baby in a small wagon and pull it if a sling makes their balance unstable. Some women lie on their back on the floor, place the baby on their chest, and scoot across the floor. The important point is not how a woman carries her baby but that she has thought through a safe and comfortable way to do this.

All parents need to make eye contact with newborns, so urge a visually challenged woman to remember to do this when talking to her infant. If she ordinarily doesn't turn on the lights in her home, encourage her to develop a habit of doing that after dinner because her infant will need light to develop vision. If her support person is also visually challenged, suggest she check with a close friend or neighbor monthly to ensure that light bulbs have not burned out.

One of the biggest worries for the woman who is hearing impaired is she will not be able to hear her baby crying. Help her plan to bring the infant's crib or bassinet close to her bed so she can feel the vibration of the baby's stirring and waking. If the baby hears, urge her to talk to her infant as she gives care so the baby is introduced to sounds and words. A woman whose speech is severely affected by her hearing disorder may be reluctant to speak to strangers. Assure her that her infant welcomes the sound of her voice and will quiet readily to the sound. The child may develop her speech pattern because of this. Being spoken to and sung to during the first year is important for overall development, however, so this is still preferable to living in a world of silence.

Some women who are cognitively challenged may have been raised in a group home and only recently moved to their own apartment. Unlike those raised at home, they may have unusual difficulty making plans for child care because they have never seen the care of young children. You have a legal obligation to investigate whether a newborn will receive safe care before hospital discharge. Be certain to ask enough questions so you are sure a woman who is severely cognitively challenged, for example, has a responsible friend or partner to help her with child care.

QSEN Checkpoint Question 22.4

PATIENT-CENTERED CARE

Mindy makes friends with another adolescent at the prenatal clinic: a 19-year-old who has a cognitive deficit.

When planning care for this patient, what would be the best way to meet this woman's educational needs?

a. Provide simple, written materials rather than providing verbal instructions.

b. Provide education to the woman's partner or another person with full cognitive function.

c. Ensure that teaching is appropriate to the woman's level of cognition.

d. Enlist the help of a social worker when teaching the woman.

Look in Appendix A for the best answer and rationale.

A Woman Who Is Substance Dependent

Substance dependence is a growing health problem in women of childbearing age, so its incidence during pregnancy is also increasing. The number of women who use illicit substances during pregnancy is unknown, but as many as 375,000 infants may be affected yearly. As many as 10% to 20% of pregnant women admit using illicit substances during pregnancy (NCHS, 2012). Common illicit substances used are marijuana, cocaine, and methamphetamine. Adolescents have an increased rate of inhalant abuse and binge drinking.

Substance abuse is defined as the inability to meet major role obligations, an increase in legal problems or risk-taking behavior, or exposure to hazardous situations because of an addicting substance. A person is **substance dependent** when he or she has withdrawal symptoms following discontinuation of the substance, combined with abandonment of important activities, spending increased time in activities related to the substance use, using substances for a longer time than planned, or continued use despite worsening problems because of substance use. Typically, substance-dependent women are late adolescents as the overall incidence of substance use is highest in this group. Any woman could be substance dependent, however, so all pregnant women need to be assessed for the possibility of substance abuse and dependency.

Many women with substance dependency come late in their pregnancy for prenatal care because they are worried their substance use will be discovered and they will be reported to authorities. If a woman is using a substance that has a short-acting effect, she can have difficulty waiting a long time to be seen for an appointment at a healthcare facility. She may also have difficulty following prenatal instructions for proper nutrition because, although she may desire to eat well, if she only has enough money to buy either drugs or food, she may choose drugs over food as her choice. She may not have money for supplemental vitamins or iron preparations for the same reason.

Illicit substances tend to be of small molecular weight and, therefore, readily cross the placenta. As a result, these substances can lead to fetal effects, and substance dependency can be responsible for fetal abnormalities or preterm birth (Slater, 2015). If a woman uses injected drugs, the risk for hepatitis B or HIV infection increases. Additionally, if a woman earns money to buy illicit substances through prostitution, this increases the risk for STI and poses yet another threat to a fetus.

 ## Nursing Diagnoses and Related Interventions

Nursing Diagnosis: Risk for injury to self and fetus related to chronic substance dependency

Outcome Evaluation: Patient states she has enrolled in a substance-dependency treatment program and consequently has reduced or is no longer abusing any substances.

Women who are substance dependent need anticipatory guidance and nursing support all during pregnancy because this is a long time to remain substance free. Many women who are substance dependent have few effective support people outside their illicit substance culture with whom they feel free to discuss problems or concerns or who could answer their questions about pregnancy. Because of their numerous needs, they require an interprofessional team approach involving both pregnancy healthcare providers and substance-dependency treatment providers. Fortunately, with good support and active participation in a substance treatment program, pregnancy can become a stimulus for substance abuse recovery and a maturing and growth experience for a woman.

If a woman is still abusing a substance by the time she begins labor, her infant may experience substance withdrawal symptoms (i.e., neonatal abstinence syndrome) shortly after birth (usually marked by nervousness, irritability or lethargy, and possibly seizures; see Chapter 26). Although it varies depending on the substance, breastfeeding is usually not encouraged for women with substance dependency because, just as all medications cross the placenta to some extent, they also are all excreted into breast milk. Women receiving methadone as part of their substance treatment can breastfeed because only a small amount of this medication is excreted in breast milk (Krans, Cochran, & Bogen, 2015). In some states, because substance dependency has the potential to seriously affect fetal health, women who test positive for illicit substances, either during pregnancy or at the time of birth, must be reported to state child protective agencies; they may be accused of child maltreatment and jailed, with their infant placed in foster care. Be certain you are familiar with agency and state policy concerning these directives (Miller, Lanham, Welsh, et al., 2014).

What If . . . 22.2

Mindy tells the nurse she is not using illicit substances anymore during pregnancy, but when she opens her purse, the nurse notices several packets of white powder inside. What should the nurse do?

COCAINE

Cocaine is derived from *Erythroxylum coca*, a plant grown almost exclusively in South America. When sniffed into the nose or smoked in a pipe, cocaine is absorbed across the mucous membranes and affects the central nervous system. As a result, sudden vasoconstriction occurs. Respiratory and cardiac rates and blood pressure all increase rapidly in response to the vasoconstriction. Alkaloidal cocaine (i.e., crack), a concentrated mixture, produces an even more rapid and intense high when inhaled—so dramatic, in fact, that immediate death may result from cardiac failure.

Cocaine is exceptionally harmful during pregnancy because the extreme vasoconstriction can severely compromise placental circulation, leading to premature separation of the placenta, which then results in preterm labor or fetal death (Box 22.8). Infants born to women who are cocaine dependent can suffer the immediate effects of intracranial hemorrhage and an abstinence syndrome of tremulousness, irritability, and muscle rigidity. Long-term effects are not well documented, but learning and social interaction defects are suspected (Messiah, Ludwig, Vidot, et al., 2015).

Because the effects of cocaine are so intense, counseling women to discontinue using it during pregnancy is often disappointing. Cocaine use can be detected by urinalysis because the metabolites of cocaine can be detected in urine up to 1 week after use.

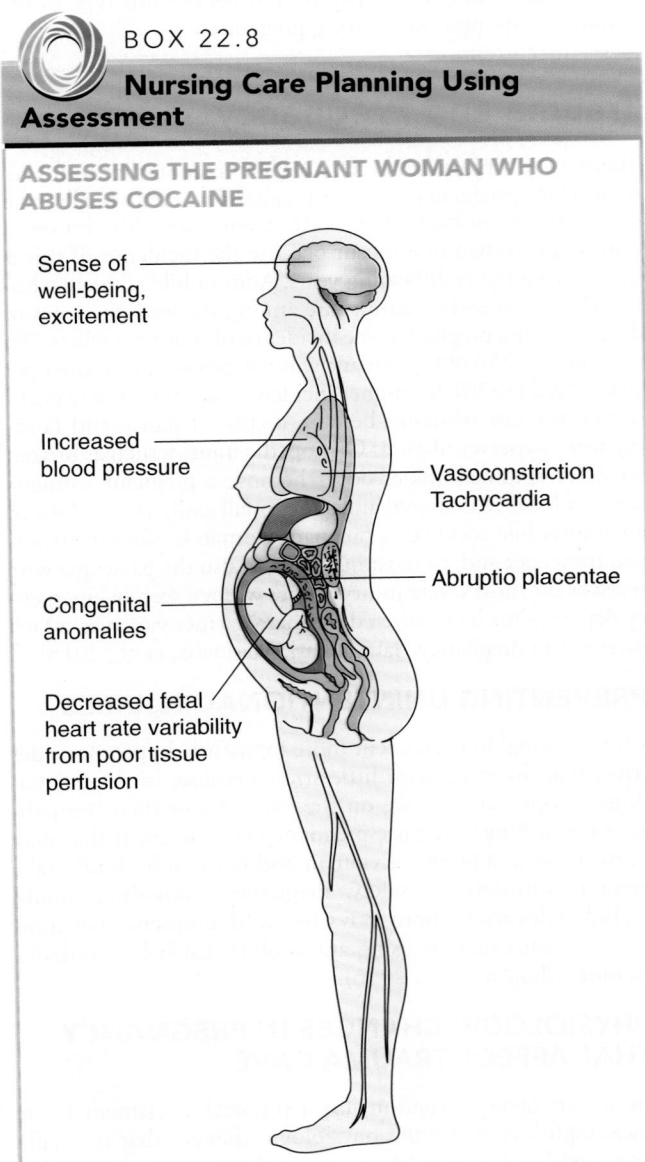

BOX 22.8
Nursing Care Planning Using Assessment

ASSESSING THE PREGNANT WOMAN WHO ABUSES COCAINE

- Sense of well-being, excitement
- Increased blood pressure
- Vasoconstriction Tachycardia
- Abruptio placentae
- Congenital anomalies
- Decreased fetal heart rate variability from poor tissue perfusion

AMPHETAMINES

Methamphetamine (i.e., speed) is a neurostimulant and neurotoxin that has a pharmacologic effect similar to cocaine and, in some communities, because it is easily and cheaply manufactured in home labs, can be more commonly used than cocaine (Wright, Schuetter, Tellei, et al., 2015). Ice, a rock type of methamphetamine that is smoked, can produce high concentrations of the substance in the maternal circulation. Women develop blackened and infected teeth. Newborns whose mothers used the substance show jitteriness and poor feeding at birth and may be growth restricted (Wachman & Schiff, 2016).

QSEN Checkpoint Question 22.5

TEAMWORK & COLLABORATION

Mindy tells the nurse she uses methamphetamine almost daily. What priority nursing intervention should the nurse perform?
a. Obtain a urine or serum sample for toxicology.
b. Emphasize the fact that meth is not good for her.
c. Advise her to stop taking the substance immediately.
d. Refer Mindy to addictions support services.

Look in Appendix A for the best answer and rationale.

MARIJUANA AND HASHISH

Both marijuana and hashish are obtained from the hemp plant, cannabis. When smoked, they produce tachycardia and a sense of well-being. Although not routinely advised, some women use marijuana to counteract nausea in early pregnancy. With the increase in the legalization of medical marijuana and the more general decriminalization of marijuana in some parts of the United States, there may be an uptick in the number of pregnant women legally using marijuana during pregnancy.

The effect of these substances on fetal development are not well documented because they are frequently part of polysubstance abuse or at the very least cigarette use (Roth, Satran, & Smith, 2015). Marijuana is associated with loss of short-term memory and an increased incidence of respiratory infection in adults. More research is needed about its possible side effects during breastfeeding. A frequent user may be advised not to breastfeed because of reduced milk production and the risk to the newborn from excretion of the substance in breast milk.

PHENCYCLIDINE

Phencyclidine (PCP) was developed in the 1950s as an intravenous anesthetic; it is no longer used that way because, although it creates a sense of euphoria, it also causes irritation and possibly long-term hallucinations (i.e., flashback episodes), and it is now seen most frequently as part of polysubstance use. Because the substance tends to leave the maternal circulation and concentrate in fetal cells, it may be particularly injurious to a fetus.

NARCOTIC AGONISTS

Narcotic agonists (i.e., opiates), used for the relief of pain, such as morphine, oxycodone, meperidine (Demerol), and codeine, are widely abused substances because they can be obtained by prescription and they have a dramatic euphoric effect. Heroin is a raw illicit opiate that is also increasing in incidence in late adolescents. It may be administered intradermally (i.e., "skin popping"), through inhalation (i.e., "snorting"), or intravenously (i.e., "shooting"). It produces an immediate and short-lived feeling of euphoria immediately followed by sedation. Pregnancy complications related to its use include gestational hypertension and—because the substance is often injected with shared needles—phlebitis, subacute bacterial endocarditis, and hepatitis B and HIV infection may occur.

Abstinence symptoms include nausea, vomiting, diarrhea, abdominal pain, shivering, insomnia, body aches, and muscle jerks. Abstinence symptoms may begin as soon as 6 hours after the last drug dose and can continue for several days. Their severity and duration depend on the amount of substance used daily and the length of the dependence period.

Heroin dependency in the pregnant woman is dangerous because it can result in fetal opiate dependence and severe abstinence symptoms in the infant after birth. Infants tend to be small for gestational age and have an increased incidence of fetal distress and meconium aspiration. They will demonstrate the same abstinence symptoms after birth as the woman would if she abruptly stopped taking the substance.

Because the fetus is exposed to substances that must be processed by the liver, the fetal liver may mature faster than usual. For this reason, newborns of women who are substance abusing can seem better able to cope with bilirubin at birth than other babies. Fetal lung tissue also appears to mature more rapidly than in other infants, apparently from the stress of the intrauterine substance exposure. This means that, although an infant is born preterm, the chance he or she will develop a condition such as respiratory distress syndrome is less than average.

If possible, a woman who is opiate dependent should be enrolled in a substance abuse program—often, a methadone maintenance or buprenorphine (Buprenex) program during pregnancy (Wilder & Winhusen, 2015). Infants of women taking methadone do not escape abstinence symptoms at birth, and some infants appear to have more severe reactions to methadone abstinence than to heroin. Because a woman is being provided an oral medication legally, however, a fetus is at least ensured better nutrition, better prenatal care, and less exposure to pathogens such as hepatitis B and HIV (Wilder & Winhusen, 2015). If a methadone program is not available, women may be treated with buprenorphine (Buprenex). Some women may already be on a buprenorphine/naloxone (Suboxone) combination to treat their substance abuse. Although some providers keep their pregnant patients on this combination, others will try to wean them to a buprenorphine monotherapy.

Narcan (Naloxone) is the medication used to reverse the effects of opioid agents in emergency situations. It is safe to it use during pregnancy to treat a pregnant woman who has a respiratory or cardiac code related to opioid overdose. It may cause withdrawal symptoms in the fetus in utero, but the alternative of not treating the pregnant woman who has overdosed is maternal, and then fetal, death. Substance abstinence symptoms in the newborn and accompanying nursing care are discussed in Chapter 26.

INHALANTS

Inhalant abuse refers to the "sniffing" or "huffing" of aerosol substances. Frequently abused by adolescents, inhalants include model airplane glue, cooking sprays, and computer keyboard cleaner. Most of these substances seem innocent; however, they contain freon as a propellant, which can lead to severe respiratory and cardiac irregularities. The effect of these substances during pregnancy is not well documented, but they appear to have effects similar to alcohol dependency (Boynukalin & Baykal, 2014). The respiratory depression they can cause could be enough to limit fetal oxygen supply to a serious level.

ALCOHOL

Although alcohol can be legally purchased and is served at social functions, it is just as detrimental to fetal growth as illicit substances. There is little documentation regarding how much alcohol must be ingested before fetal alcohol spectrum disorder, a syndrome with recognizable facial features, possible cognitive challenges, and memory deficits, occurs; therefore, women are advised to drink no alcohol during pregnancy (Green, McKnight-Eily, Tan, et al., 2016). When discussing alcohol ingestion with late adolescents, be certain to mention binge drinking (five or more alcohol drinks on one occasion) to be sure they do not believe this type of occasional drinking is safe during pregnancy.

Trauma and Pregnancy

Trauma (i.e., injury by force) is a phenomenon that seems remote from pregnancy because pregnant women usually take extra care to protect their body. Even with this, however, trauma in women does occur because the incidence of this is high during the childbearing years. Automobile accidents, homicide, and suicide attempts are among the leading causes of death. During pregnancy, the incidence of trauma is 6% to 7% (as many as 250,000 pregnant women experience trauma per year) (NCHS, 2012). Higher incidences of trauma may occur during the last trimester because of poor balance and fainting from hyperventilation. Orthopedic injuries such as broken wrists or sprained ankles occur because a pregnant woman's sense of balance is altered and she can fall easily (Box 22.9). In an automobile accident, a pregnant woman is often the front-seat passenger and, in most instances, is also the passenger who receives the most severe injury. Other women seen in emergency departments have suffered intimate partner violence, which increases in pregnancy (Jain, Chari, Maslovitz, et al., 2015).

PREVENTING UNINTENTIONAL INJURIES

Unintentional injuries occur more frequently in people under stress than in those with little stress because, in these situations, people concentrate on the stressor, not their immediate surroundings. Because pregnancy is a life event that may cause stress in a family, a woman and her family should take extra precautions for safety. Pregnancy counseling should include education about ways to avoid unintentional injuries by means such as using automobile seat belts (Auriault, Brandt, Chopin, et al., 2016).

PHYSIOLOGIC CHANGES IN PREGNANCY THAT AFFECT TRAUMA CARE

In an emergency situation, for a physical assessment to be meaningful, consider the physiologic changes that normally occur with pregnancy. A primary rule to remember is that

![BOX 22.9 icon] BOX 22.9

Nursing Care Planning to Empower a Family

PREVENTIVE MEASURES TO REDUCE UNINTENTIONAL INJURY DURING PREGNANCY

Q. Mindy tells you, "I feel so clumsy since I'm pregnant. What can I do to make sure I don't hurt my baby?"

A. The following guidelines can be helpful:

- Do not stand on stepstools or stepladders (it is difficult to maintain balance on a narrow base).
- Keep small items such as footstools out of pathways (later in pregnancy, it's difficult to see your feet).
- Avoid throw rugs without a nonskid backing so you don't slip on these.
- Use caution stepping in and out of a bathtub.
- Do not overload electrical circuits (it is difficult for a pregnant woman to escape a fire because of poor mobility).
- Do not smoke, so falling asleep with a cigarette will not be a concern.
- Do not take medicine in the dark, so you can clearly read the label.
- Avoid working to a point of fatigue, as fatigue lowers judgment.
- Avoid long periods of standing because this can lead to a drop in your blood pressure, causing you to feel dizzy and faint.
- Always use a seat belt while driving or as a passenger in an automobile.
- Refuse to ride with anyone in an automobile who has been drinking alcohol or whose judgment might be impaired in some other way.

after a traumatic injury, a woman's body will maintain her own homeostasis at the expense of the fetus. To maintain blood pressure in the face of hemorrhage, for example, a woman's body will use peripheral vasoconstriction. Because the uterus is a peripheral organ in a shock response, the blood supply to the uterus can be greatly diminished and the nutrient supply to the fetus can be greatly compromised when this happens (see Chapter 21, Fig. 21.1).

A woman's total plasma volume increases during pregnancy from approximately 2,600 to 4,000 ml at term. This increase serves as a safeguard to a woman if trauma with bleeding should occur because a woman can lose more blood than usual (up to 30% of her blood volume) before hypovolemia becomes clinically evident. This also means, however, that fluid replacement volume will undoubtedly have to be higher because a pregnant woman needs more fluid than a nonpregnant woman to restore her circulatory volume. Central venous pressure (normal is 0 to 5 cm H_2O in a nonpregnant state) is increased to 2 to 7 cm H_2O during pregnancy. Although a woman needs a large amount of replacement fluid, this increased venous pressure means it must not be given too rapidly because her circulation can be overwhelmed more easily than usual by a rapid fluid infusion.

To accommodate the increased vascular load of pregnancy, cardiac output increases from 1 L/min early in pregnancy to 6 to 7 L/min in the second trimester. This volume circulates through the placenta at a rapid rate—approximately one sixth of the total blood volume is present in the placenta at all times. This fact makes a uterine laceration always potentially serious because up to one sixth of a woman's blood volume can be quickly lost.

To move this increased blood volume adequately through the body, a woman's heart rate increases 15 to 20 beats above normal, so a pulse rate of 80 to 95 beats/min is not unusual. Based on this, do not assume a rapid pulse rate indicates hemorrhage following an unintentional injury during pregnancy. In addition, because the heart is displaced by the elevated diaphragm, an electrocardiogram may show a left-axis deviation or the pattern may look distorted from the usual during pregnancy.

Peripheral venous pressure in the pregnant woman is unchanged. However, it tends to be higher in the lower extremities because of compression by the uterus on the vena cava, which causes back pressure. As a result, lacerations of the legs or perineum bleed much more profusely in the pregnant woman. In general, peripheral blood flow is increased because of decreased peripheral vascular resistance (the effect of estrogen and decreased sympathetic activity all through pregnancy). As a result, the pregnant woman can be in severe shock; yet, her extremities will still not feel cold and clammy.

During pregnancy, the leukocyte count rises to 20,000 cells/mm^3 at term, so using this measure as a sign of infection after an open wound is yet another way an assessment can be problematic. The serum albumin level decreases during pregnancy, making the large loss that normally occurs with burns a more serious response than usual. Serum liver enzyme levels such as aspartate aminotransferase, alanine aminotransferase, and lactate dehydrogenase, remain the same during pregnancy. This means, that if these are elevated after an injury, liver trauma can still be detected. Because alkaline phosphatase, a substance also usually helpful in detecting liver trauma, is three to four times greater in the pregnant woman at term than usual (from placental origin), this marker loses its importance. Pancreatic amylase levels remain unchanged during pregnancy, so the pancreas can be evaluated as usual.

Abdominal pain is difficult to localize during pregnancy because organs are pushed aside by the growing uterus. The abdomen often feels tense during pregnancy, so the important findings of guarding and rigidity of the abdominal wall may be lost. Bleeding into the abdominal cavity with an abdominal injury is apt to be forceful and extreme because of the increased pressure in the pelvic vessels. A procedure such as a needle **paracentesis** (needle aspiration) to assess for bleeding into the abdominal cavity must be done carefully because the bowel, dislocated from its usual position, can be easily punctured. **Culdocentesis**, or needle aspiration through the posterior vaginal fornix into the peritoneal cavity, may be done instead. **Peritoneal lavage** (the process of inserting a peritoneal dialysis catheter into the abdominal cavity, adding

BOX 22.10

Nursing Care Planning Using Assessment

ASSESSING THE EFFECTS OF TRAUMA IN THE PREGNANT WOMAN

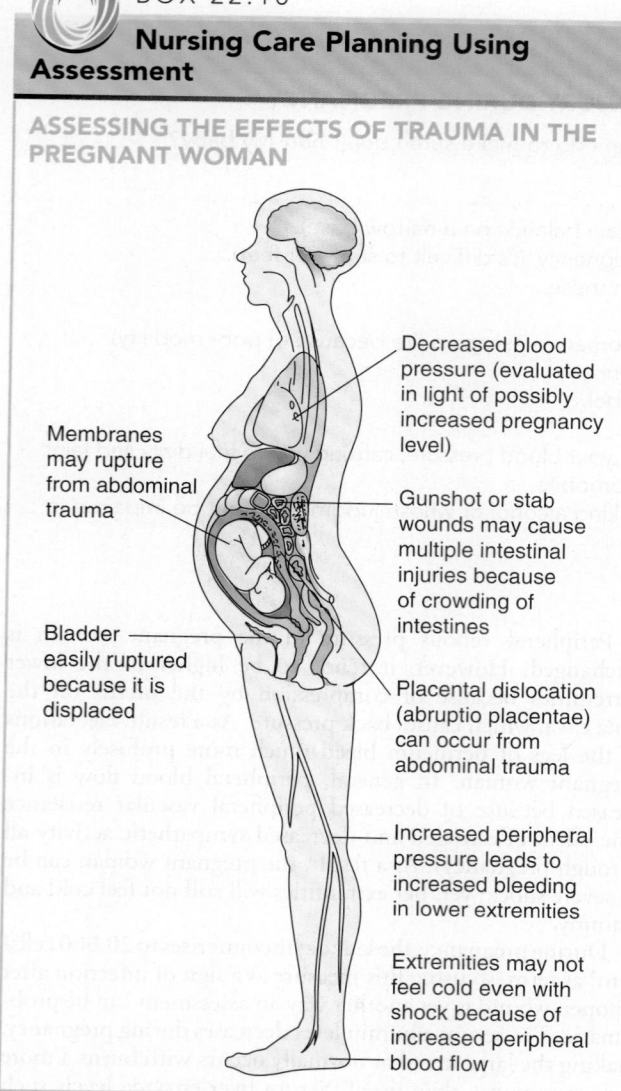

Decreased blood pressure (evaluated in light of possibly increased pregnancy level)

Membranes may rupture from abdominal trauma

Gunshot or stab wounds may cause multiple intestinal injuries because of crowding of intestines

Bladder easily ruptured because it is displaced

Placental dislocation (abruptio placentae) can occur from abdominal trauma

Increased peripheral pressure leads to increased bleeding in lower extremities

Extremities may not feel cold even with shock because of increased peripheral blood flow

---

a quantity of an isotonic solution, aspirating it again, and analyzing it for blood or urine) may reveal bleeding or bladder rupture best.

The bladder of a pregnant woman is extremely susceptible to rupture because it is the most anterior organ and is elevated abnormally (Dorairaj, Sagili, Rani, et al., 2012). After abdominal trauma, an indwelling bladder catheter is often inserted to assess for blood in the urine (Box 22.10).

PSYCHOSOCIAL CONSIDERATIONS

When a pregnant woman is seen at a healthcare facility after any type of unintentional injury, she is apt to be apprehensive and frightened, both for herself and for her fetus. She worries not only about what has happened to her but also about what could have happened (if the knife had slipped an inch farther, if the automobile had been moving faster, if she had fallen from further up the stepladder) as well as what medical care will be required. (Does she need an X-ray? Will this be safe for the fetus?)

A second emotion she may feel is guilt about her carelessness (e.g., if she were really a good mother, she would have

had her seat belt fastened or would not have tried to stand on a stepladder to hang drapes alone). A feeling of guilt lowers her self-esteem and can increase her level of stress. Remember, people under stress do not process information well and may not perceive correctly the information given to them. Always try to review information with a woman before discharge from an emergency department to be certain she has the facts of her injury and understands the necessary follow-up.

ASSESSMENT

Assessment of an injured pregnant woman must be done quickly yet thoroughly and should include both her psychological and physical status. Some women are so concerned with their fetus they do not realize they are injured. Other women might not even consider the possibility that the fetus could be injured until someone asks if she has felt the fetus move since the injury. Assessment, therefore, should be done concurrently with supportive reassurance (e.g., "Your blood pressure is low, but the fetal heartbeat sounds good") to try to relieve her fear of fetal damage. Use a Doppler to assess fetal heart tones if possible to demonstrate to a woman as well as to yourself that the fetus still appears to be well. Attaching an external monitor to record the fetal heart rate and uterine contractions may be the best way to rule out fetal distress or preterm labor.

Following a serious injury, a woman needs her support people around her. Locate them as necessary and assess their reaction to the trauma as well.

Health History

In an emergency situation, a few minutes spent attempting to calm a woman and move her past her initial fright is time well spent because reducing a woman's level of anxiety can enhance her ability to cooperate with a history and physical assessment. This is true unless symptoms of major body system disturbances require immediate efforts to be directed elsewhere.

Take a brief pregnancy history as well as a trauma history, such as the length of pregnancy or any complications. Ask specifically if fetal heart tones have been heard by an examiner during the pregnancy, if she has felt the fetus move since her injury, if she has any sensation of tightening or pain in her abdomen or back that could be uterine contractions, and if she knows what her prepregnancy and pregnancy blood pressures have been to help evaluate the extent of blood loss from the trauma.

Document the circumstances of the trauma: what happened, the time of the injury, signs and symptoms of injury she is experiencing, and actions she has taken to counteract these. If a woman fell, for example, how far was the fall? (A fall from the top of a stepladder is more likely to be serious than a fall from a low rung.) What body part did she land on? (Striking her abdomen may be very serious, although she may be in less pain than if she injured a wrist in the fall.) For an automobile accident, ask how fast the car was traveling, if she was thrown from the car, or if the windshield broke (windshields are usually broken from the impact of a head striking the windshield so the woman will need to be assessed for a head injury).

As a final measure, evaluate whether a woman's degree of injury is in proportion to the history. Injuries out of proportion (e.g., a woman states she tripped on her front steps, but you notice all her extremities are ecchymotic and her jaw is broken) suggest intimate partner violence, which is known to increase in pregnancy rather than a simple unintentional injury (Jain et al., 2015). It is important to identify such women not only to stop the abuse but also because they can have an increased incidence of postpartal depression and perhaps an increased risk of wanting to harm themselves (Burnett, Schminkey, Milburn, et al., 2016) (see Chapter 55). Also analyze whether a woman seemed to be using a sensible degree of caution for the circumstances. If not, assess how aware she is of common safety measures. In rare situations, such questions may reveal a woman who self-inflicted an injury in an attempt to end an unwanted pregnancy. A naive adolescent, for example, may attempt to fall down a flight of stairs or to poison herself, which she then reports as an unintentional injury.

Physical Examination

Unintentional injuries become fatal when lung, heart, kidney, or brain functions fail. Fetal health falls into jeopardy when uteroplacental function becomes impaired. Following trauma, therefore, it's important to evaluate these body systems first (Table 22.2). All women who receive a blow to their abdomen need to be evaluated for direct insults to fetal health, such as premature separation of the placenta, although the incidence of this occurring from abdominal injury is actually small (Jain et al., 2015).

With multiple trauma, a nasogastric tube is usually passed to empty the stomach. A Foley catheter is inserted to assess urine output and to rule out a ruptured bladder (blood would return or urine would be blood-tinged if bleeding were occurring).

To prevent supine hypotension syndrome, be certain a woman does not lie supine for an examination. If she must lie on her back, place a rolled towel or blanket under her right side to tip her body approximately 15 degrees to the side and manually displace her uterus off the vena cava. If surgery is necessary, the operating room table can be tipped to achieve this same effect.

 ## Nursing Diagnoses and Related Interventions

Planning in an emergency always involves two phases: planning for immediate care to stabilize body systems and protect the fetus and planning for ongoing care to bring the woman back to wellness. Examples of nursing diagnoses include:

- Fear related to threat of injury to the fetus
- Risk for fetal injury related to apparent self-harm attempt
- Ineffective tissue perfusion related to severed artery
- Ineffective breathing pattern related to lung laceration by gunshot wound

Once the immediate emergency phase has passed, nursing diagnoses focus on preventing additional injuries or alleviating emotional distress. Examples include:

- Risk for infection related to loss of skin integrity from knife wound
- Situational low self-esteem related to occurrence of unintentional injury
- Powerlessness related to seriousness of the injury sustained or inability to prevent an unintentional injury from occurring

TABLE 22.2 INITIAL ASSESSMENTS NECESSARY AFTER TRAUMA DURING PREGNANCY

Body System	Assessment
Respiratory system	What is the quality of respirations (labored or even)?
	What is the respiration rate?
	Are there sounds of obstruction (wheezing, retractions, coughing)?
	Does the woman have cyanosis?
	Does the woman demonstrate oxygen hunger (inability to lie flat, nasal flaring)?
Cardiovascular system	Is her color pale, which could be from hemorrhage?
	Is there gross bleeding?
	What is the pulse rate? Increased, which could identify hemorrhage?
	Or absent, which identifies heart failure?
	What is the blood pressure (decreases with hemorrhage)?
	Does the woman feel apprehensive, which can occur with altered vascular pressure?
Neurologic system	Is the woman conscious (able to answer questions coherently)?
	Are pupils equal and react to light?
	Are there bruises or bumps on the head or spinal column?
	Is there loss of motion or sensory function in a body part?
Renal system	Is there bruising over the bladder or on the back over kidneys?
	Is the urine pink or red, which could identify fresh blood in urine? Or black, which could identify old blood?
Uterine–fetal system	Is there bruising on the abdomen over the uterus?
	Is there bradycardia, tachycardia, or absence of fetal heart tones? Is there loss of variability on a fetal monitor?
	Is there evidence of vaginal bleeding?
	Is there clear fluid leaking from the vagina, which could identify ruptured membranes?

THERAPEUTIC MANAGEMENT

Implementations in emergency situations must be done quickly while always remembering a woman's primary health condition is that she is pregnant.

- For "hands only" cardiopulmonary resuscitation (CPR): Check for unresponsiveness. If the woman is not responsive and not breathing, call for help or dial 911.
- Begin heart compressions at a rate of at least 100 per minute, depressing the chest at least 2 in. each time. Cardiac massage this way may be awkward late in pregnancy because of the size of the uterus, but undue pressure should not be necessary to create heart action.
- Continue chest compressions at this rate until additional help arrives (American Heart Association [AHA], 2015).
- When help arrives, ask a person to place a rolled towel or blanket under the woman's right side to relieve uterine pressure on the vena cava and help prevent supine hypotension syndrome.

In a health agency setting, CPR should follow agency guidelines. If there has been blood loss, a central line may need to be inserted and lactated Ringer's or another isotonic solution infused to restore fluid volume as well as to provide an open line for emergency medication.

If hypotension is present, it must be corrected quickly to maintain a pressure gradient across the placenta. However, any antihypotensive agent that achieves increased blood pressure by causing peripheral vasoconstriction is contraindicated (vessels in the uterus would constrict and cut off the fetal blood supply). Ephedrine is the medication of choice for a pregnant woman to restore blood pressure because it has a minimal peripheral vasoconstrictive effect. Following emergency interventions, care depends on the specific injury or trauma present (Jeejeebhoy, Zelop, Lipman, et al., 2015).

Nursing Diagnoses and Related Interventions

Nursing Diagnosis: Risk for ineffective tissue perfusion related to blood loss from trauma

Outcome Evaluation: Patient's blood pressure remains above 100/60 mmHg, pulse rate below 100 beats/min, fetal heart rate is 120 to 160 beats/min; nonstress test shows good variability; no signs of labor contractions are present.

Open Wounds

Open wounds vary from simple lacerations to more serious puncture wounds. Because the white blood cell count is normally elevated during pregnancy, a single count is a poor indicator of the presence or extent of infection for these injuries. Serial measurements can be used, however, to assess if infection is occurring.

Lacerations

A laceration (e.g., a jagged cut) may involve only the skin layer or may penetrate to deeper subcutaneous tissue and even tendons. Lacerations generally bleed profusely. Halt bleeding by putting pressure on the edges of the laceration; this may be difficult to achieve in the lower extremities because venous

pressure is so greatly increased in the legs during pregnancy. After cleaning, the area is then sutured through each layer of tissue involved to approximate the edges. A local anesthetic such as lidocaine (Xylocaine) is necessary for suturing. Because this has only a local effect, you can assure a woman that this will be safe to use during pregnancy. If the laceration is superficial and a woman is worried about the use of an anesthetic, the edges can be approximated with a butterfly strip. This will allow it to heal, although with a slightly more noticeable scar.

QSEN Checkpoint Question 22.6

SAFETY

Mindy has a laceration on her leg from her automobile accident. What priority nursing action should the nurse initiate?

   a. Keep the laceration clean by irrigating it with hydrogen peroxide.
   b. Control bleeding by applying a pressure dressing to the wound.
   c. Administer a nonsteroidal anti-inflammatory medication for pain relief.
   d. Obtain written consent for surgery from Mindy.

Look in Appendix A for the best answer and rationale.

Puncture Wounds

A puncture wound results from the penetration of a sharp object such as a nail, splinter, nail file, or knife. Puncture wounds bleed little—an advantage in terms of minimizing blood loss but not in terms of wound cleaning. A puncture wound is usually not sutured because suturing would create a sealed, unoxygenated cavity below the sutures or a space where a tetanus bacilli infection could grow. If a woman has had a tetanus immunization within the past 10 years, tetanus toxoid (Tdap) is administered. If a woman has not had a tetanus immunization within 10 years (the usual condition), both tetanus toxoid (Tdap) and immune tetanus globulin (Tig) are administered. Both of these are safe to administer during pregnancy (Sukumaran, McCarthy, Kharbanda, et al., 2015).

Puncture wounds are usually frightening because it's difficult to tell how deep they are. They also usually occur with the added association of violence. Knife wounds cause deep penetration puncture wounds and are often directed into the abdomen. Even a paring knife may easily reach the depth of the uterus, possibly directly cutting the fetus. Most stab wounds of the abdomen, however, occur in the upper quadrants of the abdomen, above the uterus, and are more apt to strike the liver or pancreas. To determine the depth and extent of a wound, a fistulogram may be done. This is done by inserting a thin catheter into the wound and filling the wound with a radiopaque solution that outlines the depth of the wound on x-ray. If the peritoneal cavity was perforated, dye will be shown outlining the intestines. If there is a suspicion of bleeding into the abdominal cavity, a laparoscopy or celiotomy (exploratory surgical procedures into the abdominal cavity) may be performed. Although a frightening procedure for the woman, surgery this close to the uterus usually does not result in disruption of the pregnancy.

If the diaphragm was cut, the intestines may herniate into the chest cavity (diaphragmatic hernia) because of the increased abdominal pressure from the enlarged uterus, causing acute shortness of breath. After surgical repair of an injured diaphragm, cesarean birth is usually planned to avoid strain on the newly repaired diaphragm during labor. The uterus appears to have a natural resistance to infection, so even if it is punctured, infection in the uterus rarely occurs.

Animal or Snake Bites

Pregnant women are occasionally bitten by venomous snakes but are rarely bitten by any animal but a dog. Animal bites produce a form of puncture wound, so if the rabies immunization status of the dog is known to be up to date, the wound is washed and treated as a puncture wound. If the dog cannot be located or is proved to be rabid after 48 hours of observation, a woman must be administered rabies immune globulin and vaccine. Pregnancy is not a contraindication to rabies immunization because contracting the disease would be fatal (Huang, Liu, Cao, et al., 2013). It has not yet been decided if antivenom or supportive therapy is the optimal management for snake bites (Ishikawa, Ohsaka, Omori, et al., 2015).

To prevent bites, caution pregnant women to avoid contact with unfamiliar dogs. If she will be camping in a remote location, caution her to avoid feeding any wild animals such as squirrels and raccoons for the same reason.

Blunt Abdominal Trauma

Blunt trauma generally occurs from automobile accidents, when a woman's abdomen strikes the steering wheel or dashboard, or occurs from someone kicking or punching her abdomen. No visible break is present in the skin. Following the injury, however, the underlying tissue becomes edematous; broken underlying blood vessels ooze and form ecchymoses or a hematoma at the site. If the bruise is over the abdomen, to assess if there is internal bleeding, a diagnostic peritoneal lavage may be done by introducing a small amount of normal saline by a syringe into the peritoneum and then withdrawing it to see if blood is evident. Ultrasound may also be used to detect this.

Careful assessment that the pregnancy has not been harmed must be made following blunt trauma because a forceful blow to the abdomen could dislodge the placenta (i.e., abruptio placentae), which would then begin preterm labor. Palpate the uterus for any abnormal contours that would suggest edema or internal bleeding; listen and record fetal heart tones. Use a Doppler not only for easy assessment but also to help assure a woman the fetal heartbeat is good. Real-time ultrasound may also be helpful in showing that the uterus and placenta are intact. A pelvic examination is usually performed to assess for vaginal bleeding or seepage of clear fluid that would suggest rupture of the amniotic membranes. If a woman reports uterine contractions, attach uterine and fetal monitors so you can estimate the strength and effect of contractions on the fetal heart rate and determine if preterm labor has begun. A tocolytic such as terbutaline will probably be prescribed to halt preterm labor once it is established the uterine environment is still intact (see Chapter 21 for a full discussion of tocolysis).

The possibility some placental blood will enter the maternal circulation with uterine trauma is a real possibility. Rh-negative women, therefore, are typically administered Rh immune globulin after abdominal trauma. That fetal blood cells are present in the maternal bloodstream can be documented by a Kleihauer–Betke test (in a sample of maternal blood, maternal cells remain colorless on staining, whereas fetal cells turn purple-pink).

Gunshot Wounds

A woman may receive a gunshot wound because she was an intended victim or because she was an innocent bystander. Occasionally, a woman attempts to harm herself by a gunshot wound. Assessment of the wound includes inspection for the point where the bullet entered the body as well as the point where it exited (the entry wound is smaller than the exit wound because, as a bullet slows, it begins to tumble, enlarging the space it occupies). The uterine wall is so thick during pregnancy that it may trap a bullet, so there may be no exit point from a woman's body if the uterus was punctured. If the bullet entered high in the abdomen, the intestines will surely be injured because so many intestinal loops are compressed above the uterus.

Gunshot wounds are surgically cleaned and debrided, and a woman is prescribed a high dose of an antibiotic such as ampicillin. If the bullet entered the uterus, the incidence of fetal mortality is high, especially if the placenta was torn by the bullet. After providing emergency care to a woman for the injury, remember to carefully investigate the circumstances of the injury. Since President Lincoln's assassination, gunshot wounds in the United States must be reported to the police. Stay with a woman as necessary while she recounts her history of the incident for law enforcement officers.

Poisoning

Pregnant women are not apt to swallow a poison, although poisoning can occur unintentionally, for instance, from inadequately refrigerated or undercooked foods or if a woman wakes at night and attempts to take medicine in the dark. There is also the possibility a woman might poison herself as a self-harm attempt.

Poisoning in the pregnant woman is managed the same as in a nonpregnant woman. The woman should telephone the National Poison Control Center (1-800-222-1222), state she is pregnant and what she unintentionally swallowed, then follow the specific recommendation of personnel at the poison control center. When seen in an emergency department, oral activated charcoal is safe during pregnancy and so is the medication of choice to neutralize stomach poison (Karch, 2015).

After a woman has been treated and the emergency of the poisoning is over, carefully investigate the circumstances of the poisoning to help a woman learn about safety with medications or food.

Choking

If a pregnant woman chokes on a piece of food or a foreign object blocks her airway, attempting to dislodge the object with a sudden upward thrust to the upper abdomen can be difficult because there is a lack of space between the uterus and the end of the sternum. Also, the average person may not be able to reach around a woman's enlarged abdomen to perform a usual chest thrust. Box 22.11 describes how to perform chest thrusts for a pregnant woman.

BOX 22.11

Nursing Care Planning Using Procedures

CHEST THRUSTS FOR A PREGNANT WOMAN

Purpose: To relieve tracheal aspiration

Plan	Principle
For Conscious Victim in Standing Position	
1. Stand behind the woman and encircle her chest with your arms.	1. Proper positioning ensures proper placement for chest pressure and prevents inadvertent injury to underlying body structures.
2. Place the thumb side of your fist on the middle of the woman's sternum. 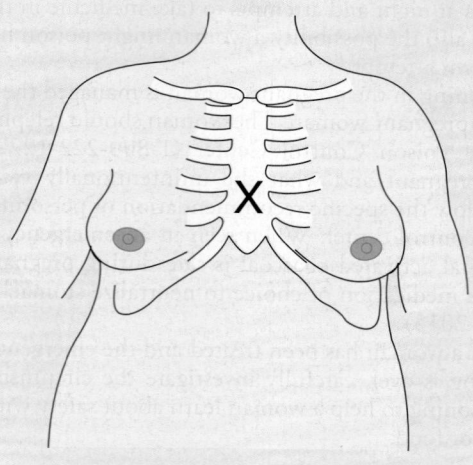	2. Placement of fist against the chest ensures a solid structure for compression.
3. Grab the fist with the other hand and perform backward thrusts until the foreign body is expelled.	3. Pressure on the chest compresses the ribs, increasing chest and lung pressure. This increased pressure forces an object lodged in the airway to move upward.

For Unconscious Victim in Supine Position

1. Place the woman in the same position as for external heart compressions (heel of the hand on the lower sternum).	1. Loss of consciousness interferes with the woman's ability to maintain an upright position.

2. Follow steps 2 and 3 as with a conscious victim.	2. Chest compression can be as effective in the supine position as in the standing position.

Orthopedic Injuries

Because women have poor balance late in pregnancy, it is easy for them to trip; when they fall, they almost automatically reach out a hand to prevent landing on their abdomen. Because of extra pregnancy weight, this can cause a serious wrist injury (a Colles fracture). Apply ice to the area to decrease swelling as an immediate first-aid measure. If limited motion is present, an X-ray may be necessary to determine whether a fracture is present. Assure a woman an X-ray of an extremity is safe during pregnancy as long as her abdomen is shielded during the procedure. Be certain to delegate someone to accompany her to the X-ray department and remain with her (outside the actual X-ray room) to ensure lead protection is offered and to remain alert for signs of preterm labor that could suddenly develop as a result of a yet undetected injury.

Because women of childbearing age are usually healthy, fractures or torn ligaments generally heal rapidly without complications. Be certain a woman can identify good calcium food sources if she has a fracture so both she and the fetus can obtain adequate calcium for new bone growth.

Because many more adolescent girls and young adult women participate in sports today than ever before, combined with the cartilage softening and extra weight caused by pregnancy, an increasing number of pregnant women suffer knee cartilage or knee ligament injuries.

Any woman who has had a previous knee injury should have it reevaluated early in the pregnancy because a support device such as a knee immobilizer may be required for the last 3 months of pregnancy to keep the joint from dislocating or the ligament from tearing again. You can assure her having a knee immobilizer in place at the time of birth will not interfere with birth.

The laxness of body cartilage may also cause separation of the symphysis pubis if a woman falls with her legs outspread.

Many women experience some nagging suprapubic joint pain during pregnancy. A suture separation is very painful, especially when walking or turning. To avoid pain and allow the cartilage to heal, a woman is usually advised to remain on bed rest at home for 4 to 6 weeks. If separation of the symphysis pubis is still present at the time of birth, this can make labor very painful, especially during the pelvic division of labor as the fetus is pushed through the pelvic ring. She may need additional analgesia at this time.

> *What If . . . 22.3*
> **Mindy tore her anterior cruciate ligament (ACL) in an automobile accident and is prescribed a knee immobilizer. She's unable to drive with this in place, and her family lives in a second floor walk-up apartment. What factors should the nurse assess with her?**

Burns

Burns are dangerous for the pregnant woman not only because of the thermal injury that occurs but also because inhalation of carbon monoxide gases from the fire can lead to extreme fetal hypoxia because carbon monoxide can cross the placenta in place of oxygen (Wu & Hueppchen, 2015).

In addition, inhaled smoke is extremely irritating to lung tissue and so can result in extensive local lung edema, which can lead to additional fetal hypoxia because of the lack of oxygen–carbon dioxide exchange space in the woman's lungs. Because fluid and electrolyte losses occur with burns, hypotension from hypovolemia or an electrolyte imbalance can occur. Yet another concern, in response to a severe trauma such as a burn, is that prostaglandins are produced, possibly causing preterm labor. The more extensive the burned area, the poorer the prognosis for both the woman and fetus. Interestingly, burn tissue heals more quickly than usual during pregnancy, probably related to the overall increased metabolism and the increased corticosteroid serum level, which prevents inflammation and damage to tissue from the pressure of edema. Care of burns is discussed in Chapter 52.

POSTMORTEM CESAREAN BIRTH

If a pregnant woman does not survive serious trauma, it may still be possible for her child to be born safely by a postmortem cesarean birth (Drukker, Hants, Sharon, et al., 2014). This is usually attempted if the fetus is past 24 weeks and less than 20 minutes has passed since the mother died (preferably 5 minutes). By general practice, no consent is necessary for the procedure because the fetus is assumed to want to live but cannot give consent. A classic cesarean incision is used. Personnel should be available to resuscitate the newborn immediately.

What If . . . 22.4
The nurse is particularly interested in exploring one of the 2020 National Health Goals with respect to women with special needs during pregnancy (see Box 22.1). Most government-sponsored money for nursing research is allotted based on these goals. What would be a possible research topic to explore pertinent to these goals that would be applicable to the Carson family and that would also advance evidence-based practice?

KEY POINTS FOR REVIEW

- Adolescent pregnancy is a major concern because although it is decreasing in incidence, it still occurs at a high rate and can interfere with the development of both an adolescent and fetus. Nursing care needs to be individualized to meet the prepartal, intrapartal, and postpartum needs of this age group. Planning nursing care that helps adolescents view a pregnancy as a growth experience not only meets QSEN competencies but can also best help a girl mature to be an effective parent.

- Women who delay childbearing until age 40 years may need additional discussion time at prenatal visits to help them incorporate a pregnancy into their lifestyle. They may need reminders to save time during the day for rest, particularly if at risk for gestational hypertension or varicosities.

- Women who are physically, cognitively, visually, mobility, or hearing challenged are apt to have special needs during pregnancy that must be addressed by healthcare providers so adjustments to ensure a safe outcome can be made during pregnancy. Providing time for discussion early in pregnancy so these needs can be identified and anticipated is an important role for nurses.

- Women who are physically or cognitively challenged may need help adjusting their usual regimen to pregnancy. Be certain they are aware of how to contact help in an emergency. Ensure all medications they are taking for their primary disorder are safe for use during pregnancy.

- A woman who is substance dependent presents a unique challenge for healthcare providers during pregnancy. Encouraging her to decrease or halt her substance intake to safeguard the health of a fetus is a short-term goal. Addressing her need to decrease her substance

intake for the remainder of her life so she can be a quality parent is a long-term goal.

- The fetus of a woman who is substance dependent is at high risk because of the direct effects of the substance and the indirect effects of an unhealthy lifestyle. Women should be encouraged to join substance reduction/maintenance programs if possible to reduce fetal risk.

- Trauma in pregnancy results from sources such as violence, automobile accidents, and falls. Women with traumatic injuries need to be carefully assessed to be certain their fetus is unhurt and to determine if intimate partner violence could have been the cause of the trauma.

CRITICAL THINKING CARE STUDY

Anifisa Alkaev is a 42-year-old Russian Catholic woman who, after several fertility treatments, is 10 weeks pregnant. She lived with her parents in Russia until 1 year ago, and she speaks almost no English. She met her partner, a U.S. citizen, approximately 1 year ago. She began living with him 6 months ago in a conservative Jewish community. In Russia, Anifisa was a lawyer but is currently not working because of her language barrier. Her partner's 90-year-old mother has just moved in with them. A 15-year-old niece whom Anifisa does not know well will also be staying with them until she finishes high school. You notice Anifisa is both hypertensive and overweight.

1. Analyzing Anifisa's situation, what needs would you identify?
2. What nursing interventions would you implement?
3. What complications of pregnancy could Anifisa be at a high risk for that you would want to especially assess for during her pregnancy?

RELATED RESOURCES

Explore these additional resources to enhance learning for this chapter:
- Student resources on thePoint, including answers to the What If . . . and Critical Thinking Care Study questions, http://thepoint.lww.com/Flagg8e
- Adaptive learning powered by PrepU, http://thepoint.lww.com/prepu

REFERENCES

Agopian, A. J., Tinker, S. C., Lupo, P. J., et al. (2013). Proportion of neural tube defects attributable to known risk factors. *Birth Defects Research. Part A, Clinical and Molecular Teratology, 97*(1), 42–46.
American Heart Association. (2015). *Highlights of the 2015 American Heart Association guidelines update for CPR and ECC.* Irving, TX: Author.
Auriault, F., Brandt, C., Chopin, A., et al. (2016). Pregnant women in vehicles: Driving habits, position and risk of injury. *Accident Analysis and Prevention, 89*, 57–61.
Bayer, R., Santelli, J., & Klitzman, R. (2015). New challenges for electronic health records: Confidentiality and access to sensitive health information about parents and adolescents. *JAMA, 313*(1), 29–30.
Ben-David, A., Glasser, S., Schiff, E., et al. (2016). Pregnancy and birth outcomes among primiparae at very advanced maternal age: At what price? *Maternal and Child Health Journal, 20*(4), 833–842.
Boynukalin, F. K., & Baykal, C. (2014). Prenatal diagnosis of multiple fetal anomalies in naphthalene-addicted pregnant women: A case report. *Clinical and Experimental Obstetrics & Gynecology, 41*(2), 217–218.
Brown, H. K., Lunsky, Y., Wilton, A. S., et al. (2016). Pregnancy in women with intellectual and developmental disabilities. *Journal of Obstetrics and Gynaecology Canada, 38*(1), 9–16.

Brown, H. L., Hughes-Bell, A., & McDuffie, A. W. (2015). Caring for patients who are deaf or hard of hearing. *Journal of the American Academy of Physician Assistants, 28*(12), 50–55.

Burnett, C., Schminkey, D., Milburn, J., et al. (2016). Negotiating peril: The lived experience of rural, low-income women exposed to IPV during pregnancy and postpartum. *Violence Against Women, 22*(8), 943–965.

Castro, J. S., Lourenço, C., & Carrilho, M. (2014). Successful pregnancy in a woman with paraplegia. *BMJ Case Reports.* Advance online publication.

Centers for Disease Control and Prevention. (2014). Vital signs: Births to teens aged 15–17 years—United States, 1991–2012. *Morbidity and Mortality Weekly Report, 63*(14), 312–318.

Cheng, E. R., Rifas-Shiman, S. L., Perkins, M. E., et al. (2016). The influence of antenatal partner support on pregnancy outcomes. *Journal of Women's Health, 25*(7), 672–679.

Conroy, K. N., Engelhart, T. G., Martins, Y., et al. (2015). The enigma of rapid repeat pregnancy: A qualitative study of teen mothers. *Journal of Pediatric and Adolescent Gynecology, 29*(3), 312–317.

Debost-Legrand, A., Rivière, O., Dossou, M., et al. (2015). Risk factors for severe secondary postpartum hemorrhages: A historical cohort study. *Birth, 42*(3), 235–241.

Dorairaj, J., Sagili, H., Rani, R., et al. (2012). Delayed presentation of intraperitoneal bladder rupture following domestic violence in pregnancy. *Journal of Obstetrics & Gynaecology Research, 38*(4), 753–756.

Drukker, L., Hants, Y., Sharon, E., et al. (2014). Perimortem cesarean section for maternal and fetal salvage: Concise review and protocol. *Acta Obstetricia et Gynecologica Scandinavica, 93*(10), 965–972.

Eggemoen, Å. R., Falk, R. S., Knutsen, K. V., et al. (2016). Vitamin D deficiency and supplementation in pregnancy in a multiethnic population-based cohort. *BMC Pregnancy and Childbirth, 16*(1), 7.

Erikson, E. (1963). *Childhood and society.* New York, NY: Norton.

Fletcher, W., & Russo, M. (2015). Preconception counseling and prenatal care. In J. L. Bienstock, H. Fox, E. E. Wallach, et al. (Eds.), *The Johns Hopkins manual of gynecology and obstetrics* (5th ed., pp. 58–77). Philadelphia, PA: Lippincott Williams & Wilkins.

Fouquier, K. F., & Camune, B. D. (2015). Meeting the reproductive needs of female adolescents with neurodevelopmental disabilities. *Journal of Obstetric, Gynecologic & Neonatal Nursing, 44*(4), 553–563.

Garfield, C. F., Duncan, G., Rutsohn, J., et al. (2014). A longitudinal study of paternal mental health during transition to fatherhood as young adults. *Pediatrics, 133*(5), 836–843.

Green, P. P., McKnight-Eily, L. R., Tan, C. H., et al. (2016). Vital signs: Alcohol-exposed pregnancies—United States, 2011-2013. *Morbidity and Mortality Weekly Report, 65*(4), 91–97.

Hamilton, B. E., Martin, J. A., Osterman, M. J. K., et al. (2015). Births: Final data for 2014. *National Vital Statistics Reports, 64*(12), 1–64.

Houde, M., Dahdouh, E. M., Mongrain, V., et al. (2015). The effect of adequate gestational weight gain among adolescents relative to adults of equivalent body mass index and the risk of preterm birth, cesarean delivery, and low birth weight. *Journal of Pediatric and Adolescent Gynecology, 28*(6), 502–507.

Huang, G., Liu, H., Cao, Q., et al. (2013). Safety of post-exposure rabies prophylaxis during pregnancy: A follow-up study from Guangzhou, China. *Human Vaccines & Immunotherapeutics, 9*(1), 177–183.

Ishikawa, K., Ohsaka, H., Omori, K., et al. (2015). Pregnant woman bitten by a Japanese mamushi (Gloydius blomhoffii). *Internal Medicine, 54*(19), 2517–2520.

Jain, V., Chari, R., Maslovitz, S., et al. (2015). Guidelines for the management of a pregnant trauma patient. *Journal of Obstetrics and Gynaecology Canada, 37*(6), 553–574.

Jeejeebhoy, F. M., Zelop, C. M., Lipman, S., et al. (2015). Cardiac arrest in pregnancy: A scientific statement from the American Heart Association. *Circulation, 132*(18), 1747–1773.

Jeha, D., Usta, I., Ghulmiyyah, L., et al. (2015). A review of the risks and consequences of adolescent pregnancy. *Journal of Neonatal-Perinatal Medicine, 8*(1), 1–8.

Karch, A. M. (2015). *Lippincott's nursing drug guide.* Philadelphia, PA: Lippincott Williams & Wilkins.

Kawakita, T., Wilson, K., Grantz, K. L., et al. (2016). Adverse maternal and neonatal outcomes in adolescent pregnancy. *Journal of Pediatric and Adolescent Gynecology, 29*(2), 130–136.

Kirbas, A., Gulerman, H. C., & Daglar, K. (2016). Pregnancy in adolescence: Is it an obstetrical risk? *Journal of Pediatric and Adolescent Gynecology, 29*(4), 367–371.

Krans, E. E., Cochran, G., & Bogen, D. L. (2015). Caring for opioid-dependent pregnant women: Prenatal and postpartum care considerations. *Clinical Obstetrics and Gynecology, 58*(2), 370–379.

Laganà, A. S., Triolo, O., D'Amico, V., et al. (2015). Management of women with epilepsy: From preconception to post-partum. *Archives of Gynecology and Obstetrics, 293*(3), 493–503.

Lumish, R. A., Young, S. L., Lee, S., et al. (2014). Gestational iron deficiency is associated with pica behaviors in adolescents. *The Journal of Nutrition, 144*(10), 1533–1539.

Martin, J. A., Hamilton, B. E., & Osterman, M. J. K. (2015). *Births in the United States, 2014* (NCHS Data Brief No. 216). Hyattsville, MD: National Center for Health Statistics.

Matthews, T. J., & Hamilton, B. E. (2016). *Mean age of mothers is on the rise: United States, 2000–2014* (NCHS Data Brief No. 232). Hyattsville, MD: National Center for Health Statistics.

Menon, K. C., Ferguson, E. L., Thomson, C. D., et al. (2016). Effects of anemia at different stages of gestation on infant outcomes. *Nutrition, 32*(1), 61–66.

Messiah, S. E., Ludwig, D. A., Vidot, D. C., et al. (2015). Prenatal cocaine exposure and cardiometabolic disease risk factors in 18- to 20-year-old African Americans. *Ethnicity & Disease, 25*(4), 419–426.

Miller, C., Lanham, A., Welsh, C., et al. (2014). Screening, testing, and reporting for drug and alcohol use on labor and delivery: A survey of Maryland birthing hospitals. *Social Work in Health Care, 53*(7), 659–669.

National Center for Health Statistics. (2012). *Trends in the health of Americans.* Hyattsville, MD: Author.

Olaiya, O., Dee, D. L., Sharma, A. J., et al. (2016). Maternity care practices and breastfeeding among adolescent mothers aged 12-19 years—United States, 2009-2011. *Morbidity and Mortality Weekly Report, 65*(2), 17–22.

Paradis, G., & Koester, L. S. (2015). Emotional availability and touch in deaf and hearing dyads. *Journal American Annals of the Deaf, 160*(30), 303–315.

Potter, J., & Santelli, J. S. (2015). Contraceptive counseling for adolescents. *Women's Health, 11*(6), 737–741.

Richards, M. K., Flanagan, M. R., Littman, A. J., et al. (2016). Primary cesarean section and adverse delivery outcomes among women of very advanced maternal age. *Journal of Perinatology, 36*(4), 272–277.

Roth, C. K., Satran, L. A., & Smith, S. M. (2015). Marijuana use in pregnancy. *Nursing for Women's Health, 19*(5), 431–437.

Santos, A. J., Daniel, J. R., Fernandes, C., et al. (2015). Affiliative subgroups in preschool classrooms: Integrating constructs and methods from social ethology and sociometric traditions. *PLoS One, 10*(7), e0130932.

Seay, D. M., Jahromi, L. B., Umaña-Taylor, A. J., et al. (2016). Intergenerational transmission of maladaptive parenting strategies in families of adolescent mothers: Effects from grandmothers to young children. *Journal of Abnormal Child Psychology, 44*(6), 1097–1109.

Slater, L. (2015). Substance use in pregnancy. *The Practising Midwife, 18*(1), 10–13.

Society for Adolescent Health and Medicine. (2016). Emergency contraception for adolescents and young adults: Guidance for health care professionals. *Journal of Adolescent Health, 58*(2), 245–248.

Sukumaran, L., McCarthy, N. L., Kharbanda, E. O., et al. (2015). Safety of tetanus toxoid, reduced diphtheria toxoid, and acellular pertussis and influenza vaccinations in pregnancy. *Obstetrics and Gynecology, 126*(5), 1069–1074.

Timofeev, J., Reddy, U. M., Huang, C. C., et al. (2013). Obstetric complications, neonatal morbidity, and indications for cesarean delivery by maternal age. *Obstetrics & Gynecology, 122*(6), 1184–1195.

U.S. Department of Health and Human Services. (2010). *Healthy people 2020.* Washington, DC: Author.

U.S. Equal Employment Opportunity Commission. (1990). *The American Disabilities Act.* Washington, DC: Author.

Wachman, E. M., & Schiff, D. M. (2016). Bringing attention to a need for a standardized treatment and weaning protocol for neonatal abstinence syndrome. *Translational Pediatrics, 5*(1), 12–15.

Waugh, J. S., & Smith, M. C. (2012). Hypertensive disorders. In D. K. Edmonds (Ed.), *Dewhurst's textbook of obstetrics & gynaecology* (8th ed., pp. 101–110). Oxford, United Kingdom: Wiley.

Wilder, C. M., & Winhusen, T. (2015). Pharmacological management of opioid use disorder in pregnant women. *CNS Drugs, 29*(8), 625–636.

Willie, T. C., Powell, A., & Kershaw, T. (2016). Stress in the city: Influence of urban social stress and violence on pregnancy and postpartum quality of life among adolescent and young mothers. *Journal of Urban Health, 93*(1), 19–35.

Wilson, E., Casanueva, C., Smith, K. R., et al. (2014). Risk of early sexual initiation and pregnancy among youth reported to the child welfare system. *Child Welfare, 93*(1), 127–147.

Wright, T. E., Schuetter, R., Tellei, J., et al. (2015). Methamphetamines and pregnancy outcomes. *Journal of Addiction Medicine, 9*(2), 111–117.

Wu, E. S., & Hueppchen, N. A. (2015). Surgical disease & trauma in pregnancy. In J. L. Bienstock, H. Fox, E. E. Wallach, et al. (Eds.), *The Johns Hopkins manual of gynecology and obstetrics* (5th ed., pp. 248–256). Philadelphia, PA: Lippincott Williams & Wilkins.

Zeiders, K. H., Umaña-Taylor, A. J., Jahromi, L. B., et al. (2015). Grandmothers' familism values, adolescent mothers' parenting efficacy, and children's well-being. *Journal of Family Psychology, 29*(4), 624–634.

23

Nursing Care of a Family Experiencing a Complication of Labor or Birth

*Y*ou admit Rosann Bigalow, a 28-year-old woman about to give birth to her first baby, to a birthing room. Her contractions have been 5 minutes apart for 10 hours. She feels more pain in her back than in her abdomen, saying it feels "like my spine is tearing apart." A contraction monitor shows contractions are hypotonic. A sonogram shows her fetus is "borderline" large for gestation and in an occipitoposterior position. Her husband asks you if the reason Rosann's labor is taking so long is because she's overweight.

Previous chapters discussed uncomplicated pregnancy and labor and birth. This chapter adds information about what happens when complications of labor occur. Nurses play a vital role in making any labor safe. They play an even greater role when a complication arises. The sooner a complication in labor is recognized, the better the chance the situation can be corrected, the concern resolved, and both fetal and maternal health can be protected.

How would you answer Mr. Bigalow?

KEY TERMS

amnioinfusion

amniotic fluid embolism

augmentation of labor

battledore placenta

dysfunctional labor

dystocia

external cephalic version

hypertonic uterine contraction

hypotonic uterine contraction

induction of labor

oxytocin

placenta accreta

placenta circumvallata

placenta marginata

placenta succenturiata

precipitate labor

umbilical cord prolapse

uterine inversion

vacuum extraction

OBJECTIVES

After mastering the contents of this chapter, you should be able to:

1. Describe the common deviations in the power (i.e., force of labor), the passage, or the passenger that can cause complications during labor or birth.

2. Identify the 2020 National Health Goals related to complications of labor that nurses can help the nation achieve.

3. Assess a woman in labor and during birth for deviations from the usual labor process.

4. Formulate nursing diagnoses related to deviations in labor and birth.

5. Identify expected outcomes associated with deviations from usual labor and birth such as induction of labor as well as help couples manage seamless transitions across differing healthcare settings.

6. Using the nursing process, plan nursing care that includes the six competencies of Quality & Safety Education for Nurses (QSEN): Patient-Centered Care, Teamwork & Collaboration, Evidence-Based Practice (EBP), Quality Improvement (QI), Safety, and Informatics.

7. Implement nursing care related to complications of labor or birth, such as preparing the family for a cesarean birth.

8. Evaluate expected outcomes for achievement and effectiveness of care.

9. Integrate knowledge of deviations from normal labor and birth with the interplay of nursing process, the six competencies of QSEN, and Family Nursing to promote quality maternal and child health nursing care.

Although labor often proceeds without any deviation from the normal, many potential complications can occur. A difficult labor—**dystocia**—can arise from any of the four main components of the labor process: (a) the power, or the force that propels the fetus (uterine contractions); (b) the passenger (the fetus); (c) the passageway (the birth canal); or (d) the psyche (the woman's and family's perception of the event) (Neal, Ryan, Lowe, et al., 2015).

Because complications can occur at any point in labor, a continuous assessment of a laboring woman and her fetus as well as providing emotional support for her and her family are essential. The hours of labor are stressful even when everything is proceeding normally. Be certain to reassure all women in labor that everything is going smoothly and both she and her fetus appear to be doing well. If a complication arises and assurances cannot be given as freely, it is doubly important that a woman has someone who is both knowledgeable about the deviation and what measures need to be taken as well as able to feel empathetic to her sense of helplessness and the necessary change in her birth plan (Zielinski, Brody, & Low, 2016). Nurses are able to play a key role in providing this type of care because they are skilled practitioners of both physical and emotional care.

The National 2020 Health Goals that relate to attempts to decrease maternal complications and prevent infant injury related to birth are shown in Box 23.1.

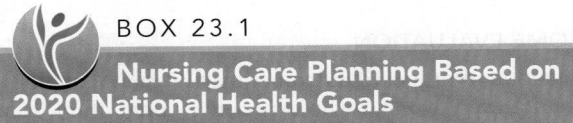

BOX 23.1

Nursing Care Planning Based on 2020 National Health Goals

A number of 2020 National Health Goals speak directly to complications of labor.

- Reduce the number of cesarean births among low-risk women to no more than 23.9 per 100 births from a baseline of 26.5 per 100 births.
- Reduce the number of cesarean births among women who have had a previous cesarean birth to no more than 61.7 per 100 births from a baseline of 90.8 per 100 births.
- Reduce the maternal mortality rate to no more than 11.4 per 100,000 live births from a baseline of 12.7 per 100,000 live births.
- Reduce the rate of maternal complications during hospitalized labor and birth to no more than 28 per 100 births from a baseline of 31.1 per 100 births (U.S. Department of Health and Human Services, 2010; see www.healthypeople.gov).

Nurses can help the nation achieve these goals by helping identify women in labor who are developing a complication; by assisting with cesarean births and careful assessment during labor; and by being alert to the preliminary symptoms of uterine rupture, which accounts for a substantial number of maternal deaths during labor.

Nursing Process Overview

FOR A WOMAN WITH A LABOR OR BIRTH COMPLICATION

ASSESSMENT

One of the major nursing roles with a woman who is having a variation in labor is a conscientious assessment of labor progress. One of the major assessment tools used to detect deviations is a fetal and uterine monitor. Because such equipment can limit a woman's ability to walk about or even turn freely, thus making labor different than anticipated, a woman in labor may not be totally accepting of technologic or pharmacologic intervention. This calls for frequent adjustment of the equipment to achieve a clear tracing. Caring for a woman with such an apparatus in place involves explaining its importance to both a woman and her partner, winning their cooperation, and using judgment in reading the various patterns.

NURSING DIAGNOSIS

Common nursing diagnoses specific to a woman experiencing a complication during labor or birth refer to specific problems. Some examples might include:

- Pain related to induction and labor procedures
- Fear related to uncertainty of pregnancy outcome
- Anxiety related to medical procedures and apparatus necessary to ensure health of woman and fetus
- Fatigue related to loss of glucose stores through work and duration of labor
- Ineffective coping related to lack of knowledge or lack of preparation for labor
- Fatigue related to prolonged labor

- Risk for ineffective tissue perfusion related to excessive loss of blood with complication of labor
- Risk for injury (maternal or fetal) related to effect on woman and fetus of a labor complication and treatment required
- Risk for injury (maternal or fetal) related to labor involving a multiple gestation pregnancy
- Anticipatory grieving related to nonviable monitoring pattern of fetus

OUTCOME IDENTIFICATION AND PLANNING

If a complication of labor or childbirth occurs, identification of expected outcomes can be difficult because an outcome that must be included in planning may not be what the woman desires. Encouraging a couple to clarify their priorities when a complication occurs is helpful. For example, early in labor, a woman's birth plan might state her chief goal is to avoid monitoring equipment or any analgesia. If fetal bradycardia occurs, however, monitoring and a cesarean birth may become necessary. If this happens, reminding the woman her primary goal is really to have a healthy baby, not to avoid specific interventions, can help her accept these changes. Refer patients and their partners to helpful websites and other resources when appropriate (see Chapter 20).

IMPLEMENTATION

If a woman develops a complication of labor or birth, actions to increase the fetal heart rate (FHR) or to strengthen uterine contractions are a priority and possibly an emergency. Interventions must be planned and performed efficiently and effectively, based on the individual circumstances. Be certain to provide psychological reassurance to accompany actions to fully safeguard both the woman and her fetus.

OUTCOME EVALUATION

An evaluation of proposed outcomes may reveal unhappiness because not every woman who experiences a deviation from the normal in labor and birth will be able to give birth to a healthy child. Some deviations will be too great; some interventions will not be maximally effective because of individual circumstances. Some infants will die; a few women may be left unable to bear future children. An evaluation may lead to a new analysis that the couple's chief need at that point is to grieve for the child or for a lifestyle that can no longer be theirs. If the outcome is more positive, evaluate the couple for signs that they are able to begin interacting with their child after their harrowing experience.

Examples of outcome achievement might include:

- Patient voices confidence she can cope with the fear she feels about her fetus's welfare.
- Patient demonstrates adequate energy during course of labor to maintain effective breathing patterns.
- Patient's blood pressure does not drop below 90/50 mmHg despite excessive blood loss with delivery of the placenta.
- Patient begins positive grieving behaviors in response to loss of newborn.

> **BOX 23.2**
>
> ## Common Causes of Dysfunctional Labor
>
> - Primigravida status
> - Pelvic bone contraction that has narrowed the pelvic diameter so a fetus cannot pass (cephalopelvic disproportion [CPD]) such as could occur in a woman with rickets
> - Posterior rather than anterior fetal position or extension rather than flexion of the fetal head
> - Failure of the uterine muscle to contract properly or overdistention of the uterus, as with a multiple pregnancy, polyhydramnios, or an excessively oversized fetus
> - A nonripe cervix
> - Presence of a full rectum or urinary bladder that impedes fetal descent
> - A woman becoming exhausted from labor
> - Inappropriate use of analgesia (excessive or too early administration)

Complications With the Power (The Force of Labor)

Inertia is a time-honored term to denote sluggishness of contractions, or that the force of labor, is less than usual. A more current term is **dysfunctional labor** (Neal, Lowe, Schorn, et al., 2015). Dysfunction can occur at any point in labor, but it is generally classified as primary (i.e., occurring at the onset of labor) or secondary (i.e., occurring later in labor). The risk of maternal postpartal infection, hemorrhage, and infant mortality is higher in women who have a prolonged labor than in those who do not. Therefore, it is vital to recognize and prevent dysfunctional labor to the extent possible (Hunt & Menticoglou, 2015).

Prolonged labor appears to result from several factors but is most likely to occur if a fetus is large or if the contractions are hypotonic, hypertonic, or uncoordinated contractions occur (Box 23.2).

INEFFECTIVE UTERINE FORCE

Uterine contractions are the basic force that moves the fetus through the birth canal. They occur because of the interplay of the contractile enzyme adenosine triphosphate and the influence of major electrolytes such as calcium, sodium, and potassium, specific contractile proteins (actin and myosin), epinephrine and norepinephrine, **oxytocin** (a posterior pituitary hormone), estrogen, progesterone, and prostaglandins. In about 95% of labors, contractions follow a predictable, efficient course. When they have less strength than usual or are rapid but ineffective, dysfunctional labor occurs (Neal, Lowe, et al., 2015).

Hypotonic Contractions

Figure 23.1A illustrates the appearance of normal uterine contractions recorded on a uterine contraction monitor. With **hypotonic uterine contractions**, the number of contractions is unusually infrequent (not more than two or three occurring in a 10-minute period). The resting tone of the uterus remains less than 10 mmHg, and the strength of contractions does not rise above 25 mmHg (Fig. 23.1B). Hypotonic contractions occur during the active phase of labor and tend to occur after the administration of analgesia, especially if the cervix is not dilated to 3 to 4 cm or if bowel or bladder distention is preventing descent or firm engagement. They also may occur in a uterus that is overstretched by a multiple gestation, a larger than usual single fetus, polyhydramnios, or in a uterus that is lax from grand multiparity. Such contractions are not exceedingly painful because of their lack of intensity. Keep in mind, however, that pain is a subjective symptom. Some women, therefore, may interpret these contractions as very painful.

Hypotonic contractions will increase the length of labor because more of them are necessary to achieve cervical dilatation. If the uterus becomes exhausted, this can cause it to not contract as effectively during the postpartal period, thus increasing a woman's chance for postpartal hemorrhage. In the first hour after birth following a labor of hypotonic contractions, it is very important to palpate the uterine fundus, obtain the woman's blood pressure, and assess the amount of lochia every 15 minutes for the first hour to ensure postpartal contractions are not also hypotonic and therefore not adequate to halt postpartal hemorrhage.

Hypertonic Contractions

Hypertonic uterine contractions are marked by an increase in resting tone to more than 15 mmHg (Fig. 23.1C). However, the intensity of the contraction may be no stronger than that associated with hypotonic contractions. In contrast to hypotonic contractions, these occur frequently and are most commonly seen in the latent phase of labor. Hypertonic contractions may occur because more than one uterine pacemaker is stimulating contractions or because the muscle fibers of the myometrium do not repolarize or relax after a contraction,

Figure 23.1   (A) Normal uterine contractions. **(B)** Hypotonic contractions; notice that the rise in pressure is no more than 10 mmHg. **(C)** Hypertonic contractions; notice the high resting pressure (35–40 mmHg).

thereby "wiping it clean" to accept a new pacemaker stimulus. They tend to be more painful than usual because the myometrium becomes tender from constant lack of relaxation and the anoxia of uterine cells that results.

A danger of hypertonic contractions is that the lack of relaxation between contractions may not allow optimal uterine artery filling; this can lead to fetal anoxia early in the latent phase of labor. Applying a uterine and a fetal external monitor to any woman whose pain seems out of proportion to the quality of her contractions will help identify that the resting phase between contractions is adequate and that the FHR is not showing late deceleration.

If decelerations in the FHR, an abnormally long first stage of labor, or lack of progress with pushing (i.e., "second-stage arrest") occurs, cesarean birth may be necessary. Although this is disappointing, be certain the woman and her support person understand that, although contractions are strong, they are ineffective and are not achieving cervical dilatation. To help identify the difference, hypotonic and hypertonic contractions are compared in Table 23.1.

Uncoordinated Contractions

Normally, all contractions are initiated at one pacemaker point high in the uterus. A contraction sweeps down over

the organ, encircling it; repolarization occurs; relaxation or a low resting tone is achieved; and another pacemaker-activated contraction begins. With uncoordinated contractions, more than one pacemaker may be initiating contractions, or receptor points in the myometrium may be acting independently of the pacemaker. Uncoordinated contractions can occur so closely together that they can interfere with the blood supply to the placenta. Because they occur so erratically, such as one on top of another and then a long period without any, it may be difficult for a woman to rest between contractions or to breathe effectively with contractions.

Applying a fetal and a uterine external monitor and assessing the rate, pattern, resting tone, and fetal response to contractions for 15 minutes (or longer if necessary in early labor) reveals the abnormal pattern. Oxytocin administration may be helpful in uncoordinated labor to stimulate a more effective and consistent pattern of contractions with a better, lower resting tone.

DYSFUNCTIONAL LABOR AND ASSOCIATED STAGES OF LABOR

For a graphic illustration of the most frequent times dysfunctional labor is apt to occur (Fig. 23.2). Regardless of when dysfunctional labor occurs, the effect on a woman and her support person will be the same: anxiety, fear, or discouragement. A woman needs good explanations of what is happening: "We're going to take an ultrasound to check the baby's position." "This is a drug to make your contractions stronger." "I know resting is the last thing you feel like doing, but that is what I want you to try to do."

Dysfunction at the First Stage of Labor

Dysfunction that occurs with the first stage of labor involves a prolonged latent phase, protracted active phase, prolonged deceleration phase, and secondary arrest of dilatation.

TABLE 23.1 COMPARISON OF HYPOTONIC AND HYPERTONIC CONTRACTIONS

Criteria	Hypertonic	Hypotonic
Most common phase of occurrence	Latent	Active
Symptoms	Painful	Limited pain
Medications used		
Oxytocin	Unfavorable reaction	Favorable reaction
Sedation	Helpful	Little value

Figure 23.2 Graph showing normal and abnormal patterns of labor. **(A)** Labor curves. **(B)** Patterns of descent.

Prolonged Latent Phase

When contractions become ineffective during the first stage of labor, a prolonged latent phase can develop. How long the stages of labor take is affected by individual circumstances and whether a woman has received analgesia or an epidural anesthesia (Eggebø, Hassan, Salvesen, et al., 2015). Usual parameters for the stages of labor that can be expected are highlighted in Table 23.2. A prolonged latent phase, as defined by Friedman (1978), is a latent phase that lasts longer than 20 hours in a nullipara or 14 hours in a multipara. This may occur if the cervix is not "ripe" at the beginning of labor. It may occur if there is excessive use of an analgesic early in labor. With a prolonged latent phase, the uterus tends to be in a hypertonic state. Relaxation between contractions is inadequate, and the contractions are only mild (less than 15 mmHg on a monitor printout) and, therefore, ineffective. One segment of the uterus may be contracting with more force than another segment.

Management of a prolonged latent phase in labor that has been caused by hypertonic contractions involves helping the uterus to rest, providing adequate fluid for hydration, and pain relief with a drug such as morphine sulfate. Changing the linen and the woman's gown, darkening room lights, and decreasing noise and stimulation can also be helpful.

TABLE 23.2 LENGTHS OF PHASES AND STAGES OF NORMAL LABOR IN HOURS

Phase	Nullipara		Multipara	
	Average	Upper Normal	Average	Upper Normal
First stage: time span from beginning of regular contractions to complete cervical dilatation				
Latent phase: onset of labor to 4 cm dilatation	8.6 hr	20.0 hr	5.3 hr	14.0 hr
Active phase: 4 cm to complete dilatation	4.9 hr; minimum rate of dilatation 1.2 cm/hr	12.0 hr	2.5 hr; minimum rate of dilatation 1.5 cm/hr	6.0 hr
Second stage: from full dilatation to birth of infant	1 hr	Under 2 hr without epidural; under 3 hr with epidural	0.5 hr	Under 1 hr without epidural; under 2 hr with epidural
Placenta stage	30 min		30 min	

These measures usually combine to allow labor to become effective and begin to progress. If it does not, a cesarean birth or amniotomy (i.e., artificial rupture of membranes) and oxytocin infusion to assist labor may be necessary.

Protracted Active Phase

A protracted active phase is usually associated with fetal malposition or cephalopelvic disproportion (CPD) (the diameter of the fetal head is larger than the woman's pelvic diameters), although it may reflect ineffective myometrial activity. This phase is prolonged if cervical dilatation does not occur at a rate of at least 1.2 cm/hr in a nullipara or 1.5 cm/hr in a multipara, or if the active phase lasts longer than 12 hours in a primigravida or 6 hours in a multigravida (see Table 23.2). If the cause of the delay in dilatation is fetal malposition or CPD, cesarean birth may be necessary. Dysfunctional labor during the dilatational division of labor tends to be hypotonic in contrast to the hypertonic action at the beginning of labor. After an ultrasound to show CPD is not present, oxytocin may be prescribed to augment labor (see later discussion on augmentation by oxytocin).

Prolonged Deceleration Phase

A deceleration phase has become prolonged when it extends beyond 3 hours in a nullipara or 1 hour in a multipara. A prolonged deceleration phase most often results from abnormal fetal head position. A cesarean birth is frequently required.

Secondary Arrest of Dilatation

A secondary arrest of dilatation has occurred if there is no progress in cervical dilatation for longer than 2 hours. Again, cesarean birth may be necessary (Hamilton, Warrick, Collins, et al., 2015).

Dysfunction at the Second Stage of Labor

Dysfunction that occurs with the second stage of labor involves prolonged descent and arrest of descent.

Prolonged Descent

Prolonged descent of the fetus occurs if the rate of descent is less than 1.0 cm/hr in a nullipara or 2.0 cm/hr in a multipara. It can be suspected if the second stage lasts over 2 hours in a multipara (Zheng, 2012).

With both a prolonged active phase of dilatation and prolonged descent, contractions have been of good quality and duration, effacement and beginning dilatation have occurred, but then the contractions become infrequent and of poor quality, and dilatation stops. If everything else is within normal limits except for the suddenly faulty contractions and CPD and poor fetal presentation have been ruled out by ultrasound, then rest and fluid intake, as advocated for hypertonic contractions, also applies. If the membranes have not ruptured, rupturing them at this point may be helpful. Intravenous (IV) oxytocin may be used to induce the uterus to contract effectively (see later discussion on induction of labor by oxytocin). A semi-Fowler's position, squatting, kneeling, or more effective pushing may speed descent.

Arrest of Descent

Arrest of descent results when no descent has occurred for 2 hours in a nullipara or 1 hour in a multipara. *Failure* of descent occurs when expected descent of the fetus does not begin or engagement or movement beyond 0 station does not occur. The most likely cause for arrest of descent during the second stage is CPD. Cesarean birth usually is necessary. If there is no contraindication to vaginal birth, oxytocin may be used to assist labor (Choubey & Werner, 2015).

Nursing Diagnoses and Related Interventions

It is impossible to prevent all dysfunctional labor, just as it is impossible to predict the functioning of any woman's hormonal system or individual response to labor. However, a number of nursing interventions can contribute to the progression of normal labor and help change a dysfunctional labor to a functional one.

Nursing Diagnosis: Fatigue and anxiety related to prolonged labor

Outcome Evaluation: Patient states she is able to continue active participation in labor; maintains effective breathing with contractions.

Because labor is work, a woman's glucose stores can deplete over hours of labor. On a woman's admission to a birthing room, assess the likelihood of glucose depletion by asking when she ate her last meal. If she ate breakfast at 8:00 AM and then began labor by 2:00 PM, it has only been 6 hours since her last full meal. However, if she last ate at 5:00 PM the preceding evening and did not eat breakfast because she awoke with labor this morning, it has been 11 hours since a full meal. Alert her primary care provider to this situation. If the woman is still in early labor, she may be encouraged to drink a high-carbohydrate fluid such as a sports drink or to eat a light meal. Sucking on a lollipop or hard candy are enjoyable ways to supply additional glucose.

Although the effect of emotion on labor is difficult to document, for many women, the cervix seems to dilate more rapidly, and therefore, labor is shortened if the woman is neither tense nor frightened. To try to identify stress, ask at a healthcare facility admission if a woman has any special concerns. Offer explanations of all procedures. Help her support person feel welcome and comfortable as well. Allow the woman and her support person as many choices as possible to give them a sense of control. Asking a question such as "Is labor what you thought it would be?" to both the woman and her support person often helps them express their concerns.

Remember that long-term pain is both depressing and exhausting. Encourage a partner to use nonpharmacologic comfort measures such as breathing with the woman, offering a back rub, changing sheets, using cool washcloths, or whatever else seems comforting. An individual woman may find a complementary therapy such as aromatherapy, acupressure, or music helpful for relaxation (Koyyalamudi, Sidhu, Cornett, et al., 2016).

Be certain that if a woman is in bed to urge her to lie on her side so that the uterus is lifted off the vena cava (to prevent hypotension syndrome). If a woman insists on lying supine, place a hip roll under one or the other of her buttocks to cause her pelvis to "tip" and, at least to some extent, move the uterus to the side.

A full bladder can slow descent of the fetus and may also impede uterine contractions. Urge a woman in labor, therefore, to void every 2 hours to keep the bladder empty so this does not add to the slow progress caused by hypotensive or hypertensive contractions.

Nursing Diagnosis: Risk for deficient fluid volume related to length and work of labor

Outcome Evaluation: Urine is free of ketones; specific gravity is between 1.003 and 1.030; skin turgor and serum electrolyte levels are within acceptable parameters.

Low levels of serum electrolytes or body fluid can occur in labor for the same reason as a decreased glucose level—there has been a long interval between eating and the end of labor. Additionally, vomiting and diarrhea occasionally accompany labor; if these occur, they can add to fluid and electrolyte losses. Ask if a woman has had any vomiting or diarrhea to determine the possible extent of these because extended vomiting or diarrhea can lead to serious dehydration and electrolyte imbalance. Profuse diaphoresis and hyperventilation that occur with labor are also factors that can further increase fluid and electrolyte loss through insensible water loss.

Test urine each time a woman voids during labor for glucose, protein, ketones, and specific gravity. Ketones in the urine suggest starvation ketosis. A concentrated specific gravity suggests a lack of fluid. Extreme dehydration not only may slow labor but also can lead to increased blood viscosity, possibly increasing the risk for thrombophlebitis during the postpartal period.

Many women react negatively to the idea of IV fluid therapy during labor to restore body fluid, possibly perceiving it as loss of control over their bodies or removal of the "naturalness" of labor and birth. Introduce the idea that IV fluid therapy has been prescribed because of her particular complication before arriving with the bag of fluid and tubing. When inserting the IV catheter, try to use an insertion site in a woman's nondominant hand and, if necessary, only a small "reminder" hand board. Use long tubing or attach extensions so that the woman can move about freely and her mobility is not limited or restricted by the short length of IV tubing. Assure a woman that being out of bed and walking, turning freely, squatting, sitting, or using whatever position she prefers during labor will not disrupt the IV line or the infusion (Fig. 23.3).

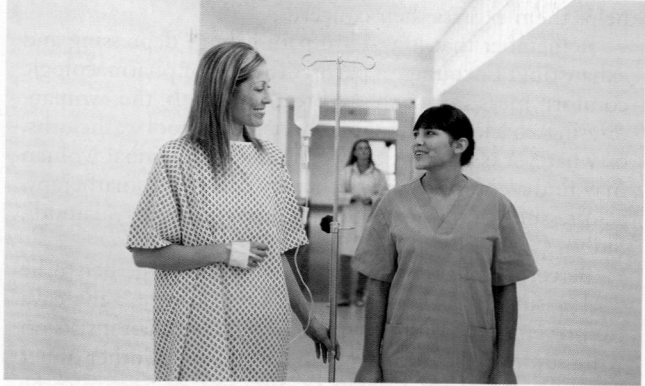

Figure 23.3 If intravenous fluid is used for women in labor, it does not need to limit mobility.

PRECIPITATE LABOR

Precipitate dilatation is cervical dilatation that occurs at a rate of 5 cm or more per hour in a primipara or 10 cm or more per hour in a multipara. *Precipitate birth* occurs when uterine contractions are so strong a woman gives birth with only a few, rapidly occurring contractions, often defined as a labor that is completed in fewer than 3 hours (Suzuki, 2016). Such rapid labor is likely to occur with grand multiparity, or it may occur after induction of labor by oxytocin. Contractions can be so forceful they lead to premature separation of the placenta or lacerations of the perineum, placing the woman at risk for hemorrhage (Kim, Kim, Kim, et al., 2014). Rapid labor also poses a risk to the fetus because subdural hemorrhage may result from the rapid release of pressure on the head. The woman and her support person can feel overwhelmed by the speed of labor.

A **precipitate labor** can be predicted from a labor graph if, during the active phase of dilatation, the rate is greater than 5 cm/hr (1 cm every 12 minutes) in a nullipara or 10 cm/hr (1 cm every 6 minutes) in a multipara.

Caution a multiparous woman by week 28 of pregnancy that because a past labor was so brief, her labor this time also may be brief so that she has time to plan for adequate transportation to the hospital or alternative birthing center. Both grand multiparas and women with histories of precipitate labor should have the birthing room converted to birth readiness before full dilatation is obtained. Then, even if a sudden birth should occur, it can be accomplished in a controlled surrounding.

What If . . . 23.1
Rosann tells the nurse her sister was only in labor 1 hour when she had her baby. Rosann is planning to spend the last days of this pregnancy camping in a mountain cabin 60 miles from the hospital. Would the nurse advise her not to go camping?

INDUCTION AND AUGMENTATION OF LABOR

When labor contractions are ineffective, several interventions, such as induction and **augmentation of labor** with oxytocin or amniotomy (artificial rupture of the membranes), may be initiated to strengthen them (Gilstrop & Sciscione, 2015). **Induction of labor** means labor is started artificially. Augmentation of labor refers to assisting labor that has started spontaneously but is not effective. Although induction may be necessary to initiate labor before the time when it would have occurred spontaneously because a fetus is in danger, it is not used as an elective procedure until the fetus is at term (over 39 weeks). At one time, induction could be completed if a fetus was proven to have adequate lung surfactant by amniocentesis at term but less than 39 weeks. However, the American College of Obstetricians and Gynecologists (ACOG) has issued a statement (ACOG, 2013) indicating that fetal lung maturity should not be used and inductions should be avoided until 39 weeks unless medically indicated. Conditions that might make induction necessary before that time include preeclampsia, eclampsia, severe hypertension, diabetes, Rh sensitization, prolonged rupture of the membranes, and intrauterine growth restriction. Postmaturity (a pregnancy lasting beyond 42 weeks) is yet another situation that makes it more potentially dangerous for a fetus to remain in utero than to be born.

Because either augmentation or initiation of labor carries a risk of uterine rupture or premature separation of the placenta, it must be used cautiously in women with multiple gestation, polyhydramnios, grand parity, who are older than 40 years, or have previous uterine scars (Norman, 2012).

Oxytocin is an effective uterine stimulant, but there is a thin line between adequate stimulation and hyperstimulation, so careful observation during the entire infusion time is an important nursing responsibility (Bor, Ledertoug, Boie, et al., 2016). Before induction of labor is begun in term and postterm pregnancies, the following conditions should be present:

- The fetus is in a longitudinal lie.
- The cervix is ripe, or ready for birth.
- The presenting part is the fetal head (vertex) and is engaged.
- There is no CPD.
- The fetus is estimated to be mature by date (over 39 weeks).

Cervical Ripening

Cervical ripening, or a change in the cervical consistency from firm to soft, is the first change of the uterus in early labor because, until this has happened, dilatation and coordination of uterine contractions will not occur. To determine whether a cervix is "ripe," or ready for dilatation, Bishop (1964) established criteria for scoring the cervix (Table 23.3). Using this scale, if a woman's total score is 8 or greater, the cervix is ready for birth and should respond to induction. To help a cervix "ripen," a number of methods can be instituted. The simplest method is known as "stripping the membranes," or separating the membranes from the lower uterine segment manually, using a gloved finger in the cervix. This is an easy procedure performed during an office visit. Possible complications of this mechanical method include bleeding from an undetected low-lying placenta, inadvertent rupture of membranes, and the possibility of infection if membranes should rupture.

For a second method, the use of hygroscopic suppositories (suppositories of seaweed that swell on contact with cervical secretions), which gradually and gently urge dilatation (laminaria technique), can be inserted. They can be held in place by gauze sponges saturated with povidone-iodine or an antifungal cream. If sponges are used, documentation of how many were placed is important so it can be documented afterward that none remain.

The most common method used to promote cervical ripening, however, is the insertion of a prostaglandin such as dinoprostone (Prepidil, Cervidil) into the posterior fornix of the vagina, by the cervix (Kunzier, Park, Cioffi, et al., 2016). If the prostaglandin is put in place in the evening, cervical ripening will usually have begun by morning. It's best if women remain in bed in a side-lying position to prevent loss or leakage of the medication. Monitor the FHR after each application and for side effects such as vomiting, fever, diarrhea, and hypertension in the mother. Oxytocin induction can be started 12 hours after the prostaglandin dose; beginning it sooner might lead to hyperstimulation of the uterus. Even with these side effects, prostaglandins are well accepted by most women as a way to aid cervical ripening (Kunzier et al., 2016). They should be used with caution in women with asthma, renal or cardiovascular disease, glaucoma, or in those who have had past cesarean births because of the danger of side effects and hyperstimulation (Karch, 2015).

Although not approved for obstetric use by the U.S. Food and Drug Administration (FDA), misoprostol is a drug you may often see used off label to assist in cervical ripening. It is as effective as dinoprostone and requires the same precautions of FHR and maternal vital sign assessments (Kunzier et al., 2016).

Induction of Labor by Oxytocin

After a cervix is "ripe," administration of oxytocin (a synthetic form of naturally occurring pituitary hormone) can be used to initiate labor contractions if a pregnancy is at term (Zheng, 2012). Oxytocin is always administered intravenously, so that, if uterine hyperstimulation should occur, it can be quickly discontinued. Because the half-life of oxytocin is approximately 3 minutes, the falling serum level and effects are apparent almost immediately after discontinuation of IV administration.

The danger of hyperstimulation is that a fetus needs 60 to 90 seconds between contractions in order to receive adequate oxygenation from placenta blood vessels. Hyperstimulation (i.e., tachysystole) is usually defined as five or more contractions in a 10-minute period or contractions lasting more than 2 minutes in duration or occurring within 60 seconds of each other, situations that have the potential to interfere with placenta filling and fetal oxygenation. If uterine hyperstimulation should occur, several

TABLE 23.3 SCORING OF THE CERVIX FOR READINESS FOR ELECTIVE INDUCTION

Rating Factor	0	1	2	3
Dilatation (cm)	0	1–2	3–4	5–6
Effacement (%)	0–30	40–50	60–70	80
Station	−3	−2	−1 to 0	+1 to +2
Consistency	Firm	Medium	Soft	
Position	Posterior	Midposition	Anterior	

A total score of 8 or higher indicates that the cervix is considered ready for birth and should respond to induction.

Adapted with permission from Bishop, E. H. (1964). Pelvic scoring for elective induction. *Obstetrics and Gynecology, 24*(2), 266.

interventions such as asking the woman to turn onto her left side to improve blood flow to the uterus, administering an IV fluid bolus to dilute the level of oxytocin in the maternal blood stream, and administering oxygen by mask at 8 to 10 L are all helpful. In addition, a primary care provider may prescribe terbutaline to relax the uterus. The surest method to relieve tachysystole, however, is to immediately discontinue the oxytocin infusion. If in doubt, err on the side of stopping the infusion when the action isn't needed (it can easily be restarted) rather than delaying stopping it so that fetal or maternal harm results.

For administration, oxytocin (Pitocin) is commonly mixed in the proportion of 10 International Units in 1,000 ml of Ringer's lactate. Ten International Units of oxytocin is the same as 10,000 milliunits, so each milliliter of this solution contains 10 milliunits of oxytocin. An alternative dilution method is to add 15 International Units of oxytocin to 250 ml of an IV solution; this yields a concentration of 60 milliunits per 1 ml.

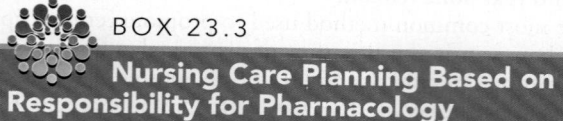

BOX 23.3

Nursing Care Planning Based on Responsibility for Pharmacology

OXYTOCIN FOR LABOR INDUCTION

Classification: Oxytocin is a synthetic form of the naturally occurring posterior pituitary hormone.

Action: used to initiate uterine contractions in a term pregnancy (over 39 weeks)

Pregnancy Risk Category: C

Dosage: initially 1–2 milliunits/min by intravenous (IV) infusion, increased at a rate no more than 1–2 milliunits/min at 30- to 60-minute intervals until a contraction pattern similar to normal labor is achieved

Possible Adverse Effects: nausea, vomiting, cardiac arrhythmias, uterine hypertonicity, tetanic contractions, uterine rupture (with excessive dosages), severe water intoxication, and fetal bradycardia

Nursing Implications

- Prepare IV solution by adding 1 ml (10 International Units) to 1,000 ml of designated IV fluid (resulting solution contains 10 milliunits/ml). Obtain an oxytocin infusion solution from pharmacy (30 units/500 ml fluid).
- Use an infusion pump to ensure accurate control of infusion rate.
- Regulate infusion rate to establish uterine contractions similar to a normal labor pattern.
- Monitor frequency, duration, and strength of contractions during infusion.
- Assess maternal pulse and blood pressure, and watch for possible hypotension. If hypotension occurs, discontinue drug and notify primary care provider.
- Continuously monitor fetal heart rate for signs of fetal distress.
- Monitor intake and output and watch for signs of possible water intoxication, such as headache or vomiting. Limit IV fluids to 150 ml/hr.
- Prepare the woman for birth (Karch, 2015).

A primary care provider's prescription for administration of oxytocin for induction usually designates the number of milliunits to be administered per minute such as 1 to 2 milliunits per minute. Be certain you know the dilution prescribed and recognize the concentration in each milliliter (Box 23.3). Don't increase the rate by more than 2 milliunits at a time.

When administering the infusion, "piggyback" the oxytocin solution to a maintenance IV solution such as Ringer's lactate and add the piggyback to the main infusion at the port closest to the woman. Then, if the oxytocin needs to be discontinued quickly during the induction, little solution remains in the tubing to still infuse and the main IV line can still be maintained. Use an infusion pump to regulate the infusion rate, so the rate will not change even if a woman changes position. In addition, a primary care provider should be immediately available during the entire procedure to ensure safety (Manjula, Bagga, Kalra, et al., 2015).

Infusions are usually begun at a rate of 1 to 2 milliunits/min. If there is no response, the infusion is gradually increased every 30 to 60 minutes by small increments of 1 to 2 milliunits/min until contractions begin. Many women respond with as little as 4 milliunits/min, and most women respond at 16 milliunits/min. Do not increase the rate to more than 30 milliunits/min without checking for further instructions because an administration rate greater than this is likely to cause tetanic contractions.

After cervical dilatation reaches 4 cm, artificial rupture of the membranes may be performed to further induce labor, and the infusion may be discontinued at that point. For other women, the infusion is continued through full dilatation.

A side effect of oxytocin is that it causes peripheral vessel dilation, and peripheral dilation can lead to extreme hypotension. To ensure safe induction, therefore, take the woman's pulse and blood pressure every hour. Monitor uterine contractions and FHR conscientiously. (See Box 23.4 for additional assessments for danger signs of oxytocin administration.)

A second side effect of oxytocin is that it can result in decreased urine flow, possibly leading to water intoxication. This is first manifested by headache and vomiting. If you observe these danger signs in a woman during induction of labor, report them immediately and halt the infusion. Water intoxication in its most severe form can lead to seizures, coma, and death because of the large shift in interstitial tissue fluid. Keep an accurate intake and output record and test and record urine specific gravity throughout oxytocin administration to detect fluid retention. Limit the amount of IV fluid being given to that prescribed (usually 150 ml/hr by ensuring the main IV fluid line is infusing at a rate not greater than 2.5 ml/min).

Contractions should occur no more often than every 2 minutes, should not be stronger than 50 mmHg pressure, and should last no longer than 70 seconds. The resting pressure between contractions should not exceed 15 mmHg by monitor (Fig. 23.4). If contractions become more frequent or longer in duration than these safe limits, or if signs of fetal distress occur, stop the IV infusion and seek help immediately. Anticipate oxygen administration may be needed to maintain fetal oxygenation. If stopping the oxytocin infusion does not stop the hyperstimulation, a tocolytic such as terbutaline may be prescribed to decrease myometrial activity. After birth, observe the infant closely for hyperbilirubinemia and jaundice because these are associated with oxytocin induction.

Nursing Care Planning Using Assessment

ASSESSING THE PREGNANT WOMAN FOR DANGER SIGNS OF OXYTOCIN ADMINISTRATION

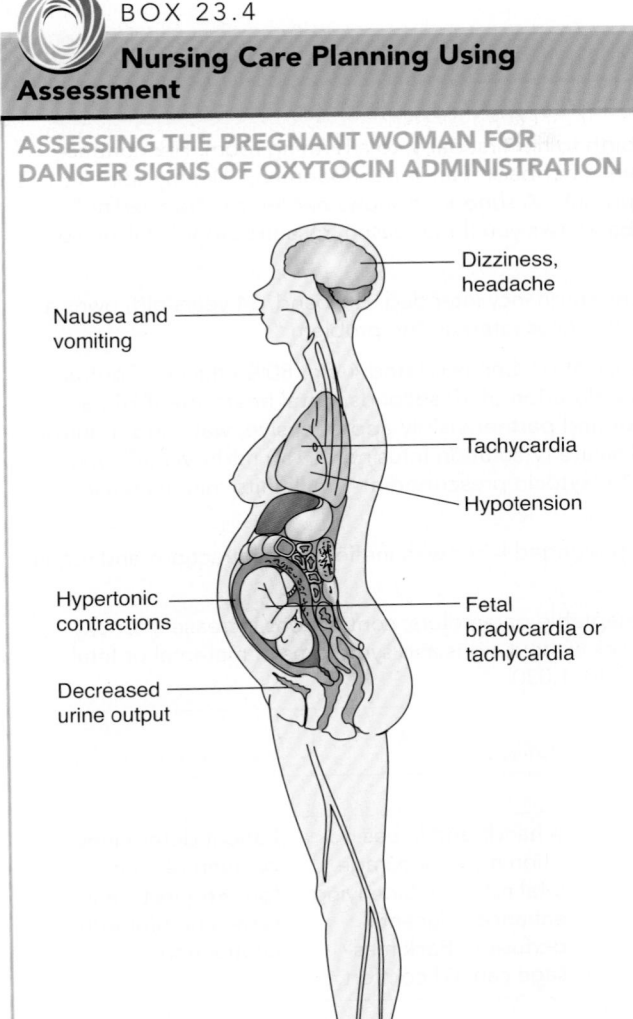

Women may worry that induced labor will be more painful or "so different" from normal labor that breathing exercises will be worthless, or that labor will progress so fast it will be harmful to the fetus. Induced labors do tend to have a slightly shorter first stage than the average unassisted labor; however, this can be an advantage not a disadvantage. Once contractions begin by this method, they are basically the same as unassisted contractions. Assure the woman of this so that she does not fight the contractions or become unnecessarily tense, which could prevent her from using her breathing techniques effectively.

Augmentation by Oxytocin

Augmentation of labor may be used if labor contractions begin spontaneously but then become weak, irregular, or ineffective (i.e., hypotonic) (Rossen, Østborg, Lindtjørn, et al., 2016).

Precautions regarding oxytocin augmentation are the same as for primary oxytocin induction of labor. Be certain the drug is increased in small increments only and that fetal heart sounds are well monitored during the procedure. Box 23.5 shows an interprofessional care map illustrating both nursing and team planning during an augmented labor.

QSEN Checkpoint Question 23.2

TEAMWORK & COLLABORATION

Rosann's primary care provider is considering whether to augment her labor with oxytocin. What would make the nurse question the care provider's use of oxytocin for her?

a. Her blood pressure is slightly elevated above normal.
b. Her membranes ruptured after only 1 hour of labor.
c. Her fetus is large for gestational age by a sonogram.
d. She had an amniocentesis performed during pregnancy.

Look in Appendix A for the best answer and rationale.

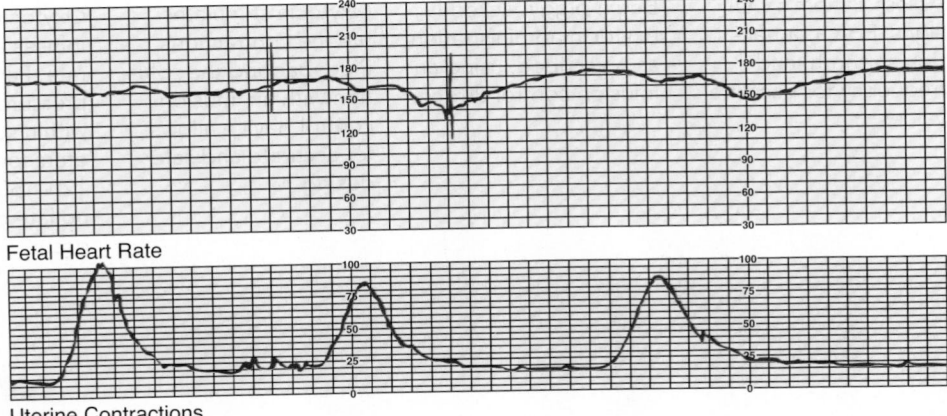

Figure 23.4 Hypertonic uterine contractions caused by an oxytocin infusion. Contractions are as high as 100 mmHg in intensity. Late decelerations and a fetal heart rate (FHR) of 170 beats/min baseline are present.

BOX 23.5

Nursing Care Planning

AN INTERPROFESSIONAL CARE MAP FOR A WOMAN EXPERIENCING AUGMENTATION OF LABOR

You admit Rosann Bigalow, a 28-year-old woman about to give birth to her first baby, to a birthing room. Her contractions have been 5 minutes apart for 10 hours. She feels more pain in her back than in her abdomen, "like my spine is tearing apart." A contraction monitor shows contractions are hypotonic. *A sonogram shows her fetus is "borderline" large for gestation and in an occipitoposterior position.* Her husband asks you if the reason Rosann's labor is taking so long is because she's overweight.

Family Assessment: Rosann has been married for 2 years. Present pregnancy intended. Husband, 34 years old, owns a car dealership. Rosann works as salesperson in dealership office. Finances rated as "no problem."

Patient Assessment: Patient, gravida 1, para 0, in latent stage of labor. Cervix dilated 4 cm, 80% effaced. Contractions every 5 minutes, with peak strength at 20–25 mmHg and a duration of 10 seconds. Fetal heart rate (FHR) at 130–140 beats/min with beat-to-beat variability present. Patient and partner visibly apprehensive, watching monitor intensely. Patient vital signs within normal parameters. Normal saline IV solution infusing at 150 ml/hr via infusion pump. Patient drinking sports beverage "to keep up strength." Oxytocin prescribed at 1 milliunits/min; increase 1 milliunits/min at 30-minute intervals.

Nursing Diagnosis: Risk for injury (maternal and fetal) related to prolonged labor with ineffective contractions and requiring oxytocin augmentation

Outcome Criteria: Patient's vital signs and FHR remain within acceptable parameters; contractions increase after oxytocin administration without becoming hypertonic; labor progresses without signs and symptoms of maternal or fetal distress. Urine output is at least 30 ml/hr; urine specific gravity, 1.010–1.030.

Team Member Responsible	Assessment	Intervention	Rationale	Expected Outcome
Activities of Daily Living, Including Safety				
Nurse	Assess what position allows patient the most comfort in light of occipitoposterior fetal position.	Encourage patient to lie on her side or on hands and knees as much as possible. Encourage partner to apply back massage.	A hands and knees position may encourage fetal rotation. Side lying enhances placental perfusion. Back massage can aid comfort.	Patient determines position of comfort. Requests massage if helpful with contractions.
Teamwork and Collaboration				
Nurse/ primary care provider	Assess whether healthcare provider coverage will be available for oxytocin administration.	Discuss need for oxytocin administration because of ineffective labor contractions.	Oxytocin administration requires a primary care provider's presence.	Healthcare provider states he or she will be available during oxytocin infusion time.
Procedures/Medications for Quality Improvement				
Nurse/ primary care provider	Assess patient's vital signs, FHR, contraction strength, and frequency for baseline values.	Begin piggybacked IV oxytocin administration as prescribed, using an infusion control device.	Oxytocin stimulates uterine contractions. Piggybacking the solution with an infusion control device allows for accurate and safe dosing.	Oxytocin solution infuses at prescribed rate. Patient's blood pressure remains within stated parameters for her; FHR is 120–160 beats/min; no late decelerations occur.

Nutrition

Nurse	Assess amount of intake and output and test urine for specific gravity.	Monitor the IV fluid infusion and adjust rate as prescribed. Monitor amount of oral fluid to help prevent water intoxication.	Intake and output and urine specific gravity are indicators of fluid volume status. Inadvertent administration of too great an amount of IV or oral fluid can increase the risk of fluid overload.	Patient shows no water intoxication symptoms: headache, lethargy, confusion, or a change in level of consciousness.

Patient-Centered Care

Nurse	Explore the meaning of prolonged labor with the couple.	Encourage couple to verbalize feelings and concerns.	Exploration, verbalization, and active questioning provide an outlet for awareness of needs and open lines of communication.	Patient and partner are able to discuss their feelings with caregivers.

Psychosocial/Spiritual/Emotional Needs

Nurse	Assess what the couple thought labor would be like.	Include couple in the treatment process; provide frequent updates about labor progress.	Frequent updates about progress help to minimize the feelings of fear about the unknown.	Couple state they feel well informed about progress in labor.

Informatics for Seamless Healthcare Planning

Nurse	Assess whether labor experience was tolerable for couple in light of a complication.	Provide time for couple to "debrief" their labor experience.	Discussing or "putting a fence around" an experience helps to integrate it into other life events.	Couple state they feel comfortable with labor outcome.

Unfolding Patient Stories: Fatime Sanogo • Part 2

Fatime Sanogo, a primiparous 23-year-old who you met in Chapter 2, is now at 41 4/7 weeks gestation and admitted to the hospital for induction of labor. What physical findings should be present before labor is induced? What nursing assessments are performed and what nursing interventions are implemented to safely manage induction of labor with an oxytocin infusion? What assessment data should be documented when artificial rupture of membranes is performed?

Care for Fatime and other patients in a realistic virtual environment: *vSim for Nursing* (thepoint.lww.com/vSimMaternityPed). Practice documenting these patients' care in DocuCare (thepoint.lww.com/DocuCareEHR).

UTERINE RUPTURE

Rupture of the uterus during labor, although rare, is always a possibility. It occurs most often in women who have a previous cesarean scar (Vachon-Marceau, Demers, Goyet, et al., 2016). Contributing factors may include prolonged labor, abnormal presentation, multiple gestation, unwise use of oxytocin, obstructed labor, and traumatic maneuvers of forceps or traction. When uterine rupture occurs, fetal death will follow unless immediate cesarean birth can be accomplished.

If a uterus should rupture, the woman experiences a sudden, severe pain during a strong labor contraction, which she may report as a "tearing" sensation. Rupture can be complete, going through the endometrium, myometrium, and peritoneum layers, or incomplete, leaving the peritoneum intact. With a complete rupture, uterine contractions will immediately stop. Two distinct swellings will be visible on the woman's abdomen: the retracted uterus and the extrauterine fetus. Hemorrhage from the torn uterine arteries floods into the abdominal cavity and possibly into the vagina. Signs of hypotensive shock begin, including a rapid, weak pulse; falling blood pressure; cold and clammy skin; and dilation of the nostrils from air starvation. Fetal heart sounds fade and then are absent (Box 23.6).

If the rupture is incomplete, the signs of rupture are less evident. With an incomplete rupture, a woman may experience only a localized tenderness and a persistent aching pain over the area of the lower uterine segment. However, fetal heart sounds, a lack of contractions, and the changes in the woman's vital signs will gradually reveal fetal and maternal distress. The rupture can be confirmed by ultrasound (Tauchi, Hasegawa, Oba, et al., 2016).

BOX 23.6

Nursing Care Planning Using Assessment

ASSESSING THE PREGNANT WOMAN WITH COMPLETE UTERINE RUPTURE

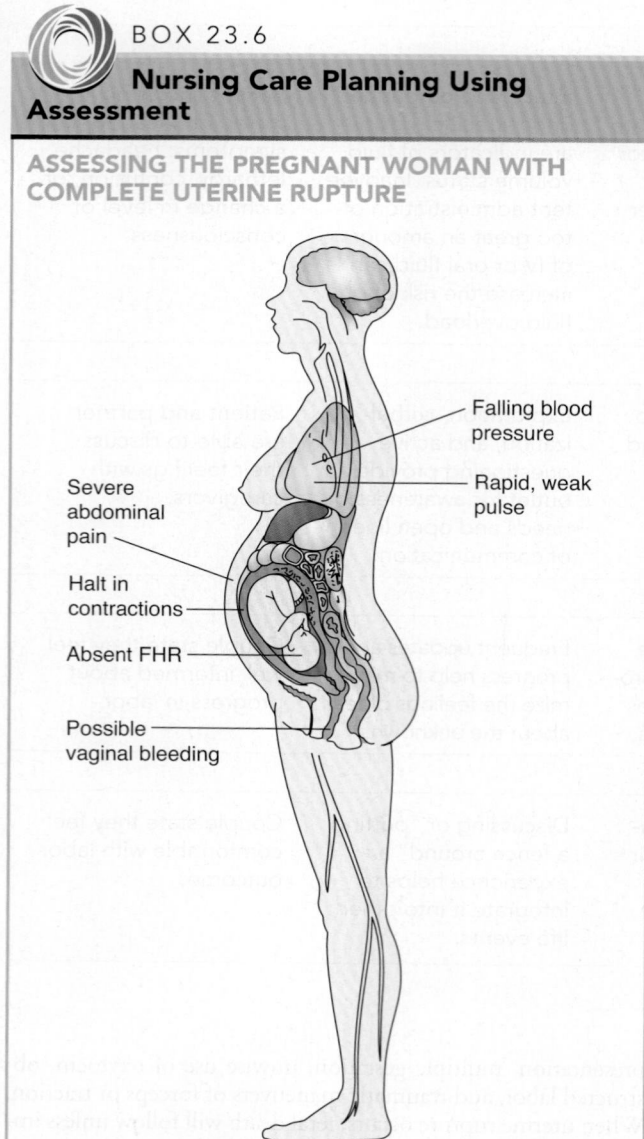

- Falling blood pressure
- Rapid, weak pulse
- Severe abdominal pain
- Halt in contractions
- Absent FHR
- Possible vaginal bleeding

blood loss was acute, she may be nonresponsive because of decreased cerebral perfusion from hypotension. If this has happened, the woman's support person must be the one who gives this consent, relying on the information provided by the primary care provider as to whether a functioning uterus can be saved (Choubey & Werner, 2015).

Be prepared to offer information to the support person and to inform him or her about fetal outcome, the extent of the surgery, and the woman's safety as soon as possible. Initially, a woman and her support person will probably be thankful her life was saved. However, they may become almost immediately angry the rupture occurred, especially if the fetus died and the woman will no longer be able to have children. Allow them time to express these emotions without feeling threatened. They may want to plan a funeral because, oftentimes, the baby is full term. Utilize clergy or counselors as needed to help the couple begin the coping process. They are not only grieving for the loss of a child but also the cost of unexpected surgery and perhaps loss of fertility.

INVERSION OF THE UTERUS

Uterine inversion refers to the uterus turning inside out with either birth of the fetus or delivery of the placenta. It is a rare phenomenon, occurring in about 1 in 20,000 births (Furukawa & Sameshima, 2015). It may occur if traction is applied to the umbilical cord to remove the placenta or if pressure is applied to the uterine fundus when the uterus is not contracted. It may also occur if the placenta is attached at the fundus so that, during birth, the passage of the fetus pulls the fundus downward (Choubey & Werner, 2015).

Because inversion occurs in various degrees, the inverted fundus may lie within the uterine cavity or the vagina, or in total inversion, it may protrude from the vagina. When an inversion occurs, a large amount of blood suddenly gushes from the vagina. The fundus is no longer palpable in the abdomen. The woman begins to show signs of blood loss: hypotension, dizziness, paleness, or diaphoresis. Because the uterus is not able to contract in this position, bleeding cannot be halted or will continue to such an extent exsanguination could occur within 10 minutes.

Never attempt to replace an inversion because handling of the uterus could increase the bleeding. Never attempt to remove the placenta if it is still attached because this would create a larger surface area for bleeding. Oxytocin, if being used, should be discontinued because it makes the uterus more tense and difficult to replace. An IV fluid line should be inserted if one is not already present (use a large-gauge needle because blood will need to be replaced). If a line is already in place, open it to achieve optimal flow of fluid to restore fluid volume. Administer oxygen by mask, and assess vital signs. Be prepared to perform cardiopulmonary resuscitation (CPR) if the woman's heart should fail from the sudden blood loss. The woman will immediately be given general anesthesia or possibly nitroglycerin or a tocolytic drug by IV to relax the uterus. The primary care provider then replaces the fundus manually. Administration of oxytocin *after* manual replacement helps the uterus to contract and remain in its natural place. Because the uterine endometrium was exposed, a woman will need antibiotic therapy to prevent infection. She needs to be informed that cesarean birth will probably be necessary in any future pregnancy to prevent the possibility of repeat inversion.

Because the uterus at the end of pregnancy is such a vascular organ, uterine rupture is an immediate emergency, comparable to splenic or hepatic rupture. Administer emergency fluid replacement therapy as prescribed. Anticipate the use of IV oxytocin to attempt to contract the uterus and minimize bleeding. Prepare the woman for a possible laparotomy as an emergency measure to control bleeding and birth the fetus. The viability of the fetus depends on the extent of the rupture and the time elapsed between rupture and abdominal extraction. A woman's prognosis depends on the extent of the rupture and the blood loss.

Most women are advised not to conceive again after a rupture of the uterus, unless the rupture occurred in the inactive lower segment. At the time of the rupture, the primary care provider, with consent, may perform a cesarean hysterectomy (i.e., removal of the damaged uterus) or tubal ligation, both of which will result in loss of childbearing ability. A woman may have difficulty giving her consent for a hysterectomy because it is unknown whether her present baby will live. If

Concept Mastery Alert

Uterine rupture occurs during labor. Contractions stop, and bleeding is primarily into the abdominal cavity. *Uterine inversion* occurs following delivery. With uterine inversion, there is a large gush of blood from the vagina, and the uterus is no longer palpable in the abdomen.

QSEN Checkpoint Question 23.3

SAFETY

The nurse notices Rosann's contractions are 70 seconds long and occur every 90 seconds when assessing the frequency of her contractions after she receives oxytocin. What would be the nurse's first action?

   a. Ask Rosann to turn onto her left side and breathe deeply.
   b. Increase the rate of Rosann's IV fluid infusion.
   c. Discontinue the administration of the oxytocin infusion.
   d. Give an emergency bolus of oxytocin to relax the uterus.

Look in Appendix A for the best answer and rationale.

AMNIOTIC FLUID EMBOLISM

Amniotic fluid embolism occurs when amniotic fluid is forced into an open maternal uterine blood sinus after a membrane rupture or partial premature separation of the placenta (Balinger, Chu Lam, Hon, et al., 2015).

Previously, it was thought particles such as meconium or shed fetal skin cells in the amniotic fluid entered the maternal circulation and reached the lungs as small emboli. A more likely cause of symptoms is a humoral or anaphylactoid response to amniotic fluid in the maternal circulation. This condition may occur during labor or in the postpartal period. The incidence is about 1 in 20,000 births, and it accounts for at least 10% of maternal deaths in the United States (Balinger et al., 2015). Although it is associated with induction of labor, multiple pregnancy, and perhaps polyhydramnios (i.e., excess amniotic fluid), it is not preventable because it cannot be predicted.

The clinical picture is dramatic. A woman, usually in the active phase of labor, sits up suddenly and grasps her chest because of sharp pain and inability to breathe as pulmonary artery constriction occurs. She becomes pale and then turns the typical bluish gray associated with a pulmonary embolism and lack of blood flow to the lungs. Within minutes, she could be unconscious, and her fetus is put in danger as placenta blood circulation halts. The immediate management is oxygen administration by face mask or cannula. Within minutes, she will need CPR; however, CPR may be ineffective because these procedures (inflating the lungs and massaging the heart) do not relieve the pulmonary constriction. Blood still cannot circulate to the lungs. Death may occur within minutes.

A woman's prognosis depends on the size of the embolism, the speed with which the emergency condition was detected, and the skill and speed of emergency interventions. Even if the woman survives the initial insult, the risk for disseminated intravascular coagulation (DIC) is high, further compounding her condition. In this event, she will need continued management, which includes endotracheal intubation to maintain pulmonary function and therapy with fibrinogen to counteract DIC. Most likely, she will be transferred to an intensive care unit (ICU). The prognosis for the fetus is guarded unless the fetus is born immediately by cesarean birth.

Problems With the Passenger

Although the fetus is basically passive during birth, complications may arise if an infant is immature or preterm or if the maternal pelvis is so undersized that its diameters are smaller than the fetal skull, such as occurs in early adolescence or in women with altered bone growth from a disease such as rickets. It also can occur if the umbilical cord prolapses, if more than one fetus is present, or if a fetus is malpositioned or too large for the birth canal.

PROLAPSE OF THE UMBILICAL CORD

In **umbilical cord prolapse**, a loop of the umbilical cord slips down in front of the presenting fetal part (Fig. 23.5). Prolapse may occur at any time after the membranes rupture

Figure 23.5 Prolapse of the umbilical cord. **(A)** The cord is prolapsed but still within the uterus. **(B)** The cord is visible at the vulva. In both instances, the fetal nutrient supply is being compromised, although only a cord such as that shown in image **B** would be visible. Both prolapses could be detected by fetal monitoring.

A   B

if the presenting fetal part is not fitted firmly into the cervix. It tends to occur most often with:

- Premature rupture of membranes
- Fetal presentation other than cephalic
- Placenta previa
- Intrauterine tumors preventing the presenting part from engaging
- A small fetus
- CPD preventing firm engagement
- Polyhydramnios
- Multiple gestation

The incidence is about 0.5% of cephalic births but can rise as high as 10% or higher with breech or transverse lies (Kaymak, Iskender, Ibanoglu, et al., 2015).

Assessment

In rare instances, the cord may be felt as the presenting part on an initial vaginal examination during labor or can be visualized on ultrasound if one of these is taken during labor. More often, however, cord prolapse is first discovered only after the membranes have ruptured, when the FHR is discovered to be unusually slow or a variable deceleration FHR pattern suddenly becomes apparent on a fetal monitor. On inspection, the cord may be visible at the vulva.

To rule out cord prolapse, always assess fetal heart sounds immediately after rupture of the membranes, whether this occurs spontaneously or by amniotomy.

Therapeutic Management

A prolapsed cord is always an emergency situation because the pressure of the fetal head against the cord at the pelvic brim leads to cord compression and decreased oxygenation to the fetus. Management is aimed, therefore, at relieving pressure on the cord, thereby relieving the compression and the resulting fetal anoxia. This may be done by placing a gloved hand in the vagina and manually elevating the fetal head off the cord, or by placing the woman in a knee–chest or Trendelenburg position, to cause the fetal head to fall back from the cord. Administering oxygen at 10 L/min by face mask to the woman is also helpful to improve oxygenation to the fetus. A tocolytic agent may be prescribed to reduce uterine activity and pressure on the fetus. Amnioinfusion (see later) is yet another way to relieve pressure on the cord (Hasegawa, Sekizawa, Ikeda, et al., 2016).

If the cord has prolapsed to the extent it is exposed to room air, drying will begin, leading to constriction and atrophy of the umbilical vessels. Do not attempt to push any exposed cord back into the vagina because this could add to the compression by causing knotting or kinking. Instead, cover any exposed portion with a sterile saline compress to prevent drying.

Because cervical dilatation is usually incomplete at the point where the cord prolapse occurred, the birth method of choice is upward pressure on the presenting part, applied by a practitioner's hand in the woman's vagina, to keep pressure off the cord until the baby can be born by cesarean birth.

Amnioinfusion

Amnioinfusion is the addition of a sterile fluid into the uterus to supplement the amniotic fluid and reduce compression on the cord. For this, a sterile double-lumen catheter is introduced through the cervix into the uterus. It is then attached to IV tubing, and a solution of warmed normal saline is rapidly infused. Initially, approximately 500 ml is infused, and then the rate is adjusted to infuse the least amount necessary to maintain an FHR monitor pattern without variable decelerations. Throughout the procedure, urge a woman to lie in a lateral recumbent position to prevent supine hypotension syndrome.

With cord compression, although amnioinfusion is used for only a short time until the cervix is fully dilated or a cesarean birth can be arranged, the procedure can also be performed daily for women with oligohydramnios. Help maintain strict aseptic technique during the catheter insertion and while it remains in place. Continuously monitor FHR and uterine contractions. Record maternal temperature hourly to detect infection. Be certain the solution is warmed to body temperature before the infusion to prevent chilling of the woman and fetus. This can be done by placing the bag of fluid on a radiant heat warmer or by using a blood/fluid warmer before administration.

Because there will be a continuous flow of the infusing solution out of the woman's vagina during the procedure, change her bed frequently. Also assess that there is constant drainage. If vaginal leakage should stop, it usually means the fetal head is firmly engaged and all fluid being infused is being held in the uterus, a potentially dangerous situation because it could lead to polyhydramnios (i.e., presence of excessive amniotic fluid) and possibly uterine rupture.

Fetal Blood Sampling

Obtaining the fetal oxygen saturation level by inserting a fetal oximeter into the uterus to rest next to the fetal cheek or obtaining a positive response to scalp stimulation usually supplies the information as to whether a fetus is becoming acidotic (see Chapter 24); however, this information can also be obtained by scalp blood or fetal blood sampling. Fetal blood sampling, obtaining a sample of blood from the fetal scalp during a vaginal exam, is gradually disappearing from practice due to the difficulty of the procedure and reasonable noninvasive alternatives, such as fetal scalp stimulation (Chandraharan, 2016).

MULTIPLE GESTATION

Multiple gestations (i.e., pregnancies with two or more fetuses) have increased substantially over the last several decades as in vitro fertilization has become more popular and often produces a multiple pregnancy (ACOG, 2014). When a woman with a multiple gestation is admitted to a birthing room, it usually causes a flurry of excitement as additional personnel are needed for the birth, including as many nurses to attend to possibly immature infants as there are infants, plus additional persons skilled in newborn resuscitation. In the middle of all the preparatory activity, it is easy to forget a woman having a multiple birth may be more frightened than excited. Be certain to focus on her needs as well as those of her babies so she isn't neglected. Twins may be born by cesarean birth to decrease the risk the second fetus will experience anoxia; often, this is also the situation in multiple gestations of three or more because of the increased incidence of cord entanglement and premature separation of the placenta (ACOG, 2014). Anemia and gestational hypertension occur at higher than usual incidences during multiple gestations. To detect these, be certain to assess the woman's hematocrit level and blood pressure closely during labor or while waiting for cesarean arrangements.

If a woman with a multiple gestation will be giving birth vaginally, she is usually instructed to come to the hospital early in labor. The first stage of labor does not differ greatly from that of a woman with a single gestation pregnancy. Coming to a hospital this early in labor, however, will make labor seem long. Urge the woman to spend the early hours of labor engaged in an activity such as playing cards or reading to make the time pass more quickly. Multiple pregnancies often end before full term, so the woman may not yet have practiced breathing exercises. The early hours of labor can be used for this as well. During labor, support the woman's breathing exercises to minimize the need for analgesia or anesthesia; this helps to minimize any respiratory difficulties the infants may have at birth because of their immaturity.

Be certain that when taking FHRs by Doppler or a fetal monitor, you are definitely hearing two separate beats as proof each infant is doing well. Because of the multiple fetuses, abnormal fetal presentation may occur. Also, because the babies are usually small, firm head engagement may not occur, thus increasing the risk for cord prolapse after rupture of the membranes. Uterine dysfunction from a long labor, an overstretched uterus, unusual presentation, and premature separation of the placenta after the birth of the first child may also be more common.

Most twin pregnancies present with both twins vertex. This is followed in frequency by vertex and breech, breech and vertex, and then breech and breech (Fig. 23.6). Multiple gestations of three or more fetuses have extremely varied presen-

tations. After the first infant is born, both ends of the baby's cord are tied or clamped permanently rather than with cord clamps, which could slip. This prevents hemorrhage through an open cord end if additional infants have shared the placenta. The first infant is identified as *A*, and newborn care is begun. In singleton pregnancies, oxytocin usually is given immediately to contract the uterus and minimize bleeding after an infant is born; with a multiple gestation woman, however, it will not be given to avoid compromising the circulation of the infants not yet born (Barrett, 2014).

After the birth of the first child, the lie of the second fetus is determined by external abdominal palpation or ultrasound. Evidence shows breech delivery of the second twin is safest if the delivery of the second twin is not imminent. Often an internal podalic version, where the feet are grasped by the delivering provider, is completed to accomplish a breech delivery of the second twin (Barrett, 2014).

Parents usually want to inspect multiple gestation infants thoroughly after birth. The time allowed for this inspection depends on the infants' weights and conditions because, if preterm, cold hypothermia is a concern. Some parents worry the hospital will confuse their infants through improper identification. Review with them the measures used, such as armbands, to ensure this will not happen.

The infants need careful assessment to determine their true gestational age and whether a phenomenon such as twin-to-twin transfusion could have occurred (see Chapter 26). Even though women have known for months they are having

Figure 23.6 Four different twin presentations. **(A)** Both infants vertex. **(B)** One infant vertex and one breech. **(C)** Both infants breech. **(D)** One infant vertex and one in a transverse lie.

multiple infants, many have difficulty believing it has really happened. They feel a need to recount over and over their surprise and to view their infants together to prove to themselves it is true. If parents are unable to inspect their infants thoroughly immediately after birth because of the infants' low birth weights and the danger of chilling, be certain they have an opportunity to do so as soon as possible to dispel any fears they had throughout pregnancy the babies would be born less than perfect.

Assess the woman carefully in the immediate postpartal period because a uterus that was overly distended because of the multiple gestation may have more difficulty contracting than usual, thus placing her at risk for hemorrhage from uterine atony (i.e., lacking normal tone). In addition, the risk for uterine infection increases if labor or birth was prolonged.

PROBLEMS WITH FETAL POSITION, PRESENTATION, OR SIZE

Occipitoposterior Position

In approximately one tenth of all labors, the fetal position is posterior rather than anterior. That is, the occiput (assuming the presentation is vertex) is directed diagonally and posteriorly, either to the right (right occipitoposterior [ROP]) or to the left (left occipitoposterior [LOP]). In these positions, during internal rotation, the fetal head must rotate not through a 90-degree arc (Fig. 23.7) but through an arc of approximately 135 degrees (Fig. 23.8). Rotation from a posterior position can be aided by having the woman assume a hands-and-knees position, squatting, or lying on her side (on her left side if the fetus is ROP or on her right side if the fetus is LOP). Theoretically, shifting the weight from right to left or "lunging" or swinging her body right to left while elevating her left foot on a chair widens the pelvic path and makes fetal rotation easier. This is not evidence-based, however, is not proven to be effective, and is tiring for women in labor. Because a high percentage of women choose epidurals for their deliveries, a peanut ball placed between the woman's legs has been found to open the pelvis and reduce total labor time (Roth, Dent, Parfitt, et al., 2016).

Posterior positions tend to occur in women with android, anthropoid, or contracted pelvises. It is suggested by a dysfunctional labor pattern such as a prolonged active phase, arrested descent, or fetal heart sounds heard best at the lateral sides of the abdomen.

A posteriorly presenting head does not fit the cervix as snugly as one in an anterior position. Because this increases the risk of umbilical cord prolapse, the position of the fetus is confirmed by vaginal examination or ultrasound. The majority of fetuses presenting in posterior positions, if they are of average size, in good flexion, and aided by forceful uterine contractions, rotate through the large arc, arrive at a good birth position for the pelvic outlet, and are born satisfactorily with only increased molding and caput formation. However, it is not unusual for the labor to be somewhat prolonged because the arc of rotation is greater (Malvasi, Bochicchio, Vaira, et al., 2014).

Because the fetal head rotates against the sacrum, a woman may experience pressure and pain in her lower back because of

Figure 23.7 Left occipitoanterior (LOA) rotation. **(A)** A fetus in a cephalic presentation, LOA position. View is from the outlet. The fetus rotates 90 degrees from this position. **(B)** Descent and flexion. **(C)** Internal rotation complete. **(D)** Extension; the face and chin are born.

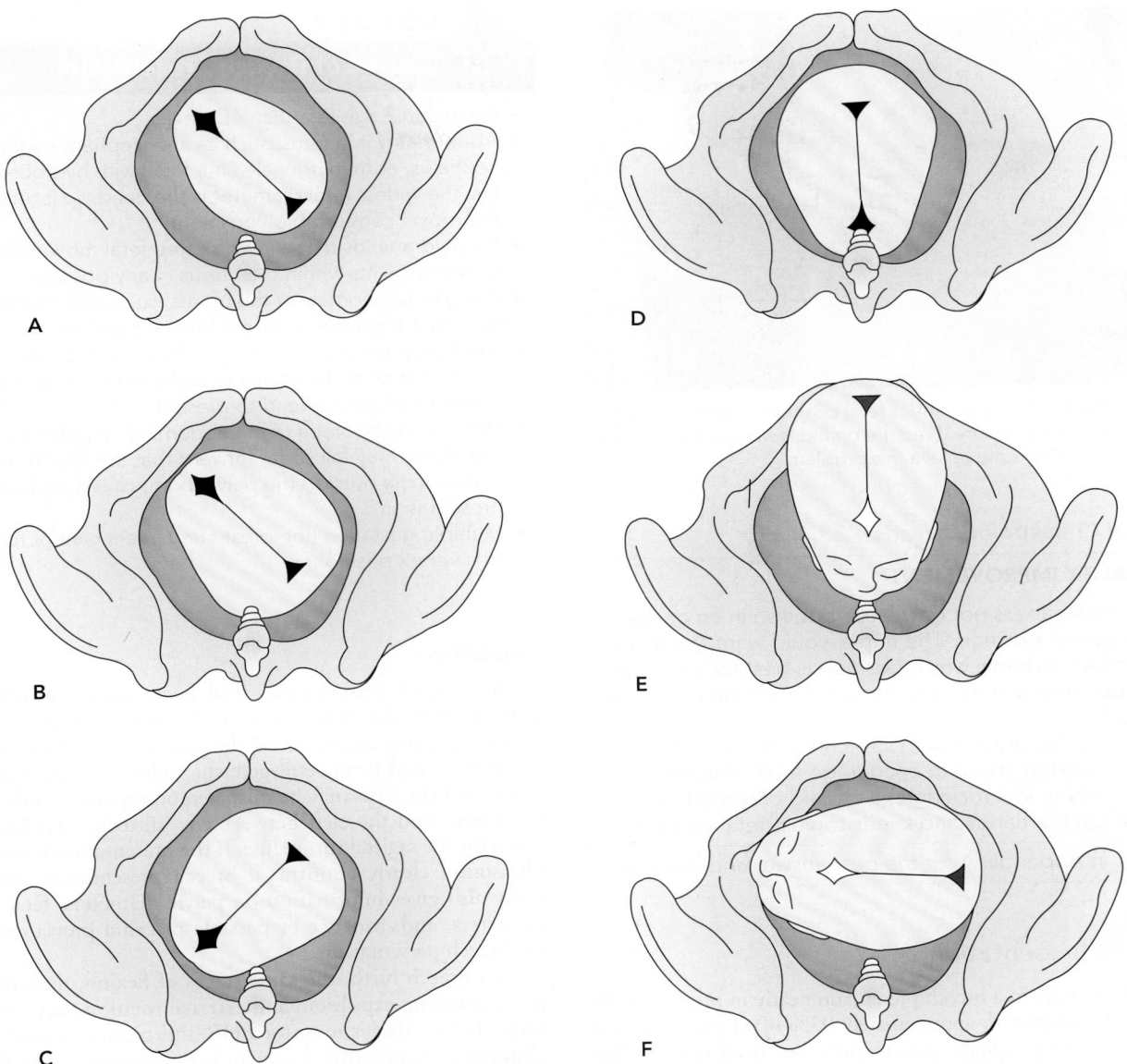

Figure 23.8   Left occipitoposterior (LOP) rotation. **(A)** Fetus in a cephalic presentation, LOP position. View is from outlet. The fetus rotates 135 degrees from this position. **(B)** Descent and flexion. **(C)** Internal rotation beginning. Because of the posterior position, the head will rotate in a longer arc than if it were in an anterior position. **(D)** Internal rotation complete. **(E)** Extension; the face and chin are born. **(F)** External rotation; the fetus rotates to place the shoulders in an anteroposterior position.

sacral nerve compression. These sensations may be so intense she asks for medication for relief, not for her contractions but for the intense back pressure and pain. Applying counterpressure on the sacrum by a back rub may be helpful in relieving a portion of the pain (Fig. 23.9). The Rebozo method of jiggling and massaging the uterus may be helpful when assisting the fetus to rotate into a better position (Cohen & Thomas, 2015). During a long labor of this type, be certain a woman voids approximately every 2 hours to keep her bladder empty because a full bladder could further impede descent of the fetus. Be aware of how long it has been since the woman last ate because she may need an oral sports drink or IV glucose solution to replace glucose stores she is using to keep active in labor.

If contractions are not effective, or if the fetus is larger than average or not in good flexion, rotation through the 135-degree

arc may not be possible. The woman may become exhausted. The fetal head may arrest in the transverse position (i.e., transverse arrest), or rotation may not occur at all (i.e., persistent occipitoposterior position). In these instances, the fetus must be born by cesarean birth. Some women are able to pass a persistent occipitoposterior position through their pelvis. The baby is then born looking at the ceiling or "sunny side up."

Most women need a great deal of support during such a long labor to prevent them from becoming worried about the length of labor or that things are not going "by the book." Provide frequent reassurance that although their pattern of labor is not "textbook," it is within safe, controlled limits. Although rare, if forceps are used to help the fetus rotate, observe a woman closely for hemorrhage from cervical lacerations or infection in the postpartum period.

Figure 23.9   With a posterior fetal position, a woman may feel extensive back pressure. Pressure on her lower back by her support person may help relieve this problem.

QSEN Checkpoint Question 23.4

QUALITY IMPROVEMENT

Rosann's baby is not only large but also in an occipitoposterior position. The nurse would want the team members to know which position is best for a woman whose baby is in the occipitoposterior position during labor?

a. On her right side to stretch the pelvic inlet
b. Walking about to encourage fetal descent
c. Sitting in a rocking chair to aid presentation
d. On her hands and knees to help fetal rotation

Look in Appendix A for the best answer and rationale.

Breech Presentation

Most fetuses are in a breech presentation early in pregnancy. By week 38, however, in approximately 97% of all pregnancies, a fetus turns to a cephalic presentation (i.e., head down). This probably happens because, although the fetal head is the widest single diameter, the buttocks (breech) plus the legs of the fetus actually take up more space. As the fundus is the largest part of the uterus, this places the bulkiest parts of the fetus in the fundus.

There are several types of breech presentations: complete, frank, and footling (see Chapter 15). Examples of why such presentations occur are shown in Box 23.7. Overall, a breech presentation is more hazardous to a fetus than a cephalic presentation because there is a higher risk of the following:

- Developing dysplasia of the hip
- Anoxia from a prolapsed cord
- Traumatic injury to the after-coming head (possibility of intracranial hemorrhage or anoxia)
- Fracture of the spine or arm
- Dysfunctional labor
- Early rupture of the membranes because of the poor fit of the presenting part
- Meconium staining

Meconium staining occurs because of cervical pressure on the buttocks and rectum, not because of fetal anoxia, and so is not a sign of fetal distress. Meconium excretion can, however, lead to meconium aspiration if the infant inhales amniotic fluid.

BOX 23.7

Causes of Breech Presentation

- Gestational age less than 40 weeks
- Abnormality in a fetus, such as anencephaly, hydrocephalus, or meningocele (in a fetus with hydrocephalus, the widest fetal diameter is the head, so it retains the most "comfortable" position)
- Polyhydramnios that allows for free fetal movement, so the fetus fits within the uterus in any position
- Congenital anomaly of the uterus, such as a midseptum, that traps the fetus in a breech position
- Any space-occupying mass in the pelvis, such as a fibroid tumor of the uterus or a placenta previa, that does not allow the head to present
- Pendulous abdomen (if the abdominal muscles are lax, the uterus may fall so far forward that the fetal head comes to lie outside the pelvic brim, causing a breech presentation)
- Multiple gestation (the presenting infant cannot turn to a vertex position)

Assessment

With a breech presentation, fetal heart sounds usually are heard high in the abdomen. Leopold maneuvers and a vaginal examination usually reveal the presentation. If the breech is complete and firmly engaged, the tightly stretched gluteal muscles of the fetus may be mistaken on vaginal examination for a head and the cleft between the buttocks may be mistaken for the sagittal suture line. If the presentation is unclear, ultrasound clearly confirms a breech presentation. Such a study also gives information on pelvic diameters, fetal skull diameters, and evidence of possible placenta previa causing the breech presentation.

In a breech birth, the same stages of flexion, descent, internal rotation, expulsion, and external rotation occur as in a vertex birth. Always monitor FHR and uterine contractions frequently because this allows for early detection of fetal distress from a complication such as prolapsed cord or arrest of descent.

Birth Technique

If the infant will be born vaginally, a woman is allowed to push after full dilatation is achieved, and the breech, trunk, and shoulders are born (Fig. 23.10A,B). As the breech spontaneously emerges from the birth canal, it is steadied and supported by a sterile towel held against the infant's inferior surface (Fig. 23.10C). The shoulders present to the outlet with their widest diameter anteroposterior. If they are not born readily, the arm of the posterior shoulder may be drawn downward by passing two fingers over the infant's shoulder and down the arm to the elbow, then sweeping the flexed arm across the infant's face and chest and out. The other arm is delivered in the same way. External rotation is then allowed to occur to bring the head into the best outlet diameter.

Birth of the head is the most hazardous part of a breech birth. Because the umbilicus precedes the head, a loop of cord passes down alongside the head. The pressure of the head against the pelvic brim automatically causes compression on this loop of cord.

Figure 23.10   Breech birth. **(A)** Position before labor; left sacroposterior. **(B)** Descent and internal rotation. **(C)** Legs being born; the shoulders turn to present to the anteroposterior diameter. **(D)** The head is born. External rotation has put the anteroposterior diameter of the head in line with the anteroposterior diameter of the woman's pelvis. The head is born by gentle pressure to flex the head fully and by gentle traction to the shoulders upward and outward. Additional pressure might be applied by an assistant to the abdominal wall to ensure head flexion.

A second danger of a breech birth is intracranial hemorrhage. With a cephalic presentation, molding to the confines of the birth canal occurs over hours. With a breech birth, pressure changes occur instantaneously, a situation that can result in tentorial tears leading to gross motor and mental incapacity or lethal damage to the fetus. A danger to the infant who is born gradually to reduce the possibility of intracranial injury is hypoxia. In contrast, the infant who is born suddenly to reduce the duration of cord compression may suffer an intracranial hemorrhage.

To aid in birth of the head, the trunk of the infant is usually straddled over the primary care provider's right forearm (Fig. 23.10D). Two fingers of the right hand are then placed in the infant's mouth. The left hand is slid into the woman's vagina, palm down, along the infant's back, and pressure is applied to the occiput to flex the head fully. Gentle traction applied to the shoulders (upward and outward) delivers the head. Because of these difficulties with birth of the head is the reason why planned cesarean birth is the usual method of birth for many infants in breech presentation (Berhan & Haileamlak, 2016).

Parents of a breech baby can be worried about their baby's outcome all during labor (Toivonen, Palomäki, Huhtala, et al., 2014). They usually inspect their child a little more

closely after birth than do parents whose babies were not breech. They, as well as the person who makes the initial physical assessment of the infant, are looking for a possible reason for the breech presentation. An infant who was born from a frank breech position tends to keep his or her legs extended and at the level of the face for the first 2 or 3 days of life. The infant who was a footling breech may tend to keep the legs extended in a footling position for the first few days. Be sure to point out to the parents that this is normal so that they do not misinterpret the unusual posture of their infant.

What If . . . 23.2
Rosann's baby was presenting as breech and the nurse noticed that when her membranes ruptured, the amniotic fluid was green stained. Is this an emergency situation?

Face Presentation

A fetal head presenting at a different angle than expected is termed *asynclitism*. Face and brow presentations are examples. Face (chin, or mentum) presentation is rare, but when it does occur, the head diameter the fetus presents to the pelvis is often too large for birth to proceed. A head that feels more prominent than normal, with no engagement apparent on Leopold maneuvers, suggests a face presentation. It is also suggested when the head and back are both felt on the same side of the uterus with Leopold maneuvers. The back is difficult to outline in this presentation because it is concave. If the back is extremely concave, fetal heart tones may be transmitted to the forward-thrust chest and heard on the side of the fetus where feet and arms can be palpated. A face presentation is confirmed by vaginal examination when the nose, mouth, or chin can be felt as the presenting part.

A fetus in a posterior position, instead of flexing the head as labor proceeds, may extend the head, resulting in a face presentation; this usually occurs in a woman with a contracted pelvis or placenta previa. It also may occur in the relaxed uterus of a multipara or with prematurity, polyhydramnios, or fetal malformation. It is a warning signal. Something abnormal is usually causing the face presentation.

When a face presentation is suspected, an ultrasound is done to confirm it; if indicated, the pelvic diameters are measured. If the chin is anterior and the pelvic diameters are within normal limits, it may be possible for the infant to be born without difficulty (perhaps after a long first stage of labor because the face does not mold well to make a firm engaging part). If the chin is posterior, cesarean birth is usually the method of choice; otherwise, it would be necessary to wait for a long posterior-to-anterior rotation to occur. Such rotation could result in uterine dysfunction or a transverse arrest.

Babies born after a face presentation have a great deal of facial edema and may be purple from ecchymotic bruising. Observe the infant closely for a patent airway. In some infants, lip edema is so severe that they are unable to suck for a day or two. Gavage feedings may be necessary to allow them to obtain enough fluid until they can suck effectively. They may be transferred to a neonatal intensive care unit (NICU) for 24 hours. Reassure the parents that the edema is transient and will disappear in a few days with no aftermath.

Brow Presentation

A brow presentation is the rarest of the presentations. It occurs in a multipara or a woman with relaxed abdominal muscles. It almost invariably results in obstructed labor because the head becomes jammed in the brim of the pelvis as the occipitomental diameter presents. Unless the presentation spontaneously corrects, cesarean birth will be necessary to birth the infant safely. Brow presentations also leave an infant with extreme ecchymotic bruising on the face. On seeing this bruising over the same area as the anterior fontanelle, or "soft spot," parents may need additional reassurance that the child is well after birth.

Transverse Lie

Transverse lie occurs in women with pendulous abdomens, with uterine fibroid tumors that obstruct the lower uterine segment, with contraction of the pelvic brim, with congenital abnormalities of the uterus, or with polyhydramnios. It may occur in infants with hydrocephalus or another abnormality that prevents the head from engaging. It may also occur in prematurity if the infant has room for free movement, in multiple gestations (particularly in a second twin), or if there is a short umbilical cord.

A transverse lie usually is obvious on inspection because the ovoid of the uterus is found to be more horizontal than vertical. The abnormal presentation can be confirmed by Leopold maneuvers. An ultrasound may be taken to further confirm the abnormal lie and to provide information on pelvic size.

A mature fetus cannot be born vaginally from this presentation. Often, the membranes rupture at the beginning of labor. Because there is no firm presenting part, the cord or an arm may prolapse, or the shoulder may obstruct the cervix. Cesarean birth is necessary.

Oversized Fetus (Macrosomia)

Size may become a problem in a fetus who weighs more than 4,000 to 4,500 g (approximately 9 to 10 lb). Babies of this size complicate up to 10% of all births and are most frequently born to women who enter pregnancy with diabetes or who develop gestational diabetes (Ray & Alhusen, 2016). Large babies are also associated with multiparity because each infant born to a woman tends to be slightly heavier and larger than the one born just before.

An oversized infant may cause uterine dysfunction during labor or at birth because of overstretching of the fibers of the myometrium. The wide shoulders may pose a problem at birth because they can cause fetal pelvic disproportion or even uterine rupture from obstruction. A woman may be left with perineal lacerations (Wang, Zhu, Zhang, et al., 2016).

If the infant is so oversized that he or she cannot be born vaginally, a cesarean birth becomes the birth method of choice. The large size of a fetus may be missed in an obese woman because the fetal contours are difficult to palpate and obesity does not necessarily indicate a larger than usual pelvis. Pelvimetry or ultrasound can be used to compare the size of the fetus with the woman's pelvic capacity.

The perinatal mortality rate of larger infants is substantially increased to about 15%, compared with the normal 4%. In addition, a large infant born vaginally has a higher than normal risk of cervical nerve palsy, diaphragmatic nerve injury, or a fractured clavicle because of shoulder dystocia. Postpartally, the woman has an increased risk of hemorrhage because the overdistended uterus may not contract as readily as usual.

Shoulder Dystocia

Shoulder dystocia is a birth problem that is increasing in incidence because the weight and therefore the size of newborns is increasing (McCarthy, Walker, Ugoni, et al., 2016). The problem occurs at the second stage of labor, when the fetal head is born but the shoulders are too broad to enter and be born through the pelvic outlet. This is hazardous to the woman because it can result in vaginal or cervical tears. It is hazardous to the fetus if the cord is compressed between the fetal body and the bony pelvis. In addition, the force of birth can result in a fractured clavicle or a brachial plexus injury for the fetus.

Shoulder dystocia is most apt to occur in women with diabetes, in multiparas, and in postdate pregnancies. The condition may be suspected earlier if the second stage of labor is prolonged, if there is arrest of descent, or if, when the head appears on the perineum (crowning), it retracts instead of protruding with each contraction (a turtle sign). The problem often is not identified, however, until the head has already been born and the wide anterior shoulder locks beneath the symphysis pubis.

Asking or assisting a woman to flex her thighs sharply on her abdomen (McRoberts maneuver) widens the pelvic outlet and may allow the anterior shoulder to be born. Applying suprapubic pressure may also help the shoulder escape from beneath the symphysis pubis and be born. These are the first two of a series of maneuvers that help resolve a shoulder dystocia (Stitely & Gherman, 2014).

QSEN Checkpoint Question 23.5

EVIDENCE-BASED PRACTICE

To determine which risk factors were associated with shoulder dystocia, researchers studied a cohort of births from 1967 to 2009 in Norway, a sample of 2,014,956 vaginal births. The results of the study found an increased incidence of shoulder dystocia associated with increased fetal weight, maternal diabetes, prolonged labor, instrumental delivery and parity (Øverland, Vatten, & Eskild, 2014).

Based on this study and the fact that a sonogram has shown Rosann's fetus to be extremely large, what assessment would the nurse want to prioritize for Rosann's baby after birth?

a. If his abdominal wall appears to be ruptured
b. If his arms feel warm and are the same length
c. If his buttocks or back have extensive bruising
d. If his eyes can focus steadily on a nearby object

Look in Appendix A for the best answer and rationale.

Fetal Anomalies

Fetal anomalies of the head such as hydrocephalus (i.e., fluid-filled ventricles) or anencephaly (i.e., absence of the cranium) are a final category of fetal factors that can complicate birth because the fetal presenting part does not engage the cervix well (see Chapter 27).

Problems With the Passage

Aside from a concern with the power of labor and the passenger, the third reason dystocia can occur is a contraction or narrowing of the passageway or birth canal. This can happen at the inlet, at the midpelvis, or at the outlet. The narrowing causes CPD, or a disproportion between the size of the fetal head and the pelvic diameters, which then results in failure to progress in labor.

INLET CONTRACTION

Inlet contraction is narrowing of the anteroposterior diameter of the pelvis to less than 11 cm, or of the transverse diameter to 12 cm or less. It usually is caused by rickets in early life or by an inherited small pelvis. Rickets is caused by a lack of calcium and is therefore rare in developed countries but can occur among immigrants who were raised where milk supplies were not plentiful. In primigravidas, the fetal head normally engages between weeks 36 and 38 of pregnancy. If this occurs any time before labor begins, it is proof the pelvic inlet is adequate as lightening, by definition, means the fetal head has sunk below the inlet. Following the general rule that "what goes in, comes out," a head that engages or proves it fits into the pelvic brim will probably also be able to pass through the midpelvis and through the outlet.

If engagement does not occur in a primigravida, then either a fetal abnormality (larger than usual head) or a pelvic abnormality (smaller than usual pelvis) should be suspected. As a rule, engagement does not occur in multigravidas until labor begins. For these women, previous vaginal birth of a full-term infant without problems is proof their birth canal is adequate.

Every primigravida should have pelvic measurements taken and recorded before week 24 of pregnancy so, based on these measurements and the assumption the fetus will be of average size, a birth decision can be made.

If CPD exists, because the fetus may not engage but instead remains "floating," the possibility of cord prolapse can lead to a secondary concern.

OUTLET CONTRACTION

Outlet contraction is a narrowing of the transverse diameter, the distance between the ischial tuberosities at the outlet, to less than 11 cm. This measurement is made by sonogram during pregnancy but can also easily be made manually at a prenatal visit or at the beginning of labor.

TRIAL LABOR

If a woman has a borderline (just adequate) inlet measurement and the fetal lie and position are good, her primary care provider may allow her a "trial" labor to determine whether labor will progress normally. The trial labor continues as long as descent of the presenting part and dilatation of the cervix continue to occur. With a trial labor, monitor fetal heart sounds and uterine contractions frequently. Urge the woman to void every 2 hours so her urinary bladder is as empty as possible, allowing the fetal head to use all the space available. If, after a definite period (6 to 12 hours), adequate progress in labor cannot be documented, or if at any time fetal distress occurs, the trial labor will be discontinued and the woman will be scheduled for a cesarean birth.

It may be difficult for women to undertake labor they know they may not be able to complete because the effort subjects them needlessly to pain. Emphasize, but do not overstress, that it is best for their baby to be born vaginally. If the trial labor fails and cesarean birth is scheduled, provide an explanation as to why cesarean birth is necessary and why it has become the best route for the birth of their baby (Box 23.8).

Some women undergoing a trial labor feel as if they themselves are on trial. When dilatation does not occur, they begin to feel discouraged and inadequate, as if they are at fault. A woman may not be aware of how much she wanted the trial labor to work until she is told it is not working. The support person may be as frightened and feel as helpless as she does and so momentarily stops being a support person. You can assure a woman and her support person that a cesarean birth is just an alternative, not an inferior, method of birth for them. Because labor is not progressing, it is the method of choice to allow them to achieve their goal of a healthy mother and healthy child.

EXTERNAL CEPHALIC VERSION

External cephalic version is the turning of a fetus from a breech to a cephalic position before birth. It may be done as early as 34 to 35 weeks, although the usual time is by

Nursing Care Planning Tips for Effective Communication

Rosann Bigalow is having her first baby. Her primary care provider has told her she has a borderline pelvis but she wants her to try a trial labor.

Tip: When communicating, avoid making any assumptions. Follow up with additional clarification to ensure the patient understands any procedure she may be having. If a woman develops a complication of pregnancy, which is referred to by a Latin name, it is generally expected that the couple will not understand the term and so will need to have the complication thoroughly explained. If a condition has a common name, such as protracted pelvis or trial labor, however, it is easy to assume little explanation of the condition is necessary. In reality, couples need explanations about all conditions because what is common to healthcare personnel may not be common to everyone. In this scenario, Rosann was not aware a trial labor might mean she would need surgery.

Nurse: Hello, Rosann. Is it all right if I attach a fetal heart rate and uterine contraction monitor so we can observe you closely during labor?

Rosann: Sure. Although I should be having this baby any minute. It's already been 10 hours.

Nurse: I thought I heard your doctor say she's thinking of this as a trial labor.

Rosann: Whatever. I told her anything but surgery would be all right.

Nurse: Let's talk about what a trial labor means.

37 to 38 weeks of pregnancy (Velzel, de Hundt, Mulder, et al., 2015). For the procedure, FHR and possibly ultrasound are recorded continuously. A tocolytic agent may be administered to help relax the uterus. The breech and vertex of the fetus are located and grasped transabdominally by the examiner's hands on the woman's abdomen. Gentle pressure is then exerted to rotate the fetus in a forward direction to a cephalic lie (Fig. 23.11). Although not always successful, the use of external version can decrease the number of cesarean births necessary from breech presentations (Velzel et al., 2015). Contraindications to the procedure include multiple gestation, severe oligohydramnios, small pelvic diameters, a cord that wraps around the fetal neck, and unexplained third-trimester bleeding, which might be a placenta previa. External version can be uncomfortable for a woman because of the feeling of pressure. Women who are Rh negative should receive Rh immunoglobulin after the procedure in case minimal bleeding occurs.

FORCEPS BIRTH

Obstetrical forceps are steel instruments constructed of two blades that slide together at their shaft to form a handle. One blade is slipped into the woman's vagina next to the fetal head, and the other is slipped into place on the other side of the head. Next, the shafts of the instrument are brought together in the midline to form the handle. The primary care provider then applies pressure on the handle to manually extract the fetus from the birth canal.

In years past, babies were routinely born with forceps. Today, the technique is rarely used (in only about 4% to 8% of births) because it can lead to rectal sphincter tears in the woman, which can lead to dyspareunia, anal incontinence, or increased urinary stress incontinence (Halscott, Reddy, Landy, et al., 2015). Although no longer

Figure 23.11 External cephalic version. The fetus is rotated by external pressure to a cephalic lie. An ultrasound helps guide a safe result.

used routinely, forceps may be necessary with any of the following conditions:

- A woman is unable to push with contractions in the pelvic division of labor such as might happen with a woman who received regional anesthesia or who has a spinal cord injury.
- Cessation of descent in the second stage of labor occurs.
- A fetus is in an abnormal position.
- A fetus is in distress from a complication such as a prolapsed cord.

Although forceps appear as if they would put forceful pressure on the fetal head, the pressure registers on the steel blades rather than the head so they can actually reduce pressure, thus avoiding a complication such as subdural hemorrhage (Halscott et al., 2015).

Before forceps are applied:

- Membranes must be ruptured.
- CPD must not be present.
- The cervix must be fully dilated.
- The woman's bladder must be empty.

Record the FHR before forceps application. Because there is a danger that the cord could be compressed between the forceps blade and the fetal head, assess FHR again immediately after application. The woman's cervix needs to be carefully assessed after forceps birth to be certain no lacerations have occurred. To rule out bladder injury, record the time and amount of the first voiding. In addition, assess the newborn to be certain no facial palsy exists from pressure. A forceps birth may leave a transient erythematous mark on the newborn's cheek (see Chapter 18). This mark will fade in 1 to 2 days with no long-term effects.

VACUUM EXTRACTION

A fetus, if positioned far enough down the birth canal, may be born by **vacuum extraction** (Fruscalzo, Londero, Calcagno, et al., 2015). With the fetal head at the perineum, a soft, disk-shaped cup is pressed against the fetal scalp and over the posterior fontanelle. When vacuum pressure is applied, air beneath the cup is suctioned out and the cup then adheres so tightly to the fetal scalp that traction on the vacuum cord leading to the cup extracts the fetus (Fig. 23.12).

To vacuum

Posterior fontanel

Figure 23.12 Vacuum extraction.

Vacuum extraction has advantages over forceps birth in that little anesthesia is necessary, thus leaving the fetus with less respiratory depression at birth. One disadvantage over natural birth is that more perineal lacerations may occur (Steinhauer, 2015). Its major disadvantage is that it causes a marked caput on the newborn head that may be noticeable as long as 7 days after birth. Tentorial tears from extreme pressure also have occurred. A woman may need reassurance that the caput swelling is harmless for her infant and will decrease rapidly. Vacuum extraction should not be used as a method of birth if fetal scalp blood sampling was used because the suction pressure can cause severe bleeding at the sampling site. Moreover, vacuum extraction is not advantageous for preterm infants because of the softness of the preterm skull.

Anomalies of the Placenta and Cord

The third stage of labor (i.e., delivery of the placenta) can also result in complications; therefore, continued careful observation of the mother is important (Begley, Gyte, Devane, et al., 2015).

ANOMALIES OF THE PLACENTA

The placenta and cord are always examined for the presence of anomalies after birth. The normal placenta weighs approximately 500 g and is 15 to 20 cm in diameter and 1.5 to 3.0 cm thick. Its weight is approximately one sixth that of the fetus. A placenta may be unusually enlarged in women with diabetes. In certain diseases, such as syphilis or erythroblastosis, the placenta may be so large that it weighs half as much as the fetus. If the uterus has scars or a septum, the placenta may be wide in diameter because it was forced to spread out to find implantation space.

Placenta Succenturiata

A **placenta succenturiata** (Fig. 23.13A) is a placenta that has one or more accessory lobes connected to the main placenta by blood vessels. No fetal abnormality is associated with this type. However, it is important it be recognized because the small lobes may be retained in the uterus after birth, leading to severe maternal hemorrhage. On inspection, the placenta appears torn at the edge, or torn blood vessels extend beyond the edge of the placenta. If the remaining lobes are recognized and removed from the uterus manually, the uterus will contract as usual with no adverse maternal effects.

Placenta Circumvallata

Ordinarily, the chorion membrane begins at the edge of the placenta and spreads to envelop the fetus; no chorion covers the fetal side of the placenta. In **placenta circumvallata**, the fetal side of the placenta is covered to some extent with chorion (Fig. 23.13B). The umbilical cord enters the placenta at the usual midpoint, and large vessels spread out from there. However, they end abruptly at the point where the chorion folds back onto the surface. (In **placenta marginata**, the fold of chorion reaches just to the edge of the placenta.) Although no abnormalities are associated with this type of placenta, its presence should be noted.

Figure 23.13 Abnormal placental formation. **(A)** Placenta succenturiata. **(B)** Placenta circumvallata. **(C)** Battledore placenta. **(D)** Velamentous cord insertion.

Battledore Placenta

In a **battledore placenta**, the cord is inserted marginally rather than centrally (Fig. 23.13C). This anomaly is rare and has no known clinical significance either.

Velamentous Insertion of the Cord

Velamentous insertion of the cord is a situation in which the cord, instead of entering the placenta directly, separates into small vessels that reach the placenta by spreading across a fold of amnion (Fig. 23.13D). This form of cord insertion is most frequently found with multiple gestations. Because the fetal blood supply may not be as generous as usual, this type of placenta is associated with fetal anomalies. An infant born with this type of placenta needs to be examined carefully at birth.

Vasa Previa

In vasa previa, the umbilical vessels of a velamentous cord insertion cross the cervical os and therefore deliver before the fetus (Suzuki & Kato, 2015). The vessels may tear with cervical dilatation, just as a placenta previa may tear. Before inserting any instrument such as an internal fetal monitor, be certain to identify structures to prevent accidental tearing of a vasa previa because tearing would result in sudden fetal blood loss. If sudden, painless bleeding occurs with the beginning of cervical dilatation, either placenta previa or vasa previa is suspected. It can be confirmed by ultrasound. If vasa previa is identified, the infant needs to be born by cesarean birth.

Placenta Accreta

Placenta accreta is an unusually deep attachment of the placenta to the uterine myometrium, so deep that the placenta will not loosen and deliver (Silver, 2015). Attempts to remove it manually may lead to extreme hemorrhage because of the deep attachment. Hysterectomy to remove the uterus or treatment with methotrexate to destroy the still-attached tissue may be necessary.

What If . . . 23.3
While inspecting the placenta, the nurse observe one edge appears torn with torn blood vessels extending beyond its edge. Would the nurse rate the placenta as normal or report its appearance as potentially serious?

ANOMALIES OF THE CORD

Two-Vessel Cord

A normal cord contains one vein and two arteries. The absence of one of the umbilical arteries is associated with congenital

heart and kidney anomalies because the insult that caused the loss of the vessel may have also affected other mesoderm germ layer structures. Inspection of the cord as to how many vessels are present must be made immediately after birth, before the cord begins to dry, because drying distorts the appearance of the vessels. Document the number of vessels conscientiously because an infant with only two vessels needs to be observed carefully for other anomalies during the newborn period.

Unusual Cord Length

Although the length of the umbilical cord rarely varies, some abnormal lengths may occur. An unusually short umbilical cord can result in premature separation of the placenta or an abnormal fetal lie. An unusually long cord may be easily compromised because of its tendency to twist or knot. Occasionally, a cord actually forms a knot, but the natural pulsations of the blood through the vessels and the muscular vessel walls usually keep the blood flow adequate. It is not unusual for a cord to wrap once around the fetal neck (nuchal cord) but, again, with no interference to fetal circulation (Zhao, Geng, Kong, et al., 2015).

What If . . . 23.4
The nurse is particularly interested in exploring one of the 2020 National Health Goals with respect to complications of labor. What would be a possible research topic to explore pertinent to this goal that would be applicable to the Bigalow family and that would also advance evidence-based practice?

KEY POINTS FOR REVIEW

- Complications of labor can arise from problems with the force of labor, the passage, the passenger (the fetus), or the woman's reaction to the experience (the psyche). Hypotonic, hypertonic, and uncoordinated contractions all can occur, resulting in ineffective first or second stages of labor.

- Supporting families who experience a complication of labor is important to not only plan nursing care that meets QSEN competencies but also that best meets a family's total needs.

- Precipitate labor is birth that is completed in less than 3 hours. It can be responsible for subdural hemorrhage in the fetus and cervical or perineal lacerations in the woman.

- Be certain a woman meets the criteria for labor induction before preparing an oxytocin solution. These criteria include engagement of the fetal head, a "ripe" cervix, and absence of CPD. Question if oxytocin should be used if these criteria are not met.

- Always prepare oxytocin as a "piggyback" solution, being extremely careful of the dose used. Both a uterine monitor and an FHR monitor should be used during labor induction to be certain uterine overstimulation does not occur. Observe that contractions occur no less than 2 minutes apart and are no longer than 70 seconds in duration.
- Uterine rupture, although rare, is a complication that is an immediate emergency because of blood loss to the mother and potential anoxia for the fetus.
- Uterine inversion is another rare but grave complication because it leads to inability to control hemorrhage. If the situation is not immediately corrected, emergency hysterectomy may be necessary to save the woman's life.
- Amniotic fluid embolism occurs when amniotic fluid is forced into an open maternal uterine blood sinus. A woman will notice chest pain and dyspnea. Administer oxygen and notify the woman's primary care provider of this emergency.
- Prolapse of the umbilical cord is an emergency situation that requires prompt action. Position a woman quickly into either a Trendelenburg or a knee–chest position to relieve cord compression, or apply manual pressure vaginally to lift the fetal head away from the cord. Notify the woman's primary caregiver of the emergency.
- A multiple gestation can complicate birth. Many infants of multiple gestations are born by cesarean birth to avoid entangled cords or arrest of descent.
- Abnormal position, presentation, or size of the fetus (such as occipitoposterior position; breech, face, or brow presentation; transverse lie) as well as problems of the passage such as inlet and outlet contraction can lead to labor complications.
- Vacuum extraction and forceps are methods that can be used to assist birth. The woman as well as the infant needs special observation after these procedures to detect head trauma or cervical or vaginal tearing.
- Anomalies of the placenta and cord (such as placenta succenturiata, velamentous cord insertion, vasa previa, and two-vessel cord) can lead to birth complications.

CRITICAL THINKING CARE STUDY

Debbie and Craig O'Hara are a married couple having their first baby. Craig works as a football coach; Debbie is a telemarketer. When you admit them to a birthing room, Debbie tells you, "I'm going to have a terrible labor because something's wrong with my baby." On examination, her cervix is 4 cm dilated, 75% effaced; contraction duration is 30 seconds; and frequency is every 5 minutes. Her fetus is in an occipitoposterior position.

1. Would you assume when Debbie said "something's wrong with my baby" she meant the posterior position? Would you assure her the baby will be fine?
2. Debbie's husband tells you he's proud he's having a boy. You notice he talks to his son all during labor with comments such as "Why aren't you following the playbook?" or "Put your head down and push. The clock is running." Would you be concerned he's coaching his son and not his wife?

3. Debbie's primary care provider wants Debbie to rest between contractions on her hands and knees in the hope that will help her fetus rotate more efficiently and avoid a cesarean birth. Craig tells you he'd rather Debbie have a cesarean than spend so long in labor. How would you respond to him?

RELATED RESOURCES

Explore these additional resources to enhance learning for this chapter:
- Student resources on thePoint, including answers to the What If . . . and Critical Thinking Care Study questions, http://thepoint.lww.com/Flagg8e
- Adaptive learning powered by PrepU, http://thepoint.lww.com/prepu

REFERENCES

American College of Obstetricians and Gynecologists. (2013). ACOG Committee Opinion No. 560: Medically indicated late-preterm and early-term deliveries. *Obstetrics and Gynecology, 121*(4), 908–910.

American College of Obstetricians and Gynecologists. (2014). ACOG Practice Bulletin No. 144: Multifetal gestations: Twin, triplet, and higher-order multifetal pregnancies. *Obstetrics and Gynecology, 123*(5), 1118–1132.

Balinger, K. J., Chu Lam, M. T., Hon, H. H., et al. (2015). Amniotic fluid embolism: Despite progress, challenges remain. *Current Opinion in Obstetrics & Gynecology, 27*(6), 398–405.

Barrett, J. F. (2014). Twin delivery: Method, timing and conduct. *Best Practice & Research. Clinical Obstetrics & Gynaecology, 28*(2), 327–338.

Begley, C. M., Gyte, G. M., Devane, D., et al. (2015). Active versus expectant management for women in the third stage of labour. *Cochrane Database of Systematic Reviews*, (3), CD007412.

Berhan, Y., & Haileamlak, A. (2016). The risks of planned vaginal breech delivery versus planned caesarean section for term breech birth: A meta-analysis including observational studies. *British Journal of Obstetrics and Gynecology, 123*(1), 49–57.

Bishop, E. H. (1964). Pelvic scoring for elective induction. *Obstetrics and Gynecology, 24*(2), 266–268.

Bor, P., Ledertoug, S., Boie, S., et al. (2016). Continuation versus discontinuation of oxytocin infusion during the active phase of labour: A randomised controlled trial. *British Journal of Obstetrics and Gynecology, 123*(1), 129–135.

Chandraharan, E. (2016). Should national guidelines continue to recommend fetal scalp blood sampling during labour? *The Journal of Maternal-Fetal & Neonatal Medicine, 29*(22), 3682–3685.

Choubey, V., & Werner, E. F. (2015). Complications of labor & delivery. In J. L. Bienstock, H. Fox, E. E. Wallach, et al. (Eds.), *The Johns Hopkins manual of gynecology and obstetrics* (5th ed., pp. 104–115). Philadelphia, PA: Wolters Kluwer.

Cohen, S. R., & Thomas, C. R. (2015). Rebozo technique for fetal malposition in labor. *Journal of Midwifery & Women's Health, 60*(4), 445–451.

Eggebø, T. M., Hassan, W. A., Salvesen, K. Å., et al. (2015). Prediction of delivery mode by ultrasound-assessed fetal position in nulliparous women with prolonged first stage of labor. *Ultrasound in Obstetrics & Gynecology, 46*(5), 606–610.

Friedman, E. (1978). *Labor, clinical evaluation and management* (2nd ed.). New York, NY: Appleton-Century-Crofts.

Fruscalzo, A., Londero, A. P., Calcagno, A., et al. (2015). Building a prediction model for vacuum-assisted operative vaginal delivery risk. *Gynecologic and Obstetric Investigation, 80*(4), 246–252.

Furukawa, S., & Sameshima, H. (2015). The importance of the monitoring of resuscitation with blood transfusion for uterine inversion in obstetrical hemorrhage. *Obstetrics and Gynecology International, 2015*, 269156.

Gilstrop, M., & Sciscione, A. (2015). Induction of labor—pharmacology methods. *Seminars in Perinatology, 39*(6), 463–465.

Halscott, T. L., Reddy, U. M., Landy, H. J., et al. (2015). Maternal and neonatal outcomes by attempted mode of operative delivery from a low station in the second stage of labor. *Obstetrics and Gynecology, 126*(6), 1265–1272.

Hamilton, E. F., Warrick, P. A., Collins, K., et al. (2015). Assessing first-stage labor progression and its relationship to complications. *American Journal of Obstetrics and Gynecology, 214*(3), 358.e1–358.e8.

Hasegawa, J., Sekizawa, A., Ikeda, T., et al. (2016). Clinical risk factors for poor neonatal outcomes in umbilical cord prolapse. *Journal of Maternal-Fetal & Neonatal Medicine, 29*(10), 1652–1656.

Hunt, J. C., & Menticoglou, S. M. (2015). Perinatal outcome in 1515 cases of prolonged second stage of labour in nulliparous women. *Journal of Obstetrics and Gynaecology, 37*(6), 508–516.

Karch, A. M. (2015). *Lippincott's nursing drug guide.* Philadelphia, PA: Lippincott Williams & Wilkins.

Kaymak, O., Iskender, C., Ibanoglu, M., et al. (2015). Retrospective evaluation of risk factors and perinatal outcome of umbilical cord prolapse during labor. *European Review for Medical and Pharmacological Sciences, 19*(13), 2336–2339.

Kim, J. W., Kim, Y. H., Kim, C. H., et al. (2014). Uterine artery pseudoaneurysm manifesting as delayed postpartum hemorrhage after precipitous delivery: Three case reports. *Gynecologic and Obstetric Investigation, 78*(2), 136–140.

Koyyalamudi, V., Sidhu, G., Cornett, E. M., et al., (2016). New labor pain treatment options. *Current Pain and Headache Reports, 20*(2), 11.

Kunzier, N. B., Park, H., Cioffi, J., et al. (2016). A comparison of obstetrical outcomes and costs between misoprostol and dinoprostone for induction of labor. *Journal of Maternal-Fetal & Neonatal Medicine, 29*(22), 3732–3736.

Malvasi, A., Bochicchio, M., Vaira, L., et al. (2014). The fetal head evaluation during labor in the occiput posterior position: The ESA (evaluation by simulation algorithm) approach. *Journal of Maternal-Fetal & Neonatal Medicine, 27*(11), 1151–1157.

Manjula, B. G., Bagga, R., Kalra, J., et al. (2015). Labour induction with an intermediate-dose oxytocin regimen has advantages over a high-dose regimen. *Journal of Obstetrics and Gynaecology, 35*(4), 362–367.

McCarthy, E. A., Walker, S. P., Ugoni, A., et al. (2016). Self-weighing and simple dietary advice for overweight and obese pregnant women to reduce obstetric complications without impact on quality of life: A randomised controlled trial. *British Journal of Obstetrics and Gynecology, 123*(6), 965–973.

Neal, J. L., Lowe, N. K., Schorn, M. N., et al. (2015). Labor dystocia: A common approach to diagnosis. *Journal of Midwifery & Women's Health, 60*(5), 499–509.

Neal, J. L., Ryan, S. L., Lowe, N. K., et al. (2015). Labor dystocia: Uses of related nomenclature. *Journal of Midwifery & Women's Health, 60*(5), 485–498.

Norman, J. E. (2012). Induction and augmentation of labour. In D. K. Edmonds (Ed.), *Dewhurst's textbook of obstetrics & gynaecology* (8th ed., pp. 287–295). Oxford, United Kingdom: Wiley.

Øverland, E. A., Vatten, L. J., & Eskild, A. (2014). Pregnancy week at delivery and the risk of shoulder dystocia: A population study of 2,014,956 deliveries. *British Journal of Obstetrics and Gynecology, 121*(1), 34–41.

Ray, E. M., & Alhusen, J. L. (2016). The suspected macrosomic fetus at term: A clinical dilemma. *Journal of Midwifery & Women's Health, 61*(2), 263–269.

Rossen, J., Østborg, T. B., Lindtjørn, E., et al. (2016). Judicious use of oxytocin augmentation for the management of prolonged labor. *Acta Obstetricia et Gynecologica Scandinavica, 95*(3), 355–361.

Roth, C., Dent, S. A., Parfitt, S. E., et al. (2016). Randomized controlled trial of use of the peanut ball during labor. *MCN. The American Journal of Maternal Child Nursing, 41*(3), 140–146.

Silver, R. M. (2015). Abnormal placentation: Placenta previa, vasa previa, and placenta accreta. *Obstetrics and Gynecology, 126*(3), 654–668.

Steinhauer, S. (2015). Perineal protection. *The Practising Midwife, 18*(7), 14–16.

Stitely, M. L., & Gherman, R. B. (2014). Shoulder dystocia: Management and documentation. *Seminars in Perinatology, 38*(4), 194–200.

Suzuki, S. (2016). Clinical significance of precipitous labor. *Journal of Clinical Medicine Research, 7*(3), 150–153.

Suzuki, S., & Kato, M. (2015). Clinical significance of pregnancies complicated by velamentous umbilical cord insertion associated with other umbilical cord/placental abnormalities. *Journal of Clinical Medicine Research, 7*(11), 853–856.

Tauchi, M., Hasegawa, J., Oba, T., et al. (2016). A case of uterine rupture diagnosed based on routine focused assessment with sonography for obstetrics. *Journal of Medical Ultrasonics, 43*(1), 129–131.

Toivonen, E., Palomäki, O., Huhtala, H., et al. (2014). Maternal experiences of vaginal breech delivery. *Birth, 41*(4), 316–322.

U.S. Department of Health and Human Services. (2010). *Healthy people 2020.* Washington, DC: Author.

Vachon-Marceau, C., Demers, S., Goyet, M., et al. (2016). Labor dystocia and the risk of uterine rupture in women with prior cesarean. *American Journal of Perinatology, 33*(6), 577–583.

Velzel, J., de Hundt, M., Mulder, F. M., et al. (2015). Prediction models for successful external cephalic version: A systematic review. *European Journal of Obstetrics & Gynecology and Reproductive Biology, 195*, 160–167.

Wang, D., Zhu, L., Zhang, S., et al. (2016). Predictive macrosomia birthweight thresholds for adverse maternal and neonatal outcomes. *The Journal of Maternal-Fetal & Neonatal Medicine, 29*(23), 3745–3750.

Zhao, F., Geng, Q., Kong, F., et al. (2015). Quantitative analysis of tightness of nuchal cord and its relationship with fetal intrauterine distress. *International Journal of Clinical and Experimental Medicine, 8*(10), 17507–17514.

Zheng, T. (2012). Labor & delivery. In T. Zheng (Ed.), *Comprehensive handbook of obstetrics and gynecology* (2nd ed., pp. 16–58). Phoenix, AZ: Phoenix Medical Press.

Zielinski, R. E., Brody, M. G., & Low, L. K. (2016). The value of the maternity care team in the promotion of physiologic birth. *Journal of Obstetric, Gynecologic & Neonatal Nursing, 45*(2), 276–284.

Nursing Care of a Family During a Surgical Intervention for Birth

*M*oja Hamma is a 29-year-old woman pregnant with her first baby. Her labor began with ruptured membranes and dark green meconium-stained amniotic fluid. Moja called her nurse-midwife, who instructed her to come to the hospital immediately. Moja drove herself and arrived in 20 minutes. Fetal heart rate (FHR) was 100 beats/min. An obstetrician was consulted, and she scheduled Moja for an immediate cesarean birth. Moja reacted calmly to the news that she needed surgery until she realized her boyfriend would not be able to get to the hospital in time to be with her in surgery. At that point, she refused to sign permission for surgery, saying, "I can't. I just can't go through this alone."

Previous chapters described the physiology of labor and the sequence of usual birth. This chapter adds information about surgical interventions for those women who must have a surgical procedure to ensure a safe outcome for themselves or their child.

Is Moja's response typical of a woman who is told she needs a surgical procedure for the birth of her baby? What would be your best action to help her accept this procedure?

KEY TERMS

amniotomy

cesarean birth

classic cesarean incision

dehiscence

elective cesarean birth

episiotomy

low segment incision

vaginal birth after cesarean (VBAC)

OBJECTIVES

After mastering the contents of this chapter, you should be able to:

1. Describe the usual indications for surgical interventions such as amniotomy, episiotomy, and cesarean birth.

2. Identify the 2020 National Health Goals related to cesarean birth that nurses can help the nation achieve.

3. Assess a woman scheduled for a surgical intervention for preoperative, intraoperative, and postoperative needs.

4. Formulate nursing diagnoses related to the family experiencing a surgical intervention for birth.

5. Establish outcomes that meet the needs of a woman requiring a surgical intervention for birth as well as help her manage seamless transitions across different healthcare settings.

6. Using the nursing process, plan nursing care that includes the six competencies of Quality & Safety Education for Nurses (QSEN): Patient-Centered Care, Teamwork & Collaboration, Evidence-Based Practice (EBP), Quality Improvement (QI), Safety, and Informatics.

7. Implement common preoperative and postoperative care for surgical interventions for birth.

8. Evaluate expected outcomes for achievement and effectiveness of care to be certain expected outcomes have been achieved.

9. Integrate knowledge of surgical birth interventions with the interplay of nursing process, the six competencies of QSEN, and Family Nursing to achieve quality maternal and child health nursing care.

BOX 24.1

Nursing Care Planning Based on 2020 National Health Goals

Two National Health Goals speak directly to cesarean birth:

- Reduce the rate of cesarean births among low-risk (full-term, singleton, vertex presentation) women having their first child to 23.9% of live births from a baseline of 26.5%.
- Reduce the rate of cesarean births among women who have had a prior cesarean birth to 81.7% of live births from a baseline of 90.8% (U.S. Department of Health and Human Services, 2010; see www.healthypeople.gov).

Nurses can help the nation achieve these goals by exploring with women who choose elective cesarean birth whether their goals are sound and by encouraging women who fulfill the criteria for vaginal birth after cesarean (VBAC) to attempt a vaginal birth with a second child.

Cesarean birth, or birth accomplished through an abdominal incision into the uterus, is slightly more hazardous than vaginal birth, but compared with other surgical procedures, it is one of the safest types of surgeries and one with few complications (Speichinger & Holschneider, 2013).

The term *cesarean birth*, rather than *cesarean delivery*, is used in nursing literature to accentuate that this is a birth more than it is a surgical procedure. The 2020 National Health Goals related to cesarean birth are shown in Box 24.1.

Nursing Process Overview

FOR A WOMAN HAVING A SURGICAL INTERVENTION FOR BIRTH

ASSESSMENT

Some women elect cesarean rather than vaginal birth. Women with smaller than usual pelvic diameters may be informed during pregnancy a cesarean birth will be necessary. Others learn only during labor that a cesarean birth will be necessary because a complication is developing. Surgical interventions such as episiotomy and amniotomy are not usually anticipated before labor. Assessment as to whether a woman will be a good candidate for surgery must include both physiologic and psychological status and the woman's preparedness for the procedure.

NURSING DIAGNOSIS

Nursing diagnoses specific to surgical interventions are often related to the prevention of common complications or patient/family concerns about the procedure. Specific examples might include:

- Fear related to impending surgery
- Pain related to a surgical incision
- Deficient fluid volume related to blood loss from surgery
- Powerlessness related to medical need for episiotomy or cesarean birth

- Risk for anxiety related to unanticipated circumstances surrounding birth
- Risk for infection related to a surgical incision
- Risk for hemorrhage related to surgical procedure
- Risk for impaired parent–infant attachment related to unplanned method of birth

OUTCOME IDENTIFICATION AND PLANNING

The same important outcome applies to a woman having a cesarean birth as to a woman giving birth vaginally: a healthy mother and a healthy baby. In either instance, decisions for a method of birth can be made so suddenly, planning is limited to only a few minutes. This means you have only a very short time to organize presurgical steps such as gastrointestinal or anesthesia preparation or to check off a presurgical checklist. Be certain plans afterward include discharge or home care instructions because a woman will remain in the healthcare facility only 2 to 4 days. Refer women who know in advance they will have a cesarean birth to helpful websites and other resources when appropriate (see Chapter 20).

IMPLEMENTATION

Every woman is aware childbirth poses some risk to health. When major surgery is superimposed on top of this, it is imperative that a woman and her support person feel confidence in the healthcare personnel who will care for them. When giving care to any woman during labor, be certain to establish early on a helping relationship with both the woman and her support person as this relationship becomes especially advantageous should the birth method need to be altered.

An important intervention includes coordination of healthcare team members such as an anesthesiologist, surgeon, pediatrician or neonatologist, and recovery room or high-risk nursery personnel.

Many interventions focus on teaching and support because the more a woman understands what is happening, the more she can accept and cooperate. After surgery, be certain to provide adequate "talk time" to allow a woman time to review what has happened and integrate the experience with what she and her partner expected would happen.

OUTCOME EVALUATION

Evaluation of expected outcomes is important in the care of a woman after a surgical intervention to ensure she is not developing a complication and is developing a positive mother–infant (or parent–infant or family–infant) relationship. Examples that would demonstrate successful achievement of outcomes include:

- Patient states she understands the reason for her cesarean birth.
- Patient states she felt well prepared for cesarean birth even in light of an emergency.
- Couple states they feel able to cope with newborn care even with mother recovering from surgery.
- Patient remains free of signs and symptoms of infection after an episiotomy.
- Patient states her incisional pain is controlled and tolerable.
- Patient states birth was a fulfilling experience even in light of the unplanned cesarean birth.

Surgical Interventions

AMNIOTOMY

Amniotomy is the artificial rupturing of membranes during labor if they do not rupture spontaneously to allow the fetal head to contact the cervix more directly, which possibly increases the efficiency of contractions and therefore increases the speed of labor. There is still conflicting evidence about the risks and benefits of amniotomy with regard to shortening labor duration and risks for cesarean section after amniotomy; therefore, practices may vary widely in how often this technique is used (Jackson & Gregory, 2015). If the procedure is scheduled, a woman is asked to assume a dorsal recumbent position; an amniohook (a long, thin crochet-like instrument) or a hemostat is passed vaginally. The membranes are torn, and amniotic fluid is allowed to escape. A disadvantage of amniotomy is that it puts a fetus momentarily at risk for cord prolapse if a loop of cord escapes into the vagina with the fluid. It is important to only perform an amniotomy if the fetal head is well applied to the cervix. Always measure the FHR immediately after the rupture of membranes to determine this did not happen (Maher & Heavey, 2015).

QSEN Checkpoint Question 24.1

SAFETY

Suppose Moja had an amniotomy during her labor. Immediately after this procedure, which nursing assessment would be most important for the nurse to make?
  a. Ask her to rate her pain level after the procedure.
  b. Assess maternal heart rate to detect possible bleeding.
  c. Assess FHR to detect possible cord prolapse.
  d. Document the amount of amniotic fluid that has been lost.

Look in Appendix A for the best answer and rationale.

EPISIOTOMY

An **episiotomy** is a surgical incision of the perineum made to prevent tearing of the perineum, release pressure on the fetal head with birth, and possibly shorten the last portion of the second stage of labor (Verghese, Champaneria, Kapoor, et al., 2016).

An episiotomy incision is made with blunt-tipped scissors in the midline of the perineum (i.e., a midline episiotomy) or is begun in the midline but directed laterally away from the rectum (i.e., a mediolateral episiotomy) (Fig. 24.1). Mediolateral incisions have the advantage over midline cuts in that, if tearing occurs beyond the incision, the tear will not be directed toward the rectum, thus creating less danger of a rectal mucosal tear, which can result in loss of sphincter function and fecal incontinence later in life (Verghese et al., 2016). Midline episiotomies, however, heal more easily, cause less blood loss, and result in less postpartal discomfort. The pressure of the fetal head against the perineum as a woman pushes just prior to birth is so intense the nerve endings in the perineum are momentarily deadened, allowing an episiotomy

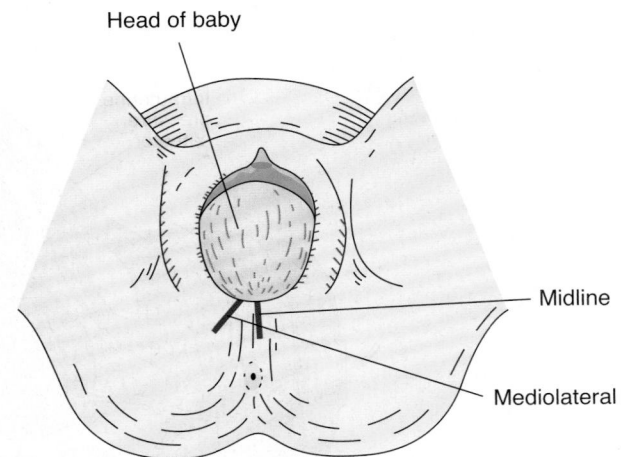

Figure 24.1 An episiotomy incision.

to be done without anesthesia. There is a slight loss of blood, but the pressure of the presenting part immediately seals the cut edges and minimizes bleeding. Episiotomies are sutured after birth.

Theoretically, if this is done immediately, a woman will still have so much natural-pressure anesthesia of the perineum that she will not require an anesthetic for the repair. In actuality, by the time the placenta is delivered (approximately 5 minutes), enough sensation has returned to the perineum that most women need an injection of a local anesthetic for comfort. Women who received epidural anesthesia will probably not need additional medication.

One instance in which episiotomy (defibulation) may be necessary is in women who have had female circumcision with perineal scarring because their perineum is unable to stretch to allow the vaginal outlet to open for birth (Abdulcadir, Dugerdil, Yaron, et al., 2016).

PROCEDURES FOR HIGH-RISK PREGNANCIES

If a woman or fetus is found to be high risk during labor, a number of procedures over and above a usual assessment can become necessary. All these procedures cause increased anxiety for the woman and her family and so need special instructions and supportive reassurance.

Internal Electronic Monitoring

Internal electronic monitoring is the most precise method for assessing FHR and uterine contractions. It is most often used to assess whether contractions are strong enough to cause cervical change in the case of a prolonged labor course. This can be done by wireless telemetry but is usually managed by a pressure-sensing catheter passed through the vagina after the membranes have ruptured, and the cervix has dilated to at least 3 cm. It is then passed into the uterine cavity and alongside the fetus (Fig. 24.2). The end of the catheter extending from the vagina is attached to a pressure recorder. As each uterine contraction puts pressure on the uterine contents, the pressure exerted on the catheter is recorded. When contractions are monitored by an internal pressure gauge in this way, the frequency, duration, baseline strength, and peak strength of contractions can all be evaluated. Contraction strength is

Figure 24.2   Internal fetal monitoring.

evaluated by the height of the peak of the contraction on the tracing. Equally important to evaluate is the return of the uterine tone to baseline strength between contractions. This ensures there is placental filling between contractions.

With contractions during the latent phase of labor, the baseline level is usually less than 5 mmHg; with active contractions, it is about 12 mmHg. During the second stage of labor, the baseline may be as high as 20 mmHg. Baseline readings that do not return to 20 mmHg or less following a contraction suggest uterine hypertonia and a possible compromise of fetal well-being.

An accurate FHR recording is obtained from a fetal scalp electrode. This type of monitoring is most useful when babies are difficult to monitor because of maternal habitus or during abnormal tracings due to FHR decelerations. Once the fetal head is engaged, the electrode is inserted vaginally and attached to the fetal scalp with a small puncture of the skin. A fetal electrocardiograph signal is obtained, amplified, and then fed into a cardiotachometer. The output from the cardiotachometer is recorded on permanent graph paper.

Although internal monitoring produces clear details of fetal heartbeats, it is invasive, carries the risk of uterine infection, and limits a woman's movement. It is, therefore, reserved for women whose fetus is at high risk during labor.

Scalp Stimulation

Although not well studied, if a fetus shows an unresponsive heartbeat during labor, vibroacoustic stimulation can be used the same as is done for nonstress tests during pregnancy to be certain a fetus is responding well to labor (Tan, Smyth, & Wei, 2013). If FHR variability appears to be depressed during labor, the welfare of a fetus can be assessed by scalp stimulation. This is done by applying pressure with the fingers to the fetal scalp through the dilated cervix (Fig. 24.3). This causes a tactile response in the fetus that momentarily increases the FHR. If the fetus is in distress and becoming acidotic,

FHR acceleration will not occur. Scalp stimulation, therefore, is an assessment of acid–base balance in a fetus in labor.

Fetal Oxygen Saturation Level

Fetal oxygen saturation may be measured by an oxygen saturation sensor introduced into the uterus and placed beside the fetus's cheek after membranes have ruptured. Because the procedure creates a small chance of uterine infection, this is generally reserved for women who already have an internal contraction or fetal monitor in place.

Fetal Blood Sampling

Although not often used anymore, monitoring of the fetal blood composition (obtained from the fetal scalp following cervical dilatation during labor) can reveal hypoxia in a fetus (Chandraharan, 2016). A small laceration will be present on

Figure 24.3   Fetal scalp stimulation. (Redrawn from *Journal of Perinatal and Neonatal Nursing*, 16[1]; with permission from Aspen Publishers, Inc.)

the newborn scalp as a result, which needs to be observed for bleeding or signs of infection following birth.

Cesarean Birth

Although cesarean birth may be elected by some women, the procedure is used most often as a prophylactic measure to alleviate problems of birth such as cephalopelvic disproportion, breech or multiple fetus births, or failure to progress in labor.

A major concern in maternal and child health nursing is the increasing number of cesarean births being performed annually (Betrán, Ye, Moller, et al., 2016). In 1970, only 5.5% of women in the United States had infants born by cesarean birth. In 2013, the rate had risen by 53% reaching 32%, the highest rate ever reported in the United States (Martin, Hamilton, Osterman, et al., 2015).

This increased rate has resulted from a combination of the increasing safety of cesarean birth, the use of fetal monitors (which provide for early detection of fetal problems), an increased incidence of obese women (Carlson, Hernandez, & Hurt, 2015), and scheduled or **elective cesarean births**, chosen by women for convenience or to prevent potential urinary or anal incontinence later in life (Tähtinen, Cartwright, Tsui, et al., 2016). The increase in rate may also be related to a healthcare provider's fears of malpractice suits should a fetus be allowed to be born vaginally and then be discovered to have suffered anoxia.

Several legal and ethical issues have arisen in recent years when women have refused to undergo cesarean birth after being advised they need one. Because women do have a right to decide whether they will undergo surgery, the right to refuse the procedure must be respected (Box 24.2). In some instances, however, a court order for the procedure has been obtained to save a fetus. Be certain you are aware of the opinion of your agency's ethics committee on this issue.

As a rule, nurse-midwifery or interprofessional birthing services have a lower incidence of cesarean births than hospital services even when controlling for a higher incidence of low-risk women in these settings (Rosenstein, Nijagal, Nakagawa, et al., 2015). Continuous support during labor by a concerned healthcare provider (such as a nurse) appears to decrease the incidence (Cox & King, 2015).

SCHEDULED CESAREAN BIRTH

Scheduled cesarean births are planned, which means there is time for thorough preparation for the experience throughout the antepartal period. Some women are even able to take a childbirth preparation class specifically for cesarean birth. Women who plan these need to be aware they will need epidural anesthesia, and the risk of injury to them from cesarean birth is higher than that from vaginal birth. Scheduling cesarean births this freely also can result in preterm birth with the accompanying threats to the fetus or newborn (Box 24.3).

In the past, many cesarean births were performed because the woman had undergone a cesarean birth with a previous child; with new surgical techniques, particularly the use of a low cervical incision, "once a cesarean, always a cesarean" no longer applies. The majority of women who have had a cesarean birth within the past 10 years are eligible to give birth vaginally in subsequent pregnancies if the circumstances are appropriate for vaginal birth (Iriye, 2015).

Yet, other reasons for scheduled cesarean births are when there is a physical indication such as transverse presentation, an infection that could be contacted by the fetus if born vaginally, or cephalopelvic disproportion (Box 24.4). For instance, cesarean birth reduces the transfer of the herpes type 2 from mother to newborn, so it is recommended for women who have this infection and an active lesion in the vaginal area at the onset of labor (Liu, Li, Chen, et al., 2014). It also can reduce mortality among infants presenting breech (Cunningham, Leveno, Bloom, et al., 2014). It may be advantageous for a preterm birth to avoid pressure on the fetal head (Delnord, Blondel, Drewniak, et al., 2014). It is generally contraindicated when there is a documented dead fetus (labor can be induced to avoid a surgical procedure).

EMERGENT CESAREAN BIRTH

Emergent cesarean births are done for reasons that arise suddenly in labor, such as placenta previa, premature separation of the placenta, fetal distress, or failure to progress. With this second type of cesarean birth, preparation must be done

---

BOX 24.2
Elective Cesarean Birth

Because about 30% of women have a baby by cesarean birth in the United States today, there is an emerging culture of women who advocate cesarean birth as superior to vaginal birth as a way to eliminate long hours of labor pain. This effect—to make birth a surgical procedure—is in sharp contrast to other efforts to make birth more natural. Because there are added risks to both the woman and her fetus from a cesarean birth, it can cause a nursing care problem if a woman who has no medical reason for a cesarean birth insists on having one. Being certain to explain that a cesarean birth is a method to be used when vaginal birth is not possible, rather than a true option, can help a woman put her choice of type of birth into perspective.

BOX 24.3
Nursing Care Planning to Respect Cultural Diversity

Several cultural issues can come into play when planning a cesarean birth. A religious family that was expecting a vaginal birth but needs cesarean birth during labor may ask for time to pray before surgery. If there is no need for an urgent or emergent delivery, it is best to give the family private time to pray. Jehovah's Witnesses cannot accept blood products as a part of their spirituality. If they are at high risk for hemorrhage such as in the case of a placenta previa, it is important for healthcare providers to consider whether this type of high-risk patient should be cared for in a setting where bloodless or transfusion-free medicine is available. These types of specialty groups can help reduce blood loss, increase a patient's ability to make more blood, and circulate a patient's blood back to her, so that she does not need to accept blood from another person.

BOX 24.4

Selected Indications for Cesarean Birth

MATERNAL FACTORS

Active genital herpes or (perhaps) human papillomavirus
AIDS or (perhaps) HIV-positive status
Cephalopelvic disproportion
Cervical cerclage
Disabling conditions, such as severe gestational hypertension, that would prevent pushing to accomplish the pelvic division of labor
Failed induction or failure to progress in labor
An obstructive benign or malignant tumor
Previous cesarean birth by classic incision
Fear of birth or wish to help prevent uterine prolapse or urinary incontinence in later years

PLACENTAL FACTORS

Placenta previa
Premature separation of the placenta
Umbilical cord prolapse

FETAL FACTORS

Compound conditions such as macrosomic fetus in a breech lie
Extreme low birth weight
Fetal distress
A major fetal anomaly, such as hydrocephalus
Multigestation or conjoined twins
Transverse fetal lie and perhaps breech presentation

rapidly but with the same concern for fully informing a woman and her support person about what circumstances created the need for the cesarean birth and how the birth will proceed. Cesarean birth is mentioned in most childbirth classes, so any woman who has taken such a class may at least understand that cesarean births are sometimes necessary.

An emergent cesarean birth carries with it the same risks of any emergent surgery: The woman may not be a prime candidate for anesthesia and may be psychologically unprepared for the experience. In addition, the woman may have a fluid and electrolyte imbalance and be both physically and emotionally exhausted from a long labor.

Effects of Surgery on a Woman

Like any surgical procedure, cesarean birth has systemic effects.

STRESS RESPONSE

Whenever the body is subjected to stress, either physical or psychosocial, it responds with measures to preserve the function of major body systems. This results in a release of epinephrine and norepinephrine from the adrenal medulla. Epinephrine increases the heart rate, causes bronchial dilatation, and elevates the blood glucose level. It also leads to peripheral vasoconstriction, which forces blood to the central circulation and increases blood pressure. In the pregnant woman, such responses may minimize blood supply to the

lower extremities. Pregnant women are already prone to thrombophlebitis from stasis of blood flow, so these responses compound or greatly increase thrombophlebitis risk.

INTERFERENCE WITH BODY DEFENSES

The skin serves as the primary line of defense against bacterial invasion, so when skin is incised for a surgical procedure, this important line of defense is lost. Strict adherence to aseptic techniques during surgery and in the days following the procedure is necessary to compensate for this impaired defense. If the cesarean birth is performed hours after the membranes rupture, a woman's risk for infection will be higher than if the membranes were still intact. Many women receive prophylactic antibiotics, such as ampicillin (Omnipen) or a cephalosporin, such as cefazolin (Ancef), to ensure protection against postsurgical endometritis, even if the membranes remained intact (Gyte, Dou, & Vazquez, 2014).

INTERFERENCE WITH CIRCULATORY FUNCTION

Although vessels that must be cut for surgery are immediately clamped and ligated, some blood loss occurs with surgery. Compared to other surgeries, the amount of blood lost in a cesarean birth is comparatively high, caused by the fact abdominal and pelvic vessels are congested with blood waiting to supply the placenta. During a vaginal birth, a woman loses 300 to 500 ml of blood. This loss increases to 500 to 1,000 ml with a cesarean birth (Graham, Gimovsky, Roman, et al., 2016).

INTERFERENCE WITH BODY ORGAN FUNCTION

When any body organ is handled, cut, or repaired in surgery, it may respond with a temporary disruption in function. Therefore, close postoperative assessment, not only of the primary organ involved but also of total body function, is necessary to determine the total degree of disruption present.

Because the uterus is handled during cesarean birth, it may not contract well afterward, which can lead to postpartum hemorrhage. For a healthcare provider to reach the uterus, the bladder must be displaced anteriorly. As a result of this handling, the bladder may not sense filling as well as usual after the procedure (Cordon, Fracchia, & Armenakas, 2014). During surgery, pressure is also felt by the intestine, so a paralytic ileus or halting of intestinal function with obstruction may occur (Sahin & Terzioglu, 2015). As mentioned previously, thrombophlebitis from impaired lower extremity blood flow is yet another possibility. After a cesarean birth, therefore, uterine, bladder, intestinal, and lower extremity circulatory function must all be carefully assessed.

INTERFERENCE WITH SELF-IMAGE OR SELF-ESTEEM

Surgery always leaves an incisional scar that is noticeable to some extent afterward, and its appearance may cause a woman to feel self-conscious. Although most women accept cesarean birth well, a woman who was intent on having a vaginal birth may feel a loss of self-esteem and depression if she believes the procedure marks her as a woman less capable than others because she was unable to give vaginal birth (Ayers, Bond, Bertullies, et al., 2016).

Nursing Care for a Woman Anticipating a Cesarean Birth

A woman who is admitted to the hospital for an anticipated cesarean birth may be more worried about the procedure (because she has had more time to worry) than a woman who is told during labor an emergent cesarean is necessary. After the woman is admitted, allow her time to talk about any fears she has. Encourage her to do as much as possible for herself preoperatively to help her feel in control and to diminish her fear (Silva, de Jesus, Merighi, et al., 2014).

Be aware that it is difficult for a woman undergoing surgery to relax as long as her support person remains nervous and worried. Make a point of including this person in all explanations and admission routines to keep his or her anxiety under control as well.

What If . . . 24.1

After learning that Moja wanted to wait for her cesarean birth to begin until her boyfriend arrives, the nurse learns the boyfriend has texted to say he cannot possibly stay with Moja in the operating room; he'll feel so nauseated he'll probably faint. Would it be best to plan on supporting Moja yourself or to try to involve the boyfriend?

PREOPERATIVE INTERVIEW

Both a woman's primary care provider and the team member who will be administering the anesthesia interview a woman preoperatively to obtain a health history and to make assessments and decisions for safety of the procedure and the use of anesthesia. In addition to these, a nursing assessment is also essential. Be certain to ask about any past surgeries, secondary illnesses, allergies to foods or drugs, reactions to anesthesia, bleeding problems, or current medications to help establish surgical risk, and any body piercings that need to be removed because of the use of electrosurgery or an arterial cauterizing machine. In addition, include questions to discover the woman's knowledge about:

- What the procedure will entail
- Length of hospitalization anticipated
- If she's been told about any postsurgical equipment to be used, such as an indwelling catheter or intravenous (IV) fluid line
- Any special precautions that are being planned for her infant such as high-risk nursery care

OPERATIVE RISK FOR A WOMAN

Women who are in less than optimal physical or psychological health are at risk for a complicated surgical outcome unless the risk factor is identified, and special precautions are taken.

Poor Nutritional Status

A woman who is obese because of poor nutrition is at added risk from surgery, because tissue that contains an abundance of fatty cells is difficult to suture, thus causing the surgical incision to take longer to heal. A prolonged healing period increases the risk for infection and rupture of the incision (**dehiscence**) (Ayres-de-Campos, 2015).

Because an obese woman's heart has an increased workload, the physiologic shock of surgery may place greater stress on the already overworked organ. In addition, an obese woman often has more difficulty turning and ambulating postoperatively than does a woman with a lower body mass index (BMI) and therefore has an increased risk for developing respiratory or circulatory complications such as pneumonia or thrombophlebitis (Quinlan & Murphy, 2015).

A woman with a protein or vitamin deficiency is also at risk for poorer healing because protein and vitamins C and D are necessary for new cell formation at the incision site. Vitamin K is necessary to ensure blood clotting after surgery. Pregnant women who are iron deficient (in particular, women with a multiple gestation or women who have not taken supplements), coupled with the blood loss from surgery, are at high risk for extreme fatigue after surgery, which could interfere with parent–child bonding (Drukker, Hants, Farkash, et al., 2015).

Age Variations

Age affects surgical risk because it can cause both decreased circulatory and renal function. Fortunately, most pregnant women fall within the young adult age group, so are excellent candidates for surgery. A woman older than 40 years falls into a category of slightly higher risk not because of surgery itself but because of associated conditions such as gestational diabetes (Inocêncio, Braga, Lima, et al., 2015).

Altered General Health

A woman who has a secondary illness such as cardiac disease, diabetes mellitus, anemia, kidney, or liver disease is at greater than usual surgical risk, depending on the extent of her primary disease, because the pathology from the secondary illness may interfere with her ability to physically adjust to the demands of surgery. Therefore, asking if the woman has a secondary illness is an essential component of a preoperative nursing history.

A general medication history also is important because some drugs increase surgical risk by interfering with the effect of an anesthetic or with healing of tissue. Examples of drugs that pregnant women might be taking and their potential complications are shown in Box 24.5.

Fluid and Electrolyte Imbalance

A woman who enters surgery with a lower than usual blood volume will experience the effect of surgical blood loss more than a woman who has a normal blood volume. A woman who has had a long labor before a cesarean birth is scheduled may fall into this category because she may have had little to eat or drink for almost 24 hours. Recent vomiting, diarrhea, or a chronic poor fluid intake compounds her risk. IV fluid replacement may need to be initiated preoperatively and continued postoperatively to prevent a serious fluid or electrolyte imbalance.

Fear

Women who are extremely worried about surgery need a very detailed explanation of the procedure in order to reduce their anxiety to a tolerable level. If a woman seems particularly anxious, inform the team member who will administer the anesthesia so that an antianxiety drug can be administered, if necessary, to make the experience less frightening for her.

BOX 24.5

Nursing Care Planning Based on Responsibility for Pharmacology

DRUGS THAT MAY RESULT IN COMPLICATIONS OF CESAREAN BIRTH

Type of Drug	Action
Antibiotics	Specific antibiotics may predispose one to renal insufficiency or increase neuromuscular blockage; can lead to opportunistic infections
Anticoagulants	May cause hemorrhage due to lack of hemostasis during surgery
Anticonvulsants	May increase liver action and metabolism of anesthetic agent
Antihypertensives	May result in hypotension after anesthesia
Corticosteroids	May block body's response to shock and so lead to lack of adrenal function
Insulin	May lead to hypoglycemia during labor or hyperglycemia if a dextrose solution is administered
Antianxiety agents	May cause hypotension after anesthesia

In many instances, just helping a woman acknowledge that her fear of surgery is a normal reaction can be helpful. This does not make the procedure any less traumatic, but the woman may then view her feelings as expected, which can help to enhance her self-esteem and lower anxiety (Silva et al., 2014).

OPERATIVE RISK TO THE NEWBORN

Cesarean birth places a newborn at a greater risk than does a vaginal birth. When a fetus is pushed through the birth canal, pressure on the chest helps rid the newborn's lungs of fluid, making it easier for the baby to take a first breath. For this reason, more infants born by cesarean birth develop some degree of respiratory difficulty for a day or two after birth than those born vaginally (Wang, Liu, Zhu, et al., 2015). See Chapter 26 for a discussion of this condition, which is often referred to as transient tachypnea of the newborn.

PREOPERATIVE DIAGNOSTIC PROCEDURES

Preoperative assessment procedures for a woman who is to have a cesarean birth include documentation of fetal status and presentation and maturity by ultrasound assessment. In addition, assessments also include circulatory and renal function and those for all presurgery patients, including:

- Vital sign determination
- Urinalysis
- Complete blood count
- Coagulation profile (prothrombin time [PT], partial thromboplastin time [PTT])
- Serum electrolytes and pH
- Blood typing and cross-matching

Remember blood values need to be evaluated in light of the changes that occur with pregnancy. During pregnancy, for example, a woman (particularly one who was in prolonged labor) can have an elevated leukocyte count (up to 20,000 cells/mm³), so this finding is not as helpful an indicator for the presence of infection in the pregnant woman as it is in others.

PREOPERATIVE TEACHING

Preoperative teaching is aimed at acquainting a woman with the cesarean procedure and any special equipment to be used so she is as informed as possible.

Before beginning teaching, assess how much a woman knows about her surgery. A woman who has had a cesarean birth for her first child and now is being admitted for a second procedure, for example, already knows many details. Even so, she will undoubtedly appreciate having her memory refreshed and recall confirmed. Answer all specific questions she has and fill in gaps in knowledge as necessary. Be certain all information you offer is accurate. Be certain not to use hospital jargon such as "NPO." People under stress do not process new information well. They cannot process information at all if they do not understand the terminology.

Be certain to explain the immediate preoperative measures that will be necessary, such as surgical skin preparation, eating nothing before the time of surgery, premedication (if this will be used), and method of transport to surgery. Review the necessity for an indwelling bladder catheter, IV fluid administration, and placement of an epidural catheter (if this will be used for postprocedure pain relief).

For scheduled cesarean births, an explanation of not only what is going to happen immediately but also what activities should be performed to help maintain respiratory and skeletal muscle function and to prevent postsurgical complications (e.g., early ambulation) should also be included in teaching. Women who practice exercises to maintain good respiratory and circulatory function postoperatively tend to experience fewer postoperative respiratory and circulatory complications than those who do not. These preventive exercises are best taught during the preoperative period, when the woman is free of pain and can concentrate on learning. Such teaching also gives a woman a positive outlook on surgery and a sense of control over her situation.

Throughout teaching, use visual aids as necessary. Draw pictures or show illustrations of anatomy, as needed. Be careful, however, not to leave textbooks about cesarean procedure techniques with a woman. Typically, these books also describe complications, and although knowledge of possible complications is necessary for informed consent, reading about complications complete with color illustrations can be overwhelming.

Deep Breathing

Periodic deep breathing exercises fully aerate the lungs and help prevent stasis of lung mucus from the prolonged time spent in the supine position during surgery. Because stasis always has the potential to cause infection, preventing this helps prevent lung infection such as pneumonia.

A typical exercise is to take 5 to 10 deep breaths every hour. The woman simply inhales as deeply as possible, holds her breath for a second or two, and then exhales as deeply as possible. Be certain she both inhales and exhales fully. Otherwise, she might experience light-headedness from hyperventilation.

Incentive Spirometry

A common device used three to four times a day postoperatively to encourage deep breathing is an incentive spirometer. These devices, which cause a small ping-pong–like ball to rise in a narrow tube or cause lights to flash, are both easy and fun to operate and give a woman a sense of reward for her effort. The initial impression of most people is that the device works by blowing into it. Because its purpose is to fully aerate lung spaces, however, most models are triggered by *inhalation*, not exhalation. A gauge can be set to monitor levels and tabs to set goals.

Turning

Be certain women understand that turning postoperatively is important to prevent both respiratory and circulatory stasis.

Ambulation

The most effective way to stimulate lower extremity circulation after a cesarean birth is by early ambulation. For this reason, most primary healthcare providers prefer a woman to be out of bed and walking as soon as the effect of the epidural anesthesia has worn off. Helping a woman ambulate this early can be difficult because she is both fatigued and has pain from her incision. Help her to understand ambulation is extremely important after cesarean birth because the edema from the low pelvic surgery compresses circulation to the lower extremities, thus increasing the risk for lower extremity circulatory stasis. Some women may be prescribed sequential compression devices (SCDs) or antiembolic stockings (thromboembolic devices [TEDs]) to support and encourage venous return in addition to ambulation.

IMMEDIATE PREOPERATIVE CARE MEASURES

A number of measures must be taken immediately before surgery to help ensure a safe outcome.

Informed Consent

Obtaining operative consent is the primary healthcare provider's responsibility, but being certain, it is obtained prior to surgery is everyone's responsibility. You may be asked to witness a woman's signature on such a form. Before signing as a witness, be certain that it was *informed* consent, or one in which the risks and benefits of the procedure were explained in terms the woman could easily understand.

The law differs from state to state with regard to who qualifies to be considered an emancipated or mature minor. Emancipated minors can sign their own permission for a cesarean birth, even though they are legally underage.

Overall Hygiene

On admission, provide a clean hospital gown. If a woman's hair is long, encourage her to braid it or put it into a ponytail, so it will more easily fit under the surgical cap she will wear; hair contained by a cap is less likely to spread microorganisms during surgery. Follow your institution's procedures with regard to removing nail polish, jewelry, contact lenses, lip or mouth piercings, or hair ornaments before surgery. A growing number of women wear acrylic fingernails and are reluctant to remove them for surgery. If this is the case, ensure that the woman's toenails are free of polish so that toenails can be used to assess capillary refill if this assessment is needed.

> ## What If . . . 24.2
> **Moja, who will have epidural anesthesia for her cesarean birth, refuses to remove her contact lenses for surgery even though it is hospital policy for anyone receiving anesthesia to do so. She tells the nurse, "I won't be able to see my baby afterward without them." Would the nurse insist she take them out or ask the anesthesia team member if she could be an exception to a rule?**

Gastrointestinal Tract Preparation

A gastric emptying agent, such as metoclopramide (Reglan), to speed stomach emptying or a histamine blocker, such as ranitidine (Zantac), to decrease stomach secretions may be prescribed prior to surgery. Yet, another possibility is an oral antacid such as citric acid and sodium citrate (Bicitra), which acts to neutralize acid stomach secretions. These precautions are necessary because the woman will be lying on her back during the procedure, making esophageal reflux and aspiration highly possible.

Baseline Intake and Output Determinations

To reduce bladder size and keep the bladder away from the surgical field, an indwelling urinary catheter may be prescribed before transport for surgery or after arrival in the surgical suite. Use good lighting so that the woman's perineum is clearly revealed. After catheter insertion, be certain urine drains freely because fetal pressure on the urethra may considerably reduce the flow of urine. During transport, be certain to keep the drainage bag below the level of the woman's bladder to prevent urine backflow and the possible introduction of microorganisms into the bladder.

If catheterization is difficult before surgery, do not traumatize the urethra by repeated attempts as catheterization can be done in the operating room (OR) after the anesthetic agent is given. If there will be a delay between the time the catheter is inserted and the time of surgery, mark the level of drainage in the bag just before surgery or empty it, so that presurgery urine output can be differentiated from postsurgery urine output. This is because one of the gravest dangers of any surgical procedure is kidney failure from the physiologic stress of surgery or lack of blood flow to the kidneys due to decreased blood pressure. All reproductive tract surgery puts ureter flow at risk as well because the edema that collects in the surgery area can press on the ureters.

Hydration

Most women have an IV fluid line begun before surgery with a fluid such as lactated Ringer's solution. Doing so helps to ensure a woman will be fully hydrated and will not experience hypotension from epidural anesthesia administration, temporary use of a supine position, or blood loss at birth. Be certain this line is begun in the woman's nondominant hand if possible so she can hold her newborn after surgery without interference. Use a large-size catheter or needle (18 or 20 gauge), so that blood replacement therapy can be administered by the same line if needed.

QSEN Checkpoint Question 24.2

TEAMWORK & COLLABORATION

The nurse gives a report to an OR nurse prior to a cesarean birth and describes actions she took to reduce the size of the patient's bladder and to keep it away from the surgical field during the procedure. Which action should the nurse describe to her colleague?

a. Inserting a Foley catheter to drain the bladder and decrease its size
b. Administering an oxytocic drug to cause the bladder to forcefully contract
c. Restricting the woman's fluids for at least 16 hours before surgery
d. Administering the woman a diuretic to reduce bladder volume

Look in Appendix A for the best answer and rationale.

Preoperative Medication

A minimum of preoperative medication is used with a woman having a cesarean birth to prevent compromising the fetal blood supply and to ensure that the newborn is wide awake at birth and can initiate respirations spontaneously. Be aware if a woman has been in labor, what medications, if any, she has already received to help prevent a drug interaction.

Patient Chart and Presurgery Checklist

Documentation of nursing care up until the time a woman leaves the nursing care unit or labor room must be completed before a woman leaves for the surgical suite. Many hospitals use an electronic preoperative checklist, such as that shown in Figure 24.4, as a reminder of all necessary measures to be taken. Checking and signing such a form indicates that the specific measures were completed.

Transport to Surgery

A woman may be transferred to surgery in her bed, or she may be helped to move to a stretcher. Urge her to lie on her left side during transport to prevent supine hypotension syndrome. Ensure additional safety by raising the side rails. Cover her with a blanket or sheet to avoid her feeling chilled. Check that her identification is secure before she leaves the patient unit. Make certain, even though steps are being completed rapidly, that her chart or electronic record remains secure and will be available to OR personnel.

Patient concerns

	Completed
Skin preparation	_____
Identification in place	_____
Temperature, pulse, respiration _____	_____
Blood pressure _____	_____
Height _____	_____
Voided _____ Time _____ Weight _____	_____
NPO after _____ Amount _____	_____
Hospital gown	_____
Hairpins removed	_____
Nail polish removed	_____
Jewelry removed	_____
Preoperative medication _____	_____
Dentures removed _____ In place _____	_____
Contact lenses removed _____	_____
Prosthetic devices removed _____	_____
Abdominal piercing removed _____	_____

Chart concerns

Addressograph plate attached	_____
Operative permit obtained	_____
Urinalysis	_____
Hematocrit or CBC	_____
Blood order of _____	_____

Signature _____ R.N.

Figure 24.4 A preoperative checklist for cesarean birth. Checklists vary from hospital to hospital.

PATIENT-CENTERED CARE

Moja Hamma needs to have an IV infusion started prior to her cesarean procedure. Which course of action would be best?

    a. Introduce the cannula into the back of either hand.
    b. Begin the IV infusion in the hand nearest to you.
    c. Ask Moja which hand she would prefer you to use.
    d. Explain that IVs are typically started in the right hand.

Look in Appendix A for the best answer and rationale.

Role of the Support Person

In most instances, a woman's family can be as involved in a cesarean birth as they would be for a vaginal birth. A support person may need more encouragement to watch a cesarean than a vaginal birth, because he or she may believe the surgery will be much bloodier than it actually is. Helping family members realize cesarean birth is little different from vaginal birth not only allows them to stay with a woman during the procedure but also helps them progress to bonding with the infant and incorporating the new member into their family more easily.

Nursing Care for a Woman Having an Emergent Cesarean Birth

Many women who will have a cesarean birth have no warning during pregnancy that a cesarean birth will be necessary. Suddenly, during labor, they develop a complication such as prolapsed cord or fetal distress, and surgery becomes necessary.

A woman who has severe pain with labor and is told an emergent procedure is necessary actually may be relieved surgery has been suggested because the surgery will alleviate the pain. In contrast, another woman might feel great disappointment when told her baby must be born by cesarean birth. In many women, both emotions intertwine.

Surgical risk in an emergent situation is determined from the baseline history and physical examination information previously obtained at the beginning of labor. Preoperative preparation measures such as vital signs, urinalysis, and blood work have also already been obtained. An immediate preparation, therefore, involves gaining an informed consent, application of SCDs or elastic stockings (if appropriate), preparing the gastrointestinal tract, adding bladder catheterization, and establishing an IV line. Because, ideally, a cesarean birth should be completed within 30 minutes from the time the procedure was documented to be necessary, teaching about postoperative measures needs to be delayed until after surgery (Lipman, Carvalho, Cohen, et al., 2013).

Available time before the surgery must be spent explaining the immediate procedures to the woman such as transfer, abdominal preparation, and anesthesia. Document carefully what was taught, so that the nurse caring for the woman postoperatively will be aware of the need for additional teaching. At birth, at least one person whose sole responsibility is neonatal resuscitation needs to be present to care for the baby. Some babies born by cesarean birth need assistance to begin breathing at birth, even at full term; about 3% of babies need extensive resuscitation to survive (Konstantelos, Ifflaender, Dinger, et al., 2014).

INFORMATICS

The nurse notices that a colleague who was helping to prepare Moja has left the room to liaise with the OR in anticipation of the cesarean birth. The nurse also notices that the colleague left Moja's electronic health record open and in view of her support people. Which course of action would be best?

    a. Immediately close the record even though all care may not yet be recorded.
    b. Locate the nurse and ask her to come back so she can close the record.
    c. Minimize the record and wait for the nurse to come back and close it.
    d. Report the nurse to the nurse manager for violating confidentiality.

Look in Appendix A for the best answer and rationale.

Intraoperative Care Measures

Cesarean birth is most similar to vaginal birth if the woman is awake during the surgery; therefore, after discussion with a woman, the anesthesia of choice is usually a regional block, such as epidural anesthesia (Box 24.6).

> ### BOX 24.6
> ### Nursing Care Planning Tips for Effective Communication

Moja Hamma has been told she will need a cesarean birth because of fetal distress that has led to meconium staining.

Tip: Be certain to ask enough questions so you can learn the importance or meaning of the event to an individual woman. Most women appreciate that cesarean births are done to prevent their infant from being harmed. Others interpret a cesarean birth as being done because the harm has already occurred. Some women interpret a cesarean birth as an announcement they are somehow not as competent as other women. Still, others are relieved labor is being interrupted.

Nurse: Moja, can I answer any questions for you?

Moja: I want something to put me to sleep so I won't know what's happening.

Nurse: Most women want an epidural.

Moja: I have to be so sound asleep I won't know what's happening.

Nurse: You're not interested in seeing your baby born?

Moja: I'm not interested in seeing him born dead.

Nurse: Let me find your doctor to explain to you again that you need surgery to prevent something from going wrong, not because something is wrong.

ADMINISTRATION OF ANESTHESIA

A surgical nurse will assist a woman to move from the transport stretcher or bed to the OR table and will remain with her while anesthesia is administered. If the woman has an epidural catheter in place from labor, be careful not to dislodge it while she is being moved. During transport and while in surgery, encourage the woman to remain on her side, or place a pillow under her right hip to keep her body slightly tilted to the side, to prevent supine hypotension syndrome. If a spinal anesthetic (which may be used in an emergency) is to be administered, the anesthesiologist usually will do this with the woman sitting up. The anesthesiologist may then ask you to help the woman curve her back to separate the vertebrae and facilitate entry of the spinal needle. Remember, though, that it is difficult for a woman having uterine contractions to remain in this position for long. Talking to her while letting her lean against you is the most effective means of helping her maintain this position. Epidural anesthesia is usually administered with the woman lying on her side. Duramorph is a form of morphine commonly used in addition to a local anesthesia in epidurals. Its effect lasts up to 24 hours, but because it can cause late occurring respiratory depression, respirations should be assessed every 2 hours postsurgery (Butwick, Blumenfeld, Brookfield, et al., 2016).

SKIN PREPARATION

Reducing the number of bacteria on the skin before surgery automatically reduces the possibility of bacteria entering the incision at the time of surgery. Shaving away abdominal hair, if indicated, and washing the skin area over the incision site with soap and water accomplishes this.

The skin preparation area for a cesarean birth varies among agencies. Be certain to follow agency policy. To avoid being shaved, some women who are scheduled for a planned cesarean birth choose to have a bikini wax done 3 or 4 days before surgery.

SURGICAL INCISION

After the anesthetic administration, a woman is positioned with a towel under her right hip to move abdominal contents away from the surgical field and to lift her uterus off the vena cava. Be sure the support person is positioned at the woman's head to provide support. Next, a screen is placed at her shoulder level and covered with a sterile drape to block the flow of bacteria from her respiratory tract to the incision site. This also helps block the woman's and the support person's lines of vision, thus preventing additional anxiety caused by the sight of the incision.

The incision area on the woman's abdomen is then scrubbed with an antiseptic such as iodine, and appropriate drapes are placed around the area so that only a small area of skin is left exposed. Sponge and instrument counts are simplified by the use of prepackaged cesarean birth components. Watching a cesarean birth is usually the first time a father or support person has ever witnessed surgery. Because of this, the person may be too overwhelmed by and interested in the procedure to be of optimum support. Prepare the woman and support person for the sights they might see or help talk them through them as they occur.

Due in part to family and nursing staff pressure, cesarean sections have started to become more family friendly.

In the past, babies were often delivered, went to the warmer for nursing assessments, and were eventually wrapped up and given to the partner to hold near the mother while surgery was finishing. More recently, several interventions have happened to make the experience more "gentle." There are special sterile drapes that allow for a clear plastic window to be exposed, so the mother and partner can watch the baby being delivered. The opaque drape is lowered just before delivery and replaced after the newborn is delivered, so that the mother and her partner avoid watching both the initial incision and the repair. Additionally, mothers often hold their babies skin to skin after delivery, and they can attempt to breastfeed, even though the position is not ideal for latching. Cesarean sections are often not the ideal solution to delivery, but these changes can help women feel more satisfied with the experience when surgery is necessary.

Types of Cesarean Incision

There are two types of cesarean incisions. The type chosen depends on the presentation of the fetus and the speed with which the procedure will be performed (Fig. 24.5).

In a **classic cesarean incision**, the incision is made vertically through both the abdominal skin and the uterus. The incision is made high on the uterus, so that it avoids cutting a possible placenta previa. A disadvantage of this type of incision is that it leaves a wide skin scar and also runs through the active contractile portion of the uterus. Because this type of scar could rupture during labor, if this type of incision is used, a woman will be advised not to have a subsequent vaginal birth.

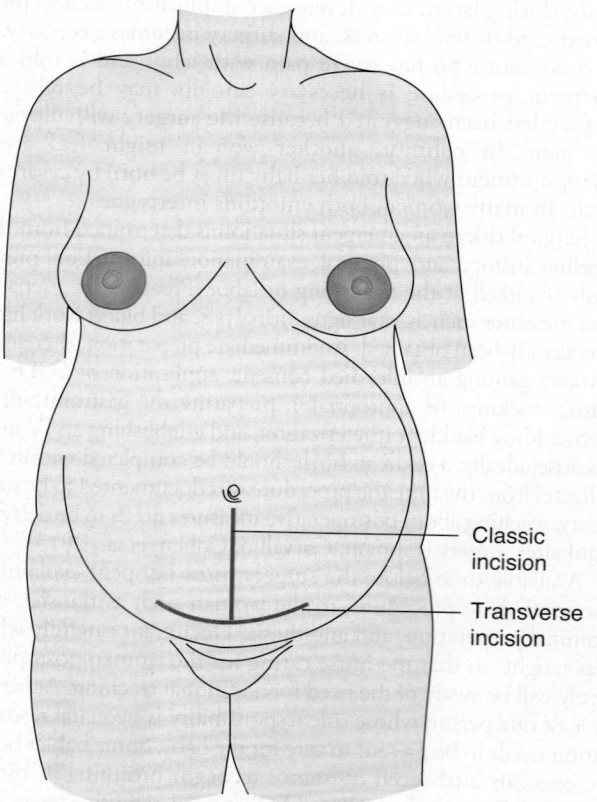

Figure 24.5 Types of cesarean incisions.

A **low segment incision** (commonly referred to as a low transverse uterine incision and a Pfannenstiel skin incision) is one made horizontally across the abdomen just over the symphysis pubis and also horizontally across the uterus just over the cervix. This is the most common type of cesarean incision used today. It is also referred to as a Misgav-Ladach or a "bikini" incision because even a low-cut bathing suit will cover the scar. Because this type of incision is through the nonactive portion of the uterus (the part that contracts minimally with labor), it is less likely to rupture in subsequent labors, making it possible for a woman to have a **vaginal birth after cesarean (VBAC)** in a subsequent pregnancy (Wu & Chou, 2015). VBAC rates have waxed and waned over the years along with its popularity among patients and providers, but with the recent focus on preventing cesarean births, many institutions are supportive of women who desire VBAC. The low segment incision is preferred because it:

- Results in less blood loss
- Is easier to suture
- Decreases postpartal uterine infections
- Is less likely to cause postpartum gastrointestinal complications (Kawakita, Reddy, Grantz, et al., 2017)

The major disadvantage of this incision is that it takes longer to perform, possibly making it impractical for an emergent cesarean birth. In a few instances, the skin incision is made horizontally (Pfannenstiel) and then the uterine incision is made vertically or vice versa. For this reason, during a future pregnancy, do not assume a woman who has a low transverse skin incision also has had a low transverse uterine incision.

QSEN Checkpoint Question 24.5

EVIDENCE-BASED PRACTICE

The majority of women who have a cesarean birth are physically eligible to future births vaginally. Researchers examined what influences a woman's choice in birth mode. They looked at 20 papers reporting views of 507 women who had a previous cesarean section. Women choosing a vaginal birth after cesarean were strongly influenced by a preconceived anticipation of vaginal birth. Women seeking repeat cesarean were often influenced by a prior traumatic birth experience. Women who were open to hearing suggestions had fewer preconceptions about the birth method and were able to hear a range of options (Black, Entwistle, Bhattacharya, et al., 2016).

Moja tells the nurse, although she knows she will be eligible, she isn't certain if she wants to have a vaginal birth for her next child. Based on the previous study findings, what would be the nurse's best assurance for her?

a. "It doesn't matter. Once a cesarean, always a cesarean is the rule."
b. "Birth is such a personal experience it's impossible to say."
c. "Let's talk about the risks and benefits of both types of deliveries to help you make your decision."
d. "My coworker had a vaginal birth after a cesarean birth and she was satisfied with her choice."

Look in Appendix A for the best answer and rationale.

BIRTH OF THE INFANT

Once the surgical incision is complete, the uterus is then cut and the child's head is born manually (Fig. 24.6). The mouth and nose of the baby may be suctioned by a bulb syringe, before the remainder of the child is born. Oxytocin (Pitocin) is administered via IV by the anesthesiologist as the child or placenta is delivered to increase uterine contraction and reduce blood loss. In many instances, a woman's partner may be allowed to cut the umbilical cord the same as in a vaginal birth. After full birth, the uterus is pulled forward onto the abdomen and covered with moist gauze or left in the abdomen for repair. The internal cavity of the uterus is then inspected, and the membranes and placenta manually removed. If the woman wishes to have a tubal ligation or an intrauterine device (IUD) inserted for contraception, either of these can be done at this time (Garcia, Richardson, Gonzalez, et al., 2015; Goldthwaite & Shaw, 2015).

The uterus, subcutaneous tissues, and skin incisions are then closed. Be sure to remind a woman and her support person that closing the incision can be a long process because many layers of tissue have to be closed so that they do not become concerned something is wrong. Either Dermabond, metal staples, or sutures can be used to close the exterior skin.

Observing the amount of abdominal manipulation that is involved with surgery helps predict how tender a woman's abdomen will be as well as why she has an overall "aching" feeling after surgery.

INTRODUCTION OF THE NEWBORN

Once it is determined the newborn is breathing spontaneously, he or she is shown to the mother and support person, just as is done after a vaginal birth (Schorn, Moore, Spetalnick, et al., 2015). Both the support person and the mother may hold the baby immediately. The mother may have some difficulty doing this. Assist her as necessary. Women are able to breastfeed after cesarean births the same as after vaginal births. However, initial breastfeeding may be delayed until the woman has been moved to a recovery room along with her infant because breastfeeding is difficult to do while still in the operating room due to position and monitors or IVs attached to the mother.

Postpartal Care Measures

Women who have a cesarean birth develop an additional care concern in the immediate postpartal period because they are not only postpartal patients but postsurgical ones. In addition to afterpains from their contracting uterus, they have postsurgical incision pain. A goal of nursing care should be to help women bond successfully with their new infant.

 Nursing Diagnoses and Related Interventions During the Immediate Postpartal Period

Immediately after surgery, a woman is transferred by stretcher from the OR table to the postanesthesia care unit (PACU) or a postpartal room. If spinal anesthesia was used, remember that her legs are fully anesthetized, and she will not be able to help move them.

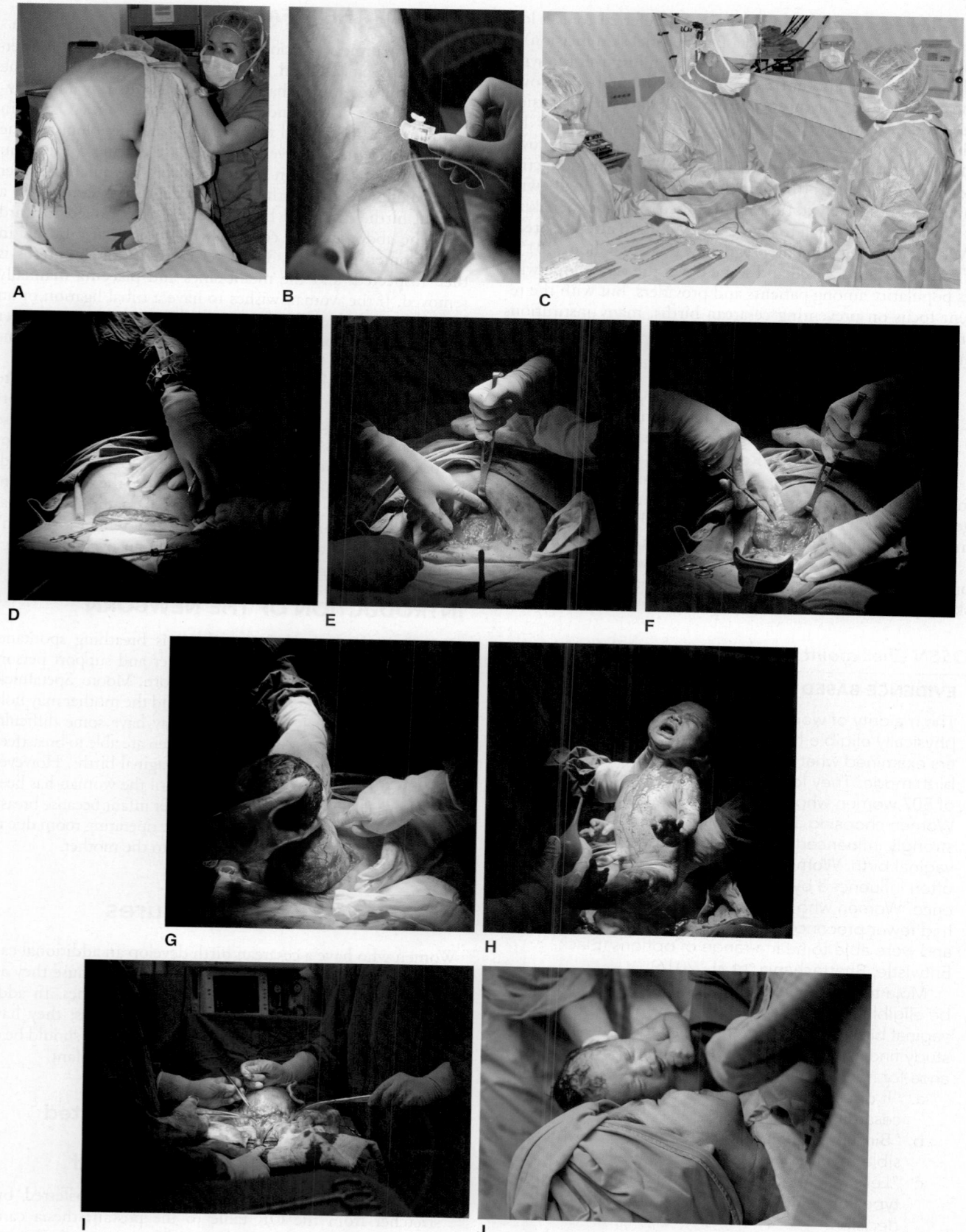

Figure 24.6 A cesarean birth. **(A)** Positioning for epidural placement. **(B)** Epidural placement. **(C)** Surgical team preparation and sterile draping. **(D–F)** Incision and retraction of skin. **(G)** Birth of the head and posterior shoulder. **(H)** The infant is born. **(I)** Skin closure. **(J)** Mother bonding with newborn. (**A and C.** From Hatfield, N. T. [2014]. *Introductory maternity & pediatric nursing* [3rd ed.]. Philadelphia, PA: Wolters Kluwer. **B.** martin81/shutterstock.com. **D–H.** Chattapat/shutterstock.com. **I.** ARZTSAMUI/shutterstock.com. **J.** VectorDoc/shutterstock.com.)

Nursing Diagnosis: Pain related to surgical incision

Outcome Evaluation: Patient verbalizes extent of pain (from 1 to 10) and need for relief; states level of pain is tolerable.

In the past, pain control was a major problem after cesarean birth because pain was so intense from either the uterine or abdominal incision that it interfered with a woman's ability to move and deeply breathe. This led to surgical complications such as pneumonia or thrombophlebitis. It also made holding an infant so painful that it threatened to impair a woman's ability to bond with her newborn. Today, a number of effective types of pain management are available, so this problem is lessened. Always use a pain rating scale to allow a woman to rate her pain. Using a specific tool helps to ensure accuracy of the assessment in light of a woman's overall excitement at having a new child.

Anxiety and fear heighten a pain response. Therefore, a woman who is concerned about her infant may rate pain higher than a woman who feels confident that her infant is doing well. In addition, a tense body posture also causes pressure on sutures. Women who had a long-action morphine epidural for labor have good pain relief up to 24 hours after birth. Others, who received a shorter acting drug for birth, need additional analgesia to be comfortable. Patient-controlled analgesia (PCA) or continued epidural injections are both effective systems for maximum pain relief. No matter what system of pain relief is used, when administering analgesics after surgery, be certain to supplement them with other comfort measures, such as urging a change of position or straightening bed linen. Always ask a woman what type of pain she is experiencing before administering a new dose of analgesia to be certain she is describing incisional or uterine pain, not pain in some other body part that would suggest a complication of surgery. Check for abdominal distention, which suggests the pain may be caused by intestinal gas rather than incision pain. If this is so, ambulation is often the most effective method to relieve this type of pain.

Urge a woman to continue to take adequate analgesia to effectively manage her pain after she returns home, so she is not so distressed that she cannot nurse her infant or ambulate. Be certain she understands not to use acetylsalicylic acid (aspirin) because this can interfere with blood clotting and uterine healing. Many women who are breastfeeding are reluctant to accept any type of analgesic, especially just before breastfeeding, for fear it will pass into breast milk and to the infant. Although it is true that most analgesics do pass into breast milk, the infant takes such a small amount of breast milk (mainly colostrum) during the first days after surgery, the amount of analgesia received is negligible. Placing a pillow over her lap while the infant nurses can deflect the weight of the infant from her suture line and lessen pain. Encourage the football hold for breastfeeding as another way to keep the infant's weight off her incision (see Chapter 19).

Patient-Controlled Analgesia. With PCA, women administer doses of IV narcotic analgesia, such as morphine, to themselves by means of an IV line as needed. To receive a dose of analgesia, the woman pushes a but-

Figure 24.7 Patient-controlled analgesia (PCA) pump. By pushing the button, a patient delivers a bolus of narcotic to herself. (LesPalenik/shutterstock.com)

ton similar to a call bell. This alerts the automatic pump to deliver a set amount of narcotic into the IV line. The pump has a "lock-out" setting that prevents a woman from administering a larger dose or doses more frequently than would be safe (e.g., every 8 minutes) (Fig. 24.7).

With PCA, a fairly constant level of pain relief can be maintained, and pain and fear of injections are eliminated. PCA works well with postcesarean women because they feel overall well and so are interested in self-care and self-administration of analgesia. Because the narcotic is injected in such small amounts, women tend to use less analgesia with a PCA system than they would receive with intramuscular injections.

Epidural Analgesia. Today, women who have epidural anesthesia for cesarean birth can have morphine (Duramorph) or fentanyl added to the epidural catheter immediately after surgery, a technique that keeps them pain free for the next 24 hours (see Chapter 16). Fentanyl creates few side effects. Although epidural morphine offers effective pain relief, side effects of administration, such as intense itching, nausea, and vomiting, can occur. An antihistamine such as diphenhydramine (Benadryl) may be needed to reduce pruritus; an antiemetic such as metoclopramide (Reglan) may be administered to counteract nausea. Even with these annoying side effects, however, epidural analgesia can be a very effective means of pain control after cesarean birth (Chen, Liu, Cherng, et al., 2014).

On the postpartal unit, an infusion pump is connected to the woman's epidural catheter, and the woman can infuse a bolus of narcotic as additional pain relief as needed. This patient-controlled epidural analgesia (PCEA) not only is an effective means of relieving pain but also omits the problem of infiltration of an IV infusion, which can occur with IV PCA.

Transcutaneous Electrical Nerve Stimulation. Transcutaneous electrical nerve stimulation (TENS) is, as the name implies, the transmission of an electrical current across the skin. Small electrodes are attached to the woman's skin near her incision; when she feels pain, she pushes a transformer button. Irritation or stimulation of large afferent nerve fibers by the electrical stimulation blocks the ability of the smaller, pain-carrying nerve fibers to transmit impulses (as predicted by gating control theory). This is the same phenomenon that rubbing or scratching skin at a point of pain achieves (see Chapter 16). The use of TENS can provide important pain relief after a cesarean birth because it gives a woman a sense of control over her situation, as does PCA or PCEA (Kayman-Kose, Arioz, Toktas, et al., 2014).

Nursing Diagnosis: Risk for deficient fluid volume related to blood loss during surgery

Outcome Evaluation: Patient's blood pressure is 100/60 mmHg; pulse remains between 60 and 100 beats/min; scant to no bleeding on surgical dressing is apparent.

The potential always exists for deficient fluid volume from surgery due to blood loss until all blood vessels that were cut and ligated during surgery have thrombosed, sclerosed, and permanently sealed closed. The risk of heavy bleeding doubles for the postpartum woman because she may not only hemorrhage vaginally from a noncontracted uterus but also internally from blood vessels not yet securely closed. This danger is most acute during the first hour after surgery; it remains an acute problem for the first 24 hours.

To detect the earliest signs of bleeding, monitor blood pressure, pulse, and respiratory rate approximately every 15 minutes for the first hour after surgery, every 30 minutes for the next 2 hours, every hour for the next 4 hours, or as specifically prescribed. Signs indicative of possible hemorrhage include:

- Falling blood pressure (more than 20 mmHg systolic), a systolic blood pressure less than 80 mmHg, or a drop of 5 to 10 mmHg over several readings
- A change in pulse rate (greater than 110 beats/min or less than 60 beats/min)
- Respirations more rapid and distressed from previous readings
- Restlessness and a sense of thirst

Inspect the dressing over the woman's surgical incision for blood staining each time vital signs are assessed to document there is no incisional bleeding. Observe the perineal pad for lochia flow and palpate the fundal height each time to document uterine contraction. Lochial discharge may be decreased in a woman after a cesarean birth because the uterus was cleaned following the birth, but some lochia will always be present. It will follow a typical rubra, serosa, and alba pattern. Be certain to help a woman turn as you assess for perineal bleeding, so you can look under her body. Blood oozing vaginally or from a surgical wound can pool considerably under a woman before it is otherwise visible.

Oxytocin (Pitocin) may be prescribed to be added to the first 1 or 2 L of IV fluid after surgery to ensure firm uterine contraction. If the rate of fluid administration should fall behind, be careful about "catch-up" administration. Because oxytocin (Pitocin) can elevate blood pressure by causing vasoconstriction, it may be safer to allow the fluid to remain behind for a time rather than risk elevating blood pressure by a more rapid infusion. Be aware that a woman is very prone to hemorrhage at the point the

oxytocin (Pitocin) is discontinued because this is the first time her uterus is asked to maintain contraction on its own. Remember, a minimal but continued change in vital signs (e.g., pulse steadily increasing, blood pressure steadily declining) is as ominous a sign of hemorrhage, as is a sudden alteration in these measurements. Notify a primary care provider of any changes in vital signs that might indicate hemorrhage so that prompt action can be taken.

A woman who has had either spinal or epidural anesthesia usually will not experience pain on uterine palpation until the anesthesia has worn off in approximately 4 to 24 hours. Therefore, uterine palpation should not increase her pain. Once the effect of the anesthesia or analgesia has decreased, palpate gently enough to not cause increased pain but thoroughly enough to determine uterine consistency.

At the same time you assess a woman's uterus for firmness, assess the remainder of her abdomen for softness. A hard, "guarded" abdomen is one of the first signs of peritonitis (i.e., peritoneal infection), a complication that may occur with any abdominal surgical procedure.

What If . . . 24.3
Moja Hamma refuses to allow the nurse to assess her fundal height after her cesarean birth because she has so much pain. How would the nurse approach this situation?

Nursing Diagnoses and Related Interventions During the Extended Postpartal Period

The average woman whose child is born by cesarean birth remains in the hospital from 48 hours to 4 days, depending on her preferences and the regulations of her insurance carrier. During this period and until she returns to have her sutures or staples removed, common concerns include pain, fatigue, interference with gastrointestinal function, and reduced activity level.

Nursing Diagnosis: Risk for deficient fluid volume related to postsurgical fluid restriction

Outcome Evaluation: Patient's urine specific gravity remains between 1.003 and 1.030; weight loss is not more than 5 to 10 lb; fluid intake equals 2 to 3 L/day.

Adequate fluid intake is important after surgery to replace blood loss from surgery and to maintain blood pressure and renal function. Because the intestine is handled during surgery, it takes approximately 24 to 48 hours before full peristaltic function is restored and oral intake is possible. It's important IV fluids be infused during this time at a rate that is not too rapid (which could lead to cardiac overload) or too slow (which could lead to inadequate circulatory compensation). Keep an accurate intake and output record for at least the first 24 hours to be certain an adequate fluid balance has been achieved.

Women are kept nothing by mouth (NPO) for a time after surgery until intestinal peristalsis has returned. To establish this is returning, assess a woman's abdomen at least once every 8 hours for bowel sounds, such as small "pinging" sounds heard on auscultation at a rate of 5 to 10 per minute, as these demonstrate air and fluid are moving through the intestines. Passage of flatus is another indication that intestinal function is again becoming active. As soon as these signs are present, IV fluid therapy is usually discontinued and the woman is allowed sips of fluid. After she begins oral intake, wait 1 hour before removing the IV line. Waiting ensures a woman is not experiencing nausea and vomiting, which might require restarting IV therapy. Introduce oral fluid slowly (e.g., ice chips for the first hour, then sips of clear fluid such as ginger ale, Jell-O, tea, or flavored frozen ice). Gradually advance her diet to a soft and then a regular diet as prescribed.

Teach women to continue to drink large quantities of fluid after they return home (at least six glasses daily), so they have adequate body fluid to make breastfeeding successful.

Nursing Diagnosis: Constipation related to effects of abdominal surgery and anesthesia

Outcome Evaluation: Woman voices she has a bowel movement every 2 to 3 days or her usual pattern.

Carefully note the time of a woman's first bowel movement following surgery. If she has had no bowel movement by the time of hospital discharge, her primary care provider may prescribe a stool softener, a suppository, or an enema to facilitate stool evacuation. You can reassure a woman who is not receiving much food yet that it is normal not to have bowel movements for 3 or 4 days postoperatively.

Keep women's water pitchers full to remind them to drink fluids. Urge them to eat a diet high in roughage and fluid and to attempt to move their bowels at least every other day to avoid constipation after they return home. Some women may need a stool softener prescribed to manage this because incisional pain interferes with their ability to use their abdominal muscles effectively. Caution them not to strain to pass stools because this puts pressure on their incision.

Nursing Diagnosis: Risk for impaired urinary elimination related to surgical procedure

Outcome Evaluation: Urinary output is more than 30 ml/hr; patient reports no pain, frequency, burning, or hesitancy on voiding.

Voiding after surgery provides evidence the woman has adequate renal and circulatory function because the kidneys must have adequate blood flow through them to function. Because the bladder was handled and displaced during surgery, its tone or ability to sense filling may be inadequate to initiate voiding for the first day postsurgery. For this reason, the indwelling catheter placed before surgery is usually left in place for 4 to 24 hours to ensure good urine drainage. Assess that the catheter is draining; a postpartal woman has a urine output of 3,000 to 5,000 ml per 24 hours, so bladder distention can occur rapidly if the catheter becomes blocked.

Before catheter removal, a urine culture may be requested to check for the possibility of a urinary tract infection. After removal of the catheter, the average woman will void in 4 to 8 more hours. Assess for bladder filling at the end of this time by palpation, pressing lightly over the symphysis pubis to assess fullness (Fig. 24.8A), and by percussion. On percussion, an empty bladder sounds

Figure 24.8 **(A)** Assessing bladder filling by palpation. **(B)** Assessing bladder filling by percussion. (© Caroline Brown, RNC, MS, DEd.)

dull; a full bladder, resonant; and an extended bladder, hyperresonant (Fig. 24.8B). If a bladder has filled to capacity but cannot empty properly or if the woman is voiding 30 to 60 ml of urine every 15 to 20 minutes, she may have retention with overflow. This voiding pattern is potentially dangerous because it means the woman's bladder is held continuously under tension. This can result in permanent bladder damage if the condition goes undetected. In addition, the constantly full bladder may prevent the uterus from contracting, possibly increasing the risk of postpartal hemorrhage. The woman will need to be catheterized or the urinary catheter to be replaced to avoid these concerns.

To help a woman void, suggest she take her prescribed analgesic to help relax abdominal musculature. In addition, assist the woman to walk to the bathroom at least every 2 hours and provide privacy. Other measures that might be effective include pouring warm water over her vulva (measure the amount of water used, so that it can be differentiated from urine) or running water from a tap within hearing distance.

Teach women to continue to drink adequate fluid (at least five to six glasses daily) to ensure an adequate fluid output and to help prevent urinary tract infection after they return home. Be certain they know to telephone their primary care provider if they should develop symptoms of a urinary tract infection, such as pain with or frequency of voiding or blood in urine.

Nursing Diagnosis: Risk for ineffective peripheral tissue perfusion related to immobility during and after surgery

Outcome Evaluation: Capillary refill is less than 5 seconds; there is absence of calf pain, redness, edema, or areas of warmth on lower extremities.

Because a woman's abdominal muscles are lax from the stretching that occurred during pregnancy, abdominal contents tend to shift forward and put pressure on the suture line when she is sitting or standing, causing pain and an uncomfortable feeling often described as "everything falling out." A woman usually feels more

comfortable turning and sitting up if she supports her abdomen with one hand or splints the incision with a pillow.

Leg exercises such as flexing and extending her knees and early ambulation are a woman's best safeguards against lower extremity circulatory problems. SCDs may be prescribed to help promote venous return and prevent venous stasis. Always allow a woman to sit on the edge of her bed for a few minutes before helping her to a standing position to prevent orthostatic hypotension (i.e., sudden low blood pressure that occurs with sudden position changes). Assessing that a woman's blood pressure is adequate before she gets out of bed for the first time is an additional safeguard. Before ambulation, also assess the lower extremities for pain in the calf on dorsiflexion of the foot (i.e., Homans sign, which may or may not be reliable) or for pain, edema, warmth, or redness in the calf, to detect the possibility of a thrombus. It is dangerous for a woman to ambulate if signs of a thrombus are present. A thrombus could shift, becoming an embolus, a potentially lethal situation.

Often, it is difficult for women to understand the importance of turning and ambulating as soon as possible after surgery (Fig. 24.9). Still experiencing the "taking in" postpartal phase, they may prefer to spend their first days after surgery just resting quietly in bed. Encourage women to use adequate analgesia during this time, so they can move and ambulate with the least amount of pain. Reinforce the need for continued activity balanced with rest after discharge. Be certain a woman understands the signs and symptoms of complications, such as thrombophlebitis.

Nursing Diagnosis: Risk for impaired parenting related to the emergent nature of birth or discomfort from surgery

Outcome Evaluation: Parents hold and feed child and voice positive comments about the infant.

When a cesarean birth is unscheduled, a woman does not have much preoperative time to think about how she will feel after surgery. Most women are surprised to realize not

A   **B**

Figure 24.9 **(A)** Teaching a women how to support her incision during movement will decrease pain after a cesarean birth. **(B)** Using an incentive spirometer will promote normal respiratory function. (From Carter, P. J. [2016]. *Lippincott textbook for nursing assistants* [4th ed.]. Philadelphia, PA: Wolters Kluwer.)

Figure 24.10 A mother holds her newborn in the recovery area after a cesarean section.

only how well they feel overall but also how quickly they become fatigued and how painful a simple surgical incision can be. Encourage women to breastfeed, although this causes temporary uterine pain as the uterus contracts with breastfeeding.

If the woman's baby was born with a complication or has been placed in an intensive care nursery or transferred to a distant hospital for tertiary care, a woman's postpartal course can be difficult, because she experiences a sense of loss in addition to the pain and fatigue of surgery. Depression, which can slow all body functions and certainly her ability to "take hold" in the postpartal period, can occur.

Unless her baby was transferred to another site, be certain to provide her with ample time to hold and feed her child; assist her to visit in the hospital's high-risk nursery if needed. The average woman can breastfeed satisfactorily after a cesarean birth. She may have some reason to think her baby is not quite perfect—after all, the baby was not born "perfectly"—so she may need additional time to inspect her baby and feel comfortable with him or her (Fig. 24.10).

Nursing Diagnosis: Fatigue related to effects of surgery

Outcome Evaluation: Patient states she is pleased with level of self-care; ambulates well by 24 hours, and sleeps restfully at night.

Although a woman needs activity and movement after surgery, she also needs adequate rest. Many women attempt to handle their own and their newborn's needs immediately after surgery because their excitement over their baby and their new role as a mother makes them unaware of their underlying fatigue. However, extreme fatigue interferes with healing and possibly increases the risk of infection. A woman can notice increased uterine bleeding leading to excessive loss of fluid and iron stores and, eventually, interfere with bonding. Help a woman plan a day, therefore, that includes care of her new child as well as periods of rest for herself. Be certain she has adequate analgesic medication at bedtime to allow her to be pain free for the night. Provide a space of time in the middle of the morning and again in the afternoon for uninterrupted rest while she's still in the hospital. Explore her plans for care at home to be certain her plans for rest seem realistic for a postsurgical/postpartal woman (Box 24.7). Once she returns home, rest is often best accomplished if it is scheduled for every time her newborn sleeps.

Nursing Diagnosis: Impaired skin integrity related to surgical incision

Outcome Evaluation: Incision line is clean, dry, and intact without erythema; oral temperature is less than 38°C (100.4°F).

Surgical incisions heal by primary intention. Assess the surgical incision once during each nursing shift while a woman is hospitalized to ensure the wound edges are approximated and there are no signs of infection, such as erythema or presence of a discharge. As soon as she can walk steadily, a woman can take a shower (after first removing the dressing) because warm, clean water on the incision feels soothing.

Teach women to continue to observe their incision at least daily at home. Instruct them in signs and symptoms of possible infection and to report any of these signs to

BOX 24.7

Nursing Care Planning Based on Family Teaching

MEASURES TO REGAIN ENERGY AFTER A CESAREAN BIRTH

Q. Moja tells you, "I am exhausted after my cesarean. What can I do to feel stronger again?"

A. Some suggestions to help regain your energy rapidly include:

- Drink adequate fluid daily (at least six glasses). This helps prevent a urinary tract infection and also helps supply all the cells in your body with adequate fluid.
- Rest twice a day for at least one-half hour each time. This helps you get adequate sleep if your baby wakes you at night.
- Do not hesitate to accept help from family and friends for tasks such as house cleaning or grocery shopping.
- Limit the number of stairs you climb daily to one flight once a day. Also limit the amount of weight you lift to the weight of your new baby.
- Do not attempt to be a social hostess as well as a new mom. Put your energy toward relaxing and enjoying your new baby.

their primary care provider. Following a cesarean birth, healing will be adequate enough by day 3 that skin sutures or clamps can be removed, although these may be left in place until the woman returns for a follow-up appointment in 2 weeks.

QSEN Checkpoint Question 24.6

QUALITY IMPROVEMENT

Moja tells the nurse she does not intend to continue breastfeeding after she returns home, stating, "My stomach's too painful." What action would the nurse add to the plan of care that is most apt to be helpful to Moja?

a. Insist Moja speak with one of the hospital's lactation consultants.

b. Instruct her to take over-the-counter analgesics just before breastfeeding.

c. Design a study to identify factors that affect breastfeeding success.

d. Explain that her uterine pain will not last more than a few more days.

Look in Appendix A for the best answer and rationale.

DISCHARGE PLANNING

A woman being discharged after cesarean birth takes home not only her new baby but also a fair amount of pain and discomfort. Be certain to discuss home care arrangements, emphasizing the need for adequate help with her newborn and other responsibilities at home. Be sure a woman is aware of any restrictions on exercise or activity she needs to follow (common restrictions are not to lift any object heavier than 10 lb or walk upstairs more than once a day for the first 2 weeks). Also teach her to recognize signs of possible complications directly related to the surgery that should be reported to her primary care provider because they may require readmission, including:

- Redness or drainage at the incision line
- Lochia heavier than a normal menstrual period
- Abdominal pain (other than suture line or afterpain discomfort)
- Temperature greater than 38°C (100.4°F)
- Frequency or burning on urination

A woman can plan on resuming coitus as soon as the act is comfortable for her. Cesarean birth does not interfere with future fertility, so be sure she has contraceptive information, if desired (Sok, Sanders, Saltzman, et al., 2016). Also ensure she has an appointment for a return visit with her healthcare provider for both herself (usually in 2 to 4 weeks) and her newborn (usually 1 to 2 days).

Unless the reason for the cesarean birth was cephalopelvic disproportion, a woman can probably have her next child vaginally (see Chapter 15). Being certain the woman is aware of this not only makes her an informed consumer of health care but also can influence whether she plans an additional pregnancy. Box 24.8 shows an interprofessional care map illustrating both nursing and team planning following an emergent cesarean birth.

 What If . . . 24.4

The nurse is interested in exploring one of the 2020 National Health Goals related to cesarean birth (see Box 24.1). Most government-sponsored money for nursing research is allotted based on these goals. What would be a possible research topic to explore, pertinent to these goals, that would be applicable to Moja and her family and that would also advance evidence-based practice?

KEY POINTS FOR REVIEW

- The term *cesarean birth* is preferred to *cesarean section* or *delivery* because it puts the focus on the childbirth rather than surgical elements of the procedure.

- Cesarean birth may be either a scheduled or an emergent procedure. Because it carries more risk for the woman and infant than does vaginal birth, it is usually undertaken only when medically necessary, although a current trend allows for elective procedures.

- The skin incision may be vertical (i.e., a classic incision), although it is usually a horizontal one just above the pubic hair. The internal incision into the uterus is also usually a horizontal incision into the lower uterine segment.

- Establishing surgical risk, including an assessment of nutritional status, age, general health, fluid and electrolyte balance, and psychological condition, not only meets QSEN competencies for safety but also best meets a woman's total needs.

- Assessment measures before surgery usually include vital sign determination; urinalysis; blood studies such as complete blood count, electrolytes, blood typing, and crossmatching; and ultrasound.

- Support people can lose a great deal of their ability to support if they feel intimidated, overwhelmed, and out of place in an OR; offer them support as needed to make this a positive experience for them as well.

- Cesarean birth is one of the safest types of surgery performed. To keep a woman safe after the procedure, remember that she is both a postsurgical and a postpartum patient. Make assessments to ensure that neither postpartum nor postsurgical complications occur.

- Adequate pain management is important to allow a woman a sense of control and comfort and bonding with her newborn.

- Women are physically exhausted after cesarean birth and may be psychologically exhausted because of the emergent nature of the experience. Provide rest time to relieve the physical strain and a chance to verbalize the experience to help relieve the psychological strain.

- A major intervention after cesarean birth is early ambulation to prevent complications. Incisional pain may make this difficult, so strong nursing support and adequate pain management are necessary.

- The old saying, "Once a cesarean, always a cesarean," is no longer true as long as cephalopelvic disproportion does not exist and the previous incision was a low transverse one.

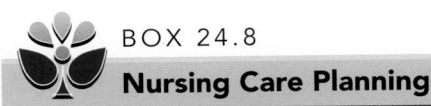 BOX 24.8

Nursing Care Planning

Moja Hamma is a 29-year-old primigravida who underwent an emergent cesarean birth with epidural anesthesia for fetal distress. She gave birth to a healthy 8-lb 2-oz baby girl who breathed immediately. She tells you, "My mouth is dry and my stomach hurts so much I can't move. Don't ask me to hold or feed my baby until the pain goes away."

Family Assessment: Patient lives with boyfriend in a westside apartment. Works as a sales clerk in a bridal salon. Boyfriend is currently unemployed. Borrowed money from a friend for hospital bill because Moja has no health insurance.

Patient Assessment: Postcesarean birth 4 hours ago. Estimated blood loss of 700 ml. Abdomen soft but tender with low transverse incision. No bowel sounds present. Incisional dressing clean, dry, and intact. Fundus of uterus firm, one fingerbreadth below umbilicus. Minimal lochia rubra vaginal drainage present. Urine output 100 ml in last hour. Skin pink, warm, and dry with good skin turgor. Ringer's lactate infusing at 100 ml/hr. Intravenous site clean, dry, without signs of infiltration. Vital signs slightly elevated above baseline: temperature, 98.4°F; pulse rate, 78 beats/min; respirations, 23 breaths/min and shallow; blood pressure, 130/76 mmHg. States she has abdominal pain, especially at incisional area. Holding hands over abdomen; barely moving in bed. Patient's mother at bedside holding her hand and stroking her forehead. Patient-controlled epidural analgesia (PCEA) pump in place but not being used by patient. When asked why she wasn't using the PCEA pump, she answered, "I don't want to take the chance of being paralyzed forever."

Nursing Diagnosis: Pain related to tissue trauma from abdominal incision of cesarean birth

Outcome Criteria: Patient identifies pain management measure of choice; reports a decrease in pain with analgesic administration; pulse, respirations, and blood pressure return to baseline.

Patient holds infant warmly, maintains eye contact with infant, and makes positive statements about the newborn prior to discharge.

Team Member Responsible	Assessment	Intervention	Rationale	Expected Outcome
Activities of Daily Living, Including Safety				
Nurse	Assess extent of patient's ability to move in bed and breastfeed infant.	Explain the importance of getting out of bed and caring for infant.	Early ambulation helps prevent thrombophlebitis; early breastfeeding helps establish an adequate milk supply.	Patient walks to chair in room and feeds infant by 4 hours' time; states chosen pain relief method is effective.
Teamwork and Collaboration				
Nurse/pain management team	Investigate whether pain management team is available for consultation.	Ask pain management team to consult with patient on a more suitable pain relief measure.	Other pain relief measures are available that would be more suitable for patient.	Pain management team discusses options for pain relief with patient; patient chooses a suitable procedure by 2 hours' time.
Procedures/Medications for Quality Improvement				
Nurse/pain management team	Assess what measures patient feels would make her most comfortable.	Institute additional comfort measures, such as changing position, splinting incision, using pillows for support.	Comfort measures help reduce stress and anxiety, elevate mood, and raise the pain threshold, thus enhancing the therapeutic effectiveness of analgesics.	Patient reports additional comfort measures aid pain relief effectively.
Nurse/lactation consultant	Assess what measures patient thinks would help her be more successful with breastfeeding.	Assist patient with handling newborn. Support breastfeeding efforts.	Breastfeeding is a new skill for a first-time mother.	Patient breastfeeds her infant successfully with support from healthcare providers.

Continued on following page

BOX 24.8

Nursing Care Planning (continued)

Team Member Responsible	Assessment	Intervention	Rationale	Expected Outcome
Nutrition				
Nurse	Assess bowel sounds to determine when oral fluid can be safely offered.	Offer ice cubes for dry mouth as soon as bowel sounds are present.	Patient should not drink full liquids or eat solid foods until bowel sounds return.	Patient states mouth discomfort is reduced by 1 hour after first fluid consumed.
Patient-Centered Care				
Nurse/pain management team	Assess patient's expectations of pain relief measures and safety of PCEA administration.	Review PCEA pump and technique with patient.	Patient cannot have realistic expectations or feel safe with system unless she understands the technique.	Patient states she will use PCEA pump on trial basis for 4 hours. Reevaluate pain relief at that time.
Psychosocial/Spiritual/Emotional Needs				
Nurse	Assess what additional measures patient needs to feel secure after frightening experience of emergent cesarean birth.	Provide reinforcement for positive coping mechanisms that patient demonstrates.	Positive reinforcement enhances self-esteem and control. Praise promotes self-esteem and confidence to manage new situations.	Patient states she feels healthcare providers are providing her support equal to her level of pain and fatigue.
Nurse	Assess patient's expectations of a newborn.	Praise patient for positive behaviors and interactions with the child in light of pain and fatigue level. Encourage patient to keep newborn in the room with her for extended periods as she is able.	Extended contact within the patient's ability to tolerate the activity encourages bonding while minimizing the risk of additional fatigue.	Patient keeps newborn with her in room for the majority of daylight hours. Feeds and interacts actively with child
Informatics for Seamless Healthcare Planning				
Nurse	Assess the level of support patient will have after she returns home.	Review with patient importance of maintaining a level of pain relief at home so she can ambulate and care for new child.	Ambulation and child care are important for both maternal and child health. Keeping pain to a minimum helps the patient achieve these activities.	Patient states she will take enough pain relief at home to allow her to be active and care for newborn. Names at least one person who will serve as her support person
Nurse	Assess whether patient understands signs and symptoms, such as pain on urination, she will need to report after discharge.	Teach signs of all complications she should report to her primary healthcare provider.	Knowing signs and symptoms of complications allows patient to be an informed healthcare consumer.	Patient repeats danger signs she will report to her primary healthcare provider.

CRITICAL THINKING CARE STUDY

Amy Whithaven is a 38-year-old gravida 4, para 3, who wants to have her fourth child as naturally as possible, the same as she did for her other three children. Her husband, Paul, the chief executive of a public relations firm, is with her in a birthing room as her support person. He assures you Amy is a "veteran" at labor, will use controlled breathing as pain management, and will have no problems. He adds they are especially looking forward to this baby because she will be their first girl. Four hours into labor, Amy experiences sharp abdominal pain and begins to have fresh vaginal bleeding. Amy's blood pressure falls to 100/55 mmHg; the FHR decreases to 80 beats/min. Amy's obstetrician diagnoses placental abruption and asks you to prepare her for an emergent cesarean birth.

1. Because having a cesarean birth is so opposite from what the couple planned for labor, Paul says he wants to investigate Amy's symptoms on the Internet using his laptop or else secure a second opinion from another doctor before surgery can proceed. Would you support him in asking for this?

2. Amy realizes immediately that something is wrong. She asks you if this has something to do with the fact she is having her first girl. Are more girl infants born by cesarean than male infants?

3. Amy is transported to surgery and, within 20 minutes, a 7-lb 3-oz girl is born. Named Honor, she needs resuscitation to breathe and is transferred immediately afterward to the neonatal intensive care nursery for care. Paul declines to visit Honor in the nursery. He says he'll wait until Amy can be "disappointed" along with him. What actions could you take to help this couple begin bonding with their new daughter?

RELATED RESOURCES

Explore these additional resources to enhance learning for this chapter:
- Student resources on thePoint, including answers to the What If . . . and Critical Thinking Care Study questions, http://thepoint.lww.com/Flagg8e
- Adaptive learning powered by PrepU, http://thepoint.lww.com/prepu

REFERENCES

Abdulcadir, J., Dugerdil, A., Yaron, M., et al. (2016). Obstetric care of women with female genital mutilation attending a specialized clinic in a tertiary center. *International Journal of Gynaecology and Obstetrics, 132*(2), 174–178.

Ayers, S., Bond, R., Bertullies, S., et al. (2016). The aetiology of post-traumatic stress following childbirth: A meta-analysis and theoretical framework. *Psychological Medicine, 46*(6), 1121–1134.

Ayres-de-Campos, D. (2015). Obesity and the challenges of caesarean delivery: Prevention and management of wound complications. *Best Practice & Research. Clinical Obstetrics & Gynaecology, 29*(3), 406–414.

Betrán, A. P., Ye, J., Moller, A. B., et al. (2016). The increasing trend in caesarean section rates: Global, regional and national estimates: 1990-2014. *PLoS One, 11*(2), e0148343.

Black, M., Entwistle, V. A., Bhattacharya, S., et al. (2016). Vaginal birth after caesarean section: Why is uptake so low? Insights from a meta-ethnographic synthesis of women's accounts of their birth choices. *BMJ Open, 6*(1), e008881.

Butwick, A. J., Blumenfeld, Y. J., Brookfield, K. F., et al. (2016). Racial and ethnic disparities in mode of anesthesia for cesarean delivery. *Anesthesia and Analgesia, 122*(2), 472–479.

Carlson, N. S., Hernandez, T. L., Hurt, K. J. (2015). Parturition dysfunction in obesity: Time to target the pathobiology. *Reproductive Biology and Endocrinology, 13*(1), 135.

Chandraharan, E. (2016). Should national guidelines continue to recommend fetal scalp blood sampling during labour? *The Journal of Maternal-Fetal & Neonatal Medicine, 29*(22), 3682–3685.

Chen, S. Y., Liu, F. L., Cherng, Y. G., et al. (2014). Patient-controlled epidural levobupivacaine with or without fentanyl for post-cesarean section pain relief. *BioMed Research International, 2014,* 965152.

Cordon, B. H., Fracchia, J. A., & Armenakas, N. A. (2014). Iatrogenic non-endoscopic bladder injuries over 24 years: 127 cases at a single institution. *Urology, 84*(1), 222–226.

Cox, K. J., & King, T. L. (2015). Preventing primary cesarean births: Midwifery care. *Clinical Obstetrics and Gynecology, 58*(2), 282–293.

Cunningham, F. G., Leveno, K., Bloom, S. L., et al. (2014). Breech delivery. In F. G. Cunningham, K. Leveno, S. L. Bloom, et al. (Eds.), *Williams obstetrics* (24th ed., pp. 558–573). New York, NY: McGraw-Hill.

Delnord, M., Blondel, B., Drewniak, N., et al. (2014). Varying gestational age patterns in cesarean delivery: An international comparison. *BMC Pregnancy and Childbirth, 14,* 321.

Drukker, L., Hants, Y., Farkash, R., et al. (2015). Iron deficiency anemia at admission for labor and delivery is associated with an increased risk for cesarean section and adverse maternal and neonatal outcomes. *Transfusion, 55*(12), 2799–2806.

Garcia, G., Richardson, D. M., Gonzales, K. L., et al. (2015). Trends and disparities in postpartum sterilization after cesarean section, 2000 through 2008. *Women's Health Issues, 25*(6), 634–640.

Goldthwaite, L. M., & Shaw, K. A. (2015). Immediate postpartum provision of long-acting reversible contraception. *Current Opinion in Obstetrics & Gynecology, 27*(6), 460–464.

Graham, N. M., Gimovsky, A. C., Roman, A., et al. (2016). Blood loss at cesarean delivery in women on magnesium sulfate for preeclampsia. *The Journal of Maternal-Fetal & Neonatal Medicine, 29*(11), 1817–1821.

Gyte, G. M., Dou, L., & Vazquez, J. C. (2014). Different classes of antibiotics given to women routinely for preventing infection at caesarean section. *Cochrane Database of Systematic Reviews,* (11), CD008726.

Inocêncio, G., Braga, A., Lima, T., et al. (2015). Which factors influence the type of delivery and cesarean section rate in women with gestational diabetes? *The Journal of Reproductive Medicine, 60*(11–12), 529–534.

Iriye, B. K. (2015). Impact of obstetrician/gynecologist hospitalists on quality of obstetric care (cesarean delivery rates, trial of labor after cesarean/vaginal birth after cesarean rates, and neonatal adverse events). *Obstetrics and Gynecology Clinics of North America, 42*(3), 477–485.

Jackson, S., & Gregory, K. D. (2015). Management of the first stage of labor: Potential strategies to lower the cesarean delivery rate. *Clinical Obstetrics and Gynecology, 58*(2), 217–226.

Kawakita, T., Reddy, U. M., Grantz, K. L., et al. (2017). Maternal outcomes associated with early preterm cesarean delivery. *American Journal of Obstetrics and Gynecology, 216*(3), 312.e1–312.e9.

Kayman-Kose, S., Arioz, D. T., Toktas, H., et al. (2014). Transcutaneous electrical nerve stimulation (TENS) for pain control after vaginal delivery and cesarean section. *The Journal of Maternal-Fetal & Neonatal Medicine, 27*(15), 1572–1575.

Konstantelos, D., Ifflaender, S., Dinger, J., et al. (2014). Analyzing support of postnatal transition in term infants after c-section. *BMC Pregnancy and Childbirth, 14,* 225.

Lipman, S. S., Carvalho, B., Cohen, S. E., et al. (2013). Response times for emergency cesarean delivery: Use of simulation drills to assess and improve obstetric team performance. *Journal of Perinatology, 33*(4), 259–263.

Liu, Y., Li, G., Chen, Y., et al. (2014). A descriptive analysis of the indications for caesarean section in mainland China. *BMC Pregnancy and Childbirth, 14,* 410.

Maher, M. D., & Heavey, E. (2015). When the cord comes first: Umbilical cord prolapse. *Nursing, 45*(7), 53–56.

Martin, J. A., Hamilton, B. E., Osterman, M. J., et al. (2015). Births: Final data for 2013. *National Vital Statistics Reports, 64*(1), 1–68.

Quinlan, J. D., & Murphy, N. J. (2015). Cesarean delivery: Counseling issues and complication management. *American Family Physician, 91*(3), 178–184.

Rosenstein, M. G., Nijagal, M., Nakagawa, S., et al. (2015). The association of expanded access to a collaborative midwifery and laborist model with cesarean delivery rates. *Obstetrics and Gynecology, 126*(4), 716–723.

Sahin, E., & Terzioglu, F. (2015). The effect of gum chewing, early oral hydration, and early mobilization on intestinal motility after cesarean birth. *Worldviews on Evidence-Based Nursing, 12*(6), 380–388.

Schorn, M. N., Moore, E., Spetalnick, B. M., et al. (2015). Implementing family-centered cesarean birth. *Journal of Midwifery & Women's Health, 60*(6), 682–690.

Silva, G. S., de Jesus, M. P., Merighi, M. B., et al. (2014). The experience of women regarding cesarean section from the perspective of social phenomenology. *Online Brazilian Journal of Nursing, 13*(1), 5–14.

Sok, C., Sanders, J. N., Saltzman, H. M., et al. (2016). Sexual behavior, satisfaction, and contraceptive use among postpartum women. *Journal of Midwifery & Women's Health, 61*(2), 158–165.

Speichinger, E., & Holschneider, C. H. (2013). Surgical disorders in pregnancy. In A. H. DeCherney, L. Nathan, T. M. Goodwin, et al. (Eds.), *Current diagnosis and treatment: Obstetrics and gynecology* (11th ed., pp. 433–453). Columbus, OH: McGraw-Hill/Lange.

Tähtinen, R. M., Cartwright, R., Tsui, J. F., et al. (2016). Long-term impact of mode of delivery on stress urinary incontinence and urgency urinary incontinence: A systematic review and meta-analysis. *European Urology, 70*(1), 148–158.

Tan, K. H., Smyth, R. M., & Wei, X. (2013). Fetal vibroacoustic stimulation for facilitation of tests of fetal wellbeing. *Cochrane Database of Systematic Reviews,* (12), CD002963.

U.S. Department of Health and Human Services. (2010). *Healthy people 2020.* Washington, DC: Author.

Verghese, T. S., Champaneria, R., Kapoor, D. S., et al. (2016). Obstetric anal sphincter injuries after episiotomy: Systematic review and meta-analysis. *International Urogynecology Journal, 27*(10), 1459–1467.

Wang, J., Liu, X., Zhu, T., et al. (2015). Analysis of neonatal respiratory distress syndrome among different gestational segments. *International Journal of Clinical and Experimental Medicine, 8*(9), 16273–16279.

Wu, J. L., & Chou, B. (2015). Normal labor & delivery, operative delivery & malpresentations. In J. L. Bienstock, H. Fox, E. E. Wallach, et al. (Eds.), *The Johns Hopkins manual of gynecology and obstetrics* (5th ed., pp. 78–94). Philadelphia, PA: Lippincott Williams & Wilkins.

Nursing Care of a Family Experiencing a Postpartum Complication

Bailey Cheshire is a 26-year-old woman who teaches chemistry at a local university. You enter her room 2 hours after she gave birth to an 8-lb girl and find her just finishing breastfeeding. Her face appears abnormally pale. You obtain her vital signs and document her pulse as 90 beats/min and her blood pressure as 90/50 mmHg. When you fold back her bedclothes, you discover her perineal pad is saturated. The capillary refill in her fingers is sluggish. You suspect she is experiencing one of the most serious complications of pregnancy: postpartum hemorrhage.

Previous chapters discussed the nursing care for a woman during the typical postpartum period. This chapter contributes information about how to care for a woman and her family when there is a deviation from normal. Comprehensive and recurring nursing care is essential when a postpartum complication develops because it can provide an early alert to conditions that can impact the health of not only the woman but also her child and family.

What immediate measures does Ms. Cheshire need? What would be your first action?

KEY TERMS

endometritis

mastitis

peritonitis

postpartum depression

postpartal psychosis

puerperal infection

subinvolution

thrombophlebitis

uterine atony

uterine inversion

OBJECTIVES

After mastering the contents of this chapter, you should be able to:

1. Describe a woman at risk for common deviations from the normal that can occur during the puerperium.

2. Identify 2020 National Health Goals related to deviations from the normal in the postpartal period that nurses can help the nation achieve.

3. Assess a woman and her family for deviations from the normal during the puerperium.

4. Formulate nursing diagnoses related to postpartum complications.

5. Establish expected outcomes for a woman and her family experiencing a postpartum complication.

6. Using the nursing process, plan nursing care that includes the six competencies of Quality & Safety Education for Nurses (QSEN): Patient-Centered Care, Teamwork & Collaboration, Evidence-Based Practice (EBP), Quality Improvement (QI), Safety, and Informatics.

7. Implement evidence-based nursing care when a woman and her family experience a postpartum complication.

8. Evaluate expected outcomes for achievement and effectiveness of care.

9. Integrate knowledge of postpartum complications with the interplay of nursing process, the six competencies of QSEN, and Family Nursing to promote quality maternal and child health nursing care.

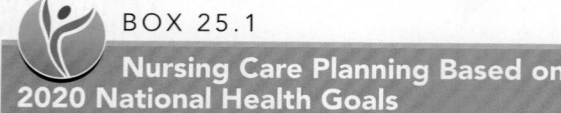

BOX 25.1

Nursing Care Planning Based on 2020 National Health Goals

The postpartal period is a time when women are very susceptible to hemorrhage and thrombophlebitis and, when these complications develop, women may choose not to breastfeed because of them. The 2020 National Health Goals that speak to this include:

- Reduce the maternal mortality rate to no more than 11.4 per 100,000 live births from a baseline of 12.7 per 100,000.
- Increase the proportion of infants who are breastfed to at least 81.9% from a baseline of 74%.
- Increase the proportion of infants who are breastfed at 6 months from a baseline of 43.5% to 60.6% (U.S. Department of Health and Human Services, 2010; see www.healthypeople.gov).

Nurses can help the nation achieve these goals by carefully monitoring uterine involution in the postpartal period and by encouraging women to breastfeed even in the face of a postpartal complication.

Although the puerperium is usually a period of health, complications can occur. It's important to be knowledgeable about predisposing factors and clinical manifestations of postpartum complications to ensure the prompt initiation of corrective measures in order to prevent long-term consequences to a woman and her family (Guntupalli, Karnad, Bandi, et al., 2015).

Postpartum complications are always potentially serious because they can impact so many people. A complication may be so serious it could cause a personal injury, leave a woman with her future fertility impaired, or even result in death. Any complication that affects the health of the mother can also affect her interactions with her newborn, such as causing her to discontinue breastfeeding (Odom, Li, Scanlon, et al., 2013). Her family can be disrupted because of an extended hospital stay or from an impairment that prevents her from performing her normal family responsibilities. Financial difficulties may arise because of her inability to maintain employment and the need for additional child and health care. Fortunately, most postpartum complications are preventable, and if they do occur, the majority can be treated effectively without long-term complications. Because the health of women and newborns is so important to a nation's health, Box 25.1 describes 2020 National Health Goals that speak to possible puerperium complications (Andrighetti, 2013).

Nursing Process Overview

FOR A WOMAN EXPERIENCING A POSTPARTUM COMPLICATION

ASSESSMENT

Women who assume they will immediately return to an active lifestyle after birth of their child may view an extended hospitalization for a postpartum complication as more unsettling than women who view the postpartum period as one in which they are expected to rest. Assess each woman holistically, therefore, to determine how the health problem a woman is experiencing is impacting her and her family.

Assessment findings associated with a postpartum complication may be subtle, such as tenderness in the calf of a leg, an increase in uterine or perineal pain, a slight elevation in temperature, or a small increase in the amount of lochia flow (Box 25.2). Because the average woman usually has no postpartum complications and the length of stay in the hospital is short, it is easy to overlook these subtle signs, but it is important to be alert to any findings that are unusual because they may be the beginning of a serious concern. To be certain, do not rely solely on a woman's report of perineal healing or amount of lochia; always inspect her perineum and lochia yourself because the report of "I feel fine" or "my bleeding was just a small amount" may be deceptive if she has no familiarity with "normal" lochia, perineal healing, or fundal height against which to accurately compare her own condition.

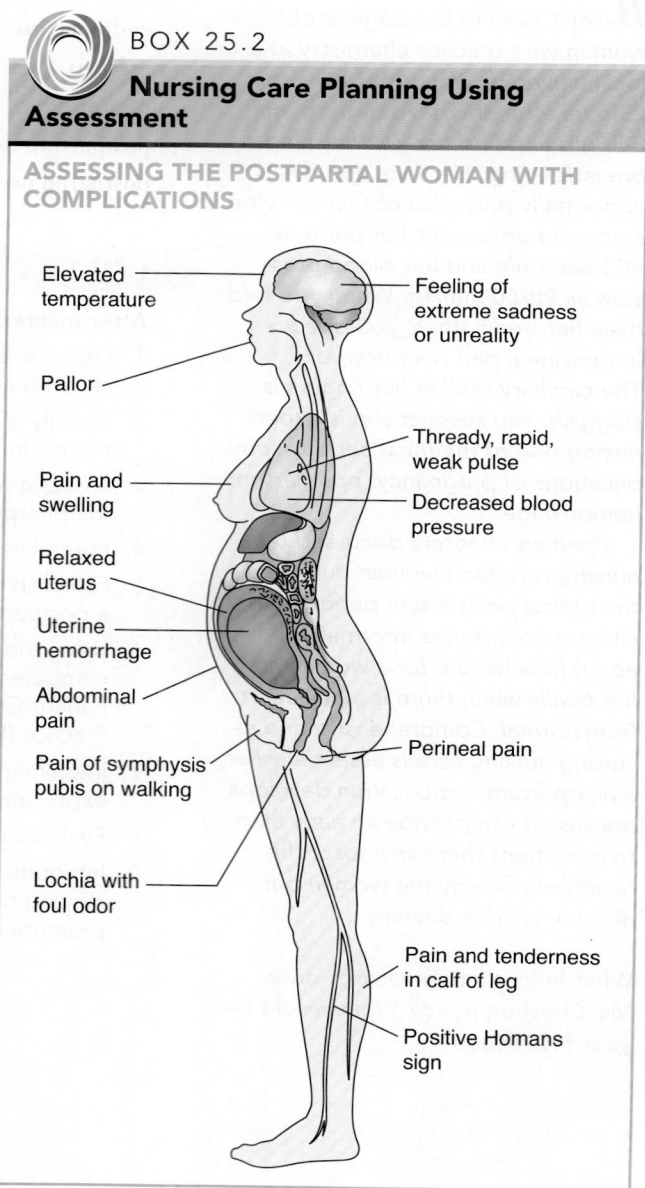

BOX 25.2

Nursing Care Planning Using Assessment

ASSESSING THE POSTPARTAL WOMAN WITH COMPLICATIONS

- Elevated temperature
- Pallor
- Pain and swelling
- Relaxed uterus
- Uterine hemorrhage
- Abdominal pain
- Pain of symphysis pubis on walking
- Lochia with foul odor
- Feeling of extreme sadness or unreality
- Thready, rapid, weak pulse
- Decreased blood pressure
- Perineal pain
- Pain and tenderness in calf of leg
- Positive Homans sign

An increased temperature except during the first 24 hours after birth is a potentially extremely serious finding. Women may try to "explain away" an increased temperature because they know if they have an elevated temperature, they may need to stay longer in the hospital for treatment of an infection. Do not be tempted to rationalize such a finding with explanations such as, "The room was warm," or "She just drank some hot coffee." Although these factors may make a slight difference in body temperature, they do not affect it enough to account for an oral temperature greater than 100.4°F (38.0°C).

NURSING DIAGNOSIS

Nursing diagnoses during this time vary depending on the postpartal complication. Some examples include:
- Deficient fluid volume related to blood loss
- Ineffective breastfeeding related to the development of mastitis
- Risk for impaired parenting related to postpartum depression
- Risk for injury to self and newborn related to postpartal psychosis
- Acute pain related to a collection of blood in traumatized tissue (hematoma) secondary to birth trauma
- Situational low self-esteem related to inability to perform regular tasks
- Social isolation related to precautions necessary to protect infant and others from infection transmission
- Ineffective peripheral tissue perfusion related to interference with circulation secondary to development of thrombophlebitis (blood clot)
- Risk for infection related to microorganism invasion of episiotomy, surgical incision site, or migration of microorganisms from the vagina to the uterus

OUTCOME IDENTIFICATION AND PLANNING

Outcome identification for a woman with a postpartum complication may be particularly difficult, because although a woman wants to do everything necessary to return to health, she also does not want anything to interfere with her ability to bond with and take care of her new child. As a rule, however, never underestimate how much a woman will endure to enable herself to "mother" her new child. This ability of a mother to overcome challenges to meet her child's needs is the essence of motherhood.

When planning care for a postpartum family, provide for measures that will restore the woman most quickly to health and promote contact among her, her child, and her primary support person. If physical contact between a mother and her newborn is not possible, give the mother frequent reports of her infant's condition and include her in planning care for her newborn. During her taking-in phase, ask the nursery staff to contact the mother at least once every nursing shift to update her on her infant's status; during her taking-hold phase, encourage her to contact the nursery. If the infant is being cared for in another facility, ask them to provide photographs of the infant. This provides something tangible to which a new mother can connect with her newborn. Many women respond well to notes written as if they were from her child, for example, "Hi, Mom. I'm drinking well but I miss you and can't wait for you to get better and take care of me.

Love, Kelsey." Such a note serves to lessen a woman's concern for her child (because she is doing well) and also helps to promote mother–infant attachment. Because childbirth is generally seen as a happy time, being faced with a postpartal complication can cause a great deal of emotional stress. The risk of both postpartal depression and postpartal psychosis increases when a complication develops. Refer patients to helpful websites and other resources when appropriate (see Chapter 20).

IMPLEMENTATION

Interventions for a woman with a postpartum complication should include instruction for both self-care and child care (if appropriate) because continuing to review these measures helps a woman accept her situation as temporary, thus reinforcing the idea she will be able to care for herself and her infant when she is healthy again.

OUTCOME EVALUATION

An evaluation of a woman with a postpartal complication should address both her and her family's health as well as her family's ability to integrate the new child into the family. The evaluation may suggest the need for home care follow-up to assist a woman in coping with both old and new responsibilities in the face of reduced energy from an illness.

Examples of expected outcomes include:
- Lochia is free of foul odor.
- Fundus remains firm and midline with progressive descent.
- Patient maintains a urinary output greater than 30 ml/hr.
- Lochia discharge amount is 6 in. or less on a perineal pad in 1 hour.
- Patient maintains vital signs and oxygen saturation within defined normal limits.
- Patient identifies signs and symptoms that should be reported.
- Patient demonstrates attachment behaviors with infant despite separation or activity restrictions.

Postpartum Hemorrhages

Hemorrhage, one of the primary causes of maternal mortality associated with childbearing, is a major threat during pregnancy, throughout labor, and continuing into the postpartum period. Traditionally, postpartum hemorrhage is defined as blood loss of 500 ml or more following a vaginal birth; this occurs in as many as 5% to 15% of postpartal women (Dahlke, Menez-Figueroa, Maggio, et al., 2015). With a cesarean birth, hemorrhage is present when there is a 1,000-ml blood loss or a 10% decrease in the hematocrit level (Pratts & Henderson, 2015). Although hemorrhage may occur either early (within the first 24 hours following birth) or late (from 24 hours to 6 weeks after birth), the greatest danger is in the first 24 hours because of the grossly denuded and unprotected uterine area left after detachment of the placenta.

The four main reasons for postpartum hemorrhage are uterine atony, trauma (lacerations, hematomas, uterine inversion, or uterine rupture), retained placental fragments, and the development of disseminated intravascular coagulation (DIC). These causes are generally referred to as the *four T's* of postpartum hemorrhage: tone, trauma, tissue, and

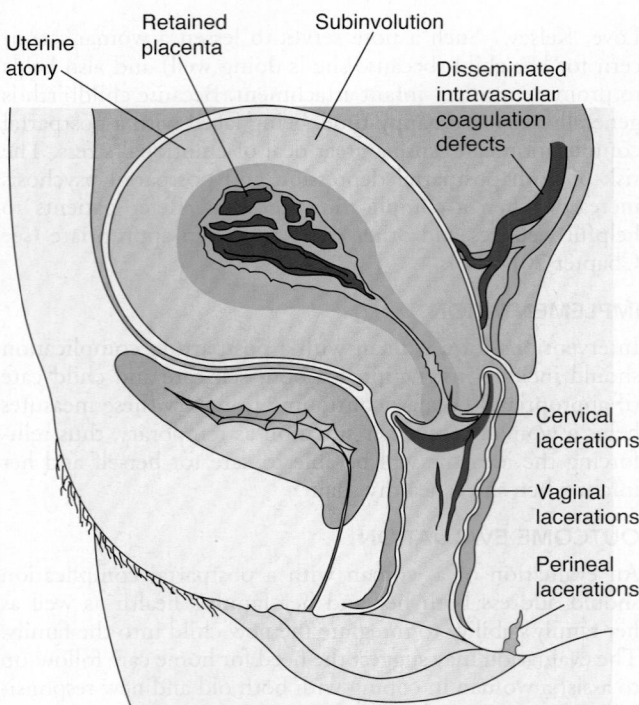

Figure 25.1 The common causes of postpartal hemorrhage.

BOX 25.3

Conditions That Increase a Woman's Risk for a Postpartal Hemorrhage

Conditions that distend the uterus beyond average capacity	Multiple gestation Polyhydramnios (excessive amount of amniotic fluid) A large baby (>9 lb) The presence of uterine myomas (fibroid tumors)
Conditions that could have caused cervical or uterine lacerations	An operative birth A rapid birth
Conditions with varied placental site or attachment	Placenta previa Placenta accreta Premature separation of the placenta Retained placental fragments
Conditions that leave the uterus unable to contract readily	Deep anesthesia or analgesia Labor initiated or assisted with an oxytocin agent High parity or maternal age over 35 years of age Previous uterine surgery Prolonged and difficult labor Chorioamnionitis or endometritis Secondary maternal illness such as anemia Prior history of postpartum hemorrhage Prolonged use of magnesium sulfate or other tocolytic therapy
Conditions that lead to inadequate blood coagulation	Fetal death Disseminated intravascular coagulation (DIC)

thrombin—a common mnemonic for the etiology of hemorrhage experienced in the puerperium (Fig. 25.1).

UTERINE ATONY

Uterine atony, or relaxation of the uterus, is the most frequent cause of postpartum hemorrhage; it tends to occur most often in Asian, Hispanic, and Black woman (Grobman, Bailit, Rice, et al., 2015). Factors that predispose a woman to poor uterine tone or the inability of her uterus to maintain a contracted state are summarized in Box 25.3. When caring for a woman in whom any of these conditions are present, be especially conscientious in your observations and be on guard for signs of uterine bleeding.

 Nursing Diagnoses and Related Interventions

Nursing Diagnosis: Deficient fluid volume related to excessive blood loss after birth.

Outcome Evaluation: Patient's blood pressure and heart rate remains within usual defined limits; lochia flow is less than one saturated perineal pad per hour.

If the uterus suddenly relaxes, there will be an abrupt gush of blood vaginally from the placental site. This can occur immediately after birth but is more likely to occur gradually, over the first postpartum hour, as the uterus slowly loses its tone. If the loss of blood is extremely copious, a woman will quickly begin to exhibit symptoms of hypovolemic shock such as a falling blood pressure; a rapid, weak, or thready pulse; increased and shallow respirations; pale, clammy skin; and increasing anxiety. If the blood loss is

unnoticed seepage, there is little change in pulse and blood pressure at first because of circulatory compensation. Suddenly, however, the system is able to compensate no more, and the pulse rate rises rapidly and becomes weak. Blood pressure then drops abruptly. With slow bleeding, a woman develops these symptoms over a period of hours; the end result of continued seepage, however, can be as life threatening as a sudden profuse loss of blood (Andrighetti, 2013).

It is difficult to estimate the amount of blood a postpartal woman is losing because it is difficult to estimate the amount of blood it takes to saturate a perineal pad (between 25 and 50 ml). By counting the number of perineal pads saturated in given lengths of time, such as half-hour intervals, a rough estimate of the amount of blood loss can be formed. Five pads saturated in half an hour is obviously a different situation from five pads saturated in 8 hours. In either situation, however, a woman will have lost approximately 250 ml of blood, and if either scenario is allowed to continue unattended, she will be in grave danger of hypovolemia. Be certain that when you are counting perineal pads, you differentiate between *saturated* and *used*. Weighing perineal pads before and after use and then subtracting the difference is an accurate technique to measure vaginal discharge: 1 g of weight is comparable to 1 ml of blood volume, so if a pad weights 50 g more after use, the woman has lost 50 ml of blood. Always be sure to turn a woman on her side when inspecting for blood loss to be certain a large amount of blood is not pooling undetected beneath her.

The best safeguard against uterine atony is to palpate a woman's fundus at frequent intervals to be assured her uterus is remaining contracted. Under usual circumstances, a well-contracted uterus feels firm and is easily recognized because it feels like no other abdominal organ. If you are unsure whether you have located a woman's fundus on palpation, it means the uterus is probably in a state of relaxation. Frequent assessments of lochia (to be certain the amount of the flow is under a saturated pad per hour and that any clots are small), as well as vital signs, particularly pulse and blood pressure, are equally important determinations.

Therapeutic Management

In the event of uterine atony, the first step in controlling hemorrhage is to attempt fundal massage to encourage contraction (Box 25.4). Unless the uterus is extremely lacking in tone, this procedure is usually effective in causing contraction, and, after a few seconds, the uterus assumes its healthy, grapefruit-like feel (World Health Organization [WHO], 2015).

With uterine atony, even if the uterus responds well to massage, the problem may not be completely resolved because, as soon as you remove your hand from the fundus, the uterus may relax and the lethal seepage will begin again. To prevent this, remain with a woman after massaging her fundus and assess to be certain her uterus is not relaxing again. Continue to assess carefully for the next 4 hours.

If a woman's uterus does not remain contracted, contact her primary care provider so interventions to increase contraction such as administering a bolus or a dilute intravenous infusion of oxytocin (Pitocin) can be prescribed to help the uterus maintain tone (Lang, Zhao, & Robertson, 2015).

When oxytocin is given intravenously (IV), its action on the uterus is immediate. Be aware, however, that oxytocin has a short duration of action, approximately 1 hour, so symptoms of uterine atony can recur quickly if it is administered only as a single dose (see Chapter 23, Box 23.3 for cautions to be aware of with an oxytocin infusion).

If oxytocin is not effective at maintaining tone, carboprost tromethamine (Hemabate), a prostaglandin F_{2a} derivative, or methylergonovine maleate (Methergine), an ergot compound, both given intramuscularly, are second possibilities. Misoprostol (Cytotec), a prostaglandin E_1 analogue, may also be administered rectally to decrease postpartum hemorrhage. Carboprost tromethamine may be repeated every 15 to 90 minutes up to 8 doses; methylergonovine maleate may be repeated every 2 to 4 hours up to 5 doses. A second dose of misoprostol should not be administered unless a minimum of 2 hours has elapsed. It's important to check that all of these drugs are readily available for use on a hospital unit in the event of postpartum hemorrhage. Because prostaglandins tend to cause diarrhea and nausea as side effect, assess for this after administration; some women will need to be administered an antiemetic to limit these side effects (Bateman, Tsen, Liu, et al., 2014).

Be aware that all of these medications can increase blood pressure and so must be used cautiously in women with hypertension. Assess blood pressure prior to administration and about 15 minutes afterward to detect this potentially dangerous side effect.

Additional measures that can be helpful to combat uterine atony include:

- Elevate the woman's lower extremities to improve circulation to essential organs.
- Offer a bedpan or assist the woman to the bathroom at least every 4 hours to be certain her bladder is emptying because a full bladder predisposes a woman to uterine atony. To reduce the possibility of bladder pressure, insertion of a urinary catheter may be prescribed.
- Administer oxygen by face mask at a rate of about 10 to 12 L/min if the woman is experiencing respiratory distress from decreasing blood volume. Position her supine (flat) to allow adequate blood flow to her brain and kidneys.
- Obtain vital signs frequently and assess them for trends such as a continually decreasing blood pressure with a continuously rising pulse rate.

When planning continuing care after sudden blood loss, remember that a woman may be so exhausted from labor and the effect of the blood loss that she resents frequent uterine and blood pressure assessments. Explain that you realize these measures are disturbing, but that they are important for her welfare. Obtain measurements as quickly and gently as possible to cause a minimum of discomfort and disruption, allowing the woman time to rest.

Bimanual Compression

If fundal massage and administration of uterotonics (drugs to contract the uterus) are not effective at stopping uterine bleeding, a sonogram may be done to detect possible retained placental fragments. The woman's primary care provider may attempt bimanual compression (Weeks & Mallaiah, 2016). With this procedure, the primary care provider inserts one hand into a woman's vagina while pushing against the fundus through the abdominal wall with the other hand. If this is ineffective, the woman may be returned to the birthing room, so that her uterine cavity can be explored manually. Under sonogram visualization, a balloon catheter may be introduced vaginally and inflated with sterile water until it puts pressure against the bleeding site. Vaginal packing is inserted during this procedure to stabilize the placement of the balloon. Be certain to document the presence of the packing so it can be removed before agency discharge because retained packing serves as a growth medium for microorganisms that could lead to postpartal infection (Vintejoux, Ulrich, Mousty, et al., 2015).

Blood Replacement

Blood transfusion to replace blood loss with postpartal hemorrhage is often necessary. In most agencies, blood typing and cross-matching is done when a woman is admitted to the labor service so blood can be rapidly cross-matched.

BOX 25.4

Nursing Care Planning Using Procedures

FUNDAL MASSAGE

Purpose: To stimulate uterine contraction, promote uterine tone and consistency, and minimize the risk of hemorrhage.

Procedure	Principle
1. Explain the necessity for the procedure and provide privacy.	1. Explanations help to decrease anxiety, and providing privacy enhances self-esteem.
2. Ask patient to void (unless bleeding is extensive and more rapid action seems necessary). Ask her to lie supine with knees flexed.	2. An empty bladder prevents displacement of the uterus and ensures accurate assessment of uterine tone. Proper positioning enhances visualization and effectiveness of procedure.
3. Put on gloves. Place one hand on the abdomen just above the symphysis pubis. Place the other hand around the top of the fundus (Fig. A).	3. This anchors the lower uterine segment and allows you to locate and assess the fundus.

| 4. Rotate the upper hand to massage the uterus until it is firm, being careful not to overmassage (Fig. B). | 4. Massage should be done only when the uterus is not firm, and aggressive massage may lead to a partial or complete uterine prolapse. |

Procedure	Principle
5. When the uterus is firm, press the fundus between the hands using slight downward pressure against the lower hand.	5. Gently squeezing with downward pressure helps to expel blood or clots collected in the uterine cavity.
6. Remove and observe the woman's perineum for the passage of clots and the amount of bleeding.	6. This helps to assess the degree of bleeding.
7. Massage the uterus one more time to be certain it remains firm, cleanse the perineum, and apply a clean perineal pad. Discard gloves and soiled pads according to agency policy.	7. This helps to promote comfort and hygiene while reducing the risk for infection.
8. Document the results of the procedure. Continue to assess the fundus and lochia according to agency policy. Notify the primary care provider if the fundus does not remain firm or if bleeding continues.	8. Documentation provides a means for evaluation. Continued assessment allows for early identification and prompt intervention with additional measures, such as oxytocin, to prevent hemorrhage.

Under usual circumstances, the average woman takes the full postpartal period to regain her strength. Women who experience postpartal hemorrhage tend to have an even longer recovery period, because the physiologic exhaustion of body systems can interfere with recovery. Iron therapy may be prescribed to ensure good hemoglobin formation. Activity level, exertion, and postpartal exercise may be somewhat restricted. Discuss with the woman the possibility of having someone stay with her at home, at least for the first week, to help with the care of her newborn and to prevent exhaustion so childbearing doesn't turn into a less than satisfying event.

Extensive blood loss is one of the precursors of postpartal infection because of the general debilitation that results. Therefore, observe any woman who has experienced more than a normal loss of blood for changes such as scant or odorous lochia discharge. Monitor her temperature closely in the postpartal period to detect the earliest signs of developing infection. Make certain the woman knows how to assess for normal lochia and temperature once she is discharged.

Hysterectomy or Suturing

Usually, uterine massage and administration of a drug to contract the uterus (uterotonic) are effective to halt bleeding. With extreme bleeding, embolization of pelvic and uterine vessels by angiographic techniques may be necessary. As a last resort, ligation of the uterine arteries or a hysterectomy (removal of the uterus) may be necessary (Ghosh & Mala, 2015). In this totally unexpected outcome of childbearing, provide comfort and support to both the woman and her support person.

After a hysterectomy, a woman usually wants to talk about what happened, why surgery was necessary, or how she feels now that she can no longer bear children so she can sort through her feelings of "Why me?" She may reveal ambivalent feelings: She wanted to have more children (or at least have the ability to have more), but she is also grateful to be alive. She is both thankful her life has been saved, but she may also feel resentful you couldn't have done more to protect her future childbearing. She may grieve for children who will not be born. If her child was born outside the hospital (although postpartum hemorrhage is lower during home births than hospital births), she may have a need to talk about her choice of location for childbirth and that she did not choose a higher resource setting for childbirth (Zielinski, Ackerson, & Kane Low, 2015).

Open lines of communication between the couple and healthcare providers that allow a family to vent their feelings are most helpful to a couple in this crisis. Referral to a grief counselor may be necessary because grieving for future children who will not be born can interfere with bonding with the present child.

QSEN Checkpoint Question 25.1

INFORMATICS

All postpartum women are at risk for uterine hemorrhage. What assessment data should the nurse first collect when appraising Ms. Cheshire's risk for hemorrhage?

    a. Ask her to describe her perineal care.
    b. Assess the skin integrity of her abdomen.
    c. Assess her oxygen saturation level.
    d. Assess her uterus for height and tone.

Look in Appendix A for the best answer and rationale.

LACERATIONS

Small lacerations or tears of the birth canal are common and may be considered a normal consequence of childbearing. Large lacerations, however, can be sources of infection or hemorrhage. They occur most often:

- With difficult or precipitate births
- In primigravidas
- With the birth of a large infant (>9 lb)
- With the use of a lithotomy position and instruments (e.g., forceps, vacuum extraction)

Lacerations may occur in the cervix, the vagina, or the perineum. After birth, anytime a uterus feels firm but bleeding persists, suspect a laceration at one of these three sites is causing the bleeding.

Cervical Lacerations

Lacerations of the cervix are usually found on the sides of the cervix, near the branches of the uterine artery. If the artery is torn, the blood loss may be so great that blood gushes from the vaginal opening. Because this is arterial bleeding, it is a brighter red than the venous blood lost with uterine atony.

Fortunately, this bleeding ordinarily occurs immediately after detachment of the placenta, when the primary care provider is still in attendance.

Therapeutic Management

The repair of a cervical laceration usually requires sutures and can be difficult because, if the bleeding is intense, this obstructs visualization of the area. A woman is not always aware of what is happening at this point, but she quickly senses something is seriously wrong. Try to maintain an air of calm and, if possible, stand beside the woman at the head of the table. She may be worried that the extra activity in the room has something to do with her baby. Assure her of her baby's condition and inform her about the need to stay in the birthing room a little longer than expected while the primary care provider places sutures or packing. Remember, the protective attitude a woman has felt toward her body all during pregnancy now turns toward her baby, so she usually is relieved to learn any problem that may be occurring is hers, not her infant's.

If the cervical laceration appears to be extensive or difficult to repair, it may be necessary for the woman to be given a regional anesthetic to relax the uterine muscle and to prevent pain. Explain the need for an anesthetic and the procedures being carried out. Be certain the primary care provider has adequate space to work, adequate sponges and suture supplies, and a good light source.

Vaginal Lacerations

Vaginal lacerations are easier to locate and assess than cervical lacerations because they are so much easier to view.

Therapeutic Management

Unfortunately, vaginal tissue is friable, making vaginal lacerations difficult to suture. A balloon tapenade similar to the type used with a uterine hemorrhage may be effective if suturing does not achieve hemostasis (Atilgan, Ozkan, Orak, et al., 2014). Some oozing often occurs after a vaginal repair, so the vagina may be packed to maintain pressure on the suture line. An indwelling urinary catheter (Foley catheter) may be placed following the repair because the packing causes such pressure on the urethra that it can interfere with voiding. Be certain to document in the woman's electronic record when and where packing was placed so you can be certain it is removed after 24 to 48 hours or before hospital discharge to prevent infection.

Perineal Lacerations

Lacerations of the perineum are more apt to occur when a woman is placed in a lithotomy position for birth rather than a supine position because a lithotomy position increases tension on the perineum. Perineal lacerations are classified by four categories, depending on the extent and depth of the tissue involved. These categories are shown in Table 25.1.

Therapeutic Management

Perineal lacerations are sutured and treated the same as an episiotomy repair. Make certain the degree of the laceration is documented because women with fourth-degree lacerations need extra precautions to avoid having sutures loosened or infected. Both sutured lacerations and episiotomy incisions tend to heal in the same length of time. A diet high in fluid and a stool softener may be prescribed for the first week after birth to prevent constipation and hard stools, which could break the new sutures. Any woman who has a third- or fourth-degree laceration should not have an enema or a rectal suppository prescribed or have her temperature taken rectally because the hard tips of equipment could open sutures near to or including those of the rectal sphincter. Although fourth-degree lacerations can lead to long-term dyspareunia, rectal incontinence, or sexual dissatisfaction, they usually heal without further complications.

RETAINED PLACENTAL FRAGMENTS

Occasionally, a placenta does not detach in its entirety; fragments of it separate and are left still attached to the uterus. Because the portion retained keeps the uterus from contracting fully, uterine bleeding occurs. Although this is most likely to happen with a succenturiate placenta—a placenta with an accessory lobe (see Chapter 23)—it can happen in any instance. Placenta accreta—a placenta that fuses with the myometrium because of an abnormal decidua basalis layer—may also be retained. This is associated with previous cesarean birth and in vitro fertilization and occurs at an incidence of about 1 out of 3,000 births; it can be identified by an ultrasound exam during pregnancy. Removing such a deeply embedded placenta can lead to severe postpartal hemorrhage (Silver, 2015). To identify the complication of a retained placenta, every placenta should be inspected carefully after birth to be certain it is complete. Retained placental fragments may also be detected by ultrasound. A blood serum sample that contains human chorionic gonadotropin (hCG) hormone also reveals that part of a placenta is still present.

Assessment

If an undetected retained fragment is large, bleeding will be apparent in the immediate postpartal period because the uterus cannot contract with the fragment in place. If the fragment is small, bleeding may not be detected until postpartum day 6 to 10, when the woman notices an abrupt discharge and a large amount of vaginal bleeding. On examination, usually the uterus is found to not be fully contracted.

Therapeutic Management

Removal of the retained placental fragment is necessary to stop the bleeding and can usually be accomplished by a dilatation and curettage (D&C). If it cannot be removed,

TABLE 25.1 CLASSIFICATION OF PERINEAL LACERATIONS

Classification	Description of Involvement
First degree	Vaginal mucous membrane and skin of the perineum to the fourchette
Second degree	Vagina, perineal skin, fascia, levator ani muscle, and perineal body
Third degree	Entire perineum, extending to reach the external sphincter of the rectum
Fourth degree	Entire perineum, rectal sphincter, and some of the mucous membrane of the rectum

methotrexate may be prescribed to destroy the retained fragment. Because the hemorrhage from retained fragments may be delayed until after a woman is at home, be certain women know to continue to observe the color of lochia and to report any tendency for the discharge to change from lochia serosa or alba back to rubra. In some instances, placenta accreta is so deeply attached that balloon occlusion and embolization of the internal iliac arteries may be necessary to minimize blood loss. In others, a hysterectomy must be performed (Silver, 2015).

QSEN Checkpoint Question 25.2 ✓

TEAMWORK & COLLABORATION

Suppose Bailey Cheshire has a retained placental fragment that is causing extensive postpartal bleeding. Which test prescribed by her primary care provider would best reveal a retained fragment is present?

a. Placental and cord blood estrogen
b. Progesterone
c. Human chorionic gonadotropin hormone
d. Oxytocin

Look in Appendix A for the best answer and rationale.

UTERINE INVERSION

Uterine inversion is a prolapse of the fundus of the uterus through the cervix so that the uterus turns inside out. This usually occurs immediately after birth and so is discussed in Chapter 23.

DISSEMINATED INTRAVASCULAR COAGULATION

DIC is a deficiency in clotting ability caused by vascular injury. It may occur in any woman in the postpartal period, but it is usually associated with premature separation of the placenta, a missed early miscarriage, or fetal death in utero. DIC is discussed in Chapter 21 along with these disorders.

SUBINVOLUTION

Subinvolution is the incomplete return of the uterus to its prepregnant size and shape. With subinvolution, at a 4- or 6-week postpartal visit, the uterus is still enlarged and soft. Lochial discharge usually is still present. Subinvolution may result from a small retained placental fragment, a mild endometritis (infection of the endometrium), or an accompanying problem such as a uterine myoma that is interfering with complete contraction.

Therapeutic Management

Oral administration of methylergonovine, 0.2 mg four times daily, is the usual prescription to improve uterine tone and complete involution. If the uterus feels tender to palpation, suggesting endometritis is present, an oral antibiotic also will be prescribed. Being certain women are able to recognize the normal process of involution and lochia discharge before hospital discharge helps women to be able to identify subinvolution and seek early care if it occurs. A chronic loss of blood from subinvolution will result in anemia and a lack of energy, conditions that possibly could interfere with infant bonding or lead to infection.

What If . . . 25.1
Bailey Cheshire tells the nurse she has a PhD in chemistry. She says that based on her background, she knows she is having a normal amount of lochia flow, so there is no need for the nurse to assess her perineum or perineal pad. Would the nurse respect her privacy or would insist the need to assess the amount of her lochia flow?

PERINEAL HEMATOMAS

A perineal hematoma is a collection of blood in the subcutaneous layer of tissue of the perineum. The overlying skin, as a rule, is intact with no noticeable trauma. Blood accumulates underneath, however, from injury to blood vessels in the perineum during birth. Hematomas are most likely to occur after rapid, spontaneous births and in women who have perineal varicosities. They may occur at the site of an episiotomy or laceration repair if a vein was punctured during suturing. Although these can cause a woman acute discomfort and concern, they usually represent only minor bleeding.

Assessment

Perineal sutures almost always give a postpartal woman some discomfort. If a woman reports severe pain in the perineal area or a feeling of pressure between her legs, inspect the perineal area to see if a hematoma could be causing this. If a hematoma is present, it appears as an area of purplish discoloration with obvious swelling. It could be as small as 2 cm or as large as 8 cm in diameter (Fig. 25.2). At first it may feel fluctuant, but as seepage into the area continues and tissue is drawn taut, it palpates as a firm globe and feels tender.

Therapeutic Management

Report the presence of a hematoma, its estimated size, and the degree of the woman's discomfort to her primary care provider. Describe a definite size such as "5 centimeters" or the size of a quarter or a half dollar rather than documenting it as "large" or "small" as this best establishes a baseline and will enable you to assess if it is growing larger.

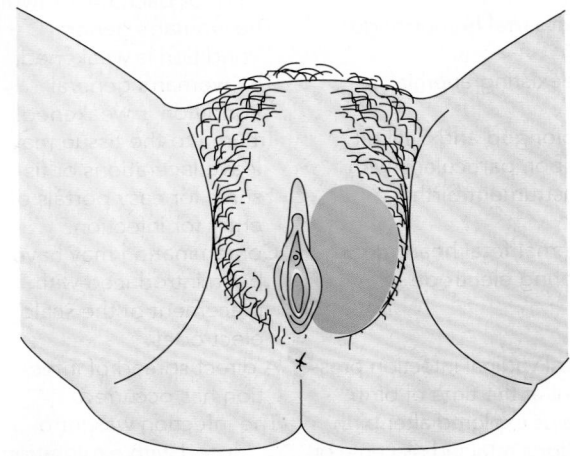

Figure 25.2 The appearance of a perineal hematoma from a bleeding subcutaneous vessel.

Administer a mild analgesic as prescribed for pain relief. Applying an ice pack (covered with a towel to prevent thermal injury to the skin) may prevent further bleeding. Usually, a hematoma is absorbed over the next 3 or 4 days. If one is large when discovered or continues to increase in size, the woman may have to be returned to the birthing room to have the site incised and the bleeding vessel ligated under local anesthesia.

You can assure the woman that even though the hematoma is causing her considerable discomfort, it is not a serious complication and will slowly reabsorb over the next 6 weeks, causing no further difficulty. If an episiotomy incision line was opened to drain a hematoma, it may be left open and packed with gauze rather than resutured. Be certain to record this packing was placed so it can be removed in 24 to 48 hours. A suture line opened this way heals by tertiary intention or from the bottom to the top, rather than side to side, so healing will occur more slowly than a usual primary intention suture line. Be certain the woman has clear instructions before discharge regarding necessary suture line care she will need to do at home, such as keeping it clean and dry and perhaps using a sitz bath once or twice a day.

Puerperal Infections

Infection of the reproductive tract in the postpartal period is another major cause of maternal mortality (Galvão, Braga, Gonçalves, et al., 2016). Factors that predispose women to infection during this time are shown in Box 25.5. When caring for a woman who has any of these circumstances, be aware that the risk for postpartal infection is greatly increased.

BOX 25.5

Conditions That Increase a Woman's Risk for Postpartal Infection

Risk Factor	Basis for Risk
Rupture of the membranes more than 24 hours before birth	Bacteria may have started to invade the uterus while the fetus was still in utero.
Retained placental fragments within the uterus	The tissue necroses and serves as an excellent bed for bacterial growth.
Postpartal hemorrhage	The woman's general condition is weakened.
Preexisting anemia	The woman's general condition is weakened.
Prolonged and difficult labor, particularly with instrument births	Trauma to the tissue may leave lacerations or fissures for easy portals of entry for infection.
Internal fetal heart monitoring electrode	Contamination may have been introduced with placement of the scalp electrodes.
Local vaginal infection present at the time of birth	A direct spread of infection has occurred.
Uterus explored after birth for a retained placenta or abnormal bleeding site	The infection was introduced with exploration.

Theoretically, the uterus is sterile during pregnancy and up until the membranes rupture. After rupture, pathogens can begin to invade; the risk of infection grows even greater if tissue edema and trauma are present. If infection should occur, the prognosis for complete recovery depends on such factors as the woman's general health, virulence of the invading organism and portal of entry, the degree of uterine involution at the time of the invasion, and the presence of lacerations in the reproductive tract.

A **puerperal infection** is always potentially serious, because, although it usually begins as only a local infection, it has the potential to spread to the peritoneum (peritonitis) or the circulatory system (septicemia), conditions that can be fatal in a woman whose body is already stressed from childbirth.

Organisms commonly cultured postpartally include group B streptococci, staphylococci, and aerobic gram-negative bacilli such as *Escherichia coli*. The management for puerperal infection focuses on the use of an appropriate antibiotic after culture and sensitivity testing of the isolated organism.

Nursing Diagnoses and Related Interventions

Nursing Diagnosis: Risk for infection related to loss of uterine sterility with childbirth

Outcome Evaluation: Patient's temperature remains below 100.4°F (38°C) orally, excluding the first 24 hours after birth; lochia is present without foul odor.

To help prevent an infection, any articles such as gloves or instruments that are introduced into the birth canal during labor, birth, and the postpartal period should be sterile. In addition, adherence to standard infection precautions is essential.

Be certain to instruct a postpartal woman in proper perineal care, including wiping from front to back so that she does not bring *E. coli* organisms forward from the rectum. Use good hand washing technique before, during, and after any patient care to prevent cross-contamination. When giving perineal care, both wash your hands and wear gloves. Each postpartal woman should have her own perineal supplies and should not share them to prevent the transfer of pathogens from one woman to another.

Intravenous antibiotics usually are prescribed for a postpartal infection. Frequently used antibiotics include ampicillin, gentamicin, and third-generation cephalosporins such as cefixime (Suprax). If the woman will be continuing drug therapy at home, stress that she must take the full course to prevent the infection from recurring. Be certain women who are breastfeeding are not prescribed antibiotics incompatible with breastfeeding. Alert them to observe for problems in their infant, such as white plaques or thrush (oral candidiasis) in their infant's mouth that can occur when a portion of the maternal antibiotic passes into breast milk and causes an overgrowth of fungal organisms (i.e., an opportunistic infection) in the infant. The infant also should be assessed for easy bruising because a decrease in microorganisms in the bowel caused by an antibiotic passed in breast milk may lead to insufficient vitamin K formation and, consequently, decreased blood-clotting ability.

Nursing Diagnosis: Social isolation related to precautions necessary to protect baby and others from exposure to infectious microorganisms

Outcome Evaluation: Patient acknowledges agency policy regarding precautions and a willingness to comply with policies. States plans for diversional activities to pass the time if separated from her newborn; demonstrates bonding behaviors, such as asking about newborn and expressing desire to see infant.

Healthcare agencies have well-defined guidelines on whether a woman who has an infection should be separated from other women or her newborn. As a general rule, the baby of a mother with an increased temperature (100.4°F [38°C]) for two consecutive 24-hour periods exclusive of the first 24 hours is kept in a closed incubator in her room until the cause of the infection is determined because she may have an upper respiratory or gastrointestinal tract infection unrelated to childbearing that is transmittable to a newborn.

If the cause of the fever is found to be related to childbirth but involves a closed infection, such as thrombophlebitis, there is no danger of the baby contracting the disease, so the woman may care for her child as long as she maintains the degree of prescribed bed rest necessary for her primary condition. If the infection involves drainage such as can occur with endometritis or a perineal abscess, the mother should wash her hands thoroughly before holding her infant and avoid placing her baby on the bottom bed sheet, where there may be some infected drainage from her perineal pad. Instead, furnish a clean sheet for her to spread over the covers.

If the woman develops a high fever, breast milk may become deficient. Fortunately, with modern antimicrobial therapy, the period of high fever usually is transient. If the mother is too ill to nurse her baby during this time or if she is receiving an anticoagulant or antibiotic that would be harmful to the baby, the infant should be fed by a supplementary milk formula. Urge her to manually express or pump breast milk during this time to maintain the production of milk. She may need support to do this because, if she fatigues easily, her energy level may not be enough to support her good intentions.

It's difficult for many women to accomplish their new role change even when things are going well. If a woman is segregated from others, frightened by her condition, and denied the pleasure of holding and feeding her newborn, her situation may seem overwhelming. Women who are isolated this way need friendly, understanding support from hospital personnel during such a stressful time.

ENDOMETRITIS

Endometritis is an infection of the endometrium, the lining of the uterus (Pratts & Henderson, 2015). Bacteria gain access to the uterus through the vagina and enter the uterus either at the time of birth or during the postpartal period. This may occur with any birth, but the infection is usually associated with chorioamnionitis and a cesarean birth (Shanks, Mehra, Gross, et al., 2016).

Assessment

A benign temperature elevation may occur on the first postpartal day, particularly if a woman is not drinking enough fluid. In contrast, the fever of endometritis usually manifests itself on the third or fourth postpartal day, suggesting that much of the invasion occurred during labor or birth (consistent with the time it takes for infectious organisms to grow).

Normally, the white blood cell count of a postpartal woman is increased to 20,000 to 30,000 cells/mm³ due to the stress of labor. Because of this increase, the conventional method of detecting infection (elevated white blood cell count) is not of great value in the puerperium. Infection is suspected, instead, in postpartal women who have a temperature over 100.4°F (38°C) for two consecutive 24-hour periods. Because women may be at home when this elevated temperature occurs, be certain they know to take their temperature if they feel it is increased and to notify their primary care provider if it is elevated.

A rise in temperature that occurs on the third or fourth day postpartum occurs coincidentally at the same time as breast filling occurs. Do not be led astray by attributing an elevated temperature at this time to breast filling. Suspect fever on the third or fourth day postpartum as possible endometritis until proven otherwise.

Depending on the severity of the infection, a woman may have accompanying chills, loss of appetite, and general malaise. Her uterus usually is not well contracted and is painful to touch. She may feel strong afterpains. Lochia usually is dark brown and has a foul odor. It may be increased in amount because of poor uterine involution, but if the infection is accompanied by high fever, lochia may, in contrast, be scant or absent. A sonogram may be prescribed to confirm the presence of placental fragments that could be a possible cause of the infection.

Therapeutic Management

When taking a culture to identify the offending organism, be certain to obtain fluid from the vagina using a sterile swab rather than from a perineal pad to ensure you are culturing the endometrial infectious organism and not an unrelated one from the pad. Treatment will consist of the administration of an appropriate antibiotic, such as clindamycin (Cleocin), as determined by the culture. An oxytocic agent such as methylergonovine may also be prescribed to encourage uterine contraction. Urge the woman to drink additional fluid to combat the fever. If strong afterpains and abdominal discomfort are present, ask if she needs an analgesic for pain relief.

Sitting in a semi-Fowler's position or walking encourages lochia drainage by gravity and helps prevent pooling of infected secretions. Because any drainage on perineal pads or bed linens is contaminated, be certain to wear gloves when helping a woman change her perineal pads and changing bed linen. In addition, be certain both you and the woman use good hand washing techniques before and after handling pads.

As with any infection, endometritis can be controlled best if it is discovered early. If you can interpret the normal color, quantity, and odor of lochia discharge and the size, consistency, and tenderness of a normal postpartal uterus, you can be the first person to recognize that an infection is present. Because a woman may be at home when signs of infection occur, be certain you've taught about the signs and symptoms of endometritis before healthcare agency discharge.

If the infection is limited to the endometrium, the course of infection will be about 7 to 10 days. If this occurs while a woman is hospitalized, she may have to make arrangements for her baby's discharge before her own or arrange for help with newborn care when she is discharged. Be certain she knows to take the full course of antibiotics prescribed so the infection is completely eradicated and does not return.

An added danger of endometritis is that it can lead to tubal scarring and interference with future fertility. At a future time, if the woman desires more children, she may need a fertility assessment (including a sonohysterosalpingogram) to determine tubal patency. With mild endometritis, this is usually not a problem, but a woman should be forewarned that it could occur.

> ### What If . . . 25.2
> Just before hospital discharge on her third postpartal day, Bailey Cheshire develops a shaking chill and a fever of 101.5°F (38.6°C). She's already dressed to go home and assures the nurse the temperature elevation is inaccurate because she just drank some hot coffee. On palpation, the nurse notices her abdomen is tender. Would the nurse agree with her that it's safe to be discharged?

INFECTION OF THE PERINEUM

If a woman has a suture line on her perineum from an episiotomy or a laceration repair, a ready portal of entry exists for bacterial invasion.

Assessment

Infections of the perineum usually remain localized. They are revealed by symptoms similar to those of any suture-line infection, such as pain, heat, and a feeling of pressure. The woman may or may not have an elevated temperature depending on the systemic effect and spread of the infection.

Inspection of the suture line will reveal inflammation. One or two stitches may have sloughed away, so an area of the suture line is open with purulent drainage present (Fig. 25.3). Notify the woman's primary care provider of the localized symptoms, and culture the discharge using a sterile cotton-tipped applicator touched to the secretions.

Therapeutic Management

Typically, either a systemic or topical antibiotic is ordered even before the culture report is returned. An analgesic may be prescribed to alleviate discomfort. It may be necessary to remove perineal sutures to open the area and allow for drainage. Sitz baths, moist warm compresses, or Hubbard tank treatments may be prescribed to hasten drainage and cleanse the area. Remind the woman to change perineal pads frequently. Because they are contaminated by drainage, if left in place too long, they might cause vaginal contamination or reinfection. Repeat again that the woman should wipe front to back after urinating or a bowel movement to prevent bringing contamination forward from the rectum onto the healing area.

With a local infection of this nature, a woman is usually discharged with a referral for home care follow-up because the incision site, once opened, must heal by tertiary rather than by primary intention. Infections of this nature are annoying and painful, but fortunately, with improved techniques during birth and the puerperium, perineal infections occur only rarely. Because they are localized, there is no need to restrict the woman from caring for her infant as long as she washes her hands well before holding her newborn. Be certain not to place the infant on the bottom bed sheet of the woman's bed where the baby could contact pathogenic bacteria. Encourage the woman to ambulate and ask for analgesia as needed. Often, the pain from an infected suture line is severe, and the woman may decrease ambulation unless she is urged to continue.

PERITONITIS

Peritonitis, or infection of the peritoneal cavity, usually occurs as an extension of endometritis. It is one of the gravest complications of childbearing and is a major cause of death from puerperal infection. The infection spreads from the uterus through the lymphatic system or directly through the fallopian tubes or uterine wall to the peritoneal cavity. An abscess may form in the cul-de-sac of Douglas because this is the lowest point of the peritoneal cavity and gravity causes infected material to localize there.

Assessment

Symptoms are the same as those of a surgical patient in whom a peritoneal infection develops: rigid abdomen, abdominal pain, high fever, rapid pulse, vomiting, and the appearance of being acutely ill. When assessing the abdomen of a postpartal woman, be sure to note not only that her uterus is well contracted but also that the remainder of her abdomen is soft because the occurrence of a rigid abdomen (i.e., guarding) is one of the first symptoms of peritonitis.

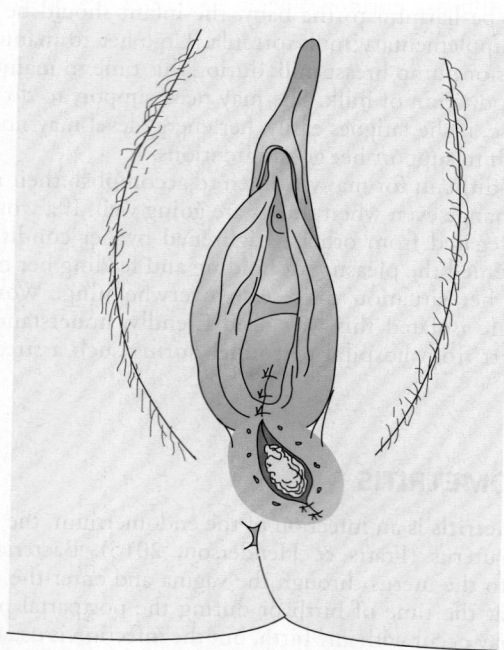

Figure 25.3 An infected suture line appears reddened and edematous and often contains infected secretions.

Therapeutic Management

Peritonitis is often accompanied by a paralytic ileus (a blockage of inflamed intestines). This requires insertion of a nasogastric tube to prevent vomiting and to rest the bowel. Intravenous fluid or total parenteral nutrition will then be necessary. A woman will need analgesics for pain relief and intravenous antibiotics to treat the infection. Her hospital stay will be extended, but with effective antibiotic therapy, the outcome should be good. Peritonitis can interfere with future fertility because it can leave scarring and adhesions in the peritoneum, which separate the fallopian tubes from the ovaries to the extent that ova can no longer easily enter the tubes.

QSEN Checkpoint Question 25.3

QUALITY IMPROVEMENT

Bailey Cheshire develops endometritis. When planning nursing care, which activity would be best to advise for Bailey?
a. Walking around her room listening to music
b. Lying supine with a cold cloth on her forehead
c. Reading while resting in a slight Trendelenburg position
d. Alternating between prone and supine positions

Look in Appendix A for the best answer and rationale.

Thrombophlebitis

Phlebitis is inflammation of the lining of a blood vessel. **Thrombophlebitis** is inflammation with the formation of blood clots. Thrombophlebitis is classified as either superficial vein disease (SVD) or deep vein thrombosis (DVT). When either type occurs in the postpartum period, it tends to occur because:

- A woman's fibrinogen level is still elevated from pregnancy, leading to increased blood clotting.
- Dilatation of lower extremity veins is still present as a result of pressure of the fetal head during pregnancy and birth so blood circulation is sluggish.

It tends to occur most often in women who:

- Are relatively inactive in labor and during the early puerperium because this increases the risk of blood clot formation
- Have spent prolonged time in a birthing room with their legs positioned in stirrups
- Have preexistent obesity and a pregnancy weight gain greater than the recommended weight gain, which can lead to inactivity and lack of exercise
- Have preexisting varicose veins
- Develop a postpartal infection
- Have a history of a previous thrombophlebitis
- Are older than age 35 years or have increased parity
- Have a high incidence of thrombophlebitis in their family
- Smoke cigarettes because nicotine causes vasoconstriction and reduces blood flow

FEMORAL THROMBOPHLEBITIS

With femoral thrombophlebitis, the femoral, saphenous, or popliteal veins are involved. Although the inflammation site in thrombophlebitis is a vein, an accompanying arterial spasm often occurs, diminishing arterial circulation to the leg as well. This decreased circulation, along with edema, gives the leg a white or drained appearance. It was formerly believed that breast milk drained into the leg, giving it its white appearance. The condition was, therefore, formerly called *milk leg* or *phlegmasia alba dolens* ("white inflammation").

Ambulation and limiting the time a woman remains in obstetric stirrups encourages circulation in the lower extremities, promotes venous return, and decreases the possibility of clot formation, thus helping to prevent thrombophlebitis. If stirrups on examining tables or birthing rooms are used, be certain that they are well padded to prevent any sharp pressure against the calves of the legs and that the woman remains in a lithotomy position for as short a period of time as possible. If a woman had varicose veins before or during pregnancy, wearing support stockings for the first 2 weeks after birth can help increase venous circulation and prevent stasis. If these are prescribed, be certain the woman knows to buy medical support stockings, not panty hose advertised as offering support, and to put them on before she rises in the morning. If she waits until she is already up and walking, venous congestion will have already occurred and the stockings will be less effective. Encourage her to remove the support stockings twice daily and assess her skin underneath for mottling or inflammation that would suggest inflammation of her veins.

Women are not normally prescribed acetylsalicylic acid (aspirin) for pain because aspirin is a mild anticoagulant, which interferes with blood clotting by preventing platelet aggregation and clot formation. However, women who are high risk for thrombophlebitis may be prescribed aspirin every 4 hours as a preventive measure. If this is so, be certain to not interpret aspirin used this way as an as needed (PRN) analgesic order and withhold it depending on the woman's level of pain. Other measures for preventing thrombophlebitis are summarized in Box 25.6.

Assessment

If a pelvic thrombophlebitis develops, a woman will generally have an elevated temperature, a systemic fever, chills, and pain. Comparatively, a woman experiencing a femoral thrombophlebitis will usually have unilateral localized symptoms such as redness, swelling, warmth, and a hard inflamed vessel in the affected leg. Symptoms for thrombophlebitis usually present about 10 days after birth. The woman's leg begins to swell below the lesion at the point at which venous circulation is blocked. Her skin may become so stretched from swelling that it appears shiny and white. A Homans sign (pain in the calf of the leg on dorsiflexion of the foot) may be positive; however, a negative Homans sign does not rule out obstruction. The diameter of the leg at thigh or calf level may be increased compared with the other leg. Doppler ultrasound or contrast venography will be prescribed to confirm the diagnosis (Al-Thani, El-Menyar, Asim, et al., 2016).

Therapeutic Management

Treatment consists of the administration of anticoagulants, the application of moist heat (to decrease inflammation), and bed rest with the affected leg elevated. A bed cradle over the leg can lift the pressure of the bedclothes off the affected leg and can both decrease the sensitivity of the leg and improve circulation. Assess the woman for risk of a pressure ulcer and

BOX 25.6

Nursing Care Planning Based on Family Teaching

PREVENTING THROMBOPHLEBITIS

Q. Bailey Cheshire tells you, "My sister developed a thrombophlebitis after the birth of her first baby. How can I prevent that from happening to me?"

A. Here are a few helpful hints:

- Ask your primary care provider if you can use a side-lying or back-lying (supine recumbent) position for birth rather than a lithotomy position because a lithotomy position can increase the tendency for pooling of blood in the lower extremities.
- If you will be using a lithotomy position, ask for padding on the stirrups to prevent pressure on the calf of your legs.
- Drink adequate fluids to be certain you're not dehydrated (6 to 8 glasses of fluid per day).
- Do not sit with your knees crossed or bent sharply and avoid wearing constricting clothing such as knee-high stockings.
- Ambulate as soon after birth as possible because walking is the best preventive measure. When resting in bed, wiggle your toes or do leg lifts to improve venous return.
- Ask your primary care provider if he or she recommends support stockings in the immediate postpartal period. Be certain to put these on before ambulating in the morning before leg veins fill.
- Quit smoking because this is associated with the development of thrombophlebitis

provide good back, buttocks, and heel care for as long as she is on bed rest.

Although simple in theory, application of moist compresses is, unfortunately, one of the most technically difficult treatments to carry out because dressings invariably dry or become cold and dampen bed clothes after only a short time. Compresses and water used in this way do not have to be sterile because with thrombophlebitis, there is no break in the skin. Because of edema in the area, be certain to test water temperature by dipping your inner wrist into it before soaking a dressing to be sure it is not so warm it could cause a burn. Cover wet, warm dressings with a plastic pad to hold in heat and moisture. In addition, position a commercial pad with circulating heating coils or chemical hot packs over the plastic to ensure soaks stay warm. Be certain the weight of a hot pack or pad does not rest on the leg, causing an obstruction to flow of blood.

Never massage the skin over the clotted area because this could loosen the clot, causing a pulmonary or cerebral embolism. Check the woman's bed frequently to be certain the mattress does not become wet from seeping water. For compresses to stay in place, a woman must lay with her leg fairly immobile. However, be certain she does not interpret this as meaning she cannot turn or move about. Help her select activities to exercise the other parts of her body or stimulate her mind such as reading a good book or information on newborn care. Women who have been discharged from the hospital may be cared for at home on bed rest or may need to return to the hospital so strict bed rest can be enforced. If infection was the underlying cause of the condition, an antibiotic to treat the initial infection will be prescribed. In order to prevent further blood clotting, an anticoagulant such as unfractionated heparin (given IV) or low–molecular-weight heparin (given subcutaneously) will be prescribed. Thrombolytics (medications that dissolve clots) may also be prescribed; these should be initiated within the first 24 hours for best results. With the use of anticoagulants, a blood coagulation study will be necessary to establish a baseline value

followed by sequential tests to determine the effectiveness of the drug therapy. Heparin therapy is usually continued until symptoms resolve and the international normalized ratio (INR) is >2 for at least 24 hours (Box 25.7). Be certain that protamine sulfate, the antagonist for heparin, and vitamin K, the antagonist for warfarin, are both readily available until the woman's anticoagulation therapy is stabilized.

Following this initial treatment with heparin, a woman will be discharged on subcutaneous heparin or oral anticoagulation therapy such as warfarin (Coumadin). If she will be doing her own subcutaneous injections at home, be certain she demonstrates good injection technique before discharge, is aware of complications associated with anticoagulant therapy, and understands the importance of required blood work so she schedules these appropriately.

The woman can continue to breastfeed while receiving heparin. She has to discontinue breastfeeding during therapy with warfarin (Coumadin) because warfarin-derived anticoagulants are passed in breast milk. If the thrombophlebitis does not seem to be severe and the woman wants to restart breastfeeding after the course of warfarin (Coumadin) (about 10 days), encourage her to manually express breast milk at the time of normal feedings so she maintains a good milk supply.

Lochia usually increases in amount in a woman who is receiving an anticoagulant. Be sure to keep a meaningful record of the amount of this discharge, so that it can be estimated; "lochia serosa with scattered pinpoint clots; three perineal pads saturated in 8 hours," for example, is far more meaningful than "large amount of lochia." Also assess for other possible signs of bleeding, such as bleeding gums, ecchymotic spots on the skin, or oozing from an episiotomy suture line.

With proper treatment, the acute symptoms of femoral thrombophlebitis last only a few days, but the full course of the disease takes 4 to 6 weeks before it is fully resolved. Anticoagulant therapy may need to be continued for as long as 3 to 6 months. The affected leg may never return to its former size and may always cause discomfort after long periods of standing.

BOX 25.7

Nursing Care Planning Based on Responsibility for Pharmacology

LOW–MOLECULAR-WEIGHT HEPARIN

Classification: Heparin is a common anticoagulant.

Action: Heparin blocks the conversion of prothrombin to thrombin and of fibrinogen to fibrin, decreasing clotting ability and resulting in the inhibition of thrombus and clot formation. It is used to prevent and treat thrombosis and pulmonary embolism (Karch, 2015).

Pregnancy Risk Category: B

Dosage: Dosage is dependent on coagulation studies. Dosage is considered therapeutic when the activated partial thromboplastin time (aPTT) is 1.5 to 3 times the control value. The drug is given by subcutaneous injection.

Possible Adverse Effects: Hemorrhage, bruising, thrombocytopenia (lowered platelet count), urticaria (hives and itching)

Nursing Implications

- Obtain coagulation studies as prescribed; *adjust dosage as necessary.*
- Heparin is usually injected into subcutaneous tissue of the abdomen. For best absorption, rotate injection sites. Do not aspirate for blood return or massage the injection site afterward to avoid bruising or hematoma formation.
- Avoid any intramuscular injection of other medications because a hematoma may form at the injection site.
- Assess a woman and alert her to self-assess for signs and symptoms of bleeding, such as oozing from the gums, nosebleeds, hematuria, or frank or occult blood in stool.
- Closely monitor patient's lochia, including amount and color. Assess pad count to determine extent of vaginal bleeding.
- Keep protamine sulfate, the antidote, readily available in case of overdose.
- Instruct the woman about antibleeding precautions such as using a soft toothbrush to minimize the risk of bleeding and in the correct injection technique and allow her to demonstrate this before health agency discharge.

PELVIC THROMBOPHLEBITIS

Pelvic thrombophlebitis involves the ovarian, uterine, or hypogastric veins. It usually follows a mild endometritis and occurs later than femoral thrombophlebitis, often around the 14th or 15th day of the puerperium. Inflammation of the blood vessels in the pelvic area causes a partial obstruction, which leads to slowed blood flow and clots in the stagnant blood in the vessel. Risk factors are the same as for femoral thrombophlebitis. The prevention of endometritis by the use of good aseptic technique during and after birth is important to help prevent the disorder (Laifer-Narin, Kwak, Kim, et al., 2014).

Assessment

With pelvic thrombophlebitis, a woman suddenly becomes extremely ill, with a high fever, chills, abdominal pain, weakness, and general malaise. Her infection can be so severe it necroses the vein and results in a pelvic abscess. In severe instances, it can become systemic and results in a lung, kidney, or heart valve abscess.

Therapeutic Management

As with femoral thrombophlebitis, therapy involves total bed rest and the administration of analgesics, antibiotics, and anticoagulants.

The disease runs a long course of 6 to 8 weeks. If an abscess forms, it can be located by sonogram and incised by laparotomy. A woman may need surgery to remove the affected vessel before she attempts to become pregnant again.

Regardless of the type of thrombophlebitis, teach women preventive measures to reduce the risk of recurrence with future pregnancies such as wearing nonconstricting clothing on their lower extremities, resting with the feet elevated, and ambulating daily. Caution a woman to tell her primary care provider before her next pregnancy of the difficulty she experienced at this time, so that extra prophylactic precautions can be taken to prevent thrombophlebitis in a future pregnancy.

QSEN Checkpoint Question 25.4

SAFETY

Ms. Cheshire has a risk for DVT during the postpartal period. What would be the best suggestion the nurse could make to help prevent this?
  a. Rest in bed as much as possible for the first several days.
  b. Assume a knee–chest position for 15 minutes every day.
  c. Increase fluid intake to reduce blood viscosity.
  d. Ambulate early and consistently to improve circulation.

Look in Appendix A for the best answer and rationale.

PULMONARY EMBOLUS

A pulmonary embolus is obstruction of the pulmonary artery by a blood clot; it usually occurs as a complication of thrombophlebitis when a blood clot moves from a leg vein to the pulmonary artery (Konkle, 2015). The signs of pulmonary embolus are sudden, sharp chest pain; tachypnea; tachycardia; orthopnea (inability to breathe except in an upright position); and cyanosis (the blood clot is blocking both blood flow to the lungs and return to the heart). This is an emergency. A woman needs oxygen administered immediately and is at high risk for cardiopulmonary arrest. Her condition is extremely guarded until the clot can be lysed or adheres to the pulmonary artery wall and is reabsorbed. Because of the seriousness of this condition, a woman with a pulmonary embolism commonly is transferred to an intensive care unit for continuing care.

Mastitis

Mastitis (infection of the breast) may occur as early as the seventh postpartal day or not until the baby is weeks or months old (Witt, Bolman, Kredit, et al., 2016). The organism causing the infection usually enters through cracked and fissured nipples. Therefore, to prevent mastitis, it's important to prevent nipples from cracking through measures such as:

- Making certain the baby is positioned correctly and grasps the nipple properly, including both the nipple and areola
- Helping a baby release a grasp on the nipple before removing the baby from the breast
- Washing hands between handling perineal pads and touching breasts
- Exposing nipples to air for at least part of every day
- Possibly using a vitamin E ointment daily to soften nipples
- Encouraging women to begin breastfeeding (when the infant sucks most forcefully) on an unaffected nipple (if a woman has one cracked nipple and one well nipple)

Occasionally, the organism that causes mastitis comes from the nasal–oral cavity of the infant. In these instances, the infant has usually acquired *Staphylococcus aureus*, a methicillin-resistant *S. aureus* infection (MRSA), or candidiasis while in the hospital. The infant introduces the organisms into the milk ducts by sucking, where they proliferate (breast milk is an excellent medium for bacterial growth). Because this spreads from one person to another, this is termed *epidemic mastitis* or *epidemic breast abscess*. When it occurs, it is usually discovered that several women discharged from the hospital at the same time have similar infections.

ASSESSMENT

Mastitis is usually unilateral, although epidemic mastitis, because it originates with the infant, may be bilateral. The affected breast feels painful and appears swollen and reddened. Fever accompanies these first symptoms within hours, and breast milk becomes scant. If the diagnosis is not clear from the typical symptoms, the woman may have a sonogram prescribed to be certain a deep lying breast abscess isn't also present (Irusen, Rohwer, Steyn, et al., 2015).

THERAPEUTIC MANAGEMENT

Treatment consists of antibiotics effective against penicillin-resistant staphylococci such as dicloxacillin or a cephalosporin, and, because symptoms often appear after a hospital discharge, it is treated on an outpatient basis (Pustotina, 2015). Breastfeeding should be continued if possible because keeping the breast emptied of milk helps to prevent the growth of bacteria. Some women find an infected breast too painful to allow their infant to suck, however, and prefer to express milk manually from the affected breast until their antibiotic has taken effect and the mastitis has diminished (about 3 days). Cold or ice compresses and a good supportive bra help with pain relief until the process improves, although warm, wet compresses can also be helpful because this reduces inflammation and edema.

If therapy is started as soon as symptoms appear, the condition runs a short course of about 2 or 3 days. If left untreated, a breast infection can become a localized abscess. If unrecognized, this can spread to involve a large portion of the breast and even rupture through the skin, with thick, purulent drainage. If an abscess forms, breastfeeding on that breast is discontinued as the abscess may need incision and drainage. Encourage women to continue to pump breast milk, if possible, until the abscess has resolved in order to preserve breastfeeding. Many women find a breast this infected too tender to do this, however, so instead choose to bottle-feed their infant. Although this is not the outcome she hoped for, you can assure a woman that formula feeding will be an acceptable alternative for this child.

Neither mastitis nor a breast abscess leaves any permanent breast disease. A woman can be assured that such an incident is not associated with the development of breast cancer and does not interfere with future breastfeeding potential. Box 25.8 shows an interprofessional care map illustrating both nursing and team planning for a woman with mastitis.

Urinary System Disorders

Because a woman's bladder is compressed by the infant's head during birth, several urinary tract disorders can occur.

URINARY RETENTION

Urinary retention occurs when the bladder is unable to empty completely (Mulder, Oude Rengerink, van der Post, et al., 2016). After childbirth, bladder sensation for voiding is decreased because of bladder edema caused by the pressure of birth. This concern is compounded during prolonged labor, perineal lacerations, and the use of epidural anesthesia. Unable to empty, the bladder fills to overdistention. When the woman does void, instead of emptying completely, the bladder empties only a small portion of its contents (retention with overflow). As a result, it quickly becomes overdistended again. If it is allowed to continue, bladder overdistention can cause permanent damage to bladder tone, leading to permanent incontinence (Mulder et al., 2016).

Assessment

In a postpartal woman, urinary retention with overflow may be more difficult to detect than primary or simple overdistention. With primary overdistention, a woman does not void at all. A longer than usual time (>8 hours) passes after birth or between voids. Assessment by percussion or palpation of the bladder reveals bladder distention.

With urinary retention and overflow, a woman is able to void. Voiding is very frequent, however, and in very small amounts, so her overall output is inadequate. Always measure the amount of a woman's first voiding after birth because with diuresis occurring, this should be large. As a rule, if this first voiding is less than 100 ml, suspect urinary retention.

Urinary retention is confirmed by catheterizing a woman immediately after she voids. If the amount of urine left in the bladder after voiding (termed *residual*) is greater than 100 ml, the woman is retaining more than the usual amount of urine. Typically, the prescription for catheterization is written as: "Catheterize for residual urine. If this is greater than 100 ml, leave indwelling catheter in place." Always use an indwelling (Foley) catheter, rather than a temporary one (straight catheter), therefore, to catheterize for residual urine so this can be inflated and left in place. Use strict antiseptic technique to prevent introducing pathogenic bacteria into the sterile urinary tract and causing a urinary tract infection.

BOX 25.8

Nursing Care Planning

AN INTERPROFESSIONAL CARE MAP FOR A WOMAN WITH MASTITIS

Bailey Cheshire calls your clinic 3 weeks after childbirth because she has a fever and swelling and pain in her right breast. She comes into the clinic for an evaluation.

Family Assessment: Patient lives in three-bedroom apartment with boyfriend. Employed as a chemistry teacher but has not returned to work. Boyfriend is a short-order cook but is currently unemployed; wants her to stop breastfeeding because of her infection.

Patient Assessment: A 30-year-old primipara woman who gave birth vaginally 3 weeks ago and is breastfeeding exclusively. Temperature 101.1°F (38.4°C). Other vital signs within acceptable parameters. Right breast reddened and edematous, tender and warm to touch. Slight fissure noted on right nipple. States, "I hurt too much to breastfeed any longer. How can I be a good mother if I don't breastfeed my baby?"

Nursing Diagnosis: Pain related to development of mastitis

Outcome Criteria: Patient states amount of pain is decreasing with prescribed therapy; describes measures used to promote comfort. Breast swelling, redness, fever, and tenderness decrease.

Team Member Responsible	Assessment	Intervention	Rationale	Expected Outcome
Activities of Daily Living, Including Safety				
Nurse/primary care provider	Assess extent of mastitis and whether patient could continue breastfeeding with additional support.	Encourage patient to continue breastfeeding on left breast. Recommend patient try continuing to breastfeed on right breast.	Milk provides a medium for bacterial growth. Emptying breasts prevents stasis of milk and reduces further infection and pain.	Patient states she will try to continue breastfeeding even though infection is present.
Teamwork and Collaboration				
Nurse/lactation specialist	Assess whether patient has a support person she uses for breastfeeding advice or if she would like one.	Suggest patient contact the local La Leche League chapter hotline for consultation and support.	Support from experts in the technique of breastfeeding can offer helpful tips to ensure success.	Patient states she will contact a support service for additional information within 2 days.
Procedures/Medications for Quality Improvement				
Nurse/primary care provider	Assess what actions patient feels will help relieve her pain best.	Instruct patient in ways to apply warm moist heat, such as with a shower or warm packs, at home.	Moist heat promotes circulation to the area, decreasing inflammation, edema, and pain.	Patient states she understands purpose and techniques of warm, moist heat.
Nurse	Review modifying breastfeeding strategies with mastitis.	Encourage patient to nurse every 2 to 3 hours, wear a support bra, and start each infant feeding on the unaffected breast.	Beginning feeding on the unaffected breast reduces discomfort on infected breast because infant will not suck as hard on affected breast.	Patient states she will try suggested techniques.
Nutrition				
Nurse	Assess whether patient understands the importance of good fluid intake for breastfeeding success.	Advise patient to drink at least 8 glasses of fluid daily.	Fluid is important for breast milk formation and to prevent dehydration with fever.	Patient states she has access to fluid and understands the importance of fluid intake.

Continued on following page

BOX 25.8

Nursing Care Planning (continued)

Team Member Responsible	Assessment	Intervention	Rationale	Expected Outcome
Patient-Centered Care				
Nurse/nurse-midwife	Assess patient's knowledge of the cause and therapy for mastitis.	Explain mastitis is not unusual postpartum and should not interfere with continued breastfeeding.	Misconceptions can negatively affect success with breastfeeding.	Patient states the infection is not her fault, and she is not a "bad mother" because of it.
Psychosocial/Spiritual/Emotional Needs				
Nurse	Attempt to identify the meaning of breastfeeding to patient.	Encourage patient to express feelings about continuing or not continuing breastfeeding because of mastitis.	Identifying the meaning of breastfeeding assists in determining the effect a diagnosis of mastitis may have on patient.	Patient states she views this event as only a minor setback to her childrearing plans.
Informatics for Seamless Healthcare Planning				
Nurse	Determine whether patient has appointment for follow-up care.	Praise for decision-making ability to foster self-esteem. Urge boyfriend to provide breastfeeding support.	Adequate self-esteem is important to make effective childrearing decisions.	Patient will discuss lack of breastfeeding support with boyfriend and keep follow-up appointment.

Catheterizing a woman during the early postpartal period can be more difficult than usual because vulvar edema often distorts the position and appearance of the urinary meatus. Use a gentle technique, remembering that a woman's perineum is apt to feel tender to touch.

Therapeutic Management

The amount of urine to remove from an overdistended bladder is controversial. There is a suggestion that removing more than 750 to 1,000 ml of urine at any one time may create such an extreme pressure change in the lower abdomen that it causes blood to flow into the area, causing supine hypotension. There is little evidence of this actually happening, however, and particularly not in the postpartal period, when a bladder is easily distended and the uterus is larger than normal. Although this shift in pressure may not be as important as usual, follow your healthcare agency's policy concerning how much urine to remove from a full bladder at catheterization.

If an indwelling catheter will be left in place, be certain to explain the rationale for its insertion, and how the inflated balloon will hold it in place so the woman does not limit activity and leave herself open to other complications, such as thrombophlebitis.

After 24 hours, the indwelling catheter is usually clamped for a short time and then removed. Encourage a woman to void by the end of 6 hours after removal of the catheter by offering fluid, administering an analgesic so she can relax, assisting her to the bathroom as necessary, and trying time-tested solutions such as running water at the sink or letting her hold her hand under warm running water. In most women, bladder and vulvar edema have decreased so much

by this time that they are able to void without further difficulty. If a woman has not voided by 8 hours after catheter removal, she may need reinsertion of the indwelling catheter for an additional 24 hours.

Difficulty with bladder function after childbirth is becoming less of a problem because less anesthesia and fewer forceps are used at birth, thus decreasing bladder and vulvar pressure. If problems do arise, they may be difficult for a woman to accept because bladder elimination is a basic step of self-care and discouraging for a woman who wants to be able to care not only for herself but also a new infant. You can assure the woman that bladder complications are not uncommon after childbirth. Fortunately, they are usually present for no longer than 48 hours and most likely do not recur.

URINARY TRACT INFECTIONS

A woman who is catheterized at the time of childbirth or during the postpartal period is prone to the development of a urinary tract infection because bacteria may be introduced into the bladder at the time of catheterization. Pushing with labor may also have allowed some secretions to enter the urinary urethra.

Assessment

If a urinary tract infection develops, the woman notices symptoms of burning on urination, possibly blood in the urine (hematuria), and a feeling of frequency or that she always has to void. The pain feels so sharp on voiding that she may resist voiding, further compounding the problem of urinary stasis. She may also have a low-grade fever and discomfort from lower abdominal pain.

Obtain a clean-catch urine specimen from any woman with symptoms of a urinary tract infection as an independent nursing action (see Nursing Care Planning Using Procedures in Chapter 11, Box 11.6). To make sure lochial discharge does not contaminate the specimen, provide a sterile cotton ball for the woman to tuck into her vagina after perineal cleansing. Be certain to ask if she removed the cotton ball after the procedure; otherwise, it could cause stasis of vaginal secretions and increase the possibility of endometritis. Mark the specimen "possibly contaminated by lochia" so that any blood in the specimen will not be overly interpreted by the laboratory technician.

Therapeutic Management

Although sulfa drugs are usually prescribed for a urinary tract infection, they are contraindicated for breastfeeding women because they can cause neonatal jaundice. Typically, therefore, a broad-spectrum antibiotic such as amoxicillin or ampicillin will be prescribed to treat a postpartal urinary tract infection. If an antibiotic contraindicated during breastfeeding is prescribed, check with a woman's primary care provider about possibly changing the antibiotic to one that is safe for breastfeeding. Otherwise, once she is home, in order to breastfeed, the woman will not take the prescribed antibiotic.

In addition to the antibiotic, encourage a woman to drink large amounts of fluid (a glass every hour) to help flush the infection from her bladder. She may need an oral analgesic, such as acetaminophen (Tylenol), to reduce the pain of urination for the next few times she voids until the antibiotic begins to have an effect and the burning sensation disappears. Otherwise, because voiding is painful, she may not drink the fluid you suggest, knowing it will increase the number of times she needs to void.

Although symptoms of a urinary tract infection decrease quickly, be certain the woman understands the importance of continuing to take the prescribed antibiotic for the full 5 to 7 days to eradicate the infection completely. Plan with the woman what will be an effective reminder system for her to use, such as a chart on her refrigerator door or a reminder signal on her smartphone because when women are busy—and a woman caring for a newborn is busy— forgetting to take medicine is easy to do. If she stops taking the antibiotic, however, bacteria in the urine will begin to multiply again and, in another week, symptoms and the active infection will recur. Discuss with the woman common methods that all women should use to prevent urinary tract infections such as voiding after intercourse as more assurance that she can remain infection free (see Chapter 46).

What If . . . 25.3

Eight hours after birth, Bailey Cheshire tells the nurse that she has frequency and burning on urination. She had a urinary tract infection during pregnancy, so she recognizes the symptoms. Because she has some medicine left from pregnancy, she tells the nurse there's no need to report her symptoms because she will take her unused medicine to cure the infection. What advice would the nurse give her?

Cardiovascular System Disorders

Because pregnancy requires major changes in the volume of blood and gestational hypertension may occur, some excess volume and pressure changes can still be present in the postpartal period.

POSTPARTAL PREECLAMPSIA

Because preeclampsia usually develops during pregnancy, it is discussed in Chapter 21. Mild preexisting hypertension from this may increase in severity during the first few hours or days after birth. Rarely, it develops for the first time in a woman who has had no prenatal or intranatal symptoms. When this happens, the cardinal symptoms are the same as those of prenatal preeclampsia: proteinuria, edema, and increased blood pressure (Takaoka, Ishii, Taguchi, et al., 2016).

The reason the condition occurs is usually retention of some placental material. The woman may be taken to surgery to have a D&C to be certain all placental fragments have been removed from her uterus. After the D&C, blood pressure often falls dramatically to normal. If not, continued treatment measures are the same as for antepartal preeclampsia: bed rest, a quiet atmosphere, frequent monitoring of vital signs and urine output, and the administration of magnesium sulfate or an antihypertensive agent. Antihypertensive therapy can be administered in higher doses than during pregnancy because there is no longer any risk of injury to a fetus.

Seizures, if they occur postpartally as a symptom of eclampsia, typically develop 6 to 24 hours after birth. Seizures occurring more than 72 hours after birth are probably not the result of eclampsia but the result of some cause unrelated to childbearing.

Women in whom postpartal preeclampsia develops may be bewildered by what has happened to them. If seizures occur, they are frightened to discover how little control they have over their body. They worry they will have a seizure after they are at home while holding their baby. You can assure them that preeclampsia, although it appears late, is a condition of pregnancy, so the symptoms will fade quickly. Women with chronic hypertension need frequent monitoring during a future pregnancy to help detect preeclampsia symptoms should these occur (Anjum, Goel, Sharma, et al., 2016).

Reproductive System Disorders

Pregnancy has the potential to leave reproductive system organs weakened or displaced, especially in women with grand multiparity or who had an instrument birth.

REPRODUCTIVE TRACT DISPLACEMENT

If the ligaments of the uterus are weakened because of pregnancy, they may no longer be able to maintain the uterus in its usual position or level after pregnancy, thus creating concerns such as retroflexion, anteflexion, retroversion, and anteversion or prolapse of the uterus. These uterine displacement disorders can interfere with future childbearing and fertility and may cause continued pain or a feeling of lower abdominal heaviness or discomfort.

If the walls of the vagina are weakened, a cystocele (outpouching of the bladder into the vaginal wall) or a rectocele (outpouching of the rectum into the vaginal wall) may occur (see Chapter 5, Figs. 5.7A and B). These are identified on pelvic exam or by sonogram (Lamblin, Delorme, Cosson, et al., 2016). If extensive, surgery to repair such conditions may be necessary. If stress incontinence (involuntary voiding on exertion) occurs, Kegel exercises to strengthen perineal muscles, injection of bulking agents, pelvic floor physical therapy, or Botox may be helpful (Vitale, Laganà, Gulino, et al., 2016).

SEPARATION OF THE SYMPHYSIS PUBIS

During pregnancy, many women feel some discomfort at the symphysis pubis because of relaxation of the joint preparatory for birth. If a fetus is unusually large or the fetal position is not optimal, the ligaments of the symphysis pubis may be so stretched by birth they actually tear. After birth, the woman experiences acute pain on turning or walking; her legs tend to rotate externally, giving her a waddling gait. A defect over the symphysis pubis can be palpated: The area is swollen and feels tender to touch (Urraca-Gesto, Plaza-Manzano, Ferragut-Garcías, et al., 2015).

Bed rest and the application of a snug pelvic binder to immobilize the joint may be necessary to relieve pain and allow healing. As with all ligament injuries, a 4- to 6-week period is necessary for healing to be complete. During this time, a woman should avoid heavy lifting; she may need to arrange for a person to help her with child care at home. She may be advised to consider a cesarean birth for any future pregnancy.

Emotional and Psychological Complications of the Puerperium

Any woman who is extremely stressed or who gives birth to an infant who in any way does not meet her expectations such as being the wrong sex, being physically or cognitively challenged, or being ill may become so depressed she has difficulty bonding with her infant. Both depression and an inability to bond is a postpartal complication with far-reaching implications, possibly affecting the future health of the entire family.

POSTPARTAL DEPRESSION

Almost every woman notices some immediate (1 to 10 days postpartum) feelings of sadness (postpartal "blues") after childbirth. This probably occurs as a response to the anticlimactic feeling after birth and also probably is related to hormonal shifts as the levels of estrogen, progesterone, and gonadotropin-releasing hormone in her body decline.

In as many as 20% of women, however, especially in women who are disappointed in some aspect of their newborn or who have poor family support, these normal feelings continue beyond the immediate postpartal period (possibly as long as 1 year) or reflect a more serious problem than usual "baby blues." They become **postpartum depression** (Box 25.9). Depression of this type, manifested by overwhelming sadness, can occur in both new mothers and fathers (Paulson, Bazemore, Goodman, et al., 2016).

The syndrome can interfere with breastfeeding, child care, and returning to a career. Both women and men may notice extreme fatigue, an inability to stop crying, increased anxiety about their own or their infant's health, insecurity (unwillingness to be left alone or inability to make decisions), psychosomatic symptoms (nausea and vomiting, diarrhea), and either depressive or extreme mood fluctuations (Paulson et al., 2016) (Table 25.2). Risk factors for postpartal depression include:

- History of depression
- Troubled childhood
- Low self-esteem
- Stress in the home or at work
- Lack of effective support
- Different expectations between partners (e.g., if a woman wants a child and her partner does not)
- Disappointment in the child (e.g., a boy instead of a girl)

It is difficult to predict which women will develop postpartal depression before birth because childbirth can result

---

BOX 25.9
Nursing Care Planning Tips for Effective Communication

Bailey Cheshire is about to be discharged from the hospital 72 hours after childbirth. You notice that although her boyfriend visited with her, left some baby clothes, and then went downstairs to complete the discharge papers, Bailey has made no attempt to change to street clothes or dress her new baby in the baseball jersey her boyfriend left for the baby.

Tip: Be sure to ask enough questions to be certain a woman's sadness is not something more serious than simple "baby blues" before she is discharged from the healthcare facility so she can be referred to the proper professional for help and support. Almost all women experience some fatigue after childbirth. As many as 70% experience a temporary feeling of sadness (baby blues). About 10%, however, develop depression severe enough to need therapy.

Nurse: Bailey? Are you ready to leave?

Bailey: I feel too tired to go home. Are you sure I can't stay?

Nurse: Tell me more about that.

Bailey: I'm so tired it feels easier for me to sit here and cry than go home, work full-time, and take care of this baby.

Nurse: Is that different from how you thought things would be?

Bailey: I thought he'd ask me to marry him if I had a baby. Bet he would have if I'd had a boy instead of a girl.

Nurse: I'd like to ask you a few more questions about how you're feeling [this would be a great time to do a depression screen like the PHQ-9 or the EPDS]. I'd also like for our social worker to see you to make sure you have all the information you need about feeling sad after having a baby before you go home.

TABLE 25.2 COMPARING POSTPARTAL BLUES, DEPRESSION, AND PSYCHOSIS

	Postpartal Blues	Postpartal Depression	Postpartal Psychosis
Onset	1–10 days after birth	1–12 months after birth	Within first year after birth
Symptoms	Sadness, tears	Anxiety, feeling of loss, sadness	Delusions or hallucinations of harming infant or self
Incidence	70% of all births	10% of all births	1%–2% of all births
Etiology (possible)	Probable hormonal changes, stress of life changes	History of previous depression, hormonal response, lack of social support	Possible activation of previous mental illness, hormonal changes, family history of bipolar disorder
Therapy	Support, empathy	Counseling, possibly drug therapy	Psychotherapy, drug therapy
Nursing role	Offer compassion and understanding	Screen for depression and refer to counseling	Refer to psychiatric care, safeguarding mother from injury to self and newborn

American Psychiatric Association. (2013). *Diagnostic and statistical manual of mental disorders* (5th ed.). Arlington, VA: Author; Feingold, S. B. (2013). *Happy endings, new beginnings: Navigating postpartum disorders*. Far Hill, NJ: New Horizon Press.

in so many varied reactions. In the postpartal period, discovery of the problem as soon as symptoms develop is a nursing priority. A number of depression scales to help detect postpartum depression are available (such as the Patient Health Questionnaire-9 (PHQ-9) or the Edinburgh Postnatal Depression Scale [EPDS]), but conscientious observation and discussion with women can reveal symptoms as well. The woman may need counseling and possibly antidepressant therapy to integrate the experience of childbirth into her life (O'Connor, Rossom, Henninger, et al., 2016). This is crucial to the development of a healthy maternal–infant bond, to the health of any other children in the family, and to overall family functioning. Ask at postpartal return visits and well-child visits about symptoms that would suggest depression and recommend an appropriate referral. Measures to help prevent depression are shown in Box 25.10.

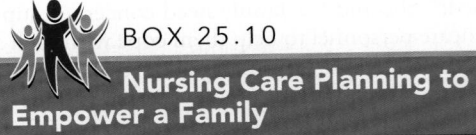

BOX 25.10

Nursing Care Planning to Empower a Family

Q. Bailey asks you, "How can I avoid becoming depressed after I return home with my new baby?"

A. Some helpful guidelines include:

- Plan a balanced program of nutrition, exercise, and sleep. Plan meals that are easy to prepare, sleep whenever your baby sleeps, and begin a program of walking daily with your baby.
- Share your feelings with a support person. Many communities have postpartum support groups to help with this.
- Take some time every day to do something for yourself (e.g., work on a scrapbook, go shopping) so you have a break from baby care.
- Do not try to be perfect. Analyze what are the important things to do and get them done. Let unimportant things go for another day.
- Do not let yourself be isolated by baby care. Use the Internet or your cell phone to keep in contact with your friends so you are not lonely.

QSEN Checkpoint Question 25.5

EVIDENCE-BASED PRACTICE

Postpartal depression affects not only the postpartum woman but also her entire family because partners can become depressed during this time as well. To assess developmental impacts on children, researchers assessed 192 fathers, 54 who met criteria for depression, and their interactions with their infants in a play session. Fathers with depression were more likely to be withdrawn in their behavior with their infants, providing less stimulation for their babies (Sethna, Murray, Netsi, et al., 2015). Based on the given study, which statement by Bailey's boyfriend would concern the nurse he might be as depressed as she seems to be?

   a. "I never guessed I'd ever really be lucky enough to be a father."
   b. "I don't like talking to the baby yet. She can't talk back yet."
   c. "I didn't really understand the reason that Bailey bled after the baby was born."
   d. "No one told me women could become depressed after birth."

Look in Appendix A for the best answer and rationale.

POSTPARTAL PSYCHOSIS

As many as 1 woman in 500 has enough symptoms during the year after the birth of a child to be considered psychiatrically ill (this statistic seems high but represents the current rate of overall mental illness in woman) (American Psychiatric Association [APA], 2013). When the illness coincides with the postpartal period or occurs during the following year, it is termed **postpartal psychosis**. Rather than being a response to the physical aspects of childbearing, it is probably a response to the crisis of childbearing. The majority of these women have had symptoms of mental illness before pregnancy. If the pregnancy had not precipitated the illness, a death in the family, loss of a job or income, divorce, or some other major life crisis might have precipitated the same recurrence.

A woman with postpartal psychosis usually appears exceptionally sad. By definition, psychosis exists when a person has lost contact with reality. Because of this break with reality, the woman may deny she has had a child and, when the child is brought to her, insist she was never pregnant. She may voice thoughts of infanticide or that her infant is possessed. If observation tells you a woman is not functioning in reality, you cannot improve her concept of reality by simple measures such as explaining what her correct perception should be because her sensory input is too disturbed to comprehend this. In addition, she may interpret your contrasting opinion as threatening and respond with anger or threats. Instead, the woman needs referral to a professional psychiatric counselor and probably antipsychotic medication (Kimmel, Lara-Cinisomo, Melvin, et al., 2016).

While waiting for such a skilled professional to arrive, do not leave the woman alone because her distorted perception might lead her to harm herself. In addition, don't leave her alone with her infant because she could harm the infant as well.

Always keep in mind when evaluating women during pregnancy or the puerperium that postpartal psychosis, although rare, does exist. Remembering childbearing can lead to this degree of mental illness helps you to put childbearing into perspective. Because it can cause such a crisis in a woman's life, it cannot be considered an everyday incident in anyone's life.

QSEN Checkpoint Question 25.6

PATIENT-CENTERED CARE

The nurse is making an effort to address Bailey Cheshire's psychosocial health in addition to her physiologic well-being. Which of Bailey's statements would be most suggestive of possible postpartal psychosis?

a. "I wish my baby had longer hair."
b. "I've felt exhausted ever since birth."
c. "I'm happy not to have any children."
d. "Breastfeeding is way harder than I thought."

Look in Appendix A for the best answer and rationale.

WOMEN WITH UNIQUE POSTPARTAL CARE NEEDS

A number of women have unique postpartal needs because of unexpected circumstances.

The Woman Whose Child Is Born With an Illness or a Physical Challenge

Immediately after birth, the average woman often has momentary difficulty believing that her pregnancy is finally over, and her child has been born. This difficulty can be compounded for a woman whose child is challenged in some way because she must not only grasp the fact that her baby has been born but also that her baby is different from the one she envisioned (Riley & Baas, 2015).

During pregnancy, most women say they do not care about the sex of their child as long as the child is born healthy. This can make them feel cheated or disappointed when this one requirement is not met. They may experience a loss of self-esteem: They have given birth to an imperfect child and so they see themselves as imperfect. A woman sometimes responds with a grief reaction, as if her child had died because the image of the "perfect" child she thought she was carrying *has* died.

Parents should be shown their child moments after birth so if a condition or problem exists, the newborn's condition, prognosis, and usual plans for care can be immediately explained to them. Although hearing such an explanation is a shock to couples, it allows them to face the problem as early as possible and while they are surrounded by professional support people. The primary care provider usually makes it her or his responsibility to tell the parents about the infant's concern. Be prepared to reinforce this information or review the explanation during the postpartum period because people who are under stress are not good listeners and may need repeated explanations before they completely understand the problem.

Encourage the parents to care for the child during the postpartal period, so they can touch, relate to, and "claim" the infant in as nearly normal a manner as possible. Many women wait until their support person is present to visit an intensive care nursery so that visiting with their ill newborn is a family activity.

Open lines of communication between the parents and the hospital staff, which allow for free discussion of feelings and fears, will do much to strengthen parent–child relationships and prepare for future hospitalizations or care of the child.

The Woman Whose Newborn Has Died

A woman whose newborn dies at birth always has questions about what happened. She is likely to feel bewildered, perhaps bitter, and perhaps resentful that despite emergency interventions, the hospital staff was not able to save her child. She asks, "Why me? Of all the women here, why was my baby the one who died?" She and her family need concerned support from healthcare personnel to help them cope with such a devastating loss (Ellis, Chebsey, Storey, et al., 2016).

Most women are interested in seeing the baby. This is generally therapeutic because it helps them begin grieving. Clean the baby, wrap the baby in an infant blanket, and bring him or her to the parents. Remain with them but give them time to handle and inspect the child as they wish. Parents may want to take a photograph or a lock of hair for a memory book. Be familiar with the forms the mother or father have to sign when a baby dies or is born dead. Know whether your state requires stillborn infants to be given a name and a burial.

Other women on the unit tend to stay away from a woman whose child has died, as if what happened to her baby is contagious. Friends and relatives may be equally unable to talk about the situation. Most women, therefore, are anxious to have a nurse approach them and say, "Do you want to talk about what's happened?" Be careful not to use trite sympathy phrases such as "one door closes, another one opens" or "God must have another purpose for you" because although these may be your beliefs, they may not be the woman's beliefs.

Provide a private room for the family to allow them an opportunity to grieve and visit freely as they begin to work through this potentially devastating event in their life. The process of grieving and the support a woman requires at this time is further discussed in Chapter 56.

What If . . . 25.4

The nurse is particularly interested in exploring one of the 2020 National Health Goals with respect to complications of the puerperium (see Box 25.1). What would be a possible research topic to explore pertinent to this goal that would be applicable to Bailey's family and that would also advance evidence-based practice?

KEY POINTS FOR REVIEW

- Hemorrhage (defined as a loss of blood greater than 500 ml within a 24-hour period) is a major potential danger in the immediate postpartal period. The most frequent causes of postpartal hemorrhage are uterine atony or a retained placental fragment. Continuous limited blood loss can be as important as sudden, intense bleeding. Administration of oxytocin or uterotonics may be necessary to initiate uterine tone and halt the bleeding.

- Other causes of hemorrhage include lacerations (vaginal, cervical, or perineal) and DIC. Lacerations are most apt to occur with an instrument birth or with the birth of a large infant.

- Puerperal infection (a temperature greater than 100.4°F [38.0°C]) after the first 24 hours is a potential complication after any birth until the denuded placental surface has healed. Retained placental fragments and the use of internal fetal monitoring leads are potential sources of infection.

- Thrombophlebitis, an inflammation of the lining of a blood vessel, occurs most often as an extension of an endometrial infection. Therapy includes bed rest with moist heat applications and anticoagulant therapy. *Never massage the leg of a woman with thrombophlebitis.* Doing so can cause the clot to move and become a pulmonary embolus, which is a possibly fatal complication.

- Mastitis is an infection of the breast. The symptoms include pain, swelling, and redness. Antibiotic therapy is necessary to promote healing.

- Postpartal "blues" are a normal accompaniment to birth. Postpartal depression (a feeling of extreme sadness) and postpartal psychosis (an actual separation from reality) are not normal and need accurate assessment so a woman can receive adequate therapy for these conditions.

- A woman whose child dies at birth or is born with a physical or cognitive challenge needs special consideration after birth. This obviously creates a time of stress, and a woman needs supportive nursing care.

- Establishing a firm family–newborn relationship may be difficult when a woman has a postpartal complication. Planning nursing care that allows a woman to care for her baby and begin her new family role not only meets QSEN competencies but also best meets a family's total needs.

CRITICAL THINKING CARE STUDY

Jonella is a 37-year-old gravida 5, para 5 who gave birth to a boy (8 lb 6 oz) last night. You enter her postpartum room because you've noticed her newborn has been crying for some time. You find Jonella lying in bed reading from an electronic reader, seemingly unaware that her baby, swaddled in a bassinette at the foot of the bed, is crying. When you ask her if she would like some help with her newborn, she sighs as if exhausted, slowly puts down her reader, and says, "I'm waiting for someone to bring him a bottle." Jonella's chart shows she's not going to breastfeed because she has four other children (10, 8, 5, and 2 years of age) at home. Her husband's occupation is listed as a maintenance man on a Gulf of Mexico oil rig. Because her labor only lasted 6 hours, he wasn't able to get home in time to be with her in labor. Her mother also couldn't come because she is watching Jonella's other children.

1. Jonella seems less than pleased to have had a new baby. Is her attitude typical for a mother having her fifth child or would you want to investigate mother–newborn bonding further?

2. Jonella had an episiotomy for birth and so has painful perineal stitches. She's had urinary retention since birth and has a Foley catheter inserted. When her husband arrives, you notice he is enthusiastic about having a boy because now he has a "basketball team of boys." He confides to you the only reason his wife consented to have another child was because she was certain this one would be the girl she always wanted. He tells you, "Guess she's pretty depressed." Could Jonella's lack of interest in her baby be the beginning of postpartal depression? What risk factors does she have for developing this?

3. Jonella will be discharged tomorrow. Her husband will be back at work in 3 days, and her mother has arthritis and so is "little help." In addition to developing postpartal depression, for what other postpartal complications is Jonella high risk?

RELATED RESOURCES

Explore these additional resources to enhance learning for this chapter:
- Student resources on thePoint, including answers to the What If . . . and Critical Thinking Care Study questions, http://thepoint.lww.com/Flagg8e
- Adaptive learning powered by PrepU, http://thepoint.lww.com/prepu

REFERENCES

Al-Thani, H., El-Menyar, A., Asim, M., et al. (2016). Clinical presentation, management, and outcomes of deep vein thrombosis based on doppler ultrasonography examination. *Angiology, 67*(6), 587–595.

American Psychiatric Association. (2013). *Diagnostic and statistical manual of mental disorders* (5th ed.). Arlington, VA: Author.

Andrighetti, T. (2013). Postpartum hemorrhage: Best practices in management. In B. A. Anderson & S. Stone (Eds.), *Best practices in midwifery: Using the evidence to implement change* (pp. 243–256). New York, NY: Springer Publishing.

Anjum, S., Goel, N., Sharma, R., et al. (2016). Maternal outcomes after 12 hours and 24 hours of magnesium sulfate therapy for eclampsia. *International Journal of Gynaecology and Obstetrics, 132*(1), 68–71.

Atilgan, R., Ozkan, Z. S., Orak, U., et al. (2014). Complete tamponade system for management of severe postpartum vaginal haemorrhage due to uterine atony. *BMJ Case Reports, 2014*, 1–2.

Bateman, B. T., Tsen, L. C., Liu, J., et al. (2014). Patterns of second-line uterotonic use in a large sample of hospitalizations for childbirth in the United States: 2007-2011. *Anesthesia and Analgesia, 119*(6), 1344–1349.

Dahlke, J. D., Mendez-Figueroa, H., Maggio, L., et al. (2015). Prevention and management of postpartum hemorrhage: A comparison of 4 national guidelines. *American Journal of Obstetrics and Gynecology, 213*(1), 76.e1–76.e10.

Ellis, A., Chebsey, C., Storey, C., et al. (2016). Systematic review to understand and improve care after stillbirth: A review of parents' and healthcare professionals' experiences. *BMC Pregnancy Childbirth, 16*(1), 16.

Galvão, A., Braga, A. C., Gonçalves, D. R., et al. (2016). Sepsis during pregnancy or the postpartum period. *Journal of Obstetrics and Gynaecology, 36*(6), 735–743.

Ghosh, S. B., & Mala, Y. M. (2015). Alternate sequential suture tightening: A novel technique for uncontrolled postpartum hemorrhage. *Obstetrics and Gynecology International, 2015,* 145178.

Grobman, W. A., Bailit, J. L., Rice, M. M., et al. (2015). Racial and ethnic disparities in maternal morbidity and obstetric care. *Obstetrics and Gynecology, 125*(6), 1460–1467.

Guntupalli, K. K., Karnad, D. R., Bandi, V., et al. (2015). Critical illness in pregnancy: Part II: Common medical conditions complicating pregnancy and puerperium. *Chest, 148*(5), 1333–1345.

Irusen, H., Rohwer, A. C., Steyn, D. W., et al. (2015). Treatments for breast abscesses in breastfeeding women. *Cochrane Database of Systematic Reviews,* (8), CD010490.

Karch, A. M. (2015). *Lippincott's nursing drug guide.* Philadelphia, PA: Lippincott Williams & Wilkins.

Kimmel, M. C., Lara-Cinisomo, S., Melvin, K., et al. (2016). Treatment of severe perinatal mood disorders on a specialized perinatal psychiatry inpatient unit. *Archives of Women's Mental Health, 19*(4), 645–653.

Konkle, B. A. (2015). Diagnosis and management of thrombosis in pregnancy. *Birth Defects Research. Part C, Embryo Today, 105*(3), 185–189.

Laifer-Narin, S. L., Kwak, E., Kim, H., et al. (2014). Multimodality imaging of the postpartum or posttermination uterus: Evaluation using ultrasound, computed tomography, and magnetic resonance imaging. *Current Problems in Diagnostic Radiology, 43*(6), 374–385.

Lamblin, G., Delorme, E., Cosson, M., et al. (2016). Cystocele and functional anatomy of the pelvic floor: Review and update of the various theories. *International Urogynecology Journal, 27*(9), 1297–1305.

Lang, D. L., Zhao, F. L., & Robertson, J. (2015). Prevention of postpartum haemorrhage: Cost consequences analysis of misoprostol in low-resource settings. *BMC Pregnancy and Childbirth, 15*(1), 305.

Mulder, F. E., Oude Rengerink, K., van der Post, J. A., et al. (2016). Delivery-related risk factors for covert postpartum urinary retention after vaginal delivery. *International Urogynecology Journal, 27*(1), 55–60.

O'Connor, E., Rossom, R. C., Henninger, M., et al. (2016). Primary care screening for and treatment of depression in pregnant and postpartum women: Evidence report and systematic review for the US preventive services task force. *JAMA, 315*(4), 388–406.

Odom, E. C., Li, R., Scanlon, K. S., et al. (2013). Reasons for earlier than desired cessation of breastfeeding. *Pediatrics, 131*(3), e726–e732.

Paulson, J. F., Bazemore, S. D., Goodman, J. H., et al. (2016). The course and interrelationship of maternal and paternal perinatal depression. *Archives of Women's Mental Health, 19*(4), 655–663.

Pratts, M. E., & Henderson, J. (2015). Gestational complications. In J. L. Bienstock, H. Fox, E. E. Wallach, et al. (Eds.), *The Johns Hopkins manual of gynecology and obstetrics* (5th ed., pp. 116–127). Philadelphia, PA: Lippincott Williams & Wilkins.

Pustotina, O. (2015). Management of mastitis and breast engorgement in breastfeeding women. *The Journal of Maternal-Fetal & Neonatal Medicine, 29*(19), 3121–3125.

Riley, C., & Baas Rubarth, L. B. (2015). Supporting families of children with disabilities. *Journal of Obstetric, Gynecologic & Neonatal Nursing, 44*(4), 536–542.

Sethna, V., Murray, L., Netsi, E., et al. (2015). Paternal depression in the postnatal period and early father-infant interactions. *Parenting, Science and Practice, 15*(1), 1–8.

Shanks, A. L., Mehra, S., Gross, G., et al. (2016). Treatment utility of postpartum antibiotics in chorioamnionitis study. *American Journal of Perinatology, 33*(8), 732–737.

Silver, R. M. (2015). Abnormal placentation: Placenta previa, vasa previa, and placenta accreta. *Obstetrics and Gynecology, 126*(3), 654–668.

Takaoka, S., Ishii, K., Taguchi, T., et al. (2016). Clinical features and antenatal risk factors for postpartum-onset hypertensive disorders. *Hypertension in Pregnancy, 35*(1), 22–31.

U.S. Department of Health and Human Services. (2010). *Healthy people 2020.* Washington, DC: Author.

Urraca-Gesto, M. A., Plaza-Manzano, G., Ferragut-Garcías, A., et al. (2015). Diastasis of symphysis pubis and labor: Systematic review. *Journal of Rehabilitation Research and Development, 52*(6), 629–640.

Vintejoux, E., Ulrich, D., Mousty, E., et al. (2015). Success factors for Bakri™ balloon usage secondary to uterine atony: A retrospective, multicentre study. *The Australian and New Zealand Journal of Obstetrics and Gynaecology, 55*(6), 572–577.

Vitale, S. G., Laganà, A. S., Gulino, F. A., et al. (2016). Prosthetic surgery versus native tissue repair of cystocele: Literature review. *Updates in Surgery, 68*(4), 325–329.

Weeks, A. D., & Mallaiah, S. (2016). Beyond MBRRACE: New developments to stem the tide of postpartum haemorrhage. *European Journal of Obstetrics & Gynecology and Reproductive Biology, 199,* 66–68.

Witt, A. M., Bolman, M., Kredit, S., et al. (2016). Therapeutic breast massage in lactation for the management of engorgement, plugged ducts, and mastitis. *Journal of Human Lactation, 32*(1), 123–131.

World Health Organization. (2015). *Pregnancy, childbirth, postpartum and newborn care: A guide for essential practice* (3rd ed.). Geneva: Switzerland.

Zielinski, R., Ackerson, K., Kane Low, L. (2015). Planned home birth: Benefits, risks, and opportunities. *International Journal of Women's Health, 7,* 361–377.

26

Nursing Care of a Family With a High-Risk Newborn

KEY TERMS

acute bilirubin encephalopathy (ABE)

apnea

apparent life-threatening event (ALTE)

appropriate for gestational age (AGA)

brown fat

developmental care

dysmature

extremely-low-birth-weight (ELBW) infant

extracorporeal membrane oxygenation (ECMO)

fetal alcohol spectrum disorder

gestational age

hemorrhagic disease of the newborn

hydrops fetalis

hyperbilirubinemia

intrauterine growth restriction (IUGR)

large for gestational age (LGA)

low–birth-weight (LBW) infant

macrosomia

ophthalmia neonatorum

periodic respirations

periventricular leukomalacia (PVL)

postterm infants

preterm infants

retinopathy of prematurity (ROP)

shoulder dystocia

small for gestational age (SGA)

term infants

very-low-birth-weight (VLBW) infant

OBJECTIVES

After mastering the contents of this chapter, you should be able to:

1. Define the common classifications of high-risk infants and describe common illnesses that occur in these classifications of newborns.

2. Identify 2020 National Health Goals related to high-risk newborns that nurses can help the nation achieve.

3. Assess a high-risk newborn to determine whether safe transition to extrauterine life has occurred.

4. Formulate nursing diagnoses related to a high-risk newborn and family.

5. Identify expected outcomes for a high-risk newborn and family to help parents manage seamless transitions across differing healthcare settings.

6. Using the nursing process, plan nursing care that includes the six competencies of Quality & Safety Education for Nurses (QSEN): Patient-Centered Care, Teamwork & Collaboration, Evidence-Based Practice (EBP), Quality Improvement (QI), Safety, and Informatics.

7. Implement nursing care for a high-risk newborn, such as monitoring body temperature.
8. Evaluate expected outcomes for achievement and effectiveness of care.
9. Integrate knowledge of the needs of a high-risk newborn with the interplay of nursing process, the six competencies of QSEN, and Family Nursing to promote quality maternal and child health nursing care.

During pregnancy, screening women for risk factors such as younger or older than average maternal age, having concurrent disease conditions such as diabetes or HIV infection, experiencing pregnancy complications such as placenta previa, or an unhealthy maternal lifestyle such as drug abuse—all of which could lead to illness in a newborn—is essential to identify infants who may need greater than usual care at birth (Eken, Tuten, Ozkaya, et al., 2016; Hoppe, 2013).

Unfortunately, not all instances of high risk can be predicted during pregnancy or birth because even a newborn from a "perfect" pregnancy may require specialized care or may develop a problem over the first few days of life, necessitating special interventions. Any infant, especially one who is born **dysmature** (a newborn whose birth weight is inappropriately low for gestational age), whether preterm, term, or postterm, is at risk for complications at birth or in the first few days of life. Parents need a thorough explanation of their baby's health because these problems may require rehospitalization or additional follow-up at home. Because preterm birth, in particular, has the potential for leading to high-risk newborns, several 2020 National Health Goals directly concern preterm births (Box 26.1).

Being able to predict if an infant is at high risk allows for advanced preparation so that specialized, skilled healthcare personnel can be present at the child's birth to perform necessary interventions, such as resuscitating a newborn who has difficulty establishing respirations. Immediate, skilled handling of any problems that occur may help to save the newborn's life and also prevent future problems, such as neurologic disorders (Wyckoff, Aziz, Escobedo, et al., 2015).

Nursing Process Overview

ASSESSMENT

All infants need to be assessed at birth for obvious congenital anomalies and **gestational age** (number of weeks the newborn remained in utero). Both determinations can be done by the nurse who first examines an infant. Be certain such a first assessment is done under a prewarmed radiant heat warmer to guard against heat loss.

Continuing assessment of high-risk infants involves the use of technology and equipment such as cardiac, apnea, oxygen saturation, and blood pressure monitoring. Regardless of how many monitors are used, they do not replace the role of frequent, close, common sense observations by a nurse who knows an infant well from having cared for the baby consistently over time because such a nurse often senses changes before a monitor or other equipment begins to put a quantitative measurement on the change. Carefully evaluate comments from fellow nurses such as an infant "isn't himself" or "breathes irregularly." These comments, although not evidence based, are the same observations that parents who know their baby well report at healthcare visits.

NURSING DIAGNOSIS

To establish nursing diagnoses for high-risk infants, it is important to be aware of the usual parameters of newborns. Examples of nursing diagnoses that center on the priority areas of care for all newborns include:

- Ineffective airway clearance related to the presence of mucus or amniotic fluid in the airway
- Ineffective tissue oxygenation related to breathing difficulty
- Ineffective thermoregulation related to immature status
- Risk for deficient fluid volume related to insensible water loss
- Risk for imbalanced nutrition, less than body requirements, related to the lack of strength for effective sucking
- Risk for infection related to lowered immune response due to prematurity
- Risk for impaired parenting related to illness in newborn at birth

---

BOX 26.1

Nursing Care Planning Based on 2020 National Health Goals

A preterm birth has the potential for leading to so many complications in newborns that several 2020 National Health Goals were written specifically concerning preterm birth:

- Reduce low birth weight (LBW) to an incidence of no more than 7.8% of live births and very low birth weight (VLBW) to an incidence of no more than 1.4% of live births from baselines of 8.2% and 1.5%, respectively.
- Increase the proportion of VLBW infants born at level III hospitals or subspecialty perinatal centers from a baseline of 76.1% to a target level of 83.7%.
- Reduce the rate of fetal and infant deaths during the perinatal period (28 weeks of gestation to 7 days or more after birth) to 5.9 per 1,000 live births from a baseline of 6.6 per 1,000 live births.
- Reduce the rate of deaths from sudden infant death syndrome (SIDS) to 0.5 per 1,000 live births from a baseline of 0.55 per 1,000 live births (U.S. Department of Health and Human Services, 2010; see www.healthypeople.gov).

Nurses can help the nation achieve these goals by teaching women the symptoms of preterm labor so that, ideally, birth can be delayed until infants reach term. Nurses also need to be prepared for resuscitation at birth for high-risk infants and to plan developmental care that can help prevent conditions such as apnea, intraventricular hemorrhage, and periventricular leukomalacia.

- Deficient diversional activity (lack of stimulation) related to illness at birth
- Readiness for developmental care to decrease overstimulation easily caused by necessary lifesaving procedures

OUTCOME IDENTIFICATION AND PLANNING

Be certain when establishing expected outcomes that they are consistent with a newborn's potential. A goal that implies complete recovery from a major illness, for example, may be unrealistic for one newborn but completely appropriate for another. Be certain plans for care are individualized considering a newborn's developmental level as well as physiologic strengths, weaknesses, and needs. Many families of a high-risk newborn will need support to care for their infant at home and therefore may need a referral to a home health care or other agency. Direct patients to helpful websites and other resources when appropriate (see Chapter 20).

IMPLEMENTATION

Interventions for any high-risk newborn are best carried out by a consistent caregiver and should focus on conserving the baby's energy and providing a thermoneutral environment to prevent exhaustion and hypothermia. Painful procedures should be kept to a minimum to help the infant achieve a sense of comfort and balance. Assisting parents to participate in care such as bathing or feeding their infant can help make the child real to them for the first time and can set the stage for effective bonding.

OUTCOME EVALUATION

High-risk newborns need long-term follow-up so any consequences of their birth status, such as minimal neurologic injury, can be identified, and arrangements for special schooling or counseling can be made. Examples of expected outcomes include:

- Infant maintains a patent airway.
- Infant demonstrates an ability to suck effectively.
- Infant tolerates procedures without accompanying apnea, bradycardia, or oxygen desaturation.
- Infant demonstrates growth and development appropriate for gestational age, birth weight, and condition.
- Infant maintains a body temperature of 98.6°F (37.0°C) in an open crib with one added blanket.
- Parents visit at least once and make three telephone calls to the neonatal nursery weekly.
- Parents demonstrate positive coping skills and behaviors in response to the newborn's condition and ability to care for their newborn.

Newborn Priorities in the First Days of Life

All newborns have a number of needs in the first few days of life that take priority. They include:

1. Initiation and maintenance of respirations
2. Establishment of extrauterine circulation
3. Maintenance of fluid and electrolyte balance
4. Control of body temperature
5. Intake of adequate nourishment
6. Establishment of waste elimination

7. Prevention of infection
8. Establishment of an infant–parent/caregiver relationship
9. Institution of developmental care or care that balances physiologic needs and stimulation for best development

These same needs are also the primary needs of high-risk newborns. Because of small size or immaturity or illness, however, fulfilling these needs may require special equipment or care measures. Not all newborns will be able to achieve full wellness because of extreme insults to their health during pregnancy or at birth or difficulty adjusting to extrauterine life. Indications a newborn is having difficulty making the immediate transition from intrauterine to extrauterine life may be first apparent by a low Apgar score rating (see Chapter 18).

INITIATING AND MAINTAINING RESPIRATIONS

Ultimately, the prognosis of a high-risk newborn depends primarily on how the first moments of life are managed because most deaths occurring during the first 48 hours after birth result from the newborn's inability to establish or maintain adequate respirations (National Vital Statistics Service [NVSS], 2011). An infant who has difficulty accomplishing effective breathing may experience residual neurologic morbidities as a result of cerebral hypoxia. Therefore, prompt, thorough, and immediate care is necessary for the best outcome.

Most infants are born with some degree of respiratory acidosis. However, this initial acidosis is rapidly corrected by the spontaneous onset of respirations. If respiratory activity does not begin immediately, respiratory acidosis not only doesn't improve but also increases in amount so much that the blood pH and bicarbonate buffer system can fail. Newborn defense mechanisms then become inadequate to reverse the process. This means the effort to establish respirations must be started immediately after birth because, by 2 minutes, the development of severe acidosis is already well under way (Dani, Bresci, Berti, et al., 2013).

Any infant who sustains any degree of asphyxia in utero, such as could occur from cord compression, maternal anesthesia, placenta previa, intrauterine growth restriction, or premature separation of the placenta, may already be experiencing acidosis at birth and may have difficulty before the first 2 minutes of life.

An additional concern that ineffective respirations creates is the failure of fetal circulatory shunts, particularly the ductus arteriosus, to close. Because left-side heart pressure is stronger than right-side pressure, blood then circulates through the patent ductus arteriosus from the left to right or from the aorta to the pulmonary artery, thus creating ineffective pump action in the heart. Struggling to breathe and circulate blood, the infant is forced to use available serum glucose quickly and so may become hypoglycemic, compounding the initial problem even further.

For all these reasons, resuscitation is important for both infants who fail to take a first breath and for those who have difficulty maintaining adequate respirations on their own (Wyckoff et al., 2015). Common factors that predispose infants to respiratory difficulty and so may require resuscitation are shown in Box 26.2.

Resuscitation

Approximately 10% of newborns require some assistance to begin breathing at birth. In order to assure newborn resuscitation can be consistent from infant to infant and one facility

BOX 26.2

Factors Predisposing Infants to Respiratory Difficulty in the First Few Days of Life

Low birth weight
Intrauterine growth restriction
Maternal history of diabetes
Premature rupture of membranes
Maternal use of barbiturates or narcotics close to birth
Meconium staining
Irregularities detected by fetal heart monitor during labor
Cord prolapse
Lowered Apgar score (<7) at 1 or 5 minutes
Postmaturity (postterm)
Small for gestational age
Breech birth
Multiple birth
Chest, heart, or respiratory tract anomalies

Figure 26.1 Suctioning a newborn with mechanical suction controlled by a finger valve. The suction is applied as the catheter is withdrawn. If the catheter is rotated as it is withdrawn, the risk of traumatizing the membrane is reduced.

to the next, the American Academy of Pediatrics (AAP) has instituted a Neonatal Resuscitation Program updated at intervals that lists steps and rationales for newborn resuscitation (Sawyer, Umoren, & Gray, 2017).

Based on these recommendations, resuscitation should follow an organized process: (a) Establish an airway, (b) expand the lungs, and (c) initiate and maintain effective ventilation. If respiratory depression becomes so severe that a newborn's heart begins to fail (heart rate is less than 60 beats/min) despite effective positive pressure ventilation, resuscitation should then also include chest compressions (Wyckoff et al., 2015).

Airway

For a well, term newborn, usually warming, drying, and stimulating the baby by rubbing the back is enough to initiate respirations. A rubber bulb syringe is a standard piece of equipment in most birthing rooms and was often used in the past to suction infants' noses and mouths, but because bradycardia can be associated with bulb suctioning, routine suctioning of the nose and mouth is no longer recommended unless there is concern that the airway is obstructed (Wyckoff et al., 2015).

If a newborn does not initiate spontaneous breathing following gentle stimulation, place the infant under a radiant heat warmer in a "sniffing" position (head slightly tipped back) and rub and dry his or her back and hair again to see if this additional stimulation initiates respirations. Assess a precordial pulse over the heart and attach a pulse oximeter to monitor oxygen saturation. It is reasonable to consider the application of a 3-lead cardiac monitor during resuscitation to obtain an accurate heart rate quickly (Wyckoff et al., 2015).

A newborn whose amniotic fluid was meconium stained at birth but is breathing does not need suctioning to clear the airway. If the newborn whose amniotic fluid was meconium stained at birth presents with poor muscle tone and inadequate breathing, it is important to begin the initial steps of resuscitation under the warmer. Positive pressure ventilation should be initiated immediately if the newborn is not breathing or the heart rate is less than 100 beats/min (Wyckoff et al., 2015). In most newborns, this degree of resuscitation will initiate responsive respirations and a strong heartbeat (over 100 beats/min).

Color, muscle tone, and reflexes will all improve. Mechanical suctioning should occur only if there is an obstruction such as a mucus plug that is interfering with effective breathing; otherwise, it may cause bradycardia (Fig. 26.1).

An infant who still makes no effort at spontaneous respirations after these initial steps may require insertion of an endotracheal tube to be certain the airway is not obstructed so air can be effectively administered. If the heart rate or oxygen saturation levels remain low with air, oxygen may be administered to achieve a preductal oxygen saturation close to the interquartile range measured in healthy term infants after vaginal delivery (Wyckoff et al., 2015).

In the first few seconds of life, a newborn this severely depressed may take several weak gasps of air and then almost immediately stop breathing; the heart rate begins to fall. This period of halted respirations is termed *primary apnea*. After 1 or 2 minutes of **apnea** (defined as a pause in respirations longer than 20 seconds with accompanying bradycardia), an infant again tries to initiate respirations with a few strong gasps. Most newborns, however, cannot maintain this effort longer than 4 or 5 minutes. After this, the respiratory effort will become weaker again and the heart rate will fall further until the newborn stops the gasping effort altogether. The infant then enters a period of *secondary apnea*. Although usually a phenomenon that occurs after birth, both types of apnea may occur in utero.

During the period of first gasps, resuscitation attempts are generally successful. Once a newborn is allowed to enter a secondary apnea period, however, resuscitation becomes difficult and may be ineffective. Because it is impossible to distinguish between the two periods simply by observation, resuscitation must always be started as if secondary apnea is the phase occurring.

A healthcare provider skilled in laryngoscope and endotracheal tube insertion should be present at the birth of all infants identified as high risk so a laryngoscope can be quickly inserted into the airway as necessary (Wyckoff et al., 2015). Laryngoscope insertion is easy in theory; in practice, the wide

Figure 26.2 Intubation. Place the head in a neutral position with a towel under the shoulders. The blade of the laryngoscope is inserted to reveal the vocal cords. An endotracheal tube for ventilation is then passed into the trachea, past the laryngoscope.

variation in the size of infants' posterior pharynges and tracheas and the emergency conditions present under which it is attempted, make it an often difficult procedure (Fig. 26.2).

Laryngoscopes are equipped with different-size blades; a size 0 or 1 should be available for newborns. Following insertion of the laryngoscope, an endotracheal tube is slid through the laryngoscope down into the trachea. Infants under 1,000 g need a 2.5-mm endotracheal tube (think of a thin coffee straw); those over 3,000 g need a 4.0-mm tube. Because preterm infants are prone to hemorrhage because of capillary fragility, gentle care during insertion is crucial.

Lung Expansion

Once an airway has been established, a newborn's lungs need to be expanded. Well newborns inflate their lungs adequately independently with a first breath. The sound of the baby crying loudly is proof that lung expansion is good because the vocal sounds are produced by a free flow of air over the vocal cords.

If an infant needs air or oxygen by bag and mask to aid lung expansion, be certain the mask covers both the mouth and the nose. However, it is important to make sure it doesn't cover the eyes because eye injury could occur from either pressure of the mask on the eyes or from drying of the cornea from air or oxygen administration. Air (or oxygen if needed) should be administered at a rate of 40 to 60 ventilations per minute. To prevent unnecessary cooling or drying, the oxygen that is administered should be both warmed (between 89.6° and 93.2°F [32° and 34°C]) and humidified (60% to 80%).

The pressure needed to open lung alveoli for the first time can be as high as 40 cm H_2O. After that, pressures of 15 to 20 cm H_2O are generally adequate to continue inflating alveoli (Wyckoff et al., 2015). The pressure from anesthesia bags is controlled solely by the pressure a healthcare provider uses when the hand squeezes against the bag. Other types of bags such as the self-inflating (Ambu) bag can be set with a blow-off valve that limits the pressure in the apparatus to be certain only gentle pressure is applied (Fig. 26.3).

It is important not to let oxygen levels in a newborn fluctuate greatly because fluctuation can cause bleeding from immature cranial vessels. In addition, applying pressure above what is necessary could rupture lung alveoli. If adequate ventilation is not achieved, however, a newborn stands little chance of survival. To be certain air is reaching the lungs with resuscitation, monitor the newborn's oxygen saturation with pulse oximetry in addition to auscultating the chest for the sounds of air movement (Wyckoff et al., 2015).

Be certain to listen to both lungs to verify both lungs are being aerated. If air can be heard on only one side or sounds are not symmetric, the endotracheal tube is probably at or below the bifurcation of the trachea (where the trachea splits into the left and right main-stem bronchi) and the tube is likely blocking the air from entering one of the main-stem bronchi. Pulling the tube back half a centimeter will usually allow oxygen to flow to both lungs. Correct placement of the endotracheal tube in the trachea and not the esophagus can be confirmed by a CO_2 monitor (no CO_2 will return if the tube is in the esophagus) immediately after insertion. An X-ray will confirm proper placement and depth in the trachea.

When air is given under pressure to a newborn this way, the stomach also quickly fills with air. If the resuscitation

Figure 26.3 Types of ventilation bags used in neonatal resuscitation. **(A)** The flow-inflating (anesthesia) bag requires a compressed gas source for inflation but is able to deliver 100% oxygen. **(B)** The self-inflating (Ambu) bag remains inflated at all times and is not dependent on a compressed gas source. It is limited to delivering oxygen concentration to about 40%.

has continued for over 2 minutes, insert an orogastric tube (through the mouth to the stomach instead of through the nose to the stomach because babies are obligate nose breathers). Leaving the distal end open helps deflate the stomach, which allows for better ventilation of the lungs and decreases the possibility that vomiting and aspiration of stomach contents from overdistention will occur.

Drug Therapy

Few medications are necessary for newborn resuscitation. Even if an infant's respiratory depression appears to be related to the administration of a narcotic such as morphine or meperidine (Demerol) to the mother during labor, naloxone (Narcan), a drug to reverse the action of narcotics, should not be routinely administered because it has little effect and may cause seizures in a newborn (Leone, Finer, & Rich, 2012). Instead, resuscitation efforts should focus on effective ventilation and airway support for the persistently apneic newborn (Wyckoff et al., 2015). If heart rate continues to be inadequate (less than 60 beats/min), epinephrine 1:10,000 may be administered intravenously (IV) to stimulate heart action. Preterm infants may receive surfactant to replace the natural surfactant that has not yet formed in their lungs.

Ventilation Maintenance

To allow a newborn to adjust to and maintain the cardiovascular changes that occur at birth, effective ventilation (continued respirations) must be maintained. Healthy newborns accomplish this task on their own. Those who have difficulty establishing respirations at birth need to be carefully observed in the first few hours after birth to be certain respirations are maintained. Use of pulse oximetry is crucial to be certain oxygen saturation remains adequate; infants this young do not have dramatic skin color changes as do older infants and can be mildly hypoxic (low in oxygen) without becoming cyanotic.

A steadily increasing respiratory rate, grunting, and nasal flaring are often the first signs of obstruction or respiratory compromise in newborns. If these are present, undress the baby's chest and look for intercostal retractions (inward sucking of the anterior chest wall on inspiration). Pulling in the chest muscle this way reflects the degree of difficulty the newborn is having in breathing in air (tugging so hard to inflate the lungs that the anterior chest muscles are pulled inward).

Place a newborn who is having difficulty with maintaining respirations under an infant radiant warmer to help prevent cooling and acidosis; under a warmer, the clothing (except diaper) should be removed to promote better respiration and observation while keeping the newborn warm. Positioning an infant on the back with the head of the mattress elevated approximately 15 degrees can also help because it allows the abdominal contents to fall away from the diaphragm, thus increasing breathing space.

If secretions accumulating in the respiratory tract appear to be creating ineffective breaths, an infant may need additional suctioning. "Bagging" the infant with a mask and positive-pressure ventilation bag for a minute before suctioning will usually improve the infant's oxygen level and prevent it from desaturating to dangerous levels during suctioning. As a final step, the cause of the respiratory distress must be determined and appropriate interventions must be undertaken to correct the difficulty (see Chapter 40).

ESTABLISHING EXTRAUTERINE CIRCULATION

Although establishing respirations is the first priority at a high-risk infant's birth, lack of cardiac function may be present concurrently or may develop if respiratory function cannot be quickly initiated and maintained. If an infant has no audible heartbeat, or if the cardiac rate is below 60 beats/min, chest compressions should be started. Hold the infant with fingers encircling the chest and wrapped around the back and depress the sternum with both thumbs on the lower third of the sternum, approximately one third of its depth (1 or 2 cm) at a rate of at least 100 times per minute (Wyckoff et al., 2015). Lung ventilation at a rate of 30 times per minute should be coordinated with chest compressions at a rate of 90 compressions per minute at a ratio of three compressions to one ventilation. If a newborn's heart rate is greater than 60 but less than 100 beats/min, chest compressions can be stopped but ventilations should be continued. Ensuring adequate ventilation is the major priority and should continue until the heart rate is greater than 100 beats/min.

Continue to monitor pulse oximetry to evaluate respiratory function and cardiac efficiency. If the pressure and the rate of chest compressions used are adequate, it should be possible, in addition, to palpate a femoral pulse. If the heartbeat is not above 60 beats/min after at least 30 seconds of coordinated positive-pressure ventilation and chest compressions, intravenous epinephrine to stimulate heart action may be prescribed (Wyckoff et al., 2015). Following cardiopulmonary resuscitation, newborns should be transferred to a transitional or high-risk nursery for continuous cardiorespiratory observation and care to be certain cardiac function is maintained.

MAINTAINING FLUID AND ELECTROLYTE BALANCE

After an initial resuscitation attempt, hypoglycemia (decreased blood glucose) often results from the effort the newborn expended to begin breathing. Dehydration may also result from increased insensible water loss caused by rapid respirations. Infants with hypoglycemia are treated initially with intravenous 10% dextrose in water to restore their blood glucose level. Fluids such as a dilute mixture of saline and dextrose in water are commonly used to maintain glucose and fluid levels and electrolytes. Sodium, additional glucose, and potassium are added as needed according to electrolyte laboratory results.

Be certain to monitor the rate of fluid administration conscientiously in high-risk newborns because a high fluid intake can lead to fluid overload, resulting in a patent ductus arteriosus or heart failure. When using a radiant warmer, remember there is a tendency for water loss from either convection or radiation. A newborn on a warmer, therefore, may require more fluid than if he or she were placed in a double-walled incubator.

Monitor fluid status both by urine output and urine specific gravity values. An output less than 2 ml/kg/hr or a specific gravity greater than 1.015 to 1.020 suggests inadequate fluid intake.

If hypovolemia is present immediately after birth, the cause is usually fetal blood loss from a condition such as placenta previa (see Chapter 21) or twin-to-twin transfusion. With hypovolemia, typically tachypnea, pallor, tachycardia, decreased arterial blood pressure, decreased central venous pressure, and decreased tissue perfusion of peripheral tissue, with a progressively developing metabolic acidosis, will develop. The hematocrit may be normal for some time after acute blood loss, however, because blood cells present are in proportion to plasma. An isotonic solution (usually normal saline) may be administered to increase blood volume. A vasopressor such as dopamine may be given to increase blood pressure and improve cell perfusion.

REGULATING TEMPERATURE

All high-risk infants may have difficulty maintaining temperature because, in addition to stress from an illness or immaturity, the infant's body is often exposed for long periods during procedures such as resuscitation.

It's important to keep newborns in a neutral-temperature environment, one that is neither too hot nor too cold because doing so places less demand on them to maintain a minimal metabolic rate necessary for effective body functioning. If their environment becomes too hot, they are forced to decrease metabolism to cool their body. If it becomes too cold, they must increase their metabolism to warm body cells. Increased metabolism can be destructive because it calls for increased oxygen, and without this oxygen available because of respiratory difficulty, body cells become hypoxic. To spare oxygen for essential body functions, vasoconstriction of peripheral blood vessels occurs so blood can be pushed into the central torso. If this process continues for too long a time, pulmonary vessels constrict and pulmonary perfusion decreases. The infant's PO_2 level will fall and PCO_2 will increase. As mentioned previously, a lowered PO_2 level causes fetal shunts such as the ductus arteriosus to remain open. Surfactant production in the lungs can halt as well, further interfering with lung function. To supply glucose to maintain increased metabolism, an infant has to resort to anaerobic glycolysis, which pours acid into the bloodstream. As the infant becomes more and more acidotic, the risk of acute bilirubin encephalopathy or *kernicterus* (the accumulation of unconjugated bilirubin into brain cells) increases as more bilirubin-binding sites are lost and more bilirubin is free to pass out of the bloodstream in brain cells. In short, because of becoming chilled, heart action, breathing, electrolytic balance, and possibly brain function all become compromised.

In addition to covering the newborn with an infant cap, wiping the body and head dry with a towel or blanket, and using a radiant warmer or prewarmed incubator (Fig. 26.4), suggest skin-to-skin contact with one of the parents. Additional measures that can be used to ensure the infant's temperature stays between 36.5°C and 37.5°C (97.8°F and 99.5°F) axillary are plastic wrap, increasing the room temperature, and warmed mattresses (Wyckoff et al., 2015). To prevent heat loss, be certain during any procedure that the infant is not placed on a cool X-ray table or scale.

A

B

Figure 26.4   A neutral thermal environment. **(A)** A neonate in an intensive care bed with overhead radiant warmer can be examined periodically with ease. **(B)** Use of an incubator allows maintenance of a neutral thermal environment for neonates not requiring minute-to-minute interventions.

Radiant Heat Sources

Radiant heat warmers are open beds that have an attached overhead source of radiant heat and provide both warmth and visibility for observation. Such units have small probes, covered by a small shield, often silver metallic, which when placed on the baby's skin, register the baby's temperature. Abdominal skin temperature, when measured this way, should be 95.9° to 97.7°F (35.5° to 36.5°C). If an infant's temperature falls below this level, an alarm on the unit can be set to sound. Be certain, with the infant laying on his or her back, you tape the probe or disk onto the infant's abdomen between the umbilicus and the xiphoid process. Do not tape it on the underside of an infant or it will register a falsely high reading. Be certain as well it is not over the liver because the heat generated by the liver can lead to false high readings or over the rib cage where the thin subcutaneous tissue and ribs are also apt to yield an inaccurate reading. When performing care or leaning over the infant, be careful your head does not block the heat from the overhead source so it no longer reaches the baby. An additional warming pad placed under an infant may be necessary for very preterm infants or for lengthy procedures to maintain body heat.

Incubators

Newborns needing both warmth and visual observation may also be cared for in incubators. By placing the baby in such a steady, warm environment, the need for clothing can be eliminated, so the observation for any respiratory difficulty, possible color changes, or unusual movements (such as seizures) can be readily observed. The temperature of incubators varies with the amount of time portholes remain open and the temperature of the area in which the incubator is placed. Placing one in direct sunlight or near a warm radiator, for example, can increase the internal temperature markedly. Placing it near a cold window can decrease the temperature. For these reasons, a newborn's temperature must be assessed at frequent intervals when in an incubator to be certain the temperature level designated is being maintained. Use of an additional acrylic shield inside the incubator helps prevent radiation and convection heat loss when portholes are opened and may be necessary for very immature infants.

Similar to radiant warmers, some incubators have servo control mechanism units that monitor the infant's temperature once the probe is placed on their abdomen and automatically changes the temperature of the incubator as needed. Portholes must remain closed to keep the servo control operating efficiently.

As infants become both medically stabile and old enough to maintain a steady body temperature, they can be weaned from an incubator. Dress the infant as if he or she were going to be in a bassinet and then set the incubator about 2°F (1.2°C) below the infant's temperature. After a half hour, assess whether the infant is able to maintain body temperature. If so, lower the incubator temperature another 2°F and continue until room temperature is reached. If an infant cannot maintain adequate temperature as the incubator temperature level is lowered, it suggests the infant is not yet ready for room-temperature air, and the weaning process should be slowed or stopped until the baby is more mature or better able to self-regulate temperature.

Skin-to-Skin Care

Originally referred to as *kangaroo care*, skin-to-skin care is the use of skin-to-skin contact with a parent to maintain body heat. Provide a quiet setting with lights dimmed. Undress the infant except for a diaper and a cap. Assist the parent to sit comfortably in a chair and hold the infant snugly against his or her unclothed chest, skin to skin. Place a blanket over the infant for added warmth. This method of care not only supplies heat but also encourages parent–child bonding (Moore, Anderson, Bergman, et al., 2012).

QSEN Checkpoint Question 26.1

EVIDENCE-BASED PRACTICE

A review of the literature was completed to examine interventions that prevent hypothermia in the premature newborn in the delivery room and that maintain core body temperature. In addition to the use of the standard thermoregulation interventions such as knit hats, the literature showed using respiratory gases during ventilation, the use of gel thermal mattresses, and the use of polyethylene wraps or bags (Fawcett, 2014). Based on the previous study, which response by Mrs. Atkins, whose infant was born prematurely, would alert the nurse she may need further teaching?

   a. "Holding my baby directly on my chest will help with warmth and temperature stability."
   b. "I like singing to him and notice that helps his temperature stay even."
   c. "I'll use this adorable little hat I was given to help him stay warm."
   d. "I'm afraid he'll suffocate if he sleeps on a warmed mattress."

Look in Appendix A for the best answer and rationale.

ESTABLISHING ADEQUATE NUTRITIONAL INTAKE

Infants who experienced severe asphyxia at birth usually receive intravenous fluids so they do not become exhausted from sucking or until necrotizing enterocolitis has been ruled out, which can result when there is a temporary reduction of oxygen to the bowel (see Chapter 45 for a discussion of necrotizing enterocolitis). If an infant's respiratory rate remains so rapid that the infant cannot suck effectively, gavage feedings may be introduced (Fig. 26.5). Others with a long-term nutrition concern may have gastrostomy tubes placed. Preterm infants should be fed breast milk if at all possible because of the immune protection this offers (Lee, Martin-Anderson, Lyndon, et al., 2013; Martin, Ling, & Blackburn, 2016). If breastfeeding is not possible because the infant is too immature to suck effectively, a mother can manually express breast milk or use a breast pump to initiate and continue her milk supply until the time the infant is mature enough or otherwise ready to breast feed. Her expressed breast milk can then be used in the infant's gavage feeding (Martin et al., 2016). Be certain when bottled breast milk is supplied by the mother that it is well marked with the infant's name, date and time it was pumped, and medical record number or breast milk errors can occur the same as medication errors (Centers for Disease Control and Prevention [CDC], 2016). It should

Figure 26.5 Infants who are ill at birth often need supplemental feedings by nasogastric or gastrostomy tube.

be stored in polycarbonate- (bisphenol A) free plastic bags or bottles, which can leech into stored milk and possibly lead to endocrine disruptions (Trasande, 2014).

Preterm infants reveal hunger by the same signs as term infants, such as rooting, crying, and sucking motions. All babies who are gavage or gastrostomy fed need oral stimulation from nonnutritive sucking and so seem to enjoy a pacifier at feeding times. In immature infants, this may actually help them develop an effective sucking reflex. In mature infants, pacifier use has also been shown to be a deterrent to sudden infant death syndrome (Alm, Wennergren, Möllborg, et al., 2016). Exceptions to pacifier use are for infants too immature to have a sucking reflex; infants who must not swallow air, such as those with a tracheoesophageal fistula awaiting surgery; or infants mature enough to breastfeed. The techniques of gavage feeding and gastrostomy feeding are both discussed in Chapter 37.

ESTABLISHING WASTE ELIMINATION

Although most immature infants void within 24 hours of birth, they may void later than term newborns because, as a result of all the procedures for resuscitation, their blood pressure may not be adequate to optimally supply their kidneys. Carefully document any voidings that occur during resuscitation because this is proof that hypotension is improving and the kidneys are being perfused. Immature infants also may pass stool later than the term infant because meconium has not yet reached the end of the intestine at birth.

PREVENTING INFECTIONS

Infections in high-risk newborns may occur from prenatal, perinatal, or postnatal causes. In some instances, such as preterm premature rupture of the membranes, the risk of adverse neurodevelopmental outcomes from the infection is what places the infant in a high-risk category (Committee on Practice Bulletins-Obstetrics, 2016). Contracting an infection has the potential to drastically complicate a high-risk newborn's ability to adjust to extrauterine life, another reason breastfeeding is good for such infants because, beginning with colostrum, it supplies important immune protection (Verardo, Gómez-Caravaca, Arráez-Román, et al., 2017). Infection, like chilling, has the detrimental effect of increasing metabolic oxygen demands as well as stressing an immature immune system, thus lowering defense mechanism protection.

Common viruses that affect infants during intrauterine life are cytomegalovirus and toxoplasmosis virus. An infant born after contracting either of these infections may be born with congenital anomalies from the virus invasion (see Chapter 12). The most prevalent perinatal infections are those contracted from the vaginal canal during birth such as herpes simplex 2 and hepatitis B. Early-onset sepsis is most commonly caused by group B streptococcus, *Escherichia coli*, *Klebsiella* (a gram-negative rod that causes pneumonia), and *Listeria monocytogenes* (a gram-positive bacteria associated with nausea, vomiting, and possibly meningitis). Late-onset, or hospital-acquired, infections are more commonly caused by *Staphylococcus aureus*, *Enterobacter*, and *Candida*. Late-onset infections are probably most commonly spread to newborns from healthcare personnel, which is the reason all persons coming in contact with or caring for infants must observe good hand washing techniques and standard precautions to reduce the risk of infection transmission. Healthcare personnel with infections have a professional and moral obligation to refrain from caring for newborns or wear protective measures such as a face mask to avoid spreading infections.

ESTABLISHING PARENT–INFANT BONDING

It is helpful if all women who are diagnosed as having a high-risk pregnancy are offered a tour of a neonatal intensive care unit (NICU) during pregnancy, so if their infant should be admitted to a NICU, they will be more comfortable in the high-tech environment.

Be certain the parents of a high-risk newborn are kept informed of what is happening during resuscitation at birth. They should be able to visit the special nursing unit where the infant is admitted as soon as possible and as often as they choose, and, after washing their hands and in some situations wearing a gown, hold and touch their infant, both of which are actions that help make the infant's birth more real to them. Should an infant not survive an initial illness, these interactions can also help make the death more real and can help parents work through their feelings to accept this event.

Most parents handle newborn babies tentatively until they have "claimed" them or have become firmly acquainted. If an infant was ill at birth, it may take days or weeks before the parents are able to handle their baby comfortably and confidently because of the number of tubes involved in care and their fear of doing something that could hurt the infant. Urge parents to spend as much time with their infant in the intensive care nursery as possible, especially as the infant is improving and is able to begin interacting with them. Be certain parents have continuing access to healthcare personnel after discharge so they can care confidently for the infant at home.

If an infant dies despite newborn resuscitation attempts, parents need to see the infant when no longer attached to equipment. Viewing the baby can help reassure them the baby was a perfect newborn in every other way except lung function or whatever was the infant's specific fatal disorder. Believing this is one way they may be able to develop confidence to plan for other children or simply to continue their lives after such a devastating experience.

ANTICIPATING DEVELOPMENTAL NEEDS

High-risk newborns need special care to ensure the amount of pain they experience during procedures is limited to the least amount possible and that they also receive adequate stimulation for growth. Most high-risk infants experience "catch-up" growth once they stabilize from the trauma of birth or whatever caused them to be considered high risk. They quickly move to playing with age-appropriate toys and interacting with parents. Some parents may need support before and after their infant is discharged home so they can begin to view their child as well and capable of doing all the things the infant is now capable of doing. Discussing usual growth and development of infants can help prepare them and look forward to the next developmental step.

Follow-Up of the High-Risk Infant at Home

Each time parents visit a special/intensive care nursery, assess their level of knowledge about their child's condition and development. For parents whose child has a complex concern, additional education and referral to a home care agency may be necessary to help them continue with the level of care required when the infant is discharged home (see Chapter 4). Before discharge, the safety of their home for the care of an infant that has healthcare needs (physical or developmental) should be evaluated. Transporting a preterm infant in a car, for example, will require special measures, including a commercial head support because a very small infant does not fit securely into a standard infant car seat.

Although not well documented regarding when or why it occurs, some preterm infants experience episodes of oxygen desaturation, apnea, or bradycardia when seated in standard car safety seats (Davis, 2015). To detect if this will occur, the AAP recommends all preterm infants be assessed for cardiorespiratory stability in their car seat prior to discharge from the healthcare facility—the "car seat challenge" (AAP, 2012).

High-Risk Infants and Child Maltreatment

When a child is born ill or preterm, the expected reaction of parents would be to protect the infant even more than the healthy infant so no further harm could occur. In actuality, particularly in reference to the preterm infant, the opposite may occur. Probably related to the feeling they are "different" or because they were separated from the parents for a long time following birth, the preterm infant may be at an increased risk for maltreatment (see Chapter 55) (Nandyal, Owora, Risch, et al., 2013).

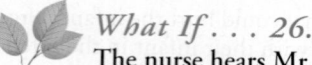
What If . . . 26.1

   The nurse hears Mr. Atkins repeat the question he first asked his wife when he heard his baby had been born prematurely, "What did you do to cause this?" Would the nurse try to intervene or allow the Atkins to work out their feelings as a couple?

The Newborn at Risk Because of Altered Gestational Age or Birth Weight

Infants need to be evaluated as soon as possible after birth to determine their weight, height, head circumference, and gestational age to determine their immediate healthcare needs and to help anticipate possible future problems. Birth weight is normally plotted on a growth chart such as the Colorado

(Lubchenco) Intrauterine Growth Chart, a special chart for newborns (available at http://thePoint.lww.com/Flagg8e).

Term infants are those born after the beginning of week 38 and before week 42 of pregnancy (calculated from the first day of the last menstrual period). Approximately 90% of all live births fall into this category. Infants born before term (before the beginning of the 38th week of pregnancy) are classified as **preterm infants** regardless of their birth weight (Quinn, Munoz, Gonik, et al., 2016). Infants born after the end of week 41 of pregnancy are classified as postterm infants or postmature (Blencowe, Cousens, Oestergaard, et al., 2012).

Normally, birth weight increases for each additional gestational week of age. Infants who fall between the 10th and 90th percentiles of weight for their gestational age, whether they are preterm, term, or postterm, are considered **appropriate for gestational age (AGA)**. Infants who fall below the 10th percentile of weight for their age are considered **small for gestational age (SGA)**. Those who fall above the 90th percentile in weight are considered **large for gestational age (LGA)**. Other terms used include:

- **Low–birth-weight (LBW) infant**: one weighing less than 2,500 g at birth
- **Very-low-birth-weight (VLBW) infant**: one weighing less than 1500 g at birth
- **Extremely-low-birth-weight (ELBW) infant**: one weighing less than 1,000 g at birth

Infants in all of these classifications have immediate needs that are different from or that are more pronounced than the needs of AGA term newborns. Each of these categories also carries its own set of potential risks.

THE PRETERM INFANT

A preterm infant is traditionally defined as a live-born infant born before the end of week 37 of gestation. In terms of the degree of care needed, they are further divided into *late preterm* (born between 34 and 37 weeks) and *early preterm* (born between 24 and 34 weeks). Neonatal assessments such as inspection for sole creases, skull firmness, ear cartilage, and neurologic development plus the mother's report of the date of her last menstrual period along with a sonographic estimation of age all can be helpful to determine gestational age. Preterm birth occurs in approximately 11% of live births worldwide, with the United States having one of the highest rates of preterm births (Blencowe et al., 2012).

Most preterm infants need intensive care from the moment of birth to give them their best chance of survival without neurologic aftereffects because they are more prone than others to hypoglycemia and intracranial hemorrhage. Lack of lung surfactant, because this does not form until about the 34th week of pregnancy, makes them extremely vulnerable to respiratory distress syndrome (Landry & Menzies, 2011).

No matter what their weight, the initial assessment needs to differentiate healthy preterm babies from SGA babies (who also may have a low birth weight but have more possibility of being unhealthy and so require more help to adjust to extrauterine life). In contrast to an SGA infant, a preterm infant appears immature and has a low birth weight but is well proportioned for age because the baby appears to have been doing well in utero. For an unexplained reason, however, the trigger that initiates labor was activated too early and birth resulted even though the baby was not yet mature. Characteristics of SGA and preterm infants are compared in Table 26.1.

TABLE 26.1 CONTRASTS BETWEEN SMALL-FOR-GESTATIONAL-AGE AND PRETERM INFANTS

Characteristic	Small-for-Gestational-Age Infant	Preterm Infant
Gestational age	24–44 wk	<37 wk
Birth weight	<10th percentile	Normal for age
Congenital malformations	Strong possibility	Possibility
Pulmonary problems most apt to occur	Meconium aspiration, pulmonary hemorrhage, pneumothorax	Respiratory distress syndrome
Hyperbilirubinemia	Possibility	Very strong possibility
Hypoglycemia	Very strong possibility	Possibility
Intracranial hemorrhage	Strong possibility	Possibility
Apnea episodes	Possibility	Very strong possibility
Feeding problems	Most likely because of accompanying problem such as hypoglycemia	Small stomach capacity; immature sucking reflex
Weight gain in nursery	Rapid	Slow
Future restricted growth	Possibly always be <10th percentile because of poor organ development	Not likely to be restricted in growth because "catch-up" growth occurs

Etiology

At least 50% of neonatal deaths are preterm (Blencowe, Cousens, Chou, et al., 2013). Infant mortality could be reduced dramatically if the causes of preterm birth could be discovered and corrected and all pregnancies could be brought to term. However, even with the examples of possible causes listed in the following, the exact cause of premature labor and early birth is rarely exactly known.

Box 26.3 summarizes factors associated with preterm birth. Important among these is a high correlation between low socioeconomic level and early birth. In women from middle and upper socioeconomic groups, for example, only 4% to 8% of pregnancies are not carried to term. In women from low socioeconomic levels, as many as 10% to 20% end

---

BOX 26.3
Common Factors Associated With Preterm Birth

- Low socioeconomic level
- Poor nutritional status
- Lack of prenatal care
- Multiple pregnancy
- Previous early birth
- Race (non-Whites have a higher incidence of prematurity than Whites)
- Cigarette smoking
- Age of the mother (highest incidence is in mothers younger than age 20 years)
- Order of birth (early birth is highest in first pregnancies and in those beyond the fourth pregnancy)
- Closely spaced pregnancies
- Abnormalities of the mother's reproductive system, such as intrauterine septum
- Infections (especially urinary tract infections)
- Pregnancy complications, such as premature rupture of membranes or premature separation of the placenta
- Early induction of labor
- Elective cesarean birth

---

before term (Joseph, Fahey, Shankardass, et al., 2014). Risk factors associated with preterm birth include inadequate nutrition and smoking or alcohol use. The increasing use of assisted fertility methods that result in multiple births, such as in vitro fertilization, is another reason preterm births can occur because more multiple pregnancies result in preterm birth than term pregnancies (Blencowe et al., 2013). Iatrogenic (health-care-caused) issues, such as elective cesarean birth or inducing labor before 39 weeks of pregnancy (which is not recommended but sometimes necessary because of maternal illness or fetal reasons), also result in early births.

Assessment

Although a detailed pregnancy history may sometimes reveal the reason for a preterm birth, the pregnancy history is often normal up to the beginning of labor. When interviewing parents of a preterm infant, be careful not to convey disapproval of reported pregnancy behaviors such as cigarette smoking that may have contributed to preterm birth. Once an infant is born, a new mother needs a high level of self-esteem and all of her inner resources to sustain her through this crisis and not be burdened by guilt over what should or could have been. An accurate but comforting answer to a direct inquiry about why preterm birth occurs is, "No one really knows what causes prematurity."

Observing a number of physical findings and reflex testing is used to differentiate between term and preterm newborns at birth (Figs. 26.6 and 26.7). On gross inspection, a preterm infant's head appears disproportionately large (≥3 cm greater than chest size). The skin is generally unusually ruddy because there is so little subcutaneous fat beneath it, making veins easily noticeable; a high degree of acrocyanosis may be present. Newborns delivered at greater than 28 weeks of gestation are typically covered with vernix caseosa. In very preterm newborns, however (less than 28 weeks of gestation), the vernix will be lacking. Lanugo is usually scant the same way in very low gestation infants but will be extensive, covering the back, forearms, forehead, and sides of the face in late preterm babies. Both anterior and posterior fontanelles will be small. There are few or no creases on the soles of the feet (Visscher & Narendran, 2014).

The eyes of most preterm infants appear small in relation to term infants. Although difficult to elicit, a pupillary reaction

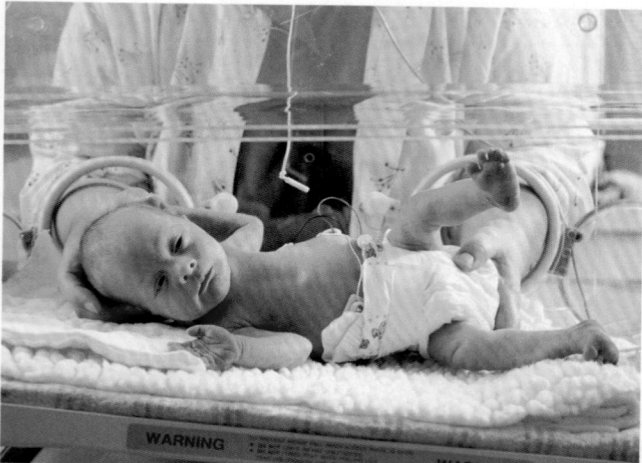

Figure 26.6 An immature newborn at birth. (Photodisc/Punch-Stock.)

is present. An ophthalmoscopic examination is extremely difficult and often uninformative because the vitreous humor may be hazy. A preterm infant has varying degrees of myopia (nearsightedness) because of a lack of eye globe depth.

The ears appear large in relation to the head. The cartilage of the ear is immature and allows the pinna to fall forward. The level of the ears should be carefully inspected to rule out chromosomal abnormalities (see Chapter 8).

Neurologic function in the preterm infant is often difficult to evaluate because the neurologic system is still immature. Observing the infant make spontaneous or provoked muscle movements can be as important as formal reflex testing. If they are tested, reflexes such as sucking with coordinated swallowing and breathing will be absent if an infant's age is below 33 weeks; deep tendon reflexes such as the Achilles tendon reflex will also be markedly diminished. During an examination, a preterm infant is much less active than a mature infant and rarely cries. If the infant does cry, the cry is weak and high pitched.

Laboratory values for a preterm infant are compared with those of the term infant at http://thePoint.lww.com/Flagg8e.

A
Premature Infant

Full-Term Infant

RESTING POSTURE *The premature infant is characterized by very little, if any, flexion in the upper extremities and only partial flexion of the lower extremities. The full-term infant exhibits flexion in all four extremities.*

B
Premature Infant, 28–32 Weeks

Full-Term Infant

WRIST FLEXION *The wrist is flexed, applying enough pressure to get the hand as close to the forearm as possible. The angle between the hypothenar eminence and the ventral aspect of the forearm is measured. (Care must be taken not to rotate an infant's wrist.) The premature infant at 28–32 weeks gestation will exhibit a 90-degree angle. With the full-term infant, it is possible to flex the hand onto the arm.*

Figure 26.7 Examples of physical examination findings and reflex tests used to judge gestational age. **(A)** A resting posture. **(B)** Wrist flexion.

Premature Infant

C

Full-Term Infant

Response in Premature Infant

Response in Full-Term Infant

RECOIL OF EXTREMITIES *Place an infant supine. To test recoil of the legs (1) flex the legs and knees fully and hold for 5 seconds (shown in top photographs), (2) extend the legs fully by pulling on the feet, (3) release. To test the arms, flex forearms and follow same procedure. In the premature infant, response is minimal or absent (bottom left); in the full-term infant, extremities return briskly to full flexion (bottom right).*

Premature Infant

D

Full-Term Infant

SCARF SIGN *Hold the baby supine, take the hand, and try to place it around the neck and above the opposite shoulder as far posteriorly as possible. Assist this maneuver by lifting the elbow across the body. See how far across the chest the elbow will go. In the premature infant, the elbow will reach near or across the midline. In the full-term infant, the elbow will not reach the midline.*

Figure 26.7   *(continued)* **(C)** Recoil of extremities (legs). **(D)** The scarf sign.

E

Premature Infant

Full-Term Infant

HEEL TO EAR *With the baby supine and the hips positioned flat on the bed, draw the baby's foot as near to the ear as it will go without forcing it. Observe the distance between the foot and head as well as the degree of extension at the knee. In the premature infant, very little resistance will be met. In the full-term infant there will be marked resistance; it will be impossible to draw the baby's foot to the ear.*

F

Premature Infant

Full-Term Infant

SOLE (PLANTAR) CREASES *The sole of the premature infant has very few or no creases. With the increasing gestation age, the number and depth of sole creases multiply, so that the full-term baby has creases involving the heel. (Wrinkles that occur after 24 hours of age can sometimes be confused with true creases.)*

G

Premature Infant

Full-Term Infant

BREAST TISSUE *In infants younger than 34 weeks gestation the areola and nipple are barely visible. After 34 weeks, the areola becomes raised. Also, an infant of less than 36 weeks gestation has no breast tissue. Breast tissue arises with increasing gestational age because of maternal hormonal stimulation. Thus, an infant of 39–40 weeks will have 5–6 mm of breast tissue, and this amount will increase with age.*

Figure 26.7 *(continued)* **(E)** Heel to ear. **(F)** Plantar creases. **(G)** Breast tissue.

Premature Infant, 34–36 Weeks

H

Full-Term Infant

EARS *At fewer than 34 weeks gestation, infants have very flat, relatively shapeless ears. Shape develops over time so that an infant between 34 and 36 weeks has a slight incurving of the superior part of the ear; the term infant is characterized by incurving of two thirds of the pinna; and in an infant older than 39 weeks the incurving continues to the lobe. If the extremely premature infant's ear is folded over, it will stay folded. Cartilage begins to appear at approximately 32 weeks so that the ear returns slowly to its original position. In an infant of more than 40 weeks gestation, there is enough ear cartilage so that the ear stands erect away from the head and returns quickly when folded. (When folding the ear over during examination, be certain that the surrounding area is wiped clean or the ear may adhere to the vernix.)*

Premature Male

I

Full-Term Male

MALE GENITALIA *In the premature male, the testes are very high in the inguinal canal, and there are very few rugae on the scrotum. The full-term infant's testes are lower in the scrotum and many rugae have developed.*

Premature Female

J

Full-Term Female

FEMALE GENITALIA *When the premature female is positioned on her back with hips abducted, the clitoris is very prominent and the labia majora are very small and widely separated. The labia minora and the clitoris are covered by the labia majora in the full-term infant.*

Figure 26.7 *(continued)* **(H)** Ears. **(I)** Male genitalia. **(J)** Female genitalia. (© Caroline Brown, RNC, MS, DEd.)

Potential Complications

Because of immaturity, preterm infants are prone to several specific conditions.

Anemia of Prematurity

Many preterm infants develop a normochromic, normocytic anemia (normal cells, just few in number), which can make infants appear pale, lethargic, and anorectic. Anemia occurs from a combination of immaturity of the hematopoietic system (the effective production of red cells with an elevated reticulocyte count may not begin until 32 weeks of pregnancy) combined with the destruction of red blood cells because of low levels of vitamin E, a substance that normally protects red blood cells against oxidation. Excessive blood drawing for electrolytes, complete blood counts, or blood gas analysis after birth can potentiate the problem. For this reason, it's important to see that blood draws in preterm infants are coordinated to the fewest possible and a record of the blood loss for these tallied. Delaying cord clamping at birth to allow a little more blood from the placenta to enter the infant may also help reduce the development of anemia (Frank, Mueller-Burke, Bullard, et al., 2015).

Acute Bilirubin Encephalopathy

Acute bilirubin encephalopathy (ABE) is the destruction of brain cells by invasion of indirect or unconjugated bilirubin (Mesić, Milas, Medimurec, et al., 2014). This invasion results from the high concentration of indirect bilirubin that forms in the bloodstream from an excessive breakdown of red blood cells at birth. Preterm infants are more prone to this condition than term infants because, with the acidosis that occurs from poor respiratory exchange, brain cells appear to be more susceptible to the effect of indirect bilirubin than usual. Preterm infants also have less serum albumin available to bind indirect bilirubin and inactivate its effect. Because of this, ABE may occur at lower levels in these infants than in term newborns (Thilo & Rosenberg, 2012). At the point that indirect bilirubin levels rise and jaundice occurs, phototherapy or exchange transfusion can be initiated to prevent excessively high indirect bilirubin levels.

Persistent Patent Ductus Arteriosus

Because preterm infants may lack surfactant, their lungs are noncompliant, so it is more difficult for them to move blood from the pulmonary artery into the lungs. This condition leads to pulmonary artery hypertension, which then interferes with closure of the ductus arteriosus. Always administer intravenous therapy cautiously to preterm infants, therefore, because increasing blood pressure could further compound this problem. In term infants, indomethacin or ibuprofen may be used to cause closure of a patent ductus arteriosus, making ventilation more efficient; however, indomethacin is given cautiously to preterm infants because it has been associated with adverse effects such as decreased renal function, decreased platelet count, and gastric irritation (Mitra, Florez, Tamayo, et al., 2014). Carefully monitor urine output and observe for bleeding, especially at injection sites, if this is prescribed.

Periventricular/Intraventricular Hemorrhage

Preterm infants are prone to periventricular hemorrhage (bleeding into the tissue surrounding the ventricles) or intraventricular hemorrhage (bleeding into the ventricles) because of fragile capillaries and immature cerebral vascular development. When there is a rapid change in cerebral blood pressure, such as could occur with hypoxia, intravenous infusion, ventilation, or pneumothorax (lung collapse), capillary rupture could occur; brain anoxia then occurs distal to the rupture.

Intraventricular hemorrhage occurs most often in VLBW infants and is classified as:

- Grade 1, bleeding in the periventricular germinal matrix regions or germinal matrix, occurring in one ventricle
- Grade 2, bleeding within the lateral ventricle without dilation of the ventricle
- Grade 3, bleeding causing enlargement of the ventricles
- Grade 4, bleeding in the ventricles and intraparenchymal hemorrhage

A long-term effect of hemorrhage may be the development of hydrocephalus if there was bleeding into the narrow aqueduct of Sylvius (Robinson, 2012). Preterm infants usually have a cranial ultrasound performed after the first few days of life and again at different intervals based on the gestational age of the infant to detect if a hemorrhage has occurred. Infants with grade 1 or 2 bleeds have a good long-term prognosis; the prognosis of those with more intense bleeds is guarded until further complications are ruled out (Shah & Wusthoff, 2016).

Other Potential Complications

Preterm infants are also particularly susceptible to several illnesses in the early postnatal period, which can also occur in term infants, including respiratory distress syndrome, apnea, and retinopathy of prematurity (all discussed later in this chapter), as well as necrotizing enterocolitis (discussed in Chapter 45).

 ## Nursing Diagnoses and Related Interventions

Because a preterm infant has few body resources, both physiologic and psychological stress must be reduced as much as possible and interventions should be initiated gently to prevent the depletion of available resources. Close observation and an analysis of findings are essential so concerns can be managed quickly.

Nursing Diagnosis: Impaired gas exchange related to immature pulmonary functioning

Outcome Evaluation: Newborn initiates breathing at birth after resuscitation; maintains normal newborn respirations of 30 to 60 breaths/min free of assisted ventilation; exhibits oxygen saturation levels of at least 95% as evidenced by pulse oximetry.

Preterm infants have great difficulty initiating respirations at birth because pulmonary capillaries are still so immature, and lung surfactant, which does not form in adequate amounts until about the 34th to 35th week of pregnancy, may not be present. Inadequate lung surfactant leads to alveolar collapse with each expiration. This collapse forces the infant to use maximum strength to inflate lung alveoli each time. Because this is so tiring, it becomes very difficult for infants to maintain effective ventilations under these stressful conditions.

Cesarean birth, although it has the advantage of reducing pressure on the immature head, may be elected with a preterm birth but also may lead to additional respiratory complications because infants born by cesarean birth retain more lung fluid than those born by vaginal birth. Giving the mother oxygen by mask during the birth can help provide a preterm infant with optimal oxygen saturation at birth (85% to 90%). Keeping maternal analgesia and anesthesia to a minimum also offers a preterm infant the best chance of initiating effective respirations.

Even term infants experience temporary respiratory acidosis until they take a first breath. Once respirations are established, however, this condition quickly clears. Because preterm infants cannot initiate effective respirations as quickly as mature infants, they are susceptible to irreversible acidosis. Birthing room teams need to be prepared with preterm-size laryngoscopes, endotracheal tubes, suction catheters, and synthetic surfactant to be administered by the endotracheal tube so resuscitation can be accomplished immediately. Be certain infants are kept warm during resuscitation so they do not have to expend extra energy to increase metabolic rate to maintain body temperature. Be certain as well that all procedures are carried out gently; a preterm infant's tissues are extremely sensitive to trauma and can be damaged or bruised easily by an oxygen mask. When blood from bruising is reabsorbed, this could yet lead to **hyperbilirubinemia** (an excess amount of bilirubin in the blood).

Many preterm babies, particularly those under 32 weeks of age, continue to have an irregular respiratory pattern (a few quick breaths, a period of 5 to 10 seconds without respiratory effort, a few quick breaths again, etc.). There is no bradycardia with this irregular pattern (sometimes termed **periodic respirations**). Although the pattern is seen in term infants as well, it seems to be intensified by immaturity. If true apnea, which needs immediate attention, is occurring, the pause in respirations is more than 20 seconds and usually results in bradycardia.

The soft rib cartilage of a preterm infant is yet another source of respiratory problems because it causes ribs to collapse on expiration. The accessory muscles of respiration may be underdeveloped as well, leaving preterm infants with no backup muscles to use when they become fatigued. Because of this, preterm infants may need continued oxygen administration after resuscitation to allow them to effectively maintain respirations.

Giving a high level of oxygen to preterm infants during resuscitation or to maintain respirations presents two additional dangers: pulmonary edema and ROP. The development of both of these conditions depends on saturation of the blood with oxygen (PO_2) of more than 100 mmHg, which usually occurs when oxygen is administered at a concentration over 70% (Abdel Ghany, Alsharany, Ali, et al., 2016).

Nursing Diagnosis: Risk for deficient fluid volume related to insensible water loss at birth and small stomach capacity

Outcome Evaluation: Plasma glucose is between 40 and 60 mg per 100 ml; specific gravity of urine is maintained at 1.003 to 1.020; urine output is maintained at a minimum of 1 ml/kg/hr; electrolyte levels are within normal limits.

A preterm newborn experiences a high insensible water loss because of a large body surface relative to total body weight. Preterm infants also cannot concentrate urine well because of immature kidney function. Because of this, a high proportion of body fluid is excreted. All these factors may make a preterm baby need a higher percentage of fluid daily than a term infant (Mohan & Jain, 2012).

Intravenous fluid should be given via a continuous infusion pump to ensure a constant infusion rate and to prevent accidental overload. Assess intravenous sites conscientiously because, if infiltration should occur, the lack of subcutaneous tissue places a preterm newborn at risk for damaged tissue. Specially designed small gauge needles are available for use on small veins. However, many preterm infants lack adequately sized peripheral veins for even this small of a needle. Therefore, they need to receive intravenous fluid by an umbilical or central venous catheter.

Monitor the baby's weight, urine output and specific gravity, and serum electrolytes to ensure adequate fluid intake because too little fluid and calories can lead to weight loss, dehydration and starvation, and increased acidosis. Overhydration may lead to nonnutritional weight gain, pulmonary edema, and heart failure.

Most preterm infants void and pass meconium within 24 hours after birth, although this is delayed in very small infants. Measure urine output by weighing diapers rather than using urine collection bags because disposable collection bags can lead to skin irritation and breakdown from frequent changing and leaking.

The amount of urine output for the first few days of life in preterm babies is high in comparison with that of the term baby because of poor urine concentration: 40 to 100 ml/kg per 24 hours, compared with 10 to 20 ml/kg per 24 hours, respectively. The specific gravity is low, rarely more than 1.012 (normal term babies may concentrate urine up to 1.030). Test urine as well for glucose and ketones because these can reveal hyperglycemia caused by the glucose infusion, which then can lead to diuresis and extreme fluid loss. If too little glucose is being supplied and body cells are using protein for metabolism, ketone bodies will appear in the urine.

Blood glucose determinations should range between 40 and 60 mg/dl. Check for blood in stools to evaluate possible bleeding from the intestinal tract because this can help determine a cause of hypovolemia if this occurs.

Nursing Diagnosis: Risk for imbalanced nutrition, less than body requirements, related to additional nutrients needed for maintenance of rapid growth, possible sucking difficulty, and small stomach

Outcome Evaluation: Infant's weight follows percentile growth curve, skin turgor is good, specific gravity of urine is maintained between 1.003 and 1.020; the infant has no more than 15% weight loss in the first 3 days of life and continues to gain weight after this point.

Nutrition problems can arise with a preterm infant because the infant's body is attempting to continue to maintain the rapid rate of intrauterine growth appropriate for the gestational age. Because of this, a preterm newborn requires a relatively larger amount of nutrients than the mature infant,

115 to 140 calories per kilogram of body weight per day compared with 100 to 110 calories per kilogram of body weight per day needed by a term infant. Protein requirements are 3 to 3.5 g per kilogram of body weight, compared with 2.0 to 2.5 g per kilogram for a term newborn. Because preterm infants have a smaller stomach capacity than term neonates, as a rule, they must be fed more frequently with smaller amounts than term infants, perhaps as small as 1 or 2 ml every 2 to 3 hours.

If these nutrients are not supplied, an infant can develop hypocalcemia (decreased serum calcium) or azotemia (low protein level in the blood). Delayed feeding and a resultant decrease in intestinal motility may also add to hyperbilirubinemia, a problem infants already are at high risk of developing when fetal red blood cells begin to be destroyed.

Digestion and absorption of nutrients in a preterm infant's stomach and intestine may be immature, making the digestion of milk difficult. Nutrition problems are further compounded by a preterm infant's immature reflexes, which make swallowing and sucking difficult. Increased activity that occurs from ineffective sucking may increase the metabolic rate and oxygen requirements; if this happens, it increases the caloric requirements even more. In addition, the preterm infant's stomach capacity is so small that feedings quickly fill the stomach. If a small stomach is distended from a full feeding, this puts pressure on the diaphragm and can lead to respiratory distress. An immature cardiac sphincter (between the stomach and esophagus) allows regurgitation to occur readily. The lack of a cough reflex may lead an infant to aspirate regurgitated formula.

Feeding Schedule. With the early administration of intravenous fluid to prevent hypoglycemia and supply fluid, feedings may be safely delayed until an infant has stabilized his or her respiratory effort from birth. Very preterm infants may be fed by total parenteral nutrition until they are stable enough for enteral feedings. Breast, gavage, or bottle feedings are then begun as soon as the infant is able to tolerate them to prevent the deterioration of the intestinal villi. Preterm infants may have a chest X-ray taken before a first feeding. The presence of air in the stomach shows that the route to the stomach is clear or that no anomaly such as a tracheoesophageal fistula exists.

Gavage Feeding. Although a sucking reflex is present earlier, the ability to coordinate sucking and swallowing is inconsistent until approximately 34 weeks of gestation. A gag reflex is not intact until 32 weeks of gestation. For this reason, for infants who are ill or experiencing respiratory distress may be started on gavage feedings; bottle feeding or breastfeeding will then be gradually introduced as the infant matures and begins to demonstrate feeding behaviors such as being awake, moving, or fussing as if hungry (Fig. 26.8). To avoid tiring, preterm nipples with a slightly larger hole than regular nipples and that are softer are used for bottle feedings.

Observe preterm infants closely after oral or gavage feeding to be certain their filled stomach is not causing respiratory distress. Offering a pacifier during gavage feeding can help strengthen the sucking reflex, better prepare

Figure 26.8   Feeding a preterm infant. Notice the small bottle used. (Fuse/PunchStock.)

an infant for bottle feeding or breastfeeding, and provide oral satisfaction.

Gavage feedings may be given intermittently every few hours or continuously via tubes passed into the stomach or intestine through the mouth or nose. This can be helpful for infants on ventilators or those who cannot tolerate intermittent feedings because of the volume. If feedings are given intermittently, stomach contents may be aspirated, measured, and replaced before each feeding. An infant who has a large amount of milk left in the stomach (volume depends on the amount of milk the infant is receiving) is not digesting the milk. Feedings should not be increased and possibly even cut back to ensure better digestion and to decrease the possibility of regurgitation and aspiration. An inability to digest in this way is also a sign that necrotizing enterocolitis, a destructive intestinal disorder that often occurs in preterm babies, may be developing (Su, Lin, Huang, et al., 2015) (see Chapter 45).

Breast Milk. There is increasing evidence that although preterm infants grow well on commercial formulas, the best milk for them, the same as with term infants, is breast milk (Briere, McGrath, Cong, et al., 2016). The immunologic properties of breast milk may play a major role in preventing neonatal necrotizing enterocolitis as well as an increase in immune defenses.

Mothers can express breast milk manually or with a breast pump for their infant's gavage feedings. If a woman cannot bring this in daily, she can freeze it for safe transport and storage. The sodium content of breast milk in a mother whose infant was born preterm is higher than that of milk in a mother whose infant has been born at term. Therefore, it is better for infants to receive their own mother's breast milk rather than banked milk if possible. This high level of sodium seems to be necessary for fluid retention in the preterm infant. Breast milk is 20 calories per ounce, so parents may be advised to add a human milk fortifier to supplemental bottles of breast milk to supply additional calories, protein, vitamins, and minerals (Brooks, Vickers, & Aryal, 2013). Urge mothers to continue to breastfeed their preterm infants after hospital discharge.

Formula. The caloric concentration of formulas used for preterm infants is usually 22 calories per ounce compared to 20 calories per ounce for a term baby (Mohan & Jain, 2012). Supplementing additional minerals such as iron, calcium, and phosphorus and electrolytes such as sodium, potassium, and chloride may be necessary, depending on the newborn's blood studies. Vitamin A is important in improving healing and possibly reducing the incidence of lung disease. Vitamin E seems to be important in preventing hemolytic anemia in preterm infants (Londhe, Nolen, Das, et al., 2013).

Nursing Diagnosis: Ineffective thermoregulation related to immaturity

Outcome Evaluation: Infant's temperature is maintained at 97.6°F (36.5°C) axillary.

Preterm newborns have a great deal of difficulty maintaining body temperature because they have a relatively large surface area per kilogram of body weight. In addition, because they do not flex their body well but remain in an extended position, rapid cooling from evaporation is more likely to occur.

A preterm infant has little subcutaneous fat for insulation and poor muscular development and so cannot move as actively as an older infant to produce body heat. A preterm infant also has a limited amount of **brown fat**, the special tissue present in newborns that helps maintain body temperature. Preterm infants also cannot shiver, a useful mechanism to increase body temperature, nor can they sweat and thereby reduce body temperature because of their immature central nervous system and hypothalamic control. This makes preterm infants dependent on the environmental temperature provided to keep warm. In a birthing room, typically kept at 62° to 68°F (16.6° to 20°C), a 1,500-g infant exposed to this low temperature loses 1°C of body heat every 3 minutes if left unprotected. Keeping preterm infants under radiant heat warmers, in incubators, or warmed by skin-to-skin contact helps to counteract this natural cooling. It is recommended that the birthing room temperature be increased to 76°F. Be certain a radiant heat warmer is prewarmed before the infant is born. Unless there are obvious abnormalities noted, a physical assessment of a preterm infant, even weighing, can be delayed until the infant can be placed in the warmth of an incubator or under a radiant warmer with a servo control. Some radiant warmers are equipped with built-in scales to weigh the newborn.

If an infant is going to be transported to a department within the hospital, such as the X-ray department, or to a regional center for specialized care, keeping the newborn warm during transport is crucial. Remember that infants lose heat by radiation as well as conduction. If a warmed incubator is placed in a cold transport ambulance, for example, the infant will lose heat to the distant source. An additional heat shield or plastic wrap may need to be placed over an infant, or a portable warming mattress can be placed under the infant to help conserve heat during transport.

Nursing Diagnosis: Risk for infection related to immature immune defenses in the preterm infant

Outcome Evaluation: Temperature is maintained at 97.6°F (36.5°C) axillary; further signs and symptoms of infection such as poor growth or a reduced temperature are absent.

The skin of a preterm infant is easily traumatized and therefore offers less resistance to infection than the skin and mucous membrane of a mature infant. In addition, preterm infants have a lowered resistance to infection because they have difficulty producing phagocytes to localize infection as well as a deficiency of immune globulin M (IgM) antibodies because of insufficient production. To help prevent infection, linen and equipment used with preterm infants must not be shared with other infants. Staff members must be free of infection, and hand washing and gowning (if indicated) regulations should be strictly enforced.

Nursing Diagnosis: Risk for impaired parenting related to interference with parent–infant attachment resulting from hospitalization of infant at birth

Outcome Evaluation: Parents visit frequently and hold the infant; parents speak of their child in positive terms.

In a preterm infant, the first and second periods of reactivity normally observed in newborns at 1 hour and 4 hours of life (see Chapter 18) may be delayed. In some infants, no period of increased activity or tachycardia may appear until 12 to 18 hours of age. If the purpose of a period of reactivity is to stimulate respiratory function, this places a preterm infant at an even greater threat of respiratory failure because respiratory efforts may not be stimulated. A second consequence of a delayed period of reactivity is the loss of an opportunity for interaction between parents and the newborn in the early postpartum period.

Although it is extremely important to conserve a preterm infant's strength by reducing sensory stimulation as much as possible and handling an infant gently, preterm infants appear to need as much attention and affection as term newborns. Rocking, singing and talking to them, and gentle holding them are measures to help preterm infants develop a sense of trust in people, which will enable them to relate satisfactorily to people in the future. Encourage parents to begin interacting with their infant as soon as possible (Box 26.4). Holding an infant with skin-to-skin contact is an effective way to begin this interaction.

Before effective bonding can be established, parents may need time to come to terms with their feelings of disappointment that the infant is so small or guilt that they were not able to prevent the preterm birth. Helping them air these feelings and develop a more positive attitude toward their preterm infant is an important nursing responsibility.

Because parents may not be psychologically ready for birth when a preterm infant is born, it may be more difficult for them to believe they have a child and to begin interacting than if the infant had been born at term. Even if an infant cannot be removed from an incubator or a radiant heat warmer, parents can still handle and stroke the infant in the incubator or warmer for interaction. Encourage the mother to come to the nursery and hold the infant before and after gavage feedings and to breast-feed or bottle feed as soon as the baby is ready for this.

BOX 26.4

Nursing Care Planning to Empower a Family

GUIDELINES FOR PARENTS OF A NEWBORN IN INTENSIVE CARE

Q. Mrs. Atkins tells you, "I'm always afraid I'll touch the wrong thing when I visit our son in the neonatal intensive care unit. What can I do to feel more comfortable there?"

A. Here are some guidelines that should be helpful:

- Learn the name of your child's primary healthcare provider and primary nurse or care manager. Make a point of talking to them when you visit so the information you receive is consistent and so these important people can get to know you.
- Discuss with your child's primary nurse the time you will usually visit so she or he can schedule your baby's procedures and rest times other than when you visit so there is time for you to hold your child and interact with him uninterrupted.
- Ask for explanations of any equipment or medications being used with your child so you understand the plan of care. Insist on being included in care decisions. The nurses are always nearby and will be happy to explain what can be touched and moved and what should be left alone for now.
- Any day you are unable to visit, call the nursery and ask to talk to your child's primary care nurse. Such telephone calls are not viewed as a bother but are welcomed as the mark of a concerned parent.
- Ask if you can supply expressed breast milk for your infant as soon as feedings are started so you can feel you're having a greater part in your baby's care.
- You might supply a tape recording of your voice so your baby can learn to recognize it, as well as supply a small toy for your baby's bed. These actions not only supply auditory and visual stimulation for your infant but also help to give you a more "normal" feeling toward infant care.
- Use your baby's name when you talk about him (not "the baby") to help you gain a firm feeling that this is your baby, not the nursery's.
- If your child is hospitalized a distance from home, ask if transfer to a local hospital in a less technical environment will be possible as soon as he's not so ill.

By feeding her infant or expressing milk for feedings, the mother is directly participating in care and learning the first steps of her new role.

If the baby is going to be transferred to a regional center, make sure the parents have an opportunity to see the infant before the transfer. A photograph of the infant for them to keep is helpful in making the birth more real. Encourage them to visit the distant site as often as possible. Sending them photos snapped with a cell phone or pasting notes as if they're messages from the baby taped to the incubator or warmer ("Hi, Mom & Dad. I'm doing well") for them to see when they visit can not only keep parents involved but also help with bonding.

On days they cannot visit, parents can still stay in touch by telephone, video, or nursery e-mail. By these means, by the time the baby is ready for discharge, the parents should be able to feel they are taking home "their" baby, one whom they know and have already begun to love.

Parents visiting a high-risk nursery often need a great deal of support from nursing personnel. Remember that, although radiant warmers, incubators, ventilators, and monitors are familiar equipment to nurses, they are unusual and frightening to parents (Box 26.5). In such a high-tech setting, a parent may want very much to touch his or her infant but is so afraid touching might set off an alarm that he or she stands with arms folded (Fig. 26.9).

Because preterm infants can be hospitalized for long periods, parents can feel baffled by receiving information from a parade of different healthcare providers or a different person every time they visit. Primary nursing or case management with one nurse as the consistent caregiver helps to reduce the number of people who contact the parents and who communicate the parents' needs to the rest of the staff.

Try to make a baby's siblings as welcome in a high-risk nursery as the baby's parents in order to build family unity. Check to be certain siblings do not have an upper respiratory infection or fever. Also, their immunizations should be up to date and they should not have been recently exposed to a communicable disease, such as chickenpox, before they visit.

Nursing Diagnosis: Deficient diversional activity (lack of stimulation) related to preterm infant's rest needs

Outcome Evaluation: Infant demonstrates interaction with caregivers by attuning to faces or voices.

Figure 26.9 Encourage families to visit with immature infants to establish bonding. (Phanie/Alamy Stock Photo)

BOX 26.5

Nursing Care Planning Tip for Effective Communication

Mrs. Atkins gave birth 2 days ago to a 2-lb boy at 30 weeks of pregnancy who has been classified as a small-for-gestational-age preterm infant. Although you have told Mrs. Atkins twice she is welcome to visit the neonatal intensive care unit (NICU) as much as she'd like, you notice her electronic record indicates she has done so only once.

Tip: Ask enough questions to determine what the patient wants without making assumptions. In this scenario, the nurse could have assumed waiting for the husband to come to the hospital was what was important, but the patient most desired another person to accompany her to the nursery—a need the nurse could meet. Visiting a NICU can be intimidating for parents, not only because of the high-tech equipment that surrounds their baby but also because their baby often appears much smaller or sicker than they imagined.

Nurse: Mrs. Atkins, I've noticed you haven't been to the nursery to see your son yet.

Mrs. Atkins: I'm waiting for my husband to get here.

Nurse: Will that be today?

Mrs. Atkins: Tomorrow. He's still out of town on business.

Nurse: Have you called the nursery and asked about your son?

Mrs. Atkins: I'm waiting for my husband. We'll do it together.

Nurse: I know it seems important for you to go as a family, but I hate to see you miss these first few days with your son. What if I go with you?

Mrs. Atkins: Could you? I absolutely can't go up there alone.

Preterm infants need rest to conserve energy for growth and respiratory function, to combat hypoglycemia and infection, to stabilize temperature, and to develop inner balance and attentiveness. To allow for this, try to organize procedures to maximize the amount of rest available to an infant. If not a coordinated effort, an infant may be awakened constantly for procedures. Preterm infants may have more difficulty blocking out stimuli than term infants do because their nervous systems are so immature. They may demonstrate they are overstimulated by such behaviors as gagging, crying, splaying fingers and toes, or going limp when exposed to bright lights, noise, pain, or overly strenuous handling. Because these infants have little strength to move away from an unwanted stimulus, it is a caregiver's responsibility to be sensitive to these cues and move the object or noise away from the infant (Silberstein & Litmanovitz, 2016). Until ready to take in stimuli, the infant may need to be shielded from noise and light and pain may need to be limited as much as possible.

Just as a preterm infant needs rest, he or she also needs planned periods of pleasing sensory stimulation. Like all newborns, preterm infants respond best to stimulation that appeals to their senses of sight, sound, and touch.

A passive face, picture, or decal may be appealing for only a short period of time.

The acrylic dome of an incubator can distort an infant's view. Also, most people view an infant in an incubator with themselves standing up and the infant lying horizontally. This means that an infant's face is rarely in the same line of vision as the adult's (an *en face* position). It is important to look directly at an infant in the straightforward position as much as possible so the infant is provided with the stimulation of a human face. As infants mature, they should have mobiles (perhaps black and white) or bright objects placed in view. As an infant's position is changed from the left side to the right side, move the object to be in line with the child's vision.

Infants in closed incubators may be able to hear nothing but the sound of the incubator motor. They may see people looking or nodding at them and may see their mouths moving, but they cannot benefit from the sound of their voices because this is obscured by the continuous hum of the motor. To help them hear better, provide some "talk time"—words spoken softly but clearly into an infant's ear during each nursing shift, perhaps while the infant is being fed out of the incubator, to offer usual sensory stimulation.

Even an infant who cannot be removed from an incubator should not suffer from lack of touch. Gently stroking an infant's back or smoothing the back of the head should not be tiring. Pulse oximetry can be used to help you recognize when an infant is comforted by handling (e.g., oxygen saturation remains steady or increases) and when the infant is growing tired (e.g., oxygen saturation falls). Be certain during every nursing shift that close interaction is provided, particularly if clinical interventions with an infant include uncomfortable procedures such as suctioning or blood drawing. As soon as infants can be out of incubators or removed from warmers, they need special time just to be rocked and held.

Nursing Diagnosis: Risk for disorganized infant behavior related to prematurity and environmental overstimulation

Outcome Evaluation: Newborn's vital signs remain within normal limits; infant demonstrates increasing ability to adapt to stimuli; demonstrates decreasing levels of irritability, crying, respiratory pauses, tachypnea, and color changes.

The amount of rest and stimulation required by preterm infants for healthy development is best individualized. **Developmental care** (care designed to meet the specific needs of each infant) can lead to increased weight gain and decreased crying and apnea spells in preterm infants (Samra, McGrath, Wehbe, et al., 2012) (Box 26.6).

Because preterm infants have an immature central nervous system, their reactions or adjustments to stimuli may be different from those of term infants. The environment of an intensive care unit is also totally different from what infants would have experienced if they had remained in utero until term. Based on these two premises, nursing care should be geared toward making the environment of infants as atraumatic as possible while helping them adjust to new experiences within their limited ability.

BOX 26.6

Developmental Care

Developmental care is care individually designed based on a preterm infant's behavioral cues to meet the special needs of a preterm or newborn infant. Common measures include:

PARENT WELCOMING PROCEDURES

- Make parents feel welcome in a neonatal intensive care environment by both words and actions.
- Provide room around incubators or warmers for rocking chairs so parents can hold their baby comfortably.
- Encourage parent participation in feeding or supplying nonnutritive sucking experiences.
- Demonstrate the infant's capabilities and how, although immature, these are correct for the infant's age or weight.
- Keep parents informed of their baby's progress and the rationale for therapies.
- Ask parents for input into their baby's rhythm of care that will best suit them and the infant after they return home.

INFANT DEVELOPMENTAL PROCEDURES

- Provide a consistent routine to help the infant develop sleep/wake cycles.
- Time infant care and feeding based on the sleep/wake cycle of the infant.
- Cluster aspects of care so the infant enjoys the longest possible sleep intervals to conserve energy.
- Provide a "nest" with blankets to offer a sense of boundaries or security.
- Position infants so they can self-soothe—curled on side, or hands near face, knees tucked near body, or whatever way each baby seems to prefer.
- Provide quiet or rest times by covering an incubator and limiting sound.
- Provide tactile stimulation by back stroking or massage.
- Provide audio and visual stimulation by the use of mobiles and music or a parent's voice.
- Halt procedures as soon as the infant evidences stress.

The usual sound level of nurseries, for example, has been documented to be about 40 to 50 dB; a radio playing raises this to 60 to 65 dB. The closing of portholes or tapping on the sides of incubators raises the sound level inside them to 80 dB or more, or a sound level that can be painful. Other abnormal stimuli are bright lights for 24 hours a day, frequent handling, and painful procedures.

Activities such as dimming the lights or covering an incubator, turning an infant to the side and containing the body with rolled towels (nesting), offering nonnutritive sucking, and maintaining a "quiet hour" to reduce sound are all ways to reduce stimuli or construct an environment conducive to healthy development (Laubach, Wilhelm, & Carter, 2014).

Nursing Diagnosis: Parental health-seeking behaviors related to preterm infant's needs for health maintenance

Outcome Evaluation: Parents describe schedule for basic immunizations and health assessments and state who will provide ongoing health care.

Discharge from a NICU is a major transition for parents as well as their infant. Before discharge, the parents of a preterm infant need to learn and practice any special methods of care necessary for their infant and interventions to help maximize their child's development. Some parents tend to overprotect preterm infants, such as not allowing visitors or not taking an infant outside. Let parents know their concern is normal, but overprotection is not necessary.

Ongoing health maintenance of a preterm infant follows the usual pattern of well-child care. Basic immunizations are given according to the chronologic age of an infant. In many communities, NICUs maintain their own well-child settings for infants who were hospitalized there. This allows for long-term follow-up studies on the effect of oxygen or drug therapy and continuity of care. Many parents prefer bringing their infant back to such a facility rather than establishing a new network of health care because they have already established trust and confidence in that healthcare team. This often also increases their self-esteem because they hear the staff's delight in the progress made by their child. However, preterm infants can be followed by any healthcare provider for well-child care.

When plotting the height and weight of preterm infants at well-child visits, remember to account for early birth on the growth chart by double charting—that is, plotting the child's weight and height according to the chronologic age (a pattern that, in the early months, probably places the child below the 10th percentile). Then, in another color, plot the height and weight according to an infant's adjusted age, or plot the weight of a baby born 2 months early 2 months earlier on the graph. A preterm baby typically gains "catch-up" weight in the first 6 months of life, so by 1 year of age, a baby plots over the 10th percentile on a growth chart without accounting for a setback age.

Evaluate growth and developmental milestones of a preterm infant in the same manner. A preterm infant can be expected to meet first-year milestones not at the chronologic age but at the setback age. To evaluate the parents' transition to having so small an infant at home, ask at health promotion visits if the parents are:

- Beginning to feel more comfortable with their infant
- Able to allow the child to stay with a babysitter or another family member
- Beginning to incorporate their infant into their family life
- Making plans for the infant beyond the immediate newborn period

QSEN Checkpoint Question 26.2

TEAMWORK & COLLABORATION

Baby Atkin's father plays in a garage band for a hobby, and his mother enjoys knitting. The nurse's care team has agreed to design a developmental care environment for Baby Atkins that will both make him feel secure and help his parents interact more with him. The care team determines which action is best?

a. Turning up the lights in his part of the nursery so he can see his parents better

b. Asking the father to bring in a recording of his band to play for the baby

c. Arranging a blanket Mrs. Atkins has knit into a circle or "nest" for the baby

d. Reminding the parents that he must stay awake for extended periods for his eyes to fully develop

Look in Appendix A for the best answer and rationale.

THE SMALL-FOR-GESTATIONAL-AGE INFANT

An infant is SGA (also called microsomia) if the birth weight is below the 10th percentile on an intrauterine growth curve for that age. Such infants may be born:

- Preterm: before week 38 of gestation
- Term: between weeks 38 and 42
- Postterm: past 42 weeks

SGA infants are small for their age because they have experienced **intrauterine growth restriction (IUGR)** or failed to grow at the expected rate in utero (Rahimian, 2013). This characteristic makes them distinctly different from infants who are born with a less weight than usual but their low weight is consistent for their gestational age.

Etiology

A woman's nutrition during pregnancy plays a major role in fetal growth, so a lack of adequate nutrition may be a major contributor to IUGR (Ota, Tobe-Gai, Mori, et al., 2012).

Adolescents are prone to having a high incidence of SGA infants because if they eat only enough to meet their own nutritional and growth needs, the needs of a growing fetus can be compromised. In still other instances, the placental supply of nutrients is adequate but an infant cannot use them because of a chromosomal abnormality or an intrauterine infection such as rubella or toxoplasmosis.

Even in light of these nutritional influences, the most common cause of IUGR is a placental issue: either the placenta did not obtain sufficient nutrients from the uterine arteries or it was inefficient at transporting nutrients to the fetus. Placental underdevelopment or damage, such as partial placental separation with bleeding is an example of a situation that would limit placental function because the area of placenta that separated infarcted and fibrosed, reducing the placental surface available for nutrient exchange. Women with systemic diseases that decrease blood flow to the placenta, such as severe diabetes mellitus or gestational hypertension (diseases in which blood vessel lumens are narrowed), are at higher risk for birthing SGA babies than others. Women who smoke heavily or use opiates also tend to have SGA infants (Ortigosa, Friguls, Joya, et al., 2012).

Assessment

The SGA infant may be detected in utero when fundal height during pregnancy becomes progressively less than expected.

However, if a woman is unsure of the date of her last menstrual period, this discrepancy can be hard to substantiate; a sonogram can then demonstrate the decreased size. A biophysical profile including a nonstress test, placental grading, amniotic fluid amount, and an ultrasound examination documents additional information on placental function and fetal growth. If poor placental function is apparent from such determinations, it can be predicted that the infant will do poorly during labor during the periods of relative hypoxia, which occur during contractions. Cesarean birth, therefore, is the birth method of choice in such circumstances.

Appearance

Generally, an infant who suffers nutritional deprivation early in pregnancy, when fetal growth consists primarily of an increase in the number of body cells, is below average in weight, length, and head circumference. An infant who suffers deprivation late in pregnancy, when growth consists primarily of an increase in cell size, may have only a reduction in weight. Regardless of when deprivation occurs, the infant tends to have an overall wasted appearance. The infant may have poor skin turgor and generally appears to have a large head because the rest of the body is so small. Skull sutures may be widely separated. Hair may be dull and lusterless. The infant may have a small liver, which can cause difficulty regulating glucose, protein, and bilirubin levels after birth. The abdomen may be sunken. The umbilical cord often appears dry and may be stained yellow.

In contrast, because an infant's age is more advanced than the weight implies, an infant may have better developed neurologic responses, sole creases, and ear cartilage than expected for a baby of that weight. The infant may also seem unusually alert and active. As a first assessment, the SGA infant needs to be examined carefully for possible congenital anomalies that occurred because of the poor nutritional intrauterine environment.

Laboratory Findings

Blood studies at birth usually show a high hematocrit level (less than normal amounts of plasma in proportion to red blood cells are present because of a lack of fluid) and an increase in the total number of red blood cells (polycythemia). The increase in red blood cells occurs because anoxia during intrauterine life stimulated excess development of them. An immediate effect of polycythemia is to cause increased blood viscosity, a condition that puts extra work on the infant's heart because it is more difficult to effectively circulate thick blood. As a consequence, acrocyanosis (blueness of the hands and feet) may be prolonged and persistently more marked than usual. If the polycythemia is extreme, vessels may actually become blocked and thrombus formation can result. If the hematocrit level is more than 65% to 70%, an exchange transfusion to dilute the blood may be necessary.

A second problem of polycythemia is hyperbilirubinemia because so many extra red blood cells break down and release bilirubin.

Because SGA infants have decreased glycogen stores, still another common problem that develops is hypoglycemia (decreased blood glucose, or a level below 45 mg/dl). Such infants may need intravenous glucose to sustain blood sugar until they are able to suck vigorously enough to take sufficient oral feedings.

Nursing Diagnoses and Related Interventions

Nursing Diagnosis: Ineffective breathing pattern related to underdeveloped body systems at birth

Outcome Evaluation: Newborn maintains respirations at a rate of 30 to 60 breaths/min after resuscitation at birth.

Birth asphyxia is a common problem for SGA infants, both because they have underdeveloped chest muscles and because they are at risk for developing meconium aspiration syndrome (MAS) as a result of meconium release, which occurs when fetal anoxia develops during labor to cause reflex relaxation of the anal sphincter. When gasping for breath in utero, the fetus draws meconium discharged from the intestine into the amniotic fluid down into the trachea and bronchi. Acting as a foreign substance, this blocks airflow into the alveoli and causes the SGA infant to need resuscitation at birth. Closely observe both respiratory rate and character in the first few hours of life as underdeveloped chest muscles not only make taking the first breath difficult but can make SGA infants unable to sustain an adequate newborn respiratory rate.

Nursing Diagnosis: Risk for ineffective thermoregulation related to lack of subcutaneous fat

Outcome Evaluation: Infant's temperature is maintained at 36.5°C (97.8°F) axillary.

SGA infants are less able to control body temperature than other newborns because they lack subcutaneous fat. A carefully controlled environment is essential to keep the infant's body temperature in a neutral zone (see Chapter 18).

Nursing Diagnosis: Risk for impaired parenting related to child's high-risk status and possible cognitive or neurologic impairment from lack of nutrients in utero

Outcome Evaluation: Parents express interest in infant and ask questions about what the child's care needs will be at home; parents hold infant warmly.

Although SGA infants may gain weight and appear to thrive in the first few days of life, their cognitive development may have been impaired because of lack of oxygen and nourishment in utero. Babies who were growing normally in utero but whose gestation was interrupted (true preterm, AGA babies) usually gain weight and height so rapidly that by the end of the first year of life they are near the 50th percentile on growth charts. SGA infants, in contrast, may always be below the usual height on standard growth charts. This inability to reach normal levels of growth and development can interfere with bonding if a child does not meet the parents' expectations. Eventually, it can interfere with the child's self-esteem if the child is never able to meet parental expectations or reach full height.

Yet, another need of an SGA infant is adequate stimulation during the infant period in order to reach normal growth and developmental milestones. Encourage parents to provide toys suitable for their child's chronologic age, not physical size. Because an infant tires easily in the first few weeks of life, urge them to space play periods with rest periods or hypoglycemia or apnea can occur. All infants with IUGR need continued follow-up after hospital discharge because they may have neurologic deficits that will interfere with learning at preschool age (Murray, Fernandes, Fazel, et al., 2015).

THE LARGE-FOR-GESTATIONAL-AGE INFANT

An infant is LGA (also termed **macrosomia**) if the birth weight is above the 90th percentile on an intrauterine growth chart for that gestational age. Such a baby appears deceptively healthy at birth because of the weight, but a gestational age examination often reveals immature development. It is important that LGA infants be identified immediately so they can be given care appropriate to their gestational age rather than being treated as term newborns (Sjaarda, Albert, Mumford, et al., 2014).

Etiology

Infants who are LGA have been subjected to an overproduction of nutrients and growth hormone in utero. This happens most often to infants of women who are obese or who have diabetes mellitus (Sjaarda et al., 2014). Multiparous women may also have large babies because with each succeeding pregnancy, babies tend to grow larger. Beckwith–Wiedemann syndrome, a rare condition characterized by general body overgrowth and congenital anomalies such as omphalocele, may also be a cause.

Assessment

A fetus is suspected of being LGA when a woman's uterus appears to be unusually large for the date of pregnancy. Abdominal size can be deceptive, however. Because a fetus lies in a flexed fetal position, he or she does not occupy significantly more space at 10 lb than at 7 lb. If a fetus does seem to be growing at an abnormally rapid rate, a sonogram can confirm the suspicion. A nonstress test to assess the placenta's ability to sustain a large fetus during labor may be prescribed. Lung maturity may be assessed by amniocentesis.

If an infant's large size was not detected during pregnancy, it may be first recognized during labor when the baby appears too large to descend through the pelvic rim. If this happens, a cesarean birth may be necessary because **shoulder dystocia** (the wide fetal shoulders cannot pass; or needs significant manipulation to pass through the outlet of the pelvis) would halt vaginal birth at that point.

Appearance

At birth, LGA infants may show immature reflexes and low scores on gestational age examinations in relation to their size. They may have extensive bruising or a birth injury such as a broken clavicle or Erb–Duchenne paralysis from trauma to the cervical nerves if they were stressed in order for the wide shoulders to be born vaginally (see Chapter 51). Because the head is large, it may have been exposed to more than the usual amount of pressure during birth, causing a prominent caput succedaneum, cephalohematoma, or molding.

TABLE 26.2 IMPORTANT ASSESSMENT CRITERIA FOR A LARGE-FOR-GESTATIONAL-AGE INFANT

Assessment	Rationale
Assess skin color for ecchymosis, jaundice, and erythema	Bruising occurs with vaginal birth because of the large size; polycythemia causes ruddiness of skin. Ecchymosis is important to document because jaundice may occur from breakdown of ecchymotic collections of blood.
Assess motion of upper extremities is spontaneous and also occurs in response to a Moro reflex to detect if clavicle fracture (crepitus or swelling may then be palpated at the fracture site) or Erb's palsy caused by edema of the cervical nerve plexus are present.	Clavicle or cervical nerve injuries may occur because of problem at birth of wider than usual shoulders.
Assess asymmetry of the anterior chest or unilateral lack of movement to detect diaphragmatic paralysis from edema of the phrenic nerve.	The cervical nerve may be stretched by birth of wide shoulders.
Assess eyes for evidence of unresponsive or dilated pupils; assess for vomiting, bulging fontanelles, or a high-pitched cry suggestive of increased intracranial pressure.	The larger than usual head can be more compressed than usual resulting in increased intracranial pressure. Compression of the third, fourth, and sixth cranial nerves limits eye response; other signs are additional signs of increased intracranial pressure.
Assess for activities such as jitteriness, lethargy, and uncoordinated eye movements that suggest seizure activity.	Seizures are yet another indication of increased intracranial pressure; hypoglycemia seizures in newborns from the result of a low glucose level often produce the more vague symptoms.

Because LGA newborn are large but often immature, they require the same cautious care necessary for a preterm infant. Specific criteria for initial or continuing assessments are shown in Table 26.2.

Cardiovascular Dysfunction

Polycythemia may occur in an LGA fetus as the fetus attempts to fully oxygenate more than the average amount of body tissue. Following birth, observe LGA infants closely for signs of hyperbilirubinemia that may result from absorption of blood from bruising and breakdown of the extra red blood cells created by polycythemia. Assess the infant's heart rate also. If cyanosis is present, it may be a sign of poor heart function, but it could also be from transposition of the great vessels, a serious heart anomaly associated with macrosomia (see Chapter 41).

Hypoglycemia

LGA infants also need to be carefully assessed for hypoglycemia in the early hours of life because large infants require large amounts of nutritional stores to sustain their weight. If the mother had diabetes that was poorly controlled (the cause of the large size), the infant would have had an increased blood glucose level in utero to match the mother's glucose level; this caused the infant to produce elevated levels of insulin. After birth, these increased insulin levels will continue for up to 24 hours of life, possibly causing rebound hypoglycemia.

Nursing Diagnoses and Related Interventions

Nursing Diagnosis: Ineffective breathing pattern related to possible birth trauma in the LGA newborn

Outcome Evaluation: Newborn initiates independent breathing at birth; maintains usual newborn respiratory rate of 30 to 60 breaths/min.

Some LGA infants have difficulty establishing respirations at birth because of birth trauma. Increased intracranial pressure from birth of the larger than usual head, for example, could have led to pressure on the respiratory center causing a decrease in respiratory function. If the infant was born vaginally, a diaphragmatic paralysis or broken clavicle, both of which can prevent effective lung function, may have occurred in order for the wide shoulders to be born. If the infant was born by cesarean birth, transient fluid can remain in the lungs and can interfere with effective gas exchange. Careful observation is needed, therefore, to detect all these conditions. Care of an infant with transient lung fluid is discussed later in this chapter.

Nursing Diagnosis: Risk for imbalanced nutrition, less than body requirements, related to additional nutrients needed to maintain weight and prevent hypoglycemia

Outcome Evaluation: Infant's weight follows percentile growth curve, skin turgor is good, specific gravity of urine is 1.003 to 1.020; serum glucose is above 45 mg/dl.

As a rule, an LGA infant needs to be fed immediately after birth (preferably by breastfeeding) to prevent hypoglycemia. Evaluate carefully the intake of LGA infants at this feeding so you don't overestimate their ability to suck effectively. Such infants may seem as if they should be able to suck well because they are already the size of a 2-month-old. However, despite their size, these infants are inexperienced newborns, and sucking may not be effective enough to obtain the larger than usual amount of milk needed.

These infants may need supplemental formula feedings after breastfeeding to supply enough fluid and glucose for the larger than normal size for the first 24 hours. Newborns who are offered bottles often have more difficulty than do others learning to breastfeed, however, so in light of this, although it seems extreme, additional glucose may be offered intravenously.

Nursing Diagnosis: Risk for impaired parenting related to high-risk status of LGA infant

Outcome Evaluation: Parents hold infant warmly; speak of the child in positive terms; state accurately why their infant needs to be closely observed in postnatal period.

Parents may also underestimate this infant's needs because of the child's large size. He or she seems so big and healthy, so it can be confusing to be told the infant needs careful observation. If they are worried the infant must be sick in some way and they are not being told about, it can interfere with bonding happening as instinctively as it might. If a woman sustained a cervical or perineal tear or required a cesarean birth, she may need some time to air any negative feelings she may be experiencing toward the infant for causing her extra pain. Otherwise, her perception that her infant is the cause of her additional distress is another factor that could interfere with her ability to bond with the child.

Note whether parents treat their baby as a newborn who needs warm nurturing care, not as a tough, big infant who has grown past that stage because the baby may miss out on usual parental comforting measures. You may need to remind parents an infant's birth weight does not correlate with the child's projected adult size. Otherwise, parents may fear their infant may grow to be a larger than usual adult.

> *What If . . . 26.2*
> Mrs. Atkins tells the nurse she wishes her baby was 11 lb like the baby in the incubator next to hers so he wouldn't have any problems. What patient education would the nurse provide?

THE POSTTERM INFANT

A **postterm infant** is one born after the 41st week of a pregnancy (Rahimian, 2013). Infants who stay in utero past week 41 are at special risk because a placenta appears to function effectively for only 40 weeks. After that time, it seems to lose its ability to carry nutrients effectively to the fetus, and the fetus begins to lose weight (postterm syndrome). Infants with this syndrome demonstrate many of the characteristics of the SGA infant: dry, cracked, almost leatherlike skin from lack of fluid, and an absence of vernix. They may be SGA, and the amount of amniotic fluid surrounding them may be less at birth than usual and it may be meconium stained. Fingernails will have grown well beyond the end of the fingertips. Because they are older than a term infant, they may demonstrate an alertness much more like a 2-week-old baby than a newborn.

When a pregnancy becomes postterm, a sonogram is usually obtained to measure the biparietal diameter of the fetus. A nonstress test or complete biophysical profile (see Chapter 9) may be done to establish whether the placenta is still functioning adequately. A cesarean birth may be indicated if a nonstress test reveals that compromised placental functioning is apt to occur during labor.

At birth, the postterm baby is likely to have difficulty establishing respirations, especially if meconium aspiration occurred. Polycythemia may have developed from decreased oxygenation in the final weeks. The hematocrit may be elevated because polycythemia and dehydration have lowered the circulating plasma level. In the first hours of life, hypoglycemia may develop because the fetus had to use stores of glycogen for nourishment in the last weeks of intrauterine life. Subcutaneous fat levels may also be low, having been used in utero. This loss of fat can make temperature regulation difficult, making it important to prevent a postterm infant from becoming chilled at birth or during transport.

Any woman is anxious when she does not have her baby on her due date. She is apt to become extremely anxious and perhaps angry when it is determined her baby is postterm. It seems that, if her baby stayed so long in utero under her protection, the baby should be extra healthy and strong. Why, then, she asks, is her baby being transferred for special care? The mother may also feel guilty for not providing well for her infant in the last few weeks of the pregnancy.

Make certain a woman spends enough time with her newborn to assure herself that although birth did not occur at the predicted time, the baby should do well with appropriate interventions to control possible hypoglycemia or meconium aspiration. All postterm infants need follow-up care until at least school age to track their developmental abilities because the lack of nutrients and oxygen in utero may have left them with neurologic symptoms that will not become apparent until they attempt fine-motor tasks.

Illnesses That Occur in Newborns

A number of illnesses occur specifically in newborns that automatically cause the infant to be classified as high risk.

RESPIRATORY DISTRESS SYNDROME

Respiratory distress syndrome (RDS) of the newborn, formerly termed *hyaline membrane disease*, is most often seen in newborns born prematurely. Other causes of RDS include newborns with meconium aspiration syndrome, sepsis, a newborn who is slow to transition to extrauterine life, and pneumonia (Hermansen & Mahajan, 2015).

The pathologic feature of RDS is a hyalinelike (fibrous) membrane formed from an exudate of an infant's blood that begins to line the terminal bronchioles, alveolar ducts, and alveoli. This membrane prevents the exchange of oxygen and carbon dioxide at the alveolar–capillary membrane, interfering with effective oxygenation. The cause of RDS is a low level or absence of surfactant, the phospholipid that normally lines the alveoli and reduces surface tension to keep the alveoli from collapsing on expiration. Because surfactant does not form until the 34th week of gestation, as many as 30% of LBW infants and as many as 50% of VLBW premature infants are susceptible to this complication.

Pathophysiology

High pressure is required to fill the lungs with air for the first time and overcome the pressure of lung fluid. For example, it takes a pressure between 40 and 70 cm H_2O to inspire a first breath but only 15 to 20 cm H_2O to maintain quiet, continued breathing. If alveoli collapse with each expiration, as happens when surfactant is deficient, forceful inspirations requiring optimum pressure are still required to inflate them.

Even very immature infants release a bolus of surfactant at birth into their lungs from the stress of birth. However, with deficient surfactant, areas of hypoinflation begin to occur and pulmonary resistance increases. Blood then shunts through the foramen ovale and the ductus arteriosus as it did during fetal life. The lungs become poorly perfused. As a result, the production of surfactant decreases even further.

The poor oxygen exchange that results leads to tissue hypoxia, which causes the release of lactic acid. This, combined with the increasing carbon dioxide level resulting from the formation of the hyaline membrane on the alveolar surface, leads to severe acidosis. Acidosis causes vasoconstriction and decreased pulmonary perfusion from vasoconstriction, which further limits surfactant production. With surfactant production almost lost, the ability to stop alveoli from collapsing with each expiration becomes more and more difficult. This vicious cycle continues until the oxygen–carbon dioxide exchange in the alveoli is no longer adequate to sustain life without ventilator support.

Assessment

Most infants who develop RDS have difficulty initiating respirations at birth. After resuscitation, they appear to have a period of hours or a day when they are free of symptoms because of an initial release of surfactant. During this time, however, subtle signs may appear, such as:

- Low body temperature
- Nasal flaring
- Sternal and subcostal retractions
- Tachypnea (more than 60 breaths/min)
- Cyanotic mucous membranes

Within several hours, expiratory grunting occurs caused by closure of the glottis as it tries to increase the pressure in alveoli on expiration in order to help to keep them from collapsing. Even with this attempt at better oxygen exchange, however, as the disease progresses, infants become cyanotic and their PO_2 and oxygen saturation levels fall in room air. On auscultation, there may be fine rales and diminished breath sounds because of poor air entry. As distress increases, an infant may exhibit:

- Seesaw respirations (on inspiration, the anterior chest wall retracts and the abdomen protrudes; on expiration, the sternum rises)
- Heart failure, evidenced by decreased urine output and edema of the extremities
- Pale gray skin
- Periods of apnea
- Bradycardia
- Pneumothorax

The diagnosis of RDS is made on the clinical signs of grunting, central cyanosis in room air, tachypnea, nasal flaring, and retractions. A chest X-ray will reveal a diffuse pattern of radiopaque areas that look like ground glass (haziness) in the lungs. Blood gas studies will reveal respiratory acidosis. A β-hemolytic, group B streptococcal infection may mimic RDS because this infection is so severe in newborns that it stops surfactant production. Cultures of blood, cerebrospinal fluid, and skin may be obtained, therefore, to rule out this condition. An antibiotic (penicillin or ampicillin) and an aminoglycoside (gentamicin or kanamycin) may be started while culture reports are pending.

Therapeutic Management

Surfactant Replacement

RDS can be largely prevented by the administration of surfactant at birth for an infant at risk because of low gestational age (Box 26.7). Immediately after birth, synthetic surfactant is administered into an endotracheal tube by a syringe or catheter (lung lavage) (Wyckoff et al., 2015).

It's important the infant is tipped to an upright position following administration and the infant's airway is not suctioned for as long as safely possible after administration of surfactant to help it reach lower lung areas and to avoid suctioning the drug away. Although there are almost no unfavorable reactions to surfactant administration, some, such as mucus plugging from the solution, do occur. An infant who is receiving surfactant and then is placed on a ventilator needs close observation because lung expansion can improve so rapidly, the ventilator pressure becomes too high. Anticipate the need to adjust ventilator settings to accommodate the vastly improved lung function.

Oxygen Administration

The administration of oxygen is often necessary to maintain correct PO_2 and pH levels following surfactant administration, and it may be administered in a variety of ways from a simple cannula or mask, continuous positive airway pressure (CPAP), or assisted ventilation with positive end-expiratory pressure (PEEP). The advantage of CPAP or PEEP is that this exerts pressure on the alveoli at the end of expiration and helps keep alveoli from collapsing in addition to supplying oxygen (Wyckoff et al., 2015). High-frequency, oscillatory, and jet ventilation are still other methods of introducing oxygen to infants with noncompliant lungs. These systems

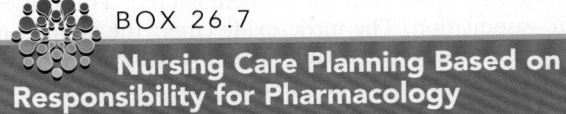

BOX 26.7

Nursing Care Planning Based on Responsibility for Pharmacology

SURFACTANT (SURVANTA)
(http://survanta.com/dosage.cfm)

Action: Surfactant restores naturally occurring lung surfactant to improve lung compliance.

Pregnancy Risk Category: X

Dosage: 4 ml/kg intratracheally; four doses in first 48 hours of life

Possible Adverse Effects: Transient bradycardia, rales

Nursing Implications
- Suction infant before administration.
- Assess infant's respiratory rate, rhythm, oxygen saturation, and color before administration.
- Ensure proper endotracheal tube placement before dosing.
- Change infant's position during administration to encourage the drug to flow to both lungs.
- Assess infant's respiratory rate, color, and pulse oximetry or arterial blood gases after administration.
- Do not suction endotracheal tube for 1 hour after administration to avoid removing the drug (Karch, 2013).

maintain airway pressure and then intermittently "jet" or oscillate an additional amount of air at a rapid rate (400 to 600 times per minute) to inflate alveoli.

A possible complication of oxygen therapy in the very immature or very ill infant is ROP (see discussion later in chapter) or bronchopulmonary dysplasia (BPD) which is also known as chronic lung disease (see Chapter 40).

Ventilation

Normally, on a ventilator, inspiration is shorter than expiration, or there is an inspiratory/expiratory (I/E) ratio of 1:2. It is difficult to deliver enough oxygen to stiff, noncompliant lungs in this usual ratio, however, without forcing the air into the lungs at such a high pressure and rapid rate that a pneumothorax becomes a constant concern (Kitsommart, Martins, Bottino, et al., 2012). Infant ventilators are therefore available with a reversed I/E ratio (2:1). These are pressure cycled to control the force with which air is delivered.

Complications of any type of ventilation are possible, such as pneumothorax and impaired cardiac output because of decreased blood flow through the pulmonary artery from increased lung pressure. There is also a possible risk of increased intracranial and arterial pressure and hemorrhage from fluctuating blood pressures. Being certain infants are not overhydrated is important to help prevent increased blood pressure and increased pulmonary artery pressure, which may delay the closure of the ductus arteriosus and interfere with both heart and lung function.

Additional Therapy: Nitric Oxide

An additional therapy that can help to oxygenate a newborn's lungs is the administration of nitric oxide, a potent vascular dilator. It causes pulmonary vasodilation without decreasing systemic vascular tone. It combines with hemoglobin in the intravascular space to form methemoglobin. This causes systemic vasodilation. The nitric oxide enters the alveoli on ventilation and redirects the pulmonary blood by dilating the pulmonary arterioles (Nair & Lakshminrusimha, 2014).

Extracorporeal Membrane Oxygenation

Extracorporeal membrane oxygenation (ECMO) was first developed as a means of oxygenating blood during cardiac surgery. Its current use has expanded to include the management of severe hypoxemia in newborns with illnesses such as meconium aspiration, RDS, pneumonia, and diaphragmatic hernia. Formerly used as a mainstay of therapy for RDS, it is now rarely needed because surfactant lavage is so effective.

What If . . . 26.3

While the nurse was caring for Baby Atkins, who is ventilator dependent and receiving the paralyzing agent pancuronium, a power failure occurred. What would be the nurse's first actions?

Supportive Care

An infant with RDS must be kept warm because cooling increases acidosis in newborns, and for the newborn with RDS, acidosis may increase to lethal levels. Keeping an infant warm also reduces the infant's metabolic oxygen demand. Provide hydration and nutrition with intravenous fluids and glucose or gavage feedings because the respiratory effort makes an infant too exhausted to suck. Box 26.8 shows an interprofessional care map illustrating both nursing and team planning for a newborn with RDS.

Prevention

RDS rarely occurs in mature infants. Dating a pregnancy by sonogram and by documenting if the level of lecithin in surfactant obtained from amniotic fluid exceeds that of sphingomyelin by a 2:1 ratio are both important ways to be certain an infant born by cesarean birth or for whom labor is induced is mature enough that RDS is not likely to occur.

Using a tocolytic agent such as magnesium sulfate can help prevent preterm birth for a few days. During this time, if a woman receives two injections of a glucocorticosteroid, such as betamethasone, it may be possible to prevent RDS in the newborn because steroids appear to quicken the formation of lecithin. The administration is most effective when given between weeks 24 and 34 of pregnancy. Unfortunately, there is often no warning that preterm birth is imminent until hours before birth. Because the steroid does not take effect before 24 to 48 hours, some labors and births will progress too rapidly for this preventive measure to be effective.

QSEN Checkpoint Question 26.3

INFORMATICS

Baby Atkins has surfactant administered at birth. When Mrs. Atkins asks why her baby had to receive surfactant, the nurse determines which response is best?

a. "Surfactant helps him raise his lung secretions by relaxing his airway."
b. "Surfactant keeps his tiny lung sacs open and this improves his breathing."
c. "Surfactant relaxes his respiratory muscles to synchronize his breathing pattern."
d. "Surfactant reduces the amount of lung secretions that he produces."

Look in Appendix A for the best answer and rationale.

TRANSIENT TACHYPNEA OF THE NEWBORN

At birth, a newborn may have a rapid rate of respirations, up to 80 breaths/min when crying, caused by retained lung fluid (Wyckoff et al., 2015).

Within 1 hour, however, this rapid rate slows to between 30 and 60 breaths/min. In about 5 or 6 out of 1,000 live births, the respiratory rate doesn't slow as a result of a delayed absorption of alveolar fluid in the lungs. The infant does not appear to be in a great deal of distress aside from the tiring effort of breathing. Mild retractions and some nasal flaring may be noticed, enough to make feeding difficult because the infant cannot suck and breathe this rapidly at the same time. A chest X-ray will reveal some fluid in the lung along with hyperexpansion. Blood gases may show some respiratory acidosis, hypercapnia, and hypoxemia (Hermansen & Mahajan, 2015).

Although transient tachypnea of the newborn (TTN) may reflect a slight decrease in the production of phosphatidylglycerol or mature surfactant, it is a direct result of retained lung fluid, which then limits the amount of alveolar surface

BOX 26.8

Nursing Care Planning

AN INTERPROFESSIONAL CARE MAP FOR A NEWBORN WITH RESPIRATORY DISTRESS SYNDROME

Mr. and Mrs. Atkins are the parents of a 30-week-old, 2-lb baby boy, born last night after a short 4-hour labor.

Family Assessment: Family consists of two parents: Mr. Atkins works as a consulting engineer; Mrs. Atkins worked before pregnancy as a home decorator. Mr. Atkins was out of town on business so was not present for the infant's birth. Mrs. Atkins has not visited the intensive care nursery. She refused to sign the birth certificate because she could not decide on a name. She said, "I don't want to give him our favorite name because he might die." Mr. Atkins telephoned early this morning and acted more upset the baby was born than relieved that the baby was receiving intensive care. He asked his wife, "What did you do to cause this?"

Patient Assessment: A 2-lb newborn, 5 hours old, born vaginally. Had difficulty establishing respirations at birth. Resuscitated by the neonatal nurse practitioner and respiratory therapist and then transported to the intensive care nursery. Temperature: 97.2°F (36.2°C). Bradycardic and tachypneic with grunting respirations. Sternal and subcostal retractions present. Skin pale and somewhat cyanotic. Chest X-ray shows "ground-glass" appearance. Arterial blood gases (ABGs) reveal respiratory acidosis. Endotracheal (ET) intubation, mechanical ventilation, supplemental oxygen, and intravenous fluid therapy initiated.

Nursing Diagnosis: Impaired gas exchange related to immaturity of newborn's lungs and lack of surfactant

Outcome Criteria: Vital signs within acceptable parameters. Temperature maintained at 97.7°F (36.5°C). Absence of cyanosis, diminished retractions, ABG values within acceptable parameters, and no sound of grunting with respirations.

Team Member Responsible	Assessment	Intervention	Rationale	Expected Outcome
Activities of Daily Living, Including Safety				
Nurse/neonatal primary care provider team	Assess respiratory rate, depth, and rhythm; auscultate lung sounds; evaluate oxygen saturation and skin color.	Maintain respiratory program as prescribed, such as oxygen by ET tube or ventilator.	Signs of increasing respiratory distress may denote lessening air exchange.	Infant maintains a stable respiratory rate and depth with assistive respiratory aids in place.
Nurse	Assess infant's axillary temperature every hour.	Maintain a neutral thermal environment so infant's temperature remains stable.	A neutral thermal environment minimizes the risk of cold stress, which increases metabolic demands for oxygen.	Infant's temperature is maintained at 97.7°F (36.5°C) axillary.
Teamwork and Collaboration				
Nurse/early intervention specialist/developmental care coordinator	Determine what developmental care resources will be available for infant care.	Consult with developmental care coordinator regarding specific developmental care measures for infant.	Developmental care or trying to reduce infant stress can improve infant's outcome.	Developmental care coordinator establishes an individualized program for infant care.
Procedures/Medications for Quality Improvement				
Nurse/neonatal nurse practitioner/primary care provider/respiratory therapist	Assess infant's response to respiratory support. Assess oxygen saturation levels via pulse oximetry.	Maintain ET tube, mechanical ventilation, and supplemental warm humidified oxygen. Anticipate the need for continuous positive airway pressure (CPAP) or positive end-expiratory pressure (PEEP).	The ET tube protects a patent airway. Mechanical ventilation with warm humidified air assists with delivering necessary air to the lungs and helps prevent drying of mucous membranes.	Respiratory support measures are in place, and infant's respiratory rate remains within designated parameters.

Continued on following page

BOX 26.8

Nursing Care Planning (continued)

Team Member Responsible	Assessment	Intervention	Rationale	Expected Outcome
Procedures/Medications for Quality Improvement				
Nurse/primary medical care provider	Assess availability of surfactant for administration.	Administer surfactant via ET tube as per protocol. Refrain from suctioning for 1 hour if possible.	Surfactant restores the naturally occurring lung surfactant to improve lung compliance. Suctioning would remove the drug from its intended site.	Surfactant lavage is administered. Ventilatory assistance is regulated as required.
Nutrition				
Nurse/nutritionist/ primary care provider	Assess infant's need for nourishment based on gestational age and exhaustion from rapid breathing.	Administer nutrition via enteral feedings: breast milk supplemented with high-calorie formula. Anticipate the need for total parenteral nutrition if weight gain is not sufficient.	Additional nutrients are necessary because stress of respiratory distress syndrome (RDS) requires increased caloric expenditure. Total parenteral nutrition may be necessary to meet these additional needs.	Infant tolerates enteral feedings without difficulty. Mother supplies breast milk for feedings.
Nurse	Assess blood glucose levels every 4 hours by heel stick.	Report hypoglycemia (blood glucose level <45 mg/dl).	Glucose is a source of energy. Monitoring glucose levels helps to determine if sufficient energy is available to meet the newborn's metabolic needs.	Infant maintains a glucose level >45 mg/dl.
Patient-Centered Care				
Nurse/primary care provider	Assess what parents know about the cause of preterm birth.	Teach parents the cause of preterm birth often cannot be identified.	Parents will need to work with healthcare team to arrange for best care for preterm infant.	Parents state they are adjusting to the shock of preterm birth based on better knowledge of cause.
Psychosocial/Spiritual/Emotional Needs				
Nurse/primary care nurse	Assess what activities parents think their very small infant can accomplish.	Invite parents to see, touch, and spend as much time as possible with newborn. Guide them in activities such as skin-to-skin contact and basic caregiving.	Seeing, touching, and caring promote attachment. Guidance in activities helps to alleviate anxiety.	Parents visit in nursery or telephone at least every other day and touch and talk to newborn.
Nurse/NICU social worker	Assess if parents have worked through shock of preterm birth.	Suggest parents bring in a mobile or toy to keep near newborn.	A mobile or toy provides visual stimulation and promotes feelings of participation in the newborn's care.	Parents state they know preterm birth is no one's fault and express interest in parenting.
Informatics for Seamless Healthcare Planning				
Nurse/NICU social worker	Assess what community organizations will be available to family for continued support.	Refer parents to helpful websites for preterm information and suggest they join local Parents of Preemies organization.	Parents may need continued support after they return home with a small infant.	Parents give examples of how they are making active plans for infant's discharge and care.

that is available for oxygen exchange. This limitation requires an infant to increase respiratory rate and depth of respirations to better use the limited surface available. TTN occurs more often in infants who are born by cesarean birth, in infants whose mothers received extensive fluid administration during labor, and in preterm infants. Infants born by cesarean birth are probably more prone to develop this form of respiratory distress because the thoracic cavity is not compressed as it is in a vaginal birth, and so less lung fluid is expelled.

Close observation of such a newborn is a priority. Watch carefully to be certain the increased effort is not tiring and other signs of respiratory distress such as nasal flaring or retractions are not occurring because a rapid respiratory rate is often the first sign of respiratory obstruction. Other signs that suggest illness are grunting and difficulty feeding. Oxygen administration may be necessary for some infants. Some infants will be prescribed a mild glucosteroid to reduce respiratory tract inflammation. TTN usually has an onset at about two hours of life and can last approximately 36 hours. The higher the respiratory rate at onset, the longer TTN lasts. Treatment is supportive and typically by 72 hours of life it resolves (Hermansen & Mahajan, 2015).

MECONIUM ASPIRATION SYNDROME

Meconium is present in the fetal bowel as early as 10 weeks of gestation. If hypoxia occurs, a vagus reflex is stimulated, resulting in relaxation of the rectal sphincter. This releases meconium into the amniotic fluid. Babies born breech may expel meconium into the amniotic fluid from pressure on the buttocks. In both instances, the appearance of the fluid at birth is green to greenish black from the staining. Meconium staining occurs in approximately 10% to 20% of all births; in 2% to 4% of these births, infants will aspirate enough meconium to cause meconium aspiration syndrome (MAS) (Wyckoff et al., 2015). Meconium aspiration does not tend to occur in ELBW infants because the substance has not passed far enough in the bowel for it to be at the rectum in these infants.

An infant may aspirate meconium either in utero or with the first breath at birth. Meconium can cause severe respiratory distress (tachypnea, retractions, and grunting). The infant may also require increased oxygen to maintain saturations in the mid to upper 90s. This oxygen requirement usually starts in the first couple hours after birth without any congenital anomalies that may cause the low oxygen saturations (Lindenskov, Castellheim, Saugstad, et al., 2015).

Assessment

Infants with meconium-stained amniotic fluid can have difficulty establishing respirations at birth (those who were not born breech have had a hypoxic episode in utero to cause the meconium to be in the amniotic fluid). The Apgar score is apt to be low. Almost immediately, tachypnea, retractions, and cyanosis begin. The infant should be placed on the warmer, and resuscitation should begin including the initiation of positive pressure ventilation as necessary (Wyckoff et al., 2015).

After the initiation of respirations, an infant's respiratory rate may remain rapid (tachypnea) and coarse bronchial sounds may be heard on auscultation. The infant may continue to have retractions because the inflammation of bronchi tends to trap air in the alveoli, limiting the entrance of oxygen. This air trapping may also cause enlargement of the anteroposterior diameter of the chest (barrel chest). Pulse oximetry or blood gases will reveal poor gas exchange evidenced by a decreased PO_2 and an increased PCO_2. A chest X-ray will show bilateral coarse infiltrates in the lungs, with spaces of hyperaeration (a peculiar honeycomb effect). The diaphragm will be pushed downward by the overexpanded lungs.

Therapeutic Management

Amnioinfusion can be used to dilute the amount of meconium in the amniotic fluid and has shown to improve the outcomes for the newborn with meconium in situations where perinatal observation is limited. The benefits may be related to dilution of the meconium or having an effect on the oligohydramnios (Hofmeyr, Xu, & Eke, 2014). If deeply stained amniotic fluid is identified during labor, the infant may be scheduled for a cesarean birth. After birth, infants may need to be treated with oxygen administration and assisted ventilation. Antibiotic therapy may be prescribed to forestall the development of pneumonia as a secondary problem. If lung compliance is poor, surfactant may be administered (Wyckoff et al., 2015). If lung noncompliance continues, this may necessitate high inspiratory pressure. Unfortunately, this can cause a pneumothorax or pneumomediastinum (air in the chest cavity). Observe the infant closely, therefore, for signs of trapping air in the alveoli because the alveoli can expand only so far and then will rupture, sending air into the pleural space (pneumothorax).

Yet, a further complication that can occur because of increased pulmonary resistance is the ductus arteriosus remaining open, causing blood to shunt from the pulmonary artery into the aorta and compromising cardiac efficiency and increasing hypoxia. To detect this, observe an infant closely for signs of heart failure such as increased heart rate or respiratory distress. Maintain a temperature-neutral environment to prevent the infant from having to increase metabolic oxygen demands. A chest physiotherapy with percussion and vibration may be helpful to encourage the removal of remnants of meconium from the lungs (see Chapter 40). Some infants may need to be administered nitric oxide or maintained on ECMO to ensure adequate oxygenation (Chettri, Bhat, & Adhisivam, 2016).

APNEA

Apnea is a cessation in respirations lasting longer than 20 seconds, sometimes accompanied by bradycardia and/or cyanosis. Many preterm infants have periods of apnea as a result of fatigue or the immaturity of their respiratory mechanisms. Babies with secondary stresses, such as infection, hyperbilirubinemia, hypoglycemia, or hypothermia, tend to have a high incidence of apnea also (Thilo & Rosenberg, 2012).

Gently stimulating an infant or flicking the sole of the foot often causes the baby to breathe again, almost as if the infant needed to be reminded to maintain this function. If an infant does not respond to these simple measures, positive-pressure ventilation and resuscitative interventions may be necessary.

Closely observe all newborns, especially preterm ones, to detect these apneic episodes. Apnea monitors that record respiratory movements are invaluable tools to detect apnea and sound a warning when an infant needs attention. Infants with frequent or difficult-to-correct episodes may be placed on respiratory support (CPAP or ventilator) until they are more mature.

To help prevent episodes of apnea, maintain a neutral thermal environment and use gentle handling to avoid excessive fatigue. Always suction gently and only when needed to minimize nasopharyngeal irritation, which can cause bradycardia because of vagal stimulation. Using indwelling nasogastric tubes rather than intermittent ones can also reduce the amount of vagal stimulation. After feeding, observe an infant carefully because a full stomach can put pressure on the diaphragm and can potentially compromise respirations. Careful burping also helps to reduce this effect. Never take rectal temperatures in infants prone to apnea because the resulting vagal stimulation can reduce the heart rate (bradycardia). Caffeine, a methylxanthine, may be prescribed for apnea of prematurity to stimulate breathing (Kreutzer & Bassler, 2014). The mechanism by which this medication reduces the incidence of apneic episodes is unclear, but they appear to increase the infant's sensitivity to carbon dioxide, which stimulates respiratory function. Infants who have had an apneic episode severe enough to require resuscitation are at a high risk for sudden infant death syndrome. Such infants may be discharged home with a monitoring device to be used for the first several months of life.

SUDDEN INFANT DEATH SYNDROME

Sudden infant death syndrome (SIDS) is a sudden unexplained death in infancy. It tends to occur at a higher than usual rate in infants of adolescent mothers, infants of closely spaced pregnancies, and underweight and preterm infants. Also prone to SIDS are infants with BPD, twins, Native American infants, Alaskan Native infants, economically disadvantaged Black infants, and infants of narcotic-dependent mothers. The peak age of incidence is 2 to 4 months of age (AAP, 2011b).

Although the cause of SIDS is unknown, in addition to prolonged but unexplained apnea, other possible contributing factors include:

- Sleeping prone rather than supine
- Viral respiratory or botulism infection
- Exposure to secondary smoke
- Pulmonary edema
- Brainstem abnormalities
- Neurotransmitter deficiencies
- Heart rate abnormalities
- Distorted familial breathing patterns
- Decreased arousal responses
- Possible lack of surfactant in alveoli
- Sleeping in a room without moving air currents (the infant rebreathes expired carbon dioxide)

Typically, affected infants are well nourished. Parents may report an infant had a slight head cold. After being put to bed at night or for a nap, the infant is then found dead a few hours later. Infants who die this way do not appear to make any sound as they die, which indicates they die with laryngospasm. Although many infants are found with blood-flecked sputum or vomitus in their mouths or on the bedclothes, this seems to occur as the result of death, not as its cause. An autopsy often reveals petechiae in the lungs and mild inflammation and congestion in the respiratory tract. However, these symptoms are not severe enough to cause sudden death. It is clear these infants do not suffocate from bedclothes or choke from overfeeding, underfeeding, or crying. Since the AAP made the recommendation to put newborns to sleep on their back, the incidence of SIDS has declined almost 50% to 60%. Other recommendations include the use of a firm sleep surface; breastfeeding; room sharing without bed sharing; routine immunizations; consideration of using a pacifier; and avoidance of soft bedding, overheating, and exposure to tobacco smoke, alcohol, and illicit drugs (Byars & Simon, 2017). Although it was once thought having infants sleep with a fan in their room to keep air moving might decrease the incidence of SIDS, the AAP has noted that, currently, there is insufficient evidence to recommend the use of a fan as a SIDS risk-reduction strategy (AAP, 2011b).

Parents have a difficult time accepting the death of any child. This can be especially difficult when it happens so suddenly and to an infant. In discussing the child, they often use both the past and present tense as if they are not yet aware of the death. Many parents experience a period of somatic symptoms that occur with acute grief, such as nausea, stomach pain, or vertigo. Parents should be counseled by someone who is trained in counseling at the time of the infant's death; it helps if they can talk to this same person periodically for however long it takes to resolve their grief. The American Sudden Infant Death Syndrome Institute, listed at the beginning of the chapter, offers suggestions for counseling.

Autopsy reports should be given to parents as soon as they are available (if toxicology tests are included in the autopsy, results will not be available for weeks). Reading that their child's death was unexplained can help to reassure parents the death was not their fault. They need this assurance if they are to plan for other children. If there are older children in the family, they also need assurance SIDS is a disease of infants and the strange phenomenon that invaded their home and killed a younger brother or sister will not also kill them. If they wished the infant dead, as some children wish siblings were dead occasionally, they need reassurance their wishes did not cause the baby's death.

When another child is born, parents can be expected to become extremely frightened at any sign of illness in their child. They need support to see them through the first few months of the second child's life, particularly until past the point at which the first child died. Some parents may need support to view a second child as an individual child and not as a replacement for the first child.

A new baby born to a family in which a SIDS infant died can be screened using a sleep assessment as a precaution within the first 2 weeks of life or, if the parents' level of anxiety is acute, before hospital discharge. The baby may then be placed on continuous apnea monitoring pending the results of the sleep assessment.

APPARENT LIFE-THREATENING EVENT

Some infants have been discovered cyanotic and limp in their beds but have survived after mouth-to-mouth resuscitation by parents. This event, also referred to as an **apparent life-threatening event (ALTE)** is characterized by a noticeable color change, some degree of apnea, and decreased tone (Sahewalla, Gupta, & Kamat, 2016). For these infants, as well as for preterm infants with a tendency toward apnea, or new babies born to a family whose child died from SIDS, apnea monitoring may be prescribed. With apnea monitoring in place, an alarm sounds when the infant experiences a period of apnea of 20 seconds or longer or a decreased heart

Figure 26.10   A home apnea monitor is used for this high-risk infant during sleep to alert the parents of any apnea episodes. (From Hatfield, N. T. [2014]. *Introductory maternity & pediatric nursing* [3rd ed.]. Philadelphia, PA: Wolters Kluwer.)

rate below 80 beats/min (or as determined by the medical provider) (Fig. 26.10). If parents are going to use an apnea monitor at home, make certain they will be able to hear it in all parts of the house or apartment. Usually, for example, the alarm is not loud enough to be heard in the basement from an upstairs bedroom. Caution parents about household noises such as a loud television, radio, vacuum cleaner, or hair dryer that may interfere with hearing the alarm. Be certain they know how to apply and reposition the apnea leads and that they are comfortable enough with the monitor to see past it to the infant. In addition, parents should be taught infant cardiopulmonary resuscitation before their infant is discharged from the hospital; reviewing the technique of this at healthcare visits is helpful (Fig. 26.11).

Caring for a child at home on an apnea monitor may be extremely stressful because parents are often reluctant to

Figure 26.11   Parents of infants with respiratory disorders need to learn cardiac massage before their infant is discharged from the hospital. Here, parents learn the technique using specialized dolls. (Ian Miles, Flashpoint Pictures/Alamy.)

leave the baby in someone else's care for even a short time or they have difficulty finding a competent babysitter. These parents can benefit from a community or home care referral so they have a second opinion regarding how well they are managing as well as a listening ear to discuss the strain of having to be constantly alert for a sound that means their infant has stopped breathing. Having someone periodically review with them what steps to take should the alarm sound (e.g., gently stimulate the baby, begin mouth-to-mouth resuscitation, call emergency response personnel) can be very comforting.

QSEN Checkpoint Question 26.4

SAFETY

Baby Atkins is at risk for having apnea and bradycardia. What initial nursing intervention should the nurse initiate during these events to maintain his vital signs in a safe range?

   a. Administer 2 drops (gtt) of oral theophylline by a small syringe into his mouth.

   b. Gently flick the sole of his foot to stimulate the baby to breathe again.

   c. Monitor rectal temperatures to prevent him from becoming cold or hot.

   d. Vigorously suction him every 2 hours to keep airway clear of secretions.

Look in Appendix A for the best answer and rationale.

PERIVENTRICULAR LEUKOMALACIA

Periventricular leukomalacia (PVL) is the result of ischemia of the white matter of the brain (Gupta, Sodhi, Saxena, et al., 2016). It is caused by an anoxic episode that interferes with circulation to a portion of the brain. Phagocytes and macrophages invade the area to clear away necrotic tissue. What is left is an abnormality in the white matter of the brain, which is revealed on a sonogram as a hollow space. PVL occurs most frequently in preterm infants who experience cerebral ischemia. Once the condition has occurred, there is no therapy. Infants may die of the original insult; they may be left with long-term effects such as learning disabilities or cerebral palsy. Any action to reduce environmental stimuli or sudden shifts in cerebral blood flow, such as avoiding rapid fluid infusions or reducing pain, is important for preventing PVL and limiting this long-term effect of prematurity (Alderliesten, Lemmers, Smarius, et al., 2013).

HEMOLYTIC DISEASE OF THE NEWBORN (HYPERBILIRUBINEMIA)

The term "hemolytic" is Latin for "destruction" (lysis) of red blood cells. A certain degree of lysis of red blood cells in the newborn results from the destruction of red blood cells by a normal physiologic process as the newborn breaks down excess red blood cells formed in utero (see Chapter 18). Hemolytic disease is present when there is excessive destruction of red blood cells, which leads to elevated bilirubin levels (hyperbilirubinemia). In the past, hemolytic disease of the newborn was most often caused by an Rh blood type incompatibility. Because the prevention of Rh antibody formation has been available for almost 50 years, the disorder is now most often caused by an ABO incompatibility. In both instances, because the fetus has a different blood type than the mother, the mother builds antibodies against the fetal red blood cells, leading to hemolysis of the cells, severe anemia, and hyperbilirubinemia.

Rh Incompatibility

In every pregnancy, a few red blood cells enter the maternal circulation. If the mother's blood type is Rh negative and the fetal blood type is Rh positive, this introduction of fetal blood causes sensitization to occur and the woman to begin to form antibodies against the specific antigen (most commonly the D antigen). Few antibodies actually form this way during pregnancy, however. Most form in the woman's bloodstream in the first 72 hours after birth because there is an active exchange of fetal–maternal blood as placental villi loosen and the placenta is delivered. Because of this surge in antibody formation after a pregnancy, in a second pregnancy, there will be a high level of antibody already circulating in the woman's bloodstream. This will then act to destroy the fetal red blood cells beginning early in the next pregnancy if the new fetus is Rh positive, leading to the fetus being severely compromised by the end of that pregnancy.

Rh incompatibility is not commonly seen today because if Rh-negative women receive Rho immune globulin (RHIG or RhoGAM) (passive Rh antibodies) within 72 hours after birth of an Rh-positive newborn, the process of antibody formation will be halted and sensitization will not occur. The possibility Rh incompatibility could exist, however, must be assessed for during pregnancy and again at birth because some women (especially those who received prenatal care in another country) may not have received RHIG following the birth or miscarriage of a former Rh-positive fetus.

ABO Incompatibility

In most instances of ABO incompatibility, the maternal blood type is O and the fetal blood type is either A or B type blood.

Hemolysis can become a problem with a first pregnancy in which there is an ABO incompatibility because the antibodies to A and B cell types are naturally occurring antibodies or are present from birth in anyone whose red cells lack these antigens. Fortunately, unlike the antibodies formed against the Rh D factor, these antibodies are of the large (IgM) class and so do not cross the placenta. An infant of an ABO incompatibility, therefore, is not born anemic, as the Rh-sensitized child could be. Hemolysis of the blood begins with birth, when blood and antibodies are exchanged during the mixing of maternal and fetal blood as the placenta is loosened; destruction may continue for as long as 2 weeks. Interestingly, preterm infants do not seem to be affected by ABO incompatibility. This may be because the receptor sites for anti-A or anti-B antibodies do not appear on red cells until late in fetal life. Even in the mature newborn, a direct Coombs test may be only weakly positive because of the few anti-A or anti-B sites present. The reticulocyte count (immature or newly formed red blood cells) is usually elevated as the infant attempts to replace destroyed cells.

Assessment

Rh incompatibility of the newborn can be predicted by finding a rising anti-Rh titer or a rising level of antibodies (indirect Coombs test) in a woman during pregnancy. It can be confirmed by detecting antibodies on the fetal erythrocytes in cord blood (positive direct Coombs test) by percutaneous umbilical blood sampling (see Chapter 9) or at birth. The mother in this situation will always have Rh-negative blood, and the baby will be Rh positive.

With Rh incompatibility, an infant may not appear pale at birth despite the red cell destruction that occurred in utero because the accelerated production of red cells during the last few months in utero compensates to some degree for the destruction. The liver and spleen may be enlarged from attempts to destroy damaged blood cells. If the number of red cells has significantly decreased, the blood in the vascular circulation may be hypotonic to interstitial fluid, causing fluid to shift from the lower to higher isotonic pressure by osmosis, resulting in extreme edema. Finally, the severe anemia can result in heart failure as the heart has to beat at a faster rate than normal to push the diluted blood forward. **Hydrops fetalis** is a Greek term that refers to a pathologic accumulation of at least two or more cavities with a collection of fluid in the fetus.

Most infants do not appear jaundiced at birth because the maternal circulation has evacuated the rising indirect bilirubin level. With birth, progressive jaundice, usually occurring within the first 24 hours of life, will begin, indicating in both Rh and ABO incompatibility that a hemolytic process is occurring. The jaundice occurs because, as red blood cells are destroyed, indirect bilirubin is released. Indirect bilirubin is fat-soluble and cannot be excreted from the body. Under usual circumstances, the liver enzyme glucuronyl transferase converts indirect bilirubin to direct bilirubin. Direct bilirubin is water-soluble and combines with bile for excretion from the body through feces. In preterm infants or those with extreme hemolysis, the liver cannot convert all of the indirect bilirubin produced into direct bilirubin fast enough, so jaundice occurs.

Normally, cord blood has a total serum bilirubin (TsB) level of 0 to 3 mg/100 ml. An increasing bilirubin level becomes dangerous if the level rises above 20 mg/dl in a term infant and perhaps as low as 12 mg/dl in a preterm infant because brain damage from bilirubin-induced neurologic dysfunction (BIND), a wide spectrum of disorders caused by increasingly severe hyperbilirubinemia ranging from mild dysfunction to acute bilirubin encephalopathy (ABE) (invasion of bilirubin into brain cells), can occur. A second concern that arises from excessive red blood cell destruction is that an infant is forced to use glucose stores to maintain metabolism in the presence of anemia. This can cause a progressive hypoglycemia, compounding the initial problem. A decrease in hemoglobin during the first week of life to a level less than that of the cord blood is a later indication of blood loss or hemolysis.

Therapeutic Management

Bilirubin levels in blood may be measured by either a blood draw (TsB) or by holding a transcutaneous meter against the infant's skin (transcutaneous bilirubin [TcB]). The initiation of early feeding (urge mothers to breastfeed 8 to

10 times a day for the first 2 days), use of phototherapy, and exchange transfusion all may be measures necessary to reduce the TsB level in an infant affected by a blood incompatibility. In infants with severe hemolytic disease, the hemoglobin concentration can continue to drop during the first 6 months of life, or their bone marrow may fail to increase production of erythrocytes in response to continuing hemolysis so they need an additional blood transfusion to correct this late anemia. Therapy with erythropoietin to stimulate red blood cell production is also possible (Wüest, Manser, Küster, et al., 2016)

The Initiation of Early Feeding

Bilirubin is removed from the body by being excreted through the feces. Therefore, the sooner bowel elimination begins, the sooner bilirubin removal begins. Early feeding (either breast milk or formula), therefore, stimulates bowel peristalsis and helps to accomplish this.

Phototherapy

A fetus's liver processes little bilirubin in utero because the mother's circulation does this for the fetus. With birth, exposure to light is believed to trigger the liver to assume this function. Additional light supplied by phototherapy appears to speed the conversion of unconjugated (fat-soluble) into conjugated (water-soluble) bilirubin. Phototherapy exposes the infant to continuous specialized light such as quartz halogen, cool white daylight, or special blue fluorescent light. The lights are placed 12 to 30 in. above the newborn's bassinet or incubator.

Term newborns are generally scheduled for phototherapy when the TsB level rises to 10 to 12 mg/dl at 24 hours of age; preterm infants may have treatment begun at levels lower than this (Bhardwaj, Locke, Biringer, et al., 2017). Although the results of the therapy are mixed, the administration of intravenous immunoglobulin (IVIG) has been used in neonates with hemolytic disease in combination with phototherapy, especially in ABO incompatibility to try and extenuate the effect of phototherapy (Keir, Dunn, & Callum, 2013).

Continuous exposure to bright lights by phototherapy may be harmful to a newborn's retina, so the infant's eyes must always be covered while under bilirubin lights. Commercial phototherapy masks or eye coverings must be used at all times when the infant is under phototherapy (with the use of bilirubin blankets, eye protection is not usually necessary if it is a full-term newborn). Check the eye covering/mask frequently to be certain it has not slipped. Infants are most apt to dislodge the eye covering when they cry as they wake for a feeding. Urge parents to respond quickly, therefore, if the infant is in their postpartum room to avoid eye damage and possible suffocation by the infant pushing the eye covering down over the nose (Fig. 26.12).

The stools of an infant under bilirubin lights are often bright green because of the excessive bilirubin being excreted as the result of the therapy. They are also frequently loose and may be irritating to the skin. Urine may be dark colored from urobilinogen formation. Monitor the infant's axillary temperature to prevent him or her from overheating under the bright lights. Assess skin turgor and intake and output to ensure dehydration is not occurring from the warm environment.

Figure 26.12 A newborn receiving phototherapy is undressed except for a diaper so he receives maximum exposure to the lights. His eyes are covered snugly to protect them from the ultraviolet light.

Infants receiving phototherapy should be removed from under the lights for feeding so they continue to have interaction with their mother. Remove the eye patches while the infant is out from under the lights for a period of visual stimulation. To prevent a lengthy hospital stay, infants may be discharged and continue therapy at home. Specialized fiber optic light systems incorporated into a fiber optic blanket also have been developed and are ideal for home care. The light generated by the blanket has the same effect on bilirubin levels as banks of overhead lights. The infant is undressed except for a diaper to protect the ovaries or testes and so as much skin surface as possible is exposed to the light. Two big advantages are that an infant can be held for long periods without interrupting the phototherapy, and eye patches are unnecessary.

Parents need an explanation of the rationale for phototherapy and why their infant needs it. Although phototherapy has not been used long enough that long-term effects can be studied, there appears to be minimal risk to an infant from the procedure, provided the infant's eyes remain covered and dehydration from increased insensitive water loss does not occur. Even though there is no evidence so far that infants who received phototherapy are at greater risk for developing skin cancer, all infants who receive phototherapy should (as should all infants) have sunscreen applied when they are in the sun and follow-up assessments in coming years to detect skin cancer that possibly could occur from the therapy (Oláh, Tóth-Molnár, Kemény, et al., 2013).

Exchange Transfusion

The use of intensive phototherapy in conjunction with hydration and close monitoring of serum bilirubin levels has greatly reduced the need for exchange transfusions. If this is done, small amounts (2 to 10 ml) of the infant's blood are drawn from the infant's umbilical vein and then replaced with equal amounts of donor blood. The therapy may be used for any condition that leads to hyperbilirubinemia or polycythemia. When used as therapy for blood incompatibility, it removes approximately 85% of sensitized red cells. It reduces the serum concentration of indirect bilirubin and can prevent heart failure in infants with severe anemia or polycythemia.

A transfusion should be done under a radiant heat warmer to keep the infant warm during what can be a lengthy procedure to prevent energy expenditure from having to maintain body temperature. Donor blood must be maintained at room temperature, or hypothermia from the cold insult could result. Use only commercial blood warmers to warm blood, not hot towels or a radiant heat warmer, to avoid destroying red cells.

The type of blood used for transfusion is O Rh-negative blood, even if an infant's blood type is positive; if Rh-positive or type A or B blood were given, the maternal antibodies that entered the infant's circulation would destroy this blood also, and the transfusion would be ineffective. If the baby will be transported to a regional center for the exchange transfusion, a sample of the mother's blood should accompany the infant, so cross-matching on the mother's serum can be done there.

After a transfusion, closely observe the infant to be certain vital signs are stable and there is no umbilical vessel bleeding or inflammation of the cord if this was the transfusion site, which would suggest infection. Report any changes in vital signs. Monitor bilirubin levels for 2 or 3 days after the transfusion to ensure the level of indirect bilirubin is not rising again and that no further phototherapy or transfusion is necessary.

TWIN-TO-TWIN TRANSFUSION

Twin-to-twin transfusion is a phenomenon that can occur if twins are monozygotic (identical; share the same placenta) and abnormal arteriovenous shunts occur that direct more blood to one twin than the other (Swiatkowska-Freund, Pankrac, & Preis, 2012). The process occurs in as many as one third of all identical twin pregnancies, although enough blood is exchanged to be clinically important in only about 15% of such pregnancies. The result of this shift of blood leads to anemia in the donor twin and polycythemia in the receiving twin. The anemic twin may also be pale and SGA because of the lack of nutrients or oxygen for growth as well as hypoglycemic from lack of glucose stores. The polycythemic twin is prone to hyperbilirubinemia as the excessive red blood cell level is broken down.

Twin-to-twin transfusion can be identified in utero by a sonogram because one twin is noticeably larger than the other. All identical twins should have hemoglobin determinations done at birth and the results should be compared. A hemoglobin difference of more than 5.0 g/100 ml is enough to suggest a transfusion between the twins has occurred. Each twin needs therapy as indicated by the extent of the blood distribution. The donor twin may need a transfusion to establish a functioning blood cell level, and the recipient twin may need an exchange transfusion to reduce the polycythemia and viscosity of the blood.

QSEN Checkpoint Question 26.5

QUALITY IMPROVEMENT

The nurse is concerned that Baby Atkins will develop hyperbilirubinemia because of his immaturity. Because the prevention of jaundice is one of the NICU's quality indicators, what priority nursing intervention would the nurse initiate to best prevent hyperbilirubinemia in Baby Atkins?
  a. Administering phenobarbital to all infants to help prevent jaundice
  b. Urging all mothers to breastfeed early to promote infants' bowel motility
  c. Placing all preterm and SGA infants in warm, dark, comforting environments
  d. Immediately placing all infants under phototherapy following birth

Look in Appendix A for the best answer and rationale.

NECROTIZING ENTEROCOLITIS

Necrotizing enterocolitis (NEC) is a gastrointestinal disease. Premature newborns are at the greatest risk for developing the disease, with approximately 5% of all infants developing it in intensive care nurseries (Pun, Jones, Wolfe, et al., 2016). The bowel develops necrotic patches, interfering with digestion and possibly leading to a paralytic ileus, perforation, and peritonitis. It occurs because of anoxia to the bowel and so may result as a complication of exchange transfusion or an episode of breathing difficulty. Because it shares common features with other gastrointestinal disorders, it is discussed in Chapter 45.

RETINOPATHY OF PREMATURITY

Retinopathy of prematurity (ROP), an acquired ocular disease that leads to partial or total blindness in children, is caused by vasoconstriction of immature retinal blood vessels. It was first recognized as an eye disorder in 1942, but only later was a high concentration of oxygen established as the causative agent (Fleck & Stenson, 2013). Immature retinal blood vessels constrict when exposed to high oxygen concentrations; endothelial cells in the periphery of the retina then proliferate, causing retinal detachment and possible blindness. Infants who are most immature and most ill (and consequently receive the most oxygen) are at the highest risk for developing ROP.

When blood PO_2 levels rise to higher than 100 mmHg, the risk of the disease increases greatly. Based on this, all preterm infants who receive oxygen must have blood oxygen levels monitored by pulse oximeter or blood gas monitoring so the blood PO_2 level can be regulated within normal limits.

In the past, once ROP occurred, there was no reversing it. Today, cryosurgery or laser therapy may be effective at preserving sight. A person experienced in recognizing ROP should examine the eyes of all babies who have received oxygen (especially LBW newborns) before discharge from a hospital nursery and again at 4 to 6 weeks of age to detect any occurrence of the syndrome. Nurses can be instrumental in limiting the occurrence of ROP by securing oxygen saturation levels and by the conscientious management of oxygen (Martínez-Castellanos, Schwartz, Hernández-Rojas, et al., 2013).

The Newborn at Risk Because of a Maternal Infection

Newborns are susceptible to infections during pregnancy and at birth because their ability to produce antibodies is immature. A number of infections in newborns, such as toxoplasmosis, rubella, syphilis, and cytomegalovirus infections, spread to the fetus across the placenta in utero and are discussed in Chapter 12 with other complications of pregnancy. Other infections, such as those discussed in the following sections, are not contracted in utero but are contracted from exposure to vaginal secretions at birth.

β-HEMOLYTIC, GROUP B STREPTOCOCCAL INFECTION

A serious cause of infection in newborns is the gram-positive β-hemolytic, group B streptococcal (GBS) organism, a natural inhabitant of the female genital tract. Between 50 and 300 infants out of every 1,000 live births display a positive culture for the organism (AAP, 2011a). It also may be spread from baby to baby if good hand washing technique is not used in caring for newborns. If a woman is found to be positive for GBS during late pregnancy (see Chapter 21), ampicillin administered IV during pregnancy and again during labor helps to reduce the possibility of newborn exposure.

Assessment

Universal screening is recommended for pregnant women at 35 to 37 weeks of gestation to see if they have GBS organisms in their vaginal secretions (Albright, MacGregor, Sutton, et al., 2017). Typically, a newborn at risk, such as one born after prolonged rupture of membranes or if the woman's vaginal culture is positive for GBS, will be screened at birth for infection by a specialized GBS blood culture.

Colonization by GBS can result in either an early-onset or a late-onset illness. With the early-onset form, signs of pneumonia such as tachypnea, apnea, extreme paleness, hypotension, or hypotonia become apparent within the first day of life. Decreased urine output can occur from the hypotension. A chest X-ray may not be diagnostic because the changes seen are almost indistinguishable from those of RDS (a ground-glass appearance). Without therapy, the disease progresses so rapidly, as many as 20% of infants who contract the infection die within 24 hours of birth.

A late-onset type occurs at 2 to 4 weeks of age. With this, instead of pneumonia being the infection focus, meningitis tends to occur. Typical signs include lethargy, fever, loss of appetite, and bulging fontanelles from increased intracranial pressure. Mortality from the late-onset type is not as high as that from the early-onset form (15% vs. 20%), but neurologic consequences can occur in up to 50% of infants who survive.

Therapeutic Management

If a newborn displays signs of infection or a blood screening test is positive, antibiotics such as penicillin, cefazolin, clindamycin, or vancomycin are all effective against the GBS organism.

Parents may have difficulty understanding how their infant could suddenly have become this ill, and they may need a great deal of support to care for their infant. This is even more important if the newborn survives the infection but is left neurologically challenged. In the future, immunization of all women of childbearing age against streptococcal B organisms could decrease the incidence of newborns infected at birth.

OPHTHALMIA NEONATORUM

Ophthalmia neonatorum is an eye infection that occurs at birth or during the first month of life (Matejcek & Goldman, 2013). The most common causative organisms are *Neisseria gonorrhoeae* and *Chlamydia trachomatis*, which are contracted from vaginal secretions. An *N. gonorrhoeae* infection is an extremely serious form of infection because, if left untreated, the infection progresses to corneal ulceration and destruction, resulting in opacity of the cornea and severe vision impairment.

Assessment

Ophthalmia neonatorum is generally bilateral. The conjunctivae become fiery red and covered with thick pus. The eyelids appear edematous. Although this usually occurs on day 1 to day 4 of life, it should be considered as a possibility when conjunctivitis occurs in any infant younger than 30 days of age.

Prevention

The prophylactic instillation of erythromycin ointment into the eyes of newborns prevents both gonococcal and chlamydial conjunctivitis. In the past, eye prophylaxis was given immediately after birth so it was never forgotten. Now it is more customary to delay the administration of the ointment until after the first reactivity period so the newborn can clearly see the parents during this important attachment period. This makes it easy for administration to be forgotten, so use some type of a checklist as a reminder of this important prophylaxis. Infants born outside the hospital also need prophylaxis to prevent ophthalmia neonatorum, the same as for infants born in a birthing room.

Therapeutic Management

If conjunctivitis occurs, therapy is individualized depending on the organism cultured from the exudate. If gonococci are identified, intravenous ceftriaxone (Rocephin) and penicillin are effective drugs. If *Chlamydia* is identified, an ophthalmic solution of erythromycin is commonly used.

Use standard and contact infection precautions when caring for this newborn. In addition to systemic antibiotic therapy, sterile saline solution lavage to clear the copious discharge from the eyes may be prescribed. When irrigating eyes, use a sterile medicine dropper or bulb syringe and use barrier protection, including goggles to avoid splashing any solution into your own eye. The solution should be at room temperature. Direct the stream of the irrigation fluid laterally so it does not enter and contaminate the other eye.

The mother of the infected infant needs treatment for gonorrhea or chlamydia before fallopian tube sterility or pelvic inflammatory disease can result. Sexual contacts of the mother should be treated also so the spread of the disease can be halted. With either infection, parents can be assured with early diagnosis and treatment that the prognosis for normal eyesight in their child is good.

HEPATITIS B VIRUS INFECTION

Hepatitis B virus (HBV) can be transmitted to the newborn through contact with infected vaginal blood at birth when the mother is positive for the virus (positive for the surface antigen of the hepatitis B virus [HBsAg+]). Hepatitis B is a destructive illness with greater than 90% of infected infants becoming chronic carriers of the virus as well as the risk of developing liver cancer later in life (Ni, 2011). To reduce the possibility of HBsAg being spread to newborns in the future, parents are asked if they would like their infant vaccinated against hepatitis B at birth (Kurosky, Davis, & Krishnarajah, 2016).

If the mother is identified as HBsAg+, her infant should be bathed as soon as possible after birth to remove HBV-infected blood and secretions. Gentle suctioning is necessary to avoid trauma to the mucous membrane, which could allow HBV invasion. To further protect against infection, the infant is administered serum hepatitis B immune globulin (HBIG) in addition to the HBV vaccination. Although the virus is transmitted in breast milk, once immune globulin has been administered, women may breastfeed without risk to an infant. Hepatitis B is further discussed in Chapter 45 because it shares common symptoms with other liver disorders and also occurs in older children.

GENERALIZED HERPESVIRUS INFECTION

A herpes simplex virus type 2 (HSV-2) infection, which is most prevalent among women with multiple sexual partners, can be contracted by a fetus across the placenta if the mother has a primary infection during pregnancy. More often, however, the virus is contracted from the vaginal secretions of a mother who has active herpetic vulvovaginitis at the time of birth. Between 15% and 30% of women of childbearing age demonstrate antibodies to this virus or have the potential to have active lesions during labor (Looker, Magaret, May, et al., 2017).

Assessment

If the infection was acquired during pregnancy, an infant may be born with vesicles covering the skin. The long-term prognosis of the child is guarded because severe neurologic damage may have occurred simultaneously with the development of the lesions. If infants don't acquire the infection until birth, by day 4 to day 7 of life, they show a loss of appetite, perhaps a low-grade fever, and lethargy. Stomatitis (ulcers of the mouth) or a few vesicles on the skin appear. Herpes vesicles always cluster, are pinpoint in size, and are surrounded by a reddened base. After the vesicles appear, infants become extremely ill. They develop dyspnea, jaundice, purpura, convulsions, and hypotension. Death may occur within hours or days. Between 25% and 70% of newborns who survive generalized herpesvirus infections have permanent central nervous system sequelae (Pinninti & Kimberlin, 2014).

To confirm the diagnosis, cultures are obtained from representative vesicles as well as from the nose, throat, anus, and umbilical cord. Blood serum is analyzed for IgM antibodies.

Therapeutic Management

An antiviral drug such as acyclovir (Zovirax), a drug that inhibits viral DNA synthesis, is effective in combating this overwhelming infection. Prevention, however, is the newborn's best protection. Antenatal antiviral prophylaxis reduces viral shedding and recurrences at birth and reduces the need for cesarean birth (Pinninti & Kimberlin, 2014). Women with active herpetic vulvar lesions are advised to have cesarean birth rather than vaginal birth to minimize the newborn's exposure. Infants with an infection should be separated from other infants in a nursery. Although transmission from this source is rare, women with herpes lesions on their face (herpes simplex I, or cold sores) need to be assessed before they hold their newborns to be sure lesions are crusted and, therefore, are no longer contagious. Healthcare personnel who have herpes simplex infections should not care for newborns until the lesions are crusted. Although facial herpes simplex lesions are probably caused by herpesvirus type 1, limiting contact does not seem excessive in light of the severity of HSV-2 disease. Urge a woman who is separated from her newborn at birth to view her infant from the nursery window and participate in planning care to aid bonding.

HIV INFECTION

HIV infection and AIDS can be caused by placental transfer or direct contact with maternal blood during birth. Because older children can also be exposed to this disease, the care of children with this infection is discussed in Chapter 42.

The Newborn at Risk Because of a Maternal Illnesses

AN INFANT OF A WOMAN WHO HAS DIABETES MELLITUS

Infants of women who have diabetes mellitus whose illness was poorly controlled during pregnancy are typically longer and weigh more than other babies (macrosomia). The baby also has a greater chance of having a congenital anomaly such as a cardiac anomaly because hyperglycemia is teratogenic to a rapidly growing fetus.

Most such babies have a cushingoid (i.e., fat and puffy) appearance. They tend to be lethargic or limp in the first days of life as a result of hyperglycemia. The macrosomia results from overstimulation of pituitary growth hormone and extra fat deposits created by high levels of insulin during pregnancy. This infant's large size is deceptive, however, because, like all LGA babies, they are often immature. RDS occurs at a higher rate than usual in these infants because they may be born preterm or, if born at term, lecithin pathways may not be mature. High fetal insulin secretion during pregnancy to counteract the hyperglycemia can interfere with cortisol release. This could block the formation of lecithin and further prevent lung maturity (Murphy, Janzen, Strehlow, et al., 2013). A term frequently used for these infants is "fragile giant."

An infant of a woman with diabetes loses a greater proportion of weight in the first few days of life than does the average newborn because of the loss of extra fluid accumulated. Observe such an infant closely to be certain this weight loss actually represents a loss of extra fluid and that dehydration is not occurring.

Complications

A macrosomic infant has a greater chance of birth injury, especially shoulder and neck injury. A cesarean birth may be necessary to avoid cephalopelvic disproportion. Immediately after birth, the infant tends to be hyperglycemic because the mother was at least slightly hyperglycemic during pregnancy and excess glucose transfused across the placenta. During pregnancy, the fetal pancreas responded to this high glucose level with islet cell hypertrophy, resulting in matching high insulin levels. After birth, as an infant's glucose level begins to fall because the mother's circulation is no longer supplying glucose, the overproduction of insulin will cause the development of severe hypoglycemia. Hyperbilirubinemia also may occur in these infants because, if immature, they cannot effectively clear bilirubin from their system. Hypocalcemia also frequently develops because parathyroid hormone levels are lower in these infants due to hypomagnesemia from excessive renal losses of magnesium.

Although infants of women with diabetes are usually LGA, an infant born to a woman with extensive blood vessel involvement may be SGA because of poor placental perfusion. The problems of hypoglycemia, hypocalcemia, and hyperbilirubinemia remain the same.

Therapeutic Management

In a newborn, hypoglycemia is defined as a serum glucose level of less than 45 mg/dl. To avoid a serum glucose level from falling this low, infants of women with diabetes need to be fed early; if they are unable to suck, a continuous infusion of glucose can be prescribed. It is important the infant not be given only a bolus of glucose; otherwise, rebound hypoglycemia (accentuating the problem) can occur. Some infants of women with diabetes have a smaller than usual left colon, apparently another effect of intrauterine hyperglycemia, which can limit the amount of oral feedings they can take in their first days of life. Signs of an inadequate colon include vomiting or abdominal distention after the first few feedings. Careful monitoring for any vomiting and normal bowel movements can help identify this condition.

QSEN Checkpoint Question 26.6

PATIENT-CENTERED CARE

Mrs. Atkins asks the nurse why the baby in the incubator next to her baby whose mother has diabetes mellitus was fed so soon after birth. Why is it important for infants of women with diabetes to be fed early?

 a. Their stomach is larger than usual due to overgrowth.
 b. This helps prevent rebound hypoglycemia from occurring.
 c. The mother probably didn't eat much during her labor.
 d. This helps clear thick mucus from the lower intestinal tract.

Look in Appendix A for the best answer and rationale.

AN INFANT OF A DRUG-DEPENDENT MOTHER

Infants of drug-dependent women tend to be SGA. If the woman took a drug close to birth, her infant may show withdrawal symptoms (neonatal abstinence syndrome) shortly after birth (Box 26.9). These include such signs as:

- Irritability
- Disturbed sleep pattern
- Constant movement, possibly leading to abrasions on the elbows, knees, or nose
- Tremors
- Frequent sneezing
- Shrill, high-pitched cry
- Possible hyperreflexia and clonus (neuromuscular irritability)
- Convulsions
- Tachypnea (rapid respirations), possibly so severe that it leads to hyperventilation and alkalosis
- Vomiting and diarrhea, leading to large fluid losses and secondary dehydration

Specific neonatal abstinence scoring tools can be used to quantify and assess an infant's status. When symptoms begin to appear and when they fade varies with the drug involved, but, on average, symptoms occur in 24 to 48 hours and last about 2 weeks. The infants of women who were on methadone maintenance during pregnancy will show the same

BOX 26.9

Nursing Care Planning Using Assessment

ASSESSING THE NEWBORN OF A DRUG-DEPENDENT MOTHER

Irritability

Frequent sneezing

Shrill, high-pitched cry

Tachypnea

Vomiting

Diarrhea

Disturbed sleep patterns

Constant movement

Tremors

Hyperreflexia, clonus

beginning and length of symptoms. The abstinence sequence for the cocaine-addicted neonate is usually milder, but factors such as maladaptive coping behaviors may be present in such newborns into preschool (Buckingham-Howes, Berger, Scaletti, et al., 2013).

Narcotic metabolites or quinine (heroin is often mixed with quinine) may be obtained from an infant's urine or meconium in the first hour after birth to establish that the drug was transferred into the infant before birth. These products are quickly cleared from the body, however, so by the time symptoms become severe, detection of narcotic substances may no longer be possible. Cocaine, in contrast, may be detected in infants' hair samples for an extended time.

Infants of drug-dependent women usually seem most comfortable when firmly swaddled. Keep them in an environment free from excessive stimuli (a small isolation nursery or the mother's room, not a large, open nursery). Some quiet best if the room is darkened. Some may suck vigorously and continuously and seem to find comfort and quiet if given a pacifier. In contrast, infants of methadone- and cocaine-addicted women may have extremely poor sucking ability and may have difficulty achieving sufficient fluid intake unless gavage fed. Unless a woman intends to remain drug free, she is usually advised not to breastfeed to avoid passing narcotics in breast milk to the infant.

Specific therapy for an infant has to be individualized according to the nature and severity of the signs. If an infant has vomiting or diarrhea, intravenous administration of fluid may be indicated. The most common medications to counteract abstinence symptoms are morphine and methadone (Bagley, Wachman, Holland, et al., 2014). Other drugs that may be used include methadone, chlorpromazine (Thorazine), and diazepam (Valium). These are typically used if the neonatal abstinence scoring system average score is elevated on three successive occasions and other nursing interventions do not reduce the score.

Once an infant has been identified as having been exposed to drugs in utero, the mother needs treatment for withdrawal symptoms and follow-up care as much as the infant. In addition, an evaluation is necessary to determine before discharge from the healthcare facility whether an environment that allowed for drug abuse will be safe for an infant at home (Bagley et al., 2014). Infants also need long-term follow-up because long-term neurologic problems may develop.

AN INFANT WITH FETAL ALCOHOL EXPOSURE

Alcohol crosses the placenta in the same concentration as is present in the maternal bloodstream so may result in fetal alcohol exposure, or **fetal alcohol spectrum disorder** (Tsai, Manchester, & Elias, 2012). The disorder appears in about 2 out of 1,000 newborns and is often more difficult to document than recreational drug exposure because alcohol abuse may be more difficult to document. Because alcohol has serious deteriorating effects on the placenta and it is unknown if there is a safe threshold of alcohol ingestion during pregnancy, all pregnant women are advised to avoid alcohol intake to prevent any teratogenic effects on their newborn (Dunney, Muldoon, & Murphy, 2015).

A newborn with fetal alcohol spectrum disorder has several possible problems at birth. Characteristics that mark the syndrome include prenatal and postnatal growth restriction; central nervous system involvement such as cognitive challenge, microcephaly, and cerebral palsy; and a distinctive facial feature of a short palpebral fissure and thin upper lip. During the neonatal period, an infant may appear tremulous, fidgety, and irritable and may demonstrate a weak sucking reflex. Sleep disturbances are common, with the baby tending to be either always awake or always asleep depending on the mother's alcohol level close to birth.

The most serious long-term effect is cognitive challenge. Behavior problems such as hyperactivity may occur in school-age children. Growth deficiencies may remain throughout life. An infant needs conscientious follow-up so any future problems can be discovered. The mother needs a follow-up to see if she can reduce her alcohol intake for better overall health (Cook, Green, Lilley, et al., 2016)

What If . . . 26.4

The nurse is interested in exploring one of the 2020 National Health Goals with respect to high-risk newborns (see Box 26.1). Most government-sponsored money for nursing research is allotted based on these goals. What would be a possible research topic to explore pertinent to these goals that would be applicable to the Atkins family and that would also advance evidence-based practice?

KEY POINTS FOR REVIEW

- Priorities for infants born with special needs, such as preterm or postterm infants, are the same as for term infants: initiation and maintenance of respirations, establishment of extrauterine circulation, control of body temperature, intake of adequate nourishment, establishment of waste elimination, establishment of an infant–parent relationship, prevention of infection, and provision of developmental care for mental and social development.

- Many high-risk infants need resuscitation at birth. Prompt action with such measures as warmth, oxygen, intubation, and suctioning are needed.

- An SGA infant is one whose birth weight is below the 10th percentile on an intrauterine growth curve for that gestational age infant. An infant could be born preterm, term, or postterm. They typically have difficulty maintaining body warmth because of low fat stores and may develop hypoglycemia from low glucose stores.

- An LGA infant is one whose birth weight is above the 90th percentile on an intrauterine growth chart for that gestational age. The infant could be born preterm, term, or postterm. They tend to be infants of women with diabetes, and they are particularly prone to hypoglycemia or birth trauma.

- An early preterm infant is one born between 24 and 34 weeks of gestation; a late preterm infant is one born between 34 and 37 weeks of gestation. Preterm infants have particular problems with respiratory function, anemia, jaundice, persistent patent ductus arteriosus, and intracranial hemorrhage.

- Infants who are born weighing less than 2,500 g at birth are termed low–birth-weight infants, those born weighing less than 1,500 g are termed very-low-birth-weight infants, and those born weighing less than 1,000 g are extremely low–birth-weight infants. Most of these infants need intensive care from the moment of birth to give them their best chance of survival.

■ A postterm infant is one who has remained in utero past week 42 of pregnancy. Postterm infants have particular problems with establishing respirations, meconium aspiration, hypoglycemia, temperature regulation, and polycythemia.

■ RDS commonly occurs in preterm infants from a deficiency or lack of surfactant in the alveoli. Without surfactant, the alveoli collapse on expiration and require extreme force for reinflation. Primary therapy is synthetic surfactant replacement at birth, followed by oxygen and ventilatory support.

■ TTN is a temporary condition caused by the slow absorption of lung fluid at birth. It is seen most often in infants born by cesarean birth. Close observation of the infant is necessary until the fluid is absorbed and respirations slow to a usual rate.

■ MAS occurs when an infant aspirates meconium-stained amniotic fluid before or during birth. Meconium is irritating to the airway and so leads to both airway spasm and pneumonia. Infants need oxygen, ventilatory support, and possibly an antibiotic until the effects of the insult to the airway subside

■ Apnea is a pause in respirations longer than 20 seconds and may be accompanied by bradycardia. It tends to occur in preterm infants who have secondary stresses such as an infection, hyperbilirubinemia, hypoglycemia, or hypothermia. Apnea monitors are used to detect this, and infants who are at high risk for apnea may be discharged with a home monitoring program.

■ SIDS is the sudden, unexplained death of an infant. It is associated with infants sleeping on their stomachs (prone) and infants born preterm. An important preventive measure is advising parents to position their infant on the back and possibly use a pacifier for sleeping.

■ Hyperbilirubinemia results from the destruction of red blood cells, owing either to a usual physiologic response or an abnormal destruction of red blood cells. Hemolytic disease of the newborn occurs from destruction of red blood cells from Rh or ABO incompatibility. The administration of RHIG (Rh antibodies) to Rh-negative mothers during pregnancy and after the birth of an Rh-positive infant to an Rh-negative mother has greatly reduced the incidence of the condition. Affected infants appear jaundiced from the release of bilirubin from injured red blood cells. Phototherapy and an exchange transfusion are used to prevent ABE (the deposition of bilirubin in brain cells, causing destruction of the cells).

■ **Hemorrhagic disease of the newborn** is a lack of clotting ability resulting from a deficiency of vitamin K at birth. This disorder is prevented by administering vitamin K to a newborn within the first hour following birth.

■ ROP is destruction of the retina caused by exposure of immature retinal capillaries to high levels of oxygen. Monitoring oxygen saturation by pulse oximetry or ABGs are important preventive measures and help in planning nursing care that not only meets QSEN competencies but that also best meets a family's total needs.

■ Severe infections acquired by infants at birth include streptococcal group B pneumonia, hepatitis B infection, ophthalmia neonatorum (gonococcal and chlamydial conjunctivitis), and

herpesvirus infections. Assessing newborns for symptoms of these infections is an important nursing responsibility.

■ Infants of women with diabetes and those of drug-abusing women are at high risk at birth for further complications. Both need a careful assessment for respiratory distress and hypoglycemia.

CRITICAL THINKING CARE STUDY

Priscilla Angelini is an unmarried 17-year-old who has just given birth via cesarean birth to her first baby, a girl, at 37 weeks of gestation because of a breech presentation. Priscilla did not receive any prenatal care. At birth, she tests positive for group B streptococcal infection. When assessing her newborn, you conclude she is SGA. At 6 hours of age, Priscilla calls you and explains her baby seems to be struggling to breathe. She wants to know if this is normal. When you assess the newborn, you find a respiratory rate of 70 breaths/min and mild subcostal retractions.

1. What possible risk factors should you look for in Baby Angelini?

2. What is the most likely explanation for Baby Angelini's respiratory rate and the subcostal retractions? What priority nursing intervention should you initiate? What should you tell Priscilla about the situation?

3. Does Priscilla's infection put Baby Angelini at risk? What nursing interventions should be in the newborn's care plan to prevent infection and what signs and symptoms of infection should you look for in the newborn?

RELATED RESOURCES

Explore these additional resources to enhance learning for this chapter:

• Student resources on thePoint, including answers to the What If . . . and Critical Thinking Care Study questions, http://thepoint.lww.com/Flagg8e

• Adaptive learning powered by PrepU, http://thepoint.lww.com/prepu

REFERENCES

Abdel Ghany, E., Alsharany, W., Ali, A., et al. (2016). Anti-oxidant profiles and markers of oxidative stress in preterm neonates. *Paediatrics and International Child Health*, 36(2), 134–140.

Albright, C., MacGregor, C., Sutton, D., et al. (2017). Group B streptococci screening before repeat cesarean delivery: A cost-effectiveness analysis. *Obstetrics & Gynecology*, 129(1), 111–119.

Alderliesten, T., Lemmers, P., Smarius, J., et al. (2013). Cerebral oxygenation, extraction, and autoregulation in very preterm infants who develop peri-intraventricular hemorrhage. *The Journal of Pediatrics*, 162(4), 698–704.e2.

Alm, B., Wennergren, G., Möllborg, P., et al. (2016). Breastfeeding and dummy use have a protective effect on sudden infant death syndrome. *Acta Paediatrica*, 105, 31–38.

American Academy of Pediatrics. (2011a). Policy statement—recommendations for the prevention of perinatal group B streptococcal (GBS) disease. *Pediatrics*, 128(3), 611–616.

American Academy of Pediatrics. (2011b). SIDS and other sleep-related infant deaths: Expansion of recommendations for a safe infant sleeping environment. *Pediatrics*, 128(5), e1341–e1367.

American Academy of Pediatrics. (2012). *Where we stand: Car seats for children*. Washington, DC: Author.

Bagley, S. M., Wachman, E. M., Holland, E., et al. (2014). Review of the assessment and management of neonatal abstinence syndrome. *Addiction Science & Clinical Practice*, 9(1), 19.

Bhardwaj, K., Locke, T., Biringer, A., et al. (2017). Newborn bilirubin screening for preventing severe hyperbilirubinemia and bilirubin encephalopathy: A rapid review. *Current Pediatric Reviews.* Advance online publication. doi:10.2174/1573396313666170110144345

Blencowe, H., Cousens, S., Chou, D., et al. (2013). Born too soon: The global epidemiology of 15 million preterm births. *Reproductive Health, 10*(Suppl. 1), S2.

Blencowe, H., Cousens, S., Oestergaard, M., et al. (2012). National, regional, and worldwide estimates of preterm birth rates in the year 2010 with time trends since 1990 for selected countries: A systematic analysis and implications. *Lancet, 379*(9832), 2162–2172.

Briere, C., McGrath, J., Cong, X., et al. (2016). Direct-breastfeeding in the neonatal intensive care unit and breastfeeding duration for premature infants. *Applied Nursing Research, 32,* 47–51.

Brooks, C., Vickers, A. M., & Aryal, S. (2013). Comparison of lipid and calorie loss from donor human milk among 3 methods of simulated gavage feeding: One-hour, 2-hour, and intermittent gravity feedings. *Advances in Neonatal Care, 13*(2), 131–138.

Buckingham-Howes, S., Berger, S. S., Scaletti, L. A., et al. (2013). Systematic review of prenatal cocaine exposure and adolescent development. *Pediatrics, 131*(6), e1917–e1936.

Byars, K. C., & Simon, S. L. (2017). American Academy of Pediatrics 2016 safe sleep practices: Implications for pediatric behavioral sleep medicine. *Behavior Sleep Medicine, 15*(3), 175–179.

Centers for Disease Control and Prevention. (2016). *Proper handling and storage of breast milk.* Atlanta, GA: Author.

Chettri, S., Bhat, B. V., & Adhisivam, B. (2016). Current concepts in the management of meconium aspiration syndrome. *Indian Journal of Pediatrics, 83,* 1125–1130.

Committee on Practice Bulletins-Obstetrics. (2016). Practice Bulletin No. 160: Premature rupture of membranes. *Obstetrics & Gynecology, 127*(1), e39–e51.

Cook, J., Green, C., Lilley, C., et al. (2016). Fetal alcohol spectrum disorder: A guideline for diagnosis across the lifespan. *Canadian Medical Association Journal, 188*(3), 191–197.

Dani, C., Bresci, C., Berti, E., et al. (2013). Short term outcome of term newborns with unexpected umbilical cord arterial pH between 7.000 and 7.100. *Early Human Development, 89*(12), 1037–1040.

Davis, N. (2015). Screening for cardiopulmonary events in neonates: A review of the infant car seat challenge. *Journal of Perinatology, 35,* 235–240.

Dunney, C., Muldoon, K., & Murphy, D. (2015). Alcohol consumption in pregnancy and its implications for breastfeeding. *British Journal of Midwifery, 23*(2), 126–134.

Eken, M., Tuten, A., Ozkaya, E., et al. (2016). Evaluation of the maternal and fetal risk factors associated with neonatal care unit hospitalization time. *The Journal of Maternal Fetal and Neonatal Medicine, 29*(21), 3553–3557.

Fawcett, K., (2014). Preventing admission hypothermia in very low birth weight neonates. *Neonatal Network, 33*(3), 143–149. Retrieved from https://search-proquest-com.ezp.welch.jhmi.edu/docview/1525750840?accountid=11752

Fleck, B., & Stenson, B. (2013). Retinopathy of prematurity and the oxygen conundrum. *Clinics in Perinatology, 40*(2), 229–240.

Frank, K. M., Mueller-Burke, D., Bullard, J., et al. (2015). Delayed cord clamping in the premature neonate: Development of an interdisciplinary guideline. *Journal of Pregnancy & Child Health, 3,* 237.

Gupta, P., Sodhi, K. S., Saxena, A. K., et al. (2016). Neonatal cranial sonography: A concise review for clinicians. *Journal of Pediatric Neurosciences, 11*(1), 7–13.

Hermansen, C., & Mahajan, A. (2015). Newborn respiratory distress. *American Family Physician, 92*(11), 994–1002.

Hofmeyr, G. J., Xu, H., & Eke, A. C. (2014). Amnioinfusion for meconium-stained liquor in labour. *Cochrane Database of Systematic Reviews,* (1), CD000014.

Hoppe, C. C. (2013). Prenatal and newborn screening for hemoglobinopathies. *International Journal of Laboratory Hematology, 35*(3), 297–305.

Joseph, K., Fahey, J., Shankardass, K., et al. (2014). Effects of socioeconomic position and clinical risk factors on spontaneous and iatrogenic preterm birth. *BMC Pregnancy and Childbirth, 14,* 117.

Karch, A. M. (2013). *Lippincott's nursing drug guide.* Philadelphia, PA: Lippincott Williams & Wilkins.

Keir, A. K., Dunn, M., & Callum, J. (2013). Should intravenous immunoglobulin be used in infants with isoimmune haemolytic disease due to ABO incompatibility? *Journal of Paediatrics & Child Health, 49*(12), 1072–1078.

Kitsommart, R., Martins, B., Bottino, M. N., et al. (2012). Expectant management of pneumothorax in preterm infants receiving assisted ventilation: Report of 4 cases and review of the literature. *Respiratory Care, 57*(5), 789–793.

Kreutzer, K., & Bassler, D. (2014). Caffeine for apnea of prematurity: A neonatal success story. *Neonatology, 105*(4), 332–336.

Kurosky, S., Davis, K., & Krishnarajah, G. (2016). Completion and compliance of childhood vaccinations in the United States. *Vaccine, 34*(3), 387–394.

Landry, J. S., & Menzies, D. (2011). Occurrence and severity of bronchopulmonary dysplasia and respiratory distress syndrome after a preterm birth. *Paediatrics & Child Health, 16*(7), 399–403.

Laubach, V., Wilhelm, P., & Carter, K. (2014). Shhh . . . I'm growing: Noise in the NICU. *Nursing Clinics of North America, 49*(3), 329–344.

Lee, H. C., Martin-Anderson, S., Lyndon, A., et al. (2013). Perspectives on promoting breastmilk feedings for premature infants during a quality improvement project. *Breastfeeding Medicine, 8*(2), 176–180.

Leone, T. A., Finer, N. N., & Rich, W. (2012). Delivery room respiratory management of the term and preterm infant. *Clinics in Perinatology, 39*(3), 431–440.

Lindenskov, P. H., Castellheim, A., Saugstad, O. D., et al. (2015). Meconium aspiration syndrome: Possible pathophysiological mechanisms and future potential therapies. *Neonatology, 107*(3), 225–230.

Londhe, V., Nolen, T., Das, A., et al. (2013). Vitamin A supplementation in extremely low-birth-weight infants: Subgroup analysis in small-for-gestational-age infants. *American Journal of Perinatology, 30*(9), 771–780.

Looker, K., Magaret, A., May, M., et al. (2017). First estimates of the global and regional incidence of neonatal herpes infection. *Lancet Global Health, 5*(3), e300–e309.

Martin, C. R., Ling, P. R., & Blackburn, G. L. (2016). Review of infant feeding: Key features of breast milk and infant formula. *Nutrients, 8*(5), 279.

Martínez-Castellanos, M. A., Schwartz, S., Hernández-Rojas, M. L., et al. (2013). Long-term effect of antiangiogenic therapy for retinopathy of prematurity. *Retina, 33*(2), 329–338.

Matejcek, A., & Goldman, R. D. (2013). Treatment and prevention of ophthalmia neonatorum. *Canadian Family Physician, 59*(11), 1187–1190.

Mesi , I., Milas, V., Medimurec, M., et al. (2014). Unconjugated pathological jaundice in newborns. *Collegium Antropologicum, 38*(1), 173–178.

Mitra, S., Florez, I., Tamayo, M., et al. (2016). Effectiveness and safety of treatments used for the management of patent ductus arteriosus (PDA) in preterm infants: A protocol for a systematic review and network meta-analysis. *BMJ Open, 6*(7), e011271.

Mohan, S. S., & Jain, L. (2012). Care of the late preterm infant. In C. A. Gleason & S. U. Devaskar (Eds.), *Avery's diseases of the newborn* (9th ed., pp. 405–416). Philadelphia, PA: Elsevier/Saunders.

Moore, E. R., Anderson, G. C., Bergman, N., et al. (2012). Early skin-to-skin contact for mothers and their healthy newborn infants. *Cochrane Database of Systematic Reviews,* (5), CD003519.

Murphy, A., Janzen, C., Strehlow, S. L., et al. (2013). Diabetes mellitus and pregnancy. In A. H. DeCherney, L. Nathan, T. M. Goodwin, et al. (Eds.), *Current diagnosis and treatment: Obstetrics and gynecology* (11th ed., pp. 509–518). Columbus, OH: McGraw-Hill/Lange.

Murray, E., Fernandes, M., Fazel, M., et al. (2015). Differential effect of intrauterine growth restriction on childhood neurodevelopment: A systematic review. *British Journal of Obstetrics and Gynaecology, 122*(8), 1062–1072.

Nair, J., & Lakshminrusimha, S. (2014). Update on PPHN: Mechanisms and treatment. *Seminars in Perinatology, 38*(2), 78–91.

Nandyal, R., Owora, A., Risch, E., et al. (2013). Special care needs and risk for child maltreatment reports among babies that graduated from the neonatal intensive care. *Child Abuse & Neglect, 37*(12), 1114–1121.

National Vital Statistics Service. (2011). *Trends in the health of Americans.* Hyattsville, MD: Author.

Ni, Y. H. (2011). Natural history of hepatitis B virus infection: Pediatric perspective. *Journal of Gastroenterology, 46*(1), 1–8.

Oláh, J., Tóth-Molnár, E., Kemény, L. et al. (2013). Long-term hazards of neonatal blue-light phototherapy. *British Journal of Dermatology, 169,* 243–249.

Ortigosa, S., Friguls, B., Joya, X., et al. (2012). Feto-placental morphological effects of prenatal exposure to drugs of abuse. *Reproductive Toxicology, 34*(1), 73–79.

Ota, E., Tobe-Gai, R., Mori, R., et al. (2012). Antenatal dietary advice and supplementation to increase energy and protein intake. *Cochrane Database of Systematic Reviews,* (9), CD000032.

Pinninti, S., & Kimberlin, D. (2014). Preventing herpes simplex virus in the newborn. *Clinics in Perinatology, 41*(4), 945–955.

Pun, P., Jones, J., Wolfe, C., et al. (2016). Changes in plasma and urinary nitrite after birth in premature infants at risk for necrotizing enterocolitis. *Pediatric Research, 79*(3), 432–437.

Quinn, J., Munoz, F., Gonik, B., et al. (2016). Preterm birth: Case definition & guidelines for collection, analysis, and presentation of immunisation safety data. *Vaccine, 34*(49), 6047–6056.

Rahimian, J. (2013). Disproportionate fetal growth. In A. H. DeCherney, L. Nathan, T. M. Goodwin, et al. (Eds.), *Current diagnosis and treatment: Obstetrics and gynecology* (11th ed., pp. 290–300). Columbus, OH: McGraw-Hill/Lange.

Robinson, S. (2012). Neonatal posthemorrhagic hydrocephalus from prematurity: Pathophysiology and current treatment concepts. *Journal of Neurosurgery Pediatrics, 9*(3), 242–258.

Sahewalla, R., Gupta, D., & Kamat, D. (2016). Apparent life-threatening events: An overview. *Clinical Pediatrics, 55*(1), 5–9.

Samra, H. A., McGrath, J. M., Wehbe, M., et al. (2012). Epigenetics and family-centered developmental care for the preterm infant. *Advances in Neonatal Care, 12*(Suppl. 5), S2–S9.

Sawyer, T., Umoren, R. A., & Gray, M. M. (2017). Neonatal resuscitation: Advances in training and practice. *Advances in Medical Education and Practice, 8*, 11–19.

Shah, N., & Wusthoff, C. (2016). Intracranial hemorrhage in the neonate. *Neonatal Network, 35*(2), 67–71.

Silberstein, D., & Litmanovitz, I. (2016). Developmental care in the neonatal intensive care unit according to Newborn Individualized Developmental Care and Assessment Program (NIDCAP). *Harefuah, 155*(1), 27–31, 67, 68.

Sjaarda, L., Albert, P., Mumford, S., et al. (2014). Customized large-for-gestational-age birthweight at term and the association with adverse perinatal outcomes. *American Journal of Obstetrics and Gynecology, 210*(1), 63.e1–63.e11.

Su, B., Lin, H., Huang, F., et al. (2015). Gastric residuals, feeding intolerance, and necrotizing enterocolitis in preterm infants. *Pediatrics & Neonatology, 56*(2), 136–137.

Swiatkowska-Freund, M., Pankrac, Z., & Preis, K. (2012). Results of laser therapy in twin-to-twin transfusion syndrome: Our experience. *Journal of Maternal-Fetal & Neonatal Medicine, 25*(10), 1917–1920.

Thilo, E. H., & Rosenberg, A. A. (2012). The newborn infant. In W. Hay, M. Levin, R. Deterding, et al. (Eds.), *Current diagnosis & treatment pediatrics* (21st ed., pp. 9–72). New York, NY: McGraw-Hill/Lange.

Trasande, L. (2014). Further limiting bisphenol A in food uses could provide health and economic benefits. *Health Affairs, 33*(2), 316–23. Retrieved from http://search.proquest.com/docview/1498231656?accountid=11752

Tsai, A., Manchester, D. K., & Elias, E. R. (2012). Genetics and dysmorphology. In W. Hay, M. Levin, R. Deterding, et al. (Eds.), *Current diagnosis & treatment pediatrics* (21st ed., pp. 1088–1123). New York, NY: McGraw-Hill/Lange.

U.S. Department of Health and Human Services. (2010). *Healthy people 2020.* Washington, DC: Author.

Verardo, V., Gómez-Caravaca, A. M., Arráez-Román, D., et al. (2017). Recent advances in phospholipids from colostrum, milk and dairy by-products. *International Journal of Molecular Sciences, 18*(1), E173.

Visscher, M., & Narendran, V. (2014). Vernix caseosa: Formation and functions. *Newborn and Infant Nursing Reviews, 14*(4), 142–146.

Wüest, A., Manser, H., Küster, H., et al. (2016). Comparison of treatment strategies for anaemia of prematurity in extremely low birthweight infants between 1997 and 2011 *Archives of Disease in Childhood Fetal and Neonatal Edition, 101*(5), F480–F481.

Wyckoff, M., Aziz, K., Escobedo, M., et al. (2015). Part 13: Neonatal resuscitation. 2015 American Heart Association guidelines update for cardiopulmonary resuscitation and emergency cardiovascular care. *Circulation, 132*(18 Suppl. 2), S543–S560.

27

Nursing Care of the Child Born With a Physical or Developmental Challenge

*M*aia Sparrow, 22 years old, is a new mother whose newborn has been admitted to the neonatal intensive care unit for care of a neural tube disorder and developmental dysplasia of the hip. Ms. Sparrow is obviously upset over the diagnosis. She has not named the baby, and her parents have not visited. She says to you, "I'm a good person. The only thing I did wrong during pregnancy was to take some cough medicine. How could this have happened to me?"

Previous chapters described the importance of assessing all newborns at birth. This chapter includes information about common congenital anomalies or structural disorders that may occur in newborns. This information serves as a basis for a newborn assessment and for health teaching for parents.

How would you answer this mother? What type of advice and support does she need?

KEY TERMS

achondroplasia	fistula	polydactyly
ankyloglossia	frenulum	spina bifida
atresia	gastroschisis	stenosis
cleft lip	glossoptosis	syndactyly
cleft palate	hydrocephalus	talipes
craniosynostosis	meconium plug	torticollis
developmental dysplasia of the hip (DDH)	omphalocele	transillumination
	pectus excavatum	volvulus

OBJECTIVES

After mastering the contents of this chapter, you should be able to:

1. Describe common physical and developmental disorders that occur in newborns, infants, and children.

2. Assess newborns who are born physically or developmentally challenged.

3. Formulate nursing diagnoses for newborns born with a physical or developmental challenge.

4. Establish expected outcomes to meet the needs of the child with a physical or developmental challenge and assist parents to manage transitions across differing healthcare settings.

5. Implement nursing interventions for care of a newborn born with a physical or developmental challenge, such as preventing infection in a child with a neural tube disorder.

6. Evaluate expected outcomes to determine achievement and effectiveness of care.

7. Integrate knowledge of congenital physical or developmental challenges with the interplay of nursing process; the six competencies of Quality & Safety Education for Nurses (QSEN), including Patient-Centered Care, Teamwork & Collaboration, Evidence-Based Practice (EBP), Quality Improvement (QI), Safety, and Informatics; and Family Nursing to promote quality maternal and child health nursing care.

8. Assist with achieving 2020 National Health Goals related to newborns born physically or developmentally challenged.

Few things can change the usually joyous tone of a birthing room faster than the birth of a baby with a physical or developmental challenge. Primary care providers who are used to saying mentioning the "perfect" boy or girl find themselves without words. The usual congratulatory remarks hang unsaid in the air.

When a newborn is born with an apparent physical or developmental challenge, nurses play a major role in supporting and educating the parents to promote bonding. With some newborns, their congenital disorder may be corrected with surgery, and they will have no long-term sequela. With other newborns, the congenital disorders may require long-term care even with surgical correction. This chapter covers physical disorders of the skeletal, gastrointestinal, and neurologic systems that are apparent at birth or recognized soon after. Congenital disorders of the cardiovascular system are addressed in Chapter 41.

Birth defects remain a major public health burden. The Centers for Disease Control and Prevention (CDC) estimates that 3% of all newborns born in the United States are affected by a birth defect and 20% of all infant deaths are attributed to birth defects (CDC, 2016). Box 27.1 shows 2020 National Health Goals related to decreasing the number of newborns born with congenital anomalies.

BOX 27.1

Nursing Care Planning Based on 2020 National Health Goals

Many congenital anomalies, such as a cleft lip, an omphalocele, and neural tube disorders, can be detected by sonogram during intrauterine life. The following 2020 National Health Goals address the importance of prevention and therapy postbirth:

- Increase the proportion of women delivering a live birth who took multivitamins/folic acid prior to pregnancy from a baseline of 30.1% to 33.1%.
- Reduce the occurrence of spina bifida from 34.2 per 100,000 live births to 30.8 per 100,000 live births per year.
- Reduce the occurrence of anencephaly from 24.6 per 100,000 live births to 22.1 per 100,000 live births per year.
- Increase the proportion of children with special healthcare needs who have access to a medical home from 47.1% to 51.8%.
- Increase the proportion of children aged 0 to 11 years with special healthcare needs who receive their care in family-centered, comprehensive, and coordinated systems from a baseline of 20.4% to 22.4%; and in children aged 12 to 17 years from 13.7% to 15.1% (U.S. Department of Health and Human Services, 2010; see www.healthypeople.gov).

Nurses can help the nation achieve these goals by urging women to enter pregnancy with an adequate folic acid level, ensuring women obtain prenatal care, and receive comprehensive advice and support after diagnosis of a fetal or newborn disorder.

Nursing Process Overview

FOR CARE OF A NEWBORN WHO IS PHYSICALLY OR DEVELOPMENTALLY CHALLENGED

ASSESSMENT

The nursing assessment of a newborn who is physically or developmentally challenged focuses on determining the infant's immediate physiologic needs required to sustain life and the parents' immediate emotional needs to promote bonding. These are not different that those of all newborns. The following eight primary needs of newborns should be assessed for signs that they are being established considering the newborn's physical and developmental challenges:

- Adequate respiration
- Extrauterine circulation
- Body temperature stabilization
- Blood sugar stabilization
- Prevention of infection
- An infant–parent bond
- Adequate stimulation
- Ability to take in adequate nutrients
- Ability to achieve waste elimination

Anomalies that affect a newborn's appearance may have the most immediate effect on the parents' ability to establish a positive bond with their child. It is important, however, not to jump to conclusions about what will be the parents' response. An assessment of the family's verbal and nonverbal responses may reveal that parents are prepared and agreeable to meet this infant's special needs. The parent's adjustment may be affected by their prior knowledge of their child's physical or developmental challenge.

NURSING DIAGNOSIS

Many nursing diagnoses established for children who are physically or developmentally challenged address the effect of the disorder on body function, including the child's primary needs and the family's coping ability (Farrell & Krahn, 2014).

Examples of possible diagnoses include:

- Imbalanced nutrition, less than body requirements, related to inability to take in adequate nutrition secondary to a physical challenge
- Impaired physical mobility related to congenital anomaly
- Risk for impaired parenting related to the birth of child with a congenital anomaly
- Anticipatory grieving (parental) related to loss of the idea of the "perfect" child

OUTCOME IDENTIFICATION AND PLANNING

Nurses play an important role in providing immediate care to high-risk newborns at birth as well as stabilizing them until the pediatric team arrives to assume care or transport the newborn to a high-risk nursery. Consideration of the family's resources, both emotional and financial, is an important aspect of planning care and establishing expected outcomes (Nes, Røysamb, Hauge, et al., 2014). It's important to consider both the short- and long-term needs of the newborn and how these needs may affect the family. Supportive family members can be a critical asset to parental adjustment (Carmichael,

Ma, Tinker, et al., 2014). Providing nursing support as part of an interdisciplinary team, including social workers, therapists, nutritionists, medical specialists, and other community resources can also help with parental adjustment. Refer parents to helpful websites and other resources when appropriate (see Chapter 20).

IMPLEMENTATION

Nursing interventions for a newborn who is physically challenged include immediate life-sustaining measures such as providing oxygen or adequate intake of nutrients when a disorder prevents the infant from establishing respirations or sucking. Encouraging skin-to-skin contact and interacting with the newborn promotes infant–parent bonding. Educating the parents about procedures the infant may undergo lessens the parental anxiety and enhances self-esteem.

Parents experience the same stages of grief: denial, anger, bargaining, depression, and adjustment as those whose child has died at birth (see Chapter 56). It is important for the nurse to provide positive role modeling when caring for the emotional and physical needs of the newborn; it helps the parents to adjust to parenting a child born with a physical or developmental challenge.

OUTCOME EVALUATION

Outcome evaluation should focus on establishing expected outcomes for the child's physical and developmental health needs as well as the family's coping ability for current and future health of the child. This includes addressing the family concerns and providing resources to support the family during and after discharge.

Examples of expected outcomes may include:

- Parent describes positive features of child by 2 weeks.
- Parents state they are comfortable with enteral feeding by 1 month.
- Child is ambulatory with walker or wheelchair by 2 years of age.

Care at Birth of the Newborn Who Is Physically or Developmentally Challenged

The pediatric provider or neonatologist typically provides the parents with medical information regarding the health status of their newborn. This information should be provided to the parents as quickly and accurately as possible. The nurse can provide support to the family by keeping them informed of their newborn's health status and facilitating their interaction with the healthcare team. It is distressing for parents, who expect to hold their newborn immediately after birth, to watch their newborn undergo a medical evaluation and medical intervention while physically separated from their newborn (Box 27.2).

When the parents are with their newborn, the nurse can begin by describing the newborn's physical condition, related to the diagnosis, to the parents. Medical equipment and its purpose should also be explained. Parents should be given the opportunity to ask questions and interact with their newborn. Comments by the nurse related to normal newborn

BOX 27.2

Nursing Care Planning to Respect Cultural Diversity

The causes of most congenital anomalies are unknown, although they probably arise from a combination of environmental and genetic factors. New parents need an explanation of their child's disorder and a chance to talk about why they believe their child's disorder occurred. Despite the evidence, many cultural myths persist around congenital anomalies. Many people persist in believing infants with congenital anomalies are born to people less deserving than others. Common beliefs include myths such as being looked on by an evil eye (*mal de ojo* in Spanish) can cause a deformity. Parents may also blame themselves for their child's condition thinking something they did or didn't do may have caused it. Common beliefs also include the idea that eating raisins causes brown birth marks and eating strawberries causes red hemangiomas. Educating parents relieves any guilt that they were the cause of the anomaly, helping them regain sufficient self-esteem to raise a child with a congenital disorder.

observations can assist the parents in relating their newborn. A typical explanation for Maia, for example, might be, "When your doctor placed your baby on your abdomen, you might have noticed that your baby's spinal cord isn't completely formed, something called a meningocele. Although that could be more extensive, at first inspection, it seems to be a problem that can be repaired. Her hips may also need some treatment. I'll bring the baby's Isolette over so you can see her. Notice how bright-eyed and alert she is for just being born." Referring to the newborn by their name is helpful to personalize the interaction.

What If . . . 27.1

The nurse notices Maia remains obviously upset at her child's appearance. She doesn't want to feed him and tells the nurse she'd like to place him for adoption. In contrast, the child's father, also a teenager, handles the baby warmly and asks questions about surgery. No grandparents visit. What interventions would the nurse want to begin with this family?

Physical and Developmental Disorders of the Skeletal System

Either genetic or environmental factors can compromise fetal physical growth to such an extent that they result in skeletal disorders in the newborn.

ABSENT OR MALFORMED EXTREMITIES

Congenital skeletal disorders can result from reasons such as maternal drug ingestion or virus invasion or amniotic band formation in utero. In most instances, however, the cause of the anomaly is unknown. Children born without an extremity or with a malformed extremity can be fitted with a prosthesis as early in life as about 6 months so the infant can learn to stand at the normal time or handle and explore objects readily. However, it may be adventitious to allow the child to grow and learn to use their altered body or limb without a prosthesis. Introducing a prosthesis early in life may prevent a child from adjusting to a missing extremity, for example, such as learning to write with their feet or sliding across the floor rather than walking. Often, parents and therapists will teach children in therapy to function both with and without a prosthesis. Children are resilient and can become so proficient at these adjustments in their born deformity that later in life they may not see any advantage to using a prosthesis. Those affected by a skeletal anomaly can choose to use a prosthesis as an adult or not.

Depending on the condition, in many children, there is a potential for better function if the malformed portion of an extremity is amputated before a prosthesis is fitted. This creates a difficult decision for parents because it is one they cannot undo later. They need assurance that hands with malformed fingers, for example, will not later grow to become normal and that a well-fitted prosthesis will allow their child a more usual childhood and adult life than if the original disorder was left unchanged (Fig. 27.1).

Learning to use a hand prosthesis takes weeks to months, and it also involves therapy. It helps if parents can think of interesting activities when introducing the prosthesis so the child can immediately see how useful it will be to use. Gait training for the use of lower extremity prostheses begins with the use of parallel bars and proceeds to independent walking and mastery of steps. Again, suggesting activities the child needs to walk to do offers motivation for trying to use the prosthesis.

Children who are born with an absent extremity may need help not only in mastering the use of a prosthesis but also in forming a positive body image of themselves as whole. If possible, in the newborn period, introduce parents to the rehabilitation team who will be following their child. Further steps will then be outlined to help them move past the helplessness they may be feeling to more positive actions. Visiting with a child who uses a prosthesis well can be a great help in convincing parents that their child can lead a normal life. Young children with a congenital extremity may not grieve over the lost extremity as do adults or older children.

FINGER AND TOE CONDITIONS

Finger or hand deformities occur in about 3% of all births. **Polydactyly** is the presence of one or more additional fingers or toes. When an entire extra finger or toe forms, the supernumerary digit is usually amputated in infancy or early childhood. These extra fingers are often just cartilage or skin tags, and removal is simple and cosmetically sound. In **syndactyly** (two fingers or toes are fused), the fusion is usually caused by a simple webbing (Fig. 27.2); separation of the digits into two sound and cosmetically appealing ones is usually successful. In other instances, the bones of the fingers or toes are also fused, and cosmetic appearance and function cannot be fully reconstructed (Sullivan & Adkinson, 2016).

These digit anomalies are always upsetting to parents (one of the first things new parents do is count the fingers and toes of newborns) and may cause them to view their infant as defective rather than being an infant with a simple anomaly. Encourage them to air their feelings and concerns as they deliver the news to family and friends. Because hands are so important for writing, self-care, or computing, they may need reassurance at health maintenance visits for the first few years of their child's life that the child is perfect in other ways so they can accept and help the child develop self-esteem. Children may need this same type of assurance as they grow older so they can think of themselves as well people. Often, identifying a skill or talent that the child excels in can provide another avenue for developing self-esteem. There are many examples of children with one limb or a deformity playing sports, such as swimming, excelling in the arts, or playing

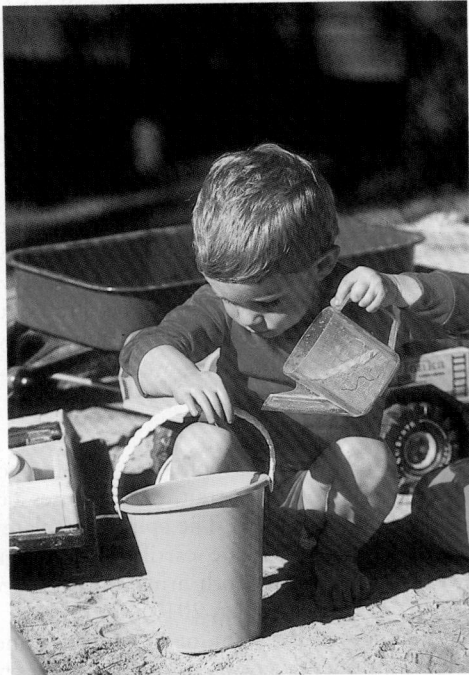

Figure 27.1 A young child learns to use a hand prosthesis during play. (M. Grecco/Stock Boston.)

Figure 27.2 Syndactyly. (JPD/Custom Medical Stock Photograph.)

musical instruments. If a child expresses a desire to learn these activities, allowing the child to participate (if medically safe and sound) typically leads to profound beneficial outcomes for all.

CHEST DEVIATIONS

Pectus excavatum, or "funnel chest," is an indentation of the lower portion of the sternum. It is the most common congenital deformity of the anterior chest, occurs in about 1 out of 500 live births, and affects boys 4 times more often than girls. The concern may not be present at birth but becomes more obvious as the child grows to school age or adolescence. As a result of the deformity, lung volume is apt to be decreased and the heart is displaced to the left. The condition can be repaired, for either cosmetic reasons or physiologic reasons, such as to expand lung volume (Abdullah & Harris, 2016). With *pectus carinatum*, the sternum is displaced anteriorly, increasing the anteroposterior diameter of the chest. This anomaly can be surgically corrected (Tikka, Kalkat, Bishay, et al., 2016).

TORTICOLLIS (WRY NECK)

Torticollis is a term derived from the terms *tortus* ("twisted") and *collum* ("neck"). Torticollis (wry neck) occurs as a congenital anomaly when the sternocleidomastoid muscle is injured and bleeds during birth (Ryu, Kim, Kim, et al., 2016). This tends to occur in newborns with wide shoulders when pressure is exerted on the head to deliver the shoulder either with a vaginal or cesarean birth. The infant holds the head tilted to the same side as the muscle that is involved; the chin rotates to the opposite side. The injury may not be noticeable in the newborn and may become evident only as the original hemorrhage recedes and fibrous contraction occurs at 1 to 2 months of age. A thick mass over the muscle can usually be palpated at that time.

To relieve torticollis, parents need to begin a program of passive stretching exercises and therapy, laying the infant on a flat surface and rotating the head through a full range of motion. Often, pediatric physical therapists are involved in the home therapy treatment for infants with torticollis. In addition, parents should always encourage the infant to look in the direction of the affected muscle. They can encourage this by holding the child to feed in such a position that the child must look in the desired direction. Placing a mobile on the child's crib can encourage the child to look toward the affected side. Speaking to and handing the child objects from the affected side is another helpful exercise.

If manual stretching is begun early and performed consistently by parents, further treatment usually is not necessary. If extreme injury to the muscle occurred, torticollis can lead to the continued elevation of one shoulder. Although a rare complication, this has the potential to lead to scoliosis later in life. Therefore, help parents to understand that their actions are important therapy, not just games. Otherwise, the exercises seem so simple parents may not take them seriously. In the few instances in which simple exercises are not effective and the condition still exists at 1 year of age, surgical correction followed by a neck immobilizer may be necessary.

CRANIOSYNOSTOSIS

Craniosynostosis is the premature closure of the sutures of the skull. This may occur in utero or early in infancy because of rickets or irregularities of calcium or phosphate metabolism; it also occurs as a dominantly inherited trait and occurs more often in boys than in girls (Children's Craniofacial Association, n.d.). Measuring the infant's head circumference during the first 18 months of life is advocated by the American Academy of Pediatrics (AAP; Mulpuri, Song, Gross, et al., 2015).

This condition needs to be detected early because premature closure of the suture line will close the fontanelles, seal the skull closed, and compromise brain growth. If the sagittal suture line is the one that closes prematurely, the child's head tends to grow anteriorly and posteriorly. If the coronal suture line fuses early, the orbits of the eyes become misshapen and the increased intracranial pressure may lead to eye disorders such as exophthalmos, nystagmus, papilledema, strabismus, and atrophy of the optic nerve with consequent loss of vision. Premature closure of the coronal suture line is associated with syndactyly. Therefore, make a point at well-child assessments to observe the head circumference for all infants, especially those with syndactyly. Cardiac anomalies, choanal atresias, or disorders of elbows and knee joints can also be associated.

Craniosynostosis is diagnosed by X-ray or ultrasound, which reveals the fused suture line. If the suture line involved is the sagittal, treatment may involve only careful observation; if the coronal suture line is involved, it will need to be surgically opened to prevent brain compression and an abnormally shaped head by 9 to 12 months (Jubbal, Agrawal, & Hollier, 2017).

ACHONDROPLASIA

Achondroplasia (chondrodystrophia) is a failure of bone growth inherited as a dominant trait, which causes a disorder in cartilage production in utero. The epiphyseal plate of long bones cannot produce adequate cartilage for longitudinal bone growth; this results in both arms and legs becoming stunted (Ornitz & Legeai-Mallet, 2017).

Because the bones of the cranium are of membranous origin, the head continues to grow normally, causing children's heads to appear unusually large in contrast to their extremities.

The forehead is particularly prominent and the bridge of the nose becomes flattened. Children's trunks are of near-normal size, but a thoracic kyphosis (outward curve) and lumbar lordosis (inward curve) of the spine may develop. Because this is a cartilage, not a brain growth concern, gross motor development may be slowed, but intelligence is not affected.

Achondroplasia can be diagnosed in utero by ultrasound or at birth by X-ray by comparing the length of extremities to the usual length (in the average child, the arms can be extended to the distance of the midthigh). An X-ray will also reveal characteristic abnormally flaring epiphyseal lines. Children with achondroplasia rarely reach a height of more than 4 ft 6 in. (140 cm). Women with this condition may have difficulty with childbearing because of a small pelvis, generally necessitating a cesarean birth.

Children with achondroplasia become aware of their appearance as early as the preschool years. They are apt to become acutely aware of their appearance during school age, when they realize they look so different from other children. In order to help them grow, they may be prescribed growth hormone, or although controversial, leg lengthening may be possible (Ornitz & Legeai-Mallet, 2017). Ideally, such children have parents who have helped them adjust well to their short stature as well as help them develop good self-esteem so they can be happy in their body, no matter what is their final height.

Children need to be informed as they reach adolescence that, as with all dominantly inherited disorders, there is a high probability their children will inherit the disorder. This can make adolescence a particularly difficult time for these children as they realize both some occupational and reproductive options may be limited for them. Continued guidance or counseling can help them to emerge from this period with feelings of high self-esteem as adults.

TALIPES DISORDERS

The word *talipes* is formed from the Latin *talus* ("ankle") and *pes* ("foot"). The **talipes** deformities, therefore, are ankle–foot disorders, popularly called clubfoot. The term "clubfoot" implies permanent crippling to many people, and because this is no longer true with effective surgery, avoid using the term when discussing talipes disorders with parents. Concerns that may remain after surgery include that the child's right and left shoe size may vary and the child may have asymmetry of leg length.

Approximately 1 child in every 1,000 is born with a talipes disorder, and it occurs more often in boys than in girls. It probably is inherited as a polygenic pattern, and it usually occurs as a unilateral problem (Sanzarello, Nanni, & Faldini, 2017).

Some newborns who appear to have a talipes disorder actually have only an unusual foot position (a pseudotalipes) that developed because of their cramped intrauterine position. In these infants, the foot can be brought into a straight position by manual manipulation. In a true disorder, the foot cannot be properly aligned without further intervention. Be certain to demonstrate to parents that, if a pseudodisorder is present, the foot can easily be brought into line or is not deformed. Otherwise, the first time parents fit booties or shoes on the infant, they may notice this odd position and worry the foot is misshapen when it is not. Stretching the foot into line every day will solve the problem in a short time.

A true talipes disorder can be one of four separate types: plantar flexion (an equinus or "horse foot" position, with the forefoot lower than the heel); dorsiflexion (the heel is held lower than the forefoot or the anterior foot is flexed toward the anterior leg); varus deviation (the foot turns in); or valgus deviation (the foot turns out). Most children with talipes deformities have a combination of these conditions or have an equinovarus (Fig. 27.3A) or a calcaneovalgus disorder (a child walks on the heel with the foot everted).

Assessment

The earlier a true disorder is recognized, the better will be the correction. Make a habit, therefore, of straightening all newborn feet to the midline as part of the initial assessment to detect this disorder. If there is a possible questionable deformity, refer to the pediatric physician and orthopedist specialist to begin the process of evaluating the infant properly.

Therapeutic Management

Correction is achieved best if it is begun in the newborn period. For correction, a series of casts or braces are applied to gradually mold the foot into good alignment (a Ponseti method) (Sanzarello et al., 2017). Although the disorder involves the ankle, the cast or brace extends above the knee to ensure a firm correction (see Fig. 27.3B). (Care of the child in a cast is discussed in Chapter 51.) Because talipes casts

Figure 27.3   (A) Talipes equinovarus. (SPL/Photo Researchers, Inc.) **(B)** Casts for bilateral equinovarus.

are high on the leg, change diapers frequently to prevent a wet diaper from touching the cast and causing it to become soaked with urine or meconium. Review with parents how to check the infant's toes for coldness or blueness and how to blanch a toenail bed and watch it turn pink to assess for good circulation. Because a newborn cannot report pain except by generalized crying, they must evaluate crying episodes in the infant carefully. Such crying may be because of colic, hunger, or wet diapers, or it might also be because of the tingling feeling of circulatory compression (as when a foot is "asleep") from too tight a cast.

Infants grow so rapidly in the neonatal period that casts or braces for talipes deformities must be changed or adjusted almost every 1 or 2 weeks. If a mother has a complication or is exhausted from childbirth, be certain she will be able to make arrangements for another family member or friend to bring the infant to the hospital for frequent cast changes or brace adjustments.

After approximately 6 weeks (the time varies depending on the extent of the problem), the final cast will be removed. Following this, the infant may have to sleep in Denis Browne splints (shoes attached to a metal bar to maintain position) or high-top shoes at night for a few more months to ensure an effective correction. Parents may need to perform passive foot exercises such as putting the infant's foot and ankle through a full range of motion several times a day for several months. These seem to be simple maneuvers, so be certain to stress their importance to the parents; otherwise, they are easy exercises to omit when people's lives are busy. Pediatric physical therapists are often part of the interprofessional therapy team to assist in rehabilitation at the hospital and at home.

Although a successful correction cannot be guaranteed, the prognosis for a full correction is good. For children who do not achieve correction by casting, additional surgery is yet another option to achieve a final correction.

DEVELOPMENTAL DYSPLASIA OF THE HIP

Developmental dysplasia of the hip (DDH) (often referred to as congenital hip dysplasia) is improper formation and function of the hip socket and is considered a spectrum of abnormalities affecting the hip joint. DDH is a fairly common musculoskeletal condition found in newborns, with the prevalence estimated to range from 1.6 to 28.5 per 1,000 infants, averaging about 5% of newborns who have some radiographic abnormality of the hip (Shaw & Segal, 2016).

DDH is a leading cause of orthopedic disability in childhood and adult life because it can lead to premature arthritis requiring hip replacement (the disorder is responsible for up to 28% of hip replacements in people under 60 years of age) (Shaw & Segal, 2016). The disorder may be evident as either subluxation or dislocation of the head of the femur (Fig. 27.4).

With the disorder, the acetabulum of the pelvis is unusually flattened or shallow. This prevents the head of the femur from remaining in the acetabulum and rotating adequately. In a subluxated hip, the femur "rides up" because of the flat acetabulum; in a dislocated hip, the femur rides so far up it actually leaves the acetabulum. Why the disorder occurs is unknown, but it may be from a polygenic inheritance pattern. It may also occur from a uterine position that causes less-than-usual pressure of the femur head on the acetabulum.

DDH is more likely to occur with breech birth, a female infant, and a mother's first pregnancy (Jackson, Runge, & Nye, 2014). It is usually unilateral and found 6 times more frequently in girls than in boys, possibly because the hips are normally more flaring in females and possibly because the maternal hormone relaxin causes the pelvic ligaments to be more relaxed during pregnancy, which causes the femur to not press as effectively into the acetabulum during intrauterine life, thus deepening the space. Additional risk

Figure 27.4 Hip dysplasia. **(A)** A normal femur head and acetabulum. **(B)** A subluxated hip. The femur head is "riding high" in the shallow acetabulum. **(C)** A dislocated hip. The femur head is not engaged in the shallow acetabulum.

factors include family history of DDH, oligohydramnios, large birth weight for gestational age, metatarsus adductus, and torticollis (Shaw & Segal, 2016). Current literature suggests that the natural history to delineate the reason for the DDH appears to be dependent both on the type and severity of the hip abnormality and may be the combination of risk factors presented (Mulpuri et al., 2015).

Assessment

All infants should be screened for DDH from birth and up until 3 months of age by performing the Ortolani & Barlow maneuver (Shaw & Segal, 2016). Detecting developmental dysplasia of the hip in the newborn is important because the longer the condition goes undetected, the more difficult it is to correct. On inspection, the affected leg may appear slightly shorter than the other because the femur head rides so high in the socket. This is most noticeable when the child is lying supine and the thighs are flexed to a 90-degree angle toward the abdomen, causing one knee to be lower than the other (a Galeazzi sign; Fig. 27.5A). An unequal number of skin folds may also be present on the posterior thighs (see Fig. 27.5B). This finding is unreliable, however, because some infants with normal hips have an uneven number of posterior thigh skin folds. Subluxated or dislocated hips are best assessed by noting whether the hips abduct (Box 27.3).

In some infants, the hip abducts properly at a newborn assessment, but at the time of a health maintenance visit at 4 to 6 weeks, a secondary shortening of the adductor muscles will have occurred, and the disorder will be first evident. Hip dysplasia may also be difficult to detect at birth in an infant who was born from a breech presentation because the knees tend to be stiff and not flex readily. Because tight adductor muscles occur in children with cerebral palsy, these children also need careful assessment. Current guidelines recommend physical exam screening of all infants up to 6 to 12 months of age at all primary care visits via hip assessment and continual screening of those with risk factors until walking age (Mulpuri et al., 2015). In regard to radiologic screening, current guidelines recommend performing an imaging study, such as a hip ultrasound, before 6 months of age only in infants with one or more of these risk factors: such as breech presentation, family history, or history of clinical hip instability (Mulpuri et al., 2015). Hip ultrasonography has a good negative predictive value (as high as 90%) for ruling out DDH (Shaw & Segal, 2016). Generally plain radiography (X-ray) is not as effective in children less than 6 months of age due to musculoskeletal immaturity and unreliability to accurately screen for DDH; in children older than 6 months, radiology may be a useful assessment evaluation tool of treatment progress.

Therapeutic Management

Current recommendations from American Academy of Orthopaedic Surgeons and the AAP (2017) suggest close monitoring in mild DDH cases because 60% to 80% of clinically identified abnormalities and 90% of ultrasonographic abnormalities spontaneously resolve without treatment in early infancy (Mulpuri et al., 2015). In contrast, severe DDH may adversely affect normal hip growth and development and may cause issues into adulthood, such as osteoarthritis of the hip (Shaw & Segal, 2016). Infants less than 6 months of age are usually treated by using flexion-abduction splinting devices. Correction of subluxated and dislocated hips involves positioning the hip into a flexed, abducted (externally rotated) position to press the femur head against the acetabulum and cause the acetabulum to deepen its contour from the pressure. Brace and splints, such as the von Rosen, Pavlik, Craig, or Frejka, may be utilized for treatment of an unstable hip, and patient–family preferences should have a substantial influence on which type is chosen (Mulpuri et al., 2015). The Pavlik harness is shown to have a high success rate in treating subluxation and reducible DDH. There will be a small number of children who do not achieve correction by noninvasive methods will have corrective and therapeutic hip surgery, which may involve having a pin inserted to stabilize the hip.

 ## Nursing Diagnoses and Related Interventions

Nursing Diagnosis: Deficient parental knowledge related to splint, halter, or cast correction for hip dysplasia

Outcome Evaluation: Parents verbalize correct technique for and correctly demonstrate application and removal of splint or halter device and care of device or cast.

A Pavlik Harness. A Pavlik harness is an adjustable chest halter that abducts the legs. It is the method of choice for therapy because it reduces the time interval for therapy to 3 to 4 weeks and simplifies care (Fig. 27.6A). Soft plastic stirrups (booties) with quick-fastening closures attach to leg extension straps and hold the hips flexed, abducted, and externally rotated. Instruct parents how to lay the infant supine, grasp the infant's thighs, and abduct them to place the femoral head into the acetabulum and then apply the harness. The harness is then worn under clothing continually except for bathing. Advise parents to assess the skin under the straps daily for irritation or redness or potential skin breakdown from the harness rubbing. Caution them also that the harness achieves its effect by gentle continual pressure; it will be ineffective if parents remove it frequently or forget to put it in place.

Figure 27.5 Signs of developmental dysplasia of the hip. **(A)** With the child in a supine position, the right knee on the side of the subluxation appears lower than the left because of malposition of the femur head. **(B)** Asymmetry of skin folds and prominence of the trochanter on the right side.

BOX 27.3

Nursing Care Planning Using Procedures

ASSESSING ORTOLANI AND BARLOW SIGNS

Purpose: To assist in detecting developmental dysplasia of the hip

Procedure	Principle
1. Lay the infant supine and flex the knees to 90 degrees at the hips.	1. Proper positioning helps ensure accurate results.
2. Place your middle fingers over the greater trochanter of the femur and your thumb on the internal side of the thigh over the lesser trochanter (Fig. A).	2. Placing your fingers in this way allows for abduction of the hips.

3. Abduct the hips while applying upward pressure over the greater trochanter and listen for a clicking sound.	3. Normally, no sound is heard. A clicking or clunking sound is a positive Ortolani sign as it occurs when a displaced femoral head reenters the acetabulum.
4. Next, with your fingers in the same position and holding the hips and knees at 90-degree flexion, apply a backward pressure (down and laterally) and adduct the hips. Note any feeling of the femoral head slipping (Fig. B).	4. Normally, the hip joint is stable. A feeling of the femur head slipping out of the socket posterolaterally is a positive Barlow sign, which is indicative of hip instability associated with the developmental dysplasia of the hip.

A

B

Figure 27.6 **(A)** A Pavlik harness (shown over clothing for illustrative purposes). **(B)** A hip abduction cast for correction of subluxation of the hip.

A Spica Cast. If a hip is fully dislocated or the subluxation is severe, an infant may be placed immediately in a frog-leg, A-line cast, or a spica cast to maintain an externally rotated hip position (see Fig. 27.6B). These casts are heavy and are so wide that dressing infants or sitting them in an infant car seat or using a bassinet can be difficult. Be certain parents have a car seat that can be modified to accommodate a large cast. Like babies with a talipes, these infants are unable to report a cast is causing circulatory constriction, so they need to be assessed hourly for circulation to the extremities for the first 24 hours the cast is in place and daily thereafter. Teach parents how to do this type of neurovascular assessment (check temperature and circulation in toes) before they take an infant home from the hospital so they can prevent circulatory compression from a rapidly growing leg outgrowing the cast. Casts will be changed as growth and casting therapy require but maintained for 6 to 9 months. Casting is a second line of correction because the child is much harder to care for because of the weight of the cast. In some cases, the joint may become compressed due to the reduction maneuver or tension in the soft tissues around the hip, blocking the blood supply to the femoral head (avascular necrosis). In its severest form, this can lead to femoral head death and loss of future growth at the proximal growth plate, causing unequal leg lengths.

General Care Guidelines. Rarely, but sometimes surgery may still be necessary for a final correction. With severe

hip involvement, some children will be 2 years old before the final cast is removed.

The child and parents will be visiting their orthopedist frequently during these early years. Assess that they also schedule general health maintenance visits for routine immunizations and overall growth and development assessment. Spend time during health maintenance visits talking with them about infant stimulation. Teach parents to hold their child for feeding and to rock and cuddle the infant, even though a large cast or a brace may be bulky and awkward. Discuss how to bring experiences to the infant because the child cannot crawl and walk toward interesting objects in the environment. A child's wagon can supply convenient and fun transportation. The child may also be able to lie prone and move about on a large skateboard. Many parents worry the child who is still in a large cast at the normal age for walking (12 months) will never learn to walk. They can be assured that this is not a problem; when the cast is removed, the child will quickly catch up with this developmental step. Children who are diagnosed with severe DDH will often have an adjunct therapy team, such as pediatric physical therapists who are assisting with gross-motor milestone development while the child is in a brace or recovering from surgery. Nurses must assess that the family is receiving any needed adjunct therapies, such as physical therapy, and assist with any referrals that are necessary.

QSEN Checkpoint Question 27.2

INFORMATICS

Because Maia's baby was born with developmental dysplasia of the hip, he has a Pavlik harness prescribed. What information would the nurse want Maia to know about his care?

a. The harness may not be effective, but she should trial it before surgery.

b. She should keep the harness on her baby for 12 hours a day.

c. Her baby should wear the harness at all times except while bathing.

d. For more advice, she should look at mothers' blogs online.

Look in Appendix A for the best answer and rationale.

Physical and Developmental Disorders of the Gastrointestinal System

Many of the most common congenital anomalies of the gastrointestinal system, such as cleft lip and cleft palate, occur because of midline closure failure extremely early in intrauterine life. Others occur because the tract first forms as a solid tube and then undergoes canalization (hollowing out). At any site where this hollowing out does not occur, a partial or complete blockage or obstruction will be present. All gastrointestinal disorders can interfere with an infant's ability to take in nourishment to some degree at birth.

ANKYLOGLOSSIA (TONGUE-TIE)

Ankyloglossia is an abnormal restriction of the tongue occurring in a small number of newborns caused by an abnormally tight **frenulum**, the membrane attached to the lower anterior tip of the tongue (Yoon, Zaghi, Weitzman, et al., 2017). Tongue-tie (ankyloglossia) is a congenital anomaly in which a tight or shortened lingual frenulum causes restricted tongue mobility and impaired tongue function (Hazelbaker, 2010). Incidence rate is estimated to range from 4% to 10% within the newborn population (Yoon et al., 2017). Normally, the frenulum appears short and is positioned near the tip of the tongue. As the anterior portion of the infant's tongue grows, the frenulum becomes located farther back. In most instances, therefore, an infant suspected of being tongue-tied has a normal tongue at birth; it just seems short to parents who are unaware of a newborn's appearance. Tongue tie is often evaluated based on the mobility and how close to the tip of the tongue the leading edge of the frenulum is attached. Types 1 and 2 are the most common, accounting for 75% of tongue-ties and are often called "classic" and "anterior ties." Types 3 and 4 account for remaining 25 % and are often referred as "posterior ties."

The Hazelbaker Assessment tool can also be used to evaluate an infant's tongue-tie. The grading levels range from Class I (least severe) to Class IV (most severe) and are based on the tongue's appearance and function (Hazelbaker, 2010). With the increased emphasis on initiating and maintaining breastfeeding, a resurgence of feeding difficulties due to tongue-tie has been identified. In addition, decreased tongue mobility may cause short- and long-term consequences including feeding, speech, orthodontic problems, mandibular abnormalities, and difficulty with oral cleanliness (Academy of Breastfeeding Medicine [ABM], 2017).

This condition may cause difficulty with breastfeeding due to difficulty with tongue mobility and the ability to latch to create a strong suction at the breast. Mother's will often note that their infants (with a tongue-tie) tend to slip off the breast and cannot maintain a long latch without falling asleep. In addition, this mislatch will often cause moderate to severe nipple pain in about 80% of breastfeeding mothers. If it does, then a frenotomy release can be performed in the newborn period, typically by a trained physician, pediatric dentist, or advanced practice registered nurse (APRN). Ankyloglossia or tongue-tie are associated with a 25% to 60% incidence of breastfeeding difficulty and contributes to 10% to 26% of early cessation of breastfeeding (Wong, Patel, Cohen, et al., 2017). Current literature supports frenotomy for treatment of clinically significant tongue-tie that is causing difficulty with breastfeeding. Early identification of tongue-tie allows for close evaluation of breastfeeding and possible difficulties that might arise and referral to a specialist for a frenotomy if indicated. The majority of infants with tongue-tie have the ability to breastfeed successfully but may require extra lactation support, guidance, and feeding assistance by additional specialists, such as a lactation consultant (ABM, 2017).

THYROGLOSSAL CYSTS

A thyroglossal cyst arises from an embryogenic fault that leaves a cyst formed at the base of the tongue, which then drains through a **fistula** (an abnormal or surgically made passage between a hollow or tubular organ and the body surface, or between two hollow or tubular organs) to the anterior surface of the neck (Gowda & Joseph, 2017). Thyroglossal cysts are congenital defects located in or around the midline of the neck, extending to the base of the tongue. This condition may occur as an autosomal dominant trait. The cyst may involve the hyoid bone (the bone at the anterior surface of the neck at the root of the tongue) and may contain aberrant thyroid gland tissue. As the cyst fills with fluid, swelling and obstruction can lead to respiratory difficulty from pressure on the trachea. If infected, the cyst often appears swollen and reddened, with drainage of mucus or pus from the anterior neck and requires antibiotic therapy.

The cyst is surgically removed to avoid future infection of the space and, if thyroid tissue is present, the possibility of developing thyroid carcinoma later in life. Observe infants closely in the immediate postoperative period for respiratory distress because the operative area will develop at least minimum edema from surgical trauma. Position infants on their sides so secretions drain freely from their mouths. Intravenous (IV) fluid therapy is given after surgery until the edema at the incision recedes somewhat and swallowing is safe once more (approximately 24 hours). If the mother is breastfeeding, encourage her to express her milk via a hospital-grade pump or manual expression during this time to preserve her milk supply. Observe infants closely the first time they take fluid orally to be certain they do not aspirate. Be certain parents have a chance to feed their infant before the infant is discharged from the surgical unit so they can be assured the infant is swallowing safely, thus allowing them to feel confident at feeding the infant at home in a relaxed and comfortable way.

OROFACIAL CLEFTS: CLEFT LIP AND CLEFT PALATE

The maxillary and median nasal processes normally fuse between weeks 5 and 8 of intrauterine life. In infants with **cleft lip**, the fusion fails to occur in varying degrees, causing this disorder to range from a small notch in the upper lip to total separation of the lip and facial structures up into the floor of the nose, with even the upper teeth and gingiva absent. The deviation may be unilateral or bilateral. The infant's nose generally appears flattened because the incomplete fusion of the upper lip has allowed it to expand in a horizontal dimension (Allori, Mulliken, Meara, et al., 2017) (Fig. 27.7A). Overall rates of cleft lip and/or palate in the United States average to 1 in 600 newborns (American Cleft Palate–Craniofacial Association, n.d.).

Cleft lip is the most common orofacial cleft. It is more prevalent among boys than girls and occurs at a rate of approximately 20 cases per day and 7,500 cases each year in the United States (Tolarova & Elluru, 2015). This incidence is highest in the Asian population at 1 out of every 500 people, moderate in the European-derived population at 1 out of 1,000 people, and significantly lower in the African-derived population at 1 out of 2,500 people. It appears to be caused by the transmission of multiple genes aided by teratogenic factors present during weeks 5 to 8 of intrauterine life, such as a viral infection, certain seizure medicines such as phenytoin, maternal smoking or binge drinking, hyperthermia, stress, and maternal obesity (Funato & Nakamura, 2017). Folic acid deficiency may also be associated with incomplete anterior midline closures (Funato & Nakamura, 2017).

Because of the genetic influence, parents of a child with a cleft lip should be referred for genetic counseling to ensure they understand they have a small increased chance of having another child with a cleft lip or palate and that any future children are at a greater risk than usual for this problem.

Figure 27.7 Appearance of **(A)** a cleft lip and **(B)** a cleft palate. (From Moore, K. L., Agur, A. M. R., & Dalley, A. F. [2013]. *Clinically oriented anatomy* [7th ed.]. Philadelphia, PA: Wolters Kluwer.)

A **cleft palate** is an opening of the palate and occurs when the palatal process does not close as usual at approximately weeks 9 to 12 of intrauterine life. The incomplete closure is usually on the midline and may involve the anterior hard palate, the posterior soft palate, or both (see Fig. 27.7B). It may occur as a separate anomaly or in conjunction with a cleft lip. As a single entity, in contrast to cleft lip, it tends to occur more frequently in girls than boys. Like cleft lip, it appears to be the result of polygenic inheritance or environmental influences. In connection with cleft lip, the incidence is approximately 1 out of every 1,000 births. As a single entity, it occurs in approximately 1 out of every 2,000 births. Almost 30% of children with both cleft lip and palate have associated birth defects, or the cleft palate occurs as only a portion of a larger syndrome (Dixon, Marazita, Beaty, et al., 2011).

Assessment

Cleft lip may be detected by a sonogram while an infant is in utero. If not detected then, it is readily apparent on inspection of the mouth at birth. When assessing newborns, be sure you have good lighting so you can visualize the palate clearly. Because cleft palate is a component of many syndromes, assess the child for other congenital anomalies as well.

Therapeutic Management

If a cleft lip is discovered while the infant is still in utero, fetal surgery can repair the condition, although this procedure is not usually attempted. If the disorder is discovered at birth, a cleft lip can be repaired surgically shortly thereafter, often at the time of the initial hospital stay or between 2 and 12 weeks of age. Because the deviation of the lip interferes with sucking, infants may be a better surgical risk as newborns than they are after a month or more of poor nourishment. Early repair also helps infants experience the pleasure of sucking as soon as possible. It is equally important from a psychological standpoint as a parent may need caring support to bond with an infant whose face is deformed in this way (Nidey, Moreno Uribe, Marazita, et al., 2016). Because facial contours change as a child grows, a revision of the original repair or a nasal rhinoplasty to straighten a deviated nasal septum may be nec-

essary when the child reaches 4 to 6 years of age. Some infants may have a nasal mold apparatus applied before surgery to shape a better nostril (Funato & Nakamura, 2017).

The optimal time for repair of a cleft palate is controversial because early repair increases speech development but may result in a necessary second-stage repair as the child's palate arch expands with growth (Taub & Piccolo, 2016). Surgery may be recommended as a two-stage palate repair, with soft palate repair at 3 to 6 months of age and hard palate repair at 6 to 18 months of age, called the Malek protocol. This type of repair results in less need for future surgery and better facial results (Taub & Piccolo, 2016). Using infant orthodontic devices and delaying hard palate closure until later has not been shown to increase speech clarity or overall wellness (Taub & Piccolo, 2016).

Currently, the results of surgical repair of cleft lip and cleft palate are excellent (Fig. 27.8). It is helpful to show parents photographs of babies with good repairs to assure them their child's outcome can also be as successful.

One issue that may remain is that because palate repair narrows the upper dental arch, a child may be left with less space in the upper jaw for the eruption of teeth, creating poor teeth alignment. All children born with a cleft palate, therefore, need follow-up treatment by a pediatric dentist skilled in children's dental problems, so that as the child grows, extractions or realignment of teeth can be done as indicated. Children also need follow-up to detect if hearing or speech difficulty occurs; because the angle of the eustachian tube may be changed in surgery, a child may develop more ear infections than usual, possibly leading to some hearing impairment. After surgical repair, about 80% of children affected by cleft palate progress to develop normal speech, yet referral to speech therapy early in infancy should always occur to ensure successful speech development (American Cleft Palate–Craniofacial Association, n.d.).

Children with cleft problems tend to receive better, more frequent, and well-coordinated care when seen in an interprofessional team setting including pediatric dentists, audiologists, speech pathologists, geneticists, and craniofacial surgeons, so referring parents to an appropriate interprofessional center before discharge is critical for these infants and their families (Taub & Piccolo, 2016).

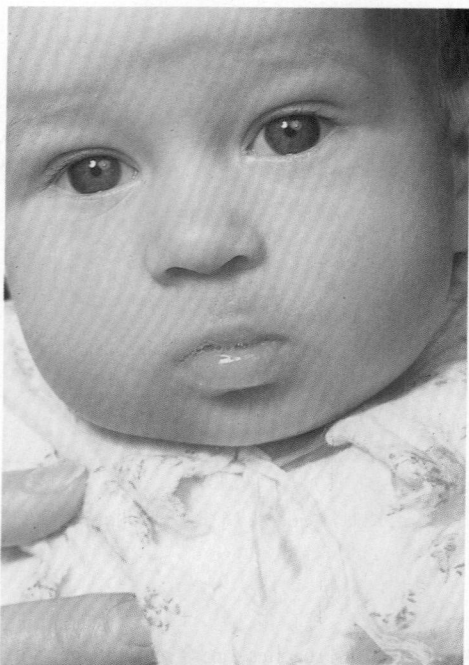

Figure 27.8 An infant showing surgical repair of cleft lip. Parents can be encouraged that the results of cleft lip repair are generally excellent. (Photo Researchers, Inc.)

Nursing Diagnoses and Related Interventions

Nursing Diagnosis: Risk for imbalanced nutrition, less than body requirements, related to feeding problem caused by cleft lip or palate

Outcome Evaluation: Newborn ingests an adequate diet of 110 kcal/kg (50 kcal/lb) in 24 hours; weight is maintained within 10% of birth weight.

Preoperative Period. Before a cleft lip or palate is repaired, feeding the infant becomes a concern because the infant has difficulty maintaining suction with a bottle or breast; there is evidence of slower growth when compared

to infants without a cleft disorder (Taub & Piccolo, 2016). In addition, it is important the child does not aspirate.

It may be possible for an infant with a cleft lip to breastfeed because the bulk of the mother's breast tends to form a seal against the incomplete upper lip. Although the baby needs the enjoyment of sucking, some surgeons do not want a baby to either breastfeed or suck on a nipple, however, before surgical correction of the disorder to avoid any local bruising of tissue. Therefore, the best feeding method for the child with cleft lip may be to support the baby in an upright position and feed the infant gently using a soft bottle and a commercial cleft lip nipple or a spoon. Breck or Haberman feeders are commercial apparatuses similar to a bulb syringe, which also can be used (Fig. 27.9). If the surgical repair for a cleft lip will be done immediately, the mother will be able to breastfeed as early as 7 to 10 days after surgery. Typically after the surgical repair and healing, the baby can latch to the breast. If there is difficulty with latching, a nipple shield can be suggested to help form a tighter seal at the breast. Review with the mother how to pump or manually express breast milk to maintain a milk supply prior to surgical correction and after, if needed. If surgery will be delayed for 1 month, the mother will need continuing support from the nursing staff to support her efforts on pumping and to remind her that her breast milk will be very beneficial to her infant and the healing process.

If a cleft extends to the nares so the nose and mouth are joined, breathing causes the oral mucous membranes and lips to become dry. Offering small sips of fluid between feedings can help keep the mucous membranes moist and prevent cracks and fissures that could lead to infection. Following a feeding, be certain an infant with a cleft lip is burped well because the inability to grasp a nipple or syringe edge securely causes the infant to swallow more air than usual.

Infants with a cleft palate cannot suck effectively either because pressing their tongue or a nipple against the roof of their mouth forces milk up into their pharynx, possibly leading to aspiration. The most successful method for feeding this infant, like the child with a cleft lip, therefore, is to use a commercial cleft palate nipple that has an extra

Figure 27.9 **(A)** Specialty feeding devices used for infants with cleft lip and cleft palate. **(B)** An infant uses a Haberman Feeder.

flange of rubber to close the roof of the mouth. If the nipple is used with a plastic bottle that can be squeezed gently to increase the flow of the feeding, this can compensate for poor sucking. A Breck feeder may also be used to feed infants with a cleft palate.

If surgery will be delayed beyond 6 months of age or the time when solid food would usually be introduced, teach parents to be certain any food they offer is soft because particles of coarse food could invade the nasopharynx and be a cause of aspiration.

Postoperative Period. After surgery for cleft lip or palate, an infant is kept nothing by mouth (NPO) for approximately 4 hours and then introduced to liquids such as plain water. Be certain to begin this process with only a small amount each time to prevent vomiting.

It's important that no tension is placed on a lip suture line because this helps keep the sutures from pulling apart and leaving a large scar. During this immediate postoperative period, therefore, the infant is usually fed using a specialized feeder because this causes less suture line tension than bottle feeding or breastfeeding.

After palate surgery, only liquids are generally given the first 3 or 4 days, and then a soft diet is followed until healing is complete. Ask parents before surgery what fluids the child prefers so they can be made available postsurgery.

When children begin to eat soft food, observe they don't use a spoon because spoons can invariably be pushed against the roof of their mouth and possibly disrupt sutures. If being fed rather than allowing the infant to use a spoon evokes an intense reaction, it is probably better to leave a child on a liquid diet until the sutures are removed. Be certain milk is not included in the first fluids offered because milk curds tend to adhere to the suture line and so are difficult to remove. After a feeding, always offer the child a sip of clear water to rinse the suture line and keep it as clean as possible. Also, educate parents to be diligent about oral health care. In infants with clefts involving the maxillary alveolar ridge (upper gum), it is common for some teeth—typically the upper incisors and cuspids on the side of the cleft—to be misshapen or turned (Cleft Palate Foundation, 2010). Prudent twice-daily gum and teeth brushing with an age appropriate toothbrush and tooth paste is crucial, as are biyearly dental visits for monitoring.

Nursing Diagnosis: Risk for ineffective airway clearance related to oral surgery

Outcome Evaluation: Child's respiratory rate remains at baseline level for age without retractions or obvious distress.

Because of the local edema that occurs after cleft lip or palate surgery, it's important to observe children closely in the immediate postoperative period for respiratory distress. Remember that before surgery, the infant with a cleft lip may have breathed through the mouth. After surgery, the infant now has to learn to breathe through the nose, possibly adding to respiratory difficulty. Generally, however, this is not a problem because newborns normally are strict nose breathers.

Following either cleft lip or cleft palate surgery, infants may need their mouth suctioned to remove mucus, blood, and unswallowed saliva. When doing this, be exceedingly gentle so you don't touch the suture line with the catheter. Place infants on their side to allow mouth secretions to drain forward. And, following a cleft lip repair, be sure a child does not turn onto his or her abdomen because this could put pressure on the suture line, possibly tearing it. Placing the child in an infant bouncy chair is another possibility.

Nursing Diagnosis: Impaired tissue integrity at incision line related to cleft lip or cleft palate surgery

Outcome Evaluation: Incision line appears clean and intact and free of erythema or drainage during postoperative period.

After cleft lip surgery, the suture line may be held in close approximation by a Logan bar (a wire bow taped to both cheeks; Fig. 27.10) or an adhesive bandage such as a Band-Aid simulating a bar that brings together the incision line but does not cover the incision. Assess the simulated or Logan bar is secure and continues to protect the suture line from tension after each feeding or cleaning of the suture line. Furnish adequate pain relief also so the infant does not cry because this puts increased tension on the sutures. To help avoid crying, try to anticipate the infant's needs by having formula ready to feed. Help the parents use whatever measures, such as rocking, carrying, or holding, that are necessary to make the infant feel secure and comfortable.

Nothing hard or sharp must come in contact with a recent cleft suture line. Observe infants after palate repair carefully, therefore, to be certain they do not put toys with sharp edges into their mouths. It's also good practice to not allow them to use a straw to drink or hold a toothbrush to clean their teeth so they don't brush the suture line accidentally. Keep elbow restraints in place as necessary so they do not put their fingers in their mouth and poke or pull at the sutures. Sutures on the lip or palate feel extremely odd, so most children not only run their tongue over their sutures but also don't respond to advice not to do this. Because this often occurs when children have nothing to think about, help the parents provide diversional activities such as reading or singing to keep the child's attention off the suture line.

Figure 27.10   A Logan bar is an apparatus that may be used to protect the surgical incision for a cleft lip repair.

If parents will be continuing to give an analgesic such as acetaminophen (Tylenol) or ibuprofen (Advil) after they return home, be certain they are aware of the correct dosage and time schedule for administration of the liquid forms. They must also continue to keep the suture line protected until healing is complete.

Nursing Diagnosis: Risk for infection related to surgical incision

Outcome Evaluation: Infant's temperature is below 98.6°F (37°C) by tympanic membrane; incision site is clean, dry, and intact without erythema or foul drainage.

An infection and subsequent scarring may result if crusts from serous drainage are allowed to form on a cleft lip suture line. Most surgeons, therefore, prescribe cleaning the suture line with sterile water or sterile saline with sterile cotton-tipped applicators after every feeding or whenever the normal serum that forms on suture lines accumulates. Do not rub the suture line; use a smooth, gentle, rolling motion to avoid loosening sutures. Gently dry the suture line with a dry sterile cotton-tipped applicator afterward. Remember that the infant has sutures on the inside of the lip that need the same meticulous care as those visible on the outside.

Nursing Diagnosis: Risk for impaired parenting related to birth of an infant who is physically challenged

Outcome Evaluation: Parents state they believe there will be a positive outcome for their child and demonstrate positive coping behaviors evidenced by holding and helping with infant care.

To promote effective bonding, parents need to hold and interact with their infant during both the preoperative and postoperative periods. Caution them the child's incision line will appear swollen in the immediate postoperative period, but its appearance will improve with time. As soon as the child's sutures have been removed, parents may breastfeed or feed with an ordinary bottle. Caution both the breastfeeding mother (who has been maintaining her milk supply through expression) and the formula-feeding mother that because the infant has never sucked before, time will be needed to learn how to suck, just like a newborn.

Observe whether parents look at their baby's face while feeding the baby. Help them to understand that any negative feelings they feel toward the child or themselves, such as sadness or anger, are normal. This assurance does not instantly make them feel better about what has happened, but the knowledge the feelings they are experiencing are normal can help them begin to deal with such emotions. Many communities have support groups for parents of children born with a cleft lip or palate. Referral to these groups can offer parents additional support. The National Cleft Palate Foundation provides parent education materials at www.cleftline.org.

Nursing Diagnosis: Risk for situational low self-esteem related to child's facial surgery

Outcome Evaluation: Child participates in normal childhood activities that involve contact with other people,

states activities he or she enjoys at healthcare visits, and demonstrates age-appropriate developmental milestones.

If a scar remains after cleft lip surgery, children may need some help adjusting to their appearance until a second cosmetic repair can be completed later in life. Reinforce children's positive attributes, stressing that the scar is only one small aspect of who they are. As children reach adolescence, you may need to review a familial inheritance pattern of cleft lip so they are aware of the possible risk for transmission to their own children.

Nursing Diagnosis: Risk for infection (ear) related to the altered angle of the eustachian tube with cleft palate surgery

Outcome Evaluation: Parents state signs and symptoms of ear infection and importance of early treatment; parents list signs of diminished hearing and appropriate agencies for support and guidance.

Changing the contour of the palate when it is repaired also changes the slope of the eustachian tube to the middle ear. This can lead to a high incidence of middle ear infection (otitis media) because organisms are able to reach this area from the oral cavity more readily than usual. Review the signs of infection such as fever, pain, pulling on an ear, or discharge from the ear with parents. Remind them of the importance of reporting pharyngeal infection to their primary care provider promptly so it can be treated before the infection spreads to the middle ear. Because the eustachian tube may remain partially closed in its changed position, serous otitis media (accumulation of fluid in the middle ear) also tends to occur more frequently in these children than in others. If this happens, myringotomy tubes may be inserted to drain middle ear fluid and to help protect hearing (see Chapter 50). Be certain parents understand the need for routine screening for hearing loss during childhood because this is a common early sign of serous otitis media.

Nursing Diagnosis: Risk for impaired verbal communication related to cleft palate

Outcome Evaluation: Family members voice satisfaction with child's speech; developmental milestone of clearly articulated two-word sentences by age 2 years is met.

Infants with a cleft palate will begin to make speech sounds at the normal time (age 2 months). This speech, however, is usually guttural and unclear as many alphabet sounds are made by touching the tongue against the roof of the mouth. Depending on the age of the cleft palate repair, some children will continue to have accompanying speech difficulty because the soft palate must function for the child to pronounce "p" and "b" sounds (Prathanee, Pumnum, Seepuaham, et al., 2016). If cleft palate surgery is going to be delayed past age 2 years (as might happen if the child has other congenital anomalies, such as heart disease), a plastic prosthesis to cover the incomplete palate may be prescribed because this allows the child to articulate more efficiency.

Altered speech patterns in children generally do not resolve spontaneously and require intervention by a speech pathologist prior to school age.

EVIDENCE-BASED PRACTICE

Maia is having difficulty caring for her new baby because he was born with a birth disorder. To investigate whether it is common for a woman whose child is born with a birth anomaly to act differently than other mothers, researchers studied maternal gaze between mothers and infants and found maternal gaze changes as infants become more social.
A decrease in gaze to the mouth area was associated with infant's with cleft lip and might affect maternal responsiveness (De Pascalis, Kkeli, Chakrabarti, et al., 2017). This decrease in maternal gaze could be the basis for interventions for mothers of infants born with oral abnormalities (De Pascalis et al., 2017).

Based on the study, what type of role modeling would the nurse demonstrate to a mother when caring for a newborn with a cleft lip?
   a. Omit picking up the infant to show the mother how uncaring her actions seem.
   b. Hold the infant warmly; smile and play and talk to him.
   c. Tactfully point out to the mother that her actions may be seen to be uncaring.
   d. Ask the mother what you could do to help her adjust better.

Look in Appendix A for the best answer and rationale.

THE PIERRE ROBIN SEQUENCE

The Pierre Robin sequence (also called Pierre Robin syndrome) is a rare triad of micrognathia (small mandible), cleft palate, and **glossoptosis** (a tongue malpositioned downward). This triad of conditions can result in severe upper airway obstruction, which then may cause secondary respiratory distress due to upper airway obstruction. Estimates of occurrence range from 1 in every 8,500 births to 1 in every 20,000 births; the primary event that leads to the syndrome tends to be unknown. More than half of the children born with Pierre Robin syndrome have associated disorders of congenital glaucoma; cataracts; cardiac disorders; or other genetic, chromosomal, or medical concerns. They need thorough physical and genetic assessments to be certain that none of these other associated disorders are present (Bütow, Zwahlen, Morkel, et al., 2016).

Monitor infants for possible airway obstruction (as a result of their small jaw, their tongue tends to drop backward and obstruct their airway). Suctioning to remove secretions may be necessary. A side-lying rather than a supine sleeping position is recommended for all newborns and infants (until they can roll over) to avoid obstruction. Occasionally, infants have such extensive airway obstruction that a suture is attached to the anterior aspect of the tongue and the mucous membrane of the lower lip to pull the tongue forward and prevent the rear of the tongue from blocking the upper airway. Maintaining positioning as the infant grows and gains mobility may be increasingly difficult, but sleep studies have shown these children have severe sleep apnea, with as many as 49 episodes of apnea leading to oxygen desaturation per hour if sleeping supine (Bütow, Naidoo, Zwahlen, et al., 2016). Nasopharyn-

geal airways (NPAs) have been shown to be effective in upper airway obstruction, and 86.5% of infants studied maintained adequate airways with positioning or temporary placement of an NPA for several months. The airways of older children can be well maintained using nasal continuous positive airway pressure (CPAP); with this, after several years of therapy, the episodes of obstructive sleep apnea decrease to about five per hour, possibly decreasing the need for more invasive surgery.

As the child grows older, the jaw will grow somewhat, although the mandible will always be small. Parents need instructions on how to feed these infants until the cleft palate can be repaired. The child may have a gastrostomy tube or button inserted to relieve feeding difficulty (see Chapter 37).

Parents of the child with this syndrome take on a great deal of responsibility when they assume their infant's care; it's best if they are referred to an interprofessional team prior to discharge from the hospital. Be certain they have the name and number of a primary healthcare provider they can call when they have questions. Many of these parents grow exhausted during the first few weeks of their child's life, afraid they may sleep so soundly at night they miss their child having respiratory difficulty. Using a respiratory monitor at night can be helpful. As parents' confidence grows in their ability to provide care, this problem lessens, but it may be months or even years before a high level of confidence is achieved.

ESOPHAGEAL ATRESIAS AND TRACHEOESOPHAGEAL FISTULAS

Between weeks 4 and 8 of intrauterine life, the laryngotracheal groove in the chest develops into the larynx, trachea, and beginning lung tissue; the esophageal lumen forms parallel to this. A number of anomalies can occur if the trachea and esophagus are affected by some teratogen that does not allow the two organs to fully form separately and possibly become connected.

Esophageal atresia is the incomplete formation of the esophageal lumen, resulting in the proximal (upper) esophagus forming a "blind pouch," which then does not connect to any other structure. *Tracheoesophageal fistula* occurs when an opening develops between the closed distal (lower) esophagus and the trachea. Five usual types of esophageal atresia that result are:
   1. The esophagus ends in a blind pouch; there is a tracheoesophageal fistula between the distal part of the esophagus and the trachea (Fig. 27.11A).
   2. The esophagus ends in a blind pouch; there is no connection to the trachea (see Fig. 27.11B).
   3. A fistula is present between an otherwise normal esophagus and trachea (see Fig. 27.11C).
   4. The esophagus ends in a blind pouch. A fistula connects the blind pouch of the proximal esophagus to the trachea (see Fig. 27.11D).
   5. There is a blind end portion of the esophagus. Fistulas are present between both widely spaced segments of the esophagus and the trachea (see Fig. 27.11E).

All of these are potentially serious disorders because, during a feeding, milk can fill the blind pouch of the upper esophagus and then overflow into the trachea, or a fistula can allow milk to enter the trachea from the esophagus, resulting in aspiration. Even if not fed, the swallowed saliva of the baby will fill the esophagus and overflow into the airway, resulting in repeated aspiration. The incidence of the disorder ranges from 1 out of 2,500 to 4,500 live births (Vergouwe, IJsselstijn, Wijnen, et al., 2015).

Figure 27.11   An esophageal atresia and a tracheoesophageal fistula. **(A)** In the most common type of esophageal atresia, the esophagus ends in a blind pouch. The trachea communicates by a fistula with the lower esophagus and stomach (approximately 90% of infants with the defect have this type). **(B)** Both upper and lower segments end in blind pouches (5% to 8% of infants with the defect have this type). **(C)** Both upper and lower segments communicate with the trachea (2% to 3% of infants with the defect have this type). **(D)** Very rarely, the upper segment ends in a blind pouch and communicates by a fistula to the trachea, or **(E)** a fistula connects to both upper and lower segments of the esophagus.

Assessment

Esophageal atresia must be ruled out in any infant born to a woman with hydramnios (excessive amniotic fluid). This is because hydramnios occurs because, normally, a fetus swallows amniotic fluid during intrauterine life. A fetus with esophageal atresia cannot effectively swallow, so the amount of amniotic fluid can grow abnormally large. Many infants with esophageal atresia are born preterm because of the accompanying hydramnios, compounding their original problem with immaturity. The infant needs to be examined carefully for other congenital anomalies that could have occurred from the teratogenic effect at the same week in gestation, such as *v*ertebral, *a*nal, *c*ardiac, *t*racheo*e*sophageal, *r*enal, and *l*imb anomalies (VACTERL syndrome) (Vergouwe et al., 2015).

If not diagnosed in utero, diagnosing a child who has an esophageal atresia/tracheoesophageal fistula before the infant is first fed is important. Otherwise, the infant will cough, become cyanotic, and have obvious difficulty breathing as fluid is aspirated. Newborns who have so much mucus in their mouths that they appear to be blowing bubbles should be suspected of having either disorder. Esophageal atresia can be diagnosed with certainty if a catheter cannot be passed through the infant's esophagus to the stomach so stomach contents can be aspirated. If helping with this, supply a firm catheter because a soft one will curl in a blind-end esophagus and appear to have passed. An X-ray will reveal a radiopaque catheter coiled in the blind end of the esophagus. A flat-plate X-ray of the abdomen or an ultrasound also may reveal a stomach distended with the air that has passed from the trachea into the esophagus and stomach, demonstrating that a fistula is present. Either a barium swallow or a bronchial endoscopy examination can also reveal the blind-end esophagus and fistula.

Therapeutic Management

Emergency actions are required for the infant with this group of esophageal disorders in order to prevent the development of pneumonia, one of the major complications that is apt to occur from leakage of oral or stomach secretions into the lungs. The best position for the infant is an upright, 60-degree angle so acid stomach fluids stay in the stomach through the use of gravity (sitting the baby in an infant chair does this). If a nasogastric tube is inserted into the distal end of the esophagus and connected to low intermittent suction, oral secretions will no longer collect in the blind pouch, decreasing aspiration risks. A gastrostomy may be inserted into the stomach (under local anesthesia) with the tube allowed to drain by gravity as another way of keeping the stomach empty of secretions and preventing reflux into the lungs. IV fluids and parenteral nutrition are begun to prevent dehydration and an electrolyte imbalance from lack of oral intake. IV medications that restrict the stomach's ability to produce acid may be prescribed, and an antibiotic may be prescribed to help prevent an infection.

When the infant has been stabilized by this sequence of measure, surgery consists of closing the fistula and anastomosing the esophageal segments. If the defect was only a simple fistula, surgery may be done by thoracoscopy to minimize the time required for surgery (Vergouwe et al., 2015). If the repair will be more complex, it may be necessary for the surgery to be completed in different stages and to use a portion of the intestine to complete the anastomosis if the esophageal segments are too far apart to join readily. After an anastomosis repair, observe infants closely at postoperative days 7 to 10 because this is the point when their internal sutures will dissolve, possibly allowing a leak from the anastomosis site to occur at this time. If such a leak occurs, fluid and air can leak out into the chest cavity, and pneumothorax (collapse of a lung) can occur.

In some infants, some stenosis or stricture at the anastomosis site remains. If this occurs, esophageal dilatation at periodic intervals to keep the repaired esophagus fully patent may be necessary. Gastroesophageal reflux may also occur after a repair, especially if the esophagus is left shorter than usual; this can lead to recurrent fistula formation and irritation from the presence of stomach acid in the esophagus (Vergouwe et al., 2015).

The ultimate prognosis for children with this disorder depends on the extent of the repair necessary, the condition of the child at the time of surgery, and the presence or absence of other congenital anomalies. Even with larger disorders, if surgery can be performed before pneumonia develops, the repair of the esophagus and trachea will be effective. The mortality rate for the condition remains high, however, because of the presence of other congenital disorders and low birth weight that often accompanies the tracheal abnormality.

 ## Nursing Diagnoses and Related Interventions

Both nursing diagnosis and outcomes established for the child with either a tracheoesophageal fistula or esophageal atresia must be realistic in terms of the extent of the disorder, the timing of anticipated surgery, and the stage of grief or readiness for decision making and planning the parents have reached.

Nursing Diagnosis: Risk for imbalanced nutrition, less than body requirements, related to inability to take in oral feedings

Outcome Evaluation: Child maintains weight within 10% of birth weight and maintains weight in same percentile on growth curve.

Before surgery, because oral fluid cannot be given until the esophagus is repaired, IV therapy or total parenteral nutrition (TPN) can be used to supply fluid and calories. Following surgery, the infant may be fed orally, may be continued on TPN, or may be started on gastrostomy feedings, depending on whether the surgery could be completed in one stage or not.

Early introduction of oral fluid may help to ensure patency of the esophagus because it helps to decrease adhesion formation at the anastomosis site and also allows the infant the enjoyment and practice of sucking. If formula is given by gastrostomy feedings, be certain to introduce it into the tube slowly and allow it to run by gravity pressure only to prevent fluid from entering the esophagus and putting pressure on the new suture line. After the feeding, the end of the tube should be elevated, covered by sterile gauze, and kept in the elevated position, *not clamped*, so any air introduced during the feeding will be released from the tube and not enter the esophagus to put pressure on the suture line. This also helps to ensure that if the infant should vomit the feeding, the vomitus will be projected into the gastrostomy tube and again will not contaminate the fresh sutures. Most newborns enjoy sucking a pacifier during gastrostomy feedings for sucking pleasure. If a mother wishes to breastfeed, she can manually express breast milk for the gastrostomy feedings.

If the child is to return home to await a second-stage operation, the gastrostomy tube will be left in place. Be certain parents are comfortable doing gastrostomy feedings as well as usual infant care, such as holding or talking to the infant in the face of this different feeding method.

Nursing Diagnosis: Risk for infection related to aspiration or seepage of stomach secretions into lungs

Outcome Evaluation: Child's temperature remains below 98.6°F (37°C) axillary; there is absence of rales on auscultation.

Preoperative Care. In addition to measures such as keeping the child in a sitting position, if surgery will be significantly delayed, an infant may have a cervical esophagostomy (the distal end of the blind esophagus is brought to the surface just over the sternum) as a method to allow oral secretions to drain. Use absorbent gauze around the opening of the site to absorb moisture and apply a protective ointment liberally to the skin to help prevent excoriation of the skin. Consult as necessary with a wound, ostomy, and continence therapy nurse to prevent further skin irritation.

Keeping the infant under a radiant heat warmer with a high-humidity oxygen source helps to maintain body heat and liquefy bronchial secretions. Try to keep the infant from crying because, with crying, air enters the stomach from the trachea, distending the stomach and possibly causing vomiting with aspiration into the lungs. A pacifier may be helpful to relax the baby and also to satisfy a sucking need.

Postoperative Care. The baby will return from final surgery with multiple tubes (e.g., chest tubes, endotracheal tube, Foley catheter, multiple IV lines, probably an arterial line, possibly a gastrostomy tube if not previously inserted), as well as blood pressure, oxygen saturation, and electrocardiography monitoring equipment. The posterior chest tube drains collecting fluid, and the anterior tube allows air to leave the chest space so the lungs can reexpand (see Chapter 41 for care of an infant with chest tubes in place).

Anticipatory teaching about how the infant will appear is important for the family at this stressful time to keep them from growing overwhelmed. Skilled nursing care of both the child and family is essential.

In the first few days after surgery, a major assessment is to observe the infant for respiratory distress. Continue to suction saliva from the mouth as prescribed because this tends to continue to accumulate in the pharynx. Suctioning must be done only shallowly, however, to prevent the suction catheter from touching the suture line in the esophagus. Turning the child frequently discourages fluid from accumulating in the lungs. Humidified oxygen helps to keep respiratory secretions moist and not become stagnant. Keep an infant laryngoscope and endotracheal tube readily available at the bedside in case extreme edema develops, which may increase the infant's risk for airway obstruction.

Nursing Diagnosis: Risk for impaired skin integrity related to gastrostomy tube insertion site

Outcome Evaluation: Skin surrounding gastrostomy tube remains clean, dry, and without erythema.

Gastric secretions, which are highly acidic, can leak onto the skin from the gastrostomy site, leading to skin irritation. Protect the skin by using a cream or commercial skin protection system. If the problem is not easily resolved, consult with a wound, ostomy, and continence therapy nurse to reduce the possibility of skin irritation and infection.

ABDOMINAL WALL DEFECTS

Abdominal wall defects, with the exception of umbilical hernia, are potentially serious disorders because they directly affect the gastrointestinal system and infant nutrition.

Umbilical Hernias

An umbilical hernia is a protrusion of a portion of the intestine through the umbilical ring, muscle, and fascia surrounding the umbilical cord (Mirza & Ali, 2016). This creates a bulging protrusion under the skin at the umbilicus. It is rarely noticeable at birth while the cord is still present but becomes increasingly noticeable at healthcare visits during the first year.

Umbilical hernias occur most frequently in Black children (seen in 30% term infants), low–birth-weight infants, and more often in girls than in boys. The structure is generally 1 to 2 cm (0.5 to 1 in.) in diameter but may be as large as an orange when children cry or strain. The size of the protruding mass is not as important as the size of the fascial ring through which the intestine protrudes. If this fascial ring is less than 2 cm, closure will usually occur spontaneously after the child begins to walk to around 2 years of age, so surgical repair is often not necessary for mild (small) cases. If the fascial ring is larger than 2 cm, ambulatory surgery repair is generally indicated to prevent herniation and intestinal obstruction or bowel strangulation. This is usually done at 1 to 2 years of age. If the small umbilical hernia has not closed by preschool age, a repair will often be done when the child is 4 to 5 years old.

Some parents believe holding an umbilical hernia in place by using "belly bands" or taping a silver dollar over the area will help reduce the hernia. These actions can actually lead to bowel strangulation and so should be avoided.

The child returns from surgery with a dressing, which remains in place until the sutures are well healed. Remind parents to sponge bathe the child until they return for a postoperative visit when the dressing is removed. If the child is not yet toilet trained, caution parents to keep diapers folded well below the dressing to prevent contaminating the suture line with stool.

Omphaloceles

An **omphalocele** is a protrusion (herniation) of abdominal contents through the abdominal wall at the point of the junction of the umbilical cord and abdomen (Fig. 27.12). The herniated organs involved are usually the intestines, but they may include the stomach and liver. Occurring about 1 out of 5,000 live births, the organs are usually covered and contained by a thin transparent layer of amnion and chorion with the

Figure 27.12 An omphalocele with a membrane sac covering the organs.

umbilical cord protruding from the exposed sac. This condition occurs because, at approximately weeks 6 to 8 of intrauterine life, the fetal abdominal contents, which grow faster than the fetal abdomen, are pushed out from the abdomen into the base of the umbilical cord. At 7 to 10 weeks, when the fetal abdomen has enlarged sufficiently, the intestine normally returns to the abdomen. An omphalocele occurs when abdominal contents fail to return in the usual way. In 67% of cases, the occurrence is associated with other congenital disorders such as cardiac, neurologic, genitourinary, skeletal, and chromosomal abnormalities (Tappero & Honeyfield, 2015).

Gastroschisis

Gastroschisis, a term derived from the Greek word for "stomach cleft" or "fissure," is a condition similar to an omphalocele, except the abdominal wall disorder is a distance from the umbilicus, usually to the right, and abdominal organs are not contained by a membrane but rather spill freely from the abdominal wall (Jones, Isenburg, Salemi, et al., 2016). Also, a greater amount of intestinal contents tends to herniate, increasing the potential for volvulus and obstruction. The condition occurs because of failure of the abdominal wall to close, usually during the fourth week of development, and its incidence is about 4 to 5 per 10,000 live births. The disorder is similar to a neural tube defect (covered later in this chapter) because both are a failure to close at about the same gestational time. Children with gastroschisis often have decreased bowel motility and, even after surgical correction, may have difficulty with absorption of nutrients and passage of stool. Long-term follow-up may be necessary to ensure that nutrition and elimination are adequate (Jones et al., 2016).

Assessment

The incidence of omphalocele remains steady, whereas the incidence of gastroschisis is steadily rising, perhaps associated with maternal obesity (Jones et al., 2016). The wall defect with the herniated organs may be identified by sonogram during intrauterine life (Jones et al., 2016). These may also be revealed by an elevated maternal serum α-fetoprotein (MAFP) examination during pregnancy, which is done at the 15th week of pregnancy; the level of MAFP will be abnormally increased if there is an open spinal or abdominal lesion. If the result is elevated, an amniocentesis is then done to assess the level of AFP in amniotic fluid. A prenatal sonogram is also helpful to determine the presence of both abdominal wall or spinal disorders (see Chapter 11 for further discussion of these prenatal assessments). If an omphalocele or gastroschisis is not identified during pregnancy, their presence is obvious on inspection at birth. When an omphalocele or gastroschisis is identified in utero, a cesarean birth may be performed to protect the exposed intestine. If this is the only disorder identified, however, a vaginal birth may be preferred. Be certain to document the general appearance of the defect and its size in centimeters at birth to serve as a baseline assessment. Both conditions can vary greatly in size, from small, where the exposed intestine is the size of a ping-pong ball, to extensive, where all of the abdominal contents are externalized.

Therapeutic Management

With both omphalocele and gastroschisis, until surgery and the bowel is effectively returned to the abdomen, the infant will be fed by TPN to supply nutrients and keep the bowel from filling with air or stool. Most infants with gastroschisis will have surgery within 24 hours to replace the bowel before the blood supply becomes hampered, the intestinal membranes dry, bowel volvulus occurs, or the bowel becomes infected. It is often difficult to replace the entire bowel with immediate surgery because the infant's abdomen, which did not need to grow to accommodate the abdominal contents, is smaller at birth than usual. Replacing the total bowel into this small abdomen could result in respiratory distress from the pressure of the visceral bulk on the diaphragm and lungs. Also, the bowel might not have room for effective peristalsis. If a gastroschisis is small, a one-stage repair may be possible. If large, one surgical approach is the use of a prosthetic patch repair that bridges the unformed gap on the abdomen with a synthetic material; the skin is then drawn tight and closed over the patch. A second approach is to replace only a portion of the bowel at one time. The remainder is contained by a Silastic pouch termed a "silo" that is suspended over the infant's bed. Over the next 5 to 7 days, the bowel is gradually returned to the abdomen by multiple surgical procedures (O'Connell, Dotters-Katz, Kuller, et al., 2016).

For an omphalocele, if the sac is ruptured, the defect is treated like gastroschisis because of the potential for infection. If unruptured, an external dressing producing mild pressure may be used over the intact membrane. This gradually compresses the abdominal contents, allows the skin to stretch between treatments, and does not appear to be a painful procedure.

Nursing Diagnoses and Related Interventions

Both nursing diagnosis and outcomes established for the infant with gastroschisis or an omphalocele, like those with esophageal disorders, must be realistic in terms of the extent of the disorder, the timing of anticipated surgery, and the stage of grief or readiness for decision making and planning the parents have reached. Gastroschisis and omphalocele defects can be an extreme shock to parents because they are conditions that are obviously severe yet also generally unknown.

Nursing Diagnosis: Risk for infection related to exposed abdominal contents

Outcome Evaluation: Child's temperature remains below 98.6°F (37°C) axillary; skin surrounding omphalocele remains clean, dry, and intact, without erythema or foul drainage.

Before surgery, it is important that the lining of the peritoneum covering an omphalocele not be ruptured or allowed to dry and crack; if this happens, infection and malrotation of the uncontained intestine can then occur, thus complicating the surgical repair. Exposure of the intestine to air also causes a rapid loss of body heat. Therefore, be certain not to leave an infant with either gastroschisis or an omphalocele under a radiant heat source in the birthing room because this will quickly dry the exposed bowel. Place the baby in a warmed incubator instead. In both instances, also cover the herniated bowel with either sterile, warm, saline-soaked gauze or a sterile plastic bowel bag until surgery can be scheduled. Because of the large amount of exposed intestinal surface, be certain the saline is at body temperature to prevent lowering the baby's body temperature.

The prognosis for a final successful surgical repair with both these conditions is good (Emil, Canvasser, Chen, et al., 2012). Except for a large abdominal scar, following surgery, the child who had gastroschisis or an omphalocele will be the child originally envisioned by parents. If the size of the scar is a problem for the child in later life, cosmetic surgery can reduce its appearance.

Nursing Diagnosis: Risk for imbalanced nutrition, less than body requirements, related to exposed abdominal contents

Outcome Evaluation: Child's weight remains within 10% of birth weight; skin turgor is good; specific gravity of urine is 1.003 to 1.030.

Infants are maintained on TPN prior to surgery. A nasogastric tube for decompression is inserted at birth to prevent intestinal distention, which would enlarge the bowel lumen and make it even more difficult to replace. Do not feed the infant orally or allow the infant to suck on a pacifier until the bowel repair is complete because doing so would distend the exposed bowel with food or air and would also make its return to the abdomen more difficult. Some infants have an accompanying **volvulus** (a twisting of the bowel causing obstruction), which is another reason to omit oral feedings. After surgery, the infant continues to be maintained on TPN until the final stage of bowel repair is complete, and breastfeedings or formula feedings can be gradually introduced. Assess infants carefully for signs of obstruction such as abdominal distention, constipation, diarrhea, or vomiting when they begin oral feedings to be certain a bowel obstruction or volvulus is not present.

Infants with extensive repairs can be hospitalized for as long as 1 or 2 months until second-stage or even a third-stage operation is complete (an average is about 30 days). Encourage parents to room-in or visit frequently because this is a critical adjustment period for both the infant and parents. Be sure the infant has age-appropriate toys available for stimulation.

Parents may voice frustration because their child's treatment is being done in such small stages. Offer support to help them accept this treatment method as the best way to manage this type of intestinal disorder and to protect the safety and long-term function of the bowel.

QSEN Checkpoint Question 27.4

SAFETY

Maia tells the nurse her baby was born on an unlucky day because the baby born before hers had his bowel outside his body. What is the most important nursing consideration at birth in the care of a baby with gastroschisis?

a. Position the infant on his or her stomach so the intestine is well contained.

b. Wrap the intestines with chilled gauze to prevent intestinal swelling.

c. Keep the infant seated upright under a radiant warmer for warmth.

d. Contain the intestine in a warmed, sterile saline–lined bowel bag.

Look in Appendix A for the best answer and rationale.

Intestinal Obstructions

If canalization of the intestine does not occur in utero at any point, an **atresia** (complete closure) or **stenosis** (narrowing) of the fetal bowel can develop, although the most common site is the duodenum.

Obstruction may also occur because the mesentery of the bowel twisted as the bowel reentered the abdomen after being contained in the base of the umbilical cord early in intrauterine life or from looseness of the intestine in the abdomen after it was returned (Juang & Snyder, 2012). This twisting pattern is termed a *volvulus* and continues to be a potential problem for the first 6 months of life until the infant develops firmer intestinal supports. Yet another reason obstruction can occur is because of thicker-than-usual meconium formation, blocking the lumen (meconium plug or meconium ileus).

Assessment

Intestinal obstruction may be anticipated if the mother had hydramnios during pregnancy (i.e., swallowed amniotic fluid could not be absorbed effectively by the fetus) or if more than 30 ml of stomach contents can be aspirated from the newborn stomach by catheter and syringe at birth (fluid is not passing freely through the tract). If the obstruction is not revealed by either of these findings, then symptoms of intestinal obstruction in the neonate are the same as at any other time in life: The infant passes no meconium or may pass one stool (meconium that formed below the obstruction) and then not pass any more; the abdomen becomes distended and tender. As the effect of the obstruction progresses, the infant will vomit. Remember, many neonates spit up feedings when burped. This rapid ejection of milk smells barely sour. True vomiting from intestinal obstruction is usually sour smelling (stomach acid has acted on it), includes bile, and occurs spontaneously without coughing or back patting. Vomitus may also be black from the color of meconium.

Bowel sounds will begin to increase in number as the bowel increases peristaltic action in an effort to push stool past the point of obstruction. Waves of peristalsis may be observable across the abdomen. The infant may reveal that abdominal pain is developing by crying—hard, forceful, indignant crying—and by pulling the legs up against the abdomen. Lastly, the child's respiratory rate will increase as the intestine fills, the diaphragm is pushed up harder and harder against the lungs, and lung capacity decreases. An abdominal X-ray, sonogram, MRI, or barium enema will reveal no air below the level of obstruction in the intestine or isolate the level of the obstruction.

Therapeutic Management

As soon as a bowel obstruction is confirmed, an orogastric or nasogastric tube is inserted and then attached to low suction or left open to the air to prevent further gastrointestinal distention (see Chapter 37). Always use low intermittent suction with decompression tubes in neonates because pressure greater than this can irritate and ulcerate their sensitive stomach lining.

IV therapy is begun to restore fluid and electrolyte balance; immediate surgery is scheduled to relieve the obstruction before pressure on the bowel causes death of the involved intestinal lining (Sundaram, Hoffenberg, Kramer, et al., 2012).

Repair of the obstruction (with the exception of meconium plug syndrome) can usually be accomplished by laparoscopy, although full abdominal surgery may be necessary.

The area of stenosis or atresia is removed, and the bowel is anastomosed. If the repair is anatomically difficult or the infant has other anomalies that interfere with overall health, a temporary colostomy may have to be constructed, and the infant discharged to home care with follow-up surgery rescheduled at 3 to 6 months of age (see Chapter 37 for care of a child with a colostomy). If a large portion of the bowel has to be removed, this can have an impact on nutrient absorption (called short bowel syndrome) as the child grows older.

Nursing Diagnoses and Related Interventions

Nursing Diagnosis: Risk for deficient fluid volume related to vomiting

Outcome Evaluation: Child's skin turgor is good; capillary refill is 1 to 2 seconds; pulse rate is at least 100 to 120 beats/min; no further vomiting occurs; urine output is at least 1 to 2 ml/kg/hour.

Once an obstruction is suspected, keep an infant NPO to prevent the bowel from filling and causing vomiting and aspiration. Vomiting is always serious in neonates not only because aspiration may occur but also because infants can become dehydrated rapidly. They also lose chloride (a component of the hydrochloric acid found in stomach contents), which then leads to metabolic alkalosis. As a way of compensating for the loss of chloride, the baby's kidneys excrete potassium, which can cause infants to become hypokalemic. Keeping an infant NPO, restoring fluid by IV therapy, and monitoring laboratory values for electrolyte balance until surgery, therefore, are crucial actions to prevent all these events. Following surgery, TPN or IV fluid will be continued until bowel sounds return; after a short postoperative course, assuming no other bowel condition such as short bowel syndrome is present, an infant should have no further problems.

Meconium Plug Syndrome

A **meconium plug** is an extremely hard portion of meconium that has completely blocked the intestinal lumen, causing bowel obstruction. The cause is unknown but probably reflects normal variations of meconium consistency. Meconium plugs usually form in the lower end of the bowel because this meconium formed early in intrauterine life and has the best chance to become dry and obstructive. The condition is associated with Hirschsprung disease, cystic fibrosis, hypothyroidism, and magnesium sulfate administration to halt preterm labor (Cuenca, Ali, Kays, et al., 2012).

Assessment

Because the obstruction is low in the intestinal tract, signs of obstruction such as abdominal distention and vomiting may not occur for at least 24 hours. Typically, the infant will be identified first as an infant who has had no meconium passage in the first 24 hours postbirth. A gentle rectal examination may reveal the presence of hardened stool, although the plug may be too high up in the bowel to be palpated. An X-ray or sonogram may reveal distended air-filled loops of bowel up to the point of obstruction. A barium enema not only reveals the level of obstruction but also may be therapeutic in loosening the plug.

Therapeutic Management

A subset of patients experiences spontaneous resolution of the meconium plug without any treatment. Of the 70% of patients requiring treatment, contrast or saline barium enema was used, with 97% success (Cuenca et al., 2012). The administration of a small (about 5 ml) saline enema (never use tap water in newborns, infants, and young children because it can lead to water intoxication) may cause enough peristalsis to expel the plug. Instillation of acetylcysteine (Mucomyst) rectally may be prescribed to soften stool. Gastrografin, a highly osmotic radiographic substance, administered as an enema, is yet another solution. Because it is hyperosmotic, the substance pulls fluid into the bowel, allowing the stool to soften and the plug to pass. Assess that the infant is well hydrated before and after the procedure because an infant can become hypovolemic from the effect of such a strong-acting medium.

Once the thickened portion of meconium has been passed, the infant should have no further difficulty and, over the next several hours, may pass a great amount of stool. Postprocedure prognosis is very good. Observe the infant for further passage of meconium (which should occur at least once daily) over the next 3 days, however, to be certain additional plugs do not exist farther up in the bowel. If an infant is going to be discharged before this time, instruct parents on the importance of observing for meconium and also about phoning their primary care provider should the infant have no further bowel movements while at home.

Occasionally, a neonate passes a small plug of hardened meconium—hard enough it would have caused an obstruction except it is so small—in the first 1 or 2 days of life. Be certain to record and report such a finding because the infant will need close observation for continued defecation, the same as for the infant who actually had an obstruction, to be certain there is not a larger and truly obstructing plug higher in the bowel.

Assess the family history of a newborn who has a meconium plug for cystic fibrosis, a recessively inherited disorder (see Chapter 40), aganglionic megacolon (Hirschsprung disease), or a polygenic inherited disorder (see Chapter 45) because, if there is a family history, the infant will need observation for these disorders. Hypothyroidism can also present with constipation or hardened stool in newborns along with signs such as a large protruding tongue, lethargy, and subnormal body temperature. Both hypothyroidism and cystic fibrosis screening are done along with phenylketonuria screening in newborns. Be certain this blood test is obtained in any newborn with a meconium plug (Levy, 2010). Infants born at home, especially, may not have had this done.

Meconium Ileus

Meconium ileus (obstruction of the intestinal lumen by hardened meconium) is a specific phenomenon that occurs almost exclusively in infants with cystic fibrosis, resulting from the abnormal pancreatic enzyme function seen with cystic fibrosis (see Chapter 40) and reflects extreme meconium plugging (Tappero & Honeyfield, 2015). The usual symptoms of bowel obstruction occur: no meconium passage, abdominal distention, and vomiting of bile-stained fluid. Meconium ileus is the only bowel obstruction that can present with abdominal distention at birth (Tappero & Honeyfield, 2015). Unlike simple meconium plugging, the obstruction point may be too high in the intestine for enemas to reduce it; instead, the bowel must be incised and the hardened meconium removed by laparotomy. Meconium ileus is so strongly associated with cystic fibrosis, the infant needs close follow-up by an interprofessional cystic fibrosis team in the following months.

What If . . . 27.2

On the second day of life you notice Maia Sparrow's baby, who was born with meconium staining, is spitting up green mucus. Would it be safe to assume this is just more meconium-stained mucus? Should the nurse consider the baby might be vomiting bile-stained vomitus?

Diaphragmatic Hernias

A diaphragmatic hernia is a weakness in the musculature that permits a portion of the abdominal organs, such as the stomach or intestine, to protrude through the chest wall. This can cause a collapse of the left lung due to cardiac displacement on the right side of the chest. It occurs in 1 to 5 per 10,000 live births, with slight increased frequency in boys and a decreased frequency in Blacks (Oluyomi-Obi, Kuret, Puligandla, et al., 2017).

The defect is caused because, early in intrauterine life, the chest and abdominal cavity are one; at approximately week 8 of intrauterine growth, the diaphragm forms and divides them. If the diaphragm does not form completely, the intestines can herniate through the diaphragm opening into the chest cavity as a diaphragmatic hernia (Fig. 27.13).

Assessment

Diaphragmatic hernia is frequently detected in utero by routine sonogram (Oluyomi-Obi et al., 2017). If not, it is apparent at birth when the newborn has extreme difficulty establishing effective respirations. It can also be indicated by a scaphoid (sunken) abdomen caused by the displacement of

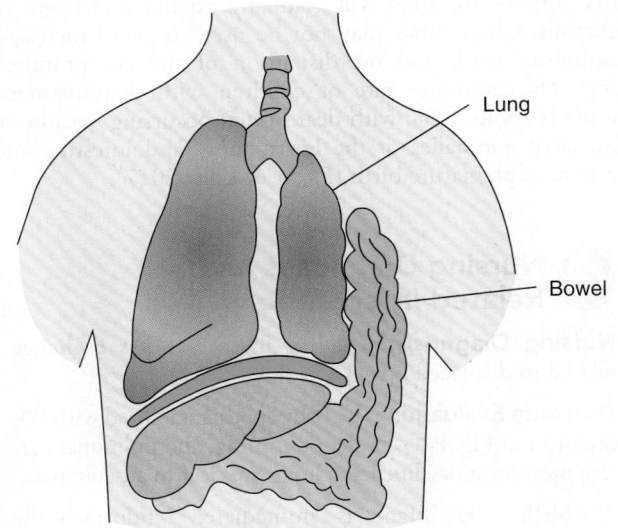

Figure 27.13 A diaphragmatic hernia. The bowel loop in the chest compresses the heart and lung on that side.

abdominal contents into the chest (Tappero & Honeyfield, 2015). Surgeons have tried fetal surgery to correct or lessen the lung compromise from this diagnosis, but multiple randomized trials comparing prenatal surgical intervention to postnatal intervention show no benefit to prenatal intervention (Hedrick, 2013).

At birth, breath sounds are usually absent on the affected side of the chest cavity because at least one of the lobes of the lungs on that side cannot expand completely (and may not have fully formed). The infant may be cyanotic with intercostal or subcostal retractions. The abdomen generally appears sunken because it is not as filled with intestine as usual. These infants have a potential for developing persistent pulmonary hypertension because blood cannot perfuse readily through the unexpanded lung. This can lead to right-to-left shunting through the foramen ovale in the heart and also causes the ductus arteriosus to remain patent. One condition, then, has led to another until heart involvement complicates an already serious lung picture. The mechanics of right-to-left heart shunts are further discussed in Chapter 41.

Therapeutic Management

Although surgical repair may be done as an imminent surgical procedure, it is usually delayed until cardiorespiratory status has been stabilized as much as possible and the baby can be transported to a high-acuity nursery for care. Surgery includes repair of the diaphragm and replacement of the herniated intestine and organs back into the abdomen, possibly requiring both thoracic and abdominal incisions. If the disorder of the diaphragm is large, an insoluble polymer (Teflon) patch may be used to reconstruct a better diaphragm shape.

The repair can be complicated if there is not enough room in the abdomen for the intestine to be returned. In these infants, the abdominal incision may not be closed. The intestine is covered by silicone elastomer (Silastic) and left to be closed at a later date after the abdomen has grown, the same as gastroschisis surgery.

If the lung that was compressed in utero is truly hypoplastic and so cannot function, it will be removed at the time of surgery. If it is developed but just deflated, over the next week after surgery, the lung will gradually expand and begin to function. Chest tubes may not be used to avoid increased respiratory work and overdistention of the compromised lung. The mortality rate of children with diaphragmatic hernia is about 40%, with death often occurring because of associated anomalies of the heart, lung, and intestine and because of premature birth (Kadir & Lilja, 2017).

Nursing Diagnoses and Related Interventions

Nursing Diagnosis: Risk for ineffective gas exchange related to displaced bowel

Outcome Evaluation: The baby appears stabilized with PO_2 over 40 mmHg, PCO_2 under 60 mmHg, and pulmonary artery pressure at baseline level; lungs are clear to auscultation.

At birth, the infant is immediately endotracheally intubated and then gently ventilated with low-pressure, high-frequency, low-intensity oxygen to aid breathing.

A nasogastric tube or a gastrostomy tube will be inserted to prevent the distention of the herniated intestine and to avoid further respiratory difficulty. Keep the infant NPO to prevent the bowel from filling and becoming distended. Be certain the suction is attached to only low intermittent suction to avoid injuring the lining of the newborn's stomach.

While they wait for surgery, infants breathe better if they are turned on their side with the compressed lung down and their head elevated because this allows the herniated intestine to fall back as far as possible into the abdomen and allows the unaffected lung to expand more completely.

Following surgery, maintain the infant in a head elevated position to keep the pressure of the replaced intestine off the repaired diaphragm. Suction the airway as necessary and keep the infant in a warmed, humidified environment to encourage lung fluid drainage from the now uncompromised lungs. Chest physiotherapy may be prescribed to ensure lung secretions do not pool and cause pneumonia. Positive-pressure ventilation may be ordered to increase lung expansion, although this pressure is kept to a minimum to prevent tearing the undeveloped or previously unopened lung tissue. Maintaining arterial oxygen (PO_2) at a lower level of 60 mmHg and permitting PCO_2 to rise to a higher level of up to 60 mmHg may help prevent damage to the immature lung, thereby improving lung function (O'Rourke-Potocki, Ali, Murthy, et al., 2016). In addition, inhaled nitric oxide, or extracorporeal membrane oxygenation (ECMO) may be used as other ways to aid respirations and increase oxygenation.

Nursing Diagnosis: Risk for imbalanced nutrition, less than body requirements, related to NPO status

Outcome Evaluation: Child's skin turgor remains good; weight is maintained within 10% of birth weight or between a percentile curve on growth chart.

After surgery, to prevent pressure on the suture line in the diaphragm by a full stomach and bowel, nutrition will be supplied with TPN. When oral feedings are started, be certain to burp the infant frequently during and after feedings to reduce the amount of swallowed air and limit bowel pressure against the diaphragm.

QSEN Checkpoint Question 27.5

QUALITY IMPROVEMENT

The nurse positions Mia's baby on his side to keep pressure off his back. She asks why the nurse isn't positioning a baby with diaphragmatic hernia in the same way. Before surgery, what would be the best position for a newborn with left-sided diaphragmatic hernia?

   a. On his left side to support his left lung
   b. On his stomach with his head turned sideways
   c. On his left side elevated in an infant chair
   d. On his right side so his left lung can expand

Look in Appendix A for the best answer and rationale.

Figure 27.14   An imperforate anus. The lower bowel ends in a blind pouch.

An Imperforate Anus

An imperforate anus (Fig. 27.14) is a stricture or the absence of the anus (Gourlay, 2013). In week 7 of intrauterine life, the upper bowel elongates to pouch and combine with a pouch invaginating from the perineum. These two sections of bowel meet, the membranes between them are absorbed, and the bowel is then patent to the outside. If this motion toward each other does not occur or if the membrane between the two surfaces does not dissolve, an imperforate anus occurs. The disorder can be relatively minor, requiring just surgical incision of the persistent membrane, or much more severe, involving sections of the bowel that are many inches apart with no anus. There may be an accompanying fistula to the bladder in boys and to the vagina in girls (retrovaginal fistula), further complicating a surgical repair. The problem occurs in approximately 1 in 5,000 live births, more commonly in boys than in girls. It may occur as an additional complication of spinal cord disorders because both the external anal canal and the spinal cord arise from the same germ tissue layer.

Assessment

The condition may be detected by a prenatal sonogram. It is discovered at birth when inspection of a newborn's anal region reveals no anus, a membrane filled with black meconium protrudes from the anus, or if it is impossible to insert a rubber catheter into the rectum. A "wink" reflex (touching the skin near the rectum should make the anus contract) cannot be elicited if sensory nerve endings in the rectum are not intact. Even with all these methods, some instances of the stricture will not be detected at birth because the anus appears as usual, and the stricture exists so far inside that it can't be seen. By 24 hours, no stool will be passed, and abdominal distention will become evident. An X-ray or sonogram will reveal the disorder if the infant is held in a slightly head-down position to allow swallowed air to rise to the end of the blind pouch of the bowel. This method is also helpful to estimate the distance the intestine is separated from the perineum or the extent of the correction that will be necessary.

Because newborns are discharged at 2 or 3 days or even a few hours after birth, it's important that follow-up care by parents includes an assessment of whether the infant is defecating. If not, they may be asked to collect a urine specimen so it can be examined for the presence of meconium to help determine whether the infant has a rectal–bladder fistula. Placing a urine collector bag over the vagina in girls may reveal a meconium-stained discharge or that a rectovaginal fistula is present.

Therapeutic Management

The degree of difficulty in repairing an imperforate anus depends on the extent of the problem. If the rectum ends close to the perineum (at or below the level of the levator ani muscle) and the anal sphincter is formed, repair involves simple laparoscopy with anastomosis of the separated bowel segments (Nam, Kim, & Kim, 2016). A repair becomes complicated if the end of the rectum is at a distance from the perineum (above the levator ani muscle), the anal sphincter exists only in an underdeveloped form, or a fistula to the bladder or vagina is present. If the repair is estimated to be extensive, the child may be given a temporary colostomy, and the final repair performed when the infant is somewhat older (6 to 12 months).

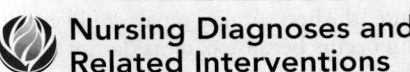

Nursing Diagnoses and Related Interventions

Nursing Diagnosis: Imbalanced nutrition, less than body requirements, related to bowel obstruction and inability to take in oral fluid

Outcome Evaluation: Child's weight remains within 10% of birth weight or is maintained on a percentile curve on a growth chart; skin turgor is good; urine output is 1 to 2 ml/kg/hour.

Preoperative Care. Before surgery, keep the infant NPO to avoid further bowel distention. A nasogastric tube attached to low intermittent suction for decompression will be inserted to relieve vomiting and prevent pressure on other abdominal organs or the diaphragm from the distended intestine. IV therapy or TPN will be started to maintain fluid and electrolyte balance.

Postoperative Care. The newborn will return from surgery with the nasogastric tube still in place. When bowel sounds can be heard so the nasogastric tube can be removed, small oral feedings of glucose water, formula, or breast milk can be started.

Infants who are scheduled for repair in a second-stage operation and who have a temporary colostomy are not permitted high-residue foods to lessen the bulk of stools. Although this is rarely a problem with infants because their diet naturally is a low-residue one, do not assume parents know what low residue means. Examples include rice cereal and strained fruits and vegetables. They should avoid unrefined rice and grains, vegetables with fibers, or fruits with peels.

Nursing Diagnosis: Impaired tissue integrity at rectum related to surgical incision

Outcome Evaluation: Incision line remains free of erythema or drainage until it heals by about day 7 after surgery.

If a rectal repair was completed, remember there is a fresh suture line at the rectum. Take axillary or tympanic temperatures rather than rectal temperatures to avoid loosening a suture. The infant also should have no enemas, suppositories, or any other intrusive rectal procedures (it might be helpful to hang a sign above the infant's crib cautioning against these). Infants may be prescribed a stool softener daily to keep stool from becoming hard and tearing the healing suture line. Placing a diaper under, not on, the infant may be helpful so bowel movements can be cleansed away as soon as they occur. Clean the suture line well after each bowel movement by irrigating it with normal saline or other prescribed solution to help guard against infections. Do not place the infant on the abdomen because, in this position, newborns tend to pull their knees under them, causing tension in the perineal area and the suture line. A side-lying or supine position is best.

Some infants may need rectal dilatation done once or twice a day for a few months after surgery to ensure proper patency of the rectal sphincter. Review this technique (gently inserting a lubricated cot-covered finger into the rectum) with the parents and document they are able to perform this procedure before the child is discharged from the hospital. Be certain they also understand the importance of the procedure (the best surgical repair could end in failure if constriction occurs because parents do not follow up with this procedure). If infants are to be discharged with a prescription for a daily stool softener, be certain parents understand how important it is to give this and have a plan for remembering the correct times and dosage.

Nursing Diagnosis: Risk for impaired parenting related to difficulty in bonding with infant ill from birth

Outcome Evaluation: Parents hold and comfort infant; and describe positive characteristics of infant.

An imperforate anus may be a difficult anomaly for a parent to accept because it deals with a body area that they may not feel comfortable discussing. If it involves a temporary (or permanent) colostomy, learning to care for their infant can be difficult. For these reasons, parents need a great deal of support following the diagnosis. If a final surgical repair can be completed, they can be assured their child will have relatively normal bowel function thereafter. If a final repair could not be surgically achieved, they have the task of caring for a child with a permanent ostomy. You can assure them children who always have ostomies accept these well as they grow older because they have never known any other method of defecation (see Chapter 37 for a discussion of care priorities for the child with an ostomy).

Physical and Developmental Disorders of the Nervous System

The most common developmental disorders of the nervous system at birth include abnormal accumulation of cerebrospinal fluid (CSF) (hydrocephalus), which has several causes, and abnormalities associated with neural tube closure (meningocele or meningomyelocele).

HYDROCEPHALUS

CSF is formed in the first and second ventricles of the brain and then passes through the aqueduct of Sylvius and the fourth ventricle to empty into the subarachnoid space of the spinal cord, where it is absorbed. **Hydrocephalus** is the accumulation of an excess amount of CSF in the ventricles or the subarachnoid space (Tappero & Honeyfield, 2015). Hydrocephalus is thought to result from aqueductal stenosis and blockage of the CSF outflow from the fourth ventricle (Tappero & Honeyfield, 2015). Because cranial sutures are not firmly knitted in infants, the pressure of this excess fluid causes enlargement of their skull. If fluid is able to reach the spinal cord, the disorder is called a communicating or extraventricular hydrocephalus. If there is a block to CSF so it cannot circulate into the subarachnoid space, the disorder is termed obstructive or intraventricular hydrocephalus.

Hydrocephalus can occur at birth (congenital) or) from an incident later in life (acquired). Although the increased fluid may occur in isolation, 90% of babies with congenital hydrocephalus have a diagnosis of meningomyelocele (discussed in the following paragraphs) (Sinha, Dhua, Mathur, et al., 2012). A preterm infant, less than 24 weeks gestation, may have acquired hydrocephalus from an intraventricular hemorrhage. The degree of blockage is directly related to the quantity of intraventricular blood, which blocks the passage of CSF (Oliveira, Teixeira, Norremose, et al., 2015).

Three main reasons explain why CSF accumulates:
- Overproduction of fluid by the choroid plexus in the first or second ventricle as could occur from a growing tumor (rare).
- Obstruction of the passage of fluid in the narrow aqueduct of Sylvius (the most common cause) or the foramina of Magendie and Luschka, the openings that allow fluid to leave the fourth ventricle: Hemorrhage from trauma, a growing tumor, or infections such as toxoplasmosis, meningitis, or encephalitis may leave adhesions behind that block fluid flow at these points. Arnold–Chiari disorder (elongation of the lower brain stem and displacement of the fourth ventricle into the upper cervical canal) or a Dandy–Walker cyst (a fluid-filled sack by one of the ventricles in the brain) are still other causes (Tappero & Honeyfield, 2015).
- Interference with the absorption of CSF from the subarachnoid space if a portion of the subarachnoid membrane has been removed, as occurs with surgery for a meningocele or after extensive subarachnoid hemorrhage, when portions of the membrane absorption surface become obscured.

Assessment

With an obstruction present, excessive fluid accumulates and dilates the system forward of the point of obstruction. If the atresia is in the aqueduct of Sylvius, the first, second, and third ventricles will dilate. If it is at the exit from the fourth ventricle, all ventricles will dilate. Symptoms may develop rapidly or slowly depending on the extent of the atresia.

Hydrocephalus detected in utero through a prenatal sonogram may be shunted prior to birth, particularly if it is associated with a meningomyelocele (Moldenhauer, 2014). Although the condition occurs in approximately 3 to 4 out of 1,000 live births, it is only overtly evident during pregnancy or at birth in 15% of newborns with the disorder because intrauterine pressure prohibits skull expansion (Sinha et al., 2012). During the first few weeks of life, the infant's fontanelles widen and appear tense, the suture lines on the skull separate, and the head diameter enlarges. As the fluid accumulation continues, the scalp becomes shiny and scalp veins become prominent. The brow bulges forward (bossing), and the eyes become "sunset eyes" (the sclera shows above the iris because of upper lid retraction). Infants begin to show symptoms of increased intracranial pressure, such as decreased pulse and respirations, increased temperature and blood pressure, hyperactive reflexes, strabismus, and optic atrophy. They may become either irritable or lethargic with a typical shrill, high-pitched cry (Box 27.4). When a patient is suspected to have hydrocephalus, neurologic, neurosurgical, urologic, and orthopedic consultations should be considered to rule out any comorbid conditions (Tappero & Honeyfield, 2015).

Treatment is most effective when the disorder is recognized early because once intracranial pressure becomes so acute that brain tissue is damaged and motor or mental deterioration results, even the best shunting procedure cannot replace and repair this damage to brain cells. To best detect hydrocephalus, measure the head circumference of all newborns within an hour of birth and again before discharge from the healthcare facility to establish a baseline. All children younger than 2 years of age should then have their head circumference recorded and plotted on an appropriate growth chart at all healthcare visits so the child whose head is growing abnormally can be detected (Scheffler, Greil, & Hermanussen, 2017).

Because it is possible for infants to develop hydrocephalus following head trauma, all infants who have suffered head trauma severe enough to be seen in a medical facility should have their head circumference noted at the time of the accident so, if other symptoms of increased intracranial pressure appear, this head circumference measurement can be a meaningful part of the store of information available concerning the child's condition (Scheffler et al., 2017).

In addition to the general enlargement of the head, note any asymmetry that is occurring because this may suggest the point of obstruction. A skull that is enlarging anteriorly with a shallow posterior fossa, for example, suggests the obstruction is in the aqueduct or third ventricle.

As the head continues to enlarge, the infant's motor function becomes impaired because of both neurologic impairment and atrophy caused by the inability to move such a heavy head. However, as long as a child has more than 1 cm of cerebral tissue present, motor function often is not impaired. Even with an extremely enlarged head, therefore, children's intelligence may also remain normal, although fine motor development may be affected.

Hydrocephalus can be demonstrated by ultrasound, computed tomography (CT), or MRI. A skull X-ray film will reveal the separating sutures and thinning of the skull. **Transillumination** (holding a bright light such as a flashlight or a specialized light [a Chun gun] against the skull with the child in a darkened room) will reveal that the skull is filled with fluid rather than solid brain tissue (Fig. 27.15). Assessing ventricular pressure will document the increased tension and presence of additional fluid.

Therapeutic Management

The treatment for hydrocephalus depends on its cause and extent. If it is caused by overproduction of fluid, acetazolamide (Diamox), a diuretic, may be prescribed to promote the excretion of this excess fluid. Destruction of a portion of the choroid plexus may be attempted by ventricular endoscopy; if a tumor in that area is responsible for

---

BOX 27.4

Nursing Care Planning Using Assessment

ASSESSING AN INFANT WITH HYDROCEPHALUS

- Enlarged fontanelles
- "Bossing" of forehead
- "Sunset" eyes
- Separated suture line
- Prominent scalp veins
- Increased head circumference
- Lethargy or irritability
- Shrill cry
- Signs of increased cranial pressure
  - ↓ pulse
  - ↑ temperature
  - ↓ respirations
  - ↑ blood pressure
- Hyperactive reflexes

Figure 27.15 An infant with a hydrocephalus. Transillumination reveals a fluid-filled skull. (© Southern Illinois University/Photo Researchers, Inc.)

the overproduction of fluid, removal of the tumor should provide a solution. Hydrocephalus is usually caused by obstruction, however, so the treatment for children that do not have other neural tube involvement (such as a meningomyelocele) usually involves laser surgery to reopen the route of flow or bypassing the point of obstruction by shunting the fluid to another point of absorption. As more and more obstructions in the third or fourth ventricles are relieved by endoscopy, the next generation of children with isolated hydrocephalus may not need artificial shunting. Children today with hydrocephalus occurring with a meningomyelocele may still undergo a shunting procedure, however, and you may care for many older children or adults who have shunts in place.

A shunting procedure involves threading a thin polyethylene catheter under the skin from the ventricles to the peritoneum (a ventriculoperitoneal shunt) (Fig. 27.16). Fluid drains by this route into the peritoneum, where it is absorbed across the peritoneal membrane into the body circulation. The shunt usually has to be replaced as the child grows or it will become too short. As another complication, it could become enclosed in a fold of peritoneum and become obstructed or it could become infected.

The ultimate prognosis for a child with hydrocephalus depends on whether brain damage occurred before shunting, whether the child develops a cerebral infection, and whether the parents can accept and recognize when a shunt needs to be replaced to prevent increased intracranial pressure (Box 27.5). Referral early in infancy for intervention services and screening is warranted to assess the infant's speech, fine, and gross motor milestones and detect any delays.

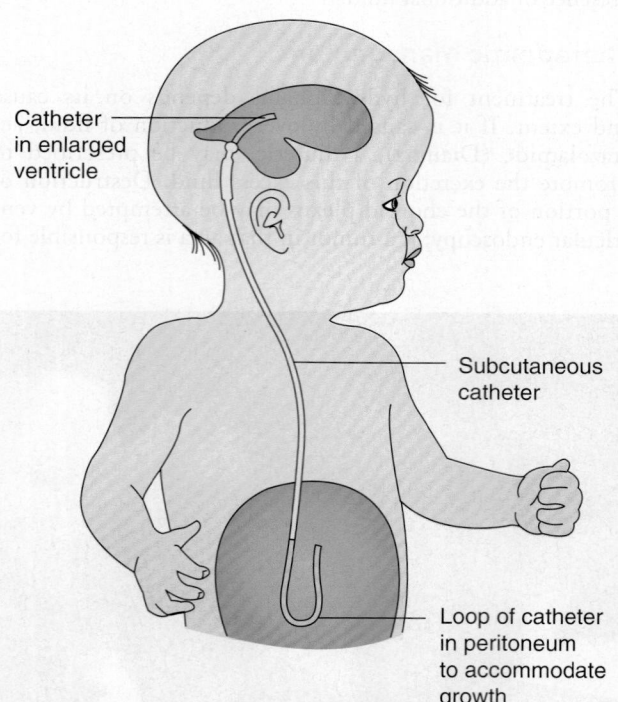

Figure 27.16 A ventriculoperitoneal shunt removes excessive cerebrospinal fluid from the ventricles and shunts it to the peritoneum. A one-way valve is present in the tubing behind the ear.

- Catheter in enlarged ventricle
- Subcutaneous catheter
- Loop of catheter in peritoneum to accommodate growth

BOX 27.5
Nursing Care Planning Tips for Effective Communication

Maia's baby is scheduled to have a ventriculoperitoneal shunt inserted this afternoon. You talk to Maia before surgery.

Tip: Offer quick reassurance alleviates a parent's concern. Better listening can also help reveal the true problem. Because surgical procedures are so safe today and the results of surgery for newborns are so successful, it is easy to begin to think of surgery as more inconvenient than serious. To a parent, however, the difference between a child born with one of these conditions and the "perfect" child the parent envisioned can be significant.

Nurse: Is there anything I can explain to you about your son's surgery, Ms. Sparrow?

Ms. Sparrow: No. I just want to see him back here with a smaller head.

Nurse: The shunt won't actually make his head smaller. Its purpose is to keep his head from growing any larger.

Ms. Sparrow: What is the chance he'll die in surgery?

Nurse: All surgery has a risk, certainly, but he should do well.

Ms. Sparrow: But there is a chance he'll die in surgery?

Nurse: You sound more worried than I'd expect. Is there something specific you're worried about?

Ms. Sparrow: I wouldn't feel bad if he died in surgery. I mean, how am I going to take care of a child with a tube in his head?

Nurse: Let's sit down and talk about this some more.

Nursing Diagnoses and Related Interventions

Nutrition and parent–child bonding are two major concerns for the infant with hydrocephalus. Box 27.6 shows an interprofessional care map illustrating both nursing and team planning for an infant with the concern.

Nursing Diagnosis: Risk for ineffective cerebral tissue perfusion related to increased intracranial pressure

Outcome Evaluation: Child shows no increased temperature or blood pressure, decreased pulse or respiratory rate or level of consciousness; PERLA (*p*upils *e*qual and *r*eactive to *l*ight and *a*ccommodation) is present; muscle strength is equal and strong bilaterally; head circumference is maintained at age-appropriate level.

Following the surgery for the initial shunt insertion, infants may have three incisions: one just behind the ear, one in the neck (done to help thread the catheter), and one in the abdomen where the end of the shunt is embedded. Their bed should be left flat or raised only about 10 degrees so their head remains level with the body so CSF does not flow too rapidly, possibly leading to tearing of cerebral arteries or signs of too rapid decompression.

BOX 27.6

Nursing Care Planning

AN INTERPROFESSIONAL CARE MAP FOR A CHILD WITH HYDROCEPHALUS

At 1 month of age, Maia's baby, still not named, has a ventriculoperitoneal shunt inserted for developing hydrocephalus.

Family Assessment: Child lives with 16-year-old mother, her parents, and four of mother's siblings. Child's father works as motorcycle mechanic; visits infant frequently. Mother no longer attending school because of child care. Mother asking many questions about the surgery. "This'll fix everything, right? I want a healthy baby."

Patient Assessment: One-month-old infant whose head circumference has continued to increase since meningomyelocele surgery at birth. Head circumference at birth was at 40th percentile, now is at 60th percentile. Mother noted infant has had increasing irritability and difficulty swallowing formula over the last few weeks.

Anterior fontanelle 4 × 4 cm; posterior fontanelle 3 × 1 cm. Sagittal suture line separated 0.25 in. Scalp veins prominent. No upward gaze. Parents report two episodes of forceful vomiting yesterday. Also, "His cry is so high pitched it hurts your ears." Cerebral perfusion pressure, 55 mmHg. Blood pressure, 100/40 mmHg; pulse, 100 beats/min; respirations, 16 breaths/min. Afebrile.

Nursing Diagnosis: Risk for ineffective cerebral tissue perfusion related to increased intracranial pressure from hydrocephalus

Outcome Criteria: Infant's vital signs are within age-appropriate parameters; head circumference is maintained at current level; infant responds to auditory stimuli; cerebral perfusion pressure remains above 50 mmHg.

Team Member Responsible	Assessment	Intervention	Rationale	Expected Outcome
Activities of Daily Living, Including Safety				
Nurse	Assess if infant is able to turn freely because of increased head size.	Provide an environment for child that is stimulating yet not tiring (e.g., mobile, soft toys). Urge parent to interact with child.	Lack of mobility can lead to pressure ulcers on head as well as insufficient 1-month development.	Child's parent plays with and feeds infant. Infant appears interested in age-appropriate toys. No irritated areas present on head.
Teamwork and Collaboration				
Nurse/primary healthcare provider	Assess if neurosurgeon is available to answer mother's questions.	Arrange for consultation for mother with neurosurgeon to discuss surgery and child's prognosis.	Viewing a child as totally disabled can cause a parent to not appreciate the child's capabilities.	Neurosurgeon meets with mother to discuss that child's IQ appears normal and that shunting will halt head growth.
Procedures/Medications for Quality Improvement				
Nurse	Assess infant's neurologic status postoperatively, including response to sound, pupillary response, increasing irritability, or lethargy.	Position infant with head of bed slightly elevated; prevent flexion, hyperextension, or rotation of the head. Record cerebral perfusion pressure as prescribed.	Elevating head of bed aids shunt functioning, helping to reduce intracranial pressure. Cerebral perfusion pressure reveals the extent of intracranial pressure.	Child's cerebral perfusion pressure remains greater than established parameter. Infant responds to sound; with no increasing irritability or lethargy.
Nurse	Assess head circumference and anterior fontanelle for tenseness every 4 hours as prescribed.	Document head circumference and appearance of anterior fontanelle.	A tense, bulging fontanelle or increasing head circumference indicates accumulating cerebrospinal fluid (CSF).	Child's head circumference does not increase in size; fontanelles no longer feel tense.

Continued on following page

BOX 27.6

Nursing Care Planning (continued)

Team Member Responsible	Assessment	Intervention	Rationale	Expected Outcome
Nutrition				
Nurse/nutritionist	Observe mother feeding the infant.	Assist mother with positioning as necessary and avoid flexion or hyperextension of head during feeding.	Proper positioning is important to avoid pressure on the shunt, which could increase intracranial pressure.	Mother states she is comfortable feeding infant following surgery.
Nurse	Monitor intake and output closely.	Administer osmotic diuretic and corticosteroids as prescribed.	Adequate hydration is necessary to ensure renal function. Osmotic diuretics decrease intracranial pressure. Corticosteroids reduce inflammation.	Child's output remains over set parameter. Diuretic and corticosteroids are administered as necessary.
Patient-Centered Care				
Nurse/nurse practitioner	Assess the parents' understanding of a hydrocephalus and treatment measures.	Review the structure and function of the brain and explain how a hydrocephalus develops. Clarify any misconceptions.	Reviewing and clarifying aid in learning and strengthen understanding.	Mother states she understands the purpose of the shunt to relieve excess CSF.
Psychosocial/Spiritual/Emotional Needs				
Nurse/nurse practitioner	Assess mother's acceptance of child in light of congenital disorders and no name for baby as yet.	Observe mother's interaction with infant and remind her that congenital disorders occur in a proportion of all births for unknown reasons.	Young mother may have had little experience with life crises; needs support from healthcare providers to master this crisis.	Mother states she understands child's condition is neither hers nor the child's fault and states she will be able to work through the present crisis.
Informatics for Seamless Healthcare Planning				
Nurse	Assess if child's parents have adequate psychological support from family members or questions about care child will need for shunt care. Explore why child has not been named as yet.	Review care of child and assure parents healthcare providers can be contacted any time if they have questions. Establish a convenient follow-up care appointment.	In crisis situations, parents may need additional support to continue care of child and form a strong parent–infant bond. Positive reinforcement enhances self-esteem and aids in coping.	Mother states the grandmother is supportive. Together, they understand future care necessary and will contact primary care provider for any questions. Mother keeps postsurgery appointment and states she has plans to name the child.
Nurse	Assess if parent would like home care follow-up.	Make referral for home care if needed. Also, refer parents to support group of other parents of children with hydrocephalus.	Support groups can decrease feelings of isolation and provide opportunities for further learning. Follow-up home care provides continuing support, guidance, and education.	Mother and grandmother state they will attend a support group at least once to evaluate benefit for them. Agree to at least one home visit for follow-up care.

A one-way valve, which is inserted into the shunt and can be palpated just behind the ear, opens when CSF has accumulated to the extent cerebral pressure has increased. It closes when enough fluid has drained to reduce the pressure. The surgeon who performed the shunting procedure prescribes how often the infant is to be turned and to what side after surgery. Often, infants are not turned to lie on the side with the shunt to prevent putting pressure on the valve, which might cause it to open and rapidly decompress CSF.

Formerly, shunts had fixed valves that allowed a set amount of CSF to be drained daily. Today, they are fitted with adjustable pressure valves. Because the valve contains a magnet, it can be readjusted to regulate the amount of CSF flow by manipulation of an external magnet, thus avoiding the problem of repeat surgery for readjustment (because shunts contain a magnet, remind parents to ask their primary care provider if it would be safe for their child to have an MRI, and also to keep toys containing magnets or electronic devices such as tablet computers away from the child) (Strahle, Selzer, Muraszko, et al., 2012).

Continue to assess for signs of increased intracranial pressure after surgery such as tense fontanelles, increasing head circumference, irritability or lethargy, decreased level of consciousness, poor sucking ability, vomiting, an increase in blood pressure (difficult to measure accurately in infants unless arterial or umbilical lines are used with Doppler instrumentation), increasing temperature, and a decrease in pulse and respiratory rates (see Chapter 49 for tips on a complete neurologic assessment). Also, assess for symptoms of infection such as increased temperature, increased pulse rate, general malaise, and signs of meningitis such as a stiff neck and marked irritability (Box 27.7). Be certain a child receives adequate pain management not only for comfort but also because crying elevates CSF pressure.

Nursing Diagnosis: Risk for imbalanced nutrition, less than body requirements, related to increased intracranial pressure

Outcome Evaluation: Child's weight remains within 5th to 95th percentile on height and weight chart; no vomiting occurs.

Because an abdominal incision is involved to thread the catheter into the peritoneum, an infant may be prescribed to be kept NPO until bowel sounds return. Introduce fluid gradually in small quantities because vomiting that results from the introduction of fluid too soon after any surgery causes increased intracranial pressure.

Like all infants, those with hydrocephalus should be held when being fed if possible. Be certain to support their heads well when moving them to avoid strain on their neck if their head appears enlarged. Help breastfeeding mothers to find a comfortable way to support the infant's head as needed. Use of a breastfeeding pillow will help to provide firm head support along with correct positioning at the breast.

Document whether the child sucks well because increasing intracranial pressure may be noted first because of poor or ineffective sucking. Vomiting after feeding without nausea (difficult to detect in a small infant) is also a common first sign of increased intracranial pressure.

Also, observe whether constipation exists because straining while passing stool is another cause of increased intracranial pressure. This is not usually a problem with young infants who are totally breastfed or formula fed. It can be a problem when children return for shunt replacement at an older age. Urge parents to offer adequate fluid and roughage in their child's diet as a preventive measure as the child grows.

Nursing Diagnosis: Risk for impaired skin integrity related to extra weight and immobility of the head

Outcome Evaluation: Child's skin remains clean, dry, and intact and without signs of erythema or ulceration.

If the infant's head has enlarged, it may be difficult for the infant to move it freely because of the extra weight. As the skin of the head stretches thin, skin breakdown can occur at the pressure point. Wash the child's head daily

---

BOX 27.7

Nursing Care Planning Based on Family Teaching

CARING FOR A CHILD WITH A VENTRICULOPERITONEAL SHUNT

Q. Following her child's ventriculoperitoneal shunt surgery, Maia asks you, "What do I need to do to care for him as he grows older?"

A. Here are some helpful things to remember:

- Be aware of the signs of increased intracranial pressure, such as drowsiness, vomiting, headache, irritability, and lack of appetite.
- Observe the site of the pump daily for any sign of swelling or redness.
- Don't allow your baby to fall asleep with his head hanging over the side of a couch or bed or in a position that could bend the shunt at the neck.
- Offer sufficient fruit, vegetables, cereal, and a generous amount of fluid so he doesn't become constipated; hard stool might press against the shunt in the abdomen and obstruct the flow of fluid. In addition, straining to pass a hard stool can increase intracranial pressure.
- Do not call attention to the pump behind your child's ear; teach him not to touch the pump when he's nervous or as an attention-getting action.
- Be certain your child wears a helmet for tricycle and bicycle riding (as all children should) to avoid injury to the shunt. Monitor his participation in roughhousing or school sports to avoid head trauma.
- If your child develops signs of infection such as an increased temperature, phone your primary care provider. This could be a simple respiratory infection but could also indicate an infected shunt that needs immediate treatment.
- Be certain to keep your regularly scheduled health assessment visits. As your child grows taller, the shunt will eventually need to be replaced for proper functioning.

and change the position of the head approximately every 2 hours so no portion of the head rests against the mattress for a long period. A synthetic sheepskin or silicon pad or an air, water, or alternating air mattress may help to reduce pressure points. If a Kling or stockinette bandage is used to hold a surgical head dressing in place, place a piece of gauze or cotton behind the child's ear before the bandage is applied to prevent skin surfaces from touching and becoming excoriated. Make certain the bandage does not become wet from backward-draining oral secretions or drainage from the shunt insertion site. The infant is also at risk for developing a flattened surface on the side or back of the head (nonsynostotic plagiocephaly) because of the inability to freely move the head, so awareness of position also becomes important from a cosmetic craniofacial aspect (De Bock, Braum, Renz-Polster, 2017).

Nursing Diagnosis: Deficient knowledge related to home care needs of child with hydrocephalus

Outcome Evaluation: Parents state fears regarding ability to provide care but voice they are able to manage this; state signs of increased intracranial pressure for which they should watch; demonstrate competence in shunt care.

Caring for a child with a shunt in place is an ongoing responsibility for parents because most children will have a shunt in place for the rest of their life. If parents do not seem to be asking many questions about the child's care after surgery, do not assume this is because they are taking the child's care in stride. They may be too frightened or do not understand neuroanatomy enough to know what questions to ask. An opening question such as "Most parents are a little nervous when they think about taking a child home with a shunt in place; do you feel that way?" gives them an opportunity to discuss how they feel and, hopefully, bring their anxiety down to a manageable level. It also offers assurance that healthcare providers are interested in helping and supporting them.

As their child grows older, remind parents to stress to their child that the strange object that can be felt behind the ear should not be continually touched. A child nervously fidgeting with a pressure pump can inadvertently evacuate CSF from the ventricles at a dangerously rapid rate.

Before an infant with a shunt in place is discharged from the hospital after surgery, be certain the parents have ample opportunity to feed and provide care so they can feel comfortable and confident they "know" their infant. Because irritability, lethargy, vomiting, and a change in the baby's cry are signs of increased intracranial pressure, be certain parents have the telephone number of their primary healthcare provider so they can report these findings immediately. A referral for home care follow-up may be appropriate to offer further support.

Parents need an appointment for the child's first checkup or who to call to make an appointment. Be certain they understand an infection of the shunt is not just a possibility but a severe complication because it can lead to meningitis; this means they need to report ear or pharyngeal infections at the first sign of illness. If meningitis should develop, in addition to being rehospitalized and receiving the usual treatment for meningitis (see Chapter 49), the child may have an extraventricular shunt placed to promote drainage and allow antibiotics to be administered directly into the CSF to prevent infected CSF from draining into the peritoneal cavity, where it could cause peritonitis.

Nursing Diagnosis: Risk for delayed growth and development related to potential neurologic challenge

Outcome Evaluation: Child demonstrates regular observable growth and achieves age-appropriate developmental milestones.

Like all children, children with hydrocephalus need intellectual and emotional stimulation such as being talked to, smiled at, and played with. Always role-model talking and singing to the child to help parents include these actions in their care. As necessary, reposition mobiles or pictures over a crib so the child can receive adequate visual stimulation without turning a heavier than usual head.

As the child reaches preschool and school age, parents need to confer with their primary healthcare provider to what sports will be safe. Usually, contact sports are contraindicated, although it may be allowed with helmet head protection. Carrying a heavy backpack or purse on the side of the shunt is also not advised to avoid breaking the shunt. Helmet use should be enforced with tricycle or bicycle riding or any other activates, such as skiing or snowboarding, where a head injury may be a concern.

QSEN Checkpoint Question 27.6

TEAMWORK & COLLABORATION

The primary healthcare provider for Maia's baby asks the nurse to observe him for signs that he is developing increased intracranial pressure while he waits for surgery. What vital sign changes should most prompt the nurse to report the findings to the primary care provider?

a. Decreased temperature and increased blood pressure
b. Increased respirations and decreased pulse rate
c. Increased temperature and decreased pulse rate
d. Decreased blood pressure and increased temperature

Look in Appendix A for the best answer and rationale.

NEURAL TUBE DISORDERS

The term "neural tube defect" (NTD) is used to describe many distinctly different malformations of the neural tube (Wallingford, Niswander, Shaw, et al., 2013). Because the neural tube forms in utero first as a flat plate and then molds to form the brain and spinal cord, it is susceptible to malformation. The term **spina bifida** (Latin for "divided spine") is most often used as a collective term for all spinal cord disorders, but there are well-defined degrees of spina bifida involvement, and not all neural tube disorders even involve the spinal cord. All of these disorders, however, occur because of a lack of fusion of the posterior surface of the embryo in early intrauterine life. They can be compared with cleft palate or cleft lip, which are also midline closure disorders.

The worldwide incidence of NTDs ranges from 1 to 10 per 1,000 births. The incidence of neural tube disorders has fallen dramatically in the United States since the inclusion of 600 μg of folic acid in prenatal vitamins and the mandatory inclusion of folic acid in all cereal and grain products, reducing the rate to 2 in 10,000 live births. In addition to folic acid deficiency, other risks identified are maternal age under 20 years or over 40 years, maternal education below 12th grade level, and low socioeconomic status (Zaganjor, Sekkarie, Tsang, et al., 2016). However, 30% to 50% of NTDs are not prevented by folate, indicating other possible environmental factors such as maternal diabetes, maternal obesity, and possibly certain drugs such as valproic acid (Wallingford et al., 2013). All women, especially those who have given birth to a first child with a spinal cord disorder, are advised to have maternal serum assay MAFP levels during a second pregnancy to determine if such a disorder could be present.

Types of Neural Disorders

Anencephaly

Anencephaly is the absence of the cerebral hemispheres. It occurs when the upper end of the neural tube fails to close in early intrauterine life. It is revealed by an elevated level of MAFP, amniocentesis, or a prenatal sonogram.

Labor with an infant with anencephaly may be prolonged because the infant may present in a breech position or the underdeveloped head may not engage the cervix well. On visual inspection at birth, the disorder is obvious (Fig. 27.17). Because the respiratory and cardiac centers are located in the intact medulla, infants may survive for several days after birth but cannot survive further because they have little or no cerebral function.

When the condition is discovered prenatally, parents are offered the option of pregnancy termination. If they elect to carry the pregnancy to term, they will need concerned support in the first few days of life as they realize the baby is as ill and incomplete as predicted. Providing culturally and spiritually sensitive care is a priority. Accommodate the needs of the family as best as possible, especially if the mother chooses to birth her baby. Allowing the parents to hold their newborn and to take photos can help with the grieving process. Many families opt to name their child and hold a funeral after the infant passes. This again can be helpful in their grieving process.

Microcephaly

Microcephaly is a disorder in which the fetal brain grows so slowly that it falls more than three standard deviations below normal on a growth chart at birth. The cause might be a disorder in brain development associated with an intrauterine infection such as rubella, cytomegalovirus, or toxoplasmosis (Russo & Beltrão-Braga, 2017). Recently, the Zika virus, which is transmitted via an infected *Aedes* species mosquito, has been linked to infantile microcephaly (CDC, 2016). A pregnant woman infected with Zika can pass the virus to her fetus, causing a range of certain birth defects, including microcephaly (CDC, 2016). More information is being learned about Zika transmission and preventative measures along with the hopes for development of a vaccine. The CDC has published guidelines, specifically for women and men of childbearing age. For more information, refer to the CDC website. Microcephaly may also result from severe malnutrition or anoxia following birth or in early infancy.

The prognosis for a normal life is guarded in children with microcephaly and depends on the extent of restriction of brain growth and on the cause. Generally, the infant is cognitively challenged because of the lack of functioning brain tissue. True microcephaly must be differentiated from *craniosynostosis* (normal brain growth but premature fusion of the cranial sutures), which also causes decreased head circumference but is curable.

Spina Bifida Occulta

Spina bifida occulta, the mildest form of all NTDs, occurs when the posterior laminae of the vertebrae fail to fuse. Spina bifida occulta is a malformation caused by nonclosure or incomplete closure of the posterior portion of the vertebrae (Tappero & Honeyfield, 2015). This occurs most commonly at the fifth lumbar or first sacral level but may occur at any point along the spinal canal. The appearance of a normal spinal cord is shown in Figure 27.18A. Spina bifida occulta may be first noticed as a dimpling at the point of poor fusion; abnormal tufts of hair or discolored skin may also be present (Ross, Mason, & Finnell, 2017). Simple spina bifida occulta is a benign disorder, and it can occur as frequently as in one out of every four children (see Fig. 27.18B).

Because the term "spina bifida" is commonly used to denote all spinal cord anomalies, parents, when told their child has a spina bifida occulta, may interpret this as meaning their child has an extremely serious disorder. Help clarify the degree of this defect for them: It simply means a surface of bone is missing, and the spinal cord is intact.

Meningocele

The spinal cord is protected by three layers of meninges or membranes: the pia mater, the arachnoid, and the dura mater. If these membranes herniate through an unformed vertebrae, they protrude as a circular mass, about the size of an orange, at the center of the back and termed a *meningocele* (see Fig. 27.18C). The protrusion generally occurs in the lower lumbar and lumbosacral region, although it might be

Figure 27.17   An infant with anencephaly. (© Joseph R. Siebert, PhD/Custom Medical Stock Photograph.)

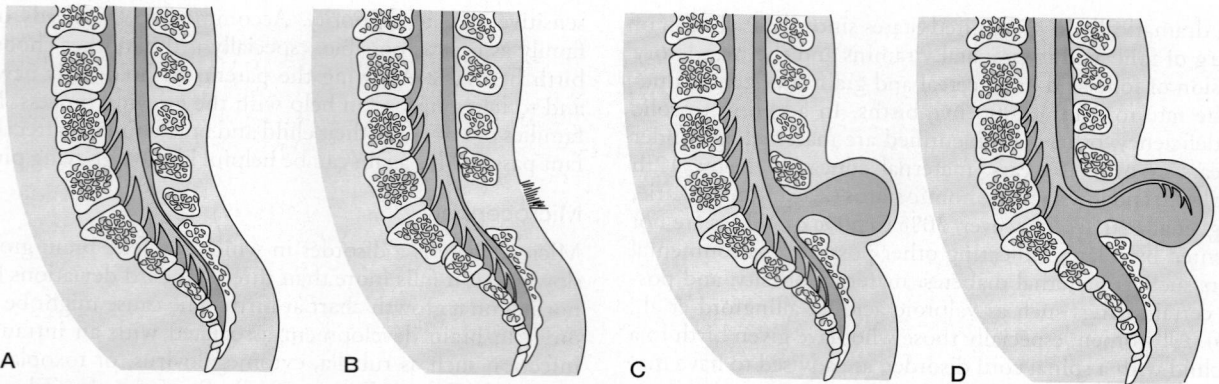

Figure 27.18   Degrees of spinal cord anomalies. **(A)** A normal spinal cord. **(B)** Spina bifida occulta. **(C)** A meningocele. **(D)** A meningomyelocele.

present anywhere along the spinal canal. The protrusion is either covered by a layer of skin or, more frequently, only the clear dura mater. No sensory or motor deficits accompany the disorder unless the membrane sac should rupture, but damage to the cord could occur or infection could enter the now unprotected CSF.

Meningomyelocele

This is the defect that most people think of when they say "spina bifida" because it is the most common birth defect affecting the central nervous system and is frequently viewed as the most complicated birth defect compatible with survival (Zaganjor et al., 2016). Lesions associated with spina bifida are called meningoceles. In a meningomyelocele, not just the meninges protrude through the vertebrae, but the spinal cord usually ends at the point of protrusion (Tappero & Honeyfield, 2015). Motor and sensory function will be decreased or absent beyond this point (see Fig. 27.18D).

Generally, the higher the defect is along the spine, the greater the degree of paralysis.

The child will have partial or complete paralysis, partial or complete lack of sensation of the lower extremities, as well as loss of bowel and bladder control. The infant's legs may appear lax because the infant cannot move them; urine and stools continually dribble because of a lack of sphincter control. Children may have an accompanying talipes (clubfoot) disorder and developmental dysplasia of the hip. A hydrocephalus develops in as many as 90% of these infants because of the lack of an adequate subarachnoid membrane for CSF absorption and obstruction of CSF circulation from the spinal deformity; the higher the meningomyelocele occurs on the cord, the more likely it is that a hydrocephalus will accompany it. Simultaneous shunting during a primary meningomyelocele repair during the first 72 hours of life has been shown to decrease hospital stay length, decrease loss of and infection rates of CSF, and lessen damage from progressive ventricular dilation (Zaganjor et al., 2016).

Encephalocele

An encephalocele is a cranial meningocele. These occur most often in the occipital area of the skull but may occur as a nasal or nasopharyngeal disorder. Encephaloceles generally are covered fully by skin, although they may be open or covered only by the dura. It is difficult to tell from the size of the encephalocele if only CSF is trapped in the protruding meninges or

whether brain tissue could also be involved. Transillumination of the sac will reveal whether brain tissue is in the sac. A CT, MRI, or ultrasound will reveal the size of the skull disorder and help predict the extent of surgery, which will be needed.

Assessment

Neural tube disorders may be discovered during intrauterine life by prenatal ultrasound, fetoscopy, amniocentesis (discovery of increased AFP in amniotic fluid), or analysis of MAFP. If the condition is discovered in utero, it may be possible to close the lesion by fetoscopic surgery. An infant may be born by cesarean birth to avoid pressure and injury to the spinal cord. It is generally difficult to tell from visual appearance whether the disorder is a meningomyelocele (Fig. 27.19) or the simpler meningocele. Observe and record whether an infant born with a neural tube disorder has spontaneous movement of the lower extremities to assess if the child has lower motor function. Also, assess the nature and pattern of voiding and defecation. The usual newborn appears to be "always wet" from voiding but actually voids in amounts of approximately 30 ml and then is dry for 2 or 3 hours before voiding again. An infant without motor or sphincter control voids continually. This pattern is the same for defecation. Observing these features aids in differentiating between a meningocele and a meningomyelocele. Differentiation will be further established by CT, ultrasound, or MRI.

Figure 27.19   A meningomyelocele. The infant also has hydrocephalus and a subluxated hip. (NMSB/Custom Medical Stock Photograph.)

TABLE 27.1 MOTOR FUNCTION ABILITY IN CHILDREN WITH MENINGOMYELOCELE

Spinal Cord Lesion	Resultant Effects
T6–T12	Complete flaccid paralysis of the lower extremities; weakened abdominal and trunk musculature in higher lesions; kyphosis and scoliosis common; ambulation with maximal support
L1–L2	Hip flexion present; paraplegia; ambulation with maximal support
L3–L4	Hip flexion, adduction, and knee extension present; hip dislocation common; some control of hip and knee movement possible; ambulation with moderate support
L5	Hip flexion, adduction, and varying degrees of abduction; knee extension and weak knee flexion; paralysis of the lower legs and feet; ambulation with moderate support
S1–S2	As previous, with preservation of some foot and ankle movement; ambulation with minimal support
S3	Mild loss of intrinsic foot muscular function possible; ambulation without support

Therapeutic Management

Children with spina bifida occulta need no surgical correction because there is no tissue extruding from the vertebrae. The parents should be made aware of the defect, however, so they are not surprised if it is revealed on a spinal X-ray taken for some reason later in life. They should also receive adequate patient education so that they can recognize more serious symptoms as the child grows such as numbness, weakness, or pain, which might indicate a need for reevaluation. Some children may eventually need surgery to prevent vertebral deterioration because of the unbalanced spinal column.

Treatment for a meningocele or encephalocele involves immediate surgery to replace the meninges and to close the gap in the skin to prevent infection. This is done as soon after birth as possible (usually within 24 to 48 hours) so an infection through the exposed meninges does not occur. The surgery is not without risk, and if a brain disorder accompanies an encephalocele, the child's cognitive potential may be impaired. If a large portion of meninges have to be removed by surgery, this can limit the rate of absorption of CSF, which can lead to a buildup of CSF and hydrocephalus.

Children with a meningomyelocele have the same surgery to return the meninges to the spinal cord and close the gap in the skin surface. The child will continue to have partial or complete paralysis of the lower extremities and loss of bowel and bladder function because, although the lesion on the back can be repaired, the absent lower cord cannot be replaced. There also is the same risk of hydrocephalus. Table 27.1 provides a classification of motor function ability, which can be anticipated according to the location of a spinal cord disruption.

Nursing Diagnoses and Related Interventions: Immediate Concerns

Although parents of an infant with a meningomyelocele were told before surgery that their child's spinal disorder is a type that means motor and sensory function are absent in the child's lower extremities, they do not necessarily "hear" this information. It is only after surgery that they begin to comprehend the extent of physical challenges their child will face. Before the child is discharged from the hospital, be certain the parents are linked with an interprofessional care team specializing in neural tube disorders to prevent them from feeling deserted when they most need support—the time when they first begin to appreciate what this problem will mean to them in the coming years, and what it will mean to their child throughout life.

Nursing Diagnosis: Risk for infection related to rupture or bacterial invasion of the meningeal sac

Outcome Evaluation: Neural tube sac remains intact; axillary temperature remains below 98.6°F (37°C).

If the exposed meningeal sac is allowed to dry, it can crack, allowing CSF to drain and microorganisms to enter. Pressure on the protruding mass is a prime reason why the sac ruptures. When this happens, it can lead to an infection such as meningitis as well as quick decompression of the CSF. Sudden compression can lead to herniation of the brain stem into the spinal cord and interference with respiratory and cardiac centers. Such pressure may also force CSF from the sac into the spinal column, thus increasing intracranial pressure. It is crucial, therefore, to prevent the drying of and pressure on the exposed membrane.

Preoperative Positioning. Before surgery, use sterile gloves and sterile linens when caring for an infant with either a meningocele or meningomyelocele. Use a sterile, wet, warm compress of saline, antiseptic, or antibiotic gauze over the lesion to keep the sac moist. Rather than remove this to wet it again and risk rupturing the sac, merely add additional warm fluid as needed.

Position infants carefully to prevent pressure on the exposed meninges, either in a prone position or supported on their side. When they are on their side, use a rolled blanket or diaper placed behind their upper back (above the disorder) and a separate one behind their lower back (below the disorder) so no pressure will be exerted on the lesion, and the infant will be protected from rolling backward onto it. Placing a folded diaper between the legs prevents skin surfaces from touching and rubbing in this position as well as helps to keep the hips from internally rotating. Positioning infants on their abdomen has the added advantage of keeping the flow of feces and urine away from the spinal defect as well as keeping the protruding meninges free from pressure (infants at home should sleep on their back but in an acute care setting with monitoring available, you can assure parents infants can be safely positioned on their abdomen). Placing a piece of plastic or sturdy plastic wrap below the protruding membranes on the child's back and taping it in place as an apron is another method of preventing feces from touching the open lesion.

A folded towel under the abdomen helps to flex the infant's hips in a prone position, reduce pressure on the sac, and ensure good leg position. Always notice if the position of the infant's legs appears comfortable because, if the infant lacks motor control, he or she cannot move them to a more comfortable position independently.

Although no pressure should be exerted on the open lesion by a top sheet or swaddling blanket, make certain the child is adequately warm. The presence of the sac adds to the amount of body surface area exposed, so heat loss will be greater than usual. Don't place the infant under a radiant heat source for warmth because the radiant heat can dry the lesion and cause cracking. An incubator both supplies a better heat source and also allows you to constantly assess and monitor the lesion. Any seepage of clear fluid from the defect should be reported promptly because this is probably escaping CSF. If you are in doubt whether the fluid is urine or CSF, check it against a glucose test strip: CSF will test positive for glucose, whereas urine or mucus will not.

Postoperative Care. After surgery, a baby is again placed on a cardiorespiratory monitor and positioned on the abdomen until the skin incision has healed (about 7 days). The same careful precautions against allowing urine or feces to touch the incision area continue.

Nursing Diagnosis: Risk for imbalanced nutrition, less than body requirements, related to difficulty assuming normal feeding position

Outcome Evaluation: Child's skin turgor is good; weight is maintained within 10% of birth weight; specific gravity of urine remains between 1.003 and 1.015.

If the defect repair was large and the risk of picking up the infant is too great, the infant may be fed while lying on the side in an incubator or prone on a specialized bed frame. Raise the infant's head slightly by slipping a folded diaper under it. Make certain your supporting arm does not press against the lesion. Remember (and remind parents) that, when burping the infant, not to pat the infant's back over the defect. Stroke the head, arms, or upper back while the infant sucks to try to give the child the same comfort and assurance at feeding time as a baby would receive if being held. Infants may enjoy a pacifier after feeding because they do not experience the same enjoyment of sucking while feeding that would be experienced if they could be held and cuddled. If a mother plans to breastfeed, urge her to pump and to provide expressed breast milk for the infant; as soon as the infant can be held, she can breastfeed (which will be as early as 3 to 4 days).

Nursing Diagnosis: Risk for ineffective cerebral tissue perfusion related to increased intracranial pressure

Outcome Evaluation: Child's head circumference remains within present percentile on growth chart; signs and symptoms of increased intracranial pressure are absent.

Preoperative Care. Increasing head size from poor absorption of CSF (hydrocephalus) is a common complication of both meningocele and meningomyelocele surgical repairs. To detect increased head size, measure head circumference as prescribed in the preoperative period to set a baseline. Head circumference measurements done by various caregivers are accurate only if the tape measure is placed on the same points of the child's head each time. Placing an indelible pen mark on the scalp above and below the tape measure over both ears and on the back of the scalp allows different people to measure the head at the same point while not leaving such a large mark that it interferes with facial features.

Postoperative Care. Head circumference measurement needs to be continued after surgery because this is the time when an increase in size most often occurs. Continue to observe the child as well for signs of increased intracranial pressure such as bulging fontanelles, vital change variations, neurologic signs such as pupillary changes, or behavioral changes such as irritability or lethargy to help detect if this is happening.

Nursing Diagnosis: Risk for impaired skin integrity related to required prone positioning

Outcome Evaluation: Infant's skin on knees remains intact, without erythema or ulceration.

Preserving skin integrity is a major problem before surgery because the constant prone position puts pressure on the infant's knees and elbows. If a hydrocephalus has developed, pressure areas at the temples can occur if the head is not repositioned about every 2 hours. After surgery, use paper tape or a stockinette for dressing changes or place a protective dressing such as Stomahesive on the skin under the area where the tape will touch. Change diapers frequently to prevent excessive contact of acidic urine with skin.

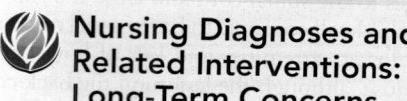

Nursing Diagnoses and Related Interventions: Long-Term Concerns

Nursing Diagnosis: Impaired physical mobility related to neural tube disorder

Outcome Evaluation: Child ambulates with the least amount of accessory equipment possible.

Parents need to begin to plan stimulation activities that their infant can accomplish with limited mobility as soon as surgery is completed. Encourage them to take the infant to the places children normally accompany parents, such as relatives' homes, shopping, or the zoo, because encouraging children to be as independent as possible as they grow helps them lead as active a life as possible (Fig. 27.20) (Deroche, Holland, McDermott, et al., 2015).

Parents will need to perform passive exercises to prevent muscle atrophy and formation of contractures if a child has impaired lower extremity motor control. The child may need leg braces to help maintain good alignment and

Figure 27.20 A child born with a neural tube disorder demonstrates her ability to walk using braces and a crutch. (Alexander Tsiara/Photo Researchers, Inc.)

enable walking with crutches. Parents are generally anxious to do something for their child and follow routines of passive exercises well if they are given sufficient support for their accomplishments at healthcare visits. As the child grows older, tendon transplants or an osteotomy may be necessary to prevent contractures and poor bone alignment. Because children with meningomyeloceles have no sensation in their lower extremities, parents should make a routine of daily inspections of the child's lower extremities and buttocks for any area of irritation or possible infection. Teach children as they grow older to do this themselves. When children are using a wheelchair, be certain they press with their arms on the armrests to raise their buttocks off the wheelchair seat at least once every hour to help provide adequate circulation to lower extremities. Often, children will have a team of rehabilitation therapists, such as occupational and physical therapists, who are involved with promoting the child's physical development, milestones, and strengths to their optimal abilities.

Nursing Diagnosis: Risk for impaired elimination related to a neural tube disorder

Outcome Evaluation: Child demonstrates ability to independently manage bowel and bladder elimination by school age.

To ensure bladder emptying, an intermittent clean urinary catheterization technique may be taught to parents (inserting a clean catheter through the urethra into the bladder every 4 hours to drain urine from the bladder; Box 27.8). An advantage of this is children who are begun on intermittent clean catheterization from birth require fewer bladder augmentation procedures as they grow older. As they reach

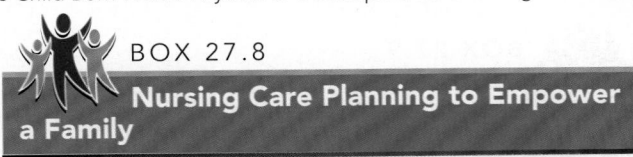

BOX 27.8

Nursing Care Planning to Empower a Family

TECHNIQUE FOR CLEAN INTERMITTENT CATHETERIZATION

Q. Maia needs to learn clean intermittent catheterization for her son (now named Marcus Tyler). She asks you, "How do I do this?"

A. Here are some helpful guidelines to follow:

1. The purpose of intermittent catheterization is to keep the bladder empty by using a clean technique and frequent emptying so microorganisms do not have time to grow in urine or the bladder. Always use clean equipment and catheterize at least every 4 hours.
2. Always carry catheterization equipment with you when away from home (e.g., a plastic bag containing a new catheter and a water-soluble lubricant). If you will be using a public lavatory, you might want to include a presoaped washcloth rather than have to use rough paper towels.
3. To begin catheterization, wash your hands well in warm, soapy water. This reduces the chance you will introduce germs from your hands into your child's bladder.
4. Next, wash around your child's urinary meatus with a clean washcloth or paper towel and warm, soapy water. Rinse the washcloth and wash again with clear water. This reduces the chance that germs on the child's skin will be pushed into the bladder.
5. Coat the tip of the catheter with a water-soluble lubricant. This reduces friction and allows the catheter to slide into the bladder easily.
6. Quickly but gently insert the catheter into the urinary meatus approximately 3 in. Urine should begin to flow immediately through the catheter. Let this drain into a collecting bag.
7. When urine stops flowing, gently remove the catheter. Most health insurance plans furnish enough clean catheters that you don't ever have to reuse one. If you should need to do this, clean the catheter with soap and water, rinse with clear water, and replace in the plastic bag with the lubricant.
8. Be certain that on special days such as family celebrations or while on vacation, you do not forget the importance of catheterization.
9. As your child reaches school age, you can teach him how to do this himself. He will need to insert the catheter about 6 in. Be certain he will be able to have access to a school bathroom every 4 hours during the day so he can successfully do this.
10. Phone your healthcare provider if urine is ever blood tinged, smells foul, or is cloudy rather than clear or if your child appears to have pain in his abdomen or lower back or has an elevated temperature. These may be symptoms of a urinary tract infection, which will need treatment.

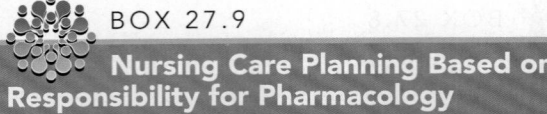

BOX 27.9

Nursing Care Planning Based on Responsibility for Pharmacology

OXYBUTYNIN CHLORIDE (DITROPAN)

Classification: Oxybutynin is an anticholinergic, urinary antispasmodic.

Action: relaxes smooth muscle to relieve symptoms of bladder instability associated with neurogenic bladder (Karch, 2013)

Pregnancy Risk Category: C

Dosage: individually prescribed depending on weight of child

Possible Adverse Effects: drowsiness, dizziness, blurred vision, decreased sweating

Nursing Implications

- Advise parents to give or have the child take the medication exactly as prescribed.
- Alert parents about the need for frequent healthcare visits during treatment to document the drug's effect.
- Ask the child to report drowsiness or blurred vision. Caution the child to not attempt activities that require balance until they adjust to taking the drug.
- Caution the child and parents that the drug causes decreased sweating, which can cause body temperature to rise. Encourage parents to keep the child's environment cool and to avoid extreme, high temperatures.

early school age, they can learn this technique for themselves. In addition to self-catheterization, a drug such as oxybutynin chloride (Ditropan) may improve bladder capacity and allow a child to need less frequent catheterizations (Box 27.9) (Karch, 2013). In some children, it is possible to place artificial bladder sphincters to help establish continence. In other children, a continent urinary reservoir or a ureterosigmoid-ostomy (see Chapter 46) can be constructed to bypass the nonfunctioning bladder. The school nurse is a key facilitator to help enable the child to achieve their highest level of self-care and voiding during school hours.

What If . . . 27.3

Maia repeats that she's too young to care for a child with so many problems so she wants to let him die rather than undergo palliative surgery to close the neural tube disorder. Whose rights should be honored, the parent's or the child's, and how should these rights be determined? What would be the nurse's role?

ARNOLD–CHIARI (CHIARI II) MALFORMATION

An Arnold–Chiari malformation is categorized as Chiari I, Chiari II, or Chiari III. Chiari Type I malformation involves the downward herniation of the caudal end of the cerebellar vermis through the foramen magnum. Chiari Type II occurs

in 0.5 to 1 per 1,000 of children with spina bifida myelome-ningocele. Children with Chiari I typically show symptoms in the second or third decade (Wallingford et al., 2013) of life, so it is referred to as an "adult type," although current sonogram scan capabilities have allowed for earlier inciden-tal diagnosis. Chiari II and the very rare Chiari III types are present at birth and so are considered primary neural tube abnormalities. The Chiari II disorder is caused by overgrowth of the neural tube in weeks 16 to 20 of fetal life. The cerebel-lum, medulla oblongata, and fourth ventricle project into the spinal canal at the cervical level, causing the upper cervical spinal cord to jackknife backward, obstructing CSF flow, and causing hydrocephalus. An accompanying lumbosacral me-ningomyelocele is also present in about 50% of children with this anomaly (Bernard, Knupp, Yang, et al., 2012).

A diagnosis is made by MRI and is sometimes accidently identified via an initial MRI because the older child is being evaluated for chronic headaches. The prognosis for the child with an Arnold–Chiari malformation depends on the extent of the disorder and the surgical repair procedure possible. Be-cause of the upper motor neuron involvement, gagging and swallowing reflexes may be absent, increasing the risk for tra-cheal aspiration. Serious levels of sleep apnea may also occur (Fuller, Sinha, Caruso, et al., 2016), which require surgical intervention. Overall prognosis is encouraging. A lumbar puncture (LP) should never be performed on a child with Arnold–Chiari malformation for risk of a brainstem hernia-tion; neurosurgery must always be consulted when necessary.

What If . . . 27.4

The nurse is interested in exploring one of the 2020 National Health Goals related to infants born with physical or developmental disorders (see Box 27.1). Most government-sponsored money for nursing research is allotted based on these goals. What would be a possible research topic to explore pertinent to these goals that would be applicable to the Sparrow family and that would also advance evidence-based practice?

KEY POINTS FOR REVIEW

- Learning about the way a child will be physically chal-lenged immediately after birth helps parents adjust most easily. Advocate for parents by helping them obtain as much information as they need about their child's condi-tion in order to help them manage transitions across dif-ferent healthcare settings.

- Parent–infant bonding can be difficult to establish when a child is hospitalized at birth. Assess family relationships at health maintenance visits to see that bonding is occur-ring while incorporating cultural and spiritual respect and customs.

- Absent or malformed extremities may range from absence of a finger to absence of an entire limb. Children may need physical therapy and teaching on how to use a prosthesis to gain full mobility and function.

- Developmental hip dysplasia is the improper formation and function of the hip socket; talipes deformities are foot and ankle deformities. Children may need extensive brac-ing and casting to correct these disorders.

- Cleft lips and cleft palates result from the failure of the maxillary process to fuse in intrauterine life. Surgical repair is possible early in life, with a good prognosis for both of these conditions.
- Esophageal atresias and tracheoesophageal fistulas occur from failure of the trachea and esophagus to completely divide and fully form independently in intrauterine life. Surgical intervention begins immediately but often needs to be performed in several stages.
- Omphaloceles are protrusions of abdominal contents through the abdominal wall at birth, protected only by a peritoneal membrane. When the membrane is not present, this is called gastroschisis. Although several stages of repair are often necessary, surgical correction has a good outcome.
- Intestinal obstructions can result from atresia (complete closure) or stenosis (narrowing) of a part of the bowel. Correction is surgical removal of the narrowed bowel portion.
- Meconium plugs occur when an extremely hard portion of meconium blocks the lumen of the intestine. Infants with meconium plug syndrome need to be observed for continuing bowel function and assessed for cystic fibrosis because a meconium plug is often the first symptom of this illness.
- Diaphragmatic hernias occur when the abdominal organs protrude through a defect in the diaphragm into the chest cavity. This prevents the lungs from fully forming in utero or expanding at birth. These infants are critically ill at birth and need extensive surgical correction.
- An imperforate anus is the incomplete formation of the anus, resulting in an inability to pass stool. The infant may have a temporary colostomy created before a final surgical correction can be completed.
- Physical developmental disorders of the nervous system include hydrocephalus (excess CSF in the ventricles) and neural tube disorders (incomplete closure of the vertebrae). Infants with hydrocephalus need surgery to relieve a ventricular obstruction or have a shunt implanted from their ventricles to the peritoneal cavity to remove excess CSF. Children with meningomyeloceles, the most severe form of neural tube disorder, face a permanent full or partial loss of lower neuron function and require continued rehabilitation.
- Planning nursing care that includes assurance not only meets QSEN guidelines but also best meets the family's total needs.

CRITICAL THINKING CARE STUDY

Cecelia Dove is a 7-lb baby born by vaginal birth to a 25-year-old mother. At birth, she appeared healthy and cried lustfully. An hour after birth, however, the first time her mother tried to breastfeed her, she coughed and choked 5 minutes into the feeding. Her primary care provider suspects Cecelia may have esophageal atresia.

1. What steps should you immediately take because of this diagnosis while you wait for diagnostic tests to be scheduled?
2. After a barium swallow is completed, Cecelia's mother is told her infant has an isolated esophageal atresia without a fistula. The mother exclaims, "I can't take home a baby who isn't normal. My mother will say it's my fault because I never should have gotten pregnant. My boyfriend will be so embarrassed, he'll leave me." How could you help this mother gain a better insight into her child's condition?
3. Cecelia returns from the operating room after successful surgery. She has a temporary gastrostomy tube in place for decompression and feedings of breast milk. When the mother asks you, "What now?" what would be your best answer?

RELATED RESOURCES

Explore these additional resources to enhance learning for this chapter:

- Student resources on thePoint, including answers to the What If . . . and Critical Thinking Care Study questions, http://thepoint.lww.com/Flagg8e
- Adaptive learning powered by PrepU, http://thepoint.lww.com/prepu

REFERENCES

Abdullah, F., & Harris, J. (2016). Pectus excavatum: More than a matter of aesthetics. *Pediatric Annals, 45*(11), e403–e406.

Academy of Breastfeeding Medicine. (2017). *Protocol #11. Guidelines for the evaluation and management of neonatal ankyloglossia and its complications in the breastfeeding dyad*. Retrieved from http://www.bfmed.org/Media/Files/Protocols/ankyloglossia.pdf

Allori, A. C., Mulliken, J. B., Meara, J. G., et al. (2017). Classification of cleft lip/palate: Then and now. *The Cleft Palate-Craniofacial Journal, 54*(2), 175–188.

American Academy of Pediatrics. (2017). Evidence and rationale. In *Bright Futures: Guidelines for health supervision of infants, children, and adolescents* (4th ed., pp. 275–302). Retrieved from http://www.aap.org/periodicityschedule

American Cleft Palate–Craniofacial Association. (n.d.). *Healthcare professional resources*. Retrieved from http://www.cleftline.org/healthcare-professionals/

Bernard, B. J., Knupp, K., Yang, M. L., et al. (2012). Neurologic & muscular disorders. In W. Hay, M. Levin, R. Deterding, et al. (Eds.), *Current diagnosis & treatment pediatrics* (21st ed., pp. 740–829). New York, NY: McGraw-Hill/Lange.

Bütow, K.-W., Naidoo, S., Zwahlen, R. A., et al. (2016). Pierre Robin sequence: Subdivision, data, theories, and treatment—part 4: Recommended management and treatment of Pierre Robin sequence and its application. *Annals of Maxillofacial Surgery, 6*(1), 44–49.

Bütow, K.-W., Zwahlen, R. A., Morkel, J. A., et al. (2016). Pierre Robin sequence: Subdivision, data, theories, and treatment—part 1: History, subdivisions, and data. *Annals of Maxillofacial Surgery, 6*(1), 31–34.

Carmichael, S. L., Ma, C., Tinker, S., et al. (2014). Maternal stressors and social support as risks for delivering babies with structural birth defects. *Paediatric and Perinatal Epidemiology, 28*(4), 338–344.

Centers for Disease Control and Prevention. (2016). *Data & statistics*. Retrieved from https://www.cdc.gov/ncbddd/birthdefects/data.html

Children's Craniofacial Association. (n.d.). *Syndromes*. Retrieved from http://www.ccakids.com/syndromes.html

Cleft Palate Foundation. (2010). *Your baby's first year*. Retrieved from http://www.cleftline.org/docs/Booklets/FYL-01.pdf

Cuenca, A. G., Ali, A. S., Kays, D. W., et al. (2012). "Pulling the plug"—management of meconium plug syndrome in neonates. *The Journal of Surgical Research, 175*(2), e43–e46.

De Bock, F., Braum, V., & Renz-Polster, H. (2017). Deformational plagiocephaly in normal infants: A systematic review of causes and hypotheses. *Archives of Disease in Childhood, 102*(6), 535–542.

De Pascalis, L., Kkeli, N., Chakrabarti, B., et al. (2017). Maternal gaze to the infant face: Effects of infant age and facial configuration during mother-infant engagement in the first nine weeks. *Infant Behavior & Development, 46*, 91–99.

Deroche, C. B., Holland, M., McDermott, S., et al. (2015). Development of a tool to describe overall health, social independence and activity limitation of adolescents and young adults with disability. *Research in Developmental Disabilities*, 38, 288–300.

Dixon, M., Marazita, M., Beaty, T., et al. (2011). Cleft lip and palate: Understanding genetic and environmental influences. *Nature Reviews: Genetics*, 12(3), 167–178.

Emil, S., Canvasser, N., Chen, T., et al. (2012). Contemporary 2-year outcomes of complex gastroschisis. *Journal of Pediatric Surgery*, 47(8), 1521–1528.

Farrell, F., & Krahn, G. L. (2014). Family life goes on: Disability in contemporary families. *Family Relations*, 63(1), 1–6.

Fuller, J. C., Sinha, S., Caruso, P. A., et al. (2016). Chiari malformations: An important cause of pediatric aspiration. *International Journal of Pediatric Otorhinolaryngology*, 88, 124–128.

Funato, N., & Nakamura, M. (2017). Identification of shared and unique gene families associated with oral clefts. *International Journal of Oral Science*. Advance online publication. doi:10.1038/ijos.2016.56

Gourlay, D. M. (2013). Colorectal considerations in pediatric patients. *The Surgical Clinics of North America*, 93(1), 251–272.

Gowda, D., & Joseph, S. (2017). Thyroglossal cyst: What is the right age to operate? *Clinical Pediatrics*. Advance online publication. doi:10.1177/0009922816687330

Hazelbaker, A. K. (2010). *Tongue-tie: Morphogenesis, impact, assessment and treatment*. Columbus, OH: Aiden and Eva Press.

Hedrick, H. L. (2013). Management of prenatally diagnosed congenital diaphragmatic hernia. *Seminars in Pediatric Surgery*, 22(1), 37–43.

Jackson, J. C., Runge, M. M., & Nye, N. S. (2014). Common questions about developmental dysplasia of the hip. *American Family Physician*, 90(12), 843–850.

Jones, A. M., Isenburg, J., Salemi, J. L., et al. (2016). Increasing prevalence of gastroschisis—14 States, 1995-2012. *Morbidity and Mortality Weekly Report*, 65(2), 23–26.

Juang, D., & Snyder, C. L. (2012). Neonatal bowel obstruction. *The Surgical Clinics of North America*, 92(3), 685–711.

Jubbal, K. T., Agrawal, N., & Hollier, L. H., Jr. (2017). Analysis of morbidity, readmission, and reoperation after craniosynostosis repair in children. *The Journal of Craniofacial Surgery*, 28(2), 401–405.

Kadir, D., & Lilja, H. E. (2017). Risk factors for postoperative mortality in congenital diaphragmatic hernia: A single-centre observational study. *Pediatric Surgery International*, 33(3), 317–323.

Karch, A. M. (2013). *2013 Lippincott's nursing drug guide*. Philadelphia, PA: Lippincott Williams & Wilkins.

Levy, P. (2010). An overview of newborn screening. *Journal of Developmental and Behavioral Pediatrics*, 31(7), 622–631.

Mirza, B., & Ali, W. (2016). Distinct presentations of hernia of umbilical cord. *Journal of Neonatal Surgery*, 5(4), 53.

Moldenhauer, J. S. (2014). In utero repair of spina bifida. *American Journal of Perinatology*, 31(7), 595–604.

Mulpuri, K., Song, K. M., Gross, R. H., et al. (2015). The American Academy of Orthopaedic Surgeons evidence-based guideline on detection and nonoperative management of pediatric developmental dysplasia of the hip in infants up to six months of age. *The Journal of Bone and Joint Surgery*, 97(20), 1717–1718.

Nam, S. H., Kim, D. Y., & Kim, S. C. (2016). Can we expect a favorable outcome after surgical treatment for an anorectal malformation? *Journal of Pediatric Surgery*, 51(3), 421–424.

Nes, R. B., Røysamb, E., Hauge, L. J., et al. (2014). Adaptation to the birth of a child with a congenital anomaly: A prospective longitudinal study of maternal well-being and psychological distress. *Developmental Psychology*, 50(6), 1827–1839.

Nidey, N., Moreno Uribe, L. M., Marazita, M. M., et al. (2016). Psychosocial well-being of parents of children with oral clefts. *Child: Care, Health and Development*, 42(1), 42–50.

O'Connell, R. V., Dotters-Katz, S. K., Kuller, J. A., et al. (2016). Gastroschisis: A review of management and outcomes. *Obstetrical & Gynecological Survey*, 71(9), 537.

Oliveira, M. F., Teixeira, M. J., Norremose, K. A., et al. (2015). Surgical technique of retrograde ventricle-sinus shunt is an option for the treatment of hydrocephalus in infants after surgical repair of myelomeningocele. *Arquivos de Neuro-Psiquiatria*, 73(12), 1019–1025.

Oluyomi-Obi, T., Kuret, V., Puligandla, P., et al. (2017). Antenatal predictors of outcome in prenatally diagnosed congenital diaphragmatic hernia (CDH). *Journal of Pediatric Surgery*, 52(5), 881–888.

Ornitz, D. M., & Legeai-Mallet, L. (2017). Achondroplasia: Development, pathogenesis, and therapy. *Developmental Dynamics*, 246(4), 291–309.

O'Rourke-Potocki, A., Ali, K., Murthy, V., et al. (2016). Resuscitation of infants with congenital diaphragmatic hernia. *Archives of Disease in Childhood*. Advance online publication. doi:10.1136/archdischild-2016 -311432

Prathanee, B., Pumnum, T., Seepuaham, C., et al. (2016). Five-year speech and language outcomes in children with cleft lip-palate. *Journal of Cranio-Maxillo-Facial Surgery*, 44(10), 1553–1560.

Ross, M. E., Mason, C. E., & Finnell, R. H. (2017). Genomic approaches to the assessment of human spina bifida risk. *Birth Defects Research*, 109(2), 120–128.

Russo, F. B., & Beltrão-Braga, P. C. (2017). The impact of Zika virus in the brain. *Biochemical and Biophysical Research Communications*. Advance online publication. doi:10.1016/j.bbrc.2017.01.074

Ryu, J. H., Kim, D. W., Kim, S. H., et al. (2016). Factors correlating outcome in young infants with congenital muscular torticollis. *Canadian Association of Radiologists Journal*, 67(1), 82–87.

Sanzarello, I., Nanni, M., & Faldini, C. (2017). The clubfoot over the centuries. *Journal of Pediatric Orthopedics. Part B*, 26(2), 143–151.

Scheffler, C., Greil, H., & Hermanussen, M. (2017). The association between weight, height, and head circumference reconsidered. *Pediatric Research*, 81(5), 825–830.

Shaw, B. A., & Segal, L. S. (2016). Evaluation and referral for developmental dysplasia of the hip in infants. *Pediatrics*, 138(6), e20163107.

Sinha, S. K., Dhua, A., Mathur, M. K., et al. (2012). Neural tube defect repair and ventriculoperitoneal shunting: Indications and outcome. *Journal of Neonatal Surgery*, 1(2), 21.

Strahle, J., Selzer, B. J., Muraszko, K. M., et al. (2012). Programmable shunt valve affected by exposure to a tablet computer. *Journal of Neurosurgery. Pediatrics*, 10(2), 118–120.

Sullivan, M. A., & Adkinson, J. M. (2016). Congenital hand differences. *Plastic Surgical Nursing*, 36(2), 84–89.

Sundaram, S. S., Hoffenberg, E. J., Kramer, R. E., et al. (2012). Gastrointestinal tract. In W. Hay, M. Levin, R. Deterding, et al. (Eds.), *Current diagnosis & treatment pediatrics* (21st ed., pp. 624–662). New York, NY: McGraw-Hill/Lange.

Tappero, E., & Honeyfield, M. (2015). *Physical assessment of the newborn: A comprehensive approach to the art of physical examination* (5th ed.). Petaluma, CA: NICU/INK.

Taub, P. J., & Piccolo, P. (2016). Cleft lip repair: Through the looking glass. *The Journal of Craniofacial Surgery*, 27(8), 2031–2035.

Tikka, T., Kalkat, M. S., Bishay, E., et al. (2016). A 20-year review of pectus surgery: An analysis of factors predictive of recurrence and outcomes. *Interactive Cardiovascular and Thoracic Surgery*, 23(6), 908–913.

Tolarova, M. M. & Elluru, R. G. (2015). *Pediatric cleft lip and palate*. Retrieved from http://emedicine.medscape.com/article/995535-overview

U.S. Department of Health and Human Services. (2010). *Healthy people 2020*. Washington, DC: Author.

Vergouwe, F. W., IJsselstijn, H., Wijnen, R. M., et al. (2015). Screening and surveillance in esophageal atresia patients: Current knowledge and future perspectives. *European Journal of Pediatric Surgery*, 25(4), 345–352.

Wallingford, J. B., Niswander, L. A., Shaw, G. M., et al. (2013). The continuing challenge of understanding, preventing, and treating neural tube defects. *Science*, 339(6123), 1222002.

Wong, K., Patel, P., Cohen, M. B., et al. (2017). Breastfeeding infants with ankyloglossia: Insight into mothers' experiences. *Breastfeeding Medicine*, 12, 86–90.

Yoon, A., Zaghi, S., Weitzman, R., et al. (2017). Toward a functional definition of ankyloglossia: Validating current grading scales for lingual frenulum length and tongue mobility in 1052 subjects. *Sleep & Breathing*. Advance online publication. doi:10.1007/s11325-016-1452-7

Zaganjor, I., Sekkarie, A., Tsang, B. L., et al. (2016). Describing the prevalence of neural tube defects worldwide: A systematic literature review. *PLoS One*, 11(4), e0151586.

UNIT 5

The Nursing Role in Health Promotion for Childrearing Family

Principles of Growth and Development

*J*ohn Olson is a 6-year-old, mildly overweight boy brought into an emergency department because his leg is broken from a bicycle accident. At 4 months of age, John was placed in foster care because his mother was not caring for him adequately. He was then moved back and forth among 12 different foster homes until he was finally adopted at age 3.5 years. His adoptive parents now have 3-year-old twins of their own in addition to John. They tell you that, although John has lived with them for 3 years, they find him cold and unloving. They ask you what they can do to change this.

Nurses are directly responsible for assessing the growth and development of children in many healthcare settings. Previous chapters discussed childbearing and what an important time the first weeks after birth can be in a child's life. This chapter adds information about growth and development that are important for a child's continuing life.

How has John's background contributed to his behavior? What stage of psychosocial development does he not seem to have achieved? How could his adoptive parents help him at this point?

KEY TERMS

abstract thought

accommodation

assimilation

autonomy versus shame or doubt

centering

cognitive development

conservation

development

developmental milestones

developmental task

growth

identity versus role confusion

industry versus inferiority

initiative versus guilt

intimacy versus isolation

maturation

permanence

reversibility

role fantasy

schemas

sensorimotor stage

temperament

trust versus mistrust

OBJECTIVES

After mastering the contents of this chapter, you should be able to:

1. Describe principles of growth and development and developmental stages according to major theorists.

2. Identify 2020 National Health Goals related to growth and development that nurses can help the nation achieve.

3. Assess a child to determine if a stage of development has been achieved.

4. Formulate nursing diagnoses that address wellness as well as both a potential for and an actual delay in growth and development.

5. Identify expected outcomes for a growing child as well as how to manage seamless transitions across differing healthcare settings.

6. Using the nursing process, plan nursing care that includes the six competencies of Quality & Safety Education for Nurses (QSEN): Patient-Centered Care, Teamwork & Collaboration, Evidence-Based Practice (EBP), Quality Improvement (QI), Safety, and Informatics.

7. Implement nursing care, such as suggesting age-appropriate play materials to support normal growth and development.

8. Evaluate outcome criteria for achievement and effectiveness of care.

9. Integrate knowledge of the principles of growth and development with the interplay of the nursing process, the six competencies of QSEN, and Family Nursing to promote quality maternal and child health nursing care.

BOX 28.1

Nursing Care Planning Based on 2020 National Health Goals

A number of 2020 National Health Goals speak to growth or development of children. They include:

- Increase the proportion of children with special health-care needs who receive their care in family-centered, comprehensive, coordinated systems from 20.4% to a target level of 22.4%.
- Reduce the proportion of children diagnosed with a disorder through newborn blood spot screening who experience a developmental delay requiring special education services from 15.1% to a target level of 13.6%.
- Increase the proportion of young children who are screened for an autism spectrum disorder (ASD) and other developmental delays by 24 months of age from 19.5% to a target level of 21.5%.
- (Developmental) Increase the proportion of children with a developmental delay who have a first evaluation by 36 months of age.
- Reduce the proportion of children 2 to 5 years of age who are considered obese from 10.7% to a target level of 9.6%; for children 6 to 11 years, from 17.4% to 15.7%; and for adolescents, from 17.9% to 16.1% (U.S. Department of Health and Human Services, 2010; see www.healthypeople.gov).

Recognizing normal growth and development patterns of children helps to determine if children are following normal development and when referrals are needed. Nurses are the healthcare providers who interact with children as they weigh and measure them or help with interviewing or examinations and so are prime people to recognize developmental delays.

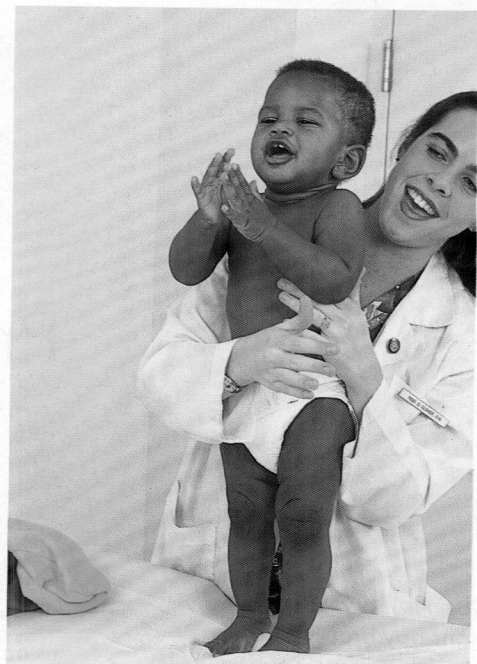

Figure 28.1 Growth and development are assessed by both observation and specific testing. Here, a 12-month-old demonstrates mastery of well-coordinated and intentional hand movements.

All children pass through predictable stages of growth and development as they mature. Parents often ask what to expect from their children regarding their developmental progress at healthcare visits. Such visits provide opportunities for you to assess growth and development and provide anticipatory guidance (Butterworth & Kovas, 2013).

For these reasons, including growth and development is essential to establish complete and effective nursing care plans for children. This chapter addresses the most important factors to assess for each age group. Later chapters supply detailed descriptions of individual age groups. Box 28.1 shows 2020 National Health Goals that speak directly to aspects of growth and development.

Nursing Process Overview

FOR PROMOTION OF NORMAL GROWTH AND DEVELOPMENT

ASSESSMENT

To assess **growth** (defined as an increase in physical size, typically measured as height, weight and head circumference), measure and plot height and weight on a standard

growth chart for children at all well-child care visits. Measurement of the head circumference is included for children age 2 years and younger. Growth charts are available through the Centers for Disease Control and Prevention (CDC; www.cdc.gov/growthcharts/) and the World Health Organization (WHO; www.who.int/childgrowth/standards). This will aid in determining if the child's growth is following the predicted pattern.

Obtain a developmental health history from both parents (if they are available) and the child (if age-appropriate). **Development** refers to the progression toward maturity in mental, physical, and social markers of normal development. Observe what specific activities the child can accomplish to establish whether **developmental milestones** (major markers of normal development) are achieved (Fig. 28.1). Document a 24-hour recall history for nutritional intake, sleep, and a description of school and play behaviors (see Chapter 34). Periodic screening tests such as the Ages & Stages Questionnaires (http://agesandstages.com/) and routine screening, including hearing and vision, should be scheduled following the periodicity schedule of the American Academy of Pediatrics (AAP at https://www.aap.org/en-us/professional-resources/practice-support/Pages/PeriodicitySchedule.aspx).

NURSING DIAGNOSIS

When an assessment is completed, a nursing diagnosis can be identified to reflect the problem. Examples of nursing diagnoses applicable to growth and development include:

- Risk for delayed growth and development related to lack of age-appropriate toys and activities
- Delayed growth and development related to prolonged illness

- Readiness for enhanced family coping related to parents seeking information about a child's growth and development
- Health-seeking behaviors related to appropriate stimulation for infants
- Imbalanced nutrition, less than body requirements, related to parental knowledge deficit regarding a child's protein needs
- Deficient knowledge related to potential long-term effects of obesity in the school-age child

OUTCOME IDENTIFICATION AND PLANNING

To provide holistic nursing care, consider all aspects of a child's health (physical, emotional, cultural, cognitive, spiritual, and social), remembering that each child's developmental progress is unique. Children achieve milestones at a predictable age range and identifying delays encourages prompt evaluation and treatment to promote the child's optimal potential.

Providing anticipatory guidance to caregivers provides them with realistic expectations for their child's achievements. Unrealistic parental expectations are factors that can lead to a child experiencing an unintentional injury (see Chapter 52). Planning should include a child's family because growth and development proceed within a family context. To develop psychosocially, children need emotional support from loved ones, just as they need nutritional support to grow physically.

Parents of a child with a developmental delay may use denial as a protective mechanism. Planning may have to initially focus on assisting parents with acceptance of the current situation. Plans for the child may have to be delayed until the parents are emotionally prepared to address the problem. It may be helpful to refer parents to online resources for further information.

ONLINE RESOURCES

Al-Anon/Alateen	www.alateen.com
American Association for Health Education	www.aahperd.org/aahe
American Academy of Pediatrics	www.aap.org
American Association of Poison Control Centers	www.aapcc.org
American Association of Suicidology	www.suicidology.org
BabyCenter	www.BabyCenter.com
Centers for Disease Control and Prevention Child Passenger Safety	www.cdc.gov/features /passengersafety and www.cdc.gov/MotorVehicle Safety/Child_Passenger _Safety/CPS-Factsheet .html
Centers for Disease Control and Prevention	www.CDC.gov/growthcharts
Cyberbullying Research Center	www.cyberbullying.us/
GLBT National Help Center	www.GLBTnationalhelp center.org or 1-888-843-4564
Healthy & Active Preschoolers	www.healthypreschoolers .com
March of Dimes	www.MarchofDimes.com /baby
National Eating Disorders Association	www.nationaleatingdisorders .org
National Poison Control Center	1-800-222-1222
Partnership for Drug-Free Kids	drugfree.org
Planned Parenthood Federation of America, Inc	www.plannedparenthood.org
Sexual Information and Education Council of the United States	www.siecus.org
Students Against Destructive Decisions	www.sadd.org
U.S. Consumer Product Safety Commission	www.CPSC.gov
World Health Organization	www.WHO.int/childgrowth

IMPLEMENTATION

Interventions to foster growth and development include encouraging age-appropriate self-care in a child and suggesting age-appropriate toys or activities to parents. Role modeling is an important ongoing intervention to help parents accept a child's delayed growth or appreciate a child who is scoring extremely high on standard scales and needs increased stimulation. Modeling, for example, can demonstrate that problem solving is a more effective approach to life's challenges than "acting out" behaviors.

OUTCOME EVALUATION

An evaluation for specific growth and developmental milestones (see Chapters 29 to 33) must be conducted throughout childhood and repeated if there are any concerns regarding a delay. The evaluation must be comprehensive and include all physical growth parameters and all aspects of development. Developmental aspects include social, language, and fine motor and gross motor skills. Expected outcomes for abnormal findings include the following examples:

- Child, 5 years of age, expresses less negativism at next clinic visit.
- At the 9-month checkup, parents describe how they have made a safe space in their home for their infant to crawl so he is not confined to a playpen.
- Parents list household tasks they believe are appropriate for a 6-year-old child by the next office visit.
- Parents describe the pattern they are using to phase out high-carbohydrate, nonnutritive snacks for their preschooler.
- Parents express confidence that they will be able to guide their toddler past the stage of the "terrible twos."

Growth and Development and the Role of the Nurse

Assessing for growth and development milestones is a nursing role in the care of both well and ill children.

HEALTH PROMOTION AND ILLNESS PREVENTION

Determining a child's developmental stage is often the primary focus of a well-child health interview and examination. For instance, during her child's 24-month checkup, a mother might ask if it is normal that her child cannot yet pedal a tricycle, a question that cannot be answered without a full understanding of average ranges of motor coordination.

Parenting style and competence are major influences on the behavioral and mental health of children (Barton & Kirtley, 2012). In addition to reassuring parents that their child is doing well, parents also need periodic anticipatory guidance regarding their child's development. For example, it would be important to discuss additional home safety with a parent when a child is approaching the age for crawling. Parents should be cautioned to think about installing a gate in front of a stairway and removing products or installing a lock on accessible cabinets where hazardous materials are stored.

Parents of the 1-year-old child will appreciate being cautioned that their child's appetite may decrease during the coming year. This information helps prevent the misinterpretation of a child's rejection of food as the beginning of a feeding problem, and it helps the parents see it as a normal developmental stage instead. Likewise, the parent of a child approaching puberty generally welcomes discussion on how to prepare a child for this challenging growth phase.

Anticipatory guidance must be provided in a timely manner. Information given too early is forgotten by the time it is needed. Given too late, parents may have already addressed the issue and possibly not in the most growth-enhancing way for their child. Recognizing the predictable stages of growth and development, from newborn through late adolescence, will enable you to provide anticipatory guidance at the appropriate stage of the child's development (Halfon, Stevens, Larson, et al., 2011; The Nemours Foundation, 2016).

HEALTH RESTORATION AND MAINTENANCE

It is equally essential to consider the developmental stage of a child when providing care during illness (both acute and chronic) and in preparation for a medical or surgical procedure. Preparing a 5-year-old child for surgery, for example, would be ineffective unless you know how much a 5-year-old child will understand (e.g., anesthesia, some body parts are necessary for life and some are not, or stitches will not stay in permanently). During the postsurgical period, you need growth and development knowledge to assess whether a child is old enough to swallow pills, whether a child will be able to accurately rate a degree of pain on a standard scale, and how to approach a child who says "no" to every suggestion.

Physical growth is another important factor to consider because disease affects children differently at various stages of growth. A 12-year-old child who has fractured a long bone, for example, has a potentially more serious fracture than an 8-year-old child who fractures the identical bone. This is because the 8-year-old must metabolize enough calcium to meet two major needs: healing the fracture site and maintaining healthy bone cells. The 12-year-old child, who is undergoing a period of rapid growth, must meet three needs: calcium for healing, maintaining existing healthy bone cells, and an additional amount for rapid bone growth. If a child does not take in adequate calcium during the healing period to supply the extra amount for growth, the affected limb could be left shorter than its mate. You can help protect against permanent disability by recommending ways the child can ingest extra calcium.

Principles of Growth and Development

Growing up is a complex phenomenon because of the many interrelated facets involved. Children do not merely grow taller and heavier as they get older; maturing also involves growth in their ability to perform skills, to think, to relate to people, and to trust or have confidence in themselves.

The terms "growth" and "development" are sometimes used interchangeably, but they are actually different terms.

- Growth is used to denote an increase in physical size or a *quantitative* change. Growth in weight, for example, is measured in pounds or kilograms; growth in height is measured in inches or centimeters.
- Development indicates an increase in skill or the ability to function (a *qualitative* change). Development is measured by observing a child's ability to perform specific tasks such as how well a child picks up small objects, by recording the parent's description of a child's progress, or by using standardized tests such as the Ages & Stages Questionnaires. **Maturation** is a synonym for development.

Psychosexual development is a specific type of development that refers to developing instincts or sensual pleasure (Freudian theory). Psychosocial development refers to Erikson's stages of personality development. Kohlberg's theory of moral development is the ability to know right from wrong and to apply these to real-life situations.

Cognitive development refers to the ability to learn or understand from experience, to acquire and retain knowledge, to respond to a new situation, and to solve problems (see the section that follows on Piaget's theory of cognitive development). It is measured by intelligence tests and by observing children's ability to function effectively in different environments.

PATTERNS

Neither physical growth nor aspects of maturation occur haphazardly but in a predictable pattern governed by several principles (Box 28.2). As shown in Figure 28.2, the pattern for general growth, such as respiratory, digestive, renal, musculoskeletal, and circulatory tissue, proceeds fairly smoothly during childhood. Certain body tissues, however, mature in spurts. Neurologic tissue (spinal cord and brain) grows so rapidly during the first 2 years that the brain reaches mature proportions by 2 to 5 years of age. Lymphoid tissue (spleen, thymus, lymph nodes, and tonsillar tissue) also grows rapidly during infancy and childhood to provide young children early protection against infection. In 5-year-olds, for example, tonsillar tissue has already reached its peak size (about twice that of an adult). On assessment, the back of the throat of young school-age children appears to be "all tonsils." Although the spleen is not usually palpable in adults, the spleen is palpable 1 or 2 cm below the left ribs in preschool children as another example of this rapid immune tissue growth. In contrast, reproductive organs (genital tissue) show little growth until puberty (Levine, 2011).

BOX 28.2

Nursing Care Planning Based on Family Teaching

Q. John's mother asks you, "Are there principles of growth and development I should know to be a better mother?"

A. Aspects of growth and development are well studied. General principles include:

- *Growth and development are continuous processes from conception until death.* Although there are highs and lows in terms of the rate at which growth and development proceed, a child is growing new cells and learning new skills at all times. An example of how the rate of growth changes is a comparison between that of the first year and later in life. An infant triples in birth weight and increases height by 50% during the first year of life. If this tremendous growth rate were to continue, a 5-year-old child, ready to begin school, would weigh 1,600 lb and be 12.5 ft tall.
- *Growth and development proceed in an orderly sequence.* Growth in height occurs in only one sequence—from smaller to larger. Development also proceeds in a predictable order. For example, the majority of children sit before they crawl, crawl before they stand, stand before they walk, and walk before they run. Occasionally, a child will skip a stage (or pass through it so quickly the parents do not observe the stage). Occasionally, a child will progress in a different order, but most children follow a predictable sequence of growth and development.
- *Children pass through the predictable stages at different rates.* All stages of development have a range of time rather than a certain point at which they are usually accomplished. Two children may pass through the motor sequence at such different rates, for example, that one begins walking at 9 months, whereas another starts at 14 months. They are both following the predictable sequence and are developing normally; they are merely developing at different rates.
- *All body systems do not develop at the same rate.* Certain body tissues mature more rapidly than others. For example, neurologic tissue experiences its peak growth during the first year of life, whereas genital tissue grows little until puberty.
- *Development is cephalocaudal.* *Cephalo* is a Greek word meaning "head"; *caudal* means "tail." Development proceeds from head to tail. Newborns can lift only their head off the bed when they lie in a prone position. By age 2 months, infants can lift both the head and chest off the bed; by 4 months, the head, chest, and part of the abdomen; by 5 months, infants have enough control to turn over; by 9 months, they can control legs enough to crawl; and by 1 year, children can stand upright and perhaps walk. Motor development has proceeded in a cephalocaudal order—from the head to the lower extremities.
- *Development proceeds from proximal to distal body parts.* This principle is closely related to cephalocaudal development. It can best be illustrated by tracing the progress of upper extremity development. A newborn makes little use of the arms or hands. Any movement, except to put a thumb in the mouth, is a flailing motion. By age 3 or 4 months, the infant has enough arm control to support the upper body weight on the forearms, and can coordinate the hand to scoop up objects. By 10 months, the infant can coordinate the arm and thumb and index fingers sufficiently to use a pincerlike grasp or to be able to pick up an object as fine as a piece of breakfast cereal on a high chair tray.
- *Development proceeds from gross to refined skills.* This principle parallels the preceding one. Once children are able to control distal body parts such as fingers, they are able to perform fine motor skills (e.g., a 3-year-old colors best with a large crayon; a 12-year-old can write with a fine pen).
- *There is an optimum time for initiation of experiences or learning.* Children cannot learn tasks until their nervous system is mature enough to allow that particular learning. A child cannot learn to sit, for example, no matter how much the child's parents have him or her practice, until the nervous system has matured enough to allow for back control. Children who are not given the opportunity to learn developmental tasks at the appropriate or "target" times for a task may have more difficulty than the usual child learning the task later on. A child who is confined to a body cast at 12 months, the time the child would normally learn to walk, may take a long time to learn this skill once free of the cast at, say, age 2 years. The child has passed the time of optimal learning for that particular skill.
- *Neonatal reflexes must be lost before development can proceed.* An infant cannot grasp an item with skill until the grasp reflex has faded nor can the infant stand steadily until the walking reflex has faded. Neonatal reflexes are replaced by purposeful movements.
- *A great deal of skill and behavior is learned by practice.* Infants practice over and over taking a first step before they accomplish this securely. If children fall behind in growth and development because of an illness, they are capable of "catch-up" growth to bring them equal again with their age group.

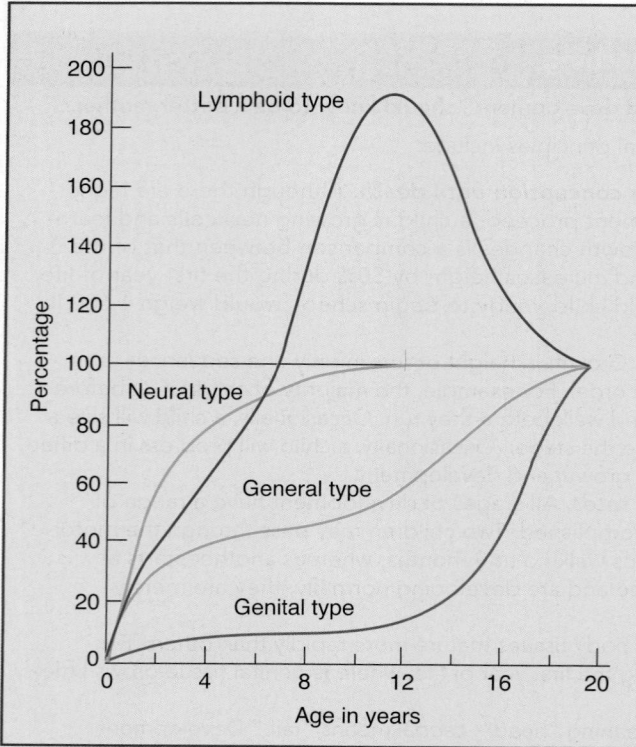

Figure 28.2 The main types of postnatal growth of various body tissue types. (Redrawn from Scammon, R. E. [1930]. The measurement of the body in childhood. In J. A. Harris, C. M. Jackson, D. G. Paterson, et al. [Eds.], *The measurement of man* [pp. 214–226]. Minneapolis, MN: University of Minnesota Press, with permission.)

QSEN Checkpoint Question 28.1

INFORMATICS

John is 6 years old. The nurse should teach his parents that which of his body systems should be reaching its peak point of development at this time?
a. His neurologic system
b. His lymphatic system
c. His respiratory system
d. His musculoskeletal system

Look in Appendix A for the best answer and rationale.

Factors Influencing Growth and Development

Genetic and environmental influences are primary factors in determining if a child will be able to reach his or her genetic potential.

Temperament—the typical way a child reacts to situations—is an example of genetic influence. Whether a fetus enjoyed a healthy uterine existence or whether the child was born into a family with sufficient funds to supply adequate health care are examples of environmental influences (Pike, Jane Pillow, & Lucas, 2012). Whether a child receives good nutrition, beginning with being breastfed, is yet another (Johnston, Landers, Noble, et al., 2012). It is the intertwining of these

or a combination of these factors that determines how each child grows and matures.

GENETICS

From the moment of conception when a sperm and ovum fuse, the basic genetic makeup of an individual is cast. In addition to physical characteristics such as eye color and height potential, inheritance determines characteristics such as learning style. A child may also inherit a genetic abnormality, which could result in disability or illness at birth or later in life and so prevent optimal growth.

GENDER

On average, girls are born lighter (by an ounce or two) and shorter (by an inch or two) than boys. Boys tend to keep this height and weight advantage until prepuberty, at which time girls surge ahead as they begin their puberty growth spurt 6 months to 1 year earlier than boys. By the end of puberty (age 14 to 16 years), boys again tend to be taller and heavier than girls. This difference in growth patterns is why different growth charts are used for boys than for girls (available at http://thePoint.lww.com/Flagg8e) (Pastor & Reuben, 2011).

HEALTH

A child who inherits a genetically transmitted disease may not grow as rapidly or develop as fully as a healthy child depending on the type of illness and the therapy or care available for the disease. Before insulin was discovered in 1922, for example, many children with type 1 diabetes mellitus died in early childhood; those who lived were left physically challenged. Currently, with good health supervision and insulin therapy, the effects of type 1 diabetes can be minimized so that children with diabetes both grow and thrive. Diabetes is still a major factor in the health of children, however. As more and more children become obese because of fast-food diets and lack of an exercise program, type 2 diabetes now has begun to occur in children as young as school age (Dea, 2011; Morgan, 2012)

INTELLIGENCE

Children with high intelligence do not generally grow faster physically than other children, but they do tend to advance faster in skills. Occasionally, children of high intelligence actually fall behind in physical skills because they spend their time with books or mental games rather than with games that develop motor skills. Intelligence begins to make major differences as children become adolescents and begin to plan future careers (Viner, Ozer, Denny, et al., 2012).

TEMPERAMENT

Temperament is the usual reaction pattern of an individual or an individual's characteristic manner of thinking, behaving, or reacting to stimuli in the environment. Unlike cognitive or moral development, temperament is not developed in stages but is an inborn characteristic set at birth. Understanding that children are not all alike (e.g., some adapt quickly to new situations, others adapt slowly, some react intensely, some react passively based on an inborn disposition) helps parents better understand why their children are different from one another and help them plan individualized care for each child.

Reaction Patterns

Chess and Thomas (1985) are the researchers who identified nine separate characteristics that define temperament, or how children react to common situations. Each child's pattern is made up of a combination of these individual elements.

Activity Level

The level of activity among children differs widely right from birth. Some babies seem to be constantly on the go and rarely are quiet. They wiggle and squirm in their crib as early as 2 weeks of age. Parents put such children to sleep in one end of a crib and find them in the other end an hour later; such children will not stay seated in bathtubs and refuse to be confined in playpens. Other babies, by contrast, move little, stay where they are placed, and appear to take in their environment in a quieter, more docile way. Both patterns are normal; they merely reflect the extremes of *activity level*, one characteristic of temperament.

Rhythmicity

A child who has *rhythmicity* manifests a regular rhythm in physiologic functions. Even as infants, such children tend to wake up at the same time each morning, are hungry at regular 4-hour periods, nap the same time every day, and have a bowel movement at the same time every day. They are predictable and easy to care for because their parents learn early on what to expect from them. On the other end of the scale are infants who rarely awaken at the same time 2 days in a row. They may go a long time without eating 1 day and the next day appear hungry almost immediately after a feeding. Such children are typically more difficult to care for because it is difficult to anticipate a schedule for them. Parents must constantly adapt their own routine to the child's routine.

Approach

Approach refers to a child's response on initial contact to a new stimulus. When introduced to a new situation, some children approach the challenge in an unruffled manner. They smile and "talk" to strangers and accept a first feeding or a new food without spitting up or fussing. They explore new toys without apprehension. Other children demonstrate withdrawal rather than approach. They cry at the sight of strangers, new toys, and new foods; they fuss the first time they are placed in a bathtub. They are difficult to take on vacation or to meet a new child-care provider because they react so fearfully to new situations.

Adaptability

Adaptability is the ability to change one's reaction to stimuli over time. Infants who are adaptable can change their first reaction to a situation without exhibiting extreme distress. The first time such children are placed in a bathtub, they might protest loudly, for example, but by the third time, they sit splashing happily. This is in contrast to infants who cry for months whenever they are put into a bathtub or who cannot seem to accustom themselves to a new bed, new car seat, or new caregiver.

Intensity of Reaction

A child who has an *intensity of reaction* meets new situations with their whole being. They cry loudly, thrash their arms, and begin temper tantrums when their diapers are wet, when they are hungry, and when their parents leave them. Other children, probably equally frustrated or angry, rarely demonstrate such overt symptoms or have a mild- or low-intensity reaction to stress.

Distractibility

Children who are easily distracted or who can easily shift their attention to a new situation (*distractibility*) are easy to care for. If they are crying over the loss of a toy, they can be appeased by the offer of a different one. If children cannot be distracted this way, their parents may describe them as stubborn, willful, or unwilling to compromise because they persistently return to an activity or refuse to adapt or change.

Attention Span and Persistence

Attention span is the ability to remain interested in a project or activity for an average length of time. Like other aspects of temperament, this can vary a great deal among children. Some play by themselves with one toy for an hour; others spend no more than 1 or 2 minutes with each toy. The degree of *persistence* also varies. Some infants keep trying to perform an activity even when they fail time after time; others stop trying after one unsuccessful attempt.

Threshold of Response

The *threshold of response* is the intensity level of stimulation necessary to evoke a reaction. Children with a low threshold need to meet little frustration before they react; those with a high threshold need intense frustration before they become upset over a situation or with a person.

Mood Quality

A child who is always happy and laughing is said to have a positive *mood quality*. Obviously, this can make a major difference in the parents' enjoyment of a child; parents tend to spend more time with a child with a positive mood quality than with a child who seems always unhappy and whining or has a negative mood quality.

Nursing Implications and Temperament

Four categories or levels of temperament are shown in Box 28.3. Children who have a usual activity level and regular rhythmicity; who approach and adapt to new situations easily; and who have a long attention span, a high level of persistence, and a positive mood quality are "ideal" or "easy" children to care for from a parent's point of view. Highly active infants are much more difficult for parents to care for, especially if they demonstrate irregular physiologic rhythms, withdrawal rather than approach, and little ability to adapt. Such children require more planning and creative distraction measures.

Bringing characteristics of temperament to parents' attention helps them better understand their child and lays the foundation for beginning to accept and respect the child as an individual, which is essential for successful childrearing (Hudson, Dodd, Lyneham, et al., 2011).

Noticing children's temperament as they are admitted to a hospital can help you anticipate their probable reactions to procedures or pain. For example, a child with an intense reactivity pattern may voice even a minor discomfort loudly; a child with a less intense pattern may barely react. Both situations make it difficult to evaluate the true level of pain the children are experiencing unless temperament is considered.

BOX 28.3

Nursing Care Planning to Empower a Family

CATEGORIES OF TEMPERAMENT

Q. Mrs. Olson asks the nurse why her children solve problems so differently.

A. Children's temperament can be a reason they approach problems differently.

The Easy Child

Children are rated as "easy to care for" if they have a predictable rhythmicity, approach and adapt to new situations readily, have a mild-to-moderate intensity of reaction, and have an overall positive mood quality. Most children are rated by their parents as being in this category.

The Intermediate Child

Some characteristics of both easy and difficult groups are present.

The Difficult Child

Children are "difficult" if they are irregular in habits, have a negative mood quality, and withdraw rather than approach new situations. Only about 10% of children fall into this category.

The Slow-to-Warm-Up Child

Children fall into this category if, overall, they are fairly inactive, respond only mildly and adapt slowly to new situations, and have a general negative mood. About 15% of children display this pattern. When discussing this temperament with parents, try to use positive terms such as "ways to find a healthy fit for your child" rather than stressing ways the child is hard to manage.

What If . . . 28.1

John's mother describes her 3-year-old twins as being "totally different" from each other. One is shy and quiet; the other is aggressive and persistent. The nurse recognizes that she probably views which child as easier to care for? What anticipatory guidance could the nurse give her to help her better understand these differences in temperament in her children?

ENVIRONMENT

Although children cannot grow taller than their genetically programmed height potential allows, their adult height can be considerably less than their genetic potential if their environment hinders their growth. For example, a child could receive inadequate nutrition because of a family's low socioeconomic status, a parent could lack childcare skills or not give a child enough attention or stimulation, or a child could contact an infectious disease and be left with a long-term disability. Illness can lower children's appetites, thus interfering with growth; others, such as certain endocrine disorders, directly alter growth rate. Having a parent who abuses alcohol or other substances can cause such inconsistency in care that it can affect mental health (Rossow & Moan, 2012).

Environmental influences, however, like genetic ones, are not always detrimental. For example, children with phenylketonuria, an inherited metabolic disease that leads to poor growth and cognitive challenge, can achieve normal growth and development in spite of their genetic makeup if their diet (a part of the environment) is properly regulated. The following environmental influences are those most likely to affect growth and development.

Socioeconomic Level

Because health care and good nutrition both cost money, children born into families of low socioeconomic means may suffer from a lack of both of these. Poor health supervision can leave them without immunization against measles or other childhood illnesses and therefore vulnerable to permanent neurologic damage (Mulholland, Griffiths, & Biellik, 2012). Poor nutrition can also leave them vulnerable to disease because antibody formation depends on a good protein intake (Whitney & Rolfes, 2012).

The Parent–Child Relationship

What a parent expects a child to become as an adult varies from culture to culture and family to family but plays a role in how much a child is guided to try to achieve in life. Cultural norms also play a role because some cultures have different perspectives on education and value different ways of contributing to society (Box 28.4).

Children who are loved and are paid attention to by their parents thrive better than those who are not (Feigelman, 2012). Luckily, for parents and children, either parent or even a nonparent may form this primary parent–child love relationship. When assessing families, don't just examine how much time parents spend with children; examine the quality of that time because it is the quality, not the quantity, that is most important (Box 28.5). Loss of love from a primary caregiver, as might occur with the death of a parent, or interruption of parental contact through hospitalization, imprisonment, or divorce can have such an effect on a child that it interferes with a desire to eat, improve, and advance. It is important to support parents' active involvement in their child's care so that a parent–child relationship is strengthened and is valued in all healthcare and childcare settings (Vicedo, 2011).

Ordinal Position in the Family

The position of a child in the family (e.g., first-born child, middle child, youngest child, only child) and the size of the family also have some bearing on a child's growth and development. An only child or the oldest child in a family, for example, generally excels in language development because conversations are mainly with adults. Youngest children, in contrast, may develop language more slowly, especially if older children talk "baby talk" with them. Children learn by watching other children, however, so a youngest child who has many examples to watch may excel in other skills, such as toilet training or writing at an early age.

Health

Diseases that come from environmental sources can have as strong an influence on growth and development as genetically inherited diseases. Infants cared for in neonatal intensive

BOX 28.4

Nursing Care Planning to Respect Cultural Diversity

Not all nations foster the growth and development of children in the same manner, in part because of cultural variations. Childhood in the United States covers a relatively long period. In other countries, childhood is short because girls are asked to assume domestic responsibilities early in life and outside or farm work is required early for boys. In some countries, the predominant theory of childrearing is protective nurturing. Children are not rushed into new experiences like toilet training or beginning school. In others, it is customary to treat children in a harsh, strict manner, using shame or corporal punishment for discipline. Praising children for learning a new skill may be viewed as unnecessary or actually harmful because this could result in a child being subject to evil forces. In some Asian cultures, an infant's personality is thought to depend not so much on genetic or environmental influences but on the year and time of birth.

What foods children receive also varies with culture. Vegetables such as jicama and chayote, for example, may not even be recognized by children in the Northeast United States but may be popular with those in the Southwest.

Asking a parent questions such as "What do you do when your baby cries?" "What kind of things do you think a 2-year-old should be able to do?" and "What do you do when your 4-year-old misbehaves?" can help you to isolate and better understand cultural differences. Recognizing cultural variations this way helps to plan care individualized to a particular child and family.

BOX 28.5

Nursing Care Planning Tips for Effective Communication

You see John's mother in clinic for a follow-up visit and ask about his socialization at meals.

Tip: Avoid asking multiple or compound questions because you might only receive incomplete answers. Ask individual questions with focused follow-up questions to obtain the information you need.

Nurse: How are you today, Mrs. Olson? How is John?

Mrs. Olson: I'm good.

Nurse: And John?

Mrs. Olson: He's the same.

Nurse: Is your family eating more meals together?

Mrs. Olson: We eat together for sure three nights a week.

Nurse: Does John seem to enjoy that?

Mrs. Olson: He never talks at the table. It's as if he isn't there.

Nurse: Let's talk about other ways you could bring John into the family.

care units, for example, may develop some decrease in hearing because of the overstimulation of sound, an example of health being directly influenced by the environment (Matook, Sullivan, Salisbury, et al., 2010). Children who have residual heart impairment as a result of contracting rheumatic fever might be limited in their ability to play an active sport. The eventual degree of disability will depend, however, not only on the damage caused by the actual disease but also on the attitudes of the people around the child (i.e., how disabled they believe the child to be) (Russell, Sinclair, Poteat, et al., 2012). When parents treat children differently after they have been critically ill (i.e., don't react warmly to them), the children are referred to as "vulnerable children" (Green & Solnit, 1964). Fortunately, if an illness does not last long and leaves no permanent disability, most children achieve catch-up growth and score well on growth measures after an illness.

Nutrition

In the past 20 years, nutrition has become a major focus of health promotion and disease prevention because the quality of a child's nutrition during the growing years (and prenatally) has such a major influence on health, weight, and stature (Whitney & Rolfes, 2012). Poor maternal nutrition may limit the growth and intelligence potential of a child by furnishing a less than desired prenatal environment. In some communities, poor nutrition has such an effect that children begin to show inadequate physical growth as early as infancy. A lack of energy and stamina prevents children from learning at their best intellectual level, which causes them to fall behind in school. In contrast, in other communities, eating too much food (or the wrong kinds of food) causes as many as 20% of children to be obese (Skinner & Skelton, 2014).

Children who become obese may develop motor skills more slowly than other children because physical movement is more tiring for them. Obese children are also likely targets of taunting by playmates and so run a risk of lacking a strong and supportive group of friends. Lack of a strong support system can lead to depression as the child reaches adolescence (Ting, Huang, Tu, et al., 2012).

Nutrition also plays a vital role in the body's susceptibility to disease because poor nutrition limits the body's ability to resist infection. Lack of calcium could leave a child prone to rickets, a disease that affects growth by causing shortening or bowing of long bones. Lack of vitamins can lead to visual impairments, poor healing, and poor bone growth. Excessive obesity is linked with the development of type 2 diabetes in children as young as 6 years of age (Sizer & Whitney, 2011) as well as being linked to hypertension and heart disease.

QSEN Checkpoint Question 28.2

EVIDENCE-BASED PRACTICE

Preventing obesity is a major healthcare goal worldwide. To determine if preschoolers are aware of what an average weight child looks like in contrast to one who is overweight, nurse researchers recruited 17 children between 4 and 5 years of age from preschool settings. Each child was weighed and measured for height so their body mass index (BMI) could be calculated and then shown images of children of various body shapes and sizes. All the children were able to correctly identify the body shape that depicted an overweight child as if they understood the concept of overweight. When asked if they liked their own body shape, however, even those who were overweight answered "yes" or apparently had difficulty applying the concept of overweight to themselves (Burgess & Broome, 2012).

John shares a similar body shape with his mother and is overweight. The nurse identifies which statement by John as typical according to the study?

a. "No one looks fat in my family."
b. "I like the way I look in my uniform."
c. "We look like the people in these pictures."
d. "People shouldn't worry about what they look like."

Look in Appendix A for the best answer and rationale.

Nutrition Guidelines for a Healthy Diet

Since 1980, a new edition of the *Dietary Guidelines for Americans* has been published every 5 years with the goal of promoting health and preventing disease (available at http://health.gov/dietaryguidelines/2015/guidelines/executive-summary/). The 2015–2020 edition of *Dietary Guidelines* focuses on healthy eating patterns. Because patterns of eating are established in early childhood and persist throughout a lifetime, it is paramount to educate parents to ensure healthy eating in children. Parents model eating patterns for their children.

Eating patterns represent the totality of all foods and beverages consumed. Nutritional needs should be met primarily from foods, especially nutrient-dense foods. Vegetables, fruits, whole grains, and dairy are associated with reduced risk of many chronic diseases and improved health in children. The new guidelines state that eating patterns can be adaptable and tailored to the individual's social-cultural and personal preferences. It is important to explore the family's preferences when providing nutrition education.

Physical activity is also a key recommendation. No specific recommendations are made for children under the age of 6 years,

but youth ages 6 to 17 years need at least 60 minutes of physical activity per day. This can include aerobic exercise as well as muscle and bone strengthening activities 2 or more days each week.

Differences in calories for males and females start at age 9 years. They range from 1,000 calories a day for a 2-year-old to 2,400 calories a day for an 18-year-old male and 1,800 calories a day for an 18-year-old female. Table 28.1 lists recommended servings for children from the five food groups. In addition, good nutrition in children should follow a number of healthy eating pattern guidelines including:

- **Eat a variety of foods.** Choices from all food groups—dairy, protein, fruits, vegetables, and grains—should be included in meals every day. It is also important to vary choices within each food group because not all foods within a group are nutritionally equivalent.
- **Balance the food you eat with physical activity and maintain or improve your weight.** Although the tendency for obesity may be inherited, being overweight in early life also seems to play a long-term role. Urge parents to be certain their infants receive all the nutrients they need for the substantial growth they are undergoing (including a percentage of fat because this is important for myelination of nerves); at the same time, it is important that infants not be overfed so they do not become obese (Kmietowicz, 2012). Physical activity, balanced with calcium intake, is the secret to strong bones and the reduction of osteoporosis (Jones, 2011).
- **Choose a diet with plenty of grain products, vegetables, and fruits.** Foods with starch and fiber are more beneficial for gastrointestinal function than more processed foods. Fiber, in particular, has been linked to the lowered incidence of a variety of illnesses such as constipation and perhaps colon cancer in later life (Brownawell, Caers, Gibson, et al., 2012). Fiber can be included as early as during preschool years in the form of whole-grain cereals and raw fruits such as apples.
- **Choose a diet low in saturated fat and trans fats.** According to the *2015-2020 Dietary Guidelines*, "Healthy eating patterns limit saturated and *trans* fats. Less than 10% of daily calories should come from saturated fats. Foods that are high in saturated fat include but-

TABLE 28.1 FOOD GROUP SERVINGS FOR CHILDREN

		Recommended Daily Amounts		
Group	Examples of Foods	Children 2–6 Years of Age	Older Children	Major Nutrients Provided By the Food Group
Grains	Cereals, rice, pasta (best if whole-grain and enriched)	6 servings	6–11 servings	Thiamine, niacin, riboflavin (if enriched), iron (if enriched), incomplete protein, carbohydrates
Vegetables	Vegetables (yellow and green)	3 servings	3–5 servings	Vitamin A, iron, calcium, carbohydrates (include vitamin A source at least every other day)
Fruit	Oranges, apples, lemons	2 servings	2–4 servings	Vitamin C (include vitamin C daily), carbohydrates
Dairy	Whole milk and other milk products such as yogurt and cheese	2 servings	2–3 servings	Calcium, phosphorus, complete protein, riboflavin, niacin, vitamin D (if vitamin D–fortified milk used), fats
Protein	Muscle meats (veal, beef, pork) dry beans, eggs, fish, poultry	2 servings	2–3 servings	Complete protein, iron, thiamine, riboflavin, niacin, vitamin B_{12}, fats

From Office of Disease Prevention and Health Promotion. (2016). *Top 10 things you need to know about the 2015–2020 Dietary Guidelines for Americans.* Retrieved from http://health.gov/news/dietary-guidelines-digital-press-kit/2016/01/top-10-things-you-need-to-know/

ter, whole milk, meats that are not labeled as lean, and tropical oils such as coconut and palm oil. Saturated fats should be replaced with unsaturated fats, such as canola or olive oil." For children, fat intake does not need to be restricted for the first 2 years of life because fat is necessary for myelination of spinal nerves. Thereafter, fat intake can be tailored to meet the guidelines of 30% of total intake (saturated fat should be less than 7% of total intake) for both children and adults.

- **Choose a diet moderate in sugars.** Too much sugar in a diet can contribute to both dental caries and obesity (Danyliw, Vatanparast, Nikpartow, et al., 2012). In addition, refined sugar such as is used in soft drinks, prepared foods, candy, and chocolate represents empty calories, or is high in calories yet provides no essential nutrients. Although children need adequate carbohydrates for energy, parents can give their children a good start by preventing excessive sugar intake.

- **Choose a diet moderate in salt and sodium.** The taste for salt is acquired and plays a role in both heart disease and hypertension. If unsalted or only lightly salted solid food is offered to infants from the time they begin solid food, they do not develop a desire for heavily salted foods. It is helpful to assess the diet of school-age children and check whether they are eating a diet heavier in salt than necessary because of the availability of many salty after-school snacks.

- **If drinking alcoholic beverages, do so in moderation.** Adolescents are at increased risk for establishing unhealthy patterns of alcohol use, particularly binge drinking, as they begin to explore adult life. Educating them about the long-term consequences, such as liver disease, from long-term alcohol use is as important as educating them on the importance of healthy nutrition to help ensure proper growth (see Chapter 33 for a discussion of adolescents).

Components of a Healthy Diet

Eating a variety of foods from all five food groups in moderation is a way of guaranteeing the intake of a balanced diet of proteins, carbohydrates, fats, vitamins, and minerals (Fig. 28.3).

Protein

Protein is the major component of bones, skin, hair, and muscle and is responsible for a wide variety of essential functions in the body. Because it is essential for growth, protein

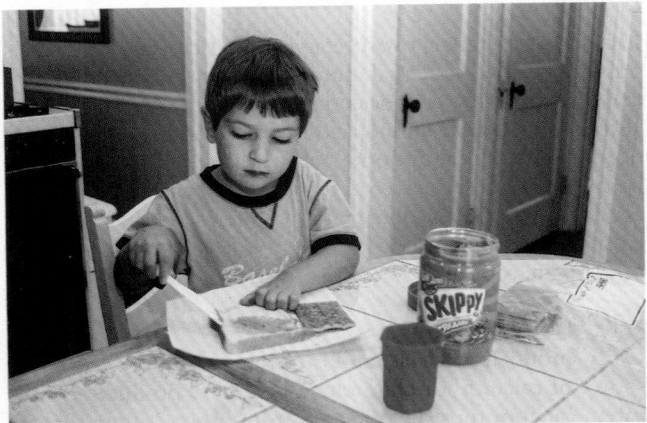

Figure 28.3 Good nutritional habits developed early in life provide a child with a health advantage.

intake is crucial for children. Complete proteins contain all amino acids; incomplete proteins do not, but combining two types of incomplete proteins (e.g., pasta and beans) allows the body to construct complete proteins.

Carbohydrate

Carbohydrates are the main and preferred fuel of the body to supply energy, so they are essential to the functioning of body systems and the neurologic system, in particular. This makes carbohydrates vitally important to infants and toddlers because their brain cells are actively growing. As all athletes learn, sugar supplies an immediate but short-term source of energy; starches, as a rule, supply sustained energy.

Fat

Dietary fat is a second source of energy for the body. It can be an immediate energy source or can be stored if not used, then released when energy is required. Some fat deposits also serve as insulating material for subcutaneous tissues; in infants, fats are necessary to ensure myelination of nerve fibers.

Vitamins

Vitamins are organic compounds essential for specific metabolic actions in cells. They do not produce energy but are needed by cells to produce energy. For children, fat-soluble vitamins (A, D, K, and E) are mainly supplied by fortified dairy products, fortified cereals, and plant or fish oils. Such vitamins are not absorbed from the gastrointestinal tract by themselves but only if accompanied by fat molecules, which is why fish and plant oils are such good sources of these. Once absorbed, they are used by the cells for growth and function or are stored in the liver or fat cells for later use. Because fat-soluble vitamins can be stored by the body this way, an infant or child can ingest too many of them, although overdosing usually occurs from overuse of supplements rather than from dietary sources.

Water-soluble vitamins (B complex and C) do not need fat for absorption and are not stored well in the body, so they must be taken daily to maintain effective levels in the body. They are found most abundantly in fruits and vegetables. Sources and functions of all the essential vitamins and results of their deficiencies are summarized in Table 28.2.

Minerals

Minerals are necessary for building new cells as well as for the regulation of body processes such as fluid and electrolyte balance, nerve transmission, and muscle contractions, making them vital for optimal health in a growing infant or child. Minerals are classified according to the amounts needed daily. If more than 100 mg is needed daily, a mineral is a *macronutrient* (a major mineral). If the amount needed is less than 100 mg, it is a minor mineral or *micronutrient*. Trace minerals refer to those needed in only extremely small amounts. Sources and functions of various minerals and results of their deficiencies are shown in Table 28.3.

Promoting Adequate Nutritional Intake in Vegetarian Diets

Increasing numbers of adults of childrearing age are vegetarians; therefore, many women during pregnancy and children during their years of most rapid growth eat such diets (Krebs & Primak, 2011). Families select vegetarian diets for many reasons, including:

- Ecologic: If everyone ate lower on the food chain, world hunger could be reduced.

TABLE 28.2 VITAMINS ESSENTIAL FOR HEALTH

Vitamin	Selected Dietary Sources	Function in Body	Results of Deficiency
Fat Soluble			
A (retinol)	Liver, carrots, spinach	Important for night vision and corneal integrity and growth	Keratinization of the eye (xerophthalmia) and blindness
D	Egg yolk, margarine, salmon, fortified milk, fortified cereals	Regulates absorption of calcium and phosphorus for bone growth	Rickets (bone deformity) in growing children
E	Margarine, corn oil, peanuts	An antioxidant that protects red blood cells from destruction by oxygen	In immature infants, severe anemia from destruction of red blood cells
K	Cabbage, spinach, pork, best source: green leafy vegetables	Aids blood clotting (synthesis of prothrombin)	Bleeding from lack of sufficient clotting action
Water Soluble			
B complex:			
Thiamine	Wheat germ, yeast, pork	Important for use of glucose in cells	Beriberi, a disease that causes nerve paralysis
Riboflavin	Beef, chicken, liver, avocados, milk	Breaks down fatty acids and amino acids for energy	Red swollen tongue, inflamed eyes, fissures of lips
Niacin	Peanuts, rice bran, liver	Converts glucose to energy; involved in carbohydrate, protein, and fat metabolism	Pellagra (diarrhea, mental confusion, dermatitis, death)
Vitamin B_6 (pyridoxine)	Liver, herring, salmon, chicken, fish, pork, eggs	Metabolizes amino acids and glucose	Neuritis, depression, nausea, vomiting
Vitamin B_{12} (cobalamin)	Lamb, beef kidney, egg yolk, animal products	Blood formation; DNA and RNA synthesis; myelin formation; carbohydrate, protein, and fat metabolism	Macrocytic, megaloblastic anemia (large, nonfunctioning red blood cells)
Folic acid (folacin)	Liver, asparagus, bran	Red and white blood cell structure	Poor red blood cell formation
C (ascorbic acid)	Broccoli, collards, citrus fruit	Collagen structure, antioxidant	Scurvy (weakness, easy bleeding, joint pain)

All fat-soluble vitamins can be absorbed only in the presence of lipids and can be transported only in the presence of protein.

- Medical or health related: Avoiding animal foods stops the ingestion of hormones and chemicals used in meat and poultry production as well as lowers serum cholesterol and saturated fat, thereby reducing the frequency of atherosclerosis and obesity.
- Philosophical: They may hold a belief that killing animals for food is unnecessary or wrong.
- Spirituality: Religions such as Hinduism and Seventh-Day Adventist promote a vegetarian lifestyle. Islam and Judaism also have some restrictions on what meat can be eaten.
- Economic: Vegetables and grains are less expensive than animal-based food.

Although a balanced vegetarian diet is sufficient during childhood, careful assessment and family education may be necessary to ensure a child's intake is adequate for growth. Urge parents to become knowledgeable about good nutrition so they are aware of ways to include essential nutrients in vegetarian diets for growing children, particularly if their children participate in active sports.

Five main types of vegetarian diets commonly seen include:
- The lacto-ovo-vegetarian diet, which includes dairy products ("lacto"), eggs ("ovo"), and plants (vegetables, fruits, and grains)
- The ovovegetarian diet, which includes eggs but excludes dairy products
- The lacto-vegetarian diet, which includes dairy products but excludes eggs
- The vegan diet, which excludes all animal products and consists of only vegetables, fruits, and grains

- The macrobiotic diet, which is a primarily vegetarian diet. Its main sources of protein are grains, seeds, and nuts, but small quantities of egg, fish, and wild game can be added.

The vegan diet is obviously the most restrictive of these diets, so it is usually recommended that parents be extremely conscientious about including a variety of foods to help ensure their children are receiving adequate nutrients. All families who eat vegetarian diets need to be conscientious that their children receive adequate amounts of several specific nutrients.

Protein

Lacto-ovo-vegetarian, ovovegetarian, and lacto-vegetarian diets provide all of the essential amino acids for growth (both eggs and dairy products provide complete proteins). Vegan diets can also supply essential amino acids by cereal and legume combinations such as peanut butter and wheat bread, corn and lima beans, pasta and beans, corn tortillas and beans, or chickpeas and sesame seeds. Complementary proteins do not have to be eaten at the same meal to be effective, as long as varied plant proteins are consumed over the course of a day.

Calcium

Dairy products such as milk and cheese supply the usual source of calcium for children. When dairy products are not eaten, calcium must be obtained from other sources such as green leafy vegetables (broccoli, spinach, or grain products) or calcium-fortified tofu or soy flour.

TABLE 28.3 MINERALS ESSENTIAL FOR HEALTH

Mineral	Selected Dietary Sources	Function in Body	Results of Deficiency or Excess
Macronutrients			
Calcium	Milk, hard cheese	Formation of bone and teeth, muscle contractility	Improper bone growth and maintenance shown by diseases such as rickets in children
Phosphorus	Milk, meats	Formation of bone and teeth, used in cell structure, aids use of glucose	Deficiency unlikely as long as calcium and protein needs are met
Sodium	Table salt	Regulates fluid volume and pH	Deficiency rare but excess leads to hypertension in genetically determined individuals
Chloride	Table salt	Formation of hydrochloric acid, regulates body fluid with sodium	Deficiency rare except with vomiting, which causes loss of hydrochloric acid
Potassium	Meats, dried fruits	Major cation of cells, essential for electrical conduction in muscle and therefore in heart action	Deficiency leading to muscle weakness and heart irritability, occurs in people taking diuretics because potassium is excreted with urine
Sulfur	Milk, meat, eggs	Essential for protein formation and cell growth	Deficiency rare as long as protein intake is adequate
Magnesium	Cocoa, nuts, green leafy vegetables	Relaxation of muscles after contraction	Deficiency leads to muscle contraction
Micronutrients			
Iodine	Seafood, dairy, iodized salt	Formation of thyroxine and regulation of metabolic rate	Reduced basal metabolic rate, goiter (enlarged thyroid gland)
Iron	Meats, fish, dried fruits, nuts, fortified cereals	Formation of hemoglobin, transport of oxygen to body cells	Deficiency leads to microcytic (small) and hypochromic (pale) red blood cells (iron-deficiency anemia); excess leads to infiltration of tissue (hemosiderosis)
Copper	Nuts, raisins, legumes	Formation of collagen and nerve fibers	Anemia, neutropenia, and severe bone demineralization
Fluoride	Fluoridated water	Reduces dental caries and demineralization from bone	Dental caries
Zinc	Meat, eggs, seafood	Formation of eyes, male reproductive organs, insulin, and taste sensation	Diabetes-like symptoms because of decreased insulin production, poor taste sensation leading to poor food intake
Manganese	Nuts, grains, legumes	Formation of enzymes	Deficiency unlikely
Molybdenum	Organ meats, grains	Mobilizes iron in body	Deficiency apparently unknown
Cobalt	Many sources	Formation of red blood cells in bone marrow	Deficiency rare as long as animal food sources are ingested
Selenium	Seafood, kidney, liver	Immunoglobulin formation and prevention of oxidation of cells	Deficiency unknown
Chromium	Meat, cheese, grains	Glucose metabolism	Deficiency seen only in severe malnutrition
Silicon	Many sources	Aids growth of connective tissue and bone	Retarded growth and bone deformity
Nickel	Many sources	Duplication of growth of cells	Has not been determined to be essential for health in humans
Vanadium	Many sources	Lipid metabolism	Has not been determined to be essential for health in humans
Tin	Many sources	Blood formation	Has not been determined to be essential for health in humans

Iron

Because there may be an association between iron-deficiency anemia and learning deficits, children need to consume good sources of iron (Black, Quigg, Hurley, et al., 2011). Meat is the richest source of iron. With meat omitted from a diet, parents should include this from foods such as legumes, whole grains, fortified cereals, dark-green leafy vegetables, or dried fruits. Vitamin C enhances the duodenal absorption of iron found in plants, so eating fruits and vegetables rich in vitamin C such as oranges or broccoli aids iron absorption.

Vitamins

Vitamin B_{12} is unique among vitamins because it is present only in animal products (Whitney & Rolfes, 2012). This includes eggs and milk. Children who totally omit animal sources need to have this vitamin supplemented daily. Reliable supplements of vitamin B_{12} include vitamin B_{12} tablets or fortified foods such as commercial breakfast cereals, soy beverages, and some brands of nutritional yeast.

Riboflavin is a B vitamin normally supplied by fortified milk. When dairy products are not eaten, it can be supplied by soy milk, vegetables, or brewer's yeast, all of which contain all the B vitamins except vitamin B$_{12}$. Good sources of riboflavin in vegan diets are whole and enriched grains and cereals, nuts, and dark-green leafy vegetables.

Vitamin D is necessary for calcium and phosphorus metabolism and is normally supplied in fortified milk. It is not present in plant foods and therefore must be supplemented in a vegan or ovovegetarian diet by vitamin D drops or tablets. Exposure to sunshine also supplies vitamin D but is generally an inadequate source (Whitney & Rolfes, 2012).

Minerals

Zinc is present primarily in animal foods but is also present in brewer's yeast, nuts, and wheat germ; therefore, zinc deficiency is not a problem with vegetarian diets. Iodine is supplied normally by seafood. In a vegan or vegetarian diet, it can be supplied by seaweed and iodized table salt. Many families add a small amount of powdered kelp (a seaweed) to food two or three times a week to ensure an adequate iodine intake. Calcium, as mentioned previously, can be supplied by green leafy vegetables or a daily supplement.

Total Calories

Plant foods have fewer total calories than meats. Generous servings of nuts and legumes are recommended to take the place of meat servings. All other recommended serving sizes for various caloric level patterns are the same as those presented in meat-containing food guidelines (available at http://thePoint.lww.com/Flagg8e).

Theories of Child Development

A *theory* is a systematic statement of principles that provides a framework for explaining a phenomenon. Developmental theories are theories that provide road maps for explaining human development.

Developmental tasks are a skill or a growth responsibility arising at a particular time in an individual's life, the achievement of which will provide a foundation for the accomplishment of future tasks. It is not so much chronologic age as the completion of the task that defines whether a child has passed from one developmental stage of childhood to another. For example, children are not toddlers just because they are 1 year plus 1 day old; they become toddlers when they have passed through the developmental stage of infancy. For reference, however, childhood is generally divided into the seven age periods shown in Table 28.4.

A number of types of developmental theories have been proposed to describe how children grow emotionally,

psychologically, and intellectually as they pass through these different periods. *Sociocultural theories* are those that stress the importance of environment on growth and development. *Learning theory* suggests children are like blank pages that can be shaped by learning. Cognitive theorists such as Piaget stress learning skills are the key to achieving success in life. *Epigenetic theories* stress that genes are the true basis for growth and development. Previously discounted as too simplistic, epigenetic theories are being revised and given new credence based on new knowledge about genes now available through the Human Genome Project and the mapping of all human genes (Naidoo, Pawitan, Soong, et al., 2011).

Still, other theories deal mainly with negative aspects of childrearing that can lead to mental illness in children, either immediately, or later when a child reaches adulthood (see discussion on Freud that follows). Erikson is a psychoanalyst who discussed positive aspects necessary for normal growth and development so that a mentally healthy and productive adult will result (Erikson, 1993).

FREUD'S PSYCHOANALYTIC THEORY

Sigmund Freud (1856–1939), an Austrian neurologist and the founder of psychoanalysis, offered the first real theory of personality development (Freud, 1962; Freud & Brill, 1995). The theory, based on Freud's observations of mentally disturbed adults, described adult behavior as being the result of instinctual drives of a primarily sexual nature (*libido*). He described child development as being a series of psychosexual stages in which a child's sexual gratification becomes focused on a particular body part at each stage. These stages are summarized in Table 28.5.

Criticisms of Freud's Theory

To construct his theory, Freud relied on his knowledge of people seen in his practice and looked at circumstances that lead to mental illness (Freud & Brill, 1995). This "looking at illness" rather than "looking at wellness" perspective limits the applicability of the theory as a health promotion measure. The theory is also criticized as being gender biased because females are viewed in a less favorable light than males. Gender bias has the potential to perpetuate gender inequality, which doesn't provide a level playing field for women (Brandt, 2011).

QSEN Checkpoint Question 28.3

TEAMWORK & COLLABORATION

John, at 6 years old, is a school-age child. What should members of the nurse's interprofessional team recognize when caring for school-age children according to Freud?

   a. It's important for parents to teach children creativity during this time.

   b. Children develop their moral compass or spirituality during school-age years.

   c. Freud saw the school-age period as a largely latent or inactive period.

   d. Every school-age child needs responsibilities in order to learn trust and integrity.

Look in Appendix A for the best answer and rationale.

TABLE 28.4 BASIC DIVISIONS OF CHILDHOOD

Stage	Age Period
Neonate	First 28 days of life
Infant	1 month–1 year
Toddler	1–3 years
Preschooler	3–5 years
School-age child	6–12 years
Adolescent	13–17 years
Late adolescent	18–21 years

TABLE 28.5 SUMMARY OF FREUD'S AND ERIKSON'S THEORIES OF PERSONALITY DEVELOPMENT

	Freud's Stages of Childhood		Erikson's Stages of Childhood	
	Psychosexual Stage	*Nursing Implications*	*Developmental Task*	*Nursing Implications*
Infant	Oral stage: Child explores the world by using the mouth.	Provide oral stimulation by giving pacifiers; do not discourage thumb sucking.	Developmental task is to form a sense of trust versus mistrust. Child learns to love and be loved.	Provide a primary caregiver. Provide experiences that add to security.
Toddler	Anal stage: Child learns to control urination and defecation.	Help children achieve bowel and bladder control without undue emphasis on its importance.	Developmental task is to form a sense of autonomy versus shame. Child learns to be independent and make decisions for self.	Provide opportunities for independent decision making, such as choosing own clothes.
Preschooler	Phallic stage: Child learns sexual identity through awareness of genital area.	Accept children's sexual interest, such as fondling his or her own genitals, as a normal area of exploration.	Developmental task is to form a sense of initiative versus guilt. Child learns how to do things (basic problem solving) and that doing things is desirable.	Provide opportunities for exploring new places or activities. Allow free-form play.
School-age child	Latent stage: Child's personality development appears to be nonactive or dormant.	Help children have positive experiences with learning so their self-esteem continues to grow.	Developmental task is to form a sense of industry versus inferiority. Child learns how to do things well.	Provide opportunities such as allowing child to assemble and complete a short project.
Adolescent	Genital stage: Adolescent develops sexual maturity and learns to establish satisfactory relationships with others.	Provide appropriate opportunities for the child to relate with opposite and own sex relationships.	Developmental task is to form a sense of identity versus role confusion. Adolescents learn who they are and what kind of person they will be.	Provide opportunities for an adolescent to discuss feelings about events important to him or her. Offer support and praise for decision making.

ERIKSON'S THEORY OF PSYCHOSOCIAL DEVELOPMENT

Erik Erikson (1902–1996) was trained in psychoanalytic theory but later developed his own theory of psychosocial development, a theory that stresses the importance of culture and society in development of the personality (Erikson, 1993). One of the main tenets of his theory, that a person's social view of self is more important than instinctual drives in determining behavior, allows for a more optimistic view of the possibilities for human growth. Whereas Freud looked at ways mental illnesses develop, Erikson looked at actions that lead to mental health. He describes eight developmental stages covering the entire life span. At each stage, there is a conflict between two opposing forces. The resolution of each conflict, or accomplishment of the developmental task of that stage, allows the individual to go on to the next phase of development. Table 28.5 summarizes Erikson's developmental stages through adolescence as compared to Freud's stages.

The Infant

According to Erikson (1993), the developmental task for infants is learning **trust versus mistrust** (other terms are "learning confidence" or "learning to love"). When an infant is hungry, a parent feeds and makes the infant comfortable again. When an infant is wet, a parent changes his or her diaper and the infant is dry again. When an infant is cold, a parent holds the baby closely. By these simple processes, infants learn to trust that when they have a need or are in distress, a parent will come and meet that need.

If care is inconsistent, inadequate, or rejecting, infants learn mistrust; they become fearful and suspicious of people and then of the world. Like a burned child who avoids fire, emotionally burned children shun the potential pain of further emotional involvement. This can cause children to be "stuck" emotionally at this stage, although they continue to grow and develop in other ways.

Fortunately, because not all children achieve developmental tasks readily, each task need not be resolved once and for all the first time it arises. The problem of trust versus mistrust, for example, is not resolved forever during the first year of life but arises again at each successive stage of development. Children who enter school with a sense of mistrust may come to trust a teacher with whom they form a close relationship; given this second chance, children can overcome early mistrust. Likewise, children who come through infancy with a sense of trust intact may have a sense of mistrust activated at a later stage if their parents divorce under unpleasant circumstances or if the child is maltreated.

The Toddler

The developmental task of the toddler is to learn **autonomy versus shame or doubt**. Autonomy (self-governance or independence) arises from a toddler's new motor and mental abilities. Children not only take pride in the new things they can accomplish but also want to do everything independently, whether it is pulling the wrapper off a piece of candy, selecting a vitamin tablet out of a bottle, flushing the toilet, or replying, "No!"

Infants appear to have difficulty differentiating between their bodies and those of others; they think of their bodies as extensions of their parents or their primary caregivers. When infants approach toddlerhood, they begin to make the differentiation. As they recognize they are separate individuals, toddlers also realize they do not always have to do what others want them to do. From this realization comes the reputation toddlers have for being negativistic, obstinate, and difficult to manage.

This reputation probably exists because parents misinterpret children's cues. For example, children's refusal to accept help putting on shoes may be seen by a parent as disobedience, whereas children may view this as insisting on performing a task they can do independently—a positive expression of autonomy.

Children who are constantly told not to try things because they will hurt themselves may be left with a stronger sense of doubt than confidence at the end of the toddler period. Children who are made to feel it is wrong to be independent may leave the toddler period with a stronger sense of shame than autonomy.

If parents recognize that toddlers need to practice those things they are capable of doing, at their own pace and in their own time, their children will develop a sense of being able to control both their muscles and impulses. However, if children leave this stage with less autonomy and shame or doubt, they can be disabled in their attempts to achieve independence and can lack confidence in their abilities to achieve well into adolescence and adulthood (Fig. 28.4).

What If . . . 28.2

John's parents repeat that they find him cold and unloving. The nurse knows he lived in a series of foster homes before he was adopted into their family. What developmental task has John been unable to complete? Could it be related to the frequent moves? What actions could the nurse recommend his new parents take to try to strengthen his unfulfilled developmental task at this point?

The Preschooler

The developmental task of the preschool period is learning **initiative versus guilt**, or learning how to do things such as drawing, building an object from blocks, or playing dress up. Children initiate motor activities of various sorts on their own or no longer merely respond to or imitate the actions of other children or their parents. The same is true for language and fantasy activities.

Another word for initiative is creativity. Whether children leave this stage with a sense of initiative outweighing a sense of guilt depends largely on how parents respond to self-initiated activities. When children are given much freedom and opportunity to initiate motor play such as running, bike riding, sliding, and wrestling or are exposed to such play materials as finger paints, sand, water, and modeling clay, their sense of initiative is reinforced. Initiative is also encouraged when parents answer a child's questions (intellectual initiative) and do not inhibit fantasy or play activity. In contrast, if children are made to feel their motor activity is bad (perhaps in a small apartment or in a hospital), their questions are a nuisance, or their play is silly, they can develop a sense of guilt over self-initiated activities that will persist in later life. Those who do not develop initiative have limited brainstorming and problem-solving skills later in life; instead, they wait for clues or guidance from others before acting. They may also be unable to use simulated learning effectively (Rutherford-Hemming, 2012).

The School-Age Child

Erikson (1993) viewed the developmental task of the school-age period as developing **industry versus inferiority**, or self-confidence rather than inferiority. During the preschool period, children learned initiative (i.e., how to do things). During school age, children learn how to do things *well*. A school-age child, while doing a project, will ask, "Am I doing this right? Is it okay to use blue?" When they are encouraged in their efforts to do practical tasks or make practical things and are praised and rewarded for the finished results, their sense of industry grows (Fig. 28.5). Parents who see their children's efforts at making and doing things as merely "busy work" or who do not show appreciation for their children's efforts may cause them to develop a sense of inferiority rather than pride and accomplishment.

Figure 28.4 A toddler enjoys active, independent exploration as part of building a sense of autonomy. Here, a boy plays outdoors on playground equipment, a setting that allows for independent decision making.

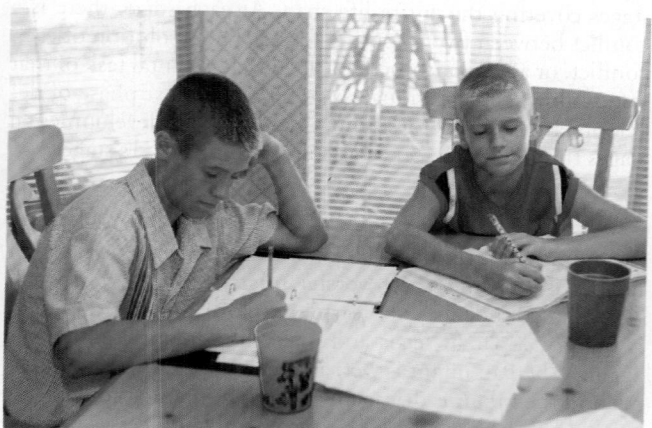

Figure 28.5 School-age children develop a sense of industry by working on projects that result in a feeling of accomplishment.

During this stage of life, a child's world grows to include the school and community; success or failure in those settings can have as lasting an impact as experiences at home. Children with an intelligence quotient of 80 or 90 (slightly below normal), for example, may have a learning style so different from the average child's that they have difficulty competing. This leads to repeated failures in their efforts to learn and reinforces a sense of inferiority even when their sense of industry has been rewarded and encouraged at home. However, children whose sense of industry has not been supported at home may have it revitalized at school through the efforts of a committed teacher. A nurse during a hospitalization could also fulfill this role.

What If . . . 28.3

John's father does not allow his 3-year-old twins to play with finger paints. If they play with crayons, he insists they color between the lines. According to Erikson, which is more important for preschoolers: allowing free-form play or teaching children that neatness and accuracy count?

The Adolescent

The new interpersonal dimension that emerges during adolescence is the development of a sense of **identity versus role confusion**. To achieve this, adolescents must bring together everything they have learned about themselves as a son or daughter, an athlete, a friend, a fast-food cook, a student, a garage band musician, and so on, and integrate these different images into a whole that makes sense. If adolescents cannot do so, they are left with role confusion or are left unsure of what kind of person they are or what kind of person they want to become. Some adolescents may seek a negative identity: being identified

Figure 28.6 Adolescents express their identity in different ways. Body piercing and tattoos makes a strong statement.

as a drug abuser or runaway is not a positive identification but may be preferable to seemingly having no identity at all. Body piercing and tattooing are ways adolescents can help establish their identity because they are outward expressions of who adolescents think they are (Fig. 28.6).

The Late Adolescent

The developmental crisis of late adolescence is achieving a sense of **intimacy versus isolation**. Intimacy is the ability to relate well with other people in preparation for developing future relationships.

A sense of intimacy grows out of earlier developmental tasks because people need a strong sense of identity before they can reach out fully and offer deep friendship or love to others. Because there is always the risk of being rejected or hurt when offering love or friendship, individuals cannot offer it if they do not have confidence that they can cope with rejection or if they did not develop a sense of trust as an infant or autonomy as a toddler. This is important for maternal and child health nursing because parents without a sense of intimacy may have more difficulty than others accepting a pregnancy and beginning to love a new child.

QSEN Checkpoint Question 28.4

QUALITY IMPROVEMENT

John, who is 6 years old, is a school-age child. According to Erikson, the nurse should identify which developmental task to integrate health promotion activities with during this period?

a. How to be creative
b. How to think abstractly
c. How to trust others
d. How to do things well

Look in Appendix A for the best answer and rationale.

A Criticism of Erikson's Theory

Erikson's main contribution to human development was the creation of stages, so that development can be broken down into separate phases for study. A criticism of his theory is that life does not occur in easily divided stages, and trying to divide it that way can create superficial divisions.

PIAGET'S THEORY OF COGNITIVE DEVELOPMENT

Jean Piaget (1896–1980), a Swiss psychologist, introduced concepts of cognitive development, or the way children learn and think. The theory has roots similar to those of both Freud and Erikson, but with differing aspects (Inhelder & Piaget, 1958). Piaget defined four stages of cognitive development, within the stages of growth, then finer units or **schemas**. To progress from one period to the next, children reorganize their thinking processes to bring them closer to adult thinking. These stages of cognitive development are summarized in Table 28.6.

The Infant

Piaget referred to the infant stage as the first four stages of the **sensorimotor stage**. Sensorimotor intelligence is practical intelligence because an infant is not yet able to use

TABLE 28.6 PIAGET'S STAGES OF COGNITIVE DEVELOPMENT

Stage of Development	Age Span	Nursing Implications
Sensorimotor		
Neonatal reflex	1 month	Stimuli are assimilated into beginning mental images. Behavior entirely reflexive.
Primary circular reaction	1–4 months	Hand–mouth and ear–eye coordination develop. Enjoyable activity for this period: a rattle or tape of parent's voice.
Secondary circular reaction	4–8 months	Infant learns to initiate, recognize, and repeat pleasurable experiences from environment. Good toy for this period: mirror; good game: peek-a-boo.
Coordination of secondary reactions	8–12 months	Infant can plan activities to attain specific goals. Good toy for this period: nesting toys (i.e., colored boxes).
Tertiary circular reaction	12–18 months	Child is able to experiment to discover new properties of objects and events. Good game for this period: throw and retrieve.
Invention of new means through mental combinations	18–24 months	Transitional phase to the preoperational thought period. Good toys for this period: those with several uses, such as blocks or colored plastic rings.
Preoperational thought	2–7 years	Thought becomes more symbolic; can arrive at answers mentally instead of through physical attempt. Comprehends simple abstractions but thinking is basically concrete and literal. Child is egocentric (unable to see the viewpoint of another). Displays static thinking (inability to remember what they started to talk about so at the end of a sentence children are talking about another topic). Concept of time is now, and concept of distance is only as far as they can see. **Centering** or focusing on a single aspect of an object causes distorted reasoning. No awareness of reversibility (for every action there is an opposite action) is present. Unable to state cause–effect relationships, categories, or abstractions. Good toy for this period: items that require imagination, such as modeling clay.
Concrete operational thought	7–12 years	Concrete operations includes systematic reasoning. Uses memory to learn broad concepts (fruit) and subgroups of concepts (apples, oranges). Classifications involve sorting objects according to attributes such as color; seriation, in which objects are ordered according to increasing or decreasing measures such as weight; and multiplication, in which objects are simultaneously classified and seriated using weight. Child is aware of reversibility, an opposite operation or continuation of reasoning back to a starting point (follows a route through a maze and then reverses steps). Understands conservation, sees constancy despite transformation (mass or quantity remains the same even if it changes shape or position). Good activity for this period: collecting and classifying natural objects such as native plants or sea shells. Expose child to other viewpoints by asking questions such as, "How do you think you'd feel if you were a nurse and had to tell a boy to stay in bed?"
Formal operational thought	12 years	Can solve hypothetical problems with scientific reasoning. Good activity for this period: "talk time" to sort through attitudes and opinions.

From Piaget, J. (1961). *The growth of logical thinking from childhood to adolescence.* New York, NY: Basic Books, with permission.

words and symbols for thinking and problem solving at this early age. At the beginning of life, babies relate to the world through their senses, using only reflex behavior. During this stage, infants learn objects in the environment—their bottle, blocks, their bed, or even a parent—are permanent and continue to exist even though they are out of sight or changed in some way. For example:

- Infants will search for a block hidden by a blanket, knowing the block still exists.

- Infants can recognize a parent remains the same person whether dressed in a robe and slippers or pants and a T-shirt.
- Infants are only ready to play peek-a-boo when they've mastered permanence because only then do they realize the person playing with them exists behind his or her hands.
- Infants identify that they are a separate entity from objects. They learn where their body stops and their bed, playthings, or parent begins.

A great deal of the mouthing and handling of objects by infants and the delight of watching a caregiver appear is part of discovering permanence.

Infants can identify their parents as different from other adults as early as 4 months of age. The world begins to make sense and the developmental task of achieving trust falls into place when the concept of **permanence** has been learned (i.e., infants know their parents exist and will return to them). Gaining a concept of permanence also contributes to separation anxiety, which can begin between 8 and 12 months of age. During this stage, infants continue to cry for their parents because they know their parents still exist even when out of sight.

The Toddler

The toddler period is one of transition as children complete the fifth and sixth stages of the sensorimotor period and begin to develop some cognitive skills of the *preoperative* period, such as symbolic thought and egocentric thinking (see Chapter 30). Children use trial and error to discover new characteristics of objects and events. A toddler sitting in a high chair who keeps dropping objects over the edge of the tray is exploring both permanence and the different actions of toys. For example, during these periods, toddlers:

- Complete their understanding of object permanence.
- Begin to be able to use symbols to represent objects.
- Start to draw conclusions only from obvious facts that they see.

The Preschooler

Preschool children move on to a substage of preoperational thought termed *intuitive thinking*. During this period, when young children look at an object, they are able to see only one of its characteristics. For example, they see a banana is yellow but do not notice that it is also long. Intuitive thinking is noticeable when children are learning about medicine (they observe it tastes bitter but cannot understand it is also good for them).

Intuitive thinking contributes to the preschooler's lack of **conservation** (the ability to discern truth, even though physical properties change) or **reversibility** (ability to retrace steps). For example, if preschoolers see water poured from a short, fat glass into a tall, thin one, they will notice only one changing characteristic. They might say there is now more water in the second glass (because the level has risen) or there is less water in the second glass (because the second glass is thinner). When the water is poured back into the first glass, they still will not understand the amount of water is unchanged, only its appearance. This immature perception leads children to make faulty conclusions as it did during the toddler period. It takes more years of development and practice for children to learn that when thought processes (i.e., knowing the amount of water did not change) and perceptions conflict, thought processes are more trustworthy.

Preschool thinking is also strongly influenced by **role fantasy** or how children would like something to turn out. Children use **assimilation** (taking in information and changing it to fit their existing ideas) as a part of this. For example, because a child wants to go outside and play, he says the outside is calling him to come and play. Children believe their wishes are as real as facts and dreams are as real as daytime happenings during this stage. They perceive animals and even inanimate objects as being capable of thought and feelings (e.g., a dog took their doll because the dog was feeling sad, a footstool meant to trip them). This phenomenon is often called "magical thinking." Magical thinking fades as, later on, children learn **accommodation** (they change their ideas to fit reality rather than the reverse).

QSEN Checkpoint Question 28.5

PATIENT-CENTERED CARE

John, who is 6 years old, says his broken leg wants to get better. When choosing an accurate and empathetic response, the nurse should be aware John is using what form of cognition?
a. Magical thinking
b. Deductive reasoning
c. Concrete operational thinking
d. Sensorial thought

Look in Appendix A for the best answer and rationale.

The School-Age Child

Piaget viewed school age as a period during which *concrete operational thought* begins because school-age children can be seen using practical solutions to everyday problems as well as begin to recognize cause-and-effect relationships. A child who understands water does not change in amount just because it is poured from one glass to another has grasped the concept of conservation. Conservation of numbers is learned as early as age 7 years, conservation of quantity at age 7 or 8 years, conservation of weight at age 9 years, and conservation of volume at age 11 years (Wadsworth, 2003). Reasoning during school age tends to be inductive or proceeds from specific to general: A school-age child holding a broken toy reasons the toy is made of plastic, and therefore, all plastic toys break easily.

The Adolescent

Adolescence is the time when cognition achieves its final form or when formal operational thought begins. When this stage is reached, adolescents are capable of thinking in terms of possibility—what could be (**abstract thought**)—rather than being limited to thinking about what already is (concrete thought). This makes it possible for adolescents to use scientific reasoning. They can use deductive reasoning in addition to the induction reasoning they used during school age or can move from the general to the specific (e.g., plastic toys break easily, the toy they are holding is plastic; therefore, it will break easily).

A Criticism of Piaget's Theory

Piaget is criticized because he used only a small sample of subjects to establish his theory (his own children). Because children today begin activities to learn counting and identifying color or reading much earlier than they did at the time the theory was devised, the age groups and norms may no longer be accurate. Playing computer games during the preschool period will probably impact the rate and type of children's cognitive developments in the future.

QSEN Checkpoint Question 28.6

SAFETY

John is a school-age child, but he still has difficulty learning Piaget's concept of conservation. The nurse recognizes this implies which statement about John?

   a. He doesn't understand why his mother insists he recycle plastic or metal soda cans.

   b. He doesn't understand that, when crossing a two-way street, he must look both right and left.

   c. He feels angry because his sister's piece of pie is long and thin where his is short and fat.

   d. He has an imaginary friend.

Look in Appendix A for the best answer and rationale.

KOHLBERG'S THEORY OF MORAL DEVELOPMENT

One more developmental theory that has relevance to maternal and child health nursing is Kohlberg's (1927–1987) theory of moral development. A German psychologist, Kohlberg (1984) studied the reasoning ability of boys and, based on Piaget's development stages, developed a theory on the way children gain knowledge of right and wrong or moral reasoning. These stages, as described by Kohlberg, are summarized in Table 28.7.

Recognizing where a child is developmentally according to these stages can help identify how children may feel about an illness such as whether they think it is fair that they are ill. Recognizing moral reasoning also helps determine whether children can be depended on to carry out self-care activities such as administering their own medicine or whether children have internalized standards of conduct so they do not cheat when away from external control. Moral stages closely approximate cognitive stages of development because children must be able to think abstractly (be able to conceptualize an idea without a concrete picture) before being able to understand how rules apply even when no one is there to enforce them (Juujärvi, Pesso, & Myyry, 2011).

A Criticism of Kohlberg's Theory

Kohlberg's (1984) theory is frequently challenged as being male-oriented because his original research was conducted entirely with boys. Carol Gilligan (1993), a sociologist, argues that there are two modes of moral reasoning: the ethic of justice that focuses on individual rights and the ethic of care that focuses on responsibilities in relationships. She suggests that girls may not score well on Kohlberg's scale because, being more concerned with relationships than are boys, they make moral decisions based on individual circumstances or the effect of their actions on others at a much younger age than boys, which skews their results on a standard male-influenced scale.

Using Growth and Development in Practice

An assessment of children's growth and development should be included in all children's nursing care plans because whether they are growing and developing within usual parameters is a significant mark of wellness. Because nurses do not work alone but as members of a healthcare team, Box 28.6 shows an interprofessional care map illustrating both nursing and team planning for supporting a child's growth and development.

TABLE 28.7 KOHLBERG'S STAGES OF MORAL DEVELOPMENT

Age (in Years)	Stage	Description	Nursing Implications
Preconventional (Level I)			
2–3	1	Punishment/obedience orientation ("heteronymous morality"). Child does right because a parent tells him or her to and to avoid punishment.	Child needs help to determine what are right actions. Give clear instructions to avoid confusion.
4–7	2	Individualism. Instrumental purpose and exchange. Carries out actions to satisfy own needs rather than society's. Will do something for another if that person does something for him or her.	Child is unable to recognize that like situations require like actions. Unable to take responsibility for self-care because meeting own needs interferes with this.
Conventional (Level II)			
7–10	3	Orientation to interpersonal relations of mutuality. Child follows rules because of a need to be a good person in own eyes and eyes of others.	Child enjoys helping others because this is nice behavior. Allow child to help with bed making and other such activities. Praise for desired behavior such as sharing.
10–12	4	Maintenance of social order, fixed rules, and authority. Child finds following rules satisfying. Follows rules of authority figures as well as parents in an effort to keep the system working.	Child often asks what the rules are and if something is right. May have difficulty modifying a procedure because one method may not be right. Follows self-care measures only if someone is there to enforce them.
Postconventional (Level III)			
Older than 12	5	Social contract, utilitarian law-making perspectives. Follows standards of society for the good of all people.	Adolescents can be responsible for self-care because they view this as a standard of adult behavior.
Older than 12	6	Universal ethical principle orientation. Follows internalized standards of conduct.	Many adults do not reach this level of moral development.

From Kohlberg, L. (1984). *The psychology of moral development.* New York, NY: Harper & Row, with permission.

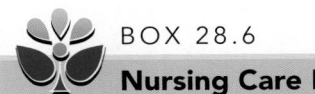

BOX 28.6

Nursing Care Planning

AN INTERPROFESSIONAL CARE MAP FOR A CHILD WITH A DEVELOPMENTAL CONCERN

John Olson is a 6-year-old, mildly overweight boy brought into an emergency department because his leg is broken from a bicycle accident. His parents tell you that although John has lived with them for 3 years, they find him cold and unloving. They ask you what they can do to change this.

Family Assessment: Family lives in a three-bedroom house in suburbs. Father works as a plumber; mother has a part-time job as a substitute grade-school teacher.

Patient Assessment: At 4 months of age, John was taken away from his mother because she was not caring for him adequately. He then moved among 12 different foster homes until he was finally adopted at age 3.5 years. His adoptive parents have 3-year-old twins of their own.

Nursing Diagnosis: Interrupted family processes related to inability of child to meet parents' developmental expectations

Outcome Criteria: Child demonstrates greater participation in family activities and improved response to parents' attempts to bond with him by 3 months' time.

Team Member Responsible	Assessment	Intervention	Rationale	Expected Outcome
Activities of Daily Living, Including Safety				
Nurse	Assess if family has thought through impact of bicycle accident on child's daily activities.	Suggest some obvious accommodations needed for cast care (e.g., no tub bathing, difficulty with stairs, no bike riding).	If a family is already under stress, an accident can compound family concerns.	Family members state they realize accidents are not anyone's "fault" and are prepared to make adjustments needed.
Teamwork and Collaboration				
Nurse/primary care provider	Assess if parents feel psychological counseling would be appropriate for child.	Assist parents with gaining a consultation if they feel they would welcome this.	Consultation with a skilled professional can offer parents information on specific actions to take.	Parents state whether they feel situation merits more skilled help at this time.
Procedures/Medications				
Nurse/primary care provider	Assess what emergency actions are necessary for a child with a fractured tibia.	Apply cast; give instructions for cast care. Keep pain or discomfort to a minimum.	Definite measures to prevent pain are important in promoting a sense of trust.	Patient states he understands cast care and states emergency department experience was at best an adventure, and at worst, not an ordeal.
Nutrition				
Nurse	Obtain a 24-hour recall dietary history to assess for usual calcium and vitamin D intake.	Suggest additional sources of calcium or vitamin D if needed.	Calcium is important for good bone healing and is absorbed best in the presence of vitamin D.	Patient states he understands calcium will help healing and is willing to ingest more if needed.
Patient-Centered Care				
Nurse	Assess what parents understand about the development of trust in early life.	Suggest ways to initiate a sense of trust by demonstrating dependability and a warm, loving relationship.	Even if a sense of trust is not achieved as an infant, it can be achieved at a later developmental stage.	Parents state they are willing to identify and begin more active steps toward improving relationship with son.

Continued on following page

BOX 28.6

Nursing Care Planning (continued)

Team Member Responsible	Assessment	Intervention	Rationale	Expected Outcome
Psychosocial/Spiritual/Emotional Needs				
Nurse	Assess what type of ideal child parents thought they were adopting.	Suggest measures that could bring parents and child closer together such as a "game night," always eating meals together, or quiet "talk times" before bed.	Identifying differences between expectations and reality can help people understand dissatisfactions.	Patient and parents state they are willing to begin an active program of shared activities.
Informatics for Seamless Healthcare Planning				
Nurse	Assess if patient or parents have "walked through a day" to identify their child's needs after returning home.	Discuss with patient and parents adjustments they recognize patient will have to make to attend school with a cast in place.	Small needs not met can grow into major needs before a return appointment and can interfere further with a sense of trust.	Patient and parents state they understand adjustments that need to be made and will work them out together with child.

What If . . . 28.4

The nurse is interested in exploring one of the 2020 National Health Goals related to growth and development (see Box 28.1). Most government-sponsored money for nursing research is allotted based on these goals. What would be a possible research topic to explore that would be applicable to the Olson family, pertinent to these goals, and advance evidence-based practice?

KEY POINTS FOR REVIEW

- Knowledge of growth and development is important in health promotion and illness prevention because it lays the basis for assessments and anticipatory guidance.
- Including growth and development guidelines in nursing care helps to achieve care that not only meets QSEN competencies but also best meets a family's total needs.
- Genetic factors that influence growth and development are gender, ethnicity, intelligence, and health.
- Environmental influences include quality of nutrition, socioeconomic level, the parent–child relationship, ordinal position in the family, and environmental health.
- To meet growth and development milestones, children (like adults) need to follow basic guidelines for a healthy diet, such as eating a variety of foods, maintaining an ideal weight, avoiding extreme levels of saturated fat, eating foods with adequate starch and fiber, and avoiding too much sugar.
- Temperament is a child's characteristic manner of thinking, behaving, or reacting. Helping parents understand the effect of temperament is a nursing role.
- Common theories of development are Freud's psychoanalytic theory and Erikson's theory of psychosocial development. Both of these theories describe specific tasks

children must complete at each stage of development to become a well-adapted adult.
- Piaget's theory of cognitive development describes ways children learn.
- Kohlberg advanced a theory of moral development or how children use moral reasoning to solve problems.
- Although growth and development occur in known patterns, the rate that a child develops and grows varies from child to child. Caution parents not to be concerned that two siblings are very different as long as they both fit within usual parameters.

CRITICAL THINKING CARE STUDY

Andrew is a preschooler who "hates" his first days at preschool. He lives with his mother Berkley, a calculus teacher; his father Edgar, a physicist; and Molly, his 5-day-old baby sister. His mother is disappointed at his reaction to school. She tells you, "We worked so hard to prepare him for school. Taught him his whole alphabet and how to count to 100. He's so excited about learning he wanted to practice writing his name rather than go to a friend's birthday party." She asks you what could be wrong. How can she make his first school experience better?

1. What additional information would you like to know before you advise his mother? What are some reasons you can think of as to why he might not be enjoying preschool?
2. Could temperament be playing a role in why Andrew is not fitting in well at preschool? Are there other indications he doesn't approach new situations well?
3. As a preschooler, should Andrew be interested in exploring new things and going new places? Is there a reason he doesn't want to leave his house to go to school just now?

RELATED RESOURCES

Explore these additional resources to enhance learning for this chapter:

- Student resources on thePoint, including answers to the What If . . . and Critical Thinking Care Study questions, http://thepoint.lww.com/Flagg8e
- Adaptive learning powered by PrepU, http://thepoint.lww.com/prepu

REFERENCES

Barton, A. L., & Kirtley, M. S. (2012). Gender differences in the relationships among parenting styles and college student mental health. *Journal of American College Health, 60*(1), 21–26.

Black, M. M., Quigg, A. M., Hurley, K. M., et al. (2011). Iron deficiency and iron-deficiency anemia in the first two years of life: Strategies to prevent loss of developmental potential. *Nutrition Reviews, 69*(Suppl. 1), S64–S70.

Brandt, M. J. (2011). Sexism and gender inequality across 57 societies. *Psychological Science, 22*(11), 1413–1418.

Brownawell, A. M., Caers, W., Gibson, G. R., et al. (2012). Prebiotics and the health benefits of fiber: Current regulatory status, future research, and goals. *Journal of Nutrition, 142*(5), 962–974.

Burgess, J. N., & Broome, M. E. (2012). Perceptions of weight and body image among preschool children: A pilot study. *Pediatric Nursing, 38*(3), 147–152.

Butterworth, B., & Kovas, Y. (2013). Understanding neurocognitive developmental disorders can improve education for all. *Science, 340*(6130), 300–305.

Chess, S., & Thomas, A. (1985). Temperamental differences: A critical concept in child health care. *Pediatric Nursing, 11*(3), 167–171.

Danyliw, A. D., Vatanparast, H., Nikpartow, N., et al. (2012). Beverage patterns among Canadian children and relationship to overweight and obesity. *Applied Physiology, Nutrition, & Metabolism, 37*(5), 900–906.

Dea, T. L. (2011). Pediatric obesity & type 2 diabetes. *MCN: American Journal of Maternal Child Nursing, 36*(1), 42–48.

Erikson, E. H. (1993). *Childhood and society.* New York, NY: W. W. Norton.

Feigelman, S. (2012). Overview and assessment of variability. In R. M. Kliegman, B. F. Stanton, J. W. Geme, et al. (Eds.), *Nelson textbook of pediatrics: Extra consult edition* (19th ed., pp. 192–212). Philadelphia, PA: Elsevier/Saunders.

Freud, S. (1962). *Three essays on the theory of sexuality.* New York, NY: Hearst.

Freud, S., & Brill, A. A. (1995). *The basic writings of Sigmund Freud.* New York, NY: Random House.

Gilligan, C. (1993). *In a different voice: Psychological theory and women's development.* Cambridge, MA: Harvard University Press.

Green, M., & Solnit, A. (1964). Reactions to the threatened loss of a child: A vulnerable child syndrome. *Pediatrics, 34,* 58–66.

Halfon, N., Stevens, G. D., Larson, K., et al. (2011). Duration of a well-child visit: Association with content, family-centeredness, and satisfaction. *Pediatrics, 128*(4), 657–664.

Hudson, J. L., Dodd, H. F., Lyneham, H. J., et al. (2011). Temperament and family environment in the development of anxiety disorder: Two-year follow-up. *Journal of the American Academy of Child & Adolescent Psychiatry, 50*(12), 1255–1264.

Johnston, M., Landers, S., Noble, L., et al. (2012). Breastfeeding and the use of human milk. *Pediatrics, 129*(3), e827–e841.

Jones, G. (2011). Early life nutrition and bone development in children. *Nestle Nutrition Workshop Series: Pediatric Programme, 68,* 227–233.

Juujärvi, S., Pesso, K., & Myyry, L. (2011). Care-based ethical reasoning among first-year nursing and social services students. *Journal of Advanced Nursing, 67*(2), 418–427.

Kmietowicz, Z. (2012). Study identifies behaviours in young children that might prevent obesity. *BMJ, 344*(4), e2608.

Kohlberg, L. (1984). *The psychology of moral development.* New York, NY: Harper & Row.

Krebs, N. F., & Primak, L. E. (2011). Pediatric nutrition and nutritional disorders. In K. J. Marcdante, R. M. Kliegman, H. B. Jenson, et al. (Eds.), *Nelson essentials of pediatrics* (6th ed., pp. 103–122). Philadelphia, PA: Saunders/Elsevier.

Levine, D. A. (2011). Growth & development. In K. J. Marcdante, R. M. Kliegman, H. B. Jenson, et al. (Eds.), *Nelson essentials of pediatrics* (6th ed., pp. 13–44). Philadelphia, PA: Saunders/Elsevier.

Matook, S. A., Sullivan, M. C., Salisbury, A., et al. (2010). Variations of NICU sound by location and time of day. *Neonatal Network, 29*(2), 87–95.

Morgan, A. R. (2012). Determining genetic risk factors for pediatric type 2 diabetes. *Current Diabetes Reports, 12*(1), 88–92.

Mulholland, E. K., Griffiths, U. K., & Biellik, R. (2012). Measles in the 21st century. *The New England Journal of Medicine, 366*(19), 1755–1757.

Naidoo, N., Pawitan, Y., Soong, R., et al. (2011). Human genetics and genomics a decade after the release of the draft sequence of the human genome. *Human Genomics, 5*(6), 577–622.

Pastor, P. N., & Reuben, C. A. (2011). Emotional/behavioral difficulties and adolescent obesity: Effect of sex and Hispanic origin/race. *International Journal of Pediatric Obesity, 6*(5–6), 462–466.

Inhelder, B., & Piaget, J. (1958). *The growth of logical thinking from childhood to adolescence: An essay on the construction of formal operational structures.* New York, NY: Basic Books.

Pike, K., Jane Pillow, J., & Lucas, J. S. (2012). Long term respiratory consequences of intrauterine growth restriction. *Seminars in Fetal & Neonatal Medicine, 17*(2), 92–98.

Rossow, I., & Moan, I. S. (2012). Parental intoxication and adolescent suicidal behavior. *Archives of Suicide Research, 16*(1), 73–84.

Russell, S. T., Sinclair, K. O., Poteat, V. P., et al. (2012). Adolescent health and harassment based on discriminatory bias. *American Journal of Public Health, 102*(3), 493–495.

Rutherford-Hemming, T. (2012). Learning in simulated environments: Effect on learning transfer and clinical skill acquisition in nurse practitioner students. *Journal of Nursing Education, 51*(7), 403–406.

Sizer, F., & Whitney, E. (2011). The vitamins. In F. Sizer & E. Whitney (Eds.), *Nutrition: Concepts & controversies* (12th ed., pp. 228–277). Belmont, CA: Wadsworth Cengage Learning.

Skinner, A. C., & Skelton, J. A. (2014). Prevalence and trends in obesity and severe obesity among children in the United States, 1999-2012. *JAMA Pediatrics, 168*(6), 561–566.

The Nemours Foundation. (2016). *KidsHealth: Growth & development.* Retrieved from http://kidshealth.org/en/parents/growth/

Ting, W. H., Huang, C. Y., Tu, Y. K., et al. (2012). Association between weight status and depressive symptoms in adolescents: Role of weight perception, weight concern, and dietary restraint. *European Journal of Pediatrics, 171*(8), 1247–1255.

U.S. Department of Health and Human Services. (2010). *Healthy people 2020.* Washington, DC: Author.

Vicedo, M. (2011). The social nature of the mother's tie to her child: John Bowlby's theory of attachment in post-war America. *British Journal for the History of Science, 44*(162, Pt. 3), 401–426.

Viner, R. M., Ozer, E. M., Denny, S., et al. (2012). Adolescence and the social determinants of health. *Lancet, 379*(9826), 1641–1652.

Wadsworth, B. J. (2003). *Piaget's theory of cognitive and affective development: Foundations of constructivism* (5th ed.). New York, NY: Longman.

Whitney, E. N., & Rolfes, S. R. (2012). Life cycle nutrition: Pregnancy and lactation. In E. N. Whitney & S. R. Rolfes (Eds.), *Understanding nutrition* (13th ed., pp. 468–497). Belmont, CA: Wadsworth Publishing.

29

Nursing Care of a Family With an Infant

*Y*ou meet Ms. Simpson, 19 years old, at a pediatric clinic when she brings in her 2-month-old son, Bryan. She looks tired and tells you she is exhausted because her baby is "awake all night, crying constantly." She stopped breastfeeding and changed to formula to see if that would help. It didn't. She also began giving him cereal. That didn't help either. She tells you his bowel movements are normal. When you weigh Bryan, you find he has gained weight well. When you talk to him, he demonstrates a social smile.

Previous chapters described the newborn and the capabilities with which children are born. This chapter adds information about the dramatic changes, both physical and psychosocial, that occur during the first year. Such information can build a base for care and health teaching for the age group.

What condition common to early infancy might Ms. Simpson be describing? What factors might be playing a role? What suggestions could you make to help her enjoy caring for Bryan more?

KEY TERMS

baby-bottle syndrome

binocular vision

deciduous teeth

eighth-month anxiety

extrusion reflex

hand regard

natal teeth

neck-righting reflex

neonatal teeth

object permanence

pincer grasp

seborrhea

social smile

thumb opposition

OBJECTIVES

After mastering the contents of this chapter, you should be able to:

1. Describe normal infant growth and development and associated parental concerns.

2. Identify 2020 National Health Goals related to infant growth and development that nurses can help the nation achieve.

3. Assess an infant for normal growth and development milestones.

4. Formulate nursing diagnoses related to infant growth and development and associated parental concerns.

5. Identify expected outcomes to promote optimal infant growth and developmental needs as well as manage seamless transitions across differing healthcare settings.

6. Using the nursing process, plan nursing care that includes the six competencies of Quality & Safety Education for Nurses (QSEN): Patient-Centered Care, Teamwork & Collaboration, Evidence-Based Practice (EBP), Quality Improvement (QI), Safety, and Informatics.

7. Implement nursing care related to normal growth and development of an infant, such as encouraging eye–hand coordination.

8. Evaluate expected outcomes for achievement and effectiveness of care.

9. Integrate knowledge of infant growth and development with the interplay of the nursing process, the six competencies of QSEN, and Family Nursing to promote quality maternal and child health nursing care.

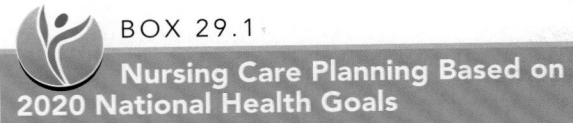

BOX 29.1

Nursing Care Planning Based on 2020 National Health Goals

A number of 2020 National Health Goals focus on the promotion of health during the infant year. These include:

- Increase the proportion of mothers who exclusively breastfeed until 6 months of age from a baseline of 14.1% to 25.5%.
- Reduce the rate of infant deaths from a baseline of 6.9 out of 1,000 live births to 6.7 out of 1,000 live births.
- Increase immunization levels for universally recommended vaccines among young children for such diseases as diphtheria, tetanus, poliomyelitis, pertussis, measles, mumps, rubella, and varicella (chickenpox) from varying actual levels to the target level of 90%.
- Increase age-appropriate vehicle restraint system use in children aged 0 to 12 months from 86% to 95%.
- Decrease the number of infants who die from sudden infant death syndrome (SIDS) from 0.55 out of 1,000 live births to 0.50 out of 1,000 live births (U.S. Department of Health and Human Services, 2010; see www.healthypeople.gov).

Nurses can help the nation achieve these goals by educating parents about the importance of using infant car seats, continuing exclusive breastfeeding for 6 months, and instigating measures to prevent SIDS such as placing infants to sleep on their backs.

Traditionally, infancy is designated as the period of time from 1 month to 1 year of age. In these important months, an infant undergoes such rapid development that parents sometimes believe their baby looks different and demonstrates new abilities every day. During this time, an infant typically triples birth weight and increases length by 50%. Babies' senses sharpen, and with the process of attachment to a primary caregiver, they form a first social relationship. Because of the growth and learning potential that occurs, this first year is a crucial one.

Without proper nutrition, a baby will not grow and physically thrive; without proper stimulation and nurturing care by a consistent caregiver, an infant may not develop a healthy interest in life or a feeling of security essential for future development (Olusanya & Renner, 2013). Box 29.1 highlights 2020 National Health Goals addressing this important developmental stage.

Nursing Process Overview

FOR HEALTHY DEVELOPMENT OF AN INFANT

ASSESSMENT

Nursing assessment of an infant begins with an interview with the primary caregiver. Important areas to discuss include nutrition, elimination, growth patterns, and development.

An infant's height, weight, and head circumference are important indicators of growth, so they should be measured and plotted on standard growth charts (see Chapter 28) (Parsons, George, & Innis, 2011).

Typical infant appearance is shown in Box 29.2. The physical assessment of an infant must be done quickly yet thoroughly because a baby can tire or become hungry, making it difficult to judge overall behavior and temperament. It's best if a parent is present to make the infant feel comfortable. Using a calm, unhurried approach helps an infant feel safe enough to accept your interventions.

NURSING DIAGNOSIS

Much of your assessment of an infant and family will focus on basic needs such as sleep, nutrition, and activity and the parents' adjustment to their new role. Examples of nursing diagnoses include:

- Ineffective breastfeeding related to maternal fatigue
- Disturbed sleep pattern (maternal) related to baby's need to nurse every 2 hours
- Deficient knowledge related to normal infant growth and development
- Imbalanced nutrition, less than body requirements, related to infant's difficulty sucking
- Health-seeking behaviors related to adjusting to parenthood
- Delayed growth and development related to lack of stimulating environment
- Risk for impaired parenting related to long hospitalization of infant
- Readiness for enhanced family coping related to increased financial support
- Social isolation (maternal) related to lack of adequate social support
- Ineffective role performance related to new responsibilities within the family

OUTCOME IDENTIFICATION AND PLANNING

Outcomes established for infant care need to be realistic based on the family's new circumstances. Parents of infants, especially first-time parents, must do a lot of adjusting, and this takes time. Try to suggest activities that can be easily incorporated into the family's lifestyle.

If your assessment data indicate that a child needs more exposure to language and you know both parents work during the day, for example, you might suggest the parents ask their child's caretaker to talk to their infant more. Encourage parents to spend additional time each evening reading or reciting nursery rhymes to their baby. Working together, these combined actions should increase the baby's language skills. Parents also might find it helpful to be referred to online resources for further information (see Chapter 28).

IMPLEMENTATION

One of the most important interventions of the infant period is teaching new parents about normal growth and development milestones, such as the age range for rolling over or reaching for objects. Whenever possible, this information should be anticipatory so parents are not surprised by a new

> **BOX 29.2**
>
> ## Nursing Care Planning Using Assessment
>
> **APPEARANCE OF THE AVERAGE INFANT**
>
> - Follow across midline at 3 months
> - Social smile at 2 months; first tooth erupts at 6 months
> - Respiratory rate slows to 20 to 30 breaths/min by end of year
> - Heart rate slows to 100–120 beats/min by end of first year
> - Pincer grasp at 10 months
> - Abdomen protuberant
> - Liver remains immature
> - Triples weight by 1 year
> - Legs may appear short and bowed
> - Grows in height by 50% (from 20 to 30 in.)

skill and instead are prepared for changes and developments before they occur.

OUTCOME EVALUATION

Evaluate expected outcomes at each visit to detect that changes in growth and development are occurring. Helping parents understand the total developmental profile, not just a single element, provides the most important description of their child. Variation is so much the rule rather than the exception that a 2-month variation from the average during the infant year is considered normal. Many 4-month-old infants, for example, have mastered most of the 4-month skills and some of the 5-month skills, yet they may still be at a 3-month level on one or two other criteria.

Examples of expected outcomes include:

- Mother states she feels fatigued but able to cope with sleep disturbance from night waking.
- Parents state five actions they are taking daily to encourage bonding.
- Father states both he and spouse are adjusting to new role as parents.
- Parents verbalize appropriate techniques they use to stimulate infant.
- Infant demonstrates age-appropriate growth and development.
- Infant exhibits weight, height, and head and chest circumference within usual norms.

Growth and Development of an Infant

Infants grow rapidly both in size and in their ability to perform tasks during their first year. A standard schedule for healthcare visits is for 2-week, 2-month, 4-month, 6-month, 9-month, and 12-month visits (American Academy of Pediatrics [AAP], 2017). These visits are important for the infant because they provide time for immunizations and health assessments; they are also important for parents because they provide an opportunity for parents to ask questions about their child's growth pattern and developmental progress. They provide opportunities for healthcare providers to assess for potential problems as they first appear.

Anticipatory guidance offered at these visits can help parents prepare for the rapid changes that mark the first year of life. When appropriate, encouraging parents to join clubs or networking groups is another way to help increase their knowledge base and confidence level to care for their rapidly growing infant. Table 29.1 details the usual procedures done at infant health maintenance visits. The vaccines administered during the first year are discussed in Chapter 34 (also available at http://thePoint.lww.com /Flagg8e).

PHYSICAL GROWTH

The physiologic changes that occur in the infant year reflect both the increasing maturity and growth of body organs.

TABLE 29.1 HEALTH MAINTENANCE SCHEDULE, INFANT PERIOD

Physical Health	Physical Examination	Frequency
Developmental milestones including psychosocial interaction	History, observation Ages and Stages Questionnaire	Every visit At 9 months
Growth milestones	Height, weight, head circumference plotted on standard growth chart; physical examination	Every visit
Vision and hearing	History, observation	Every visit
Physical examination		Every visit
Nutritional adequacy	History, observation	Every visit
Parent–child relationship	History, observation	Every visit
Sleep positioning counseling	Discussion of placing infants on back to sleep; using "tummy time" for play periods during the day	Every visit up to 9 months
Unintentional injury counseling	Discussion of safety measures to take with infants	Every visit
Dental health	History, physical examination Fluoride varnish	Every visit after teeth erupt Recommended every visit starting at 6 months with tooth eruption
Anemia	Hematocrit, hemoglobin	12-month visit
Lead screening	Point of Care rapid lead screening	12-month visit
Tuberculosis screening	Purified protein derivative (PPD) test (if warranted)	If indicated based on risk
Newborn screening	Heel blood sample	At 2-week visit

Immunizations

Review of history and health record; teaching parent about any risks and side effects; administering immunization in accordance with healthcare agency policies

Haemophilus influenzae type B	Hib	2-, 4-, 6-, and 12-month visits
Varicella	VAR	12-month visit
Inactivated poliomyelitis	IPV	2-, 4-, and 6-month visits
Pneumococcal disease	PCV	2-, 4-, 6-, and 12-month visits
Diphtheria, tetanus and pertussis (whooping cough)	DTaP	2-, 4-, 6-, and 12–15 months
Hepatitis B	HepB	Birth, 2-month, and 6- or 12-month visits
Rotavirus	RV	2-, 4-, and possibly at 6-month visit depending on manufacturer
Influenza	IIV	Yearly at 6-month or later visit
Mumps, measles, and rubella	MMR	12- or 15-month visit
Varicella	Var	12- or 15-month visit
Hepatitis A	HepA	12- or 15-month visit

Anticipatory Guidance

Infant care	Active listening and health teaching	Every visit
Expected growth and developmental milestones before next visit	Health teaching	Every visit
Poison and unintentional injury prevention	Educate parents about infant safety, such as using car seats and locking up poisons; provide telephone number of national poison control center (800-122-1222)	Every visit

Problem Solving

Any problems expressed by parent during course of the visit	Active listening and health teaching regarding nutrition, exercise, language development	Every visit

Centers for Disease Control and Prevention. (2013). *Recommended immunizations for children (birth through 6 years) United States, 2013.* Washington, DC: Author

Weight

As a rule, most infants double their birth weight by 4 to 6 months and triple it by 1 year. During the first 6 months, infants typically average a weight gain of 2 lb per month. During the second 6 months, weight gain is approximately 1 lb per month. The average 1-year-old boy weighs 10 kg (22 lb); the average girl weighs 9.5 kg (21 lb). An infant's weight, however, is relevant only when plotted on a standard growth chart and compared to that child's own growth curve (available at http://thePoint.lww.com/Flagg8e).

Height

An infant increases in height during the first year by 50%, or grows from the average birth length of 20 in. to about 30 in. (50.8 to 76.2 cm). Height, like weight, is best assessed if it is plotted on a standard growth chart. Infant growth is most apparent in the trunk during the early months. During the second half of the first year, it becomes more apparent as lengthening of the legs occurs. At the end of the first year, the child's legs may still appear disproportionately short, however, and perhaps bowed. For accuracy, measure infants lying supine on a measuring board even if they are beginning to be able to stand (see Chapter 34, Box 34.9).

Head Circumference

By the end of the first year, the brain already reaches two thirds of its adult size. Head circumference increases rapidly during the infant period to reflect this rapid brain growth.

Some infants' heads appear asymmetric until the second half of the first year, especially if they are always placed on their back to sleep (which they should be), causing the skull bones to flatten in the back. Suggest to parents they continue to place the infant on the back to sleep but to spend "tummy time" daily with the infant placed in a prone position to prevent this flattening. This early head distortion will gradually correct itself as the child sleeps less and spends more time with the head in an erect position. Persistence of asymmetry suggests an infant is not receiving enough stimulation or is spending the majority of time lying in bed.

Body Proportion

Body proportion changes during the first year from that of a newborn to a more typical infant appearance. By the end of the infant period, the lower jaw is definitely prominent and remains that way throughout life.

The circumference of the chest is generally less than that of the head at birth by about 2 cm. It is even with the head circumference in some infants as early as 6 months and in most by 12 months. The abdomen remains protuberant until the child has been walking well for some time, generally well into the toddler period. Cervical, thoracic, and lumbar vertebral curves develop as infants hold up their head, sit, and walk. Lengthening of the lower extremities during the last 6 months of infancy readies the child for walking and often is the final growth that changes the appearance from "babylike" to "toddlerlike."

Body Systems

In the cardiovascular system, heart rate slows from 110 to 160 beats/min to 100 to 120 beats/min by the end of the first year. The heart continues to occupy a little over half the width of the chest. Pulse rate may slow with inhalation (sinus arrhythmia), but this does not become marked until preschool age. That the heart is becoming more efficient is shown by a decreasing pulse rate and a slightly elevated blood pressure (from an average of 80/40 to 100/60 mmHg).

Infants are prone to develop a physiologic anemia at 2 to 3 months of age. This occurs because the life of a typical red cell is 4 months, so the cells the child had at birth begin to disintegrate at that time, yet new cells are not yet being produced in adequate replacement numbers. Hemoglobin in an infant becomes totally converted from fetal to adult hemoglobin at 5 to 6 months of age. Infants may experience a decrease in serum iron levels at 6 to 9 months as the last of iron stores established in utero are used.

The respiratory rate of an infant slows from 30 to 60 breaths/min to 20 to 30 breaths/min by the end of the first year. Because the lumens of the respiratory tract remain small and mucus production by the tract to clear invading microorganisms is still inefficient, upper respiratory infections occur readily and tend to be more severe than in adults.

At birth, the gastrointestinal tract is immature in its ability to digest food and mechanically move it along. These functions mature gradually during the infant year. Although the ability to digest protein is present and effective at birth, the amount of amylase, which is necessary for the digestion of complex carbohydrates, is deficient until approximately the third month. Lipase, necessary for the digestion of saturated fat, is decreased in amount during the entire first year.

The liver of an infant remains immature, possibly causing an inadequate conjugation of drugs (if a drug should be necessary for treatment of illness) and the inefficient formation of carbohydrate, protein, and vitamins for storage. Until age 3 or 4 months, an **extrusion reflex** (food placed on an infant's tongue is thrust forward and out of the mouth) prevents some infants from eating effectively if they are offered solid food this early (not recommended). Newborns can drink from a cup as long as a parent controls the fluid flow. An infant can independently drink from a cup by age 8 or 10 months.

The kidneys remain immature and not as efficient at eliminating body wastes as in an adult. The endocrine system remains particularly immature in response to pituitary stimulation, such as adrenocorticotropic hormone, or insulin production from the pancreas. Without these hormones functioning effectively, an infant may not be able to respond to stress as effectively as an adult.

An infant's immune system becomes functional by at least 2 months of age; an infant can actively produce both immune globulin (Ig)G and IgM antibodies by 1 year. The levels of other immunoglobulins (IgA, IgE, and IgD) are not plentiful until preschool age, which is the reason why infants continue to need protection from infection (Goldson & Reynolds, 2011).

The ability to adjust to cold is mature by age 6 months. By this age, an infant can shiver in response to cold (which increases muscle activity and provides warmth) and has developed additional adipose tissue to serve as insulation. The amount of brown fat, which protected the newborn from cold, decreases during the first year as subcutaneous fat increases.

Although the fluid in body compartments shifts to some extent, extracellular fluid accounts for approximately 35% of an infant's body weight, with intracellular fluid accounting for approximately 40% by the end of the first year, in contrast to adult proportions of 20% and 40%, respectively. This proportional difference increases an infant's susceptibility to dehydration from illnesses, such as diarrhea, because loss of extracellular fluid could result in loss of over a third of an infant's body fluid.

Teeth

The first baby tooth (typically a central incisor) usually erupts at age 6 months, followed by a new one monthly. Fluoride supplementation should be administered at 6 months of age (AAP, 2017). However, teething patterns can vary greatly among children. Figure 29.1 illustrates the usual ages of deciduous (baby teeth) eruption by tooth type.

Some newborns (about 1 in 2,000) may be born with teeth (**natal teeth**) or have teeth erupt in the first 4 weeks of life (**neonatal teeth**). The lower central incisors (see Fig. 29.1) are the teeth most frequently involved in this early growth. These very early teeth may be membranous and so may be reabsorbed (supernumerary or extra teeth). If they are loosely attached, they are usually removed before they loosen spontaneously and are aspirated by the infant. In most infants, natal or neonatal teeth are deciduous or are fixed firmly. These should not be removed because no other teeth will grow to replace them until the permanent teeth erupt at age 6 or 7 years. **Deciduous teeth** are essential for allowing proper growth of the dental arch. If they are injured, children need conscientious follow-up to be certain there is space for permanent teeth to erupt effectively or that permanent teeth are not discolored (de Amorim Lde, Estrela, & da Costa, 2011).

UPPER

Central incisor
8–12 months

Lateral incisor
9–13 months

Cuspid
16–22 months

First molar
13–19 months

Second molar
25–33 months

LOWER

Second molar
23–31 months

First molar
14–18 months

Cuspid
17–23 months

Lateral incisor
10–16 months

Central incisor
6–10 months

Figure 29.1 A typical eruption pattern of deciduous teeth.

MOTOR DEVELOPMENT

An average infant progresses through systematic motor growth during the first year, strongly reflecting the principles of cephalocaudal (head to toe) and gross-to-fine motor development. Control proceeds from head to trunk to lower extremities in a progressive, predictable sequence. As different infants show individual variations in accomplishing different tasks, the ages given here are only averages.

To assess motor development, both *gross motor development* (ability to accomplish large body movements) and *fine motor development*, measured by observing or testing *prehensile ability* (ability to coordinate hand movements), are evaluated.

Gross Motor Development

Four positions—ventral suspension, prone, sitting, and standing—are used to assess gross motor development.

Ventral Suspension Position

Ventral suspension refers to an infant's appearance when held in midair on a horizontal plane and supported by a hand under the abdomen (Fig. 29.2A). In this position, the newborn allows the head to hang down with little effort at control. One-month-old infants lift their head momentarily and then drop it again. Two-month-old infants hold their head in the same plane as the rest of their body, a major advance in muscle control. By 3 months, infants lift and maintain their head well above the plane of the rest of the body in ventral suspension.

A *Landau reflex* is a new reflex that develops at 3 months. When held in ventral suspension, the infant's head, legs, and spine extend. When the head is depressed, the hips, knees, and elbows flex. This reflex continues to be present in most infants during the second 6 months of life, but then it becomes increasingly difficult to demonstrate. It is an important reflex to assess because a child with motor weakness, cerebral palsy, or other neuromuscular defects will not be able to demonstrate the reflex.

At 6 to 9 months, an infant also demonstrates a *parachute reaction* from a ventral suspension position. This means that when infants are suddenly lowered toward an examining table, the arms extend as if to protect themselves from falling. Children with cerebral palsy do not demonstrate this response because they flex their extremities too tightly.

Prone Position

When lying on their stomach, newborns can turn their head to move it out of a position where breathing is impaired, but they cannot hold their head raised for an extended time (see Fig. 29.2B). By 1 month of age, they lift their head and turn it easily to the side. They still tend to keep their knees tucked under their abdomen, however, as they did as a newborn. Two-month-old infants can raise their head and maintain the position, but they cannot raise their chest high enough to look around yet. Their head is still held facing downward.

A 3-month-old child lifts the head and shoulders well off the table and looks around when prone. The pelvis is flat on the table, no longer elevated. Some children can turn from a prone to a side-lying position at this age.

Four-month-old infants lift their chests off the bed and look around actively, turning their head from side to side. They are able to turn from front to back. The first time, this tends to occur as an extension of lifting the chest combined

Figure 29.2 **(A)** The ventral suspension position. **(B)** The prone position.

with a **neck-righting reflex**, which begins at this age. This reflex causes babies to lose their balance and roll sideways when lifting the head up. The baby is frightened by the sudden feeling of rolling free and probably cries. After this happens a few more times, however, a baby begins to delight in this new accomplishment.

Most babies turn front to back first and then, 1 month later, back to front. When taking a health history, ask which way a child turned first. Those with spasticity may turn first back to front. This is not necessarily an indication of spasticity because some healthy babies turn back to front first also.

Five-month-old infants are able to rest weight on their forearms when prone. They can turn completely over, front to back and back to front. By 6 months, infants can raise their chests and the upper part of their abdomens off the table.

By 9 months, a child can creep from the prone position. Creeping means the child has the abdomen off the floor and moves one hand and one leg and then the other hand and leg, using the knees on the floor to locomote (Fig. 29.3).

Sitting Position

When placed on his or her back and then pulled to a sitting position, a newborn has extreme head lag; this lag is present until about 1 month (Fig. 29.4). In a sitting position, the back appears rounded and an infant demonstrates only momentary head control.

By 2 months, infants can hold their head fairly steady when sitting up, although their head does tend to bob forward and will still show head lag when pulled to a sitting position. A 4-month-old child reaches an important milestone by no longer demonstrating head lag when pulled to a sitting position.

A 5-month-old infant can be seen to straighten his or her back when held or propped in a sitting position. By 6 months, infants can sit momentarily without support. They anticipate being picked up and reach up with their hands from this position. Some parents expect a child this age to be able to sit securely and may be worried because their sitting posture is still extremely shaky when it is normal (Fig. 29.5). Infants are capable of movement by hitching or sliding backward from this position. Alert parents that an infant this young is capable of moving from one spot to another in this way so they are prepared for this and can prevent unintentional injuries.

Figure 29.3 Creeping. When infants creep, they move forward with one arm and leg and then the other arm and leg, carrying the torso above and parallel to the floor. (leungchopan/Shutterstock.com)

Figure 29.4 An infant is pulled to a sitting position to demonstrate head lag. Notice how evident this is in the very young infant.

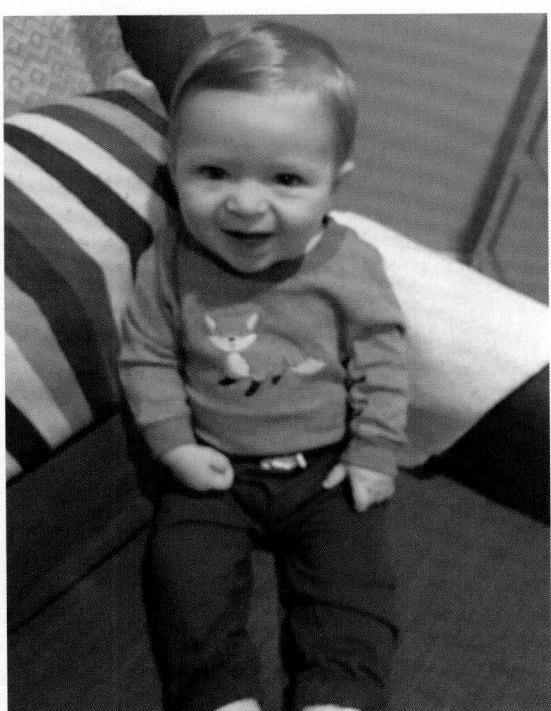

Figure 29.5 A 6-month-old infant not quite ready to sit on his own. Notice how he is propped with pillows to maintain the position.

A 7-month-old child can sit alone but only when the hands are held forward for balance. An 8-month-old child can sit securely without any additional support (Fig. 29.6). This is a major milestone in development that should always be considered in an assessment. Children with delayed cognitive or motor development may not accomplish this step at this time. At 9 months, infants sit so steadily that they can lean forward and regain their balance. They may still lose their balance if they lean sideways, which is a skill not achieved for another month.

Standing Position

A newborn stepping reflex can still be demonstrated at 1 month of age. In a standing position, the infant's knees and hips flex rather than support more than momentary weight. At 3 months, infants try to support part of their weight on their feet.

At 4 months, infants are able to support their weight on their legs. They are successful at doing this because the stepping reflex has faded. By 5 months, the tonic neck reflex should be extinguished, and the Moro reflex should be fading.

By 6 months, infants nearly support their full weight when in a standing position. A 7-month-old child bounces with enjoyment in a standing position. Nine-month-olds can stand holding onto a coffee table if they are placed in that position. Ten-month-olds can pull themselves to a standing position by holding onto the side of a playpen or a low table, but they cannot let themselves down again as yet.

At around 11 months, an infant learns to "cruise" or move about the crib or room by holding onto objects such as the crib rails, chairs, walls, and low tables (Fig. 29.7). At 12 months, the child can stand alone at least momentarily. Some parents expect children to walk at this time and may be disappointed to see their child is merely standing still. A child has until about 22 months of age to walk and still be within the normal limit, however (Fig. 29.8).

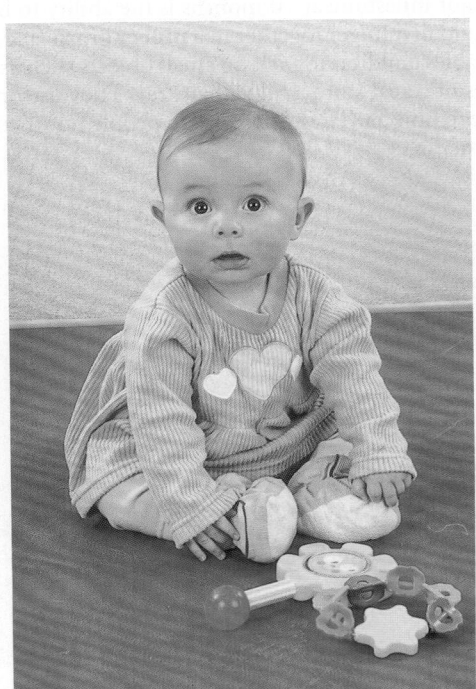

Figure 29.6 At 8 months of age, an infant sits independently.

Figure 29.7 An 11-month-old child cruising along the walls. Further childproofing of the house will be necessary to keep the child safe. (Photo Researchers, Inc.)

Figure 29.8 There is a wide variation in the age at which children take a first step, typically ranging from 8 to 15 months. Here, a child has mastered walking.

QSEN Checkpoint Question 29.1

TEAMWORK & COLLABORATION

Bryan is 2 months old, and the nurse is collaborating with the occupational therapist in his care. When planning care, the nurse identifies that John should sit securely at what age?

a. 2.5 months
b. 6 months
c. 8 months
d. 12 months

Look in Appendix A for the best answer and rationale.

Fine Motor Development

One-month-old infants still have a strong grasp reflex so they hold their hands in fists so tightly that it is difficult to extend their fingers. As the grasp reflex fades, a 2-month-old infant will hold an object for a few minutes before dropping it. The hands are held open, not closed in fists.

By 3 months, infants reach for attractive objects in front of them. Their grasp is unpracticed so they usually miss them. You can assure parents this is part of normal development so they do not think their child is nearsighted or farsighted or has poor coordination.

When they reach 4 months, infants bring their hands together and pull at their clothes. They will shake a rattle placed in their hand. **Thumb opposition** (ability to bring the thumb and fingers together) begins, but the motion is a scooping or raking one, not a picking-up one, and is not very accurate. This limits the infant to handling large objects (Fig. 29.9). Palmar and plantar grasp reflexes have disappeared.

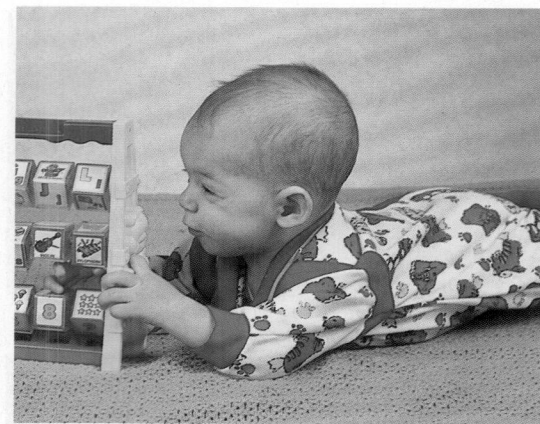

Figure 29.9 By age 4 months, an infant is able to manipulate large objects.

Five-month-old children can accept objects that are handed to them by grasping with the whole hand. They can reach and pick up objects without the object being offered and often play with their toes as objects. Fisting that persists beyond 5 months suggests a delay in motor development. Unilateral fisting suggests hemiparesis or paralysis on that side.

By 6 months, grasping has advanced to a point where a child can hold objects in both hands. Infants at this age will drop one toy when a second one is offered, however. They can hold a spoon and start to feed themselves (with much spilling). The Moro, the palmar grasp, and the tonic neck reflexes have completely faded. A Moro reflex that persists beyond this point should arouse suspicion of neurologic disease.

Seven-month-old infants can transfer toys from one hand to the other. They hold a first object when a second one is offered. By 8 months, random reaching and ineffective grasping disappear as a result of advanced eye–hand coordination.

A major milestone at 10 months is the ability to bring the thumb and first finger together in a **pincer grasp** (Fig. 29.10). This enables children to pick up small objects such as crumbs or pieces of cereal from a high chair tray. They use one finger to point to objects. They offer toys to people but then cannot release them.

Figure 29.10 An infant almost ready to demonstrate a pincer grasp.

At 12 months, infants can hold a crayon well enough to draw a semi-straight line. They enjoy putting objects such as small blocks in containers and taking them out again. They can hold a cup and spoon to feed themselves fairly well (if they have been allowed to practice) and can take off socks and push their hands into sleeves (again, if they have been allowed to practice). They can offer toys and release them.

DEVELOPMENTAL MILESTONES

In addition to the gross and fine motor skills developing at this time, language and play behavior also reach major milestones. For easy reference, motor and cognitive development and play throughout this year are summarized in Table 29.2.

Language Development

Language develops step by step the same as motor development. Infants begin to make small, cooing (dovelike) sounds by the end of the first month. By 2 months, they can differentiate their cry. For example, parents can begin to distinguish a cry that means "hungry" from one that means "wet" or from one that means "lonely." This is an important milestone in development for an infant; asking if a parent can tell the difference in crying is a good way to assess how far a parent has progressed in the task of parenting (Mesman, Oster, & Camras, 2012). A first-time parent usually has more difficulty making the distinction in crying than one who has experienced this before.

TABLE 29.2 SUMMARY OF INFANT GROWTH AND DEVELOPMENTAL MILESTONES

Month	Motor Development	Fine Motor Development	Socialization and Language	Time Reflexes Fade	Play
0–1	Largely reflex actions	Keeps hands fisted; able to follow object to midline with eyes			Enjoys watching face of primary caregiver; needs play time in prone position
2	Holds head up when prone	Demonstrates social smile	Makes cooing sounds; differentiates cry	Grasp reflex fading	Enjoys bright-colored mobiles
3	Holds head and chest up when prone	Follows object past midline with eyes	Laughs out loud	Landau reflex is strong	Spends time looking at hands (hand regard); "tummy time" important during the day
4	Turns back to front; no longer has head lag; bears partial weight on feet			Stepping, tonic neck, extrusion reflexes are fading	Needs space to practice turning
5	Should turn readily front to back and back to front			Tonic neck reflex fading	Handles rattles well
6	Beginning to show ability to sit	Uses palmar grasp	May say vowel sounds (*oh-oh*)	Moro and tonic neck reflex have faded	Enjoys bathtub toys, rubber ring for teething
7	Reaches out to be picked up; first tooth (central incisor) erupts	Transfers objects hand to hand	Shows beginning fear of strangers		Likes objects that are good size for transferring
8	Sits securely without support		Fear of strangers peaks		Enjoys manipulation, rattles, and toys of different textures
9	Creeps or crawls (abdomen off floor)		Says first word (*da-da*)		Needs safe space for creeping
10	Pulls self to standing	Uses pincer grasp (thumb and finger) to pick up small objects			Plays games like patty-cake and peek-a-boo
11	Cruises (walks with support)				Cruising can be main activity
12	Stands alone; some infants take first step	Holds cup and spoon well; helps to dress (pushes arm into sleeve)	Says two words plus *ma-ma* and *da-da*	Landau reflex fades	Likes toys that fit inside each other (pots and pans); nursery rhymes; will like pull toys as soon as walking

In response to a nodding, smiling face, or a friendly tone of voice, a 3-month-old infant will squeal with pleasure or laugh out loud. The same as with differentiating a cry, this is an important step in development because it makes a baby even more fun to be with. Parents spend increased time with infants at this age, not just to care for them but because they enjoy watching them smile at attention.

By 4 months, infants are very talkative, cooing, babbling, and gurgling when spoken to. They definitely laugh out loud. By 5 months, an infant says some simple vowel sounds (e.g., "goo-goo," "gah-gah").

At 6 months, infants learn the art of imitating. They may imitate a parent's cough, for example, or say "Oh!" as a way of attracting attention. The amount of talking infants do increases still more at 7 months. They can imitate vowel sounds well (e.g., "oh-oh," "ah-ah," "oo-oo"). By 9 months, an infant usually speaks a first word: "da-da" or "ba-ba." Occasionally, a mother may need reassurance that "da-da" for daddy is an easier syllable to pronounce than "ma-ma" for mommy. German mothers report the first word their babies say is "here," which is "da" in German. By 10 months, an infant masters another word such as "bye-bye" or "no." By 12 months, infants can generally say two words in addition to "ma-ma" and "da-da," and they use those two words with meaning.

QSEN Checkpoint Question 29.2

INFORMATICS

Beginning verbal communication is one of the most important tasks that infants need to achieve. The nurse teaches Bryan's mother that by 12 months of age he should display which characteristics?

a. "Children this age can usually say around two words, plus 'ma-ma' and 'da-da.'"
b. "One-year-olds can usually say more words than they are able to understand."
c. "A 12-month-old child can express his or her basic needs verbally."
d. "An infant who is this age usually can't understand spoken words."

Look in Appendix A for the best answer and rationale.

Play

Parents often ask what toys their infant would enjoy. Because 1-month-olds can fix their eyes on an object, they are interested in watching a mobile over their crib or playpen. Mobiles are best if they are black and white or brightly colored and light enough in weight so they move when someone walks by. Be sure they face down toward the infant, not toward the adult standing beside the crib. Musical mobiles provide extra stimulation. One-month-old children also spend a great deal of time watching their parents' faces, appearing to enjoy this activity so much a face may become their favorite toy. Help parents understand they are not spoiling infants by sitting and holding them for long periods of time, just studying each other, in these early months. Parents will enjoy recalling such calm moments later, when they are stacking blocks, winding up toys, or playing table games with their growing child.

Hearing is a second sense that is a source of pleasure for children in early infancy. Even newborns listen to the sound of a music box or a musical rattle. They stir and seem apprehensive at the sound of a raucous rattle. Two-month-old infants will hold light, small rattles for a short period of time but then drop them. They are attuned to mobiles or cradle gyms strung across their crib. They continue to spend a great deal of time just watching the people around them.

Three-month-old infants can handle small blocks or small rattles. Four-month-olds need a playpen or a sheet spread on the floor so they have an opportunity to exercise their new skill of rolling over. Rolling over may be so intriguing that it can serve as a toy for the entire month.

Five-month-old infants are ready for a variety of objects to handle, such as plastic rings, blocks, squeeze toys, clothespins, rattles, and plastic keys. Check that all of these are small enough that an infant can lift them with one hand, yet big enough that he or she cannot possibly swallow them.

A 6-month-old child can sit steadily enough to be ready for bathtub toys such as rubber ducks or plastic boats if carefully supervised. Because they are starting to teethe, most at this age enjoy a teething ring to chew on.

Because 7-month-old infants can transfer toys, they are interested in items such as blocks, rattles, or plastic keys that are small enough to be transferred easily. As their mobility increases, they begin to be more interested in brightly colored balls or toys that previously rolled out of reach.

Eight-month-old infants are sensitive to differences in texture. They enjoy having toys with different feels to them, such as velvet, fur, and fuzzy, smooth, or rough items.

The 9-month-old infant needs the experience of creeping. This means time out of a crib or playpen so there is room to maneuver. Many 9-month-olds begin to enjoy toys that go inside one another, such as a nest of blocks or rings of assorted sizes that fit on a center post. Some are more interested in pots and pans that stack rather than toys.

By 10 months, infants are ready for peek-a-boo and will spend a long time playing the game with their hands or with a cloth over their head that they can easily reach and remove. They can clap, so they are also ready to play patty-cake. These games have a positive value, just as laughing out loud did for the 3-month-old. They make the baby feel like an active part of the household. A family feeling begins to grow as the baby begins to actively participate in this type of game.

By 11 months, children have learned to cruise or walk by holding on to low tables. They often find this so absorbing that they spend little time doing anything else during the month. Twelve-month-old infants enjoy putting things in and taking things out of containers. They like little boxes that fit inside one another or dropping small blocks into a larger box. As soon as they can walk, they will be interested in pull toys. A lot of time may be spent listening to someone saying nursery rhymes or listening to music.

Although there is an advantage to television watching for children during the preschool age because it can help them learn language, the AAP recommends infants not be exposed to television (AAP, 2012b). They don't need exposure to the amount of violence seen on TV (remember children's cartoons may be the worst offenders of this), and interaction with real people (their parents or siblings) is less confusing and a better experience for them without it.

DEVELOPMENT OF SENSES

Like other facets of development, maturation of the senses proceeds progressively during the infant year.

Vision

One-month-old infants are able to regard an object in the midline of their vision (something directly in front of themselves) as soon as it is brought in as close as about 18 in. (46 cm). They follow the object a short distance if it moves but not across the midline as yet. They study or regard a human face with a fixed stare. Two-month-old infants focus well (from about age 6 weeks) and so are able to follow moving objects with the eyes (although still not past the midline). The ability to follow and focus in this way is a major milestone in development, indicating that an infant has achieved **binocular vision**, or the ability to fuse two images into one (Fig. 29.11). Teach parents to make a point of initiating eye-to-eye contact with newborns right from birth as a method of stimulating vision as well as a way of promoting socialization.

Three-month-old infants can follow an object across their midline. They typically hold their hands in front of their face and study their fingers for long periods of time (**hand regard**). Blind children also demonstrate this phenomenon, however, so it may not be so much a test of vision as of cognitive or exploratory development. Up until 6 months of age, it is not unusual for infants to experience some difficulty with establishing eye coordination. After 3 months, however, an infant whose eyes still cross the majority of the time should be examined by a primary care provider to be certain the muscles that control side-to-side vision are not impaired.

Four-month-old infants are able to recognize familiar objects, such as a frequently seen bottle, rattle, or toy animal. They eagerly follow their parents' movements with their eyes. By 6 months, infants are capable of organized depth perception. This increases the accuracy of their reach for objects as they begin to perceive distances correctly.

Seven-month-olds pat their own image in a mirror. Their depth perception has matured to the extent that they can perform such tasks as transferring toys from hand to hand. By 10 months, an infant looks under a towel or around a corner for a concealed object (the beginning of **object permanence**, or an awareness that an object out of sight still exists).

Most parents are aware that infants enjoy mobiles and also a crib mirror. Occasionally, parents supply so many of these that they can overwhelm the infant with too many patterns and objects dangling above the crib. Ask parents to consider how all these trappings must appear from an infant's viewpoint.

In a hospital environment, because hospital walls tend to be bland, assess that infants receive adequate visual stimulation (Fig. 29.12). If a child's movement is restricted in any way, such as by a cast, move the position of a mobile or mirror from time to time to provide a new view. Photos of family members or pictures drawn by older brothers or sisters can be posted near the crib. Ask parents if there are any items from home that the infant would normally see during the course of the day while being fed, changed, or bathed. Bringing those items into the hospital, if possible, could help visual stimulation.

Hearing

That an infant can hear can be demonstrated at birth by the way a newborn quiets momentarily at a distinctive sound such as a bell or a squeaky rubber toy. By 1 month, this reaction is even more marked. Hearing awareness becomes so acute by 2 months of age that infants will stop an activity at the sound of spoken words. Many 3-month-old infants turn their head to attempt to locate a sound. At 4 months of age, when infants hear a distinctive sound, they turn and look in that direction.

By 5 months of age, infants demonstrate they can localize sounds downward and to the side, by turning their head and looking down. Six-month-olds have progressed to being able to locate sounds made above them. By 10 months, infants can recognize their name and listen acutely when spoken to.

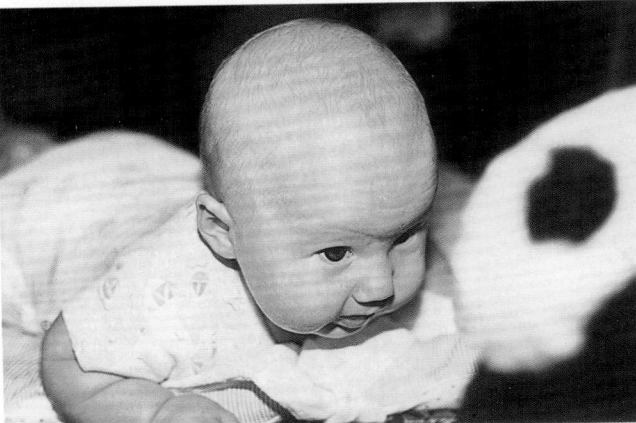

Figure 29.11 A 2-month-old infant focuses steadily and lifts her head up while prone. Note her interest in the stuffed bear.

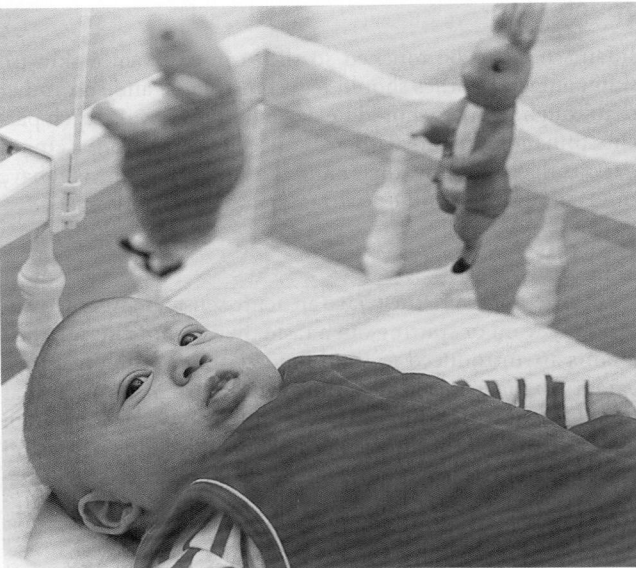

Figure 29.12 A 2-month-old infant enjoys watching a simple mobile.

BOX 29.3

Nursing Care Planning Tips for Effective Communication

A healthcare visit for Bryan is over, and you dress him while his mother talks to her healthcare provider.

Tip: Role model effective communication with infants to help parents learn to incorporate language development as they give care. Infants appreciate someone talking to them even if they don't understand the words. Use language that involves the infant and promotes vocabulary development, such as the naming of colors.

Nurse: Are you ready to go home? Your mother said you're going to pick up Daddy and then go shopping. Do you know about shopping? That's when you ride in a buggy while your mother buys things. Look what a cute yellow sweater you have. It matches the yellow duck on your shirt. Ducks say quack, quack, quack when they talk. Okay. You look ready. Let's find your mother.

By 12 months, infants can easily locate sounds in any direction and turn toward them. A vocabulary of two words plus "ma-ma" and "da-da" also demonstrates that an infant can hear.

During the first year, infants appear to enjoy soft, musical sounds or cooing voices (Box 29.3); they are startled by harsh, raucous rattles or loud bangs. Urge parents to choose for an infant's first toys ones that make these types of welcoming sounds. Recordings of maternal heart sounds can be soothing to very young infants. For the hospitalized infant, a recording of family voices might be a soothing reminder of their presence. Encourage parents to read to their child daily from the beginning of life through the early school-age years, not only because the sound of the parent's voice is comforting but also because this increases language development dramatically.

Touch

Infants need to be touched so they can experience skin-to-skin contact. Clothes should feel comfortable and soft rather than rough; diapers should be dry rather than wet. Teach parents to handle infants with assurance yet gentleness. Remind parents that right now their child is a baby; he or she will have time enough to become a strong man or woman later.

Taste

Infants demonstrate they have an acute sense of taste by turning away from or spitting out a taste they do not enjoy. When infants are introduced to solid food at about 6 months, urge parents to make mealtime a time for fostering trust as well as supplying nutrition by being certain feedings are done at an infant's pace and the amount offered fits the child's needs and not the parent's idea of how much should be eaten.

Smell

Infants can smell accurately within 1 or 2 hours after birth. They respond to an irritating smell by turning their head away from it. They appear to enjoy pleasant odors and learn early in life to identify the familiar smell of breast milk. Teach parents to be alert to substances that cause sneezing when sprayed into the air, such as room deodorizers or cleaning compounds, and to keep irritating odors of this nature out of their child's environment.

EMOTIONAL DEVELOPMENT

Socialization, or learning how to interact with others, is an extensive phenomenon. One-month-old infants show they can differentiate between faces and other objects by studying a face or the picture of a face longer than other objects. They are calm and feed well for the person who has been their primary caregiver.

When an interested person nods and smiles at a 6-week-old infant, the infant smiles in return. This is a **social smile** and is a definite response to the interaction, not the faint, quick smile that younger infants, even newborns, demonstrate. It is a major milestone because it reflects growing maturity in a number of areas, most notably vision, motor control, and intelligence. Cognitively challenged children or children with spasticity may not demonstrate a social smile until much later in the infant year.

By 3 months, infants demonstrate increased social awareness by readily smiling at the sight of a parent's face (Fig. 29.13). Three-month-old infants laugh out loud at the sight of a funny face. By 4 months, when a person who has been playing with and entertaining an infant leaves, the infant is likely to cry or show that the interaction was enjoyable. Infants at this age recognize their primary caregiver and prefer that person's presence to others. By 5 months, infants may show displeasure when an object is taken away from them. This is a step beyond showing displeasure when a person leaves.

By 6 months, infants are increasingly aware of the difference between people who regularly care for them and strangers. They may begin to draw back from unfamiliar people. Seven-month-old infants begin to show obvious fear of strangers. They may cry when taken from their parent, attempt to cling to the parent, and reach out to be taken back. Parents may view this as a bad trait or a regression in socialization. Help them appreciate that it is actually a big step forward because it shows that their infant can differentiate between people and also can recognize the difference between persons to trust and others.

Figure 29.13 A 3-month-old smiles delightedly at her father's happy face. This indicates increased social awareness.

Fear of strangers reaches its height during the eighth month, so much so that this phenomenon is often termed **eighth-month anxiety**, or stranger anxiety (Levine, 2011). Remember that an infant at the height of this phase will not go willingly from a parent's arms to a nurse's arms. Taking a few minutes to talk to the child and parent first so you are perceived as a friend, not a stranger, is time well spent.

Nine-month-old infants are very aware of changes in tone of voice. They cry when scolded not because they understand what is being said but because they sense their parent's displeasure. By 12 months, most children have overcome their fear of strangers and are alert and responsive again when approached. They like to play interactive nursery rhymes and rhythm games and "dance" with others. They also like being at the table for meals and joining in family activities.

COGNITIVE DEVELOPMENT

In the first month of life, an infant mainly uses simple reflex activity. There is little evidence infants at this early age see themselves as separate from their environment. However, this does not mean they cannot respond actively or interact with people. They demonstrate they are very people oriented moments after birth by cuddling against an adult's chest.

Primary and Secondary Circular Reaction

By the third month of life, a child enters a cognitive stage identified by Piaget (1952) as *primary circular reaction*. During this time, the infant explores objects by grasping them with the hands or by mouthing them (Fig. 29.14). Infants appear to be unaware of what actions they can cause or what actions occur independently, however. For example, if an infant's hand should accidentally strike a mobile across the crib, the infant appears to enjoy watching the brightly colored birds move in front of him but makes no attempt to hit the mobile again because he does not realize his hand caused the movement.

Figure 29.14 Infants explore the world by mouthing objects or fingering them. This also helps them separate self from environment.

At about 6 months of age, infants pass into a stage Piaget (1952) called *secondary circular reaction*. Now when infants reach for a mobile above the crib, hit it, and watch it move, they realize it was their hand that initiated the motion, and so they hit it again.

By 10 months, infants discover object permanence. Infants are ready for peek-a-boo once they have gained this concept. They know their parent still exists even when hiding behind a hand or blanket and wait excitedly for the parent to reappear.

As infants reach 1 year of age, they are capable of reproducing new events (they deliberately hit a mobile once, it moves, and they hit it again). They drop objects from a high chair or playpen and watch where they fall or roll. This is a frustrating activity for parents because it involves a great deal of reaching and picking up. It is an important activity for infants, however because it confirms their awareness of the permanence of objects and how they are able to control events in their world.

QSEN Checkpoint Question 29.3

QUALITY IMPROVEMENT

The nurse is discussing object permanence with Bryan's mother. Which action by her infant best illustrates that he understands object permanence?

   a. The child looks for the mother after she walks away.
   b. The child cries when either hungry or lonely.
   c. The child prefers a large yellow ball to a small red one.
   d. The child smiles when the mobile on the crib jingles.

Look in Appendix A for the best answer and rationale.

The Nursing Role in Health Promotion of an Infant and Family

The nursing role with infants is wide ranging because infants are so dependent on their caregivers for safety, learning, and emotional development.

PROMOTING ACHIEVEMENT OF THE DEVELOPMENTAL TASK: TRUST VERSUS MISTRUST

Erikson (1993) proposed that the developmental task of the infant period is to form a sense of trust (see Chapter 28). Infants who have numerous caregivers, who may be fed 1 day on a rigid schedule and the next only when they are hungry, who sometimes are treated roughly and sometimes gently, or who don't always have their needs met can have difficulty learning to trust. Cultures can vary in how they address care of an infant and promote trust. Variations in cultural influences for the same infant should be explored, so the infant is provided with consistency of care and can anticipate an expected response (Box 29.4).

BOX 29.4

Nursing Care Planning to Respect Cultural Diversity

Although development follows set patterns during the infant year, the care of them is more dependent on cultural factors. One difference is in the way mothers carry their infants. Western mothers tend to carry infants in their arms and so have to put them down to work or into a stroller to shop. South American women carry their infants in shoulder slings or on their hips, positions that allow a woman to continue to work or walk while holding an infant close. Infants who are held with their legs outspread that way tend to develop deeper hip sockets and have less hip dysplasia (see Chapter 27).

The amount of infant bathing that is done is also inconsistent across cultures. In the United States, most infants are bathed daily. In colder climates or countries where warm, clean water is not readily available, infant bathing is more limited. The use of diapers varies also. In hot climates, infants are often not diapered. Being aware of these cultural differences leads to better understanding of the reasons for an individual woman's particular method of childrearing.

Figure 29.15 An infant's sense of trust develops through warm interpersonal relationships. Here, a mother and infant share a bonding moment.

It is important for infants to establish the ability to love, or trust, early in life in this way because development is sequential. If a first developmental step is inadequate, this inadequacy can pervade all future steps. In reference to trust, the end result could be an adult unable to instill a sense of trust in his or her own child, perpetuating the inadequacy from generation to generation.

How do parents (or a nurse) encourage a sense of trust in an infant? Trust arises primarily from a sense of confidence that one can predict what is coming next. This does not mean parents should set up a rigid schedule of care for their infant. However, it does imply that parents should study their infant's reaction to activities and then establish a workable schedule based on that (e.g., breakfast, bath, playtime, nap, lunch, walk outside, quiet playtime, dinner, story, and bedtime). This gentle rhythm of care gives infants a sense of being able to predict what is going to happen and gives life consistency.

All little children thrive on routine such as the same story read over and over again, the same bedtime rituals, or the same spoon every day for lunch. Infancy is not too early for children to learn family traditions such as decorating for a holiday because this type of repetition can help them feel secure in their world. Some parents have difficulty accepting routine as important to a child. They may be so tired of their own work schedules that they want to raise their children as free spirits. Do not discourage this philosophy; however, you might suggest a few modifications to instill some order into infants' lives.

Just as it is important that there is a rhythm to the care, it is also important that the care is mainly given by one person (Fig. 29.15). This person can be the mother, father, grandparent, a conscientious babysitter, a foster parent, or anyone who can give consistent care. For infants ill at birth who are

hospitalized for months, this person is often a primary nurse or case manager. You may have to encourage parents who are reluctant at first to interact with their infant not to feel self-conscious about talking to a baby who does not talk back. Pointing out the importance of such interactions and role modeling them while caring for children help parents use this type of stimulation as they care for their baby's physical needs.

Women who work outside their home during the first year of a baby's life (at least 90% of women) should try to arrange for one person to care for their child while they are away from home or choose a day care center that will provide a consistent caregiver. Urge them to discuss their methods of child care with alternative caregivers to prevent disrupting an infant's routine. When a child is admitted to a hospital, document and list this information on an infant's electronic record.

Urge parents to make certain that not only will the number of caretakers for their child be limited but also that caretakers will be actively interacting with their child. Passively caring for infants—not talking to them or touching or stroking them while feeding or changing them—amounts to little more than not being with them at all. An increasing number of parents are installing video cameras to make sure a caretaker is actively interacting with their baby to instill a sense of trust in their child. Nursing actions designed to help an ill infant develop a sense of trust in addition to individual caretaking are detailed in Table 29.3.

PROMOTING INFANT SAFETY

Unintentional injuries are a leading cause of death in children from 1 month through 24 years of age. These are second only to acute infections as a cause of acute morbidity and primary care provider visits (Centers for Disease Control and Prevention [CDC], 2011).

Most unintentional injuries in infancy occur because parents either underestimate or overestimate a child's ability. Nursing interventions that help parents become sensitive to their infant's developmental progress, therefore, not only help

TABLE 29.3 WAYS FOR NURSES TO HELP AN ILL INFANT DEVELOP A SENSE OF TRUST

Area of Care	Nursing Actions
Nutrition	Encourage mothers to continue to breastfeed if possible while their infant is hospitalized; provide privacy and support as necessary.
	If a parent is not present to do so, hold the infant no matter what feeding method is used (e.g., gavage, total parenteral, oral, enteral). If this is not possible, hold infants for a time after or between feedings so they receive holding equal to what they would ordinarily receive with being fed.
	If infant feeding is not oral, provide a pacifier (medical condition and parent preference considered) five or six times daily for sucking pleasure.
Dressing change	Use nonallergenic tape to avoid irritation while it is applied and reduce pain when removed.
	Use stockinette, rolled gauze, or Kling gauze to hold a bandage in place rather than tape if possible.
	To prevent chilling, be certain irrigation solutions are warm; keep exposure during dressing changes to a minimum.
	Restrain only those body parts necessary for safety.
	Describe what you are doing in a nonthreatening tone of voice as you give care to give comfort.
Medicine administration	Flavor oral medicine to disguise disagreeable taste. Never add medicine to formula to prevent changing the formula's taste.
	Comfort the infant after injections or intravenous insertion by holding and rocking or immediately give the infant to a parent. Check intravenous sites frequently for infiltration and pain. Role model for parents how to hold the infant despite tubing and restraints.
Rest	Encourage parents to rock infants to sleep. Do this yourself if no parent is present.
	Always wake infants gently because it is frightening (for anyone) to be awakened by a stranger.
	If bed rest is necessary, check for irritated elbows, heels, and knees from rubbing against sheets; protect with long sleeves or pants or a Kling bandage.
Hygiene	Check the temperature of bath water for comfort and to prevent chilling or burning.
	Change diapers frequently to reduce discomfort from irritation.
	To avoid caries, begin toothbrushing with first tooth.
Pain	Hold and comfort an infant in pain.
	Do not ask parents to restrain a child for a painful procedure. Allow parents to comfort the child afterward because that is a better parent role.
	Reduce painful procedures to a minimum (e.g., combine blood drawing so only one puncture is necessary for many tests).
Stimulation	Remember that infants focus longest on a human face. Face them directly to talk to them.
	Provide a crib mirror or a mobile because visual stimulation seems satisfying to an infant.
	If no mobile is available, create one from string or strips of adhesive tape, colored paper, cotton balls, or colored tongue blades. For safety, hang the mobile high enough for the infant to see but not reach.
	During the second half of the first year, infants need to try to crawl. Put a pad or sheet on the floor and encourage them to come to you while you stand by to offer reassurance. If contagion or immunosuppression is not a problem, bring the infant's crib to the nursing desk where the infant can still interact with you while you do necessary paperwork.

establish sound parent–child relationships but also guard infant safety (Box 29.5).

Aspiration Prevention

Aspiration is a chief injury threat to infants throughout the first year. Round, cylindrical objects are more dangerous than square or flexible objects in this regard. A 1-in. (3.2-cm) cylinder, such as a carrot or hot dog, is particularly dangerous because it can totally obstruct an infant's airway. A deflated balloon can be sucked into the mouth, obstructing the airway in the same way. Educate parents who feed their infant formula not to prop bottles. By doing this, they are overestimating their infant's ability to push the bottle away, sit up, turn the head to the side, cough, and clear the airway if milk should flow too rapidly into the mouth, allowing an infant to aspirate.

Other instances of aspiration occur because parents underestimate their infant's ability to grasp and place objects in their mouth. Even a newborn can wiggle to a new position to reach an attractive object such as a teddy bear with small button eyes. Newborns' grasp and sucking reflexes automatically cause them to grasp and pull the object into their mouth. Caution parents to be certain nothing comes within an infant's reach that would not be safe to put into the mouth. Using clothing without decorative buttons and checking toys and rattles to ensure they have no small parts that could snap off or fall out are good steps for parents to follow.

A test of whether a toy could be dangerous if an infant puts it inside the mouth is whether it fits inside a toilet paper roll. If it does, it is small enough to be aspirated. When solid foods are introduced, encourage parents to offer small pieces of hot dogs or grapes, not large chunks for this reason. Children under about 5 years of age should not be offered popcorn or peanuts because of the danger of aspiration.

As infants become more adept at handling toys, parents need to reassess toys for loose pieces or parts. If parents are going to offer an infant a pacifier, they should use one that has a one-piece construction with a flange large enough to keep it from completely entering the child's mouth (Fig. 29.16).

BOX 29.5

Nursing Care Planning Based on Family Teaching

UNINTENTIONAL INJURY PREVENTION MEASURES FOR INFANTS

Q. Bryan's mother is worried about keeping him safe. She asks, "How can I prevent accidents at this age?"

A. Here are some tips to help prevent specific types of unintentional injuries:

Potential Unintended Injury	Prevention Measures
General	Be aware that the frequency of injury is increased when parents are under stress. Take special precautions at these times. Choose babysitters carefully and explain and enforce all precautions when sitters are in charge.
Aspiration	Be certain any object an infant can grasp and bring to the mouth is either safe to eat or too big to fit in the mouth. Do not offer foods such as popcorn or peanuts because these are easily aspirated. Store baby powder out of reach; inspect toys and pacifiers for small parts that could be aspirated if broken off.
Falls	Never leave an infant on an unprotected surface, such as a bed or couch, even if the infant is in an infant seat. Place a gate at the top and bottom of stairways; do not allow your infant to walk with a sharp object in the hands or mouth. Raise crib rails and make sure they are locked before walking away from the crib. Do not leave a child unattended in a high chair; avoid using an infant walker near a stairway.
Motor vehicle	Never transport an infant in an automobile unless the infant is buckled into an age-appropriate seat in the back seat of the car. Be aware of the proper technique for tethering the car seat to the car. Do not be distracted by an infant while driving. Do not leave an infant unattended in a parked car (the infant can become dehydrated from excess heat, can move the gear shift, or be abducted).
Suffocation	Allow no plastic bags within infant's reach; don't use pillows in cribs. Store unused appliances such as refrigerators or stoves with the doors removed. Buy a crib that is approved for safety (spacing of rails is not over 2 3/8 in. [6 cm] apart). Remove constricting clothing such as a bib or pacifier string from neck at bedtime.
Drowning	Do not leave infants alone in a bathtub or unsupervised near water (even buckets of cleaning water).
Animal bites	Do not allow an infant to approach a strange dog; supervise play with family pets.
Poisoning	Never present medication as a candy; buy medications in containers with safety caps; put away in a high cabinet immediately after use; never leave medication in a pocket or handbag. Never take medication in front of infants. Place all medication and poisons in locked cabinets or overhead shelves. Do not use lead-based paint in any area of the home. Hang plants or set on high surfaces. Post telephone number of the national poison control center by the telephone (1-222-1222).
Burns	Test warmth of formula and food before feeding (use extra precaution with microwave warming). Do not smoke or drink hot liquids while holding or caring for an infant. Buy flame-retardant clothing for infants; turn handles of pans toward back of stove. Use a sunscreen on a child over 6 months when out in direct or indirect sunlight and limit the child's sun exposure to less than 30 minutes at a time. If a vaporizer is used, use a cool-mist, not a hot-mist type; remain in room to monitor so child cannot reach vaporizer. Monitor infants carefully near candles. Do not leave infants unsupervised near hot-water faucets. Keep a screen in front of a fireplace or heater. Do not allow infants to blow out matches or candles (don't teach infants that fire is fun). Keep electric wires and cords out of reach; cover electrical outlets with safety plugs.
General	Be aware some infants are more active, curious, and impulsive and therefore more vulnerable to unintentional injury than others.

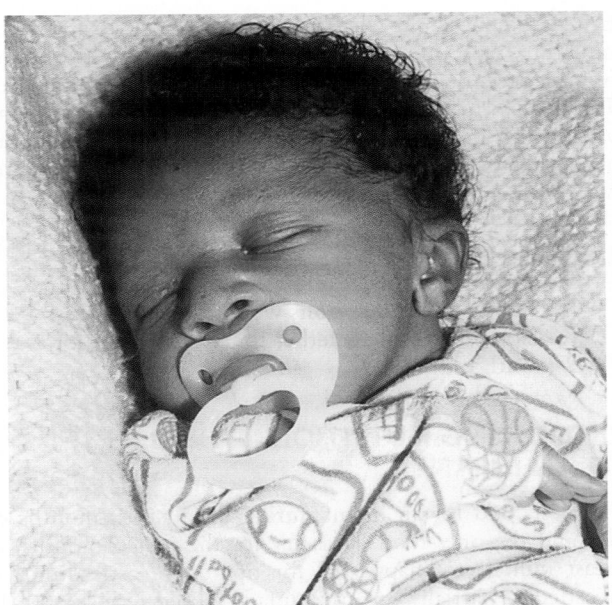

Figure 29.16 Many infants enjoy sucking on a pacifier to help them fall asleep. This may also help prevent sudden infant death syndrome.

QSEN Checkpoint Question 29.4

EVIDENCE-BASED PRACTICE

Scalding injuries occur in infants when caretakers spill hot beverages while holding them in their lap or, toward the end of the first year, the infant is able to pull a pan of hot liquid off the stove. To confirm the incidence of this type of injury, researchers studied the admission records of an urban pediatric emergency department in Ireland. Of 280 children seen for burns, 161 (57%) were scalds. Of these, 79% occurred in children under 5 years of age, 65% were caused by hot beverages, 16% were caused by hot water, and 16% by hot food. The areas of children most affected were upper limbs and upper trunks. The researchers concluded that more parent education as to the danger of scalding is needed to reduce the number of these very painful injuries in young children (Yates, McKay, & Nicholson, 2011).

Based on the study, the nurse is most concerned about which remark by Bryan's mother?
- a. "I never drive without a cup of coffee in my cup holder."
- b. "I'm going to switch to drinking tea to reduce my caffeine intake."
- c. "I drank coffee during Bryan's pregnancy; it's why he's so high strung."
- d. "I'm a coffee addict; I always have a fresh cup in my hand."

Look in Appendix A for the best answer and rationale.

Fall Prevention

Falls are a second major cause of infant injuries. As a preventive measure, no infant, beginning with a newborn, should be left unattended on a raised surface. Normal wiggling can bring even a newborn to the edge of a bed, couch, or table top, resulting in a fall.

Teach parents to be prepared for their infant to turn over by 2 months of age. From that time on, they must be especially vigilant not to leave the baby unattended on a changing table or counter. If the child sleeps in a crib, the mattress should be lowered to its bottom position so the height of the side rails increases; rails should be no more than $2\frac{3}{8}$ in. apart, narrow enough so children cannot put their head between them. Two months is about the maximum length of time infants can safely sleep in a bassinet; they need the protection of a crib and high side rails before they turn over.

All of these safety precautions apply to the hospital environment as well as to the home. Be sure crib sides are raised and secure before you walk away from a crib, even for just a moment. Also ensure the space between the mattress and headboard is small enough that an infant's head could not become trapped. Make sure cords from nursing call bells or other equipment are out of an infant's reach.

Car Safety

Teaching car safety for infants (as well as for the whole family) is an important protective health measure. The use of car seats for newborns is discussed in Chapter 18. Infants should be placed in backward facing seats in the back seat because an inflating front seat airbag could suffocate an infant (AAP, 2012a). Backward-facing car seats should continue to be used without interruption until age 2 years or until the child reaches the highest weight or height allowed by the car safety seat's manufacturer. If parents are firm about keeping infants in car seats even when they are fussy or impatient, children will eventually become more comfortable and accepting of car seats.

QSEN Checkpoint Question 29.5

SAFETY

The nurse reviews infant safety with Bryan's mother. It is most important to teach his mother about preventing which common injuries among infants?
- a. Drowning and hypersensitivities
- b. Poisoning and suffocation
- c. Auto accidents and burns
- d. Aspiration and falls

Look in Appendix A for the best answer and rationale.

Safety With Siblings

As infants become more fun to play with at about 3 months of age, older brothers and sisters grow more interested in interacting with them. You may need to remind parents that children under about 5 years of age, as a group, are not responsible enough or knowledgeable enough about infants to be left unattended with them. They might introduce an unsafe toy or engage in play that is too rough for an infant. Some preschoolers may be so jealous of a new baby they will physically harm an infant if left alone.

Bathing and Swimming Safety

As babies begin to develop good back support, many parents begin to bathe them in an adult tub. Caution parents to never leave an infant unattended in a tub, even when propped up out of the water or sitting in a bath ring or bath seat. Normal wiggling can easily cause a baby to slip down under the water. This applies to a hospital setting as well.

Many communities offer infant swim programs for babies as young as 6 months. If an infant is enrolled in one of these programs, parents may become overconfident about their infant's ability to operate safely in water. Urge them to think carefully before enrolling their infant in such a program, because, although infants can dog paddle momentarily in a swimming pool, this action does not mean they can sustain that position for any length of time in a bathtub or pool by themselves. As a second danger, being able to swim momentarily may cause children to lose their instinctive fear of water and so be in more danger when around water than children who are still naturally more cautious. Such programs can also cause hypothermia and spread microorganisms because infants this age are not yet toilet trained. Exposure to chlorinated water might damage lung epithelium, which then has the possibility to become a precursor to childhood asthma (Klootwijk & Krul, 2011).

Childproofing

Toward the end of pregnancy, parents need to begin preparing for their infant's arrival by childproofing their home. As soon as infants begin teething at 5 to 6 months, they chew on any object within reach to lessen gumline pain. Remind parents to thoroughly check for possible sources of lead paint, such as painted cribs, playpen rails, or windowsills before this time to avoid lead poisoning (CDC, 2014). Paints safe for baby furniture should be marked "Safe for use on surfaces that might be chewed by children." If an infant is going to play on the floor, urge parents to move furniture in front of electrical fixtures or buy protective caps for outlets. Infants are especially fascinated by the holes in electric outlets and will probe them with (often wet) fingers. Parents may need to install safety gates at the top and bottom of stairways as additional safety measures before the infant crawls.

Urge parents to move all potentially poisonous substances from bottom cupboards and store them well out of their infant's reach. Infants of any age should not be left unattended in carriages, high chairs, grocery shopping carts, or strollers. Baby walkers are extremely dangerous because infants can maneuver them near stairways and fall the length of the stairs.

When infants begin creeping, remind parents to recheck bottom cupboards and stairways for safety. When the child begins to walk, higher areas, such as coffee tables, need to be cleared of dangerous items. In a hospital setting, assess low counter areas for dangerous objects. Do not leave possibly dangerous supplies in an infant's room.

By 10 months, achievement of a pincer grasp makes infants able to pick up very small objects. Remind parents to check play areas or areas such as tabletops for pins or other sharp objects that could be swallowed. At this point, some of an infant's toys may now be 10 months old and need to be checked to be certain they are still intact and safe.

Although infants can seem very independent and able to take care of themselves toward the end of the infant year, their judgment about what situations could be dangerous is immature. As soon as they can walk, they're able to venture into the street or a swimming pool if not carefully supervised (Fig. 29.17). In a hospital setting, a 12-month-old child can wander into an elevator, out of the hospital, into a laboratory area, or fall down a flight of stairs if not supervised (Ibrahim, Wood, Margulies, et al., 2011).

What If . . . 29.2
Bryan's mother is interested in "childproofing" her house. What questions would the nurse want to ask to determine whether the house is safe for a 2-month-old?

PROMOTING NUTRITIONAL HEALTH OF AN INFANT

The best food for an infant during the first 12 months of life (and the only food necessary for the first 6 months) is breast milk (see Chapter 19 for tips on breastfeeding). A breastfed or partially breastfed infant should receive 400 IU of vitamin D supplement starting at 2 weeks of age (AAP, 2017). How long mothers continue to breastfeed is an individual choice, although it is recommended that infants be exclusively breastfed for 6 months. It is optimal if breastfeeding is then continued through the entire first year (Whitney & Rolfes, 2012). There is some research indicating early weaning from breastfeeding can lead to an increased incidence of obesity (Townsend & Pitchford, 2012). For infants whose mothers choose not to or are unable to breastfeed, a commercial iron-fortified formula will supply adequate nutrition for the infant year (Krebs & Primak, 2011) (for types of commercial formulas, see http://thePoint.lww.com/Flagg8e).

Figure 29.17 Once walking begins, the extended range of activities brings an infant in contact with potentially dangerous places or objects unless the house is childproofed. The bathroom is an important room in which to begin childproofing.

Supplementation is generally unnecessary with iron-fortified commercial formula. Although after 6 months, if the water supply does not contain fluoride, fluoride may need to be supplemented. Infants who are changed to cow's milk before 1 year of age should receive a supplementary form of vitamin C and iron and possibly fluoride to make up for the deficiency of these components in cow's milk. However, the practice of switching to cow's milk is not recommended because the protein in it is difficult for an infant to digest, possibly leading to such intestinal irritation that slight but continuous gastrointestinal bleeding occurs, which results in anemia.

Recommended Dietary Allowances for Infants

Because children's nutritional needs vary so much from infancy through adolescence, the recommended allowances of calories, protein, vitamins, and minerals also vary with each period of development (see Chapter 28).

The entire first year of life is one of extremely rapid growth, so a high-protein, high-calorie intake is necessary. Calorie allowances can be gradually reduced during the first year from a level of 120 calories per kilogram of body weight (50 to 55 calories per pound) at birth to approximately 100 calories per kilogram (45 calories per pound) of body weight at the end of the first year to prevent babies from becoming overweight.

Although heredity plays a role, a baby who is overweight during the first year of life is more likely to become an adult who is obese than one whose weight is within normal limits. Such long-term effects occur because overfeeding in early life may produce large numbers of excess fat cells (adipocytes) used to store fat. Because these cells are permanent and remain filled with fat, once they are present, weight regulation can become difficult throughout life. Breastfed infants gain less weight than those who are formula fed and so usually tend to be somewhat lighter in weight and have less risk of becoming overweight (Thilo & Rosenberg, 2011).

Introduction of Solid Food

From a nutritional standpoint, a normal full-term infant can thrive on breast milk or a commercial iron-fortified formula without the addition of any solid food until 6 months (Conti, Patel, & Bhat, 2011). Delaying solid food until this time also helps prevent overwhelming an infant's kidneys with a heavy solute load. Although difficult to document, it also may delay the development of food allergies in susceptible infants and be yet another way to help prevent future obesity (Gaffney, Kitsantas, & Cheema, 2012).

Most parents are eager to begin feeding their infant solid food, hoping this will help their child sleep through the night. So eager, in fact, some parents do begin food before the recommended time without apparent ill effects, possibly because much of the food is not processed by the gastrointestinal tract, but rather passes through undigested because of the immaturity of the digestive system, and decreased amounts of amylase and lipase (digestive enzymes).

Generally speaking, parents can tell infants are physiologically ready for solid food when they are nursing vigorously every 3 to 4 hours and do not seem satisfied or when they are taking more than 32 oz (960 ml) of formula a day and do not seem satisfied.

Introducing Solid Food

Infants are not ready to digest complex starches until amylase is present in saliva at approximately 2 to 3 months. Biting movements begin at approximately 3 months. Chewing movements do not begin until 7 to 9 months. Therefore, foods that require chewing should not be given until this age.

In addition to these cautions, the extrusion reflex needs to fade before infants accept food readily. With the extrusion reflex intact, when anything is placed on the anterior third of an infant's tongue, it is automatically extruded or thrust out of the mouth by the tongue (Fig. 29.18). This is a lifesaving reflex in early infancy because it prevents infants from swallowing or aspirating foreign objects that touch the mouth. The reflex fades at 3 to 4 months at about the same time the gastrointestinal tract has matured to be ready to digest solid food.

Techniques for Feeding Solid Food

The introduction of solid food begins a new type of interaction between parents and their infant and can require a period of adjustment (AAP, 2017). A typical pattern for the introduction of solid food beginning at 6 months includes:

- Iron-fortified infant cereal mixed with breast milk, orange juice, or formula; it aids in preventing iron-deficiency anemia, is the least allergenic type of food, and is the most easily digested so it is usually the first food offered.
- Vegetables; these are a good source of vitamin A and add new texture and flavors to the diet.
- Fruit; these are the best sources of vitamin C and a good source of vitamin A.
- Meat is a good source of protein, iron, and B vitamins.
- By 6 months of age, egg yolk, a good source of iron, can be added.

Commercial jar food is used in the hospital environment, but the appropriate consistency table food is recommend for home use. Caution parents to omit wheat, tomatoes, oranges, fish, and egg whites if there are allergies in the family because these foods are those most likely to cause allergies. Also, parents should never use honey as a sweetener because it may

Figure 29.18 A 3-month-old baby demonstrates an extrusion reflex. Caution parents not to interpret this action as a food dislike but recognize it as the reflex action that it is.

contain botulism spores and never use cow's milk because it can cause microscopic intestinal bleeding.

Teach parents to offer new foods one at a time and to allow their child to eat that item for about 3 to 7 days before introducing another new food. This system helps parents to detect a possible food allergy in addition to allowing the infant to get used to the new experience.

A newborn's stomach can hold approximately 2 tablespoons (30 ml). By 1 year, a stomach can hold no more than about 1 cup (240 ml). For this reason, when they begin eating solid food, infants rarely take more than 2 tablespoons (30 ml) at a time.

For the first solid food feeding, it is best if an infant is held in the parent's arms as if for breastfeeding or bottle feeding. This reduces the newness of the experience and minimizes the amount of stress associated with it. Some infants accept new experiences of this type readily, whereas other infants resist heartily. If an infant does not take readily to solid food, advise parents to wait a few days and then try again. Remind them this is not a contest to see whose child takes cereal, vegetables, or fruit first.

Babies have distinct taste preferences even at young ages and may spit out a food because they do not like the taste. Even after the extrusion reflex has faded, some infants continue to spit out food. This is because, when infants drink from a bottle or breast, they press their tongue and the nipple against their hard palate. When an infant tries to eat solid food using the same technique, it appears the child is spitting out the food. A parent who knows an infant's cues will be able to distinguish taste preferences from inadequate management of solid food. Box 29.6 lists pointers to help make the introduction of solid foods a positive experience.

If a parent is going to prepare baby food, the parent needs to avoid preparing spinach, carrots, beets, green beans, and squash because these can contain excessive amounts of nitrates that are not processed well by infants. Commercial baby food has the nitrates removed and so does not present this problem.

Cereal

Infant cereal is fortified with B vitamins and iron. It is supplied as a precooked, fine dry powder to which expressed breast milk, infant formula, or juice is added. Adding sugar to cereal is unnecessary. Extra sugar in the diet can lead to diarrhea in young infants and beginning caries in older infants.

Fortified cereal costs no more than unfortified cereal, so remind parents to buy the fortified product. The first cereal introduced is usually rice cereal because fewer children are allergic to rice products than to wheat and corn products. Usually, this is offered twice a day, in the morning and evening. Once the child has taken rice cereal for 1 week, if they wish, parents can try another kind.

Caution parents not to mix cereal into the infant's bottle because, as it is necessary to cut a larger hole in the bottle nipple for the cereal and milk mixture to flow freely, there is a danger an infant may aspirate if the hole cut is too big or if the parent then uses that nipple for formula without cereal added. This practice also denies the child the opportunity of learning to eat from a spoon and experiencing different food tastes and textures.

Infant cereal is so rich in iron that parents should continue feeding it at least through the first year. Ideally, children should eat infant cereal until age 3 or 4 years because few popularly advertised products can match the nutrients of fortified infant cereal.

Vegetables and Fruit

Because the iron content in vegetables is generally higher than that of fruits, vegetables are usually the second food added to the diet (after 6 months of age). To prepare their own, a parent simply cooks a vegetable and then blends or processes it, so it does not have to be chewed. Caution parents not to add butter, sugar, or salt to the preparation because infants have difficulty digesting fats until almost the end of the first year, and the added salt or sugar is unnecessary. By filling ice-cube trays with the blended vegetables, parents can make a 1-week supply and defrost a cube at a time. An ice cube is approximately 1 oz, or one fourth the size of a jar of baby food.

If parents use commercial baby food, they should begin with level 1 types (single ingredient and pureed) and feed from a dish rather than directly from the jar. This is because, if the spoon carries salivary enzymes from an infant's mouth

---

 BOX 29.6

Nursing Care Planning to Empower a Family

TIPS TO HELP INTRODUCE SOLID FOODS TO INFANTS

Q. Bryan's mother has already started feeding him solid food. She asks, "When and how should I have begun food?"

A. It's best if infants are exclusively breastfed for 4 months so infants typically are ready for solid food at 4 to 6 months of age. Usual guidelines to help introduce solid foods include:

- Introduce one food at a time, waiting 3 to 7 days between new items.
- Introduce the food before formula or breastfeeding when the infant is hungry.
- Introduce small amounts of a new food (1 or 2 teaspoons) at a time.
- Respect infant food preferences; a child cannot be expected to like all new tastes equally well.
- Use only minimal to no salt and sugar on solid food to minimize the number of additives.
- Remember that the extrusion reflex is present for the first 4 to 6 months of life, so any food placed on an infant's tongue will be pushed forward and extruded.
- To prevent aspiration, *do not* place food in bottles to drink with formula.
- Even though you don't like a particular food, introduce it with a positive, "You'll like this" attitude. It could be your child's favorite.

back to the food jar, the enzymes will quickly liquefy what remains in the jar. Also, there is a danger of transferring bacteria (principally streptococci) from an infant's mouth to the jar. Then, if the parent keeps the jar for another feeding in the next 24 hours, bacteria will multiply rapidly because the contents serve as a culture medium. Baby food jars should be refrigerated once they are opened, and manufacturers recommend they be used no longer than 48 hours after they were first opened.

When vegetables are added to the diet, they are usually offered at lunch. Remind parents to offer both green and yellow vegetables. Help them to remember that their own dislike of a particular vegetable does not mean their child will feel the same way about it. If they do convey distaste for a food, their child will pick up on the feeling and may not like the vegetable either.

Fruit is usually offered 1 week after beginning vegetables (after 6 months of age). It can be given in addition to cereal for breakfast and dinner. Raw mashed banana is easy to prepare with just a fork; peaches are easily prepared in a blender. As with vegetables, parents should offer a selection so an infant is exposed to different tastes and textures.

Meat and Eggs

Meat is usually introduced at 9 months of age because this is the time an infant's iron stores are beginning to be depleted. Parents can grind a portion of the meat they have prepared for their own meal so it is tender, or they can use commercially prepared baby food. If they use commercial baby meat, remind them to use the plain meat preparations, not vegetable and meat dinners because these contain mostly vegetables. Chicken has the advantage of being low in cholesterol, but this is not a priority with infants. Beef and pork have more iron than chicken, so encourage parents to offer a variety. When meat is added to an infant's diet, it is usually added as part of the evening meal in place of cereal.

Egg yolks are offered after 6 months of age. Egg yolks contain the bulk of the iron content of eggs; the white contains the bulk of protein. Egg yolk alone should be given at first because the protein of the egg white can lead to allergy or can be difficult for an infant to digest. Eggs may be hard-boiled (then a little formula or breast milk can be added to the mashed yolk to make it more liquid) or purchased as commercial baby food. Soft boiling or poaching is not usually recommended because salmonella, the chief offending microorganism that may be in eggs, may not be killed by these methods. Also, thorough cooking makes protein easier to digest.

Table Food

With the introduction of solid food, encourage parents to establish a three-meal-a-day pattern, if that is the family's lifestyle, and to have the infant join the family at the table. If an individual infant is too distracted by the activity at a family table to eat well, parents may find the infant eats more if fed first and then given a cracker to chew on while just sitting at the table and being with the family.

Commercial junior foods are now prepared without excessive additives and are convenient for parents who have little time to prepare food. Generally, however, encourage parents to use homemade foods rather than relying on commercially prepared junior or toddler foods (often labeled as level 4 foods) as much as possible so the infant will have less difficulty switching to a parent's cooking when older.

Mashed potatoes or peas and cut-up meatloaf are examples of table foods that infants older than 6 months of age like to eat and busy parents can prepare quickly. If hot dogs are offered, caution parents to cut them into small bite-size portions; otherwise, their shape is dangerous if aspirated. As infants begin teething, they may enjoy dried bread or teething biscuits.

Remind parents that high chairs are one of the most dangerous pieces of baby equipment they own. Urge them to always fasten the restraint and never leave an infant unattended in a high chair because even a 6-month-old can squirm out of a chair with little effort. This is important to keep in mind as well when feeding infants in a hospital setting.

Establishment of Healthy Eating Patterns

Some parents may need to be reminded that there are no hard-and-fast rules for infant feeding. The rules are only guidelines based on what seems to work well with most infants. Encourage them to individualize their approach according to the cues their child is giving them for readiness and to understand that refusing a teaspoonful of carrots is refusing a teaspoonful of carrots and nothing more.

Most infants, however, eat hungrily, so feeding problems tend to be reported more frequently as a second-year or toddler problem than as an infant concern. If an infant does refuse to eat, ask the parents what foods they are offering. Have them list exactly the types and amounts of foods the child ate the day before (a 24-hour dietary recall history). It may be apparent from this that enough is being eaten in a day's time and the parents' expectations are unrealistic for the child's size and age.

If intake is inadequate and the child is, indeed, a fussy eater, ask about the parents' methods of feeding. For example, infants generally accept the new experience of eating from a spoon better when they are hungry, not when their stomach is full. Some babies, however, particularly those with an intense temperament, may be so hungry at mealtime that they cannot tolerate the frustration of spoon feeding until some of their hunger is relieved. They may need to drink 2 or 3 oz of formula or nurse at the breast for a few minutes before they will eat a spoonful of food.

If infants are fatigued or overstimulated, they also may not eat well. Providing a quiet environment away from older brothers or sisters or other distractions before mealtime might be a solution to this problem.

Encourage parents not to force infants to eat if they do not seem hungry. Healthy, happy infants will be hungry at mealtime and will eat. Those who refuse a meal may be tired, distracted, or perhaps ill. Forcing only leads to regurgitation or, if they are ill, vomiting. Infants who are eating and not thriving or not eating and therefore are not thriving should be examined by their primary care provider to determine if a cause such as a metabolic disorder or failure to thrive exists (see Chapters 48 and 55).

Weaning

Mothers are advised to exclusively breastfeed for the first 6 months and continue breastfeeding for the full first year with complementary solids. Infants are capable of approximating their lips to a cup, and they can drink effectively from one at about 9 months of age. The sucking reflex begins to diminish in intensity between 6 and 9 months, which makes this the time to consider weaning from a bottle.

To wean from either formula or breast milk, the parent needs to choose one feeding a day and begin offering fluid by the new method at that feeding. Choosing a time of day that is not an infant's fussy period is helpful; other than that, the time is unimportant. After 3 days to 1 week, when an infant has become acclimated to the one change, the parent then changes a second feeding and so on. Should an illness such as an upper respiratory infection occur or should the child have teething discomfort, there will be setbacks. Infants also usually need more fluid during hot weather than cold weather because of increased perspiration. No set number of weeks should be prescribed to complete weaning.

Self-Feeding

At approximately 6 months of age, infants become interested in handling a spoon and beginning to feed themselves. Their coordination, unfortunately, has not developed enough for them to use a spoon without a great deal of spilling, so they are much more adept at feeding themselves with their fingers (Fig. 29.19). Parents concerned with neatness can spread newspapers, a plastic tablecloth, or a towel on the floor around a high chair to catch most of the dropped food, and then let the child practice. When an infant becomes fatigued or frustrated at attempts of self-feeding, a parent can then quietly help without making an issue of it.

When infants play with their food by squeezing it through their fingers or dabbing it in their hair, it is time to end the meal. Infants who are hungry eat; those who are full, play.

A Vegetarian Diet

An infant eating a vegetarian diet should continue to be breastfed or ingest an iron-fortified commercial formula for the entire first year. If a milk allergy is present, a soy-based

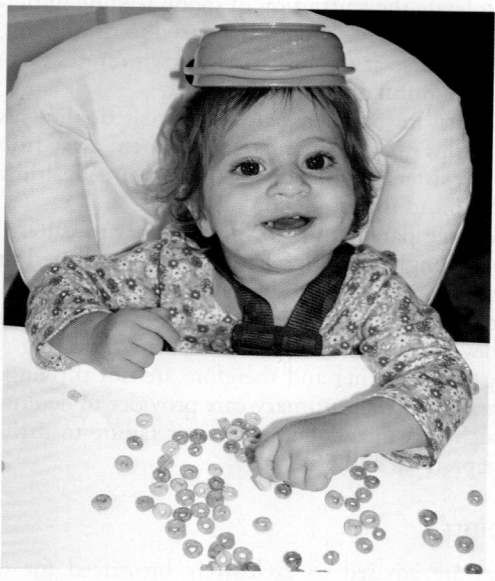

Figure 29.19 Self-feeding is not always a neat process for young children.

formula can be substituted. As soon as they are introduced to solid food, they can begin vegetarian foods (Amit, 2010). As with all infants, an assortment of foods should be provided, including vegetables such as peas, potatoes, and carrots; fruits such as apples, prunes (which are high in iron), and bananas; infant cereal; tofu; wheat germ; legumes; brewer's yeast; and synthetic vitamin D. Feeding fortified cereal throughout the first year will ensure that iron stores are built. If the diet is to include dairy products, these can be added toward the end of the first year as usual.

Because vegetarian diets are high in fiber, infants who eat them may have more frequent and looser than usual bowel movements. Teach parents to change diapers frequently to avoid skin irritation. Using less fibrous, more concentrated forms of protein, such as tofu and powdered nuts rather than green vegetables, can minimize this problem.

A sound vegetarian diet can be easily designed for the older infant who prefers finger foods because many vegetables, fruits, and grains such as pieces of oranges, peaches, tomatoes, and crackers are easily eaten this way.

PROMOTING INFANT DEVELOPMENT IN DAILY ACTIVITIES

In the first year, caring for an infant—feeding, bathing, dressing, and so forth—occupies what may seem like nearly all of the parents' waking hours. All of these basic care-related activities provide important opportunities for parents and infants to get to know one another and to become used to each other's unique personalities and patterns. Nurses can play a key role in teaching parents about these activities and stressing their importance.

Bathing

Except in very hot weather, an infant does not need a bath every day. If a parent is tired and would not enjoy bath time or if some days are just too rushed, a complete bath can be omitted, with only the infant's face, hands, and diaper area washed. Some infants do need their head and scalp washed frequently (i.e., every day or every other day) to prevent **seborrhea**, a scaly scalp condition often called cradle cap (Lyon, 2011).

If seborrhea lesions do develop, they adhere to the scalp in yellow, crusty patches. The skin beneath them may be slightly erythematous. The patches can be softened by oiling the scalp with mineral oil or petroleum jelly and leaving it on overnight. The crusts can then be removed by shampooing the hair the next morning. A soft toothbrush or fine-toothed comb can be used to help remove them.

Bath time should be enjoyable for an infant and can serve many functions other than just the obvious one of cleanliness (Fig. 29.20). Especially during the second half of the first year, a child enjoys poking at soap bubbles on the surface of the water or playing with bath toys. Bath time also helps an infant learn different textures and sensations and provides an opportunity to exercise and kick as well as a good opportunity for a parent to touch and communicate with the child. Teach parents never to leave infants alone in a tub even if they are supported by an infant seat because they could easily slip under the water and drown.

Diaper-Area Care

The most effective means of promoting good diaper-area hygiene is to change diapers frequently, about every 2 to

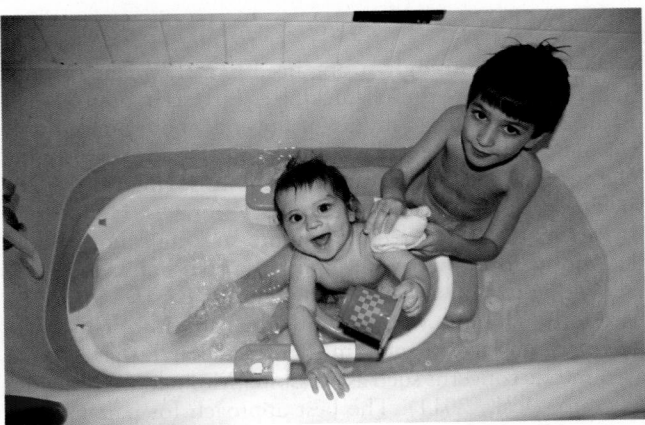

Figure 29.20 An infant enjoys bath time with his big brother. Parents should always watch carefully while infants and toddlers are in the tub.

4 hours. However, it is rarely good practice to interrupt the child's sleep to change diapers. If an infant develops a rash from sleeping in wet diapers, air drying or sleeping without a diaper may be a solution.

At each diaper change, parents should wash the skin with clear water or a commercial alcohol-free (and perfume-free if an infant has sensitive skin) diaper wipe and then pat or allow the skin to air dry. Routinely using an ointment such as zinc oxide or petroleum ointment to keep urine and feces away from an infant's skin is good prophylaxis. Parents should not use baby powder, as it is a potential source of aspiration. Following a diaper change, remind parents to wash their hands to reduce the possibility of spreading infection.

Dental Care

It is well accepted that exposing developing teeth to fluoride is one of the most effective ways to promote healthy tooth formation and prevent tooth decay. A water level of 0.3 ppm fluoride in water is recommended because this is the level that protects tooth enamel best yet does not lead to staining of teeth. In communities where the water supply does not provide enough fluoride or where parents prefer to drink un-fluoridated bottled water or use unfluoridated well water, the use of an oral fluoride supplement (fluoride drops) beginning at 6 months of age or the use of fluoride toothpaste or rinses after tooth eruption is recommended (AAP, 2011a). Urge parents to ask about the presence of fluoride in the drinking water in their community and help them to determine what, if any, supplementation is necessary.

Toothbrushing can begin even before teeth erupt by rubbing a soft washcloth over the gum pads. This eliminates plaque and reduces the presence of bacteria, creating a clean environment for the arrival of first teeth. Once teeth erupt, all surfaces should be brushed with a soft brush or washcloth once or twice a day. Children lack the coordination to brush effectively until they are school age, so parents must be responsible for this activity well past infancy (Milgrom & Chi, 2011). Toothpaste is not necessary for an infant because it is the scrubbing that removes the plaque. An initial dental checkup should be made before 2 years of age, and checkups should continue at 6-month intervals until adulthood.

Dressing

Clothing for infants should be easy to launder and simply constructed, so neither dressing nor undressing are a struggle. When they begin to creep, infants need long pants to protect their knees. Until they begin to walk, they need only soft-soled shoes or merely socks or booties to keep their feet warm. Even when they begin walking, the soles of their shoes need only be firm enough to protect their feet against rough surfaces. Extremely hard soles and high ankle sides are unnecessary.

Sleep

Sleep needs and habits vary greatly among infants, but most require 10 to 12 hours of sleep at night and one or several naps during the day. Parents are advised to let a baby sleep in a separate space close by rather than in their bed so the parents do not awaken at every toss and squeak and possibly avoid infant suffocation. Doing so also allows infants to learn to quiet themselves and go back to sleep should they awaken briefly. Caution parents not to place pillows in an infant's crib. Always place an infant on his or her back to sleep because this position markedly reduces the incidence of sudden infant death syndrome (SIDS) (AAP, 2011b). In addition to supine positioning, use of a firm sleep surface, breastfeeding, room sharing without bed sharing, routine immunizations as shown in Table 29.1, considering the use of a pacifier, and avoidance of overheating, closed spaces, and exposure to tobacco smoke are other suggestions for helping to prevent the syndrome (Scollan-Koliopoulos & Koliopoulos, 2010) (see Chapter 26 for a further discussion of SIDS).

Exercise

Infants benefit from outings in a carriage or stroller because sunlight provides a natural source of vitamin D. In hot weather, caution parents to protect an infant from sunburn by exposing the child to the sun for only very short periods, beginning with 3 to 5 minutes the first day, a little more the next day, and so on up to 15 to 20 minutes at a time. The sun is most intense between 10 AM and 3 PM, so early mornings and late afternoons are the best times for infants to be outside. These short time spans are necessary because the use of sunscreen is not recommended in children until they are at least 6 months old.

Toward the end of the first year, infants need space to crawl and then to walk, such as in an enclosed outdoor play space. In addition to providing fresh air, going for leisurely walks while pointing out the sights of the world—trees, birds, dogs, houses, neighbors—helps children develop language and allows for quality time with a parent. Parents can judge how much outdoor clothing to put on an infant by how much they need themselves.

Caution parents to supervise infants using walkers because they can be seriously injured if they maneuver the walker too near a stairway and fall the length of the steps.

PROMOTING HEALTHY FAMILY FUNCTIONING

A primary task of parents during the infant year is to learn to interpret infants' cues so they can better decipher their needs. This becomes an easier task by 2 months of age, when infants can indicate by their particular cry whether they are feeling cold, hungry, wet, or lonely.

Parental Concerns and Problems Related to Normal Infant Development

Some of the difficulties parents are apt to have in evaluating the health of infants are shown in Table 29.4. Both new and experienced parents may need reassurance and answers to questions about child care procedures or health during the infant period because they have not yet learned to interpret infant cues. The unique characteristics of each child require at least some adjustment from parents.

Teething

Most infants have little difficulty with teething, but some appear very distressed by the process. Generally, gums are sore and tender before a new tooth breaks the surface. As soon as the tooth is through, the tenderness passes (Kiran, Swati, Kamala, et al., 2011).

Because of this pain, infants can be resistant to chewing for a day or two and be slightly cranky, possibly because they are a little hungry from not eating as much as usual. High fever, seizures, vomiting or diarrhea, as well as earache are never normal signs of teething. An infant with any of these symptoms has an underlying infection or disease process that requires further evaluation.

Rubbing the gumline with a finger or a soft cloth can help a new tooth erupt and so can be effective (Plutzer, Spencer, & Keirse, 2011). Teething rings that can be placed in the refrigerator or freezer provide soothing coolness against tender gums. Remind parents that an infant who is teething will place almost any object in the mouth to chew on, so parents must screen articles within the baby's reach to be certain they are edible or safe to chew on.

Many over-the-counter medicines are sold for teething pain. As a rule, these should be discouraged, especially if they contain benzocaine, a topical anesthetic. If applied too far back in the throat, this could interfere with a gag reflex. Infant's or children's liquid acetaminophen (Tylenol) may be given for teething discomfort after parents check with their primary care provider for the correct dose. As a rule, they always need to check with their infant's healthcare provider before giving any over-the-counter drug this way to be certain that pain enough to warrant an analgesic is simple teething discomfort.

Thumb-Sucking

Sucking is a surprisingly strong need in early infancy: Sonograms demonstrate thumb-sucking as early as in utero. Many infants begin to suck a thumb or finger at about 3 months of age and continue the habit through the first few years of life. The sucking reflex peaks at 6 to 8 months, whereas thumb-sucking peaks at about 18 months.

Parents can be assured that thumb-sucking is normal and does not deform the jaw in infancy. It does not cause "baby talk" or any of the other speech concerns commonly attributed to it. Children who continue the habit into school age, however, can have changes in their dental arch that leads to asymmetric concerns such as crossbite (Montaldo, Montaldo, Cuccaro, et al., 2011). The best approach for parents is to be certain an infant has adequate sucking pleasure and then to ignore thumb-sucking. Making an issue of it rarely causes a child to stop; if anything, it may intensify and prolong it.

Use of Pacifiers

Whether to use pacifiers is a question that parents must settle for themselves depending on how they feel about them and their infant's needs. Benefits of pacifiers include the following: They appear to be comforting to an infant, they may aid in pain relief, and there is a decreased risk of SIDS. Risks associated with them are an increased incidence of acute otitis media (ear infection), possibly a negative impact on breastfeeding, and dental malocclusion, particularly if usage is greater than 2 to 3 years (Nelson, 2012).

An infant who completes a feeding and still seems restless and discontent, who actively searches for something to put into the mouth, or who sucks on hands and clothes may need a pacifier. Babies who have colic crave sucking and enjoy pacifiers because their abdomen hurts, and they interpret this as a hunger sensation. If a child is formula fed, parents should check nipples to be certain the holes are small and the rubber is sturdy so their infant can suck hard enough to derive pleasure. If the nipples are satisfactory, parents could offer a pacifier after feeding for more sucking. Theoretically, a child whose sucking needs are met in infancy will not crave as much oral stimulation later in life and is less likely to become a pencil chewer, cigarette smoker, nail biter, or the like.

TABLE 29.4 COMMON DIFFICULTIES PARENTS EXPERIENCE IN EVALUATING THE HEALTH OF INFANTS

Difficulty	Suggestions for Improving Assessment
Evaluating pain	Infants manifest pain by fussiness or crying if it is sharp pain. They reveal arm and leg pain by immobility of the body part, ear pain by brushing or tugging at the ear, and stomach pain by pulling up the legs against the abdomen.
Evaluating degree of reduced activity	Infant has lack of interest in smiling or interaction; may lie supine with legs nonflexed (frog-legged) as if exhausted.
Evaluating infant temperature	All parents should learn how to take an axillary or tympanic temperature so they can report a specific degree of fever rather than a subjective finding, such as "feels hot."
Evaluating amount of vomiting or diarrhea	Count the number of times vomiting and/or diarrhea has occurred. Estimating amount in comparison with what the child ate is helpful as well as estimating an amount (e.g., a cupful). Knowing whether diapers are soaked or stained with stool helps to estimate severity of diarrhea. Caution parents that vomiting and diarrhea are always serious in infants; if these occur, they should alert their primary healthcare provider and ask for advice.

A major drawback of pacifiers is the problem of cleanliness. They tend to fall on the floor or sidewalk and are then put back into an infant's mouth. If not well constructed, they may come apart and the nipple part may be aspirated. Hanging a pacifier on a string around an infant's neck could cause strangulation.

Parents should attempt to wean a child from a pacifier any time after 3 months of age and certainly during the time the sucking reflex is fading at 6 to 9 months. Weaning after this age is difficult because a pacifier becomes a comfort mechanism, like a warm blanket or fuzzy toy to which a child may continue to cling.

Head Banging

Some infants rhythmically bang their head against the bars of a crib for a period of time before they fall asleep, an action that can be a distressing behavior for parents. Besides fearing their children will hurt themselves, they may have heard blind children or those with mental illness or an autism spectrum disorder do this and worry their child is ill in some way.

Head banging in this limited fashion—beginning during the second half of the first year of life and continuing through to the preschool period, associated with naptime or bedtime, and lasting under 15 minutes—can be considered normal. Children use this measure to relax and fall asleep. Investigating stress factors operating in the house may be helpful. If some of the stress can be relieved (such as the parents' overestimation of the child's development, marital discord, illness in another family member), the head banging may decrease or it may have already become such an engrained habit that it will persist for months or even years.

Advise parents to pad the rails of cribs so infants cannot hurt themselves and reassure them this is a normal mechanism for the relief of tension in children of this age. No therapy should be necessary. Excessive head banging done to the exclusion of normal development or activity, head banging past the preschool period, or if associated with other symptoms suggests a pathologic basis; such children need a referral for further evaluation (Singer, 2011).

Sleep Concerns

Infants should be placed on their backs to sleep until they are able to roll over on their own at around 4 months of age. Co-sleeping is discouraged due to safety concerns. Breastfed babies tend to wake more often than those who are formula fed because breast milk is more easily digested, and so infants become hungry sooner. In late infancy, the problem of waking at night and remaining awake for an hour or more can become common. Although an infant may be content and not cry during this time, parents are reluctant to sleep while a child is awake, so they may become extremely fatigued. Suggestions for eliminating or at least coping with night waking include delaying bedtime by 1 hour, shortening afternoon naps, not responding immediately to infants at night so infants can have time to fall back to sleep on their own, and providing soft toys or music to allow infants to play quietly alone during this wakeful time.

Reassuring parents that infants take varying lengths of time to adjust to night sleeping is helpful in assuring them their child is not ill. Suggesting parents use the time they are awake at night to do things such as solve a problem at work, watch a late show, or plan a shopping list may help them view the situation as a constructive time rather than a concern. If infants have difficulty falling or staying asleep, this is not correlated with long-term sleep disorders (Price, Wake, Ukoumunne, et al., 2012).

Constipation

Breastfed infants are rarely constipated because their stools tend to be naturally loose. Constipation may occur in formula-fed infants from something as simple as if their diet is deficient in fluid. This can be corrected simply by offering more fluid.

Some parents misinterpret the normal pushing with bowel movements of a newborn and report that their infant is constipated. When infants defecate, their faces do turn red, and they grimace and grunt. As long as stools are not hard and contain no evidence of fresh blood (as might occur with a rectal fissure), this is not constipation but normal infant behavior.

If hard bowel movements are present beyond 5 or 6 months of age, encourage parents to check with the infant's primary healthcare provider about measures to relieve this. Adding foods with bulk, such as fruits or vegetables, and increasing fluid intake generally relieves the problem. Apple juice (3 or 4 oz) or prune juice (0.5 to 1 oz daily) may be given as a temporary measure.

All infants with a history of true constipation (exceedingly hard or no bowel movements) should be examined for an anal fissure or tight anal sphincter. Softening stools and thereby relieving the pain of defecation often solves the problem and helps the fissure to heal. If an unusually tight anal sphincter exists, parents will be given instructions to manually dilate the sphincter two or three times daily until it dilates sufficiently.

Hirschsprung disease (aganglionic megacolon, or lack of nerve innervation to a portion of the colon) may be manifested early in life as constipation. If no stool is present in the rectum of a constipated infant on rectal examination, this disease is suggested (Sundaram, Hoffenberg, Kramer, et al., 2011). A careful history must then be taken to assess for other symptoms of Hirschsprung disease: ribbonlike stools, bouts of diarrhea, and a distended abdomen (see Chapter 45).

Chronic constipation also may occur in children with congenital hypothyroidism (decreased functioning of the thyroid gland). An infant with constipation should be carefully observed for characteristic signs of hypothyroidism, such as lethargy, protruding tongue, and failure to meet developmental milestones (see Chapter 48). Infants with either of these disorders need therapy to correct the disorder.

Loose Stools

Many new parents are unfamiliar with the consistency or color of normal newborn stools, so they mistakenly report normal stooling as diarrhea. Stools of breastfed infants are generally softer than those of formula-fed infants. If a mother takes a laxative while breastfeeding, an infant's stools may be very loose. An infant who is formula fed can have loose stools if the formula is not diluted properly. Occasionally, loose stools may begin with the introduction of vegetables or fruit.

A serious reason for loose stools is celiac disease or the inability to process gluten (sometimes termed malabsorption syndrome) (see Chapter 45). The inability to digest fat and fat-soluble vitamins, accompanied by a distended abdomen, are other common symptoms of celiac disease; an infant needs a referral to a primary care provider for this.

When talking to a parent about loose stools, ask them how long the infant has been having them, the number of stools per day, their color and consistency, and whether there is any mucus or blood in them. Also, is there associated fever, cramping, or vomiting? Does an infant continue to eat well? Appear well? Seem to be thriving? Is an infant wetting at least six diapers daily?

Infants with associated signs and symptoms such as fever, cramping, vomiting, loss of appetite, a decrease in voiding, and weight loss should be examined by their healthcare provider because this suggests an infectious process. If in doubt as to whether their child is ill, teach parents to err on the side of phoning their healthcare provider. Dehydration occurs rapidly in a small infant who is not eating and is losing body fluid through loose stools (Mehal, Esposito, Holman, et al., 2012).

Colic

Colic is paroxysmal abdominal pain that generally occurs in infants under 3 months of age and is marked by loud, intense crying (Shergill-Bonner, 2010). Infants pull their legs up against their abdomen, their faces become red and flushed, their fists clench, and their abdomens become tense. If offered a bottle, an infant with colic will suck vigorously for a few minutes as if starved and then stop as another wave of intestinal pain occurs.

The cause of colic is unclear and probably results for several reasons. It may occur in susceptible infants from overfeeding or from swallowing too much air while feeding. Formula-fed babies tend to have more symptoms than breastfed babies, possibly because they swallow more air while drinking or because formula is harder to digest.

Although infants continue to thrive despite colic, the condition should not be dismissed as unimportant. It is a distressing and frightening problem for parents because their infant is not only in acute pain but also the distress persists for hours, usually into the middle of the night, allowing no one in the family to get adequate rest. This creates a difficult beginning to a parent–child relationship, which needs to be strong and binding for parents to enjoy parenting and for an infant to thrive in their care.

Take a thorough history of an infant with signs of colic because an intestinal obstruction or infection can mimic an attack of colic and be misinterpreted by the casual interviewer. With colic, symptoms of abdominal pain typically last up to 3 hours a day and occur at least 3 days every week; bowel movements are normal. Constipation; narrow, ribbonlike stools; and the presence of blood or mucus suggest other problems.

If the infant is bottle fed, ask about the type of formula used, how it is prepared, and if parents hold the baby upright and burp the infant adequately after feeding. For a breastfed baby, ask about the mother's diet (Is she avoiding "gassy" food such as cabbage?).

A number of interventions can be helpful to recommend to relieve colic symptoms. For example, both breastfed and formula-fed infants may feel more comfortable with small, frequent feedings to prevent distention and discomfort. Offering a pacifier can be comforting. Reducing stimuli, taking infants for car rides, or playing a music box that simulates the sound of a heartbeat are often reported as being helpful (Gahagan, 2011). Dietary changes have little effect, although there is some evidence using hydrolyzed protein, probiotics or prebiotics, or a soy-based formula for bottle-fed babies may be helpful (Iacovou, Ralston, Muir, et al., 2011; Thomas & Greer, 2010).

Some parents try placing a hot water bottle on their infant's stomach for comfort, but this should be discouraged. A basic rule for any abdominal discomfort is to avoid heat in case appendicitis is developing. This is highly unlikely in so young an infant, but parents will remember they once used heat and may use it again when the child is older. Hot water bottles and heating pads also might burn the delicate skin of infants.

Caution parents to check with their primary care provider before using herbs or home remedies such as star anise to be certain what they have heard to be effective is safe for infants (Madden, Schmitz, & Fullerton, 2012). They should use the same precaution for chiropractic or acupressure therapy.

As a final measure, it is important to think of colic as a family problem or else a vicious circle may gradually begin. An infant cries and the parents may become tense and unsure of themselves. An infant then senses the tension and develops more colic. Some parents benefit from planning relief time from infant care to relieve their stress level and prevent this cycle. Box 29.7 shows an interprofessional care map illustrating both nursing and team planning to address such a problem as infant colic.

In about 85% of infants, colic disappears almost magically at 3 months of age, probably because it becomes easier to digest food and an infant maintains a more upright position by this time, which allows less gas to form.

What If . . . 29.3

Bryan's mother asks the nurse if changing her work shift so that her mother cares for Bryan during his awake time would help solve her problem. Would the nurse agree with her?

Spitting Up

Almost all infants spit up, although formula-fed babies appear to do this more than breastfed babies, possibly due to overfeeding. Ask parents to carefully describe what they mean by "spitting up." How long has the baby been doing it? How frequently? What is the appearance of the spit-up milk? Almost all milk that is spit up smells at least faintly sour, but it should not contain blood or bile.

The baby who spits up a mouthful of milk (rolling down the chin) two or three times a day (or sometimes after every meal) is experiencing normal, early-infancy spitting up. Associated signs such as diarrhea, abdominal cramps, fever, cough, cold, or loss of activity suggest illness. If an infant is spitting up so forcefully that milk is projected 3 or 4 ft away, it may be the beginning of pyloric stenosis (an abnormally tight valve between the stomach and duodenum), which requires surgical intervention. If the spitting up is a large amount with each feeding, parents may be describing gastroesophageal reflux, in which a lax cardiac sphincter and esophagus allow for the regurgitation of gastric contents

---

BOX 29.7

Nursing Care Planning (continued)

Team Member Responsible	Assessment	Intervention	Rationale	Expected Outcome
Psychosocial/Spiritual/Emotional Needs				
Nurse/nurse practitioner	Assess why parent is taking the fact the infant cries only during her care time personally.	Reassure parent it's a coincidence colic occurs at the time she is giving care.	Reassurance that the problem is not the mother's fault can aid in objective problem solving.	Parent states she understands the problem is not a personal one.
Nurse	Assess parent's level of stress about constant crying.	Caution parent that crying in infants produces frustration in adults. Help plan respite time if necessary.	Acknowledging frustration helps to validate feelings. Time away can help relieve tension.	Parent states she is frustrated but also ready to work on solving the problem.
Informatics for Seamless Healthcare Planning				
Nurse	Urge the parent to call for further suggestions if needed. Stress that colic usually resolves by 3 months of age.	Advise parent to contact clinic if measures are ineffective by 1 week.	Assurance that continuing support will be available can help relieve stress.	Parent agrees to call in 1 week if crying has not improved.

into the esophagus. This also requires medical attention (see Chapter 45).

Burping the baby thoroughly after a feeding often limits spitting up. Parents may try sitting an infant in an infant chair for half an hour after feeding. Changing formulas generally is of little value. Reassure parents spitting up decreases in amount as the baby becomes better at coordinating swallowing and digestive processes (the cardiac sphincter matures). In the meantime, a bib can protect the baby's clothing and the parent. After a few months, the child will naturally stay in an upright position longer, and gravity will help to correct the problem.

Diaper Dermatitis

Some infants have such sensitive skin that diaper dermatitis (diaper rash) is a problem from the first few days of life. It occurs for a number of reasons.

When parents do not change a child's diapers frequently, feces is left in contact with skin, and irritation may result in the perianal area. Urine that is left in diapers too long breaks down into ammonia, a chemical extremely irritating to infant skin. Ammonia dermatitis of this type is generally a problem in the second half of the first year of life, when an infant is producing a larger quantity of urine than before. For some infants, however, it is a problem from the first week.

Frequent diaper changing, applying an ointment, and exposing the diaper area to air may relieve the problem. Some infants may have to sleep without diapers at night to solve the problem. If a diaper area is covered with lesions that are bright red, with or without oozing, that last longer than 3 days, and appear as red pinpoint lesions, suspect a fungal (monilial or candidiasis) infection that will also need therapy (an antifungal medicine such as Nystatin). Fungal infections of this type are discussed in Chapter 43.

Whenever the entire diaper area is erythematous and irritated so the outline of the diaper on the skin can be identified, an allergy to the material in the diaper or to laundry products if a commercially washed or home-washed diaper is being used is suggested. Changing the brand or type of diaper or washing solution usually alleviates this problem.

Miliaria

Miliaria, or prickly heat rash, occurs most often in warm weather or when babies are overdressed or sleep in overheated rooms. Clusters of pinpoint, reddened papules with occasional vesicles and pustules surrounded by erythema usually appear on the neck first and may spread upward to around the ears and onto the face or down onto the trunk.

Bathing an infant twice a day during hot weather, particularly if a small amount of baking soda is added to the bath water, may improve the rash. Eliminating sweating by reducing the amount of clothing on an infant or lowering the room temperature should bring almost immediate improvement and prevent further eruptions.

Baby-Bottle Tooth Decay Syndrome

Putting an infant to bed with a bottle can result in decay of all the upper teeth and the lower posterior teeth (Bishop, 2011) (Fig. 29.21). Decay occurs because, while an infant sleeps, liquid from the propped bottle continuously soaks the upper front teeth and lower back teeth (the lower front teeth are protected by the tongue). The problem, called **baby-bottle syndrome**, is most serious when the bottle is filled with sugar water, formula, milk, or fruit juice. The carbohydrate in these solutions ferments to organic acids that demineralize the tooth enamel until it decays.

Figure 29.21 Baby-bottle syndrome. Notice the extensive decay in the upper teeth. (From K. L. Boyd, DDS/Custom Medical Stock Photograph.)

To prevent this problem, advise parents never to put their baby to bed with a bottle. If parents insist a bottle is necessary to allow a baby to fall asleep, encourage them to fill it with water and use a nipple with a small hole to prevent the baby from receiving a large amount of fluid. If the baby refuses to drink anything but milk, the parents might dilute the milk with water more and more each night until the bottle contains water only.

Obesity in Infants

Obesity in infants is defined as a weight greater than the 90th to 95th percentile on a standardized height/weight chart. Obesity occurs when there is an abnormal increase in the number of fat cells because of excessive calorie intake. Preventing obesity in infants is important because the extra fat cells formed at this time are likely to remain throughout childhood and even into adulthood. If a child becomes obese because of over-ingesting milk, iron-deficiency anemia may also be present because of the low iron content of both breast and commercial milk. Once infant obesity begins, it is difficult to reverse, so prevention is the key (Taylor, Heath, Galland, et al., 2011).

Overfeeding in infancy often occurs because parents were taught to eat everything on their plate, and they continue to instill this concept in their children. This appears to be the case most often with formula-fed infants whose parents urge them to empty their bottle or finish a cereal serving. It can occur any time parents automatically feed an infant when the child cries rather than investigating what the cry might really mean. As a general rule, an infant should take no more than 32 oz of formula daily and shouldn't be breastfeeding more often than every 2 hours. When solid food is introduced, a bottle of water can be substituted for formula at one feeding to reduce calories. Nonfat milk should not be given because it contains so little fat that essential fatty acid requirements may not be sufficient to ensure cell growth.

Another way to help prevent obesity is to add a source of fiber, such as whole-grain cereal and raw fruit, to an infant's diet. These prolong the stomach-emptying time, so they can help reduce food intake. Caution parents about giving infants who are obese foods with high amounts of refined sugars, such as pudding, cake, cookies, and candy. Encourage parents to learn more about balanced nutrition and to provide this for their entire family.

Concerns of the Family With an Infant With Unique Needs

An infant born with a cognitive or physical challenge is usually hospitalized immediately after birth for diagnosis and treatment. This can result in delayed bonding because the newborn is separated from the parents during this critical time. Encourage parents to regularly visit an intensive care nursery to help form a strong parent–child attachment. If parents cannot visit, urge them to telephone the hospital as frequently as they can to ask about their child. E-mailing them photographs or posting them by the infant's crib for parents to take home are other ways to encourage bonding.

Many of the developmental events of the infant year (e.g., social smile, laughing out loud, reaching for an object, uttering the first word, sitting, talking) are activities that encourage parent–child interaction because they make an infant fun to be with and naturally make a parent want to spend more time with the child. Children who are cognitively challenged may not reach these milestones. Children who are physically challenged may be unable to achieve them as well if they cannot reach up and pat their mother's face or hold out arms to be picked up by the father. If infants leave the hospital with a cast or other equipment such as a ventilator for care, parents may be so concerned with these items that they cannot initiate normal singing and playing activities with their children.

To encourage a good parent–child relationship, point out the positive things the infant can do. Perhaps the child's facial expression says, "Pick me up," even though he doesn't reach up with his hands, or perhaps his eyes follow his mother's actions even though he can't yet call to her.

Helping parents to interact more fully with their infants this way helps to build a sense of trust in the infant. Keeping painful procedures to a minimum when infants are ill is also important in helping infants achieve a positive outlook on the world (Stevens, Abbott, Yamada, et al., 2011).

Without this sense of trust, children have difficulty expressing themselves to others, and they may not believe they are lovable or that people would want to interact with them. Individuals who are physically challenged, no matter what their ages, need people around them to give them help at whatever point they cannot meet their own needs. It is unfortunate when children who are physically challenged cannot reach out for help because they have difficulty developing a sense of trust.

Infants who are cognitively or physically challenged or chronically ill experience the same health and growth problems as other infants such as colic or diaper rash. Parents may be reluctant to mention these concerns at healthcare visits because they believe such problems pale in comparison to the child's primary illness or condition. When taking the health histories of children with chronic or long-standing medical problems, ask parents about these secondary concerns. "What about everyday things? Any problems there?" Treat these concerns seriously, so parents can feel confident about bringing them to your attention at future healthcare visits. Also mention they are part of normal infant development so parents can begin to view their child apart from his or her illness.

Discomfort from diaper rash and colic may actually occur more frequently in babies with other illnesses than those who are well because a parent may not want to bother an ill infant with physical care or burp the infant as long or as often as they would a well child. The bowel movements of children who are physically disabled or chronically ill may be looser than normal because of a liquid diet or medicine. Their urine may be more concentrated because of reduced intake. These conditions make diaper rash more apt to occur. Offering anticipatory guidance to parents can go a long way toward helping them avoid these special concerns of infancy.

QSEN Checkpoint Question 29.6

PATIENT-CENTERED CARE

When planning care for an infant who has unique needs, the nurse best promotes the parents' psychosocial well-being by which means?

a. Lowering the family's expectations around their infant's skills

b. Clearly describing the etiology of the infant's development deficits

c. Encouraging the family to have more children

d. Emphasizing what the infant can do more than what he or she cannot do

Look in Appendix A for the best answer and rationale.

Nutrition for the Infant With Unique Needs

Ill infants may tire too easily to suck long enough to take in adequate feedings. If any degree of neurologic involvement exists, sucking and swallowing reflexes may not be coordinated. If an infant has some gastrointestinal disorders, feeding may be impossible.

To ensure adequate calorie and protein intake, infants may need to be maintained on nasogastric tube or gastrostomy feedings, or total parenteral nutrition. Because these methods limit the amount of sucking that is possible and sucking provides pleasure as well as satisfying thirst, this is a major loss. Provide an infant with nonnutritive sucking experiences such as a pacifier if possible (which is acceptable with the parent's and the infant's condition) to fill this need. Help parents find time each day to hold the infant equal to the time they would have held the child if fed by breast or bottle to make parenting more satisfying and more like the role they planned (Wilken, 2012).

Infants who are ill for a long time may not eat solid foods eagerly once they are introduced because they are not hungry enough to be interested in a new eating method. Help parents to experiment with different foods to find a taste that does appeal to ill children or teach them to limit foods to only those that the child appears to like most from all five food groups.

What If . . . 29.4

The nurse is particularly interested in exploring one of the 2020 National Health Goals with respect to infant care (see Box 29.1). What would be a possible research topic to explore pertinent to this goal that would be applicable to Bryan and his family and that would also advance evidence-based practice?

KEY POINTS FOR REVIEW

■ The infant period is from 1 month to 12 months of age. Children typically double their birth weight at 4 to 6 months and triple it at 1 year.

■ Infants develop their first tooth at about 6 months; by 12 months, they have six to eight teeth.

■ Important gross motor milestones during the infant year are lifting the chest off a bed at 2 months, sitting at 6 to 8 months, creeping at 9 months, cruising at 10 to 11 months, and walking at 12 months.

■ Important fine motor accomplishments are the ability to pass an object from one hand to the other (7 months of age) and a pincer grasp (10 months of age).

■ Important milestones of language development during the first year are differentiating a cry (2 months of age), making simple vowel sounds (5 to 6 months of age), and saying two words besides "ma-ma" and "da-da" (12 months of age). The more infants are spoken to, the easier it is for them to acquire language.

■ Providing infants with proper toys for play helps development. All infant toys need to be checked to be certain they are too large to be aspirated (wider than a toilet paper roll).

■ Important milestones of vision development are the ability to follow a moving object past the midline (3 months of age) and ability to focus securely without eyes crossing (6 months of age).

■ According to Erikson (1993), the developmental task of the infant year is the development of a sense of trust versus mistrust. Helping parents spend quality time with their infant helps a sense of trust to develop and helps in planning nursing care that not only meets QSEN competencies but that also best meets the family's total needs.

■ Safety is important. Infants must be protected from falls and the aspiration of small objects. Skills an infant cannot accomplish one day, such as crawling (which can lead to danger), may be accomplished the next.

■ Solid food is generally introduced into an infant's diet at 6 months of age. Before infants can eat solid food, they must lose their extrusion reflex.

■ Common concerns related to infant development include teething, thumb-sucking, use of pacifiers, sleep problems, constipation, colic, diaper dermatitis, baby-bottle syndrome (decayed teeth from sucking on a bottle of formula while they sleep), and obesity. Nurses play a key role in teaching parents about these problems and suggestions to deal with them.

■ Remember that parent–infant attachment is critical to mental health. Urge parents to continue to give as much care as possible to ill infants to maintain this important relationship.

CRITICAL THINKING CARE STUDY

Alicia Scinta is a 3-month-old you meet in an emergency room because she has mild diarrhea. Her mother tells you Alicia is a "picky eater," and "no wonder she's sick."

Her mother works weekends as a drugstore clerk so Alicia is cared for at a child care center on the weekends. Her father, a university professor, tells you he'll watch her weekends "later on, when she's more fun."

1. Alicia's mother said she was a "picky eater." What questions would you want to ask to discover why she says that?

2. Alicia is cared for at a child care center every weekend. What questions would you want to ask about the center to evaluate if they are encouraging Alicia's infancy developmental task?

3. Mr. Scinta says he'll watch Alicia later "when she's more fun." What features of a 3-month-old could you point out to him to help convince him she is fun to care for now?

RELATED RESOURCES

Explore these additional resources to enhance learning for this chapter:
- Student resources on thePoint, including answers to the What If . . . and Critical Thinking Care Study questions, http://thepoint .lww.com/Flagg8e
- Adaptive learning powered by PrepU, http://thepoint.lww.com/prepu

REFERENCES

American Academy of Pediatrics. (2011a). *Fluoride supplements.* Washington, DC: Author.

American Academy of Pediatrics. (2011b). SIDS and other sleep-related infant deaths. *Pediatrics, 128*(5), e1341–e1367.

American Academy of Pediatrics. (2012a). *Where we stand: Car seats for children.* Washington, DC: Author.

American Academy of Pediatrics. (2012b). *Where we stand: TV viewing time.* Washington, DC: Author.

American Academy of Pediatrics. (2017). *Bright futures: Guidelines for health supervision of infants, children and adolescents* (4th ed.). Elk Grove Village, IL: Author.

Amit, M. (2010). Vegetarian diets in children and adolescents. *Paediatric Child Health, 5*(5), 303–314.

Bishop, W. P. (2011). Oral cavity. In K. J. Marcdante, R. M. Kliegman, H. B. Jenson, et al. (Eds.), *Nelson essentials of pediatrics* (6th ed., pp. 475–476). Philadelphia, PA: Saunders/Elsevier.

Centers for Disease Control and Prevention. (2011). Ten great public health achievements—United States, 2001–2010. *Morbidity & Mortality Weekly Report, 60*(19), 619–623.

Centers for Disease Control and Prevention. (2014). *10 Leading causes of death by age group, United States - 2014.* Retrieved from https://www.cdc .gov/injury/images/lc-charts/leading_causes_of_death_age_group_2014 _1050w760h.gif.

Conti, T. D., Patel, M., & Bhat, S. (2011). Breast-feeding & infant nutrition. In J. E. South-Paul, S. C. Matheny, & E. L. Lewis (Eds.), *Current diagnosis & treatment in family medicine* (3rd ed., pp. 28–35). Columbus, OH: McGraw-Hill.

de Amorim Lde, F., Estrela, C., & da Costa, L. R. (2011). Effects of traumatic dental injuries to primary teeth on permanent teeth. *Dental Traumatology, 27*(2), 117–121.

Erikson, E. (1993). *Childhood and society* (3rd ed.). New York, NY: W. W. Norton.

Gaffney, K. F., Kitsantas, P., & Cheema, J. (2012). Clinical practice guidelines for feeding behaviors and weight-for-age at 12 months. *Worldviews on Evidence Based Nursing, 9*(4), 234–242.

Gahagan, S. (2011). Crying and colic. In K. J. Marcdante, R. M. Kliegman, H. B. Jenson, et al. (Eds.), *Nelson essentials of pediatrics* (6th ed., pp. 45–47). Philadelphia, PA: Saunders/Elsevier.

Goldson, E., & Reynolds, A. (2011). Child development & behavior. In W. W. Hay, M. J. Levine, J. M. Sondheimer, et al. (Eds.), *Current pediatric diagnosis & treatment* (20th ed., pp. 64–103). Columbus, OH: McGraw-Hill.

Iacovou, M., Ralston, R. A., Muir, J., et al. (2011). Dietary management of infantile colic: A systematic review. *Maternal Child Health Journal, 16*(6), 1319–1331.

Ibrahim, N. G., Wood, J., Margulies, S. S., et al. (2011). Influence of age and fall type on head injuries in infants and toddlers. *International Journal of Development & Neuroscience, 30*(3), 201–206.

Kiran, K., Swati, T., Kamala, B. K., et al. (2011). Prevalence of systemic and local disturbances in infants during primary teeth eruption. *European Journal of Paediatric Dentistry, 12*(4), 249–252.

Klootwijk, T., & Krul, M. (2011). Some concerns remain about the proposed association between swimming and asthma. *American Journal of Respiratory Critical Care Medicine, 184*(12), 1419–1420.

Krebs, N. F., & Primak, L. E. (2011). Pediatric nutrition & nutritional disorders. In K. J. Marcdante, R. M. Kliegman, H. B. Jenson, et al. (Eds.), *Nelson essentials of pediatrics* (6th ed., pp. 103–107). Philadelphia, PA: Saunders/Elsevier.

Levine, D. A. (2011). Normal development. In K. J. Marcdante, R. M. Kliegman, H. B. Jenson, et al. (Eds.), *Nelson essentials of pediatrics* (6th ed., pp. 16–18). Philadelphia, PA: Saunders/Elsevier.

Lyon, V. B. (2011). Dermatology. In K. J. Marcdante, R. M. Kliegman, H. B. Jenson, et al. (Eds.), *Nelson essentials of pediatrics* (6th ed., pp. 713–734). Philadelphia, PA: Saunders/Elsevier.

Madden, G. R., Schmitz, K. H., & Fullerton, K. (2012). A case of infantile star anise toxicity. *Pediatric Emergency Care, 28*(3), 284–285.

Mehal, J. M., Esposito, D. H., Holman, R. C., et al. (2012). Risk factors for diarrhea-associated infant mortality in the United States, 2005–2007. *Pediatric Infectious Disease Journal, 31*(7), 717–721.

Mesman, J., Oster, H., & Camras, L. (2012). Parental sensitivity to infant distress: What do discrete negative emotions have to do with it? *Attachment & Human Development, 14*(4), 337–348.

Milgrom, P., & Chi, D. L. (2011). Prevention-centered caries management strategies during critical periods in early childhood. *Journal of the California Dental Association, 39*(10), 735–741.

Montaldo, L., Montaldo, P., Cuccaro, P., et al. (2011). Effects of feeding on non-nutritive sucking habits and implications on occlusion in mixed dentition. *International Journal of Paediatric Dentistry, 21*(1), 68–73.

Nelson, A. M. (2012). A comprehensive review of evidence and current recommendations related to pacifier usage. *Journal of Pediatric Nursing, 27*(6), 690–699.

Olusanya, B. O., & Renner, J. K. (2013). Pattern and characteristics of growth faltering in early infancy in an urban Sub-Saharan African setting. *Pediatrics & Neonatology, 54*(2), 119–127.

Parsons, H. G., George, M. A., & Innis, S. M. (2011). Growth assessment in clinical practice: Whose growth curve? *Current Gastroenterology Reports, 13*(3), 286–292.

Piaget, J. (1952). *The origins of intelligence in children.* New York, NY: International University Press.

Plutzer, K., Spencer, A. J., & Keirse, M. J. (2011). How first-time mothers perceive and deal with teething symptoms: A randomized controlled trial. *Child: Care, Health and Development, 38*(2), 292–299.

Price, A. M., Wake, M., Ukoumunne, O. C., et al. (2012). Outcomes at six years of age for children with infant sleep problems: Longitudinal community-based study. *Sleep Medicine, 13*(8), 991–998.

Scollan-Koliopoulos, M., & Koliopoulos, J. S. (2010). Evaluation and management of apparent life-threatening events in infants. *Pediatric Nursing, 36*(2), 77–79.

Shergill-Bonner, R. (2010). Infantile colic: Practicalities of management, including dietary aspects. *Journal of Family Health Care, 20*(6), 206–209.

Singer, H. S. (2011). Stereotypic movement disorders. *Handbook of Clinical Neurology, 100*(1), 631–639.

Stevens, B. J., Abbott, L. K., Yamada, J., et al. (2011). Epidemiology and management of painful procedures in children in Canadian hospitals. *Canadian Medical Association Journal, 183*(7), E403–E410.

Sundaram, S., Hoffenberg, E., Kramer, R., et al. (2011). Gastrointestinal tract. In W. W. Hay, M. J. Levine, J. M. Sondheimer, et al. (Eds.), *Current pediatric diagnosis & treatment* (20th ed., pp. 595–630). Columbus, OH: McGraw-Hill.

Taylor, B. J., Heath, A. L., Galland, B. C., et al. (2011). Prevention of overweight in infancy. *BMC Public Health, 11*(1), 942.

Thilo, E. H., & Rosenberg, A. A. (2011). The newborn infant. In W. W. Hay, M. J. Levine, J. M. Sondheimer, et al. (Eds.), *Current pediatric diagnosis & treatment* (20th ed., pp. 1–63). Columbus, OH: McGraw-Hill.

Thomas, D. W., & Greer, F. R. (2010). Probiotics and prebiotics in pediatrics. *Pediatrics, 126*(6), 1217–1231.

Townsend, E., & Pitchford, N. J. (2012). Baby knows best? The impact of weaning style on food preferences and body mass index in early childhood in a case-controlled sample. *BMJ Open, 2*(1), e000298.

U.S. Department of Health and Human Services. (2010). *Healthy people 2020.* Washington, DC: Author.

Whitney, E. N., & Rolfes, S. R. (2012). Life cycle nutrition: Infant, childhood & adolescence. In E. N. Whitney & S. R. Rolfes (Eds.), *Understanding nutrition* (pp. 528–573). Belmont, CA: Wadsworth Publishing.

Wilken, M. (2012). The impact of child tube feeding on maternal emotional state and identity: A qualitative meta-analysis. *Journal of Pediatric Nursing, 27*(3), 248–255.

Yates, J., McKay, M., & Nicholson, A. J. (2011). Patterns of scald injuries in children—has anything changed? *Irish Medical Journal, 104*(9), 263–265.

30

Nursing Care of a Family With a Toddler

*J*ason is a 2.5-year-old boy you see at a pediatric clinic. His mother tells you he has changed completely in the past 6 months from an easy-to-care-for baby into a "monster" who refuses to do anything she asks. The only word he says anymore is "no." He has a temper tantrum every night at dinner over some type of food. She tells you this has changed parenting from "fun" to "a real chore."

The previous chapter discussed the growth and development of infants and the abilities that infants develop in the first year. This chapter adds information about the dramatic changes, both physical and psychosocial, that occur during the toddler years and that form the basis for care and health teaching for this age group.

What advice could you give Jason's mother to help her regain a positive view of parenting?

OBJECTIVES

After mastering the contents of this chapter, you should be able to:

1. Describe normal growth and development of a toddler as well as common parental concerns.

2. Identify 2020 National Health Goals related to the toddler age group that nurses can help the nation achieve.

3. Assess a toddler for normal growth and development milestones.

4. Formulate nursing diagnoses related to toddler growth and development or parental concerns regarding growth and development.

5. Identify expected outcomes for nursing care of a toddler as well as help parents manage seamless transitions across differing healthcare settings.

6. Using the nursing process, plan nursing care that includes the six competencies of Quality & Safety Education for Nurses (QSEN): Patient-Centered Care, Teamwork & Collaboration, Evidence-Based Practice (EBP), Quality Improvement (QI), Safety, and Informatics.

7. Implement nursing care to promote normal growth and development of a toddler, such as discussing toddler developmental milestones with parents.

8. Evaluate expected outcomes for achievement and effectiveness of care.

9. Integrate knowledge of toddler growth and development with the interplay of the nursing process, the six competencies of QSEN, and Family Nursing to promote quality maternal and child health nursing care.

During the toddler period, the age span from 1 to 3 years, enormous changes take place in a child and, consequently, in a family. During this period, children accomplish a wide array of developmental tasks and change from largely immobile and preverbal infants who are dependent on caregivers for the fulfillment of most needs to walking, talking young children with a growing sense of **autonomy** (independence). To match this growth, parents must also change during this period.

If parents enjoyed caring for an infant because time could be spent rocking or singing to the child, they may not enjoy being the parents of a toddler because now their task is to support their child's growing independence by letting the child experiment with toys or other activities. In contrast, some parents thrive during this time as they enjoy playing with this more active child. Because healthy children and families are constantly being challenged by the process of normal development this way, parents often have questions about how to guide their child in different situations and how to cope with special needs and concerns relevant to this age (Nelson, 2013). Box 30.1 shows 2020 National Health Goals that speak to the toddler age group.

Nursing Process Overview

FOR HEALTHY DEVELOPMENT OF A TODDLER

ASSESSMENT

Whether a child is seen for a routine checkup or has come to a healthcare center because of a specific health concern, assessment begins with a careful health history. Asking parents about a toddler's ability to carry out activities of daily living offers assessment information not only on the child's developmental progress but also offers important clues about the child–parent relationship. Because parents see their children daily, they are the best source of information and opinion on when a child seems to be acting "out of sorts" or "different" (a typical sign a child may not be feeling well).

Careful observation is another crucial element of the nursing assessment of a toddler, although toddlers may not show typical behavior at a healthcare visit (e.g., may not talk, may cling to a parent instead of demonstrating walking).

NURSING DIAGNOSIS

Nursing diagnoses related to growth and development of toddlers usually focus on the parents' eagerness to learn more about the parameters of normal growth and development or issues of safety or care. Examples include:

- Health-seeking behaviors related to normal toddler development
- Deficient knowledge related to the best method of toilet training
- Risk for injury related to impulsiveness of the toddler
- Interrupted family process related to need for close supervision of a 2-year-old
- Readiness for enhanced family coping related to the parents' ability to adjust to the new needs of the child

---

BOX 30.1

Nursing Care Planning Based on 2020 National Health Goals

A number of 2020 National Health Goals relate specifically to safety during the toddler years. These include:

- Increase the use of child automotive restraints in children 3 years of age and under from a baseline of 72% to 79%.
- Eliminate or improve elevated blood lead levels in children from a target level of 0.9% of children to a target level of 0%.
- Increase the percentage of persons 2 years of age and older who have had a dental visit in the past 12 months from a baseline of 44.5% to 49%.
- Maintain the rate of deaths caused by poisonings from a baseline at 13.1 out of 100,000 (U.S. Department of Health and Human Services, 2010; see www.healthypeople.gov).

Nurses can help the nation achieve these goals by continuing to educate parents about the importance of using car seats and childproofing their homes against household and lead poisoning.

- Risk for imbalanced nutrition, more than body requirements, related to fast food choices
- Disturbed sleep pattern related to lack of bedtime routine

OUTCOME IDENTIFICATION AND PLANNING

To help parents resolve a concern during the toddler period, focus largely on family education and anticipatory guidance. Urge them to establish realistic goals and outcomes so they can meet the rapidly changing needs of their toddler and learn to cope with typical toddler behaviors. Otherwise, parents can expect too much of a toddler and grow frustrated instead of enjoying being a parent of a child this age.

IMPLEMENTATION

When teaching about typical toddler behavior, teach parents that a good rule is to think of a toddler as a visitor from a foreign land who wants to participate in everything the family is doing but doesn't know the customs or the language.

Also teach parents not only how to approach a current problem but also how to learn adequate methods for resolving similar situations that are sure to arise in the future. If parents do not learn methods that can be applied throughout their child's growing years, they may win battles but lose wars. For instance, parents may find that if they promise a child a treat when the child is in the middle of a temper tantrum, that will stop the tantrum, but it will not prevent other tantrums from occurring in the future (and, in fact, may encourage them). Health visits provide opportunities to help parents learn healthier coping techniques as well as a time to demonstrate effective communication skills so parents can improve their interactions with their child.

OUTCOME EVALUATION

Expected outcomes must be evaluated frequently during the toddler period because children change so much and learn so many new skills during this time that their abilities and associated parental concerns can change from day to day. Examples of expected outcomes include:

- Parents state the child maintains a consistent bedtime routine within the next 2 weeks.
- Parents state they have childproofed their home by putting a lock on kitchen cupboards by the next clinic visit.
- Grandmother states she has modified usual activities to conserve strength to care for toddler granddaughter by 1 week's time.

Nursing Assessment of a Toddler's Growth and Development

An assessment of a toddler begins with the child's physical growth and skill development. Box 30.2 describes a typical toddler appearance. Table 30.1 provides some guidelines to help parents evaluate illness at this age.

BOX 30.2

Nursing Care Planning Using Assessment

APPEARANCE OF THE AVERAGE TODDLER

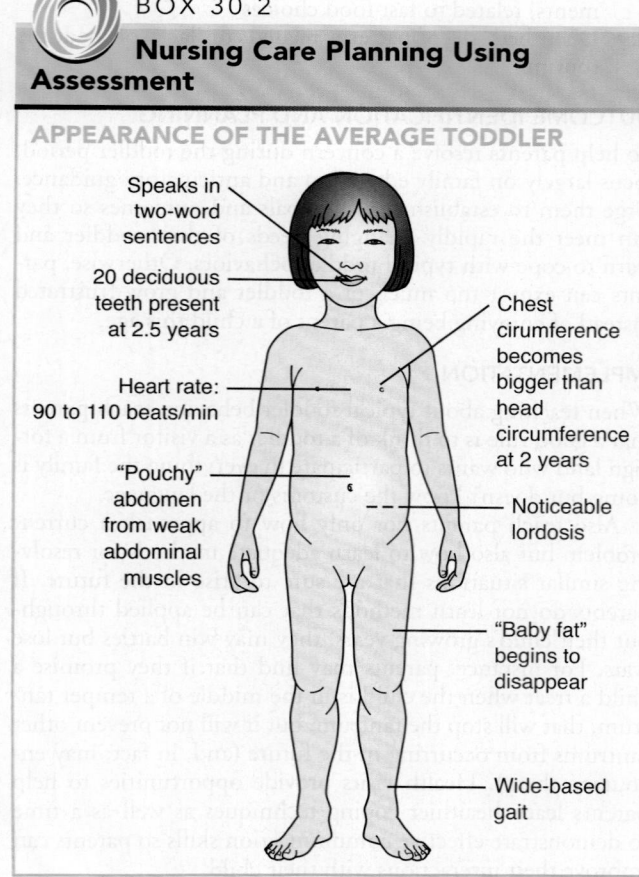

- Speaks in two-word sentences
- 20 deciduous teeth present at 2.5 years
- Heart rate: 90 to 110 beats/min
- "Pouchy" abdomen from weak abdominal muscles
- Chest cirumference becomes bigger than head circumference at 2 years
- Noticeable lordosis
- "Baby fat" begins to disappear
- Wide-based gait

PHYSICAL GROWTH

Although toddlers are making great strides developmentally, their physical growth begins to slow.

Weight, Height, Head Circumference, and Body Mass Index

Plot weight and height on a standard growth chart for toddlers (available at http://thePoint.lww.com/Flagg8e) at each healthcare visit to determine if progress is normal for that particular child. If a child is not yet walking, continue to measure height with the child lying down. A child gains only about 5 to 6 lb (2.5 kg) and 5 in. (12 cm) a year during the toddler period, much less than the rate of growth during the infant year. As subcutaneous tissue, or baby fat, begins to disappear toward the end of the second year, the child changes from a plump baby into a leaner, more muscular little girl or boy. A toddler's appetite decreases accordingly, yet adequate intake of all nutrients is still essential to meet energy needs (Whitney & Rolfes, 2013).

Head circumference increases only about 2 cm during the second year compared to about 12 cm during the first year. Head circumference equals chest circumference at 6 months to 1 year of age. By 2 years, chest circumference should have grown greater than that of the head.

Body mass index (BMI) screening is completed at 24 months to identify toddlers who are overweight or underweight. A good website to use to calculate a child's BMI is the one available via the Centers for Disease Control and Prevention (CDC) website (https://nccd.cdc.gov/dnpabmi/calculator.aspx).

Body Contour

Toddlers tend to have a prominent abdomen because, although they are walking well, their abdominal muscles are not yet strong enough to support abdominal contents as well as they will be able to do later (Fig. 30.1A). They also have a forward curve of the spine at the sacral area (**lordosis**). As they become more experienced at walking, this will correct itself naturally. In addition, many toddlers waddle or walk with a wide stance (see Fig. 30.1B). This stance seems to increase the lordotic curve, but it keeps them on their feet.

Body Systems

Body systems continue to mature during this time.

- Respirations slow slightly but continue to be mainly abdominal.
- Heart rate slows from 110 to 90 beats/min.
- Blood pressure increases to about 99/64 mmHg.
- The brain develops to about 90% of its adult size.
- In the respiratory system, the lumens of vessels enlarge progressively so the threat of lower respiratory infection lessens.
- Stomach secretions become more acid; therefore, gastrointestinal infections also become less common.
- Stomach capacity increases to the point a child can eat three meals a day.
- Control of the urinary and anal sphincters becomes possible with complete myelination of the spinal cord so toilet training is possible.

TABLE 30.1 PARENTAL DIFFICULTIES IN EVALUATING ILLNESS IN TODDLERS

Problem	Guidelines for Parents
Evaluating seriousness of illness	Toddlers typically answer "no" to almost all questions; therefore, a question such as "Does your arm hurt?" may bring a "no" response even if an arm does hurt. Observing children for indications of illness (e.g., holding an arm stiffly, rubbing abdomen, crying when they void) is more helpful. Many toddlers do not know the words to describe a feeling of nausea or a sore throat. They reveal these symptoms by not eating. If the child is normally a light eater, as many are, it is difficult for a parent to appreciate these signs.
Differentiating tiredness from illness	Toddlers tend to whine or sleep when they are either tired or ill. Reviewing the child's day and activities often helps to evaluate what is happening. If the child is not tired (it is not nap or bedtime) or if there is not a break in usual routine, crying and whining or temper tantrums suggest illness.
Evaluating nutritional intake	Toddlers are normally fussy eaters compared to infants. Evaluating children as to whether they are active and growing is better than assessing any one day's food intake.
Age-specific diseases to be aware of	The toddler period is an important age to assess speech development; children should be further evaluated if they cannot use simple sentences composed of a noun or pronoun and verb ("me go") by 2 years of age.
	As children begin to walk, they should be observed for an abnormal gait. Osteomyelitis (bone infection) occurs with a high frequency in toddlers; symptoms of limping, swollen joints, or arm or leg pain should be regarded as serious until ruled otherwise.
	Toddlers contract 10–12 mild upper respiratory infections a year. Otitis media (middle ear infection) may occur as a complication of these. The child with an upper respiratory infection who suddenly develops a high fever and pulls or manipulates his or her ears should be seen by a primary care provider.
	Children who attend day care programs have a high incidence of hepatitis A, *Giardia*, and *Shigella* infections. Teach parents to report jaundice or diarrhea promptly to a healthcare provider to detect these infections.

A · · · · B

Figure 30.1 The physical characteristics of toddlers. **(A)** Toddlers typically have a prominent abdomen. **(B)** Toddlers typically walk with an unsteady gait for better stability.

• Immune globulin (Ig)G and IgM antibody production becomes mature at 2 years of age. The passive immunity obtained during intrauterine life is no longer operative.

QSEN Checkpoint Question 30.1

QUALITY IMPROVEMENT

The nurse provides patient education to Jason's father who had asked if it is normal for his 2-year-old son to spread his feet wide apart when he walks. Which of his statements suggests that he received accurate teaching?

- a. "Jason may be all right, but toddlers with dislocated hips also walk that way."
- b. "A wide-spaced gait is a common characteristic of toddlers."
- c. "Most toddlers walk with feet close together to better stabilize themselves."
- d. "His shoes may not have a good arch and this could be causing him to walk unsteadily."

Look in Appendix A for the best answer and rationale.

Teeth

Eight new teeth (the canines and the first molars) erupt during the second year. All 20 deciduous teeth are generally present by 2.5 to 3 years of age (Bishop, 2011).

DEVELOPMENTAL MILESTONES

The developmental milestones of the toddler years are less numerous but no less dramatic than those of the infant year because this is a period of slow and steady, not sudden, growth. Toddler development is influenced to some extent by the amount of social contact and the number of opportunities children have to explore and experience new degrees of independence. It is strongly influenced by individual readiness for a new skill. Table 30.2 highlights growth and development milestones of gross and fine motor skills, language, and play during the toddler years.

Language Development

Toddlerhood is a critical time for language development, although even this varies among children because to master language, children need practice time. A child who is 2 years old and does not talk in two-word, noun–verb simple sentences needs a careful assessment to determine the cause because this implies underdevelopment. Parents are often worried a lack of language means their child has an autism spectrum disorder (ASD) (Barbaro & Dissanayake, 2012). It is true that a delay in language can represent the first symptom of autism, but it also may only be a temporary phenomenon until the child fully grasps the essence of speech.

A word that is used frequently by toddlers and that is a manifestation of their developing autonomy is "no." Toddlers may use the word to mean they are refusing a task, that they do not understand it, or they may only be practicing a sound they have noticed has potent effects on those around them.

To learn other words, children needs to be exposed to words through conversation and having books read to them. Language develops quickest if parents respect what toddlers have to say so children grasp the use and purpose of language. Watching television promotes little learning in toddlers because the activity is passive, and it is difficult to discern how language causes action. The American Academy of Pediatrics (APP, 2012) recommends severely limiting television viewing until at least 2 years of age.

Urge parents to encourage language development by naming objects (e.g., ball, block, music box, doll) as they play

TABLE 30.2 MILESTONES OF TODDLER GROWTH AND DEVELOPMENT

Age (in Months)	Fine Motor	Gross Motor	Language	Play
15	Puts small pellets into small bottles; scribbles voluntarily with a pencil or crayon; holds a spoon well but may still turn it upside down on the way to mouth	Walks alone well; can seat self in chair; can creep up stairs	4–6 words	Can stack two blocks; enjoys being read to; drops toys for adult to recover (exploring sense of permanence)
18	No longer rotates a spoon to bring it to mouth	Can run and jump in place; can walk up and down stairs holding onto a person's hand or railing; typically places both feet on one step before advancing	7–20 words; uses jargoning; names one body part	Imitates household chores such as dusting; begins parallel play (playing beside, not with, another child)
24	Can open doors by turning doorknobs; unscrew lids	Walks up stairs alone, still using both feet on same step at same time	50 words; two-word sentences (noun or pronoun and verb), such as "Daddy go," "Dog talks"	Parallel play evident
30	Makes simple lines or strokes for crosses with a pencil	Can jump down from chairs	Verbal language increasing steadily; knows full name; can name one color and holds up fingers to show age	Spends time playing house, imitating parents' actions; play is "roughhousing" or active

with their child or when they give the toddler something ("Here is your drink of water," "Let's put on these pajamas," etc.). This helps children grasp the fact that words are not meaningless sounds but that they apply to people and objects and have uses.

Always answering a child's questions is another good way to do this. Be certain answers for toddlers are simple and brief because they have such a short attention span.

Still, other toddlers do not develop language readily because they are not called on to use it. When they point at an object, someone hands it to them; when they climb into their high chair, someone places a meal in front of them. To assess whether parents are encouraging language development, ask them what happens when the child wants something. Do they provide opportunities for the child to ask for things? Children should not be made to name an object before they can have it because their vocabulary is so limited, but parents can reinforce language by voicing the request (e.g., "You want the ball?"). Reading aloud is another effective way to strengthen vocabulary. Reading the exact words in a book is not as important at this age as is pointing to the pictures and describing what the picture shows, such as "See Jane throwing the ball?" "Look, that dog took that ball!" Reading this way can also have the additional benefit of strengthening parent–child bonds and offering respite for parents who are tired of more active games (Landry, Smith, Swank, et al., 2011).

Children who are very active may use fewer words than children who are less active because active children are too busy doing things to describe what it is they are doing. Such children probably have a large unexpressed vocabulary, however, or understand more words (comprehensive vocabulary) than can be expressed (expressive vocabulary).

Because children learn language from imitating what they hear, if they are spoken to in baby talk, their enunciation of words can be poor; if they hear examples of bad grammar, they will not use good grammar. Remind parents that pronouns are difficult for children to use correctly; many children are 3.5 or 4 years of age before they can separate the different uses of "I," "me," "him," and "her." Bilingual children often interchange words from both languages.

QSEN Checkpoint Question 30.2

INFORMATICS

Toddlers learn a great deal about oral communication in the course of their development. The nurse expects Jason, a 2-year-old, to have mastered which statement?

a. "Red tomatoes."
b. "Daddy come."
c. "Old MacDonald."
d. "Please, please."

Look in Appendix A for the best answer and rationale.

Emotional Development

Children change a great deal in their ability to understand the world and how they relate to people during the toddler years.

Autonomy

The developmental task of the toddler years according to Erikson (1993) is the development of a *sense of autonomy*

versus shame or doubt (see Chapter 28). Children who have learned to trust themselves and others during the infant year are better prepared to do this than those who have not learned to trust themselves or others.

To develop a sense of autonomy is to develop a sense of independence. A healthy level of autonomy is achieved when parents are able to balance independence with consistently sound rules for safety.

Socialization

Once toddlers are walking well, they become resistant to sitting in laps and being cuddled. This is not lack of a desire for socialization but a function of being independent. At 15 months, children are still enthusiastic about interacting with people, providing those people are willing to follow them where they want to go. By 18 months, toddlers imitate the things they see a parent doing, such as "study" or "sweep," so they seek out parents to observe and imitate. By 2 or more years of age, children become aware of gender differences and may point to other children and identify them as "boy" or "girl."

Play Behavior

All during the toddler period, children play beside other children, not with them. This side-by-side play (**parallel play**) is not unfriendly but is a normal developmental sequence that occurs during the toddler period (Fig. 30.2). Caution parents that if two toddlers are going to play together, they must provide similar toys because an argument over one toy is likely to occur (Levine, 2011).

The toys toddlers enjoy most are those they can play with by themselves and that require action. Trucks they can make go, squeaky frogs they can squeeze, rocking horses they can ride, pegs they can pound, and a toy telephone they can talk into are all favorites. These are all toys children can control, giving them a sense of power in manipulation, which is an expression of autonomy (Fig. 30.3).

Some parents are not prepared for this change in play habits in their child. They wonder why a child who used to play quietly in his crib is now more interested in banging trucks together. However, they need only watch a toddler tug a pull toy, stop to see if it is following, walk again, and stop and

Figure 30.2 Toddlers play beside, but not with, other children (parallel play).

Figure 30.3 Toddlers enjoy toys they can manipulate. (India Picture/Shutterstock.com)

look to see if it is still following to understand the feeling of accomplishment involved in manipulating toys.

At 15 months of age, children are still in a put-in, take-out stage, so they continue to enjoy stacks of boxes that fit inside each other. They enjoy throwing toys out of a playpen or from a high chair tray as long as someone will pick them up and return them again and again.

The 18-month-old child walks securely enough to enjoy pull toys. Toys should be strong enough to take a great deal of abuse because children this age may use toys in ways other than those for which they were designed. For example, an infant will sit and softly stroke a stuffed cat; however, a toddler will pick it up by the tail and swing it, pound it, or pull at it. There is no need for parents to correct children about the way they are using a toy as long as it is safe and appears to give satisfaction. If toddlers find a toy frustrating because they are holding or using it incorrectly, showing them the right way will ease frustration.

By age 2 years, when toddlers begin to spend time imitating adult actions in their play such as wrapping a doll and putting it to bed or "driving the car," they begin to use fewer toys than before. The act of imitating has become their play. By the end of the toddler period, both boys and girls begin to like roughhousing and spend at least part of every day in this

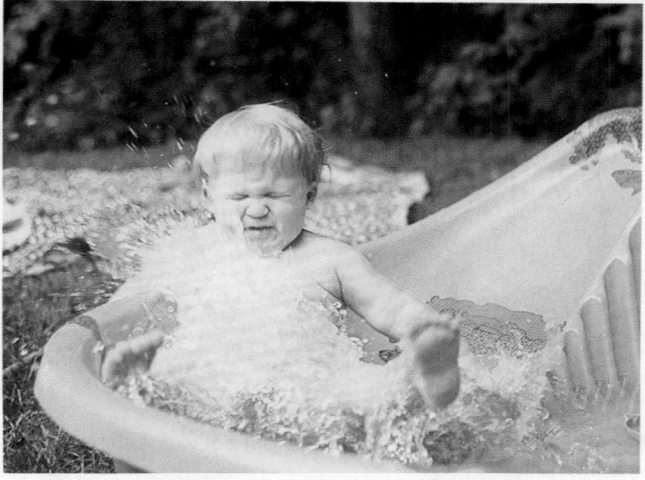

Figure 30.4 Toddlers usually enjoy rough and tumble play.

very active, stimulating type of play (Fig. 30.4). Encouraging parents to schedule this type of play outdoors, where vases or other prized possessions cannot be broken, makes it more acceptable.

A child who feels a need for active play is notably not easy to get to sit down and eat, fall asleep, or play quiet games and so may be described as "trouble." It is good to explore with parents the amount of outside or roughhousing time they allow a child each day. Stroller walks are good because they provide fresh air and sunshine, but toddlers also need opportunities to engage in strenuous activity such as running and jumping (Hodges, Smith, Tidwell, et al., 2012). Because of this rough activity, most toddlers have at least one black-and-blue mark on their legs at all times from tripping over their feet while trying to run too fast or from jumping or bumping into a chair or doorway. Examine these and document their presence but don't mistake them for child maltreatment (Hooker, Ward, & Verrinder, 2012).

What If . . . 30.1
Jason's mother tells the nurse, "I arrange play dates for Jason but he never shares his toys. How can I make him do that?" How would the nurse best answer her?

Cognitive Development

As a toddler, a child enters the final stages of Piaget's sensorimotor thought and the beginning of the preoperative period at approximately 12 months (see Chapter 28) (Piaget, 1952). During the fifth and sixth stages of the sensorimotor phase, toddlers are described as "little scientists" because of their interest in trying to discover new ways to handle objects or new results that different actions can achieve. For instance, by trial and error, toddlers discover that cats do not like baths and cookies on the center of a table can be reached by pulling them down using the tablecloth. Obviously, toddlers need supervision for these types of scientific investigations because they can lead to errors or injury.

Infants, when they want to retrieve a ball that rolled under a chair, crawl under the chair or along the same path the ball took. Many children at 15 months of age are able to follow a different path (walk in back of the chair) to obtain the object because they can project where it will stop rolling. This results from increased awareness that the ball is permanent and, even if it follows a different direction from the one the child must take, it will be there to retrieve.

By stage 6 of cognitive development (between 18 and 24 months of age), toddlers are able to try out various actions mentally rather than having to actually perform them—the beginning of problem solving or symbolic thought. They may have difficulty viewing one object as being different from another, however. On a walk through a department store decorated with teddy bears, for example, children are not sure whether they are seeing a succession of bears or if the same bear keeps reappearing as if it is following them through the store, asking to be taken home.

Children at this stage have a type of faulty reasoning (prelogical reasoning) that can lead them to wrong conclusions and faulty judgment. Daddy is shaving; therefore, he must be going to work because he went to work after he shaved yesterday. If you made a toddler's bed yesterday and he was taken to surgery afterward, he may cry at the sight of you approaching his crib with clean sheets today, thinking he will have to go to surgery again.

Children at this stage are also able to remember an action and imitate it later (**deferred imitation**); they can do such things as pretend to drive a car or put a baby to sleep because they have seen this previously and not just in the recent past. Object permanence becomes complete.

At the end of the toddler period, children enter a second major period of cognitive development termed **preoperational thought** and begin to use a process termed **assimilation**. Because they are not able to change their thoughts to fit a situation, they learn to change the situation (or how they perceive it). This ability is what causes toddlers to use toys in the "wrong" way. For example, if a child is given a toy hammer, instead of pounding with it, she may shake it to see if it rattles (i.e., the child has changed the toy's use to fit her thoughts, or used assimilation).

Planning and Implementation for Health Promotion of a Toddler and Family

Toddlers tend to develop many upper respiratory and ear infections but otherwise come to healthcare facilities most often for health maintenance visits (recommended at 15, 18, and 24 months of age) and for important immunizations. These visits allow you to focus on health promotion and provide the opportunity for early detection of any growth and development delays. Table 30.3 lists specific areas to assess during these visits.

Routine health maintenance visits also provide opportunities to support parents through the normal crises of the toddler period. Ways to encourage parents to promote healthy development of independence in their toddler include listening carefully to their concerns, asking questions to help separate the objective circumstances surrounding a problem from the parents' possible emotional biases, and providing guidelines on how to handle specific problems.

PROMOTING TODDLER SAFETY

Accidents (unintentional injuries) are the major cause of death in infants through late adolescents in the United States (CDC, 2012a). Unintentional ingestions (poisoning) and auto accidents are the types of unintentional injuries that occur most frequently in toddlers (Beirens, van Beeck, Brug, et al., 2010).

Although poisoning can involve medicine such as acetaminophen (and there is a growing concern of illegal or prescription drug ingestions even in toddlers), it most often occurs from ingestion of cleaning products. Aspiration or ingestion of small objects such as watch or hearing aid batteries, pencil erasers, or parts of crayons is also a major danger for children of this age (Litovitz, Whitaker, & Clark, 2010). Urge parents to childproof their home by putting all poisonous products, drugs, and small objects out of reach by the time their infant is crawling, and certainly by the time their infant is walking, to avoid these problems (Lee & Marcdante, 2011).

Other unintentional injuries that occur frequently in toddlers include motor vehicle accidents, burns, falls, drowning, and playground injuries. These occur because toddlers' motor ability jumps ahead of their judgment. To prevent serious injury, teach parents to be alert as to what their toddler is doing at all times.

By the end of the toddler period, children can walk surely; if they are left outside to play, they can very quickly travel a block away. Because they have no judgment concerning moving cars, they walk across streets with no regard for oncoming cars. Because they cannot swim well, parents need to check whether backyard pools—another area prone to unintended injury—are securely fenced (Bowman, Aitken, Robbins, et al., 2012).

For safety in automobiles, parents should keep their toddlers in rear-facing seats until age 2 years, or until the child reaches the maximum height and weight for their particular seat. Following that, children need to ride in a car seat with a five-point restraint (Fig. 30.5). Car seats should be placed in the back seat so the child is not struck by the passenger seat airbag (AAP, 2013). Remind parents that it is unsafe to leave a toddler alone in a car. One way for a parent to be reminded that the child is in the back seat is to always place a purse or briefcase in the back seat alongside the child's car seat.

Toddlers need to wear a helmet as soon as they begin riding a tricycle. Although parents are becoming conscientious about using car seats, they are not as conscientious about using toddler or booster car seats or helmets for bicycle riding, so these are areas where health teaching is necessary (Macy, Clark, Freed, et al., 2012).

Some 15-month-old children are able to climb over the side rails of their cribs and enjoy exploring the house early in the morning before anyone else is awake. Parents might have to move their child to a regular bed with a side rail as early as this time to keep the child from falling when climbing out of a crib. A safety gate on the door of his or her room is another way to keep a toddler contained and safe.

As the child reaches 2 years of age and begins to imitate housework or repairing a car, parents must be sure the child does not use real cleaning compounds or sharp tools. Box 30.3 summarizes unintentional injury prevention measures to encourage parents to take with their toddler.

QSEN Checkpoint Question 30.3

EVIDENCE-BASED PRACTICE

As television sets become larger and thinner, viewing becomes easier. To investigate if television sets can also be a threat to young children, researchers reviewed a Canadian trauma database over a 15-year period as to how many emergency room visits were caused by a television set falling onto a young child. They identified a total of 179 injuries (20 to 24 per year). Toddlers were the most frequently injured age group, and head and neck injuries were the most common consequences of a television pulled down onto a young child (Mills, Grushka, & Butterworth, 2012).

Based on the study and the AAP recommendations on television viewing, the nurse advises Jason's parents to take which action?

   a. Encourage Jason to watch television in his room where the television set is smaller.
   b. Teach Jason to always watch television from a distance of no less than 12 feet.
   c. Teach Jason to use the remote control so he can watch television safely by himself.
   d. Allow Jason to watch television only when a parent is free to supervise his actions.

Look in Appendix A for the best answer and rationale.

TABLE 30.3 HEALTH MAINTENANCE SCHEDULE, TODDLER PERIOD

Well-Child Visits (Typically Scheduled at 15, 18, 24, and 30 Months)

Area of Focus	Methods	Frequency
Health history	Health interview	Every visit
Physical health	Physical examination	Every visit
Developmental milestones	History and observation	Every visit
	Ages & Stages Questionnaire	18- and 24-month visits
Autism spectrum disorder screening	Observation and language assessment	18- and 24-month visits
Growth milestones	Height and weight plotted on standard growth chart	Every visit
	Head circumference	15-, 18-, and 24-month visits
	Body mass index	Beginning at 24-month visit
Nutrition	History, observation; height and weight information	Every visit
Parent–child relationship	History and observation	Every visit
Social/behavior assessment	History and observation	Every visit
Vision and hearing	History and observation	Every visit
Dental health	History and physical examination	18- or 34-month visit
	Dental appointment	Every 6 months
	Fluoride varnish	Recommended each visit
Anemia	Hematocrit/hemoglobin	Risk assessment at 15 and 30 months
Lead screening	Point-of-care rapid lead screening	24 months and more frequently if at elevated risk
Tuberculosis	Purified protein derivative (PPD) test	If indicated based on risk
Urinalysis	Clean-catch urine	Based on symptoms
Dyslipidemia	Cholesterol level	24-month visit if indicated based on risk

Immunizations

(Administer immunization in accordance with healthcare agency policies. Check history and past records and inform caregiver about any risks and side effects before administration [www.cdc.gov/vaccines/schedules].)

Diphtheria, tetanus, and pertussis	DTaP	15-month visit (4th)
Haemophilus influenzae type B	HiB	15-month visit (4th)
Pneumococcal vaccine	PVC	15-month visit if not previously immunized
Hepatitis A	HepA	12- or 18-month visit (1st and 2nd)
Hepatitis B	HepB	15- or 18-month visit (3rd)
Influenza	IIV	Yearly
Measles, mumps, and rubella	MMR	12- or 15-month visit (1st)
Inactivated poliomyelitis	IPV	12- or 15-month visit (3rd)
Varicella vaccine	VAR	12- or 15-month visit (1st)

Anticipatory Guidance

Area of Focus	Methods	Frequency
Toddler care	Active listening and health teaching	Every visit
Expected growth and developmental milestones before next visit	Health teaching	Every visit
Poison and unintentional injury prevention	Educate parents about toddler safety, such as using car seats and bicycle helmets, locking up poisons, and such precautions as removing drawstrings from hooded clothing to prevent strangulation; provide telephone number of national poison control center (1-800-222-1222).	Every visit

Problem Solving

Any problems expressed by caregiver during course of the visit	Active listening and health teaching regarding temper tantrums, toilet training, negativity	Every visit

Source: American Academy of Pediatrics, Committee on Practice and Ambulatory Medicine. (2012). *Recommendations for preventive pediatric health care.* Washington, DC: Author; Centers for Disease Control and Prevention. (2013). *Birth–18 years & "catch up" immunization schedules.* Washington, DC: Author.

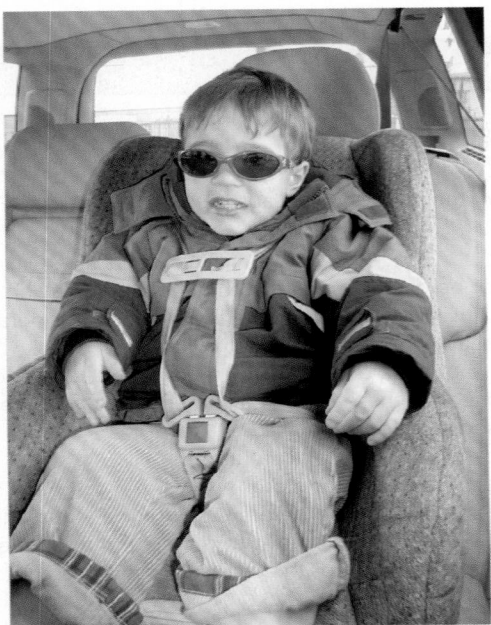

Figure 30.5 Toddlers should use a car seat with a five-point restraint while riding in an automobile until they are 2 years of age.

Lead Screening

The CDC has set as a goal the elimination of elevated blood lead levels in children (CDC, 2012b). All children between the ages of 6 months and 6 years who live in communities with buildings built before 1950 and immigrant children who might have been exposed to sources of lead in another country should be tested for the presence of lead in their body (lead poisoning). Elevated lead levels are caused by eating, chewing, or sucking on objects (e.g., windowsills, paint chips, furniture) that are covered with lead-based paint. Although federal law has prohibited the use of lead in the manufacture of both interior and exterior paints since the mid-1970s, many older houses are still coated with lead-based paint. Additional sources of lead poisoning can include:

- Toys manufactured in countries where restrictions on lead are not enforced or cribs that were painted with lead-based paint
- Soil around the exterior of the house and contaminated food grown there
- Dust or fumes created by home renovation
- Pottery made with lead glazes or jewelry made from lead or lead alloys
- Colored print in newspapers or older lead-based water pipes
- Lead dust brought home on the clothing of parents who work with lead products such as batteries

Lead-based gasoline used to be a concern but is no longer available in the United States. Because lead is toxic to body tissue, ingestion of it leads to serious damage to the brain and nervous system, kidneys, and red blood cells. Levels as low as 5 µg/dl can cause learning and behavioral problems (CDC, 2012b). High levels may result in seizures, cognitive challenges, coma, and even death. Although 10 µg/dl was the standard to define lead toxicity for the past decade, the new lower level of 5 µg is proposed as the best way to help prevent minimal damage (Kuehn, 2012).

Beginning symptoms of lead poisoning include irritability, headache, fatigue, and abdominal pain. Often, however, there are no symptoms before damage occurs, which is why blood screening is essential. The CDC (2012b) recommends screening for all children between the ages of 9 and 12 months at least once and again at 18 or 24 months of age. A small amount of blood taken by a finger prick is analyzed. A positive result (over 5 µg/dl) must be confirmed by further testing. The long-term effects of lead poisoning and therapy are discussed in Chapter 52.

QSEN Checkpoint Question 30.4

SAFETY

Jason's grandmother often visits the family. When she does, she brings a number of medications with her. The nurse teaches the family to follow which precautions about unintentional poisoning?

a. Advise the grandmother to keep her medicine in her purse and stress that no one should open her purse but her.
b. Show Jason his grandmother's pills and emphasize that he is not permitted to touch them.
c. Assure the grandmother that as long as her vials of medicine have childproof caps, there is no danger.
d. Buy the grandmother a medicine case that locks and place it on a high shelf when she visits.

Look in Appendix A for the best answer and rationale.

PROMOTING NUTRITIONAL HEALTH IN TODDLERS

Because growth slows abruptly after the first year of life, a toddler's appetite is usually less than an infant's. Children who ate hungrily 2 months earlier now may sit and play with their food. It is important to educate parents that, while the child is still an infant, this decline in food intake will occur, so they will not be concerned when it happens. Because the actual amount of food eaten daily varies from one child to another, teach parents to place a small amount of food on a plate and allow their child to eat it and ask for more rather than serve a large portion that the child cannot finish. One tablespoonful of each food served is a good start. Also, cleaning a plate gives a child a feeling of independent functioning, whereas leaving food uneaten suggests that parents expected something more.

Because mothers are urged to breastfeed for the entire first year, many mothers begin weaning from breastfeeding or bottle feeding during the toddler years. Recommend that mothers do this gradually in order to avoid confrontation. Additional tips for weaning are discussed in Chapter 29.

Allowing self-feeding is a major way to both strengthen independence in a toddler and improve the amount of food consumed. Offering finger foods such as pieces of chicken, slices of banana, pieces of cheese, and crackers and allowing a choice between two types of food helps promote independence while exposing children to varied foods (Whitney & Rolfes, 2013). Toddlers usually prefer to eat the same type of food over and over because of the sense of security this offers.

BOX 30.3

Nursing Care Planning Based on Family Teaching

UNINTENTIONAL INJURY PREVENTION MEASURES FOR TODDLERS

Q. Jason's mother tells you, "My toddler is constantly on the go. How can I keep him safe?"

A. Injury prevention has to be constant while your child is a toddler. Try the following precautions:

Potential Unintended Injury	Prevention Measure
Motor vehicles	Maintain your child in a car seat; do not be distracted by the child from safe driving.
	Do not allow the child to play outside unsupervised. Do not allow the child to operate electronic garage doors or play near lawn mowers or snow blowers.
	Supervise toddlers with pedaling toys (e.g., look before crossing driveways, do not cross streets) but do not expect toddler will obey these rules at all times (i.e., stay close by).
Falls	Keep house windows closed or keep secure screens in place.
	Place gates at top and bottom of stairs. Supervise at playgrounds.
	Do not allow child to walk with sharp object in hand or mouth.
	Raise crib rails and check to make sure they are locked before walking away from crib.
Aspiration	Examine toys for small parts that could be aspirated; remove toys that appear dangerous.
	Do not feed toddler popcorn or nuts; caution child not to eat while running. Do not leave toddler alone with a balloon.
Drowning	Do not leave toddler alone in a bathtub or near water (including buckets of cleaning water). Fence pools; insist toddlers wear safety "floats" or life vests; supervise at all times when near water.
Animal bites	Do not allow toddler to approach strange dogs.
	Supervise child's play with family pets.
Poisoning	Never present medication as candy. Buy medications with childproof caps; put away immediately after use.
	Never take medication in front of child.
	Place all medication and poisons in locked cabinets or overhead shelves where child cannot reach them.
	Never leave medication in parents' purse or pocket where child can reach it.
	Always store food or substances in their original containers.
	Know the names of houseplants and find out if they are poisonous. (Call national poison control center for information: 800-222-1222.)
	If unsure if plants are safe, hang them or set them on high surfaces beyond toddler's grasp.
	Be certain small batteries or magnets are out of reach.
	Post telephone number of national poison control center by the telephone or add as a contact on a cell phone: (800-222-1222).
	Inspect toys to be certain if they were manufactured in another country that they are free of lead-based paint.
Burns	Cook on the back burners of stove if possible; turn handles of pots toward back of stove to prevent toddler from reaching up and pulling them down.
	If a vaporizer is used, use a cool-mist type rather than a steam vaporizer so child cannot be scalded.
	Keep screen in front of fireplace or heater.
	Monitor toddlers carefully when they are near lit candles.
	Do not leave toddlers unsupervised near hot-water faucets; check temperature setting for hot-water heater so thermostat is not over 125°F.
	Do not leave coffee/tea pots on a table where child can reach them.
	Never drink hot beverages when a child is sitting on your lap or playing within reach. Buy flame-retardant clothing.
	Do not allow toddlers to blow out matches (teach fire is not fun); store matches out of reach.
	Keep electric wires and cords out of toddlers' reach; cover electrical outlets with safety plugs.
General	Know whereabouts of toddlers at all times. Toddlers can climb onto chairs or high stools they could not manage before, can turn door knobs and go places they could not go before, and are able to pull a television set over on top of themselves.
	Be aware the frequency of injuries increases when the family is under stress and therefore less attentive to children. Special precautions must be taken at these times.
	Be aware some children are more active, curious, and impulsive and therefore more vulnerable to unintentional injury than others.

Most toddlers insist on feeding themselves and generally will resist eating if a parent insists on feeding them. An independent child may react to repeated attempts at being fed by refusing to eat at all.

Toddler Nutrition Requirements

Parents may become frustrated when trying to provide adequate nutrition for their toddler because of a toddler's varying and unpredictable appetite and food preferences. Although a toddler's daily food consumption may vary greatly, energy needs are generally met when sufficient food is supplied in a positive environment.

- Sedentary children ages 1 to 3 years should consume 1,000 kcal daily; active children in this age group may need up to 1,400 kcal daily (U.S. Department of Agriculture, 2012).
- Calories are best supplied by a variety of foods spaced into three meals a day.
- Protein and carbohydrate needs are often those most easily met during the toddler period; diets high in sugar should be avoided to help prevent toddler obesity.
- Fats should generally not be restricted for children under 2 years old; however, children over 2 years old should have a total fat intake between 30% and 35% of calories, with most fat coming from sources of polyunsaturated and monounsaturated fatty acids, such as fish, nuts, and vegetable oils, the same as adults.
- Trans fats should be kept to a minimum.
- Adequate calcium and phosphorus intake is important for bone mineralization. Milk should be whole milk until age 2 years, after which 2% milk can be introduced (Whitney & Rolfes, 2013).

A Vegetarian Diet

Vegetarian diets are adequate for toddlers if parents are well informed about needed vitamins and minerals (Chisholm, 2011). A vegetarian diet can be easily designed for a toddler who prefers finger foods because many vegetables, fruits, and grains such as pieces of oranges, peaches, raisins, chickpeas, and crackers are easily eaten this way. The use of fortified soy milk prevents fluid, protein, vitamin B_{12}, and calcium deficiencies. Tofu should be served often to supply protein.

PROMOTING TODDLER DEVELOPMENT IN DAILY ACTIVITIES

A toddler's new independence and developing abilities in self-care, such as dressing, eating, and to a limited extent hygiene, present special challenges for parents. Learning how to promote autonomy yet maintain a safe, healthful environment should be a major goal for the family.

Dressing

By the end of the toddler period, most children can put on their own socks and underpants (Fig. 30.6). Some may also be able to pull on slacks, pullover shirts (the sleeves of a shirt often confuse a toddler), or simple dresses. Parents may be reluctant to encourage toddlers to dress themselves because it is easier and quicker for a parent to do so. Also, a toddler who is dressed by parents will (usually) be wearing clothes in the correct way. When toddlers dress themselves, they invariably

Figure 30.6 Getting dressed by himself is a fun morning activity for this older toddler.

put shoes on the wrong feet and shirt and pants on backward. Encourage parents to give up perfection for the benefit of the child's developing sense of autonomy. If they feel they must change the child's clothes, urge them to begin with a positive statement, such as "You did a good job," before making the switch.

Don't judge whether the parents encourage self-dressing by what they do at a healthcare-setting visit. In this setting, parents may dress a child quickly to show the child that the examination is over, or they may simply be in a hurry to get home.

As soon as children are up on their feet and walking, they need shoe soles that are firm enough to provide protection from rough surfaces. However, toddlers do not need extremely firm or ankle-high shoes. Because a toddler's arches are still developing, it is better for their arches to provide foot support rather than having it provided by shoes. Sneakers are an ideal toddler shoe because the soles are hard enough for rough surfaces and arch support is limited.

Sleep

The amount of sleep children need gradually decreases as they grow older (Gahagan, 2011). They may begin the toddler period napping twice a day and sleeping 12 hours each night and end it with one nap a day and only 8 hours of sleep at night. Parents who are not aware that the need for sleep declines at this time may view a child's disinterest in sleeping as a problem (about 10% of parents report toddler-age sleep problems (Byars, Yolton, Rausch, et al., 2012). If a child has difficulty falling asleep at night, it may be time to omit or shorten an afternoon nap. If a child is so short tempered at dinnertime that eating is impossible, perhaps the child needs two naps a day. Some toddlers begin having night terrors or awake crying from a bad dream and so may receive little sleep because they are reluctant to fall back asleep (Bhargava, 2011). Night terrors are further discussed in Chapter 31.

When toddlers are tired, they naturally fall asleep. They may begin to resist naps, however, as well as nighttime sleep as they become aware for the first time that activities go on while they sleep. Caution parents when they say, "We'll do this after naptime," that they wait until then to do it. Otherwise, a child may be reluctant to nap the next day for fear of missing another activity. Also, parents must be sure older siblings do not point out to a toddler all the exciting things a toddler missed while napping.

Other toddlers resist naptime as part of their developing negativism. Parents might minimize this by including a nap as part of lunchtime routine, not as a separate activity (i.e., the child always goes from the table directly to bed as if the two things are connected). The parent can state simply, "It's naptime now," and then give a secondary choice: "Do you want to sleep with your teddy bear or your rag doll?" Toward the end of the toddler period, when children are ready to omit their afternoon naps, they may still be agreeable to a "shoes off" or "quiet play" period until they begin to attend school full-time.

As with any other activity of this period, a toddler loves a bedtime routine: bath, pajamas, a story, toothbrushing, being tucked into bed, having a drink of water, choosing a toy to sleep with, and turning out the lights. Parents must be careful, however, not to let a child maneuver them into such a long procedure that sleep is delayed considerably past the time initially set. Although toddlers need to be independent, they also need a feeling of security. Just as adults like to know there are guardrails along steep mountain roads, toddlers like to see parents as firm, consistent people who can be counted on to be reliable over and over, especially when they're tired.

Many toddlers are ready to be moved out of a crib into a youth bed or regular bed with protective side rails or a chair strategically placed beside it by the end of the toddler period. Remind parents to stress that sleeping in a regular bed does not give children the right to get in and out of bed as they choose. Some toddlers do well if they are allowed to sleep in a regular bed and a folding gate is placed across the door to their room. This arrangement gives them a feeling of independence but still keeps them safe. When first moved to a bed without side rails, many children are found sleeping on the floor of the room in the morning. There is no harm in this unless it is cold or drafty. Dressing the child in warm pajamas or putting a blanket on the floor might be solutions to help parents accept this.

Bathing

The time for a toddler's bath should depend on the parents' and the child's wishes and schedule. Some parents prefer to bathe a toddler before the evening meal because it has a quieting effect and prepares the child for eating; others prefer to give it at bedtime because it has a relaxing effect and helps a child sleep. However, the time is not as important as the attempt to establish a sense of routine and a sense that life has order. Learning to be independent is sometimes frightening, and there is security in knowing that certain events are predictable.

Toddlers usually enjoy bath time, and parents should make an effort to make it fun by providing a toy, such as a rubber duck or plastic fish. Bath time is usually so enjoyable for toddlers that parents can use it as a recreational activity or something to do on a rainy day when they can find nothing else to interest their child. Remind parents that although toddlers can sit well in a bathtub, it is still not safe to leave them unsupervised. They might slip and get their head under water or reach and turn on the hot-water faucet and scald themselves (Hutchings, Barnes, Maddocks, et al., 2010). Parents

shouldn't add bubble bath to the water because its use is associated with vulvovaginitis and possibly urinary tract infections, especially in girls (S. Smith, 2011).

Dental Care

Toddlers often need between-meal snacks. To help prevent dental caries from frequent snacking, encourage parents to offer fruit (e.g., bananas, pieces of apple, orange slices) or protein foods (e.g., cheese, pieces of chicken) for snacks rather than high-carbohydrate items such as cookies to limit exposure of the child's teeth to carbohydrate (G. A. Smith & Riedford, 2012). Calcium (found in large amounts in milk, cheese, and yogurt) is especially important for the development of strong teeth and so are other good snack foods. In addition, children should continue to drink fluoridated water or, if not available, receive fluoride supplements so all new teeth form with cavity-resistant enamel (Tubert-Jeannin, Auclair, Amsallem, et al., 2011).

Remind parents not to put a child to bed with a bottle of milk or juice to help prevent the development of caries. Toddlers need a toothbrush they recognize as their own. Toward the end of the toddler period, they can begin to do the brushing themselves under supervision (almost all children need some supervision until about age 8 years). Remind parents that it is better for a child to brush thoroughly once a day, probably at bedtime, than to do it poorly many times a day. After brushing, parents can use dental floss to clean between their child's teeth and remove plaque.

Urge parents to schedule a first dental visit with a dentist skilled in pediatric dental care by 12 months of age. Screenings and assessment of dentition can begin as early as 6 months of age but should occur no later than 24 months of age. Dental services can begin by age 3 years (Hoeft, Barker, & Masterson, 2011).

Parents can prepare their child for this first visit and subsequent visits by reading a story about a dentist visit, maintaining a positive attitude about the visit, avoiding the use of frightening words such as "drill" or "shot," and answering their child's questions honestly without going into too much detail. Because children rarely have cavities this early, the visit is usually painless and sets a positive stage for future dental supervision visits.

PROMOTING HEALTHY FAMILY FUNCTIONING

Because learning self-reliance is the primary goal of a child during the toddler period, some parents who enjoyed caring for their child as an infant may find it difficult to have their authority challenged by a toddler. Help parents to understand their responses to these attempts at independence are crucial to the healthy development of their child. Although the child still needs firm limits to feel secure, a child must be given room to make independent decisions in areas the parents feel they do not need to control. Someone outside of the family, such as a nurse, can provide an important perspective on this issue.

At bedtime, naptime, or anytime they are tired, toddlers may become much more like their old selves, wanting to sit on a parent's lap and be rocked or picked up and carried. This does not signal babyish behavior or regression in a toddler; it is a natural state between infant and preschool ages.

PARENTAL CONCERNS ASSOCIATED WITH THE TODDLER PERIOD

Parental concerns of the toddler period usually arise because of a conflict over autonomy.

Toilet Training

Toilet training is one of the biggest tasks a toddler tries to achieve. There are so many theories concerning toilet training that understanding the procedure can become one of the biggest tasks of this period for parents. Most first-time parents ask when to start, when training should be completed, and how to go about it (Box 30.4). You can explain to parents that toilet training is an individualized task for each child. It should begin and be completed according to a child's ability to accomplish it, not according to a set schedule (Kiddoo, 2012).

Before children can begin toilet training, they must have reached three important developmental levels, one physiologic and the other two cognitive:

- They must have control of rectal and urethral sphincters, usually achieved by the time they walk well.
- They must have a cognitive understanding of what it means to hold urine and stools until they can release them at a certain place and time.
- They must have a desire to delay immediate gratification for a more socially accepted action.

Because physiologic development is cephalocaudal, the rectal and urethral sphincters are not mature enough for control in most children until at least the end of the first year, when tracts of the spinal cord are myelinated to the anal level. A good way for a parent to know a child's development has reached this point is to wait until the child can walk well independently.

Toilet training need not start this early, however, because cognitively and socially, many children do not understand what is being asked of them until they are 2 or even 3 years old. The markers of readiness are subtle, but as a rule, children are ready for toilet training when they begin to be uncomfortable in wet diapers. They demonstrate this by pulling

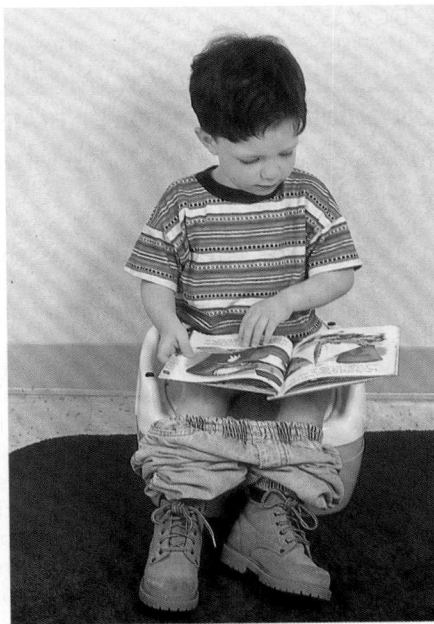

Figure 30.7 Toddlers are interested in toilet training as an expression of autonomy.

or tugging at soiled diapers, or they may bring a parent a clean diaper after they have soiled so they can be changed (Fig. 30.7).

Teach parents not to underestimate the difficulty of the task they are expecting their child to achieve. Toddlers live by a pleasure principle: They want what they want when they want it. Before they can complete toilet training, they must be able to give up an immediate pleasure—relieving themselves whenever they have the urge—to gain other pleasure later on—improved physical comfort and another step in growing up. Guidelines for how to toilet train a toddler are shown in Box 30.5.

Some toddlers smear or play with feces, often at about the same time that toilet training is started. This occurs because they have become fully aware of body excretions but have no adult values toward them; stools seem little different from the modeling clay they play with. This activity can be minimized by providing toddlers with play substances of similar texture and by changing diapers immediately after defecation. Teach parents to accept this behavior for what it is: enjoyment of the body and of the self and the discovery of a new substance. After a child is fully toilet trained, this activity rarely persists.

Ritualistic Behavior

Although toddlers spend a great deal of time every day investigating new ways to do things and trying activities they have never done before, they also enjoy ritualistic patterns. They will use only "their" spoon at mealtime or only "their" blanket at bedtime. They will not go outside unless a mother or father locates their favorite cap.

The child who seems to need an excessive number of objects to cling to or an excessive number of routines, however, may be trying to say, "I need more guidelines, more rules. Don't let me be quite so independent."

BOX 30.4

Nursing Care Planning to Respect Cultural Diversity

In the United States, toilet training is usually introduced during the toddler period. Like so many other aspects of childrearing, however, the time when parents begin these activities is culturally determined. In other countries, toilet training may be started as soon as a child can sit—at about 6 months. Although praise is used in the United States as a common means of encouraging toddlers to learn new tasks, other cultures believe praise could bring a child harm by attracting evil spirits; instead, strategies of shame or strict discipline are used. Being aware that childrearing practices are not consistent across the world is a help in understanding why parents approach childrearing problems differently and why childrearing advice must be individualized.

BOX 30.5

Nursing Care Planning to Empower a Family

COMMON GUIDELINES FOR TOILET TRAINING

Q. Jason's mother asks you, "How can I tell if my 2-year-old is ready for potty training? And if he is, how do I start?"

A. Try the following suggestions:

1. Children are physically ready for toilet training when they can walk securely. Plan 1 or 2 weeks of psychological "readiness" activities such as showing your child "grown up" pants and how other family members use the toilet, activities that will help him realize the task of toilet training is a step toward growing up, not something only toddlers do.
2. Check that training pants pull down readily and slacks are free of complicated buttons or grippers; otherwise, your child will have accidents because he cannot undress quickly enough.
3. Purchase either a potty chair that sits on the floor or an infant seat that is placed on the regular toilet. If you choose a toilet seat, place a footstool in front of the toilet so your child has some support for his feet.
4. Begin with defecation training because this is so much easier to grasp than urination. Sit your child on the potty chair or toilet at the time he usually defecates, such as when he wakes up in the morning.
5. Praise your child if he does defecate. Remind him to wash his hands afterward.
6. Be careful not to flush the toilet while your child is sitting on it because 2-year-old children are unable to realize they will not be flushed away. Encourage your child to flush the toilet independently after you have helped him get redressed.
7. Do not allow a child to remain on a potty chair for much longer than 10 minutes (less than that if he is resistant). Also, do not allow your child to use the chair to eat or as a play table, so he doesn't become confused as to its purpose.
8. If your child does not seem ready on a day-to-day basis, return him to diapers for a short period. Be careful not to make this feel like failure or equate "good" with being dry and "bad" with being wet. Continue with readiness activities. Reintroduce training pants and attempt toilet training again when your child seems more ready.
9. When children have mastered defecation, it's time to include urination. Boys enjoy standing to urinate and aiming at objects in a toilet bowl, such as pieces of breakfast cereal.
10. Some toddlers have difficulty remaining dry at night until they are 3 to 4 years old. Do not pressure your child to accomplish nighttime dryness but assume he is doing the best he can. Change him to training pants for the night by explaining (not punitively) that it is hard to keep dry while he sleeps. After your child has been dry during the night for about 1 month, he has probably mastered nighttime dryness.
11. Do not wake your child during the night and carry him to the bathroom to void. This system may keep him dry during the night, but it does not help him stay dry for long periods. It may even prolong nighttime wetness because it conditions him to void every 4 hours instead of retaining urine for 8 hours while he sleeps.

What If . . . 30.2

Jason's mother tells the nurse he is toilet trained, but when he's admitted to the hospital for minor surgery, he refuses to use the toilet. How would the nurse best respond?

Negativism

As part of establishing their identities as separate individuals, toddlers typically go through a period of extreme negativism. They do not want to do anything a parent wants them to do. Their reply to every request is a very definite "no."

It is easy for parents to believe their authority is being questioned when this happens and to worry children are becoming so disrespectful they will have difficulty getting along in the world. They can be baffled by the extreme change from happy, cooperative infants who lived to please them to irritating, uncooperative toddlers. They may need some help to realize that this is not only a normal phenomenon of toddlerhood but also a positive stage in development.

This change indicates toddlers have learned that they are separate individuals with separate needs. It is important toddlers do this if they are to grow up to be persons who are independent and able to take care of their own needs and desires.

Parents who went away from home for the first time for college or camp might remember they behaved similarly. They may recall they rarely slept or ate sensibly; they tried, in effect, to break every rule their parents used to enforce on them. Most regained their equilibrium in time to find a midpoint between irresponsible independence and common sense. If parents can recall such circumstances, it helps them to understand that this behavior in their toddler is not specific to the age but to the first feeling of independence. They can also remember they meant no vindictiveness by their behavior, so they can realize their child means none either. This understanding can help to put the child's "no" into a better light.

Once it runs its course, extreme negativism will pass. In the meantime, the more parents try to make children obey them, the more children are likely to resist. Some long-term parent–child interaction problems begin during this period because parents insist on being obeyed totally or are inconsistent in their approach.

A toddler's "no" can best be reduced by limiting the number of questions asked of the child. A father does not really mean, for example, "Are you ready for dinner?" He means, "Come to the table. It's dinnertime." A mother asks, "Will you come take a bath now?" She means, "It's time for your bath." Making a statement instead of asking a question in this way can avoid a great many negative responses.

A toddler needs experience in making choices, however. To provide the opportunity to do this, a parent could give a secondary choice. "No" is not allowed for the major task, so the parent states, "It's bath time now" but then says, "Do you want to take your duck or your toy boat into the tub with you?" Other example is "It's lunchtime. Do you want to use a big or little plate?" or "It's time to go shopping. Do you want to wear your jacket or your sweater?" Although this solution is simple, it is one parents may not arrive at by themselves because finding a solution to a problem is always more difficult for the person in the middle of the problem than it is for an objective observer. Once they are helped to practice this approach, however, parents usually find it helpful in smoothing out the friction caused by the negativism of the toddler period (Box 30.6).

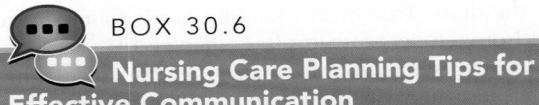

BOX 30.6
Nursing Care Planning Tips for Effective Communication

Jason's mother has brought 2-year-old Jason to the clinic for a health maintenance visit.

Jason is rambunctious and uncooperative. His mother is obviously frustrated.

Tip: Use positive language and encourage patient involvement. Offer focused choices that minimize "no" responses. Avoid commands and attempts to bribe the child.

Nurse: Jason, I need to listen to your heart so you must be very quiet. Would you rather sit quietly on the chair or the table?

Jason: Table.

Nurse: All right, Jason, jump up.
Jason climbs onto the table and starts to fidget.

Ms. Matthis: Jason, sit still for the nurse.

Jason: No!

Nurse: If you'd like, you can use the stethoscope for a few seconds. Do you want to listen to your mom's heart or my heart?

Jason: Mom's.

Nurse: Great, now we will both be very quiet so you can hear.
Jason listens to his mother's heart.

Nurse: Good, now it's my turn.

Jason: Okay. (Jason hands back the stethoscope.)
The nurse listens to Jason's heart.

Discipline

Some parents ask during the last part of the infant year or the early toddler period when they should start to discipline their child, or when toddlers are old enough for punishment to be acceptable. Remind parents that discipline and punishment are not interchangeable terms. **Discipline** means setting rules or road signs so children know what is expected of them. **Punishment** is a consequence that results from a breakdown in discipline or the child's disregard of the rules that were learned.

Parents should begin to instill some sense of discipline early in life because part of it involves setting safety limits and protecting others or property (e.g., a child must stay away from the fireplace or heater, she must not go into the street, she must not hit other children). Enforcing most limits of this type arises out of the day-to-day interactions with the child and out of the rhythm of child care, not out of a set procedure such as "Today, I'm going to teach discipline." Two general rules to follow include:

1. Parents need to be consistent.
2. Rules are learned best if correct behavior is praised rather than wrong behavior punished.

A "time-out" is a technique to help children learn that actions have consequences. To use a time-out effectively, parents first need to be certain their child understands the rule they are trying to enforce (e.g., "You can't hit people. If you hit your brother, you'll have time-out."). Parents should give one warning. If the child repeats the behavior, parents select an area that is nonstimulating, such as a corner of a room or a hallway. The child is directed to go immediately to the time-out space. The child then sits there for a specified period of time. If the child cries or shows any other disruptive behavior, the time-out period doesn't begin until there is quiet. When the specified time has passed, the child can return to the family. A guide as to how long children should remain in their time-out chair is 1 minute per year of age (e.g., a 2-year-old would stay in the corner for 2 minutes). Using a timer that rings when time is up is an effective way to let children know when they can return to the family.

QSEN Checkpoint Question 30.5

TEAMWORK & COLLABORATION

Jason's mother would prefer to use a time-out for punishment. What should the nurse teach Jason's mother or his daycare setting caregivers about the use of this technique?

 a. The child should sit still for as many minutes as his age.
 b. The child should sit still for as many minutes as he misbehaved.
 c. Time-out activities can include quiet play or reading books.
 d. Children are not ready for time-outs until school age.

Look in Appendix A for the best answer and rationale.

Separation Anxiety

As discussed in Chapter 29, fear of being separated from parents begins at about 6 months of age and persists throughout the preschool period. This universal fear in this age group is known as separation anxiety. Toddlers who have separation anxiety have difficulty accepting being separated from their primary caregiver to spend the day at a day care center or if they or their primary caregiver is hospitalized. Chapter 36 discusses nursing responsibility for care of toddlers in the hospital as well as the reactions of toddlers to the separation caused by hospitalization and the methods used to minimize these reactions.

Parents may ask what they can do about this problem. They believe they have a right to leave their child in a baby-sitter's or center's care, but how can they tolerate the crying at the door? Most toddlers react best to separation if a regular babysitter is employed or if the day care center has consistent caregivers. It helps if toddlers have fair warning they will have a babysitter. For example, they could be told, "Mommy is fixing dinner early because Mommy and Daddy are going to visit some friends tonight. Marsha is going to come and baby-sit for you. She'll put you to bed. When you wake up in the morning, Mommy and Daddy will be here again."

No matter how well prepared toddlers are, they may cry when the babysitter actually appears or may greet the babysit-ter warmly only to cry when the parents reach for their coats. It helps if parents say goodbye firmly, repeat the explanation they will be there when the child wakes in the morning, and then leave. Prolonged goodbyes only lead to more crying. Sneaking out prevents crying and may ease the parents' guilt, but it can strengthen a child's fear of abandonment and so should be discouraged. This applies to leaving after hospital visits as well.

QSEN Checkpoint Question 30.6

PATIENT-CENTERED CARE

Jason replies to every request by his mother with, "No!" His mother admits that she is exasperated and embarrassed by this, and she states that she is desperate to change this behavior. How can the nurse best meet the mother's expressed learning needs?

   a. Have her tell Jason she doesn't want him to say no anymore.

   b. Instruct her to answer all Jason's questions by saying, "No!"

   c. Encourage her to reduce the number of questions she asks Jason.

   d. Tell her to explain he is not using good commu-nication skills.

Look in Appendix A for the best answer and rationale.

TEMPER TANTRUMS

Almost every toddler has a temper tantrum at one time or another. The child may kick; scream; stomp feet; shout, "No, no, no"; flail arms and legs; bite; or bang his or her head against the floor.

Temper tantrums occur as a natural consequence of tod-dlers' development. They occur because toddlers are inde-pendent enough to know what they want, but they do not have the vocabulary or the wisdom to express their feelings

in a more socially acceptable way (J. A. Green, Whitney, & Potegal, 2011). For example, temper tantrums occur most often when children are tired, just before naptime or bed-time, or during a long shopping trip or visit. They may be a response to an unrealistic request by a parent, such as asking a child to comb her hair before she is coordinated enough to do so, asking her to pick up toys before she has a feel-ing of family responsibility, or asking her to share before she can understand what that means. Tantrums may also occur if parents are saying "no" too frequently with regard to such things as touching the coffee table, using a spoon, or running and jumping, thus making children feel constantly thwarted. A tantrum may also be a response to difficulty making choices or decisions or to pressure from activities such as toi-let training. Such children need to express feelings in some way and do so with temper tantrums. These episodes are not only taxing for the parents but are also energy consuming for children.

Some children hold their breath as part of a temper tan-trum until they become cyanotic. This occurs when a child is provoked; the child develops a distended chest (a halt after in-spiration), often has air-filled cheeks, and shows increasing dis-tress as the body registers oxygen want. Ignoring the child will make it an ineffective technique for expressing frustration or getting what is wanted. True breath holding is an unprovoked neurologic problem in which children, under stress, appear to "forget" to breathe in or halt breathing after expiration, usu-ally at the peak of anger. They become so short of breath they slump to the floor. True breath holding needs follow-up to separate it from temper tantrums (see Chapter 49).

Box 30.7 offers suggestions for managing temper tantrums. Probably the best approach is for parents to simply tell a child that they disapprove of the tantrum and then ignore it. They might say, "I'll be in the bedroom. When you're done kicking, you come into the bedroom, too." Children who are left alone in a kitchen this way will usually not continue a tantrum but will stop after 1 or 2 minutes and rejoin their parents. Parents should then accept the child warmly and proceed as if the tantrum had not occurred. This same approach works well for nurses caring for hospitalized toddlers.

 ### Nursing Diagnoses and Related Interventions

Nursing Diagnosis: Risk for compromised family coping related to toddler behavior

Outcome Evaluation: Family states temper tantrums now occur less than two times daily.

Helping parents correct problems early may limit the number of tantrums they must deal with; however, it will not prevent them because parents cannot anticipate all the circumstances that will cause this reaction. In fact, parents should not feel they must prevent all of them; after all, they are parents, not mind readers. As the child matures, increases his or her vocabulary, and is capable of better responses to stress situations, tantrums begin to fade by themselves. Box 30.8 shows an interprofessional care map illustrating both nursing and team planning to address such a problem as temper tantrums.

BOX 30.7

Nursing Care Planning Based on Family Teaching

MANAGING TODDLER'S TEMPER TANTRUMS

Q. Jason's mother tells you, "I've had it with temper tantrums. I can't stand to watch another one."

A. Here are suggestions to prevent them:

Try to determine the reason for the behavior:

- Do tantrums always occur just before bedtime? If so, you might schedule an earlier bedtime or an afternoon nap.
- Do tantrums occur every time you go shopping? If so, perhaps it would help to schedule two shorter trips each week rather than one long one.
- Do tantrums occur whenever you ask the child to do something? If so, is the child being asked to perform tasks that are not age appropriate?
- Do tantrums occur in response to not being able to make a decision? If so, you may have to limit the number of choices you are asking of the child.

Next, be certain it seems like a tantrum, not something more:

- Is there a possibility you are mistaking seizure activity for temper tantrums?
- Could you be confusing neurologic breath holding with a temper tantrum?

Lastly, think through what you do when the child has a tantrum:

- Do you give either material or emotional bribes (e.g., "Come and get a cookie")? This method is rarely effective because, by acceding to the child's wishes, you are encouraging your child to have more tantrums because they are so rewarding.
- Do you punish the child? Toddlers have a right to express opinions; they just need to be guided to learn a more controlled and mature way of doing that.
- Do you role model adult behavior in managing anger or frustration? For example, if your child shouts or kicks, do you respond, "I can shout as loud as you"? Instead of showing the child a better way to express feelings, this reinforces the way the child is responding.

What If . . . 30.3

Although the nurse is caring for Jason in the hospital, he has a temper tantrum in the middle of a busy hallway. Would the nurse ignore it or move him to a quieter place?

CONCERNS OF THE FAMILY WITH A TODDLER WHO HAS UNIQUE NEEDS

It may be difficult for children with handicaps or disabilities to achieve a sense of autonomy or independence because they may never be totally independent. However, it is important for these children to develop as strong a sense of autonomy as possible so they see themselves as independent and can work to become increasingly self-sufficient as they grow older.

Nursing actions designed to help the challenged or chronically ill child develop a sense of autonomy are outlined in Table 30.4. Most important are such actions that allow toddlers to do as much for themselves as possible. If toddlers have physical limitations, for example, they may be unable to explore freely or may not have the physical ability to pound and manipulate toys as the average toddler does. They do, however, have the ability to work at a project while they sit in a chair at a table.

A toddler with a long-term illness or who is physically challenged can be expected to exhibit normal toddler behaviors, such as temper tantrums, and to have normal outlooks, such as negativism. Parents whose child is uncoordinated or has a neurologic disease may mistake temper tantrums for seizure activity. Investigate such activity carefully and explain to parents the difference between the two. Parents may also mistake particular toddlers' insistence on having their own way as a manifestation of illness. Remind these parents the behavior is more often an indication of age and development rather than of illness so that they can respond appropriately.

Toilet training is difficult for a child who is hospitalized at periodic intervals because success usually requires a consistent caregiver; in addition, hospitalization can result in regressive behaviors. If a chronically ill child has difficulty with ambulation, soiling accidents may occur beyond the usual age because of an inability to reach a bathroom easily.

Children who survive a long-term illness are sometimes referred to as medically fragile or vulnerable children (M. Green & Solnit, 1964). Some parents tend to protect and shelter such a child, and you may have to remind them that, even though the toddler is chronically ill, he or she will demand independence and has the right to explore. A child who uses a lower extremity prosthesis, for example, might prefer to crawl somewhere rather than wait for help to put the prosthesis in place. Although this degree of independence is good, parents may have to limit how it is expressed so the child will learn how to use the prosthesis (e.g., they could make a rule the child must use the prosthesis to walk but can choose whether to use a spoon when eating).

BOX 30.8

Nursing Care Planning

AN INTERPROFESSIONAL CARE MAP FOR A TODDLER WITH TEMPER TANTRUMS

Jason is a 2.5-year-old boy you see at a pediatric clinic. His mother tells you he has changed completely in the past 6 months from an easy-to-care-for baby into a "monster" who refuses to do anything she asks. The only word he says anymore is "no." He has a temper tantrum every night at dinner over some type of food. She tells you this has changed parenting from "fun" to "a real chore."

Family Assessment: Child lives with two parents in three-bedroom home. Father is a ferry boat captain; works 6 days a week. Mother works as a secretary at local university. Finances are "good. We've worked hard to get where we are."

Patient Assessment: Well-nourished 2-year-old boy. Physical findings within normal limits. Mother reports the child is having temper tantrums "at least 20 times a day. He throws himself on the floor and pounds his head and fists." Mother unable to describe any precipitating factors for the tantrums. She states, "He seems to have them just when I start to do something. I could be playing with him one minute, and then I get up to do something, like answer the phone or start dinner, and he starts." Mother reports picking up the child immediately because she fears he will hurt himself. "I just don't know what to do anymore."

Nursing Diagnosis: Health-seeking behaviors related to measures for dealing with and reducing the number of temper tantrums.

Outcome Criteria: Mother describes measures to manage tantrums and reports tantrums have decreased to fewer than four a day by end of 1 week.

Team Member Responsible	Assessment	Intervention	Rationale	Expected Outcome
Activities of Daily Living, Including Safety				
Nurse	Ask mother to describe a typical day; document when tantrums occur and situations that seem to provoke them.	Make suggestions to eliminate cause of distress as revealed by assessment.	Temper tantrums can increase with stress and inability of child to feel independent.	Mother reviews a typical day and identifies times when tantrums are most apt to occur.
Teamwork and Collaboration				
Nurse/primary healthcare provider	Assess if child has possible neurologic symptoms.	Refer child for full neurologic workup if physical exam suggests the need.	Temper tantrums can be confused with seizures if a careful history is not taken.	Mother agrees to further neurologic testing if suggested.
Procedures/Medications for Quality Improvement				
Nurse/nurse practitioner	Assess what measures mother thinks would prevent temper tantrums best.	Work with the mother to develop actions such as ignoring the tantrum and encouraging the mother not to pick up child unless there is actual danger of injury.	Temper tantrums are a method to express emotion. Rewarding the behavior prevents the child from learning more mature methods of coping with frustration.	Mother voices agreement to try suggested solutions and to telephone clinic in 3 days if there is no improvement.
Nutrition				
Nurse practitioner	Assess if child appears well nourished and assess usual dietary pattern.	Because tantrums occur at meal time, review with mother if her actions are different at this time than others.	Eating is an area in which children want to express independence.	Mother lists foods that allow child independent eating, which she will try to serve, to keep meals tantrum-free.

Patient-Centered Care

Nurse	Assess mother's knowledge of toddler behavior and temper tantrums.	Review normal toddler growth and development, explaining that some temper tantrums during this period are natural occurrences.	Information about normal toddler growth and development provides a foundation for further teaching and instruction.	Mother states she understands tantrums occur because of toddler's limited capabilities to express desires.
Nurse	Assess why mother is so fearful her child will hurt himself during a tantrum.	Inform the mother that children rarely hurt themselves during tantrums.	Increased knowledge about the minimal risk of injury during tantrums should help to alleviate the mother's anxiety.	Mother states she has increased understanding about the danger of tantrums.

Psychosocial/Spiritual/Emotional Needs

Nurse/nurse practitioner	Assess what mother feels would be most helpful to relieve her degree of stress and frustration.	Suggest she arrange for "time out" breaks for herself by having husband or friend relieve her.	Short periods away from the child can allow her to regroup her thinking.	Mother describes a plan to receive more help with child care from friend because husband is home only 1 day per week.

Informatics for Seamless Healthcare Planning

Nurse/nurse practitioner	Review with mother the plan for added support and interventions.	Instruct the mother to keep a diary of the child's behavior and measures used during the next week. Set up an appointment for a telephone conference next week to review the diary and discuss the child's behavior.	Keeping and reviewing a diary aids in evaluating the child's behavior and the effectiveness of the methods used. A follow-up telephone call provides an additional opportunity for feedback, teaching, and support.	Mother states she will follow suggestions for managing tantrums and will keep telephone and clinic appointments for follow-up care.

Autism Spectrum Disorder

Classic ASD is a complex range of neurodevelopment disorders characterized by communication difficulties, poor social interaction, and frequent repetitive and stereotyped movements (Fountain, Winter, & Bearman, 2012). It occurs in all ethnic and socioeconomic groups, as frequently as 1 in 88 children, and more frequently in boys than in girls. Milder forms of the disorder are termed Asperger syndrome, Rett syndrome, childhood disintegrative disorder, or pervasive developmental disorder not otherwise specified (usually referred to as PDD-NOS).

Symptoms begin to appear slightly in infancy but are usually obvious enough during the toddler years for parents to become concerned because their child tends not to speak any words, does not make eye contact with others, and has difficulty interacting with playmates, preferring instead to watch a spinning toy, water swirling down the toilet, or repeating sing-song repetitive phrases.

Children need to be screened for autism symptoms by 12 months of age and again at 18 and 24 months of age by observation and parent report. Additional symptoms and therapy for autism are discussed in Chapter 54.

Nutrition and the Physically Challenged or Chronically Ill Toddler

All toddlers need experience feeding themselves if at all possible, but allowing a child with neurologic deficits do this can be difficult for parents. Help them accept the accidents that occur, and suggest finger foods if possible.

If children are on a special diet, it may be difficult to prepare finger foods. If they are tube fed, they receive no experience at all with finger foods. For these children, parents should try to provide other, comparable experiences in independence, such as letting them choose what toy to take to bed or what clothing to wear.

What If . . . 30.4

The nurse is particularly interested in exploring one of the 2020 National Health Goals with respect to toddler growth and development (see Box 30.1). What would be a possible research topic to explore pertinent to this goal that would be applicable to Jason's family and that would also advance evidence-based practice?

TABLE 30.4 NURSING INTERVENTIONS TO HELP A PHYSICALLY CHALLENGED OR CHRONICALLY ILL CHILD DEVELOP A SENSE OF AUTONOMY

Area	Nursing Action
Nutrition	A special diet may limit typical finger foods. Use imagination to offer other foods not usually eaten this way as finger foods. Allow child to help pour liquid diet for a tube feeding. Toddlers are frightened by vomiting because they have no control over it. Comfort afterward. Check for possibility that child is nauseated. Toddlers have no way to express this other than by not eating.
Dressing changes	A child can hold pieces of tape or put tape in place to maintain sense of control. The child can remove an old bandage if it is not contaminated. Allow the child to view his or her incision and watch dressing changes, explaining each step of a procedure as you perform it helps the child maintain control. Restrain only those body parts necessary during a procedure to allow a child a sense of control. Remove all supplies after a procedure or the child may "redo" the dressing.
Medication	Allow children no choice as to whether a medicine will be taken. Do allow a child to choose a "chaser," such as milk or juice, after oral medicine. Do not ask a toddler to indicate a choice of site for an injection or intravenous insertion. This is too advanced a decision for a toddler to handle.
Rest	Locate or create a ritual for bedtime (e.g., put child into bed, tuck him in, say, "Goodnight, Bobby." Tuck in bear. Say, "Goodnight, Bear"). Allow a choice of toy or cover but not a choice of bedtime or naptime hour.
Hygiene	Allow a child a choice of bathtub toy or clothing. Allow a child to wash face and hands to gain control of the situation. Allow the child to put toothpaste on a brush, but you should brush or "touch up" teeth afterward to ensure all plaque has been removed.
Pain	Encourage a child to express pain (e.g., "Say 'ouch' when I pull off the tape"). Help channel a child's self-expression to what is acceptable (the child may shout, for example, but may not kick).
Stimulation	Provide a toddler with a toy that can be manipulated, such as boxes that fit inside one another and can be taken out again, trucks that can be pushed, and pegs that can be pounded. In a healthcare setting, items can usually be found that fit together (e.g., boxes from central supply, plastic vials from the pharmacy). Another action toy: Buy a nonlatex balloon and tie it to the crib side to be used as a punching bag; another one tied to the foot of the crib can serve as a leg exerciser.
Elimination	A child who is toilet trained needs to be encouraged to continue to use a potty chair or toilet during an illness. Help children with ureter or bowel stomas to help with changing bags so they are as independent in bowel function as possible.

KEY POINTS FOR REVIEW

- Erikson's developmental task for the toddler period is to form a sense of autonomy or independence versus shame or doubt.
- Toddlers make great strides forward in development, but their physical growth slows.
- A critical milestone of toddler development is being able to form two-word sentences (a noun and a verb) by 2 years of age.
- Toddlers are capable of preoperational thought or are able to deal much more constructively with symbols than they could while infants.
- Important aspects of toddler care are promoting safety, toddler development, and healthy family functioning because all three of these facets help in planning nursing care that not only meets QSEN competencies but that also best meets a family's total needs.
- Toddler appetites decrease from those of the infant, so children eat proportionally less than they did as infants.
- Common concerns of parents during the toddler period are toilet training, ritualistic behavior, negativism, temper tantrums, discipline, and separation anxiety.
- Promoting autonomy in the child who is physically challenged or chronically ill calls for creative planning because there may be many tasks that must be done for the child to be certain they are done safely.

CRITICAL THINKING CARE STUDY

Bobby is a 2.5-year-old boy you meet at a pediatric clinic because he has a "tummy ache." He lives with his single mother in a one-bedroom apartment on the third floor of a rent-controlled building. His mother tells you he doesn't get outside much because she's afraid to walk to the local park because it is "owned" by a street gang. Bobby sleeps with her in a double bed. Yesterday, he got up before her; she found him sitting on a kitchen counter near the stove. She adds, "His father wants him to be a baseball player. I just want him to learn enough words so he can say when he needs to use a bathroom."

1. What are some safety precautions you would want to discuss with Bobby's mother?

2. The walls of this family's apartment are painted with automobile paint his father secured from his job as a car painter. Would you be concerned with the use of such paint?

3. Bobby does not yet speak in sentences. What questions would you want to ask his mother to help determine if his development is delayed?

RELATED RESOURCES

Explore these additional resources to enhance learning for this chapter:

- Student resources on thePoint, including answers to the What If . . . and Critical Thinking Care Study questions, http://thepoint.lww.com/Flagg8e
- Adaptive learning powered by PrepU, http://thepoint.lww.com/prepu

REFERENCES

American Academy of Pediatrics. (2012). *Where we stand: TV viewing time.* Washington, DC: Author.

American Academy of Pediatrics. (2013). *Where we stand: Car seats for children.* Washington, DC: Author.

Barbaro, J., & Dissanayake, C. (2012). Developmental profiles of infants and toddlers with autism spectrum disorders identified prospectively in a community-based setting. *Journal of Autism & Developmental Disorders, 42*(9), 1939–1948.

Beirens, T. M., van Beeck, E. F., Brug, J., et al. (2010). Why do parents with toddlers store poisonous products safely? *International Journal of Pediatrics, 2010*(2010), 702827.

Bhargava, S. (2011). Diagnosis and management of common sleep problems in children. *Pediatric Review, 32*(3), 91–98.

Bishop, W. P. (2011). The oral cavity. In K. J. Marcdante, R. M. Kliegman, H. B. Jenson, et al. (Eds.), *Nelson essentials of pediatrics* (6th ed., pp. 475–476). Philadelphia, PA: Saunders/Elsevier.

Bowman, S. M., Aitken, M. E., Robbins, J. M., et al. (2012). Trends in U.S. pediatric drowning hospitalizations, 1993–2008. *Pediatrics, 129*(2), 275–281.

Byars, K. C., Yolton, K., Rausch, J., et al. (2012). Prevalence, patterns, and persistence of sleep problems in the first 3 years of life. *Pediatrics, 129*(2), 276–284.

Centers for Disease Control and Prevention. (2012a). *10 Leading causes of death by age group, United States.* Atlanta, GA: Author.

Centers for Disease Control and Prevention. (2012b). *Childhood lead poisoning prevention program.* Atlanta, GA: Author.

Chisholm, K. (2011). Vegetarian diets in children. *Advance for NPs & PAs, 2*(1), 39–41.

Erikson, E. H. (1993). *Childhood and society.* New York, NY: W. W. Norton.

Fountain, C., Winter, A. S., & Bearman, P. S. (2012). Six developmental trajectories characterize children with autism. *Pediatrics, 129*(5), e1112–e1120.

Gahagan, S. (2011). Normal sleep and pediatric sleep disorders. In K. J. Marcdante, R. M. Kliegman, H. B. Jenson, et al. (Eds.), *Nelson essentials of pediatrics* (6th ed., pp. 57–62). Philadelphia, PA: Saunders/Elsevier.

Green, J. A., Whitney, P. G., & Potegal, M. (2011). Screaming, yelling, whining, and crying: Categorical and intensity differences in vocal expressions of anger and sadness in children's tantrums. *Emotion, 11*(5), 1124–1133.

Green, M., & Solnit, A. A. (1964). Reactions to the threatened loss of a child: A vulnerable child syndrome. *Pediatrics, 34*(2), 56–66.

Hodges, E. A., Smith, C., Tidwell, S., et al. (2012). Promoting physical activity in preschoolers to prevent obesity: A review of the literature. *Journal of Pediatric Nursing, 28*(1), 3–19.

Hoeft, K. S., Barker, J. C., & Masterson, E. E. (2011). Maternal beliefs and motivations for first dental visit by low-income Mexican American children in California. *Pediatric Dentistry, 33*(5), 392–398.

Hooker, L., Ward, B., & Verrinder, G. (2012). Domestic violence screening in maternal and child health nursing practice. *Contemporary Nurse, 42*(2), 198–215.

Hutchings, H., Barnes, P. M., Maddocks, A., et al. (2010). Burns in young children: A retrospective matched cohort study of health and developmental outcomes. *Child Care Health & Development, 36*(6), 787–794.

Kiddoo, D. A. (2012). Toilet training children: When to start and how to train. *Canadian Medical Association Journal, 184*(5), 511–512.

Kuehn, B. M. (2012). Panel advises tougher limits on lead exposure. *JAMA, 307*(5), 445.

Landry, S. H., Smith, K. E., Swank, P. R., et al. (2011). The effects of a responsive parenting intervention on parent–child interactions during shared book reading. *Developmental Psychology, 48*(4), 969–986.

Lee, K. J., & Marcdante, K. J. (2011). Poisoning. In W. W. Hay, M. J. Levine, J. M. Sondheimer, et al. (Eds.), *Current pediatric diagnosis & treatment* (20th ed., pp. 158–163). Columbus, OH: McGraw-Hill.

Levine, D. A. (2011). Normal development. In K. J. Marcdante, R. M. Kliegman, H. B. Jenson, et al. (Eds.), *Nelson essentials of pediatrics* (6th ed., pp. 16–18). Philadelphia, PA: Saunders/Elsevier.

Litovitz, T., Whitaker, N., & Clark, L. (2010). Preventing battery ingestions: An analysis of 8648 cases. *Pediatrics, 125*(6), 1178–1183.

Macy, M. L., Clark, S. J., Freed, G. L., et al. (2012). Carpooling and booster seats: A national survey of parents. *Pediatrics, 129*(2), 290–298.

Mills, J., Grushka, J., & Butterworth, S. (2012). Television-related injuries in children—the British Columbia experience. *Journal of Pediatric Surgery, 47*(5), 991–995.

Nelson, T. (2013). The continuum of behavior guidance. *Dental Clinics of North America, 57*(1), 129–143.

Piaget, J. (1952). *The origins of intelligence in children.* New York, NY: International University Press.

Smith, G. A., & Riedford, K. (2013). Epidemiology of early childhood caries: Clinical application. *Journal of Pediatric Nursing, 28*(4), 369–373.

Smith, S. (2011). Vulvovaginitis. In K. J. Marcdante, R. M. Kliegman, H. B. Jenson, et al. (Eds.), *Nelson essentials of pediatrics* (6th ed., pp. 415–446). Philadelphia, PA: Saunders/Elsevier.

Tubert-Jeannin, S., Auclair, C., Amsallem, E., et al. (2011). Fluoride supplements (tablets, drops, lozenges or chewing gums) for preventing dental caries in children. *Cochrane Database of Systematic Reviews,* (12), CD007592.

U.S. Department of Agriculture. (2012). *Choose my plate: A guide to daily food choices.* Washington, DC: Author.

U.S. Department of Health and Human Services. (2010). *Healthy people 2020.* Washington, DC: Author.

Whitney, E. N., & Rolfes, S. R. (2013). Life cycle nutrition: Infancy, childhood and adolescence. In E. N. Whitey & S. R. Rolfes, *Understanding nutrition* (13th ed., pp. 504–550). New York, NY: Wadsworth/Cengage Learning.

31

Nursing Care of a Family With a Preschool Child

*C*athy Edwards is a 3-year-old you meet at a health maintenance visit. Her father cares for her at present because her mother is hospitalized with preterm labor for a second pregnancy. Her father tells you he is concerned because Cathy talks constantly with an imaginary friend named Emma. She makes up stories about events that can't possibly be true. When corrected, Cathy stutters so badly no one can understand her. Her father is also concerned because his daughter cries when he leaves her at daycare.

The previous chapter described toddler growth and development and the abilities children develop during that period. This chapter adds information about the changes, both physical and psychosocial, that occur during the preschool years. Such information builds a base for care and health teaching for this age group.

Is Cathy's father describing typical preschool behavior, or does Cathy need a referral to a child care specialist?

KEY TERMS

broken fluency

bruxism

conservation

ectomorphic body build

egocentrism

Electra complex

endomorphic body build

genu valgus

intuitional thought

Oedipus complex

secondary stuttering

OBJECTIVES

After mastering the contents of this chapter, you should be able to:

1. Describe normal growth and development as well as common parental concerns of the preschool period.

2. Identify 2020 National Health Goals related to the preschool period that nurses can help the nation achieve.

3. Assess a preschooler for normal growth and developmental milestones.

4. Formulate nursing diagnoses related to preschool growth and development or common parental concerns.

5. Identify expected outcomes for nursing care of a preschooler as well as help parents manage seamless transitions across differing healthcare settings.

6. Using the nursing process, plan nursing care that includes the six competencies of Quality & Safety Education for Nurses (QSEN): Patient-Centered Care, Teamwork & Collaboration, Evidence-Based Practice (EBP), Quality Improvement (QI), Safety, and Informatics.

7. Implement nursing care related to normal growth and development of a preschooler, such as preparing a preschooler for an invasive procedure.

8. Evaluate expected outcomes for achievement and effectiveness of care.

9. Integrate knowledge of preschool growth and development with the interplay of nursing process, the six competencies of QSEN, and Family Nursing to promote quality maternal and child health nursing care.

The preschool period traditionally includes the years 3, 4, and 5. Although physical growth slows considerably during this period, personality and cognitive growth continue at a rapid rate. Therefore, this is also an important period of growth for parents because they may be unsure how much independence and responsibility for self-care they should allow their rapidly maturing child. Most children of this age want to do things for themselves—choose their own clothing and dress themselves, feed themselves independently, wash their own hair, and so forth. As a result, parents of a preschooler may find their child dressed in one red and one green sock, going to preschool with unwashed ears, or trying to eat soup with a fork. They need reassurance that this behavior is typical because it is the way children explore and learn about new experiences (Fergusson, Boden, & Horwood, 2013).

Parents may also need some guidance in separating those tasks that a preschooler can accomplish independently from those that still require some adult supervision so they can set sensible limits. Setting limits protects children from harming themselves or others while participating in all the interesting experiences available to them. Box 31.1 lists 2020 National Health Goals related to this in-between toddler and school-age period.

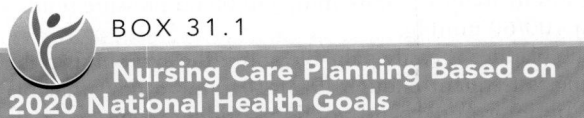

BOX 31.1

Nursing Care Planning Based on 2020 National Health Goals

A number of 2020 National Health Goals are designed to target the preschool population. They include:

- Increase the number of states and the District of Columbia with laws requiring helmets for bicycle riders under 15 years of age, from 19 states to 27 states.
- Decrease acute middle ear infections (otitis media) among children from 246 out of 1,000 to 221 out of 1,000.
- Increase the proportion of children aged 19 to 35 months who receive the recommended doses of diphtheria, tetanus, and pertussis (DTaP); polio; MMR; Haemophilus influenzae type B (HiB); hepatitis B; varicella; and PCVs from 44.3% to 90%.
- Increase the rate of use of forward-facing child car seats among children age 1 to 3 years from a baseline of 72% to 79%.
- Reduce the proportion of children 3 to 11 years exposed to secondhand smoke from 52.2% to 47% (U.S. Department of Health and Human Services, 2010; see www.healthypeople.gov).

Nurses can help the nation achieve these goals by alerting parents to these concerns as well as by serving as consultants at child care and preschool settings to be certain that preschoolers are protected against secondhand smoke, that recommended automobile restraints are used, and that children are fitted with helmets before beginning bicycle riding.

Nursing Process Overview

FOR HEALTHY DEVELOPMENT OF A PRESCHOOLER

ASSESSMENT

Regular assessment of a preschooler includes obtaining a health history and performing both a physical and developmental evaluation at healthcare visits. Preschoolers may speak very little during a health assessment; they may even revert to baby talk or infantile actions such as thumb-sucking if they find a health visit stressful. A history that details their usual performance level is therefore important for accurate evaluation.

Assess a child's weight, height, and body mass index (BMI) according to standard growth charts (available at http://thePoint.lww.com/Flagg8e). Keep in mind that these charts are based on average weights and heights of white American children, so children from other racial backgrounds may not completely conform with these norms (i.e., they may fall into the lower or upper percentiles). Also assess a child for general appearance. Does the child appear alert? Happy? Active? Preschoolers typically have 6 to 12 respiratory infections per year; therefore, many of them will have one at the time of a health assessment.

NURSING DIAGNOSIS

Nursing diagnoses for preschoolers typically center on health promotion or unintentional injury prevention. Examples include:

- Health-seeking behaviors related to developmental expectations
- Risk for injury related to increased independence outside the home
- Delayed growth and development related to frequent illness
- Risk for imbalanced nutrition, more than body requirements, related to fast food choices
- Risk for poisoning related to maturational age of the child
- Parental anxiety related to lack of understanding of childhood development

OUTCOME IDENTIFICATION AND PLANNING

For many parents, preschool is a difficult time because a child is at an in-between stage—no longer an infant, although not yet ready for formal school. Planning and establishing expected outcomes for care of children at this age often begin with establishing a schedule for discussing normal preschool development with the parents. Planning for unintentional injury prevention such as how to cross streets safely becomes increasingly critical as children begin to enjoy experiences away from home. It is also important to plan opportunities for adventurous activities and interaction with other children. Parents may find it helpful to be referred to online resources for further information (see Chapter 28).

IMPLEMENTATION

Preschool children imitate moods as well as actions. An important nursing intervention, therefore, is role-playing a mood or attitude you would like a child to learn. To project an attitude that a health assessment is an enjoyable activity, you might suggest preschoolers participate by listening to their heart or coloring the table paper. Unintentional injury prevention is also best taught by role modeling (e.g., a parent always crosses streets at the corner, a parent doesn't start the car until seatbelts are in place).

OUTCOME EVALUATION

An evaluation of expected outcomes needs to be continuous and frequent. Because growth during this period is more cognitive and emotional than physical, parents may report little growth. Evaluating specific areas can help them appreciate that progress has occurred. Examples of expected outcomes might include:

- Child states importance of holding parent's hand while crossing streets.
- Parent states realistic expectations of 3-year-old child's motor ability by next visit.
- Mother reports she has prepared her 4-year-old for new baby by next visit.

Nursing Assessment of a Preschooler's Growth and Development

An assessment of preschoolers needs to include physical, cognitive, and developmental growth (Box 31.2).

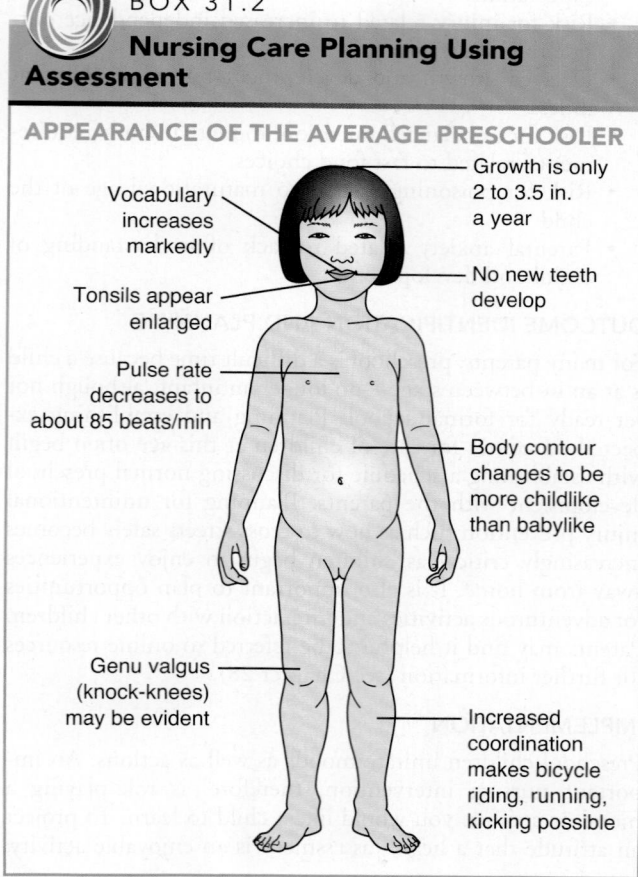

BOX 31.2

Nursing Care Planning Using Assessment

APPEARANCE OF THE AVERAGE PRESCHOOLER

- Vocabulary increases markedly
- Tonsils appear enlarged
- Pulse rate decreases to about 85 beats/min
- Genu valgus (knock-knees) may be evident
- Growth is only 2 to 3.5 in. a year
- No new teeth develop
- Body contour changes to be more childlike than babylike
- Increased coordination makes bicycle riding, running, kicking possible

PHYSICAL GROWTH

A definite change in body contour occurs during the preschool years. The wide-legged gait, prominent lordosis, and protuberant abdomen of the toddler change to slimmer, taller, and much more childlike proportions. Contour changes are so definite that future body type—**ectomorphic body build** (slim body build) or **endomorphic body build** (large body build)—becomes apparent. Handedness also begins to be obvious. A major step forward is a child's ability to learn extended language, which is achieved not only by motor development but also by cognitive development. Children of this age who are exposed to more than one language or who live in a bilingual family have a unique opportunity to master two languages with relative ease because of this increased cognitive ability.

Lymphatic tissue begins to increase in size, particularly the tonsils; levels of immune globulin (Ig)G and IgA antibodies increase. These changes tend to make preschool illnesses more localized (e.g., an upper respiratory infection remains localized to the nose with little systemic fever).

Physiologic splitting of heart sounds may be present for the first time on auscultation; innocent heart murmurs may also be heard for the first time. This type of murmur occurs because of the changing size of the heart in reference to the thorax because the anteroposterior and transverse diameters of the chest have not yet reached adult proportions. Pulse rate decreases to about 85 beats/min, and blood pressure holds at about 100/60 mmHg.

The bladder is easily palpable above the symphysis pubis; voiding is frequent enough (9 or 10 times a day) that play must be interrupted, and voiding accidents may occur if a child becomes absorbed in an activity.

A child who earlier in life had an indeterminate longitudinal arch in the foot generally demonstrates a well-formed arch now. Muscles are noticeably stronger, so activities such as gymnastics become possible. Many children at the beginning of the period exhibit **genu valgus** (knock-knees); this disappears with increased skeletal growth at the end of the preschool period.

Weight, Height, Body Mass Index, and Head Circumference

Weight gain is slight during the preschool years; the average child gains only about 4.5 lb (2 kg) a year. During these years, appetite remains the same as it was during the toddler years, a level perhaps considerably less than some parents would like or expect.

Height gain is also minimal during this period: only 2 to 3.5 in. (6 to 8 cm) a year on average. Head circumference is not routinely measured at physical assessments on children over 2 years of age because it changes little after this time.

Teeth

Children generally have all 20 of their deciduous teeth by 3 years of age; permanent teeth don't replace these until school age. Preserving these teeth is important because they hold the position for the permanent teeth as the child's jaw grows larger. If a deciduous tooth has to be removed, children need conscientious follow-up to be certain a space for

Figure 31.1 Preschoolers like to imitate the roles of adults as they learn about the world around them.

BOX 31.3

Nursing Care Planning to Respect Cultural Diversity

Whether children are allowed to ask questions is culturally determined and can make a difference in how much vocabulary a child uses. In a society in which children are expected to be seen and not heard, a preschool child may not have the same expressive vocabulary as a child who has been encouraged to ask questions. Recognition that differences among cultures can affect levels of development means assessments must be individualized and meaningful in terms of the cultural milieu.

a permanent tooth remains (de Amorim Lde, Estrela, & da Costa, 2011).

DEVELOPMENTAL MILESTONES

Each year during the preschool period marks a major step forward in gross motor, fine motor, and language development. Play activities change focus dramatically as the preschooler learns new skills and understands more about the world (Fig. 31.1). Table 31.1 summarizes major milestones of the period.

Language Development

The extent of a 3-year-old child's vocabulary varies depending on how much the child has been encouraged to ask questions or participate in conversations (Box 31.3). A child typically, however, has a vocabulary of about 900 words and uses it to ask questions constantly, up to 400 a day, such as "Why is snow cold?" "How do worms hear?" and "What does your tongue do?" A child needs simple answers to such questions to encourage curiosity, vocabulary building, and questioning. Words that sound alike but mean different things such as "whether" and "weather" can be confounding to children of this age. If a parent tells a child her shoes should go on with the buckles on the outside, she may seem to understand but return in a few minutes to ask, "Why do I have to go outside to put on my shoes?"

Egocentrism, or perceiving that one's thoughts and needs are better or more important than those of others, is also strong during the preschool period. Preschoolers cannot believe that not everyone knows facts they know; if asked, "What is your name?" they may reply, "Don't you know it?" As a part of egocentrism, preschoolers define objects mainly in relation to themselves, so a spoon is "what I eat with," not a curved metal object; a crayon is "what I write with," not an orange wax object.

Four- and 5-year-old children enjoy participating in mealtime conversation and can describe an incident from their day in great detail. Remember that preschoolers tend to imitate language exactly, so if they hear less-than-perfect language, this is the language pattern they adopt. They may imitate and use "bathroom language" because of the attention from adults this generates.

Preschoolers are egocentric, so they define objects in relation to themselves (e.g., a key is not a metal object but "what I use to open a door," a car is not a means of transportation but "what Mom uses to take me to school").

Play

Preschoolers do not need many toys because, with an imagination keener than it will be at any other time in life, they enjoy games that use imitation such as pretending they are a teacher, cowboy or cowgirl, firefighter, or store clerk. Many preschoolers have imaginary friends at this stage (Nielsen, 2012), which often exist until children formally begin school.

Four- and 5-year-olds divide their time between roughhousing and imitative play. Five-year-olds become interested in group games or reciting songs they have learned in kindergarten or preschool.

TABLE 31.1 SUMMARY OF PRESCHOOL GROWTH AND DEVELOPMENT

Age (in Years)	Fine Motor Skills	Gross Motor Skills	Language	Play
3	Undresses self; stacks tower of blocks; draws a cross	Runs; alternates feet on stairs; rides tricycle; stands on one foot	Vocabulary of 900 words	Able to take turns; very imaginative
4	Can do simple buttons	Constantly in motion; jumps; skips	Vocabulary of 1,500 words	Pretending is major activity
5	Can draw a six-part figure; can lace shoes	Throws overhand	Vocabulary of 2,100 words	Likes games with numbers or letters

EMOTIONAL DEVELOPMENT

Children change a great deal in their ability to understand their world and how they relate to other people during the preschool years.

Initiative

The developmental task for the preschool-age child is to achieve a sense of initiative versus guilt (Erikson, 1993). Children with a well-developed sense of initiative like to explore because they have discovered that learning new things is fun.

If children are criticized or punished for attempts at initiative, they can develop a sense of guilt for wanting to try new activities or to have new experiences. Those who leave the preschool period with a sense of guilt can carry it with them into school situations. They may even have difficulty later in life making decisions about everything from changing jobs to choosing an apartment because they cannot envision that they are capable of solving the associated problems that will come with change.

To gain a sense of initiative, preschoolers need exposure to a wide variety of experiences and play materials so they can learn as much about how things work as possible. They are ready to explore outside their homes such as enjoying a trip to the zoo or an amusement park (Fig. 31.2). They enjoy going with their family on vacation. These types of experiences lead to increased vocabulary (e.g., at the zoo, words such as giraffe, elephant, and bear come alive because they are transferred from abstract concepts to the actual animals).

Urge parents to provide play materials that encourage creative play, such as finger paints, soapy water to splash or blow into bubbles, sand to build castles, and modeling clay or homemade dough to mold into figures or make into pretend cookies. These are messy activities, so some parents prefer not to allow a child to indulge in them more than once a week, but any experience with free-form play is helpful.

Preschoolers tend to have such active imaginations that they need little guidance in this type of play. They smear both hands into clay or finger paint and create instinctively. What they make may not be recognizable; it is the enjoyment of feeling the material and how they can manipulate it that captures the experience.

Imitation

Imitating the actions of the people around them peaks during preschool age. Role modeling this way should be fun and

does not have to be accurate. If a child is pretending to be a police officer who is busy putting out fires or a firefighter who is stopping playmates from speeding, the fact that the child is freely imitating a role is more important than getting the role absolutely correct. If a parent is concerned that a child should recognize these roles more accurately, it is usually best to suggest that the parent not to stop the play but rather to explain where firefighters work and that their job is to put out fires the next time they drive past the fire station.

Children generally imitate those activities best that they see their parents performing at home. A young girl will set the table for breakfast, eat with her "spouse," help clean off the table, and leave for work. A young boy might work on his computer, pretend to feed a doll, and put the doll to bed as he has seen his father do with a younger sibling. In addition to learning what activities adults carry out at home, preschoolers should also be introduced to their parents' work environments. Such visits not only provide a visual context for the parent's job but also let a child learn such words as photocopier, assembly line, legal brief, or fax machine.

Fantasy

Toddlers cannot differentiate between fantasy and reality; they believe cartoon characters they see on television are real. Preschoolers, however, begin to make this differentiation. They may become so engrossed in a fantasy role that they fear they are "stuck" in the fantasy and are no longer themselves. Such intense involvement in play is part of "magical thinking," which is active at this age (i.e., believing thoughts and wishes can come true).

Parents sometimes strengthen this feeling without realizing it, so they (and you) need to be careful in this regard. A preschooler, like Cathy for example, whom you care for in the hospital might be pretending she is a white rabbit. When you walk into her room, you are aware of the game, so you might say, "That's strange; I don't see Cathy anywhere. All I

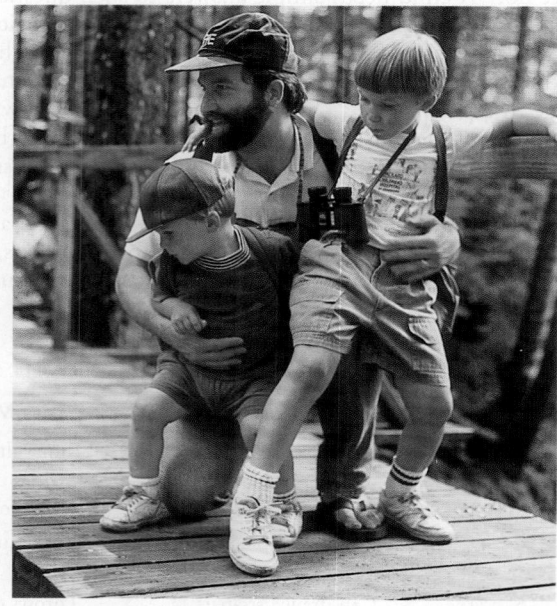

Figure 31.2 Preschoolers like exposure to new events and places. Here, a 3-year-old child is eager to explore the woods during a hike with the family.

see is a white rabbit." Cathy may be frightened that she has actually become a white rabbit; how will she ever get home again? A better response from you would be to support the imitation—this is age-appropriate behavior and a good way to explore roles—by saying instead, "What a nice white rabbit you're pretending to be." This both supports the fantasy and yet reassures the child she is still herself.

Oedipus and Electra Complexes

Although the development of Oedipus and Electra complexes may have been overstated by Freud—possibly because of gender bias—many children do seem to manifest such behavior (Erreich, 2011). An **Oedipus complex** refers to the strong emotional attachment a preschool boy demonstrates toward his mother; an **Electra complex** is the attachment of a preschool girl to her father. A daughter demonstrating this complex might prefer to always sit beside her father at the table, or she may ask for her father to tuck her in at night. She makes a point that she is "Daddy's girl." A mother who is not prepared for this behavior may feel hurt and cut off from family interaction. A father may feel the same way when his son wants to sit beside his mother and prefers her to be the one to tuck him in for the night.

Parents can be assured this phenomenon of competition and romance in preschoolers is a normal part of maturing. Some parents may need help in handling feelings of jealousy and anger, however, particularly if a child is vocal in expressing feelings toward a parent.

Gender Roles

Preschoolers begin to be aware of the difference between sexes and so need to be introduced to both gender roles. Encourage single parents to plan opportunities for their children to spend some time with adults other than themselves, such as a grandparent, a friend, or a relative of the opposite sex, for this experience. If a child is hospitalized during the preschool period, a nurse could readily fill this role.

Many parents do not want their child to grow up as they did, with a fixed gender role as a result of stereotyping. Help them understand that parents reinforce such attitudes by their actions as well as by their words. For example, a father may tell his son it is important for both boys and girls to do housework, but if the father never does dishes, he is teaching his son that managing a household is not a man's job.

Socialization

Because 3-year-olds are capable of sharing, they play with other children their age much more agreeably than do toddlers, which makes the preschool period a sensitive and critical time for socialization. Preschoolers who are exposed to other playmates have an easier time learning to relate to people than those raised in an environment where they rarely see other children of the same age (Paulus & Moore, 2012) (Fig. 31.3).

Although 4-year-olds continue to enjoy play groups, they may become involved in arguments more than they did at 3 years of age, especially as they become more certain of their role in the group. This development, like so many others, may make parents worry that a child is regressing. However, it is really forward movement that involves some testing and identification of their group role.

Figure 31.3 The preschool child moves past parallel play to make new friendships.

Five-year-olds begin to develop "best" friendships, perhaps on the basis of who they walk to school with or who lives closest to them. The elementary rule that an odd number of children will have difficulty playing well together generally pertains to children at this age: two or four will play, but three or five will quarrel.

Cognitive Development

According to Piaget (1969), cognitive development is still preoperational by 3 years of age, although children during this period also enter a second phase called **intuitional thought**. During this second phase of development, children learn by asking questions such as "How come?" and "Why?" Piaget named this stage "intuitive thought" because he believed that children tend to be so certain of their knowledge and understanding that they are unaware of how they gained this knowledge initially. Children in the intuitive substage may still demonstrate many advances in cognitive skills. They may shift from using only magical beliefs to using rational beliefs to explain situations or events that they had not experienced previously. Very young children may explain that a new building "grew out of the ground," whereas older children understand it was built.

Intuitive children show a style of thinking he called "centration." These children typically are focused on the characteristic of an object or person, and they base their decisions or judgment on that one characteristic (as opposed to considering multiple characteristics). For example, a 4-year-old who was asked to put toys into groups might focus his or her attention on the color of the toy instead of the shape or the material from which they are constructed. Centration also means that preschoolers cannot make mental substitutions and often feel they are always right. It's important to remember this when explaining procedures to preschoolers. They cannot see your side of the situation, they cannot hurry because you must have something done by 10 o'clock, and they cannot hold still just because you want them to.

Preschoolers are not yet aware of the property of **conservation**. This means that if they have two balls of clay of equal size, but one is squashed flatter and wider than the other, they will insist the flatter one is bigger (because it is wider) or the intact one is bigger (because it is taller). They cannot see that only the form, not the amount, has changed. This inability to appreciate conservation has implications for nursing care because it means preschoolers are not able to comprehend that a procedure performed two separate ways is the same procedure. If the nurse before you, for example, told a child to turn on his right side and then his left side while his bed was made, you may have to allow him to turn those same ways or he will insist you are making his bed wrong. Decentering, combined with the concept of conservation, appear prior to more sophisticated logical thinking abilities.

Moral and Spiritual Development

Children of preschool age determine right from wrong based on their parents' rules because they have little understanding of the rationale for these rules or even whether the rules are consistent. If asked the question, "Why is it wrong to hit other children?" the average preschooler answers, "Because my mother says so." Because preschoolers depend on their parents to supply rules for them, when faced with a new situation, they may have difficulty understanding the rules they know also apply to the new situation such as a hospital.

Preschoolers begin to have an elemental concept of spirituality if they have been provided some form of religious training. Belief in an outside force aids in the development of conscience; however, preschoolers tend to do good out of self-interest rather than because of strong spiritual motivation (Kohlberg, 1984). Children at this age enjoy the security of religious holidays and religious rituals such as prayer before meals because these rituals offer them the same reassurance and security as a familiar nursery rhyme read over and over.

What If . . . 31.1
Cathy, 3 years old, understands the rule "Don't steal from a store." Would she also understand "Don't steal from a hospital"?

Planning and Implementation for the Health Promotion of a Preschooler and Family

Preschoolers are old enough to begin to take responsibility for their own actions. Children's safety, nutritional health, daily activities, and family functioning are all affected by this increased responsibility.

PROMOTING PRESCHOOLER SAFETY

As preschoolers broaden their horizons, safety issues must also widen. By age 4 years, children may project an attitude of independence and the ability to take care of their own needs. However, they still need supervision to be certain they do not injure themselves or other children while roughhousing and to ensure they do not stray too far from home. Their interest in learning adult roles may lead them to exploring the blades of a lawn mower or an electric saw or a neighbor's

pool (Bowman, Aitken, Robbins, et al., 2012). Because they imitate adult roles so well, they may imitate taking medicine if they see family members doing so. It's also not too early to think about gun safety or being certain any gun in their home is locked away separate from its ammunition (Senger, Keijzer, Smith, et al., 2011).

A final area to consider is automobile safety. Preschoolers must be reminded repeatedly to buckle their booster seat and not to walk in back of or in front of automobiles. Otherwise, a preschooler's thought "I want to play with Mary across the street" can be so quick and so intense that the child will run into the middle of the street before remembering street safety rules. Additional safety points for the preschool period are summarized in Box 31.4.

Keeping Children Safe, Strong, and Free

The preschool years are not too early a time to educate children about the potential threat of harm from strangers or how to address bullying behavior (from children or adults) at preschool or at play (Jonson-Reid, Kohl, & Drake, 2012) through such measures as:

- Cautioning a child never to talk with or accept a ride from a stranger
- Teaching a child how to call for help in an emergency (yelling or running to a designated neighbor's house if outside, or dialing 911 if near a phone)
- Describing what police officers look like and explaining that police can help in an emergency situation
- Explaining that if children or adults ask them to keep secrets about anything that has made them uncomfortable, they should tell their parents or another trusted adult, even if they have promised to keep the secret
- Explaining that bullying behavior from other children is not to be tolerated and should be reported so they can receive help managing it

It is often difficult for parents to impart this type of information to preschoolers because they don't want to terrify their child about the world. They also can't imagine their child will ever be in a situation in which the information will be needed. If the information is presented in a calm and everyday manner, however, children can use it to begin to build safe habits that will help them later when they are old enough to walk home from school alone or play with their friends unsupervised.

Motor Vehicle and Bicycle Safety

Because of front seat airbags, preschoolers need to be buckled into car seats or booster seats in the back seat (American Academy of Pediatrics, 2012). Urge parents to stress the important role of seat belts in preventing injury and to make a rule that the car does not move until seat belts are fastened. Many preschoolers outgrow their car seats during this period (when they reach about 40 lb) and need to graduate to a booster-type seat. Remind parents to check the position of the shoulder harness in both types of seat so the belt doesn't cross a child's face or throat.

Preschool is also the right age to promote bicycle safety because falls off bicycles are a major cause of severe head injuries in this age group (Agarwal & Pruthi, 2010). To prevent such injuries, preschoolers need a safety helmet approved for children their age and size. Encourage parents who ride

BOX 31.4

Nursing Care Planning to Empower a Family

COMMON SAFETY MEASURES TO PREVENT UNINTENTIONAL INJURIES TO PRESCHOOLERS

Q. Cathy's father says to you, "My preschooler is so active! How can I keep her safe?"

A. All of the safety measures that apply to toddlers also apply to preschoolers. In addition, try these tips:

Possible Unintentional Injury	Prevention Measure
Motor vehicles	Teach safety with tricycles (e.g., look before crossing driveways, do not cross streets).
	Teach the child to always hold hands with an adult before crossing a street.
	Teach parking lot safety (e.g., hold hands with an adult, do not run behind cars that could be backing up).
	Teach children to consistently wear helmets when beginning bicycle riding.
Falls	Always supervise a preschooler at a playground.
	Remove drawstrings from hooded clothing.
	Help the child to judge safe distances for jumping or safe heights for climbing.
Drowning	Teach beginning swimming.
Animal bites	Do not allow the child to approach strange dogs.
	Supervise the child's play with family pets.
Poisoning	Never present medication as a candy.
	Never take medication in front of a child.
	Never store food or substances in containers other than their own.
	Post the telephone number of the poison control center by the telephone or as a cell phone contact number (1-800-222-1222).
	Teach the child that medications are a serious substance and not for play.
Burns	Store matches in closed containers.
	Do not allow the preschooler to help light birthday candles or fireplaces; fire is not fun or a treat.
Community safety	Teach the preschooler that not all people are friends (e.g., "Do not talk to strangers or take candy from strangers").
	Define a stranger as someone the child does not know, not someone odd looking.
	Teach the child to say "no" to people whose touching he or she does not enjoy, including family members. (When a child is sexually maltreated, the offender is usually a family member or close family friend.)
General	Know the whereabouts of the preschooler at all times.
	Be aware the frequency of unintentional injuries increases when parents are under stress. Special precautions must be taken at these times.
	Some children are more active, curious, and impulsive and therefore more vulnerable to unintentional injuries than others.

bicycles to demonstrate safe riding habits by wearing helmets as well. Seeing a parent routinely wearing a helmet may well be the most compelling reason for a preschooler to wear one.

What If . . . 31.2

Cathy tells the nurse she knows to not leave preschool with anyone who is strange. Is that the same as knowing not to leave with a stranger?

PROMOTING THE NUTRITIONAL HEALTH OF A PRESCHOOLER

Like the toddler period, the preschool years are not a time of fast growth, so preschool children are not likely to have ravenous appetites (Raman, 2011). Being certain they get

enough daily exercise helps to improve this. A sense of initiative, or learning how to do things, can be strengthened by allowing a child to prepare simple foods, such as making a sandwich or spreading jelly on toast.

Most children are hungry after preschool and enjoy a snack when they arrive home. Because sugary foods can dull a child's appetite for dinner and it is not too soon to begin measures to prevent childhood obesity, urge parents to offer snacks such as fruit, cheese, or milk rather than cookies and a soft drink or juice (Bevan & Reilly, 2011).

Preschool Nutrition Requirements

As with all age groups, foods selected for preschoolers should include variety (U.S. Department of Agriculture, 2012) and be based on MyPlate (www.choosemyplate.gov) recommendations.

Preschoolers may not eat a great deal of meat because it can be hard to chew. Many parents ask whether their preschooler needs to take supplementary vitamins to make up for this. As long as a child is eating foods from all five food groups and meets the criteria for a healthy child such as being alert and active with height and weight within normal averages, additional vitamins are probably unnecessary.

If parents do give vitamins, remind them that a child will undoubtedly view a vitamin as candy rather than medicine because of the attractive shapes and colors of preschool vitamins, so they must be stored out of reach. Caution parents not to give more vitamins than the recommended daily amount, or poisoning from high doses of fat-soluble vitamins or iron can result.

A Vegetarian Diet

A vegetarian diet is usually colorful and therefore appeals to preschoolers. Vegetables, fruits, and grains are also healthy snack foods.

If vegetarian diets are deficient in any aspects, it is usually in calcium, vitamin B_{12}, and vitamin D. Check to be sure a child is ingesting a variety of calcium sources (e.g., green leafy vegetables, milk products) because calcium is very important for bone growth. Vitamin D is found in fortified cereals and milk. Vitamin B_{12} is found almost exclusively in animal products, so a child on a vegetarian intake may need a supplemental source (Whitney & Rolfes, 2013).

PROMOTING THE DEVELOPMENT OF THE PRESCHOOLER IN DAILY ACTIVITIES

The preschooler has often mastered the basic skills needed for most self-care activities, including feeding, dressing, washing (with supervision), and toothbrushing (again, with supervision).

Dressing

Many 3-year-olds and most 4-year-olds can dress themselves except for difficult buttons, although conflict may occur over what the child will wear. Preschoolers prefer bright colors or prints and so may select items that are appealing in color rather than matching. As with other preschool activities, however, children need the experience of choosing their own clothes. One way for parents to solve the problem of mismatching is to fold together matching shirts and slacks so a child sees them as a set rather than individual pieces. If children insist on wearing mismatched clothing, urge parents to make no apologies for their appearance. A simple statement, "Mark chose his own clothes today" explains the situation. Anyone who understands preschoolers appreciates that the experience children gain in being able to select their own clothing is worth more than a perfect appearance by adult standards.

Sleep

Many toddlers, who go through a typical negative phase, resist taking naps no matter how tired they are. Preschoolers, however, are more aware of their needs; when they are tired, they often curl up on a couch or soft chair and fall asleep. Many, particularly those who attend afternoon child care or preschool, give up afternoon naps. If they nap at preschool,

they may have some difficulty going to sleep at the usual bedtime established at home.

On some occasions, even though they may be tired, children in this age group may refuse to go to sleep because of fear of the dark and may wake at night terrified by a bad dream (Byars, Yolton, Rausch, et al., 2012). This means that preschoolers may need a night-light turned on, although they did not need one before. A helpful suggestion for parents is to screen out frightening stories or TV watching just prior to bedtime and to be certain when the light in their bedroom is dimmed, it has a soothing atmosphere (no staring teddy bears or evil smiling dolls). Box 31.5 is an interprofessional care map for a child with preschool fears.

QSEN Checkpoint Question 31.2

EVIDENCE-BASED PRACTICE

Many preschoolers have difficulty falling asleep or wake during the night with nightmares. To see if changes in the type of television watched could improve preschooler's sleep, researchers encouraged half of a group of families studied to replace television watching with quality educational and prosocial video content through use of an initial home visit and follow-up telephone calls over 6 months. Among the 565 children studied, the most common sleep problem was delayed sleep onset (38%). Results at the end of 18 months showed that children in the intervention group had significantly lower odds of any sleep problems (Garrison & Christakis, 2012).

Based on the study, what is the best advice the nurse could give the Edwards family?

a. Don't allow Cathy to watch television until she is 5 years of age.
b. Encourage Cathy to watch specific DVDs that her parents choose for her.
c. Discuss with Cathy that TV does not necessarily reflect reality.
d. Allow her to only watch cartoons so she won't be seeing violence.

Look in Appendix A for the best answer and rationale.

Exercise

The preschool period is an active phase, so preschool play tends to be vigorous. Roughhousing helps relieve tension and should be allowed as long as it does not become destructive. In addition, preschoolers love time-honored games such as ring-around-the-rosy, London Bridge, or other more structured games they were not ready for as toddlers. Promoting these types of active games and reducing television watching can be steps toward helping children develop motor skills as well as prevent childhood obesity (Hodges, Smith, Tidwell, et al., 2012; Mitka, 2012).

Hygiene

Preschoolers can wash and dry their hands adequately if the faucet is regulated for them (so they do not scald themselves with hot water). When possible, parents should turn down the temperature of the water heater in their home to under 120°F to help prevent scalds.

BOX 31.5

Nursing Care Planning

Cathy Edwards is a 3-year-old whom you meet at a health maintenance visit. Her father tells you he is concerned because Cathy talks constantly with an imaginary friend named Emma. She makes up stories about events that can't possibly be true. When corrected, Cathy stutters so badly that no one can understand her. Her father is also concerned because his daughter cries when he leaves her at child care.

Family Assessment: The family lives in a rented apartment in the inner city. The mother, a stay-at-home mom, is hospitalized with complications of a second pregnancy. The father works as a city police detective.

Patient Assessment: A 3-year-old girl within normal limits for height, weight, and development. The child is currently enrolled in an all-day preschool program while the mother is hospitalized. The father picks the child up after his work. The father arrived late to pick the child up from preschool last week. She states, "He forgot me." The child refuses to return to preschool. When he tries to drop her off now, she cries, sticks her finger in her mouth to make herself vomit, and complains her stomach hurts.

Nursing Diagnosis: Fear related to separation and abandonment during preschool period.

Outcome Criteria: The child verbalizes fear. The father demonstrates measures to minimize the child's fears; reports by 2 weeks that crying episodes at school have decreased.

Team Member Responsible	Assessment	Intervention	Rationale	Expected Outcome
Activities of Daily Living, Including Safety				
Nurse	Ask father to detail a 24-hour day for the family to gain clear picture of child's role and capabilities.	Father describes differences in family life since wife has been hospitalized and strain it causes on Cathy.	People are unable to solve a problem until the extent of the problem is clear.	Father details a typical day and expresses his wish to continue or not continue the preschool experience for Cathy.
Teamwork and Collaboration				
Nurse/nurse practitioner	Assess if father feels referral to child guidance service is necessary to help reduce fear.	Encourage the father to talk with the preschool staff about the problem and common methods to decrease a child's fear.	Discussion with care providers can help reinforce the measures used by the father to provide consistency and thereby help to minimize a child's fears.	Father states he will consult with preschool staff to help solve the problem.
Procedures/Medications for Quality Improvement				
Nurse	Assess what father knows about measures to reduce fear in preschoolers.	Instruct the father in measures to help reduce child's fear, such as reinforcing the time he will return, calling if he's running late, and posting memo to self to pick her up.	Reassurance helps to reduce a child's fear of abandonment.	Father describes steps he will take to be certain he will not be late again at preschool for pickup.
Nutrition				
Nurse	Assess if child uses threat of vomiting at any other time.	Stress that effect of eating disorders is potentially dangerous.	Frequent vomiting in young children can lead to fluid and electrolyte imbalances.	Father states whether he has ever seen pseudovomiting before.
Patient-Centered Care				
Nurse/nurse practitioner	Assess father's knowledge of typical preschool fears such as abandonment and fear of the dark.	Review with the father the typical fears experienced by the preschooler, including those of separation and abandonment.	Knowledge of normal growth and development helps to reduce the father's anxiety about the behavior and possible causes.	Father acknowledges he deals mainly with adults in his business; expresses desire to learn more about preschool period.

Continued on following page

BOX 31.5

Nursing Care Planning (continued)

Team Member Responsible	Assessment	Intervention	Rationale	Expected Outcome
Psychosocial/Spiritual/Emotional Needs				
Nurse	Explore with child why she is so fearful her father will not return for her.	Encourage the father to set up a special time for himself and his daughter in the evening or on weekends so they have a consistent close time.	Special time for a father and daughter enhances the parent–child relationship. Consistently adhering to this time helps to foster a sense of trust and security and shows he is dependable.	Father states he will plan for a special time each week, even if it is difficult to arrange because of wife's hospitalization and his irregular work schedule.
Informatics for Seamless Healthcare Planning				
Nurse	Assess if father would find a follow-up telephone call helpful.	Arrange for a follow-up telephone call (if desired) in 1 week.	Follow-up provides additional support and means for evaluating the effectiveness of the methods used.	Father states he is receptive to follow-up care.

Although preschoolers certainly sit well in bathtubs, they should still not be left unsupervised at bath time in case they decide to add more hot water or to practice swimming and then be unable to get their head out of the water again. Some girls develop vulvar irritation (and perhaps bladder infections) from exposure to bubble bath so parents shouldn't add such products to the water (S. Smith, 2011). Although not well studied, cranberry juice may help prevent these infections the same as in adult women (Goldman, 2012).

Children this age are not paragons of neatness and may not clean their hands thoroughly. Preschoolers do not clean their fingernails or ears well, either, so these areas often need "touching up" by a parent or older sibling. Using a nonirritating shampoo and hanging a mobile over the tub so they have a reason to look up while their hair is rinsed helps make hair washing a fun procedure.

Care of Teeth

If independent toothbrushing was not started as a daily practice during the toddler years, it should be started during preschool (G. A. Smith & Riedford, 2012). One good toothbrushing period a day is often more effective than more frequent half-hearted attempts. Electric or battery-operated toothbrushes are favorites of preschoolers and can be used safely if the child is taught not to use it or any other electrical appliance near a basin of water. Although many preschoolers do well brushing their own teeth, parents must check that all tooth surfaces have been cleaned. Parents should also floss the child's teeth because this is a skill beyond a preschooler's motor ability.

Preschoolers should continue to drink fluoridated water or receive a prescribed oral fluoride supplement if fluoride is not provided in the water supply (Tubert-Jeannin, Auclair, Amsallem, et al., 2011). Encouraging children to eat apples, carrots, chicken, or cheese for snacks rather than candy or sweets is yet another way to prevent tooth decay. If a child is allowed to chew gum, it should be the sugar-free variety.

A first visit to a dentist should be arranged no later than 2 years of age for an evaluation of tooth formation because

deciduous (baby) teeth must be preserved to protect the dental arch. Dental services can be performed at 3 years of age. If a tooth has to be pulled for any reason, this can cause the permanent teeth to drift out of position or the jaw not to grow enough to accommodate them (Merlino & Gigli, 2012). Because initial visits usually reveal no cavities, this should be a pain-free experience and should help implant the idea that dentists like to help rather than hurt.

Teeth grinding (**bruxism**) may begin at this age as a way of "letting go," similar to body rocking, which children do for a short time each night before falling asleep. Children who grind their teeth extensively may have greater than average anxiety. Children who have cerebral palsy may do this because of the spasticity of jaw muscles. If grinding is extensive, the crowns of the teeth can actually become abraded. The condition can advance to such an extent that tooth nerves become exposed and painful. If damage is evident, refer the family to a pediatric dentist so the teeth can be evaluated, repaired (capped), and conserved.

What If . . . 31.3

Cathy's father tells the nurse she hates to take a bath and brush her teeth. What suggestions could the nurse make to help Cathy enjoy these bedtime activities more?

PROMOTING HEALTHY FAMILY FUNCTIONING

An important role of preschooler parents is to respect creativity. Some who enjoyed maintaining a gentle rhythm of care for an infant can have difficulty being the parents of a preschooler because more flexibility and creativity are required. Other parents come into their own as their child reaches 3 years; they delight in encouraging imaginative games and play.

Part of encouraging creativity is encouraging vocabulary building. One way for parents to do this is to read aloud to their child; another is to answer questions so the child sees language as an organized system of communication. Answering a preschooler's questions can be difficult, because the questions are frequently philosophical, not fact finding such as, "Why is grass green?" A child may listen to an explanation of chlorophyll but then repeat the question, regardless of the clarity of the explanation, because the parent underestimated the depth of the question. The child did not want to know what makes grass green but why, philosophically, it is not red, blue, or yellow. The obvious answer to that is "I don't know." Parents who are confident can give this answer without feeling threatened. Parents who are less sure of themselves may feel extremely uncomfortable when they realize they do not know the answer to what a 4-year-old is asking (Box 31.6).

Discipline

Preschoolers have definite opinions on things such as what they want to eat, where they want to go, and what they want to wear, and these opinions may bring them into opposition with parents. A major parental responsibility when this happens is to guide a child through these struggles without discouraging the child's right to have an opinion. A "time-out" is a useful technique for parents to correct behavior throughout the preschool years (see Chapter 30). Although the technique has some critics, it allows parents to discipline without using physical punishment and allows a child to learn a new way of behavior without extreme stress. Time-out periods should be

---

BOX 31.6

Nursing Care Planning Tips for Effective Communication

Cathy is being seen for a health maintenance visit. You overhear her father talking to his daughter in the waiting room.

Tip: Preschoolers ask 300 to 400 questions a day as they explore their world. Encourage parents to more completely answer their child's questions by explaining they are helping to build their child's vocabulary. Parents sometimes try to discourage questions by offering minimal answers, and discouraging questions can become the habitual method of interaction.

Cathy: Why do we have to wait so long?

Mr. Edwards: It's how things work here.

Cathy: Why?

Mr. Edwards: People have to take turns. We're waiting for our turn.

Cathy: Why is that girl here? Is she sick?

Mr. Edwards: She might be. Some children are here because they're sick and some are just here for a checkup like you.

Cathy: When are we going home?

Mr. Edwards: As soon as the nurse practitioner checks you over.

Cathy: What's that girl's name?

Mr. Edwards: I don't know. Do you want to ask her?

---

as many minutes long as the child is old, so 3 to 5 minutes is appropriate for preschoolers.

PARENTAL CONCERNS ASSOCIATED WITH THE PRESCHOOL PERIOD

A number of common health problems and fears usually arise during the preschool years.

Common Health Problems of the Preschooler

The mortality of children during the preschool years is low and becoming lower every year as more infectious diseases are preventable. This results in the major cause of death being automobile accidents, followed by poisoning and falls (Centers for Disease Control and Prevention [CDC], 2012).

Even though the number of major illnesses is few in this age group, the number of minor illnesses, such as common colds and ear infections, are high. Children who live in homes in which parents smoke have a higher incidence of ear (otitis media) and respiratory infections than others (Yilmaz, Caylan, & Karacan, 2012). Children who attend child care or preschool programs also have an increased incidence of gastrointestinal disturbances (vomiting and diarrhea) and upper respiratory infections from the exposure to other children unless frequent hand washing is stressed at the setting (Sun & Sundell, 2011).

Children may demonstrate frequent whining or clinging behavior because of this parade of constant minor infections. Assess to be certain such constant illness is not causing parents to perceive a child as sickly or not able to cope with everyday life so they don't begin to discourage independence in favor of overprotection. As parents become more experienced in handling these conditions, their perception of whether an illness is serious or not and their ability to cope with them will change.

Table 31.2 shows the recommended health maintenance schedule for preschoolers. Table 31.3 lists common problems parents may have in evaluating a preschooler's illness.

Common Fears of the Preschooler

Because preschoolers' imaginations are so active, this leads to a number of fears such as fear of the dark, mutilation, and separation or abandonment. These can rise in incidence when combined with the stress of an illness, hospitalization, or unsafe conditions in the child's community (Kushnir & Sadeh, 2011). Although most of these fears can be handled by comforting from parents, in some children, fears are so intense that they need therapy such as desensitization in order for the fear to be conquered.

Fear of the Dark

The tendency to fear the dark is an example of a fear heightened by a child's vivid imagination: a stuffed toy by daylight becomes a threatening monster at night. Children awaken screaming because of nightmares. They may be reluctant to go to bed or go back to sleep by themselves unless a light is left turned on or a parent sits nearby.

If parents are prepared for this fear and understand it is a phase of growth, they are better able to cope with it. It is generally helpful if they monitor the stimuli their children are exposed to, especially around bedtime. This includes television, adult discussions, and frightening stories. Parents are

TABLE 31.2 HEALTH MAINTENANCE SCHEDULE, PRESCHOOL PERIOD

Area of Focus	Methods	Frequency
Assessment		
Health history	Health interview	Every visit
Physical health	Physical examination	Every visit
Developmental milestones	History, observation	Every visit
	Formal Denver Developmental Screening Test (DDST-II)	Before start of school
Growth milestones	Height and weight plotted on standard growth chart; body mass index (BMI) and physical examination	Every visit
Hypertension	Blood pressure	Every visit
Nutrition	History, observation; height and weight information	Every visit
Parent–child relationship	History and observation	Every visit
Social behavior	History and observation	Every visit
Vision and hearing defects	History and observation	Every visit
	Preschool E stereo and audiometer testing	Before start of school
Autism spectrum disorder screening	History and observation	At 18 and 24 months
Dental health	History, physical examination	Every visit
	Dental visit	Every 6 months
	Fluoride varnish	Recommended each visit
Dyslipidemia	Cholesterol, triglycerides	If indicated by risk
Lead	Blood analysis (depending on risk in area)	If indicated by risk
Tuberculosis	Purified protein derivative (PPD) test (if there are high-risk factors)	If indicated by risk
Immunizations		
(Administer immunization in accordance with healthcare agency policies. Check history and past records and inform caregiver about any risks and side effects before administration [www.cdc.gov/vaccines/schedules].)		
Diphtheria, pertussis, and tetanus	DTaP 5	Before start of school
Measles, mumps, and rubella (MMR)	MMR #2	Before start of school
Poliomyelitis (inactivated)	IPV #4	Before start of school
Varicella	VAR #2	Before start of school
Influenza	IIV	Yearly
Pneumococcal	Pneumococcal conjugate vaccine (PCV)	May be indicated before school in susceptible children
Anticipatory Guidance		
Preschool care	Active listening and health teaching	Every visit
Expected growth and developmental milestones before next visit	Active listening and health teaching	Every visit
Unintentional injury prevention	Counseling about street and personal safety	Every visit
Problem Solving		
Any problems expressed by caregiver during course of the visit	Active listening and health teaching regarding preschool illnesses and imaginative play	Every visit

Source: American Academy of Pediatrics, Committee on Practice and Ambulatory Medicine. (2012). *Recommendations for preventive pediatric health care.* Washington, DC: Author; Centers for Disease Control and Prevention. (2013). *Birth–18 years and "catch up" immunization schedules.* Washington, DC: Author.

sometimes reluctant to leave a child's light on at night because they do not want to cater to the fear. Leaving on a dim night-light, however, can solve the problem and costs only pennies. Children who awake terrified and screaming need reassurance that they are safe and that whatever was chasing them was a dream and is not in their room (Fig. 31.4). Most preschoolers do not remember in the morning that they had such a dream; however, they remember for a lifetime that they received comfort when they needed it.

If parents take sensible precautions against fear of the dark or nightmares and a child continues to have this kind of disturbance every night, it may be a reaction to undue stress, which needs to be investigated and eliminated. Giving sleep medication to counteract the sleep disturbance does not solve the basic problem, so this is rarely recommended. Fear of the dark and sleep disturbances both can become intensified in a hospital setting and require careful planning to relieve (Linder & Christian, 2011).

TABLE 31.3 PARENTAL DIFFICULTIES EVALUATING HEALTH PROBLEMS IN THE PRESCHOOL CHILD

Difficulty	Helpful Suggestions for Parents
Evaluating seriousness of illness or condition	Preschoolers are eager to please and tend to answer all questions such as "Does your stomach hurt?" with a yes. Observing the child for signs of illness (e.g., refusing to eat, holding an arm stiffly, having to go to the bathroom frequently) is often more productive as an evaluation technique.
Evaluating bowel and bladder problems	Preschoolers are independent in toilet habits for the first time, so parents do not have diaper contents to evaluate. Frequent trips to the bathroom, rubbing the abdomen, and holding genitals are the usual signs of bowel or bladder dysfunction.
Evaluating nutritional intake	Preschoolers begin to eat away from home at friends' houses or at child care, or stay overnight with grandparents for the first time, so parents have less opportunities to observe daily food intake as accurately as before. Observing whether a child is growing and is active is better than monitoring any one day's intake.
Evaluating bed-wetting	Many preschoolers continue to have occasional enuresis at night until school age. If other signs are present (e.g., pain, low-grade fever, listlessness), a child should have a urine culture because persistent bed-wetting can indicate a low-grade urinary tract infection.
Evaluating activity versus hyperactivity	Many lay magazines have articles on hyperactivity in children. Parents wonder whether their active child could be hyperactive. As a rule of thumb, if a child can sit through a meal (when he is hungry), watch a half-hour television show (that is his favorite), or sit still while his favorite story is read to him, he is not hyperactive.
Age-specific diseases to be aware of	Preschool age is a time for vision and hearing assessment because, for the first time, a child is able to be tested by a standard chart or by audiometry tests. Urinary tract infections tend to occur with a high frequency in preschool-age girls. A language assessment should be done if a child is not able to make wants known by complete, articulated sentences by age 3 years (exceptions are transposing *w* for *r* and broken fluency: "I want-want-want to go").

Fear of Mutilation

Fear of mutilation is also significant during the preschool age, as revealed by the intense reaction of a preschooler to even a simple injury such as falling and scraping a knee or having a needle inserted for an immunization. A child cries afterward not only from the pain but also from the intrusiveness of the injury or procedure. Part of this fear arises because preschoolers do not know which body parts are essential and which ones—like an inch of scraped skin—can be easily replaced. According to Freud, boys develop a fear of castration because, developmentally, they are more in tune with their body parts and are starting to identify with the same-sex parent as they go through the Oedipal phase (Zepf, Ullrich, & Seel, 2016).

Preschoolers can be worried that if some blood is taken out of their bodies, all of their blood will leak out. They often lift a bandage to peek at an incision or cut to see if their body is still intact underneath. They dislike procedures such as needlesticks, rectal temperature assessments, otoscopic examinations, or having a nasogastric tube passed into their stomach. They need good explanations of the limits of healthcare procedures, such as clarifying a tympanic thermometer does not hurt or a finger prick heals quickly as well as distraction techniques in order to feel safe.

QSEN Checkpoint Question 31.3

PATIENT-CENTERED CARE

Cathy keeps her entire family awake at night because she is so afraid of the dark. The nurse teaches Cathy's parent to take which action to help overcome this fear?

a. Assure Cathy the room's window is locked so no one can kidnap her.
b. Suggest Cathy temporarily sleep in the living room in front of the television set for safety.
c. Buy a night-light for Cathy's room and inspect the room to be certain it appears safe.
d. Teach Cathy that her fear is not grounded in reality.

Look in Appendix A for the best answer and rationale.

Fear of Separation or Abandonment

Fear of separation is yet another major concern for preschoolers. Their sense of time is still so distorted that they cannot be comforted by assurances such as "Mommy will pick you up from preschool at noon." Their sense of distance is also limited, so making a statement such as "I work only a block away"

Figure 31.4 Having mom close by after a bad dream is a comfort to a preschooler.

is not reassuring. Relating time and space to something a child knows better, such as meals, television shows, or a friend's house, is more effective. For example, stating, "Mommy will pick you up from preschool after you have had your snack" is apt to be more comforting than "Mommy will pick you up at 3 PM."

Caution parents to be sensitive to such fears when they talk about missing children or if they have their preschooler's photo or fingerprints taken for identification. Children whose chief fear is that they will be abandoned or kidnapped might be alarmed someone will take them away from their parents and not understand their fingerprints are being taken to keep them safe.

A hospital admission or going to a new school often brings a child's fear of separation to the forefront. Help parents thoroughly prepare preschoolers for these experiences so they can survive them in sound mental health (see Chapter 35). Help them give clear instructions on when they will visit the child in the hospital.

Behavior Variations

A combination of a keen imagination and immature reasoning results in a number of other common behavior variations in preschoolers.

Telling Tall Tales

Stretching stories to make them seem more interesting is a phenomenon frequently encountered in preschoolers. For example, after a trip to the zoo, if you ask a preschooler, "What happened today?" a child perceives you want something exciting to have happened, and so might answer, "A bear jumped out of his cage and ate the boy next to me." This is not lying, but merely supplying an expected answer. Parents may be concerned that tall tales of this nature can lead to chronic lying if supported. Caution them not to encourage this kind of storytelling but instead help the child separate fact from fiction by saying, "That's a good story, but now, tell me what really happened." This conveys the idea that the child has not told the truth, yet does not squash imagination or initiative (Talwar & Crossman, 2011). On the other hand, parents must be alert to not dismiss important information inadvertently such as children reporting an adult molesting them.

QSEN Checkpoint Question 31.4

SAFETY

Cathy's father, a police detective, says that he and his wife wish to take measures to prevent Cathy from being kidnapped. What action should the nurse recommend to this family?

a. Limit playdates to Cathy's own home.
b. Withdraw Cathy from daycare to limit her exposure to other adults.
c. Describe common kidnapping culprits the father knows.
d. Be certain Cathy understands not to leave daycare with anyone but her parents.

Look in Appendix A for the best answer and rationale.

Imaginary Friends

Many preschoolers have an imaginary friend who plays with them (Nielsen, 2012). They tell a parent to "wait for Eric" or to "set a place at the table for Lucy." Although imaginary friends are a normal, creative part of the preschool years and can be invented by children who are surrounded by real playmates as well as by those who have few friends, parents may find them disconcerting. If so, let parents know that as long as their child has exposure to real playmates and imaginary playmates do not take center stage in children's lives or prevent them from socializing with other children, they should not pose a problem and often leave as quickly as they come. In the meantime, pretend friends can encourage language development, may provide an outlet for a child to express innermost feelings, or serve as a handy scapegoat for behavior about which a child has some conflict.

Parents can help their preschooler separate fact from fantasy about their imaginary friend by saying, "I know Eric isn't real, but if you want to pretend, I'll set a place for him." This response helps a child understand what is real and what fantasy is without restricting imagination or creativity.

Difficulty Sharing

Sharing is a concept that first comes to be understood around the age of 3 years. Before this, children engage in parallel play (two children need two toys and two spaces to play because they cannot pass one toy back and forth or play together). Around 3 years of age, children begin to understand some things are theirs, some belong to others, and some can belong to both. For the first time, they can stand in line to wait for a drink, take turns using a shovel at a sandbox, and share a box of crayons. Sharing does not come easily, however; children who are ill or under stress have greater difficulty with it than usual.

Assure parents that sharing is a difficult concept to grasp, and, as with most skills, preschoolers need practice to understand and learn it (Sutherland & Friedman, 2012). Parents may need to help a child learn property rights as part of learning to share, such as "This is my private drawer and no one touches what is in it but me." "That is your private box, and no one touches the things in it but you." "A shovel is ours and can be used by everyone playing in the sand pile." Defining limits and exposing children to these three categories (i.e., mine, yours, ours) helps them determine which objects belong to which category.

Regression

Some preschoolers, generally in relation to stress, revert to behavior they previously outgrew, such as thumb-sucking, negativism, loss of bladder control, and inability to separate from their parents. Although the stress that causes this may take many forms, it is usually the result of such things as a new baby in the family, a new school experience, seeing frightening and graphic television news or programming, stress in the home from financial or marital difficulties, or separation caused by hospitalization.

Help parents understand that regression in these circumstances is normal, and a child's thumb-sucking is a little different from the parents' reaction to stress (e.g., smoking many cigarettes, nail biting, overeating), so it's easier for them to accept and understand. Obviously, removing the stress is the best way to help a child discontinue this behavior. The stresses mentioned, however, are not ones that are easily controlled. New babies cannot be returned, irreparable marriages cannot be patched together, frightening news happens every day, and hospitalizations do occur.

Techniques for minimizing the stress of hospitalization for preschoolers are discussed in Chapter 35. Children's reactions to severe and prolonged stress are discussed in Chapter 54. Children undergoing less severe stress can be assured that although situations are changing, the important aspect of their life—that someone still loves them and will continue to take care of them—is not. The manifestations of stress, such as thumb-sucking, are best ignored; calling them to a child's attention merely causes more stress because, in addition to experiencing the primary stress, it makes children aware they are not pleasing their parents.

Sibling Rivalry

Jealousy of a brother or sister may first become evident during the preschool period because this is the first time children have enough vocabulary to express how they feel (i.e., know a name to call) and partly because preschoolers are more aware of family roles and how responsibilities at home are divided (Snowling, 2011). For many children, this is also the time when a new brother or sister is born.

A firstborn child is rarely allowed the privileges of a second child. The parents are untried, unsure of how far they should let a first child venture or what level of responsibility a child could accept, allowing the firstborn to serve as the "trial run" for all children who come after. Children as young as preschool can tell when a younger sibling is allowed behavior that is not tolerated in them. They are little appeased by the explanation, "Your brother is just a baby."

To help preschoolers feel secure and to promote self-esteem during this time, reminding them that there are things they can do that a younger sibling is not allowed to do and supplying them with a private drawer or box for their things that parents or other children do not touch can be helpful. A private box serves as a defense against younger children who do not yet appreciate property rights.

Preparing for a New Sibling

Introduction of a new sibling is such a major happening that parents need to take special steps to be certain their preschooler will be prepared (Volling, 2012). There is no rule as to when this preparation should begin, but it should be before the time the child begins to feel the difference the new baby will make. This is perhaps when the mother first begins to look pregnant. It is certainly before parents begin to make physical preparations for the new child. It is always less frightening to understand why things are happening, no matter how distasteful they may be rather than hear people whispering or having people obviously evading the issue. The unknown is always more fearful than a definite event because those can be faced and conquered.

Help parents not to underestimate the significance of a bed to a preschool child because it is security, consistency, and

"home." If their preschooler is sleeping in the crib that will be used for the new baby, it's usually best if the preschooler can be moved to a bed about 3 months in advance of the birth. Parents might explain, "It's time to sleep in a new bed now because you're a big girl." The fact that the child is growing is a better reason for such a move than because a new brother or sister needs their bed. The latter may be a direct route to sibling rivalry and jealousy.

If children are to start preschool or child care, it's also best if they can do so either before the new baby is born or 2 or 3 months afterward. That way, children can perceive starting school as a result of maturity and not of being pushed out of the house by the new child.

If the mother will be hospitalized for the birth, parents should be certain their child is prepared for this separation. Because the mother is likely to go to the hospital during the night, it is unrealistic to expect a child to be happy to learn in the morning about the arrival of a new sibling when he realizes the new baby has taken away his mother. Some communities offer preparation for birth classes for preschoolers, the same as for parents, or to include children in adult preparation courses to help them master this new experience.

Encourage women to maintain contact with their preschooler during the short time they are hospitalized for the new birth. Some preschoolers may react very coldly to their mothers, turning their head away and refusing to come to them after even a few days of separation when they return home. This is a reaction not to the new baby but to the separation, and the same phenomenon that may occur when a child returns home after being hospitalized (see Chapter 35). Allowing the child to visit in the hospital can help relieve this type of separation anxiety.

Ask pregnant women or couples what kind of preparation they are making for older children and ask the mother of a new baby how everything is working out. Most parents find the problem of jealousy is bigger than they anticipated and welcome a few suggestions about how to provide more time for their preschooler during the day or which activities a preschooler would especially enjoy (Fig. 31.5 and Box 31.7).

Figure 31.5 A preschooler greets a new baby sister. She feels special as dad explains how important it is to be a big sister.

BOX 31.7

Nursing Care Planning Based on Family Teaching

ANTICIPATORY GUIDANCE TO HELP MINIMIZE SIBLING RIVALRY

Q. Cathy's father says to you, "Cathy's acting jealous of her new sister and she's not even born yet. What can we do to reduce sibling jealousy?"

A. This isn't a simple problem, but the following suggestions might be helpful:

- After returning home from the hospital with the baby, devote attention to your preschooler and spend some special time together after the baby has gone to bed.
- When friends and family visit, encourage them to spend time with the preschooler as well as the baby. If they bring gifts for the baby, it is often wise for them to bring a small present for the preschooler as well.
- So your preschooler doesn't come to expect gifts (promoting sibling rivalry), teach her to help open the baby's gifts. Explain it is the baby's birthday and on her birthday she will receive gifts, too.
- Don't ask your preschooler a question such as "Do you like your new sister?" It is better to express feelings of empathy such as "New babies cry a lot. It's hard to get used to that, isn't it?"
- Provide special time for your preschooler during each day, so when you say, "Mommy and Daddy love you just the same," it seems real. This might be a quiet time for talking or reading.
- While feeding the baby, read or tell a story to your preschooler. Some children enjoy feeding a doll while a parent feeds the baby or giving a doll a bath while the baby has one.

Concept Mastery Alert

A new baby makes a significant difference in a child's life. To reduce the child's feeling of being "replaced" by the new baby, significant changes, such as starting preschool, should be done either well before the new baby is born or 3 to 4 months afterward.

QSEN Checkpoint Question 31.5

TEAMWORK & COLLABORATION

Cathy's family is expecting a new baby. When Cathy is visiting the birthing center, the nurse should promote which behavior as a means of fostering family bonding during this time of transition?

a. Take action to help Cathy spend as much time with her mother and the infant as possible.
b. Teach Cathy about the ways that her life might change after the birth of the baby.
c. Remind Cathy that her parents love her very much.
d. Explain to Cathy that she's very lucky because sisters grow up to become best friends.

Look in Appendix A for the best answer and rationale.

Sex Education

During the preschool age, children become acutely aware of the difference between boys and girls. Possibly, this is a normal progression in development, and, possibly, this may be the first time they are exposed to the genitalia of the opposite sex as they watch while a new brother or sister has a diaper changed, they see other children using the bathroom at a preschool, or they see a parent nude.

Preschoolers' questions about genital organs are simple and fact finding; for example, "Why does James look like that?" or "How does Jasmine pee?" Explanations should be just as

simple: "Boys look different from girls. The different part is called a penis." It is important that parents do not convey that these body parts are never to be talked about so they leave an open line of communication for sexual questions. Occasionally, girls attempt to void standing up as they have seen boys doing, and boys may try to void sitting down as they try to use this new body knowledge.

It is common for preschoolers to engage in masturbation while watching TV or before they fall asleep at night. The frequency of this may increase under stress, as does thumbsucking. If observing a child doing this bothers parents, suggest they explain certain things are done in some places but not in others. Children can relate to this kind of direction without feeling inhibited, just as they can accept the fact they use a bathroom in private or eat only at the table. Calling unnecessary attention to the act can increase anxiety and cause increased, not decreased, activity.

Because this may be the time a new brother or sister comes into the family, it is also the most likely time for questions such as "Where do babies come from?" Because a child is asking a simple fact-finding question, parents usually find a simple, factual answer to this type of question is best, such as "Babies grow in a special place in a mother's body called a uterus." Saying "uterus" rather than "tummy" prevents children from envisioning babies and food all mixed together in their mother's stomach (Fig. 31.6).

It is so natural for preschoolers to ask about where babies come from that those who do not ask are exceptions and may not be asking because they sense from a preliminary exploratory question that the subject is closed. A parent could introduce the subject by visiting a new baby in the neighborhood with the child or pointing out a neighbor who is pregnant. Visiting new kittens or puppies can also offer the chance to introduce the subject. If a new brother or sister will be born at a birthing center or at home, many parents may want their preschooler to be present at the birth. Encourage parents to prepare children thoroughly for this experience, or else the sight of their mother in pain and the wonder of birth

Figure 31.6 Preschool children have the beginnings of sexual awareness and are interested in learning where babies grow. (Taeke Henstra/Science Source/Photo Researchers, Inc.)

can become an overwhelming and negative experience rather than a positive one for them (see Chapter 14).

Preschool children generally do not ask how babies get inside mothers to start growing or how babies get out at the end of the process.

Many books for children explain the birth process, same-sex parenting, and adoption. These are helpful for parents to read to a child to increase understanding if they feel the child is ready for longer explanations. Correct terminology should be used when providing an explanation to a child.

QSEN Checkpoint Question 31.6

QUALITY IMPROVEMENT

The nurse is drafting an educational handout for parents of preschoolers that addresses the topic of sex education. What guideline should be included in this educational material?

   a. Tell your child that you will explain these matters when they are old enough to start kindergarten.
   b. Emphasize the fact that sexual intercourse between adults must always be consensual.
   c. Describe some of the differences between boys and girls in clear and accurate terms.
   d. Distract your child from questions about sexuality for as long as possible.

Look in Appendix A for the best answer and rationale.

Another important part of sex education for preschoolers is teaching them to avoid sexual maltreatment, such as not allowing anyone to touch their body unless they and their parents agree that it is all right (Pérez-Fuentes, Olfson, Villegas, et al., 2012). Because children have been taught this, remember to ask permission before giving nursing care

that involves touching, especially before procedures such as catheterization or clean catch urines (see Chapter 32, Box 32.4).

Choosing a Preschool or Child Care Center

A school or child care experience is helpful for preschoolers because peer exposure seems to have a positive effect on social development (Gubbels, Van Kann, & Jansen, 2013). Children who have learned to be comfortable in a preschool group, for example, approach school comfortably and ready to learn; children who have played only infrequently in groups during the preschool age can be so busy adjusting to this new concept that they are left behind in learning new skills in kindergarten or first grade. Most parents enroll their child in a child care program because both parents work outside their home. A parent who is at home full-time has to weigh whether it would be best for a child to have socialization experiences or to not diminish the family time.

The terms "child care center" and "preschool" are often used interchangeably, so parents cannot depend on the name of a school to define its structure. Traditionally, the main purpose of a child care center is to provide child care while parents work or are otherwise occupied. A preschool is dedicated to stimulating children's sense of creativity and initiative and introducing them to new experiences and social contacts that they would not ordinarily receive at home. Head Start programs and many modern child care centers fulfill both functions (Wrobel, 2012).

If there are other 3- or 4-year-old children in a neighborhood with whom a child has almost daily contact and if a parent can supervise organized play dates and projects (providing peer interaction, in which working together is the key), a preschool program may not be necessary. However, if all the neighborhood children are either older or younger or there is only one other child available to play with during the day, a preschool experience will probably be beneficial. Parents with large families point out that their child gets ample exposure to groups because every meal is a "group session." This is not a peer group, however, so this situation does not offer the same experience as does preschool.

Be sure parents investigate preschools or child care centers carefully before they enroll their child to be certain their child will not only be safe there but also that the child will have an enjoyable experience. Guidelines to aid parents in this assessment are shown in Table 31.4.

To continue to evaluate their child's school experience, urge parents to make a habit of asking children what happened at school, what they learned, and the names of any new friends. For the remainder of the growing years, school will have important influences on their child's development. By taking an active role in education, parents influence what and how their child learns.

Child care centers may be responsible for the spread of infectious disease among those age 5 years and under because bringing together children from so many different homes to one setting each day increases the risk of spreading contagious disease. Preschoolers in child care settings may develop frequent upper respiratory infections or gastrointestinal illnesses. Outbreaks of cytomegalovirus and human parvovirus (fifth disease) make working in such centers a particular hazard to pregnant women because such illnesses are potentially teratogenic. To prevent the spread of infection,

TABLE 31.4 QUESTIONS TO USE IN EVALUATING CHILD CARE CENTERS

Question	Finding
Management	
How long has the center been in operation?	Length of operation does not necessarily indicate quality, but it allows you to locate other parents who have used the center to ask about their experience there.
Is the center licensed, registered, approved, or inspected by the appropriate agency?	Ask in your local community what agency has the responsibility for licensing child care centers. If not licensed, its quality is suspect.
What are the qualifications of staff members?	If staff members are teachers, more learning activities will be provided; staff should be qualified to perform cardiopulmonary resuscitation.
Is there a fast turnover rate of staff?	A fast turnover rate means little continuity of care will be provided (and probably suggests dissatisfaction with center administration).
What is the child–staff ratio?	A ratio of three or four children to one staff member provides time for quality interaction.
What is the center's policy on parental visits?	Parents should be able to drop in at any time. Be wary of facilities that restrict parental visiting in any way.
Physical Environment	
Is there adequate space in the center?	There should be opportunities for rough-and-tumble and imaginative play in addition to naptime areas and table activities.
Does the space appear safe?	Stairways should be fenced. No paint should be peeling.
Can children get in and out of the building easily?	A first-floor plan is safest. Fire exits should be well marked. An evacuation plan should be practiced.
Is there a safe play area for children outside?	Find out how often children are taken outside: once or twice a day, or only occasionally for "outings"?
Is there a quiet place for naps?	Ask if a child can nap if tired or has to wait until a set naptime.
Can the bathroom be reached easily?	Both potty chairs and small toilet seats should be available.
If food is provided, does it meet preschool recommendations?	Food should be preschool friendly and healthy, not just high-fat snacks.
Is there adequate refrigeration?	Food poisoning is a concern without refrigeration.
Staff Philosophy	
Are the caregivers warm and affectionate toward children?	Watch how they greet children. They should ask questions and listen to answers.
Do caregivers spend most of their time performing janitorial tasks (cleaning) or devoting their time to children?	It is best if the cleaning staff are separate from the care staff.
Is each child assigned to a particular caregiver on a continuing basis?	Ask caregivers to describe their care pattern; if this is not planned, little continuity of care results.
Are the children provided stimulating toys and equipment?	Imaginative items, such as a puppet theater, finger paint, and water play, should be included.
How do caregivers discipline children? Do they yell or treat the children roughly?	The method should reflect the parents' philosophy. Staff should be able to talk to children calmly without raising their voices in anger.
Is there a planned curriculum?	There should be specific goals the caregivers hope to accomplish.
Can the child pursue an individual interest?	Play or learning activities should be individualized.
Healthcare Protocols	
How does the center care for an ill child?	There should be access to a nurse. Staff should be able to evaluate for illness. They should know actions to take in an emergency.
What precautions do caregivers take to prevent the spread of infection?	The counter where diapers are changed should be wiped with a disinfectant; tissues and hand-washing facilities should be present.
Does the center follow good sanitary practices?	Be sure the center requires waterproof disposable diapers to minimize contamination of the environment and other children and separates diaper-changing areas from other activities, especially anything related to food handling. Observe caregivers changing diapers. Do they wash hands after each change? Are children encouraged to wash their hands before eating?
Under what conditions are children not allowed to attend the center?	A center should have a very specific policy on what illness symptoms require a child to be kept home, and they should enforce this policy strictly. For instance, a runny nose may be acceptable, but a fever is not, and children with chickenpox should be kept at home until the lesions are covered with scabs. Children with special needs should be integrated into usual activities.
Children's Behavior	
Do the children appear happy and relaxed?	Observe for at least one morning.
Do children rush to greet any new visitors?	This could be a sign of boredom with their center's activities and a strong need for adult attention.

children need to wash their hands frequently and cover their mouths with their sleeve when coughing. Child care centers where infants are enrolled need to take special precautions against hepatitis A or parasitic infections because these can be spread by caregivers not washing their hands or not washing tables after changing diapers. Hepatitis may be subclinical in the preschooler, but other members of the preschooler's family can develop overt symptoms as the illness spreads through the family, making vaccinations important (CDC, 2011).

Preparing a Child for School

At the end of the preschool period, children begin a formal school experience as they enter kindergarten. Parents may wonder whether their child is old enough for this, especially if a child's birthday is in the late summer or early fall. If this is a concern, urge parents to discuss their concern with school officials to determine whether their child should be registered for kindergarten or delayed for a year. Because school involves a great deal of children's time and influences their future greatly, it's important for parents to take time to prepare preschoolers not only physically, by being certain their immunizations are up-to-date (see Table 31.2), but also emotionally.

Essential to this preparation is the parents' attitude. If school is discussed as something to look forward to, as an adventure that will be satisfying and rewarding, a child comes to look forward to it as a positive experience. If school is presented as a punishment ("Wait until you get into first grade—your teacher will make you behave"), there can be little delight in anticipating it.

If a child was not attending preschool, some parents may have to change their child's daily routine a few months in advance of beginning school to accustom the child to waking earlier or going to bed earlier. School has so many new components that it's wise for parents to try to eliminate as many distractions as possible.

If a child is to ride a bus to school, a parent might take a child on a municipal bus as an introduction to this form of transportation. If a child is to walk to school, a trial walk is in order. In either instance, safety should be stressed such as "Don't walk behind the bus because the driver can't see you" and "Wait for the crossing guard to help you cross the street."

If a child will be required to take a lunch to school, a parent can introduce this new experience by preparing a bagged lunch at home. If a child is to purchase lunch at school, the parent can play "cafeteria" at home by serving a buffet-style meal and letting the child practice walking from one dish to another to select food.

Some kindergartens suggest that children should know how to tie their shoes, name basic colors, and print their name before they begin. Parents should familiarize themselves with any such suggestions from the school, but the wisdom of requiring these skills can be questioned. Identifying colors should be established by this age, but some children are not coordinated enough at 4 to 5 years of age to tie their shoes or to print. A better contribution for parents to make toward their children's achievement in school is to instill in their children the concept that learning is fun, and that their child may not always be able to do all the things other children can do, but trying to do one's best is what is important. Trying to make children complete fine motor tasks for which they are not developmentally prepared does not instill that concept.

For children to do well in a formal school setting, they must be able to follow instructions and sit at a table and chair for a short work period. When some parents examine their child's day, they are surprised to realize how few instructions they give the child in a day. They put on the child's coat, pick up the child's toys, and lead the child to the table for dinner. Similarly, they never encourage their child to spend any time in a chair, which is something the child will have to do for at least short periods in school. Coloring at a table rather than on the floor will introduce this situation without any problem.

Finally, going to school is a form of separation and a new experience if a child has not attended child care or preschool, so parents must make preparations for this. It might be good to arrange to have a child stay with another caregiver such as a grandparent for part of a day. Staying at school can then be compared with that successful event.

These are minimum preparations parents can complete to ready their child for school. Caution both parents and children that no matter how hard they try, not everything can be anticipated; school will bring some new happenings that are not expected. If a child has been led to believe learning is fun and new experiences are enjoyable (creating a strong sense of initiative), solving these unpredictable problems is good preparation for the thousands of surprise experiences ahead.

Broken Fluency

Developing language is such a complicated process that children from 2 to 6 years of age typically have some speech difficulty. A child may begin to repeat words or syllables, saying, "I-I-I want a n-n-new spoon-spoon-spoon." This is called **broken fluency** (repetition and prolongation of sounds, syllables, and words). It is often referred to as **secondary stuttering** because the child began to speak without this problem and then, during the preschool years, develops it. Unlike the adult who stutters, children are unaware that they are not being fluent unless it is called to their attention. You may need to remind parents that this is a part of normal development and, if accepted as such, will pass (Nippold & Packman, 2012). It is resolved most quickly if parents follow a few simple rules, including:

- Do not discuss in the child's presence that he or she is having difficulty with speech because this can make the child conscious of speech patterns and compound the problem.
- Listen with patience rather than interrupt or ask the child to speak more slowly or to start over. These actions make the child aware speech is repetitious, and broken fluency increases.
- Always talk to the child in a calm, simple way to role model slow speech. If adults talk quickly, the child imitates this pattern and has difficulty speaking clearly.
- Protect space for the child to talk if there are other children in the family. Rushing to say something before a second child interrupts is the same as rushing to conform to adult speech.
- Do not force a child to speak if he or she does not want to. Do not ask preschoolers to recite or sing for strangers.
- Do not reward a child for fluent speech or punish for nonfluent speech. Broken fluency is a developmental stage in language formation, not an indication of regression or a chronic speech pattern.

"Bathroom Language"

Many preschoolers imitate the vocabularies of their parents or older children in the family so well during this time that they incorporate swear words into their vocabularies if they hear these used. Parents may have to be reminded that children do not necessarily understand what the word they are using means; they have simply heard it, just as they have heard hundreds of other words and have decided to use it. Correction should be unemotional such as, "That's not a word I like to hear you say. When you're angry, why don't you say 'fudge' [or whatever]?" The correcting is no different from that involved when a child uses poor grammar. If parents become emotional, a child realizes the value of such a word and may continue using it for the attention it creates.

CONCERNS OF THE FAMILY WITH A PRESCHOOLER WITH UNIQUE NEEDS

Learning how to do things when you have physical or cognitive limitations can be very frustrating. A preschooler with a disability has a greater need for problem-solving skills than the average child because even simple procedures such as eating or getting dressed can be difficult if their physical challenge limits the options (see Chapter 54).

Physically challenged or chronically ill preschoolers should attend a preschool program if at all possible because of the socialization benefits. If a child must remain in bed, parents may be reluctant to offer potentially messy experiences like finger paint. A large tray of dry oatmeal or other breakfast cereal with sand shovels or cars and trucks is a neater substitute activity for such a child. Although not necessarily tidy, these substances (which are available even in a hospital setting) can be vacuumed away easily at the finish of play. Table 31.5 lists nursing actions that can aid a chronically challenged child to solve problems and develop a sense of initiative.

Nutrition and the Preschooler With Special Needs

Experiences with eating help to reinforce a sense of initiative in preschoolers. Chronically ill preschoolers who are limited in the foods they can eat (e.g., perhaps they can eat only soft foods) or in their ability to help with food preparation may miss this reinforcement. If their appetite is diminished because of illness to the point where they take little or nothing orally, it is still important that they continue to join the family at meals if at all possible. In most households, this is a time for socialization, and preschoolers are ripe for the learning that goes with this type of daily interaction.

TABLE 31.5 NURSING INTERVENTIONS TO ENCOURAGE A SENSE OF INITIATIVE IN THE PRESCHOOLER WITH SPECIAL NEEDS

Consideration	Nursing Actions
Nutrition	Serving toast or sandwiches cut into animal shapes with cookie cutters, cereal in the form of alphabet characters, or food arranged on a plate to make a face appeals to the imagination and may make a preschooler with a limited appetite more interested in eating.
	Respect the child's food preferences because trying to eat a nonfavorite food is difficult for everyone.
Dressing changes	Allow preschoolers to measure and cut tape or draw a face on it.
	Allow child to see the incision site. Explain the steps of dressing change as you work to reduce unknowns and areas of fear.
	Provide extra bandages to put on a doll so the child can see that bandages are not to be feared.
Medicine	Allow the child to choose a "chaser" such as juice or milk after oral medicine.
	Choosing a site for injection or intravenous line is too advanced for the preschooler; do not suggest such choices.
Rest	Provide a light in the room or bring the child's bed into the hallway so fear of the dark is reduced and the child can deal solely with problems based in the real world.
	Identify sounds the preschooler might hear in the hospital, such as an air conditioner turning on, and explain what these are.
Hygiene	Allow the child to choose bathtub toys and clothing to wear after a bath.
	Allow the child to wash his or her own hands and face.
	Allow the child to splash in water as a play activity as well as for cleanliness.
Pain	Encourage the preschooler to express pain.
	Allow the child to handle a syringe or suction catheter, and give "shots" or suction to a doll to alleviate anger or fear.
	Encourage the child to ask for analgesic if necessary.
Stimulation	Guessing games encourage a sense of initiative. Draw a dog or a house and ask the child to close his or her eyes while you add one more detail to the drawing, such as an ear or a chimney, then ask the child to identify the new item. Reverse the game and ask the child what you erased from the drawing, or allow the child to do his or her own drawing.
	Provide manipulative toys, such as finger paint, soapy water, clay, or dry cereal to use as sand.
	Allow the preschooler to accompany you to other departments is a way of teaching more about the hospital.
	Use "Simon Says" games not only for socialization but also to urge treatments, such as deep-breathing exercises.
	Encourage use of the playroom for socialization.
	Encourage the child to interact with his or her family by drawing pictures for siblings or telephoning home.

What If . . . 31.4

The nurse is particularly interested in exploring one of the 2020 National Health Goals with respect to preschool growth and development (see Box 31.1). What would be a possible research topic to explore pertinent to this goal that would be applicable to Cathy's family and that would also advance evidence-based practice?

Unfolding Patient Stories: Jackson Webber • Part 1

Jackson Webber, age 3, is diagnosed with generalized seizures and started on phenobarbital. His mother is single and employed full time. The mother is concerned about his recent developmental regression and how that will affect his return to child care. What education can the nurse provide on normal growth and development for a 3 year old and the relationship between developmental milestones and the new onset of an illness? What questions can the nurse ask to evaluate the adequacy and safety of the child care center that Jackson attends when considering his new diagnosis of seizures? (Jackson Webber's story continues in Chapter 49.)

Care for Jackson and other patients in a realistic virtual environment: **vSim** *for Nursing* (thepoint.lww.com/vSimMaternityPed). Practice documenting these patients' care in DocuCare (thepoint.lww.com/DocuCareEHR).

KEY POINTS FOR REVIEW

- Although preschoolers grow only slightly and gain just a little weight, they seem much taller than when they were toddlers because their contour changes to more childlike proportions.
- Erikson's developmental task for the preschool period is to gain a sense of initiative versus guilt, or to learn how to do things. Play materials ideal for this age group are those that stimulate creativity, such as modeling clay or colored markers.
- Promoting childhood safety is a major role because preschoolers' active imaginations can lead them into dangerous situations; stressing this helps in planning nursing care that not only meets QSEN competencies but that also best meets a family's total needs.
- Common parental concerns during the preschool period are broken fluency, imaginary friends, difficulty sharing, and sibling rivalry. Preschoolers may develop a number of universal fears, such as fear of the dark, mutilation, and abandonment.
- The preschool age is often the time when a new sibling is born. Helping parents offer good preparation for this is necessary to prevent intense sibling rivalry.
- Preschoolers are still operating at a cognitive level that prevents them from understanding conservation (objects have not changed substance even if they have changed appearance).
- Preschoolers are self-centered (egocentric) so it is difficult for them to share and view someone else's side of a problem. They need good explanations of how a procedure will benefit them before they can agree to it.

- Many preschoolers begin preschool programs or child care. Late in the preschool period, they may be enrolled in kindergarten. Parents often appreciate guidance on how to prepare their children for these new experiences.
- Preschoolers who have special needs may have difficulty achieving a sense of initiative because they may be limited in their ability to participate in activities that stimulate initiative. They may need special playtimes set aside for stimulation and learning.

CRITICAL THINKING CARE STUDY

Calvin Saunders is a 4-year-old who lives with his single mom and 6-year-old brother, David. Calvin stays with his grandmother 2 days a week and with his father 3 days a week because his mother works full-time in a local grocery store. His BMI is 27 (overweight).

1. At preschool, Calvin pushes and shoves other children rather than plays well with them. What suggestions could you make to his mother to improve his social relationships?
2. Calvin speaks with broken fluency. His mother jokes, "If he yelled 'fire,' we'd all burn to death before we understood him." She saw a movie where a king learned not to stutter by singing so, although it's expensive, she has enrolled Calvin in a boy's chorus. Is this her best approach to helping Calvin speak clearly?
3. Calvin's mother doesn't supervise Calvin or his older brother while they warm up snacks in the microwave. Is Calvin mature enough to do this independently?

RELATED RESOURCES

Explore these additional resources to enhance learning for this chapter:
- Student resources on thePoint, including answers to the What If . . . and Critical Thinking Care Study questions, http://thepoint.lww.com/Flagg8e
- Adaptive learning powered by PrepU, http://thepoint.lww.com/prepu

REFERENCES

Agarwal, A., & Pruthi, M. (2010). Bicycle-spoke injuries of the foot in children. *Journal of Orthopedic Surgery, 18*(3), 338–341.
American Academy of Pediatrics. (2012). *Where we stand: Car seats for children.* Washington, DC: Author.
Bevan, A. L., & Reilly, S. M. (2011). Mothers' efforts to promote healthy nutrition and physical activity for their preschool children. *Nursing, 26*(5), 395–403.
Bowman, S. M., Aitken, M. E., Robbins, J. M., et al. (2012). Trends in US pediatric drowning hospitalizations, 1993–2008. *Pediatrics, 129*(2), 275–281.
Byars, K. C., Yolton, K., Rausch, J., et al. (2012). Prevalence, patterns, and persistence of sleep problems in the first 3 years of life. *Pediatrics, 129*(2), 276–284.
Centers for Disease Control and Prevention. (2011). National and state vaccination coverage among children aged 19–35 months—United States, 2010. *MMWR: Morbidity & Mortality Weekly Report, 60*(34), 1157–1163.
Centers for Disease Control and Prevention. (2012). *Injuries among children and adolescents.* Atlanta, GA: Author.
de Amorim Lde, F., Estrela, C., & da Costa, L. R. (2011). Effects of traumatic dental injuries to primary teeth on permanent teeth. *Dental Traumatology, 27*(2), 117–121.
Erikson, E. H. (1993). *Childhood & society.* New York, NY: W. W. Norton.
Erreich, A. (2011). More than enough guilt to go around: Oedipal guilt, survival guilt, separation guilt. *Journal of the American Psychoanalytical Association, 59*(1), 131–151.

Fergusson, D. M., Boden, J. M., & Horwood, L. J. (2013). Nine-year follow-up of a home-visitation program: A randomized trial. *Pediatrics, 131*(2), 297–303.

Garrison, M. M., & Christakis, D. A. (2012). The impact of a healthy media use intervention on sleep in preschool children. *Pediatrics, 130*(3), 492–499.

Goldman, R. D. (2012). Cranberry juice for urinary tract infection in children. *Canadian Family Physician, 58*(4), 398–401.

Gubbels, J. S., Van Kann, D. H., & Jansen, M. W. (2013). Play equipment, physical activity opportunities, and children's activity levels at childcare. *Journal of Environmental & Public Health, 2012*(2012), 326520.

Hodges, E. A., Smith, C., Tidwell, S., et al. (2012). Promoting physical activity in preschoolers to prevent obesity. *Journal of Pediatric Nursing, 28*(1), 3–19.

Jonson-Reid, M., Kohl, P. L., & Drake, B. (2012). Child and adult outcomes of chronic child maltreatment. *Pediatrics, 129*(5), 839–845.

Kohlberg, L. (1984). *The psychology of moral development.* New York, NY: Harper & Row.

Kushnir, J., & Sadeh, A. (2011). Sleep of preschool children with night-time fears. *Sleep Medicine, 12*(9), 870–874.

Linder, L. A., & Christian, B. J. (2011). Characteristics of the nighttime hospital bedside care environment (sound, light, and temperature) for children with cancer. *Cancer Nursing, 34*(3), 176–184.

Merlino, G., & Gigli, G. I. (2012). Sleep related movement disorders. *Neurological Sciences, 33*(3), 491–513.

Mitka, M. (2012). Programs to reduce childhood obesity seem to work, say Cochrane reviewers. *JAMA, 307*(5), 444–445.

Nielsen, M. (2012). Imitation, pretend play, and childhood: Essential elements in the evolution of human culture? *Journal of Comparative Psychology, 126*(2), 170–181.

Nippold, M. A., & Packman, A. (2012). Managing stuttering beyond the preschool years. *Language, Speech & Hearing Services in Schools, 43*(3), 338–343.

Paulus, M., & Moore, C. (2012). Producing and understanding prosocial actions in early childhood. *Advances in Child Development & Behavior, 42*(8), 271–305.

Pérez-Fuentes, G., Olfson, M., Villegas, L., et al. (2012). Prevalence and correlates of child sexual abuse: A national study. *Comprehensive Psychiatry, 54*(1), 16–27.

Piaget, J. (1969). *The theory of stages in cognitive development.* New York, NY: McGraw-Hill.

Raman, L. (2011). Why do we eat? Children's and adults' understanding of why we eat different meals. *Journal of Genetic Psychology, 172*(4), 401–413.

Senger, C., Keijzer, R., Smith, G., et al. (2011). Pediatric firearm injuries: A 10-year single-center experience of 194 patients. *Journal of Pediatric Surgery, 46*(5), 927–932.

Smith, G. A., & Riedford, K. (2013). Epidemiology of early childhood caries: Clinical application. *Journal of Pediatric Nursing, 28*(4), 369–373.

Smith, S. (2011). Vulvovaginitis. In K. J. Marcdante, R. M. Kliegman, H. B. Jenson, et al. (Eds.), *Nelson essentials of pediatrics* (6th ed., pp. 415–416). Philadelphia, PA: Saunders/Elsevier.

Snowling, M. J. (2011). Editorial: What's behind sibling rivalry: Checks and balances in the sibling relationship. *Journal of Child Psychology & Psychiatry & Allied Disciplines, 52*(6), 629–630.

Sun, Y., & Sundell, J. (2011). Early daycare attendance increases the risk for respiratory infections and asthma of children. *Journal of Asthma, 48*(8), 790–796.

Sutherland, S. L., & Friedman, O. (2012). Preschoolers acquire general knowledge by sharing in pretense. *Child Development, 83*(3), 1064–1071.

Talwar, V., & Crossman, A. (2011). From little white lies to filthy liars: The evolution of honesty and deception in young children. *Advances in Child Development & Behavior, 40*(4), 139–179.

Tubert-Jeannin, S., Auclair, C., Amsallem, E., et al. (2011). Fluoride supplements (tablets, drops, lozenges or chewing gums) for preventing dental caries in children. *Cochrane Database of Systematic Reviews,* (12), CD007592.

U.S. Department of Agriculture. (2012). *Choose my plate: A guide to daily food choices.* Washington, DC: Author.

U.S. Department of Health and Human Services. (2010). *Healthy people 2020.* Washington, DC: Author.

Volling, B. L. (2012). Family transitions following the birth of a sibling: An empirical review of changes in the firstborn's adjustment. *Psychology Bulletin, 138*(3), 497–528.

Whitney, E. N., & Rolfes, S. R. (2013). Life cycle nutrition: Infancy, childhood and adolescence. In E. N. Whitney & S. R. Rolfes (Eds.), *Understanding nutrition* (13th ed., pp. 504–550). New York, NY: Wadsworth/Cengage Learning.

Wrobel, S. (2012). From threat to opportunity: A Head Start program's response to state-funded pre-K. *Journal of Health & Human Services Administration, 35*(1), 74–105.

Yilmaz, G., Caylan, N. D., & Karacan, C. D. (2012). Effects of active and passive smoking on ear infections. *Current Infectious Disease Reports, 14*(2), 166–174

Zepf, S., Ullrich, B., & Seel, D. (2016). Oedipus and the Oedipus complex: A revision. *International Journal of Psycho-Analysis, 97*(3), 685–707.

Nursing Care of a Family With a School-Age Child

KEY TERMS

accommodation	conservation
caries	malocclusion
class inclusion	nocturnal emissions

OBJECTIVES

After mastering the contents of this chapter, you should be able to:

1. Describe the normal growth and development pattern and common parental concerns of the school-age period.
2. Identify 2020 National Health Goals related to school-age children that nurses can help the nation achieve.
3. Assess a school-age child for normal growth and developmental milestones.
4. Formulate nursing diagnoses related to both school-age children and their families.
5. Establish expected outcomes for nursing care of school-age children to help children and parents manage seamless transitions across differing healthcare settings.
6. Using the nursing process, plan nursing care that includes the six competencies of Quality & Safety Education for Nurses (QSEN): Patient-Centered Care, Teamwork & Collaboration, Evidence-Based Practice (EBP), Quality Improvement (QI), Safety, and Informatics.
7. Implement nursing care to promote normal growth and development of a school-age child, such as counseling parents about helping their child adjust to a new school.
8. Evaluate expected outcomes for achievement and effectiveness of care.
9. Integrate knowledge of growth and development in school-age children with the interplay of nursing process, the six competencies of QSEN, and Family Nursing to promote quality maternal and child health nursing care.

The term "school age" refers to children between the ages of 6 and 12 years. Although these years represent a time of slow physical growth, the school-age child's cognitive growth and development continue to proceed at rapid rates. There are many differences among children at each year of this age group. For example, 7- and 10-year-old children have very different needs and outlooks than do 11- and 12-year-old children. Because of these big differences, always assess children as individuals to understand the particular developmental needs of each child based on what developmental status has been achieved, not on what stage you think the child should have reached (Lowe, Godoy, Rhodes, et al., 2013).

Unlike the infant or toddler periods, when progress is marked by obvious new abilities and skills such as the ability to sit up or roll over or the ability to speak a full sentence, the development of a school-age child is much more subtle. In addition, the child may demonstrate contradictory responses. For example, what the child enjoys on one occasion may change over time. It is not uncommon for a child to ask his or her parents for a guitar and lessons and subsequently lose interest in music and prefer another activity. School-age children become increasingly more influenced by the attitudes of their friends. They may select activities based on the interests of their peers. Parents who don't understand this normal aspect of development may engage in excessive conflicts with their child. The school-age period is the initiation of independent decision making. Parents unprepared for this may experience conflicts with their child. Box 32.1 lists 2020 National Health Goals related to the school-age period.

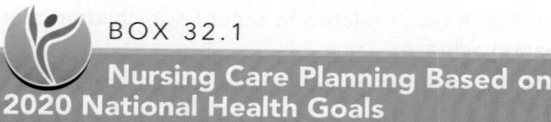

BOX 32.1

Nursing Care Planning Based on 2020 National Health Goals

A number of 2020 National Health Goals address the health of the school-age population:

- Increase the proportion of public and private schools that require daily physical education for elementary school students from a baseline of 3.8% to a target of 4.2%; for middle school students, from 7.9% to 8.6%.
- Increase the proportion of public and private schools that require students to wear appropriate protective gear when engaged in school-sponsored physical activities from 76.8% to 84.5%.
- Reduce the proportion of children who have dental caries (in permanent or primary teeth) to no more than 49% from a baseline of 54.4%.
- Increase age-appropriate vehicle restraint system use in children from 78% to 86%.
- Increase the number of states that require helmet use by bicyclists from 19 to 27 states (U.S. Department of Health and Human Services, 2010; see www.healthypeople.gov).

Nurses can help the nation achieve these goals by urging children to begin and maintain a consistent exercise program, to brush teeth and go for dental checkups regularly, and to follow safety rules for bicycles and automobiles.

Nursing Process Overview

FOR HEALTHY DEVELOPMENT OF A SCHOOL-AGE CHILD

ASSESSMENT

History and physical examination are used to assess growth and development of school-age children. History questions include school progress and extracurricular activities. School-age children are interested and able to contribute to their own health history. The school-age child may be interviewed with his or her parent and separately depending on the circumstances. During a physical examination, be attentive to the school age child's need for privacy when undressed. Parents of school-age children often mention behavioral issues or conflicts during yearly health visits. This is a time period where children begin to express their own opinions and beliefs.

School personnel may be involved in a child's health care as optimal school functioning has the greatest potential when a child is healthy physically, emotionally, and socially.

NURSING DIAGNOSIS

Common nursing diagnoses pertinent to growth and development during the school-age period include:

- Health-seeking behaviors related to normal school-age growth and development
- Readiness for enhanced parenting related to improved family living conditions
- Anxiety related to slow growth pattern of child
- Risk for injury related to deficient parental knowledge about safety precautions for a school-age child

OUTCOME IDENTIFICATION AND PLANNING

When identifying expected outcomes and planning care, keep in mind that school-age children tend to enjoy small or short-term projects rather than long, involved ones. In her early school years, a child with diabetes, for example, may gain a feeling of achievement by learning to assess her own serum glucose level, but she may have difficulty continuing glucose assessments on a regular basis.

Behavior problems need to be well defined before outcomes are identified and interventions planned. Often, it is enough for parents to accept the problem as one consistent with normal growth and development. Refer parents to helpful websites and other resources when appropriate (see Chapter 28).

IMPLEMENTATION

School-age children are interested in learning about adult roles, so this means they will watch you to note your attitude as well as your actions in a given situation. When giving care, keep in mind that children this age feel more comfortable if they know the "hows" and "whys" of actions. This means that they may not cooperate with a procedure until they are given a satisfactory explanation of why it must be done.

OUTCOME EVALUATION

Yearly health visits covering both physical and psychosocial development are important at this age (American Academy of Pediatrics [AAP], 2016). Examples of expected outcomes include:

- Parent states that he permits the child to make his own age-related decisions.
- Child identifies books he has read together with parents in the past 2 weeks.
- Child states he understands the variations of growth as related to the growth chart.
- Child does not sustain injuries from sports activities.

Growth and Development of a School-Age Child

The school-age period is a relatively long time span, and even though growth is slow, children grow and develop extensively during this time period.

PHYSICAL GROWTH

The average annual weight gain for a school-age child is approximately 3 to 5 lb (1.3 to 2.2 kg); the increase in height is 1 to 2 in. (2.5 to 5 cm). Children who did not lose a lordosis and knock-kneed appearance during the preschool period lose this now.

By 10 years of age, brain growth is complete, so fine motor coordination becomes refined. As the eye globe reaches its final shape at about this same time, an adult vision level is achieved. If the eruption of permanent teeth and growth of the jaw do not correlate with final head growth, malocclusion with teeth malalignment may be present (Massignan, Cardoso, Porporatti, et al., 2016).

The immune globulins IgG and IgA each reach adult levels, and lymphatic tissue continues to grow in size until about age 9 years. The resulting abundance of tonsillar and adenoid tissue in early school children is often mistaken for disease because the tonsils seem to fill the entire back of the throat. This may also result in temporary conduction deafness from eustachian tube obstruction until the tissue recedes normally. The appendix is also lined with lymphatic tissue, so swelling of this tissue in the narrow tube can lead to trapped fecal material and inflammation (appendicitis) in the early school-age child (Bishop, 2011). Frontal sinuses develop at about 6 years, so

sinus headaches become a possibility (before then, a headache in children is rarely caused by a sinus infection) (Smith, 2011).

The left ventricle of the heart enlarges to be strong enough to pump blood to the growing body. Innocent heart murmurs may become apparent due to this extra blood crossing heart valves. The pulse rate decreases to 70 to 80 beats/min; blood pressure rises to about 112/60 mmHg. Maturation of the respiratory system leads to increased oxygen–carbon dioxide exchange, which increases exertion ability and stamina. Scoliosis may become apparent for the first time in late childhood (Fletcher & Bruce, 2012). All school-age children older than 8 years should be screened for this at all health appraisals (see Chapter 51).

Sexual Maturation

At a set point in brain maturity, the hypothalamus transmits an enzyme to the anterior pituitary gland to begin production of gonadotropic hormones, which then activate changes in the testes and ovaries to cause puberty. Hormone changes that occur with puberty are discussed in detail in Chapter 5. Table 32.1 describes the usual order in which secondary sex characteristics develop.

Timing of the onset of puberty varies widely, between 8 and 14 years of age (Edmonds, 2012), partly due to genetic and cultural differences, and is rated according to Tanner stages (shown in Chapter 33). The length of time it takes to pass through puberty until sexual maturity is complete also varies. Sexual maturation in girls usually occurs between the years of 12 and 18; in boys, between 14 and 20 years. Puberty is occurring increasingly earlier, however, and in a class of 11-year-old sixth graders, it is not unusual to discover more than half of the girls are already menstruating. This change in the onset of puberty is important because it means, for sex education to be effective, parents or schools must introduce this material as early as when their children are in grade school. Precocious puberty is an abnormal onset of puberty and is discussed in Chapter 47.

Sexual and Physical Concerns

The changes in physical appearance that come with puberty can lead to concerns for both children and their parents. The school-age period is a time for parents to discuss with children the physical changes that will occur and the sexual responsibility these changes dictate. This is also a time to reinforce

TABLE 32.1 CHRONOLOGIC DEVELOPMENT OF SECONDARY SEX CHARACTERISTICS

Age (in Years)	Boys	Girls
9–11	Prepubertal weight gain occurs.	Breasts: elevation of papilla with breast bud formation; areolar diameter enlarges.
11–12	Sparse growth of straight, downy, slightly pigmented hair at base of penis.	Straight hair along the labia; vaginal epithelium becomes cornified.
	Scrotum becomes textured; growth of penis and testes begins.	pH of vaginal secretions becomes acidic; slight mucous vaginal discharge is present.
	Sebaceous gland secretion increases.	Sebaceous gland secretion increases.
	Perspiration increases.	Perspiration increases.
		Dramatic growth spurt.
12–13	Pubic hair present across pubis.	Pubic hair grows darker; spreads over entire pubis.
	Penis lengthens.	Breasts enlarge, still no protrusion of nipples.
	Dramatic linear growth spurt.	Axillary hair present.
	Breast enlargement may occur.	Menarche occurs.

previous teaching with children that their body is their own, to be used only in the way they choose. Specific measures for children to help prevent sexual maltreatment are discussed later in this chapter. Nurses can play a major role in this type of education (Breuner & Mattson, 2016).

In both sexes, puberty brings changes in the sebaceous glands. Under the influence of androgen, glands become more active, setting the stage for acne (see Chapter 33). Vasomotor instability commonly leads to blushing; perspiration also increases.

Concerns of Girls

Prepubertal girls are usually taller by about 2 in. (5 cm) or more than preadolescent boys because their typical growth spurt begins earlier. In a culture in which boys are expected to be taller than girls, this can cause concern. Sometimes, a girl notices the change in her pelvic contour when she tries on a skirt or dress from the year before and realizes her hips are becoming broader. She may misinterpret this finding as a gain in weight and attempt a crash diet. You can assure her that broad bone structure of the hips is part of an adult female profile.

Girls are usually conscious of breast development. A girl who develops ahead of her peers may tend to slouch or wear loose clothing to hide the size of her breasts. Another girl studies herself in a mirror and wonders whether her breasts are going to develop enough. Breast development is not always symmetrical, so it is not unusual for a girl to have breasts of slightly different sizes. After the condition has been checked during a physical examination to assure her that no tumors are present to make one breast larger or that the other is diseased in some way to make it smaller, she can be reassured this development is normal. Supernumerary (additional) nipples may darken or increase in size at puberty. Be sure girls understand that a supernumerary nipple is affected by the hormones in her body in the same way as other breast tissue, so she isn't concerned by the accessory nipple enlarging with puberty or in a future pregnancy.

Early preparation for menstruation is an important preparation for future childbearing and for a girl's concept of herself as a woman (AAP, 2016) (Box 32.2). A girl who is told menstruation is a normal function that occurs every month in all healthy women has a different attitude toward her body than a girl who wakes up one morning to find blood on her pajamas and is told bluntly, "You'd better get used to that. You'll have to put up with it for the rest of your life." In the first instance, the girl can trust her body: It is doing what every woman's body does. In the second instance, the girl may feel her body is out of control. How can she accept and enjoy growing up if it involves something so unpredictable?

In addition to an explanation of the reason for menstrual flow, girls need an explanation of proper hygiene and reassurance they can bathe, shower, and swim during their periods. They can use either sanitary napkins or tampons; if they choose tampons, they must take precautions to avoid toxic shock syndrome (see Chapter 47).

Girls also need to know that vaginal secretions will begin to be present. If this is not explained, a girl may fear needlessly she has contracted an infection. Explain that any secretions that cause vulvar irritation should be evaluated by a healthcare provider because this does suggest infection.

Most girls have some menstrual irregularity during the first year or two after menarche (the start of menstruation). This occurs primarily because a girl's cycles are at first anovulatory. With added maturity and the onset of ovulation, cycles become more regular.

BOX 32.2

Nursing Care Planning Tips for Effective Communication

Shelly, 11 years old, comes into the nurse's office at her school in her gym clothes. She was sent to the office because she refused to change into her school clothes. She asks to go home because she needs to change her clothes. She is crying and asking the nurse to call her mother.

Tip: Through effective communication and listening, you can help them talk about their problems and concerns. In the past, when topics such as menstruation were discussed only in whispers, and neither television nor magazines advertised tampons or medicine for menstrual discomfort, most 11-year-old children had little idea about what to expect at puberty. Today, with this information readily available, it is easy to forget that preadolescents still may not know much about what to expect at puberty.

Nurse: Hello, Shelly. What can I do for you?

Shelly: I'm having cramps.

Nurse: Are you having your period?

Shelly: No. I haven't started them yet.

Nurse: Can you describe your cramps to me?

Shelly: Both my sisters started their periods when they were 10.

Nurse: Are you sick to your stomach?

Shelly: I'm the only girl in my gym class who doesn't have her period yet.

Nurse: You sound as if you're more worried about that than what you came in for.

Shelly: I need to know why I'm so different. Will I be able to have children?

Nurse: Let's talk about that.

Irregular periods can cause concern because girls need to know when their periods will occur so they can get used to this new phenomenon and learn to trust their bodies (AAP, 2016). A girl in college can explain matter-of-factly that she prefers not to go to the beach because she is having her period, but for a preadolescent, this topic may be too sophisticated and too emotionally charged to discuss openly. Preteenagers want to be able to plan activities to avoid having to make such explanations.

This means that menstrual irregularity can be a significant concern for preadolescents. A girl may fear that irregular periods indicate a hormone imbalance. She may worry about her future ability to conceive, or she may be ill informed about how conception occurs and may fear irregularity of her periods means that she is pregnant. Both malnourishment and obesity possibly influence menstrual regularity. Emotions can also affect consistent cycles. If irregularity continues beyond the first year, a careful history of the girl's nutrition; overall health; and school, social, and home adjustment should be taken. Dysmenorrhea, or painful menstruation, is discussed in Chapter 47.

For a nominal charge, manufacturers of sanitary napkins or tampons will mail an introductory kit of their products, together with well-illustrated, factual booklets, to introduce girls to menstruation. Such kits are useful if they supplement a parent's or a nurse's discussion, but they should not take the place of individual discussions.

Concerns of Boys

Boys who are not prepared for the physical changes of puberty worry about them in the same way as girls. Just as girls become keenly aware of breast development, boys become aware of increasing genital size. If they do not know testicular development precedes penis growth, they can worry that their growth will be inadequate.

Hypertrophy of breast tissue (gynecomastia) can occur in prepubescent boys, most often in those who are obese. A youth with this condition may be concerned a breast tumor is present or may feel embarrassed about his growing breasts. He can be assured that this is a transitory phenomenon and, although it makes him self-conscious, will fade as soon as his male hormones become more mature and active.

Some boys can also become concerned because although they have pubic hair, they cannot yet grow a beard or do not have chest hair, which are outward, easily recognized signs of maturity. You can assure them that pubic hair normally appears first and that chest and facial hair may not grow until several years later.

As increased seminal fluid begins to be produced, boys begin to notice ejaculation during sleep, termed **nocturnal emissions** (Widaman & Helm, 2012). Preadolescent boys may believe the old myth that loss of seminal fluid is debilitating; also, boys may have heard the term "premature ejaculation" and worry this is a forewarning of a problem in years to come. Both are fallacies.

Concerns for Transgender Children

Transgender children identify with the gender that is not their natal (sex assigned at birth) sex. Studies on the mental health of transgender children reported a higher incidence of psychosocial disorders such as depression and anxiety (Olson, Durwood, DeMeules, et al., 2015). Children who are supported by their family may experience less anxiety and depression. A study by Olson et al. (2015) sought to compare the difference in anxiety and depression scores, as rated by their parents, between transgender children (ages 3 to 12 years) and a control group. Seventy-three children were recruited in each group, including 49 siblings in the control group. The mean age was 7.5 years. The children were recruited from support groups, a website, conferences, and word of mouth. The results of the depression scores between the transgender children and the control group were not statistically different. The results of the anxiety scores were slightly higher in the transgender children compared with the control group but not in the preclinical or clinical range. The findings may be difficult to generalize to all children as the family income was $125,000 or more in 50% or more of each group. The majority of the children in the study were self-identified by the parents as White/non-Hispanic. The study was promising in supporting the premise that family and community support is a protective factor for transgender children. All children benefit from being treated as unique individuals unrelated to their gender preference. Transgender children are no different in this respect. In the past, it was thought that gender preference was fluid until the child reached late adolescence. It is now known that gender preferences are often identified in early childhood (Sherer, 2016).

This would indicate that support for transgender children should begin early in childhood. It is important that children are not ridiculed or isolated secondary to their gender preference because exposure to positive interaction with adults regardless of gender preference is helpful in promoting healthy child development.

Teeth

Deciduous teeth are lost and permanent teeth erupt during the school-age period (Fig. 32.1). Because of this, the average child gains 28 teeth between 6 and 12 years of age: the central and lateral incisors; first, second, and third cuspids; and first and second molars (Fig. 32.2).

DEVELOPMENTAL MILESTONES

As with all ages, you can measure school-age children's progress by whether they meet typical developmental milestones.

Gross Motor Development

School-age development is summarized in Table 32.2. At the beginning of the school-age period (age 6 years), children endlessly jump, tumble, skip, and hop. They have enough coordination to walk a straight line, many can ride a bicycle, and they learn to skip rope with practice.

A 7-year-old child appears quiet compared with the more active 6-year-old. Gender differences usually begin to manifest themselves in play: where girls may gravitate to more traditional female roles and activities and boys may gravitate to more traditional male roles and activities.

The movements of 8-year-olds are more graceful than those of younger children, although, as their arms and legs grow, they may appear awkward in their play and eating habits. They ride a bicycle well and enjoy sports such as gymnastics, soccer, and hockey.

Nine-year-olds are on the go constantly, as if they always have a deadline to meet. They have enough eye–hand coordination to enjoy baseball, basketball, and volleyball. By 10 years of age, children are more interested in perfecting their athletic skills than they were previously.

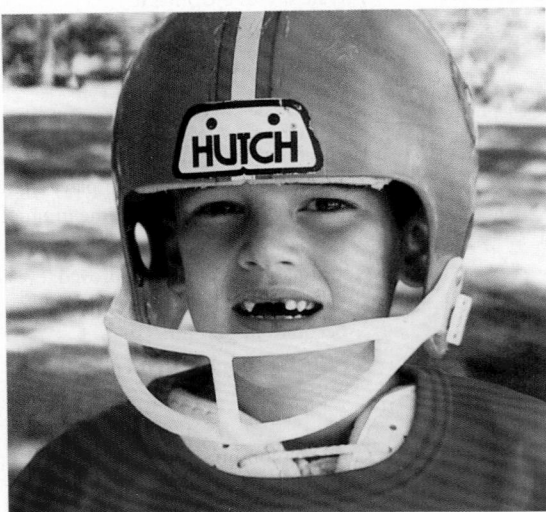

Figure 32.1 Early school-age children typically have a missing upper incisor as deciduous teeth are replaced by permanent teeth.

UPPER

Central incisor
7–8 years

Lateral incisor
8–9 years

Cuspid
11–12 years

First bicuspid
10–11 years

Second bicuspid
10–12 years

First molar
6–7 years

Second molar
12–13 years

Third molar
17–21 years

LOWER

Third molar
17–21 years

Second molar
11–13 years

First molar
6–7 years

Second bicuspid
11–12 years

First bicuspid
10–12 years

Cuspid
9–10 years

Lateral incisor
7–8 years

Central incisor
6–7 years

Figure 32.2   The eruption pattern of permanent teeth.

TABLE 32.2 SUMMARY OF SCHOOL-AGE DEVELOPMENT

Age (in Years)	Physical Development	Psychosocial and Cognitive Development
6	A year of constant motion; skipping is a new skill; first molars erupt.	First-grade teacher becomes authority figure; adjustment to all-day school may be difficult and may lead to nervous manifestations of fingernail biting, etc. Defines words by their use (e.g., a key is to unlock a door, not a metal object).
7	Central incisors erupt; difference between sexes becomes apparent in play (e.g., video games vs. dolls); spends time in quiet play.	A quiet year; striving for perfection leads to this year being called an eraser year. Learns conservation (e.g., water poured from tall container to a wide, flat one is the same amount of water); can tell time; can make simple change.
8	Coordination definitely improved; eyesight fully develops; playing with friends becomes important.	"Best friends" develop; whispering and giggling begin; can write in cursive as well as print; understands concepts of past, present, and future.
9	All activities done with friends	Friend or club age; a 9-year-old club is formed to spite someone, has secret codes, is all boy or all girl; clubs disband and reform quickly.
10	Coordination improves.	Ready for camp away from home; collecting age; likes rules; ready for competitive games.
11	Active, but awkward and ungainly	Insecure with members of opposite sex; repeats off-color jokes.
12	Coordination improves.	A sense of humor is present; is social and cooperative.

At 11 years of age, many children feel awkward because of their growth spurt and drop out of sports activities rather than look ungainly attempting them. They may channel their energy into constant motion instead: drumming fingers and tapping pencils or feet. This fall in sports participation may bother parents who see sports as the key to popularity, self-esteem, fitness, and teamwork.

Twelve-year-olds plunge into activities with intensity and concentration. They often enjoy participating in sports events for charities such as walkathons. They may be refreshingly cooperative around the house, able to handle a great deal of responsibility and complete given tasks.

Fine Motor Development

Six-year-olds can easily tie their shoelaces. They can cut and paste well and draw a person with good detail. They can print, although they may routinely reverse letters. Seven-year-olds concentrate on fine motor skills even more than they did the year before. This has been called the "eraser year" because children are never quite content with what they have done. They set too high a standard for themselves and then have difficulty performing at that level.

By 8 years of age, children's eyes are developed enough so they can read regular-size type. This can make reading a greater pleasure and school more enjoyable (Fig. 32.3). Eight-year-olds are able to write script in addition to print. They enjoy showing off this new skill in cards, letters, or projects. By age 9 years, their writing begins to look mature and less awkward.

Older school-age children begin to evaluate their teachers' ability and may perform at varying levels depending on each teacher's expectations. The middle school curriculum involves more challenging science and mathematics courses than previously and includes good literature. This may be a child's first exposure to reading as a fulfilling and worthwhile experience rather than just as an assignment and may be the time a child is "turned on" to reading.

Play

Play continues to be active at age 6 years; however, when children discover reading as an enjoyable activity that opens doors to other worlds, they can begin to spend quiet time with books. Many children spend hours playing increasingly challenging video games, an activity that can either foster a healthy sense of competition or create isolation from others.

By 7 years of age, children require more props for play than when they were younger. To be a police officer, for example, a 7-year-old may need a badge and gun, whereas before, a pointed finger sufficed. This is the start of a decline in imaginative play, which will continue unless a child receives adequate encouragement to use imagination. At age 7 years, children begin to prefer teenage dolls if they play with dolls, and their coordination is good enough that they can button the miniature dresses and pull on the tiny boots.

Around 7 years of age, children also develop an interest in collecting items such as baseball cards, dolls, rocks, or marbles. The type of item is not as important as the quantity. These collections become structured as a child reaches 8 years of age; time is spent sorting and cataloging. Most girls and boys of this age also enjoy helping in the kitchen with jobs such as making cookies and salads or frosting cakes. They start to be more involved in simple science projects and experiments. Eight-year-olds also like table games but hate to lose, so they tend to avoid competitive games. They may change the rules in the middle of a game to keep from losing.

Nine-year-olds play hard. They wake in the morning, squeeze in some activity before school, and plan something the moment they arrive home again. They may have difficulty going to bed at night because they want to play just one more game. Play is rough; children are not as interested in perfecting their skills as they will be in another year. Some parents or coaches expect children of this age to be more interested in perfecting their skills, so conflicts can arise.

Many schools begin music lessons for children at about 9 years of age. Children do well if others in their group are taking similar lessons. Talent for music or art becomes evident, and children respond with new interest in school or wherever they are exposed to these arts. Nine years of age is also a time when children use social media. This is an activity parents need to supervise as they may not realize that their accounts are available to the public and potential child predators.

Many 10-year-olds spend most of their time playing screen games. Boys and girls play separately at age 10 years, although interest in the opposite sex is apparent. Boys show off as girls pass their group; girls talk loudly or giggle at the sight of a familiar boy. Girls become more interested in the way they look and dress. Slumber parties and campouts become increasingly popular.

During their 10th year, children become very interested in rules and fairness. Before this time, they gave younger children breaks in games, allowing extra turns or hints. Now, they strictly enforce rules (Fig. 32.4). Club activities become structured, with a president, a secretary, and rules of order.

Children age 11 and 12 years enjoy dancing and playing table games; they are accommodating enough again to be able to play with younger siblings who need the rules modified to their advantage. Time with friends is often spent just talking. Twelve-year-olds typically like to do jobs around the house or babysitting for money. State laws vary on when a child may care for younger children without adult supervision. Both boys and girls seem to feel they are on the verge of something great and anxiously wait to turn 13 years old and become teenagers. The website www.healthychildren.org provides guidance for parents on developmental norms.

Figure 32.3 One of the biggest discoveries of childhood is that reading and writing are fun. These are activities that can help a child pass the hours during an illness.

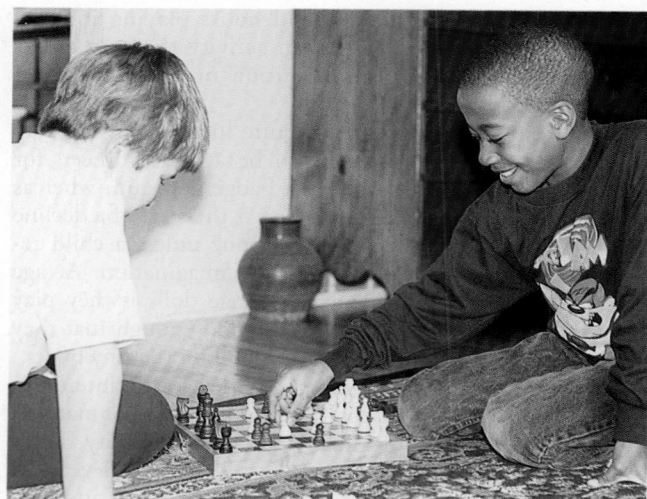

Figure 32.4 By 10 years of age, children are ready for competition. These two children enjoy a game of chess.

LANGUAGE DEVELOPMENT

Six-year-olds talk in full sentences, using language easily and with meaning. They no longer sound as though talking is an experiment but appear to have incorporated language permanently. They still define objects by their use (e.g., a key is to unlock a door, a fork is to eat with).

Most 7-year-olds can tell the time in hours, but they may have trouble with concepts such as "half past" and "quarter to," especially with the prevalence of digital clocks. They know the months of the year and can name the months in which holidays fall. They can add and subtract and make simple change (if they have had experience), so they can go with a parent to a store and make simple purchases. Much of children's talk is concerned with these concepts as they practice them and show them off for family or friends.

Because children discover "dirty" jokes at about age 9 years, they like to tell them to friends or try to understand those told by adults. They use swear words to express anger or just to show other children that they are growing up. They may have a short period of intense fascination with "bathroom language," as they did during the preschool years. As before, if parents want to discourage this, it should be made clear that they find such language unacceptable, and they refrain from using it themselves in their child's presence.

By 12 years of age, children can carry on an adult conversation, although stories are limited because of a lack of experience.

EMOTIONAL DEVELOPMENT

Ideally, children enter the school-age period with the ability to trust others and with a sense of respect for their own worth. They can accomplish small tasks independently because they have gained a sense of autonomy. They should have practiced or mimicked adult roles, learned to share, discovered that learning is an adventure, and grasped the idea that doing things is more important and more rewarding than watching things being done (a sense of initiative).

Developmental Task: Industry Versus Inferiority

During the early school years, children attempt to master their new developmental step: learning a sense of industry or accomplishment (Erikson, 1993). If gaining a sense of initiative can be defined as learning how to do things, then gaining a sense of industry is learning how to do things well.

If children are prevented from achieving a sense of industry or do not receive rewards for accomplishment, they can develop a feeling of inferiority or become convinced they cannot do things they actually can do. These children can have difficulty tackling new situations later in life (e.g., new job, new school, new responsibility) because they cannot envision how they will be successful in handling them. This can result in frustration in school or work activities.

The questions a preschool child asks reflect curiosity, such as "how," "why," and "what." During the early school years, children concentrate their questions on the "how" of tasks: "Is this the right way to do this?" "Am I making this right?" and "Is this good?" Often, school-age children will comment, "I can't do anything right" because their craft project falls short of expectations. School-age children need reassurance that they are doing things correctly, and this reassurance is best if it comes immediately after a task is completed.

 Concept Mastery Alert

Children benefit from honest praise and are quick to identify praise that is undeserved. Situations in which the child can be successful—and for which they can receive honest and deserved recognition—are vital to the development of confidence.

The books preferred by school-age children have many short chapters; children experience a sense of accomplishment as they finish each chapter. Small chores that can be completed quickly also give this type of reward. Children can survey their finished work and see they have done a good job. A child may dislike vacuuming, for instance, because the rug may not look very different when the task is complete. Picking up the scattered contents of a toy box, however, is a task that clearly makes a difference in the appearance of the room and so offers a reward.

Hobbies and projects also are enjoyed best if they are small and can be finished within a short time. Most school-age children, for example, prefer putting together two or three fairly simple model-car kits to assembling one extremely complicated kit. The three kits offer three rewards, whereas the involved one delays the reward so long that the child may become bored and never complete it. With adolescence will come more respect for quality. Teenagers realize that if they want the better model, they will have to spend the extra energy and attention and that quality products involve quality work (Fig. 32.5).

Home as a Setting to Learn Industry

Parents of a school-age child may need to take a step forward in development along with their child. For the first time, they realize their child has begun to look to other role models than themselves. Parents who enjoyed fostering imagination in a preschooler may feel frustrated when a school-age child they can provide hours of constructive activity and strengthen a sense of industry. Merit badge systems are geared to the needs of school-age children, offering small but frequent rewards. As with school activities, parents should determine the worth of each organization for their individual child.

Urge parents to evaluate competitive sports programs as well. Before children can compete successfully in these, they must be able to lose a game without feeling devastated—in other words, be able to say, "I lost because I played badly," not "I lost because I am a bad person." Children do not usually develop sufficient ego strength to do this until they are about 10 years old.

Another problem to consider with organized contact sports is the possibility of athletic injuries. Encourage parents to consider their child's maturity and the risk of injury (see Chapter 52) before they decide whether team competition is right for their child (Theisen, Frisch, Malisoux, et al., 2012). Parents should encourage children to vary the type of sport throughout the year to avoid repetitive use injuries by using the same muscle groups.

Problem Solving

An important part of developing a sense of industry is learning how to solve problems. Parents and teachers can help children develop this skill by encouraging practice. When a child asks, "Is this the right way to do this?" a parent can encourage problem solving by saying, "Let's talk about possible ways of doing it" rather than offering a quick solution.

The world depends on machinery, so mishaps and breakdowns (and therefore sudden changes) do occur. A child who can create an indoor playhouse with a card table and blanket when it is too wet or cold to use an outdoor one will be able, as an adult, to problem solve another solution to a data distribution problem when a computer malfunctions. This attitude of optimism rather than pessimism toward problem solving produces adults who rarely say, "It can't be done." Just as important, it leaves these adults with confidence, a sense of pride, and feeling good about themselves because they have control of their environment and abilities.

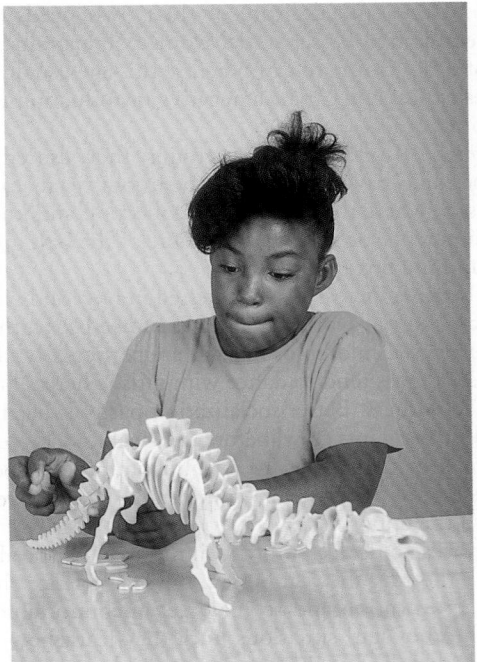

Figure 32.5 Assembling this simple model in a short time helps a school-age child gain a sense of industry. (© Stephen Frisch/Stock Boston.)

chooses to conform to rules and insists on the "right way" to do things. They may feel they have failed to encourage the child's creativity, but conformity is vital to children at this age. It is how they learn more about their world's rules (Weisleder, Cates, Dreyer, et al., 2016).

Children 8 or 9 years of age begin to spend more and more time with their peers and less time with their family. They forget to do household chores they once enjoyed, such as setting the table or mowing the lawn, or they may do the work sloppily so they have more time to spend with their friends. Although this may seem like a regression in behavior, it is actually a step of independence away from the parents and into the larger world, a developmental step toward helping them become emotionally mature. This is an example of a new role the child is trying out, one of many that will be tried in the process of reaching maturity, when an eventual "right fit" is found.

School as a Setting to Learn Industry

Adjusting to and achieving in school are two of the major tasks for this age group. Ideally, a child's teacher will think of learning as fun and will encourage a child to plunge into new experiences.

Schools are increasingly assuming responsibility for education about sex, safety, avoidance of substances of abuse, and preparation for family living. These discussions are generally superficial, however, and, if the classes are large, may raise more questions than they answer. Although learning these skills with peers helps children learn other people's opinions in these areas, such classes should not replace parental teaching.

Structured Activities

The Girl Scouts, the Boy Scouts, the Camp Fire Girls, and 4-H clubs are respected school-age activities. If the local chapters are well run by leaders who understand children's needs,

QSEN Checkpoint Question 32.1

QUALITY IMPROVEMENT

According to Erikson, a sense of industry or accomplishment is the developmental task of the school-age period. When planning care, what would be the best activity to introduce to Shelly to help her achieve this?
a. Encourage her to establish a new club.
b. Suggest she begin a diary in which she records her secret thoughts.
c. Help her with spelling so over a year's time she becomes an expert at this.
d. Locate small projects she could complete in 1 day and feel rewarded.

Look in Appendix A for the best answer and rationale.

Learning to Live With Others

School-age children are sometimes so interested in tasks and in accomplishing physical projects that they forget they must work with people to achieve these goals. A good time to urge children to learn compassion and thoughtfulness toward others is during the early school years, when children are first exposed to large groups of other youngsters. Writing thank you letters or shoveling an older neighbor's sidewalk are examples of activities that can help children develop empathy toward others.

Learning to give a present without receiving one in return or doing a favor without expecting a reward is also a part of this process, and this can be taught by example. Children should see their parents doing such things with an attitude not of "What will I get out of this?" but "What can I contribute?"

Children may show empathy toward others as early as 20 months, but cognitively, they cannot relate others' experiences to their own until about 6 years of age. Therefore, it is usually ineffective to lecture a child by saying, "That was cruel to call Mary names." The child may feel she had every right to do so. A better technique is to ask children to put themselves in Mary's place for a minute and imagine how they would feel if they were Mary. A school-age child will generally be able to do this and understand why name-calling hurts. Following this, a simple statement such as "It doesn't feel good to be called names, does it?" may suffice.

Socialization

Six-year-old children play in groups, but when they are tired or under stress, they usually prefer one-to-one contact. In a first-grade classroom, for example, students compete actively for a few minutes of special time with their teacher. At the end of a day, they enjoy spending individual time with parents. You may have to remind parents that this is not babyish behavior but that of a typical 6-year-old.

Seven-year-olds are increasingly aware of family roles and responsibility. Promises must be kept because 7-year-olds view them as definite, firm commitments. Children this age tattle because they have such a strong sense of justice (Loke, Heyman, Forgie, et al., 2011).

Eight-year-olds actively seek the company of other children. Most 8-year-old girls have a close girlfriend; boys have a close boyfriend. Girls begin to whisper among themselves as they share secrets with close friends, annoying both parents and teachers.

Nine-year-olds take the values of their peer group very seriously. They are much more interested in how other children dress than in what their parents want them to wear. This is typically the friend or club age because children form groups, usually "spite clubs." This means if there are four girls on the block, three form a club and exclude the fourth. The reason for exclusion is often unclear; it might be that the fourth child has a chronic disease, she has more or less money than the others, she was at the dentist's the day the club was formed, or simply that the club cannot exist unless there is someone to exclude. Such clubs typically have a secret password and secret meeting place. Membership is generally all girls or all boys.

If an excluded child does not react badly to being shut out, the club will probably disband after a few days because its purpose is lost. The next day, the excluded member may meet with two others and snub a different child. Parents need to use caution deciding whether to intervene with this type of play because loyalties shift quickly: The child who is club president today may be the excluded one tomorrow.

Because they are so ready for social interaction, 9-year-olds are ready for activities away from home, such as a week at camp. They can take care of their own needs and are mature enough to be separated from their parents for this length of time. Going to camp before this age usually results in homesickness and can be a negative introduction to being away from home.

Although 10-year-olds enjoy groups, they also enjoy privacy. They like having their own bedroom or at least their own dresser, where they can store a collection and know it is free from parents' or siblings' eyes. One of the best gifts for a 10-year-old is a box that locks.

Girls become increasingly interested in boys and vice versa by 11 years of age. Favorite activities are mixed-sex rather than single-sex ones. Children of this age are particularly insecure, however, and girls tend to dance with girls, whereas boys talk together in corners. Better socialization patterns need not be rushed. Just as infants crawl before they walk, so 11-year-olds must attempt many awkward and uncomfortable social experiences before they become comfortable forming relationships with the opposite sex.

Twelve-year-olds feel more comfortable in social situations than they did the year before. Boys experience erections on small provocation and so may feel uncomfortable being pushed into boy–girl situations until they learn how to better control their bodies. Because some children develop faster than others, every group has some members who are almost adolescent and some who are still children, making social interactions sometimes difficult.

QSEN Checkpoint Question 32.2

INFORMATICS

Shelly belonged to a series of clubs when she was 9 years old. How would the school nurse describe the typical characteristic of a 9-year-old's club to the nursing student?
  a. Clubs have formal rules and regulations.
  b. Clubs are designed to help shy children get outside of their "comfort zone."
  c. Clubs invariably exclude one or more children.
  d. Clubs always include both boys and girls.

Look in Appendix A for the best answer and rationale.

COGNITIVE DEVELOPMENT

The age from 5 to 11 years is a transitional stage where children undergo a shift from the preoperational thought they used as preschoolers to concrete operational thought or the ability to reason through any problem they can actually visualize (Piaget, 1969) (Fig. 32.6).

Children can use concrete operational thought because they learn several new concepts during school age, such as:
- Decentering, the ability to project one's self into other people's situations and see the world from their viewpoint rather than focusing only on their own view.
- **Accommodation**, the ability to adapt thought processes to fit what is perceived such as understanding that there can be more than one reason for other people's actions. A preschooler might expect to see the same nurse in the morning who was there the evening before, whereas a school-age child will understand that different nurses work different shifts.

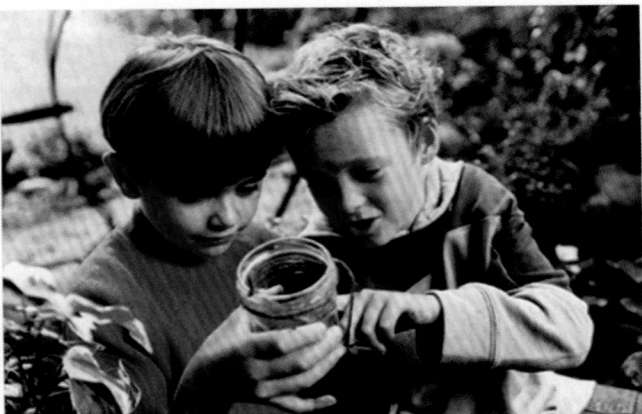

Figure 32.6 School-age children learn concrete operational thought or concentrate on phenomena they can actually see occurring. For example, children may have closely catalogued collections of action figures, science specimens, sports materials, or books and spend much time attending to and enhancing such collections.

- **Conservation**, the ability to appreciate that a change in shape does not necessarily mean a change in size. If you pour 30 ml of cough medicine from a thin glass to a wide one, the preschooler will say that one glass holds more than the other; a school-age child will know that both glasses hold an equal amount.
- **Class inclusion**, the ability to understand that objects can belong to more than one classification. A preschooler is able to categorize items in only one way, for example, stones and shells are found at the beach; a school-age child can categorize them in many ways such as by different materials or by a difference in sizes and shapes, not just that they are found at the beach.

These cognitive developments lead to some of the typical changes and characteristics of the school-age period. Decentering enables a school-age child to feel compassion for others, which was not possible in younger years. Because understanding the principle of conservation is possible, a school-age child is not fooled by perceptions as often as before. The ability to classify objects leads to the collecting activities of the school-age period. Class inclusion is also necessary for learning mathematics and reading, systems that categorize numbers and words.

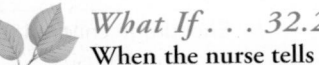

What If . . . 32.1
The nurse makes Shelly's hospital bed one day and then gives her an injection. What if the next day she begins to cry while the nurse is making her bed because she "doesn't want a shot"? The lack of what cognitive process led her to believe the nurse's actions would be exactly the same the second day?

MORAL AND SPIRITUAL DEVELOPMENT

School-age children begin to mature in terms of moral development as they enter a stage of *preconventional reasoning*, sometimes as early as 5 years of age (Kohlberg, 1984). During this stage, if asked, "Why is it wrong to steal from your neighbor?" school-age children will answer, "The police say it's wrong," or "Because if you do, you'll go to jail."

They concentrate on "niceness" or "fairness" and cannot see yet that stealing hurts their neighbor, the highest level of moral reasoning. Because they are still limited in their ability to understand others' views, they may interpret something as being right because it is good for them, not because it is right for humanity as a whole.

Remember that school-age children are rule oriented; when they ask for something, because they were good, they expect to receive what they are asking.

What If . . . 32.2
When the nurse tells Shelly it would be good if she lost some weight, she says the nurse isn't being fair. Is this a typical school-age response?

Health Promotion for a School-Age Child and Family

Because of still limited judgment, school-age children need guidelines in reference to safety, nutrition, and daily care. These are always excellent topics for discussion at healthcare visits.

PROMOTING SCHOOL-AGE SAFETY

School-age children are ready for time on their own without direct adult supervision. This means that they need good education on safety practices (Box 32.3). As with adults, unintentional injuries tend to occur when children are under stress or when they are distracted.

QSEN Checkpoint Question 32.3

SAFETY
Teaching safety is an important area to consider for school-age children. Which advice would be best?
a. "Keep your backpack filled to capacity to avoid falling on frequent trips back to your locker."
b. "As soon as you no longer need an automobile booster seat, you'll no longer need a seatbelt either."
c. "Gaining weight isn't serious in the school-age years; it only becomes a real problem after age 18 years."
d. "You're old enough to tell if you are sick or not; your mother's opinion isn't as important as when you were younger."

Look in Appendix A for the best answer and rationale.

School age is not too early for parents to look at the effect of carrying heavy backpacks on children's posture. A backpack that weighs more than 10% of the child's body weight is enough to cause a child to have to lean forward chronically to bear the weight. This can lead to chronic back pain (Kistner, Fiebert, & Roach, 2012).

Sexual maltreatment is an unfortunate and all-too-common hazard for children. Teaching points to help children avoid sexual maltreatment are summarized in Box 32.4 (see also Chapter 55).

BOX 32.3

Nursing Care Planning Based on Family Teaching

COMMON SAFETY MEASURES TO PREVENT UNINTENTIONAL INJURIES DURING THE SCHOOL YEARS

Q. Shelly's mother tells you, "She's constantly on the go. How can I keep her free from accidents when I'm not always with her?"

A. Putting preventive steps in place, such the ones that follow, is the key.

Source of Unintentional Injury	Preventive Measure
Motor vehicle	Encourage children to use seat belts and a booster seat if needed; role model seat belt use. Teach street-crossing safety; stress that streets are no place for roughhousing, pushing, or shoving. Teach parking lot and school bus safety (e.g., do not walk in back of parked cars, wait for crossing guard).
Bicycle	Teach bicycle safety, including wearing a helmet and not giving "passengers" rides.
Community	Teach to avoid unsafe areas, such as train yards, grain silos, and back alleys. Stress to not go with strangers (parents can establish a code word with child; child does not leave school with anyone who does not know the word). Teach children to say "no" to anyone who touches them if they do not wish it, including family members (most sexual maltreatment is by a family member, not a stranger). Teach children not to arrange a meeting with people they meet on the Internet. For older school-age children, teach rules of safer sex so they know these rules before they need to use them a first time.
Burns	Teach safety with candles, matches, and campfires and that fire is not fun. Also teach safety with beginning cooking skills (e.g., be certain to include microwave oven safety, such as closing firmly before turning on oven; not using metal containers). Teach safety with sun exposure; use sun block. Teach to not climb electric poles.
Falls	Educate that roughhousing on fences or climbing on roofs is hazardous. Teach skateboard, scooter, and skating safety.
Sports injuries	Teach that wearing appropriate equipment for sports (e.g., face masks for hockey; mouthpiece and cup for football; helmet for bicycle riding, skateboarding, or in-line skating; batting helmets for baseball) is not babyish but smart management. Stress not to play to a point of exhaustion or in a sport beyond physical capability (no pitching baseballs or toe ballet for an early grade-school child). Use trampolines only with adult supervision to avoid serious neck injury.
Drowning	Teach how to swim; dares and roughhousing when diving or swimming are not appropriate. Stress not to swim beyond limits of capabilities.
Drugs	Help your child avoid all recreational drugs; prescription medicine should only be taken as directed. Teach to avoid tobacco and alcohol.
Firearms	Teach firearm safety. Keep firearms in locked cabinets with bullets separate from gun.
General	School-age children should keep adults informed as to where they are and what they are doing; cell phones can help with this. Be aware the frequency of unintentional injures increases when parents are under stress and therefore less attentive. Special precautions must be taken at these times. Caution that some children are more active, curious, and impulsive and therefore more vulnerable to unintentional injuries than others.

Nursing Care Planning Based on Family Teaching

TEACHING POINTS TO HELP CHILDREN AVOID SEXUAL MALTREATMENT

Q. Shelly's mother wants to protect her daughter from being abused sexually. She asks you, "What are good rules to teach children without scaring them?"

A. A number of suggestions include:

1. Your body is your property and you can decide who looks at it or touches it.
2. Secrets are fun things to keep. If a person asks you not to tell about something that was done to you that you didn't like, however, it's not a secret. It's all right to tell someone about it.
3. Don't go anywhere with a stranger (a stranger is someone you do not know, not someone "strange"). Don't be fooled by people asking you to give them directions or to go with them because your mother is sick or hurt or because they have lost a pet.
4. Being touched by someone you like is a good feeling. You don't have to allow anyone to touch you in a way you don't like. Don't allow yourself to be left alone with a person you are uncomfortable with because that person touches you in a way you don't like.
5. Avoid meeting with people you talk with on social media and the Internet because they may not be the age or the person whom they say they are.
6. A "private part" is the part of you a bathing suit touches. If anyone asks you to show them a private part or touches a private part, tell them to stop, and tell someone what happened.
7. If the person you tell doesn't believe you, keep telling people until someone does believe you.

Figure 32.7 School lunch programs are being modified to better provide nutritious meals to school-age children.

Many children qualify for a free or reduced-price school lunch and breakfast (Hirschman & Chriqui, 2012). A government-regulated school lunch provides milk (8 oz), protein (2 oz), one starch serving, a vegetable (¾ cup), and fruit (¾ cup). Serving sizes vary according to age to provide one third of a child's nutrition requirements for a day (Fig. 32.7). Children with food allergies should be provided with alternative foods. Depending on the severity of the allergy, such as peanuts, they may need to sit at an allergy-free table at school.

Nutritious after-school snacks are important in this age group.

Poor eating habits developed in the school-age years may last through adulthood and lead to an increased risk of health-related diseases, such as type 2 diabetes, hypertension, cardiovascular disease, and obesity.

Fostering Industry and Nutrition

As a part of fostering industry, school-age children usually enjoy helping to plan meals. They can prepare simple meals with healthy ingredients. They can assist with the preparation of more complex meals and learn the safe use of kitchen appliances such as the microwave and stove.

The development of proper etiquette is important in the school-age years. Parents can model this behavior for their child and encourage meals to be eaten at the table rather than while watching television. Meals eaten while watching television or performing another activity is a risk factor for obesity.

Recommended Dietary Intakes

Although parents may have less to say about what a school-age child eats, it is important that the increasing energy requirements that come with this age (often in spurts) are met daily with foods of high nutritional value.

During the late school years, the recommended dietary intakes for children begin to be separated into different categories for girls then for boys because boys require more calories and other nutrients at this time. Both girls and boys require more iron in prepuberty than they did between the ages of 7 and 10 years. Adequate calcium and fluoride intake remains important to ensure good teeth and bone growth. A major deficit may be fiber because school-age children typically dislike vegetables.

PROMOTING NUTRITIONAL HEALTH OF A SCHOOL-AGE CHILD

Most school-age children have good appetites, although meals may be influenced by the day's activity. If children have had a full day of active play, they may come to the dinner table ready to eat anything. If a day was filled with frustration—a child received a poor mark in school, had an argument with a friend, or has a big game to think about—the child's appetite may be affected. This is no different from the way adults feel at times and so should be respected.

Establishing Healthy Eating Patterns

School-age children should be encouraged to eat a healthy breakfast to ensure the ability to concentrate during the school day. It is helpful if parents model this behavior.

School-age children can help prepare a nutritious lunch to take to school. If they purchase lunch at school, healthy choices should be discussed with the child. Healthcare personnel can play an active role in nutrition education at health maintenance visits.

A Vegetarian Diet

School-age children who are vegetarians or vegans need to learn how to obtain essential nutrients whether they pack their lunch or purchase it at school. The consumption of adequate protein and calcium is important for muscle, bone, and dental development.

Foods highest in calcium are green leafy vegetables such as spinach and turnip greens, enriched bread, and cereals. Soybeans, legumes, grains, and immature seeds such as green beans, lima beans, and corn are relatively high in protein. Encourage outside activities for sun exposure to increase vitamin D. Iron may need to be supplemented as well, especially in girls with heavy menstrual flows (Whitney & Rolfes, 2012).

PROMOTING DEVELOPMENT OF A SCHOOL-AGE CHILD IN DAILY ACTIVITIES

With life centered on school activities and friends, a school-age child still needs parental guidance for most daily activities because the habits and lifestyle patterns gained during this period will form the basis for the patterns of living later in life. Figure 32.8 shows a day in the life of a family with school-age children. Along with nutritional needs, areas of concern for a school-age child and family include dressing, sleep needs, exercise, hygiene, and dental care.

Dress

Although school-age children can fully dress themselves, they are not skilled at taking care of their clothes until late in the school-age years. This is the right age, however (if not started already), to teach children the importance of caring for their own belongings. School-age children have definite opinions about clothing styles, often based on the likes of their friends, a popular sport, or a popular musician rather than the preferences of their parents. Help parents be aware that a child who wears different clothing than others may become the object of exclusion from a school club or group. In schools with a gang or bullying culture, children may not be able to wear a certain color or style lest they be mistaken for a gang member or become a bully's victim (White & Mason, 2011). A number of schools require uniforms or have a dress code to eliminate such concerns.

Sleep

Sleep needs vary among individual children. Younger school-age children typically require 10 to 12 hours of sleep each night, whereas older children require about 8 to 10 hours. Most 6-year-olds are too old for naps but do require a quiet time after school to get them through the remainder of the day. Nighttime terrors may continue during the early school years and may actually increase during the first-grade year as a child reacts to the stress of beginning school.

During early school years, many children enjoy a quiet talk or a reading time at bedtime. At about age 9 years, when friends become important, children generally are ready to give up bedtime talks with parents in preference to phoning or text messaging a friend. Some parents may need some help to take at face value their child's statement, "I'm tired. I'd rather go to sleep," rather than feel rejected.

Children with television sets, electronic games, or smartphones in their bedrooms not only have shorter sleep times at night but also are more likely to be obese (Chahal, Fung, Kuhle, et al., 2013).

Exercise

School-age children need daily exercise. Although they go to school all day, they do not automatically receive much exercise because school is basically a sit-down activity. Children who are bused or driven by a parent to school may therefore return home without having spent much time in active exercise.

Increasing time spent in exercise need not involve organized sports. It can come from neighborhood games, walking with parents or a dog, or bicycle riding. As children enter preadolescence, those with poor coordination may become reluctant to exercise. Urge them to participate in some form of daily exercise, however, or obesity or osteoporosis can result later in life (Eagle, Sheetz, Gurm, et al., 2012; Gunter, Almstedt, & Janz, 2012).

Hygiene

Children 6 or 7 years of age still need help in regulating bath water temperature and in cleaning their ears and fingernails. By age 8 years, children are generally capable of bathing themselves but may not do it well because they are too busy to take the time or because they do not find bathing as important as do their parents.

Both boys and girls become interested in showering as they approach their teen years. This can be encouraged because perspiration increases with puberty, along with sebaceous gland activity. When girls begin to menstruate, they may be afraid to take baths or wash their hair during their period if they have heard this is not safe. They need information that both of these practices are safe during their menses. Boys who are uncircumcised may develop inflammation under the foreskin from increased secretions if they do not wash regularly (Meng & Tanagho, 2013).

QSEN Checkpoint Question 32.4

EVIDENCE-BASED PRACTICE

Shelly has told the nurse she wants to try out for cheerleading when she gets to high school. This is a sport appealing to school-age children and adolescents because of its combinations of dance and gymnastics, the friendships that can develop, and the school status it almost automatically creates. To investigate what type of injuries typically occur with cheerleading, researchers reviewed all cheerleading injuries (over 4,000) presented to U.S. emergency departments during a 5-year period. The types of injuries most often seen were sprains/strains (44%), fractures (16%), and contusions (16%). The activities resulting in the most injuries were body collisions (29%), stunting (19%), tumbling (11%), and tossing (2.5%) (Currie, Fields, Patterson, et al., 2016).

Based on the study, how would the nurse best advise Shelly?

a. Cheerleading will be good for her because she is likely to lose weight from the exercise.
b. She will need to drink an extra source of calcium every day to avoid broken bones.
c. She should pursue a sport or activity that is safer.
d. She should be aware that cheerleading may be beneficial to her but does carry some risks.

Look in Appendix A for the best answer and rationale.

7:00 AM: The family sits down to a healthy breakfast. Claudia helps Laura with the butter.

7:30 AM: John walks Marc to school, emphasizing safety when crossing the street.

10:00 AM: Claudia and Laura bake a cake for the night's dessert. Four-year-old Laura enjoys practicing adult roles.

3:00 PM: Marc and Laura play together after Marc gets home from school. Their cooperative play is punctuated by an occasional argument.

Figure 32.8   A day in the life of a family with young children.

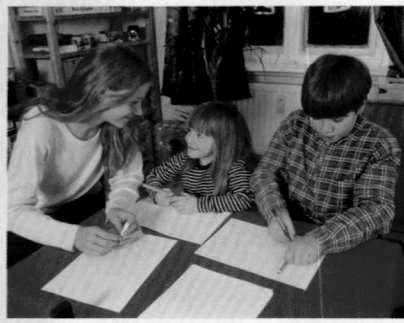

4:00 PM: Claudia helps Marc with his homework. Laura likes to draw alongside her big brother.

5:00 PM: The family greets John as he comes home from work.

5:30 PM: John and Marc go rollerblading before dinner. John makes sure Marc's protective gear is in place.

7:00 PM: After dinner, Marc helps with the dishes, then the family spends time together playing a game.

8:30 PM: Time to get ready for bed! Claudia helps the kids clean up and brush their teeth. And there's always time to read them a story.

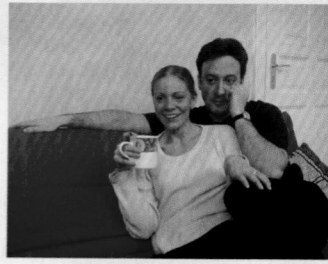

9:00 PM: John and Claudia relax together at the end of the day.

Figure 32.8 (continued)

Care of Teeth

With proper dental care, the average child today can expect to grow up cavity free. To ensure this happening, school-age children should visit a dentist at least twice yearly for a checkup, cleaning, and possibly a fluoride treatment to strengthen and harden the tooth enamel or sealants on secondary teeth (Tubert-Jeannin, Auclair, Amsallem, et al., 2011) (Fig. 32.9). Remind them that not all bottled water is fluoridated, so they don't want this to be their main source of drinking water. Some children develop a fear of dentists and, if a dentist visit was painful, want to avoid going at all. The advantage of frequent visits permits problems to be addressed early and familiarizes the child with the dental visit. Pedodontists specialize in caring for children's teeth and understand the developmental level of their patients. The parents of children who tend to develop caries might be encouraged to visit a pedodontist if one is available and affordable.

School-age children have to be reminded to brush their teeth daily. For effective brushing, a child should use a soft toothbrush, fluoride-based toothpaste, and dental floss to clean between teeth to help remove plaque. Electric toothbrushes can be used safely by school-age children.

Snacks are best limited to high-protein foods such as chicken and cheese rather than candy. Fruits, vegetables, and cereals fortified with minerals and vitamins (not empty calorie ones) can all be fun after-school snacks for school-age children. If the child does eat candy, a type that is eaten quickly and dissolves quickly is better than slowly dissolving or sticky candy because these types stay in contact with the teeth longer.

Figure 32.9 Dental caries are the number one health problem in school-age children. Stress to parents that good dental health is important and encourage school-age children to visit a dentist twice a year.

QSEN Checkpoint Question 32.5

TEAMWORK & COLLABORATION

Shelly tells the nurse she collected "a ton of candy on Halloween. Because of how common this phenomenon is, in consultation with a dental hygienist, you would teach children that what type of candy is less likely to cause dental caries?

a. Salt water taffy
b. A chocolate bar
c. Chewy caramels
d. Hard candy

Look in Appendix A for the best answer and rationale.

PROMOTING HEALTH FAMILY FUNCTIONING

To their parents' annoyance, many 6-year-olds often quote their teacher as the final authority on all subjects. This may be the first time the parents see someone surpassing them in their child's eyes, and accepting the situation can be painful. Children also cite their friends as guides for behavior; for example, "Mary Jane doesn't have to go to bed until 10 o'clock" or "Carlos's mother lets him go to the movies every Saturday." Parents may require help to realize these remarks are a normal consequence of being exposed to other adults and children. A simple statement such as "There are all kinds of ways to do things, but in our house, the rule is this" shows no criticism of Carlos's or Mary Jane's family yet conveys a special and secure "our house" feeling.

Parents may also need to be reminded that even the simplest tasks of everyday life require repeated practice before they can be accomplished well. The way parents correct children as they learn these tasks influences children's opinions of themselves and their ability to continue learning. "Putting all the silverware in a pile is one way of putting it away; another way would be to divide spoons, forks, and knives separately" is always preferable to "What a silly way to put away silverware!" Comments such as "Can't you do anything right?" or "Why don't you ever do what I say?" should always be avoided because children will rise only to the level expected of them.

If parents have difficulty telling what a child's completed project is supposed to be, the time-honored "Tell me about it" is preferable to "What is it?" It is good for parents to find a redeeming characteristic in a project, no matter how shakily it is put together: "I like the bright color you painted it" or "That must have been fun to make." Displaying and using children's gifts are part of having school-age children in a family. A finger painting hung on the refrigerator door enhances, not detracts from, the most elegant home.

In talking to parents of school-age children, good questions to ask to estimate the degree of interaction that occurs in the home and whether parents are strengthening a child's sense of accomplishment include:

- How do they correct the child when he or she does something wrong?
- Do they display school projects?
- Does the child have chores that are his or hers to accomplish?
- Do they ask the child to participate in family decision making?

COMMON HEALTH PROBLEMS OF THE SCHOOL-AGE PERIOD

Children in their early school years may have many small health concerns such as head lice or ringworm (see Chapter 43). At the same time, they have one of the lowest rates of death and serious illness of any age group. The two causes of death seen most frequently are from unintentional injury and cancer. Minor illnesses are largely due to dental caries, gastrointestinal disturbances, and upper respiratory infections (Heron, 2012).

Because learning difficulties such as attention deficit hyperactivity disorder (ADHD) and autism spectrum disorders (ASDs) are identified during the school-age years, they are important parental concerns (see Chapter 54). Table 32.3 shows the usual health maintenance pattern for a school-age child (AAP, Committee on Practice and Ambulatory Medicine, 2012). Table 32.4 lists problems that parents may have in evaluating illnesses in school-age children.

Dental Caries

Caries (cavities) are progressive, destructive lesions or decalcification of the tooth enamel and dentin. When the pH of the tooth surface drops to 5.6 or below (which happens after children eat readily fermented carbohydrates, such as table sugar), acid microorganisms (acidogenic lactobacilli and aciduric streptococci) found in dental plaque attack the cementing medium of teeth and destroy it. Plaque tends to accumulate in deep grooves of the teeth and contact areas between teeth, making these areas most susceptible to dental decay. The enamel on primary teeth is thinner than on permanent teeth, so these are even more susceptible to destruction than permanent teeth. The distance from the enamel to the pulp is shorter also, so invasion of the tooth nerve can occur quickly. Neglected caries result in poor chewing and therefore poor digestion, abscesses and pain, and sometimes osteomyelitis (bone infection) if the jaw bone is involved.

As stated earlier, dental caries are largely preventable with proper brushing and use of fluoridated water or fluoride application. When caries do occur, it's important they be treated quickly and the child's dental hygiene practices be evaluated and improved if necessary. Most importantly, children must believe that they have a stake in the health of their teeth, so even though they are cavity free, they willingly undertake the self-care measures necessary to ensure healthy teeth with parental support rather than parental command (Wen, Goldberg, Marrs, et al., 2012). Dental visits are recommended every 6 months. With the eruption of the permanent teeth, sealants can be applied at dental visits to lessen the development of dental decay.

Malocclusion

The upper jaw in children matures during early childhood along with skull growth; the lower jaw reaches maturity more slowly, forcing teeth to make a prolonged series of changes until they reach their final adult alignment and position. Good tooth occlusion, in which the upper teeth overlap the lower teeth by a small amount and teeth are evenly spaced and in good alignment, is necessary for optimal formation of teeth, health of the supporting tissue, optimal speech development, and what most people view as a pleasant physical appearance. **Malocclusion** (a deviation of tooth position from the normal) may be congenital due to conditions such as cleft palate, a small lower jaw, or familial traits tending toward malocclusion. The condition can result later on from constant mouth breathing or abnormal tongue position (tongue thrusting). Thumb-sucking is still another possibility if it persists past the time of eruption of the permanent front teeth (6 to 7 years) (Sandler, Madahar, & Murray, 2011). The loss of teeth due to extraction or an unintentional injury may lead to malocclusion if not properly treated so that alignment is maintained.

Malocclusion may be either crossbite (sideways) or anterior or posterior. Children with a malocclusion should be evaluated by an orthodontist to see if orthodontic braces or other therapy is necessary. The time to begin correction varies with the extent of the malocclusion and jaw size. Braces are painful when they are first applied and at periodic visits when they are tightened to maintain pressure for further straightening. Some children develop mild, shallow ulcerations (canker sores) on the buccal membrane from friction of metal wires. Rubbing the offending wire with dental wax dulls the surface and gives relief. Oral acetaminophen or an agent such as Orajel (an over-the-counter drug) rubbed on the ulceration may also offer relief.

All children who wear braces need to brush their teeth well and be assessed periodically to see that they are brushing properly around the braces (a Waterpik is often recommended for thorough cleaning). They should use dental floss to remove plaque from around wires.

After the removal of braces, many children usually wear retainers to maintain the correction the braces achieved. Although braces are wired into place, retainers are not. Loss of a retainer can be a problem if it must be removed when eating; check bedside food trays of school-age children before removing them to be certain a child has not placed a retainer on the tray.

Show appropriate sympathy and help children problem solve if they are bothered by the appearance of braces or wearing a retainer. Once thought of as implements to be made fun of, teeth braces have become such a common feature of life for schoolchildren that most children who wear them find comfort in not being the only one to suffer this indignity and, once used to their own appliances, experience little reluctance in letting their classmates see them. Some even view them as a mark of pride or a status symbol (Hamdan, Singh, & Rock, 2012).

CONCERNS AND PROBLEMS OF THE SCHOOL-AGE PERIOD

Two of the most important disorders of the school-age period are ADHD and ASDs because these interfere so dramatically with school progress (see Chapter 54). Other problems concern language, fears, and responsibility.

 Nursing Diagnoses and Related Interventions

Nursing Diagnosis: Parental anxiety related to less-than-expected behavior of a school-age child

Outcome Evaluation: Parent states undesired behavior has decreased in frequency; parent feels less stress about the child's health or future.

TABLE 32.3 HEALTH MAINTENANCE SCHEDULE, SCHOOL-AGE PERIOD

Area of Focus	Methods	Frequency
Assessment		
Health history	Health interview	Every visit
Physical health	Physical examination	Every visit
Developmental milestones	History and observation	Every visit
Growth milestones	Height and weight plotted on standard growth chart; body mass index (BMI) and physical examination	Every visit
Hypertension	Blood pressure	Every visit
Nutrition	History and observation; height and weight information	Every visit
Parent–child relationship	History and observation	Every visit
Behavior or school problems	History and observation	Every visit
Vision and hearing disorders	History and observation	Every visit
	Formal Snellen or Titmus testing	At 7–9 years and 10–12 years
	Audiometer testing	At 7–9 years and 10–12 years
Dental health	History and physical examination	Every visit
Scoliosis	Physical examination	Yearly after age 8 years
Thyroid	Physical examination and history	Every visit after age 10 years
Dyslipidemia	Cholesterol and triglycerides	6–8 years and 10–12 years
Tuberculosis	Purified protein derivative (PPD) skin test	Depending on prevalence of tuberculosis in community
Bacteriuria	Clean-catch urine	At 6–7 years
Anemia	Hematocrit and hemoglobin	At 7–8 years and 11–12 years
Immunizations		
Check history and past records, inform caregiver about any risks and side effects, and administer immunization in accordance with healthcare agency policies.		
Diphtheria, tetanus, and pertussis vaccine	(DTaP)	11–12 years
Hepatitis A vaccine	(HepA)	If not previously administered
Hepatitis B vaccine	(HepB)	If not administered in infancy or three injections were not completed
Human papillomavirus vaccine	(HPV or HPV4)	11 or 12 years; second injection 2 months later; third injection 6 months after first dose
Inactivated poliomyelitis vaccine	(IPV)	If four doses not previously administered
Influenza vaccine	(IIV)	Yearly
Meningococcal conjugate vaccine	(MCV4)	11–12 years
Pneumococcal vaccine	(PPSV)	To children at high risk
Measles, mumps, rubella vaccine	(MMR)	If two doses not previously administered
Varicella vaccine	(VAR)	At any age after 1 year if not previously immunized, or at 11–12 years if lacking reliable history of chickenpox
Anticipatory Guidance		
School-age care	Active listening and health teaching	Every visit
Expected growth and developmental milestones before next visit	Active listening and health teaching	Every visit
Unintentional injury prevention	Counseling about street and personal safety	Every visit
Problem Solving		
Any problems expressed by caregiver during course of the visit	Active listening and health teaching regarding cigarette smoking, substance abuse, sex education, school adjustment, etc.	Every visit

American Academy of Pediatrics, Committee on Practice and Ambulatory Medicine. (2012). *Recommendations for preventive pediatric health care*. Washington, DC: Author; and Centers for Disease Control and Prevention. *Birth–18 years & "catch up" immunization schedules*. Washington, DC: Author.

TABLE 32.4 PARENTAL DIFFICULTIES EVALUATING HEALTH PROBLEMS IN THE SCHOOL-AGE CHILD

Difficulty	Helpful Suggestions for Parents
Evaluating seriousness of illness	For the first time, a school-age child may view illness as a way to avoid unpleasant activities (e.g., school, a coach who asks too much, household chores). Evaluating whether the child has symptoms when asked to do a favorite thing often reveals the difference between exaggeration and an ill child (e.g., too sick to eat spinach, not too sick to eat ice cream; too sick to go to school, not too sick to go ice skating). If the child uses symptoms of illness as a means of avoiding situations, parents must evaluate what it is about the situation they could improve or see if some change should be made in their expectations.
Evaluating nutritional intake	Many school-age children eat lunch at school, and they may spend weekends away from home and weeks away at camp. As with all ages, noting whether they are growing and active is better than monitoring any one day's food intake.
Evaluating puberty changes	There is a wide variation in the time secondary sex characteristics occur (8–17 years for girls; 10–20 years for boys). Children should be examined if and when they or their parents are concerned pubertal changes are delayed or appearing too early.
Age-specific diseases to be aware of	School age is a time to evaluate vision because vision changes occur with increased maturity of the eye globe. Squinting, rubbing the eyes, or poor marks in school may be signs of poor vision. Streptococcal sore throats occur frequently in early school-age children. Those with sore throats should be examined by a healthcare provider to prevent complications, such as glomerulonephritis or rheumatic fever, from developing. Girls, in particular, must be evaluated for scoliosis (curvature of the spine). Parents may detect this by noticing that a girl's skirt hangs unevenly or bra straps are uneven. Parents may need to be cautioned that vomiting or a headache in the morning that passes fairly quickly (at about the same time the school bus leaves) may be a symptom of school phobia, but a physical examination is in order because these are also symptoms of other conditions. Absence seizures, a neurologic condition that typically arises in the school-age years, can be confused with behavior problems if observation is not thorough (see Chapter 49). Attention deficit hyperactivity disorder (ADHD) (see Chapter 54) can also lead to behavior or inattention disorders.

Problems Associated With Language Development

The common speech problem of the preschool years is broken fluency; the most common problem of a school-age child is articulation. The child has difficulty pronouncing s, z, th, l, r, and w or substitutes w for r ("westroom" instead of "restroom") or r for l ("radies' room" instead of "ladies' room"). This is most noticeable during the first and second grades; it usually disappears by the third grade. Unless it persists, speech therapy for this normal developmental stage is not necessary.

Common Fears and Anxieties of a School-Age Child

School-age children are old enough to experience adult reactions to problems at home or school.

Anxiety Related to Beginning School

Adjusting to grade school is a big task for 6-year-olds (AAP, Council on Early Childhood, Council on School Health, 2016). Even if they attended preschool, grade school is different: The rules are firmer, and the elective feeling (e.g., "If I don't like it, I can quit") no longer applies. School is for keeps until age 16 years or longer, a time span too long for a young child to even imagine. Also, where preschool learning was carried out through fun activities, part of every day in grade school involves obvious work (Box 32.5 shows an interprofessional care map for a child with school concerns). Some instances of anxiety may be a reflection of a parent's anxiety (Pass, Arteche, Cooper, et al., 2012).

Because school requires an adjustment, a health assessment of all school-age children should include an inquiry about progress in school by a question such as "How is Shelly doing in school?" followed by a second question "How does her teacher say she is doing?" If there is a discrepancy between those two answers, the situation bears study. Some parents may have to alter their expectations of how much their child should be achieving to conform to their child's actual ability. This can obviously be difficult.

One of the biggest tasks of the first year of school is learning to read. It is best if parents have prepared children for this by reading to them since infancy, pointing to the words and pictures as they read. This helps children realize that sentences flow from left to right and that the words, not the pictures, tell the story. Box 32.6 offers some useful hints to help parents encourage reading in their young school-age child.

Many first graders are capable of mature action at school but appear less mature when they return home. They may bite their fingernails, suck their thumb, or talk baby talk. Some develop tics (irregular movements of isolated muscle groups), such as wrinkling the forehead, shrugging the shoulders, clearing the throat, or frequently blinking. Such movements may occasionally be confused with seizure activity. Tics, however, disappear during sleep and occur mainly when the child is subjected to stress or anxiety. Scolding, nagging, threatening, or punishing does not stop either tics or nail biting and invariably makes these problems worse. Methods such as using bad-flavored nail polish and restraining the child's hands to prevent nail biting are also ineffective.

These behaviors stop when the underlying stress is discovered and alleviated. Urge parents to spend some time with the child after school or in the evening so the child continues to feel secure in the family and does not feel pushed out by being sent to school. If such behavior manifestations persist despite attempts to eliminate their cause, the family might

BOX 32.5

Nursing Care Planning

AN INTERPROFESSIONAL CARE MAP FOR A SCHOOL-AGE CHILD BEGINNING MIDDLE SCHOOL

Shelly Lewis is an 11-year-old girl who recently started middle school. Her mother tells you that, although Shelly, who is overweight, says she likes school and wants to try out for cheerleading, she has developed a lot of nervous habits such as nail biting since school started.

Family Assessment: Child lives with mother, stepfather, and three younger stepsisters in a four-bedroom home. Family owns a boarding kennel for dogs; both parents work full-time at business. Mother describes finances as "Okay. It's hard with a big family."

Patient Assessment Child: Child has been "chubby" since preschool. States she likes to read rather than play sports. Is in seventh grade (age appropriate). Observed to be restless in chair during conversation with mother about the new school. Mother states, "Her sisters have no trouble with change; she always does. Don't you think if she lost weight she'd fit in better?"

Nursing Diagnosis: Anxiety related to beginning a new school.

Outcome Criteria: Child states she feels more comfortable with new school setting; nail biting has decreased in intensity; child agrees to begin weight-reduction program.

Team Member Responsible	Assessment	Intervention	Rationale	Expected Outcome
Activities of Daily Living, Including Safety				
Nurse	Assess what activities patient enjoys.	Review with patient the advantages of participating in activities that involve more exercise than reading. Support cheerleading; suggest walking with a friend.	Effective weight reduction calls for increased exercise. Books on tape can supply reading enjoyment while walking.	Child states she will try some active activity for at least 20 minutes each day.
Teamwork and Collaboration				
Nurse/nurse practitioner	Assess if child would be interested in a weight-reduction class at the health center.	Suggest different options available such as a weight-loss group or a commercial weight-reduction program.	Children respond well to group activities. Other group members supply friendship as well as increase motivation.	Child states whether she would like to join a weight-reduction group.
Procedures/Medications for Quality Improvement				
Nurse	Ask child to try to identify if she feels something is upsetting about the new school; if so, ask what it is.	Help child "walk through" a day at school and discuss how small changes could affect her fitting in to school.	Talking with the child allows her to share feelings and concerns openly and safely, possibly increasing her awareness of them and their impact on her.	Child describes a typical day and points she would like to see change.
Nutrition				
Nurse/nutritionist	Assess child's intake by 24-hour recall history.	Review with child changes that would reduce calories, yet maintain her lifestyle.	Eleven-year-old children are old enough to take responsibility for what and when they eat.	Patient reviews her dietary intake and makes at least three suggestions on things she will attempt to change.
Patient-Centered Care				
Nurse	Assess if family members appreciate the stress a new school setting can create.	Review with mother and child ways to reduce stress when encountering new situations, such as equating them with something already known.	It is easy for parents to view 11-year-olds as able to handle new situations better than they can because of pseudomaturity.	Mother states she may have been taking the change in school too lightly and agrees to offer more support.

Continued on following page

BOX 32.5

Nursing Care Planning (continued)

Team Member Responsible	Assessment	Intervention	Rationale	Expected Outcome
Psychosocial/Spiritual/Emotional Needs				
Nurse/nurse practitioner	Assess family functioning with child's mother.	Stress that all children are individuals and what works for her stepsisters may not work for the patient.	Being constantly compared to siblings can create feelings of low self-esteem, which can lead to difficulty solving problems.	Mother states she will try to reduce comparisons to stepsisters to help reduce stress at home.
Informatics for Seamless Healthcare Planning				
Nurse	Assess if child or mother thinks an early follow-up appointment would be helpful.	Arrange for a follow-up clinic appointment within 1 month with the mother and daughter if desired.	It is difficult for a family to make internal changes if they are too emotionally involved to be objective.	Mother and child express their preferences based on their future plans.

benefit from formal counseling, cognitive behavioral therapy, and possibly pharmacology support for the child (Pringsheim, Doja, Gorman, et al., 2012).

School Refusal or Phobia

School refusal is a fear of attending school. It is a type of "social phobia" similar to agoraphobia (fear of going outside

BOX 32.6

Nursing Care Planning to Respect Cultural Diversity

With the activities of children in modern cultures turning more toward electronic games than opening books, reading for pleasure is threatened with becoming a lost art. A number of tips for making reading more enjoyable and increase cultural understanding for children include:

- Read books yourself to set an example so your child thinks of reading as an adult activity. If you spend most of your free time watching television, your child will think reading is mainly for children and assume that it is not important.
- Make reading more fun by encouraging your child to make practical use of what he or she reads. Ask the child to read culturally different recipes while you cook or to read road signs during a car trip.
- Play a treasure hunt game where you hide a small object, such as a favorite toy, and then write simple clues on slips of paper: "Look under a lamp," "Look in a book," and so on until your child has been led to the hidden object. Your child can develop writing skills by playing the same game for you to follow.
- Suggest to relatives that a gift certificate from a bookstore would be a good present. Let your child browse the store to select the book.
- Talk about books the child has read—what was good, what was bad, or what the child learned while reading.
- Read a book together as a bedtime family activity.

the home) or separation anxiety disorder (SAD). Children who resist attending school this way develop physical signs of illness, such as vomiting, diarrhea, headache, or abdominal pain on school days. This lasts until after the school bus has left or the child is given permission to stay home for the day.

A particular child may be reacting to a situation such as a harsh teacher, having to shower in gym class, or facing a class bully every day. In these instances, counseling may help the child manage the situation better. School refusal may also occur if the child is overly dependent on the parents or may be reluctant to leave home because of worry that younger siblings will usurp the parents' affection. The anxiety of separation may also result because the parent is overprotective of the child or is the one having the most difficulty separating.

Because the problem of school refusal is usually only partly the child's, the entire family generally requires counseling to resolve the issue. As a rule, once it has been established that the child is free of any illness and the resistance stems from separation anxiety or phobia, the child should be made to attend school. Reinforcement by parents to go to school this way helps to prevent problems such as school failure, peer ridicule, or a pattern of avoiding difficulties. Some children may benefit from a gradual program of school involvement, such as walking to school but not going in for one day, then going to school but staying for only 1 hour the next day, then staying for half a day, and so on until the child can stay all day every day. Give support to parents so they can matter-of-factly treat the child's illness symptoms (a great deal of reassurance that these symptoms are not major will be necessary) so they can take the child firmly to the bus or to the classroom.

Managing school refusal requires coordination among the school, the school nurse, and the healthcare provider who identifies the problem. A nurse is the ideal person to coordinate such efforts and to help parents allow the child some independence not only in going to school but also in other activities. A few children have such difficulty that they require formal counseling and pharmacologic therapy to overcome school refusal (Scheffer, 2011).

What If . . . 32.3

Shelly's mother tells the nurse that the many nervous habits she began since starting middle school are increasing. What suggestions would the nurse make to her mother regarding this?

Homeschooling

Because of religious or personal preference or because of disillusionment with the school system, a growing number of children are homeschooled today (Anthony & Burroughs, 2010). Because their main contact has been with well-educated parents at home, the vocabulary of homeschooled children may be advanced or may suggest they are older than their actual age. When discussing homeschooling with parents, assess if children have peer experiences, perhaps through participation in community sports teams or clubs. Ask if they receive exposure to other cultures or families, so they can better adjust to people different from themselves later on at college or at a job.

Children Who Spend Time Independently

Children whose parents both work outside the home may spend time alone without adult supervision for a part of each weekday. Such children have become a prominent concern because, in as many as 90% of families today in the United States, both parents work at least part time outside of the home. Few parents have work hours so flexible that they can always be at home when a child leaves for or returns from school. Extended family members who once watched children after school are often working as well or may no longer be close at hand; many communities are no longer close-knit enough to have neighbors who can be depended on to help out with informal child care.

A major concern of children staying home alone is that they will experience an increased number of unintentional injuries, delinquent behavior, alcohol or substance abuse, or decreased school performance from a lack of adult supervision. For children who are responsible and feel safe in their community, however, a short period of independence every day may actually be beneficial because it encourages problem solving in self-care (Mack, Dellinger, & West, 2012).

Suggestions for parents whose children must spend time alone before or after school are shown in Box 32.7. Many communities and schools offer special after-school programs so children do not have to be home alone. Nurses are in a position to educate parents about such services so their children can feel both safe and stimulated creatively during this time. Both Boy and Girl Scouts, the Boys & Girls Clubs of America, and Camp Fire USA are examples of organizations that offer programs in many neighborhoods to help children adjust to being home alone. Many communities also organize hotline numbers that a child who is alone can call if a problem arises. At health visits, assess whether parents and a child appear to have a concern with or are uncomfortable about after-school arrangements. For a child who is extremely fearful or impulsive or who finds problem solving difficult, time alone after school may not be appropriate. Determine the individual circumstances and recommend changes as appropriate. State laws vary as to when children can provide self-supervision.

Sex Education

It is important that school-age children be educated about pubertal changes and responsible sexual practices. Also, preteens should have adults they can turn to for answers to questions about sex. Ideally, these should be their parents, but because sex is an emotionally charged topic, some parents may be extremely uncomfortable discussing it with their children. As a result, healthcare personnel often become resource persons.

It's best if sex education is incorporated into health education classes throughout the school years in a manner that is appropriate to age and development. Topics to teach and discuss in a sex education course for both preadolescent boys and girls include:

- Reproductive organ function and physiology of reproduction, so children understand what menstruation is and why it occurs
- Secondary sexual characteristics, so children will understand what is happening in their bodies
- Male sexual functioning, including why the production of increased amounts of seminal fluid leads to nocturnal emissions
- The physiology of pregnancy and the possibility for unintended pregnancies, which will come with sexual maturity
- Responsibilities of sexual maturity
- Reproductive life planning measures and the principles of safer sex if appropriate to the cultural setting (see Chapters 5 and 6). Sexual orientation questions and concerns may arise at this time, and questions should be addressed honestly and openly.

Lesbian, gay, bisexual, and transgender (LGBT) youth may not obtain the same levels of care due to fear of discrimination. They may choose not to disclose their sexual orientation or gender identity to healthcare providers or they may avoid care completely. Nurses can take steps to improve health outcomes for LGBT youth by providing care that is affirming and inclusive (Hadland, Yehia, & Makadon, 2016).

A sex education course that includes films and discussions is helpful for preadolescents but never answers all of a preteen's questions (most youngsters would rather avoid asking a question than risk appearing ignorant in front of their peers in such a setting). Using an anonymous question box is one method to address questions and lessens the embarrassment that may occur with more a more public forum of asking questions. Urge parents or other health educators to watch films or read booklets with children to show they are truly available to answer questions.

Stealing

During early school age, most children go through a period during which they steal loose change from their mother's purse or father's dresser. This usually happens at around 7 years of age, when children first learn how to make change and also discover the importance of money. Stealing occurs because, although a child is gaining an appreciation for money, this appreciation is not yet balanced by strong moral principles or an understanding of ownership.

Parents should explore the reason for the stealing, including:

- Do other children on the block receive an allowance and so have money for small items?
- Did their child make a bet that must be paid?

BOX 32.7

Nursing Care Planning to Empower a Family

TIPS FOR CHILDREN WHO SPEND TIME INDEPENDENTLY AND THEIR PARENTS

Q. Shelly stays by herself after school for a half hour each week day. Her mother asks you, "What are good tips for being sure it's safe to let her do that?"

A. Think in a number of areas:

Safety Points for Children

Always lock doors and never show keys to others or indicate you stay home alone.

When answering the telephone, say a parent is busy, not absent from home.

Have a plan in the event you lose your key (e.g., stay with a neighbor).

Don't go into the house if the door is open or a window is broken.

Learn fire safety (practice a fire drill from all rooms of the house).

Check in with parents by telephone or laptop when you first arrive home.

Identify a caller before opening the door. Agree on a secret code word; you should not open the door or go with a person unless the person knows the word.

Learn how to change light bulbs safely if it will be dark before parents return home. If appropriate, learn how to change fuses or reset circuit breaker switches.

Learn how to report a fire and telephone police (practice this with your parents).

Safety Responsibilities for Parents

Prepare a safety kit with bandages and such; include a flashlight in case of a power failure so children do not need to light candles.

Plan after-school snacks that do not require cooking to prevent burns.

Keep firearms locked, with the key in a place unknown to child.

Keep a list of emergency telephone numbers (including parents' work numbers) by the telephone.

Arrange with a neighbor who is usually home during the late afternoon for the child to stay there in an emergency.

If an older child will be watching a younger one, be certain both children understand the rules laid down and the degree of responsibility expected.

Be certain the child understands the rules that apply during other times also apply during independent time (e.g., never swim alone, do not play by the railroad tracks).

Parental Actions to Prevent Loneliness

Leave messages on the refrigerator or in the bathroom that just say "hi."

Leave a tape- or video-recorded message for the child to play when he or she first arrives home (make sure it is not full of tasks to do but is a welcoming message).

Be certain to make parent–child time available after work to allow for quality relationship time.

Each morning, help the child plan an activity for that day so he or she has something purposeful to look forward to during the time alone.

Allow special privileges such as listening to music other members of the family do not like; consider allowing extra television hours during this time.

Consider getting a pet. Even a caged animal, such as a hamster or a bird, offers companionship in a quiet house.

Call the child if there will be a delay in arriving home; unexpected time alone is very frightening.

Encourage the child to read; fictional characters can serve as friends as well as help to pass time.

Urge the child to network with other children who spend time alone as to how they use time effectively; talking on the telephone or e-mailing another child reduces loneliness for both.

Parental Actions to Increase Socialization

Help the child plan after-school activities such as joining a science club for one afternoon a week.

Explore sports programs at school or in the community because these often are held after school.

Explore after-school programs at the school the child attends, or at a public library, a church, or a temple.

Network with other parents or ask for flex time so child supervision can be alternated after school.

Be certain the child has opportunities to socialize with friends on weekends or on days when either parent is home.

Parental Actions to Increase Self-Esteem

Praise the child for the ability to take care of himself or herself for short time intervals (e.g., rather than scold him or her that there are cracker crumbs on the carpet).

Walk with the child through the empty house and together identify sounds (e.g., the click of the furnace turning on, the refrigerator starting to defrost), so they can determine the cause of sounds when home alone and not be frightened.

Help the child to view the quiet as a beneficial time in which they can do some things more efficiently, such as homework, than at noisy times.

Do not allow the child to use their time alone role to provoke parental guilt. Allow children to have some say in family spending so they can see how their time alone (which allows both parents to work) contributes to family unity and progress.

- Is a child buying a bully's friendship by purchasing gum or candy for that child?
- Does a child need more security and view money as security?

As a rule, early childhood stealing is best handled without a great deal of emotion. A parent should tell the child the money is missing. The importance of property rights should be reviewed: Mother's and father's money is theirs, the child's money is the child's, and they are not interchangeable. Youngsters who continue to steal past 8 years of age may require counseling because they should have progressed beyond this normal developmental step by this age (Sourander, Fossum, Rønning, et al., 2012).

Some shoplifting occurs with early school-age children, but the major problem with this arises during preadolescence. Some of this happens for the same reason that past generations tipped over outhouses or untied the preacher's horse and buggy: It is a public act of rebellion against authority, a "coming of age" ritual. It usually occurs because of peer pressure such as when children believe they must have a certain type of clothing to belong to the "in" crowd. It can also be an initiation ritual for gang membership.

Shoplifting must be taken seriously by parents because it is a punishable crime, not a prank. Just as money missing from a purse should not be ignored, shoplifting should be confronted immediately to prevent children who succeed once from taking something even bigger the second time. Children should be asked how they came to possess the article and they should not be allowed to use it. Children should then be denied access to stores until they demonstrate more responsibility. A child who shoplifts more than once may need counseling because it reflects more than simple confusion about property rights.

As an overall principle, parents should set good examples if they expect their child to be honest. If one parent takes money from the other without permission, neither should be surprised to find their child attempting to do the same. If a parent unwraps items and eats them without paying for them in the supermarket, a parent cannot expect a child to do otherwise.

Violence or Terrorism

Children basically view their world as safe, so it is a shock when violence such as a school shooting or reports of terrorists enter their lives (Dowdell, 2012). Common recommendations for parents to help children feel safe when they hear of these instances include:

- Assure children they are safe; even if the violence is in their community, their parents are actively involved in being certain they are not in danger.
- Observe for signs of stress such as sleep disturbances, fatigue, lack of pleasure in activities, or signs of beginning substance abuse.
- Do not allow children or adolescents to view footage of traumatic events over and over because this decreases their ability to feel safe.
- Watch news programs with children so it can be explained that the situation portrayed is not near them and that their child is safe.
- Explain that there are bad people in the world, and bad people do bad things, but not all people in a particular group or who look a particular way are bad. Lashing out at people who resemble them only causes more harm.

- Prepare a family disaster plan, including such things as bottled water, blankets, toiletries, pet supplies, appropriate clothing, flashlights, and information such as what immunizations their children have had (particularly tetanus) and, if a child is ill, a history of medical needs or care so that such items are ready in an emergency.
- Designate a "rally point" where the family will meet if ever separated by a disaster or evacuation (AAP, 2012b).

Some parents may be reluctant to talk to their children about a disaster plan for the family, believing that these preparations will frighten children unnecessarily, but such preparations should have the major effect of increasing a feeling of safety, not decreasing it. Fear of the unknown is always more intense than a fear of something tangible.

Bullying

A frequent reason school-age children cite for feeling so unhappy that they turn guns on classmates or commit suicide is because they were ridiculed or bullied to the point they could no longer take such abuse (Cooper, Clements, & Holt, 2012). Alert parents that Internet or texting bullying are both also possible and that a bully doesn't have to be in fact-to-face contact with their child to be harmful (D'Auria, 2014).

Traits commonly associated with school-age bullies include:
- Advanced physical size and strength for their age
- Aggressive temperament (both male and female)
- Parents who are indifferent to the problem or are permissive with an aggressive child
- Parents who typically resort to physical punishment
- There is the presence of a child who is a "natural victim" (e.g., small, insecure, with low self-esteem).

Bullying can be done face to face or through social media and/or texting. Suggestions for school personnel to deal with bullies include:
- Supervise recreation periods closely.
- Intervene immediately to stop bullying.
- Insist if such behavior does not stop, both the school and parents will become involved.
- Advise parents to discuss bullying with their school-age child and help them understand that it should be reported to allow adults to intervene.
- Parents should monitor their child's social media and texting interactions.

If bullying behavior is ingrained, therapy may be needed to correct the behavior. Stopping bullying helps not only the victim but also the bully because statistics show that children with this type of aggressive behavior in grade school are more apt to be incarcerated as adults than others (AAP, 2012a).

Recreational Drug Use

Once considered a college or high school problem, illegal drugs such as marijuana, cocaine, and amphetamines are now available to children as early as elementary school and certainly by the time they reach the seventh and eighth grades. Because they are available in so many homes, alcohol, inhalants, and prescription drugs have also become commonly abused by this age group (Blake & Davis, 2011; Young, Glover, & Havens, 2012). Parents should be particularly aware of children who may be taking adult antidepressant drugs from home medicine cabinets because this is associated with suicide in young children (Adegbite-Adeniyi, Gron, Rowles, et al., 2012).

The use of hard drugs and alcohol and ways to encourage children to avoid their use are discussed in Chapter 33. Inhalants, which are easily available to school-age children for abuse, include airplane glue (toluene) and aerosolized cooking oil. Children do not become physically addicted to glue but do become psychologically dependent on it. To achieve the desired effect, they drop quantities of the glue into a paper bag and then sniff the fumes to experience a feeling of exhilaration or giddiness. This may seem like a harmless procedure, but, in high concentrations, glue fumes can cause extensive liver damage or enough pulmonary edema to be fatal. Cooking spray or computer keyboard cleaner gives this same effect. Because these products contain Freon, they can cause severe respiratory and cardiac irregularity (Baydala, 2010).

Children who report being happy and are able to communicate with their family are less likely to be regular users than others (Farmer & Hanratty, 2012). Parents should suspect recreational drug use if their child regularly appears irritable, inattentive, or drowsy.

Abuse of androgenic steroids or human growth hormone to enhance sports performance are yet other drugs that can be found in preteen children. Counsel children against this because abuse of steroids can lead to cardiovascular irregularities, uncontrollable aggressiveness, and possible cancer in later life (Oberlander & Henderson, 2012).

Cigarette smoking also begins in school-age children. With the sure knowledge that cigarette smoking plays a large part in the development of lung cancer and other serious respiratory illnesses, many parents assume their children will know better than to begin smoking. Smoking is viewed as an adult activity, however, so adopting the habit can be considered a giant step on the road to adulthood. Although the amount of cigarette advertising targeting young people as consumers has decreased, school-age children should still be taught to recognize advertising manipulation aimed at them. Caution children against experimenting with smokeless tobacco as well because this can lead to mouth and throat cancer, the same as smoking (Kamboj, Spiller, Casavant, et al., 2016). The use of e-cigarettes and vaping has increased, and the health risks of these products are still being uncovered (Duderstadt, 2015).

To discourage use of tobacco by school-age children, healthcare professionals and parents need to be role models of excellent nonsmoking health behavior in hope that children will follow their good examples.

QSEN Checkpoint Question 32.6

PATIENT-CENTERED CARE

The school-age period is the time when many young people begin smoking. To design interventions that are effective and patient-centered, the nurse should begin by acknowledging which of the following?

a. Most children who try smoking do not like it.
b. The media have occasionally exaggerated the risks of smoking.
c. Many people view smoking as being an "adult" activity.
d. Children under puberty cannot become addicted to smoking.

Look in Appendix A for the best answer and rationale.

CONCERNS OF THE SCHOOL-AGE CHILD AND FAMILY WITH UNIQUE NEEDS

A number of situations cause school-age children to have additional needs or concerns.

The Child of Alcoholic Parents

Children who live with an alcoholic parent are at greater risk for having emotional problems than others because of the frequent disruption in their lives (Allen, Garcia-Huidobro, Porta, et al., 2016). In addition, because alcoholism may have a genetic base, children of alcoholics may be more likely to become alcoholics as adults. This makes it imperative for such children to learn effective coping behaviors. Immediate problems that can occur with children of alcoholic parents include:

- A feeling of guilt that they are the cause of the parent's drinking
- Constant worry that the alcoholic parent will become sick or die, leaving the child alone; at the same time, the child may fear the alcoholic parent and wish the parent would leave
- A feeling of shame that prevents the child from inviting friends home or asking for help
- Decreased ability to trust adults because the parent has been unreliable so many times
- Poor nutrition and decreasing grades in school because the alcoholic parent's behavior is so erratic that no regular schedule of bedtime or meals exists
- Anger at the alcoholic parent for drinking and at the non-alcoholic parent for not doing more to correct things
- Helplessness to change the situation

Such fears may be revealed by not only failing marks in school but also withdrawal from friends or social activities and delinquent behavior such as stealing. With adolescence may come depression, suicidal thoughts, or abuse of drugs or alcohol. School nurses are in an excellent position to identify such children, monitor their school progress, and refer them to organizations such as Al-Anon or Alateen (www.al-anon.alateen.org) for support.

The Child With a Long-Term Illness or Physical Cognitive Challenge

One of the biggest problems facing school-age children with a long-term illness or physical challenges is time lost from school. This threatens not only their academic achievement but also their relationships with peers because it may make the child the "odd person out" with respect to making friends or joining clubs. Whether children are on home care or hospitalized, helping them to keep in contact with friends by texting, e-mail, or letters can help foster the socialization that is so important for continued development. Keeping up with schooling, whether it is homeschool or a distant learning option, is also important and an area where school nurses can play an important role (AAP, Council on School Health, 2016; Singer, 2013).

If at all possible, children with physical or cognitive challenges should attend regular schools and classes (inclusion) based on federal law (Public Law 99-457), which stipulates that all children have the right to equal education in the least restrictive environment possible (Sass-Lehrer & Bodner-Johnson,

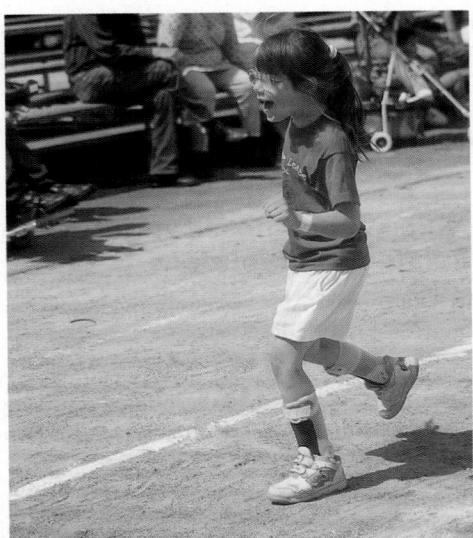

Figure 32.10 A school-age child who is physically challenged is elated at a finish line. This accomplishment can go far toward her developing a sense of industry. (© Jose Carillo/Stock Boston.)

1989). The decision as to which classroom would be best for an individual child is determined by a committee in each school system. You may need to advocate for a child with such a committee to demonstrate, for example, that although a child uses a wheelchair or needs continuous oxygen, the child will be able to contribute to regular classroom activities. It may be necessary to meet with a school nurse, teacher, or the child's classmates (with the parents' permission) to increase their understanding and acceptance of a child's illness or to help arrange a period each day with a special resource teacher.

Urge parents of children with physical or cognitive challenges to assign them household chores just like other children and to allow them to participate in peer activities, such as Girl or Boy Scouts, in which accomplishment is encouraged. It is important for such children to develop a sense of industry or accomplishment so they can persevere in measures that will help them to be as independent as possible in the future (Fig. 32.10).

When you are caring for a school-age child who is chronically ill or physically challenged, choose short-term activities that can be completed independently, as with all school-age children. Conversely, be careful not to insult a child with tasks that are obviously not age appropriate. Table 32.5 describes some nursing actions to help foster a sense of industry in children who are physically challenged or chronically ill.

Nutrition and the School-Age Child With a Challenge

Food preparation and washing the dishes are times for socializing in most households. A school-age child who cannot be involved in these activities because of a physical challenge may need extra time during the day to make up for these lost socializing experiences, such as a specific hour set aside for talking or sharing a project that can be accomplished in one sitting.

When eating in cafeterias or at a friend's home, children who must eat special diets are usually tempted to select the same food as everyone else rather than limit what they choose.

TABLE 32.5 NURSING ACTIONS THAT ENCOURAGE A SENSE OF INDUSTRY IN THE PHYSICALLY CHALLENGED OR CHRONICALLY ILL SCHOOL-AGE CHILD

Category	Actions
Nutrition	Allow choices of food when possible and respect food preferences.
	Provide small food servings that child can finish, which encourages a sense of accomplishment.
Dressing	Ask for suggestions as to how bulky the child wants the dressing and where to apply tape.
Medicine	Teach the child the name and action of medicine.
	Encourage the child to keep track of medication times by clock or record.
	The child may feel more in control of injections or intravenous insertions if allowed to choose the site from among options offered.
	Allow the child to choose oral medicine form (capsules or liquid) if possible.
Rest	Establish clear rules for rest periods (e.g., reading or watching television is all right; playing a game is not).
Hygiene	Respect the modesty of a school-age child at an adult level.
	Allow as much choice as possible such as own clothing and timing of self-care.
Pain	Encourage the child to express and rate pain.
	Encourage the child to use distraction techniques, such as counting backward from 100 or imagery, during episodes of pain.
	Explain the source and cause of pain to give the child sense of mastery.
Stimulation	Encourage school work.
	Encourage activities that end in a product (e.g., putting together a picture puzzle rather than listening to a CD).
	Encourage paper-and-pencil games, such as connect the dots or tic-tac-toe.
	Card games provide social interaction and also encourage simple addition skills (make a deck from paper if one is not available).
	Don't suggest competitive games for children younger than age 10 years.
	Encourage using the playroom for socialization.
	Encourage the child to keep in contact with school friends by texting or e-mailing them.

They may decline invitations rather than admit to requiring a special diet or needing help with eating. Ask at healthcare visits if any of these problems are present. Help children with special diets to plan ways they could be comfortable in social food-based settings such as bringing a party snack that is appropriate and can be easily eaten, or how to politely decline particular foods. Help children who are hospitalized to select a diet that is enjoyable as well as nutritious.

The Child Who Is Overweight or Obese

In some communities, as many as 50% of school-age children are obese by body mass index guidelines. Some of these children have been overweight since infancy, and the natural prepubertal weight gain makes them become obese. Children with an endomorphic build (a natural tendency to accumulate body fat) are more likely to be obese at any time in life than those with a mesomorphic (normal) or ectomorphic (slender) build. Many families rely on fast-food meals several times a week, and such foods tend to be high in calories and fat and can lead to obesity. The lack of nutritional food in school lunches and the availability of foods of poor nutritional values available in vending machines compound the problem. Children of obese parents are also more apt to become obese, probably related to both genetic and environmental influences (E. Robinson & Sutin, 2016).

By preteen years, children who are obese begin to develop many of the same health problems as adults who are obese, such as hypertension, type 2 diabetes, and an elevated total cholesterol level, with possible atherosclerosis. They also may be ridiculed or bullied for their size and may be unable to participate on sports teams. This is strong evidence of the need for active measures to help preteens regulate their weight (Schantz, 2012). Children are influenced by promotional advertisements that influence food selection (Emond, Smith, Mathur, et al., 2015)

Those who become so obese that friends leave them out of activities or they cannot play sports because they tire so quickly may develop such a poor self-image they have little motivation for self-improvement. The type of weight-reduction program that will probably work best is one that emphasizes long-term lifestyle changes and contains features such as:

- An intake of about 1,200 calories a day (no more than 30% as fat), with lifestyle changes such as a structured family meal, eliminating eating or snacking in front of the television, decreasing portion sizes, and eliminating sugar-rich drinks.
- An active exercise program, including monitoring and limiting time spent in physical inactivity (e.g., watching television, playing computer and video games, surfing the Internet, texting).
- A counseling program to discuss aspects such as self-image and motivation to reduce weight.

Total caloric intake should not be reduced too drastically in children because they need calories to form new body tissue for continued growth. Caution children not to try faddish high-protein diets (as most adults should not) because such diets do not supply enough carbohydrates and may produce a heavy renal solute load (the breakdown product of proteins) to the kidneys. It helps if children aim to lose 5 lb over a short time rather than 50 lb over a year. This short-term goal coincides better with the task of developing industry.

Surgical techniques such as an intestinal bypass or lap band surgery are obviously extreme measures and inappropriate for children. Children who are obese might request one, however, in an attempt to avoid the not insignificant difficulty of long-term weight loss.

 ## Nursing Diagnoses and Related Interventions

Nursing Diagnosis: Altered family dynamics related to lack of motivation to reduce weight

Outcome Evaluation: Child states reasonable weight loss and exercise goals; discusses feelings about being overweight and reactions from schoolmates; expresses positive feelings about self-worth.

Motivating preteens to lose weight can be very difficult because they are not concerned when told that people who are obese do not live as long as average weight persons or that they have more heart attacks because this will happen so far in the future. They do, however, have a great respect for adults who are sympathetic to their problems. They follow better dietary regimens, therefore, if they are asked to do so by a respected adult, such as a nurse, or if they fear being left out of social interactions.

Overweight school-age children often do well if a healthy eating club is formed; they are not too young to participate in formal weight-control organizations. Having tangible support from other group members helps them follow tedious and monotonous nutrition patterns. As a way of increasing daily activity, preadolescents do well with formal exercise classes because, again, they enjoy the support from other children. In addition, encourage them to increase informal exercise, such as walking to and from school or walking a dog. Encourage coaches of childhood sports to accept children who are obese as part of a team, not because the child will necessarily benefit the team but because the exercise will benefit the child. Not only does exercise burn up calories but also if children's daylight hours are filled with activities and friends, they have less time to eat and spend less time in sedentary activities.

Lifestyle change is the ultimate goal for the entire family because obesity is usually a family problem. Rather than preparing special meals for just the child who is obese, the entire family probably needs to eat in a healthier manner. Because preadolescents do not generally prepare their own food, the person in the home who prepares meals requires as much information on the planned weight loss as the child. The old concepts that used to hold ("A clean plate is good" and "How can you leave food when people in other countries are starving?") may have to be changed so children and other family members reduce their intake appropriately. The importance of exercise should also be reflected in the home. Family members should not only encourage the child who is obese to exercise, but they should also partake in some form of daily activity with them. The encouragement of adequate fruit and vegetable consumption is helpful in achieving healthy eating patterns (Herrick, Rossen, Nielsen, et al., 2015).

There is some danger in pointing out to preadolescents that they are overweight because some children can become so obsessed with losing weight that they develop eating disorders (see Chapter 54). Stressing that children should "become healthier" or "improve stamina" may be better advice than talking about losing weight (Field, Sonneville, Micali, et al., 2012).

What If . . . 32.4

The nurse is particularly interested in exploring one of the 2020 National Health Goals with respect to school-age growth and development (see Box 32.1). What would be a possible research topic to explore pertinent to this goal that would be applicable to Shelly's family and that would also advance evidence-based practice?

KEY POINTS FOR REVIEW

■ School-age children mature slowly but steadily. Their average annual weight gain is 3 to 5 lb; their increase in height is 1 to 2 in.

■ At about age 10 years, children begin to develop secondary sex characteristics. Preparation for this helps them accept these changes positively.

■ Deciduous teeth are lost, and permanent teeth erupt during the school-age period.

■ Erikson's developmental task for the school-age period is to gain a sense of industry or how to do things well.

■ Common health problems during the school-age period include minor respiratory and gastrointestinal infections as well as dental caries and malocclusion.

■ Common parental concerns during this period are language development, fears and anxieties, and behavior problems such as stealing and exposure to recreational drugs. Treating preventive strategies regarding these helps in planning nursing care that not only meets QSEN competencies but also best meets a family's total needs.

■ As many as 90% of parents of school-age children are dual-earner families. This means that many school-age children return home before their parents. Counseling families on ways to turn this independent time into a positive experience is helpful.

■ Children in a concrete stage of operational thought are limited to understanding concepts that they can actually see. When health teaching, use concrete examples (actually let them hold a syringe, don't just talk about it) to increase their understanding.

■ School-age children thrive on rules. It is confusing for them when rules are changed (e.g., medicine will now be taken four rather than three times a day) unless they have a clear explanation of why the change is occurring.

■ School-age children look for good adult role models; it is hard for them to feel confidence in an adult who isn't honest with them or who fails to live up to their expectations by not following through on promises.

■ School-age children with a family tendency toward obesity may become overweight. Helping the family learn a healthier lifestyle is important.

CRITICAL THINKING CARE STUDY

Georgia is a 6-year-old girl in the first grade whom you meet when working as a school nurse. She lives with her 10-year-old sister and her parents in a three-bedroom home. Her father works long shifts as a coal miner, and her mother cleans houses for a commercial housecleaning firm.

1. Georgia's mother tells you she received a note from her teacher asking her to help Georgia "speak more clearly." Is this a common concern with early school-age children? What further information do you need to know to evaluate whether this is a concern?

2. Georgia's teacher is also concerned because Georgia does not share well. Is this a developmental step that Georgia should have already mastered?

3. Georgia's mother wants her to be popular and so has enrolled her in dance classes two times per week, a school soccer club four times per week, violin lessons once per week, and a gymnastics class twice per week. Despite all the effort she puts in driving her daughter to all these sessions, the mother tells you Georgia doesn't act grateful. She asks you why Georgia isn't interested in making friends.

RELATED RESOURCES

Explore these additional resources to enhance learning for this chapter:

• Student resources on thePoint, including answers to the What If . . . and Critical Thinking Care Study questions, http://thepoint.lww.com/Flagg8e

• Adaptive learning powered by PrepU, http://thepoint.lww.com/prepu

REFERENCES

Adegbite-Adeniyi, C., Gron, B., Rowles, B. M., et al. (2012). An update on antidepressant use and suicidality in pediatric depression. *Expert Opinion on Pharmacotherapy, 13*(15), 2119–2130.

Allen, M. L., Garcia-Huidobro, D., Porta, C., et al. (2016). Effective parenting interventions to reduce youth substance use: A systematic review. *Pediatrics, 138*(2), e20154425.

American Academy of Pediatrics. (2012a). *Bullying: It's not okay.* Evanston, IL: Author.

American Academy of Pediatrics. (2012b). *Terrorism disaster fact sheet.* Evanston, IL: Author.

American Academy of Pediatrics. (2016). Menstruation in girls and adolescents: Using the menstrual cycle as a vital sign. *Pediatrics, 137*(3), e20154480.

American Academy of Pediatrics, Committee on Practice and Ambulatory Medicine. (2012). *Recommendations for preventive pediatric health care.* Evanston, IL: Author.

American Academy of Pediatrics, Council on Early Childhood, Council on School Health. (2016). The pediatrician's role in optimizing school readiness. *Pediatrics, 138*(3), e20162293.

American Academy of Pediatrics, Council on School Health. (2016). Role of the school nurse in providing school health services. *Pediatrics, 137*(6), e20160852.

Anthony, K. V., & Burroughs, S. (2010). Making the transition from traditional to home schooling: Home school family motivations. *Current Issues in Education, 13*(4), 1–30

Baydala, L. (2010). Inhalant abuse. *Paediatrics & Child Health, 15*(7), 443–454.

Bishop, W. P. (2011). The digestive system. In K. J. Marcdante, R. M. Kliegman, H. B. Jenson, et al. (Eds.), *Nelson essentials of pediatrics* (6th ed., pp. 463–498). Philadelphia, PA: Saunders/Elsevier.

Blake, K., & Davis, V. (2011). Substance abuse. In K. J. Marcdante, R. M. Kliegman, H. B. Jenson, et al. (Eds.), *Nelson essentials of pediatrics* (6th ed., pp. 281–284). Philadelphia, PA: Saunders/Elsevier.

Breuner, C. C., & Mattson, G. (2016). Sexuality education for children and adolescents. *Pediatrics, 138*(2), e20161348.

Chahal, H., Fung, C., Kuhle, S., et al. (2013). Availability and night-time use of electronic entertainment and communication devices are associated with short sleep duration and obesity among Canadian children. *Pediatric Obesity, 8*(1), 42–51.

Cooper, G. D., Clements, P. T., & Holt, K. E. (2012). Examining childhood bullying and adolescent suicide: Implications for school nurses. *The Journal of School Nursing, 28*(4), 275–283.

Currie, D. W., Fields, S. K., Patterson, M. J., et al. (2016). Cheerleading injuries in United States high schools. *Pediatrics, 137*(1), e20152447.

D'Auria, J. P. (2014). Cyberbullying resources for youth and their families. *Journal of Pediatric Health Care, 28*(2), e19–e22.

Dowdell, E. B. (2012). Urban seventh grade students: A report of health risk behaviors and exposure to violence. *Journal of School Nursing, 28*(2), 130–137.

Duderstadt, K. G. (2015). E-cigarettes: Youth and trends in vaping. *Journal of Pediatric Health Care, 29*(6), 555–557.

Eagle, T. F., Sheetz, A., Gurm, R., et al. (2012). Understanding childhood obesity in America: Linkages between household income, community resources, and children's behaviors. *American Heart Journal, 163*(5), 836–843.

Edmonds, D. K. (2012). Puberty and its disorders. In D. K. Edmonds (Ed.), *Dewhurst's textbook of obstetrics & gynaecology* (8th ed., pp. 471–489). Oxford, United Kingdom: Wiley.

Emond, J. A., Smith, M. E., Mathur, S. J., et al. (2015). Children's food and beverage promotion on television to parents. *Pediatrics, 136*(6), 1095–1102.

Erikson, E. H. (1993). *Childhood and society*. New York, NY: W. W. Norton.

Farmer, S., & Hanratty, B. (2012). The relationship between subjective wellbeing, low income and substance use among schoolchildren in the north west of England: A cross-sectional study. *Journal of Public Health (Oxford), 34*(4), 512–522.

Field, A. E., Sonneville, K. R., Micali, N., et al. (2012). Prospective association of common eating disorders and adverse outcomes. *Pediatrics, 130*(2), e289–e295.

Fletcher, N. D., & Bruce, R. W. (2012). Early onset scoliosis: Current concepts and controversies. *Current Reviews in Musculoskeletal Medicine, 5*(2), 102–110.

Gunter, K. B., Almstedt, H. C., & Janz, K. F. (2012). Physical activity in childhood may be the key to optimizing lifespan skeletal health. *Exercise & Sport Science Reviews, 40*(1), 13–21.

Hadland, S. E., Yehia, B. R., & Makadon, H. J. (2016). Caring for lesbian, gay, bisexual, transgender, and questioning youth in inclusive and affirmative environments. *Pediatric Clinic of North America, 63*, 955–969.

Hamdan, A. M., Singh, V., & Rock, W. P. (2012). Assessment of the relationship between perceptions of dental aesthetics and demand for orthodontic treatment in 10–11 year old school children in Birmingham, UK. *Community Dental Health, 29*(1), 124–128.

Heron, M. (2012). Deaths: Leading causes. *National Vital Statistics Reports, 60*(6), 1–90.

Herrick, K. A., Rossen, L. M., Nielsen, S. J., et al. (2015). Fruit consumption by youth in the United States. *Pediatrics, 136*(4), 664–671.

Hirschman, J., & Chriqui, J. F. (2012). School food and nutrition policy, monitoring and evaluation in the USA. *Public Health Nutrition, 25*(9), 1–7.

Kamboj, A., Spiller, H. A., Casavant, M. J., et al. (2016). Pediatric exposure to e-cigarettes, nicotine, and tobacco products in the United States. *Pediatrics, 137*(6), e20160041.

Kistner, F., Fiebert, I., & Roach, K. (2012). Effect of backpack load carriage on cervical posture in primary schoolchildren. *Work, 41*(1), 99–108.

Kohlberg, L. (1984). *The psychology of moral development*. New York, NY: Harper & Row.

Loke, I. C., Heyman, G. D., Forgie, J., et al. (2011). Children's moral evaluations of reporting the transgressions of peers: Age differences in evaluations of tattling. *Developmental Psychology, 47*(6), 1757–1762.

Lowe, S. R., Godoy, L., Rhodes, J. E., et al. (2013). Predicting mothers' reports of children's mental health three years after hurricane Katrina. *Journal of Applied Developmental Psychology, 34*(1), 17–27.

Mack, K. A., Dellinger, A., & West, B. A. (2012). Adult opinions about the age at which children can be left home alone, bathe alone, or bike alone: Second Injury Control and Risk Survey (ICARIS-2). *Journal of Safety Research, 43*(3), 223–226.

Massignan, C., Cardoso, M., Poporatti, A. L., et al. (2016). Signs and symptoms of primary tooth eruption: A meta-analysis. *Pediatrics, 137*(3), e20153501.

Meng, M. V., & Tanagho, E. A. (2013). Physical examination of the urinary tract. In J. McAninch & T. F. Lue (Eds.), *Smith & Tanagho's general urology* (18th ed., pp. 41–47). New York, NY: McGraw-Hill.

Oberlander, J. G., & Henderson, L. P. (2012). The Sturm und Drang of anabolic steroid use: Angst, anxiety, and aggression. *Trends in Neurosciences, 35*(6), 382–392.

Olson, K. R., Durwood, L., DeMeules, M., et al. (2015). Mental health of transgender children who are supported in their identities. *Pediatrics, 137*(3), e20153223.

Pass, L., Arteche, A., Cooper, P., et al. (2012). Doll play narratives about starting school in children of socially anxious mothers, and their relation to subsequent child school-based anxiety. *Journal of Abnormal Child Psychology, 40*(8), 1375–1384.

Piaget, J. (1969). *The theory of stages in cognitive development*. New York, NY: McGraw-Hill.

Pringsheim, T., Doja, A., Gorman, D., et al. (2012). Canadian guidelines for the evidence-based treatment of tic disorders: Pharmacotherapy. *Canadian Journal of Psychiatry, 57*(3), 133–143.

Robinson, E., & Sutin, A. R. (2016). Parental perception of weight status and weight gain across childhood. *Pediatrics, 137*(5), e20153957.

Sandler, P. J., Madahar, A. K., & Murray, A. (2011). Anterior open bite: Aetiology and management. *Dental Update, 38*(8), 522–524.

Sass-Lehrer, M., & Bodner-Johnson, B. (1989). Public Law 99-457: A new challenge to early intervention. *American Annals of the Deaf, 134*(2), 71–77.

Schantz, S. (2012). Overweight and obesity in youth. *Journal of School Nursing, 28*(6), 167–168.

Scheffer, R. (2011). Anxiety and phobias. In K. J. Marcdante, R. M. Kliegman, H. B. Jenson, et al. (Eds.), *Nelson essentials of pediatrics* (6th ed., pp. 67–71). Philadelphia, PA: Saunders/Elsevier.

Sherer, I. (2016). Social transition: Supporting our youngest transgender children. *Pediatrics, 137*(3), e20154358.

Singer, B. (2013). Perceptions of school nurses in the care of students with disabilities. *The Journal of School Nursing, 29*(5), 329–336.

Smith, S. (2011). Sinusitis. In K. J. Marcdante, R. M. Kliegman, H. B. Jenson, et al. (Eds.), *Nelson essentials of pediatrics* (6th ed., pp. 389–390). Philadelphia, PA: Saunders/Elsevier.

Sourander, A., Fossum, S., Rønning, J. A., et al. (2012). What is the long-term outcome of boys who steal at age eight? *Social Psychiatry & Psychiatric Epidemiology, 47*(9), 1391–1400.

Theisen, D., Frisch, A., Malisoux, L., et al. (2012). Injury risk is different in team and individual youth sport. *Journal of Science and Medicine in Sport, 16*(3), 200–204.

Tubert-Jeannin, S., Auclair, C., Amsallem, E., et al. (2011). Fluoride supplements (tablets, drops, lozenges or chewing gums) for preventing dental caries in children. *Cochrane Database of Systematic Reviews*, (12), CD007592.

U.S. Department of Health and Human Services. (2010). *Healthy people 2020*. Washington, DC: Author.

Weisleder, A., Cates, C. B., Dreyer, B. P., et al. (2016). Promotion of positive parenting and prevention of socioemotional disparities. *Pediatrics, 137*(2), e20153239.

Wen, A., Goldberg, D., Marrs, C. F., et al. (2012). Caries resistance as a function of age in an initially caries-free population. *Journal of Dental Research, 91*(7), 671–675.

White, R., & Mason, R. (2011). Bullying and gangs. *International Journal of Adolescent Medicine & Health, 24*(1), 57–62.

Whitney, E. N., & Rolfes, S. R. (2012). Life cycle nutrition: Infancy, childhood & adolescence. In E. N. Whitney & S. R. Rolfes (Eds.), *Understanding nutrition* (pp. 528–573). Belmont, CA: Wadsworth.

Widaman, K. F., & Helm, J. L. (2012). Nocturnal emissions: A failure to replicate. *The American Journal of Psychology, 125*(1), 39–50.

Young, A. M., Glover, N., & Havens, J. R. (2012). Nonmedical use of prescription medications among adolescents in the United States: A systematic review. *The Journal of Adolescent Health, 51*(1), 6–17.

33

Nursing Care of a Family With an Adolescent

*R*aul is a 15-year-old teenager you meet at an adolescent clinic. His chief concern is a head cold. He has numerous acne lesions on his forehead and cheeks. His parents tell you Raul seemed depressed for a long time after his girlfriend broke up with him but now seems happy again. They are pleased to see him maturing so much that he recently gave away his collection of baseball cards to a young neighbor. You mention to Raul a decongestant would probably make him feel better. He asks you how many pills it would take to kill someone and then jokes he was kidding. His healthcare provider prescribes a decongestant and suggests Raul return in 6 months.

The previous chapter discussed school-age children and the capabilities children develop during that time period. This chapter adds information about the changes, both physical and psychosocial, which occur during adolescence. Such information builds a base for care and health teaching for this age group.

Did Raul have some needs that were not met by his clinic visit?

KEY TERMS

adolescence

comedones

formal operational thought

glycogen loading

identity

puberty

role confusion

stalking

substance use disorder

OBJECTIVES

After mastering the contents of this chapter, you should be able to:

1. Describe normal growth and development and common parental concerns of the adolescent period.
2. Identify 2020 National Health Goals related to adolescents that nurses could help the nation achieve.
3. Assess an adolescent for normal growth and development milestones.
4. Formulate nursing diagnoses related to adolescent growth and development or common parental concerns.
5. Identify expected outcomes for nursing care of an adolescent as well as help parents manage seamless transitions across differing healthcare settings.
6. Using the nursing process, plan nursing care that includes the six competencies of Quality & Safety Education for Nurses (QSEN): Patient-Centered Care, Teamwork & Collaboration, Evidence-Based Practice (EBP), Quality Improvement (QI), Safety, and Informatics.
7. Implement nursing care related to growth and development or special needs of an adolescent, such as organizing a discussion group on ways to prevent substance use disorders.
8. Evaluate expected outcomes for achievement and effectiveness of care.
9. Integrate knowledge of adolescent growth and development with the interplay of nursing process, the six competencies of QSEN, and Family Nursing to promote quality maternal and child health nursing care.

Adolescence is generally defined as the period between ages 13 and up to 20 years, a time that serves as a transition between childhood and becoming a late adolescent. It can be divided into an early period (13 to 14 years), a middle period (15 to 16 years), and a late period (17 to 20 years). During all periods, adolescence is defined not so much by chronologic age as by physiologic, psychological, and sociologic changes. The drastic change in physical appearance and the change in expectations of others (especially parents) that occur during the period can lead to both emotional and physical health concerns (Sass & Kaplan, 2016).

Adolescents invariably feel a sense of pressure throughout this period because they are mature in some respects but still young in others. For example, an adolescent's sexual interests are awakening, yet personal or parental pressures discourage sexual exploration. An adolescent may not feel mature enough to live away from home, yet parents and teachers may urge the adolescent to apply for an out-of-town college. This duality causes a major dilemma or conflict for an adolescent, leading to many of the growth and developmental concerns of the age (Ahern & Norris, 2011). The 2020 National Health Goals related to adolescence are shown in Box 33.1.

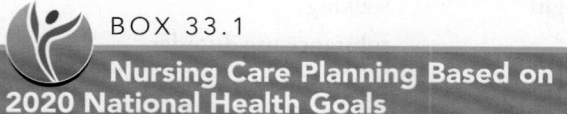

BOX 33.1

Nursing Care Planning Based on 2020 National Health Goals

Health teaching in the adolescent years is important because healthy habits begun at this time can influence health over a lifetime. For this reason, a number of 2020 National Health Goals relate to adolescent health, including:

- Reduce the number of adolescents who are obese from a prevalence of 17.9% to 16.1%.
- Reduce the proportion of high school students engaging in binge drinking from 25.2% to 22.7%.
- Reduce cigarette use by adolescents from 19.5% to 16%.
- Reduce the rate of smokeless tobacco use by adolescents from 8.9% to 6.9%.
- Reduce the proportion of adolescents who are offered, sold, or given an illegal drug on school property from 22.7% to 20.4%.
- Reduce the proportion of adolescents who report they rode, during the previous 30 days, with a driver who was drinking alcohol from 28.3% to 25.5%.
- Reduce the rate of suicide attempts by adolescents from 1.9% to 1.7%.
- Increase the proportion of adolescents who meet current federal physical activity guidelines for aerobic physical activity from 18.4% to 20.2% (U.S. Department of Health and Human Services, 2010; see www.healthypeople.gov).

Nurses can help the nation achieve these goals by educating adolescents about the use of cigarettes, smokeless tobacco, alcohol, and substance use disorder and by acting as support people for adolescents during times of crisis to help prevent self-injury or suicide.

Nursing Process Overview

FOR HEALTHY DEVELOPMENT OF AN ADOLESCENT

ASSESSMENT

Health maintenance visits during adolescence may become more irregular because adolescents may not seek care from healthcare facilities on their own unless they are ill. Until adolescents need a physical examination for athletic or some other clearance, they are often not seen for health assessments. When adolescents are accompanied by their parents at health visits, it is best to obtain a health history separately from the adolescent to promote independence and responsibility for self-care. When performing physical examinations on adolescents, be aware they may be very self-conscious of their body. They need health assurance and appreciate comments such as "Your blood pressure is 120/70, which is healthy," so they can learn more about their rapidly changing bodies.

NURSING DIAGNOSIS

Nursing diagnoses for adolescents can cover a wide range of topics. Frequently used diagnoses related to adolescents and their families include:

- Health-seeking behaviors related to normal growth and development
- Low self-esteem related to facial acne
- Anxiety related to concerns about normal growth and development
- Risk for injury related to peer pressure to use alcohol and drugs
- Risk for disease related to sexual activity
- Readiness for enhanced parenting related to increased knowledge of teenage years

OUTCOME IDENTIFICATION AND PLANNING

When planning care with adolescents, respect the fact that they have a strong desire to exert independence or do things their own way. This means they are not likely to adhere to a plan of care that disrupts their lifestyle or makes them appear different from others their age. Because of this, including them in planning is essential so the plan will be agreeable and accepted. Establishing a contract, such as asking an adolescent to agree to take medication daily, may be the most effective means to reach a mutual understanding.

Remember that adolescents are very oriented to the present, so a program that provides immediate results, such as increased respiratory function, will usually be carried out well. In contrast, a regimen oriented toward the future, with long-term goals such as preventing hypertension at middle age, may not be as successful. This does not mean it is not important to teach adolescents about the necessity of reducing future health risks—by eating well, not smoking, and generally taking care of their bodies—but that information will be best accepted if geared as much as possible to specific, short-term benefits to their health. Refer patients and families to helpful websites and other resources when appropriate (see Chapter 28).

IMPLEMENTATION

Adolescents tend to do poorly with tasks someone tells them they *must* do. Integrating the adolescents in their plan of care typically helps them be successful. Adolescents have little patience with adults who do not demonstrate the behavior they are being asked to achieve; a parent or nurse who smokes and asks an adolescent not to smoke, for example, will probably not be successful. For best results, evaluate how an intervention appears from an adolescent's standpoint before beginning teaching.

OUTCOME EVALUATION

An evaluation of expected outcomes should include not only whether desired outcomes have been achieved but also whether adolescents are pleased with the outcome. Individuals will have difficulty accomplishing desired goals as adults unless they have high self-esteem that includes feeling secure in their new body image.

Examples of outcome criteria that might be established include:

- Patient states she feels good about herself even though she is the shortest girl in her class.
- Patient states he has not consumed alcohol in 2 weeks.
- Parents state they feel more confident about their ability to parent an adolescent.
- Patient states she feels high self-esteem despite persistent facial acne.

Growth and Development of an Adolescent

Adolescents both grow rapidly and mature dramatically during the period from age 13 to 18 to 20 years.

PHYSICAL GROWTH

The major milestones of physical development in the adolescent period are the onset of puberty at 8 to 12 years of age and the cessation of body growth around 16 to 20 years (Sass & Kaplan, 2013). Between these milestones, physiologic growth and development of adult coordination occur. At first, the gain in physical growth is mostly in weight, leading to the stocky, slightly obese appearance of prepubescence; later comes the thin, gangly appearance of late adolescence.

Most girls are 1 to 2 in. (2.4 to 5 cm) taller than boys coming into adolescence but generally stop growing within 3 years from menarche and so are shorter than boys by the end of adolescence. Boys typically grow about 4 to 12 in. (10 to 30 cm) in height and gain about 15 to 65 lb (7 to 30 kg) during their teenage years. Girls grow 2 to 8 in. (5 to 20 cm) in height and gain 15 to 55 lb (7 to 25 kg). Growth stops with closure of the epiphyseal lines of the long bones, which occurs at about 16 or 17 years of age in females and about 18 to 20 years of age in males.

Because the heart and lungs increase in size more slowly than the rest of the body, adolescents may have insufficient energy and become fatigued trying to finish the various activities that interest them. Pulse rate and respiratory rate decrease slightly (to 70 beats/min and 20 breaths/min, respectively), and blood pressure increases slightly (to 120/70 mmHg) by late adolescence. With adulthood, blood pressure becomes slightly higher in males than in females because more force is necessary to distribute blood to the larger male body mass.

All during adolescence, androgen stimulates sebaceous glands to extreme activity, sometimes resulting in acne, a common adolescent skin problem. Apocrine sweat glands (i.e., glands present in the axillae and genital area, which produce a strong odor in response to emotional stimulation) form shortly after puberty. Adolescents begin to notice they must shower or bathe more frequently than when they were younger in order to be free of body odor because of this change.

Teeth

Adolescents gain their second molars at about 13 years of age and their third molars (wisdom teeth) between 18 and 21 years of age. Third molars may erupt as early as 14 to 15 years of age. The jaw reaches adult size only toward the end of adolescence, however. As a result, adolescents whose third molars erupt before the lengthening of the jaw is complete may experience pain and may need these molars extracted because they do not fit their jawline (Marciani, 2012).

> ### What If . . . 33.1
> Raul, a 15-year-old male, asks the nurse if he's going to grow some more; being the shortest boy in his gym class makes him feel "left out." Also, he asks if his teeth are white enough. Are these common concerns of adolescents?

Puberty

Puberty is the time at which an individual first becomes capable of sexual reproduction. A girl has entered puberty when she begins to menstruate; a boy enters puberty when he begins to produce spermatozoa. These events usually occur between ages 11 and 14 years. The age of first menstruation in girls is gradually decreasing from a mean of 13 years to 12.4 years, which is probably related to more weight gain in girls (Ledger, 2012). Puberty creates many questions for early teenagers about what is normal and what is not (Marván & Molina-Abolnik, 2012).

Secondary Sex Changes

Secondary sex characteristics, such as body hair configuration and breast growth, are those characteristics that distinguish the sexes from each other but that play no direct part in reproduction. The secondary sex characteristics that began in the late school-age period (see Chapter 32) continue to develop during adolescence. Typical stages of sexual maturation are shown in Table 33.1.

Sexual maturity in males and females is classified according to Tanner stages, named after the original researcher on sexual maturity (Tanner, 1962). Tanner stages of female

TABLE 33.1 SEXUAL MATURATION IN ADOLESCENTS

Age (years)	Males	Females
13–15	Growth spurt continuing; pubic hair abundant and curly; testes, scrotum, and penis enlarging further; axillary hair present; facial hair fine and downy; voice changes happen with annoying frequency	Pubic hair thick and curly, triangular in distribution; breast areola and papilla form secondary mound; menstruation is ovulatory, making pregnancy possible
15–16	Genitalia adult; scrotum dark and heavily rugated; facial and body hair present; sperm production mature	Pubic hair curly and abundant; may extend onto medial aspect of thighs; breast tissue appears adult; nipples protrude; areolas no longer project as separate ridges from breasts; may have some degree of facial acne
16–17	Pubic hair may extend along medial aspect of thighs; testes, scrotum, and penis adult in size; may have some degree of facial acne; gynecomastia (enlarged breast tissue), if present, fades	End of skeletal growth
17–18	End of skeletal growth	

From Tanner, J. M. (1962). *Growth at adolescence* (2nd ed.). Oxford, United Kingdom: Blackwell.

sexual development are shown in Figure 33.1, and stages of male genital growth are shown in Figure 33.2.

QSEN Checkpoint Question 33.1

INFORMATICS

The nurse realizes Raul is concerned about developing body odor and that he has consulted some websites that address this problem. The nurse recognizes a valid and reliable website would cite which aspect is true of body odor in adolescents?

a. It is largely dependent on ethnicity and body type.
b. It is caused by an increase in the activity of apocrine glands.
c. Poor hygiene is the main cause of adolescent body odor.
d. Body odor can result from clogged sebaceous glands.

Look in Appendix A for the best answer and rationale.

DEVELOPMENTAL MILESTONES

The same assessment categories of younger children continue to apply to adolescents.

Play or Recreation

Thirteen-year-old children change from school-age activities of active games to more adult forms of recreation such as listening to music, texting or chatting, or following a sports team's wins and losses. Team (or school) loyalty becomes intense and following a coach's instructions becomes mandatory, similar to the loyalty 6-year-old children showed toward their first-grade teacher. Overuse injuries from athletics occur in early adolescence until adolescents learn more about their

limits and begin to respect the advice of adults on being well prepared and trained for sports participation.

Most adolescents spend a great deal of time just talking with peers as social interaction, either face-to-face or through electronic media. Conflict can arise if parents disapprove of the number of hours spent in this activity, afraid their children are wasting important hours, or at least exchanging a great deal of trivial conversation. For an adolescent, however, talking is no more a waste of time than was imaginative play as a preschooler. It is a major way they learn about values and responsibilities (Box 33.2).

Beginning at age 16 years, most adolescents want part-time jobs to earn money. Such jobs can teach young people how to work with others, accept responsibility, and how to save and spend money wisely. For their own sake and that of the children they will care for, if adolescents plan to babysit, they first need to learn basic rules of childcare and safety. In most communities, schools or Red Cross organizations offer courses in babysitting just for the teenager.

Many adolescents engage in charitable endeavors during middle to late adolescence as a form of recreation. They do well organizing and supervising swimming or gym programs for physically challenged children or participating in marathons. A high school club may be organized to send money to children overseas. These activities fulfill an adolescent's need for satisfying interaction with others as well as indicators of maturity and willingness to accept adult roles.

EMOTIONAL DEVELOPMENT

According to Erikson (Dunkel & Harbke, 2017), the developmental task in early and mid-adolescence is to form a sense of identity versus role confusion. In late adolescence, it is to form a sense of intimacy versus isolation.

Early Adolescent Developmental Task: Identity Versus Role Confusion

The task of forming a sense of **identity** is for adolescents to decide whom they are and what kind of person they will be.

Figure 33.1 **(A)** Female breast development. *Sex maturity rating 1* (not shown): Prepubertal; elevation of papilla only. *Sex maturity rating 2*: Breast buds appear; areola is slightly widened and projects as a small mound. *Sex maturity rating 3*: Enlargement of the entire breast with no protrusion of the papilla or the nipple. *Sex maturity rating 4*: Enlargement of the breast and projection of areola and papilla as a secondary mound. *Sex maturity rating 5*: Adult configuration of the breast with protrusion of the nipple; areola no longer projects separately from remainder of breast. **(B)** Female pubic hair development. *Sex maturity rating 1*: Prepubertal; no pubic hair. *Sex maturity rating 2*: Straight hair extends along the labia and, between rating 2 and 3, begins on the pubis. *Sex maturity rating 3*: Pubic hair increases in quantity, becomes darker, and is present in the typical female triangle but in a smaller quantity. *Sex maturity rating 4*: Pubic hair more dense, curled, and adult in distribution but less abundant. *Sex maturity rating 5*: Abundant, adult-type pattern; hair may extend onto the medial part of the thighs. (Adapted from Tanner, J. M. [1962]. *Growth at adolescence* [2nd ed.]. Oxford, United Kingdom: Blackwell.)

Figure 33.2 Male genital and pubic hair development. Ratings for pubic hair and for genital development can differ in a typical boy at any given time because pubic hair and genitalia do not necessarily develop at the same rate. *Sex maturity rating 1*: Prepubertal; no pubic hair; genitalia unchanged from early childhood. *Sex maturity rating 2*: Light, downy hair develops laterally and later becomes dark; penis and testes may be slightly larger; scrotum becomes more textured. *Sex maturity rating 3*: Pubic hair extends across the pubis; testes and scrotum are further enlarged; penis is larger, especially in length. *Sex maturity rating 4*: More abundant pubic hair with curling; genitalia resemble those of an adult; glans has become larger and broader; scrotum is darker. *Sex maturity rating 5*: Adult quantity and pattern of pubic hair, with hair present along inner borders of thighs; testes and scrotum are adult in size. (Adapted from Tanner, J. M. [1962]. *Growth at adolescence* [2nd ed.]. Oxford, United Kingdom: Blackwell.)

BOX 33.2

Nursing Care Planning to Respect Cultural Diversity

In the United States, as in most developed countries, adolescence covers a long time span. In developing countries, in contrast, adolescence tends to be much shorter because children must take full-time jobs early in life to help support their families. Socioeconomic factors also influence the length of adolescence across all cultures. Recognizing that adolescents may have differing responsibilities and life experiences based on cultural expectations can be useful when making a progress assessment. In a family in which an adolescent is expected to begin working full-time or marry at an early age, you may need to include in health teaching factors such as occupational hazards or the effects of a job, family, and financial stress on an adolescent. Readiness for early childbearing may also be important.

The four main areas in which they must make gains to achieve a sense of identity include:

1. Accepting their changed body image
2. Establishing a value system or what kind of person they want to be
3. Making a career decision
4. Becoming emancipated from parents

If young people do not achieve a sense of identity, they can have little idea what kind of person they are or may develop a sense of **role confusion** (Dunkel & Harbke, 2017). This can lead to difficulty functioning effectively as adults because they are unable, for example, to decide what stand to take on a particular issue or how to approach new challenges or situations. This can lead them to exhibit acting-out (attention-getting) behaviors because they believe it is better to have a negative image than to have none at all.

Body Image

Adolescents who were able to develop a strong sense of industry during their school-age years learned to solve problems and are best equipped to adjust to the changing body image that comes with adolescence. This adjustment to changes is not always easy, however, because adolescents can feel disappointed with their final height or general appearance.

As adolescents are usually their own worst critics with regard to their bodies, they may need help from healthcare providers to realize the characteristics that make someone creative, compassionate, and fun to be with, not one's physical appearance, are the qualities on which lasting relationships are built.

Self-Esteem

Like body image, self-esteem may undergo major changes during the adolescent years and can be challenged by all the changes that occur during adolescence (Garzon & Dunn, 2013). Help parents understand how important it is for adolescents to have immediate successes such as making the high school basketball team or having a date for the senior prom. Parental comments, such as "When you're older, these things won't be so important," are not likely to erase the hurt that comes from being 16 years old and not being included in such major events. Compassionate understanding ("It's hard to be left out") is a better communication technique.

In recent years, a number of researchers have looked at the differences in the way boys and girls handle these emotional crises of adolescence. Several researchers have proposed that adolescence is a period of particular crisis for girls who are trying to find a place in a male-dominated society. The sociologist Carol Gilligan and her colleagues interviewed more than 500 girls between the ages of 7 and 16 years over a 5-year period and found many girls who, at age 11 years, were feisty, confident, and eager to speak their minds became hesitant to voice their opinions aloud by early adolescence, having pushed their earlier resistance "underground" (Gilligan, 1982; Taylor, Gilligan, & Sullivan, 1995). Gilligan (Gilligan, 1982; Taylor et al., 1995) tied this change to a growing realization among girls that their forthrightness may not be appealing to boys. They begin to self-censor, hoping to become more popular. Girls also struggle with a tug of war between valuing academic (or athletic) success (i.e., men's values) over maintaining close friendships (i.e., women's values).

Although the turmoil of adolescence can be just as confusing to boys as it is to girls, Gilligan (Gilligan, 1982; Taylor et al., 1995) hypothesized boys may feel less pressure as they become adults because they learn more easily to be competitive, independent, and separated from feelings. Girls, because they are encouraged to maintain their concern for people throughout their lives, are caught in a conflict between that and being independent and competitive. This makes girls at risk for more conflicting feelings throughout adolescence.

Long-term psychological problems, notably eating disorders, which occur in both boys and girls, may be one unfortunate result of repressing inborn feelings in order to conform. Parents can help both girls and boys deal with these conflicts by encouraging them to maintain their honesty and integrity.

Value System

Adolescents develop their values throughout their childhood as they interact with their family. As they increase the amount of time they spend with their peer group, they may question these values and participate in experiences that may put them at risk for physical and/or psychological harm. Identifying risk-taking behaviors and offering guidance and support is important in promoting the health of the adolescent.

Figure 33.3 Adolescents have a need to interact with peers to learn more about themselves and others.

Social Coupling

In early adolescence, individuals tend to dress and behave similarly to other members of their peer group (Fig. 33.3). Bullying behavior may be directed at individuals who don't conform to or associate with a peer group. Bullying behaviors should be identified, and the appropriate interventions should be initiated.

During adolescence, individuals begin to explore their sexual preferences and may question their gender identity. Encourage an open dialogue with adolescents to assist them to process their feelings and establish their own identity. Counseling may be helpful to assist with family communication if the family is not accepting.

Career Decisions

The adolescent may identify an educational and career trajectory during self-discovery of personal positive attributes. This process may take several years to achieve, and it varies for each individual. It is common for adolescents to seek and experiment with multiple roles before reaching a decision that is rewarding. Some school-age children do poorly in school during preadolescence but, as soon as they choose a career, show increased interest in learning as they come to see education as relevant to their future.

Emancipation From Parents

Emancipation from parents can become a major issue during the middle and late adolescent years for two reasons. Some parents may not yet be ready for their child to be totally independent, and some adolescents may not yet be sure they want to be on their own. They may fight bitterly for a right—for example, to stay out until midnight or later on a weekend—and then never use the privilege once they have gained it. Winning the battle may be more important than exercising the newly won right.

In many instances, the closer the tie adolescents feel with their parents, the more severe can be their struggle. As long as parents are reasonable in their restrictions, the amount of noise being made may be proof the ties are strong and separation or emancipation is not easy.

Encourage parents to give adolescents more freedom in areas such as choosing their own clothes or after-school activities; at the same time, help parents continue to place some restrictions on adolescent behavior ("You must drive the car safely," "We must know where you go after school"). These are not unreasonable rules and actually help adolescents accept the responsibility that comes with independence.

Both parents and adolescents may need help to understand that emancipation does not mean severance of a relationship but rather a change in a relationship because people who are independent of one another can have even better relationships than those who are dependent on one another. It can be helpful to remind parents this step is actually no different from the one children accomplished when they grew from infants to toddlers, when they changed from wanting to be held and rocked to wanting to run. If parents can think of it in this light, they will gain a better perspective and may realize they will not lose the children because they become adults. There are ex-wives and ex-husbands. There are no ex-children.

Late Adolescent Developmental Task: Intimacy Versus Isolation

Developing a sense of intimacy means a late adolescent is able to form long-term, meaningful relationships with persons of the opposite as well as their same sex (Erikson, 1950, 1968). Those who do not develop a sense of intimacy are left feeling isolated; in a crisis situation, they have no one to whom they feel they can turn to for help or support. A sense of intimacy is closely related to the sense of trust learned in the first year of life because, without the feeling that one can trust others, building a sense of intimacy is difficult.

Some adolescents require help from parents or other adults to differentiate between sound relationships and those that are based only on sexual attraction. Never do adolescents need an adult to listen to them more than when they are struggling with the heart-rending feelings of young love or wondering whether a particular love relationship is temporary or lasting.

Some parents may not be able to listen to their adolescent without interjecting their own opinions because they worry that relationships based on infatuation will lead to a sexual relationship. Parents should feel an obligation to inform their children of their feelings about early sexual relationships. At the same time, they have to be realistic that some adolescents will not follow their advice as shown by the rising rates of teenage pregnancy and sexually transmitted diseases, including HIV (Centers for Disease Control and Prevention [CDC], 2012c). If parents suspect their adolescent is sexually active, counsel them to be certain their child is knowledgeable about safer sex practices (see Chapter 22 for a discussion of adolescent pregnancy).

Some adolescents may believe intense sexual yearnings or peer pressure can be alleviated only by a sexual act. They can be reassured that they are pleasant people to be with because of the many fine qualities they possess and that sexual intercourse can be delayed until two persons have come to know these qualities in each other and have made a mutual commitment based on a deeper level than simply physical passion.

In our busy modern society in which adolescents engage in such a variety of activities, they may need help learning how to project themselves into another person's situation and to ask themselves how the world looks from that position. This concept, *empathy*, is the ability to understand the feelings of another, or, in other words, a developed sense of intimacy in its finest form.

Socialization

Early teenagers may feel more self-doubt than self-confidence when they meet another adolescent with whom they would like to begin a lasting relationship. The voices of most boys have not yet dependably deepened; this makes them unable to trust their voices to carry the serious tone they wish to convey. Most girls' bodies have not yet fully developed; they may look at themselves in a mirror, compare their profiles with those of models in popular magazines, and feel inadequate.

Both male and female early adolescents tend to be loud and boisterous, particularly when someone whose attention they would like to attract is nearby. They are impulsive and very much like 2-year-old children in that they want what they want immediately, not when it is convenient for others.

Many 13-year-olds begin to experience "crushes," or infatuations with schoolmates. At this age, however, they may spend more time longing for someone than they do instituting an in-depth and rewarding relationship. They have too little experience with life and too limited a frame of reference yet to know how to offer a deep commitment to another or accept one from that person.

By age 14 years, teenagers have become quieter and more introspective. They are becoming used to their changing bodies, have more confidence in themselves, and feel more self-esteem.

Adolescents watch adults carefully during this period, searching for good role models with whom they can identify. They usually have a hero—a film star, writer, scientist, or athlete—whom they want to grow up to be like. They may form a friendship with an older adolescent, trying to imitate that person in everything from thoughts to clothing. If the older adolescent has dropped out of school or plays a particular sport, the younger person may express a wish to drop out or train for that sport, too.

Idolization of famous people or older adolescents of this nature fades as adolescents become more interested in forming reciprocal friendships. Attachments to older adolescents are often severed abruptly and painfully as older teenagers make it clear they are more interested in being with people their own age. Rejection by an older member of a pair forces the younger member to turn to his or her own-age friends and ends the intense hero worship so typical of early adolescence.

Most 15-year-olds fall "in love" five or six times a year. However, many of these relationships are based on attraction because of physical appearance, not because of inner qualities or characteristics that are compatible with their own. Because infatuation is fleeting, it can lead to extremely intense but brief attachments that fade once the two young people discover they have little in common. Beginning romantic attachments this often, however, does not mean their feelings are any less strong or that they feel any less pain when the relationship ends (Fig. 33.4).

By age 16 years, boys are becoming sexually mature (although they continue to grow taller until about 18 years of age). Both sexes are better able to trust their bodies than they were the year before. By age 17 years, they tend to have adult values and responses to events. They have left behind the childish behaviors they used in early adolescence—shoving and punching—to get the attention of others.

Figure 33.4 Although infatuation or love can be fleeting, adolescents may feel intensely for another.

COGNITIVE DEVELOPMENT

The final stage of cognitive development, the stage of **formal operational thought**, begins at age 12 or 13 years and grows in depth over the adolescent years, although it may not be complete until about age 25 years (Piaget, 1969). This step involves the ability to think in abstract terms and use the scientific method (i.e., deductive reasoning) to arrive at conclusions. The problems that adolescents are asked to solve in school depend on this type of thought. Problem solving in any situation depends on the ability to think abstractly and logically.

With the ability to use scientific reasoning, adolescents can plan their future. They can create a hypothesis (What if I go to college? What if I don't?) and think through the probable consequences (In the long run, I'll earn more money, or I could begin earning money immediately).

MORAL AND SPIRITUAL DEVELOPMENT

Because adolescents enlarge their thought processes to include formal reasoning, they are able to respond to the question "Why is it wrong to steal from your neighbor's house?" with "It would hurt my neighbor by requiring him to spend money to replace what I stole," rather than with the immature response of the school-age child, "The police will punish me." Some adolescents, however, may have difficulty envisioning a department store or a large corporation as capable of suffering economic loss from stealing, a concept that can contribute to the frequent practice of petty shoplifting at this age.

Almost all adolescents question the existence of God and any religious practices they have been taught (Kohlberg, 1984). This questioning is a natural part of forming a sense of identity and establishing a value system at a time in life when they draw away from their families.

Health Promotion for an Adolescent and Family

Because their judgments are still limited, adolescents still need guidelines in reference to safety, nutrition, and daily care. These are always excellent topics for discussion at healthcare visits.

PROMOTING ADOLESCENT SAFETY

Unintentional injuries, most commonly those involving motor vehicles, are the leading cause of death among adolescents. Although teenagers are at the peak of physical and sensorimotor functioning, their need to rebel against authority or to gain attention through risk-taking leads them to take careless actions, such as speeding or driving while intoxicated.

In the interest of an adolescent's safety and that of others, parents need to have the courage to insist on emotional maturity rather than age as the qualification for obtaining a driver's license. Adolescents need to take seriously the graduated licensing requirements for their state so they not only learn the techniques of safe driving but also learn a sense of responsibility toward others (Williams, McCartt, & Sims, 2016).

Some adolescents dismiss seat belts as childish and so need extra instruction that it is wise to use every safety precaution available when in a motor vehicle (Chen, Cao, & Logan, 2012). Equally dangerous for adolescents are motorcycles, motorbikes, and motor scooters, which are appealing because of their low cost and convenience in parking. Both drivers and riders should wear safety helmets to prevent head injury, long pants to prevent leg burns from exhaust pipes, and a full body covering to prevent abrasions in case of an accident. Advise adolescents who choose these forms of transportation to be as familiar with safety rules as automobile drivers and to wait until they are emotionally mature enough to use sound driving judgment.

Although drowning tends to occur in younger children, it does occur in adolescents when good swimmers go beyond their capabilities on dares or in hopes of impressing friends. Teaching water safety, such as not swimming alone or when tired, is as important as teaching the mechanics of swimming (CDC, 2012b).

BOX 33.3

Nursing Care Planning to Empower a Family

MEASURES TO PREVENT UNINTENTIONAL INJURIES IN ADOLESCENTS

Q. Raul's mother tells you, "My son doesn't always use mature judgment. How can I keep him safe from accidents?"

A. Teaching the following points can be helpful to him:

Unintentional Injury	Health Teaching Measure
Motor vehicle	Always use a seat belt whether a driver or a passenger. Never use a cell phone or text while driving.
	Do not drink alcohol while driving and always refuse to ride with anyone who has been drinking (name a designated driver or arrange with your parents to be picked up or provide money for a taxi).
	Wear a helmet and long trousers as driver or passenger on a motorcycle.
	Accepting dares has no place in safe driving.
	Take graduated driver programs seriously so you learn safe driving habits for both two-wheel and four-wheel vehicles.
Firearms	Always consider all guns loaded and potentially lethal.
	Learn safe gun handling before attempting to clean a gun or hunt.
Drowning	Learn how to swim. Follow safe water rules, such as never swimming alone, no diving into the shallow end of swimming pools, no hyperventilating before swimming underwater, and no swimming beyond one's own limit.
	Taking dares has no place in water safety.
Sports	Use protective equipment, such as facemasks for hockey and pads and a helmet for football.
	Do not attempt to participate beyond physical limits.
	Keep well hydrated by drinking fluid before and after play.
	Careful preparation for sports through training is essential to safety.
	Recognize and set one's own limit for sports participation.

Other common causes of death in adolescents are homicide and self-harm (i.e., suicide) (Swahn, Ali, Bossarte, et al., 2012). These are related to the easy accessibility of guns when added to depression, binge drinking, and impulsivity. Gang violence and the desire to protect themselves are additional factors. Unintentional gunshot injuries increase in early adolescence, often for the same reason that drowning increases: Youngsters want to impress friends by showing they can handle guns. Be certain that firearm safety is taught creatively through problem solving rather than lecturing because teenagers tend to rebel against such lectures or claim that they have heard it all before.

Athletic injuries, especially overuse injuries from poor conditioning, tend to increase in number during adolescence because of the vigorous level of competition that occurs in organized sports (Khan, Thompson, Blair, et al., 2012). Types of athletic injuries are discussed in Chapter 52. Health teaching measures to prevent unintentional injuries, especially while participating in athletics, are summarized in Box 33.3.

PROMOTING NUTRITIONAL HEALTH FOR AN ADOLESCENT

Adolescents experience such rapid growth that they may always feel hungry (Fig. 33.5). If their eating habits are unsupervised, because of peer pressure and when in a hurry to get to other activities, they tend to eat faddish or quick snack foods rather than more nutritionally sound ones. Some adolescents turn away from the basic MyPlate food groups to eat sweets, soft drinks, or empty-calorie snacks and so are left poorly nourished. This type of eating pattern, combined with a lack of exercise, also leads to obesity (Wengle, Hamilton, Manlhiot, et al., 2012).

One form of adolescent rebellion is to refuse to eat foods that parents stress as important. Parents who stock their kitchens with healthy snacks such as fruit and vegetables and who are willing to meet their adolescents halfway in terms of food preferences can be more certain their child is eating nutritious foods than if such food aren't available. Giving an adolescent

Figure 33.5 Adolescents experience rapid physical growth, so typically, they eat frequently. (© Billy Barnes/Stock Boston.)

some responsibility for food planning or meals, such as making dinner every Wednesday night, can teach some important lessons about nutrition without conflict.

Adolescents who are slightly obese because of prepubertal changes may begin low-calorie or starvation diets during adolescence to lose weight. Some diet so excessively they develop eating disorders such as bulimia or anorexia nervosa (see Chapter 54). A weight-loss diet is appropriate during adolescence, but it must be supervised to ensure the adolescent is consuming sufficient calories and nutrients for growth. For example, many adolescents entirely omit breads and cereals to lose weight rather than just reducing the amounts they eat. Diets such as these can be deficient in vitamins B_1 (thiamine) and B_2 (riboflavin), which are necessary for growth.

Recommended Dietary Reference Intakes

An adolescent needs an increased number of calories over that needed previously to support the rapid body growth that occurs. Foods must come from a variety of sources to supply necessary amounts of carbohydrates, vitamins, protein, and minerals.

The nutrients that are most apt to be deficient in both male and female adolescent diets are iron, calcium, and zinc. Iron is necessary to meet expanding blood volume requirements. Females require a high iron intake not only because of this increasing blood volume but also because iron begins to be lost with menstruation. Girls with a heavy menstrual flow (i.e., menorrhagia) and especially those who participate in strenuous athletics may need to take an additional iron supplement to prevent iron-deficiency anemia (Bruinvels, Burden, Brown, et al., 2016).

Increased calcium and vitamin D plus physical exercise are necessary for rapid skeletal growth as well as to "stockpile" calcium to prevent osteoporosis later in life (Chouinard, Randall Simpson, & Buchholz, 2012). Zinc is necessary for sexual maturation and final body growth. Good sources of iron are meat and green vegetables, calcium is abundant in milk and milk products, and meat and milk are also high in zinc.

Promoting Nutritional Health With a Varied Diet

Vegetarian Diets

Because vegetables generally contain fewer calories than meat, adolescents need to consume large amounts of them to achieve an adequate caloric intake from a vegetarian diet. Textured vegetable protein or tofu can be added to meals to increase the amount of protein supplied and help meet adolescent growth needs (Case, 2016). Some adolescents may find it difficult to follow a vegetarian diet because it makes them different from their peers and limits the foods they can eat at parties or at school, such as pizza, meat tortillas, or hot dogs. Whether to continue to follow this type of diet is a decision an adolescent must make as part of achieving a sense of identity. Be certain that adolescents who have become semi-vegetarians in order to lose weight add enough protein to their food intake to sustain their rapid body growth (Timko, Hormes, & Chubski, 2012).

Glycogen Loading

Athletes need more carbohydrate or energy than those who do not engage in strenuous activity; the source of carbohydrate that best sustains athletes comes from the breakdown of glycogen because this supplies a slow and steady release of glucose. **Glycogen loading** is a procedure used to ensure there is adequate glycogen to sustain energy through an athletic event. Several days before a sports event, athletes lower their carbohydrate intake and exercise heavily to deplete muscle glycogen stores. They then switch to a diet high in carbohydrate. With the renewed carbohydrate intake, muscle glycogen is stored at two to three times the usual level, which supplies them with up to twice the glucose needed for sustained energy (Bagnulo, 2006).

Although used by many high school athletes, the effects of frequent glycogen loading in this age group are not well studied and so should be done cautiously. As a rule, the goals of nutrition that are best for everyone, such as eating a well-balanced diet rather than a diet that interferes with carbohydrate, fluid, or fat intake, are also the best rules for athletes.

PROMOTING DEVELOPMENT OF AN ADOLESCENT IN DAILY ACTIVITIES

Adequate sleep, hygiene, and exercise are important health education topics for adolescents as these become an adolescent's responsibility rather than the responsibility of the parents.

Dress and Hygiene

Adolescents are capable of total self-care and, because of their body awareness, may even be overly conscientious about personal hygiene and appearance. Both sexes try many types of shampoo, deodorant, breath fresheners, and toothpaste. They may take seriously (without admitting it) the content of ads showing that toothpastes or deodorants can help win an attractive person or gain instant success. Remember that when caring for hospitalized adolescents, providing time for self-care, such as shampooing hair, is important to include in an adolescent's nursing care plan.

Adolescents can be acutely aware of how their peers dress. When hospitalized, most teenagers seem to improve markedly when allowed to wear their own clothing rather than a hospital gown. Needing to look like everyone else is undoubtedly a factor in adolescent shoplifting. Only during late adolescence do teenagers discover that who they really are shows through their clothing.

Care of Teeth

Adolescents are generally very conscientious about tooth brushing because of a fear of developing bad breath. They should continue to use a fluoride paste rather than a brand advertised as providing white teeth. They should also continue to drink fluoridated water to ensure firm enamel growth (Armfield, Spencer, Roberts-Thomson, et al., 2013), but they should also be careful to not use so much fluoride through the use of mouth rinses or toothpaste that they develop fluorosis (i.e., a blue discoloration of teeth). Teens with braces must be extremely conscientious about tooth brushing to prevent plaque buildup on hidden tooth surfaces. If they snack a great deal, and so their teeth are always exposed to bacterial erosion, some may develop a cavity for the first time during this period.

Sleep

Although it is widely believed everyone needs 8 hours of sleep a night, some need more and others can adjust to considerably less. Because protein synthesis occurs most readily during sleep and adolescents are building so many new cells, this age group may need proportionately more sleep than any other age group (Short, Gradisar, Lack, et al., 2013). In addition, because this is a busy time with extracurricular activities and also a stressful period similar to first grade, adolescents may sleep restlessly as their mind reworks the day's tensions. Even long periods of sleep, therefore, may not leave them feeling refreshed. This is why adolescents, admitted to a hospital for even a minor illness, for example, may sleep as if exhausted. Even though frequent lack of sleep can lead to chronic fatigue or depression, medication is not usually recommended for adolescents; instead, they are urged to reduce activity to get more sleep (Frost & Burns, 2012).

Exercise

Just as with younger children, adolescents need exercise every day both to maintain muscle tone and to provide an outlet for tension. Unlike younger children, however, and although they are constantly on the go, adolescents often receive very little real exercise. They may ride a bus to school, sit for classes, and sit at a mall after school and talk to friends. They have put in a full day, yet most of their time was spent sitting. Because of this, adolescents who have had an injury and must learn an activity such as crutch walking usually need to do muscle-strengthening exercises at first, just as adults must.

Adolescents who are involved in structured athletic activities do receive daily exercise. If they have not participated in competitive sports before, however, they may need advice on increasing exercise gradually so they do not overdo it and consequently develop muscle sprains or other overuse injuries (Hoang, Coel, Vidal, et al., 2012).

Sun Exposure

Because some adolescents spend a great deal of time outdoors participating in athletics, it is a critical time for them to avoid excessive sun exposure so they don't develop skin cancer (i.e., melanoma) from ultraviolet rays. Encourage teenagers to use sunscreen, avoid tanning beds, and report to their primary healthcare provider any skin mole that changes in shape or color. Do this as creatively as possible because teenagers have difficulty looking to the future and imagining how drastically the development of melanoma could affect their lives (Cohen, Brown, Haukness, et al., 2013).

PROMOTING HEALTHY FAMILY FUNCTIONING

Early adolescents may have many disagreements with parents that stem partly from wanting more independence and partly from being so disappointed in their bodies. It may be helpful to counsel parents to appreciate that although it is not easy to live with a teenager, it is equally difficult to be the teenager.

When a child reaches about age 15 years, parent–child friction tends to peak. By this age, adolescents have discovered from careful observation that most adults are far from perfect. Teachers they previously thought were all knowing are revealed to have very human shortcomings. School marks may slump as a reflection of this "fallen angel" syndrome.

Adolescents discover even more faults in their parents and wonder, for instance, how they can exist with such outdated ideas. Adolescents may follow health advice poorly because they view healthcare personnel in the same light.

By the time they are 16 years old, adolescents generally become more willing to listen and talk about problems. As a result, they may learn adults are not as inadequate as they previously thought. This changed perception does not mean an adolescent of 16 years is calm and quiet and free of parent–child discord. Adolescents may comprehend how hard it was for parents to get where they are, but they may not understand, for example, why they themselves are not allowed to stay out later than midnight on weekends.

Most 17-year-old adolescents, who have stayed in school, are usually high school seniors; for most of them, this year is likely to be stormy. Looking ahead to leaving a school system with which they may have been involved since they were very young may give them a feeling of losing security. Even if going away to college or beginning a full-time job seems exciting, it can also be an unwelcome change from the people and routines they feel so comfortable with to new contacts and new regulations that appear strange and even hostile.

The ambivalence that such feelings create makes some 17-year-olds enjoy having parents perpetuating family traditions such as the house decorated for a holiday in the same way as usual or being served a traditional birthday meal. This clinging to security is not a step backward but a preliminary working through to a time of separation that will be a major milestone in reaching maturity.

Unfortunately, as another way to prove they are old enough to leave high school and enter into a more mature college or work world, older adolescents may begin to experiment with drugs or alcohol, interpreting the use of these as the mark of being an adult (Lewis & Hession, 2012).

COMMON HEALTH PROBLEMS OF AN ADOLESCENT

A health maintenance schedule for the adolescent period and the assessments to be included at visits are shown in Table 33.2.

Hypertension

Hypertension is present if blood pressure is above the 95th percentile, or 127/81 mmHg for 16-year-old girls and 131/81 for 16-year-old boys for two consecutive readings in different settings. (Pulse, respiration, and blood pressure value charts are available at http://thePoint.lww.com/Flagg8e.) Adolescents who are obese, who are Black, who eat a diet high in salt, or who have a family history of hypertension are most susceptible to developing the condition. All children older than 3 years of age should have their blood pressure routinely taken at all health assessments to detect this (Hagan, Shaw, & Duncan, 2017). This is particularly important for adolescents because new medications plus education can help to greatly reduce the incidence of cardiovascular disease as they reach adulthood (Flynn & Falkner, 2011). Prevention and management of hypertension in children and adolescents are discussed in Chapter 41.

Poor Posture

Many adolescents, particularly those who reach adult height before their peers, demonstrate poor posture, a tendency to round shoulders and a shambling, slouchy walk to not be taller than those around them. This is also due to the imbalance of growth that arises from the skeletal system growing a little more rapidly than the muscles attached to it. Girls, especially, may slouch so as not to appear taller than boys

TABLE 33.2 HEALTH MAINTENANCE SCHEDULE, ADOLESCENT PERIOD

Area of Focus	Methods	Frequency
Assessment		
Developmental milestones	History, observation	Every visit
Growth milestones	Height, weight plotted on standard growth chart; body mass index (BMI), physical examination	Every visit
Hypertension	Blood pressure	Every visit
Nutrition	History, observation; height/weight, BMI information	Every visit
Dyslipidemia	Total cholesterol and triglycerides	At 18 years of age; earlier screening for children who have family members with the disorder
Parent–child relationship	History, observation	Every visit
Behavior or school problems	History, observation	Every visit
Substance use disorder	History, observation	Every visit
Vision and hearing disorders	History, observation	Every visit
	Formal Snellen or Titmus testing	At 15 and 18 years of age
	Audiometer testing	If concern or high risk is present
Dental health	History, physical examination	Every visit; recommend a yearly checkup with dental health provider
Cervical dysplasia (scoliosis)	Physical examination	Every visit at least to 16 years of age
Thyroid disease	Physical examination, history	Every visit
Tuberculosis	Purified protein derivative (PPD) test	Depending on prevalence of tuberculosis in community
Bacteriuria	Dipstick	Annually if sexually active
Anemia	Hematocrit or hemoglobin	Annually for menstruating females
Cervical or vaginal cancer	Pap test, pelvic examination	Three years after first coitus, or at age 21 years
Sexually transmitted diseases	History, observation	Every visit if sexually active
Immunizations		
	Check history and past records; inform caregiver about any risks and side effects; administer vaccine in accordance with healthcare agency policies.	
Hepatitis A vaccine	HepA	If not previously immunized
Hepatitis B vaccine	HepB	If not previously immunized
Human papillomavirus vaccine	HPV	If not previously vaccinated
Influenza vaccine	TIV (trivalent influenza vaccine) or LAIV	Yearly
Measles, mumps, rubella vaccine	MMR	If not previously vaccinated; do not give to pregnant adolescents
Meningococcal vaccine	MPV4 (meningococcal polysaccharide vaccine)	Booster at 16 years
Pneumococcal vaccine	PCV (pneumococcal conjugate vaccine)	To high-risk groups if not previously vaccinated
Tetanus and diphtheria vaccine	Tdap	If not previously immunized
Varicella vaccine	VAR	If not previously vaccinated
Anticipatory Guidance		
Adolescent care including violence and nutrition counseling	Active listening and health teaching	Every visit
Expected growth and developmental milestones before next visit	Active listening and health teaching	Every visit
Unintentional injury prevention	Counseling about street and personal safety	Every visit
Any problems expressed by caregiver or adolescent during visit	Active listening and health teaching	Every visit

LAIV, live attenuated influenza vaccine.
From American Academy of Pediatrics. (2012). *Recommendations for preventive pediatric health care*. Evanston, IL: Author.

or to diminish the appearance of their breast size if they are developing more rapidly than their friends. Yet another reason may be related to carrying backpacks that are too heavy (Kistner, Fiebert, & Roach, 2012).

Urge children of both sexes to use good posture during these rapid-growth years. Assess posture at all adolescent health appraisals to detect the difference between simple poor posture and the beginning of spinal dysplasia or scoliosis (i.e., lateral curvature of the spine) (see Chapters 34 and 51).

Body Piercing and Tattoos

Body piercing and tattoos are a strong mark of adolescence (Stein & Jordan, 2012). Both sexes may have ears, lips, chins, navels, and breasts pierced and filled with studs or tattoos applied to arms, legs, or their central body. Body piercings and tattoos have become a way for adolescents to make a statement of who they are and that they are different from their parents. Be certain they know the symptoms of infection at a piercing or tattoo site (e.g., redness, warmness, drainage, swelling, mild pain) and to report these to their healthcare provider if they occur because serious staphylococcal or streptococcal infections can occur at piercing sites. It is important to caution adolescents that sharing needles for piercing or tattooing carries the same risk for contacting a blood-borne disease as sharing needles for intravenous drug use.

Fatigue

Because so many adolescents comment that they feel fatigued to some degree, it can be considered normal for the age group. However, fatigue may also be a beginning symptom of disease, so it is important that it is not underestimated as a concern. Always assess the diet, sleep patterns, and activity schedules of fatigued adolescents. Be aware that if the fatigue began as a short period of extreme tiredness, it suggests disease more so than a long, ill-defined report of always feeling tired.

If an adolescent's sleep and diet appear to be adequate, his or her activity schedule is reasonable, and a physical assessment suggests no illness, then the fatigue may be of emotional origin. It can be a means of avoiding school, conflict with parents (e.g., when children appear ill, parents are more sympathetic), or social situations (e.g., too tired to go to the mall). Those who are under stimulated by school may develop fatigue as a sign of boredom.

Blood tests may be indicated to rule out anemia and common infections in adolescents, such as infectious mononucleosis (see Chapter 43). Chronic fatigue syndrome, although not seen as often in this age group as in adults, may also need to be ruled out (Lloyd, Chalder, & Rimes, 2012). If tests for these categories of conditions are normal, teenagers can be assured they are healthy and should be offered guidance to solve the problem with better diet, more sleep, fewer activities, and better problem-solving techniques to relieve tension.

Menstrual Irregularities

Menstrual irregularities can be a major health concern of adolescent girls as they learn to adjust to their individual body cycles. Chapter 47 discusses these problems in detail.

Acne

Acne is a self-limiting inflammatory disease that involves the sebaceous glands, which empty into hair shafts (the pilosebaceous unit). It is the most common skin disorder of adolescence, occurring in as many as 80% to 95% of adolescents (Morelli & Prok, 2016). It occurs slightly more frequently in boys than in girls. The peak age for the lesions occurring in girls is 14 to 17 years of age; for boys, 16 to 19 years of age. Although not proven, genetic factors may play a part in their development.

Changes associated with puberty that cause acne to develop include:

- As androgen levels rise in both sexes, sebaceous glands become active.
- The output of sebum, which is largely composed of lipids, mainly triglycerides, increases.
- Trapped sebum causes whiteheads, or closed comedones.
- As trapped sebum darkens from accumulation of melanin and oxidation of the fatty acid component on exposure to air, blackheads, or open comedones, form. Leakage of fatty acids causes a dermal inflammatory reaction.
- Bacteria (generally, *Propionibacterium acnes*) lodge and thrive in the retained secretions and ducts.

Acne is categorized as mild (i.e., **comedones** or blocked hair follicle), moderate (i.e., papules and pustules are also present), or severe (i.e., cysts are present). The most common locations of acne lesions are the face, neck, back, upper arms, and chest (Fig. 33.6). Flare-ups are associated with emotional stress, menstrual periods, or the use of greasy hair creams or makeup that can further plug gland ducts. Lesions are less noticeable in summer months, probably because of increased exposure to the sun, which increases epidermal peeling, or because of a reduction in stress as a result of being out of school.

Assessment

Always ask adolescents at health assessments if they are troubled with acne and to what extent it interferes with their self-image because this can be a major cause of stress in adolescents. Inspect for facial, chest, and back lesions on physical examination.

Therapeutic Management

The goal of therapy for acne is threefold: (a) decrease sebum formation, (b) prevent comedones, and (c) control bacterial proliferation.

External Medication

Medications that are applied externally peel away the superficial skin layer to prevent sebum plugs from forming and

Figure 33.6 Facial acne in an adolescent.

are sufficient if only comedones are present. A common prescription medication is tretinoin (Retin-A cream). This reduces keratin formation and plugging of ducts. Caution adolescents using a vitamin A cream to avoid prolonged sun exposure and to use a sunblock of SPF 15 or higher because the preparation makes their skin more susceptible to ultraviolet rays (Karch, 2013). Additional creams frequently prescribed contain benzoyl peroxide or azelaic acid. Caution adolescents that for the first week or two of therapy, peeling or oxidizing agents may make the complexion appear worse. If the adolescent has inflammatory lesions, topical antibiotic creams such as dapsone, tetracycline, or doxycycline may be prescribed to reduce the bacterial level on the skin. Tetracycline is not prescribed for children under age 12 years because it can cause permanent staining of teeth and may possibly interfere with growth of long bones. It is contraindicated for adolescents who are or may become pregnant as it is teratogenic (Simonart, 2012).

Systemic Medication

In pustular and cystic acne, systemic (i.e., oral) antibiotics can be helpful. Systemic antibiotics have anti-inflammatory properties, and they are effective against *P. acnes*. Tetracycline (500 mg twice daily the first week and then tapered to 250 mg daily for maintenance) is effective against the anaerobic bacteria that break down sebum to form irritating acids. However, the more lipophilic antibiotics, such as doxycycline and minocycline, are generally more effective than tetracycline (Zaenglein, Pathy, Schlosser, et al., 2016). Improvement is not generally seen for 2 to 4 weeks, so you may need to support adolescents to continue to take the medication during the waiting period. Without noticeable improvement, adolescents have a tendency to continue taking the higher dose or even increase the dose, hoping to initiate a faster effect.

Food impairs the absorption of oral tetracycline so the drug should be taken on an empty stomach (2 hours before or after eating). Adolescents must be certain of the date of expiration of the drug; outdated tetracycline breaks down into an extremely toxic composition. Females taking systemic antibiotics for long periods of time become susceptible to developing candidal vaginitis and need to be instructed about the symptoms of this: a white, pruritic vaginal discharge. As yet another precaution, because antibiotic use may interfere with oral contraceptives, adolescent girls who are sexually active should use another method of birth control while taking the antibiotic. Alternative antibiotics prescribed are erythromycin or clindamycin. Although these drugs avoid the complications of tetracycline, they may not produce the same effective results.

Other Treatment Methods

Estrogen, alone or in combination with progesterone, suppresses sebaceous gland activity and, therefore, oral contraceptives are useful therapy in some girls with acne (Neuhaus, Nagler, & Orlow, 2017). Oral contraceptives taken for this reason carry the same precautions as when they are prescribed as a reproductive planning method: Estrogen tends to close epiphyseal centers of long bones, causing bone growth to halt, and long-term therapy does have potential side effects, including embolism and thrombophlebitis. A last resort is administration of isotretinoin (a retinoid or vitamin A compound) for a short time (Lyon, 1978; Rathi, 2011). Isotretinoin must be taken with caution, however, because it is extremely teratogenic and also has been linked to inflammatory bowel disease. It should

not be taken at the same time as tetracycline or it can lead to brain edema. Many adolescents are left with some degree of scarring following teenage acne lesions. Laser therapy is a follow-up possibility to reduce the effect of scarring.

 Nursing Diagnoses and Related Interventions

Nursing Diagnosis: Risk for low self-esteem related to the development of acne during adolescence and lack of knowledge regarding treatment possibilities

Outcome Evaluation: Adolescent verbalizes positive aspects of self; states acne does not affect self-image, or if patient admits to feelings of negative self-esteem, is able to discuss feelings and concerns about condition; describes ways to prevent or reduce acne outbreaks and states realistic short- and long-term goals of treatment.

It is necessary to respect how devastating acne can be to some adolescents. The actual extent of the condition often is not as important as an adolescent's feelings about it. With a face constantly covered by red marks, it may be extremely difficult for adolescents to feel good about themselves.

When carrying out interventions, remember that acne is a potentially destructive disease; if left untreated, it can cause irreparable physical and emotional scarring. Therefore, advise parents and adolescents to seek medical treatment rather than self-medicate if the condition is severe. At the same time, being overly concerned may lead to becoming unduly self-conscious, which may affect performance in school and the establishment of social relationships. Common health teaching measures for the prevention and treatment of acne are summarized in Box 33.4.

QSEN Checkpoint Question 33.3

PATIENT-CENTERED CARE

Raul is prescribed both a topical cream and oral tetracycline to treat his acne. The nurse identifies that he needs additional health information from which statements (list all that apply)?
 a. "I know acne is not contagious even though all my friends seem to have it."
 b. "My girlfriend wants to borrow my tetracycline; I don't mind sharing it."
 c. "I know not to take hot showers as hot water can create new lesions."
 d. "I know not to eat chocolate because that always makes lesions worse."

Look in Appendix A for the best answer and rationale.

Obesity

Most overweight adolescents have obese parents, suggesting that both inheritance and environment play a part in the development of adolescent obesity. Obesity can interfere with developing a sense of identity if it is difficult for adolescents to like their reflection in a mirror or if they are always excluded from groups because of their weight. Because of stress related to weight, the attempted suicide rate for obese female adoles-

BOX 33.4

Nursing Care Planning Based on Family Teaching

GUIDELINES FOR THE PREVENTION AND TREATMENT OF ACNE

Q. Raul says to you, "I've had acne for the last 3 months. How can I make this go away?"

A. Most adolescents have some acne lesions. Try the following suggestions:

- Do not pick or squeeze acne lesions, which ruptures glands and spreads sebum into the skin, thus increasing inflammation. The times you are most likely to do this are during periods of stress, such as when you are taking a test. When you find your hand on your face, distract yourself with some other motion, such as interlocking your fingers.
- Greasy hair preparations or tight sweatbands can both plug ducts of glands and increase comedone formation, so avoid these, if possible. For girls, makeup can plug ducts; using medicated makeup both covers and helps lesions heal.
- Topical acne preparations work by unplugging glands, so you must use them consistently for them to be effective. Plan enough time in the morning before school and a time in the evening to apply these. Post a chart by your bathroom mirror to remind yourself.
- Washing daily to remove irritating fatty acids is helpful. Excessive washing is not necessary and, in fact, can actually harm healing by rupturing glands.
- Oral medications work by reducing sebum secretions or preventing bacterial invasion. Again, these work only if you take them conscientiously. Make a chart to post in your bathroom or kitchen to remind you to take these. Remember, tetracycline must be taken on an empty stomach or it is not effective.
- Both topical and oral vitamin A makes your skin very sensitive to sunlight. Avoid long exposures to sunlight, or you will sunburn readily.
- Although diet does not influence the development of acne lesions, you should eat a healthy, well-balanced diet for good general health.
- No acne medication works immediately. While you are waiting for lesions to heal, keep yourself occupied with a new activity (e.g., join a school club, try dancing lessons). When your skin is clear, these experiences will help make you an interesting person as well as one with clear skin.

cents is higher than for non-obese adolescents (Perera, Eisen, Dennis, et al., 2016).

Some adolescents may be unaware that their food intake is excessive because they have been told they need excess nutrients for healthy adolescent growth and everyone in their family eats large portions. Health teaching with these adolescents may need to begin with a discussion of "normal" weight and standard food portions because, if they do not begin to own this problem as adolescents, they run a high risk of becoming obese adults.

If adolescents eat a diet too low in protein for any length of time, they can develop a faulty nitrogen balance, which can lead to seriously impaired growth. Therefore, a diet of fewer than 1,400 to 1,600 calories per day can rarely be tolerated by adolescents. They generally do better and will stick with a diet closer to 1,800 calories per day.

 Nursing Diagnoses and Related Interventions

Nursing Diagnosis: Ineffective individual coping by overeating related to stresses of the adolescent period, which has led to obesity

Outcome Evaluation: Adolescent identifies stressful situations that lead to overeating; describes ways to avoid those situations or methods that would help coping with them.

Adolescents who are overweight because of stress need support until their pleasure in eating diminishes and their satisfaction with themselves as a "new" person or until their friends' satisfaction with them can sustain them. They may need to visit a healthcare facility once or twice a week for encouragement and praise for their efforts. National weight-control organizations are good to use if other adolescents also attend the meetings. They tend to be less effective if all the other members are adults because adolescents generally cannot relate to adult concerns. It's important an adolescent's self-esteem is maintained while losing weight or an adolescent may switch to binge eating or such severe dieting that the opposite—extreme weight loss—can occur (Sánchez-Carracedo, Neumark-Sztainer, & López-Guimerà, 2012).

In addition to reducing calories consumed, encourage activities that burn calories, such as swimming, gym classes, or walking their dog (Loprinzi, Cardinal, Loprinzi, et al., 2012). These activities are generally preferable to formal exercises, such as sit-ups and push-ups, which may be viewed as punishment.

Adolescents who use overeating as their main reaction to stress may require psychological counseling rather than diet counseling if they are to develop a more mature emotional response to stress. Behavior modification is sometimes successful with adolescents as a means of helping them lose weight, but it is rarely recommended for obesity alone (see Chapter 35).

General measures to help adolescents decrease overeating include:

- Making a detailed log of the amount they eat, the time, and the circumstances (including how they felt while they were eating) and then changing those circumstances
- Always eating in one place (the kitchen table) instead of while walking home from school or watching television
- Slowing the process of eating by counting mouthfuls and putting the fork down between bites, or being served food on small plates so helpings look larger

These measures may be of little use, however, unless they are combined with a suitable diet and adequate exercise. Despite all these interventions, weight reduction may not always be effective with adolescents. For some, a more realistic goal might be to prevent additional weight gain until they reach adulthood.

CONCERNS REGARDING SEXUALITY AND SEXUAL ACTIVITY

Adolescents who engage in sexual risk behaviors can have unintended health outcomes, including unplanned pregnancies and sexually transmitted infections (STIs) such as HIV. During routine health assessments of adolescents and preadolescents, this topic should be explored.

According to a 2015 CDC survey report, 41% of U.S. high school students have had sexual intercourse, and of that number, 30% was in the previous 3 months. The survey also reported 43% did not use a condom the last time they had sex. Only 10% had ever been tested for HIV. Yet, those age 13 to 24 years accounted for an estimated 22% of all new HIV diagnoses in the United States in 2014, and within this group, 80% were gay and bisexual males. Half of the nearly 20 million new STIs reported each year were among adolescents and late adolescents age 15 to 24 years in 2014. Pregnancy in adolescence, although decreasing, is still a concern. Nearly 250,000 births were to girls ages 15 to 24 years in 2014 (CDC, 2017d).

When discussing sexuality with adolescents, the nurse should avoid assumptions about the gender of the adolescent's partner. Ask open-ended questions when providing education on health promoting behaviors. This will also help the adolescent feel more open to asking questions.

Counseling can assist adolescents improve their perspective and also learn how to say no. For adolescents who agree to have intercourse but who do not really want to, the primary reasons given are peer pressure, curiosity, and affection for their partner (Fuzzell, Fedesco, Alexander, et al., 2016; Katsufrakis & Nusbaum, 2011).

According to the CDC (2017b), most lesbian, gay, bisexual, and transgender (LGBT) youth are well adjusted during their adolescent years. The nurse should explore the school and home environment, as adjustment can be promoted by a supportive learning environment and caring and accepting parents (CDC, 2017b). If the adolescent is not provided with this environment, they may have difficulties in their lives and possibly be at risk for violence from bullying behaviors. Bullying is described in more detail in this chapter.

Adolescents may seek a healthcare appointment for an unrelated health concern as a reason to discuss a sexual health question with a healthcare professional. During routine health visits, it is important to obtain a complete sexual health history and offer health related education appropriate to the adolescent's individualized history. General guidelines on counseling an adolescent with respect to sexual activity are summarized in Box 33.5.

Information on date rape and rape prevention should be provided as adolescents are in a high-risk age group for date rape (Makin-Byrd & Bierman, 2013) (see Chapter 55). One form of date rape occurs when flunitrazepam (Rohypnol) (i.e., the "date-rape drug"), a colorless, odorless, and flavorless benzodiazepine drug, is dropped into a drink, causing drowsiness, impaired motor skills, and amnesia for a time (Karch, 2013). Adolescents who are seen for sexual assault who appear intoxicated or have amnesia for the event should be suspected of unknowingly ingesting flunitrazepam or another drug such as ketamine. In these instances, a urine specimen analysis will reveal the drug's metabolites or that the drug was ingested (D'Aloise & Chen, 2012).

BOX 33.5

Nursing Care Planning Based on Family Teaching

HEALTH TEACHING GUIDELINES FOR ADOLESCENTS REGARDING SEXUALITY

Q. Raul asks you, "How will I know when I'm ready for sex?"

A. Here are a few common guidelines:

- It is your choice whether to participate in sexual relations. Do not be influenced by friends who may be exaggerating stories to impress you or who ask you to do something you do not want to do. When you say no, be firm and clear about your wishes.
- There is no 100% method to prevent pregnancy or a sexually transmitted infection (STI) except abstinence. Be direct with a sexual partner in discussing abstinence or reproductive and infection prevention measures.
- Sexual relations neither add to nor detract from your physical strength or general wellness.
- The mark of an adult sexual relationship is that the activity is pleasurable to both partners. If sexual partners are not interested in your enjoyment as well as their own, you should reconsider the relationship.
- There is no "normal" mode of sexual expression. Any activity that is pleasurable to both partners is "normal."
- Learn about safer sex techniques and practice them.

Stalking

Stalking refers to repetitive, intrusive, and unwanted actions such as constant and threatening pursuit directed at an individual to gain the individual's attention or to evoke fear. Electronic media can be used for cyberstalking, Internet harassment, and Internet bullying to embarrass, harass, or threaten adolescents (CDC, 2017c). The overall term for these methods is electronic aggression (CDC, 2017c). It can result in the same victim responses as that from aggression that is not inflicted electronically. To avoid stalking, adolescents should be aware of and avoid situations where they will be vulnerable to being alone with a stalker and, with assistance, report stalking to law enforcement.

QSEN Checkpoint Question 33.4

SAFETY

Raul is depressed because his girlfriend broke up with him. Which of his statements could be interpreted as stalking?

- a. "I keep her photo on my bedside stand so I can kiss her goodnight."
- b. "We take the same route to school every day so I often still see her."
- c. "I e-mail her every night to tell her what a huge mistake she's made."
- d. "I took down her photo from Facebook but wish I could put it back."

Look in Appendix A for the best answer and rationale.

CONCERNS REGARDING HAZING OR BULLYING

Bullying, which began during school age (see Chapter 32), can easily continue into adolescence and actually becomes more serious because this can be the time the bullied child has the ability to retaliate through self-destructive behavior or school violence.

Hazing, a form of organized bullying, refers to demeaning or humiliating rituals that prospective members have to undergo to join sororities, fraternities, adolescent gangs, or sports teams (Diamond, Callahan, Chain, et al., 2016). Most rituals are secret and in the past were accepted as "rites of passage." In recent years, hazing has become so extreme the practice has moved out of the "just fun" category into activities that can cause physical and certainly psychological harm, such as being forced to wear demeaning clothing or engaging in crude or lewd skits. They can be extended to such an extreme that adolescents may be punched or kicked, sodomized, left out in the cold so long that frostbite develops, or forced to drink alcohol until they vomit, pass out, or even die from alcohol intoxication. Initiation for street gangs can require prospective members to steal or destroy property or even kill another person.

To help prevent this from happening to their child, urge parents to be aware of what clubs or organizations their adolescent joins and what the requirements for membership are. Help adolescents make sound decisions about what type of hazing their organization advocates by asking them about the subject at health assessments.

CONCERNS REGARDING SUBSTANCE USE DISORDER

Substance use disorder (formerly referred to as substance abuse disorder) refers to the use of chemicals to improve a mental state or induce euphoria. This is so common among adolescents that as many as 50% of high school seniors report having experimented with some form of drug (CDC, 2012a). Use of drugs occurs in adolescence from a desire to expand consciousness, peer pressure, or a desire to feel more confident and mature; it also can be a form of adolescent rebellion related to childhood adversity or violence. Stages of drug use range from experimentation where teenagers try drugs to enhance social acceptance to regular use, where they actively seek the effect of drugs to relieve everyday stress (Benjet, Borges, Medina-Mora, et al., 2012).

Types of Abused Substances

Because adolescents may not have a large source of money, the drugs they most frequently abuse are those they can obtain on a limited budget and through limited contacts.

Prescription and Over-the-Counter Drugs

Adolescents may first begin drug experimentation by taking drugs prescribed for another family member or a pet such as sedatives, pain medication, ketamine (an anesthetic used in veterinary medicine), or cough syrup containing codeine or dextromethorphan (DXM). Called "pharming," adolescents who use drugs this way can easily overdose because they are unaware of usual dosages (Storck, Black, & Liddell, 2016).

Methylphenidate (Ritalin) is a drug frequently prescribed for attention deficit hyperactivity disorder. Because methylphenidate (Ritalin) is a stimulant, when oral tablets are crushed and injected intravenously, they produce a feeling of giddiness and extreme well-being. Unfortunately, because they do not completely dissolve, the resultant small particles remaining in the bloodstream can result in complications such as pulmonary embolus or emphysema, so this is a very dangerous practice. Every house has a number of inhalants, such as oil-based cooking spray, gas, butane, or lighter fluid, which may be abused by adolescents. Inhalants can lead to cardiac failure from suffocation. Mephedrone, commonly called "bath salts," is a stimulant that creates an enjoyable "high" and is available for purchase online and so is easily obtained by adolescents (Nguyen, O'Brien, & Schapp, 2016). The effect of using it is seen more regularly in emergency departments as the cause of reckless driving or unconsciousness (Baumann, Partilla, & Lehner, 2013). Listed as a schedule 1 drug, it is now illegal to obtain.

Alcohol

As many as 90% of high school seniors report having consumed alcohol, and as many as 25% of high school students report having engaged in episodic heavy or binge drinking. At least 10% of high school students report driving a car or other vehicle when they had been drinking alcohol. Nearly 30% of students report having ridden in a car or other vehicle driven by someone who had been drinking alcohol (CDC, 2012a).

Although alcohol use is correlated with motor vehicle accidents, homicide, and suicide in adolescents, it has never carried the social stigma of other drugs. Some parents are actually relieved when they learn their child's strange behavior on returning home from a party was caused by drunkenness and not illegal drugs. Alcohol use cannot be taken lightly, however, because it can cause diseases such as cirrhosis and is linked to destructive behaviors such as addiction, depression, and vulnerability to date rape.

Heredity has a definite role in the use of alcohol, but environment plays an equal part in whether an adolescent becomes a frequent user (Maimon & Browning, 2012). Remind parents they have a responsibility to set good examples for adolescents in the use of alcohol by not drinking indiscriminately.

Most adolescents will admit they use alcohol if asked two specific questions: "Do you drink alcohol?" and "When was your last drink?" Adolescents who answer yes to the first and "within the last 24 hours" to the second are candidates for further assessment.

Once adolescents admit they have come to rely on alcohol as a way to feel popular or reduce stress, an organization such as Alcoholics Anonymous can be invaluable in helping them stop drinking; innovative online programs geared especially for adolescents are also available. Encourage the remainder of their family to join Al-Anon, the organization for families of alcoholics, so both children and their families can restructure their lives to find satisfaction without the use of this drug.

Many adolescents are not the primary alcohol abuser in a family but are the children of alcoholic parents. Make an effort to identify this group of children as well, not only to prevent them from becoming users of alcohol but also to help them build self-esteem and coping abilities for the difficulties they face living in a possibly disorganized household.

QSEN Checkpoint Question 33.5

EVIDENCE-BASED PRACTICE

It has long been theorized there may be a "gateway" drug or one that, when used first, leads to further and more dangerous substance use disorders. To determine whether alcohol, tobacco, or marijuana was the gateway drug, researchers obtained information on the drug use of a nationally representative sample of high school seniors. Results of the study showed alcohol was the gateway drug, leading to tobacco, marijuana, and then other illicit substances (Barry, King, Sears, et al., 2016).

Based on the previous study, which statement by Raul would give you the most concern?

a. "Some of my friends got hammered last weekend but I decided not to stick around."

b. "Some of my friends use weed; they tell me it really helps them relax."

c. "My parents said I could celebrate my next birthday by drinking my first beer."

d. "My mother eats some kind of chocolate almost every day. Is that hereditary?"

Look in Appendix A for the best answer and rationale.

Tobacco

Although it is well documented that cigarette smoking leads to increased cardiovascular and respiratory illnesses by middle age, every day, approximately 4,000 American youth aged 12 to 17 years try their first cigarette. As many as 20% of high school students report current cigarette use, and about 14% report current cigar use. Eight percent of high school students report current smokeless tobacco use (CDC, 2012d).

Adolescents usually begin smoking because the habit conveys a stamp of maturity; those who are having difficulty demonstrating maturity in other areas may view smoking as especially desirable. Although at one time, proportionately more males than females smoked, adolescent girls now are the population most likely to begin smoking. One of the strongest determinants of whether adolescents will smoke a first cigarette is whether their friends smoke.

As cigar smoking is becoming more popular with adults, it also is becoming more popular with adolescents. "Smokeless tobacco" or chewing tobacco is also becoming more popular (Kozlowski & Sweanor, 2017). Although chewing tobacco does not have the potential dangers of smoking tobacco in relation to lung disease, it can cause gingival recession and lip and mouth cancer, and it can be just as habit forming as cigarettes.

It has been well documented that adolescents are influenced to begin smoking by advertising (Widome, Brock, Noble, et al., 2013). Most school systems have extensive programs as early as grade school to caution children not to listen to cigarette advertising. Unfortunately, the ultimate danger of illness or death in middle age is not a strong threat to young persons who are interested only in the present.

More effective campaigns, therefore, might be those that point out that cigarette smoking causes foul-smelling hair, clothes, and breath, which detracts from physical appearance (i.e., "now" concerns). Helping adolescents find other methods to demonstrate their maturity, such as allowing them opportunities for increased decision making and emphasizing that being able to *not* smoke is a sign of true maturity, needs to be investigated. Urge adolescents who want to quit cigarette smoking to enroll in a group cigarette or online withdrawal program. Nicotine gum and nicotine patches have both been successfully used with adolescents (Harvey & Chadi, 2016).

Additionally, in recent years, the use of e-cigarettes and vaping has increased significantly among adolescents. Their use has been demonstrated to actually increase the use of cigarette consumption. This is because they become addicted to the nicotine in the e-cigarette (Gostin & Glasner, 2014). The lack of regulations regarding the sale of vaping products causes additional problems for their use among adolescents. To purchase cigarettes, all persons must show identification and be older than 18 years of age. However, less than half of the states require identification to purchase e-cigarettes (Gostin & Glasner, 2014).

Adolescents are very reluctant to follow instructions that are given from a "do as I say, not as I do" standpoint. Nurses who smoke, therefore, can have extreme difficulty launching an effective campaign against the habit with adolescents. Stopping smoking can be especially difficult during periods of stress or inactivity. Trying to introduce such an action during exam week, for example, is not good planning. During an illness is also a bad time, unless not feeling well has reduced the urge to smoke. A return visit for follow-up and health maintenance care might be a better time to introduce the topic.

What If . . . 33.2

Raul tells the nurse during a history assessment that he does not smoke, but the nurse smells cigarette smoke on his clothing. Although he says he doesn't use drugs, a number of blue-and-white capsules fall out of his shirt pocket when he unbuttons his shirt. What questions would the nurse want to ask him to determine if he is smoking cigarettes or using drugs? What would be the nurse's next action if he does admit he is not only heavily into drugs but also does not intend to stop using them?

Performance-Enhancing Substance Use Disorder

Anabolic steroids are derivatives of the natural hormone testosterone. Common names are stanozolol, an oral compound, and testosterone propionate, an injectable form. Adolescents take steroids (obtained illegally) to enhance lean body mass and muscular development and so improve their athletic ability or appearance. These substances have side effects of euphoria and lessened fatigue, which make them doubly appealing.

Unfortunately, steroid use can lead to early closure of the epiphyseal line of long bones, acne, elevated triglyceride levels, hypertension, aggressiveness, possibly psychosis, abnormal liver function, and perhaps liver cancer. In addition, athletes using them and paying vigorous sports can die from ventricular hypertrophy (Montisci, El Mazloum, Cecchetto, et al., 2012).

Students using anabolic steroids need to be identified so they can be cautioned that the use of such drugs is illegal in sports competitions as well as being detrimental to their health.

If needles are shared for administration, they additionally run the risk of acquiring hepatitis B or HIV infections.

Human growth hormone is a second drug used to enhance athletic performance. This increases muscle strength and stamina and is more difficult to detect than steroid use and so is also becoming a commonly abused substance in athletes (Albertson, Chenoweth, Colby, et al., 2016). It's dangerous in adolescents because side effects are joint pain and swelling and the development of diabetes.

Marijuana

Marijuana (widely known as "pot," "grass," or "weed"), derived from the leaves and stems of the Indian hemp plant *Cannabis sativa*, is the most frequently abused illicit substance, next to alcohol, used by adolescents (Kaul, 2016). It is generally rolled into cigarettes ("joints" or "reefers") and smoked, although it can also be mixed with food or sniffed. Scraping the resin from the flowering leaves produces a much stronger substance called hashish. Sinsemilla is a seedless form that is even more potent.

Breakdown products of marijuana are not readily eliminated from the body and remain in the fatty cells of the brain. This residue can create synaptic gaps that interfere with electrical brain waves and memory storage, especially for short-term memory. Physical and psychological effects of all forms of marijuana are euphoria and a sense of well-being, temporary impairment of coordination, rapid mood swings, decreased attention span, and loss of memory for recent events (up to 1 hour's time). Withdrawal symptoms include irritability, drowsiness, and cravings for high-carbohydrate snacks.

Long-term side effects can include pulmonary disorders such as sinusitis, bronchitis, emphysema, and perhaps lung cancer (which can develop after only 1 year of continual use compared with 20 years of cigarette use) as well as lack of sperm formation or subfertility in males (Fronczak, Kim, & Barqawi, 2012).

Because the drug is prescribed to relieve nausea and vomiting, adolescents may view it as harmless. Help them to realize marijuana is more than an amusing leisure activity or a way to relieve stress so they can put its long-term effects into perspective.

Amphetamines

Amphetamines are a group of drugs used in the treatment of hyperactivity and narcolepsy, among other central nervous system disorders. They are easily manufactured in "meth labs" in people's homes and so may be readily available to adolescents. Amphetamines are called "uppers" or "speed" because they give the user a false sense of well-being, alertness, or self-esteem. A newer, stronger form that produces intense symptoms is known as "ice." Some of the side effects of either form are aggressive or demanding behavior, paranoia, and extreme restlessness. Chronic methamphetamine abuse results in destruction of teeth enamel or blackened, crumbling teeth (Auten, Matteucci, Gaspary, et al., 2012). Amphetamines can be especially appealing to obese adolescents as they suppress the appetite and result in weight loss.

Cocaine

Cocaine is one of the most popular drugs of abuse for late adolescents; its use can begin in adolescents. The drug may be sniffed into the nose (snorted), smoked, or injected intravenously. Occasionally, it is combined with heroin (termed a "speedball") and injected. Common street names for cocaine are "snow" and "white lady" because of its fine, white powder. A stronger form, called "crack," is manufactured by heating cocaine powder with baking soda and water. This preparation process is dangerous in itself because it involves using volatile solvents that can ignite or explode. The resulting drug, often called "freebase" or "rock," is so strong it can cause immediate cardiac and respiratory arrhythmias (Paczynski & Gold, 2011).

It is difficult to document how many adolescents use cocaine, but estimates range from 3% to 9%. After absorption, blood levels rise rapidly for the first 20 minutes, peak at 60 minutes, and then decline over the next 3 hours. Although a toxic dose of cocaine is usually considered to be 600 to 700 mg, toxicity has been reported in as low as a 20 mg dose (a single line).

Cocaine produces the physical effects of increased pulse and respiration rates, increased temperature, increased blood pressure, and decreased appetite. Psychological effects produced are euphoria, excitement and restlessness, increased sociability, and possible hallucinations.

Toxic symptoms include seizures, tachyarrhythmias, tachypnea, hypertension, nausea and vomiting, abdominal pain, headaches, chills, and fever. It can be a major cause of cardiovascular arrest in late adolescents (Eisendrath & Lichtmacher, 2013). It may be a cause of adolescent automobile accidents because it creates such a sense of well-being and safety (Stoduto, Mann, Ialomiteanu, et al., 2012).

Cocaine is rarely ingested orally, but occasionally, adolescents swallow it when trying to hide a supply from parents or school personnel. Gastric acid destroys the action of cocaine, so unless the amount is extremely large, it is potentially harmless when swallowed in this way.

Teach adolescents that although cocaine sniffing may be fascinating and offer temporary pleasure and relief from stress, it also causes psychological dependency and is potentially extremely dangerous because of its cardiac and respiratory effects. Chronic inhalation of cocaine can cause ulceration in the mucous membrane of the nose, and injection of the substance exposes an adolescent to the risk of HIV and AIDS or hepatitis B. During pregnancy, it can cause separation of the placenta with potential fetal and maternal death (Mbah, Alio, Fombo, et al., 2012).

Hallucinogens

Examples of hallucinogenic drugs used by adolescents are lysergic acid diethylamide (LSD), dimethyltryptamine (DMT), 2,5-dimethoxy-4-methylamphetamine (STP), phencyclidine (PCP) hydrochloride, *Salvia divinorum*, mephedrone ("bath salts"), and methaqualone (Quaalude). The use of LSD has substantially increased in popularity since the 1960s when it first became available because it is a drug that can be manufactured by an informed adolescent in a "kitchen lab." 3,4-Methylenedioxymethamphetamine (MDMA), also known as Molly/Ecstasy, is similar to both stimulants and hallucinogens. It gives users feelings of euphoria, pleasure, distorted time, and sensory perception. It is popular at dance clubs and "raves." Usually, this drug is taken in tablet or capsule form; however, it can be snorted as well. MDMA affects typically last 3 to 6 hours, and side effects may include irritability, aggression, depression, anxiety, decreased appetite, and memory problems. There is still some disagreement as to whether MDMA is addictive because research results had demonstrated varying results.

All of these drugs cause bizarre mind reactions such as distortion in vision, smell, or hearing. Adolescents report seeing colors more vividly than they have ever seen them before, hearing sounds so clear they cause physical pain, or perceiving themselves as being totally impervious to harm leading to "good trips" or "bad trips."

Recurrences or flashbacks of drug-induced experiences may, unfortunately, recur at unpredictable times and in unexpected places. Such flashbacks are not only disconcerting but also can be dangerous, especially if they occur while a person is driving a motor vehicle. They can be so frightening that some users believe they are becoming mentally deranged.

QSEN Checkpoint Question 33.6

TEAMWORK & COLLABORATION

At the conclusion of a long conversation, Raul admits he has experimented with cocaine. Which assessment finding would most strongly warrant a referral to addiction services?

    a. Raul has frown lines in his forehead.
    b. Raul has thin, fissured lips.
    c. Raul's eyebrows appear thin.
    d. Raul lacks nasal hair.

Look in Appendix A for the best answer and rationale.

Opiates

Opiates include drugs such as heroin, meperidine (Demerol), and morphine. At one time, these were not typically used by adolescents because they are expensive, but their use has increased with staggering health effects. According to the CDC (2017a), drug overdose involving heroin increased from 1.2 to 2.8 per 100,000 for those 15 to 24 years old between 2010 and 2015.

The American Academy of Pediatrics recommends screening adolescents for substance use disorders. Screening, Brief Intervention, and Referral to Treatment (SBIRT) is a model used to help prevent substance use disorders and to limit the progression to riskier drugs, such as heroin (Harris, 2016). The nurse should discuss the use of opiates with the adolescent and encourage an open dialogue to identify whether they are at risk for substance use consequences.

Opiates can be extremely dangerous because of their tendency to decrease one's respiratory rate. The increase in overdose deaths has prompted the training of first responders in the use of naloxone to reverse the respiratory depression effects and to decrease the rate of deaths from overdoses. Adolescents should be encouraged to seek care for themselves or others whenever an overdose situation is apparent as prompt treatment can be lifesaving.

Assessment of Substance Use Disorders

If adolescents form a trusting relationship with healthcare providers, they will generally disclose high-risk behaviors (Box 33.6). Increased school absences and a decrease in school achievement are important to note. Diagnosis of hepatitis B, HIV positive, or appearing to receive no benefit from usual analgesic agents are later indicators of high-risk behaviors. Physical symptoms that indicate specific substance use disorder are summarized in Table 33.3.

Nursing Diagnoses and Related Interventions

Nursing Diagnosis: Risk for injury related to the use of alcohol or addictive chemical substances

Outcome Evaluation: Adolescent states he is not experimenting with drugs; can describe a way to respond to peers who encourage such use; shows no evidence of drug use such as lethargy, confusion, positive urine drug screen, or parental suspicion.

One of the greatest dangers of early drug experimentation is that it affects an adolescent's ability to solve problems, which creates a delay in maturity. Because adolescents may avoid adults who might detect their drug use, they remove themselves from exposure to adult role models.

Important teaching points for avoiding drug use include:

- Whether a drug is inhaled, swallowed, or injected, it still is absorbed, enters your body, and is therefore potentially harmful.
- Relying on drugs to give you courage to solve problems (or to help you forget you have problems) prevents you from learning to handle life situations and maturing.
- The bottom line of substance use disorder is that you have the final say: You are the only one who can stop chemical dependency from happening.
- Despite their social acceptability, alcohol and nicotine are drugs. A short span of daily use of either can make you addicted.

Therapeutic communities or 24-hour facilities in which adolescents can live while they recover from chemical dependency may be necessary for some adolescents. The aim of all these programs is to increase adolescents' sense of self-esteem, improve problem-solving ability, realign them

BOX 33.6

Nursing Care Planning Tips for Effective Communication

You talk to Raul, age 15 years, in an adolescent clinic and provide patient education on substance use.

Tip: Sometimes, adolescents repeat the same answer to questions even when different questions are asked in conversations. Asking them about their friends and their drug use may encourage the adolescent to respond more fully to questions.

Nurse: Some adolescents find it useful to read about drug use among their peers. Here's a pamphlet about adolescents and drug use.

Raul: Okay, thanks.

Nurse: Sometimes, it's difficult to talk to parents or other adults about such things.

Raul: That's true.

Nurse: Do any of your friends use drugs?

Raul: Some people in my class have tried drugs. I never would because I am on the baseball team and I would be kicked off if I did any drugs.

TABLE 33.3 SYMPTOMS TO HELP IDENTIFY SUBSTANCE USE DISORDERS

Drugs Used	Symptoms of Use	Dangers
Glue	Violence, drunken appearance, dreamy or blank expression; glue smears on clothing or fingers; tubes of glue, paper bags in possession	Lung, brain, or liver damage; death through suffocation or choking; anemia
Heroin, morphine, codeine	Stupor, drowsiness, needle marks on body, watery eyes, loss of appetite, bloodstains on shirt sleeve, runny nose; possession of needles or hypodermic syringes, cotton, tourniquet strings, burnt bottle caps or spoons, glassine envelopes	Death from overdose; addiction; liver and other infections due to unsterile needles
Cough medicines containing codeine	Drunken appearance, lack of coordination, confusion, excessive itching; possession of empty bottles of cough medicine	Addiction
Marijuana	Sleepiness, wandering mind, enlarged pupils, lack of coordination; discolored fingers, strong odor of burnt leaves; possession of small seeds in pocket lining, cigarette papers	Psychological dependence
Hallucinogens (LSD, DMT, PCP)	Severe hallucinations, feelings of detachment, incoherent speech, cold hands and feet, laughing and crying, vomiting, strong body odor; possession of cube sugar with discoloration in center	Suicidal tendencies, unpredictable behavior; chronic exposure may have neurologic effects
Stimulants (methamphetamine, cocaine)	Aggressive behavior, giggling, silliness, rapid speech, confused thinking, no appetite, extreme fatigue, black caries, dry mouth, shakiness, insomnia, absence of nasal hair; possession of pills or capsules of varying colors, possession of a glass pipe	Death from overdose; hallucinations; psychosis
Depressants (barbiturates, alcohol)	Drowsiness, stupor, dullness, slurred speech, drunken appearance, vomiting, odor of alcohol on breath; possession of pills or capsules of varying colors	Death or unconsciousness from overdose; addiction; seizures from withdrawal
Steroids	Aggressive behavior, increase in muscle strength and mass	Violent actions; possibly tumor growth

LSD, lysergic acid diethylamide; DMT, dimethyltryptamine; PCP, phencyclidine.

with society's values, and increase their self-awareness so they can function effectively without the aid of substances of abuse. Unfortunately, campaigns against substance use disorder for adolescents have not been very successful, so the problem continues.

Adolescents who are no longer chemically dependent should be evaluated by a history and physical examination at all healthcare visits because, if the circumstances that initially caused them to become chemically dependent recur, they may return to a dependency pattern. A continuing relationship with healthcare personnel not only allows time for this evaluation but also provides concrete role models of nonchemical, productive behavior.

CONCERNS REGARDING DEPRESSION AND SELF-INJURY

Self-injury includes a range of self-destructive actions from cutting to suicide, the planned intent to end one's life. Cutting is found more frequently in girls than boys and can begin as early as grade school (Barrocas, Hankin, Young, et al., 2012).

Successful suicide occurs more frequently in males than in females, although more females apparently attempt suicide than males (a ratio of about 8:1). Adolescent suicides tend to be attempted most often in the spring or the fall, reflecting school stress at these times of year, and between 3 PM and midnight, reflecting depression that increases with

the dark. Suicide is so common in adolescents it ranks in the top four causes of death in the 10- to 24-year-old age group. The top four causes of death are motor vehicle crashes (23%), other intentional injuries (17%), homicide (14%), and suicide (17%) (Kann, McManus, Harris, et al., 2016). This statistic may actually be underestimated as they may be reported as unintentional injuries. Injuries or deaths that are due to high-risk behaviors in adolescents, such as motor vehicle accidents, may mask a suicide attempt. Some degree of depression is present in most adolescents because they are losing not only their parents while they grow apart from them but also their carefree childhood (Fried, Williams, Cabral, et al., 2013). If school failure, loss of a girlfriend or boyfriend, loss of a competition with loss of self-esteem, or rejection by a peer group is superimposed on existing depression, the pressure may be great enough to cause some adolescents to attempt suicide. This makes the reasons for adolescent suicide varied: Incest, maltreatment, increased chemical dependency, marital instability in the family, and poor problem-solving ability are all reasons that may lead an adolescent to decide death may be easier than coping with overwhelming problems.

Yet, other reasons may involve anger with others, trying to get even, and manipulation (e.g., psychological blackmail) as a way of having one's needs met. Because some adolescents may be unable to believe a parent was at fault in the case of divorce, they may instead believe they somehow caused the parent to leave.

Assessment

Adolescents need to have thorough physical examinations at health maintenance visits to assure them they are in good physical health. Assess at these visits signs of depression such as anorexia, insomnia, excessive fatigue, or weight loss (Gampetro, Wojciechowski, & Amer, 2012). In younger adolescents, depression may be manifested not so much by appearing sad, but by behavior problems such as disobedience, temper tantrums, truancy, and running away. Self-destructive behavior or injury proneness; difficulties in school; acting out with chemicals, alcohol, or sexual promiscuity; or trouble with legal authorities may be further clues.

Occasionally, depressed adolescents find it so hard to be alone that they seek constant activity as a means of escape. Others may withdraw from contact with other people and become completely isolated. Either behavior needs to be detected through assessing activity and interaction levels.

Adolescents who attempt suicide do not fall into any one category, although many tend to be loners or have difficulty expressing their feelings to others and, therefore, do not receive emotional support from friends or family. Others appear to be "perfect" students, so friends or family do not see a need to counsel them. The stress of trying to continually achieve at a high level, however, is the trigger that provokes suicide. LGBT youths appear to have higher levels of suicide than others, reflecting the level of stress they may be experiencing. Assess for LGBTs as well (Shields, Whitaker, Glassman, et al., 2012).

If another member of a family or a close friend commits suicide, the chance an adolescent will also do so is greater than usual. The anniversary of a family member's suicide is an especially vulnerable time because wishing to join the dead family member may appear attractive. Adolescent suicide rates may actually reach epidemic proportions after a popular student's suicide. Students who have Internet contacts may arrange a group suicide as a method of making a statement or gaining support.

Because suicide usually reflects a problem in family interaction, a family assessment is helpful. A thorough family history may reveal conflict with one or both parents or reveal how little support the adolescent receives at home. School friends may often be the ones who are first aware that an adolescent is contemplating suicide. Caution parents not to discount reports from their child's friends who tell them they are concerned.

Close to the chosen time of suicide, some adolescents demonstrate characteristic behaviors that show they are making preparations to end their life. Teach family and friends these typical danger signs (Box 33.7).

When caring for a child after a suicide attempt, ask enough questions on a health history so you can help to analyze whether an adolescent made a detailed suicide plan. For example, a young person who took four aspirins and left the empty aspirin container conspicuously on the kitchen counter just before his mother was due to arrive home from work is more likely to be only making a cry for help; one who took 100 aspirins and hid the container under the bed just after his mother left for 8 hours of work is much more apt to be making a serious attempt.

As you care for an adolescent in a healthcare facility, you may be the first to realize the boy or girl is not "just talking" about suicide (it is a fallacy that people who talk about suicide do not attempt it) but is someone with a definite,

---

BOX 33.7

Nursing Care Planning Based on Family Teaching

SUICIDE WARNING SIGNS

Q. Raul's father says to you, "Our neighbor's son recently committed suicide. What are warning signs of this to look for in our son?"

A. The following are commonly seen clues:

- Giving away prized possessions
- Organ donation questions, such as "How do you leave your body to a medical school?"
- Sudden, unexplained elevation of mood, which may indicate the individual has reached a decision about the suicide and feels relief
- Injury proneness, carelessness, and death wishes
- Decrease in verbal communication or a statement such as "This is the last time you will see me"
- Withdrawal from peer activities or previously enjoyed events
- Previous attempt (80% of all completed suicides have been preceded by a failed attempt)
- Preference for art, music, and literature with themes of death
- Recent increase in interpersonal conflict with significant others
- Running away from home
- Recent experience of a friend or famous person committing suicide
- Inquiring about the hereafter
- Asking for information (supposedly for a friend) about suicide prevention and intervention
- Almost any sustained deviation from the normal pattern of behavior

---

well-thought-out plan to accomplish it. An adolescent who has been admitted to a hospital unit after a serious suicide attempt may formulate a new plan that will be successful the next time unless some action is taken and the adolescent's life can be changed in some way (see Box 33.8 for an interprofessional care map for an adolescent with possible suicide intent).

Nursing Diagnoses and Related Interventions

Nursing Diagnosis: Risk for violence, self-directed, related to symptoms of depression or expressed desire to hurt oneself

Outcome Evaluation: Patient expresses feelings of depression to healthcare providers or other adults; states he will contact support person should the desire to commit suicide become overwhelming.

Crisis intervention for adolescents who are contemplating suicide includes trying to alleviate their pain and depression and counseling them in an effort to help them change their perspective on the value of life. Be aware that

BOX 33.8

Nursing Care Planning

AN INTERPROFESSIONAL CARE MAP FOR AN ADOLESCENT WITH POSSIBLE SUICIDE INTENT

Raul is a 15-year-old boy you meet at an adolescent clinic. His chief concern is a head cold. He has numerous acne lesions on his forehead and cheeks. His parents tell you Raul seemed depressed for a long time after his girlfriend broke up with him but now seems happy again. They are pleased to see him maturing so much; for example, he recently gave away his collection of baseball cards to a young neighbor. You mention to Raul a decongestant would probably make him feel better. He asks you how many pills it would take to kill someone and then jokes he was kidding.

Family Assessment: Patient lives with both parents and two younger siblings. Father manages a funeral parlor; mother works as a beautician for funeral parlor. Patient describes finances as "All right, if you think burying people is a good way to earn money."

Patient Assessment: Fifteen-year-old male with history of acne for the last 6 months. Reports washing his face approximately five or six times a day with abrasive soap and covering lesions with cocoa butter cream twice a day. He states, "Look at me. I look terrible." Physical examination reveals scattered pustules and comedones on forehead and face. Two lesions on right cheek with large erythematous base and tender to touch. Remainder of physical examination unremarkable.

Nursing Diagnosis: Risk for self-injury related to disappointing appearance because of acne lesions and lack of friendships

Outcome Criteria: Adolescent states causes of acne; identifies measures for prevention and treatment; agrees to counseling to reestablish self-esteem.

Team Member Responsible	Assessment	Intervention	Rationale	Expected Outcome
Activities of Daily Living, Including Safety				
Nurse/nurse practitioner	Assess adolescent's understanding of acne and its causes.	Instruct adolescent in measures to prevent and control acne.	Gentle washing removes irritating fatty acids. Omit greasy creams.	Patient states intent to follow recommendations to decrease acne symptoms.
Teamwork and Collaboration				
Nurse/primary healthcare provider/mental health counselor	Evaluate if patient was joking or was serious about a self-injury attempt.	Schedule consultation if patient may be contemplating self-injury.	Patient shows typical signs of self-injury behavior.	Mental health counselor meets with patient to make recommendations on patient safety.
Procedures/Medications for Quality Improvement				
Nurse/nurse practitioner	Assess what measures patient has been using to self-treat acne.	Discuss treatment options available.	Discussion provides the adolescent with correct information on acne therapy.	Patient describes full range of therapies available and what new measures he would be willing to try.
Nutrition				
Nurse/nutritionist	Assess patient's understanding of the effect of nutrition on acne.	Counsel patient to follow a well-balanced diet.	No particular food is associated with development of acne, despite old beliefs.	Patient states he understands food intake is not the major cause of acne.
Patient-Centered Care				
Nurse	Assess family's communication level, overall coping techniques, and abilities.	Discuss how better communication can aid in helping adolescent cope with life changes.	Better communication among family members provides support for all family members.	Parents discuss family communication pattern and make suggestions for better patterns.

Psychosocial/Spiritual/Emotional Needs

Nurse	Assess how acne affects patient's self-esteem.	Review and reinforce with adolescent positive attributes about self.	Positive attributes provide a foundation for rebuilding self-esteem.	Patient states he knows that others value his friendship above his appearance.

Informatics for Seamless Healthcare Planning

Nurse/nurse practitioner/ mental health counselor	Assess with mental health counselor if it will be safe for patient to return home.	Give patient hotline telephone number and instruct to use as needed.	Knowing a support source is available can be as valuable as actually contacting the source.	Patient assures staff he has the hotline number available and will call if needed.

establishing expected outcomes with adolescents who are contemplating suicide or who have made an attempt will be difficult because they are often too depressed to come up with alternative solutions to their problems (their goal was to kill themselves, not solve problems).

It is important not to underestimate adolescents' determination and capability to end their own life. In most instances, adolescents at this point need referral to a consultant who is well versed in suicide prevention to improve self-image and offer alternative solutions to problems.

As another measure, try to find out the things in the child's life that are still viewed as important; build a plan that will help view life as worth living enough to work through difficulties. Show them how no one can change everything, but everyone can make one or two changes that can make a difference. After these small changes are made, a domino effect can be created to change more and more of one's circumstances.

Because adolescents resort to suicide as a method of solving problems, helping all adolescents learn better problem-solving skills is a prime intervention strategy. Ask "what would happen if" questions such as "Suppose you did fail a course; what would be the worst that could happen?" Your help in this area is important because, generally, persons who are depressed do not have strong support people around them or do not believe anyone cares enough about them to help.

For an adolescent's safety, a period of observation on an adolescent or a psychiatric service is desirable after a suicide attempt to prevent the adolescent from inflicting personal injury again and to allow an assessment in a neutral setting, away from the stress that precipitated the attempt. Evidence for the effectiveness of selective serotonin reuptake inhibitors, as are used with adults, is limited with children; these medications have a black box warning to use with caution in persons under 25 years of age as some have been associated with elevating the mood of depressed children enough that they then are able to formulate a plan and commit suicide after taking them (Gibbons, Brown, Hur, et al., 2012).

The continuing evaluation by both history taking and physical examination should be ongoing because the young person who has attempted suicide once may attempt it again if support people and better problem-solving abilities are not available.

What If . . . 33.3

Raul seems unusually happy at a clinic visit when usually he is sad because of loss of his girlfriend. The nurse knows he recently gave away his collection of baseball cards to a neighborhood boy because "I won't need them where I'm going." Would the nurse be concerned about him? If the nurse learned he is about to leave to be an exchange student in England, would this affect your assessment?

CONCERNS OF THE ADOLESCENT AND FAMILY WITH UNIQUE NEEDS

Homeless youth (i.e., runaways) and adolescents who are disabled have specific concerns that need special attention.

Homeless or Runaway Youth

A *runaway* is commonly defined as an adolescent between the ages of 10 and 17 years who has been absent from home at least overnight without permission of a parent or guardian. Fortunately, most teenagers who run away do not go far or stay away long (under 1 week); about 1 in 20 adolescent runaways stays away as long as 1 year, and some never return home and become homeless youth. Runaway adolescents are most likely to be from either low- or high-income families. Stress factors such as family unemployment, alcoholism, sexual maltreatment, incest, attempted suicide, and poverty are frequent characteristics in their families (Moskowitz, Stein, & Lightfoot, 2012). They are slightly more likely to be male than female.

Assessment

Running away is usually preceded by an argument with parents that is often the last straw after a number of long-term disagreements. Other reasons may be personal concerns such as loneliness; pregnancy; and problems with friends, school, or the police. A school history often reveals frequent truancy, failing grades, possible drug use, and runaway behavior by friends. It is a sad fact that some adolescents are "throwaways" or cannot remain at home because they have been rejected by their families.

Common health reasons for which runaway adolescents are seen at healthcare facilities are sexually transmitted diseases, including HIV and AIDS, rape, pregnancy, substance use disorders, hepatitis, and vaginitis. They also have a high incidence of suicide attempts (Palepu, Hubley, Russell, et al., 2012).

When caring for adolescents with these concerns, be certain to secure a thorough history so the fact that they are no longer living at home will not be overlooked. Do not reveal you are shocked by a report such as an adolescent has been sleeping on a park bench for 2 months, has been robbed, or steals to obtain money because this could prevent you from learning even greater concerns, such as having a sexually transmitted disease, being pregnant, or using drugs.

As they lack references for jobs and do not necessarily qualify for public assistance programs, homeless adolescents generally have no secure source of income. This can cause both males and females to resort to stealing or prostitution to support themselves. Legally, they are considered to be juvenile delinquents, so police are required to return them to their homes if discovered.

Because many adolescents who run away are not good problem solvers, setting goals with them may be difficult. A short-term goal to stay home through a holiday rather than a long-term one of finishing high school may be all you can achieve. Try to imagine yourself in the adolescent's circumstances to determine whether your health instructions or goals will be sensible for their lifestyle. As they have no money for food, giving them an instruction to eat iron-rich foods to prevent anemia, for example, may be ludicrous. If they do not have a source of running water, telling them to soak a lesion or change a dressing may be impossible. If they don't have a means of transportation, they may be unable to return to the healthcare facility for frequent follow-up visits so try to meet as many of the runaway's needs as possible at one visit. Remember that many runaways have associated school failure and so have poor health literacy; discuss the information with them as well as give them a pamphlet or written instructions.

Be certain, also, to ask if an adolescent wants to return home. Even though being homeless is high stress, and many adolescent runaways want to take the first step back toward their parents, they may not know how to begin the process or be certain they will be welcomed back at home. Check if they are familiar with the National Youth Crisis Hotline, which they can telephone day or night when they want to return home (1-800-448-4663 [1-800-HIT HOME]). Remember also they are runaways because, for some reason, their home was intolerable. Although they agree to return home, they may not remain there unless circumstances have been or can be changed.

A Physically Challenged or Chronically Ill Adolescent

Achieving a sense of identity may be difficult for adolescents who have a chronic illness or other challenges. It is vital, however, for such individuals to learn to look past their particular condition to their real selves. For example, a 16-year-old girl in a wheelchair must learn to perceive herself as a teenager who is intelligent, is a good conversationalist, has a good sense of humor, enjoys watching football, and only incidentally uses a wheelchair to ambulate.

Some of the biggest problems of chronically ill adolescents are likely to be difficulties in being as independent as they would like to be, achieving in school, and establishing intimate relationships. Those who cannot learn to drive when their friends are learning to do so, who are not invited to dances and parties because of a unique concern, or who are too hesitant to ask someone to go with them may feel acute loneliness and loss of self-esteem. Moreover, the loss of many hours of school due to illness or frequent hospitalization may result in the inability to pursue a desired career, at least a delay in doing so. Adolescence may be the first time these individuals realize certain occupations or opportunities, such as a military career, may be closed to them. As they prepare to leave the security of a familiar school system, it may be the first time they examine just how they will be able to function on their own. Some may come to realize they will never be able to do so with complete independence.

Chronic hospitalization or the realization they will never be free of symptoms can cause depression in such adolescents, placing them at high risk for substance use disorders or self-injury. Helping these adolescents realize that even completely well people must compromise life decisions for other reasons such as lack of money, lack of qualifications, or other personal responsibilities helps them feel they are not so different from others. The fact an adult is willing to make a time commitment to discuss their future with them can be enough to give these adolescents the self-esteem they need to alter aspirations and plans and find a future role consistent with their capabilities. Nursing actions to encourage a sense of identity in an adolescent with a long-term illness or who is physically challenged are summarized in Table 33.4.

Nutrition and the Chronically Ill Adolescent

Adolescents who are not fully mobile must be cautious of their total calorie intake because, as growth needs decline at the end of adolescence, they may become obese. They should also be knowledgeable about good nutrition, so they can participate in meal planning, an action that can help them feel a sense of control over this area of their life. Assess how often they have a chance to eat at fast-food restaurants; although this is not a source of excellent nutrition, eating there occasionally can provide an important social experience and a chance to be like their peers.

What If . . . 33.4

The nurse is particularly interested in exploring one of the 2020 National Health Goals with respect to adolescent growth and development (see Box 33.1). What would be a possible research topic to explore that is pertinent to this goal that would be applicable to Raul's family and that would also advance evidence-based practice?

KEY POINTS FOR REVIEW

- The major milestones of development in the adolescent period are the onset of puberty and the cessation of body growth. Between these milestones, physical growth is rapid, although the development of adult coordination and thought processes is slow.

- The development of secondary sex characteristics is completed during adolescence. These are rated according to Tanner stages.

- The developmental task of an adolescent according to Erikson (Dunkel & Harbke, 2017) is to establish inde-

TABLE 33.4 NURSING ACTIONS THAT ENCOURAGE A SENSE OF IDENTITY IN THE PHYSICALLY CHALLENGED OR CHRONICALLY ILL ADOLESCENT

Category	Actions
Nutrition	If adolescent is on special diet, discuss role of food preferences with dietitian (e.g., hot dogs, pizza).
	Respect food preferences in all ways possible.
Dressing change	Allow adolescent to order supplies.
	Ask for suggestions as to final appearance of dressing.
	If soaks are included, have adolescent time the treatment.
	Allow adolescent to choose time for dressing change.
Medicine	Offer the adolescent a choice of site for injection or intravenous insertion to encourage a sense of control.
	Teach name, action, and possible side effects of medicine.
Rest	Contract with adolescent for time and length of rest periods.
Hygiene	Respect modesty as you would with an adult.
	Contract with adolescent for extent of self-care (e.g., will give own bath and make bed, not medicate self).
Pain	Encourage adolescent to express pain and teach distraction technique for sharp pain, such as deep breathing and counting backward from 100.
	Encourage adolescent to ask for analgesics as needed.
Stimulation	Provide favorite music with earphones.
	Provide a radio to listen to talk shows to foster active involvement.
	Encourage schoolwork (you may need to help adolescents divide up school assignments so they do not become overly fatigued and frustrated).
	Provide crossword puzzles or card games to increase socialization (make or have the adolescent make a card deck from pieces of paper if one is not available).
	Encourage adolescents to network with one another.
	Encourage adolescents to keep in contact with friends through texting, e-mail, or writing notes.

pendence from parents by gaining a sense of identity versus role confusion. Therefore, adolescents usually respond best to healthcare personnel who respect their attempts at independence and who allow them as many choices as possible in care.

- Adolescents reach a point of cognitive development termed *formal operational thought*. With this gained, they are able to think in abstract terms and use rational thinking to arrive at conclusions.
- Adolescents need to consume adequate calories and especially protein, iron, calcium, and zinc to meet their increased growth needs, but at the same time, be certain they don't become overweight.
- Being an adolescent is difficult in today's world. Be aware that to reduce stress, some adolescents may begin to abuse substances. Asking about an adolescent's drug experiences during a health assessment is not intruding on privacy. Rather, it is a method of safe health interviewing and helps in planning nursing care that not only meets QSEN competencies but also best meets a family's total needs.
- Promoting adolescent safety is an important nursing role. Motor vehicle accidents, homicide, and suicide are leading causes of death in this age group.
- Common health problems in an adolescent are sometimes minor and include poor posture, fatigue, or acne; they can also be serious, such as beginning hypertension, substance use disorders, and scoliosis. Identifying these problems and referring an adolescent for help are important nursing actions.

CRITICAL THINKING CARE STUDY

Genève is a 14-year-old who lives with her parents and an 8-year-old brother. They take a vacation for 2 weeks every summer at the beach.

1. Genève has asked her parents if she can bring her best friend, a 24-year-old neighbor, with her on vacation. Her parents ask you whether that would be a good idea. How would you respond?
2. Genève was stopped by security at a department store for shoplifting a red sweater she said she needed to wear to a party that evening. Her father paid for the sweater so she was not charged with shoplifting. Would you suggest her parents let her wear the sweater to the party?
3. Genève has her own television in her bedroom. Her parents tell you she often stays awake until 2 in the morning watching programs. Her parents ask you if they should monitor what she watches or if she is old enough to do this for herself.

RELATED RESOURCES

Explore these additional resources to enhance learning for this chapter:
- Student resources on thePoint, including answers to the What If . . . and Critical Thinking Care Study questions, http://thepoint.lww.com/Flagg8e
- Adaptive learning powered by PrepU, http://thepoint.lww.com/prepu

REFERENCES

Ahern, N. R., & Norris, A. E. (2011). Examining factors that increase and decrease stress in adolescent community college students. *Journal of Pediatric Nursing, 26*(6), 530–540.

Albertson, T. E., Chenoweth, J. A., Colby, D. K., et al. (2016). The changing drug culture: Use and misuse of appearance- and performance-enhancing drugs. *FP Essentials, 441*, 30–43.

Armfield, J., Spencer, J., Roberts-Thomson, K., et al. (2013). Water fluoridation and the association of sugar-sweetened beverage consumption and dental caries in Australian children. *American Journal of Public Health, 103*(3), 494–500.

Auten, J. D., Matteucci, M. J., Gaspary, M. J., et al. (2012). Psychiatric implications of adolescent methamphetamine exposures. *Pediatric Emergency Care, 28*(1), 26–29.

Bagnulo, J. D. (2006). Carbohydrate. In I. Kohlstadt (Ed.), *Scientific evidence for musculoskeletal, bariatric, and sports nutrition* (pp. 81–94). Boca Raton, FL: Taylor & Francis.

Barrocas, A. L., Hankin, B. L., Young, J. F., et al. (2012). Rates of nonsuicidal self-injury in youth: Age, sex, and behavioral methods in a community sample. *Pediatrics, 130*(1), 39–45.

Barry, A. E., King, J., Sears, C., et al. (2016). Prioritizing alcohol prevention: Establishing alcohol as the gateway drug and linking age of first drink with illicit drug use. *Journal of School Health, 86*(1), 31–38.

Baumann, M. H., Partilla, J. S., & Lehner, K. R. (2013). Psychoactive "bath salts": Not so soothing. *European Journal of Pharmacology, 698*(1–3), 1–5.

Benjet, C., Borges, G., Medina-Mora, M. E., et al. (2012). Chronic childhood adversity and stages of substance use involvement in adolescents. *Drug & Alcohol Dependence, 131*(1–2), 85–91.

Bruinvels, G., Burden, R., Brown, N. et al. (2016). The prevalence and impact of heavy menstrual bleeding (menorrhagia) in elite and non-elite athletes. *PLoS One, 11*(2), e0149881.

Case, P. (2016). Nutrition through the life cycle. *Journal of Nutrition Education and Behavior, 48*(1), 84.

Centers for Disease Control and Prevention. (2012a). *Alcohol & drug use.* Atlanta, GA: Author.

Centers for Disease Control and Prevention. (2012b). Drowning—United States, 2005–2009. *Morbidity & Mortality Weekly Report, 61*(19), 344–347.

Centers for Disease Control and Prevention. (2012c). *Sexually transmitted disease surveillance.* Atlanta, GA: Author.

Centers for Disease Control and Prevention. (2012d). *Youth & tobacco use: Fact sheet.* Atlanta, GA: Author.

Centers for Disease Control and Prevention. (2017a). *Heroin overdose data.* Retrieved from https://www.cdc.gov/drugoverdose/data/heroin.html

Centers for Disease Control and Prevention. (2017b). *LGBT youth.* Retrieved from https://www.cdc.gov/lgbthealth/youth.htm

Centers for Disease Control and Prevention. (2017c). *Prevent bullying.* Retrieved from https://www.cdc.gov/features/prevent-bullying/index.html

Centers for Disease Control and Prevention. (2017d). *Reproductive health: Teen pregnancy.* Retrieved from https://www.cdc.gov/teenpregnancy/index.htm

Chen, H., Cao, L., & Logan, D. B. (2012). Analysis of risk factors affecting the severity of intersection crashes by logistic regression. *Traffic Injury Prevention, 13*(3), 300–307.

Chouinard, L. E., Randall Simpson, J., & Buchholz, A. C. (2012). Predictors of bone mineral density in a convenience sample of young Caucasian adults living in Southern Ontario. *Applied Physiology, Nutrition, and Metabolism, 37*(4), 706–714.

Cohen, L., Brown, J., Haukness, H., et al. (2013). Sun protection counseling by pediatricians has little effect on parent and child sun protection behavior. *Journal of Pediatrics, 162*(2), 381–386.

D'Aloise, P., & Chen, H. (2012). Rapid determination of flunitrazepam in alcoholic beverages by desorption electrospray ionization-mass spectrometry. *Science & Justice, 52*(1), 2–8.

Diamond, A. B., Callahan, S. T., Chain, K. F., et al. (2016). Qualitative review of hazing in collegiate and school sports: Consequences from a lack of culture, knowledge and responsiveness. *British Journal of Sports Medicine, 50*(3), 149–153.

Dunkel, C. S., & Harbke, C. A. (2017). Review of measures of Erikson's stages of psychosocial development: Evidence for a general factor. *Journal of Adult Development, 24*(1), 58–76.

Eisendrath, S. J., & Lichtmacher, J. E. (2013). Substance use disorders. In M. Papadakis & S. J. McPhee (Eds.), *Current medical diagnosis & treatment, 2013* (52nd ed., pp. 1079–1087). New York, NY: McGraw-Hill/Lange.

Erikson, E. H. (1950). *Childhood and Society.* New York, NY: Norton.

Erikson, E. H. (1968). *Identity: Youth and crisis.* New York, NY: Norton.

Flynn, J. T., & Falkner, B. (2011). Obesity hypertension in adolescents: Epidemiology, evaluation, and management. *Journal of Clinical Hypertension, 13*(5), 323–331.

Fried, L. E., Williams, S., Cabral, H., et al. (2013). Differences in risk factors for suicide attempts among 9th and 11th grade youth: A longitudinal perspective. *Journal of School Nursing, 29*(2), 113–122.

Fronczak, C. M., Kim, E. D., & Barqawi, A. B. (2012). The insults of illicit drug use on male fertility. *Journal of Andrology, 33*(4), 515–528.

Frost, L. A., & Burns, C. E. (2012). Sleep and rest. In C. E. Burns, A. M. Dunn, M. A. Brady, et al. (Eds.), *Pediatric primary care* (5th ed., pp. 256–273). Philadelphia, PA: Elsevier/Saunders.

Fuzzell, L., Fedesco, H., Alexander, S., et al. (2016). "I just think that doctors need to ask more questions": Sexual minority and majority adolescents' experiences talking about sexuality with healthcare providers. *Patient Education and Counseling, 99*(90), 1467–1472.

Gampetro, P., Wojciechowski, E. A., & Amer, E. S. (2012). Life concerns and perceptions of care in adolescents with mental health care needs: A qualitative study in a school-based health clinic. *Pediatric Nursing, 38*(1), 23–30.

Garzon, D. L., & Dunn, A. M. (2013). Developmental management of adolescents. In C. E. Burns, A. M. Dunn, M. A. Brady, et al. (Eds.), *Pediatric primary care* (5th ed., pp. 110–131). Philadelphia, PA: Elsevier/Saunders.

Gibbons, R. D., Brown, C. H., Hur, K., et al. (2012). Suicidal thoughts and behavior with antidepressant treatment: Reanalysis of the randomized placebo-controlled studies of fluoxetine and venlafaxine. *Archives of General Psychiatry, 69*(6), 580–587.

Gilligan, C. (1982). *In a different voice: Psychological theory and women's development.* Cambridge, MA: Harvard University Press.

Gostin, L., & Glasner, A. (2014). E-cigarettes, vaping, and youth. *JAMA, 312*(6), 595–596.

Hagan, J. F., Shaw, J. S., & Duncan, P. M. (Eds.). (2017). *Bright futures: Guidelines for health supervision of infants, children, and adolescents* (4th ed.). Elk Grove Village, IL American Academy of Pediatrics.

Harris, B. R. (2016). Talking about screening, brief intervention, and referral to treatment for adolescents: An upstream intervention to address the heroin and prescription opioid epidemic. *Preventive Medicine, 91*, 397–399.

Harvey, J., & Chadi, N. (2016). Strategies to promote smoking cessation among adolescents. *Paediatrics & Child Health, 21*(4), 201–208.

Hoang, Q. B., Coel, R. A., Vidal, A., et al. (2012). Sports medicine. In W. Hay, M. Levin, R. Deterding, et al. (Eds.), *Current diagnosis & treatment pediatrics* (21st ed., pp. 849–880). New York, NY: McGraw-Hill/Lange.

Kann, L., McManus, T., Harris, W. A., et al. (2016). Youth risk behavior surveillance—United States, 2015. *Morbidity & Mortality Weekly Report, 65*(6), 1–180.

Karch, A. M. (2013). *2013 Lippincott's nursing drug guide.* Philadelphia, PA: Lippincott Williams & Wilkins.

Katsufrakis, P., & Nusbaum, M. (2011). Adolescent sexuality. In J. South-Paul, S. Matheny, & E. Lewis (Eds.), *Current diagnosis and treatment: Family medicine* (3rd ed., pp. 122–130). New York, NY: McGraw-Hill/Lange.

Kaul, P. (2016). Adolescent substance abuse. In W. Hay, M. Levin, R. Deterding, et al. (Eds.), *Current diagnosis & treatment pediatrics* (23rd ed., pp. 145–158). New York, NY: McGraw-Hill/Lange.

Khan, K. M., Thompson, A. M., Blair, S. N., et al. (2012). Sport and exercise as contributors to the health of nations. *Lancet, 380*(9836), 59–64.

Kistner, F., Fiebert, I., & Roach, K. (2012). Effect of backpack load carriage on cervical posture in primary schoolchildren. *Work, 41*(1), 99–108.

Kohlberg, L. (1984). *The psychology of moral development: The nature and validity of moral stages.* New York, NY: Harper & Row.

Kozlowski, L. T., & Sweanor, D. T. (2017). Young or adult users of multiple tobacco/nicotine products urgently need to be informed of meaningful differences in product risks. *Addictive Behavior.* Advance online publication. doi:10.1016/j.addbeh.2017.01.026

Ledger, W. L. (2012). The menstrual cycle. In D. K. Edmonds (Ed.), *Dewhurst's textbook of obstetrics & gynaecology* (8th ed., pp. 487–494). Oxford, United Kingdom: Wiley.

Lewis, T. P., & Hession, C. (2012). Alcohol use: From childhood through adolescence. *Journal of Pediatric Nursing, 27*(5), e50–e58.

Lloyd, S., Chalder, T., & Rimes, K. A. (2012). Family-focused cognitive behaviour therapy versus psycho-education for adolescents with chronic fatigue syndrome: Long-term follow-up of an RCT. *Behavior Research & Therapy, 50*(11), 719–725.

Loprinzi, P. D., Cardinal, B. J., Loprinzi, K. L., et al. (2012). Benefits and environmental determinants of physical activity in children and adolescents. *Obesity Facts, 5*(4), 597–610.

Lyon, R. E. (1978). Comparative effectiveness of benzoyl peroxide and treti-noin in acne vulgaris. *International Journal of Dermatology, 17,* 246–251.

Maimon, D., & Browning, C. R. (2012). Underage drinking, alcohol sales and collective efficacy: Informal control and opportunity in the study of alcohol use. *Social Science Research, 41*(4), 977–990.

Makin-Byrd, K., & Bierman, K. L. (2013). Individual and family predictors of the perpetration of dating violence and victimization in late adoles-cence. *Journal of Youth & Adolescence, 42*(4), 536–550.

Marciani, R. D. (2012). Complications of third molar surgery and their management. *Atlas of the Oral & Maxillofacial Surgery Clinics of North America, 20*(2), 233–251.

Marván, M. L., & Molina-Abolnik, M. (2012). Mexican adolescents' experi-ence of menarche and attitudes toward menstruation: Role of communi-cation between mothers and daughters. *Journal of Pediatric & Adolescent Gynecology, 25*(6), 358–363.

Mbah, A. K., Alio, A. P., Fombo, D. W., et al. (2012). Association between cocaine abuse in pregnancy and placenta-associated syndromes using propensity score matching approach. *Early Human Development, 88*(6), 333–337.

Montisci, M., El Mazloum, R., Cecchetto, G., et al. (2012). Anabolic an-drogenic steroids abuse and cardiac death in athletes: Morphological and toxicological findings in four fatal cases. *Forensic Science International, 217*(1–3), e13–e18.

Morelli, J. G., & Prok, L. D. (2016). Acne. In W. Hay, M. Levin, R. Deter-ding, et al. (Eds.), *Current diagnosis & treatment pediatrics* (23rd ed., pp. 404–406). New York, NY: McGraw-Hill/Lange.

Moskowitz, A., Stein, J. A., & Lightfoot, M. (2012). The mediating roles of stress and maladaptive behaviors on self-harm and suicide attempts among runaway and homeless youth. *Journal of Youth and Adolescence, 42*(7), 1015–1027.

Neuhaus, C. P., Nagler, A. R., & Orlow, S. J. (2017). Teens, acne, and oral contraceptive pills: The need for greater clarity on when teens can con-sent. *JAMA Dermatology, 153*(4), 249–250.

Nguyen, J., O'Brien, C., & Schapp, S. (2016). Adolescent inhalant use pre-vention, assessment, and treatment: A literature synthesis. *International Journal on Drug Policy, 31,* 15–24.

Paczynski, R. P., & Gold, M. S. (2011). Cocaine and crack. In P. Ruiz & E. Strain (Eds.), *Lowinson and Ruiz's substance abuse: A comprehensive textbook* (5th ed., pp. 191–213). Philadelphia, PA: Lippincott Williams & Wilkins.

Palepu, A., Hubley, A. M., Russell, L. B., et al. (2012). Quality of life themes in Canadian adults and street youth who are homeless or hard-to-house: A multi-site focus group study. *Health & Quality of Life Outcomes, 10*(8), 93.

Perera, S., Eisen, R. B., Dennis, B. B., et al. (2016). Body mass index is an important predictor for suicide: Results from a systematic review and meta-analysis. *Suicide & Life-Threatening Behavior, 46*(6), 697–736.

Piaget, J. (1969). *The theory of stages in cognitive development.* New York, NY: McGraw-Hill.

Rathi, S. K. (2011). Acne vulgaris treatment: The current scenario. *Indian Journal of Dermatology, 56*(1), 7–13.

Sánchez-Carracedo, D., Neumark-Sztainer, D., & López-Guimerà, G. (2012). Integrated prevention of obesity and eating disorders: Barri-ers, developments and opportunities. *Public Health Nutrition, 15*(12), 2295–2309.

Shields, J. P., Whitaker, K., Glassman, J., et al. (2012). Impact of victim-ization on risk of suicide among lesbian, gay, and bisexual high school students in San Francisco. *Journal of Adolescent Health, 50*(4), 418–420.

Short, M. A., Gradisar, M., Lack, L. C., et al. (2013). A cross-cultural com-parison of sleep duration between U.S. and Australian adolescents: The effect of school start time, parent-set bedtimes, and extracurricular load. *Health Education & Behavior, 40*(3), 323–330.

Simonart, T. (2012). Newer approaches to the treatment of acne vulgaris. *American Journal of Clinical Dermatology, 13*(6), 357–364.

Stein, T., & Jordan, J. D. (2012). Health considerations for oral piercing and the policies that influence them. *Texas Dental Journal, 129*(7), 687–693.

Stoduto, G., Mann, R. E., Ialomiteanu, A., et al. (2012). Examining the link between collision involvement and cocaine use. *Drug & Alcohol Depen-dence, 123*(1–3), 260–263.

Storck, M., Black, L., & Liddell, M. (2016). Inhalant abuse and dextro-methorphan. *Child and Adolescent Psychiatric Clinics of North America, 25*(3), 497–508.

Swahn, M. H., Ali, B., Bossarte, R. M., et al. (2012). Self-harm and suicide attempts among high-risk, urban youth in the U.S.: Shared and unique risk and protective factors. *International Journal of Environmental Research & Public Health, 9*(1), 178–191.

Tanner, J. M. (1962). *Growth at adolescence* (2nd ed.). Oxford, United Kingdom: Blackwell.

Taylor, J. M., Gilligan, C., & Sullivan, A. M. (1995). *Between the voice and silence: Women and girls, race and relationship.* Cambridge, MA: Harvard University Press.

Timko, C. A., Hormes, J. M., & Chubski, J. (2012). Will the real veg-etarian please stand up? An investigation of dietary restraint and eating disorder symptoms in vegetarians versus non-vegetarians. *Appetite, 58*(3), 982–990.

U.S. Department of Health and Human Services. (2010). *Healthy people 2020.* Washington, DC: Author.

Wengle, J. G., Hamilton, J. K., Manlhiot, C., et al. (2012). The 'Golden Keys' to health—a healthy lifestyle intervention with randomized indi-vidual mentorship for overweight and obesity in adolescents. *Paediatrics & Child Health, 16*(8), 473–478.

Widome, R., Brock, B., Noble, P., et al. (2013). The relationship of neigh-borhood demographic characteristics to point-of-scale tobacco advertis-ing and marketing. *Ethnicity & Health, 18*(2), 136–151.

Williams, A. F., McCartt, A. T., & Sims, L. B. (2016). History and current status of state graduated driver licensing (GDL) laws in the United States. *Journal of Safety Research, 56,* 9–15.

Zaenglein, A. L., Pathy, A. L., Schlosser, B. J., et al. (2016). Guidelines of care for the management of acne vulgaris. *Journal of the American Academy of Dermatology, 74*(5), 945 .e33–973.e33.

34

Child Health Assessment

Keoto Wiser is a 13-year-old you meet in an ambulatory clinic. Her father has brought both her and her 2-year-old sister, Candy, for health assessment before Keoto begins seventh grade. He knows they both need an immunization update. Her father is worried Keoto doesn't see well because she always sits close to the television set. He's concerned that if glasses are prescribed, his daughter won't be able to play on her school's soccer team.

Previous chapters described the normal growth and development of children. This chapter adds information about techniques for assessing the health of children, including history taking; physical examination; related screening procedures for hearing, vision, and development; and recommended immunizations. This information builds a base for care and health teaching for differing age groups throughout childhood.

What questions would you want to ask Keoto? What screening tests for vision would be best for this 13-year-old? What could you do to help her adjust to wearing glasses if they are prescribed?

KEY TERMS

antitoxins

audiogram

auscultation

bruit

chief concern

conjunctivitis

deep tendon reflexes

diaphragmatic excursion

epispadias

esotropia

exotropia

gamma globulin

geographic tongue

hordeolum

hydrocele

hypospadias

inspection

intelligence

intercostal spaces

kwashiorkor

palpation

percussion

physiologic splitting

point of maximum impulse (PMI)

ptosis

retractions

review of systems

sinus arrhythmia

strabismus

temperament

toxoid

turgor

varicocele

OBJECTIVES

After mastering the contents of this chapter, you should be able to:

1. Describe the purposes and techniques of health assessment in children of all ages.

2. Identify 2020 National Health Goals related to health assessment of children that nurses can help the nation achieve.

3. Assess a child and family by health interview, physical examination, and developmental screening.

4. Formulate nursing diagnoses based on health assessment findings.

5. Identify expected outcomes based on health assessment findings as well as help parents manage seamless transitions across differing healthcare settings.

6. Using the nursing process, plan nursing care that includes the six competencies of Quality & Safety Education for Nurses (QSEN): Patient-Centered Care, Teamwork & Collaboration, Evidence-Based Practice (EBP), Quality Improvement (QI), Safety, and Informatics.

7. Implement nursing care, such as conducting an age-appropriate health interview or physical examination by modifying techniques based on the child's age.

8. Evaluate expected outcomes for achievement and effectiveness of care.

9. Integrate knowledge of health assessment with the interplay of nursing process, the six competencies of QSEN, and Family Nursing to promote quality maternal and child health nursing care.

A nursing assessment is not only the first step in the nursing process but also the fundamental means by which healthcare personnel establish and maintain contact with children and their families throughout childhood. Child health assessment is especially important as an opportunity to provide families with information about health promotion, signs of health and illness, and expected developmental progress in children. This anticipatory guidance can have a long-lasting and positive impact on the health of children and their families (Cameron, Rice, Sparkman, et al., 2013).

An effective assessment for the maternal–child population first requires you to be familiar with health maintenance standards and usual findings because this knowledge is essential to the ability to recognize illness. Most health screening procedures are performed in ambulatory settings such as pediatric clinics, healthcare offices, community clinics, and schools, but they can be used to evaluate children in all settings, including during hospitalizations.

Sometimes, it is necessary to complete just a partial history or a partial physical examination, such as when a child is referred for a vision examination. This chapter, however, covers all aspects of physical examination, so when necessary, a complete examination can be performed. Assessment procedures specific to particular illnesses are discussed in later chapters with the illness they detect. Box 34.1 lists 2020 National Health Goals related to health assessment in children.

Nursing Process Overview

FOR HEALTH ASSESSMENT OF THE CHILD AND FAMILY

ASSESSMENT

Health assessment can be a positive, educational experience for the child and family if time is taken to listen carefully to the family's concerns and responses to questions. Never rush either an interview or a physical examination. Be sure children have time to familiarize themselves with the environment and the equipment that will be used. The recommendations for standard preventive child health care for the United States are available at http://thePoint.lww.com/Flagg8e.

NURSING DIAGNOSIS

Nursing diagnoses related to health assessment most commonly speak to a health concern identified at the time of

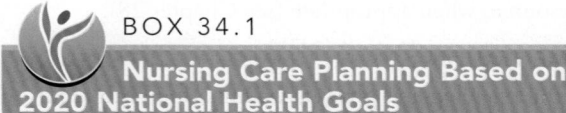

BOX 34.1

Nursing Care Planning Based on 2020 National Health Goals

A number of 2020 National Health Goals directly relate to health assessment of children:

- Developmental: Increase the proportion of children with a diagnosed condition identified through newborn screening who have an annual assessment of services needed and received.
- Increase the proportion of children and youth, 17 years of age and younger, who have a specific source of ongoing care from a baseline of 94.3% to a target of 100%.
- Increase the proportion of adolescents aged 12 to 19 years who have had a hearing examination in the past 5 years from a baseline of 79.3% to 87.2%.
- Increase the proportion of preschool children aged 5 years and under who receive vision screening from a baseline of 40.1% to a target of 44.1%.
- Achieve and maintain effective vaccination coverage levels for universally recommended vaccines among young children from baselines of 85% (DTaP), 94% (hepatitis B), 57% (*Haemophilus influenzae* type b), 94% (poliomyelitis), 91% (varicella), and 92% (MMR) to a target level of 90% (U.S. Department of Health and Human Services, 2010; see www.healthypeople.gov).

Nurses can help the nation achieve these goals by actively participating in health assessment, including vision and hearing, and conscientiously screening for and administering vaccines.

the assessment. When establishing nursing diagnoses, however, be certain not to overlook diagnoses that accentuate the healthy functioning of a child and family in addition to addressing any specific problems that have been identified. These wellness diagnoses are crucial components of the entire assessment picture. For instance, the nursing diagnosis of "Impaired social interaction related to lack of self-esteem secondary to disability" would be appropriate for a 4-year-old child who ambulates by wheelchair who, according to the parents, feels uncomfortable around other children. If the parents have difficulty adapting to their child's disability but are eager to accept advice from healthcare experts on how to provide the most stimulating environment for their child, the diagnosis "Readiness for enhanced family coping" would also be appropriate. Using both these diagnoses allows the development of a plan of care that takes advantage in the best way of this family's strengths.

OUTCOME IDENTIFICATION AND PLANNING

Health promotion and illness prevention are vital parts of outcome identification following a health assessment. Helping parents plan for their child's next developmental stage or keeping them aware of important safety measures is also important. Remind parents about future immunizations that will be needed and be certain they know when to schedule the next healthcare visit. Refer parents to helpful websites and other resources when appropriate (see Chapter 28).

IMPLEMENTATION

Health interviewing and physical examination both require a great deal of skill—skills that can only be perfected through practice. To perfect skills and judgment with children of different ages, take advantage of every opportunity by practicing interviewing and physical examination techniques with them.

OUTCOME EVALUATION

Health assessment of children is an ongoing process that does not end when the first database is created. Because children change so much, data must be added at all future interactions so the database remains current and meaningful. Examples suggesting expected outcomes have been achieved include:

- After a health examination, parents state they are satisfied with their child's motor development.
- After Snellen test, the child states she is aware her vision needs correction.
- The parents state they will continue to assess their child's growth by weighing the child weekly.

Health History: Establishing a Database

The assessment of a young child begins with an interview of the child's parents. An adolescent or preadolescent may choose to be interviewed without the parents present, although many preadolescents and adolescents still prefer to have a parent with them for support.

The purpose of a health interview is to gather information that will direct physical or laboratory examinations to complete a thorough health evaluation. An extensive interview not only elicits facts such as parental problems in childrearing or detection of future health problems but also lays a foundation for health education and health promotion. Important principles of child health interviewing include establishing a conducive interview setting, formulating the right types of questions to ask, and organizing the information collected.

INTERVIEW SETTING

An interview is best conducted in a private room with all parties seated comfortably (Fig. 34.1); if not seated, a healthcare provider can appear rushed and is also unable to interact at

Figure 34.1 Maintaining good eye contact and allowing children to play as active a part as possible in the assessment process are important for good health interviewing.

eye level. During the interview, be certain to call the parents by their names. This lets them know that their input and opinions about how their child is developing are valued. A question such as "Does Candy speak in sentences yet, Mr. Wiser?" is far more personal and a better form than "Does baby sit up yet?" As children grow, they are able to answer questions themselves.

TYPES OF QUESTIONS ASKED

The phrasing of questions varies depending on the type of answer desired. Closed-ended and open-ended questions are two types of effective questions; compound, expansive, and leading questions, in contrast, are three types of questions to avoid.

Closed-Ended Questions

This simplest form of question directly asks for a fact, such as "Did you take Candy's temperature?" This is an effective type of question if a particular point is being sought. It is limited in scope, however, because the response usually will be a "yes" or a "no," with no further elaboration.

Open-Ended Questions

An open-ended question allows for elaboration. In contrast to the closed-ended question, "What did you do for Candy?" is open ended. The parent will answer with a list of all the things he did, such as he took Candy's temperature, had her lie on the couch, gave her extra fluid, and so on. It is important to ask open-ended questions with school-age children and adolescents so they are encouraged to fully describe a problem (Box 34.2).

Compound Questions

Compound questions should be avoided if all possible because the information they elicit is often inaccurate and must be followed by a clarifying question. An example is "Did Candy have nausea and vomiting?" The parent answers "yes," but it remains unknown whether Candy had vomiting and nausea, just vomiting, or just nausea because the question included multiple possibilities.

BOX 34.2

Nursing Care Planning Tips for Effective Communication

A second reason Keoto's father has brought her to your ambulatory clinic is because she has noticed frequency and burning on urination.

Tip: At about 10 years of age, children are able to supply much of a health history by themselves. As children become teenagers, it is increasingly important for them to do this because they may not have shared a total history with a parent. If a parent provides initial intake information, ask follow-up questions and make sure children have the opportunity to give a history in their own words.

In this scenario, when asked directly for information, Keoto's father responds before Keoto can respond. Some urinary tract infections occur in girls following sexual intercourse, making it important to ask if she is sexually active. If she is sexually active, it is also critical to provide anticipatory guidance regarding pregnancy prevention and safer sex practices.

Nurse: Hello, Keoto. What's the reason you've come into clinic today?

Mr. Wiser: It hurts when she urinates.

Nurse: I am going to ask Keoto more questions about this. Some of these questions may be of a personal nature and possibly embarrassing for her to share. Mr. Wiser, would you like to share any additional information before I ask you to have a seat in the waiting room while Keoto and I talk privately? I will come get you when we are finished.

Mr. Wiser: Oh, I didn't think of that. Sure. She is old enough to answer questions.

Nurse: [turning to Keoto after Mr. Wiser leaves] Anything we discuss now is confidential, and I would ask your permission before sharing with your parent. Can you tell me more about your symptoms?

Keoto: It hurts when I go to the bathroom.

Nurse: When did you first notice that?

Keoto: About an hour after I came in from my date last night.

Nurse: I'm going to ask you some questions of a personal nature because it will help guide me to the source of the problem. We'll also do some tests such as a urine test.

Expansive Questions

Expansive questions are open-ended questions gone wrong because the question being asked is too vague to answer. "What can you tell me about Candy?" leaves a parent wondering where to start. "How has Candy been since her last visit?" limits the question and makes it answerable.

Leading Questions

Leading questions supply their own answers and so they should also be avoided. "Candy has had all her immunizations, hasn't she?" implies that Candy should have had them and perhaps implies that the parent is a poor caregiver if he responds with anything other than "yes." The result of such an exchange could be a child left vulnerable to disease.

CONTENTS OF A HEALTH INTERVIEW

Data gathering for an initial health assessment can be divided into nine sections:
1. Introduction and explanation
2. Demographic data
3. Chief concern
4. History of chief concern
5. Health and family profile
6. Day history
7. Past health history, including pregnancy history
8. Family health history
9. Review of systems

At return visits, the categories used generally include only introduction and explanation, chief concern, health and family profile, interval history, and day history.

Using Transition Statements

While conducting a health interview, be certain to make a transition statement before shifting from one section of an interview to another because, without a transition, a parent can possibly misinterpret a question's significance. For instance, if a parent has been providing information on the family's hospital insurance policy and, without a transition, is asked whether the child has been vomiting, a parent may think the interviewer believes the child needs hospitalization when that is not the intent at all. A statement such as "Before we talk about Keoto's current symptoms, let me ask you some general questions about your family so I can get to know you better" is an example of a good transition statement.

Introductions and Explanations

As a matter of courtesy, you should introduce yourself to parents and children and introduce what topics you will be discussing. "Hello, Mr. Wiser, I'm Janet Dickson, a nurse here in the One-Day Surgery Department. I'd like to ask you some questions about Candy" is an example of a suitable introduction. Because some families have never had the benefit of in-depth health care, it is also helpful to include a statement about the subjects that will be discussed during the interview. For example, "So I can get a picture of Candy's overall health, I'd like to ask you questions about not just why you've brought her here today but also her birth history and any past concerns you've had" would be appropriate. Hearing that, parents begin to concentrate on those areas because they realize healthcare providers in this setting are interested not just in Candy's health on this particular day but also in her total health.

Demographic Data

Demographic data refers to data such as a child's name, address, gender, social security number, and the name of the person who will be providing information. To provide culturally competent care and make provisions for special needs, a child's culture, ethnicity, place of birth, religious or spiritual practices, and primary and secondary language should also be identified (Box 34.3).

BOX 34.3

Nursing Care Planning to Respect Cultural Diversity

Health assessment findings in children differ depending on racial and ethnic characteristics. Whether people establish eye contact with an interviewer, for example, is a characteristic that is may be culturally related. In Vietnam, touching the head of a child during a physical assessment is thought to be harmful because the head is considered to be the seat of the soul. Asking the parent and/or child permission before examining any part of the body that may elicit a negative response is helpful.

Because height and weight charts are standardized on middle-class White children, measurements of children who do not fit this description may not plot well on these charts.

To establish rapport with children and their families and to make a health assessment more thorough and meaningful, it is important to recognize that people may hold different cultural expectations and have different characteristics.

Some cultures advocate for all children to be immunized against childhood communicable disease. In other cultures, even if awareness about the danger of disease exists, it does not mean all people in a community are conscientious about having their children immunized or agree that it is important. Other factors, such as cost and convenience, religious beliefs, and safety concerns, are also important. The Amish is an example of a group who do not encourage immunization. Being aware immunization rates are not consistent from place to place aids in understanding the importance of planning health education and health surveillance based on findings gained from health assessment.

Be certain to identify the child's primary caregiver. If the parents are divorced or deceased, it is especially important to identify who has custody of the child or who has the right to sign a consent for healthcare treatment.

Chief Concerns

The first topic parents want to talk about is the reason they have brought their child to the healthcare agency on this day or the **chief concern**. An effective way to elicit this information is to ask directly "Why did you bring Candy to the clinic today, Mr. Wiser?" Such an opening allows the parent freedom to answer in a number of areas of concern: physical, emotional, nutritional, or developmental. If asked "How is Candy feeling today?" or "Is Candy ill?" a parent is left to think about only physical aspects and may not voice the biggest concern: Candy's teething difficulty or frequent temper tantrums. Record the chief concern in the child's electronic record exactly as it is stated ("She has constant headaches," not, "Headache") because the parent's description often not only reveals information about a disease condition but also the depth of the parent's concern about the symptom (Levine, 2011).

History of Chief Concerns

Once a parent has voiced a chief concern, ask him or her to describe at least six aspects of the problem, including:

1. Duration
2. Intensity
3. Frequency
4. Description
5. Associated symptoms
6. Actions taken

Duration refers to the length of time a specific symptom such as vomiting or the parent's concern about the child's symptom has been present. The intensity, in this example, refers to the kind of vomiting the child is having (e.g., drooling, spitting up, actual vomiting). The description is the amount (e.g., a cupful, a mouthful) and color (e.g., whether it contains blood, bile, mucus). Associated symptoms might include fever, abdominal pain, difficulty eating, or signs of respiratory illness. A good question to use to obtain associated symptoms is "Is Candy ill in any other way?"

Knowing the parent's actions helps to establish ineffective actions or whether anything a parent has been doing, such as offering a great deal of fluid to replace that which was vomited, has actually made the illness worse. This information also reveals the parent's response to caring for an ill child. The parent who says, "I tucked her into bed and gave her a little tea to drink" is different from one who replies, "Nothing. I fall apart when my child is ill." If the child is going to return home under the parents' care, the parents in the second example need more instructions and support before they leave the healthcare setting than the first parents.

During this phase of the interview, it is also important to gather information to see if a parent has other related or additional health concerns. "Is there anything else that worries you about Candy?" is a good way to elicit this information. Unless asked about a second concern this way (e.g., the parent is also concerned about frequent temper tantrums; as soon as he arrives home and he knows Candy will begin stomping her feet in the car, unwilling to go into the house), the parent will feel that the health care Candy received was less than adequate because he did not receive help with this concern.

Do not assume parents will always reveal their most important concern in the initial minute of an interview; discussing certain symptoms such as constipation can be embarrassing for parents. It also can be frightening to put a fear that their child has a serious illness into words. As long as a concern hangs as a nebulous thought in the mind, it is easy to tell oneself it may not be true. Only when a parent voices the thought ("Do you think Candy is mentally handicapped?" "Do you think this is leukemia?" "Could this be inherited?") does the fear become real. Before parents dare to speak openly this way, they must trust healthcare providers not to treat their statement lightly. For this reason, it is helpful to repeat the question about a second concern once more at the very end of the interview to be certain other concerns were not missed.

Health and Family Profiles

A family profile includes documentation of the circumstances in which the child lives. A good introduction to a health and family profile is a sentence such as "Before we talk about any past illnesses or happenings with Candy, let me ask you some questions about your family as a whole."

Important information concerning the family includes:

- Is the parent married, single, or divorced? If divorced, who has legal custody?
- What is the family type (e.g., nuclear, extended, blended)?
- How many children are in the family?
- What are the family's living arrangements?
- What are the parents' occupations? (This helps establish the family's socioeconomic level and time available for childcare.)
- If both parents work outside the home, how do they manage childcare?

Obtaining a family profile is sometimes delayed by medical interviewers until the end of the interview, when, theoretically, a parent or child is more comfortable and will answer these personal questions more readily. However, by following a nursing model and obtaining the information earlier in the interview, you can better assess the child and evaluate data.

Day Histories

The child's current skills, sleep patterns, hygiene practices, eating habits, and interactions with the family can all be elicited by asking a parent to describe a typical day. Day histories are fun to obtain because most parents are eager to describe their day with their child and information gained this way is surprisingly rich and pertinent, much more so than if parents are just asked how their child sleeps, eats, or plays.

Begin by asking, "Was yesterday a fairly typical day?" (The parent says, "Yes, it was.") "Describe for me everything Candy did yesterday, beginning with when she first woke up." Some parents offer this information in great detail; with others, it is necessary to backtrack for particular details, such as "What did she eat for breakfast? Does she use a fork and spoon? Does she sit in a high chair or on your lap?"

Play

Play is the work of children and so reveals a great deal about a child's development and overall well-being. Important questions to ask about play include:

- Is the child kept in a playpen or given room to run?
- What is the child's favorite toy?
- Does she play active, chasing games or engage in quiet, pretending types of activities?
- Is she able to sit and play quietly or does she act as if driven by a motor?
- Do you (the parent) read to the child?
- Do you (the parent) play with the child or let the child play alone? (This allows for an estimation of the quality of interaction during the day.)

Sleep

Every child needs adequate rest for healthy growth and development. Poor sleep patterns can often reveal a psychosocial or physical health problem. Important questions regarding sleep include:

- What time does the child go to sleep at night?
- How long does the child sleep at night?
- What time does the child wake up?
- Does the child wake independently or do you need to wake the child?

- How long does the child nap (if appropriate for age)?
- Does the child share a room? With whom? Does the child share a bed? Is falling asleep a problem?
- Where does the child sleep? Does the child have night terrors or nightmares?
- Does the child sleepwalk?
- Does the child wet the bed (if the child is toilet trained)?

Hygiene

Good hygiene practices promote healthy teeth, gums, and skin; prevent infections; and improve self-esteem. Poor hygiene may reflect neglect, depression, substance abuse, or inability of the household to have hot water. Important questions regarding hygiene include:

- How much self-care does the child do?
- Can the child shower or bathe independently?
- Does the child brush her teeth? How often? Does she floss regularly? (Responses depend on the age of the child.)
- Does the child wash her hands before snacks and meals?
- Has there been a recent change in hygiene practices?

Nutrition

Nutritional assessment is an important portion of a health assessment because it strongly influences health (Whitney & Rolfes, 2015). Characteristics of a nutritionally healthy child that can be revealed by assessment are summarized in Table 34.1. Food and nutrient intake risk factors are summarized in Box 34.4.

Taking a history of a child's food intake can help determine whether there are any foods missing in a typical meal plan or if any quantities seem inadequate or excessive. Be certain to assess not only the quantity of food taken but also the quality; for example, for an infant, cereal should be iron-fortified.

TABLE 34.1 PHYSICAL SIGNS OF ADEQUATE NUTRITION

Assessment	Finding
Overall impression	Alert, with good energy level; positive mood
Hair	Shiny, strong, with good body
Eyes	Good eyesight, particularly at night; conjunctiva moist and not pale
Mouth	No cavities in teeth; no swollen or inflamed gingivae; no cracks or fissures at corners of mouth; mucous membrane moist and pink; tongue smooth and nontender
Neck	Normal contour of thyroid gland
Skin	Smooth; normal color and turgor; no ecchymotic or petechial areas present
Extremities	Normal muscle mass and circumference; normal strength and mobility; normal reflexes; legs not bowed; no tender joints or edema present
Gastrointestinal	No diarrhea or constipation present
Finger and toenails	Smooth, pink; not cracked or broken
Height and weight	Within normal limits on growth chart and body mass index (BMI)
Blood pressure	Normal for age

BOX 34.4

Food and Nutrient Intake Risk Factors

History or evidence of any of the following may pose a potential nutritional risk:

- Intake less or greater than standard for age, for calories, protein, vitamins, or minerals
- Unusual food habits, such as pica, faddism, and meal skipping
- Inappropriate use of supplements (excessive vitamins, minerals, fortified food products)
- A healthcare provider's prescription for nothing by mouth (NPO) or a clear liquid diet for more than 3 days without enteral or parenteral nutrition
- Minimal or no intake from a major food group
- Fluid intake less than output
- Eating disorders such as bulimia
- Food allergies
- Restricted diet, such as a restricted potassium diet for kidney disease

Food intake is best obtained by including this as part of a typical day (24-hour recall) history, listing what the child ate for each meal and between meals as well. With an older child, the 24-hour recall can be a joint parent–child venture. Providing this history can be difficult for parents if the child consumes some meals at home and others at day care or school. It may be necessary to ask for a weekend history to get a complete picture.

When assessing an adolescent, take a 24-hour recall nutritional history without a parent present, if possible. In front of a parent, adolescents may add nutritional foods to a food intake history or leave out foods they have eaten such as milkshakes, potato chips, or pizza to avoid a lecture later; however, they may also leave out healthy items or add less desirable ones because they may enjoy the obvious parental disapproval, indicative of their rebellion against adult authority.

After taking a history of a child's food intake, determine whether the child is receiving foods that comply with the MyPlate recommendations (U.S. Department of Agriculture, 2015; www.ChooseMyPlate.gov). If whole food groups are absent or grossly inadequate, a follow-up evaluation should include a food frequency record as a verification to see if the 24-hour recall was truly representative of a usual day. Remember, children do not have to eat food from all groups at every meal as long as they eat from them every day. If parents think in terms of days rather than meals, it allows them to exert less pressure regarding what the child eats at each meal.

Be certain to consider the role of food preferences and cultural, lifestyle, religious, and financial variations when assessing food intake as well as the number of meals eaten at home versus outside the home, how traditional meals are cooked, and the pattern of meals. Do not appear critical of a child's diet as you record a history. If you convey dismay at erratic eating habits, parents or older children (especially adolescents) may begin to fabricate a food history to make it seem more acceptable to you.

Past Health Histories

For a past health history, ask whether a child has ever had any serious illnesses. Parents do not generally think of childhood diseases such as measles, chickenpox, and mumps as serious illnesses; inquire about these separately. Also, inquire about the child's immunization history and whether immunizations are up to date for the child's age (see the discussion of immunizations later in this chapter). Has a child had any accidents (unintentional injuries)? Any surgery? Parents may not think of a tonsillectomy as surgery because there were no stitches; ask about that separately. Did a child ever ingest anything inedible or harmful? Has a child been hospitalized for any reason? If so, for how long? How many times has a child been seen in an emergency room? What was the child seen for? These last questions provide information about the degree of adult supervision and possibly clues to maltreatment (Khan, McCormack, Bolger, et al., 2015). Information about the outcomes of past illnesses is as important to obtain as information about the illnesses themselves. If the child had otitis media (i.e., middle ear infection) at age 2 years and recovered without complications, the parent has every reason to be confident the child will also get better from a present illness because there is confidence in healthcare personnel. If the child was left with a hearing difficulty from the previous illness, parents may not be as trustful of the care being given to their child now; they may need extra support to follow instructions. A child who had had frequent ear infections may need referral to an audiologist or an ear, nose, and throat (ENT) specialist. This is important information to gain before planning care.

QSEN Checkpoint Question 34.1

EVIDENCE-BASED PRACTICE

Over 300 children (from birth through age 19 years) in the United States are seen in the emergency room due to ingestion of poisonous substances. Substances include common household products and medications. It is important to provide guidance and injury prevention information to parents to prevent unintentional ingestions by children (CDC, 2016c). Based on this information, which would be the most important question to ask Candy's father?

- a. "Has Candy tried to drink something that you're drinking?"
- b. "Do you keep all your prescription drugs securely locked?"
- c. "What do you keep in the cupboards below your sinks?"
- d. "Where do you store the alcoholic beverages in your house?"

Look in Appendix A for the best answer and rationale.

Pregnancy Histories

The health of children is affected by their mother's health during pregnancy. For children younger than 5 years of age, therefore, a pregnancy history is usually obtained. Document which pregnancy this was for the mother. Were there complications in any of her pregnancies? Induced abortions or miscarriages? Stillbirths? Children born prematurely?

A history of the pregnancy of the child being assessed can begin with a question such as "How was your pregnancy with Candy?" This allows the mother to answer in both physical and emotional areas. After exploring details mentioned by the mother, ask about specific events that are known to occur with pregnancy that may have had an effect on a fetus, such as:

- Did the mother have any complications such as bleeding, falls, swelling of hands and feet, high blood pressure, or unusual weight gain or loss?
- Did she take any medication?
- Were any X-ray films or sonograms taken other than a routine one to date the pregnancy?
- Did she smoke cigarettes, drink alcohol, or use recreational drugs while she was pregnant?
- Did the pregnancy end early or late?

Because life contingencies such as loss of finances or illness in the family during a pregnancy may affect a parent's ability to form a bond with a child, the emotional experiences of a woman during pregnancy are also important to obtain. Ask if the pregnancy was intentional. A question such as "A lot of pregnancies come as a sort of surprise. Is that how it was with Candy?" or "Some women want to have children and some don't. How was it with you?" lets parents know you will nonjudgmentally accept any answer they give.

Next, review the labor and birth by including such questions as:

- How long was labor? Was it spontaneous or induced? Did it go according to expectations?
- Were there any complications? Was the birth vaginal or cesarean?
- Was anesthesia used for birth?
- Was the baby born vertex (i.e., head first) or breech?

Then, ask about the health of the child immediately after birth, including:

- Did the baby cry right away?
- Did the infant room in or need care in a special nursery?
- Did the infant need special procedures or equipment?
- Was there cyanosis or jaundice?
- Was the infant discharged from the birth setting with the mother?
- How did the parents feel about having a boy or a girl?
- How did it feel for them to be new parents?
- Was the infant breastfed or formula fed?

Family Health Histories

Because some diseases are inherited or familial, it is important to know which ones tend to occur in a family. Ask if any family member has a condition, such as cardiac disease (childhood or adult type), kidney disease, congenital anomalies, seizures, diabetes (type 1 or 2), tuberculosis, cancer, hypertension, a sexually transmitted infection (STI), allergies, or mental health issues, or is cognitively challenged.

Review of Systems

The last step in a health interview is a summary of body symptoms or a **review of systems**. Once more, make certain to introduce this part of the history with a transition

statement. Otherwise, parents may think the local problem they were describing (e.g., vomiting) has spread to other body systems. A statement such as "I'd like to ask about different parts of Candy's body, from her head down to her toes, just to be certain I didn't miss anything" provides such a transition.

Although the important items to be covered in a review of systems differ according to the age of the child, a basic list is shown in Box 34.5.

A review of systems covers a lot of ground, but it generally takes no more than 5 minutes. However, do not rush through the questions so quickly that a parent does not have time to answer or begins to believe this part of the interview is only an unimportant exercise ("Has Candy ever had nausea/vomiting/diarrhea/painful joints/broken bones?") Each question is important. If a child has any of the symptoms described, an entirely new area of the child's health needs to be explored.

Conclusion

A quick review of the information you have gathered during the health history will help clarify any misunderstandings or fill in areas forgotten by the patient. It should close with one last open-ended question: "Is there anything more we should know?" or "Is there anything I didn't mention you want to ask about?" A parent may have been reluctant to bring up something earlier. Asking this final question gives a parent a final opportunity to reveal a concern.

QSEN Checkpoint Question 34.2

QUALITY IMPROVEMENT

With the participation of her father, the nurse obtains a health history from Keoto. What question should the nurse ask at the end of this and every interview?

    a. "Where do you think we should go from here?"
    b. "Is there anything else you'd like to discuss?"
    c. "Are you still feeling okay?"
    d. "Am I a good interviewer? I'm trying hard."

Look in Appendix A for the best answer and rationale.

Physical Assessment

Mastery of physical examination technique is essential to incorporating physical assessment data into the assessment step of the nursing process, so a physical assessment, along with health interviewing, is one of the most frequently practiced skills of a nurse. The scope and extent of a pediatric physical assessment will vary, like health interviewing, depending on the circumstances of each health contact. At a first healthcare encounter, for example, children usually receive a complete physical examination. Later on, only a single focus may be required to obtain the information needed. If a child has a gastrointestinal disorder, for example, an assessment might be only a brief, multisystem examination followed by concentration on the gastrointestinal system (i.e., mouth, abdomen, rectum, fluid status).

BOX 34.5

Review of Systems

The following questions provide a guide when completing a review of systems:

Overall health
- *What is the general state of health?*
- Is the child taking any prescription medications? Over-the-counter medications? Home or folk remedies, such as herbal remedies?

Neuropsychiatric symptoms
- Has the child ever had a head injury? Seizures?
- Attention problems?
- Depression?
- Aggressive behavior?
- Has the parent ever had such difficulty rousing the child that the parent believed the child was unconscious?
- Is there any concern about suspected substance abuse?

Eye
- Has the child ever had difficulty with eyes not focusing?
- Eye infection?
- Does the parent have any reason to believe the child does not see well?
- Does the child wear eyeglasses or contact lenses?

Ears
- Ear infections?
- Drainage from the ears?
- Ear aches?
- Tubes in ears?
- Any infection from piercing?
- Reason to believe the child does not hear well?

Nose
- Frequent drainage or cold symptoms?
- Difficulty breathing?
- Nosebleeds?

Mouth
- Difficulty with teeth or teething?
- Mouth infections?
- Has the child seen a dentist (if older than 2 years of age)?
- Does the child chew tobacco?

Throat
- Throat infections?
- Difficulty swallowing?

Neck
- Masses or swelling?
- Stiffness?
- Does the child hold the head and neck straight? (Torticollis or wry neck will make a child hold the head crookedly; children with poor vision also may cock their heads to the side to try to see better.)

Chest
- Is breast development in girls appropriate for age?
- Any pain in breasts?

Lungs
- Breathing problems?
- Infections?
- Pneumonia?
- Asthma?
- Does the child smoke any substance?

Heart
- Has a healthcare provider ever said there was difficulty? What exactly was said?

Gastrointestinal system
- Has there been an eating problem?
- Frequent nausea?
- Vomiting?
- Diarrhea?
- Constipation?
- Is the child toilet trained? Any difficulty with this?

Genitourinary system
- Pain or burning on urination? Blood in urine? Does the child have a good urine stream?
- If a girl is age 10 years or older, has she started menstruation? Any concerns with menstruation?
- If an adolescent male, has he begun testicular self-examination?
- If an adolescent, is the child sexually active? Knows safer sex practices? Uses contraception? Wants more information on contraception? Ever had a sexually transmitted infection (STI)? (To protect privacy, it is essential to ask the adolescent, not the parents, questions regarding sexuality.)

Extremities
- Painful or swollen joints?
- Broken bones?
- Muscle sprains?
- Is the parent pleased with the child's coordination?

Skin
- Rashes?
- Lesions such as warts?

Immunizations
- What immunizations has the child received to date? Are they up to date?

PURPOSE AND TECHNIQUES

The actual process of a physical examination involves four separate techniques:

1. Inspection
2. Palpation
3. Percussion
4. Auscultation

These techniques are usually carried out in the listed order in each area of the body except the abdomen. **Auscultation** (a stethoscope examination) should follow **inspection** (a visual examination) and precede **palpation** (a hands-on examination) of the abdomen because handling the abdomen may obliterate bowel sounds. The findings from these techniques strengthen or validate history findings and help determine whether a concern requires immediate action (Box 34.6).

Effective use of physical assessment skills takes practice. Palpating an abdomen, for example, is a simple procedure; recognizing abdominal pathology through palpation is a more complicated skill. It is difficult to distinguish between normal liver tissue and a distended liver, for example, until both these conditions have been felt many times.

EQUIPMENT, SETTING, AND APPROACH

When performing a complete physical assessment, you'll need the following equipment: a thermometer, a stethoscope, a tongue depressor, an ophthalmoscope, an otoscope, disposable otoscope covers, a sphygmomanometer, a tape measure, a tuning fork, a reflex (**percussion**) hammer, examination gloves, and perhaps a patient drape or gown. Nurses who work in community settings or patients' homes must be sure to carry with them any equipment that may be needed.

Be certain to provide privacy and that the temperature in an examining room is comfortable. Change paper table covers between children to avoid possible spread of illness. During a complete physical examination, every part of the child's body should be exposed for inspection. To protect against chilling and to provide for modesty, expose body parts individually and only for the amount of time necessary for the examination. Because examining body parts such as the mouth or an open lesion exposes your hands to body fluids, as part of infection control precautions, wear gloves as appropriate during an examination.

People have the right not to have another person touch their body unless they permit them to do so. It is essential, therefore, to inform children that it is necessary to touch them for a physical examination and tell them what is happening at each step during the examination so they know when they will be touched. For instance, say "Next I want to look at your throat" to prevent surprises. Giving the child an option of what to examine first allows the child to feel in control. Never ask permission to exam a body part. If you proceed with the examination anyway, you will lose trust if the child had said "no." If some action will cause discomfort, such as deep palpation of the abdomen, offer fair warning such as "You'll feel pressure for a minute."

Assume that adolescents will cooperate in placing themselves in whatever position is required to inspect body parts unless they are short of breath or in some other way unable to cooperate. Small children may not cooperate readily and so may need to be restrained during an examination of such body parts as the nose, throat, and ears. Proper restraint enables an examiner to see well and also to ensure an instrument such as an otoscope will not accidentally cause injury. As a rule, do not ask parents to restrain during any procedure in which the child will feel threatened or feel pain; parents are best used as protectors and comforters after the procedure. If a parent does volunteer to restrain a child, urge them to do this with a positive approach such as "I'll help you keep your head still."

VARIATIONS FOR AGE AND DEVELOPMENTAL STAGE

Techniques of physical examination need to be tailored to the age and developmental stage of the individual child being assessed. Expected findings also depend on the child's age and developmental stage.

The Newborn

All newborns receive a physical examination immediately after birth and again after the first 24 hours of life. When examining newborns, cover body areas that are not being

BOX 34.6
Techniques of Physical Examination

Inspection:	Examining a child or adolescent initially with your eyes or nose and being alert to visual indications or odors that may point to a health problem.
Palpation:	Examining by touch, either light or deep. Use light palpation before deep palpation so the child or adolescent does not tense muscles and make light palpation difficult. The tips of your fingers are most sensitive to texture, vibration, consistency, and contour; the back of your hand is most sensitive to warmth. *If a child has a sensitive or painful body part, palpate that area last.* Otherwise, the child may be unwilling to allow you to touch other parts for fear of additional pain.
Percussion:	The assessment of a body structure by determining the sound you hear in response to striking the part with an examining finger and then interpreting the sound. Dense body areas such as bone have a dull, flat sound; those filled with air, such as lungs, are resonant. If an organ is stretched (e.g., a distended bladder), it has a hyperresonant or low and hollow sound. An organ stretched to an even greater point of distention has a tympanic or extremely hollow, ringing sound.
Auscultation:	Listening to sounds that are either discernible to the ear (e.g., wheezing or heavy breathing) or, as in most instances, made louder by means of a stethoscope. Always listen for four qualities of sound: duration, frequency, intensity (i.e., loudness), and pitch (i.e., high or low).

directly examined or perform the exam under a radiant heat warmer because maintaining body temperature is difficult for the newborn (Gupta, Patel, Murty, et al., 2015). Take axillary or tympanic temperatures to prevent rupture of rectal mucosa. Assess the heart rate apically because peripheral pulses may be too faint to be counted accurately. Be certain to obtain femoral pulses in newborns to rule out coarctation of the aorta. Include newborn reflexes, head circumference, and an assessment of gestational age (see Chapter 18) as routine parts of the examination. Taking blood pressure is not necessary because this value is unreliable in newborns. If possible, examine newborns with the parents present and use this assessment time to teach them about normal appearance and development.

The Infant

Infants are usually examined most effectively if a parent holds them during most of the examination. Use an "Isn't this fun?" or "This is a game" approach with the infant. As a rule, assess heart and lung function first; do intrusive procedures such as ear and throat assessment last so an infant does not cry and complicate the remainder of the examination. Blood pressure is still not taken routinely. Temperatures can be taken temporally. Include assessment of newborn reflexes until 6 months of age; continue to take the heart rate apically and the temperature in the axilla or by tympanic membrane. Measure head circumference for a full 24 months.

Between 7 and 12 months, children become fearful of strangers. Taking an extra minute to become well acquainted with an infant at the beginning of an examination can help to counteract this problem. Remember, infants calm to the tone of your voice as much as they do to what you actually say. They can be distracted by brightly colored toys while you listen to their heart or lungs. Offering a bottle of water or pacifier may be necessary during a heart assessment.

The Toddler and Preschooler

Ask parents to remove clothing or allow a toddler or preschooler to do this independently so it is less threatening. Children this age may be very afraid of examining equipment. To alleviate their fears, allow them to sit on their parent's lap for most of the exam and let them handle items such as stethoscopes, otoscopes, and blood pressure cuffs before the examination (Fig. 34.2).

Figure 34.2 Children need the opportunity to play with examining equipment so they become more familiar with and less frightened by it. (© Fotosearch.com)

BOX 34.7

Nursing Care Planning to Empower a Family

SUGGESTIONS FOR PREPARING A CHILD FOR A HEALTH ASSESSMENT

Q. Candy's father asks you, "How can I best prepare my 2-year-old for a preschool health exam?"

A. Here are some suggestions to help prepare a child for a health assessment:

- Promote the attitude that a health visit will be a positive experience.
- Bring a comfort item from home (e.g., a favorite doll or toy).
- Never threaten the child that if she is not good, a healthcare provider will punish her.
- Review with your daughter what she can expect during an assessment, such as a healthcare provider will ask questions of her parent; she or he will then look at the child's head, hands, etc.
- If she has been taught not to let strangers touch her body (as she should have been taught), reassure her it is all right for the healthcare provider to examine her.
- Dress your daughter in clothing that is easy to remove and replace so you can dress her quickly after an examination to rapidly assure her that the examination is over.

Leave intrusive procedures such as assessment of the genitalia, ears, and throat until last. Give generous praise for cooperation (anything short of hysterical screaming or kicking is good cooperation for intrusive procedures in this age group). Box 34.7 describes ways parents can prepare children of this age for assessment.

Begin to include blood pressure as part of routine assessment at 3 years of age; take a temporal temperature by an electronic thermometer rather than a tympanic temperature. Children up to school age often need to be restrained for ear and throat examinations because they grow fearful about procedures performed on a part of the body they cannot see (e.g., ears) or about a throat examination that may be uncomfortable. Before beginning an examination, establish a good rapport with the child's parents because children this age sense parental trust or suspicion.

The School-Age Child and Adolescent

Some children of this age may still be unaware of what a physical examination includes and whether it will cause discomfort. Offer good explanations so they are not frightened by the unknown. Provide older children with a choice about having a parent with them during the examination. Comment on body parts as you examine them to teach about good health such as "Your heart sounds good. And your ears look fine." Sometimes, adolescents are so concerned with a part of their body (e.g., a supernumerary nipple) that they are unable to voice this concern. A comment such as "This is a supernumerary (extra) nipple. Does it ever worry you that you have that?" may help an adolescent talk about what has indeed been a concern for years. Use a head-to-toe procedure; leave genitalia for last. Be certain to assess height and weight because more children in this age group are obese than ever before.

It is increasingly important to take blood pressure beginning in early school age also because as more children are overweight, more have elevated blood pressure (Spagnolo, Giussani, Ambruzzi, et al., 2013). Because obesity in school-age children and adolescents is associated with the development of type 2 diabetes mellitus and future cardiovascular disorders (Ayers, Charakidah, Deanfield, et al., 2015) and because there is also an association between being overweight and self-harm (Perera, Eisen, Bawor, et al., 2015), signs of these conditions need to be assessed as well.

School-age children and adolescents are particularly modest. Respect this by using gowns or drapes. Include a breast exam for adolescent girls and testicular exam for boys and teach testicular self-examination for boys beginning at about age 13 years.

QSEN Checkpoint Question 34.3

PATIENT-CENTERED CARE

Keoto's sister is 2 years old and appears fearful of medical equipment. To preserve her comfort, the nurse can exclude blood pressure measurement from assessment until what age?

a. 2.5 years
b. 3 years
c. 5 years
d. 7 years

Look in Appendix A for the best answer and rationale.

COMPONENTS OF PHYSICAL EXAMINATIONS

Presented here are the components of routine or general physical assessment. It is important to recognize what a "general" physical examination entails so you can interpret the extent of the assessment a child has received when the parent states, "He had a routine physical." The physical examination may be done in any order, but traditionally, the order proceeds from head to toe, examining each body part thoroughly before moving on to the next. Infants and young children are the exception, however, because if the infant cries, findings in a specific area become difficult to assess.

If abnormalities are discovered during an examination, a further assessment will be necessary. A complete neurologic examination, for example, is not routine and so is not included here (see Chapter 49 for details of a complete neurologic examination).

Vital Signs Assessment

Vital signs refer to temperature, pulse, respiration, blood pressure, and whether the child has pain (i.e., the state of vital bodily functions including heart and lung function, metabolic rate, and comfort level). Temperature is

an important assessment in children because it can reveal a subtle infection not as obvious yet by other signs. Because of the important information these provide, measurements of vital signs are recorded not only with complete physical examinations but also in many other instances of care. Techniques of these measurements and the nursing responsibilities that accompany them are discussed in Chapter 37. Remember, blood pressure in children can be elevated if they are anxious in a medical setting, the same as happens to adults and so needs to be evaluated in light of that (Spagnolo et al., 2013).

General Appearance

General appearance establishes an overall impression of a child's health as well as reveals specific body areas that will need a detailed assessment (Fig. 34.3 and Box 34.8). Be certain to include such areas as:

- Does the child appear well or ill overall?
- Is the child's height and weight proportional?
- Does the child appear well nourished? Appear underweight or overweight?
- What is the child's color? Pale? Yellow (jaundiced)? Cyanotic (blue)?
- Is posture normal? (Children who are in pain often assume an abnormal posture for relief.)
- What is the child's hygiene level? (Fatigue or illness can cause poor hygiene.)
- Is the child dressed appropriately for temperature and climate?
- Are lesions or symptoms of a specific illness present?
- Are there any significant body odors (Table 34.2)?
- Does the child appear relaxed or distressed? Lethargic or active?
- Is breathing easy or distressed?

Figure 34.3 A general appearance assessment reveals that this child is well proportioned and active.

BOX 34.8

Nursing Care Planning Using Assessment

ASSESSING THE CHILD FOR GENERAL WELL HEALTH

History
→Demographic data
→Chief concern
→History of chief concern
→Health and family profile

→Past health history
→Family health history
→Review of systems

Physical examination
→General appearance
→Vital signs

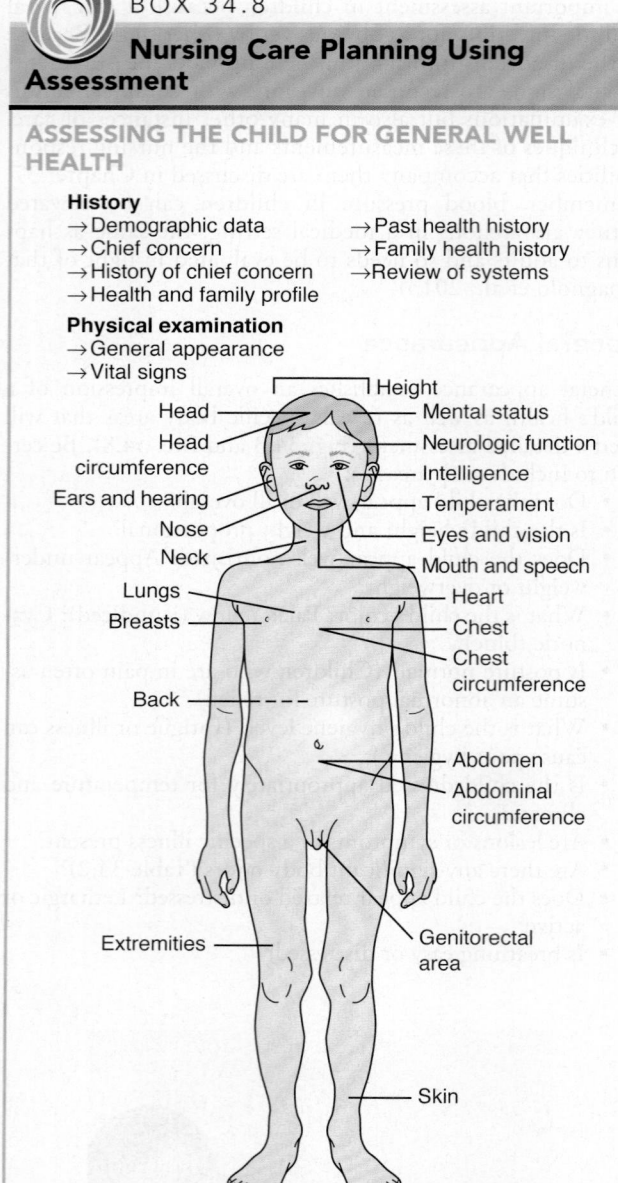

TABLE 34.2 SIGNIFICANT BODY ODORS

Source of Odor	Possible Cause
Breath	
Alcohol	Possible recent ingestion (important if coma or neurologic symptoms are present as cause of abnormal functioning)
Camphor	Mothball ingestion
Halitosis (bad breath)	Poor dental hygiene, lung infection; foreign body in respiratory tract
Burnt rope	Marijuana use
Sweet	Acidosis (seen in a child in diabetic coma)
Body	
Stale urine	Incontinence; poor kidney function leading to uremia; infrequently changed diapers; neglect
Sweat	May imply child is too fatigued or stressed to maintain hygiene
"Spoiled fruit"	Wound infection
Sweet	*Pseudomonas* infection
Urine	
Maple syrup	Protein metabolic condition
Musty or mousy	Phenylketonuria or a protein metabolism disorder
Ammonia	Urinary tract infection or poor hydration leading to concentrated urine
Stool	
Putrid	Fat in stool from inadequate absorption

surroundings? Assess the appropriateness of behavior and mood (e.g., Is a child hostile, frightened, shy, relaxed?). At some point in the examination of children older than preschool age, ask questions that test recent memory (e.g., what they ate for breakfast) and distant memory (e.g., the name of their first-grade teacher).

Body Measurements

Body measurements are important determinants of health in children because, with chronic illness, the body expends so many nutrients combating the destructive process of the disease that normal height and weight cannot be maintained. Conversely, being overweight (i.e., obesity) needs to be documented because this can lead to illnesses such as heart, endocrine, and lung disease later in life.

Weight

Until they can stand well, infants are weighed nude lying or sitting on an infant scale (diapers can be heavy in proportion to total body weight). Always keep a protective hand over an infant on an infant scale (hovering but not touching) because infants squirm readily and there is danger of them falling (Fig. 34.4A,B). Cover both infant scales and adult scales with scale paper before weighing to prevent the spread of infection from one child to another.

If the child appears to have pain, ask the child to rate it on a child-appropriate pain scale, such as the Faces scale, to better determine the degree of pain (Ely, Chen-Lim, Zarnowsky, et al., 2012).

Mental Status Assessment

A mental status assessment is also made early in an examination as a complement to general appearance. As with general appearance, additional information is gained on mental status throughout the entire examination.

Begin by assessing a child's level of consciousness: Is the child alert? Next, assess orientation, or if the child is aware of person, place, and time (i.e., awareness of who they are, where they are, and the date) if the child is over preschool age. If an infant, does the child "attune" or look aware of

Figure 34.4 (A,B) Weighing an infant. Note the protective hand to ensure the infant's safety. **(C)** Weighing an older child.

Children older than 2 years of age are weighed on standing scales, in street clothes (no shoes), or, if in a hospital, in a gown or pajamas (Fig. 34.4C). If children are going to have serial weights (i.e., weighed every day), be sure they wear the same clothing every time they are weighed so any discrepancy in weight is truly a difference in body weight and not due to more or less clothing. Also, take serial weights at the same time each day (preferably before breakfast) on the same scale for greatest accuracy.

Most children and their parents want to know their weight. To convert from kilograms to pounds, multiply the kilogram amount by 2.2 (50 kg × 2.2 = 110 lb). To assess whether weight is average for height, compare the child's weight with a standardized height/weight graph (available at http://thePoint .lww.com/Flagg8e). On these standardized graphs, all weights between the 10th and 90th percentiles are considered normal (statistically, a range of weights that includes two standard deviations from the mean or the 50th percentile). All children with weight below the 25th or above the 75th percentiles need close examination because they are moving close to the end points of the usual weight continuum. There are also specific graphs for premature infants and those with Trisomy 21. (These graphs are available at www.ncbi.nlm.nih.com.)

As important as it is for children's weight to fall between the 10th and 90th percentile on growth charts, it is also important that, over time, the weight follows one of the percentile curves; in other words, children should not be at the 70th percentile the first time they are weighed, and a month later, at the 80th or 40th percentile. Although both readings are within the normal range, they reflect a weight change that would need investigation. A child is defined as "failing to thrive" if height or weight drops below the third percentile on a standardized growth chart (Jaffe, 2011). Any height or weight in this category definitely needs to be reported so its cause can be investigated. Identifying that one is overweight is equally important because this can lead to so many illnesses later on in life (Ward, Welker, Choate, et al., 2017).

U.S. growth charts were compiled by the Centers for Disease Control and Prevention (CDC) in the 1960s when almost all infants were formula fed, not breastfed, so breastfed infants tend to score lower on these charts than might be expected (often at the 25th percentile). The World Health Organization (WHO) has published growth charts that better reflect the weight of breastfed infants. It can be helpful to plot infant weight on these alternative growth charts to reassure parents that their breastfed infant is thriving (de Onis, 2015).

Another method to determine whether a child's weight is consistent with height is to compute his or her body mass index (BMI) by using a website such as www.cdc.gov. Many electronic medical records now record and graph BMI.

Height

In children, height is as good a determinant of health and normal nutrition as is weight. For tips on accurately measuring the height of infants and older children, see Box 34.9.

Following a measurement, plot the height of children on a standard graph, the same as for weight. Height and weight should follow the same percentiles. Remember that height/weight charts have been standardized for middle-class White American children, so there will be variations among children from different ethnic and socioeconomic backgrounds. The important thing to look for is consistency in measurements over time (i.e., always at the same percentile).

What If . . . 34.1
Keoto, 13 years old, weighs 93 lb. Would the nurse be concerned? What if 6 months earlier she weighed 110 lb and a year earlier she weighed 105 lb?

BOX 34.9

Nursing Care Planning Using Procedures

MEASURING A CHILD'S HEIGHT

Purpose: To assess for optimal growth

Procedure	Principle
Infant	
1. Until they can stand securely (at approximately age 2 years), measure infants lying down on a measuring frame or an examining table.	1. Promotes accuracy
2. Align the infant's head snugly against the top bar of the measuring frame and ask an assistant to secure it there. Parents can help you restrain infants for height measurements because it is a painless procedure.	2. Provides a starting point for measurement
3. Straighten the infant's body (Fig. A).	3. Knees are difficult to straighten in infants because they usually keep them flexed.

A

Procedure	Principle
4. Hold the infant's feet in a vertical position. Bring the foot board up snugly against the bottom of the foot.	4. Completes measurement
5. If an examining table is used instead of a measuring frame, mark the spots at the top of the child's head and bottom of the feet on the table paper and then measure between the marks with a tape measure.	5. Provides for an alternative approach
6. Plot height measurements on a standard graph.	6. Allows for interpretation of findings
Older Child	
1. Have the child remove shoes and step onto the scale.	1. Promotes accuracy
2. Ask the child to stand straight with head held level.	2. Puts the child in the proper position for accurate measurement
3. Align the measuring bar of a standing scale with the top of the child's head.	3. Determines the measurement
4. If a scale with a measuring bar is not available, place a flat object such as a clipboard on the child's head in a horizontal position and read the height at the point at which the object touches a measuring tape on the back of the scale or a flat wall surface (Fig. B).	4. Provides for an alternative approach
5. Plot height measurement on a standard graph.	5. Allows for interpretation of findings

MEASURING A CHILD'S HEIGHT

B

Head Circumference

Head circumference is measured at birth and routinely on physical assessment until 1 or 2 years of age. Head growth occurs because the brain is growing, so head circumference reflects brain growth and potential neurologic function. The measurement is made by placing a tape measure around the infant's head just above the eyebrows and around the most prominent portion of the back of the head (i.e., the occipital prominence) (Fig. 34.5). Babies generally push any object away from their head, so it may be more difficult than it seems to carry out this simple procedure. Plot measurements on a standardized graph (see "Growth Charts" available at http://thePoint.lww.com/Flagg8e). Head circumference should correlate with the child's length; that is, if length is in the 40th percentile, head circumference also should be. If measurements of head circumference plot at different percentiles over time, this should be reported because it implies brain or skull growth is in some way abnormal and needs to be investigated.

Chest and Abdominal Circumference

Measurements of chest and abdominal circumference are not done routinely but rather only when specific pathology warrants. Chest circumference is measured at the nipple line, and the abdominal circumference is measured at the level of the umbilicus.

Skin

Skin is assessed in conjunction with the examination of each body region. Always assess temperature, color, dryness, texture, **turgor** (i.e., amount of fluid in body tissue), and the presence of any lesions such as a rash that might reveal a communicable illness. Table 34.3 summarizes various findings that may be detected on skin examination. Be

certain there is adequate lighting, especially when assessing dark-skinned children. Also, be certain to examine a child's total skin surface at some point during an examination. If necessary, remove and replace adhesive bandages or other dressings that could hide important findings (e.g., possible maltreatment).

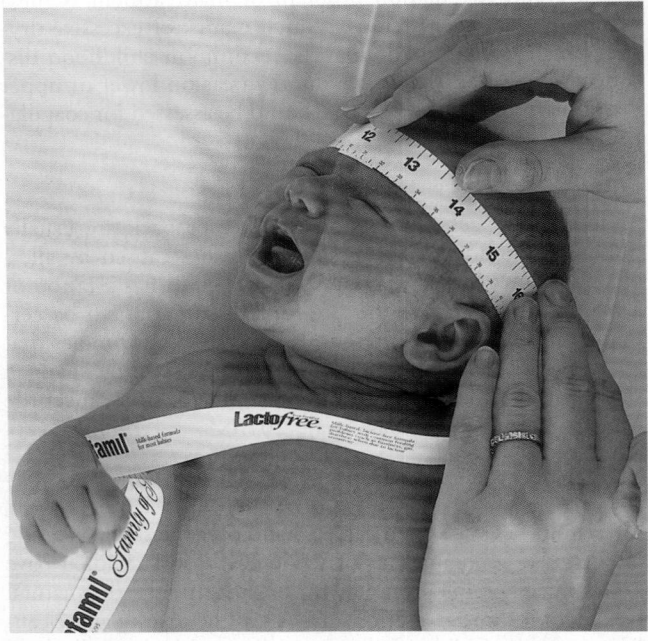

Figure 34.5 Measuring head circumference. The measuring tape passes just above the eyebrows and around the prominent posterior aspect of the head.

TABLE 34.3 SKIN FINDINGS IN CHILDREN THAT SUGGEST ILLNESS

Finding	Indication
Central bluish color	Cyanosis from decreased respiratory function or cyanotic heart disease; acrocyanosis (blue hands and feet) is normal in newborns for first 48 hours.
White color	Edema (accumulated subcutaneous fluid is stretching the skin)
Pale color	Anemia or decreased circulation to a body part
Reddened area	Local inflammation or increased systemic temperature
Linear abrasion	Scratch marks from local irritation from an insect bite or allergic reaction
Ecchymoses (black and blue marks)	Recent injury to skin
Petechiae (pinpoint blood marks)	Blood dyscrasia (poor clotting ability)
Yellow color	Jaundice from increased bilirubin in subcutaneous tissue; carotenemia (excess carotene in skin)
Moistness	Excess perspiration from elevated temperature
Localized cold temperature	Decreased circulation to particular body part
Warm temperature	Local irritation or elevated systemic temperature
Poor turgor	Dehydration
Rash	Infectious childhood illness, excessive heat, or allergy

The Newborn and Infant

Newborns may appear ruddy because, as their layer of subcutaneous fat is thin, the intense redness of their blood circulation is visible. Erythema toxicum (i.e., newborn rash) or birthmarks (e.g., hemangiomas, Mongolian spots, nevi) may be present (see Chapter 18). After the first few days of life, a diaper rash may be present.

The Toddler, Preschooler, and School-Age Child

Many children this age have minor lesions from mosquito bites or from fleabites if they own a pet. They also typically have a number of ecchymotic spots on their lower extremities from bumping into objects during active play. Ecchymotic spots on upper extremities are less common and may suggest a blood coagulation problem or maltreatment (Chiesa & Sirotnak, 2014). Lesions, scratch marks, or excessive dryness can reveal atopic dermatitis, a common childhood disorder (Spiewak, 2012). Ecchymotic areas on lower or upper extremities not typical of a fall should be assessed for coagulation disorders or abuse.

The Adolescent

At least a few acne lesions on the face or back are usually present in an adolescent. Lesions or rashes caused by allergies to cosmetics also may be seen. If a child has a tattoo or a body piercing, assess the site for inflammation to be certain an infection is not present. Look carefully for moles that are very dark, have uneven borders, or have recently changed shape because these are signs of melanoma or skin cancer (de Maleissye, Beauchet, Saiag, et al., 2013).

The Head

To examine a child's head, slide a hand over the skull, assessing for irregular configurations or tenderness. Most children have a prominent occipital outgrowth; do not mistake this natural head contour for an abnormality. Assess the texture and cleanliness of hair. Children who are well nourished usually have hair of good texture; poorly nourished children tend to have dry, brittle, or limp hair. If hair is exceptionally oily, it may suggest a lack of adequate hygiene, possibly from fatigue due to

an unidentified illness. If a serious protein deficiency such as **kwashiorkor** is present, the hair becomes striped with dark and light color because dark hair forms during periods of good protein intake and the light color forms during periods of protein deficiency. Patches of hair loss (i.e., alopecia) suggest a fungal infection (e.g., tinea capitis), child maltreatment, or a possible drug reaction (chemotherapy will cause total hair loss, not patches).

The Newborn and Infant

In a newborn, the head usually shows molding (i.e., an elongated shape due to pressure against the cervix before birth). A caput succedaneum or cephalohematoma from the pressure of birth may be present (see Chapter 18). Skull suture lines are palpable. In both newborns and infants, sit the child upright and palpate the skull for the presence of fontanelles (i.e., the places where the skull bones fuse). The anterior fontanelle is diamond-shaped and measures 2 to 3 cm (0.8 to 1.2 in.) in width and 3 to 4 cm (1.2 to 1.6 in.) in length. The posterior fontanelle is triangular and measures approximately 1 cm (0.5 in.) in length (see Chapter 15, Fig. 15.2).

With the infant sitting, fontanelles should be felt as soft spots but should not appear indented (a sign of dehydration) or bulging (a sign of increased intracranial pressure). When an infant cries, cerebral pressure increases, so with crying, the fontanelles may feel tense, and sometimes, the fluctuation of a pulse can even be observed. The anterior fontanelle normally closes at 12 to 18 months and the posterior fontanelle by the end of 2 months so should not be palpable after these times. The closing of fontanelles too early or too late can indicate decreased or increased brain or ventricle growth and is, therefore, a serious finding.

Because of the campaign to encourage "back" sleeping for infants, many infants have a flat occiput "plagiocephaly." Infants should start with "tummy time" when they are discharged from the hospital. By 3 to 4 months, they should be getting 20 minutes of tummy time per day. A scalp problem commonly encountered in infants is seborrhea (i.e., scaling, greasy-appearing, salmon-colored patches) or "cradle cap." You can advise parents that increasing the frequency of hair washing to once a day and applying baby oil to the scalp typically reduces this problem.

The Toddler, Preschooler, and School-Age Child

Examine the hair of children who attend school or day care carefully for small white-yellow, sand-sized particles attached to hair strands, which are the eggs (i.e., nits) of pediculi (i.e., head lice). Pediculi can spread easily in school-age children due to sharing of combs and towels in school. Nits cling and cannot be readily removed from the hair by running fingers the length of the hair (Devore & Schutze, 2015). The child may have recent scratch marks on the scalp or state that the scalp feels itchy.

Also examine the scalp carefully for round circular areas (perhaps weeping in the center, crusting and scaling on the edges) that would suggest tinea capitis (i.e., ringworm, which is a fungal infection). Like pediculi, fungal infections can easily spread among school-age children; a prescription medication is necessary to best cure tinea capitis (see Chapter 43). Both over-the-counter and prescription medications are available for pediculosis.

The Adolescent

Adolescents may streak their hair with dye or arrange it in a way that requires gel, hair extensions, or use of a curling iron. Inspect to see that their scalp and hair are healthy underneath the styling. Tight cornrows and weaves can cause hair to break, resulting in areas of baldness.

The Eyes

Observe eyes for symmetry and signs of redness (i.e., erythema), frequent blinking, crusting, squinting, or rubbing because these are signs of **conjunctivitis**, an infection of the thin conjunctiva covering the eye globe (Braverman, 2016). Also, observe lids and lashes for redness or abnormalities to detect a **hordeolum** or stye (i.e., an infection of the gland that lubricates an eyelash). Both conditions require an antibiotic for therapy (see Chapter 50).

Assess the location of eyes in relation to the nose (i.e., not unusually wide or narrow spaced) and the relationship of the globe to the socket (i.e., neither sunken nor protruding from the socket [exophthalmos]). Abnormalities in these areas occur in chromosomal or metabolic illnesses such as hyperthyroidism. Inspect the sclera of the eye for spots of hemorrhage (i.e., subconjunctival hemorrhage) or yellowing. Black children often have a slight yellowing of the sclera and small black spots on the sclera; do not mistake these for abnormal findings. Assess that no sclera shows above the pupil (if it does, this is termed a *sunset sign*, a possible indication of increased intracranial pressure or trisomy 21).

Palpate each eye globe with the eyelid closed to assess for tenseness, a finding suggesting glaucoma (although this is rare in children). Determine whether the eyelids completely close; edema or neurologic illnesses may shorten eyelids so they cannot close. Lastly, determine whether the lids retract far enough so they do not obscure vision when the child opens his or her eyes. When a lid obscures vision (**ptosis**), it generally denotes neurologic involvement. The difference in Western and Eastern eye creases is shown in Figure 34.6.

Examine the inner lining of the lower eyelid (i.e., the conjunctiva) by pulling the lid down slightly with your fingertip. Here, the mucous membrane should appear moist and not pale. In children with anemia, it often appears pale; for a child with an allergy or infection, it may appear unusually red

Figure 34.6 Differences in eye formation. **(A)** Western. **(B)** Eastern. The extra inner fold of tissue is an epicanthal fold.

and irritated. Do not initiate a blink reflex by touching the cornea with a wisp of cotton, as is done in adults, because this is momentarily painful and frightening for children.

In addition, observe whether the eyes appear to be in good alignment. **Strabismus** refers to eyes that are not evenly aligned. If an eye is always turning in, the condition is termed **esotropia**; if it always turns out, this is termed **exotropia**. Two screening procedures for straight eye alignment include the Hirschberg test and the cover test. During a Hirschberg test, the light of an otoscope should reflect evenly off both pupils if they are in equal alignment (Fig. 34.7).

Figure 34.7 Testing good eye alignment by the Hirschberg test. The child is asked to look directly at the light of the otoscope. The light reflex on the pupils of both eyes will be equal if the eyes are in straight alignment.

Figure 34.8 The cover test. **(A)** The child's eyes appear to be in good alignment. **(B)** The left eye is covered for 5 seconds. **(C)** When the card is removed, the left eye is seen to move perceptibly back to good alignment. This movement indicates it "drifted" into a deviant position while covered; that is, an exophoria (misalignment) is present.

To perform a cover test (Fig. 34.8), perform the following steps:

- Have children look at an attractive object approximately 4 ft in front of them.
- Hold a 3 × 5 in. card over the left eye for a count of five. If any degree of strabismus is present, the eye will wander to its misaligned position while covered.
- Remove the card and observe the eye for movement.
- As the child again fixes vision on the specified object, the eye will move back into line, revealing the misalignment.
- Repeat the process with the right eye.

Some children, particularly preschoolers with wide epicanthic folds, may appear at a quick glance, to show misalignment. A cover test is helpful in these children because there will be no eye movement after removal of the card, demonstrating no actual misalignment, only the temporary appearance of that. Reasons for true misalignment are discussed in Chapter 50.

To test the eyes for their ability to focus in all fields of vision:

- Ask the child to follow a moving light (or catch the attention of an infant with a moving light) while holding the child's chin stationary.
- Move the light out to the side, then up, and then down.
- Cross to the opposite side and move it up and down.
- Bring the light back to the midline and observe whether the child's eyes converge (follow the light in to the nose). Infants younger than 3 months of age cannot follow past the midline; the eyes of children under school age do not converge well.

If the pupil constricts (i.e., reduces in size) in response to the light, it is confirmation the third cranial nerve is intact. For this test, it is best to approach the child's eye from the forehead so the light suddenly appears on the pupil rather than advancing it toward the child slowly because this makes the pupil constrict more dramatically. When one pupil constricts in response to a bright light, this is termed *direct constriction*; constriction should also occur in the opposite eye

(i.e., *consensual constriction*). Record pupils are equal in size and react to light as PERL (pupils equal, react to light). If the pupil converges (i.e., moves to follow a light in toward the nose), this is charted as PEARL or PERLA (pupils equal, react to light, accommodate).

For a final step, shine a flashlight or ophthalmoscope light into the pupil. A red reflex or the red pupil that occurs with a flash photo should appear. This is evidence the retina is intact and the lens and cornea are clear (i.e., no tumor, cataract, scarring, or infection is present).

The Newborn and Infant

Newborns often have a small, bright-red spot on the sclera (i.e., a subconjunctival hemorrhage) because the pressure of birth ruptured a small conjunctival blood vessel. This is normal and will fade in 7 to 10 days as the blood is absorbed.

Newborns and infants can easily be tested for a red reflex, but until they are about 3 months, they cannot follow an object or light across the midline or follow a light into all six positions of gaze. Assessing for a red reflex is especially important in newborns because a congenital cataract can lead to a loss of central vision if not discovered early.

The Toddler and Preschooler

Most young children are reluctant to let someone look into their eyes. Explaining what will happen during an eye examination is important to reduce the child's anxiety about this part of the assessment.

The School-Age Child and Adolescent

Many older children wear contact lenses (a red reflex is visible with a contact lens in place), and others may be nervous about having their eyes examined because they know they should be wearing prescribed eyeglasses but are not wearing them because they do not like their appearance. Observe carefully for pupillary appearance and ability to constrict in adolescents to rule out drug abuse. Many adolescent girls are anemic and so have pale conjunctiva.

The Nose

Observe the nose for flaring of the nostrils (a sign of a need for oxygen). Using an otoscope light, observe the mucous membrane of the nose for color—it should be pink; pale suggests allergies, and redness suggests infection. Note and describe any discharge. Document the septum is in the midline because a displaced septa such as those that occur after facial injuries can interfere with respiration and make nasal intubation in emergencies difficult. Gently press one nostril closed and ask the child to inhale. Repeat on the opposite side to ensure both sides of the nose are patent; that is, no choanal atresia or membrane obstructing the posterior nares exists. Sinuses do not fully develop until about 6 years. For children 6 years or older, palpate the areas over the frontal and maxillary sinuses for tenderness, which is a symptom of sinus infection. Assess the sense of smell in school-age children and adolescents by asking them to identify a familiar odor such as chocolate or an orange.

The Newborn and Infant

Infants are obligate nose breathers. They cannot coordinate mouth breathing, so they become disturbed when the nose is temporarily blocked to check for patency; do this only momentarily to avoid discomfort. Most newborns have milia (i.e., small white papules) on the surface of the nose, which are of no consequence and disappear without treatment.

The Older Child

Many children preschool age and older have upper respiratory infections that cause reddened nasal mucous membranes and a purulent discharge. In contrast, allergies cause a clear discharge and pale mucous membranes. Children who have dry mucosa due to dry air, which leads to cracking and nosebleeds, may be reluctant to allow inspection of their nose. Adolescents who sniff cocaine lose nasal hair and may have excoriations or abscesses in the mucous membrane as well as holes in the septum. If the child has a nose piercing, inspect the site for redness or drainage.

Ears

Observe ears for proper alignment. In the average child, a line drawn from the inner canthus of the eye to the outer canthus and then to the ear will touch the top of the pinna of the ear (Fig. 34.9). Ears set lower than this are associated with chromosomal disorders such as trisomy 13. Observe the opening to the ear canal for any discharge. Touch the pinna and watch for evidence of pain, which is a sign of external canal infections.

Figure 34.10   An otoscopic examination. Note how the nurse's hand rests between the otoscope and the child's head. Should the child move, no injury to the tympanic membrane will be sustained with this technique because the otoscope will move with the child's head.

Observe the area immediately in front of the ear for a dermal sinus or skin tag, findings that are usually innocent but may be associated with kidney abnormalities. Observe the ear lobes for redness or drainage from infected piercing sites, if applicable.

To examine the ear canal:

- Select the smallest size otoscope tip possible that will still give adequate visibility.
- Straighten the ear canal by pulling the pinna gently down and back in the child under 2 years of age and up and back in the older child.
- Insert an otoscope tip into the external canal.
- Be certain to rest the instrument on your hand, not on the child's head (Fig. 34.10). In this position, the otoscope will move with the child, avoiding the danger the plastic tip will scratch the canal if the child should move suddenly.
- Inspect the sides of the ear canal and then locate landmarks on the surface of the tympanic membrane.

The outline of the malleus of the inner ear should be visible through the translucent membrane and is a key landmark to visualize (Fig. 34.11). The color of the membrane should be pinkish gray; usually, if the tension of the membrane is normal, a cone of light (i.e., the light reflex) should

Figure 34.9   Normal ear alignment. When a line is drawn from the inner canthus through the outer canthus of the eye to the ear, the top of the ear pinna should meet the line **(A)**. Abnormal ear alignment **(B)** is associated with certain chromosomal abnormalities.

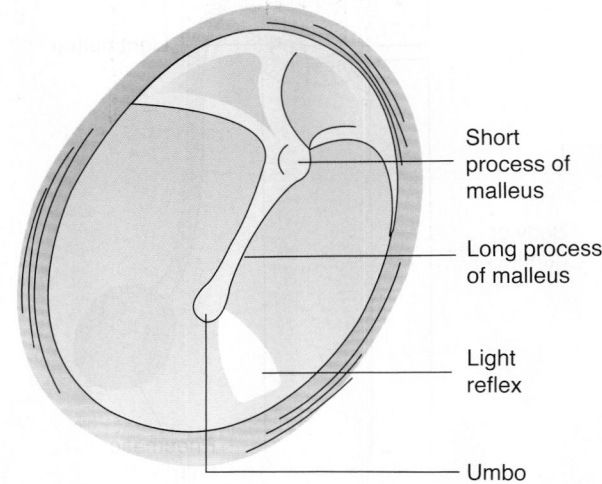

Short process of malleus

Long process of malleus

Light reflex

Umbo

Figure 34.11   A tympanic membrane as viewed with an otoscope.

be present in one of the lower corners (at either the 5 o'clock in the right ear or the 7 o'clock position in the left ear).

Although many children have wax (i.e., cerumen) in their ear canals, which appears as a dark-brown, glistening substance or flaky amber, viewing the tympanic membrane past the wax is almost always possible.

If an ear infection is present, the tympanic membrane will appear reddened and will often bulge forward so the malleus is no longer discernible and the cone of light is absent (Yoon, Kelley, & Friedman, 2016).

If there is fluid in the middle ear, it may be possible to see bubbles of air through the membrane. With chronic middle ear disease (i.e., serous otitis media), the tympanic membrane may be retracted, the malleus will then be extremely prominent, and the cone of light will be missing. If the membrane has been torn from trauma or rupture, the jagged edge and opening to the middle ear are discernible and may have purulent discharge. Inspect also for any ulcerated areas that could be a cholesteatoma or an ingrowing tumor, most often seen on the upper part of the membrane (see Chapter 50).

Although not a routine procedure, the mobility of the eardrum can be tested by injecting a column of air into the ear canal against the drum by a pneumatic attachment on an otoscope, which looks like the bulb of a blood pressure cuff (Fig. 34.12). A normal drum is freely mobile and can be seen to move with pressure on the bulb; one with fluid behind it has decreased mobility. Before introducing air, warn the child air against the membrane will tickle. A tympanogram can also assess for fluid behind the eardrum.

Finally, appraise hearing. Appraisal for this can be done grossly in older children by assessing their response to your questions. Distract an infant with a toy and then make a sound behind the infant's back, out of peripheral vision, and watch if there is a response. Hearing infants will show some noticeable reaction, although they have difficulty looking directly toward or locating the sound until about 4 months of age.

The Newborn and Infant

Many newborns still have amniotic fluid or vernix caseosa in their ear canal, so inspecting the ear canal is ineffective. Be certain to assess for ear level and normal pinna contour. Assess gross hearing ability, for example, by watching the infant startle to a sudden sound or quiet to the calming effect of quiet talking.

The Older Child

Middle ear infection (i.e., otitis media) is a common childhood illness. This causes the ear to be painful when examined. An external ear infection (often called swimmer's ear) causes any movement of the pinna to be painful. Explaining what is happening during the examination helps to allay a child's fear of having an instrument pressed into the ear. Beginning with preschool age, children may have myringotomy tubes (i.e., small circular plastic tubes placed into the tympanic membrane) to relieve chronic fluid collected in the middle ear. Inspect that the area surrounding the tube is not inflamed and the tube is not merely lying in the external canal and no longer inserted into the membrane (see Chapter 50).

The Mouth

Assess the external appearance of the lips for symmetry and color. Ask the child to smile and frown to evaluate the mobility of facial muscles. Count the number of teeth present and assess their condition (e.g., number missing or cavities present). Inspect the gum line (i.e., gingivae) for redness, tenderness, and edema, symptoms of periodontal disease. Inspect the buccal membrane and palate for color (e.g., pink) and the presence of any lesions. Ask the child to stick out his or her tongue and assess for midline position and no fasciculations (i.e., trembling). Inspect the area under the tongue for lesions in school-age children and adolescents who smoke or chew tobacco because this is the most common first site for oral cancer.

A child's tongue is normally smooth and moist. With dehydration present, it often appears roughened and dry. **Geographic tongue** is the term for the rough-appearing tongue surface that often accompanies general symptoms of illness such as fever; it may also normally occur. If a child has a pierced tongue, inspect for redness at the site. Assess that the object is secure so there is little chance of aspiration and that it is not striking and wearing down the tooth enamel.

Use a tongue blade to press down and forward on the back of the tongue to inspect the uvula in midline (Fig. 34.13).

Figure 34.12 An otoscope with pneumatic attachment.

Figure 34.13 Inspecting the pharynx in a school-age child.

The epiglottis can usually be observed with the tongue depressed. Observe for abnormal enlargement, palatine redness, or drainage of tonsils. Although tonsillar tissue differs greatly in size, it should not be reddened or have pus in the crypts (i.e., indentations). After initiating a gag reflex in infants to view the back of their throat, always turn their head to the side so they do not choke on any saliva that accumulated in the mouth during the throat examination because infants are less able to manage this than are adults.

Do not depress the tongue of any child who is suspected to have epiglottitis or whose glottis is inflamed. Symptoms of this condition are a sore throat, drooling, high fever, difficulty with respiration, dysphagia, and a barking cough. If a swollen, inflamed epiglottis rises with the pressure of a tongue blade, it can obstruct the respiratory tract so completely that the child is immediately unable to breathe.

The Newborn and Infant

Many newborns have considerable mucus in their mouths because they are less able to handle swallowing due to immature muscle coordination. If a newborn has teeth, evaluate them for stability; if teeth are loose, they may need to be removed to prevent aspiration. Assess for white patches that do not scrape away from the buccal membrane or tongue (i.e., thrush), a common but abnormal finding in infants that requires antifungal therapy (see Chapter 43). White patches that scrape away easily are usually caused by an accumulation of formula or breast milk.

The Older Child

Tonsillar tissue in children reaches its maximum growth at early school age, making many preschool children appear to be "all tonsils." As long as the tissue does not appear reddened or tender, you can assume it to be normal for the age. Many children with enlarged tonsils snore at night and wake feeling tired. These children should be assessed by an ENT specialist for sleep apnea. Many children have irregular, pale-pink, and elevated projections on the posterior pharynx as a normal finding. A stream of mucopurulent discharge in the posterior pharynx, however, is not usual and suggests an upper respiratory infection and that a "postnasal" flow of secretions is present. For a child with orthodontic appliances such as braces, assess carefully for pinpoint ulcers on the gum line to be certain the wires are not causing undue discomfort or infection. Cavities appear as dark-brown areas on the tooth enamel. Many school-age children or adolescents have at least one present and will need a dental care referral.

QSEN Checkpoint Question 34.4

TEAMWORK & COLLABORATION

Pressing a tongue blade against the back of the throat causes a gag reflex. When would the nurse want the team members to know it is important *not* to elicit a gag reflex?
a. When a child is under 5 years of age
b. When a child has symptoms of epiglottitis
c. When a boy has a possible inguinal hernia
d. When a girl has a geographic tongue

Look in Appendix A for the best answer and rationale.

The Neck

Assess the neck for symmetry (the trachea should be in the midline; any deviation suggests lung or thyroid pathology). Observe the outline of the thyroid gland (barely noticeable before puberty) because it is obscured by the sternocleidomastoid muscle, on the anterior neck, to be certain it is not swollen or tender. Palpate the area in front of the ear, which is the location of the parotid gland, and smooth a hand over the location of lymph nodes at the sides of the neck and under the chin to palpate for swelling. Figure 34.14 shows the location of lymph node chains of the head and neck. Because children have so many upper respiratory infections, a few nodes that are freely movable, about the size of peas, termed "shotty" nodes because they simulate the feel of buckshot under the skin, are often present. Commonly, preauricular and postauricular nodes are palpable after ear infections, and postoccipital nodes are palpable after a scalp infection. Submental nodes generally denote a tooth abscess. Palpable submaxillary, anterior, and posterior cervical nodes follow throat infections.

Ask the child to move the head (or move it for the child) through flexion (i.e., touch chin to chest) and extension (i.e., raise chin as high as possible) and turn it right and left (i.e., rotation) to see that a child does all of these movements easily. Pain on forward flexion is an important sign because it can be caused by neurologic (i.e., meningeal) irritation or is a sign of meningitis.

The Newborn and Infant

With infants, always assess the ability to control the head by laying the infant supine and pulling the child to a sitting position. Babies younger than 4 months of age will let their heads lag backward as they are pulled up this way, and they will right their heads only as they reach a sitting position. After 4 months, infants should bring their head up with no head lag if their neuromuscular coordination is adequate for their age. This simple but important test yields information about overall neuromuscular control as well as neck strength.

The Adolescent

In adolescents, be certain to palpate the thyroid gland for both symmetry and possible nodes. To do this, have the adolescent tilt their head slightly forward and press on the right

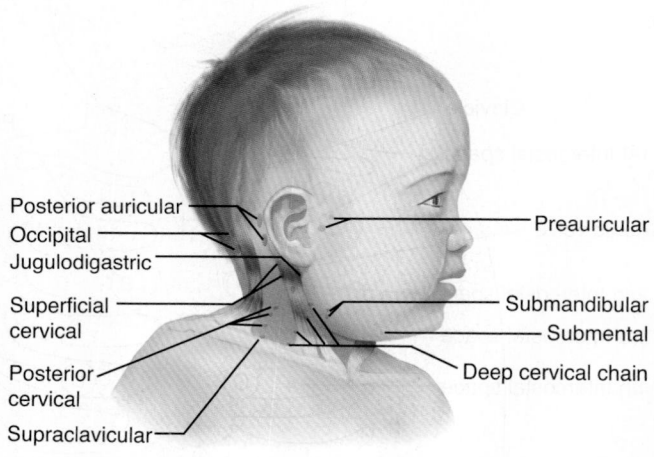

Figure 34.14 The location of lymph node chains in the head and neck.

side of the gland, which will cause it to be more prominent on the left side. Palpate the left half to discern any irregularities (areas of hardness). Repeat on the right side. A finding of a thyroid node needs to be investigated because it may be only an innocent transient cyst or it may be the first indication of thyroid malignancy. Many adolescents have a normal increase in the size of the thyroid at puberty; this hypertrophy should not be accompanied by any nodes.

The Chest

For ease in specifying the location of chest pathology, the chest is divided into sections by imaginary lines drawn through the midclavicle, midmammary, and midsternum points on the front; the midaxilla on the side; and the midscapula on the back. Pathology is described in terms of these lines such as "abnormal lung sound heard at left midaxillary line." Other helpful means of locating pathology is by the suprasternal notch, the ribs, and the spaces between them (**intercostal spaces**). Intercostal spaces are numbered according to the ribs immediately above them (Fig. 34.15). Inspect both front and back surfaces of the chest for symmetry of appearance and motion. Inspect for **retractions** or indentation of intercostal spaces or the suprasternal and substernal areas reflect in difficult respirations. Assess the proportion of the anteroposterior to the lateral diameter (normally 1:2). Children with chronic lung disease develop a broad (i.e., barrel) chest or a chest more rounded than usual. This and other chest abnormalities are shown in Figure 34.16. An infant with a diaphragmatic hernia (i.e., intestine herniated into the chest cavity) may have a chest enlarged on that side. An infant with atelectasis (i.e., collapsed lung) may have a chest smaller on the affected side. If a child has an enlarged heart, the left side of the chest may appear larger.

The Breasts

The degree of breast assessment depends on the child's age and development. As part of a usual breast assessment, inspect and palpate the breasts of all children to detect any abnormalities.

The Newborn

Both male and female newborns may have breast edema from the influence of maternal hormones. A few drops of clear fluid may be present from the nipples. This is normal and will fade in a few days' time. Do not squeeze the nipple to remove the fluid. Document if a supernumerary nipple is present for baseline data.

The School-Age Child and Adolescent

Do a breast examination on all girls past puberty. If a girl younger than 8 years is beginning breast development, precocious puberty (see Chapter 48) should be suspected. Often, one breast starts to develop before the other. Young girls who are starting to develop breast tissue may complain of discomfort in the developing breast. Many preadolescent boys develop hypertrophy of breast tissue due to increased hormonal influences (i.e., gynecomastia); such boys may be concerned and will need reassurance that this is normal for their age and will fade as soon as androgen becomes their dominant hormone. Adolescent girls may be concerned their breast tissue is inadequate or that breast growth is uneven. They can be assured many women do not have completely symmetric breasts.

Inspection of breast tissue is easiest if the child sits on the examining table, arms at the sides, with both breasts exposed. Inspect for symmetry. As mentioned, it is not unusual for a girl to have breasts of slightly unequal size.

Inspect next for edema, erythema (i.e., redness), wrinkling, retraction, or dimpling of the skin because all suggest a tumor may be growing in deeper layers of the breast. Edema, resulting from blockage of lymph channels, makes the skin appear not only swollen but also pitted (an orange-peel effect). Note any nipple discharge or "pulled" nipple placement as another way to detect edema.

With the girl's arms at her sides to take pressure off breast tissue, palpate well into each axilla (breast tissue extends that far) and also to assess axillary lymph nodes. Normally, no nodes under the arm should be felt. Next, ask the girl to lie down and place a folded towel under her near shoulder.

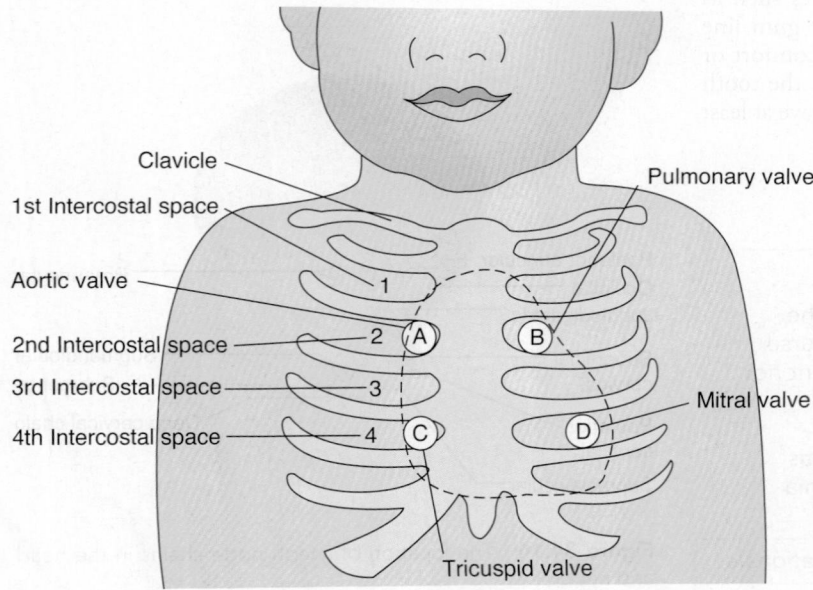

Figure 34.15 Intercostal (between rib) spaces are numbered according to the ribs immediately above them. The points (*A, B, C, D*) are the locations where the sounds of the heart valves radiate or where they can be heard best.

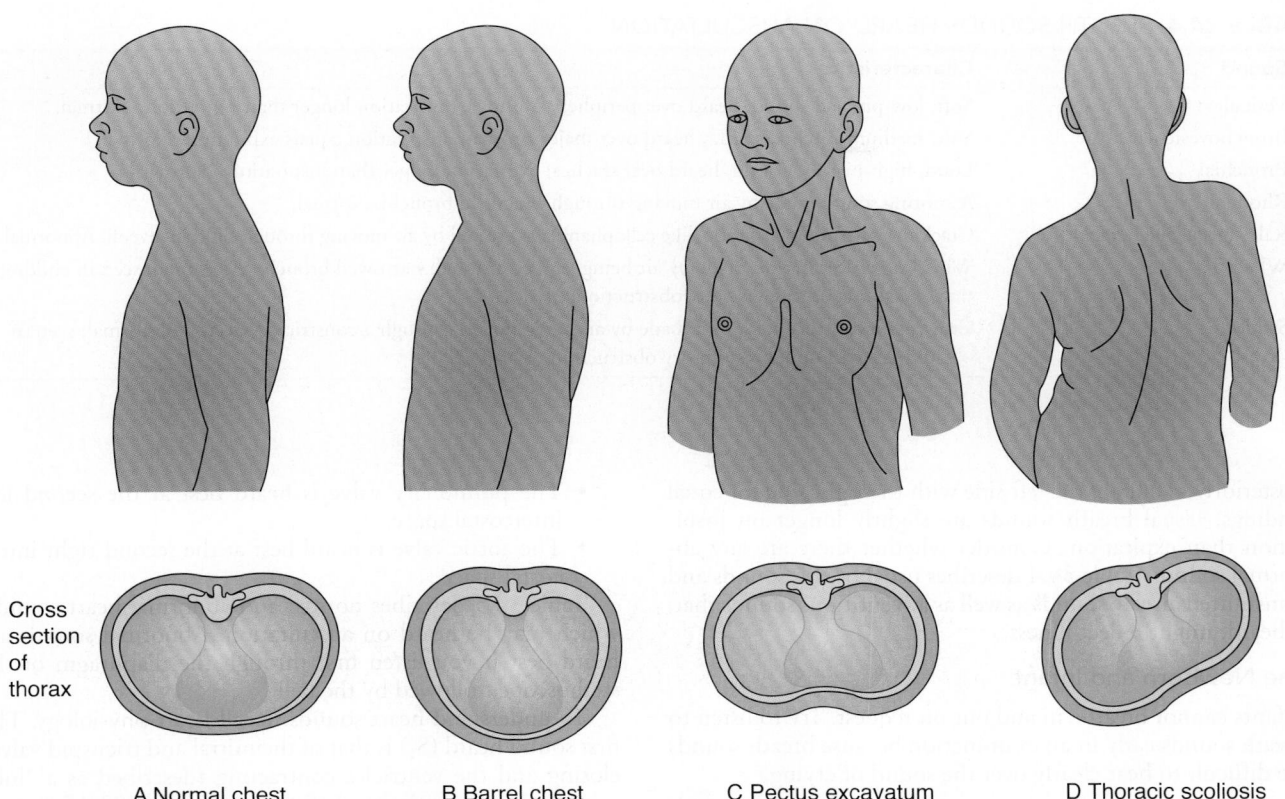

Cross
section
of
thorax

A Normal chest   B Barrel chest   C Pectus excavatum   D Thoracic scoliosis

Figure 34.16 Chest contours that can be assessed by inspection. **(A)** Normal chest. **(B)** Barrel chest. **(C)** Funnel chest (pectus excavatum). **(D)** Thoracic kyphoscoliosis.

Palpate the near breast with her arm raised and placed under her head because this spreads out breast tissue; begin at the nipple and palpate outward in a circular motion. The lower edge of each breast feels hard; do not mistake this or rib prominences underneath for a tumor. Repeat on the other side. Although breast self-exams are no longer recommended, it's good to teach adolescents breast awareness or to know what their breasts normally feel like so if a condition such as fibrocystic breast disease should develop, they will be able to recognize this and report it to their primary healthcare provider.

The Lungs

Various findings reveal respiratory distress in children. Assess the rate of respirations and whether respirations seem easy and relaxed or stressed. Assessment related to skin tone can affect findings such as jaundice in a newborn or cyanosis in a child in respiratory distress. Assessing for cyanosis is different in dark-skinned than in fair-skinned children (the mucous membrane is the best place to detect this). Note if it's necessary for a child to use accessory muscles to achieve effective ventilation. Palpate over the lung area for vibrations that suggest air is having difficulty moving through small air passages.

On the anterior chest, lung tissue extends from above the clavicles to the sixth or eighth rib. On the posterior chest, lung tissue extends as low as the 10th to 12th thoracic vertebrae. The right lung has three lobes; the left, only two. Attempt to evaluate all five lobes during lung assessment because lung disease can be specific for a lobe rather than involve the entire lung.

Following palpation, percuss lung tissue. Normal lung sounds are resonant in older children; in infants and younger children, sounds are hyperresonant due to the thinness of the chest wall. Overexpanded lungs will sound hyperresonant in older children, and lungs filled with fluid sound dull in older children and less resonant in younger children. The lower anterior lobe of the right lung will sound dull because the liver covers it on the anterior surface below the fourth or fifth intercostal space. The space over the heart will also percuss as dull.

Diaphragmatic excursion (i.e., the distance the diaphragm descends with inhalation) is an estimation of lung volume. To establish this, perform the following steps:
- Ask the child to take a deep breath and hold it.
- Percuss downward to locate the bottom of the lungs (the percussion note changes from resonant to flat at that point).
- Ask the child to expire fully and momentarily hold that position.
- Percuss upward to locate the expired or empty lung position (the percussion note changes from flat to resonant).

The difference between these two points is the diaphragmatic excursion. Children who have overexpanded lungs from obstructive disease have little diaphragmatic excursion in relation to others.

Auscultate breath sounds by listening through one full cycle at each auscultatory site with the diaphragm of a stethoscope over each lung lobe while a child inhales and exhales (preferably with the mouth open). Listen both anteriorly and

TABLE 34.4 BREATH SOUNDS HEARD ON AUSCULTATION

Sound	Characteristics
Vesicular	Soft, low-pitched sound, heard over periphery of lungs; inspiration longer than expiration. Normal.
Bronchovesicular	Soft, medium-pitched sound, heard over major bronchi; inspiration equals expiration. Normal.
Bronchial	Loud, high-pitched sound, heard over trachea; expiration longer than inspiration. Normal.
Rhonchi	A snoring sound made by air moving through mucus in bronchi. Normal.
Rales (also called crackles)	Crackling or crinkling sounds (like cellophane) are created by air moving through fluid in alveoli. Abnormal.
Wheezing	Whistling on expiration made by air being pushed through narrowed bronchi. Abnormal; seen in children with asthma or foreign body obstruction.
Stridor	Crowing or rooster-like sound made by air being pulled through a constricted larynx. Abnormal; seen in children with upper respiratory obstruction.

posteriorly; compare the left side with the right side for equal findings. Usual breath sounds are slightly longer on inspiration than expiration. Consider whether there are any abnormal sounds. Table 34.4 describes usual breath sounds and transmitted airway sounds as well as adventitious sounds that, if heard, might reflect illness.

The Newborn and Infant

Infants cannot breathe in and out on request. Try to listen to breath sounds early in an examination because breath sounds are difficult to hear clearly over the sound of crying.

The Heart

Heart assessment begins with asking children if they have ever noticed any cardiac symptoms such as pain. Visual inspection to see if there is a point on the chest where the heartbeat can be observed follows this. This point represents the location of the left ventricle or the point where the apical heartbeat can be heard best. In children younger than 7 years of age, this point is generally lateral to the nipple line and at the fourth intercostal space. In children older than 4 years, it is at the nipple line or just medial to it and at the fifth intercostal space. This point is termed the **point of maximum impulse (PMI)** and is observable in approximately 50% of children.

Percuss the left side of the chest to discern the left side of the heart. Percussing in from the axilla, the sound will become dull as the heart is identified. Normally, the percussion note changes from resonant (i.e., percussing over lung) to flat (i.e., percussing over heart) midway between the midaxillary and midmammary line. A heart located further to the left than this suggests enlargement.

Heart Sounds

To assess heart function, first listen over the heart and record the rate (Fig. 34.17). Compare this to the child's age to determine if it is normal. To hear differences in first and second heart sounds, auscultate at the four main points in the following bullets. Although these are not the anatomic locations of heart valves, they are the sites to which the sounds of the valves radiate and can be heard best in children (see Fig. 34.15).

- The mitral valve is heard best at the fourth or fifth left intercostal space at the nipple line.
- The tricuspid valve is heard best near the base of the sternum (fourth or fifth right intercostal space).
- The pulmonary valve is heard best at the second left intercostal space.
- The aortic valve is heard best at the second right intercostal space.

Table 34.5 describes normal and abnormal heart sounds, which may be heard on auscultation. Abnormal sounds are heard best if you listen first through the diaphragm of the stethoscope, followed by the bell.

To understand heart sounds, recall heart physiology. The first sound heard (S_1) is that of the mitral and tricuspid valves closing and the ventricles contracting (described as a "lub" sound). The second sound (S_2; described as a "dub" sound) is made by the closure of the aortic and pulmonary valves and atrial contraction. The first sound is generally longer and lower pitched than the second. Over the heart ventricles, it is louder but at other sites tends to be slightly quieter.

The rhythm of the heart sounds should be regular. **Sinus arrhythmia** is a normal but marked heart rate increase that occurs as a child inspires and a marked decrease in heart rate as the child expires and is frequently noted in school-age children and adolescents. Ask a child to take and hold a breath, and the rhythm of the heart should remain steady.

Another variation in heart sounds occurs because with inspiration and the resulting increase of pressure in the lungs, the pulmonary valve closes slightly later than the aortic valve. This is termed **physiologic splitting** and is heard as a

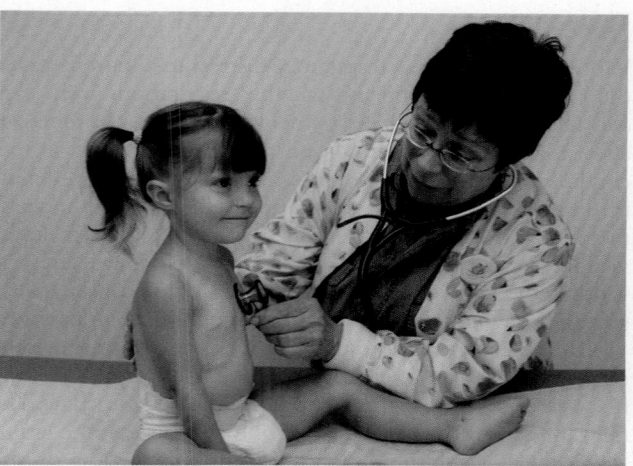

Figure 34.17 Auscultating heart sounds.

TABLE 34.5 HEART SOUNDS HEARD ON AUSCULTATION

Sound	Cause
S_1 (first heart sound)	Closure of tricuspid and mitral valves with beginning of ventricular contraction (systole)
S_2 (second heart sound)	Closure of pulmonary and aortic valves with beginning of atrial contraction (diastole)
S_3 (third heart sound)	Rapid ventricular filling
S_4 (fourth heart sound)	Abnormal filling of ventricles

"lub d-dub" sound. As long as this is associated with inspiration, it is a normal finding. Splitting that is always present implies there is difficulty with the pulmonary valve closing and suggests pathology.

At times, a distinct third heart sound (S_3) may be heard due to rapid filling of the ventricles. Although this is not necessarily a serious finding, further investigation is warranted. The presence of a fourth heart sound (S_4) generally signifies heart pathology because this sound (a gallop rhythm) is caused by an abnormal filling of the ventricles, which causes increased pressure on values.

Lastly, listen for heart murmurs. These are caused by the sound of blood flowing with difficulty or in an abnormal pathway within the heart (sounds like a swishing sound) and can be either innocent (i.e., functional) or pathogenic (i.e., organic). If a heart is pumping with abnormal force, there may be a palpable vibration, termed a *thrill*, on the chest wall. Palpate the precordium (i.e., area over the heart) for evidence of this (feels like a cat purring) or a heave (a definite outward chest movement), which also denotes a struggling heart. On hearing or palpating any accessory heart sounds or movements, describe them with reference to Table 34.6.

All unusual heart sounds need further identification and investigation as to their cause. The skills of listening to and identifying normal and abnormal heart sounds require considerable practice. Determining the cause of an abnormal heart sound requires a cardiac specialist. However, determining that an abnormal sound exists and securing proper referral is an important nursing role.

The Newborn, Infant, and Toddler

Listen to heart sounds in young children early in an examination, before a child begins to cry, because it is almost impossible to evaluate heart sounds over the sound of crying. Allowing a parent to hold a child while listening to the heart helps reduce fear.

The School-Age Child and Adolescent

Listen carefully for sounds of murmurs in children of school age and older. Be particularly conscientious with student athletes; it seems paradoxical that they could have heart disease, but if present, this could be fatal to them during athletic events (Harmon, Asif, Maleszewski, et al., 2016). Refer them to their primary healthcare provider for further evaluation if any abnormalities are detected. Parents are always frightened by an unusual heart sound, but unless the child has other symptoms, they can be assured that although you are referring them, most murmurs are innocent (i.e., functional) and caused only by the normal flow of blood across valves.

QSEN Checkpoint Question 34.5

INFORMATICS

The nurse is using a stethoscope to auscultate the sound of Keoto's mitral heart valve closing. When determining where to listen, the nurse identifies which location as best?
 a. Over the anterior sternum
 b. The right 9th or 10th intercostal space
 c. The left interior rim of the left clavicle
 d. The fourth or fifth left intercostal space at the nipple line

Look in Appendix A for the best answer and rationale.

TABLE 34.6 DESCRIPTION OF ACCESSORY HEART SOUNDS

Assessment	Information to Be Gathered
Location	At which listening post is the sound most distinct?
Quality	Can sound be described as blowing, rubbing, rasping, or musical?
Intensity	*Murmurs* are graded according to the following criteria: • Grade 6: so loud it can be heard with stethoscope not touching the chest wall; has a thrill (palpable vibration) • Grade 5: very loud but must touch stethoscope to chest to hear; has a thrill • Grade 4: loud; may or may not have a thrill • Grade 3: moderately loud; no thrill • Grade 2: quiet, but easily discernible • Grade 1: very quiet; difficult to hear
Timing	When in relation to S_1 and S_2, did you hear the murmur? A sound superimposed between S_1 and S_2 is a *systolic murmur*; one between S_2 and the next S_1 is a *diastolic murmur*. Innocent murmurs (functional, denoting no pathology) are usually systolic, although there are exceptions to this. Pathologic murmurs are more likely to be diastolic.
Pitch	Can the sound be described as high pitched or low pitched?
Radiation and thrills	Is there an accompanying thrill? Does sound radiate so it can be heard at another location, such as the back of the chest?

The Abdomen

The abdomen is anatomically divided into four quadrants. The quadrants and the organs that lie within them are shown in Figure 34.18. To assess an abdomen, first inspect the surface for symmetry and contour. It will be slightly protuberant in infants and scaphoid in older children. Note any skin lesions or scars.

Auscultate the abdomen for bowel sounds before palpating because palpating may alter bowel action (i.e., peristalsis) and therefore disturb bowel sounds. Bowel sounds can normally be heard in all quadrants of the abdomen. They are high "pinging" sounds that occur normally at intervals of approximately 5 to 10 seconds and, because they are high-pitched sounds, are heard best with the bell of a stethoscope. If the bowel is distended, the sounds occur more frequently; if the bowel is blocked, so there is no movement of contents, sounds will be absent below the obstruction. Listen for 3 to 5 minutes before concluding that no bowel sounds are present to be certain they are not just widely spaced.

Next, listen along the middle of the abdomen over the aorta for irregular sounds. A **bruit** is a swishing or blowing sound occurring if there is an outpouching of the aorta (i.e., an aneurysm), a condition that can be congenital, although it usually occurs with aging.

Palpate the abdomen in a systematic manner (e.g., the lower left quadrant, upper left quadrant, upper right quadrant, lower left quadrant) to include all four quadrants. First, palpate lightly and then deeply. Ascertain whether any area is tender by watching the child's face while palpating; observe for guarding or the child tensing the abdominal muscles to keep you from pressing deeply at that point. If a child indicates any portion of the abdomen is tender, begin assessment at the farthest point and work toward the tender area. If no tenderness is present, the order of palpation is unimportant

as long as it is thorough. Note any hard areas or masses. If a tender area is detected, attempt to elicit rebound tenderness to determine its cause. To do this, press on the abdomen and then lift your hand suddenly. This causes internal organs to vibrate. Although all children do not show this sign, the occurrence of more pain with the vibration than with the original pressure is one of the standard diagnostic criteria for appendicitis (Santillanes, Simms, Gausche-Hill, et al., 2012).

When palpating from the right lower quadrant to the right upper quadrant, the hand will bump against the lower edge of the liver 1 to 2 cm below the right ribs. On the left side, the lower edge of the spleen may be discernible in the same way. A liver or spleen larger than this is suggestive of disease. Lastly, palpate the umbilicus to try to identify the presence of an umbilical hernia. A fascial ring at the umbilicus of more than 2 cm in diameter in an infant denotes a ring of fascia larger than will normally close spontaneously; when this is present, the child will generally need surgery to prevent an umbilical hernia. Liver, spleen, and bladder size can all be documented further by percussion.

The Newborn and Infant

Kidneys may be located by deep abdominal palpation in newborns and infants. The right kidney is slightly lower than the left and so is easier to locate. The optimal time to palpate the kidney of a newborn is during the first few hours of life, before the bowel begins to fill with air and obscures palpation. To palpate for kidneys, perform the following:

- Place a hand under an infant's back just below the 12th rib.
- Press upward.
- Place the other hand on that side of the abdomen just below the umbilicus.
- Press deeply with your upper hand.
- Locate the kidney, which can be felt as a firm mass approximately the size of a walnut, between the hands.

The Preschooler and the School-Age Child

Children's abdomens at this age are often ticklish, and children may tense or guard their abdominal muscles when touched, making it difficult to palpate. Distract a child by asking a question about home or school or let a child place his or her hand under your hand to help relax (Fig. 34.19).

Right Upper Quadrant (RUQ)
Liver
Gallbladder
Duodenum
Pancreas
Right kidney
Hepatic flexure
of colon

Left Upper Quadrant (LUQ)
Stomach
Spleen
Left kidney
Pancreas
Splenic flexure
of colon

Right Lower Quadrant (RLQ)
Rectum
Appendix
Right ovary
and tube

Left Lower Quadrant (LLQ)
Sigmoid colon
Left ovary
and tube

Uterus

Bladder

Figure 34.18 The quadrants of the abdomen and underlying structures.

Figure 34.19 Decrease ticklishness during abdominal palpation by placing the child's hand under yours.

The Genitorectal Area

In both sexes, the rectum should be inspected for any protruding hemorrhoidal tissue (rare in children) or fissures. Fissures may signify chronic constipation, intra-abdominal pressure, or sexual maltreatment.

The Female Genitalia

Inspection of the external genitalia and an assessment of femoral nodes are included in every complete health assessment in girls (American College of Obstetricians and Gynecologists, 2014). An external examination consists of inspecting for the Tanner stage of pubic hair growth and configuration (i.e., an inverted triangle) and inspection of external genitalia (i.e., clitoris, labia majora, and labia minora) for normal contours. Look for signs of discharge or irritation. A vaginal discharge that suggests infection or a fourchette tear in a young child may be an indication of sexual maltreatment, and in an adolescent, this can be an indication of rape (Peterson, Nurre, & Dunn, 2017).

A pelvic examination is usually scheduled at the time the girl becomes sexually active, at 21 years of age, or at the first sign of a gynecologic disorder (American Academy of Pediatrics [AAP], 2016). The technique for internal pelvic examinations is discussed in Chapter 11.

The Male Genitalia

Inspection of male genitalia consists of observing:
- The distribution and the Tanner stage of pubic hair, which has a diamond shape
- The penis, for lesions that might suggest an STI
- Appearance and placement of the urethral opening, which should be slit-like and centered at the penis tip. Note whether the boy is circumcised because boys who are uncircumcised have more urinary tract infections than those who are circumcised (Stein, Dogan, Hoebeke, et al., 2015); repeated urinary tract infections can cause scarring of the meatal opening, making it small and round.
- The ability to retract the foreskin, if a boy is uncircumcised. *Phimosis* exists when the foreskin of a child older than 6 to 12 months is too tight to retract. Do not retract a tight foreskin over the corona of the penis.

Hypospadias means the urethral opening is located on the inferior or ventral (i.e., under) surface of the penis; **epispadias** denotes a urethral opening on the superior or dorsal (i.e., upper) surface. Both these conditions need to be identified. If more than a slight deviation is present, repair is usually initiated before school age because such a urethral placement may interfere with self-image if not corrected. During adulthood, it can interfere with fertility.

Inspect the scrotum for size and the presence of testes. In most boys, the left testicle is slightly lower than the right, so the scrotum does not appear truly symmetric. Palpate to check that both testes are present by placing one hand at the top of the scrotum over the inguinal ring and then palpating the testis on that side (see Chapter 18, Fig. 18.21). This hand position prevents the testis from slipping up into the inguinal ring and appearing to be absent on palpation. If the testis cannot be palpated with the boy lying supine, have him sit upright with his legs crossed while palpating. Gravity often will help the testicle fall into place. Any swelling or mass in the scrotum needs to be identified. The most likely cause of such

BOX 34.10

Nursing Care Planning Based on Family Teaching

TESTICULAR SELF-EXAMINATION

Q. Keoto's father asks you, "What is the best technique for testicular self-examination?"

A. Starting in their adolescent years, all males need to perform testicular self-examination once a month. Follow these guidelines:

- Select a certain day each month (e.g., first day, last day) to perform the examination.
- Perform the examination in or immediately after a shower because warmth makes scrotal skin relaxed.
- Gently roll each testicle between your thumb and fingers, feeling for any hard lumps or nodules, a change in consistency, or a difference in size.
- Also, feel for the epididymis found at the rear of the testes. It should feel like a strong cord.
- Remember that for most males, one testicle is slightly larger than the other and hangs a little lower in the scrotal sac.
- If you notice any changes in size, tenderness, or unusual mass, call or visit your healthcare provider.

a condition is a **hydrocele** (i.e., a fluid-filled sac), but it could represent a serious finding such as testicular cancer in adolescents. Hydroceles can be transilluminated; when a flashlight is held in back of the scrotum, the fluid-filled cyst glows. A **varicocele** (i.e., enlarged veins of the epididymis) may be palpated. These are not important findings in young boys, but they could possibly interfere with fertility later in life.

Assess the urethral meatus for any discharge that could reveal an STI, such as gonorrhea, or any lesions that would suggest herpes simplex type 2 infection or syphilis (see Chapter 47). Palpate femoral nodes (located in the groin and on the inner surface of the upper thigh) for any swelling, which suggests infection. Beginning at puberty, teach boys to do testicular palpations every month. The technique for this is described in Box 34.10.

To assess for the presence of an inguinal hernia in an infant, simply observe the groin area for any bulging, especially while the infant is crying. In the school-age child or adolescent, with the child standing, place a fingertip against the inguinal ring in the groin area and ask the child to cough. If the tendency for a hernia is present, coughing tightens the abdominal muscles and forces the abdominal contents to bulge against the finger.

The Extremities

Observe the upper extremities for good color and warmth. Because changes in fingernails can be a sign of overall ill health, inspect them for color, contour, and shape (Chernoff & Scher, 2016). Normally, nails are pink (or deeply pigmented in darker skinned children), smooth, and convex. They should feel hard to the touch but not so brittle they break readily. Signs of bitten fingernails in the school-age

Figure 34.20 Clubbed fingers are a sign of cyanosis from heart or respiratory disease. (NMSB/Custom Medical Stock Photo.)

child may reflect a high level of stress. A blue or purple tinge denotes cyanosis; a yellow tinge denotes jaundice. Children who have decreased respiratory function or heart disease develop clubbed fingers (Fig. 34.20); children with endocarditis often have characteristic linear hemorrhages under the nails.

Iron-deficiency anemia may cause extremely concave surfaces of fingernails (spoon-shaped). Press against a fingernail, release the pressure, and time the refilling interval (should be under 5 seconds). Count the fingers and check for webbing between fingers. Examine that fingerprints are present. Distinctive dermatoglyphics are present on fingertips from the third month of intrauterine life; these are unique to every person and show patterns of circular grooves. Abnormal fingerprints may occur with chromosomal anomalies. Check also for normal palmar creases. Children with chromosomal abnormalities may have only one central palm crease (i.e., a simian line) on each hand rather than the normal three (see Chapter 7). Check the wrist, elbow, and shoulder joints for movement and for normal range of motion; palpate joints for swelling or warmth. Palpate to be certain no lymph nodes are present in the antecubital space; palpate to check a radial pulse is present.

Inspect the lower extremities for color and warmth. Count the toes and check for webbing between toes. Check the ankle, knee, and hip joints for normal range of motion. Check for developmental hip dysplasia in infants by attempting to abduct the hips fully (see Chapter 18, Fig. 18.22). Palpate to ensure no enlarged lymph nodes are present in the groin or popliteal areas and femoral pulses are present and equal bilaterally. Ask the older child to walk and observe for ease of gait, limping, or any foot displacement such as toeing in or out. Toddlers typically walk with a wide-based gait; they walk best if allowed to walk toward their parent (a safe action) rather than away. Remember many adolescents are self-conscious and slouch or amble rather than present their true, natural gait. Children who limp need a further evaluation. A limp can be due to something as simple as a blister on the foot from wearing new shoes or can be a sign of a serious hip or bone condition (Lyons, 2015).

The Back

Inspect the back for symmetry and the spinal column for any deviation. Inspect the base of the spine for a dermal sinus (i.e., a pinpoint opening) or a tuft of hair or a hemangioma that might reveal spina bifida occulta (i.e., a defect of the bony structure of the canal). Also inspect for any dimpling that might denote a dermal cyst (i.e., pilonidal cyst). This is an innocent finding unless it becomes infected or connects to deeper tissue layers. Assess for tenderness along the spinal column by palpating each vertebra because chronic lower back pain can be present as early as school age (Spiteri, Busuttil, Aquilina, et al., 2017).

A routine assessment of the school-age child beginning at 10 years of age and through adolescence should include screening for scoliosis (i.e., sideways curvature of the spine) (Walter, 2011). Box 34.11 details the steps to follow for a scoliosis screening exam (see Chapter 51 for more details on scoliosis).

Neurologic Function

A full neurologic examination takes at least 20 minutes to complete, so this is not included in a routine physical examination. It is important, however, to assess for **deep tendon reflexes** (such as triceps, biceps, patellar, and Achilles reflexes) to test for motor and sensory function and balance and coordination. Techniques for eliciting deep tendon reflexes are shown in Figure 34.21. Grade reflexes according to the scale is shown in Table 34.7. The biceps reflex tests the fifth and sixth cervical nerves; the triceps reflex tests the seventh and eighth cervical; the patellar reflex tests the second, third, and fourth lumbar; and the Achilles reflex tests the first and second sacral. Test the sole of the foot for a Babinski reflex (see Chapter 18, Fig. 18.9). Fanning of the toes will occur in an infant younger than 3 months of age; a downward reflex of the toes will occur beyond 3 months of age. (Some normal infants demonstrate a flaring Babinski response until they are 2 years of age, and in the absence of other neurologic findings, this is not significant.)

Test for superficial reflexes: abdominal reflexes in both sexes and a cremasteric reflex in boys. An abdominal reflex is elicited by lightly stroking each quadrant of the abdomen. Normally, the umbilicus moves perceptibly toward the stroke. Presence of the reflex indicates integrity of the 10th thoracic nerve and the first lumbar nerve of the spinal cord. A cremasteric reflex is elicited by stroking the medial aspect of the thigh in boys. With this, the testes move perceptibly upward. The presence of this reflex indicates integrity of the first and second lumbar nerves.

Motor and Sensory Function

Test general facial nerve function by asking a child to make a face. The child's ability to grasp with the hands and push against a surface with the feet establishes general motor ability. Recall whether the child's gait was adequate when observed walking to assess for balance and coordination.

To test sensory function, ask children to close their eyes and identify the location where you touch them at (at least) six points on different body parts.

> *What If . . . 34.2*
> Although the nurse knows children should be completely undressed for physical examinations so all body surfaces can be inspected, Candy's father says he doesn't want Candy undressed because the exam room is too cold. How would the nurse best respond if not wanting to remove a Band-Aid from Candy's back?

BOX 34.11

Nursing Care Planning Using Procedures

SCOLIOSIS SCREENING

Purpose: To assess for scoliosis (sideways curvature of the spine)

Procedure	Principle
1. Have the child remove clothing except for undergarments. Ask the child to stand up straight, with feet together and arms at sides. Observe the child from a posterior view.	1. Promotes optimal view of back
2. To inspect for a curved spinal column (Fig. A), observe: • Is one shoulder higher than the other? • Is one shoulder blade more prominent than the other? • Does one hip seem higher or more prominent than the other? • Does the child seem to lean to one side? • Does the spinal column appear curved?	2. Denotes signs of spinal curvature

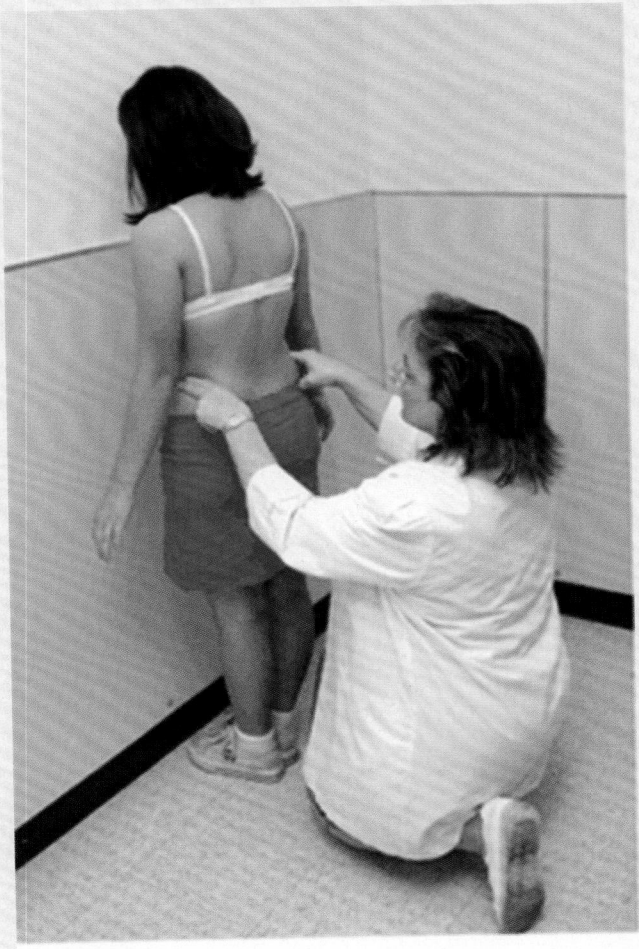

A

Continued on following page

BOX 34.11

Nursing Care Planning Using Procedures (continued)

Procedure	Principle
3. With the child's arms hanging down at his or her sides, compare the level of the elbows in relation to the iliac crests: • Are the elbows held at the same level? • Do the elbows fall at the level of the crest or closer to the crest on one side? (Normally, elbows fall above the iliac crest.)	3. Helps to determine uneven posture because it will affect level of elbows
4. Ask the child to bend over and touch toes while you continue to observe the back (Fig. B). • Is there a hump in the back? • Does the spinal column appear to curve? • Is one shoulder blade more prominent than the other?	4. Provides evidence of spinal rotation. As the child bends, the rotation of the spine accompanying scoliosis becomes more prominent.

B

| 5. Refer the child to his or her primary healthcare provider for further examination if any of the previous observations are noted. | 5. Provides for proper referral |
| 6. Educate the child to inform parents or healthcare providers if signs of scoliosis, such as a skirt hanging unevenly or bra straps need to be adjusted, begin to develop. | 6. Encourages health promotion |

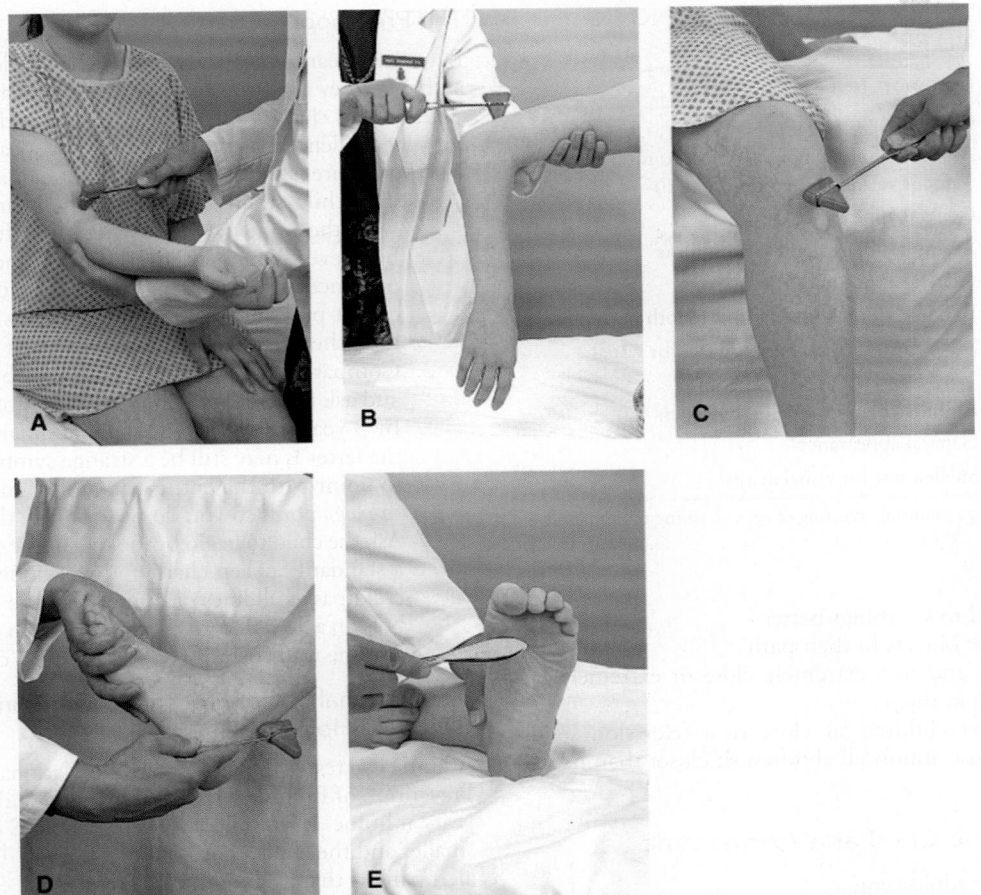

Figure 34.21 Techniques for eliciting major reflexes. **(A)** The biceps reflex. **(B)** The triceps reflex. **(C)** The patellar reflex. **(D)** The ankle or Achilles reflex. **(E)** The Babinski response. (From Weber, J., & Kelley, J. [2003]. Health assessment in nursing [2nd ed.]. Philadelphia, PA: Lippincott Williams & Wilkins. Images © B. Proud.)

Vision Assessment

Assessing vision is an important part of a physical assessment because good vision is so important to childhood development. The extent and type of testing depends on the age of the child.

Any child with congenital anomalies, low birth weight, or fetal alcohol syndrome is at risk for eye abnormalities, as is a child who received oxygen at birth. During an assessment, if you notice an unreported eye injury or infection or signs of neglected vision, make a special note. Because the average parent is careful of a child's eyes, these findings may be indicative of child neglect.

TABLE 34.7 GRADING OF DEEP TENDON REFLEXES

Grade	Interpretation
4+	Hyperactive; extremely marked reaction; abnormal
3+	Stronger than average but within normal range
2+	Average response
1+	Less than average response but within normal range
0	No response; abnormal

VISION SCREENING

Routine vision screening can begin as early as 6 to 12 months of age. Parents can provide important clues to possible problems; therefore, listen carefully any time a parent expresses concern about or questions a child's ability to see well. Common vision screening, indicators, and techniques for children of different ages are summarized in Table 34.8.

Newborn and Infant

Newborns should be able to focus on a moving object such as a finger and follow it to the midline. Infants see black and white objects better than they do colored objects. They seem to see objects that are at a distance of about 19 cm [8 to 10 in.]) best. Ask parents if an infant's eyes follow them as they move around the room. Does an infant who is older than 6 weeks return their smile? Do the parents have any reason to think their child has difficulty seeing?

The Toddler and Preschooler

Ask parents if their children do any of the following, which may be signs of vision problems:
- Rub their eyes, blink frequently, squint, or frown
- Cover one eye to look at objects

TABLE 34.8 COMMON VISION SCREENING INDICATORS AND PROCEDURES

Age	Common Test
Newborn	General appearance*
	Ability to follow moving object to midline; focus steadily on an object at 10–12 in.
Infant and toddler	General appearance*
	Ability to follow light past midline
Age 3 years to school age	General appearance*
	Random dot E for stereopsis (depth perception)
	Allen cards or preschool E chart for visual acuity
	Ishihara's plates for color awareness
School age to adult	General appearance*
	Snellen test for visual acuity

*Note redness, blinking, squinting, crusting of eyes, or tilting of head.

- Tilt the head to see things better
- Stumble over objects in their path
- Hold books and toys extremely close or extremely far away to look at them

Asking whether children sit close to a television set is meaningless because almost all children sit closer than necessary if allowed.

The School-Age Child and Adolescent

Ask if the child or adolescent:
- Reports difficulty seeing
- Reports frequent headaches
- Does poorly with class work
- Avoids sports that require long-distance vision, such as baseball or softball
- Avoids watching movies
- Skips over words when reading aloud
- Reports blurriness or double vision
- Has reddened conjunctivae or drainage from the eyes
- Blinks at bright light

Techniques of Vision Testing

Vision is tested by asking a child to read a standardized eye chart. All children need good orientation to such testing so they can appreciate that this is not a test in the usual sense of the word; otherwise, they may be unusually anxious or try to "pass" it by cheating. Vision testing needs to be started in the preschool period, so children with amblyopia (i.e., lazy eye; see Chapter 50), a potentially serious vision disorder, can be identified while the condition is still correctable (Taylor & Elliot, 2014). In addition to usual testing, a digital photo of the child's face can be used to help identify strabismus (i.e., uneven gaze or eyes not symmetrically aligned).

The Snellen Chart

As soon as children can identify letters of the alphabet (i.e., early school age), their vision can be tested by use of a Snellen eye chart. Because this chart is standardized, set procedures must be followed when using it to test vision (Box 34.12).

The Preschool E Chart

Between 3 years of age and the age when children can read the alphabet, they can be tested by use of a preschool E chart (Fig. 34.22). This chart is also helpful to test children who are cognitively challenged or those who do not speak fluent English. The procedure is similar to that of the standard Snellen chart:

1. The child stands 20 ft from the chart and reads first with the right eye, then with the left, and then with both eyes. Young children do not understand the importance of not pressing the card against their eye and of not peeking, so a second person is often needed to hold the occluder card for children of this age.

2. Compare the E on the chart with a table with three legs and ask the child which way the legs of the table point. By 3 years of age, children are familiar with tables, but the letter E may still be a strange symbol. Tell the child to point with the entire arm and hand in the direction the legs point so you do not confuse the hand motion.

3. Ask the child to begin by looking at the 40-ft line, as with a standard Snellen chart, and work downward until the child passes all lines or cannot read the majority of symbols on a line. Record the distance from the chart and the last line read correctly (20 over the last correct line).

The National Society for the Prevention of Blindness Home Test

A home eye test is available from the National Society for the Prevention of Blindness for parents to test children ages 3 to 6 years at home. It is similar to the preschool E chart except it is smaller and the child stands only 10 ft away. The test can help alert parents that a child needs a professional eye examination. Home tests can be given or suggested to parents whose child is tired or who, for some other reason, does not test well in a healthcare facility (Prevent Blindness America [PBA], 2016).

Allen Cards

Allen cards consist of pictures of common objects such as a horse and rider, a car, a house, and a birthday cake. The cards are shown to the child at a 15-ft distance, and the child is asked to identify the pictures (proof the child sees them). Be certain children have time to examine the cards before the test so you're sure they know the names of the objects.

STYCAR Cards

For this test, a child is given cards with nine letters: H, C, O, L, U, T, X, V, and A. The child holds up the card that matches the one you point to on a STYCAR chart.

Titmus Vision Tester

Another useful method for testing the vision of children is the Titmus Vision Tester, the same instrument used by many motor vehicle licensing offices. As the child looks into the eyepieces of the machine, alphabet letters, or preschool Es are projected onto a screen for the child to identify. Closed vision testers such as the Titmus have an advantage over wall charts in that a child is less easily distracted during testing. Also, because children cannot see the vision chart beforehand, they cannot memorize the letters while waiting to be tested.

Vision Color Awareness Testing

The inability to discern colors is a sex-linked recessive characteristic that occurs in males rather than in females, although

BOX 34.12

Nursing Care Planning Using Procedures

SNELLEN EYE CHART ASSESSMENT

Purpose: To assess vision

Procedure	Principle
1. Hang the chart so the 20-ft line is at the child's eye level.	1. The child who has to look up or down must look farther than the child who is looking straight across at the chart. A possible solution to avoid moving the chart is to have smaller children stand and taller children sit. To accommodate children in wheelchairs, the chart needs to be lowered (or have all children sit for the test).
2. Provide a good light for the chart and place it so there is no glare. A light intensity of 20-ft candles is recommended.	2. Appropriate lighting provides for optimal test conditions.
3. Measure a distance of 20 ft from the chart. Mark the floor at this point with a piece of masking tape or other similar mark. For younger children, it is helpful to cut out paper footprints and paste them to the floor with the heels of the footprints touching the 20-ft line. If the child sits in a chair, the back legs of the chair should touch the 20-ft line.	3. Twenty feet is the optimal distance from the chart for testing.
4. Provide the child being examined with a 3 × 5 in. card to cover the eye not being tested.	4. Covering the other eye allows for one eye to be tested at a time.
5. If the child wears glasses, screen first with the glasses in place. Do not screen the child first without glasses and then with them because this forces the child to strain to read the chart.	5. Testing with corrective lenses screens for corrected eyesight. After squinting, a child may have difficulty readjusting to reading with glasses, and this makes the prescription appear too weak or too strong.
6. To begin testing, tell the child to stand with shoes on the footprints (heels against the line), keep both eyes open and cover the left eye with the occluding card. Be certain the child does not press the card against the eye (instead, the edge of the card should rest across the child's nose).	6. Covering the eye not being tested provides one eye to be tested at a time. Pressure will cause blurred vision when the child removes the card to test that eye.
7. Begin at the 40-ft line of the chart and, using a pointer or pencil, point to each symbol on the line from left to right (the order in which children are taught to read). If the child reads the majority of symbols in a line, the line is passed satisfactorily.	7. Starting at the 40-ft line is the standardized testing procedure.

Continued on following page

BOX 34.12

Nursing Care Planning Using Procedures (continued)

Procedure	Principle
8. If the child "passes" the 40-ft line, have the child read the 30- and 20-ft lines or the last line the child can read. Record the last line read. If the child fails to read the 40-ft line satisfactorily, then begin at the top of the chart and move downward to identify the last line the child can read. Record this reading. Because the 200-ft, 100-ft, and 70-ft lines have so few symbols, the child must read all the symbols on them to have read them satisfactorily.	8. Moving to the 30-ft line or less reflects use of the standardized testing procedure.
9. Visual acuity is always stated as a fraction. The top number is the distance in feet the child stands from the chart (always 20). The bottom of the fraction represents the last line the child read correctly. The adult with good (average) vision can read the 20-ft line from 20 ft away and thus is said to have 20/20 vision.	9. Using a fraction for visual acuity is the standardized reporting procedure.
10. It is important to test the eyes separately and then together. For example, suppose Keoto reads all the symbols on the 40-ft line with her right eye but she misses three out of four on the 30-ft line. Her visual acuity for her right eye is 20/40 (the distance from the chart/the last line she read correctly). With her left eye, she reads the 40-ft, 30-ft, and 20-ft lines correctly. Her vision in that eye is 20/20. With both eyes, Keoto reads the 40-ft, 30-ft, and 20-ft lines correctly. Her visual acuity for both eyes is therefore 20/20.	10. If only this last reading were taken, the right eye weakness (a symptom of amblyopia or "lazy eye") would be missed.
11. Observe children for straining or squinting as they read the chart.	11. By squinting and changing the shape of the eyeball, children can improve vision and will score higher; therefore, children will appear to see better than they actually do in everyday situations.

Figure 34.22 An astigmatic and preschool E chart. (American Optical Company August 1935 Catalog. "Ophthalmological Instruments and Equipment." Courtesy of the Optical Heritage Museum.)

females carry the recessive gene for the disorder. All male children should be screened once for the disorder during their early school years.

To test a child for color awareness, ask the child to identify the colored stripes at the top of a Snellen eye chart or show the child a series of colored diagrams (i.e., Ishihara plates). With the latter, a person with color vision is able to see hidden figures such as butterflies, but people with red-green or yellow-blue color vision deficits cannot. Detecting a color vision deficit in children is important because many educational materials and some occupations depend on the ability to identify color. Even such a simple childhood pleasure as riding a bicycle safely on city streets depends on being able to distinguish colors, such as deciphering red from green on a traffic light.

Vision Referrals

Always screen children twice before referring them to their primary care provider. Some children do not perform well on eye tests because they are too easily distracted or do not know their alphabet as well as they pretend (e.g., they may say they do not see a letter when they really mean they do not know or remember its name). Testing twice helps eliminate or identify this type of misleading result.

After a second screening, the following children generally require a vision referral:

- Preschool children (3 to 5 years of age) who have 20/50 vision or less in one or both eyes
- Children 6 years of age or older who have 20/40 vision or less in one or both eyes
- Any child with a two-line difference between the eyes, as this might be a beginning of amblyopia
- Any child who states or shows other symptoms of visual difficulty (PBA, 2016)

What If . . . 34.3

Keoto's father expresses concern she may have a vision problem because she always sits very close to a television set. Keoto doesn't want to be tested because she "will not wear glasses." What questions would the nurse identify as important to ask her on history? What type of eye chart would the nurse use with Keoto to assess her vision?

Hearing Assessment

A thorough health assessment should also include an evaluation of hearing, including both history and observation, because good hearing is so important for the development of age-appropriate skills. Parents and grandparents are usually attuned to hearing difficulty in children and may be suspicious of it in advance of its official detection. When taking an auditory history, therefore, be certain to ask the accompanying adult or parent an overall question such as "Do you have any reason to believe your child doesn't hear as well as other children?"

AUDITORY SCREENING

Routine screening for adequate hearing levels is usually begun at 3 years of age. Testing requires knowledge of the technique, use of an audiometer, and a quiet, undistracted setting.

Newborn and Infant

All infants should be screened at birth. Those most apt to be born with a hearing difficulty are those with:

- A history of childhood hearing impairment in the family
- Perinatal infection, such as cytomegalovirus, rubella, herpes, toxoplasmosis, or syphilis
- Anatomic malformations involving the head or neck
- Birth weight less than 1,500 g
- Hyperbilirubinemia at a level exceeding indication for exchange transfusion
- Bacterial meningitis, especially when caused by *Haemophilus influenzae*
- Severe birth asphyxia: infants with an Apgar score of 0 to 3, those who failed to breathe spontaneously within 10 minutes of birth, or those with hypotonia persisting to 2 hours of age

A newborn's hearing is assessed through simple response testing—observing whether an infant stirs or responds to a sound delivered to the child with a commercial sound device (CDC, 2012).

It can also be done by brain stem auditory-evoked response (BAER) testing. For this method, an earphone is placed on the infant and an electrode is attached to the scalp. When sound is transmitted to the child's ear through the earphone, the electrical potential created as the sound is processed by the brain stem is read by the scalp electrode, processed by a microcomputer, and plotted on a graph. This type of testing may be used at any age and is successful even in children who are comatose or anesthetized. Smaller units using transient evoked otoacoustic emissions (TEOAEs) are also available. With these, a click stimulus delivered to a normal ear produces an echo from the cochlea. This can be detected by a miniature microphone to reveal the presence of even minor hearing loss. Although newborn hearing screening can lead to false-positive results because many infants of this age are still sleepy from birth analgesia and may have fluid- or vernix-filled ear canals, a repeat test usually decreases the incidence of false-positive results.

The Older Child

Older children who are at risk for hearing loss are those who have been exposed to loud noises such as an explosion or loud music, were of low birth weight, have congenital anomalies, have a repaired cleft palate, or have had repeated ear infections. During history taking, ask children if they ever worry if they have difficulty hearing. Be certain not to confuse difficulty hearing with shyness or recalcitrance in answering. Also, ask them how they are doing in school. Some children with a minimal hearing impairment are considered to have behavioral problems in school because they do not follow directions well, when in fact, they may be unable to hear the instruction. Children with an ear infection (i.e., otitis media) or allergies should be tested after the fluid in their ears clears because their hearing may be temporarily affected by these conditions. Almost all children have some cerumen (i.e., ear wax) in their ear canals; only when this becomes impacted it is a cause of hearing loss (Krug, Cieza, Chadha, et al., 2016).

Principles of Audiometric Assessment

With proper instruction in technique, nurses conduct audiometric testing in schools and other ambulatory settings.

Frequency

Sound is the result of vibration; the frequency of sound is the number of vibrations a sound creates per second. When frequency is increased, the pitch of the sound increases. For audiometric testing, frequency is measured in hertz units. Normal speech sounds fall into a narrow range of 500 to 2,000 Hz; so, to function adequately and speak effectively, a child must be able to hear in this range. Children are tested for a wider frequency range than this, however, from 500 to 6,000 Hz, on a routine screening assessment.

Loudness

Decibels are an expression of the intensity or loudness of a sound (or vigor of the vibrations). A decibel level of 0 dB is the softest sound that can be heard. Normal conversation is held at approximately 50 to 60 dB. The sound level at which inner ear damage can occur is about 90 dB. Sound levels of 140 dB are so intense they actually cause pain. Screening audiometry is done at 25 dB.

Hearing Loss

Table 34.9 lists levels of hearing loss and the effect of hearing loss on conversation and speech. If children can hear all frequencies at the 25-dB level, they have passed an audiometric screening check. If a child fails to hear two or more frequencies

TABLE 34.9 LEVELS OF HEARING LOSS

Hearing Loss (dB Level)	Hearing Level Present
Slight (less than 30 dB)	Inability to hear whispered words or faint speech
	No speech challenge present
	Possible lack of awareness of hearing difficulty
Mild (30–50 dB)	Achievement in school and home is attained by leaning forward, speaking loudly
	Beginning speech challenge may be present
Moderate (55–70 dB)	Difficulty hearing if not facing speaker; some difficulty with hearing normal conversation
	Speech challenge present, possibly requiring speech therapy
	Difficulty hearing normal conversation
Severe (70–90 dB)	Difficulty hearing any but nearby loud voice
	Vowels easier to hear than consonants
	Speech therapy required for clear speech
	Possible ability to still hear loud sounds such as jets or whistle of train
Profound (more than 90 dB)	Almost no sound heard

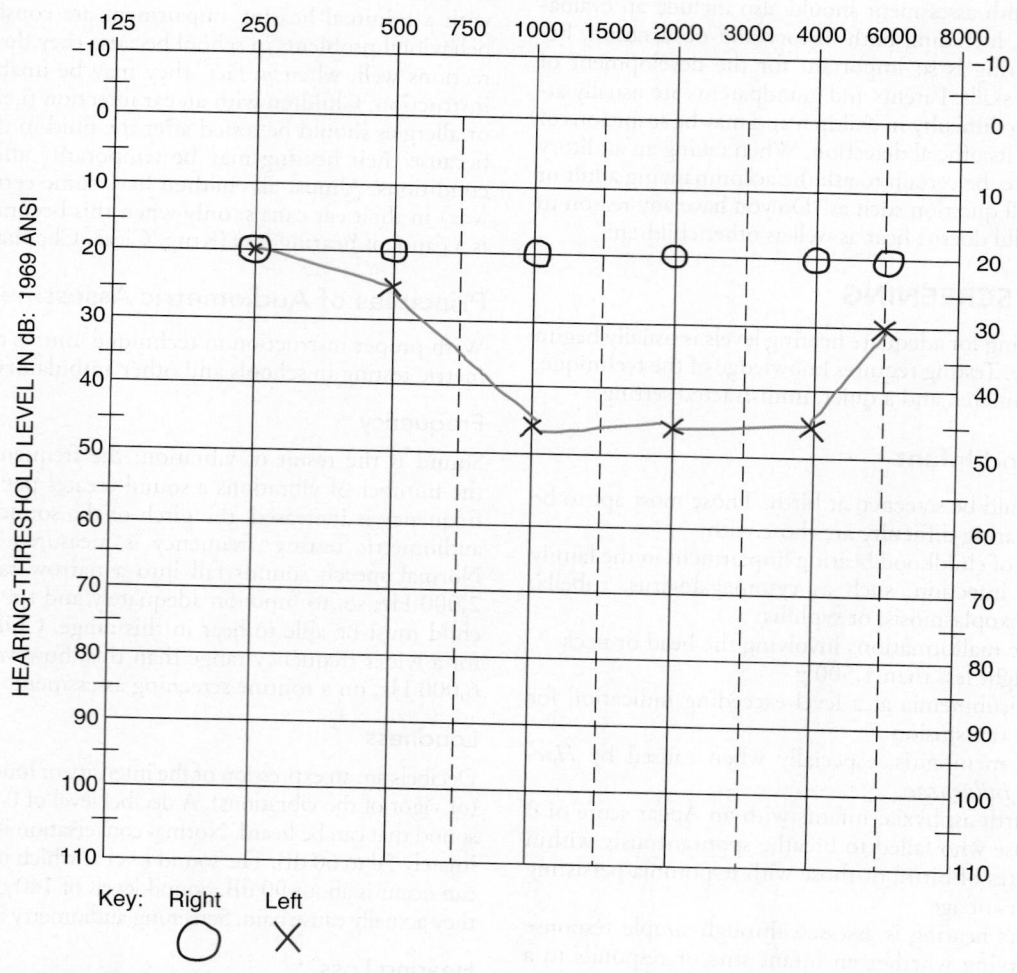

Figure 34.23 An audiogram done as a screening procedure. Notice that hearing is normal in the right ear (all frequencies are heard at the 20-dB level). In the left ear, there is hearing loss (the frequencies 1,000, 2,000, and 4,000 Hz are heard only at the 45-dB level). (Courtesy of Dr. H. Schill, Speech Pathology and Audiology Department, Boston University.)

at 25 dB, in either or both ears, the child has failed and should be referred to the primary care provider or an otologist. An **audiogram** is a record of audiometric testing. Figure 34.23 shows an audiogram of a child with normal hearing in the right ear (the child heard all frequencies at the 20-dB level), but with an inability to hear sounds softer than 45 dB in the left ear at frequencies of 1,000, 2,000, and 4,000 Hz.

Acoustic Impedance Testing

Acoustic impedance testing is based on the principle that sound entering the ear canal meets resistance at the tympanic membrane. If the middle ear is functioning normally, there will be a symmetric pattern of resistance on a tympanogram printout. If the middle ear is not functioning normally, the level of resistance will be greater or less, and so the pattern will be abnormal.

Acoustic impedance testing is performed by audiologists. For the assessment, the ear to be tested is plugged with a rubber disc. Sound is then administered to the ear through the center of the disc. The resistance met at the eardrum is registered and recorded as a graph. Tympanograms are inaccurate in children younger than 7 months of age because the tympanic membrane is too compliant under that age to register normal impedance.

Conduction Loss Testing

Both the Rinne and the Weber tests are used to perform assessments that can be used to identify conduction loss in older children (Box 34.13).

Speech Assessment

Speech problems are directly related to hearing problems: Infants who do not hear will make preliminary babbling sounds but then will not develop intelligible speech because they cannot hear speech sounds to repeat. Speech difficulties may also be related to:

- Motor development, such as when a child does not have enough control of tongue and facial muscles to be able to form words properly
- Cognitive development, such as when a cognitively challenged child cannot grasp the concept of speech or word use until later than usual, or possibly not at all
- Cultural influences, such as when parents speak two languages, making it difficult for a child to accurately learn and articulate either language or if parents spoke "baby

BOX 34.13
Rinne and Weber Tests

Rinne and Weber tests are assessments for air and bone conduction.

RINNE TEST

Strike a 500-Hz tuning fork and hold the stem of it against the child's mastoid bone. Ask the child to say when the tuning fork's ringing sound can no longer be heard. When the child says it is no longer audible, move the fork forward so it is at the auditory meatus (Fig. A). Because air conduction is normally better than bone conduction, the child should hear it when it is held in front of the meatus, although it can no longer be heard when it was held against the bone. If the child does not hear it when it is brought forward, then the child's air conduction is probably reduced.

WEBER TEST

Strike a 500-Hz tuning fork and hold the stem of it against the top of the child's head (Fig. B). The child with normal hearing in both ears will hear the sound equally well with both ears. If the child has an air conduction loss in one ear, the child will hear the sound better in that ear than in the good ear. The test must be used in conjunction with other evaluation tools because if the sound is intensified in one ear, it may mean that there is no hearing perception (i.e., there is nerve loss) in the opposite ear.

talk" for so long that the child mimicked that instead of pronouncing words clearly

Speech screening begins by asking children a few simple questions to determine their language pattern. Also, ask parents if they have noticed any difficulties with their child's pronunciation or comprehension. Standardized tests, such as the Denver Articulation Screening Examination (DASE), may also be administered.

DENVER ARTICULATION SCREENING EXAMINATION

The DASE is designed to detect significant developmental delays as well as normal variations in the acquisition of speech sounds. Because it is a standardized test, its directions must be followed precisely. The test is only standardized for use with English-speaking children.

Administration

Before the test, explain that the child will need to repeat the words he or she hears you speak. Give enough examples so you are certain the child understands what he or she is to do: "When I say 'boat,' then you say 'boat.'" When you are certain the child understands the directions, say each of the 22 words shown on the DASE form (Fig. 34.24A). Convey the impression there are no right or wrong answers. Give the child approval for responding and following directions correctly, no matter how inaccurately the child repeats the word.

Scoring

The DASE is designed for use with children between the ages of 2.5 and 6 years. In scoring, consider the child's age to be the closest previous age shown on the percentile rank

A

```
    DENVER ARTICULATION SCREENING EXAM          NAME
    for children 2 1/2 to 6 years of age
                                                 HOSP. NO.
    Instructions:  Have child repeat each word after
    you.  Circle the underlined sounds that he pro-  ADDRESS
    nounces correctly.  Total correct sounds is the
    Raw Score.  Use charts on reverse side to score
    results.
```

Date: _____ Child's Age: _____ Examiner: _____ Raw Score: _____
Percentile: _____ Intelligibility: _____ Result: _____

1. table   6. zipper   11. sock   16. wagon   21. leaf
2. shirt   7. grapes   12. vacuum   17. gum   22. carrot
3. door   8. flag   13. yarn   18. house
4. trunk   9. thumb   14. mother   19. pencil
5. jumping   10. toothbrush 15. twinkle   20. fish

Intelligibility: (circle one) 1. Easy to understand   3. Not understandable
                                2. Understandable 1/2   4. Can't evaluate
                                   the time.

Comments:

Date: _____ Child's Age: _____ Examiner: _____ Raw Score _____
Percentile: _____ Intelligibility: _____ Result: _____

1. table   6. zipper   11. sock   16. wagon   21. leaf
2. shirt   7. grapes   12. vacuum   17. gum   22. carrot
3. door   8. flag   13. yarn   18. house
4. trunk   9. thumb   14. mother   19. pencil
5. jumping   10. toothbrush 15. twinkle   20. fish

Intelligibility: (circle one) 1. Easy to understand   3. Not understandable
                                2. Understandable 1/2   4. Can't evaluate
                                   the time.

Comments:

Date: _____ Child's Age: _____ Examiner: _____ Raw Score _____
Percentile: _____ Intelligibility: _____ Result: _____

1. table   6. zipper   11. sock   16. wagon   21. leaf
2. shirt   7. grapes   12. vacuum   17. gum   22. carrot
3. door   8. flag   13. yarn   18. house
4. trunk   9. thumb   14. mother   19. pencil
5. jumping   10. toothbrush 15. twinkle   20. fish

Intelligibility: (circle one) 1. Easy to understand   3. Not understandable
                                2. Understandable 1/2   4. Can't evaluate
                                   the time.

Comments:

Figure 34.24 The Denver Articulation Screening Exam (DASE). **(A)** The test form. *(continued)* chart (Fig. 34.24B). Score the child's pronunciation of the underlined sounds or blends in each word on the test form. A perfect raw score is 30 correctly articulated sounds. Match this raw score on the percentile rank chart with the column representing the child's age. The number at which the raw score line and the age column meet is the percentile rank of the child (how the child compares with other children of that age). Percentiles shown above the heavy line are abnormal; those below the line are normal. For example, a 3-year-old who says only 12 sounds correctly ranks in the ninth percentile (abnormal ranking); a 3-year-old who scores 20 sounds correctly ranks in the 58th percentile (normal ranking).

In addition to determining the percentile ranking, rate the child's spontaneous speech in terms of intelligibility as 1, easy to understand; 2, understandable half the time; 3, not understandable; or 4, cannot evaluate (e.g., maybe the child did not speak in sentences or phrases during your contact time). Score intelligibility according to the chart in Figure 34.24B. For a final score, rate the child's total test result (e.g., normal or abnormal on the DASE or intelligibility).

Children who score abnormally on this screening test should be retested in about 2 weeks. If they still score abnormally, they should be referred for a complete speech evaluation.

Developmental Appraisal

It would be ideal if children demonstrated all the developmental skills they are capable of every time they are asked to demonstrate them. Rarely, however, do they accomplish this. Infants become hungry, sleepy, or upset during testing. Older children may become shy. Therefore, a portion of developmental

B

To score DASE words: Note Raw Score for child's performance. Match raw score line (extreme left of chart) with column representing child's age (to the closest previous age group). Where raw score line and age column meet number in that square denotes percentile rank of child's performance when compared to other children that age. Percentiles above heavy line are ABNORMAL percentiles, below heavy line are NORMAL.

PERCENTILE RANK

Raw Score	2.5 yr.	3.0	3.5	4.0	4.5	5.0	5.5	6 years
2	1							
3	2							
4	5							
5	9							
6	16							
7	23							
8	31	2						
9	37	4	1					
10	42	6	2					
11	48	7	4					
12	54	9	6	1	1			
13	58	12	9	2	3	1	1	
14	62	17	11	5	4	2	2	
15	68	23	15	9	5	3	2	
16	75	31	19	12	5	4	3	
17	79	38	25	15	6	6	4	
18	83	46	31	19	8	7	4	
19	86	51	38	24	10	9	5	1
20	89	58	45	30	12	11	7	3
21	92	65	52	36	15	15	9	4
22	94	72	58	43	18	19	12	5
23	96	77	63	50	22	24	15	7
24	97	82	70	58	29	29	20	15
25	99	87	78	66	36	34	26	17
26	99	91	84	75	46	43	34	24
27		94	89	82	57	54	44	34
28		96	94	88	70	68	59	47
29		98	98	94	84	84	77	68
30		100	100	100	100	100	100	100

To Score intelligibility:

		NORMAL	ABNORMAL
	2 1/2 years	Understandable 1/2 the time, or, "easy"	Not Understandable
	3 years and older	Easy to understand	Understandable 1/2 time Not understandable

Test Result: 1. NORMAL on Dase and Intelligibility = NORMAL

2. ABNORMAL on Dase and/or Intelligibility = ABNORMAL

* If abnormal on initial screening rescreen within 2 weeks. If abnormal again child should be referred for complete speech evaluation.

Figure 34.24 *(continued)* **(B)** The percentile rank form. (Reprinted by permission. Denver Developmental Materials, Inc.)

information, especially developmental milestones, on almost all health assessment must be elicited by history taking.

DEVELOPMENTAL HISTORIES

Many parents keep careful records of their first child's development, a less careful record of their second, a scanty record of the third, and so on. Information, therefore, generally depends on parents' memories.

If parents cannot recall the month during which a skill was first demonstrated, ask them to try to remember in terms of holidays or seasons when they first saw the child performing the skill. They may not recall, for example, at which month their infant first used a pincer grasp (grasped cleanly with index finger and thumb) but do recall the child pinched the ear of the family dog at a summer picnic.

If parents seem to have no recall at all of developmental milestones and these are important to the child's present evaluation, suggest they ask other family members or look through family photographs to jog their memories and to call back with as much information as they can gather.

The CDC has developmental norms listed on their website (www.cdc.gov) that parents can use to compare their child's progress (CDC, 2016a). In addition to getting the parents' descriptions of whether their child has mastered these skills, it is helpful to watch a child perform skills and rate them according to standard criteria.

Denver II Developmental Screening Test

The Denver II Developmental Screening Test (available at http://thePoint.lww.com/Flagg8e) is the most widely used tool to assess early childhood development (Frankenburg, 1994). Four categories are rated:
1. Personal–social
2. Fine motor–adaptive
3. Language
4. Gross motor skills

Administration

The Denver II should ideally be administered when a child is approximately 3 or 4 months of age, again at about 10 months, and again at 3 years. It is a supplement to the developmental evaluation by history that should be a part of every well-child assessment.

The materials to administer the test must be purchased as a kit. They include a skein of red wool, a box of raisins, a small bottle, a bell, a rattle with a narrow handle, a tennis ball, ten 1-in. brightly colored blocks, a small plastic doll, a toy baby bottle, a plastic cup, and a pencil.

Although administration of the Denver II is not difficult, it should not be attempted except by healthcare providers trained specifically in its procedures and interpretation. This precaution is necessary to ensure the validity of its developmental norms. Periodic retraining and proficiency testing are recommended, so administrators sustain a high degree of accuracy in administration.

Caution a parent before administration that this is not a test of intelligence but of the child's level of development or ability to perform age-appropriate tasks.

The child's inability to perform a task most children of the same age can accomplish indicates a delay in that area. Further evaluation is then needed to determine the reason for this delay.

Scoring

The child is scored P (passed), F (failed), R (refused), or N.O. (no opportunity) on each item according to guidelines in the instruction manual. Each item is represented on the Denver II test form by a bar showing the ages by which 25%, 50%, 75%, and 90% of children normally have mastered that item. For example, on the form, 25% of children are expected to demonstrate the task "plays pat-a-cake" at 7 months, 50% perform this between 9 and 10 months, 75% between 10 and 11 months, and 90% by ages 11 to 12 months. A description of each task and an interpretation of performance are detailed in the manual.

Prescreening Test

A Revised Denver Prescreening Developmental Questionnaire (R-PDQII) is available in addition to the Denver II. The PDQII is a questionnaire completed by the parents addressing 10 developmental items. A child who scores 8 out of 10 or fewer should be retested in approximately 2 weeks. If the initial score is under 6 or the retest score is 8 or below, the child should be referred for Denver II testing. Encouraging parents to complete a questionnaire this way is helpful because it can detect developmental delays otherwise missed in a busy office or clinic.

Intelligence

Children must learn many important concepts or ideas such as near and far, number sequences, how to judge time intervals, how to reason and solve problems, and how to judge weight before they can function effectively in the world.

This type of learning—gaining concepts—is cognitive learning and is measured by intelligence tests. **Intelligence** can be defined as the ability to think abstractly, to adjust to new situations, and to profit from experience. Almost everyone has their IQ rated at some point in a school career. Although intelligence tests are not part of routine health appraisals, it is helpful to be familiar with those that are used for childhood measurements because these findings can help predict a child's school success.

The IQ is the ratio of mental age as measured by an intelligence test to chronologic age. To determine IQ, the formula is

$$(\text{mental age} \div \text{chronologic age}) \times 100$$

A child aged 9 years old (i.e., chronologic age) who passes all the items on an intelligence test that an average 9-year-old child is expected to pass would be

$$(9\ [\text{mental age}] \div 9\ [\text{chronologic age}]) \times 100 = 100\ (\text{child's IQ})$$

If a child passes no more items than the average 5-year-old child would pass, the IQ would be

$$(5\ [\text{mental age}] \div 9\ [\text{chronologic age}]) \times 100 = 55$$

If a child passed all the items that a 12-year-old child normally passes, the IQ would be

$$(12\ [\text{mental age}] \div 9\ [\text{chronologic age}]) \times 100 = 133$$

Intelligence scores are not always accurate; for instance, children may score poorly because of test anxiety. Cultural bias and past experience can also affect scores. Labeling children by IQ and classifying them into divisions based on IQ is no longer used as extensively as in the past. It must be done with considerable thought and study.

It is difficult to test very young children with any degree of accuracy because they lack the ability to complete tasks in the areas used for scoring intelligence tests, including comprehension, imagination, reasoning, memory, and vocabulary. The most common tests used with infants include the Cattell Infant Intelligence Scale, the Bayley Mental Scale, and the Gesell Developmental Schedule. These tests rely heavily on perceptual and motor skills as rating devices.

The two most frequently used tests for older children are the Wechsler Intelligence Scale for Children and the Stanford–Binet test. The results of these can be made available, with parental permission, to child healthcare teams if they can demonstrate to school officials that such information is necessary for total health care or planning. If the information is unavailable, the child can be referred to a psychologist or a psychological testing clinic for assessment at the time of a disease diagnosis.

GOODENOUGH-HARRIS DRAWING TEST

A Goodenough-Harris Drawing Test is a quick intelligence measurement that can be administered without special training to children between 3 and 10 years of age (Goodenough, 1926). To administer this, give a child a pencil and paper and tell the child to draw a person. Urge the child to draw carefully and take enough time to do it well.

The child receives 1 point for each of the items listed in Box 34.14 that are demonstrated in the drawing. For each 4 points scored, 1 year is added to a base age of 3 years to calculate the child's mental age. The picture shown in Figure 34.25, for example, was drawn by a 4.5-year-old: It received 8 points. The child's IQ level is therefore

$$(5.0 \text{ [mental age]} \div 4.5 \text{ [chronologic age]}) \times 100 = 111$$

Scores on the test are reasonably reliable, correlating well with a Stanford–Binet test, although results may not be as reliable with children who are mentally ill. A child who scores significantly lower than chronologic age (after allowing for fatigue, illness, strange surroundings, nervousness, physical ability to use a pencil, and previous practice using a pencil and paper) should be referred for more refined testing.

Temperament

Temperament refers to a child's innate behavioral characteristics, such as activity level, rhythmicity, tendency to approach or withdraw, and adaptability to situations (see Chapter 28).

BOX 34.14

Goodenough-Harris Drawing Test

Score 1 point for each characteristic listed as follows that is present on the drawing. For every 4 points scored, add 1 year to a base mental age of 3 years.

1. Head present
2. Legs present
3. Arms present
4a. Trunk present
4b. Length of trunk greater than breadth
4c. Shoulders indicated
5a. Both arms and legs attached to trunk
5b. Legs attached to trunk; arms attached to trunk at correct point
6a. Neck present
6b. Neck outline continuous with head, trunk, or both
7a. Eyes present
7b. Nose present
7c. Mouth present
7d. Nose and mouth in two dimensions; two lips shown
7e. Nostrils indicated
8a. Hair shown
8b. Hair nontransparent, over more than circumference
9a. Clothing present
9b. Two articles of clothing nontransparent
9c. No transparencies, both sleeves and trousers shown
9d. Four or more articles of clothing definitely indicated
9e. Costume complete, without incongruities
10a. Fingers shown
10b. Correct number of fingers shown

10c. Fingers in two dimensions; length greater than breadth, angle less than 180°
10d. Opposition of thumb shown
10e. Hand shown distinct from fingers or arms
11a. Arm joint shown, either elbow, shoulder, or both
11b. Leg joint shown, either knee, hip, or both
12a. Head in proportion
12b. Arms in proportion
12c. Legs in proportion
12d. Feet in proportion
12e. Both arms and legs in two dimensions
13. Heel shown
14a. Firm lines without overlapping at junctions
14b. Firm lines with correct joining
14c. Head outline more than circle
14d. Trunk outline more than circle
14e. Outline of arms and legs without narrowing at point of junction with body
14f. Features symmetric, correct position
15a. Ears present
15b. Ears in correct position and proportion
16a. Eye detail: brow and lashes shown
16b. Eye detail: pupil shown
16c. Eye detail: proportion correct
16d. Eye detail: glance directed to front in profile drawing
17a. Both chin and forehead present
17b. Projection of chin shown

From Goodenough, F. L. (1926). *Measurement of intelligence by drawings.* New York, NY: World Book Company. Revised Harris, D. B. (1963). *Children's drawings as measures of intellectual maturity.* New York, NY: Harcourt, Brace & World. Reprinted with permission from Estate of Dale B. Harris.

Figure 34.25 An 8-point drawing, as scored on the Goodenough-Harris Drawing Test.

A child with an "easy" temperament is generally adaptable and easy to care for; in contrast, a child with a "difficult" temperament will almost invariably create childrearing concerns. Helping parents assess their child's temperament helps them, in turn, recognize their child's uniqueness and so anticipate and ideally prevent personality conflicts as a child grows older and expresses identified reactions to situations. If a behavior or parent–child interaction problem is already present, a nursing assessment can be useful to determine whether temperament is a factor in the problem and to assist parents with constructive solutions (Thomas & Chess, 1977).

Immunizations

One of the most important health assessment and promotion measures for children is to verify their immunization status is up to date (see "Recommended Childhood and Adolescent Immunization Schedule" available at http://thePoint.lww.com/Flagg8e).

Teach parents about the importance of having their children immunized and the need to be able to describe the number and type of immunizations a child has received. If gaps are present in a child's number of immunizations, remind the child's primary care provider about this lack in protection and prepare to administer the necessary vaccines.

Help parents understand that although diseases such as measles and mumps are referred to as common childhood illnesses, they are potentially serious and possibly lead to complications such as pneumonia and encephalitis (see Chapter 43).

TYPES OF IMMUNIZATIONS

Vaccines are the solutions used to immunize children in order to provide artificially acquired active or passive immunity (Box 34.15) for the definition of active and passive immunity).

Vaccines are prepared in a number of forms. Attenuated vaccines are made from live organisms reduced in virulence to a point where they will not cause active disease but will ensure a good antibody response. Because they are strong solutions, a single dose usually provides a good degree of active immunity.

Because some bacteria, such as diphtheria, cause disease by producing a toxin, the vaccine against such a disease, a **toxoid**, is actually an extract of the toxin with reduced virulence. The antibodies produced against toxin-producing bacteria are called **antitoxins**.

Gamma globulin is serum obtained from the pooled blood of many people. Because it combines the serum of many people, it probably has antibody protection against measles,

BOX 34.15

Active Versus Passive Immunity

Immunity, the ability to combat a particular antigen, may be either active or passive.

Active Immunity. When a child produces antibodies after the natural invasion of a pathogen (e.g., the child has measles), the child develops *naturally acquired active immunity.* Active antibodies (or the child's ability to produce antibodies rapidly should the specific antigen [measles] invade again) last a lifetime. When pathogens are artificially injected into the child by immunization, the child receives *artificially acquired active immunity.* If the specific antigen should enter again, antibodies will be produced against the pathogen that are just as lasting as those produced in naturally acquired active immunity.

Passive Immunity. Immunoglobulin G (IgG) antibodies a woman possesses either through immunization or through having had a disease are transferred across the placenta to a fetus in utero. Because the fetus does not make these antibodies but merely receives them, this is termed *naturally acquired passive immunity.* Passive immunity usually lasts only a few months, although some antibodies transferred across the placenta, such as those for measles, have been isolated up to age 1 year (which is why measles immunization must be delayed until 15 months of age).

When children are exposed to a disease against which they have no antibodies, antibodies made synthetically or obtained from animal serum may be injected into the child to give rapid immunity (*artificially acquired passive immunity*). Like naturally acquired passive antibodies, these last only approximately 6 weeks. A child who is susceptible to tetanus, for example, would receive tetanus antibodies after a stab wound to ensure she has protection against the tetanus virus.

rubella, poliomyelitis, varicella, and hepatitis B, among many other infectious diseases. When administered, it offers artificially acquired passive immunity.

Immune serums are serums available against specific diseases such as diphtheria, tetanus, the pit viper snake, the black widow spider, and respiratory syncytial virus. Like general immune globulin, these provide passive immunity.

CHILDHOOD IMMUNIZATIONS

The AAP and the CDC both issue specific recommendations for childhood immunization (available at http://thePoint.lww.com/Flagg8e).

The Diphtheria, Tetanus, and Pertussis Vaccine

Diphtheria, tetanus toxoid, and acellular pertussis (i.e., whooping cough) (DTaP) vaccines are supplied in a single vial as DTaP and given in one intramuscular injection. It is recommended that children receive a primary series of four immunizations with the vaccine (at 2, 4, 6, and 15 to 18 months of age). A booster is then given between 4 and 6 years of age or before entry into school. Because whooping cough outbreaks have occurred in the teenage and late adolescent population, a combined injection of the DTaP vaccine is recommended at 11 to 12 years of age. Teenagers who did not receive the booster at 11 to 12 years of age or who received only a diphtheria/tetanus (Td) injection at that time are encouraged to receive one dose of DTaP 5 years after the last Td/DTaP dose. It is recommended that late adolescents continue with tetanus prophylaxis every 10 years throughout life to keep their tetanus immunizations current.

Side effects to these vaccines include drowsiness, fretfulness, low-grade fever, and redness and pain at the injection site. A pertussis vaccination may not be recommended for children who have a progressive or unstable neurologic disorder. A Td vaccine can be substituted for these children.

The Polio Vaccine

Inactivated polio vaccine (IPV) contains all three strains of poliovirus and is the preferred type for routine immunization. It is administered in a primary series of three doses and given along with DTaP at 2, 4, and 6 to 18 months of age with a fourth booster dose given between the ages of 4 and 6 years or before school entry (CDC, 2016b).

The Measles, Mumps, and Rubella Vaccine

The measles, mumps, and rubella (MMR) vaccine is furnished in one injection and routinely administered between 12 and 15 months of age. A second dose of MMR is generally given between the ages of 4 and 6 years, or if the child did not receive this dose at 4 to 6 years of age, it is given at 11 to 12 years of age. The first dose is delayed until the end of the first year because children receive a great deal of passive immunity to measles from their mothers while they are in utero. Until this passive immunity has faded, the injected vaccine would be neutralized by passive antibodies and no immunity would result. For the same reason, children who have recently received immune globulin or other blood products that contain antibodies should not receive an MMR vaccination for about 3 months because the passively acquired antibodies could interfere with the child's immune response to the vaccine.

Side effects to the vaccine include transient rash and a fever, which may begin 5 to 12 days after vaccination and last several days. Adverse reactions include joint pain, low-grade fever, rash, and lymphadenopathy 5 to 12 days after vaccination.

Before the vaccine is administered, children who are at risk should be skin tested for tuberculosis because the measles virus can cause tuberculosis to become systemic. Tuberculosis skin tests also may show false-negative reactions if given shortly after a measles immunization (i.e., a child who has active tuberculosis would be wrongly identified as not having the illness).

Formerly, there was a concern the administration of the MMR vaccine was associated with the development of autism in children, as symptoms of autism often begin to be apparent during the second year or close to the time of MMR vaccine administration. Further research has shown there to be no causal relationship between the vaccine and autism (Uno, Uchiyama, Kurosawa, et al., 2015). Parents may ask about this association, however, or may refuse to have their child immunized against MMR for this reason (Salmon, Dudley, Glanz, et al., 2015).

The Hepatitis B Vaccine

The vaccine for hepatitis B virus (HBV) is recommended for all infants in the United States because hepatitis B is associated with liver cancer later in life. Three doses are required. Those infants born to hepatitis B surface antigen (HBsAg)-negative mothers should receive the first dose in the newborn period before hospital discharge, a second dose at 1 or 2 months, and a third dose at 6 or 18 months. Those born to HBsAg-positive mothers should receive hepatitis B immune globulin within 12 hours of birth plus HBV vaccine. A second dose of HBV vaccine is then recommended at 1 to 2 months of age and a third dose at 6 months.

If the mother's HBsAg status is unknown, infants should receive the vaccine within 12 hours of birth, the second dose at 1 month of age, and the third dose at 6 months of age. Children who did not receive the vaccine at birth may begin a two- or three-injection series, depending on the vaccine used at any well-child visit.

In addition, the HBV immunization is recommended for populations at increased risk for contracting hepatitis B infection, including healthcare providers with significant exposure to blood, patients receiving hemodialysis, those with hemophilia or who receive clotting factor concentrates, those who take illicit injectable drugs, and sexually active individuals with multiple sexual partners.

The Hepatitis A Vaccine

Two doses of hepatitis A vaccine, administered 6 months apart, are recommended for all children between 1 and 2 years of age. Children who did not receive this as toddlers can be vaccinated against hepatitis A at any time.

The Rotavirus Vaccine

Rotaviruses are responsible for the majority of severe gastrointestinal disease in infants, so immunization against these viruses is important for preventing outbreaks of diarrhea in infants, particularly those who attend a day care setting. The vaccine is given at 2, 4, and 6 months of age. No doses should be given after children reach 32 weeks of age.

Haemophilus influenzae Type B Vaccine

Haemophilus influenzae type B conjugate vaccine (Hib) protects against *H. influenzae* bacteria, a major cause of meningitis in children. You may need to explain the difference between *H. influenzae* (a bacteria) and the influenza virus so that parents do not think a "flu shot" protects against this. Several formulations of this vaccine are available; depending on the individual vaccine, they are administered in a two-dose (at age 2 and 4 months of age) or a three-dose regimen (at 2, 4, and 6 months of age, with an additional booster at 12 months of age). Local reactions include tenderness at the injection site. Reactions such as crying and fever may occur (CDC, 2016b).

The Varicella Vaccine

The varicella (i.e., chickenpox) vaccine was a difficult vaccine to develop because of the complex structure of the herpes zoster virus. It's an important vaccine because once a generation of children has been successfully immunized, it should mark the end of an epidemic childhood illness. Infants may receive varicella vaccine at any visit after their first birthday (usually scheduled at 12 to 18 months of age) and again at 4 to 6 years of age. Those who did not receive the vaccine as infants and who lack a reliable history of chickenpox should be immunized during adolescence with two doses of vaccine administered at least 1 month apart.

The Pneumococcal Pneumonia Vaccine

The pneumococcal vaccine is recommended for all children between 2 and 23 months of age. The vaccine is administered at 2, 4, 6, and 12 months of age and provides protection for 6 to 10 years (AAP, 2013). It is especially recommended for children (and adults) who would be prone to a pneumococcal infection (e.g., those with pulmonary or cardiac disease, those without a spleen, those who are immunosuppressed).

The Human Papillomavirus Vaccine

The human papillomavirus (HPV) is associated with the development of cervical cancer in women. It is recommended that all preteens (male and female) receive three injections of this vaccine beginning at 11 to 12 years of age. The second dose should be administered 2 months after the first dose, and the third dose should be given 6 months after the first dose. Those who did not receive the vaccine in early adolescence can receive it at any time, with the proper monthly intervals for administration. Some teenagers who have taken abstinence pledges not to have sexual relations until they are married may state they do not need the vaccine. Counseling them about the safety of being immunized in case they change their mind about abstinence or to be protected when they become sexually active may be necessary.

The Meningococcal Vaccine

Children who have immunologic deficiencies or have had their spleen removed due to trauma or those receiving therapy for a blood dyscrasia are prone to develop meningitis caused by meningococcal bacteria. Children in these high-risk groups are, therefore, advised to receive a meningococcal vaccine between 2 and 10 years of age. Administer a single dose of meningococcal vaccine at age 11 through 12 years, with a booster dose at age 16 years. If the first dose of meningococcal vaccine is administered at age 16 years or older, a booster dose is not needed.

The Lyme Disease Vaccine

Lyme disease is a serious and debilitating infection caused by *Borrelia burgdorferi* and transmitted by the bite of a deer tick. A vaccine to guard against it is no longer available. Children who contract the disease can be successfully treated with antibiotics to minimize the disease. Tips for preventing Lyme disease are shown in Chapter 43.

The Influenza Vaccine

Influenza is caused by A, B, or C retroviruses, which mutate so easily that it has been impossible to design a vaccine that is effective for more than 1 year. All children—infants 6 months of age through adolescents—and particularly those who have chronic pulmonary or cardiovascular disorders or are immunosuppressed should receive a yearly injection of the vaccine (CDC, 2016b). For most healthy children age 2 years and older, the live attenuated influenza vaccine (LAIV) can be administered. Children 6 months through 8 years who have never received the influenza vaccine before will require two doses at least 1 month apart.

The Anthrax and Smallpox Vaccines

Anthrax is a potentially fatal disease caused by a gram-positive, spore-forming *Bacillus anthracis* and spread by farm animal feces. It is extremely rare, but parents may ask about a vaccine for it because of the threat of biologic warfare associated with terrorism. A vaccine is available for people in high-risk occupations, such as hunters, taxidermists, or veterinarians, but it is not recommended for children.

Smallpox is an extremely infectious disease caused by the smallpox virus and transmitted by direct or indirect contact. Smallpox vaccination has not been required in the United States for over 30 years because the disease is theoretically extinct across the world. As with anthrax, parents may ask about a smallpox vaccination because it is a disease associated with biologic warfare and terrorism. Both a vaccine (active artificial immunity) and passive artificial immunity are available should a child be exposed to the virus. In some high-risk communities, healthcare providers are asked to be immunized to be certain they will not contract the virus if a terrorist attack should occur (Frey, Winokur, Salata, et al., 2013).

ADMINISTRATION OF IMMUNIZATIONS

Current immunization recommendations are available at http://thePoint.lww.com/Flagg8e. Assess both well children at health maintenance visits and ill children at clinic or hospital admission to identify those who need their immunizations updated according to this schedule. Children who are seriously ill should not receive immunizations, but a slight upper respiratory tract infection (e.g., a stuffy nose with no fever) is not a contraindication. So many infants and preschoolers have common cold symptoms (the average toddler has 10 to 12 colds a year); if children were not immunized at health maintenance visits when they have slight cold symptoms, many would never receive basic immunizations. Catch-up schedules for children who did not receive primary immunizations or who are behind in an immunization schedule are also available at http://thePoint.lww.com/Flagg8e. Because these schedules change yearly based on the introduction of new vaccines or new potential health threats, consult the AAP website (www.aap.org) or the CDC website (www.cdc.gov) for up-to-date information before immunizing a specific child.

When preparing to administer an immunization, be certain to follow the manufacturer's recommendations for storage and handling of vaccines, such as whether the vaccine should not be exposed to light or whether it needs refrigeration. Failure to follow these precautions may significantly reduce the potency and effectiveness of vaccines.

CHILDREN WITH UNIQUE NEEDS

Children with chronic illnesses may be hospitalized at the time an immunization is due and so fall behind schedule. Children who miss the scheduled time for an immunization do not need to have the series started over but rather should simply continue at the point they left off. Primary care providers may choose to alter the sequence of immunization schedules if specific infections are prevalent at the time. For example, the measles vaccine might be given on a first health maintenance visit (providing a child is older than 12 months of age) if an epidemic was underway in the community at the time.

Children who are immunosuppressed, receiving corticosteroids, or receiving chemotherapy or radiation therapy should not receive live virus vaccines. The live attenuated viruses such as measles, rubella, oral polio vaccine (OPV), and mumps must not be given to girls who are pregnant because these vaccines could cross the placenta, thus causing disease in the fetus. Before traveling internationally, parents should consult their local public health service to see what additional vaccines are required for children for overseas travel.

Although MMR vaccines are prepared from chick embryo cultures, egg sensitivities are not likely to occur because egg albumin and yolk components of the egg are absent from the culture. The minute quantity of egg proteins contained in the MMR vaccine seems to be insufficient to cause an allergic reaction in egg-allergic people. Therefore, no allergy testing needs to be completed prior to the administration of the vaccine.

PARENTAL EDUCATION

A major reason parents do not bring children for routine immunizations is they do not know what is required or have misconceptions about immunity. Fully inform parents and, when old enough, children about what immunizations are recommended. When vaccines are given, be certain parents know what is being given and what side effects may be expected. Because children may develop a low-grade fever after any immunization, counsel parents that they may need to give acetaminophen (Tylenol) or children's ibuprofen for a fever higher than 101°F (38.4°C).

Unfavorable reactions are most likely to occur within a few hours or days of administration. With live attenuated virus vaccines, viruses can multiply, so reactions may occur up to 30 days later. With the rubella vaccine, a reaction (serum sickness) may occur up to 60 days later. Ask parents to report any untoward symptoms of immunization.

When giving a vaccine, record the date, type of vaccine, vaccine manufacturer, lot number, and name and address of the vaccine provider so that if a vaccine reaction should occur, the instance can be investigated. Make a copy of the child's immunization record for the parents and urge them to keep good track of such a record. They will need this information to admit their child to school and to feel safe in the event an epidemic of a particular disease occurs. They will need to know their child's record of tetanus immunizations if the child should receive a puncture wound so that the correct therapy can be given for this.

QSEN Checkpoint Question 34.6

SAFETY

Keoto's father wants to be sure Keoto's immunizations are up to date. The nurse determines the immunization for HPV is recommended by which age?

- a. At 12 to 18 months of age
- b. Before kindergarten entrance
- c. At 16 years of age
- d. At 11 to 12 years of age

Look in Appendix A for the best answer and rationale.

Concluding a Health Assessment

At every health maintenance visit, inform parents and the child (or ask the child's primary care provider to inform them, depending on agency policy) of any available results of screening procedures performed. After learning the results, some parents may require counseling to assist them with health or behavior concerns. Box 34.16 shows an interprofessional care map illustrating both nursing and team planning for a child in need of a pre-sports health assessment. Ask parents if they have any other remaining questions. If the health assessment revealed some health concerns and follow-up procedures are planned, be certain parents understand the reason for the upcoming tests. Suggest to parents that follow-up phone calls are welcome after they return home from a health assessment so additional questions can be answered. Provide parents with the best hours to call so someone will be available to answer questions for them. Many providers now have patient portals families can use to ask additional questions or download physical forms and immunization records.

What If . . . 34.4

The nurse is particularly interested in exploring one of the 2020 National Health Goals with respect to health assessment (see Box 34.1). What would be a possible research topic to explore that is pertinent to this goal, applicable to Keoto's family, and that would also advance evidence-based practice?

Unfolding Patient Stories: Eva Madison • Part 1

Eva Madison, a 5-year-old female, is at the clinic with her mother for a routine checkup. How can the nurse create an environment that is conducive to obtaining health information? How can the nurse prepare the child and the mother for the physical exam? What key areas of the health history and physical assessment should the nurse evaluate in this 5-year-old female? (Eva Madison's story continues in Chapter 36.)

Care for Eva and other patients in a realistic virtual environment: *vSim for Nursing* (thepoint.lww.com/vSim MaternityPed). Practice documenting these patients' care in DocuCare (thepoint.lww.com/DocuCareEHR).

KEY POINTS FOR REVIEW

- Health assessment always causes some degree of apprehension for both parents and children because of the worry that an illness will be detected. Giving reassurance of wellness during examinations helps to alleviate this worry.

- A health history is an important part of an assessment. The purpose is to gather information that will supplement physical or laboratory examinations to provide a more thorough health evaluation.

- A health history includes an introduction, chief concern, family profile, history of past illnesses, day history, family health history, and review of systems.

BOX 34.16

Nursing Care Planning

AN INTERPROFESSIONAL CARE MAP FOR A CHILD IN NEED OF A PRE-SPORTS HEALTH ASSESSMENT

Keoto Wiser is a 13-year-old you meet in an ambulatory clinic. Her father has brought her for health assessment before Keoto begins seventh grade.

Family Assessment: Child lives with two parents and 2-year-old sister, Candy. Father works as a paramedic for the fire department; mother is a notary public employed by a bank. Father rates finances as "good."

Child Assessment: Keoto was born with a lung cyst that required removal not only of the cyst but also a portion of her left upper lung lobe at 6 months of age. Her father is concerned her lessened lung size may make her ineligible for competitive sports participation. He asks if carbohydrate loading would give her enough energy to make up for any decreased lung function. He's also concerned she may need eyeglasses because she always sits close to the television set. He asks you if wearing glasses could decrease her chance of being chosen for a sports team.

Nursing Diagnosis: Anxiety related to ability to participate in school sports program

Outcome Criteria: Patient participates in school sports program to the degree dictated by physical findings.

Team Member Responsible	Assessment	Intervention	Rationale	Expected Outcome
Activities of Daily Living, Including Safety				
Nurse	Assess child's development by taking a 24-hour day history.	Discuss with parent and child any areas that cause concern.	Parents can "get behind" in expectations of child, as pre-teenage children grow and develop rapidly.	Parent or child gives day history and discusses any areas seen as problematic.
Teamwork and Collaboration				
Nurse/primary healthcare provider	Determine name of healthcare provider who determines eligibility for sports teams at child's school.	Consult with identified healthcare provider to determine eligibility rules for sports.	Schools may have restrictions on children who do not have both pairs of duplicate organs such as lungs.	Qualifications for sports participation are obtained and outlined for parents and child.
Procedures/Medications for Quality Improvement				
Nurse/primary healthcare provider	Obtain health assessment, particularly with regard to stamina and past ability to participate in sports activities.	Perform complete physical examination focusing on heart, lung, and muscle status.	Physical examination can reveal additional findings regarding lung capacity and stamina.	A physical examination yields information on child's overall health.
Nurse	Assess whether child is familiar with Snellen vision testing.	Assess child's eyesight using a Snellen eye chart.	A Snellen eye chart is a standardized test for vision appraisal.	Child completes eye exam and is told results.
Nutrition				
Nurse/nutritionist	Assess what parents and child know about carbohydrate loading.	Counsel regarding disadvantages of carbohydrate loading for children.	Children and parents who are well informed can make better choices for nutrition practices.	Parent and child state they understand carbohydrate loading is not recommended for children.
Patient-Centered Care				
Nurse	Assess past health history and recommended immunizations.	Review with parents and child the child's current immunization status and any immunizations needed.	Parents are often unfamiliar with required immunizations and so need to be reminded of recommended schedules.	Parents and child agree to any immunization necessary before child returns to school.

Psychosocial/Spiritual/Emotional Needs

Nurse	Assess what will be child's likely reaction if she cannot participate in her school's sports program or needs to wear eyeglasses.	If child is unable to participate in school sports, review with child other options: joining a club, petition school sports committee, etc. Discuss advantage of clear vision.	Planning ahead can help child adjust to less-than-desired results if these occur.	Child lists alternate ways to participate with other children at school, if sports are not an option, or describes a sensible plan for petitioning for an exception to rules.

Informatics for Seamless Healthcare Planning

Nurse	Assess if parents or child have had questions answered during the health assessment.	Answer remaining questions, if any; schedule a return visit as needed.	If questions remain unanswered at the health assessment, needs haven't been fully met.	Parents and child state they have no further questions; describe plans for next action.

- A physical examination involves four techniques: inspection, palpation, percussion, and auscultation. Techniques and approaches must be varied according to the child's age.

- Be certain to use examining instruments safely, such as supporting an otoscope base so that if a child moves, the otoscope moves with the child. Be certain young children are not left unsupervised on an examining table because this could cause a fall.

- The components of a physical examination include vital sign assessment, general appearance, mental status assessment, body measurements, and an assessment from head to toes.

- Adolescent boys can be taught testicular self-examination at the time of a health appraisal. Breast self-examinations for females should be done by the examiner but is no longer thought to reveal enough information to be practical as a preventive measure.

- A vision assessment consists of asking children to read a standardized chart such as a Snellen or preschool E chart, cover testing, or color discrimination assessment.

- A hearing assessment consists of such assessments as audiometric testing and Rinne and Weber tests.

- Determining a child's development is an important part of total assessment. The Denver II Developmental Screening Test and the DASE are specific development tests used.

- The Goodenough-Harris Drawing Test correlates well with IQ and is an easy test to administer to children between the ages of 3 and 10 years to assess intelligence.

- An assessment of immunization status is included as part of a health assessment. Childhood immunizations are a major safeguard for children against common childhood illnesses; being certain they receive what is needed at each healthcare visit not only helps in planning nursing care that meets QSEN guidelines but also helps to keep a child safe.

CRITICAL THINKING CARE STUDY

Suzanne is a 6-year-old you meet at a school-based clinic. You notice from her attendance record that she misses about 4 days of school every month for "constipation." As she walks down the hallway, you notice she walks on her tiptoes.

1. Suzanne's mother tells you Suzanne walks on her tiptoes because she learned to do that so her father, who works nights, won't be awakened during the day. Would you want to examine Suzanne's gait any further?

2. Suzanne's mother confirms Suzanne has almost "constant constipation." Her mother explains it is because Suzanne never eats vegetables. On examination, you locate a hard mass in her upper right quadrant. Would you want to ask more questions about Suzanne's constipation?

3. Suzanne tells you she often doesn't eat lunch at school because she forgets her lunch money. Would you want to assess Suzanne's short-term or long-term memory?

RELATED RESOURCES

Explore these additional resources to enhance learning for this chapter:
- Student resources on thePoint, including answers to the What If . . . and Critical Thinking Care Study questions, http://thepoint.lww.com/Flagg8e
- Adaptive learning powered by PrepU, http://thepoint.lww.com/prepu

REFERENCES

American Academy of Pediatrics. (2013). *Your teen's yearly checkup.* Evanston, IL: Author.

American Academy of Pediatrics. (2016). *Recommendations for preventive pediatric health care.* Evanston, IL: Author.

American College of Obstetricians and Gynecologists. (2014). Committee Opinion No. 598: The initial reproductive health care visit. *Obstetrics & Gynecology, 123*(5), 1143–1147.

Ayers, J., Charakidah, M., Deanfield, J. E., et al. (2015). Lifetime risk: Childhood obesity and cardiovascular risk. *European Heart Journal, 36*(22), 1371–1376.

Braverman, R. S. (2016). The eye. In W. W. Hay Jr., M. J. Levin, R. R. Deterding, et al. (Eds.), *Current diagnosis & treatment: Pediatrics* (21st ed., pp. 424–464). Columbus, OH: McGraw-Hill/Lange.

Cameron, J. R., Rice, D. C., Sparkman, G., et al. (2013). Childhood temperament-based anticipatory guidance in an HMO setting: A longitudinal study. *Journal of Community Psychology, 41*(2), 236–248.

Centers for Disease Control and Prevention. (2012). CDC grand rounds: Newborn screening and improved outcomes. *Morbidity and Mortality Weekly Report, 61*(21), 390–393.

Centers for Disease Control and Prevention. (2016a). *Developmental milestones.* Washington, DC: Author.

Centers for Disease Control and Prevention. (2016b). *Immunization schedules.* Washington, DC: Author.

Centers for Disease Control and Prevention. (2016c). *Poisoning prevention.* Retrieved from https://www.cdc.gov/safechild/poisoning/index.html

Chernoff, K., & Scher, R. (2016). Nail disorders: Kids are not just little people. *Clinics in Dermatology, 34*(6), 736–741.

Chiesa, A., & Sirotnak, A. (2014). Child abuse & neglect. In W. W. Hay Jr., M. J. Levin, R. R. Deterding (Eds.), *Current diagnosis & treatment: Pediatrics* (22nd ed., pp. 239–247). New York, NY: McGraw-Hill/Lange.

de Maleissye, M. F., Beauchet, A., Saiag, P., et al. (2013). Sunscreen use and melanocytic nevi in children: A systematic review. *Pediatric Dermatology, 30*(1), 51–59.

de Onis, M. (2015). The WHO Child Growth Standards. *World Review of Nutrition and Dietetics, 113*, 278–294.

Devore, C., & Schutze, G. (2015). Head lice. *Pediatrics, 135*(5), e1355–e1365.

Ely, E., Chen-Lim, M. L., Zarnowsky, C., et al. (2012). Finding the evidence to change practice for assessing pain in children who are cognitively impaired. *Journal of Pediatric Nursing, 27*, 402–410.

Frankenburg, W. K. (1994). Preventing developmental delays: Is developmental screening sufficient? *Pediatrics, 93*(4), 586–589.

Frey, S., Winokur, P., Salata, R., et al. (2013). Safety and immunogenicity of IMVAMUNE® smallpox vaccine using different strategies for a post event scenario. *Vaccine, 31*(29), 3025–3033.

Goodenough, F. L. (1926). *Measurement of intelligence by drawings.* New York, NY: World Book Company.

Gupta, R., Patel, R., Murty, N., et al. (2015). Developing sustainable global health technologies: Insight from an initiative to address neonatal hypothermia. *Journal of Public Health Policy, 36*(1), 24–40.

Harmon, K., Asif, I. M., Maleszewski, J., et al. (2016). Incidence and etiology of sudden cardiac arrest and death in high school athletes in the United States. *Mayo Clinic Proceedings, 91*(11), 1493–1502.

Jaffe, A. C. (2011). Failure to thrive: Current clinical concepts. *Pediatrics in Review, 32*(3), 100–107.

Khan, A., McCormack, H., Bolger, E., et al. (2015). Childhood maltreatment, depression, and suicidal ideation: Critical importance of parental and peer emotional abuse during developmental sensitive periods in males and females. *Frontiers in Psychiatry, 6*, 42.

Krug, E., Cieza, A., Chadha, S., et al. (2016). *Childhood hearing loss: Strategies for prevention and Care.* Geneva, Switzerland: World Health Organization.

Levine, D. A. (2011). Evaluation of the well child. In K. J. Marcdante, R. M. Kliegman, H. B. Jenson, et al. (Eds.), *Nelson essentials of pediatrics* (6th ed., pp. 24–30). Philadelphia, PA: Saunders/Elsevier.

Lyons, R. (2015). Acute limping in a young child: Evaluation and management review. *The Journal for Nurse Practitioners, 11*(10), 1004–1010.

Perera, S., Eisen, R., Bawor, M., et al. (2015). Association between body mass index and suicidal behaviors: A systematic review protocol. *Systematic Reviews, 4*, 52.

Peterson, G. M., Nurre, N., & Dunn, A. M. (2017). Role relationships. In C. E. Burns, A. M. Dunn, M. A. Brady, et al. (Eds.), *Pediatric primary care* (6th ed., pp. 311–338). St. Louis, MO: Elsevier.

Prevent Blindness America. (2012). *Distant vision test for younger children.* Chicago, IL: Author.

Salmon, D., Dudley, M., Glanz, J., et al. (2015). Vaccine hesitancy: Causes, consequences, and a call to action. *Vaccine, 33*(Suppl. 4), D66–D71.

Santillanes, G., Simms, S., Gausche-Hill, M., et al. (2012). Prospective evaluation of a clinical practice guideline for diagnosis of appendicitis in children. *Academy of Emergency Medicine, 19*(8), 886–893.

Spagnolo, A., Giussani, M., Ambruzzi, A., et al. (2013). Focus on prevention, diagnosis and treatment of hypertension in children and adolescents. *Italian Journal of Pediatrics, 39*, 20.

Spiewak, R. (2012). Contact dermatitis in atopic individuals. *Current Opinion in Allergy and Clinical Immunology, 12*, 491–497.

Spiteri, K., Busuttil, M. L., Aquilina, S., et al. (2017). Schoolbags and back pain in children between 8 and 13 years: A national study. *British Journal of Pain, 11*(2), 81–86.

Stein, R., Dogan, H., Hoebeke, P., et al. (2015). Urinary tract infections in children: EAU/ESPU guidelines. *European Urology, 67*(3), 546–548.

Taylor, K., & Elliot, S. (2014). Interventions for strabismic amblyopia. *Cochrane Database of Systematic Reviews,* (7), CD006461.

Thomas, A., & Chess, S. (1977). *Temperament and development.* Oxford, United Kingdom: Brunner/Mazel.

Uno, Y., Uchiyama, T., Kurosawa, M., et al. (2015). Early exposure to the combined measles-mumps-rubella vaccine and thimerosal-containing vaccines and risk of autism spectrum disorder. *Vaccine, 33*(21), 2511–2516.

U.S. Department of Agriculture. (2015). *Choose MyPlate: A guide to daily food choices.* Washington, DC: Author.

U.S. Department of Health and Human Services. (2010). *Healthy people 2020.* Washington, DC: Author.

Walter, K. D. (2011). Orthopedic assessment. In K. J. Marcdante, R. M. Kliegman, H. B. Jenson, et al. (Eds.), *Nelson essentials of pediatrics* (6th ed., pp. 735–737). Philadelphia, PA: Saunders/Elsevier.

Ward, D., Welker, E., Choate, A., et al. (2017). Strength of obesity prevention interventions in early care and education settings: A systematic review. *Preventive Medicine, 95*(Suppl.), S37–S52.

Whitney, E. N., & Rolfes, S. R. (2015). Life cycle nutrition: Infancy, childhood & adolescence. In E. N. Whitney & S. R. Rolfes (Eds.), *Understanding nutrition* (pp. 509–541). Belmont, CA: Wadsworth.

Yoon, P. J., Kelley, P. E., & Friedman, N. R. (2016). Ear, nose, & throat. In W. W. Hay Jr., M. J. Levine, M. J. Abzug, et al. (Eds.), *Current diagnosis & treatment: Pediatrics* (21st ed., pp. 477–509). Columbus, OH: McGraw-Hill/Lange.

35

Communication and Teaching With Children and Families

*Y*ou meet two patients of very different ages in an outpatient clinic. Wolf Whitefeather is a 3-year-old boy who is scheduled for repair of syndactyly (webbed fingers) next week. His mother tells you his favorite activity is coloring. She is concerned he will be hard to entertain after surgery because the large pressure bandage he will have afterward will prevent him from using that hand. "I don't even want to begin to talk to him about surgery," she tells you.

Barry Sandoz is a 16-year-old with a recurring peptic ulcer. His mother tells you health teaching with Barry will be ineffective because he never listens to a thing adults say.

Previous chapters discussed normal growth and development and how children's understanding increases with age. This chapter adds information about techniques for effective communication and health teaching with children and adolescents. This type of information is what builds a successful base for disease prevention and health promotion as well as increases health literacy.

What would be a good strategy for teaching 3-year-old Wolf about his surgery? Would you try to teach Barry more about his condition, or not? How would your communication with these children vary because of their age difference?

KEY TERMS

affective learning

behavioral therapy

clarifying

cognitive learning

communication

demonstration

empathy

feedback

focusing

health literacy

nontherapeutic communication

paraphrasing

perception checking

positive reinforcement

psychomotor learning

redemonstration

reflecting

therapeutic communication

OBJECTIVES

After mastering the contents of this chapter, you should be able to:

1. Describe principles of effective communication as well as teaching and learning as they relate to health teaching with children.

2. Identify 2020 National Health Goals related to communication and teaching with children that nurses can help the nation achieve.

3. Assess children for their ability to communicate and their readiness to learn.

4. Formulate nursing diagnoses related to communication and health teaching with children.

5. Identify expected outcomes for a specific child based on the child's age, developmental maturity, emotional needs, and communication or learning style to better enable parents to manage seamless transitions across differing healthcare settings.

6. Using the nursing process, plan nursing care that includes the six competencies of Quality & Safety Education for Nurses (QSEN): Patient-Centered Care, Teamwork & Collaboration, Evidence-Based Practice (EBP), Quality Improvement (QI), Safety, and Informatics.

7. Implement health teaching, such as creating a puppet show, using principles of effective communication and teaching and learning.

8. Evaluate expected outcomes for achievement and effectiveness of care.

9. Integrate knowledge of communication and teaching with the interplay of nursing process, the six competencies of QSEN, and Family Nursing to promote quality maternal and child health nursing care.

Health literacy is an individual's ability to read, understand, and use healthcare information to make decisions and follow instructions (Taylor, Nicolle, & Maguire, 2013). Both communication and health teaching are independent nursing actions that are important for increasing health literacy, helping children learn more about their illness, and providing better measures to use to stay well. Increasing health literacy is especially important when preparing a child for surgery or some other healthcare procedure.

Communication is fundamental to social interaction and is one of the first and most important skills children learn (Cruz, Quittner, Marker, et al., 2013). It can be either a formal or an informal exchange. Health teaching can also be both formal, such as teaching a group of preschoolers about hospitalization, or informal, such as assuring a parent a child is getting enough nutrition even though the child snacks rather than sits down to regular meals. It may be offered to an individual child or to a group of children with similar learning needs. Health teaching is so important that a number of 2020 National Health Goals speak to it (Box 35.1).

Nursing Process Overview

FOR HEALTH TEACHING WITH CHILDREN

ASSESSMENT

Communication and health teaching are best accomplished when they are placed within the context of the nursing process. Learner needs and characteristics, teacher characteristics, available support people, and the level of content are all factors that affect learning and whether communication will be received. Assessing these allows for nursing diagnoses that clearly state the specific health needs to be formulated.

NURSING DIAGNOSIS

Common examples of nursing diagnoses related to communication or health teaching include:

- Risk for impaired verbal communication related to use of Russian as primary language
- Deficient knowledge related to importance of taking medicine daily
- Health-seeking behaviors related to ways to improve the child's nutritional intake
- Impaired verbal communication related to placement of endotracheal tube
- Anxiety related to perceived amount of material needed to be learned for home care of child

OUTCOME IDENTIFICATION AND PLANNING

After formulating a nursing diagnosis, an individualized plan for communication or teaching should be constructed. The plan should detail not only what is to be communicated or learned but also methods to accomplish this and how it can be evaluated. The most effective way to ensure expected outcomes are achieved is to ask a child or family to join in the planning. Be certain outcomes are concrete and measurable (not "Child will discuss general aspects of his disease" but "Child will list three steps to help prevent disease reoccurrence"). Refer families to helpful websites and other resources when appropriate (see Chapter 28).

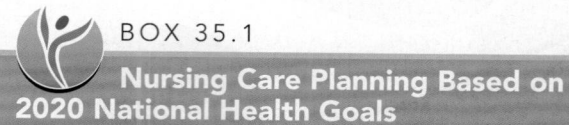

BOX 35.1

Nursing Care Planning Based on 2020 National Health Goals

A number of 2020 National Health Goals address good communication and health teaching because it is such an important mechanism of preventive health care.

- Increase the proportion of schools that provide school health education from a baseline of 35.2% to 38.7% for elementary school, from 56.9% to 62.2% for middle school, and from 76.8% to 84.5% for high school.
- Increase the health literacy of the population by increasing the proportion of persons who report their healthcare provider always gave them easy-to-understand instructions about what to do to take care of their illness or health condition (developmental).
- Increase the proportion of persons who report their healthcare providers have satisfactory communication skills by increasing the proportion of persons who report their healthcare provider always explained things so they could understand them from 60% to 66%.
- Increase the proportion of local health departments that have established culturally appropriate and linguistically competent community health-promotion and disease-prevention programs (developmental) (U.S. Department of Health and Human Services, 2010; see www.healthypeople.gov).

Nurses can help the nation achieve these goals by consulting with schools and healthcare organizations to develop what health teaching programs are needed, and then teaching in such programs.

IMPLEMENTATION

The step of implementation involves the actual carrying out of the communication or teaching. Teaching children is not always easy and requires practice and knowledge of each child's particular developmental level and needs.

OUTCOME EVALUATION

As a final step of communication or teaching, what was communicated or learned must be evaluated to be certain learning occurred. A new plan may need to be developed and teaching continued if communication or learning proves to be less than optimal. Examples of outcome criteria include:

- Child demonstrates good technique for self-injection of insulin.
- Child demonstrates anger using language rather than punching wall.
- Child lists five foods to include in a high-protein diet.
- Family demonstrates improved family communication techniques by next clinic visit.
- Parents/guardians demonstrate effective cardiopulmonary resuscitation technique at home visit.

Communication

Communication is the exchange of ideas between two or more persons. It can be verbal (i.e., using words) or nonverbal (i.e., using actions, such as touch or eye contact, or a remote system, such as mail or e-mail). Communication is important in the care of children because it can make or break an effective relationship. As a process, communication is divided into two major categories: *nontherapeutic* (i.e., casual, everyday conversation) and *therapeutic* (i.e., helpful, constructive interchanges).

NONTHERAPEUTIC COMMUNICATION

Nontherapeutic communication is identified by its lack of structure or planning; that is, it lacks deliberate purpose other than socializing. Dinner conversation is an example of nontherapeutic communication.

THERAPEUTIC COMMUNICATION

Therapeutic communication is a face-to-face process of interaction focusing on advancing the physical and emotional well-being of patients. It is an interaction between two people that is planned (e.g., you deliberately intend to determine how a child truly feels), has structure (e.g., you use specific wording techniques that will encourage a truthful response), and is helpful and constructive (e.g., at the end of the exchange you will know more about the child than you did at the beginning, and ideally, the child will know more about a particular problem or concern) (Roberts, Fenton, & Barnard, 2015).

In some instances, there is no cure for a child you care for—no surgery, no medication, and no pain relief. If you practice therapeutic communication, however, you still have something to offer this child and family: support by your words or nonverbal communication such as touch. In perspective, this is often the most valued, most appreciated, and most helpful aspect of care (Leathers & Eaves, 2015).

COMPONENTS OF GOOD COMMUNICATION

Communication can be broken down and diagrammed according to its essential components: the encoder, the code, the decoder, and response or feedback (Arnold, 2015) (Fig. 35.1).

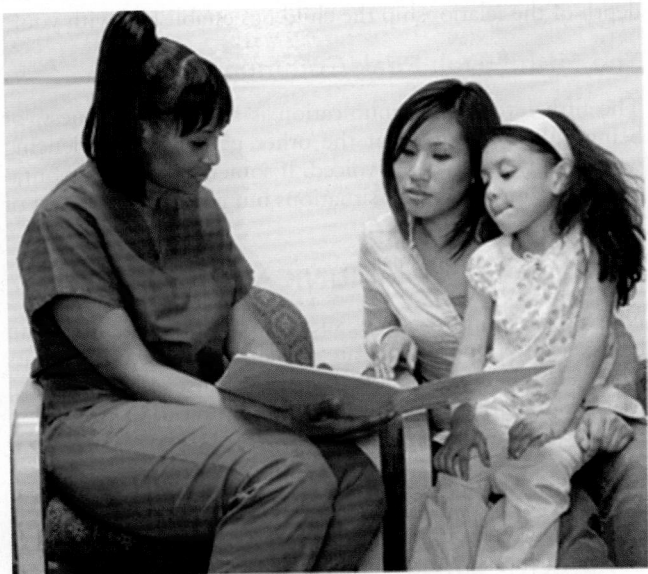

Figure 35.1 Health teaching is an interactive process, in which both a teacher and a learner share in the learning experience.

The Encoder

The encoder is a person who desires to share a thought or feeling with someone else and so originates a message. This person molds this thought into a form suitable for transferring to another person (i.e., a code). Communication can be ineffective if a person omits cognitive processing or speaks without thinking; chooses the wrong words for the message; or accompanies the spoken words with a facial expression, tone of voice, or gesture that is inappropriate for the message.

The Code

The code is the message conveyed and includes the medium or system used to convey it. Although this usually involves a simple spoken system, messages can also be conveyed by such methods as a painting, writing a poem or novel, Morse code, Braille, by electronic devices such as through text messaging, a movie projector, or over the telephone. Communication can be ineffective when a person chooses the wrong medium for a message; for instance, delivering a lecture with many technical words when a drawing would have made the message much clearer, or e-mailing when confronting a person directly would have had more impact.

The Decoder

The receiver (decoder) is the person who not only receives the message (i.e., hears it, reads it, views it) but also interprets or decodes its meaning (i.e., cognitive processing). Messages are interpreted in light of the receiver's previous knowledge. They may be misinterpreted if a receiver's store of knowledge is too different from that of the sender or if the receiver misses part of the transmission, such as a wink accompanying the spoken words that would have let the receiver know the sender was joking. Under stress, children tend to narrow their ability to receive information to a small area of concern (i.e., they center). Children who are extremely anxious, therefore, may not receive or be unable to interpret a message because of anxiety, even though both the sender and the message components of the communication were adequate.

Feedback or Response

Feedback is the reply the decoder returns to the sender to acknowledge the message has been received and interpreted. This could be a spoken statement, a nod of the head, a facial grimace or smile, a hand gesture, a return e-mail, or the sudden slamming of a telephone receiver. With feedback, the roles of sender and receiver become reversed and another communication cycle is begun. Communication can be ineffective if children do not offer feedback (i.e., the message was neither received nor understood) or if they offer feedback before the message is fully interpreted (i.e., acting before thinking). When you are caring for children with sensory challenges such as vision or hearing, you may need to change your usual feedback mechanisms in order to be understood because a nod of the head or quiet response may not be received. When a child is from a culture different than yours, it may require sensitive adaptation to be fully heard or to hear and understand.

THE DEVELOPMENT OF LANGUAGE

The development of language involves not only physically being able to form and voice words but also the comprehension of what they mean and how they are used (Box 35.2). One of the first responses an infant makes at birth is to cry. This first cry is important because it both signals that the infant is breathing well and also announces to the parents the birth is real, therefore stimulating the beginning of parent–child interactions.

By 2 years of age, children have mastered language well enough to be able to put two-word sentences (a noun and a verb) together. By preschool age, they not only have a vocabulary of about 900 words but also can code them into simple jokes or stories (Levine, 2014). Even children with cognitive challenges, although they may interpret jokes differently, still appreciate them (Briggs, Schuitema, & Vorhaus, 2016).

School-age children enlarge their ability to communicate from oral exchanges to use of the telephone and various electronic devices. They can write poetry and, by the end of the period, show an adult sense of humor by the jokes they create. Adolescents progress to a new phase in which they originate new words for objects or feelings ("cool" and "whatever" as responses). This form of communication helps them separate their world from adults and keep their adolescent culture separate.

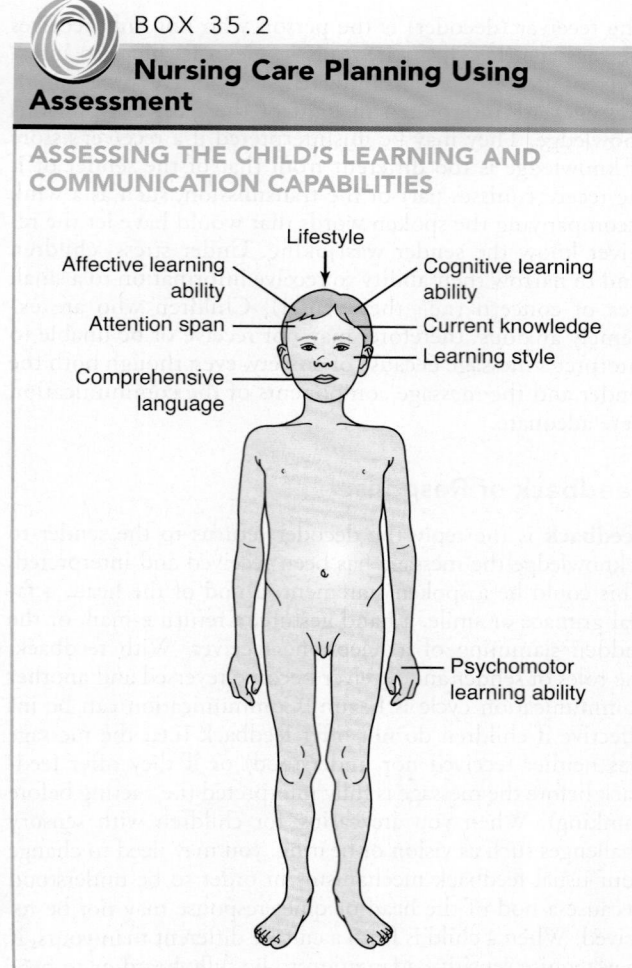

BOX 35.2
Nursing Care Planning Using Assessment

ASSESSING THE CHILD'S LEARNING AND COMMUNICATION CAPABILITIES

Lifestyle
Affective learning ability
Attention span
Comprehensive language
Cognitive learning ability
Current knowledge
Learning style
Psychomotor learning ability

LEVELS OF COMMUNICATION

Not every conversation you engage in has the same depth level, nor should it. Throughout the day, a person may use as many as five levels, from clichés to peak communication.

The First Level: Cliché Conversation

Cliché conversation is pleasant chatting or comments such as "Have a nice day" between people who do not intend for their relationship to extend beyond a superficial level. It is important when meeting a child for the first time that you introduce yourself not only with your name but also with your position and function (e.g., "I'm a student nurse who is going to take care of you"; "I'm a nurse who will be visiting you in your home"). This information leads the family to move the conversation from the cliché level to a more meaningful one.

The Second Level: Fact Reporting

Fact reporting is simply stating facts about oneself (a child says, "I'm 12; I'm in sixth grade"). Fact reporting is necessary for you to understand children, but it does not tell you anything about their feelings or needs. Children can move from this level to a higher level of communication only when they feel they can trust you with more information.

The Third Level: Shared Personal Ideas and Judgments

When children know you well, they are able to share ideas such as "I always wanted to be an astronaut" and judgments such as "This is too hard for me." This level of communication exposes them to a loss of self-esteem if their views are not respected. It is the level that is the beginning of therapeutic interactions.

The Fourth Level: Shared Feelings

It is difficult to share feelings until you truly trust another person because feelings are fragile concepts, easily destroyed and crushed by inept or uncaring comments. Listen carefully for an expression of feeling from children such as "I hate always being sick." These admissions are telling you much more than how a child feels today; they represent trust in you and the depth of the relationship the child has established with you.

The Fifth Level: Peak Communication

The fifth level of communication is a sense of oneness, or being able to know what the other person is experiencing without any words being voiced. It sometimes occurs spontaneously in high-intensity situations but generally arises out of long-term relationships.

NONVERBAL COMMUNICATION

Nonverbal communication, such as wrinkling the nose, can be especially important in areas such as intensive care units when a child may be unable to speak because of endotracheal tubes and ventilators. Nonverbal communication can be expressed in a number of ways.

General Appearance

Children who have high self-esteem tend to maintain good body hygiene and care about their appearance. Those who are depressed may not feel the effort involved in grooming is worthwhile. Personal hygiene varies, however, and it is difficult to assess on your first contact with a child. What you see as ill-kempt may be neat and trim for that particular child; what you think of as well groomed may be comparatively sloppy for the child on that day.

Be aware that your impression of how children look or dress registers very strongly in your subconscious. Do not let an unconscious dislike for something such as body piercings or tattoos cause you to draw back. Preparing to give nursing care is not the same kind of activity as evaluating whether you wish to invite that person to dinner.

Body Posture and Gait

Children who feel good about themselves usually assume an upright body posture and walk rapidly, and surely, those who are depressed or insecure tend to slouch and move more timidly, and those who are threatened tend to either draw back or act aggressively. Children who are in agreement with you usually maintain eye contact with you as you speak to them. Very depressed or insecure children do not do that (they feel too inferior), nor do children who are very angry. Remember that children from some cultures may not meet your gaze because it is not culturally appropriate (Box 35.3).

Humor

Some people have a natural knack for finding humor in any situation; others do not instinctively have this quality and so must cultivate it. Those who can laugh at their own mistakes are usually enjoyable people to have around because their laughter at themselves suggests, when you make a mistake, they will be able to accept it the same way (or at least not be angry about it).

Be careful of the use of humor with children, however, because they are usually school age before they appreciate most adult jokes. If they are fatigued or ill, they may be looking

BOX 35.3

Nursing Care Planning to Respect Cultural Diversity

Cultural differences between a teacher and a learner can complicate techniques of health teaching and the evaluation of its effectiveness. Even when language is not a barrier, the way children show they are listening or comprehending may vary from culture to culture. Looking directly at a speaker, for example, is considered disrespectful in some Asian countries. The "Ok" sign traditional in the United States can be interpreted as vulgar, not positive, in Spain. In South Africa and some Middle Eastern countries, a "thumbs up" sign is insulting. In India, the way people move their head to express yes and no can be opposite to those used in the United States. A hand raised in a "stop" position may not be interpreted as halt by a child from a Middle Eastern culture but as a "go ahead" direction.

Being aware of these cultural differences is important when planning health teaching for diverse cultural groups so neither teaching nor reactions to teaching are misinterpreted.

for a support person to be with them more than one who is amusing. You can often measure the fall in a child's anxiety after a procedure by noting the first time the child responds to you with a humorous statement. Remember, though, laughter and joking can also be signs of increasing anxiety. Ascertain whether a child really finds a situation amusing or would rather have a serious caregiver.

Drawings

A useful nonverbal technique to learn how children feel about a frightening experience is to ask them to draw a picture of what happened or a picture of themselves. A child hospitalized for heart surgery, for example, might draw her heart prominently. She's revealing that she realizes she cannot survive if something happens to such an important body part.

A child's use of color may be a clue as to mood (happy children tend to use bright colors; depressed children use black or dark colors). A child with high self-esteem usually fills the full page with a drawing; one with less self-esteem crowds a drawing into a corner. These observations are quite variable, however, as a child may have had only a black crayon with which to color or may be saving the rest of the paper for a second drawing.

Music

The type of music to which children listen often also conveys their mood. The better they feel about themselves, the more likely they are to choose lively music; if they are sad, they often choose a quieter, more comforting type. Children enjoy repetition, however, and so may play the same music over and over, independent of their mood.

TECHNIQUES TO ENCOURAGE THERAPEUTIC COMMUNICATION

Several techniques are effective at deepening communication patterns and relationships. These techniques can be learned if they are not a spontaneous part of your present communication pattern (Avegno & DeBlieux, 2013).

Distance

Although it is affected by cultural and personal variables, the distance at which you position yourself from the person you are talking to can indicate your feelings or the type of conversation you want to initiate. People generally consider the space directly surrounding them (up to 18 in.) as *intimate* space to be crossed only by people who know them well or with whom they are comfortable having close body contact. Those from Middle Eastern cultures may define a wider space as intimate space than those from Western cultures. Sometimes, you will notice, in a heated discussion, one person moves aggressively into this space; the other will automatically step back to protect it. People in elevators usually separate themselves from others by this much space if the car is not full.

Whenever you touch a child, you violate intimate space, so always tell them when you are about to touch them ("I'm going change your bandage now"). If a child agrees to let you enter this space, it means they see you as safe, protective, and helpful.

The space between 18 in. to 4 ft is sensed by most people as *personal* space. This is the distance people usually stand apart from each other for casual conversation or hand shaking. When you stand by the side of a crib or bed or sit next to a person at home, you are within this space. It is a concerned, I-care-about-you distance but does not invade intimate space.

The distance between 4 ft and 12 ft is *social* space, the usual distance used to conduct business or to teach a class. Conversation spoken at this distance is readily heard by others. Do not use social space to ask a personal question. If you ask a child, "How are you feeling?" as you pass by in a hallway, for example, the child will probably answer, "Fine, thank you," a programmed reply almost everyone is taught in early childhood. In contrast, if you ask that same question from a personal or intimate distance, in a more private setting, the answer might be, "I'm scared I'm never going home again."

Although it is carried out miles apart, most people perceive texting, speaking on the telephone, or using mail or e-mail as either social or personal space. The tone of voice or the words used help to differentiate which area it appears to be. A message such as "Have I got news for you!" suggests social space. "Can you keep a secret?" brings it into personal space.

The distance beyond 12 ft is *public* space. To communicate from this distance, you need to shout and privacy is not respected. Waving to a friend in a hallway or across a parking lot is an example of public space communication.

QSEN Checkpoint Question 35.1

PATIENT-CENTERED CARE

The nurse wants to review some health educational materials with Barry, age 16 years. To maximize his learning and his comfort level, this activity should take place in which type of physical space?
   a. Intimate space
   b. Social space
   c. Public space
   d. Personal space

Look in Appendix A for the best answer and rationale.

Genuineness and Truthfulness

Genuineness is a quality of projecting sincerity or being yourself. Children can have difficulty trusting you and therefore may be unable to move to a deep relationship with you if you change your behavior from one day to the next, such as from maximum patience one day to short-tempered the next, because this causes them to have to spend energy testing to see who you are on that particular day. The way to achieve a feeling of genuineness is being true to yourself, not trying to be what you are not, as the insecurity that comes from pretending can manifest itself as negative feelings such as aggressiveness or a bored attitude.

Warmth

Warmth is an innate quality some people manifest more spontaneously than others. Basic ways in which warmth is demonstrated are direct eye contact, use of a gentle tone of voice, listening attentively, approaching a child within a comfortable space of 1 to 4 ft, and using touch appropriately. Warmth is a quality you display best when you know

another person well. Therefore, any action that helps you to know a person better (e.g., taking a health history, talking about school or family or how a child feels about the present situation) not only lets you plan care but also allows you to become increasingly comfortable with the child and creates opportunities to deepen the warmth of your relationship.

Empathy

Empathy is the ability to put yourself in another person's place and understand and be sensitive to the feelings of another (DalSanto, Pohl, Saiani, et al., 2014). People who are capable of empathy are the best support people because they can anticipate a child's reactions or fears. Feeling empathy is emotionally draining because when you assume another person's emotions, you experience them at the same depth as that person. Nurses who are capable of empathy need to surround themselves with good support people so they have refueling resources when they need them.

Gestures

Children vary a great deal in the gestures they use to accompany their spoken words. Although gestures are culturally influenced, it is also an individual trait. Be careful not to assess emotion only by a child's gestures. Some children wave their arms wildly describing an everyday occurrence; others would use that degree of expression only when in extreme distress. Be aware also that your own gestures are not always read well by children. A verbal statement that you approve of something is contradicted by placing your arms across your chest in a disapproving, stern manner.

Facial Expressions

Facial expressions are an important accompanying gesture to words. Clenched teeth, frowns, and smiles are easily interpreted by most people. The degree of pain a child is experiencing may be more evident by distressed facial expressions than words. Your approval or disapproval of an action may be more evident in your face than in your words.

Touch

Touch is the most intimate and meaningful of nonverbal techniques. When words are inadequate, touch rarely is. Learn to use touch such as clapping a child's shoulder or squeezing a hand to accompany reassuring words or in place of words as a strong support signal (e.g., I'm here; I understand; it's all right to be afraid). Be aware, however, some children enjoy being touched more than others. Due to individual preferences or cultural variations, some children are not used to being touched or hugged. Assess individually for the appropriateness of using touch.

Attentive Listening

No one likes to talk to someone who does not appear to be listening or responding. Good listening, therefore, like speaking, is not passive but active. Be aware your posture reveals to a great extent whether you are listening (e.g., sitting, not standing, to convey you are not on the run; leaning forward, not backward; stooping to meet a child's level). Nodding, maintaining eye contact, and stopping all other activities are strong indicators you are attuned to what is being said. Making it clear you are attentively listening indicates you value what the other person is saying. Children who feel valued are much more likely to confide feelings and concerns than those who sense you do not consider them important.

In some instances, it is necessary to repeat a part of what a child said, interject an appropriate "uh-huh" or "m-m-m," or make a direct statement ("I'm listening. Go on") to indicate you are listening. Be certain, when you are listening to the 20th child on any given day, you do not exhibit "end-of-the-day" behavior. To be therapeutic, you have to give everyone's concerns the same alert attention (Box 35.4).

Reflecting

Reflecting is a technique, like attentive listening, that is so simple that its importance is easy to discount. Reflecting is restating the last word or phrase a child has said when there is a pause in the communication. A child says, "I'm worried," and then stops. You repeat the last word. "Worried?" The child, assured you are listening and interested, will generally enlarge on the first statement: "I'm worried I'll be too short of breath to make the football team this year." In contrast, adolescents may not respond well to reflection; they may interpret it as imitating them, not seeking information.

Clarifying

Clarifying consists of repeating statements others have made so you can be certain you understood them. This is particularly helpful if a child has been describing a set of symptoms or series of actions. A statement such as "Let me see if I understand this. You said you always get the pain first

in your stomach. Then, it spreads to your chest" clarifies or makes clear what you have heard. If you are not quoting correctly, the child will interrupt and restate the problem: "No, the chest pain comes first."

Paraphrasing

Paraphrasing is restating what the child has said not only to assure the child you have heard correctly (as in clarifying) but also to help the child explain a thought. In clarifying, you repeat a child's exact words; in paraphrasing, you retain the meaning of the words but repeat them in a clearer or more condensed form. The child says, for example, "I don't talk about my problems with my parents." A paraphrasing statement might be, "You're telling me you and your parents haven't discussed home care. Is that right?" When paraphrasing, ask for confirmation your interpretation is correct; otherwise, you may find yourself putting words in children's mouths.

When the topic is embarrassing or emotionally charged (e.g., an adolescent discussing sexual orientation), the child might use such vague terms that the explanation becomes difficult to follow. Paraphrasing using basic terms would let him or her know not only that you understand him but also that if he or she can describe the problem better with such words than with medical terminology, it is all right to do that.

Perception Checking

Perception checking documents a feeling or emotion reported to you. This makes it a step deeper than paraphrasing. In paraphrasing, you document a statement or fact; in perception checking, you document a feeling or emotion. The child says for the second time, "I'm not at all worried about surgery. I mean, what could happen?" You say, "You're telling me you're not worried, but the number of times you've said it makes me wonder if you really are worried. Are you?"

Always ask for validation that your perception is correct so you do not make false assumptions. Perception checking is helpful because, as a rule, children are not ready to deal with emotions until they can admit they are experiencing them. When you bring an emotion out in this way, it allows them to confront it and deal with it for the first time. They may also lose their reluctance to admit other worries because you have implied worrying is acceptable.

What If . . . 35.1

Because Barry Sandoz's family has hypercholesterolemia, Barry, 16 years old, needs to begin a low-cholesterol diet. He needs to learn more about foods so he can eat safely in the school cafeteria. The nurse determines it is most important to provide patient education about Barry's diet to which person? Barry? His mother who prepares his food? Or his father who does the grocery shopping?

Focusing

Focusing helps children to center on a subject you suspect is causing them anxiety because they comment about it indirectly or else completely avoid it. It is done by repeating something they said ("You mentioned you feel tired all the time") or by mentioning the avoided topic ("You haven't said a word about how you feel about this surgery"). Once a

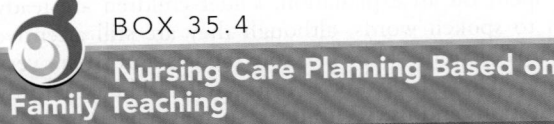

BOX 35.4
Nursing Care Planning Based on Family Teaching

LISTENING TO CHILDREN

Q. Barry's mother says to you, "My son always tells me I don't listen to him. How can I be a better listener?"

A. Try the following tips:

1. Stop talking. You cannot listen if you are talking.
2. Look and act interested. Don't read or write while he talks. Listen to understand rather than to reply.
3. Remove distractions. Do not doodle, tap, or shuffle papers. Turn off the television or put down your cell phone.
4. Empathize. Try to put yourself in your child's place so you can appreciate his point of view.
5. Be patient. Allow plenty of time. Do not interrupt. Do not edge toward the door as if you're about to walk away.
6. Hold your temper, argument, or criticism. An angry person can easily misinterpret the meaning of words.
7. Ask questions. This is proof that you have been listening.
8. Stop talking. This is the first and last suggestion, because all others depend on it.

subject is brought up for discussion, most children respond to it. As long as it can be avoided, however, they do not have to face the problem and won't begin to solve it.

Supportive Statements

Supportive statements let children know you accept their behavior or at least appreciate they have dealt well with unfortunate circumstances. For example, an adolescent says, "My girlfriend dumped me while I've been here in the hospital." Such a statement deserves a supportive reply such as "That must not feel good." The adolescent will take this response to mean you want to discuss the topic and, encouraged by your support, may elaborate on it because it still affects him.

Silence

If you ask a question and a child does not respond immediately, it is natural to ask another question or perhaps change the subject, assuming the child is not interested in the topic. This is a social custom that prevents you from putting someone into the awkward position of having to discuss a sensitive topic. Silence, however, can be an effective therapeutic technique. If you ask an emotion-laden question (e.g., "Are you worried?") and the child does not answer immediately, allow a period of silence to pass. Because you do not hurry to fill in the silence, the child is likely to respond (by hurrying an answer). When this happens, the answer is usually spontaneous and often open and uninhibited. In other instances, a child may answer the question deliberately and cautiously and, because you have provided a period of time to answer, may offer additional information.

Do not overdo silence, however, either by the number of times you use it or the length of time you allow it to extend. In this era of constant noise, many individuals are extremely uncomfortable with silence. Too much silence can also indicate to a child that you are not interested enough to maintain the conversation.

Process Recording

Process recording is a method to examine how effective you are at therapeutic communication. After your next interaction with a child, draw three columns on a sheet of paper. Take a few minutes to write down in the left column a statement the child made to you. In the middle column, write what you thought on hearing the statement. In a third column, write your response. Try to record both statements and responses verbatim or as close to the actual words used as possible. The average person can accurately recall about 3 minutes of communication this way.

Next, examine your responses to each statement by asking: Did I encourage the child to tell me more by my response, or did I block communication? Were my responses supportive, critical, or trite? Did I check perceptions, or did I just assume I understood correctly what was told to me? See Box 35.5 for an example of a process recording with an adolescent.

QSEN Checkpoint Question 35.2

INFORMATICS

The nurse has heard from a colleague that Barry, 16 years old, hates school. When considering the use of informatics to respond to this statement, which principle should guide the nurse's actions?
a. Communication is most effective when it is enhanced by cutting-edge technology.
b. Referral to an appropriate, evidence-based website can likely resolve this issue.
c. Technology cannot usually substitute for skilled interpersonal communication.
d. Communication skills are being replaced by technologic innovation in nursing.

Look in Appendix A for the best answer and rationale.

FACTORS THAT CAN INTERFERE WITH EFFECTIVE COMMUNICATION

Because so much of nursing care is influenced by verbal communication, it is important to avoid miscalculations in communication and to recognize common situations in which meanings can easily be distorted.

Age and Developmental Level

Age and developmental levels are important to communication abilities because they influence vocabulary and reading ability so greatly. Newborns and infants are amazingly perceptive regarding nonverbal communication. They quiet readily at a gentle tone of voice, and they show discomfort if an adult shouts or handles them roughly. Toddlers and preschoolers remain just as adept at reading nonverbal communication signals. They much prefer a happy approach (e.g., "Isn't this fun?") rather than a stern one. Because of their short attention span, their concentration wanders after about 5 minutes of time spent on an explanation. Older children are ready to listen to spoken words, although they are still attentive to nonverbal actions. They like role models and so are very opposed to "Do as I say, not as I do" advice. They are ready to ask questions and use techniques, such as reflection, to be certain they understand what you have just said.

Intellectual or Behavioral Level

Intellectual level, like age, affects vocabulary and ability both to encode and decode messages. It influences the number of languages a child speaks, reading ability, and the depth of explanation a child is capable of understanding. Children with cognitive challenges or autism spectrum disorder can have difficulty both receiving and transmitting messages (Bal, Katz, Bishop, et al., 2016)

Physical Factors

Physical factors, such as speech impairments and hearing or vision challenges, interfere with the transmission and reception of messages (Harris & Lord, 2016). When children are distracted by such sensations as fatigue or pain, they also may have a reduced ability to transmit or receive messages correctly.

Technical Terminology

Adults have heard common medical words and so usually have little difficulty understanding an explanation of one. Children, in contrast, have not heard many medical words. Listen to the

BOX 35.5

A Process Recording

The following is a record of an interaction between a nursing student and Barry Sandoz, a 16-year-old who is hospitalized. Barry has been diagnosed as having a recurrent peptic ulcer.

What Patient Said and Did	What I Thought and Felt	What I Said and Did
	I felt anxious meeting a new patient, although I thought he'd be friendly because he was so close to my own age.	I walked into his room and said, "Good morning."
He was sitting up in bed holding his hands on his abdomen. He asked, "When are you going to get me my purple pill?"	I felt attacked. As if he thought I should have done something sooner, but I had just arrived.	I asked, "What kind of pain are you having?"
He said, "Hydrochloric acid is carving a hole in my stomach lining. Is that enough explanation?"	I felt angry he insisted on putting me down so.	I said, "It certainly is," and left to find my instructor. I returned in 15 minutes with omeprazole (Prilosec) (his "purple pill").
He asked, "Did you have to take so long to do that?"	I was getting really angry at his threatening tone.	I checked his ID band and handed him the pill. I asked him, "Are you always so demanding?"
He turned on his side so his back was to me, clenched his teeth, and pushed his hands into his abdomen again.	I realized my criticism was unfair because he was in pain. But it was too late to take it back.	I said, "I'm sorry. I know you're uncomfortable."
He said, "Hand me that book on the chair over there before you leave, will you? If I don't get to it today, I might as well cash it in."	Getting angry again but also "hearing" what he had said for the first time.	I said, "Cash it in?"
He said, "I can't go back to school with pain like this. If I don't get better soon, I'll fail out."	I was surprised how one quick response on my part had brought out so much emotion. I also knew I was in over my head again (but in a good way).	

EVALUATION

My overall interaction with Barry would have been better if I hadn't been caught so off guard in the beginning by assuming he was going to be someone who had a lot in common with me (student–student, close age group). His initial response to me seemed so much more intense because I had stereotyped him that way.

In the final interaction, I was so concerned with my own needs (to get my work done); I completely missed why a book would be important to him. Fortunately, at the last minute, I got my mind off my problem and onto his and was able to produce a therapeutic response for him. He shouldn't have had to describe something with the impact of driving a truck over me before he caught my attention, though. Better listening (and thinking while I'm listening) would make me hear better and be more helpful sooner in this type of interaction.

---

explanations you give them to be certain they understand the concepts. You may want to ask yourself if you would have understood terms such as "lung rales" or "colostomy" at their age.

Showing Disapproval

Parents and children do not come for health care to be criticized; they come to learn more about how to stay well or how to recover from an illness. If you criticize them, they may not reveal any further information to you because they do not want you to react in the same way you did to their preliminary statements.

Be aware that nonverbal disapproval signs (e.g., frowning, sighing) can be just as disapproving as spoken words. On the other hand, this does not mean you should show approval of wrong actions. Merely listen to them with no action or

comment and make a mental note. At the end of your interaction, introduce the change in behavior you'd like to see (e.g., "Let's plan some ways you can include more calcium in your meals every day").

Not Showing Approval When Warranted

Every student has had the experience of completing a difficult assignment and receiving only criticism from a teacher (i.e., no other comments that, aside from the part that was not satisfactory, the rest of the assignment was well done). This happens because the instructor assumed the student would do a good job; no reward was given for meeting minimum criteria. From the other side of the desk, however, it would have been satisfying—and would have offered motivation to continue to do well—to have heard the words "good job."

When discussing healthcare problems with children, it is easy to forget what you accept as standard behavior may take a great deal of effort for an ill child to accomplish, such as coughing and deep breathing after surgery. Giving children praise for what they do well encourages them to continue what they're doing and to try more advanced things. If a topic is difficult for them to talk about, saying you realize it is a sensitive topic may help them continue to discuss it.

Growing Defensive

In the same way children who request health care do not enjoy being criticized, neither does the average healthcare provider. If a child makes a critical remark, therefore, it is easy to respond with a defensive or protective comment rather than a therapeutic one. An adolescent might say, for example, "We have to wait so long here; this is a really dumb clinic." It is easy to reply, "Don't say that. This is a good clinic." This type of response implies any complaint is out of line. Try to respond instead with a supportive comment such as "I know it makes a long day for you." No healthcare agency is so good that there is nothing to criticize.

Cliché Advice

Cliché advice (i.e., advice given from a formula, not individualized to the situation) is meaningless because it is too general to be helpful. Statements such as "Rome wasn't built in a day" and "You have to walk before you can run" are examples of this kind of advice. Use it guardedly because children consider their problem unique and resent being given advice that could apply to anyone.

Topping Up

"Topping up" is minimizing a child's views by telling a better story. A child tells you, for example, she has a problem. You say, "You want to know what problems really are? Come and work here." This implies that their problems are inconsequential, at least in respect to yours. They will not be likely to tell you any more about themselves after such a response.

COMMUNICATION SITUATIONS THAT REQUIRE UNIQUE SKILLS

Some communication situations require special skills in addition to the usual therapeutic communication techniques to promote understanding.

The Shy Child

Shy children, as a rule, have much more difficulty talking to people they meet for the first time and establishing peer relationships than others (Coplan, Rose-Krasnor, Weeks, et al., 2013). A reluctance to express their needs to others can leave their needs unrecognized and unmet. If they do not give you much verbal feedback, it's easy to believe they do not have a concern. That leaves them without support people when they most need them.

Fortunately, in most instances, once children know you and realize they can trust you, shyness fades. A therapeutic response, therefore, would be to not leave them alone but to maintain an active relationship despite the lack of feedback. This does not necessarily involve talking to the child but may involve checking on them frequently, remaining in the room while their primary healthcare provider completes an examination, helping secure the adhesive strip after a technician obtains a blood sample, or sitting with them for a few minutes while a medication takes effect.

The Angry Child

All children grow angry at some time, although boys may express anger more openly than girls (Olino, Durbin, Klein, et al., 2013). They also express it differently, using more controlled than uncontrolled responses (Sears, Repetti, Reynolds, et al., 2014). It is difficult to work with angry children because you may feel yourself being pulled into their anger. The typical response at hearing an angry outburst is to imitate it (e.g., a child is radiating anger as tight-lipped silence, so you say nothing as well; a child shouts at you, and you shout back). This is not therapeutic, however, so make a point of not allowing yourself to be drawn into children's anger. At the same time, acknowledge that it is all right to be angry (e.g., "I understand that you're angry but please don't shout"). Help them to focus their anger if at all possible, so they can better identify why they are angry and can begin to deal with it.

To encourage focusing, ask children to detail why they are angry. An adolescent who says he is angry at the entire healthcare delivery system, for example, may be feeling highly frustrated because he cannot begin to fight a huge bureaucracy. Establishing what he is really angry about is one nursing action that can build a base for resolving the problem. If a child uses silence as a method of maintaining anger, suggesting possible reasons for the anger can be helpful (e.g., "I know your mother was just talking to you. Are you angry about something she said?" or "I know you were asking about crutch walking before. Does it have something to do with that?"). Once the subject is out in the open, few children can resist describing the extent of or the reason for their anger. Be aware, too, that when you ask someone to explain why he or she is angry, you ask for all the emotion and all the distress that goes with it to be expressed as well. Even if you are the object of the anger, at that point, you are committed to listening to the child's views. Keep anger from affecting you by reacting to the explanation, not the tone or force of it. Keep any response on your part a tone gentler and quieter than that used toward you.

The Demanding Child

Nursing has few equals in job satisfaction (provided salary and other working conditions are adequate) because the majority of people you care for are grateful for what you do for them. It can be upsetting, therefore, to discover a particular child who is not grateful for or even satisfied with anything you do. This type of child is easy to back away from or avoid.

Demanding behavior generally stems from insecurity or fear (e.g., they're so afraid something will happen to them while you are out of the room they constantly find reasons to keep you in the room; they're so afraid of unplanned events they structure things so nothing unexpected can happen). Give more of yourself, not less, to counteract this response. When you have proven you are dependably there for them, children do not feel so insecure, and the need to be demanding usually fades. Withdrawing from them has the opposite effect if it increases the child's insecurity and the demanding behavior. Ask, "Is there anything else I can do for you?" instead of "Haven't I already done enough?"

The Bullying or Sexually Aggressive Adolescent

Both bullying and sexually aggressive behavior can cause friction in a nurse/child relationship (Espelage, Basile, De La Rue, et al., 2015). As these are similar behaviors, they both probably stem from the same cause as demanding behavior: insecurity. Aggression can be manifested as telling unwelcome, off-color jokes or participating in inappropriate physical touching. This may be most pronounced in adolescents who worry that their illness or surgery will interfere with sexual function. Adolescents with this degree of insecurity may benefit from counseling to help them channel coping responses into more socially acceptable behaviors. Be certain they have factual information as to the extent or effect of their illness. Set limits, as necessary, to make giving care acceptable to you. Always censor the action, not the adolescent. Be aware sexually aggressive behavior can occur with both males and females.

The Child Who Is Not Proficient in English

It is not unusual in any nursing care setting to encounter children who have a different primary language from yours; in other instances, a child's speech may be limited or difficult to understand because of an accent, dialect, or speech impairment. Still, other children may speak your language but their use of words is so different from yours the words appear to have different meanings (Kirk, Prusick, French, et al., 2012). Most children who speak another language have a support person who can serve as an interpreter. Anticipate the instructions you will need to give the child (e.g., cough, breathe deeply, save urine) and ask the interpreter to write them out in the child's language for when the interpreter may not be present. Post them conspicuously in the room or in the child's care plan so everyone giving care can be familiar with them.

Most healthcare facilities have a list of people who serve as translators as needed. Generally, you can contact such a person by telephone to ask for a specific word you want to know. If you have to give instructions and no translator is present, do not be self-conscious about using hand gestures or drawing a picture to express the action you want the child to perform (e.g., a child lying in bed, an arrow pointing to a chair, and a child sitting in a chair for, "I'm going to help you get out of bed."). Allow children ample paper to draw pictures to show you what they want you to know. Supply pictures for preschool children so they can select the one that applies.

Everyone has a tendency to shout at children who speak a different language as if loudness will increase understanding; try to avoid this. When using an interpreter, be certain to speak slowly and use common words that can be translated literally (e.g., "I need to stick Mary's arm for blood" could be interpreted literally to mean putting a stick in the child's arm).

The Unconscious Child

Be aware that because a child is unconscious, it does not mean he or she cannot hear (Tapson, Sierotowicz, Marks-Maran, et al., 2015). This means you always need to be aware that children who do not respond to you may still be able to hear and interpret anything you say. Never say anything to unconscious children or within their hearing you would not say if they were fully alert. Continue to use nonverbal communication such as touch to help convey a message.

The Child With Hearing Impairment

It's difficult for children with hearing impairment to enunciate words clearly because they're not aware the sounds they are forming are not clear (Lund & Douglas, 2016). When communicating with children with hearing impairment, check whether they use a hearing aid; if so, be certain it is turned on. Face them when you speak so they can follow your lip movements. Use hand gestures as necessary to convey your message, or write out instructions. If you have difficulty understanding what they are trying to say, ask them to write it down if they're old enough. Use common sense about how loud to raise your voice to facilitate communication. As a rule, at the point privacy is lost, it is time to resort to written words or sign language. Children who use sign language to communicate have a right to have an interpreter present to facilitate communication, the same as children who do not use English as their primary language.

The Child With Vision Impairment

Children with vision impairment are capable of understanding spoken instructions well if the instruction does not require an accompanying visual image such as "Take a piece of gauze about this long" (you then indicate the length with your hand) (McLinden & McCall, 2016). Never touch children who cannot see you without asking their permission or warning them first so you do not startle them.

Health Teaching in a Changing Healthcare Environment

In the past, when children were admitted to hospitals well in advance of surgery and then remained in the hospital after surgery or therapy until they were almost totally well, there was a wide window of time for health teaching. Today, when surgery is often a 1-day experience, the window for teaching is narrowed to hours (Farber, Curie, Brown, et al., 2015). This means that nurses must use more creative approaches to achieve the same health education results. Discharge instructions must also be quickly explained, requiring both verbal and written approaches (Wu, Tyler, Logsdon, et al., 2016).

Children's sophistication about learning techniques has also changed. Because children today are exposed to such a rich diet of clever animation on TV or in movies, a simple lecture on good nutrition can seem dull and uninteresting. Children who are adept at arcade or electronic games, where dexterity is a requirement, may no longer find handling a syringe or a feeding tube a challenging feat. Before beginning health teaching, assess each child to find out what he or she expects to learn, to identify individual learning styles, and to determine what teaching techniques would best suit the individual child.

THE ART OF TEACHING

Teaching is more than presenting information; it is presenting information to increase someone's knowledge or insight. Before teaching can be considered effective, learning has to have occurred. Conversely, before learning occurs, teaching must have been present in some form. Common principles of teaching are summarized in Table 35.1.

TABLE 35.1 PRINCIPLES OF TEACHING

Principle	Rationale
Know the subject.	To effectively teach children, you must be able to not only present material but also answer questions about it. Children's questions can be as probing as an adult's, and they can often be more frequent because children are used to asking questions of a teacher or a parent.
Know the audience.	Children vary a great deal in cognitive development depending on their age group. To teach preschoolers about oral health, you might choose to teach how to brush teeth using puppets as a teaching aid. The same clever puppet and tooth brushing presentation likely would not be well received by adolescents.
Know yourself.	Analyze which teaching techniques (e.g., lecture, role-playing, small group discussion, audiovisual aids) fit your teaching style. Using techniques that are comfortable allows teaching to be most effective.
Assess individual learning styles.	Most children respond well to visual images (e.g., a demonstration, a drawing) to complement learning. Assessing individual learning styles helps to meet each child's best way of learning.
Define expected outcomes.	Expected outcomes serve as guidelines to help you select from all you know about a subject that part which is most pertinent to an individual child. Outcomes should be realistic, measurable, and mutually established. Instructions on how to walk using crutches for an early school-age child might include how to carry school books while using crutches; for an adolescent, instruction might include how to board a city bus so he or she can get to and from a part-time job.
Provide an environment conducive for learning.	Children are easily distracted from learning. Divide material into segments to keep teaching sessions short; avoid competing factors such as television or mealtime.
Be consistent.	Nothing is more confusing to a person learning a new skill than to be told two different ways to do it. Choose one method you anticipate will work best for a child and then consistently stress that method. After a child has learned one method, you then could suggest alternative methods if the child is interested.
Recognize that actions teach as much as or sometimes more so than verbal statements.	Children watch facial expressions and nonverbal gestures as much as they listen. Be certain that a nonverbal statement is not contradicting a verbal one.
Teach from the simple to the complex.	Fundamentals must be grasped before advanced learning can proceed. Because many children have little idea of body anatomy, you often need to begin with the basics. When these are mastered, you can proceed to teach about more complicated aspects.
Teach principles.	Teaching children the principle behind a procedure makes the reason for the procedure make sense. This also allows children to modify and change to an alternative method as long as the principle is fulfilled.
Emphasize what the child should do; mention, but do not emphasize, what the child should not do.	Teaching from a positive standpoint makes learning more enjoyable. Because healthcare information should last a lifetime, thinking of it in a positive way makes it more applicable to lifetime use.
Include evaluation as a final step.	The only way to determine the effectiveness of teaching is to test or evaluate if learning has occurred. Structure the time and method of evaluation when first establishing a teaching plan.

The Teacher–Learner Relationship

Effective teaching and learning depend a great deal on the teacher–learner relationship because if such a relationship is based on mutual sharing, it empowers and motivates an individual to learn more readily than a relationship in which a teacher maintains ultimate control and authority. Finally, the teacher–learner relationship is best if it is interactive or the teacher and learner both actively participate in the process and modify the teaching plan as they learn from one another.

THE ART OF LEARNING

Learning is a two-step process involving both the acquisition of knowledge and a change in behavior based on the new knowledge. Learning has not really occurred unless the change in behavior is measurable. For example, a parent teaching a child about the need to brush teeth daily must not only elicit the child's statement that daily brushing is important but also see that the child is, in fact, brushing her teeth every day. Principles of effective learning are summarized in Table 35.2.

TYPES OF LEARNING

There are a number of different types of learning. For example, learning the mathematical formula necessary to change pounds to kilograms (i.e., a cognitive task) is different from learning how to fill a syringe (i.e., a psychomotor task). Learning to be

TABLE 35.2 PRINCIPLES OF LEARNING

Principle	Rationale
Learning occurs best when children are ready to learn.	Interferences with learning may be physical (e.g., pain, hunger) or psychological (e.g., fear, anxiety). The first time children are told that they must inject insulin daily, for example, they may be too anxious to learn about it.
Learning occurs most quickly if children can see how the new information will benefit them directly.	Sixteen-year-old children learn how to drive a car quickly because they readily grasp that being able to drive will immediately enlarge their world. Children are only ready to learn how to perform an insulin injection when they can see how it will benefit them.
Learning occurs best if rewards, not penalties, are offered.	Notice the amount of shoulder patting and back slapping high school coaches engage in (i.e., rewarding by praise). Giving positive reinforcement immediately like this makes it more effective than if such reinforcement is delayed. If you must criticize the way a task was done, first compliment children on some aspect they did well and then explain the part that needs improvement. This increases self-esteem and allows children to feel good enough about themselves that they can accept the criticism. Never be reluctant to praise in public; always criticize in private.
Children learn best by actively participating in learning.	Active participation requires involvement in learning. Ask questions to involve participation; allow children to touch and handle equipment to increase participation.
Learning occurs best in a nonstressful and accepting environment.	No one wants to take a chance redemonstrating a procedure or asking a question if they believe that actions or opinions will not be respected. People do learn from "top sergeants," but the learning experience has so many unpleasant memories attached to it that they may not retain the learning. Health teaching is too important to be presented in a way that will lead to it being quickly discarded.
Children learn best those things that hold a particular interest for them.	Most people have specific interests. A child with diabetes mellitus who enjoys dancing might be most interested in learning regulation of insulin for exercise. A child anxious to leave for college might be most interested in learning how to select a diabetic diet from a cafeteria.
Learning occurs best when ability plateaus are recognized.	Children learn to the point of saturation; learning and interest in learning halt at that point and do not continue until the material learned is thoroughly digested and understood. Wait until information is processed, and at that point, the child will be interested once more.

kind to a brother with a chronic illness is yet another type (i.e., an affective task). For best results, before you begin teaching, analyze the type of learning you want to see take place because this helps in setting goals and designing teaching strategies.

Cognitive Learning

Cognitive learning involves a change in the individual's level of understanding or knowledge (Barrouillet, 2015). Learning the principle behind why a particular medicine must be injected into a muscle, as opposed to subcutaneous tissue, is an example. Cognitive learning requires adequate development, intelligence, and attention span. It can be gained through exposure to any teaching technique but is usually learned through lecture, reading, and audiovisual aids. It's important for techniques for teaching when cognitive learning is the goal to be consistent with the learner's cognitive ability (Singer, 2012).

During the school-age years, learning capability is concrete (e.g., children have difficulty picturing body parts functioning unless they can actually see them doing this); during the adolescent years, it becomes possible to learn abstract concepts, so adolescents can accept that liver enzymes are released with liver damage even though they never see that occur (Piaget, 1952).

Psychomotor Learning

Psychomotor learning requires a change in a person's ability to perform a skill. Learning to hold a syringe, fill the syringe with medicine, and inject it into a muscle is an example of

psychomotor learning. Acquiring psychomotor skills depends on muscle and neurologic coordination. It is best mastered through demonstration and redemonstration.

Affective Learning

Affective learning involves a change in a person's attitude and is the most difficult area in which to bring about change. For example, to teach a child the reason for and the skill of giving a self-injection may be easy; teaching the child to *like* giving a self-injection may never be possible. The best goal accomplished could be that the child will *value* the procedure because it will prevent him from developing hyperglycemia. Affective learning is gained best though role modeling, roleplaying, or shared-experience discussion.

INFLUENCE OF AGE AND STAGE ON ABILITY TO LEARN

Learning ability varies a great deal depending on a child's stage of development and the past experiences the child has had in the specific area of learning.

The Infant

Infants learn by exploring the environment with their senses (i.e., psychomotor learning). They learn best from a primary caregiver because that is whom infants most want to please. Any healthcare points taught must be presented not as a structured activity but as a game or an amusing or attractive activity. For example, you could teach an infant to exercise a leg by hanging a ball next to his foot and encouraging the infant to kick it.

The Toddler

Toddlers are developing a sense of autonomy or learning to be independent (Erikson, 1993). That means, trying to teach toddlers a new activity such as eating a new food or brushing their teeth may be met with a sharp "No!" This retort does not mean the activity is unappealing to a child; however, only that the child is aware he does not have to do everything he is told to do. Toddlers also sometimes resist a change in routine because they need rituals to feel secure. If an activity will allow children to increase a level of independent functioning, they will usually learn it rapidly. Teaching activities such as exercise or deep breathing by having children imitate the action is an effective teaching method because it presents the activity as a game (i.e., there is nothing to be resisted). Parents can be instrumental in maintaining a new skill their child has learned by incorporating it into a daily routine or a ritual.

The Preschooler

Preschool children are interested in learning because developing a sense of initiative is the main developmental task of the period. Provided that instructions are geared to their small vocabularies, they "soak up" new methods of doing things. Because they are so imaginative and uninhibited, they have few reservations about the "right" way to do things. They watch a demonstration eagerly and freely redemonstrate a skill; they ask many questions about equipment and procedures. Keep explanations short and words simple; a preschooler's attention span rarely exceeds 5 minutes.

In terms of cognitive development, preschool children "center" or notice only one characteristic of an object. This can limit their ability to learn all aspects of care or more than one method of doing something on any one day (Piaget, 1952).

Preschoolers tend to be frightened of intrusive procedures such as rectal temperature taking, bladder catheterization, or nasopharyngeal suction. They typically remove adhesive bandages minutes after application to check on the condition of their skin underneath (that it has not disappeared); they worry any blood removed may be the last they have. Teaching this type of procedure or explaining to children why it is necessary calls for clear explanations and praise for learning. Use dolls or puppets to help children visualize details whenever possible because pointing to a place on a puppet's body is not as intrusive as pointing to the child's own body (Fig. 35.2 and Box 35.6).

The School-Age Child

School-age children enjoy short projects that offer an immediate reward. Therefore, they learn best if a procedure is broken down into different stages and presented as separate short steps. Because they enjoy games, playing "Simon Says" may be an effective way to have school-age children learn deep breathing.

School-age children are used to learning things and accept learning a new procedure or new information as just another experience in a busy day. The "staying power" of school-age children is notoriously short; however, the ability to continue

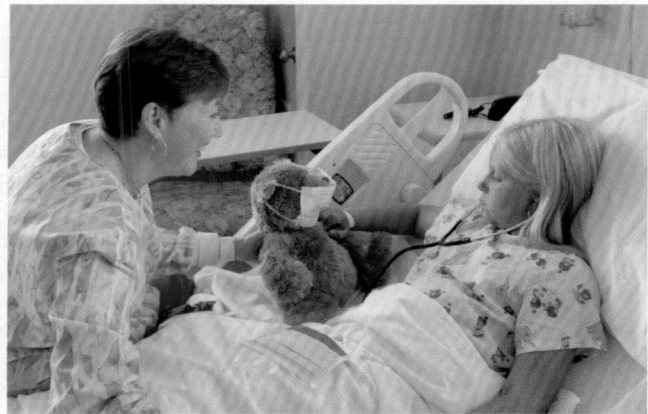

Figure 35.2 Teaching with dolls or toys can help to make an intrusive procedure seem less frightening for a preschooler.

to perform at the level taught tends to decrease sharply if learning is not reinforced. Be certain, therefore, that a support person in the home knows the healthcare information as well as the child so that person can reinforce it or carry out the procedure if necessary.

Toward the end of the school-age period, children become interested in doing only those things their friends are doing. Children may interpret as unreasonable, therefore, a request to do something after school (e.g., taking medication), whereas their friends are stopping at the playground or mall. Modify a teaching plan as necessary to help children fit what they must learn into their school and social schedule. Otherwise, the teaching may be very short lived.

As part of moral development, school-age children thrive on rules, or the "right way" to do things (Kohlberg, 1984).

BOX 35.6

Nursing Care Planning Tips for Effective Communication

Wolf Whitefeather is a 3-year-old boy scheduled for a syndactyly (webbed fingers) repair next week. You speak with him through a puppet at a clinic visit to assess his understanding of the surgery.

Tip: It is important to ask children about what they expect to have happen during surgery.

Nurse: Hello. I'm Nancy Nurse. Could you tell me what the little boy named Wolf is going to have done in surgery?

Wolf: His fingers got sick when he was born.

Nurse: When is he going to have them fixed?

Wolf: The day after we go to church.

Nurse: Is his surgery going to hurt?

Wolf: No. His fingers are going to be asleep.

Nurse: Will he have a big bandage afterward?

Wolf: So big he can't see how his fingers got cut off.

Nurse: Cut off?

Wolf: That's what happens to bad kids.

This means that if two or more people are going to be involved in teaching, they must be consistent in their approach because it is frustrating for school-age children to not have a "right way" to do something. Parents who have been supervising their child's school learning through checking homework easily assume a role in supervising health learning also. Parents who haven't been previously monitoring learning may need support to fulfill this role.

The Adolescent

Adolescents, struggling for identity, like to learn things separately from their parents. As a rule, they can be responsible for their own self-care if they understand how the new action they have been taught will directly benefit them and, unlike school-age children, they will continue to carry out those actions conscientiously. Adolescents have a strong need to be exactly like their friends, however. This means they rarely continue any action that makes them different or conspicuous in front of their peers.

Remember, adolescents are also very present-oriented; they learn procedures and new information best if they can see how it will immediately benefit them. They learn poorly if the only benefit of new information presented to them is something that will affect them at some future date. Not rotating insulin injection sites, for example, will cause "pockmark" formations (*lipoatrophy*) in the skin by the time the child reaches adulthood. Given this information, adolescents tend not to rotate injection sites because the benefit is not relevant to them at that moment. An explanation such as "Rotating injection sites will ensure insulin absorption and allow you to play basketball this semester," which is an equally true statement, is a better adolescent motivator.

For the first time, adolescents are able to think abstractly or use scientific reasoning. This means they can create hypotheses ("what if" questions) and think through what will be the consequences of an action (Piaget, 1952). This allows them to understand the principle of what they are being taught and enforces the reason for the learning. Parents may find they are not as effective with teaching their child as they were when the child was younger. They may need to "step aside" and let you introduce a subject until a phase of adolescent rebellion passes.

QSEN Checkpoint Question 35.3

QUALITY IMPROVEMENT

The nurse wants Barry, age 16 years, to increase his cognitive understanding of his condition. After teaching sessions, which statement from him would best show that his cognitive knowledge has increased?

a. "I feel so much better now about the care I need."
b. "I understand I have to take two types of medicine."
c. "I've finally learned how to swallow big capsules."
d. "I hate having to take medicine but will take it."

Look in Appendix A for the best answer and rationale.

Developing and Implementing a Teaching Plan

A teaching plan is a design of the content to be taught, the teaching/learning techniques to be used, and the evaluation method and tools to be used.

ASSESSING TEACHING/LEARNING NEEDS

Designing a plan begins with assessment of the individual child's needs and how the new knowledge will meld with the child's and family's lifestyle, the child's intellectual and language level, current knowledge level, physical/cognitive capabilities, sociocultural values, and attention span.

FORMULATING THE PLAN

Formulating a teaching plan begins with establishing expected outcomes and techniques of teaching. It may need to include communication strategies for parents as well as children.

Identifying Personal Strengths and Limitations

When formulating a teaching plan, be honest about your capabilities. If you feel uncomfortable teaching a child about surgery with clever puppets dressed in scrub suits, it might be better to avoid that approach because, in the wrong hands, such a method can sound so flat or complicated a child is left feeling more confused than comforted by the presentation.

Some health teaching involves giving instructions in areas of care that may be personally embarrassing, such as instructing a member of the opposite sex how to obtain a clean-catch urine specimen. Proceeding blindly may not result in effective teaching because the child may be so embarrassed by your discomfort that concentrating on instructions becomes difficult. In doing this type of teaching (as in any contact with a child), nothing serves you as well as honesty. Admit to children you are not used to giving this type of instruction. This approach will probably evoke a response from children that they are not used to having anyone talk about it either. Once you have found common ground, you have formed a basis for effective health teaching. Honesty also allows a child to recognize your discomfort is not from lack of knowledge on the subject (i.e., the child can trust what is being said) and is also not the child's fault (the subject, not the child, is the disturbing factor).

Preparing Expected Outcomes

Planning outcomes is most effective when they are planned collaboratively with a child and family. They should reflect the type of learning desired: cognitive, psychomotor, or affective. They should help to establish both content and time guidelines based on both the child's cognitive ability to learn and the time frame available for teaching. It is unnecessary (and often overwhelming) for a child to learn everything about an illness in the first day or week after a diagnosis. Likewise, information on how to stay well does not need to be presented in one setting. In many instances, it is effective to teach only part of the information needed; another nurse in another setting, such as in an ambulatory clinic or in the child's home, can teach the remainder. For best results, state outcomes as behavioral objectives or as the activity the child is expected to demonstrate when the child has learned the new knowledge (i.e., not "Tim understands the importance of deep-breathing exercises daily" but "Tim does deep-breathing exercises daily").

Identifying Teaching Formats

Teaching techniques vary with the content to be covered, teacher/learner characteristics, and the environment for teaching.

Formal Versus Informal Teaching

Because both formal and informal teaching formats can be effective in health education, careful consideration is necessary to determine which format would be the best technique to use for a given situation. An example of formal teaching would be conducting a class on healthy eating as part of a health education course. An example of informal teaching would be explaining to a child who refuses to eat that he needs to at least drink something because, to get better, his body needs more fluids. Sometimes, informal teaching occurs so spontaneously, it is easy to be unaware it is happening. In response to a question such as "How long will I have to take this medicine?" If you answer "For 2 weeks," you are just answering a question. If you answer, "For 2 weeks because . . . ," you are health teaching.

Informal teaching, although communicated in a less structured way, requires the same teaching/learning principles as formal teaching—that is, knowing the subject, recognizing individual learning styles, providing an effective environment, and limiting time span. Table 35.3 lists suggestions for incorporating informal teaching into care.

Group Versus Individual Teaching

Although most health teaching with children is done on an individual basis, teaching groups of children can be effective in some situations. Individual instruction more directly addresses a child's unique needs; group teaching can add depth to learning as children share information within the group. For many children, learning they are not the only person with their particular problem is very important to hear. Listening to a peer discuss how to solve a problem may be more meaningful than hearing the same information explained by an adult. Peer learning, therefore, not only improves knowledge but may also improve the child's attitude and motivation to learn (Deibel & Wagner, 2013).

Important guidelines for group teaching include:
1. Assess for common interests and goals so the information presented will appeal to as many in the group as possible.
2. Be certain all members of the group can see and hear all others and you.
3. Encourage all members of the group to participate by calling on individual members if necessary; use a question such as "Juan, you've been quiet. What do you think about that?"
4. Limit any one person from dominating the group by a statement such as "That's a good point, Reneé. Has anyone else had a similar experience?"
5. Avoid competition in the group. No one is always right; no one is always wrong.
6. Ask group members to evaluate the experience afterward to be certain it met the group's needs.

TABLE 35.3 WAYS TO INCORPORATE INFORMAL TEACHING INTO NURSING CARE

Activity	Type of Teaching
Medication administration	Children as young as early school age should know the type, action, and any expected side effects of all medication they are taking. Present medicine not by saying "Here is your pill" but rather "Here is your [name of medication]. It should help your temperature come back to normal. After you take this, you might feel yourself start to sweat. That means it's working."
Vital sign measurement	When taking vital signs such as blood pressure, temperature, and pulse, tell children what normal levels are, such as "Your blood pressure is 100/70 mmHg. That's normal." If the child is in a high-risk category for hypertension, add some prevention measures to teaching.
Any procedure	Always tell children the purpose and principle of procedures. For instance, do not say "You need to drink a lot of fluid" but rather "You need to drink a lot of fluid because . . . "
Dressing changes	Dressing changes provide an opportunity to teach the danger of introducing infection into an open wound. The parents or child may not change this dressing, but they will apply bandages to small cuts in the future and so will benefit from teaching.
Mealtime	Provide information about nutrition, such as "I know you're not hungry enough to eat the entire sandwich, but could you try the meat? Meat is high in protein and that's important for healing."
Hygiene	Emphasize the necessity for covering the mouth with a shirt sleeve to prevent the spread of upper respiratory infections or good perineal hygiene (i.e., wiping front to back in girls) to decrease the possibility of urinary tract infections.
Physical assessment	Assure children that their body parts are healthy as you examine them (e.g., "Your hair feels squeaky clean and strong") as both education and reassurance. Explain the importance and technique of self-testicular examination.
Positioning	Don't just reposition children in bed. Teach the hazards of immobility and how a change of position and ambulation increases circulation and respiratory function.
Sleep	Teach that sleep is a healing therapy and so should not be considered a waste of time.
Bowel elimination	Teach children elimination patterns vary and that occasional variations in their elimination patterns are normal but stools should not be loose or black or painful.

Alternative Settings Versus Institutional Teaching

Health teaching in a healthcare agency usually focuses on immediate, acute care concerns. Teaching in a school may focus on topics such as basic health promotion and hygiene, reproductive and sex education, and drug abuse prevention. Teaching in the home may focus on medication regimens, dressing changes, or measures to prevent complications of a particular illness. It may also involve helping a child and parents adapt a procedure to the home setting, such as accommodating a wheelchair or oxygen therapy. Be certain parents know how to obtain the supplies they will need to learn and perform the procedure in the home.

Teaching in the home offers the advantage of being able to assess a child's environment, interactions with other family members, and overall family functioning. This may yield data that prove useful to further planning and implementation of care. It may also provide an opportunity to include other family members—siblings, grandparents, and so forth—in the teaching plan; this can strengthen the impact of teaching and ensure all family members understand the procedures in the same way. Always include evaluation as a step of teaching in all settings so you can feel confident that learning has occurred.

What If . . . 35.2

The nurse organizes a discussion group of adolescents on special diets so they can learn more about healthy nutrition in general. Barry, who needs to follow a low-cholesterol diet, says he won't participate in the group because nutrition is a "childish" subject. Would the nurse insist he come to the meetings, or take the extra time to teach good nutrition to Barry at his bedside?

Determining Teaching Strategies

Because children's knowledge base, capabilities, learning styles, and attention spans vary so much, teaching strategies are most effective when they are both intermixed and selected in response to the individual child to be taught. The more interactive the method, the more appealing it is apt to be.

Lecture

Lecture (or directly explaining information) is the most efficient and time-saving method of offering information to both individual children and to groups. A lecture, however, does not allow for much participation, and it is effective only in short, well-structured periods. It is rarely effective for children who are not yet school age.

Demonstration

Demonstration is actually performing a procedure, such as a dressing change or instillation of eye drops, so the child can clearly see how the procedure should be done. Do not demonstrate a procedure unless you have all the necessary equipment to do it. If you have to stop in the middle of a demonstration to say, "Be sure to use a sterile syringe, not what I'm using," the poor technique demonstrated may be the lesson learned, not the good technique. The purpose of demonstration is to show how the procedure is actually done; having to imagine steps is little different than reading about it. School-age children, because of their stage of cognitive development (i.e., concrete operations), learn best by demonstration.

Figure 35.3 A school-age child redemonstrates blood glucose monitoring.

Redemonstration

To determine whether a child has truly grasped a demonstration, ask the child to perform a **redemonstration**, or an exact imitation of the procedure (Fig. 35.3). This is best if it immediately follows demonstration. Praise the effort to redemonstrate even if the redemonstration was not of the quality desired. No one likes to be put on the spot, and children may be unwilling to expose themselves again by a second redemonstration if criticized. Children do not have to follow your motions exactly because there are many different ways to do almost everything as long as their technique accomplishes the same goal. An effective way to correct a wrong action is to say, "That's one way of doing that; you might find it easier, though, to . . . ." This type of criticism is nonthreatening because it acknowledges the child's effort in a positive way before offering a correction.

Discussion

Discussion is a shared learning experience in which children ask questions about particular concerns and you answer based on the child's individual circumstances. At the end of the discussion, hopefully all questions are answered and the problems are solved. The first time children are introduced to a subject, they tend to ask few questions because they do not know enough about the illness or health issue as yet to anticipate concerns. As their knowledge increases, so does their ability to project and modify information to fit their own lifestyle. Remember, children tend to think in the present: A problem that will arise once tomorrow is usually viewed as more important than one that can be predicted will arise repeatedly in years to come. Because this technique recognizes and respects their opinions, school-age children and adolescents enjoy discussion.

Role Modeling

Role modeling is demonstrating a certain attitude or behavior that you want a child to learn. Be certain when health teaching not only to present facts but also to radiate a positive role-modeling attitude because children pick up on role modeling cues as readily as a spoken message. Showing annoyance at getting a bubble out of a syringe demonstrates, for example, that giving injections is frustrating; showing a bored attitude toward nutrition implies eating well is boring.

Role modeling is an important technique used to teach new parents newborn care; as they watch a nurse hold, comfort, and talk to their newborn, they quickly learn to model these behaviors.

Behavioral Therapy

Typically, learning occurs best with **positive reinforcement** (e.g., a child tries to understand a new procedure, is praised for the effort, and tries even harder). **Behavioral therapy**, also called *behavior modification*, is a term used for a system aimed at *erasing* some form of behavior that interferes with healthy functioning. It was originally designed to help people who are cognitively challenged erase socially unacceptable behavior. Currently, it has many uses, including as a way to control disruptive classroom behavior. The basic premise of behavior modification is that a child is rewarded for healthful behavior, whereas unhealthful behavior is ignored or unrewarded. For example, a child who are cognitively challenged may have a socially unacceptable habit of constantly rocking back and forth. The child is not scolded or criticized for rocking, but the action is ignored. The preferred behavior (e.g., sitting for 5 minutes without rocking), however, is praised. Children respond best to behavior modification if, in addition to praise, they receive a tangible reward such as a star on a chart or an extra privilege for good behavior.

A behavior modification program must be discussed with the child before it is begun because no behavior can be modified—just as no new behavior can be learned—until a child truly wants a change to occur. It might be necessary to ask older children to sign a learning contract to be certain both teacher and learner agree on the method to be used. Many older children are able to use self-rewards to reinforce a behavior modification program such as rewarding themselves by playing a video game or going to a movie after an afternoon of efficient studying or an hour of doing breathing exercises.

Behavior modification must be used with common sense and concern so children are not being manipulated more than they are being helped to achieve a more healthful lifestyle. It is a legitimate device to use to encourage children to do as much self-care as possible or to reduce anxiety disorders (Wergeland, Fjermestad, Marin, et al., 2016).

Trying to modify beliefs or values, not actions, by behavior modification is considered unethical and is one reason why behavior modification is often criticized as a learning technique for children. However, some behavior changes also require a change in values to be effective and long term. For example, a child's behavior of talking back to parents can be extinguished by ignoring or not responding to the behavior and by praising polite communication. This method teaches the child to value improved communication and parental approval in order to meet his or her needs.

Selecting Teaching Tools

Teaching tools are the mechanical devices used to present content. They vary based on content, teacher/learner characteristics, and environment.

Visual Aids

"A picture is worth a thousand words" is not an idle quotation but a realistic one. Because small children know little about their bodies or where body organs are located, using visual aids such as drawings or photographs of anatomy can be very helpful to explain disease. Figure 35.4 shows abdominal contents as an example of such a drawing. You could use such an illustration to show a preschooler how food moves through the body. Figure 35.5 is an example of a good tool to use while naming body parts. Pointing to a figure drawing and saying, "This is the part of your tummy you're going to have fixed," is less threatening than actually pointing to the child's abdomen. Clarifying body parts this way is important because young children may have no clear understanding of where a body part such as a hand ends and an arm begins.

Do not be afraid to draw a picture of a heart, a kidney, a bladder, or any other organ to make a point about anatomic structure. Children are more interested in understanding procedures or the reason for a health maintenance measure than criticizing your artwork because they likely do not know anatomy well enough to be able to tell if a drawing is distorted.

Pamphlets

Pamphlets or information sheets are helpful teaching aids with school-age children, adolescents, and parents (Pile, 2013). These usually contain brief, easy to read, and easily understood information and are often cleverly illustrated with cartoon characters to make them enjoyable for a wide age range. Be certain to read any pamphlet before you offer it to a child to be certain the information included in it is accurate. Medical advances occur so quickly that a 1-year-old pamphlet may contain a gross inaccuracy in the light of subsequent knowledge.

If a pamphlet contains some statements that are inaccurate or do not apply to a child, do not simply cross out the information that would be contradictory before offering it (most

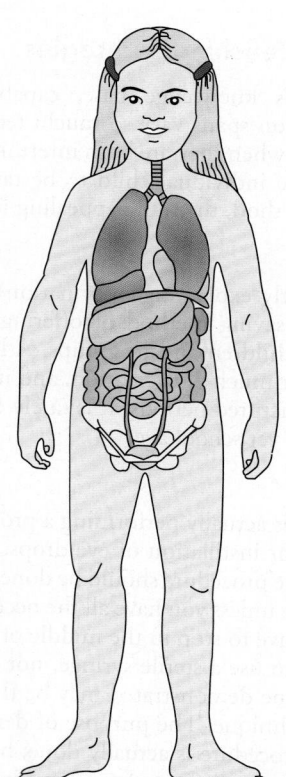

Figure 35.4   Anatomic drawings are helpful to illustrate basic health education topics and healthcare procedures.

Figure 35.5 Simple line drawings such as these can be used to explain to a child exactly what part of his or her body will be "fixed" in surgery. For many children, having this pointed out on a drawing seems much less intrusive than having it pointed to on their own bodies.

children deliberately read what they have been told not to read). Instead, take the time to explain why it doesn't apply. Also, do not be misled into believing that because children are given clever pamphlets, they will necessarily read them and learn from them. Sit with a school-age child and read the pamphlet together. Talk with an adolescent about the pamphlet's contents later to ensure it was not just tossed aside.

Learning Games

For memorizing certain kinds of information, such as what foods are high or low in potassium or sodium, flash cards can be a helpful learning tool. Many children older than 10 years of age (the age the average child is ready for competition) enjoy playing trivia-type board games. For health teaching, instead of using the game's categories of information, make up new cards with questions such as "Where is insulin produced in your body?" Children learn information quickly this way because the reward for learning is immediate (e.g., they get to move their token on the board). Having parents play the game with their child can effectively educate parents at the same time.

Word scrambles are easy games to develop. Crossword puzzles are fairly easy to design; one might be developed to address the important activities for a child to do after surgery such as deep breathing, exercising legs, and not eating immediately.

Videos

Many healthcare agencies, homes, schools, and community centers have video playback equipment, such as a DVD player, that can be used to show a short video or PowerPoint presentation as part of a health education program. Most households have CD or DVD players, so discs can be sent home for families to view. Viewing such programs can offer children a sense of power in that the program seems to be talking directly to them. Such a program can also be used over and over to refresh children's knowledge of the steps they need to take to remain well (Aljafari, Rice, Gallagher, et al., 2015). As with pamphlets, view the material first before showing it to a child and be certain the vocabulary used will be appropriate for an individual child or family.

Playing video or electronic games can be used to urge children to exercise, although the worth of these must be carefully compared to more traditional forms of exercise such as walking or joining a sports team (Gao, Chen, Pasco, et al., 2015).

QSEN Checkpoint Question 35.4

SAFETY

The nurse wants to teach Barry more about his hypercholesterolemia, and he has expressed a preference for video resources. To ensure that such videos are safe, age-appropriate, and accurate, the nurse should do which action?

 a. Preview any potential video resources before referring them to Barry.
 b. Encourage Barry to search YouTube and then report back to you.
 c. Emphasize the fact that written materials are usually preferable to video materials.
 d. Refer Barry to his local public library and have him liaise with a librarian.

Look in Appendix A for the best answer and rationale.

Puppets and Dolls

Many children are shy about talking to strangers. This shyness, in addition to their concern about what will happen to them, may make it difficult for them to discuss or explain what they know about their health, illness, or intended surgery. However, they may be able to open up to an uncritical puppet or doll because they see this as a usual part of play (Sposito, Silva-Rodrigues, de Cássia Sparapani, et al., 2015). Box 35.7 shows an interprofessional care map illustrating both nursing and team planning for a preschooler having surgery. Preschool children are particularly receptive to puppets and dolls because, with their imagination at its peak, they believe the puppet or doll is actually talking to them.

Teaching preschool children about what to expect from a hospital experience is often taught by using a series of puppets or dolls to represent different hospital personnel such as a surgeon, a nurse, and a nurse's assistant. Children can

BOX 35.7

Nursing Care Planning

AN INTERPROFESSIONAL CARE MAP FOR A PRESCHOOLER HAVING SURGERY

Wolf Whitefeather is a 3-year-old boy who is scheduled for repair of syndactyly (webbed fingers) next week.

Family Assessment: Patient lives with mother in two-bedroom mobile home. Parents separated. Mother works at local hospital in medical billing. Grandmother does child care 4 hours a day; child attends Head Start program in afternoon. Mother describes finances as "I'm making it." Father will visit after surgery; mother has custodial authority.

Patient Assessment: Favorite activity: coloring. His mother is concerned Wolf will be hard to entertain after surgery because the large pressure bandage he will have in place will prevent him from using that hand. "I don't even want to begin to talk to him about surgery," she added. When nervous or frightened, child has a habit of biting his hand; he has done this constantly since admission.

Nursing Diagnosis: Deficient knowledge related to what to expect in surgery

Outcome Criteria: Child describes expected outcomes of surgery. Demonstrates a minimum of nervous behaviors such as biting hand, can play "Simon Says" for hand exercises postsurgery, and describes how pain will be relieved by a "special button" (patient-controlled analgesia).

Teaching Points: Child is shy with strangers; mother states he learns best by "hands-on" experiences; "cocks head" when puzzled. Also learns better from his mother than from his father (father tends to be authoritarian).

Cognitive Learning to Be Taught: Why surgery is necessary

Psychomotor Skills to Be Taught: To keep hand in elevated position after surgery

Affective Aspects to Be Taught: Accepts surgery as a growth experience

Team Member Responsible	Assessment	Intervention	Rationale	Expected Outcome
Activities of Daily Living, Including Safety				
Nurse	Assess what child and parent understand about care necessary postoperatively.	Introduce postoperative hand exercises child will need to do by playing "Simon Says."	Games are an appealing way to keep the preschooler interested and motivated in doing exercises.	Child demonstrates opening and closing hand to help prevent contractions postprocedure.
Teamwork and Collaboration				
Nurse/surgical healthcare provider	Assess which anesthesia team member will be available for operating room and postoperative pain management.	Request anesthesia/analgesia consult.	Child is too young to be cooperative during surgery; needs pain relief afterward.	Anesthesia service meets with child and parent; determines best form of pain management and anesthesia.
Procedures/Medications for Quality Improvement				
Nurse/surgical healthcare provider	Assess health history.	Complete the physical exam.	Health assessment helps ensure readiness for surgery.	Child cooperates with the history and exam.
Nurse	Assess Wolf's and parent's knowledge of surgery and postoperative procedures.	Introduce dressing and show how child's hand will be suspended postoperatively by letting Wolf dress and suspend puppet's hand.	Therapeutic play provides an excellent medium for teaching and learning with toddlers and preschoolers.	Child demonstrates he understands how hand will be positioned by showing position with puppet.
Nutrition				
Nurse	Assess if child and parent know child will be nothing by mouth (NPO) for general anesthesia for surgery.	Teach parent importance of NPO preoperatively and immediately postoperatively.	Maintaining NPO status helps prevent aspiration with anesthesia.	Child and parent state they understand need for NPO status and will adhere to requirement.

Patient-Centered Care				
Nurse	Assess child's cognitive level and ability to learn and who is child's main support person.	Using puppets, teach that the child's hand will be washed with antiseptic solution before surgery.	Reducing skin bacteria prior to surgery can help prevent osteomyelitis.	Child cooperates with preprocedure washes. Names mother as person he wants with him.
Psychosocial/Spiritual/Emotional Needs				
Nurse/pain management team member	Assess what past experiences, if any, the child has had with pain.	Teach child he will have pain after surgery, but it can be relieved by a "special button" on his intravenous pump.	Explaining how pain will be relieved before surgery can help reduce amount of stress after surgery.	Child and parent state they know there will be pain and understand method to be used for control.
Informatics for Seamless Healthcare Planning				
Nurse	Assess if child and parent feel equipped to change bandages, carry out hand exercises at home, and have return appointment.	Review with parent a schedule of care based on Head Start and grandmother involvement.	Helping a parent walk through how postprocedure activities can be managed helps ensure adherence.	Mother states she has a plan for how to consistently arrange care given by three caregivers and will keep return appointment.

practice giving the doll "shots" or submitting it to the procedures they will experience (see Chapter 36 for a discussion of therapeutic play).

Mass Media

Television and radio are examples of effective mass media that are used to teach many children about self-help or self-care. Consulting on the topics to present or helping develop the material used in these types of health messages can be an important role for nurses. Messages originated for these media must be attention getting and brief to compete with the programs and commercial messages that precede or follow them.

Computers and Internet

Many children learn to solve problems using computers as early as preschool age. Using an Internet application to answer questions about an illness or prepare children for surgery is effective because this type of activity can be both entertaining and informative (Kain, Fortier, Chorney, et al., 2015). Caution children not all information posted on the Web is reliable, and participating in chat rooms can lead not only to the information they were seeking but also to exposure to Internet predators (Briggs, Simon, & Simonsen, 2011). Giving the family a list of appropriate YouTube videos or website addresses can also support learning at home.

Preparing Teaching Supplies

To avoid having to reorganize equipment or instructions each time a procedure is taught, put together a basket or box containing all the information and equipment needed to teach a particular task. This helps ensure that teaching will not only be organized but also economical in that everyone on a hospital unit is not opening new equipment for demonstrations. It also helps to ensure everyone is teaching the same information. Nothing is more confusing to someone learning a new skill than to be taught two different principles or techniques for doing something.

IMPLEMENTING THE PLAN

Health teaching can begin immediately after contact with a child and should flow easily if goals have been well developed and strategies for teaching have been carefully designed.

Using Designated Teachers

Many healthcare agencies, including home care agencies, have specific people who are available for health teaching about specific subjects such as diabetes, stomal care, respiratory exercises, or drug abuse prevention. Using such people is helpful because they know all the "tricks of the trade" for teaching that particular subject.

Some children do not learn as well from such designated teachers, however, because they see them only infrequently, unlike a primary nurse, whom they may see daily. Some parents react badly to the thought that if it takes an expert to tell them about the care needed, how can they possibly learn it? They may also find it inconvenient to be told their questions cannot be answered until the following day when the designated teacher is available to answer them. Be certain if a designated teacher does teach a subject, you coordinate your teaching with that person. Make a point of introducing the person to the child so the child does not view the person as a suspicious stranger.

QSEN Checkpoint Question 35.5

EVIDENCE-BASED PRACTICE

Preparing children, through the use of parental preparation, for surgery can vary in effectiveness depending on the method of education. A study was conducted to determine if a preoperative DVD instructional program could have an effect on parental knowledge, participation, and anxiety and thereby reduce the distress, pain, analgesic requirements, and length of recovery in a child undergoing same day surgery. The DVD intervention was provided to 123 parent–children (ages 3 to 10 years) dyads undergoing same-day surgery, whereas the control group received standard care. Parents in the intervention group demonstrated an increase in knowledge, provided more positive reinforcement, and increased their use of distraction and relaxation methods toward their child as compared with the control group. The children's postoperative pain was significantly lower in the intervention group as compared with the intervention group (Chartrand, Tourigny, & MacCormick, 2017).

Based on the previous study, what does the nurse determine for Wolf, 3 years old, if he seemed exceptionally anxious before surgery?
a. Face-to-face instruction is preferable because it is most effective.
b. He has no reason to feel anxious because 1-day surgery is finished so quickly.
c. He should be given the choice between a Web-based/DVD program or face-to-face instruction.
d. He, like most preschoolers, is too young to understand an explanation of his surgery.

Look in Appendix A for the best answer and rationale.

Parent Education

With very young children, parents as well as children need teaching. It's good practice with all children to be certain at least one adult in the household has the necessary information or can perform the required skill as well as the child. If at all possible, allowing for cultural beliefs that may dictate child care responsibilities in the family, let the child choose this person because the individual who everyone assumes is a child's chief support person may not be the person the child perceives as the most reliable choice for a healthcare backup. This person, when identified, needs as much information as the child about why the health measure is important.

What If . . . 35.3
Wolf, 3 years old, refuses to tell the nurse whether he has pain because the nurse is a "stranger" and he doesn't talk to strangers. How would the nurse best respond?

EVALUATING THE EFFECTIVENESS OF TEACHING

Evaluation, or assessing whether teaching has been effective, is the final step in teaching. It is optimum if evaluation occurs not only after the teaching plan has been implemented but also throughout the entire learning process. This ongoing evaluation helps both teacher and learner modify the teaching plan to better meet changing needs.

There is some advantage in asking children questions before and after teaching to prove teaching was effective and the child has safely learned a new healthcare measure. Demonstration of a change of behavior or attitude, however, is the real proof learning has occurred.

TEAMWORK & COLLABORATION

The nurse wants Wolf, 3 years of age, to know how to do the hand exercises he will need to do after surgery. When collaborating with the physiotherapist, which technique below would probably be most effective with Wolf?
a. A pamphlet you read together
b. A lecture from a sports hero
c. Playing a game of Simon Says
d. A group discussion on hand pain

Look in Appendix A for the best answer and rationale.

Health Teaching for a Surgical Experience

Teaching to prepare a child for surgery is an example of teaching that requires planning for several stages of learning. The child and the child's parents often feel anxious about surgery because this is always a potentially frightening experience. Therefore, teaching must first address this anxiety. Such preparation differs according to the type of surgery being performed, but certain activities apply to all surgery and all children.

A psychological preparation of both the child and the parents is aimed at reducing a child's fears about the procedure and consists primarily of providing health teaching and opportunities for therapeutic play. A physical preparation includes providing for restrictions on food and fluid intake before surgery, preparing the incision site on the child's skin, and arranging for transportation of the child to surgery. Because many children's surgical procedures are done on an ambulatory basis, parents often perform a part of physical preparation in preparation for the surgery as well as postoperative care and so must have clear instructions as to their responsibility. Do not downplay a family's fears but allow the child and family opportunities to express their concerns as part of the teaching/learning process.

ASSESSING CURRENT LEVEL OF KNOWLEDGE

On admission to the healthcare setting, whether the surgery will include a 1-day or longer hospitalization experience, elicit from parents what preparation they have made for this experience and what specifically they have told their child about what will happen. It's good to also ask whether a child's concerns about the experience seem more or less than the parents had anticipated. To see if the child is emotionally prepared, ask if there has been an unpleasant surgery or hospitalization in the family recently the child might have heard discussed or if the child has seen anything recently on a medical show on TV that might have been upsetting?

Emotional Preparation

Preparing a child emotionally for surgery requires minimizing fears common to all children such as fear of separation, fear of mutilation, or fear of death. Give careful explanations of what the procedure will entail and describe any specific equipment or techniques that will be used, such as anesthesia, eye bandages, nasogastric tubes, sutures, or special aftercare. Be certain all preparation is appropriate to the child's age. Most children who need surgery receive a general anesthetic rather than a local or regional anesthetic, as might be used with adults, because this minimizes their fears of intrusive or mutilating procedures, and because children who are not yet adolescent are not mature enough to cooperate adequately during surgery if they are not fully anesthetized.

It is best to prepare a child for a major experience like this in stages rather than all at once because it is difficult to absorb so much information in a short time span. However, contact before surgery may be limited to only one office or clinic visit, or the morning of surgery, so time constraints can force information to be more compacted.

Be certain to discuss presurgery preparations such as necessary blood work and not eating in the morning of surgery. If the child will have general anesthesia, it is important to emphasize that anesthetized sleep is "special" sleep. Otherwise, toddlers or preschoolers may be reluctant to fall asleep after surgery for fear people will come and do strange things to them. Do not say a child will be "put to sleep" (dogs and cats that are "put to sleep" are never seen again). To help prepare a young child for surgery, a doll's abdomen could be washed, a hospital gown put on, and an injection given to make the doll sleepy. It could be carried to a cart made from a cardboard box. After saying goodbye to its parents, the doll could be wheeled to surgery by a puppet nurse.

The surgery procedure should be discussed but minimized. "After you're asleep, the doctor will fix your tummy. You won't feel anything because of the special sleep. When you wake up, you'll be in a room called a recovery room where you'll stay until you're wide awake." Be honest concerning pain: "Your tummy will feel sore afterward, but I'll give you something to make it feel better" is a fair statement.

It is important to alert children that personnel in surgery wear surgical masks. Assure toddlers and preschoolers the persons behind the masks are doctors and nurses, some of whom the child has probably already met, not superheroes or bandits.

It is also good to mention recovery rooms in preparation because this is often an area parents neglect to mention. In fact, parents may not be aware that in some institutions, they will not be allowed in the recovery room and may have

promised the child, "As soon as you wake up, I'll be there." Clarify the parents' misconceptions about recovery rooms and reiterate the child will get to see his parents back in his own room once he is fully awake. This both makes the parents' preparation correct and saves the child from feeling deceived.

Explain postsurgery items, such as the use of oxygen, monitors, bedpans, bandages, or intravenous equipment. Furnishing a doll with such equipment is especially helpful in preparing younger children (Fig. 35.6). This play level is less stressful for preschoolers rather than being taken to an intensive care unit where they can feel overwhelmed by the sight of actual monitors and ventilators. After surgery, be certain to evaluate whether a child's preparation was adequate, both to document the experience was as trauma free as it could have been and to evaluate your expertise in teaching children.

What If . . . 35.4

The nurse is particularly interested in exploring one of the 2020 National Health Goals with respect to communication and teaching with children (see Box 35.1). What would be a possible research topic to explore pertinent to this goal that would be applicable to Barry's or Wolf's family and that would also advance evidence-based practice?

Unfolding Patient Stories: Sabina Vasquez • Part 1

Sabina Vasquez is 5 years old and was diagnosed with asthma at age 3 while living in Mexico. Now living in the United States, she is at her first visit to the primary care provider's office with asthma symptoms, and the mother shows the nurse Sabina's albuterol inhaler. The family is learning English, but Spanish is the primary language spoken at home. What decision making by the nurse determines if an interpreter is needed to assess the family's knowledge of asthma and to provide asthma-related patient education? What appropriate age-related strategies should be used in planning asthma education for this patient and her family? (Sabina Vasquez's story continues in Chapter 40.)

Care for Sabina and other patients in a realistic virtual environment: *vSim for Nursing* (thepoint.lww.com/vSimMaternityPed). Practice documenting these patients' care in DocuCare (thepoint.lww.com/DocuCareEHR).

KEY POINTS FOR REVIEW

- Communication is the exchange of ideas between two or more persons. It can be verbal or nonverbal.

- Therapeutic communication is a planned interaction, has structure, and is constructive. Nontherapeutic communication lacks deliberate purpose other than socializing.

- Successful communication requires an encoder, a code, a decoder, and feedback or a response.

- Levels of communication include: (1) cliché, (2) fact reporting, (3) shared ideas, (4) shared feelings, and (5) peak communication.

Figure 35.6 Pretending to be a pirate helps this young child prepare for having to wear an eye patch after surgery.

- Typical methods of nonverbal communication are using distance, gestures, body posture, touch, use of drawings, and empathy.
- Techniques that encourage therapeutic communication are attentive listening, open-ended questions, reflecting, clarifying, paraphrasing, perception checking, focusing, supportive statements, and silence.
- Some situations require special communication techniques such as interacting with demanding or shy children, children who are visually or hearing challenged, or children who are not proficient in English.
- Establishing a teacher–learner relationship based on mutual input and setting expected outcomes are effective ways to meet the unique needs and goals of a child and family as well as to help in planning nursing care that meets QSEN competencies.
- There are three types of learning: cognitive, psychomotor, and affective. For something to be learned well, all of these areas may need to be involved.
- To individualize a teaching program for a child, assess the child's attention span, cognitive or intellectual capability, lifestyle, and learning style and your own teaching strengths and limitations.
- In many instances, there is a great deal of material a child must learn about an illness. If possible, divide material into lessons that can be taught immediately and lessons that can be taught at return health visits.
- The format and strategies of teaching used with children vary depending on a child's age and developmental level. Various types to consider are formal versus informal, single or group teaching, lecture, discussion, and role-playing.
- Behavior modification is a special technique aimed at erasing some form of behavior that interferes with good health.
- Children learn many other things besides health information every day. This may make the retention of information not as great as you would like. You may need to schedule frequent reviews and updates to keep information current.

CRITICAL THINKING CARE STUDY

Lucy is a 7-year-old who is scheduled to have her tonsils removed. She lives with her mother and father in a central city apartment. Her father works as a taxi driver. Her mother is a stay-at-home mom. Lucy is home schooled because she is cognitively challenged due to a birth injury and because she doesn't want other children to "laugh at her because she's in a special class." Her mother does not know her exact developmental age but says, "She can't begin to comprehend" second-grade work. Because Lucy is becoming overweight, you'd like to teach her more about the importance of exercise, so hopefully she can include some every day into her home schooling schedule.

1. You schedule a hospital tour every week for children who will have a tonsillectomy the following week. Lucy's mother replies she doesn't want to take advantage of this learning opportunity. Are you surprised by this? Is declining the tour in Lucy's best interest?
2. Following Lucy's tonsillectomy, you bring your teaching basket about exercise to her bedside. Lucy refuses to look at anything you show her; instead, she just concentrates on putting shoes on her doll. Would you continue teaching?
3. Lucy's mother has told you she doesn't know Lucy's developmental age. Would it be important for her to have a psychology consult prior to surgery so you could be certain your preparation for surgery will be effective?

RELATED RESOURCES

Explore these additional resources to enhance learning for this chapter:
- Student resources on thePoint, including answers to the What If . . . and Critical Thinking Care Study questions, http://thepoint.lww.com/Flagg8e
- Adaptive learning powered by PrepU, http://thepoint.lww.com/prepu

REFERENCES

Aljafari, A., Rice, C., Gallagher, J. E., et al. (2015). An oral health education video game for high caries risk children: Study protocol for a randomized controlled trial. *Trials, 16*(1), 237.

Arnold, E. C. (2015). Theoretical perspectives and contemporary dynamics. In E. C. Arnold & K. U. Boggs (Eds.), *Interpersonal relationships: Professional communication skills for nurses* (7th ed., pp. 1–21). Philadelphia, PA: Elsevier/Saunders.

Avegno, J., & DeBlieux, P. M. C. (2013). Characteristics of great teachers. In R. L. Rogers, A. Mattu, M. Winters, et al. (Eds.), *Practical teaching in emergency medicine* (pp. 159–167). Hoboken, NJ: Wiley.

Bal, V. H., Katz, D., Bishop, S. L., et al. (2016). Understanding definitions of minimally verbal across instruments: Evidence for subgroups within minimally verbal children and adolescents with autism spectrum disorder. *Journal of Child Psychology and Psychiatry, and Allied Disciplines, 57*(12), 1424–1433.

Barrouillet, P. (2015). Theories of cognitive development: From Piaget to today. *Developmental Review, 38*, 1–12.

Briggs, G., Schuitema, K., & Vorhaus, J. (2016). Children with profound and multiple learning difficulties: Laughter, capability and relating to others. *Disability and Society*, 1–15.

Briggs, P., Simon, W. T., & Simonsen, S. (2011). An exploratory study of Internet-initiated sexual offences and the chat room sex offender: Has the Internet enabled a new typology of sex offender? *Sexual Abuse, 23*(1), 72–91.

Chartrand, J., Tourigny, J., & MacCormick, J. (2017). The effect of an educational pre-operative DVD on parents' and children's outcomes after same-day-surgery: A randomized controlled trial. *Journal of Advanced Nursing, 73*(3), 599–611.

Coplan, R. J., Rose-Krasnor, L., Weeks, M., et al. (2013). Alone is a crowd: Social motivations, social withdrawal, and socioemotional functioning in later childhood. *Developmental Psychology, 49*(5), 861–875.

Cruz, I., Quittner, A. L., Marker, C., et al. (2013). Identification of effective strategies to promote language in deaf children with cochlear implants. *Child Development, 84*(2), 543–559.

DalSanto, L., Pohl, S., Saiani, L., et al. (2014). Empathy in the emotional interactions with patients: Is it positive for nurses too? *Journal of Nursing Education and Practice, 4*(2), 74–81.

Deibel, M. D., & Wagner, M. J. (2013). Small group discussion skills. In R. L. Rogers, A. Mattu, M. Winters, et al. (Eds.), *Practical teaching in emergency medicine* (pp. 180–191). Hoboken, NJ: Wiley.

Erikson, E. H. (1993). *Childhood and society*. New York, NY: W. W. Norton.

Espelage, D. L., Basile, K. C., De La Rue, L., et al. (2015). Longitudinal associations among bullying, homophobic teasing, and sexual violence perpetration among middle school students. *Journal of Interpersonal Violence, 30*(14). 2541–2561

Farber, H. J., Curie, N. L., Brown, T., et al. (2015, May). *Process, evaluation and family participation to improve the preoperative evaluation of neuromuscular patients receiving general anesthesia*. Paper presented at the American Thoracic Society 2015 International Conference, Denver, CO.

Gao, Z., Chen, S., Pasco, D., et al. (2015). A meta-analysis of active video games on health outcomes among children and adolescents. *Obesity Reviews, 16*(9), 783–794.

Harris, J., & Lord, C. (2016). Mental health of children with vision impairment at 11 years of age. *Developmental Medicine and Child Neurology, 58*(7), 774–779.

Kain, Z. N., Fortier, M. A., Chorney, J. M., et al. (2015). Web-base tailored intervention for preparation of parents and children for outpatient surgery (WebTIPS): Development. *Anesthesia and Analgesia, 120*(4), 905–914.

Kirk, K. I., Prusick, L., French, B., et al. (2012). Assessing spoken word recognition in children who are deaf or hard of hearing: A translational approach. *Journal of the American Academy of Audiology, 23*(6), 464–475.

Kohlberg, L. (1984). *The psychology of moral development: Moral stages and the life cycle.* San Francisco, CA: Harper & Row.

Leathers, D. G., & Eaves, M. (2015). *Successful nonverbal communication: Principles and applications* (4th ed.). New York, NY: Routledge.

Levine, D. A. (2014). Growth & development. In K. J. Marcdante, R. M. Kliegman, H. B. Jenson, et al. (Eds.), *Nelson essentials of pediatrics* (7th ed., pp. 13–44). Philadelphia, PA: Elsevier/Saunders.

Lund, E., & Douglas, W. M. (2016). Teaching vocabulary to preschool children with hearing loss. *Exceptional Children, 83*(1), 26–41.

McLinden, M., & McCall, S. (2016). *Learning through touch: Supporting children with visual impairment and additional difficulties.* New York, NY: Routledge.

Olino, T. M., Durbin, C. E., Klein, D. N., et al. (2013). Gender differences in young children's temperament traits: Comparisons across observational and parent-report methods. *Journal of Personality, 81*(2), 119–129.

Piaget, J. (1952). *The origins of intelligence in children.* New York, NY: International Universities Press.

Pile, D. (2013). Does using an asthma prompting form improve asthma care in a pediatric office? *Journal of Pediatric Nursing, 28*(3), 275–281.

Roberts, J. F., Fenton, G., & Barnard, M. C. (2015). Developing effective therapeutic relationships with children, young people and their families. *Nursing Children and Young People, 27*(4), 30–35.

Sears, M. S., Repetti, R. L., Reynolds, B. M., et al. (2014). A naturalistic observational study of children's expressions of anger in the family context. *Emotion, 14*(2), 272–283.

Singer, B. (2012). Perceptions of school nurses in the care of students with disabilities. *The Journal of School Nursing, 29*(5), 329–336.

Sposito, A. M., Silva-Rodrigues, F. M., de Cássia Sparapani, V., et al. (2015). Coping strategies used by hospitalized children with cancer undergoing chemotherapy. *Journal of Nursing Scholarship, 47*(2), 143–151.

Tapson, K., Sierotowicz, W., Marks-Maran, D., et al. (2015). "It's the hearing that is last to go": A case of traumatic head injury. *British Journal of Nursing, 24*(5), 277–281.

Taylor, S. P., Nicolle, C., & Maguire, M. (2013). Cross-cultural communication barriers in health care. *Nursing Standard, 27*(31), 35–43.

U.S. Department of Health and Human Services. (2010). *Healthy people 2020.* Washington, DC: Author.

Wergeland, G. J. H., Fjermestad, K. W., Marin, C. E., et al. (2016). Predictors of treatment outcome in an effectiveness trial of cognitive behavioral therapy for children with anxiety disorders. *Behaviour Research and Therapy, 76*, 1–12.

Wu, S., Tyler, A., Logsdon, T., et al. (2016). A quality improvement collaborative to improve the discharge process for hospitalized children. *Pediatrics, 138*(2), e20143604.

UNIT 6

The Nursing Role in Supporting the Health of Ill Children and Their Families

36

Nursing Care of a Family With an Ill Child

OBJECTIVES

After mastering the contents of this chapter, you should be able to:

1. Describe illness and illness experiences as they must appear to children.
2. Identify 2020 National Health Goals related to the care of ill children that nurses can help the nation achieve.
3. Assess the impact of an illness, especially one requiring a hospital stay, on a child.
4. Formulate nursing diagnoses related to the stress of illness in children.
5. Establish expected outcomes for an ill child to help manage a childhood illness as well as manage seamless transitions across differing healthcare settings.
6. Plan nursing care to reduce the stress of illness, such as helping parents plan for ambulatory care or therapeutic play.
7. Using the nursing process, plan nursing care that includes the six competencies of Quality & Safety Education for Nurses (QSEN): Patient-Centered Care, Teamwork & Collaboration, Evidence-Based Practice (EBP), Quality Improvement (QI), Safety, and Informatics.
8. Evaluate expected outcomes for achievement and effectiveness of care.
9. Integrate knowledge of a child's response to illness with the interplay of nursing process, the six competencies of QSEN, and Family Nursing to promote quality maternal and child health nursing care.

Becky is a 7-year-old whose foot was unintentionally burned by a campfire. She is going to be admitted to the hospital for a 1-day surgery to have the wound debrided. Becky's parents tell you that Becky "hasn't been herself" since the injury. She has reverted to temper tantrums and sulking, more like a 3-year-old than one of school age. Even though she has been told eating meat is important because it provides protein for healing, she refuses to eat anything but Jell-O or soup. In the admission suite of the hospital, she picked up a doll and twisted its leg off. "How can we get our old daughter back again?" her mother asks you.

Previous chapters described the normal growth and development of children and their special needs at each stage of development. This chapter adds information about the additional needs of children when they become ill. Such information builds a basis for nursing care and health teaching.

Becky is obviously showing some effects of her unintentional injury. What type of additional explanation might be helpful to her? What advice would you give her mother to help her better prepare Becky for the upcoming debridement procedure?

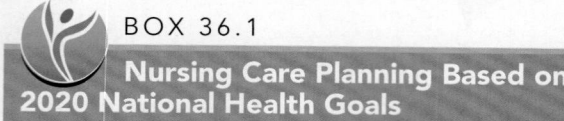

Illness and hospitalization can be major stressors for children; therefore, three 2020 National Health Goals address this:

- Increase the proportion of children with special health-care needs who have access to a medical home from 47.1% to 51.8%.
- Increase the proportion of children aged 0 to 11 years with special healthcare needs who receive their care in family-centered, comprehensive, and coordinated systems from 20.4% to 22.4%.
- Increase the proportion of children aged 0 to 11 years with special healthcare needs who receive their care in family-centered, comprehensive, and coordinated systems from 20.4% to 22.4% (U.S. Department of Health and Human Services, 2010; see www.healthypeople.gov).

Nurses can help the nation achieve these goals by helping reduce the stress of hospitalization or health care so families use preventive services to help children stay well rather than totally use emergent or ill child care services.

Illnesses that require the attention of healthcare professionals are outside the usual occurrences of childhood, so most children typically have little knowledge about them. Helping a child and family prepare for or adjust to such an experience is a fundamental nursing role. This role goes well beyond just providing information on what to expect throughout an illness. It involves providing emotional support as well.

Studies from the 1980s and 1990s found that family visitation was associated with lower anxiety levels among adult postanesthesia care unit (PACU) patients, and similar results have been found among pediatric patients. The literature has repeatedly shown that unrestricted visitation in healthcare settings increases family satisfaction, improves children's morale, and can improve communication among the staff, the patient, and the family (Houle, Belew, & Miller, 2015). In response to this, children and families should be enrolled in orientation programs before hospital admission, and nurses should advocate for the use of therapeutic play and be more open to parental visiting and overnight stay policies, even in intensive care areas, if these are not already in effect (Zempsky, Palermo, Corsi, et al., 2013). In addition, nurses can help families establish a therapeutic environment for the care of an ill child in the home after a hospitalization. Box 36.1 shows 2020 National Health Goals concerned with children and illness.

Nursing Process Overview

FOR AN ILL CHILD

ASSESSMENT

An assessment for a child diagnosed with an illness that requires hospitalization begins with an interview of the child and parents to identify ways they think the illness will change

their lives. This could include a wide range of situations such as increased expenses, changes in schedules to visit or stay with a hospitalized child, the need for one parent to take a leave from work to care for an ill child at home, the need to schedule frequent ambulatory visits, consultation to handle body image changes, and the need to arrange for child care for other children. Because these needs change as the course of an illness changes, the assessment must be ongoing.

NURSING DIAGNOSIS

Nursing diagnoses vary greatly depending on the extent of a child's illness, the care needed, and the age of the child. Those often used with families of children seen in ambulatory and in-hospital settings include:

- Health-seeking behaviors related to lack of knowledge regarding illness
- Anxiety related to pending hospital admission
- Risk for social isolation related to hospitalization
- Fear related to being away from home for the first time
- Activity intolerance related to fatigue from illness
- Potential for unintentional injury related to high-tech therapy equipment

OUTCOME IDENTIFICATION AND PLANNING

Planning for the care of an ill child requires consideration of all aspects of the child's and the family's life: financial, social, and personal. When children become ill, many of their needs, such as those for nutrition, play, and family support, change. If a child will need long-term care or hospitalization, the entire family may find their priorities changing. Identifying additional needs and putting in place necessary services or interventions is an important nursing role.

Helpful resources and support programs that address the needs of the ill child and their families are available. Refer families to online resources for further information when appropriate.

ONLINE RESOURCES

American Academy of Pediatrics (AAP): offers information on general medicine administration, tips on how to read medicine labels, and suggestions for pain management — www.aap.org

Association for Early Learning Leaders: provides helpful information on the hospitalization of children for both parents and healthcare providers — www.earlylearningleaders.org

KidsHealth: assists parents in preparing their children for procedures — www.kidshealth.org

Mayo Clinic: educates and instructs parents on procedure preparation — www.mayoclinic.com

IMPLEMENTATION

Five hazards that may occur with children with all illnesses are (1) experiencing harm or injury, such as physical discomfort, pain, mutilation, and death; (2) being separated from routines, parents, peers, and respected adults; (3) facing the unknown (new and strange sights and sounds and happenings); (4) facing uncertain limits (unclear definition of acceptable and expected behavior); and (5) experiencing a loss of control (loss of competence or loss of the ability to make decisions).

Being aware of these potential concerns is important to guard against those that are preventable and to reduce a child's concern associated with those that cannot be prevented (such as facing new sights and sounds). Discussing these hazards with children based on their developmental age is important so that implementations to reduce their impact can be tailored to each child. Based on the child's developmental age, methods for assessing these potential concerns and introducing effective strategies to help the child cope may include reading to a child, role-playing, and puppetry.

OUTCOME EVALUATION

An evaluation of expected outcomes for ill children should include specific measures such as whether discomfort was kept to a minimum during the experience. Indicators to evaluate outcomes that are long term should include whether children were able to return to usual behaviors after the experience. The following are examples that suggest achievement of outcomes regarding a hospital experience:

- Parents state their level of anxiety regarding hospitalization of their infant is now at a tolerable level.
- Parents have effectively changed work schedules to be able to stay with their child in the hospital.
- Social isolation of a toddler is minimized through a case manager nursing assignment.

The Meaning of Illness to Children

The response of children to illness depends on their cognitive ability, past experiences, and level of knowledge. It parallels cognitive development (see Chapter 28). From early school age, children generally know quite a bit about the workings of their major body parts. As general guidelines, early grade-school children are usually able to name the function of the heart, lungs, and stomach. However, children are not able to see the body as a system until the age of 10 to 11 years (Bibace & Walsh, 1980).

Younger children may think the cause of illness is magical or that it occurs as a consequence of breaking a rule. With this perspective, they may also think getting well again is possible only if they follow another set of rules, such as staying in bed and taking medicine. By fourth grade, children are generally aware of the role germs play in illness but may be fooled by thinking that all illnesses are caused by germs. Because of this, they may see a passive role for themselves in getting well because illness comes from outside influences. At about eighth grade, children are able to voice an understanding that illnesses can occur from several causes, such as being susceptible to chickenpox because they did not get a vaccine. This understanding is due to the formal logical stage that Piaget (1930) described. Where there is differentiation between self and other.

An illness in a child is a stress, especially if it includes hospitalization (Foster, Whitehead, & Maybee, 2016). Knowing how children of each age view illnesses affects the planning of nursing care and influences how explanations should be worded. For example, saying you are going to "stick" a child for blood work could be interpreted by young children as meaning you are actually going to put a stick in their arm. Saying a child will receive dye for a test could be interpreted as meaning the child will "die" during the procedure. Explanations of procedures can sound confusing if words sound alike or have double meanings (e.g., "drawing" as in making a picture vs. "drawing" blood). Because of these distorted perceptions, explanations of procedures do not always relieve children's stress.

DIFFERENCES IN RESPONSES OF CHILDREN AND ADULTS TO ILLNESS

Keeping in mind that children are not just small adults is important when evaluating how children react to illness, perceive an illness, or react to health care (Fig. 36.1). Their body images, for example, as evidenced in their drawings, are different from those of adults. They may have difficulty telling which body parts are indispensable and which are not (this is why it is wise to talk to preschool and early school-age children about "fixing" body parts, such as tonsils, rather than "taking them out").

Inability to Communicate

Very young children do not have the vocabulary to describe symptoms. Children younger than 5 years of age have a great deal of difficulty describing a headache. Dizziness and nausea can be equally bewildering because young children do not know the words to express these phenomena.

By the time children reach school age, most can describe symptoms with accuracy. They may intensify their concerns if they believe someone expects symptoms to be more serious. They may minimize symptoms if they are afraid that an illness will interfere with an activity they want to do; thus, it is important to evaluate a child's symptoms as much by observation as by a child's report. A crying, whining preschooler who is "just not herself" probably has a symptom she cannot describe. A school-age child who guards her abdomen (i.e., keeps abdominal muscles rigid) is in pain just as clearly as a child who verbalizes a source of discomfort.

Figure 36.1 Illness is potentially traumatic because of the unknown and because of the pain and discomfort that may be involved. Children need extra attention and reassurance to calm their fears.

Inability to Monitor Own Care and Manage Fear

Adults who are ill often ask questions about medications prescribed for them or procedures they are scheduled to undergo. If a hospitalized adult knows he is to receive a diuretic three times a day and by 10 AM has not been offered it as yet, he usually reminds someone of the oversight. School-age and younger children cannot monitor their own care this way because they may not know which medicine or procedures they are scheduled to receive. If they do know, they may be confused about the time. In addition, children have fears that adults do not experience. For example, by 8 to 9 months, the infant fears separation above all else; the toddler and preschooler enlarge their fears to include separation, the dark, intrusive procedures, and mutilation of body parts. The school-age child and adolescent may be concerned about the loss of body parts, loss of life, and loss of friends. Adults have fears also, but most have prior experiences to draw from, making coping easier. Children in a strange environment, such as a hospital, have not learned coping skills as yet and so require proportionally more support and active intervention to manage their stress and fears. Otherwise, hospitalization, particularly if it follows trauma from unintentional injury, can result in posttraumatic stress disorder (PTSD) or the development of characteristic symptoms, such as difficulty falling asleep, outbursts of anger, difficulty concentrating, difficulty completing tasks, or experiencing symptoms such as stomach aches or headaches (Franck, Wray, Gay, et al., 2015).

Nutritional Needs

Children differ from adults in many ways. In addition to psychological differences, there are major physiologic differences in the way illnesses affect children compared with adults. Children have greater metabolic demand, breathe in more air per pound of body weight than adults do, have a higher surface to body mass ratio (Centers for Disease Control and Prevention [CDC], 2015a), and are at greater risk for insensible fluid loss when they are sick.

For example, children need more nutrients (calories, protein, minerals, and vitamins) per pound of body weight than adults because their basic metabolic rate is faster, and they must take in not only enough to maintain body tissues but also enough to allow for growth. The infant, for example, requires 120 kcal/kg of body weight per day; the adult requires only 30 to 35 kcal/kg of body weight per day. An ill child who must limit food intake because of nausea or vomiting, therefore, may require hospitalization for intravenous therapy, even though this might not be necessary for an adult under the same circumstances.

Fluid and Electrolyte Balance

In the adult, extracellular water (the water held in plasma and outside body cells) represents approximately 23% of total body water; in a newborn, extracellular water is closer to 40%. This means that an infant does not have as much water stored in the cells as an adult and so is more likely to lose a devastating amount of body water with diarrhea or vomiting. The full implications of both vomiting and diarrhea are discussed in Chapter 45.

Systemic Response to Illness

Because a child's body is continually growing, young children tend to respond to disease systemically rather than locally.

The child with pneumonia, for example, may be brought to an emergency department not because of a cough (although the child may have one) but because of accompanying systemic symptoms such as fever, vomiting, and diarrhea. In fact, nausea and vomiting occur so frequently in children with any type of illness that these symptoms do not have the diagnostic value that they may have in adults. Systemic reactions of these kinds can delay diagnosis and therapy and can cause increased fluid and nutrient loss, circumstances that compound the initial illness.

Age-Specific Diseases

Most adults have achieved immunity to common infectious diseases; children, however, are very susceptible to illnesses such as measles, mumps, and chickenpox. Febrile children between the ages 6 and 60 months who do not have an intracranial infection or metabolic disturbance are typically diagnosed with "febrile seizure" (Steering Committee on Quality Improvement and Management & Subcommittee on Febrile Seizures, American Academy of Pediatrics, 2008).

Care of the Ill Child and Family in the Hospital

Research has raised awareness about the psychological trauma children and their parents face when hospitalized. This trauma can have lasting effects after discharge, undermining the child's recovery and the overall well-being of the family (Franck et al., 2015). The caregivers of a child admitted to an intensive care unit (ICU), neonatal intensive care unit (NICU), or general pediatric unit are likely to experience a high degree of stress during their child's hospitalization both because of the severity of their child's illness and the high-tech pediatric ICU (PICU) or NICU setting. The child in an acute care setting is much more apt to have invasive procedures compared with children on a general pediatric floor, which can also increase anxiety not only for the child but also the parent. A child's type of surgery is also related to parental anxiety and should be taken into consideration when speaking with the family (Woolf, Muscara, Anderson, et al., 2016).

THE EFFECT OF HOSPITAL SEPARATION AND CHILDREN: DECREASING SEPARATION ANXIETY

Social/emotional development begins early in infancy. Babies display sadness, happiness, and anger at a young age, and they begin to change their facial expressions to register changes in their emotions around 5 months. During this period, infants also become attached to parents and caregivers. When in the presence of strangers, infants fix their eyes on them, become restless, perhaps thrash arms or legs, and begin to cry. This activity peaks at approximately 9 months of age. It is a developmental milestone that shows that an infant is able to distinguish a primary caregiver from other persons. The timing of separation anxiety can vary widely from child to child. Within the hospital setting, that anxiety may be relieved by establishing a primary nurse.

In many instances, toddlers and preschoolers can be as affected by separation as infants and even express their feelings better, louder, and longer. Although many toddlers and preschoolers attend day care and have had prior experiences with separation, others may have had only limited experiences being away from their parents. Being hospitalized may be the first time they are away from parents in a strange setting or away from home overnight. The effect of separation can become especially intense in young children before they are able to understand time, because statements such as "Mom will visit again tomorrow" or "Dad will be here by 6 o'clock" are meaningless unless they know what "tomorrow" or "6 o'clock" means.

School-age children and adolescents react better than younger children to the separation imposed by hospitalization because they have experiences they can use for comparison. They have been to school for whole days, perhaps they have stayed with a grandparent or a friend overnight, and they may have been to a summer camp. This can make hospitalization a time for developing self-esteem and confidence in their ability to be independent. Even in light of this, ill school-age children and adolescents appreciate their parents being near them and reassurance that their parents will be there to support them through this crisis.

Remember that being separated may create an equally difficult time for parents. You may need to spend time with them, assuring them that their child will receive comprehensive, evidence-based care at all times, even if they have to leave for a commitment or to care for other children at home.

To appreciate why preventing separation is so important, it is helpful to review the research that provided the foundation for this method of care. Spitz (1945) was one of the first researchers who documented the effects of separation on children. He observed children in a penal nursery and in a foundling home who had been separated from their mothers for both short and long periods of time. From this observation, he was able to document that infant's growth and development slowed the longer they were away from their parent. Bowlby (1951) conducted additional studies with children separated from their parents during World War II. Building on Spitz's and Bowlby's work, Robertson (1958) applied these effects to the hospitalization of children and supplied labels for separation effects. Although defined over 50 years ago, these findings are still applicable to children today.

Reducing the ill effects of separation and hospitalization to the extent possible should be a high priority for all healthcare providers (Hilton, 2014). Nurses play a major role in this on both direct care and management levels. Unfortunately, even despite the best preparation by parents or nurses, not all of these effects of hospitalization can be prevented.

QSEN Checkpoint Question 36.1

TEAMWORK & COLLABORATION

The nurse collaborates with an interprofessional team to care for Becky, age 7 years. The social worker believes that Becky is showing the first signs of separation anxiety. The nurse determines which symptoms of anxiety corroborate the social worker's assessment?

    a. Loud, demanding crying
    b. Silent, sullen protesting
    c. Quiet, introspective thought
    d. Inability to respond verbally

Look in Appendix A for the best answer and rationale.

PREPARING THE ILL CHILD AND FAMILY FOR HOSPITALIZATION

Preparing for hospitalization involves disseminating developmentally appropriate information, facilitating communication and developing trusting relationships with healthcare professionals (Koller, 2008). Many childhood illnesses such as febrile seizures, appendicitis, poisonings, and asthma exacerbations are acute, making advance preparation for hospital admission impossible. However, when hospitalizations such as elective surgeries are scheduled, advance preparation is possible with programs such as preoperative orientation. The preparations parents make for a child obviously vary depending on the child's developmental age and experiences.

Depending on the age of the child, there may be anxiety if the child is told about an approaching hospitalization too far in advance. Conversely, few things are more frightening for children than to hear a conversation halt as they enter a room or to hear adults spelling out unknown words. As a rule, therefore, children between 2 and 7 years of age should be told about a scheduled ambulatory or inpatient hospitalization as many days before the procedure as the child's age in years. For example, a 2-year-old should be informed 2 days before hospitalization; a 4-year-old, 4 days before; and so forth. Children older than 7 years of age can be told as soon as the parents are aware of it.

On the day of hospital admission, it is important for you to ask the parents what preparation they have done to ensure the child and family accurately understand the child's condition and upcoming procedures. Based on that, you can provide further health teaching and clear up any misunderstandings as necessary (Box 36.2).

Many hospitals sponsor hospital orientation programs for children's groups or school groups during which hospitalization is discussed. These programs are beneficial because they lay a foundation for all children about what to expect during a hospitalization; then, if they must be admitted on an

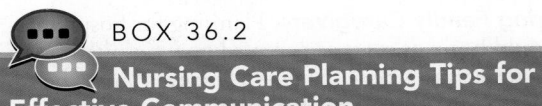
BOX 36.2
Nursing Care Planning Tips for Effective Communication

Becky, 7 years old, is admitted to your ambulatory surgery unit for burn debridement.

Becky and her mother arrive together on the unit.

Tip: Ask direct questions and be careful not to assume anything regarding the level of patient knowledge or preparation.

Nurse: Hello, Becky. How are you?

Becky: Good.

Nurse: Do you know why you're coming into the hospital?

Mrs. Miller: We've talked about surgery. She knows that's why she's here.

Nurse: Tell me why you're here yourself, Becky.

Becky: To read a book. I brought a book.

Nurse: Let's talk about everything you told her, Mrs. Miller.

Mrs. Miller: Well, I didn't want to introduce anything scary.

Nurse: Let's take some time and talk about the whole procedure.

Figure 36.2 Children learn what to expect from hospitalization by becoming familiar with some of the equipment that might be used.

emergency basis, they may not be so frightened. Programs are offered by nurses at the hospital or on visits to children's groups or schools (Fig. 36.2). Box 36.3 provides guidelines for setting up hospital tours or discussions for early school-age children.

 Nursing Diagnoses and Related Interventions

Nursing Diagnosis: Deficient knowledge related to preparation for hospitalization

Outcome Evaluation: Parents and child both state they feel prepared for hospitalization; child has brought some personal item important to self. Child describes with accuracy and detail appropriate to age the reason for hospital stay; asks questions and expresses feelings appropriate to age about hospitalization.

Preparing Family Caregivers. Planning for hospitalization should begin as soon as parents know hospitalization will be necessary. Some parents, however, may be so concerned about the reason for hospitalization that they cannot begin to prepare their child until they are better prepared themselves. Easing parental concerns regarding illness and hospitalization is particularly important because children may be able to sense a parent's stress. Even though a parent says, "Don't worry, everything will be all right," a child can sense if parents really do not believe everything will be all right.

As part of preparation, urge parents to ask questions about things such as what diagnostic procedures will be necessary, how long the hospital stay will be, and what kind of dressings or other equipment will be used, so they can be as familiar as possible with what will happen. Informing parents can help allay anxiety and will also keep them abreast of what the plan is so that they can be active in shared decision making. This is important as they are an integral part of their child's care.

Depending on your practice setting, familiarize yourself with available resources to help caregivers navigate what is available to them before, during, and after a hospital stay.

BOX 36.3

Guidelines for Conducting Hospital Tours With Early School-Age Children

1. Keep groups small (about 10 children per group) so individual reactions to the presentation can be assessed.
2. Allow or encourage parents to join the tour so their concerns about the hospital can also be relieved.
3. Conduct the tour for only 20 to 30 minutes to meet the short attention span of children.
4. Use an indirect method to present various aspects of a hospital that would be exceptionally anxiety producing such as the intensive care unit (ICU) or an operating room by using puppets, films, or a PowerPoint slide show. Include nonthreatening features such as a hospital playroom.
5. Present explanations about hospitalization in concrete terms and at the child's level of understanding. Include only what the child will see, hear, and feel.
6. Avoid dwelling on unpleasant and threatening events or intrusive procedures, such as blood drawing or anesthesia, that may create apprehension.
7. Allow children opportunities to ask questions.
8. Allow children opportunities to play with dolls and hospital equipment to decrease anxiety and satisfy curiosity.

Many parents ask a nurse to repeat their primary care provider's explanation for a procedure or to have instructions clarified to be certain they have understood everything correctly. If parents arrive at a hospital unit with questions still unanswered, continue to keep them informed and educate as new questions or concerns arise.

Preparing an Infant. Because an infant cannot understand explanations of surgery or treatments, verbal preparation is minimal. Remind parents to pack special items such as a favorite toy, blanket, or pacifier because these objects provide a special kind of security for which there is no substitute.

The infant's primary caregiver should plan to spend a great deal of time in the hospital with the infant. Ask whether the parent who will be staying with the infant has made plans for other children, a spouse, work, or other obligations ahead of time. If a parent cannot arrange to stay with the child during the hospital stay, attempt to have a consistent nurse assigned to the infant, which may help to lessen caregiver anxiety and minimize separation anxiety in the infant.

Preparing a Toddler or Preschooler. Three chief fears of toddlers or preschoolers are fear of the unknown, fear of abandonment or separation, and fear of mutilation. Preparation for children of this age, therefore, should clearly aim at alleviating these three fears. Bringing a favorite toy or personal item such as a blanket can help. Referred to as "transitional objects," these items are reminders about something familiar from home.

When making hospital beds or changing paper on examining tables, be alert for ragged blankets and threadbare stuffed animals because it is easy for these to cling to sheets and be easily discarded. Throw nothing away in a child's room without first asking a child or parent if it is important. What looks like a useless alphabet block to you may mean security and home to a 2-year-old.

Several helpful books about hospitalization are available for parents to read with children and to also learn more about children's health care (Box 36.4). These can be obtained from local bookstores, libraries, or websites and may also be found in the hospital library. For preschool preparation, parents could read one of these books to a child, adapting the story to include information specific to their child.

Because the imagination of preschoolers is at a peak, role-playing can be an effective means of preparing a child of this age for a new experience. To do this, a parent could encourage a child to act out a hospitalization experience with puppets or dolls. Or the child could change into pajamas and get into bed and have a meal in bed. Due to their developmental stage, children often apply literal meaning to spoken words. Be cautious of using common phrases for procedures, such as "put you to sleep" or "taking your blood" as these phrases can be interpreted as literal, leaving the child scared or confused. For example, a child may realize that animals that are put to sleep are not seen again. Talking to another child who has undergone the same experience and come through it intact is yet another helpful way to introduce children and adolescents to hospitalization. Although parents cannot usually supply such a person in advance, upon admission to the hospital, a visit to a recovering patient is often possible and is a constructive way to give reassurance.

If hospitalization is to be more than 1 week long, parents need to think about how their child will continue schooling. Advise them to ask their care provider at what point the child will be able to do homework. Many school systems provide tutors, and children's hospitals often have their own teachers from the local school system to carry out this service so children do not fall behind due to hospitalization (Steinke, Elam, Irwin, et al., 2016).

Preparing a School-Age Child or Adolescent.
School-age children enjoy reading and visual media; thus, books or videos about surgery and hospitalization can be helpful for preparation. Be sure both school-age children and adolescents receive factual explanations of what will happen during surgery.

If parents do not have enough information to be able to answer a school-age child's questions, remind them that few people know everything and caution them that their best response may be "I don't know, but I will find out."

Preparing a Child With a Different Cultural Background.
Perhaps the most important aspect to consider when preparing a child from a different culture for hospitalization is to identify if there are traditions or practices that will be in opposition to usual healthcare facility practices. Ask enough questions and practice good listening skills to gain information about the particular needs of a

child and his or her family. When cultural differences do exist, be prepared to act as a liaison between the family and the healthcare team. If a different language is interfering with communication, a medical translator may be necessary in this preparation phase. Provide the opportunity for parents to voice their fears and ask questions and allow time and opportunity for discussion and effective communication.

Preparing a Child With Unique Concerns or Who Is Chronically Ill.
Children with unique physical concerns or those who are chronically ill frequently come to ambulatory healthcare settings for care; they also are often admitted to the hospital for care and possibly remain in the hospital for an extended time followed by continuing care at home. Children with chronic illness are likely to have been admitted to the hospital in the past, draw upon past experiences, and may be able to let you know how they like certain things (e.g., taking medications a certain way). A child with a chronic illness is still at risk for the same type of anxiety that a child with an acute illness requiring hospitalization has. To decrease anxiety, help children to maintain contact with their families and school friends during a long hospitalization by encouraging telephone calls, social media use, e-mails, text messaging, letters, and visits.

BOX 36.4

Books on Hospitalization for Children and Parents

Bourgeois, P., & Clark, B. (2000). *Franklin goes to the hospital*. New York, NY: Scholastic Publishers. (Grades pre-K to 3)

Bridwell, N. (2011). *Clifford visits the hospital*. New York, NY: Scholastic Publishers. (Grades pre-K to 3)

Civardi, A. (2005). *Going to the hospital*. Tulsa, OK: Usborne Publishers. (Infant to preschool)

Keen, N. (2015). *Your child in the hospital: A practical guide for parents*. (3rd ed.). Bellingham, WA: Childhood Cancer Guides.

Mills, J. C., & Sebern, B. (2003). *Little tree: A story for children with serious medical illness*. Washington, DC: Magination Press. (Early school age)

Rey, H. A. (1999). *Curious George goes to the hospital*. Boston, MA: Houghton Mifflin Co. (Grades 2 to 3)

Ross, T. (2013). *I don't want to go to the hospital!* London, United Kingdom: Andersen Press Picture Books. (Early school age)

Slanina, A. M. (2011). *The adventures of Annie Mouse: Baby brother goes to the hospital*. Harrisville, PA: Anna Mouse Books Publishing. (School age)

What If . . . 36.1

The nurse notices the mother of Becky's roommate, a 2-year-old, brought pots and pans to the hospital as her child's favorite play items. Would the nurse suggest that she bring an actual toy?

QSEN Checkpoint Question 36.2

EVIDENCE-BASED PRACTICE

Preparing children and their families for surgery is crucial and also challenging. Prior to elective surgery, children and their families are often invited to visit the hospital, whereby the child is allowed to learn about the procedure in age-appropriate terms and express his or her concerns through play. Studies have investigated the use of providing age-appropriate preparatory information about procedures, through board games (Fernandes, Arriaga, & Esteves, 2014), interactive puppet shows (Cuzzocrea, Gugliandolo, Larcan, et al., 2013), or web-based programs. Utilizing different platforms not only informs and prepares the child but also reduces anxiety for the child and their caregiver(s).

Based on the study, what would be the best outcome to establish after teaching Becky and her family about surgical process and her anticipated course of recovery?

a. Becky and her family will adhere to preoperative and postoperative instructions.
b. Becky will be able to describe the reasons why a surgical intervention is necessary.
c. Becky will state that she understands the basic principles of asepsis better than before the teaching.
d. Becky will state that she feels less anxious about the prospect of having her foot debrided.

Look in Appendix A for the best answer and rationale.

Unfolding Patient Stories: Eva Madison • Part 2

Recall **Eva Madison**, the 5-year-old child you met in Chapter 34. She is diagnosed with bacterial gastroenteritis. How would the nurse prepare Eva and her parents for hospitalization? What nursing actions can promote a more favorable hospital experience in this age group?

Care for Eva and other patients in a realistic virtual environment: *vSim for Nursing* (thepoint.lww.com /vSimMaternityPed). Practice documenting these patients' care in DocuCare (thepoint.lww.com /DocuCareEHR).

ADMITTING THE ILL CHILD AND FAMILY

Whether an ambulatory or inpatient hospital unit admission, children and parents need to be admitted as a single entity to encourage parents to feel that they are true partners in care (Fig. 36.3). A child coming to a hospital for an elective admission generally arrives at a reception area where demographics are obtained, such as name, age, address, and hospital insurance coverage. The child and parents are then brought to the hospital unit. Remember that first impressions count. If parents are left standing at a counter without being addressed, they can easily feel that no one appreciates their concern and that possibly their child will not receive optimal

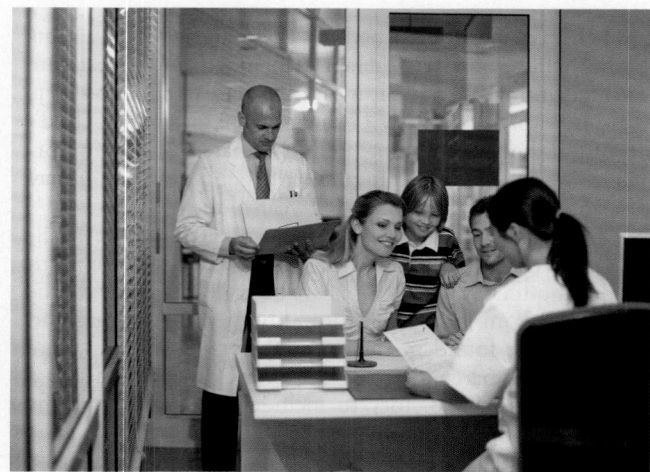

Figure 36.3 A child is admitted to a hospital unit. Notice how the nurse engages all the family's members. (© F1online digitale Bildagentur GmbH/Alamy.)

care. Introduce yourself, explain your role to the parents and child, and find a comfortable place for the family to wait until someone is available to orient them to the unit. When introducing yourself to children, stoop down so that your face is level with the child's face. Call the child by his or her name or ask for a nickname.

All children should have an armband attached which lists their name, date of birth, and hospital medical record number. Because their hands are not much larger than their wrists, and their feet are not much larger than their ankles, small infants often need two bands in place as an extra safeguard. If a band should fall off, verify the patient's identity using at least two patient identifiers (acceptable identifiers may be the individual's name, an assigned identification number, telephone number, or other person-specific identifier) (Joint Commission on Accreditation of Healthcare Organizations, 2015) and secure it back onto the child; never tape it to the crib or bedside stand because this will not properly identify the patient, and the child could be given a wrong medication or have an unintentional procedure.

Assessment on Admission

Assess each child's level of preparation for a hospitalization on admission (Box 36.5). Be aware of not only what the child describes verbally but also note any facial expressions or nervous manifestations.

Interview parents upon hospital admission for a nursing history to obtain the information needed to plan nursing care (see Chapter 34 for a description of a full child database interview history). Many hospitals have information checklists for parents to bring with them. Obtaining information in this way is highly efficient; however, the nurse should review the checklist and ask caregivers if they have any questions and/or concerns. Typical information that is necessary to obtain about a child and that should be included in a plan of care is shown in Table 36.1. Box 36.6 shows an interprofessional care map illustrating both nursing and team planning for a child admitted for 1-day surgery.

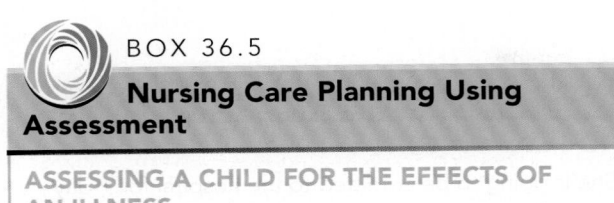

ASSESSING A CHILD FOR THE EFFECTS OF AN ILLNESS

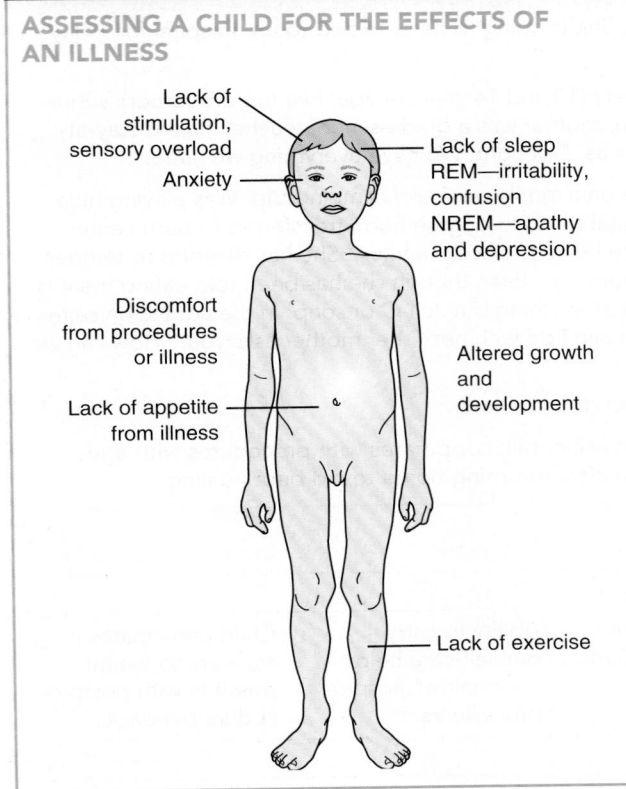

Make a note of any medication or food allergy on the child's plan of care and, if pertinent, post this information in the child's chart and per hospital protocol such as with a specific identification bracelet/band. Unlike an adult, a child cannot call these things to the attention of healthcare personnel when food or medication is offered.

Based on hospital's protocol, the timing of a child's vital signs varies. Initial vital signs include temperature, pulse, and respirations. Measurement of height and weight to determine overall growth and to allow for the determination of safe medication dosages is also warranted. Dependent on the age of the child and diagnosis, blood pressure should be taken using the appropriate size cuff (usually obtained in children over 3 years of age). Review any orders for routine labs and obtain a specimen. Be sure to explain all equipment used and allow the child to touch and handle the equipment as much as possible to help reduce fear.

Inspect for gross motor ability when weighing a child and measuring height. Listen for language ability. Perform a physical examination (see Chapter 34) to gain the information necessary for nursing diagnosis and planning.

The way children deal with hospitalization is based on the same factors that determine how they deal with any crisis: perception of the event, whether support people are available, and effectiveness of past coping experiences or skills. After an assessment, analyze whether a child's coping ability seems to be enough to balance the hazards of inpatient or ambulatory care hospitalization.

TABLE 36.1 INFORMATION NECESSARY FOR THE CHILD'S PLAN OF CARE ON ADMISSION

Area of Information	Specific Knowledge
Chief concern	Determine what the parents' understanding is of why the child is being admitted. (This view may differ widely from the family care provider's view regarding the reason the child is being admitted.) What has the child been told about the reason for hospitalization?
Family profile	Obtain child's name and birthday. Who lives at home (including pets)? Ask about the parents' occupation and education levels. Who is the child's primary caregiver? Have there been any disruptive happenings lately in the child's life, such as a move or a divorce, that would make the child particularly insecure at this time? Will a parent be staying with the child? If parents are separated or divorced, what will the visiting arrangements be? Who has legal authority to sign medical permission?
Past experience with illness or separation	Ask about previous hospital experiences and how the child feels about them. Has there been a recent hospitalization for anyone in the family that resulted in a bad outcome? Has the child been away from the parents before? Overnight at a grandparent's? Summer camp? What is the child's past experience with taking medicine? Has the child swallowed pills before? Does the child have any known allergies to food or medications? (Document these by asking for exact symptoms and happenings.)
Daily routines	Ask about the child's regular bedtime and sleep times. Does the child nap? Is there an important bedtime ritual? What type of bed does the child sleep in at home? Does the child sleep with a favorite toy or blanket? What is the bath time routine? Does the child need help brushing teeth or combing hair or is this done independently? What words does the child use for voiding and defecating? Is the child completely toilet trained? If a preschooler, is the child accustomed to using a potty chair or toilet? Does the child have enuresis (bed-wetting)? What is the child's usual meal plan? Are there foods the child does not eat? Did the child pack a favorite toy for the hospital? What are the child's favorite games and hobbies or interests? Are there television programs the parents especially like the child to see or not see?
Developmental survey	Ascertain the child's developmental level. Does child feed self? Use a spoon, cup, bottle? Dress self? If school age, what grade in school?
Special information	Obtain any special information about the child the parents think would make him or her more comfortable in the hospital.

BOX 36.6

Nursing Care Planning

AN INTERPROFESSIONAL CARE MAP FOR A CHILD HAVING 1-DAY SURGERY

Becky is a 7-year-old who burned her foot in a campfire accident. She is going to be admitted to the hospital for 1-day surgery to have the wound debrided.

Family Assessment: Child lives with parents and two older brothers (10 and 14 years of age) in a three-bedroom suburban home. Father works as sound technician at a recording studio; mother was a grade-school teacher, now is stay-at-home mom; home schools all three children. Father rates finances as, "All right. We have everything we need."

Patient Assessment: Patient burned left foot on a campfire while on a family weekend camping trip. Was playing hide and seek with brothers and ran into the fire. Treated at local hospital for third-degree burn; transferred to burn center for follow-up care. Becky's parents tell you that Becky "hasn't been herself" since the injury. She has reverted to temper tantrums and sulking, more like a 3-year-old than one of early school age. Even though she has been told eating meat is important because it provides protein for healing, she refuses to eat anything but Jell-O or soup. In the admission suite of the hospital, she picked up a doll and twisted its leg off. "What can I do with her?" her mother asks you. "How can we get our old daughter back again?"

Nursing Diagnosis: Anxiety related to hospital admission and burn debridement

Outcome Criteria: Child accurately describes what debridement will entail; cooperates with procedures with age-appropriate responses. Describes measures she will need to take after returning home to aid burn healing.

Team Member Responsible	Assessment	Intervention	Rationale	Expected Outcome
Activities of Daily Living, Including Safety				
Nurse	Assess the degree of self-care child usually carries out.	Allow child maximum inclusion in procedures.	Ability to carry out self-care helps "normalize" hospital procedures.	Child participates in self-care to extent possible with postprocedure bandage.
Teamwork and Consultation				
Nurse/child life specialist	Consult with child life service on what type of therapeutic play would be most beneficial.	Conduct therapeutic play with child before and after debridement procedure.	Therapeutic play can be helpful to children to relieve their anxiety about a painful procedure.	Child participates in therapeutic play and demonstrates less anxious behaviors following debridement.
Procedures/Medications for Quality Improvement				
Nurse	Assess what is the child's greatest concern about the debridement procedure.	Prepare child for surgery, stressing anesthesia will be used to relieve pain during procedure and analgesia will be available after procedure.	A clear understanding of what is to happen helps relieve concern, and knowing pain relief is available is invaluable to well-being.	Child and parent state they understand what procedure will entail, and child cooperates in age-appropriate ways.
Nutrition				
Nurse/nutritionist	Assess what are child's favorite foods.	Suggest ways mother could incorporate protein into soup (meat or beans) to increase protein in child's diet.	Jell-O is a protein source, and adding meat to what child eats will provide protein yet respect the child's choice of food.	Mother details ways she can increase child's protein intake without opposing child's food preferences.
Patient-Centered Care				
Nurse/nurse practitioner	Assess what child and parent understand about debridement procedure.	Educate family about procedure and pre- and postoperative care.	Well-prepared child and the family can better cooperate with care to make the experience a positive one for child.	Child and parents ask questions about the procedure; state they understand what it will entail.

Psychosocial/Spiritual/Emotional Needs

Nurse/nurse practitioner	Take history about unintentional injury resulting in severe burn.	Review with mother what she believes has caused the change in child's attitude. Does she think the child or parents feel guilty about the child's injury?	Children can believe they are being punished by procedures if they believe an injury was their fault; guilt can also influence parent's relationship with child.	Child and parent state they both should have been more diligent to avoid the unintentional injury, but these do happen even in the best circumstances.

Informatics for Seamless Healthcare Planning

Nurse	Assess what will be a typical day for the child after returning home.	Plan with parent what measures child will need to carry out to keep the bandage clean, to exercise the foot, and to return to home schooling.	Prospective planning can help avoid problems in home care.	Child and parent review a typical day and decide on actions that will promote healing.
Nurse/primary healthcare provider	Assess when follow-up visit will be necessary.	Schedule follow-up visit as determined by primary healthcare provider.	A follow-up visit will help ensure the burn is healing without further complications.	Child and parent state they understand importance of follow-up visit and will keep appointment.

 Nursing Diagnoses and Related Interventions

Nursing Diagnosis: Parental and child anxiety related to the need for the child's hospitalization

Outcome Evaluation: Parents and child accurately state the reason for the child's hospital admission and therapy the child will receive; state that although worried, they feel confident they can manage their apprehension.

To help reduce family anxiety regarding hospitalization, assess whether a family is oriented to a hospital stay by discussing the need for hospitalization and what they can expect when the hospitalization is first suggested to them in an ambulatory care setting. When children are admitted for emergency care, this type of orientation must be completed immediately, as soon as their physical needs are met.

On admission, both parents and the child need at least basic information. If the child's diagnosis is uncertain, tell them what steps are being taken to confirm it. It helps if these steps are named specifically (e.g., blood work, X-ray studies, observation, recording of vital signs, calling in a consultant). Ascertain whether they know the tentative plan for the child (e.g., complete bed rest, infection control procedures until the results of blood work or cultures are back, special diet, special procedures). If the plan of care changes, inform the parents and/or child as soon as possible. If the plan of care is uncertain, explain to the family that you are in communication with the healthcare team to obtain it.

If a child is admitted from the emergency room, parents may have little understanding of their child's condition or the treatment plan. Conversely, someone might have taken a great deal of time to explain what was happening while the child was being cared for in the emergency department. Ask them what they have been told and if they have any further questions about their child's condition or the course of treatment they want to discuss with the inpatient facility's healthcare team.

Ideally, a parent or caregiver should be prepared to stay with the child, but if the admission was an emergency, a parent may have to leave rather than remain because of other obligations. If this happens, be certain the parent sees the child's room before leaving because it is important for children to feel confident that their parents know where they can be found when the parents return. If there are other children in the room, introduce the new child to them. Let children wear their own clothes if possible rather than change into hospital gowns for a greater sense of control.

PROMOTING A POSITIVE HOSPITAL STAY

Several nursing actions lay an important foundation for creating a successful, rather than an unsuccessful, hospital experience.

Providing Continuity of Care

To ensure that children are exposed to as few caregivers as possible and to maintain the consistency and quality of care, nursing assignments are best if one nurse gives as much care to the same child as possible (**primary nursing**) (Fig. 36.4). "Primary nursing promotes ongoing communication between the patient, family, nurses, and physicians by building rapport and facilitating discharge planning beginning on admission" (Baynton, 2015). These staffing patterns allow the same nurse to admit the child, take the nursing history, establish nursing diagnoses, set goals for care in cooperation with the parents and the child, and evaluate progress toward achieving goals.

Figure 36.4 Hospitalized children should have one nurse who is "theirs" to minimize the effect of separation from parents (primary care nursing).

Figure 36.5 Rooming-in helps alleviate separation anxiety for both the child and the parent.

It allows children to have one main nurse to call their own. It is also helpful to parents because it allows them to establish a meaningful contact with the hospital staff and maintains continuity of care, planning, and implementation.

 ## Nursing Diagnoses and Related Interventions

Nursing Diagnosis: Anxiety of child related to separation during hospitalization

Outcome Evaluation: The child will have the ability to eliminate or reduce feelings of apprehension and tension from an identified source. The child will express their feelings and remain calm.

Promoting Open Parent Visiting. When possible, young children should have a parent room-in with them when they are in the hospital (Fig. 36.5). Even children 10 to 12 years of age enjoy short time spans alone but also continue to enjoy the feeling of security rooming-in provides. Because a parent will be sleeping alongside the child, check the room has a parent as well as a child bed. When parents were first allowed to sleep over in children's units, it was thought their presence would reduce the need for nursing care. In many instances, because so much parental education is needed, requirements for healthcare personnel actually increase.

If parents cannot stay continuously, they may ask for help in smoothing the transition of coming or going. You may need to remind them that it is not uncommon for this age group to go through three different phases: protest, despair, and detachment. Initially, if a child is left alone by his or her parent, they may scream and cry in protest. Explain to the parents that this is normal and to not feel guilty leaving their child if they need to attend to other commit-

ments. Once the crying stops, children will act depressed and withdraw themselves from the parent and healthcare providers. During the detachment phase, children often become more interested in their surroundings than in visitors. This is a coping mechanism only and is not a sign that they have accepted separation from their parent. It is not unusual that when a toddler first sees parents after being separated, a common reaction might be to ignore them (a sign of despair). This is a defense mechanism: "I won't show you I love you until you show me you love me; that way I won't be hurt again." If a parent's reaction to being treated this way causes the parent to play with a child in the next bed—a "well, be that way then" reaction—the toddler's worst fears are fulfilled: a parent has forgotten about him. To avoid this type of interaction, urge parents to speak to the child for a few minutes or try to interest the child in a toy despite the child's "cold shoulder"; after a short time, a child will generally reach out to be comforted and will act relieved the parents are there.

Parents often need help in saying goodbye when it is time to leave a child so they can eat a meal or go home for the night (if the parent is not sleeping in). Assure parents that although someone will not be in their child's room every minute while they are gone, the child will be well cared for. When the parents of an infant are leaving, go into the room a few minutes before they leave and hold or play with the infant. Help a parent to say once, "I have to go now," and then leave. Prolonged departures only delay the process and do not reduce the amount of crying that may occur. After parents leave, hold and rock infants to let them know that they are safe even though their preferred caregiver is no longer present.

If the parents of a toddler or preschooler have to leave, urge them first to give a warning they will soon have to go: "I have to leave in a minute to fix dinner for Daddy." When the time to go has come, the parent should say firmly that it is time to go and then explain the time he or she will return. Time for a preschooler is best measured in terms of events rather than clock hours. "I'll be back after you've eaten supper," is better than "I'll be back at seven"; and "after you wake up tomorrow," is better than 8 AM as these times give the child a concrete event by which to measure time. Like infants, toddlers need someone with them when their parents leave; they like to be held or played with so they know they are not alone.

When parents leave a school-age child or adolescent, urge them to provide definite times when they will return and to leave suggestions for activities a child could do to occupy the time (e.g., "Why don't you finish your book? Get a start on your homework and I'll check it when I come back"). Remind them it is more comforting to name a specific time, "I'll be back around 9 tomorrow morning" rather than a vague time period such as "I'll be back sometime tomorrow."

When a child has to leave the patient unit for surgery, it may be especially difficult for parents to separate. Reminding them that the surgery is important and helping them manage this is an important part of preoperative nursing care.

Providing Opportunities for Parents to Participate in Child's Care.
One of the most stressful parts of a child's hospitalization is the parents feeling that their parental role is diminished (Foster et al., 2016). Participating in their child's care can make parents feel more in control, thereby reducing their unease, which then hopefully transmits to reducing anxiety in their child. Encourage parents, therefore, to give as much care as possible during a hospital stay, such as bathing or feeding their child, giving oral medicine, helping with procedures such as warm soaks, or assessing that their child is awake from anesthesia. Most parents are eager to help and do these things spontaneously. Be certain they have proper instruction on the tasks they will be able to do. Be sure parents who change diapers or feed children know whether the number of diaper changes or the amount of food intake needs to be recorded; ask them to report when they do these things or write them down on a flow sheet attached to the child's door or crib. Do not ask them to restrain children for a procedure that will be painful because their main job should be to comfort. Occasionally, parents may be reluctant to give care for fear of being judged inadequate. You can assure them they are the persons from whom their child would most like to receive care.

Because children may be especially apprehensive about undergoing a procedure without a parent present, there is rarely any reason a parent cannot accompany a child into a treatment room to help with undressing, measuring weight and height, and taking a temperature or accompanying a child to another department for a procedure such as an ultrasound or blood work. Most importantly, the mother or father can continue to comfort the child in these strange surroundings.

Patient- and family-centered care includes the whole family, whereby the family has an integral part in shared decision making. Patient- and family-centered care is an approach to the planning, delivery, and evaluation of healthcare that is grounded in mutually beneficial partnerships among healthcare providers, patients, and families. It redefines the relationships in health care (Institute for Patient- and Family-Centered Care, 2016).

Promoting patient- and family-centered care is essential and allows parents and caregivers to participate in their child's care. Family-centered care opportunities include allowing caregivers to be active in patient rounds, which include decision making regarding clinical management and communication among the team members and serve as a venue for teaching and discussion (Blankenship, Harrison, Brandt, et al., 2015).

What If . . . 36.2
Becky's father does not call the nurse when her intravenous pump alarms that it is finished. Instead, he resets the pump himself. How would the nurse best respond?

Supporting Sibling Visitations.
Children in a family are under considerable stress while a sibling is hospitalized because their world changes as much as the parents' world does (Ivany, LeBlanc, Grisdale, et al., 2016). Incorporating family-centered care supports the need for sibling visitation. Sibling visitation refers to allowing the brothers and sisters of a hospitalized child to visit the ill child along with parents. Allowing this alleviates loneliness on both sides, helps prevent other children at home from imagining the ill child is sicker than is true, and helps the ill child continue to feel a part of the family. Check with parents that siblings who visit are free of communicable disease. During a visit, you may need to help parents divide their time between the ill child and siblings (short, frequent visits may be better for young children than long ones).

Minimizing Negative Effects of Procedures.
Children often undergo numerous diagnostic and therapeutic procedures that have the potential to cause pain, fear, and anxiety. Details related to specific procedures are discussed in Chapter 37. General guidelines designed to make any procedure less painful or frightening are discussed in the following sections.

Nursing Diagnosis: Fear related to diagnostic or therapeutic procedures

Outcome Evaluation: Child voices satisfaction with comfort measures; describes self-participation in a procedure; rates experience as no less than "tolerable" after the procedure.

Reducing or Eliminating Pain.
Some pain and discomfort are unavoidable in association with health care. Limit this whenever possible, however, by such measures as advocating for the use of intermittent infusion devices such as heparin locks (see Chapter 38) to eliminate multiple punctures for intravenous medication or blood sampling, providing traditional comforts such as a change of clothing or position, or talking about a favorite subject. Children respond well to alternative therapy techniques, such as distraction or imagery, to divert attention from painful stimuli, lessening pain and distress. Music, video, breathing exercises and storytelling are examples of distraction techniques that have been effective (Al-Yateem, Brenner, Shorrab, et al., 2016). Children may not always express discomfort as freely as adults; thus, age-appropriate assessments before and after a procedure are necessary to assess their pain.

Maintaining the Child's Bed as a Safe Area. To assure children that their bed is an area that is safe, all painful procedures should be done in a treatment room or another department, away from the child's bed. Decreasing painful procedures at the bedside promotes a child's feeling of safety. Remember that finger punctures for blood work, although done quickly, can cause as much pain and stress as a venipuncture. In addition, dressing changes, although not necessarily painful, can cause worry and also should be done in a treatment or procedure room, when applicable.

Helping Children Maintain Control. Events are always more frightening if they seem to be beyond our control. Based on the child's *developmental age*, explaining to children what will happen, including what they will feel or what they will see, and helping them to make choices whenever possible limits this type of fear because these actions offer a sense of control (Fig. 36.6). In almost any procedure, there is some choice a child can make (e.g., whether or not to use a straw to drink, deciding what size of tape to use on a bandage, or deciding which direction to walk down the hallway).

Providing Adequate Play Facilities

Play is often described as the work of children because it is the medium through which they learn. Play is often an indicator of how the child is coping with the stressors of hospitalization and may act as way to control their environment (Potasz, Varela, Carvalho, et al., 2013). Children need to be able to play as much as possible not only to aid in distraction but also to encourage emotional well-being. Most children's hospital units are equipped with a playroom or play space that is maintained as a "pain-free" zone. No medical procedures, not even painless ones, should be performed in this area because the child may then perceive the space as frightening. Children who are on bed rest need age-appropriate activities supplied for them to prevent boredom and a loss of control, which can lead to depression or behavioral regression.

Therapeutic play is play designed to help children express their feelings about painful or frightening procedures (He, Zhu, Chan, et al., 2015); however, play needs are different for each child. A child's characteristics, such as temperament,

Figure 36.6 Include children in procedures whenever possible to offer them a feeling of control. (gpointstudio/Shutterstock.com)

coping style, and cognitive abilities; family variables such as parental anxiety, presence, and involvement; and diagnosis/treatment variables are known to affect psychosocial vulnerability and thus influence the child's particular needs in terms of play (Brown, Chitkara, Percelay, et al., 2014; Koller, 2008). The uses of therapeutic play and guidelines for providing this are discussed later in this chapter.

Setting Limits on Behavior

Setting limits on behavior can help promote a positive hospital stay because it can help to provide a sense of security and safety. Children who refuse to cooperate for procedures generally do so out of fear of the unknown rather than deliberate misbehavior. The better prepared a child is for a procedure, the more apt the child is to accept it (Raleting, 2015). If limit setting is necessary, such as with a child who hits or bites other children, confer with the child's parents about the need for limit setting and what measures they would suggest. Gain their cooperation and approval so that what you do is consistent with their usual care. Using "time-out" periods or removing the child to a nonstimulating area for a short time could be an effective measure. Be certain a child understands time-out rules (e.g., if the child bites or hits again, sitting alone for a designated period will be necessary). The next time the child does misbehave, give one warning that the behavior is against the rules; if the behavior continues, take the child to the time-out spot. If the child is disruptive, begin timing the period from when the child quiets down. When the child has been quiet for the specified duration (usually 1 minute per year of age), the child can leave the time-out place and rejoin activities.

DISCHARGE PLANNING

Discharge planning is not only an important link between the hospital and the home, but it is also a final way to create a satisfying hospital experience.

> **Nursing Diagnoses and Related Interventions**
>
> **Nursing Diagnosis:** Parental health-seeking behaviors related to care for child at home after hospital discharge
>
> **Outcome Evaluation:** Parents state accurately the care their child will need at home; describe and demonstrate any procedures they will need to perform with child.

Discharge from the hospital involves education, even if the hospitalization lasted a few hours (e.g., same-day surgery). It is vitally important that nurses anticipate the family's and child's discharge needs so the discharge process is one of continuity with hospital care. It is important to collaborate with the interdisciplinary team and assess the family's resources (physical and emotional) for the ability to provide continued care before the child is discharged home. Discharge planners can be indispensable in helping to ready parents for home care. Often, discharge follow-up instructions include referrals to services such as physical therapy, mental health, and visiting nurses. Communicating with the family through verbal and written instructions is essential for maintaining comprehensive care. Electronic communication, in the form of e-mail, text messaging, and mobile apps, are being utilized for follow-up care (Holland, Conlon, Rohlik, et al., 2015).

If a child has been admitted to an ambulatory care unit, preparation for discharge should begin at almost the same time as admission. If caregivers are instructed to continue a procedure at home, allow them to demonstrate that skill in the hospital; this allows for education and guidance before a parent is to perform independently at home. For example, if a parent is to continue changing sterile dressings, where can they buy dressings? Will they be able to afford them? Allowing communication between the nurse and parent is essential for transition of care to the home.

It is not uncommon for preschool children to manifest regression in behavior, such as thumb-sucking, bedwetting, temper tantrums, and nightmares, after returning home from a hospital stay; school-age children may manifest these behaviors to a lesser extent. Reassure parents that this regression in behavior is often temporary. More serious manifestations after hospital discharge include posttraumatic stress and are often seen after a stay in a PICU. "Parents describe decreases in children's self-esteem and emotional well-being, increased anxiety, and negative behavioral changes, e.g., sleep disturbances, social isolation" (Rennick, Dougherty, Chambers, et al., 2014).

Nursing Responsibilities for Care of the Ill Child and Family

Nursing responsibilities will vary, naturally, with the type, extent, and seriousness of a child's illness, age, care setting, and individual circumstances. Chapter 37 discusses specific responsibilities related to diagnostic tests or interventions. Chapter 39 discusses the important role of promoting comfort in an ill child. A number of responsibilities such as promotion of normal growth and development, sleep, stimulation, and play are more global, cross all ages and phases of care, and are discussed here.

PROMOTING GROWTH AND DEVELOPMENT OF THE ILL CHILD

It is easy for children to fall behind in growth and development because of an illness unless healthcare providers monitor for and strengthen this.

 Nursing Diagnoses and Related Interventions

Nursing Diagnosis: Risk for delayed growth and development related to the effects of illness

Outcome Evaluation: Child demonstrates only limited signs of regression to previous stage; is able to continue doing the activities most recently accomplished.

Illness represents a crisis event, and, in a crisis state, children, like adults, can grow from the experience or, in contrast, can be overwhelmed and regress.

The Ill Infant. To promote optimal growth and development in infants, maintain their at-home schedule when possible. Sameness provides security to an infant and encourages the development of trust. An infant who is used to sleeping in a bassinet, for example, may feel loose and insecure in a large crib. Swaddling such a child in a receiving blanket in a large crib would help to offer the same close, bound feeling of a smaller sleeping area. Providing a singular room in a NICU has been shown to improve parent satisfaction with care because it removes the parents from the noise and tension of the larger, unstructured room (Caldwell, 2015).

Unless a child is diagnosed with failure to thrive or is obviously underweight, illness is not an ideal period in which to introduce new foods or formula. Breastfeeding should be continued if at all possible. If a mother cannot be at the hospital constantly, urge her to pump milk, freeze it, and bring it in so her child can continue to receive the immunologic protection of breast milk. Overall, because infants cannot begin to understand the strange feelings accompanying illness, they need increased swaddling and comforting. As their condition improves, provide stimulation and play opportunities suitable for their developmental age.

The Ill Toddler and Preschooler. Because illness can limit autonomy and prevent children from learning how to do new things, try to find opportunities to promote both autonomy in toddlers and initiative in preschoolers. One way to accomplish this is to encourage children to make choices about their care whenever possible. For instance, taking medications is not a choice, so never ask "Do you want to take your medicine now?" unless there's really a choice—almost all children will say "NO!" Instead ask, "Which do you want to take first, the white medicine or the pink?" Toddlers and preschoolers who are not used to sleeping in cribs at home may resent being placed in a crib in a hospital unless you explain to them, "All our beds here have side rails." Watch energetic toddlers closely to be certain they do not attempt to climb over crib rails to get out of bed. A child who does try to climb out of a crib might be safer sleeping in a bed or may need a safety crib cover when a parent is not in the room.

As with infants, illness is a poor time to change the eating habits of toddlers and preschoolers. Because children of this age insist on self-feeding, they often eat better at a small table than using a tray in bed. Many child care units organize "toddler tables" so children this age can eat together. Supervise children carefully if they are eating with others to be certain they eat only their own food, not food belonging to someone else. Also be certain they are not so distracted by other children that they do not eat. All children may eat better when a parent joins them for a meal.

Illness is also a poor time to introduce toilet training, even if this is an appropriate activity for the child's age. However, if parents have already begun toilet training, continue this if possible, so you maintain a usual routine.

The Ill School-Age Child. Ill school-age children need to continue to work on a sense of industry or learning more about how and why things are done. Explaining specific procedures and involving them as much as possible in planning their care allows school-age children to have some semblance of independence and control, which in turn promotes self-care. Self-care attributes the practice of activities that an individual initiates and performs on his or her own behalf to maintain life, health, and well-being (Orem, 2001).

School-age children (and adolescents) who are hospitalized for the short or long term become socially isolated from their families, classmates, and friends and from the normalcy of everyday life (Hopkins, Green, Henry, et al., 2014). They need to continue schooling, provided their condition allows it. Maintaining that routine, everyday activity provides security to an otherwise insecure day. With increased, readily available technologies providing access, communication and interaction, and with a variety of tools and software applications, the use of technology may offer opportunities for learning for children in hospitals who otherwise will not be able to connect to their original schools (Maor & Mitchem, 2015).

Remember, school-age children also are developing moral responsibility and so may find comfort in spiritual practices. Ways to assist with spiritual needs during a hospitalization are shown in Table 36.2.

Encourage school-age children to carry out as much self-care as usual, and, if being cared for at home, to continue to contribute to household routines, such as helping with dishes or picking up after themselves as much as they are able. This not only takes some burden off caregivers but also sends a signal that people expect this illness to pass and the child to become a full family member again.

The Ill Adolescent. An adolescent who is struggling to develop a sense of identity may find it difficult to be ill because the limitations imposed by an illness make the development of a sense of identity so difficult. If possible, help adolescents to continue to participate in activities they did before becoming hospitalized to help them feel that their world is not totally changing. Encourage them to maintain self-care activities and good hygiene practices to help preserve self-esteem.

Illness can be especially difficult for adolescents also because peer relationships are so important to them and a hospitalization automatically interferes with those. They may miss acting in a school play, being chosen for a sports team, or competing for a scholarship. A girlfriend or boyfriend may break off a relationship. To help avoid feelings of exclusion and hurt, urge them to welcome visitors from their peer group. Suggest electronic communication formats such as texting or e-mailing as easy ways to keep in contact with friends and maintain relationships with individuals who are important to them while separated from them.

Adolescents usually appreciate being hospitalized in a special adolescent unit or at least in a room free of childish decor. Consider that parents of an adolescent have the same anxiety and concerns as parents with younger children. Fear of procedures and pain of separation are not limited to the younger than 13 years of age set. Although many adolescents enjoy having parents stay overnight because it is reassuring to know that they are concerned, they may also enjoy being separated (assuming everything is going well) and may not want their parents present all day and night.

Often, adolescents convey a blasé attitude toward procedures (e.g., having an X-ray taken is nothing, surgery is a cinch, a cast change is a snap). Listen carefully to make certain adolescents really feel this way and are not trying to convince themselves that a procedure is harmless. Remember that adolescents are extremely worried about their body image. Explain to them what is going to happen in surgery or in other departments because it is easy to assume from their attitude they know more than they do.

TABLE 36.2 NURSING INTERVENTIONS TO MEET CHILDREN'S SPIRITUAL NEEDS

Action	Implementation
Rituals/religious/ spiritual practice	Ask on hospital admission whether a child follows rituals or a religious/ spiritual practice. Write it on the plan of care so all health care providers know to provide time for this.
Services	Include time for children and their families to attend religious and/or spiritual services. When warranted, ensure transportation by wheelchair or other means available.
Spiritual support	Allow volunteers representing different faith communities or congregations to be providers of spiritual care.
Religious articles	A child's parent may wish to attach a religious article to the child's clothing or pillow or to post it over the bed. Be careful when changing linen or gowns so that you do not throw away such articles. Mark their presence and importance on the child's plan of care.

PROMOTING NUTRITIONAL HEALTH OF THE ILL CHILD

Nursing responsibilities related to nutrition for ill children include maintaining optimal nutritional status in the face of an illness or therapy that interferes with adequate intake, correcting nutritional deficiencies or otherwise aiding children and families to follow the nutritional care plan devised by the healthcare team, and educating a child and family regarding specific nutritional needs as well as overall sound nutritional health. Specific procedures for promoting nutrition such as measuring fluid intake and output and providing enteral feedings, gastrostomy tube feedings, and total parenteral nutrition are described in Chapter 37.

 Nursing Diagnoses and Related Interventions

Nursing Diagnosis: Risk for imbalanced nutrition, less than body requirements, related to lack of appetite

Outcome Evaluation: Child will exhibit no further weight loss and, if malnourished, will gain 2.2 lb (1 kg) per week. The child will maintain adequate nutritional status as evidenced by weight within the normal range for age.

An acute illness in a child, such as pneumonia, is often accompanied by a loss of appetite; gastrointestinal illnesses frequently cause nausea, vomiting, and diarrhea, making hydration difficult to maintain. Because most acute illnesses last only a few days, there is no need for children to eat more than a small amount during this time as long as they can drink fluid. Trying to force them to eat only increases nausea and vomiting, which increases the possibility of creating an electrolyte imbalance. The need for IV hydration is discussed in Chapters 38 and 45. When an illness lasts for more than a few days, however, providing adequate nutrition becomes increasingly important because children need nutrients not only to repair ill or diseased tissue but also to maintain normal childhood growth.

Important points to address when planning nutrition for ill children are summarized in Table 36.3. Children who are hospitalized often tolerate hospital-prepared food, which can be repetitive and bland, better than adults. Provided that it is the kind of food they like, such as chicken fingers or pizza, these may appeal to children more than the elaborate dishes with spices and sauces preferred by adults. Children who are receiving care at home need as much nursing supervision of their nutrition as those in healthcare agencies (possibly more) because they may not have a dietitian planning meals to ensure adequate nutrition. Assess not only the quantity but also the quality of food to ensure that intake is optimal. If prescribed, ask whether nutrition supplements are being offered to increase intake.

Encouraging Fluid Intake: Increasing oral fluid intake when a child is at risk for dehydration is important. A primary care provider's instruction should state in detail the amount of fluid a child is to receive during 24 hours because the amount differs from age to age.

- Offer small, full glasses frequently rather than larger, half-full glasses; children are mid–school age before they

evaluate the amount of fluid in a container rather than the size of the container.
- Determine the child's favorite fluid and then offer it, if appropriate.
- Popsicles and Jell-O count as fluids.
- Children can drink more of a clear fluid (e.g., ginger ale, water) than a thicker fluid (e.g., milk shakes, cream soups) because thicker fluids are absorbed from the stomach much more slowly.
- Suggest soothing beverages such as milk or Pedialyte popsicles for children with mouth lesions. Avoid carbonated beverages and citrus or acidic fruit juices because the acid content and/or carbonation sting their mouths.
- Ice melts to one half its volume. Count a glass of ice chips as only a half-full glass of fluid.
- Encourage breast feeding whenever possible.
- Unless contraindicated, let children drink fluids with a straw; this is a novelty to many who do not normally use these and so encourages intake.
- Introduce a game, such as Simon Says (Simon says, "Drink") or a board game in which a child takes turns and with each turn has to take a drink. Use play as a method of teaching nutrition and sound dietary habits to children (Hayes, Spano, Donnelly, et al., 2014).

Encouraging Food Intake. **Calorie counting**, as the name implies, involves counting the number of calories that children ingest each day. To do this, record all the foods that a child eats during each 24-hour period, being certain to include snacks, candy, or gum. A dietitian then will analyze the list and determine the caloric intake. Be certain when doing this that you describe the types of food and amounts (i.e., not "some toast," but "half a slice of whole wheat toast"). Make sure that everyone caring for the child (including parents) is aware that calories are being counted so that they also record this information accurately.

TABLE 36.3 AREAS TO CONSIDER WHEN PLANNING NUTRITION FOR ILL CHILDREN

Area	Importance
Meaning of food	Early in life, infants learn to associate eating with being held and loved; if they cannot eat for some reason, such as while waiting for surgery, they may view the restriction as punishment or a restriction of love. Encourage a parent to sit and rock them or read to them to lessen this uncomfortable time.
Opportunity for socialization	Mealtime is an ideal time for family members to socialize and share their day; being separated from family for meals can create loneliness and, consequently, a poor appetite. Urge parents to visit at mealtime if possible, so "sharing a day" can continue.
Level of stress	Children under stress may either feel a loss of appetite or experience a need to snack frequently; this can make it necessary to be certain children maintain adequate intake if not hungry and that, when hungry, their snacks are nutritious.
Custom and culture	Food customs are important; for example, many children like foods served separately and resist eating them if they are mixed into a casserole. They like best the foods they typically eat at home. If possible, ask if a parent could bring in a favorite food treat to stimulate appetite.
Environment	Hunger is associated with the sight and smell of food; many children are normally in the kitchen and help prepare meals; they may not feel as hungry, therefore, when food is served to them without their having seen and smelled it being prepared. Allowing them to pick what foods they want for meals, if possible, gives them at least some sense of food preparation and selection.

QSEN Checkpoint Question 36.3

QUALITY IMPROVEMENT

The nurse wants to encourage Becky to drink a lot of water to promote hydration. During the most recent rounds, Becky drank an entire 10-oz glass at once and vomited several minutes later. Considering the failed attempt to encourage oral hydration, what would be the nurse's best next course of action?

a. Teach Becky about the consequences of failing to drink sufficient water.
b. Set up a plan with Becky and her parents to provide small glasses of water frequently.
c. Continue to offer her large glasses of water so she does not have to drink so often.
d. Alert her that if she does not increase her fluid intake she will likely have to receive IV fluids.

Look in Appendix A for the best answer and rationale.

Promoting Safety for the Ill Child

A prime consideration of nursing interventions is to keep children safe during illness care.

Nursing Diagnoses and Related Interventions

Nursing Diagnosis: Risk for injury related to procedures or therapy necessary for care

Outcome Evaluation: Child remains free of injury, such as a fall from bed or injury from medical equipment.

Promoting safety for children is a responsibility for all healthcare providers. Care of a child who is ill and being cared for at home includes assessing the safety of the house and providing family teaching. It also includes making provisions for emergencies. For example, a family may need to install a counter-level telephone or purchase a cell phone so a child in a wheelchair can call for emergency help. Parents might also need to make a plan for how to evacuate an ill child from the home in an emergency such as a fire.

Safety on a children's unit or clinic is the responsibility of all healthcare providers, from the administrator of the institution to part-time healthcare personnel. Important steps to follow to make a child healthcare environment a safer place include:

- Always be sure of the location of all children in your care.
- Ensure that doors or gates are provided near stairways or elevators.
- Ensure that doors of healthcare facilities have working alarms to prevent children from going out and to prevent strangers from coming in.
- Be sure windows are covered by screens or guards so children cannot climb up on sills and fall out.
- Check that the side rails of beds and cribs are in good repair, raised appropriately, and locked.
- Always raise bedside rails after a child has received preoperative or sedative medication.

- Test a crib rail after it is raised to ensure the lock has caught so the rail will remain raised.
- Push bedside tables or stands away from cribs so a child cannot climb over the railing and use the stand as a step down.
- Be certain crib caps are available for small children to prevent them from climbing out of bed.
- Fasten the seat belt restraint for infants in high chairs. Never leave an infant in a high chair (at home or in a hospital) without someone close enough to reach the child because infants can easily squirm out of a high chair restraint.
- Ensure that electrical cords or appliances such as hair dryers are not used in bathrooms, where they could come in contact with water.
- Be careful of the placement of television/call cords or window blind cords so they cannot lead to strangulation.
- Never leave children alone in a bathtub; they could turn on the hot water and scald themselves or slip under the water and drown.
- Never leave equipment or items that would be harmful to eat within the reach of children.
- Adhere to all fire precaution measures.
- Closely follow standard infection precautions to prevent the spread of infections.

Promoting Fire Safety. Fire precautions both in the home and in the hospital are essential in preserving the safety of children. Adults can usually take responsibility for removing themselves from a burning structure, but children depend on care providers. Ensure that there is a plan of action in case of a fire and that everyone in the home, in the clinic, or on a hospital unit knows it. To be certain a home is safe, having a smoke detector on each floor is a wise precaution. A downstairs bedroom is not only safest in case of a fire but also allows a child more self-care ability. Fire departments supply free decals for the bedroom windows of children or those with a unique concern so they can be easily located in a fire. Parents can contact their local fire department for this safety measure.

Electrical equipment such as respiratory and cardiac monitors, radiant heat warmers, special-care equipment, and electrical heating pads are often used in the care of children. Do not use equipment with frayed cords or equipment that is not properly grounded. Plugs should be three pronged for extra safety; do not overload circuits with additional plugs. Electrical outlets should have safety caps to cover them when they are not in use so toddlers cannot poke objects into them and electrocute themselves.

Adhering to Standard Infection Precautions. In every healthcare setting, closely follow standard infection precautions to protect ill children, the family, and staff from infections (CDC, 2015b). With a compromised immune system, ill children may be more susceptible to repeat or secondary infections than usual, especially drug-resistant strains of bacteria such as methicillin-resistant *Staphylococcus aureus* (MRSA), which can spread easily if not everyone is conscientious about precautions. A proper hand washing technique, disposal of tissues and waste materials, and efforts to minimize exposure of other ill children or adults are all effective methods to decrease the risk of infection. For more details on infection control, see Chapter 43.

Promoting Adequate Sleep for the Ill Child

Ill children need adequate rest and sleep so their body tissues can effectively use nutrients for repair and normal growth can continue (Stremler, Adams, & Dryden-Palmer, 2015). Children may not sleep well when they are ill because of discomfort, pain, the administration of medications, or intensified symptoms of chronic sleep problems. They may not sleep well in a hospital because it is a strange setting; they may have to undergo so many procedures that they also do not nap or rest as much during the day as usual. Children who are recovering from trauma such as injuries from a car accident or burns may be unable to sleep because of nightmares about the accident. These nightmares can cause them to suffer sleep deprivation in the same way as a child who is frequently awakened for procedures during the night. Encourage parents to stay with these children for support and comfort. Remember, though, that parents who sleep in hospital rooms do not obtain adequate sleep either. Although their presence is healthy for children, it can limit the parents' capacity to meet the child's needs (Angelhoff, Edéll-Gustafsson, & Mörelius, 2015).

SLEEP PATTERNS

Sleep is influenced by apprehension level, state of health, habit, medication, and environment at the time of sleep. Stages of sleep are summarized in Table 36.4. Figure 36.7A shows a pattern of normal sleep. According to the National Sleep Foundation (2017), as a sleep cycle begins, children first enter **non–rapid eye movement (NREM) sleep**. This type of sleep occurs in up to 80% of total sleep time. As children fall deeper and deeper asleep, they pass from stage I to stages II, III, and IV of NREM sleep over a period of 20 to 30 minutes. **Rapid eye movement (REM) sleep** follows. In infants, most of sleep time is REM sleep, whereas late adolescents have the least amount of this type of sleep. The sleep pattern of a child who is awakened frequently during the night for procedures would resemble that shown in Figure 36.7B.

The purpose of NREM sleep, the first phase of sleep, is rest and restoration of the body; this stage keeps body cells functioning and healthy. During the periods of stages III and IV NREM sleep, the secretion of growth hormone (somatotropic hormone) from the pituitary is at its highest level. Growth hormone is necessary for protein synthesis, for the growth of new cells, and for the repair and maintenance of all cells. Corticosteroids and adrenaline from the adrenal gland, which are instrumental in the catabolism or breakdown of cells, are at their lowest levels. This balance of hormones produces the ideal combination for protein synthesis and cell growth and repair.

The purpose of REM sleep is less clear. The REMs may serve to coordinate binocular vision. Dreams that occur during this time apparently serve as a release of tension or help to integrate new knowledge and experiences with the old in the brain's memory system. Vital signs may fall during NREM sleep. During REM sleep, vital signs rise to near normal levels. These periods of REM sleep interspersed with NREM sleep, therefore, may be a fail-safe measure to prevent vital signs from falling too low during sleep.

SLEEP DEPRIVATION

Infants are dependent on sleep to promote brain development. Deprivation of sleep from 2 to 4 hours in healthy infants has been studied and thought to lead to short-term variations in cardiac function as well as an increase in apneic events (Allen, 2012). Children who do not receive enough sleep can suffer **sleep deprivation**, just as adults do. After approximately 4 days of poor sleep, this can cause them to experience difficulty in concentrating and episodes of disorientation and misperception.

TABLE 36.4 STAGES OF SLEEP IN CHILDREN

Stage	Description	Nursing Implications
Non–rapid eye movement (NREM) stage I	A feeling of drifting or falling. Often described as twilight sleep. Temperature and heart rate decrease slightly; electroencephalogram (EEG) waves show peaked, frequent (alpha) waves.	A child can be roused easily from this early sleep by the slightest noise or silent presence of another person in the room. Reduce noise level in room to promote sleep.
NREM stage II	Sleep deepens. Temperature and heart rate decrease slightly more.	It is more difficult to wake a child from sleep when this point is reached.
NREM stage III	Sleep deepens still further. An EEG tracing reveals mixed spindle and slow (delta) waves. Temperature and heart rate decrease further. This period lasts about 10 min.	It is very difficult to wake a child from stage III sleep. Use patience to wake a child fully to offer medicine.
NREM stage IV	Approximately 20–30 min after beginning to fall asleep, a child enters stage IV sleep. Respirations and heart rate slow even more, and blood pressure and temperature decrease; EEG shows slow, steady (delta) waves. Children remain at a stage IV sleep level for approximately 30 min and then progress back through stages III and II until they then pass into a phase of REM sleep.	Children may be confused and unable to orient themselves readily if awakened from stage IV sleep. Use patience until a child is fully awake, particularly if asking a question.
Rapid eye movement (REM)	Eyes move in rapid, involuntary motions. Respirations are irregular; body turnings, movements, and penile erections may occur. Lasts 10 to 30 min and then a new sleep cycle with NREM sleep begins.	Dreaming occurs during REM sleep. Although children appear to be close to waking because of the active eye movements, they are really very soundly asleep. Children may wake afraid and crying, disturbed by a frightening dream.

Figure 36.7 Sleep patterns. **(A)** A normal sleep pattern. Notice how the periods of rapid eye movement (REM) sleep increase in length during the last half of the night. **(B)** The sleep pattern of a child who has been awakened frequently during the night. Notice how little REM sleep is present.

If the sleep loss is mainly REM deprivation, children show symptoms of irritability and difficulty concentrating. Lack of stage IV NREM sleep, in contrast, tends to cause apathy, physical fatigue, and depression and can slow recovery. This is the same phenomenon that can happen in adolescents if they are studying for exams. It easily occurs in younger children during illness if they are awakened frequently for treatments.

 Nursing Diagnoses and Related Interventions

Nursing Diagnosis: Disturbed sleep pattern related to timing of medication, discomfort, or sleep disorder

Outcome Evaluation: Child sleeps through the night without interruption (when therapeutic regimen allows); is alert and active during the day; is able to take nap during the day if that is part of his or her usual sleep schedule.

Because sleep is so important for ill children, you need to take special steps to ensure that children are able to sleep during an illness. Be certain children are as free of pain and worry as possible. Try to let them maintain as normal a bedtime routine as possible (e.g., bath, change to nightclothes, nighttime story, prayers). Provide an atmosphere conducive to sleep (e.g., lights out, quiet surroundings, reassuring support people). Children who are bored with bed rest may catnap constantly during the day and then be wide awake at night. Providing more interesting activities for them during the day can help reduce their naps and increase nighttime sleep.

Managing Chronic Sleep Problems. Some children may have chronic sleep problems such as night terrors, nocturnal enuresis, somnambulism (sleepwalking), sleep talking, and sleep apnea. These sleep problems can intensify with illness and can increase sleep deprivation in ill children.

Somnambulism is a common sleep problem in children. It apparently occurs during NREM sleep, probably during the deepest part of stage IV. It is frightening for children to wake and realize they have been sleepwalking. Sleepwalking can be potentially dangerous when children are ill because, while getting out of bed, they could dislodge intravenous tubing or oxygen equipment. It is untrue that sleepwalkers should not be wakened; instead, wake them gently, help them get reoriented, and then return them to bed after reassuring them they are safe. Be certain that the side rails are raised on the bed of a child who tends to sleepwalk. In a hospital, it may be necessary to move a child's bed out into the hallway at night near the nurses' desk if a parent will not be sleeping over so the child can be observed for sleepwalking.

Sleeptalking seems to occur during REM sleep. Dreaming of some frightening or puzzling situation, a child calls out a name or instruction such as "Stop!" Because illness is a stressful situation that increases anxiety, sleeptalking may also occur at an increased rate during this time. It is unnecessary to wake a child who is sleeptalking unless the child is thrashing about and would dislodge equipment such as intravenous tubing. However, because sleeptalking usually results from a frightening dream, waking the child gently can be comforting. Parents may need to be assured that sleeptalking is harmless and will probably subside when their child is well again.

Some children are prone to night terrors, or wake up screaming approximately 20 minutes after they fall asleep. The condition tends to be familial. Waking children and comforting them helps everyone in the house or hospital unit return to sleep. In the morning, children rarely remember the incident.

Sleep apnea is the cessation of respirations during sleep for 20 seconds or more. It tends to occur more frequently in obese children, possibly because of the increased weight of their chest. It may contribute to sudden infant death syndrome or failure to thrive (Qubty, Mrelashvili, Kotagal, et al., 2014) (see Chapters 26 and 55). Infants who are diagnosed with sleep apnea may be prescribed respiratory monitors to evaluate their breathing pattern and warn against any cessation of respirations.

Promoting Adequate Stimulation for the Ill Child

Children are in constant interaction with both their internal environment (body) and their external environment (surroundings) by means of their five senses and the central nervous system. This makes them capable of responding to changes in the environment and, by so doing, meets basic needs. Any illness that changes their ability to respond to their environment can cause either sensory deprivation or sensory overstimulation.

SENSORY DEPRIVATION

Sensory deprivation is the condition of being deprived of, or lacking, adequate sensory, social, physical, or cognitive stimulation. When this happens, children tend to lose the ability to make decisions and become easily confused and depressed. Some children are more prone to sensory deprivation than others.

Ill children may have sensory deprivation because they are confined to their homes or hospital rooms and their varied activities such as school, sports, and clubs are replaced with hours of watching television or playing video games. Hospitalized children respond best to a diversity of readily available, independently accessible, age-appropriate, gender-appropriate, and developmentally appropriate leisure and entertainment facilities seamlessly integrated throughout the hospital environment (Lambert, Coad, Hicks, et al., 2014).

Children with hearing or visual deficits are more prone than others to sensory deprivation. Children with forms of sensory nerve loss or those receiving chemotherapy may lose their sense of touch, taste, or proprioception (the sense of where they are in space). After losing these forms of perception, children may draw back from interacting with other people because they are self-conscious about the loss, so they may be further deprived of social and cognitive stimulation. Techniques for interacting with sensory-deprived children are discussed in Chapter 50.

Some children receive medication to lessen awareness of the stimulating factors in their environment. To ensure they do not suffer sensory deprivation, give them definite orientation measures, such as always mentioning the time of day and the day of the week in conversations with them.

 Nursing Diagnoses and Related Interventions

Nursing Diagnosis: Deficient stimulation from (or interest or engagement in) recreational or leisure activities

Outcome Evaluation: Child demonstrates alert and interested attitude toward self-care and play activities.

Providing Stimulation for the Child on Bed Rest. Children on bed rest cannot secure materials for cognitive stimulation by themselves or participate in physical activities, except to a limited degree. A room where walls and windows offer no visual appeal and therapeutic equipment provides the only sound offers them little sensory stimulation. If no one comes into the room, they may suffer from social deprivation. When possible, encourage a child with restricted mobility to move out of bed into a wheelchair; this can provide some mobility and transportation to a place of interest, such as near a window or, in a hospital, near the nurses' desk. Watching television, playing with tablets/phones, and engaging in social media are all common activities for children on and off bed rest; however, these activities can actually overstimulate the infant or child's brain and can decrease executive function. Executive function comprises the cognitive skills that undergird self-regulation. In other words, it helps us plan, focus attention, remember instructions, and perform multiple tasks at the same time (Lillard, Drell, Richey, et al., 2015).

Occasionally, a child must remain in bed, depending on the diagnosis (e.g., a liver or spleen injury). When possible, other stimulation, such as a favorite toy, games, books, or simply talking with someone, must be provided for these children to help them maintain physical bed rest; otherwise, they become bored and irritable and thrash and turn instead of lying still (Fig. 36.8).

If a child is home on bed rest and the bedroom is away from the main activities of the home, encourage family members to include the ill child in as many family activities as possible (e.g., bring the television set into the child's bedroom so the entire family gathers there, set up a card table in the room so everyone can eat there) or encourage the child to join the rest of the family for activities by resting on the couch in the living room, a lounge chair in the backyard, or a chair in the kitchen. This principle applies to hospitalized children as well.

Figure 36.8 Children on bed rest need stimulation. Here, a young child enjoys coloring. (sonya etchison/Shutterstock.com)

A toddler, for example, may rest in a parent's lap rather than in a bed.

Providing Stimulation for Children on Transmission-Based Precautions. Children who are placed on transmission-based precautions because of the possibility of contagious illness may experience severe sensory deprivation if everyone who enters the room must wear a gown and mask or if the number of visitors must be kept to a minimum. If gloves are part of precautions, a child can experience a significant loss of skin-to-skin contact as well. Transmission-based precautions are discussed in Chapter 43. Careful planning must be done to ensure that a child who is isolated this way is not psychologically isolated and that every possible measure is carried out to maintain sensory, social, physical, and cognitive stimulation. For example, try to visit with a child at a time other than those times in which you must perform procedures so you can simply talk, place the bed so the child can see out of the room, encourage the child to text message or video chat friends, make posters to decorate their room, or encourage interactive play with electronic games. For ideas on providing stimulation to children in specific age groups, refer to Chapters 29 to 33.

Providing safe, reliable Internet resources for immunosuppressed adolescents with chronic conditions wanting to socialize with peers can be an alternative to direct socialization and also decreases the risk of contracting a communicable illness (Maor & Mitchem, 2015).

SENSORY OVERLOAD

Sensory overload, in contrast to deprivation, occurs when children receive more stimulation than they can tolerate or process. Children with sensory overload react similarly to those with sensory deprivation or feel confused, unable to make decisions, and feel severely fatigued. Sometimes, it is difficult to determine the cause of these symptoms (whether they are caused by sensory deprivation or overload) unless assessed carefully.

The lights in ICUs, for example, are never turned out. Although children may find this comforting, it can also result in excessive stimulation. In addition to constant light, there is excessive sound such as the whir of machines, the buzzing of ventilators, the ringing of alarms, or the mix of voices in consultation. Excessive noise levels in the NICU have been studied as a factor influencing the function of a premature infant's brain through alterations of cortisol levels, apnea, decreased oxygen saturation and perfusion from exaggerated startle response. and abrupt fluctuations in heart rate (Campbell, 2016). The U.S. Environmental Protection Agency (EPA), Office of Noise Abatement and Control (1974) and American Academy of Pediatrics (1997) recommend that hospital noise not exceed 45 dB during daytime hours and 35 dB at night. Using indirect lighting whenever possible, implementing the national recommended safe sound level (NRL) of 45 dB in infants' rooms, reducing unnecessary conversations, and covering incubators for "quiet times" are all measures used to reduce these types of stimulation (Laubach, Wilhelm, & Carter, 2014).

QSEN Checkpoint Question 36.4

PATIENT-CENTERED CARE

Becky's mother is worried Becky will have a traumatic hospital experience. Which of the following would the nurse advise her to do to help make Becky's hospitalization less traumatic?

a. Suggest she keep her visits short so Becky can spend time with her nurse.
b. After visiting, don't tell Becky she is leaving. Just try to slip quietly away.
c. Insist Becky have blood drawn by her bed because she fears the treatment room.
d. Take Becky to the playroom, a place where she can feel free from being hurt.

Look in Appendix A for the best answer and rationale.

Promoting Play for the Ill Child

Play, often described as "the work of children," is an invaluable component of child health care. Providing a space and opportunity for play can help children feel more comfortable and allow for an important release of energy for children who are confined to a room or bed. Play also may be used to help assess children's level of knowledge and feelings about their condition so that more individualized nursing care can be planned. Depending on a child's age, play can also be a useful tool in health teaching (see Chapter 35). Children enjoy making friends with other children, talking to other children in nearby beds, and being in the playroom where they can talk to and get to know other children (Lambert et al., 2014).

Defining play is not a simple task because play activities vary greatly from child to child and among different developmental age, cultural, and socioeconomic groups. A common definition is that play is any voluntary activity engaged in for the purpose of enjoyment. If a child views an activity as enjoyment, therefore, no matter what it is and whether it would be fun or not for an adult, it is play.

Play is clearly the means by which children develop increasing cognitive, psychomotor, and social capabilities. Touching a soft toy, passing colored blocks from one hand to the other, pounding with a plastic hammer, feeding a doll, and playing board games are all ways in which children are exposed to and learn about different textures and colors, experience the feeling of possessing and owning, and learn about competition, winning, and losing as well as develop fine motor skills. Colored blocks reveal how parts can join to make a whole, how things stacked too high will fall (there are limits one cannot go beyond), and practice makes perfect. As children talk with playmates during play, they develop both language and social skills. The repetitive acts involved in most games encourage the development of musculoskeletal skills. Therefore, play is not something children do when they have nothing else to do, but rather, it is something children *have* to do. During illness, it provides a feeling of security because it is an activity that has continuity with everyday life.

The manner in which children play differs as they mature. Types of play and the developmental age groups in which these types are seen most frequently are shown in Box 36.7.

BOX 36.7

Nursing Care Planning Based on Family Teaching

UNDERSTANDING DIFFERENT PLAY TYPES

Q. Becky's mother tells you, "When Becky was younger, she didn't like toys as much as the boxes they came in. What's normal for children and play?"

A. Children play differently at different ages. Examples of typical play patterns include:

Type of Play/Age	Description	Example
Observation/infant	Child watches particular play intently, although not actively engaged in it.	Watching a mobile
Parallel/toddler	Two children play side by side but seldom attempt to interact with each other.	Playing separately with a similar push toy
Associative/preschooler	Children play together in a similar activity; there is little organization of responsibilities.	Engaging in typical backyard play
Cooperative/school age	Children play with an organized structure or compete for desired goal or outcome.	Playing organized games with rules

ASSESSING CHILD HEALTH THROUGH PLAY

Children who are acutely ill do not play or play very little because they do not have the strength, the attention span, or the interest in activities required for play. They continue to enjoy being read to, and they find comfort in holding a favorite toy even if they do not actively manipulate it. Once children are over the acute phase of an illness, interest in play returns. Therefore, whether a child is spontaneously playing is a good index of health. The toys children use at play are a good indication of their growth and development level and emotional state.

Parents typically know a child's play preferences and current favorite game or toy. Asking for this information during a health interview helps to assess a child's developmental level and helps to assess the quality of parenting (if parents view play as important or are familiar with the child's activities).

PROVIDING PLAY IN AMBULATORY SETTINGS

Children and families in ambulatory department may be under a great deal of stress as they sit in a waiting room, waiting for their name to be called. This anxiety for the family may be diverted with the use of child life services, if available, or toys/books/games that the child may redirect their focus to.

It is best if ambulatory departments are stocked with toys that can be played with quickly and by single children. There should be a low table and chairs so a parent can come to a table and play with a child. Examining rooms should have toys, which may be used to distract a child while a procedure such as an ear examination is performed, and because the wait in an examining room may be as long as the wait in a waiting room. Well siblings who accompany a parent and sick child to the facility can play with toys to distract them as well so that a parent can concentrate on the ailing child. Some hospitals furnish computer games for older children for this reason. Examples of ways that play can be used in an ambulatory care setting are shown in Table 36.5.

PROVIDING PLAY IN THE HOSPITAL

Ideally, all hospital units in which children are cared for should have a play space big enough for most of the children on the unit to come to. There should be enough space to accommodate children who are not fully ambulatory, such as those with casts or who are in wheelchairs (Fig. 36.9). Tables for board games and play materials such as crayons and paints should be available. Children can release a great deal of anger or tension by splashing water, squeezing or pouring sand, or smearing finger paint.

School-age children can play games and create objects with arts and crafts. Adolescents enjoy table tennis and pool tables. A great deal of "play" by older school-age children and adolescents centers on conversation with peers they meet in the playroom.

TABLE 36.5 WAYS TO INCORPORATE PLAY INTO NURSING CARE

Nursing Care	Play Activity
Aid with physical assessment	Distract child's attention with puppet during respiratory and cardiac assessment.
	Play Simon Says to encourage child to take deep breaths for respiratory assessment.
	Allow child to listen to own heart with a stethoscope.
	Play Follow the Leader to assess gait.
	Draw a face on the tongue blade used to assess the throat.
	Show child how to "blow out" the otoscope light.
	Draw child's outline on the table examining paper and give it to the child to take home to color.
Health teaching	Use puppets as a teacher.
	Create word scrambles or crossword puzzles.

Figure 36.9 Children enjoying themselves in a hospital playroom, which is spacious and well equipped with age-appropriate toys and activities.

PROVIDING PLAY FOR CHILDREN ON BED REST

Children who are on bed rest, at home or in a hospital, need to have play periods built into their day. The length of time for play and the toys individual children can play with depend on their developmental age and physical and emotional states. Suggestions for play activities for children on bed rest are shown in Table 36.6.

Infants need toys in their cribs, such as mobiles, blocks, soft toys, and rattles. They also need to be out of cribs, sitting on a parent's or a healthcare provider's lap, or securely sitting in strollers or swings. As soon as they are able, they need some time on the floor (with a sheet or other covering under them) to practice crawling or walking. At about 3 months, when infants discover their hands, those become that month's "toys." For a child learning to crawl, "cruise," or walk, that activity is the toy or interest for the month.

Toddlers need put-in and take-out types of toys such as blocks that can be repeatedly dropped into a box or that can be stacked to play with in bed. They enjoy listening to songs and nursery rhymes. Toddlers are in constant motion. They need to be out of bed as much as their physical condition allows, playing with take-apart, put-together, or pull-and-push toys. Preschoolers need creative materials such as modeling clay or sand. School-age children need quiet games such as books or crayons or markers by their bedside. They also enjoy electronic devices such as tablets, iPads, or iPods. Most activities for hospitalized children must be short-term projects because children are called away for treatments or procedures, and because, when they are ill, their attention span is shorter than usual. Short-term projects always appeal to the school-age child because they help a child of this age achieve a sense of industry.

Watching television is a nonparticipant activity, so it is not the best activity for children. There is some value, however, in watching nature programs or specials on television that depict school-age children in real-life situations coping with problems common to the child's age group. Encouraging parents or friends to watch a game show with a school-age child and help the child guess the solution to a puzzle or watch "Sesame Street" with a preschooler can make the activity a participatory one. Watching a DVD or video download with an adolescent and then discussing the people and their problems can also turn television watching into active participation.

SAFETY WITH PLAY

Inspect all toys for safety. They should be washable to prevent spreading disease, without sharp edges and small parts that could

TABLE 36.6 PLAY ACTIVITIES FOR CHILDREN ON BED REST

Care Measure	Play Activities
Bathing	Allow children to play in bath water with water toys.
Encouraging fluid	Hold a pretend "tea party" for a preschooler and drink "tea" with important but imaginary guests.
	Play a board game with a school-age child in which each turn starts with taking a drink.
	Draw a circle and let the child color in a section each time a drink is taken.
	Play Simon Says, in which Simon says, "Drink."
Deep breathing exercises	Have child blow soap bubbles in a glass of soapy water with a straw.
	Have child blow a cotton ball across the surface of a bedside table.
	Play Simon Says, in which Simon says, "Take a deep breath."
	Allow the child to score points for reaching a high number on an incentive spirometer.
Muscle-strengthening exercises	Have children throw bean bags or large wads of paper (computer waste) at a wastebasket.
	Play Simon Says, in which Simon says, "Raise your arms," and so forth.
	Have children throw and catch a ball.
	Have children squeeze and mold modeling clay.
	Help preschoolers pretend they are butterflies, airplanes, and so forth.
Procedures such as blood transfusion	Save a favorite game or activity only for these times.
Health teaching	Use puppets as teacher.
	Make up board games, word scrambles, and crossword puzzles.

be swallowed or aspirated. Toys should be at least 1¼ in. (3 cm) in diameter and 2¼ in. (6 cm) in length to prevent aspiration and choking. A cylinder 1 in. in diameter, such as a rubber hot dog, is the most dangerous size for a toy because it totally occludes the trachea if it is aspirated. A toy smaller than this would cause only partial obstruction; something larger could not be inhaled into the trachea. As a rule, if a toy can fit through the center of a toilet tissue tube, it is too small for safe play.

Consider the type of toy for a specific patient. Tossing a ball to a child on bed rest is generally a safe activity. One who has a large cast in place, however, might lean over to retrieve a dropped ball and fall out of bed. Chasing a ball could lead to collisions with door frames or other equipment.

If children become bored with an activity or toy because it is not stimulating enough or they have had it for too long a time, they may begin to use the toy in an unsafe way. After toddlers grow tired of stacking blocks, for example, they may begin to throw them. Children who normally play safely with modeling clay but who are on a restricted diet may eat it because they are hungry. Knowing where children are and what activity they are engaged in at all times is the best prevention against unsafe play.

For the child cared for at home, parents may need to purchase new toys. This is especially true if the bulk of the toys they furnished previously were for outside play such as balls, in-line skates, or skateboards. Because of an illness, they may now need to provide more "sit-down" toys such as markers, puzzles, or board games.

CHILD SUPPORT PROGRAMS

Child support programs, such as child life services, are incorporated into major children's hospitals and are an integral feature of child health care (Brown et al., 2014). As part of a child support program, a specialist offers children the opportunity to reenact and thereby master the unease associated with illness. Through therapeutic play, child specialists provide programs that prepare children for hospitalization and, once hospitalized, prepare children for surgery or for procedures that could be painful. They consult with parents about good toys to choose for home care. These specialists also help children air their frustration about painful or intrusive procedures, prevent social isolation of children by means of an active recreation program, and ensure that the total healthcare environment is conducive to children's well-being.

Such a program not only aids in promoting children's mental health but also leads to more cooperative responses of children to treatments or procedures. It is complementary to play programs initiated by nurses.

QSEN Checkpoint Question 36.5

SAFETY

The nurse is worried Becky's 2-year-old roommate might aspirate a toy the family friend brought in for her. Which of the following items is most likely to be aspirated and therefore poses the greatest risk to safety?

   a. Puzzle pieces
   b. Clothing for a baby doll
   c. Crayons
   d. Blocks that are 1-in. square

Look in Appendix A for the best answer and rationale.

THERAPEUTIC PLAY

Anything almost automatically becomes less threatening when a person can talk about it. Many children cannot talk about what is happening to them during illness because of fear or because their vocabulary is so limited they cannot describe their feelings.

Because play is the language of children, children who have difficulty voicing their thoughts in words can often speak clearly through play. Play that involves specialized activities that are developmentally supportive and facilitate the emotional well-being of a pediatric patient is considered therapeutic play. It should be noted that therapeutic play and play therapy are different. **Play therapy** addresses basic and persistent psychological issues associated with how a child may interact with his or her world (Koller, 2008).

For therapeutic play, only the child's verbal cues are used as responses. Therapeutic play can be divided into three types:
   1. Energy release
   2. Dramatic play
   3. Creative play

Energy Release

Children release energy by pounding, hitting, running, punching, or shouting. Furnishing children with materials that allow them to do these things helps them release anxiety as well. Toddlers enjoy pounding pegs with a plastic hammer or pretending to cut wood with a toy saw. Other examples include giving modeling clay to a preschooler (an anxious child often pounds it flat; a relaxed child, however, will build it into shapes). The overall goal is to maintain a sense of empowerment and self-efficacy during hospitalization (Teksoz, Bilgin, Madzwamuse, et al., 2017).

Dramatic Play

Dramatic play is acting out an anxiety-producing situation. It is most effective with preschool children because they are at the peak of imagination. During illness, the situations about which children need to express feelings are illness related, and therefore, the equipment needed for therapeutic play is common healthcare equipment, such as dolls, doll beds, play stethoscopes, IV equipment, syringes, masks, and gowns. Puppets of doctors, nurses, mothers, fathers, and children help young children express their feelings. Anatomically correct dolls are used to help children describe their feelings about sexual maltreatment.

It is good to have a play session with a child near the beginning of an illness to see whether the child communicates any fears about this experience through play. This initial session also serves as a way of preparing the child for events that will occur during the illness (Fig. 36.10). Repeat a play session after any painful or traumatic procedure such as surgery so that the child can express new feelings. A list of procedures that fall into this category is shown in Table 36.7. If such play sessions reveal fears, a child should be scheduled for other play sessions, perhaps once daily.

Furnish children with a wide range of equipment and then let them choose those items with which they wish to play. Children invariably choose a piece of equipment that has been used with them. They poke at a doll with a syringe without a needle or with a small rubber tube attached to simulate a needle or enjoy giving it a "shot." They wrap the

Figure 36.10 Therapeutic play allows children the opportunity to voice their fears of illness and procedures. (Ivolodina/Shutterstock.com)

doll in bandages or put tubes into its mouth or stomach, acting out things that were done to them or that they saw done to other children on a nursing unit or at a clinic visit they fear will be done to them. Allow play to be nondirective (let children proceed at their own pace, choosing freely what equipment to play with and what they want to do with equipment). As a child works through an experience this way, the experience becomes less fearful and the child gains increased control over it.

Observe for children who may be using equipment in an unusual way, such as hitting dolls with stethoscopes or poking them in the eye with a thermometer (suggesting they are confused about the purpose of such equipment or are acting out for another reason). Such behavior can alert you to the importance of explaining the purpose of equipment to children. Listen to what children say as they play. A comment such as "I'm giving shots to all the bad dolls" suggests the child thinks injections are punishment. It would be important to stress the next time the child needs an injection that medicine is to make the child feel well again. A comment such as "They are going to put you to sleep" when explaining anesthesia could infer that she will never wake up (she may have had a pet that needed to be put to sleep). Do not be surprised about the force with which children insert nasogastric tubes into dolls. In part, this reflects how they perceive these procedures, but it also represents energy or nervous release, in the way that pounding or hitting releases anger.

To better understand how a child feels, repeat what the child says verbally: "You are giving the bad dolls shots?" or ask the child to tell you more about the activity: "Do you think that's the only kind of children who get shots—bad children?" Do not rush to reassure ("Do not worry, that is not going to happen to you"). Quick reassurance tells children they should not ask any more questions or that the topic is not open for discussion.

Sometimes, even children who seem well prepared may be taken by surprise during a procedure. For example, 7-year-old Tanya, seen in an ambulatory setting for a diagnostic workup after a urinary tract infection, showed little interest in dolls and syringes and tubing in the playroom. She had been prepared by her mother for the experience and seemed to understand what would happen during her X-ray procedure. After returning from the X-ray room, where she had a voiding cystourethrogram; however, she was obviously upset.

TABLE 36.7 THERAPEUTIC PLAY TECHNIQUES FOR CHILDREN AFTER PROCEDURES

Procedure	Play Activity (Provide a doll and . . .)
X-ray	A table and box labeled "X-ray machine"; children sometimes worry X-rays will injure them, just as laser rays in science fiction shows do. Handling a "machine" can reduce anxiety.
Blood drawing	Syringe, alcohol wipes, tourniquet, or finger lancets; remember that finger sticks are as frightening for children as needles.
Clean-catch urine	Alcohol wipes and a collection cup; children are often more embarrassed by urine collection than adults realize.
Intravenous therapy	Intravenous tubing, as well as tape and an armboard; some children are as angry about being restrained as having the needle inserted.
Endoscopy such as bronchoscopy, cystoscopy	Catheters or a penlight to simulate an endoscope.
Scans	Intravenous fluid and tubing because scans usually require the intravenous injection of isotopes
Bone marrow	Alcohol wipes, syringe
Electroencephalogram (EEG), electrocardiogram (ECG)	Electrode leads that attach to a box; children might be afraid of these procedures because of their fear of electricity.
Surgery	An anesthesia mask and a blunt kitchen knife; watch and listen for where the child cuts and how the experience is described.
Dental examination	Suction catheter, a penlight to simulate a drill, and a 4 in. × 4 in. piece of plastic to simulate a dental dam; some children are angered by the use of plastic in their mouth.
Dressing changes	Gauze and paper adhesive tape
Cast application or removal	Provide plaster to soak and apply; simulate a cast cutter with an electric razor or hair dryer.
Nasogastric tube insertion, enema, catheterization	Appropriate tubes
Temperature assessment	Thermometer

Her nurse brought her a rag doll, a doctor and a nurse figure, a play X-ray machine, and some tubing that could simulate a urinary catheter and encouraged Tanya to play with them. Tanya picked up the girl doll and put her under the X-ray machine. She imitated the doctor doll shouting, "Pee in front of everybody!" Tanya's mother had not realized that she would have to void during a cystourethrogram and so had not prepared her for that. Tanya felt betrayed by not really being prepared for this embarrassing situation. Her play brought her emotion out in the open, where it could be talked about and handled. When Tanya was scheduled the next day for ureteral reflux surgery, her nurse was alerted to make the preparation absolutely thorough.

Children older than 9 or 10 years of age may find playing with dolls too childish to be of benefit. They would rather handle equipment such as nasogastric tubes in advance of them being inserted. Active handling helps to eliminate fear because it identifies exactly what the child has to face, and it meets their concrete-level learning needs.

Creative Play

Some children are too angry to be able to act out their feelings through dramatic play. However, they may be able to draw a picture that expresses their emotions or conveys the extent of their knowledge. To encourage this, give a child a blank paper and crayons or markers. If a child seems reluctant to draw something spontaneously, suggest a topic: "Why don't you draw a picture of yourself?"

Some children are so concerned with particular parts of their bodies that when asked to draw pictures of themselves, they draw only the body part about which they are worried.

Such children generally are saying they need to talk about that part of their body to be given reassurance that it is going to be all right. Figure 36.11A shows a picture drawn by Becky when she was admitted to the hospital for 1-day surgery for debridement of a campfire burn on her left foot. She stated on admission that she was being admitted to have the burn on her foot "cleaned out." This sounds like a child who understands what debridement involves. Note, however, that the figure she drew has no left leg. One has to wonder whether she was concerned that she was going to surgery to have more than debridement. After the word "debridement" was explained to her, she drew the picture in Figure 36.11B. The child in the drawing now has a left and a right leg, with the left leg covered by a bandage. Through a drawing, this child was able to say something she could not express without this help.

Many ill children draw pictures that reflect punitive images: a boy or girl tied to a bed or shut behind bars, or doctors and nurses frowning at them, obviously unhappy with them (Fig. 36.12). Such children may need assurance that they are not being punished but rather that they need to stay in bed or are being cared for by doctors and nurses to be made well. Other children draw pictures that are symbolic of death: airplanes crashing, boats sinking, buildings on fire, or children in graveyards. They need assurance that they will not die.

Other concerns such as fear of abandonment and loss of independence may also be manifested in drawings. For example, preschoolers may draw a child in one corner of a picture and an adult in a far corner. They may comment that the parent cannot find the child because she's gone to the hospital. They need to be reassured that their parents know where they are and, although they're not there constantly, they will visit them each day after work.

Figure 36.11 (A) Children who are concerned about body parts may draw pictures with that part missing or exaggerated. Note the missing left leg here. **(B)** After reassurance that her leg will be all right, the girl who did the drawing in **A** now draws a girl with two legs.

Figure 36.12 A picture drawn by a hospitalized child. Note the prison like appearance of the crib. (Courtesy of Rita Crever.)

Older school-age children and adolescents may not be interested in drawing but can be interested in making a list of procedures or experiences they like and dislike. Examine the dislike list for procedures such as "shots" or "chemo." Mark the nursing care plan for nurses to take special time to explain these procedures and to offer special support when they must be done.

BOX 36.8

Guidelines for Therapeutic Play

1. Allow children to choose the articles with which they want to play (something may be too frightening for a child to play with immediately, or more time may be needed to work up to the activity).
2. Provide the materials specific to the child's experiences of which you are aware, such as a nasogastric tube, syringe, or bandages but do not supply only those things; a child may have misunderstandings and fears of situations you cannot know about.
3. Allow play to be unstructured; let children use the materials however they wish. If a child seems uninterested in materials, initiate play such as giving a doll an injection to see if this reduces the child's fear enough to be able to handle items.
4. If a child cannot manipulate materials for some reason such as a large cast or traction, ask the child what would be good for you to do with an item.
5. Reflect only what the child expresses (verbal expression).
6. Do not criticize play; this inhibits further expression.
7. Use a therapeutic response; not "Don't worry, that won't happen," but "Are you worried that could happen?"
8. Ask children to describe paintings; not "That's a good picture of yourself," but "Tell me about your picture."
9. Do not be reluctant to use real equipment such as real catheters and blood lancets. Handling real equipment best helps to reduce stress.
10. Supervise therapeutic play because some equipment could cause an injury (and therapeutically responding to the child's comments is necessary).

What If . . . 36.3
While the nurse is playing with Becky, Becky draws a purple person with only three body parts. Would this worry the nurse? Why or why not?

Guidelines for Conducting Therapeutic Play

Use common sense when conducting therapeutic play. For example, try not to interpret a child's black and gloomy drawing as meaning the child is depressed when a black marker was the only one available. Many children 4 to 5 years of age draw a person lacking many body parts because, from a developmental standpoint, that is how they start to draw (usually just a head and no body, with lines representing arms and/or legs coming out of the head).

Remember, too, that all children occasionally treat dolls badly. A 2-year-old who pounds and bangs a rag doll may not be expressing anger toward the doll image at all but may be intent on discovering the feel of a new texture and is unaware for the moment that the object is a doll.

A conference with healthcare team members, including a psychologist or a psychiatric nurse specialist, may be needed if a child continues to express mutilating behavior after normal reassurance. Guidelines for conducting therapeutic play are summarized in Box 36.8.

What If . . . 36.4
The nurse is interested in exploring one of the 2020 National Health Goals related to illness in children (see Box 36.1). Most government-sponsored money for nursing research is allotted based on these goals. What would be a possible research topic to explore pertinent to these goals that would be applicable to the Miller family and that would also advance evidence-based practice?

QSEN Checkpoint Question 36.6

INFORMATICS

Becky's mother and father ask the nurse what type of therapeutic play would be best for Becky. Which type of therapeutic play would best meet Becky's needs if she will have a large bandage on her foot after surgery?
   a. Letting her hold and handle a syringe (with no needle attached)
   b. Giving her a doll and a bandage to change
   c. Supplying a video tape of a child having surgery for her to watch
   d. Giving her a book to read about a child's hospitalization experience

Look in Appendix A for the best answer and rationale.

KEY POINTS FOR REVIEW

■ Illnesses may be more traumatic for children than for adults because of children's inability to communicate and monitor their own care and because they have different nutrition, fluid, and electrolyte needs. The stress of hospitalization can be so acute that it can result in PTSD.

- Separation from parents because of hospitalization can have permanent psychological effects on children. Methods to reduce this include keeping hospital stays as brief as possible, promoting open parent and sibling visiting, and providing primary or case management nursing. **Case management nursing** is a collaborative approach of applying the nursing process to meet the needs of patient and their family.

- Currently, many medical procedures can be done on an ambulatory basis. Advocating for care to be done in such settings is a nursing responsibility.

- The presence of parents during health care can help reduce trauma to children. Making parents as welcome as possible in healthcare facilities makes it possible for them to room-in. Include parents in both the planning and the implementation of care. Parents reinfect children with fear if their own fear is not reduced.

- Preschoolers may have the most difficult time during hospitalization because they have so many fears. Preparation and promotion of therapeutic play may be essential to reduce trauma to a tolerable level.

- Because hospitalizations currently are so brief, parents need good discharge instructions to continue to care for children safely at home. Providing clear instructions, including suggestions for play or how to avoid sleep deprivation, is important to help plan nursing care that not only meets QSEN competencies but also best meets a family's total needs.

CRITICAL THINKING CARE STUDY

Timothy, a 10-year-old child, has been in the hospital for 10 days due to a nephrectomy because of a malignant tumor. He has been having significant difficulty sleeping because of pain. His mother is a single parent who works days. She spent several days with him but then needed to return to work.

When his mother comes to visit in the evenings, you notice he is irritable and acts rude to her. He tells her not to visit and then throws books at the wall when she leaves. His mother is distraught and does not know how she can cope with his subsequent hospitalizations for future chemotherapy.

1. What is a likely cause of Timothy's behavior?
2. What could you do to help Timothy adjust to hospitalization better?
3. What could you do to assist Timothy's mother?

RELATED RESOURCES

Explore these additional resources to enhance learning for this chapter:
- Student resources on thePoint, including answers to the What If . . . and Critical Thinking Care Study questions, http://thepoint.lww.com/Flagg8e
- Adaptive learning powered by PrepU, http://thepoint.lww.com/prepu

REFERENCES

Allen, K. (2012). Promoting and protecting infant sleep. *Advances in Neonatal Care, 12*(5), 288–291.

Al-Yateem, N., Brenner, M., Shorrab, A. A., et al. (2016). Play distraction versus pharmacological treatment to reduce anxiety levels in children undergoing day surgery: A randomized controlled non-inferiority trial. *Child: Care, Health & Development, 42*(4), 572–581.

American Academy of Pediatrics. (1997). Committee on Environmental Health. Noise: A hazard for the fetus and Newborn. *Pediatrics, 100*(4), 724–727.

Angelhoff, C., Edéll-Gustafsson, U., & Mörelius, E. (2015). Sleep of parents living with a child receiving hospital-based home care: A phenomenographical study. *Nursing Research, 64*(5), 372–380.

Baynton, J. (2015). Primary nursing in a short-stay unit. *Creative Nursing, 21*(1), 26–29.

Bibace, R., & Walsh, M. E. (1980). Development of children's concepts of illness. *Pediatrics, 66*(6), 912–917.

Blankenship, A. Harrison, S., Brandt, S., et al. (2015). Decision making regarding clinical management, communication among the team members, and serving as a venue for teaching and discussion. *American Journal of Critical Care, 24*,532–538.

Bowlby, J. (1951). Maternal care and mental health. *Bulletin of the World Health Organization, 3*, 355–534.

Brown, C., Chitkara, M., Percelay, J., et al. (2014). Child life services. *Pediatrics, 133*(5), E1471–E1478.

Caldwell, C. D. (2015). Single-family room NICUs and neurodevelopmental outcomes. *Neonatal Network, 34*(2), 137–138.

Campbell, C. (2016). Quieting the NICU: How a Sonicu solution stabilizes NICU noise environments and calms babies to better outcomes. *Neonatal Intensive Care, 29*(1), 36–39.

Centers for Disease Control and Prevention. (2015a). *Caring for children in a disaster. How are children different from adults?* Retrieved from https://www.cdc.gov/childrenindisasters/differences.html

Centers for Disease Control and Prevention. (2015b). *Guide to infection prevention for outpatient settings: Minimum expectations for safe care.* Retrieved from https://www.cdc.gov/infectioncontrol/pdf/outpatient/guide.pdf

Cuzzocrea, F., Gugliandolo, M. C., Larcan, R., et al. (2013). A psychological preoperative program: Effects on anxiety and cooperative behaviors. *Pediatric Anesthesia, 23*, 139–143.

Fernandes, S. C., Arriaga, P., & Esteves, F. (2014). Providing preoperative information for children undergoing surgery: A randomized study testing different types of educational material to reduce children's preoperative worries. *Health Education Research, 29*, 1058–1076.

Foster, M., Whitehead, L., & Maybee, P. (2016). The parents', hospitalized child's, and health care providers' perceptions and experiences of family-centered care within a pediatric critical care setting: A synthesis of quantitative research. *Journal of Family Nursing, 22*(1), 6–73.

Franck, L. S., Wray, J., Gay, C., et al. (2015). Predictors of parent post-traumatic stress symptoms after child hospitalization on general pediatric wards: A prospective cohort study. *International Journal of Nursing Studies, 52*, 10–21.

Hayes, D., Spano, M., Donnelly, J. E., et al. (2014). Proceedings of the learning connection summit: Nutrition, physical activity, and student achievement. *Nutrition Today, 49*, 18–25.

He, H., Zhu, L., Chan, S. W., et al. (2015). The effectiveness of therapeutic play intervention in reducing perioperative anxiety, negative behaviors, and postoperative pain in children undergoing elective surgery: A systematic review. *Pain Management Nursing, 16*, 425–439.

Hilton, L. (2014). Calming kids' hospital anxieties. *Contemporary Pediatrics, 31*(6), 18–21.

Holland, D., Conlon, P., Rohlik, G., et al. (2015). Identifying hospitalized pediatric patients for early discharge planning: A feasibility study. *Journal of Pediatric Nursing, 30*(3), 454–462.

Hopkins, L., Green, J., Henry, J., et al. (2014). Staying engaged: The role of teachers and schools in keeping young people with health conditions engaged in education. *Australian Educational Researcher, 41*(1), 25–41.

Houle, K. E., Belew, J., & Miller, B. (2015). Implementation of a Phase I Caregiver Visitation Program for a Specialized Pediatric Population. *Journal of Perianesthesia Nursing, 30*(4), 301–307.

Institute for Patient- and Family-Centered Care. (2016). *Advancing the practice of patient- and family-centered care: How to get started.* Bethesda, MD: Author. Retrieved from http://www.ipfcc.org/resources/getting_started.pdf

Ivany, A., LeBlanc, C., Grisdale, M., et al. (2016). Reducing infection transmission in the playroom: Balancing patient safety and family-centered care. *American Journal of Infection Control, 44*(1), 61–65.

Joint Commission on Accreditation of Healthcare Organizations. (2015). *National patient safety goals.* Retrieved from http://www.jointcommission.org/assets/1/6/2015_npsg_hap.pdf

Koller, D. (2008). *Child Life Council evidence-based practice statement: Child life assessment: Variables associated with a child's ability to cope with hospitalization.* Rockville, MD: Child Life Council. Retrieved from https://www.childlife.org/files/EBPAssessmentStatement-Complete.pdf

Lambert, V., Coad, J., Hicks, P., et al. (2014). Social spaces for young children in hospital. *Child: Care, Health & Development, 40*(2), 195–204.

Laubach, V., Wilhelm, P., & Carter, K. (2014). Shhh . . . I'm growing: Noise in the NICU. *Nursing Clinics of North America, 49*(3), 329–344.

Lillard, A., Drell, M., Richey, E., et al. (2015). Further examination of the immediate impact of television on children's executive function. *Developmental Psychology, 51*(6), 792–805.

Maor, D., & Mitchem, K. J. (2015). Can technologies make a difference for hospitalized youth: Findings from research. *Journal of Computer Assisted Learning, 31*(6), 690–705.

National Sleep Foundation. (2017). *Children and sleep.* Retrieved from https://sleepfoundation.org/sleep-topics/children-and-sleep

Orem, D. E. (2001). *Nursing: Concepts and practice* (6th ed.). St. Louis, MO: Mosby.

Piaget, J. (1930). *The child's conception of physical causality.* London, United Kingdom: Kegan Paul.

Potasz, C., Varela, M., Carvalho, L. D., et al. (2013). Effect of play activities on hospitalized children's stress: A randomized clinical trial. *Scandinavian Journal of Occupational Therapy, 20*, 71–79.

Qubty, W., Mrelashvili, A., Kotagal, S., et al. (2014). Comorbidities in infants with obstructive sleep apnea. *Journal of Clinical Sleep Medicine, 10*(11), 1213–1216.

Raleting, P. (2015). Preparing children and caregivers for medical treatment procedures. *Pediatric Blood & Cancer, 62*, S199–S200.

Rennick, J. E., Dougherty, G., Chambers, C., et al. (2014). Children's psychological and behavioral responses following pediatric intensive care unit hospitalization: The caring intensively study. *BMC Pediatrics, 14*, 276.

Robertson, J. (1958). *Young children in hospitals.* London, United Kingdom: Tavistock.

Spitz, R. A. (1945). Hospitalism; An inquiry into the genesis of psychiatric conditions in early childhood. *The Psychoanalytic Study of the Child, 1*, 53–74.

Steering Committee on Quality Improvement and Management & Subcommittee on Febrile Seizures, American Academy of Pediatrics. (2008). Febrile seizures: Clinical practice guideline for the long-term management of the child with simple febrile seizures. *Pediatrics, 121*, 1281–1286.

Steinke, S. M., Elam, M., Irwin, M. K., et al. (2016). Pediatric hospital school programming: An examination of educational services for students who are hospitalized. *Physical Disabilities: Education and Related Services, 35*(1), 28–45.

Stremler, R., Adams, S., & Dryden-Palmer, K. (2015). Nurses' views of factors affecting sleep for hospitalized children and their families: A focus group study. *Research in Nursing & Health, 38*(4), 311–322.

Teksoz, E., Bilgin, I., Madzwamuse, S. E., et al. (2017). The impact of a creative play intervention on satisfaction with nursing care: A mixed-methods study. *Journal for Specialists in Pediatric Nursing, 22*(1), e12169.

U.S. Department of Health and Human Services. (2010). *Healthy people 2020.* Washington, DC: Author.

U.S. Environmental Protection Agency, Office of Noise Abatement and Control. (1974). *Information on levels of environmental noise requisite to protect public health and welfare with an adequate margin of safety.* Washington, DC: Author. Retrieved from http://www.nonoise.org/library/levels74/levels74.html

Woolf, C., Muscara, F., Anderson, V., et al. (2016). Early traumatic stress responses in parents following a serious illness in their child: A systematic review. *Journal of Clinical Psychology in Medical Settings, 23*, 53–66.

Zempsky, W. T., Palermo, T. M., Corsi, J. M., et al. (2013). Daily changes in pain, mood and physical function in children hospitalized for sickle cell disease pain. *Pain Research & Management, 18*, 33–38.

37

Nursing Care of a Family When a Child Needs Diagnostic or Therapeutic Modalities

*F*elipe Ramos is a preschooler who is about to undergo computed tomography (CT) of his brain because he was pushed off a 6-ft-high slide at a playground and hit his head, causing a brief loss of consciousness. Felipe's mother asks you through an interpreter, "He's upset because of being bullied at school and he's afraid of the dark, how can I allow him to be put inside a long dark machine that way? What will this exam be like and how can we make sure he will be safe?"

Previous chapters described the growth and development of well children. This chapter adds information about how to care for children who are having diagnostic or therapeutic procedures. This is important information because it builds a base for both care and health teaching.

How would you explain the CT scan to Felipe and his mother?

KEY TERMS

aspiration studies

bronchoscopy

clean-catch urine specimen

colonoscopy

computed tomography (CT)

electrical impulse studies

endoscopy

magnetic resonance imaging (MRI)

positron emission tomography (PET)

radiopharmaceuticals

single-photon emission computed tomography (SPECT)

total parenteral nutrition (TPN)

ultrasound

OBJECTIVES

After mastering the contents of this chapter, you should be able to:

1. Describe common nursing interventions used in the health care of children to aid diagnosis and therapy.

2. Identify 2020 National Health Goals related to diagnostic and therapeutic procedures for children that nurses can help the nation achieve.

3. Assess children regarding their developmental stage and knowledge level before beginning diagnostic or therapeutic procedures.

4. Formulate nursing diagnoses related to common diagnostic or therapeutic procedures used with children.

5. Identify expected outcomes for a child who needs a diagnostic or therapeutic procedure as well as help families manage seamless transitions across differing healthcare settings.

6. Using the nursing process, plan nursing care that includes the six competencies of Quality & Safety Education for Nurses (QSEN): Patient-Centered Care, Teamwork & Collaboration, Evidence-Based Practice (EBP), Quality Improvement (QI), Safety, and Informatics.

7. Implement nursing care relevant to diagnostic or therapeutic procedures, such as preparing a child for magnetic resonance imaging.

8. Evaluate expected outcomes for achievement and effectiveness of care.

9. Integrate knowledge of common diagnostic and therapeutic procedures with the interplay of nursing process, the six competencies of QSEN, and Family Nursing to promote quality maternal and child health nursing care.

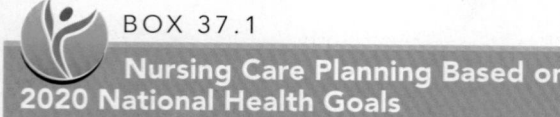

BOX 37.1

Nursing Care Planning Based on 2020 National Health Goals

2020 National Health Goals speak to efforts to keep children well so they need a minimal number of diagnostic or therapy procedures.

- Reduce hospitalizations for asthma among children under age 5 years from a baseline of 41.4% to a target level of 18.1%.
- Increase age-appropriate vehicle restraint systems in children aged 4 to 7 years from a baseline of 43% to a target level of 47%.
- Increase the number of adolescents who have had a wellness checkup in the past 12 months from 68.7% to 75.6%. (U.S. Department of Health and Human Services, 2014; see www.healthypeople.gov).

Nurses can help the nation achieve these goals by providing health counseling to parents and children to help prevent children from becoming ill and subsequently requiring hospitalization, such as teaching sound nutrition and common practices on avoiding unintentional injury.

Illness can be particularly stressful. When illness requires diagnostic and therapeutic procedures, that stress can worsen. In today's healthcare climate, time is crucial for teaching and preparation, so detailed planning and evaluation of understanding are essential when procedures are scheduled. Chapter 36 described measures to make an illness experience, inpatient and outpatient, more positive. Health teaching, discussed in Chapter 35, is also a cornerstone in this process.

Many nursing actions offer an opportunity to accomplish several goals. Supporting a child and family during a diagnostic procedure, for instance, not only aids in an efficient diagnosis but also may help establish a trusting relationship between the family and healthcare providers that will make all future interactions more successful. This chapter describes the most common diagnostic and therapeutic techniques used in the care of ill children, including modifications needed to make these procedures safe and to reduce associated stress, depending on the child's age and condition. Box 37.1 shows 2020 National Health Goals that address this area of child health practice.

Nursing Process Overview

FOR A CHILD WHO NEEDS DIAGNOSTIC OR THERAPEUTIC PROCEDURES

ASSESSMENT

Before performing procedures such as assisting with a diagnostic test or collecting laboratory specimens, first carefully evaluate a child's age and developmental stage as well as any special needs a child may have. Even the most common and painless procedures create a certain amount of stress for children and parents. During complex diagnostic procedures, this stress level is almost certain to increase even further due to fear of the unknown. Unfamiliar people (e.g., doctors, nurses, other health team members), high-tech supplies and equipment, and strange surroundings all add up to a frightening experience for most adults; imagine how frightening they are to children.

It is important to acknowledge that many procedures that involve highly technologic equipment may be painful or uncomfortable for a child, especially if the child has a chronic disease. Assess a child's level of anxiety associated with a procedure as well as the child's knowledge concerning a technique before initiating the procedure or beginning health teaching. Pointing out a child's past experience with similar procedures can lay a foundation for increased cooperation.

NURSING DIAGNOSIS

Common nursing diagnoses related to diagnostic and therapeutic procedures are as varied as the procedures themselves. Some examples include:

- Fear related to new and strange surroundings of the procedure room
- Pain related to a lumbar puncture procedure
- Deficient knowledge related to the technique for 24-hour urine collection
- Deficient diversionary activity related to hospitalization and lengthy procedures
- Imbalanced nutrition, less than body requirements, related to need for food restriction preprocedure and postprocedure
- Risk of injury related to need for intrusive procedures

OUTCOME IDENTIFICATION AND PLANNING

Procedures can produce stress in addition to the anxiety caused by a primary illness. An important nursing goal, therefore, is to perform procedures and complete interventions with the least amount of anxiety possible. To achieve this goal, plan specific ways to prepare children in advance and apply the best communication techniques possible to explain a procedure at the level of understanding and developmental stage appropriate for each child. Consideration should be given to the number of diagnostic or therapeutic procedures and the time frame in which they are performed. Some children may have less anxiety if diagnostic tests are scheduled over several days to preserve the child's coping ability. Conversely, some older children (and parents) do better if they can complete all necessary tests in 1 day to reduce the anxiety produced by the anticipation of more testing still to come. Refer families to online resources for further information when appropriate (see Chapter 36).

IMPLEMENTATION

Whether assisting with a procedure or performing a therapeutic intervention, it is necessary to function in several roles simultaneously: organizing supplies, performing (or assisting with) the procedure, providing active support to the child and parents, and observing and then documenting the child's reactions. As a final follow-through step, plan for introducing therapeutic play techniques that would be helpful in relieving stress caused by the procedure.

OUTCOME EVALUATION

Evaluating expected outcomes related to diagnostic and therapeutic procedures is not only helpful in determining the effect of the procedure on a child but also aids in future planning should other procedures be required. Recording that a particular child who did not appear nervous during a procedure later admitted to being "more scared than I've ever been before," for example, can help another nurse provide reassurance to this child, even if the child is successful at masking emotions the next time the procedure is performed. Examples suggesting achievement of expected outcomes include:

- The child reports the ability to cope with a second bone marrow aspiration.
- The child lists steps for successful 24-hour urine collection at home.
- The child participates in 1 hour of active exercise daily.
- The child eats a minimum of 1,000 calories per day.
- The child experiences minimal loss of blood, less than 10 ml, during a diagnostic procedure.
- The parent outlines plan to use alternative therapies to reduce the child's anxiety.

Nursing Responsibilities With Diagnostic and Therapeutic Techniques

Stress related to hospitalization occurs across the life span. A greater awareness regarding psychological trauma for children and their parents that can occur with hospitalization and that can undermine the child's recovery is a major focus of research (Franck, Wray, Gay, et al., 2015). Reducing the number of hospitalizations is likely to reduce the overall stress; however, when this cannot be accomplished, the next step is aimed at reducing the number of diagnostic or therapeutic procedures children have to undergo. Despite these attempts, some children, such as those who are chronically ill or are dependent on technology such as a ventilator, require 24-hour care in either a healthcare setting or their home. Children who show initial symptoms of a progressive illness likely require diagnostic procedures in order for their condition to be confirmed and effective therapy initiated.

When hospitalization is indicated, the stress of the experience can be reduced for both the child and parents if procedures are carried out in the least stressful way possible. The use of new information technology devices (NITDs) allows healthcare providers to engage, educate, and communicate with patients and families and reduce anxiety related to hospitalization (Kompany, Luis, Manganaro, et al., 2016). When performing or assisting with procedures on children, remember to maintain safety and legal responsibilities for care such as:

- Verify that an informed consent is obtained, as needed.
- Utilize the electronic health record to verify the prescription for the procedure.
- Explain the procedure to the child and parents to ensure both are well informed.
- Schedule the procedure.
- Prepare the child physically and psychologically.
- Obtain necessary equipment for the procedure.
- Accompany a child to a treatment room or hospital department where the procedure will be performed.
- Coordinate and collaborate with other healthcare providers to ensure the safety and efficacy of all procedures.
- Provide support during the procedure, using the least amount of restraint possible.
- Ensure adherence to standard infection precautions.
- Assess a child's response to the procedure.
- Provide care to a child and specimens obtained once the procedure is completed.
- Document the outcome of the procedure and the child's reaction to the procedure.

OBTAINING INFORMED CONSENT

Informed consent is a process in which the healthcare provider discloses or explains a proposed medical treatment, along with the risk(s), benefit(s), and alternative(s) for that treatment. Informed consent is legally required and must be obtained before any procedure or treatment that has a risk of causing injury to the child is performed. Each procedure or treatment must have a documented consent. The benefits and risks of the treatment or procedure must be discussed along with the risks if the treatment or procedure was not performed. Although obtaining consent is the provider's responsibility, ensuring that it is obtained is a nursing responsibility. Acting as an advocate for a family if they do not understand the consent form, the procedure, or the risks of the procedure is an important nursing role.

According to Katz and Webb (2016), informed consent is valid when the following criteria are met:

- Disclosure of information to patients or their surrogates
- Assessment of patient and surrogate understanding of the information and their capacity for medical decision making
- Obtaining informed consent before treatments and interventions

A minor who is emancipated by the state is considered to have the same legal rights as an adult and may consent to treatment. Adolescents who are living on their own, are married, and/or serving with the armed forces are generally considered legally emancipated and able to provide informed consent or refusal for their own medical care (Katz & Webb, 2016). All 50 states recognize an adolescent's right to consent for healthcare needs related to sexual activity, including treatment of sexually transmitted infections, contraceptive services, and prenatal care (Katz & Webb, 2016); however, consenting to these services does not always guarantee confidentiality.

In emergent or life-threatening situations, when a legal guardian or parent is unavailable to consent, the Emergency Medical Treatment and Active Labor Act mandates that a medical screening examination and delivery of appropriate medical care for the pediatric patient are never withheld or delayed.

When a legal guardian refuses to consent to medical care or transport that is necessary to save the child's life, law enforcement may be needed. When feasible, it is always better to discuss why the legal guardian is refusing treatment so that an ameliorable plan for the child's health can take place.

The pediatric population is considered vulnerable; thus, parents must consent on the child's behalf prior to a procedure or involvement in research. To maintain the child's autonomy, assent is also often obtained much like consent is. The American Academy of Pediatrics (AAP) Policy Statement (Katz & Webb, 2016) states that assent must have at least the following four elements: (a) helping the patient achieve a developmentally appropriate awareness of the nature of his or her condition, (b) telling the patient what he or she can expect with tests and treatment(s), (c) making a clinical assessment of the patient's understanding of the situation and the factors influencing how he or she is responding (including whether there is inappropriate pressure to accept testing or therapy), and (d) soliciting an expression of the patient's willingness to accept the proposed care.

According the regulations at 45 CFR 46.408(a), assent may be waived if (U.S. Department of Health and Human Services, 2010):

1. The capability of some or all of the children is so limited that they cannot reasonably be consulted.
2. The intervention or procedure involved in the research holds out the prospect of direct benefit to the health or

well-being of the children and is available only in the context of the research.

3. The research meets the same conditions as those for waiver or alteration of informed consent in research involving adults, as specified in the regulations.

EXPLAINING PROCEDURES

To be able to explain procedures clearly and answer questions about them appropriately, try to observe as many procedures as you can. After any procedure, asking children to describe what sensations they experienced can help them work through possibly frightening situations (often called "debriefing") and can also increase your knowledge of common procedures.

As a general guide, before a procedure, a child needs a detailed description of what to expect, such as "I'll clean your finger. You will feel a small pinprick" as well as an explanation of:

- Why the procedure is being performed (e.g., "Your doctor needs to look at your blood to see why you're so sick")
- Where the procedure will be done (e.g., the X-ray department, a treatment room)
- Any unusual sensations to be expected during the procedure (e.g., "The alcohol I use to clean your skin will feel cold")
- Any pain involved (e.g., "The needle will sting, although I'll put some cream on first to dull the feeling")
- Any equipment that will be unfamiliar such as a magnetic resonance imaging machine
- The approximate length of time the procedure will take
- Any special care after the procedure (e.g., "You will need to lie quietly for 15 minutes afterward")

Use age-appropriate language when explaining procedures and be careful not to use words that might be confusing during an explanation, such as "transducer" or "electrode," without defining them in age-appropriate terms. Try to associate the procedure with something you know the child is already familiar and comfortable with, such as describing an X-ray machine as "a big camera." Try not to use the word *test* in explanations because school-age children associate the word *test* with a pass/fail situation. Wondering if they "passed" a procedure can make them unduly worried afterward.

If you are unfamiliar with what a procedure entails, do not guess the answers to a child's questions because nothing is more confusing than being told two different versions of an answer to the same question. Familiarize yourself with the procedure and explain to the child and/or parent in terms that are understandable. When possible, encourage parents to stay with their child during the procedure, if possible, as they can be extremely helpful in reducing the threatening aspects of a procedure.

SCHEDULING

If a child is having more than one diagnostic procedure in a day, try to arrange for the child to have time for meals and some free play time between the procedures. If food or fluid must be restricted, monitor the child's degree of discomfort and physiologic needs related to the restriction. Advocate as necessary for sufficient periods of time between examinations so a child can eat or for decreased time between procedures so the time spent without food or fluid is limited.

PREPARING A CHILD AND FAMILY PHYSICALLY AND PSYCHOLOGICALLY

Physical preparation varies with each procedure to be performed. In many instances, preparing a child for an examination, such as a barium enema, involves another procedure such as a saline enema, so that physical preparation also becomes education for the actual examination. In all instances, explain both the preparative and actual procedures and allow the child to ask questions because appropriate explanations aid in reducing anxiety and fear (Box 37.2).

Before a procedure, children may be given an anxiolytic, such as midazolam (Versed), to both relieve apprehension and allow them to be mildly sedated. For painful procedures or those that demand extreme cooperation, such as a bronchoscopy (see section on Direct Visualization Procedures) or closed fracture reduction, children may be administered moderate sedation. Used in both ambulatory and inpatient settings, moderate sedation results in a depressed level of consciousness induced by the intravenous administration of a sedative such as midazolam in combination with a dissociative anesthetic, such as ketamine. It is administered by an anesthesiologist, a physician, or a nurse specially prepared in the technique.

While under moderate sedation, children are able to maintain their ability to breathe independently and also respond appropriately to verbal commands such as "Lift your head." They feel minimal pain, however, because of the analgesic administered. Before the technique is started, emergency equipment, including respiratory and pharmacologic measures for medication reversal, must be on hand. The child's level of consciousness and ability to respond, heart rate, respiratory rate, blood pressure, oxygen saturation, and end tidal CO_2 must be monitored throughout the procedure. Using moderate sedation is an excellent technique to allow children to accept a potentially painful procedure both emotionally and physically. Preparation is essential for both the child and the family in terms of medication and possible side effects that may occur.

ACCOMPANYING THE CHILD

Parental presence is essential when a child is undergoing a procedure because it reduces the child's stress (Matziou, Chrysostomou, Vlahioti, et al., 2013). However, if the parents are unable to be present during a procedure, allow them

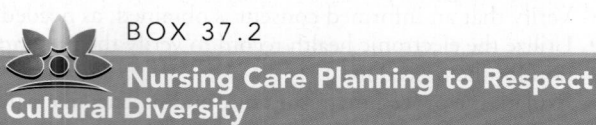

BOX 37.2

Nursing Care Planning to Respect Cultural Diversity

Professional nursing practice must continually adapt to the changing values and beliefs of the population it serves. The diversity of the population is reflected in pediatric patients and their families, many of whom are from various cultural backgrounds, have a language other than English as their primary language, have difficulty reading English so have questionable health or reading literacy, and may be overwhelmed by the information and expectations of adaptation to a new healthcare system. Translators should be available to comply with The Joint Commission (TJC) standards in health care to ensure effective communication. Prior to educating parents and children on certain procedures or handing out written instructions, first assess the child's and parent's ability to understand English.

to remain close by, such as a waiting room, so that they can be called once the procedure is completed. Ideally, a nurse whom the child knows should accompany the child to the procedure and remain with the child throughout the procedure, or at least until the child has met a primary person who will be responsible for the procedure. Check for any medication or specific baseline assessment procedures such as vital signs that should be performed before leaving the unit for another department, in case the child will be away from the primary unit for an extended time. If a child is an inpatient, also check that the identification band is securely in place and readily visible despite any intravenous equipment. In most healthcare settings, variations of the SBAR (Situation, Background, Assessment, Recommendation) or ISBAR (Introduction, Situation, Background, Assessment, Recommendation) format is implemented for interdisciplinary/interdepartmental communication to safeguard preparation procedures follow The Joint Commission standards on communication (The Joint Commission, 2014). If there will be a considerable wait in another department, ask children if they would like to bring along an activity such as a game or book. In addition, hallways can be cool. Provide adequate blankets for comfort, especially for infants; because their temperature-control mechanisms are underdeveloped, their temperature can decrease quickly. Always use cart straps and side rails for safety because safety is a priority during all procedures performed on children (Jain, Petrillo-Albarano, & Parks, et al., 2013).

PROVIDING SUPPORT

Children do well with diagnostic and evaluative procedures as long as they have adequate support from a familiar provider or parent with them. Try to provide support both verbally (i.e., explain what is going to happen in age-appropriate terms) and nonverbally (e.g., a hand on the arm or a nearby presence).

MODIFYING PROCEDURES ACCORDING TO A CHILD'S AGE AND DEVELOPMENTAL STAGE

It is important to consider a child's age and potential understanding of procedures when planning the number and order of tests and the way they will be performed.

The Infant

The number of painful or uncomfortable procedures done on infants should be kept to an absolute minimum to avoid interfering with an infant's developing sense of trust. Advocate for limitation of unnecessary procedures and always keep parents informed of what type of procedure the infant may need to undergo.

Advocate for parents to remain during procedures to offer support. Some parents may ask to hold their child during a procedure that causes pain, but do not ask parents to restrain the child during such a procedure. Their role should be supportive and comforting, not one that causes pain.

Infants become dehydrated quickly, so the time they can remain nothing by mouth (NPO) for procedures should not exceed 6 hours (4 hours for breast milk and 6 hours for formula; Academy of Breastfeeding Medicine, 2012). You may need to advocate time for breastfeeding before and after a procedure for the comfort of both the infant and mother. If a procedure continues for longer than 3 to 4 hours, provide the mother a room in which to use a breast pump, if needed. Assess the

infant's temperature to guard against extremes. Have a blanket available to prevent chilling.

After procedures, allow parents to pick up infants and actively comfort them.

The Toddler and Preschooler

Toddlers and preschoolers resist any diagnostic testing that involves any degree of discomfort or pain or any procedure that is unfamiliar to them. Give children of this age short explanations of what to expect close to the time of the procedure so that little time can be spent worrying. Try to associate any new equipment with things that they are already familiar, such as comparing a magnetic resonance imaging to a giant cell phone camera. If possible, introduce any equipment that will be used in procedures such as a nasogastric tube in a play session with a doll so the child can handle the new object and see that the doll is not injured or minds having the tube inserted.

The School-Age Child and Adolescent

School-age children are concrete thinkers and so are interested in the theory and reason for procedures. They can often be persuaded to cooperate for a procedure by being promised a look at their X-ray or a point-of-care meter readout afterward. Be careful, however, to ensure that viewing the results is actually possible before promising this to children; otherwise, it can be difficult to obtain any further cooperation. Adolescents may project an air of maturity or sophistication beyond their years to remain in control of themselves in the face of frightening procedures. Do not be misled into thinking an adolescent would not appreciate an explanation or a comforting hand on a shoulder during a procedure.

What If . . . 37.1

Felipe, who is scheduled for a cranial MRI, puts his hands over his ears and refuses to listen to the nurse's explanation of what will happen during the MRI. How could the nurse give an explanation to him? Why do you think he is acting this way?

PROMOTING SAFETY DURING PROCEDURES

Whether a procedure will be safe depends a great deal on the nursing planning and support that accompanies the procedure. Children are unable to guard their own safety because they are unable to form mature judgments, a situation that leaves them vulnerable to harm unless their caregivers give special consideration to promoting safety during procedures.

Nursing Diagnoses and Related Interventions

Nursing Diagnosis: Risk for injury related to diagnostic procedure

Outcome Evaluation: Child remains free of injury from diagnostic equipment; voices afterward that procedure was not as frightening as anticipated.

As the first safety measure, before performing any procedure, and even before offering food or a medication, read the name on a child's identification armband. If an armband must be removed because it interferes with an intravenous infusion site, cut it away but immediately anchor it to another extremity with adhesive tape. Ask the registrar to provide a new armband as soon as possible. Do not leave the old one off while waiting for a replacement band because this leaves the child susceptible to the danger of mistaken identity during the waiting period.

Because of their natural curiosity, children tend to fuss with equipment to see what will happen if they turn a knob or spin a dial. This means they need close monitoring while procedures are performed to ensure they do not touch any buttons or in other way unintentionally harm themselves. After a procedure, remove all equipment from a room. Syringes and needles can cause puncture wounds. Infants and young children can choke on small objects such as needle covers.

Use of Restraints

The purpose of a restraint (physical or chemical) during a procedure is to keep a child safe from injury. Whenever possible, healthcare providers should use alternative means of keeping a child safe. Alternative methods include "family member presence, the use of sitters, distraction, and placing the

patient near the nurses' station. When alternative methods are deemed ineffective or the actions of the patient indicate immediate need for restraints, the least restrictive type of restraint should be utilized and only as a last resort. Additionally, restraints should be removed at the earliest opportunity" (Longo & Miller-Hoover, 2016).

Patients who are restrained must be continuously monitored in accordance with federal, state, and regulatory agency guidelines (American Psychiatric Nurses Association, 2014). No part of a child's body other than that which is necessary should be restrained. When infants have scalp vein infusions in place, such as for injection of a radioactive isotope for a nuclear medicine scan, for example, their arms may need to be immobilized so they do not touch the infusion site. Their trunk may need to be immobilized so they do not turn. Their lower extremities, however, do not need to be restrained so they can still actively kick and exercise. When a nurse or a parent is with a child, in most instances, all restraints can be removed. Various types of restraints commonly used are described in Table 37.1 and shown in Figure 37.1.

PROVIDING CARE AFTER PROCEDURES

After a procedure, assess how well a child reacted to the procedure by both observation and history. Allowing children to

TABLE 37.1 SAFETY WITH RESTRAINTS

Type of Restraint	Purpose	Method
Wheelchairs and carts	Promote safety while transporting children to and from a healthcare facility procedure department.	For a wheelchair, use a vest restraint. Attach straps to the frame of the wheelchair with enough slack so the child has some mobility. For a cart, fasten a restraining belt and raise the side rails.
		Even with restraints in place, never leave a child unattended in hallways outside departments in a wheelchair or on a cart. Not only is this unsafe because the child may attempt to get down from the cart or wheelchair but also the anxiety of waiting in a strange department for a procedure without a support person with them may be too acute for young children to handle.
Clove-hitch restraints	Secure one arm or leg for a procedure, such as an intravenous infusion.	Use disposable restraints, gauze, or soft muslin tape. Soft muslin tape "gives" a little if the child exerts pressure against it so it will not pull too tight and reduce circulation or cause pain. Tie the restraint as shown in Figure 37.1A.
		If a child struggles against restraints, fold several layers of soft gauze around the wrist or ankle under the restraint. Secure the restraint to the underpart of the bed. Never tie restraints to side rails; when a side rail is lowered, it will jerk the child's arm or leg and possibly cause an injury.
		Release arm and leg restraints whenever someone can be with the child to keep the limb in the desired position.
Jacket restraints	Restrain children younger than 6 months in a supine position.	Fasten the ties at the back of the jacket. Tie strips attached to the sides of the jacket under the mattress to keep the child in one position (see Fig. 37.1B). Assess that the restraint is not pressing against the neck or could be causing interference with a child's airway.
Elbow restraints	Prevent children from touching the head or face (e.g., following facial surgery).	Dress the baby in a long-sleeved shirt to prevent irritation from the restraint. Slip a commercial restraint such a NoNoSleeve up over the infant's arm and secure it by the Velcro strips (see Fig. 37.1C). Assess the infant's fingers to ensure the sleeve is not too tight that it interferes with circulation.
Mummy or blanket restraints	Temporarily immobilize young children for a procedure involving the head, neck, or throat (e.g., during insertion of a nasogastric tube or blood drawing).	Use this only for the duration of the procedure because it is a total body restraint. Follow the steps shown in Figure 37.1D.
		If the child is exceptionally strong, a few safety pins can be used to hold the restraint even more firmly in place.
		For the infant who needs continuous observation for respiratory function, fold the mummy restraint so the chest is exposed. For newborns or infants, use a Papoose Board, a commercial restraint used in the same way as a full or mummy restraint (see Fig. 37.1E).

Figure 37.1 Types of restraints. **(A)** A clove-hitch restraint. **(B)** A jacket restraint. **(C)** A NoNoSleeve or commercial elbow restraint. **(D)** A mummy restraint. **(E)** A Papoose Board.

explain what happened helps them retrace the procedure in their mind so they can conquer their fear of it. Fill in gaps in information as necessary to improve a child's perception of the procedure. Provide therapeutic play, as necessary, to help reduce anxiety (see Chapter 36).

If tissue samples are obtained during a procedure, such as bone marrow aspiration, send the specimen to the proper laboratory for analysis as soon as possible. Guard against specimens being dropped or improperly labeled.

If moderate sedation was used, children may be discharged home or to an inpatient hospital unit as early as 30 minutes

after the procedure if they are awake and oriented; have a patent airway; respiratory status is without retraction, stridor, or wheezing; and oxygen saturation is 95% or greater on room air. Blood pressure, heart rate, and respiratory rates should be age-appropriate, and the child should be reasonably free of pain. Using a postanesthesia score sheet (Fig. 37.2) is an effective method to rate recovery from anesthesia and to document that all criteria are met.

Parents often have questions about what care their child will need after they return home after having moderate sedation. Tips for parents about this are highlighted in Box 37.3.

Postanesthesia Assessment

Activity:	Description:	Score:
Activity	Able to move four extremities	2
	Able to move two extremities	1
	Able to move no extremities	0
Respiration	Regular, able to deep breathe/cough	2
	Dyspnea, limited and obstructed breathing	1
	Apneic	0
Circulation	BP within 20 mmHg of preprocedure	2
	BP within 20–25 mmHg of preprocedure	1
	BP 25 mmHg above or below preprocedure level	0
Level of consciousness	Awake, alert	5
	Drowsy, but easily aroused	4
	Stupor, aroused by vigorous stimuli	2
	Responds to pain only	1
	No response to pain	0
Skin color	Preprocedure color, warm, dry	2
	Pale, dusky, blotchy, clammy	1
	Cyanotic, diaphoretic, cold	0
Ambulation	Ambulates with minimum help	5
	Ambulates with minimum support	4
	Unable to ambulate	2

Figure 37.2 A postanesthesia recovery score. A passing score is at least 10 with a level of consciousness score no lower than 4. (From Tolia, V., Peters, J. M., & Gilger, M. A. [2000]. Sedation for pediatric endoscopic procedures. *Journal of Pediatric Gastroenterology and Nutrition, 30*[5], 477–485.)

BOX 37.3

Nursing Care Planning Based on Family Teaching

CARE AFTER MODERATE SEDATION

Q. Felipe's mother says to you, "If my son receives moderate sedation for his MRI, what special care will he need when he comes home?"

A. Here are some tips to help you:

- Most children sleep for at least an hour after leaving the healthcare facility. Some feel sleepy for the remainder of the day.
- Do not allow the child to walk alone for at least 4 hours. The child may suddenly feel dizzy and fall without warning.
- Wait until getting home to give the child something to eat or drink to avoid car sickness because moderate sedation may cause children to feel nauseated more easily than usual.
- For the first 12 hours, do not ask him to do any activity that requires alertness, coordination, or balance, such as riding a bicycle, swimming, or doing homework because the sedative can affect coordination and balance.
- Remember that the child may forget things readily for the rest of the day. This forgetfulness should go away, however, after a night's sleep.
- Moderate sedation may cause children to behave in unexpected ways, such as losing self-control or becoming very emotional. By the next day, the child's usual behavior should return.
- Give infants clear liquids (e.g., water, apple juice, tea) after getting home. Wait approximately 30 minutes to make sure the child does not choke or vomit. Then, breast milk, formula, or other foods may be given.
- Wait approximately 30 minutes after the child is able to tolerate oral fluids. If there is no vomiting or choking, the child can be given food.
- Call your primary care provider if the child has pain or recurrent vomiting or if any of the effects mentioned last for more than 12 hours.

Measuring Vital Signs

Vital signs for children consist of temperature, pulse, respiratory rate, blood pressure, and pain assessment. All vital signs need to be recorded conscientiously and with knowledge of the child's underlying condition so they can be meaningfully analyzed. Be especially alert that assessing any of these measures is not enough; if they are abnormal or if a child has pain, a measure to relieve the problem needs to be initiated. Average pulse rates, respiration rates, and blood pressures for children of different ages, because these differ according to the size and age of the child, can be viewed at http://thePoint.lww.com/Flagg8e. Pain assessment and management is discussed in Chapter 39.

TEMPERATURE

A normal temperature is not a specific number but instead can range from 97° to 100.4°F (Wycoff, 2009). Common temperature values in children are the same as in adults: axillary, 97.6°F (36.5°C); oral or tympanic, 98.6°F (37.0°C); and rectal, 99.6°F (37.6°C). Thermometers that assess the temporal artery temperature are ideal for assessment in children because they register within 2 seconds and therefore cause less fear. Kemp (2013) put forth a position statement that "temperatures taken with temporal artery thermometers correlated with rectal temperatures better than axillary and tympanic membrane thermometry" (Batra & Goyal, 2013) (Fig. 37.3A).

In newborns, take the temperature using the temporal artery thermometer instead. Taking a temperature rectally increases the risk of damaging their fragile rectal mucosa with a thermometer (Fig. 37.3B). Children receiving chemotherapy have fragile rectal mucosa as well and so should not have their temperature routinely assessed using the rectum.

For temporal artery thermometer use, gently position the probe flush (flat) on the center of the forehead, midway between the eyebrow and the hairline. Press and hold the SCAN button. Lightly slide the thermometer across the forehead keeping the sensor flat and in contact with the skin until you reach the hairline (Exergen, 2014).

For a tympanic temperature recording, straighten the ear canal by pulling down on the earlobe in a child younger than age 2 years and pulling up on the pinna of the child older than age 2 years. Insert the tip of the tympanic thermometer gently into the child's ear canal directing the sensor beam toward the center of the tympanic membrane. Even if the child has earwax, tympanic membrane temperature is not affected, so the reading is consistently accurate within seconds. By 4 years of age, children are usually old enough to close their mouth sufficiently for oral temperature recording by use of an electronic thermometer.

Figure 37.3   Temperature taking. **(A)** Temporal artery thermometer. (Image Point Fr/Shutterstock.com) **(B)** Axillary temperature.

For an axillary recording, place the tip of an electronic thermometer in the axilla and hold the child's arm down to the side to keep the thermometer firmly in place until it registers. For the rare occasions when a rectal temperature must be taken, insert the electronic thermometer only to the length of the tip (0.5 in.) in infants, and not over 1 in. in older children, and hold it in place for 5 minutes.

PULSE RATE

As children grow older, the heart rate slows and the range of normal values narrows. If possible, measure a child's pulse rate while the child is at rest. An apical pulse (i.e., listening at the heart apex through a stethoscope) is taken in children younger than 1 year of age because their radial (i.e., wrist) pulse is too faint to be palpated accurately. In an infant, the point of maximum intensity, or the point on the chest wall where the heartbeat can be heard most distinctly, is just above and outside the left nipple (i.e., just lateral to the midclavicular line at the third or fourth intercostal space). This point gradually becomes more medial and slightly lower up to 7 years of age. By 7 years of age, it is at the fourth or fifth interspace at the midclavicular line as in adults. For greatest accuracy, count the pulse rate for 1 full minute.

Concept Mastery Alert

By the time a child reaches school age, the radial pulse may be used for measuring pulse. In infants younger than 1 year of age, the apical pulse is used.

RESPIRATORY RATE

Respirations also should be measured before an infant is disturbed because the respiratory rate increases with crying. If possible, count the infant's respirations while the infant is being held by their parent or lying quietly in a crib before lowering the side rail. For a child, count the respirations when they are seated in a parent's lap. Infants tend to breathe with their abdominal muscles so it is just as accurate to take respirations by counting movements of the abdomen as it is to count chest movements. Again, for greatest accuracy, count respirations for 1 full minute.

BLOOD PRESSURE

Beginning at 3 years of age, children should have their blood pressure measured at every office visit (National Heart, Lung, and Blood Institute, 2005). Offer an age-appropriate explanation of the procedure, especially to young children, because wrapping their arm and feeling the pressure applied can be frightening if they are not prepared for it.

Systolic pressure in children is read as the manometer pressure is dropping and at the point where the first sound is heard. The point at which the sound disappears is considered the diastolic pressure. Blood pressure can be difficult to measure in infants because the cuff used must be no more than two thirds and not less than one half the length of their upper arm; a wider cuff gives a lower reading and a narrower cuff gives a higher reading (Fig. 37.4). Doppler ultrasound blood pressure, which bounces high-frequency sound waves off blood moving through a vein, is especially effective when continuous monitoring is necessary for infants because it can be set to record at specified times and the result is obtained so much faster. If a Doppler lead is placed over an artery, either the movement of the blood (i.e., pulse wave) or its tension (i.e., blood pressure) can be registered on a digital readout or monitor print or the sound of the pulse waves can be broadcast for auscultatory assessment.

Preschoolers and school-age children enjoy watching the digital readout numbers, so digital recording also works well with these age groups. Direct measurement (i.e., intraarterial monitoring by an indwelling catheter into the radial or femoral artery) is used with children who are critically ill and is described in Chapter 41.

If a child's arms are not free for blood pressure recording, blood pressure may be recorded by wrapping a cuff over the thigh and palpating or auscultating the popliteal pulse behind

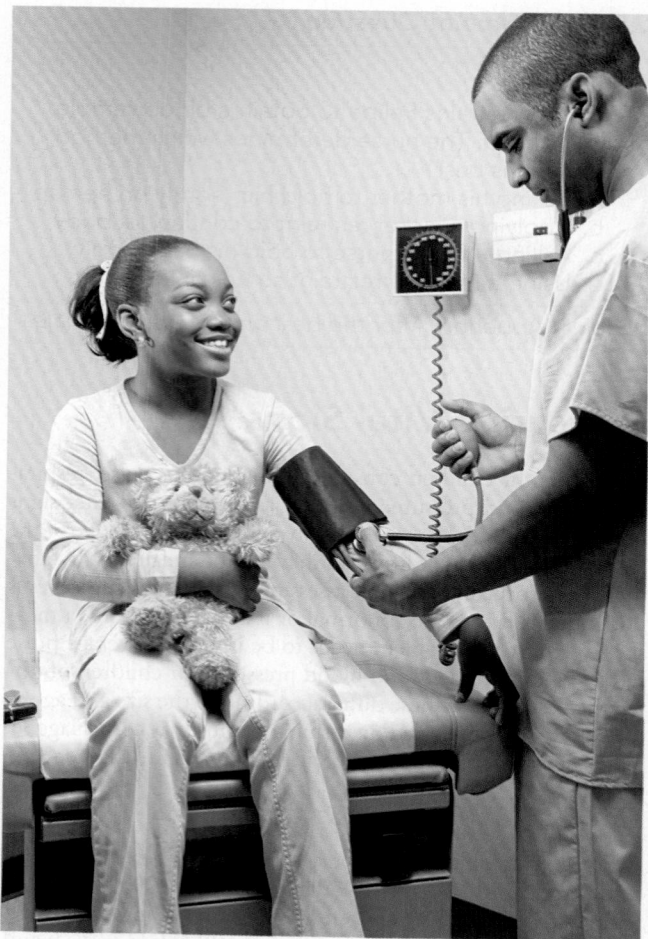
Figure 37.4   Blood pressure measurements are essential during routine health assessments and before diagnostic or therapeutic procedures. Here, a nurse assesses a child's blood pressure during a routine examination. (XiXinXing/Shutterstock.com)

the knee or at the ankle. In infants younger than 1 year of age, the thigh and arm blood pressure should be equal. In children older than 1 year of age, the systolic pressure in the thigh tends to be 10 to 40 mmHg higher, whereas diastolic pressure remains the same. If the thigh blood pressure reading is lower than that in the arm, coarctation of the aorta or an interference with circulation to the lower extremities may be the cause and should be addressed immediately.

When assessing blood pressure, pay attention to the pulse pressure—the difference between systolic and diastolic readings—in addition to the actual numbers because both an unusually wide (more than 50 mmHg) or narrow (less than 10 mmHg) range may suggest congenital heart disease. An abnormally narrow pulse pressure, for instance, is a sign of aortic stenosis. An abnormally low diastolic pressure (causing a wide pulse pressure) occurs with patent ductus arteriosus.

Reducing Elevated Temperature in Children

Fever is such a common symptom in children that reducing temperature, or giving a parent instructions on how to reduce a child's temperature at home, is a common intervention with children.

Nursing Diagnoses and Related Interventions

Nursing Diagnosis: Risk for hyperthermia related to illness or interference with temperature regulation from medication or surgery

Outcome Evaluation: Child's tympanic temperature returns to 98.6°F (37°C) within 2 hours.

Because the temperature-regulating mechanism in children is immature, fever tends to be more marked than in adults, and may even be out of proportion to the seriousness or extent of their disease. A high temperature occurs because a child's temperature-regulating point (set point) has been elevated. The child's temperature, therefore, cannot be reduced until the set point returns (or is returned) to normal.

Acetaminophen (Tylenol) and ibuprofen (Motrin or Advil) are excellent antipyretics and are often initiated when a child has a fever of more than 101°F (38.3°C). It is important to counsel parents that fever in children does not typically last long and is a means by which the body tries to protect itself by fighting off illness (Box 37.4).

Acetaminophen in a dosage of 10 to 15 mg/kg every 4 to 6 hours to treat fever in children is safe and effective. It is estimated that 80% of children will have a decrease in temperature within the first 30 to 60 minutes after administration. Ibuprofen in a dosage of 10 mg/kg every 6 to 8 hours is as effective as acetaminophen and may have a longer effect on lowering body temperature; however, ibuprofen should not be given to infants younger than 6 months of age (Sullivan & Farrar, 2011).

Caution parents also to never give acetylsalicylic acid (aspirin) to children with fever because aspirin is associated with Reye syndrome, a severe neurologic disorder (see Chapter 49).

Many parents dress febrile children warmly in flannel pajamas to keep them from "getting a chill." This actually increases the child's temperature and does not prevent the shaking, trembling reaction that comes with a high fever. In addition to antipyretic administration, suggest parents dress children with a fever in lightweight clothing. They can remove all clothing but the diaper from an infant. Placing a cool cloth (not ice) on a child's forehead often feels comforting and can help prevent a headache. Sponging children with ice water used to be prescribed on a routine basis to reduce fever, but the practice may lead to extreme chilling and shock to an immature nervous system and has little advantage over the use of oral antipyretics.

Common Diagnostic Procedures

Diagnostic and therapeutic procedures used with children vary depending on a child's condition and age but are similar to those used with adults. Blood, urine, and stool studies are commonly prescribed. Respiratory illnesses require special procedures and are discussed in Chapter 40. Biopsies (i.e., surgical procedures to remove tissue for examination) are done to detect malignancy and are discussed in Chapter 53. Stress or exercise testing for cardiovascular pathology is discussed in Chapter 41.

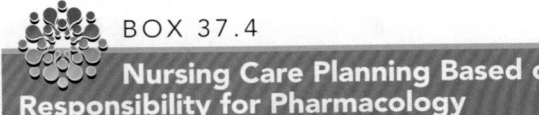

IBUPROFEN (ADVIL, MOTRIN)

Action: used to reduce inflammation, fever, and mild-to-moderate pain

Pregnancy Risk Category: B; D if used in last trimester

Dosage: (for fever or pain) individually based on child's weight, not over four doses in 24 hours

Possible Adverse Effects: gastric upset, headache, dizziness, nausea, occult blood loss, prolonged bleeding, peptic ulceration (Karch, 2015)

Nursing Implications

- Use with caution in children who have gastrointestinal irritation because ibuprofen causes gastric irritation.
- Encourage fluid intake; ibuprofen may cause renal failure if child becomes dehydrated.
- Administer this medication with food or drink to minimize gastrointestinal irritation.
- Do not give to infants younger than 6 months of age without healthcare provider's approval.
- Always use the measuring device supplied by the manufacturer, not a kitchen spoon, for dosage accuracy.

ELECTRICAL IMPULSE STUDIES

As their name implies, **electrical impulse studies** are those that include electrical conduction. Children need special preparation for studies such as electrocardiograms (ECGs) (Fig. 37.5) or electroencephalograms (EEGs) because they have been warned not to play with electric wires and so may worry about being burned or electrocuted. You can assure a child the electricity passes from their body to the machine, not the other way around. Except for electromyelograms (i.e., study of the conduction paths of the spinal cord), you can also assure them these tests are painless. The electrodes are attached to the body by paste or sticky tape, which is easily removed afterward.

X-RAY STUDIES

A variety of X-ray studies are used to inspect internal aspects of the body, such as bony structures. These range from simple

Figure 37.5 Administering an electrocardiogram (ECG). Children can be assured this is a painless procedure. (© Fotosearch.com.)

Figure 37.6   Positioning of a child for an X-ray. (iStock.com/ xavierarnau)

flat-plate views to more complicated computed tomography scan or studies using contrast dye.

Flat-Plate X-Rays

X-rays are used to diagnose and evaluate the progress of illnesses as well as assess the placement of apparatuses such as gastrointestinal feeding tubes. As a rule, children accept X-rays without protest because the X-ray machine can be compared with a camera, an instrument with which they are familiar (Fig. 37.6). A lead apron and thyroid shield are used on portions of the body where X-ray exposure is not needed. Parents and healthcare providers who remain in the room during an X-ray should be provided with safety equipment such as a lead apron. Remove any objects that contain metal because they may obscure the image.

Dye Contrast Studies

To visualize a body cavity, radiopaque dye may be swallowed, instilled by enema, or administered intravenously and then revealed by X-ray. Caution the child who is asked to drink barium for a gastrointestinal study that even if flavored, it does not taste terribly good (more like warm thick milk). Always check the child's allergy status before administering anything that they have to ingest or be injected with. Evidence exists of a nonspecific cross-reactivity between contrast material sensitivity and allergy to seafood as well as other foods (Harrison, 2013). The frequency of allergic-like and physiologic adverse events related to the intravascular administration of iodinated contrast media (ICM) is low and has decreased considerably with changes in the use of ionic high-osmolality contrast media (HOCM) to nonionic low-osmolality contrast media (LOCM) (American College of Radiology, 2016). As the contrast dye is injected, the child may feel a hot flush, a sensation that can be frightening if the child is unprepared for this. Try not to use the word *dye* when describing a contrast medium to prevent young children from worrying they will be dyed like an Easter egg or will *die*. Use the phrase *special medicine* instead.

Children easily grow bored during this type of procedure because of the time involved waiting for the contrast medium to reach and outline the specific organ to be studied. Have the child take along an activity to the exam room to make the time pass faster. Maintaining NPO status may also be difficult for lengthy procedures. Ensure that parents understand children do not "radiate" X-rays or radioactivity after the procedure, so they will not be afraid to hold a child closely for comfort.

Computed Tomography

Computed tomography (CT), more commonly known as a CT or CAT scan, is an X-ray procedure in which many views of an organ or body part are obtained to represent what the organ would look like if it were cut into thin slices. As with any X-ray, dense structures appear white and less dense structures appear gray to black on the films.

The procedure may include injection of an iodine-based radioisotope contrast medium. If this is necessary, the study may be referred to as **positron emission tomography (PET)** or **single-photon emission computed tomography (SPECT)**.

A CT scanner is a large machine with a hole, or short tunnel, in the center. A moveable examination table slides into and out of this tunnel. In the center of the machine, the X-ray tube and electronic X-ray detectors are located opposite each other on a ring, called a gantry, which rotates around the patient (Fig. 37.7A). It's important for children to lie still during the procedure to avoid creating artifacts on the film. Sedation may be needed to aid in the procedure. You can assure parents that although the radiation exposure from CT scans occurs over a long period of time, such low doses are used that the actual

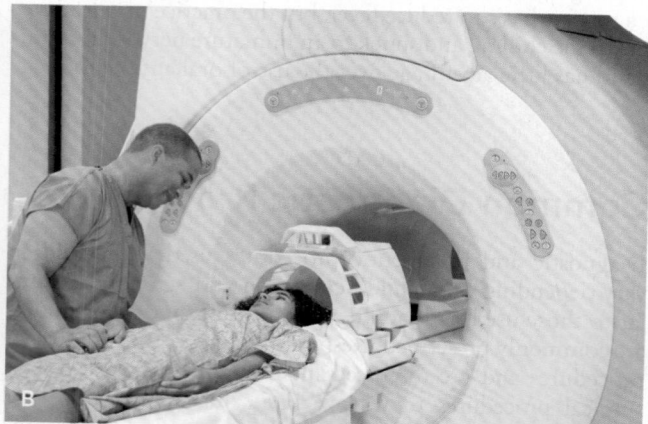

Figure 37.7   Some procedures are potentially frightening because of the size of the machinery used. **(A)** A computed tomography (CT) scanner. (From Michelle Del Guercio/Photo Researchers, Inc.) **(B)** A magnetic resonance imaging (MRI) scanner. (© Fotosearch.com.)

exposure is comparable to a regular X-ray. Radiation dose from CT procedures varies from patient to patient. The particular radiation dose will depend on the size of the body part examined, the type of procedure, and the type of CT equipment and its operation (U.S. Food and Drug Administration, 2016).

QSEN Checkpoint Question 37.2

INFORMATICS

Felipe's mother is relieved that he does not need an MRI because she tells the nurse she "would not have not allowed that." What would be the nurse's best response to her?

a. "MRIs are almost never used for children under 4 years so you don't have to worry."

b. "Aren't you prepared to take some risks to ensure Felipe's well-being?"

c. "If, at any point, Felipe does need an MRI, be prepared to change your mind."

d. "What is the reason you wouldn't have allowed an MRI for your son?"

Look in Appendix A for the best answer and rationale.

Magnetic Resonance Imaging

Magnetic resonance imaging (MRI) combines a magnetic field, radio frequency, and computer technology to produce diagnostic images that aid in the diagnosis of disorders such as the cause of renal or brain pathology. The child lies on a moving pallet that is pushed into the core of the machine, where the magnet is housed (Fig. 37.7B). When the magnetic field surrounding the child is turned on, it causes tissue atoms to line up in a parallel fashion. As radio waves are turned on and off, the atoms change position. This change is sensed and converted into a visual display on a computer screen (Delso, Ter Voert, & Veit-Haibach, 2015).

The procedure has an advantage over X-rays in that it has no apparent ill effects, it can reveal astonishingly clear structural defects in soft tissue, and, if a contrast medium is required, it is not iodine based, so the danger of a reaction is minimal. Because metal may deflect the magnetic waves, children with a metal prosthesis or metal dental braces are poor candidates for the procedure. Hairpins and eye makeup (which often has a metallic base), watches, or other jewelry should be removed. Remove any metal from the child's hospital gown, which may include metal snaps.

When the radio waves are turned on and off during the procedure, a booming noise can be heard. Prepare children for this sound (which is often compared with the sound of drums) as well as the feeling of claustrophobia they may experience. Except for cranial exams, headphones can be provided to decrease the noise. Because the total procedure (excluding cranial examinations) may take up to 45 minutes, sedation may be indicated so they can lie quietly for this length of time and not skew the images recorded. Box 37.5 depicts an interprofessional care map for a child having a cranial MRI exam.

What If . . . 37.2

Felipe's mother repeats to the nurse that he is very frightened of dark places. Knowing this, how would the nurse best prepare him for a CT scan?

ULTRASOUND

Ultrasound is a painless procedure in which images of internal tissue and organs, such as the appendix, are produced by the use of sound waves (RadiologyInfo.org, 2015). Because it is noninvasive, children accept ultrasound easily and may even enjoy watching the oscilloscope screen during the procedure. Alert a child that the clear gel, which is applied to the skin over the body part to be studied, may feel cool and sticky. Compare the transducer that is used on the body surface to pick up internal images to a television camera so it is not viewed as something strange (Fig. 37.8). Explain that the ultrasound procedure is not an X-ray, so they can remain in the room to comfort their child during the procedure. Because ultrasound appears to have no long-term effects, it can be repeated over and over for serial determinations.

NUCLEAR MEDICINE STUDIES

Radiopharmaceuticals are radioactive-combined substances that when given orally or by injection, flow to designated body organs. When a scintillation machine (a form of Geiger counter) is passed over the organ where the radiopharmaceutical has collected, the pattern of the collected material outlines the organ. The pattern can then be reproduced as a screen image or a photograph.

Parents may worry that a child will be harmed by exposure to a radioactive substance (Adelstein, 2014), and although this procedure exposes the patient to low levels of ionizing radiation, the risk is minimal when used judiciously. Within the media are a number of reports about the medical use of radiation and the risk of neoplasm development. It is important to effectively communicate with families and patients about the medical use of radiation, the level of radiation exposure, and its potential risks (World Health Organization [WHO], 2016).

DIRECT VISUALIZATION PROCEDURES

Direct visualization procedures involve the observation of an internal body cavity by way of a thin tube inserted through a body surface opening. Types of direct visualization include endoscopy, bronchoscopy, and colonoscopy.

Endoscopy

Endoscopy involves the use of an endoscope, which is passed through the mouth, to examine the gastrointestinal tract and has become a common method of diagnosis for gastrointestinal disorders in children. The procedure is also used as an emergency measure to remove foreign objects such as quarters or toys swallowed by children. When first developed, endoscopes were straight and stiff metal instruments, so their use was limited. Currently, they are made up of fiberscopes, which are extremely flexible and easily maneuvered, so these examinations are not nearly as uncomfortable as before.

The thought of having a tube passed down the throat can be very frightening. Even after children understand what the procedure will consist of, they can still be very uncomfortable at the thought of a tube being passed into them. Before the procedure, children must remain on an NPO status for between 4 and 6 hours. They will need a sedative or moderate sedation so they can lie quietly for the time required. Good support during both the anxious time waiting for the procedure and during the procedure is crucial. Ask whether the child can have a digital photograph taken during the procedure to keep as a scrapbook souvenir.

BOX 37.5

Nursing Care Planning

AN INTERPROFESSIONAL CARE MAP FOR A CHILD IN NEED OF DIAGNOSTIC TESTS

Felipe is a preschooler who is scheduled to have a computed tomography study for a possible head injury.

Family Assessment: Child lives with single-parent mother and younger sibling in two-bedroom loft in refurbished inner city warehouse. Mother is a commercial artist. Rates finances as "healthy."

Patient Assessment: Child was playing at community playground with day care staff. Was pushed off top of slide by another child. Fell approximately 6 ft onto his head and sustained brief loss of consciousness. Brought to emergency department by rescue. Temperature (T) = 100.6°F tympanic; Pulse (P) = 90; Blood pressure (BP) = 100/65 mmHg. Crying from pain in neck and upper back.

  "He's upset because of being bullied at school and he's afraid of the dark. What will this exam be like and how can we make sure he will be safe?"

Nursing Diagnosis: Anxiety (child and parent) related to necessary diagnostic procedure

Outcome Criteria: Mother listens to explanation of advantages of computed tomography (CT) scan for diagnosis of brain, neck, or spine injury. Voices agreement to allow procedure. Helps prepare child for anxiety-filled experience.

Team Member Responsible	Assessment	Intervention	Rationale	Expected Outcome
Activities of Daily Living, Including Safety				
Nurse	Take history to assess if child has change of behavior from usual.	Review with parent that traumatic events can affect all body systems.	Head injury, if severe, can affect vital signs and cognitive processing.	Parent states she feels child is reacting as usual except for neck pain.
Teamwork and Collaboration				
Nurse/primary care provider	Assess if further neurologic consultation will be necessary following physical and neurologic exam.	Consult as necessary with neurologist about child's condition and continued care based on CT findings.	A 6-ft fall could cause considerable intracranial swelling or bleeding.	Neurologist on call completes necessary consult and any needed additional procedures.
Procedures/Medications for Quality Improvement				
Nurse/pain management team	Ask child to rate pain using faces scale.	Explain CT procedure to parent and child. Assist with moderate sedation.	Moderate sedation will allow child to sleep during an otherwise frightening procedure.	Consent for moderate sedation is obtained. Sedation is used during procedure without complications.
Nutrition				
Nurse	Assess last time child ate or drank.	Keep child nothing by mouth (NPO) prior to procedure.	Moderate sedation can cause aspiration in children with a full stomach.	Child remains NPO until postprocedure.
Patient-Centered Care				
Nurse/nurse practitioner	Assess parent's understanding of the need and technique of CT scan.	Fill in gaps of knowledge for parent about procedure.	A well-informed parent is able to make well-informed decisions about care.	Mother states she understands why procedure is needed.
Psychosocial/Spiritual/Emotional Needs				
Nurse	Assess if child is still frightened from bullying episode at playground.	Review with child that bad things can happen to good people.	Discussion of an injury can help to relieve guilt and increase self-esteem.	Child discusses what happened; states he knows incident was not his fault.

Informatics for Seamless Healthcare Planning

Nurse/primary care provider	Assess if parent understands importance of assessing child's respirations and pulse every 4 hours after return home.	Review with parent technique for respiration and pulse assessment.	A decreasing pulse or respiratory rate can indicate increased intracranial pressure.	Parent confirms she will be able to take vital signs accurately; will notify emergency department if vital signs vary from norms given to her

Because the endoscope is passed through the throat, edema of the throat may occur from the pressure on the esophagus and pharynx. This means that the child requires close observation afterward for at least an hour to confirm that the edema is not interfering with respirations or causing discomfort. Observe closely the first time the child drinks after the procedure to ensure that the gag reflex is intact despite throat edema or the effect of a local pharyngeal anesthetic that may have been sprayed into the throat before the procedure.

Bronchoscopy

Bronchoscopy is the direct visualization of the larynx, trachea, and bronchi through a lit, flexible, fiberoptic tube (i.e., a bronchofiberscope) that is passed through the naris or trachea. The procedure is used with children who have aspirated a foreign object, to instill certain medications, or to take culture and or biopsy specimens (Singh & Singhal, 2015). Typically, the throat is sprayed with a local pharyngeal anesthetic to numb the area. Moderate sedation is then administered, and continuous monitoring of vital signs is standard care. Different types of bronchoscopes are used depending on the age of the child and/or the size of the endotracheal tube being used. Procedural complications are not common but may include compromise to the airway such as hemorrhage, pneumothorax and airway edema. After the procedure, continue to assess the child's respiratory function and airway patency. Postprocedure complications may include bronchospasm, stridor, desaturation, or respiratory distress. Observe children carefully the first time they drink after the procedure to assess that their gag reflex is intact and they do not choke.

Figure 37.8 Ultrasound can be potentially frightening for children unless they receive good preparation because they don't understand the concept of sound waves. (© iStockphoto/Thinkstock.)

Colonoscopy

Colonoscopy is an endoscopic examination of the large intestine with a flexible fiberscope that is inserted through the anus and advanced as far as the ileocecal valve. Air is then infused to expand the bowel walls for good visualization. The technique allows the colon walls to be visualized; if abnormalities are found, photographs can be taken for analysis. It is used to diagnose inflammatory bowel disease or to obtain biopsies if a malignancy is suspected.

Before the procedure, children are given a clear liquid diet for about 24 hours and then they are asked to drink an isotonic saline laxative that causes fluid diarrhea so their bowel is clean for the procedure. It can be difficult for younger children to drink as much of the laxative solution as is needed so their bowel is cleared completely of stool (Elitsur, Butcher, Vicki, et al., 2013). Playing games such as Simon Says can be helpful to gain their cooperation. If a child cannot swallow all the laxative, a saline enema may be necessary. Moderate sedation is used during the procedure to reduce discomfort.

Postprocedure, children may pass a great deal of flatus in the first 12 hours because of the air introduced during the procedure. If the procedure was done on an ambulatory basis, children are discharged about 2 hours after the procedure (but they are kept NPO during that time to allow the bowel to have a brief rest). Provide parents with instructions on what observations they should make and report if they occur after they return home, such as abdominal pain, blood in stool, weakness, or pallor (signs of bowel bleeding) especially if a polyp was removed or a biopsy specimen was obtained. Even with moderate sedation, colonoscopies are difficult procedures for children to accept. Give generous praise afterward for their cooperation with both the preparation for the procedure and the actual procedure.

ASPIRATION STUDIES

Aspiration studies, which are the removal of body fluids by such techniques as lumbar puncture or bone marrow aspiration, are always anxiety-causing procedures. The size of the needle that will be used can be frightening to parents and children alike. Children may need a sedative or moderate sedation so that they remain still during the procedure. Support and restrain children by talking and using touch as appropriate. Assess for bleeding at the puncture site after the procedure and apply pressure as needed to halt bleeding completely. After a lumbar puncture, remind children to remain quiet and with their head flat to help prevent a postdural puncture headache (see Chapter 49 for specific procedural details).

Collecting Specimens for Analysis

The collection of body fluids, secretions, and excretions is a collaborative nursing function essential to the complete assessment of a child. Elements of these fluids are measured by a variety of means; findings can be used to help diagnose an illness, evaluate the progress of a condition, or evaluate a child's response to therapy. As with all procedures, use standard infection precautions regardless of the source from which the sample is taken. Ensure precautions are maintained through the entire process, from obtaining, transporting, discarding, or storing specimens.

OBTAINING BLOOD SPECIMENS

Having a blood specimen taken can be terrifying for a child. For many children, their past experience with losing blood has involved a nosebleed or a cut knee and the discomfort or pain they felt. They have also had injections for immunizations, so they know that injections sting. Putting the two experiences together makes collecting a blood specimen an extremely terrifying process. For these reasons, prepare children both before and during the procedure. Patient immobilization is crucial to the safety of pediatric and neonatal patients undergoing phlebotomy (WHO, 2010). When feasible, blood specimens should always be obtained away from a child's bedside to keep the room and bed as a "safe" area. Applying a Band-Aid afterward to cover the needle site provides physical as well as psychological support.

Venipuncture

For very small infants, the usual sites for venipuncture (entrance into a vein) are the same as for adults: the superficial veins of the dorsal surface of the hand or the antecubital fossa. In a few instances, the jugular or femoral vein can also be used. In nonemergent situations, apply an anesthetic cream such as EMLA (eutectic mixture of local anesthesia) before venipuncture to reduce pain (see Chapter 39) and liberally use distraction techniques such as using toys with flashing lights, blowing bubbles, or playing a game for toddlers and asking distraction questions or playing a movie for school-age children (Stevens & Marvicsin, 2016).

Offer children a simple explanation of the procedure in terms they can understand: "I need to take some blood from your hand. First, I'll put some cream on your skin so when I come back to take the blood in a little while, you'll feel only a pinprick because of the cream." Let the child know you understand how difficult it is to agree to the procedure. Try not to say "drawing blood" because this sounds as if you're proposing an activity with crayons, not a procedure that will cause discomfort (Box 37.6).

Preschoolers may worry that they will lose all their blood during the procedure because they have no concept of how much blood their body contains. Many children younger than school age may have to be restrained for blood sampling because no matter how cooperative or brave they might be initially, the minute they see the needle, they can be too overwhelmed with fear to hold still.

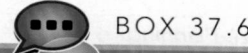

BOX 37.6

Nursing Care Planning Tips for Effective Communication

Felipe is a 4-year-old who is going to have several diagnostic studies. He's coloring a picture when you approach him to obtain a blood specimen for electrolyte levels.

Tip: Carefully explain what you need to do and why it is important. It is easy to forget that what a word means to you may not be interpreted the same way by a young child.

Nurse: Hi, Felipe. I see you are coloring a picture, can you tell me about it?

Felipe: It is a birthday card for my grandma.

Nurse: I am sure she will like it. Remember when we used this syringe and tubing to check on your blood last week? I need to do another check today. We can't see inside your body, and by checking your blood, we can see if you are getting better. Which arm would you like me to use today?

Felipe: Use this one [holds out left arm]. I need this one [indicates right arm] to color with.

Nurse: You can squeeze this ball with your other hand while I clean off your arm with the (alcohol) pad. Let's count to 10 together. If you hold real still I will be finished by the time we get to 10 [counts to 10 together]. You did great. I know it hurt for a second. Would you like to pick out a sticker?

QSEN Checkpoint Question 37.3

EVIDENCE-BASED PRACTICE

One of the biggest problems with trying to reduce pain from a procedure such as a venipuncture or an injection is that anesthetic creams do not take effect until 30 minutes to an hour. To test whether commercial devices called a J-tip (a needle-free device for subcutaneous delivery of lidocaine) and the Buzzy (a cooled, vibrating device that uses gate control to minimize procedural pain) could serve as an effective distraction technique to immediately reduce pain, researchers prospectively investigated patients aged 1 month to 21 years. Participants were enrolled in phase 1 (J-tip only) and then phase 2 (Buzzy and J-tip) for analgesia prior to venipuncture or IV start. Results revealed that patients who received either intervention reported lower scores on pain scales during venipuncture or IV start than the group receiving no analgesia (Kearl, Yanger, Montero, et al., 2015).

Based on this study, the next time Felipe needs to have blood drawn, the nurse's best action would be which of the following?

a. Assessing Felipe's pain and anxiety levels before and after venipuncture

b. Explaining that venipuncture feels much the same as a mild bee sting

c. Planning a distraction technique for him that his mother thinks would be effective

d. Explaining to Felipe that an attempt will be made to distract him before performing the procedure

Look in Appendix A for the best answer and rationale.

Capillary Puncture

Capillary blood heel or fingertip punctures are often obtained for glucose and hematocrit determinations. Apply an anesthetic cream before the procedure to reduce discomfort if needed; however, be careful when applying this to a finger that the child doesn't lick this off and anesthetize their tongue or throat. Use the side of the finger, not the center, for the puncture to reduce discomfort afterward; for heel punctures, use the lateral aspect of the heel to avoid striking the medial plantar artery or the periosteum of the bone (Fig. 37.9). Comfort the child afterward because fingertip punctures seem minor but can be more painful than a venipuncture afterward.

In many settings, laboratory analysis such as glucose level can then be completed immediately using a commercial meter (a point-of-care test).

Figure 37.9 Sites for a capillary blood heel puncture. Choose a site to the right or left on the heel to avoid the medial artery.

QSEN Checkpoint Question 37.4

PATIENT-CENTERED CARE

Felipe will be having a fingertip puncture for serum glucose. The nurse determines which instruction is best to empower him before the procedure.

a. "It won't hurt a bit; it's only a small finger prick."

b. "Why don't you choose which finger you'd like me to use."

c. "Most other boys your age don't mind this at all."

d. "Make sure you hold still, otherwise you won't get a special treat."

Look in Appendix A for the best answer and rationale.

OBTAINING URINE SPECIMENS

Depending on the type of test required, urine may be collected with a usual voiding, after the external meatus has been cleaned (i.e., a clean-catch specimen), by catheterization, or suprapubic aspiration. A specimen may require a single specimen or collection of all the urine voided within a 24-hour period.

Routine Urinalysis

Routine urinalysis requires only a single voided specimen. The specimen will then be analyzed for appearance, glucose, specific gravity, and microscopic analysis. Specimens must always be collected in sterile containers to prevent contamination.

The Infant and Toddler

An infant or a child who has not been toilet trained cannot be expected to urinate on command; thus, a collecting device must be attached to the genitalia to collect their next voiding. Contamination rates for bagged specimens are high; thus, a bagged specimen should not be used for urinary tract infection (UTI) diagnosis. If the bagged specimen is negative for bacteria, the possibility of a UTI diagnosis is low (Kim & Koo, 2015).

For girls, wash the perineum to remove any fecal matter and then rinse with water and dry the site where the collecting device will be attached to ensure good adherence. For boys, wash the penis and rinse and thoroughly dry the same way. Maintain dry skin that is free from powder, lotions, and oils (Fig. 37.10A). Apply the adhesive side of the collection device firmly and smoothly to the skin (any folds or wrinkling will cause leakage) to cover the urethral opening.

If an infant attempts to loosen the collector, cover the device with a diaper to keep it out of reach. Otherwise, leave the device visible so that it can be observed for urine output. Offer the child something to drink to encourage voiding. Most infants void shortly after a feeding, so if the collector is applied just before a regular feeding, voiding will probably result soon afterward. Remove the collector as soon as the infant voids and transfer the specimen to a specimen cup by cutting a bottom corner of the bag.

Urine may be aspirated from diapers for tests such as specific gravity, dipstick protein, pH, or glucose (Fig. 37.10B). Current disposable diapers, however, are designed to trap urine in the material so effectively, they can make it impossible to squeeze out a specimen. Placing cotton balls inside the diaper can be a help because these can be squeezed for additional urine.

The Preschooler and School-Age Child

It may be difficult to obtain routine urine specimens from preschoolers or toilet-trained toddlers because they can void only when they feel a definite urge to do so, not on command. Another problem is language. It is not unprofessional to use words such as "pee-pee" if this is what the child will understand. Provide a potty chair if one is available; if not, put a urine collection cap device on a toilet. A generally successful approach with a child this age is to act as if voiding is not a difficult procedure. Offer the child a glass of water or

Figure 37.10 (A) A urine collector for infants. The trick to making the collector adhere is to make certain the child's skin is dry. **(B)** Testing specific gravity of urine with a refractometer. The advantage of this is that only one drop of urine is required.

other fluid and ask a parent to reinforce the request to void so that the child knows a parent approves. A school-age child is usually able to void when asked, although the child may find it more difficult than the adult.

The Adolescent

Adolescents are usually knowledgeable and cooperative about providing urine specimens. As with adults, give them a clean specimen container and tell them what is needed. Unless they have voided recently, they usually are able to void on command. Remember, however, that adolescents are concerned and self-conscious about body functions and therefore are often reluctant to carry a urine specimen through a crowded waiting room to the desk area. They may be too self-conscious to void if they know someone is nearby, for example, just outside a curtain waiting for them. Send them to a nearby bathroom with a closed door, or leave the area to give them privacy. Collect the specimen from them immediately so they do not have to carry it themselves.

Some adolescents are suspicious that a urine specimen is being requested for drug testing. Providing a good explanation of its actual purpose relieves this fear. If you are in doubt regarding whether the fluid returned to you is urine, not water, assess its specific gravity. Water has a specific gravity of 1.000; urine will have a specific gravity more than this (1.003 to 1.030).

Adolescent girls may be embarrassed to mention they are menstruating so be sure to ask an adolescent girl about this before she voids. To prevent having a urine specimen contaminated by menstrual blood, which changes the specific gravity,

protein, and red blood cell analysis, ask the girl who is menstruating to wash her perineum well with soap and water and rinse and dry it to remove menstrual blood.

Twenty-Four–Hour Urine Specimens

Although a urinalysis of a single urine specimen will indicate the presence of substances such as protein or glucose, a 24-hour urine specimen may be necessary to determine how much of a substance is excreted during a full day (quantitative analysis). To begin a 24-hour urine collection, ask a child to void (with an infant, attach a collecting bag and wait for the child to void). This specimen (i.e., the discard specimen) is discarded so that a specific time for the ensuing collection is known. If the urine collection was started early in the morning and this first specimen was counted as part of the collection, the urine collected during the next 24 hours would include urine that had been forming all night, resulting in an approximately 32-hour collection period that would distort the analysis.

Record the start of the collection period as the time of the discarded urine. Save all urine voided for the next 24 hours and place it in one collection bottle. Have the child void (or watch for an infant to void) at the end of the 24-hour period and add the final specimen to the collection bottle. Record the time of the collection as being from the time of the discarded urine to the final specimen added to the collection.

For an infant, use a 24-hour rather than a single specimen urine collector. These types of collectors, however, will adhere for this length of time only if a child's perineum is thoroughly dry at the time of application. Also, before applying the collector, apply tincture of benzoin or a commercial product to make the skin somewhat tacky and to help the collector firmly adhere to the skin. After the collector is applied, place the infant in a semi-Fowler's position, if possible, to encourage urine to flow freely into the collector. It may be necessary to place a diaper on the infant to keep the apparatus out of sight. Make certain the tubing from the collector is pinned out of the infant's reach or the infant may pull the collector free. Provide activities for the child and make sure the parents understand they can pick up infants and hold them during this time as long as they take care not to kink or pull the tubing.

To keep the bacterial count to a minimum, 24-hour collection containers are generally kept on ice; after each voiding, pour the new specimen into the larger container, which is kept refrigerated for the 24-hour period and until it can be transported to the laboratory for analysis. Because a preservative (considered a hazardous chemical) is added to the large container for some types of collections, instruct older children to void into a smaller container and then add their urine to the large container, or never void directly into the chemical-added container. Appropriate warning labels should be visible on the container to alert anyone handling the container. The Material Safety Data Sheet (MSDS) should be included with the handling instructions.

With active infants, fitting them with a colostomy bag applied to cover the urinary meatus may be more effective than using a collector with tubing because this allows them more mobility (Fig. 37.11). For this, puncture a small hole in the corner of the top of the colostomy bag. Insert a small feeding tube through this into the bottom of the bag and then apply the bag to the child's perineum. When the child voids, attach a syringe to the feeding tube and aspirate the urine. Transfer the specimen to the collection bottle. For the active toddler, this collector may be the only type that is acceptable to obtain a day-long specimen.

Clean-Catch Specimens

A **clean-catch urine specimen** is ordered when urine is needed for urinalysis and culture. The objective is to obtain

Figure 37.11 A 24-hour urine collector made from a colostomy bag. When the infant voids, the bag fills with urine, which can be aspirated from the bag by the inserted feeding tube.

urine that is uncontaminated by external organisms, such as skin flora, which would increase the organism count of the urine. Specimens used for protein or blood analysis may be ordered as clean-catch specimens because this careful cleaning also reduces the possibility that vaginal or foreskin (in uncircumcised males) secretions, which contain protein or blood, could be added to the specimen.

The technique for obtaining a clean-catch urine specimen from an older child is the same as that for an adult (see Chapter 11, Box 11.6). Some modifications are necessary for the young child or infant because it is not always possible to obtain a midstream urine specimen from young children. For girls, clean the labia from front to back using a cleansing pad or cotton balls saturated with the agency's designated cleaning solution. For boys, clean the tip of the penis using a cleansing pad or cotton balls saturated with the agency's designated cleaning solution.

To collect a specimen from a young child, ask the child to void. During the child's voiding, ask the parent to collect a "midstream" sample into a sterile container provided.

Clean-catch urine specimens have a major advantage over bladder catheterized specimens: They are not invasive, so they carry no risk of introducing a bladder infection, and if clean-catch specimens are obtained with care, they practically eliminate the need for catheterization. A clean-catch specimen with a bacterial colony count of more than 50,000 colony-forming units per milliliter is considered a positive specimen, or evidence that a UTI exists (AAP, 2011).

To confirm that school-age children and adolescents understand the procedure, have them repeat the instructions you gave to them and then send them to a nearby bathroom to carry out the procedure by themselves.

Suprapubic Aspiration

Suprapubic aspiration is the withdrawal of urine from the bladder of a child who is not old enough or in some other way cannot cooperate enough so that a clean-catch or catheterized specimen can be obtained. Suprapubic aspiration has an advantage for uncircumcised boys with phimosis, or girls with labial adhesions in whom catheterized specimens are more technically challenging to obtain (Schmidt & Copp, 2015). The procedure is done by inserting a sterile needle into the bladder through the anterior wall of the abdomen. Suprapubic aspiration is usually done by primary care providers, although nurses in specialty units may also perform this procedure. A successful suprapubic aspiration depends on the following steps:

1. Apply EMLA cream to lessen the discomfort 30 minutes to 1 hour before the procedure.
2. Secure a sterile syringe and needle and designated antiseptic solution.
3. Clean the anterior abdominal wall with the antiseptic.
4. Block the urinary meatus by pressure from a gloved finger to confine urine in the bladder.
5. Insert the needle on the syringe just above the pubis into the bladder.
6. Aspirate urine through the needle into the syringe, then withdraw the syringe and needle.
7. Comfort the infant or child afterward because the sight of the needle is frightening, it may cause some pain, and some restraint is necessary.

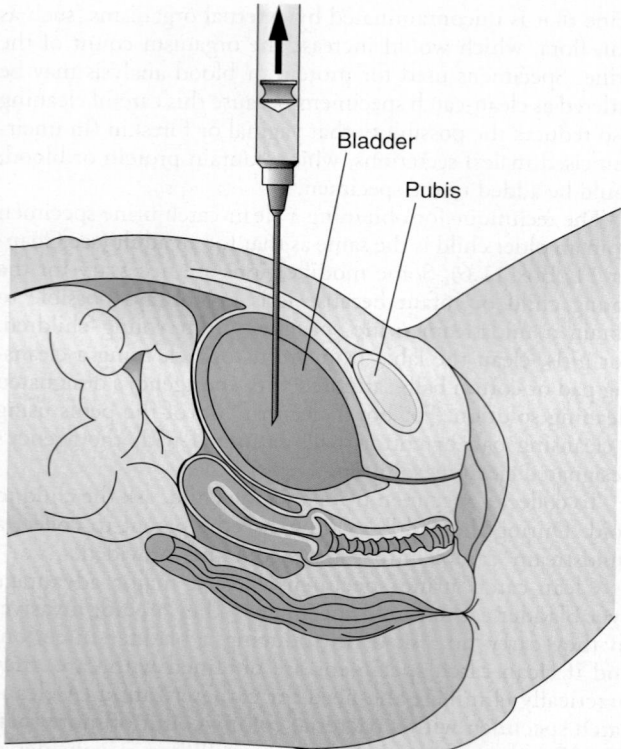

Figure 37.12 A suprapubic bladder aspiration. The full bladder is easily accessible by an abdominal puncture.

Withdrawal of urine by suprapubic aspiration is effective because the bladder is the most anterior of abdominal organs and, when distended with urine, is easily accessible just under the abdominal wall (Fig. 37.12). However, the needle can cause a bladder spasm and can produce a moment of sharp discomfort as the needle is inserted. Explain the necessity of the procedure to parents, specifically why the urine specimen is needed and the reason for the method being used, as they may not be familiar with this procedure. A suprapubic or catheterized urine sample with greater than 50,000 colony-forming units per milliliter indicates the presence of a UTI.

Catheterization

Bladder catheterization is accomplished most easily in infants and young children if a small (#5 or #8) feeding tube is used instead of a urinary catheter because such a thin tube passes readily through the meatus of even an infant. Before beginning catheterization, assess the urinary meatus in girls as it is not as readily observable in infants and young children as it is in adult women. For uncircumcised boys, gently retract the foreskin until the urinary meatus is visualized. Like any invasive procedure, explain to parents how it is performed and why the procedure is needed. If a parent is present, ask the parent to assure the child it is all right for you to touch his or her perineum or penis because he or she may have been told many times not to allow strangers to touch these areas. Distraction techniques such as blowing bubbles or imagery may help the child to relax. Offer support and praise to the child for submitting to the procedure and, afterward, for their cooperation (even if they were not cooperative).

OBTAINING STOOL SPECIMENS

Stool specimens are frequently obtained to be analyzed for blood, bacterial or viral infections, or ova and parasites. Ask children who are toilet trained to use a potty seat or to place a collector cap device on a toilet. Transfer the specimen to a laboratory collection cup using tongue depressor blades. To obtain a specimen from a child who is not toilet trained, scrape stool from a diaper using tongue depressor blades and place it in a stool collection cup. Some stool specimens need a preservative added to the container. If it is important to keep urine from contaminating the stool specimen, place a separate urine collector bag on the infant. Ask an older child to void first into the toilet and then defecate into the potty seat or collection device.

Specimens should be sent to the laboratory promptly so they do not dry and have to be collected a second time because most children need at least 24 more hours to produce a stool specimen. If the stool specimen is for ova and parasites, do not refrigerate it because refrigeration destroys the organisms to be analyzed.

QSEN Checkpoint Question 37.5

TEAMWORK & COLLABORATION

Felipe needs to have a 24-hour urine specimen collected and this will require the nurse to coordinate care with nurses on subsequent shifts. To ensure accurately timed collection, when would the nurse identify the collection's start point?
   a. The time you discard the first void
   b. The first time he voids in the morning
   c. A set time, which is most often 0700
   d. At the time of his first void after the discarded urine

Look in Appendix A for the best answer and rationale.

Assistance With Elimination

Two aspects of intestinal elimination that require special care are administration of enemas and ostomy care.

ADMINISTERING ENEMAS

Enemas are rarely used with children unless they are used as therapy for fecal impaction, Hirschsprung disease, a part of preparation for surgery, or a diagnostic test. If an enema is necessary, offer a careful explanation of what the child can expect.

Commercial enemas, such as Fleet enemas, are not routinely administered to children younger than 2 years of age because of the harsh action of the sodium biphosphate and sodium phosphate they contain. Tap water is not used either because, as it is not isotonic, it causes a rapid shift of fluid in body compartments, possibly leading to water intoxication. Although a solution of milk and molasses may be used in an emergency department to relieve a fecal impaction, normal saline (0.9% sodium chloride) is the usual solution used. It can be made by parents at home by adding 1 teaspoonful of salt to 1 pint (500 ml) of water.

As the sizes of children's bowels vary greatly, the usual amounts of enema solutions used are:

- Infant: less than 250 ml (exact amount should be stipulated by primary care provider's prescription)
- Preschooler: 250 to 350 ml
- School-age child: 300 to 500 ml
- Adolescent: 500 ml

For an infant, use a small, soft catheter (#10 to #12 French) in place of an enema tip to prevent rectal trauma. Lubricate the catheter generously with a water-soluble lubricant and insert it only 2 to 3 in. (5 to 7 cm) in children and only 1 in. (2.5 cm) in infants. If using an enema bag, hold the solution container no more than 1 ft above the level of the sigmoid colon (12 to 15 in. above the bed surface) so the solution flows at a controlled rate. If a child experiences intestinal cramping, clamp the tubing to halt the flow temporarily and wait until the cramping passes before instilling any more fluid. An older child can be instructed to take deep breaths to reduce guarding of abdominal muscles and to help the cramping sensation pass. The amount of solution used in infants is so small that this is not usually a problem.

Until late school age, children cannot retain an enema as adults can (rarely more than 5 to 10 minutes). For this reason, ensure that the bathroom the child will use is available before administering the enema.

Infants and children up to ages 3 or 4 years cannot retain enema solutions at all, so hold the buttocks together for a short time to prevent immediate expulsion of the solution, or pad the edge of a bedpan so it is not cold or sharp, and rest their pelvis on it following the procedure. Elevate the child's upper body by placing a pillow under the upper body for better positioning and comfort. If the enema solution is to be retained, such as an oil solution, hold the child's buttocks together for a count of 10 after administration.

After any type of enema administration, praise a child for cooperating. Allow a preschooler an opportunity for therapeutic play because this is a frightening, intrusive procedure.

PROVIDING OSTOMY CARE

An ostomy is a surgically formed opening from an internal structure to the surface of the body. Ostomies in newborns are created in the gastrointestinal system to relieve bowel obstruction caused by conditions such as ileal atresia, necrotizing enterocolitis, and imperforate anus. In older children, gastrointestinal ostomies are constructed for conditions such as inflammatory bowel disease, Crohn disease, and ulcerative colitis (Crohn's & Colitis Foundation of America, 2014). If an ostomy is created in the ileum (i.e., an ileostomy), the stoma is located on the right side of the abdomen and drains liquid stool, which is extremely irritating to the skin because of the digestive enzymes it contains. If an ostomy is created in the sigmoid portion of the bowel (i.e., a colostomy), the stoma is on the left lower abdomen and passes normally formed stool (Fig. 37.13).

An ileostomy requires the use of a collecting ostomy appliance to contain acid stool and to prevent excoriation of the abdominal skin. Older children also may use an appliance with a colostomy. For an infant with a colostomy, parents may choose (with support and advice) to use an appliance or just apply a diaper.

Two basic problems commonly arise when using an ostomy appliance with an infant: It may be difficult to locate one small enough to contain liquid drainage without leaking, and the skin under the appliance may become extremely irritated. Consulting with a wound ostomy continence nurse (WOCN) can be helpful to resolve these problems. As a rule, clear plastic, ringless colostomy bags are more easily cut to fit the size of the stoma and the contour and size of an infant's abdomen than bags with a ring attached. When using a commercial skin sealant to harden the skin surrounding the stoma, apply it according to the brand directions and allow it to dry. If a spray is used, protect the infant's face so that the infant does not inhale the solution. Tuck the chosen stoma collection appliance inside the diaper to help keep the infant from pulling it loose.

Check the appliance or bag for collecting stool at least every 4 hours. To protect the underlying skin, do not remove a self-adhering bag if it is full but drain collected stool from the bottom of the appliance into a basin or paper cup for disposal. To reduce odor, flush the appliance bag with a warm water and soap solution, using a bulb-type syringe (an Asepto syringe), and rinse with clear water. The collection bag may stay in place for as long as 1 week if properly secured. To remove a bag that was placed with a sealant, use the designated solvent to prevent pulling or harming the underlying skin. After removal, wash the skin with soap and water or the

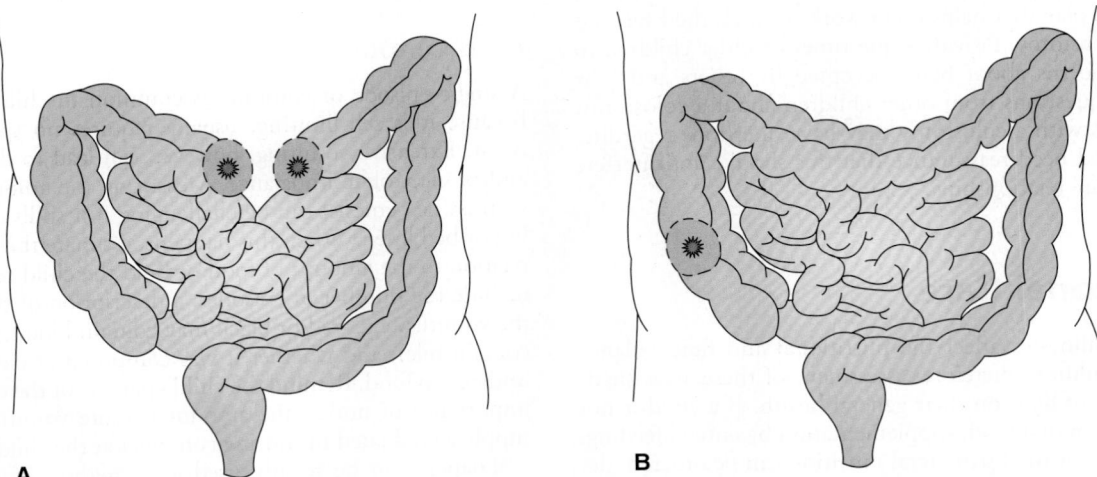

A   **B**

Figure 37.13   Different sites for ostomies. **(A)** A double-barrel colostomy. **(B)** A single-barrel colostomy.

solvent can become an irritant. Because most infants enjoy tub bathing, a long, soaking bath is an excellent way to loosen an adherent appliance.

If a parent chooses not to use an appliance, stool will be discharged onto the abdomen three or four times a day, similarly to the usual newborn or infant stool pattern. Wash and dry the stoma and surrounding skin area well after defecation. Follow your agency's protocol for skin care, such as applying karaya powder or a skin protection cream. Apply ample absorbent gauze (fluffed) and an absorbent pad over the stoma. Secure in place with nonadhesive tape or a binder. Without an appliance in place, stool is kept from touching the skin only by the protection of the ointment and frequent changing of the dressing, so assess for stool about every 4 hours. Turning an infant from side to side after every feeding can be helpful in keeping stool from flowing continuously to one side. Leaving the abdominal skin exposed to air for at least 1 hour per day also helps protect skin integrity.

Reassure parents caring for an infant with an ostomy that little is different from usual because all parents must change their infant's diapers frequently and clean the diapered area. Discuss with parents that the stoma has no nerves, so a parent can feel free to wash it without hurting the child and that compression against the stoma will not cause a child pain so the parent can feel comfortable placing an infant on the abdomen or holding the infant closely against his or her body for comfort.

Colostomies are rarely irrigated in children. On occasion, to prepare a child for second-stage abdominal surgery, irrigation of the "blind-end" bowel (i.e., the bowel between the rectum and colostomy) of a double-barreled colostomy may be prescribed daily to keep it lubricated and to maintain bowel tone. The exact amount of fluid to be used should be specified by the primary care provider; typically, the amount is small in infants, only 40 to 100 ml. Normal saline (0.9% sodium chloride) should be used in place of tap water, which could lead to water intoxication because tap water is not isotonic.

Children who have had a colostomy since infancy adapt well to having it because they have never known another method of defecation. Suggest that parents begin toilet training for urine control at the usual time (2 to 3 years of age). In contrast, school-age children often have a great deal of difficulty adjusting to a new colostomy. Encourage children to perform complete self-care as soon as possible to develop early independence. Preschool children usually benefit from therapeutic play that helps them work through their feelings about a colostomy. Provide some time for older children to discuss concerns about being accepted by others and how to answer questions from other children about a colostomy. Adolescents with a colostomy may have questions regarding sexuality and need reassurance that this should not interfere with intimate relationships.

Nutritional Care

Almost all illnesses affect the nutritional and fluid balance status of children; therefore, assessment of these areas sheds a great deal of light on their general health. If a child is not able to take in oral food, supplementation by enteral feeding, gastrostomy, or total parenteral nutrition can be ordered, depending on the child's need for nutrients.

 ## Nursing Diagnoses and Related Interventions

Nursing Diagnosis: Risk for imbalanced nutrition, less than body requirements, related to chronic illness

Outcome Evaluation: Skin turgor remains good; no signs of dehydration are present; child gains a minimum of 1 lb weekly as evidence that nutritional need is being met.

Supplying adequate nutrition includes a variety of measures such as measuring fluid intake and output and administering supplemental methods of feeding.

MEASURING FLUID INTAKE AND OUTPUT

Fluid is an essential element of nutrition because it cannot only supply water but also be a source of calories and vitamins. Children with a myriad of conditions such as vomiting, diarrhea, burns, hemorrhage, dehydration, cardiac and kidney disease, draining wounds, gastrointestinal suction, edema, or receiving diuretic or intravenous therapy need to have fluid intake and output measured and recorded in order to assess for fluid balance.

Fluid Intake

Estimating the intake of infants who are formula fed is simply a matter of estimating the kind and amount of fluids that were swallowed. Intake in breastfed infants is merely recorded as "breastfed for however minutes." If it is necessary to estimate the amount more closely than this, an infant can be weighed before and after a feeding. The difference in weight (measured in grams) is calculated to establish the number of milliliters of breast milk ingested (1 g = 1 ml).

With preschool children, record fluids ingested during snacks as well as meals because children this age may drink more with snacks than with meals. At approximately 10 years of age, children can be depended on to record their own intake as long as they have a list of how many milliliters are contained in each glass or cup they swallow (an average cup is 150 ml; a glass, 180 ml). Remind them that soup, flavored frozen ice such as popsicles, gelatin, sherbet, and ice cream are liquids (they liquefy at room temperature so should be counted as fluid).

Fluid Output

A single episode of vomiting is common in childhood and, because it is self-limiting, usually requires no special treatment. Extensive vomiting, however, can lead to dehydration and/or electrolyte imbalance. Measuring the amount a child vomits (i.e., emesis) can be challenging if it spills onto clothing or bed linen. When this happens, estimate the amount in relation to the amount of food or fluid the child recently ate; include the number of episodes, a description of the color of the vomitus (e.g., red or black may contain blood; green may contain bile), and whether it was composed of clear fluid or undigested food. Remind the child's parents or the child of the importance of noting the amount if more vomiting occurs; supply a graduated measuring container at the child's bedside.

Diapers can be readily used as a method of measuring urine output. Weigh a diaper before it is placed on an infant and record this weight conspicuously (e.g., mark it on the front of the plastic covering with a ballpoint pen). Reweigh the diaper after it is wet and subtract the difference to determine the amount of urine present. This difference will be in grams but because 1 g = 1 ml, the amount can be recorded in milliliters. In infants who have liquid stools, it is difficult to separate stool from urine because these blend together in a diaper. Separate urine from stool by applying a urine collector to the infant; check it frequently for filling.

Girls often void along with bowel movements when they use a toilet, which means that a urine specimen is easily lost or a stool specimen is contaminated with urine. To separate urine from bowel movements, teach older children to void first before trying to move their bowels.

ENTERAL FEEDINGS

Enteral feedings, also called nasogastric or orogastric tube feedings, are a common means of supplying adequate nutrition to an infant who is unable to suck (or who tires too easily when sucking) or to an older child who cannot chew or swallow. Enteral feedings have the advantage over parenteral (i.e., intravenous) nutrition because they preserve the stomach mucosa and also decrease the risk of intravenous infiltration or infection. Parents who care for children at home find them easy to manage and so express high satisfaction with the method (López, Pedrón-Giner, Martínez-Costa, et al., 2015). In infants, such feedings may be referred to as *gavage feedings* (Box 37.7 and Table 37.2).

Whether enteral catheters should be passed through the nares or the mouth is controversial. Because newborns are obligate nasal breathers, passing a catheter through the nose may obstruct their breathing space, and repeated insertion of a nasal gastric tube can cause inflammation and obstruction of the nose; thus, most tubes are inserted orally in small infants (Vermilyea & Goh, 2015).

Orogastric insertion can also decrease the possibility of striking the vagal nerve in the back of the throat and causing bradycardia. For older children, insertion through a nostril is often more comfortable. To prevent irritation or ulcer formation from the tube rubbing against the tip of the nose, always tape nasogastric tubes to the child's cheek rather than the forehead to secure it in place.

Because tubes are radiopaque, their placement or that they extend into the stomach can be confirmed by X-ray. Table 37.2 describes other methods to use before a feeding, verifying that the tube is not in the trachea or has pulled out so is actually just resting in the back of the throat.

Although children with long-term neurologic disabilities may have enteral tubes left in place for continuous feedings administered by an enteric feeding pump, most children are generally offered bolus or intermittent feedings at what would be a usual meal time, rather than continuous infusions, to more closely mimic a normal feeding pattern. The nutrition formula infused should be at room temperature to prevent chilling the child. Before a feeding, elevate the child's upper trunk 30 to 40 degrees (i.e., a semi-Fowler's position), so the fluid will flow downward into the stomach and not upward into the esophagus, possibly causing aspiration into the trachea. For infants, you can do this by holding the infant in your lap or placing the infant in an infant seat. For an older child, use pillows or elevate the head of the bed. For small infants, it is often necessary to aspirate stomach contents before a feeding because this reveals whether an infant is absorbing the quantity of fluid given as well as confirms the tube's placement is in the stomach. After noting the amount and type of fluid aspirated, unless prescribed otherwise, replace this fluid so the child does not lose the electrolytes or stomach enzymes it contains.

Following this, to administer a feeding, attach a syringe to the tube and allow the specified amount of nutrition formula to flow by gravity into the tube. Do not use the barrel of the syringe to force the feeding forward in order to prevent reflux and possible aspiration. Most infants enjoy having a pacifier for nonnutritive sucking during a feeding. This action helps to maintain or strengthen the sucking reflex for later when the child returns to oral feedings.

At the end of the feeding, flush the tube with 1 to 5 ml of water to clear it of the feeding solution, prevent blockage, and maintain patency. Keep the child's head elevated for at least 1 hour after a feeding to help prevent esophageal reflux. Provide mouth care at least twice a day to encourage salivation in children who are receiving nasogastric tube feedings; otherwise, their mouths can become dry and prone to the formation of mucosal ulcers.

GASTROSTOMY TUBE FEEDINGS

A gastrostomy tube is one inserted under regional anesthesia through an abdominal puncture site into the stomach and used for nutritional formula feedings (Fig. 37.14). The method may be necessary for children who cannot swallow, have an esophageal stricture, or who need long-term enteral feedings (Vermilyea & Goh, 2015). The tube used in children is usually an indwelling urinary catheter (i.e., a Foley catheter) rather than a true gastrostomy tube because these are smaller in size, can be removed easily, and changed should they become plugged. In addition, the balloon used to secure the tube is small enough so it does not obscure and fill the small stomach space. As with nasogastric feedings, gastrostomy feedings should be at room temperature to prevent chilling and given at spaced times to simulate meal times. Aspirate for stomach secretions to assess absorption and placement before the feeding and then allow the formula to flow by gravity only, not forced. If a child has had esophageal surgery, suspend the unclamped tube in an elevated position after the feeding because leaving the tube unclamped and elevated this way ensures that if the child should vomit, vomitus will be evacuated from the stomach by the tube rather than past new sutures in the esophagus. Cover the open end of the tube with a clean piece of porous gauze to reduce bacterial colonization.

Because infants who are fed by gastrostomy tube miss the pleasure of sucking the same as those fed by nasogastric tubes, offer a pacifier to suck on during the procedure unless contraindicated.

The biggest problem with managing gastrostomy tubes is they may not fit snugly, so formula or irritating gastric secretions can leak around the tube onto the abdominal skin. At least daily, wash skin around the tube with soap and warm water, removing any drainage and/or crusting. Once clean, make sure site remains clean and dry. A dry gauze dressing may be used. If a gastrostomy tube remains in place for a long period of time, the tube can move into the duodenum through the pyloric sphincter and cause obstruction. Observe and report any vomiting, abdominal distention, or brown or green tube drainage, which could be duodenal secretions that

BOX 37.7

Nursing Care Planning Using Procedures

INITIATING AN ENTERAL FEEDING FOR AN INFANT

Purpose: To supply nutrition by an enteral tube

Procedure	Principle
1. Loosely swaddle the infant using a mummy restraint.	1. Mummy or blanket restraints effectively contain arms and legs without causing any unwarranted pressure on the infant.
2. Measure the space from the bridge of the infant's nose to the earlobe then to a point halfway between the xiphoid process and the umbilicus using a #8 or #10 feeding tube. If the child is older than 1 year of age, measure from the bridge of the nose to the earlobe to the xiphoid process (Fig. A).	2. Measuring the tube ensures it will be long enough to enter the stomach. If a tube is passed too far, it will curl and end up in the esophagus; if not passed far enough, it will also be in the esophagus. Both situations could lead to aspiration of the feeding.

Procedure	Principle
3. Mark the tube at the measured point with a small clamp or piece of tape. Lubricate the tip of the catheter with water.	3. Water lubrication helps the tube pass through the esophagus without trauma. Don't use an oil lubricant because, although the tube is going to be passed into the stomach, occasionally it can unintentionally pass into the trachea. Oil left in the trachea could lead to lipoid pneumonia, a complication an infant already burdened with a disease may not be able to tolerate.
4. Pass the catheter with gentle pressure to the point of the clamp or tape. If the catheter is inadvertently passed into the trachea rather than the esophagus, the infant usually will cough and become dyspneic. If this happens, withdraw and replace the catheter.	4. Using gentle pressure helps to ensure comfort and safety.
5. Assess the catheter for position (confirm that it is not in the trachea) before administering a feeding (see Table 37.2).	5. Assessing for proper placement helps to ensure the feeding will enter the stomach, not the infant's respiratory tract.

Procedure	Principle
6. Aspirate stomach contents to assess amount. If the amount aspirated is small (a few milliliters), merely replace it at the beginning of the feeding. If large (large is determined by comparing it to the care provider's nutrition prescription), replace it through the tubing and reduce the amount of the feeding by that amount.	6. Assessing stomach content amount aids in determining if the previous feeding was absorbed. Replacing stomach secretions rather than discarding them helps prevent electrolyte loss.
7. After being certain the catheter is in the stomach, attach a syringe or special feeding funnel to the tube. Elevate the infant's head and chest slightly to encourage fluid to flow downward into the stomach.	7. Elevating the infant's upper body allows the feeding to flow by gravity.
8. Add the specific kind and amount of feeding prescribed to the syringe or funnel and allow it to flow by gravity into the infant's stomach. Don't elevate the syringe end of the tube more than 12 in. above the infant's abdomen (Fig. B).	8. Excessive elevation can cause the feeding to flow too quickly, filling the esophagus and increasing the risk for aspiration. Hurrying feedings by using the plunger of the syringe or a bulb attachment for more pressure also can lead to aspiration.

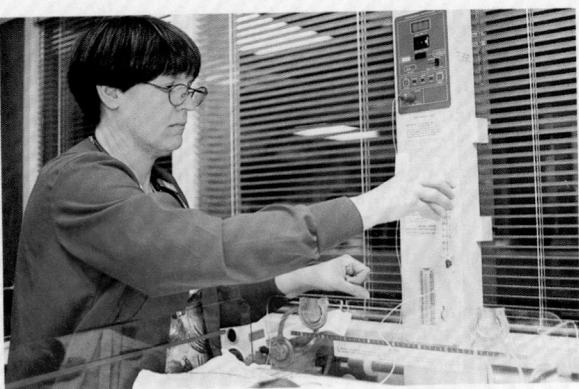

Procedure	Principle
9. Offer a pacifier (nonnutrient sucking) during the feeding if the infant appears to enjoy this.	9. Nonnutrient sucking can help satisfy the infant's normal need to suck, which would otherwise go unsatisfied with enteral feedings.
10. When the feeding has passed through the tube, reclamp the tube securely and gently and rapidly withdraw it.	10. Clamping the tube before it is withdrawn is important to prevent any milk remaining in the tube from flowing out as the tube is removed, thereby reducing the risk of aspiration.
11. If the tube is to remain in place, flush it with 1 to 5 ml of clear water and cap it.	11. Flushing a tube helps prevent plugging of the tube with the feeding solution. Capping a tube helps to prevent air and bacteria from entering.
12. If the tube is to be left in place, tape it below the nose and to the cheek. Do not tape it to the forehead.	12. Taping a tube to the forehead can put pressure on the anterior naris, leading to ulceration.
13. Burp the baby after an enteral feeding the same as you would after bottle or breastfeeding. If a parent is present, encourage him or her to do this.	13. Burping helps to prevent air accumulation and regurgitation of the feeding. Encouraging parental participation aids in promoting close contact, which is essential to the baby's development.
14. Unswaddle and place the infant on the right side with the head slightly elevated or hold and rock the infant in this position.	14. Placing on the right side helps the feeding solution enter the pyloric valve, thus promoting stomach emptying.
15. Assess that the infant appears comfortable. If a parent observed the procedure, answer any questions or concerns.	15. Assessing the infant after the feeding aids in outcome evaluation. Helping parents feel comfortable with alternative feeding methods can promote bonding with the infant.

TABLE 37.2 METHODS TO DETERMINE FEEDING TUBE PLACEMENT

Method	Considerations
1. If an X-ray is obtained to document correct tube placement, measure the length of the tube evident at that time. Remeasure the length of tube before a feeding to document that the tube has not pulled out or advanced further.	This system has inherent problems because it requires an X-ray and does not verify that the tube is actually in the stomach, but it can be used if it is healthcare policy.
2. Attach a syringe to the end of the tube and aspirate stomach contents. Test for pH (below 7 is acidic), which reveals the tube is in the stomach.	In most instances, stomach contents aspirated this way are returned to the stomach before the feeding; in small infants, the amount of stomach contents is subtracted from the prescribed amount of feeding. Because stomach contents are highly acid, discarding them at each feeding could lead to alkalosis.
3. Inject 5 ml air into the feeding tube and listen over the stomach with a stethoscope to the sound of injected air.	The injected air is heard as a whistling or growling sound. Do not use an adult-size stethoscope on small infants to listen for it; the diaphragm of the stethoscope will be partially over lung, and where one is hearing the air injection is unknown.

Gastrostomy tube

Stomach

Abdominal wall

A

B

Figure 37.14   Children who are ill often need supplemental feedings by nasogastric or gastrostomy tube feedings. **(A)** Internal placement of a gastrostomy tube. **(B)** An infant with a gastrostomy tube in place. (From W. McIntyre/Photo Researchers, Inc.)

would suggest the tube has moved. Stomach secretions are acidic, and duodenal secretions are alkaline. Therefore, testing residual aspiration fluid before a feeding to see that it is acid is a guarantee the tube is in the stomach. Also, putting a mark on the tube with an indelible pen lets you check that the tube has not migrated further into the gastrointestinal tract but is remaining securely in place.

Tubes are replaced approximately every 6 weeks. To replace a tube, deflate the catheter balloon by withdrawing the water in it and then gently pull the tube free. Insert a clean catheter into the stomach opening approximately 1 in. beyond the balloon and then inflate the balloon with 2 to 4 ml water. Apply skin protection and tape the tube into place.

Help parents to view gastrostomy feeding as merely an alternative way of feeding rather than a totally different one. Provide opportunities for parents and caregivers to participate and learn the feeding procedure. Assess whether they are comfortable with the procedure before the child is discharged from the hospital. Reinforce with them the understanding that it does not hurt their child to have pressure put against the tube so they do not worry about holding their child snugly.

If a child is going to need gastrostomy feedings for an extended time, a gastrostomy button will usually be implanted for easier stomach access, to prevent skin irritation, and to prevent ulceration of the stomach mucosa from the internal balloon (Fig. 37.15). For feeding with a button in place, a catheter is inserted through the device for a feeding and removed following the feeding. Advantages of gastrostomy buttons are the cosmetic benefit because only a small access device is visible instead of a bulky tube, and there is a lessened incidence of skin irritation.

What If . . . 37.3

The child in the hospital room next to Felipe has a gastrostomy button in place, with which she will be discharged. Her mother tells the nurse she's going to take her daughter to a restaurant as soon as they are discharged because she thinks "eating out" is an excellent way to teach table manners. What patient education would the nurse provide?

Figure 37.15   Placement of a gastrostomy button.

TOTAL PARENTERAL NUTRITION

Total parenteral nutrition (TPN), or nutrition administered intravenously, has become one of the most important therapies for children who have gastrointestinal illnesses that prevent proper absorption of basic caloric or fluid requirements or respiratory illnesses that make infants too exhausted to suck.

 ## Nursing Diagnoses and Related Interventions

Nursing Diagnosis: Imbalanced nutrition, less than body requirements, related to malabsorption of nutrients

Outcome Evaluation: Skin turgor is supple; signs of dehydration are not present; child loses no weight during therapy; intestinal cramps and distention lessen.

Traditional intravenous therapy contains fluid, electrolytes, and sugars but not protein and fat, ingredients which are essential for the maintenance and growth of body tissues. With TPN, all of a child's nutritional needs can be met by a concentrated hypertonic solution containing glucose, vitamins, electrolytes, trace minerals, and protein. An intralipid solution (emulsified fat able to be administered intravenously), given once or twice per week, supplies needed fatty acids. Children with chronic diarrhea or vomiting, inflammatory bowel disease, bowel obstruction, anorexia, or extreme immaturity are examples of children who benefit greatly from TPN.

TPN solutions may be administered via a central intravenous access site or via a peripherally inserted central venous catheter (PICC line) (Corkins, Griggs, Groh-Wargo, et al., 2013). If a central access site is chosen, a catheter is inserted through the right external jugular vein into the superior vena cava, or directly into the subclavian vein under strict aseptic conditions (see Chapter 38). The catheter is secured at the site of insertion with sutures and covered with a sterile dressing to help reduce bacterial invasion. A major vein of this type is chosen to avoid inflammation reactions and resulting venous thrombosis from the high-caloric and high-osmotic fluid that will be infused.

The TPN solution is prepared by the pharmacy under sterile conditions according to prescription. A Millipore filter, which removes small particles in the solution that might cause an embolus to form, is inserted into the tubing. Because the solution is concentrated, it is administered by means of a constant infusion pump so the rate can be governed. As a general rule, if the rate should fall behind, do not increase it the next hour to make up the amount of fluid, as serious cardiovascular overload could result because the fluid is so concentrated.

Infection is a major danger of TPN because the solution is a perfect medium for the growth of bacteria or *Candida* organisms. The dressing over the insertion site and the intravenous tubing need to be changed every 48 hours or as needed according to the Centers for Disease Control and Prevention (CDC) *Guidelines for Prevention of Intravascular Catheter-Related Infections* (O'Grady, Alexander, Burns, et al., 2011). Do not use the tubing for obtaining blood or for adding medications (unless a double-barreled tube is used) because such processes have the potential to introduce infection. Use sterile technique to change both the bags of solution and the dressing so infection is not introduced. Inspect the insertion site at the time of a dressing change for indications of local infection, such as redness, tenderness, or discharge because infection at the insertion site can lead to a serious sepsis or thrombosis.

A second major problem that can occur with TPN is dehydration. This occurs because a TPN solution contains approximately twice the amount of glucose normally administered in an intravenous solution to ensure that the amino acids in the solution will be used for protein synthesis, not for energy. Dehydration can occur when the kidneys recognize the amount of glucose in the bloodstream as excessive and begin to reduce it by excreting it (the same phenomenon that leads to high urine output in persons with diabetes mellitus). Before TPN is started and during the administration, test urine for glucose and specific gravity with each voiding. If two or more consecutive samples indicate a 3+ or 4+ glucose level, either the rate of the infusion or the amount of glucose in the solution may need to be decreased or insulin may need to be added to the solution to counteract the excess glucose. Generally, decreasing the concentration of glucose and then gradually increasing it again allows the child's body to adjust to the glucose overload without problems.

After the first few days of TPN, a rebound effect (e.g., the child's body produces increased insulin) may cause hypoglycemia. A urine sample that suddenly is negative for glucose after several serial specimens have been highly positive and, therefore, is not necessarily an encouraging sign; rather, it may be a warning the child's glucose level has become dangerously low. The TPN solution should never be discontinued abruptly but rather should be gradually tapered, or hypoglycemia could also occur. If a TPN catheter is accidentally pulled out by a child, notify the child's primary healthcare provider immediately and apply pressure to the insertion site to halt bleeding. The child must be immediately assessed for the effect of loss of blood and closely observed for signs of hypoglycemia (e.g., lethargy, lack of motor coordination, fidgeting, seizures). Parents need to be alerted to these steps if managing a child with parenteral nutrition on home care.

Remember that, to a child, eating is more than a means of receiving nourishment; it is also a means of receiving comfort and love. Even though children are able to voice the reason they must have TPN and appear to understand they are receiving all the needed nutrients by infusion, they still may miss eating food and the natural social interaction that comes with it. While in a hospital, they may be upset by the smell of food from a hospital unit kitchen or by the fact playmates have to leave to eat a meal. Finding an activity for a child receiving TPN while other children eat, such as helping to check unit supplies or stamping laboratory slips, can be helpful to supply the interaction a child misses. When feasible, help parents arrange for special times each day with the child to make up for the time normally spent interacting at meals.

Some children tolerate TPN better if they can be allowed chewing gum or occasional hard candy; advocate for these as necessary. Remind the child to continue tooth brushing twice a day to keep oral mucous membrane healthy because he or she is not chewing. An infant may enjoy the sucking pleasure from a pacifier.

QSEN Checkpoint Question 37.6

QUALITY IMPROVEMENT

Felipe's primary healthcare provider asks the nurse to keep as accurate a record as possible of Felipe's intake and output while he is undergoing diagnostic testing. Felipe vomits without warning on his gown and the floor. How should the nurse document this form of output to ensure an accurate assessment?

a. Estimating the amount of emesis and describe the character in his health record
b. Describing the event in Felipe's health record and note that it was not possible to gauge the quantity
c. Weighing his soiled gown and compare the weight to a clean gown of the same size
d. Asking his mother to approximate the amount that he vomited

Look in Appendix A for the best answer and rationale.

Hot and Cold Therapy

Children who sustain muscle sprains or undergo procedures such as bronchoscopy or tonsillectomy may have cold applications prescribed to prevent swelling or edema, help control hemorrhage, or provide an analgesic effect. Ice packs are left in place for about 20 minutes. To prevent frostbite, never place an ice pack directly on the skin; instead, insert a towel between the pack and the skin. Document the type of application, duration of the therapy, and the condition of the skin before and after the treatment.

Local application of heat may be prescribed to relieve congestion and pain by increasing circulation through vasodilation and muscle relaxation (Box 37.8). Heat may also be prescribed

BOX 37.8

Nursing Care Planning to Empower a Family

GUIDELINES FOR HOT AND COLD APPLICATIONS WITH CHILDREN

Q. Felipe's mother tells you, "I need to apply cold compresses to my child's head to help with his headache. How do I do this?"

A. When applying any type of hot or cold therapy such as cold or warm compresses, use the following guidelines:

- Apply neither heat nor cold for longer than 20 minutes unless prescribed because after that time, the vasoconstriction caused by cold and the vasodilatation caused by heat begins to reverse.
- When using electrical sources of heat with toddlers and preschoolers, never make a game of plugging in and pulling out the apparatus that makes the light come on or a dial glow. Otherwise, the child may play with it after you leave.
- Supply a special activity for a child to enjoy while a hot or cold application is in place (e.g., playing a board game, reading a story to the child), so that the procedure is not viewed as a chore but as a pleasant time to look forward to.
- Put tape on the gauge of an electric appliance at the point where you want it, so that you will be able to tell if the child changes the setting.
- To determine that solutions or heat sources are not too hot, always test them with your inner wrist or the dorsal surface of your hand before applying them to the child.
- Do not apply ice packs or ice directly to the skin. Cover the pack or ice with a towel or other cover such as dish towel to prevent frostbite and cell damage from cold.
- Be cautious using heat or cold applications with a child who is receiving an analgesic because the child's perception of heat or cold may be reduced and the site could easily be burned.

to help resolve superficial inflammation and hasten the formation and drainage of abscesses or absorption from subcutaneous tissue if IV fluid infiltrated. It is important to not leave either hot or cold compresses in place continuously or a rebound effect that blocks their effectiveness may occur. Always assess the skin before and after the treatment to determine that tissue damage (e.g., a burn) did not occur from treatment. If you are using a heating pad to maintain warmth in a young child, set the temperature dial and then tape it in place so the child cannot spin the dial and increase the temperature beyond a safe level.

Wound Care

Children frequently have a dressing or bandage put in place to cover a surgical incision or sutured laceration. Such dressings are the same as those used with adults except in size, material, and methods used to secure them. Keeping a dressing dry to avoid introducing infection to the wound in infants and toddlers who are not toilet trained can be a major problem if the dressing is near the diaper area. In many instances after surgery, collodion (i.e., a clear substance similar to nail polish) or other commercially available "wound glues" are used to cover the incision because these solutions not only replace stitches but also keep the incision line from coming in contact with urine or feces. These materials allow good visualization of the healing surface as well because they are clear. Assure parents that such a covering is adequate and actually preferable if the incision is in the groin such as from a hernia repair. They are also preferable if an incision or laceration is on the face because they tend to heal with less scarring than if sutures were used.

If a gauze dressing is used near the diaper area, it can be covered with plastic and held in place with nonadhesive, waterproof tape to protect it from becoming soiled. When cutting plastic to cover a dressing, do not to leave an extra piece behind in the crib because a child could pull this over the head and suffocate.

Occlusive dressings (e.g., hydrogel sheets, hydrocolloids, polyurethane films) are dressings especially designed to keep a healing surface clean and dry. Apply and remove these according to each product's directions or agency policy to protect irritating the skin underneath.

Apply Band-Aids generously after venipuncture or finger punctures because young children find bandages comforting and accept them as a "badge of courage."

Use nonadhesive tape (e.g., silk, paper) or secure a dressing with a nonadhering bandage (Kling) or roller gauze instead of adhesive tape to protect sensitive skin. Don't be surprised to see a young child pull a dressing loose and inspect what is underneath. Do not discourage children from looking at their incision during dressing changes. Even if the area looks raw and unhealed, it may look better than what the child envisioned was under the dressing.

What If . . . 37.4
The nurse is particularly interested in exploring one of the 2020 National Health Goals with respect to diagnostic or therapeutic procedures in children (see Box 37.1). Most government-sponsored money for nursing research is allotted based on these goals. What would be a possible research topic to explore pertinent to these goals that would be applicable to Felipe's family and that would advance evidence-based practice?

KEY POINTS FOR REVIEW

- Preparing children for procedures reduces anxiety. Prepare a child and parents by trying to relate a procedure to something a child is already familiar with, such as comparing an X-ray machine to a camera.
- Include parents in both the planning and implementation of care because parents can reinfect children with fear if their own fear is uncontrolled. Try to give explanations on two levels: "I'm going to change the dressing on her suture line" for a parent; "I'm going to put a clean bandage on your tummy" for the child.
- Minimize the number of painful procedures; for instance, combine blood sampling procedures, if possible.
- Perform any procedures that will cause pain in a treatment room or away from the child's bedside so the bed remains a "safe" place.
- Perform treatments without chilling or exposure. Respect modesty even in very young children.
- Allow a child to voice anger or fear of a procedure. Provide therapeutic play after a procedure to help reduce these reactions.
- Children feel more secure with adults who are confident in their actions. Practice as necessary the steps of a procedure before you begin so you can demonstrate confidence and skill.
- Once you have announced that a procedure needs to be done, proceed to do it; waiting for something to happen is often as stressful as actually having it done.
- Involve children in procedures to implement care that not only meets QSEN competencies but also best meets a family's total needs. Allow a child to examine electrodes or apply gel for electrode contact before a procedure, for example. Give children a portion of an ECG strip as a badge of courage after the procedure, or let children apply their own adhesive bandage.
- Praise children for cooperation even if none was visibly obvious. For painful procedures, any behavior short of hysterical screaming counts as cooperation.
- Following the use of moderate sedation, observe children carefully until they are fully awake. Check for the return of the child's gag reflex before offering any fluids to minimize the risk of aspiration.
- Help make feeding by a route such as a gastrostomy tube as close to normal as possible by talking to the child to simulate mealtime conversation and socialization.

CRITICAL THINKING CARE STUDY

Donald Kohl is an 8-year-old whose father has brought him to the emergency room because he has been vomiting all morning and, over the past hour, has developed sharp pain in his right lower abdomen. You need to schedule him for an ultrasound to rule out appendicitis. Because Donald's parents are divorced and the father is not the custodial parent, he phones Donald's mother. She screams at him for being completely incompetent at child care and tells him, "Don't you dare sign anything until I can get there."

1. Because it will take a minimum of 45 minutes for Donald's mother to arrive, you are concerned that a long delay in having the ultrasound could be a significant

threat to Donald's health because, if he has appendicitis, his appendix could rupture during that time. Would you ask the father to sign the permission despite his wife's opinion or wait for the mother to arrive?

2. Donald has had three X-rays over the past year because he broke his right tibia in an auto accident due to a combination of him not having his seatbelt fastened and his father's unsafe driving. His father asks you, in light of the radiation Donald has already received over the past year, whether an ultrasound will be safe for him.

3. You talk to Mrs. Kohl on her cell phone while she is in her car and she says it will be all right if you draw blood for a white blood count on Donald. As he's already anxious, would it be more important to apply anesthetic cream to his venipuncture site to help reduce pain or obtain the blood sample immediately?

RELATED RESOURCES

Explore these additional resources to enhance learning for this chapter:
- Student resources on thePoint, including answers to the What If . . . and Critical Thinking Care Study questions, http://thepoint.lww.com/Flagg8e
- Adaptive learning powered by PrepU, http://thepoint.lww.com/prepu

REFERENCES

Academy of Breastfeeding Medicine. (2012). ABM Clinical Protocol #25: Recommendations for preprocedural fasting for the breastfed infant: "NPO" guidelines. *Breastfeeding Medicine, 3*, 197–202.

Adelstein, S. J. (2014). Radiation risk in nuclear medicine. *Seminars in Nuclear Medicine, 44*, 187–192.

American Academy of Pediatrics. (2011). Urinary tract infection: Clinical practice guideline for the diagnosis and management of the initial UTI in febrile infants and children 2 to 24 months. *Pediatrics, 128*, 595–610.

American College of Radiology. (2016). *ACR Manual on Contrast Media: Version 10.2.* Retrieved from http://www.acr.org/~/media/37D84428BF1D4E1B9A3A2918DA9E27A3.pdf

American Psychiatric Nurses Association. (2014). *Seclusion and restraints standards of practice APNA position on the use of seclusion & restraint.* Retrieved from http://www.apna.org/i4a/pages/index.cfm?pageid=3730

Batra, P., & Goyal, S. (2013). Comparison of rectal, axillary, tympanic, and temporal artery thermometry in the pediatric emergency room. *Pediatric Emergency Care, 29*, 63–66.

Corkins, M. R., Griggs, K. C., Groh-Wargo, S., et al. (2013). Standards for nutrition support: Pediatric hospitalized patients. *Nutrition in Clinical Practice, 28*(2), 263–276.

Crohn's & Colitis Foundation of America. (2014). *Diagnosing and managing IBD.* Retrieved from http://www.ccfa.org

Delso, G., Ter Voert, E., & Veit-Haibach, P. (2015). How does PET/MR work? Basic physics for physicians. *Abdominal Imaging, 40*(6), 1352–1357.

Elitsur, R., Butcher, L., Vicki, L., et al. (2013). Polyethylene glycol 3350 based colon cleaning protocol: 2 d vs 4 d head to head comparison. *World Journal of Gastrointestinal Endoscopy, 5*, 165–168.

Exergen. (2014). *Temporal artery thermometer: Instructions for use.* Retrieved from http://www.exergen.com/medical/PDFs/tat2000cmanual.pdf

Franck, L. S., Wray, J., Gay, C., et al. (2015). Predictors of parent post-traumatic stress symptoms after child hospitalization on general pediatric wards: A prospective cohort study. *International Journal of Nursing Studies, 52*, 10–21.

Harrison, P. (2013). *Shellfish allergy doesn't predict reaction to imaging agents.* Retrieved from http://www.medscape.com/viewarticle/781031

Jain, R., Petrillo-Albarano, T., Parks, W. J., et al. (2013). Efficacy and safety of deep sedation by non-anesthesiologists for cardiac MRI in children. *Pediatric Radiology, 43*(5), 605–611.

Karch, A. M. (2015). *Lippincott's nursing drug guide.* Philadelphia, PA: Lippincott Williams & Wilkins.

Katz, A. L., & Webb, S. A. (2016). Informed consent in decision-making in pediatric practice. *Pediatrics, 138*(2), e1–e16.

Kearl, Y., Yanger, S., Montero, S., et al. (2015). Does combined use of the J-tip (R) and Buzzy (R) device decrease the pain of venipuncture in a pediatric population? *Journal of Pediatric Nursing, 30*(6), 829–833.

Kemp, C. (2013). Temporal artery thermometers may rival rectal thermometers in ED. *AAP News, 34*, 2. Retrieved from http://www.aappublications.org/content/34/4/2.1

Kim, G. A., & Koo, J. W. (2015). Validity of bag urine culture for predicting urinary tract infections in febrile infants: A paired comparison of urine collection methods. *Korean Journal of Pediatrics, 58*(5), 183–189.

Kompany, L., Luis, K., Manganaro, J., et al. (2016). Items of interest. Children's Specialized Hospital and Get Well Network™ collaborate to improve patient education and outcomes using an innovative approach. *Pediatric Nursing, 42*(2), 95–99.

Longo, M., & Miller-Hoover, S. (2016). Effective decision making in the use of pediatric restraints. *Journal of Pediatric Nursing, 31*(2), 217–221.

López, L. G., Pedrón-Giner, C. C., Martínez-Costa, C., et al. (2015). Home enteral nutrition. In R. Rajendram, V. R. Preedy, & V. B. Patel (Eds.), *Diet and Nutrition in Critical Care* (pp. 1255–1267). New York, NY: Springer Publishing.

Matziou, V., Chrysostomou, A., Vlahioti, E., et al. (2013). Parental presence and distraction during painful childhood procedures. *British Journal of Nursing, 22*(8), 470–475.

National Heart, Lung, and Blood Institute. (2005). Measurement of blood pressure in children. In *The fourth report on the diagnosis, evaluation, and treatment of high blood pressure in children and adolescents* (pp. 5–6). Washington, DC: U.S. Department of Health. Retrieved from https://www.nhlbi.nih.gov/files/docs/resources/heart/hbp_ped.pdf

O'Grady, N. P., Alexander, M., Burns, L. A., et al. (2011). Guidelines for the prevention of intravascular catheter-related infections. *Clinical Infectious Diseases, 52*(9), e162–e193.

RadiologyInfo.org. (2015). *Children's (pediatric) ultrasound—abdomen.* Retrieved from http://www.radiologyinfo.org/en/info.cfm?pg=abdomus-pdi

Schmidt, B., & Copp, H. (2015). Work-up of pediatric urinary tract infection. *Urologic Clinics of North America, 42*(4), 519–526.

Singh, V., & Singhal, K. (2015). The tools of the trade—uses of flexible bronchoscopy. *Indian Journal of Pediatrics, 82*(10), 932–937.

Stevens, K. E., & Marvicsin, D. J. (2016). Evidence-based recommendations for reducing pediatric distress during vaccination. *Pediatric Nursing, 42*(6), 267–274.

Sullivan, J. E., & Farrar, H. C. (2011). Fever and antipyretic use in children. *Pediatrics, 127*, 580–587.

The Joint Commission. (2014). *Advancing effective communication, cultural competence, and patient- and family-centered care: A roadmap for hospitals.* Oakbrook Terrace, IL: Author. Retrieved from http://www.jointcommission.org/roadmap_for_hospitals/

U.S. Department of Health and Human Services. (2010). *Code of federal regulations; title 45 and 46.* Retrieved from http://www.hhs.gov/ohrp/humansubjects/guidance/45cfr46.html

U.S. Department of Health and Human Services. (2014). *Increase the proportion of adolescents who have had a wellness checkup in the past 12 months.* Retrieved from https://www.healthypeople.gov/node/3936/data_details

U.S. Food and Drug Administration. (2016). *What are the radiation risks from CT?* Retrieved from http://www.fda.gov/Radiation-EmittingProducts/RadiationEmittingProductsandProcedures/MedicalImaging/MedicalX-Rays/ucm115329.htm

Vermilyea, S., & Goh, V. L. (2015). Enteral feedings in children: Sorting out tubes, buttons, and formulas. *Nutrition in Clinical Practice, 31*, 59–67.

World Health Organization. (2010). Pediatric and neonatal blood sampling. In *WHO guidelines on drawing blood: Best practices in phlebotomy* (pp. 35–37). Geneva, Switzerland: Author. Retrieved from https://www.ncbi.nlm.nih.gov/books/NBK138647/

World Health Organization. (2016). *Communicating radiation risks in paediatric imaging information to support healthcare discussions about benefit and risk.* Retrieved from http://www.who.int/ionizing_radiation/pub_meet/radiation-risks-paediatric-imaging/en/

Wycoff, A. S.. (2009). Thermometer use 101. *AAP News, 30*(11), 29. Retrieved from http://www.aappublications.org/content/aapnews/30/11/29.2.full.pdf

Nursing Care of a Family When a Child Needs Medication Administration or Intravenous Therapy

KEY TERMS

absorption
distribution
excretion
intermittent infusion devices

intracath
metabolism
pharmacokinetics
vascular access ports (VAPs)

*T*erry, an 8-year-old with Down syndrome, is brought to the emergency department by her parents because she has pain in her ankle. She is diagnosed with osteomyelitis, a bone infection. When you give her a tablet of acetaminophen (Tylenol) for pain, she spits it out. She does the same when you repeat with a second tablet. Her mother tells you Terry can't swallow pills. Her father tells you, "You'll have to give her an IV."

Previous chapters described the difficulty children may have adjusting to illness and also diagnostic and therapeutic procedures that are frequently used with children. This chapter adds information about techniques for administering medication and intravenous (IV) therapy to children. Because therapy for almost all illnesses today involves some form of medicine or IV administration, and safe medication administration is one of the most important parts of a child health nurse's role, this information is pertinent to the care of almost all children.

What would be an effective method of administering acetaminophen (Tylenol) to Terry if she cannot swallow pills?

OBJECTIVES

After mastering the contents of this chapter, you should be able to:

1. Describe common methods of medication and intravenous (IV) therapy used in the health care of children.

2. Identify nursing contributions in achieving Healthy People 2020 goals related to medication and IV therapy.

3. Assess the developmental stage and knowledge level of children and adolescents before beginning administration of medication or IV therapy.

4. Formulate nursing diagnoses related to medication or IV therapy with children.

5. Identify expected outcomes to meet the needs of children receiving medication or IV therapy as well as manage seamless transitions across healthcare settings.

6. Using the nursing process, plan nursing care that includes the six competencies of Quality & Safety Education for Nurses (QSEN): Patient-Centered Care, Teamwork & Collaboration, Evidence-Based Practice (EBP), Quality Improvement (QI), Safety, and Informatics.

7. Implement nursing interventions specific to pediatrics related to medication and IV therapy and children.

8. Evaluate the effectiveness and achievement of expected outcomes for a child receiving medications and/or IV therapy.

9. Integrate knowledge of medication and IV therapy using the nursing process, the six competencies of QSEN, and Family Nursing to promote quality maternal and child health nursing care.

Most adults immediately grasp that taking a medicine you offer them will be important to relieve whatever symptoms they are experiencing from an illness. Because children do not necessarily have this same level of understanding, they may resist taking medicine unless its importance is thoroughly explained to them and the medication is given to them by a method that best meets their preference and developmental stage. Many children do not have enough coordination to swallow tablets or pills until they are 6 or 7 years of age, and many adolescents still "don't like pills." This might mean getting a child to agree to try an oral medication only if it is furnished in a liquid or meltaway form. Almost all children fear intrusive procedures. This can make them forcibly resist accepting medication given by a rectal, nasal, intramuscular (IM), or IV route. Cognitive impairment, physical challenges, or developmental delay in a child may further complicate medication administration. Because children range in size from as small as 1 lb (0.5 kg) if preterm to more than 200 lb (90.9 kg) by late adolescence, there is no "standard" dose of medicine for children. Therefore, medications in children are dosed according to body weight (milligrams per kilogram) or body surface area (BSA) (milligrams per square meter). Before calculating the dose, weight must be converted from pounds to kilograms (1 lb = 2.2 kg). In addition, children have differing abilities to metabolize and excrete medications and have difficulty reporting adverse effects of medicine as accurately as adults. This can make it difficult to determine whether side effects or adverse effects are occurring. All these things make medicine administration for children one of the most challenging interventions in nursing (Walsh, Mazor, Roblin, et al., 2013). The 2020 National Health Goals that address this area of child health practice are shown in Box 38.1.

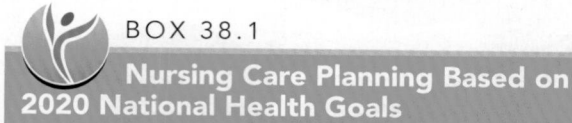

BOX 38.1

Nursing Care Planning Based on 2020 National Health Goals

When administering medicine to children or teaching children and parents how to take or give medicine, remember that medicines can be as dangerous in overdoses as they are helpful in the correct doses. They can be ineffective if a dose is inadequate or missed. Drugs also must be stored safely to avoid poisoning. National Health Goals that speak to medicine administration include:

- Reduce emergency department (ED) visits for medication overdoses among children less than 5 years of age from 32.8% to a target level of 29.5%.
- Increase the proportion of at-risk adolescents aged 12 to 17 years who, in the past year, refrained from using alcohol for the first time from 85.8% to a target level of 94.4%.
- Reduce the proportion of adolescents reporting the use of alcohol or any illicit drugs during the past 30 days from 18.4% to 16.6%.
- Reduce the past year nonmedical use of any psychotherapeutic drug (including pain relievers, tranquilizers, stimulants, and sedatives) from 6.1% of persons aged 12 years and older to 5.5% (U.S. Department of Health and Human Services, 2010; see www.healthypeople.gov).

Nurses can help the nation achieve these goals by educating parents about safe drug storage (locked in elevated cabinets) and teaching children and parents about effective nonpharmacologic ways to relieve stress or anxiety to help reduce drug dependence.

Nursing Process Overview

FOR A CHILD NEEDING MEDICATION/INTRAVENOUS THERAPY

ASSESSMENT

Because children vary so greatly in size and individual need, administering medication to children begins by assessing the child's weight in kilograms so that weight-based dosing can occur. For some medications, such as chemotherapy, height and weight are both used to calculate dosage (body surface area dosage). Also crucial to the assessment is the child's developmental age. This is important because it reveals if a child can swallow oral medicine or will be able to use such self-medication methods as patient-controlled analgesia (PCA); in addition, it will help you determine which site would be best for an IM or IV injection. Also assess the child's chronologic age and cognitive level to aid in planning the level of explanation that will be needed. An assessment of the child's past experience with taking medicine will help to determine the child's response to medication administration. The family's access to care and financial means to purchase the medicine can help predict whether the child will actually receive the medicine. Following the administration of the medicine, careful observation must continue to determine whether the medication is having its desired effect or whether any adverse effects are occurring (Yin, Dreyer, Moreira, et al., 2014).

NURSING DIAGNOSIS

Common nursing diagnoses related to medicine administration vary widely. Some examples include:

- Disturbed sleep pattern related to timing of medication administration
- Deficient knowledge related to action and side effects of medicine
- Fear related to IV administration of medicine
- Discomfort related to side effects of medicine
- Health-seeking behaviors by parent related to desire to learn more about different types of medicine available for the child's illness

OUTCOME IDENTIFICATION AND PLANNING

Planning the administration of medicine for children involves the same safe rules of administration as those for adults. Additional consideration is necessary at each step because determining the right form and route of medicine, such as liquid or capsule and oral or IM, varies so widely. Establishing a dose that is accurate for the size of the child can involve recalculating the dose using a milligram per kilogram formula or a nomogram that shows body surface area. The schedule for administration must be not only one that is effective for the drug's action but also one that will not interfere with school activities, eating, or sleep.

Explain to children the effects that can be expected from any medicine. Be certain to give this explanation at an age-appropriate level and be sure it is consistent with any prior explanation that a parent or other healthcare provider has supplied. Refer families to online resources for further information when appropriate (see Chapter 36).

IMPLEMENTATION

Interventions related to medication and IV therapy with children include both administering medicine to ill children as well as teaching parents and children how to continue to take the medicine when at home or at school. As long as the child is uncomfortable or has definite disease symptoms, parents tend to give medicine conscientiously. However, when symptoms fade, a child returns to school, or the family returns to its busy everyday schedule, it is easy for parents to forget to give medicine. This can leave children open to a recurrence of the condition or symptoms, such as pain or recurrent infection, because the organisms causing the illness were only suppressed, not killed. The classic example is strep throat—the child feels better, the medicine is stopped before completed, and, in the worst case scenario, rheumatic fever may result, possibly causing damage to the heart valves (see Chapter 41). Helping parents fill out administration schedules to post in a readily visible location, such as on the refrigerator or a bathroom mirror, or leaving reminder messages on their smartphones can be as important as explaining the drug's action to help ensure all doses of medicine will be given.

OUTCOME EVALUATION

Expected outcomes associated with medication administration should ensure that a child receives the medicine as prescribed and that the medicine has the desired effect. Specific examples suggesting outcome achievement include:

- Child states she understands she must continue to take thyroid hormone for a lifetime.
- Parents list the adverse effects of prescribed drug and state the telephone number they will call if adverse symptoms occur.
- Parents demonstrate the correct dose using the medication delivery device (oral syringe) that they will use at home.
- Adolescent describes an administration program that includes four doses daily but allows time for sports activities after school.
- Adolescent states he realizes his prescribed medicine is for his illness alone so it or other medicines in the family medicine cabinet are not to be shared with friends.

Medication Administration

Medications in children are given by a variety of routes: orally, intranasally, transdermally, topically, rectally, and via injection (subcutaneous, intradermal, IM, IV, intraosseous, or epidural) or by inhalation. Epidural administration is described in Chapter 16 because this route is also frequently used with women in labor. Inhalation techniques are discussed in Chapter 40 with respiratory illnesses.

Administering drugs safely requires knowledge of **pharmacokinetics**, or the way drugs are absorbed, distributed throughout the body, metabolized, inactivated, and excreted.

PHARMACOKINETICS IN CHILDREN

The four basic processes of absorption, distribution, metabolism, and excretion determine the intensity and duration of a drug's action. The immaturity of body systems in children (and especially in newborns) plays a major role in drug action throughout each of these processes (Reed & Bestic, 2014).

Absorption

Drug **absorption** (the transfer of the drug from its point of entry in the body into the bloodstream) is influenced by the route of administration as well as by the concentration and acidity of the drug. Some routes of administration in children are limited and so are rarely used. For example, children younger than school age usually cannot hold tablets under their tongue for sublingual administration; they tend to swallow them instead. The small muscle size of young children limits sites for IM injection. Transdermal patches can be easily removed by infants. The gastrointestinal system may be so immature at birth that gastrointestinal absorption can be ineffective. Vomiting and diarrhea, frequent symptoms of childhood illnesses, also interfere with absorption because a drug does not remain in the gastrointestinal tract long enough to be absorbed.

Distribution

Distribution refers to the movement of the drug through the bloodstream to a specific site of action. Children tend to have more fluid held in interstitial spaces and less in intracellular spaces than adults, so drugs may not be distributed as quickly as in adults. Many drugs are distributed bound to serum albumin (which is manufactured by the liver), so adequate albumen must be present for the drug to reach its site of action. This binding action limits the amount of free drug in the circulation, thereby providing protection against toxic levels of a drug. As free drug is used, the bound drug is released to maintain a therapeutic level. Newborns with immature liver function may not have enough serum albumin to transport drugs readily. This is particularly true if elevated bilirubin levels are present because bilirubin is also carried by serum albumin. Bound to serum albumin this way, bilirubin is harmless. In free form, however, it can leave the bloodstream and enter other body tissues. If it enters the brain cells, it destroys their ability to function (acute bilirubin encephalopathy). If a newborn who has a high level of bilirubin from destruction of fetal hemoglobin receives a drug such as a sulfonamide that competes for albumin binding sites, a large quantity of bilirubin may be left unbound and the infant may develop acute bilirubin encephalopathy or may not receive benefit from the sulfonamide because it cannot be carried to the infection site. In addition, newborns have sluggish peripheral circulation, so distribution to arms or legs in children this young may not be effective. Any child with cardiovascular disease also may have limited distribution of drugs because of general poor circulation.

Metabolism

Metabolism involves conversion of the drug into an active form (biotransformation) or into an inactive form (inactivation). Because a child's basic metabolic rate is faster than that of an adult, certain drugs are metabolized more rapidly in children. This means that the drug must be administered more frequently to a child to maintain effective drug levels than it would be in adults. Whether drugs are coadministered can also make a difference because this could cause the drugs to metabolize more quickly or more slowly than usual. Some drugs, such as the salicylates and chloramphenicol, are metabolized directly by liver enzymes. Because liver enzymes are not fully developed in newborns, these drugs cannot be metabolized and so can reach toxic levels rapidly. Older children with liver disease who have impaired liver enzymes also have a decreased ability to inactivate or transform drugs (Thakkar, Salerno, Hornik, et al., 2017).

Excretion

Excretion (the elimination of raw drug or drug metabolites, a process that largely prevents properly administered drugs from becoming toxic) is potentially limited until about 12 months of age, when kidney function becomes mature. If a child has kidney disease, excretion potential is limited at any age. A few drugs, such as digitoxin, are excreted in bile. Most newborns have sluggish bile formation, so excretion of these drugs is questionable. Monitoring intake and output is important in children receiving drugs to be certain urine excretion or an outlet for drug metabolites is adequate.

QSEN Checkpoint Question 38.1

INFORMATICS

After Terry receives an antibiotic, her body must distribute it to the site where it will act. Which assessment parameter addresses her body's ability to distribute a drug?
a. Terry's renal function
b. Terry's arterial blood gases
c. Terry's plasma protein levels
d. Terry's gallbladder function

Look in Appendix A for the best answer and rationale.

ADVERSE DRUG EFFECTS IN CHILDREN

Children respond to drugs in much the same way as adults, but they may experience unique or exaggerated side effects because of immature liver function or rapid metabolism during periods of rapid growth. The newborn may suffer adverse effects from drugs taken by the mother prenatally or from drugs transferred in breast milk.

SAFE STORAGE OF DRUGS

Because young children do not appreciate that overdoses of medicine can be serious and even fatal, they may self-administer additional doses of medicine resulting in toxic levels of medications. This can occur with prescription medications, over-the-counter medication, and even alternative/complementary medications (Schoenewald, Ross, Bloom, et al., 2013).

Adolescents can deliberately take extra doses of drugs such as steroids or pain medicine, hoping for an added effect. Oxycodone (OxyContin), for example, is an analgesic that may be prescribed for adolescents and also is frequently abused by them. Methylphenidate (Ritalin), administered to children

with attention deficit hyperactivity disorder, is a second prescription drug that may also be frequently abused (Albertson, Chenoweth, Colby, et al., 2016).

Adults always need to be certain to store medicine in a safe place. Because poisoning from medicine is a frequent type of poisoning in preschool children, children's medicine—whether prescription, over-the-counter, or alternative/complimentary—should be secured in a *locked* and safe place.

In most homes, this is in a locked medicine cabinet or a locked drawer above the height their child can reach; a motivated toddler can climb so well that just placing medicines "out of reach" is not sufficient. Remind parents that most childhood poisonings occur when a family is under stress because, during these times, the family may forget usual procedures and leave medications unlocked or within reach. Be certain to teach parents that they should never take medicine in front of children; children may imitate this action with the parent's medication when the parents are out of sight. Another caution is not to pour or prepare medicine in the dark. Because almost all medicine bottles dispensed from local pharmacies look and feel the same, it is easy to pour the wrong liquid, extract the wrong pills, or read the bottle instructions incorrectly without adequate light. Teaching parents the importance of reading over-the-counter medication labels for proper dosing and frequency is critical.

Remember that these same rules apply in a healthcare setting. Medications left at a bedside table in the hospital or on a medication cart could be easily accessible to an unsupervised toddler or preschool child walking around.

THE SAFE ADMINISTRATION OF DRUGS

Administering drugs safely to children requires that you first determine that you are giving the right drug (and right drug form) to the right child, in the right dosage, and by the right route, at the right time, for the right action. Afterward, you observe for the right response and use the right documentation. You also need to ensure that the parents or child have the right information about the medicine.

Right Medication/Right Drug Form

Most medication errors are made in situations where multiple medications are being administered in a fast-paced environment. Intensive care units and emergency departments, therefore, are the highest areas at risk for medication errors, often because of interruptions during the medication administration process (Frith, 2013). Errors can occur because prescribers may write a prescription using either generic or trade names. It is the responsibility of the person administering the medication to identify the correct brand or generic equivalent. As the number of medicines available increases yearly, so does the possibility that two drugs will have similar names. These factors make identifying the correct drug and form critical.

What If . . . 38.1
Terry's father tells the nurse that Terry is such a "picky eater" that she rarely eats a full meal. When should he give Terry a medicine that should be taken with a meal?

Right Patient

When asked what is their name, children cannot be depended on to reply with their correct name. Anxious to please, a preschooler will answer the question, "Are you Johnny Jones?" with "yes." He may also, however, agree with any other name you propose. School-age children who want to avoid taking a medicine may deny they are the person whose name you called. To prevent these types of errors, never ask children their names for identification. Instead, read or scan the bar code on their identification arm bands and compare them with the medication sheet or electronic record. In ambulatory care settings or homes, ask a parent to confirm the child's identity; to include the child, ask for their date of birth (or their age for younger children).

Right Dosage

The correct dosage of most drugs for children is based on weight. However, for drugs such as chemotherapy, the dosage is based on a body surface, which requires height and weight (Fig. 38.1). To calculate surface area using such a chart, find the child's height in the left column (e.g., 40 cm); next, find the child's weight in the right column (e.g., 20 kg). Hold a ruler or straightedge to connect the two points. The mark at which the ruler crosses the center column is the child's body surface area (e.g., 0.38 m^2). Before administering any medication to a child, confirm that the dose prescribed is correct for the child's weight or the child's body surface area. Take and record height and weight measurements conscientiously at health visits or on hospital admission (or daily, if important, during an admission) to obtain this information for dose calculation.

Adult patient providers often use the *Physicians' Desk Reference* (PDR Staff, 2013), but child health nurses need to use drug manuals made specifically for children's dosing. Every child health unit or clinic should have a pediatric drug reference, such as *The Harriett Lane Handbook* (Branden & Flerlage, 2014) to help determine safe drug doses. Neonatal units often use a manual, especially for neonates and premature infants, called *Neofax* (Thompson Reuters Clinical Editorial Staff, 2013).

Using child or neonatal references that are weight based rather than age based is important because a 3-year-old

Figure 38.1 A nomogram to estimate body surface area. To use such a chart, draw a line from the child's height to the child's weight. The point at which it crosses the middle line is the child's surface area.

BOX 38.2

Nursing Care Planning Based on Responsibility for Pharmacology

To calculate a fractional drug dose use the formula:

$$\frac{\text{Strength Desired (D)}}{\text{Strength You Have (H)}} \times \frac{\text{Quantity Desired (QD)}}{\text{Quantity You Have (QH)}} = \text{Answer}$$

For example, you have a prescription for 90 mg acetaminophen. Acetaminophen is supplied as 125 mg drug in 5 ml liquid. Using the formula:

$$\frac{90 \text{ mg (D)}}{125 \text{ mg (H)}} \times \frac{\text{QD (what you are asking)}}{5 \text{ ml (QH)}} = ?$$

Cross multiply: 125 QD = 450 (5 × 90)

Dose ordered = 90 mg divided by what you have on hand (how the medication is available) 125 mg times quantity (5 ml)

$$\frac{90 \text{ mg}}{125 \text{ mg}} \times 5 \text{ ml} = 3.6 \text{ ml}$$

who weighs only as much as a 1-year-old needs a dose of an antibiotic consistent with that given to a 1-year-old (not the child's actual age); a 12-year-old who is obese may need a dose greater than the average 12-year-old. This is exactly why weight-based dosing is used. If a prescribed dose does not conform to a child's weight, recheck the dose for accuracy with the prescriber before it is administered because preventing medication errors in children is everyone's responsibility (Lan, Wang, Yu, et al., 2014).

Although most medication on hospital units is supplied by the pharmacy in unit doses, nurses may still need to occasionally calculate fractional dosages (Box 38.2). When talking to parents about giving medicine, stress that if a medicine comes supplied with a dosing cup, it is best to use that to measure the correct dose. If there is no dosing cup, then an oral medicine syringe or dropper are the next best methods to measure liquid medicine because the "teaspoons" in their kitchen drawer are rarely exactly 5 ml. If they do not have any of these measuring devices, encourage them to use cooking measuring spoons for more accurate dosing (Yin et al., 2014).

Right Route and Time

Possible routes of administration for medicine in children are discussed in the following sections. Each of these methods requires special techniques because most children do not enjoy taking medicine and need support during administration. Proper spacing of time between doses is also necessary for accurate medication uptake, but choosing the right time of day for parents to give medicine (e.g., planning doses for 11 PM and 7 AM instead of 8 PM and 4 AM) can positively impact the ability of a family to successfully complete the medication as prescribed.

Right Information and Documentation

Because so many medications are advertised on television or in magazines, many parents and children are already aware of drug names and the action of individual drugs before they are prescribed. However, because the information provided may be limited, they also may have misconceptions about a particular drug. Be certain when giving medicine to a child or handing a prescription to a parent that you review the drug's purpose and action, when and how it should be taken, and any side or adverse effects the parent or child should be aware of. Ask them if they have any questions (Box 38.3).

BOX 38.3

Nursing Care Planning to Respect Cultural Diversity

Assessing children's and families' health beliefs and attitudes toward Western medicine is important because attitudes are not consistent across cultures. In some cultures, it is more acceptable to utilize an herb or a home remedy than a prescribed medicine. Because of this, a family may accept a prescription but then not fill it or hesitate to administer the medicine. An herbal remedy they use may duplicate or counteract a prescribed medicine's effect. Socioeconomic factors affect medicine administration as well because medicine is expensive and difficult to afford for many families who do not have health insurance.

As part of health histories, always ask if a child commonly takes any type of herbal or home remedy or if the child has been given anything specific for the present illness. Because medicine is expensive, when discussing a prescription with parents, ask them whether they have insurance and can fill their child's medications in a timely manner. Educate the family on the action and side effects of the medication and explain to them to contact their provider if the child's condition does not improve or if the child experiences any side effects or complications. Such inquiries allow parents to say they have questions about the medicine or are uncertain whether they should give it because of a cultural belief.

Remember that people under stress do not retain information easily, so although the prescriber may have reviewed this information with parents when the prescription was written, reinforcement may be necessary. Children as young as 5 or 6 years of age are able to identify adverse or side effects, so be certain your explanation of drug action includes them as well. Correct documentation assures other healthcare providers that a drug was administered and allows for continuity of care (Buchholz, 2016).

QSEN Checkpoint Question 38.2

SAFETY

The nurse gives acetaminophen (Tylenol) to Terry in the emergency department and she has no ID band currently in place. The nurse determines which identification method is best?

  a. Asking her what her name is
  b. Stating a need to know her name
  c. Asking a parent to provide two identifiers (name and date of birth)
  d. Asking to see her school student card

Look in Appendix A for the best answer and rationale.

ORAL ADMINISTRATION

Children younger than 3 years of age are unable to swallow pills. However, the ability of children to swallow pills varies from one child to the next and is not age-dependent. Typically, children older than 9 years of age can be offered tablets; however, some adolescents are not capable of swallowing tablets. The best practice is to ask the child and parent whether they are able to swallow tablets before offering the tablet form of the medication. Most oral medications for young children are available in liquid, chewable, or meltaway forms (Buchholz, 2016).

In infants, oral medication can be given with a medicine dropper or a unit-dose oral syringe (without a needle). Never give medicine with the child lying completely flat; otherwise, a child could choke and aspirate. Instead, gently restrain the child's arms and head by holding the child against your body with the head raised. A crying child is already opening his or her mouth for you; otherwise, gently open the mouth by pressing on the child's chin or gently squeezing the child's cheeks. Be certain the end of the syringe or dropper rests at the side of the infant's mouth to help prevent aspiration (Fig. 38.2). Press the bulb of the medicine dropper or use the plunger of the syringe so that the fluid flows slowly into the side of the child's mouth. An infant also may be given fluid from a small spoon. Allow the fluid to flow a little at a time so that the child has time to swallow between small sips. Because oral solutions are pleasantly flavored, most infants resist the first drop but then suck the remainder of the medicine into their mouth.

Restraining the child while giving a medicine may cause them to be frightened afterward or for future administration. Take the time to sit and comfort the child afterward (or let a parent do this). These actions are as important as checking the correct dosage of the drug because promoting the child's psychological well-being is crucial.

Figure 38.2 To administer oral medicine with a syringe, place the medicine at the side of the child's mouth. Note that infants should be positioned at least at a 45-degree angle.

Preschoolers and early school-age children respond well to rewards such as stickers or small prizes each time they take their medicine. For older children, hand them the cup of liquid or tablet medicine and offer them a favorite fluid to swallow (Box 38.4). If a child has difficulty swallowing tablets, some pills can be crushed or added to a teaspoonful of applesauce or a flavored syrup. If pills are not to be chewed (e.g., capsules, enteric coated tablets), be certain to tell the child not to chew them.

Some children may be old enough to swallow tablets but have never done it before. To let them practice learning how to do this, give them small bits of ice to use for practice; these melt rapidly and so do not stick in the back of the throat or esophagus. Tell the child to put the ice on the back of the tongue, tip the head slightly to the side, take a sip of water, and swallow the water. Give generous praise for learning this new skill. Another useful technique to help the child learn to swallow pills is to push them into a teaspoonful of ice cream or pudding. Children tend not to chew this type of food; rather, as they swallow the pudding, they also swallow the pill. If using this technique, push the pill into the ice cream or pudding in front of the child so it's obvious what you're doing. The intent is not to hide the pill or fool the child but to help the child learn to swallow the medicine (Box 38.5).

BOX 38.4

Nursing Care Planning to Empower a Family

GUIDELINES FOR ADMINISTERING ORAL MEDICATION

Q. Terry's mother tells you, "All my children fight me anytime they need to take medicine. How can I get them to take medicine without a battle?"

A. The following guidelines can often help make the task a bit easier:

- Do not say, "*Can* you drink this for me?" If an adult seems unsure whether children can do a task, children can develop grave doubts themselves or they may just not want to and say "No."
- Do not say, "*Will* you drink this for me?" This leaves a child the opportunity to say no and creates the awkward position of having to admit the child really does not have a choice in the matter; the child must take the medicine.
- State firmly, "It's time for you to drink your medicine now." Give the child a secondary choice to allow a sense of control: "It's time to drink your medicine now; do you want milk or water to swallow after it?" is a suitable choice, assuming both milk and water are compatible with the medication.
- Never refer to medicine as candy. If they think it is candy, children may help themselves to fatal amounts of medicine when everyone's back is turned.
- Do not use reward systems to persuade children to take medicine. Bribing may work for one dose, but when a second dose is due, the child will ask for a bigger bribe; for a third dose, an even bigger one. At some point (generally reached quickly), it is impossible to supply such large bribes, and therefore, it is impossible to gain the child's cooperation.
- Do not threaten. Statements such as "Take this quickly or I'll ask the doctor to make it into a shot" are not appropriate or therapeutic.
- Children expect honesty from adults; therefore, do not lie about the taste of medicine. If in doubt about the taste, taste it (with the obvious exception of drugs such as digoxin). Most children's medicines are artificially flavored with raspberry, orange, or cherry syrup, so they do not taste bad.
- If a medicine tastes bitter, mix it with a spoonful of strained applesauce or a teaspoonful of flavored syrup. Do not mix medicine with a full jar of baby food or put it into a bottle of milk or juice because the child will then have to eat the entire jar of food or drink the entire bottle to get all of the medicine. As a rule, encourage children to take liquid medicine straight and then follow it with a pleasant-tasting drink to take away any bitter taste. You could offer the choice of taking it in a syringe or a medicine cup to provide some control.
- If a medicine is supplied in tablet form, you could crush or dissolve it in with syrup or applesauce for a better taste if appropriate. Be certain before removing the particles from a capsule that the medicine will work properly when not in capsule form: Some are encapsulated to keep them from dissolving in the stomach and to bring them into the intestine, where they have a therapeutic effect. The same precaution must be followed when giving enteric coated tablets.
- Never leave medicine by a child's bed or chair for the child to take "in a minute" or "after your shower." The child may become involved with another activity "in a minute" and will not take it or a smaller child could find the medicine appealing and swallow it.

BOX 38.5

Nursing Care Planning Tips for Effective Communication

You want to give acetaminophen (Tylenol) to Terry, 8 years old, to help relieve her pain.

Tip: In this scenario, the nurse explains the advantage of taking the medicine and conveys an expectation of cooperation. Avoid making requests, commands, or threats. Instead, allow a secondary choice (such as a choice of beverage) by offering the child a sense of control while at the same time preventing the child from saying "no" to the primary request.

Nurse: I have your medicine, Terry. Swallow these for me.

Terry: No. My ankle is too sore.

Nurse: That's why I want you to swallow the pills. It'll take away the hurt.

Terry: I'd rather get a shot; my ankle is so sore.

Nurse: This type of medicine has to be swallowed. Do you want orange juice or apple juice to drink with them?

Terry: Orange juice.

Nurse: Good. Take a big swallow and they'll be gone.

TEAMWORK & COLLABORATION

Although Terry is 8 years old, she doesn't know how to swallow pills. If the nurse needs to delegate the administration of an oral medication to a licensed practical nurse, what instruction would the nurse provide to her colleague?

    a. "Draw a picture of a child swallowing medicine and talk about it."

    b. "Tell the child that all medicines taste sweet so she'll take it readily."

    c. "Give the child a small ice chip to use to practice swallowing."

    d. "Tip the child's head forward to avoid the possibility of choking."

Look in Appendix A for the best answer and rationale.

INTRANASAL ADMINISTRATION

Because nasal drops and sprays are easy to administer, more medications are supplied in these forms every year (Del Pizzo & Callahan, 2014).

Drugs are well absorbed across the nasal mucosa, so this route is an effective means of drug administration and can be a route for important and even life-sustaining drugs. Having medication sprayed or dropped into the nose can feel very uncomfortable and frightening for a child. The child's developmental stage will determine how to best approach administration of an intranasal medicine. Utilizing resources such as parents, Child Life (specialists trained to support children in hospitals), or the child's nurses can make the experience less traumatic.

The following suggested techniques can be used: Turn the child or ask the child to turn onto his or her back. A school-age child can extend the head over the side of the bed so that it is lower than the trunk. Preschoolers generally are too frightened by this strange position and do better with a pillow under their shoulders so that their head extends over the pillow and rests downward. Infant may need to be restrained in a mummy restraint for nose drop administration if they struggle to keep the syringe or dropper away from their nose (see Chapter 37 for a discussion of appropriate restraints).

Instill the appropriate number of drops into one nostril. Turn the child's head to the side—to the left after the left nostril, to the right after the right nostril—so that the medicine stays in the nose longer. If the child is a preschooler or older, ask him or her to further "sniff" the medicine so that it goes far back into their nose. If a child gets up immediately, the medicine will flow out and will be less effective. Therefore, have the child remain in the head-flat position for at least 1 minute to be certain the medicine remains in contact with the mucous membrane of the nose. Praise the child even if the child did not cooperate fully because it lets child know that you understand how hard it was for the child to stay still while the medicine was instilled. Children over about age 6 years may be able to use nasal sprays competently after they have been introduced to the technique. Acknowledge that spraying a liquid into the nose is uncomfortable because it tickles or causes a sneezing sensation. Have the child sit or stand upright, hold the spray bottle upright with the tip just inside one side of the nose, and gently squeeze the spray bottle. In most instances, a child should then tip the head to the side (the right side for the right nostril, the left side for the left nostril) or sniff, depending on the bottle instructions, for best absorption. The administration is then repeated for the second nostril.

Spray bottles should be individually prescribed for children and should not be used by any other child to prevent the spread of disease organisms.

OPHTHALMIC ADMINISTRATION

Eye medications, in particular, antibiotics to treat eye infections, are administered by being dropped into the conjunctival sac of the eye (Shaw, 2016). This type of administration, like nose drops, is frightening for children because the eyes are a sensitive area and a natural reflex occurs to avoid contact with the eyes. Also, children know that getting something such as dust in their eye can be very painful. As a result, infants and preschoolers generally may need to be restrained for eye drop administration. Always prepare the child first, with a developmentally appropriate explanation. Place the child on his or her back. Open the eyes of infants and preschoolers by gently but firmly pressing on the lower lid with the thumb and on the upper lid with the index finger. A school-age child or adolescent will open their eyes cooperatively, but you may need to rest a hand on the eyelid to keep the eye open long enough for the drug to be administered (Fig. 38.3). Be certain your fingernails are cut short to avoid scratching the child's cornea.

Instill the correct number of drops into the conjunctiva of the lower lid. Allow the eyelid to close. Avoid placing the drops directly on the cornea because that can be painful. To prevent the conjunctiva from drying, do not hold the eyelids apart any longer than necessary. After the child has blinked two or three times, allow the child to sit up. Do not forget to give praise for his or her cooperation after administration is complete.

To instill an ophthalmic ointment, apply a fine line of the ointment along the inside rim of the conjunctival sac, working from the inner to the outer eye canthus; be careful not to touch the tube to the eye. Always work from the inner to the outer canthus because if the eye is pus filled, applying

Figure 38.3 Administering eye drops.

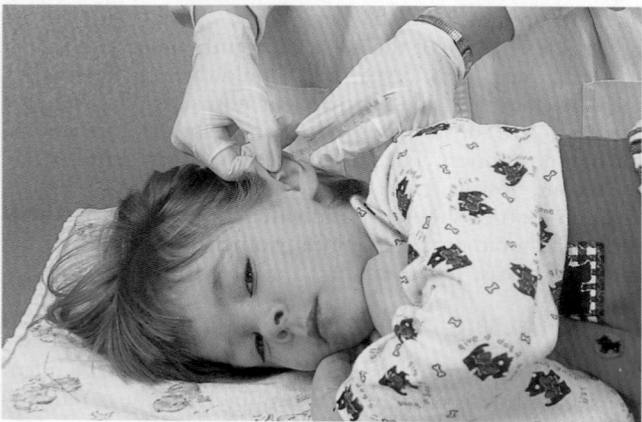

Figure 38.4   Administering ear drops. For the child older than 2 years old of age, the pinna of the ear is pulled up and back.

medication under pressure toward the midline could force pus across to the other eye or down into the lacrimal duct. Eye medicine should be individually prescribed and not used by other children because if even the tip of the dropper or tube touches the conjunctival sac, it is contaminated with body fluid or microorganisms.

OTIC ADMINISTRATION

Otic administration refers to administering medicine, primarily drops, into the ear canal. Like other forms of medicine, this is difficult for children to accept because they have been told many times not to put anything into their ears. Also, because ear drops are generally administered for an earache, which is sharp, excruciating pain, a child may worry having medicine put into the ear will make the pain even worse. In addition, a child's inability to watch what is happening may contribute to the child's fear. It is important to be honest with the child and provide information that is developmentally appropriate.

Ear drops must always be used at room temperature or warmed slightly because cold fluid may exacerbate pain and may also cause severe vertigo as it touches the tympanic membrane.

Turn the child or ask the child to turn onto his or her back or use restraint as necessary. Turn the child's head to one side (Fig. 38.4). The slant of the ear canal in children is shown in Chapter 50. If the child is younger than 2 years of age, straighten the external ear canal by pulling the pinna down and back. If the child is older than 2 years of age, pull the pinna of the ear up and back. Instill the specified number of drops into the ear canal. Hold the child's head in the sideways position to ensure the medication fills the entire ear canal. Praise the child for cooperating during this difficult procedure (AAP, n.d.).

Concept Mastery Alert

In order to straighten the ear canal in children older than age 2 years, the pinna of the ear is pulled *upward* and back. In children younger than age 2 years, the pinna is pulled *downward* and back.

RECTAL ADMINISTRATION

In certain circumstances, administering medication to children through the rectum is recommended. Rectal administration not only assist in absorption across the mucous membrane of the intestine but also avoids the danger of aspiration in certain situations such as seizures or when a patient is unconscious (Jannin, Lemagnen, Gueroult, et al., 2014). Rectal administration may also be used to give a drug such as acetaminophen (Tylenol) to young children who are unable to swallow oral medicine or to those who are vomiting. This method may be difficult for children due to its invasive nature; therefore, it is not a major route of administration. Moreover, absorption rates vary widely, so dosing is inconsistent. Because the child cannot see what is happening during rectal administration, and what parents discuss with them about "safe touching" and private body parts, a child can be easily frightened by this procedure. Show the child the medication so the child can be certain that it is not an injection.

Also given by this route are rectal suppositories and retention enemas. Many suppositories are supplied already lubricated. If not, add a drop of water-based lubricant such as K-Y Jelly to the tip. Use a glove and insert the suppository gently but quickly beyond the rectal sphincters (approximately 0.5 in. or as far as the first knuckle of your little finger for infants and approximately 1 in. or as far as the first knuckle of your index finger for older children). Withdraw your finger and press the child's buttocks together and hold for a count of approximately 10 or until the child's urge to evacuate the suppository passes.

If the medication is to be administered by a retention enema to a young child, follow enema administration procedure and volume ordered by the prescriber. Press and hold the child's buttocks together to prevent the expulsion of the medication, using a distraction technique or any developmentally appropriate method while administering an enema. Keep in mind that any invasive procedure is particularly threatening to a child.

What If . . . 38.2
Terry's mother tells the nurse her child's school has a "no drug" policy, so Terry will not be able to take her oral antibiotic at school. What would the nurse advise her to do?

TRANSDERMAL/TOPICAL ADMINISTRATION

Children sometimes require administration of topical creams or lotions for skin irritation or to relieve itching or dryness. Most children are more tolerant of this type of application because it may provide immediate relief of symptoms. Older children may be able to assist with topical applications with your supervision. Be certain they wash their hands afterward so they do not lick any extra off their fingers and inadvertently take it orally.

Transdermal patches are an effective and pain-free route of administration of medication absorbed through the skin. The child's skin should be dry and intact at the site where the patch will be applied. Apply a patch over the trunk or a major muscle, not on distal extremities, for best absorption. Assess the skin under the patch every time a patch is changed to be certain the site is not becoming irritated because an irritated

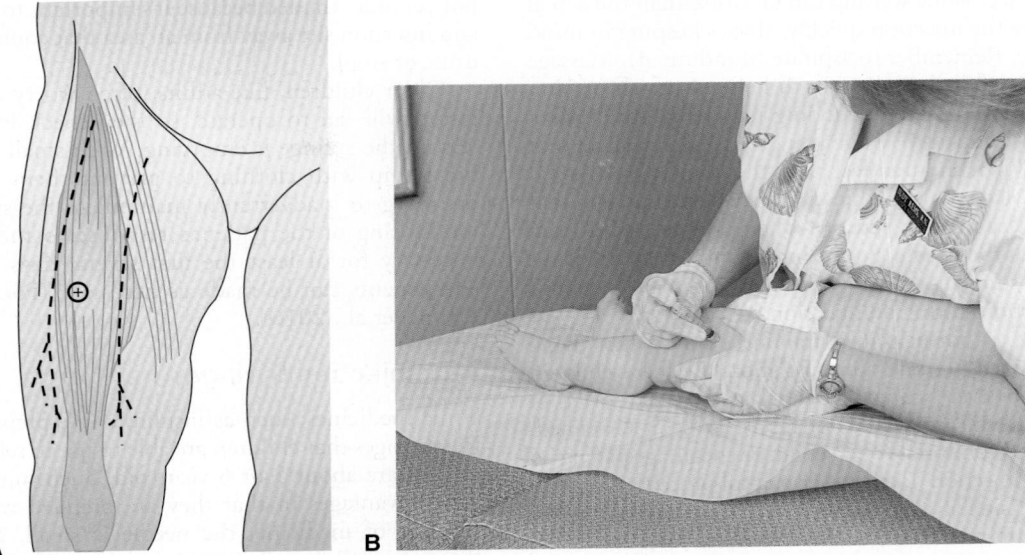

Figure 38.5 **(A)** For infants under walking age, use the vastus lateralis muscle for intramuscular injections. **(B)** The technique for administering an intramuscular injection to an infant. Note the way the nurse uses her body to restrain and stabilize the infant.

site might alter absorption. If possible, change the site every time a new patch is applied to decrease the possibility of irritation to the skin from the patch and clean the area of the skin before application.

Young children tend to remove transdermal patches the same as they do Band-Aids because of normal curiosity about what is underneath. Putting clothes on the young child immediately so the patch is out of sight is helpful. Assess infants carefully to be certain they have not pulled off the patch and are chewing on it because this can lead to drug toxicity. Be certain as well that patches applied to children wearing diapers are not placed where a leaking diaper could wet the patch and irritate the skin or dilute the medicine.

INTRAMUSCULAR AND SUBCUTANEOUS ADMINISTRATION

IM injections are rarely prescribed for children admitted to the hospital because many children do not have sufficient muscle mass for easy deposition of medication and they are also painful. However, IM injections may be used in an emergency department and are commonly used for immunization. For IM injections in infants, the preferred site for administration is the vastus lateralis muscle of the anterior thigh (Fig. 38.5). Use the lateral aspect rather than the medial portion because this site is not as tender and should cause less pain. Using the gluteal muscle in children younger than 1 year of age is to be avoided due to the risk of damage to the sciatic nerve. Figure 38.5 shows an effective restraining technique for giving injections to infants. In older children, as in adults, the deltoid muscle (Fig. 38.6A) or a ventrogluteal site (Fig. 38.6B) should be used.

Injecting an infant or child while he or she is sleeping should be avoided because they will be awaken and may be terrified of being attacked. Instead, play with the infant until they are awake, and depending on the developmental stage of young children, you may provide a short explanation

immediately prior to injection. Be honest and do not make promises you cannot keep, such as telling the child it will not hurt. To reduce pain, ask for a prescription anesthetic cream to be applied to the injection site 30 minutes before the injection (see Chapter 39).

When giving injections, once you have described to the caregiver the drug's purpose and what you are going to do, do not delay the injection further because the anticipation

Figure 38.6 Sites for intramuscular injection. **(A)** In older children, the deltoid muscle is an acceptable site. **(B)** A ventrogluteal site may also be used in older children. Place the heel of the hand on the greater trochanter and the index finger angled toward the child's anterosuperior iliac crest, spreading the middle finger along the crest posteriorly. The triangle formed by the space between the index and middle fingers is the correct site.

the child may feel while waiting can be worse than the actual injection. Give the injection quickly, always keeping in mind safe technique. Remember to aspirate (if indicated). Massage the area briefly after the injection to help ensure absorption of the medication, although rubbing may be painful. Statements such as "Don't cry" while you give an injection are not therapeutic. When children feel pain, they should be allowed to cry. Acknowledge that an injection may be painful and that it is "okay to cry or even scream" when they feel pain from the insertion of the needle. Squeezing a hand or a stuffed animal, singing a song, or counting may help with pain tolerance and/or distraction during an injection.

If necessary, ask for help in restraining a child when giving an injection to ensure safe administration. Evaluate children individually, however; school-age children may take pride in their ability to lie still and would not appreciate being restrained. Always hold and comfort a young child, or encourage parents to do so, after an injection or any other painful procedure.

Record the site of any injection while documenting the medication administration, so that sites can be rotated for better absorption. For subcutaneous injections, use the same injection sites, the lateral aspect of the thigh or upper arm, and inject the vaccine at a 45-degree angle.

If children are going to receive a series of injections, you can teach them distraction techniques, for example, imagery (e.g., thinking of the needle as a long thin rocket ship landing on their arm to help reduce apprehension). The distraction techniques used will depend on the developmental stage of the child (see Chapter 39).

Subcutaneous Pump Infusion

Continuous subcutaneous pump infusion using a medication pump is the administration of a medication by the constant infusion into the subcutaneous tissue (Peters, Mount, Huggins, et al., 2013). Continuous pump infusions supply a constant level of medicine to sustain consistent blood levels. The disadvantage of the technique is that a child must be careful to protect the catheter at the insertion site from being dislodged.

With a subcutaneous infusion pump, the drug is delivered by the pump via a medicine-filled syringe. The site chosen is usually the abdomen because this both protects the pump and allows it to be out of sight. Insulin (see Chapter 48), heparin, and deferoxamine (Desferal), a chelating agent to remove stored iron from children with hematology disorders (see Chapter 44), are drugs often prescribed for use with infusion pumps.

The hub of the medicine-filled syringe is attached to a small tube with the needle attached at the distal end. The syringe is then clamped to the pump, the skin site is cleaned with alcohol, and the needle is inserted at a 45-degree angle (the usual subcutaneous insertion technique). The needle is typically retracted, leaving a small catheter in the subcutaneous tissue, which is taped in place before the pump is turned on (see Chapter 20, Fig. 20.5).

The insertion site should be changed every 3 days to reduce the possibility of infection. The pump should be removed before showering so it doesn't get wet, although the catheter can remain in the subcutaneous tissue. For swimming or tub bathing, the entire pump, syringe, tubing, and catheter should be removed and then replaced again immediately. Pumps may not be advocated for children who are not yet toilet trained because it's important to keep the pump and insertion site away from an area that could be soiled with urine or stool.

Older children, like adults, often worry at first that the pump will fail to operate, so they check frequently to be certain the syringe is emptying. With small children, cover the pump with clothing to prevent them from touching or trying to inadvertently manipulate the syringe. Careful monitoring of the patient's response to the medication is necessary for at least the first several days so that dosage adjustments can be made as necessary (Pozzilli, Battelino, Danne, et al., 2016).

Autoinjection Syringes

Some medicines, such as insulin, come prepared in autoinject syringes that children are able to use to self-inject as soon as they are about 5 or 6 years old. Such injectable syringes have advantages in that they are prefilled with the correct amount of medicine, the needle is small, and the spring that causes the needle to inject the medication acts quickly, reducing pain during injection. You may need to remind preschool children not to play with the syringe or school-age children not to use it as a weapon against their friends or they could unintentionally inject them with the medicine. The use of EpiPens, which are filled with epinephrine (used to counteract anaphylactic reactions to allergens), is described in Chapter 42.

QSEN Checkpoint Question 38.4

QUALITY IMPROVEMENT

Suppose Terry, 8 years old, needs to have ear drops administered. If the nurse consults the unit's policies and procedures, the nurse should expect which directive?

  a. Have the child self-administer the drops to give the child a sense of control.
  b. Refrigerate the drug for at least 30 minutes so it numbs the ear canal.
  c. Pull the pinna of the child's ear down to straighten the canal.
  d. Keep the child's head turned to the side to help retain the drops.

Look in Appendix A for the best answer and rationale.

Intravenous Therapy

In the past, IV therapy was used extensively as a rapid means of hydrating children who were dehydrated as a result of diarrhea. Today, oral rehydration therapy is most often used in this case (Powers, 2015). IV therapy is a fast and effective means of maintaining fluid and electrolyte balance, producing therapeutic levels of drugs quickly, to provide nutritional support and offer blood or blood product replacement, so it still has a common place in children's care. The amount, type, and rate of IV fluids for children are prescribed carefully to prevent fluid overload. IV fluid may be infused into a peripheral vein, a central venous access device, or a peripherally inserted central venous catheter (McNab, 2016).

Despite its common use, IV therapy with children is not without problems. Because children move about a great deal and tend to remove bandages, all IV access sites must be assessed at least hourly for signs of infiltration. With movement, peripheral IV catheters can poke through fragile veins, central access devices can become dislodged, and ports can disconnect from the internal tubing, especially with the activity level of most children. Carefully inspect sites in order to identify any swelling or disconnections.

Infection is another problem associated with IV access. If a line becomes infected, it is usually removed, which may involve surgery for a centrally placed device. To avoid infection, insertion sites must be changed using a sterile technique as well as be carefully monitored. Keeping an IV site wrapped with something such as Kling gauze may help protect a curious toddler from removing the dressing and disrupting the site. However, remain vigilant about removing the gauze to inspect the site frequently if the gauze covers the insertion site.

DETERMINING FLUID AND CALORIC NEEDS OF THE CHILD

IV fluid administered to children and infants must be isotonic (exerts the same osmotic pressure as their bloodstream) to prevent the destruction of red blood cells or the development of water intoxication. The use of isotonic fluid prevents fluid shifting from the bloodstream into interstitial tissue (as would happen if the IV fluid were hypotonic) or fluid shifting from interstitial tissue into the bloodstream (as would happen if the IV fluid were hypertonic). A 0.9% sodium chloride (0.9% sodium chloride is normal saline solution) is the IV fluid most commonly used in children because it is isotonic (Powers, 2015). Dextrose 10% in 0.9% sodium chloride or mannitol solution are examples of a hypertonic solution that might be used to cause fluid to shift into the bloodstream to relieve cerebral edema for a child with a head injury.

It is important to understand the principles of IV therapy, including the fluid and caloric needs of children (which differ significantly from those of the adult), to protect against overhydration, underhydration, or electrolyte imbalances such as hyponatremia (Powers, 2015).

Table 38.1 shows a typical method of calculating fluid requirements for children. Fluids administered using this table should ideally contain at least 5% dextrose, 0.9% saline, and 20 mEq potassium per liter so nutrients for energy and electrolytes are also replaced. For example, according to Table 38.1, a child weighing 45 kg would need 2,000 ml of a maintenance solution. A flow rate would be calculated for this amount (2,000 ml fluid in 24 hours = 83 ml/hr).

TABLE 38.1 CALCULATING FLUID REQUIREMENTS FOR CHILDREN

Body Weight	Fluid Requirement per 24 Hours
Up to 10 kg	100 ml/kg
11–20 kg	1,000 ml + 50 ml/kg for each additional kilogram over 10 kg
More than 20 kg	1,500 ml + 20 ml/kg for each additional kilogram over 20 kg

OBTAINING VENOUS ACCESS

The needle size for IV therapy varies depending on the solution and the rate at which it will be administered. Commonly used needle sizes include 22 gauge, 24 gauge, 25 gauge, or 27 gauge.

Sites frequently used for IV insertion in young children or infants include the veins on the dorsal surface of the hand or on the flexor surface of the wrist. Leg and foot veins also may be used. In infants, another site is a scalp vein over the temporal area. Seeing IV fluid infusing into a scalp vein can be frightening for parents because it looks like a much more serious procedure than an infusion administered into a hand. You can explain to parents that scalp vein infusion is just another site to use to administer fluid or medicine to infants and ultimately might cause the least discomfort for their child because needles there do not infiltrate readily (Box 38.6). If any hair will be shaved away to place such a needle, ask parents if they wish to save the child's hair because this may be baby's first haircut.

Preschoolers and older children often express a preference regarding where they want an IV inserted. Offer a choice, if possible, or suggest the nondominant hand. Advocate for the child to ensure their wishes are respected.

Children who have IV infusions for long periods may require the placement of an **intracath** (a slim, pliable catheter threaded into a vein). The advantage of this type of device is that it cannot be dislodged as easily as a normally inserted IV needle, allowing a child the ability to move about more freely. For all children (including adolescents), IV infusions are sometimes secured in place with a small arm board. Without an arm board, it is easy to unintentionally and accidentally pull the catheter.

DETERMINING THE RATE AND AMOUNT OF FLUID ADMINISTRATION

Because children's hearts and circulatory systems are smaller than those of adults, IV fluid must be infused at a slower rate to keep the child's cardiovascular system from becoming quickly overloaded. Therefore, just as in medication administration, supervising the amount of solution infused is critical. Infusion pumps are required in most settings for infants and children receiving IV fluids and when giving potent medications and always for small children because they regulate the flow accurately to a few drops per minute (Fig. 38.7). Overloading of IV fluid in infants and children can also be prevented by use of fluid chambers, devices that allow only 50 to 100 ml of fluid into the drip chamber at a time. With these in place, even if the pump fails, only the amount of fluid in the drip chamber will be infused.

Another safety measure is the use of programmable infusion pumps that can be programmed to infuse fluids and medications in a prescribed rate. This allows for flow to be easily regulated and provides more accurate IV administration.

Keep a careful record of both the rate and amount of IV fluid administered to guard against fluid overload. At least once an hour, record the type and amount of fluid and the rate of flow (including the number of drops per minute). Signs of fluid overload are those of congestive heart failure and include coarse breath sounds and increased pulse rate and blood pressure. As the heart becomes overwhelmed by excessive fluid, blood pressure falls and signs of edema develop.

BOX 38.6

Nursing Care Planning Using Procedures

INITIATING A SCALP VEIN INFUSION IN AN INFANT

Purpose: To provide a route for intravenous therapy

© Lesha Photography

Procedure	Principle
1. Apply an anesthetic cream to the chosen site.	1. An anesthetic cream decreases discomfort.
2. In about 30 minutes (the time for the anesthetic cream to take effect), adequately restrain the infant using a mummy restraint.	2. Restraining the infant promotes safety. Trying to hold the infant's arms and legs still without a restraint can be exhausting. Utilize Child Life, if available, to assist with the procedure.
3. Press the child's head to the side and hold it firmly in that position, with one hand on the occiput and the other securing the front of the head. Be certain the hand resting over the child's face does not obstruct the child's breathing.	3. This positions the child without interfering with respirations.
4. Lather the site over the temporal bone with a cleaning solution and carefully shave the hair. Ask parents if they want to save the clippings of hair if it is their child's first haircut. Assure them the hair will grow back in quickly.	4. The cleaning solution potentially reduces the possibility of nicks to the scalp. Hair removal allows a clear view of the insertion site and possibly reduces the risk of infection.
5. Place a rubber band around the infant's head at the level of the forehead.	5. A tourniquet is needed to dilate scalp veins.
6. Wash the shaved area with an antiseptic solution.	6. Washing the scalp further reduces the possibility of infection.
7. Insert a special small scalp vein needle or polytetrafluoroethylene (Teflon) catheter into a vein on her temple.	7. Use of an appropriate insertion device establishes a fluid route.
8. Continue to hold the infant firmly until the needle is securely taped in place and until satisfied the infusion is running well.	8. Securing the infant and device ensures an effective insertion site.
9. Cover the infusion needle with a clear dressing such as Tegaderm or OPSITE. Use a protective device, such as plastic shield, as needed to further protect the IV site from trauma.	9. Covering the site keeps the infant from dislodging the needle when the infant turns her head.
10. If necessary, use hand mitts to prevent the infant from touching the insertion site.	10. Using hand mitts to protect the site is advised. Restraints are not recommended and only used as a last resort.
11. Spend some time comforting the child, talking and smiling, or lightly touching and stroking. Many infants enjoy sucking a pacifier or a bottle of glucose water during or after painful procedures; being held and rocked is the best comfort. Elicit the parents' support and institute principles of a traumatic care.	11. The infant may be frightened by the pinprick of the needle insertion as well as by having been held so firmly for a length of time.

Figure 38.7 An infusion pump and calibrated infusion chamber are safety features used with children's intravenous infusions.

In addition to observing for changes in vital signs such as these, assess intake and output per the following guidelines:

Infants = 2 ml/kg/hr

Children = 0.5 to 1 ml/kg/hr

Adolescents and adults = 40 to 80 ml/hr

It is difficult for children to lie still and wait for an IV infusion to finish (see Box 38.7, an interprofessional care map for a child receiving intravenous medication). Try to provide children with quiet activities that will not interfere with the infusion. If a child will have medicine administration daily, help the child plan a special activity such as play a board game, listen to special music, or watch a favorite TV program, an activity reserved for only that time so IV infusion time is not seen as a dreaded activity. Be sure parents understand the importance of the IV therapy and help guard the infusion site while they are with their child. Infants who receive total fluids by IV infusion may enjoy sucking on a pacifier to fulfill their oral needs, ask the infant's mother if she would allow this, especially if the infant will return to breastfeeding soon.

QSEN Checkpoint Question 38.5 ✔️

EVIDENCE-BASED PRACTICE

To investigate whether the viewing of cartoons can reduce the perception of pain in pediatric patients, younger children who presented to a major emergency department were randomized to watch a Barney cartoon in Spanish or English, and older children were randomized to view a Tarzan cartoon in either of the same two languages during painful procedures. Younger children were assessed 5 minutes before the procedure, during the procedure, and 5 minutes after the procedure using either a Poker Chip Tool or FACES Pain Scale. Older children were assessed at the same time interval using self-reporting and a visual analog scale. Results revealed children who watched the cartoons rated their pain as significantly lower than those who did not watch the cartoons (Sahiner & Bal, 2016).

Based on the previous study, if Terry were watching television as the nurse approached her to insert an IV cannula, what would be the nurse's best action?

a. Temporarily turning off the TV so she can clearly hear instructions

b. Asking Terry's mother to turn the TV set to the cartoon channel

c. Putting on an age-appropriate movie for Terry to watch

d. Allowing Terry to continue to watch the current channel

Look in Appendix A for the best answer and rationale.

Intravenous Medication Administration

Medications may be added to an IV line as a small, one-time administration (bolus), a fluid chamber infusion, or by piggyback for larger children. As with any medication administration, identify the child before adding medicine to an IV line. Also ensure that the drug to be injected is compatible with the IV fluid being infused.

To administer medicine using a bolus technique, depending on what is available and the protocol at your facility, you may use a syringe pump for administering a medication or, if giving an IV push medication, clamp the IV tubing above the medicine port in the IV line, clean the port with alcohol, insert the needleless syringe filled with the prescribed medicine into the port, and inject the medicine slowly and gently based on the manufacturer's instructions. Once the medication has been given, remove the syringe and reopen the IV line immediately to allow the IV solution to flush the medicine into the child.

Currently, most intravenous fluids and medications are delivered using an infusion pump to ensure patient safety. Smart infusion pumps (SIPs) are equipped with safety features such as guardrails to alert nurses to specified parameters designated to prevent overdosing or to alert them of adverse drug interactions (Mason, Roberts-Turner, Amendola, et al., 2014).

For a piggyback infusion of medicine, medication is provided by the pharmacy prepared and diluted in small fluid-filled plastic bags. To begin a piggyback infusion, hang the piggyback bag, clean the medicine port on the IV line, and insert the piggyback system into the port. Lower the level of the main infusion bag and adjust the flow rate to that desired to allow the piggyback system to operate. As soon as the piggyback bag has emptied, elevate the maintenance bag of fluid again and make certain the IV line is flowing well and at the proper rate.

Analgesics are commonly administered to children either by intermittent IV administration or PCA pumps (Anghelescu, Faughnan, Oakes, et al., 2012; DiGiusto, Bhalla, Martin, et al., 2014). PCAs are set with lockout time intervals and are safe to use with children (see Chapter 39). When programmed, such pumps help protect against medication errors, but they still need to be monitored.

🌿 *What If . . . 38.3*

Terry's mother tells the nurse she does not believe in introducing any "foreign" substance into her child's body, so she does not want her to have IV medicine. How would the nurse counsel her?

BOX 38.7

Nursing Care Planning

AN INTERPROFESSIONAL CARE MAP FOR A CHILD RECEIVING MEDICATION

Terry is an 8-year-old with Down syndrome whom you meet in the emergency room. She has been diagnosed with osteomyelitis, a bone infection at her ankle. When you gave her a tablet of acetaminophen (Tylenol) for pain, she spit it out. Her mother tells you Terry cannot swallow pills. Her father tells you, "You'll have to give her an IV."

Family Assessment: Child is the youngest of four siblings. Lives with parents and other siblings in five-bedroom home on dairy farm. When asked about finances, parents state, "Fine, as long as people keep drinking milk."

Patient Assessment: Child diagnosed with Down syndrome at birth; IQ approximately 60. Lacerated right foot on farm equipment in fall from hay loft 2 weeks ago. Laceration cleaned and bandaged by mother; not seen by healthcare provider. Today, wound has not healed, is open and erythematous; foot swollen; pain radiates up leg from foot. X-ray reveals abscess in bone. Child is so frightened by injections; she screams at the sight of any kind of needle. Placed on bed rest and prescribed an intravenous (IV) antibiotic and acetaminophen (Tylenol) and oxycodone for pain.

Nursing Diagnosis: Pain related to disease process (infection) in foot

Outcome Evaluation: Child rates pain on pain scale as 2 or below; cooperates with IV medication therapy to supply antibiotic and pain relief.

Team Member Responsible	Assessment	Intervention	Rationale	Expected Outcome
Activities of Daily Living, Including Safety				
Nurse	Assess what self-care measures child is able to complete by herself while on bed rest.	Explain to family that resting foot and maintaining IV therapy are crucial measures. Provide child with comfort and safety measures, age-appropriate diversional activities, and appropriate coverage of IV site to prevent dislodging.	Non–weight-bearing and antibiotic therapy will best cure the condition and relieve pain.	Child, nurse, and parent agree on plan of care for activities of daily living.
Teamwork and Collaboration				
Nurse/primary care provider	Assess if pain management team advice will be necessary.	Meet with pain consultant to discuss problem: Child is in pain but needs to remain still for IV therapy.	Sustained antibiotic therapy is necessary to treat bone infection; consultation can help avoid infiltration.	Pain management consultant meets with child and parent as appropriate; agrees on pain management plan.
Procedures/Medications for Quality Improvement				
Nurse	Assess if child has a preference for IV therapy site.	Begin IV therapy in nondominant hand if possible.	Allowing a child as much choice as possible helps to prevent a feeling of entrapment.	Parent will assist in keeping the child calm during the procedure.
Nutrition				
Nurse	Assess the child's food preferences to encourage eating.	Discuss with child and parent the importance of continuing nutrition while on bed rest. Suggest taking pain medication before meals.	Hospitalization can be a major stress to children. Pain can interfere with nutrition.	Child helps to choose foods from hospital menu that she would like to eat.
Patient-Centered Care				
Nurse	Assess if child has had experience with IV therapy in the past.	Review importance and plan for IV therapy with child and parents. Include child life as well as medical play as appropriate for development.	Knowledgeable patients and parents can aid in the success of therapy.	Child and parents state they understand why antibiotic and analgesia are needed and why administration method is required.

Psychosocial/Spiritual/Emotional Needs				
Nurse	Ask child to rate pain by FACES Pain Scale hourly.	Discuss with family typical behaviors their child exhibits when in pain.	Important to ask the parent about their child's reaction to pain and specific behaviors that child displays. Pain relief can be adapted to child's specific needs.	Child and parent are satisfied with pain level. Pain is managed and child can participate in activities such as playing, eating, and sleeping.
Informatics for Seamless Healthcare Planning				
Nurse	Assess if parents have questions about child's care at home.	Explain the importance of continuing IV and then oral antibiotic. Practice swallowing pills with ice chips to ready child for oral administration.	Continuing antibiotic administration will be necessary to combat deep-seated infection.	Parents state they understand importance of continuing medicine administration. Keep follow-up visit for evaluation.

USING INTERMITTENT INFUSION DEVICES

Intermittent infusion devices, sometimes called saline locks, are devices that maintain open venous access for medicine administration while allowing children to be free to move about without being restricted by IV tubing and pumps (Fig. 38.8). A vein on the back of the hand is generally chosen as the IV site. The saline lock is flushed as frequently as hospital policy requires to keep it patent. Be certain the tubing and stopper are both firmly secured to the wrist and, if necessary, an arm board is taped in place to remind the child to protect the site from trauma.

Children who are hospitalized or receiving home care for a long time and who need only IV medication, not additional fluid, are good candidates for such devices because IV medicine can be added to the site as needed without further venipunctures. Intermittent infusion devices also can be used if frequent venous blood samples are required because they can be used for blood draws. Similar devices may be inserted into arteries when arterial blood is required,

Figure 38.8 An intermittent infusion device in place. Advocating for this type of apparatus increases mobility for parent and child. (From Ricci, S. S. [2017]. *Essentials of maternity, newborn, and women's health nursing* [4th ed.]. Philadelphia, PA: Wolters Kluwer.)

for example, for the child who is having blood gases monitored frequently.

USING CENTRAL VENOUS ACCESS CATHETERS AND DEVICES

Venous access for long-term IV therapy can be obtained using a tunneled catheter inserted into the vena cava just outside the right atrium; the catheter then exits the chest just under the clavicle for easy access (Fig. 38.9). Typical catheters used in this way include Broviac, Hickman, and Groshong types. Such catheters have a wrinkle-resistant fabric (Dacron) cuff that adheres to the subcutaneous tissue and helps to seal the catheter in place and keep out infection. These catheters are usually inserted in the operating room because tunneling under the skin is required and general anesthesia is preferred. These semipermanent catheters are used to administer bolus or continuous infusions of medications and fluid (Crocoli, Tornesello, Pittiruti, et al., 2015). Care of the catheter (depending on agency policy) consists of dressing changes over the exit site and periodically flushing the line with heparin or saline to ensure patency.

Such catheters are advantageous because discomfort from further skin punctures is avoided. One disadvantage is that the catheter could become snagged on something and accidentally be pulled out. If this happens, it is an emergency situation because the child could lose an appreciable amount of blood from the point of entrance into the vena cava. Unless there is a waterproof dressing covering the insertion site, children with central venous catheters in place are usually not allowed to swim or take showers to avoid infection. Another disadvantage is the potential for profuse bleeding or air embolus if the IV tubing becomes disconnected from the catheter. Connections should be carefully secured and monitored. Infections must be prevented or the catheter will likely need to be removed.

Vascular access ports (VAPs), also known as Infusaports or PORT-A-CATHs, are small plastic infusion devices that are implanted under the skin, usually on the anterior chest just under the clavicle, for long-term fluid or medication administration via bolus or continuous administration (see Fig. 38.9D). A small catheter threads from the port internally into a central vein. After skin cleansing, blood

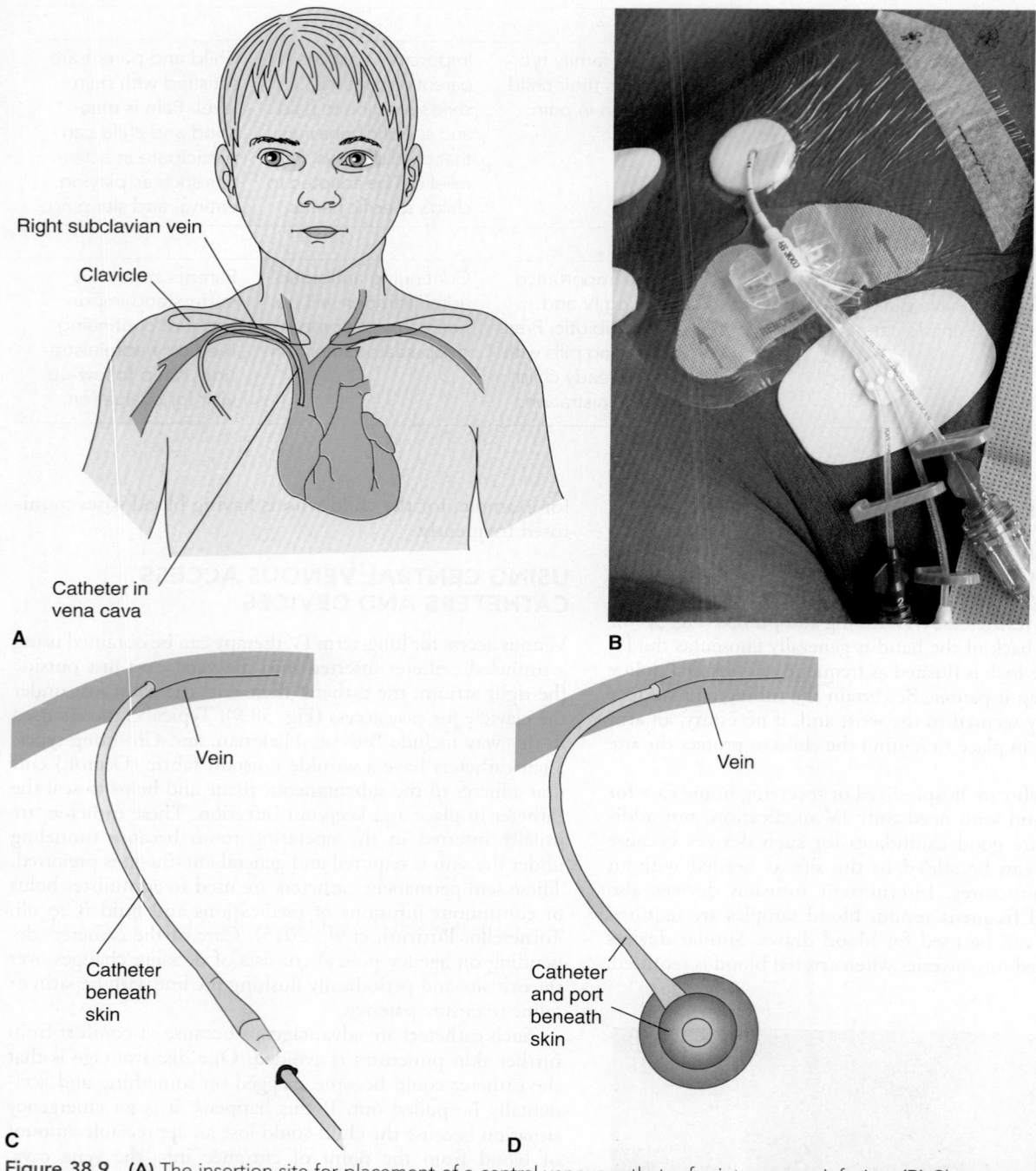

Figure 38.9 **(A)** The insertion site for placement of a central venous catheter for intravenous infusion. **(B)** Changing a dressing for a central venous catheter. (From Lippincott Solutions. [n.d.]. *Critical Care* [online module]. Retrieved from http://lippincottsolutions.com/specialties/critical-care). **(C)** The central venous catheter beneath the skin. **(D)** A vascular access port (VAP) device beneath the skin.

samples can be removed or medication can be injected by a needle inserted through the chest into the port. Puncturing the chest causes pain, so advocate for the child to receive a topical anesthetic at least 30 minutes prior to inserting the needle. Unlike the other types of central venous catheter that are visible outside of the chest, no dressing is required for these ports when they are not accessed with a needle. This allows for a full range of activities, such as showering and swimming. Be certain when accessing these ports to use only the needle supplied by the manufacturer because a regular needle tends to "core" or remove a small circle of

the membrane over the port and destroy the integrity of the device. As with central lines, air emboli, bleeding from a disconnected line, and infection are major concerns with VAPs also.

Another type of IV access is peripherally inserted central catheters (PICC lines) for therapy (Xiang, Li, Yi, et al., 2016). These are advantageous particularly for home care because they can remain in place for up to 4 months without being changed. For this, a catheter is inserted into an arm vein (usually at the antecubital space into the median, cephalic, or basilic vein) and advanced until the tip rests in the superior vena cava. If a shorter catheter is used, the tip will rest closer to the head of the clavicle (a midline insertion).

Drugs commonly administered via PICC lines are antibiotics and analgesics. After medication is administered, the line is flushed with a small amount of a solution such as normal saline. The dressing over the insertion site is changed periodically according to agency policy.

Many parents seem more comfortable with this type of insertion than with a central venous catheter because it appears so much more like a routine IV. Newborns can also have a catheter inserted into an umbilical vessel, with fluid and medications being administered by that route (see Chapter 26).

Remember that when caring for children with any type of central venous access systems, they all have the potential for hemorrhage, infection, air embolism, and thrombosis. Be certain to use strict aseptic techniques when changing the dressing covering the insertion site to prevent infections (Cesaro, Cavaliere, Pegoraro, et al., 2016).

QSEN Checkpoint Question 38.6

PATIENT-CENTERED CARE

Terry has her IV site changed to her dominant hand. Terry becomes agitated and begins to pull at her IV site. The nurse identifies which activity as best for her while her medication infuses?

a. Listening to a story
b. Playing kick ball in the hallway
c. Playing Simon Says with her parents
d. Building a tower in the play area with another child

Look in Appendix A for the best answer and rationale.

ADMINISTERING AN INTRAOSSEOUS INFUSION

Intraosseous infusion is the infusion of fluid into the bone marrow cavity of a long bone, usually the distal or proximal tibia, the distal femur, or the iliac crest (Reuter-Rice, Patrick, Kantor, et al., 2015). Because the bone marrow communicates directly with the circulatory system, fluid reaches the bloodstream as quickly by this route as if it were administered intravenously. All fluids that can be administered intravenously, including whole blood or medication, can also be administered by this route.

Intraosseous infusion is used in an emergency when it is difficult to establish usual IV access or in a child with such extensive burns that the usual sites for IV infusion are not available. It is a temporary measure until a usual route of administration can be obtained because of the danger of osteomyelitis, a devastating infection with long-term effects to bone marrow. Intraosseous infusion is painful as the needle enters the bone marrow cavity. Prepare the child for this and offer support to both the child and caregiver.

The intraosseous needle may be inserted manually or using a power-assisted device, which is the preferred method for intraosseous insertion. Either way, identifying the correct anatomical landmarks for insertion is necessary. The following steps are used to initiate an intraosseous infusion:

1. The skin over the chosen site is cleaned as per protocol and anesthetized with a local anesthetic.
2. A small incision is made into the skin with a scalpel blade.

3. A large hypodermic or bone marrow needle is inserted through the incision into the cavity of the bone.
4. To ensure the needle tip has reached the bone marrow cavity, a syringe is attached to the needle and bone marrow is aspirated.
5. When bone marrow is obtained, the syringe is removed and IV tubing, including a filter and the fluid to be administered, is attached to the needle and opened to a gravity flow.
6. A dressing with additional antiseptic is then applied over the needle site.
7. A restraint is applied to the leg to help the child hold the leg still.

Tubing and dressings must be changed as per protocol (approximately every 48 hours for the tubing and approximately every 24 hours for the dressing), again, to reduce the possibility of infection. Assess for a distal pulse and adequate temperature and color of the leg every hour throughout the infusion to ensure there is adequate circulation to the extremity. To optimize assessment, place a pulse oximeter on a toe distal to the infusion and monitor waveform. If the needle should become dislodged, symptoms of circulatory impairment or pain and taut skin over the site occur.

Occasionally during fluid administration, a bone chip or thick marrow will occlude an intraosseous needle and slow the infusion. If this occurs, a stylet passed through the needle clears it and allows for continued fluid administration.

What If . . . 38.4

The nurse is interested in exploring one of the 2020 National Health Goals with respect to the administration of medicine in children (see Box 38.1). Most government-sponsored money for nursing research is allotted based on these goals. What would be a possible research topic to explore pertinent to these goals that would be applicable to Terry and her family and that would also advance evidence-based practice?

Unfolding Patient Stories: Brittany Long • Part 1

Brittany Long, a 5-year-old Black diagnosed with sickle cell anemia, is having an acute pain crisis, and her mother brings her to the emergency department (ED). Her last visit to the ED was 1 year ago when she was hospitalized for a vaso-occlusive crisis episode. How would the nurse prepare Brittany for insertion of an intravenous line and administration of intravenous fluids? How would the explanation differ for her mother? What nursing interventions safeguard the intravenous line and administration of fluids? (Brittany Long's story continues in Chapter 56.)

Care for Brittany and other patients in a realistic virtual environment: **vSim** *for Nursing* (thepoint.lww.com /vSimMaternityPed). Practice documenting these patients' care in DocuCare (thepoint.lww.com /DocuCareEHR).

KEY POINTS FOR REVIEW

- The effectiveness of medicines varies depending on the pharmacokinetics (absorption, distribution, metabolism, and excretion) of the drug.

- The principles of safe medicine administration for adults also apply to children: right medicine, right child, right dose, right route, right time, and right patient instructions.

- The correct drug dose in children is usually calculated according to the child's body weight. Body surface area, determined by using a nomogram or BSA formula, may also be used. The body surface area formula is based on height and weight for calculating medication dosages.

- Use adequate restraints as needed when giving medicine to be certain children will not inadvertently be harmed in the process.

- In children, the majority of medications are given orally or intravenously to avoid the discomfort of other routes. Subcutaneous pumps infuse medicine such as insulin.

- IV therapy may be administered peripherally or via a central venous access site. A scalp vein is a common IV site used for infants.

- An intraosseous infusion is used in an emergency when it is difficult to establish usual IV access or in a child with such extensive burns that the usual sites for IV infusion are not available.

- Teach parents safe actions for giving medicine at home so children can continue to receive accurate doses after hospital discharge and ensure they understand the importance of storing medications in a locked area; such thoroughness helps in planning care that not only meets QSEN competencies but also best meets a family's total needs.

CRITICAL THINKING CARE STUDY

Casey is a previously healthy 4-year-old boy brought to the pediatric emergency room by his parents because he has diarrhea and has been refusing to eat today. He says his throat hurts too much for him to swallow and wants something to "stop the pain." Upon examination, Casey is found to be mildly to moderately dehydrated. Pain medication (acetaminophen) and an oral rehydration solution (Pedialyte) are prescribed. His throat swab reveals he has a "strep throat," so he is also started on a course of oral antibiotics.

1. Casey has been prescribed two oral medications plus an oral rehydration solution, yet one of his chief concerns is that his throat hurts too much for him to swallow. How would you approach this problem?

2. Suppose Casey vomits the rehydration solution so his primary care provider asks you to begin an IV infusion with him. How would you approach him to do this?

3. Casey has 2-year-old twin sisters and a new baby brother, 6 months old, at home. What would be important safety precautions to remind his parents about before he is discharged from the emergency room?

RELATED RESOURCES

Explore these additional resources to enhance learning for this chapter:
- Student resources on thePoint, including answers to the What If . . . and Critical Thinking Care Study questions, http://thepoint.lww.com/Flagg8e
- Adaptive learning powered by PrepU, http://thepoint.lww.com/prepu

REFERENCES

Albertson, T. E., Chenoweth, J. A., Colby, D. K., et al. (2016). The changing drug culture: Use and misuse of cognition-enhancing drugs. *FP Essentials, 441*, 25–29.

American Academy of Pediatrics. (n.d.). *Medication safety.* Retrieved from https://healthychildren.org/english/safety-prevention/at-home/medication-safety/Pages/default.aspx

Anghelescu, D. L., Faughnan, L. G., Oakes, L. L., et al. (2012). Parent-controlled PCA for pain management in pediatric oncology: Is it safe? *Journal of Pediatric Hematology/Oncology, 34*(6), 416–420.

Branden, E., & Flerlage, J. (2014). *The Harriett Lane handbook* (20th ed.). Philadelphia, PA: Elsevier Health Sciences.

Buchholz, S. (2016). *Henke's med-math: Dosage calculation, preparation, and administration* (8th ed.). Philadelphia, PA: Wolters Kluwer.

Cesaro, S., Cavaliere, M., Pegoraro, A., et al. (2016). A comprehensive approach to the prevention of central venous catheter complications: Results of 10-year prospective surveillance in pediatric hematology-oncology patients. *Annals of Hematology, 95*(5), 817–825.

Crocoli, A., Tornesello, A., Pittiruti, M., et al. (2015). Central venous access devices in pediatric malignancies: A position paper of Italian Association of Pediatric Hematology and Oncology. *The Journal of Vascular Access, 16*(2), 130–136.

Del Pizzo, J., & Callahan, J. M. (2014). Intranasal medications in pediatric emergency medicine. *Pediatric Emergency Care, 30*(7), 496–501.

DiGiusto, M., Bhalla, T., Martin, D., et al. (2014). Patient-controlled analgesia in the pediatric population: Morphine versus hydromorphone. *Journal of Pain Research, 7*, 471–475.

Frith, K. H. (2013). Medication errors in the intensive care unit: Literature review using the SEIPS model. *AACN Advanced Critical Care, 24*(4), 389–404.

Jannin, V., Lemagnen, G., Gueroult, P., et al. (2014). Rectal route in the 21st century to treat children. *Advanced Drug Delivery Reviews, 73*(30), 34–49.

Lan, Y.-H., Wang, K.-W. K., Yu, S., et al. (2014). Medication errors in pediatric nursing: Assessment of nurses' knowledge and analysis of the consequences of errors. *Nurse Education Today, 34*(5), 821–828.

Mason, J. J., Roberts-Turner, R., Amendola, V., et al. (2014). Patient safety, error reduction, and pediatric nurses' perceptions of smart pump technology. *Journal of Pediatric Nursing, 29*(2), 143–151.

McNab, S. (2016). Intravenous maintenance fluid therapy in children. *Journal of Paediatrics and Child Health, 52*(2), 137–140.

PDR Staff. (2013). *Physicians' desk reference* (67th ed.). Montvale, NJ: PDR Network.

Peters, J. E., Mount, E., Huggins, C. E., et al. (2013). Insulin pump therapy in children and adolescents: Changes in dietary habits, composition and quality of life. *Journal of Paediatrics and Child Health, 49*(4), E300–E305.

Powers, K. S. (2015). Dehydration: Isonatremic, hyponatremic, and hypernatremic recognition and management. *Pediatrics in Review, 36*(7), 274–285.

Pozzilli, P., Battelino, T., Danne, T., et al. (2016). Continuous subcutaneous insulin infusion in diabetes: Patient populations, safety, efficacy, and pharmacoeconomics. *Diabetes/Metabolism Research and Reviews, 32*, 21–39.

Reed, M. D., & Bestic, M. L. (2014). Developmental pharmacokinetics: Drug disposition relative to age. In K. Gordon (Ed.), *Bone drugs in pediatrics: Efficacy and challenges* (pp. 5–22). New York, NY: Springer Publishing.

Reuter-Rice, K., Patrick, D., Kantor, E., et al. (2015). Characteristics of children who undergo intraosseous needle placement. *Advanced Emergency Nursing Journal, 37*(4), 301–307.

Sahiner, N. C., & Bal, M. D. (2016). The effects of three different distraction methods on pain and anxiety in children. *Journal of Child Health Care, 20*(3), 277–285.

Schoenewald, S., Ross, S., Bloom, L., et al. (2013). New insights into root causes of pediatric accidental unsupervised ingestions of over-the-counter medications. *Clinical Toxicology, 51*(10), 930–936.

Shaw, M. (2016). How to administer eye drops and eye ointment. *Nursing Standard, 30*(39), 34–36.

Thakkar, N., Salerno, S., Hornik, C. P., et al. (2017). Clinical pharmacology studies in critically ill children. *Pharmaceutical Research, 34*(1), 7–24.

Thompson Reuters Clinical Editorial Staff. (2013). *Neofax* (26th ed.). Montvale, NJ: PDR Network.

U.S. Department of Health and Human Services. (2010). *Healthy people 2020*. Washington, DC: Author.

Walsh, K. E., Mazor, K. M., Roblin, D., et al. (2013). Multisite parent-centered risk assessment to reduce pediatric oral chemotherapy errors. *Journal of Oncology Practice, 9*(1), e1–e7.

Xiang, M., Li, N., Yi, L., et al. (2016). Causes and nursing countermeasures in pediatric PICC catheter complications. *Pakistan Journal of Pharmaceutical Sciences, 29*(1 Suppl.), 335–337.

Yin, H. S., Dreyer, B. P., Moreira, H. A., et al. (2014). Liquid medication dosing errors in children: Role of provider counseling strategies. *Academic Pediatrics, 14*(3), 262–270.

39

Pain Management in Children

Robin Harvey is a 3-year-old girl who was admitted to your hospital unit and has just returned from a bone marrow aspiration to rule out the possibility of leukemia. Robin received intravenous (IV) morphine sulfate during the procedure. Her mother asks you if Robin could have some more. "I know she's not having pain yet," her mother tells you, "But I want her to have something before the pain comes back."

Previous chapters described the growth and development of children and general care of ill children. This chapter adds information about the care of children when they need pain management. Such information builds a base for care and health teaching in a crucial area.

Is this mother's assessment or Robin's pain apt to be accurate or should you ask Robin herself about pain? Would anticipating pain in this way be the best intervention for Robin?

KEY TERMS

acute pain

chronic pain

conscious sedation

cutaneous pain

distraction

epidural analgesia

gate control theory

hyperalgesia

pain

pain threshold

pain tolerance

patient-controlled analgesia (PCA)

referred pain

somatic pain

substitution of meaning

thought stopping

transcutaneous electrical nerve stimulation (TENS)

visceral pain

OBJECTIVES

After mastering the contents of this chapter, you should be able to:

1. Describe the major methods and techniques of pain management for children.

2. Identify 2020 National Health Goals related to pain management in children that nurses can help the nation achieve.

3. Assess a child regarding whether pain management is needed or adequate.

4. Formulate nursing diagnoses for a child in pain.

5. Identify expected outcomes associated with management of pain in children as well as help families manage seamless transitions across differing healthcare settings.

6. Using the nursing process, plan nursing care that includes the six competencies of Quality & Safety Education for Nurses (QSEN): Patient-Centered Care, Teamwork & Collaboration, Evidence-Based Practice (EBP), Quality Improvement (QI), Safety, and Informatics.

7. Implement nursing care related to a child in pain, such as suggesting an alternative therapy.

8. Evaluate outcomes for achievement and effectiveness of care for a child in pain.

9. Integrate knowledge of pain management in children with the interplay of nursing process, the six competencies of QSEN, and Family Nursing to promote quality maternal and child health nursing care.

Pain is a difficult concept to define because it is a subjective symptom (experienced by the person), not an objective one (able to be determined using an objective scale), and is unique to each person. Because it respects children's opinion of where and how much pain they feel, McCaffery's (1979) classic description of **pain** is the one most useful to use with children: "The sensation of pain is whatever the person experiencing it says it is, and it exists whenever the person says it does."

For children, because pain is such a different sensation than usual, pain is not only a hurting sensation but it can also be a very confusing one—the child did not anticipate the pain, does not have words to explain how it feels, and cannot always understand its cause. In addition, preschoolers and younger children lack an understanding of time, which makes it difficult to explain to them when the pain will go away. This can leave them feeling frustrated or angry while they wait for someone to give them relief.

Children's perception of the situation influences their response to how much pain they feel. This means that children experiencing procedures that are less intrusive but who feel maximum anxiety from them may describe the degree of pain felt as more intense than they otherwise might have because of the accompanying anxiety (Vervoort, Eccleston, Goubert, et al., 2010).

Both helping children describe the type and extent of pain they are feeling and performing active interventions to relieve pain are some of the most important nursing roles in children's care. Assessing for pain is so important that pain is often considered the "fifth vital sign" (Harrison, Elia, Royle, et al., 2013).

The 2020 National Health Goals that speak to pain management are shown in Box 39.1.

Nursing Process Overview

FOR A CHILD IN PAIN

ASSESSMENT

Children, like adults, experience pain individually depending on the type and cause of the pain, their temperament, their previous experience with pain, and their expectation of relief. Infants and young children cannot verbalize what they are feeling and so have the most difficulty communicating how they feel.

Beginning as young as 3 years of age, children can indicate by pointing to a body part where they feel pain. They can also learn to express the degree of pain through a system such as comparing its intensity to a number of poker chips or drawings of faces. Older school-age children and adolescents can rate their pain on a scale of 0 to 10. Be aware that some children may be reluctant to admit pain because they are trying to be brave. Some may be reluctant to say they have pain because they are afraid they will receive a "shot" to relieve it, which will cause more pain. As a rule, it is most efficient to assess pain levels using an appropriate scoring tool along with a vital sign measurement.

NURSING DIAGNOSIS

Nursing diagnoses for children with pain focus not only on the pain but also on the stress, fear, or anxiety that pain produces. Examples of nursing diagnoses include:

- Pain related to an invasive procedure
- Fear related to anticipation of painful procedure

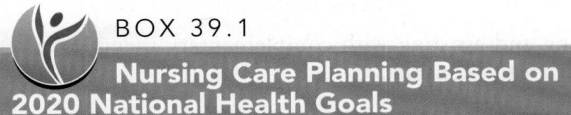

BOX 39.1

Nursing Care Planning Based on 2020 National Health Goals

Several 2020 National Health Goals speak directly to alleviating pain in several different areas:

- Reduce the proportion of patients suffering from untreated pain due to a lack of access to pain treatment.
- Reduce serious injuries from the use of pain medicines.
- Reduce the number of non–U.S. Food and Drug Administration (FDA)-approved pain medications on the market.
- Reduce deaths from the use of pain medicines (U.S. Department of Health and Human Services, 2010; see www.healthypeople.gov).

Nurses can help the nation reduce pain among children by active management of pain as well as by teaching children about the importance of avoiding painful unintentional injuries by the use of safety belts and bicycle helmets.

- Disturbed sleep pattern related to chronic pain
- Anxiety related to planned dressing changes that cause pain

OUTCOME IDENTIFICATION AND PLANNING

The mark of efficient pain control is to anticipate when pain will occur and plan interventions to prevent it rather than let it occur and then relieve it. Three common reasons why nurses and other pediatric providers may not provide adequate pain relief to children include a belief that infants and young children do not experience pain, a fear children will become addicted to pain relief medications, and a fear of causing respiratory depression from analgesics. Infants and young children do experience pain, and there is little chance that children receiving opioids during a short hospital stay will become opioid dependent or that opiates cause greater respiratory depression in children than in adults (Fanning, Stucke, Christensen, et al., 2012). Refer parents to online resources for further information when appropriate (see Chapter 36).

IMPLEMENTATION

Implementation for pain relief includes choosing the specific method of pain relief that is best for each child. Everyone involved in a child's care needs to be aware of the signs and symptoms that an individual child uses to express pain and specific ways that will help the child manage pain. If children are reluctant to admit they have pain because of the fear of receiving an injection, advocate for an oral form of analgesia or an intermittent IV infusion device or patient-controlled analgesia as appropriate options. Many parents are unsure about the safety of using strong analgesics for pain relief and so may give less than the prescribed dose. Therefore, regardless of whether they verbalize their concerns, educating parents about the need for pain relief, complications from undertreated pain, proper doses, and taking actions to involve them in the assessment and evaluation process are essential.

Planning and assisting with complementary therapies is yet another area to consider.

OUTCOME EVALUATION

An evaluation of expected outcomes is a key aspect of managing pain because no one pain relief measure is effective for everyone. After a child is given an analgesic, look for nonverbal clues, assess vital signs, and listen to the child's statements about pain to determine whether a drug was effective. Based on these findings, it may become clear that the technique of pain management being used may need to be modified or increased. A new technique may need to be added to the regimen so a child receives maximum pain relief.

Possible examples indicating achievement of expected outcomes include:

- Child states pain is now at a tolerable level that will not interfere with activity or sleep.
- Adolescent says she has managed her fear through imagery.
- Child rates pain less than previously rated.
- Child describes ways he will help reduce pain when it returns.
- Child resumes age-appropriate behaviors following analgesia administration.

The Physiology of Pain

As in adults, acute pain in children usually occurs for one of four reasons: reduced pH alterations which cause depletion of oxygen in tissues, pressure on tissue, external injury, or overstretching of body cavities with fluid or air. Chronic pain often involves irritation of nerves and/or tissue, which can occur with the pain of shingles, fibromyalgia, or other long-term injuries and irritations. The stimulus causing pain is not always visible or measurable. In addition, anxiety can lead to increased pain regardless of the physical stimuli.

Pain conduction consists of four major steps: transduction (sensing the pain sensation), transmission (routing the pain sensation to the spinal cord), perception (the brain interprets the sensation as pain), and modulation (steps the body takes to relieve pain).

Pain impulses join central nervous system (CNS) fibers in the dorsal horn of the spinal cord. Here, the impulses are projected upward to the brain, where they will be perceived as pain.

- **Acute pain** means sharp pain. It generally occurs abruptly after an injury. The pain of a pinprick is an example.
- **Chronic pain** is pain that lasts for a prolonged period or beyond the time span anticipated for healing. Acute pain usually causes extreme distress and anxiety; chronic pain can lead to depression and decrease patient's ability to achieve relief as the threshold to sense pain lowers and creates a "feedback loop" (Palermo, Eccleston, Lewandowski, et al., 2010). This is also referred to as **hyperalgesia** which is defined as an increased sensitivity to pain and is seen when patients have a heightened response to minimal painful stimuli.
- **Cutaneous pain** is pain that arises from superficial structures such as the skin and mucous membrane. A paper cut is an example.
- **Somatic pain** is pain that originates from deep body structures such as muscles or bones. The pain of a sprained ankle is somatic pain.
- **Visceral pain** involves sensations that arise from internal organs such as the intestines. The pain of appendicitis is visceral pain.
- **Referred pain** is pain that is perceived at a site distant from its point of origin. The pain of right lower lobe pneumonia, for example, is often first thought to be abdominal pain because the pain is referred or felt in the abdomen.

A child's **pain threshold** refers to the point at which the child first senses pain. This varies greatly from person to person and is probably most influenced by heredity. All people also have a point above which they are not willing to bear any additional pain. This is a person's **pain tolerance**. Pain tolerance levels are probably most affected by cultural influences.

When pain is felt, the pituitary and hypothalamus glands both respond reflexively by releasing *endorphins* or polypeptide compounds that simulate opiates in their ability to produce analgesia and a sense of well-being. Children also consciously try to modify pain by physical actions such as shifting position or rubbing the body part.

Several theories have been proposed to explain the transmission of pain and how pain can best be managed. Of these, the gate control theory is the best known.

QSEN Checkpoint Question 39.1

INFORMATICS

Robin, 3 years of age, has just returned from having a bone marrow biopsy. The nurse documents the presence of which type of pain in Robin's electronic health record?

  a. Cutaneous pain
  b. Somatic pain
  c. Visceral pain
  d. Neuropathic pain

Look in Appendix A for the best answer and rationale.

GATE CONTROL THEORY OF PAIN

The **gate control theory** of pain (Melzack & Wall, 1965) attempts to explain how pain impulses travel from a site of injury to the brain, where the impulse is registered. This theory envisions gating mechanisms in the substantia gelatinosa of the dorsal horn of the spinal cord that, when activated, can halt an impulse at that level of the cord. This prevents the pain impulse from being received at the brain level and interpreted as pain. Gating mechanisms can be stimulated by four techniques:

1. Cutaneous stimulation
2. Distraction
3. Anxiety reduction
4. Nerve blocks

Cutaneous stimulation (skin stimulation) has an effect because, when the peripheral nerves next to an injury site are stimulated, the ability of the A-δ or C fiber nerves at the injury site responsible for transmitting pain impulses appears to decrease. Rubbing an injured part such as a stubbed toe and applying heat or cold to the site are types of maneuvers that suppress pain because these actions activate the nearby peripheral fibers. This technique is especially effective with children because the rubbing is not only comforting from a physical standpoint but also conveys psychological warmth.

Distraction allows the cells of the brain stem that register an impulse as pain to be preoccupied with other stimuli so a pain impulse cannot register. Having a child focus intently on an action or a thought or telling a child to say "ouch" while an injection is administered are common uses of this technique. For a child in pain after a procedure, a gift of a Mylar balloon or their favorite toy to hug can be wonderful distractions.

Pain impulses are perceived more quickly by the brain if anxiety is present. Therefore, any attempt to reduce a child's anxiety as much as possible, such as teaching a school-age child what to expect with a procedure so there are no surprises, can help reduce the intensity of pain. In addition to teaching when something is going to happen, be certain you also teach when nothing is going to happen. Being told a clinic visit is just for a checkup and so will not involve painful procedures allows a child to relax and feel less anxiety.

The effectiveness of gate control theory techniques varies with a child's age, ability to cooperate, degree of pain, and time allowed for learning and applying pain management techniques. Because memory may influence the sensation of pain (expecting to have pain produces anxiety, which increases pain), these techniques are best taught to children before they begin to have pain. In all instances, children should know to use them just before or at the moment they first feel the pain. If they wait until pain is intense, the pain may be so distracting that they cannot concentrate on using a technique. Children who were able to use a distraction technique in the past but can no longer do so need to be evaluated for what has changed. Is it their ability to cope with the pain or is the pain increasing in intensity?

Assessing the Type and Degree of Pain

Pain assessment can be difficult with children not only because children have difficulty describing pain but also because some children will suffer with pain rather than report it, unaware that someone could make it go away. Other children

may distract themselves by methods such as concentrating on play. Others may sleep, not from comfort but from the exhaustion caused by the pain. Cultural differences also influence how pain is expressed (Box 39.2). All of these factors can make using only subjective measures to assess pain, such as observation, misleading.

Parents may be unclear and don't intervene with pain assessment or control because they assume healthcare providers are experts on pain control. Healthcare providers, on the other hand, may depend on parents to speak up if their child is in pain. Discussing how pain will be assessed, everyone's role, and what is available for pain relief clearly and openly early in a treatment program help ensure that these misunderstandings do not occur. Be certain that you also frequently reassess pain to be certain interventions such as the administration of an analgesic, distraction, or improved positioning are effective.

Keeping in mind each child's developmental level as well as chronologic age are important when assessing pain because assessment varies widely from that of a nonverbal infant to a very verbal adolescent (Box 39.3).

THE INFANT

In the past, it was believed that infants do not feel pain because of incomplete myelination of peripheral nerves. Evidence-based practice has shown this not to be true because myelination is not necessary for pain perception.

BOX 39.2

Nursing Care Planning to Respect Cultural Diversity

Because children may have difficulty describing pain in a manner that adults can understand, it is difficult to assess the extent of their discomfort. Also, because pain is an individualized sensation, it may be experienced and expressed differently by different children. In some families, for example, pain may be expressed very openly and freely. In others, children are expected to be stoic about pain. The expression of pain is culturally determined in this way; therefore, two children who have the same degree of pain may express it very differently and it is important to be aware of these differences when taking care of any patient.

BOX 39.3

Nursing Care Planning Using Assessment

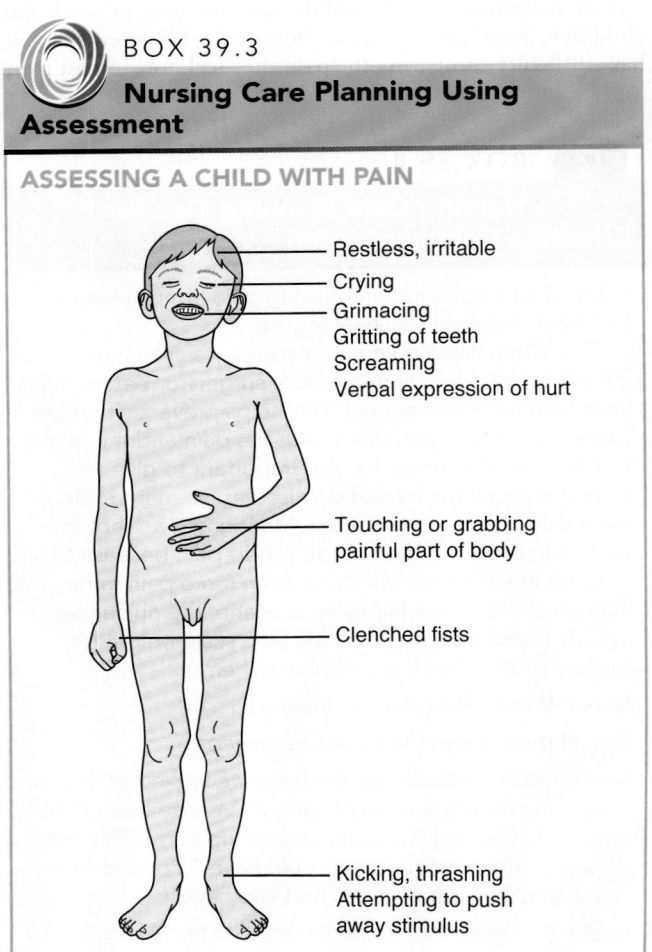

ASSESSING A CHILD WITH PAIN

- Restless, irritable
- Crying
- Grimacing
- Gritting of teeth
- Screaming
- Verbal expression of hurt
- Touching or grabbing painful part of body
- Clenched fists
- Kicking, thrashing Attempting to push away stimulus

A second argument in the past against needing to provide pain relief for infants was that they have no memory. It can be shown, however, that physiologic changes occur with pain even in preterm infants, so even with a lack of memory, it is clear that pain is experienced. Even newborns instinctively guard a body part by holding an extremity still or tensing the abdomen. Other clues are diffuse body movements; tears; a high-pitched, harsh cry; a stiff posture; alterations in facial expression such as eyes squeezed shut; a quivering chin; lack of play; and fisting (Schiavenato, Butler-O'Hara, & Scovanner, 2011). Perhaps, the chief mark in infants, however, is that when pain is present, they cannot be comforted completely. Preterm neonates particularly may have a difficult time organizing a distress response to cue a healthcare provider to the presence of pain. When working with any infant, be sensitive to situations that could cause pain and try to reduce them to the maximum extent possible.

THE TODDLER AND THE PRESCHOOLER

Determining when and how much pain is present continues to be difficult with toddlers and preschoolers because they may not have a word in their limited vocabularies to describe the sensation they feel because words such as "sharp," "nagging," or "aching" have little meaning until a child has experienced each type (Box 39.4). Parents often encourage children of this age to refer to pain as "my boo-boo" or to use other word such as "hurt" or "ouchie," so children often are not sure if what you mean by the word "pain" (to be most accurate in assessment, use the child's term for pain or teach the child that "pain" is the same as "boo-boo"). Children also can have difficulty comparing the pain they feel now to past pain

(e.g., Is it better or worse?) because they have had so little experience with pain. For some toddlers, pain is such a strange sensation that aside from crying in response to it, they may react aggressively (e.g., pounding, rocking) as if to fight it off. They also may avoid being touched or held.

Preschool children can describe that they have pain but continue to have difficulty describing its intensity. They begin to use comforting mechanisms, such as gritting teeth, pressing a hand against a forehead, pulling on their ear, holding their throat, rubbing an arm, or grimacing, to control or express pain. Some preschoolers do not think to mention they have pain because they believe it is something to be expected or, because of their egocentric thinking, they assume adults are already aware of their pain. They also may think pain is punishment for some act, so this is what they deserve. It is sometimes difficult to comfort children of this age during painful procedures by a statement such as "It's only for a minute" because they do not yet have a perception of time.

Still, other behavior changes you may see in preschoolers are regression or withdrawal. To help evaluate if they have pain, ask yourself, "What would this child normally be doing?" (e.g., playing, eating, sleeping). Input from parents on how their child usually behaves can be valuable in an evaluation. If a trial dose of analgesia is used, you can then evaluate behavior changes after the dose is given. Children who resume their usual behavior after analgesia were probably in pain before the analgesia took effect.

THE SCHOOL-AGE CHILD AND THE ADOLESCENT

Children who think concretely can have difficulty envisioning that a word like "sharp" applies both to knives and to the feeling in their abdomen. Because of this, they continue to have difficulty describing pain. They may also assume, like preschoolers, that you, as an authority figure, already know they have pain. In school-age children, guarding (tensing of body parts) is common. Sometimes, children can report they are fine while looking uncomfortable and being unwilling to move; as a nurse, you cannot always rely on what a child says; you have to read their body language, too.

Some children of school age will regress with pain such as returning to baby talk or lying in a fetal position. If pain will last only an instant, such as with an injection, children this age are old enough to control the pain through nonpharmacologic activities such as distraction techniques.

Children may be in middle school before they can understand how to use a numerical pain rating scale or that the scale intensifies from left to right. Doing preassessment work with them, such as giving them 10 different-sized triangles and asking them to arrange them from smallest to largest, is a good way to evaluate if they understand incremental measurements or "least to most" and are primed to describe pain intensity in a measurable way. A scale of 1 to 5 can be used in younger children if 1 to 10 seems overwhelming. If it seems clearer, you can turn a pain rating scale vertically so it measures bottom (little pain) to top (a lot of pain) to help a child learn incremental measurement.

Adolescents are able to use adult pain scales for assessment and also commonly use adult mechanisms for controlling pain such as grimacing or verbal outbursts. Some try to be stoic or not show pain in order to avoid stereotypes of

---

💬 **BOX 39.4**

Nursing Care Planning Tips for Effective Communication

Robin, 3 years old, has chronic leg pain from leukemia. You want to assess her level of pain.

Tip: When using pain rating scales, it's critical to introduce them to children before surgery or before they have pain from procedures. This helps prevent situations where the child experiences both the pain and the rating tool as new all at once. It's also important to give the correct instructions for standardized assessment tools, or the results will not be accurate. Mentioning a "shot for pain" can cause children not to report pain because they imagine the injection will cause even more pain rather than relieve it. In the following scenario, the nurse had already introduced Robin to the pain scale before her surgery so that that it wasn't new to her.

Nurse: Robin? How are you feeling?

Mrs. Harvey: I don't think she has any pain.

Nurse: Robin? Remember the faces we looked at this morning before surgery? I want you to use them to tell me how you feel. This one means "no hurt." This one means "the most hurt you could have." Point to the one that shows how much hurt you have.

Robin: (Points to the first face—the "no hurt" face.)

"crybaby" or "chicken." This tendency makes an assessment for body motions that could indicate pain, such as clenched hands, clenched teeth, rapid breathing, and guarding of body parts, doubly important to observe. This is also the age when concerns about addiction may begin to appear. A nurse can use this opportunity to discuss what it is adolescents may have heard about pain medications, preconceived ideas about pain, and their risk for abuse of pain medications (see Chapter 33). It is important for a nurse to read both verbal and nonverbal cues from the patient when having these discussions.

Pain Assessment

Common fallacies about pain in children are shown in Table 39.1. Although monitoring for physiologic findings such as a change in pulse or blood pressure may give some indication that a child is under stress, these are not the most dependable indicators of pain because pain is a subjective symptom. Once children can speak, asking them to tell you about their pain (self-reporting or using a pain rating scale) becomes the most accurate method for assessment (Downey & Zun, 2012).

A variety of pain rating scales have been devised to use with children. None have been proven to be consistently better than the others, mainly because both children and the type of pain they can be experiencing vary so much. As a rule, pick a well-documented effective scale and urge your care team to use that consistently for each child rather than asking a child to adapt to different assessment techniques. Be sure to follow the specific instructions for that scale.

THE PAIN EXPERIENCE INVENTORY

The Pain Experience Inventory is a tool consisting of eight questions for children and eight questions for the child's parents. It is designed to elicit the terms a child uses to denote pain and what actions a child thinks will best alleviate pain. Such a form can be used when a child is admitted to an acute care facility or on an initial home care visit (Box 39.5). If possible, it should be used before the child has pain.

BOX 39.5
Pain Experience Inventory

QUESTIONS FOR THE CHILD

Tell me what pain is.
Tell me about any hurt you have had before.
What do you do when you hurt?
Do you tell others when you hurt?
What do you want others to do for you when you hurt?
What do you *not* want others to do for you when you hurt?
What helps the most to take away your hurt?
Is there anything special you would like me to know about you when you hurt? (If yes, have the child describe.)

QUESTIONS FOR PARENTS

Describe any pain your child has had before.
How does your child usually react to pain?
Does your child tell you or others when pain is experienced?
How do you know when your child is in pain?
What do you do for your child when your child is hurting?
What does your child do to help relieve pain?
Which of these actions work best to decrease or take away your child's pain?
Is there anything special that you would like me to know about your child and pain? (If yes, have the parents describe.) (Hester & Barcus, 1986)

THE CRIES NEONATAL POSTOPERATIVE PAIN MEASUREMENT SCALE

The CRIES Neonatal Postoperative Pain Measurement Scale is a 10-point scale named for five physiologic and behavioral variables commonly associated with neonatal pain: C = crying; R = requires increased oxygen administration; I = increased vital signs; E = expression; S = sleeplessness (Krechel & Bildner, 1995) (Table 39.2).

Each area of concern is scored from 0 to 2. Infants with a total score of 4 or more are most likely to be in pain and need interventions to reduce discomfort. The scale cannot be used

TABLE 39.1 COMMON FALLACIES ABOUT PAIN IN CHILDREN

Fallacy	Fact
Nurses can accurately estimate children's pain from their actions and so do not need to rely on children's self-reports.	Nurses commonly underestimate children's pain from physical appearance or activity.
Young children, particularly newborns, do not feel pain.	Newborns and children do feel pain.
A child who resumes usual activity or who sleeps cannot be in pain.	Some children distract themselves with play or music while in pain. They may sleep from exhaustion from the pain.
Because of the possible adverse effects, narcotic analgesics are too dangerous for young children.	In the proper dose, narcotics can be used safely with children, including low–birth-weight infants.
Experiencing pain will not harm an infant or young child.	Newborns with pain can become cyanotic and bradycardic; no one knows the psychological stress of pain at this age.
If children deny they are feeling pain, you should believe them.	Children may deny pain to avoid a procedure, such as an injection, which they view as more painful. They may be afraid, fearing that they are being punished, or believe others know how they feel.

TABLE 39.2 THE CRIES NEONATAL POSTOPERATIVE PAIN MEASUREMENT SCALE

Assessment	Infant's Score		
	0	1	2
Crying	No cry or cry is not high pitched.	Cry is high pitched but baby is easily consolable.	Cry is high pitched and baby is inconsolable.
Oxygen required for SpO₂ <95%	No oxygen required.	≤30% oxygen required.	>30% oxygen required.
Increased vital signs	Heart rate and blood pressure unchanged or less than baseline.	Baseline heart rate or blood pressure increased <20% of baseline.	Baseline heart rate or blood pressure increased ≥20% of baseline.
Expression	No grimace present.	Grimace alone is present.	Grimace and noncry vocalization grunt is present.
Sleepless	Infant has been continually asleep for past hour.	Infant has wakened at frequent intervals for past hour.	Infant has been awake constantly.
Total infant score			

SpO₂ = oxygen saturation.
From Krechel, S. W., & Bildner, J. (1995). CRIES: A new neonatal postoperative pain management score. Initial testing of validity and reliability. *Pediatric Anesthesia*, 5(1), 53.

with infants who are intubated or paralyzed for ventilatory assistance because they would have no score for crying and because, if their faces are obscured, it is difficult to rate them for facial expression.

THE COMFORT BEHAVIOR SCALE

The COMFORT Behavior Scale is a pain rating scale devised by nurses to rate pain in very young infants (Boerlage, Ista, de Jong, et al., 2012; van Dijk, Peters, van Deventer, et al., 2005). On the first part of the scale, six different categories (alertness, calmness/agitation, crying, physical movement, muscle tone, and facial expression) are rated from 1 to 5. The lowest score is 6 (no pain), and 30 is the highest (a great deal of pain). In addition to rating physical parameters, the infant is then observed for 2 minutes and the evaluation of the baby's pain is documented on an analog (1 to 10) visual scale.

THE FLACC PAIN ASSESSMENT TOOL

The FLACC Pain Assessment Tool is a scale by which healthcare providers can rate a young child's pain when a child cannot give input, there is a language barrier, or the child has a developmental delay. It incorporates five types of behaviors that can be used to rate pain: facial expression, leg movement, activity, cry, and consolability. Because a child does not provide active input, older children may prefer a pain rating system in which they actively participate.

THE POKER CHIP TOOL

The Poker Chip Tool (Hester & Barcus, 1986) uses four red poker chips placed in a horizontal line in front of the child. The technique can be used with children as young as 4 years of age, provided the child has some concept of "more" or "less." To use the tool, tell the child, "These are pieces of hurt." Beginning at the chip nearest the child's left hand and ending at the one nearest the child's right hand, point to the chips and say, "This is a little bit of hurt, this is a little more hurt, this is more hurt, and this [the fourth chip] is the most hurt you could ever have." Then, ask the child, "How many pieces of hurt do you have right now?" Children without pain will reply they don't

hurt; others will point to one of the poker chips. To gain more understanding of how much pain the child is feeling, clarify the child's answer by a follow-up question such as "Oh, you have a little hurt? Tell me about that." This is an effective tool for young children because the poker chips are concrete items and children are concrete thinkers (Fig. 39.1).

WONG-BAKER FACES PAIN RATING SCALE

This scale consists of six cartoonlike faces ranging from smiling to tearful (Fig. 39.2). Explain to the child that each face from left to right corresponds to a person who has no hurt up to a lot of hurt (Wong & Baker, 1996). Use the words under each face to describe the amount of pain the face represents. Next, ask the child to choose the face that best describes the child's pain and record the number under the face the child chooses. The scale is popular with young children and can be used for those as young as 3 years of age (Pagé, Katz, Stinson, et al., 2012). The scale is widely used by healthcare providers because this appeal to children makes the evidence-based tool easy to use in practice.

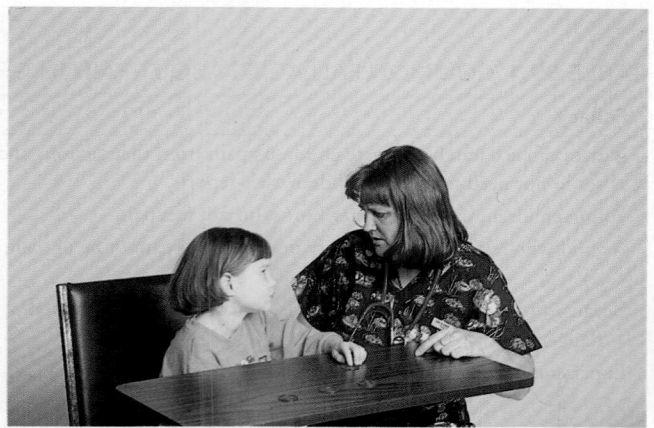

Figure 39.1 Use a pain rating tool to assess children's pain. Here, a child points to the face on the circle that represents the degree of pain she is experiencing.

0	1	2	3	4	5
No Hurt	Hurts Little Bit	Hurts Little More	Hurts Even More	Hurts Whole Lot	Hurts Worst

Figure 39.2 Wong-Baker FACES Pain Rating Scale. (Copyright 1983, Wong Baker FACES Foundation, www.WongBakerFACES.org. Used with permission. Originally published in Whaley & Wong's Nursing Care of Infants and Children. © Elsevier, Inc.)

THE OUCHER PAIN RATING SCALE

The Oucher Pain Rating Scale (Beyer, Denyes, & Villarruel, 1992) consists of six photographs of children's faces representing "no hurt" to "biggest hurt you could ever have." Also included is a vertical scale with numbers from 0 to 100. To use the photograph portion, point to each photograph and explain what each photo represents. Ask the child to point to the photo that best represents the child's degree of hurt.

To use the numbered scale portion, point to each section of the scale and explain that 0 means "no hurt," 1 to 29 means "a little hurt," 30 to 69 means "middle hurt," 70 to 99 means "big hurt," and 100 means "the biggest hurt you could ever have." Ask the child to point to the section of the scale that represents the present level of hurt. Children as young as 3 years of age can use the tool by pointing to the photograph that best describes their level of pain. If the child can count to 100 by ones and understands the concept of increasing value, the numbered scale can be used. The Oucher scale has White, Black, and Hispanic American photograph versions.

If children are most comfortable with the tool, allow them to select the version they want to use or present the version that most closely matches the cultural characteristics of the child.

THE NUMERICAL OR VISUAL ANALOG SCALE

The numerical or visual analog scale (Fig. 39.3) uses a line with end points marked "0 = no pain" on the left and "10 = worst pain" on the right. Divisions along the line are marked in units from 1 to 9. Explain to children that the left end of the line (0) means that a person feels no pain. At the other end is a 10, which means that a person feels the worst pain possible. The numbers 1 to 9 in the middle are for "a little pain" to "a lot of pain." Ask children to choose a number that best describes their pain. As soon as they can count and have a concept of "less to more," children are ready to use a numerical scale. Be certain to show school-age children the scale; do not just say score your pain from 0 to 10. Until children reach late adolescence, they use concrete thought processes and so need the help of seeing the line to rate their pain best.

THE ADOLESCENT PEDIATRIC PAIN TOOL

The Adolescent Pediatric Pain Tool (APPT) combines a visual activity and a numerical scale (Savedra, Tesler, Holzemer, et al., 1992). On one half of the form (Fig. 39.4) is an outline figure showing the anterior and posterior view of a child. To use the tool, tell a child to color in the figure drawing at the point where pain is felt. In addition, on the right side of the form, tell the child to rate the present pain in reference to "no pain," "little pain," "medium pain," "large pain," and "worst possible pain." For a third activity, tell children to point to or circle as many words as possible on the form that describe their pain (words such as horrible, pounding, cutting, and stinging). The scale is suggested for use in children 8 through 17 years of age. Because many children younger than this age group need so much help reading and interpreting the multitude of words that describe pain, it makes the form impractical for them. This is a useful tool for involving parents to talk with their child about pain. Reading the words together helps children examine the type, location, and level of pain they are experiencing. It also helps parents to better understand what their child is experiencing.

LOGS AND DIARIES

Having children keep logs or diaries in which they note when pain occurs and the intensity of the pain each time it occurs can be useful for assessing children with chronic but intermittent pain. Examining such a diary not only reveals when

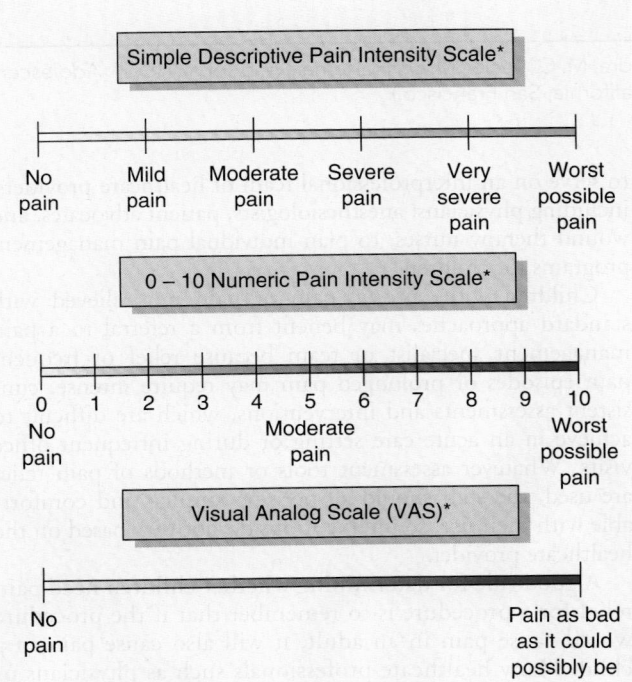

Simple Descriptive Pain Intensity Scale*

| No pain | Mild pain | Moderate pain | Severe pain | Very severe pain | Worst possible pain |

0 – 10 Numeric Pain Intensity Scale*

| 0 | 1 | 2 | 3 | 4 | 5 | 6 | 7 | 8 | 9 | 10 |
| No pain | | | | | Moderate pain | | | | | Worst possible pain |

Visual Analog Scale (VAS)*

No pain — Pain as bad as it could possibly be

*If used as a graphic rating scale, a 10-cm baseline is recommended.

Figure 39.3 Numerical and visual analog scales.

CODE _____

DATE _____

Adolescent and Pediatric Pain Tool (APPT)

1. INSTRUCTIONS

Color in the areas on these drawings to show where you have pain. Make the marks as big or as small as the place where the pain is.

Right   Left   Left   Right

2. Place a straight, up and down mark on this line to show how much pain you have.

| No pain | Little pain | Medium pain | Large pain | Worst possible pain |

3. Point to or circle as many of these words that describe your pain

1	5	10	15
annoying	blistering	awful	off and on
bad	burning	deadly	once in a while
horrible	hot	dying	sneaks up
miserable	**6**	killing	sometimes
terrible	cramping	**11**	steady
uncomfortable	crushing	crying	
2	like a pinch	frightening	If you like
aching	pinching	screaming	you may add
hurting	pressure	terrifying	other words:
like an ache	**7**	**12**	_____
like a hurt	itching	dizzy	_____
sore	like a scratch	sickening	_____
3	like a sting	suffocating	
beating	scratching	**13**	
hitting	stinging	never goes away	
pounding	**8**	uncontrollable	
punching	shocking	**14**	
throbbing	shooting	always	
4	splitting	comes and goes	
biting	**9**	comes on all of	For office use only
cutting	numb	a sudden	
like a pin	stiff	constant	BSA: _____
like a sharp knife	swollen	continuous	IS: _____
pin like	tight	forever	#S (2-9) ____ /37= ____ %
sharp			#A (10-12) ____ /11= ____ %
stabbing			#E (1,13) ____ /8= ____ %
			#T (14,15) ____ /11= ____ %
			Total ____ /67= ____ %

Figure 39.4 The Adolescent Pediatric Pain Tool (APPT). (From Savedra, M. C., Tesler, M. D., Holzemer, W. L., et al. [1992]. *Adolescent pediatric pain tool: User's manual.* San Francisco, CA: University of California, San Francisco.)

pain occurs but also provides direction for pain management. For example, if the diary shows the child always awakens with pain in the morning, the child may need a longer acting analgesic to take at bedtime; if pain is worse during weekends spent at a grandparent's house, investigate whether something different is happening in that setting than at home that could be causing increased pain.

What If . . . 39.1

The nurse asked Robin to color in a face on the FACES Pain Rating Scale that best describes her pain, and she colored in all the faces. How would the nurse best assess Robin's pain?

Pain Management

Pain management techniques, like assessment techniques, vary greatly depending on the age of a child and the degree and type of pain a child is experiencing. Many healthcare agencies employ nurses specially prepared in pain management

to serve on an interprofessional team of healthcare providers, including physicians, anesthesiologists, patient advocates, and wound therapy nurses, to plan individual pain management programs for children.

Children with chronic pain or pain not relieved with standard approaches may benefit from a referral to a pain management specialist or team because relief of frequent pain episodes or prolonged pain may require intense, consistent assessments and interventions, which are difficult to achieve in an acute care setting or during infrequent office visits. Whatever assessment tools or methods of pain relief are used, the staff should all become familiar and comfortable with their use, so interventions do not vary based on the healthcare provider.

A good rule for determining whether children need pain relief for a procedure is to remember that if the procedure would cause pain in an adult, it will also cause pain in a child. Many healthcare professionals such as physicians or X-ray or endoscopic assistants perform procedures with a child that could cause pain. Assist these team members in scheduling procedures at times when a child can be administered optimal pain relief. Help them institute nonpharmacologic measures of pain management such as distraction because often a combination of nonpharmacologic and pharmacologic methods work best (Pillai Riddell, Racine, Turcotte, et al., 2012).

General measures to alleviate pain based primarily on the gate control theory of pain management are summarized in Box 39.6. Box 39.7 shows an interprofessional care map for a child requiring pain management based on these guidelines.

What If . . . 39.2

A colleague who works with the nurse says she doesn't want to use a self-report tool with Robin because she feels that such tools replace her nursing judgment. The nurse would like her to use one. How would the nurse best justify this view to her? What are the pros and cons of pain assessment tools?

Pharmacologic Pain Relief

Pharmacologic pain relief refers to the administration of a wide variety of analgesic medications. Many children need analgesic agents in addition to nonpharmacologic techniques for pain relief, especially for acute pain. Medications can be applied topically or given orally, intramuscularly, intravenously, or by epidural injection. As a rule, intramuscularly administered analgesia should be avoided in children because children dislike injections and have a limited number of adequate injection sites. Be certain children understand that it is acceptable to ask for medication for pain because they may not know they can do so unless this is stressed by healthcare providers. Be very careful when administering pain medications to children that even if you are hurrying to provide pain relief, you use all the usual medication safeguards because mistakes can have a very serious outcome. Always check medication doses in a pharmacology reference designed specifically for children or neonates (see Chapter 38).

TOPICAL ANESTHETIC CREAM

To reduce the pain of procedures such as venipuncture, lumbar puncture, and bone marrow aspiration, a local anesthetic cream that contains 4% lidocaine can be used (Jorge, Feres, & Teles, 2011; Poonai, Alawi, Rieder, et al., 2012).

The cream is applied to the skin, and the site is then covered with an occlusive dressing or plastic wrap to keep young children from wiping away or tasting the cream. The time needed for effect between different brands varies from 30 minutes to 1 hour and so must be applied within that time frame before an expected procedure (Box 39.8). Parents can apply anesthetic cream at home before bringing a child to a clinic visit for a procedure such as bone marrow aspiration to avoid a long waiting time (Fig. 39.5). Caution them not to allow their child to remove the dressing because the cream could anesthetize the gag reflex if eaten or cause eye damage if rubbed into the eyes. They are effective with procedures such as venipuncture, intramuscular (IM), or subcutaneous injections. They also can be used effectively for pain relief with circumcision (Rosen, 2010). EMLA cream, a combination of local anesthetics, is a popular cream used but has to be applied at least 1 hour before the procedure; however, it can be applied up to 3 hours before a procedure and still be effective. A newer compound, ELA-MAX (LMX), containing only lidocaine, takes effect in 30 minutes or less (Crowley, Storer, Heaton, et al., 2011). It can be purchased without a prescription but, as an over-the-counter medication, is often not reimbursed by insurance companies.

BOX 39.6

Nursing Care Planning Based on Family Teaching

PAIN MANAGEMENT WITH CHILDREN

Q. Mrs. Harvey asks you, "How can I be sure I can keep my daughter pain free after we return home?"

A. Here are some tips on ways to offer pain relief in addition to just giving medicine:

- Let the child know you want very much to try to take away the pain and so are happy to work with her to relieve it. Use a positive approach: "This medicine will take away your pain," not "Take this and let's hope it works."
- Administer pain medication before pain becomes intense to help *prevent* pain rather than just relieve it. If a child is in the hospital, inform the staff if a particular approach works or does not work.
- Never just give an analgesic. Make the child comfortable in ways such as straightening the sheets or offering a back rub.
- Ask your child about measures she thinks will be helpful, such as an additional pillow, the television turned on, or a favorite toy nearby.
- Help your child talk about and describe the pain she is experiencing. This can help make it more concrete and not as psychologically frightening.
- Relieve anxiety about other phases of life, if possible. Relaxation reduces muscle strain and tension that can add to pain.
- Offer emotional support. Pain never seems as bad when a support person is present. Reassuring your child that she is loved and that you will be there for her can be very comforting.
- Try not to use such statements as "Be a big girl" or "Stop crying" when a child is in pain from a procedure such as an injection. Say instead, "It's all right to cry. I know it hurts," to avoid shaming a child who cannot stop crying.

BOX 39.7

Nursing Care Planning

AN INTERPROFESSIONAL CARE MAP FOR A CHILD REQUIRING PAIN MANAGEMENT

Robin Harvey, a 3-year-old girl admitted to your hospital unit, has just returned from a bone marrow aspiration to rule out the possibility of leukemia. Robin received IV morphine sulfate during the procedure. Unfortunately, the bone marrow obtained for analysis is not adequate, so a repeat procedure is scheduled for 3 hours from now.

Family Assessment: Child is only daughter of two parents. Father works as a welder in a local steel mill; mother works part-time at a local convenience store. Family rates finances as "Doing good."

Patient Assessment: A 3-year-old girl with a history of frequent nosebleeds, petechiae, and bruising admitted for diagnostic testing. First experience with hospitalization. Screams at the sight of a syringe and needle. Both parents at bedside talking with child. Child upset and crying, "Don't let them hurt me!"

Nursing Diagnoses: Anxiety related to fear of the unknown and anticipation of painful procedure.

Outcome Criteria: Child identifies pain as no higher than 1 with Oucher Pain Rating Scale; exhibits few to no nonverbal indicators of pain; exhibits age-appropriate coping behaviors, including the use of one nonpharmacologic pain relief technique.

Team Member Responsible	Assessment	Intervention	Rationale	Expected Outcome
Activities of Daily Living, Including Safety				
Nurse	Assess if IV morphine provided adequate pain relief for last procedure.	Review with parents the necessity for the repeat procedure and possible methods to help child with pain.	Being prepared for coming procedure can reduce anxiety in both parents and child.	Parents state they understand why repeat procedure must be done; are satisfied with repeat pain relief measures to be used.
Nurse	Assess vital signs and the child's present pain rating.	Engage the child in quiet activities for the first hour postprocedure.	The child is at risk for bleeding from the puncture site. Quiet activities reduce the risk for bleeding and also provide distraction.	Vital signs remain stable; pain rating is not more than 1 on child rating scale. Child colors quietly.
Teamwork and Collaboration				
Nurse/primary healthcare provider	Assess if pain management team member is available for consultation.	Consult with pain management team member for best pain relief for frightened preschool child.	Well-planned pain relief can best meet the needs of an anxious child.	Pain management team member meets with parents and child; determines best method of pain relief.
Procedures/Medications for Quality Improvement				
Nurse	Assess if repeat bone aspiration site is free of inflammation.	Apply anesthetic cream to aspiration site and cover with an occlusive dressing 1 hour before scheduled procedure.	Anesthetic cream helps reduce pain. An occlusive dressing enhances absorption and tissue penetration.	The child cooperates with application procedure. Occlusive dressing remains in place preprocedure.
Nutrition				
Nurse	Assess when the child last ate.	Keep the child nothing by mouth (NPO) for 30 minutes preprocedure.	Nausea from heavy analgesia can lead to aspiration if stomach is full.	Parents state they understand temporary restriction for fluid.

Patient-Centered Care

Nurse	Assess what the child and parents believe was most traumatic aspect of previous bone marrow aspiration.	Review with the child that a feeling of pressure with needle insertion will occur.	Anticipatory knowledge of events and feelings helps to prepare the child and aids in coping.	Parents state they feel prepared for new procedure; will support child through the procedure.
Nurse	Assess if pain assessment tool was used with child during previous procedure.	Introduce the child to Oucher Pain Rating Scale.	Introducing the child to the tool prior to the onset of pain minimizes anxiety and so can increase the tool's usefulness and accuracy in determining the level of pain.	Child rates her pain preprocedure to demonstrate she understands how to use the scale. Number sets a baseline for comparison postprocedure.

Psychosocial/Spiritual/Emotional Needs

Nurse	Assess if the child has had experience with therapeutic play.	Provide opportunities for therapeutic play with a doll and syringe before and after the procedure.	Therapeutic play helps the child express her feelings about painful procedures and possibly reduces anxiety.	The child plays with doll and syringe under nurse supervision; does not demonstrate behavior suggestive of extreme anxiety or fright.

Informatics for Seamless Healthcare Planning

Nurse	Assess if the child is free of pain postprocedure and if parents received adequate information on the outcome of the procedure.	Ask the child to rate pain on the Oucher Pain Rating Scale; ask parents if they have received a procedure report and understand the results.	A postprocedure evaluation helps to meet further needs of the child and parents and improves skills of healthcare providers.	Child rates pain as 1 or below on a pain rating scale. Parents state they have results of the procedure and they understand the next step needed for diagnosis and treatment.

What If . . . 39.3

Robin is scheduled to have blood drawn at 10 AM and, to prepare her for this, the nurse applies an anesthetic cream, which takes an hour to be effective, at 9 AM. However, the technician who will take the blood arrives early. Would the nurse ask the technician to wait, or explain to Robin that the cream is not going to work?

ORAL ANALGESIA

Oral analgesia is advantageous because it is cost-effective and relatively easy to administer. Many analgesics are supplied in liquid form and flavored with cherry or grape syrup to disguise unpleasant tastes. Caution parents that even though such drugs taste sweet, they should never refer to them as "candy." Reinforce with parents the need for proper storage (locked in a cabinet or out of the child's reach) because, otherwise, children may help themselves to more of the pleasantly flavored "candy" when the parent leaves the room. Toxicity from too frequent or overly large doses of acetaminophen is the number one reason for poisoning in small children and can lead to severe liver damage in children (Karch, 2013). If swallowing pills or large volume of liquids

is not an option, enterally dosed opioids can also be given sublingually or rectally, if appropriate.

Nonsteroidal anti-inflammatory drugs (NSAIDs) such as ibuprofen or naproxen are excellent for reducing pain because, as their name implies, they reduce inflammation as well as pain in conditions such as sprained ankles or rheumatic conditions. Long-term administration of any NSAID can lead to severe gastric irritation, so this category of analgesics should not be used longer than prescribed. Help parents giving any analgesia around the clock for several days to make out a medication sheet to hang on their refrigerator door or some other method to remind them when the next dose will be due and alert them not to give drug doses too close together.

Children should not receive acetylsalicylic acid (aspirin) for pain relief, especially in the presence of flulike symptoms, because there is an association between aspirin administration and the development of Reye syndrome, a severe neurologic disorder (see Chapter 49).

For managing severe or acute pain, such as postoperative pain or the pain of a sickle-cell crisis, opioids, such as morphine, oxycodone, and hydromorphone (Dilaudid), are frequently prescribed. Because this class of drugs is also referred to as narcotics or opioids, parents may be reluctant to give their children these medications out of concern that

BOX 39.8

Nursing Care Planning Based on Responsibility for Pharmacology

EMLA CREAM

Classification: EMLA (eutectic mixture of local anesthetics) is a topical anesthetic cream containing lidocaine and prilocaine.

Action: acts to anesthetize skin before potentially painful procedures (Karch, 2013)

Pregnancy Risk Category: B

Dosage: dollop of cream to intended skin site for at least 1 hour before procedure (2 to 3 hours before deeper procedures such as lumbar puncture or bone marrow aspiration)

Possible Adverse Effects: hypersensitivity and itching

Nursing Implications

- Explain to the child that the cream will help prevent pain during a procedure.
- Wash the site with soap and water; don't use alcohol because this removes body oil, which is necessary for the effective action of the anesthetic.
- Apply a dollop of cream to the intended site and cover with a transparent occlusive dressing at least 1 hour before the procedure. Do not rub cream into the skin.
- If the cream is to be applied at home, instruct the parents how to apply the cream and the occlusive dressing. Suggest the parents use plastic wrap for the occlusive dressing.
- Instruct the child not to touch the dressing while it is in place. If necessary, cover the occlusive dressing with an opaque material to prevent the child from touching or playing with it.
- Just before the procedure, remove the dressing and then wipe the skin to remove the cream.
- Observe the skin. Look for reddened or blanched skin, which indicates that the drug has penetrated the skin.
- Do not use the drug for a child with a known history of sensitivity or allergy to local anesthetics such as lidocaine.
- The drug is not approved for use in infants younger than 1 month, although it is frequently used for circumcisions after research showed it was tolerated well by neonates for that procedure (Rosen, 2010).

Figure 39.5 The local anesthetic cream can be applied to a child's hand and held in place with a transparent dressing at home prior to surgery. (© Sheldon Levis/Alamy.)

QSEN Checkpoint Question 39.2

SAFETY

Robin's primary healthcare provider has prescribed both an oral analgesic and an IV antibiotic for her. What is the most important thing the nurse needs to know before safely administering these medications?
a. Which medicine Robin's mother prefers
b. Robin's weight and the recommended doses based on her weight
c. Robin's precise age because some medications are not prescribed for infants
d. Robin's ability to participate in nonpharmacologic interventions

Look in Appendix A for the best answer and rationale.

INTRAMUSCULAR INJECTION

Although opiates are available as IM injections, analgesia for children is rarely given by this route because the number of suitable injection sites in children is limited, injections are associated with pain on administration, and such an injection can produce great fear in children. An IM injection also can lead to several risks, including uneven absorption, unpredictable onset of action, and nerve and tissue damage. As a rule, other routes are used whenever possible.

INTRAVENOUS ADMINISTRATION

IV administration of analgesia, the most rapid-acting route, is the method of choice in emergency situations, in the child with acute pain, and in a child requiring frequent doses of analgesia but in whom the gastrointestinal tract cannot be used. Common opioids given by this route include morphine (no common brand name), fentanyl (Sublimaze), hydromorphone (Dilaudid), and methadone (no common brand name). In equianalgesic doses, they act very similarly. Fentanyl has a shorter duration of action than the others but works quickly and produces less side effects such as pruritus and vasodilatation. These features make it an ideal drug to use for short, painful procedures, such as debriding a burn or inserting a chest tube to relieve a pneumothorax.

their child will become addicted. Acknowledge their concern but reassure them the risk for addiction during short-term use is remote. Reinforce that the main concern is supplying adequate pain relief for their child. A reminder about the consequences of undertreated pain and a discussion about how anxiety can increase levels of pain may be helpful in the discussion as well.

Opiate analgesics can be given by bolus injection or by continuous infusion. If doses will be given periodically by an IV line, advocate for the use of an intermittent infusion device to avoid repeated venipunctures with each dose or the need for a confining IV line to be in place. If a child's pain is frequent or constant so a continuous IV line is necessary, advocate for a patient-controlled pump to offer the child a sense of control and rapid analgesia. As the child becomes able to take medications by mouth, oral forms of analgesics will then be administered. When switching from IV to oral medications, be certain the oral medication is supplied in an equianalgesic dose.

All opioids have the potential to decrease respiratory rate. Other side effects include nausea, pruritus, vasodilatation, cough suppression, urinary retention, and constipation. If toxicity with opioids should occur, low-dose naloxone (Narcan), an opiate antagonist, can be administered to counteract the effects. This low dose for side effect management is a different dose than the rescue dose needed for respiratory complications.

PATIENT-CONTROLLED ANALGESIA

Patient-controlled analgesia (PCA) allows a child or a parent to self-administer boluses of medication, usually opioids, with an IV medication pump (see also Chapter 16). Children as young as 5 or 6 years of age are able to assess when they need a bolus of medicine and press the button on the pump to deliver the new dose through an established IV line. Parents or a nurse are able to administer a new dose to children younger than this as long as the child is awake. Morphine is a common analgesic used for PCA administration (Anghelescu, Faughnan, Oakes, et al., 2012). The pump is set with a lockout time so that after each dose, the pump will not release further medication even if the button is pushed again; because of this, children cannot overmedicate themselves. If pain is constant, a continuous infusion should be used so that pain relief continues even while the child sleeps. The pump can still be programmed for bolus dosing to cover episodes of increased pain.

Figure 39.6 A nurse monitors the vital signs of a child who has received conscious sedation.

free and sedated for a procedure. Unlike the use of general anesthesia, protective reflexes are left intact and a child can respond to instructions during the procedure. The technique is used for painful procedures such as dental extractions, wound care, and bone marrow aspiration, as well as for magnetic resonance imaging and endoscopy, both of which require a child to lie still for a long period of time and can be potentially frightening. Drugs used for conscious sedation can be something as common as chloral hydrate or as involved as a sedative-hypnotic-analgesic combination, which relieves both anxiety and pain and depresses the child's memory of the event. In many healthcare settings, conscious sedation is administered and monitored by nurses specially prepared in the technique (Fig. 39.6).

QSEN Checkpoint Question 39.3

PATIENT-CENTERED CARE

Robin, 3 years old, received analgesia intravenously. Her mother has asked the care team if she would possibly be a candidate for PCA. What advantage of PCA would the nurse discuss with this mother?

a. The child can gain a sense of control over his or her pain.
b. The child can have his or her pain relieved without the risk of adverse effects.
c. The child requires less nursing care in order to have his or her pain relieved.
d. The child's pain will change from acute pain to chronic pain.

Look in Appendix A for the best answer and rationale.

QSEN Checkpoint Question 39.4

TEAMWORK & COLLABORATION

Robin is scheduled for conscious sedation to have a repeat bone marrow aspiration. The nurse's colleague will accompany Robin and her mother to the procedure, and the nurse will subsequently join them and the other members of the care team. How should the nurse instruct colleagues to explain conscious sedation to Robin?

a. "You'll be given a special medicine to knock you out."
b. "I'll give you some medicine, but you will still be awake and feel everything."
c. "Conscious sedation is an analgesic, not an anesthetic, method of pain relief."
d. "I'll give you medicine so you'll be very sleepy but can still talk to me."

Look in Appendix A for the best answer and rationale.

CONSCIOUS SEDATION

Conscious sedation refers to a state of depressed consciousness usually obtained through IV analgesia therapy (Havidich & Cravero, 2012). The technique allows a child to be both pain

INTRANASAL ADMINISTRATION

Intranasal administration is becoming an attractive way to dispense medicine for children because it's easy for parents to administer and the medicine absorbs well from the nasal mucous membrane. Influenza vaccine, for example, is now available in an intranasal form (Flood, Ryan, Rousculp, et al., 2011; Wolfe & Braude, 2010). Midazolam (Versed) is a short-acting adjuvant sedative that can be administered intranasally by nasal drops or nasal spray before surgery or procedures such as nuclear medicine scanning (Karch, 2013). Because it has a very short duration of action, it may require repeat administration. Because it has no analgesic action, an analgesic should be administered concurrently if the procedure will be painful.

LOCAL ANESTHESIA INJECTION

Local anesthetics stop pain transmission by blocking nerve conduction of the impulse at the site of pain. Children receive local anesthetic injections, such as lidocaine, before procedures such as bone marrow aspiration, peritoneal dialysis, or suturing of lacerations. For many children, the sight of the anesthetic needle is so frightening that they cannot listen to the assurance that the momentary needlestick will actually prevent further pain. The use of an anesthetic cream before the injection can be helpful to relieve the needlestick pain and allow the anesthetic to numb the tissues to prevent pain (Crowley et al., 2011).

EPIDURAL ANALGESIA

Epidural analgesia, an injection of an analgesic agent into the epidural space just outside the spinal canal, can be used to provide analgesia to the lower chest, abdomen, and lower body for 12 to 24 hours or longer if needed. An opioid, often combined with a long-acting anesthetic, is instilled continuously or administered intermittently by a catheter into the epidural space. Children who have orthopedic or chest surgery, for example, may have an epidural catheter inserted in the operating room and then continue to receive analgesia by this method to relieve postsurgical pain (Wu & Raja, 2011). This is a very effective route of analgesia for the postoperative child in the first few days after surgery. Because it is commonly used for childbirth, it is discussed further in Chapter 16.

Some parents may be reluctant to allow this type of analgesia because they equate it with spinal anesthesia, which they know can cause severe headaches. You can assure them that an epidural needle does not enter the cerebrospinal fluid, so spinal headaches are extremely rare.

Nonpharmacologic Pain Management for Children

Nonpharmacologic pain relief measures (often called alternative or complementary therapies) can be used either independently or as complements to pharmacologic pain relief.

DISTRACTION

Distraction techniques aim at shifting a child's focus from pain to another activity or interest (Fig. 39.7). Blowing soap bubbles, for example, could be used during an injection to accomplish this. If oral glucose is offered to infants during painful procedures, the pain they experience appears to be significantly less (Kassab, Sheehy, King, et al., 2011). It is hypothesized that drinking glucose not only serves as a distraction technique but also activates endorphins and

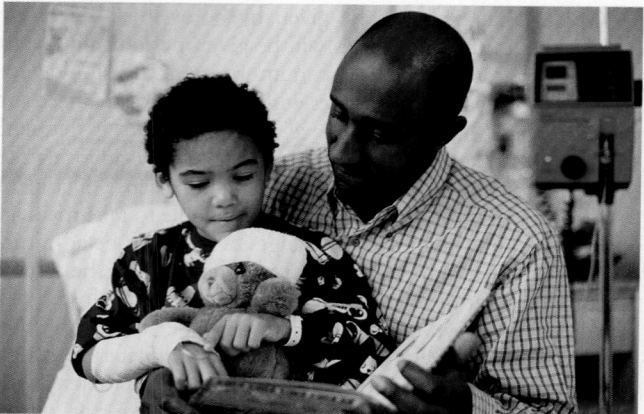

Figure 39.7 A parent using distraction (reading a book) as a pain management technique.

produces a central analgesic effect (Harrison, Beggs, & Stevens, 2012). Breastfeeding may also be used in this way but is not advised to avoid the infant making an association between breastfeeding and pain. When helping parents choose a distraction technique such as blowing soap bubbles with their child, be certain they do not interpret "distraction" as just talking to the child or suggesting a video game to divert attention. Although these are distractions, a distraction activity must require concentration; simple distractions can allow pain to break through.

SUBSTITUTION OF MEANING OR IMAGERY

Substitution of meaning or guided imagery is a distraction technique to help a child place another meaning (a nonpainful one) on a painful procedure (Kline, Turnbull, & Labruna, 2010). Children are often more adept at imagery than adults because their imagination is less inhibited. This technique works well with both quick, simple procedures such as venipunctures and chronic pain. Success with this technique requires practice, however, so it may have limited application in an acute care setting. As an example, a child could imagine a venipuncture needle as a silver rocket ship probing the moon or a submarine diving under the water to escape a torpedo just in time. Be certain a child thinks of a specific image. Help the child elaborate on the image to make it more concrete each time it is used by asking questions such as "What color is the rocket ship?" "Are there stripes on the sides?" and "What does the pilot look like?" This helps the child's mind stay on the image and not the venipuncture pain.

QSEN Checkpoint Question 39.5

EVIDENCE-BASED PRACTICE

Parents who are anxious may increase anxiety in their child during a painful procedure. To investigate whether parental anxiety affected their children, Evans, Payne, Seidman, et al. (2016) conducted a study involving 80 children, ages 8 to 29 years, experiencing pain. The study sought to identify whether variables such as solicitousness or overprotectiveness of the mother had an effect on the child's pain.

The children completed questionnaires measuring their pain and their parents' solicitousness. Maternal anxiety predicted the boys' anticipatory anxiety and pain intensity. The same results were not conclusive for girls in relation to their mother's anxiety (Evans et al., 2016).

Based on the previous study, the nurse determines which action is best when Robert has his next bone marrow biopsy?

a. Ask his mother if she and her husband would step outside the room.
b. Suggest his mother just nod her head but not talk during the procedure.
c. Ask his mother how best to draw Robert's attention elsewhere.
d. Suggest that Robert's parents avoid the words "Don't worry" when talking.

Look in Appendix A for the best answer and rationale.

THOUGHT STOPPING

Thought stopping is a technique in which children learn to stop anxious thoughts by substituting a positive or relaxing thought in its place. As with imagery, this technique requires practice before it can be used in a painful situation. It may be most helpful in relieving anticipatory anxiety, a negative force that not only increases a pain experience during a procedure but also makes the time before it full of anxiety as well. For this technique, help children think of a set of positive things about the approaching feared procedure. For a bone marrow aspiration, for example, this might include "It doesn't take long; my father will be with me; it's important to help me get better." Whenever children start to think about the impending procedure, they should stop whatever they are doing and recite the list of positive thoughts to themselves if others are present or out loud if they are alone or only important support people are present. Children can then return to a usual activity. Every time the anxious thoughts appear, however, a child should stop and recite the list again (Curtis, Wingert, & Ali, 2012).

Thought stopping is different from merely saying "Don't think about it." because the technique does not suppress thoughts; rather, it changes them into positive ones. It also gives children a feeling of control. The secret for success is for the child to use the technique every time the disturbing, anxious thoughts appear even if, at first, such thoughts crowd in as frequently as every few minutes.

HYPNOSIS

Hypnosis is not a common pain management technique with children but can be effective if a child is properly trained in the technique (Kuttner, 2012). For best results, a child needs to train with a therapist before anticipated pain, so at the time of the pain, the child can produce a trancelike state to effectively avoid sensing pain.

AROMATHERAPY AND ESSENTIAL OILS

Aromatherapy is based on the principle that the sense of smell plays a significant role in overall health. When an essential oil is inhaled, its molecules are transported via the olfactory system to the limbic system in the brain. The brain then responds to particular aromas with emotional responses. When applied externally, the oils are absorbed by the skin and then carried throughout the body. Essential oils may be able to penetrate cell walls and transport nutrients or oxygen to the inside of cells. Jasmine and lavender are oils thought to be responsible for relieving pain (Miller, Jacob, & Hockenberry, 2011).

MAGNET THERAPY

Magnet therapy is based on the belief that magnets can control or shift body energy lines to restore health or relieve pain. Magnets can be applied as jewelry or sewn into clothing or shoes. Although many people find relief from magnet therapy, the relief may be more of a placebo effect than an actual change in pain level (Lee & Raja, 2011). Copper also is believed to have pain-relieving ability and is often incorporated into rings and bracelets for this reason.

MUSIC THERAPY

The use of music for calming or improving well-being can be effective for all ages of children or adolescents, even as young as preterm infants. It works to relieve pain because it can be relaxing and also serves as a distraction (Nguyen, Nilsson, Hellstrom, et al., 2010). A child who is "blasting" music from a phone or iPad may not actually enjoy hearing the music that loud but needs that level of distraction to feel free of pain.

YOGA AND MEDITATION

Yoga, a term derived from the Sanskrit word for "union," involves a series of exercises that were originally designed to bring people who practice it closer to spirituality. It offers a significant variety of proven health benefits, such as increasing the efficiency of the heart, slowing the respiratory rate, lowering blood pressure, promoting relaxation, reducing stress, and allaying anxiety. Exercises consist of deep-breathing exercises, body postures to stretch and strengthen muscles, and meditation to focus the mind and relax the body. Yoga may be helpful at reducing pain through its ability to create total relaxation and possibly through distraction or the release of endorphins (Evans, Moieni, Sternlieb, et al., 2012).

ACUPUNCTURE AND ACUPRESSURE

Acupuncture involves the insertion of needles into critical positions (meridian lines) in the body to achieve pain relief (Chiou & Nurko, 2010). Acupressure involves applying deep pressure at the same points. Although acupuncture is almost painless, children can be very afraid of it at first because of the sight of the needles. This level of stress can make it not as attractive an option for pain management with children as acupressure. Children who consent to either technique, however, particularly those with chronic pain, report that the overall process is pleasant and the method offers relief from stress (Das, Nayak, & Margaret, 2011).

CRYSTAL OR GEMSTONE THERAPY

Some people believe gemstones or crystals have healing powers when they are arranged in certain positions around the body. If these are being used, be careful when changing bedding or rearranging equipment in a child's room that you do not tip them over or move them. A child may feel they may lose their pain-relieving powers if placed in a different position (Zuzak, Bonková, Careddu, et al., 2013).

HERBAL THERAPIES

Specific herbs are frequently used for relieving pain or for generally improving children's health. Some examples include chamomile tea (inflammation reduction), garlic (anti-inflammatory reduction, anticancer prevention), ginger (nausea or vomiting reduction), goldenrod (urinary tract inflammation reduction), or peppermint (abdominal pain relief) (Hunt & Ernst, 2011). Always ask when taking health histories if a child is being given any herbs to be informed about common herbs and to be certain what the child is receiving will complement, and not interfere with, the effects of prescribed pain medication.

BIOFEEDBACK

Biofeedback is based on the theory people can regulate internal events such as heart rate and pain in response to a stimulus (Myrvik, Campbell, & Butcher, 2012). A biofeedback apparatus is used to measure muscle tone or the child's ability to relax. Biofeedback can be effective with adolescents but is less effective with school-age and younger children because they tend to resist the biofeedback information or cannot concentrate for long enough for training to be optimal. Although some children grasp the technique in one demonstration session, most need to attend several sessions to condition themselves to adequately regulate their pain response.

THERAPEUTIC TOUCH AND MASSAGE

Massage is the use of rubbing or kneading of body parts to aid circulation and relax muscles. Therapeutic touch is the use of touch to provide comfort and relieve pain (Hall, 2012). Therapeutic touch is based on the principle that the body contains energy fields. When these are plentiful and arranged correctly, they lead to health; when they are in lesser supply, ill health results. Although therapeutic touch may serve as a form of distraction, proponents believe it is possible to redirect energy fields to increase the supply and the release of endorphins.

TRANSCUTANEOUS ELECTRICAL NERVE STIMULATION

Transcutaneous electrical nerve stimulation (TENS) involves applying small electrodes to the dermatomes that supply the body portion where pain is experienced (Ali, Drendel, Kircher, et al., 2010). When children sense pain, they push a button on a control box, which then delivers a small electrical current to the skin. The principle underlying this technique is the same as rubbing an injured part or acupressure—the current interferes with the transmission of the pain impulse across small nerve fibers.

TENS can be used to manage either acute or chronic pain. Some children (and parents) dislike TENS therapy because they are nervous about the electric current. Assure them that the current is a very mild one and will not harm their child. TENS is not recommended if the child is incontinent or has a wound that is likely to cause the electrodes to get wet. Skin should also be monitored for irritation from the TENS pads.

HEAT OR COLD APPLICATION

Cold reduces pain by constricting capillaries and therefore reducing vessel permeability and edema and pressure at an injured site. After the first 24 hours of an injury, applying heat may be more helpful because this dilates capillaries, increases blood flow to the area, and again helps reduce edema.

QSEN Checkpoint Question 39.6

QUALITY IMPROVEMENT

The algorithm on the pediatric unit for addressing pain in children includes teaching Robin guided imagery to help reduce pain. What is the rationale for using this technique to manage children's pain?
   a. Children's pain is generally not as acute as that of adults.
   b. IV pain relief is poorly distributed in children.
   c. Children's imaginations are at their peak in life.
   d. Children are typically more relaxed than adults.

Look in Appendix A for the best answer and rationale.

Ongoing Pain Relief

Because of early discharge and the increased use of ambulatory surgery, many children return home on a pain management routine. Be certain children (and parents) are provided with support and follow-up to the extent necessary to continue adequate pain management in the home. Otherwise, the lack of pain relief at home can be overwhelming.

Either oral or IV analgesia can be administered by parents in a home setting. Be certain that parents have instructions on dosing, administration, frequency, expected outcomes, and expected level of relief. Provide them with the name and telephone number of a healthcare professional whom they can call if they have questions about pain management (Johnston, Barrington, Taddio, et al., 2011).

What If . . . 39.4
The nurse is interested in exploring one of the 2020 National Health Goals related to pain management and children (see Box 39.1). Most government-sponsored money for nursing research is allotted based on these goals. What would be a possible research topic to explore pertinent to these goals that would be applicable to the Harvey family and that would also advance evidence-based practice?

KEY POINTS FOR REVIEW

- Many children and infants are undermedicated for pain relief because of common misperceptions by healthcare personnel, such as infants do not feel or remember pain. Infants do experience pain and so need pain management the same as all other groups.

- Inviting parents and the child, if preschool age or older, to participate in assessment and pain management is an important aspect of pain therapy. It not only helps in planning nursing care that meets QSEN competencies but also best meets the family's total needs.

■ Pain in children is best assessed by means of a standardized self-report tool such as the Poker Chip or Wong-Baker FACES Pain Rating Scale tools. Without self-report forms, both nurses and parents may underestimate children's pain.

■ Many nonpharmacologic pain relief measures such as imagery, distraction, and TENS are available for children based on the gate control theory of pain management.

■ Many children benefit from a combination of nonpharmacologic and pharmacologic methods of pain management such as an oral analgesic followed by a distraction technique.

■ Anesthetic cream to help dull the pain of injections or other brief procedures can be helpful to allow for suturing or venipunctures. Think ahead to use these because a child has to wait 30 to 60 minutes to feel the anesthetic effect.

■ Few analgesics are administered intramuscularly to children. For acute pain, IV administration has become the method of choice. PCA, a technique that gives a child a sense of control, can be used effectively with children.

■ Conscious sedation is useful with potentially frightening procedures. With this, protective reflexes are left intact, and the child can respond to instructions during the procedure.

CRITICAL THINKING CARE STUDY

Robert is a full-term male newborn. His parents are considering circumcision but are unsure of the procedure and the level of pain it will cause. Robert is a healthy newborn with no health issues that would contraindicate the procedure.

1. Suppose the doctor who comes to circumcise Robert doesn't like to use an anesthetic for the procedure because it requires additional time. "I've done over a thousand of these," she tells you. "Not one complained to me afterward about how much it hurt." Because she supervises the births of only a few babies a year at your healthcare facility, would you try to change her opinion?

2. Suppose your healthcare setting policy requires an anesthetic cream to be used. What could you do for comfort for Robert over and above that?

3. Nurses often sit on institutional review boards (IRBs) to approve research protocols to be certain research respects patient safety and well-being. If you were a member of a hospital IRB, would you approve a study to investigate whether a new anesthetic cream or a placebo caused less pain in newborns having circumcisions?

RELATED RESOURCES

Explore these additional resources to enhance learning for this chapter:
• Student resources on thePoint, including answers to the What If . . . and Critical Thinking Care Study questions, http://thepoint.lww.com/Flagg8e
• Adaptive learning powered by PrepU, http://thepoint.lww.com /prepu

REFERENCES

Ali, S., Drendel, A. L., Kircher, J., et al. (2010). Pain management of musculoskeletal injuries in children: Current state and future directions. *Pediatric Emergency Care, 26*(7), 518–524.

Anghelescu, D. L., Faughnan, L. G., Oakes, L. L., et al. (2012). Parent-controlled PCA for pain management in pediatric oncology: Is it safe? *Journal of Pediatric Hematology/Oncology, 34*(6), 416–420.

Beyer, J. E., Denyes, M. J., & Villarruel, A. M. (1992). The creation, validation, and continuing development of the Oucher: A measure of pain intensity in children. *Journal of Pediatric Nursing, 7*(5), 335–346.

Boerlage, A. A., Ista, E., de Jong, M., et al. (2012). The COMFORT Behavior Scale: Is a shorter observation period feasible? *Pediatric Critical Care Medicine, 13*(2), e124–e125.

Chiou, E., & Nurko, S. (2010). Management of functional abdominal pain and irritable bowel syndrome in children and adolescents. *Expert Review of Gastroenterology & Hepatology, 4*(3), 293–304.

Crowley, M. A., Storer, A., Heaton, K., et al. (2011). Emergency nursing resource: Needle-related procedural pain in pediatric patients in the emergency department. *Journal of Emergency Nursing, 37*(3), 246–251.

Curtis, S., Wingert, A., & Ali, S. (2012). The Cochrane Library and procedural pain in children: An overview of reviews. *Evidence-Based Child Health, 7*(5), 1363–1399.

Das, R., Nayak, B. S., & Margaret, B. (2011). Acupressure and physical stress among high school students. *Holistic Nursing Practice, 25*(2), 97–104.

Downey, L. V., & Zun, L. S. (2012). The impact of watching cartoons for distraction during painful procedures in the emergency department. *Pediatric Emergency Care, 28*(10), 1033–1035.

Evans, S., Moieni, M., Sternlieb, B., et al. (2012). Yoga for youth in pain: The UCLA pediatric pain program model. *Holistic Nursing Practice, 26*(5), 262–271.

Evans, S., Payne, L. A., Seidman, L., et al. (2016). Maternal anxiety and children's laboratory pain: The mediating role of solicitousness. *Children (Basel), 3*(2), 10.

Fanning, J. J., Stucke, A. G., Christensen, M. A., et al. (2012). Perioperative opiate requirements in children with previous opiate infusion. *Paediatric Anaesthesia, 22*(3), 203–208.

Flood, E. M., Ryan, K. J., Rousculp, M. D., et al. (2011). A survey of children's preferences for influenza vaccine attributes. *Vaccine, 29*(26), 4334–4340.

Hall, R. W. (2012). Anesthesia and analgesia in the NICU. *Clinical Perinatology, 39*(1), 239–254.

Harrison, D., Beggs, S., & Stevens, B. (2012). Sucrose for procedural pain management in infants. *Pediatrics, 130*(5), 918–925.

Harrison, D., Elia, S., Royle, J., et al. (2013). Pain management strategies used during early childhood immunisation in Victoria. *Journal of Paediatric Child Health, 49*(4), 313–318.

Havidich, J. E., & Cravero, J. P. (2012). The current status of procedural sedation for pediatric patients in out-of-operating room locations. *Current Opinion in Anaesthesiology, 25*(4), 453–460.

Hester, N. O., & Barcus, C. S. (1986). Assessment and management of pain in children. *Pediatrics: Nursing Update, 1*(14), 1–8.

Hunt, K., & Ernst, E. (2011). The evidence-base for complementary medicine in children: A critical overview of systematic reviews. *Archives of Disease in Childhood, 96*(8), 769–776.

Johnston, C., Barrington, K. J., Taddio, A., et al. (2011). Pain in Canadian NICUs: Have we improved over the past 12 years? *Clinical Journal of Pain, 27*(3), 225–232.

Jorge, L. L., Feres, C. C., & Teles, V. E. P. (2011). Topical preparations for pain relief: Efficacy and patient adherence. *Journal of Pain Research, 20*(4), 11–24.

Karch, A. M. (2013). *2013 Lippincott's nursing drug guide.* Philadelphia, PA: Lippincott Williams & Wilkins.

Kassab, M., Sheehy, A., King, M., et al. (2011). A double-blind randomized controlled trial of 25% oral glucose for pain relief in 2-month old infants undergoing immunisation. *International Journal of Nursing Studies, 49*(3), 249–256.

Kline, W. H., Turnbull, A., Labruna, V. E., et al. (2010). Enhancing pain management in the PICU by teaching guided mental imagery: A quality-improvement project. *Journal of Pediatric Psychology, 35*(1), 25–31.

Krechel, S. W., & Bildner, J. (1995). CRIES: A new neonatal postoperative pain measurement score. Initial testing of validity and reliability. *Paediatric Anaesthesia, 5*(1), 53–61.

Kuttner, L. (2012). Pediatric hypnosis: Pre-, peri-, and post-anesthesia. *Paediatric Anaesthesia, 22*(6), 573–577.

Lee, F. H., & Raja, S. N. (2011). Complementary and alternative medicine in chronic pain. *Pain, 152*(1), 28–30.

McCaffery, M. (1979). *Nursing management of the patient with pain* (2nd ed.). New York, NY: J.B. Lippincott.

Melzack, R., & Wall, P. D. (1965). Pain mechanisms: A new theory. *Science, 150*(3699), 971–976.

Miller, E., Jacob, E., & Hockenberry, M. J. (2011). Nausea, pain, fatigue, and multiple symptoms in hospitalized children with cancer. *Oncology Nursing Forum, 38*(5), e382–e393.

Myrvik, M. P., Campbell, A. D., & Butcher, J. L. (2012). Single-session biofeedback-assisted relaxation training in children with sickle cell disease. *Journal of Pediatric Hematology/Oncology, 34*(5), 340–343.

Nguyen, T. N., Nilsson, S., Hellstrom, A., et al. (2010). Music therapy to reduce pain and anxiety in children with cancer undergoing lumbar puncture: A randomized clinical trial. *Journal of Pediatric Oncology Nursing, 27*(3), 146–155.

Pagé, M. G., Katz, J., Stinson, J., et al. (2012). Validation of the numerical rating scale for pain intensity and unpleasantness in pediatric acute postoperative pain: Sensitivity to change over time. *Journal of Pain, 13*(4), 359–369.

Palermo, T. N., Eccleston, C., Lewandowski, A. S., et al. (2010). Randomized controlled trials of psychological therapies for management of chronic pain in children and adolescents: An updated meta-analytic review. *Pain, 148*(3), 387–397.

Pillai Riddell, P., Racine, N. M., Turcotte, K., et al. (2012). Non-pharmacological management of infant and young child procedural pain. *Evidence-Based Child Health, 7*(6), 1905–2121.

Poonai, N., Alawi, K., Rieder, M., et al. (2012). A comparison of amethocaine and liposomal lidocaine cream as a pain reliever before venipuncture in children: A randomized control trial. *Pediatric Emergency Care, 28*(2), 104–108.

Rosen, M. (2010). Anesthesia for ritual circumcision in neonates. *Pediatric Anesthesia, 20*(12), 1124–1127.

Savedra, M. C., Tesler, M. D., Holzemer, W. L., et al. (1992). *Adolescent pediatric pain tool: User's manual.* San Francisco, CA: University of California, San Francisco.

Schiavenato, M., Butler-O'Hara, M., & Scovanner, P. (2011). Exploring the association between pain intensity and facial display in term newborns. *Pain Research and Management, 16*(1), 10–12.

U.S. Department of Health and Human Services. (2010). *Healthy people 2020.* Washington, DC: Author.

van Dijk, M., Peters, J. W., van Deventer, P., et al. (2005). The COMFORT Behavior Scale: A tool for assessing pain and sedation in infants. *American Journal of Nursing, 105*(1), 33–36.

Vervoort, T., Eccleston, C., Goubert, L., et al. (2010). Children's catastrophic thinking about their pain predicts pain and disability 6 months later. *European Journal of Pain, 14*(1), 90–96.

Wolfe, T. R., & Braude, D. A. (2010). Intranasal medication delivery for children: A brief update. *Pediatrics, 126*(3), 532–537.

Wong, D., & Baker, C. (1996). *Reference manual for the Wong-Baker FACES Pain Rating Scale.* Duarte, CA: Children's National Medical Center.

Wu, C. L., & Raja, S. N. (2011). Treatment of acute postoperative pain. *Lancet, 377*(9784), 2215–2225.

Zuzak, T. J., Bonková, J., Careddu, D. A., et al. (2013). Use of complementary and alternative medicine by children in Europe: Published data and expert perspectives. *Complementary Therapies in Medicine, 21*(Suppl. 1), S34–S47.

UNIT 7

The Nursing Role in Restoring and Maintaining the Health of Children and Families With Physiologic Disorders

40

Nursing Care of a Family When a Child Has a Respiratory Disorder

Michael is a 6-year-old who is brought to the emergency department by paramedics who responded to an emergency call by his parents. The child is in respiratory distress, with obvious retractions, and he appears anxious. His parents say he has asthma and was petting a dog, to which he has a known allergy. He had several treatments with his rescue inhaler but is not improving. Michael is diagnosed with an asthma exacerbation and is treated in the emergency department.

Previous chapters described the growth and development of well children. This chapter adds information about the dramatic changes, both physical and psychosocial, that occur when children develop respiratory disorders.

What emergency care does Michael need?

KEY TERMS

adventitious breath sounds
aspiration
atelectasis
clubbing
cyanosis
expiration
hypoxemia
hypoxia
inspiration
paroxysmal coughing
percussion

pneumothorax
rales
retractions
steatorrhea
stridor
tachypnea
tracheostomy
tracheotomy
vibrations
wheezing

OBJECTIVES

After mastering the contents of this chapter, you should be able to:

1. Describe common respiratory disorders in children.
2. Identify 2020 National Health Goals related to children with respiratory disorders that nurses can help the nation achieve.
3. Assess a child with a respiratory disorder.
4. Formulate nursing diagnoses related to respiratory disorders in children.
5. Identify expected outcomes that address the priority needs of a child with a respiratory disorder to help him or her manage seamless transitions across differing healthcare settings.
6. Using the nursing process, plan nursing care that includes the six competencies of Quality & Safety Education for Nurses (QSEN): Patient-Centered Care, Teamwork & Collaboration, Evidence-Based Practice (EBP), Quality Improvement (QI), Safety, and Informatics.
7. Implement nursing care for a child with a respiratory disorder.
8. Evaluate expected outcomes for achievement and effectiveness of care.
9. Integrate knowledge of respiratory disorders in children with the interplay of nursing process, the six competencies of QSEN, and Family Nursing to achieve quality maternal and child health nursing care.

Respiratory disorders are among the most common causes of illness and hospitalization in children (Witt, Weiss, & Elixhauser, 2014). Respiratory disorders range from minor illnesses, such as a viral upper respiratory tract infection (a common cold), to life-threatening respiratory tract disease. Because the level of acuity can change quickly, respiratory deterioration or compromise must be recognized and be responded to immediately.

Because respiratory disorders are such a common cause of childhood illness and hospitalization, 2020 National Health Goals have been established for children with respiratory illnesses (Box 40.1).

Nursing Process Overview

FOR A CHILD WITH A RESPIRATORY DISORDER

ASSESSMENT

Respiratory illness can begin as early as moments after birth if a neonate has difficulty initiating a first breath or establishing regular respirations. Rating a neonate using an Apgar score can help to quickly identify a newborn who may be experiencing respiratory difficulty at this early stage.

It is important to establish both the onset and duration of the problem so that its seriousness can be determined quickly. An infant who is having difficulty feeding because of nasal congestion or a child who cannot run with other children because of shortness of breath may be having complications from a respiratory problem.

A child admitted to the hospital with a respiratory disorder is usually in an acute stage of illness. A child's condition may worsen rapidly in the first few hours until a prescribed medication, such as an antibiotic or steroid bronchodilator, begins to take effect. Nursing assessment findings that show a child is developing tachypnea or retractions may be the first indication of a child's worsening condition.

NURSING DIAGNOSIS

Nursing diagnoses established for children with respiratory disorders focus both on the alteration in mechanisms of breathing and on the emotional distress such problems can create. "Ineffective airway clearance" is a common diagnostic category used in this area. The problem may be characterized through presentations such as an ineffective/absent cough, nasal flaring, excessive sputum, or **adventitious breath sounds** (extra or abnormal breathing sounds) (Pascoal, Lopes, da Silva, et al., 2016).

Examples of nursing diagnoses include:

- Activity intolerance related to insufficient oxygenation
- Fatigue related to impaired gas exchange
- Fear related to inability to breathe without effort
- Impaired gas exchange related to excessive mucus production
- Impaired social interaction related to difficulty in keeping up with physical activities of peers
- Ineffective breathing pattern related to decreased energy and fatigue
- Deficient knowledge related to the need for continued treatment

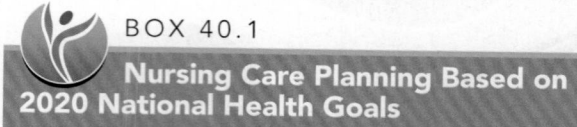

BOX 40.1

Nursing Care Planning Based on 2020 National Health Goals

Because reducing the incidence of respiratory illness in children could greatly reduce the number of emergency room visits and school days missed, a number of 2020 National Health Goals focus on respiratory illness prevention:

- Reduce hospitalizations for asthma in children under 5 years of age from a baseline of 41.4 out of 10,000 children to a target level of 18.1 out of 10,000 children.
- Reduce invasive pneumococcal infections in children younger than 5 years from 20.3 out of 100,000 children to 12.0 out of 100,000 children.
- Reduce the number of courses of antibiotics prescribed solely for the common cold from 1,728 out of 100,000 children to 864 out of 100,000 children.
- Increase the proportion of children 6 months to 2 years of age who are immunized yearly against seasonal influenza from 25% to 80%.
- Increase the proportion of children 2 to 4 years of age who are immunized yearly against seasonal influenza from 23% to 80% (U.S. Department of Health and Human Services, 2010; see www.healthypeople.gov).

Nurses can help achieve these goals by teaching children ways to help avoid respiratory infections. Prevention strategies may include good hand washing and maintaining up-to-date immunizations.

OUTCOME IDENTIFICATION AND PLANNING

If a child is experiencing an acute respiratory problem, the expected outcomes and plan of care will focus on supporting the child and family through prescribed therapy and keeping caregivers informed about their child's health status and response to treatment. Caregivers of children with chronic respiratory conditions need to learn how to continue therapy at home. Helping families plan exercise programs and learn proper medication administration use and techniques are important nursing activities. Parents also need to understand that their approach to these programs must change as their child grows older. For example, with an infant, parents simply need to perform the prescribed procedures. As a child gets older, play can be incorporated to increase the child's engagement in and compliance with respiratory treatments. Adolescents should be involved in their own plans of care to increase compliance and engagement that are appropriate for their developmental level. School needs to be considered, developing plans of care that take into consideration the available resources (i.e., school nurses) and potential limitations posed by the school day.

IMPLEMENTATION

Collaborative nursing interventions in the care of a child with respiratory dysfunction include suctioning to remove respiratory secretions, administering oxygen, and providing humidification. Various independent nursing interventions may be beneficial:

- Placing a child in an upright position to help the child cough more effectively and maintain a comfortable position
- Suctioning to remove nasal secretions

- Providing an interesting game to teach a child the importance of strengthening chest muscles
- Supporting a child and family through the anxiety created when a child is not breathing normally
- Teaching parents of a child with chronic respiratory dysfunction the basics of respiratory treatments such as percussion or chest physiotherapy techniques

All of these interventions require sound nursing judgment and skill to carry out or teach effectively.

OUTCOME EVALUATION

An acute respiratory illness can be extremely frightening for parents as well as the child. Support, reassurance, and education are important components in successful home management.

Expected outcomes for a child with chronic respiratory disease will change as a child grows and develops and may be dependent on the diagnosis and prognosis of their illness. No matter what the specific concerns are, however, evaluation should always include examination of how well an individual child and his or her family as a whole have adapted to managing the limitations imposed by the disorder while maintaining a lifestyle that fosters growth and development for all family members.

Examples of expected outcomes that would indicate achievement of goals include:

- Infant, at 3 months of age, maintains respiratory rate of at least 30 breaths/min.
- Child describes a simplified program of school activities he or she will maintain to reduce fatigue.
- Child lists steps he or she will take if breathing becomes impaired while at school.
- Parents demonstrate correct techniques for performing respiratory therapy at home.
- For the allergic/asthmatic child, the child's pulse oximetry is maintained at 94% or above with minimal wheezing.

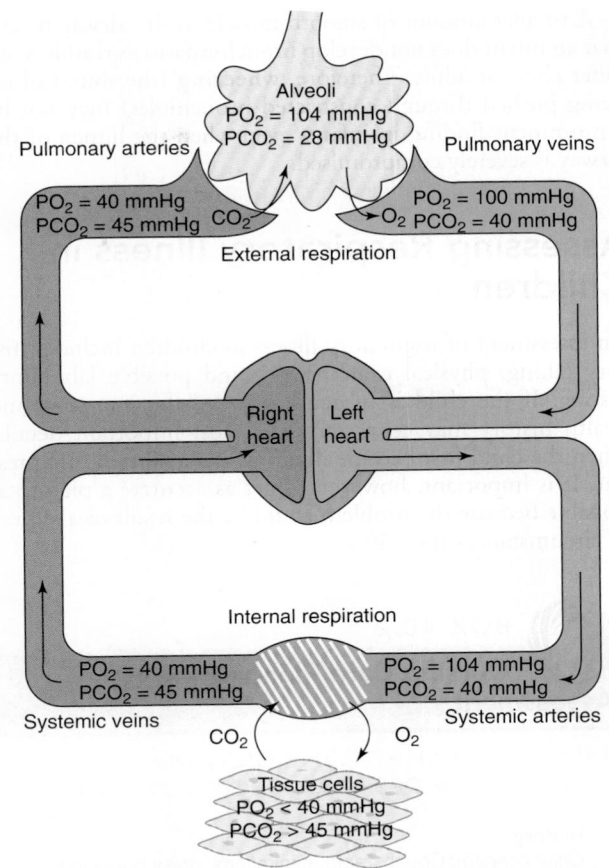

Figure 40.1 Partial pressure of gas (millimeter of mercury [mmHg]) as measured in peripheral and systemic circulation. Because of the differences in partial pressure of the gases in the different areas, O_2 moves from alveoli to pulmonary capillaries (i.e., the gas moves from the area of greater concentration to one of a lesser concentration). When it reaches the tissue capillaries, O_2 partial pressure in cells is less, so O_2 goes into the tissues and CO_2 moves out.

Anatomy and Physiology of the Respiratory System

The respiratory system can be separated into two divisions: the upper respiratory tract, composed of the nose, paranasal sinuses, pharynx, larynx, and epiglottis, and the lower tract, composed of the bronchi, bronchioles, and alveoli. Through **inspiration** (breathing in), the respiratory system delivers warmed and moistened air to the alveoli, transports oxygen across the alveolar membrane to hemoglobin-laden red blood cells, and allows carbon dioxide to diffuse from red blood cells back into the alveoli. Through **expiration** (breathing out), carbon dioxide–filled air is discharged to the outside. Levels of oxygen and carbon dioxide in the lungs, blood, and body cells are shown in Figure 40.1.

RESPIRATORY TRACT DIFFERENCES IN CHILDREN

Because the respiratory tract continues to mature during childhood, children have several important differences in respiratory anatomy and physiology from adults. The ethmoidal

and maxillary sinuses are present at birth, but the frontal sinuses (the sinuses most frequently involved in sinus infection) and the sphenoidal sinuses do not develop until 6 to 8 years of age. Because there is such rapid growth of lymphoid tissue, tonsillar tissue becomes normally enlarged in early school-age children.

An infant's airway is shaped like a funnel, with the narrowest portion at the cricoid cartilage rather than the vocal cords, as in an adult. The airway is narrower than in adults, increasing resistance if obstruction or swelling occurs, even with only small changes in the airway diameter. Infants have large occiputs when compared with an adult, which can obstruct the airway. Lying flat can put their head in a flexed position. Their tongues are large in proportion to the mouth and can more easily obstruct the airway. Infants have small nares and are obligate nose breathers until around 6 months of age. Therefore, nasal obstruction can contribute to significant respiratory distress.

The airway structures have greater laxity because of underdeveloped cartilage in the airway and a compliant chest wall that can contribute to airway obstruction and collapse.

A smaller amount of smooth muscle in the airway means that an infant does not develop bronchospasm as readily as an older child or adult. Therefore, **wheezing** (the sound of air being pushed through constricted bronchioles) may not be a prominent finding in infants even when the lumen of the airway is severely compromised.

Assessing Respiratory Illness in Children

An assessment of respiratory illness in children includes history taking, physical examination, and possible laboratory testing. If the child is in acute distress, the interview and health history may cover only the most important details: when the child first became ill and what symptoms are present. It is important, however, to get as accurate a picture as possible because the problem could be the result of a variety of circumstances (Box 40.2).

BOX 40.2

Nursing Care Planning Using Assessment

ASSESSING A CHILD FOR SIGNS AND SYMPTOMS OF RESPIRATORY DYSFUNCTION

History
Chief concern: Cough, rapid respirations, noisy breathing, rhinitis, reddened sore throat, lethargy, cyanosis, difficulty sucking, fever.
Past medical history: Poor weight gain, difficulty with respirations at birth, prematurity.
Family history: History of family member with asthma; other family members with respiratory infection.

Physical examination

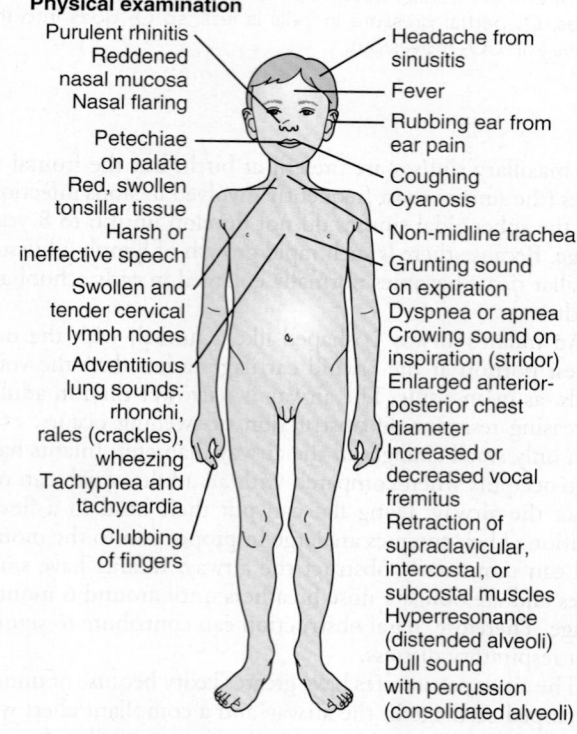

Purulent rhinitis
Reddened nasal mucosa
Nasal flaring
Petechiae on palate
Red, swollen tonsillar tissue
Harsh or ineffective speech
Swollen and tender cervical lymph nodes
Adventitious lung sounds: rhonchi, rales (crackles), wheezing
Tachypnea and tachycardia
Clubbing of fingers

Headache from sinusitis
Fever
Rubbing ear from ear pain
Coughing
Cyanosis
Non-midline trachea
Grunting sound on expiration
Dyspnea or apnea
Crowing sound on inspiration (stridor)
Enlarged anterior-posterior chest diameter
Increased or decreased vocal fremitus
Retraction of supraclavicular, intercostal, or subcostal muscles
Hyperresonance (distended alveoli)
Dull sound with percussion (consolidated alveoli)

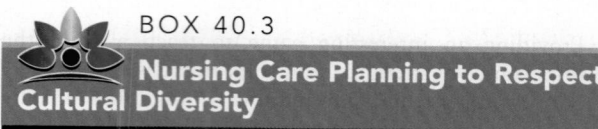

BOX 40.3

Nursing Care Planning to Respect Cultural Diversity

Upper respiratory illnesses occur universally, making them a concern of parents the world over. Home remedies for such illnesses vary greatly, however. Hanging garlic around a child's neck is a frequent therapy in Mediterranean countries. "Cupping" or applying pressure to the back to "draw out" an infection (which leaves red circular ecchymotic marks on the child's back) may be used in Asian cultures. Although the therapeutic value of these remedies may not be proved, it is important to the nurse–patient and nurse–family relationships to respect family traditions unless potential harm may be caused.

Symptoms of **hypoxemia** (deficient oxygenation of the blood), for example, are often insidious but can present with tachypnea (increased respiratory rate), decreased alertness, and decreased activity. Inability to feed because an infant cannot suck and breathe rapidly at the same time may be one of the first signs noted in the infant. Always ask about medication or homeopathic remedies used when obtaining a nursing history (Box 40.3).

PHYSICAL ASSESSMENT

A physical assessment of a child with a respiratory disorder includes generally observing the infant or child. Is he or she interactive, consolable, limp, or pale? This is followed by assessing the work of breathing. What is the child's position? Does he or she appear anxious? Does the breathing seem fast or slow? Do you see signs of respiratory distress such as retractions, nasal flaring, grunting, or gasping for breath? Breath sounds are best heard if a child is asleep or relaxed and is best done at the beginning of the physical exam, when he or she is most likely to be calm.

Cough

A cough reflex is initiated by stimulation of the nerves of the respiratory tract mucosa by the presence of dust, chemicals, mucus, or inflammation. The sound of coughing is caused by rapid expiratory air movement past the glottis. Coughing is a useful procedure to clear excess mucus or foreign bodies from the respiratory tract or as a response to gastric contents refluxed into the airway. **Paroxysmal coughing** refers to a series of expiratory coughs after a deep inspiration. Commonly, this occurs in children with pertussis (whooping cough) or in those who have aspirated a foreign body or a liquid they attempted to drink. Coughing can also be a symptom of underlying lung disease such as asthma or cystic fibrosis among others.

Some children vomit after coughing episodes (posttussive emesis), and this may be initially attributed to a gastrointestinal illness.

Rate and Depth of Respirations

Tachypnea (an increased respiratory rate) often is the first indicator of respiratory distress in young children. Assess not only the rate but also the depth and quality of respirations and other vital signs such as saturations, heart rate, and temperature.

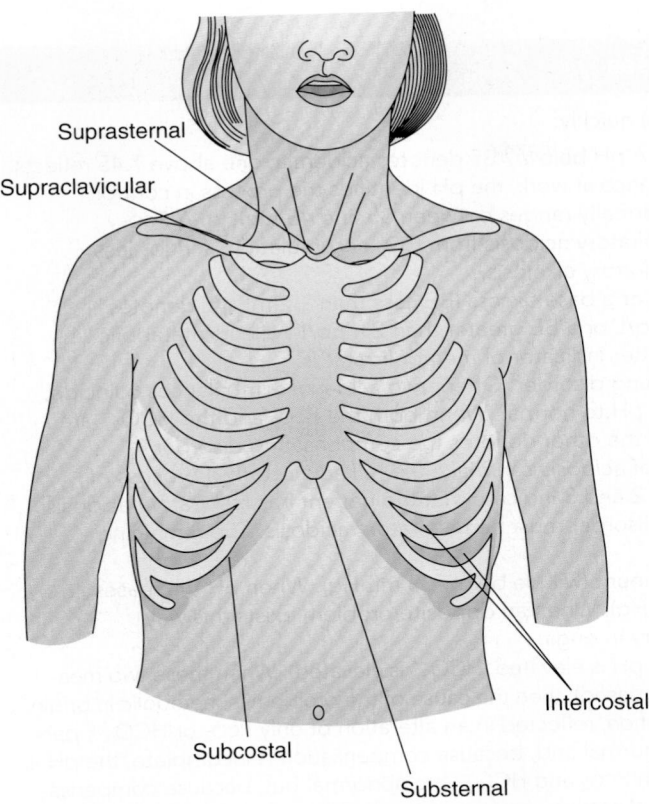

Figure 40.2 Sites of respiratory retractions.

Labels: Suprasternal, Supraclavicular, Intercostal, Subcostal, Substernal

Retractions

When children must inspire more forcefully than normal to inflate their lungs because of an airway obstruction or stiff, noncompliant lungs, intrapleural pressure is decreased to the point that the intercostal spaces draw inward, creating **retractions** (Fig. 40.2).

Restlessness

When children or infants have decreased oxygen in body cells (**hypoxia**), they can become anxious and restless. Be careful not to interpret the excessive movements of infants with respiratory distress as a sign that they are improving. Anxious or restless stirring may be a signal that respiratory obstruction is becoming acute or it may be one of the first signs of airway obstruction.

Cyanosis

Cyanosis (a blue tinge to the skin) can indicate hypoxia. If children have a low unoxygenated red blood cell count (below 5 g/100 ml), cyanosis may not be apparent because there are not enough unoxygenated red blood cells to give the arterial blood its blue tinge. The degree of cyanosis present, therefore, is not always an accurate indication of the degree of airway difficulty.

Children increase respiratory effort in an attempt to supply more oxygen to tissues.

Clubbing of Fingers

Children with chronic respiratory illnesses can develop **clubbing** of the fingers, a change in the angle between the fingernail and nail bed because of increased capillary growth in the fingertips (Fig. 40.3). The increased capillary growth occurs as the body attempts to supply more oxygen routes (more capillaries) to distal body cells.

Adventitious Sounds

Normal breath sounds are reviewed in Chapter 34. Pathologic conditions cause adventitious breath sounds (extra or abnormal breathing sounds), which can be heard on lung assessment in children with respiratory disorders.

The **vibrations** produced as air is forced past an obstruction, such as mucus in the nose or pharynx, cause a snoring sound (*rhonchi*). If the obstruction is at the base of the tongue or in the larynx, a harsher, strident sound on inspiration (**stridor**) occurs. If an obstruction is in the lower trachea or bronchioles, an expiratory whistle sound (*wheezing*) occurs. If alveoli become fluid filled, fine crackling sounds (**rales**) are heard. Diminished or absent breath sounds occur when the alveoli are so fluid filled that little or no air can enter them.

Chest Diameter

With chronic obstructive lung disease, children may be unable to exhale completely, thus allowing air to be chronically trapped in lung alveoli (hyperinflation). This produces an elongated anteroposterior diameter of the chest, sometimes termed a "pigeon breast." There is an accompanying tympanic or hyperresonant (loud and hollow) sound heard on percussion (see later discussion on chest physiotherapy) over lung spaces.

LABORATORY TESTS

Several laboratory tests can be used to confirm or rule out the presence of a respiratory disorder and to help identify the cause

Normal   Early clubbing   Advanced clubbing

Figure 40.3 Clubbing of the fingers. (*Left*) The angle between the nail and digit is normally about 20 degrees in a child. (*Center*) Flattened angle represents early stage of clubbing. (*Right*) In advanced clubbing, the nail is rounded over the end of the finger. Note also that the distal phalanx is bulbous and of greater depth than the proximal portion of the finger (interphalangeal depth).

BOX 40.4

A Quick Assessment of Arterial Blood Gases

Use a systematic format to assess arterial blood gases (ABGs) quickly:

1. Evaluate the pH: Normally, pH falls between 7.35 and 7.45. A pH below 7.35 denotes acidemia; one above 7.45 reflects alkalemia. If the patient has more than one acid–base imbalance at work, the pH identifies the process in control.

2. Evaluate P_{CO_2}: The partial pressure of arterial CO_2 (P_{CO_2}) normally ranges between 35 and 45 mmHg. A P_{CO_2} greater than 45 mmHg indicates ventilatory failure and respiratory acidosis from CO_2 accumulation. A P_{CO_2} less than 35 mmHg indicates alveolar hyperventilation and respiratory alkalosis.

3. Evaluate HCO_3: A bicarbonate (HCO_3^-) less than 22 mEq/L or a base excess (BE) less than −2 mEq/L denotes metabolic acidosis. A bicarbonate level greater than 26 mEq/L or a BE greater than 2 mEq/L reflects metabolic alkalosis. If the two measurements conflict, the BE is the better indicator of metabolic status.

4. Determine which is the primary and which is the compensating disorder: Often, two acid–base imbalances coincide; one is primary, the other is the body's attempt to return the pH to normal. When both the P_{CO_2} and the HCO_3^- are abnormal, one denotes the primary acid–base disorder and the other denotes the compensating disorder.

   a. To decide which is which, check the pH. *Only a process of acidosis can make the pH acidic; only a process of alkalosis can make the pH alkaline.* For example, if steps 2 and 3 indicate that the patient has respiratory acidosis and metabolic alkalosis and the pH is 7.25, the primary disorder must be respiratory acidosis. The remaining disorder is compensating for the primary problem.

   b. When pH rises (becomes alkalotic), P_{CO_2} decreases in amount (will be below 35 mmHg). When pH decreases (becomes acidotic), P_{CO_2} increases (will be above 45 mmHg). When an opposite problem exists this way (pH increased; P_{CO_2} decreased), the problem is respiratory in origin.

   c. pH and HCO_3^- normally move in the same direction (when pH is elevated, HCO_3^- is elevated). When these two measurements correspond this way (pH decreased, HCO_3^- decreased), then the cause of the problem is metabolic in origin.

   d. Three states of compensation are possible: *noncompensation*, reflected in an alteration of only P_{CO_2} or HCO_3^-; *partial compensation*, in which both P_{CO_2} and HCO_3^- are abnormal and, because compensation is incomplete, the pH is also abnormal; and *complete compensation*, in which both P_{CO_2} and HCO_3^- are abnormal but, because compensation is complete, the pH is normal. To identify the primary disorder when compensation is complete, consider a pH between 7.35 and 7.40 indicative of primary acidosis and a pH between 7.40 and 7.45 indicative of primary alkalosis.

5. Evaluate oxygenation: Normally, P_{O_2} remains between 80 and 100 mmHg. A P_{O_2} between 60 and 80 mmHg reflects mild hypoxemia; between 40 and 60 mmHg, moderate hypoxemia; and below 40 mmHg, severe hypoxemia.

6. Interpret the findings: Your final analysis should include the degree of compensation, the primary disorder, and the oxygenation status (e.g., "partially compensated respiratory acidosis with moderate hypoxemia").

and severity of the problem. These may include an analysis of arterial blood gases (Box 40.4), radiographs, nasopharyngeal culture, pulmonary function testing, or sputum analysis.

Pulse Oximetry

Pulse oximetry (SpO_2) is a noninvasive technique for estimating arterial oxygen saturation (SaO_2) either as a single measurement or via continuous monitoring. For the measurement, a sensor and a photodetector are placed around a vascular bed, most often a finger for a child or a foot for an infant (Fig. 40.4). Infrared light is directed through the finger from the sensor to the photodetector. Because hemoglobin absorbs light waves differently when it is bound to oxygen than when it is not, the oximeter can estimate the degree of oxygen saturation (SaO_2) (Fig. 40.5) in the hemoglobin.

One advantage of pulse oximetry is that it is noninvasive. A second advantage is that the continuous monitoring provided by a pulse oximeter allows you to modify your care appropriately. If an oxygen saturation level begins to fall while you are handling an infant, for example, you could immediately stop care until the infant's SpO_2 again returns to normal. Inaccurate pulse oximetry readings can occur because of excess ambient light in the room, dark skin pigmentation, tissue perfusion, the child's movement, and various medical conditions. It is important to remember to always monitor a

child's clinical condition, as normal pulse oximeter readings do not exclude the possibility of gas exchange problems or inadequate ventilation (Chan & Chan, 2013).

Pulse oximetry screening is recommended for all newborns prior to hospital discharge in order to increase the early detection of critical congenital heart disease.

QSEN Checkpoint Question 40.1

EVIDENCE-BASED PRACTICE

Epistaxis is a common condition encountered in pediatrics in children over the age of 2 years. Nasal infection and inflammation can be a common cause. Neoplasms and hematologic conditions are less common. In the initial assessment, if the child's airway, breathing, circulation, and neurologic status are normal and there is no trauma, treatment can be provided at home. Just like with a wound that involves bleeding, pressure on the area will facilitate clotting and prevent further bleeding. Blood allowed to enter the stomach will most likely cause vomiting (Record, 2015). Improper home care can lead to continued epistaxis or repeated episodes.

Figure 40.4 Types of pulse oximetry probes include **(A)** infant continuous, **(B)** finger continuous, and **(C)** finger intermittent.

Michael, a 6-year-old, has a nosebleed, and his parents cannot get it to stop. It has been on and off for the past 30 minutes. The child has congestion and a history of seasonal allergies. The parents have called their pediatric provider for assistance, and the advice nurse answered the call. Which action by nurse is best?

a. Advise the parent to pinch the lower part of the nose (alae nasi) for 10 minutes without releasing pressure.

b. Have Michael lean his head back to allow the blood to drain down the back of the throat.

c. Have Michael blow his nose to remove any congestion and clotted blood.

d. Have Michael stop the bleeding with ice packs applied to the face.

Look in Appendix A for the best answer and rationale.

Nasopharyngeal Culture

When done efficiently, nasopharyngeal cultures can provide valuable information about the microorganisms causing a disease. However, most children are terribly frightened by having something placed in their noses or throats and so may resist accordingly. Firm, calm support during the procedure is essential. Nose and throat cultures can reveal only the organisms present in the upper respiratory tract. As a result, they may not show organisms causing a lower respiratory tract infection. A throat culture will miss pathogenic organisms if the culture tip is not touched to the infected aspect of the pharynx.

Sputum Analysis

Because they cannot raise sputum with a cough, sputum collection is rarely feasible in children younger than school age, unless collected from an artificial airway or tracheostomy tube. Older children, however, are able to cough and expectorate sputum. Teach them exactly what you want (a specimen of what they are coughing up, not just clearing from the back of their throat). Then, ask them to breathe in and out several times, cough deeply, and spit mucus they have raised into a sterile specimen container.

DIAGNOSTIC PROCEDURES

In addition to cultures, several other diagnostic procedures are used to identify respiratory disorders in children. Many of these procedures are also used with adults, with modifications to account for the physical and developmental differences of children. Bronchoscopy (visualization of the bronchi through a bronchoscope) is discussed in Chapter 37.

Chest Radiograph

Chest X-rays will show areas of infiltration or consolidation in the lungs; if a foreign body is opaque, an X-ray study will show its location. Chest X-rays are more limited in infants than in older children because infants cannot take a breath and hold it when instructed. It is therefore difficult to picture the lungs at their most expanded position. Many other modalities are available for evaluation of the respiratory tract, such as computed tomography (CT) and magnetic resonance

Figure 40.5 The oxyhemoglobin dissociation curve.

imaging (MRI). Many factors need to be considered when deciding on other modalities, including cost, availability, and risks, such as the high amount of radiation exposure with CT and the potential need for sedation with MRI.

Pulmonary Function Studies

The process of ventilation, or the work of breathing, involves three main forces: (a) an inertial force that must be overcome to change the speed and direction of air when the lungs change from exhalation to inhalation, (b) an elastic force to help the lungs expand with inhalation, and (c) the flow resistance force or resistance to the movement of air through the bronchial tree that must be overcome. Flow resistance must be at a minimum for best ventilation. It becomes increased when the bronchioles are narrowed or plugged with mucus. Pulmonary function tests measure the forces of inertia, elasticity, and flow resistance.

The alveoli of the lungs are never completely empty at the end of expiration because as the bronchioles collapse, they trap a residual amount of air in the alveoli. In contrast, alveoli are never completely filled on inspiration because their potential for expansion exceeds that necessary for good respiratory function. Children with obstructive respiratory conditions such as asthma or bronchiolitis have some difficulty moving air into the lungs, but they have even more difficulty moving air out of the lungs so greatly expand the size of the alveoli. Even if they do expire the same amount of air as the average child, they expire it over a longer period. Children with restrictive ventilatory disorders, such as neuromuscular disorders, have equal difficulty with inspiration and expiration.

Several lung capacity studies can be done to determine the degree of obstruction or restricted ventilation ability. For these studies, the child breathes into a spirometer, a device that records the force of air exchange.

Children younger than 6 years of age are usually unable to participate in pulmonary function tests because these tests require their cooperation and understanding of the test in order to get accurate results. This limits its use in young or early school-age children. Spirometry is the most common test of lung function in children and can be done in an office or specialty setting. It measures the amount of air that can be forced out of the lungs (peak expiratory flow) in a forceful breath. Peak flow is often measured using a handheld device (peak flow meter) and is a common way to measure respiratory impairment in the office and at home. It is commonly used in children with asthma to assess impairment.

Health Promotion and Risk Management

Several ways to promote respiratory health are available for parents and children. The common cold is the most frequent respiratory disorder seen in children and is spread through families easily. Teach children as young as toddlers to help avoid spreading colds by washing their hands, properly disposing of tissues, and blocking a cough by their shirt. Yearly influenza vaccination is recommended for all infants 6 months of age and older, ideally prior to the onset of active influenza in the community. Reducing respiratory irritation by reducing exposure to secondhand smoke can help prevent upper respiratory infections and can reduce the incidence of asthma attacks as well as otitis media (middle ear infections).

Therapeutic Techniques Used in the Treatment of Respiratory Illness in Children

The primary goal of nursing interventions in the care of children with respiratory disorders is to maintain or reestablish adequate oxygenation, ventilation, and hydration. This may involve interventions aimed at clearing the airway, removing or loosening secretions. Particularly in young children, respiratory conditions may contribute to dehydration due to the inability to eat or drink due to fatigue, obstruction, or being obligate nose breathers.

HOME TREATMENTS

Any irritation of the respiratory tract causes the production of large amounts of mucus. The amount produced can become so great that the natural mechanisms for clearing it (coughing and upward cilia action) are no longer adequate. If a child is breathing rapidly because of respiratory distress, the frequent passage of air over the mucus tends to dry it and make it more viscous, thus compounding the removal problem. Instilling saline nose drops or using saline nasal sprays can be effective at moistening and loosening dried mucus in the nose (Sylvester, Carr, & Nix, 2013).

Humidification

Humidifiers are commonly used in homes for symptomatic relief of many common respiratory illnesses, although no research evidence supports their use. Humidifiers add moisture to a room by emitting a stream of fine droplets of water into the air, providing either a cool or a warm mist to the entire room. Caution parents when using a warm mist that a serious scald burn can result if children come into direct contact with the heated mist, so it should be kept out of a child's reach. Caution parents to clean humidifiers thoroughly after use to prevent the growth of mold and other contaminants in the device. Humidifiers should not be used with children with asthma because this can cause symptoms to worsen.

Inhalation Devices

Different types of inhalation devices can be used to deliver medication to the lower respiratory tract. Medication can be liquid or powder and delivered by pressure, nebulization, metered-dose inhaler, or breath actuation, depending on the illness being treated, the treatment setting, and the child's age.

Nebulizers are mechanical devices that provide a stream of moistened air directly into the respiratory tract. Most are handheld masks that fit over the nose and mouth and are attached to an electrical pump as a power source (Fig. 40.6). Metered-dose inhalers with valve holding chambers (also known as "spacers") are at least as equally effective as nebulizers in the delivery of aerosolized medications (Mudd,

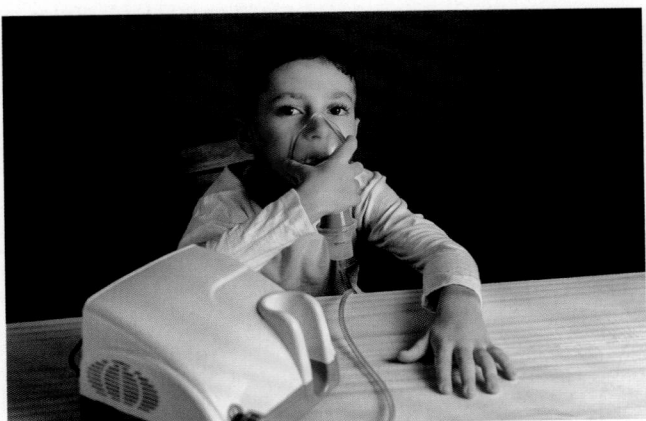

Figure 40.6 A child using a nebulizer. (Kleber Cordeiro /shutterstock.com)

Leu, Sloand, et al., 2015) and can be used with a mask or mouthpiece. Ultrasonic nebulization delivers minuscule droplets into the respiratory tract to moisten even the smallest bronchioles. Nebulizers also serve as an important means for the delivery of respiratory tract medications; medications such as antibiotics or bronchodilators can be combined with the nebulized mist and sprayed into the lungs. Young children often resist medication administration because of the need for a mask over the face. Distraction can be beneficial. It is important to monitor a child's respiratory status frequently and watch for common side effects of bronchodilators, such as tachycardia, nausea, and jitteriness.

Coughing

As a rule, encourage coughing rather than suppress it in children because it is an effective method of raising mucus. Changing a child's position and suggesting mild exercise or deep breathing are helpful techniques to initiate coughing. Cough and cold preparations are not recommended in children less than 6 years of age because of both the lack of evidence of their effectiveness and their potential harmful side effects.

Mucus-Clearing Devices

A mucus-clearing device (a Flutter device) can be used to aid in the removal of mucus. This device looks like a small plastic pipe. A stainless-steel ball inside the device moves when the child breathes out, causing vibrations in the lungs (Fig. 40.7). This vibration helps loosen mucus so that it can be moved up the airway and expectorated. This device is used most frequently with children who have cystic fibrosis or pneumonia to help remove mucus from the lungs.

Chest Physiotherapy

Simply changing a child's position helps mucus to move, initiate a cough reflex, and be expelled and to prevent mucus from pooling in certain lung areas. If a child has a localized mucus problem, lying predominantly in one position can encourage drainage of that lung segment. When the child is repositioned and the mucus drains into new bronchi, this will often result in a cough from irritation caused by this new drainage.

Three techniques are involved with chest physiotherapy (CPT) to further loosen mucus for expectoration: postural drainage, percussion, and vibration. Each technique can be used alone, but they are usually more effective at moving mucus toward the main stem bronchus when performed together.

Although CPT is usually done by respiratory therapists, you will need to integrate the activity into care because CPT is best scheduled before meals or at least an hour after a meal so the subsequent coughing does not cause vomiting.

Common postural drainage positions for the infant are shown in Figure 40.8. An infant may be positioned on your lap, whereas a slant board or other surface is needed for postural drainage with an older child. **Percussion** involves striking a cupped or curved palm against the chest to determine the consistency of tissue beneath the surface area. This technique causes a loud, thumping noise that sounds as if it hurts, but you can assure a child or parents it does not. In infants and some small children, a specialized device, a nipple, or a small oxygen mask may be used if the palm of the hand is too big (Fig. 40.9). These devices concentrate the motion and may increase the amount of mucus removed.

Vibration is done by pressing a vibrating hand against a child's chest during exhalation. Like percussion, it mechanically

Figure 40.7 (A) Flutter device. The metal ball (shown) is enclosed in the chamber and causes the vibration. **(B)** An adolescent using a flutter device.

Figure 40.8 Positions for bronchial drainage for major segments of all lobes in infants. This procedure is most readily performed with the infant in your lap, with your hand on the chest over the area to be cupped or vibrated. **(A)** The apical segment of left upper lobe. **(B)** The posterior segment of left upper lobe. **(C)** The anterior segment of left upper lobe. **(D)** The superior segment of right lower lobe. **(E)** The posterior basal segment of right lower lobe. **(F)** The lateral basal segment of right lower lobe. **(G)** The anterior basal segment of right lower lobe. **(H)** The medial and lateral segments of right middle lobe. **(I)** The lingular segments (superior and inferior) of left upper lobe.

loosens and helps move tenacious secretions upward. Vibration also may be accomplished by a mechanical vibrator or a vibrating vest.

If a child is going to need continued CPT at home, one or both parents will need to learn the technique before their child is discharged so that it can be continued conscientiously. The technique is used most frequently with children with bronchiolitis or cystic fibrosis.

What If . . . 40.1
Michael needs to cough to expectorate bronchial mucus but he refuses to try to cough. What are possible ways the nurse can encourage Michael to expectorate effectively?

THERAPY TO IMPROVE OXYGENATION

Improving oxygenation almost automatically relieves breathing distress.

Oxygen Administration

Oxygen administration elevates the arterial oxygen saturation level by supplying more oxygen to red blood cells through the respiratory tract.

Nasal cannulas provide a concentration of approximately 50%, with an oxygen flow of 4 L/min. Most children do not like nasal prongs or catheters because they are intrusive. Assess their nostrils carefully when using these as the pressure of prongs can cause areas of necrosis, particularly on the nasal septum.

Figure 40.9 Alternative percussion device. To assist with percussing an infant or small child, a nipple or mask such as that from a manual resuscitation bag may be used.

A snug-fitting oxygen mask (non-rebreather mask) is a method for supplying nearly 100% oxygen and is used in emergencies (Fig. 40.10). Masks, like prongs or catheters, are often not well tolerated by children because they tend to slip and obstruct their view.

Without proper humidification, oxygen dries mucous membranes and thickens secretions, compounding breathing difficulty. Oxygen, like any other drug, requires careful administration and a follow-up assessment. If concentrations are too low, oxygen is not therapeutic; in concentrations greater than those desired, it can be toxic. If newborns are subjected to oxygen concentrations over 100 mmHg for an extended time, retinopathy of prematurity can occur (see Chapter 26). In any child, administering oxygen concentrations of 70% to 80% for an extended period may lead to a thickening of the lung alveoli and a loss of lung pliancy (i.e., oxygen toxicity or bronchopulmonary dysplasia). For these

reasons, oxygen should not be given in high concentrations for long periods without careful monitoring.

When caring for a child with any form of oxygen equipment, follow safety rules. Because oxygen supports combustion, keep open flames away from oxygen and minimize the risks of sparks. Because oxygen is humidified, the equipment is a good source of microbial contaminants and so should be changed according to your agency's policy to keep bacterial counts within safe limits.

Pharmacologic Therapy

Children experience difficulty with exchange of air when their airways become obstructed because of unusual mucus production, bronchoconstriction, or inflammation. Several drugs may be used in children to reverse these processes. Nasal sprays such as normal saline can be administered to moisten and loosen nasal secretions. Antihistamines can reduce mucus production in the presence of allergies. Corticosteroids taken either orally or by inhalation can reduce airway inflammation. Brief use of nasal decongestants may be advised, but no data support the use of oral decongestants in children. Bronchodilators such as albuterol (Ventolin), terbutaline (Brethine), and levalbuterol (Xopenex) are examples of drugs used to open the lower airway. Antibiotics may be ordered if the illness is caused by a bacterial infection. Because so many different approaches are available to aid breathing, parents can be confused about the action of each medicine their child is prescribed. Caution them it is unsafe to give cough and cold medications to children younger than 4 years of age unless specifically prescribed by their healthcare provider because of the decreased breathing efforts these may cause (Centers for Disease Control and Prevention, 2012).

Metered-Dose Inhalers

A metered-dose inhaler (MDI) is a handheld device that provides a route for medication administration directly to the respiratory tract. The child inhales while depressing a trigger

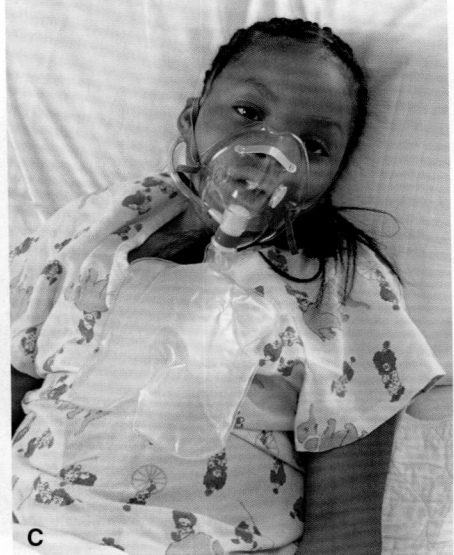

Figure 40.10 Types of oxygen administration include **(A)** simple oxygen mask, **(B)** nasal cannula, and **(C)** a rebreather mask (oxygen trapped in the bag increases the amount of oxygen available to the child).

Figure 40.11 **(A)** Many children use a metered-dose inhaler to administer a bronchodilator to themselves. Be certain children respect such medicine as medicine so they use sensible precautions. **(B)** Children need a "spacer" with inhalers.

on the apparatus. For successful use, children need to follow five general rules: shake the canister, exhale deeply, activate the inhaler and place it in their mouth as they begin to inhale, take a long slow inhalation, and then hold their breath for 5 to 10 seconds. Caution them to take only one puff at a time, with a 1-minute wait between puffs (Berlinski, 2017). Coordinating inhalation with MDI use can be difficult; therefore, use of an aerochamber (spacer) is generally recommended to prevent deposition on the posterior pharynx (National Heart, Lung, and Blood Institute [NHLBI], 2007) (Fig. 40.11). Younger children can use an MDI attached to an aerochamber with a mask. All children using inhaled corticosteroids need an aerochamber to prevent deposition of the medication in the mucous membranes of the mouth and pharynx, which can contribute to the development of thrush.

Incentive Spirometry

Incentive spirometers are devices that encourage children to inhale deeply to aerate the lungs fully or to move mucus. Although manufactured in different configurations, a common type consists of a hollow plastic tube containing a brightly colored ball or dome-shaped disk that will rise in the tube when a child inhales through the attached mouthpiece and tubing. The deeper the inhalation, the higher the ball rises in the tube.

Children need instruction on how to use this type of device because their first impression is that they should blow out against the mouthpiece rather than inhale (Fig. 40.12A). Incentive spirometry can be very effective with children because the device and procedure resemble a game more than an actual treatment.

Figure 40.12 **(A)** Incentive spirometry is an appealing method to encourage children to aerate their lungs. **(B)** Encouraging children to take a deep breath and try to blow a cotton ball across the table is also an entertaining way to help them fully expand their lungs.

Breathing Techniques

Some children need exercises prescribed to help them better inflate or more fully empty alveoli. Blowing a piece of cotton or a plastic ball across a table, blowing through a straw, or blowing out with the lips pursed are effective techniques for better emptying alveoli (Fig. 40.12B). For best results, make these activities a game or contest rather than an exercise.

Endotracheal Intubation

Endotracheal intubation (nasal or oral intubation) is a means of securing an airway in a child who is unable to oxygenate and/or ventilate adequately on his or her own. A tube is inserted into the trachea. The technique for this is discussed in Chapter 26, as this is the method used for newborn resuscitation. Because of risks of infection, injury, and impairment of mobility, endotracheal tubes (ETTs) cannot be left in place as a permanent solution. Children cannot speak while intubated and may need sedation. Supply those old enough to write with a pencil and paper for effective communication. Preschoolers can point to pictures to indicate what they need. Providing simple drawings or photos (a blanket, the television turned on, a urinal) to make needs known is helpful. ETTs are held in place by being taped to the face. Make sure tubes are carefully secured; otherwise, children can easily dislodge them.

ETTs may need to be suctioned using sterile technique in order to remove accumulated airway secretions. This should be done only as needed because it can have negative effects on children, including pain, infection, neurologic changes (due to increased intracranial pressure), bradycardia, and others.

A capnometer is a device that uses infrared technology and is attached to the distal end of the tube to measure the amount of CO_2 in exhaled breaths. By measuring the percentage of CO_2 in expired air, the arterial CO_2 (PCO_2) can be estimated. This can help ensure correct placement of an ETT at the time of placement and for ongoing monitoring.

Tracheostomy

A **tracheostomy** is an opening into the trachea to create an artificial airway. It is most often performed in infants who require prolonged ventilation but can provide a more stable airway in older children as well (Mitchell, Hussey, Setzen, et al., 2013). The procedure to create the airway is called a **tracheotomy**, and the resultant artificial airway is called the tracheostomy. Except in rare emergency situations, it is performed in a controlled setting in an operating room (Mitchell et al., 2013). Tracheostomy tubes come in different lengths and diameters (Fig. 40.13). Selection is based on a number of factors including the child's size, lung compliance, and developmental needs (such as talking) (Mitchell et al., 2013).

Humidification may be needed for some children and can be done with a tracheostomy collar or through the ventilator tubing, if a child needs mechanical ventilation. Parent education for tracheostomy care should start prior to placement and be reassessed prior to discharge. Tracheostomy tube ties should be used to prevent accidental dislodgment, the most common complication with tracheostomies (Mitchell et al., 2013). Stoma care is needed during the postoperative period. Cleaning is generally done with a cotton-tipped applicator and saline. Children will need reassurance after tracheostomy tube placement.

Figure 40.13 (A) Tracheostomy tubes: (*left*) a plastic tube, inner cannula, and obturator; (*right*) a plastic, cuffed tube. **(B)** The tracheostomy collar allows for humidification of inspired air or supplemental oxygen.

Suctioning Technique

Most tracheostomy tubes used with children today are plastic and have an inflatable cuff that helps to prevent dislodgment. Suctioning may be needed if secretions are seen or heard. The nurse should be prepared with appropriate equipment prior to suctioning, including a suction catheter, an appropriately sized bag-valve mask, an oxygen source, and a tracheostomy kit. Use sterile technique to prevent introducing microorganisms, although clean technique is generally taught to caregivers for home suctioning.

Tracheostomy tubes are held in place by cloth ties that fasten at the back of the child's neck. Change ties when they become soiled or loose and check them frequently to be certain they remain tied. Children may fuss with and untie such things, whereas adults will not. Assess that the ties not only fit snugly but also allow for one finger to be inserted underneath them so they do not rub and cause pain. For preschoolers or younger children, it is a good idea to cover the tracheostomy opening with a gauze square tied to the child's neck like a bib while they eat to prevent crumbs or spilled liquids from entering the tracheostomy opening.

Caution parents:
- Not to give their child small toys that could fit into the lumen of the tube and cause obstruction
- To keep the use of sprays such as room fresheners to a minimum so they won't be irritating to the exposed trachea
- To keep cold air from blowing against the tracheostomy opening because this can cause tracheal spasm (e.g., cover the child's throat with a loose fleece scarf when outside in cold weather)

- To inspect stuffed toys to be certain they are intact and do not shed (e.g., fur or stuffing could enter the tube)
- To supervise play with other children so they don't place anything in the tube. Stay with the child in the bathtub to be certain water does not splash into the tube.

When caring for children with tracheostomies, check on them frequently to assess for possible respiratory difficulty. Spend time playing with them or just sitting and rocking them so they can think of you in ways other than as the person who comes to suction them. If parents cannot stay with the child, assure them that you check on their child more frequently than what is necessary for suctioning alone, so they can feel confident if the child should have another episode of acute obstruction, someone will be nearby. If the tracheostomy tube is to be left in place after discharge from the hospital, be certain parents have enough experience with changing tubes if that will be necessary or suctioning so they can safely care for their child at home (Peacock & Stanik-Hutt, 2013).

Each child is considered individually with regard to when it is time to remove a tracheostomy tube.

Occasionally, a tracheostomy tube becomes dislodged. This can be a medical emergency in the immediate postoperative period, when the tract is not well formed, but not necessarily so after a tract is well established. Always keep a new tube and inserter (obturator) at the bedside so these are available if replacement is necessary. Slide the obturator into the tube and gently replace it in the tracheal opening. Remove the obturator and secure the new tube in place.

Assisted Ventilation

When children cannot oxygenate and/or ventilate effectively, assisted ventilation may be necessary. Positive-pressure machines deliver moistened or nebulized air or oxygen to the lungs under enough pressure and with appropriate timing to produce artificial, periodic inflation of alveoli, and they rely on the elastic recoil of the lungs to empty the alveoli.

Noninvasive ventilation is the preferred method of ventilation with children, although if ventilation will be used for a prolonged period, children will usually require either a tracheotomy or endotracheal intubation (Fig. 40.14). Infants need a nasogastric tube inserted to prevent stomach distention from air entering the esophagus with a ventilator in place. Providing adequate nutrition may be a challenge, but enteric (nasogastric) feedings or total parenteral nutrition solves this concern. Providing a balance of rest, stimulation, and assurance for the child is a challenge for nursing personnel and parents.

Figure 40.14 An infant with an endotracheal tube receiving assisted ventilation.

LUNG TRANSPLANTATION

Lung transplantation is a possibility for children with a chronic respiratory illness such as cystic fibrosis (Vandemheen, Aaron, Poirier, et al., 2010). The transplant may involve a single lung or both lungs, or it can be done in conjunction with heart transplantation if chronic respiratory disease has caused ventricular hypertrophy of the heart. The donor lung can be from a live donor or a cadaver.

As with any organ transplantation, children need continued immunosuppression therapy following a lung transplant to decrease cell-mediated immunity. Although this level of immunosuppression is the key to successful transplantation, it also makes posttransplant children susceptible to fungal, bacterial, and viral lung infections. In addition, families experience a tremendous psychosocial toll as they wait to see whether the new transplant will be rejected. With the transplanted lung in place, children may need to have CPT or use a portable spirometry device daily to help mobilize secretions resulting from loss of nerve innervation or a reaction to accumulating mucus in the transplant.

Disorders of the Upper Respiratory Tract

The upper respiratory tract warms, humidifies, and filters the air that enters the body (Fig. 40.15). Because the structures of the upper respiratory tract constantly come into contact with a barrage of foreign organisms, including pathogens, this can lead to airway irritation and infection. Congenital malformations of respiratory structures also cause some upper respiratory tract disorders.

CHOANAL ATRESIA

Choanal atresia is congenital obstruction of the posterior nares by an obstructing membrane or bony growth, which prevents a newborn from drawing air through the nose and

Figure 40.15 Structures of the upper respiratory tract.

down into the nasopharynx (Eladl, 2010). It may occur either unilaterally or bilaterally.

Newborns up to approximately 3 months of age are naturally nose breathers, so infants born with choanal atresia almost immediately develop signs of respiratory distress after birth as they attempt to breathe through their nose for the first time. Passing a soft #8 or #10 French catheter through the posterior nares to the stomach is a part of birthing room procedure in many healthcare facilities and confirms immediately that no atresia is present.

Choanal atresia can also be assessed by holding the newborn's mouth closed and then gently compressing first one nostril and then the other. If atresia is present, infants will struggle as they experience air hunger when their mouth is closed. Their color improves when they open their mouth to cry. Atresia is also suggested if infants struggle and become cyanotic at feedings because they cannot suck and breathe through the mouth simultaneously.

The treatment for choanal atresia is either local piercing of the obstructing membrane or surgical removal of the bony growth. Because infants with choanal atresia have such difficulty with feeding, they may receive intravenous (IV) fluid to maintain their glucose and fluid level until surgery can be performed.

ACUTE NASOPHARYNGITIS (COMMON COLD)

The common cold is the most frequent infectious disease in children. Toddlers can have as many as 10 to 12 colds a year. School-age children and adolescents have as many as 8 to 10 yearly because infection is spread so readily in classrooms. The incubation period for the common cold is typically 2 to 3 days, and most occur in the fall and winter, when respiratory viruses circulate.

Upper respiratory infections are caused by several viruses, most predominantly rhinovirus, respiratory syncytial virus (RSV), adenovirus, parainfluenza viruses, and influenza viruses. Children who are in ill health from some other cause, or who have a compromised immune system, are more susceptible than others to viral infection.

Assessment

Symptoms begin with nasal congestion, a watery rhinitis, and a low-grade fever. The mucous membrane of the nose becomes edematous and inflamed, constricting airway space and causing difficulty breathing. Posterior rhinitis, plus local irritation, leads to pharyngitis (sore throat). As upper airway secretions drain into the trachea, this leads to a cough. Cervical lymph nodes may be swollen and palpable. Although fever typically lasts only a few days, respiratory symptoms generally last for about a week. Previous viral upper respiratory infections can be a precursor to development of a secondary bacterial infection in young children, such as ear infections.

Therapeutic Management

No specific treatment is available for a common cold. Antibiotics are not effective against viral illnesses, unless a secondary bacterial infection is present. If a child has a fever that is causing discomfort, it can be alleviated by an antipyretic such as acetaminophen or ibuprofen. Help parents understand these drugs are effective only in controlling pain, discomfort, and fever symptoms; they do not reduce congestion or "cure" the cold. Children younger than 18 years of age should not be given acetylsalicylic acid (aspirin) because this is associated with the development of Reye syndrome, a potentially fatal neurologic disorder (see Chapter 49).

If infants have difficulty nursing because of nasal congestion, saline nose drops or nasal spray may be prescribed to liquefy nasal secretions and help them drain. Removing nasal mucus via a bulb syringe before feedings also allows infants to breathe more freely and be able to suck more efficiently.

Children's cough and cold preparations are generally not recommended. Little evidence indicates that oral decongestants relieve congestion to an appreciable degree with the common cold. Parents may use a cool mist vaporizer to help loosen nasal secretions if they wish. The efficiency of home vaporizers is questionable, however, and safe use of a vaporizer, including proper cleaning, must be stressed, or it can serve as a reservoir for microorganisms.

 ## Nursing Diagnoses and Related Interventions

Nursing Diagnosis: Parental health-seeking behaviors related to management of child's upper respiratory symptoms

Outcome Evaluation: Parents state intention to use cool mist vaporizer to loosen secretions, to encourage oral fluid, to administer an antipyretic to provide comfort, and to avoid cough medicine.

Care of the child with a cold is primarily supportive until the infection runs its course. Because they may have a loss of appetite, children may prefer simple liquids to solid food for the first few days of the illness. Parents generally ask whether children should remain on bed rest. Children characteristically restrict their activity when ill, so with acute cold symptoms, children often naturally curl up on the couch and sleep. One of the best ways parents can judge when children are improving is to note they have begun to increase their activity or are "acting like themselves" again.

A possible complication of a cold is otitis media (middle ear infection) because the common precursor for otitis media is a viral upper respiratory tract infection. Instruct parents about this possibility and the need to report symptoms suggestive of this infection, such as fussiness, irritability, sudden elevated temperature, and ear pain.

QSEN Checkpoint Question 40.2

QUALITY IMPROVEMENT

Michael's history reveals he was born with choanal atresia. What assessment may be performed at birth to determine whether a newborn has this condition?
 a. Observe if the infant can breathe well while lying in a prone position.
 b. Close the infant's mouth and observe if he can breathe through his nose.
 c. Assess if the infant's palatine tonsils are blocking the back of the throat.
 d. Listen for the sound of either stridor or wheezing upon inhalation.

Look in Appendix A for the best answer and rationale.

PHARYNGITIS

Pharyngitis is infection and inflammation of the throat. The peak incidence occurs between 5 and 15 years of age in winter and spring, with an incubation period of 2 to 5 days. It may be either bacterial or viral in origin. It may occur as a result of a chronic allergy in which there is constant postnasal discharge that results in a throat irritation.

Viral Pharyngitis

The causative agent of pharyngitis is usually a virus. The symptoms are generally mild: a sore throat, fever, rhinorrhea, cough, and general malaise. On a physical assessment, regional lymph nodes may be enlarged. Erythema will be present in the back of the pharynx and the palatine arch. Exudate may or may not appear on the tonsils. Laboratory studies are generally not indicated.

If the inflammation is mild, children rarely need more than an oral analgesic such as acetaminophen or ibuprofen for comfort. By school age, children are capable of gargling with a solution such as warm water to help reduce the pain. Before this age, children tend to swallow the solution unless the procedure is well explained and demonstrated to them.

Because of throat pain, food intake may be diminished, so focus needs to be on adequate oral hydration.

Streptococcal Pharyngitis

Group A β-hemolytic streptococcus is the organism most frequently involved in bacterial pharyngitis in children, particularly those between the ages of 5 and 15 years.

Assessment

Streptococcal infections are generally more severe and present more suddenly than viral infections. The back of the throat and palatine tonsils are usually markedly erythematous (bright red); the tonsils are enlarged, and there may be a white exudate in the tonsillar crypts. Petechiae may be present on the palate. A child typically appears ill, with a fever, sore throat, headache, stomach ache, and difficulty swallowing. Other respiratory symptoms are generally absent, such as cough, congestion, rhinorrhea, or conjunctivitis. A rapid antigen test and/or throat culture should be done to confirm the presence of the *Streptococcus* bacteria. These findings may vary depending on the child's age and make it difficult to distinguish it from a viral illness. Some children may develop a sandpaper-like rash (scarlatiniform rash) on the body.

Therapeutic Management

Streptococcal pharyngitis is treated with antibiotics, such as a penicillin or cephalosporin, along with supportive treatments such as those discussed for viral pharyngitis. Although rare, streptococcal infections can lead to acute rheumatic fever and glomerulonephritis if not treated. Antibiotic treatment may help decrease the occurrence of these diseases and shorten the duration of symptoms.

QSEN Checkpoint Question 40.3

TEAMWORK & COLLABORATION

Michael has had two recent streptococcal pharyngitis infections. Education on the importance of completing

the full course of prescribed antibiotics is necessary to prevent which complication?
   a. Epiglottitis
   b. Dental abscesses
   c. Rheumatic fever
   d. Emphysema

Look in Appendix A for the best answer and rationale.

Retropharyngeal Abscess

The retropharyngeal lymph nodes, which drain the nasopharynx, are located just behind the posterior pharynx wall. Although uncommon, an abscess can form in these lymph nodes and may constitute a medical emergency as it may impact the airway.

Assessment

The presentation may be a high fever, refusal to eat, and may drool because they cannot swallow saliva past the obstruction in the back of their throat. They begin to "snore" with respirations as the pharynx becomes further occluded. To allow themselves more breathing space, they may hyperextend the head, which is a very unusual position for infants.

A physical assessment may reveal swelling on one side of the neck but may require further evaluation with radiographs to further evaluate.

Therapeutic Management

IV antibiotic treatment and hospitalization is needed for these infants to monitor hydration and their respiratory status. Although some retropharyngeal abscesses will resolve with antibiotic treatment, some will need surgical drainage.

Tonsillectomy

Tonsillectomy is removal of the palatine tonsils. *Adenoidectomy* is removal of the pharyngeal tonsils. Frequent throat infections or tonsillar hypertrophy that cause breathing problems are common reasons for removal of the tonsils. Adenoids may be removed if they are so hypertrophied they cause obstruction or sleep apnea.

During a tonsillectomy, tonsillar tissue is removed by ligation or by laser surgery. Because sutures are not usually placed, the chance for hemorrhage after this type of surgery is higher than after surgery involving a closed incision. The danger of aspiration of blood at the time of surgery and the danger of a general anesthetic also compound the risk.

Nursing Diagnoses and Related Interventions

Nursing Diagnosis: Risk for fluid volume deficit related to blood loss from surgery

Outcome Evaluation: Child's pulse and blood pressure remain normal for age; there is an absence of extensive bleeding; intake and output are within acceptable parameters.

Tonsillectomies are done as ambulatory or 1-day surgery following completion of a history and physical examination and laboratory tests, including bleeding and clotting times, complete blood count, and urinalysis. An important aspect of the presurgery assessment is to observe for loose teeth because, if present, these could be dislodged during surgery and aspirated. Make certain the presence of loose teeth is noted in the child's electronic record so the anesthesia provider can be aware of this.

Following surgery, observe vital signs carefully to make certain the child is not bleeding from the surgical site.

If hemorrhage should occur after tonsillectomy, it can be acute and intense. Because children swallow any blood that is oozing from the surgical site, a child can be bleeding heavily, however, and yet, little blood will be apparent. To detect if the child is bleeding, assess for subtle signs of hemorrhage, such as an increasing pulse or respiratory rate, frequent swallowing, throat clearing, or a feeling of anxiety. If you find that the surgical site is bleeding, elevate the child's head to reduce vascular pressure on the operative site and notify the child's primary care provider.

If children have no complications from surgery, are able to swallow fluids, and have voided, they are discharged later the same day of surgery. Be certain parents have received careful instructions concerning the danger signs to watch for during the first day home (e.g., frequent swallowing, clearing the throat, bleeding, increasing restlessness, severe pain). They are usually also advised to restrict their child's activity for a set period of time or until surgical follow-up (e.g., no gymnastics, no competitive sports).

Nursing Diagnosis: Pain related to surgical procedure

Outcome Evaluation: Child states level of pain is tolerable.

A tonsillectomy is an uncomfortable and painful procedure. Be certain children receive good preparation for both the procedure and for the sensations they will experience afterward. Some children develop a mild earache after surgery for the first week in addition to a painful throat, probably caused by shifting pressure on the eustachian tube.

Liquid analgesics are better tolerated than pills or tablets following surgery because they are easier to swallow. Rectal administration is a possibility for very young children. Offer instead frequent sips of clear liquid, popsicles, or ice chips. Avoid acidic and citric juices because these sting the denuded tissue. Carbonated beverages also can irritate unless they stand for a time to become "flat." Avoid red fluid such as Kool-Aid, which, if vomited, could be mistaken for swallowed blood.

Children are then gradually advanced after 24 to 48 hours to a diet of soft foods such as gelatin, mashed potatoes, soups, and cooked fruits. Alert parents they should continue to eat only soft foods during the initial postoperative period (e.g., no toast crusts or other foods that could cause pharyngeal irritation if not chewed well). Be certain parents know whom they should call (clinic, hospital, or primary care provider) if they have a question or concern about their child's condition or care.

Figure 40.16 Emergency therapy for a nosebleed is to sit the child up and apply pressure to the sides of the nose. (From Bowden, V. R., & Greenberg, C. S. [2014]. *Children and their families: The continuum of nursing care* [3rd ed.]. Philadelphia, PA: Wolters Kluwer.)

EPISTAXIS

Epistaxis (nosebleed) is extremely common in children and usually occurs from trauma, such as picking at the nose or trauma. Dry air can cause mucous membranes to become dry and be susceptible to cracking and bleeding. Nosebleeds may also occur after strenuous exercise, with hemolytic disorders, or may be associated with nasal polyps, sinusitis, or allergic rhinitis. Some families appear to show a familial predisposition to them.

Nosebleeds can be frightening. The fear, however, and the amount of blood that can be seen is generally out of proportion to the seriousness of the bleeding.

Keep children with nosebleeds in an upright position with their head tilted slightly forward to minimize the amount of blood pressure in nasal vessels and to keep blood moving forward, not back into the nasopharynx. Apply pressure to the cartilage on the sides of the nose with your fingers for about 10 minutes (Fig. 40.16). Make every effort to quiet the child and to help stop crying because crying increases pressure in the blood vessels of the head and prolongs bleeding. Discourage putting tissue in the nose or blowing the nose, as this may disrupt a clot that has formed. Prolonged or severe bleeding may need emergency intervention and packing. Chronic nasal bleeding may need investigation to rule out a systemic disease or blood disorder.

QSEN Checkpoint Question 40.4

PATIENT-CENTERED CARE

Michael's 4-year-old roommate in the care unit is scheduled for a tonsillectomy later today. The caregiver wants to know what types of food they can have at home for him after his tonsillectomy. Which of the following would be appropriate?

    a. Grilled cheese sandwich
    b. Tomato juice and pretzels
    c. Potato chips and dip
    d. An ice pop

Look in Appendix A for the best answer and rationale.

SINUSITIS

Sinusitis is infection and inflammation of the sinus cavities. It rarely occurs in children younger than 6 years of age because the frontal sinuses do not develop fully until that age. It can occur either as a primary infection or as a secondary bacterial infection from a viral upper respiratory illness. Children with bacterial sinusitis often have a preceding upper respiratory illness but have persistent or worsening symptoms of fever, nasal discharge, and cough that generally last for over 10 days (Wald, Applegate, Bordley, et al., 2013). Treatment for acute bacterial sinusitis consists of an analgesic for pain and an antibiotic for the specific organism involved.

LARYNGITIS

Laryngitis is inflammation of the larynx, which results in brassy, hoarse voice sounds or the inability to make audible voice sounds. It may occur as a complication of pharyngitis or from excessive use of the voice, as in shouting or loud cheering. Sips of fluid (either warm or cold, whichever feels best) offer relief from the annoying tickling sensation often present.

CONGENITAL LARYNGOMALACIA/TRACHEOMALACIA

Congenital laryngomalacia means that an infant's laryngeal structure is weaker than normal and collapses more than usual on inspiration (Adil, Rager, & Carr, 2012). This produces laryngeal stridor (a high-pitched crowing sound on inspiration) present from birth and possibly intensified when the infant is in a supine position or when sucking.

Assessment

The infant's sternum and intercostal spaces may retract on inspiration because of the increased effort needed to pull air into the trachea past the collapsed cartilage rings. Many infants with this condition must stop sucking frequently during a feeding to maintain adequate ventilation and to rest from their exhausting respiratory effort.

Therapeutic Management

Most children with congenital laryngomalacia need no routine therapy other than to have parents feed them slowly and provide rest periods as needed. The condition improves as infants mature and cartilage in the larynx becomes stronger at about 1 year of age. When parents wake at night and listen in a quiet house to the sound of stridor, it seems unbearably loud and can make it difficult for them to believe it is safe for them to care for the infant at home.

Be certain that parents know the importance of bringing the child for early care if signs of an upper respiratory tract infection should develop because, with this, laryngeal collapse will be even more intense and a complete obstruction of the trachea could occur.

CROUP (LARYNGOTRACHEOBRONCHITIS)

Croup (inflammation of the larynx, trachea, and major bronchi) is a frightening illness in childhood, although complications are rare for caregivers. In children between 6 months and 3 years of age, the cause of croup is usually a viral infection such as parainfluenza virus.

Assessment

With croup, children typically have only minimal signs at bedtime. Temperature is normal or only mildly elevated. They may develop a barking cough (croupy cough), inspiratory stridor, and marked retractions from inflammation of the larynx, trachea, and major bronchi.

Therapeutic Management

Cool moist air combined with a corticosteroid, such as dexamethasone, or racemic epinephrine, given by nebulizer, usually reduces inflammation and produces effective bronchodilation to open the airway. The provider may prescribe dexamethasone for home administration but racemic epinephrine needs to be administered in a healthcare setting.

Nursing Diagnoses and Related Interventions

Nursing Diagnosis: Ineffective airway clearance related to edema and constriction of airway

Outcome Evaluation: Respiratory rate is not above 22 breaths/min; no cyanosis is present; PO_2 is 80 to 100 mmHg; and SaO_2 is over 95%.

Provide measures for a child to remain calm using distraction, toys, etc., while monitoring for respiratory changes through pulse oximetry monitoring and respiratory assessment.

Laryngospasm with total occlusion of the airway can occur if a child's gag reflex is elicited or when the child is crying. Therefore, *do not elicit a gag reflex in any child with a croupy, barking cough* and provide comfort to prevent crying.

Box 40.5 shows an interprofessional care map illustrating both nursing and team planning for a child with laryngotracheobronchitis.

What If . . . 40.2

Michael had loud stridor on admission. After oxygenation, suddenly no stridor is heard. How should the nurse respond?

EPIGLOTTITIS

Epiglottitis is inflammation of the epiglottis, which is the flap of cartilage that covers the opening to the larynx to keep out food and fluid during swallowing. Although it is rare, inflammation of the epiglottis is an emergency because the swollen epiglottis cannot rise and allow the airway to open. It occurs most frequently in children from 2 to about 8 years of age.

Epiglottitis can be either bacterial or viral in origin. *Haemophilus influenzae* type B has been replaced as the most common bacterial cause of the disorder followed by pneumococci, streptococci, or staphylococci. Echovirus and RSV also can cause the disorder. The incidence of epiglottitis has greatly decreased with the introduction of the *H. influenzae* type B vaccine.

BOX 40.5

Nursing Care Planning

AN INTERPROFESSIONAL CARE MAP FOR A CHILD WITH LARYNGOTRACHEOBRONCHITIS (CROUP)

Michael's 2-year-old neighbor is brought to the emergency department in respiratory distress. He has a sharp, barking cough and inspiratory stridor at rest. His breathing appears labored. He appears frightened and is tachypneic. His oxygen saturations are 85%. He is diagnosed with laryngotracheobronchitis (croup) and is admitted to the hospital for further monitoring and treatment.

Past Medical History: Mother received regular prenatal care beginning at 6 weeks; uncomplicated pregnancy. Full-term, spontaneous vaginal delivery, 38 weeks, birth weight 7 lb. Discharged at 2 weeks of age after surgical repair of choanal atresia. No hospitalizations following newborn discharge; no known allergies to medicine. Allergic to seafood (hives) and has received all routine immunizations.

Family Assessment: The child lives with his parents in a four-bedroom home. He has two older siblings. Both parents work and are at the child's bedside. No smokers in household.

History of the Present Illness: 2 days of congestion and rhinorrhea. A fever started in the morning with decreased appetite and hoarse voice; no treatment tried; fussy and clingy.

Physical Assessment: Ill-appearing child with increased work of breathing; audible inspiratory stridor at rest. Temperature: 102.2°F (39.0°C), heart rate: 130 beats/min, respirations: 32 breaths/min, nasal flaring, and decreased air movement to bases of lungs. Barky sounding cough in room.

Team Member Responsible	Assessment	Intervention	Rationale	Expected Outcome
Activities of Daily Living, Including Safety				
Nurse	Assess ability to maintain respiratory effort.	Place child in semi-upright position.	Upright position will facilitate optimal lung expansion.	Improved respiratory effort
Nurse	Assess degree of stridor/respiratory compromise.	Keep child calm; utilize distraction and decrease intervention.	Stridor can be worsened with agitation.	Decreased stridor; improved respiratory status
Teamwork and Collaboration				
NP/MD/PA	Assess ability to maintain ventilation and perfusion.	Supplemental oxygen, steroids, inhaled medications	May improve oxygenation, decrease airway inflammation	Maintain/improved ventilation and perfusion
Procedures/Medications for Quality Improvement				
Nurse	Assess vital signs.	Antipyretics as needed	May decrease metabolic demand	Increased comfort, decreased heart rate
NP/MD/PA	Assess respiratory status.	Inhaled racemic epinephrine and/or oral/intramuscular/intravenous steroids as indicated	Decreased airway inflammation	Decreased work of breathing, improved oxygenation and ventilation

NP, nurse practitioner; MD, medical doctor; PA, physician's assistant.

Assessment

Symptoms begin as those of a mild upper respiratory tract infection. After 1 or 2 days, as inflammation spreads to the epiglottis, the child suddenly develops severe inspiratory stridor, a high fever, hoarseness, and a very sore throat. Children may have such difficulty swallowing that they drool saliva. They may protrude their tongue to increase free movement in the pharynx.

If a child's gag reflex is stimulated with a tongue blade, the swollen and inflamed epiglottis can be seen to rise in the back of the throat as a cherry-red structure. It can be so edematous, however, that the gagging procedure causes complete obstruction of the glottis and shuts off the ability of the child to inhale. Therefore, in children with symptoms of epiglottitis (e.g., dysphagia, inspiratory stridor, cough, fever, and hoarseness), *never attempt to visualize the epiglottis directly with a tongue blade or obtain a throat culture* unless a means of providing an artificial airway, such as tracheostomy or endotracheal intubation, is immediately available. This is especially important for the nurse who functions in an expanded role and performs physical assessments and routinely elicits gag reflexes.

Therapeutic Management

If cyanosis or respiratory distress is present, they need oxygen. IV fluids, an antibiotic, and establishment of an endotracheal airway are required to treat infection and maintain hydration.

QSEN Checkpoint Question 40.5

SAFETY

Michael has a barking cough, sore throat, and fever. The nurse wants to see whether his throat looks sore and swollen. What is the safest and most accurate way of performing this assessment?

   a. Gag Michael with a tongue blade so you can inspect his tonsils.
   b. Ask Michael to press down on his tongue with one of his fingers.
   c. Elicit a gag reflex using only one gloved finger.
   d. Ask Michael to open his mouth and then visually inspect his throat.

Look in Appendix A for the best answer and rationale.

ASPIRATION

Aspiration (inhalation of a foreign object into the airway) occurs most frequently in infants and toddlers. When a child aspirates a foreign object such as a coin or a peanut, the immediate reaction is choking and hard, forceful coughing. Usually, this dislodges the object. However, if the airway becomes so obstructed and no coughing or speech is possible, intervention is essential. A series of back blows or subdiaphragmatic abdominal thrusts may be used with children (Figs. 40.17 and 40.18).

BRONCHIAL OBSTRUCTION

The right main bronchus is straighter and has a larger lumen than the left bronchus in children older than 2 years of age. For this reason, an aspirated foreign object that is not large enough to obstruct the trachea may lodge in the right bronchus, obstructing a portion or all of the right lung. The alveoli distal to the obstruction will collapse as the air remaining in them becomes absorbed (atelectasis), or hyperinflation and pneumothorax may occur if the foreign body serves as a ball valve, allowing air to enter but not leave the alveoli (see later discussion on disorders of the lower respiratory tract).

Assessment

After aspirating a small foreign body, the child generally coughs violently and may become dyspneic. If the article is not expelled, hemoptysis, fever, purulent sputum, and leukocytosis will generally result as infection develops. Localized wheezing

Figure 40.17 A subdiaphragmatic abdominal thrust on a school-age child used if back blows are not successful.

Figure 40.18 (A) Back blows and (B) chest thrusts to relieve complete foreign body airway obstruction in an infant.

(a high whistling sound on expiration made by air passing through the narrowed lumen) may occur. Because this is localized, it is different from the generalized wheezing of a child with asthma.

A chest X-ray will reveal the presence of an object if it is radiopaque. Objects most frequently aspirated include buttons, bones, popcorn, nuts, and coins. Because objects such as those made of plastic, nuts, or popcorn cannot be visualized well on X-ray film, an X-ray study may be inconclusive. Foreign bodies may also lodge in the esophagus and cause respiratory distress because of compression on the trachea. Care must be taken when feeding young children to avoid potential choking/aspiration hazards. Popcorn, grapes, nuts, etc., can pose hazards. Additionally, children may aspirate on nonfood items such as toys, coins, etc.

Therapeutic Management

A bronchoscopy may be necessary to remove the foreign body in the operating room. After a bronchoscopy, assess the child closely for signs of bronchial edema and airway obstruction that occur from mucus accumulation because of the bronchus manipulation. Obtain frequent vital signs (increasing pulse and respiratory rates suggest increased edema and obstruction).

Keep a child nothing by mouth (NPO) for at least an hour. Once a gag reflex is present, offer the first fluid cautiously to prevent additional aspiration. Cool fluid may feel more soothing than warm fluid and also can help reduce the soreness in the throat. Breathing cool, moist air or having an ice collar applied may further reduce edema.

Disorders of the Lower Respiratory Tract

The structures of the lower respiratory tract are subject to infection by the same pathogens that attack the upper respiratory tract.

INFLUENZA

Influenza involves inflammation and infection of the major airways. It is caused by the orthomyxovirus influenza type A, B, or C. It is marked by a cough and fever but may be accompanied by fatigue, body aches, a sore throat, and gastrointestinal symptoms such as vomiting or diarrhea. The disease spreads readily through a home or a classroom because children are contagious on the day before symptoms appear and for about the next 5 days. Young children are at highest risk of complications from the flu, in particular, children with chronic health conditions.

Oseltamivir (Tamiflu) may be prescribed for young children or children with risk factors such as cardiac or respiratory disease. To prevent the infection, children over 6 months of age should receive either the inactivated vaccine (given by injection) or the activated vaccine (given by a nasal spray). Because the influenza virus mutates yearly, the influenza vaccine is specific for only that year and must be readministered yearly.

BRONCHITIS

Bronchitis (inflammation of the major bronchi and trachea) is one of the more common illnesses affecting preschool- and school-age children.

It is characterized by fever and cough, usually in conjunction with nasal congestion. Causative agents include the influenza viruses, adenovirus, and *Mycoplasma pneumoniae*, among others.

Assessment

Children usually have a mild upper respiratory tract infection for 1 or 2 days, after which they develop a fever and a dry, hacking cough, which is hoarse and mildly productive and serious enough to wake a child from sleep. These symptoms may last for a week, although full recovery sometimes takes as long as 2 weeks.

On auscultation, rhonchi and coarse crackles (the sound of rales) can be heard. A chest X-ray will reveal diffuse alveolar hyperinflation and some markings at the hilus of the lung.

Therapeutic Management

Therapy is aimed at relieving respiratory symptoms, reducing fever, and maintaining adequate hydration. An antibiotic will be prescribed if bacterial infection is suspected.

BRONCHIOLITIS

Bronchiolitis is inflammation and edema of the fine bronchioles and small bronchi, usually due to a viral illness. The most common cause of bronchiolitis is the RSV, although a number of other viruses may also cause bronchiolitis (Florin, Plint, & Zorc, 2017). The infection occurs most often in the winter and spring and is the most common lower respiratory illness in children younger than 2 years of age, peaking in incidence between 3 and 6 months of age (Florin et al., 2017). It is the most common reason for hospitalization in infancy (Mahant & Parkin, 2016).

Assessment

Typically, infants have several days of symptoms of a viral respiratory infection, such as congestion, rhinorrhea, and fever. This can progress to lower respiratory symptoms, including a cough, wheezing, and retractions. Infants can have variable presentation of respiratory distress. The diagnosis of bronchiolitis is typically made by a provider based on the history and clinical symptoms. Routine testing and radiographs are not indicated in typical cases (Florin et al., 2017).

Therapeutic Management

For children with less severe symptoms, antipyretics, adequate hydration, nasal suctioning, nasal saline, avoidance of tobacco exposure, and home monitoring are adequate. Hospitalization is warranted for children with severe illness, such as apnea, hypoxia, or dehydration, which may occur due to difficulty feeding.

Because RSV infection spreads readily from person to person and can survive on surfaces for extended time periods (>6 hours), infection control and hand hygiene is important to reduce the risk of transmission (Ralston, Lieberthal, Meissner, et al., 2014). Although fevers generally last for only the first several days of illness, respiratory symptoms can last for about 2 weeks (Florin et al., 2017).

Palivizumab, a monoclonal antibody, is recommended as prophylactic injection to prevent RSV during RSV season. Infants eligible for palivizumab are defined by specific qualifying criteria, generally defined by gestational age less than 29 weeks or less than 1 year of age with preexisting health conditions, such as chronic lung disease of prematurity or congenital heart disease (Ralston et al., 2014). Injections are given monthly during RSV season.

 Nursing Diagnoses and Related Interventions

Nursing Diagnosis: Caregiver anxiety related to respiratory distress in child

Outcome Evaluation: Caregivers state their anxiety level is tolerable as signs and symptoms of disease decrease.

Education as to the course of illness is important. Understanding signs that could indicate worsening illness, such as respiratory distress and dehydration are critical during care. Additionally, caregivers need to understand that the symptoms of bronchiolitis can continue for an extended period of time, although worsening symptoms (such as recurrence of fever after the first few days of illness) should be brought to medical attention to evaluate for secondary infection. Caregivers should understand that medications, such as antibiotics, have no role in treatment of viral illnesses.

ASTHMA

Asthma is a chronic inflammatory disorder of the respiratory track and is the most common chronic illness in children (NHLBI, 2007). Typically, asthma presents before 5 years of age, although it may be difficult to make a definitive diagnosis in these early years. Many viral illnesses can present with symptoms that are similar and asthma and viral illnesses can trigger asthma symptoms, adding to the complexity of diagnosis. Asthma symptoms can be variable with each child with different triggers and clinical presentations. The severity of asthma in a child is dependent on risk factors, which include genetics as well as environmental exposures, such as allergens, stress, pollution, etc., that affect the body's immune responses (NHLBI, 2007).

When an allergen invades, mast cells release histamine and leukotrienes that result in diffuse obstructive and restrictive changes in the airway because of a triad of inflammation, bronchoconstriction, and increased mucus production. Most children with asthma can be shown to have allergy triggers. A primary irritant is environmental tobacco smoke. Other indoor allergens, such as mice and cockroaches, are common irritants. Outdoor irritants can include pollens, grasses, and pollution, among others. Viral respiratory illnesses are a common trigger for asthma exacerbations in children.

Mechanism of Disease

Asthma primarily affects the small airways. The relationship of inflammation to airway hyperresponsiveness and airway obstruction contributes to clinical symptoms. This complex interplay of factors presents as recurrent wheezing, breathlessness, chest tightness, and coughing (NHLBI, 2007, p. 14).

Assessment

The word *asthma* is derived from the Greek word for "panting," a description of the child's distress. Typically, an episode begins with a dry cough. Children then develop increasing difficulty exhaling as it becomes more and more difficult for them to force air through the narrowed lumen of the bronchioles that are not only inflamed and swollen but also filled with mucus. Typical dyspnea and wheezing (the sound caused by air being pushed forcibly past obstructed bronchioles) associated with the disorder begin. Wheezing is heard primarily upon expiration because the lumen of bronchioles are narrower during exhalation than inhalation, but it may be absent with severe asthma exacerbations.

History

An assessment should include a thorough history of the development of a child's symptoms; for example, what the child was doing at the time symptoms began, the child's known asthma triggers, and what treatments were given. After the acute attack has passed, take time to ask a parent or the child to describe the home environment, including any pets, the child's bedroom, outdoor play space, classroom environment, and type of heating in the house, to see whether more environmental control could reduce allergen triggers and future occurrences.

Physical Assessment

In some children, the initial wheezing is evident only by stethoscope auscultation; in others, it is so loud it can be heard by simply listening.

Air-filled lungs are hyperresonant to percussion or they make a louder, more hollow noise on percussion than usual. With normal respiration, the inspiration phase of breathing is longer than the expiration phase. During an asthma attack, however, a child must work so hard to exhale due to air trapping that the expiration phase becomes longer than the inspiration phase. Time the two phases to demonstrate this. Also, observe for retractions (the chest wall is drawn inward with breaths) because children have to use intercostal accessory muscles to achieve full breaths.

As constriction becomes acute, the sound of wheezing may decrease because so little air can leave the alveoli.

During attacks, children with asthma are generally more comfortable in a sitting or standing position rather than lying down and should be allowed to be in a position of comfort. If seated in a chair, they lean forward and raise their shoulders to give themselves more breathing space. Children who do agree to lie down are either at the end of an attack and beginning to feel less threatened by the dyspnea or are so exhausted by the paroxysms of coughing that they no longer have the strength to sit upright.

Pulmonary Function Studies

Pulmonary function studies or spirometry can be helpful in evaluating children for asthma. Good pulmonary function depends on good ventilation (both drawing adequate air into the lungs and expelling it again), adequate transfer of gases across the alveolar capillary membranes, and adequate volume and distribution of pulmonary capillary blood flow to transport oxygen to body cells. In children with asthma, the

Figure 40.19 A child with asthma receives instructions on using a peak flow meter to track his peak expiratory flow readings on a daily basis. (From Lippincott Professional Development Collection. [n.d.]. *Pediatric Nursing Program* [online module]. Retrieved from http://lippincottsolutions.com)

vital capacity (i.e., the air that they are able to exhale) may be low or the capacity may be normal but because of narrowed bronchioles as a result of bronchospasm, the expiratory rate will be abnormally long (more than 10 seconds rather than the normal 2 or 3 seconds). This is often difficult to perform in young children because good understanding and effort is needed to effectively perform.

Peak Expiratory Flow Rate Monitoring

Children with asthma may use a home peak flow meter daily to measure gross changes in peak expiratory flow and to help in planning an appropriate therapeutic regimen (Fig. 40.19). Children with asthma should be able to tell you their usual reading and personal best score.

To use a peak flow meter, a child places the indicator on the apparatus at the bottom of the numbered scale and takes a deep breath. The child then places the meter in his or her mouth and blows out as hard and fast as possible. The child then repeats this two more times and records the highest number achieved as the peak flow meter result. During a 2-week period when a child feels well, this should be done daily. The highest number achieved during this time is recorded as the child's personal best.

Children are assigned "zones" to help determine the level of severity of their symptoms at home. Each zone (green, yellow, or red) is associated with treatment recommendations. These may include options for inhaler use and guidelines for when to call their provider or seek emergency care.

Therapeutic Management

According to the Expert Panel report (NHLBI, 2007, p. 35), the diagnosis and management of asthma involves four components: (a) measure of asthma assessment and monitoring, which involves history and physical examination and objective testing to determine asthma severity and control; (b) education for home self-management; (c) control of environmental factors that contribute to symptoms (i.e., allergens); and (d) pharmacologic therapy, defined as quick relief and long acting medications (see Chapter 42).

The primary goal in asthma management is the prevention of airway inflammation. A child with mild intermittent asthma

---

BOX 40.6

Nursing Care Planning Based on Responsibility for Pharmacology

FLUTICASONE PROPIONATE

Classification: Fluticasone propionate is a corticosteroid used as an oral inhalation for prevention of asthma symptoms.

Action: anti-inflammatory (bronchodilator)

Pregnancy Risk Category: C

Dosage: Dosages are based on asthma severity and whether a child has had previous bronchodilators or corticosteroid use; given via a metered dose inhaler with a valve holding chamber (spacer), twice a day.

Possible Adverse Effects: Dizziness, dysphonia, oral thrush, and dermatitis; potential for decrease in linear growth, headache, nausea, dry and irritated throat, cough, nasal congestion, epistaxis, sneezing

Nursing Implications

- Instruct parents and child that this drug is not effective in an acute attack.
- Advise parent to have child rinse their mouth (or take a drink if too young to rinse) after administration to prevent thrush.
- Caution child and parents to take the drug exactly as prescribed and to continue other prescribed medications.
- Instruct child and parents in the use of metered-dose inhaler for administration.
- Advise parent to continue this daily to prevent asthma exacerbations.
- Instruct parents and child to watch for a possible recurrence of asthma symptoms if dosage is decreased.

---

may be prescribed an inhaled short-acting β-agonist, such as albuterol, to take as needed, whereas children with persistent or severe symptoms will need an inhaled corticosteroid to take daily in order to prevent exacerbations (Box 40.6).

Other medications, such as leukotriene receptor agonists (e.g., montelukast), inhaled long-acting β-agonists, immunomodulators, and mast cell stabilizers, may be used for children with more severe asthma symptoms. Short courses (generally 2 to 5 days) or an oral corticosteroid may be prescribed during an acute exacerbation.

Nursing Diagnoses and Related Interventions

Nursing Diagnosis: Fear related to sudden onset of asthma attack

Outcome Evaluation: Parents and child express confidence in their ability to prevent, recognize asthma symptoms, and intervene appropriately.

Asthma is a frightening disease and can have great impact on the child and family. Ongoing education is needed to recognize triggers, minimize exposure to triggers, manage medications, and ensure proper technique and use of inhaler.

Nursing Diagnosis: Health-seeking behaviors related to prevention of and treatment for asthma attacks

Outcome Evaluation: Parents and child accurately state triggers that cause an attack; and child correctly demonstrates breathing exercises, use of inhaler, and peak expiratory flow meter.

Children need to learn how to avoid possible triggers through environmental control. If foods are a trigger, children need to learn to be responsible for their own diets so they can avoid these foods. Children as young as 6 years of age can learn what foods they cannot eat and can take responsibility for telling a friend's parent or a schoolteacher that they must not eat certain foods. They must learn to use a metered-dose inhaler or nebulizer if prescribed. The goal of asthma management is to have symptom-free periods that allow optimal quality of life.

QSEN Checkpoint Question 40.6

INFORMATICS

The nurse wants to teach Michael's 3-year-old roommate about peak flow testing. During this diagnostic test, what instruction should the nurse provide?

   a. "Hold your breath until I say and then cough forcefully."
   b. "When I put the meter in your mouth, take a big, deep breath."
   c. "I need you to blow out through the meter as hard and fast as you can."
   d. "Breathe like you usually do when I put the meter against your mouth."

Look in Appendix A for the best answer and rationale.

Unfolding Patient Stories: Sabina Vasquez • Part 2

 Recall **Sabina Vasquez** from Chapter 35, a 5-year-old diagnosed with asthma who uses an albuterol inhaler. What questions and assessments help the nurse evaluate her current respiratory status during a routine clinic visit? What methods can the nurse use to guide asthma management and determine how well Sabina's asthma is managed at home?

Care for Sabina and other patients in a realistic virtual environment: *vSim* for Nursing (thepoint.lww.com/vSimMaternityPed). Practice documenting these patients' care in DocuCare (thepoint.lww.com/DocuCareEHR).

STATUS ASTHMATICUS

Status asthmaticus is a severe and prolonged asthma attack that is not responsive to asthma therapy. It requires hospital evaluation and close cardiopulmonary monitoring.

Assessment

A child with status asthmaticus is in acute respiratory distress. By definition, a child in status asthmaticus has failed to respond to first-line therapy (Pardue Jones, Fleming, Otillio, et al., 2015). Both heart rate and respiratory rate are elevated. The child's level of alertness and responsiveness may be altered, and they may appear anxious. Both oxygen saturation and PO_2 are low; PCO_2 is elevated because the bronchi are so constricted the child cannot exhale, resulting in CO_2 accumulation. The rising PCO_2 rapidly leads to acidosis. In contrast to the loud wheezing initially heard in an asthma attack, children with status asthmaticus may have so little air passing in or out of their lungs that breath sounds may be limited.

Therapeutic Management

Continuous nebulization with an inhaled β_2 agonist and IV corticosteroids may be necessary to reduce symptoms, along with oral or IV steroids, smooth muscle relaxers, and others. In severe attacks, endotracheal intubation and mechanical ventilation may be necessary to maintain effective ventilation and perfusion.

PNEUMONIA

Pneumonia is an infection and inflammation of alveoli. It often has a bacterial or viral origin and is categorized as hospital- or community-acquired (Box 40.7). Pneumonia occurs most often in late winter and early spring. The differences between bronchiolitis, asthma, and pneumonia are summarized in Table 40.1. *Pneumocystis carinii* pneumonia, seen almost exclusively with HIV/AIDS infection, is discussed in Chapter 42.

Pneumococcal Pneumonia

The onset of pneumococcal pneumonia is generally abrupt and follows an upper respiratory tract infection. In infants,

---

💬 BOX 40.7

Nursing Care Planning Tips for Effective Communication

Michael's 3-year-old hospital roommate, B. J. Silver, has pneumonia, and you notice that his mother is visibly upset.

Tip: Be sure to explain to parents that pneumonia is serious, but with antibiotic treatment, it is not the fatal diagnosis it was years ago. Ask enough questions to be certain parents understand the probable outcomes.

Nurse: Is something wrong, Mrs. Silver? You seem upset.

Mrs. Silver: I didn't realize pneumonia was so serious until I talked to my mother.

Nurse: Pneumonia can be serious, but we are monitoring B. J. very closely.

Mrs. Silver: My mother told me my brother had pneumonia when he was a baby. Is this oxygen? My mother said to make sure B. J. is receiving oxygen.

Nurse: I know that pneumonia can be a scary diagnosis. Would you like to talk about B. J.'s treatment plan?

TABLE 40.1 COMPARISON OF BRONCHIOLITIS, PNEUMONIA, AND ASTHMA

Assessment	Bronchiolitis	Pneumonia	Asthma
Cause	Usually respiratory syncytial virus	Possibly bacterial (pneumococcal, or *Haemophilus influenzae*), viral, or mycoplasmal; possibly secondary to aspiration	Hypersensitivity type I immune response
Age of child	Under 2 years	All through childhood	Onset: 1–5 years
Onset pattern	Follows an upper respiratory infection	Often follows an upper respiratory infection	Often triggered by respiratory infection; follows initiation by an allergen
Appearance	Fatigued, anxious, shallow respirations, increasing anteroposterior diameter of chest	Fatigued, anxious, shallow respirations	Wheezing, exhausted, frightened
Cough	Paroxysmal, dry	Productive, harsh cough	Paroxysmal, with thick mucus production
Fever	Low grade	Elevated	None
Auscultatory sounds	Barely audible breath sounds, rales, wheezing	Decreased breath sounds, rales	Wheezing, decreased breath sounds

the infection tends to be bronchopneumonia with poor consolidation. In older children, pneumonia often localizes in a single lobe with full consolidation. During the initial 24 to 48 hours of infection, children may have blood-tinged sputum that transitions to a thick, purulent sputum.

Assessment

Children may often appear acutely ill, with high fever, tachycardia, chest or abdominal pain, chills, and signs of respiratory distress. Breath sounds are often diminished, and crackles (rales) may be present. Dullness on percussion indicates total consolidation. Chest radiography will often reveal consolidation, and laboratory studies will indicate leukocytosis.

Therapeutic Management

Pharmacologic management may include IV fluid therapy, antibiotics, and antipyretics (Bradley, Byington, Shah, et al., 2011). Oxygen saturation levels should be assessed frequently. Humidified oxygen may help labored breathing and prevent hypoxemia. CPT may be used to encourage the movement of mucus and prevent obstruction. Repositioning the child will prevent pooling of secretions.

Chlamydial Pneumonia

Chlamydia trachomatis pneumonia, typically seen in newborns up to 12 weeks of age, is often contracted from contact with the mother's vagina during birth. Symptoms begin gradually with nasal congestion, a sharp cough, and poor weight gain. These progress to tachypnea and wheezing and rales on auscultation. A laboratory assessment will show elevated levels of IgG and IgM antibodies, peripheral eosinophilia, and antibodies to *C. trachomatis*. Antibiotics are often used for pharmacologic treatment.

Viral Pneumonia

Viral pneumonia is generally caused by viral infections of the upper respiratory tract. Symptoms begin as an upper respiratory tract infection and may progress to diminished breath sounds and fine rales on auscultation. Antibiotic therapy is

not effective against viral infections. Rest and antipyretics are used for treatment. Similar to bacterial pneumonia, fatigue often occurs following the acute phase of illness.

Mycoplasmal Pneumonia

Mycoplasmal pneumonia occurs more frequently in children over 5 years of age during winter months. Fever, cough, cervical lymphadenopathy, and rhinitis are common symptoms. Mycoplasmal organisms are generally sensitive to erythromycin or tetracycline.

ATELECTASIS

Atelectasis, the collapse of lung alveoli, may be a primary or secondary condition.

Primary Atelectasis

Primary atelectasis is seen in preterm newborns with limited surfactant and poor respiratory strength or mucus or meconium plugs in the trachea (Dargaville, 2012).

Respirations become irregular, with nasal flaring and apnea. Respiratory grunting, caused by the glottis closing upon expiration, increases pressure in the respiratory tract and keeps alveoli from collapsing. Grunting may also be tiring to the newborn, resulting in hypoxemia, hypotonicity, and flaccidity. Therapy must be directed at the cause of atelectasis. Crying and administration of oxygen may aerate the alveoli and may decrease cyanosis.

Secondary Atelectasis

Secondary atelectasis often occurs from a respiratory tract obstruction that prevents air from entering a portion of the alveoli (Federico, Kirby, Deterding, et al., 2011). As residual air in the alveoli is absorbed, the alveoli collapse. Causes of obstruction may include mucus plugs associated with chronic respiratory disease, foreign object aspiration, or pressure on lung tissue from outside forces, such as compression from a diaphragmatic hernia, scoliosis, or enlarged thoracic lymph nodes (Fig. 40.20).

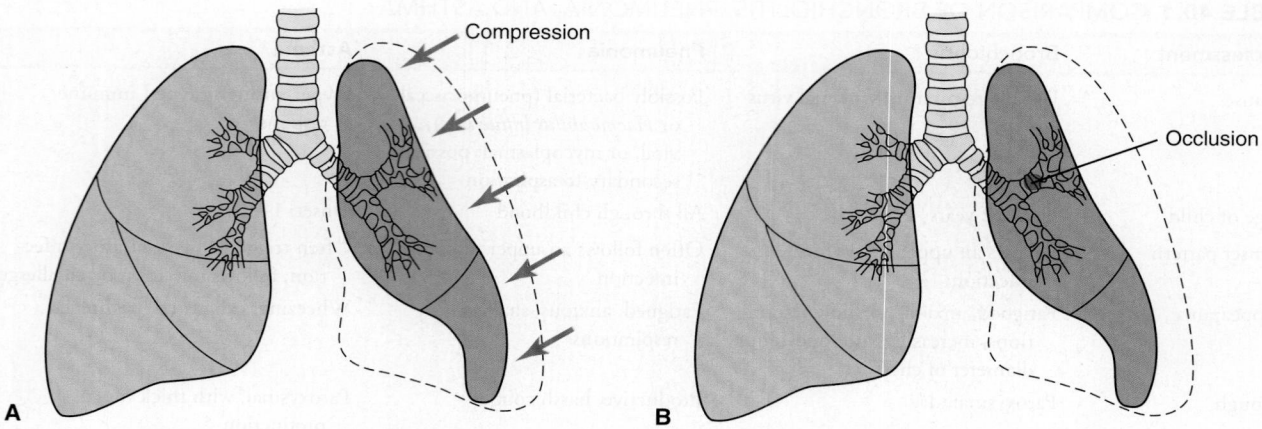

Figure 40.20 **(A)** Atelectasis caused by compression of lung tissue. **(B)** Atelectasis caused by obstruction.

Signs of secondary atelectasis depend on the degree of collapse. Asymmetry of the chest may be noticed as well as diminished breath sounds on the affected side. Tachypnea and cyanosis may be present. Chest radiography will show collapsed alveoli. Children with atelectasis are prone to secondary infection because mucus, which provides a good medium for bacteria, becomes stagnant without air exchange.

Therapeutic Management

Atelectasis caused by inspiration of a foreign object will not be relieved until the object is removed by bronchoscopy. Atelectasis caused by a mucus plug will resolve when the plug clears up. The chest of a child with atelectasis should be kept free from pressure for optimal lung expansion.

A semi-Fowler's position generally allows for the best lung expansion because it lowers abdominal contents and increases chest space. Suction, CPT, and increased humidity may prevent further bronchial plugging.

PNEUMOTHORAX

Pneumothorax is the presence of atmospheric air in the pleural space, causing atelectasis (Fig. 40.21). It can occur when external puncture wounds allow air to enter the chest (Janssen & Cardillo, 2011).

Pneumothorax occurs in approximately 1% of newborns often because of rupture of the alveoli from the extreme intrathoracic pressure needed to initiate a first inspiration. The infant will develop signs of respiratory distress. Auscultation reveals absent or decreased breath sounds on the affected side. Percussion may not be revealing. Despite the hollow air space, the chest may be hyperresonant because of the presence of increased air. A more revealing sign may be the shift of the apical pulse (mediastinal shift) away from the site of the pneumothorax. Chest radiography will show a darkened area of the air-filled pleural space.

A child with a pneumothorax needs oxygen therapy to relieve respiratory distress. A thoracotomy catheter or needle may be placed through the chest wall into the pleural space to remove accumulated air. In most children with pneumothorax, symptoms are relieved within 24 hours after suction initiation. The use of water-seal drainage with children is discussed in Chapter 41.

If air in the pleural space is from a puncture wound such as a stab wound, cover the chest wound immediately with an impervious material, such as petrolatum gauze, to prevent

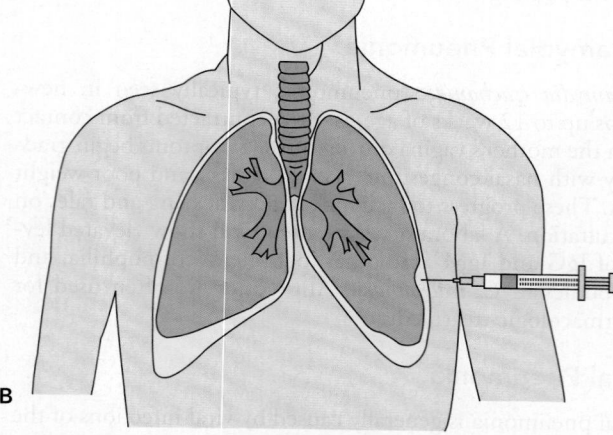

Figure 40.21 **(A)** A pneumothorax. A tear in the tracheobronchial tree has caused air to move into the pleural space; the lung collapses and the mediastinum shifts to the unaffected side. **(B)** Aspiration of air from the pleural space allows lung to reexpand after a pneumothorax.

further air from entering and to decrease the risk of atelectasis. The extent of symptoms and the outcome will depend on the cause of entry of air into the pleural space and its removal.

BRONCHOPULMONARY DYSPLASIA

Bronchopulmonary dysplasia (BPD) is chronic lung condition that can occur in infants. The condition, frequently found in preterm infants who received mechanical ventilation for respiratory distress syndrome at birth, is thought to occur from a combination of surfactant deficiency, barotrauma, oxygen toxicity, and inflammation.

Infants may develop tachypnea, retractions, nasal flaring, tachycardia, and oxygen dependence. Auscultation reveals decreased air movement. Chest radiography may show areas of overinflation, inflammation, and atelectasis. As inflamed surfaces heal, the infant is left with fibrotic scarring.

The clinical course ranges from a mild need for increased oxygen, which gradually resolves over a few months, to a severe disease requiring chronic tracheostomy and mechanical ventilation during the first few years of life.

Administration of a corticosteroid to reduce inflammation and a bronchodilator by nebulizer can improve respiratory function. Infants need to be monitored carefully for nutrition and fluid intake, especially if they are ventilator-dependent.

TUBERCULOSIS

Tuberculosis, caused by the bacterium *Mycobacterium tuberculosis*, is a highly contagious pulmonary disease that affects children worldwide (Winston & Menzies, 2012).

Children who are homeless, immunocompromised, or adopted internationally are at increased risk (Raviglione, Marais, Floyd, et al., 2012). The mode of transmission is inhalation of infected droplets, and the incubation period is 2 to 10 weeks.

In initial stages of infection, primary inflammation occurs and a slight cough develops. As the disease progresses, anorexia, weight loss, night sweats, and a low-grade fever may be present.

Leukocytes and lymphocytes invade the lung area to attack the tuberculosis organism and wall off the primary infection. The wall surrounding the bacteria then calcifies and confines the organism permanently. If the infection is unable to be contained, tuberculosis may spread to other parts of the body (miliary tuberculosis), such as bones, lymph nodes, kidneys, and the subarachnoid space (tuberculous meningitis).

Assessment

All children living in high-risk areas should have a tuberculin test as part of basic preventive healthcare screening at 9 to 12 months of age and yearly thereafter. A Mantoux test, also known as a purified protein derivative (PPD) test, is administered by injecting 5 units of protein derivative vaccine intradermally, usually in the left lower arm. Assessment of the area 72 hours after administration is necessary to evaluate the level of reaction. A positive reaction, the formation of a 5- to 15-mm reddened induration, indicates the child has been exposed to tuberculosis or has developed antibodies to the foreign products of the tuberculosis organism. Children with positive reactions need a follow-up chest radiograph. Skin testing should not be done on children who have a history of tuberculosis diagnosis because of the risk of intense reaction at the testing site. Additionally, a tuberculosis screening test should not be done immediately after administration

of the measles, mumps, and rubella (MMR) vaccine because of the possibility of a false-negative result.

Tuberculosis may not be immediately evident on chest radiography. As local inflammation occurs, however, calcification and cloudiness in the inflamed area will be noticeable.

Sputum analysis, typically done for 3 consecutive days, is needed to confirm a diagnosis of active disease. Mucus should be expectorated from the lungs. Infants and children younger than 5 years of age do not expectorate sputum but swallow it; therefore, a gastric lavage may be necessary to obtain the specimen. Therapeutic play and support are helpful throughout the procedure.

Therapeutic Management

Antituberculosis drugs include isoniazid, rifampin, pyrazinamide, and ethambutol (Getahun, Sculier, Sismanidis, et al., 2012). Dosage and frequency of pharmacologic therapy vary with history and clinical presentation and are often determined in consultation with an infectious disease specialist. In addition to drug therapy, children should ingest a diet high in protein and calcium. Children should have periodic chest radiographs to ensure the disease does not reactivate. Up-to-date vaccination is encouraged. Children may return to regular activities, including school, when drug therapy has been initiated and treatment compliance has been established.

What If . . . 40.3
Michael has a PPD test with a positive result. Would the nurse prevent him from playing with other children on the hospital unit? Why or why not?

CYSTIC FIBROSIS

Cystic fibrosis (CF) is an inherited disease of the secretory glands. The disease is characterized by a thick mucus secretions, particularly in the pancreas and the lungs, as well as electrolyte abnormalities in sweat gland secretions. An abnormality of the long arm of chromosome 7 results in the inability to transport small molecules across cell membranes, leading to dehydration of epithelial cells in the airway and pancreas.

CF is inherited from an autosomal recessive trait. It occurs in approximately 1 in 2,500 live births and is most often found in White children. Chorionic villi sampling or amniocentesis can be performed during pregnancy for early detection. Additionally, all newborns can be screened at birth (Laguna, Lin, Wang, et al., 2012).

Affected males may be unable to reproduce secondary to persistent plugging and blocking of the vas deferens by tenacious seminal fluid. Affected females may have thick cervical secretions that limit sperm motility. Alternative insemination and in vitro fertilization are options for patients who desire to become pregnant.

Pancreas Involvement

The acinar cells of the pancreas normally produce lipase, trypsin, and amylase—enzymes that flow into the duodenum to digest fat, protein, and carbohydrate. In patients with CF, these enzyme secretions may be so thick that they plug ducts, resulting in atrophy of the acinar cells and an inability to produce enzymes. The islets of Langerhans and insulin production are influenced much later because of their endocrine (ductless) activity.

An absence of pancreatic enzymes in the duodenum results in an inability to digest fat, protein, and some sugars. Bowel movements become large, bulky, and greasy (**steatorrhea**). An increase in intestinal flora and fat results in an extremely foul odor, and the increased bulk of feces often leads to a protuberant abdomen. Malnutrition occurs without therapy and may include emaciated extremities and loose skin folds on the buttocks. Fat-soluble vitamins, particularly vitamins A, D, and E, cannot be absorbed in the absence of fat absorption, resulting in vitamin deficiency

Meconium in a newborn is normally thick and tenacious. In approximately 10% of children with CF, it may be so thick that it obstructs the intestine, known as meconium ileus. A newborn who develops abdominal distention with no passage of stool within 24 hours of birth should be evaluated further (Wainwright, 2011).

Lung Involvement

The anteroposterior diameter of the chest becomes enlarged in CF. Thickened mucus pools in bronchioles and often results in frequent infections. Organisms most frequently cultured are *Staphylococcus aureus*, *Pseudomonas aeruginosa*, and *H. influenzae*. Atelectasis may occur as a result of absorption of air from alveoli behind blocked bronchioles. Clubbed fingers may occur because of inadequate peripheral tissue perfusion.

Sweat Gland Involvement

Although sweat glands are not changed in structure, the level of chloride to sodium in perspiration is increased 2 to 5 times above normal, resulting in "salty" perspiration.

Assessment

CF is typically detected at birth through screening tests. It may also be detected by documentation of chromosomal abnormality, abnormal chloride concentration in perspiration, absence of pancreatic enzymes in the duodenum, the presence of immunoreactive trypsinogen in the blood secondary to pancreatic obstruction, and pulmonary involvement.

CF may be suspected in a newborn who fails to regain normal birth weight within 7 to 10 days after birth. This occurs secondary to the infant's inability to absorb milk fat. Nurses should be concerned with poor weight gain or meconium ileus in a newborn. Children undiagnosed at birth may present with complaints of increased hunger and steatorrheic stools because these stool changes are inconsistent with simple colic.

Respiratory infections develop around 4 to 6 months of age, and wheezing and rhonchi are often heard on chest auscultation. The chest may be hyperresonant with percussion. Cough is a prominent finding by preschool, and clubbing of fingers may also be present during this time.

Sweat Testing

Sweat testing detects abnormal salt concentrations. In this procedure, the paper is analyzed for sodium chloride content. A normal concentration of sodium chloride in sweat is 20 mEq/L; more than 60 mEq/L of sodium chloride is diagnostic of CF. Sweat tests are often not necessary because of advanced chromosomal testing.

Duodenal Analysis

Duodenal secretions may be used to detect pancreatic enzymes and reveal the extent of pancreatic involvement. This is done by passing a nasogastric tube into the duodenum; secretions are then aspirated for analysis. The tube placement can be determined by pH levels. Secretions from the duodenum are sent to the laboratory for analysis of trypsin content, the easiest pancreatic enzyme to assay.

Stool Analysis

Stool may be collected and analyzed for fat content and lack of trypsin of the stool.

Pulmonary Testing

A chest X-ray generally confirms the extent of pulmonary involvement. Pulmonary function may be tested to determine the extent of atelectasis and emphysema.

Therapeutic Management

Therapeutic management is a collaborative process to reduce the involvement of the pancreas, lungs, and sweat glands.

 ## Nursing Diagnoses and Related Interventions

Nursing Diagnosis: Imbalanced nutrition, less than body requirements, related to inability to digest fat

Outcome Evaluation:

1. Adequate height and weight growth percentiles
2. Decrease in stool quantity
3. Absence of vitamin deficiency

Children are placed on a high-calorie, high-protein, and moderate-fat diet and receive supplementation with vitamins A, D, and E. Medium-chain triglycerides are more readily digested than other oils. During hot months of the year, extra salt may be added to food to replace that lost through perspiration.

Generally, infants with CF may be breastfed and also use supplementary formula. A high-protein formula is generally recommended as a supplement.

Children should take a synthetic pancreatic enzyme, pancreatic lipase, to replace the enzyme they cannot produce (Box 40.8). These synthetic enzymes are supplied in large capsules that must be opened for young children and added to a small amount of food. Enzymes should not be added to hot food because a large portion of enzyme activity can be destroyed. Additionally, enzymes should not be added to a bottle of formula. If the infant doesn't drink the entire bottle, they will not receive the total benefit of the enzyme. The use of pancreatic enzymes may decrease the size and foul odor of stool and also aid in weight gain. Adolescents may have difficulty eating adequate amounts to maintain weight because their growth requires additional caloric intake.

Children should be monitored for overheating because excessive loss of sodium and chloride may result in dehydration. Monitor heat exposure and offer water frequently.

BOX 40.8

Nursing Care Planning Based on Responsibility for Pharmacology

PANCRELIPASE (COTAZYM)

Classification: Pancrelipase is an enzyme replacement.

Action: used to aid digestion in children with cystic fibrosis (Berlinski, 2017)

Pregnancy Risk Category: C

Dosage:

- Children 6 months to 1 year of age: 2,000 units orally per meal
- Children 1 to 6 years of age: 4,000 to 8,000 units orally with each meal and 4,000 units with snacks
- Children 7 to 12 years of age: 4,000 to 12,000 units orally with each meal and with snacks

Possible Adverse Effects: nausea, abdominal cramps, diarrhea, hypersensitivity

Nursing Implications

- Administer the drug before or with meals and snacks. Instruct parents and child to do the same.
- Caution child and parents to avoid inhaling powder or spilling it on the hands because it may irritate the skin or mucous membranes.
- Do not crush or let the child chew the enteric form of the drug. Break open the capsule and mix with 1 teaspoon of food.
- Instruct the child and parents about possible adverse effects and encourage them to contact their healthcare provider should any become severe.

Nursing Diagnosis: Ineffective airway clearance related to inability to clear mucus from the respiratory tract

Outcome Evaluation:

1. Child's temperature is below 100.4°F (38.0°C).
2. PO_2 is 80 to 90 mmHg.
3. PCO_2 is less than 40 mmHg.
4. Oxygen saturation is 92% to 100%.

Pulmonary infection from plugged airways is common. It is important to keep bronchial secretions moist and flowing freely to encourage draining from the bronchial tree. This is done by frequent nebulization or aerosol therapy followed by chest physiotherapy. Frequent observation is necessary to monitor for respiratory distress. If a portion of a lung becomes obstructed from a mucus plug, a child can quickly experience respiratory distress.

The right side of the heart tends to enlarge in children with chronic respiratory disease because congestion in the lungs increases pressure in the pulmonary artery and right ventricle. After a period of stress or exercise, children may begin to show signs of cardiac failure because their already enlarged heart has inadequate compensation.

Humidified Oxygen. Oxygen is supplied to children by mask, prongs, ventilators, or nebulizer. Mist can be supplied by an ultrasonic compressor and delivered through a nebulizer mask.

Aerosol Therapy. Children may be given aerosol therapy by means of a nebulizer to provide antibiotics or bronchodilators. A mucolytic can be added to the mist to aid in diluting and liquefying secretions. Cough suppressants and codeine should be avoided because secretions must be removed to promote effective air exchange and prevent infection.

Chest Physiotherapy. Bronchial secretions may be so tenacious that children are unable to expectorate, even with liquefaction by mist or aerosol therapy. Chest physiotherapy, as often as three or four times a day, may aid in drainage secretion.

Activity. Encourage normal activities as tolerated. Children confined to a bed need frequent position changes to encourage lung drainage and prevent skin breakdown over bony prominences. A superior position will encourage lung lobes to drain.

Respiratory Hygiene. Sputum may have a disagreeable taste or odor. Encourage adequate dental hygiene.

Nursing Diagnosis: Risk for impaired skin integrity related to stool acidity

Outcome Evaluation: Skin breakdown is not present. Rectal prolapse is not present.

Stool may be irritating because of high fat content. Children who are not toilet trained should have diapers changed immediately to prevent skin breakdown.

Monitor for rectal prolapse due to weak musculature of the rectal area. Rectal prolapse appears as a bright-red mass protruding from the anal sphincter and should be replaced promptly to prevent a compromised blood supply. Prolapse occurs much less frequently in children who are receiving pancreatic enzymes than in those who are not because the incidence of rectal prolapse decreases with improved nutrition.

Nursing Diagnosis: Risk for compromised family coping related to chronic illness in a child

Outcome Evaluation: Family members state they have adequate resources to cope with diagnosis.

Family members assume a great deal of responsibility for the care of their child. Begin discharge planning and teaching when a child is first admitted to a hospital. Discuss changes that may be needed to successfully accommodate the child's therapeutic regimen. Encourage quarterly communication with the healthcare team to review individualized care plans and address barriers to CF care (Lahiri, Hempstead, Brady, et al., 2016).

Adequate Rest and Comfort. Any child with compromised lung function may have a degree of dyspnea that leads to exhaustion. Encourage periods of rest during the day, including before meals and prior to chest physiotherapy.

Growth and Development. Encourage age-appropriate activities. Children should attend regular school and participate in physical fitness, as much as possible, to encourage socialization with other children.

Continuing Care. Periodic health assessments and routine childhood immunizations, including annual influenza vaccination, are necessary. Children should receive the first dose of pneumococcal polysaccharide vaccine (PPSV23) at least 8 weeks after the last dose of pneumococcal conjugate vaccine (PCV13) (Lahiri et al., 2016).

Children with CF often report feelings of vulnerability and loss of independence due to their disease. Treatment management should include opportunities for shared decision making, control, and self-efficacy (Jamieson, Fitzgeral, Singh-Grewal, et al., 2014).

Adolescents with CF are candidates for lung transplants. Some of these are done as lower lobe transplants from a living donor. A lung transplant is advantageous for children with CF because the new lung does not possess the defective gene, greatly improving life expectancy.

What If . . . 40.4
A nurse is particularly interested in exploring one of the 2020 National Health Goals with respect to respiratory disorders and children (see Box 40.1). What would be a possible research topic pertinent to these goals that would be applicable to Michael and his family and that would also advance evidence-based practice?

KEY POINTS FOR REVIEW

- Respiratory tract disorders tend to occur more frequently in children than adults because the lumens of children's bronchi are narrow and obstruction and infection are more likely to occur. Planning nursing care that includes assurance not only meets Quality & Safety Education for Nurses (QSEN) competencies but also best meets the family's total needs.
- Acute nasopharyngitis (the common cold) is the most common infectious disease in children. Treatment should include comfort measures.
- Tonsillitis is infection and inflammation of the palatine tonsils. Adenitis is infection and inflammation of the adenoid tonsils. Children with recurring infections may have their tonsils surgically removed.
- Laryngotracheobronchitis (croup) is inflammation of the larynx, trachea, and major bronchi. Epiglottitis is inflammation of the epiglottis. Both of these conditions can severely impair the airway. Children with epiglottitis should never be assessed for a gag reflex using a tongue blade because the elevated epiglottis can occlude the airway.
- Bronchiolitis is inflammation of the fine bronchioles.
- Respiratory syncytial virus (RSV) accounts for the majority of lower respiratory tract infections in young children. Infants with RSV infections must be observed closely for signs of increased respiratory distress.

- Asthma, a type I hypersensitivity reaction, is a diffuse and obstructive airway disease with wheezing as the most common symptom. Newer drugs such as leukotriene receptor antagonists and careful environmental control have aided in the management of asthma.
- Cystic fibrosis is a disease in which there is generalized dysfunction of the exocrine glands. This results in malabsorption and tenacious pulmonary secretions, leading to infections and poor nutrition. Lung transplantation may be used to replace the diseased lung tissue and to increase the child's life span.

CRITICAL THINKING CARE STUDY

Amanda is a 14-year-old with chronic asthma whom you meet in the emergency room. She is allergic to cats, goldenrod, and tomatoes. She lives with her mother; her parents have been divorced for the past 6 months. This afternoon, she attended a birthday party for a school friend. As soon as she returned home, her respiratory rate increased, she gasped for breath, and she began wheezing. Her father, a fireman, whom she's been staying with for the weekend, came home from work still in his rubber coat and boots to bring her to the hospital. While you talk to him to obtain a history, he keeps glancing at his watch.

1. Amanda's father keeps looking at his watch while he waits for you to take vital signs on Amanda. When you ask Amanda if anything happened at the party she could identify as an asthma "trigger," she shakes her head rapidly. Would you want to ask her any more questions?
2. Amanda admits she doesn't take her medications regularly because it isn't "cool." What suggestions could you give her to make her feel better about taking medicine?
3. Amanda was suspended from school last month because she rang the fire alarm, and she is banned from entering her local convenience store because she was caught stealing candy from there. When you ask her why these things happened, she answers, "Because I have asthma." What questions would you want to ask her to see if she's using her illness as an excuse for bad behavior?

RELATED RESOURCES

Explore these additional resources to enhance learning for this chapter:
- Student resources on thePoint, including answers to the What If . . . and Critical Thinking Care Study questions, http://thepoint.lww.com/Flagg8e
- Adaptive learning powered by PrepU, http://thepoint.lww.com/prepu

REFERENCES

Adil, E., Rager, T., & Carr, M. (2012). Location of airway obstruction in term and preterm infants with laryngomalacia. *American Journal of Otolaryngology, 33*(4), 437–440.
Bradley, J., Byington, C., Shah, S., et al. (2011). Executive summary: The management of community-acquired pneumonia in infants and children older than 3 months of age: Clinical practice guidelines by the Pediatric Infectious Diseases Society and the Infectious Diseases Society of America. *Clinical Infectious Diseases, 53*(7), 617–630.
Berlinski, A. (2017). Pediatric aerosol therapy. *Respiratory Care, 62*(6), 662–677.

Centers for Disease Control and Prevention. (2012). *Cold and cough medicines*. Atlanta, GA: Author.

Chan, E. D., & Chan, M. M. (2013). Pulse oximetry: Understanding its basic principles facilitates appreciation of its limitation. *Respiratory Medicine, 107*(6), 789–799.

Dargaville, P. A. (2012). Respiratory support in meconium aspiration syndrome: A practical guide. *International Journal of Pediatrics, 2012,* 965159.

Eladl, H. M. (2010). Transnasal endoscopic repair of bilateral congenital choanal atresia: Controversies. *The Journal of Laryngology & Otology, 124*(4), 387–392.

Federico, M. J., Kirby, G. S., Deterding, R. R., et al. (2011). Respiratory tract & mediastinum. In W. Hay, M. Levin, R. Deterding, et al. (Eds.), *Current diagnosis & treatment pediatrics* (21st ed., pp. 487–584). New York, NY: McGraw-Hill/Lange.

Florin, T. A., Plint, A. C., & Zorc, J. J. (2017). Viral bronchiolitis. *Lancet, 389*(10065), 211–214.

Getahun, H., Sculier, D., Sismanidis, C., et al. (2012). Prevention, diagnosis, and treatment of tuberculosis in children and mothers: Evidence for action for maternal, neonatal and child health services. *The Journal of Infectious Disease, 205,* S216–S227.

Jamieson, N., Fitzgeral, D., Singh-Grewal, D., et al. (2014). Children's experiences of cystic fibrosis: A systematic review of qualitative studies. *Pediatrics, 133*(6), e1683–e1697.

Janssen, J., & Cardillo, G. (2011). Primary spontaneous pneumothorax: Towards outpatient treatment and abandoning chest tube drainage. *Respiration, 82*(2), 201–203.

Laguna, T. A., Lin, N., Wang, Q., et al. (2012). Comparison of quantitative sweat chloride methods after positive newborn screen for cystic fibrosis. *Pediatric Pulmonology, 47*(8), 736–742.

Lahiri, T., Hempstead, S. E., Brady, C., et al. (2016). Clinical practice guidelines from the Cystic Fibrosis Foundation for preschoolers with cystic fibrosis. *Pediatrics, 137*(4), e20151784.

Mahant, S., & Parkin, P. C. (2016). Apnea in bronchiolitis: Challenges of studying an uncommon complication of a common condition. *The Journal of Pediatrics, 177,* 11–12.

Mitchell, R. B., Hussey, H. M., Setzen, G., et al. (2013). Clinical consensus statement: Tracheostomy care. *Otolaryngology—Head & Neck Surgery, 148*(1), 6–20.

Mudd, S. S., Leu, K., Sloand, E. D., et al. (2015). Pediatric asthma and the used of metered dose inhalers with valve holding chambers: Barriers to the implementation of evidence-based practice. *Journal of Emergency Nursing, 41*(1), 13–18.

National Heart, Lung, and Blood Institute. (2007). *Expert Panel Report 3: Guidelines for the diagnosis and management of asthma* (Report No. 07-4051). Bethesda, MD: Author.

Pardue Jones, B., Fleming, G. M., Otillio, J. K., et al. (2015). Pediatric acute asthma exacerbations: Evaluation and management from emergency department to intensive care unit. *The Journal of Asthma, 53*(6), 607–617.

Pascoal, L. M., Lopes, M. V., da Silva, V. M., et al. (2016). Clinical differentiation of respiratory nursing diagnoses among children with acute respiratory infection. *Journal of Pediatric Nursing, 31*(1), 85–91.

Peacock, J., & Stanik-Hutt, J. (2013). Translating best care practices to improve nursing documentation regarding pediatric patients dependent on home mechanical ventilation and tracheostomy tube support: A quality improvement initiative. *Home Healthcare Nurse, 31*(1), 10–17.

Ralston, S. L., Lieberthal, A. S., Meissner, H. C., et al. (2014). Clinical practice guideline: The diagnosis, management, and prevention of bronchiolitis. *Pediatrics, 134*(5), e1474–e1502.

Raviglione, M., Marais, B., Floyd, K., et al. (2012). Scaling up interventions to achieve global tuberculosis control: Progress and new developments. *Lancet, 379*(9829), 1902–1913.

Record, S. (2015). Practice guideline: Epistaxis in children. *Journal of Pediatric Healthcare, 29*(5), 484–488.

Sylvester, D. C., Carr, S., & Nix, P. (2013). Maximal medical therapy for chronic rhinosinusitis: A survey of otolaryngology consultants in the United Kingdom. *International Forum of Allergy & Rhinology, 3*(2), 129–132.

U.S. Department of Health and Human Services. (2010). *Healthy people 2020*. Washington, DC: Author.

Vandemheen, K. L., Aaron, S. D., Poirier, C., et al. (2010). Development of a decision aid for adult cystic fibrosis patients considering referral for lung transplantation. *Progress in Transplantation, 20*(1), 81–87.

Wainwright, C. E. (2011). Treatment of cystic fibrosis following infant screening. *Therapy, 8*(6), 613–622.

Wald, E. R., Applegate, K. E., Bordley, C., et al. (2013). Clinical practice guideline for the diagnosis and management of acute bacterial sinusitis in children aged 1 to 18 years. *Pediatrics, 132*(1), e262–e280.

Winston, C. A., & Menzies, H. J. (2012). Pediatric and adolescent tuberculosis in the United States, 2008–2010. *Pediatrics, 130*(6), e1425–e1432.

Witt, W. P., Weiss, A. J., & Elixhauser, A. (2014). *Overview of hospital stays for children in the United States, 2012* (HCUP Statistical Brief No. 187). Rockville, MD: Agency for Healthcare Research and Quality. Retrieved from http://www.hcup-us.ahrq.gov/reports/statbriefs/sb187-Hospital-Stays-Children-2012.pdf

41

Nursing Care of a Family When a Child Has a Cardiovascular Disorder

*M*egan is a newborn who was born with a moderate-sized ventricular septal defect. Megan's parents will be taking her home this afternoon with follow-up in the pediatric cardiology office in 1 month. They tell you the cardiologist instructed them to "watch her carefully" during that time. "What does that mean?" they ask you. "Exactly what should we watch for?"

Previous chapters described the growth and development of well infants and children and care of children when ill. This chapter adds information about the child who is ill with a cardiovascular disorder and the stress that such a serious diagnosis places on families. Such information builds a base for care and health teaching for children with these disorders.

What advice would you offer Megan's parents?

KEY TERMS

acyanotic heart disease	cyanotic heart disease
afterload	diastole
cardiac catheterization	heart murmur
cardiomyopathy	preload
congestive heart failure (CHF)	systole
contractility	vasculitis

OBJECTIVES

After mastering the contents of this chapter, you should be able to:

1. Describe common cardiovascular disorders of childhood.
2. Identify 2020 National Health Goals related to children with cardiovascular disorders that nurses can help the nation achieve.
3. Assess a child with a cardiovascular dysfunction.
4. Formulate nursing diagnoses for a child with a cardiovascular disorder.
5. Establish outcomes based on the priority needs of a child with a cardiovascular disorder that can help the family manage seamless transitions across different healthcare settings.
6. Using the nursing process, plan nursing care that includes the six competencies of Quality & Safety Education for Nurses (QSEN): Patient-Centered Care, Teamwork & Collaboration, Evidence-Based Practice (EBP), Quality Improvement (QI), Safety, and Informatics.
7. Implement nursing care for a child with a cardiovascular disorder, such as teaching about the importance of taking prescribed medication.
8. Evaluate expected outcomes for achievement and effectiveness of care.
9. Integrate knowledge of cardiovascular disorders with the interplay of nursing process, the six competencies of QSEN, and Family Nursing to promote quality maternal and child health nursing care.

Cardiovascular issues in children are complex, spanning the spectrum from congenital defects that may present at birth to acquired heart disease or late-onset inherited disorders. Severity, complexity, and presentation vary depending on the disorder and the child's age. The disorders may require episodic care or mandate life-long medical management by a specialist. Managing a child with a cardiovascular disorder is very challenging and requires the nurse to have an in-depth understanding of a multitude of disease processes, congenital heart defects, and treatment regimens as well as the ability to work with children of any age and families in varying states of emotional health.

BOX 41.1

Nursing Care Planning Based on 2020 National Health Goals

Cardiovascular illness is a major health problem in adults. Because the illness and its effects can be prevented or at least minimized by instituting measures early in childhood, a number of 2020 National Health Goals address ways parents and children can modify nutrition or exercise to achieve better cardiovascular health:

- Increase the proportion of adolescents who meet current federal physical activity guidelines for aerobic physical activity (7 days/week) and for muscle-strengthening activity (≥3 days/week) from a baseline of 21.9% to a target of 24.1%.
- Reduce the proportion of children age 2 to 19 years who are considered obese from 16.1% to 14.5%.
- Reduce consumption of calories from solid fats in the population aged 2 years and older from a mean 16.6% of total daily calorie intake to 14.2%.
- Reduce consumption of calories from added sugars from a mean 15.1% of total daily calories to 9.7% in the population aged 2 years and older.
- Increase consumption of dark green vegetables, red and orange vegetables, beans, and peas to the diets of the population aged 2 years and older from a mean 0.29 cups per 1,000 calories/day to 0.53 cup equivalent.
- Reduce the proportion of children and adolescents (ages 8 to 17 years old) with hypertension from 3.5% to 3.2% (U.S. Department of Health and Human Services, 2010; see www.healthypeople.gov).

There are many more goals at the Healthy People 2020 website that are specific to the health of children. Nurses can help the nation achieve these goals by educating parents and children at every encounter about the importance of reducing obesity and implementing exercise and nutrition programs for sound cardiovascular health. These are frequently difficult lifestyle choices, so the information must be reinforced with every encounter. Encourage families to make any changes as an entire family, not just make the changes only for the child. Although encouraging a low-fat diet, it is important for nurses to caution parents not to start their children on reduced-fat diets until they are 2 years old to allow for myelination of nerve cells. Children should also not be placed on a diet or limited caloric intake unless under the direction of a healthcare provider.

Healthcare providers are not just better today at managing children with cardiovascular disorders, but they are also better at diagnosing these disorders. Genetic testing has allowed for families to test even asymptomatic children for an identified genetic syndrome based on familial patterns, including dysrhythmias, cardiomyopathies, Marfan syndrome, or long-QT syndrome. This ability to provide early diagnoses allows for enhanced therapeutic management and risk-reducing interventions, which may improve survival and provide a sense of empowerment for patients and their families.

Many heart-related problems can be prevented. Healthy People 2020 has identified several National Goals that address children's risk for preventable heart disease and other disorders secondary to hypertension, overweight, and obesity. Although it is not possible to prevent congenital heart disease, we can provide children and families with education and guidance in an effort to prevent disorders such as hypertension, obesity, and dyslipidemia, which are documented to have a negative impact on cardiovascular health. Even in families with a predisposition for these disorders, education is imperative in guiding families to incorporate lifestyle changes into their daily routine.

Box 41.1 depicts 2020 National Health Goals that address achieving cardiovascular health through health promotion and disease prevention, measures that can begin in childhood and adolescence.

An important factor affecting the health care of children with cardiovascular issues today is the increased life expectancies for children born with complex congenital heart disease and the decreased mortality experienced by children with a variety of disorders, including single-ventricle heart disease, cardiomyopathies, and dysrhythmias. Not only are traditional therapies more successful in children, but also pediatric patients of all ages now have greater access to a wide range of treatment options, including heart transplant, ventricular assistive devices, extracorporeal membrane oxygenation (ECMO), and nonsurgical catheter-based interventions. The ensuing pages provide a greater understanding of the pediatric cardiovascular system, the disease states that most frequently affect children, and management strategies to afford these children the best health possible.

Nursing Process Overview

FOR CARE OF A CHILD WITH CARDIOVASCULAR DISORDER

ASSESSMENT

Assessment of a child with a cardiovascular disorder includes both careful history taking and physical examination because many signs and symptoms of cardiac complications in children can be subtle. A variety of studies such as echocardiography, electrocardiography, cardiac catheterization, and diagnostic imaging may be used to confirm a diagnosis, guide therapy, or determine the need for surgical intervention.

Although the diagnosis, management, and treatment of cardiovascular disorders in children has progressed exceptionally far in recent decades, these therapies and survival rates do not come without consequences. Children are living longer, but their lives can be very complicated. They can have health deficits that require long-term monitoring, and they frequently have many comorbidities such as poor feeding, reactive airway disease, or diminished cognitive abilities, all of which may require other medical treatments, medications, and intervention. When assessing children with an underlying cardiovascular disorder, you must incorporate a multisystem assessment into practice, as other systems may be directly or indirectly affected by the cardiac disorder.

Cardiovascular disorders are frightening for both children and parents, as even small children realize the importance of their heart to sustain life. For the families of children with a cardiovascular disorder, understanding the functioning of the heart and circulation is an important first step toward coping with the illness. You will need to be comfortable teaching about the underlying disorder, explaining diagnostic tests, and providing emotional support to children and their families throughout the assessment process.

NURSING DIAGNOSIS

Nursing diagnoses associated with heart disease in children usually address the effect of compromised cardiac function or the impact a serious disorder can have on the child or parents. Examples include:

- Risk for ineffective peripheral tissue perfusion related to impaired myocardial function
- Decreased cardiac output related to altered cardiac anatomy, physiology, or altered cardiac rhythm
- Imbalanced nutrition, less than body requirements, related to increased metabolic demands of the disordered heart
- Deficient knowledge related to care of the child with a cardiac disorder
- Anxiety related to lack of knowledge about child's illness
- Anxiety related to lack of knowledge about caring for a child after surgery or a cardiac catheterization
- Risk for activity intolerance due to altered cardiopulmonary physiology
- Interrupted family processes related to stresses of diagnosis and care responsibilities
- Ineffective coping related to lack of adequate support people
- Impaired parenting related to inability to bond with a critically ill newborn

If the concerns in the latter three diagnoses are not identified at the time of diagnosis or when a child is ill, they may continue long after a child is treated and returns home. This can have negative consequences on the entire family and may affect parent–child bonding.

OUTCOME IDENTIFICATION AND PLANNING

Nursing planning is essential to help parents and children understand heart anatomy because a sound knowledge base can help them understand the need for diagnostic testing, medication compliance, and ongoing follow-up. Additional teaching is necessary to prepare parents and children for procedures or surgery and recovery at home. Teaching parents to conscientiously administer cardiac medications is another area where planning plays an important role. Organizations that are helpful for referral are the American Heart Association (AHA; www.heart.org), the Cardiovascular Disease Foundation (www.cvdf.org), and the Congenital Heart Information Network (www.tchin.org).

IMPLEMENTATION

Nursing interventions in the care of children with a cardiovascular disorder include teaching, providing an opportunity for children and their families to express fears about a child's illness and treatment plan, providing physiologic and psychological support such as comfort measures after surgery, and caring for a child during acute hospitalizations. An equally important role is teaching prevention of heart disease such as promoting a home environment free from smoke and encouraging a healthy lifestyle through exercise, maintaining an appropriate weight, and eating a low-fat diet.

OUTCOME EVALUATION

Outcome evaluation should include both immediate and future outcomes for the child and family because cardiac disorders may be long term. Important short-term outcomes involve receiving adequate support during procedures and treatment. If long-term care becomes necessary, evaluating the family's ability to think of their child not in terms of illness but in terms of wellness and providing opportunities for parents to express their concerns about their child's status are important.

The following examples suggest achievement of outcomes:
- The child demonstrates age-appropriate coping skills related to diagnosis and possible intervention.
- The parents demonstrate competence with procedures required for care of their child.
- The parents exhibit positive coping skills related to their child's diagnosis and the care required to foster optimal growth and development in their child.
- The parents verbalize positive thoughts about their child's future.

Health Promotion and Risk Management

Because the risk factors that lead to adult heart disease (e.g., obesity, high cholesterol levels, and lack of consistent exercise) involve health habits that begin in childhood, prevention of cardiac disease has shifted from an adult focus to a child focus in the hope that early interventions will have a major impact on reducing the incidence of preventable heart disease in the next generation.

RISK MANAGEMENT FOR CONGENITAL HEART DISEASE

The cause of congenital heart disease often cannot be documented, although some associations are seen with familial patterns of inheritance. Women need to enter pregnancy fully immunized to help prevent infection during pregnancy. Parents who have a family member who was born with a heart disorder need to be aware that other children born to them need to be carefully screened prenatally and at birth for a similar disorder.

RISK MANAGEMENT FOR ACQUIRED HEART DISEASE

Acquired heart diseases in children that have identified risk factors include rheumatic fever, hypertension, and hyperlipidemia. Rheumatic fever is an autoimmune response that follows a group A β-hemolytic streptococcal infection. Ensuring that all children who have a streptococcal infection such as streptococcal pharyngitis receive adequate antibiotic therapy is essential in preventing the complication of rheumatic fever.

Although hypertension (elevated blood pressure) is associated with a genetic predisposition, other factors such as a high intake of sodium, lack of exercise, and obesity increase the chances a susceptible child will develop the disorder by late childhood (Riley & Bluhm, 2012). Hypertension leads to changes in the left ventricle if not well managed. Urging families to reduce their intake of processed foods and snacks can reduce salt intake in children. School nurses can play an important role in this effort by monitoring the foods served daily in school cafeterias and advocating for more nutritious menus. Beginning when a child is 3 years of age, blood pressure should be included as part of routine assessment to detect as early as possible the development of prehypertension or hypertension (Expert Panel on Integrated Guidelines for Cardiovascular Health and Risk Reduction in Children and Adolescents, 2011).

Although the tendency toward hyperlipidemia is also inherited, a diet high in saturated fat has been implicated in the development of the metabolic syndrome. It is important that fat intake not be restricted in infants and toddlers because they need the fat for brain development. School-age children and adolescents, however, should reduce their fat intake to 30% of total calories (the same recommendation as for adults). Children from high-risk families (in which a family member has had an early [before the age of 50 years] myocardial infarction or hyperlipidemia) should be regularly screened for elevated cholesterol and triglyceride levels at routine healthcare visits (Expert Panel on Integrated Guidelines for Cardiovascular Health and Risk Reduction in Children and Adolescents, 2011). All families and children should be encouraged to participate in routine aerobic physical activity with daily limits on the amount of screen time, including television, phone, computer, social media, and/or games.

Nursing Care of the Child With a Cardiac Disorder

Caring for a child with a cardiovascular disorder not only requires the nurse to have a strong understanding of the cardiac anatomy and various disease states but also requires a strong understanding of developmental levels and being comfortable working with children and families as they progress through a very stressful time, emotionally, socially, psychologically, and financially.

Most parents have many questions about how to care for a child born with heart disease. Encourage them to learn as much as possible about their child's disorder and give care to their newborn or child whenever they can while in the hospital, so they will feel more secure in caring for that child at home when there are limited resources. Be certain parents are aware that children with heart disease are different from adults with heart disease. They will not have the same degree of activity or intake restrictions, so parents should not unnecessarily limit their infant's activities or types of food. Caring for an older child who has any form of heart disease is equally challenging, as the children themselves can be very stressed or anxious. Offer support at all healthcare visits to help parents feel confident that they know the child's medication regimen and reinforce any signs or symptoms they should report immediately to the child's cardiologist or primary healthcare provider.

It has been noted that many of these children have an altered quality of life. Factors that affect quality of life most are parental support, lower socioeconomic status, limitations due to physical impairment, as well as the level of a child's baseline anxiety and depression (Drakouli, Petsios, Giannakopoulou, et al., 2015). These can not only affect that child's ability to live a "normal" life but also affect the family. Recent studies have found the impact of an infant's congenital heart disease on the family is determined by both the child's medical condition and the family's psychosocial factors. Families with a poor social support network may have the greatest need for intervention. The financial burden can also be quite significant for families of children with a cardiac disorder, specifically complex congenital heart disease.

 ## Nursing Diagnoses and Related Interventions

Nursing diagnoses for children with cardiac disease need to address both physical and psychosocial care.

Nursing Diagnosis: Parental health-seeking behaviors related to desire to be informed about child's cardiac disorder

Outcome Evaluation: Parents accurately state the nature of their child's illness and unique needs of their child; parents state they will telephone or e-mail the child's cardiologist or primary healthcare provider if they have any questions or concerns.

Provide or Review Information About Care. Parents generally ask questions such as "Is it safe to let a baby with heart disease cry?" Crying for a few minutes while a parent warms a bottle or fully awakens at night to breastfeed will not harm the baby. If the child has no immediate needs to be met, such as hunger, cold, or a wet diaper, the child should be allowed to fuss so they can learn to self-soothe and do not become dependent on being held.

Another common question is "Does our child need special nutrition?" As with all newborns, breastfeeding is the preferred method of feeding, and the average infant with heart disease can be successful at this. Because some infants with congenital heart disease tire easily, they may require frequent small feeds or feeding with increased caloric density. Breastfeeding can be more tiring for an infant and may require a mother to pump breast milk so it can be fortified if necessary and fed with a bottle. Infrequently, a child may require a nasogastric or nasojejunal tube for feedings.

"How much activity can we allow the baby?" is another question that is often asked. Again, the answer to this depends on the type and extent of the heart disorder, but, as a rule, infants and young children naturally limit their own activity and stop when they are fatigued. Parents may need some guidance, however, in knowing when to set sensible limits. Encourage parents to observe their infant carefully so they can recognize the signs of respiratory distress or easy fatigability. Older children are usually encouraged to play as they desire and participate in physical education class, but varsity-level competition may require some restrictions, based on the cardiac disorder.

Although children with congenital heart disorders are usually followed by a cardiologist for health supervision, it's important they are also followed by a primary care provider so they receive routine childhood immunizations and health guidance. As a rule, parents need to bring infants and children with heart disorders for prompt treatment for minor illnesses, especially upper respiratory infections, as this may compromise their respiratory status to a greater degree than in children without underlying disease. Hydration must be closely monitored so dehydration does not occur. Baseline tachypnea will increase insensible water loss, so any changes to fluid intake due to illness or changes in metabolic demand may cause excessive fluid loss and dehydration.

Review Steps for Follow-Up Care and Emergencies.

Before parents leave the hospital with a newborn with a congenital heart disorder, be certain they have the name and number of the healthcare professional to call if they have a question about their infant's health. Be certain they also have an appointment for a first well-child visit with their primary care provider and an appointment with their specialist(s) so they can feel assured that the responsibility of caring for this child will not be theirs alone but will be shared with other healthcare personnel. If they are ever unsure of whether their child is ill or in distress, urge them to err on the side of caution by telephoning or bringing the child to their primary care setting. Everyone who cares for infants or children with heart disease appreciates the responsibility parents feel and the difficulty they can have in making health judgments about their child.

If you have any concerns, you should check with the family about transportation concerns; other persons to support the parents with providing care, especially when a parent must return to work; or financial concerns. Referring a family to a social worker or case manager before they are discharged may help ensure the child attends all necessary appointments, receives medications or special formulas, or receives home care support if needed.

Parents of newborns are frequently taught cardiopulmonary resuscitation (CPR) before they leave the hospital. Make sure all household members have an understanding of the newborn or child's needs, including feeding regimen, medications, and signs of distress. It is helpful if all adult household members can also learn CPR.

The Cardiovascular System

The cardiovascular system consists of the heart, which acts as a pump; the blood, which provides the fluid and cells for transport of oxygen, nutrients, regulatory substances, antibodies, and the evacuation of waste products; and the blood vessels, which provide the means and routes for transport throughout the body. The system has a great capacity to adapt to changing body needs.

A thorough understanding of the fetal, newborn, and older child's cardiac anatomy and physiology is essential when caring for children with a variety of heart diseases. It is necessary not only to provide optimal care but also to educate both the child and family so they understand the disease process and management strategies.

ANATOMY REVIEW

Embryologic development of the heart is described in Chapter 9; cardiac adaptations at birth are described in Chapter 18. After the infant transitions from fetal circulation, the heart can be thought of as consisting of two pumps: one on the right side that pumps blood to the lungs, where it is oxygenated before returning to the left side of the heart, and one on the left side that moves the oxygenated blood to peripheral tissues through systemic arteries. After supplying nutrients and collecting wastes, the blood returns through the veins to the right side of the heart, where the cycle begins again.

Review of Normal Heart Circulation

Deoxygenated blood returning from the upper body travels through the superior vena cava (SVC); that returning from the lower body travels through the inferior vena cava (IVC). This blood mixes in the right atrium and then goes through the tricuspid valve into the right ventricle. It then goes through the pulmonic valve and out the main pulmonary artery, continuing out the right- and left-branch pulmonary arteries to the lungs. Once the blood is oxygenated, it returns to the left atrium by way of four pulmonary veins. It then travels through the mitral valve, to the left ventricle, through the aortic valve, and out the ascending aorta (Fig. 41.1). It con-

Figure 41.1 Anatomy of the normal heart. (From Troiano, N. H., Harvey, C. J., & Chez, B. F. [2012]. *AWHONN high-risk & critical care obstetrics* [3rd ed.]. Ambler, PA: Lippincott Williams & Wilkins.)

tinues across the transverse arch and to the descending aorta. As it passes through the transverse arch, three vessels come from this area: the brachiocephalic (which branches into the right subclavian artery and the right common carotid artery), the left common carotid artery, and the left subclavian artery. When blood leaves the heart, it is fully oxygenated; when it returns, it has an average saturation of 75%.

The coronary arteries come off the root of the aorta. Two coronary origins exist: the right coronary artery and the left coronary artery. The left coronary artery branches into the left anterior descending and the circumflex coronary artery. These vessels are perfused during diastole and provide oxygenated blood to the heart itself. This blood, once deoxygenated, returns to the right atrium by the coronary sinus vessels.

A strong understanding of fetal circulation is important to understanding congenital heart defects. While in utero, the lungs exhibit high resistance to blood flow due to their fluid-filled status and constricted pulmonary arterioles. The lungs do not perform normal gas exchange functions; rather, the placenta performs the actions of oxygenation and carbon dioxide removal for the fetus. Therefore, the fetus requires blood to be mixed in the heart in order to provide oxygenated blood to the body. Three fetal shunts exist to facilitate this circulation: the foramen ovale, the ductus arteriosus, and the ductus venosus.

As the highly oxygenated blood returns from the placenta through the IVC, 40% of the flow is directed across the foramen ovale into the left atria. The foramen ovale is a flapped opening between the atria that allows for this oxygenated blood to bypass the lungs and continue from the left atrium to the left ventricle and out the ascending aorta to the coronaries and upper body, which includes the brain.

The remaining IVC blood mixes in the right atrium with the deoxygenated blood that has returned from the head and upper extremities via the SVC. This blood then passes through the tricuspid valve, to the right ventricle, and out the pulmonary artery. But because of the higher pulmonary pressures in comparison with the lower systemic pressures, almost 90% of blood flowing from the right ventricle bypasses the lungs via the ductus arteriosus. The ductus is a conduit connecting the pulmonary artery to the aorta at the level of the pulmonary artery bifurcation. It allows blood to bypass the high-pressure pulmonary system and travel directly out the aorta to the body. Only 10% or less of blood ejected from the right ventricle actually passes to the lungs for growth and development.

These two shunts, the foramen ovale and ductus arteriosus, are what allow most of the poorly saturated blood from the upper and lower body to reach the right ventricle and the more highly saturated umbilical venous return to reach the left ventricle.

The final fetal shunt is the ductus venosus. As blood returns from the placenta through the umbilical vein, some goes into the hepatic veins to the liver and slightly more than half passes though the ductus venosus into the IVC. This highly oxygenated blood that is directed to the ductus venosus is then preferentially guided to the foramen ovale, allowing this oxygenated blood to go directly to the left side of the heart and out to the body (Fig. 41.2).

The changes that occur at birth, including hormonal levels, oxygen tension changes, pressure changes, and blood flow, precipitate closure of these three shunts.

As amniotic fluid is absorbed in the lungs and they become a gas-filled system, pressures on the left side of the heart are now higher than on the right. As well, the volume of blood returning from the pulmonary veins directly to the left atrium significantly increases. These changes in volume and pressure allow for the flap of the foramen ovale to be pressed closed against the atrial septum immediately; over the ensuing weeks, the flap will become permanently closed.

The ductus arteriosus will begin to constrict immediately at birth due to changing oxygen tension levels, decreasing prostaglandin levels, and a drop in pressure within the lumen of the ductus caused by changes in pulmonary vascular resistance, ultimately closing completely within a few days at the latest. Factors such as prematurity, congenital heart defects, or persistent pulmonary hypertension can change the expected closure times for these two shunts.

Although the final shunt, the ductus venosus, will immediately see a significant reduction in flow with the elimination of umbilical–placental circulation, some portal venous flow continues through this vessel and will vary over time. Permanent structural closure is thought to occur within 2 to 3 weeks after birth.

Within a few days after birth and with no confounding factors, circulation will follow the same pattern as in an adult. It is important to note though that the pulmonary pressures in a newborn, although lower than systemic pressures immediately after birth, will continue to drop to their lowest level by approximately 4 to 6 weeks of age.

ASSESSMENT

The heart is intricately involved with all other organs. Changes in the heart's function can affect multiple organ systems, and changes in other organs can be manifested in the cardiac system as well. Therefore, a cardiac assessment must begin with a complete health history and include a thorough physical examination.

Health History

As a result of technologic advances in prenatal care, heart disease may be recognized early in fetal life. Used during pregnancy, fetal echocardiography can reveal details about heart anomalies as early as 18 weeks into a pregnancy, allowing providers to be prepared with appropriate personnel for safe, effective management of the child's disorder at the time of birth.

If heart disease was undetected in utero, some murmurs associated with abnormal circulation may not be detected until several weeks after birth as pulmonary pressures continue to drop. Half of all newborns with critical congenital heart disease, particularly those with ductal-dependent defects, have no distinctive murmur, and in many cases, the symptoms of heart disease do not present until after hospital discharge. Universal screening with pulse oximetry testing in the newborn nursery is becoming the standard of care for newborns in the United States, with the goal of increasing the early identification of previously undiagnosed cyanotic heart disease.

A thorough child and family history is important to obtain. The history must include birth history with maternal and newborn issues noted. The pregnancy history will determine whether an intrauterine insult such as infections, medications, or drug use could have led to poor fetal formation. It is important, though, to understand that congenital heart

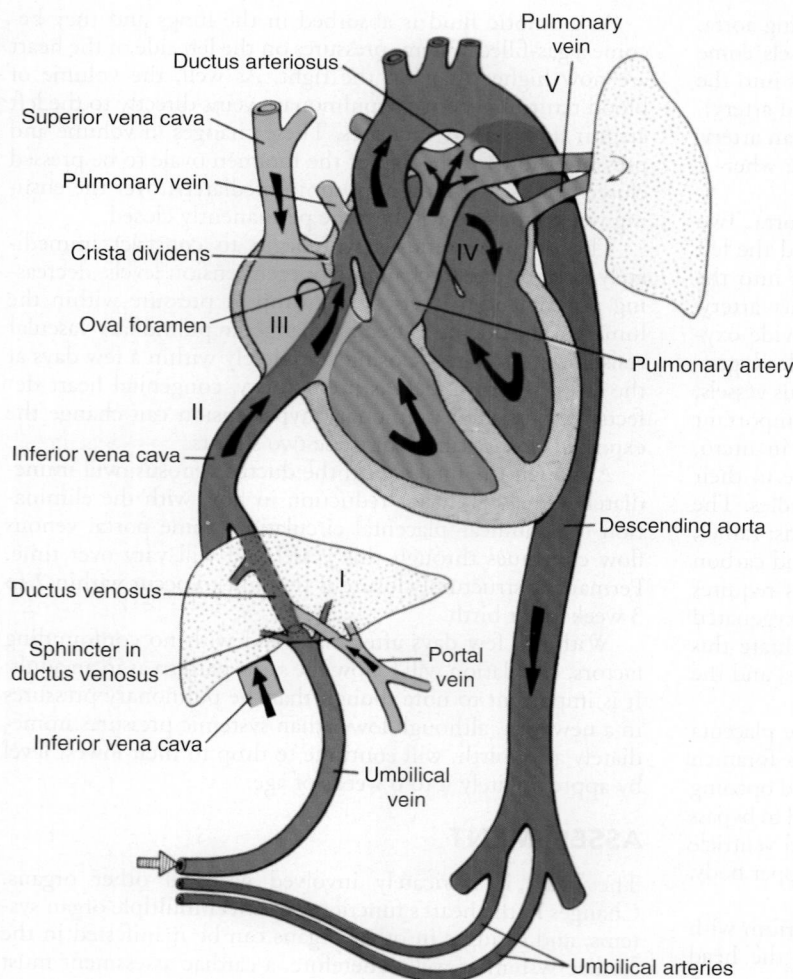

Figure 41.2   Fetal circulation. (From Sadler, T. W. [2010]. *Langman's medical embryology* [11th ed.]. Baltimore, MD: Lippincott Williams & Wilkins.)

disease has no one identified cause; many mothers who lead healthy lives and have healthy pregnancies may have a child with a cardiac disorder. The nurse must support the family and ensure they feel no guilt for the birth of a child with an anomaly.

Pertinent family history relative to the cardiac examination includes family members with cardiac disease before the age of 55 years, any episodes of sudden death, any other children born with heart problems, and any dysrhythmias. A family history is important for assessment because some heart disorders may have a polygenic inheritance pattern. Heart disorders also occur as an anomaly in chromosomal disorders such as Down syndrome, Turner syndrome, William syndrome, and DiGeorge syndrome. Therefore, if certain genetic disorders are noted, investigation into associated cardiac anomalies is necessary.

The child's current health status is important—not only their medical and surgical status, prior hospital admissions, and current medications but also their developmental level and timeline for attaining milestones. Some children may not be able to meet milestones on time because of their easy fatigability or extended hospital stays. Specific questions that indicate cardiac function focus on activity level, weight gain, and events such as chest pain or syncope. Remember, an infant's "activity level" is evaluated by how they feed: How long does

it take? Do they take frequent rests? Do they become tachypneic, diaphoretic or show other signs of distress while feeding? These are indicators of an inability to meet the metabolic demands incurred while feeding and could be related to poor cardiac function. Older children will be assessed based on their ability to keep up with their peers during times of activity such as recess, gym class, or participation in sports.

It is important to note the child's height, weight, and body mass index (BMI), as well as their vital signs, specifically heart rate, respiratory rate, blood pressure, and oxygen saturation. You will plot the child's growth parameters on the appropriate growth charts and note any deviations from their standard curve. Many children with underlying cardiac diseases may not grow on a "normal" curve but will maintain their own version of a normal curve.

You must also know the normal ranges for vital signs for children of all ages in order to perform an accurate assessment.

General Appearance

Once you have done a thorough review of the child's and family's history, you can perform a cardiac assessment. Upon entering a child's room, you should do a brief visual assessment. Does the child appear calm and comfortable? Is he lethargic? Is she in distress? What color are the child's extremities?

You should also take time to interact with the child at a developmentally appropriate level before actually performing the physical examination. Taking a few minutes to play or talk with a child can gain the child's trust and allow for a more accurate, complete examination. Infants can sit with their caregiver to feel safe and comfortable. If they are sleeping, attempts should be made to not disturb them while performing as much of the physical exam as possible. Feeding infants while performing an exam may also help to keep them from becoming upset. Older children can be distracted with noises, songs, bubbles, or videos. They too should be allowed to stay with a caregiver to keep them feeling safe and unafraid.

Be certain to inspect the distal extremities for color and measure capillary refill time, as these are indicators of poor tissue perfusion. When pressure is applied to a nail bed, it will blanch white and then quickly return to pink in a child with good circulation and oxygenation. Normal capillary refill time is less than 2 to 3 seconds. In a child with poor tissue perfusion, the pink color returns more slowly.

The mucous membranes of the mouth are the most accurate site to assess for cyanosis, so always assess the buccal membrane and lips for a blue color as these are less likely to be affected by environmental temperature. Cool, cyanotic extremities in newborns is termed *acrocyanosis* and is a normal finding in the first 24 to 48 hours of life that should not be confused with cyanosis related to heart disease. Measuring an oxygen saturation will give a more accurate measurement of circulating oxygen levels.

Physical Examination

Before actually placing your stethoscope on the patient's chest, you should place your hand on the left side of the chest to evaluate for the apical impulse, thrills, lifts, or heaves. The apical point of maximal impulse (PMI) is normally located at the fourth or fifth intercostal space, on the midclavicular line in infants and children. Deviations in the PMI can be indicators of an enlarged heart due to illness, heart failure, or congenital heart defects.

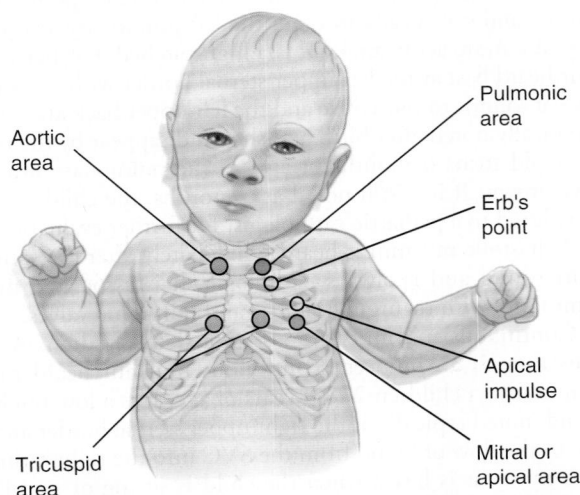

Figure 41.3 Sites for cardiac auscultation. (From Stephen, T. C., Skillen, D. L., Day, R. A., et al. [2013]. *Canadian Jensen's nursing health assessment: A best practice approach.* Philadelphia, PA: Lippincott Williams & Wilkins.)

A thrill is a vibration felt secondary to significant cardiac murmurs. It feels like the throat of a purring cat and occurs because of turbulent blood flow. A lift is a forceful cardiac contraction that causes the hand to move up. A heave is a very forceful cardiac contraction that actually causes the hand to move up and laterally.

Cardiac auscultation can be challenging in infants and young children because of their dislike of cold environments and strangers as well as fear of painful procedures such as immunizations that they come to associate with healthcare providers. A child who is ill is also more likely to be irritable and uncooperative. It is important for the room to be quiet and for the child to not speak during the examination. A pediatric-size stethoscope is necessary in order to differentiate where abnormal sounds are heard. The stethoscope has a diaphragm for hearing high-frequency sounds and a bell to detect low-frequency sounds. As you are listening to heart sounds, focus on the "normal" sounds of S1 and S2, the opening and closing of the valves. Then, listen for other sounds beside those two. You must try to block out respirations and listen for several heart beats at each location. Auscultation should be performed in a systematic manner (Fig. 41.3). With the child in a sitting position (either alone or in a parent's lap), you should start your assessment with the diaphragm of your stethoscope at the second intercostal space, at the right upper sternal border, then proceed to the second intercostal space at the left upper sternal border, and then continue listening down the left sternal border until you reach the fifth intercostal space. Once at this point, you should begin moving your stethoscope laterally, to the midclavicular line and out to the midaxillary line. After you have completed listening to the child's chest, you should then listen to their left back, along the spine, starting at the scapula and progressing halfway down the back. Finally, the chest assessment should be completed once again with the child supine.

All children may not participate with such a thorough examination, but this is the ideal technique.

First Heart Sound

The first heart sound (S1) is produced by the mitral and tricuspid valve closing. Blood fills the ventricles, and as ventricular pressure exceeds atrial pressure due to the volume within, the mitral and tricuspid valves are forced close. At this time, the aortic and pulmonic valves are forced open and the ventricles contract, ejecting blood out the aorta and pulmonary artery. This action is termed **systole**.

Second Heart Sound

The second heart sound (S2) is produced by closure of the aortic and pulmonic (semilunar) valves. After the ventricles contract and empty, the aortic and pulmonic valves close during ventricular relaxation. Relaxation of the heart is termed **diastole**.

The pulmonary valve normally closes after the aortic valve. During inspiration, the aortic and pulmonary valve components close approximately 0.05 seconds apart. This is termed a split-S2 and is a normal finding. Inspiration causes the intrathoracic pressure to become more negative which leads to an increase in venous return to the right heart and lowers pulmonary resistance. These actions prolong right ventricular systole and shorten left ventricular systole by reducing pulmonary venous return to the left heart. During expiration, the reverse occurs, so the S2 is noted as a single sound. A split-S2 can be very difficult to detect, especially in an infant with a rapid heartbeat or in an uncooperative child. On auscultation, the S2 component is not as crisp as S1; there is a subtle difference to the heart sound as the valves close at different times.

A very noticeable split-S2 or one that does not change with inspiration and expiration can be indicative of right heart volume overload, as seen with an atrial septal defect (ASD); this is termed a *fixed split-S2*.

Third Heart Sound

The third heart sound (S3) is produced from the rapid filling of the ventricles in early diastole and is best heard with the bell of the stethoscope. This can be a normal sound in children and is likened to the rhythm of "Ken-tuc-ky" with the last syllable being the S3 sound. Some cardiac diseases are associated with this sound as well, especially those associated with myocardial dysfunction or volume overload conditions.

Fourth Heart Sound

The fourth sound (S4) is produced by atrial contraction in late diastole and is always pathologic. It is heard best with the bell of the stethoscope and produces a gallop rhythm likened to "Ten-ne-see" with the first syllable being the S4 sound. This sound is noted in conditions associated with decreased ventricular compliance.

Murmurs

Heart murmurs are defined as turbulent flow through an abnormal valve, vessel, or chamber. A murmur can be either innocent or pathologic. Innocent murmurs are not associated with any intracardiac disease, whereas pathologic murmurs are always associated with a cardiac anomaly or altered cardiac function. Increased metabolic states that occur with anemia, fever, pregnancy, or anxiety can alter the characteristics of an innocent murmur.

When noting a murmur, you need to assess and document:
- Its position in the cardiac cycle (systole, diastole, continuous)
- Quality (harsh, soft, blowing)
- Pitch (high- or low-sounding noise)
- Intensity (loudness)
- Location (where it is heard best or the point of maximum intensity)
- Radiation (do you hear it elsewhere beside the maximum intensity area)
- Presence of a thrill (a palpable purring sensation)
- The response of the murmur to exercise or change of position

Systolic murmurs are graded on a scale of I to VI (Levine scale), whereas diastolic murmurs are graded on a scale of I to IV. Table 41.1 notes this systolic grading scale. Grading a murmur as II or III is subjective based on the loudness of the murmur. You cannot give a murmur a grade of IV/VI just because it is exceptionally loud. To be graded IV/VI, the murmur must be associated with a palpable thrill. Murmurs graded at V/VI or VI/VI are fairly rare in pediatric patients.

A systolic murmur can be either innocent or pathologic. A systolic murmur is heard immediately after the first heart sound and can continue for varying lengths of time depending on the defect. Common innocent systolic murmurs include the vibratory or "Still's" murmur. This murmur is thought to

TABLE 41.1 LEVINE GRADING SCALE FOR SYSTOLIC MURMURS

Murmur Grade	Characteristic
Grade I	Lowest intensity, difficult to hear
Grade II	Immediately audible but lower intensity
Grade III	Audible and louder than grade II
Grade IV	Murmur is readily noted; has an associated palpable thrill
Grade V	Palpable thrill; murmur can be heard with stethoscope partially lifted off the chest
Grade VI	Palpable thrill; loudest intensity; murmur can be heard with stethoscope raised above the chest

be secondary to the blood coming into contact with bands of muscle in the left ventricle. This contact causes a low-frequency sound that has a musical quality to it. It is typically noted at the left mid-sternal area or left lower sternal border and does not radiate. It can be louder or heard for the first time if a patient is febrile or anemic, and it will change in intensity with position changes of the child (sitting to supine). This murmur is heard in 75% of all children but is typically heard from 3 years old to adolescence.

Although innocent murmurs are of no consequence, parents need to be told when their child has one because this finding will undoubtedly be discovered again at a future health assessment or during periods of increased metabolic rate, such as a febrile illness or anxiety. Activities need not be restricted when a child has an innocent murmur, and the child does not require more frequent health appraisals. Be certain that parents understand that innocent murmurs do not turn into serious murmurs so parents do not view them as a prelude to heart disease. A murmur also does not mean their child has a "hole in their heart." At future health assessments, parents may need to be reassured again that the murmur is innocent.

Another common innocent murmur of infancy is a pulmonary flow murmur. This murmur is secondary to the turbulent flow of blood through the slightly smaller branch pulmonary arteries and specifically through the left pulmonary artery by way of a more acute angle. It is a high-pitched, harsher murmur heard best at the left upper sternal border with transmission of sounds to the axillae and the left upper back area. This is typically noted after birth and should disappear by the time the child turns 6 months of age, as the pulmonary arteries have grown. If it is still noted at 6 months, the child should be referred to a pediatric cardiologist for further evaluation.

A diastolic murmur is heard immediately after the second heart sound and is always pathologic. It is associated most commonly with regurgitant aortic and pulmonic valves.

Continuous murmurs are also noted in children. A venous hum is an innocent continuous murmur heard most commonly in children 2 to 8 years of age. It is a low-pitched sound, noted typically at the right upper sternal border and is due to the flow of blood from the SVC into the right atrium. This murmur is heard when the child is sitting or standing but will change in quality if the child's head is turned to the opposite side and will disappear completely if the child lies supine. A persistent patent ductus arteriosus will cause a continuous murmur that is considered pathologic. It is noted

TABLE 41.2 COMPARISON OF INNOCENT AND PATHOLOGIC MURMURS

Characteristic	Innocent	Pathologic
Timing	Systolic	Systolic or diastolic
Duration	Short	Longer
Quality	Soft, musical, twangy	Harsh, blowing, to and fro
Intensity	Soft	Soft or loud
Position in which heard	Can change in intensity with position changes	Does not change with position changes

at the left upper sternal border or out to the left clavicular area and will not change in quality when the child changes position. See Table 41.2 for a summary of innocent murmurs compared with pathologic murmurs.

Diagnostic Tests

Many diagnostic tools can provide you with data regarding the heart and its function, health state, or structure. The diagnostic studies performed on a child with suspected heart disease vary with the specific disorder under investigation.

Teaching about tests such as an echocardiogram, electrocardiography, or cardiac catheterization, and providing psychological support to children and their families are two major responsibilities of nurses throughout the assessment process.

Chest X-ray

Chest X-rays (CXRs) provide an understanding of the heart's size and orientation, pulmonary blood flow, and any associated lung disorders, including fluid collections (effusions).

Laboratory Testing

Basic lab work such as chemistry and hematology tests will provide insight into the child's electrolyte balance, hematologic state, and acid–base balance. Alterations in these can affect myocardial function. Specifically, potassium is lost with most diuretics; calcium is necessary for myocardial contractility and to prevent dysrhythmias; sodium is an indicator of fluid status; hemoglobin and hematocrit determine the need for blood transfusions; and coagulation studies (prothrombin time [PT], partial thromboplastin time [PTT], international normalized ratio [INR]) are imperative before and after cardiac surgery to prevent unnecessary bleeding.

If there are concerns for myocardial damage due to arrhythmia, inflammation, or infection, a specific isoenzyme of creatine kinase (CK), CK-MB, can be tested for along with troponin levels. These lab tests are specific for myocardial injury or damage.

It should be noted that cyanotic children may develop a degree of polycythemia over time as the body develops a greater number of red blood cells in an effort to provide more oxygen carrying capacity to the body. Newborns born at term may have elevated hemoglobin and hematocrit levels at birth and progress to their nadir (lowest blood count level) at 8 to 12 weeks of life as they transition from fetal hemoglobin production to adult hemoglobin production (Kett, 2012).

C-reactive protein (CRP) is an indicator of an active infectious process, and erythrocyte sedimentation rate (ESR) is

an indicator of inflammation such as occurs with rheumatic fever, Kawasaki syndrome, or myocarditis (Xiu-Yu, Jia-Yu, Qiang, et al., 2010).

B-Type natriuretic peptide (BNP) is a substance secreted from the ventricles in response to changes in pressure that occur when heart failure develops and worsens. The level of BNP in the blood increases when heart failure symptoms worsen and decreases when the heart failure condition is stable. No heart failure is indicated by a level less than 100 pg/ml. This marker shows promise for the ongoing evaluation of a child's cardiac status.

Arterial blood gas testing provides information regarding the child's arterial acid–base balance (pH and base status), carbon dioxide, oxygen, and bicarbonate levels. This test requires access to an artery and is usually only performed in acute settings such as an emergency department or intensive care unit.

Electrocardiogram

An *electrocardiogram* (ECG) is a written record of the electrical activity generated by the heart and provides information about heart rate, rhythm, state of the myocardium, presence or absence of hypertrophy (thickening of the heart walls), ischemia or necrosis due to inadequate cardiac circulation, abnormalities of conduction, or the effect of various drugs and electrolyte imbalances on the heart. Changes in the size or shape of the various waveforms may indicate chamber enlargement or poor function. If a child is experiencing an actual arrhythmia, it will be documented, but it will not capture intermittent events consistently. Details regarding ECG waveforms will be discussed with dysrhythmias later in this chapter.

Holter/Event Monitor

A Holter monitor is worn for 24 hours and gives a complete account of every heart beat the child experiences. This allows for evaluation of average rate, rhythm, and frequency of ectopic beats. An event monitor is kept by the child for at least 30 days and can be triggered to record either automatically or manually, if the child experiences a sensation such as chest pain or palpitations. This allows for documentation of potential intermittent dysrhythmias such as supraventricular tachycardia. This data is then transmitted to a cardiologist for interpretation.

Transthoracic Echocardiogram

An echocardiogram is a noninvasive ultrasound of the heart that gives detailed information about heart structure and function. For this, high-frequency sound waves, directed toward the heart, are used to locate and study the movement and dimensions of cardiac structures, such as the size of chambers; thickness of walls; relationship of major vessels to chambers; and the thickness, motion, and pressure gradients across valves. It can also evaluate velocity of blood flow through the heart, estimate pressures in the heart chambers and lungs, and provide three-dimensional images of structures. You can remind parents that echocardiography does not use X-rays, so it can be repeated at frequent intervals without exposing their child to the possible risk of radiation.

The use of a transesophageal echocardiogram (TEE) is another option to better evaluate the heart anatomy. In this imaging option, the TEE probe hangs in the esophagus immediately posterior to the heart and provides high-quality images of intracardiac structures because of the absence of interfering structures such as lung and bone. If a TEE is necessary, it will be done under moderate sedation or general anesthesia because children will not tolerate a probe being placed down their esophagus while awake.

Computed Tomography/Magnetic Resonance Imaging

These noninvasive imaging modalities provide very detailed images of the heart and chest structures and are typically used as an adjunct to echocardiography. Computed tomography angiography (CTA) of the cardiovascular system provides excellent anatomic imaging of the chest structures, including the coronary arteries, through the use of radiation. Although computed tomography (CT) is very brief, it does require a slower heart rate, and breath holding may be necessary to produce the best images. CT can be reconstructed to provide 3D images. Cardiac magnetic resonance imaging (MRI) can provide information regarding cardiac anatomy and function, blood flow measurement, tissue characterization, myocardial perfusion, and viability. An MRI does not provide radiation but is a much longer test and requires near stillness to be accurate. Many young children will require moderate sedation to successfully complete an MRI.

Exercise Stress Testing

Exercise stress testing (EST) is used to evaluate a child's clinical condition during periods of increased myocardial demand, such as with exercise. Exercise testing can be accomplished with a treadmill, bicycle, or a 6-minute walk to increase the child's heart rate. The child's heart rate and rhythm are continuously monitored, and blood pressure is measured intermittently. It is also possible to perform pulmonary function testing before and immediately after exercise to evaluate lung capacity. Many children referred for an exercise stress test have complaints of shortness of breath, chest pain, or palpitations with exercise. EST is performed in an effort to recreate these symptoms and evaluate for any true cardiac involvement in producing these symptoms. Very young children (less than approximately 8 years old) may have difficulty performing an EST on a bicycle or treadmill because of the size of the equipment and reference values for the 6-minute walk continue to be validated for children and adolescents.

Cardiac Catheterization

This procedure is invasive; catheters are inserted through a large vein and artery and floated into the heart. A cardiac catheterization allows for direct measurements of pressure as well as visualization of the heart and all blood vessels with the aid of a contrast medium. Cardiac catheterization uses fluoroscopy, which is a form of imaging that uses radiation to generate real-time moving images of structures.

Many corrective procedures can also be performed in the catheterization lab, such as atrial and ventricular septal defect closure, patent ductus arteriosus closure, or valve replacement. Care of a child after a cardiac catheterization will be discussed in greater detail later in this chapter.

Systemic Assessment

As previously stated, a cardiac assessment cannot be performed isolated from other systems. The child's respiratory status must be evaluated for increased rate or work of breathing, which could be secondary to increased pulmonary blood flow due to a defect or congestive heart failure. Frequent upper respiratory tract infections can also occur and may be an indication of the need for corrective surgery. The abdomen should be palpated for liver size, as hepatomegaly is an indicator of poor right heart function. Urine output and feeding tolerance are also indicators of cardiac output. An infant should have approximately 6 to 8 wet diapers per day; older children should void several times daily, and the urine should be light in color. Edema from retained or excess fluid is a late sign of heart disease in children. If edema does occur, periorbital edema generally occurs first.

A child's neurologic status should be considered as a possible indicator of cardiac output. If a child is lethargic or not interactive, they may be fatigued or be experiencing poor tissue perfusion. Finally, distal extremities must be evaluated for capillary refill time, presence of palpable pulses, temperature, and color—all indicators of adequacy of cardiac output.

Performing an accurate, thorough cardiac history and examination of a child is imperative to understanding the child's health state, evaluating the effectiveness of treatment regimens, and educating families. You will need to practice these assessments, but in time, you will become confident and proficient.

Congestive Heart Failure

Many cardiac disorders, including congenital heart defects, or acquired disorders such as cardiomyopathy or Kawasaki disease can manifest with either very subtle physical symptoms or symptoms of congestive heart failure with varying degrees of severity. It is important for you to understand the physiology behind the concept of heart failure and how children present when they are experiencing heart failure. Therefore, congestive heart failure is presented before further discussions about specific disorders because any myocardial dysfunction, regardless of etiology, can present with some degree of congestive heart failure.

To understand congestive heart failure, the nurse must first understand the components of adequate cardiac function. Cardiac output is the volume of blood pumped by the ventricles each minute. The formula for calculating cardiac output is heart rate multiplied by stroke volume. Stroke volume is affected by the following factors:

- **Preload**: the volume of blood in the ventricles at the point just before contraction; it is an indicator of circulating blood volume.
- **Contractility**: ability to modulate the rate and force of fiber shortening
- **Afterload**: amount of resistance met by the ventricles upon ejection
- Compliance: the ability of the ventricles to stretch and fill

Infants and children can easily modify their heart rate in an effort to increase cardiac output, but they are not as able to change their stroke volume. Much of the therapy for pediatric heart failure is aimed at altering those factors that affect stroke volume, in particular, reducing preload and afterload and increasing contractility to promote better cardiac output.

Congestive heart failure (CHF) is defined as the inability of the heart to supply adequate oxygenated blood to meet the metabolic demands of the body. Heart failure is a cluster of symptoms and physical examination findings that are secondary to an underlying process. The primary processes can be systemic or directly related to the heart. The most common causes of CHF in children are congenital heart defects that produce an excessive workload on the myocardium, cardiomyopathies due to metabolic disorders, infectious diseases, drugs, Kawasaki disease, and myocardial dysfunction after heart surgery. Regardless of the underlying etiology (inability to meet metabolic demands, decreased filling, or obstruction of flow), the outcomes are the same: Either one side or both sides of the heart are unable to pump effectively and will eventually fail if the root problem is not corrected.

When the heart begins to perform inadequately, several physiologic responses occur. The initial neurohormonal response to decreased cardiac output is peripheral vasoconstriction and fluid retention. The sympathetic nervous system provides a rapid response by increasing heart rate (chronotropy), stimulates myocardial contractility (inotropy), and promotes regional vasoconstriction. A longer term mechanism will occur with activation of the renin–angiotensin–aldosterone system (RAAS), which stimulates renal fluid retention to expand vascular volume. The body's goal is to maintain adequate blood pressure and circulating blood volume. Stroke volume and cardiac output initially improve, but because the underlying etiology of the poor cardiac output has not been addressed, the heart eventually becomes overloaded from the extra volume and cannot maintain adequate contractility against the increased afterload. In addition, the vasoconstriction and redistribution of blood flow to ensure adequate perfusion of vital organs (brain and heart) occur at the expense of skin, intestinal, and renal blood flow. This leads to lactic acidosis secondary to anaerobic metabolism, fatigue, an intolerance to oral intake, decreased urine output, and electrolyte imbalance.

ASSESSMENT

Children in a state of heart failure, regardless of the underlying etiology, will initially present with similar clinical symptoms, such as tachycardia and tachypnea. Infants and young children may present with poor feeding and failure to thrive, whereas older children may complain of fatigue, exercise intolerance, and breathlessness. CHF is more difficult to detect in infants because it may be more subtle. The infant may be noted to have rapid respirations and to use accessory muscles of respiration. The infant will tire easily, may be diaphoretic, or may have difficulty sucking because of the dyspnea and the energy required to eat. A child may gain weight from fluid overload, but more frequently, an infant will lose weight because their caloric expenditure is greater than the caloric intake.

Right-sided failure leads to hepatomegaly, increased venous pressure noted in jugular venous distention in older children, or periorbital edema. Left-sided failure results in increased pulmonary pressures, rales, tachypnea, and shortness of breath.

Regardless of age, but depending on the degree of heart failure and the amount of time the child has experienced the failure, the clinical examination may reveal hepatomegaly, a cardiac gallop, or an enlarged heart on chest radiograph, with or without pulmonary edema.

With left-sided heart failure, back pressure causes blood to accumulate in the pulmonary system, causing orthopnea (difficulty breathing except in an upright position because of increased pulmonary congestion). The child may demonstrate

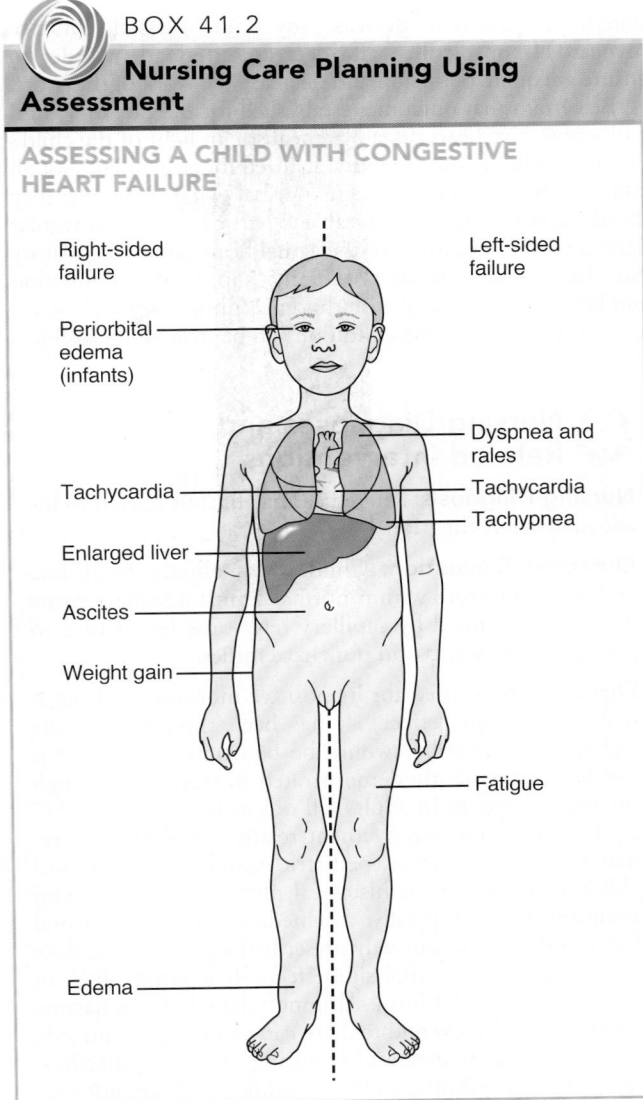

BOX 41.2

Nursing Care Planning Using Assessment

ASSESSING A CHILD WITH CONGESTIVE HEART FAILURE

Right-sided failure

Periorbital edema (infants)

Tachycardia

Enlarged liver

Ascites

Weight gain

Edema

Left-sided failure

Dyspnea and rales

Tachycardia

Tachypnea

Fatigue

use of accessory muscles to support their breathing, which causes intercostal, substernal, and/or suprasternal retractions. The sound of rales (crackles) can be heard on auscultation. Left-sided CHF can ultimately lead to right-sided failure, as excessive pressure in the pulmonary system prevents blood from leaving the right ventricle.

Right-sided heart failure manifests with an enlarged liver, which is palpable below the costal margin. Periorbital edema may be noted as well as jugular venous distention in older children. Generalized edema may be noted, but this is uncommon in children (Box 41.2).

THERAPEUTIC MANAGEMENT

Management of heart failure is twofold: (a) symptomatically manage the patient and (b) treat the underlying cause of the heart failure. Management in children is difficult because all therapies are based on adult heart failure studies and extrapolated to pediatric patients. It is difficult to study heart failure in children because of the heterogeneity of the patients and underlying disorders. Nevertheless, several pharmacologic agents are staples in heart failure management. As previously stated, the goal is to decrease any fluid overload, enhance myocardial contractility, and decrease afterload in order to ensure adequate perfusion and decrease the work of the heart.

Be certain that outcomes established for the care of a child with congestive heart disease are realistic in light of the child's overall condition and are individualized for each child. Not all children may be able to attain "normal" vital signs, but they should be comfortable and be able to participate in their regular daily activities, regardless of the actual heart rate or respiratory rate. Interventions focus on helping support heart function and helping parents deal with this crisis until the child is stabilized and the underlying condition can be treated, if possible.

 ## Nursing Diagnoses and Related Interventions

Nursing Diagnosis: Altered cardiac output related to inadequate heart function

Outcome Evaluation: Child will maintain heart rate and blood pressure within normal limits; adequate tissue perfusion, as noted by capillary refill time less than 2 to 3 seconds and warm and pink extremities.

Digoxin may be used for its positive inotropic and negative chronotropic effects. It has been thought that the increased contractility would be beneficial, but this has not been consistently demonstrated in studies. Although the use of digoxin in adults fell out of favor after a 1997 study showed no improvement relative to placebo, it remains common in many pediatric centers for infants and children because of its historical physiologic benefit and symptom relief. Typically, the medication is used in oral form, and it is not routinely prescribed with a loading dose because of the potential side effects. It is rarely given in an intravenous (IV) form. Although digoxin has a narrow therapeutic window and toxicity can cause significant side effects, such as nausea and vomiting, dizziness, diarrhea, headache, arrhythmia, and bradycardia, levels are not routinely monitored. If dosing is appropriate for a patient's weight and electrolyte status (specifically potassium level) is normal, the digoxin is considered to be therapeutic. If a child is bradycardic for their age and the heart rate is not their normal baseline value, a provider should be consulted before giving the medication.

Many children are discharged to home on digoxin. Be certain that parents understand the drug's correct dose and frequency of administration, typically twice a day in young children and infants (Box 41.3). Have them demonstrate drawing up the correct amount of oral solution into a syringe. Make sure they understand they must use the same size syringe each time, as many parents may not understand the different volumes held by different syringes. Help them choose a specific time for administration to which they can adhere faithfully. Support them by making out a medication calendar or urge them to leave a reminder on their phone to help them remember to give the drug. Parents must also be reminded to call for a refill *before* the medication actually runs out. As with all oral solutions, they are encouraged to draw up the medication away from the infant or child to prevent the bottle from getting knocked over and medication being lost.

BOX 41.3

Nursing Care Planning to Empower a Family

GIVING DIGOXIN SAFELY AT HOME

Q. Megan's mother says to you, "The doctor has prescribed our daughter digoxin to take at home. Are there any special things we should do?"

A. Use the following guidelines to ensure safe digoxin administration at home:

- Always use only a clearly marked syringe so the dose given is accurate and consistent.
- Do not change the amount or timing of the dose without specific instructions from your cardiologist.
- If you miss a single dose, give the next dose on time as prescribed. If you miss more than one dose, telephone your cardiologist for further instructions.
- Give digoxin 1 hour before or 2 hours after feeding to ensure complete absorption and to avoid a dose being lost if the infant spits up.
- If a dose is vomited, do not repeat the dose. Give the next dose at the scheduled time. If the child vomits the next dose, call your cardiologist as this could be a sign of toxicity.
- Keep the medication bottle away from the child. Draw up the dose away from the child and recap the bottle to prevent it from being knocked over and medicine being lost.
- Call your cardiology office for a refill several days before you actually run out of medicine so there is no lapse in medication availability.
- Direct the parents to NOT give their child any herbal supplements or other over-the-counter medications unless directed by their provider. Many supplements interact negatively with prescribed medications or we do not completely understand the interactions. Simple over-the-counter (OTC) medications such as acetaminophen or diphenhydramine (Benadryl) are typically safe, but it may be best to clear it with the provider before giving the first time.

Angiotensin-converting enzyme (ACE) inhibitors are another medication used in the traditional triad of pharmacologic management of pediatric heart failure. ACE inhibitors reduce afterload by blocking the conversion of angiotensin I to angiotensin II, a potent vasoconstrictor. They also block the activation of the RAAS and decrease adrenergic activity. This causes vasodilation, improves tissue perfusion, and reduces congestion by natriuresis. They have also been shown to reduce cardiac myocyte remodeling by preventing fibrosis. Examples of such medications are captopril, lisinopril, and enalapril. All three are available as an oral solution. Care must be taken when planning a medication schedule for a patient on a diuretic and an ACE inhibitor. If the two medications reach peak effect at the same time, the child is at risk for hypotension. Therefore, the nurse must ensure the medications are given 1 to 2 hours apart in order to prevent this complication. ACE inhibitors can also cause a cough, which can be irritating and prevent further use of this category of medications.

Although evidence is lacking that beta-blockers reduce mortality in children with heart failure, the therapy continues to be used in an effort to affect the counterregulatory features of CHF, specifically the activation of the sympathetic nervous system and the RAAS. Reduction in the RAAS reduces preload and then reduces ventricular wall stress and cardiomyocyte remodeling. Studies in children with a cardiomyopathy have shown an improvement in left ventricular function, improved exercise tolerance, and decreased need for heart transplantation with beta-blocker use.

Angiotensin II receptor blockers (ARBs) are a new group of agents being used very successfully in adults, with some sporadic use in the pediatric population. They act by inhibiting the RAAS, which decreases afterload and promotes reversal of ventricular remodeling with longterm use. Few data are available on the use of ARBs in children, so ACE inhibitors remain the preferred agent unless they are not tolerated. The use of one specific ARB, losartan, is noted in the literature, specifically in patients with Marfan syndrome or hypertension. Evidence in the adult literature show that losartan slows and reverses the dilation of the aortic root in this group of patients, but these results have not been consistently proven in the pediatric literature.

Other groups of medications belong to a category of inotropic agents that work directly on the heart and vasculature. These medications are administered through continuous IV infusions and are limited to intensive care settings. Common medications used in CHF include milrinone and dobutamine.

Nursing Diagnosis: Altered fluid balance, greater than body requirements due to poor myocardial function and fluid retention

Outcome Evaluation: Clear bilateral breath sounds, no clinical symptoms of respiratory distress (tachypnea, retractions), no peripheral edema, adequate urine output

Diuretics are routinely used to manage pediatric heart failure. The purpose of the diuretic is to increase the excretion of sodium and water, which in turn relieves the symptoms of fluid overload and congestion. Loop diuretics such as furosemide are usually first-line choice, as they block a large proportion of sodium reabsorption. The main complication associated with loop diuretics is hypokalemia. If the dose or frequency of the loop diuretic is significant and hypokalemia is a concern, either potassium supplements can be added, although they are not always well tolerated orally and can cause nausea or vomiting, or a potassium-sparing diuretic can be used, such as spironolactone, which by itself is not a potent diuretic but works synergistically with a loop diuretic. Spironolactone is categorized as an aldosterone receptor antagonist that has been associated with improved mortality in adult studies. This effect is independent of the diuretic effect.

If a child has dyspnea, hypoxemia, or cyanosis, supplemental oxygen by way of mask or nasal cannula may be necessary. But oxygen is a medication and has a significant vasodilatory effect on the pulmonary vasculature. If a child has a cardiac defect that increases pulmonary blood flow, the use of oxygen will dilate the pulmonary bed further, leading to more pulmonary blood flow and worsening of respiratory compromise. Oxygen should not always be the initial response to low oxygen saturation in many children with congenital heart defects and symptoms of respiratory distress or compromise.

Nursing Diagnosis: Risk for imbalanced nutrition, less than body requirements, related to easy fatigability

Outcome Evaluation: Child maintains appropriate daily weight gain and percentile curve on individual growth chart.

Maintaining proper nutrition may be a problem for children with CHF because they tire so easily. Eating several small, high-calorie, high-fat meals daily is often less tiring than eating three large meals and still provides adequate nutrition. Calorie requirements may also be supplemented with protein shakes. It should be noted that the act of breastfeeding demands a significant amount of energy. Children with moderate heart failure may need for their mothers to manually express breast milk so they can feed by a bottle to conserve energy and allow for calorie concentration.

Regardless of fatigue, a child in heart failure has increased metabolic demands and calorie consumption and may require daily increased calories to meet those demands and ensure adequate weight gain.

Nursing Diagnosis: Fear related to child's ill appearance and possible disease outcome

Outcome Evaluation: Parents and child openly discuss fears and concerns, actively question, and express confidence in treatment plan and healthcare team.

Offer time to talk or use therapeutic play so the child can express his or her fears.

Parents of a child with CHF need assurance because they are typically very worried by their child's ill appearance, lack of weight gain, or inability to keep up with others. It is often helpful to point out subtle signs of improvement that they may not notice on their own, such as a slower, less distressed respirations or an increase in daily weight.

If the child will be cared for at home, review CPR to be certain parents know how to use this in an emergency. If a parent will be making more concentrated feeds for the child, be very thorough in reviewing this technique with them. Write out the directions; ensure they have the tools necessary such as measuring cups and are very comfortable making the feed. Alterations in the prescribed concentration of the feed can cause serious complications such as seizures from hyponatremia or hypernatremia. Be certain they have a follow-up appointment with the cardiologist scheduled and a telephone number they can call if they have any concerns about their child's condition.

Box 41.4 shows an interprofessional care map illustrating both nursing and team planning for an infant with CHF.

BOX 41.4

Nursing Care Planning

AN INTERPROFESSIONAL CARE MAP FOR AN INFANT WITH CONGESTIVE HEART FAILURE

Megan is a newborn who was born with an AVSD and Down syndrome. She does not appear to have other medical issues. The family was not aware of this diagnosis prior to birth. The child is now 2 days old and is being prepared for discharge, but the parents have several questions.

Family Assessment: Child's parents were divorced 1 month ago; dual custody of infant granted. Child will spend weekdays with mother, weekends with father. Father is a city bus driver; mother is a paralegal. Father to pay child support; with child support, mother rates finances as "workable."

Patient Criteria: Two-day-old infant girl who appears pale, tachycardic, and tachypneic. Child born by vaginal birth; Apgar scores 9 and 8. Afebrile; heart rate is 150 beats/min; respirations are 36 breaths/min. Oxygen saturation via pulse oximetry is 96%. S3 heart sound noted. Lungs with mild rhonchi.

Nursing Diagnosis: Risk for activity intolerance due to altered cardiac physiology
Risk for altered nutrition due to increased pulmonary blood flow and increased metabolic demands

Outcome Evaluation: Child's vital signs remain within age-acceptable parameters; skin color pink and warm; breathing is comfortable with limited use of accessory muscles, lungs clear to auscultation, appropriate weight gain is followed.

Team Member Responsible	Assessment	Intervention	Rationale	Expected Outcome
Activities of Daily Living, Including Safety				
Nurse	Assess vital signs and heart and lung sounds, as prescribed. Monitor daily weight. Evaluate for increased work of breathing.	Frequent auscultation of breath sounds (BS) and evaluation of heart rate (HR), respiratory rate (RR), saturation Daily weight compared to previous day	The child's response to feeding and medications may vary as she grows so frequent evaluation is necessary. Daily weights ensure adequate weight gain despite increased metabolic needs.	Child's vital signs remain within prescribed parameters. Oxygen saturation is at 95%. Daily weight gain is 25 g/day on average.
Teamwork and Collaboration				
Cardiologist	Assess cardiac anatomy and function. Evaluate need for new or altered doses of medications.	Perform electrocardiogram (ECG) and echocardiogram routinely; assess child. Based on test results and assessment, determine need for medications to manage congestive heart failure (CHF).	Cardiac function may decrease over time if pulmonary pressures elevate or left heart dilates. Child may outgrow medications if weight gain is good.	Function remains within normal limits (WNL); CHF is well managed with medications as evidenced by minimal work of breathing, clear BS, adequate weight gain.
Procedures/Medications for Quality Improvement				
Pharmacist/nurse	Ensure medications are being given routinely and on schedule. Ensure timing and dosing of medications is safe.	Review all medications with family and confirm times given.	Managing CHF while the child grows and waits for surgery is dependent on the medications prescribed. Diuretics and angiotensin-converting enzyme (ACE) inhibitors should be scheduled several hours apart to prevent drops in blood pressure.	Family confirms medications are being given correctly. Family does not run out of medications without refills. Child experiences no periods of hypotension.

Procedures/Medications for Quality Improvement

Nutritionist/ cardiologist/nurse	Monitor weight gain. Assess electrolytes for hypokalemia.	Monitor weight daily at same time. Administer diuretics as prescribed.	Weight is an indicator of caloric intake and balance. Diuretics reduce edema which decreases respiratory effort. High or frequent doses of loop diuretics can cause potassium losses.	Infant weight gain is consistent and follows an individual curve. BS are clear; work of breathing is minimal. Potassium level is WNL.
Nurse/respiratory therapist	Evaluate BS and work of breathing.	Assess BS and observe for increased work of breathing.	Atrioventricular septal defect (AVSD) can cause an increase in pulmonary blood flow which can cause congestion, rales, and ultimately changes in pulmonary pressures.	Infant's oxygen saturation remains at 95% or above. Infant's RR is only mildly elevated with minimal increase in work of breathing (WOB).

Nutrition

Nurse/nutritionist	Assess child's intake for adequacy. Monitor weight gain.	Assist family with concentration of breast milk if necessary, as directed by nutritionist and provider. Encourage family to allow infant to rest during feedings.	By concentrating the feeds, the infant can gain more calories in less volume which will then require less time feeding and less energy expenditure.	Infant takes feed without significant distress or reflux. Adequate daily weight gain. Minimal respiratory distress/fatigue while feeding.

Patient-Centered Care

Nurse	Assess parents' understanding of child's condition.	Educate parents as needed about congenital heart disease and CHF. Ensure both parents have adequate quantities of medications and supplies.	Parents need an understanding of child's illness to respect need for rest and medications.	Parents both state that they understand child's condition. They both meet with cardiologist and surgeon as possible; both have supplies and are comfortable with medications and feedings.

Psychosocial/Spiritual/Emotional Needs

Social worker/ nurse	Assess whether parents feel they have enough emotional support to care for an ill infant at home while waiting for cardiac surgery in a few months.	Discuss necessity for vigilance and keeping infant free of infection.	Respiratory infection could quickly worsen child's condition.	Parents state they understand the strain caring for an ill infant can cause. Have made arrangements for continuous care. Have identified resources for daily and emergency support.

Informatics for Seamless Healthcare Planning

Nurse	Assess whether parents are familiar with cardiopulmonary resuscitation (CPR) technique for infants. Ensure all providers have contact information for parents.	Parents will watch CPR video and be trained in CPR per institution protocols. Obtain all phone numbers and e-mail addresses for parents to ensure successful communication.	Well-prepared parents can be lifesaving for a child with heart disease. Communication with providers is imperative for safety of the infant.	Parents correctly demonstrate infant CPR technique on CPR mannequin. State they understand importance of follow-up visits and will keep appointments.

QUALITY IMPROVEMENT

Children with CHF are often prescribed digoxin (Lanoxin). Knowing that this drug possesses a high risk of adverse effects if given incorrectly, the nurse provides educational materials to Megan's parents. Which statement by Megan's mother would alert the nurse that she has *not* received all the education that she needs?

   a. "I know the drug is thought to help Megan's heart pump better."
   b. "It's important I give the exact dose every time."
   c. "If I happen to miss a dose, I will not give double the dose at the next time."
   d. "Nausea and vomiting are expected side effects for the first few weeks of treatment."

Look in Appendix A for the best answer and rationale.

Congenital Heart Defects

About 8% of term newborns and 9% to 10% of preterm infants are born with a congenital cardiovascular abnormality (Darst, Collins, & Miyamoto, 2012). Approximately 25% of defects can be considered complex, and one third will require intervention during infancy. Twenty-five percent of neonates with congenital heart defects have other associated congenital anomalies. However, as a result of the advances in evaluation and treatment of these children, up to 85% of neonates born with congenital heart disease are expected to survive to adulthood.

Congenital heart defects can be classified in many ways based on embryologic formation, structure, or physiology. The defects in this chapter are categorized by physiology; this will help you understand the impact on the child, the symptoms that may be present, and the therapeutic regimens used. Defects are classified as "increasing pulmonary blood flow," "decreasing pulmonary blood flow," or "obstruction to systemic blood flow." The final type of defect discussed is single-ventricle defects such as hypoplastic left heart syndrome. It is an extremely unique defect with very complex physiology and is discussed independent of the other defects.

When caring for a child with a congenital heart defect, it is important to remember normal physiology, as this influences blood flow. The right side of the heart is a lower pressure system than the left side of the heart. This pressure difference allows blood to flow from one chamber to another, specifically from an area of high pressure to an area of low pressure; the blood will always follow the "path of least resistance." When venous blood from the right side of the heart mixes with blood on the left side, this is a "right-to-left" shunt that delivers deoxygenated blood to the body. Heart defects with this type of blood flow are termed **cyanotic heart disease**. If the blood shunts left to right, then oxygenated blood from the left side mixes with blood in the right side of the heart and goes back to the lungs again. This is called **acyanotic heart disease**.

DEFECTS THAT INCREASE PULMONARY BLOOD FLOW

Patent Ductus Arteriosus

A patent ductus arteriosus (PDA) occurs when this fetal shunt fails to close after several days of life. This remnant of fetal circulation remaining patent occurs more frequently in children born prematurely, with an incidence ranging from 20% to 60%. If a ductus arteriosus does not close after birth, it allows blood to flow from the aorta (area of high pressure) through the PDA and into the main pulmonary artery (area of low pressure). The shunted blood then returns to the left atrium of the heart and repeats the cycle. This extra blood flow increases pulmonary circulation. This is an acyanotic defect, as the blood flowing from the aorta is fully oxygenated (Fig. 41.4).

Assessment

This defect produces a systolic murmur early in life and a continuous murmur as the child ages. The murmur is noted at the second intercostal space, left upper sternal border, or out to the left clavicular area. If the defect is large enough, the flow to the lungs will be significant and can cause rales, congestion, increased work of breathing, difficulty feeding, or failure to thrive. Over time, the left heart can become dilated. The severity of the symptoms depends on the amount of blood shunting to the lungs. A PDA is confirmed with an echocardiogram.

Management

Treatment for a PDA varies. Medical management of a PDA involves addressing the symptoms of the increased blood flow by prescribing a diuretic such as furosemide. The caloric concentration of the infant's feeds may need to be increased in an effort to help the child gain weight. If the child is experiencing significant manifestations of the increased pulmonary blood

Figure 41.4 Patent ductus arteriosus. (Asset provided by Anatomical Chart Co.)

flow or if left heart dilation is noted from the extra blood flow returning to the left side of the heart, the child will be referred for PDA closure.

If the PDA is noted immediately after birth, indomethacin, a nonsteroidal anti-inflammatory and prostaglandin inhibitor, can be utilized to facilitate closure. This is usually given in three separate IV doses in the newborn nursery. In older children, a PDA can be closed in the cardiac catheterization lab with a device placed in the duct to occlude flow. Occasionally, a duct needs to be closed surgically either for a premature baby who is too small to undergo closure in the catheterization lab or due to other confounding factors. Surgical closure of a PDA is done via a left-sided thoracotomy incision and does not require cardiopulmonary bypass.

Atrial Septal Defect

An ASD is created when a portion of the atrial septal tissue does not completely form. The defect can occur in any location along the septum, but most common is the *secundum* type defect that is located in the center of the atrial septum (Fig. 41.5). Other deficiencies of the atrial septum include a *primum defect* that is found low in the atrial septum near the IVC. Defects in this area are frequently associated with atrioventricular septal defects (AVSD) (discussed in detail later in this chapter). Another atrial defect is found high in the septum where the pulmonary veins enter the left atrium. These are *sinus venosus defects* and allow communication of one or more of the pulmonary veins with the right atrium.

Regardless of where the defect is located, the physiology is consistent. This is an acyanotic defect that allows blood to flow from the high-pressure left atrium to the low-pressure right atrium and continue out to the lungs. But because the atria overall have a lower pressure than the ventricles, the amount of blood flow through this defect is significantly limited. This means an ASD may not have a murmur associated with

it; therefore, it may go unnoticed if no clinical symptoms exist. Regardless of the presence of a murmur, an ASD may have a fixed split-S2 heart sound.

Assessment

If the defect is small, it may go undetected or, if noted, may cause no clinical concern and require no intervention. If the defect is large enough, a child may show symptoms of the ASD. The child will present with symptoms of pulmonary overcirculation, such as rales, congestion, tiring with activity, or poor weight gain. Over time, the right heart may also dilate as a result of the increased volume. Murmurs associated with an ASD are not related to flow through the actual defect, as the velocity through the defect is low. Instead, the murmur is related to the relative increased blood volume traveling across the pulmonary valve. The turbulence created by the increased pulmonary blood flow produces a systolic murmur heard best at the left upper sternal border. An ASD is confirmed with an echocardiogram.

Management

If an ASD was incidentally noted, is less than 5 mm, and is producing no clinical symptoms, it will not be closed. For clinically significant defects, management will be based on the child's age and the size of the defect. Medical management of the symptoms with diuretics will be attempted first in an effort to allow the defect to close spontaneously. Defects that remain 5 mm or greater with persistent shunting after an observation period should be referred for closure to decrease the incidence of supraventricular dysrhythmias and prevent pulmonary vascular disease. If the defect is 8 mm or larger with evidence of increased pulmonary blood flow, the child will be referred for closure immediately.

A secundum ASD is typically closed in the catheterization lab with a device that sits in the defect space. Sinus venosus and primum defects typically cannot be closed in the catheterization lab because of their anatomy and are referred for surgical closure. Surgical closure involves a median sternotomy incision and cardiopulmonary bypass. These children are typically home within 2 to 3 days of cardiac surgery.

Ventricular Septal Defect

Ventricular septal defects (VSDs) are the most common defect found in children, either in isolation or combined with other defects. A VSD occurs when a portion of the ventricular septum does not completely close. VSDs may be single or multiple and are defined based on their anatomical location within the septum (Fig. 41.6).

Assessment

Regardless of the location or classification of the VSD, it is an acyanotic defect that allows oxygenated blood to flow from the left side of the heart to the right side of the heart. This increases pulmonary blood flow and ultimately increases the volume of blood returning to the left heart, causing left heart dilation over time. A murmur is always associated with a VSD because of the high velocity of flow through the defect, producing a harsh, holosystolic murmur noted at the left lower sternal border. The typical murmur of a VSD may not be heard at birth because the pulmonary vascular resistance is still high, which limits blood flow across the

Figure 41.5 Atrial septal defect. (Asset provided by Anatomical Chart Co.)

Figure 41.6 A ventricular septal defect. (Asset provided by Anatomical Chart Co.)

defect. As pulmonary resistance decreases over the first 4 to 6 weeks of life, the amount of shunted blood increases and produces an audible murmur. Symptoms associated with a VSD are similar to those found with a PDA or ASD and are determined by the size of the defect. A small defect may have a murmur but produce no clinical symptoms. If the defect is large enough, the increased pulmonary blood flow manifests as symptoms of CHF, such as tachypnea, poor feeding, or failure to thrive. The defect is confirmed with an echocardiogram.

Management

The child may be medically managed to allow for spontaneous closure of the defect as the child grows. Some children will have an audible murmur but no symptoms of pulmonary overcirculation. These may be very small defects that will close spontaneously. If the child does exhibit signs of pulmonary overload, such as tachypnea, retractions, or rales, management will include use of a diuretic such as furosemide and possibly an increase in the caloric density of the child's formula or breast milk if there are concerns for poor weight gain. As previously stated, breastfeeding demands a significant amount of energy from the child, and mothers may need to manually express the breast milk so it can be fed through a bottle or nasogastric tube.

If closure does not occur over time in a symptomatic child, or if the child experiences persistent failure to thrive, depressed myocardial function, or dilation of the left heart, they will be referred for closure. Some types of VSDs can be closed in the catheterization lab; others are closed surgically. If a child has a small defect that is causing no clinical concerns, the defect does not need to be closed. VSDs are surgically closed through a median sternotomy (entering the chest cavity through the sternum). VSD repairs can be high risk for heart block depending on the location.

What If . . . 41.1
The nurse notices Henry, a 2-month-old with a VSD, is using his accessory muscles while breathing. His mother states he is always breathing like that and sometimes it gets worse when he eats, but she is not concerned because he is not turning blue. What reasons for concern might the nurse identify?

Atrioventricular Septal Defect

This defect comprises several congenital heart defects: a primum ASD, a high VSD, and failure of the tricuspid and mitral valves to develop and attach correctly (Fig. 41.7). Varying degrees of abnormality occur with this lesion, from mild septal defects to a complete lack of central septa with incompetent valves on both sides. In a complete AVSD, blood freely mixes between the right and left sides. As with other septal defects, pulmonary blood flow can be significantly increased, but a complete AVSD also allows for right-to-left shunting, which may lead to desaturation. This is not typically noted, though, as the blood will preferentially flow to the lungs (left-to-right shunting). The atria can become dilated through regurgitation of blood through the incompetent valves. Although rare in the general population, as many as 20% of children with trisomy 21 (Down syndrome) who have heart disease, have this type of congenital cardiac disorder (Kucik, Shin, Siffel, et al., 2013).

Assessment

The child can present with symptoms of CHF similar to those seen in other defects that increase pulmonary blood flow. Because the degree of increased pulmonary blood flow is excessive, these children can present with significant symptoms early on and are at risk for developing increased pulmonary vascular resistance that can be irreversible if it persists too long.

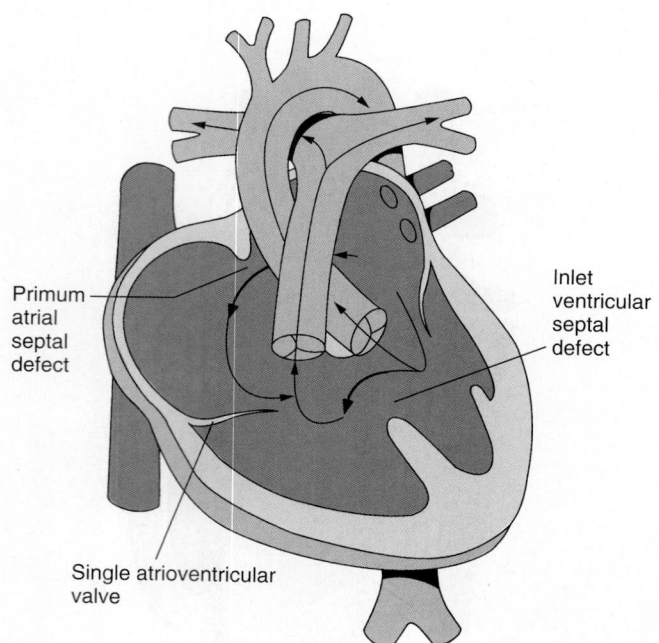

Primum atrial septal defect

Inlet ventricular septal defect

Single atrioventricular valve

Figure 41.7 Atrioventricular septal defect. (From Marino, B. S., & Fine, K. S. [2013]. *Blueprints pediatrics* [6th ed.]. Baltimore, MD: Lippincott Williams & Wilkins.)

The development of increased pulmonary resistance has been noted to occur more rapidly in children with Down syndrome, necessitating earlier repair in these children. Diagnosis is confirmed with echocardiography. A cardiac catheterization may be performed before surgical correction to measure pulmonary pressures and confirm reactivity with the administration of oxygen or nitric oxide, both of which should cause pulmonary pressures to decrease.

Management

Management typically includes medications such as furosemide, digoxin, and an ACE inhibitor like captopril or enalapril. These children may also require concentrated feeds to help maintain weight. Children with Down syndrome experience complications from the increased pulmonary blood flow earlier than children without Down syndrome, so they are typically referred for surgical correction by 3 months of age or earlier if the transthoracic echocardiogram demonstrates signs of increased pulmonary pressures. Children without Down syndrome are referred for repair by 5 or 6 months of age or as clinically necessary.

If the surgical repair needs to be delayed, a temporary measure to decrease the amount of pulmonary blood flow can be performed. This is called a pulmonary artery band, which is a band surgically placed around the pulmonary artery that constricts it to increase the resistance within the pulmonary artery, thus decreasing some of the overall pulmonary blood flow and preventing too much pulmonary circulation and long-term pulmonary vascular changes.

Surgical repair of an AVSD consists of closing atrial and VSDs and repairing the mitral and tricuspid valves to make them functional. It is important that the mitral valve be high functioning, as left-sided valve leakage is not tolerated by children; right-sided leakage is better tolerated. These children are at high risk for heart block after surgical repair. They will have a right bundle branch block on ECG with the VSD repair and may have persistent mitral valve dysfunction (stenosis or regurgitation) after surgery. If this progresses to severe dysfunction, further surgical intervention will be required. The goal is to repair the mitral valve so no stenosis and minimal regurgitation exist. If this cannot be achieved, an artificial valve will be placed.

Transposition of the Great Arteries

This is the second most common congenital defect and is described as reversal of the great arteries. The exact etiology is not completely understood. All other intracardiac structures are normal, with VSDs noted in 50% of these infants. The resultant anatomy has the aorta coming off of the right ventricle and the pulmonary artery arising from the left ventricle. This results in essentially two separate circulations whereby the oxygenated blood returns from the lungs to the left atrium, to the left ventricle, and then proceeds back through the pulmonary artery and to the lungs again, whereas the deoxygenated blood returns from the body to the right atrium, the right ventricle, and proceeds back out the aorta, supplying deoxygenated blood to the systemic circulation (Fig. 41.8). The coronary arteries are positioned on the aorta coming off the right ventricle. Although not typically thought of as a defect that increases pulmonary blood flow, if the defect is undetected or monitored for a longer time, and there is an area that allows for mixing of oxygenated and deoxygenated blood, it is possible for the child to experience increased pulmonary blood flow.

Assessment

Transposition of the great arteries is a cyanotic defect noted immediately after birth. The infant is typically tachypneic, and a murmur may not be noted. Blood must mix to provide oxygenated blood to the systemic circulation. A prostaglandin E1 (PGE1) infusion is started immediately after birth to maintain patency of the ductus arteriosus and encourage mixing of blood. Side effects of a PGE1 infusion can include apnea and hypotension. Apnea occurs in 10% to 20% of

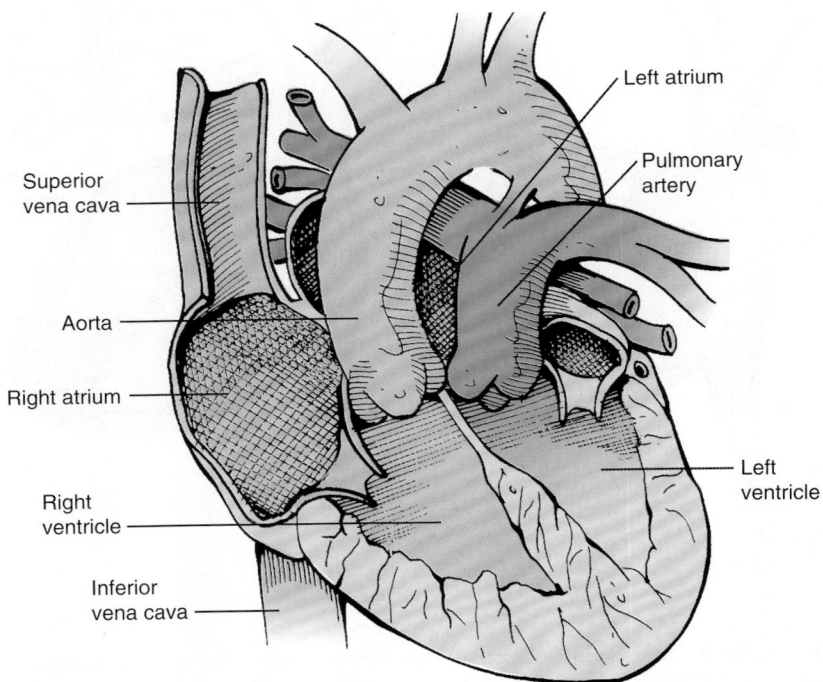

Figure 41.8 Transposition of the great arteries. (From Perrino, A. C., & Reeves, S. T. [2014]. *A practical approach to transesophageal echocardiography* [3rd ed.]. Philadelphia, PA: Wolters Kluwer.)

patients with congenital heart disease and is more common in children weighing less than 2 kg. It is typically noted within the first hour of the infusion. The goal is to use the smallest amount of medication that keeps the duct open and has minimal side effects. It is best for the child to remain on room air, spontaneously breathing, but the staff must be prepared to offer ventilator support should a child stop breathing.

However, more effective mixing occurs through a patent foramen ovale (PFO). If the PFO is in any way restrictive at birth, the opening will have to be enlarged at the bedside or in the catheterization lab through a balloon atrial septostomy. This entails a catheter being placed through the IVC up to the right atrium and floated across the foramen ovale. Once the catheter has crossed into the left atrium, a balloon is inflated at the end of that catheter, and the catheter is vigorously pulled back through the septum, effectively creating a larger ASD.

An echocardiogram will confirm this diagnosis. The echocardiogram will also delineate the coronary artery anatomy. Any deviations in this anatomy will impact surgical correction. A cardiac catheterization is not necessary for diagnosis unless the coronary arteries cannot be visualized by echocardiogram.

Management

This defect requires surgical correction within the first 14 days of life to ensure the most positive outcomes. The repair, termed an *arterial switch or Jatene procedure*, includes dissecting both the pulmonary artery and aorta above their respective valves and switching the vessels to the appropriate location. The final component of the surgical repair is removing the coronary arteries from the base of the original aorta and surgically placing them in an appropriate spot on the new aortic root, now coming off of the left ventricle.

This surgery requires cardiopulmonary bypass, and the postoperative complications are similar to other surgeries. Reimplantation of the coronary arteries, however, produces other potential complications. If any narrowing or obstruction occurs at the site of the implantation, coronary blood flow to the heart can be compromised and produce ischemia. Infants may either manifest very poor myocardial function or S-T segment changes in leads V5 or V6 on the ECG. As well, any obstruction at the great artery suture sites may cause decreased cardiac output and impair ventricular function. This may occur immediately but is also seen frequently as a long-term complication for these children as they grow and the suture line narrows. They may also experience long-segment narrowing of the pulmonary artery as a result of manipulation of the vessel in the original surgery.

These children remain in an intensive care setting from birth until they undergo their corrective surgery. Nursing care before surgery includes ensuring their oxygen saturation remains normal for this defect, which is 75% to 85%; monitoring for signs of increased pulmonary blood flow; and supporting the family as they wait for their newborn to undergo heart surgery.

Anomalous Pulmonary Venous Return and Truncus Arteriosus

Two rare, uncommon cyanotic defects are anomalous pulmonary venous return (APVR) and truncus arteriosus (TA). APVR is a result of failure of the pulmonary venous connections to unite with the left atrium in utero. Instead, they return to another vessel (left innominate, portal, or coronary sinus vein) or directly to the right atrium, and the oxygenated pulmonary blood return drains back into the right side of the heart. This can be seen with one, two, or three of the veins (partial APVR), or all four veins (total APVR) (Fig. 41.9),

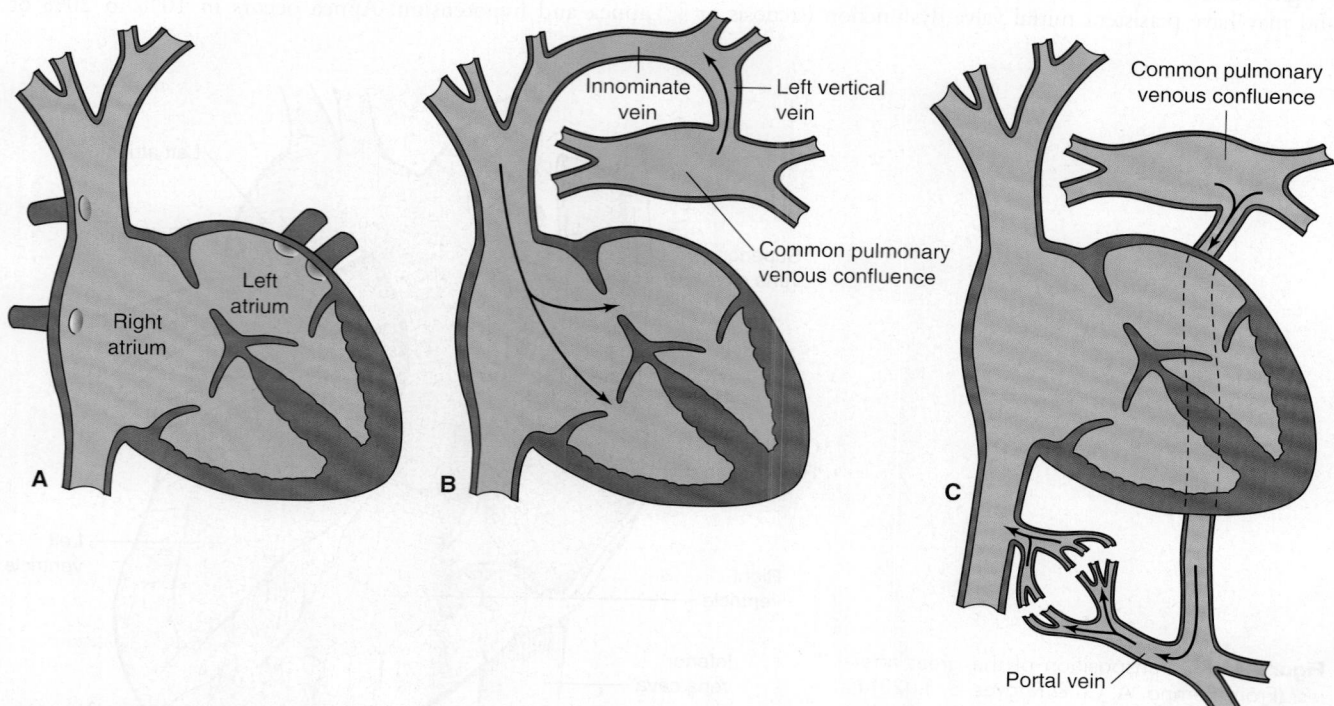

Figure 41.9 Total anomalous pulmonary venous return. **(A)** Partial anomalous pulmonary venous return (PAPVR). **(B)** TAPVR (supracardiac). **(C)** TAPVR (infradiaphragmatic). (From Nichols, D. G., & Shaffner, D. H. [2015]. *Rogers' textbook of pediatric intensive care* [5th ed.]. Philadelphia, PA: Wolters Kluwer.)

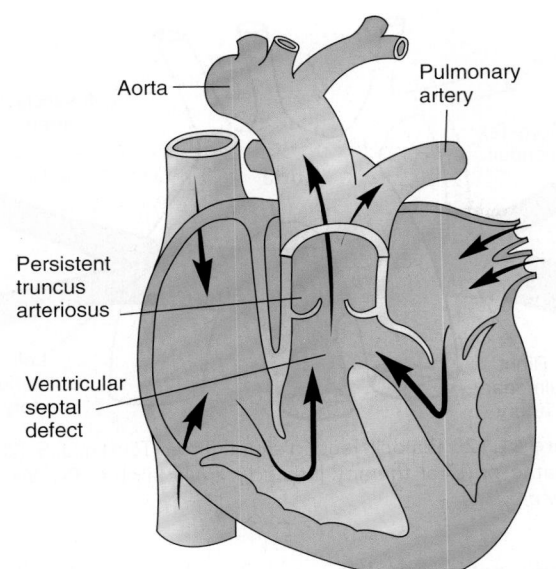

Figure 41.10 Truncus arteriosus. (From Muscari, M. [2015]. *Lippincott review: Pediatric nursing* [5th ed.]. Philadelphia, PA: Wolters Kluwer.)

draining to the venous side. Total APVR requires urgent surgical intervention. Partial PVR, if only one vessel, can be missed because it may cause no significant clinical effects.

TA is characterized by a single arterial vessel that originates from the heart, overrides the ventricular septum, and supplies all of the systemic, coronary, and pulmonary blood flow (Fig. 41.10). The branch pulmonary arteries arise at some point along this large vessel. Truncus has four classifications,

depending on where the pulmonary arteries arise from the truncal vessel. It occurs as a result of the great artery failing to divide in utero into two vessels, the pulmonary artery and the aorta. After birth, the truncus vessel arises from the ventricles; blood ejects and follows the path of least resistance to the pulmonary bed. This is a cyanotic lesion that also requires urgent surgery.

DEFECTS THAT DECREASE PULMONARY BLOOD FLOW

Tetralogy of Fallot

The prevalence of tetralogy of Fallot (TOF) in the United States is approximately 4 to 5 per 10,000 live births. This defect accounts for about 7% to 10% of cases of congenital heart disease and is one of the most common congenital heart lesions requiring intervention in the first year of life. TOF occurs equally among males and females.

This typically cyanotic defect is defined by four components: pulmonary artery stenosis, VSD, overriding aorta, and right ventricular hypertrophy (Fig. 41.11). The right ventricular hypertrophy is not an isolated problem but occurs secondary to the pulmonary stenosis.

The degree of cyanosis is directly proportional to the degree of pulmonary stenosis. Pulmonary stenosis can be noted at several sites along this right ventricular outflow tract; most typical is subpulmonary valve stenosis with anomalies of the actual pulmonary valve also seen. Significant narrowing produces increased resistance to blood flowing through the pulmonary valve and out to the lungs. Because of this increased resistance, the blood will shunt right to left through the VSD because the VSD provides less resistance, and this deoxygenated blood travels directly out through the aorta into

Tetralogy of Fallot

Figure 41.11 Tetralogy of Fallot. (From Kline-Tilford, A. M., & Haut, C. [2015]. *Lippincott certification review: Pediatric acute care nurse practitioner.* Philadelphia, PA: Wolters Kluwer.)

the systemic circulation. Children with minimal obstruction through right ventricular outflow tract may have normal systemic arterial oxygen saturations and are termed "pink" tetralogy patients.

Assessment

These children will have a systolic murmur noted at the left upper sternal border; this murmur is due to the turbulent flow out the right ventricular outflow tract. The VSD murmur may not be noticed if the defect is large. Echocardiography will confirm the diagnosis. A cardiac catheterization may be necessary if the coronary arteries are not well visualized. There have been instances where one of the coronary arteries crosses directly over the pulmonary artery. If this occurs, the surgical plan will be altered so as not to damage the coronary artery.

Occasionally, the area below the pulmonary valve may spasm, thereby increasing the resistance to flow through this area even more. This will cause a greater than usual amount of blood to shunt from right to left across the VSD, and the child will be more deoxygenated. This is termed a *hypercyanotic spell*, or a "tet spell." The exact etiology of these episodes is unclear, although a number of mechanisms have been proposed, including increased infundibular contractility, peripheral vasodilatation, hyperventilation, and stimulation of right ventricular mechanoreceptors.

During a spell, the child becomes distressed and irritable, possibly without reason. This period of lower saturations is temporary and can be managed by the family by soothing the child if he or she is upset and bringing the child's knees tightly to the chest in an effort to increase systemic vascular resistance. This increase in the pressure on the left side of the heart (the systemic side) will help force blood back through the pulmonic valve, thereby oxygenating more blood.

In a hospital setting, along with knee-to-chest positioning, blow-by oxygen can be beneficial to enhance circulating oxygen and possibly dilate the distal pulmonary bed. It will have no effect on subpulmonary spasm. The use of sedatives is controversial because they will dilate the systemic circulation, which may enhance right-to-left shunting, worsening the cyanosis. If needed, the use of alpha adrenergic agonists such as phenylephrine causes vasoconstriction and may facilitate more flow out the pulmonary artery.

If a child experiences a true hypercyanotic spell, the parents must notify their cardiologist, as this may be an indication that the child requires corrective surgery soon.

It is possible for children with a "pink" tetralogy anatomy to experience pulmonary overcirculation due to the VSD and have clinical symptoms similar to those previously discussed.

Management

Children with TOF are generally medically managed and followed by a pediatric cardiologist. If they have trouble gaining weight or experience hypercyanotic spells, they will be referred for surgery. Repair is usually performed by approximately 3 to 6 months of age, regardless of the occurrence of spells. Surgical repair of this defect includes closure of the VSD and repair of the stenotic pulmonary valve and any associated right ventricular outflow tract anomalies. Postoperative concerns center on right ventricular function, adequacy of the pulmonary valve, and flow through the pulmonary artery. In some instances, the pulmonary valve cannot be saved and is completely removed. This creates a continuous, to-and-fro

Figure 41.12 Blalock-Taussig shunt. (From Tecklin, J. S. [2014]. *Pediatric physical therapy* [5th ed.]. Philadelphia, PA: Wolters Kluwer.)

murmur noted at the left upper sternal border, with radiation throughout the chest. The valve will have to be replaced, typically during the child's school-age years.

If the right ventricular outflow tract narrowing was extremely severe at birth, a child may be referred for a palliative procedure, which will allow for adequate pulmonary blood flow until the complete surgical repair can be performed. This palliative procedure is typically a modified Blalock-Taussig (BT) shunt, which is placement of a conduit (synthetic tube) between the subclavian artery and the pulmonary artery (Fig. 41.12). This allows for a stable source of pulmonary blood flow as blood flowing out of the aorta travels through the shunt and into the lower pressure pulmonary system to become oxygenated. This ultimately increases the amount of oxygenated blood mixing with the deoxygenated blood and increases saturation. These conduits are not made of viable human tissue, however, and will not grow with the child. This is a temporary measure until it is safe for the child to undergo open heart surgery.

DEFECTS WITH OBSTRUCTION TO SYSTEMIC BLOOD FLOW

Coarctation of the Aorta

This defect is typically located at the level of the ductus arteriosus insertion; the mechanism is thought to be migration or extension of ductal tissue into the wall of the fetal thoracic aorta, causing the tissue to constrict (Fig. 41.13). Aortic narrowing occurs across a spectrum that encompasses discrete thoracic lesions, long-segmental defects, tubular hypoplasia, and, rarely, coarctation in the abdominal aorta. Coarctation accounts for 4% to 6% of all congenital heart defects, with a reported prevalence of about 4 per 10,000 live births. It occurs more commonly in males than in females.

Assessment

The common coarctation of the aorta (CoAo) typically causes a discrete narrowing of the aorta. Frequently, children are not diagnosed with a coarctation until they grow and are noted to be hypertensive. The narrowed area is most frequently distal to the right subclavian artery, so the pressures before that area increase and refer out these vessels. This causes elevated blood pressures to be noted in the right arm. Occasionally, a

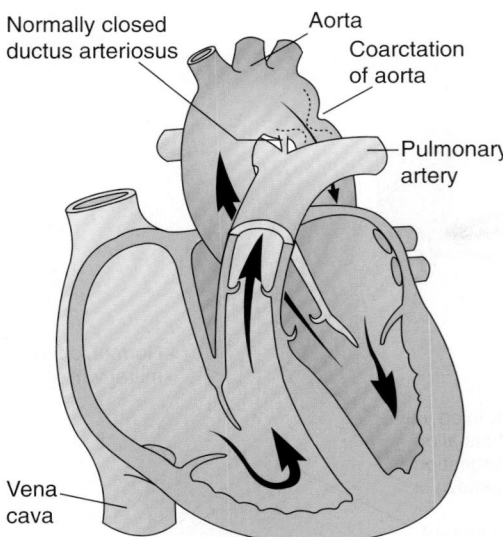

Figure 41.13   Coarctation of the aorta.

murmur may be noted in these children. If the narrowing is significant, it can cause a systolic murmur heard along the left sternal border and the left midscapular area. This narrowing increases the resistance to the left ventricle and can lead to left ventricular hypertension and hypertrophy over time.

Coarctation noted in infancy is usually more critical and can produce heart failure within weeks of birth. These emergencies require immediate surgical intervention.

To further identify the presence of a coarctation defect, you must assess the patient for the presence of pulse equality in the upper and lower extremities. While a child is lying supine, the right radial and femoral pulses are palpated concurrently. The pulses in both areas should be felt simultaneously without delay. There should be no absence or weakness in the femoral pulses compared with the radial or brachial pulse.

Another method to evaluate for the presence of a significant coarctation is to obtain blood pressures in the right arm and either leg. If the correct cuff size is used for each extremity and the child is demonstrating a similar behavior during both measurements (not crying for either reading), the pressures should be fairly equal, with the systolic pressure in the lower extremity reading slightly higher than that in the upper extremity. If the systolic pressure reading in the right upper extremity is 10 mmHg higher than that in the lower extremity, this is an indicator of potential CoAo and requires further evaluation. The exact location of the coarctation can vary but is rarely before the right subclavian branch off of the aorta. This is why using the right arm and any leg for blood pressure comparison is effective.

Management

Echocardiographic evidence of a significant gradient across the narrowing, or any signs of left ventricular hypertrophy due to the increased resistance, are indicators for correction either by balloon angioplasty in the cardiac catheterization lab or by surgical intervention. Initial repair of a coarctation defect in the catheterization lab can be controversial, as some data do not support a long-term repair of the defect by this method. CoAo is surgically repaired through a left thoracotomy incision, usually with resection of the narrowed tissue and the remaining ends of the aorta sutured together (end-to-end anastomosis). Depending on the age of the child at the initial repair, recurrent narrowing frequently occurs at the surgical area as the child continues to grow. Future interventions with balloon dilation or stent placement are typically performed in the catheterization lab.

Aortic Stenosis

Obstruction out the left ventricle can occur below the aortic valve (subvalvar), at the valve (valvar), or above the valve (supravalvar). These can be isolated abnormalities or occur with other defects. Regardless of the location of the restriction, the resultant physiology is the same. The narrowing prevents blood from passing freely from the left ventricle of the heart into the aorta. Because the heart must work harder to pass blood through the narrowed area, increased pressure and hypertrophy occur in the left ventricle (Fig. 41.14). If this pressure becomes severe, pressure in the left atrium will increase as well, resulting in back pressure through the pulmonary veins to the lungs, possibly causing pulmonary edema. Aortic stenosis accounts for about 10% of congenital cardiac abnormalities (Darst et al., 2012).

The most common location for obstruction is valvar aortic stenosis, which is typically associated with an abnormal, bicuspid aortic valve. In a bicuspid aortic valve, the leaflets are not properly divided into three. This allows for stenosis of the valve that progresses in severity in about 33% of cases. Bicuspid valves are frequently seen with other left-sided cardiac anomalies, especially CoAo.

Assessment

Aortic stenosis eventually presents with a systolic heart murmur at the right second intercostal space, but the child may be otherwise asymptomatic. If the obstruction is severe, the child may experience chest pain with exercise. Aortic regurgitation is frequently associated with stenosis, so a diastolic murmur may also be noted. ECG may note left ventricular hypertrophy if the stenosis has been ongoing. Echocardiography will determine the exact location and severity of the narrowing as well as any impact on ventricular size and function.

Management

Management of aortic stenosis is difficult and requires frequent and meticulous evaluation by a pediatric cardiologist. Stabilization with a beta-blocker or a calcium channel blocker may be necessary to reduce or prevent further ventricular hypertrophy. These children require routine echocardiograms and possibly cardiac catheterizations to best quantify the pressure gradient across the valve. More aggressive intervention is based on these pressure gradients. Typically, initial intervention is through balloon dilation in the cardiac catheterization laboratory. Surgical intervention may be necessary for recurrent stenosis or ineffective balloon dilation.

SINGLE-VENTRICLE DEFECTS

A variety of congenital abnormalities such as mitral atresia, aortic atresia, or pulmonary atresia with an intact ventricular septum result in a single-ventricle physiology. The resultant physiology and management strategies vary given each child's specific anatomy; it is not possible to address all of these

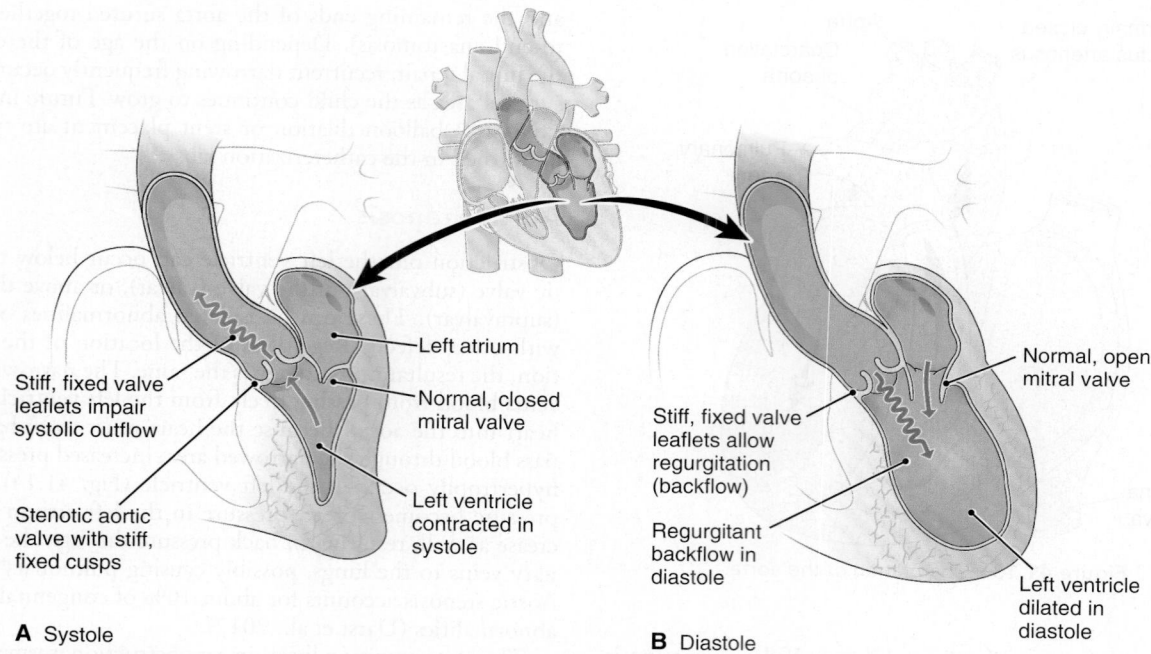

A Systole

Left atrium

Normal, closed mitral valve

Left ventricle contracted in systole

Stiff, fixed valve leaflets impair systolic outflow

Stenotic aortic valve with stiff, fixed cusps

B Diastole

Normal, open mitral valve

Stiff, fixed valve leaflets allow regurgitation (backflow)

Regurgitant backflow in diastole

Left ventricle dilated in diastole

Figure 41.14 Aortic stenosis. (From McConnell, T. H. [2014]. *Nature of disease: Pathology for the health professions* [2nd ed.]. Baltimore, MD: Wolters Kluwer.)

permutations, but the basic conceptual understanding and management of single-ventricle defects is grossly the same.

This section discusses specifically hypoplastic left heart syndrome (HLHS), its anatomy, physiology, and management strategies (Fig. 41.15). HLHS is a rare disorder, accounting for only 1% to 3% of congenital heart disease, and is detectable on prenatal ultrasound. HLHS results when there is poor or no flow to the left ventricle, typically secondary to mitral or aortic stenosis or atresia. Because of the limited amount of blood in the left ventricle, it does not develop appropriately. The ascending aorta is also hypoplas-

tic, and the coronary arteries are perfused through retrograde flow down the ascending aorta. A PFO will occur, although the atrial septum is thickened. In utero, the circulation is adequate to meet the needs of the developing fetus. But at birth, survival is dependent on a PDA. Infants are typically male, rarely premature, and have no other associated cardiac anomalies.

At birth, this cyanotic defect has normal right-sided flow out to the lungs. Oxygenated blood returning to the left atrium mixes across the PFO. This blood mixes with the deoxygenated blood returning from the systemic circulation, and the resultant oxygen saturation is approximately 75%. When this blood is ejected from the right ventricle, it travels to the lungs, with a portion of it traveling through the PDA and down the descending aorta to supply the systemic and coronary circulation.

This is a ductal-dependent lesion; these children cannot survive without their ductus remaining patent until surgery can occur. For this reason, a PGE1 infusion is initiated immediately at birth to keep the duct from closing.

A balanced circulation must be maintained while the child awaits surgical palliation. When the right ventricle contracts, it is best for the blood to distribute evenly to the lungs and the systemic circulation. If resistance in the lungs decreases, this would increase the blood flow to the pulmonary circulation but effectively "steal" from the systemic circulation. Although the saturations would read as being higher, the child would begin to experience decreased cardiac output and tissue perfusion, which would lead to a state of metabolic acidosis. It is very difficult for these children to recover from a stressor such as this. Therefore, it is extremely important that you always recognize and understand that a saturation of 70% to 80% is normal for these children. Interventions such as oxygen aimed at raising the saturation would be detrimental to the child, as oxygen is a potent pulmonary vasodilator.

ASD = Atrial Septal Defect
IVC = Inferior Vena Cava
LA = Left Atrium
LV = Left Ventricle
PA = Pulmonary Artery

PDA = Patent Ductus Arteriosus
PV = Pulmonary Vein
RA = Right Atrium
RV = Right Ventricle
SVC = Superior Vena Cava

Figure 41.15 Hypoplastic left heart defect. (From Bucklin, B. A., Baysinger, C. L., & Gambling, D. [2016]. *A practical approach to obstetric anesthesia* [2nd ed.]. Philadelphia, PA: Wolters Kluwer.)

Surgical Management of a Hypoplastic Left Heart Syndrome Defect

Norwood Procedure

This surgery, which includes several components, is done within a few days of birth once the child is hemodynamically stable (Fig. 41.16).

- Dissection of the main pulmonary artery from the branch pulmonary arteries, which is then attached to the hypoplastic ascending aorta so there is one great vessel taking blood out of the heart (right ventricle) to the body and providing blood flow to the coronary arteries.
- Shunt placement, typically either a BT shunt or a Sano shunt. The BT shunt (as discussed previously for TOF) directs blood from the right subclavian artery to the branch pulmonary artery, whereas a Sano shunt is a conduit from the right ventricle to the branch pulmonary arteries. The purpose of both shunts is to allow for stable blood flow to the lungs.
- Ligation of the PDA
- Ensuring a widely patent atrial septum

Once this surgery is complete, all blood ejected from the right ventricle travels to the systemic circulation, with some blood shunted through the BT shunt or Sano shunt (Fig. 41.17) to the lungs to get oxygenated.

The time period before the Glenn shunt is performed has a high morbidity and mortality rate. These children are at high risk for sudden death due to dysrhythmias, inability to fight infection, or metabolic imbalance. These children must receive antiviral therapy for prophylaxis against respiratory syncytial virus (RSV) monthly during the season. An RSV infection can be lethal for these children.

Bidirectional Glenn Shunt

This surgery is usually performed at approximately 4 to 6 months of age or when the child outgrows their previously placed BT or Sano shunt. The purpose of the shunt is to relieve the volume load on the single right ventricle, which is accommodating all of the circulating blood flow (Fig. 41.18). At this surgery, two procedures are performed:

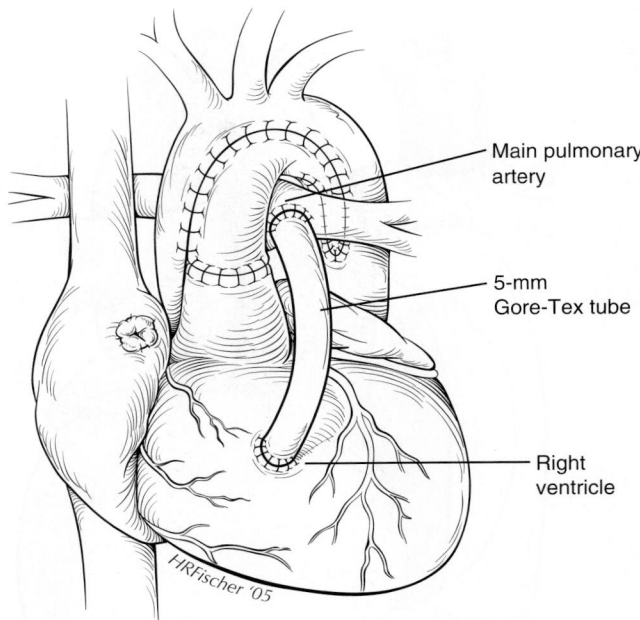

Figure 41.17 Sano shunt. (From Kaiser, L., Kron, I. L., & Spray, T. L. [2013]. *Mastery of cardiothoracic surgery* [3rd ed.]. Philadelphia, PA: Wolters Kluwer.)

1. Ligation of the previously placed BT or Sano shunt
2. Dissection of the SVC at its insertion to the right atrium and attachment of the SVC directly to the branch pulmonary artery. This allows deoxygenated blood returning from the head and upper body to flow directly but passively to the lungs to get oxygenated. Normal saturations after this surgery are approximately 85%.

Fontan Procedure

The final stage is performed when the child weighs approximately 15 kg or is 3 years old. At this time, the IVC is dissected from the right atrium, and flow from there is directed through an artificial conduit directly to the branch pulmonary artery. At this time, all of the patient's deoxygenated blood (except for coronary sinus return) flows directly but passively, to the

ASD = Atrial Septal Defect	*PA = Pulmonary Artery*
BT = Blalock-Taussig	*PV = Pulmonary Vein*
IVC = Inferior Vena Cava	*RA = Right Atrium*
LA = Left Atrium	*RV = Right Ventricle*
LV = Left Ventricle	*SVC = Superior Vena Cava*

Figure 41.16 Modified Blalock-Taussig (BT) shunt with Norwood procedure. (From Bucklin, B. A., Baysinger, C. L., & Gambling, D. [2016]. *A practical approach to obstetric anesthesia* [2nd ed.]. Philadelphia, PA: Wolters Kluwer.)

ASD = Atrial Septal Defect	*PA = Pulmonary Artery*
BDG = Bidirectional Glenn anastomosis	*PV = Pulmonary Vein*
IVC = Inferior Vena Cava	*RA = Right Atrium*
LA = Left Atrium	*RV = Right Ventricle*
LV = Left Ventricle	*SVC = Superior Vena Cava*

Figure 41.18 Bidirectional Glenn shunt. (From Bucklin, B. A., Baysinger, C. L., & Gambling, D. [2016]. *A practical approach to obstetric anesthesia* [2nd ed.]. Philadelphia, PA: Wolters Kluwer.)

Figure 41.19 Extracardiac conduit Fontan surgery. (From Kaiser, L., Kron, I. L., & Spray, T. L. [2013]. *Mastery of cardiothoracic surgery* [3rd ed.]. Philadelphia, PA: Wolters Kluwer.)

lungs, and all of the blood returning to the left atrium flows across the ASD, to the right atrium, right ventricle, and out the augmented aorta to the body. Normal saturation values after this surgery range near 90% (Fig. 41.19).

Cardiac transplantation is an alternative form of therapy, but the availability of donor hearts, rejection problems, and the need for retransplantation make this a secondary choice for most infants.

Cardiac Surgery

Pediatric cardiac surgery is relatively young in experience, but the advances made in the past decades have allowed for tremendous increases in survival rates. An effective method of implementing cardiopulmonary bypass allowing intracardiac repairs did not occur until the 1950s. Not only have techniques and experience advanced, so have palliative and bridge measures such as ventricular assistive devices, balloon pumps, and ECMO, all of which have contributed to better outcomes for children with heart disease.

In pediatrics, repair of cardiac defects varies, as each defect can differ in actual anatomy and complexity. This section focuses briefly on the care of the child in the immediate postoperative period and provides more details for care of children in a later convalescent phase.

PREOPERATIVE CARE

A child must be healthy before cardiac surgery. They must exhibit no signs of an upper respiratory tract infection or

have a fever. Vital signs (blood pressure, temperature, pulse, respirations, and oxygen saturation) will be noted to establish baseline values. An accurate height and weight are also recorded. Weight must be documented in kilograms as all medication calculations in children are based on this unit of measure. Laboratory values must be checked, specifically chemistry, hematology, and coagulation values. Blood products must also be typed and cross-matched. Pregnancy testing, either urine or serum, must be performed for any girl who has begun menstruating. It is also important to ensure that consents for surgery and anesthesia have been signed by the family and the appropriate provider.

Nursing Diagnoses and Related Interventions: Preoperative Phase

Nursing Diagnosis: Deficient knowledge related to cardiac surgery and its outcome

Outcome Evaluation: Parents and child accurately state the reason for surgery and expected outcome.

Agreeing to cardiac surgery is a difficult choice for parents because although they want their child to feel better, they are also aware there is a definite risk from this surgery. As parents, they may have been protecting and guarding their child for months or years; they feel no less protective the morning of surgery. Parents usually appreciate a visit to the intensive care unit (ICU) before surgery and meeting the ICU staff who will care for their child later. Be certain to prepare them for the amount of equipment that will surround their child after surgery, such as a cardiac monitor, oxygen, IV equipment, chest tubes, and a ventilator, as well as all of the noises associated with an intensive care environment (Fig. 41.20).

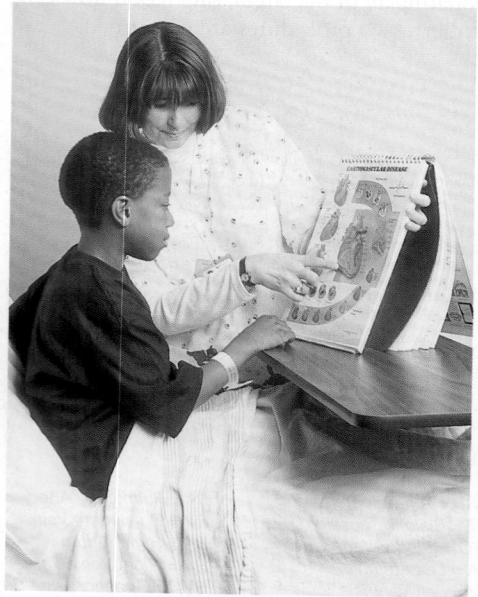

Figure 41.20 Orientation for cardiac surgery includes time for talking and learning more about the heart and why equipment such as chest tubes is necessary. (© Lesha Photography.)

It is important to include the child in developmentally appropriate discussions regarding the planned surgical procedure and postoperative course. By speaking with both the child and parents, the parents will be able to reinforce your teaching. This also demonstrates to children that their parents approve and feel secure with these surgery plans. Because many children scheduled for cardiac surgery have already had a cardiac catheterization, talking to them about their previous hospitalization experience can be helpful to reveal things they are worrying about. Any misconceptions they have can then be discussed and clarified. Be certain to explain that anesthesia is a "special sleep" from which they will have no difficulty waking. After the child is fully prepared, ask parents whether they need additional time to discuss the surgical procedure and ask questions they might not have wished to ask in front of their child.

Because the child will need to cough, breathe deeply, and use incentive spirometry to help the lungs expand after surgery, introduce these exercises and the idea of chest tubes and supplemental oxygen preoperatively so a child can learn that these will be expected. Including child life specialists in these discussions, especially for younger children, can be very beneficial to the child.

When discussing postoperative care, parents and older children can be taken to the ICU where they will return after surgery and be shown the equipment that will surround them. For younger children, it may be helpful to use pictures of the equipment so it's not so overwhelming.

POSTOPERATIVE CARE OF THE CHILD AFTER CARDIAC SURGERY

Initial management of a child after cardiac surgery occurs in an intensive care unit until the child is hemodynamically stable and invasive lines are removed. Potential complications after cardiac surgery vary given the nature of the defect and surgical repair, so it is important that you have a strong understanding of both (Fig. 41.21).

Most surgical repairs for congenital heart defects require the use of cardiopulmonary bypass (CPB), which allows the surgeon to manipulate the heart in a bloodless field while maintaining perfusion and oxygenation to the body. Briefly, it accomplishes this by placing a cannula in the right atrium, where blood is removed from the body, run through a machine that oxygenates the blood, and then returned to the body via a cannula placed in the ascending aorta. In this way, the oxygenation circuit is maintained but the actual heart is avoided. When a child undergoes surgery with CPB, he or she is cooled to decrease metabolic demand and oxygen consumption, thereby protecting the brain and other organs during the low circulatory flow that occurs with CPB. The heart itself is protected from injury during this time using hypothermia and chemical preservation.

CPB is not without secondary effects after surgery. Because of the nature of the bypass machine and the tubing the blood passes through, the body responds by releasing mediators, which cause inflammatory responses, capillary leak, and hematologic abnormalities. This can lead to acute complications such as fluid shifting out of the intravascular space into

Figure 41.21 Because children after cardiac surgery typically have a myriad of wires and tubes attached to monitors, pumps, and equipment, parents need to be prepared for how their child will look. As the child's condition improves, use of the equipment is discontinued. Here, an infant is 2 days postcardiac surgery. Note his level of alertness and the use of only a few monitoring devices and equipment. (© Caroline Brown, RNC, MS, DEd.)

the tissues, poor urine output, edema, and poor circulating volume. Anemia and altered coagulation status can also occur. These effects will be greater if the bypass run time was long.

The surgery itself can lead to potential complications depending on length of time and the complexity of the repair. Tissue perfusion is dependent on adequate cardiac output, which can be affected by many factors in the postoperative period. Poor tissue perfusion can be a result of decreased ventricular contractility from CPB, acidosis, or electrolyte imbalance; decreased intravascular volume from excessive losses, inadequate replacement, or fluid shifts; increased resistance to ventricular ejection caused by changes in pulmonary or systemic vascular resistance from vasoconstriction or hypertension; or alterations in heart rate or rhythm. All of these potential complications must be watched for and treated immediately. They should dissipate over time but can cause significant periods of hemodynamic compromise.

 Nursing Diagnoses and Related Interventions: Postoperative Phase

Nursing Diagnosis: Risk for ineffective cardiopulmonary tissue perfusion related to depressed myocardial function after surgery

Outcome Evaluation: Vital signs remain within normal limits; physical examination demonstrates adequate cardiac output.

Taking accurate vital signs is essential in the immediate postoperative period. Continuous cardiac monitoring will occur, and assisted ventilation with endotracheal intubation is frequently necessary. Blood pressure will be monitored directly by means of an intra-arterial catheter or indirectly with an automated blood pressure recording device. Hemodynamic monitoring through a central venous catheter monitors the central venous pressure (CVP) from immediately above the right atrium as an indicator of preload. Pulse oximetry is continuous, and many children will also have near-infrared spectrometry (NIRS) monitoring.

IV fluids may be ordered at less than maintenance value to prevent fluid overload. An indwelling urinary catheter is inserted at the time of surgery so urine output can be carefully measured and recorded postoperatively. Be certain to document the amount of urine drainage present when the child first returns from surgery and hourly so that diminished urinary output will not be missed. Subtle changes in cardiac output can be noted by following urine output. Preferred urine output after surgery is approximately 0.5 to 1 ml/kg/hr for infants and will be weight based for older children. If a child is voiding well after surgery, it indicates the kidneys are receiving an adequate blood flow and the heart is working effectively.

Laboratory tests such as arterial blood gases, hemoglobin, hematocrit, clotting time, and electrolytes (particularly sodium, potassium, calcium, and magnesium) must also be monitored closely to assess postoperative hemodynamic status. IV inotropic agents such as milrinone (Primacor) or dopamine may be added to enhance cardiac output and decrease afterload.

Sternal closure can be delayed after cardiac surgery, usually in small infants with complex cardiac surgical repairs. Allowing the sternum to remain open, until tissue swelling resolves, prevents compression of the heart that would occur with closure of the chest, which would impact cardiac contractility. A sterile occlusive dressing is applied to help shield the open incision from potential infection. After swelling and edema have decreased, the sternum will be closed (usually about 24 to 72 hours after surgery) either in the ICU or the operating room. The nursing care for a child with an open chest includes the same monitoring as for all children who have had cardiac surgery, plus extreme diligence in caring for the site and monitoring for infection.

Nursing Diagnosis: Risk for excess or deficient fluid volume related to fluid shifts accompanying cardiac surgery

Outcome Evaluation: Child maintains weight; skin turgor is good; urine output is normal.

Children tend to develop relative hypovolemia after cardiac surgery because of increased production of aldosterone by the adrenal glands and an increase in antidiuretic hormone secretion by the pituitary gland in response to stress. Also, cardiopulmonary bypass causes fluids to shift from the intravascular system to the interstitial spaces because of an inflammatory response that causes leaky capillaries. After surgery, as this fluid returns by osmosis to the vessels and is excreted with the help of diuretics, balance is restored.

Monitoring central venous pressures carefully to evaluate preload will help determine which type of therapy is necessary. IV volume may be given if the circulating volume is low as indicated by a low CVP. It is usually preferred that the product given have a high oncotic pressure, as with red blood cells or albumin, in order to prevent further leakage across dilated capillaries. If the CVP is high, diuretics and restricted IV fluid intake will be necessary. Oral intake is typically not restricted in children; they will self-limit their intake.

Nursing Diagnosis: Impaired gas exchange related to atelectasis and/or collection of fluid in the chest cavity (pleural effusions)

Outcome Evaluation: Child's respiratory rate remains within age-appropriate parameters; there are no rales, crackles, or other adventitious breath sounds; chest tubes function effectively.

Measures to Prevent Impaired Gas Exchange. Endotracheal suctioning is necessary while a child is receiving ventilatory assistance to prevent secretion accumulation in the lungs or obstruction of the endotracheal tube. Assist with chest physiotherapy (percussion and vibration) as needed to help keep lung secretions mobile. As soon as the endotracheal tube and ventilator are removed, encourage the child to cough and breathe deeply or use an incentive spirometer at hourly intervals as a way to mobilize secretions. Although children may have practiced such procedures preoperatively, they may have difficulty carrying them out postoperatively because coughing and deep breathing after cardiac surgery can be very painful. To minimize pain, administer prescribed analgesia or alert the child to use the patient-controlled analgesia (PCA) pump 10 to 15 minutes before it is time to breathe deeply. Teach children how to use a pillow as a splint while coughing and deep breathing. Be certain parents understand that games such as blowing cotton balls or bubbles, or using the incentive spirometer, are important exercises to help achieve lung expansion. Encourage them to work with the child throughout the day to perform these exercises.

Chest tube drainage systems are used after complex cardiac surgeries to collect air from the pleural space, and fluid, typically blood, from the mediastinum, but may be used in other situations such as isolated pleural effusions, chylothorax, or pneumothorax. After surgery, typically one tube in the mediastinal space collects blood and another in the pleural space collects air.

The drainage systems are designed not only to allow the drainage and collection of fluid or air from the chest but also to prevent air or fluid from returning to the chest. This system is based on a three-chamber concept that allows for drainage into one section, application of a water seal to prevent air from reentering the pleural cavity or mediastinum, and a third chamber to allow the continuous, controlled application of suction (Fig. 41.22). Suction can be applied in two ways: either through water or "dry" suction.

Jackson-Pratt drains can also be used postoperatively if the volume of drainage is not expected to be excessive. These tubes are much smaller and more flexible so they cause less pain. They are also significantly less cumbersome.

Nursing concerns when working with a child who has a chest drainage system include:

- Keeping the system closed and below chest level
- Ensuring suction control chambers are filled or set for the ordered amount of suction. If a fluid-filled system, ensure bubbles are in the chamber.
- Making sure the water seal chamber is filled to manufacturer's recommended level
- Monitoring for bubbles in the water seal chamber, which can indicate either a leak in the drainage system or an air leak from the patient's lungs

Figure 41.22 Pleur-Evac system for chest tube drainage.

- Assessing and documenting the amount, color, and consistency in the drainage system routinely and as ordered. Report any drainage that changes in volume, color, or bloodiness.
- NOT aggressively milking or stripping chest tubes, as this can cause very high levels of negative pressure. But it is important to keep the tubes freely draining, which can be difficult if the drainage is frank blood, which may have clots in it.
- Ensuring adequate pain control. Chest tubes can be very uncomfortable, but it is important for the child to get out of bed, ambulate, cough, or perform pulmonary toilet maneuvers. It is important to obtain a level of pain control that allows the child to be awake and interactive.

Nursing Diagnosis: Risk for ineffective peripheral tissue perfusion related to dysrhythmias.

Outcome Evaluation: Patient will remain free of postoperative dysrhythmias; any dysrhythmias will be readily identified and treated to maintain adequate cardiac output.

When children return from the operating room after complex cardiac surgery, they are at risk for dysrhythmias due to damage to the conduction system, inflammation of or injury to the heart itself, or electrolyte imbalance. In anticipation of possible dysrhythmias, children may have two pacing wires attached to the surface of the heart and brought out through the chest wall. These are temporary pacemaker wires that can be attached to a pacemaker at the bedside in the event the child experiences a dysrhythmia or heart block. If no evidence of abnormal rhythms has been seen after several days, the pacing wires will be pulled out. If a child is dependent on the pacemaker due to heart block and normal conduction does not spontaneously return after 14 days, the child is typically taken to the operating room for placement of a permanent pacemaker. The pacemaker is placed in the abdominal cavity in infants and small children. For older children and adolescents, the pacemaker is placed in the left shoulder area, and the wires are threaded transvenously to the

right heart. Currently, permanent pacemaker batteries last approximately 5 years. Having a permanent pacemaker requires monthly transmissions to document pacemaker function and will limit the child's ability to participate in contact sports.

Once a child has progressed to a less critical status and is hemodynamically stable, the child may be moved from the ICU to a routine patient care unit. This is a major step toward recovery but also may be a difficult move for both the child and the parents because they have developed confidence in the ICU staff and are reluctant to move to an area with less monitoring and entrust their child to new personnel. It helps the transition if the concept of transferring to a step-down or floor location is broached early in the postoperative phase. Visits from the floor nursing staff while the child is still in the ICU will also help. Allow parents the opportunity to voice their concern over the changes in personnel and monitoring. Understanding that their child is ready for this change and will be safe can help prepare them for the day of hospital discharge, when they will be observing and caring for their child on their own.

Once on the floor, general nursing care includes the following:

- Watching for blood loss
- Preventing infection
- Preventing/managing pain
- Maintaining lung expansion
- Encouraging mobility
- Encouraging healthy eating
- Including the family in care

Nursing Diagnosis: Risk for infection related to surgical incision

Outcome Evaluation: Child's temperature remains at or below 100.4°F (38.0°C); incision site is clean, dry, and without evidence of erythema or drainage.

Antibiotic therapy is continued for 24 to 48 hours after chest closure. To detect whether infection could be beginning, frequently monitor the temperature and assess the surgical incision site and the points of insertion of the thoracotomy tubes or central catheters for drainage and erythema.

Infants must wear shirts and bibs when feeding to prevent formula from dropping on the incision site. Older children should wear T-shirts at all times. This not only helps with food but also keeps them from scratching the site or pulling at the butterfly closures (if used).

Nursing Diagnosis: Parental anxiety related to lack of knowledge of postoperative routine and exercises

Outcome Evaluation: Family members accurately state plans for child's postoperative recovery; family members relate less anxiety after teaching and support.

Most children recover very quickly from heart surgery. Children are encouraged to be out of bed and ambulating once they are hemodynamically stable and free from cumbersome equipment. Encourage parents to participate as much as they want to in their child's care during this period. Parents can encourage their child to routinely perform breathing exercises, eat and drink throughout the day, and get out of bed.

Caution parents not to pick up an infant under the arms to move or hold the child because this pulls on the chest incision. Show them how to lift an infant by placing their hands behind the neck and scooping under the buttocks instead. Teach parents to help an older child out of bed by wrapping their arms around the child's chest. To prevent pain, they should not pull on the child's arms. Despite the sternal wound, all children should use seat belts or car seats as directed to ensure safety. Infants should not be placed prone for "tummy time" for approximately 2 to 3 weeks after surgery. If the infant rolls over independently, their own body weight will not hurt the sternal site (Box 41.5).

QSEN Checkpoint Question 41.2

EVIDENCE-BASED PRACTICE

Surgical closure of a ventricular septal defect (VSD) is the most commonly performed procedure in cardiac surgery. Although considerably safe, complication can occur. Schipper, Slieker, Schoof, et al. (2017) performed a retrospective study of all VSD closures at their single center to evaluate for risk factors for a complicated postoperative course. Of 243 patients that underwent a VSD surgical repair, there were no deaths, 0.8% required a pacemaker for heart block, and 2.1% required reoperation for hemodynamically significant residual VSD. Multivariate analysis identified a genetic syndrome, long bypass time, and low weight at operation as independent risk factors for a prolonged intensive care stay and prolonged ventilation times. None of these were associated with major adverse events.

Henry is a 2-month-old with Down syndrome and a VSD. He is in CHF and has been having difficulty gaining weight so surgery has been scheduled. Based on this study, what will you include in your preoperative discussions with his family?

 a. VSDs are very difficult to repair and children can have many complications after surgery.
 b. Because Henry has Down syndrome and his weight is less than expected for his age, he may need a few extra days on the ventilator or in the ICU, but overall, he should do fine.
 c. Henry's age, being less than 12 months old, puts him at greater risk for complications after VSD surgery.
 d. A VSD repair is not done with cardiopulmonary bypass so the risk of complications is significantly less than for other defects.

Look in Appendix A for the best answer and rationale.

DISCHARGING A CHILD AFTER CARDIAC SURGERY

There are several restrictions when a child is ready to be discharged home. Children, especially infants, are at higher risk for infection and should avoid any actively sick contacts while they are recuperating at home. Good hand washing techniques should be used by all visitors. Children are usually kept home from school for several weeks after their surgery but should return once they are cleared by the cardiologist or surgeon.

BOX 41.5
Nursing Care Planning Tips for Effective Communication

Megan is a 2-month-old infant who is being discharged after cardiac surgery. You stop at her hospital room to give discharge instructions to her mother.

Tip: Because cardiac surgery is such serious surgery, most parents assume it will take their child a long time to recover from it. Listen closely when reviewing discharge instructions and ask follow-up questions to ensure the patient fully comprehends the instructions. In the following scenario, the nurse recognizes that Megan's mother has not heard the first instruction—to let the child return to normal activities as she is able. Older children will have more activity restrictions (sports, PE class) but should still return to normal activities of daily living within 1 to 2 weeks.

Nurse: Good morning, Mrs. Carver. Let me review a few instructions with you before you go home with Megan.

Mrs. Carver: The most important thing you can tell me is how to keep a baby on bed rest.

Nurse: Most infants are more tired than usual from surgery, but just let her assume her usual activities as she likes.

Mrs. Carver: She likes to kick a mobile in bed. It'll be hard to keep her from doing that.

Nurse: And that's okay for her to do that. She won't do anything if it hurts. Infants and children don't need to be confined to bed, they just need to be allowed to rest when needed, which will be more frequently for awhile. They also need adults to pick them up carefully to prevent any pain or damage to the healing breastbone.

Mrs. Carver: So it's okay if she sits in her car seat or if I hold her? I don't want to hurt her or cause other problems.

Nurse: Absolutely! We want your family to return to their normal routine, you just need to modify how she is handled, allow her to rest, and keep her in a healthy environment.

Mrs. Carver: We can do that. Thank you, I just couldn't imagine how to keep a baby on bed rest.

Nurse: I'm glad we could clarify that for you. I would like to speak with you about a few other items before you go home. Are you okay to go on?

Mrs. Carver: Yes, I'm ready.

Continue with medication and infection control instructions.

Children who have undergone a median sternotomy must be restricted from physical activity, including physical education class and any sports activities, for 6 weeks from the time of sternal closure. They should be assigned a helper in school because these restrictions include lifting heavy backpacks or other heavy items. They should also not drive a car during this time to allow for healing of the sternum. They must be cleared by the cardiologist or surgeon before they can return to these activities.

Immediately after surgery, the child will have limited range of motion of their arms. They may be provided exercises to help with movement and to decrease pain. They will need assistance with dressing and bathing for several weeks but will soon be independent again. Children may typically undergo a sponge bath or a shower when they are discharged from the hospital. However, to prevent infection, they should not submerge their wound in a tub or pool until the wound is completely healed, and it has been evaluated by a practitioner.

Studies have been done to evaluate the neurodevelopmental outcomes of the child with congenital heart disease. A significant number of children with coronary heart disease (CHD) will manifest neurodevelopmental impairments affecting cognition, motor and language development, and higher order cognitive functions (Ringle & Wernovsky, 2016). These impairments may be mild to moderate in severity but may also occur in conjunction with other developmental or behavioral problems and significantly affect school performance and academic achievement. Risk factors for worse outcomes include:

- Genetic disorders
- Single-ventricle patients
- Complicated and extensive postoperative intensive care unit (ICU) course
- Lower socioeconomic status (Forbess, Visconti, Hancock-Friesen, et al., 2002; Latal, 2016)

It is important for families to follow through with neurologic and behavioral specialists as they are referred and to seek early intervention to assure maximum success for their child. It is important for the family to understand that other than simple ASD or VSD surgical repairs, all children will need to follow-up with a cardiologist for life. Although they have undergone a corrective procedure, they are at risk for future complications related to their growth, development of scar tissue, or long-term effects of the disorder. As children with CHD continue to survive and thrive, they have progressed to adulthood. These adult survivors of congenital heart disease have long-term medical needs that healthcare providers are only now beginning to understand. Many institutions have developed *Adult Congenital Programs* to address the needs of adults who have survived congenital heart disease as a child but now have adult medical issues and yet still require cardiology follow-up for the CHD. They require specialists who understand the anatomy and physiology of congenital heart disease as well as the normal progress of these diseases after surgery and how all of this is impacted by routine aging.

QSEN Checkpoint Question 41.3

SAFETY

After cardiac surgery, infants and children have limitations to their activity and handling. When teaching parents how to help their children with daily activities, the nurse recognizes it is most important to emphasize which statement?

a. Children are very resilient and recover quickly after cardiac surgery. Parents don't need to do anything different when handling their children when they go home.

b. Infants and children should remain in bed or on the couch at home and not be allowed to perform any activities other than go to the bathroom to prevent pain and injury until they have at least two follow-up visits with their cardiologist.

c. Infants and children should be restricted from all physical activity for 6 months from the time

of their surgery. They should not lift their arms over their head or be lifted under their arms for the same time period.

d. Infants and children should not be lifted under their arms for 6 weeks from the time of sternal closure. They should also not participate in physical activity or lift heavy items for this same time period.

Look in Appendix A for the best answer and rationale.

Cardiac Catheterization

A **cardiac catheterization** is a diagnostic or interventional procedure where one or more small catheters are passed through a large vein and/or artery into the heart. Access for a catheterization is frequently obtained in the femoral vein and artery but radial and neck access can also be used. With catheters in the heart or major vessels, the cardiologist can obtain blood samples to evaluate oxygen content, measure direct pressures in all chambers and vessels, and inject a contrast dye to define anatomy. Cardiac output, cardiac index, and systemic and pulmonary vascular resistance can be calculated. Many interventions can be performed in the catheterization laboratory including PDA and septal defect closure, dilation of narrowed valves or vessels, stent placement in narrowed vessels, closure of collateral or abnormal vessels, placement of artificial valves, and myocardial biopsy. Although cardiac catheterizations are relatively safe, potential complications can include:

- Dysrhythmias
- Inadvertent perforation of the heart or major blood vessel
- Bleeding
- Valve or vessel damage
- Stroke
- Seizures
- Death

Children are usually deeply sedated for a catheterization procedure with an anesthesiologist providing the necessary level of sedation. Depth of sedation decisions is based on the child's age, developmental status, and the extent of the proposed catheterization procedure.

 Nursing Diagnoses and Related Interventions: Preprocedure Phase

Cardiac catheterization is a stress-filled procedure for parents and children.

Nursing Diagnosis: Anxiety related to cardiac catheterization procedure.

Outcome Evaluation: Parents state goal of procedure and reasons for preparation and aftercare measures; parents state they are able to manage anxiety while waiting for results.

Try to provide an explanation of the procedure to the child with the parents present so that the parents can reinforce the information as needed. After the explanation, provide parents with a more detailed explanation if desired, allowing time for questions they did not want to ask in the child's presence.

Older children enjoy a tour of the cardiac catheterization area if possible and the opportunity to meet the personnel. Because small children can become overwhelmed by seeing the actual room, the use of developmentally appropriate play with a puppet or small doll may be helpful. Dress puppets in surgery suits and masks and have them act out what the child can expect to experience.

Do not underestimate what children know about their heart's purpose and function; even preschoolers know their heart is vital to their body. Reassure them that people are only taking pictures of their heart during this procedure, not cutting it or removing any part of it.

Let children know that after the procedure, a pressure dressing will be placed over the catheter insertion site to reduce the risk of bleeding. They will need to keep that extremity flat and straight to prevent bleeding.

POST–CARDIAC CATHETERIZATION NURSING CARE

Once the catheterization is completed and the access catheters are removed, the child is at risk for bleeding from the insertion site. Children typically remain supine with their legs straight for 2 to 4 hours after the procedure to ensure hemostasis at the site. If the access points were in the neck or arm, the activity restrictions will be less.

It is imperative that you understand the child's underlying cardiac anatomy and physiology as well as the purpose of the catheterization before the child returns from the procedure. Recovery of a child after a catheterization must include monitoring of the respiratory status including the airway, rate, and depth of respirations as well as monitoring for the hemodynamic effects of sedative agents and the catheterization process itself. Children will have frequent vital signs initially that will include heart rate, rhythm, respiratory rate, oxygen saturation, blood pressure, and temperature. With each set of vital signs, distal perfusion to the effected extremity should be included.

Oxygen may be continued for a period of time after the procedure as the child recovers from the sedation or anesthesia. Once the child has been observed and is deemed stable, oxygen may be weaned off as long as oxygen saturations remain normal for the child.

The child will have activity restrictions upon discharge. They will typically need to miss a day or two of school while the leg site continues to heal. Depending on the procedure performed, they may be restricted from physical activities for several months after device closure of a septal defect.

 Nursing Diagnoses and Related Interventions

Nursing Diagnosis: Risk for bleeding related to lack of hemostasis at insertion site(s)

Outcome Evaluation: The child's dressing will remain clean, dry, and intact, and there will be no clinical symptoms of internal bleeding.

When a child returns from the procedure, assess the pressure dressing over the catheter insertion site to be certain the dressing is snug and intact and no bleeding is present. Assess the site frequently to verify that there is no bleeding. The entire surrounding area must also be assessed for internal bleeding that has accumulated in other tissue areas such as the genitalia. The child must remain supine for several hours if the femoral site was used to prevent bleeding or hematoma formation. This is particularly important when an artery was used for catheterization because a loose dressing on an artery can cause a large blood loss in a very short time. If there is bleeding at the insertion site, apply firm, continuous pressure and notify the provider who performed the procedure immediately.

Nursing Diagnosis: Risk for ineffective peripheral tissue perfusion related to thrombus formation at catheter insertion site

Outcome Evaluation: Child's vital signs remain within established parameters; pulse is palpable distal to catheter insertion site.

Thrombus formation at the femoral site is necessary for hemostasis but can also cause compromised flow distal to that site. Vasospasm of the arterial vessels can also occur, especially in smaller children. For this reason, distal pulses (pedal and posterior tibia) are checked routinely upon arrival from the catheterization lab if the femoral artery was accessed. If a pulse cannot be palpated, a Doppler should be used in an effort to find the pulse. If no pulses are found in the foot, popliteal pulses should be obtained. A provider should be notified immediately for any loss or change in pulses. The child will need to remain flat in bed for 2 to 4 hours (although some providers may require a longer period of time supine) in an effort to prevent bleeding from the site and obstruction of flow through the femoral vessel.

The child will typically be monitored for several hours but if pulses do not return within a certain time frame (approximately 4 hours), an anticoagulant such as heparin may be initiated. The heparin will prevent further thrombosis formation at the site of the vasospasm or current thrombus formation.

Nursing Diagnosis: Risk for infection related to presence of cardiac catheterization incision site

Outcome Evaluation: The child's temperature remains less than 100.4°F (38.0°C) tympanic; the catheter insertion site appears free of erythema or drainage.

If the dressing for a cardiac catheterization is over the femoral artery or vein in a non–toilet-trained child, be certain to keep it clean of stool and urine. If the dressing becomes soiled, the site should be cleaned well with soap and water.

Although there is a risk for infection at the catheter site after a catheterization, it will most likely be noted by the family once the child is home. Detailed education regarding the symptoms of an infection must be provided to the family and child (age-dependent) prior to discharge. They should omit tub baths or other water submersion such as pools or hot tubs until the site is completely healed to prevent infection. The child may receive a sponge bath or take a shower.

What If . . . 41.2

The nurse is caring for Cara, an 8-year-old otherwise healthy female who is scheduled for a cardiac catheterization to close an ASD. The nurse will also care for her after Cara's catheterization is complete. Why is it important for the nurse to assess Cara's baseline ECG and lower extremity pulses before her catheterization? What teaching points can the nurse review with Cara and her parents about her care after the catheterization is complete?

Cardiac Transplantation

Pediatric heart transplantation is uncommon but important and successful management technique for heart failure. Diagnoses leading to the need for a heart transplant vary with the age of the child. Congenital heart disease remains the most common indication for pediatric heart transplant in infants but as children age, cardiomyopathy becomes the more common indication. According to the registry of the International Society for Heart and Lung Transplantation, in 11- to 17-year-olds, the percentage of recipients with a diagnosis of CHD decrease to 23%, whereas the percentage of myopathy increases to 65% (Schweiger, Stiasny, Dave, et al., 2015).

The choice to pursue transplantation does not occur easily. Success is not guaranteed, and this choice requires a life-long commitment to ongoing medical evaluations, medications, and the probable need for future retransplantation. Candidates and their families will experience significant stressors in their lives that will impact the entire family structure. Given these impacts, healthcare professionals will continue to medically manage a patient with a failing heart as long as possible. If transplant is unavoidable, there are options to facilitate success as the child waits for a suitable organ. These include intensive care management with IV inotropic support, typically milrinone (Primacor). Ventricular assist devices (VADs) may be used as a bridge to transplant and offer long-term support. ECMO can offer a short-term bridge to transplant.

Outcomes after transplant vary, depending on many factors including age, donor heart, wait-list management, surgery, etc. Typically, infants survive for a longer period of time than older children. In the early stages, outcome is linked to operative mortality as well as graft (heart) function. Immediate rejection remains an important cause of mortality despite immunosuppressant agents. The use of immunosuppressants places the child at risk for infection with the greatest risk of death from an infection highest during the first year after transplant. Infection remains a significant source of mortality and morbidity in the long term.

Acute rejection continues to be a serious concern, accounting for 5% of deaths even 10 years posttransplant. Chronic graft failure is a main risk factor for death (26% more than 10 years posttransplant). There is also a risk of malignancy, specifically posttransplant lymphoproliferative disease which has a high association with Epstein-Barr virus.

Although pediatric heart transplant patients thrive and can have excellent long-term outcomes, there are many risks and challenges involved with this process that patients and families must understand.

Dysrhythmias

The overall incidence of clinically significant dysrhythmias in children without underlying congenital heart disease is low. A 2012 review at a single center pediatric emergency department (ED) found an incidence of 11.5 of 10,000 ED presentations were for a diagnosis of "arrhythmias" and supraventricular dysrhythmias were the most frequently identified rhythm disturbance (56% of all encounters). Of all children diagnosed with a dysrhythmia, 13% of these children had an underlying CHD (Clausen, Theophilos, Jackno, et al., 2012). This data demonstrates that outside of an ICU or postoperative setting, dysrhythmia incidence is low, and rhythm disturbances that are noted do not routinely require defibrillator use and have low mortality.

There are differences in the structure and function of the pediatric heart that predispose it to nonlethal dysrhythmias such as sinus bradycardia or sinus tachycardia, including:

- Greater parasympathetic innervation
- Deficiency of mitochondria
- Decreased amounts of actin and myosin
- Increased intracellular water content
- Myofibrils in less parallel array, not allowing for adequate contractility

The structural differences are greatest in the neonatal and infancy periods. Some conduction abnormalities are inherited and have a defined genetic component as seen with long QT syndrome or atrial flutter, others such as supraventricular tachycardia can occur randomly.

Figure 41.23 shows the normal conduction cycle. All electrical impulses in the heart originate from the sinoatrial (SA) node. These impulses travel down the right atrium and across the internodal tracts to the left atrium. The impulse on the right side terminates at the atrioventricular (AV) node where it slows to allow for complete filling of the ventricles. It then continues to the Bundle of His and down the right and left bundle branches, terminating in the Purkinje fibers, which ultimately cause ventricular contraction.

A usual ECG wave form consists of a P wave (denoting atrial contraction), a brief period of isoelectricity depicted as a flat line, and then a prominent QRS wave as the ventricles contract. This is followed by the T wave which is a result of

Figure 41.23 Normal conduction pathway. (From Jensen, S. [2015]. *Nursing health assessment: A best practice approach* [2nd ed.]. Philadelphia, PA: Wolters Kluwer.)

Figure 41.24 A normal ECG waveform. (From Shargel, L., Mutnick, A. H., Sourney, P. F., et al. [2013]. *Comprehensive pharmacy review for NAPLEX: Practice exams, cases, and test prep* [8th ed.]. Baltimore, MD: Lippincott Williams & Wilkins.)

ventricular repolarization (Fig. 41.24). Some children may have an incompletely understood additional slow wave (the U wave). A U-wave is considered normal in children.

A rhythm is considered sinus (originating from the SA node) if in Lead II there is an upright P wave before an upright QRS complex followed by a T wave immediately afterward.

SINUS ARRHYTHMIA

Sinus arrhythmia is a common occurrence in children and decreases with age. This is a normal variation in the child's heart rhythm based on their respiratory pattern. As they breathe in, you will notice the heart rate slow down and as they exhale, there is a slight increase in rate. This is thought to be due to changes in autonomic tone during respirations. The ECG pattern itself is completely normal. There is no need for concern, and there is no intervention.

SINUS BRADYCARDIA

Sinus bradycardia is defined as a heart rate that is less than the stated normal for a child's age. Sinus bradycardia may be physiologically normal as seen in athletes, may be secondary to medications such as beta-blockers, or may be an indicator of a pathologic state.

SINUS TACHYCARDIA

Sinus tachycardia is defined as a heart rate that is greater than the stated normal for a child's age. Sinus tachycardia may be expected as with a fever, anxiety, or pain may be secondary to medications such as albuterol or may be an indicator of a pathologic state such as dehydration, anemia, or infection.

SUPRAVENTRICULAR TACHYCARDIA

This is the most common symptomatic dysrhythmia in infants and children with a frequency of 1 in 250 to 1,000 patients and a peak incidence occurring in the first 2 months of life (Lewis, Arora, Tudorascu, et al., 2017). Supraventricular tachycardia (SVT) is defined as a heart rate greater than 220 beats/min in an infant and greater than 160 beats/min in a child (Fig. 41.25). The rhythm is a narrow complex with no discernible P waves and no variability in the rate with changes in the child's activity level (i.e., crying, playing, sleeping). If noted in infancy, it may regress by the time the child turns 1 year of age but then is likely to reappear later in childhood. It can be associated with a Wolff-Parkinson-White (WPW) reentry type pattern. In WPW, the patient has an extra connection in the heart called an accessory pathway that allows the electrical impulse to bypass the AV node and move from the atria to the ventricles faster than usual. WPW produces a specific pattern to the ECG and can be associated with an Ebstein's anomaly of the heart where the tricuspid valve is abnormal.

Assessment

If a child experiences an SVT event, their response will be dictated by their age. An infant may simply be irritable but, if it continues for hours without breaking, may not take oral feeds well or have changes in the level of consciousness. An older child may describe their heart as a "racing" or having a "pounding out of their chest" sensation. If the event lasts long enough (at least 20 to 30 minutes), older children may experience a light-headed sensation that may continue to a syncopal event. You will have a difficult time counting an apical or radial pulse rate as the heart rate is so high.

Management

Treatment for an SVT event may be nonpharmacologic or pharmacologic and may include long-term treatment options.

Noninvasive Treatment

Vagal maneuvers are a noninvasive means of increasing intrathoracic pressure for a brief period, thus stimulating baroreceptor activity in the aortic arch and carotid bodies, resulting in increased vagal tone. The goal is to block the reentry conduction and allow the normal conduction pathway to dominate. In infants, a bag of ice water can be placed on the forehead

Figure 41.25 Supraventricular tachycardia. (From Kyle, T., & Carman, S. [2016]. *Essentials of pediatric nursing* [3rd ed.]. Philadelphia, PA: Wolters Kluwer.)

at the nasal bridge in an effort to stimulate the diving reflex (diving reflex is a complex cardiovascular-respiratory response to immersion). Older children can be taught vagal maneuvers such as blowing through a pinched straw, bearing down as with a bowel movement, coughing, or gagging.

Antiarrhythmic Therapy

In a hospital setting, if none of these maneuvers is effective, management would proceed to either administration of adenosine (Adenocard) or the use of synchronized cardioversion. If the child is hemodynamically stable and they either have IV access or there is time to obtain it, adenosine is preferred. If the child is not hemodynamically stable, has lost consciousness, or IV access is not obtainable, then synchronized cardioversion should be used.

If adenosine is administered, it must be given rapidly by IV push, closest to the central circulation with a large flush of normal saline (NS) immediately after. Once adenosine is given, it has a very short half-life (6 to 10 seconds) and will block at the AV node to reestablish a normal conduction pattern. With the effect of the medication, you will note a brief period of asystole on the monitor. This is transient; the child will return to either SVT or sinus rhythm within seconds. You should ensure that there are ECG strips of the rhythm before, during, and after medication administration.

Long-Term Management

Long-term management of known SVT may include medications such as digoxin or a beta-blocker such as propranolol (Inderal). Of note, if the child has a WPW pattern associated with their SVT rhythm, digoxin cannot be used as it will slow AV node conduction which will accelerate conduction across the accessory pathway, placing the child at risk for atrial fibrillation. Verapamil, a calcium channel blocker, is contraindicated in children less than 1 year of age and can cause accessory pathway acceleration and is also not often used in WPW. Other medications that can be used if initial therapies fail are amiodarone, flecainide, and sotalol. Although these medications are antiarrhythmic in nature, they are also proarrhythmic and have other side effects. They should only be prescribed and managed by a pediatric cardiologist. If medications do not provide good coverage or the child is older, they may choose to pursue radiofrequency ablation in the electrophysiology laboratory as a more permanent solution.

Children with well-managed SVT, not associated with structural heart disease, do not have any activity restrictions other than to be aware of their dysrhythmia, and if they feel they are in SVT, they should stop their activity, rest, and attempt to stop the rhythm with vagal maneuvers as possible. If the dysrhythmia is associated with WPW syndrome, those children should be evaluated by a cardiologist for risk stratification before participating in competitive sporting activities. Children and families should also be advised to restrict the intake of products that may increase their heart rate such as caffeinated beverages and energy drinks. Herbal supplements should be avoided and families should contact a healthcare provider before giving their child over-the-counter cold medications as some can be contraindicated.

ATRIAL FLUTTER

This rhythm disturbance is more rare in children but can be seen after ASD surgery or with inflammatory states. It can also be genetically inherited. If a child presents with palpitations and atrial flutter is diagnosed, it must be determined if the rhythm has been present for greater than 24 hours. If so, an echocardiogram (frequently transesophageal) is performed to evaluate for the presence of thrombus in the atria. If they are noted, the child is started on an anticoagulant such as a heparin infusion. If there are no thrombus noted, or if it has been deemed safe to proceed with conversion, synchronized cardioversion will be used to break the rhythm.

Long-term therapy for this rhythm may include antiarrhythmics. Ablation or surgical correction through a Maze procedure may be pursued if the situation is severe.

LETHAL DYSRHYTHMIAS (VENTRICULAR TACHYCARDIA, VENTRICULAR FIBRILLATION, TORSADES DE POINTES)

Life-threatening dysrhythmias in children are rare. They may be seen after cardiac surgery or during a life-threatening event. Torsades de pointes is the terminal rhythm associated with long QT syndrome (LQTS). LQTS is a disorder of delayed ventricular repolarization characterized by prolongation of the QT interval. This may be hereditary or acquired due to medications.

Pulseless ventricular tachycardia and ventricular fibrillation are rare in children and are usually seen late in a child suffering cardiopulmonary arrest. Both are treated with defibrillation.

QSEN Checkpoint Question 41.4

INFORMATICS

Marcus is a 12-year-old boy who presents to the emergency department complaining of chest pain and a racing heart that started suddenly about 1 hour earlier. He says he feels a little tired and dizzy, but otherwise, he is appropriate for age. The nurse notices during the assessment that his heart rate is 185 beats/min, and the ECG demonstrates a very narrow complex with P waves that are not visible. The heart rate does not change when Marcus is talking or resting. His blood pressure is 95/70 mmHg, his respiratory rate is 22 breaths/min, and his oxygen saturation is 98% on room air. Based on this assessment and data, the nurse recognizes Marcus is experiencing which of the following?

a. Sinus tachycardia
b. Supraventricular tachycardia
c. Torsades de pointes
d. Ventricular tachycardia

Look in Appendix A for the best answer and rationale.

Acquired Heart Disease

Acquired heart disease is a term used to define heart disorders that develop after birth. Kawasaki disease is the leading cause of acquired heart disease in children.

KAWASAKI DISEASE

Kawasaki disease (mucocutaneous lymph node syndrome) is defined as an acute febrile syndrome associated with generalized **vasculitis** (inflammation of blood vessels) affecting all blood vessels throughout the body, including the coronary arteries. The vasculitis is a principal and life-threatening symptom because it can lead to the formation of coronary aneurysms which will predispose the child to thrombus formation and a high risk of myocardial infarction.

It has an unknown etiology. Although there does seem to be a genetic predisposition to the syndrome, there is also a strong suggestion of an infectious precursor. It occurs more commonly in winter and spring, with males affected more than females; 76% of children affected are less than 5 years old. It is more common among Americans of Asian or Pacific Island descent.

Kawasaki disease is a diagnosis of exclusion as there is no imaging or laboratory test that can diagnose it. Clinical criteria have been established to help with the diagnosis of Kawasaki disease.

Assessment

Kawasaki disease can be divided into an acute phase (week 1) and subacute phase (weeks 2 and 3). There are certain criteria that a child must meet for this diagnosis, including:

- Prolonged fever (>100.4°F [39°C]) of 5 or more days
- Four or more of the following symptoms:
  - Changes in hands and feet (erythema, edema, peeling)
  - Polymorphous exanthema (diffuse maculopapular rash of the trunk and extremities)
  - Bilateral conjunctivitis without exudates
  - Changes in lips and mouth (erythema, strawberry tongue, dry, cracked lips)
  - Cervical lymphadenopathy (>1.5 cm diameter, usually unilateral) (Box 41.6)

Changes in laboratory data may also be noted such as thrombocytosis, leukocytosis, elevated ESR and CRP, elevated liver enzymes, and mild anemia. The changes in these infectious and inflammatory markers mandate a thorough investigation into possible causes for the child's symptoms including viral infections, scarlet fever, staphylococcal scalded skin syndrome, juvenile rheumatoid arthritis, or Rocky Mountain spotted fever to name a few. If no definitive cause is determined and the child's symptoms fit the criteria listed, the child is given the diagnosis of Kawasaki disease.

During the acute phase, children are very irritable and uncomfortable from the fever and inflammatory process that causes joint pain. After approximately 10 days, a subacute phase begins. The skin desquamates, particularly on the palms and soles. The platelet count rises, increasing the possibility of clot formation. If an aneurysm forms in a coronary artery, accumulating thrombi can dislodge and lead to obstructed blood flow distally in the coronary artery which will lead to myocardial ischemia and infarction.

Therapeutic Management

Treatment for Kawasaki disease is focused on addressing the immediate symptoms and preventing any long-term consequences. Primarily, supportive measures are necessary as these children are irritable and not taking adequate oral intake so antipyretics for the fever as well as IV fluids are necessary. Kawasaki disease also causes dilation of the coronary arteries and coronary artery aneurysms in 15% to 25% of untreated children, and these coronary changes can be fatal. Evidence has shown that treating these children within the first 7 to 10 days of the fever with high-dose intravenous

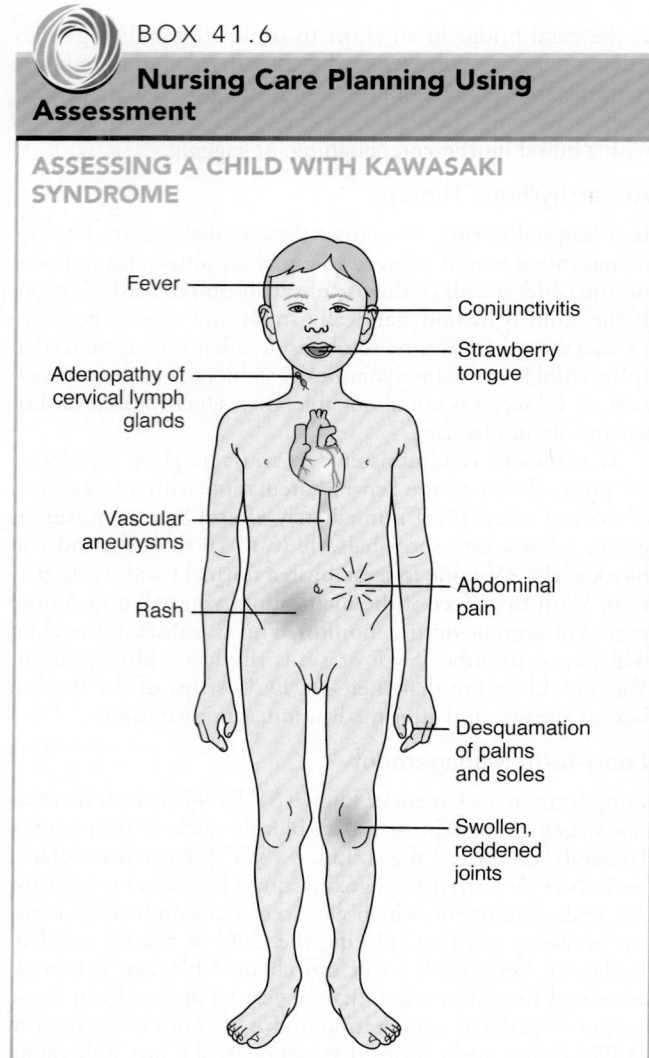

BOX 41.6

Nursing Care Planning Using Assessment

ASSESSING A CHILD WITH KAWASAKI SYNDROME

- Fever
- Conjunctivitis
- Strawberry tongue
- Adenopathy of cervical lymph glands
- Vascular aneurysms
- Abdominal pain
- Rash
- Desquamation of palms and soles
- Swollen, reddened joints

immunoglobulin (IVIG) and high-dose aspirin therapy has demonstrated a reduction in the appearance of coronary artery ectasia and aneurysms due to their anti-inflammatory properties. Children are treated with 2 g/kg of IVIG. This dose may be repeated if the fever does not break. High-dose aspirin at 80 to 100 mg/kg divided four times a day is also continued for 48 to 72 hours after the fever breaks. The aspirin is then continued at a low dose of 3 to 5 mg/kg/day once a day for 6 to 8 weeks with no evidence of coronary artery abnormalities. If abnormalities occur, aspirin may be continued indefinitely.

Nursing Diagnoses and Related Interventions

Nursing Diagnosis: Parental anxiety related to a lack of knowledge regarding Kawasaki disease

Outcome Evaluation: Parents will understand the course of this disease process and the necessary follow-up evaluations to assure their child's optimal health state.

Kawasaki disease is a frightening illness due to the danger of coronary artery aneurysm formation. Because they may never have heard of the illness before their child's diagnosis, parents need both information about and support throughout the lengthy disease process. An echocardiogram is performed at initial diagnosis to provide baseline coronary imaging, although coronary artery changes are not usually apparent at that time. Follow-up echocardiograms at 2 weeks and at 6 to 8 weeks are performed to continually evaluate for the development of any dilation or aneurysms. If there are no coronary changes at this time, it is unlikely that they will occur. It is important to explain this ongoing monitoring process to parents to help reduce parental anxiety.

Coronary images are difficult to obtain by echocardiogram, especially if the child is uncooperative. Children with Kawasaki disease are very uncomfortable and are frequently not cooperative with this test. Moderate sedation may be required to achieve accurate diagnostic imaging.

Nursing Diagnosis: Discomfort related to swelling of lymph nodes and inflammation of joints

Outcome Evaluation: Child states or demonstrates a tolerable level of discomfort, is able to participate in activities of daily living (ADLs), and maintains adequate oral intake.

A child with Kawasaki disease is uncomfortable from the joint involvement, edema, pruritic rash, and abdominal discomfort. The high fever can lead to dry, cracked lips. Antipyretics such as acetaminophen help reduce both the pain and fever. Providing additional comfort measures such as rocking and holding or distraction may help. Try to protect edematous areas from pressure; make certain clothing is not constricting and irritating areas of rash. Applying lip balm helps protect lips from drying and cracking.

Because the child's fever remains high, offer extra fluid to help maintain hydration and reduce mouth tenderness.

Children with Kawasaki disease lose their appetite and generally eat poorly because of the systemic illness, mouth soreness from cracks and fissures, and abdominal pressure from swollen lymph nodes. Carefully monitor and record the child's intake and output to be certain intake is adequate. Encourage the child to continue brushing his or her teeth (use a soft toothbrush or a commercial swab), even though the oral mucous membrane is tender, to prevent tooth decay or ulcer formation. Soft, nonirritating foods such as gelatin may be better tolerated than foods that require chewing or acidic fluids, such as orange juice, which might sting.

What If . . . 41.3

The nurse cares for Steven, a 3-year-old boy diagnosed with Kawasaki syndrome. He is irritable and continues to be febrile on day 2 of his admission. He is receiving 25 mg/kg of aspirin four times a day. His mother asks if she should be using aspirin to manage her other children when they have fevers at home. How would the nurse best respond to the mother's question?

RHEUMATIC FEVER

Although acute rheumatic fever has declined in incidence in Europe and North America over the past 50 years, it remains one of the most important causes of cardiovascular morbidity and mortality among socially and economically disadvantaged populations worldwide. Rheumatic fever is an autoimmune disease that occurs as a reaction to a group A β-hemolytic streptococcal infection, specifically, a pharyngitis. Inflammation from the immune response leads to inflammatory lesions being found in the heart, blood vessels, brain, and joints.

It occurs most often in children 6 to 15 years of age, with a peak incidence at 8 years. It has not been documented in infants, even those that have had a streptococcal infection. Because children do not develop immunity to streptococcal infections, they can recur. It is thought that in genetically susceptible individuals, the sensitized child will eventually have a group A β-hemolytic streptococcal pharyngitis that sets off an unusually high antibody response. Approximately 10 days after recovery from the pharyngitis, the autoimmune response begins, lasts many weeks and gradually damages the left heart valves.

Assessment

The signs and symptoms of rheumatic fever are divided into major and minor symptoms according to the Jones criteria which were recently revised in 2015 (Box 41.7). As noted, to have a diagnosis of rheumatic fever, children must have two major manifestations or one major and two minor manifestations documented. Of these, the heart involvement is the most serious.

Children will present with polyarthritis as multiple joints are inflamed and possibly have fluid accumulation. Fifty percent of the children present with carditis, usually as an apical systolic murmur from mitral insufficiency. This murmur is characteristically blowing and high frequency and transmits to the axilla. Sydenham chorea (sudden involuntary movement of the limbs) is a striking symptom that occurs in up to 10% of children and is exacerbated by stress. This loss of voluntary muscle control, which results in dysfunctional speech, facial grimacing, and poor hand control, occurs more often in younger children between 7 and 14 years of age.

Erythema marginatum, a macular rash found predominantly on the trunk is an infrequent symptom but if seen is a virtually definitive sign of rheumatic fever. Subcutaneous nodules on hard bony surfaces of the joints are noted during subsequent rheumatic fever attacks with well-established heart disease.

Important laboratory findings include the presence of an elevated antistreptolysin-O (ASO) titer which is evidence that the child had a recent streptococcal infection. The child will have a fever >38.5°C, and inflammatory markers such as ESR and CRP will also be elevated. ECG and CXR are not particularly helpful in diagnosing this disease. Echocardiogram is imperative to evaluate the extent of cardiac involvement. If a child meets the Jones diagnostic criteria and all other potential diagnoses have been ruled out, the child should be treated for rheumatic fever.

Therapeutic Management

If rheumatic fever diagnosis is entertained, penicillin therapy is immediately begun once throat cultures and blood work have been obtained. Therapeutic doses of intramuscular (IM)

BOX 41.7

Nursing Care Planning Using Assessment

ASSESSING A CHILD WITH RHEUMATIC FEVER

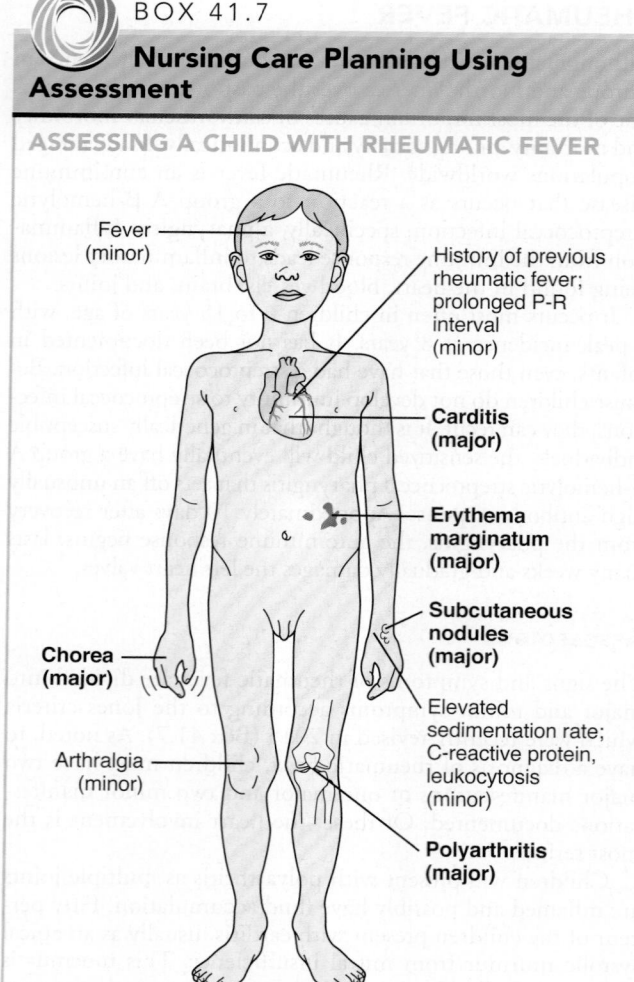

Fever (minor)

History of previous rheumatic fever; prolonged P-R interval (minor)

Carditis (major)

Erythema marginatum (major)

Subcutaneous nodules (major)

Chorea (major)

Elevated sedimentation rate; C-reactive protein, leukocytosis (minor)

Arthralgia (minor)

Polyarthritis (major)

Nursing Diagnosis: Risk for nonadherence to drug therapy related to knowledge deficit about importance of long-term therapy

Outcome Evaluation: Parents understand risk of recurrence; child takes oral penicillin daily or presents for monthly injections.

Preventive maintenance doses of penicillin are started once initial treatment is completed. These doses are given either as a monthly IM injection of penicillin G benzathine or twice-daily oral tablets of penicillin V potassium. Although the IM injection is more painful and necessitates a trip to the provider's office, it is considered more effective due to the potential lack of compliance with twice-daily oral medications. Preventive therapy continues until the child is at least 21 years of age as patients who have had acute rheumatic fever are highly susceptible to recurrent rheumatic fever. If the child incurred valve damage, preventive therapy will continue until at least 40 years of age.

CARDIOMYOPATHY

Cardiomyopathy is a disorder of the heart muscle and although rare, is a common cause of heart failure in children and the most common cause of heart transplantation in children older than 1 year of age (Wilkinson, Landy, Colan, et al., 2010). Most children have either a dilated or hypertrophic form of cardiomyopathy, although there are a variety of functional types. The estimated annual incidence of pediatric cardiomyopathy is 1.13 cases per 100,000 children aged 18 years or younger.

Based on data from the Pediatric Cardiomyopathy Registry, there is a higher incidence in boys than in girls and higher in Blacks than in Whites, and the annual incidence of dilated cardiomyopathy (DCM) and hypertrophic cardiomyopathy (HCM) was 0.58 cases per 100,000 children and 0.47 per 100,000 children, respectively. The following discussion will review dilated and HCM as well as arrhythmogenic right ventricular cardiomyopathy (ARVC), a form of cardiomyopathy that is the second most common cause of sudden cardiac death in young people after HCM (Romero, Mejia-Lopez, Manrique, et al., 2013; Soni & Oade, 2011).

Dilated Cardiomyopathy

DCM is defined as a severe disease of the heart muscle that is characterized by dilation of the left ventricle with reduced left ventricle systolic function and normal ventricular wall thickness. This is the most common cardiomyopathy noted in children, and its incidence is higher in the first year of life. Genetic causes of DCM account for 40% of cases with the remaining etiologies remaining largely unknown and considered idiopathic. Myocarditis is the most common, nongenetic, identifiable cause of DCM.

Children typically present with exercise intolerance, dyspnea on exertion, palpitations, chest pain, syncope, or possible cardiovascular collapse. Infants have more vague symptoms such as respiratory distress, poor feeding, or easy fatigability. Their physical examination may range from no significant changes except altered heart and respiratory rates to complete CHF with poor cardiac output. Cardiomegaly,

or oral penicillin are prescribed for a full 10-day course. Oral nonsteroidal anti-inflammatory agents may be prescribed to reduce inflammation and joint pain. The use of steroids is controversial and thought to be utilized only in children with severe carditis and valve damage. Phenobarbital and diazepam (Valium) are both effective in reducing the purposeless movements of chorea.

The prognosis for the child with rheumatic fever depends on the extent of myocardial involvement. Valve damage may continue over time, and some children with no initial presentation of valve damage will have it occur later in life. These children will be followed for life by a cardiologist and may require surgical intervention to repair or replace the valve.

Nursing Diagnoses and Related Interventions

Because rheumatic fever can be a severe threat to heart health, nursing diagnoses need to address both physical care and the parents' and child's reaction to the serious diagnosis.

pulmonary venous congestion, pulmonary edema, and pleural effusions may be noted on CXR. An ECG typically shows sinus tachycardia and other nonspecific changes. Echocardiogram will define the actual presence of a dilated ventricle with poor systolic function.

If no identifiable, treatable cause is found for the cardiomyopathy, treatment is supportive and nonspecific, aimed at controlling symptoms of CHF and ventricular dysfunction. This will include ACE inhibitors, beta-blockers, and inhibition of the renin–angiotensin system. If a child does not respond to supportive therapies and progressively declines, heart transplantation is an option with ECMO or VADs as a bridge if necessary.

In general, outcomes for a child diagnosed with DCM are quite varied. Recovery of function, if it will occur, will be within the first year. This will be approximately 50% of those that survive the initial presentation. In the remaining 50%, 25% will have improved but abnormal function, and 25% will have persistently severely depressed function. One- and 5-year rates of death or transplantation are 31% and 46%, respectively (Wilkinson et al., 2010).

Hypertrophic Cardiomyopathy

HCM is characterized by hypertrophy of the left ventricle, a nondilated left ventricle cavity, systolic hypercontractility, diastolic dysfunction, and, in approximately 20% of the cases, obstruction of left ventricle outflow secondary to mitral–septal contact during systole (hypertrophic obstructive cardiomyopathy). This is the most common cardiovascular disorder with an autosomal dominant genetic etiology and is the most common cause of sudden cardiac death in otherwise healthy children.

Patients typically present with limited exercise capacity as their primary symptom due to either dyspnea or chest pain. Infants will present with the typical congestive CHF clinical symptoms. Chest pain is also very common with HCM, occurring at rest or with activity. The coronary arteries have been reported to be abnormal with increased size of arteries, thickened walls, and narrowed lumens in a high percentage of children with familial HCM. Both atrial and ventricular arrhythmias are less frequent in children than in adults, and although thought to be the mechanism of sudden death in adults, this theory is not supported in children. Adolescents have the highest incidence of sudden death but are rarely found to have arrhythmias. Echocardiogram will confirm this diagnosis.

Management is aimed at reducing symptoms and prolonging survival. Beta-blocker therapy (i.e., metoprolol) is the primary pharmacologic agent used. Beta-blockers decrease the contractile force, the left ventricular outflow tract (LVOT) gradient, and the overall myocardial workload and oxygen demand. They also increase diastolic filling by slowing the heart rate and allowing for more passive filling of the left ventricle. This therapy relieves chest pain and dyspnea, but it does not improve exercise capacity. Calcium channel blockers, specifically verapamil, have a negative chronotropic effect which increases the diastolic relaxation time which increases preload and allows for symptomatic improvement. More definitive therapy such as pacemakers and surgical removal of any LVOT obstruction are patient dependent. The use of antiarrhythmics has not been effective in reducing arrhythmias associated with HCM.

Nursing Diagnoses and Related Interventions

Nursing Diagnosis: Risk for disturbed personal identity due to inability to participate in physical exercise

Outcome Measures: Child and family understand the importance of the exercise restrictions; child finds other activities that allow him or her to interact with peers.

Exercise restriction is necessary for children diagnosed with HCM. The incidence of sudden death is high in patients with HCM with one third of those deaths occurring during activity. Therefore, patients diagnosed with HCM through genetic testing or who have presented with clinical symptoms of HCM must abide by activity restrictions. They may not participate in highly aerobic activities or high school–level competitive sports. If the child does not manifest arrhythmias or exercise-induced arrhythmias, he or she may participate in mild to moderate types of exercise. Isometric activities such as weight lifting and rope climbing are prohibited because they are associated with high levels of circulating catecholamines that can predispose them to arrhythmias.

Restrictive Cardiomyopathy

Restrictive cardiomyopathy is characterized by restrictive filling and reduced diastolic volume of either or both ventricles with normal or near-normal systolic function and wall thickness. It may be idiopathic or associated with another disease process. This type of cardiomyopathy is fairly rare and accounts for only 2.5% to 5% of all diagnosed cardiomyopathies. The restrictive physiology results from increased myocardial stiffness with decreased compliance, causing a marked ventricular pressure increase with small changes in volume. This leads to poor cardiac output and ultimately symptoms of heart failure. Prognosis is poor with half of the children dying within 2 years of diagnosis.

Arrhythmogenic Right Ventricular Cardiomyopathy

ARVC is a rare inherited disease of the heart that causes ventricular tachyarrhythmias and sudden death in young people and athletes. It results in fibro-fatty replacement of the right ventricle and the subepicardial region of the left ventricle. Ultimately, certain cardiac proteins are defective and cannot keep the myocytes together when under stress such as with exercise. As the damaged and dead cells get replaced with fatty and fibrous tissue, the electrical system is impaired and ventricular dysrhythmias result.

ARVC presentation can be variable from palpitations and syncope to sudden cardiac arrest occurring during exercise. Any clinical symptom such as chest pain, palpitations, or syncope that occurs during exercise should always be noted as a red flag and further evaluated. Diagnosis of ARVC is made through patient and family history, 12-lead ECG evaluation, and an echocardiogram. Unfortunately, there is no treatment for this disorder, only management through restriction of physical exercise, antiarrhythmic drugs, beta-blocker therapy, and an implantable cardioverter defibrillator (ICD).

INFLAMMATORY PROCESSES

Inflammatory processes that impact the heart can be secondary to an infectious process (viral or bacterial) but can also be due to toxins, hypersensitivity reactions, systemic disorders, trauma, or be idiopathic. This inflammation can affect any layer of the heart, and presentation, management and outcomes vary with each form.

Myocarditis

Myocarditis is an acute or chronic inflammatory process affecting the myocardium. Specifically, there is an inflammation of the myocardium with necrosis or degeneration of adjacent myocytes. This disease can be caused by a wide variety of toxins, drugs, or infectious agents, most commonly viral agents such as coxsackievirus, adenovirus, or parvovirus. It is rare for a child to be diagnosed with myocarditis during the initial infectious event. The next phase is an acute phase where there is extensive interstitial inflammation and injury with direct myocardial damage. This appears to be initiated by an autoimmunity triggered by the initial injury. At this time, the patient presents with overt symptoms of CHF, but the presence of an actual infection is rare. Although the acute inflammatory phase may resolve, there is a third, chronic phase that is mediated by T cells. During this phase, fibroblasts replace normal myofibers with resultant scar tissue formation. This creates an electrically unstable myocardium, predisposed to the development of ventricular tachydysrhythmias.

Diagnosis of myocarditis is difficult with only clinical data. Patient presentation such as chest pain, exertional dyspnea, fatigue, syncope, or palpitations in association with acute CHF associated with left ventricle dilation and/or segmental wall abnormalities may indicate a possible myocarditis diagnosis. If suspected, an endomyocardial biopsy may be performed in an effort to provide a definitive diagnosis, but this is not completely accurate either. More recently, cardiovascular MRI has emerged as an important noninvasive tool for the diagnosis and monitoring of myocarditis. In addition to providing reliable measurements of ventricular size and function, MRI myocardial tissue characterization techniques can assess for inflammatory changes such as edema, hyperemia, capillary leak, and myocyte necrosis (Banka, Robinson, Uppu, et al., 2015).

Management of myocarditis is symptomatic, typically following heart failure management protocols. The use of steroids or immunosuppressants is not well established in the literature for global treatment of myocarditis but has been shown to be beneficial with certain types of myocarditis. For fulminant myocarditis that does not improve with pharmacologic therapy, the use of mechanical circulatory support devices (i.e., VAD or ECMO) may be necessary as a bridge to transplant or recovery.

Pericarditis

Acute pericarditis is an inflammation of the pericardial membrane with or without accumulation of excess pericardial fluid. There are a multitude of potential causes, but most are idiopathic and thought to be viral or postviral in origin. Idiopathic pericarditis accounts for 37% to 68% of inpatient admissions for pericardial effusions or acute pericarditis in children. Presentation frequently includes chest pain which can be sharp, precordial, radiating, and worse with inspiration or cough. It is characteristically positional, and patients feel better when sitting up and leaning forward. Fever is also common. Physical examination reveals an uncomfortable child, typically with a pericardial friction rub. A pericardial friction rub is a superficial scratchy or squeaking sound that is best heard with the diaphragm of the stethoscope. The rub may be localized or widespread but is usually loudest over the left sternal border.

Diagnosis of pericarditis may begin with a 12-lead ECG and CXR. The CXR may be normal if there is not an appreciable effusion. An echocardiogram may be normal but typically shows at least a small collection of pericardial fluid. Laboratory analysis will only note an infectious process and not be specific to pericarditis. If the effusion is large or there appears to be restricted myocardial contractility, a pericardiocentesis must be performed. This fluid may be sent for cultures to further investigate for causative organism or malignancy.

Treatment of pericarditis involves anti-inflammatory agents such as ibuprofen to relieve symptoms and accelerate resolution. Corticosteroids may be used if nonsteroidal anti-inflammatory drugs (NSAIDs) are not successful. Colchicine use has been reported in children to treat refractory pericarditis. Pericarditis can recur. Recurrences develop in up to 36% of children after the first episode of idiopathic acute pericarditis and in 50% of children after pericardial injury that would occur with certain cardiac surgeries such as repair of an ASD. Relapses may occur up to 2 months after the injury. Treatment remains the same and should follow a stepwise approach.

QSEN Checkpoint Question 41.5

TEAMWORK & COLLABORATION

The nurse is caring for James, a 2-year-old boy who has been admitted to the pediatric floor after his parents noted a fever of 103°F (39.4°C) for 2 days. He had an ASD repaired approximately 4 weeks earlier and has since developed a pericardial effusion. The effusion was drained, and the fluid was purulent. He is now being treated with IV antibiotics. The nurse enters the room and notes that James is only breathing about 5 breaths/min and his heart rate on the monitor is 40 beats/min. What is the nurse's first action?

a. Call for help and wait for direction when the arrest team arrives.

b. Run from the room and get the defibrillator, calling for help as you go.

c. Call the pediatric cardiologist to perform an echocardiogram and evaluate for reaccumulation of the pericardial fluid.

d. Call for help and begin providing compressions per basic life support (BLS) protocol (CPR).

Look in Appendix A for the best answer and rationale.

Infective Endocarditis

Infective endocarditis is inflammation and infection of the endocardium or valves of the heart. It is noted in children with and without heart disease. The incidence of infective endocarditis in children is rare but may be increasing due to the increased survival of children with congenital heart disease. The high-velocity blood stream of some defects creates forces thought to damage the endothelium. Indwelling catheters such as peripherally inserted central catheters (PICCs) similarly may injure the endocardial or endothelial layer allowing for the deposition of red blood cells, platelets, and fibrin. Bacteria then can adhere to the damaged endothelial layer, with further fibrin and platelet deposition trapping the bacteria in the evolving vegetation. This results in localized endocardial injury and valvulitis.

The infection is generally caused by *Streptococcus viridans* and *Staphylococcus aureus*, although fungal organisms have also been noted.

Assessment

Presentation can be acute or subacute. Acute presentation includes a systemic response to the infection and can be rapidly progressive. Children have high-spiking fevers and are severely ill and toxic in appearance. Symptoms of CHF may be present. Murmurs are frequently noted due to destruction of the cardiac valve tissue.

Subacute presentation is associated with persistent low-grade fever, malaise, weight loss, arthralgias, fatigue, rigors, and diaphoresis.

Diagnostic testing will include laboratory analysis and imaging studies. Positive blood cultures are necessary for a diagnosis of infective endocarditis. Echocardiogram is extremely helpful in allowing for visualization of the vegetations as well as the damage to the heart itself such as valve destruction and perforation, rupture of chordae, and development of valvar leaks. Other laboratory studies will reveal proteinuria or hematuria, a normochromic, leukocytosis, and an increased ESR.

Treatment

Treatment is aimed at the underlying bacterial infection but an extended course of antibiotics is necessary as the organisms are imbedded in a fibrin platelet matrix in high concentrations. Once sensitivity is determined, treatment is typically for 4 to 6 weeks of IV therapy. This will necessitate the insertion of a PICC in children so they may go home and receive home nursing services to administer their antibiotic therapy. Lesions will heal, but children may be left with long-term sequelae such as renal dysfunction from thrombi or leaky cardiac valves from primary damage.

All children diagnosed with endocarditis must receive prophylactic antibiotics prior to some invasive procedures including dental work. The 2007 recommendations from the AHA state prophylaxis prior to dental work for children with underlying cardiac disease is appropriate only if the child has:

- Prosthetic cardiac valve or prosthetic material used for cardiac valve repair
- Previous infective endocarditis
- Congenital heart disease, specifically:
  - Unrepaired cyanotic CHD, including palliative shunts and conduits
  - Completely repaired CHD with prosthetic material or device, whether placed by surgery or by catheter intervention, during the first 6 months after the procedure
  - Repaired CHD with residual defects at the site or adjacent to the site of a prosthetic patch or prosthetic device (which inhibit endothelialization)
- Cardiac transplantation recipients who develop cardiac valvulopathy

Preventive Heart Disease

Although much of the heart disease previously discussed cannot be prevented, there is a great deal that can be done to help children avert the development of cardiovascular heart disease in adulthood, typically related to hypertension or atherosclerosis. Hypertension in children is rising and is thought to be connected to the increasing numbers of children who are overweight or obese. Healthcare professionals must take on the responsibility of providing heart-healthy guidance at all encounters with children and their families to ensure these children lead long, healthy lives.

HYPERTENSION

High blood pressure in children is a growing health problem in the United States. If a child presents with hypertension, it is important to differentiate primary from secondary. Evaluating for an underlying etiology includes a thorough medical and family history and a physical examination. Diagnostic testing may be ordered based on the results of the history and physical exam. Common causes of hypertension in children can be renal (renal artery stenosis, renovascular disease, neurofibromatosis), hormonal (primary aldosteronism, adrenal insufficiency, pheochromocytoma, neuroblastoma) or cardiac (CoAo).

Management of secondary hypertension will be focused on the underlying disorder.

Assessment

Hypertension can begin in childhood and contributes to the early development of cardiovascular disease. When evaluating children for or with hypertension, it is important to follow published guidelines. Blood pressure percentile tables in the United States have been developed and are based on gender, age, and height and distributed by the National Heart, Lung, and Blood Institute (NHLBI). It is important to evaluate both the systolic and diastolic values. There are three categories (Table 41.3):

- Normal
- Prehypertension
- Hypertension (including Stage 1 and Stage 2).

TABLE 41.3 NATIONAL HIGH BLOOD PRESSURE EDUCATION PROGRAM CLASSIFICATION OF PREHYPERTENSION AND HYPERTENSION IN CHILDREN AND ADOLESCENTS

Classification	Systolic or Diastolic Blood Pressure*
Normal	<90th percentile for both values
Prehypertension	≥90th percentile or if BP >120/80**
Hypertension	≥95th percentile
Hypertension— Stage 1	Between 95th percentile and 5 mmHg above 99th
Stage 2	≥99th percentile plus 5 mmHg

BP, blood pressure.

*Based on age, gender, and height. Must be measured with correct size cuff on three separate occasions.

**If the blood pressure reads greater than 120/80 mmHg, a diagnosis of prehypertension is given, regardless of whether it is less than 90th percentile for age/gender/height.

When measuring blood pressure in children, it is important to use the correct size blood pressure cuff. The cuff should cover approximately 40% of the child's upper arm and the length of the cuff must completely cover the circumference of the arm. If a cuff is too small, it may result in a falsely elevated reading. Although a too large cuff may provide a reading that is lower, a larger cuff should be chosen if the child is in-between sizes. Blood pressure should be measured in the right arm with the child's arm supported at heart level. If an automatic blood pressure device is used and the reading is elevated, the measurement should be repeated with a manual cuff and auscultation. A diagnosis of hypertension cannot be given to a child unless the blood pressure reading is elevated on three separate readings at three different visits. Providers ask the school systems to help with blood pressure measurements to avoid the stress of going to a provider's office, which can cause a false increase in blood pressure readings.

Therapeutic Management

If there is no indication of a secondary etiology to the hypertension, the child must be managed for primary hypertension. Primary hypertension is associated with overweight or a positive family history of hypertension. Recent data also suggests an association between sleep disordered breathing and hypertension. Management of children with prehypertension or hypertension includes therapeutic lifestyle changes. These include weight reduction if necessary, regular physical activity, a healthy diet, and healthy habits including no smoking or alcohol. Family-based interventions have been shown to improve success rates. High blood pressure in childhood commonly leads to hypertension in adulthood, and adult hypertension is the leading cause of premature death around the world (Riley & Bluhm, 2012).

In adolescents, increasing the amount of sleep may also be helpful in reducing stress and development of hypertension. Adolescent girls are advised to use another reproductive life planning choice than estrogen-based oral contraceptives because these can elevate blood pressure (Narang, Manlhiot, Davies-Shaw, et al., 2012). Unfortunately, because mild hypertension produces few symptoms, often children and their family members do not adhere to nutritional suggestions or recommended exercise programs so their hypertension does not decrease.

If hypertension persists despite these interventions, antihypertensive medications may be warranted. There are multiple medications that can be used including ACE inhibitors, ARBs, beta-blockers, calcium channel blockers, diuretics, and vasodilators. It is imperative for the nurse to understand the side effects of the chosen medications when evaluating and managing these patients.

QSEN Checkpoint Question 41.6

PATIENT-CENTERED CARE

Charlene is a 15-year-old female with a family history of hypertension. She is overweight and is being evaluated because she has had four separate blood pressure readings that are higher than 95% for her gender, age, and height. Her mother is with her and wants to know what she can do to get her daughter's blood pressure down. Which response by the nurse is best?
a. Explain to Charlene's mother that the high blood pressure is genetic and her daughter can only take medications to treat the problem.
b. Tell her mother that Charlene should decrease her salt intake.
c. Discuss with Charlene and her mother heart-healthy changes such as increasing her activity level, increasing her vegetable intake, and decreasing her sodium intake.
d. Develop an exercise plan and review it with Charlene's mother to implement with her daughter in the coming months.

Look in Appendix A for the best answer and rationale.

DYSLIPIDEMIA

Atherosclerotic cardiovascular disease remains the leading cause of death in North Americans, but it is rare to see this disease in children or adolescents. Risk factors and risk behaviors that accelerate the development of atherosclerosis begin in childhood and evidence suggests that decreasing risk factors will delay progression toward clinical disease (Expert Panel on Integrated Guidelines for Cardiovascular Health and Risk Reduction in Children and Adolescents, 2011). It is important that all pediatric healthcare providers understand the risks that predispose to early atherosclerotic heart disease and the recommendations for monitoring and treating children of all ages.

The NHLBI published guidelines on reducing cardiovascular disease in children and adolescents in 2011 (Expert Panel on Integrated Guidelines for Cardiovascular Health and Risk Reduction in Children and Adolescents, 2011). These guidelines have been endorsed by the American Academy of Pediatrics. They recommend universal lipid screening once between the ages of 9 and 11 years and again between 17 and 21 years. For children with a family history of dyslipidemia or atherosclerotic disease less than 55 years of age (male) or less than 65 years of age (female), it is recommended that children be screened twice between 2 and 8 years of age with the results averaged. This testing is also recommended if the child has diabetes, hypertension, or a BMI greater than 95th percentile.

Management for children with elevated lipid or cholesterol levels initially focuses on dietary and lifestyle changes. There are recommendations for an initial specific diet that focuses on a low-fat/low–saturated fat/low-cholesterol diet. This is termed the *Cardiovascular Health Integrated Lifestyle Diet* (CHILD-1); details on this diet can be found in the NHLBI guidelines and its implementation should be guided by a registered dietitian if possible. Increased activity for obese children is also among the initial recommendations. Younger children are not placed on low-fat diets because they need calories for growth. Infants younger than 2 years of age need fat for myelinization of nerve tissue so they must continue with whole fat milk.

If no change is noted on a fasting lipid profile after a 3-month trial, then a more restrictive diet (CHILD-2) may be used. If after another 3 months, no changes are noted and if the child is 10 years of age or older, a statin medication may be prescribed.

Children taking a statin should have routine clinical monitoring for symptoms of muscle toxicity and assessment of hepatic transaminases and CK.

Because hypercholesterolemia has no symptoms, it is difficult to motivate children to continue a special diet and take medication unless the entire family changes to a lower fat diet and exercises more. Children need continued counseling at healthcare visits so they understand the damage that excess lipids can cause to coronary arteries (Lipshultz, Schaechter, Carillo, et al., 2012).

OVERWEIGHT CHILDREN AND OBESITY

One in three children in the United States is overweight or obese, which results in physical and psychological comorbidities that often persist into adulthood (National Association of Pediatric Nurse Practitioners [NAPNAP], 2015). It is a multifactorial condition with lifelong physical, emotional, social, and economic implications. Obesity is defined as a BMI at or above the 95th percentile, being overweight is ≥85th percentile BMI. Over the past 30 years, the prevalence of obesity has nearly tripled for children 2 to 5 years of age and 12 to 19 years of age and quadrupled for children 6 to 11 years old. The increasing prevalence and severity rates have resulted in a higher prevalence of hypertension, type 2 diabetes mellitus, and the development of atherosclerosis (Daniels, Jacobson, McCrindle, et al., 2009). Nurses must use every opportunity to provide education for children and their families by encouraging them to choose healthy lifestyle behaviors such as:

• Consuming low-fat diets
• Eliminating sweetened beverages and other sugary foods
• Increasing physical activity
• Decreasing screen time

It is important for these behaviors to be implemented by the entire family. It is also important to note that restricting calories is not a first-line management choice for children because they have significant metabolic needs as they grow. Childhood obesity and its risk factors must be addressed early to prevent premature cardiovascular disease in adulthood.

What If . . . 41.4

The nurse is particularly interested in exploring one of the 2020 National Health Goals related to achieving cardiovascular health in childhood (see Box 41.1). The nurse identifies which possible research topic to explore pertinent to this goal that would be applicable to Megan's family and also advance evidence-based practice? (Megan is the newborn with Down syndrome and an atrioventricular septal defect that will be surgically repaired.)

KEY POINTS FOR REVIEW

■ Cardiovascular disorders in children may be either structural, such as congenital heart disease, or acquired, such as Kawasaki syndrome, rheumatic fever, or cardiomyopathy. Assessment of children with heart disease includes history and physical examination. Echocardiogram, MRI, and cardiac catheterization are procedures used frequently to aid with diagnosis and management.

■ Congenital heart disorders are classified as those associated with increased pulmonary blood flow, decreased pulmonary blood flow, and obstruction to blood flow. Single-ventricle defects are classified separately due to their complex anatomy and physiology.

■ Common signs of CHF seen in children include tachycardia, tachypnea, enlarged liver, dyspnea, and poor weight gain. Signs tend to be subtle in infants and may be manifested chiefly by difficulties with feeding and gaining weight due to increased caloric consumption due to tachypnea and increased work of breathing.

■ Cardiac catheterization and surgery both offer palliative and corrective options for children born with congenital heart disease. Catheterization also can provide diagnostic information to ensure optimal management of heart disease.

■ The families of children undergoing cardiac surgery need a great deal of support from healthcare personnel so they can cope with this major event and provide effective support to their child and other family members.

■ SVT is the most common dysrhythmia in children, can be well tolerated, and does not typically cause any activity restrictions. If the SVT is associated with WPW, a cardiologist should perform risk stratification before the child participates in competitive sports. Many dysrhythmias can be addressed with an electrophysiologic study and ablation later in childhood if necessary.

■ Kawasaki syndrome is a diagnosis of exclusion. If diagnosed, it is imperative that the child receive IV immunoglobulin and high-dose aspirin therapy within 10 days of fever in an effort to prevent coronary artery aneurysms.

■ Hypertension in children usually occurs as a result of a secondary disorder. Helping families limit saturated fat intake and follow a consistent exercise program to help children avoid obesity and heart disease in later life is a strategy that not only meets QSEN competencies but also best meets the family's total needs.

CRITICAL THINKING CARE STUDY

Dwight is a full-term, first-born child and is 2 hours old. His respiratory rate is 68 breaths/min, and his oxygen saturation is 82%. He has a heart rate of 160 beats/min with mild cyanosis around his mouth. An echocardiogram indicates that Dwight has been born with transposition of the great arteries. Dwight's parents did not have consistent prenatal care due to transportation problems.

1. Dwight's father is concerned because he realizes a prenatal sonogram might have revealed his son's heart disorder during the pregnancy. He asks you whether he and his wife are at fault for their child being born with this heart disorder. Could they have prevented this with more routine prenatal care? How should you respond?

2. You are preparing to start a prostaglandin E1 infusion for Dwight. How would you explain to the father the purpose of this infusion?

3. Dwight's father tells you he is worried his health insurance will not cover the two surgeries described by the cardiac surgeon. "Is he trying to make money off of us?" he asks you. "Are two procedures really necessary?" How should you respond?

REFERENCES

Banka, P., Robinson, J. D., Uppu, S. C., et al. (2015). Cardiovascular magnetic resonance techniques and findings in children with myocarditis: A multicenter retrospective study. *Journal of Cardiovascular Magnetic Resonance, 17*, 96.

Clausen, H., Theophilos, T., Jackno, K., et al. (2012). Paediatric arrhythmias in the emergency department. *Emergency Medicine Journal, 29*(9), 732–737.

Daniels, S. R., Jacobson, M. S., McCrindle, B. W., et al. (2009). American Heart Association childhood obesity research summit: Executive summary. *Circulation, 119*, 2114–2123.

Darst, J. R., Collins, K. K., & Miyamoto, S. D. (2012). Cardiovascular diseases. In W. Hay, M. Levin, R. Deterding, et al. (Eds.), *Current diagnosis & treatment pediatrics* (21st ed., pp. 561–622). New York, NY: McGraw-Hill/Lange.

Drakouli, M., Petsios, K., Giannakopoulou, M., et al. (2015). Determinants of quality of life in children and adolescents with CHD: A systematic review. *Cardiology in the Young, 25*(6), 1027–1036.

Expert Panel on Integrated Guidelines for Cardiovascular Health and Risk Reduction in Children and Adolescents. (2011). Expert Panel on Integrated Guidelines for Cardiovascular Health and Risk Reduction in Children and Adolescents: Summary report. *Pediatrics, 128*(Suppl. 5), S213–S256.

Forbess, J. M., Visconti, K. J., Hancock-Friesen, C., et al. (2002). Neurodevelopmental outcome after congenital heart surgery: Results from an institutional registry. *Circulation, 106*(12 Suppl. 1), I95–I102.

Kett, J. C. (2012). Anemia in infancy. *Pediatrics in Review, 33*(4), 186–187.

Kucik, J. E., Shin, M., Siffel, C., et al. (2013). Trends in survival among children with Down syndrome in 10 regions of the United States. *Pediatrics, 131*(1), e27–e36.

Latal, B. (2016). Neurodevelopmental outcomes of the child with congenital heart disease. *Clinics in Perinatology, 43*(1), 173–185.

Lewis, J., Arora, G., Tudorascu, D. L., et al. (2017). Acute management of refractory and unstable pediatric supraventricular tachycardia. *The Journal of Pediatrics, 181*, 177–182.

Lipshultz, S. E., Schaechter, J., Carillo, A., et al. (2012). Can the consequences of universal cholesterol screening during childhood prevent cardiovascular disease and thus reduce long-term health care costs? *Pediatric Endocrinology Review, 9*(4), 698–705.

Narang, I., Manlhiot, C., Davies-Shaw, J., et al. (2012). Sleep disturbance and cardiovascular risk in adolescents. *Canadian Medical Association Journal, 184*(17), E913–E920.

National Association of Pediatric Nurse Practitioners. (2015). Position statement on the prevention and identification of overweight and obesity in the pediatric population. *Journal of Pediatric Healthcare, 29*, 13A–15A.

Riley, M., & Bluhm, B. (2012). High blood pressure in children and adolescents. *American Family Physician, 85*(7), 693–700.

Ringle, M. L., & Wernovsky, G. (2016). Functional, quality of life and neurodevelopmental outcomes after congenital cardiac heart surgery. *Seminars in Perinatology, 40*(8), 556–570.

Romero, J., Mejia-Lopez, E., Manrique, C., et al. (2013). Arrhythmogenic right ventricular cardiomyopathy (ARVC/D): A systematic literature review. *Clinical Medicine Insights. Cardiology, 7*, 97–114.

Schipper, M., Slieker, M. G., Schoof, P. H., et al. (2017). Surgical repair of ventricular septal defect: Contemporary results and risk factors for a complicated course. *Pediatric Cardiology, 38*, 264–270.

Schweiger, M., Stiasny, B., Dave, H., et al. (2015). Pediatric heart transplantation. *Journal of Thoracic Disease, 7*(3), 552–559.

Soni, R., & Oade, Y. (2011). Arrhythmogenic right ventricular cardiomyopathy. *BMJ Case Reports, 2011*, bcr0520114242.

U.S. Department of Health and Human Services. (2010). *Healthy people 2020*. Washington, DC: Author.

Wilkinson, J. D., Landy, D. C., Colan, S. D., et al. (2010). The pediatric cardiomyopathy registry and heart failure: Key results from the first 15 years. *Heart Failure Clinics, 6*(4), 401–413.

Xiu-Yu, S., Jia-Yu, H., Qiang, H., et al. (2010). Platelet count and erythrocyte sedimentation rate are good predictors of Kawasaki disease: ROC analysis. *Journal of Clinical Laboratory Analysis, 24*(6), 385–388.

42

Nursing Care of a Family When a Child Has an Immune Disorder

*D*exter Goodenough is a 6-year-old boy you meet in an ambulatory clinic. He had atopic dermatitis (infantile eczema) as an infant. Today, his eyes look red and are watering; his nose is draining a clear discharge. His mother tells you he is constantly listless, and other children have started to bully him because of his appearance and the fact he has a peanut allergy. His grades are "terrible" because his rhinitis symptoms begin the minute he gets to school. Dexter is diagnosed as having allergic rhinitis. His mother responds, "Are you sure it's just another allergy? He has a cold all of the time. I think there is something wrong with his immune system."

Previous chapters described normal growth and development of children. This chapter adds information about the dramatic changes, both physical and psychosocial, that can occur when a child is born with or develops a disorder of the immune system.

In light of the effect this condition is having on Dexter's life, is this "just" an allergy? What additional information would you want his mother to know about his condition? Knowing his problem is worse at school, what environmental control measures would you want to suggest for Dexter?

KEY TERMS

allergen
anaphylaxis
antigen
atopic dermatitis
autoimmunity
cell-mediated immunity
chemotaxis
complement

cytotoxic response
delayed hypersensitivity
environmental control
humoral immunity
hypersensitivity response
hyposensitization
immune response

immunity
immunogen
immunoglobulins
lymphokines
lysis
macrophages
phagocytosis
tolerance

OBJECTIVES

After mastering the contents of this chapter, you should be able to:

1. Describe the effects of an underactive or overactive immune response as it relates to childhood illnesses.
2. Identify the 2020 National Health Goals that nurses can help the nation achieve as related to immune disorders.
3. Assess a child with a disorder of the immune system.
4. Formulate nursing diagnoses for a child with a disorder of the immune system.
5. Establish outcomes for a child with a disorder of the immune system that can help the family manage seamless transitions across different healthcare settings.
6. Using the nursing process, plan nursing care that includes the six competencies of Quality & Safety Education for Nurses (QSEN): Patient-Centered Care, Teamwork & Collaboration, Evidence-Based Practice (EBP), Quality Improvement (QI), Safety, and Informatics.
7. Implement nursing care for a child with an immune disorder.
8. Evaluate expected outcomes for achievement and effectiveness of care.
9. Integrate knowledge of immune disorders with the interplay of nursing process, the six competencies of QSEN, and Family Nursing to promote quality maternal and child health nursing care.

The immune system is made up of a variety of proteins and cell types, which work together to protect the body against invasion by foreign substances. The study of the immune system is a growing field as more diseases and genetic mutations are identified, making it important to have an understanding of how the immune system works in health and disease in order to provide safe nursing care (Hellmann & Imboden, 2013).

Disorders of the immune system can be the result of an underactive or nonfunctional system (immunodeficiency), an overactive or poorly regulated system (allergy or hypersensitivity), or an abnormal or excessive response against one's own cells (autoimmune disease). Immunodeficiencies and allergic disorders are described in this chapter. Autoimmune disorders include a wide range of diseases and often affect a particular body system. These are described in the chapter that discusses the affected system (e.g., juvenile arthritis, which affects the joints, is discussed in Chapter 51). The 2020 National Health Goals related to immune disorders and children are shown in Box 42.1.

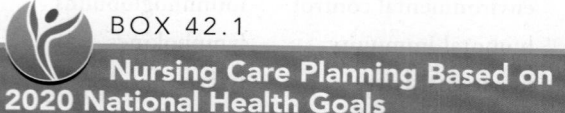

BOX 42.1

Nursing Care Planning Based on 2020 National Health Goals

Allergies affect at least 25% of the population; therefore, efforts to reduce them are reflected in several 2020 National Health Goals:

- Reduce indoor allergen levels such as cockroach allergens in settled dust from a baseline of 0.51 units to 0.46 units.
- Increase the proportion of the nation's elementary, middle, and high schools that have an indoor air quality management program to promote a healthy and safe physical school environment from a baseline of 51.4% to a target level of 56.5%.
- Reduce new cases of perinatally acquired AIDS from a baseline of 28 cases yearly to 25 new cases yearly.
- Reduce new AIDS cases among adolescents and adults from a baseline of 14.4 new cases per 100,000 to a target level of 13.0 new cases per 100,000.
- Increase the proportion of sexually active unmarried females aged 15 to 44 years who use condoms from a baseline of 34.5% to a target level of 38% (U.S. Department of Health and Human Services, 2010; see www.healthypeople.gov).

Nurses can help the nation achieve these goals by advocating for improved air quality in schools and initiating educational programs for children and adolescents that includes teaching about the way HIV is transmitted (sexual relations and unclean intravenous needles) and protective measures they can take to avoid contracting the disease (using safer sex practices and not using intravenous drugs).

Nursing Process Overview

FOR A CHILD WITH AN IMMUNE DISORDER

ASSESSMENT

The purpose of the immune system is to provide protection to the body from invading organisms or antigens. A deficiency in any of the components of the immune system or alteration in function can limit this protection. An assessment focuses on the types of illnesses or problems the child is having in order to target the part of the immune system which is mal- or nonfunctioning. A thorough history and analysis of presenting symptoms is the best way to identify the problem and to develop appropriate interventions.

NURSING DIAGNOSES

Examples of nursing diagnoses associated with immune disorders include:

- Risk for infection related to altered immune response
- Impaired skin integrity and risk for infection related to atopy
- Activity intolerance related to chronic illness
- Risk for delayed or altered growth and development related to chronicity of immune disorder

Nursing diagnoses specific to the child with allergies focus on the specific symptom. Examples include:

- Situational low self-esteem related to symptoms of contact dermatitis or atopy
- Ineffective breathing pattern related to bronchospasm of allergic response or anaphylaxis
- Anxiety related to continuing or uncontrolled allergic response
- Powerlessness related to difficulty determining cause of allergy

OUTCOME IDENTIFICATION AND PLANNING

Outcome identification and planning for a child with an immune disorder should focus both on present and future concerns. Relief of immediate symptoms is the first priority followed by planning for long-term care and infection prevention. Examples of organizations helpful for supplying information to parents or children are the National Eczema Association (www.nationaleczema.org), the Asthma and Allergy Foundation of America (www.aafa.org), American Academy of Allergy Asthma and Immunology (www.AAAAI.org), the Jeffrey Modell Foundation (www.info4pi.org), and the Immune Deficiency Foundation (www.primaryimmune.org). Other allergy-specific resources include the PRACTALL program, which is a common initiative of the European Academy of Allergy and Clinical Immunology and the American Academy of Allergy Asthma and Immunology. It focuses on practical aspects of allergy to deliver updated and evidence-based recommendations for clinicians. Several PRACTALL publications are referenced in the chapter.

IMPLEMENTATION

A major nursing intervention in the care of children with immune disorders is child and family teaching. The family of a child with an immunodeficiency may need help in identifying ways to keep the child from contracting life-threatening infections while at the same time providing enough stimulation and social contact to promote normal growth and development.

The family of a child with a chronic allergic disorder needs to learn ways to help their child avoid triggers or situations that provoke the allergic response but at the same time not keep the child so isolated or fearful that the child misses out on important socialization and life experiences.

OUTCOME EVALUATION

Outcome evaluation with immune disorders must be ongoing because these diseases are not static. Children with allergies can develop new allergic triggers at any time. Children with immunodeficiencies can similarly develop infections or related comorbidities at any time. New therapies for disease processes are constantly being investigated. Because the field of immunology is continually evolving, theories about immune diseases and associated treatments change year to year. This means that healthcare providers need to keep abreast of the latest developments. Emphasize to parents that they need to know the latest technologic information as well, especially as it relates to providing a safe environment for their child. Examples of outcomes suggesting the achievement of goals include:

- The child voices high self-esteem despite altered skin integrity related to atopy.
- The child and parents are able to adhere to the plan of care.
- The child lists three actions he takes daily to help feel a greater sense of control and well-being.
- The child demonstrates achievement of developmental milestones within age-acceptable parameters despite chronic illness.

The Immune System

The immune system is composed of a variety of cell types and proteins. The cells either recognize or react against foreign substances (**antigens**); some cells both recognize and react against antigens. Antigens include pathogens (bacteria, fungi, or viruses), food proteins, and pollens. There is significant redundancy in the immune system so that if one part does not function properly, another component may serve as a backup to take over some or all of the role of the malfunctioning part. The immune system response includes host defenses, nonspecific responses, and specific responses.

Host defenses include physical protective barriers including the skin, mucous membranes, cilia, and normal flora. Nonspecific responses include complement, phagocytes, and natural killer cells. Specific responses include antibody production and cellular immunity. All these components work together to protect the system from foreign invasion. If an invading pathogen does get through the physical, protective barrier, **phagocytosis**, or the destruction of the invaders, begins. **Macrophages** (mature white blood cells) engulf, ingest, and neutralize the pathogen. At the same time, an inflammatory response creates vascular and cellular changes that help to rid the body of dead tissue and the inactivated antigens. The immune system maintains cells ready to attack this way whenever necessary, directing the efforts of macrophages and supplementing the inflammatory response as necessary. It also singles out specific antigens for interactions (*antibody–antigen reactions*). This immune response not only furnishes

immediate protection but also creates a template for how to destroy that particular antigen again in the future.

IMMUNE RESPONSE

The **immune response** is the body's action plan devised to combat invading organisms or substances by leukocyte and antibody activity. An antigen is any foreign substance capable of stimulating an immune response. Most antigens are proteins, but other large molecules such as polysaccharides may also function the same way. Penicillin, although not antigenic by itself, can become antigenic when it combines with a higher weight molecule, usually a protein (a process called *hapten formation*). If an antigen is one that can be readily destroyed by an immune response, and **immunity** (the ability to destroy like antigens) results, the antigen may be referred to as an **immunogen**.

If, during the immune response, mediating substances are released that cause tissue injury and allergic symptoms, the antigen is termed an **allergen**. Allergens can enter the body through a variety of routes. They may be ingested (foods such as milk, egg, or peanut), inhaled (pollen, dust, or mold spores), injected (drugs), or absorbed across the skin or mucous membranes (poison ivy).

IMMUNE SYSTEM ORGANS AND CELLS

The major organs of the immune system are the thymus, liver, bone marrow, spleen, tonsils, lymph nodes, and blood. All of the cells of the immune system originate in the bone marrow where they develop from stem cells. Lymphocytes, produced in the bone marrow travel to different parts of the body, where they function. In the thymus, lymphocytes mature into T cells (Fig. 42.1). In other organs, such as the tonsils and spleen, lymphocytes collect and communicate with each other. The liver synthesizes the proteins of the complement system and contains large numbers of phagocytes to ingest and destroy bacteria.

B Lymphocytes

B Cells originate in the bone marrow where they develop from plasma or memory cells. Their major function is to produce antibodies or **immunoglobulins**. These immunoglobulins bind to and destroy specific antigens. When an antibody is formed in response to a particular antigen, it is specific to that antigen. For example, an antibody against the pertussis antigen, for instance, will not have any effect on the tetanus antigen. *Memory cells* are responsible for retaining the formula or ability to produce specific immunoglobulins. Immunoglobulins are classified as IgG, IgA, IgM, IgD, and IgE. Those involved in immunity include IgG, IgA, and IgM.

IgE is primarily responsible for allergic or hypersensitivity responses and is present at proportions capable of extreme response early in infancy. The functions of immunoglobulins are summarized in Table 42.1.

T Lymphocytes

T Lymphocytes account for 70% to 80% of blood lymphocytes and are responsible for *cell-mediated immunity*. They are produced by the bone marrow but mature under the influence of the thymus gland (hence their name). When mature, T lymphocytes leave the thymus to enter specific body regions

Figure 42.1 Lymphocyte production. From the bone marrow stem cell, T and B lymphocytes are formed. T-Lymphocyte action leads to cell-mediated immunity. B-Lymphocyte action results in humoral immunity. Ig, immunoglobulin.

(thymus-dependent zones), mostly in the lymph nodes and spleen; there, they react specifically to viruses, fungi, and parasites but have an effect on all antigens. T cells can be differentiated into three subtypes.

The first type, *cytotoxic (killer) T cells*, are T lymphocytes that have a specific ability to bind to the surface of antigens and directly destroy the cell membrane and, therefore, the cell. As a part of this process, cytotoxic cells secrete **lymphokines**, the purpose of which is to contain or prevent the migration of antigens as well as to call other lymphocytes into the area (the property of chemotaxis). *Interferon* is an example of a lymphokine widely discussed because it is important in preventing viral infections.

The second type, *helper T cells* (CD4 cells), serve the purpose of stimulating B lymphocytes to divide and mature into plasma cells so the B cells can begin secreting immunoglobulins. The IgA antibody response, especially, depends on stimulation by helper T cells. Helper T cells can be identified in blood because of specific markers on their surfaces. In patients with HIV/AIDS, analysis of these (CD4 counts) is an important assessment criteria used to determine if antiretroviral therapy is beginning to be effective (Boyd, 2011).

The third type, *suppressor T cells*, are specific cells that reduce the production of immunoglobulins against a specific antigen and prevent their overproduction.

TYPES OF IMMUNITY

The action of B and T lymphocytes leads to two different types of immunity: humoral and cell mediated.

Humoral Immunity

Humoral immunity refers to immunity created by antibody production or B-lymphocyte involvement. The process begins when helper T cells recognize an antigen and cause activation of B lymphocytes (possibly by an intermediary macrophage). B lymphocytes differentiate into plasma cells and begin the creation of specific immunoglobulins that mark the antigen for destruction (Fig. 42.2). A few antigens (e.g., *Escherichia coli*) are capable of activating a B-lymphocyte response without recognition by T lymphocytes.

The first time a specific antigen enters the body and is identified by T lymphocytes, B-cell differentiate and growth

TABLE 42.1 LOCATIONS AND FUNCTIONS OF IMMUNOGLOBULINS

Immunoglobulin	Description
IgM	Effective in agglutinating antigens as well as lysing cell walls; discovered early in the course of an infection in the bloodstream as it is the first response to pathogenic antigens.
IgG	Most frequently occurring antibody in plasma; during secondary response, it is the major immunoglobulin to be synthesized. It freely diffuses into extravascular spaces to contact antigens. In prenatal life, it diffuses across the placenta to supply passive immune protection to the fetus until the infant can effectively produce immunoglobulins. It has the major responsibility for neutralizing bacterial toxins and in activating phagocytosis (destruction of bacteria).
IgA	Found in external body secretions such as saliva, sweat, tears, mucus, bile, and colostrum. It provides defense against pathogens on exposed mucosal surfaces, especially those of the gastrointestinal tract and respiratory tract, and works, apparently, by preventing adherence of pathogens to mucosal cells.
IgD	Found in plasma. It may be the receptor that binds antigens to lymphocyte surfaces but its true function is unclear.
IgE	Involved in immediate hypersensitivity reactions. It exists bound to mast cells on tissue surfaces. When contacted by an antigen, cellular granules are released. It is associated with allergy and parasitic infections.

begins rapidly. Within 6 days, IgM antibodies specific to the antigen can be measured in the bloodstream. This level peaks at 14 days and then declines until, within a few weeks, little IgM can be measured. At approximately day 10, antigen-specific IgG production begins and remains high for several weeks (Fig. 42.3). When a specific antigen enters the body an additional time, antibody production is able to begin again immediately because of the presence of memory cells which develop after the first exposure. The main type of immunoglobulin produced in a secondary response is IgG (see Fig. 42.3). This secondary response is why immunocompetent people do not get the same disease twice.

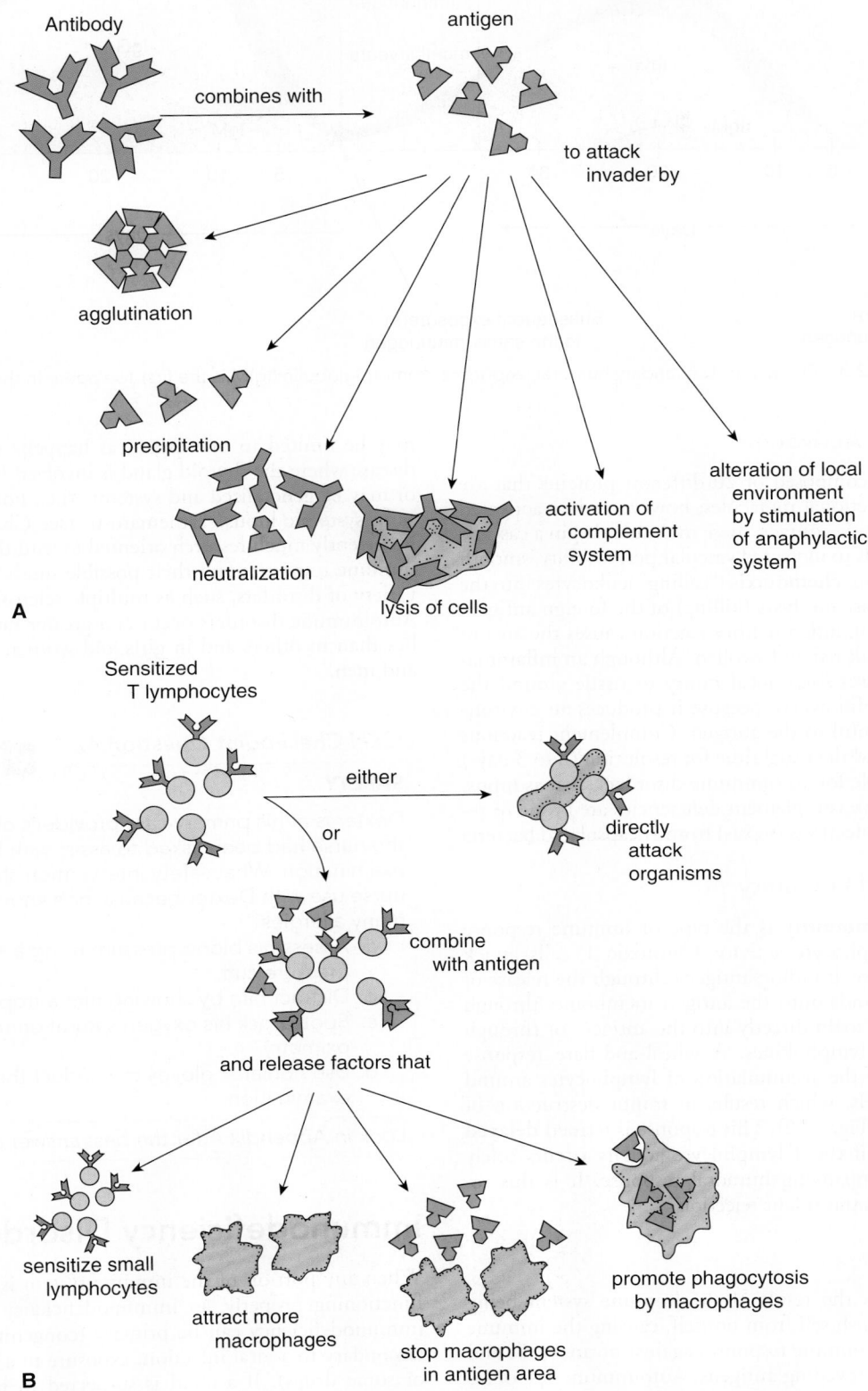

Figure 42.2   Mechanism of immunity response. **(A)** Humoral immunity. **(B)** Cell-mediated immunity.

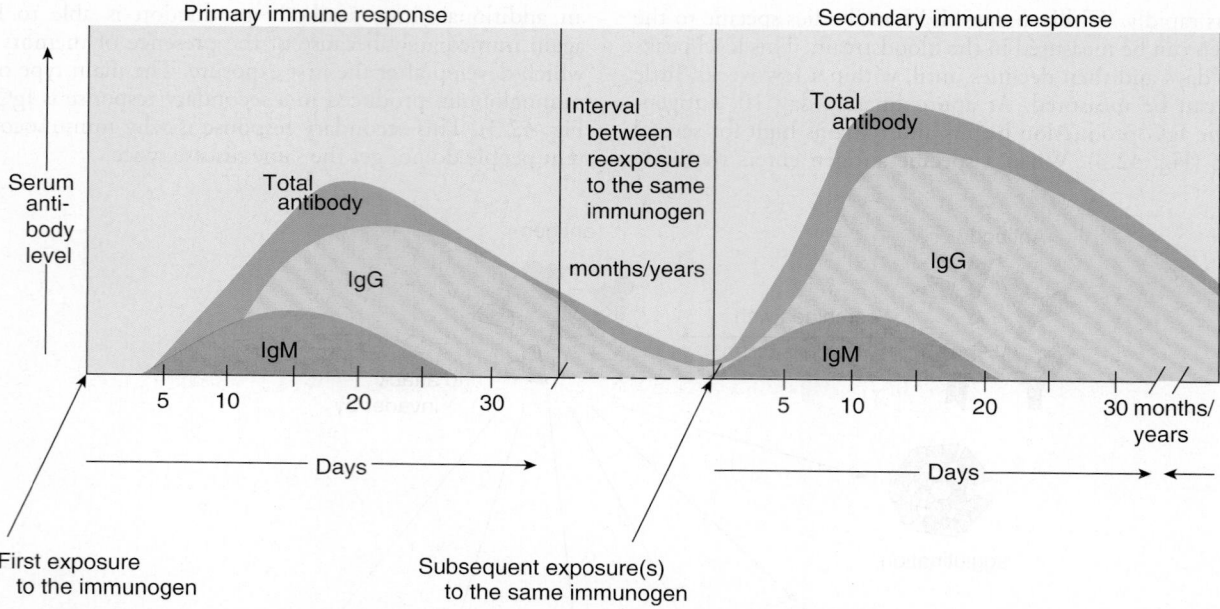

Figure 42.3 Primary and secondary humoral responses. Immunoglobulin (Ig)M is the first to appear in the serum.

Complement Activation

Complement is composed of 20 different proteins that are normally nonfunctional molecules; however, when activated by antigen–antibody contact, these molecules begin a cascade response that leads to increased vascular permeability, smooth muscle contraction, **chemotaxis** ("calling" leukocytes into the area), phagocytosis, and **lysis** (killing) of the foreign antigen. The accompanying inflammatory reaction causes the area to feel warm and look red and swollen. Although an inflammatory reaction causes some local injury to tissue around the antigen, it is helpful overall because it produces an environment that is harmful to the antigen. Complement reactions that persist beyond the usual time for resolution (2 to 3 days) may be responsible for autoimmune disorders such as lupus. Children who have complement deficiencies are prone to repeated systemic infections (sepsis) from encapsulated bacteria

Cell-Mediated Immunity

Cell-mediated immunity is the type of immune response caused by T-lymphocyte activity. Cytotoxic T cells attack and directly destroy invading antigens through the release of chemical compounds onto the antigen membrane, through the injection of a toxin directly into the antigen, or through the secretion of lymphokines. A wheal-and-flare response occurs because of the accumulation of lymphocytes around small blood vessels, which results in minor destruction of blood vessels (see Fig. 42.2). This response is termed **delayed hypersensitivity** if the T-lymphocyte activity occurs solely without an accompanying humoral response. It is this response that causes transplant rejection.

Autoimmunity

Autoimmunity is the result of the immune system being unable to distinguish self from nonself, causing the immune system to trigger immune responses against normal cells and tissue rather than invading antigens. Autoimmune responses

may be limited to one organ, as happens with Hashimoto disease where the thyroid gland is involved (see Chapter 48), or may be generalized and systemic (i.e., not organ specific), as in systemic lupus erythematosus (see Chapter 20). There is currently much research oriented toward the study of autoimmune responses and their possible implications in a wide variety of disorders, such as multiple sclerosis (Spiro, 2012). Autoimmune disorders occur at a greater rate in some families than in others and in girls and women more than boys and men.

QSEN Checkpoint Question 42.1

SAFETY

Dexter is at his primary care provider's office and the nurse had been asked to assist with his physical examination. What safety intervention should the nurse use with Dexter because he's known to have many allergies?

a. Assess his blood pressure using a new blood pressure cuff.
b. Distract him by showing him a tropical fish tank.
c. Spot-check his oxygen saturation using pulse oximetry.
d. Use nonlatex gloves to conduct the examination.

Look in Appendix A for the best answer and rationale.

Immunodeficiency Disorders

When any portion of the immune system is missing or not functioning properly, an immunodeficiency can result. An immunodeficiency can be primary (congenital) or acquired (secondary to a viral infection, exposure to a toxic substance or some drugs). If a child is suspected to have a humoral immunodeficiency, live viral vaccines are contraindicated, and all blood products should be irradiated.

PRIMARY IMMUNODEFICIENCY

Primary immunodeficiencies comprise over 150 inherited disorders. They can present and be diagnosed at various ages and affect all parts of the immune system, including humoral defects, cell-mediated defects, complement deficiencies, and phagocyte disorders (Younger, Epland, Zampelli, et al., 2015).

Humoral Deficiencies

Children with humoral defects are generally well until 4 to 6 months of age because of the presence of maternal antibody which crosses the placenta. As this antibody wanes and the child fails to produce his or her own antibody, infections can begin to present. Selective IgA deficiency, agammaglobulin-emia (either X-linked or autosomal recessive), and common variable immunodeficiency (CVID) are the most common humoral defects. In X-linked agammaglobulinemia, male children lack the enzyme necessary for B cells to mature; the B cells are incapable of maturing into antibody, and patients are susceptible to infection from a wide variety of pathogens. In patients with CVID, the levels of immunoglobulins are low but usually not absent, and antibody development is impaired. The cellular or T-lymphocyte response remains adequate in CVID, protecting the child from some pathogens.

Agammaglobulinemia and CVID are treated with the regular infusion of pooled human immunoglobulin, synthesized from human plasma. Immunoglobulin can be delivered intravenously every 3 to 4 weeks or subcutaneously every 1 to 2 weeks. The importance of early recognition of signs and symptoms of infection needs to be emphasized to both children and parents. Children with these immunodeficiencies may need longer courses of antibiotic treatment than immunocompetent children with the same infection. There is also an association with a higher prevalence of autoimmune diseases and lymphoreticular cancers in children with CVID. Healthcare providers and families must be taught to be aware of the signs of these illnesses.

Selective IgA deficiency is the most common of the humoral immunodeficiencies. The clinical definition for this disorder is an undetectable level of IgA, not merely a low level. The disorder can occur in as frequently as 1:500 people. Most people who lack IgA are completely asymptomatic, and the deficiency is noted when the person is being evaluated for another illness, such as celiac disease. IgA deficiency may result from an increase in IgA suppressor cells or defect in helper T-cells necessary for IgA production. IgA is normally found on mucosal surfaces, so in patients who are symptomatic, it is possible to see upper respiratory infections or inflammatory bowel disease. IgA deficiency is also associated with atopic diseases (allergies) because without IgA on the surface mucosa, many more antigens than usual can enter the body, thus permitting more antigens to interact with IgE and produce allergic symptoms. There is no treatment specific for IgA deficiency because there is no way to provide IgA to the body.

T-Lymphocyte Deficiencies

T-Lymphocyte immunodeficiencies involve inadequate numbers or inadequate functioning of one or more types of T lymphocytes; this affects cell-mediated immunity and, because of helper T-lymphocyte function, possibly humoral immunity as well. An example of one of these types of illnesses is DiGeorge syndrome. DiGeorge syndrome is a chromosomal deletion syndrome with tremendous phenotypic variability. Manifestations include congenital heart disease, abnormal facies, aplastic or hypoplastic thymus, hypocalcemia, and cleft lip and/or palate (Woo & Bahna, 2011).

Combined T- and B-Lymphocyte Deficiency

Severe combined immunodeficiencies (SCID) are a group of inherited rare disorders associated with large defects in T- and B-cell immunity (Hellmann & Imboden, 2013). SCID is caused by a developmental abnormality (sometimes but not always related to the absence of a particular enzyme), which prevents the formation of T lymphocytes (a stem cell abnormality). This, in turn, prevents the maturation of both T and B lymphocytes. Children cannot respond directly to antigen invasion, and no antibodies are produced. The definitive treatment for children with SCID is correction of the immunologic defect by hematopoietic stem cell transplantation, possibly from cord blood (Accetta Pedersen, Verbsky, & Routes, 2011).

In many states, newborns with SCID can be identified via a T-cell receptor excision circle (TREC) assay done at the same time as other routine newborn screening via dried blood spots. Low TREC numbers indicates a low number of lymphocytes and indicates further testing. This is critically important because SCID is 100% fatal if untreated, and early recognition is key to early treatment and survival (Kwan & Puck, 2015).

SECONDARY (ACQUIRED) IMMUNODEFICIENCY

Secondary immunodeficiency, or loss of immune system response, can occur from factors such as severe systemic infection, cancer, radiation therapy, severe stress, malnutrition, monoclonal antibody therapy targeted at B cells, other immunosuppressive therapy, and aging. Anything that causes the body to lose protein such as renal disease or protein-losing enteropathies may also cause a secondary immunodeficiency. There can be complete or partial loss of both B- and T-lymphocyte response.

Stress appears to alter the immune response by stimulating the release of corticosteroids from the adrenal gland. This suppresses the inflammatory response by inhibiting macrophage action. Immunosuppressive drugs, such as prednisone, also act to suppress the inflammatory response. The action of radiation or chemotherapy limits the function of or destroys rapidly growing cells and so destroys both T and B lymphocytes as these are rapidly growing and dividing cells. Extreme infection is yet another cause for a decreased immune response because the body's continued ability to combat infection becomes exhausted over time.

HIV Infection and AIDS

HIV is a slowly replicating retrovirus and has at least two main divisions, HIV-1 and HIV-2, followed by a variety of further subtypes. The virus acts by attacking the lymphoreticular system, in particular CD4-bearing helper T lymphocytes. The virus enters the cell, substitutes its own RNA and DNA for the cell's DNA, and begins to replicate, destroying the lymphocytes in the process as well as their ability to initiate an effective B-lymphocyte response.

There is no effective way to destroy the HIV, so it remains in the body for life and can activate if the immune system becomes depressed. When monocytes and macrophages become affected, the person with HIV infection cannot resist usual infections such as the common cold. When the CD4 count falls below 500 cells/mm³ or the viral load rises above 5,000 copies/ml, it is difficult for infected individuals to resist opportunistic infections such as fungal infections. The final result is that both the immune response and the ability to screen and remove malignant cells from the body are lost (Smith, 2011).

Transmission

HIV infection is spread by exposure to blood and/or other body secretions through sexual contact, the sharing of contaminated needles for injection, the transfusion of contaminated blood or blood products, perinatally from mother to fetus, and possibly through breastfeeding. Children can also acquire the infection because of sexual maltreatment. Healthcare providers must maintain vigilance to guard against needle punctures, as these injuries can be a direct source of blood transfer and, potentially, infection.

Although it is decreasing in incidence, the transmission of HIV from mother to child by placental spread is still the most common reason for childhood HIV infection in the United States. Transmission of HIV through sexual activity is a growing concern for adolescents and an important area where health education is needed (Sawyer, Afifi, Bearinger, et al., 2012). HIV is not transmitted by animals or through usual, casual contact, such as shaking hands or kissing.

Assessment

HIV has a long incubation period of about 10 years in adults. The disorder appears to progress more rapidly in children and infants, however, who receive the virus via placental transmission (if mothers do not receive treatment). These children are usually HIV positive by 6 months and develop clinical signs of the disease by 1 to 3 years of age. Children who receive the virus from another source usually convert to HIV positivity by 2 to 6 weeks or at least by 6 months after exposure. During this preconversion time, a child may display preliminary symptoms such as poor resistance to infection, fever, swollen lymph nodes, respiratory tract infections, and oral candidiasis.

All infants born to infected mothers test positive for antibodies to the virus at birth because of passive antibody transmission (which persists for about 18 months). The disease is diagnosed, therefore, by recovery of the HIV antigen in children under this age and antibodies to the virus in children over this age. Tests to detect the antigen are termed *polymerase chain reaction* (PCR) tests; those for the antibody are termed *enzyme-linked immunosorbent assay* (ELISA) or Western blot confirmation. CD4 counts are used to document the disease status and predict disease progression. Normal counts vary somewhat according to age because the lymphocyte count normally varies by age, but generally, a CD4 count of 500 cells/mm³ to 1,500 cells/mm³ is a healthy count.

The Centers for Disease Control and Prevention (CDC, 1994) classification of HIV infection in children has three categories:

- Category A, *mildly symptomatic*: Two or more symptoms such as enlarged lymph nodes, hepatomegaly and/or splenomegaly, or recurrent or persistent upper respiratory infections, sinusitis, or otitis media are present.
- Category B, *moderately symptomatic*: More serious illnesses such as oropharyngeal candidiasis, bacterial meningitis, pneumonia, sepsis, cardiomyopathy, cytomegalovirus (CMV) infection, hepatitis, herpes simplex virus (HSV), bronchitis, pneumonitis, esophagitis, herpes zoster (shingles), lymphoid interstitial pneumonia (LIP), pulmonary lymphoid hyperplasia complex, or toxoplasmosis are present.
- Category C, *severely symptomatic (AIDS)*: Serious bacterial infections such as septicemia, mycobacterial pneumonia, meningitis, bone or joint infection, abscess of an internal organ or body cavity, candidiasis (esophageal or pulmonary), encephalopathy, herpes simplex lasting over 1 month, histoplasmosis, lymphoma, tuberculosis, *Pneumocystis jiroveci* pneumonia (PCP; a form of pneumonia caused by a yeast-like fungus), and Kaposi sarcoma (a malignancy that causes large purple/blue tumors to grow from the lining of capillaries) have occurred.

Therapeutic Management

Because of advances in general health care, increased birth control education focused on the needs of women who are HIV positive as well as the availability of antiretroviral medications, the number of infants born with HIV infection is decreasing (Gay, Hardee, & Croce-Galis, 2011). Those infants who are born with HIV, once thought to have a short life expectancy, now have an opportunity for long-term survival.

 Nursing Diagnoses and Related Interventions

Nursing Diagnosis: Risk for infection related to decreased immune function

Outcome Evaluation: Child's temperature is within normal parameters; no signs of infection are present.

Combating HIV infection and maintaining an effective CD4 count requires continuous specific antiretroviral medications to prevent progressive deterioration of the immune system and to provide prophylactic measures against opportunistic infections. The introduction of highly active antiretroviral therapy (HAART) in pediatric HIV/AIDS treatment has made the difference between an acute disease where 60% of children died by age 6 years to a life expectancy of 40 to 50 years (Shulman, Yogev, & Murphy, 2011). Four classes of drugs are the mainstay of therapy: nucleoside reverse transcriptase inhibitors (NRTIs), nonnucleoside reverse transcriptase inhibitors (NNRTIs), protease inhibitors (PIs), and integrase strand transfer inhibitors (ISTIs). NRTIs are designed to block the production of viral DNA, limiting the ability of the virus to infect cells; zidovudine is an example (Box 42.2).

BOX 42.2

Nursing Care Planning Based on Responsibility for Pharmacology

ZIDOVUDINE

Classification: a nucleoside analog reverse-transcriptase inhibitor (NRTI)

Action: Zidovudine (ZDV) inhibits the replication of some retroviruses, including HIV. It reduces the possibility of maternal–fetal transmission of HIV (Commins, 2017).

Pregnancy Risk Category: C

Dosage: Individually determined based on the infant's or child's weight and whether it is administered twice or three times a day. Making certain the infant takes the full dose is an important nursing responsibility.

Possible Adverse Effects: nausea, loss of appetite, change in taste, paresthesia (tingling or numbness), headache, fever, agranulocytopenia, and rash

Nursing Implications

- When administering the drug intravenously, infuse the drug over 60 minutes to avoid too rapid infusion.
- Administer the drug around the clock for maximum effectiveness.
- Monitor blood studies frequently for change.
- Advise child to eat or feed child frequent, small meals to counteract change in taste and loss of appetite.
- If the child experiences paresthesias, institute safety precautions and instruct child and parents in measures to prevent injury related to loss of feeling.
- Caution child and parents that ZDV does not reduce the risk of HIV transmission except placentally. Reinforce the importance of hygiene and infection control measures.

NNRTIs also inhibit the DNA synthesis of viruses but act at different sites on the viral enzyme; nevirapine and efavirenz are examples. Children are prescribed a regimen involving multiple drugs, such as one PI plus two NRTIs.

In addition, many children are given prophylactic therapy for PCP (such as trimethoprim-sulfamethoxazole [TMP-SMZ]) beginning at 6 months of age. Children with HIV infection are more susceptible to tuberculosis than other children, so they also must be safeguarded against contracting this (Getahun, Raviglione, Varma, et al., 2012). If a child develops tuberculosis, a combination of antituberculosis drugs, such as isoniazid or rifampin, is used.

Children with HIV should receive routine immunizations according to the usual schedule including pneumococcal and human papillomavirus (HPV) vaccines. Attenuated live vaccines such as varicella and measles, mumps, and rubella (MMR) should be used with caution in children who are symptomatic or who have low CD4 counts. If a child is exposed to varicella, intravenous varicella zoster immune globulin (VZIG) can be prescribed in an attempt to prevent disease.

In addition to these measures, children with HIV infection and their families must maintain strict personal hygiene by measures such as frequent hand washing and avoiding close contact between the child and anyone who is ill to try to prevent the child from contracting dangerous opportunistic infections such as yeast and herpes infections. If a viral or fungal infection does occur, antiviral and antifungal treatment should be prompt and aggressive. The same is true of bacterial infections.

Nursing Diagnosis: Risk for compromised family coping related to the diagnosis of HIV infection in child

Outcome Evaluation: Parents state an ability to continue providing child's physical and emotional care; identify outside resources for help with care and decision making as needed.

The diagnosis of HIV infection in an infant or child can prove devastating for a family. When the infection is transmitted maternally, this diagnosis may be the first indication of the existence of HIV infection in the mother; as such, this signals tremendous stress for the whole family. When it occurs in an adolescent, parents may blame themselves for not supervising the child's activities more closely or providing better safe sex information. In any instance, the family's coping skills are certain to be stressed. Siblings may feel left out of the family circle because of the many healthcare appointments needed for the ill child. The siblings may fear contracting the infection themselves. One of the first nursing priorities in the care of such a family should be to help the family establish an appropriate level of functioning so they can focus on their child's emotional and physical care needs and to total family needs as well.

Physical care requirements for the child with HIV infection can be extensive depending on the child's symptoms and disease progression. No matter what the child's physical needs, love and emotional support continue to be essential to the child's well-being and psychological health. To continue to offer this support for such a long-term illness, parents need extensive support, education, and anticipatory guidance from healthcare providers. Telehealthcare (information received by electronic means such as laptops or smartphones) is an emerging phenomenon whereby healthcare personnel can provide support to families and patients; a caution is that this should always be supplemental support and should not take the place of "hands-on" care (McLean, Chandler, Nurmatov, et al., 2011).

A Pregnant Woman With HIV Infection

One fourth of the nearly 1 million people in the United States infected with this virus are female; a number of them become pregnant each year through intended or unintended conception (Hoyt, Storm, Aaron, et al., 2012). If the disorder is first discovered during pregnancy, pregnancy does not appear to accelerate the progression of the disease. It occurs more often in women who have bisexual or multiple sexual partners or when women or their partners use intravenous drugs.

Assessment

Unlike other sexually transmitted infections (STIs), HIV infection rarely begins with reproductive tract lesions. Instead, early symptoms are more subtle and often difficult to differentiate from those of other diseases or even from the symptoms of early pregnancy such as fatigue, anemia, diarrhea, and weight loss.

Without therapy, HIV infection progresses more slowly in adults than it does in children, and so the pregnant woman can be seen passing through a number of stages:

- The initial invasion of the virus, which may be accompanied by mild, flu-like symptoms
- Seroconversion, in which a woman converts from having no HIV antibodies in her blood serum (HIV serum negative) to having antibodies against HIV (HIV serum positive). Seroconversion happens 6 weeks to 1 year after exposure.
- An asymptomatic period during which the woman appears to be disease free except for symptoms such as weight loss and fatigue. She is not free of the disease, however, because the virus continues to replicate during this time. The length of this period varies but averages 3 to 11 years.
- A symptomatic period during which a woman develops opportunistic infections and possibly malignancies including oral and vaginal candidiasis, gastrointestinal illness, herpes simplex, PCP, *Candida* esophagitis, Kaposi sarcoma, and HIV-associated dementia. At this point, the CD4 count is usually below 200 cells/mm^3.

Although women are not as yet routinely screened for HIV during pregnancy, women who practice high-risk sexual behaviors should be asked if they want to be screened. A woman with HIV infection may also have contracted other diseases and STIs such as syphilis, gonorrhea, chlamydia, and hepatitis B and so should be screened for these diseases as well as tuberculosis. Because they are also at higher risk for developing toxoplasmosis and CMV infections, a health history should include questions about cat ownership, ingestion of raw meat, and recent mild, flu-like symptoms (see Chapter 12).

If a woman is found to be HIV positive during pregnancy (i.e., has developed antibodies from having been exposed to the virus) through an ELISA antibody reaction or a Western blot analysis, the issues of safer sex practices, testing of sexual contacts, and treatment during pregnancy need to be addressed. If a woman is not treated, as many as 20% to 50% of infants contract the virus and develop AIDS in the first year of their life. HIV infection is associated with both preterm births and low–birth-weight infants. The use of rapid HIV testing for all women in labor who did not receive prenatal care is being encouraged throughout the United States in order to identify women in need of specialized care and to help identify those infants in need of immediate antiviral therapy (Levison, Williams, Moore, et al., 2011).

Therapeutic Management

Women who are identified as HIV positive need education about reproductive life planning so they can effectively prevent pregnancy if they so desire. Often, however, the existence of HIV is discovered only after the affected woman is already pregnant. Progression of the disease is assessed by frequent CD4 cell counts and viral load levels during the pregnancy.

A goal of therapy during pregnancy is to maintain the CD4 cell count at greater than 500 cells/mm^3 by administering oral zidovudine, which helps to dramatically halt maternal–fetal transmission (see Box 42.2) along with one or more PIs, such as ritonavir (Norvir) or indinavir (Crixivan), in conjunction with an NRTI.

If PCP develops, a woman is treated with TMP-SMZ (Bactrim, Septra), a combination drug not without consequences, because trimethoprim may be teratogenic in early pregnancy and sulfamethoxazole may lead to increased bilirubin levels in the newborn if administered late in pregnancy. Although not well studied, pentamidine (Pentam), the drug of choice for PCP in nonpregnant women, is yet another option.

Kaposi sarcoma is normally treated with chemotherapy. Chemotherapy is contraindicated during early pregnancy, however, because of the potential for fetal injury. It can be used later in pregnancy to halt these malignant growths.

Thrombocytopenia (low platelet counts) may be present as a part of HIV disease pathology or as a response to zidovudine therapy. Women may need a platelet transfusion close to birth. This may make a woman a poor candidate for an epidural injection for anesthesia during labor or for an episiotomy. To reduce the risk of mother-to-newborn transmission, affected women should be offered the option of a cesarean birth.

Follow-up testing of newborns being treated with zidovudine for the first 6 weeks of life is important because if the child has two negative HIV tests by 4 months of age, HIV infection can be reasonably excluded.

 ## Nursing Diagnoses and Related Interventions

Nursing Diagnosis: Risk for infection (opportunistic) related to dysfunction of the immune system secondary to invasion of HIV

Outcome Evaluation: CD4 counts remain above 500 cells/mm^3; viral load less than 5,000 copies/ml; no symptoms of lung, vaginal, esophageal, or central nervous system infections are present.

Pregnant women who have CD4 counts below 200 cells/mm^3 may be prescribed drugs to help prevent opportunistic infections. Such drugs include acyclovir (Zovirax) for herpes simplex, clotrimazole troches (Mycelex) for oral candidiasis, pyrimethamine (Daraprim) and sulfadiazine for toxoplasmosis, and trimethoprim and sulfamethoxazole (Bactrim) for PCP. They may be immunized against pneumonia, influenza, and hepatitis B.

During pregnancy and at birth, active interventions are necessary to reduce the possibility of fetal exposure to maternal blood, often the mode of transmission to the fetus. Amniocentesis, for example, presents a risk of exposure to maternal blood and therefore is avoided if at all possible. During labor, internal fetal monitors, scalp blood sampling, forceps, and vacuum extraction are avoided to prevent the creation of a source of bleeding (i.e., an open lesion on the fetal scalp). Episiotomy also is avoided to limit this as a possible blood source. Although the risk may be lower than previously believed, breast milk can transmit HIV and breastfeeding can be exhausting for a debilitated woman; in nations where safe infant formula is not available, however, the advantages of breastfeeding may outweigh the risk of HIV transmission (Natchu, Liu, Duggan, et al., 2012).

Women who are HIV positive need to be aware that they can spread their illness to others through unprotected sexual relations or unintentional contamination by blood, even though they are being treated with zidovudine or other antiviral drugs. Nurses can help reduce this risk by providing patient education about the mode of HIV transmission and safer sex practices.

In addition, healthcare providers must be conscientious in their use of standard infection precautions (see Chapter 43) to protect against the spread of all infections, including HIV. This includes the use of gloves when there is a possibility of contact with body secretions, cover gowns if clothing will be exposed to secretions, and goggles worn at birth when there may be splashing of amniotic fluid. Gloves should be worn when handling the newborn until all maternal blood has been removed by a first bath. Also, no blood sampling or injections should be completed on the neonate until after a first bath and the removal of maternal blood.

Caring for a woman who is HIV positive during pregnancy and childbirth calls for great sensitivity in order to respect the woman as a patient with a possibly fatal disease while at the same time encouraging her to continue with prenatal care and bond with her newborn. Research into the cause and treatment of this disease is ongoing, and as a result, recommendations constantly change. Because of this, nurses need to remain current on recommendations for therapy or prevention.

QSEN Checkpoint Question 42.2

INFORMATICS

When Dexter's mother heard he had another allergic diagnosis, she wanted Dexter worked up for an immune system disorder "because he has colds all of the time." When reviewing the blood work of a child with allergic rhinitis, what results are most helpful? Select all that apply.

a. Specific IgE levels to cat, dog, tree, grass, and weed mix
b. Serum immunoglobulins (IgG, IgA, and IgM)
c. Complete blood count with differential
d. Basic metabolic panel

Look in Appendix A for the best answer and rationale.

Allergy

Allergic diseases occur as a result of abnormal antigen–antibody responses. Symptoms can be chronic and minor, such as those that occur with seasonal rhinitis, or acute and severe, as in an anaphylactic reaction. Because they can be constant, they can disrupt a child's life and development and the life of the family. When the cause of an allergic response

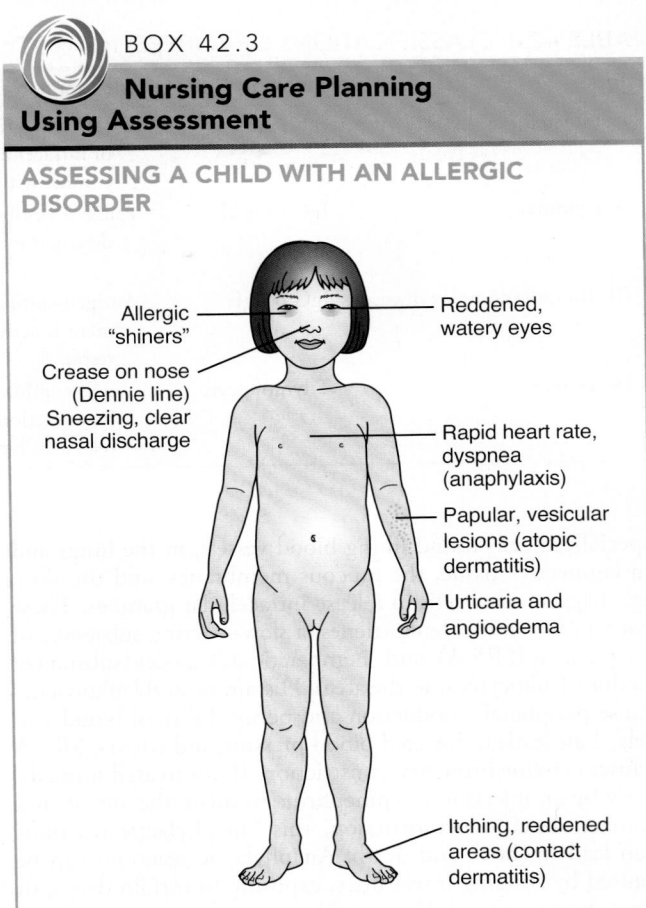

BOX 42.3

Nursing Care Planning Using Assessment

ASSESSING A CHILD WITH AN ALLERGIC DISORDER

- Allergic "shiners"
- Crease on nose (Dennie line) Sneezing, clear nasal discharge
- Reddened, watery eyes
- Rapid heart rate, dyspnea (anaphylaxis)
- Papular, vesicular lesions (atopic dermatitis)
- Urticaria and angioedema
- Itching, reddened areas (contact dermatitis)

---

is difficult to pinpoint, it is easy for the child and parents to become frustrated. Even when the child has a known allergy, symptoms can vary from minor to acute without warning, ultimately disrupting family functioning (Box 42.3).

What If . . . 42.1

Dexter tells the nurse that his symptoms always increase at school or that school "is making him sick." He's being bullied at school and acting out both in school and at home. How could the nurse explain Dexter's disease process to him in language he can understand?

HYPERSENSITIVITY

The underlying cause of all allergic disorders appears to be an excessive antigen–antibody response when the invading organism is an allergen rather than an immunogen. This is termed a type I response, or a **hypersensitivity response**, when it happens immediately. It can also occur as a type II, III, or IV response (Table 42.2). Types I, II, and III are mediated by antibodies (humoral response), whereas type IV is mediated by the T lymphocytes (cell-mediated response).

Type I: Immediate

With an immediate or type I allergic response, IgE receptor sites attached to the surface of mast cells bind to IgE antibodies responding to the presence of an antigen. Mast cells are

TABLE 42.2 CLASSIFICATIONS OF HYPERSENSITIVITY REACTIONS

Type	Involved Cell	Mechanism	Effect
I: Immediate	IgE	IgE attached to surface of mast cell triggers release of intracellular granules from mast cells on contact with antigens.	Allergies, asthma, atopic dermatitis, anaphylaxis
II: Cytotoxic	IgG or IgM	Antigen–antibody reaction leading to antigen destruction; complement is activated.	Hemolytic anemia, transfusion reaction, erythroblastosis fetalis
III: Immune complex disease	IgG or IgE	Antigen–antibody complexes precipitate; complement is activated, leading to inflammatory response.	Rheumatoid arthritis, systemic lupus erythematosus
IV: Delayed	T lymphocyte	T cells combine with antigen to induce inflammatory reactions by direct cell involvement or the release of lymphokines.	Contact dermatitis, transplant graft reaction

specialized cells found lining blood vessels, in the lungs and in connective tissue, the mucous membranes, and the skin. IgE triggers mast cells to release intracellular granules. These contain histamine, leukotrienes, a slow-reacting substance of anaphylaxis (SRS-A), and chemotactic substances (substances to draw leukocytes into the area). Histamine and leukotrienes cause peripheral vasodilation and permeability of blood vessels. This leads to lowered blood pressure and edema. SRS-A causes extreme bronchial constriction. If not treated immediately by an injection of epinephrine to dilate the airway and initiate vessel vasoconstriction, this "anaphylactic reaction" can lead to shock and death. Anaphylactic reactions can be caused by stinging insect bites, exposure to certain drugs, or latex; however, food allergy is the most common cause of anaphylaxis seen in hospital emergency rooms in both children and adults (Robison & Pongracic, 2012).

Type II: Cytotoxic Response

In a **cytotoxic response**, cells are detected as foreign and immunoglobulins directly attack and destroy them without harming surrounding tissue. Foreign red blood cells that are introduced to an Rh-negative woman by an Rh-positive fetus are destroyed by this process (see Chapter 26). Tumor cells may be destroyed by this process. Why this immune response fails when malignant cells begin to proliferate is not understood. Current research is attempting to devise ways to activate this natural immune response as a method of destroying malignant cells. Care of the child with a malignancy (neoplasm) and immunotherapy is discussed in Chapter 53.

Type III: Immune Complex

A type III response is an IgG- or IgE-mediated antigen–antibody complex reaction that involves complement and initiates the inflammatory response. Complement reactions that persist beyond the usual inhibition may serve as the basis for many autoimmune illnesses and serum sickness.

Type IV: Cell-Mediated Hypersensitivity

In a delayed hypersensitivity response, T lymphocytes react with antigens and release lymphokines to call macrophages into the area. An inflammatory response occurs that helps to destroy the foreign tissue. A Mantoux or purified protein derivative (PPD) tuberculin test is an example of this.

Redness and induration of the site do not begin initially but only approximately 12 hours after the injection. The reaction peaks in 24 to 72 hours (a delayed response).

Contact dermatitis is another example of a delayed hypersensitivity response. Certain substances, such as cosmetics, household products, or cured leather, alter the protein of skin cells so that the skin cells become an antigen or the foreign substance combines with the protein (hapten formation) to become an antigenic protein. Lymphocytes and macrophages infiltrate the area and attempt to destroy the offending protein. Redness and vesicles develop, and pruritus may be intense.

ASSESSMENT OF ALLERGIES IN CHILDREN

History

Taking a health history of a child with an allergy can be time-consuming because many factors have to be considered. A family history is important because there seem to be familial tendencies with allergic diseases. Obtaining the exact symptoms of the allergy is important to help identify the allergen: Rhinitis, for example, can be related to an airborne antigen; urticaria (swelling and itching) is often caused by ingested antigens; and contact dermatitis (often a rash) is usually related to something that contacts the skin in that area of the rash. The time of the year the allergy occurs also may give a clue to its cause. If the child's allergy exists all year, the antigen is likely one that is present all year (e.g., house dust mites or pet dander). If it occurs in the spring, it may be due to a tree pollen; in the early summer, a grass pollen; and if it occurs just in the fall, ragweed is a prime suspect.

Children with allergic rhinitis develop common symptoms such as a horizontal crease across the nose (called a Dennie line) from their habit of constantly wiping away nasal secretions. They also may develop dark patches ("allergic shiners") under their eyes secondary to back pressure from nasal congestion (see Box 42.3).

Many symptoms of allergy are vague, described as "colds all winter," "itching," or "runny nose." Listen carefully: Even though no one symptom is acute, together, such symptoms can interfere with a child's comfort, school experience, and long-term health. Children are often poor reporters of when they have symptoms. Sometimes, they cannot remember clearly whether they had the same rhinitis and watery eye symptoms last summer as they do this summer. Having the parents and the child keep a chart or diary of when symptoms are worse and better often helps identify a specific allergen. Children with allergic rhinitis, for example, may have more symptoms on a windy day when pollens are being blown around and fewer after a rainstorm when the pollen is washed out of the air. A record that details when symptoms start— on arising, or only after the child reaches school, as another example—also can help identify an allergen.

Laboratory Testing

Clinical laboratory testing is important in the diagnosis and management of allergic disorders. The presence of IgE antibodies detected either in serum or via skin testing are useful biomarkers. It is important to note that although the presence of allergen-specific IgE is necessary to diagnose type I sensitivity, the mere presence of allergen-specific IgE is not sufficient to diagnose type I sensitivity. Lab-based serologic analysis for IgE antibodies such as ImmunoCAP, Immulite, and HYTEC 288 are only useful in the context of a thorough clinical history. Because allergies tend to raise an eosinophil count, most children with allergies have 5% or more eosinophils on a differential white blood cell count and a total eosinophil count of ≥ 250 cells/mm^3. Another cause of an increased eosinophil count, however, is invasion by ova or parasites, which is why a stool specimen for ova and parasites may be collected to rule out these problems as the cause of the increased eosinophil count in the absence of any atopic symptoms.

Skin Testing

Skin testing is done to determine potential triggers for atopic symptoms by detecting the presence of IgE to specific allergens. When an allergen is introduced into the child's skin and the child is sensitive to that allergen, a wheal (a small, raised bump that looks like a mosquito bite) and flare (erythema that surrounds the wheal) response will appear at the site of the test from the release of histamine by the local mast cells. Because this reaction appears quickly, the test should be read within 15 to 20 minutes. Systemic administration of an antihistamine will suppress the response, so the child must be off of antihistamines for five half-lives of the antihistamine (usually 5 to 7 days before testing). Corticosteroid therapy does not affect immediate skin reactivity and so may be continued during skin testing.

Scratch, prick, or puncture skin testing is done to detect sensitivity to aeroallergens, foods, stinging insects, and some drugs. Skin testing is done by placing a drop of allergen solution on the skin of the upper back or volar aspect of the arm and then scratching/pricking or puncturing through the drop of liquid with a sharp device (needle, lancet, or multihead device). In order to be valid, both a positive (histamine) and negative (saline) control must be included in the panel tested. The average diameter of the negative control should be less than 3 mm, and the positive control must be at least 3 mm larger than the negative control for the testing to be interpreted.

Skin testing interpretation has limitations. The sensitivity and specificity for aeroallergens are acceptable, but there is a high false-positive rate for skin testing to foods. All skin testing results should be interpreted in terms of clinical history.

Intracutaneous testing to allergens is done when a sensitivity to aeroallergens, some drugs (primarily penicillin),

Figure 42.4 Allergy skin testing. Note the positive reactions. (© SPL/Custom Medical Stock Photograph.)

or stinging insects is suspected but not confirmed by prick/puncture/scratch skin tests. Intracutaneous testing is done by injecting a small amount of a solution of allergen below the epidermis of the skin of the forearm or back. The forearm is usually preferred to allow for the application of a tourniquet if a systemic reaction occurs. Solutions used for intracutaneous injections are 100 to 1,000 times more dilute than those used for scratch testing. The extracts are not interchangeable from a group prepared for scratch testing to a group prepared for intracutaneous injections or vice versa. Intracutaneous testing is never done with food allergens because of the potential for the intracutaneous testing to cause an anaphylactic reaction. With all forms of skin testing, if the child is sensitive to the test solution, a wheal and flare will occur at the test site (Fig. 42.4). The size of the reaction is then measured and graded as 1+ to 4+ or as slight, moderate, or marked response in comparison to the wheal and flare response to the positive control.

Always have a syringe filled with 0.3 ml epinephrine (Adrenalin) 1:1,000 on hand to counteract an unexpected anaphylactic reaction from skin testing (Box 42.4). Epinephrine is given intramuscularly in doses of 0.01 mg/kg, up to 0.3 mg. Children should be observed in the healthcare setting for at least 30 minutes after skin testing to ensure anaphylaxis management is available in the event of a reaction.

The allergens chosen for any IgE testing (serum IgE, prick/puncture/scratch skin testing or intracutaneous testing) is always done in context of the clinical history. Determining the seasonality or timing of the symptoms may eliminate or identify potential triggers. Clinical history is especially critical when dealing with suspected food allergies.

THERAPEUTIC MANAGEMENT

No matter what the symptoms of a child's allergy are, the goals for therapy are to reduce the child's exposure to the allergen and modify the child's response to the allergen with a pharmacologic agent. If symptoms persist, immunotherapy to produce a state of increased clinical **tolerance** or "sustained unresponsiveness" should be considered.

Reducing the child's exposure to the allergen is possible when the offending allergen is a drug, food, or irritant. Reducing exposure can be much more difficult when the allergic trigger is ubiquitous in the environment.

BOX 42.4

Nursing Care Planning Based on Responsibility for Pharmacology

EPINEPHRINE HYDROCHLORIDE (ADRENALIN)

Classification: Epinephrine is a sympathomimetic drug.

Action: Acts on both α- and β-receptor sites of sympathetic receptor cells to cause increased blood pressure and heart rate. It also relaxes the smooth muscles of the bronchi. It is used to counteract the symptoms of anaphylaxis (Commins, 2017).

Pregnancy Risk Category: C

Dosage: 0.01 mg/kg, up to 0.3 mg of a 1:1,000 solution intramuscularly into the vastus lateralis of the thigh every 20 minutes for up to four doses. This may be followed by an individualized intravenous bolus if symptoms still persist.

Possible Adverse Effects: Anxiety, restlessness, headache, nausea, arrhythmias, hypertension, palpitations, pallor

Nursing Implications

- Be sure to calculate the drug dosage and check the solution strength carefully; solution is available in different concentrations, and epinephrine is a very potent drug.
- Obtain blood pressure, pulse, and respirations and auscultate breath sounds before and immediately after administration. Assess the child for signs indicating the resolution of anaphylaxis.
- Rotate injection sites to prevent necrosis at the site.
- Have a rapidly acting α-adrenergic blocking agent or vasodilator readily available in case of a hypertensive reaction or have a β-adrenergic blocking agent readily available in case of arrhythmias.
- Protect the drug from light and heat. Use only solutions that are clear and colorless.

Environmental Control

Environmental control involves limiting exposure to allergens in a child's environment. Common measures of environmental control are shown in Table 42.3 and Box 42.5. Some control measures such as dust mite covers on mattresses and pillows are inexpensive and very effective. Others measures, such as replacing carpeting with hardwood in the bedroom or removing the family pet from the house are expensive or just not feasible for every family. Help parents understand that goal of environmental controls measures are to decrease exposure to allergic triggers and reduce their child's symptoms and decrease the need for medications or immunotherapy (Krouse, 2014).

Concept Mastery Alert

Environmental control of allergens works to remove as many allergens and reservoirs for allergens as possible from the child's environment. For items that cannot be removed, it is best to encase them in a hypoallergenic covering.

Pharmacologic Therapy

A number of pharmacologic preparations can be used to reduce the symptoms of childhood allergies. Intranasal steroids can be used prophylactically to prevent inflammation (de Souza Campos Fernandes, Ribeiro de Andrade, & da Cunha Ibiapina, 2014). Second- and third-generation antihistamines, such as cetirizine (Zyrtec) and loratadine (Claritin), cause little drowsiness yet effectively block histamine release and, as a result, control itching, sneezing, and rhinorrhea (Nayak, Berger, LaForce, et al., 2017). Decongestants, such as pseudoephedrine (Sudafed), decrease nasal edema and can help enlarge breathing space and so may also be recommended.

Immunotherapy

Immunotherapy, or **hyposensitization**, is done when the child's allergy symptoms cannot be controlled by avoidance of an allergen or conventional drug therapy. It can be accomplished by subcutaneous immunotherapy (SCIT) or by tablets that are given sublingually.

Immunotherapy works by increasing the plasma concentration of IgG antibodies, which then act to prevent or block IgE antibodies from coming in contact with an allergen. For the injection method, after specific environmental allergens have been determined with skin testing, small amounts of allergy extracts, which are dilute enough to be clinically subreactive, are injected subcutaneously at weekly intervals. The dose of antigen is increased in strength each time until the peak concentration, called "maintenance," is reached. Following immunotherapy, the child's allergy symptoms should be greatly reduced. Unfortunately, the child then needs periodic injections every 3 to 4 weeks to maintain maintenance to the allergen. This approach is not currently approved by the U.S. Food and Drug Administration (FDA) for treatment of food allergy because of the real threat of significant anaphylaxis.

Sublingual immunotherapy (SLIT) administration of chosen allergen solutions is growing in use because it has the advantage of being painless, can be self- or parent-administered, and produces results equal to that of other therapies. The liquid form of SLIT is widely used in Europe, but, currently, the only FDA-approved SLIT are tablets directed at two types of grass and short ragweed.

If children are going to have an anaphylactic reaction to an injected or sublingual allergen, it generally occurs within 30 to 60 minutes after the injection. Therefore, children must be observed for a minimum of 30 minutes after an allergy shot. Caution parents to observe their child for anaphylaxis after sublingual administration.

Immunotherapy is generally continued for 3 to 5 years because the longer it is used, the longer the period of relief from symptoms occurs after it is stopped. Be certain parents know from the beginning of treatment that this therapy will not "cure" their child. However, it can reduce allergy symptoms for a length of time. It may also prevent a mild atopic disorder such as allergic rhinitis from turning into a severe atopic disorder such as asthma (Tsabouri, Mavroudi, Feketea, et al., 2017) (see Chapter 40). Be certain children have adequate education and preparation if injection procedures are used. Help them understand the importance of returning for additional injections and remaining under observation after the administration of immunotherapy.

TABLE 42.3 COMMON MEASURES FOR ENVIRONMENTAL CONTROL OF ALLERGENS

Area of Concern	Measures	Rationale
Child's bedroom	Encase mattress and pillow in allergy encasements that are impervious to house mites.	Reduces dust and dust mites
	Cover the zipper of plastic pillow and mattress case with adhesive tape.	Keeps dust confined
	Use blankets or quilts made of or stuffed with smooth, synthetic material; avoid wool.	Minimizes dust; wool is a good dust collector or may be an allergen itself.
	Wash bed linens including mattress pads, sheets, blankets, and comforters in hot water every 2 weeks. Dry thoroughly in a hot dryer.	The heat from the hot water and hot dryer kills dust mites.
	Take down any ornamental items, such as a bed canopy.	Prevents dust collection
	Remove stuffed chairs and replace with wooden ones.	Removes dust collectors
	Remove venetian blinds and curtains that need to be dry cleaned; replace with easily laundered types.	Removes dust collectors
	Remove stuffed toys unless filled with synthetic material.	Removes dust collectors and possible sources of allergens
	Remove aquariums and plants.	Removes mold spores
	Clean closet, so it contains only currently used items.	Eliminates dust collectors
	Remove any fur or woolen items from the child's wardrobe.	Removes possible allergens
Living or television room	Remove all carpets. If a rug is necessary, vacuum at least weekly; replace an animal hair pad with a foam rubber one.	Avoids containers for dust collection
	Provide a wooden chair, not a stuffed one, for sitting.	Provides space free from allergens
	Vacuum floor surfaces frequently.	Minimizes dust collection
	Use a piece of linoleum or plastic laminate surface on top of carpet if the child sits on the floor.	Provides space free from allergens
Bathroom	Use nonscented toilet paper, soaps, and cleaners.	Minimizes exposure to potential irritants
School room	Have child sit away from blackboard, caged animals, or fish tanks.	Minimizes exposure to chalk, mold spores, and animal dander, which are allergens
	Keep locker free of collectibles.	Reduces dust collection
General	Purchase a dehumidifier; add compounds to paint to decrease mold spores.	Reduces mold spores
	Use high-efficiency particulate air (HEPA) filters on furnaces and vacuums.	Filters air of possible allergens
	Keep a favorite pet but do not purchase a new pet.	Reduces exposure to animal dander
	Dust daily with a moist cloth.	Controls dust better than dry dusting

BOX 42.5

Nursing Care Planning Tips for Effective Communication

The Goodenough family has been instructed on environmental control measures because Dexter has severe allergic rhinitis. Despite this, Dexter's symptoms have not improved. You meet with his parents to confirm they are carrying out recommended measures.

Tip: Be careful not to make assumptions by taking patient or caregiver responses to questions at face value. Ask follow-up questions and review patient education when needed.

Nurse: Have you been able to make any of the needed changes around your house to reduce dust?

Mrs. Goodenough: As many as we can.

Nurse: What about Dexter's bedroom? Do you have the mattress covered? Any frilly curtains taken down? His stuffed animals taken out?

Mrs. Goodenough: I've done everything I can.

Nurse: Let's discuss what changes you've been able to make.

Mrs. Goodenough: I covered the mattress. I had to leave the curtains up, though, because they match the rug. I took out a lot of the toys but had to leave the stuffed bears because they were gifts from his grandmother.

Nurse: Getting the mattress covered is a good start. Our goal is to decrease Dexter's exposure as much as possible to improve his symptoms. Let's discuss any other possible measures we could take.

Look in Appendix A for the best answer and rationale.

QSEN Checkpoint Question 42.3

PATIENT-CENTERED CARE

Dexter's mother asks the nurse about the potential risks and benefits of immunotherapy, stating that some websites she has consulted convey dire warnings against the practice. What potential benefit could the nurse describe to Dexter's mother to alleviate her anxiety?

   a. Dexter will recover more quickly from infections.
   b. Dexter will be protected against secondary infections.
   c. Dexter's level of helpful immunoglobulins will be increased.
   d. The overall health of Dexter's immune system will be increased.

Common Allergic Reactions

ANAPHYLACTIC SHOCK

Anaphylactic shock is an immediate, life-threatening, type I hypersensitivity reaction that occurs after exposure to an allergen in a previously sensitized child. **Anaphylaxis** can be caused by exposure to foods such as milk, egg, peanut, and tree nuts; stinging insects including yellow jackets, honeybees, paper wasps, hornets, and fire ants; certain drugs, primarily antibiotics, nonsteroidal anti-inflammatory drugs (NSAIDs), and neuromuscular blocking agents; and latex. Anaphylactic shock must be recognized and treated immediately because it can be fatal (Simons, Ardusso, Bilò, et al., 2014).

Assessment of Anaphylaxis

Symptoms of anaphylaxis may include:
- Breathing: wheezing, shortness of breath, throat tightness, cough, hoarse voice, chest pain/tightness, trouble swallowing, itchy mouth/throat, nasal stuffiness/congestion
- Circulation: pale/blue color, low pulse, dizziness, lightheadedness/passing out, low blood pressure, shock, loss of consciousness
- Skin: hives, swelling, itch, warmth, redness, rash
- Stomach: nausea, pain/cramps, vomiting, diarrhea
- Other: anxiety, feeling of impending doom, itchy/red/watery eyes, headache, cramping of the uterus

Therapeutic Management of Anaphylaxis

Preventing and recognizing anaphylaxis are as important as knowing how to respond when it occurs. Exposure to certain food, stinging insects, medications, and latex are the most common triggers of anaphylaxis. Avoiding offending foods is extremely difficult because of the presence of unexpected food proteins in prepared foods and significant issues with cross-contamination during food preparation and packaging. Avoiding stinging insects is easier given the seasonality of insect exposure, but insect stings are unpredictable. Exposure to offending drugs and latex is manageable if a thorough history has been obtained.

Epinephrine, injected intramuscularly, is the standard of care for the treatment of anaphylaxis regardless of the cause (Muraro, Lemanske, Castells, et al., 2017). Epinephrine is the only treatment for anaphylaxis that reduces the risk of prolonged hospitalization and death. For maximum effectiveness, if anaphylaxis follows an injection or an insect sting, inject the epinephrine into the vastus lateralis muscle of the thigh or the unaffected arm. Additional emergency interventions to take in a healthcare setting are summarized in Box 42.6.

Administering antihistamines, steroids, and/or albuterol to treat the symptoms of anaphylaxis does nothing to address the immediate cause of the symptoms, thus allowing the anaphylactic event to progress. The vasoconstrictor effects of epinephrine prevent/relieve airway edema, hypotension, and shock and the beta-agonist effects increase the effectiveness of cardiac contractions and lead to bronchodilation (Simons, Ebisawa, Sanchez-Borges, et al., 2015).

Every child with a history of anaphylaxis needs a written anaphylaxis treatment plan such as the one in Figure 42.5. When a sensitized child reacts, parents, teachers, coaches, day-care providers, and family members all must know the proper procedure to follow for anaphylactic shock so they can give the child immediate help. All children with a history of anaphylaxis need to carry an epinephrine auto-injector

---

BOX 42.6

Emergency Measures for Anaphylactic Shock

Anaphylaxis is a true emergency, so fast interventions are necessary.

- Administer aqueous epinephrine (Adrenalin) 1:1,000 intramuscularly at a dosage of 0.01 mg/kg of body weight up to 0.3 mg. This relieves laryngeal edema and severe bronchospasm by widening the airway.
- Initiate 911 emergency or notify the cardiac arrest team because both respiratory and cardiac arrest may occur.
- If hypoxia is present, administer oxygen by mask or nasal cannula.
- Anticipate the need for an intravenous (IV) fluid line as a route for a vasopressor such as dopamine and fluid to help restore blood pressure.
- If an insect sting was the cause of the condition, a tourniquet, applied above the site of the bite, may be prescribed to limit absorption of the insect venom into the bloodstream.
- Anticipate use of a nebulized bronchodilator such as albuterol to halt wheezing or diphenhydramine (Benadryl) intramuscularly or IV if urticaria (itching and swelling) is present.
- If the child is experiencing seizures, turn the child onto his or her side and prepare to administer an antiseizure medication such as phenobarbital or diazepam.
- A corticosteroid may be administered as a second-line drug. This does not act immediately but does reduce inflammation. IV methylprednisolone is a typical drug given.
- Keep the child and family members calm; anxiety adds to bronchospasm and decreases breathing ability.

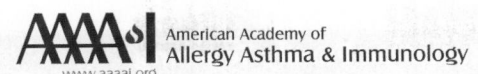

American Academy of
Allergy Asthma & Immunology
www.aaaai.org

Anaphylaxis Emergency Action Plan

Patient Name: _____ Age: _____

Allergies: _____

Asthma ☐ Yes *(high risk for severe reaction)*   ☐ No

Additional health problems besides anaphylaxis: _____
_____

Concurrent medications: _____
_____

Symptoms of Anaphylaxis

MOUTH	itching, swelling of lips and/or tongue
THROAT*	itching, tightness/closure, hoarseness
SKIN	itching, hives, redness, swelling
GUT	vomiting, diarrhea, cramps
LUNG*	shortness of breath, cough, wheeze
HEART*	weak pulse, dizziness, passing out

Only a few symptoms may be present. Severity of symptoms can change quickly.
**Some symptoms can be life-threatening. ACT FAST!*

Emergency Action Steps - DO NOT HESITATE TO GIVE EPINEPHRINE!
1. Inject epinephrine in thigh using (check one):
☐ Adrenaclick (0.15 mg)   ☐ Adrenaclick (0.3 mg)
☐ Auvi-Q (0.15 mg)   ☐ Auvi-Q (0.3 mg)
☐ EpiPen Jr (0.15 mg)   ☐ EpiPen (0.3 mg)

Epinephrine Injection, USP Auto-injector- authorized generic
☐ (0.15 mg)   ☐ (0.3 mg)
☐ Other (0.15 mg)   ☐ Other (0.3 mg)

Specify others: _____

IMPORTANT: ASTHMA INHALERS AND/OR ANTIHISTAMINES CAN'T BE DEPENDED ON IN ANAPHYLAXIS.

2. Call 911 or rescue squad (before calling contact)

3. Emergency contact #1: home_____ work_____ cell_____
   Emergency contact #2: home_____ work_____ cell_____
   Emergency contact #3: home_____ work_____ cell_____

Comments: _____
_____
_____

Doctor's Signature/Date/Phone Number

Parent's Signature (for individuals under age 18 yrs)/Date

This information is for general purposes and is not intended to replace the advice of a qualified health professional. For more information, visit www.aaaai.org. © 2017 American Academy of Allergy, Asthma & Immunology   4/2017

Figure 42.5 Sample anaphylaxis emergency action plan form. (Reprinted with permission from The American Academy of Allergy, Asthma & Immunology – aaaai.org.)

(Box 42.7). Anyone who has responsibility for a child with history of anaphylaxis needs to know how to recognize the symptoms of anaphylaxis and how to administer epinephrine using the auto-injector device. Responsible adults and children need practice using the epinephrine auto-injector correctly. There are reports of people using the auto-injectors incorrectly and accidentally puncturing their thumb, thus creating circulation problems in their own hand (Sheikh, Simons, Barbour, et al., 2012).

Once epinephrine has been administered, the emergency response system (911) must be activated. An anaphylactic event can be stopped with a single dose of epinephrine, but in some cases, the epinephrine only stops the reaction temporarily, and once the dose of epinephrine has been metabolized, the reaction come roaring back. In addition, some anaphylactic reactions are biphasic and involve a second wave of symptoms several hours later. Children who have had an anaphylactic reaction need to be observed for a minimum of 4 hours to ensure that a reaction has subsided. An evaluation of the child after an anaphylactic reaction involves not only a physical examination but also an evaluation of the exposure and the implementation of the anaphylaxis treatment plan to determine appropriate avoidance measures as well as potential improvements in the response to anaphylaxis.

BOX 42.7

Nursing Care Planning Based on Family Teaching

GUIDELINES FOR USING AN EPINEPHRINE AUTO-INJECTOR

Q. Dexter's father says to you, "If my child is stung by a bee, I'm supposed to inject epinephrine. How do I do that?"

A. It is important you think about this in advance because from the moment your child is stung, it will be an emergency situation.

- Obtain a prescription for an epinephrine auto-injector, which is a preloaded syringe with a designated dose of epinephrine for use in emergencies.
- Epinephrine auto-injectors need to be available at home and at your child's school/day care. You or your child needs to carry an epinephrine auto-injector with you at all times.
- Store epinephrine auto-injectors at room temperature; don't refrigerate or allow epinephrine to be exposed to heat.
- Inspect the color of the epinephrine solution and replace it if it is cloudy or discolored.
- If your child exhibits symptoms of a severe allergic reaction, see your anaphylaxis plan for a description of symptoms that constitute a severe allergic reaction. Administer the epinephrine by removing the safety cap, grasping the auto-injector by the barrel (avoid placing your thumb over the end), and, using firm pressure, applying the auto-injector to the outer aspect of the thigh until the auto-injector "clicks."
- If necessary, the device can inject through clothing. The needle is long enough to pass through clothing and into your child's skin.
- Be careful before injecting that you are holding the auto-injector by the barrel with the needle toward your child. If not, you will accidentally inject your own thumb (a serious circumstance because the dose of epinephrine could seriously injure your thumb).
- Keep in mind that not all the solution in the auto-injector will be ejected. Do not try to give the remainder of the solution.
- Call 911 for transportation assistance or transport your child to an emergency facility for further care.

QSEN Checkpoint Question 42.4

TEAMWORK & COLLABORATION

Any child can have an anaphylactic reaction to a food, drug, or insect sting, and Dexter is at risk because of his allergy history. If Dexter, who weighs 48 kg, had an anaphylactic reaction after a beesting, what is the correct dose of epinephrine for a school nurse or staff member to give him?

  a. 0.03 mg
  b. 0.15 mg
  c. 0.3 mg
  d. 3.0 mg

Look in Appendix A for the best answer and rationale.

URTICARIA AND ANGIOEDEMA

Urticaria, or hives, refers to macular wheals surrounded by erythema arising from the chorion layer of skin; they are intensely pruritic (often described as having a burning sensation). Hives may occur so closely together that they tend to coalesce (blend together); dilatation of capillaries and venules with increased permeability occurs around the lesions. The cause of urticaria is a type I or immediate hypersensitivity reaction created by the release of histamine from an antibody–antigen reaction, similar to but of lesser intensity than anaphylaxis. In chronic urticaria, it is possible that no causative allergen can be found.

Angioedema is edema of the skin and subcutaneous tissue. This occurs most frequently on the eyelids, hands, feet, genitalia, and lips—areas where skin is loosely bound by subcutaneous tissue. Angioedema can be distinguished from other edemas because it is not dependent, is generally asymmetrically distributed, and usually occurs in conjunction with urticaria. With severe angioedema, the larynx may be involved. This is a serious problem because laryngeal edema could be so extreme that it leads to airway obstruction and, subsequently, asphyxiation and death.

The allergens that most frequently cause urticaria and angioedema include drugs, foods, and insect stings. In some children, exposure to hot or cold can also cause these reactions. All children need the causative agent be identified so it can be avoided. Although a rare event, children who have a reaction to hot or cold especially must be identified because, if they swim in cold water, the sudden release of histamine could cause dizziness so severe that they could drown. Immediate therapy for urticaria or angioedema is an intramuscular epinephrine injection or the administration of an oral antihistamine. For long-term therapy, corticosteroids may be prescribed; cyclosporine (an immunosuppressant) and omalizumab (Xolair), a monoclonal antibody, are usually reserved for older adolescents or adults (Kaplan, 2012).

Atopic Disorders

Individuals with atopic disease are prone to all types of allergic responses. Three disorders occur most frequently: allergic rhinitis, eczema (**atopic dermatitis**), and asthma (discussed with other respiratory diseases in Chapter 40).

The gene responsible for an immune response is located near the human leukocyte antigen that is responsible for graft rejections. In certain children, a tendency for sensitivity to antigens or abnormality of this gene is apparently inherited. These children have a higher-than-normal production of IgE antibodies, which makes them more responsive to allergens than other people. There are familial tendencies with these diseases, but not all family members manifest the symptoms in the same way. In one family, for example, the father may have allergic rhinitis, one child may have asthma, and another may have atopic dermatitis.

ALLERGIC RHINITIS

Allergic rhinitis is associated with an IgE-mediated inflammatory response to allergen exposure. It is a risk factor for the development of asthma. Rhinitis can a have major impact on quality of life, including sleep impairment and decreased work and school performance. It is also one of the most common chronic conditions affecting people in the United States with estimates of 35 to 50 million people affected; incidences are increasing, especially among the pediatric population (Muraro, Lemanske, Hellings, et al., 2016).

Assessment

Common symptoms of allergic rhinitis include congestion, sneezing, nasal engorgement, and profuse watery nasal discharge. The mucous membrane of the nose is generally paler than normal. It may be edematous, adding to nasal congestion. The eyes tend to water. The conjunctivae may be pruritic, often with a distinctive pebbly appearance, called cobblestoning. Children constantly rub their noses in an upward motion, termed an "allergic salute." Over a long period, rubbing the nose this way leads to a horizontal crease across the tip of the nose, called an allergic crease or Dennie line. Because of congestion in the nose, there tends to be back pressure to the blood circulation around the eye orbit,

which leads to blackened areas under the eyes, termed "allergic shiners" (Fig. 42.6).

Children older than 6 years of age (when frontal sinuses develop) may report full frontal headaches that become even more marked with adolescence. Some children have many symptoms—they feel exhausted and lethargic and do not function well in school. Recurrent otitis media may occur because of swollen pharyngeal tissue causing eustachian tube blockage. A smear of the nasal discharge will reveal an increased eosinophil count (more than 10% of the white cell count). Children with allergic rhinitis are also prone to allergic conjunctivitis.

The triggers that usually cause allergic rhinitis are pollens, molds, or irritants rather than foods or drugs. Many children are brought to a healthcare setting during peak pollen months because parents think they have a constant "summer cold." However, with an upper respiratory infection, the mucous membrane of the nose is more apt to be reddened than pale and the secretions draining from the nose are apt to be thick white or yellow rather than the thin, watery secretions of allergic rhinitis. With an upper respiratory infection, a sore throat and cervical adenopathy may also be present, whereas these rarely accompany allergic rhinitis.

Therapeutic Management

Allergic rhinitis is managed by a three-pronged program: avoidance of offending allergens, use of pharmacologic agents (antihistamines, leukotriene inhibitors, or corticosteroids), and/or immunotherapy. It may be impossible for some children to avoid all the allergens that cause symptoms because the child has sensitivity to so many allergens. If children always show symptoms at one particular time of the year, parents may be able to carry out environmental control for that period of the year to limit symptoms.

Parents usually ask how sick children should be before they need to see an allergist about skin testing and definitive treatment. As a rule, if the child's symptoms are increasing in intensity, if there is associated lower respiratory tract involvement, or if the condition interferes with activities in which the child wants to participate, the child needs testing and treatment. Those children with minor symptoms can be managed by environmental control and medications such as antihistamines and/or intranasal steroids to reduce symptoms.

It is helpful if children and parents choose an antihistamine that causes the least amount of drowsiness so the medication does not interfere with schoolwork or, if an adolescent, with safe driving. Review with parents that if nasal antihistamine sprays are given for more than 3 days, a rebound effect can occur (the nasal mucosa becomes more edematous rather than less edematous) and symptoms will appear to worsen rather than improve.

Allergic rhinitis is often considered a minor illness by parents, something children will outgrow. However, although the condition exists, it may not be a minor illness for the child if it keeps the child from interacting with peers because going outside intensifies symptoms. Box 42.8 shows an interprofessional care map illustrating both nursing and team planning for a child with allergic rhinitis.

Figure 42.6 Back pressure to the blood circulation around the eye orbit from allergic rhinitis may lead to dark areas under the eyes (allergic shiners). The frequent rubbing of the nose in an upward direction can lead to a peculiar horizontal crease (Dennie line).

BOX 42.8

Nursing Care Planning

AN INTERPROFESSIONAL CARE MAP FOR A CHILD WITH ALLERGIC RHINITIS

Dexter Goodenough is a 6-year-old boy you meet in an ambulatory setting. His mother has just been told he has allergic rhinitis (hay fever). "Thank heavens," his mother exclaims. "I thought when I heard he had an immune system disease he had AIDS. What a relief it's only an allergy."

Family Assessment: Child lives with his mother and stepfather in a beachfront cottage. Also in the family is a brother, 8 years old; a stepbrother, 16 years old; and a paternal grandmother. His stepfather owns a jewelry store. His mother is a stay-at-home mom. Finances are rated as "not a problem."

Patient Assessment: Child has documented peanut allergy. Child's eyes are reddened and watery; nose drains a clear discharge. His mother tells you he frequently has a headache and is constantly listless. Other children at school have started to bully him because of his appearance. His grades are "terrible" because the minute he gets to school, his symptoms begin. Dexter is prescribed an antihistamine and environmental control.

Nursing Diagnosis: Situational low self-esteem related to feelings of inadequacy and embarrassment

Outcome Criteria: Patient states he is able to function in school despite allergy symptoms and discomfort; is taking active measures to avoid allergens; will report bullying to school official.

Team Member Responsible	Assessment	Intervention	Rationale	Expected Outcome
Activities of Daily Living, Including Safety				
Nurse	Assess if Dexter has an epinephrine auto-injector to manage his peanut allergy at home, at school, and during day-care or after-school events.	Obtain a prescription for epinephrine auto-injectors and ensure that the family has the resources to obtain the devices. Demonstrate the proper use of the auto-injector and provide the family and school with a written anaphylaxis management plan.	Epinephrine is necessary to maintain a safe environment for food-allergic children.	Dexter has access to epinephrine at home, at school, and during activities outside his home. All of the adults responsible for Dexter's care throughout his day will know when and how to administer epinephrine in the case of an allergic reaction.
Nurse	Assess what Dexter's classroom is like to identify potential allergens because child's symptoms are most intense when he is at school.	Discuss potential source of allergens with mother; ask her to meet with teacher to see if modifications could be made.	Environmental control can reduce the number of allergens that cause symptoms.	Mother visits classroom as necessary to suggest changes such as moving Dexter's seat further away from the hamster cage.
Teamwork and Collaboration				
Nurse/primary healthcare provider	Assess if child's symptoms could be reduced with hyposensitization.	Arrange a consultation with allergist about the possibility of hyposensitization.	Hyposensitization can greatly reduce allergy symptoms if specific allergens can be identified.	Parent and child meet with allergist to discuss the possibility of sublingual hyposensitization if antihistamine is not effective.
Procedures/Medications for Quality Improvement				
Nurse	Assess if child has had experience with taking medicine.	Help mother set up a medicine chart that will help with antihistamine adherence.	Allergy medicine is most effective when it is taken conscientiously.	Parent states she will be conscientious about antihistamine administration.

Nutrition

Nurse/nutritionist	Ask the child how he manages the peanut allergy.	Review with the mother how to read labels to detect the presence of peanut in foods. Review potential hidden sources of peanut allergen in baked goods, restaurant, and prepared foods.	Most food reactions are the result of accidental exposure to offending allergens.	Mother and child describe how to read a food label for the presence of peanut allergen as well as ways to avoid accidental exposure to peanut ingestion.

Patient-Centered Care

Nurse	Assess environmental aspects at home that could be causing the child's symptoms.	Discuss environmental control with parents.	Reducing allergens in the home can also aid in reducing the child's symptoms.	Parents agree to any modifications necessary in their home.
Nurse	Assess if the child is exposed to secondary smoke in the home.	Educate family on the damage that secondary smoke can cause.	Secondary smoke is a potent allergen that also contributes to lung and heart disease.	Parents agree to make their home smoke free.

Psychosocial/Spiritual/Emotional Needs

Nurse/social work counselor	Assess the extent of ridicule the child undergoes at school.	Discuss coping measures with child; urge mother to report bullying to school authorities.	Psychological health is as important as physical health.	Child describes experiences at school are improving; states he is no longer bullied about allergy symptoms.

Informatics for Seamless Healthcare Planning

Nurse	Assess if parent has other questions about child's allergies.	Schedule a follow-up visit for reevaluation of new medication.	A range of medicine types are available for allergy control; therefore, if one isn't effective, another can be selected and prescribed.	Mother states she understands the importance of a follow-up visit and will keep appointment.

QSEN Checkpoint Question 42.5

QUALITY IMPROVEMENT

Dexter is prone to allergies. When planning his care, what desired outcome should the nurse prioritize?
  a. Dexter states that his symptoms do not interfere with being able to play with his friends.
  b. Dexter is able to describe the cause of his allergic response.
  c. Dexter states that he no longer has allergies.
  d. Dexter states he enjoys taking medicine to prevent his allergy symptoms.

Look in Appendix A for the best answer and rationale.

PERENNIAL ALLERGIC RHINITIS

Allergic rhinitis becomes perennial (year round) when the allergen is one that is present in the environment year round, such as house dust mites or pet hair. Although the child's symptoms may not result in the obvious distress associated with seasonal allergic rhinitis, the child needs treatment just as much because the symptoms otherwise may never go away. In addition, serous otitis media can accompany the disorder as a long-term consequence (see Chapter 50). Because the agent that causes perennial allergic rhinitis is often something in the house, environmental control as well as SLIT can play a big role in the control of the allergic symptoms (Papadopoulos, Bernstein, Demoly, et al., 2015).

ATOPIC DERMATITIS (INFANTILE ECZEMA)

Atopic dermatitis is a highly pruritic, chronic inflammatory skin disease that is often the first manifestation of allergic disease. Many children with atopic dermatitis will go on to develop allergic rhinitis and asthma. Food allergy is a major trigger of atopic dermatitis in infants. Any infant who presents with atopic dermatitis needs to have a thorough food allergy evaluation. Atopic dermatitis can have a significant impact on quality of life for children and their families. This disorder involves intense pruritus and associated scratching that disturbs sleep. Sweating, heat, tight clothing, and contact irritants such as soap tend to increase the pruritus associated with eczema. Symptoms may be more annoying in the winter when the skin dries out and heavier clothing is worn. Other children have eczema triggered by sweating and find the humid, summer months more difficult (Muraro et al., 2016).

Assessment

Atopic dermatitis is a complex inflammatory process that involves an epidermal barrier defect. Children develop papular and vesicular skin eruptions with surrounding erythema. The vesicles rupture and exude yellow, sticky secretions that form crusts on the skin as they dry. Because the lesions are extremely pruritic, the child scratches and further irritates the lesions, causing linear excoriations. Secondary infections of open lesions may then occur. As the infected lesions heal, the skin becomes depigmented and lichenified (shiny), and dry, flaky scales form. If a secondary infection occurs, the infant may have a low-grade fever and pus-filled lesions, and local lymph nodes may be enlarged.

The common sites for lesions change as the child grows and develops dexterity. Infants usually present with rash on the face, neck, and extensor surfaces (Fig. 42.7). Infants with atopic dermatitis will rub their face, arms, and legs to relieve the intense itching. As children develop dexterity, they focus on flexural folds of the extremities and neck. Because the lesions feel so uncomfortable, children with infantile atopic dermatitis become fussy and irritable. They may not eat well because of this generalized discomfort. The combination of poor sleep patterns, poor intake, and an increase need of energy to repair damaged skin can result in a decrease in nutritional status.

Although infantile atopic dermatitis is generally diagnosed based on a family history (by considering other allergic individuals in the family) and noticing the characteristic lesions and their patterns, it is sometimes difficult to distinguish from seborrheic dermatitis (cradle cap; see Chapter 29). The findings in seborrheic dermatitis and infantile atopic dermatitis are contrasted in Table 42.4. A child with seborrheic dermatitis needs little therapy than soaking the scales in mineral oil and then lifting them away; infants with infantile atopic dermatitis must be referred for long-term therapy.

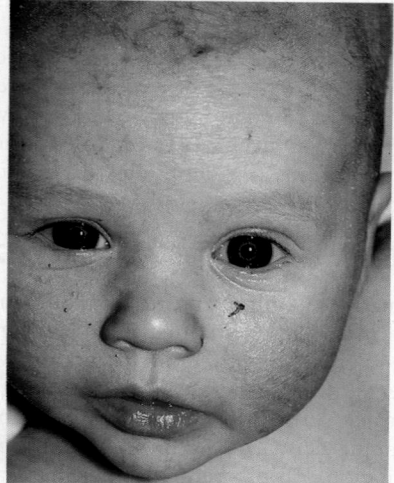

Figure 42.7   An infant with atopic dermatitis. (From Goodheart, H. P. [2003]. *Goodheart's photoguide of common skin disorders* [2nd ed.]. Philadelphia, PA: Lippincott Williams & Wilkins.)

TABLE 42.4 COMPARISON OF SEBORRHEIC DERMATITIS AND ATOPIC DERMATITIS

Finding	Seborrheic Dermatitis	Atopic Dermatitis
Age at onset	0–6 months	2–6 months
Length of disease	Rarely 1 year	2–3 years
Mood of child	Happy; parents happy	Irritable; parents tired
Location of lesions	Scalp, behind ears, near umbilicus	Cheeks, extensor surfaces, some flexor surfaces
Types of lesions	Salmon-colored erythematous lesions with greasy scales	Papulovesicular erythematous lesions with weeping and crusting
Itching	No	Severe
Depigmentation	No	Yes
Lichenification	No	Yes
White dermographism	No	Yes
Eosinophilia	No nasal mucus or blood eosinophilia	Nasal mucus or blood eosinophilia
IgE serum levels	Low	High

Therapeutic Management

The treatment of atopic dermatitis is aimed at reducing the amount of allergen exposure, if such allergens can be identified. The most likely foods to which infants are allergic are milk, eggs, and peanuts. The use of elimination diets to identify food allergens is discussed later in this chapter. A second major consideration in treatment is aimed at reducing pruritus so children do not irritate lesions and cause secondary infections by scratching. Microbial colonization and superinfection increase pruritus contributing to the scratch-itch-scratch cycle and can justify additional antimicrobial treatment. Hydrating the skin by bathing or applying wet dressings (moistened with tap water or Burow's solution) for 15 to 20 minutes, followed by the application of a barrier to seal in the moisture is helpful. In children who develop frequent secondary infections, weekly use of dilute bleach baths can be very effective (Schneider, Tilles, Lio, et al., 2013).

Regardless of the mode of hydration, the skin should still be wet or moist when applying lubricants. While infants are having wet dressings applied, be conscientious that they don't become chilled, especially if a large portion of the body is to be covered with the dressings. Use a stockinette dressing with holes cut out for the eyes, nose, and mouth pulled over the head to hold wet dressings in place so you don't have to use any form of tape. To prevent corneal irritation, be careful that dressings don't come in contact with the eyes. Antihistamine can be useful to reduce itching. Low potency steroids can be used for maintenance with intermittent and high-dose topical steroids for exacerbations. Intermittent and high-dose topical steroids should not be applied to face, eyelids, or genitalia, and they need to be used sparingly in young infants. Although absorption with topical application is limited, some absorption does occur with the intermittent and high-dose topical steroids and can suppress adrenal gland functioning. Topical calcineurin inhibitors tacrolimus and pimecrolimus are also useful in atopic dermatitis management. Relapsing atopic dermatitis and severe refractory cases of atopic dermatitis may require long-term, anti-inflammatory therapy with intermittent use of systemic anti-inflammatory or immunosuppressive treatment (Wollenberg, Oranje, Deleuran, et al., 2016).

Nursing Diagnoses and Related Interventions

Nursing Diagnosis: Risk for impaired parenting related to feelings of inadequacy secondary to infant's chronic atopic dermatitis

Outcome Evaluation: Parents express confidence in their ability to follow recommended therapy; express positive aspects of infant; hold and interact with infant warmly.

Parents of children with infantile atopic dermatitis need a great deal of support through the course of the disease because infants can become extremely irritable from the constant pruritus. No matter how hard parents try, they do not seem to be able to make their child happy. Parents need a listening ear so they can vent these concerns and maintain their self-esteem as parents. Attending support groups with other parents also can help meet this need.

Nursing Diagnosis: Impaired skin integrity related to infantile atopic dermatitis

Outcome Evaluation: Infant does not scratch lesions; parents state infant is less irritable and easier to care for; lesions show signs of healing.

Skin hydration with liberal use of moisturizers is essential to prevent excessive skin dryness. Be certain that parents know that the infant should soak in the bath for approximately 15 to 30 minutes and then be patted dry, not rubbed, so lesions are not aggravated. The moisture must immediately be applied to seal in the moisture to help prevent dryness and avoid evaporation which contributes to pruritus. Caution them not to use soap for bathing because it can be drying.

Suggest that parents trim the infant's fingernails short or cover the hands with cotton socks to prevent scratching. Let them know that exposure to the herpes virus can cause a generalized reaction. This means that they should screen babysitters and/or alert childcare personnel with active herpes lesions not to care for the infant while atopic dermatitis is active.

In most infants, the lesions of infantile atopic dermatitis clear by the time they are 3 years old. Unless secondary infection with scarring has occurred, the skin surface will not be marked. Many of these children go on to develop other allergies, however. In the preschool years, parents may report that the child has "one cold after another" (allergic rhinitis). By early school years, the child may show signs of asthma.

ATOPIC DERMATITIS IN THE OLDER CHILD

Atopic dermatitis that occurs at later ages is prominent on the flexor surface of the extremities and on the dorsal surfaces of the wrists and ankles. It often occurs in the eyebrows; if the child scratches the lesions, hair loss and scant eyebrows can result. Depigmentation or hyperpigmentation is usually noticed as lesions fade; lichenification can be marked. Often, the child's fingernails have a glossy sheen caused by the buffing action of constant rubbing and scratching. In some children, an "itch–scratch cycle" occurs as a response to stress and leads to an exacerbation of symptoms. For example, children, who feel pressured in school to achieve or who are upset because their parents are about to be divorced, rub their skin, a nervous, comforting mannerism; the rubbing or scratching leads to irritation of lesions. The lesions itch intensely, and the child scratches even more vigorously because of the increased discomfort. The accelerated scratching leads to an increased number of lesions, the increased number of lesions leads to more scratching, and so on.

Therapeutic Management

Atopic dermatitis is a difficult disease for older children because they realize the scratching leads to depigmentation or lichenification, but they are unable to stop scratching because the itching is so intense. Adolescents, especially, are acutely aware of their appearance, so this can be an especially difficult illness for them. Suggest that adolescents use only a prescription soap (or none at all) to prevent skin drying. Swimming in chlorinated pools may also help for those who experience chronic secondary infections. When children swim in chlorinated pools, encourage them to shower well afterward to remove chlorine from the skin as well as to apply a skin emollient and moisturizer after the shower. After a period of activity in which sweating occurs, such as gymnastics, suggest the child take a shower to remove perspiration so this doesn't irritate the skin. Avoiding tight clothing at the flexor portions of the extremities is also important.

Medical treatment for older children is basically the same as for the infant with atopic dermatitis: keeping the skin hydrated and identifying allergens and any psychological problems that are initiating an itch–scratch cycle. The application of hydrocortisones or phototherapy with ultraviolet light both can make a big difference in helping lesions improve.

An evaluation for the older child with atopic dermatitis should include an assessment of not only how well the lesions are healing but also how well the child is adjusting to school and family in light of having this irritating disorder.

What If . . . 42.2

When Dexter had atopic dermatitis (infantile eczema) as an infant, almost his entire face was covered with weeping, crusting lesions and his forehead was lined with scratch marks. His mother was exhausted because Dexter never slept because of the constant itching. What suggestions could the nurse have made to Dexter's mother for making him more comfortable? What could the nurse suggest his mother do for herself?

Drug and Food Allergies

DRUG ALLERGIES

One of the hazards of giving any medication is the risk that a child may experience a reaction to it or exhibit allergic symptoms (Muraro et al., 2017). Because reactions to drugs differ, it is important to be familiar with the differences between an allergic reaction, a toxic reaction, or a known side effect to a drug.

A *toxic reaction* is one that occurs when a child has received too much of a drug. *Side effects* of drugs are those that are known to occur in addition to a therapeutic effect. When an *allergic effect* occurs, a range of unpredictable symptoms occurs. With the exception of antibiotics, acetylsalicylic acid (aspirin), and NSAIDs, allergies rarely occur to orally administered drugs. Children with atopic diseases appear to be most prone to allergic drug reactions, although anyone can have such a reaction.

A drug itself may not be an allergen, but when the drug combines with body protein, it becomes an allergen, which is why allergic responses occur not with the initial administration of a drug but only after the protein interaction (hapten formation or sensitivity) has occurred.

Skin manifestations seen frequently include urticaria, angioedema, allergic contact dermatitis, flushing, pruritus, and/or purpura. Respiratory symptoms include wheezing or rhinitis. Thrombocytopenia and hemolytic anemia may develop. Anaphylactic shock may occur. Children with a known drug allergy should wear a medical identification bracelet stating the drug to which they are sensitive.

Injectable drugs that are most frequently involved in allergic reactions are cephalosporins and penicillin. In most instances, discontinuing the drug or never again administering the drug or vaccine is the only therapy needed. If urticaria, an antihistamine such as diphenhydramine hydrochloride (Benadryl) may be helpful in relieving the symptoms. If anaphylaxis results, the treatment would be the administration of epinephrine.

FOOD ALLERGIES

Food allergies are an abnormal immune response caused by exposure to a particular food protein. They can be IgE-mediated, cell-mediated, or mixed reactions, although IgE-mediated (type I hypersensitivity) reactions account for most food reactions (Robison & Pongracic, 2012). Symptoms of food allergies vary greatly among children, but cutaneous reactions to foods including urticaria, angioedema, flushing, and pruritus are some of the most common presentations of food allergy (Sampson, Aceves, Bock, et al., 2014).

Type I hypersensitivity reactions can manifest themselves only seconds after an offending food is eaten. Additional symptoms may develop over a period of 2 hours, often making the offending food difficult to recognize. Symptoms can begin gradually and crescendo to a full blown anaphylactic event. Although not every food allergic reaction develops into anaphylaxis, food is the number 1 cause of anaphylaxis, and prior reaction severity does not predict future reactions. Every child with a history of significant symptoms with a food trigger needs an epinephrine auto-injector and an anaphylaxis action plan. The most common foods that cause immediate allergy symptoms include peanut, egg whites, milk, wheat, soy, seafood, and tree nuts. If children are allergic to milk, caution them that they are allergic to milk products such as ice cream, yogurt, and cheese as well. Children who are allergic to eggs often cannot eat any foods that contain eggs, such as egg noodles or mayonnaise.

Children with milk and egg allergy may be able to tolerate baked good that contain milk and/or egg. Because the exposure to high heat destroys the conformational epitopes, about 70% of children with a diagnosed milk or egg allergy tolerate those proteins after they have been baked in foods such as muffins and cakes (Bloom, Huang, Bencharitiwong, et al., 2014). Because milk and egg avoidance present a major challenge to families and eliminates important dietary proteins, children who are avoiding milk or egg should be evaluated for tolerance to baked milk and baked egg.

Assessment

For some children, the food allergy diagnosis is clear. Sensitization can occur as food protein cross the placenta or via breast milk. For some children, the first "known" exposure to milk, egg, or peanut causes an immediate type I response such hives, swelling, and vomiting. These reactions can be anaphylactic. Other reactions are less intense and may involve things such as an increase in atopic dermatitis. Young children may not be able to describe why they do not enjoy eating a particular food, but they do tend to avoid foods that affect them, which often earns them the reputation of being "fussy eaters." This is not diagnostic of food allergies, however, because children may refuse to eat foods as a form of toddler rebellion or may be reported as fussy eaters because parents are expecting them to eat more than their small size requires.

Encouraging a child or the parents to keep a food diary or a record of everything a child eats each day and then documenting if any symptoms occur is often the best way to spot offending foods that don't present with immediate reactions. A food that is found on lists when symptoms were few but not on days when the child is in distress is not an offending food. A food that appears only on "bad days," however, can be strongly suspected as being an allergen.

An elimination diet can be an effective tool to detect mild food allergies. The suspect food is eliminated from the child's diet to see if symptoms resolve. If the symptoms reoccur when the suspect food is added back to the diet, the food is the likely culprit. Because most of the foods that are implicated in food allergy are major food proteins such as milk or egg, eliminating foods has significant implications to the child's nutrition. For example, milk is a major source of vitamin D and calcium. Children who are forced to avoid all milk and milk products need a vitamin D and calcium supplement. To establish whether the problem is truly a milk allergy, milk can be reintroduced under medical observation every 6 to 12 months. If the problem is a true milk allergy, symptoms will recur.

Therapeutic Management

The easiest treatment for a food allergy is to eliminate offending foods from the child's diet. This is difficult when the foods are great in number or if, like milk, wheat, or eggs, are found in many products. If many foods are involved, the child's nutrition status (whether the child is growing adequately and increasing in weight) needs to be assessed at healthcare visits.

Urge parents to become conscientious shoppers and read labels carefully to be certain the foods they are buying do not contain products to which their child is sensitive. Help school-age children learn to choose foods they can safely eat at the school cafeteria or at summer camp to avoid reactions. The National Institutes of Health expert panel has created guidelines for the diagnosis and management of food allergy. The guidelines are available at https://www.niaid.nih.gov /diseases-conditions/guidelines-clinicians-and-patients-food -allergy.

VACCINES

Mild local reactions and fever after vaccinations are common and do not contraindicate future doses. Anaphylactic reactions to vaccines are rare. Children who are egg allergic can and should receive injectable influenza vaccine (Kelso, Greenhawt, & Li, 2013) as well as the MMR vaccine. The yellow fever vaccine requires special precautions for children with egg allergy.

MILK INTOLERANCE

Milk is one of the leading causes of type I reactions to foods. However, not all milk reactions are IgE-mediated reactions. Milk intolerance usually presents in infancy and is typified by failure to gain weight, diarrhea, perhaps vomiting, and abdominal pain. Because these symptoms also occur in gastrointestinal disorders, infants with colic (characterized by abdominal pain, no change in stools, and no failure to gain weight), those with lactase deficiency, or those with a gastroenteritis infection (have nausea and vomiting) may be incorrectly diagnosed as having a milk allergy. Most infants can tolerate breast milk, even if the mother consumes milk in her diet. Supplementing with a hydrolyzed protein-based formula usually decreases symptoms dramatically.

PEANUT HYPERSENSITIVITY

Peanut and tree nut ingestions are the cause of more than 85% of fatalities caused by food anaphylaxis in the United States (Robison & Pongracic, 2012). Adults who care for children who are food allergic including day-care providers, coaches, grandparents, and school personnel need to be very aware of this danger and need anaphylaxis action plans and epinephrine auto-injectors available at all times (Pistiner & Lee, 2012).

Because peanut allergy affects 1% to 3% of children, and peanut is a major contributor to food allergic reactions and anaphylaxis, there is significant interest in preventing peanut allergy rather than dealing with the consequences once the allergy has developed. In the past, recommendations to prevent peanut allergy included avoiding peanut allergen through the first 3 years of life. There is emerging evidence to contradict this and support early rather than delayed introduction of peanut, especially in "high-risk" infants. Children at "high risk" for developing peanut allergy include those 4 to 11 months old diagnosed with egg allergy and/or those with severe eczema. High-risk infants require skin testing and possible observed ingestion of peanut prior to home introduction (Du Toit, Roberts, Sayre, et al., 2015; Togias, Cooper, Acebal, et al., 2017).

QSEN Checkpoint Question 42.6

EVIDENCE-BASED PRACTICE

Food allergies are an important concern for nurses working in childcare or preschool settings because such sites may be where a child eats allergenic food and experiences a possibly fatal reaction. Early, appropriate administration of epinephrine for the treatment of the symptoms of anaphylaxis can significantly reduce the likelihood of anaphylaxis-related hospital admission. Delayed administration of epinephrine contributes to anaphylaxis-related fatalities. Epinephrine is significantly less likely to be injected in food-induced anaphylaxis than in venom-induced anaphylaxis. Reasons for failure to administer epinephrine include poor perception of the severity of symptoms or patient refusal (Simons et al., 2015). Based on the previous study and the fact that Dexter is allergic to peanuts, which statement by Dexter's mother should cause a nurse the most concern?

a. "I pack his lunch every day so I'll know what he eats."
b. "He doesn't need one of those EpiPen things. They are too expensive, and it's not like he has a beesting allergy. If he goes to a party, I'll ask if peanuts will be served."
c. "I know how to read food labels to limit Dexter's food to things I know are safe."

Look in Appendix A for the best answer and rationale.

Stinging Insect Hypersensitivity

Children may have severe hypersensitivity reactions to stings from bees, wasps, hornets, or yellow jackets (Yavuz, Sahiner, Buyuktiryaki, et al., 2013). Although a serum sickness reaction may occur, the usual reaction to these stings is an immediate type I hypersensitivity reaction (anaphylaxis).

THERAPEUTIC MANAGEMENT

The best way to protect children with allergies to stinging insects is to begin hyposensitization by immunotherapy against insect stings after the first reaction. An extract of wasp, yellow jacket, hornet, and honeybee venom accomplishes this.

The child who has not been hyposensitized must be treated immediately after a sting by an injection of epinephrine. If children are going on a hiking or camping expedition away from parents, caution parents that their child needs to learn to self-administer epinephrine or be certain that a responsible adult accompanying them will be able to do it. Someone at school should be given the responsibility of administering epinephrine if a child is stung during recess or an outside gym period. If a school nurse is in attendance, this certainly is the nurse's responsibility. In schools where there is no full-time nurse, however, another person must be designated and taught how to give the injection. If the child has an antihistamine medication in addition to epinephrine, antihistamine should never be taken in place of epinephrine. Ice applied to the site minimizes the amount of venom absorbed. After the initial epinephrine administration, the child should be transported to a healthcare setting in case additional epinephrine is needed (the initial injection will be effective for only approximately 20 minutes).

Teach children who are allergic to stinging insects ways to avoid them such as not using scented preparations such as hair spray, deodorants, lotions, or perfume because these attract insects. They also should not go outside barefoot because bees are often found in ground clover. They should not be assigned household chores such as mowing the lawn or weeding the garden, actions that might stir up bees. Because insects tend to cluster around garbage containers, taking out the trash is also an inappropriate chore for these children. Whenever they are out of doors, they should have a fast-acting insecticide handy to use on flying insects. Encourage them to refrain from drinking out of open soda cans at outside activities because bees and wasps are drawn to the sugar in the soda, but the child may be unaware that an insect has entered the open can.

🍃 *What If . . . 42.3*

Dexter's school does not have a plan for managing students with immune disorders. After obtaining a parent's permission to discuss his care with the school nurse, how could the nurse involve the school nurse more in Dexter's plan of care?

Contact Dermatitis

Contact dermatitis is an example of a delayed or type IV hypersensitivity response; it is a reaction to skin contact with an allergen (a substance irritating to the child only with prior sensitization). The first reaction is generally erythema, followed by the development of intensely pruritic papules and then vesicles. The allergen causing the irritation is often suggested by the part of the child's body that is affected. For example, dermatitis from a diaper-washing compound appears in the diaper area. Allergy to cosmetics appears on the face. Oozing at the site of pierced ears suggests an allergy to the nickel used in earring posts. Poison ivy appears on the hands and arms where the child brushed against the plant (Fig. 42.8). Children who have had repeated surgeries such as those with spina bifida are at high risk of developing allergies to latex and will have lesions where the latex touches them (Martin, 2015).

ASSESSMENT

Patch testing may be used to identify contact dermatitis allergens. A child should not be taking a corticosteroid at the time of patch testing because these drugs reduce delayed hypersensitivity reactions. However, a child may continue to take antihistamines or sympathomimetic drugs because these do not interfere with this testing. After 48 hours, the patches used for testing are removed and the reactions are graded 1+ to 4+, the same as in regular skin testing.

THERAPEUTIC MANAGEMENT

Treatment for contact dermatitis consists of removing the identified allergen from the child's environment. In children, this is generally not difficult to do. In adults, because allergens may be work related, this is much more difficult.

Dressings moistened with water, saline, or Burow's solution relieve itching. Calamine and Caladryl lotions are also

Figure 42.8   Poison ivy on a child's hand. (© Beckman/Custom Medical Stock Photograph.)

generally effective. Hydrocortisone lotions or creams reduce itching and also promote healing. Baths with baking soda or oatmeal in the water may be helpful if a large area of the body is involved. Some children may need a sedative to relieve their discomfort during the period of intense pruritus. As with all allergies, nurses need to document contact allergies on health records so all healthcare providers can be aware of them and guard against a reaction.

🍃 *What If . . . 42.4*

A nurse is particularly interested in exploring one of the 2020 National Health Goals with respect to immune disorders and children (see Box 42.1). What would be a possible research topic pertinent to this goal that would be applicable to Dexter and his family and that would also advance evidence-based practice?

Unfolding Patient Stories: Charlie Snow • Part 1

Charlie Snow, a 6-year-old with a known hypersensitivity to perfumes and dyes and an allergy to peanuts, comes for a routine clinic visit accompanied by his aunt. He is living with his aunt and uncle while his parents are serving in the military. The nurse discovers a rash in multiple areas underneath his clothing. What questions should the nurse ask to determine the cause of the rash? What education should the nurse provide for the aunt, who has limited knowledge of allergies and childcare experience? (Charlie Snow's story continues in Chapter 55.)

Care for Charlie and other patients in a realistic virtual environment: *vSim for Nursing* (thepoint.lww.com /vSimMaternityPed). Practice documenting these patients' care in DocuCare (thepoint.lww.com/DocuCareEHR).

KEY POINTS FOR REVIEW

- An antigen is a foreign substance capable of stimulating an immune response. The immune system protects the body from invasion by such substances.

- Humoral immunity refers to immunity created by antibody production originated by B lymphocytes. Cell-mediated immunity refers to T-lymphocyte involvement.

- Autoimmunity results from an inability to distinguish self from nonself, causing the immune system to carry out immune responses against normal cells.

- HIV/AIDS is spread by the retrovirus HIV through blood and body secretions. Conscientious use of standard infection precautions is essential to prevent transmission.

- Allergic disorders occur as a result of an abnormal antigen–antibody response. These generally are long-term disorders, and children must participate in their own care to remain well, such as avoiding allergens or conscientiously taking a medication to suppress reactions. Involving children from the start both helps them play an active role in their own care and helps to plan nursing care that not only meets Quality & Safety Education for Nurses (QSEN) competencies but that also best meets a family's total needs.

- Anaphylactic shock is an acute type I hypersensitivity reaction characterized by extreme vasodilation and bronchoconstriction. If action is not taken immediately, the reaction can be fatal. Epinephrine is the standard of care for treatment.

- Atopic disorders include allergic rhinitis, atopic dermatitis, and asthma.

- Environmental control refers to ways to reduce the number of allergens to which children are exposed.

- Hyposensitization by subcutaneous or sublingual immunotherapy is a method to increase the plasma concentration of IgG antibodies to prevent or block IgE antibody formation and allergic symptoms.

CRITICAL THINKING CARE STUDY

Kayla is a 14-year-old girl with a diagnosis of multiple allergies, among them eggs, shellfish, and cats. Although she admits she doesn't take her prescribed antihistamine on a regular basis (it wouldn't be "cool" for her friends to see it in her purse), she's concerned because her runny nose and frequent cough have been growing worse over the last 6 months. Because she finds her family "old fashioned," she spends a lot of time at her new best friend's house. The community where she lives is a coastal one where shellfish is a popular food; her best friend's mother is a waitress at a seafood restaurant. Kayla had an episode last month when she was taken to the local emergency room with sudden shortness of breath because she was eating at the restaurant with a group of friends and "forgot" about her allergy.

1. What may be a reason that Kayla's allergy symptoms are worsening?

2. How can you work with Kayla to create a plan of care that minimizes the impact of her allergies on her social life and development and that creates a safe environment for her as well?

3. Kayla has been advised to carry an epinephrine auto-injector with her at all times. She usually "forgets," however, and leaves it at home. How would you approach Kayla to teach her the importance of having the epinephrine auto-injector with her at all times? What facts or safety concerns would you want to discuss with Kayla?

RELATED RESOURCES

Explore these additional resources to enhance learning for this chapter:

- Student resources on thePoint, including answers to the What If . . . and Critical Thinking Care Study questions, http://thepoint.lww.com/Flagg8e
- Adaptive learning powered by PrepU, http://thepoint.lww.com/prepu

REFERENCES

Accetta Pedersen, D., Verbsky, J., & Routes, J. (2011). Screening newborns for primary T-cell immunodeficiencies: Consensus and controversy. *Expert Review of Clinical Immunology, 7*(6), 761–768.

Bloom, K. A., Huang, F. R., Bencharitiwong, R., et al. (2014). Effect of heat treatment on milk and egg proteins allergenicity. *Pediatric Allergy and Immunology, 25*(8), 740–746.

Boyd, S. (2011). Management of HIV infection in treatment-naive patients: A review of the most current recommendations. *American Journal of Health-System Pharmacy, 68*(11), 991–1001.

Centers for Disease Control and Prevention. (1994). 1994 Revised classification system of human immunodeficiency virus infection in children less than 13 years of age. *Morbidity & Mortality Weekly Report, 43*(RR-12), 1–10.

Commins, S. P. (2017). Outpatient emergencies: Anaphylaxis. *The Medical Clinics of North America, 101*(3), 521–536.

de Souza Campos Fernandes, S., Ribeiro de Andrade, C., & da Cunha Ibiapina, C. (2014). Application of Peak Nasal Inspiratory Flow reference values in the treatment of allergic rhinitis. *Rhinology, 52*(2), 133–136.

Du Toit, G., Roberts, G., Sayre, P. H., et al. (2015). Randomized trial of peanut consumption in infants at risk for peanut allergy. *The New England Journal of Medicine, 372*(9), 803–813.

Gay, J., Hardee, K., Croce-Galis, M., et al. (2011). What works to meet the sexual and reproductive health needs of women living with HIV/AIDS. *Journal of the International AIDS Society, 14*(1), 56.

Getahun, H., Raviglione, M., Varma, J., et al. (2012). CDC Grand Rounds: The TB/HIV syndemic. *Morbidity and Mortality Weekly Report, 61*(26), 484–489.

Hellmann, D. B., & Imboden, J. B., Jr. (2013). Musculoskeletal & immunological disorders. In M. Papadakis & S. J. McPhee (Eds.), *Current medical diagnosis & treatment* (52nd ed., pp. 809–869). New York, NY: McGraw-Hill/Lange.

Hoyt, M. J., Storm, D. S., Aaron, E., et al. (2012). Preconception and contraceptive care for women living with HIV. *Infectious Diseases in Obstetrics & Gynecology, 2012*, 604183.

Kaplan, A. P. (2012). Treatment of chronic spontaneous urticaria. *Allergy, Asthma & Immunology Research, 4*(6), 326–331.

Kelso, J. M., Greenhawt, M. J., & Li, J. T. (2013). Update on influenza vaccine of egg allergic patients. *Annals of Allergy, Asthma & Immunology, 111*(4), 301–302.

Krouse, H. (2014). Environmental controls and avoidance measures. *International Forum of Allergy & Rhinology, 4*(Suppl. 2), S32–S34.

Kwan, A., & Puck, J. M. (2015). History and current status of newborn screening for severe combined immunodeficiency. *Seminars in Perinatology, 39*(3), 194–205.

Levison, J., Williams, L., Moore, A., et al. (2011). Increasing use of rapid HIV testing in labor and delivery among women with no prenatal care: A local initiative. *Maternal and Child Health Journal, 15*(6), 822–826.

Martin, S. F. (2015). New concepts in cutaneous allergy. *Contact Dermatitis, 72*, 2–10.

McLean, S., Chandler, D., Nurmatov, U., et al. (2011). Telehealthcare for asthma: A Cochrane review. *Canadian Medical Association Journal, 183*(11), E733–E742.

Muraro, A., Lemanske, R. F., Jr., Castells, M., et al. (2017). Precision medicine in allergic disease-food allergy, drug allergy, and anaphylaxis-PRACTALL document of the European Academy of Allergy and Clinical Immunology and the American Academy of Allergy, Asthma and Immunology. *Allergy, 72*(7), 1006–1021.

Muraro, A., Lemanske, R. F., Jr., Hellings, P. W., et al. (2016). Precision medicine in patients with allergic diseases: Airway diseases and atopic dermatitis—PRACTALL document of the European Academy of Allergy and Clinical Immunology and the American Academy of Allergy, Asthma, & Immunology. *The Journal of Allergy and Clinical Immunology, 137*(5), 1347–1358.

Natchu, U. C., Liu, E., Duggan, C., et al. (2012). Exclusive breastfeeding reduces risk of mortality in infants up to 6 mo of age born to HIV-positive Tanzanian women. *The American Journal of Clinical Nutrition*, *96*(5), 1071–1078.

Nayak, A. S., Berger, W. E., LaForce, C. F., et al. (2017). Randomized, placebo-controlled study of cetirizine and loratadine in children with seasonal allergic rhinitis. *Allergy and Asthma Proceedings, 38*(3), 222–230.

Papadopoulos, N. G., Bernstein, J. A., Demoly, P., et al. (2015). Phenotypes and endotypes of rhinitis and their impact on management: A PRACTALL report. *Allergy, 70*(5), 474–494.

Pistiner, M., & Lee, J. J. (2012). Creating a new community of support for students with food allergies. *NASN School Nurse, 27*(5), 260–266.

Robison, R., & Pongracic, J. (2012). Food allergy. *Allergy and Asthma Proceedings, 33*(Suppl. 1), S77–S79.

Sampson, H. A., Aceves, S., Bock, S. A., et al. (2014). Food allergy: A practice parameter update—2014. *The Journal of Allergy and Clinical Immunology, 134*(5), 1016–1025.

Sawyer, S., Afifi, R., Bearinger, L., et al. (2012). Adolescence: A foundation for future health. *Lancet, 379*(9826), 1630–1640.

Schneider, L., Tilles, S., Lio, P., et al. (2013). Atopic dermatitis: A practice parameter update 2012. *The Journal of Allergy and Clinical Immunology, 131*(2), 295–299.

Sheikh, A., Simons, F. E., Barbour, V., et al. (2012). Adrenaline auto-injectors for the treatment of anaphylaxis with and without cardiovascular collapse in the community. *Cochrane Database of Systematic Reviews*, (8), CD008935.

Shulman, S., Yogev, R., & Murphy, S. B. (2011). 30 Years of pediatric HIV/AIDS treatment: A time of breakthroughs, innovation. *Pediatrics Annals, 40*(7), 340–341.

Simons, F. E., Ardusso, L. R., Bilò, M. B., et al. (2014). International consensus on (ICON) anaphylaxis. *The World Allergy Organization Journal, 7*, 9.

Simons, F. E., Ebisawa, M., Sanchez-Borges, M., et al. (2015). 2015 Update of the evidence base: World Allergy Organization anaphylaxis guidelines. *The World Allergy Organization Journal, 8*(1), 32.

Smith, S. (2011). Infectious diseases. In K. J. Marcdante, R. M. Kliegman, H. B. Jenson, et al. (Eds.), *Nelson essentials of pediatrics* (6th ed., pp. 355–462). Philadelphia, PA: Saunders/Elsevier.

Spiro, D. B. (2012). Early onset multiple sclerosis: A review for nurse practitioners. *Journal of Pediatric Health Care, 26*(6), 399–408.

Togias, A., Cooper, S. F., Acebal, M. L., et al. (2017). Addendum guidelines for the prevention of peanut allergy in the United States: Report of the National Institute of Allergy and Infectious Diseases-sponsored expert panel. *The Journal of Allergy and Clinical Immunology, 139*(1), 29–44.

Tsabouri, S., Mavroudi, A., Feketea, G., et al. (2017). Subcutaneous and sublingual immunotherapy in allergic asthma in children. *Frontiers in Pediatrics, 5*, 82.

U.S. Department of Health and Human Services. (2010). *Healthy people 2020.* Washington, DC: Author.

Wollenberg, A., Oranje, A., Deleuran, M., et al. (2016). ETFAD/EADV Eczema task force 2015 position paper on diagnosis and treatment of atopic dermatitis in adult and paediatric patients. *Journal of the European Academy of Dermatology and Venereology, 30*(5), 729–747.

Woo, C., & Bahna, S. (2011). Evaluation of the child with immune deficiency disorder. *Pediatric Annals, 40*(4), 205–211.

Yavuz, S. T., Sahiner, U. M., Buyuktiryaki, B., et al. (2013). Clinical features of children with venom allergy and risk factors for severe systemic reactions. *International Archives of Allergy and Immunology, 160*(3), 313–321.

Younger, E. M., Epland, K., Zampelli, A., et al. (2015). Primary immunodeficiency disease: A primer for PCP's. *The Nurse Practitioner, 40*(2), 1–7.

43

Nursing Care of a Family When a Child Has an Infectious Disorder

KEY TERMS

catarrhal stage
chain of infection
convalescent period
enanthem
exanthem
exotoxin
fomites
health care–associated infections
incubation period
Koplik spots

mode of transmission
nosocomial infections
portal of entry
portal of exit
prodromal period
reservoir
septicemia
susceptible host
vectors

Jack Noma, a 10-year-old boy, was admitted to the hospital yesterday for appendicitis. The morning after surgery, he broke out in a papular rash with some vesicles. He was diagnosed with varicella. His family works as migrant farm workers. His mother is not sure whether he received all of his vaccines because she did not feel comfortable giving some of them to him. "His sister is home with mono," his mother tells you. "How could our family get two infections plus appendicitis all in 1 week?"

Previous chapters described the growth and development of well children. This chapter will address the physical and psychosocial changes that can occur when children contract an infectious disorder. The clinical presentation of childhood infection varies from an asymptomatic viral infection confirmed through diagnostic testing to a critical life-threatening illness (Alter, Bennett, Koranyi, et al., 2015). It's important to know about the spread and care of these diseases to limit spread to other people.

How would you respond to Jack's mother? Is it most likely that Jack contracted this new disease while he was in the hospital or before he was admitted? What is a measure you would recommend to help reduce the household transmission of infection?

OBJECTIVES

After mastering the contents of this chapter, you should be able to:

1. Describe the causes and course of common infectious disorders of childhood.
2. Identify 2020 National Health Goals related to infectious disorders in children that nurses could help the nation achieve.
3. Assess a child with an infectious disorder.
4. Formulate nursing diagnoses for a child with an infectious disorder.
5. Establish outcomes to help a family manage an infectious disorder as well as manage seamless transitions across differing healthcare settings.
6. Using the nursing process, plan nursing care that includes the six competencies of Quality & Safety Education for Nurses (QSEN): Patient-Centered Care, Teamwork & Collaboration, Evidence-Based Practice (EBP), Quality Improvement (QI), Safety, and Informatics.
7. Plan nursing care for a child with an infectious disorder, such as helping them understand infectious precautions.
8. Evaluate expected outcomes for the achievement and effectiveness of care.
9. Integrate knowledge of infectious diseases with the interplay of nursing process, the six competencies of QSEN, and Family Nursing to achieve quality maternal and child health nursing care.

BOX 43.1

Nursing Care Planning Based on 2020 National Health Goals

Several 2020 National Health Goals address ways to prevent and reduce the incidence of infectious disease in children.

- Reduce, eliminate, or maintain elimination of vaccine-preventable diseases such as measles from 115 infected children per year to a target of 30 children per year.
- Achieve and maintain effective vaccination coverage levels for universally recommended vaccines such as the diphtheria, tetanus, and acellular pertussis (DTaP) vaccine among young children from 84% to 90%.
- Increase the number of states that use electronic data from rabies surveillance to inform public health prevention programs from 8 states to 29 states.
- Reduce central-line–associated bloodstream infections (developmental).
- Reduce invasive health care–associated methicillin-resistant *Staphylococcus aureus* (HA-MRSA) infections from 26 per 100,000 people to 6.5 per 100,000 people (U.S. Department of Health and Human Services, 2010; see www.healthypeople.gov).

Nurses can help the nation achieve these goals by educating parents about the importance of immunizations and ways to avoid infections. They can also help prevent the spread of infection in hospital units by scrupulously adhering to infection control precautions.

Although immunizations have protected an increasing number of children against infections, infectious diseases remain a leading cause of morbidity in children (Alter et al., 2015). Nurses can play a key role in reducing the incidence of these disorders by educating parents about the importance of household infection control measures and how infectious diseases are spread. Prevention measures can be successful in controlling the spread of infectious diseases, but vaccination programs have been the most effective in reducing infectious diseases in children. Nurses should understand the signs and symptoms of a variety of infections to properly triage children to reduce transmission to others. Several 2020 National Health Goals, shown in Box 43.1, relate to the prevention of infectious disorders in children.

Nursing Process Overview

FOR A CHILD WITH AN INFECTIOUS DISORDER

ASSESSMENT

Many infectious diseases have an insidious onset, whereas others present acutely with high fever and rapid deterioration. With the insidious onset of an infection, parents note behavioral, sleep, elimination, or appetite changes. They may comment, "He doesn't act like himself" or "She's not eating as well." Fever, malaise, myalgia, and arthralgia are common

associations with infectious diseases due to an increase in cytokines—leukotrienes and interleukins. The child can be contagious only before the onset of the infection, as with parvovirus B19, or may be contagious until the lesions start to dry, as with varicella. In other cases of infectious diseases, such as sepsis of the newborn or toxic shock syndrome, there is an acute onset of high fever with rapid deterioration of vital signs and organ failure. These patients are not contagious.

NURSING DIAGNOSIS

Common nursing diagnoses used with children directly related to the infectious process include:

- Pain related to pruritus from skin lesions
- Impaired skin integrity related to rash, pruritus, and scratching
- Risk for infection related to presence of infective organism in sibling or family member
- Altered body temperature (fever) related to systemic infection
- Fluid volume deficit related to insensible fluid loss from increased body temperature
- Knowledge deficit (learning) related to disease prognosis, prevention, and treatment

Additional diagnoses when children must be separated from others to prevent infection transmission might include:

- Social isolation related to precautions required to prevent infection transmission
- Deficient diversional activity related to activity restriction and precautions to prevent disease transmission

OUTCOME IDENTIFICATION AND PLANNING

Nursing outcomes for care of children with infectious disorders center around preventing disease through immunization, treating the current infection, and preventing further spread by practicing good infection control measures in the household or the medical setting. Educating parents about infection control measures and teaching them about how the particular infectious agent is spread remains critical to preventing the spread of disease in the community. There are several websites to educate families about the reduction of infectious disease including the National Foundation for Infectious Diseases (www.nfid.org), Immunization Action Coalition (http://www.immunize.org), World Health Organization (WHO) (http://www.WHO.org), and the Centers for Disease Control and Prevention (CDC) (www.cdc.gov).

IMPLEMENTATION

Nursing responsibilities when caring for a child with an infectious disorder always includes patient education regarding the disease, its management, possible complications, when to seek health care, and modes of disease transmission. Patients can use a variety of new technologies (including secure text messages, e-mail, and Skype) to transmit pictures of rashes for evaluation and management. Counseling parents about techniques to relieve the irritation of rashes and managing mild symptoms can be done over the telephone, through secure text messages, or by secure e-mail programs. The use of these technologies can allow for children with mild self-limiting illnesses to be cared for at home; however, children who are sicker and/or who appear toxic need to be brought in for a more complete evaluation. The nurse doing telephone triage must use standardized protocols to avoid missing key points in the history. Nursing responsibilities include getting a complete history including immunization status, evaluating vital signs, obtaining a history, and doing a physical assessment in order to appropriately triage patients as they arrive in the medical setting. In addition, the nurse must monitor for changes in the patient's condition, relieve symptoms such as fever, promote rest, and administer medications including antipyretics and anti-infectious agents. In the inpatient setting, planning care for a child who requires restrictions to prevent disease transmission requires thoughtful consideration to prevent boredom and promote development.

OUTCOME EVALUATION

An evaluation of outcomes for a child with an infectious disease promote a return to the child's previous state of wellness, prevent complications, prevent transmission to the family and community members, and promote the importance of hand washing in disease prevention. If one member of the family has a decreased immune response due to chemotherapy or steroid therapy, prevention of transmission takes on even greater importance.

Examples of expected outcomes that would indicate achievement of goals include:

- Child indicates relief from pruritus and pain.
- All family members remain free of signs and symptoms of the infectious disorder.
- Parent identifies appropriate diversional activities for distracting the child.
- Parent verbalizes how to prevent transmission of infectious disease to other family members and understands the importance of proper hand washing.

The Infectious Process

Pathogens are any organism that causes disease and can be classified into five types of microorganisms: viruses, bacteria, rickettsia, helminths, and fungi. The properties of these organisms are discussed in conjunction with the common diseases that they cause.

STAGES OF INFECTIOUS DISEASE

Infectious diseases follow certain stages, during which the communicability (i.e., ability to be spread to others) or severity of the illness can be predicted (Fig. 43.1).

- The **incubation period** is the time between the invasion of an organism and the onset of symptoms of infection. During this time, microorganisms grow and multiply. Incubation periods vary widely depending on the virulence of the organism, the mechanism of spread, and the host. The incubation period for tetanus, for example, is 2 to 21 days.
- A **prodromal period** is the time between the beginning of nonspecific symptoms such as malaise, low-grade fever, fatigue, and arthralgia to the onset of disease-specific symptoms such as a rash, diarrhea, and vomiting. Depending on the organism, children may be infectious (capable of spreading the microorganisms to others) during the prodromal period. During the prodromal period, therefore, infectious diseases spread readily through

Figure 43.1 The time frame for infectious diseases. Period of communicability is the time during which the disease can be transmitted to other people.

communities from a person with the disease to any susceptible individual. Fortunately, prodromal stages are generally short, ranging from hours to a few days.

- *Illness* is the stage during which specific symptoms occur. It is important to keep in mind that the body's response to infectious agents causes a variety of symptoms including fever, myalgia (muscle aches), arthralgia (joint pain without swelling), malaise, increased need for sleep, and headache, which is usually secondary to fever. There is also a site-specific reaction such as coughing, runny nose, and sore throat when a respiratory virus like rhinovirus or respiratory syncytial virus infects the respiratory tract (Mauskopf, Margulis, Samuel, et al., 2016) or diarrhea and/or vomiting when rotavirus infects the gastrointestinal tract.
- Some childhood infections will manifest with a specific rash on the skin (**exanthem**) or mucous membrane (**enanthem**) (Box 43.2).
- The **convalescent period** is the interval between when symptoms first begin to fade and when the child returns to a healthy baseline. The return to baseline will vary from child to child depending on the host, other underlying illnesses, and the type and severity of infection.

CHAIN OF INFECTION

The **chain of infection** is the method by which organisms are spread and enter a new individual to cause disease. Breaking the chain at one of its susceptible points is the most efficient way to prevent infection from spreading (Chusid & Rotar, 2016). Nurses are instrumental in doing this by teaching parents the importance of infection control measures such as good hand washing and asking them to monitor that every person that touches their child also washes their hands. In practicing hand washing and teaching parents to act as advocates for their child, nurses can prevent **nosocomial infections** (infections transmitted in healthcare facilities).

Reservoir

The **reservoir** is the container or place in which an organism grows and reproduces. The reservoir would be another person with the disease, a contaminated object such as a kitchen counter, or an animal or insect. Not all infectious agents can live on fomites. **Fomites** are inanimate objects that can also transmit infections from one person to another without direct contact with a human vector.

Nursing Care Planning Using Assessment

ASSESSING A CHILD FOR COMMON SIGNS AND SYMPTOMS OF INFECTIOUS DISORDERS

History
Chief concern: Does child have a fever, general malaise, vomiting, or diarrhea? Was child recently exposed to someone with an infection?
Past medical history: Are child's immunizations current?

Physical examination

Mouth: lesions on mucous membrane (*Koplik spots*)
White plaques on mucous membrane (*thrush*)
Skin: warm and dry from fever; rash present
Reddened, swollen pharynx (*infectious mononucleosis, pharyngitis*)
Gray membrane in pharynx (*diphtheria*)
Circular, scaly ring (*tinea corporis*)
Flesh-colored papule (*plantar wart*)

Linear abrasions on scalp; sandlike particles on hair shafts (*pediculosis*)
Nose: watery discharge (*prodromal symptoms of measles*)
Swollen parotid gland (*mumps*)
Pinpoint papules on an erythematous base (*herpes simplex*)
Paroxysmal cough (*whooping cough*)
Oozing, honey-colored, crusty lesions of face and hands (*impetigo*)
Crusty lesions between fingers (*scabies*)

Portal of Exit

The **portal of exit** is the route by which an organism leaves an infected child's body to be spread to others. Organisms can be carried out of the body by upper respiratory excretions, feces, vomitus, saliva, urine, vaginal secretions, blood, or lesion secretions (Table 43.1). Depending on the way an organism is spread, it may be necessary to wear gowns, gloves, or mask and/or face shield to care for the child. In some cases, nothing more than standard precautions are needed even though the child has an infectious disease. Washing after contact with any body secretions and covering a cough and/or sneeze with tissue can limit droplet or airborne spread. Hand washing is the most effective way to prevent the spread of infection (Chusid & Rotar, 2016).

QSEN Checkpoint Question 43.1

EVIDENCE-BASED PRACTICE

Multiple studies reported the effectiveness of hand hygiene in the reduction of infection. As a result, the WHO and the CDC have endorsed the importance of hand hygiene to reduce infection (WHO, 2016a). A study Chittleborough, Nicholson, Basker, et al. (2012) conducted in the primary school setting found that proper hand hygiene correlated positively with student observations of teaching practicing hand hygiene. Based on this study, the nurse determines which action is most effective to ensure Jack, a 10-year-old, consistently washes his hands before meals?

a. Continue to remind him to wash his hands as often as possible.
b. Talk to Jack's mother about the importance of modeling good hand hygiene practices.
c. Explain to Jack the role that bacteria play in the transmission of illness.
d. Stress that washing his hands makes him look grown-up and responsible.

Look in Appendix A for the best answer and rationale.

TABLE 43.1 METHODS BY WHICH INFECTIONS SPREAD

Portal of Exit	Means of Transmission	Portal of Entry	Prevention Measures
Blood	Arthropod vectors	Injection into the bloodstream	Decreasing exposure to vectors
	Blood sampling		Careful handling of blood sampling equipment
	Transfusion		Prescreening of blood for organisms such as HIV or hepatitis B
Respiratory secretions	Airborne droplets	Respiratory tract	Wearing a mask
	Fomites		Droplet and airborne precautions
			Hand washing
Feces	Water, food	Gastrointestinal tract	Hand washing before eating, after using bathroom, or after handling diapers
	Fomites		
	Vectors such as flies		
Exudate from lesions	Direct contact	Skin, mucous membranes	Contact precautions
	Contact with soiled dressings		Self-screening for sexual contacts
			Gloves

Means of Transmission

The **mode of transmission** refers to whether the infection is spread by *direct* or *indirect* contact. Sexually transmitted infections, for example, are spread by mucous membrane to mucous membrane or direct contact. Other infections are spread indirectly by fomites—inanimate objects such as soil, food, water, bedding, towels, combs, nonrefrigerated food, or drinking glasses. Infections can also be spread by **vectors** such as insects, rats, or other vermin—who may not be ill but are carriers of a human disease.

The most common means of indirect contact is the spread of mouth and nose secretions (droplet infection) through talking, sneezing, coughing, breathing, kissing, and sharing drinking glasses or straws. Some droplets containing pathogenic organisms are spread immediately to another individual in this way. Some droplets fall to the ground, where the organisms dry and then are spread by dust. If small, the organisms become suspended in the air (airborne transmission) and can move with the wind to infect people at a distance. A common respiratory tract infection is an example of an illness spread by indirect contact.

To break a chain of infection at this point, use transmission-based precautions as appropriate and wash hands before, between, and after patient care. Household measures such as using paper bathroom cups, separating toothbrushes, and using different towels for different people can help prevent house reinfection.

Portal of Entry

The **portal of entry** refers to the opening through which a pathogen can enter a child's body such as by inhalation, ingestion, or breaks in the skin from bites, abrasions, or burns. To break a chain of infection at this point, teach children to wash their hands after sneezing or coughing, before eating, and after using the bathroom. It is important to teach girls to wipe their perineum from front to back after defecating or voiding to prevent organisms from spreading from the rectum to the urethra. Parents need to wash dirt from cuts with soap and water and avoid hydrogen peroxide as a cleaning agent as this interferes with fibroblast production, delaying wound healing (Totoraitis, Cohen, & Friedman, 2017; Wilkins & Unverdorben, 2012).

Susceptible Host

For infection to occur, one more step must be present: The child must be susceptible to the infection (**susceptible host**). Certain characteristics make some individuals more prone to infection than others, including:

- Age: Infection occurs most readily in the very young and the very old.
- Gender: Girls, for example, have more urinary tract infections than boys.
- Virulence: Some organisms are stronger than others or cause disease more readily.
- Body defenses: Physical, chemical, and immune responses all protect against foreign invaders. Children with immunosuppression are more susceptible than others. Infants who are breastfed are less susceptible to infection than formula-fed infants.

THE BODY'S IMMUNE RESPONSE TO ORGANISMS

The immune system has two lines of defense—innate immunity, which is a nonspecific response, and adaptive immunity, which is more specific to the infective organism. Because of the innate response, when a foreign organism (antigen like a bacteria, virus, or fungi) enters the body, it is first met by neutrophils, phagocytic (cell-engulfing) white blood cells (WBCs). Neutrophils are the first line of defense and will activate another WBC, a monocyte, to become a macrophage. Macrophages have two roles—to clean cellular debris and kill the infecting organism. These cells do not need to have a previous exposure to the infecting antigen. The neutrophils, macrophages, complements, and cytokines (such as leukotrienes, interferons, and tumor necrosis factor alpha) provide a host defense to help ward off infection. The different actions of all the WBCs are summarized in Table 43.2.

Complement and cytokines signal specific cellular and humeral immunity to add in host defenses. Complement amplifies the innate immune response by enhancing phagocytosis via opsonin and attracting white cells to the site of inflammation (chemoattractive quality). The vascular response to antigens or breaks in the skin brings the plasma protein (clotting factors), WBCs, and platelets to the area.

TABLE 43.2 TYPES AND FUNCTIONS OF WHITE BLOOD CELLS (LEUKOCYTES)

Type	Percentage of Total Count	Origin	Function
Granular Forms			
Neutrophils	60% at birth; 33% at 2 years of age; 60% thereafter	Bone marrow	Active in acute bacterial infections
Eosinophils	1%–4%	Bone marrow	Increased in parasitic infection
Basophils	0.0%–0.5%	Bone marrow	Increased with inflammation
Nongranular Forms			
Lymphocytes	30% at birth; 50% at 2 years of age; 30% thereafter	Bone marrow	T lymphocytes (stored in the thymus gland) directly react with invading antigens; B lymphocytes from bone marrow produce antibodies that inactivate antigens
Monocytes	5%–10%	Bone marrow	Serve as a backup for neutrophils in acute infection; macrophages are mature form

The initial adaptive response is linked to adaptive immunity. In terms of adaptive immunity, the T lymphocyte has a twofold role. The T lymphocyte differentiates into TH1 cell. The TH1 promotes cellular immunity by activating microphages, enhancing cytotoxic T cell function, producing cytokines, and recognizing the infecting agent. TH2 cells release cytokines, which enhance antibody formation (immunoglobulins) by B cells and mediating eosinophil recruitment and activation (Nayak & Sant, 2011). The immunoglobulins can be specific to the particular infecting organism. (See Chapter 42 for a more detailed discussion of the immune response and Chapter 34 for a discussion of immunizations.)

The action of phagocytes on organisms produces a small amount of pus (remnants of the organisms, phagocytes, and destroyed tissue) and indicates phagocytosis is occurring and the infection is resolving. A large amount of pus may indicate that the infecting organism is overwhelming the immune response. When an infecting organism is overwhelming the immune response, the bacteria can enter the blood and lymphatic system and infect other organ systems such as the bone causing a bone infection (osteomyelitis), or an infection of the blood stream.

Pathogenic organisms in the bloodstream can cause a nonspecific bacteremia without any signs of organ failure in which the person can clear the bacteria. This is called a blood infection. When the organism leads to a more serious systemic inflammatory response syndrome, it can present in three ways: (1) sepsis syndrome or infection with some alteration of body temperature, respiratory rate, heart rate, or WBC; (2) septic shock with organ dysfunction, hypotension, and hypoperfusion; or (3) severe sepsis with hypotension despite vigorous treatment (Randolph & McCulloh, 2014). A systemic inflammatory response is always serious as it can progress, leading to organ failure and death.

Health Promotion and Risk Management

Preventing infectious diseases is important due to the risk of death (mortality) and complications (morbidity) secondary to the infection. An assessment of overall health status includes that the child has basic needs met as defined by Maslow (1943). A second important step is to be certain all parents are aware of the need for their children to be immunized. Nurses need to ensure immunizations are offered to children at healthcare visits to avoid missed opportunities and maintain the immunization schedule (Restrepo-Méndez, Barros, Wong, et al., 2016). A recent review showed a relationship between vaccine refusal and reoccurrence of vaccine-preventable disease (Phadke, Bednarczyk, Salmon, et al., 2016). Continual education about the effectiveness of vaccines to prevent serious diseases need to be done at every visit whether the family is refusing to vaccinate or regularly vaccinating. The nurse should educate guardians that common childhood illness such as scarlet fever, chickenpox (varicella), and mumps (infectious parotitis) have the potential to be serious and can be complicated by secondary infections such as pneumonia and toxic shock syndrome. Prompt evaluation and treatment for any changes in the expected course of an illness can prevent mortality.

Prevention of transmission of infectious disease is a public health issue with advice for prevention and treatment coming from the CDC in the United States and the WHO internationally. Federal, state, and local departments of health play an active role in case finding as well as making sure that immunizations are available for all children in the United States. Parents are expected to obtain such immunizations for children by school age. Schools and school nurses, as well as the school system's frontline health officers, take an active role in enforcing these regulations. Community health nurses serve an important role in educating families about immunizations and administering immunizations. Nurses also should educate families about vaccine resources that provide accurate information about the possible side effects of vaccines. In 2007, Andrew Wakefield authored an article published in *Lancet* that linked the measles, mumps, and rubella (MMR) vaccine to autism (Chittleborough et al., 2012). Despite the fact that the research was proven to be false, resulting in both the loss of Andrew Wakefield's license and withdrawal of the article, the information continues to be spread via the Internet by members of the anti-vaccine movement (Haberman, 2015). A recent meta-analysis showed no association between autism spectrum disorder and vaccines (Taylor, Swerdfeger, & Eslick, 2014.)

Developing countries use the immunization schedule recommended by WHO. This schedule is different from the United States, and therefore, vaccines for diseases such as varicella, meningococcal, and hepatitis A may not be recommended for the child's country of origin (WHO, 2016b). When caring for children from families of newly arrived immigrants, the child may need the missing immunizations. The family may question this need for further immunizations.

PREVENTING THE SPREAD OF INFECTIONS

Nosocomial or **health care–associated infections** (HAIs) are infections that are contracted while in a hospital or other healthcare setting. At present, there is a three-pronged approach to prevent HAIs that center around prevention of infection with surgery or catheter placement, prevent spread of infection between patients, and appropriate antibiotic use (CDC, 2016c). These kinds of infections are a major threat to hospitalized children. Antibiotic misuse is the chief reason for the emergence of resistant bacteria (Goldman & Newland, 2015). At the present time, HAIs include six antibiotic-resistant bacteria that are identified by the CDC as either urgent or serious infections. They include carbapenem-resistant Enterobacteriaceae (CRE), methicillin-resistant *Staphylococcus aureus* (MRSA), extended-spectrum β-lactamases (ESBL)-producing Enterobacteriaceae, vancomycin-resistant enterococci (VRE), multidrug-resistant pseudomonas, and multidrug-resistant *Acinetobacter* (CDC, 2016c). It is important for nurses to know about antibiotic-resistant infections in their workplace and use dedicated equipment for a patient who has resistant bacteria (CDC, 2016c).

The children at highest risk for contracting an HAI include children younger than 2 years of age, children with a nutritional deficit, those who are immunosuppressed, those who have indwelling vascular lines or catheters, are receiving multiple antibiotic therapy, or who remain in the hospital for longer than 72 hours. Nurses should follow hand hygiene protocols, use appropriate isolation required for the patient's infection, and make sure that device and cleaning practices follow protocols (CDC, 2016c). Summaries of standard infection precautions and transmission-based infection control precautions are available at http://thePoint.lww.com/Flagg8e and in Box 43.3.

What If . . . 43.1

The nurse realizes that Jack, who was diagnosed as having scarlet fever a day after surgery for appendicitis, must have been infectious while he was in surgery because that was his prodromal period. What can the nurse do to make sure other people do not contract the infection?

Caring for the Child With an Infectious Disease

Most all childhood infectious diseases include one of the following symptoms: fever, malaise, arthralgia, or myalgia. Nursing care must address identification and relief of these symptoms.

Nursing Diagnoses and Related Interventions

Nursing Diagnosis: Pain related to infection

Outcome Evaluation: Child states he is more comfortable; several simple remedies are available for reducing discomfort (Box 43.4).

Nursing Diagnosis: Fever related to infection

Some infectious diseases also involve fever. Measures to combat fever in children are discussed in Chapter 37.

Nursing Diagnosis: Social isolation related to required activity restriction associated with precautions to prevent disease transmission

Outcome Evaluation: Child states reasons for restrictions; expresses interest in activities proposed by nurses or parents.

A child who is restricted from others because of infection control precautions can begin to feel lonely and depressed unless stimulation and social needs are met. The nurse should try to have a child life specialist therapist visit the child on a daily basis and encourage families to play games with the children during the day. It is important to plan nursing care appropriately to avoid excessive exposure to infection by coming in and out of the room.

Parents must be educated on the type of precautions that their child needs to avoid infecting themselves and other patients on the unit. Helping the family feel comfortable with these procedures so they continue to visit is a nursing responsibility. Remember that when children are admitted to a hospital, parents may not hear everything said to them during admission because of their anxiety. Reeducation and reinforcement of infection control measures is key to prevent the spread of disease.

Parents may be reluctant to give children who require transmission-based precautions their favorite toy, thinking it will have to be destroyed after contagious precautions are discontinued. There are few toys, however, that cannot be cleaned with soap and water, so there is no reason to restrict such items. A child should always have an activity or toy to play with to promote development and keep them occupied for the length of time they will be alone. See Chapter 36 for a discussion of interventions that can be used to promote adequate stimulation for a child requiring transmission-based precautions as well as the role of a child life specialist to help locate and provide stimulating activities for children.

Viral Infections

In children, infections by viral agents are the majority of recognized infectious diseases (Alter et al., 2015). Most viral infections are treated based on symptoms with only a small number of viral infections treated with antiviral agents. Viruses are the smallest infectious agents known and are so small that they cannot be seen through an ordinary microscope. They actually are not true cells because they contain either RNA or DNA but not both. As a result, viruses cannot replicate on their own but only by invading bacteria, plant, animal, or human cells and using the biochemical products of those cells to function. Although body cells may not look to be outwardly altered by a viral invasion, they can fail to function or die because of lysis of internal components or rupture. Symptoms usually do not become apparent until many cells have been invaded in this way, creating a long incubation period. Some viruses are capable of invading only specific cells. The Epstein–Barr virus, for example, resides in the B lymphocytes (Pinninti, Hough-Telford, Pati, et al., 2016), HIV viruses invade CD4 T lymphocytes, and influenza viruses affect specific receptor sites in tracheal cells. Most viral agents have a site-specific organ or cell that they infect, but the systemic manifestations are due to cytokines release as discussed above.

VIRAL EXANTHEMS

Viruses cause childhood exanthems (skin rashes). Each of these diseases has specific symptoms, characteristic lesions, and a specific distribution or pattern to the rash that allows it to be identified (Figs. 43.2 and 43.3). There are several vaccine-preventable viral infections: rubeola (regular measles), rubella (German measles), mumps, varicella, rotavirus, hepatitis A, hepatitis B, polio, influenza, and human papillomavirus.

Exanthem Subitum (Roseola Infantum)

- Causative agent: human herpesvirus 6 (HHV-6)
- Incubation period: 9 to 10 days
- Period of communicability: during febrile period
- Mode of transmission: unknown
- Immunity: Contracting the disease offers lasting natural immunity; no vaccine is available (American Academy of Pediatrics [AAP], 2015).

BOX 43.3

Standard and Transmission-Based Precautions for Infection Control

To decrease the transmission of infectious agents in the healthcare setting:

1. Wash hands for at least 20 seconds immediately with a non-antimicrobial soap and water or alcohol-based hand sanitizers before and after examining patients and after any contact with blood, body fluids, excretions, secretions, and contaminated items despite the use of gloves (AAP, 2015). Soap and water is always used if the hands are visibly dirty or contaminated.
2. Wear clean, nonsterile gloves anytime contact with blood, body fluids, mucous membranes, or broken skin is likely. Hand hygiene should be done before and after glove use. Change gloves between tasks or procedures on the same patient. Before going to another patient, remove gloves, wash hands, and then put on new gloves.
3. Wear a mask, protective eyewear, gowns, and face shields during any patient care activity when splashes or sprays of body fluids, excretions, secretions, or blood are likely. Remove the soiled gown and wash hands as soon as possible. Remove the gown and gloves in the room of the patient before moving to the next patient (CDC, 2016b).
4. Make sure contaminated nondisposable equipment is not reused with another patient until it has been cleaned, disinfected, and sterilized properly. Do not recap needles. Dispose of nonreusable needles, syringes, and other sharp patient care instruments in puncture-resistant containers.
5. Ensure housekeeping routinely clean and disinfect frequently touched surfaces including beds, bed rails, examination tables, and bedside tables.
6. Do not touch linens soiled with blood or body fluids with bare hands. Use plastic bags to transport soiled linen.
7. Place a patient whose blood or body fluids are likely to contaminate surfaces or other patients in an isolation room or area.
8. Minimize the use of invasive procedures to avoid the potential for injury and accidental exposure. Use oral rather than injectable medications whenever possible.
9. When a specific diagnosis is made, find out how the disease is transmitted. Use precautions according to the transmission risk (AAP, 2015)

AIRBORNE PRECAUTIONS

Airborne precautions reduce the risk of small-particle organisms being transmitted through the air as microorganisms carried by this route can be carried widely. If airborne transmission is possible:

1. Place the patient in a single-patient isolation room that is not air-conditioned or where air is not circulated to the rest of the healthcare facility. Make sure the room has a door that can be closed.
2. Wear a high-efficiency particulate air (HEPA) or other biosafety mask when in the patient's room.
3. Limit movement of the patient from the room to other areas. Place a surgical mask on a patient who must be moved.

DROPLET PRECAUTIONS

Droplet precautions reduce the risk of pathogens being spread through large-particle droplet contact by acts such as coughing, sneezing, and talking or through procedures such as suctioning or bronchoscopy. Large droplets do not remain suspended in the air for long periods and generally travel only short distances, so close proximity is required for the spread of disease. Respiratory viruses, *Bordetella pertussis*, and patients within the first 24 hours of meningococcal infections or group A streptococcal infections can be transmitted by droplets. If droplet transmission is possible:

1. Place the patient in a single-patient isolation room.
2. Wear a HEPA or other biosafety mask when caring for the patient.
3. Limit movement of the patient from the room to other areas. If the patient must be moved, place a surgical mask on the patient.

CONTACT PRECAUTIONS

Contact precautions reduce the risk of transmission of pathogens by direct contact such as skin-to-skin contact (shaking hands) or indirect contact through an intermediate object such as a comb or soiled dressing. If contact transmission is possible:

1. Place the patient in an isolation room and limit access.
2. Wear gloves during contact with the patient and with infectious body fluids or contaminated items.
3. Wear a disposable gown when in the patient's room.
4. Limit movement of the patient from the isolation room to other areas.
5. Avoid sharing equipment between patients. Designate equipment for each patient if supplies allow. If sharing equipment is unavoidable, clean and disinfect it before use with the next patient.

From Centers for Disease Control and Prevention. (2016). *Guidelines to infection prevention for outpatient settings: Expectations for safe care.* Retrieved from https://www.cdc.gov/infectioncontrol/pdf/outpatient/guide.pdf; Centers for Disease Control and Prevention. (2017). *Guideline for isolation precautions: Preventing transmission of infectious agents in healthcare settings.* Retrieved from https://www.cdc.gov/infectioncontrol/guidelines/isolation/updates.html

BOX 43.4

Nursing Care Planning Based on Family Teaching

RELIEVING THE ITCHINESS OF A RASH

Q. Jack's mother says to you, "Our son is miserable because his rash is so itchy. What can we do to help him?"

A. Itching is a very uncomfortable sensation. Use the following to help relieve the itch of a rash:

- Dress your child in light cotton clothing so overheating and perspiration do not occur. Perspiration can make itching worse.
- Avoid wool clothing because it can irritate the skin and increase itching.
- Offer adequate fluid to maintain good hydration because dry skin increases discomfort.
- Keep your child's fingernails short to avoid injury to the skin from scratching.
- Teach your child to press on an itchy area rather than scratching to relieve discomfort; cold cloths or compresses applied to an area can also be helpful.
- Administer an analgesic, such as acetaminophen, as needed for comfort.
- Adding a few teaspoons of baking soda to bath water can be soothing. Use lukewarm rather than hot water.
- Keep in mind that some children need an antihistamine such as diphenhydramine (Benadryl) to reduce itching. Ask your primary care provider about using this medication.

Assessment

Roseola is a disease with fever followed by a defervescence. HHV-6 is the causative viral agent, and nearly all humans develop this infection with 77% of children acquiring roseola by age 2 years (Alter et al., 2015). The first symptom is fever (101° to 105°F [38.3° to 40.6°C]). Infants may be cranky due to the fever, but they will be playful and alert when the fever is done. There may be associated cervical adenopathy with mild injection of the pharynx. The fever will fall abruptly after 3 to 5 days (Alter et al., 2015), and a distinctive rash of discrete, rose-pink macules approximately 2 to 3 mm in size appears (see Fig. 43.3). The lesions occur most prominently on the trunk, fade on pressure, and last 1 to 2 days. The children have no accompanying coryza (upper respiratory symptoms), conjunctivitis, or cough. Not all children who seroconvert from infection with the virus will develop clinical symptoms. The condition is diagnosed based on the history with the hallmark appearance of a rash appearing immediately after the sharp decline in fever (AAP, 2015).

Roseola is a cause of febrile seizure in up to 10% to 15% of children. Other rare complications of roseola include encephalitis, encephalopathy, and bulging fontanels (AAP, 2015).

Therapeutic Management

Treatment focuses on measures to reduce the fever with acetaminophen (Tylenol) or ibuprofen (Motrin) if the child is over 6 months. Management of this type of seizure is discussed in Chapter 49.

There are no long-term effects of roseola. If an infant should develop this exanthem in the hospital, follow standard infection precautions.

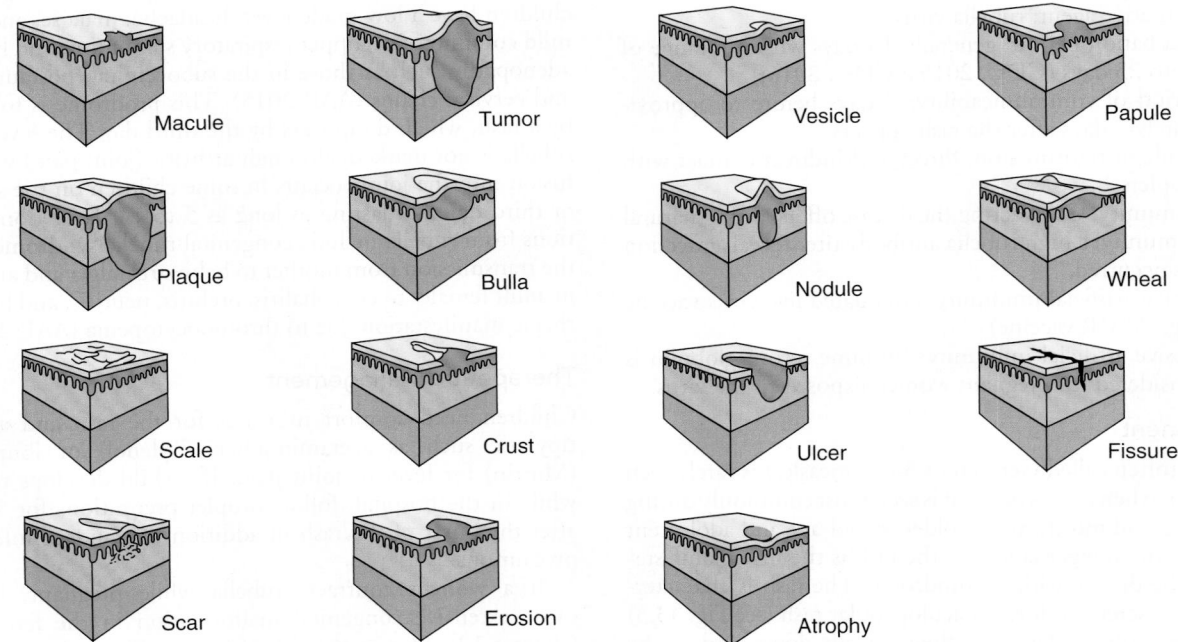

Figure 43.2 Primary and secondary skin lesions and their characteristics.

Figure 43.3 The differences between five acute exanthems characterized by rash.

Rubella (German Measles)

- Causative agent: rubella virus
- Incubation period: generally 14 days within a range of 12 to 23 days (CDC, 2015a; CDC, 2016j)
- Period of communicability: 7 days before to approximately 7 days after the rash appears
- Mode of transmission: direct and indirect contact with droplets
- Immunity: Contracting the disease offers lasting natural immunity; a high rubella antibody titer reveals infection has occurred.
- Active artificial immunity: attenuated live virus vaccine (e.g., MMR vaccine)
- Passive artificial immunity: Immune serum globulin is considered for pregnant women exposed to the virus.

Assessment

Rubella (often called German or 3-day measles) is rarely seen today, but when it does occur, it is seen most commonly during the spring and mostly affects older school-age and adolescent children. In younger children, the rash is the first manifestation of the disease with no prodrome. The rash is characterized by a discrete pink-red maculopapular rash (see Fig. 43.3) that begins on the face and then spreads downward to the trunk and extremities. In older children and adolescents,

the disease has a 1- to 5-day prodromal period, during which children have a low-grade fever, headache, malaise, anorexia, mild conjunctivitis, upper respiratory symptoms, and lymphadenopathy such as those in the suboccipital, postauricular, and cervical chains (AAP, 2015). This prodrome is followed by a rash, which disappears by the third day. The fever with rubella is not marked, although arthritis (joint pain) with effusion into the joints occurs in some children on the second or third day and lasting as long as 5 to 10 days. Complications from rubella include congenital rubella syndrome from the transmission from mother to baby, arthralgia and arthritis in adult females to encephalitis, orchitis, neuritis, and hemorrhagic manifestation due to thrombocytopenia (AAP, 2015).

Therapeutic Management

Children need comfort measures for the rash and an antipyretic such as acetaminophen (Tylenol) or ibuprofen (Motrin) for fever or joint pain. If a child develops rubella while in the hospital, follow droplet precautions for 7 days after the onset of the rash in addition to standard infection precautions.

If a woman contracts rubella while pregnant, it can cause extensive congenital malformation in the fetus (see Chapter 12). Due to the risk of fetal malformations as a result of exposure to rubella virus in utero, this disease is not considered a simple disease. It is important that girls are immunized against rubella before they reach childbearing age. Therefore, the MMR vaccine is administered at age 1 year and again at age 4 years to expand protection. MMR vaccine is not recommended in pregnancy because it is a live viral vaccine (CDC, 2016j).

QSEN Checkpoint Question 43.2

SAFETY

A nurse is preparing to enter Jack's room. Because his infection involves potential airborne transmission, what isolation precautions should the nurse use?
  a. Goggles and nonsterile gloves
  b. Gown and nonsterile gloves
  c. Mask, gown, and nonsterile gloves
  d. No precautions provided Jack wears a mask

Look in Appendix A for the best answer and rationale.

Measles (Rubeola)

- Causative agent: measles virus
- Incubation period: 8 to 12 days from time of exposure to onset of any symptoms (AAP, 2015) with a range from 7 to 21 days (Goodson & Seward, 2015)
- Period of communicability: 4 days before the rash to 4 days after the rash appears (AAP, 2015)
- Mode of transmission: direct contact with droplets or airborne spread (AAP, 2015)
- Immunity: Contracting the disease offers lasting natural immunity.
- Active artificial immunity: attenuated live measles vaccine (e.g., MMR)
- Passive artificial immunity: immune serum globulin

Assessment

Measles is an acute febrile viral illness associated with cough, coryza (clear nasal discharge), and conjunctivitis (the "three Cs") with a confluent maculopapular, erythematous rash, which starts behind the ear and spreads to the feet over a course of 3 to 6 days. **Koplik spots**, or small white spots with a bluish white center on an erythematous background, are seen in the oral mucosa opposite the buccal mucosa before symptoms appear (AAP, 2015; Goodson & Seward, 2015).

Globally, measles is still seen because funding shortfalls have affected immunization programs (Shibeshi, Masresha, Smith, et al., 2014). Recent outbreaks of measles in the United States have occurred with a peak of 667 cases in 2014 (CDC, 2016d) due to declining rates of immunizations. When it does occur, it can be a devastating illness because of the serious complications that can occur.

During the prodromal period, postauricular, cervical, and occipital lymph nodes become enlarged, and the child develops a low-grade fever along with malaise, photophobia, cough, coryza, and mild gastrointestinal symptoms. The child may look like they are developing an upper respiratory infection (Drutz, 2016). Koplik spots then develop on the buccal mucosa and are a hallmark symptom because they are unique to measles (Fig. 43.4). Koplik spots look like raised papules on an erythematous base (Drutz, 2016). Any rash on mucosa surfaces is called an enanthem.

Figure 43.4 Koplik spots on the oral mucous membrane. (© SPL/Custom Medical Stock Photograph.)

As this enanthem fades, the fever rises to as high as 104°F (40°C) and a viral exanthem develops on the skin, gradually spreading down over the body as described earlier (AAP, 2015; Drutz, 2016). This maculopapular coalescing rash develops over the entire body and eventually turns from red to brown desquamation over a few days (Fig. 43.5). While the rash is red, it fades on pressure; when it is brown, it does not fade. This differentiates it from the rash of scarlet fever, which always fades on pressure. After 5 to 6 days, the rash fades, leaving a fine desquamation of skin cells behind.

The complications of measles can involve multiple systems (Goodson & Seward, 2015) and includes otitis media, pneumonia, croup, and diarrhea. Pneumonia is the most common complication and can be from the measles virus or a secondary bacterial infection (Goodson & Seward, 2015). A rare subacute sclerosing panencephalitis leading to central nervous system degeneration, behavioral changes, and seizures can occur 7 to 11 years after the initial measles infection (Goodson & Seward, 2015). Fever that lasts beyond the third or fourth day of a rash or coughing that continues generally

Figure 43.5 The typical rash of measles on a child's upper body. (© NMSB/Custom Medical Stock Photograph.)

suggests one of the complications of measles, such as pneumonia, has occurred.

Therapeutic Management

Children with measles need comfort measures for the rash and an antipyretic for the fever. Applying a lubricating jelly or an emollient (e.g., A&D ointment) to the area below the nose may help prevent excoriation. The use of buckwheat honey in children older than 1 year of age may be helpful with the cough (Paul, Beiler, McMonagle, et al., 2007). Photophobia is an accompanying symptom, so drawing the curtains or wearing sunglass is a comfort measure. When children are seen for diagnosis and management, office staff should be aware that the child may have measles and the child should be seen after office hours. If a child is hospitalized, follow airborne precautions for the duration of the illness in addition to standard infection precautions (AAP, 2015).

Chickenpox (Varicella)

- Causative agent: varicella-zoster virus (VZV)
- Incubation period: 10 to 21 days with the most common incidence at 14 to 16 days following exposure (Kroger, 2015)
- Period of communicability: 1 day before the rash to 5 to 6 days after its initial appearance, when all the vesicles have crusted
- Mode of transmission: highly contagious; spread by direct or indirect contact of saliva or open vesicles
- Immunity: contracting the disease offers lasting natural immunity to chickenpox; however, because VZV is latent, it causes herpes zoster (shingles) when it is reactivated at a later time
- Active artificial immunity: attenuated live virus vaccine
- Passive artificial immunity: children who are immunosuppressed, such as those with leukemia or HIV/AIDS, or those who are being treated with corticosteroids are offered varicella-zoster immune globulin (VZIG) within 72 hours of exposure to help prevent or modify disease symptoms.

Assessment

Chickenpox is a common and highly contagious childhood infection caused by the VZV with a household attack rate approaching 90% (Alter et al., 2015). It has a decreasing incidence due to the varicella vaccine (Alter et al., 2015). In children, the rash occurs first accompanied by a low-grade fever and malaise (Kroger, 2015) (see Fig. 43.3). The lesions of varicella present as a macule, papule, and vesicle all appearing at the same time, starting on the trunk and progressing outward to the arms, face, legs, and mucosal surfaces including the genitalia. When the lesion is in the healing stage, there is a characteristic black crust. The hallmark is a 2- to 3-mm vesicle on an erythematous base. The lesions appear in crops, with each new lesion moving through progressive stages (Fig. 43.6). Usually, all four stages of lesions (macule, papule, vesicle, and crust) may be present at the same time. The fever has a wide range depending on the severity of the infection and is worse in immunocompromised patients such as patients undergoing chemotherapy or with an underlying immune deficiency. Secondary soft tissue infections can also occur with the common organisms of staphylococcus and streptococcal causing mild to severe secondary infections (Gershon, Breuer, Cohen, et al., 2015).

Figure 43.6 An older school-age boy with varicella. (© Martin/Custom Medical Stock Photograph.)

Therapeutic Management

The rash of varicella is very pruritic and so it is important to decrease scratching to reduce infection. Topical oatmeal-based creams along with an antihistamine such as diphenhydramine (Benadryl) can reduce the pruritus, and an antipyretic such as acetaminophen (Tylenol) can reduce the fever. The development of Reye syndrome (see Chapter 49) has been associated with aspirin use during varicella and influenza viral illnesses, so caution parents to avoid aspirin and instead use acetaminophen or ibuprofen to control fever. In high-risk patients (such as those on steroids or chemotherapy and those who are immunodeficient or older than 13 years of age), acyclovir (Zovirax), an antiviral, may be prescribed to reduce the number of lesions and shorten the course of the illness (AAP, 2015).

During hospitalization due to a complication of varicella infection, standard infection precautions along with airborne and contact precautions are adhered to until all lesions are crusted. Children may return to school as soon as all the lesions are crusted as the crusted lesions are not infectious. Complications include secondary infections of the lesions, pneumonia, and encephalitis.

Herpes Zoster

Herpes zoster is a reactivation of the VZV. The herpes viral family has viral latency, which means that once you develop varicella, the virus lies latent in the posterior dorsal root ganglia (Alter et al., 2015). The reactivation of the VZV occurs during aging as well as during times of immunosuppression.

The first manifestations are paresthesia and pain with subsequent groups of vesicular lesions in different stages of healing along a dermatomal distribution (Fig. 43.7). The course in the elderly and immunocompromised can be protracted,

Figure 43.7 Herpes zoster on a child's back. (© Dr. P. Marazzi/ SPL/Science Source/Photo Researchers.)

and today, there is a varicella-zoster vaccine for patients older than 50 years of age (Keighley, Saunderson, Kok, et al., 2015).

Treatment for herpes zoster includes analgesia for pain and measures to reduce pruritus. Acyclovir, which inhibits viral DNA synthesis, may be effective at limiting the disease but should be started within 72 hours of the start of the rash. Administration of VZIG within 96 hours can be used for immunocompromised children and may minimize symptoms.

Smallpox (Variola)

- Causative agent: smallpox virus
- Incubation period: 7 to 17 days with a mean of 12 days
- Period of communicability: The child is contagious for 24 hours before the onset of the rash and remains contagious until all lesions are dried which can take up to 4 weeks.
- Mode of transmission: airborne transmission (Kroger, 2015)

There are distinct differences between smallpox and varicella. In general, patients with smallpox develop a febrile prodrome not seen in varicella (AAP, 2015). Although the lesions of smallpox may resemble those of varicella, the lesions of smallpox are similar in the same stage of disease and all the smallpox lesions progress at the same rate. Unlike varicella, smallpox has a pustular stage. These pustular lesions are firm and deeply embedded in the skin dermal layer (AAP, 2015). In the crusting phase, the lesions of smallpox are contagious, whereas the crusted varicella lesions are not contagious

Smallpox is a serious illness; its mortality rate is greater than 30% (AAP, 2015), and it can be spread readily by direct contact with an infected person or indirect contact with a fomite (AAP, 2015). Disease symptoms can be modified by administration of disease specific vaccinia immune globulin (VIG) with experimental drugs in development (Damon, Damaso, & McFadden, 2014). Antibiotics may be used to prevent secondary infection of lesions. Oxygen or

other measures to support respiratory and cardiac function should be provided as necessary, or these systems can fail.

The last case of smallpox occurred in Somalia in 1977 (AAP, 2015), and the United States decided to stop vaccinating children in 1972. However, the chief concern in the United States is the possibility of the use of the smallpox virus as weapon of bioterrorism.

The causative agent is the smallpox virus. The lesions are similar, but the VZV has superficial vesicles as the primary lesion, whereas smallpox lesions on one part of the body do not vary and are deeper in the dermis. VIG is available through the CDC.

There is a severe prodrome phase for this disease with a high fever from 102° to 104°F (38.9° to 40.0°C) and symptoms that include headache, abdominal pain, malaise, and severe fatigue. Within 24 hours of symptoms starting, skin lesions develop on the face, spreading down the body to the forearms, trunk, and legs. The face and distal extremities are the most frequently affected (AAP, 2015). The lesions start as macules and then progress to papules, vesicles, and firm pustules by the seventh day. Eventually, the lesions become umbilicated and more confluent.

QSEN Checkpoint Question 43.3

PATIENT-CENTERED CARE

Jack's rash is causing him to scratch his skin. To maintain skin integrity and promote comfort, which action should the nurse prioritize in his plan of care?
   a. Allow him to keep his nails long.
   b. Administer an antihistamine as prescribed.
   c. Instruct Jack not to ever scratch the lesions.
   d. Cover his hands and fingernails with mittens.

Look in Appendix A for the best answer and rationale.

Erythema Infectiosum ("Fifth Disease")

- Causative agent: parvovirus B19
- Incubation period: most common between 4 to 14 days, with an outside window of 21 days (AAP, 2015)
- Period of communicability: uncertain
- Mode of transmission: respiratory tract secretion, blood transfusion, vertical transmission from mother to baby (AAP, 2015)
- Immunity: none

Assessment

Erythema infectiosum is more common in late winter through the spring and can occur at any time during the life span. The virus has several clinical features. Because the virus causes a relative aplasia of the red cell (erythrocyte) line for 7 to 10 days, the patient with a hemolytic anemia such as sickle cell disease can develop dangerously low hemoglobin, leading to cardiac failure. In patients with an HIV infection, the child can also develop a symptomatic anemia. In the pregnant woman, infected with parvovirus B19, fetal death may occur in 2% to 6% or the child may be smaller than expected (intrauterine growth restriction); however, in the well child, the infection can be asymptomatic and may not manifest as a clinical illness. The classic presentation starts with mild systemic symptoms, which can include a fever in

Figure 43.8 The "slapped face" appearance of fifth disease. (© Dr. P. Marazzi/SPL/Science Source/Photo Researchers.)

15% to 30%, headache, and malaise. This is present for 7 to 10 days before the child develops a "slapped cheek" appearance with erythema of the cheeks with circumoral pallor (Fig 43.8). Following this rash, a maculopapular, lacy-appearing rash on the arms, thigh, and buttocks may appear. This can fade and become more intense depending on the child's activity level and environmental changes, which includes sunlight and ambient room temperature.

Other presentations of this virus include a petechial, papular purpuric stocking and glove distribution or a mild respiratory illness without rash. Occasionally, the child will develop arthralgia and arthritis secondary to infection with parvovirus B19 (AAP, 2015).

Therapeutic Management

Treatment is typically supportive, with antipyretics and analgesics and comfort measures for the rash (see Box 43.4). There are no known complications of fifth disease for a child; children with a known parvovirus B19 infection should avoid contact with pregnant women. Use droplet precautions in a hospital. Children can return to school as soon as the rash appears because they are no longer infectious after this point.

NONPOLIO ENTEROVIRUSES

- Causative agent: member of the enteroviral family
- Incubation period: most common is between 3 to 6 days, with hemorrhagic conjunctivitis having a shorter incubation of 24 to 72 hours (AAP, 2015)
- Period of communicability: uncertain
- Mode of transmission: respiratory tract secretion, fecal–oral, vertical transmission from mother to baby at the time of birth; possibly breastfeeding (AAP, 2015)
- Immunity: none

There are over 90 serotypes (members of the same viral family) with three members of enteroviral family: numbered enteroviruses, echoviruses, and coxsackievirus (Alter et al., 2015). More recently, the virus was reclassified into enterovirus A, B, C, and D based on their genetics and their phenotypes (Lugo & Krogstad, 2016). As a group, there are several common manifestations from these viruses including:
- Nonspecific viral illness
- Respiratory illness (coryza, pharyngitis, stomatitis, pneumonia, pleurodynia, bronchitis)

- Skin infections (hand, foot, and mouth disease)
- Gastrointestinal illness (gastroenteritis, pancreatitis, and hepatitis)
- Eye infections (hemorrhagic conjunctivitis, uveitis)
- Neurologic disease (aseptic meningitis, encephalitis, acute flaccid paralysis)
- Genitourinary illness (orchiditis)
- Heart disease (myocarditis)
- Muscular manifestations (myositis) (AAP, 2015)

Numbered Enterovirus and Echovirus Infections

These echoviruses and numbered enteroviruses are responsible for a number of childhood diseases, including aseptic meningitis, diarrhea, acute respiratory illness, and maculopapular rashes. Although potentially serious, such infections are usually benign and self-limiting. Treatment involves supportive measures such as an antipyretic for fever and comfort measures for the rash. If a child is hospitalized, follow contact precautions for the duration of the illness in addition to standard infection precautions.

Coxsackievirus Infections

The coxsackievirus groups are also responsible for a variety of diseases. Coxsackievirus A6 and A16 are associated with hand-foot-mouth disease with distinctive erythematous papules mainly on the hands and feet but occasionally on the buttocks and oral ulcers in the pharynx. It is associated with high fever and anorexia, which can lead to dehydration. Herpangina is also caused by a coxsackie virus and is associated with fever, anorexia, difficulty swallowing, sore throat, headache, abdominal pain, and vomiting. The small lesions associated with herpangina are generally discrete pinpoint grayish vesicles or ulcers appear on the tonsillar fauces, soft palate, and uvula (Simões, 2016). After a few more days, they disappear and the temperature returns to normal. There are generally no complications.

Children need a bland, soft diet or nonirritating liquids when they have the mouth lesions. Analgesia with acetaminophen (Tylenol) dosed at 10 mg/kg/dose to 15 mg/kg/dose every 4 to 6 hours but no more than five doses per day is important prior to feeding the child. If a child is hospitalized, follow contact precautions for the duration of the illness in addition to standard infection precautions.

Poliovirus Infections: Poliomyelitis (Infantile Paralysis)

- Causative agent: poliovirus
- Incubation period: Nonparalytic polio—3 to 6 days. Paralytic polio is commonly 7 to 21 days with a range of 3 to 35 days.
- Period of communicability: greatest shortly before and after onset of clinical symptoms, when virus is present in the throat (1 to 2 weeks after the onset of illness and in feces (3 to 6 weeks); however, the virus is contagious as long as it is present in the feces.
- Mode of transmission: respiratory secretions and feces (AAP, 2015)
- Immunity: Contracting the disease causes active immunity against the one strain of virus causing the illness.

- Active artificial immunity: inactivated polio virus (IPV) vaccine
- Passive artificial immunity: none

The last outbreak of polio caused by a wild polio virus in the United States was in 1979 (CDC, 2016g). From 1980 to 1997, the cases of polio in the United States were acquired through the use of the live attenuated trivalent (three strains) oral vaccine. In 1997, the United States changed to using the inactivated vaccine to prevent any additional cases of polio (CDC, 2016g). The illness may be caused by any of the three strains of poliovirus.

Assessment

It is important to recognize that 72% of infections with the polio virus do not produce a paralysis and is asymptomatic. A nonspecific fever with a sore throat occurs in approximately 24% of children infected with polio. This means that only 4% of children develop more symptoms after the poliovirus enters the child's gastrointestinal tract, where it multiplies. The symptoms of paralytic polio include fever, headache, nausea, vomiting, abdominal pain, constipation, and malaise initially followed by a period of no symptoms. Less than 1% will go on to paralysis with areflexia and bulbar symptoms such as difficulty swallowing and respiratory muscle involvement (AAP, 2015). Sensation remains intact and the disease is a motor paralysis.

In 25% to 40% of patients, a postpolio syndrome can occur 15 to 40 years after polio infection, presenting as weakness and pain affecting the muscles and joints that were most affected with the original infection.

Therapeutic Management

Treatment for nonparalytic poliomyelitis is bed rest with antipyretics. There is no antiviral known to treat any form of polio. Supportive care is given depending on symptoms. If the respiratory muscles are involved, long-term ventilation may be necessary. Physical therapy is needed to prevent contracture and promote strength during the recovery period.

VIRAL INFECTIONS OF THE INTEGUMENTARY SYSTEM

Viral infections of the skin include herpes infections and warts (verrucae).

Herpesvirus Infections

Herpesviruses (HSV) infections are common, potentially life threatening, and are caused by both HSV-1 and HSV-2 (James & Kimberlin, 2015). They can be found as primary mucocutaneous infection, an acute infection of the ganglia, or in a latent form, reactivated form or a recurrent infection. They are responsible for mucocutaneous lesions in children and adolescents that can occur anywhere on the skin. HSV-1 is more commonly found acutely in the oral region as herpetic gingivostomatitis and in the chronic recurrent form as herpes labialis. HSV-2 is more commonly found in the genital region as both an acute or recurrent infection. However, both viruses can be found in either location (Stanberry, 2016).

- Causative agent: herpes simplex, type 1 or type 2 virus
- Incubation period: 2 days to 2 weeks (AAP, 2015), average of 6 days (Simos, Flynn, Peicuch, et al., 2009)

- Period of communicability: greatest early in the course of the infection
- Mode of transmission: direct contact with persons with active lesions or persons shedding the virus asymptomatically
- Immunity: Herpes viruses like VZV have viral latency, so patients can have recurrent infections. There is currently no vaccine available (Stanberry, 2016).

Acute Herpetic Gingivostomatitis

Acute herpetic gingivostomatitis is most common in children from 6 months to 5 years but can be seen in older children. In the initial infection, there is a sudden onset of pain, drooling, anorexia, and a significant fever as high as 105°F (40.6°C) (Stanberry, 2016). Their gumline is also swollen, reddened, and bleeds easily. White, shallow ulcers with red borders appear on the gum, lips, buccal mucosa, tongue, palate, perioral skin, and, less commonly, on the tonsillar pillars. The anterior cervical lymph nodes are usually enlarged and tender. The disease runs its course in 5 to 14 days.

Children will need an antipyretic to reduce fever and soft, nonirritating, acid-free foods to reduce irritation. Popsicles, ice milk, and Jell-O are soothing against inflamed mucous membranes. Oral acyclovir can be used to shorten the course of illness. Use contact precautions with hospitalized children to avoid contact with lesions. Although usually mild, the disease can become serious, especially in infants and children where the lack of fluid intake leads to dehydration.

Herpes Simplex (Herpes Labialis)

Herpes labialis, popularly known as a cold sore or fever blister, is the recurrent form of HSV. In the case of herpes labialis, the HSV remains dormant in the ganglia of the trigeminal or fifth cranial nerve. Herpes simplex typically appears as a cluster of painful, grouped vesicles surrounded by an erythematous base on the border of the lips (vermillion border) (Stanberry, 2016). Initially, there is tingling, burning, itching, or pain for about 6 to 48 hours prior to the eruption of erythematous papules that rapidly progress to grouped vesicles. Complete healing without scar formation occurs within 6 to 10 days (Stanberry, 2016). Although topical acyclovir (Zovirax cream/ointment) has mild effectiveness in shortening the course of herpes labialis, oral acyclovir reaches a higher plasma concentration. Children may feel conspicuous about the appearance of the lesion and need reassurance that these lesions will go away and are not as conspicuous as they think.

Acute Herpetic Vulvovaginitis (Genital Herpes)

Genital herpes is caused primarily by HSV type 2, which remains dormant in the ganglia of the sacral nerves. Genital herpes is spread primarily by sexual contact and is discussed in Chapter 47 with other sexually transmitted infections. The occurrence of HSV in children is suggestive of child sexual maltreatment and should be reported (Frieden, Jaffe, Cono, et al., 2014).

Warts (Verrucae)

There are over 100 types of human papillomaviruses (HPV), which are members of the virus family *Papillomaviridae* (Moscicki, 2016). The papillomavirus most commonly cause skin manifestation but can cause both genital and oral malignancies (Moscicki, 2016). HPV infect the conjunctiva, oral cavity, respiratory tract, genital tract, and the skin (Gerlero & Hernández-Martínb, 2016). The incubation period varies from 3 weeks to 8 months, but the average is 3 months (Gerlero & Hernández-Martínb, 2016). The mode of transmission is likely direct contact as there is little evidence to suggest indirect transmission by fomites (Moscicki, 2016).

Warts appear as flesh-colored, dirty-appearing papules that generally occur on the dorsal surface of the hands. Plantar warts on the soles of the feet can be differentiated from calluses in that they obliterate skin lines as they grow and are generally painful.

Warts on the hands or the face generally are removed if they are cosmetically unattractive to children. Plantar warts may have to be removed due to pain. There are several treatment options including over-the-counter preparations with a salicylic acid solution. Carbon dioxide snow, liquid nitrogen, electrodessication, laser, and cryotherapy are other methods also available for removal, but these methods are painful and rarely necessary (Gerlero & Hernández-Martínb, 2016).

The myth that people catch warts from frogs or toads needs to be dispelled. Anogenital warts in young children, like HSV lesions, can be a mark of sexual maltreatment. Certain strains of HPV can cause vaginal, vulvar, and cervical cancer in women, penile cancer in men, as well as anal or oropharyngeal cancers in both sexes. The Gardasil 9 vaccine is protective against cancer caused by nine strains of HPV (6, 11, 16, 18, 31, 33, 45, 52, and 58). It is recommended for all children at 11 to 12 years of age as well as males from 13 to 21 years and females from 13 to 26 years who have not yet received the vaccine (Petrosky, Bocchini, Hariri, et al., 2015).

VIRUSES CAUSING CENTRAL NERVOUS SYSTEM DISEASES

Viruses are the causative agent for central nervous system disorders such as rabies, encephalitis, and meningitis. Encephalitis and meningitis are discussed in Chapter 49.

Rabies

Rabies causes an acute encephalitis that is fatal and caused by *Lyssavirus* genus, which includes rabies virus (RABV) (Caicedo, Paez, Kuzmin, et al., 2015). RABV infections number over 59,000 people worldwide (Hampson, Coudeville, Lembo, et al., 2015) and is most common in poor countries. The domestic dog causes most rabies worldwide due to lack of vaccination (Hampson et al., 2015).

- Causative agent: RABV
- Incubation period: average is 1 to 3 months but can range from days to years
- Period of communicability: 3 to 5 days before the onset of symptoms through the course of the disease
- Mode of transmission: the bite of a rabid animal; rarely through saliva from an infected animal being transferred to an open lesion on a child's skin
- Immunity: Contracting the disease apparently offers active immunity, but few people have ever survived the illness to verify this.
- Active artificial immunity: human diploid cell rabies vaccine
- Passive artificial immunity: rabies immune globulin (RIG) (AAP, 2015)

Any warm-blooded animal can contract rabies. Although worldwide unvaccinated dogs are the most common source of RABV infection, in the United States the most common cause is the bat (AAP, 2015). Dogs bite children more often, and therefore, more children are treated for possible rabies due to dog bites. Any mammal can be infected with the virus and unprovoked attacks are suggestive of a rabid animal (AAP, 2015). Rodents (squirrels, mice, or rats) seldom carry the RABV virus. Infection with RABV causes a rapidly progressive central nervous system infection.

Assessment

After the long incubation period of the virus, children begin to show prodromal signs of malaise, fever, anorexia, nausea, sore throat, drowsiness, irritability, and restlessness. The clinical manifestations include anxiety, radicular pain pruritus, hydrophobia, dysautonomia, and in some patients, paralysis. The disease almost always leads to death (AAP, 2015) with a history of only four survivors of rabies (Caicedo et al., 2015). When children try to drink, they experience violent contractions of the muscles of the mouth leading to drooling of saliva. This phenomenon gives the disease its former name: hydrophobia ("water fear") (Jackson, 2016). As symptoms progress, children will become comatose. Peripheral vascular collapse and death can follow as quickly as 5 or 6 days later.

Therapeutic Management

Once the disease process begins, rabies is almost invariably fatal, so the key is prevention of the active process. A healthcare provider, paying close attention to the circumstances and kind of animal, should evaluate the child's animal bite. In taking a history from a child, it is important to avoid naming different kinds of animals. To gain a more accurate history, ask the child what the animal looked like or show pictures of different animals asking them to point to the one that bit them. Rabid animals will bite under unprovoked circumstances so this history is key. The child needs to be assured that they will not be punished if they provoked the bite. The immunity status of the animal is key in deciding whether treatment will be necessary. The healthcare provider must know if there have been rabid animals found in the community; however, if the bite seems unprovoked, rabies vaccine and RIG should be given. The decision to immunize and use prophylaxis should be done after contact with the local department of health and/or an infectious disease specialist. In cases where a bat has been present in the room of a child, the bite or scratch may be small and not evident. Therefore, postexposure prophylaxis may be indicated if the bat is in the room (AAP, 2015). Following any bite or close exposure to bats, prophylaxis should be initiated as soon as possible and, if the animal is unknown, or suspected to have rabies, there should be no delay in prophylaxis treatment (AAP, 2015).

Prophylaxis is twofold. The child receives human rabies vaccine immediately along with the administration of RIG (20 IU/kg) into the area of the bite with the remainder of the RIG administered in an intramuscular (IM) injection. Following this day 0 administration of rabies vaccine and RIG, the rabies vaccine is given again on days 3, 7, and 14 (AAP, 2015; Rupprecht, Briggs, Brown, et al., 2010).

The immediate administration of RIG provides antibodies against the RABV while administering the rabies vaccine allows the child to begin additional antibody formation so that by the time the RABV from the bite begins to have an effect (2 to 6 weeks after the bite), the child has developed sufficient antibodies to combat it and prevent the illness.

OTHER INFECTIONS TRANSMITTED BY ANIMAL VECTORS

Animal vectors can transmit viruses and bacteria to human hosts. For example, mice and rats are reservoirs of the bacteria *Leptospira*. The bacteria can be transmitted to humans by the infected animal's urine, and it can pass to humans via damaged skin or mucosa (Gomes-Solecki, Santecchia, & Werts, 2017). The transmission of viruses and bacteria by animal vectors is not uncommon, and it is important to take a careful travel history as well as a history of any exposure to animals.

Hantavirus Pulmonary Syndrome Infection

The hantavirus is a member of the arbovirus group and can cause two different diseases—hantavirus pulmonary syndrome (HPS), with a mortality rate of 60%, and hemorrhagic fever with renal syndrome (HFRS), with a mortality rate of 12% (Jonsson, Figueiredo, & Vapalahti, 2010). The virus infects rodents. There are over 22 different types of hantavirus, divided into old world and new world viruses. The "new world" viruses started infecting humans in the United States in 1993 with the initial outbreak occurring in the four corners of the Southwest. This virus was different from those that had previously been recognized in other parts of the world and became known as HPS.

HPS has an incubation period between 1 to 6 weeks. In HPS, there is prodrome of no more than 5 days, characterized by fever, chills, cough, myalgia, gastrointestinal symptoms of diarrhea, and vomiting and headache (Jonsson et al., 2010). One to 3 days after the onset of respiratory symptoms, capillary leak develops in the lung resulting in pulmonary edema and hypoxemia after cough and dyspnea. Hypotension leads to cardiac dysfunction and subsequent death (Jonsson et al., 2010).

In contrast, HFRS has an incubation of 3 weeks with a range of 10 days to 6 weeks. The clinical manifestations depend on the type of hantavirus. There are usually five phases: (a) febrile phase, (b) hypotension, (c) oliguria, (d) polyuria, and (e) convalescence (Jonsson et al., 2010).

At present, no antiviral medication immunotherapy or vaccines are approved for the treatment of hantavirus. The treatment is supportive, but prevention is key. Rodent control is the best prevention, and rodents should be kept out of the house. Campers need to avoid rodent-infested areas.

QSEN Checkpoint Question 43.4

QUALITY IMPROVEMENT

Jack's sister is home with "mono," or infectious mononucleosis. In the event that she requires hospital care, assessment protocols should emphasize what action?
a. Lymph nodes should be palpated before being percussed.
b. The spleen should be evaluated by nontouching maneuvers using the scratch test.
c. Lymph nodes should be assessed by Doppler.
d. Petechiae should be lightly massaged.

Look in Appendix A for the best answer and rationale.

Zika Virus Disease

The yellow fever mosquito is one of the world's most deadly animals, causing yellow fever, Zika virus, dengue, and chikungunya viral infections. These mosquitos lay their eggs in any containers that can hold water, including cups, tree holes, bowls, discarded tires, flower pots, cans, and clogged rain gutters. They are daytime biters with peak feeding activity 2 hours before sunrise and 2 hours after sunset (Higgs & Vanlandingham, 2016). *Aedes aegypti* is the main vector, but transmission of the virus via the *Aedes albopictus* appears possible. The Zika virus was first known to cause infection in 1947 when it was isolated in Uganda, but there have been several outbreaks recently across the globe. Nonmosquito transmission has been known to occur via sexual contact, blood products, and from mother to fetus. The relationship of microcephaly to active Zika viral infection in pregnant women has been established, and the CDC recommends testing of all pregnant women who have traveled to counties with active infection. Because Zika virus is new, the long-term sequelae is yet to be determined (Karwowski, Nelson, Staples, et al., 2016).

The incubation period is thought to be less than 1 week (Petersen, Jamieson, Powers, et al., 2016). The symptoms of Zika virus infection include fever, arthralgia, conjunctivitis, eye pain, myalgia, rash, and headache (Karwowski et al., 2016). Guillain-Barré syndrome is now a rare complication of Zika infection (Petersen et al., 2016).

To prevent infection with Zika virus, the nurse should screen potential blood donors and advise the use of condoms after travel to countries with known Zika viral infections. Stress that the use of insect repellants with a maximum of 30% N, N-diethyl-meta-toluamide (DEET) for infants and children can help prevent mosquito bites, but to avoid over use of DEET; the use of products that combine DEET with a sunscreen should not be used in children (CDC, 2015b).

West Nile Virus Disease

West Nile virus is the most common arboviral disease in the United States (Lindsey, Lehman, Staples, et al., 2015). The transmission of arbovirus occurs between arthropods and their hosts, which are usually small mammals or birds. Infected mosquitoes or ticks transmit the virus to humans, with person-to-person transmission occurring from organ transplant or blood transmission.

The majority of clinical disease is asymptomatic. The symptomatic manifestations include fever, arthralgia, and myalgia. The neuroinvasive form of West Nile virus is uncommon and includes encephalitis, meningitis, and acute flaccid paralysis. The symptoms of encephalitis and meningitis include mental confusion, lethargy, photophobia, headache, muscle weakness, and coma, leading to death. Encephalitis or meningitis may not be present in cases of acute flaccid paralysis. West Nile virus disease is diagnosed when antibodies to the virus are recovered from blood serum. There is no evidence-based therapy for the disorder, except for supportive measures to maintain function; however, ribavirin and intravenous immunoglobulin (IVIG) have been used to reduce symptoms.

Commercially available West Nile virus–specific immunoglobulin M (IgM) antibodies in either serum or cerebrospinal fluid is the current way to establish the diagnosis. The antibodies can be found 3 to 8 days after illness onset and persists for 1 to 3 months at the minimum. Therefore, positive results may reflect past rather than current infection. If the testing was done before 8 days of illness, there may be an absence of West Nile virus–specific IgM antibodies and repeat testing may be needed.

There is also currently no vaccine for this condition. It is important to follow the guidelines for mosquito bite prevention previously discussed.

OTHER VIRAL INFECTIONS

Viruses are the most common causes of infectious diseases in children. There can be isolated outbreaks of viral infections in a community even if there are vaccines for the virus available. This may be due to lack of vaccination or waning immunity.

Mumps (Epidemic Parotitis)

- Causative agent: mumps virus
- Incubation period: usually 16 to 18 days with an outside range from 12 to 25 days (AAP, 2015)
- Period of communicability: communicable for 5 days from onset of the swollen parotid gland (CDC, 2016e)
- Mode of transmission: direct contact with respiratory droplets (AAP, 2015; Rubin, Kennedy, & Poland, 2016)
- Immunity: Contracting the disease gives lasting natural immunity.
- Active artificial immunity: attenuated live mumps vaccine in combination with measles and rubella (MMR)
- Passive artificial immunity: mumps immune globulin

Assessment

Mumps is one of the oldest infectious diseases and is now uncommon in the United States due to the MMR vaccine (Rubin et al., 2016). Outbreaks have occurred in recent years on college campuses and in religious communities where immunizations are spotty (CDC, 2016e). If the disease occurs, it begins with fever, headache, anorexia, and malaise. About one third of infections are subclinical, and therefore,

no swelling of the parotid gland is noted. Humans are the only host for the mumps virus.

Mumps cause a parotid gland enlargement without skin erythema in the majority of patients. This enlargement will obscure the angle of jaw and therefore is helpful from differentiating it from submaxillary adenitis (inflammation of lymph nodes). The best method of differentiation is to place a hand along the child's jawline. If the major amount of swelling is above the hand, it is probably mumps (Fig. 43.9). Fever typically occurs early and is accompanied by anorexia and inability to open the mouth (trismus). The swelling will resolve in 5 to 7 days (Alter et al., 2015).

Boys may also develop testicular pain and swelling (orchitis) after puberty, and this complication is more likely as an adult or adolescent. Sterility is a rare complication of the orchitis.

 Concept Mastery Alert

In a patient with mumps, most of the associated swelling occurs above the jawline. If the swelling is primarily below the jawline, the patient likely has adenitis.

Therapeutic Management

Supportive care is key including pain control and fever control with acetaminophen or nonsteroidal anti-inflammatory and a soft bland diet. If a child is hospitalized, follow droplet precautions in addition to standard infection precautions (Alter et al., 2015).

Some parents worry that because their child had swelling only on one side, their child will develop mumps on the opposite side in the future. One attack of mumps gives lasting immunity, so the child will not contract the disease again. If a child does appear to have contracted mumps twice, the diagnosis was probably confused with cervical adenitis at one occurrence.

Figure 43.9 Epidemic parotitis. **(A)** The parotid gland is located just in front of the ear. **(B)** A boy with parotitis (mumps). (© Morris Huberland/Science Source/Photo Researchers.)

Parotid gland

TEAMWORK & COLLABORATION

A nurse on the care team calls off work because she's worried she has contracted mumps (infectious parotitis). Which of the following symptoms is most associated with mumps?
  a. A productive cough and a severe runny nose
  b. Pronounced swelling behind both of her ears
  c. Swelling above the jaw line in front of the ear, obscuring the jaw line
  d. Adenoid tonsils are reddened and swollen and hurt

Look in Appendix A for the best answer and rationale.

Epstein–Barr Infectious Mononucleosis

- Causative agent: Epstein–Barr virus (EBV)
- Incubation period: Incubation period in adults and adolescents is 30 to 50 days with a shorter incubation period in children (Pinninti et al., 2016)
- Period of communicability: occurs during direct contact with saliva by individuals who are symptomatic or asymptomatic but shedding the virus (Pinninti et al., 2016)
- Mode of transmission: direct contact and through blood transfusions
- Immunity: Most of the time, one episode gives lasting immunity; however, EBV is latent and can reactivate and cause a milder clinical presentation. No vaccination is available.

Infectious mononucleosis is the most common manifestation of Epstein–Barr infection (AAP, 2015). It is also known as glandular fever or because it was first discovered as a disease that is transferred readily from one person to another by kissing, the *kissing disease* due the presence of the virus in saliva. The highest incidence of EBV is between 15 and 24 years old, but 50% of children seroconvert before 5 years of age (Pinninti et al., 2016). Central nervous system manifestations include meningitis, encephalitis, cranial nerve palsies, myelitis, transverse myelitis, Guillain-Barré syndrome, and Alice in Wonderland syndrome. Hematologic manifestations include agranulocytosis, hematologic complications, splenic rupture, hemolytic anemia, thrombocytosis, and hemophagocytic lymphohistiocytosis.

Assessment

The classic symptoms of EBV infection include several days of prodromal symptoms of anorexia, chills, and malaise with fever in 90% and enlargement of the cervical nodes and tonsils. Pharyngitis with palatal petechial and periorbital edema and found with splenomegaly is present in about 5% (Pinninti et al., 2016) (Fig. 43.10). If the mesenteric lymph nodes enlarge, children may experience abdominal pain so sharp that it simulates appendicitis.

On a blood smear, atypical lymphocytosis is seen and a total elevation of the lymphocyte count peaks between 2 and 3 weeks of illness (Pinninti et al., 2016). A positive Monospot test, which can be reported in minutes, or a heterophile antibody test is positive in 80% of children older than 4 years of age and are more accurate in older adolescents. The Monospot or heterophile antibody tests in children less than 4 years

Figure 43.10 The appearance of the tonsils in a child with infectious mononucleosis. Note the degree of erythema, enlargement, and purulent covering. (© Dr. P. Marazzi/SPL/Science Source/Photo Researchers.)

tend to be negative. There are several antibodies against the EBV that will be positive at different times during the disease and a positive IgM antibody against viral capsid antigen (VCA) is diagnostic of primary infection.

Therapeutic Management

Children with infectious mononucleosis should be treated for pain and fever with acetaminophen or nonsteroidal anti-inflammatory agents. The child should be encouraged to rest when fatigued, and all contact sports should be avoided for at least 4 weeks after the onset of infection (AAP, 2015; Pinninti et al., 2016).

It can take 3 months for the child to return to his or her baseline fitness. The nurse should stress fluid intake with cool, nonacidic fluids and soft, nonirritating foods. It can interfere with the completion of school work and normal activities. The nurse can support the child or adolescent by listening to them about talk about the effect this illness has on their lives.

Bacterial Infections

Bacteria are independent, living organisms with a nucleus that contains both DNA and RNA. They reproduce by fission, in which one cell enlarges and duplicates itself and then divides into two equal parts. They occur in three main shapes: spheres (cocci), rods (bacilli), and spirals (spirochetes).

Types of bacteria can be distinguished after they are fixed onto a laboratory slide and then stained. Bacteria that stain violet are said to be gram-positive organisms and those that stain red are gram-negative organisms. Those that cannot be decolorized with acid after being stained are acid-fast. Different bacteria from the same family can act differently. In the case of streptococcus, they have an M protein surrounding their cell wall. Some of the M protein produce pyogenic **exotoxins**, which are toxins that act as super antigens (Silva-Costa, Carriço, Ramirez, et al., 2014). When this happens, disease symptoms arise from the bacteria and the effect of the exotoxins on the body. Tetanus, botulism, exotoxin producing staphylococcus and streptococcus, and diphtheria are examples of diseases caused by the systemic spread of toxins produced by bacteria.

STREPTOCOCCAL DISEASES

Streptococci, which are gram-positive organisms, are found normally in the respiratory, alimentary, and female genital tracts. There are more than 120 serotypes or genotypes of group A β-hemolytic streptococci or *Streptococcus pyogenes*. *S. pyogenes* or Lancefield group A streptococcus are responsible for mild infections like impetigo, tonsillitis, or scarlet fever; however, they can also produce severe infections such as toxic shock syndrome or necrotizing fasciitis (Silva-Costa et al., 2014). *S. pyogenes* (β-hemolytic streptococci, group A) is responsible for strep throat and scarlet fever, and this is treated due to the risk of nonsuppurative complications of rheumatic fever and glomerulonephritis. A β-hemolytic, group B streptococcal infection can be contracted from vaginal secretions at birth (see Chapter 26); when newborns become infected with this bacteria, they can die from sepsis, pneumonia, or meningitis.

The manifestations of group A streptococcal infections include erysipelas, cellulitis, pneumonia, endocarditis, pericarditis, osteomyelitis, sepsis, bacteremia, and toxic shock syndrome (Silva-Costa et al., 2014).

Streptococcal pharyngeal infections are discussed in Chapter 40 with other throat infections. Rheumatic fever and glomerulonephritis, conditions that may result as an autoimmune response to streptococci, are discussed in Chapters 41 and 46, respectively.

Scarlet Fever

- Causative agent: β-hemolytic streptococci, group A
- Incubation period: 2 to 5 days for streptococcal pharyngitis (AAP, 2015)
- Period of communicability: greatest during acute phase of respiratory illness; 1 to 7 days
- Mode of transmission: direct contact from a person with the disease and large droplets, not fomites or household pets (AAP, 2015)
- Immunity: One episode of disease gives lasting immunity to scarlet fever toxin. No vaccination is available.

Assessment

Scarlet fever occurs most commonly in school-age children, peaking in the 7- to 8-year-old age group (AAP, 2015). The incidence is highest in temperate climates, and the disease occurs usually in late autumn, winter, and early spring (AAP, 2015).

Symptoms of streptococcal pharyngitis begin abruptly and include fever, sore throat, headache, chills, a rapid pulse, and malaise. As the disease progresses, the production of exotoxins SpeA, SpeC, and SSA causes a rash that appears 12 to 48 hours after the onset of the pharyngeal symptoms (Silva-Costa et al., 2014).

The skin rash typically is red with pinpoint lesions that blanch on pressure and feel as rough as sandpaper (see Fig. 43.3). They tend to be densest on the trunk and very prominent in skin folds (Pastia's sign). The rash persists for approximately 1 week. It desquamates or peels off in fine flakes (AAP, 2015).

In addition to the rash, the tonsils appear inflamed and enlarged and are usually covered with white exudate. The palate may be covered with reddened punctiform (pinpoint) lesions and perhaps scattered petechiae. The tongue, during the first 2 days of the illness, is white and appears furry. By day 3, papillae enlarge and protrude through the white coat, giving the tongue a "white strawberry" appearance. By day 4 or 5, the white coat disappears and the prominent papillae of the tongue give it a "red strawberry" appearance. A "strawberry tongue" is a hallmark symptom of scarlet fever and helps to differentiate the disease from other rashes or pharyngeal infections. A positive rapid strep test or positive throat culture is the diagnostic test of choice.

Therapeutic Management

Children with scarlet fever usually recover without sequela once penicillin is administered. Penicillin V is the drug of choice, but the American Heart Association guidelines and the Pediatric Infectious Disease Society guidelines all endorse orally administered once a day amoxicillin at 50 mg/kg up to 1,200 mg as a daily dose for 10 days (Lennon, Stewart, & Anderson, 2016; Shulman, Bisno, Clegg, et al., 2012; Wilson, Taubert, Gewitz, et al., 2007). IM penicillin G benzathine is an alternative therapy if there is a history of noncompliance. Children may need an analgesic and antipyretic, such as acetaminophen (Tylenol) or children's ibuprofen (Motrin) for pain and fever. They need a soft or liquid diet until the pain from the pharyngitis improves. Comfort measures are important for the rash. Because the underlying cause of the illness is a streptococcal infection, a course of antibiotics is prescribed (AAP, 2015). Caution parents to give the full amount prescribed for the full course to prevent the complications of β-hemolytic, group A streptococcal infections (acute glomerulonephritis or rheumatic fever); however, poststreptococcal reactive arthritis can also occur (AAP, 2015). Box 43.5 describes a one of the disorders previously discussed (varicella) that presents with a rash.

QSEN Checkpoint Question 43.6

INFORMATICS

Jack, who has varicella, is missing his school friends so is eager to return to school. When should the nurse inform the school nurse that it would be safe for Jack to return to school?
- a. Whenever he feels that he is strong enough
- b. When all the lesions have dried and there are no new lesions
- c. As soon as his fever is within normal range
- d. One week after he began the antibiotic

Look in Appendix A for the best answer and rationale.

Impetigo

- Causative agent: β-hemolytic streptococcus, group A or *S. aureus* including MRSA
- Incubation period: 7 to 10 days for impetigo (AAP, 2015)
- Period of communicability: from outbreak of lesions until lesions are healed
- Mode of transmission: direct contact with lesions
- Immunity: none

It is common to see several children in a family with identical impetigo lesions because it is spread by direct contact. An underlying scabies infection can cause impetigo due to infection from scratching with nails (Tasani, Tong, Andrews, et al., 2016).

BOX 43.5

Nursing Care Planning

AN INTERPROFESSIONAL CARE MAP FOR A CHILD WITH VARICELLA

Jack, a 10-year-old boy, was admitted to the hospital yesterday for appendicitis. This morning after surgery, he breaks out in varicella. "His sister is home with mono," his mother tells you. "How could our family get two infections plus appendicitis all in 1 week?"

Family Assessment: Child has three siblings: a 16-year-old sister and two brothers, 6 years and 10 days old. Parents are migrant crop workers. Family moves yearly from Florida to Connecticut to follow crops. Mother rates finances as "We have no money."

Patient Assessment: Multiple papular and vesicular lesions over the body centered on the trunk. Temperature: 103°F (39.5°C). There are several papular lesions on the palate and oral mucosa. Other physical examination findings within normal limits for postoperative course. Child upset and crying, saying, "I wish my mom was here to stay with me. I can't even go to the playroom." Mother usually visits once a day in the late afternoon.

Nursing Diagnosis: Social isolation related to required restrictions associated with infection control precautions

Outcome Evaluation: Child states reason for restrictions, identifies time when restrictions will be lifted, and expresses interest in activities proposed.

Team Member Responsible	Assessment	Intervention	Rationale	Expected Outcome
Activities of Daily Living, Including Safety				
Nurse	Assess what child understands about how communicable diseases are spread.	Review the reason for restrictions and infection control precautions. Institute droplet precautions.	Child may associate precautions and restrictions with feelings of being punished. Droplet precautions help reduce the spread of the disease.	Child states he understands reason for isolation; cooperates to maintain infection precautions.
Nurse	Assess what play activity would provide stimulation.	Visit the child frequently and provide him with opportunities for therapeutic play.	Frequent visits help to decrease feelings of being alone. Therapeutic play helps the child deal with resentment about condition.	Child states that although he wants to go to playroom, he has found an enjoyable activity to occupy his time in his hospital room.
Teamwork & Collaboration				
Nurse/primary healthcare provider	Determine whether hospital infection control committee is aware of contagious illness in a postoperative patient.	Consult with infection control members on the possibility that surgical personnel may have been exposed to varicella.	Varicella is contagious for 1 to 2 days prior to the outbreak of a rash (AAP, 2015).	Infection control officer states she is aware of possible spread of illness and the need for varicella vaccine for exposed unimmunized healthcare personnel and family members.
Procedures/Medications for Quality Improvement				
Nurse	Determine whether child has ever had a reaction to acyclovir.	Begin acyclovir (Zovirax) therapy as prescribed.	Acyclovir is effective for varicella-zoster, the causative organism of varicella.	Child's parents are contacted and report child has not had a previous reaction to acyclovir. Child should take oral acyclovir as prescribed.
Nurse	Ask child to rate pain of postoperative site and itchiness of rash on scale of 1 to 10.	Administer analgesia and antihistamine prescribed. Caution child that antihistamine may make him feel sleepy.	An antihistamine such as diphenhydramine (Benadryl) can greatly reduce the pruritus of a rash.	Child states the itchiness of rash and pain of operative site have decreased to tolerable levels.

Continued on following page

BOX 43.5

Nursing Care Planning (continued)

Team Member Responsible	Assessment	Intervention	Rationale	Expected Outcome
Nutrition				
Nurse/nutritionist	Assess what fluid child would find most appealing to drink.	Provide frequent oral fluids. When soft diet is begun (child is post-op appendicitis), provide soft foods.	Adequate fluid intake is important to prevent skin dryness, which increases discomfort. A soft or liquid diet is less irritating to the child's mouth.	Child identifies favorite fluid to drink; states he is able to eat soft foods even with mouth lesions
Patient-Centered Care				
Nurse/primary care provider	Determine whether other members of family will need a varicella vaccine.	Explain the purpose of varicella immunization for susceptible family members.	Because family members were near the child during the prodromal period, they are susceptible to also contracting the disease.	Parent identifies susceptible family members; she will get them immunized today.
Psychosocial/Spiritual/Emotional Needs				
Nurse	Assess whether child and parent understand the cause of scarlet fever.	Discuss that the spread of infectious diseases is not related to "good or bad" values.	Mother voiced she was concerned because two diseases happened to her child at the same time.	Mother and child state they understand diseases are caused by infectious organisms, not moral status.
Informatics for Seamless Healthcare Planning				
Nurse	Assess if parent is aware the child's rash will be itchy for about 1 week.	Discuss possible measures the parent can take to reduce pruritus (e.g., loose clothing, cool compresses) and measures to reduce pain of sore throat (e.g., analgesic).	If children scratch pruritic lesions, they can cause a secondary infection. Mouth lesions interfere with comfort and an ability to eat well.	Parent states she understands common measures to reduce pruritus and will begin them.

Assessment

Impetigo involves the top layer or epidermal layer of the skin and is generally characterized by honey-colored crusts with local erythema (Fig. 43.11). It is usually caused by either *S. aureus* or by group A hemolytic streptococci. The lesions are found most commonly on the face and extremities. They are often seen as secondary infections of insect bites or in children who have body piercings. If the impetigo is extensive, children may have local lymph node enlargement.

Therapeutic Management

Localized disease is treated with mupirocin (Bactroban) ointment for 7 to 10 days (Box 43.6) or with retapamulin (Altabax) for children over 9 months twice a day (bid) for 5 days. The use of oral antibiotic that cover both staphylococcus and streptococcus is reserved for extensive impetigo.

Although rare, complications of rheumatic fever or acute glomerulonephritis may occur as a sequelae to impetigo.

Cat-Scratch Disease

- Causative agent: *Bartonella henselae* bacteria which is slow growing
- Incubation period: usually 1 to 2 weeks with a range of 7 to 60 days
- Period of communicability: unknown
- Mode of transmission: bite or scratch from more commonly a kitten rather than a cat
- Immunity: one episode of disease gives lasting immunity; no passive artificial immunity

Cat-scratch disease occurs most commonly in preschool children because children at that age play roughly with cats or pick them up and so receive scratches. At the time, the child contracts the disease, the cat does not appear ill.

The first symptom is a single skin papule or pustule at the site of inoculation which precedes the lymphadenopathy by 1 to 2 weeks (range of 5 to 50 days). A Bartonella-infected lymph node will usually resolve over a period of 4 to 6 weeks

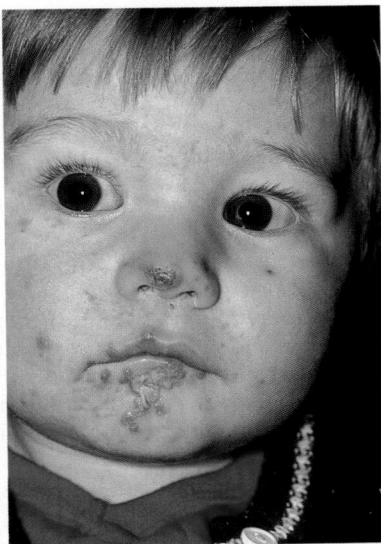

Figure 43.11 Impetigo in a toddler. Note the honey-colored crust appearance of some of the lesions. (© Dr. P. Marazzi/SPL/ Science Source/Photo Researchers.)

without treatment, and 10% to 25% will eventually drain spontaneously. Other forms of this disease includes Parinaud oculoglandular syndrome, which presents clinically with preauricular lymphadenitis and a follicular conjunctivitis as well as 1 to 2 weeks of fever with nonspecific symptoms. Less common presentations include neuroretinitis, endocarditis,

osteolytic lesions, pneumonia, thrombocytopenia purpura, and encephalopathy (AAP, 2015).

The diagnostic test is an indirect immunofluorescent antibody (IFA) for antibody detection to serum antigens of the Bartonella species. Culture is difficult because it is such a slow-growing organism. Although enzyme immunoassays (EIAs) for antibody detection have been developed, more research is needed about their specificity and sensitivity.

Treatment is symptomatic, although azithromycin may be prescribed to decrease the lymph node size. With more severe disease, treatment with antimicrobials for several weeks will be initiated (AAP, 2015). Children may need an analgesic to relieve pain from the swollen lymph node.

Parents may ask if the cat should be destroyed. Because an attack of cat-scratch disease gives lifetime immunity and fewer than 10% of children scratched by the same cat contract cat-scratch disease, there is no need to destroy the cat for an act it may have seen as defending its safety.

STAPHYLOCOCCAL INFECTIONS

Gram-positive *S. aureus* is the most common infecting organism for pyogenic infections of the skin as well as soft tissue (Gaensbauer & Todd, 2016). Staphylococci are normally found on the skin surface; therefore, they are commonly the organisms involved in skin infections (pyodermas). Because the organisms grow rapidly in cream foods that are not well refrigerated, such as potato salad or cream pies, they are also often the organisms involved in summer food poisoning episodes. Because food poisoning produces gastrointestinal symptoms, these infections are discussed in Chapter 45.

 BOX 43.6
Nursing Care Planning Based on Responsibility for Pharmacology

MUPIROCIN (BACTROBAN)

Classification: Mupirocin is a topical antibiotic.

Action: Mupirocin is used to treat impetigo caused by *Staphylococcus aureus* and *Streptococcus pyogenes*.

Pregnancy Risk Category: B

Dosage: small amount applied three times a day to the affected areas for 10 days duration

Possible Adverse Effects: local irritation including erythema, dry skin, pruritus, burning, stinging (Taketomo, 2015)

RETAPAMULIN OINTMENT 1% (ALTABAX)

Classification: Retapamulin ointment 1% is a topical antibiotic.

Action: Retapamulin ointment 1% is used to treat impetigo caused by *S. aureus* and *S. pyogenes*.

Pregnancy Risk Category: B

Dosage: small amount applied twice times a day to the affected areas for 5 days duration

Possible Adverse Effects: local irritation including erythema, pruritus, burning, stinging (Taketomo, 2015)

Nursing Implications
- Advise parents to wash the lesions with soap and water and pat dry before applying ointment to soften crusts for better absorption.
- Caution parents that causative organisms are infectious by direct contact. Instruct them to wash their own hands before and after applying the ointment.
- Although the lesions may begin to improve before 10 days have elapsed, urge parents to continue to use the ointment to ensure eradication of the causative bacteria.
- Instruct parents to use caution if applying the ointment around the eyes because the ointment is irritating to the eyes.

Furunculosis/Carbunculosis (Abscesses or Boils)

A furuncle is a staphylococcal infection of a single hair follicle, and a carbuncle has multiple hair follicles with openings. A single or multiple yellow pustule forms at the site. There is localized redness, pain, and edema of the surrounding skin. As these enlarge, they may need an incision and drainage to drain the pus. The nurse should educate the family and child to never press an abscess to rupture the lesions. The use of antibiotics after an incision and drainage is controversial and depends on the size of carbuncle.

Cellulitis

Cellulitis is staphylococcal inflammation of the dermal and subcutaneous layers of skin. It can occur anywhere on the body and there will be warmth, tenderness, and erythema at the area of cellulitis. The treatment is a systemic antibiotic that will cover both staphylococci and streptococci.

Methicillin-Resistant *Staphylococcus aureus*

MRSA is a strain of staphylococcus that causes skin infections and has become resistant to common broad-spectrum antibiotics. When an infection occurs in a healthcare setting, it is referred to as health care–associated MRSA or HA-MRSA. If it occurs in a community setting, it is termed community-associated MRSA (CA-MRSA). Children with weakened immune systems are at greatest risk for contracting the infection. A recent retrospective research review found the rates of MRSA are falling in the pediatric population (Sutter, Milburn, Chukwuma, et al., 2016).

Vancomycin is the drug of choice for treatment of hospital-based lesions because the bacteria are still susceptible to its design. Clindamycin or trimethoprim-sulfamethoxazole is commonly used with community infections. Use strict standard infection precaution measures when caring for a child with an MRSA infection.

Prevention centered on nasal, skin, and household decolonization is important because most children with a *S. aureus* skin or soft tissue infection will have a recurrence within 1 year (Creech, Al-Zubeidi, & Fritz, 2015).

Good hand washing and reporting skin wounds to a healthcare provider before an open wound can become infected can help prevent these infections.

Scalded Skin Disease

Staphylococcal scalded skin syndrome (Ritter disease) is a staphylococcal infection seen in infants. Newborns develop rough-textured skin and general erythema, especially on areas that encounter friction. Large bullae (vesicles) filled with clear fluid form. The epidermis separates in large sheets and desquamates, leaving a raw, red, glistening, and scalded-looking surface. This is called Nikolsky sign.

OTHER BACTERIAL INFECTIONS

S. aureus and streptococcal infections are the most common bacterial infections in children, but other bacteria are also responsible for infections in pediatric patients. Although vaccines are available to protect against *Haemophilus influenzae*, *Strepto-* *coccus pneumoniae*, *Clostridium tetani*, and diphtheria, children can still get infections with other serotypes due to lack of vaccination, waning immunity, or be infected with a serotype that vaccines do not protect against.

Diphtheria

- Causative agent: *Corynebacterium diphtheriae* (Klebs–Löffler bacillus)
- Incubation period: 2 to 5 days with a range of 1 to 10 days (AAP, 2015)
- Period of communicability: In untreated persons, the organism is contagious from nares, throat, skin, and eyes for 2 to 6 weeks following infection; 48 hours after initiation of antibiotics in treated children and adults.
- Mode of transmission: direct contact or indirect contact droplets
- Immunity: Contracting the disease gives lasting natural immunity.
- Active artificial immunity: diphtheria toxin given as part of diphtheria, tetanus, and pertussis (DTaP) vaccine
- Passive artificial immunity: diphtheria antitoxin

Assessment

Diphtheria is a rare illness due to available immunizations with only 2 cases in the United States since 2004 and under 8,000 cases reported to WHO worldwide (CDC, 2016a). Diphtheria bacilli invade and grow in the nasopharynx of children and produce an exotoxin that causes massive cell necrosis and inflammation. The endotoxin promotes bacilli growth and causes the infected cells form a characteristic gray membrane on the nasopharynx. This may extend up into the nose and down into the major bronchi, causing a purulent nasal discharge and a brassy cough. The toxin is absorbed from the membrane surface and spreads systemically by the bloodstream to affect major organs, such as the heart and nervous system. If untreated, myocarditis with heart failure and conduction disturbances may occur. Central nervous system involvement can include severe neuritis with paralysis of the diaphragm and pharyngeal and laryngeal muscles. Diphtheria can also form skin lesions aside from the usual presentation of respiratory infections. As a result, the diagnosis of diphtheria is made based on clinical appearance and culture from the nose, throat, or any mucosal or cutaneous lesion, and it must be placed on special media so the lab must be notified that there is a suspicion of diphtheria bacilli (AAP, 2015).

Therapeutic Management

Treatment involves a single dose of equine antitoxin based on clinical suspicion, and this can be obtained through the CDC (AAP, 2015). In addition, children are given penicillin or erythromycin intravenously. Complete bed rest is crucial during the acute stage of the illness. Droplet precautions must be followed until cultures are negative. Children need careful observation at all times to prevent airway obstruction. If obstruction occurs, endotracheal intubation may be necessary.

Due to the vaccine, the disease is almost extinct, but in cases of travel, this disease should be considered in a sick child with a classic gray membrane on the tonsils. Prompt recognition and treatment are necessary to avoid death.

Whooping Cough (Pertussis)

- Causative agent: *Bordetella pertussis*
- Incubation period: 5 to 21 days
- Mode of transmission: highly contagious by direct or indirect contact
- Period of communicability: greatest in catarrhal (respiratory illness) stage; eliminates contagiousness within 5 to 7 days of treatment, but it continues for weeks in the untreated patient (Gabutti, Azzari, Bonanni, et al., 2015)
- Immunity: contracting the disease offers lasting natural immunity
- Active artificial immunity: pertussis vaccine given as part of DTaP vaccine
- Passive artificial immunity: pertussis immune serum globulin

Pertussis has been increasing in the United States despite an active vaccine program (Faulkner, Skoff, Tondella, et al., 2016). This is due to healthcare providers' awareness, improved diagnostic lab tests, waning immunity from the acellular vaccine, and decreases in immunization rates in certain parts of the United States (Faulkner et al., 2016).

Assessment

The disease can primarily manifest as a mild rhinitis with a mild cough to persistent cough illness or to the classic pertussis disease. Classic pertussis manifests itself in three steps: the catarrhal stage, the paroxysmal stage, and the convalescent stage. The **catarrhal stage** begins with upper respiratory symptoms such as coryza, sneezing, lacrimation, cough, and a low-grade fever, symptoms subtle enough they may at first be mistaken for those of a common cold. This first period lasts 1 to 2 weeks.

The paroxysmal stage lasts from 2 to 6 weeks (Long, 2016). During this time, the cough changes from a mild one to paroxysmal, involving 5 to 10 short, rapid coughs, followed by a rapid inspiration, which causes the hallmark "whoop" or high-pitched crowing sound of whooping cough. Children are in obvious distress while coughing. They may become cyanotic or red faced, and their nose may drain thick, tenacious mucus. They often vomit after a paroxysm of coughing, and they feel exhausted afterward from the effort. Immunized children and adolescents have shortened phases in the classic presentation.

During the convalescent stage, there is a gradual cessation of the coughing and vomiting.

Pertussis is diagnosed by its striking symptoms, although in children younger than 6 months of age, the "whoop" of the cough may be absent, making it more difficult to diagnose. Current diagnostics available include culture, direct fluorescent antibody (DFA) testing, polymerase chain reactions (PCR), and serology; however, PCR is the primary method of diagnosis early in the disease with serology more commonly used later in the disease and in adults (Faulkner et al., 2016; Heininger, 2012). The serology tests are poorly standardized from lab to lab (Heininger, 2012). The WBC count, particularly the lymphocyte count, is markedly increased to as high as 20,000 to 30,000/mm^3 (normal levels are 5,000 to 10,000/mm^3).

Therapeutic Management

Infants younger than 3 months with pertussis are generally admitted to the hospital for at least 48 hours to see how the disease course is progressing and to monitor for complications from paroxysms, particularly nutritional intake and oxygen levels (Long, 2016). The child may need oxygen if the pertussis is severe. The family must keep children with pertussis secluded from environmental factors, such as cigarette smoke and dust, and to avoid strenuous activities because these initiate coughing episodes. Nutrition may become a problem if the child is constantly coughing and vomiting. As a rule, frequent small meals are vomited less than larger meals and so should be encouraged.

A full 10-day course of erythromycin or azithromycin may be prescribed because these drugs have the potential to shorten the period of communicability and may shorten the duration of symptoms. Droplet precautions are used until 5 days after a child starts antibiotic therapy. Complications of pertussis include alkalosis and dehydration caused by vomiting and pneumonia, atelectasis, or emphysema from plugged bronchioles. Epistaxis, subconjunctival and subarachnoid bleeding, or seizures from asphyxia as a result of severe paroxysms of coughing may also occur. Infants with pertussis may be admitted to a healthcare facility for observation because they become dehydrated or may have such tenacious secretions that they need airway suction. For safety, place an intercom in the infant's room so you can identify severe coughing even when not in the room.

Prevention

The current recommendation is to immunize the pregnant woman from 27 weeks to 36 weeks of gestation to maximize maternal antibody transfer to the fetus and reduce the risk of pertussis to the newborn (Kroger, 2015). Cohorting of young infants and making sure that all caretakers are immunized is another method of risk reduction to the young infant. All children should be immunized in infancy with DTaP and a booster dose given at 11 to 12 years of age (Kroger, 2015).

What If . . . 43.2
An adolescent who has pertussis vomits after an episode of coughing. Should the nurse urge him to try to eat again immediately, or would he be too nauseated to do so?

Anthrax

- Causative agent: *Bacillus anthracis*, a bacteria
- Incubation period: 1 to 7 days (inhalational), 1 to 12 days (cutaneous), 1 to 7 days (gastrointestinal)
- Mode of transmission: originally contracted from contact with the feces of infected cows or sheep; not transmissible from person to person
- Types of immunity: unstudied
  - Active artificial immunity: At present, the anthrax vaccine is not used in children but is available for adults 18 to 65 years of age who work with anthrax in the lab, certain vets who handle animals or animal products contaminated with anthrax, and only some members of the military (CDC, 2016i).
  - Passive artificial immunity: not available

Anthrax is an acute infectious disease that is contracted from exposure to the anthrax bacteria or its spores. As the organism grows inside the human body, a toxin is produced that causes the bulk of the symptoms. Children may present with any of the three clinical forms: cutaneous, inhalational, or gastrointestinal.

Inhalational anthrax has a mortality rate of over 90%. It begins with a brief prodromal period of flulike symptoms, followed shortly by dyspnea, severe systemic shock, and marked evidence of mediastinal widening and pleural effusion on X-ray. Because it can be fatal and spreads through coughing, anthrax has been proposed as bacteria that could be used in bioterrorism (AAP, 2015).

Cutaneous anthrax is characterized by a skin lesion that begins as a papule and then passes through a vesicle stage, to a painless depressed black eschar. Fever, malaise, headache, and regional swollen lymph nodes may accompany the skin lesion. The mortality of cutaneous anthrax is as low as 1% with antibiotic therapy.

Gastrointestinal anthrax is contracted by eating undercooked meat infected with the organism. The child develops severe abdominal pain, fever, bloody diarrhea, and **septicemia** (blood infection). The mortality rate for this form is about 25%.

If exposed to anthrax, prophylaxis with ciprofloxacin (Cipro) for those older than 18 years of age and doxycycline for younger patients are the drugs of choice. Drug therapy is continued for 60 days because of the potential persistence of and difficulty in killing spores.

Tetanus (Lockjaw)

- Causative agent: *C. tetani*
- Incubation period: 3 days to 3 weeks
- Period of communicability: none
- Mode of transmission: direct or indirect contamination of a closed wound
- Immunity: development of the disease gives lasting natural immunity
- Active artificial immunity: tetanus toxoid contained in DTaP vaccine
- Passive artificial immunity: TIG

Tetanus occurs worldwide causing an acute, spastic paralytic illness caused by neurotoxin produced by *Clostridium* (Arnon, 2016). It is a highly fatal disease if untreated and is caused by an anaerobic, spore-forming bacillus found in soil and the excretions of animals. It enters the body through an open wound. If the wound is deep, such as a stab wound, where the distal end of the wound is shut off from an oxygen source, tetanus bacilli begin to reproduce. The organism may also enter through a burn site, which crusts, thus creating an anaerobic environment. As the bacilli grow, they produce exotoxins that cause the disease symptoms by affecting the motor nuclei of the central nervous system (Arnon, 2016). The onset of the disease occurs gradually over 1 to 7 days with severe muscle spasm stimulated by external stimuli and autonomic dysfunction causing arrhythmias, tachycardia, and diaphoresis (AAP, 2015).

The entrance site of the bacillus does not appear infected (no pus or reddened area is present unless a secondary infection also exists). After the incubation period, the exotoxins have developed to such an extent, however, that they are capable of disrupting the nervous system. In the United States, most children are vaccinated against tetanus. In developing countries, it continues to have a high incidence, caused by infection of an entry point such as the umbilical cord at birth (AAP, 2015).

Assessment

The first symptoms that are noticeable are stiffness of the neck and jaw (lockjaw). Within 24 to 48 hours, muscular rigidity of the trunk and extremities develops. The back becomes arched (opisthotonos), the abdominal muscles are stiff and board-like, and the face assumes an unusual appearance, with wrinkling of the forehead and distortion of the corners of the mouth (a "sardonic grin" sign). Any stimulation, such as a sudden noise, a bright light, or a touch, causes painful, paroxysmal spasms. The sensorium is clear throughout the course of the disease, so the child is aware of the pain associated with the muscle spasms. As these spasms begin to include the larynx, respiratory obstruction and death by asphyxiation can occur.

Therapeutic Management

A child needs to be cared for in a quiet, stimulation-free room with total parenteral nutrition, sedation, and a muscle relaxant to prevent aspiration from muscle spasms. If the wound is filled with necrotic tissue, it may be debrided to ensure no secondary infections arise. The first line of treatment is human tetanus immune globulin (TIG) with parenteral penicillin G or oral or intravenous metronidazole (Flagyl) administration to decrease the vegetative forms of *C. tetani*. A child may need to be intubated and mechanical ventilation begun to maintain respiratory function.

Prevention

Tetanus is a serious disease, but it can be prevented through active immunization and suitable booster immunizations. Children routinely receive tetanus immunization as part of routine DTaP immunization with a booster dose at school age; thereafter, they should receive a booster dose every 10 years. At the time of a wound, the wound site should be cleaned well with soap and water and a suitable antiseptic. It should not be sutured but should be left open to heal by secondary intention to reduce the possibility of an anaerobic pocket forming in the wound. If the child received basic immunization against tetanus and it has been fewer than 10 years since the last injection, no booster or antitoxin management is needed at the time of the wound.

If a child's immunization record cannot be obtained or is fewer than three doses, a child will be treated with a booster injection and TIG. The booster injection provides tetanus antigen to the child. If the child has received three or more DTaP, Td, or Tdap vaccines, and the wound is clean and it has been less than 10 years since the child received a vaccine, no immunization is needed; however, if the wound is dirty and it has been more than 5 years, then a Td is needed.

Lyme Disease

- Causative agent: *Borrelia burgdorferi*, a spirochete
- Incubation period: 3 to 30 days
- Period of communicability: not communicable from one person to another
- Mode of transmission: deer tick
- Active artificial immunity: none available; Lyme vaccine discontinued
- Passive artificial immunity: immune globulin

Lyme disease is caused by a spirochete, *B. burgdorferi*, which is transmitted by a tick frequently carried on deer (Choi, Pyzocha, & Maurer, 2016). The disease is the most frequently reported vector-borne infection in the United States, occurring most often in the summer and early fall and on the east coast (it is named after the city in Connecticut where it was first identified). A vaccine for the disease is not

Figure 43.12 The rash of Lyme disease. (© Larry Mulvehill/ Science Source/Photo Researchers.)

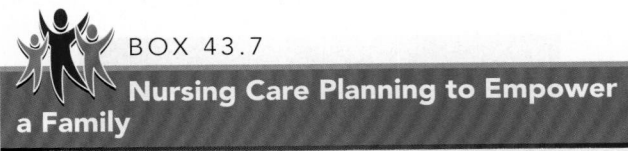

BOX 43.7

Nursing Care Planning to Empower a Family

TIPS FOR AVOIDING EXPOSURE TO LYME DISEASE

Q. Jack's father tells you, "My children love to play in the woods, but I'm so afraid they'll get Lyme disease. What can I do to protect them?"

A. Here are some suggestions to help reduce the risk of exposure:

- Wear protective clothing when hiking or playing in wooded areas, such as long sleeves, high necklines, and long slacks. Tuck bottom of slacks into socks or boots.
- Wear light-colored clothing so any tick present on clothing can be readily observed.
- Inspect the skin daily and thoroughly for ticks after hiking or playing in wooded areas.
- Remove any ticks found with tweezers placed at the head of the tick, pulling gently and steadily for several seconds. The tick mouth takes a while to release their hold.
- Report any area of inflammation that might be a tick bite to a healthcare provider for early diagnosis.

currently available because the manufacturer ceased production in 2002 due to low demand (CDC, 2015c).

Almost immediately after a tick bite, an erythematous papule is noticeable at the site, which spreads over the next 3 to 30 days (the incubation period) to become a large, round ring with a raised swollen border (erythema chronicum migrans) (Fig. 43.12). This is followed by systemic involvement that can lead to cardiac, musculoskeletal, and neurologic symptoms. Cardiac involvement may be so severe that it includes heart block from atrioventricular conduction abnormalities. Neurologic symptoms commonly include stiff neck, headache, and cranial nerve palsy. Musculoskeletal symptoms include painful swollen arthritic joints, particularly in the knee.

Amoxicillin is administered to symptomatic children less than 8 years old, whereas doxycycline is given to those older than 8 years of age. Encourage parents to inspect the skin of children who have been playing in wooded areas for tick bites to help identify the disorder before debilitating symptoms occur (CDC, 2016h). Other suggestions for avoiding Lyme disease are shown in Box 43.7.

Other Infectious Pathogens

RICKETTSIAL DISEASES

Rickettsiae are organisms that resemble viruses both in size and in their inability to reproduce except inside the cells of a host organism. They reproduce by fission, however, as bacteria do; like bacteria, they are complete organisms containing both RNA and DNA. They multiply inside ticks, lice, mites, or fleas (arthropods) without causing disease. They are transmitted to humans through the bite or feces of the infected arthropod. An exception is Q fever, which is spread by droplet infection. All rickettsial diseases include fever, trigger an immune response, and almost all include a rash caused by rickettsial multiplication in the endothelial cells of small blood vessels.

What If . . . 43.3
Jack's mother tells the nurse that she's always been afraid her children would contact Lyme disease because, in the winter, the family picks both limes and lemons in Florida. Can the nurse assure her Jack will never contract Lyme disease while in an orchard picking fruit?

Rocky Mountain Spotted Fever

- Causative agent: *Rickettsia rickettsii*
- Incubation period: 3 to 12 days
- Period of communicability: not communicable from one person to another
- Mode of transmission: wood, dog, or rabbit tick
- Active artificial immunity: Rocky Mountain spotted fever (RMSF) vaccine is not available.

RMSF is transmitted by ticks and is a common rickettsial disease seen in the United States (Biggs, Behravesh, Bradley, et al., 2016).

Most tick infections occur between April and October; however, ticks can bite in the winter with 9% of infections in New York, New Jersey, and Pennsylvania reported in the winter (Mukkada & Buckingham, 2015). The initial presentation is nonspecific and includes malaise, nausea, vomiting, and myalgia. The reported clinical presentation of RMSF is a triad rash, fever, and tick bite history; however, this occurs in fewer than 60% of children (Mukkada & Buckingham, 2015). The others reported a prominent reddened area at the site of the tick bite. In 2 to 8 days, a blanching pink macular rash on the ankles, wrists, or forearms develops, eventually spreading to the palms, soles, arms, legs, and trunk but tending to spare the face (Biggs et al., 2016). The classic petechial rash will develop by 5 to 6 days and is a sign of advanced disease (Fig. 43.13).

Approximately 50% of patients have no rash in the first 3 days of illness (Biggs et al., 2016). The child will also have abdominal pain that mimics appendicitis, diarrhea, gastroenteritis, conjunctiva redness, and periorbital and peripheral edema (Biggs et al., 2016). A persistent headache and fever (as high as 104°F [40°C]) with mental confusion can also occur.

Figure 43.13 The typical rash of Rocky Mountain spotted fever. (Courtesy of Stuart Starr, MD, The Children's Hospital of Philadelphia.)

In late-stage disease, untreated children will develop central nervous system involvement including a meningoencephalitis (stiff neck and seizures) and renal failure, with signs of cardiac and pulmonary failure including pneumonia.

RMSF is the most common fatal rickettsial disease in the United States (Kellen & Berlin, 2016) and was a serious childhood illness before antibiotic therapy was available. First-line therapy is with doxycycline for 7 to 10 days and should be initiated within the first 5 days of the appearance of symptoms. Children are generally admitted for initiation of treatment and as they improve are discharged home. Caution parents to finish the full course of therapy to ensure disease eradication and to prevent the risk of complications.

PSITTACOSIS

Psittacosis, caused by *Chlamydophila psittaci*, is a respiratory disease transmitted to children through the inhalation of aerosolized excrement or respiratory sections from the eyes or beaks of birds that are infected with the bacteria (AAP, 2015). Although the bird does not appear ill, children develop symptoms of a respiratory infection with cough, fever, pharyn-

gitis, headache, malaise, or diarrhea. An extensive interstitial pneumonia can develop. More serious complications include myocarditis, endocarditis, nephritis, hepatitis, or encephalitis. The course of the disease is as long as 3 to 4 weeks. The treatment of choice is either tetracycline or doxycycline for children older than 8 years or erythromycin or azithromycin for younger children or pregnant teens (AAP, 2015).

PARASITIC INFECTIONS

Parasites are organisms that live on and obtain their food supply from other organisms. Although many of these can cause illness, ones frequently associated with children include head lice and scabies (Table 43.3). Parents are often embarrassed when they learn their child has one of these illnesses. You can reassure them that these infestations could happen to any child (Box 43.8).

HELMINTHIC INFECTIONS

Helminths are pathogenic or parasitic worms. They include roundworms (nematodes), flukes (trematodes), or tapeworms (cestodes). Most helminths begin life when the eggs or larvae are eliminated in the feces or urine of humans. They are then transmitted to the oral cavity by contaminated foods or hands. Because children tend to be careless about washing their hands before eating or tend to suck their thumbs, it makes them prone to these infections.

Roundworms (Ascariasis)

Ascaris lumbricoides are generally asymptomatic infections but when there is an extensive parasite load, malnutrition and gastrointestinal symptoms result (AAP, 2015). With an incubation period of 8 weeks, the nurse must obtain a history of travel to underdeveloped countries. The roundworm parasite lives in the intestinal tract. Larvae, which hatch from the ingested eggs, penetrate the intestinal wall and enter the circulation. From there, they may migrate to any body tissue. Children develop a loss of appetite and nausea and vomiting. Intestinal obstruction may occur from a mass of roundworms in the intestine. Ascariasis can be prevented by the sanitary disposal of feces to prevent contamination of the soil. There are several treatment options: (a) a single dose of albendazole with food, (b) nitazoxanide twice a day for 3 days,

TABLE 43.3 COMMON PARASITIC INFECTIONS

Infection	Organism	Symptoms	Treatment
Pediculosis capitis	Head lice	Small, white flecks on hair shaft (nits or eggs of lice); extreme pruritus	Wash hair with one of several approved products, starting with an over-the-counter permethrin-based or pyrethrin-based shampoo (AAP, 2015) and comb nits from hair with fine-toothed comb. Wash bed sheets and recently worn clothes; vacuum pillows, mattresses, or other items unable to be washed. Teach children not to exchange combs, hair barrettes, or other personal items.
Pediculosis	Pubic lice	Same as for head lice except on pubic hair	Same as head lice
Scabies	Female mite (*Acarus scabiei*)	Black burrow filled with mite feces 1–2 in. long, usually between fingers and toes, on palms, or in axilla or groin	Caution that adolescent groin infestations might be spread by physical intimacy. Topical permethrin 5% cream is the drug of choice with two doses of oral ivermectin (off-label use) 1 week apart, also being an effective drug (AAP, 2015).

BOX 43.8

Nursing Care Planning Tips for Effective Communication

When Jack's 6-year-old brother Joshua visits him, you notice Joshua has scratch marks on his neck and forehead. His hair shafts are covered by sand-like particles. You suspect he has pediculosis capitis or head lice.

Tip: Ask follow-up questions and provide appropriate patient education. The following scenario is an example of what can happen if people believe the myth that communicable diseases are always associated with poor hygiene or poverty. Head lice can spread easily in locker rooms or classrooms, so any child can contract them.

Nurse: I am noticing sand-like particles in your son's hair.

Mrs. Noma: Well, you know boys. They don't always wash well.

Nurse: They resemble the eggs of head lice.

Mrs. Noma: We're not that poor. Don't insult us.

Nurse: I apologize if you think I am insulting you. People from all walks of life get head lice. Let's talk about head lice and how easy it is for anyone to get them.

or (c) a single dose of ivermectin (off-label use and not to be used in children less than 15 kg) (AAP, 2015).

Hookworms

Hookworm infections tend to be asymptomatic and are more common in children living in tropical climates with poor sanitation. Hookworm eggs, like roundworm eggs, are found in human feces. They enter children's bodies through the skin and then migrate to the intestinal tract, where they attach themselves onto the intestinal villi and suck blood from the intestinal wall to sustain themselves. Abdominal pain which is colicky in nature, nausea, and diarrhea with marked eosinophilia can be a presenting sign 4 to 6 weeks after exposure. If a great number of hookworms are present, severe anemia may result. Treatment is with albendazole (Albenza), mebendazole (Vermox), and pyrantel pamoate (Pin X) are effective (AAP, 2015). Children may also need therapy for the anemia.

Enterobiasis (Pinworms)

Pinworms are small, white, threadlike worms that live in the cecum. After ingestion of the egg either by ingestion or breathing, the mature worms develop over a period of 2 months in the cecum. The mature female pinworm then migrates out of the anus to deposit eggs on the skin in the anal and perianal region (CDC, 2016f). The movement of the worms causes the anal area to itch, and the child will awaken at night crying and scratching. Some of the eggs are then carried from the child's fingernails to the mouth. After being ingested, they hatch in the child's intestinal tract, and the cycle is repeated (CDC, 2016f).

The worms are large enough that they can be seen if the child's buttocks are separated. Pressing a piece of cellophane tape against the anus and then inspecting it under a microscope will generally reveal pinworm eggs.

Treatment is with a single dose of mebendazole (Vermox) or pyrantel pamoate (antihelminthic) (CDC, 2016f). Underclothing, bedding, towels, and nightclothes should be washed before reuse. In addition, all family members need to be treated for pinworm infestation because the worms are easily transmitted from person to person. Teach children to avoid nail biting and to wash their hands before food preparation or eating to avoid transfer of pinworm eggs and to prevent this type of infection.

PROTOZOAN INFECTIONS

Protozoa are unicellular organisms. They absorb fluid through their cell membrane and can move from place to place by pseudopod, flagella, or cilia action. They are most pathogenic in the gastrointestinal, genitourinary, and circulatory systems. Some protozoa reproduce by simple binary fission, whereas other forms have complex life cycles. They have the ability to form cysts or surround themselves with a membrane, which makes them resistant to destruction.

Giardiasis

Giardia lamblia, a flagellated protozoa, is the most common intestinal parasitic infection in the United States with transmission occurring from ground water contamination and untreated surfaces that are contaminated (Painter, Gargano, Collier, et al., 2015). The peak of the disease occurs in the early summer through the fall (AAP, 2015).

Transmission occurs through the fecal–oral route and occurs from fecal contaminated water and stool. Transmission can occur from person to person or from person to animal. The child ingests the cysts of the organism, and the cysts develop in the intestine into the mature form of the organism. Ingestion of as little as 10 cysts has been associated with illness (Painter et al., 2015). It is contagious as long as the infected person still has excreted cysts (AAP, 2015).

The disease can be asymptomatic or, in symptomatic people, associated with diarrhea, weight loss, abdominal cramps, bloating, and weight loss. The diagnosis is made through DFA assays as well as specific EIA (AAP, 2015, Painter et al., 2015) with DFA being the recommended test by the CDC (Painter et al., 2015). According to the 2015 *Red Book*, metronidazole (Flagyl), nitazoxanide (Alinia, Nizonide), and tinidazole (Tindamax) are the drugs of choice in pediatric patients, with metronidazole being the least expensive (AAP, 2015). Nitazoxanide is approved over 1 year of age, whereas tinidazole is approved over 3 years of age. Treatment of asymptomatic carriers is not recommended for well children living in a household with well people (AAP, 2015).

Prevention measures include hand washing for more than 20 seconds (CDC, 2017), improved sanitation at day care, adequate chlorination of pool and drinking water, and camping water decontamination.

FUNGAL INFECTIONS

Fungi are larger than bacteria; some are unicellular (yeasts), but generally, they are multicellular (molds). Deep mycoses invade internal organs. Respiratory transmission is by the inhalation of spores. Subcutaneous mycoses invade the skin, subcutaneous tissue, and bone. Infections usually occur from introduction of the fungi into a wound. Superficial mycoses invade only the hair, skin, or nails.

Superficial Fungal Infections

Four superficial fungal infections seen frequently in children are tinea cruris, pedis, capitis, and corporis.

Tinea Cruris

Tinea cruris (jock itch) is a brownish to erythematous, well-demarcated patch on the groin, inner thighs, and scrotum. The patch can sometimes have central clearing and may have a papular or vesiculopapular border. The area is pruritic and may result from moisture, close-fitting garments, and obesity. The incubation period is from 1 to 3 weeks (AAP, 2015). Local application of an antifungal agent for 4 to 6 weeks is needed, and the use of corticosteroids in the area should be avoided.

Tinea Pedis

Tinea pedis (athlete's foot) produces pruritic, pinpoint vesicles with fissuring between the toes and on the plantar surface of the foot. It is treated with antifungal agent such as clotrimazole (Lotrimin).

Tinea Capitis

Tinea capitis is a dermatophytic fungal infection of the scalp which can present one of four ways: (a) a patchy alopecia with short 2 to 4 mm broken-off hair shafts, (b) a well demarcated scaling erythematous patch in circular area, (c) a yellow crusting, perifollicular erythema of scalp which has heavy hair loss, or (d) a kerion or boggy circular area of hair loss which is the result of an inflammatory response to the fungus. The child must be treated with oral antifungal such as griseofulvin (Gris-PEG) or terbinafine (Lamisil) and topical shampoo such as selenium sulfide (Selsun Shampoo), ketoconazole (Nizoral shampoo), and ciclopirox (Loprox Shampoo) applied two to three times a week (AAP, 2015).

Adolescents should be cautioned not to consume alcohol while taking any oral antifungal medications as they are metabolized by the liver and can cause nausea and vomiting. Safety of the drug during pregnancy is not established. Caution children to avoid strong sunlight during griseofulvin therapy because photosensitivity may occur (AAP, 2015).

Tinea Corporis

Tinea corporis is a superficial, well-demarcated, mildly erythematous, ring-like infection of the epidermal layer of the skin characterized by slightly scaly central clearing and raised papular borders. It starts as a papular lesion and spreads over several days. It is called ringworm due to its circular shape (Fig. 43.14). The incubation period is 1 to 3 weeks. The lesions are confused with granuloma annulare and nummular eczema. Topical antifungal treatment should be applied to the affected area for 1 week following complete clearing of the lesion.

Candidiasis

Candida albicans is a yeast that reproduces by budding and, in well infants, causes oral and skin monilial or candida infections (AAP, 2015). *Candida* is common normal flora of the vagina and infants acquire this during the birth process (see Chapter 47).

Figure 43.14 Ringworm (tinea corporis). The fungus spreads rapidly, producing a circular, ringlike lesion. (© SPL/Science Source/Photo Researchers.)

The common clinical presentation in well infants is mild and easily treated, with person to person transmission being rare. Oral candidiasis, or thrush, is characterized by white plaques on an erythematous base on the buccal membrane and the surface of the tongue. It resembles a milk curd left from a recent milk feeding; however, unlike milk curds, the thrush plaques do not scrape away. The underlying surface is erythematous and therefore may be painful. On the skin *C. albicans* can also cause a severe, bright red, sharply circumscribed rash, most commonly in the diaper area (Fig. 43.15). The diaper rash is marked by intense erythema with a well-demarcated border surrounded by satellite lesions and goes into the folds. It fails to improve with usual diaper rash measures, such as application of a protective ointment, frequent changing of diapers, or exposure to air.

Figure 43.15 Monilial (candidiasis) diaper rash. Note the intense red color of the rash and the satellite lesions. (© Custom Medical Stock Photograph.)

Skin infections are treated with antifungal drugs like nystatin (Mycostatin), clotrimazole (Lotrimin), naftifine (Naftin), ketoconazole (Nizoral), econazole (Spectazole), ciclopirox (Ciclodan), or miconazole (Zeasorb); however, nystatin (Mycostatin) is the cheapest agent (AAP, 2015). For oral candidiasis, nystatin is generally administered by mouth approximately four times a day. The lesions need to be cleaned prior to the application of the nystatin and it should be administered after feeding. Oral candidiasis or thrush is common.

What If . . . 43.4

A nurse is particularly interested in exploring one of the 2020 National Health Goals related to infectious diseases in children (see Box 43.1). What would be a possible research topic pertinent to this goal that would be applicable to Jack and his family and that would also advance evidence-based practice?

KEY POINTS FOR REVIEW

- The incubation period of an infectious disease is the time between the invasion of an organism and the onset of symptoms. The prodromal period is the time between the beginning of nonspecific symptoms and specific ones and the time when children are most infectious. Illness is the stage during which specific symptoms are evident. The convalescent period is the period from when the symptoms fade and the child returns to baseline.

- The chain of infection depends on the presence of a reservoir, a portal of exit, a mode of transmission, a portal of entry, and a susceptible host. To reduce the spread of infection, use standard infection precautions to break the chain of infection. Transmission-based precautions—airborne, droplet, and contact—also may be necessary.

- Common viral infections of childhood include exanthem subitum (roseola), rubella (German measles), measles (rubeola), chickenpox (varicella), herpes zoster, erythema infectiosum (fifth disease), mumps (epidemic parotitis), infectious mononucleosis, and cat-scratch disease. Other important viral infections include poliomyelitis (now almost extinct), herpesvirus infections, verrucae (warts), rabies, West Nile virus disease, and Zika virus.

- Common streptococcal diseases include streptococcal pharyngitis, scarlet fever, and impetigo. Staphylococcal infections include impetigo, furunculosis (boils), cellulitis, and staphylococcal scalded skin syndrome. There has been a resurgence of pertussis in the United States due to immunization refusal and waning of efficacy. Outbreaks of diphtheria and tetanus (lockjaw) are rare.

- Common examples of tick-borne diseases are Rocky Mountain spotted fever and Lyme disease. Parasitic infections are pediculosis capitis (head lice), pediculosis pubis, and scabies. Helminthic infections include roundworms, hookworms, and pinworms. Fungal infections are tinea capitis and tinea corporis, both of which are forms of ringworm.

- Teaching parents and children about infection control measures and the need for keeping immunizations up to date is essential not only for reducing the risk of infectious disorders in children but also for meeting QSEN competencies and best meeting the family's total needs.

CRITICAL THINKING CARE STUDY

While working as a nurse at a residential summer camp, you meet Madison, a 10-year-old. Both her forearms and lower legs have several crusted erythematous superficial lesions with some. Four days ago was "sleep out" day, so she spent the night in a tent with three friends but didn't sleep well because "mosquitoes bit me all night." Madison's parents return from their vacation, and when they learn of the lesions comment, "Look at her; she'll probably end up with scars from this."

1. What do you suspect is the cause of the scattered lesions?

2. Given how impetigo is transmitted to others, what implications does its presence have for infection control practices in the camp setting?

3. What if you learn Madison has never had more immunizations than those she received as an infant because her mother believes the danger of vaccines is higher than contracting "simple childhood infections"? Would immunization have prevented Madison from contracting impetigo? Would you recommend she receive routine immunizations now or, at 10 years of age, is she no longer in much danger from common contagious illnesses?

RELATED RESOURCES

Explore these additional resources to enhance learning for this chapter:
- Student resources on thePoint, including answers to the What If . . . and Critical Thinking Care Study questions, http://thepoint.lww.com/Flagg8e
- Adaptive learning powered by PrepU, http://thepoint.lww.com/prepu

REFERENCES

Alter, S. J., Bennett, J. S., Koranyi, K., et al. (2015). Common childhood viral infections. *Current Problems in Pediatric and Adolescent Health Care, 45*, 21–53.

American Academy of Pediatrics. (2015). Summaries of infectious diseases. In D. W. Kimberline, M. T. Brady, M. A. Jackson, et al. (Eds.), *Red book: 2015 Report of the committee on infectious disease* (30th ed., pp. 225–868). Elk Grove Village, IL: Author.

Arnon, S. (2016). Tetanus (*Clostridium tetani*). In R. M. Kliegman, B. Stanton, N. Schor, et al. (Eds.), *Nelson's textbook of pediatrics* (20th ed., pp. 1432–1434). Philadelphia, PA: Elsevier.

Biggs, H., Behravesh, C., Bradley, K., et al. (2016). Diagnosis and management of tickborne Rickettsial disease: Rocky mountain spotted fever and other spotted fever group rickettsioses, Ehrlichioses, and Anaplasmosis—United States: A practice guide for health care and public health professionals. *Morbidity and Mortality Weekly Report, 65*(RR-02), 1–44. Retrieved from http://www.cdc.gov/mmwr/volumes/65/rr/rr6502a1.htm

Caicedo, Y., Paez, A., Kuzmin, I., et al. (2015). Virology, immunology, and pathology of human rabies during treatment. *The Infectious Disease Journal, 34*(5), 520–528.

Centers for Disease Control and Prevention. (2015a). *Epidemiology and prevention of vaccine-preventable diseases* (13th ed.). Washington, DC: Public Health Foundation.

Centers for Disease Control and Prevention. (2015b). *Insect repellent use & safety: Which mosquito repellents work best*. Retrieved from https://www.cdc.gov/westnile/faq/repellent.html

Centers for Disease Control and Prevention. (2015c). *Lyme disease vaccine*. Retrieved from https://www.cdc.gov/lyme/prev/vaccine.html

Centers for Disease Control and Prevention. (2016a). *Diphtheria: Clinical features*. Retrieved from http://www.cdc.gov/diphtheria/clinicians.html

Centers for Disease Control and Prevention. (2016b). *Guide to infection prevention for outpatient settings: Minimum expectations for safe care*. Retrieved from https://www.cdc.gov/infectioncontrol/pdf/outpatient/guide.pdf

Centers for Disease Control and Prevention. (2016c). *Making health care safer: Protecting patients from antibiotic resistance.* Retrieved from http://www.cdc.gov/vitalsigns/pdf/2016-03-vitalsigns.pdf

Centers for Disease Control and Prevention. (2016d). *Measles: Cases and outbreaks.* Retrieved from http://www.cdc.gov/measles/cases-outbreaks.html

Centers for Disease Control and Prevention. (2016e). *Mumps: Cases and outbreaks.* Retrieved from http://www.cdc.gov/mumps/outbreaks.html

Centers for Disease Control and Prevention. (2016f). *Parasites—Enterobiasis.* Retrieved from http://www.cdc.gov/parasites/pinworm/epi.html

Centers for Disease Control and Prevention. (2016g). *Polio.* Retrieved from http://www.cdc.gov/ticks/avoid/on_people.html

Centers for Disease Control and Prevention. (2016h). *Preventing tick bites.* Retrieved from http://www.cdc.gov/ticks/avoid/on_people.html

Centers for Disease Control and Prevention. (2016i). *Prevention: Anthrax.* Retrieved from http://www.cdc.gov/anthrax/medical-care/prevention.html

Centers for Disease Control and Prevention. (2016j). *Rubella in the United States.* Retrieved from http://www.cdc.gov/rubella/about/in-the-us.html

Centers for Disease Control and Prevention. (2017). *Wash your hands.* Retrieved from https://www.cdc.gov/features/handwashing/

Chittleborough, C. R., Nicholson, A. L., Basker, E., et al. (2012). Factors influencing hand washing behavior in primary schools: Process evaluation within a randomized controlled trial. *Health Education Research, 27*(6), 1055–1068.

Choi, E., Pyzocha, N., & Maurer, D. (2016). Tick-borne illnesses. *Current Sports Medicine Reports, 15*(2), 98–104.

Chusid, M. J., & Rotar, M. M. (2016). Infection prevention and control. In R. M. Kliegman, B. Stanton, N. Schor, et al. (Eds.), *Nelson's textbook of pediatrics* (20th ed., pp. 1260–1264). Philadelphia, PA: Elsevier.

Creech, C. B., Al-Zubeidi, D. N., & Fritz, S. A. (2015). Prevention of recurrent staphylococcal skin infections. *Infectious Disease Clinics of North America, 29*(3), 429–464.

Damon, I., Damaso, C., & McFadden, G. (2014). Are we there yet? The smallpox research agenda using variola virus. *PLoS Pathogens, 10*(5), e1004108. Retrieved from https://www.ncbi.nlm.nih.gov/pmc/articles/PMC4006926/

Drutz, J. (2016). Measles. *Pediatrics in Review, 37*, 220–221.

Faulkner, A., Skoff, T., Tondella, M. L., et al. (2016). Trends in pertussis diagnostic testing in the United States, 1990–2012. *The Infectious Disease Journal, 35*(1), 39–44.

Frieden, T., Jaffe, H. W., Cono, J., et al. (2014). *Youth risk behavior surveillance—United States, 2013 surveillance summaries.* Atlanta, GA: Centers for Disease Control and Prevention.

Gabutti, G., Azzari, C., Bonanni, P., et al. (2015). Pertussis: Current perspectives on epidemiology and prevention. *Human Vaccines & Immunotherapeutics, 11*(1), 108–117. Retrieved from https://www.ncbi.nlm.nih.gov/pmc/articles/PMC4514233/

Gaensbauer, J. T., & Todd, J. K. (2016). Staphylococcus aureus. In R. M. Kliegman, B. M. D. Stanton, J. St Geme, et al. (Eds.), *Nelson textbook of pediatrics* (20th ed., pp. 1315–1319). Philadelphia, PA: Elsevier.

Gerlero, P., & Hernández-Martínb, A. (2016). Treatment of warts in children: An update. *Actas Dermo-Sifiliographicas, 107*(7), 551–558.

Gershon, A., Breuer, J., Cohen, J., et al. (2015). Varicella zoster viral infections. *Nature Review: Disease Primers, 1*, 15016. Retrieved from https://www.ncbi.nlm.nih.gov/pmc/articles/PMC5381807/pdf/nihms854463.pdf

Goldman, J. L., & Newland, J. G. (2015). New horizons for pediatric antibiotic stewardship. *Infectious Disease Clinics of North America, 29*, 503–511.

Goodson, J. L., & Seward, J. F. (2015). Measles 50 years after use of the measles vaccine. *Infectious Disease Clinics of North America, 29*, 725–743.

Gomes-Solecki, M., Santecchia, I., & Werts, C. (2017). Animal models of leptospirosis: Of mice and hamsters. *Frontiers in Immunology, 8*, 58. Retrieved from http://journal.frontiersin.org/article/10.3389/fimmu.2017.00058/full

Haberman, C. (2015, February 1). A discredited study continuing impact on public health. *The New York Times.* Retrieved from https://www.nytimes.com/2015/02/02/us/a-discredited-vaccine-studys-continuing-impact-on-public-health.html?_r=0

Hampson, K., Coudeville, L., Lembo, T., et al. (2015). Estimating the global burden of endemic canine rabies. *PLoS Neglected Tropical Diseases, 9*(4), e0003709. https://dx.doi.org/10.1371/journal.pntd.0003709

Heininger, U. (2012). Pertussis: What the pediatric infectious disease specialist should know. *The Pediatric Infectious Disease Journal, 31*(1), 78–79.

Higgs, S., & Vanlandingham, D. L. (2016). Search and one will find: Zika virus everywhere. *Transactions of the Royal Society of Tropical Medicine and Hygiene, 110*, 207–208.

Jackson, A. C. (2016). Human rabies: A 2016 update. *Current Infectious Disease Reports, 18*(11), 38.

James, S. H., & Kimberlin, D. (2015). Neonatal herpes simplex virus infection. *Infectious Disease Clinics of North America, 29*, 391–400.

Jonsson, C., Figueiredo, L. T., & Vapalahti, O. (2010). A global perspective on hantavirus ecology, epidemiology, and disease. *Clinical Microbiology Reviews, 23*, 412–441.

Karwowski, M. P., Nelson, J. M., Staples, J. E., et al. (2016). Zika virus disease: A CDC update for pediatric health care providers. *Pediatrics, 137*(5), 1–13.

Keighley, K. L., Saunderson, R. B., Kok, J., et al. (2015). Viral exanthems. *Current Opinion in Infectious Diseases, 28*, 139–150.

Kellen, R., & Berlin, J. M. (2016). Dermatology emergencies. *Journal of the Dermatology Nurse's Association, 8*(3), 193–202.

Kroger, A. (2015). *Epidemiology and prevention of vaccine-preventable diseases* (13th ed.). Washington, DC: Public Health Foundation.

Lennon, D., Stewart, J., & Anderson, P. (2016). Primary prevention of rheumatic fever. *Pediatric Infectious Disease Journal, 35*(7), 820.

Lindsey, N. P., Lehman, J., Staples, J. E., et al. (2015). West Nile virus and other nationally notifiable arboviral diseases—United States, 2014. *Morbidity and Mortality Weekly Review, 64*(34), 929–934.

Long, S. (2016). Pertussis (*Bordetella pertussis* and *Bordetella parapertussis*). In R. M. Kliegman, B. Stanton, N. Schor, et al. (Eds.), *Nelson's textbook of pediatrics* (20th ed., pp. 1377–1382). Philadelphia, PA: Elsevier.

Lugo, D., & Krogstad, P. (2016). Enteroviruses in the early 21st century: New manifestations and challenges. *Current Opinion in Pediatrics, 28*(1), 107–113.

Maslow, A. H. (1943). A theory of human motivation. *Psychological Review, 50*, 370–396.

Mauskopf, J., Margulis, A. V., Samuel, M., et al. (2016). Respiratory syncytial virus hospitalizations in healthy preterm infants: Systematic review. *The Pediatric Infectious Disease Journal, 35*(7), e229–e238.

Moscicki, A. (2016). Human papillomaviruses. In R. M. Kliegman, B. Stanton, N. Schor, et al. (Eds.), *Nelson's textbook of pediatrics* (20th ed., pp. 1618–1622). Philadelphia, PA: Elsevier.

Mukkada, S., & Buckingham, S. (2015). Recognition of and prompt treatment for tick-borne infections in children. *Infectious Disease Clinics of North America, 29*, 539–555.

Nayak, J. L., & Sant, A. (2011). T cell immunology for the clinician. *Pediatric Infectious Disease Journal, 30*, 248–250.

Painter, J., Gargano, J., Collier, S., et al. (2015). Giardiasis surveillance—United States, 2011–2012. *Morbidity and Mortality Weekly Report, 64*(SS-03), 15–25.

Paul, I. M., Beiler, J., McMonagle, A., et al. (2007). Effects of honey, dextromethorphan, and no treatment on nocturnal cough and sleep quality for coughing children and their parents. *Archives of Pediatrics & Adolescent Medicine, 161*(12), 1140–1146.

Petersen, L. R., Jamieson, D., Powers, A., et al. (2016). Zika virus. *The New England Journal of Medicine, 374*, 1552–1563.

Petrosky, E., Bocchini, J., Hariri, S., et al. (2015). Use of 9-valent human papillomavirus (HPV) vaccine: Updated HPV vaccination recommendations of the advisory committee on immunization practices. *Morbidity and Mortality Weekly Report, 64*(11), 300–304.

Phadke, V. K., Bednarczyk, R. A., Salmon, D. A., et al. (2016). Association between vaccine refusal and vaccine-preventable diseases in the United States: A review of measles and pertussis. *JAMA, 315*(11), 1149–1158.

Pinninti, S., Hough-Telford, C., Pati, S., et al. (2016). Cytomegalovirus and Epstein–Barr virus infections. *Pediatrics in Review, 37*, 223–234.

Randolph, A., & McCulloh, R. (2014). Pediatric sepsis: Important considerations for diagnosing and managing severe infections in infants, children, and adolescents. *Virulence, 5*(1), 179–189.

Restrepo-Méndez, M., Barros, A., Wong, K. L., et al. (2016). Missed opportunities in full immunization coverage: Findings from low- and lower-middle-income countries. *Global Health Action, 9*, 30963. Retrieved from http://www.globalhealthaction.net/index.php/gha/article/view/30963

Rubin, S., Kennedy, R., & Poland, G. (2016). Emerging mumps infection. *The Pediatric Infectious Disease Journal, 35*(7), 799–801.

Rupprecht, C., Briggs, D., Brown, C., et al. (2010). Use of a reduced (4-dose) vaccine schedule for post exposure prophylaxis to prevent human rabies: Recommendations of the Advisory Committee on Immunization Practices. *Morbidity and Mortality Weekly Report, 59*(RR-02), 1–9.

Shibeshi, M. E., Masresha, B. G., Smith, S. B., et al. (2014). Measles resurgence in southern Africa: Challenges to measles elimination. *Vaccine, 32*(16), 1798–1807.

Shulman, S. T., Bisno, A. L., Clegg, H. W., et al. (2012). Clinical practice guideline for the diagnosis and management of group A streptococcal pharyngitis: 2012 update by the Infectious Diseases Society of America. *Clinical Infectious Diseases, 55*(10), e86–e102.

Silva-Costa, C., Carriço, J., Ramirez, M., et al. (2014). Scarlet fever is caused by a limited number of *Streptococcus pyogenes* lineage and is associated with the exotoxin gene ssa, speA and speC. *The Pediatric Infectious Disease Journal, 33*(3), 306–310.

Simões, E. (2016). Poliovirus. In R. M. Kliegman, B. Stanton, N. Schor, et al. (Eds.), *Nelson's textbook of pediatrics* (20th ed., pp. 1554–1561). Philadelphia, PA: Elsevier.

Simos, C., Flynn, T., Piecuch, J., et al. (2009). Infections of the oral cavity. In R. D. Feigin & J. Cherry (Eds.), *Feigin & Cherry's textbook of pediatric infectious diseases* (6th ed., pp. 146–160). Philadelphia, PA: Saunders/ Elsevier.

Stanberry, L. R. (2016). Herpes simplex virus. In R. M. Kliegman, B. Stanton, N. Schor, et al. (Eds.), *Nelson's textbook of pediatrics* (20th ed., pp. 1572–1579). Philadelphia, PA: Elsevier.

Sutter, D. E., Milburn, E., Chukwuma, U., et al. (2016). Changing susceptibility of *Staphylococcus aureus* in a US pediatric population. *Pediatrics, 137*(4), e20153099.

Taketomo, C. K. (2015). *Pediatric & neonatal dosage handbook* (22nd ed.). Hudson, OH: Lexi-Comp.

Tasani, M., Tong, S., Andrews, R., et al. (2016). The importance of scabies coinfection in the treatment considerations for impetigo. *The Pediatric Infectious Disease Journal, 35*(4), 374–378.

Taylor, L. E., Swerdfeger, A. L., & Eslick, G. D. (2014). Vaccines are not associated with autism: An evidence-based meta-analysis of case-control and cohort studies. *Vaccine, 32*(29), 3623–3629.

Totoraitis, K., Cohen, J. L., & Friedman, A. (2017). Topical approaches to improve surgical outcomes and wound healing: A review of efficacy and safety. *Journal of Drugs in Dermatology, 16*(3), 209–212.

U.S. Department of Health and Human Services. (2010). *Healthy people 2020*. Washington, DC: Author.

Wilkins, R. G., & Unverdorben, M. (2012). Wound cleaning and wound healing: A concise review. *Advances in Skin & Wound Care, 26*(4), 160–163.

Wilson, W., Taubert, K. A., Gewitz, M., et al. (2007). Prevention of infective endocarditis: Guidelines from the American Heart Association: A guideline from the American Heart Association Rheumatic Fever, Endocarditis, and Kawasaki Disease Committee, Council on Cardiovascular Disease in the Young, and the Council on Clinical Cardiology, Council on Cardiovascular Surgery and Anesthesia, and the Quality of Care and Outcomes Research Interdisciplinary Working Group. *Circulation, 116*, 1736–1754.

World Health Organization. (2016a). *Evidence of hand hygiene to reduce transmission and infection by multi-resistant organisms in a healthcare setting.* Retrieved from http://www.who.int/gpsc/5may/MDRO_literature-review .pdf

World Health Organization. (2016b). *Summary of the WHO position papers— recommendations for routine immunization.* Retrieved from http://www .who.int/immunization/policy/Immunization_routine_table1.pdf?ua=1

44

Nursing Care of a Family When a Child Has a Hematologic Disorder

*L*ana is a 4-year-old girl diagnosed with thalassemia major whom you meet at a pediatric clinic. She has a prominent mandible and wide-spaced upper front teeth from overgrowth of bone marrow centers. Joey is a 7-year-old with sickle-cell anemia who attends the same clinic. His growth is only in the fifth percentile, and he's had two vaso-occlusive crises in the past year. "Why did this happen to our families?" Lana's mother asks you. "What can we do to help our children have better lives?"

Previous chapters described the growth and development of well children. This chapter adds information about the dramatic changes, both physical and psychosocial, that occur when children have a hematologic disorder.

What additional health teaching does Lana's mother need so she can better understand hematologic diseases?

KEY TERMS

allogeneic transplantation	leukocytes
aplastic crisis	megakaryocytes
autologous transplantation	pancytopenia
blood dyscrasias	petechiae
erythroblasts	plethora
erythrocytes	poikilocytic
erythropoietin	priapism
granulocytes	purpura
hemochromatosis	reticulocyte
hemolysis	syngeneic transplantation
hemosiderosis	thrombocytes
ischemia	thrombocytopenia

OBJECTIVES

After mastering the contents of this chapter, you should be able to:

1. Describe the major hematologic disorders of childhood.
2. Identify 2020 National Health Goals related to children with hematologic disorders that nurses could help the nation achieve.
3. Assess a child with a hematologic disorder such as sickle-cell anemia.
4. Formulate nursing diagnoses related to a child with a hematologic disorder.
5. Identify expected outcomes for a child with a hematologic disorder to help parents manage seamless transitions across differing healthcare settings.
6. Using the nursing process, plan nursing care that includes the six competencies of Quality & Safety Education for Nurses (QSEN): Patient-Centered Care, Teamwork & Collaboration, Evidence-Based Practice (EBP), Quality Improvement (QI), Safety, and Informatics.
7. Implement nursing care related to a child with a hematologic disorder, such as reducing the possibility of infection.
8. Evaluate expected outcomes for achievement and effectiveness of care.
9. Integrate knowledge of childhood disorders of the blood with the interplay of nursing process and Family Nursing to promote quality maternal and child health nursing care.

The blood and blood-forming tissues that make up the hematologic system play a vital role in body metabolism because they transport oxygen and nutrients to body cells, remove carbon dioxide from cells, and initiate blood coagulation when vessels are injured. As a result of all of these functions, any alteration in the substance or function of blood can have immediate and life-threatening effects on the functioning of all body systems (Zempsky, Palermo, Corsi, et al., 2013).

Hematologic disorders, often called **blood dyscrasias**, occur when components of the blood are formed incorrectly or either increase or decrease in amount beyond normal ranges. Most blood dyscrasias in children originate in the bone marrow, where blood cells are formed. They do not occur at equal rates in all countries because many of these disorders are inherited. Sickle-cell anemia, for example, occurs mainly in Blacks; thalassemia occurs in children of Mediterranean heritage. Being aware of the differences in the incidence of blood dyscrasias this way can be helpful in planning care and providing healthcare services for children and communities. Treatment for blood disorders vary as well based on cultural influences. Families who are Jehovah's Witnesses, for example, may refuse blood transfusions, a common therapy for blood disorders, on religious grounds (Campbell, Machan, & Fisher, 2016). Box 44.1 shows 2020 National Health Goals related to blood disorders.

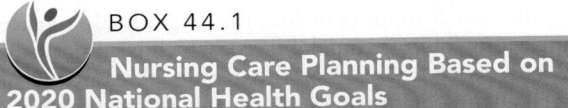

BOX 44.1

Nursing Care Planning Based on 2020 National Health Goals

2020 National Health Goals speak to ways to improve children's health. Because both iron-deficiency and sickle-cell anemia are seen worldwide, improving care in these areas could have a dramatic effect on both national and world health.

- Reduce the incidence of iron deficiency among children aged 1 to 2 years from a baseline of 15.9% to a target level of 14.3%; in children aged 3 to 4 years, from 5.3% to 4.3%.
- Reduce the incidence of iron deficiency among adolescents 12 to 18 years of age from 10.4% to 9.4%.
- Reduce the proportion of persons with hemophilia who develop reduced joint mobility due to bleeding into joints from 82.9% to 74.6%.
- (Developmental) Reduce hospitalization due to preventable complications of sickle-cell disease yearly among children aged 9 years and younger.
- Increase the proportion of children with special healthcare needs who have access to a medical home from 47.1% to 51.8% (U.S. Department of Health and Human Services, 2010; see www.healthypeople.gov).

Nurses can help the nation achieve these goals by educating parents about the importance of women taking an iron supplement during pregnancy, encouraging iron-rich food sources for young children, and educating adolescents about healthy diets. Being certain that parents are well informed about preventive measures for children with all types of hematologic disorders could help reduce hospital admissions.

Nursing Process Overview

FOR A CHILD WITH A HEMATOLOGIC DISORDER

ASSESSMENT

Many of the symptoms of hematologic disorders begin insidiously, with symptoms such as pallor, lethargy, and bruising. These are such minor symptoms that parents may not bring their children to a healthcare facility for some time. When they do, they are surprised to learn such subtle symptoms signify the presence of a serious illness.

Children with iron deficiency, for example, aside from appearing pale and irritable, look plump and "healthy." It takes careful history taking to reveal the possibility of an iron deficiency.

NURSING DIAGNOSIS

When a child is diagnosed with an inherited disorder, parents may feel guilty or blame themselves or their partner for their child's disease. This can make it difficult for a family to act together to support a child during an illness when members need intensive support themselves. Examples of nursing diagnoses that address the entire family include:

- Deficient knowledge related to the cause of the child's illness
- Imbalanced nutrition, less than body requirements, related to family pattern of not eating iron-rich foods
- Anxiety related to frequent blood-sampling procedures
- Pain related to tissue **ischemia** (inadequate blood supply to a local area due to blockage)
- Compromised family coping related to long-term care needs of child with a chronic hematologic disorder

OUTCOME IDENTIFICATION AND PLANNING

When helping parents plan outcomes, be certain that the outcomes planned are realistic for both the child and family. It may not be possible to reduce the number of blood-sampling procedures, for example, but fear, pain, and anxiety related to the procedures can be addressed with distraction techniques.

Children with hematologic disorders often are prescribed a long-term medication such as a corticosteroid. When a child appears very ill, parents are usually very conscientious about giving such medicine. When a child has a disorder with few symptoms, however, like a blood dyscrasia, it is easy for parents to forget to give the medication. In addition, a child may refuse to take the medication for a long time because it tastes bad or upsets the stomach. Planning, therefore, includes helping parents devise ways to disguise the taste and to remember to give medication over the long term. If a child will be restricted in activity for long periods because the immune system is compromised as a part of the illness, planning must include ways to keep the child engaged with friends to promote development. Parents may need help investigating possible resources for education and support to do this.

Some organizations helpful for referral are the Aplastic Anemia and MDS International Foundation (http://www.aamds.org), the Sickle Cell Disease Association of America (www.sicklecelldisease.org), the American Society of Pediatric Hematology/Oncology (www.aspho.org), and the National Hemophilia Foundation (www.hemophilia.org).

IMPLEMENTATION

Nursing interventions for children with hematologic disorders range from obtaining blood specimens for testing to assisting with blood or hematopoietic stem (bone marrow) cell transfusions. Remember that a fingertip puncture for blood is often as painful as a venipuncture. Suggesting that blood be drawn by means of an intermittent device and applying an anesthetic cream (mixtures of lidocaine and prilocaine) before finger punctures or venipunctures are effective measures to help reduce pain and improve cooperation with these procedures. Even so, children may need some therapeutic playtime with a syringe and a doll to express their anger about constant invasion by needles.

OUTCOME EVALUATION

An evaluation focuses on whether short-term outcomes such as moderation of pain or elimination of anxiety in a child undergoing diagnosis or treatment were achieved. The focus also includes assessing the achievement of long-term outcomes such as improving the ability of the family to manage the stress of raising a child with a chronic illness or dealing with frequently occurring health crises.

Examples of expected outcomes that suggest goals were achieved include:

- Parents correctly state the most frequent causes of iron-deficiency anemia.
- Child states she feels better able to cope with blood-sampling procedures through the use of imagery.
- Parents describe realistic plans to ensure adherence to long-term medication administration.
- Parents voice that they understand the importance of preventing dehydration in their school-age child with sickle-cell anemia.

Anatomy and Physiology of the Hematopoietic System

Blood components originate in the bone marrow, circulate through blood vessels, and ultimately are destroyed by the spleen.

BLOOD FORMATION AND COMPONENTS

The total volume of blood in the human body is roughly proportional to body weight: 85 ml/kg at birth, 75 ml/kg at 6 months of age, and 70 ml/kg after the first year. Although the *blood plasma* is important in diseases that cause vomiting and diarrhea (when this fluid may become depleted, leading to dehydration), plasma is not a major site of hematologic disease. The formed elements—the erythrocytes (red blood cells [RBCs]), leukocytes (white blood cells [WBCs]), and thrombocytes (platelets)—are the portions most affected by hematologic disorders in children.

Erythrocytes (Red Blood Cells)

Erythrocytes (RBCs) function chiefly to transport oxygen to and carry carbon dioxide away from body cells. They are formed in the bone marrow under the stimulation of **erythropoietin**, a hormone formed by the kidneys that is produced whenever a child has tissue hypoxia. Children with kidney disease often have a low number of RBCs because erythropoietin secretion is inadequate in diseased kidneys. *Polycythemia*, which is displayed as an elevated hematocrit, often occurs when a child has impaired tissue oxygenation and increased erythropoietin (Jeevasankar, Agarwal, Chawla, et al., 2008).

At birth, an infant has approximately 5 million RBCs per cubic millimeter of blood. This concentration diminishes rapidly in the first months, reaching a low of approximately 4.1 million/mm^3 at 3 to 4 months of age. The number then slowly increases until adolescence, when the adult value of approximately 4.9 million/mm^3 is reached.

RBCs form first as **erythroblasts** (large, nucleated cells), then mature through normoblast and reticulocyte stages, to mature, nonnucleated erythrocytes. An elevated **reticulocyte** (immature red blood cell) count (more than 1% of the total count) indicates that rapid production of new RBCs is occurring. At the end of their life span (about 120 days), erythrocytes are destroyed through phagocytosis by reticuloendothelial cells, found in the highest proportion in the spleen.

Hemoglobin

The component of RBCs that allows them to carry out the transport of oxygen is *hemoglobin*, composed of globin, a protein, and heme, an iron-containing pigment. It is the heme portion that combines with oxygen and carbon dioxide for transport.

The hemoglobin in erythrocytes during fetal life differs from that formed after birth. Fetal hemoglobin is composed of two α and two γ polypeptide chains. At birth, 40% to 70% of the infant's hemoglobin is this type (hemoglobin F). During the first 6 months of life, this is gradually replaced by adult hemoglobin (hemoglobin A), which is composed of two α and two β chains. For this reason, diseases such as sickle-cell anemia or the thalassemias, which are disorders of the β chains, do not become apparent clinically until this hemoglobin change has occurred (at approximately 6 months of age). Because some hemoglobin A is present, however, even in early intrauterine life, they can be diagnosed prenatally by hemoglobin analysis or electrophoresis in fetal or newborn life (Hartung, Olson, & Bessler, 2013).

Hemoglobin levels are highest at birth (13.7 to 20.1 g/100 ml); they reach a low at approximately 3 months of age (9.5 to 14.5 g/100 ml) and then gradually rise again until adult values are reached at puberty (11 to 16 g/100 ml).

Bilirubin

After an RBC reaches its life span of approximately 120 days, it disintegrates and its protein component is preserved by the reticuloendothelial cells of the liver and spleen for further use. Iron is reused by the bone marrow to construct new RBCs. As the heme portion is degraded, it is converted into protoporphyrin; protoporphyrin is then further broken down into indirect bilirubin. Indirect bilirubin is fat-soluble and so cannot be excreted by the kidneys. It is therefore converted by the liver enzyme glucuronyl transferase into *direct bilirubin*, which is water-soluble and excreted in bile.

In the newborn, generally, liver function is so immature that the conversion from indirect to direct bilirubin is difficult, allowing a portion of bilirubin to remain in the indirect form. When the level of indirect bilirubin in the blood rises to more than 7 mg/100 ml, it permeates outside the circulatory system, and the infant begins to show signs of yellowing or jaundice from the color of bilirubin. At any point in life, if excessive **hemolysis** (destruction) of RBCs occurs from other than usual causes, a child will also show signs of jaundice.

Stage 1   Platelets adhere to each other

Stage 2   Platelet phospholipid → Complete thromboplastin (III)

Stage 3   Prothrombin (II) → Thrombin

Stage 4   Fibrinogen (I) → Fibrin

(Coagulation factors involved): VIII, IX, X, XI, XII, IV, IV, V, VII, X, XIII

Figure 44.1 The steps in blood coagulation.

Leukocytes (White Blood Cells)

Leukocytes (WBCs) are nucleated cells and few in number compared with RBCs (there is approximately only 1 WBC to every 500 RBCs). Their primary function is defense against antigen invasion; their life span varies from approximately 6 hours to unknown intervals. With the exception of neutropenia (a reduced number of WBCs), leukocytes are not major hematologic concerns; because they are important in immune disorders and malignancies, they are further discussed in Chapters 42 and 53.

Thrombocytes (Platelets)

Thrombocytes are round, nonnucleated bodies formed by the bone marrow; their function is capillary hemostasis and primary coagulation. The usual number is 150,000 to 300,000/mm³ after the first year. Immature thrombocytes are termed **megakaryocytes**. If large numbers of these are present in serum, it indicates that a rapid production of platelets is occurring.

BLOOD COAGULATION

Effective blood coagulation depends on a complex series of four events, including a combination of blood and tissue factors released from the plasma (the intrinsic pathway) and from injured tissue (the extrinsic pathway) (Overbey, Jones, & Robinson, 2014). The numbers of coagulation factors refer to the order in which factors were discovered, not to the order of action in coagulation. The plasma-released factors include factors VIII, IX, and XII. Factors released from injured tissues are a tissue factor (an incomplete thromboplastin or factor III), plus factors VII and X. Together, these pathways unite to form factor V.

When a vessel is injured, vasoconstriction occurs in the area proximal to the injury, thus narrowing the vessel lumen and reducing the amount of blood that can flow to the injured area. Platelets begin to adhere to the damaged vessel site and to one another, forming a platelet plug and initiating the first stage of clotting (Fig. 44.1).

In the second stage, factors from either the intrinsic or the extrinsic system combine with platelet phospholipids to form complete thromboplastin. In the third stage, thromboplastin converts prothrombin (factor II) to thrombin if ionized calcium is present. The production of prothrombin and factors VII, IX, and X all depend on the presence of vitamin K. This stage will be incomplete, therefore, if levels of any of factors VIII through XII, vitamin K, or calcium are deficient.

In the fourth stage, thrombin converts fibrinogen (factor I) to fibrin. Fibrin strands form a mesh incorporating RBCs, WBCs, and platelets to form a permanent protective seal at the site of injury. Factor XIII (fibrin stabilizing factor) then acts to make the fibrin clot insoluble and permanent.

To prevent too much coagulation after the seal is complete, plasminogen is then converted to plasmin (a fibrinolysin) near the injury to halt the clotting sequence. Common tests for blood coagulation are described in Table 44.1.

TABLE 44.1 COMMON TESTS FOR BLOOD COAGULATION

Test	Definition	Normal Value
Prothrombin time (PT)	Measures the action of prothrombin; reveals deficiencies in prothrombin, factors V, VII, and X	11–13 s (PT) or 2.0–3.0 international normalized ratio (INR)
Partial thromboplastin time (PTT)	Measures activity of thromboplastin; reveals deficiencies in thromboplastin, factors VIII to XII	30–45 s
Bleeding time	Measures the time required for bleeding at a stab wound on the earlobe to stop; reveals deficiencies in platelet formation and vasoconstrictive ability	3–10 min
Clot retraction	Measures platelet function; interval from placement of blood in a tube to the point clot shrinks and expels serum	Retraction at side of test tube should be present by 1 hr; complete in 24 hr
Tourniquet	Measures capillary fragility and platelet function; response of tissue to application of tourniquet to forearm for 5–10 min	0–2 petechiae per 2-cm area
Prothrombin consumption time	Evaluates thromboplastin function; if clot formation used a great deal of prothrombin (as it should), serum prothrombin time will be brief; prolongation denotes defects in thromboplastin function	Approximately 20 s
Thromboplastin generation time	Tests basic ability to form thromboplastin; distinguishes factor VIII from factor IX disorders	12 s or less
Plasma fibrinogen	Measures stage 4 clotting process or level of fibrinogen in blood	200–400 mg/100 ml plasma
Venous clotting time (Lee-White clotting time)	Measures factor deficits in stages 2 and 4	9–12 min

Assessment and Therapeutic Techniques for Hematologic Disorders

An assessment of children with hematologic disorders begins with a complete history, including family history, to identify inherited disorders. For a specific diagnosis, children generally require several diagnostic procedures such as blood cell or bone marrow analysis.

BONE MARROW ASPIRATION AND BIOPSY

Bone marrow aspiration provides samples of bone marrow so the type and quantity of cells being produced can be determined (Ambruso, Nuss, & Wang, 2016). In children, the aspiration sites used are the iliac crests or spines (rather than the sternum, which is commonly used in adults) because performing the test at these sites is usually less frightening for children (Fig. 44.2). These sites also have the largest marrow compartments during childhood. In neonates, the anterior tibia can be used as an additional site.

For a bone marrow aspiration, following conscious sedation, a child lies prone on a hard surface such as a treatment table because pressure is needed to insert the needle through the surface of the bone into the marrow compartment. Topical anesthesia may be applied to help reduce pain (Kato, Maeda, Aoki, et al., 2014).

The area of the aspiration is cleaned with an antiseptic solution and draped. The overlying skin is infiltrated with a local anesthetic and then a large-bore needle and stylus is introduced through the overlying tissue into the bone. When the marrow cavity is reached, the stylus is removed, a syringe is attached to the needle, and bone marrow is aspirated (which appears as thick blood in the syringe). The syringe is then removed, and the marrow obtained is expelled onto a slide, sprayed with a preservative, and taken to a laboratory for analysis. Pressure must be applied to the puncture site for 5 to 10 minutes immediately afterward to prevent bleeding. A pressure dressing is then applied to maintain pressure and to continue to halt bleeding.

Figure 44.2 A common site used for bone marrow aspiration in children is the iliac crest. In neonates, the anterior tibia may be used.

A child will feel pain from the local anesthetic injection and uncomfortable pressure while the needle is inserted. Some report a sharp pain when the marrow is actually aspirated. If conscious sedation is used, monitor vital signs until the child is fully awake. Monitor pulse and blood pressure and observe the dressing every 15 minutes for the first hour after the procedure to be certain no bleeding is occurring. Keep the child fairly quiet for the first hour by playing a quiet game or other activity. Because bone marrow aspiration is a painful and invasive procedure, allow young children an opportunity for therapeutic play with a doll and syringe to help them express their feelings about the procedure. If the procedure was done as an ambulatory one, instruct parents to take the child's temperature 12 and 24 hours after the procedure to detect infection.

BLOOD TRANSFUSION

Transfusions of blood or its products are commonly used in the treatment of blood disorders, and may include whole blood, packed RBCs, washed RBCs (as much "foreign" matter is removed as possible to reduce the possibility of an antagonistic reaction), plasma, plasma factors, platelets, WBCs, and albumin. No matter what type of blood product is used, it is important that it has been carefully matched with the child's blood type and is infused with a solution as nearly isotonic as possible (normal saline). If blood should be given with a hypertonic solution, this will cause fluid to be drawn out of the transfused RBCs, causing them to shrink and be useless; if blood is infused with a hypotonic solution, fluid will be drawn into the cells, causing them to burst, and again, be destroyed.

Packed RBCs are the most common form of transfusion used with children because they help minimize the risk of fluid overload. The usual amount of blood transfused is typically 15 ml/kg of body weight. The commonly accepted rate for transfusions in a child is 10 ml/kg/hr unless the child has hypovolemic shock and volume equilibrium needs to be established quickly. An infusion of packed RBCs at a proportion of 10 ml/kg will raise the hematocrit level 5 points. A transfusion of platelets will elevate the platelet count by approximately 10,000 cells. Because platelet life span may be shortened after transfusion as a result of increased platelet destruction, frequent transfusions may be necessary (Ambruso et al., 2016).

Even if given slowly, a blood transfusion is always a strain on a child's circulation beyond that of a regular intravenous infusion because the circulatory system must accommodate such a thick, difficult-to-mobilize fluid.

Before any transfusion, ensure a signed consent form is obtained that respects sociocultural or religious beliefs. Obtain vital signs to establish a baseline and monitor these about every 15 minutes during the first hour and about every half hour for the remainder of the transfusion. Keep the infusion rate slow for the first 15 minutes; then, if no reaction occurs, increase the rate to about 10 ml/kg/hr or as otherwise prescribed. Common symptoms of blood transfusion reactions that may occur are shown in Table 44.2.

To prevent children from becoming bored or attempting to increase the infusion rate to speed up the process, think of and provide an enjoyable activity for children during transfusions.

TABLE 44.2 COMMON SYMPTOMS OF BLOOD TRANSFUSION REACTIONS

Symptoms	Cause	Time of Occurrence	Nursing Interventions
Headache, chills, back pain, dyspnea, hypotension, hemoglobinuria (blood in urine)	Anaphylactic reaction to incompatible blood; agglutination of red blood cells occurs; kidney tubules may become blocked, resulting in kidney failure	Immediately after start of transfusion	Discontinue transfusion. Maintain normal saline infusion for accessible intravenous (IV) line. Administer oxygen as necessary. Anticipate administration of a diuretic to increase renal tubule flow and reduce tubule plugging and/or heparin to reduce IV coagulation.
Pruritus, urticaria (hives), wheezing	Allergy to protein components of transfusion	Within first hour after start of transfusion	Discontinue transfusion temporarily. Give oxygen as needed. Anticipate administration for antihistamine to reduce symptoms.
Increased temperature	Possible contaminant in transfused blood	Approximately 1 hr after start of transfusion	Discontinue transfusion. Obtain blood culture to rule out or identify bacterial invasion.
Increased pulse, dyspnea	Circulatory overload	During course of transfusion	Discontinue transfusion; give oxygen as needed. Provide supportive care for pulmonary edema or congestive heart failure, which may develop. Anticipate administration of diuretic to increase excretion of excess fluid.
Muscle cramping, twitching of extremities, seizure	Acid-citrate-dextrose anticoagulant in transfusion combines with serum calcium and causes hypocalcemia	During course of transfusion	Discontinue transfusion. Anticipate administration of calcium gluconate intravenously to restore calcium level.
Fever, jaundice, lethargy, tenderness over liver	Hepatitis from contaminated transfusion	Weeks or months after transfusion	Obtain transfusion history of any child with hepatitis symptoms. Refer for care of hepatitis.
Bronze-colored skin	Hemosiderosis or deposition of iron in skin from transfusion	After repeated transfusions	Support self-esteem with altered body image. Administer iron-chelating agent (deferoxamine) as prescribed to help reduce level of accumulating iron.

HEMATOPOIETIC STEM CELL TRANSPLANTATION

Stem cell transplantation is the intravenous infusion of hematopoietic stem cells from bone marrow obtained by marrow aspiration or from peripheral or umbilical cord blood drawn from a compatible donor to reestablish marrow function in a child with deficient or nonfunctioning bone marrow.

Stem cell transplantation has become a relatively common procedure for children with blood disorders such as acquired aplastic anemia, sickle-cell disease, thalassemia, leukemia, and some forms of immune dysfunction diseases. Although a stressful procedure to undertake, it offers children the opportunity for a complete reversal of symptoms. However, there is no guarantee that the grafted cells will be accepted by the recipient or that improvement will occur, but with good tissue compatibility in the absence of infection, it can be effective in most children.

Stem cell transplantation can be allogeneic, syngeneic, or autologous. **Allogeneic transplantation** is the transfer of stem cells from an immune-compatible (histocompatible) donor, usually a sibling, or from a national cord blood bank or national volunteer donor registry (Petrini, 2013). **Syngeneic transplantation** (which is rare) involves a donor and recipient who are genetically identical (i.e., identical twins). **Autologous transplantation** involves use of the child's own stem cells removed from cord blood banked at the time of the child's birth. If this is not available, in some instances, stem cells can be aspirated from the child's bone marrow or

obtained from circulating blood, treated to remove abnormal cells and then reinfused.

Hematopoietic stem cells are recovered from a donor's circulating peripheral blood after the stimulation of stem cell production by a cytokine or stem cell colony-stimulating factor. Success is most likely if the recipient has not already received multiple blood transfusions that have sensitized the child to blood products and the donated stem cells are a close human leukocyte antigen (HLA) match to the child's blood. Siblings have about a 25% chance of being HLA compatible with the ill child.

To prevent a child's T lymphocytes from rejecting the newly transplanted donor stem cells, total body irradiation to destroy the child's marrow or an immunosuppressive drug such as cyclophosphamide (Cytoxan) is administered intravenously to the child before the procedure. This is a difficult time for the child because even with antiemetic therapy, both total body irradiation and the immunosuppressive drug cause extreme nausea, vomiting, and diarrhea.

If the marrow will be taken directly from a donor rather than from peripheral blood, on the day of the procedure, the donor is admitted to the hospital for a 1-day stay and receives epidural anesthesia or conscious sedation because multiple bone marrow aspirations from the posterior iliac crests are necessary for retrieval. The marrow is strained to remove fat and bone particles and any other unwanted cells. An anticoagulant is added to prevent clotting, and it is then infused intravenously into the recipient's bloodstream.

Because an infused hematopoietic stem cell solution is fairly thick, the infusion takes 60 to 90 minutes. The filter normally used with the infusion of blood products should not be used because it would filter out the marrow tissue. Monitor the child's cardiac rate and rhythm during the infusion to detect circulatory overload or pulmonary emboli from unfiltered particles.

Fever and chills are common reactions to a hematopoietic stem cell transplant infusion. Acetaminophen (Tylenol) or diphenhydramine hydrochloride (Benadryl) may be prescribed to reduce this reaction. After the infusion, take the child's temperature at 1 hour and then about every 4 hours to detect an infection that could occur because the child's WBCs are nonfunctional from radiation or immunosuppression. Reinforce strict hand washing and limit the child's diet to cooked foods to reduce exposure to bacteria.

Almost immediately after the infusion, stem cells begin to migrate from the child's bloodstream into the marrow. If *engraftment* occurs (the transplant is accepted), new RBCs can be detected in the peripheral blood in approximately 3 weeks. The WBC count will be measured daily to be certain WBCs are regenerating, although WBCs and platelet cells may not return to normal for up to 1 year after the transplant. Bone marrow aspirations or venous blood samples are then scheduled at regular intervals over the next year to assess the growth of the new marrow.

What If . . . 44.1
Lana's 12-year-old sister donates hematopoietic stem cells to Lana, but the transplant is not successful. The sister tells the nurse she knew it wouldn't be successful because she and Lana are more rivals than compatible sisters. How would the nurse best provide patient education for Lana's sister?

Nursing Diagnoses and Related Interventions

Because it takes a long time for the success or failure of stem cell transplantation to be documented, the procedure almost always produces anxiety not just in the child but also in the donor and the entire family.

Nursing Diagnosis: Anxiety related to long period of waiting to receive results of hematopoietic stem cell transplant and necessary extended restrictions and infection control precautions in hospital or at home.

Outcome Evaluation: Parents state they are managing their level of anxiety, are carrying out infection restrictions as prescribed, and are expressing satisfaction with child's ongoing development.

Be certain when discussing the risks of a stem cell transplant that both the child who received the transplant and the donor understand they are not responsible for the outcome of the procedure because its success does not depend on their behavior or what kind of person they are but on immunologic factors over which they have no control.

Because not all hematopoietic stem cell transplants are successful, some children will die of the original disease that necessitated the transplant. And, even if the transplant

was successful, another risk is that a child will develop an infection despite all precautions and die of sepsis in the weeks immediately after the transplant.

To prevent the child from contracting an infection until the WBC count returns to a safe range, children are restricted from interacting with other children either by remaining in the hospital or by employing visiting restrictions at home. Be certain to visit the room of an isolated child frequently and provide sterilized play materials the child can enjoy as appropriate. Because raw vegetables and fruits have the potential to carry germs, thick-skinned fruits such as bananas and oranges can be given soon after the procedure, but unwashed foods are typically avoided because these are foods most likely to carry bacteria.

Be certain children are well prepared for all procedures. Allow them to make as many choices as they can about their care to help them preserve a sense of control over their lives. Encourage periods of therapeutic play into their care so they can begin to express their anger and frustration at the number of intravenous therapies or follow-up bone marrow aspirations they require. Frequent visits by their parents and measures to help the child cope with pain, such as imagery, can help them accept one more painful procedure.

Ask the parents if they have made provisions for schoolwork as soon as the child has a return of RBCs in the peripheral blood (about 3 weeks). This can be accomplished by assisting parents with setting up a meeting with the child's teachers and school principal to devise an individualized education plan. Help them locate a support group in their community if they feel this will be helpful. Be certain they feel free to call the transplant center after discharge to discuss any problems. Once the danger of infection has passed and the restrictions can be discontinued, some parents may still be reluctant to allow their child outside or to interact with other children. This makes frequent follow-ups by e-mail or texting for the next year necessary to not only ensure that the child is free of infection but also assess whether the parents allow their child to pursue age-appropriate activities to encourage growth and development.

Graft-Versus-Host Disease

Graft-versus-host disease (GVHD) is a potentially lethal immunologic response of donor T cells to the tissue of the bone marrow recipient (Alousi, Bolaños-Meade, & Lee, 2013). The symptoms range from mild to severe and generally include a rash and general malaise beginning 7 to 14 days after the transplant. Severe symptoms include high fever, diarrhea, and liver and spleen enlargement.

Because there is no known cure for GVHD, prevention is essential. Careful tissue typing, intravenous administration of a corticosteroid and an immunosuppressant before transplant, and irradiation of blood products (which helps to inactivate mature T lymphocytes) before the infusion all can help reduce the incidence of this complication. Immunosuppressant drugs such as methotrexate or cyclosporine work by killing all rapidly growing cells, including WBCs and T lymphocytes, so administration of these drugs after transplantation cannot be continued or they would also interfere with the growth of the host's new stem cells. Prophylactic antibiotics and intravenous immune globulin are prescribed to decrease the risk of infection, and should be given consistently (Graham, Craddock, Quinones, et al., 2016).

QSEN Checkpoint Question 44.1

PATIENT-CENTERED CARE

Lana, who has thalassemia major, is scheduled for a bone marrow transplant, and her mother is highly anxious about this upcoming procedure. The nurse recognizes which statement is most accurate and best exemplifies patient-centered care?

  a. "If you can hold her still during the procedure, the pain will pass more quickly for her."
  b. "We will go to great lengths to make sure Lana doesn't develop an infection."
  c. "Lana will need to lie still while the new bone marrow infuses into her bones."
  d. "She will not need any further bone marrow aspirations after this."

Look in Appendix A for the best answer and rationale.

SPLENECTOMY

One of the purposes of the spleen is to remove damaged or aged blood cells. This poses a problem with diseases such as sickle-cell anemia and the thalassemias because the spleen interprets the typical cells of these diseases as damaged and destroys them. This causes children with these disorders to have a continuous anemia, with hemoglobin levels as low as 5 to 9 g/ml. In some children, therefore, removal of the spleen (splenectomy) will not cure the basic defect of the blood cells but will limit the degree of anemia. Splenectomy formerly required a large abdominal incision, but today, it can be performed by laparoscopy so, although still a procedure with risks, it does not require as long a recovery period.

A second function of the spleen is to strain blood particles that might lead to blood clots, as well as invading microorganisms, from the blood plasma so phagocytes and lymphocytes can destroy them. Children who have their spleen removed are more susceptible to pneumococcal infections and other bacterial infections because the spleen is no longer present to remove invading microorganisms from the body (Ambruso et al., 2016). After surgery, oral penicillin is typically given as a prophylactic antibiotic for a year or two to guard against infection. Assess to be certain the child also receives *Haemophilus influenzae* type b (Hib) and pneumococcal and meningococcal vaccines for further protection. Review with parents the signs of infection (e.g., cough, fever, general malaise) and encourage them to report any such signs immediately to their primary care provider.

Health Promotion and Risk Management

Hematologic disorders cover a wide range of diseases, both inherited and as an immunosuppressive response to infection, so they produce multiple symptoms in children (Box 44.2). Health promotion and disease prevention, therefore, begins

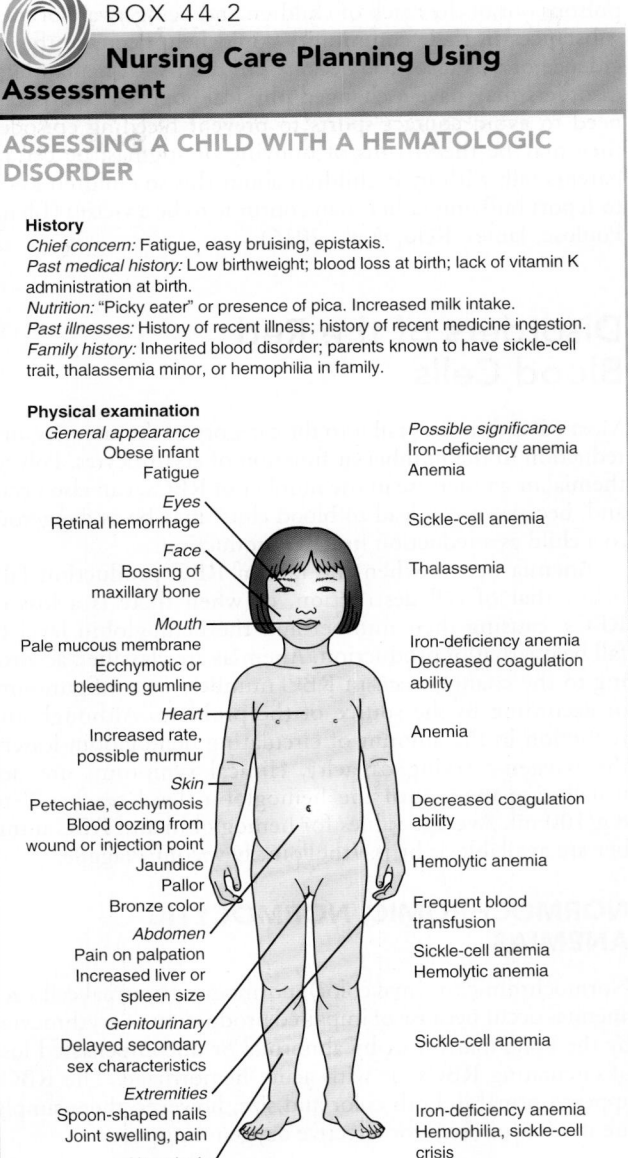

BOX 44.2

Nursing Care Planning Using Assessment

ASSESSING A CHILD WITH A HEMATOLOGIC DISORDER

History
Chief concern: Fatigue, easy bruising, epistaxis.
Past medical history: Low birthweight; blood loss at birth; lack of vitamin K administration at birth.
Nutrition: "Picky eater" or presence of pica. Increased milk intake.
Past illnesses: History of recent illness; history of recent medicine ingestion.
Family history: Inherited blood disorder; parents known to have sickle-cell trait, thalassemia minor, or hemophilia in family.

Physical examination

	Possible significance
General appearance	
Obese infant	Iron-deficiency anemia
Fatigue	Anemia
Eyes	
Retinal hemorrhage	Sickle-cell anemia
Face	
Bossing of maxillary bone	Thalassemia
Mouth	
Pale mucous membrane	Iron-deficiency anemia
Ecchymotic or bleeding gumline	Decreased coagulation ability
Heart	
Increased rate, possible murmur	Anemia
Skin	
Petechiae, ecchymosis Blood oozing from wound or injection point	Decreased coagulation ability
Jaundice	Hemolytic anemia
Pallor	
Bronze color	Frequent blood transfusion
Abdomen	
Pain on palpation Increased liver or spleen size	Sickle-cell anemia Hemolytic anemia
Genitourinary	
Delayed secondary sex characteristics	Sickle-cell anemia
Extremities	
Spoon-shaped nails	Iron-deficiency anemia
Joint swelling, pain	Hemophilia, sickle-cell crisis
Neurologic	
Weak muscle tone	Iron-deficiency anemia

with ensuring families have access to genetic counseling so they can be aware of the incidence of a disorder in their family and the potential for the disease to develop in their child.

The most frequently occurring anemia in children, iron-deficiency anemia, could be virtually eliminated if all infants were breastfed and those infants who are formula fed were fed iron-fortified formula for the full first year. The disorder occurs again with a high incidence in adolescents because adolescent diets tend to be low in meat and green vegetables, the chief dietary sources of iron. Adolescents who begin pseudo-vegetarian diets are another group especially prone to developing the disorder. Counseling parents of young children to maintain well-child healthcare visits and urging adolescents to ingest iron-rich foods could have a major impact on decreasing the incidence of the disorder.

Aplastic anemia, or the inability to form blood elements, can be acquired if a child is exposed to a toxic drug or chemical. Educating parents about the importance of keeping poisons out of the reach of children and being aware of toxic substances in their community could help decrease the incidence of this disorder. Because children with hematologic disorders may have a changed physical appearance and also need to avoid contact sports to prevent bleeding episodes, they may be the victims of bullying or stigmas; be certain parents talk with their children about this so children know to report bullying rather than continue to be a victim (Bhatt-Poulose, James, Reid, et al., 2016).

Disorders of the Red Blood Cells

Most RBC disorders fall into the category of the anemias, or a reduction in the number or function of erythrocytes. Polycythemia, or an increase in the number of RBCs, can also occur and, because it can lead to blood clots, may be as dangerous to a child as a reduction in RBC production.

Anemia occurs when the rate of RBC production falls below that of cell destruction, or when there is a loss of RBCs, causing their number and the hemoglobin level to fall below that of production. Anemias are classified according to the changes seen in RBC numbers or configuration, or according to the source of the problem. Although any reduction in the amount of circulating hemoglobin lessens the oxygen-carrying capacity, clinical symptoms are not usually apparent until the hemoglobin level reaches 7 to 8 g/100 ml. Average values for hemoglobin and RBC number are available at http://thePoint.lww.com/Flagg8e.

NORMOCHROMIC, NORMOCYTIC ANEMIAS

Normochromic (normal color), normocytic (normal cell size) anemias occur because of impaired production of erythrocytes by the bone marrow or by abnormal or uncompensated loss of circulating RBCs, as with acute hemorrhage. The RBCs appear normal in both color and size; however, there simply are too few of them for effective oxygen transport.

Acute Blood-Loss Anemia

Blood loss that is sufficient to cause anemia can occur from trauma such as an automobile accident with internal bleeding; from acute nephritis in which blood is lost in the urine; or in the newborn from disorders such as placenta previa, premature separation of the placenta, maternal–fetal or twin-to-twin transfusion, or trauma to the cord or placenta. In childhood, it can occur from the action of long-term intestinal parasites such as a tapeworm or hookworm or, in small infants, bedbug bites.

With sudden blood loss, children immediately appear pale. Because their heart must push the reduced amount of blood through their body more rapidly than usual, tachycardia will occur. Children will also begin to breathe rapidly because body cells are still not able to receive adequate oxygen. Newborns may have gasping respirations, intercostal retractions, and cyanosis. Children with rapid heart and respiratory rates due to this do not respond well to oxygen therapy because they lack RBCs to transport and use the oxygen. They become listless and inactive, dizzy, and, possibly, comatose.

This type of acute blood-loss anemia generally is transitory because the sudden reduction in available oxygen stimulates the release of erythropoietin from the kidney and a regeneration response in the bone marrow. The reticulocyte count rises, which is evidence that the bone marrow is trying to increase production of erythrocytes to meet the sudden shortage.

Treatment involves control of bleeding by addressing its underlying cause and transfusing additional RBCs. Lay the child flat to provide as much circulation as possible to brain cells. Keep the child warm with blankets; place the infant in an incubator or under a radiant heat warmer. Until blood is available for transfusion, a blood expander such as plasma or intravenous fluid such as normal saline or lactated Ringer's may be given to expand blood volume and improve blood pressure. With such emergency steps, the situation should be transitory with no long-term consequences.

Anemia of Acute Infection

Acute infection or inflammation, especially in infants, can cause increased destruction or decreased production of erythrocytes. Common conditions that do this include osteomyelitis and ulcerative colitis. Management involves treatment of the underlying condition. When the condition is reversed, blood values will return to normal.

Anemia of Renal Disease

Either acute or chronic renal disease can cause loss of function in kidney cells, which causes an accompanying decrease in erythropoietin production, resulting in a normocytic, normochromic anemia. Administration of recombinant human erythropoietin can increase RBC production and correct the anemia, but not the renal disease.

Anemia of Neoplastic Disease

Malignant growths such as leukemia or lymphoma (common neoplasms of childhood) result in normochromic, normocytic anemias because the invasion of bone marrow by proliferating neoplastic cells impairs RBC production. There may be accompanying blood loss if platelet formation also is decreased. The treatment of such an anemia involves measures designed to achieve remission of the neoplastic process and transfusion to increase the erythrocyte count.

Hypersplenism

Under usual conditions, blood filters rapidly through the spleen. If the spleen becomes enlarged, however, blood cells pass through more slowly, with more cells being destroyed in the process. The overactive spleen then leads to increased destruction of RBCs which can cause anemia and may lead to **pancytopenia** (deficiency of all cell elements of blood). Virtually any underlying splenic condition can cause this syndrome.

Therapeutic management consists of treating the underlying splenic disorder and includes a possible splenectomy.

Aplastic Anemias

Aplastic anemias result from depression of hematopoietic activity in the bone marrow. The formation and development of WBCs, platelets, and RBCs can all be affected (Ambruso et al., 2016).

Congenital aplastic anemia (Fanconi syndrome) is inherited as an autosomal recessive trait. A child is born with several congenital anomalies, such as skeletal and renal abnormalities, hypogenitalism, and short stature. Within 10 years, most of these children develop bone marrow failure as well as thrombocytopenia and neutropenia (Ambruso et al., 2016).

Acquired aplastic anemia is a decrease in bone marrow production, which occurs if a child is excessively exposed to radiation, drugs, or chemicals known to cause bone marrow damage. Exposure to insecticides and chemotherapeutic drugs temporarily causes this. Other examples of drugs that cause acquired aplastic anemia include chloramphenicol, sulfonamides, arsenic (contained in rat poison, sometimes eaten by children), hydantoin, benzene, or quinine. A serious infection such as meningococcal pneumonia might cause autoimmunologic suppression of the bone marrow, which then also results in this condition.

Assessment

When symptoms begin, a child appears pale, fatigues easily, and has anorexia from the lowered RBC count and tissue hypoxia. Because of reduced platelet formation (**thrombocytopenia**), the child bruises easily or develops **petechiae** (pinpoint, macular, purplish-red spots caused by an intradermal or submucous hemorrhage). A child may have excessive nosebleeds or gastrointestinal bleeding. As a result of a decrease in WBCs (neutropenia), a child may contract an increased number of infections and respond poorly to antibiotic therapy. Observe closely for signs of cardiac decompensation such as tachycardia, tachypnea, shortness of breath, or cyanosis from the long-term increased workload of all these effects on the heart. Bone marrow samples will show a reduced number of blood elements, and blood-forming spaces will be infiltrated by fatty tissue (Ambruso et al., 2016).

The child is apt to be irritable because of the fatigue and recurring symptoms. Parents may feel distressed if the illness originated from exposure to a chemical they should have kept away from their child, such as an insecticide. This can cause parents to have less confidence in healthcare personnel if the illness followed treatment with a drug such as chloramphenicol. They may wonder how they can trust in a drug to cure the illness if they believe a prescribed drug caused the illness.

Therapeutic Management

The first step in therapy is to immediately discontinue any drug or chemical suspected of causing the bone marrow dysfunction and removing the substance from the child's environment to avoid exposure. The ultimate therapy for both congenital and acquired aplastic anemia is hematopoietic stem cell transplantation (Korthof, Békássy, & Hussein, 2013). If a donor cannot be located, the disease is managed by a variety of procedures to supplement blood or to suppress T lymphocyte–dependent autoimmune responses while waiting for a histocompatible donor. Packed RBCs, platelet transfusions, cyclosporine, antithymocyte globulin (ATG), and an RBC-stimulating factor such as erythropoietin are generally necessary to maintain adequate blood elements. Some children show improvement with a course of an oral corticosteroid (prednisone) to further decrease the immune response or a course of testosterone to stimulate RBC growth. Be certain to observe a child well when administering ATG intravenously because of the high risk for anaphylaxis.

BOX 44.3

Nursing Care Planning to Empower a Family

TECHNIQUES FOR REDUCING BLEEDING WITH THROMBOCYTOPENIA

Q. Lana's mother asks you, "What precautions do you take to limit black and blue spots on Lana when her platelet count is low?"

A. "We try, as a team, to do the following."

- Limit the number of blood-drawing procedures; combine samples whenever possible.
- Use a blood pressure cuff instead of a tourniquet to reduce the number of petechiae.
- Apply pressure to any puncture site for a full 5 minutes before applying a bandage.
- Minimize the use of adhesive tape to the skin (pulling for removal may tear the skin and cause petechiae).
- Pad side and crib rails to prevent bruising. Assess the need for routine blood pressure determinations because tight cuffs can lead to petechiae.
- Protect intravenous sites to avoid numerous reinsertions.
- Administer medication orally or by intravenous infusion when appropriate to minimize the number of subcutaneous or intramuscular injection sites.
- Assess that the child is using a soft toothbrush and is offered foods that can be chewed without irritation (e.g., avoid toast crusts).
- Check toys for sharp corners, which may cause scratches. Urge the child to be careful with paper because paper cuts can bleed out of proportion to their size.
- Distract the child from rough play; suggest stimulating but quiet activities to minimize risk of injury.

For children who receive a hematopoietic stem cell transplant, chances of complete recovery are good. For others, the course will be uncertain. A decreased WBC count leaves the child open to infection. The decreased platelet count may persist for years after other blood elements have returned to normal, producing long-term problems of bleeding, especially petechiae or purpura (Box 44.3).

Nursing Diagnoses and Related Interventions

Nursing diagnoses need to speak to not only the physical symptoms of aplastic anemia but also the continual stress the parents feel if laboratory reports do not reveal a dramatic change in their child's blood cell production. It may be helpful to urge them to deal with this problem by facing only one day or one blood test at a time rather than trying to dwell on the outcomes of all the blood tests to come.

Nursing Diagnosis: Risk for disturbed body image related to changed appearance occurring as medication side effects

Outcome Evaluation: Child views self as a worthwhile person; does not appear to be excessively shy or reluctant to interact with peers.

Children who receive corticosteroids such as prednisone to suppress the immune response almost always experience some of the drug's side effects, such as a cushingoid appearance, hirsutism, hypertension, and marked weight gain. Long-term therapy with testosterone can result in masculinizing effects, such as growth of facial and body hair, the development of acne, and deepening of the voice. Be certain both children and their parents know these effects are related to the medication and will fade when the medication is withdrawn.

Adolescents may have an especially difficult time accepting weight gain and increased acne and so need a chance to express their feelings about their changed appearance. Reinforce and emphasize things they are doing well such as how well they are managing this unexpected turn in their life.

Hypoplastic Anemias

Hypoplastic anemias also result from depression of hematopoietic activity in bone marrow and can also be either congenital or acquired. Unlike aplastic anemias, however, in which WBCs, RBCs, and platelets are all affected, with hypoplastic anemias, only RBCs are affected.

Congenital hypoplastic anemia (Blackfan–Diamond syndrome) is a rare disorder apparently caused by an inherent defect in RBC formation that affects both sexes and shows symptoms as early as the first 6 to 8 months of life (Sakaguchi, Nakanishi, & Kojima, 2013). An acquired form of this can be caused by infection with parvovirus B19, the infectious agent that causes fifth disease.

The onset of a hypoplastic anemia is insidious, and at first, it may be difficult to differentiate from iron-deficiency anemia. With iron-deficiency anemia, blood cells appear hypochromic and microcytic and are few in number; however, in hypoplastic anemia, they are not only few in number but also their structure is normochromic and normocytic.

With the acquired type, the reduction of RBCs is transient, so no therapy other than monitoring is necessary. Children with the congenital form receive corticosteroid therapy along with transfusions of packed RBCs to raise erythrocyte levels. As a result of the necessary number of transfusions, **hemosiderosis** (a deposition of iron in body tissue) can occur. An iron chelation program such as subcutaneous infusion of deferoxamine (Desferal) may be started concurrently with transfusions to bind with iron and aid its excretion from the body in urine. Although an oral form is available for children over 10 years of age, this is usually given by a subcutaneous infusion pump over an 8-hour period for 5 or 6 nights a week. Remind the parent to assess that the child is voiding as usual and that his or her specific gravity is normal (1.003 to 1.030) before beginning an infusion so iron removed from tissues can be excreted (Karch, 2013).

To begin such an infusion, an area beside the scapula or on the thigh is cleaned with alcohol and a short 25-gauge needle is inserted at a low angle into the subcutaneous tissue and attached to an infusion pump by intravenous tubing. In addition to the assessments of voiding and specific gravity, periodic slit-lamp eye examinations should be scheduled to check for cataract formation, a possible adverse effect of deferoxamine.

Although congenital hypoplastic anemia has to be thought of as a chronic condition, about one fourth of affected children will undergo spontaneous permanent remission before the age of 13 years. If not, they are candidates for hematopoietic stem cell transplantation. As with aplastic anemia, both the child and the parents need support from healthcare personnel to help them accept the many procedures and tests required before full remission is finally achieved.

QSEN Checkpoint Question 44.2

INFORMATICS

Lana has received iron chelation therapy by deferoxamine in the past. Which statement by her mother would best assure the nurse she understands the use and action of iron chelation therapy?
a. "I know the drug acts to remove excess iron from my child."
b. "I have to check Lana's pulse before I turn on the pump."
c. "The drug is used to increase the level of iron in bone cells."
d. "The drug has minimal side effects, so I can't really give it wrong."

Look in Appendix A for the best answer and rationale.

HYPOCHROMIC ANEMIAS

When hemoglobin production is inadequate, erythrocytes appear pale (hypochromia) and are also usually reduced in diameter (microcytic).

Iron-Deficiency Anemia

Although the incidence of iron-deficiency anemia is decreasing in the United States due to improved infant nutrition, it is still the most common anemia of infancy and childhood, occurring whenever the intake of dietary iron is inadequate. Without adequate iron, hemoglobin cannot be incorporated into RBCs.

Children are at a higher risk for iron-deficiency anemia than adults because they need more daily iron in proportion to their body weight to maintain an adequate iron level than do adults—a daily intake of 11 to 15 mg of iron. This type of anemia occurs most often between the ages of 9 months and 3 years from infants drinking more milk than they are eating iron-rich foods. Its frequency rises again in adolescence, when iron requirements increase, especially for girls who are menstruating. It is also found at a high incidence in overweight teenagers if they ingest most of their calories from high-carbohydrate, not iron-rich, foods.

The Infant

A newborn usually has enough iron in reserve to last for the first 6 months of life. After that, the infant needs iron incorporated into the diet. Because iron stores are laid down near the end of gestation, infants born preterm will have fewer iron stores than those born at term and so tend to develop iron-deficiency anemia before 5 to 6 months. Women with iron deficiency during pregnancy tend to give birth to iron-deficient babies because the babies do not receive iron stores. As a preventive measure, preterm infants and those whose mother was iron deficient during pregnancy may be given an iron supplement beginning at about 2 months of age.

Infants born with structural defects of the gastrointestinal system, such as gastroesophageal reflux or chalasia (where an immature valve exists between the esophagus and stomach resulting in regurgitation) or pyloric stenosis (narrowing between the stomach and duodenum, resulting in vomiting), are particularly prone to iron-deficiency anemia because iron is not adequately digested. Infants with chronic diarrhea may not be able to make use of iron due to inadequate absorption. If infants are fed cow's milk rather than breast milk, so much minimal gastrointestinal bleeding may occur that iron deficiency anemia may develop.

Urging parents to breastfeed or use iron-fortified formula as well as introduce iron-fortified cereal as a "first food" are important health teaching measures to prevent this form of anemia. Occasionally, infants can become constipated while ingesting iron-rich formula, but this is the exception rather than the rule.

Older Children

In children older than 2 years of age, chronic blood loss is the most frequent cause of iron-deficiency anemia caused by gastrointestinal tract lesions such as polyps, ulcerative colitis, Crohn disease, protein-induced enteropathies, parasitic infestation, or frequent epistaxis. Adolescent girls with heavy menstrual periods can become iron deficient when this is combined with frequent attempts to diet or with overconsumption of snack foods that are low in iron.

Assessment

Common symptoms of iron-deficiency anemia are shown in Box 44.4. The mark of iron-deficiency anemia is pale conjunctiva. Because this pallor develops slowly, however, parents may describe their child as "fair skinned" especially when their face develops the same pale appearance.

With extended iron deficiency, infants develop poor muscle tone and reduced activity. Their heart may enlarge and, on auscultation, demonstrate a soft systolic precordial murmur as the heart beats faster in an attempt to supply body cells with more oxygen. The spleen may be slightly enlarged. Fingernails typically become spoon-shaped or depressed in contour.

As a rule, infants should not ingest more than 32 oz of milk a day. A 24-hour dietary history of an iron-deficient infant generally reveals a much higher milk intake than this, perhaps as high as 50 oz a day. Parents also report the child resists or parents do not offer iron-fortified cereal (1 quart of milk provides only about 0.5 mg of iron; in contrast, 1 tablespoon of iron-fortified baby cereal supplies 2.5 to 5.0 mg of iron).

Laboratory studies will reveal a decreased hemoglobin level (a level less than 11 g/100 ml of blood) and reduced hematocrit level (below 33%). The RBCs are not only microcytic and hypochromic but possibly also **poikilocytic** (irregular in shape). The mean corpuscular volume, the mean corpuscular hemoglobin, and serum iron levels are all low. Monoamine oxidase (MAO) is an enzyme important for central nervous system maturation. Because iron is a basic component of MAO, without available iron, this necessary enzyme will be absent, possibly affecting central nervous system maturation.

In school-age children, there is an association between iron-deficiency anemia and poor school achievement, probably related to the chronic fatigue children experience. It is also associated with pica (the craving for ice cubes or the eating of inedible substances such as dirt and paper). Until the

BOX 44.4

Nursing Care Planning Using Assessment

ASSESSING A CHILD WITH IRON-DEFICIENCY ANEMIA

anemia is corrected, parents need to supervise their child's environment to keep inedible materials out of his or her reach (Rabel, Leitman, & Miller, 2016).

Therapeutic Management

Therapy for iron-deficiency anemia focuses on treatment of the underlying cause: the lack of iron. An iron compound such as ferrous sulfate for 4 to 6 weeks is the drug of choice to improve RBC formation and replace iron stores (Box 44.5) (Ambruso et al., 2016). In addition, the diet of the child must be changed to one rich in iron and vitamin C, which enhances iron absorption.

 Concept Mastery Alert

Ferrous sulfate will stain the teeth, and a simple rinse with water will not remove drug left in the mouth after swallowing. The patient should be reminded to brush teeth thoroughly after administration.

 ## Nursing Diagnoses and Related Interventions

Nursing Diagnosis: Imbalanced nutrition, less than body requirements, related to inadequate ingestion of iron

Outcome Evaluation: Parents report child's dietary intake includes iron-rich foods; parents administer ferrous sulfate as prescribed; serum iron levels increase to normal by 6 months.

FERROUS SULFATE (FEOSOL)

Classification: Ferrous sulfate is an iron salt.

Action: Supplies iron for red cell production. It elevates the serum iron concentration and then is converted to hemoglobin or trapped in the reticuloendothelial cells for storage and eventual conversion to a usable form of iron (Karch, 2013).

Pregnancy Risk Category: A

Dosage: For severe iron-deficiency anemia: 4 to 6 mg/kg/d in three divided doses. For mild iron-deficiency anemia: 3 mg/kg/d in two divided doses.

Possible Adverse Effects: Gastrointestinal upset, anorexia, nausea, vomiting, constipation, dark stools, stained teeth (liquid preparations)

Nursing Implications

- Instruct parents to administer the drug on an empty stomach with water to enhance absorption. If this causes gastrointestinal irritation, administer it after meals. Avoid giving it with milk or tea because these interfere with absorption.
- If the liquid preparation is ordered, advise parents to mix it with water or juice to mask the taste. Have the child drink the medication through a straw to avoid staining the teeth.
- Remember that iron is absorbed best in the presence of an acid. Suggest parents give the iron with a citrus juice such as orange juice to help absorption. Some children may be prescribed vitamin C to take concurrently to increase absorption.
- Inform the child and parents that iron may turn stools black.
- Encourage parents to include high-fiber foods in the child's diet to minimize the risk of constipation.
- Reinforce the need for thorough brushing of teeth to prevent staining.
- Remind parents about the need for follow-up blood studies to evaluate the effectiveness of the drug.

When planning care for an infant with iron-deficiency anemia, it is helpful to minimize the child's activities to prevent fatigue, particularly at mealtime because a fatigued child is more reluctant to eat any food, let alone iron-rich foods.

Counsel parents on measures to improve their infant's nutrition, such as adding iron-rich foods while decreasing formula or breast milk intake. If the child is not fond of meat, suggest parents substitute cheese, eggs, green vegetables, or fortified cereal. Because iron-rich foods are often expensive, remind parents that these items are important and they should not substitute less expensive, high-carbohydrate foods for them. Help them also devise a reminder system so they can manage to give the iron supplement

over a long period of time. Alert parents to possible side effects, such as stomach irritation, constipation, and that liquid iron preparations can stain teeth if not taken through a straw. Iron is absorbed best with an accompanying acid medium, so ascorbic acid may also be prescribed (or the parent should be advised to give the iron medication with orange juice) to increase absorption. To avoid constipation, the child may need additional fiber like that supplied by green leafy vegetables. If oral iron is not tolerated or if there is a doubt the child will take it, an iron–dextran injection (Imferon) can be given intramuscularly, although this is extremely irritating and stains the skin unless it is given by deep Z-track intramuscular injection.

Of all age groups, adolescents tend to do the least well with taking medicine consistently. Help them plan a daily time for taking their iron supplement with a medication reminder chart. At first, they may reject this as childish, but assure them that everyone needs some sort of aid to remember such things. Review with them the iron-rich foods they will need to eat daily and that an iron supplement is only a supplement if taken with iron-rich foods.

After 7 days of iron therapy, a reticulocyte count is usually obtained. If elevated, this means the child is now receiving enough iron that erythrocytes are now proliferating and correcting the anemia. Iron medication is taken for at least 4 to 6 weeks after the RBC count has returned to normal so iron stores are rebuilt as well. In some children, maintenance therapy may continue for as long as a year.

Chronic Infection Anemia

Acute infection interferes with RBC production, producing a normochromic, normocytic anemia. When infections are chronic, however, anemia of a hypochromic, microcytic type occurs, which is probably caused by impaired iron metabolism. The degree of anemia is directly related to the severity of the underlying disease; treatment of the underlying cause will usually result in increased hemoglobin levels (Ambruso et al., 2016).

MACROCYTIC (MEGALOBLASTIC) ANEMIAS

A macrocytic anemia is one in which the RBCs appear abnormally large (Wang, 2016). Such cells are actually immature erythrocytes or megaloblasts (nucleated immature red cells), so these anemias are often also referred to as megaloblastic anemias. Because these anemias are caused by nutritional deficiencies, they occur most often in developing countries.

Anemia of Folic Acid Deficiency

A deficiency of folic acid combined with vitamin C deficiency produces an anemia in which the erythrocytes grow abnormally large. There is often accompanying neutropenia and thrombocytopenia. Although the mean corpuscular hemoglobin concentration will be normal, the mean corpuscular volume and mean corpuscular hemoglobin will both be increased. Bone marrow contains megaloblasts, indicating inhibition of the production of erythrocytes at an early stage. Megaloblastic arrest, or inability of RBCs to mature past this early stage, may occur in the first year of life from the continued use of infant food containing too little folic acid or from an infant drinking goat's milk, which tends to be deficient in folic acid. Treatment is daily oral administration of folic acid. With this treatment, the response is dramatic.

Pernicious Anemia (Vitamin B_{12} Deficiency)

Vitamin B_{12} is necessary for the maturation of RBCs. Pernicious anemia results from a deficiency in vitamin B_{12}, either from inadequate intake or malabsorption (Sun, Chang, Wang, et al., 2016).

In children, the cause is more often a lack of ingestion of vitamin B_{12} rather than poor absorption. Adolescents may be deficient in vitamin B_{12} if they are ingesting a long-term, poorly formulated vegetarian diet because the vitamin is found primarily in foods of animal origin (Stredny, Frosch, Singhi, et al., 2016).

For vitamin B_{12} to be absorbed from the intestine, an intrinsic factor must be present in the gastric mucosa. If a child is born with an intrinsic factor deficiency, symptoms occur as early as the first 2 years of life. The child appears pale, anorexic, and irritable, with chronic diarrhea. The tongue appears smooth and beefy red due to papillary atrophy. If not identified and treated at that point, neuropathologic findings such as ataxia, hyporeflexia, paresthesia, and a positive Babinski reflex will develop.

The rate and efficiency of absorption of vitamin B_{12} can be tested by the ingestion of the radioactively tagged vitamin when a dose of intrinsic factor is also measured. If the anemia is identified as being caused by a vitamin B_{12}–deficient diet, temporary injections of vitamin B_{12} will reverse the symptoms. If the anemia is caused by lack of the intrinsic factor, lifelong monthly intramuscular injections of vitamin B_{12} may be necessary.

HEMOLYTIC ANEMIAS

Hemolytic anemias are those in which the number of erythrocytes is low because there is increased erythrocyte destruction. The destruction may be caused by fundamental abnormalities in erythrocyte structure or by extracellular destruction forces.

Congenital Spherocytosis

Congenital spherocytosis is a hemolytic anemia that occurs most frequently in the White Northern European population and is inherited as an autosomal dominant trait. RBCs are small and have a short life span apparently due to abnormalities of the protein of the cell membrane (Ambruso et al., 2016).

The anemia can be noticeable shortly after birth, although symptoms may not be recognized until later in the first year as the abnormal cells swell, rupture, and then are destroyed by the spleen creating a severe anemia. Chronic jaundice and splenomegaly also develop. Because the cells are so small, the mean corpuscular hemoglobin concentration will be increased. Gallstones may be present in older school-age children and adolescents because of the continuous hemolysis, bilirubin release, and incorporation of bilirubin into gallstones.

Infections can precipitate a crisis or cause bone marrow failure. During such a period, the anemia increases rapidly as the hemolysis continues. Blood transfusion will be necessary to maintain a sufficient number of circulating erythrocytes until the crisis passes.

The diagnosis of the disease is based on family history, the obvious hemolysis, and the presence of the abnormal spherocytes. The treatment generally is a splenectomy at approximately 5 to 6 years. This measure will increase the number of RBCs present but will not alter their abnormal structure.

Glucose-6-Phosphate Dehydrogenase Deficiency

The enzyme glucose-6-phosphate dehydrogenase (G6PD) is necessary for maintenance of RBC life; lack of the enzyme results in premature destruction of RBCs. The disease is an X-linked recessive trait inheritance and is found most often in persons of African, Mediterranean, or Asian decent (Ambruso et al., 2016).

G6PD disease occurs in two identifiable forms. Children with a congenital nonspherocytic type develop hemolysis, jaundice, and splenomegaly and may have aplastic crises. Other children have a drug-induced form in which the blood pattern is normal until the child is exposed to fava beans or drugs such as antipyretics, sulfonamides, antimalarials, and naphthoquinones (the most common drug in these groups is acetylsalicylic acid [aspirin]). Approximately 2 days after ingestion of such an oxidant drug, the child begins to show evidence of hemolysis, a low-grade fever, and perhaps back pain. A blood smear will show *Heinz bodies* (oddly shaped particles in RBCs).

The degree of RBC destruction depends on the drug and the extent of exposure to it. Occasionally, a newborn is seen with marked hemolysis because the mother ingested an initiating drug during pregnancy.

G6PD deficiency may be diagnosed by a rapid enzyme screening test or electrophoretic analysis of RBCs. The drug-induced type usually is self-limiting, and if a child is not exposed to substances that cause hemolysis, blood transfusions are rarely necessary. Be certain that both parents and children know about the abnormality in the child's metabolism so they can avoid common drugs such as acetylsalicylic acid.

Sickle-Cell Anemia

Sickle-cell anemia is an autosomal recessive inherited disorder carried on the β chain of hemoglobin; the amino acid valine takes the place of the normally appearing glutamic acid. With this, the erythrocytes become characteristically elongated and crescent shaped (sickled) when they are submitted to low oxygen tension (less than 60% to 70%), a low blood pH (acidosis), or increased blood viscosity, such as occurs with dehydration or hypoxia. When RBCs sickle or change to an elongated shape, they cannot move freely through vessels. Stasis and further sickling occurs (a *sickle-cell crisis*). Blood flow halts and tissue distal to the blockage becomes ischemic, resulting in acute pain and cell destruction (Ambruso et al., 2016).

Because fetal hemoglobin contains a γ, not a β, chain, the disease usually will not result in clinical symptoms until a child's hemoglobin changes from the fetal to the adult form at approximately 6 months. However, the disease can be diagnosed prenatally by chorionic villi sampling or from cord blood during amniocentesis. If these were not done, it will be identified at birth by neonatal screening (Forman, Coye, Levy-Fisch, et al., 2013).

Sickle-cell disease occurs in about 1 out of every 400 Black infants in the United States. The sickle-cell trait (a child carries a gene for the disease but does not have active symptoms) occurs in approximately 1 in 12 Blacks in the United States (Housten, Abel, Dadekian, et al., 2015).

The form of hemoglobin in this disorder is designated hemoglobin S. A child with sickle-cell disease is said to have hemoglobin SS (homozygous involvement). Both parents of the child with the disease will have a combination of usual adult and hemoglobin S types or be carriers (heterozygous) of the *sickle-cell trait* (hemoglobin AS). People with the trait produce enough normal hemoglobin to compensate for any hemoglobin that is sickled and therefore show no symptoms. A child with the disease (homozygous) produces no normal hemoglobin and so will demonstrate characteristic symptoms of sickle-cell anemia. A small number of children have combinations of hemoglobin S and hemoglobin C or E, which leads to chronic mild anemia.

QSEN Checkpoint Question 44.3

EVIDENCE-BASED PRACTICE

The sickle-cell trait (hemoglobin AS) occurs in about 8% of Blacks, and although typically benign, there is some concern that intense physical exercise in such individuals could lead to cardiac deaths from occlusive crises. It has been reported that patients with sickle-cell disease are more prone to kidney and renal failure as well as rhabdomyolysis during times of extreme exertion. Controversies as to whether testing of athletes for sickle cell should be mandatory continue to exist. Although occurrences of death associated with sickle cell and exertion are rare, the National Collegiate Athletic Association (NCAA) has mandated testing for athletes (Lawrence, 2014).

Based on the previous study, which would be the best exercise for Joey, who has sickle-cell disease, and his father who has the sickle-cell trait?
a. Playing video games with each other
b. Joining a swimming program at their local YMCA
c. Watching sports together on TV each evening
d. Organizing a touch (no contact) football game each weekend

Look in Appendix A for the best answer and rationale.

Sickle-Cell Crisis

Sickle-cell crisis is the term used to denote a sudden, severe onset of sickling. There is pooling of many new sickled cells in blood vessels causing consequent tissue hypoxia beyond the blockage (a *vaso-occlusive crisis*). Such a crisis is most apt to occur when a child has a gastrointestinal illness causing dehydration, a respiratory infection that results in lowered oxygen exchange and a lowered arterial oxygen level, or after extremely strenuous exercise (enough to lead to tissue hypoxia); however, sometimes, no obvious cause of a crisis can be found (Boxes 44.6 and 44.7). Symptoms are sudden, severe, and painful (Box 44.8, an interprofessional care map for the child with sickle-cell anemia). A laboratory report will reveal a hemoglobin level of only 6 to

BOX 44.6

Nursing Care Planning Using Assessment

ASSESSING A CHILD WITH SICKLE-CELL CRISIS

BOX 44.7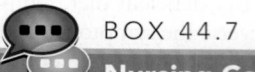

Nursing Care Planning Tips for Effective Communication

Joey, who has sickle-cell disease, is seen in the emergency department with a new vaso-occlusive crisis. His right knee is discolored by a large brush burn. He's crying from pain.

Tip: In an emergency room, it's important that both children and parents recognize the first priority of the nurse is to obtain an accurate history and not to blame anyone for breaking the treatment plan. The nurse will work to find ways to actively assist parents to move past a broken rule so that therapy can be started.

Children with sickle-cell anemia have to follow what seems like a great many rules to avoid clotting or bleeding episodes, such as not playing contact sports or playing too hard in the sun. The following is an example of how to facilitate a conversation when a patient has not followed the treatment plan and the caregiver is upset.

Nurse: Hello, Mr. Harrow. I need to ask some questions to see if anything triggered this new crisis.

Mr. Harrow: He better not have been doing something he's not allowed to do.

Nurse: His knee looks like he may have fallen. Were you running, Joey? So you got dehydrated?

Mr. Harrow: He better not say he was doing that.

Nurse: Mr. Harrow, why don't we let Joey tell us how he thinks the accident happened? Then later on, we can talk about what are good rules for him to be following.

BOX 44.8
Nursing Care Planning

AN INTERPROFESSIONAL CARE MAP FOR A CHILD WITH SICKLE-CELL ANEMIA

Joey is a 7-year-old with sickle-cell anemia you see in the emergency room for a vaso-occlusive crisis.

Family Assessment: Child lives with two older brothers (10 and 12 years of age) and both parents in a three-bedroom home. Father works as a distributor for a local water bottling company. Mother, an X-ray technician, is temporarily on duty with the National Guard in the Middle East. Father rates finances as, "Not good. Medical bills are killing us."

Patient Assessment: Thin, early school-age child with weight at 5th percentile for age. Was screened and diagnosed with sickle-cell anemia at birth. Described as "picky eater"; has eaten little since mother was deployed because he doesn't like father's cooking. Has a history of two former vaso-occlusive crises. Missed last regularly scheduled health assessment 2 weeks ago because father had difficulty taking off from work. Was playing "tag" with older brothers this afternoon. Sclera was jaundiced and child was crying from pain by time father returned from work. Hemoglobin 6 g/100 ml; hematocrit 31%.

Nursing Diagnosis: Altered tissue perfusion related to vaso-occlusive crisis

Outcome Criteria: Oxygen saturation level is maintained at 95% or higher, pain decreases to tolerable level, and symptoms of hemolytic crisis decrease.

Team Member Responsible	Assessment	Intervention	Rationale	Expected Outcome
Activities of Daily Living, Including Safety				
Nurse	Assess if child understands he will need to remain in bed.	Admit child to hospital unit; restrict to bed rest.	Bed rest reduces the need for oxygen in body cells.	Child complies with bed rest; plays nonaction games with parent or healthcare personnel.
Teamwork and Collaboration				
Nurse/primary care provider	Assess if hematology service is needed for consult.	Meet with hematology service as needed for emergency and long-range planning.	Repeated vaso-occlusive crises suggest family needs better management strategies.	Hematology service meets with parent and child as indicated.
Procedures/Medications for Quality Improvement				
Nurse/nurse practitioner	Assess degree of child's pain by use of FACES Pain Scale.	Administer prescribed analgesic as needed.	Vaso-occlusive crises can cause sharp pain that requires strong analgesia.	Child rates pain as no higher than 2 following analgesia administration.
Nurse	Assess oxygen saturation level by continuous pulse oximetry.	Administer oxygen by nasal prongs to keep oxygen saturation above 95% or as prescribed.	Oxygen saturation decreases because sickled cells are unable to carry a full complement of oxygen.	Child cooperates with pulse oximetry and oxygen administration. Oxygen saturation remains above 95%.
Nurse	Determine whether child has been taking folic acid and hydroxyurea at home.	Administer medications to initiate red blood cell (RBC) production as prescribed.	Folic acid and hydroxyurea help to build new RBCs to replace those that have been hemolyzed.	Child takes medication cooperatively.
Nutrition				
Nurse	Assess child's intake and output.	Begin oral rehydration or intravenous (IV) therapy as prescribed.	Restoring hydration reduces sickle-cell clotting.	Child names best hand to start IV infusion; drinks prescribed fluid.
Nurse/nutritionist	Assess child's usual nutrition intake by 24-hour dietary recall history.	Demonstrate child's reduced weight to parent. Plan ways to increase calorie intake.	Even "picky eaters" need to take in enough food daily to meet growth and maintenance needs.	Father states he will try harder to serve foods the child likes; child voices intent to eat at least one meat helping daily.

Continued on following page

BOX 44.8

Nursing Care Planning (continued)

Team Member Responsible	Assessment	Intervention	Rationale	Expected Outcome
Patient-Centered Care				
Nurse	Assess family members' understanding of the causes of sickle-cell vaso-occlusive crises.	Review with family members the importance of child avoiding dehydration and oxygen deficiency.	Dehydration leads to clumping of sickled cells, cutting off circulation in distant body parts.	Family members state they are aware they must be as responsible as the child for avoiding sickling circumstances.
Psychosocial/Spiritual/Emotional Needs				
Nurse	Assess the stress level of family in light of absent mother and child with chronic illness.	Review with family ways to maintain a tight knit family unit (e.g., game night, common activities) to maintain family unity until mother returns.	When families miss a support person, they need to rally together to devise other support methods.	Father states he will try harder to meet children's needs, although worrying about keeping his job and his wife's safety are major concerns.
Informatics for Seamless Healthcare Planning				
Nurse	Determine whether parent has any questions about care of his or her child.	Schedule a follow-up visit in 3 days following hospital discharge for evaluation as prescribed.	Care of a chronically ill child can be a major strain on a family. Follow-up visits help share responsibility for care.	Father states he understands importance of follow-up visit and will keep appointment with child.

8 g/100 ml. A peripheral blood smear will demonstrate sickled cells. Bilirubin and reticulocyte levels will be increased and the WBC count is often elevated to 12,000 to 20,000/mm³.

Further complications that may occur are aseptic necrosis of the head of the femur or humerus causing sharp joint pain or a cerebrovascular accident that occurs from a blocked artery, resulting in loss of motor function, coma, seizures, or even death. If there is renal involvement, hematuria or flank pain may be present.

Other types of crisis that may occur include:

- A *sequestration crisis* occurs when there is splenic sequestration of RBCs or severe anemia occurs due to pooling and increased destruction of sickled cells in the liver and spleen. Shock symptoms occur from hypovolemia. The spleen is enlarged and tender.
- A *hyperhemolytic crisis* occurs when there is increased destruction of RBCs.
- A *megaloblastic crisis* occurs if the child has folic acid or vitamin B deficiency (new RBCs cannot be fully formed due to lack of these ingredients).
- An **aplastic crisis** (temporary cessation of RBC production) occurs when there is a sudden decrease in RBC production. This form usually occurs with infection. It creates a severe anemia.

Assessment for Sickle-Cell Anemia

Sickle-cell anemia is diagnosed at birth because of required blood-spot screening. At approximately 6 months of age, children begin to show initial signs of fever and anemia. Stasis of blood and infarction may occur in a body part, leading to local pain. Some infants have swelling of the hands and feet (a hand–foot syndrome) probably caused by aseptic infarction of the bones of the hands and feet. As they grow, children tend

to have a slight, thin build and characteristically long arms and legs. They may have a protruding abdomen because of an enlarged spleen and liver. In adolescence, the spleen size may decrease in size from repeated infarction and atrophy, leaving the teenager more susceptible to infection than usual because the spleen can no longer filter bacteria. *Streptococcus pneumoniae* and *meningococcus* are two common bacterial agents that frequently cause illness; the child with sickle-cell anemia needs prophylactic antibiotics and age-appropriate vaccines to prevent these and other infections (Obaro & Iroh Tam, 2016).

During late childhood or adolescence, an acute chest syndrome with symptoms of fever, tachypnea, wheezing, or cough that leads to pneumonia may begin to occur (Novelli & Gladwin, 2016). The syndrome develops because when areas of the lung become inflamed and hypoxic, sickle cells adhere to the irritated endothelium and then fail to be reoxygenated. Blood transfusion is used to increase the oxygen-carrying capacity of the blood, and broad-spectrum antibiotics are given to resolve the pneumonia.

Another change that may occur is stasis of blood flow because of cirrhosis of the liver (fibrotic degeneration), which will eventually occur from infarcts and tissue scarring. The kidneys may have subsequent scarring also, so kidney function may be decreased. Eye sclera become icteric (yellowed) from release of bilirubin from destruction of the sickled cells; small retinal occlusions may lead to decreased vision. **Priapism**, a persistent painful erection, is a clinical manifestation of sickle cell caused by vaso-occlusion in the penis (Ambruso et al., 2016).

Therapeutic Management

The child in a sickle-cell crisis has three primary needs: pain relief, adequate hydration, and oxygenation to prevent further sickling and halt the crisis.

Acetaminophen (Tylenol) may be adequate pain relief for some children; for others, a narcotic analgesic such as intravenous morphine may be necessary. Once children are pain free and able to relax, the metabolic demand for oxygen is reduced and sickling begins to end. Hydration is generally accomplished with intensive intravenous fluid replacement therapy. The acidosis that develops from tissue hypoxia must be corrected by electrolyte replacement. As a rule, because some kidney infarction may have occurred, do not administer potassium intravenously until kidney function has been determined (e.g., the child voids). Otherwise, excessive potassium levels can lead to cardiac arrhythmias. If infection appears to be the precipitator for a sickling crisis, blood and urine cultures, a chest X-ray, and a complete blood count will be taken and the infection will be treated with antibiotics. Blood transfusion (usually packed RBCs) may be necessary to prevent life-threatening complications and maintain a normal hemoglobin count (Novelli & Gladwin, 2016).

Hydroxyurea, an antineoplastic agent, has the potential to increase the strength and oxygenation capacity of sickled cells (Ponnampalam & Thalange, 2013). Given orally, a side effect of the drug is anorexia, so children need their nutrition intake monitored while taking the drug to be certain it is adequate.

If none of the previous measures appears to be effective, children may be given an exchange transfusion to remove most of the sickled cells and replace them with normal cells. Hematopoietic stem cell transplantation is a permanent solution to the disorder and is advocated for the child who does not respond to usual therapies.

QSEN Checkpoint Question 44.4

QUALITY IMPROVEMENT

Joey, who has sickle-cell anemia, is being treated for sickle-cell crisis. Which statement by his father would best assure the nurse that Joey is receiving adequate nursing care?

   a. "He never used to understand why he had these crises, but now, he can describe the reason."
   b. "He says that his pain is actually quite manageable now."
   c. "He says that the nurses he's met so far are such nice people."
   d. "He's looking forward to getting home, but he really doesn't mind it here."

Look in Appendix A for the best answer and rationale.

Nursing Diagnoses and Related Interventions

Because, like most anemias, sickle-cell disease is a chronic process, nursing diagnoses need to consider both short- and long-term goals.

Nursing Diagnosis: Ineffective tissue perfusion related to generalized infarcts due to sickling

Outcome Evaluation: Child's respiratory rate is 16 to 20 breaths/min; cyanosis is absent; arterial blood gases within acceptable parameters, including $PCO_2 = 40$ mmHg, PO_2 = 80 to 90 mmHg, oxygen saturation of 95%; urine output greater than 1 ml/kg/hr.

Oxygen may be administered by either nasal cannula or mask if arterial blood gases reveal a low PO_2 level. High concentrations of oxygen are used with caution because hypoxia is a stimulant to erythrocyte production, which is badly needed to replace damaged cells. Monitor the flow rate carefully, therefore, and use pulse oximetry to evaluate oxygen saturation levels for changes. Encourage bed rest to reduce oxygen expenditure.

Nursing Diagnosis: Ineffective health maintenance related to lack of knowledge regarding long-term needs of child with sickle-cell anemia

Outcome Evaluation: Parents accurately describe disease process and identify special precautions necessary to prevent a sickle-cell crisis.

In many children, episodes of sickling grow less severe as the child reaches adolescence. Other children experience such devastating episodes in early childhood that without a stem cell transplant, the disease becomes fatal at an early age.

Between crises, parents need to focus care on preventing recurring crises. Although the hemoglobin level of children may remain as low as 6 to 9 g/100 ml, children adjust well to this chronic state. Caution parents that children who receive frequent blood transfusions should not be given supplementary iron or iron-fortified formula or vitamins because they may receive too much iron; high levels of excess iron are deposited in body tissues (**hemochromatosis**) to a point of staining body tissue or being incorporated into body tissue with fibrotic scarring (hemosiderosis). Oral folic acid may be prescribed to help rebuild hemolyzed RBCs. They need to monitor urine output and may be asked to test urine for specific gravity and hematuria to detect the extent or presence of kidney damage occurring from minor infarcts. Some children who have had kidney infarcts and a lessened ability to concentrate urine have chronic nocturnal enuresis (bedwetting).

Be certain that children receive childhood immunizations so they are not vulnerable to common childhood infections such as measles or pertussis and receive meningococcal, pneumococcal, and Hib vaccines to prevent those specific infections. If children are prescribed oral penicillin as prophylaxis against infection, help the parents determine a method to remember or remind conscientious administration of this.

Caution parents to bring their child to a healthcare facility at the first indication of infection. Some parents are reluctant to do this, afraid that they will be labeled overprotective. Assure them that healthcare personnel are knowledgeable about sickle-cell anemia and that they know that a child with even a minor infection could become very ill.

Children should attend regular school and should be allowed to participate in all school activities except contact sports (such as football), which could result in rupture of an enlarged spleen or liver. Long-distance running is also inadvisable because it can lead to dehydration. During the summer, parents need to offer the child frequent drinks to prevent dehydration, especially on long hikes and at the beach. Caution parents against taking the child on board an unpressurized aircraft in which the oxygen concentration may fall during flight.

Children with sickle-cell disease are at high risk if they need surgery because the hours of being held on nothing-by-mouth status, as well as being unable to eat afterward, may lead to dehydration; anesthesia may cause a transient hypoxia leading to sickling. Caution parents that even for a simple operation such as tooth extraction, they must alert healthcare personnel about their child's condition.

Because puberty is delayed in some children, both parents and children may need counseling to accept this; although they can be assured once puberty changes do occur, they are adequate and just appear later than usual. Children may need support and positive reinforcement during their growth years to enhance their self-esteem as they learn how to deal with the results of a chronic hematologic disorder (Box 44.9).

What If . . . 44.2

Joey's father tells the nurse he restricts Joey, who has sickle-cell anemia, from drinking any fluid after 4 PM to prevent bed-wetting. What patient education would the nurse provide for this parent?

THALASSEMIAS

The thalassemias are autosomal recessive anemias associated with abnormalities of the b chain of adult hemoglobin (hemoglobin A). Although these anemias occur most frequently in the Mediterranean population, they also occur in children of African and Asian heritage (Ponnampalam & Thalange, 2013).

Thalassemia Minor (Heterozygous β-Thalassemia)

Children with thalassemia minor, a mild form of this anemia, produce a combination of both defective β hemoglobin and normal hemoglobin. The condition represents the heterozygous form of the disorder and can be compared with children having the sickle-cell trait. Because there is some normal production, the RBC count is usually normal, but the hemoglobin concentration will be decreased by 2 to 3 g/100 ml below usual levels. The blood cells are moderately hypochromic and microcytic because of the poor hemoglobin formation.

Children may have no symptoms other than pallor. They require no treatment, and life expectancy is normal. They should not receive a routine iron supplement because their inability to incorporate it well into hemoglobin may cause them to accumulate too much iron.

Thalassemia Major (Homozygous β-Thalassemia)

Thalassemia major is also called Cooley anemia or Mediterranean anemia. It is diagnosed at birth by a blood spot test. Because this is a β-chain hemoglobin defect, symptoms do not become apparent until a child's fetal hemoglobin has largely been replaced by adult hemoglobin during the second half of the first year of life. Effects of thalassemia major on body systems are summarized in Table 44.3. Unable to produce normal β hemoglobin, the child shows symptoms of anemia, including pallor, irritability, and anorexia (DeLeo & Geraghty, 2016).

RBCs are both hypochromic and microcytic. Fragmented poikilocytes (abnormally shaped RBCs) and basophilic stippling (unevenness of hemoglobin concentration) are also usually present. The hemoglobin level is less than 5 g/100

BOX 44.9

Nursing Care Planning Based on Family Teaching

SCHOOL SAFETY PRECAUTIONS FOR CHILDREN WITH SICKLE-CELL DISEASE

Q. Joey's father says to you, "What precautions should I discuss with my son's teacher so I know he's safe at school?"

A. Some common suggestions include:

- Be certain your child either takes fluid with him or buys adequate fluid for lunch because he needs to maintain a high fluid intake to prevent blood from becoming thick.
- Provide additional fluid in the summer, when dehydration is more apt to happen. Anticipate ways to provide fluid during long hikes or school trips; time spent on a hot beach may need to be limited.
- Learn about sources high in folic acid, such as vegetables and fruit, and be certain these foods are included in your son's packed lunch or selected from a cafeteria every day.
- With the exception of contact sports (to avoid damage to an enlarged spleen) and long-distance running (to prevent dehydration), encourage your son to participate in normal school activities.
- Know that bed-wetting may occur as part of the illness. Encourage your son to take baths in the morning if this occurs so his clothes don't smell of urine.
- Maintain routine health care such as immunizations to prevent common childhood illnesses such as measles and mumps, which cause fever and dehydration.
- Have the school nurse call you for any sign of illness, such as an upper respiratory infection, so therapy can be started immediately.

TABLE 44.3 EFFECTS OF THALASSEMIA MAJOR

Body Organ or System	Effect of Abnormal Cell Production
Bone marrow	Overstimulation of bone marrow leads to bone widening, especially in the face and skull.
Skin	Bronze-colored from hemosiderosis and jaundice
Spleen	Splenomegaly
Liver and gallbladder	Cirrhosis and cholelithiasis
Pancreas	Destruction of islet cells and diabetes mellitus
Heart	Failure from circulatory overload

ml. The serum iron level is high because iron is not being incorporated into hemoglobin; iron saturation will be 100%.

Assessment

To maintain a functional level of hemoglobin, the bone marrow hypertrophies in an attempt to produce more RBCs, causing bone pain and the formation of target cells or large macrocytes that are short lived and nonfunctional. The hyperactivity of the bone marrow results in characteristic changes in the shape of the skull (parietal and frontal bossing) and protrusion of the upper teeth, with marked malocclusion. The base of the nose may be broad and flattened; the eyes may be slanted with an epicanthal fold, as in Down syndrome. An X-ray of the bone shows marked osteoporotic (of lessened density) tissue, which can lead to fractures. The child may have both an enlarged spleen and liver due to excessive iron deposits and fibrotic scarring in the liver and the spleen from increased attempts to destroy defective RBCs. Abdominal pressure from the enlarged spleen may cause anorexia and vomiting. Epistaxis is common, diabetes mellitus may result from pancreatic hemosiderosis (deposition of iron), and cardiac dilatation with arrhythmias and heart failure may result in myocardial fibrosis caused by invasion of iron.

Therapeutic Management

Stem cell transplantation is the ultimate cure for the disorder. While waiting for a matched donor, digitalis, diuretics, and a low-sodium diet may be prescribed to prevent heart failure. Transfusion of packed RBCs every 2 to 4 weeks (hypertransfusion therapy) can be used to maintain hemoglobin between 10 and 12 g/100 ml because with this level of hemoglobin, erythropoiesis is suppressed and cosmetic facial alterations, osteoporosis, and cardiac dilatation are minimized. Hypertransfusion therapy also reduces the possibility that a splenectomy will be necessary. Frequent blood transfusions, unfortunately, increase the risk of blood-borne diseases, such as hepatitis B, and hemosiderosis, so children need an oral iron-chelating agent to remove this excessive store of iron, such as deferasirox or deferoxamine.

A splenectomy may become necessary to reduce discomfort and also to reduce the rate of RBC hemolysis and the number of transfusions needed. Bone marrow stem cell transplantation can offer a cure. Even without stem cell transplantation, the overall prognosis of thalassemia is improving, although it is still grave. Most children with the disease die of cardiac failure during adolescence or as late adolescents if they do not receive a hematopoietic stem cell transplant.

Nursing Diagnoses and Related Interventions

Nursing Diagnosis: Risk for situational low self-esteem related to changed physical appearance

Outcome Evaluation: Child states she can accept altered appearance and interacts with peers.

Children with thalassemia major may have delayed growth and sexual maturation. They may develop a marked change in facial appearance because of the overgrowth of marrow-producing centers of the facial bones, which will be permanent. In addition, the child who receives frequent blood transfusions may develop such hemosiderosis that skin color appears bronze.

Children should be allowed as much activity as possible and should attend regular school to maintain a nearly normal childhood. Discussions about other children's reactions to their changing facial appearance and how people are evaluated by who they are and not what they look like can be helpful.

What If . . . 44.3

The last time the nurse saw Lana she was fair skinned, but at a clinic visit today, the nurse notices her skin looks a lot darker. She tells the nurse she and her mother both spent time at a tanning salon to get ready for a vacation in the sun. What concerns would the nurse have about Lana using a tanning bed and vacationing in the sun?

Autoimmune Acquired Hemolytic Anemia

Occasionally, autoimmune antibodies (abnormal antibodies of the immunoglobulin [Ig]G class) attach themselves to RBCs, destroying them or causing hemolysis. This can occur at any age, and its origin is generally unknown, although the disorder is associated with malignancy, viral infections, or collagen diseases such as rheumatoid arthritis or systemic lupus erythematosus. A child may recently have had an upper respiratory infection, measles, or varicella virus infection (chickenpox). The disorder may occur after the administration of drugs such as quinine, phenacetin, sulfonamides, or penicillin (Ambruso et al., 2016).

Assessment

The onset of symptoms is insidious. Children usually develop a low-grade fever, anorexia, lethargy, pallor, and icterus from release of indirect bilirubin from the hemolyzed cells. Both urine and stools appear dark as the excess bilirubin is excreted. In a few children, the illness begins abruptly with high fever, hemoglobinuria, marked jaundice, and enlarged liver and spleen.

Laboratory findings reveal RBCs have become extremely small and round (spherocytosis). The reticulocyte count will be increased as the body attempts to form replacement RBCs. A direct Coombs test result is positive, indicating the presence of antibodies attached to red cells. Hemoglobin levels may fall as low as 6 g/100 ml.

Therapeutic Management

In some children, the disease process runs a limited course and no treatment is necessary. In others, a single blood transfusion may correct the disturbance. It is difficult to cross-match blood for transfusion for these children, however, because the red cell antibody tends to clump or agglutinate all blood tested. If cross-matching is impossible, the child may be given type O, Rh-negative blood, which doesn't need to match. Carefully observe the child especially during any transfusion for signs of transfusion reaction.

If anemia is persistent, corticosteroid therapy (oral prednisone) to reduce the immune response is generally effective, increasing the RBC count and hemoglobin concentration in a short period. If this is not effective, splenectomy or stronger immunosuppressive agents such as cyclophosphamide (Cytoxan) or azathioprine (Imuran) are necessary to reduce antibody formation.

Often, it is difficult for parents to understand the process causing their child's condition. How could their child's body turn on itself this way? How long will this last? What will stop it from happening again? Because there are no certain answers to these questions, provide parents and children with support as they wait for this unexplainable process to run its course and for their child to be well again.

QSEN Checkpoint Question 44.5

> **TEAMWORK & COLLABORATION**
>
> Autoimmune acquired hemolytic anemia can occur in any child. The nurse identifies which usual cause of this disorder as important for team members to know?
> a. Allergy to the protein found in fish or shrimp
> b. A mutant gene similar to sickle-cell anemia
> c. An elevated (increased) eosinophil cell count
> d. Antibody production against red blood cells
>
> *Look in Appendix A for the best answer and rationale.*

POLYCYTHEMIA

Polycythemia is an increase in the number of RBCs. The condition results from increased erythropoiesis, which occurs as a compensatory response to insufficient oxygenation of the blood in order to help supply more oxygen to body cells. Although this may occur as a hereditary form, chronic pulmonary disease and congenital heart disease are the usual causes of polycythemia in childhood. Also, it may occur from the lower oxygen level maintained during intrauterine life in newborns or with twin transfusion at birth (one twin receives excess blood, whereas a second twin is anemic).

Plethora (marked reddened appearance of the skin) occurs because of the increase in total RBC volume. Erythrocytes are usually macrocytic (large), and the hemoglobin content is high. This means the mean corpuscular hemoglobin will be elevated; the mean corpuscular hemoglobin concentration, however, will be normal, indicating that although many in number, each erythrocyte is normally saturated with hemoglobin. The RBC count may be as high as 7 million/mm³. Hemoglobin levels may be as high as 23 g/100 ml.

Treatment of polycythemia involves treatment of the underlying cause. Because of the high blood viscosity from so many crowded blood cells, cerebrovascular accident or emboli may occur. The risk increases particularly if the child becomes dehydrated, such as with fever or during surgery. A program of low-dose aspirin to help prevent clotting or exchange transfusion or phlebotomy to reduce the RBC count may be necessary.

Disorders of Blood Coagulation

Platelets are necessary for blood coagulation, so disorders that limit the number of platelets limit the effectiveness of this process. A normal platelet level is 150,000/mm³. Thrombocytopenia (decreased platelet count) is defined as a platelet count of less than 40,000/mm³. Thrombocytopenia often leads to purpura or blood seeping from vessels into the skin. In one rare disorder, children are born with thrombocytopenia and are also missing the radius bone in the forearm (thrombocytopenia-absent radius [TAR] syndrome).

PURPURAS

Purpura refers to a hemorrhagic rash or small hemorrhages in the superficial layer of skin. Two main types of purpura occur in children: idiopathic thrombocytopenic purpura and Henoch–Schönlein syndrome.

Idiopathic Thrombocytopenic Purpura

Idiopathic thrombocytopenic purpura (ITP) is the result of a decrease in the number of circulating platelets in the presence of adequate megakaryocytes (precursors to platelets). The cause is unknown, but it is thought to result from an increased rate of platelet destruction due to an antiplatelet antibody that destroys platelets, making this an autoimmune illness.

In most instances, ITP occurs approximately 2 weeks after a viral infection such as rubella, rubeola, varicella, or an upper respiratory tract infection. Congenital ITP may occur in the newborn of a woman who has had ITP during pregnancy. An antiplatelet factor apparently crosses the placenta and causes platelet destruction in the newborn in the same way that Rh incompatibility or hemolytic disease of the newborn develops (see Chapter 26). However, in ITP, the platelets, not the RBCs, are sensitized.

Assessment

Manifestations often begin abruptly, first evidenced as miniature petechiae or as large areas of asymmetric ecchymosis most prominent over the legs, although they may occur anywhere on the body (Fig. 44.3). Epistaxis or bleeding into joints may be present.

Laboratory studies reveal marked thrombocytopenia. The platelet count may be as low as 20,000/mm³. Bone marrow examination reveals a normal number of megakaryocytes.

Therapeutic Management

Oral prednisone to reduce the immune response and intravenous immunoglobulin (IVIG) or, in Rh-positive children, anti-D immunoglobulin to supply anti-ITP antibodies are used to treat ITP. Platelet transfusion will temporarily increase the platelet count, but because the life span of platelets

Figure 44.3 An infant with idiopathic thrombocytopenic purpura (ITP). Notice the tiny petechiae and larger ecchymotic areas. (From Zitelli, B. J., & Davis, H. W. [1997]. *Atlas of pediatric physical diagnosis* [3rd ed.]. St. Louis, MO: Mosby–Year Book.)

is relatively short, a platelet transfusion has only limited effect. Children with central nervous system bleeding may require a splenectomy, although this is rarely necessary.

If the child experiences joint pain from bleeding, acetaminophen (Tylenol) rather than salicylates or ibuprofen is prescribed for pain because both salicylates and ibuprofen increase the chance for bleeding as they prevent the aggregation of platelets at wound sites.

In most children, ITP runs a limited, 1- to 3-month course. A few children develop chronic ITP. A course of immunosuppressive drugs may be attempted if the chronic state persists. All children need to be vaccinated against the viral diseases of childhood so that diseases such as rubella, rubeola, and varicella are eradicated and can no longer lead to this defective coagulation process.

 ## Nursing Diagnoses and Related Interventions

Nursing Diagnosis: Health-seeking behaviors related to injury-prevention measures

Outcome Evaluation: Parents state precautions they will take to reduce possibility of bleeding, repeat correct dose and timing of medication therapy, child's skin is free of ecchymotic areas, and platelet count rises to normal values.

The techniques for reducing bleeding described earlier in the chapter, such as padding surfaces where the child plays (see Box 44.3), can be used to reduce the possibility of bleeding for the child with ITP. Parents cannot eliminate the possibility of a serious bleeding injury, however, until the platelet count returns to normal. The chief danger to the child from ITP, aside from the psychological stress of a perplexing illness, is intracranial hemorrhage. Although this is rare, be alert for signs such as persistent headache with vomiting, lethargy, slurred speech, weakness on one side of the body, and new onset of seizure.

Nursing Diagnosis: Risk for compromised family coping related to diagnosis of child's illness

Outcome Evaluation: Parents state that they understand the nature of their child's illness and have identified ways to carry out daily activities despite the illness.

Because symptoms such as the easy bruising of ITP mimics the beginning signs of leukemia, parents may be extremely frightened when symptoms first occur. You can assure them after the diagnosis is made that this bruising is not and will not lead to leukemia. A child may have so many bruises that the parents are initially suspected of child maltreatment. This can cause them to become very defensive and angry at healthcare personnel. Allow them time to express their anger and regain confidence in their healthcare team.

It is always bewildering for parents to be told that no one knows exactly what is causing their child's illness. To feel comfortable that healthcare personnel can manage their child's care without knowing the exact cause, parents need careful explanations of all procedures.

Henoch–Schönlein Syndrome

Henoch–Schönlein purpura (also called anaphylactoid purpura) is caused by increased vessel permeability, which leads to bleeding in the small blood vessels. Although no definite allergic correlation can be identified, it is generally considered to be a hypersensitivity reaction to an invading allergen. It occurs most frequently in children between 2 and 8 years of age and more frequently in boys than girls (Bluman & Goldman, 2014). Usually, there is a history of a mild infection before the outbreak of symptoms. The syndrome presents (because of the purpura) as a possible platelet disorder until a differential diagnosis is made.

Assessment

The purpural rash occurs typically on the buttocks, posterior thighs, and extensor surface of the arms and legs (Fig. 44.4). The tips of the ears may be involved. The rash begins as a crop of urticarial lesions that change to pink maculopapules. These become hemorrhagic (bright red) and then fade, leaving brown macular spots that remain for several weeks. The child's joints are tender and swollen. The child may have gastrointestinal symptoms such as abdominal pain, vomiting, or blood in stools. Gross or microscopic hematuria may be present from kidney involvement. A biopsy shows **granulocytes** (WBCs) in the walls of small arterioles.

Laboratory studies show a normal platelet count. The child's sedimentation rate, WBC count, and eosinophil count are elevated.

Therapeutic Management

Treatment involves oral corticosteroid therapy (prednisone) and mild analgesics for a short period. Nose and throat cultures rule out continuing bacterial involvement. Urine should be assessed for protein and glucose to detect kidney involvement. Typically, the disease runs a course of 4 to 6 weeks. A few children develop mildly severe chronic nephritis as a complication (Tudorache, Azema, Hogan, et al., 2015).

Figure 44.4   The distinctive purpural rash of Henoch–Schönlein syndrome appearing on the legs and buttocks of a young child. (From Fleisher, G. R., Ludwig, S., & Baskin, M. N. [2004]. *Atlas of pediatric emergency medicine.* Philadelphia, PA: Lippincott Williams & Wilkins.)

HEMOPHILIAS

Hemophilias are inherited disorders of blood coagulation. There are numerous types, each involving a deficiency of a different blood coagulation factor.

Hemophilia A (Factor VIII Deficiency)

The classic form of hemophilia is caused by deficiency of the coagulation component factor VIII, the antihemophilic factor, and transmitted as a sex-linked recessive trait. In the United States, the incidence is approximately 1 in 5,000 White males. A female carrier may have slightly lowered but sufficient levels of the factor VIII component so that she does not manifest a bleeding disorder. The baseline level of factor determines the occurrence of bleeding episodes and can range from mild to severe (Gupta, Garg, & Singh, 2015).

Factor VIII is an intrinsic factor of coagulation; its absence causes the intrinsic system for manufacturing thromboplastin to be incomplete. The child's coagulation ability is not totally absent because the extrinsic or tissue system remains intact. Because of this system, the child's blood will eventually coagulate after an injury.

Assessment

Hemophilia often is recognized first in the infant who bleeds excessively after circumcision. If the disease has not shown itself for several generations in a family, the parents may be unaware of its existence. For this reason, all infants need careful and thoughtful observation after circumcision. Because infants do not receive many injuries, children's bleeding tendencies may not become apparent until they become active (e.g., crawling, climbing, or walking).

Suddenly, the lower extremities (where the child bumps things) become heavily bruised. There is soft tissue bleeding and painful hemorrhage into joints, which become swollen and warm. Repeated bleeding into a joint this way causes damage to the synovial membrane (hemarthrosis), possibly resulting in severe loss of joint mobility (Merono-Gallut & Cuesta-Barriuso, 2016).

Severe bleeding may also occur into the gastrointestinal tract, peritoneal cavity, or central nervous system. Although nosebleeds are common, they are not as severe as with the platelet deficiency syndromes. The platelet count and prothrombin time are both normal; the whole blood clotting time is either markedly prolonged or normal, depending on the level of factor VIII present. A thromboplastin generation test will be abnormal. Partial thromboplastin time (PTT) is the test that best reveals the low levels of factor VIII. It's important that children with hemophilia be identified by such tests before surgery; otherwise, fatal bleeding could occur.

Therapeutic Management

With even minor abrasions, bleeding can be controlled by the administration of factor VIII supplied by fresh whole blood, fresh or frozen plasma, or a concentrate of factor VIII. The concentrate is supplied as a powdered form that can be stored at home and reconstituted as needed. For most bleeding episodes, one bag of concentrate per 5 kg of body weight is usually sufficient to provide protection for approximately 12 hours; another transfusion may be necessary after that time. In some children, the administration of desmopressin (DDAVP), which stimulates the release of factor VIII, may also help prevent bleeding.

In a few children, antibodies (termed *inhibitors*) to factor VIII develop, rendering the factor ineffective. If this happens, ε-aminocaproic acid, a fibrinolytic enzyme that helps to stabilize clot formation and promote wound healing, can be self-administered every 6 hours if needed. Children with inhibitors to factor VIII can also be given a factor IX concentrate (Proplex or Konyne). This concentrate enters the coagulation cascade after factor VIII and halts bleeding at that point.

Nursing Diagnoses and Related Interventions

Nursing Diagnosis: Parental health-seeking behaviors related to strategies for protecting child from injury

Outcome Evaluation: Child's skin is free of ecchymotic areas, frequent epistaxis is absent, blood pressure is within age-appropriate parameters, and swelling or warmth at joints is absent.

Parents need information both about how to prevent bleeding episodes and how to respond when one does occur. To help prevent injuries, help parents set appropriate limits for activity. An active infant, for example, may need to have crib sides padded and all toys should be inspected for sharp edges or parts. Older children need to self-monitor activities such as roughhousing, and sports participation needs to be evaluated as to whether it will be safe. On the other hand, parents need to be certain their child is not so inactive that obesity occurs.

Parents (and the child at about age 10 years) can be taught to reconstruct and administer a replacement factor intravenously to prevent bleeding immediately after an injury. Although the child needs to be assessed by a healthcare provider, this action, combined with pressure applied to the bleeding site, immobilization of the injured extremity, and an ice pack applied locally, almost always eliminates the need for hospital admission. "Butterfly bandages" are used in place of suturing for lacerations whenever possible because sutures create additional puncture sites that could bleed.

Nursing Diagnosis: Pain related to joint infiltration by blood

Outcome Evaluation: Child states pain is at a tolerable level.

The child with hemophiliac bleeding experiences discomfort because of the bleeding into joints and may be frightened because his parents are so frightened. Acetaminophen (Tylenol) rather than ibuprofen is ordered as an analgesic because ibuprofen may prolong bleeding. As soon as effective levels of factor VIII have been provided, the pain in the bleeding joint is generally relieved, despite the continued heat or swelling. Be certain that when joints are immobilized, they are in good alignment. As soon as the acute bleeding episode has halted (approximately 48 hours), help the child perform passive range of motion as prescribed to maintain function.

Nursing Diagnosis: Risk for interrupted family processes related to fears regarding child's prognosis and long-term nature of illness

Outcome Evaluation: Family members voice their fear regarding illness, state they are able to cope despite stress level, and demonstrate positive coping responses.

Parents of children with hemophilia are frightened during a time of acute bleeding, not just because of what is currently happening but also because they may have seen other family members or even a previous child die of the disease. Be certain to give them a chance to talk about how the bleeding began (e.g., "I should have noticed that toy had a sharp edge," "He fell from his bike. I should have watched him more closely"). Parents often blame themselves, so it is important to be sensitive and nonjudgmental. It is extremely important for parents to allow the child to lead a normal life, so remind them when they do this that it is impossible to prevent all injuries.

von Willebrand Disease

von Willebrand disease, an inherited autosomal dominant disorder, affects both sexes and is most common among Whites (Ambruso et al., 2016). Along with a factor VIII defect, there is also an inability of the platelets to aggregate and the blood vessels to constrict to aid in coagulation. Bleeding time is prolonged, with most hemorrhages occurring from mucous membrane sites.

Epistaxis is a major problem, because all children tend to rub or pick at their nose as a nervous mechanism. In girls, menstrual flow is unusually heavy and may cause embarrassment from stained clothing. Childbirth is obviously a risk for women with von Willebrand disease, so women must be monitored closely for 9 months and again during the postpartal period (Committee on Adolescent Health Care, 2013). Bleeding is controlled with factor VIII replenishment as with hemophilia, or by administration of desmopressin (DDAVP), which stimulates factor VIII release.

Christmas Disease (Hemophilia B, Factor IX Deficiency)

Christmas disease, first noted in 1952 in a patient by the name of Stephen Christmas, is caused by factor IX deficiency.

It is transmitted as a sex-linked recessive trait, and only approximately 15% of people with hemophilia have this form. Treatment is with a concentrate of factor IX, which is available for home administration (Ambruso et al., 2016).

Hemophilia C (Factor XI Deficiency)

Hemophilia C, or plasma thromboplastin antecedent deficiency, is caused by factor XI deficiency, is transmitted as an autosomal recessive trait, and occurs in both sexes. The symptoms are generally mild compared with those in children with factor VIII or factor IX deficiencies. Bleeding episodes are treated with administration of desmopressin (DDAVP) or transfusion of fresh blood or plasma.

Disseminated Intravascular Coagulation

Disseminated intravascular coagulation (DIC) is an acquired disorder of blood clotting that results from excessive trauma or some similar underlying stimulus, such as an acute infection or trauma.

A child begins to develop petechiae or have uncontrolled bleeding from puncture sites from injections or intravenous therapy. Ecchymoses and petechiae form on the skin. Observe all children with a serious illness carefully for signs such as these of increased bleeding to help identify that this is happening. DIC is also discussed in Chapter 21 as a frequent complication of bleeding disorders in pregnancy.

What If . . . 44.4
The nurse is particularly interested in exploring one of the 2020 National Health Goals with respect to hematologic disorders and children (see Box 44.1). What would be a possible research topic to explore pertinent to this goal that would be applicable to Lana's or Joey's family and that would also advance evidence-based practice?

KEY POINTS FOR REVIEW

- Hematopoietic stem cell transplantation is the main therapy for numerous blood dyscrasias. Transplantation can be allogeneic (from a histocompatible donor), autologous (using the child's own marrow or umbilical cord blood), or syngeneic (the donor and recipient are identical twins).
- Splenectomy, another possible treatment, may increase a child's susceptibility to pneumococcal infections. Assess whether a child has received pneumococcal vaccine after a splenectomy.
- Disorders of the RBCs that commonly occur in children include acute blood loss anemia and anemia of acute infection. Aplastic and hypoplastic anemias occur from depression of hematopoietic activity in bone marrow. These anemias can be congenital or acquired.
- A major hypochromic anemia that develops in children is iron-deficiency anemia. Children invariably fatigue easily because they cannot oxygenate body cells well. Their care must include measures to keep them from tiring; oxygen administration may be necessary.
- Macrocytic anemias occur from folic acid deficiency and pernicious anemia (vitamin B_{12} deficiency).

■ Hemolytic anemias include congenital spherocytosis, G6PD, sickle-cell anemia, thalassemia, and autoimmune acquired hemolytic anemia. Sickle-cell anemia occurs most often in Black children.

■ Disorders of blood coagulation include the purpuras (ITP and Henoch–Schönlein syndrome), DIC, and the hemophilias.

■ Children with blood coagulation disorders must carefully guard against injury. This includes monitoring types of toys and activities. It may also include padding a crib or side rail.

■ Disorders of the blood tend to be long-term illnesses. Education of the parents and child is important to promote adaptation to the condition and enhance long-term medication therapy that not only meets QSEN competencies but also best meets a family's total needs.

CRITICAL THINKING CARE STUDY

Tooley James is a 12-year-old you meet at an emergent care clinic. Tooley has sickle-cell anemia and is awaiting a stem cell transplant. He had a splenectomy 2 years ago. He lives with his older sister Michele (18 years of age), his mother (32 years of age), and his grandmother (76 years of age). Tooley's mother works two jobs to support the family (as an assembly line worker making paper products during the day and as a waitress at a local restaurant in the evening). Tooley is responsible for taking his folic acid and his hydroxyurea daily as well as "staying clear of infections" independently.

1. He's at the clinic today because "a kid shoved him" on his way home from school. His sister offered to bring him to the hospital, but because she has a cold, Tooley refused to ride in the car with her. By the time his mother returned home from her second job his right knee was visibly swollen, he had pain "all over," and was gasping for breath. Tooley knows it's important to avoid infections, but did he make a good decision about his care?

2. Tooley needs some emergency measures in your clinic. What are the three main measures you anticipate he will need? Should you explore further how his injury happened?

3. Tooley's mother tells you Tooley's school grades have fallen from Bs to Cs and Ds over the past year. When you ask him why this is happening, he tells you, "If I don't get a transplant, how will it matter what my grades are?" Is that a typical preadolescent attitude or would you worry Tooley is becoming depressed about his situation?

RELATED RESOURCES

Explore these additional resources to enhance learning for this chapter:

• Student resources on thePoint, including answers to the What If . . . and Critical Thinking Care Study questions, http://thepoint.lww.com/Flagg8e

• Adaptive learning powered by PrepU, http://thepoint.lww.com/prepu

REFERENCES

Alousi, A. M., Bolaños-Meade, J., & Lee, S. J. (2013). Graft-versus-host disease: State of the science. *Biology of Blood & Marrow Transplantation*, *19*(1 Suppl.), S102–S108.

Ambruso, D. R., Nuss, R., & Wang, M. (2016). Hematologic disorders. In W. W. Hay, M. J. Levin, R. R. Deterding, & M. J. Abzug (Eds.), *Current diagnosis & treatment pediatrics* (23rd ed.). New York, NY: McGraw-Hill.

Bhatt-Poulose, K., James, K., Reid, M., et al. (2016). Increased rates of body dissatisfaction, depressive symptoms, and suicide attempts in Jamaican teens with sickle cell disease. *Pediatric Blood & Cancer*, *63*(12), 2159–2166. http://dx.doi.org/10.1002/pbc.26091

Bluman, J., & Goldman, R. D. (2014). Henoch-Schönlein purpura in children: Limited benefits of corticosteroids. *Canadian Family Physician*, *60*(11), 1007–1010.

Campbell, Y. N., Machan, M. D., & Fisher, M. D. (2016). The Jehovah's Witness population: Considerations for preoperative optimization of hemoglobin. *AANA Journal*, *84*(3), 173–178.

Committee on Adolescent Health Care. (2013). Committee Opinion No. 580: Von Willebrand disease in women. *Obstetrics and Gynecology*, *122*(6), 1368–1373.

DeLeo, A., & Geraghty, S. (2016). Thalassaemia in pregnancy: Contemporary care for a timeless disease. *British Journal of Midwifery*, *24*(8), 567–572.

Forman, J., Coyle, F., Levy-Fisch, J., et al. (2013). Screening criteria: The need to deal with new developments and ethical issues in newborn metabolic screening. *Journal of Community Genetics*, *4*(1), 59–67.

Graham, D. K., Craddock, J. A., Quinones, R. R., et al. (2016). Neoplastic disease. In W. W. Hay, M. J. Levin, R. R. Deterding, et al. (Eds.), *Current diagnosis & treatment pediatrics* (23rd ed.). New York, NY: McGraw-Hill.

Gupta, S., Garg, K., & Singh, J. (2015). Assessment of musculoskeletal function and its correlation with radiological joint score in children with hemophilia A. *Indian Journal of Pediatrics*, *82*(12), 1101–1106.

Hartung, H. D., Olson, T. S., & Bessler, M. (2013). Acquired aplastic anemia in children. *Pediatric Clinics of North America*, *60*(6), 1311–1336. http://dx.doi.org/10.1016/j.pcl.2013.08.011

Housten, A. J., Abel, R. A., Dadekian, J., et al. (2015). Youth with sickle cell disease: Genetic and sexual health education needs. *American Journal of Health Behavior*, *39*(6), 856–865. http://dx.doi.org/10.5993/AJHB.39.6.13

Jeevasankar, M., Agarwal, R., Chawla, D., et al. (2008). Polycythemia in the newborn. *Indian Journal of Pediatrics*, *75*(1), 68–72.

Karch, A. M. (2013). *2013 Lippincott's nursing drug guide*. Philadelphia, PA: Lippincott Williams & Wilkins.

Kato, Y., Maeda, M., Aoki, Y., et al. (2014). Pain management during bone marrow aspiration and biopsy in pediatric cancer patients. *Pediatrics International*, *56*, 354–359. http://dx.doi.org/10.1111/ped.12283

Korthof, E. T., Békássy, A. N., & Hussein, A. A. (2013). Management of acquired aplastic anemia in children. *Bone Marrow Transplantation*, *48*(2), 191–195.

Lawrence, R. H., & Shah, G. H. (2014). Athlete's perceptions of National Collegiate Athletic Association–mandated sickle cell trait screening: Insight for academic institutions and college health professionals. *Journal of American College Health*, *62*(5), 343–350. http://dx.doi.org/10.1080/07448481.2014.902840

Merono-Gallut, J., & Cuesta-Barriuso, R. (2016). Design of a myofascial therapy protocol for the treatment of hemophilic arthropathy of the knee and ankle. *Alternative and Complementary Therapies*, *22*(4), 148–152. http://dx.doi.org/10.1089/act.2016.29065

Novelli, E. M., & Gladwin, M. T. (2016). Crises in sickle cell disease. *Chest*, *149*(4), 1082–1093. http://dx.doi.org/10.1016/j.chest.2015.12.016

Obaro, S. K., & Iroh Tam, P. Y. (2016). Preventing infections in sickle cell disease: The unfinished business. *Pediatric Blood & Cancer*, *63*(5), 781–785. http://dx.doi.org/10.1002/pbc.25911

Overbey, D. M., Jones, E. L., & Robinson, T. N. (2014). How hemostatic agents interact with the coagulation cascade. *AORN Journal*, *100*(2), 148–159. http://dx.doi.org/10.1016/j.aorn.2013.12.012

Petrini, C. (2013). Ethical issues in umbilical cord blood banking: A comparative analysis of documents from national and international institutions. *Transfusion*, *53*(4), 902–910.

Ponnampalam, J., & Thalange, N. (2013). Blood & cancer. In N. Thalange, R. Beach, D. Booth, et al. (Eds.), *Essentials of paediatrics* (2nd ed., pp. 59–78). Philadelphia, PA: Elsevier/Saunders.

Rabel, A, Leitman, S. F., & Miller, J. L. (2016). Ask about ice, then consider iron. *Journal of the American Association of Nurse Practitioners*, *28*(2), 116–120. http://dx.doi.org/10.1002/2327-6924.12268

Sakaguchi, H., Nakanishi, K., & Kojima, S. (2013). Inherited bone marrow failure syndromes in 2012. *International Journal of Hematology, 97*(1), 20–29.

Stredny, C. M., Frosch, O., Singhi, S., et al. (2016). Vitamin B12 deficiency presenting with neurological dysfunction in an adolescent. *Pediatric Neurology, 62,* 66–70. http://dx.doi.org/10.1016/j.pediatrneurol.2016.03.022

Sun, A., Chang, J., Wang, Y., et al. (2016). Do all patients with vitamin B12 deficiency have pernicious anemia? *Journal of Oral Pathology & Medicine, 45,* 23–27. http://dx.doi.org/10.1111/jop.12330

Tudorache, E., Azema, C., Hogan, J., et al. (2015). Even mild cases of paediatric Henoch-Schönlein purpura nephritis show significant long-term proteinuria. *Acta Paediatrica, 104*(8), 843–848. http://dx.doi.org/10.1111/apa.12723

U.S. Department of Health and Human Services. (2010). *Healthy people 2020.* Washington, DC: Author.

Wang, M. (2016). Iron deficiency and other types of anemia in infants and children. *American Family Physician, 93*(4), 270–278.

Zempsky, W. T., Palermo, T. M., Corsi, J. M., et al. (2013). Daily changes in pain, mood and physical function in children hospitalized for sickle cell disease pain. *Pain Research & Management, 18*(1), 33–38.

45

Nursing Care of a Family When a Child Has a Gastrointestinal Disorder

Barry Abraham is a 2-year-old boy with poor growth recently diagnosed with celiac disease. You see him at a birthday party, where he is having a temper tantrum because he wants to eat birthday cake like the other children. His mother gives in and says, "Well, I guess it won't hurt him to eat a piece this one time."

Previous chapters described the growth and development of well children and the nursing care for children with disorders of other systems. This chapter adds information about the dramatic changes, both physical and psychosocial, that can occur when children develop gastrointestinal disorders. Such information builds a base for care and health teaching for children with these disorders.

Does Barry's mother understand her son's disease? What could she have done differently in this situation to help him adhere to a gluten-free diet?

KEY TERMS

beriberi

dehydration

gastroesophageal reflux

inguinal hernia

insensible loss

intussusception

keratomalacia

kwashiorkor

liver transplantation

McBurney's point

Meckel's diverticulum

necrotizing enterocolitis

nutritional marasmus

overhydration

pellagra

rickets

scurvy

steatorrhea

volvulus

xerophthalmia

OBJECTIVES

After mastering the contents of this chapter, you should be able to:

1. Describe common gastrointestinal disorders seen in children.

2. Identify 2020 National Health Goals related to gastrointestinal disorders in children that nurses can help the nation achieve.

3. Assess a child with a gastrointestinal disorder.

4. Formulate nursing diagnoses for a child with a gastrointestinal disorder.

5. Identify expected outcomes for a child with a gastrointestinal disorder as well as how to manage seamless transitions across differing healthcare settings.

6. Using the nursing process, plan nursing care that includes the six competencies of Quality & Safety Education for Nurses (QSEN): Patient-Centered Care, Teamwork & Collaboration, Evidence-Based Practice (EBP), Quality Improvement (QI), Safety, and Informatics.

7. Implement nursing care for a child with a gastrointestinal disorder, such as preparing the child for surgery.

8. Evaluate expected outcomes for achievement and effectiveness of care.

9. Integrate knowledge of gastrointestinal disorders in children with the interplay of nursing process, the six competencies of QSEN, and Family Nursing to promote quality maternal and child health nursing care.

Because the gastrointestinal (GI) system is so long and so diverse, a multitude of possible disorders can occur along the tract, including both congenital disorders and acquired illnesses. Also, because the GI system is responsible for taking in and processing nutrients for all parts of the body, any problem with the system can quickly affect other body systems and, if not adequately treated, can affect overall health, growth, and development.

Because it can be difficult to appreciate the seriousness of a GI illness, parents often are surprised to learn that what they thought was a simple "stomach flu" has caused a serious electrolyte imbalance and possibly a life-threatening state for their child. Some GI disorders require both parents and the child to learn new nutritional patterns. As children grow older, counseling to help them maintain self-esteem and learn nutritional requirements so they can become independent is vital. Food poisoning and hepatitis are examples of GI illnesses that are so pervasive that 2020 National Health Goals have been set to limit their incidence (Box 45.1).

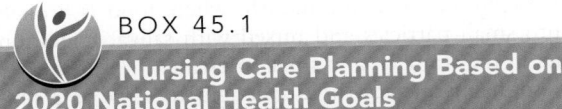

BOX 45.1

Nursing Care Planning Based on 2020 National Health Goals

Nutrition deficiencies, unsafe food preparation, and hepatitis are three areas that could be reduced in incidence if people knew more about them and took active interventions to reduce their occurrence or spread. The 2020 National Health Goals addressing these include:

- Increase the contribution of fruits and vegetables to the diets of the population aged 2 years from 0.5 cup of fruits per 1,000 calories to 0.9 cup per 1,000 calories.
- Achieve and maintain effective vaccination coverage levels for universally recommended vaccines among young children and older (three doses of hepatitis B vaccine and two doses of hepatitis A vaccine by 19 to 35 months of age).
- Reduce infections caused by key pathogens transmitted commonly through food (including *Escherichia coli* [from 200 to 180 cases per year], *Listeria* [from 0.3 to 0.2 cases per 100,000 population per year], and *Salmonella* [from 15.2 to 11.4 cases per 100,000 population per year]).
- Increase the proportion of consumers who follow key food safety practices of "Chill: refrigerate promptly" from 88.1% to 91.1% (U.S. Department of Health and Human Services, 2010; see www.healthypeople.gov).

Nurses can help the nation achieve these goals by counseling parents about safe food preparation and the need for children to ingest adequate fiber from fruit and vegetables for sound bowel function, by serving as consultants to day care providers to reduce the spread of stool contamination and by actively administering hepatitis A and B vaccines to infants and adolescents to eradicate these forms of the illness in another generation.

Nursing Process Overview

FOR A CHILD WITH A GASTROINTESTINAL DISORDER

ASSESSMENT

Children with GI disorders quickly need to be assessed for signs of fluid loss, such as poor skin turgor, dry mucous membranes, or lack of tearing. When talking to parents about a child's symptoms, ask exactly what they mean when they say "spitting up" or "a little vomiting" to be certain you're talking about the same amount. Also, ask how many times a child has voided or how many diapers have been wet in the past 24 hours and whether this is less than usual. Compare the child's current weight with past weight measurements, if available. Unless the child is an adolescent who has been actively dieting, there is rarely a normal reason for weight loss in children.

Most children with diarrhea have self-limited viral illness and can be treated at home. Children with severe diarrhea, especially small children, need to be seen by a healthcare provider because fluid and electrolyte changes occur rapidly in children because of the greater percentage of fluid held extracellularly rather than intracellularly increasing the risk of dehydration.

For many children, a GI tract disorder is largely diagnosed by presenting symptoms such as those just described. In other instances, X-ray studies with a contrast medium (barium) or an endoscopic examination may be needed to confirm the presence of an anomaly. Ultrasound or magnetic resonance imaging (MRI) also may be helpful. Another important assessment area is laboratory testing for electrolyte balance through serum analysis or fluid concentration through urinalysis.

NURSING DIAGNOSIS

Nursing diagnoses relevant to children with GI disorders invariably center on imbalanced nutrition because most GI diseases alter the kind and amount of nutrients ingested or absorbed into the body in some way. In addition, because feeding is one of the primary ways mothers bond with their newborns, and the process of eating and the types of food eaten are integral components of family life and culture, any disruption caused by an illness can place a strain on the entire family. Examples of nursing diagnoses include:

- Impaired parenting related to interference with establishing the parent–infant bond
- Interrupted family processes related to a chronic illness in child
- Risk for deficient fluid volume related to chronic diarrhea
- Imbalanced nutrition, less than body requirements, related to malabsorption of necessary nutrients
- Situational low self-esteem related to feelings of being different resulting from special dietary restrictions

OUTCOME IDENTIFICATION AND PLANNING

Be certain when helping plan a new nutritional pattern for a child that you include the person who actually prepares or supervises the child's nutrition. In many instances, some of the foods that a child eats are prepared by a babysitter, day care center staff, the child's other parent, or a grandparent. Many children eat breakfast and lunch at school cafeterias. That means it may be necessary to contact school staff to ask them to make meal exceptions for a child or to supervise a choice of foods (or to see that a child eats only the packaged lunch brought to school, not extra items the child trades for with friends).

Some parents are unfamiliar with basic food categories and the importance of providing food from the MyPlate nutrition guidelines (www.ChooseMyPlate.gov). When a special diet is requested, parents may have little understanding of which foods have high or low fiber content, or which foods are "bland" or "clear." Many parents have difficulty keeping children restricted to nothing by mouth (NPO) for tests or to rest the GI tract because they know dehydration happens quickly in infants (which is true). They need support to follow the necessary restrictions when this action is so opposed to basic parenting, such as giving food.

If feedings will be given by nasogastric or gastrostomy tube, parents need enough practice to be proficient with the equipment and the technique before they are given the responsibility of doing it alone at home. If a child is going to gag or become distressed when a new oral or nasal tube is passed, parents need to have this happen where there are calm, supportive people nearby, not when they are by themselves at home.

Agencies that might be helpful for referral to parents are the Celiac Disease Foundation (www.celiac.org), the Crohn's & Colitis Foundation (www.crohncolitisfoundation.org), the International Foundation for Functional Gastrointestinal Disorders (www.iffgd.org), and the North American Society for Pediatric Gastroenterology, Hepatology and Nutrition (www.naspghan.org).

IMPLEMENTATION

Never underestimate the difficulty family members may experience adapting to alternative nutrition methods such as total parenteral nutrition, enteric or gastrostomy feedings, or caring for a child with a colostomy. Parents need a great deal of support to adapt their busy life to these alternative methods of feeding or care.

GI disorders that occur at birth are discussed in Chapter 27. Insertion of a nasogastric tube, enteral and parenteral nutrition, and administration of an enema are discussed in Chapter 37. Be certain to give clear, simple explanations and praise both parents and child after they demonstrate these procedures. Children can easily interpret enemas as punishment because of the extreme intrusiveness. Provide therapeutic play before and after these procedures to reduce children's anxiety.

OUTCOME EVALUATION

Recording children's height and weight is a primary method to evaluate nutritional outcomes. Even if a diet is limited in a special way, if it is adequate, children should gain weight and maintain growth.

Because children will ultimately be responsible for their own nutrition, expected outcomes should include making certain children gradually learn more about their specific nutritional measures so they can become increasingly responsible for their own intake. Often, only when they are at this stage can their parents feel secure enough to let them stay overnight with a friend, visit a relative in a distant city, or go to summer camp—activities that become important to children as they reach school age.

Children who require special nutritional plans need to be evaluated for self-esteem at periodic health visits. Do children think of themselves as inferior to or different from others because of food restrictions? What kind of positive experiences can be offered to such children, or what can parents do to provide children with experiences that would improve self-esteem?

Some examples of expected outcomes include:
- Child lists examples of gluten-free foods to select for lunch from the school cafeteria menu.
- Parent states steps she will take to seek medical care if her child has a second episode of severe diarrhea.
- Family members state they have adjusted to care of their child with liver disease.

Anatomy and Physiology of the Gastrointestinal System

Digestion occurs the same in children and infants as it does in adults beginning with the mouth, where food is broken down into small particles and mixed with saliva. Digestion continues in the stomach and small intestine.

The esophagus pierces the diaphragm to serve as a passageway to the stomach (Fig. 45.1). At the junction of the esophagus and the stomach is the gastroesophageal (cardiac) sphincter. A sphincter is a section of circular muscle. In newborns, this sphincter is immature and allows fluid to regurgitate into the esophagus (gastroesophageal reflux). At the distal end of the stomach is the pyloric sphincter. In some infants, this muscular channel becomes narrowed (stenosed), preventing food from flowing out of the stomach freely (pyloric stenosis). Originally, it was believed that the stomach was sterile because the action of hydrochloric acid could easily kill invading organisms and limit infections. However, since the discovery that a bacterium, *Helicobacter pylori*, is the cause of peptic ulcer disease, it is now obvious that organisms can and do survive in the stomach. The small intestine is divided into three sections: the duodenum, the jejunum, and the ileum. The large intestine is divided into the cecum, the ascending colon, the transverse colon, the descending colon, the sigmoid colon, and the rectum. The appendix, which frequently becomes diseased in children, is attached to the cecum.

Diagnostic and Therapeutic Techniques

Several typical procedures, such as a endoscopy, small intestine wireless enteroscopy (capsule endoscopy), colonoscopy, and radiology studies, are used in the diagnosis and therapy of GI disorders. Children need good preparation for all of these procedures because they are all potentially frightening (Hardee, 2012). If children receive conscious sedation or anesthesia for a procedure, they need preparation for this as well as for the actual procedure. They should receive a clear and simple explanation of what will occur and be reassured that the parent can remain with them until they fall asleep. Involvement of child life specialists can be helpful for anxious children (Ortiz, O'Connor, Carey, et al., 2017).

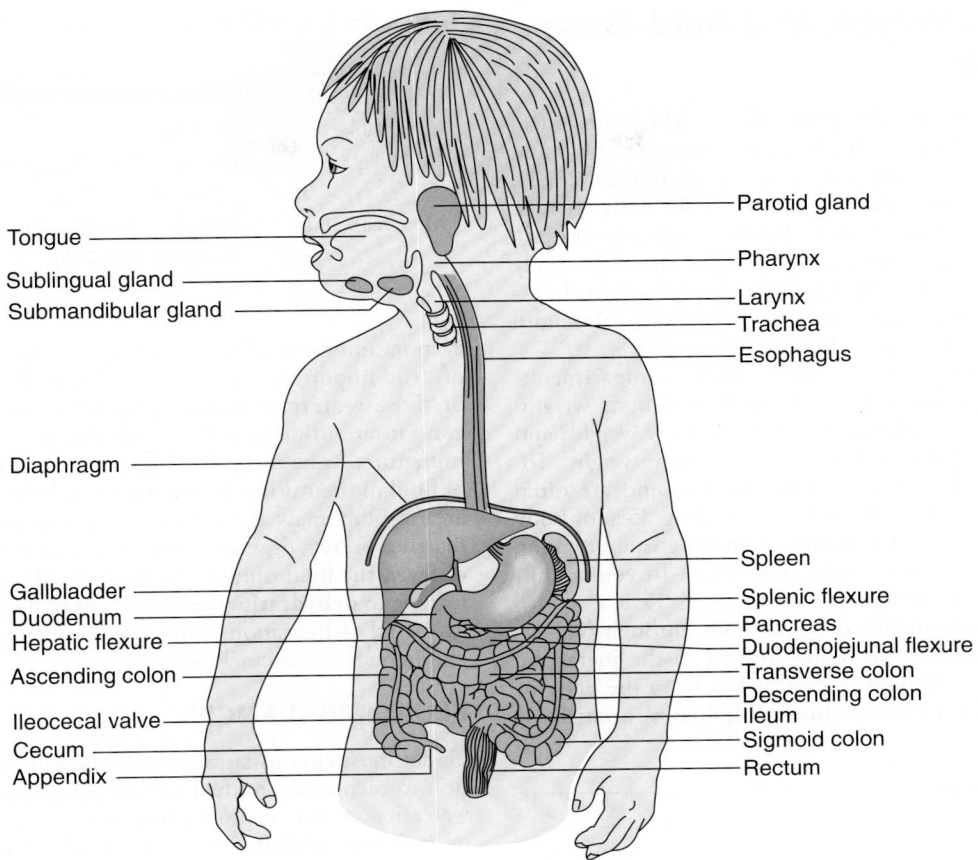

Figure 45.1   The gastrointestinal tract.

Therapy may include alternative methods of feeding such as enteral (nasogastric or gastrostomy tube feedings) or nutrition sources such as total parenteral nutrition and intravenous (IV) therapy to rest the GI tract. A colostomy or ileostomy may be created to further rest the GI tract. Because these are used for other disorders as well, these procedures, their meaning, their impact on children, and nursing responsibilities are discussed in Chapters 37 and 38.

Health Promotion and Risk Management

Health promotion related to GI disorders focuses on a wide area because the causes of these disorders cover a wide range. Some disorders, such as appendicitis, cannot be prevented because they occur from unpredictable causes. Other disorders, such as celiac disease (sensitivity or abnormal immunologic response to gluten), involve genetic aspects that cannot be changed. Still others, such as Crohn disease and ulcerative colitis, are associated with an autoimmune response. Other conditions, such as vomiting and diarrhea, are often caused by foods that were refrigerated improperly or are spread through improper hand washing and so can be prevented. Hepatitis can be prevented through good hand washing (for hepatitis A) and immunization (for both hepatitis A and B). Vitamin and protein deficiency disorders can be prevented by educating parents about the importance of a consistently healthy diet. A vaccine to prevent rotavirus infections (taken by mouth so it

is painless) is recommended for infants (Centers for Disease Control and Prevention [CDC], 2016a).

Because any interference in nutrition pervades many aspects of children's lives, families often need help with planning care. Help families plan the necessary adaptations to their lifestyle to prevent the disease from interfering with family functioning (e.g., Will day care center personnel do gastrostomy feedings? Will a nursery school accept a child with a colostomy? Can a child select a gluten-free diet at the school cafeteria?). All families should be encouraged to eat at least one meal a day together so they can have time to share experiences and "touch base" with each other. For the family with a child who has a feeding problem that requires gastrostomy feeding or total parenteral nutrition, this can be difficult. Urge such families to bring the child to the table for a social time even if the child cannot eat with the family. If watching family members eat while the child cannot eat is too difficult, urge the family to provide a "together" time in some other way so the child does not miss out on this valuable family activity.

Some GI disorders in children, such as esophagitis due to allergic disease or acid reflux, are diagnosed late because parents think the child's refusal to eat is just the sign of being a "picky eater" or a manifestation of 2-year-old autonomy. Educating parents about normal nutrition and how to distinguish things such as vomiting from illness from normal "spitting up," or severe diarrhea from a simple GI upset, helps parents bring their children for care at the earliest possible time. Early intervention prevents the child from becoming dehydrated and seriously ill.

Fluid, Electrolyte, and Acid–Base Imbalances

Because the GI system is the main route by which substances are taken into the body, it can be a major source of fluid and electrolyte loss if vomiting or diarrhea occurs (Smith, 2011). Retaining fluid is of greater importance in the body chemistry of infants than that of adults because fluid constitutes a greater fraction of the infant's total weight. In adults, body water accounts for approximately 60% of total weight. In infants, it accounts for as much as 75% to 80% of total weight; in children, it averages approximately 65% to 70%.

Fluid is distributed in three body compartments: (a) intracellular (within cells), 35% to 40% of body weight; (b) interstitial (surrounding cells), 20% of body weight; and (c) intravascular (blood plasma), 5% of body weight. Together, the interstitial and the intravascular fluid are often referred to as *extracellular fluid* (ECF), totaling 25% of body weight. In infants, the ECF portion is much greater, totaling up to 45% of total body weight (Fig. 45.2). In young children, this amount is 30%; in adolescents, it is 25%.

Fluid is normally obtained by the body through oral ingestion of fluid and by the water formed in the metabolic breakdown of food. Primarily, fluid is lost from the body in urine and feces. Minor losses (**insensible losses**) occur from

TABLE 45.1 A METHOD TO CALCULATE FLUID REQUIREMENT

Body Weight	Fluid Requirement per 24 Hours
Up to 10 kg	100 ml/kg
11–20 kg	1,000 ml + 50 ml/kg for each additional kilogram over 10 kg
More than 20 kg	1,500 ml + 20 ml/kg for each additional kilogram over 20 kg

evaporation from skin and lungs and from saliva, which is of little importance except in children with tracheostomies or those requiring nasopharyngeal suction. Infants do not concentrate urine as well as adults because their kidneys are immature. As a result, they have a proportionally greater loss of fluid in their urine. In infants, the relatively greater surface area to body mass also causes a greater insensible loss. When diarrhea occurs, or when a child becomes diaphoretic because of fever, the fluid output can be markedly increased, quickly leading to **dehydration** (excessive loss of fluid) (Porth, 2011). To avoid dehydration, fluid requirements for infants and children are shown in Table 45.1.

FLUID IMBALANCES

Under most circumstances, water and salt are lost in proportion to each other, termed *isotonic dehydration*. Occasionally, water is lost out of proportion to salt, and water depletion or *hypertonic dehydration* occurs. If electrolytes are lost out of proportion to water, this is termed *hypotonic dehydration*. Each of these abnormal states produces specific symptoms.

Isotonic Dehydration

Isotonic dehydration occurs when a child's body loses more water than it absorbs (as with diarrhea) or absorbs less fluid than it excretes (as with nausea and vomiting). The main result of isotonic dehydration is a decrease in the volume of blood serum. Typical signs and symptoms of isotonic dehydration are summarized in Table 45.2.

What If . . . 45.1
Barry's mother tells the nurse her primary care provider has told her to "force fluids" for Barry whenever he has diarrhea. She asks how much she should force the child to drink. How would the nurse best answer her?

= Adult

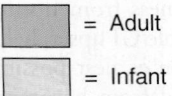 = Infant

Figure 45.2 The distribution of fluid in body compartments.

TABLE 45.2 SIGNS AND SYMPTOMS OF DEHYDRATION

	Isotonic	Hypotonic	Hypertonic
Thirst	Mild	Moderate	Extreme
Skin turgor	Poor	Very poor	Moderate
Skin consistency	Dry	Clammy	Moderate
Skin temperature	Cool	Cool	Warm
Urine output	Decreased	Decreased	Decreased
Activity	Irritable	Lethargic	Very lethargic
Serum sodium level	Normal	Reduced	Increased

Hypertonic Dehydration

When water is lost in a greater proportion than electrolytes, hypertonic dehydration occurs. This might occur in a child with nausea (thus preventing fluid intake) and fever (which increases fluid loss through perspiration); profuse diarrhea, where there is a greater loss of fluid than salt; or renal disease associated with polyuria such as nephrosis with diuresis. Electrolytes such as sodium, chloride, and bicarbonate concentrate in the blood. The red blood cell count and hematocrit will be elevated because the blood is more concentrated than usual. Additional signs and symptoms are summarized in Table 45.2.

Hypotonic Dehydration

With hypotonic dehydration, there is a disproportionately high loss of electrolytes in proportion to fluid loss. The plasma concentration of sodium and chloride are low. This could result from excessive loss of electrolytes by vomiting, from an increased loss of salt from diuresis, or from diseases such as adrenocortical insufficiency or diabetic acidosis. In order to achieve an electrolyte balance, the kidneys begin to excrete more fluid to bring the proportion of electrolytes and fluid back in balance, leading to a secondary extracellular dehydration (see Table 45.2).

Overhydration

Overhydration, or excessive body fluid intake, can be as serious as dehydration. It generally occurs in children who are receiving IV fluid and can lead to cardiovascular and cardiac failure.

When large quantities of salt-poor fluid (hypotonic solutions) such as tap water are ingested or are given by enema, the body transfers water from the extracellular space into the intracellular space to restore normal osmotic relationships. This transfer results in intracellular edema manifested by a headache, nausea, vomiting, dimness and blurring of vision, cramps, muscle twitching, and seizures. A situation in which intracellular edema may occur is when tap water enemas are given to a child with aganglionic disease of the intestine.

ACID–BASE IMBALANCE

When vomiting or diarrhea occurs, the GI system often is involved with two severe acid–base imbalances: metabolic acidosis and metabolic alkalosis. Whether body serum is becoming acidotic is determined by analyzing a sample of arterial blood for blood gases. The pH of blood is normally slightly alkaline, ranging from 7.35 to 7.45. The amount of dissolved carbon dioxide in arterial blood (P_{CO_2}) is normally 35 to 45 mmHg. The level of bicarbonate (HCO_3) in arterial blood is normally 22 to 26 mEq/L.

Metabolic Acidosis

Metabolic acidosis results from diarrhea because a great deal of sodium is lost with stool. This excessive loss of Na^+ causes the body to conserve H^+ ions in an attempt to keep the total number of positive and negative ions in serum balanced. With metabolic acidosis, an arterial blood gas analysis will reveal a decreased pH (under 7.35) and a low HCO_3 value (near or below 22 mEq/L). The lower the HCO_3 value is, the more Na^+ ions that have presumably been lost or the more extensive the diarrhea has been. The child breathes rapidly (hyperpnea) to "blow off" CO_2 to prevent it from combining with H_2O and reforming HCO_3. Urine becomes more acidic as ammonia formation in the urine is increased.

Metabolic Alkalosis

With vomiting, a great deal of hydrochloric acid is lost. When Cl^- ions are lost this way, the body has to decrease the number of H^+ ions present so the number of positive and negative charges remains balanced. This causes the child to become alkalotic because the number of H^+ ions becomes proportionately lower than the number of OH^- ions present. The lungs attempt to conserve CO_2 and water by slowing respirations (hypopnea). The excessive CO_2 retained by this maneuver dissolves in the blood as carbonic acid and then is converted into excessive H^+ and HCO_3^-. With metabolic alkalosis, therefore, the serum HCO_3 will invariably be high. The higher the value, presumably the more Cl^- ions have been lost or the more extensive the vomiting has been. The child will breathe slowly and shallowly; pH will be elevated (near or above 7.45), and HCO_3 level will be near or above 28 mEq/L.

When alkalosis occurs from vomiting, a secondary electrolyte problem often occurs. As the kidneys begin to help conserve H^+ ions, K^+ ions are exchanged for H^+ ions—that is, K^+ ions are excreted in order to retain H^+ ions. As a result of this loss of K^+ into the urine, low K^+ levels (hypokalemia) invariably accompany metabolic alkalosis.

QSEN Checkpoint Question 45.1

INFORMATICS

Barry has frequent bouts of vomiting. If the nurse is caring for Barry in a hospital setting after repeated bouts of vomiting, the nurse would expect the diagnostic testing to reveal which health problem?
   a. Respiratory acidosis
   b. Fluid volume excess
   c. Metabolic alkalosis
   d. Hyperchlorosis

Look in Appendix A for the best answer and rationale.

Common Gastrointestinal Symptoms of Illness in Children

Vomiting and diarrhea in children commonly occur as symptoms of a GI tract disease as well as symptoms of disease in other body systems (Box 45.2). Pneumonia or otitis media, for example, may present first with vomiting or diarrhea. A danger of this is that either can lead to a disturbance in hydration, electrolyte, or acid–base balance. In many infants, vomiting and diarrhea can be more threatening to the child than the primary disease.

VOMITING

Most children with vomiting are suffering from a mild gastroenteritis (infection) due to a viral or bacterial organism, but other causes of vomiting should be considered, such as obstruction, increased intracranial pressure, and metabolic disease. The adolescent who is pregnant may mistake the

BOX 45.2

Nursing Care Planning Using Assessment

ASSESSING A CHILD WITH ALTERED GASTROINTESTINAL FUNCTION

History

Chief concern: Vomiting, diarrhea, constipation, abdominal pain, abdominal distention, weight below normal standard, lethargy, paleness.

Past medical history: History of past vomiting or diarrhea or abdominal pain; hydramnios in pregnancy.

Family history: Relatives have a similar disorder; high stress level because of home or school environment.

Physical examination

Signs of dehydration (dry mucous membranes)

Caries, malocclusion, inflamed gumline (periodontal disease)

Enlarged liver (cirrhosis, hepatitis)

Visible peristalsis (pyloric stenosis)

Increased bowel sounds (diarrhea)

Tender abdomen (appendicitis)

Mass at umbilicus or by inguinal ring (hernia)

Distended veins from pressure in portal circulation (liver disease)

Hair: Brittle; loss of pigment (decreased protein intake)

Jaundice (liver involvement)

Lethargy and paleness (anemia)

Displaced heart sounds (diaphragmatic hernia)

Edema (kwashiorkor)

Distended abdomen (Hirschsprung disease)

Weight below 10th percentile

---

normal nausea and vomiting of pregnancy for an illness. Some children develop persistent or cyclic vomiting (Lee, Abbott, Mahlangu, et al., 2012).

Assessment

In describing symptoms of vomiting, be certain to differentiate between the various terms that are used (Table 45.3). It is important that vomiting be thoroughly described this way because different conditions are marked by different forms of vomiting, and a correct description of the child's actions can aid greatly in a diagnosis.

Therapeutic Management

The treatment for vomiting related to gastroenteritis is to give small amounts of fluid frequently as soon as tolerated to prevent dehydration and electrolyte imbalance. Clear liquids such as ginger ale, tea, and sports drinks can be used to maintain hydration, but they are not suitable for rehydration. Oral rehydration solutions (ORS) such as Pedialyte should be used for infants and younger children as well as older children with dehydration. Children with intractable vomiting or severe dehydration will require IV fluids.

Nursing Diagnoses and Related Interventions

Nursing Diagnosis: Risk for deficient fluid volume related to vomiting

Outcome Evaluation: Skin turgor remains good; specific gravity of urine is 1.003 to 1.030, urine output is more than 1 ml/kg/hour; episodes of vomiting decrease in frequency and amount.

For the older child, start by offering a few ice chips and then water in small amounts—approximately 1 tablespoon every 15 minutes, four times, and then 2 tablespoons every half hour, four times. Popsicles can be substituted for water. If this is retained, children can be given small sips of clear liquids, such as tea, ginger ale, or an ORS. Parents are not advised to make ORS solutions at home as the recipe needs to be exact (Barros, Victoria, Forsberg, et al., 1991).

Children may become hungry and want whole glasses of fluid, but keeping the quantity to small sips prevents vomiting. Once the child is able to retain sips of clear liquids, the child can be offered portions of broth, clear soup, and skim milk in addition to clear liquids. Dry crackers or toast will help assuage hunger. By the second day, children can take a soft diet; by the third day, they should be back to their regular diet. Young infants with vomiting should be evaluated by a healthcare professional. Maintain hydration by giving 5 to 10 ml ORS every 5 to 10 minutes and gradually increase as tolerated. Once tolerating the ORS, the infant should return to breastfeeding or bottle feeding. Infants should be monitored closely for signs of dehydration.

TABLE 45.3 DIFFERENTIATION BETWEEN REGURGITATION AND VOMITING

Characteristic	Regurgitation	Vomiting
Timing	Occurs with feeding	Timing unrelated to feeding
Forcefulness	Runs out of mouth with *little force*	Forceful: often projected 1 ft away from the infant; *projectile vomiting*: projected as much as 4 ft (most often associated with pyloric stenosis)
Description	Smells barely sour; only slightly curdled	Extremely sour smelling and curdled, yellow, green, clear or watery, or black or blood tinged
Distress	Nonpainful; no appearance of distress; may even smile as if sensation is enjoyable	Possible crying just before vomiting as if abdominal pain is present and after vomiting as if the force of action is frightening
Duration	Occurs once per feeding	Continuing until stomach is empty; followed by dry retching
Amount	1–2 teaspoons	Full stomach contents

A decrease in wet diapers to one within a 6-hour period, dry mouth, and increased thirst are signs of mild dehydration. If vomiting is prolonged, infants may need IV therapy to restore hydration (Moritz & Ayus, 2011).

Assure parents that if children receive a small amount of fluid and do not vomit it, they will ultimately receive more fluid than if they take a large amount, but because of gastroenteritis, they vomit that amount. Stress that stomach secretions are lost along with vomitus each time, and the preservation of these stomach secretions is equally important. Antiemetic medicine is rarely necessary for children because acute gastroenteritis is a self-limiting condition and vomiting may actually be helpful if it rids the child's body of toxic substances. If vomiting is severe, however, an antiemetic such as promethazine (Phenergan) or ondansetron (Zofran) may be prescribed. Always ask parents if they have used an herbal remedy to stop vomiting to be certain that any medication prescribed will be safe with the alternative treatment (Box 45.3).

DIARRHEA

Diarrhea that is acute is usually associated with infection; chronic diarrhea is more likely related to a malabsorptive or inflammatory cause. *Giardia lamblia* is a frequent protozoan infection that causes diarrhea. The most common viral pathogens that invade the GI tract include rotaviruses and adenoviruses. The most common bacterial pathogens include *Campylobacter jejuni*, *Salmonella*, *Clostridium difficile*, and *Escherichia coli* (Porth, 2011). Both viral and bacterial infections are easily spread in common diaper changing areas in day care centers or in public restrooms (Rimon & Freedman, 2010).

Diarrhea in infants is always serious because infants have such a small ECF reserve that sudden losses of water quickly exhaust the supply. Breastfeeding may actively prevent diarrhea by providing more antibodies and possibly an intestinal environment less friendly to invading organisms.

Mild Diarrhea

Assessment

Normal and diarrheal stool characteristics are compared in Table 45.4. Children usually are anorectic, irritable, and appear unwell; a fever of 101° to 102°F (38.4° to 39.0°C) may be present. The episodes of diarrhea consist of 2 to 10 loose, watery bowel movements per day.

The mucous membrane of the mouth appears dry and the skin feels warm, although skin turgor will not yet be decreased. The pulse may be rapid and out of proportion to the low-grade fever. Urine output is usually normal.

Therapeutic Management

At this stage, diarrhea is not yet serious, and children can be cared for at home. Parents can begin to offer an ORS such as Pedialyte in small amounts on a regimen similar to that for vomiting (Smith, 2011). For breastfed infants, breastfeeding should continue. Probiotics (dietary supplements containing potentially beneficial bacteria or yeasts) to change the bacterial flora of the intestine may be administered (Guarino, Ashkenazi, Gendrel, et al., 2014). Children also may need measures to reduce their elevated temperature.

Caution parents to contact their healthcare provider prior to initiating over-the-counter drugs such as loperamide (Imodium) or bismuth subsalicylate (Kaopectate) to halt diarrhea because, as a rule, toxic levels of these can occur quickly (Karch, 2013). Caution parents to wash their hands after changing diapers to prevent the spread of infection to themselves and to notify their healthcare provider if fever, pain, or diarrhea worsens.

Infants may develop a temporary lactase deficiency after diarrhea that leads to lactose intolerance. Lactase is the enzyme that digests lactose, the sugar in milk. Lactase deficiency results in gas and diarrhea. It may appear as though the initial diarrheal illness is persisting when this occurs. It may be necessary to try a using a lactose-free formula or to try having the mother withdraw dairy products from her own diet if the infant is breastfed.

BOX 45.3

Nursing Care Planning to Respect Cultural Diversity

The incidence of gastrointestinal (GI) illnesses varies among communities. Vomiting and diarrhea, for example, tend to occur because of food poisoning in communities where refrigeration is less than optimal and from eating raw meat or unprocessed cheese. Celiac disease occurs most frequently in children of Northern European ancestry. Because constipation, vomiting, and diarrhea are so common, every culture has home remedies for these symptoms: cascara for constipation; psyllium for diarrhea; and ginger, peppermint, licorice, or chamomile tea for nausea or vomiting. To be certain that a child seen in a healthcare facility does not receive two forms of the same drug (one prescribed and one given in an herb form by a parent), always ask what alternative therapies or home remedies have been given and document these on the child's plan of care.

TABLE 45.4 DIFFERENTIATION BETWEEN NORMAL STOOL AND DIARRHEAL STOOL IN AN INFANT

Characteristic	Infant Normal Stool	Diarrheal Stool
Frequency	One to three daily	Unlimited number
Color	Yellow	Green
Effort of expulsion	Some pushing effort	Effortless; may be explosive
pH	More than 7.0 (alkaline)	Less than 7.0 (acidic)
Odor	Odorless	Sweet or foul smelling
Occult blood	Negative	Positive; blood may be overt
Reducing substances	Negative	Positive

Severe Diarrhea

Severe diarrhea may result in dehydration and the need for hospitalization.

Assessment

Infants with severe diarrhea appear obviously ill. Rectal temperature is often as high as 103° to 104°F (39.5° to 40.0°C). Both pulse and respirations are weak and rapid, and the skin is pale and cool. Infants may be apprehensive, listless, and lethargic. Obvious signs of dehydration such as a depressed fontanelle, sunken eyes, and poor skin turgor are usually present. The episodes of diarrhea usually consist of a movement of liquid green stool perhaps mixed with mucus and blood, passed with explosive force every few minutes. Urine output will be scanty and concentrated. Laboratory findings will show elevated hematocrit, hemoglobin, and serum protein levels because of the dehydration. Electrolyte determinations will indicate a metabolic acidosis (Huether, 2012).

It is difficult to measure the amount of fluid a child has lost with diarrhea, but an estimate can be derived from the loss in body weight, if known. For example, if a child weighed 10.4 kg yesterday at a health maintenance visit and today weighs 8.9 kg, the child has lost more than 10% of body weight. A loss of 2.5% to 5% of body weight suggests mild dehydration. Severe diarrhea quickly causes a 5% to 15% loss of body weight, which suggests severe dehydration. Any infant who has lost 10% or more of body weight requires immediate treatment.

Therapeutic Management

Treatment focuses on regulating electrolyte and fluid balance by initiating oral or IV rehydration therapy and on discovering the organism responsible for the diarrhea.

All children with severe diarrhea or diarrhea that persists longer than 24 hours should have a stool culture taken to determine if infection is causing the diarrhea, and if appropriate, a definite antibiotic therapy can be prescribed. Because a side effect of many antibiotics is diarrhea, antibiotics should not routinely be used to treat diarrhea without an identifiable bacterial cause. Stool cultures may be taken from the rectum or from stool in a diaper or a bedpan.

Blood serum specimens need to be drawn for a hemoglobin level (an estimation of hydration as well as anemia); white blood cell and differential counts (to attempt to establish whether infection is present); and determinations of PCO_2, Cl^-, Na^+, K^+, and pH (to establish electrolyte needs). If a child can drink, the most effective way to replace fluid is by offering oral rehydration therapy. For a child who will not drink, an IV solution such as normal saline or 5% glucose in normal saline is begun to provide replacement of fluid, sodium, and calories.

Although infants usually have a potassium depletion, potassium is not given until it is established that the child is not in renal failure because giving a potassium IV when the body has no outlet for excessive potassium can lead to excessively high potassium levels and heart block. *Before this initial IV fluid is changed to a potassium solution, therefore, be certain the infant or child has voided—proof that the kidneys are functioning.*

Enough fluid must be given not only to replace the deficit that has occurred but also to replace the continuing loss until the diarrhea improves. If an infant has lost less than 5% of total body weight, his or her fluid deficit is approximately 50 ml/kg of body weight. If an infant has lost 10% of body weight, he or she needs approximately 100 ml/kg of body weight to replace the fluid deficit. If the weight loss suggests a 12% to 15% loss of body fluid, the infant requires 125 ml/kg of body weight to replace the fluid lost. This fluid will be given rapidly in the first 3 to 6 hours, and then it will be slowed to a maintenance rate. Once infants void, a potassium additive can be prescribed to restore serum potassium.

 Nursing Diagnoses and Related Interventions

Nursing Diagnosis: Deficient fluid volume related to loss of fluid through diarrhea

Outcome Evaluation: Skin turgor remains good; specific gravity of urine is 1.003 to 1.030; urine output is more than 1 ml/kg/hour; and bowel movements are formed and fewer than four per day. Stool tests negative for reducing substances and blood pH is 7.41.

Promote Hydration and Comfort. During the time an infant is NPO, wet the infant's lips with a moisturizing cream or jelly such as Vaseline if they appear to be dry. Offer a pacifier to suck if this seems to comfort him or her. (Infants want to suck because they are very thirsty and, if they have intestinal cramping with the diarrhea, they interpret this as hunger.) As the infant's condition improves, oral intake can be increased, changing to a soft then a regular diet.

If the child with severe diarrhea also has a fever, measures to reduce the fever will be necessary (see Chapter 37). Do not obtain rectal temperatures to assess fever because stimulating the anal sphincter could initiate more diarrhea. Change diapers frequently, assess perianal skin for irritation from liquid stools, and keep the skin clean and dry.

Record Fluid Intake and Output. Much of the nursing care of children with diarrhea focuses on careful recording of fluid intake and output. For children with severe dehydration, oral rehydration or IV therapy serves as their lifeline. Be certain to maintain proper functioning of an IV infusion and site if this is used by use of an arm board or soft restraints to prevent catheter dislodgment or interference with the infusion. If soft restraints are used, remember to release them every hour and passively exercise the child's extremities. Be certain parents understand why the IV infusion is important so they will understand the need for the soft restraints.

In children who are not toilet trained, it is important to separate urine from stool so the appearance of the stool can be accurately described and measured. Because current diapers contain a gel that quickly absorbs urine, apply a disposable urine collection bag to the infant so you can be assured the infant is voiding, thus confirming kidney function.

For each stool passed, record its color, consistency, odor, size, and the presence of any blood or mucus. Weigh soiled diapers to reveal the number of grams of stool in the diaper (1 g = 1 ml fluid). Testing the stool for acidity and for reducing substances (e.g., sugars) indicates how quickly the stool has passed through the irritated tract. A stool that is both positive for sugar and with a pH below

7.0 (acid) indicates diarrhea is acute because so little absorption of sugar has occurred (sugar is normally absorbed rapidly from ingested food). Diarrheal stools appear green from lack of time for bile to be modified in the intestine. As diarrhea improves and stool remains in the intestine for a longer period, the stool deepens in color, and the acid and sugar contents fade.

Nursing Diagnosis: Risk for impaired skin integrity related to presence of diarrheal stool on skin

Outcome Evaluation: Skin in diaper area is not erythematous or ulcerated.

Because diarrheal stool is extremely irritating to the skin, change diapers immediately after infants pass any stool. Wash the skin of the diaper area well after each stool, and, if agency policy advises, cover it with a barrier ointment to protect it from further irritation. If the child is older, caution the child to wipe away stool thoroughly.

If infants already have skin excoriation from the number of stools they have had at home, a zinc oxide cream may help soothe the irritated skin. Exposing infants' buttocks to air also is generally helpful in healing irritations. Assure older children that a stool "accident" because of diarrhea is not "shameful" or "babyish" but to be expected because they are so ill.

Nursing Diagnosis: Anxiety related to traumatic experience

Outcome Evaluation: Child interacts with parents in age-appropriate way; can be comforted after painful procedures.

All children with diarrhea are assumed to have an infectious form of gastroenteritis and therefore need contact and standard infection precautions until their condition is ruled otherwise. To counteract the discomfort of diarrhea, children need the security of someone to stay with them. Be sure to take time during initial procedures to touch and soothe children and talk to them; once the initial admission procedures are done, sit by the bed and hold the child or gently stroke the child's head. Encourage parents to give as much care as possible. Children need this support to counteract the strange world into which they have suddenly been plunged.

BACTERIAL INFECTIOUS DISEASES THAT CAUSE DIARRHEA AND VOMITING

A number of common microorganisms are responsible for the majority of diarrheal infections in children. Common methods to prevent contracting an infection from these organisms are shown in Box 45.4.

Salmonellosis

- Causative agent: one of the *Salmonella* bacteria
- Incubation period: 6 to 72 hours for intraluminal type; 7 to 14 days for extraluminal type
- Period of communicability: as long as organisms are being excreted (may be as long as 3 months)
- Mode of transmission: ingestion of contaminated food, especially chicken and raw eggs

 BOX 45.4

Nursing Care Planning to Empower a Family

PREVENTING SALMONELLA- OR LISTERIA-CAUSED GASTROENTERITIS

Q. Barry's mother says to you, "I hear so much about food poisoning. How can I protect my family against that?"

A. Anyone can get food poisoning. However, it can be prevented by using the following measures:

- Wash your hands well before preparing any foods, especially chicken and eggs.
- Remember that chicken may have been contaminated with *Salmonella* at the factory where it was prepared. Wash your hands well after handling raw chicken to prevent the spread of infection to other foods being prepared.
- Clean cutting boards or food preparation surfaces with hot, soapy water and dry thoroughly after use to prevent them from becoming reservoirs of infection. Use plastic cutting boards and avoid wooden cutting boards because they may be more difficult to clean.
- Make a habit of preparing chicken last, after other foods are prepared.
- Cook eggs well (do not use raw eggs in milkshakes; cook soft-boiled or poached eggs for at least 3 minutes).
- Refrigerate chicken and eggs after preparation.
- Wash hands well after playing with or feeding a pet turtle or changing the turtle's water because turtles can also transmit *Salmonella*.
- Wash raw vegetables thoroughly before eating.
- Avoid soft cheeses such as feta, Brie, Camembert, blue-veined, and Mexican queso fresco cheese. Hard cheeses; processed cheeses, including sliced cheese, cream cheese, cheese spreads, and cottage cheese; and yogurt need not be avoided.
- Cook leftover foods or ready-to-eat foods such as hot dogs until steaming hot before eating.
- Avoid foods from delicatessen counters such as prepared salads, meats, and cheeses or heat/reheat these foods until steaming before eating.
- Avoid refrigerated pâtés and other meat spreads or heat and/or reheat these foods before eating; canned or shelf-stable pâté and meat spreads need not be avoided.
- Avoid raw or unpasteurized milk, including goat's milk, or milk products or foods that contain unpasteurized milk or milk products.

Listeriosis

- Causative agent: *Listeria monocytogenes*
- Incubation period: variable, ranging from 1 day to more than 3 weeks
- Mode of transmission: ingestion of unpasteurized milk or cheeses or vegetables grown in contaminated soil. The infection is particularly important to avoid during pregnancy because infections during pregnancy can lead to miscarriage or stillbirth, prematurity, or infection of the newborn.

Shigellosis (Dysentery)

- Causative agent: organisms of the genus *Shigella*
- Incubation period: 1 to 7 days
- Period of communicability: approximately 1 to 4 weeks
- Mode of transmission: contaminated food, water, or milk products

Staphylococcal Food Poisoning

- Causative agent: staphylococcal enterotoxin produced by some strains of *Staphylococcus aureus*
- Incubation period: 1 to 7 hours
- Period of communicability: Carriers may contaminate food as long as they harbor the organism.
- Mode of transmission: ingestion of contaminated food such as poultry, creamed foods (e.g., potato salad), and inadequate cooking

---

QSEN Checkpoint Question 45.2

PATIENT-CENTERED CARE

Barry's mother tells that the nurse she is anxious about the possibility of "food poisoning" and that she particularly wants to prevent *Salmonella* poisoning in her family. Which actions would the nurse suggest?

a. Urge family members to keep their immunizations up to date.
b. Avoid excessive intake of dairy products.
c. Don't cut vegetables on a cutting board used to cut raw chicken.
d. Wash fruits such as strawberries and grapes with soap and water before eating.

Look in Appendix A for the best answer and rationale.

PROTOZOAN OR VIRAL DIARRHEA

Most protozoan or viral diarrhea results in loose, watery stools. The chief therapy for these is ORS. Children who are cultured with *G. lamblia* may be prescribed metronidazole (Flagyl).

Common Disorders of the Stomach and Duodenum

Disorders of the upper GI tract in children tend to involve inadequate function of the gastroesophageal valve or infection.

GASTROESOPHAGEAL REFLUX

Gastroesophageal reflux is the regurgitation of stomach secretions into the esophagus through the lower esophageal (cardiac) sphincter. It is a normal physiologic process that occurs throughout the day in infants, children, and adults.

Gastroesophageal Reflux in Infants

Gastroesophageal reflux in infants occurs due to the immaturity of the lower esophageal sphincter, which allows easy regurgitation of gastric contents into the esophagus. It is very common during infancy, with about 70% of infants affected, and it usually requires no treatment. It usually starts within 1 week after birth and may be associated with a hiatal hernia. The emesis occurs after eating, is effortless, and most often consists of 1 to 2 oz of undigested milk.

Gastroesophageal reflux disease (GERD) may be diagnosed when infants develop complications from reflux such as irritability, failure to thrive, esophagitis, and, in severe cases, aspiration pneumonia, wheezing, and apnea. Children with cerebral palsy or other neurologic involvement are at particular risk (Vandenplas, Rudolf, Di Lorenzo, et al., 2009). Reflux is occasionally due to cow's milk protein intolerance.

Assessment

Diagnosis is informed by patient history, and therefore, diagnostic testing is not necessary for uncomplicated reflux. In patients with GERD, diagnostic workup may include the following:

- Upper GI series to look for anatomical abnormalities such as intestinal malrotation
- pH probe (catheter inserted through the nose into the lower esophagus) to calculate the amount of acidic reflux into the esophagus in a 24-hour period
- Esophageal manometry to assess esophageal motility to ensure there is normal esophageal peristalsis
- Endoscopy to obtain biopsies to assess the degree of esophagitis

Therapeutic Management

Therapeutic management options for gastroesophageal reflux in infants include conservative treatment, medication, and surgery. Conservative treatment has been shown to reduce reflux symptoms by about 60% (Orenstein & McGowan, 2008).

The traditional treatment of GI reflux is to feed infants small frequent feedings of formula thickened with rice cereal (1 tablespoon of cereal per 1 oz of breast milk or formula). The infant should be held in an upright position for 30 minutes after feedings if possible (e.g., on the parent's shoulder). The infant should not be placed in the car seat at home as this puts pressure on the stomach, making emesis more likely. Tight clothing and diapers should be avoided. Cigarette smoke should be avoided as exposure to nicotine worsens reflux. Asking the breastfeeding mother to eliminate dairy from her diet or a trial of a hypoallergenic formula for 2 weeks may be indicated (Orenstein & McGowan, 2008).

Medication is not indicated for uncomplicated reflux, but for infants experiencing irritability and poor feeding due to esophagitis, an H_2-receptor antagonist such as ranitidine (Zantac) or a proton pump inhibitor such as omeprazole (Prilosec) may be prescribed daily to reduce the possibility of the stomach acid contents irritating the esophagus.

In infants, gastroesophageal reflux is usually a self-limiting condition. As the esophageal sphincter matures and the child begins to eat solid food or is maintained in a more upright position, the problem disappears.

If such medical therapy is ineffective, a laparoscopic or surgical fundoplication may be performed. The fundoplication procedure involves wrapping the upper portion of the stomach (fundus) around the lower esophagus to prevent regurgitation of stomach contents. After this procedure, the child will temporarily have a nasogastric tube attached to intermittent low suction. Assess nasogastric tube drainage and any vomitus for coffee-colored drainage after the first 24 hours (it is a normal finding in the first 24 hours), which would indicate bleeding from the surgical site. When infants are first fed after surgery, they may display signs of abdominal discomfort, such as gagging, retching, and distention, because food can no longer reflux into the esophagus as readily as it previously could. As the stomach adjusts, however, symptoms will fade. Before this happens, the distention may be so extreme that it leads to bradycardia and dyspnea. Be alert for the development of these important signs and symptoms.

Gastrointestinal Reflux in Children and Adolescents

GERD affects about 20% of adults; few population-based studies have been done in children, but the incidence is thought to be between 1.8 and 8% (Nelson, Chen, Syniar, et al., 2000). Young children with reflux may present with vomiting. Older children and adolescents will have similar symptoms to adults. Certain groups of children are at higher risk for reflux. These include children with cerebral palsy, Down syndrome, cystic fibrosis, and obesity. Chronic reflux is potentially dangerous because it can lead to erosion of the esophagus with perforation or stricture and is associated with the development of esophageal cancer in later life (Wang & Souza, 2011).

The typical symptoms are heartburn that occurs 30 to 60 minutes after a meal and regurgitation. Diagnosis is based on history and, if symptoms are severe, an endoscopy to reveal the irritated esophagus (esophagitis). The goal of treatment is to provide symptomatic relief and to heal any esophagitis identified. Treatment includes lifestyle changes and medication.

Therapeutic Management

To prevent reflux, the child should avoid lying down until 3 hours after a meal and should sleep at night with their upper body elevated on a foam wedge or extra pillow. They should avoid acidic foods such as tomato products, citrus fruits, or spicy foods. Avoiding foods that delay gastric emptying such as fatty foods, chocolate, or alcohol and eating smaller portions may also be helpful. Generally, losing some weight if overweight, avoiding bending over after meals, and removing tight belts are also recommended steps.

Taking an over-the-counter antacid relieves pain immediately by decreasing the concentration of the stomach acid. H_2-receptor antagonists such as famotidine (Pepcid) or ranitidine (Zantac) are also available over the counter and can be taken before meals to prevent heartburn. Proton pump inhibitors (PPIs) such as omeprazole (Prilosec) (both over-the-counter and prescription) or rabeprazole (AcipHex) (prescription), drugs that halt the release of stomach acids, offer the best long-term relief. PPIs are best taken about 30 minutes before breakfast and are generally prescribed for 8 to 12 weeks, which is usually sufficient to heal the lining of the esophagus.

As with adults, esophageal reflux in adolescents may return. Some adults require surgery in later life to relieve esophageal strictures or to prevent persistent esophagitis, which can lead to cancer if untreated.

Nursing Diagnoses and Related Interventions

Nursing Diagnosis: Risk for imbalanced nutrition, less than body requirements, related to regurgitation of food with infant esophageal reflux

Outcome Evaluation: Skin fold returns to place quickly when turgor is assessed, specific gravity of urine is 1.003 to 1.030; intake is appropriate for age and weight.

Teach parents the importance of monitoring intake, output (urination), and weight. Also, reinforce the need to keep the infant upright after a feeding. Be certain parents understand how much cereal to mix with formula or breast milk. Encourage parents to feed the infant during the short time that the infant remains in the hospital after surgery so that they can regain their confidence as parents.

PYLORIC STENOSIS

The pyloric sphincter is the opening between the lower portion of the stomach and the beginning portion of the intestine (the duodenum). If hypertrophy or hyperplasia of the muscle surrounding the sphincter occurs, it is difficult for the stomach to empty, a condition called *pyloric stenosis* (Fig. 45.3). The incidence is high, approximately 1:150 in males and 1:750 in females. It tends to occur most frequently in first-born White male infants. The exact cause is unknown, but multifactorial inheritance is the likely cause.

Assessment

With this condition, at 4 to 6 weeks of age, infants typically begin to vomit almost immediately after each feeding. The vomiting grows increasingly forceful until it is projectile, possibly projecting as much as 3 to 4 ft (Pandya & Heiss, 2012).

Figure 45.3 Pyloric stenosis. Fluid is unable to pass easily through the stenosed and hypertrophied pyloric valve.

Pyloric stenosis occurs less frequently in breastfed infants than in formula-fed infants. Breastfed infants begin having symptoms at 6 weeks, whereas formula-fed infants typically begin having symptoms at closer to 4 weeks of age because the curd of breast milk is smaller than that of cow's milk, and it passes through a hypertrophied muscle more easily.

Vomitus usually smells sour because it has reached the stomach and has been in contact with digestive enzymes. There will never be bile in the vomitus because the feeding does not reach the duodenum to become mixed with bile. Infants are usually hungry immediately after vomiting because they are not nauseated. Although it is difficult to assess whether nausea is present in infants, signs such as a disinterest in eating, excessive drooling, or chewing on the tongue may suggest this.

Many infants have signs of dehydration such as dry mucous membrane of the mouth, sunken fontanelles, fever, decreased urine output, poor skin turgor, and weight loss from the vomiting when they are first seen. Alkalosis may be present because of the excessive loss of chloride from the loss of stomach fluid, along with accompanying hypochloremia, hypokalemia, and starvation. Hypopnea (slowed respirations) occurs as the body attempts to compensate for the alkalosis. This will cause the HCO_3 content of plasma generally to be above 30 mEq/L (normal levels are 22 to 28 mEq/L). Tetany may occur with alkalosis because the increased HCO_3^- ions may combine with Ca^{2+} ions in trying to affect homeostasis and thereby lowering the level of ionized calcium.

A definitive diagnosis can be made by watching the infant drink. If a pyloric stenosis is present, the sphincter feels round and firm, approximately the size of an olive in the right abdomen. As the infant drinks, gastric peristaltic waves pass from left to right across the abdomen. The olive-size lump becomes more prominent, and the infant vomits with projectile emesis. If the diagnosis is still in doubt, an ultrasound will show a hypertrophied sphincter (Iqbal, Rivard, Mortellaro, et al., 2012). An endoscopy also may be used for diagnosis by directly visualizing the hypertrophied sphincter.

Therapeutic Management

Treatment is surgical or laparoscopic correction (a pyloromyotomy), which is performed before electrolyte imbalance occurs from the vomiting or before hypoglycemia occurs from the lack of food. Before surgery, if electrolyte imbalance, dehydration, and starvation have already occurred, these must be corrected by administration of IV fluid, usually isotonic saline or 5% glucose in saline. Oral feedings are withheld to prevent further electrolyte depletion. An infant who is receiving only IV fluid generally needs a pacifier to meet nonnutritive sucking needs and be comfortable. If tetany is present, verified by a low calcium level on blood analysis, IV calcium also must be administered. The infant usually needs additional potassium, but as a rule, this cannot be administered until it is determined the child's kidneys are functioning (e.g., the child is voiding). Otherwise, the potassium buildup could cause cardiac arrhythmias.

For surgical correction, the muscle of the pylorus is split down to the mucosa, allowing for a larger lumen. Although the procedure sounds simple, it is technically difficult to perform, and there is a high risk of infection following surgery because the abdominal incision is near the diaper area.

The overall prognosis for infants with pyloric stenosis is excellent if the condition is discovered before an electrolyte imbalance occurs.

 Nursing Diagnoses and Related Interventions

Nursing Diagnosis: Risk for deficient fluid volume related to inability to retain food

Outcome Evaluation: Skin turgor remains good; specific gravity of urine is 1.003 to 1.030; vomiting episodes have ceased; weight is within acceptable, age-appropriate parameters.

Preoperative Care. Preoperative management for pyloric stenosis consists of fluid and electrolyte replacement based on laboratory determinations. Carefully note the frequency of urination, the specific gravity of the urine, and the number of stools passed to help assess dehydration and starvation. Parents may be impatient with preoperative management because it may take 24 hours or more to restore a severe fluid imbalance. They ask why their child can't have immediate surgery. Explaining that infants cannot go to surgery with an electrolyte imbalance is helpful so parents know the hours before surgery are as important to the welfare of their child as the operation itself.

Postoperative Care. Infants will return from surgery or laparoscopy with an IV line in place. The postoperative feeding regimen differs from one surgeon to another but usually involves frequent feedings of small amounts of fluid that are gradually increased over time as tolerated. Approximately 4 to 6 hours after surgery, infants are started on a small amount of an oral rehydrating solution by bottle. If no vomiting occurs, the amount is increased or half-strength formula or breastfeeding is begun. Finally, by 24 to 48 hours, infants can take their full formula diet or can be fully breastfed. They are usually discharged from the hospital at the end of 48 hours.

Postoperatively, it is important that infants ingest a small amount of fluid because fluid passing through the sphincter helps to keep adhesions of the sphincter from forming. At the same time, it is important that infants not be given any more than the amount of fluid prescribed at any given time so the surgical repair site is not stretched from an overdistended stomach. As the amount taken orally increases, the IV fluid will be decreased and then discontinued. Infants should be burped well after a feeding so there is no pressure from air in the stomach. Lay them on their right side after feeding so that if vomiting does occur, there is little chance of aspiration, and the flow of fluid through the pyloric valve is aided by gravity. Continue to monitor daily weights to confirm the child is receiving adequate intake. Although postoperative vomiting is commonly experienced, it should be reported immediately because the physiologic cause of the vomiting may be related to delayed gastric emptying, advancing feedings too rapidly, or edema at the operative site, all of which need to be corrected. A few infants develop short-term diarrhea (dumping syndrome) after surgery because of rapid functioning of the pyloric sphincter, but this tends to resolve without additional therapy.

Nursing Diagnosis: Risk for infection at site of surgical incision related to danger of contamination from feces because of proximity of incision to diaper area

Outcome Evaluation: Infant's temperature is not above 98.6°F (37.0°C) tympanic; incision is clean, dry, and intact without erythema or drainage.

The surgical incision for pyloric stenosis may be covered with collodion, a solution similar to clear nail polish, or a similar commercial compound to help keep urine and feces from touching it. Keep diapers folded low to prevent the incision line from being contaminated, and change diapers frequently. If the incision is exposed to feces, wash the collodion thoroughly with soap and water.

Nursing Diagnosis: Risk for impaired parenting related to infant's feeding difficulty and illness

Outcome Evaluation: Parents hold and feed infant; express positive characteristics about infant.

Encourage the parents to "room-in" with their child so they can grow comfortable and confident in caring for the child again. When the child first began vomiting so forcefully, parents may have felt they were doing something wrong and so may have lost confidence in themselves as parents. Explain to them that the vomiting was caused by a physical problem and not by anything they did.

Hospitalization often occurs near the infant's second month, when the child would normally receive diphtheria-tetanus-pertussis, rotavirus, pneumococcal, oral poliomyelitis, and *Haemophilus influenzae* immunizations. If the child is otherwise healthy, ask if they could be administered before discharge so the child's immunization status remains current. This also might serve to remind parents that getting back to normal means regular healthcare visits for vaccines and checkups.

PEPTIC ULCER DISEASE

A *peptic ulcer* is a shallow excavation formed in the mucosal wall of the stomach, the pylorus, or the duodenum. They are rare occurring in only 1% to 2% of children and more frequently in males than females. *Peptic ulcer disease* includes gastritis (irritation of the lining of the stomach or duodenum) and is more commonly seen in childhood.

In infants, ulcers tend to occur in the stomach; in adolescents, they are usually duodenal. Such ulcers occur in a primary form caused by infection with *H. pylori* bacteria and a secondary form that follows severe stress such as burns or chronic ingestion of medications such as aspirin, nonsteroidal anti-inflammatory drugs (NSAIDs), alcohol, caffeine, and smoking cigarettes (Garrow & Delegge, 2010).

The small ulceration of the gastric or duodenal lining leads to pain, blood in the stool, and vomiting (with blood). If left uncorrected, peptic ulcer disease can lead to bowel or stomach perforation with acute hemorrhage or pyloric obstruction. A chronic ulcer condition may lead to anemia from the constant, gradual blood loss.

Assessment

An ulcer occurring in a neonate usually presents with hematemesis (blood in vomitus) or melena (blood in the stool). Such ulcers are usually superficial and heal rapidly, although they can lead to rupture, with symptoms of respiratory distress, abdominal distention, vomiting, and, if extensive, cardiovascular collapse. If an ulcer occurs in a toddler, the first symptoms are usually anorexia or vomiting. Bleeding follows in several weeks. If an ulcer begins when children are of preschool or early school age, pain may be the presenting symptom. The child may report pain as mild, severe, colicky, or continuous. It is often poorly localized, although it may be in the epigastric area as in adults. If the pain occurs in the right lower quadrant, it may be confused with appendicitis.

In school-age children and adolescents, symptoms are generally those of the adult—a gnawing or aching pain in the epigastric area before meals that is relieved by eating. Vomiting (because of spasm and edema of the pylorus) occurs in a small number of children. On abdominal palpation, epigastric tenderness is present.

Endoscopy is the most reliable diagnostic test to confirm the diagnosis of peptic ulcer disease; it allows for visual inspection and biopsies for *H. pylori*. Children with this condition must have blood tests done periodically to be monitored for blood loss anemia.

Therapeutic Management

Children with peptic ulcer disease due to *H. pylori* infection are treated with triple therapy, a combination of medications that is given to attempt to eradicate the bacteria from the stomach. This treatment consists of two antibiotics, usually amoxicillin and clarithromycin (Biaxin), and a PPI such as omeprazole (Prilosec). Bismuth subsalicylate (Pepto-Bismol) is soothing and mildly antibiotic and so may be prescribed concurrently. Stool can be sent for *H. pylori* stool antigen to check if the infection has cleared (Koletzko, Jones, Goodman, et al., 2011). Children with stress ulcers can be treated with a PPI alone.

 ## Nursing Diagnoses and Related Interventions

Having peptic ulcer disease can be difficult for children because it is painful, and remembering to take medicine daily can be a problem.

Nursing Diagnosis: Pain related to ulceration in intestinal tract

Outcome Evaluation: Child exhibits verbal and nonverbal signs of decreased pain; appears comfortable and without excessive crying.

Children with peptic ulcer disease should be able to eat a usual diet while avoiding heavily spiced food such as pizza or sausage if such food causes discomfort. Work with them to devise a schedule so they can remember to take their medications.

Be certain the outcomes planned are realistic because it may not be possible to relieve symptoms of peptic ulcers immediately. However, children can be helped immediately to understand why the pain occurs and what they can do to help relieve it.

Hepatic Disorders

Hepatic disorders include both congenital disorders, such as obstruction or atresia of the biliary duct, and acquired disorders, such as hepatitis or cirrhosis.

LIVER FUNCTION

In infants, 1 or 2 cm of liver is readily and normally palpable under the diaphragm on the right side of their abdomen. An organ essential for the normal metabolism of carbohydrates, proteins, and fats, the liver plays a major role in the maintenance of normal blood sugar levels by changing glucose to glycogen and storing it until needed by body cells. It then reverses the process and changes glycogen back to glucose and releases it into the blood when cells need it (Huether, 2012). It assists in the catabolism of fatty acids and protein and serves as a temporary storage space for both fat and protein.

By the means of the enzyme glucuronosyltransferase, the liver is responsible for converting indirect (or unconjugated) bilirubin into direct (or conjugated) bilirubin so it can be excreted in bile and eliminated from the body. This is an important function in the newborn, and jaundice can result if the level of glucuronosyltransferase is low because of immaturity.

Lastly, the liver manufactures bile, a secretion necessary for the digestion of fat; fibrinogen and prothrombin, substances essential for blood clotting; heparin, a substance necessary to keep blood from clotting in intact vessels; and blood proteins, which are necessary for cell growth and repair. It destroys red blood cells and detoxifies many harmful absorbed substances, such as drugs. The liver is a life-sustaining organ because of all these functions; therefore, any disorder involving the liver is always serious.

HEPATITIS

Hepatitis (inflammation and infection of the liver) is caused by invasion of the hepatitis A, B, C, D, or E virus (CDC, 2016b).

Hepatitis A

- Causative agent: a picornavirus, hepatitis A virus (HAV)
- Incubation period: 25 days on average
- Period of communicability: highest during 2 weeks preceding onset of symptoms
- Mode of transmission: in children, ingestion of fecally contaminated water or shellfish; day care center spread from contaminated changing tables

- Immunity:
  Natural immunity: one episode induces immunity for the specific type of virus.
  Active artificial immunity: HAV vaccine (recommended for all children 12 to 23 months of age, workers in day care centers, and certain international travelers)
  Passive artificial immunity: immune globulin

Hepatitis B

- Causative agent: a hepadnavirus; hepatitis B virus (HBV)
- Incubation period: 120 days on average
- Period of communicability: later part of incubation period and during the acute stage
- Mode of transmission: transfusion of contaminated blood and plasma or semen; inoculation by a contaminated syringe or needle through IV drug use; may be spread to fetus if mother has infection in third trimester of pregnancy
- Immunity:
  Natural immunity: one episode induces immunity for the specific type of virus.
  Active artificial immunity: HBV vaccine (recommended for routine immunization beginning at birth and also to all healthcare providers) (CDC, 2016b)
  Passive artificial immunity: specific hepatitis B immune serum globulin

Hepatitis C, D, and E

Although hepatitis A and B are the viruses that most frequently cause hepatitis, hepatitis C, D, and E viruses may also be involved. Hepatitis C virus (HCV) is a single-strand RNA virus. Transmission, as with HBV, is primarily by blood or blood products, IV drug use, maternal–fetal transfer, or sexual contact. The virus produces mild symptoms of disease, but there is a high incidence of chronic infection with the virus.

Hepatitis D virus (HDV), or the delta form, is similar to HBV in transmission, although it apparently requires a coexisting HBV infection to be activated. Disease symptoms are mild, but there is a high incidence of fulminant hepatitis after the initial infection.

The E form of hepatitis is enterically transmitted similarly to hepatitis A (e.g., fecally contaminated water). Disease symptoms from the E virus can range from asymptomatic to mild to chronic liver disease (Faramawi, Johnson, Chen, et al., 2011).

Assessment

No matter which virus is involved, acute hepatitis is a generalized body infection with specific and intense liver effects. Type A occurs in children of all ages and accounts for approximately 30% of instances. Hepatitis B and C tend to occur in newborns from placental–fetal transfer and in adolescents after intimate contact or the use of contaminated syringes for drug injection.

Clinically, it is impossible to differentiate the type of hepatitis from the signs that are present. All hepatitis viruses cause liver cell destruction, leading to increased serum aspartate aminotransferase (AST), alanine aminotransferase (ALT), and alkaline phosphatase levels. Albumin synthesis decreases, and bile formation and excretion are impaired. The type of virus causing the disease can be determined by the recognition of a specific antibody against the virus such as anti-HAV immunoglobulin M (IgM) or anti-HBV IgM.

Hepatitis A is an acute self-limited illness and spread via the fecal–oral route. Symptoms include headache, fever, and anorexia. Jaundice occurs as liver function slows. This lasts for approximately 1 week and then symptoms fade with a full recovery. Rarely, children may develop fulminant liver failure. Symptoms of hepatitis B are more marked. Children report generalized aching, right upper quadrant pain, and a headache. They may have a low-grade fever. They feel ill and become fretful from pruritus (itching). After 3 to 7 days of such symptoms, the color of the urine becomes darker (brown) because of the excretion of bilirubin. In another 2 days, the sclerae of the eyes become jaundiced; soon, the child has generalized jaundice. With generalized jaundice, there is little excretion of bilirubin into the stool, so the stools become white or gray. This icteric (jaundiced) phase lasts for a few days to 2 weeks. Some children have an anicteric form of infection, in which they develop the beginning symptoms but then never develop the jaundice. However, they are as infectious as children with overt jaundice. The majority of those infected with hepatitis C will be asymptomatic, but those who become acutely ill will have similar symptoms to someone with hepatitis B.

Laboratory studies will show elevations of the liver enzymes AST (SGOT) and ALT (SGPT). Levels of bilirubin are increased in the urine. Bile pigments in the stool are decreased. Serum bilirubin levels are increased.

QSEN Checkpoint Question 45.4

SAFETY

Barry's family likes to celebrate family events by eating crab, lobster, and shrimp. The nurse recognizes which form of hepatitis is most apt to be contracted by eating contaminated shellfish?
  a. Hepatitis B
  b. Hepatitis A
  c. Hepatitis E
  d. Hepatitis C

Look in Appendix A for the best answer and rationale.

Therapeutic Management

All healthcare providers should receive prophylaxis against hepatitis with the hepatitis B vaccine. Newborns should also receive routine immunization against HBV. All women should be screened during pregnancy for hepatitis B surface antigen (HBsAg). Infants born to mothers who are hepatitis B positive should receive both hepatitis B immune globulin (HBIG) and active immunization at birth to prevent them from contracting the disease (Roznovsky, Orsagova, Kloudova, et al., 2010). Hepatitis A vaccine is available for healthcare providers and included in routine immunization programs for infants beginning at 1 year of age (CDC, 2016b). The incidence of both hepatitis A and B has fallen dramatically since the introduction of routine vaccination (Daniels, Grytdal, & Wasley, 2009). Unfortunately, no vaccine for hepatitis C is yet available.

Strict hand washing and infection control precautions are mandatory when caring for children with hepatitis. Feces must be disposed of carefully because the type A virus can be cultured from feces. Syringes and needles must be disposed of with caution because the types B and C virus can be transmitted by blood. Contacts should receive immune globulin (hepatitis A) or HBIG as appropriate.

The treatment for hepatitis A is increased rest and maintenance of a good caloric intake. A low-fat diet, once recommended, is not required and, in any event, is difficult to enforce. Children are generally hungrier at breakfast than later in the day, so encourage them to eat a healthy breakfast. They should not return to school or a day care center until 2 weeks after the onset of symptoms to guard against spreading the infection. Treatment for acute hepatitis B is also supportive, as no medication is available for this stage. About 10% of children will develop chronic hepatitis B. Antiviral medications, such as interferon, entecavir, and lamivudine, have been developed for use against chronic hepatitis B and have success in eradicating the virus in some patients. Interferon and ribavirin are approved for treating hepatitis C in children. Hepatitis B is always potentially serious because newborns who contract the disease at birth have an increased risk for liver carcinoma later in life (Bailey, Shiau, Zola, et al., 2011). Because hepatitis B is a sexually transmitted disease, preadolescent children with the infection need to be screened for the possibility of sexual maltreatment (Leder, 2012).

Nursing Diagnoses and Related Interventions

Nursing Diagnosis: Pain related to pruritus of jaundice and liver inflammation

Outcome Evaluation: Child states level of itching is tolerable, no scratch marks on skin; reports right upper quadrant pain is minimal.

Pruritus from jaundice results in extreme discomfort for some children. A cool bath and being certain a child is not overheated and not perspiring usually reduces the itching. Skin moisturizers such as Eucerin or an antihistamine may also be helpful. Cholestyramine (Questran) is a bile acid sequestrant, which binds bile in the GI tract to prevent its reabsorption and so may be prescribed. Teaching a child distraction techniques such as putting pressure on a pruritic area or trying imagery to lessen the urge to scratch are also helpful measures.

Chronic Hepatitis

Hepatitis is considered chronic when it persists for longer than 6 months. This is most often the result of a hepatitis B, D, or C infection. Abnormal liver enzyme levels and a liver biopsy establish the diagnosis and can also predict the severity. With chronic hepatitis, fatty infiltration and bile duct damage can occur. The disease may progress to cirrhosis and eventually liver failure. Therapy is supportive to compensate for decreased liver function (Sundaram, Hoffenberg, Kramer, et al., 2011).

Fulminant Hepatic Failure

Fulminant hepatic failure is present when acute, massive necrosis or sudden, severe impairment of liver function occurs, leading to liver failure and hepatic encephalopathy. It can be due to infection or toxicity. Acetaminophen (Tylenol) overdose is the most likely etiology. Hepatic encephalopathy, or invasion of brain cells by ammonia, occurs because of the inability of the liver to detoxify the ammonia being constantly produced by the intestine in the process of digestion (Gluud, Vilstrup, & Morgan, 2016).

Children may show mental aberrations such as confusion, drowsiness, or disorientation. Treatment involves reducing protein intake and administering lactulose to prevent absorption of ammonia in the colon or administering nonabsorbable antibiotics such as neomycin to decrease the production of ammonia by the intestinal bacteria. **Liver transplantation** (surgical replacement of a malfunctioning liver by a donor liver) may be necessary. If a cadaver liver is not available, a lobe can be removed from a living donor such as a parent and transplanted into a child. The donor is then able to regenerate the lost lobe of the liver without long-term effects.

OBSTRUCTION OF THE BILE DUCTS

Obstruction of the bile ducts in children generally occurs from congenital biliary atresia, stenosis, or absence of the duct. It also can occur from the plugging of biliary secretions, although this is rare. When the bile duct is obstructed, bile, unable to enter the intestinal tract, accumulates in the liver. Bile pigments (direct bilirubin) enter the bloodstream and jaundice occurs, which increases in intensity daily.

Assessment

Although bile duct obstruction is a congenital disorder, the chief sign (jaundice) does not develop until between 2 and 6 weeks of age. This delay differentiates it clinically from physiologic jaundice, which occurs in almost all newborns on the third day of life, or the jaundice of Rh or ABO isoimmunization, which typically occurs during the first 24 hours of life. Laboratory findings will also distinguish this type of jaundice from other types because, with physiologic and isoimmunization jaundice, there is a rise in indirect bilirubin; in the jaundice of bile duct obstruction, there is a rise in direct bilirubin. Alkaline phosphatase levels will also be elevated. The AST (SGOT) level is normal in the early phase but later becomes abnormal, when prolonged obstruction and back pressure cause liver cell damage. In addition, because bile salts, which are necessary for fat and fat-soluble vitamin absorption, are not reaching the intestine, absorption of fat and fat-soluble vitamins (vitamins A, D, E, and K) becomes poor. Calcium absorption, which depends on vitamin D absorption, will fail as well. The infant's stools appear light in color from a lack of bile pigments. The pressure on the liver from the obstruction becomes so acute with time that cell destruction or cirrhosis occurs. Ultimately, without liver transplantation, death from liver failure will result (Kaido, Mori, Ogura, et al., 2012).

Therapeutic Management

Before treatment is begun, appropriate blood work and a liver biopsy under local anesthesia may be obtained to rule out hepatitis. Duodenal secretions may be collected by endoscopy to assess for bile. Radionuclide imaging to show that bile ducts are not patent may confirm the diagnosis. If atresia of the bile duct is the problem, surgical correction is the treatment (a Kasai procedure). With this surgery, a Roux-en-Y loop of bowel is sutured directly onto the hilum of the liver so that the remaining small bile ducts will drain into the bowel. If successful, stools will become darker in color, and the jaundice will gradually resolve. Surgical correction may not be possible in all infants because the atresia may occur too far back in the liver to be in an operable area. Liver transplantation is then needed for children with extensive involvement or in whom a Kasai procedure is not successful.

Nursing Diagnoses and Related Interventions

Nursing Diagnosis: Risk for imbalanced nutrition, less than body requirements, related to inability to digest fat

Outcome Evaluation: Infant's weight remains in same percentile on standardized growth curve; absence of signs of vitamin deficiency such as cracked lips or altered bone growth; dietary record reflects intake of adequate nutrients.

Preoperative Care. Infants who are admitted for surgery for bile duct obstruction are placed on a low-fat, high-carbohydrate diet preoperatively. They are given water-soluble forms of vitamins A, D, and K to improve vitamin levels. If the vitamin K level is too low, coagulation may be affected, so vitamin K may be administered parenterally until prothrombin levels rise to normal limits. Infants will also be well hydrated with parenteral fluids.

Postoperative Care. Following surgery, infants return with a nasogastric tube in place attached to low intermittent suction. Observe carefully for abdominal distention because paralytic ileus, or bowel dysfunction, is a frequent complication of this type of surgery. The nasogastric tube will be left in place until peristalsis has returned. Gradually, children will be introduced to oral fluids and, eventually, to a normal diet. If the repair is successful, the child's stools change to a yellow and then brown (normal stool) color after surgery. Therefore, a description of stools is an important postoperative observation.

If bile flow is inadequate after surgery, infants will remain on a medium-fat, high-carbohydrate diet or receive total parenteral nutrition while they await transplantation surgery.

NONALCOHOLIC FATTY LIVER DISEASE AND CIRRHOSIS

Nonalcoholic fatty liver disease (NAFLD) is the accumulation of fatty deposits in the liver and is usually associated with obesity. As obesity is increasing in school-age children and adolescents, this condition is also increasing in incidence (Vajro, Lenta, Socha, et al., 2012). NAFLD can progress to cirrhosis in rare cases.

Cirrhosis is fibrotic scarring of the liver. Cirrhosis means "yellow," or the typical color of hepatic scar tissue. It rarely occurs in children, although it may be seen as a result of congenital biliary atresia or as a complication of chronic illnesses such as protracted hepatitis, sickle-cell anemia, or cystic fibrosis.

When fibrotic infiltrates replace normal liver cells, total liver function becomes impaired, resulting in a decreased ability to detoxify toxic substances, decreased protein synthesis, inability to produce prothrombin, decreased ability to

Figure 45.4 A distended abdomen due to ascites results in prominent veins along the abdomen. The underlying cause in this child is portal hypertension due to cirrhosis of the liver (From Salimpour, R. R., Salimpour, P., & Salimpour, P. [2013]. *Photographic atlas of pediatric disorders and diagnosis*. Philadelphia, PA: Lippincott Williams & Wilkins.)

produce bile, and, possibly, hypoglycemia. Children will have large, fatty stools resulting from the decrease in bile production; avitaminosis of fat-soluble vitamins; symptoms of hemorrhage from decreased clotting ability; and anemia.

Portal hypertension occurs from back pressure of blood that cannot flow readily through the scarred organ (Fig. 45.4). This leads to compromised heart action, *ascites* (an exudate of fluid into the abdomen), possibly esophageal varices (back pressure causes them to dilate), and hypersplenism (D'Antiga, 2012).

Cholestyramine (Questran) may be prescribed to reduce reabsorption of bile into the circulation to minimize itching from cholestasis. Once fatty or fibrotic infiltration begins, however, there is no way to reverse the changes. Nursing care focuses on promoting comfort, providing adequate nutrition by a high-carbohydrate, medium-chain–triglyceride diet, and preventing further involvement until liver transplantation can be scheduled.

Esophageal Varices

Esophageal varices (distended veins in the esophagus) are a frequent complication of liver disorders such as cirrhosis. They generally form at the distal end of the esophagus near the stomach because of back pressure on the veins resulting from increased portal circulation blood pressure. Varices may bleed if children cough vigorously or strain to pass stool. Gastric reflux into the distal esophagus may irritate and erode the fine covering of the distended vessels, causing rupture.

A rupture of esophageal varices is an emergency because children can lose a large quantity of blood quickly from the engorged vessels. Octreotide or vasopressin may be given by IV to decrease blood flow to the esophagus and reduce the hemorrhage. Endoscopic variceal band ligation is the preferred method of treatment. A tight rubber band is placed around the varix, creating a clot that prevents further bleeding (Hwang, Shergill, Acosta, et al., 2014). Balloon tamponade may be used to prevent bleeding until more effective treatment can be given.

A Sengstaken–Blakemore tube or Linton-Nachlas catheter may be passed into the stomach. After insertion, balloons on the sides of these catheters are inflated to apply pressure against the bleeding vessels. As with an external tourniquet, the compression must be reduced for 5 to 10 minutes every 6 to 8 hours, or tissue necrosis can result.

Following one episode of bleeding, children must be monitored for future bleeding episodes. Frequent vital sign measurements and testing of stool and any vomitus for the presence of blood will indicate if new bleeding is occurring.

LIVER TRANSPLANTATION

Liver transplantation is the surgical replacement of a malfunctioning liver by a donor liver. Child-size donor livers are not readily available, so the waiting time for surgery may be months. Adult livers can be reduced in size for transplantation or a lobe of a liver from a living donor can be used. Often, the child is extremely ill with ascites, GI bleeding, extreme pruritus, hepatic encephalopathy, or renal dysfunction before the surgery. This makes nursing care after liver transplantation in a child complex because it involves taking care of a child who has had major surgery and who normally would be categorized as too ill to undergo surgery.

Despite the severity of illness and the length of surgery, however, children tend to recover quickly after liver transplantation. Both children and parents must have thorough preoperative preparation, so they understand the seriousness of the surgery and the possibility that the graft will be rejected. It helps to introduce the parents to others whose children have successfully undergone the procedure so they have support people available for this critical time.

Preoperative Management

Preoperative management consists of keeping the child in the best physiologic condition possible so that when a liver is available, the transplantation can be performed.

Surgical Procedure

Liver transplantation is a time-consuming procedure and requires a wide subcostal incision. The vena cava is temporarily clamped during the removal of the natural liver to prevent bleeding, which means that all IV lines must be placed in the upper extremities.

Postoperative Management

Rejection of a liver transplant is most often because of the function of T lymphocytes. Careful tissue matching (human leukocyte antigen [HLA] matching) is necessary to reduce the possibility of stimulating T-cell rejection. To further reduce the action of T lymphocytes, children are given an immunosuppressive drug such as mycophenolate mofetil (CellCept), cyclosporine (Sandimmune), or tacrolimus (Prograf) before the transplantation.

Children may need assisted ventilation for approximately 24 hours postoperatively to prevent pulmonary complications such as atelectasis and pneumonia because the large abdominal incision makes coughing and deep breathing difficult. In addition, ascites places pressure against the diaphragm, interfering with lung expansion, and preoperative pulmonary edema may be present. After discontinuation of mechanical ventilation and extubation, chest physiotherapy may be started to mobilize lung secretions.

Advocate for adequate pain control. Frequently assess blood pressure, capillary refill, peripheral pulses, and skin color to ensure adequate cardiovascular function, which is important for good tissue perfusion of the transplanted liver. The child may have a central venous pressure line or an arterial line such as a Swan-Ganz catheter inserted to assess hemodynamic status. Assess neurologic status hourly using a modified Glasgow Coma Scale (see Chapter 52).

Usually, a child is positioned flat for the first 24 hours to prevent cerebral air emboli, which may result from any air remaining in the transplanted liver. Typically, children have a nasogastric tube inserted during surgery that is attached to low intermittent suction postoperatively. Irrigate the tube according to agency policy to maintain patency. Assess the gastric pH by aspirating stomach contents every 4 hours; based on this assessment, administer antacids or H_2-receptor antagonists such as cimetidine or mucosal protectants as prescribed to help prevent a stress ulcer. If preoperative esophageal varices are present, assess nasogastric drainage carefully for frank or occult blood.

A T-tube inserted into the bile duct for drainage allows the amount of bile being produced by the new liver to be evaluated. Once bowel sounds become active, nasogastric suction and the T-tube are usually discontinued and liquids and then solid foods are introduced gradually. If vomiting occurs and is persistent, total parenteral nutrition may be used for 3 or 4 days to rest the intestinal tract before fluid is reintroduced.

Hypoglycemia is a major danger postoperatively because glucose levels are regulated by the liver, and the transplanted organ may not function efficiently at first. Assess serum glucose levels hourly by finger-stick puncture. A 10% solution of dextrose IV may be necessary to prevent hypoglycemia.

Sodium, potassium, chloride, and calcium levels are evaluated approximately every 6 to 8 hours to be certain electrolyte balance is maintained. Even if a low potassium level is detected, potassium is rarely added to IV solutions because of the risk that renal failure has occurred because of the stress of surgery. In addition, if the graft begins to become necrotic, the breakdown of cells will release potassium, elevating the level even more. Continuous cardiac monitoring is usually necessary to detect hyperkalemia (hyperkalemia causes elevation of T waves or ventricular fibrillation), hypokalemia (causes small T waves and a U wave), or other arrhythmias.

Many children develop hypertension within 72 hours after surgery. This occurs because of alterations in the renin–angiotensin system because of the not yet fully functioning transplanted liver or as a side effect of cyclosporine, tacrolimus, and steroid therapy, which is continued postoperatively to guard against transplant rejection. IV therapy with hypotensive agents such as hydralazine (Apresoline) and nitroprusside may be needed to reduce hypertension. In contrast, hypotension will occur if the transplanted liver becomes dysfunctional or if there is bleeding caused by poor blood coagulation. To help detect bleeding, observe and record abdominal girth, the incision line, and drainage from any catheters or tubes placed in the incision to allow peritoneal secretions to drain.

A warming blanket may be required postoperatively to maintain normal body temperature after the long exposure of surgery. Take axillary or tympanic, not rectal, temperatures because many children with liver damage have hemorrhoids that could rupture from the trauma of a thermometer insertion. Prevent the child from unnecessary exposure during procedures and care to help restore and maintain normal body temperature.

 Nursing Diagnoses and Related Interventions

Nursing Diagnosis: Risk for infection related to administration of immunosuppressive medication

Outcome Evaluation: Temperature remains within normal range; no exudate or inflammation around abdominal incision is present.

Liver transplantation is possible because of the preoperative administration of an immunosuppressive agent that suppresses T lymphocytes, the lymphocytes responsible for rejecting transplanted organs. Because children are prone to infection while receiving immunosuppressive therapy, be certain to use strict aseptic technique, standard infection precautions, and careful hand washing while giving care. Clean the skin around any abdominal drains every 4 hours to avoid skin breakdown and to prevent a portal of entry for microorganisms.

Serum transaminases (AST [SGOT] and ALT [SGPT]), alkaline phosphatase, serum bilirubin, and ammonia levels are assessed at least daily to detect rejection, although children usually do not show signs of liver rejection until 5 to 7 days after surgery. In addition to changes in these laboratory values, with liver rejection, the child also may develop fever and increasing abdominal girth. Also, the urine turns orange from increased urobilinogen excretion. If signs of rejection appear to be occurring, doses of cyclosporine, tacrolimus, and a corticosteroid such as methylprednisolone are increased to maximum levels.

Nursing Diagnosis: Interrupted family processes related to stress of surgery and uncertainty of transplantation outcome

Outcome Evaluation: Child and family state that although waiting is difficult, they are able to do so; family identifies ways they have changed family life at home to accommodate child's illness and surgery.

Children and parents need continued support during the postoperative period while they wait to see if the graft will be rejected. They also need continued contact with healthcare personnel through telephone calls and clinic visits.

After successful liver transplantation, a child should be able to function with few limitations, attending school and enjoying age-appropriate activities. Be certain on hospital discharge parents have a return appointment for evaluation and are aware of the symptoms of graft rejection, such as jaundice, lethargy, and fever. Contact sports may be limited to prevent injury to the new liver, and adolescents need to be cautioned to avoid alcohol to prevent liver damage from this source.

Intestinal Disorders

Because the intestines are a lengthy body system, several disorders, either congenital or acquired, can occur.

INTUSSUSCEPTION

Intussusception, the invagination of one portion of the intestine into another (Fig. 45.5), most frequently occurs in the second half of the first year of life (Mandeville, Chien, Willyerd, et al., 2012) with 90% of cases occurring by 2 years of age. About 75% of intussusception occurs for idiopathic reasons where there is no clear cause. In other cases, a "lead point" on the intestine likely cues the invagination. Such a point might be a Meckel's diverticulum, a polyp, hypertrophy of *Peyer patches* (lymphatic tissue of the bowel that increases in size with viral diseases), or bowel tumors. The point of the invagination is generally at the juncture of the distal ileum and proximal colon.

Assessment

Children with this disorder suddenly draw up their legs and cry as if they are in severe pain, and they may also vomit. After the peristaltic wave that caused the discomfort passes, they are symptom free and play happily. In approximately 15 minutes, however, the same phenomenon of intense abdominal pain strikes again. Vomitus, which contains bile because the obstruction is invariably below the ampulla of Vater, the point in the intestine where bile empties into the duodenum, will begin. In approximately 70% of cases, frank or occult blood is seen in the stool. The stool is described as having a "red currant jelly" appearance due to the blood and

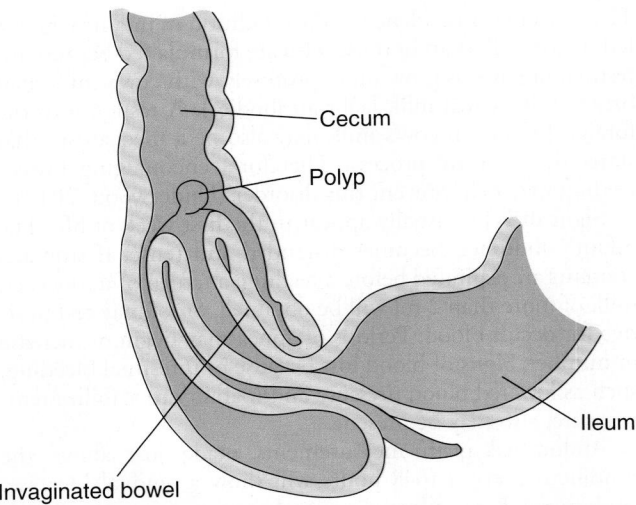

Figure 45.5 Intussusception. The distal ileal segment of bowel has invaginated into the cecum. A polyp serves as a lead point.

mucus it contains. The abdomen becomes distended as the bowel above the intussusception distends.

If necrosis occurs in the invaginated bowel, children generally develop an elevated temperature, peritoneal irritation (their abdomen feels tender and they may "guard" it by tightening their abdominal muscles), an increased white blood cell count, and often a rapid pulse.

Diagnosis is suggested by the history. Any time a parent is describing a child who is crying, be certain to ask enough questions to recognize the possibility of intussusception. Episodes of crying are for a short time but repeat every 15 to 20 minutes; the stomach feels "full" and vomitus and diarrhea with blood may occur. The presence of the intussusception is confirmed by an abdominal X-ray, or ultrasound (Rogers, 2017).

Therapeutic Management

The condition is a surgical emergency. Reduction of the intussusception must be done promptly by either instillation of a water-soluble solution, barium enema, or air (pneumatic insufflation) into the bowel or surgery to reduce the invagination before necrosis of the affected portion of the bowel occurs. If there is no lead point, just the pressure of the nonsurgical techniques may reduce the intussusception. After this type of reduction, children are observed for 24 hours because some children will have a recurrence of the intussusception within this time. If this occurs, children will be scheduled for an additional reduction or surgery.

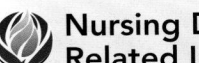

Nursing Diagnoses and Related Interventions

Nursing Diagnosis: Pain related to abnormal abdominal peristalsis

Outcome Evaluation: Child can be comforted between spasms of pain; demonstrates interest in toys or social interactions.

Infants with intussusception are bewildered by this type of episodic pain because it is so different from any pain they have experienced before. Ordinarily, if they pinch a finger on a toy and it hurts, a parent picks them up, kisses their fingers, and the pain goes away. A parent picks them up now and the pain goes away, but it returns repeatedly. Infants need to be held, rocked, and comforted in an attempt to relieve their fright at this strange happening.

Nursing Diagnosis: Risk for deficient fluid volume related to bowel obstruction

Outcome Evaluation: Infant's skin turgor is good, pulse is 90 to 100 beats/min, amount of diarrhea and blood loss in stool are minimal; episodes of vomiting decrease in frequency.

Infants are kept on NPO status before surgery or nonsurgical reduction. Because they have abdominal pain, they may find comfort in sucking a pacifier. Because they have been vomiting, IV fluid therapy may be started to reestablish their electrolyte balance and to supply adequate fluid to hydrate them.

Following a nonsurgical reduction, infants are kept NPO for a few hours and then introduced gradually to regular feedings. Infants who have surgery will return with a nasogastric tube attached to low intermittent suction and an IV infusion in place. The nasogastric tube will remain in place until the suture line is healing, and peristaltic function has returned. Once bowel sounds are present, oral feedings can be started gradually. Encourage the parents to participate with this aspect of care because it provides them with an opportunity to regain confidence in themselves as parents. Urge them to continue to hold and be with the child as recovery proceeds to reassure themselves that the child is now once again well.

VOLVULUS WITH MALROTATION

A **volvulus** is a twisting of the intestine (Fig. 45.6). The twist leads to obstruction of the passage of feces and to compromise of the blood supply to the loop of intestine involved. Volvulus occurs due to intestinal malrotation and may be associated with other congenital anomalies. In fetal life, a portion of the

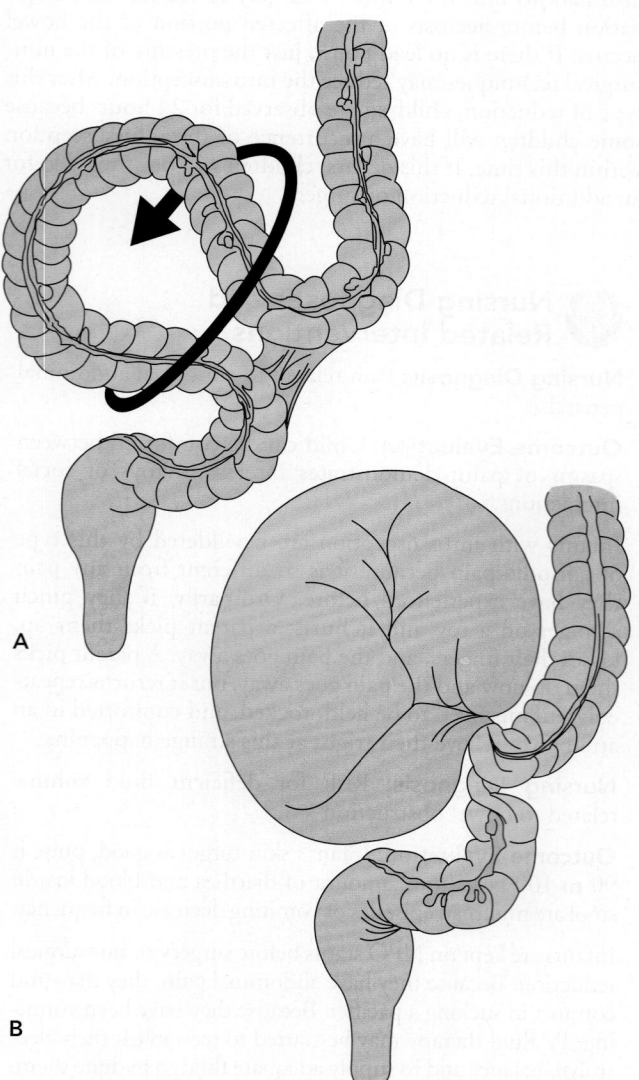

Figure 45.6 Volvulus of the sigmoid colon. **(A)** The unattached loop of bowel twists. **(B)** The bowel lumen is obstructed, leading to inability of stool to pass and compression of the blood supply to the looped bowel segment.

intestine first protrudes into the base of the umbilical cord at approximately 6 weeks of intrauterine life. At approximately 10 weeks of intrauterine life, it returns to the abdominal cavity. As the intestine returns, it rotates to its permanent position. After the rotation, the mesentery becomes fixed in this position. With a volvulus, this action is incomplete and the mesentery does not attach in a normal position. The bowel is left free to move and twist (Laurence & Pollock, 2012).

Usually, the symptoms occur during the first 6 months of life and are those of intestinal obstruction such as intense crying and pain, pulling up the legs, abdominal distention, and vomiting. A volvulus can be differentiated from pyloric stenosis because vomiting with pyloric stenosis occurs immediately after feeding, whereas pain and vomiting from a volvulus is unrelated to feeding. The diagnosis is made based on the history and an abdominal examination, which reveals an abdominal mass. It is confirmed by an ultrasound or lower barium X-ray. Surgery is an emergency and should be performed before necrosis of the intestine occurs from a lack of blood supply to the involved loop of bowel. Preoperative and postoperative care will be the same as for infants with intussusception.

NECROTIZING ENTEROCOLITIS

Necrotizing enterocolitis (NEC) is a condition that develops in approximately 5% of all infants in neonatal intensive care nurseries, with premature and low–birth-weight infants at highest risk. Necrotic areas develop in the bowel that interfere with digestion and can lead to paralytic ileus, perforation, and peritonitis (Huether, 2012).

The cause of NEC is unknown and thought to be due to a variety of factors. The necrosis appears to result from ischemia or poor perfusion of blood vessels in the entire bowel or in isolated sections of the bowel. The ischemic process tends to occur from hypovolemic shock or hypoxia in which there is vasoconstriction of blood vessels to organs such as the bowel. The incidence is highest in immature infants, those who have suffered anoxia or shock, and those fed by enteral feedings. Infants with infections may develop it as a further complication of their already stressed state.

Assessment

There is a lower incidence of the condition in infants who are fed breast milk than in those who are formula fed because intestinal organisms grow more profusely with cow's milk than breast milk (cow's milk lacks antibodies). A response to the foreign protein in cow's milk may also be a mechanism that starts the necrotic process. Therefore, encouraging breastfeeding may help prevent this disorder (Underwood, 2013).

Signs of NEC usually appear in the first week of life. The infant's abdomen becomes distended and tense. If stomach contents are aspirated before a feeding, a return of undigested milk of more than 2 ml will be obtained. Stool may test positive for occult blood. Periods of apnea may begin or increase in number. Signs of blood loss because of intestinal bleeding, such as lowered blood pressure and inability to stabilize temperature, also may be present.

Abdominal girth measurements made just above the umbilicus every 4 to 8 hours will show a gradual increase. Abdominal X-ray films show a characteristic picture of air invading the intestinal wall; if perforation has occurred, there will be air in the abdominal cavity.

Therapeutic Management

As soon as the condition is recognized, breastfeedings or formula feedings are discontinued, and the infant is maintained on IV or total parenteral nutrition solutions to rest the GI tract except for additional supplements of enteral probiotics (Vongbhavit & Underwood, 2016). An antibiotic may be given to limit secondary infection. Handle the infant's abdomen gently to lessen the possibility of a bowel perforation.

If the area of necrosis appears to be localized, surgery to remove that portion of the bowel may be successful. If a large portion of the bowel is removed, the infant may be prone to "short-bowel" syndrome or may have a problem with digestion of nutrients in the future. If the bowel perforates, peritoneal drainage or a laparotomy will be necessary to help remove fecal secretions from the abdomen. An infant may need a temporary colostomy performed to allow for bowel function.

NEC is a grave insult to an infant already stressed by immaturity. The prognosis is guarded until the infant can again take oral feedings without bowel complications.

SHORT-BOWEL/SHORT-GUT SYNDROME

Short-bowel or short-gut syndrome is an absorptive disorder in which there is not sufficient bowel surface area in the small intestine for proper nutrient absorption. The condition has several causes, including surgery for NEC, volvulus, and GI tract trauma, which resulted in a large portion of the intestine being removed. The treatment includes ensuring adequate hydration and proper intake of essential vitamins and minerals. Following bowel resection surgery, total parenteral nutrition, including lipids, may be used initially until the bowel can tolerate enteral feedings. Oral or enteral feedings are then given as tolerated. If gastrostomy or nasogastric feedings are used, nonnutritive sucking should be facilitated to preserve the suck–swallow reflex. Because long-term use of total parenteral nutrition may cause liver damage, liver transplantation may be needed in the future (Bhatia, Gates, & Parish, 2010).

APPENDICITIS

Appendicitis (inflammation of the appendix) is the most common cause of abdominal surgery in children. It occurs most frequently in school-age children and adolescents, although it can occur in preschoolers and even in newborns (Ladd, Neff, Becher, et al., 2012). The *appendix*, a blind-ended pouch attached to the cecum, may become inflamed because of an upper respiratory or other body infection, but the cause of appendicitis is generally obscure. In most instances, fecal material apparently enters the appendix, hardens, and obstructs the appendiceal lumen. Inflammation and edema develop, leading to compression of blood vessels and cellular malnutrition. Necrosis and pain result. If the condition is not discovered early enough, the necrotic area will rupture and fecal material will spill into the abdomen, causing peritonitis, a potentially fatal condition.

Assessment

Most parents assume appendicitis begins with sharp pain, so they may dismiss a child's early symptoms for some time as simple gastroenteritis. In actuality, pain is a late symptom. Diagnosis is made on a cluster of symptoms: anorexia, pain or tenderness in the right lower quadrant, nausea or vomiting, elevation of temperature, and leukocytosis (Wheeler, 2011).

The history typically begins with anorexia for 12 to 24 hours. Children do not eat and do not act like their usual selves. Nausea and vomiting may then occur. The abdominal pain, when it does start, is at first diffuse. Gradually, it becomes localized to the right lower quadrant. The point of sharpest pain is often one third of the way between the anterior superior iliac crest and the umbilicus (**McBurney's point**). If the child's appendix is displaced from this usual position, the pain will not be at this typical point, so pain at any other point does not rule out appendicitis. Pregnant adolescents are apt to have displaced pain. Fever is a late symptom.

Until the pain becomes localized, appendicitis is difficult to distinguish from acute gastroenteritis. Often, it is difficult to palpate children's abdomens because they may guard their abdomen or make abdominal muscles stiff and hard by tensing them. Although this interferes with an abdominal examination, it is in itself an important sign that children have abdominal pain. To assist in a diagnosis of a painful abdomen, always palpate the anticipated tender area last.

Rebound tenderness is a phenomenon in which a child feels relatively mild pain when the area over the appendix is palpated, but, once an examiner's hand is withdrawn, the child experiences acute pain caused by abdominal contents shifting. This is diagnostic for appendicitis, but it should be done with children only when necessary because it does cause acute pain. If, on auscultation, bowel sounds are reduced (hypoactive), this suggests peritonitis or that the appendix has already ruptured.

Laboratory findings usually indicate leukocytosis (white blood cell count between 10,000 and 18,000/mm^3), which is actually low for the extent of the infection that may be present. Ketone levels in the urine are inordinately elevated as a symptom of starvation from poor intestinal absorption.

An ultrasound or CT scan will reveal the swollen appendix. Pain in the right lower quadrant may also occur as a manifestation of right lower lobe pneumonia. Therefore, children may have a chest X-ray taken to rule this out as the source of pain. Because, in the past, an assessment of appendicitis depended on being able to detect abdominal pain, both parents and healthcare providers may be reluctant to administer analgesia to children with abdominal pain. Because ultrasound can successfully reveal appendicitis, however, analgesia to make the child comfortable can be given (Bansal, Banever, Karrer, et al., 2012).

Therapeutic Management

Therapy for appendicitis is surgical removal of the appendix by laparoscopy before it ruptures. Achieving this is easier in older than younger children because they are more capable of relating the progression of symptoms. Also, the wall of the appendix is thinner and perforates more readily in young children.

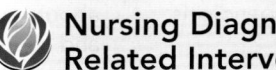

Nursing Diagnoses and Related Interventions

Priorities for nursing care must be established quickly because this is an emergency, and the child must be prepared immediately for surgery. Box 45.5 shows an interprofessional care map illustrating both nursing and team planning for a child with appendicitis.

BOX 45.5

Nursing Care Planning

AN INTERPROFESSIONAL CARE MAP FOR A CHILD WITH APPENDICITIS

Barry's parents bring his older sister, 10-year-old Addie, to the emergency department because of nausea, vomiting, and abdominal pain since yesterday. Father states, "We thought it was just an upset stomach, but it isn't getting any better, and the pain is much worse now."

Family Assessment: Child lives with two younger siblings (2 years and 12 months of age) and both parents on a rural horse farm. Father works as a newspaper printer in town; mother cares for horses and stable. Mother reports finances as, "Good. We're enjoying this time of life."

Patient Assessment: Thin-appearing 10-year-old female with a history of inflammatory bowel disease. Temperature, 101.2°F; pulse rate, 100 beats/min; respirations, 24 breaths/min. Mother reports that yesterday the child stated she was not feeling well. "She wasn't eating, and she had pains in her stomach. Last night, the pain got worse, and she started vomiting." Pain now localized in right lower quadrant. Legs drawn up against abdomen. Bowel sounds sluggish. Rebound tenderness present. White blood cell count of 17,000/mm^3. Ultrasound confirms appendicitis. Child is scheduled for emergency appendectomy.

Nursing Diagnosis: Pain related to presence of appendicitis

Outcome Criteria: Child states pain is not above a 2 on 1–10 numeric pain scale.

Team Member Responsible	Assessment	Intervention	Rationale	Expected Outcome
Activities of Daily Living, Including Safety				
Nurse	Assess what is child's most comfortable position.	Do not palpate child's abdomen.	Palpating could rupture inflamed appendix.	Child states she knows not to put pressure on abdomen.
Teamwork and Collaboration				
Nurse/primary care provider	Assess what anesthetist is available for emergency surgery.	Consult with anesthetist about emergency surgery.	Emergency surgery has added risks because of lack of preparation.	Anesthesiology service consults and readies for surgery.
Procedures/Medications for Quality Improvement				
Nurse	Assess if child has ever had surgery before. Assess if child's armband is in place.	Wash abdomen from nipple line to groin. Complete preoperative checklist.	Removing abdominal hair helps prevent infection. Safety precautions are important to prevent misidentification during surgery.	Abdominal preparation is completed prior to surgery. Child's armband is in place; preoperative checklist is completed and signed.
Nutrition				
Nurse	Assess when was the last time child ate or drank. Assess skin turgor.	Keep child nothing by mouth (NPO) while awaiting surgery. Begin intravenous (IV) fluid as prescribed.	Eating could evoke vomiting with aspiration during surgery. IV fluid can help prevent dehydration while NPO.	Child cooperates to remain NPO until surgery. Understands why IV is prescribed; protects infusion site from trauma.
Patient-Centered Care				
Nurse	Assess what child and parents understand about appendicitis.	Teach child and parents as needed about cause and course of appendicitis.	Better understanding of a child's condition can help child and parents accept the necessary procedures.	Child and parents state they have no questions about cause or course of appendicitis.

Psychosocial/Spiritual/Emotional Needs

Nurse	Assess child's level of pain using a 1–10 pain scale. Assess if child has experience with nonpharmacologic pain relief measures.	Discuss surgeon's preference to not prescribe analgesic as child will soon be anesthetized in the operating room. Teach child a nonpharmacologic pain relief method such as imagery.	Pain relief may be delayed until appendicitis is diagnosed. Nonpharmacologic pain relief can be very effective for abdominal pain in children.	Child states she understands her pain will be relieved as soon as anesthesia is begun. Uses imagery as nonpharmacologic pain relief technique.
Nurse	Assess child and parents' level of apprehension about emergency situation.	Discuss positive aspects of parents' actions.	Reinforcing that parents acted with good judgment can increase self-esteem and ability to accept new developments.	Child and parents state that although their stress level is high, they are able to cope with new developments.

Informatics for Seamless Healthcare Planning

Nurse	Assess if child and parents have any questions prior to leaving for operating room.	Review what will happen in the operating room and immediate postoperative course.	The better informed child and parents are of happenings, the better they will be able to cooperate.	Child and parents state they feel prepared for next step in treatment for child's condition.

Nursing Diagnosis: Fear related to pain and the emergency nature of disorder and immediate surgery

Outcome Evaluation: Parents and child state that they understand what interventions are necessary and cooperate as necessary; child states level of pain is tolerable.

Admission to a hospital for appendicitis often occurs rapidly. A parent telephones a primary care provider, who recommends the child be seen in the emergency room. Surgery is scheduled as soon as it can be arranged or a mere 30 minutes may have passed from the time of the first phone call to when the child is wheeled into surgery. During this time, the parent and child both need to be told exactly what is happening (e.g., "I'm going to take some blood; I'm putting your name tag on your arm") and who the people are who are caring for them (e.g., "This is Dr. Brown, the anesthesiologist. I'm Ms. Henry, a registered nurse."). Remember, parents may not think clearly in this type of emergency so their reactions to situations may not be their usual ones (e.g., they leave food cooking on the stove, they leave their car in the middle of the street, which causes a traffic jam, rather than pulling it into the parking lot). Explain that the procedures being done for their child, such as blood studies, or the short wait while an operating room is prepared are necessary for safe surgery, and the danger of the appendix rupturing is not as acute a danger as they may have believed under these controlled circumstances. Praise them for the things they did well, such as recognizing that the child was ill and bringing the child immediately for care, to help offer a sense of control.

Once a diagnosis is made by ultrasound, a child needs an analgesic for pain. Cathartics and heat to the abdomen are contraindicated to relieve pain because these increase the possibility of rupture of the appendix. If you are assisting with washing the abdomen with an antiseptic solution immediately before surgery, be certain to do this gently because the abdomen is tender, and compression could cause the appendix to rupture. Likewise, use lukewarm, not hot water, because heat can increase the possibility of appendix rupture by increasing edema in the appendix. Urge the child to find the best position of comfort and assure both parents and the child that surgery is being scheduled as soon as possible.

Nursing Diagnosis: Risk for deficient fluid volume related to NPO status presurgery and postsurgery

Outcome Evaluation: Child's skin fold returns to place quickly when turgor is assessed, pulse and blood pressure are within normal age limits; weight is maintained.

Preoperatively, obtain a urine sample for urinalysis and blood for a complete blood count. IV fluid therapy may be initiated to hydrate a child who has been vomiting a great deal. Postoperatively, children may have a nasogastric tube in place, and they will be maintained on IV fluids until they can take adequate oral feedings (approximately 24 hours). With unruptured appendicitis, the postoperative course is uneventful and children are up a few hours after surgery and discharged within several days. They generally return to school in another week.

EVIDENCE-BASED PRACTICE

The onset of appendicitis is sudden and parents may be unable to arrange to room-in with their hospitalized child. Despite being encouraged and often included in medical rounds as a means to improve communication and increase their knowledge of and participation in their child's care, work responsibilities, care of siblings, a long commute to the hospital, and other types of situations may prevent parents from being with their child during the entire stay. Having daily interaction with the healthcare team lessens parental anxiety about their child's health (Yager, Clark, Cummings, et al., 2017). A study conducted by Yager et al. (2017) found that providing access to medical rounds through telemedicine to parents had a positive effect. It offered them reassurance regarding their child's care and increased their communication with the healthcare team.

Based on this study, the nurse determines which strategy is most effective to decrease parental anxiety when parents are unable to stay with their child for several hours during the day?

a. Offer to take notes on the medical rounds and verbally provide them to the parents when they arrive.
b. Offer to call them during medical team rounds, so they can participate.
c. Reassure them their child may receive more attentive care than a child whose parent is present.
d. Ensure the parents their child will be well cared for and they can call anytime to check on them.

Look in Appendix A for the best answer and rationale.

Ruptured Appendix

If a child's appendix has already ruptured when the child is seen in the emergency department, the potential for peritonitis increases greatly. Children generally appear severely ill. Their white blood cell count is apt to be more than 20,000/mm³. Position the child in a semi-Fowler's position, if possible, so that infected drainage from the cecum drains downward into the pelvis rather than upward toward the lungs. The child needs an IV fluid line inserted for hydration. Antibiotics will be begun preoperatively or as soon as the ruptured appendix is confirmed (Hung, Lin, & Chen, 2012).

During surgery, the child will have drains placed beside the surgery incision so any infectious material in the abdomen can continue to drain. Warm soaks to the incision line may be prescribed three or four times a day to encourage drainage. Examine the wound carefully at each dressing change. Be certain not to dislodge drains while removing soiled dressings. Report immediately any drain that is expelled because the surgeon may want to replace it to ensure a patent drainage route. Often, drains are shortened with each dressing change to encourage initially deep areas, then areas closer to the skin to drain. IV fluid and antibiotic therapy are continued until full bowel function is restored.

When changing dressings, also assess for signs of peritonitis such as a boardlike (rigid) abdomen, generally shallow respirations (because deep breathing puts pressure on the abdomen and causes pain), and increased temperature. Although the postoperative course is slower (approximately 3 weeks) after a ruptured appendix, the prognosis is still good. A local abscess or intestinal adhesions may result. Adhesion formation, a long-term effect, could interfere with fertility in girls or cause bowel obstruction in both sexes later in life.

What If . . . 45.2
Barry's older sister develops appendicitis, and the nurse meets them in the emergency room. Her parent tells the nurse she "dropped everything" to rush her there. What questions would the nurse want to ask to see if she has thought through the situation?

MECKEL'S DIVERTICULUM

In embryonic life, the intestine is attached to the umbilicus by the omphalomesenteric (vitelline) duct. This duct becomes a vestigial ligament as infants reach term. In 2% or 3% of all infants, however, a small pouch of this duct remains, located off the ileum, approximately 18 in. from the ileum–colon junction: a **Meckel's diverticulum** (Kloss, Bronton, & Sullivan, 2010). The structure often contains some misplaced gastric mucosa, which secretes gastric acids that flow into the intestine and irritate the bowel wall, leading to ulceration and bleeding. Children will have painless, tarry (black) stools or grossly bloody stools. On occasion, the diverticulum may serve as the lead point, causing an intussusception. In some instances, a fibrous band extending from the diverticulum pouch to the umbilicus acts as a constricting band, causing bowel obstruction.

The history of the child suggests the diagnosis. Because the pouch is small, it does not fill, and therefore, it may not be evident on X-ray or ultrasound. A nuclear medicine test called a Meckel's scan is used to identify the area of gastric mucosa in the intestine. Treatment is laparoscopy exploration and removal of the vestigial structure.

CELIAC DISEASE (MALABSORPTION SYNDROME, GLUTEN-INDUCED ENTEROPATHY, CELIAC SPRUE)

Celiac disease is an immune-mediated abnormal response to gluten, the protein in wheat, and related proteins in rye, barley and possibly oats, in a genetically susceptible individual. When children with the disorder ingest gluten, flattening of the fingerlike projections (villi) of the small intestine occurs, preventing the absorption of foods, especially fat, into the body. If the disease goes undiagnosed, children develop **steatorrhea** (bulky, foul-smelling, fatty stools), failure to thrive, and malnutrition. The classic picture of a child with celiac disease—a thin child with a distended abdomen (Fig. 45.7)—is rarely seen today as testing has improved and children are being diagnosed more promptly.

The illness occurs most frequently in children of a Northern European background, those with a first-degree relative with celiac disease, and those who have type 1 diabetes mellitus, IgA deficiency, and Down syndrome, suggesting an associated immune response. In Europe and the United States,

Therapeutic Management

Treatment is to continue the gluten-free diet for life because there is an associated slightly increased risk of malignancy in those who are diagnosed with celiac disease as adults. There does not appear to be the same risk in those diagnosed in childhood, possibly due to early introduction of a gluten-free diet (Hill et al., 2005). Correction of any vitamin and mineral deficiencies may be necessary.

 ## Nursing Diagnoses and Related Interventions

Nursing Diagnosis: Imbalanced nutrition, less than body requirements, related to malabsorption of food

Outcome Evaluation: Child's weight is maintained on a percentile curve on a growth chart, skin turgor is good, stool pattern and consistency is normal; parents verbalize appropriate gluten-free food choices.

Parents need a great deal of nutritional counseling when their child is first placed on a gluten-free diet so they can recognize foods that contain gluten (e.g., wheat, rye, oats, and barley products) and if possible, they should meet with a registered dietitian. They need to recognize that because gluten is a part of wheat flour, gravy, soups, and sauces as well as packaged and frozen foods. Because children are anorectic when they are first introduced to the new diet, getting them to eat it may be a problem. Remember that toddlers often eat small servings more readily than larger ones. Help parents create incentives to eat, such as inviting dolls to "tea" or having a picnic outside.

As children reach school age, preparing a gluten-free diet grows more and more difficult because favorite school-age foods such as spaghetti, pizza, hot dogs, cake, and cookies are not allowed. Selecting a diet in a school cafeteria may be tricky. Holidays pose additional problems as wheat-based birthday cakes, turkey stuffing, and holiday cookies are prohibited. Parents can learn to prepare gluten-free foods, and gluten-free foods have become more available in supermarkets and on restaurant menus. A Pavlova (made with meringue) can be substituted for a birthday cake and crushed potato chips are a good substitute for flour in many recipes. Until children can recognize which foods they can or cannot eat, parents often find it difficult to let them stay at friends' houses or go to summer camp, activities that are important to children learning independence. Eating gluten-free foods is a current food fad, so parents need to make it clear to school officials and friends that their child is not eating gluten free as a fad but because a gluten-free diet is lifesaving for their child (Pietzak, 2012).

Figure 45.7 A child with celiac disease. Typically, the child's abdomen will be distended from the fat, bulky stools. A wasted appearance (often of the buttocks) is no longer commonly seen.

prevalence estimates range from 1:80 to 1:300 children (Hill, Dirks, Liptak, et al., 2005). Although it is a relatively rare condition, early recognition is essential so treatment can be provided, along with early support and nutritional guidance for the parents.

Assessment

The diagnosis is based on the history; clinical symptoms such as poor growth, bulky stools, malnutrition, distended abdomen, and anemia, which usually become noticeable between 6 and 18 months of age, after the introduction of gluten into the diet. However, celiac disease can be diagnosed at any age. Serum analysis of antibodies against gluten (endomysial antibody, tissue transglutaminase is obtained) and biopsies of the small intestinal mucosa (done by endoscopy), which are the gold standards, establish the typical changes in intestinal villi. In addition, the child's response to gluten is observed by placing the child on a gluten-free diet. In most instances, the response to this diet is dramatic: The child begins to gain weight, steatorrhea improves, and irritability fades.

Disorders of the Lower Bowel

In children, disorders of the lower bowel mainly create problems with evacuation.

CONSTIPATION

Functional constipation, or constipation without an underlying medical disease, is a very common problem in childhood,

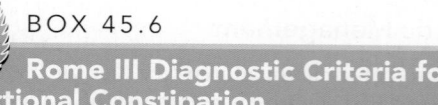

BOX 45.6

Rome III Diagnostic Criteria for Functional Constipation

In the absence of organic pathology, ≥2 of the following must occur:

FOR A CHILD WITH A DEVELOPMENTAL AGE <4 YEARS*

1. ≤2 defecations per week
2. At least 1 episode of incontinence per week after the acquisition of toileting skills
3. History of excessive stool retention
4. History of painful or hard bowel movements
5. Presence of a large fecal mass in the rectum
6. History of large-diameter stools that may obstruct the toilet

Accompanying symptoms may include irritability, decreased appetite, and/or early satiety, which may disappear immediately following passage of a large stool

FOR A CHILD WITH A DEVELOPMENTAL AGE ≥4 YEARS WITH INSUFFICIENT CRITERIA FOR IRRITABLE BOWEL SYNDROME†

1. ≤2 defecations in the toilet per week
2. At least 1 episode of fecal incontinence per week
3. History of retentive posturing or excessive volitional stool retention
4. History of painful or hard bowel movements
5. Presence of a large fecal mass in the rectum
6. History of large-diameter stools that may obstruct the toilet

*Criteria fulfilled for at least 1 month. Adapted from Hyman, P. E., Milla, P. J., Benninga, M. A., et al. (2006). Childhood functional gastrointestinal disorders: Neonate/toddler. *Gastroenterology*, 130(5), 1519–1526.
†Criteria fulfilled at least once per week for at least 2 months before diagnosis. Adapted from Rasquin, A., Di Lorenzo, C., Forbes, D., et al. (2006). Childhood functional gastrointestinal disorders: Child/adolescent. *Gastroenterology*, 130(5), 1527–1537.
Source: Tabbers, M. M., Dilorenzo, C., Berger, M. Y., et al. (2014). Evaluation and treatment of functional constipation in infants and children: Evidence-based recommendations from ESPGHAN and NASPGHAN. *Journal of Pediatric Gastroenterology and Nutrition*, 58(2), 258–274.

often starting in the first year of life. The definition of constipation is based on the Rome III Criteria (Box 45.6) and differs with the child's age (Tabbers, Dilorenzo, Berger, et al., 2014), but it is generally defined as either two or less bowel movements per week that cause distress to the child. Stools are often large, hard, and painful to pass. Anal fissures may develop. As passing stool is painful, the child represses the next urge to defecate to avoid pain. This is known as stool holding. The rectum gradually becomes distended and adjusts to the ever-present bulk of stool, and the urge to defecate becomes less frequent. When the child does pass stool, it is larger and even more firm than before and causes even more anal pain. This vicious cycle continues until the child becomes severely constipated. Children may have leakage of liquid stool or *encopresis* (involuntary release of stool) when their rectum can

hold no more (see Chapter 54). This is sometimes confused with diarrhea. The child may complain of abdominal pain and may have a decreased appetite.

Some children begin holding stool for psychological reasons. Once the process begins, however, the hardened stool, the anal fissures, and the pain on defecation soon occur, and what began for an emotional reason becomes a physical ailment. This is important to understand because with such children, therapy involves both counseling to correct the initial problem and treatment of the physical symptoms.

Assessment

When taking a history, be certain to have parents describe what they mean by constipation. Some children normally pass stool only every other day or every 3 days. As long as the stool is not hard and there is no discomfort associated with passing stool, it is not considered constipation. Examine the circumstances that may have led to constipation (e.g., diet low in fiber, little privacy in bathroom, family stress). It is also important to know the age of onset of the constipation, whether or not they are toilet trained, and if they exhibit stool withholding behaviors. Young children may hide when they need to defecate and may cry and turn red in the face with the effort of holding back the stool. In children who failed to pass meconium within the 48 hours of life, it is important to differentiate constipation from Hirschsprung disease. Other indications of an underlying problem include poor growth, congenital abnormalities, and a family history of GI disorders.

Therapeutic Management

Treatment of chronic constipation is aimed at softening stool so it will pass painlessly. Bowel cleansing to remove retained stool with weight-appropriate doses of polyethylene glycol is recommended before beginning daily treatment. Enemas are avoided if possible (Tabbers et al., 2014). After this, a stool softener such as polyethylene glycol is prescribed daily. Polyethylene glycol (Miralax) has been found to be the most effective medication for treating constipation. Normal fiber intake is recommended. There is no evidence that a high-fiber diet improves stool frequency in children (Chmielewska, Horvath, Dziechciarz, et al., 2011). Children should be encouraged to sit on the toilet after meals to attempt defecation. Young children respond well to positive reinforcement, and parents can use a sticker chart or other small rewards as motivation.

INGUINAL HERNIA

Inguinal hernia is a protrusion of a section of the bowel into the inguinal ring. It usually occurs in boys (9:1) because, as the testes descend from the abdominal cavity into the scrotum late in fetal life, a fold of parietal peritoneum also descends, forming a tube from the abdomen to the scrotum (García-Hernández, Carvajal-Figueroa, Suarez-Gutiérrez, et al., 2012). In most infants, this tube closes completely. If it fails to close, intestinal descent into it (hernia) may occur at any time when there is an increase in intra-abdominal pressure. In girls, the round ligament extends from the uterus into the inguinal canal to its attachment on the abdominal wall. In girls, an inguinal hernia may occur because of a weakness of the muscle surrounding the round ligament.

Assessment

A hernia appears as a lump in the left or right groin. In some instances, the hernia is apparent only on crying (when abdominal pressure increases) and not when children are less active. Inguinal hernias are painless. Pain at the site implies that the bowel has become incarcerated in the sac, which is an emergency that requires immediate action to prevent bowel obstruction and ischemia.

The diagnosis is established by a history and physical appearance. When taking a history of a well child, be certain to ask parents whether they have ever noticed any lumps in the child's groin area. The hernia may not be noticeable at the time of a healthcare visit, so, unless asked specifically, parents may not mention it. If present, the herniated intestine can be palpated in the inguinal ring on physical examination.

Therapeutic Management

Treatment of inguinal hernia is laparoscopy surgery. The bowel is returned to the abdominal cavity and retained there by sealing the inguinal ring. Pneumoperitoneum (instillation of carbon dioxide into the perineal cavity) during surgery may be performed to reveal the presence of an enlarged inguinal ring on the opposite side. If this is present, both sides may be repaired, and the child will return from surgery with dressings on both groins.

Formerly, surgery for inguinal hernia was delayed until the child was 3 or 4 years of age. Today, to prevent the complication of bowel strangulation—a surgical emergency—infants with inguinal hernia may have surgery before 1 year of age. If surgery is proposed as a prophylactic measure, setting outcomes may be difficult for parents as they weigh the value of surgical repair against the risk of anesthesia and surgery.

After surgery, keep the suture line dry and free of urine or feces to prevent infection. Most incisions in this area are closed by a tissue adhesive, which is waterproof and seals the incision from urine and feces. Even so, the infant will need frequent diaper changes and good diaper-area care. Assess circulation in the leg on the side of the surgical repair to be certain that edema of the groin is not compressing blood vessels and obstructing blood flow to the leg.

HIRSCHSPRUNG DISEASE (AGANGLIONIC MEGACOLON)

Hirschsprung disease, or *aganglionic megacolon*, is an absence of ganglionic innervation to the muscle of a section of the bowel—in most instances, the lower portion of the sigmoid colon just above the anus (Pakarinen, Kurvinen, Koivusalo, et al., 2013). The absence of nerve cells means there are no peristaltic waves in this section to move fecal material through the segment of intestine. This results in chronic constipation or ribbonlike stools (stools passing through such a small, narrow segment look like ribbons). The portion of the bowel proximal to the obstruction dilates, thus distending the abdomen (Fig. 45.8).

The incidence of aganglionic disease is higher in the siblings of a child with the disorder than in other children. It also occurs more often in males than in females. It is caused by an abnormal gene on chromosome 10. The incidence is approximately 1 in 5,000 live births (Stensrud, Emblem, & Bjørnland, 2012).

Assessment

Occasionally, infants are born with such an extensive section of bowel involved that even meconium cannot pass. Because newborn stools are normally soft, however, symptoms of aganglionic megacolon generally do not become apparent until 6 to 12 months of age. By this time, children appear thin and undernourished (sometimes deceptively so because

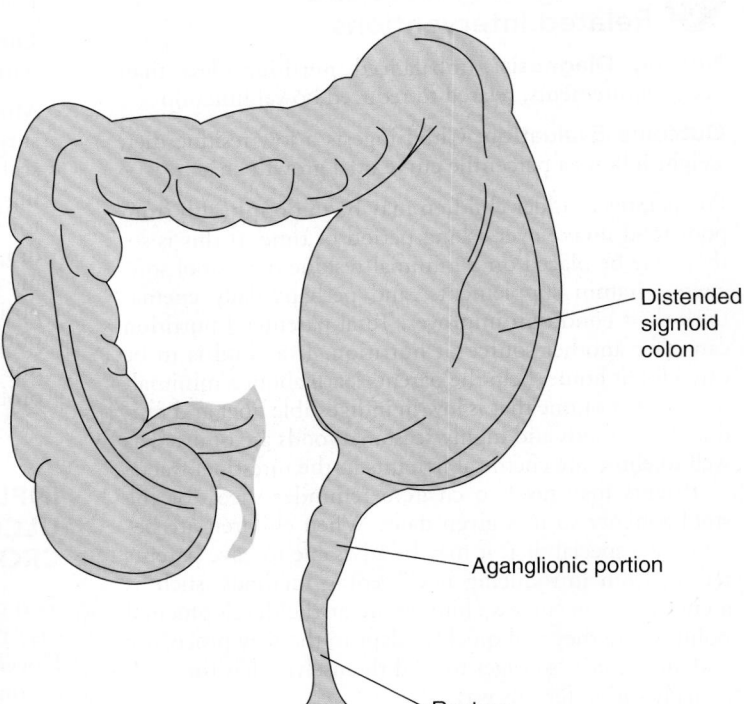

Figure 45.8 Aganglionic megacolon (Hirschsprung disease). The distal portion of the bowel lacks nerve innervation. Because there is no peristalsis in this narrowed segment, the bowel proximal to it distends markedly.

Distended sigmoid colon

Aganglionic portion

Rectum

their abdomen is large and distended) and have a history of not having a bowel movement more than once a week of ribbonlike or watery stools.

The diagnosis is suggested by a rectal exam; if a gloved finger is inserted into the rectum of a child with true constipation, the examining finger will touch hard, caked stool. With aganglionic colon disease, the rectum is empty because fecal material cannot pass into the rectum through the obstructed portion. A barium enema or ultrasound with contrast medium is generally prescribed to substantiate the diagnosis. The contrast mediums will outline the narrow, nerveless portion and the large proximal distended portion of the bowel. Enemas must be used cautiously, however, because children cannot expel this afterward any more effectively than they can stool. A definitive diagnosis is by a biopsy of the affected segment to show the lack of innervation or by anorectal manometry, a technique that tests the strength or innervation of the internal rectal sphincter by inserting a balloon catheter into the rectum and measuring the pressure exerted against it.

Therapeutic Management

Repair of aganglionic megacolon involves dissection and removal of the affected section, with anastomosis of the intestine (termed a pull-through operation). Because this is a technically difficult operation to perform in a small abdomen, the condition is generally treated in infants by two-stage surgery: First, a temporary colostomy is established, followed by bowel repair at 12 to 18 months of age. After the final surgery, children should have a functioning, normal bowel. In the few instances in which the anus is deprived of nerve endings, a permanent colostomy will need to be established.

🌀 Nursing Diagnoses and Related Interventions

Nursing Diagnosis: Imbalanced nutrition, less than body requirements, related to reduced bowel function

Outcome Evaluation: Child ingests a low-residue diet; weight follows a percentile curve on a growth chart.

Preoperatively, older children may be in poor health from poor food intake over a long period of time. If this is so, they may be placed on a minimal-residue diet, stool softeners, vitamin supplements, and perhaps daily enemas until their condition improves. Total parenteral nutrition can offer another source of nutrition. If a child is to be cared for at home, help the parents learn about a minimal-residue diet or one that is low in indigestible fiber and residue. Fried foods and highly seasoned foods are omitted as well to eliminate chemical irritants in the intestinal tract.

Parents may need to create a reminder sheet for the stool softener so it is given daily. When children are beginning a special diet, it may be advisable to have parents refrain from introducing new feeding methods, such as a cup or spoon, unless children are at the developmental point where they will quickly adapt to the new procedure and are, in fact, so eager to feed themselves that they will actually eat better this way.

Postoperatively, after removal of the aganglionic portion and anastomosis of the colon at the second step of the repair, infants will return with a nasogastric tube in place attached to low suction, an IV infusion, and probably an indwelling urinary (Foley) catheter. Observe the infant for abdominal distention. Assess bowel sounds and observe also for passage of flatus and stools. As soon as peristalsis has returned (approximately 24 hours after surgery), the nasogastric tube can be removed, and the child can be offered small, frequent feedings of fluids, such as water or gelatin. The child is then gradually introduced to full fluids, a soft diet, a minimal-residue diet, and, finally, a normal diet for age. Caring for a child with a colostomy is discussed in Chapter 37.

Nursing Diagnosis: Constipation related to reduced bowel function

Outcome Evaluation: Child has a daily bowel movement through either a colostomy or by enema.

Before surgery, the child may be prescribed daily enemas to achieve bowel movements. Remind parents that the fluid used for enemas must be normal saline (0.9% NaCl) and not tap water. Because tap water is hypotonic, if it is instilled into the bowel, it moves rapidly across the intestinal wall into interstitial and intravascular fluid compartments to equalize osmotic pressure. This has led to death of infants from cardiac congestion or cerebral edema (water intoxication). To use for enemas, parents can buy a ready-made saline preparation at a pharmacy, or they can prepare their own by mixing 2 teaspoon of noniodized salt to 1 qt of water. Although adding salt to water does not seem important, be certain parents understand the rationale for doing this so they consciously add the right proportion of salt to water.

Nursing Diagnosis: Risk for compromised family coping related to chronic illness in child

Outcome Evaluation: Parents state they are able to cope with the level of stress present from their child's condition.

Most parents feel tremendous relief after the second-stage surgery is complete. Caution parents that the child may still remain a "fussy eater" for a few months because feeding problems that begin for physical reasons can continue for emotional or psychological reasons. Help parents to diminish the importance of meals gradually; to schedule periods during the day when they give their full and positive attention to the child, such as reading a story or putting a puzzle together; and to offer praise for pleasant, not difficult, behavior. These measures will help mealtime problems gradually diminish.

INFLAMMATORY BOWEL DISEASE: ULCERATIVE COLITIS AND CROHN DISEASE

Two conditions are categorized as inflammatory bowel disease (IBD): *ulcerative colitis* and *Crohn disease* (Danese & Fiocchi, 2011). These disorders have some separate as well as some overlapping characteristics. Both involve the development of inflammation in the intestine. Ulcerative colitis

(UC) affects only the mucosal lining of the colon, whereas Crohn disease (CD) can affect any part of the GI tract from the mouth to the anus. The area most commonly involved in CD is the last part of the small intestine known as the terminal ileum. The inflammation in CD can extend through the wall of the intestine and cause abscesses and fistulae. About 25% of IBD cases are diagnosed in children younger than 20 years of age. The incidence in United States has been increasing (Kappelman, Moore, Allen, et al., 2013). The cause of IBD is unknown but thought to be multifactorial and due to an abnormal response by the immune system to an environmental trigger in a genetically susceptible individual.

Psychological factors have not been supported as a primary contributory factor to IBD, but psychological problems often occur secondary to the disease, possibly intensifying symptoms. Smoking has been shown to be a precipitating factor in CD (Ananthakrishnan, 2013).

Ulcerative Colitis

Children with UC develop crampy abdominal pain, urgency, tenesmus, and frequent bloody stools. Anemia and hypoalbuminemia due to losses in the stool may be present. It is treated with oral and sometimes IV medications such as infliximab (Remicade). If it does not respond to medical therapy, surgery to remove the colon is performed, which is curative for UC. There is an association between UC and colon carcinoma if the disease persists over 10 years. Yearly colonoscopy should be performed once the patient has reached 8 to 10 years from the date of diagnosis (Sengupta, Yee, & Feuerstein, 2016).

Crohn Disease

The symptoms of CD depend on the severity and location of the inflammation. Abdominal pain, diarrhea with or without blood, and weight loss may be present. The inflamed area may become narrowed causing a stricture of the bowel, and a bowel obstruction may develop if this goes untreated. Fistulae, small tunnels that run either from the bowel to the skin or to another organ, can develop. These most commonly involve the perianal area. CD is also treated with oral and IV medications depending on the severity of the disease. Remission has also been achieved with exclusive enteral feeding (Gupta, Nobel, Kachelries, et al., 2013). Surgery may be necessary to remove strictures or repair fistulae, but the disease can redevelop in other areas or the bowel. There are periods of exacerbations and remissions in both disorders. As inflammation becomes acute, children develop abdominal pain. Because the inflamed areas do not absorb nutrients or fluid well, diarrhea and malnutrition develop. To reduce abdominal pain, which is most acute after eating, when the bowel becomes active, children begin to skip meals. This can cause them to become malnourished and develop a vitamin or iron deficiency.

Assessment

In both conditions, diarrhea and steatorrhea develop from the irritation and the unabsorbed fluid. If inflamed portions ulcerate, there will be blood in the stool. Weight loss occurs; in prepubertal children, growth failure can occur. A recurring fever may be present (Table 45.5).

TABLE 45.5 COMPARISON OF CROHN DISEASE AND ULCERATIVE COLITIS

Comparison Factor	Crohn Disease	Ulcerative Colitis
Part of bowel affected	Ileum	Colon and rectum
Nature of lesions	Intermittent	Continuous
Diarrhea	Moderate	Severe and bloody
Anorexia	Severe	Mild
Weight loss	Severe	Mild
Growth retardation	Marked	Mild
Anal and perianal lesions	Common	None
Association with carcinoma	Rare	Common

Diagnosis is established by endoscopy and colonoscopy. Small biopsies with very low risk of bleeding are taken from multiple areas in the upper and lower GI tract. Inflammation, friability, and bleeding may be seen. The histology report shows chronic inflammation and sometimes granulomas in CD. A radiology study such as an MRI is usually obtained to examine the parts of the small bowel that can't be reached with an endoscope.

Therapeutic Management

In mild to moderate cases, oral medications are usually sufficient to control the symptoms. Vitamin and mineral deficiencies should be corrected. In more severe cases, bowel rest may be indicated to allow the bowel to heal. Enteral or total parenteral nutrition, therefore, is usually provided for nutrition during the resting period. A child can remain home during this period as long as parents have thorough education about the child's nutritional needs (see Chapter 37).

When food is reintroduced after the resting period, a high-protein, high-carbohydrate, and high-vitamin diet is prescribed to replace nutrients. Children may eat cautiously at first to avoid reintroducing diarrhea, so assess intake and output carefully. The treatment regimen depends on the child's condition. In more severe cases, remission is usually achieved with corticosteroids or infliximab (Remicade), an antibody to the inflammatory cytokine tumor necrosis factor alpha. Maintenance therapy may be with infliximab or mercaptopurine (immunomodulator) or mesalamine alone or a combination of medications (Box 45.7). If surgery for UC becomes necessary, the procedure is performed in two stages. During the first stage, total colectomy is performed and an ileostomy created. Several months later, an ileoanal pouch is created and the ileostomy is taken down (Fig. 45.9). This allows the child to be continent of stool.

Bowel surgery is always a serious step, but because it reduces the possibility of the child developing colon cancer in association with UC, it may be necessary in children whose disease is running a long-term, debilitating course that does not improve (Danese & Fiocchi, 2011). Caution parents, although they want their children to be independent with regard to bathroom use, to always report if change in the color or consistency of bowel movements does occur so a relapse can be detected.

BOX 45.7

Nursing Care Planning Based on Responsibility for Pharmacology

5-AMINOSALICYLATES (MESALAMINE, SULFASALAZINE, BALSALAZIDE)

Classification: anti-inflammatory agent

Mechanism of Action: Unknown, but it is thought that it acts topically in the bowel to reduce inflammation.

Pregnancy Risk Category: C (D at term)

Dosage: 50 mg/kg/day given either divided into two to four doses. Rectal formulation usually given 1–2 times daily.

Possible Adverse Effects: sensitivity to sunlight, dizziness, drowsiness, nausea, abdominal pains, crystalluria, and hematuria

Nursing Implications

- Caution the parents and child that the drug may turn urine orange-red and soft contact lenses yellow.
- Advise children to take with or just after meals to avoid GI irritation.
- Ensure adequate fluid intake to avoid crystallization of sulfa component in urine.
- Anticipate prescription for folic acid concurrently if sulfasalazine used. Drug decreases folic acid absorption.
- Instruct the child and parents about the need to use sunscreens and protective clothing while outside.

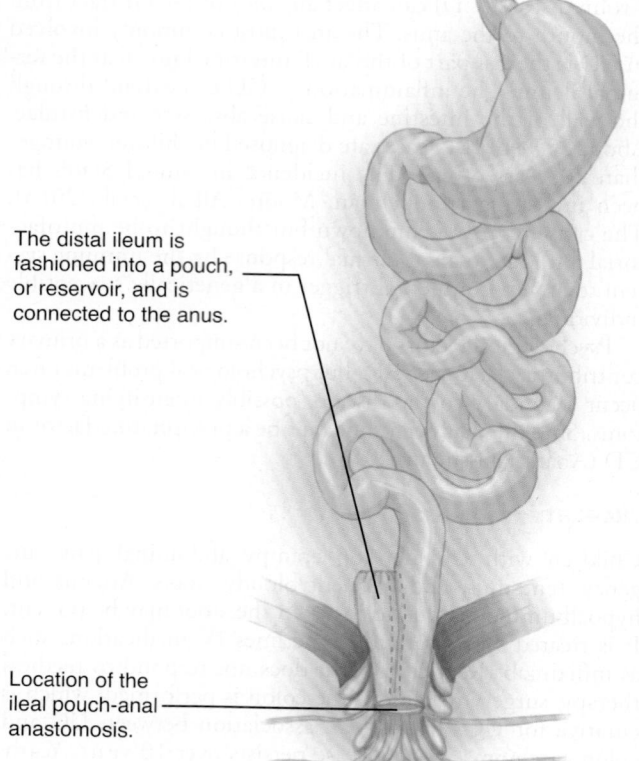

The distal ileum is fashioned into a pouch, or reservoir, and is connected to the anus.

Location of the ileal pouch-anal anastomosis.

Figure 45.9   Ileoanal pouch. (From Craven, R. F., Hirnle, C. J., & Henshaw, C. M. [2017]. *Fundamentals of nursing: Human health and function* [8th ed.]. Philadelphia, PA: Wolters Kluwer.)

Nursing Diagnoses and Related Interventions

Nursing Diagnosis: Imbalanced nutrition related to poor absorption because of disease process

Outcome Evaluation: Child's weight follows a percentile growth curve; urine specific gravity is 1.003 to 1.030; child states that alternative feeding method is tolerable.

Nutrition is a priority concern for children with IBD, especially those with CD, because malnutrition can occur from the combination of poor intestinal absorption and chronic diarrhea. If the disease is not well controlled and inflammation persists, children can be left both short in stature and light in weight. Treatment with steroids can also cause growth retardation. The advent of biologic medications such as infliximab has greatly decreased the need to use long courses of prednisone. Active disease can result in protein, vitamin, fat, and mineral deficiencies.

When nutrition is supplied by enteral or total parenteral nutrition solutions, allowing the enteral infusion to flow during the night and removing the tube during the day can make feedings more tolerable. Remember that food provides social experiences as well as nutrition. Help parents provide opportunities for usual mealtime stimulation in other ways.

Nursing Diagnosis: Risk for ineffective coping related to chronic illness

Outcome Evaluation: Child expresses feelings, states she understands the disease and therapy; suggests ways to minimize stress.

Caution children about possible side effects, such as excessive weight gain, a round facial appearance, and facial acne, which may occur if corticosteroid therapy, such as prednisone, is used so they are not surprised by this. Assess blood pressure, intake and output, weight, and sleep patterns for any child taking steroids. Provide time to listen so children have someone outside their family to talk to about their symptoms and family or stress problems (Box 45.8). The disorder follows a chronic course and can involve embarrassing episodes of diarrhea or acute abdominal pain.

What If . . . 45.3

Barry's older sister, who has Crohn disease, is being cared for at home with total parenteral nutrition. How can the nurse help her keep pace with her friends at school? How can the nurse help her maintain a sense of high self-esteem in light of her many hospitalizations, total parenteral nutrition, and home care?

BOX 45.8
Nursing Care Planning Tips for Effective Communication

Barry's older sister Addie has Crohn disease. Her primary care provider has informed her parents she won't need surgery but will need long-term treatment that will include both medical and nutritional therapy. You see Mrs. Abraham filling out forms by Addie's bedside.

Tip: Explore the parents' understanding of any instructions and help them receive more accurate information when needed. People under stress often do not hear instructions well. When this happens, they may need instructions repeated several times before they truly comprehend what was said.

Be careful not to ignore situations that arise where a parent may not have heard everything they were told about their child's condition and the full implications. In the following scenario, Mrs. Abraham does not realize Addie will need ongoing treatment.

Nurse: Mrs. Abraham, can I help you with anything?

Mrs. Abraham: No. I'm filling out forms for Addie to go back to school since she'll be well again in a short time.

Nurse: Do you mean Addie doesn't need parenteral nutrition?

Mrs. Abraham: She needs to eat, sure. But no surgery.

Nurse: Addie needs to regain her strength before she goes back to school. Do you know what is meant by parenteral nutrition?

IRRITABLE BOWEL SYNDROME

Irritable bowel syndrome (IBS) is a functional bowel disorder that typically causes symptoms of abdominal pain and altered bowel habits with no underlying organic cause. It should not be confused with IBD. It may be either constipation or diarrhea predominant or there may be a mixed picture (Chiou & Nurko, 2010). Diagnosis is based on the Rome III Criteria (see Box 45.6). It is a common disorder in adolescents and adults and thought to affect 15% of the population with a 2:1 female to male predominance (Brandt, Chey, Foxx-Orenstein, et al., 2009). The symptoms can adversely affect quality of life and cause children to miss school (Youssef, Murphy, Langseder, et al., 2006).

The cause is unknown. The onset of loose stools can follow an infection and may be due to an alteration in the intestinal flora. Other studies have looked at intestinal bacterial overgrowth, food sensitivities, visceral hyperalgesia (heightened sensitivity to bowel distension), and psychosocial factors.

Antidepressants, anticholinergics, and antibiotics that work to reduce bacteria in the gut such as rifaximin may be prescribed to treat the symptoms of IBS (Chiou & Nurko, 2010).

CHRONIC RECURRENT ABDOMINAL PAIN

Chronic recurrent abdominal pain is also a functional disorder. The pain is episodic to continuous, and the cause is unknown (Collins & Lin, 2010). Children who experience this are commonly 6 or 7 years of age or in prepuberty (11 to 12 years of age). The pain is not accompanied by a change in bowel habits. There is no association with meals. It is also generally poorly localized, although children may point to the umbilicus as the primary site. On physical examination, there is no abdominal tenderness, distention, guarding, or muscle spasm. Symptoms of stress such as sleep disturbances, fears, or eating problems may be present. A family history may indicate problems in the family such as marital discord, financial problems, or physical illness in parents or siblings.

Although the cause of the pain cannot be identified, the pain is real. Treatment for functional abdominal pain and IBS are similar and includes dietary changes such as increased fiber and probiotics, medications, behavioral, and complementary therapy (Chiou & Nurko, 2010). Cognitive behavioral therapy teaches the child coping strategies, such as distraction techniques and relaxation, and has been shown to reduce abdominal pain in at least 70% of children (Duarte, Penna, Andrade, et al., 2006). Parents are trained to redirect the child after pain complaints and use positive reinforcement. Hypnosis has also been shown to be an effective adjunct therapy (Vlieger, Menko-Frankenhuis, Wolfkamp, et al., 2007).

Disorders Caused by Food, Vitamin, and Mineral Deficiencies

There are many underfed and malnourished children in every part of the world. Although extreme diseases of food or vitamin deprivation are rare in the United States, they do exist. Such children need early identification so they can receive better nutrition before permanent damage occurs.

The average child does not develop a deficient intake of essential nutrients because, even if the child is occasionally a fussy eater, over the space of a week, a child does ingest foods containing the necessary nutrients. Carefully assess any child who has an interference in nutrition such as a GI illness or a child is receiving enteric feedings or total parenteral nutrition to make sure that nutrient deficiencies do not exist. Assess children who have been maltreated or neglected closely for nutritional deficiencies because they may not have been given adequate food.

KWASHIORKOR

Kwashiorkor, a disease caused by protein deficiency, occurs most frequently in children ages 1 to 3 years because this age group requires a high-protein intake. It is a disease found almost exclusively in developing countries in Africa, Asia, and Latin America, although it does occur in the United States (Boyd, Andea, & Hughey, 2013). It tends to occur after weaning, when children change from breast milk to a diet consisting mainly of carbohydrates. Growth failure is a major symptom. Because edema is also a symptom, however, children may not appear light in weight until the edema is relieved. There is a severe wasting of muscles, but, again, this is masked by the edema.

Edema results from hypoproteinemia, which causes a shift of body fluid from the intravascular compartments to the interstitial space, causing ascites. The edema tends to be dependent, so it is first noted in the lower extremities. Children are generally irritable and uninterested in their surroundings. They fall behind other children of the same age in motor development.

If the child had a period of good protein intake, then poor protein intake, and then good intake again, hair shafts develop a striped appearance of brown, then white, and so on—a "zebra sign." Children also have diarrhea, iron-deficiency anemia, and enlarged livers.

Without treatment, kwashiorkor is fatal. For therapy, a diet rich in protein is essential. Even so, there is evidence to suggest that protein malnutrition early in life, even if corrected later, may result in failure of children to reach their full potential of intellectual and psychological development.

QSEN Checkpoint Question 45.6 ✔

TEAMWORK & COLLABORATION

Barry's aunt and uncle adopted a toddler from a developing country. The nurse learns that a dietitian has been working with the family because of the child's history of kwashiorkor. The nurse would expect the dietitian to prioritize what nutrient in this child's diet?

a. Water-soluble vitamins
b. Fats and triglycerides
c. Quality protein
d. Vitamin K

Look in Appendix A for the best answer and rationale.

NUTRITIONAL MARASMUS

Nutritional marasmus is caused by a deficiency of all food groups—basically, a form of starvation. Although it is seen most commonly in developing countries where food supplies are scarce, it can be seen in the United States in grossly neglected children or those with failure to thrive (see Chapter 55). These children are most commonly younger than 1 year of age. They have many of the same symptoms as children with kwashiorkor, including growth failure, muscle wasting, irritability, iron-deficiency anemia, and diarrhea. Whereas children with kwashiorkor are anorectic, children with nutritional marasmus are invariably hungry (starving) and will suck at any object offered to them, such as a finger or their clothing. Treatment is a diet rich in all nutrients. Like children with kwashiorkor, they may suffer cognitive challenges that persist throughout life (Galler, Bryce, Waber, et al., 2012).

VITAMIN AND MINERAL DEFICIENCIES

Both vitamin and mineral deficiencies occur at a low rate in children of the United States because so many foods are enriched (restoration of ingredients removed by processing) or fortified (additional vitamins and minerals not normally present have been added). Milk, for example, is fortified with vitamins D and A. Orange juice is fortified with calcium. White bread is enriched with B vitamins. Vitamin deficiency diseases are summarized in Table 45.6.

What If . . . 45.4
The nurse is particularly interested in exploring one of the 2020 National Health Goals with respect to GI disorders in children (see Box 45.1). What would be a possible research topic to explore pertinent to this goal that would be applicable to the Abraham family and that would also advance evidence-based practice?

TABLE 45.6 VITAMIN DEFICIENCY DISORDERS

Vitamin	Cause of Deficiency	Signs and Symptoms
Vitamin A	Lack of yellow vegetables in diet	Tender tongue, cracks at corners of mouth, night blindness
		Xerophthalmia (dry and lusterless conjunctivae)
		Keratomalacia (necrosis of the cornea with perforation, loss of ocular fluid, and blindness)
Vitamin B_1	Most common in children who eat polished rice as dietary staple because B_1 is contained in hull of rice	**Beriberi** (tingling and numbness of extremities, heart palpitations, exhaustion)
		Diarrhea and vomiting
		Aphonia (crying without sound)
		Anesthesia of feet
Niacin	Common in children who eat corn as dietary staple because corn is low in niacin	**Pellagra** (dermatitis, resembles a sunburn), diarrhea, mental confusion (dementia)
Vitamin C	Lack of fresh fruits in diet	**Scurvy** (muscle tenderness, petechiae)
Vitamin D	Lack of sunlight	Poor muscle tone, delayed tooth formation
		Rickets (poor bone formation)
		Craniotabes (softening of the skull)
		Swelling at joints, particularly of wrists and cartilage of ribs
		Bowed legs, tetany (muscle spasms)

KEY POINTS FOR REVIEW

- Some GI disorders lead to long-term therapies such as colostomy or gastrostomy feedings. Because these disorders interfere with common body functions such as eating and elimination, they are difficult for children to accept without the support of concerned healthcare providers.

- Children lose proportionately more fluid with vomiting and diarrhea than adults, so they need rapid assessment and interventions to avoid dehydration.

- Fluid, electrolyte, and acid–base imbalances tend to occur rapidly with vomiting and diarrhea. Vomiting leads to alkalosis. Diarrhea leads to acidosis.

- GI disorders almost always interfere with nutrition to some degree. This is a greater problem in children than adults because children need to ingest adequate nutrients and fluid daily for growth as well as body maintenance.

- Gastroesophageal reflux is the passage of gastric contents into the esophagus with or without regurgitation and vomiting. In infants, it is treated by feeding a thickened formula and keeping the infant upright after feedings. Adolescents are prescribed a proton pump inhibitor and advised to sleep with two pillows.

- Pyloric stenosis is hypertrophy of the valve between the stomach and duodenum. It impedes the passage of feedings, leading to vomiting, and is repaired by surgery.

- Peptic ulcer disease may occur in children of all ages. The disorder causes a shallow excavation to form in the mucosal wall of the stomach. It is treated, like adult ulcers, with antibiotics and agents to suppress gastric acidity.

- Forms of hepatitis seen in children include hepatitis A (fecal–oral transmission) and hepatitis B, C, D, and E (caused by contaminated blood or body fluids and IV drug use). Vaccines to hepatitis A and B are available and are routinely given to children.

- Biliary atresia is an obliterative disorder of the extrahepatic biliary tree that occurs within the first 2 months of life. This can lead to fibrotic scarring of the liver (cirrhosis). Most of these children need a liver transplant to restore liver function.

- Intussusception is the invagination of one portion of the intestine into another. Volvulus is a twisting of intestine. Both may lead to bowel obstruction.

- Necrotizing enterocolitis is the development of necrotic patches in the intestine. It occurs almost exclusively in preterm infants.

- Appendicitis is inflammation of the appendix. It is always an emergency and is the most common reason for abdominal surgery in children. A laparoscopy is done to remove the appendix, ideally before it ruptures.

- Celiac disease (gluten-induced enteropathy) is a change in the ability of the intestinal villi to absorb nutrients. Children must follow a gluten-free diet for life.

- Inguinal hernia can occur in children. It is surgically corrected when recognized.

- Hirschsprung disease (aganglionic megacolon) is absence of ganglionic innervation in a section of the lower bowel. Therapy may involve a temporary colostomy followed by surgery in 6 to 12 months to remove the affected bowel portion.

- Inflammatory bowel disease can occur as either ulcerative colitis or Crohn disease, both chronic conditions. Therapy is long term. If medical therapy is unsuccessful, portions of the bowel may be surgically removed. Ulcerative colitis is associated with the development of colon cancer later in life.

- Kwashiorkor (protein deficiency), nutritional marasmus (starvation), vitamins A and D (rickets), vitamin B_1 (beriberi), and vitamin C (scurvy) deficiencies occur in children when they are not provided or cannot absorb adequate nutrients. Although more common in developing countries, they can occur in a child in any community.

- Children with GI disorders should join the family for mealtimes if possible. Even if they cannot eat the same foods as other family members, this helps not only meet QSEN competencies but also allows children to benefit from the social interaction.

CRITICAL THINKING CARE STUDY

Shanita is a 3-year-old you see in the emergency room because she has had 12 diarrheal stools in the past 8 hours. She lives with her single mother in a rented apartment in the inner city. Her mother works in the local potato chip factory. Because it was such a hot day, Shanita spent the day at the park with a playmate (Dwight, also 2 years of age) and his mother Iris. Iris called Shanita's mother at 2 PM to come home because Shanita was feeding their new puppy some hard dog food and Iris was afraid Shanita might have eaten some herself because she began to have diarrhea.

1. Shanita's mother is worried that because her clothes always smell of hot grease, this has made Shanita sick. Is it more likely the smell of grease; possibly eating some hard dog food; or eating a packed lunch of a hotdog, potato salad, and a soda is the main cause of the diarrhea?

2. Shanita is not yet toilet trained. If you need to separate Shanita's urine from stool so you can better evaluate the consistency of her stool, would you ask her to void frequently or try not to void when she has a bowel movement?

3. What point of care tests could you do to evaluate whether Shanita's diarrhea is improving?

RELATED RESOURCES

Explore these additional resources to enhance learning for this chapter:
- Student resources on thePoint, including answers to the What If . . . and Critical Thinking Care Study questions, http://thepoint.lww.com/Flagg8e
- Adaptive learning powered by PrepU, http://thepoint.lww.com/prepu

REFERENCES

Ananthakrishnan, A. N. (2013). Environmental triggers for inflammatory bowel disease. *Current Gastroenterology Reports, 15*(1), 302.

Bailey, M. B., Shiau, R., Zola, J., et al. (2011). San Francisco hep B free: A grassroots community coalition to prevent hepatitis B and liver cancer. *Journal of Community Health, 36*(4), 538–551.

Bansal, S., Banever, G. T., Karrer, F. M., et al. (2012). Appendicitis in children less than 5 years old: Influence of age on presentation and outcome. *American Journal of Surgery, 204*(6), 1031–1035.

Barros, F. C., Victora, C. G., Forsberg, B., et al. (1991). Management of childhood diarrhoea at the household level: A population-based survey in north-east Brazil. *Bulletin of the World Health Organization, 69*(1), 59–65.

Bhatia, J., Gates, A., & Parish, A. (2010). Medical management of short gut syndrome. *Journal of Perinatology, 30*(Suppl. 1), S2–S5.

Boyd, K. P., Andea, A., & Hughey, L. C. (2013). Acute inpatient presentation of kwashiorkor: Not just a diagnosis of the developing world. *Pediatric Dermatology, 30*(6), e240–e241.

Brandt, L. J., Chey, W. D., Foxx-Orenstein, A. E., et al. (2009). An evidence-based position statement on the management of irritable bowel syndrome. *The American Journal of Gastroenterology, 104*(Suppl. 1), S1–S35.

Centers for Disease Control and Prevention. (2016a). *Rotavirus prevention.* Retrieved from https://www.cdc.gov/rotavirus/about/prevention.html

Centers for Disease Control and Prevention. (2016b). *What is viral hepatitis?* Retrieved form https://www.cdc.gov/hepatitis/abc/index.htm

Chiou, E., & Nurko, S. (2010). Management of functional abdominal pain and irritable bowel syndrome in children and adolescents. *Expert Review of Gastroenterology & Hepatology, 4*(3), 293–304.

Chmielewska, A., Horvath, A., Dziechciarz, P., et al. (2011). Glucomannan is not effective for the treatment of functional constipation in children: A double-blind, placebo-controlled, randomized trial. *Clinical Nutrition, 30*, 462–468.

Collins, B., & Lin, H. (2010). Chronic abdominal pain in children is associated with high prevalence of abnormal microbial fermentation. *Digestive Diseases and Sciences, 55*(1), 124–130.

Danese, S., & Fiocchi, C. (2011). Ulcerative colitis. *The New England Journal of Medicine, 365*(18), 1713–1725.

Daniels, D., Grytdal, S., & Wasley, A. (2009). Surveillance for acute viral hepatitis—United States, 2007. *Morbidity and Mortality Weekly Report, 58*(3), 1.

D'Antiga, L. (2012). Medical management of esophageal varices and portal hypertension in children. *Seminars in Pediatric Surgery, 21*(3), 211–218.

Duarte, M. A., Penna, F. J., Andrade, E. M., et al. (2006). Treatment of nonorganic recurrent abdominal pain: Cognitive-behavioral family intervention. *Journal of Pediatric Gastroenterology and Nutrition, 43*(1), 59–64.

Faramawi, M. F., Johnson, E., Chen, S., et al. (2011). The incidence of hepatitis E virus infection in the general population of the USA. *Epidemiology and Infection, 139*(8), 1145–1150.

Galler, J. R., Bryce, C., Waber, D. P., et al. (2012). Socioeconomic outcomes in adults malnourished in the first year of life: A 40-year study. *Pediatrics, 130*(1), e1–e7.

García-Hernández, C., Carvajal-Figueroa, L., Suarez-Gutiérrez, R., et al. (2012). Laparoscopic approach for inguinal hernia in children: Resection without suture. *Journal of Pediatric Surgery, 47*(11), 2093–2095.

Garrow, D., & Delegge, M. H. (2010). Risk factors for gastrointestinal ulcer disease in the US population. *Digestive Diseases and Sciences, 55*(1), 66–72.

Gluud, L., Vilstrup, H., & Morgan, M. (2016). Non-absorbable disaccharides versus placebo/no intervention and lactulose versus lactitol for the prevention and treatment of hepatic encephalopathy in people with cirrhosis. *Cochrane Database of Systematic Reviews,* (5), CD003044.

Guarino, A., Ashkenazi, S., Gendrel, D., et al. (2014). European Society for Pediatric Gastroenterology, Hepatology, and Nutrition/European Society for Pediatric Infectious Diseases evidence-based guidelines for the management of acute gastroenteritis in children in Europe: Update 2014. *Journal of Pediatric Gastroenterology and Nutrition, 59*(1), 132–152.

Gupta, K., Noble, A., Kachelries, K. E., et al. (2013). A novel enteral nutrition protocol for the treatment of pediatric Crohn's disease. *Inflammatory Bowel Diseases, 19*(7), 1374–1378.

Hardee, L. K. (2012). Quality improvement: Universal protocol use in office-based gastrointestinal procedure units. *Gastroenterology Nursing, 35*(6), 380–382.

Hill, I. D., Dirks, M. H., Liptak, G. S., et al. (2005). Guidelines for the diagnosis and treatment of celiac disease in children: Recommendations of the North American Society for Pediatric Gastroenterology, Hepatology and Nutrition. *Journal of Pediatric Gastroenterology and Nutrition, 40*(1), 1–19.

Huether, S. E. (2012). Alterations of digestive function in children. In S. E. Huether & K. L. McCance (Eds.), *Understanding pathophysiology* (5th ed., pp. 938–953). Philadelphia, PA: Elsevier Mosby.

Hung, M. H., Lin, L. H., & Chen, D. F. (2012). Clinical manifestations in children with ruptured appendicitis. *Pediatric Emergency Care, 28*(5), 433–435.

Hwang, J. H., Shergill, A. K., Acosta, R. D., et al. (2014). The role of endoscopy in the management of variceal hemorrhage. *Gastrointestinal Endoscopy, 80*(2), 221–227.

Iqbal, C. W., Rivard, D. C., Mortellaro, V. E., et al. (2012). Evaluation of ultrasonographic parameters in the diagnosis of pyloric stenosis relative to patient age and size. *Journal of Pediatric Surgery, 47*(8), 1542–1547.

Kaido, T., Mori, A., Ogura, Y., et al. (2012). Pre- and perioperative factors affecting infection after living donor liver transplantation. *Nutrition, 28*(11–12), 1104–1108.

Kappelman, M. D., Moore, K. R., Allen, J. K., et al. (2013). Recent trends in the prevalence of Crohn's disease and ulcerative colitis in a commercially insured US population. *Digestive Diseases and Sciences, 58*(2), 519–525.

Karch, A. M. (2013). *2013 Lippincott's nursing drug guide.* Philadelphia: PA: Lippincott Williams & Wilkins.

Kloss, B. T., Bronton, C. E., & Sullivan, A. M. (2010). Perforated Meckel diverticulum. *International Journal of Emergency Medicine, 3*(4), 455–457.

Koletzko, S., Jones, N. L., Goodman, K. J., et al. (2011). Evidence-based guidelines from ESPGHAN and NASPGHAN for Helicobacter pylori infection in children. *Journal of Pediatric Gastroenterology and Nutrition, 53*(2), 230–243.

Ladd, M. R., Neff, L. P., Becher, R. D., et al. (2012). Computerized tomography in the workup of pediatric appendicitis: Why are children scanned? *The America Surgeon, 78*(6), 716–721.

Laurence, N., & Pollock, A. N. (2012). Malrotation with midgut volvulus. *Pediatric Emergency Care, 28*(1), 87–89.

Leder, M. R. (2012). Acute sexual assault and evidence collection in the DNA era. *Clinical Pediatric Emergency Medicine, 13*(3), 194–201.

Lee, L. Y., Abbott, L., Mahlangu, B., et al. (2012). The management of cyclic vomiting syndrome: A systematic review. *European Journal of Gastroenterology & Hepatology, 24*(9), 1001–1006.

Mandeville, K., Chien, M., Willyerd, F. A., et al. (2012). Intussusception: Clinical presentations and imaging characteristics. *Pediatric Emergency Care, 28*(9), 842–844.

Moritz, M. L., & Ayus, J. C. (2011). Intravenous fluid management for the acutely ill child. *Current Opinion in Pediatrics, 23*(2), 186–193.

Nelson, S. P., Chen, E. H., Syniar, G. M., et al. (2000). Prevalence of gastroesophageal reflux during childhood: A pediatric practice-based survey. *Archives of Pediatrics & Adolescent Medicine, 154*(2), 150.

Orenstein, S. R., & McGowan, J. D. (2008). Efficacy of conservative therapy as taught in the primary care setting for symptoms suggesting infant gastroesophageal reflux. *The Journal of Pediatrics, 152*(3), 310–314.

Ortiz, G. S., O'Connor, T., Carey J., et al. (2017). Impact of a child life and music therapy procedural support intervention on parental perception of their child's distress during intravenous placement. *Pediatric Emergency Care.* Advance online publication. doi:10.1097/PEC.0000000000001065

Pakarinen, M. P., Kurvinen, A., Koivusalo, A. I., et al. (2013). Surgical treatment and outcomes of severe pediatric intestinal motility disorders requiring parenteral nutrition. *Journal of Pediatric Surgery, 48*(2), 333–338.

Pandya, S., & Heiss, K. (2012). Pyloric stenosis in pediatric surgery: An evidence-based review. *The Surgical Clinics of North America, 92*(3), 527–539.

Pietzak, M. (2012). Celiac disease, wheat allergy, and gluten sensitivity: When gluten free is not a fad. *Journal of Parenteral and Enteral Nutrition, 36*(1 Suppl.), 68S–75S.

Porth, C. M. (2011). Gastrointestinal & hepatobiliary function. In C. M. Porth (Ed.), *Essentials of pathophysiology* (3rd ed., pp. 164–184). Philadelphia, PA: Lippincott Williams & Wilkins.

Rimon, A., & Freedman, S. B. (2010). Recent advances in the treatment of gastroenteritis. *Clinical Pediatric Emergency Medicine, 11*(3), 163–170.

Rogers, K. L. (2017). Radiology. In H. K. Hughes & L. Kahl (Eds.), *The Harriet Lane handbook* (21st ed., pp. 663–687). Philadelphia, PA: Elsevier.

Roznovsky, L., Orsagova, I., Kloudova, A., et al. (2010). Long-term protection against hepatitis B after newborn vaccination: 20-year follow-up. *Infection, 38*(5), 395–400.

Sengupta, N., Yee, E., & Feuerstein, J. D. (2016). Colorectal cancer screening in inflammatory bowel disease. *Digestive Diseases and Sciences, 61*(4), 980–989.

Smith, S. (2011). Infectious diseases. In K. J. Marcdante, R. M. Kliegman, H. B. Jenson, et al. (Eds.), *Nelson essentials of pediatrics* (6th ed., pp. 355–462). Philadelphia, PA: Saunders/Elsevier.

Stensrud, K. J., Emblem, R., & Bjørnland, K. (2012). Late diagnosis of Hirschsprung disease—patient characteristics and results. *Journal of Pediatric Surgery, 47*(10), 1874–1879.

Sundaram, S., Hoffenberg, E., Kramer, R., et al. (2011). Gastrointestinal tract. In W. Hay, M. Levin, R. Deterding, et al. (Eds.), *Current diagnosis & treatment: Pediatrics* (21st ed., pp. 595–630). New York, NY: McGraw-Hill/Lange.

Tabbers, M. M., Dilorenzo, C., Berger, M. Y., et al. (2014). Evaluation and treatment of functional constipation in infants and children: Evidence-based recommendations from ESPGHAN and NASPHGAN. *Journal of Pediatric Gastroenterology and Nutrition, 58*(2) 258–274.

Underwood, M. A. (2013). Human milk for the premature infant. *Pediatric Clinics of North America, 60*(1), 189–207.

U.S. Department of Health and Human Services. (2010). *Healthy people 2020.* Washington, DC: Author.

Vajro, P., Lenta, S., Socha, P., et al. (2012). Diagnosis of nonalcoholic fatty liver disease in children and adolescents. *Journal of Pediatric Gastroenterology Nutrition, 54*(5), 700–713.

Vandenplas, Y., Rudolph, C. D., Di Lorenzo, C., et al. (2009). Pediatric gastroesophageal reflux clinical practice guidelines: joint recommendations of the North American Society for Pediatric Gastroenterology, Hepatology, and Nutrition (NASPGHAN) and the European Society for Pediatric Gastroenterology, Hepatology, and Nutrition (ESPGHAN). *Journal of Pediatric Gastroenterology and Nutrition, 49*(4), 498–547.

Vlieger, A., Menko-Frankenhuis, C., Wolfkamp, S., et al. (2007). Hypnotherapy for children with functional abdominal pain or irritable bowel syndrome. *Gastroenterology, 133*(5), 1430–1436.

Vongbhavit, K., & Underwood, M. A. (2016). Prevention of necrotizing enterocolitis through manipulation of the intestinal microbiota of the premature infant. *Clinical Therapeutics, 38*(4), 716–732

Wang, D. H., & Souza, R. F. (2011). Biology of Barrett's esophagus and esophageal adenocarcinoma. *Gastrointestinal Endoscopy Clinics of North America, 21*(1), 25–38.

Wheeler, R. A. (2011). Appendicitis in children and young people. *Clinical Risk, 17*(1), 126–129.

Yager, P. H., Clark, M., Cummings, B. M., et al. (2017). Parent participation in pediatric intensive care unit rounds via telemedicine: Feasibility and impact. *The Journal of Pediatrics.* Advance online publication. doi:10.1016/j.jpeds.2017.02.054

Youssef, N. N., Murphy, T. G., Langseder, A. L., et al. (2006). Quality of life for children with functional abdominal pain: A comparison study of patients' and parents' perceptions. *Pediatrics, 117*(1), 54–59.

46

Nursing Care of a Family When a Child Has a Renal or Urinary Tract Disorder

Carey Hendricks is a 4-year-old girl admitted to the hospital with marked ascites and edema from nephrotic syndrome. She lives with her grandparents because her mother is incarcerated on a drug charge. "She's been gaining weight yet doesn't eat anything," her grandmother tells you. "She drank part of a beer I left on the coffee table last week. Could that be what caused this? What if she needs a kidney transplant? Will I be allowed to give a kidney to her?"

Previous chapters described the growth and development of well children and the nursing care of children with disorders of other systems. This chapter adds information about the dramatic changes, both physical and psychosocial, that occur when children develop urinary tract or renal disorders. This information builds a base for assessment, care, and health teaching.

How would you answer Carey's grandmother? What information does she need to better understand her grandchild's condition?

OBJECTIVES

After mastering the contents of this chapter, you should be able to:

1. Describe common renal and urinary disorders that occur in children.

2. Identify 2020 National Health Goals related to renal or urinary tract disorders in children that nurses can help the nation achieve.

3. Assess a child for a renal or urinary tract disorder.

4. Formulate nursing diagnoses related to renal or urinary disorders in children.

5. Understand expected outcomes for a child with a renal or urinary tract disorder in order to most effectively assist families in managing transitions throughout their child's healthcare experience.

6. Using the nursing process, plan nursing care that includes the six competencies of Quality & Safety Education for Nurses (QSEN): Patient-Centered Care, Teamwork & Collaboration, Evidence-Based Practice (EBP), Quality Improvement (QI), Safety, and Informatics.

7. Describe the process of implementation of nursing care for a child with a renal, bladder, or urinary tract disorder.

8. Evaluate expected outcomes for achievement and effectiveness of care.

9. Integrate knowledge of renal and urinary tract disorders with the interplay of nursing process, the six competencies of QSEN, and Family Nursing to promote quality maternal and child health nursing care.

BOX 46.1

Nursing Care Planning Based on 2020 National Health Goals

Renal disease can lead to long-term illness, so preventing it is important to improving the health of the nation. 2020 National Health Goals that address this concern are:

- Reduce the rate of new cases of end-stage renal disease from a baseline of 300 per 1 million population to a target rate of 221 per 1 million population.
- Increase the proportion of patients with treated chronic kidney failure who receive a transplant within 3 years of end-stage renal disease from a baseline of 17.1% to 18.8% (U.S. Department of Health and Human Services, 2010; see www.healthypeople.gov).

Nurses can help the nation achieve these goals by educating parents to give antibiotics conscientiously for streptococcal throat infections and being active advocates for organ transplant procedures.

Normally, the urinary system maintains the proper balance of fluid and electrolytes in the blood. When disease occurs, such as with structural abnormalities or kidney malfunction, children may be left with excessive amounts of fluid in the body or with an imbalance of electrolytes essential to body functioning that becomes long term (Ring & Huether, 2013).

Unfortunately, because symptoms may be vague, or because children or parents do not realize the seriousness of urinary tract disease (or are embarrassed to discuss it), children may not be evaluated at the first sign of illness. Therefore, health education aimed at increasing awareness of symptoms of urinary tract and kidney disorders is an important area of family health teaching. Box 46.1 shows 2020 National Health Goals related to renal disorders and children.

Nursing Process Overview

FOR CARE OF A CHILD WITH A RENAL OR URINARY TRACT DISORDER

ASSESSMENT

Because the symptoms of many urinary tract and renal disorders, such as mild abdominal pain, slowly increasing edema, or low-grade fever, are subtle, school nurses play an important role in recognizing the seriousness of such minor symptoms and making referrals for care.

Pain can be, but is not always, a symptom of kidney or bladder infection. Be sure to assess the degree of any pain, including its location and intensity, before administering an analgesic or antispasmodic to aid with diagnosis or prognosis. Assisting patients with properly procuring a urine specimen is another important means of ensuring accurate assessment of the patient.

NURSING DIAGNOSIS

Nursing diagnoses used with children with urinary tract or renal disorders are related to the symptoms these disorders

cause plus the effect chronic disease can have on a family. Some examples include:

- Pain related to bladder irritation from urinary tract infection
- Excess fluid volume related to decreased kidney function and fluid accumulation
- Fear related to renal transplantation
- Imbalanced nutrition, less than body requirements, related to effects of dietary restrictions
- Social isolation related to immunosuppressant therapy
- Interrupted family processes related to the stress of a child's chronic illness
- Compromised family coping related to the chronic nature of a child's illness

OUTCOME IDENTIFICATION AND PLANNING

Be certain that outcomes established for care are relevant to a child's age and condition. If renal disease becomes chronic, expected outcomes may need to be modified frequently to meet the evolving needs of both the child and the family unit.

Planning for a child with a urinary tract or renal disorder often involves helping parents develop a reliable system to remember to give medicine. A child with nephrotic syndrome or a renal transplant, for example, may need to take three or four different types of medicine every day, often at different times. Be certain parents understand the types of medicine prescribed and the expected action and side effects of each. Parents should receive this information both verbally and in written form so that they have easy-to-access information at home. If the school a child attends has a zero tolerance policy for taking medication at school, the child will need proper documentation from his or her medical provider in order for the school to make accommodations.

It is important to assist parents in scheduling times for hemodialysis or peritoneal dialysis as well as planning for care of their other children and around their work schedules. This should help them achieve balance among all tasks that need to be done. If a child develops severe renal impairment, parents may be asked to make a decision regarding kidney removal and transplantation. Provide them with ample time and resources for discussion about this because offering to be a living kidney donor is a major life step. Examples of organizations that are helpful for referral include the National Kidney Foundation (www.kidney.org), the Polycystic Kidney Disease Foundation (www.pkdcure.org), the Urology Care Foundation (www.urologyhealth.org), and the Kidney Dialysis Foundation (www.kdf.org.sg).

IMPLEMENTATION

Neither parents nor children may fully understand the function of the urinary system because it is not a system that receives much discussion. For example, they may confuse the words "ureter" and "urethra." Nurses should be knowledgeable resources, explaining anatomy, tests and procedures, and the rationale for various testing. In addition, nurses should be patient advocates and facilitate opportunities for family/provider discussions when indicated.

Many children with kidney disease take a corticosteroid for immunosuppression and so develop a typical cushingoid appearance with edema or ascites, making them appear obese. This can lead to teasing or bullying by classmates because of their "different" appearance. Contacting the school (with the child's and parents' permission) to assist with appropriate education of classmates can facilitate peer understanding and foster support in the school environment. Frequent contact and discussion with the child's siblings is also important to help them understand their sibling's medical situation, the reasons for so many tests and healthcare visits, and why their sibling is receiving so much attention. It is important to recognize that a chronic health condition affects the entire family, and each member of the family unit deserves care and understanding.

If kidney damage becomes extensive and the child's kidneys fail or a transplant is rejected, nursing care needs to be refocused on helping the family to face the possibility of the child's death. Caring for children with a near-fatal or fatal diagnosis is discussed in Chapter 56.

OUTCOME EVALUATION

Children with urinary or renal disease often require long-term follow-up care after their acute illness to monitor their renal and bladder function. Even though their child is being followed by a specialty renal group or clinic, remind parents that routine health maintenance such as routine childhood immunizations (although children taking steroids or other immunosuppressive therapy should not receive live-virus vaccines) remains important.

Examples suggesting achievement of outcomes are:
- Child reports that pain is at a tolerable level and decreasing in intensity after treatment.
- Family members state they are able to cope with long-term illness in their child.
- Child states the purpose of a low-sodium diet and lists the ingredients of a low-sodium meal.
- Child states he or she can accept the need for kidney transplantation.
- Child states the precautions he or she must follow to reduce possibility of infection while on immunosuppressive therapy.

Anatomy and Physiology of the Kidneys

Embryonic development of the urinary tract is discussed in Chapter 9. Figure 46.1 identifies the structures of the tract. Kidneys in children are located slightly lower in relation to the ribs than in adults. They also do not have as much perinephric fat to pad them, making their kidneys more vulnerable to trauma than in an adult.

KIDNEY FILTRATION

The glomeruli in the kidney filter water and solutes from the blood. The process is only effective, however, if the blood pressure is higher in the arteries going into the kidneys than in the internal tubular arteries. Urine production is also dependent on the blood pressure being lower in the arteries leaving the kidneys than in the internal tubular arteries. For this reason, renal function must be assessed carefully in children who present with either decreased or increased blood pressure.

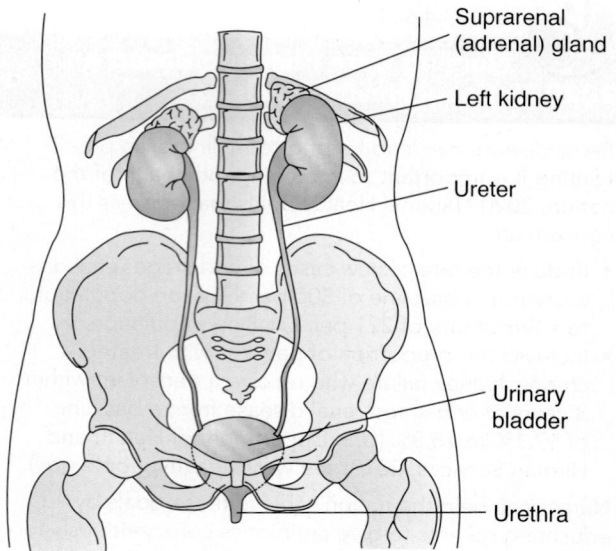

Figure 46.1 The urinary system.

Whereas hypertension in adults is most often associated with cardiac dysfunction or disease, in pediatric patients, hypertension is most often associated with renal dysfunction.

URINE

Approximate urine output from different age groups is shown in Table 46.1. A significant decrease in urine production is *oliguria*; absence of urine production is *anuria*.

When renal disease occurs and glomerular or tubular function becomes impaired, nonprotein nitrogenous substances such as creatinine, urea, ammonia, and purine bodies are retained in the blood rather than being excreted. The amount of urea in urine is an indirect indication of kidney and liver function.

Creatinine is a product released during muscle cell metabolism. The amount excreted in urine normally remains constant regardless of the amount of protein in the diet or body processes. When it is less in amount, therefore, it means kidneys are not functioning as well as usual. *Casts* are formed when there is an abnormal condition that causes the kidney tubule to become lined with protein formed from red and white blood cells, epithelial cells, or fatty cells that harden into the shape of the tubule. After urine washes the casts out, they can be detected by microscopic examination of urine. Because protein deposits in this way only when fluid is slow-moving, their presence suggests slow filtration.

TABLE 46.1 CHILD'S AVERAGE URINE OUTPUT IN 24 HOURS

Age	Amount of Urine (ml)
6 months–2 years	540–600
2–5 years	500–780
5–8 years	600–1,200
8–14 years	1,000–1,500
Over 14 years	1,500

Assessment of Renal and Urinary Tract Dysfunction

Assessment of urinary or renal tract disorders is based on history, physical examination, and laboratory/diagnostic tests (Box 46.2). Remember when taking the history of a child with a urinary or renal disorder that discussing this area of the body may not be comfortable for the child or parents (Box 46.3).

LABORATORY/DIAGNOSTIC TESTS

A variety of diagnostic tests may be performed, either in an ambulatory department or in an inpatient basis, to document renal or urinary tract disease.

Urinalysis

Urinalysis is not only one of the most revealing tests of kidney function but also one of the simplest. For best results, specimens collected should be fresh because urine that stands

BOX 46.3

Nursing Care Planning to Respect Cultural Diversity

As a general rule, because elimination functions are typically regarded as private, this is not a body system that all people discuss as comfortably as they do illnesses of other body systems. The more modesty is stressed in a culture, the more difficult it may be for people to ask questions about this system's disorders. By being aware that this is a difficult area for parents to discuss, health-care personnel can better observe whether added health education is needed when caring for a child with one of these disorders.

at room temperature for any length of time changes composition. Techniques for obtaining urine samples such as clean-catch, catheterization, 24-hour collections, and suprapubic aspiration are described in Chapter 37. A chemical reagent strip can be used to detect glucose, protein, and occult blood and to measure pH. Specific gravity is best determined by use of a refractometer (requires only a single drop; see Chapter 37).

Urine Culture

A urinary tract infection (UTI), or the presence of bacteria in urine, is diagnosed by urine culture. Urine for culture can be obtained by several techniques including midstream clean-catch, catheterization, or sterile suprapubic aspiration (see Chapter 37). The technique used should be determined by the provider and will be influenced by the patient's age, medical history, toilet training status, and cooperation. The test result interpretation varies depending on the technique. For example, a positive result from a clean-catch sample is >50,000 CFU/ml, whereas the positive threshold for a sterile catheterized sample or suprapubic aspirate is >10,000 CFU/ml (Roberts, Downs, Finnell, et al., 2011).

Radioisotope Scanning

The administration of radioisotopes (a technetium scan) is another way to assess glomeruli filtration ability. For this, radioactively tagged substances are given intravenously; the rate at which these substances flow through the kidney and are excreted in urine is then determined. The level of radioisotopes used in these studies is small, and urinating removes the substance from the body immediately afterward. You can assure parents that children do not remain radioactive after the procedure so that parents are not afraid to stay near their children or to hold them.

Blood Studies

A blood urea nitrogen (BUN) test measures the level of urea in blood or how well the kidneys can clear urea from the bloodstream. A normal value is 5 to 20 mg/100 ml.

Glomerular filtration rate is the rate at which substances are filtered from the blood to the urine. It is measured by the amount of creatinine (the breakdown product of creatine from muscle contraction) in blood serum or excreted in 24 hours as determined by a 24-hour urine sample. A normal creatinine clearance rate is 100 ml/min. A normal urine

BOX 46.2

Nursing Care Planning Using Assessment

ASSESSING A CHILD FOR RENAL AND URINARY TRACT DYSFUNCTION

History
Chief concern: Child reports burning or cries on urination; bloody or "dark" urine, frequency of urination; abdominal pain, flank pain, enuresis. Parents report increase in size of abdomen, periorbital edema, poor appetite, frequent thirst, weight gain, strong odor to urine; diaper rash in infants. A school-age child may be described as a behavior problem because he or she frequently asks to use the bathroom.
Family history: History of renal disease, such as polycystic kidney, enuresis; hypertension.
Pregnancy history: Exposure to nephrotoxic drugs (antibiotics) during pregnancy. Oligohydramnios at birth.
Past illness history: Child recently had a throat or skin infection.

Physical assessment
General appearance
Fatigue, paleness
Growth restriction
Low-grade temperature

Mouth
Pale mucous membrane, caries

Cardiovascular
Hypertension

Respiratory
Rapid respirations

Back
Pain over kidney area

Genitals
Reddened urethra
Diaper area rash in infants
Constant dripping of urine
A stronger than usual arc of urine in males
Displaced urethral opening

Skin
Poor skin turgor
White crystals on skin
Edema

Head
Swelling around eyes
Odd facies; beaklike nose, small chin, prominent epicanthal folds, low-set ears

Chest
Gynecomastia

Abdomen
Tenderness over bladder area
Abdominal mass
Slack abdominal muscles
Protuberant abdomen

Extremities
Bowed legs

Neurologic
Confusion, muscle twitching

creatinine level is 0.7 to 1.5 mg/100 ml; creatinine in blood serum rarely exceeds 1 mg/dl (Huether, 2013).

Ultrasonography and Magnetic Resonance Imaging

Either a *sonogram* or *magnetic resonance imaging* (MRI) can show differing sizes of kidneys or ureters and illustrate the difference between solid or cystic kidney masses. Because they do not involve X-rays, both ultrasound and MRI may be repeated at frequent intervals for follow-up without danger of radiation exposure (Nelson, Chow, Rosoklija, et al., 2012). When explaining ultrasound and MRI tests, compare the machines used to a camera so it's an object familiar to children and not as frightening.

X-Ray Studies

A flat-plate abdominal radiograph can provide information about the size and contour of the kidneys and may be referred to as a *KUB* (*k*idney, *u*reters, and *b*ladder). *Computed tomography* (CT) scans of the kidneys reveal both the size and density of kidney structures and adequacy of urine flow. Conscious sedation may be given before a CT scan because the size of a CT scanner can be frightening and a child must lie still for an extended time during the procedure. However, many children's hospitals are now staffed by child life specialists who can often prepare and support a child through a CT scan without sedation. If a contrast medium will be injected to better outline urine flow, be certain to ask about allergy to iodine before the study because the injected medium is iodine based and is therefore contraindicated in a person with an iodine allergy. As with MRI, explaining to the child that the machine used is much like a large camera can help reduce fear. When preparing a child for a test with an injected medium, caution children that they may experience flushing of the face, warmth, and a salty taste in their mouth after the injection of the "medicine."

Intravenous Pyelogram

An *intravenous pyelogram* (IVP) is an X-ray study of the upper urinary tract. For the procedure, a radiopaque dye is injected into a peripheral vein, circulates through the bloodstream, and is almost immediately identified as a foreign substance by the kidneys and filtered out into the urine by the glomeruli. Radiographs taken at frequent intervals during the test show the outline of collecting systems in the kidney and of the ureters as the radiopaque dye passes through them.

Voiding Cystourethrogram

A *voiding cystourethrogram* (VCUG), a study of the lower urinary tract, reveals the structure of the urethra and bladder and the presence of reflux into the ureters (Lum, 2012). After bladder catheterization, a radiopaque dye is injected into the bladder, and the catheter is then removed. The child is asked to void into a bedpan while serial X-ray films are taken. Although the catheterization can be unpleasant, being asked to void while supine and being observed may be the most stressful part of the procedure for children because they have been taught that voiding is a private act. Be sure children are told in advance that they will be asked to do this and that it is all right if a stranger watches them (something they have been taught to avoid as well). The first void after catheterization

may be painful, but you can assure the child that this is usually only a one-time occurrence and that drinking plenty of water following the test dilutes the urine and decreases dysuria. Pouring warm water over the perineal area while sitting on a toilet or sitting in a bathtub of warm water and voiding into the water can also be helpful but is rarely necessary.

A VCUG should not be done if a child has an active UTI because there is danger the radiopaque material injected into the bladder could spread bacteria from the bladder, up the ureters to the kidneys, causing pyelonephritis. Therefore, report any symptoms of a UTI, such as urinary frequency, dysuria, or low-back pain, to the radiologic service before the procedure so that the child can be properly evaluated and the test rescheduled if necessary.

Cystoscopy

Cystoscopy, or examination of the bladder and ureter openings by direct examination with a cystoscope introduced into the bladder through the urethra, may be done to evaluate for possible vesicoureteral reflux or urethral stenosis. Radiopaque dye may be introduced into the bladder at the time of cystoscopy so the bladder can be visualized on X-ray. During the procedure, small catheters can be threaded into the ureters for the introduction of dye to outline them (retrograde pyelography). Because the procedure is painful and requires a child to lie still, it is usually done under anesthesia. As with catheterization for VCUG, the first void after cystoscopy may be uncomfortable, and the child should be adequately prepared for this.

QSEN Checkpoint Question 46.1

TEAMWORK & COLLABORATION

Carey is undergoing a VCUG to help diagnose whether she has vesicoureteral reflux. A nurse collaborates with the radiology technician to ensure an accurate test that does not cause distress for Carey. What should the nurse emphasize in order to achieve these goals?

   a. The technician will have to read the instructions for the test to Carey.
   b. Lying in a large, metal tube is frightening for most children.
   c. Children often feel uncomfortable voiding in public.
   d. The dye capsules may be too large for Carey to swallow.

Look in Appendix A for the best answer and rationale.

Renal Biopsy

Renal biopsy involves passing a thin biopsy needle into the kidney through the skin over the kidney. The procedure is used to diagnose the extent of renal disease and thereby predict disease outcome or progress or reveal beginning rejection of a transplanted kidney (Tse, Yadav, Herrema, et al., 2013).

Renal biopsy may be done in an older child under only local anesthesia, but conscious sedation may be necessary for a younger child who cannot cooperate easily. The kidney is located first by ultrasound to accurately locate the best place for the biopsy. The child lies prone with a sandbag under the abdomen for firmness. If the procedure is done under a local anesthetic, prepare children for the feel of a pinprick as the local anesthetic is injected; after this, they should not feel any further pain. They will feel pressure, however, as the biopsy needle is inserted. Caution children they need to lie still while the biopsy specimen is taken (if the child moves suddenly, the needle might puncture a renal artery or vein or tear vital glomeruli). Be certain children have support people to remain with them for this procedure, so they have someone to hold their hand or comfort them when they feel the pressure of the needle.

After the biopsy, press a sterile square gauze against the biopsy site for approximately 15 minutes to halt bleeding and then apply a pressure dressing. Caution parents beforehand that a large dressing will be used, so they don't think the size of the dressing reflects the size of the specimen taken (the amount of tissue removed is actually no more than the lumen of the needle used, or about the size of a pencil lead).

Measure vital signs and observe the biopsy site every 15 minutes for at least the first hour afterward. Do not lift the dressing to assess bleeding because doing so destroys the protective function of the pressure dressing. If the procedure is done on an ambulatory basis, children can be discharged 2 to 4 hours after the procedure if vital signs are stable and they have voided. Encourage children to drink a considerable amount of fluid (a glass every hour while awake) during the first 24 hours to keep urine flowing freely and prevent blood from clotting in the kidney tubules and blocking urine flow. Play games with the child, if necessary, to encourage a high fluid intake (the child must take a drink each time before a turn at a game, or play "Simon Says" and have Simon frequently say, "Drink").

The first void after renal biopsy is invariably tinged with blood. Advise parents to restrict their child's activity for 24 hours or until no more blood (hematuria) is present. Instruct parents how to properly obtain and view serial urine samples, comparing each specimen with the previous one, to detect whether hematuria is increasing or decreasing. When urine no longer appears bloody, they can test it for occult blood a final time to confirm that all bleeding has stopped. The treating provider may order hematocrit to be tested 24 hours after the procedure in order to confirm that bleeding has ceased.

🌿 *What If . . . 46.1*

Carey's grandmother telephones the nurse after a kidney biopsy and says Carey is voiding black urine. She asks whether there is a possibility Carey is voiding blood. What recommendations should the nurse make to the grandmother?

Therapeutic Measures for the Management of Renal Disease

Because kidney function is necessary for life, if it deteriorates, therapies to replace renal function must be instituted.

PERITONEAL DIALYSIS

Dialysis is the separation and removal of solutes from body fluid by diffusion through a semipermeable membrane. *Peritoneal dialysis* uses the membrane of the peritoneal cavity to do this. Hemodialysis circulates blood through an outside

synthetic membrane to do this. Unlike hemodialysis, peritoneal dialysis does not require elaborate equipment or expense, but it does take more time. Peritoneal dialysis may be used as a temporary measure for children who experience sudden renal failure caused by trauma or shock. It is also used for fairly long periods with children with chronic renal disease to allow them to live until kidney transplantation can be arranged (Issa, Lankireddy, & Kukla, 2012).

It is usually begun when the serum creatinine level reaches 10 mg/100 ml. Other indications are congestive heart failure, BUN of more than 100 mg/100 ml, hyperkalemia (potassium level of more than 6 mEq/L), and uremic encephalopathy (confusion or coma). Continuous peritoneal dialysis allows the procedure to be done at home because less rigorous monitoring of the procedure is necessary.

Performing Peritoneal Dialysis

Before peritoneal dialysis begins, a child's weight and vital signs need to be obtained to provide baseline information. Ask the child to void to reduce bladder size, so the bladder occupies as little anterior space as possible; if a child cannot void, catheterization may be necessary. Following this, the child's abdomen is cleaned just below the umbilicus with an antiseptic solution and covered with a sterile drape; a local anesthetic is injected into the abdominal wall, and a large-bore needle is inserted into the peritoneal cavity. If ascites fluid is present, a quantity of this fluid is removed and then a warmed hypertonic glucose solution (approximately 50 to 100 ml/kg of body weight) or a commercial dialysis solution is infused by gravity flow into the peritoneal cavity. This distends the abdominal wall and allows safe insertion of a peritoneal catheter, which is sutured into place and covered with a sterile dressing (Fig. 46.2). This catheter will remain in place for the duration of dialysis.

As for any procedure, children need to be well prepared for peritoneal dialysis, but if the procedure is presented in a matter-of-fact way, children usually accept it with no more apprehension than IV therapy as both procedures involve a needle penetration. Caution children they will feel the initial prick of the needle that administers the local anesthetic but then will feel only pressure after that as the peritoneal needle or catheter is inserted. The procedure is intrusive, however, and can therefore be frightening. Provide opportunities for therapeutic play such as letting the child handle a cloth doll, a dialysis tube, IV tubing, a doll's bed, or syringes as they become familiar with the procedure.

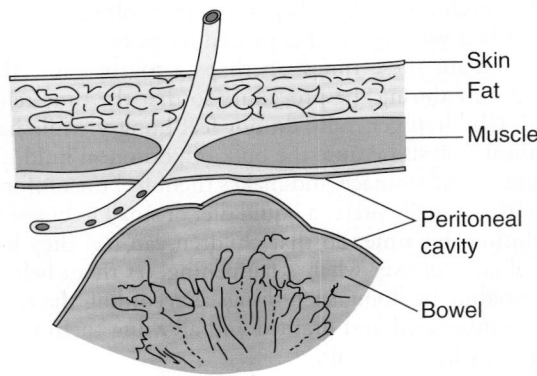

Figure 46.2 Insertion site for a peritoneal dialysis catheter.

With the dialysis tube in place, a prescribed amount of dialysis solution is infused into the peritoneal cavity by gravity drainage. This takes approximately 10 minutes and is recorded as *inflow* time. Be certain the infusion fluid is warmed to room temperature to prevent the child from becoming chilled; warming the solution in a basin of warm water or with the use of commercial warm packs so it is near body temperature also appears to improve diffusion efficiency. Heparin may be added to the first infusion to keep any initial bleeding from the abdominal puncture from plugging the tube.

The infused fluid is allowed to remain in the child's peritoneal cavity for 15 to 60 minutes (called the *equilibrium* or *dwell time*) while fluid, urea, and electrolytes move by osmosis from extracellular spaces into the hypertonic solution. After the designated equilibrium time has passed, drain the fluid from the peritoneal catheter into a collecting bottle (this takes approximately 10 minutes and is recorded as *outflow* time). More fluid generally drains from the peritoneal cavity than was infused because excessive fluid has diffused across the peritoneum, reducing accumulated peritoneal or ascitic fluid.

Peritoneal dialysis may be conducted continuously for periods of 12 to 72 hours, depending on the effectiveness of the procedure in restoring serum creatinine and BUN levels to normal.

Monitor vital signs at least every hour, or per the provider's order, while children are undergoing peritoneal dialysis. Frequent blood studies are necessary during periods of peritoneal dialysis to determine electrolyte concentrations. If electrolyte imbalances occur, electrolytes may be added to the infusion solution or administered IV. During each new infusion period and while the solution is in the abdomen, carefully observe for shortness of breath because the fluid exerts upward pressure on the diaphragm. Elevating the head of the bed a little usually helps to increase breathing space and ease respirations. If either tachycardia or hypotension occurs, this suggests that hypovolemia is occurring or fluid is moving too rapidly into the peritoneal cavity. An increasing temperature (after 24 hours) suggests peritoneal infection (Sayed, Abu-Aisha, Ahmed, et al., 2013).

Follow the agency's policy for cleaning and covering the end of the peritoneal catheter if there are periods when dialysis is halted (Fig. 46.3). The longer the peritoneal catheter remains in place, the greater is the risk of infection. Always assess the tube insertion site daily for redness or drainage. Use palpation to assess the abdomen for guarding or tenderness (rigidity suggest peritonitis or infection). Ask children to report any abdominal pain or diarrhea.

Once cycles of dialysis begin, children often grow bored lying in bed waiting for this procedure to be finished. Plan interaction for these times—perhaps a toy or game that is allowed only during the procedure so that the time remains special. Children generally do not feel hungry while having peritoneal dialysis because the bulk of peritoneal fluid causes pressure on the stomach and makes them feel uncomfortably full, so they usually prefer a liquid diet or small frequent feedings during this time. So that children can feel they have a sense of control over what is happening, let them help with the procedure by doing such things as recording the amount of solution infused and drained and allowing them to select liquids they like for meals.

Peritoneal dialysis is a simple yet important procedure. Help parents understand its importance for their child, so

Figure 46.3 Peritoneal catheter inserted into a child's abdomen. A secure dressing surrounds the insertion site to prevent infection. (Courtesy of Karen M. Polise, MSN, RN, Division of Nephrology, The Children's Hospital of Philadelphia.)

they can demonstrate a positive attitude toward it because their acceptance of the procedure helps the child accept it as well.

Continuous Cycling Peritoneal Dialysis

Continuous cycling peritoneal dialysis (CCPD) allows a child to go to school or participate in other activities while receiving dialysis (Davenport, 2012). With CCPD, a permanent dialysis catheter is inserted and sutured into place at the abdomen. Although commercial devices may be used, for the simplest method, the child or parent attaches a bag of dialysis fluid and tubing to this and infuses a prescribed dialysis solution by gravity drainage; the bag and tubing are then rolled into a compact square under the child's clothes. The infused solution remains in the child for 4 to 6 hours during the day (8 hours at night); the dialysate bag is then lowered, and the solution drains from the peritoneal cavity into it. The bag and fluid are then discarded and a new bag of dialysate solution is attached and raised, and new solution is infused.

CCPD requires careful monitoring and attention by the child or family, so there is a record of the amount of fluid infused. Children on CCPD can participate in gym programs but should not participate in contact sports or swimming. Teach parents to think ahead for holidays or family trips so they do not run short of supplies.

Because CCPD is continuous, electrolytes in the bloodstream are maintained at more constant levels than when intermittent dialysis is used. A great deal of potassium is removed, however, so caution is needed or children may become hypokalemic (Lum, 2012). The main advantage is that CCPD allows greater freedom for children to attend school. There are disadvantages, however, such as infection resulting from the long-term placement of the catheter and dehydration or hypernatremia resulting from excess fluid removal. Because the tube remains in place at all times and the peritoneal solution constantly distends the abdomen, the child appears obese and clothing is difficult to fit, frequently reminding the child of the illness. Possible complications of CCPD are summarized in Table 46.2.

TABLE 46.2 POSSIBLE COMPLICATIONS OF CONTINUOUS CYCLING PERITONEAL DIALYSIS

Assessment	Problem	Interventions
Redness, pain, or swelling at tube insertion site	Infection	Report findings; take culture of site; administer antibiotics or other site care as prescribed.
Abdominal pain, increased temperature, nausea and vomiting, cloudy return in drainage solution	Peritonitis	Report findings; administer antibiotics as prescribed; auscultate for bowel sounds with vital sign assessment.
Cramps as fluid is infused	Irritation of peritoneal cavity	Infuse solutions more slowly; warm temperature of solution to body temperature.
Difficulty with infusion or drainage of fluid	Kinked or clotted tubing; malpositioned catheter	Assess tubing for kinking; change position of child; ask child to cough to increase abdominal pressure; add prescribed amount of heparin to dialysate bag (prevents clotting).
Weight increase; moist cough, shortness of breath	Fluid overload	Assess blood pressure and weight; decrease sodium and fluid oral intake as prescribed; possibly decrease strength of dialysis fluid as prescribed.
Weight loss, hypotension, poor skin turgor, tachycardia	Fluid loss	Assess blood pressure and weight; increase fluid and sodium intake as prescribed.
Blood-tinged dialysis return	Ruptured capillary vessel	Report findings; assess pulse and blood pressure; observe for further bleeding in drainage; flush catheter with prescribed amount of heparin to keep clots from forming.

What If . . . 46.2
Carey, who receives CCPD, wants to go to her church camp this summer. Her grandmother asks the nurse whether this would be a good experience for Carey. What factors would the nurse want to know about the camp? About Carey? About her dialysis regimen?

HEMODIALYSIS

Hemodialysis removes body wastes by using an external membrane as the diffusion surface. For hemodialysis, a catheter is inserted into an artery and blood is removed from the child and circulated through a dialysis coil. Urea and electrolytes in the blood diffuse into the surrounding fluid bath as the blood passes through the coil (Hothi, Stronach, & Harvey, 2013). After diffusion is complete, the blood is returned to the child's venous circulation (Fig. 46.4).

Hemodialysis can be done as a continuous process, but it is so effective that 3 hours of hemodialysis accomplish as much as 12 hours of peritoneal dialysis. Children who have renal failure or whose kidneys have been removed while they await a kidney transplant can be maintained almost indefinitely by hemodialysis sessions two or three times a week or by continuous ultrafiltration or continuous arteriovenous hemofiltration. It can be used in infants as well as older children (Quinlan, Bates, Sheils, et al., 2013).

To establish a site for initial blood removal, children may have a double-lumen central catheter inserted into a central vein, such as the subclavian or internal jugular vein. A permanent technique is subcutaneous anastomosis of a vein and artery, creating an arteriovenous fistula (usually the brachial artery and brachiocephalic vein; Fig. 46.5A) or internal anastomosis of the artery and vein using a subcutaneous graft (see Fig. 46.5B). The possibility of infection is reduced with internal anastomosis, although, unfortunately, two venipunctures, one from a low point in the shunt to remove blood and one high in the shunt to return it, are necessary for dialysis (use an anesthetic cream beforehand to reduce pain). The ability to feel a thrill (vibration) or hear a bruit over the fistula or graft site is proof that the connection is patent.

The risks of hemodialysis include infection introduced by venipuncture (severe because the infection immediately causes septicemia) and clotting of the access site, which can lead to emboli. During hemodialysis, if too much sodium is removed, muscle cramping may occur. A "first use" syndrome or symptoms such as dizziness or muscle cramping can occur from a reaction to the fibers in the dialysis machine coil. If urea is moved from the blood at too rapid rate—faster than urea can be shifted from the brain into the blood—children may begin to show signs of confusion, vomiting, dizziness, visual blurring, or hallucinations from a *dialysis disequilibrium syndrome*.

Figure 46.4 A nurse preparing a 10-year-old girl for a hemodialysis session. A subclavian catheter from the child is connected to the hemodialysis equipment (in the background). Blood flows from the child through the catheter to the hemodialysis equipment and is then returned to the child's venous circulation. (© Life in View/Science Source.)

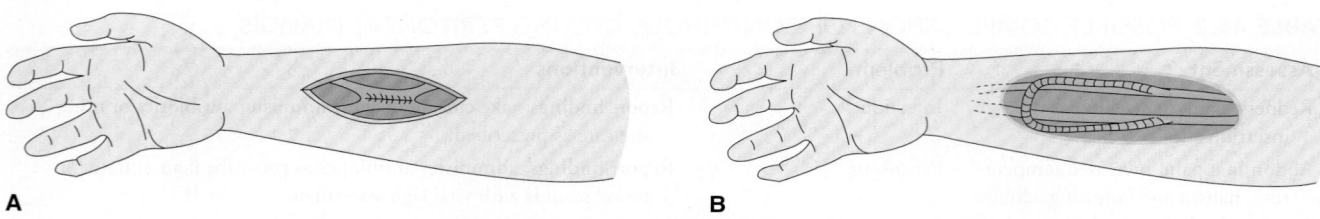

A   **B**

Figure 46.5   **(A)** An internal arteriovenous fistula. **(B)** An internal arteriovenous graft.

This occurs because, as osmotic pressure is greater in the brain than the blood, fluid shifts into the brain, resulting in cerebral edema. Hemodialysis must be temporarily halted if these symptoms occur to allow equalization.

Children grow as bored during hemodialysis as they do during peritoneal dialysis. Help parents provide stimulating activities such as a playing a board game or reading a favorite story, which are only used during that time period. When children's kidneys are removed prior to transplantation, they must remain on a continuous program of hemodialysis. These children may come to resent a machine as "owning" or "controlling" them as they become aware they cannot exist apart from it (Bayhakki & Hatthakit, 2012). Allowing them to plan special activities to do during hemodialysis time can help not only to pass the time but also to give them a feeling of control.

Health Promotion and Risk Management

Several important interventions can help prevent urinary and renal disease in children. The first intervention is to educate parents and caregivers about wiping from front to back when changing diapers of female infants. The second intervention is to prevent UTI in girls by beginning education about perineal hygiene measures from the time they are first toilet trained. Remind parents of simple ways to prevent UTI, such as not allowing children to bathe with bubble bath. Teach parents to recognize that abnormally colored urine (red, black, or cloudy) should not be dismissed because this could be the beginning of a UTI or kidney disease.

Educating parents about the importance of giving the full course of antibiotics prescribed for UTIs can help prevent return reinfection; giving the full course of antibiotics after a streptococcal infection can help prevent acute glomerulonephritis.

Structural Abnormalities of the Urinary Tract

Because the urinary tract is a system of hollow tubes, congenital disorders can rise from faulty recanalization in intrauterine life.

PATENT URACHUS

When the bladder first forms in utero, it is joined to the umbilicus by a narrow tube, the *urachus*. If this fails to close during embryologic development, a fistula is left between the bladder and umbilicus (**patent urachus**). This occurs more commonly in males than in females. Nurses are frequently the ones to discover this condition as they notice clear fluid draining from the base of the umbilical cord while changing a newborn's diaper. If you test the fluid with Nitrazine paper for pH, its acid content will identify it as urine. An ultrasound will confirm the patent connection.

A few patent urachus abnormalities heal spontaneously, but most require surgical correction to prevent pathogens from entering the fistula site and causing persistent bladder infection. This is done in the immediate neonatal period using only a small subumbilical incision (M. S. Tsai & Yeh, 2011).

EXSTROPHY OF THE BLADDER

Exstrophy of the bladder is a midline closure defect that occurs during the 10th week of pregnancy. As a result, at birth, the bladder lies exposed on the anterior abdominal wall. The latest population-based studies have shown the incidence to be between 2 and 3 per 100,000 live births, with almost identical incidence between males and females (Purves & Gearhart, 2010).

Assessment

Exstrophy is often, but not always, detected by fetal ultrasound, which reveals the lack of an anterior wall of the bladder and a lack of anterior skin covering the lower anterior abdomen (Fig. 46.6A). A skilled ultrasonographer may pick up on possible exstrophy when they do not observe a typical bladder-filling cycle during the prenatal ultrasound. At birth, the bladder appears bright red and continually drains urine from the open surface. In both sexes, pelvic bone defects, particularly a wide pubic diastasis, are a hallmark of exstrophy. In males, the genital defect is severe because the anterior corporal length is 50% shorter, and the diameter of the posterior corporal segment is 40% larger than in males without exstrophy. This leads to the appearance of a dramatically short, wide penis. In females, the urethra may be abnormally formed, and the vagina is approximately 50% shorter and 30% wider than females without exstrophy, frequently requiring vaginoplasty after puberty in order to allow sexual intercourse and tampon use without pain (Purves & Gearhart, 2010). Urethral defects in males, such as **epispadias**—the opening of the urinary meatus on the dorsal or superior surface of the penis—are also common. The skin around the bladder quickly becomes excoriated because of constant exposure to acid urine. Kidney infection can occur from ascending organisms from the open bladder. When children with this disorder begin to walk, they may demonstrate a "waddling" gait caused by the wide pubic diastasis.

Therapeutic Management

The treatment of bladder exstrophy begins with surgical closure of the bladder and the anterior abdominal wall, and construction of a urethra (see Fig. 46.6B). Because of the severe

Figure 46.6 Bladder exstrophy. **(A)** Prior to surgical reconstruction. Note the bright-red color of the bladder. **(B)** Following surgical reconstruction. (Courtesy of Karen M. Polise, MSN, RN, Division of Nephrology, The Children's Hospital of Philadelphia.)

nature of the defect and the high potential for initial closure failure, and the lifelong negative sequelae of such a failure, children born with bladder exstrophy should immediately be referred to a pediatric urologist at a major children's center who has undergone fellowship training in bladder exstrophy treatment. If the bladder is of suitable size and quality, an ideal timeline for closure is in the first 24 to 72 hours of life. If the bladder template is too small, however, the bladder can be left to grow for 3 to 6 months before closure. In such instances, the bladder mucosa should be kept moist and covered with plastic wrap to prevent the bladder surface both from drying out and from adhering to bedclothes or diapers and being injured. To prevent the skin of the abdomen from excoriation, consult a wound, ostomy, and continence nurse for the best approach, which usually involves a protective topical application such as A&D Ointment, Karaya Gum, or Maalox. If this is done, do not separate the infant's legs to apply diapers; just place them under the child instead. Be certain to change diapers promptly after defecation so feces are not brought forward to the open bladder. Position the infant on the back so urine drains freely. Sponge bathe rather than tub bathe the infant to prevent water from entering the ureters and becoming a source of infection.

It is important to help parents to view their child as healthy in every aspect other than his or her bladder defect. When a child with bladder exstrophy is received into your care, remember to

congratulate the parents on the birth of their baby. Bladder exstrophy affects only urinary elimination, and in most cases, these children are otherwise extremely healthy. With modern-day surgical approaches, these children can lead normal, healthy lives, and it is important for the emotional well-being of the family to focus on these positive aspects. In instances when the bladder closure is to be delayed, teaching the parents to properly care for the bladder at home is imperative.

Postoperative

Surgery is completed as either a one-step or staged repair. After bladder closure, a suprapubic tube is placed for urine drainage and will typically remain in place for 4 to 6 weeks to allow the bladder to drain continuously and the surgical anastomoses to heal. The infant should be positioned on the back with the legs raised in traction at 90 degrees. This position is maintained for 4 to 6 weeks after surgery and is essential to prevent failure of the closure. Approximately 30% of patients with bladder exstrophy at children's medical centers worldwide also undergo osteotomy at the time of their bladder closure. Immediately after surgery, urine draining from the catheter may be tinged with blood, but this should clear after the first few days. Children may experience sharp, painful bladder spasms after surgery. Such spasms are often the most painful and prominent source of discomfort for the recovering child. Working with the pain team to provide adequate analgesia and anticholinergic therapy is imperative for both the comfort of the child and the proper healing of the bladder.

For some children, so little bladder tissue is present that surgical reconstruction isn't possible, and a *continent urinary reservoir* (or artificial neobladder) is constructed (Purves & Gearhart, 2010) (Fig. 46.7).

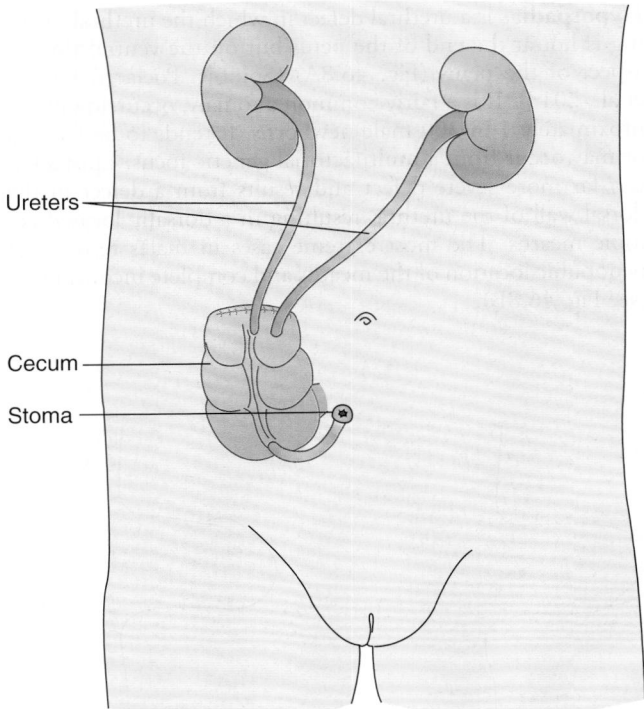

Figure 46.7 A continent urine reservoir. A portion of intestine is isolated; the attached ureters drain into it. The appendix creates an abdominal stoma for catheterization.

For continent urinary diversion, a small segment of the intestine is separated from the intestinal tract. The intestinal tract is then reanastomosed so the gastrointestinal tract is unaffected. The separated segment is made into a bladder-like reservoir, and then the appendix is tubularized to create a continent channel extending from the dome of the bladder reservoir to a continent stoma at the site where the umbilicus would normally lie.

Urine drains from the kidneys into the ureters and then into the collecting bowel segment. The parent or child catheterizes the abdominal stoma every 3 to 4 hours throughout the day to empty urine. The procedure is theoretically simple, but it is technically difficult to accomplish. Parents need a good review of anatomy to aid their understanding of the procedure. As the child reaches school age and begins school activities that expose the condition to others, such as showering, adjusting to a continent urinary reservoir can be difficult. Ensure that the child has a plan and support for peer disclosure, maintenance, and follow-up care during the school years and adolescence so the function of the reservoir and also the child's adjustment can continue to be assessed and supported.

For children who have a successful initial closure, adequate bladder capacity, pelvic floor function, and bladder contractility, an alternate continence procedure, called a bladder neck reconstruction (BNR), may be an option. This is ideally undertaken in the mid to late elementary school years or later and requires significant preparation that often takes place over a number of months or years under a specialist's care. A BNR reconstructs the bladder neck and urethra and allows the child to void via the urethra and achieve continence.

HYPOSPADIAS

Hypospadias is a urethral defect in which the urethral opening is not at the end of the penis but on the ventral (lower) aspect of the penis (Fig. 46.8A) (Spinoit, Poelaert, Groen, et al., 2013). It is a fairly common anomaly, occurring in approximately 1 in 300 male newborns. It tends to be familial or may occur from a multifactorial genetic focus. Epispadias is a far more severe defect and results from a defect in the dorsal wall of the urethra, resulting in a dorsally located ectopic meatus. The most extreme cases in males result in a penopubic location of the meatus and complete incontinence (see Fig. 46.8B).

Assessment

Be certain to inspect all male newborns at birth for hypospadias or epispadias as part of a routine physical examination. The degree of hypospadias may be minimal (on the glans but inferior in site) or maximal (at the midshaft or at the penal-scrotal junction). Many newborns with hypospadias have an accompanying short *chordee*—a fibrous band that causes the penis to curve downward (often called a cobra-head appearance; see Fig. 46.8C). Also inspect carefully for *cryptorchidism* (undescended testes), which is often found in conjunction with hypospadias.

If the penis defect is so extensive that sex determination is unclear, sex cell karyotyping or DNA analysis (see Chapter 8) should be done. Parents may have difficulty discussing this condition with relatives or healthcare personnel because it is a sensitive topic for them. Help parents work through these feelings by allowing them to talk about the disorder, by answering honestly and openly their questions about what the condition includes, and by assisting the family in receiving professional support when necessary.

Therapeutic Management

Children with hypospadias should not be circumcised because, at the time of the repair, the surgeon may wish to use a portion of the foreskin for the repair. In the newborn, the surgical procedure may be a *meatotomy*—a procedure in which the urethra is extended to a usual position—to establish better urinary function. When the child is older (age 12 to 18 months), adherent chordee can be released. If the repair will be extensive, all surgery may be delayed until the child is 3 to 4 years of age. To encourage penis growth and make the procedure easier, the child may have testosterone cream applied to the penis or receive testosterone injections until surgery. It's important that hypospadias be corrected before school age if at all possible so the child looks and feels like other males. If left uncorrected, in later years, a meatal opening at an inferior penile site may interfere with fertility because it does not allow sperm to be deposited close to the female cervix during coitus (Vidal, Gorduza, Haraux, et al., 2010).

After surgical repair, a urethral urinary drainage catheter will be inserted to allow urine output without putting tension against the urethral sutures. The child may notice painful bladder spasms as long as the catheter is in place (3 to 7 days), so an analgesic such as acetaminophen (Tylenol) and an

A

B

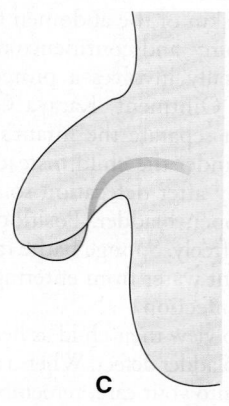

C

Figure 46.8 Urethral defects. **(A)** Hypospadias. **(B)** Epispadias. **(C)** Hypospadias with chordee.

anticholinergic medication such as oxybutynin (Ditropan) may be prescribed for pain relief. After hypospadias repair, children can be expected to have usual urinary and reproductive function unless accompanying anomalies of the penis are present.

Infections of the Urinary System and Related Disorders

As the urinary system drains to the outside of the body, infection can easily spread to the bladder or kidneys.

URINARY TRACT INFECTION

UTI occurs more often in females than in males: about 8% in girls and 2% in boys (Lum, 2012). Urinary pathogens seem to enter the urinary tract most often as an ascending infection from the perineum and are gram-negative rods such as *Escherichia coli*. UTIs also occur as a health care–acquired infection in children who have urinary catheters.

UTIs occur more often in girls than boys because the urethra is shorter in girls, and because it is located close to the vagina and anus, vulvovaginitis or rectal bacteria can easily spread to the urethra. Changing diapers frequently can help reduce the risk for infection in infants. Girls should be taught early (when they are toilet-trained) to wipe themselves from front to back after voiding and defecating to avoid contaminating the urethra. There is a suggested correlation between the use of products such as bubble bath, feminine hygiene sprays, and hot tubs and UTI in girls, so use of these should be discouraged or minimized (Gaylord & Peterson-Smith, 2012). Additional measures to prevent UTIs are summarized in Box 46.4.

It's important that UTIs are treated so they do not damage the bladder lining and/or spread to involve the kidneys (pyelonephritis) and cause permanent damage. Girls who have one UTI should be thoughtfully assessed and, if a second UTI occurs, should be referred to a fellowship-trained pediatric urologist to determine whether any congenital urologic anomaly such as an urethral stenosis or vesicoureteral reflux exists. Any male older than the age of 3 months who presents with UTI should also be evaluated by a pediatric urologist.

Assessment

Although it may be possible to locate a UTI precisely as urethritis, cystitis, ureteritis, or pyelonephritis, the signs and symptoms in young children often are not clear-cut, so all types are lumped together and referred to as UTIs. The typical symptoms that occur in older children or in adults—pain on urination, frequency, burning, and hematuria—may not be present in young children, so UTI is suspected when a child has a fever with no demonstrable cause on physical examination. If the infection is confined to the bladder (cystitis), the child may have a low-grade fever, mild abdominal pain, and day- or nighttime enuresis. If the infection progresses to pyelonephritis, the symptoms are generally more acute, with high fever, abdominal or flank pain, vomiting, and malaise.

Urine for culture can be collected using a clean-catch technique, suprapubic aspiration, or catheterization, so bacteria from the vulva or foreskin do not contaminate the sample and give a false result. Suprapubic aspiration is generally limited to infants. Catheterization, also frightening and a potential source of infection, is limited in children of all ages.

Urine obtained from suprapubic aspiration is generally sterile, so any growth from this source is significant. A clean-catch urine specimen is said to be positive for bacteriuria if the bacterial colony count is more than 100,000 per milliliter. A count of less than 10,000 per milliliter is considered a

 BOX 46.4

Nursing Care Planning to Empower a Family

PREVENTING URINARY TRACT INFECTION IN FEMALES

Q. Carey's grandmother tells you, "Carey had two urinary tract infections last year. How can we prevent that from happening again?"

A. Here are some important tips to help prevent urinary tract infection (UTI):

- Encourage your granddaughter to drink fluid periodically during the day, especially in warm weather or during exercise, to keep urine flowing freely and prevent stasis of urine in bladder.
- Urge her to urinate at least every 2 to 3 hours to prevent stasis of urine in the bladder.
- Teach her not to bathe with bubble bath; this can cause vulvar and urethral irritation.
- Help your granddaughter learn to wipe from front to back after moving her bowels or urinating to prevent moving rectal contamination forward to the urethra.
- Have your granddaughter wear cotton, not synthetic, underwear to decrease perineal irritation.
- Instruct your granddaughter to wash her vulva daily to lower the bacterial count on the perineum.
- When your granddaughter begins menstruating, encourage her to change sanitary pads at least every 4 hours to reduce the possible growth of bacteria near the urethra.
- If symptoms of UTI should occur (pain on urination, frequency, blood in urine), call your primary healthcare provider. If an antibiotic is prescribed, make sure that your granddaughter takes it for the full prescribed course, so all bacteria are completely eradicated. Otherwise, after a short time, bacteria will grow stronger, and the infection will recur and be more difficult to treat.
- When your granddaughter becomes sexually active, teach her to urinate immediately after intercourse to flush out any bacteria introduced into the urethra during intercourse.

negative culture. If the count is between 10,000 and 100,000 per milliliter or if the urine is positive for proteinuria (which could happen because of the presence of bacteria), the count is usually repeated. In addition to identifying the responsible organism, microscopic examination of the urine specimen may indicate the presence of red blood cells (hematuria) caused by bacterial irritation of the bladder mucosa. The presence of either red or white blood cells or bacteria tends to make urine more alkaline, so the pH of the sample will be elevated (>7). Surveillance urine cultures, once a common practice, are no longer recommended. The American Academy of Pediatrics (AAP) released in 2011 its updated guidelines for UTI management in children aged 2 to 24 months and encourage providers to make careful assessments and culture only in symptomatic patients (Roberts et al., 2011).

Therapeutic Management

The medical treatment for UTI is the oral administration of a broad-spectrum antibiotic such as sulfamethoxazole-trimethoprim (Bactrim) or amoxicillin, or an antibiotic specific to the causative organism that is cultured (Paintsil, 2013). Nitrofurantoin is also a good choice for UTIs because it is a broad-spectrum antibiotic that concentrates in the urine and can be used for both treatment and prophylaxis. In addition to the antibiotic, a child needs to drink a large quantity of fluid to "flush" the infection out of the urinary tract, particularly if a sulfa drug is prescribed because these can cause urinary crystals in concentrated urine. Cranberry juice is often recommended as being highly effective in acidifying urine and making it more resistant to bacterial growth. In actual practice, little evidence of its effectiveness exists, so water is the best choice; fluids with artificial coloring and carbonation should be avoided because they irritate the bladder and can cause further discomfort. If the child experiences moderate to severe pain on urination that interferes with the ability to void, suggest the child sit in a bathtub of warm water and void into the water. A mild analgesic, such as acetaminophen (Tylenol), may help reduce pain enough to allow voiding.

Remind parents that with a UTI, treatment with antibiotics must be continued for the full prescription or the infection will return. Help parents create a reminder system, such as a sheet of paper for the refrigerator door or a reminder on their smartphone, to help ensure adherence. A repeat clean-catch urine sample obtained after approximately 7 days of antibiotic dosing is indicated for some children who have had multiple recurrent UTIs. This is referred to as a "test of cure," and the goal is to confirm that the bacterial infection has been obliterated and is not simply being partially suppressed while the child is on antibiotics and will surge back to culture-positive levels when the antibiotics are discontinued.

After recurrent UTIs, children may be prescribed a prophylactic antibiotic for 6 months while measures are taken to optimize voiding habits and hydration.

"HONEYMOON" CYSTITIS

Honeymoon cystitis refers to UTI seen in young women shortly after they initiate a first sexual relationship caused by the local irritation and inflammation that results from coitus.

Like most UTIs, these respond quickly to antibiotic therapy. Voiding as soon as possible after coitus may help to flush

pathogenic organisms from the urethra and prevent such infections. When cystitis first occurs in an adolescent girl, it is an alert that she may be sexually active. In addition to the need for counseling about personal hygiene measures to prevent UTI, the girl may need information about safer sex, reproductive planning, and symptoms of sexually transmitted infections. Recurrent UTIs in a school-age or preschool girl may suggest sexual maltreatment (Beck, Bekker, & Van Driel, 2010).

QSEN Checkpoint Question 46.2

QUALITY IMPROVEMENT

Carey's grandmother is concerned because Carey had two UTIs last year. Which of the following statements best shows that Carey's grandmother received adequate patient education on the prevention of UTIs?

 a. "I won't allow Carey to drink too much milk or eat foods like yogurt."
 b. "I'll try to have Carey bathe with bath salts to discourage bacteria in her groin area."
 c. "I'll be certain to administer all of the antibiotic pills that the doctor prescribes."
 d. "I'll make sure that Carey doesn't overexert herself when she's playing with her friends."

Look in Appendix A for the best answer and rationale.

VESICOURETERAL REFLUX

Normally, urine flows from the ureters into the bladder, with almost no flow reentering the ureters from the bladder because the ureters enter the bladder obliquely and a bladder skin flap or "valve" obscures the end of the ureter, preventing backflow. **Vesicoureteral reflux** refers to retrograde flow of urine from the bladder into the ureters (Batinic, Milošević, Topalovic-Grkovic, et al., 2013). This reflux of urine occurs with micturition (voiding) when the bladder contracts (Fig. 46.9) because the valve that guards the entrance from the bladder to the ureter is defective either from birth or because of scarring from repeated UTIs; bladder pressure is stronger than usual; or ureters are implanted at unusual angles or too low on the bladder wall.

Reflux has the potential to lead to bladder infection because urine is retained in the ureters after voiding and then drains back into the bladder after the child is finished voiding where it remains. Stasis of any fluid is subject to infection. The capacity for normal bladder tissue to lyse bacteria also becomes reduced because of the large residual urine volume that is always present. If the reflex is enough that it leads to back pressure on the kidneys, it has the potential to lead to nephron destruction and, subsequently, hydronephrosis or dilatation of the renal pelvis. As the condition tends to appear in families, it is most likely caused by a heterogeneous gene disorder (Hunziker & Puri, 2012).

Assessment

A child with reflux is usually first seen by healthcare personnel because of a history of repeated UTIs. A VCUG, CT scan, MRI, cystoscopy, or cystography with contrast material

Figure 46.9   Vesicoureteral reflux. **(A)** Normal voiding pattern. **(B)** Reflux into ureters with voiding.

will show the ureteral reflux. Based on diagnostic studies, reflux is graded from I to V by degree of reflux, with grade V being the most serious.

Therapeutic Management

The majority of instances of vesicoureteral reflux resolve with maturity without a need for surgery. Until this normal growth occurs, however, the condition must be treated to decrease the possibility of glomerular scarring from infection or back pressure (Passamaneck, 2011). Teaching double voiding (having the child void and then in a few minutes attempt to void again) may help to empty the bladder more fully and prevent recurrent infection from urinary stasis. Some girls need to remain on prophylactic antibiotics for a lengthy time to prevent bladder infection from reoccurring.

If continuous antibiotic therapy does not prevent recurrent UTIs or the reflux is initially identified as severe, it can be corrected by cystoscopy. Under general anesthesia or conscious sedation, a cystoscope is passed into the bladder through the urethra and an agent such as dextranomer–hyaluronic acid (Deflux) is injected to stabilize the ureter valves (Puri, Kutasy, Colhoun, et al., 2012). To correct the implantation site of ureters, laparoscopic surgery can be scheduled to reinsert the ureters at a more oblique angle.

After surgery, a suprapubic catheter will remain in place to keep the bladder empty and prevent pressure against the surgical area. Two ureteral catheters (stents), threaded into the ureters to drain urine directly from the kidney pelvis, also exit at the suprapubic tube site. All three tubes are attached to a

closed drainage system. Sterile gauze dressings and antibiotic cream are placed around the tube insertion site to keep it free of infection.

In preparing children for this type of surgery, be certain to prepare them for the number of tubes they will have afterward. Explain that even with the tubes in place, the child will be allowed to walk and move about soon after the operation (and should do so). Be sure that the child and parents understand the importance of not raising the collection system above the child's bladder level when helping the child out of bed. This helps prevent potentially contaminated urine from flowing from the tubes back into the bladder or ureters.

Urine will drain primarily from the kidney stents for approximately the first 3 days after surgery; thereafter, drainage will flow around the stents and will be mainly from the suprapubic tube. As long as they are in place, it's important to assess that both stents are draining to ensure kidney production is equal on both sides. Observe the suprapubic tube and stent drainage closely for color or clots (should not be over pinpoint in size) and measure the amount and record it every hour for the first 24 hours and then about every 4 hours following that. Initially, drainage from the bladder catheter will be bloody, but this should clear in 2 to 3 days. To show that urine is clear of blood, obtain serial urine specimens each time collecting bags are emptied and label them with the time of removal. Comparing the color of these samples will show that urine is clearing of blood. School-age children can help label the containers, which can help add to their sense of accomplishment and control over the situation.

To help keep the ends of stents or the suprapubic tube from becoming contaminated, care should be taken to maintain aseptic technique when emptying drainage bags. Once drainage occurs primarily from the suprapubic tube, and renal status and good drainage are ensured, the stents are removed. In most cases, this is done before discharge from the hospital, but the process varies by both technique and provider. Many children are frightened because they worry this will be painful. You can assure them this is a simple procedure, and most children are not even aware when the stent is removed. This is done easily and without the need for anesthesia.

Incisional pain and painful bladder spasms may be present for the first 3 days after surgery, so antispasmodics are usually prescribed to reduce bladder spasm. Not touching or moving the suprapubic tube also helps to reduce spasms because this limits bladder irritation. The suprapubic tube is typically removed between 4 and 7 days after surgery (again, a nearly painless procedure). There may be slight urine leakage from the puncture site of the tube for 1 or 2 days after removal of the tube. Keep a sterile dressing in place to absorb the leaking urine. Remind the child and parents to avoid tub baths until the suprapubic tube site has closed completely.

A few children continue to have bladder reflux after ureter reimplantation. All children need follow-up care such as repeat VCUG and/or ultrasound at a later date in order to establish that surgery was effective in halting the reflux.

HYDRONEPHROSIS

Hydronephrosis is enlargement of the pelvis of the kidney with urine as a result of back pressure in the ureter. The backpressure is generally caused by obstruction, either of the ureter or of the point where the ureter joins the bladder, as with vesicoureteral reflux. Although this may occur at any age, it occurs most often in the first 6 months of life and is often diagnosed by ultrasound during intrauterine life (Yamaçake & Nguyen, 2013).

The condition is usually asymptomatic. The infant may have repeated UTIs caused by urinary stasis (difficult to detect in a young child except as general irritability or crying on voiding). Elevated blood pressure caused by increasing tubular pressure (which activates the renin–angiotensin system) may be detected on a routine health assessment, although blood pressure is not taken routinely in infants. With severe back pressure, the infant will eventually experience flank or abdominal pain. Abdominal palpation may reveal an abdominal mass (the dilated kidney pelvis). An IVP or ultrasound will reveal the enlarged pelvis and the point of obstruction.

Hydronephrosis is a serious disorder because if the pressure in the pelvis becomes too acute, back pressure on the kidney can interfere with tubular function or destroy the nephrons. The treatment is surgical correction of the obstruction before glomerular or tubular destruction occurs.

Disorders Affecting Normal Urinary Elimination

Common disorders can interfere with urine elimination, such as **dysfunctional elimination syndrome (DES)**, including enuresis, and rarer disorders such as kidney agenesis. DES is an abnormal pattern of elimination of unknown cause, characterized by both urine and stool and by bladder and/or bowel incontinence. It occurs in a previously toilet trained child without anatomic or neurologic abnormalities.

ENURESIS

Enuresis is involuntary passage of urine past the age when a child should be expected to have attained bladder control (Fleming, 2012). Because this is expected at 2 to 3 years of age for daytime and age 4 to 6 years for nighttime, enuresis is said to occur at approximately 7 years. Enuresis may be nocturnal (occurs only at night), diurnal (occurs during the day), or both. It is primary if bladder training was never achieved and is considered acquired or secondary if control was established but has now been lost.

Most enuresis is nocturnal; however, many children who present for treatment of nocturnal enuresis are also found to have some diurnal enuresis or DES as well. These factors are often the root cause of the nocturnal issues. Voiding dysfunction should be managed in an interdisciplinary setting that includes medicine, nursing, behavioral psychology, and nutrition, as indicated. Single treatment modalities are rarely successful long term, and management should include a multimodal approach, including bowel management, timed voiding, hydration management, improved fiber intake, behavioral management, biofeedback (when appropriate), and drug therapy when necessary (Eldridge & Lakshmanan, 2011). It occurs more frequently in boys than in girls. It also tends to be familial (if it is present in a child, one of the parents probably experienced it, too).

Assessment

Children with enuresis who are older than 5 years of age need an evaluation to determine whether there is an organic cause for the disorder. During history taking, ask how parents have tried to correct the problem; identify whether it is primarily a problem for the child or the parents (treatment will be most effective if the child wants the situation corrected). Assess whether there are stresses in the family, such as parents who expect more mature behavior of a child than the child can manage, the introduction of a new brother or sister, an uncomfortable school situation such as bullying, or marital discord.

If children wet only on nights when they are exceptionally tired or troubled, a functional rather than an organic cause is suggested. If children wet only when they are engrossed in an interesting activity, they may simply need more reminders to empty their bladder. If children have symptoms other than bed-wetting, such as abdominal pain, burning, or frequency, UTI is suggested. It is a common practice for many parents to lift children out of bed every night and take them to the bathroom so they don't wet the bed. This can be a stop gap and is not harmful. However, it does not help develop the child's arousal response, which will improve the situation long term. For this practice to be meaningful and purposeful, the child should be brought to full awareness when they are woken up at night. They should walk to the bathroom under their own power (a parent can assist to avoid any accidents given their fatigued state) and should be told that they are going to sit on the toilet because their bladder is full and the toilet is the proper place to empty.

Some children with enuresis have abnormal electroencephalographic patterns. Other children with the same abnormal patterns do not have enuresis, however, so this by itself is not a sufficiently specific finding to be helpful. In others, bed-wetting seems to occur as children pass from a period of rapid eye movement sleep pattern to a type IV level, or it is primarily a sleep disorder. It may be associated with small bladder capacity (which would explain why the condition is familial).

Although usually not necessary to aid diagnosis, an ultrasound, pre–post bladder scan, or urodynamic testing may be prescribed to rule out organic disease, and a clean-catch urine specimen may be prescribed to rule out bacteriuria if other possible symptoms are present. Assess specific gravity, protein, and glucose of urine to rule out a defect in urine concentration or reveal evidence of nephron disease.

Therapeutic Management

The treatment of enuresis can be complex because the cause is often unknown. If stress factors have been identified, not all of these can be eliminated because certain circumstances, such as the birth of a new sibling, cannot be changed, but frank discussion with children regarding what causes the stress and attempts to help them cope better with their daytime activities may lessen incidents.

In many children, it helps to limit fluids during the 2 hours before bed. Remind parents, however, that not all children are able to go without a drink from dinner until breakfast. For instance, for a child with sickle-cell anemia, restricting fluid in this way may cause increased sickling of cells as a result of dehydration and should be avoided.

Alarm bells that ring when children wet at night can be effective in some children. This type of system does not actually stop bed-wetting, but a sensor registers wetness and wakes the child and then the child stops voiding and gets up and uses the bathroom. Over time, this type of conditioning may be effective, but once the urine alarm is removed, children may relapse.

Nursing Care Planning Based on Responsibility for Pharmacology

DESMOPRESSIN ACETATE (DDAVP)

Classification: a synthetic form of human antidiuretic hormone

Action: promotes resorption of water in the renal tubule or decreases bladder filling; drug of choice for primary nocturnal enuresis (Karch, 2013)

Pregnancy Risk Category: B

Dosage: In children 6 years of age and older, 0.2 mg orally at bedtime, titrated up to 0.6 mg to obtain the desired response. Intranasal preparations are no longer recommended.

Possible Adverse Effects: transient headache, nausea, flushing, mild abdominal cramps, fluid retention

Nursing Implications

- Instruct parents and child that child should restrict fluid after dinnertime in addition to taking medication.

Bladder-stretching exercises—drinking a large quantity of water and then refraining from voiding as long as possible—to increase the functional size of the bladder are contraindicated and can cause both dysfunctional voiding and renal damage. Parents should be strongly cautioned against this.

In some cases, a synthetic antidiuretic hormone (desmopressin [DDAVP]) administered orally is the drug of choice to reduce urinary output and nocturnal enuresis in cases of primary nocturnal enuresis (Deshpande, Caldwell, & Sureshkumar, 2012). However, most children who wet at night do not have primary nocturnal enuresis and have some daytime symptoms of habits that are causing the nighttime problems. Children should be evaluated and treated in a clinic focused on DES and voiding dysfunction (Box 46.5).

Enuresis can become a major problem for children as well as family dynamics and deserves appropriate medical attention in a child after the seventh birthday. As a general measure, children who wet their beds need to take baths in the morning rather than at bedtime to minimize urine odor and avoid bullying. Parents may find planning a vacation with hotel stays difficult. They may resent the daily linen washing. Children may exclude themselves from activities such as slumber parties or camping trips with friends to avoid embarrassment.

Enuresis may occur in hospitalized children because of the stress of their new surroundings. Preschool children may experience it because they are uncomfortable using strange bathrooms or do not understand which bathroom is theirs to use. As a rule, place as little stress or importance on enuresis as possible during an illness and encourage parents to do the same.

POSTURAL (ORTHOSTATIC) PROTEINURIA

A few children will spill albumin into the urine when they stand upright for an extended period (**postural proteinuria**, also called postural albuminuria). The amount of spilling decreases when they rest in a supine position. To identify a possible cause for the condition, an MRI of kidneys and ureters may be prescribed. To document that the proteinuria is related to posture, collect urine after the child has been recumbent during the night (a first-voided specimen) and then again after the child has been up and active for several hours. Make certain when collecting these urine specimens to record the child's activity accurately. If the child stood by the crib rail crying for a parent or was held in a nurse's lap for most of the night, the urine may show protein in the morning specimen because it is not truly a "resting specimen." Likewise, the "active" specimen should be collected after the child was truly active, not lying in a supine position reading a book for most of the time. Play a game if necessary, such as follow the leader, so the child is active.

Unless the MRI reveals an obstructive cause, postural proteinuria apparently results from the effect of gravity and thus needs no therapy. However, be certain to document the condition because some of these children do have obstructive disorders that need further identification (Milani, Mazzoni, Burdick, et al., 2010).

KIDNEY AGENESIS

Agenesis means lack of growth (literally, lack of a beginning) or that no organ formed in utero. Absence of kidneys in a newborn is suggested when the volume of amniotic fluid on ultrasound or at birth is severely less than usual (oligohydramnios), indicating that fetal urine was not added to the volume of amniotic fluid. The infant often has *Potter syndrome* or accompanying misshapen, low-set ears and hypoplastic (stiff, inflexible) lungs from compression caused by the lack of amniotic fluid in utero (A. C. Tsai, Manchester, & Elias, 2012). Bilateral absence of kidneys is obviously incompatible with life unless a renal transplantation can be accomplished; the associated condition of nonfunctioning lungs, however, lessens the infant's eligibility for a successful transplantation.

POLYCYSTIC KIDNEY

Polycystic kidney implies that large, fluid-filled cysts have formed in place of normal kidney tissue. The most frequent type of polycystic kidney seen in children is inherited as an autosomal recessive trait. A more rare form is inherited as an autosomal dominant trait (Mahan, 2011). With either type, there is abnormal development of the collecting tubules. The kidneys grow large and feel soft and spongy. If the disorder is bilateral, an infant will not be able to pass urine so the mother will develop oligohydramnios during pregnancy. The newborn can have a flattened nose or *micrognathia* (small jaw), findings of Potter syndrome. A sonogram during pregnancy or at birth will reveal the fluid-filled cysts.

If the condition is unilateral, urine production will be decreased (oliguria), not absent. For this reason and because kidneys are difficult to locate in newborns, a unilateral polycystic kidney may be missed until later in life, when, with increased kidney growth, an abdominal mass can be palpated. The cystic growth offers such resistance to blood circulation that systemic hypertension often results by school age.

In many children, the condition is associated with a cerebral aneurysm, and the liver is filled with identical cysts. This is most evident later in life when increased difficulty with portal circulation occurs (blood cannot perfuse the cystic liver structures either).

The treatment for polycystic formation is surgical removal of the diseased kidney if only one is cystic. If both kidneys are cystic, treatment is renal transplantation (difficult in the young child because few infant kidneys are available for transplantation and because of the technical challenge presented by such small blood vessels). Because this kidney disease is inherited, parents and children at adolescence need genetic counseling to inform them that future children may have this problem.

RENAL HYPOPLASIA

Hypoplasia means reduced growth, so hypoplastic kidneys are small and underdeveloped and contain fewer lobes than usual. In addition to having poor kidney function, hypertension from stenosis of the renal arteries may develop. If hypoplasia is bilateral, the child may need a kidney transplant in later life to maintain kidney function and prevent extreme hypertension.

PRUNE BELLY SYNDROME

Prune belly syndrome (PBS) is a syndrome with a broad spectrum of severity. The most common abnormalities associated with PBS are cardiac, pulmonary, orthopedic, and urologic. Renal dysplasia occurs in about 50% of cases (Hassett, Smith, & Holland, 2012). Occurring mainly in boys, the severe dilation of ureters and the bladder causes back pressure and destruction of kidneys.

The condition is typically marked by the presence of three main urologic symptoms: bilateral undescended testes, the dilated faulty development of the bladder and upper urinary tract, and renal dysplasia. The infant's abdomen appears wrinkled (like a prune) because of the poorly developed abdominal muscles (Fig. 46.10). Without surgical remodeling, the infant will develop repeated UTIs, leading eventually to end-stage renal disease. Teach parents to protect their child's abdomen from trauma, such as can happen from lap belts or baby walkers because their child lacks abdominal support, while waiting for muscle transplant procedures to create more abdominal support (Fearon & Varkarakis, 2012). Some children need kidney transplants as they reach school age because of destruction of glomeruli from continual back pressure of urine on nephrons.

Figure 46.10 Prune belly syndrome. (Courtesy of Karen M. Polise, MSN, RN, Division of Nephrology, The Children's Hospital of Philadelphia.)

ACUTE POSTSTREPTOCOCCAL GLOMERULONEPHRITIS

Glomerulonephritis, inflammation of the glomeruli of the kidney, may occur as a separate entity but usually occurs in children as an immune complex disease after infection with nephritogenic streptococci (most commonly subtypes of group A beta-hemolytic streptococci) where complement, a cascade of proteins activated by antigen–antibody reactions, plugs or obstructs glomeruli. Immunoglobulin G (IgG) antibodies against streptococci can be detected in the bloodstream of children with acute glomerulonephritis, proof the illness follows a streptococcal infection (Kambham, 2012).

Intravascular coagulation occurs in the minute renal vessels; ischemic damage from this leads to scarring and decreased glomerular function. The glomerular filtration rate decreases, leading to an accumulation of sodium and water in the bloodstream. The inflammation of the glomeruli allows protein molecules to escape into the urine.

Assessment

Acute glomerulonephritis is most common in children between the ages of 5 and 10 years, the age group most susceptible to streptococcal infections. Boys appear to develop the disease more often than girls; it occurs more often during the winter and spring, as do pharyngeal streptococcal infections. The child typically has a history of a recent respiratory infection (within 7 to 14 days) or impetigo (within 3 weeks). All children who have had a "strep" throat, tonsillitis, otitis media, or impetigo caused by a streptococcal infection, ideally, should have a urinalysis 2 weeks after the infection to evaluate that glomerulonephritis is not occurring. Many children do not receive this follow-up step, however, because of lack of health insurance coverage or compliance.

The disorder is announced by a sudden onset of hematuria and proteinuria. Urinary sediment will contain white blood cells, epithelial cells, and hyaline, granular, and red blood cell casts. Testing a single specimen of urine will show 1+ to 4+ protein; a 24-hour urine specimen may contain as much as 1 g of protein (normally, urine contains none).

The hematuria is usually so extreme that the child's urine appears tea-colored, reddish-brown, or smoky. After these initial urine changes, the child develops oliguria. Specific gravity of urine becomes elevated. Hypertension from hypervolemia occurs. The child may have abdominal pain, a low-grade fever, edema, anorexia, vomiting, or headache. There may be cardiac involvement such as orthopnea, cardiac enlargement, enlarged liver, pulmonary edema, a galloping heart rhythm, or heart failure because of the difficulty in managing the excessive plasma fluid.

Blood analysis will indicate a lowered blood protein level (hypoalbuminemia) caused by the massive proteinuria. As the child's blood volume expands, a mild anemia will also develop. As in all inflammatory diseases, the erythrocyte sedimentation rate will increase. Because the glomeruli cannot filter properly, concentrations of urea, nonprotein nitrogen (BUN), and creatinine in blood will increase.

If blood pressure reaches 160/100 mmHg as part of the expanding circulatory volume, encephalopathy may occur, with symptoms of headache, irritability, seizures, vomiting, coma or lethargy, and perhaps transitory paralysis, symptoms all caused by *cerebral ischemia* (vasoconstriction of cerebral vessels that occurs to reduce cranial pressure).

Therapeutic Management

In most children, acute glomerulonephritis runs a limited, short-term, 1- to 2-week, benign course, and during this time, there is little specific therapy other than to alleviate symptoms of the disorder. A course of antibiotics may be prescribed to be certain all streptococci are removed from the child's system. Diuretics are of little value because obstructed glomeruli cannot be made to function, although a course of ethacrynic acid or furosemide (Lasix) may be tried. If heart failure occurs, keeping the child in a semi-Fowler's position, digitalization, and oxygen administration are helpful. If diastolic blood pressure rises to more than 90 mmHg, antihypertensive therapy with an antihypertensive such as labetalol will be prescribed. Phosphate binders, such as aluminum hydroxide to reduce phosphate absorption in the gastrointestinal tract, or a potassium-removing resin agent, such as sodium polystyrene sulfonate (Kayexalate), may be necessary in children who have rising phosphate and potassium levels because the kidneys are unable to clear these from the circulation.

Diet is controversial. Although restricting salt may limit edema and limiting protein intake may reduce the amount of protein lost in urine, most children who are losing large quantities of protein actually need more protein to supplement this loss. Most children do well, therefore, on a usual diet for their age. Weighing the child every day and calculating intake and output are important assessments to follow the course and extent of the disease.

Bed rest is unnecessary, although it's good to encourage children to participate in quiet play activities rather than active exercise. After 1 or 2 weeks, they can attend school and engage in their usual activities, although competitive activity is limited until kidney function has returned to normal (about 2 months). Caution parents that the results of a urine protein test may remain abnormal for up to a year, so if their child has this test done as a routine screening procedure at a health checkup, they don't worry that the finding means reinfection or the beginning of further disease.

A few children will not completely recover from acute glomerulonephritis but will develop chronic nephritis. These children apparently suffer destruction from the initial inflammation that destroys renal function (Praga & Morales, 2013).

Nursing Diagnoses and Related Interventions

Nursing care for the child with glomerulonephritis centers on helping alleviate symptoms and allowing the child to adjust to his or her sudden change in appearance.

Nursing Diagnosis: Situational low self-esteem, related to feelings of responsibility for onset of serious illness

Outcome Evaluation: Child (parent) admits feeling guilty about inadequate treatment of initial infection; discusses plans and ways to maintain health at this point; participates in care.

Glomerulonephritis is a frightening disease for both children and their parents because it begins so abruptly. Children may be frightened by the initial hematuria and upset at the appearance of periorbital edema, which makes their reflection in the mirror seem strange and often frightening

to them. Children as young as early school age are aware that kidneys are necessary for life and thus appreciate the seriousness of kidney disease.

If children were prescribed penicillin for pharyngitis 2 weeks before the development of the condition but refused to take it, they and their parents often need to talk about their feelings. To help them understand that the outcome of the original neglected therapy does not have to result in a bad outcome, provide frequent reports of subtle positive changes in the child's condition, such as "Her blood pressure is not as high as before; she doesn't need medicine for that anymore." or "She weighs 2 pounds less today than 4 days ago; that generally means her kidneys are beginning to function more efficiently."

Be certain that parents know the date and place of a return visit for follow-up care. Because this is a perplexing disease, be certain they have a telephone number to call if they have questions about their child's care or condition. Acute glomerulonephritis tends not to recur with subsequent streptococcal infections, so prophylactic penicillin to prevent further streptococcal infections is not necessary.

QSEN Checkpoint Question 46.3

PATIENT-CENTERED CARE

Carey's grandmother tells the nurse that Carey had symptoms of acute glomerulonephritis last week that were greatly distressing. The nurse identifies which reported symptom as a typical first symptom of glomerulonephritis?

a. Carey said her left knee hurt, although she didn't remember bumping it.
b. Carey asked her grandmother why there was blood in the toilet bowl.
c. Carey cried because she was starting to experience cramps.
d. Carey told her grandmother her stomach hurt after using the bathroom.

Look in Appendix A for the best answer and rationale.

CHRONIC GLOMERULONEPHRITIS

Although chronic glomerulonephritis occasionally follows acute glomerulonephritis or nephrotic syndrome, it also occurs as a primary disease (or after acute glomerulonephritis that was clinically so mild it was undiagnosed). The child is found to have proteinuria at a routine health assessment. Further investigation indicates hypertension and the presence of red cell or white cell casts and occult blood in urine with low specific gravity (below 1.003). Blood studies may indicate an increased BUN or creatinine levels. An MRI or a renal biopsy will reveal permanent destruction of glomerular membranes.

The disorder may result in either diffuse or local nephron damage. In both instances, the undamaged nephrons increase their glomerular filtration rate to compensate for the damaged nephrons. At some point in this chronic disease destruction process, however, compensatory mechanisms begin to fail, and renal insufficiency or failure results. **Alport syndrome**, which also includes hearing loss and ocular changes, is progressive chronic glomerulonephritis inherited as an X-linked or autosomal recessive disorder (Kruegel, Rubel, & Gross, 2013).

With chronic glomerulonephritis, if the child has acute symptoms of edema, hematuria, hypertension, or oliguria, bed rest may be necessary. If children have only a chronic manifestation, such as proteinuria, and continue to feel well, they can maintain normal activity, including school attendance. Children should not engage in competitive activities such as contact sports, however, because of the risk of kidney injury.

Therapy is nonspecific and directed at symptom relief rather than the disease process or its cause, which is unknown. Therapy with antihypertensive drugs such as hydralazine (Apresoline) or with diuretics to increase urine output such as ethacrynic acid (Edecrin) can be helpful. Corticosteroid therapy may reduce or halt the progress of the disorder by reducing inflammation. Children have difficulty accepting long-term corticosteroid therapy because of the side effects, in particular the typical "moon face" and extra body hair (Cushing syndrome) that develop. Talk with them about these body changes and assure them that these changes will reverse when the drug is discontinued.

Children receiving corticosteroids are at an increased risk for developing infections because of the immunosuppressive activity of these drugs. Be certain parents know how to take their child's temperature and to report the earliest signs of infection as well as shield their child from other children (and healthcare personnel) with infections.

Generally, the prognosis for children with chronic glomerulonephritis is not encouraging because, although the illness runs a long-term course, eventually it leads to renal insufficiency and renal failure (Kraut, 2013). Kidney transplantation is a possibility to replace a diseased kidney. Children can be maintained for long periods by peritoneal dialysis or hemodialysis while waiting for a transplant.

Although most children are adolescents or young adults before the disease runs its ultimate course, because children as young as early school age are aware of the importance of kidney function, most are aware of the likely outcome of their disease at an early age. They indicate that they appreciate having healthcare personnel face this outcome with them honestly while they wait for kidney transplantation to prolong their life.

NEPHROTIC SYNDROME (NEPHROSIS)

Nephrosis is altered glomerular permeability apparently due to an autoimmune process or a T-lymphocyte dysfunction that results in fusion of the glomeruli membrane surfaces, which, in turn, leads to abnormal loss of protein in urine. The highest incidence is at 3 years of age, and it occurs more often in boys than in girls (Mahan, 2011).

Nephrotic syndrome occurs in three forms: (a) congenital, as an autosomal recessive disorder; (b) secondary, as a progression of glomerulonephritis or in connection with systemic diseases such as sickle-cell anemia or systemic lupus erythematosus (SLE); and (c) idiopathic (primary). The congenital form is rare; the idiopathic form is most common (Praga & Morales, 2013).

Nephrosis can be further classified according to the amount of membrane destruction: minimal change nephrotic syndrome (MCNS), focal glomerulosclerosis (FGS), and membranoproliferative glomerulonephritis (MPGN). MCNS is the type most often seen in children (80%). As the name implies, with this type, little scarring of glomeruli occurs. Both

Figure 46.11 The process that results in the signs and symptoms of nephrotic syndrome.

of the other types involve scarring of glomeruli, and these children will have a poorer response to therapy (Hodson & Craig, 2013).

The four characteristic symptoms of nephrotic syndrome are proteinuria, edema, hypoalbuminemia (low serum albumin level), and hyperlipidemia (increased blood lipid level) (Richardson, 2012). Proteinuria occurs because increased glomerular permeability leads to protein loss in the urine and, subsequently, hypoalbuminemia. With a low level of protein in the bloodstream, osmotic pressure causes fluid to shift from the bloodstream into interstitial tissue, causing the edema. As the blood volume decreases, the kidneys begin to conserve sodium and water, adding to the potential for edema. The hyperlipidemia occurs because the liver increases production of lipoproteins to try to compensate for protein loss. Lipids are too large to be lost in urine, so they rise to high levels in the blood serum. Some children have such high lipid levels that, when blood is drawn and placed into a test tube, a circle of white fat forms across the top. Figure 46.11 illustrates the process that leads to these usual symptoms.

Assessment

Symptoms invariably begin insidiously. Edema tends to be dependent or occur in the lower parts of the body. Children develop swelling around the eyes (periorbital edema) upon waking in the morning after sleeping with their head flat on a bed. Parents may notice that clothing no longer fits a child around the waist because edematous fluid is beginning to collect in the abdominal cavity (ascites). It is easy for parents to dismiss these first symptoms as those of an upper respiratory tract infection and the normal "paunchy" belly of a toddler or preschooler. As edema progresses, however, the child's skin becomes pale, stretched, and taut. In boys, scrotal edema becomes extremely marked. Ascites may become so extensive that the resultant pressure on the stomach and intestine leads to anorexia, vomiting, or diarrhea. Because of poor nutrition, the child's growth may decline, and the child may become malnourished, yet the child will appear deceptively obese because of the extensive abdominal edema. When the abdominal ascites presses against the diaphragm, children may develop difficulty breathing. Parents report that children are irritable and fussy, probably from the feeling of abdominal fullness and generalized edema (Fig. 46.12). In addition, an increased risk for clotting can occur from the decreased intravascular fluid volume.

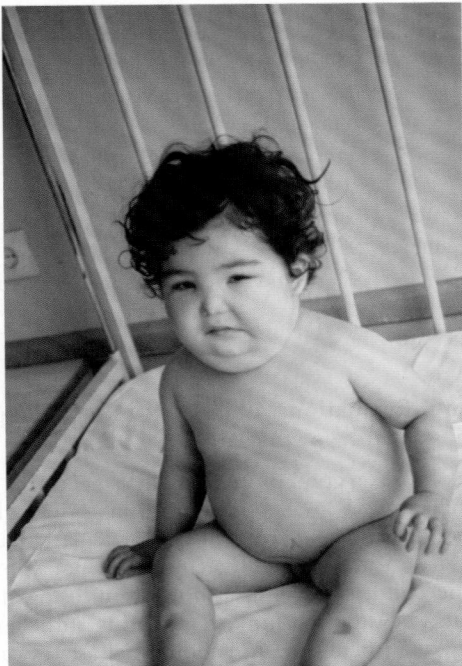

Figure 46.12 A young child with edema of the face and abdomen due to nephrotic syndrome. (From Salimpour, R. R., Salimpour, P., & Salimpour, P. [2013]. *Photographic atlas of pediatric disorders and diagnosis.* Philadelphia, PA: Lippincott Williams & Wilkins.)

Laboratory studies will reveal marked proteinuria. A single test will show a 1+ to 4+ protein; a 24-hour total urine test will show up to 15 g of protein (normally, urine contains no protein). The protein loss with nephrotic syndrome is almost entirely albumin, differentiating it from the proteinuria of glomerulonephritis, in which protein loss tends to be nonspecific. Some children with nephrotic syndrome exhibit hematuria at the onset, but it is minimal in contrast to that seen with acute glomerulonephritis. The erythrocyte sedimentation rate (demonstrating the inflammation of the glomeruli membrane) is elevated. Features of acute glomerulonephritis and nephrotic syndrome are compared in Table 46.3. An MRI or renal biopsy may be done to determine whether there is scarring of the glomerular membrane and to document the type of nephrotic syndrome present.

Therapeutic Management

Therapy for nephrotic syndrome is directed toward reducing the proteinuria and subsequent edema. This is typically achieved through a course of corticosteroids, such as IV methylprednisolone or oral prednisone, and keeping the child free of infection while the immune system is suppressed by these drugs. An initial dose of prednisone is given until diuresis without protein loss is accomplished; the dosage is then reduced for maintenance and continued for as long as 1 to 2 months.

Instruct parents to test the first urine specimen of the day for protein with a chemical reagent strip and keep an accurate chart showing the pattern of protein loss. Approximately once a week, parents are usually asked to collect a 24-hour urine specimen so total protein loss can be measured.

After an initial 4 weeks of therapy, prednisone is generally given every other day rather than every day. This is because prednisone has the potential to halt growth and to suppress adrenal gland secretion, side effects which can be reduced if the drug is given on alternate days, resulting in less alteration of adrenal steroid production (Karch, 2013). Parents may need to be assured that alternate-day therapy is best to keep them from changing the schedule to every day or giving twice the calculated dose by adding extra tablets on alternate days as an attempt to make their child well sooner. Prednisone tastes bitter, so parents may welcome suggestions regarding how to disguise the taste, such as by mixing it with applesauce or flavored syrup.

Be certain that both the parents and the child are aware long-term administration of prednisone will cause a cushingoid appearance or a "moon face," extra fat at the base of the neck, and increased body hair. Be certain also that parents know to plan ahead for pharmacy refills so prednisone therapy is not stopped abruptly because an abrupt stop can lead to adrenal insufficiency.

Diuretics are not commonly used to reduce the edema of nephrosis because they tend to decrease blood volume, which is already decreased, possibly leading to acute renal failure. Children who respond poorly to prednisone alone, however, may need diuretic therapy with a drug such as furosemide (Lasix) to initiate more kidney function. When children are taking furosemide for extended periods, there is always a danger that too much potassium will be excreted, causing hypokalemia. Children on long-term diuretic therapy, therefore, usually need frequent blood studies to determine that

TABLE 46.3 COMPARISON OF FEATURES OF ACUTE GLOMERULONEPHRITIS AND NEPHROTIC SYNDROME

Factor	Acute Glomerulonephritis	Nephrotic Syndrome
Cause	Immune reaction to group A beta-hemolytic streptococcal infection	Idiopathic or an autoimmune process or a congenital inherited type
Onset	Abrupt	Insidious
Hematuria	Profuse	Rare
Edema	Mild	Extreme
Hypertension	Marked	Mild
Hyperlipidemia	Rare or mild	Marked
Peak age frequency	5–10 years	2–3 years
Interventions	Limited activity; antihypertensives as needed; symptomatic therapy for congestive heart failure	Corticosteroid and cyclophosphamide administration; possibly diuretic and potassium supplements
Diet	Normal for age	Normal for age with some salt restriction
Prevention	Prevention or thorough treatment of group A beta-hemolytic streptococcal infections	None known

their electrolyte levels, especially potassium, are adequate. They may need supplemental potassium and should eat foods high in potassium such as bananas and milk. IV albumin may be administered to temporarily correct hypoalbuminemia. This causes edema to lessen because, as the serum albumin level rises, fluid shifts from subcutaneous spaces into the bloodstream. If the child is then administered a rapid-acting diuretic, the extra fluid in the bloodstream will be removed as urine. It's important that the diuretic be administered after the albumin infusion or the child could develop a fluid overload and, subsequently, heart failure.

Some children are prednisone-resistant or do not respond to corticosteroid therapy. With these children, a course of a cytotoxic agent, such as cyclophosphamide (Cytoxan) or cyclosporine (Sandimmune), or a stronger immunosuppressant agent, such as mycophenolate mofetil, may be effective in reducing symptoms or preventing further relapses of the disease (Banaszak & Banaszak, 2012). It is important to ensure children take in an adequate fluid intake with these drugs to prevent bladder irritation and bleeding. Cyclophosphamide is also used in chemotherapy for malignancy (see Chapter 53), so be certain parents are not misled into believing their child has cancer because their child is receiving a chemotherapeutic drug.

The prognosis for children with nephrotic syndrome varies. Almost all children with MCNS respond initially to steroid therapy and remain free of the disease. Those with FGS and MPGN types tend to have relapses at frequent or infrequent intervals over the next several years. Children who have frequent relapses this way have a relatively poorer chance of ever being free of the disorder, and many will require renal transplant later in life. All children and families need and deserve emotional support while the disease runs a long-term course.

QSEN Checkpoint Question 46.4

SAFETY

Carey is subsequently diagnosed with nephrotic syndrome. The nurse determines which action is best to provide patient education for the grandmother?

a. Caution her grandmother to not feed her foods high in salt because salt irritates glomeruli.
b. Encourage her to walk to school daily for exercise.
c. Teach her grandmother to test Carey's urine for protein using a dipstick.
d. Teach her grandmother how to take Carey's tympanic temperature daily.

Look in Appendix A for the best answer and rationale.

 ## Nursing Diagnoses and Related Interventions

Nursing interventions with nephrotic syndrome center on diminishing symptoms such as edema and proteinuria.

Nursing Diagnosis: Imbalanced nutrition, less than body requirements, related to poor appetite, restricted diet, and protein loss

TABLE 46.4 FOODS HIGH IN POTASSIUM

Food Group	Examples
Fruits	Bananas, peaches, prunes, raisins, oranges, orange juice
Vegetables	Carrots, celery, lima beans, potatoes, collards, dandelion greens, spinach
Protein	Nuts, peanuts, red meat
Dairy products	Milk, whole or skim; low-sodium milk
Miscellaneous	Salt substitutes, chocolate and cocoa, bran

Outcome Evaluation: Child follows normal growth curve on standard growth chart.

With nephrosis, a good protein intake is necessary to offset protein loss. A good potassium intake through consumption of fruits and fruit juices, particularly bananas, is necessary to maintain sufficient serum potassium levels, if the child is receiving a potassium-losing diuretic (Table 46.4). Although important, eating sufficient protein may be difficult because abdominal ascites can lead to a poor appetite. During acute phases of the disease, fluid or sodium may be temporarily restricted. If this is so, most children are happiest with many small glasses of fluid spaced throughout the day rather than several large drinks. It may help to make a chart showing the amount of fluid a child can drink each day. As fluid is given, color in a portion of the chart corresponding to the amount given to allow the child to tell from the uncolored portion how much more fluid is allowed that day, a much easier method for toddlers and preschoolers (the age group usually affected by this disease) to understand rather than hearing fluid measured in milliliters or even glassfuls.

Children need to be weighed daily to detect if fluid accumulation is continuing (caution parents to use the same scale with the child in the same clothing and measure at the same time of day for best accuracy). Review with them how to measure intake and output as well. If the child is hospitalized, taking pulse rate and blood pressure every 4 hours will help detect hypovolemia from excessive fluid shifts to interstitial tissue.

Nursing Diagnosis: Risk for impaired skin integrity related to edema

Outcome Evaluation: Child's skin is intact without erythema.

Edematous skin tends to break down easily, so children with nephrotic syndrome need frequent position changes while in bed. Check clothing to make certain an elastic band at the waist of pajamas or other constricting parts is not too tight. Place soft gauze between skin surfaces, especially around the scrotum, to help prevent skin irritation. Remember edematous tissue does not heal well, so breaks in the skin can easily become secondarily infected. Change frequently the diapers of children who are not toilet-trained and thoroughly clean their skin with each change to prevent skin breakdown and infection in the diaper area. Because medications are poorly absorbed from edematous skin areas, keep intramuscular or subcutaneous injections to a minimum. Advocate for oral

BOX 46.6

Nursing Care Planning

AN INTERPROFESSIONAL CARE MAP FOR A CHILD WITH NEPHROTIC SYNDROME

Carey is a 4-year-old girl admitted to the hospital with nephrotic syndrome. Her grandmother asks you, "Could this have happened because she drank part of a beer I left on the coffee table?"

Family Assessment: Child lives with grandparents in a trailer park while mother is incarcerated on a drug charge. Grandparents are both retired. Grandfather rates finances as, "Okay. I saved some money, and we both get Social Security."

Patient Assessment: Child began "gaining weight" and becoming irritable a week ago. Yesterday, her face appeared "very puffy." Appetite has declined sharply in last 2 weeks. States she's "always full." Marked dependent edema (4+ over tibia) present. Urine tested and found to be 4+ for protein.

Nursing Diagnosis: Excess fluid volume related to decreased kidney function and fluid accumulation

Outcome Criteria: Child's edema decreases; urine proteinuria is less than 2+.

Team Member Responsible	Assessment	Intervention	Rationale	Expected Outcome
Activities of Daily Living, Including Safety				
Nurse	Assess whether child is able to carry out routine activities with extensive ascites or edema.	Review with grandparents advantage of allowing child to continue usual activities.	Child's mobility may interfere with physical tasks; other children may make fun of her.	Child and grandparents state that child is able to continue with usual activities; will report bullying.
Teamwork and Collaboration				
Nurse/primary care provider	Assess whether grandparents have legal guardianship for child and can give permission for health care.	Contact renal service to evaluate whether child should be admitted to service for evaluation.	Nephrotic syndrome is a chronic disorder that requires conscientious, specialized health supervision.	Grandparents state they have legal guardianship; renal service personnel meet with child and grandparents for consultation.
Procedures/Medications for Quality Improvement				
Nurse	Assess if child has experience with oral medication; if grandparents will be able to do dipstick urine testing and 24-hour urine collection.	Administer oral prednisone as prescribed. Review techniques for dipstick urine testing and urine collection.	Prednisone, a corticosteroid, reduces immune response and proteinuria. Urine testing measures extent of protein loss.	Child accepts oral prednisone. Grandparents demonstrate technique of urine testing and urine collection.
Nutrition				
Nurse/nutritionist	Assess child's food intake for last 24 hours.	Suggest ways grandmother can include all food groups in child's diet even though child takes in a reduced amount.	Ascites crowds stomach, so it can give a feeling of fullness and cause undernutrition.	Child describes yesterday's intake; grandmother voices intent to devise a way to ensure child's intake remains nutritious.
Patient-Centered Care				
Nurse	Assess grandparents' knowledge about kidney function and kidney disease.	Teach grandparents about kidney function and disease process as needed.	Understanding disease process can help grandparents to better carry out therapy.	Grandparents state they understand why edema has occurred and describe action of medicine to reverse this.

Continued on following page

BOX 46.6

Nursing Care Planning (continued)

Team Member Responsible	Assessment	Intervention	Rationale	Expected Outcome
Psychosocial/Spiritual/Emotional Needs				
Nurse	Assess whether grandparents are having childrearing concerns.	Review natural inquisitiveness of preschool children, which can lead them into unsafe areas.	Grandparent states she didn't supervise child well so child drank beer off coffee table.	Grandparent states that although caring for a preschooler is difficult, she feels adequate to give care.
Informatics for Seamless Healthcare Planning				
Nurse	Assess if grandparents have transportation to return for follow-up appointment.	Schedule return appointment for 1 week at kidney clinic.	Because nephrotic syndrome is a long-term disorder, child will need continued follow-up for months to come.	Grandparents state they are aware of long-term nature of disorder and will keep follow-up appointments.

medication if at all possible (see Box 46.6, an interprofessional care map illustrating both nursing and team planning for a child with nephrotic syndrome).

Children are generally more comfortable if they sleep with their head elevated in a semi-Fowler's position rather than a supine or prone position because this reduces periorbital edema. If children do sleep in a head-flat position, edema can be so severe in the morning, their eyes are swollen completely shut or their tongues are so swollen that they cannot speak. Suggest ways parents can provide a semi-Fowler's position at home, such as by placing extra pillows on the child's bed or slipping a cardboard box under the head of the mattress to raise that end of the mattress.

What If . . . 46.3

A nurse needs to give an intramuscular injection to Carey, who has extensive dependent edema from nephrotic syndrome. Would it be best to inject into a thigh or deltoid muscle? Why?

HENOCH–SCHÖNLEIN SYNDROME NEPHRITIS

Henoch–Schönlein purpura is discussed in Chapter 44. Approximately one quarter of the children who develop this type of purpura develop renal disease as a secondary complication. The renal involvement becomes apparent within a few days after the manifestations of purpuric symptoms. Children will show either urinary abnormalities such as proteinuria or a rapidly progressing glomerulonephritis. Most children recover completely. A few will develop chronic symptoms and long-term kidney disease (Jauhola, Ronkainen, Koskimies, et al., 2012).

SYSTEMIC LUPUS ERYTHEMATOSUS

SLE is an autoimmune disease in which, when autoantibodies and antigens meet, they cause deposits of complement in the kidney glomerulus (see Chapter 20). As a result, some children with SLE develop symptoms of acute or chronic glomerulonephritis; glomerulonephritis or heart disease is the ultimate cause of death in many adults with SLE (Lateef & Petri, 2012). Therapy with corticosteroids or cytotoxic agents may be effective to stop the renal destruction. If kidney transplantation is required, the transplant should be successful because the same damage rarely occurs in the transplanted kidney.

HEMOLYTIC-UREMIC SYNDROME

With hemolytic-uremic syndrome, the lining of glomerular arterioles becomes inflamed, swollen, and occluded with particles of platelets and fibrin. The child's red blood cells and platelets become damaged as they flow through the partially occluded blood vessels. As the damaged cells reach the spleen, they are destroyed by the spleen and removed from circulation, leading to a hemolytic anemia.

Ninety percent of children who develop this syndrome have recently experienced an *E. coli* gastrointestinal infection from a source such as undercooked hamburger (*E. coli* is found in the intestine of beef cattle). Whether to treat *E. coli* infections with antibiotics is controversial because some children who have their initial *E. coli* infection treated with an antibiotic appear to have a more serious form of anemia than those not treated (Geerdes-Fenge, Löbermann, Nürnberg, et al., 2013).

Assessment

The syndrome occurs most often during the summer months and in children 6 months to 4 years of age. Children usually develop only a transient diarrhea from the *E. coli* infection, although this can progress to severe fluid loss and bowel wall necrosis. Fever may become so elevated that the child experiences stupor and hallucinations. Oliguria accompanied by proteinuria, hematuria, and urinary casts in urine follows. The oliguria will lead to increased serum creatinine and BUN and extensive edema. Children appear pale from anemia; easy bruising or petechiae may be present from *thrombocytopenia* (reduced platelet level). Laboratory studies will show fibrin split products in the serum as the fibrin deposits in glomerular vessels are degraded. Thrombocytopenia will be present because platelets are damaged by the irregular blood vessels.

Therapeutic Management

The child needs renal replacement therapy (supportive therapy) to maintain kidney and heart function. The extreme oliguria can be treated with peritoneal dialysis; anemia can be corrected by careful transfusion of packed red cells.

Ensure that parents understand the importance of follow-up care and have an appointment for this. Help them begin to view the child as well again so they do not continue to shelter the child unnecessarily but allow for normal growth and development.

Despite the extent of the illness, most infants with hemolytic-uremic syndrome recover completely. Some children, however, die of the acute illness or continue to have chronic renal involvement.

ACUTE RENAL FAILURE

Renal failure occurs in either an acute or chronic form. The acute form most often occurs because of a sudden body insult, such as severe dehydration. The chronic form results from extensive kidney disease, such as hemolytic-uremic syndrome or glomerulonephritis (Lum, 2012).

Other causes of acute renal failure include prolonged anesthesia, hemorrhage, shock, severe diarrhea, or sudden traumatic injury. It also can occur in children who are placed on cardiopulmonary bypass while undergoing heart surgery, who receive common antibiotics (aminoglycosides, penicillin, cephalosporins, and sulfonamides), who swallow a poison such as arsenic (found in rat poison), or who are exposed to industrial wastes such as mercury. All of these conditions appear to lead to renal ischemia, which ultimately leads to acute renal failure.

Assessment

One of the first symptoms noted with acute renal failure is *oliguria*, a urine output of less than 1 ml/kg of the child's body weight per hour. An indwelling urinary catheter may be inserted to rule out the possibility that urinary retention in the bladder, rather than kidney dysfunction, is causing the severe oliguria.

Both **azotemia** (accumulation of nitrogen waste from the breakdown of protein in the bloodstream) and *uremia* (extra accumulation of nitrogen wastes in the blood, with additional toxic symptoms such as cerebral irritation) will occur because of the oliguria. The BUN level rises progressively as renal insufficiency continues and fewer and fewer breakdown products of protein can be excreted. As the kidneys become unable to dilute or concentrate urine, the specific gravity of urine often becomes "fixed" at 1.010. A BUN level greater than 80 to 100 mg/100 ml is a toxic level and needs correction, usually by dialysis. Urine creatinine is another measure that can be used as an indicator of function because it is normally excreted at a uniform rate. A rate of less than 10 mg/100 ml indicates severe renal failure.

Hyperkalemia (elevated potassium level), manifested by a weak, irregular pulse, abdominal cramps, lowered blood pressure, and muscle weakness, begins to occur as potassium can no longer be excreted. Acidosis will follow shortly from the inability of H^+ ions to be excreted. As the total output decreases, phosphorus levels rise in the bloodstream. A high serum phosphorus level leads to a low calcium serum level because phosphorus and calcium have an inverse proportional relationship. Severe hypocalcemia leads to muscle twitching and seizures (*tetany*); chronic hypocalcemia leads to withdrawal of calcium from bones (*osteodystrophy*) (Wesseling-Perry, 2013).

An IVP, MRI, or radioactive uptake scan is used to substantiate the lack of kidney function. Parents and children need support for this type of study because the results may be disappointing and so different from what they hoped they would be.

Therapeutic Management

Because acute renal failure is a reaction to body stress caused by acute disease or insult, attempts to treat it focus on supporting the child's body systems while correcting the underlying condition. If the child is dehydrated (as with diarrhea or hemorrhage), IV fluid is needed to replace plasma volume. Administer such fluid slowly, however, to avoid heart failure because extra fluid cannot be removed by the nonfunctioning kidneys. Be certain the fluid prescribed does not contain potassium until it is established that kidney function is adequate; otherwise, the buildup of potassium could cause heart block. Potassium levels greater than 6 mEq/L are corrected by the IV administration of calcium gluconate (as the glucose moves into cells, it carries potassium with it), by the oral administration of a cation exchange resin such as sodium polystyrene (Kayexalate), or by dialysis. Administering sodium bicarbonate is another method for causing a shift of potassium from the bloodstream into cells, temporarily reducing the circulating potassium level. Administration of a combination of IV glucose and insulin may also be effective (insulin helps glucose move into cells and potassium is carried with it).

A diuretic such as furosemide (Lasix) may be prescribed in an attempt to increase urine production. The child's diet should be low in protein, potassium, and sodium and high in carbohydrate to supply enough calories for metabolism yet limit urea production and control serum potassium levels. Oral fluid intake may be limited to prevent heart failure due to accumulating fluid that cannot be excreted. Weigh children daily (same scale, same clothing, same time of day) and maintain accurate intake and output recordings to help evaluate fluid status. If children are so ill they cannot eat, total parenteral nutrition may be necessary. Again, regulate amounts carefully to prevent fluid overload (see Chapter 37 for administration techniques).

When recovery from acute renal failure begins, children generally have a degree of diuresis as the extra fluid accumulated by the body begins to clear. It's important that this increase in urine production is noted because children may need additional fluid intake at this point to prevent hypovolemia, which could lead once more to renal failure. Being told their child has acute renal failure is a harrowing time for parents. They usually remain anxious for an extended period after an episode of acute renal failure because they fear that the restoration of kidney function is only temporary. Reassure them that urine output is remaining at a normal level so they can relax and interact effectively with their child.

CHRONIC KIDNEY DISEASE (END-STAGE KIDNEY DISEASE)

Chronic renal failure results from developmental abnormalities, when acute failure becomes long term, or when chronic kidney disease has caused extensive nephron destruction (Braun, Sood, Hogue, et al., 2012). The nephrons that are not destroyed appear to function as usual; they simply are inadequate in number to sustain kidney function. Beginning approximately when 50% of nephrons are destroyed, kidney function diminishes by degree until the child develops end-stage kidney disease (the point when kidneys can no longer effectively evacuate waste products from the body).

Assessment

With loss of nephron function, the ability to concentrate urine halts, resulting in polyuria, possibly manifested as enuresis. The few functioning nephrons present cannot reabsorb enough sodium to maintain a functioning serum level of body fluid, so dehydration occurs. As additional nephrons are lost, the polyuria decreases, and oliguria and anuria occur. Inability to excrete H^+ ions leads to acidosis. Hypocalcemia and hyperphosphatemia occur from the kidney's inability to excrete phosphate. Osteodystrophy occurs as calcium is withdrawn from bones to compensate for the low level of calcium. In addition, because kidneys are responsible for synthesizing vitamin D to its active form, vitamin D cannot be produced. Without this, calcium cannot be absorbed from the gastrointestinal tract and deposited in bones. Bones become so calcium depleted that growth halts and the bones lose strength (renal rickets).

Erythropoietin, formed by the kidneys, stimulates red cell production. With decreased erythropoietin production, anemia develops. Pruritus may be present from skin irritation due to excretion of nitrogenous wastes. These changes are summarized in Figure 46.13.

Therapeutic Management

Children with chronic renal failure are generally placed on a low-protein, low-phosphorus, low-potassium diet to prevent rapid urea and phosphate buildup. Children may be prescribed aluminum hydroxide gel to take with meals to bind phosphorus in the intestines and prevent absorption. Milk usually is not given because it is high in sodium, potassium, and phosphate—electrolytes children may have difficulty clearing. Meat is restricted, and even beans are high enough in protein to be eliminated, making this a difficult diet for children to follow over an extended period. Letting children have some choice about what foods they eat each day helps to promote adjustment to such a restricted diet. Whoever will be preparing meals at home needs good instructions on selecting low-protein foods. Low-electrolyte, low-protein formulas are commercially available for infants with renal failure.

Total daily fluid intake may need to be restricted, although restriction should be as minimal as possible, or it can present an area of tremendous conflict between the child and parents. Many children need sodium intake restricted, and others need a normal sodium intake (but no excessively salty foods such as lunch meats, potato chips, or pretzels). In contrast, other children may actually need additional salt because, due to poor tubular reabsorption, they dump sodium in urine. Low-sodium formulas such as Lonalac are recommended for children with heart failure who need a low-sodium intake. These must be used cautiously in children with renal insufficiency, however, because their high-potassium content can lead to toxic potassium blood levels. Diuretics may be prescribed to help children regulate sodium and fluid levels and prevent edema.

As renal failure becomes prolonged, a child needs supplemental calcium to prevent muscle cramping, rickets, tetany, or seizures. As hypertension becomes more and more acute from the accumulating blood volume, a daily antihypertensive drug may be prescribed. Recombinant human erythropoietin to stimulate red blood cell formation or packed red cells may be needed to correct anemia. Like all fluid, administer blood transfusions cautiously so volume overload does not occur. Dialysis is the answer to effective excretion of urea while children wait for a kidney transplant to replace their nonfunctioning kidneys.

Nursing Diagnoses and Related Interventions

Nursing diagnoses with chronic or end-stage kidney disease must address both the physical and psychological aspects of the illness and long-term care.

Nursing Diagnosis: Risk for interrupted family processes related to chronically ill family member

Outcome Evaluation: Family members express feelings about illness to each other and to healthcare providers; participate in care of ill member.

It is easy for children to become depressed because of chronic fatigue and an unappetizing diet (Tong, Henning, Wong, et al., 2013). They begin to grow poorly because of the alteration in calcium metabolism, and if they are taking corticosteroids or other immunosuppressive drugs because of glomerulonephritis, they may be angry or disheartened about their change in appearance from taller and thin to shorter and heavier. Help them stay as active as possible to discourage boredom by suggesting age-appropriate activities. Because adolescence is an age at

Destruction of glomeruli

Retention of blood urea nitrogen, creatinine, potassium, phosphorus

Hyperkalemia and hypocalcemia

Bone growth arrest

Body growth arrest

Retention of urine

Edema

Hypertension

Decreased red blood cell production

Anemia

Figure 46.13 Pathology of chronic renal failure.

which recreational drug use is common, ask if teenagers are using a recreational drug as a method to relieve their anxiety or boredom (Steele, Belostotsky, & Lau, 2012).

Caring for a child with chronic renal disease is time-consuming and can be financially and socially devastating for parents. Parents caring for such children at home need opportunities at periodic health assessments to voice their frustrations, fears, and anxieties. They need time to do those things important to them as individuals whether taking a weekend trip or attending an evening movie. Ask parents at clinic or follow-up visits, "Do you ever get out of the house or have the opportunity to do anything for yourself?" "What can we do for *you*?" Help of this kind ultimately improves children's care because it improves the lives and mental attitudes of those around them.

QSEN Checkpoint Question 46.5

INFORMATICS

Carey's grandmother is deeply concerned that Carey will develop chronic kidney disease later in life. What findings in Carey's laboratory workup would suggest that her kidneys are failing? (Select all that apply.)

   a. She has an elevated serum phosphorus level.
   b. She is developing a normocytic anemia.
   c. Her serum vitamin D level is below normal.
   d. Her serum creatinine level is steadily falling.
   e. Her blood pressure is steadily increasing.

Look in Appendix A for the best answer and rationale.

Kidney Transplantation

The ultimate possibility for prolonging the life of children with renal failure is kidney transplantation. With complete renal failure, children who have extensive hypertension may have their damaged kidneys removed and be placed on hemodialysis or CCPD to await kidney transplantation. Kidney removal this way is an important step for both the parents and the child because although parents realize their child's kidneys are no longer functioning, this step removes all hope that a miracle might make them function once more. Parents may ask whether it is possible to leave one of the child's kidneys because only one kidney will be transplanted (not recommended because the hypertension would continue). Be certain that parents have a thorough explanation of why hypertension is destructive and that it could lead to a cerebrovascular accident or coronary artery disease. Help them understand that their child's renal biopsy shows that, short of a miracle, their child's kidneys will not function again, and so their removal is not a loss but only recognition of a loss.

PREOPERATIVE CARE

Kidney transplantation is most effective (the kidney is less likely to be rejected) if the kidney is taken from a living twin, parent, or sibling (Butani, Troppmann, & Perez, 2013). Rejection occurs at a higher incidence if a kidney comes from a cadaver or recently deceased child. Most people consider

that children should be of legal age to give consent to supply a kidney for transplantation, so few children have a sibling who is eligible to donate a kidney. Transplanted kidneys are placed in the abdomen, not the usual kidney space. Transplantation of a kidney from an adult into a child who weighs less than 10 kg can be difficult because of the difference in the size of the arteries and veins, which must be matched, and because of the possibility of hypertension, excessive diuresis, and abdominal complications (from the lack of space).

Many children anticipate that the characteristics of the donor will be transmitted to them by the kidney, so they are reluctant to accept the kidney of a family member with a character trait they do not like (perhaps a bad temper). You can assure them that transplanted organs do not transplant character traits with them.

People who are ineligible to donate a kidney include those with multiple bilateral small renal arteries, bilateral renal disease, renal infection, advanced medical illness, severe obesity, or hypertension. Although kidney removal can be done by laparoscopy, donors must understand that removal of a kidney involves major surgery. Tests kidney donors can expect to have preoperatively include human leukocyte antigen (HLA) typing, electrolyte blood analysis, complete blood count, bleeding time, urinalysis and urine culture, 24-hour urine sample for protein, a renal arteriogram, and IV pyelography. Donors will have urine samples collected after surgery to assess that their remaining kidney is capable of maintaining full function and that they are still in good health.

Before surgery, children who are to receive a transplant may be dialyzed to clear their body of excessive potassium and fluid. If the donated kidney will be from a relative, there is adequate time for thorough preoperative preparation of this type. If the donor kidney is from a cadaver, the announcement of surgery will be sudden, and time for preoperative instruction and procedures may be limited. The family should be prepared for this possibility well in advance, and teaching should occur before a cadaver kidney becomes available.

QSEN Checkpoint Question 46.6

EVIDENCE-BASED PRACTICE

When kidney disease becomes chronic, it places a great burden on caregivers' energy and finances. To investigate how parents feel about caring for a child with chronic kidney disease, researchers interviewed parents of 20 children with chronic kidney disease recruited from two pediatric hospitals. Results of the study revealed four major themes: parents had to struggle to accept the diagnosis and permanence of their child's disorder; parents found continuous caregiving stressful, exhausting, and overwhelming; spousal tension and sibling neglect occurred; and parents felt they needed support from their healthcare providers (Tong, Lowe, Sainsbury, et al., 2010). In addition, a recent first-of-its-kind meta-analysis examining caregiver stress in pediatric chronic conditions indicates that caregivers of children with chronic illness endorse greater general parenting stress than caregivers of healthy children (Cousino & Hazen, 2013).

Based on these studies, if Carey developed chronic kidney disease, which action by a nurse would be most helpful?

a. Assure the grandmother she can call the clinic at any time if she has a concern.

b. Ask the grandmother to keep a daily record of conversations she has with Carey.

c. Review with the grandmother ways that Carey will require even more care in the future.

d. Help the grandmother learn to say "no" when other family members ask her to help them.

Look in Appendix A for the best answer and rationale.

Human Leukocyte Antigen Typing

HLAs are a group of antigens found on the surfaces of all cells with a nucleus, including blood components such as leukocytes and platelets. The name is derived from the fact they were first identified on white blood cells. Such antigens are inherited from both parents and are specific for each individual. They are carried on the short arm of chromosome 6 in each cell and denote tissue type or determine which tissue the immune system will identify as foreign tissue. They also serve as the basis for paternity typing and may cause reactions to blood product transfusions and bone marrow and organ transplants.

When two people have the same, or mostly the same, HLA antigens, they are said to be *histocompatible*. Identical twins have complete histocompatibility; family members have partial histocompatibility; any two people can have histocompatibility on at least one antigen site.

Children who are awaiting kidney transplantation are HLA typed, and this information is circulated to major medical centers. When a kidney is available for transplantation, the child's tissue type is compared with the donor kidney, and factors such as "best match," general condition, size of the child, and length of time the child has been on the waiting list are considered. The chance of receiving a kidney is increased today because, with new immunosuppressive drugs, even donor kidneys that are not fully matched have a chance to successfully graft.

POSTOPERATIVE CARE

After renal transplantation, children are cared for in an environment that is as sterile as possible as they are placed on immunosuppressive therapy such as cyclosporine, azathioprine (Imuran), and methylprednisolone (Solu-Medrol), and possibly antilymphocyte globulin and antithymocyte globulin to reduce the possibility of kidney rejection. Although some transplanted kidneys begin to function immediately, hemodialysis may be continued until the implanted kidney can fully function after recovering from the initial insult of transplantation.

Children may pass through a "honeymoon" period after the transplantation or a period during which a child models perfect behavior on the belief the success of the transplant depends on good behavior rather than the condition of renal veins and arteries, the transplanted kidney, or antigen–antibody formation (Box 46.7).

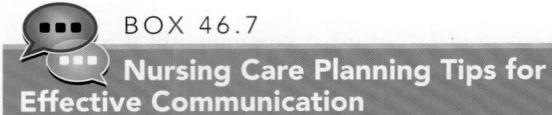

BOX 46.7

Nursing Care Planning Tips for Effective Communication

Carey's grandmother tells you Carey has "changed completely" since she became ill with acute glomerulonephritis.

Tip: Use therapeutic communication and ask specific follow-up questions. In the following scenario, the grandmother describes a "honeymoon" period that children may pass through after being told their kidneys are injured because they know how important kidneys are for life. Parents often need help seeing this for what it is, so they can begin to reassure children that behaving perfectly will not influence the outcome of their illness and that, because they loved them as they were, they will continue to love them regardless.

Nurse: Mrs. Hendricks, in what way has Carey changed?

Mrs. Hendricks: She used to whine all the time and constantly ask for things. Now, she entertains herself. It's like heaven.

Nurse: Do you think she's acting a little too perfect?

Mrs. Hendricks: Well, it does seem a bit strange.

Nurse: Do you think she feels responsible for being sick? Could she be worrying that if she misbehaves, her medicine will stop working?

Mrs. Hendricks: I never thought of that. I would feel better if she started to act like her old self.

Children with end-stage renal disease are usually behind in growth at the time of a transplant. Although the rate of growth will be improved after kidney transplantation, they may never reach full height, related to the already lost growth plus need for corticosteroid maintenance therapy to continue immunosuppression long term.

Transplant Rejection

Acute transplant rejection, if it occurs, usually develops within the first 3 months after transplantation. Children begin to develop fever, proteinuria, oliguria, weight gain, hypertension, and tenderness over the kidney. Serum creatinine and BUN levels will rise. Increasing the dose of immunosuppressants may be effective in stopping this type of rejection.

Rejection may also be *chronic*, in which the transplanted kidney gradually loses function after the first 6 months. Hypertension and anemia result. An MRI or a biopsy will show vascular changes such as narrowing of arterial lumens and interstitial changes such as fibrosis and tubular atrophy. This type of rejection is difficult to halt, although it may be such a slow, steady process that it will be 2 or 3 years before the kidney actually fails. If a kidney is rejected, it is removed, and a child is returned to a program of hemodialysis. Because one kidney was rejected does not mean a second transplant will also be rejected. Unfortunately, because the number of kidneys available for transplantation is limited, kidney rejection of this type becomes an ominous sign for the child's long-term survival.

Malignant disease is more common in transplantation recipients than in the normal population probably because of the long-term immunosuppression (Ponticelli & Graziani, 2012). The original disease for which the child underwent transplantation, such as glomerulonephritis, may also recur in the transplanted kidney. During adolescence, typically an age of poor adherence to medication regimens, monitor kidney recipients closely to be certain they are taking their immunosuppressive therapy. Parents cannot help but overprotect the child after a kidney transplant; they worry a roughhousing session with a sibling or playing a game such as baseball may injure the transplanted kidney. The child may be afraid to engage in any activity for the same reason. Ask at healthcare visits if the family needs help to return to a healthy lifestyle after this major life change.

What If . . . 46.4

A nurse is particularly interested in exploring one of the 2020 National Health Goals regarding renal disorders of children (see Box 46.1). What would be a possible research topic pertinent to this goal that would be applicable to Carey's family and also advance evidence-based practice?

KEY POINTS FOR REVIEW

- Many urinary tract disorders, such as polycystic kidneys, urethral obstruction, and bladder exstrophy, are often evident on a prenatal ultrasound. Early identification on fetal ultrasound allows therapy to begin in utero or immediately after birth.

- Many urinary tract disorders, such as polycystic kidneys or chronic renal failure, are long-term conditions requiring years of therapy. Be certain parents are well informed about their child's condition so they can continue to participate in planning their child's care that not only meets QSEN competencies but also best meets the family's total needs.

- Congenital structural abnormalities of the urinary tract include patent urachus, exstrophy of the bladder, hypospadias, and epispadias. Surgical correction is required for all of these, but the outcome should be favorable. In the case of epispadias and exstrophy, referral to a pediatric urologist trained in these conditions through a fellowship should be facilitated to support the best possible outcome.

- UTI tends to occur more often in girls than boys. "Honeymoon cystitis" refers to a UTI occurring after the first instance of sexual intercourse. Preventing recurrent infections is important in order to prevent damage to the lining of the bladder, bacterial colonization of the bladder, and long-term renal damage.

- Vesicoureteral reflux is the backflow of urine into one or both ureters with voiding because the valve that guards the entrance to the ureters is lax or the ureters insert too low in the bladder. Surgical correction may be necessary to prevent renal damage, but proper voiding habits, constipation management, and hydration should be emphasized because optimization of these key factors often decreases or, in some cases, abates vesicoureteral reflux.

- Kidney dysfunction can occur for structural reasons such as kidney agenesis, polycystic kidney, and renal hypoplasia, all conditions that limit kidney function.

- Acute poststreptococcal glomerulonephritis is inflammation of the glomeruli after a streptococcal infection. It is characterized by an acute episode of hematuria and proteinuria but typically runs a short-term course.

- Nephrotic syndrome is an immunologic process that results in altered glomerular permeability and can lead to a self-limiting or long-term course.

- Diminished kidney function leads to both fluid and electrolyte imbalances. Creative techniques are necessary to encourage children to continue to ingest a restricted-protein diet.

- When renal failure is either acute or chronic, peritoneal dialysis or hemodialysis may be used to remove body wastes until kidney function can be restored.

- Kidney transplantation is often the only long-term option for children with kidney failure. It requires extensive surgery and requires the child to remain on immunosuppressive therapy long term in order to prevent transplant rejection.

CRITICAL THINKING CARE STUDY

Jamie is a 16-year-old teenager with chronic kidney disease. He lives with his mother and a younger sister, 10 years old. He's homeschooled because he has to miss 3 days of school each week for hemodialysis.

1. You notice that although Jamie is supposed to limit the amount of potassium he ingests, when offered a choice between popcorn with orange juice or raisins and milk for an afternoon snack he chose the raisins and milk. Was that his best choice?

2. Jamie appears obese because of the long-term use of immunosuppressants. You hear him brag to his girlfriend that he has lost more weight than her as part of a New Year's resolution pact. You also notice, according to Jamie's medicine reminder sheet, that he has missed taking two doses of prednisone. Would omitting taking prednisone cause him to lose weight? What could be the effect of omitting his prescribed prednisone?

3. Jamie's mother wants him to learn to drive so he can travel to the dialysis center by himself. Jamie says he can't do that because dialysis makes him feel dizzy and nauseated. Are those common symptoms of dialysis? As his dialysis nurse, what could you do to reduce his symptoms?

RELATED RESOURCES

Explore these additional resources to enhance learning for this chapter:
- Student resources on thePoint, including answers to the What If . . . and Critical Thinking Care Study questions, http://thepoint.lww.com/Flagg8e
- Adaptive learning powered by PrepU, http://thepoint.lww.com/prepu

REFERENCES

Banaszak, B., & Banaszak, P. (2012). The increasing incidence of initial steroid resistance in childhood nephrotic syndrome. *Pediatric Nephrology, 27*(6), 927–932.

Batinic, D., Milošević, D., Topalovic-Grkovic, M., et al. (2013). Vesicoureteral reflux and urodynamic dysfunction. *Urology International, 90*(4), 480–483.

Bayhakki, A., & Hatthakit, U. (2012). Lived experiences of patients on hemodialysis: A meta-synthesis. *Nephrology Nursing Journal, 39*(4), 295–304.

Beck, J., Bekker, M., Van Driel, M., et al. (2010). Female sexual abuse evaluation in the urological practice: Results of a Dutch survey. *The Journal of Sexual Medicine, 7*(4, Pt. 1), 1464–1468.

Braun, L., Sood, V., Hogue, S., et al. (2012). High burden and unmet patient needs in chronic kidney disease. *International Journal of Nephrology Renovascular Disease, 5*, 151–163.

Butani, L., Troppmann, C., & Perez, R. V. (2013). Outcomes of children receiving en bloc renal transplants from small pediatric donors. *Pediatric Transplantation, 17*(1), 55–58.

Cousino, M., & Hazen, R. (2013). Parenting stress among caregivers of children with chronic illness: A systematic review. *Journal of Pediatric Psychology, 38*(8), 809–828.

Davenport, A. (2012). Portable or wearable peritoneal devices—the next step forward for peritoneal dialysis? *Advances in Peritoneal Dialysis, 28*(3), 97–101.

Deshpande, A. V., Caldwell, P. H. Y., & Sureshkumar, P. (2012). Drugs for nocturnal enuresis in children (other than desmopressin and tricyclics). *Cochrane Database of Systematic Reviews*, (12), CD002238.

Eldridge, M., & Lakshmanan, Y. (2011). Voiding dysfunction. In D. H. Chand & R. P. Valentini (Eds.), *Clinician's manual of pediatric nephrology* (pp. 381–395). Singapore: World Scientific.

Elshal, A. M., Abdelhalim, A., Hafez, A. T., et al. (2012). Ileal urinary reservoir in pediatric population: Objective assessment of long-term sequelae with time-to-event analysis. *Urology, 79*(5), 1126–1131.

Fearon, J. A., & Varkarakis, G. (2012). Dynamic abdominoplasty for the treatment of prune belly syndrome. *Plastic Reconstructive Surgery, 130*(3), 648–657.

Fleming, E. (2012). Supporting children with nocturnal enuresis. *Nursing Times, 108*(41), 22–25.

Gaylord, N. M., & Peterson-Smith, A. M. (2012). Genitourinary disorders. In C. E. Burns, A. M. Dunn, M. A. Brady, et al. (Eds.), *Pediatric primary care* (5th ed., pp. 809–843). Philadelphia, PA: Elsevier/Saunders.

Geerdes-Fenge, H. F., Löbermann, M., Nürnberg, M., et al. (2013). Ciprofloxacin reduces the risk of hemolytic uremic syndrome in patients with *Escherichia coli* O104:H4-associated diarrhea. *Infection, 41*(3), 669–673.

Hassett, S., Smith, G. H., & Holland, A. J. (2012). Prune belly syndrome. *Pediatric Surgery International, 28*(3), 219–228.

Hodson, E. M., & Craig, J. C. (2013). Corticosteroid therapy for steroid-sensitive nephrotic syndrome in children: Dose or duration? *Journal of the American Society of Nephrology, 24*(1), 7–9.

Hothi, D. K., Stronach, L., & Harvey, E. (2013). Home haemodialysis. *Pediatric Nephrology, 28*(5), 721–730.

Huether, S. E. (2013). Structure and function of the renal and urologic systems. In S. E. Huether & K. L. McCance (Eds.), *Understanding pathophysiology* (5th ed., pp. 724–764). New York, NY: Elsevier.

Hunziker, M., & Puri, P. (2012). Familial vesicoureteral reflux and reflux related morbidity in relatives of index patients with high grade vesicoureteral reflux. *The Journal of Urology, 188*(4 Suppl.), 1463–1466.

Issa, N., Lankireddy, S., & Kukla, A. (2012). Should peritoneal dialysis be the preferred therapy pre-kidney transplantation? *Advances in Peritoneal Dialysis, 28*(1), 89–93.

Jauhola, O., Ronkainen, J., Koskimies, O., et al. (2012). Outcome of Henoch-Schönlein purpura 8 years after treatment with a placebo or prednisone at disease onset. *Pediatric Nephrology, 27*(6), 933–939.

Kambham, N. (2012). Postinfectious glomerulonephritis. *Advances in Anatomic Pathology, 19*(5), 338–347.

Karch, A. M. (2013). *2013 Lippincott's nursing drug guide*. Philadelphia, PA: Lippincott Williams & Wilkins.

Kraut, J. A. (2013). Chronic kidney failure. In E. T. Bope & R. D. Kellerman (Eds.), *Conn's current therapy* (pp. 877–881). Philadelphia, PA: Elsevier/Saunders.

Kruegel, J., Rubel, D., & Gross, O. (2013). Alport syndrome—insights from basic and clinical research. *Nature Reviews. Nephrology, 9*(3), 170–178.

Lateef, A., & Petri, M. (2012). Unmet medical needs in systemic lupus erythematosus. *Arthritis Research Therapy, 14*(Suppl. 4), S4.

Lum, G. M. (2012). Kidney and urinary tract. In W. Hay, M. Levin, R. Deterding, et al. (Eds.), *Current diagnosis & treatment pediatrics* (21st ed., pp. 717–739). New York, NY: McGraw-Hill/Lange.

Mahan, J. D. (2011). Nephrology and urology. In K. J. Marcdante, R. M. Kliegman, H. B. Jenson, et al. (Eds.), *Nelson essentials of pediatrics* (6th ed., pp. 607–624). Philadelphia, PA: Elsevier/Saunders.

Milani, G. P., Mazzoni, M. B., Burdick, L., et al. (2010). Postural proteinuria associated with left renal vein entrapment: A follow-up evaluation. *American Journal of Kidney Disease, 55*(6), e29–e31.

Nelson, C. P., Chow, J. S., Rosoklija, I., et al. (2012). Patient and family impact of pediatric genitourinary diagnostic imaging tests. *The Journal of Urology, 188*(4 Suppl.), 1601–1607.

Paintsil, E. (2013). Update on recent guidelines for the management of urinary tract infections in children: The shifting paradigm. *Current Opinion in Pediatrics, 25*(1), 88–94.

Passamaneck, M. (2011). The changing paradigm for the management of pediatric vesicoureteral reflux. *Urologic Nursing, 31*(6), 363–366.

Ponticelli, C., & Graziani, G. (2012). Education and counseling of renal transplant recipients. *Journal of Nephrology, 25*(6), 879–889.

Praga, M., & Morales, E. (2013). Primary glomerular disease. In E. T. Bope & R. D. Kellerman (Eds.), *Conn's current therapy* (pp. 891–894). Philadelphia, PA: Elsevier/Saunders.

Puri, P., Kutasy, B., Colhoun, E., et al. (2012). Single center experience with endoscopic subureteral dextranomer/hyaluronic acid injection as first line treatment in 1,551 children with intermediate and high grade vesicoureteral reflux. *The Journal of Urology, 188*(4 Suppl.), 1485–1489.

Purves, T., & Gearhart, J. P. (2010). The bladder exstrophy-epispadias-cloacal exstrophy complex. In J. P. Gearhart, R. Rink, & P. Mouriquand (Eds.), *Pediatric urology* (2nd ed., pp. 386–415). Philadelphia, PA: Elsevier/Saunders.

Quinlan, C., Bates, M., Sheils, A., et al. (2013). Chronic hemodialysis in children weighing less than 10 kg. *Pediatric Nephrology, 28*(5), 803–809.

Richardson, M. A. (2012). The many faces of minimal change nephrotic syndrome: An overview and case study. *Nephrology Nursing Journal, 39*(5), 365–374.

Ring, P., & Huether, S. E. (2013). Alternations of renal and urinary tract function in children. In S. E. Huether & K. L. McCance (Eds.), *Understanding pathophysiology* (5th ed., pp. 764–773). New York, NY: Elsevier.

Roberts, K., Downs, S., Finnell, S., et al. (2011). Urinary tract infection: Clinical practice guideline for the diagnosis and management of the initial UTI in febrile infants and children 2 to 24 months. *Pediatrics, 128*(3), 595–610.

Sayed, S. A., Abu-Aisha, H., Ahmed, M. E., et al. (2013). Effect of the patient's knowledge on peritonitis rates in peritoneal dialysis. *Peritoneal Dialysis International, 33*(4), 362–366.

Spinoit, A. F., Poelaert, F., Groen, L. A., et al. (2013). Hypospadias repair in a single reference centre: Long term follow-up is mandatory to detect the real complication rate. *The Journal of Urology, 189*(6), 2276–2281.

Steele, M. R., Belostotsky, V., & Lau, K. K. (2012). The dangers of substance abuse in adolescents with chronic kidney disease: A review of the literature. *CANNT Journal, 22*(1), 15–22.

Tong, A., Henning, P., Wong, G., et al. (2013). Experiences and perspectives of adolescents and young adults with advanced CKD. *American Journal of Kidney Disease, 61*(3), 375–384.

Tong, A., Lowe, A., Sainsbury, P., et al. (2010). Parental perspectives on caring for a child with chronic kidney disease: An in-depth interview study. *Child: Care, Health & Development, 36*(4), 549–557.

Tsai, A. C., Manchester, D. K., & Elias, E. R. (2012). Genetics and dysmorphology. In W. Hay, M. Levin, R. Deterding, et al. (Eds.), *Current diagnosis & treatment pediatrics* (21st ed., pp. 1088–1122). New York, NY: McGraw-Hill/Lange.

Tsai, M. S., & Yeh, M. L. (2011). Images in clinical medicine. Patent urachus. *The New England Journal of Medicine, 365*(14), 1328.

Tse, Y., Yadav, P., Herrema, I., et al. (2013). Performing renal biopsies in children under general anesthesia in the lateral position. *Pediatric Nephrology, 28*(4), 671–673.

U.S. Department of Health and Human Services. (2010). *Healthy people 2020*. Washington, DC: Author.

Vidal, I., Gorduza, D. B., Haraux, E., et al. (2010). Surgical options in disorders of sex development (DSD) with ambiguous genitalia. *Best Practice & Research. Clinical Endocrinology & Metabolism, 24*(2), 311–324.

Wesseling-Perry, K. (2013). Bone disease in pediatric chronic kidney disease. *Pediatric Nephrology, 28*(4), 569–576.

Yamaçake, K. G., & Nguyen, H. T. (2013). Current management of antenatal hydronephrosis. *Pediatric Nephrology, 28*(2), 237–243.

47

Nursing Care of a Family When a Child Has a Reproductive Disorder

Navi is a 15-year-old girl you meet in a pediatric clinic. She has a purulent vaginal discharge and burning on urination; she is diagnosed with gonorrhea. When you ask her if she is sexually active, she says no; she thinks she contracted the infection from sharing a towel in a locker room. As she leaves the clinic, you hear her tell the receptionist, "I'm glad I got this early in life. Now I won't have to worry about getting it again."

Previous chapters described the growth and development of well children and health concerns that occur in other body systems. This chapter adds information about the dramatic changes, both physical and psychosocial, that occur when children develop reproductive disorders. Such information forms the basis for care and health teaching in this area.

What kind of health education does Navi need?

KEY TERMS

amenorrhea

anovulatory

cryptorchidism

dysmenorrhea

endometriosis

fibrocystic breast disease

gynecomastia

hydrocele

intersexed

menorrhagia

metrorrhagia

mittelschmerz

orchiectomy

orchiopexy

pelvic inflammatory disease (PID)

premenstrual dysphoric disorder (PDD)

sexually transmitted infection (STI)

varicocele

vulvovaginitis

OBJECTIVES

After mastering the contents of this chapter, you should be able to:

1. Describe common reproductive disorders in children.
2. Identify 2020 National Health Goals related to reproductive disorders that nurses can help the nation achieve.
3. Assess a child with a reproductive disorder.
4. Formulate nursing diagnoses for a child with a reproductive disorder.
5. Establish expected outcomes for a child with a reproductive disorder that help children and parents manage seamless transitions across differing healthcare settings.
6. Using the nursing process, plan nursing care that includes the six competencies of Quality & Safety Education for Nurses (QSEN): Patient-Centered Care, Teamwork & Collaboration, Evidence-Based Practice (EBP), Quality Improvement (QI), Safety, and Informatics.
7. Implement nursing care for a child with a reproductive disorder, such as teaching about normal menstruation.
8. Evaluate expected outcomes for achievement and effectiveness of care.
9. Integrate knowledge of children's reproductive disorders with the interplay of nursing process, the six competencies of QSEN, and Family Nursing to promote quality maternal and child health nursing care.

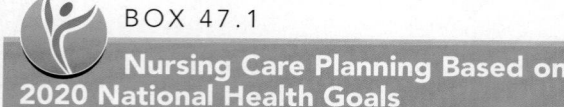

BOX 47.1

Nursing Care Planning Based on 2020 National Health Goals

Because sexually transmitted infections (STIs) not only cause short-term distress as a result of painful lesions but also can have long-term implications for fertility and future childbearing, several 2020 National Health Goals specifically address these and include:

- Reduce the proportion of adolescents with *Chlamydia trachomatis* infections seen in family planning clinics from a baseline of 7.4% to a target of 6.7%.
- Reduce the annual incidence of new cases of gonorrhea in adolescent females from a baseline of 285/100,000 cases to no more than 257/100,000 cases and in adolescent males from 220/100,000 cases to 198/100,000 cases.
- Reduce the incidence of primary syphilis in adolescent females from a baseline of 1.5/100,000 cases to no more than 1.4/100,000 cases and in adolescent males from 7.6/100,000 cases to 6.8/100,000 cases.
- Reduce the incidence of congenital syphilis from a baseline of 10.1/100,000 live births to 9.1/100,000 live births.
- Reduce the incidence of genital herpes from a baseline of 10.5% to no more than 9.5%.
- Reduce the proportion of females with human papillomavirus (HPV) infection (developmental).
- Reduce the incidence of pelvic inflammatory disease among women aged 15 through 44 years from a baseline of 3.9% to no more than 3.5% (U.S. Department of Health and Human Services, 2010; see www.healthypeople.gov).

Nurses can help the nation achieve these goals by educating adolescents about effective ways to prevent STIs and how to recognize the signs and symptoms of these illnesses.

Reproductive disorders in children range from mild infections to serious anatomic malformations. All of these disorders require prompt and careful treatment so children can reach adulthood in good reproductive health, with unaltered fertility, and with a positive sense of sexuality. Reproductive infections may suggest child maltreatment, so children with these also need careful assessment to rule out this possibility (Dubowitz, 2013) (see Chapter 55). The 2020 National Health Goals related to reproductive disorders in children are highlighted in Box 47.1.

Nursing Process Overview

FOR CARE OF A CHILD WITH A REPRODUCTIVE DISORDER

ASSESSMENT

Assessment of reproductive health begins with the first physical examination at birth and continues at health assessments throughout childhood and adolescence. Because this is a sensitive area for many people to discuss, parents may not be as comfortable inquiring about or describing disorders of the reproductive tract as they are about discussing other areas. Unless they have clear, thorough explanations of the condition and prescribed therapy, their reluctance to pursue the subject may leave them confused or misinformed. Even young children can sense that a health problem affecting genitalia is viewed by some adults as different from other disorders and so may not ask as many questions as they do about other concerns.

NURSING DIAGNOSIS

Nursing diagnoses formulated for reproductive illnesses in children focus not only on the result of the disease symptoms but also on the anxiety this type of disorder can cause. Examples of nursing diagnoses include:

- Risk for infection transmission related to lack of knowledge of safer sex practices
- Pain related to symptoms of vaginal infection
- Disturbed body image related to fibrocystic breast disease
- Anxiety related to absence or irregularity of menstrual periods in adolescent
- Fear related to surgery on genital organs

OUTCOME IDENTIFICATION AND PLANNING

An assessment of a child's knowledge about the reproductive system and ways illness can affect reproductive and sexual functioning forms the foundation for developing appropriate outcomes. Educating the child about reproductive health may be one of the first areas to plan. When establishing expected outcomes with adolescents, work with them to establish a plan that will involve them in the decision-making process.

Organizations helpful for referral to parents or adolescents include the National Women's Health Network (www.nwhn.org), the National Adolescent and Young Adult Health Information Center (nahic.ucsf.edu), the Office of Adolescent Health (www.hhs.gov/ash/oah/), and the Centers for Disease Control and Prevention (www.cdc.gov).

IMPLEMENTATION

Interventions for children with reproductive disorders should always include education about reproductive functioning and measures for maintaining reproductive and sexual health. Health education regarding the importance of testicular self-examination for adolescent males should be stressed at healthcare visits (see Chapter 34). Guidelines for teaching about menstrual health and safer sex to protect against unintended pregnancy or sexually transmitted infections (STIs) (covered in Chapter 5) are also important.

Essential nursing interventions also include supporting parents and children through difficult decisions about procedures and providing close observation and empathic counseling after surgery. For example, surgery for undescended testes is a procedure that can be traumatic for a child, especially if it is performed during a developmental stage in which a boy views such surgery as castrating (a psychological reason in addition to a physical reason as to why it is done early in life). As all children with any reproductive disorder reach puberty, they need honest explanations about any effect such a condition will have on interpersonal relationships, sexual functioning, or childbearing.

OUTCOME EVALUATION

The responses of children to reproductive dysfunction vary both with the severity of the condition and with the specific age and fears of the child. It is safe to assume, however, that children who have experienced such a health problem are at risk for a loss of self-esteem or confusion about their body image. Therefore, outcome evaluation should include a long-term evaluation of the child's coping abilities and self-image. If a child contracts an STI, the evaluation should also address the child's knowledge about avoiding STIs in the future and willingness to seek help should an infection recur.

The following are examples suggesting achievement of outcomes:

- Adolescent states discomfort from vaginal infection is tolerable after beginning medication.
- Adolescent states she is able to view self as competent despite fibrocystic breast disease.
- Child states that she is able to wait 6 months without worrying about not yet beginning her menstrual periods.
- Child states he feels less fearful about impending surgery after talking with his healthcare provider.

Assessing Reproductive Disorders in Children

Reproductive disorders in children may be congenital or acquired, so assessments for these must be ongoing throughout childhood (Box 47.2).

As with other parts of a health interview, questions regarding reproductive health are generally addressed to the parents until the child is able to answer history questions reliably and independently. Once a girl has reached adolescence, a gynecologic history (Box 47.3) should be included in the health assessment. To preserve their privacy, adolescents of both genders may prefer to not be accompanied by a parent during a physical examination for a reproductive disorder. It is also appropriate to ask the parent to step out of the room during the assessment; however, the parent has to leave willingly and cannot be made to leave.

Adolescents who are worried that they may have contracted a sexually transmitted infection or suspect they have become pregnant often visit healthcare facilities without parents. Before they can admit this chief concern, however, they may "test" a healthcare provider by eliciting a reaction to a minor problem. Be aware that an adolescent who consults a healthcare provider with a seemingly minor concern may be simply misinterpreting symptoms, and the adolescent actually may be seeking help for another problem. Asking the adolescent "Is there anything else that worries you? Is there any other way we can help you today?" may help you elicit the adolescent's primary concern (Box 47.4).

A pelvic examination is unnecessary for girls who have not yet reached adolescence. However, if vaginal walls need to be inspected (because of an inflammation, infection, or the suspicion of sexual maltreatment), an otoscope and ear tip can be used in place of a speculum. Cotton-tipped applicators can be used to take culture specimens without causing discomfort.

BOX 47.2

Nursing Care Planning Using Assessment

ASSESSING A CHILD WITH A REPRODUCTIVE DISORDER

Gynecomastia in males
Breast lumps in females
Early breast growth in females (precocious puberty)
Accessory nipples

No breast or genital changes (delayed puberty)

Abdominal pain

Early pubic hair growth (precocious puberty)

Undescended testes in males
Vulvar or vaginal discharge or pruritus in females

Abnormal genitalia
Lesion on genitalia

For adolescent girls, a pelvic examination should become part of routine health care around the age of 18 to 20 years or at the point when she becomes sexually active. Because the first pelvic examination can be stressful, spend time with the girl before the procedure to teach her about what is being assessed. A three-dimensional model of internal organs and some representative instruments may be more useful when describing the examination than a verbal description of anatomy.

Healthcare facilities should have a small speculum for examining young girls. For their comfort, warm the speculum first. Let the girl look at and handle a speculum before one is used. Remember that different cultures have different attitudes toward reproductive disorders. Adolescents from Middle Eastern countries, for example, are extremely modest, and so may be extremely uncomfortable having pelvic examinations. Girls from these countries may be more comfortable if the examiner is a woman. Remaining beside an adolescent as a support person also helps to reduce the stress the teen may be experiencing. To protect her self-esteem, be sure she meets the person who will examine her before she is placed in a lithotomy position.

If a young adolescent is uncomfortable in a lithotomy position, she can be examined in a dorsal recumbent position instead (see Chapter 11 for information on assisting with a pelvic examination). Allow an adolescent to choose whether she wants a parent to remain in the room with her.

BOX 47.3
Taking a Gynecologic History

When assessing an adolescent for a gynecologic health history, be especially conscious of an adolescent's sense of modesty and need for privacy.

MENSTRUAL HISTORY

At what age did you begin menstruating? When was your last menstrual period?

How often do your menstrual periods occur? How long do they usually last?

What is the amount of menstrual flow? (Document by number of pads or tampons used.)

Do you experience discomfort? (Document if discomfort occurs on first day or all days and action taken to relieve it.)

Do any sisters or your mother have discomfort or pain during their menstrual periods (endometriosis is familial)?

Do you experience any symptoms of irritability, moodiness, headache, or diarrhea (premenstrual dysphoric disorder) 1 or 2 days before menses?

REPRODUCTIVE TRACT HISTORY

Have you or do you have a vaginal discharge? (Document amount and whether pad is necessary; include duration, frequency, description, associated symptoms, and actions taken.)

Is there vaginal itching (pruritus)? Or vaginal odor?

Have you had reproductive tract surgery? Have you ever been pregnant? Have you ever had an abortion or miscarriage?

SEXUAL HISTORY

Are you currently sexually active (oral or vaginal)? What is the gender of your partner?

Have you had a sexually transmitted infection such as herpes, gonorrhea, or syphilis?

Do you experience any discomfort during sexual activity (dyspareunia) or any spotting afterward (postcoital spotting)?

Do you have any concerns about frequency, position, or partner's satisfaction with coitus? Do you experience orgasm?

CONTRACEPTION HISTORY

Do you use any type of birth control? If so, what contraceptive do you use? (Document length of time used, satisfaction, and any problems.)

BREAST HEALTH

Have you ever noticed any abnormality such as a lump, discharge, or pain in your breasts?

Have you ever had breast surgery?

Have you breastfed a child?

Do you have a yearly breast examination by a healthcare provider?

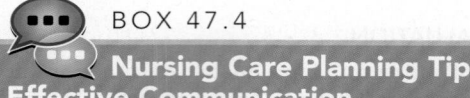

BOX 47.4
Nursing Care Planning Tips for Effective Communication

Navi, age 15 years, is seen at your pediatric clinic. She has mild symptoms of an upper respiratory tract infection.

Tip: Adolescents can have difficulty discussing symptoms of a reproductive tract infection. In this scenario, an adolescent tries to obtain an antibiotic by describing respiratory or abdominal symptoms. Be alert to this possibility to aid in recognizing a "growing" history of this type.

Nurse: Navi? Doctor Jensen doesn't believe you need anything for your cold. Just drink a little extra fluid and take it easy for a couple days.

Navi: Don't I need a prescription? Some penicillin or something?

Nurse: No. Colds are caused by viruses. Penicillin isn't necessary.

Navi: I want to be sure I get over this. I'd really like an antibiotic of some kind.

Nurse: One really isn't necessary.

Navi: I have a bad cough. I don't think I mentioned that.

Nurse: Doctor Jensen listened to your chest. You don't have anything serious there.

Navi: My stomach doesn't feel very good either. Can't I have something?

Nurse: It seems you're having more symptoms than you originally mentioned. Are you worried about something other than cold symptoms?

Navi: Well, I have this rash and . . .

Nurse: And . . . ?

Navi: I'm scared I might have a sex disease.

Health Promotion and Risk Management

Newborns need a thorough examination at birth to rule out congenital reproductive disorders so these can be diagnosed and management can begin. All children need education about how to make sexually healthy decisions and how to care for their bodies (Bakke, 2016). Adolescents may state they are not interested in this information because they are choosing abstinence. It is still important to provide the education with regard to making sexually healthy decisions and reward positive choices for staying healthy. School-health nurses are located in high schools and are considered effective at delivering preventive reproductive health education to adolescents (Smith & Stepanov, 2014).

Disorders Caused by Altered Reproductive Development

Sex chromosomes (XX or XY) develop at conception. However, development of the reproductive system, including external genitalia, occurs over two distinct periods.

Reproductive organs and genitalia begin to differentiate in utero by the eighth week, with growth and refinement occurring over the next several months. A second phase occurs with specific endocrine changes triggered during puberty and is the period of maturation of primary and secondary sexual characteristics.

Ambiguous genitalia, a rare condition that occurs during fetal development, is an example of a first-stage disorder; precocious puberty or delayed puberty are examples of second-phase disorders.

AMBIGUOUS GENITALIA

Ambiguous genitalia refers to genitalia that are not defined as male or female and the presence or absence of gonadal tissue is unknown (Lathrop, Cheney, & Hayman, 2014). Although external sexual structures generally follow from the presence of the XX or XY chromosomes, a diagnosis of ambiguous genitalia means external sexual organs in the child did not follow this normal course of development, so that, at birth, they are so incompletely or abnormally formed that it is impossible to clearly determine the child's gender by simple observation. For instance, a male infant with *hypospadias* (urethral opening on the underside of the penis) and cryptorchidism (undescended testes) may appear more female than male on first inspection (see Chapter 46 for a discussion of hypospadias).

A female fetus can become "masculinized" if exposed to androgen in utero. The most common cause of this is *congenital adrenocortical syndrome*. The adrenal gland produces androgen instead of adequate cortisone, causing the clitoris to become the size of a typical newborn male's penis (Marcdante & Kliegman, 2015c) (see Chapter 48).

If testosterone was produced in utero but development of the müllerian duct (female) was not suppressed, a child may be **intersexed** (formerly termed *hermaphrodite*), with both ovaries and testes and either male or female external genitalia. Children with ambiguous genitalia are often termed *pseudointersexed* because, as infants, they have some external features of both sexes, although only either ovaries or testes (or neither) are present.

Assessment

If there is any question about a child's gender, karyotyping or a DNA analysis establishes whether the child is genetically male or female (see Chapter 8). *Laparoscopy* (introduction of a narrow laparoscope into the abdominal cavity through a half-inch incision under the umbilicus) or possibly exploratory surgery may be necessary to determine if ovaries or undescended testes are present. Intravenous pyelography or ultrasound can be used to establish whether a complete urinary tract is present.

Therapeutic Management

Once the child's true chromosomal gender has been documented by chromosome or DNA analysis, the extent of necessary reconstructive surgery is determined in consultation with the parents. This may involve correction of a hypospadias or cryptorchidism, removal of labial adhesions, or surgical removal of an enlarged clitoris. If removal of an enlarged clitoris seems necessary, parents must consider what the absence of this organ will mean to the girl in terms of later sexual enjoyment. Parents are well advised to delay this

type of surgery until adolescence when the girl can decide for herself whether she wants this done. If a vagina will be constructed, surgery for this is usually delayed until the child is well adjusted and psychologically stable as well as when growth is complete (Lathrop et al., 2014).

If an infant is chromosomally male but does not have an adequate penis, a decision to raise the child as a female might be made, although construction of an artificial penis is more likely. Nonfunctioning ovaries or testes are generally removed to prevent malignancy later in life.

 Nursing Diagnoses and Related Interventions

The birth of a child with a perplexing disorder produces a particularly high level of stress, possibly hampering parents' ability to think calmly about their situation and make plans.

Nursing Diagnosis: Anxiety related to ambiguous gender of child at birth

Outcome Evaluation: Parents voice willingness to support treatment plan, including additional necessary tests, and state they are prepared to make decisions with guidance from healthcare team.

If the gender of a child is unclear, the parents should be told this immediately. If first told their child is a boy, only to be told 24 hours later that the child is chromosomally a girl, then parents may find this difficult to accept. During this period when the baby's gender is yet to be determined, avoid calling the baby "it." Rather, say "the baby" or "your child." Explain how sexual organs form in utero and that every child has the potential to be externally female or male.

To promote bonding, help parents understand that their child is otherwise perfect (assuming this is true). As the child grows, additional counseling may be needed for both the parents and the child to provide education about the full meaning of the congenital disorder.

PRECOCIOUS PUBERTY

Although precocious puberty (the development of breasts or pubic hair before 8 years of age in girls and 9 years of age in boys) can occur in both sexes, the condition is most often seen in girls. Such early development may be only a reflection of early maturation but is traditionally considered precocious sexual development (Marcdante & Kliegman, 2015b). Development may be limited to just breast tissue but can proceed to complete secondary sex characteristics, spermatogenesis, or menstrual function.

The condition is caused by the early production of gonadotropins by the pituitary gland; gonadotropins then stimulate the ovaries or testes to produce sex hormones. Such stimulation can occur because of a pituitary tumor, cyst, or traumatic injury to the third ventricle next to the pituitary gland. It also can occur because of estrogen-secreting cysts or tumors of the ovary or testosterone-secreting cysts of the testes. In rare instances, it occurs because of an estrogen- or testosterone-secreting adrenal tumor. In girls, ingestion of a mother's oral contraceptive pills can initiate menarche-like changes. Exogenous androgen exposure, typically through medications, and central nervous system infections are also common causes (Menon & Vijayakumar, 2014).

In children with precocious puberty, a pituitary tumor must be ruled out. If no physical cause, such as a tumor, is detected, the phenomenon appears to occur only because the *gonadostat* of the hypothalamus (the trigger that begins the development of secondary sex characteristics) has turned on several years too early.

Assessment

With precocious puberty, children have accelerated skeletal maturation as well as increased breast and genital development. Girls have menstrual bleeding yet have little pubic or axillary hair because of still low androgen secretion. Boys have obvious genital growth. The diagnosis of early puberty is confirmed by serum analysis for estrogen or androgen, which will be at adult levels.

Therapeutic Management

Children need therapy not only because of their outward appearance but also because if epiphyseal lines of long bones close early, they will be left unnecessarily short in stature. A synthetic analog to gonadotropin-releasing hormone (GnRH) is available as leuprolide acetate (Lupron) (Box 47.5). Administration of this analog desensitizes GnRH receptors, making stimulation by GnRH ineffective and halting sexual maturation at the point to which it has advanced (Karch, 2013). Therapy may also include medroxyprogesterone or cyproterone acetate during the initial 3 months to prevent flare up response from the GnRH (Menon & Vijayakumar, 2014).

BOX 47.5

Nursing Care Planning Based on Responsibility for Pharmacology

LEUPROLIDE ACETATE (LUPRON DEPOT-PED)

Classification: Leuprolide is a hormonal agent, specifically a luteinizing hormone–releasing hormone (LH-RH) agonist.

Action: occupies pituitary gonadotropin-releasing hormone (GnRH) receptors, preventing GnRH from functioning, thereby reducing the level of testosterone or estrogen in the body (Karch, 2013)

Pregnancy Risk Category: X

Dosage: intramuscular (IM) injection every 3 months

Possible Adverse Effects: nausea, vomiting, anorexia, hot flashes, headache, pain at injection site

Nursing Implications

- Administer only with the syringe supplied with the drug.
- Vary injection sites to decrease local irritation.
- Monitor injection sites for bruising and rash.
- Because injections are given only every 3 months, assist parents with preparing a calendar so they know when the next injection will be due.

 Nursing Diagnoses and Related Interventions

Nursing Diagnosis: Disturbed body image related to precocious puberty

Outcome Evaluation: Child voices an understanding of what is happening and does not evidence excessive shyness or reluctance to interact with peers.

Children who develop precociously may have difficulty interacting with peers because they appear so different from other members of their age group. Parents may worry about a child becoming sexually active and particularly about girls becoming pregnant. Both parents and children need reassurance that, after reaching the age of normal puberty, the child will maintain normal growth, development, and appearance.

Help parents to understand that their child is fully fertile and able to inseminate or conceive. Oral contraceptives, however, are not advisable for girls this young because the estrogen in them also causes early closure of epiphyseal lines, possibly stunting the child's growth further.

Parents may need to be reminded also that, although their child appears to be much older, the changes are only in sexual characteristics. Household tasks, responsibility, and expectations must be geared to the child's chronologic age, not to his or her outward appearance.

DELAYED PUBERTY

Secondary sex characteristics are normally present by age 14 years in girls and 15 years in boys. Delayed puberty, as the name implies, is the failure of pubertal changes to occur at the usual age. The family history of many of these children reveals a family tendency for late maturation. If so, the child needs a thorough physical examination to disclose whether some secondary sex characteristics are present or endocrine stimulation is beginning.

Most girls worry considerably about delayed menstruation, but, once reassured that their development is merely delayed, they are usually willing to wait for menarche to occur on its own. If girls have not begun to menstruate by age 17 years and pathology has been ruled out, menstrual cycles can be initiated by administering estrogen. Similarly, boys who are distressed by their lack of development may receive testosterone supplements to stimulate pubic hair and genital growth, but again, patience may allow usual maturation to occur.

QSEN Checkpoint Question 47.1

INFORMATICS

Suppose Navi, 15 years of age, had undergone diagnostic testing and been diagnosed with precocious puberty. What advice would a nurse give her parents?
  a. Restrict the amount of physical and mental stimulation she receives daily to halt abnormal growth.
  b. Although her sexual appearance is advanced, she is not able to conceive.
  c. Treat her appropriately for her chronologic age rather than her physical appearance.
  d. Do not allow her to eat processed meats, which contain growth hormones.

Look in Appendix A for the best answer and rationale.

Reproductive Disorders in Males

Common reproductive disorders in males include structural alterations in the penis or testes such as phimosis and cryptorchidism, inflammation such as balanoposthitis, and, in adolescents, testicular cancer.

BALANITIS (BALANOPOSTHITIS)

Balanoposthitis is inflammation of the glans and prepuce of the penis. It tends to occur in uncircumcised boys, is usually caused by poor hygiene, or may accompany a urethritis or a regional dermatitis (Morris, Waskett, Banerjee, et al., 2012).

Assessment

The prepuce and glans appear red and swollen, and there may be a purulent discharge. The boy may have difficulty voiding because of crusting at the meatal opening and because acidic urine touching the denuded surface of the glans causes pain.

Therapeutic Management

Any discharge should be cultured to rule out a sexually transmitted infection such as gonorrhea. Medical treatment involves local application of heat by warm wet soaks or warm baths. A local antibiotic ointment may be prescribed. If *phimosis* (a tight foreskin) appears to be contributing to the condition, circumcision may be advocated after the inflammation subsides to prevent the condition from recurring.

Although balanoposthitis is painful, a boy may tolerate the discomfort for several days because he may be worried it was caused by masturbation (which can contribute to the irritation) or by sexual activity and may be reluctant to seek help for fear of being criticized. He can be reassured that the problem is local and will have no long-range effect.

PHIMOSIS AND PARAPHIMOSIS

Phimosis is the inability to retract the foreskin from the glans of the penis. The foreskin is tight at birth and may even be held fast by adhesions and so, in newborns, cannot (and should not) be retracted. After a few months, the adhesions dissolve and the foreskin becomes retractable; if it does not, the infant has phimosis (Shahid, 2012). If a foreskin is extremely tight, it can interfere with voiding. Balanoposthitis may develop because the foreskin cannot be retracted for cleaning. Circumcision of newborns (discussed in Chapter 18) is no longer routinely advised but is used to relieve phimosis. Paraphimosis is the inability to replace the prepuce over the glans once it has been retracted. This is an emergency situation to address before circulation to the glans is impaired.

CRYPTORCHIDISM

Cryptorchidism is failure of one or both testes to descend from the abdominal cavity into the scrotum (Braga & Lorenzo, 2017). Normally, testes descend into the scrotal sac during months 7 to 9 of intrauterine life. They may descend any time up to 6 months after birth, but they rarely descend after that time and a referral to specialist is warranted (Fantasia, Aidlen, Lathrop, et al., 2015).

The cause of undescended testes is unclear. Testes apparently descend because of stimulation by testosterone; hence, a lower than usual level of testosterone production may prevent descent. Fibrous bands at the inguinal ring or inadequate length of spermatic vessels may prevent descent. The condition is found in about 3 out of every 1,000 male newborns; it occurs most often in premature or low–birth-weight babies (Gaylord & Petersen-Smith, 2013).

Assessment

Early detection of undescended testes is important because the warmth of the abdominal cavity may inhibit development of the testes, ultimately affecting spermatogenesis. After the age of 1 year, sperm production deteriorates rapidly in undescended testes, and the testes may even undergo a malignant change (Braga & Lorenzo, 2017). Anchoring the testes in the scrotal sac does not guarantee malignancy can be prevented, but it will allow the boy to perform preventive measures such as testicular self-examination.

Some boys may be diagnosed with undescended testes when, if an examining room is chilly, the testes have retracted to make palpation assessment difficult. Excessive palpation or stroking of the inner thigh may also stimulate the cremasteric reflex and cause retraction. In these instances, testes descend when the child is standing or after a warm bath.

Laparoscopy is effective at identifying whether an undescended testis is at the inguinal ring (true undescended testis) or ectopic (still in the abdomen). Because testes arise from the same germ tissue as the kidneys, the kidney function of a child with ectopic testes is usually evaluated as well. If undescended testes and other factors such as ambiguous genitals pose questions about the child's gender, a *karyotype* may be done to determine the child's true gender.

Therapeutic Management

Because the testes sometimes descend spontaneously during the first year of life, treatment is usually delayed for 1 year, possibly 2 years. Boys may be given a short course of chorionic gonadotropin hormone for about 5 days to see if testicular descent can be stimulated. If this is not successful, surgery (**orchiopexy**) by laparoscopy will then correct the condition (McIntosh, Scrimgeour, Youngson, et al., 2013).

 Nursing Diagnoses and Related Interventions

If an orchiopexy is scheduled, the focus is on parent and child teaching, preoperative preparation, and postoperative care.

Nursing Diagnosis: Deficient knowledge related to parents' and child's inexperience with surgical procedure and postoperative treatment plan

Outcome Evaluation: Parents (and child, if old enough) accurately describe what will be accomplished by surgery.

Boys who are old enough to understand why they need surgery need good preparation for this. Use an anatomically correct picture to point out the exact site where surgery will be performed. Reassure the boy that the penis itself will not be cut. Although the child may not voice a fear of mutilation, you can assume it exists, especially in preschool children.

During surgery, internal sutures may be inserted to hold the testis in place. Although the child may be discharged from the hospital on the same day, his activity will be limited until approximately the second day after surgery to ensure the internal suture line remains intact.

Nursing Diagnosis: Disturbed body image related to change in physical appearance

Outcome Evaluation: Child (if verbal) states he views himself as a whole person and interacts with peers without excessive shyness or hesitancy.

The postoperative evaluation should reveal that the suture line is healing well and that both testes can be palpated in the scrotum. It should also address the boy's feelings about the surgery and the changes in his body. He may need an opportunity to express his fears about mutilation or castration by playing with puppets or dolls after surgery. In years to come, even after a repair, boys who had bilateral cryptorchidism may be less fertile. When boys reach puberty, teach testicular self-examination to assess any early symptoms of malignancy, such as nodules or abnormal growth (see Chapter 34).

HYDROCELE

When a testis descends into the scrotum in utero, it is preceded by a fold of tissue, the *processus vaginalis*. Occasionally, fluid (termed a **hydrocele**) collects in this fold. In utero, the fluid can be revealed by ultrasound. At birth, the fluid causes the scrotum of the newborn to appear enlarged (Panabokke, Clifford, Craig, et al., 2016). Its presence can be revealed by ultrasound or *transillumination* (the shining of a light through the scrotal sac causes the area to glow). If the hydrocele is uncomplicated, the fluid will gradually be reabsorbed, so no treatment is necessary. The child's parents can be assured that the hydrocele is only excess fluid and the scrotal enlargement is not caused by an abnormal testis, tumor, or hernia.

Hydroceles may form later in life due to *inguinal hernias* (abdominal contents extruding into the scrotum through the inguinal ring, with accompanying fluid). If this happens, when the hernia is repaired, the hydrocele will be reabsorbed (see Chapter 45). Injection of a drug to decrease fluid production (*sclerotherapy*) may also be effective for older youths.

VARICOCELE

A **varicocele** is abnormal dilation of the veins of the spermatic cord (Fig. 47.1). It is important to identify varicoceles in adolescents because, although it may not cause a difference, the increased heat and congestion in the testicles is a possible cause of subfertility (Fine & Poppas, 2012). If fertility becomes a concern, the varicocele can be surgically removed. The adolescent will experience some local tenderness and edema for a few days after surgery. This can be minimized by applying ice for the first few hours postoperatively.

🌿 *What If . . . 47.1*
    Ryan, Navi's boyfriend, was born with undescended testes. He had surgery for this when he was 2 years old. He's concerned now that he is at high risk for testicular cancer. What patient education would the nurse best provide?

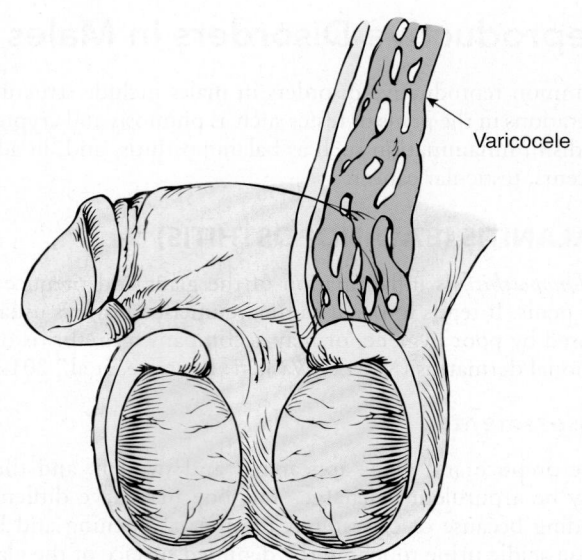

Figure 47.1   A varicocele. Identifying a varicocele in adolescent males is important because the condition may be associated with subfertility.

TESTICULAR TORSION

Testicular torsion (twisting of the spermatic cord) is a surgical emergency. Although it can be present in newborns, it occurs most frequently during early adolescence (Colaco, Heavner, Sunaryo, et al., 2015). Less than normal testicular support apparently allows the spermatic cord to twist.

The boy experiences immediate severe scrotal pain and perhaps nausea and vomiting from the extent of the pain. The testis feels tender to palpation, and edema begins to develop. If the condition is not recognized promptly (within 4 hours), irreversible change in the testis can occur from lack of circulation to the organ. Boys need to be educated about the phenomenon so that they report symptoms promptly. Fortunately, the torsion can usually be reduced manually under ultrasound guidance (Sung, Setty, & Castro-Aragon, 2012). Laparoscopic surgery, however, may be necessary to reduce the torsion and to reestablish circulation.

TESTICULAR CANCER

Testicular cancer is rare (only 1% of all malignancies) but can be an adolescent concern because it tends to occur between ages 15 and 35 years (Russell, 2014). Symptoms include painless testicular enlargement and a feeling of heaviness in the scrotum. The disease metastasizes rapidly, leading to abdominal and back pain due to retroperitoneal node extension as well as weight loss and general weakness. Human chorionic gonadotropin (hCG) and α-fetoprotein (AFP), tumor markers, will be detected in blood serum. **Gynecomastia** (enlargement of the breasts) may arise because of hCG produced by the tumor.

Therapy for testicular malignancy is **orchiectomy** (removal of the testis) followed by radiation or chemotherapy (Haugnes, Bosl, Boer, et al., 2012). At the time of surgery, a gel-filled prosthesis is inserted to provide a symmetric appearance to the scrotum. "Sperm banking," or preserving frozen sperm before the procedure, can be presented as an option for future family planning (Kelvin, 2015). Teaching all males to perform testicular self-examination for early cancer detection is important to help detect signs and symptoms of testicular cancer at an early point when the prognosis will be favorable (see Chapter 34).

Reproductive Disorders in Females

The most frequent reproductive disorders in females involve vaginal or menstrual irregularities. Other disorders are caused by physiologic or structural alterations of the reproductive organs such as imperforate hymen, pelvic inflammatory disease, or infections caused by sexually transmitted infections.

MENSTRUAL DISORDERS

Because menstruation is an ongoing process throughout half of a woman's life, an irregularity such as painful cycles can exert a major influence on her daily activities and life plans. Menstrual disorders in adolescents fall into two categories: (a) menstruation that is painful or uncomfortable and (b) infrequent or too frequent cycles (Gerlt & Starr, 2013).

Mittelschmerz

Some adolescents experience abdominal pain during ovulation from the release of accompanying prostaglandins. Pain at this time may also be caused by a drop or two of follicular fluid or blood spilling into the abdominal cavity. Called **mittelschmerz**, the pain can range from a few sharp cramps to several hours of discomfort. It is typically felt on one side of the abdomen (near an ovary) and may be accompanied by scant vaginal spotting.

An advantage of mittelschmerz is that it clearly marks ovulation. If pain is felt in the right lower quadrant, it should be differentiated from appendicitis; a lack of associated appendicitis symptoms such as nausea, vomiting, fever, abdominal guarding, and rebound tenderness does this. Mittelschmerz can be relieved by a mild analgesic such as acetaminophen.

Dysmenorrhea

Dysmenorrhea is painful menstruation (Munro, 2012). The pain is caused by the release of prostaglandins in response to tissue destruction during the ischemic phase of the menstrual cycle, which leads to smooth muscle contraction and uterine pain.

Although dysmenorrhea is exceedingly common, it needs to be investigated because it can also be a preliminary symptom of an underlying disorder such as pelvic inflammatory disease, uterine myomas (tumors), or endometriosis (abnormal formation of endometrial tissue).

Assessment

During the first year or two of menstruation, dysmenorrhea rarely occurs because early menstrual cycles are usually **anovulatory** (without ovulation). As ovulation begins, typical menstrual discomfort also begins. The actual percentage of adolescents affected by dysmenorrhea is between 64% and 93%; however, the majority of adolescents experience pain with menstruation periodically (Aktaş, 2015).

It is categorized as *primary* if it occurs in the absence of organic disease; it is *secondary* if it occurs as a result of organic disease. Symptoms each month may begin with a "bloated" feeling and light cramping 24 hours before a menstrual flow. Colicky (sharp) pain is superimposed on a dull, nagging pain across the lower abdomen, and an "aching, pulling" sensation of the vulva and inner thighs when the flow begins. Some adolescents have mild diarrhea as well. Mild breast tenderness, abdominal distention, nausea, vomiting, and headache are other symptoms that may also be present.

Therapeutic Management

Dysmenorrhea can usually be controlled by a nonsteroidal anti-inflammatory drug (NSAID) such as ibuprofen (Advil, Motrin). Be certain girls know not to take these drugs on an empty stomach because they can be extremely irritating to gastric mucosa. If symptoms do not respond to NSAIDs, hormonal treatment, such as combined estrogen and progestin oral contraceptive pills (COCs), can be tried. These prevent pain by preventing ovulation, which was the cause of the pain. If preferred, adolescents can choose to be prescribed long-acting oral contraceptives so that they have menstrual periods only every 3 months. One disadvantage of COC therapy is the possible adverse effects of long-term estrogen administration such as thrombophlebitis or early closure of epiphyseal lines of long bones.

A patient with dysmenorrhea that does not improve with the use of NSAIDs and COCs should be further evaluated for endometriosis, which is characterized by dysmenorrhea and non-menstrual pelvic pain (Facchin, Barbara, Saita, et al., 2015).

 Nursing Diagnoses and Related Interventions

Nursing Diagnosis: Pain related to menstrual period

Outcome Evaluation: Patient states she feels some control over pain through nonpharmacologic or pharmacologic methods.

Several nonpharmacologic solutions such as yoga and exercise may help relieve dysmenorrhea (Chien, Chang, & Liu, 2013). Decreasing sodium intake for a few days before an expected menstrual flow by omitting salty foods such as potato chips and luncheon meats may help reduce "bloated" feelings. Abdominal breathing (breathing in and out slowly, allowing the abdominal wall to rise with each inhalation) may also be helpful. Applying heat to the abdomen with a heating pad or taking a hot shower or bath may relax muscle tension and relieve pain (Navvabi Rigi, Kermansaravi, Navidian, et al., 2012). Abdominal massages (effleurage or light massage) or acupressures are still other options (Gharloghi, Torkzahrani, Akbarzadeh, et al., 2012). Adolescents who remain sexually active during their menses may discover an orgasm helps relieve pelvic engorgement and cramping.

If girls are going to apply heat to their abdomen, caution them not to do this until their menstrual flow actually begins because if the pain is actually from an inflamed appendix, heat could cause rupture of the appendix and life-threatening peritonitis.

Menorrhagia

Menorrhagia is an abnormally heavy menstrual flow, usually defined as greater than 80 ml per menses or a flow that soaks more than one pad or tampon an hour. It tends to occur in girls close to puberty because, without ovulation and subsequent progesterone secretion, estrogen secretion causes extreme proliferation of endometrium. There is often also an unusual amount of menstrual flow in girls using intrauterine devices (IUDs). With oral contraceptives, the flow is often light; for this reason, it may seem alarmingly heavy once pills are discontinued, when this is just a return of the adolescent's normal flow.

Heavy flows need to be investigated, however, because they also can indicate endometriosis (see later discussion), a systemic disease (anemia), a blood dyscrasia such as a clotting defect, or a uterine abnormality such as a myoma (fibroid) tumor. It can be a symptom of infection such as pelvic inflammatory disease, an indication of early pregnancy loss that is coincidentally occurring at the time of an expected menstrual period, or can occur from breakthrough bleeding from an oral contraceptive.

Assessment and Therapy

It is difficult to determine when a menstrual flow is abnormally heavy, but because a sanitary pad or tampon holds approximately 25 ml of fluid, if a pad or tampon is saturated in less than 1 hour, the flow is heavier than usual.

The adolescent who is losing excessive blood because of anovulatory cycles may be prescribed progesterone during the luteal phase to prevent proliferative growth during this phase of the cycle; if the ability to conceive is unimportant, adolescents may be prescribed a low-dose oral contraceptive or GnRH inhibitor to decrease the flow. If anemia is occurring from the heavy blood loss, an iron supplementation may be necessary to restore sufficient hemoglobin formation (Rydz & Jamieson, 2013).

Metrorrhagia

Metrorrhagia is abnormal uterine bleeding (AUB) between menstrual periods (Matteson, Raker, Clark, et al., 2013). This is normal in some adolescents who have spotting at the time of ovulation ("mittelstaining"). It may also occur in teenagers taking oral contraceptives (breakthrough bleeding) during the first 3 or 4 months of use. It also can occur from vaginal irritation caused by infection or spotting from a temporarily low level of progesterone production, which leads to endometrial sloughing (dysfunctional uterine bleeding or a luteal phase defect), although this condition most often occurs near the end of the reproductive years, not the beginning.

If AUB occurs for more than one menstrual cycle in a teenager who is not taking oral contraceptives, she needs to be referred to her primary care provider for examination because abnormal vaginal bleeding is an early sign of uterine or cervical carcinoma or an ovarian cyst (Twiss, 2013). Prescription of a COC and NSAIDs that will reduce the amount of a menstrual flow is recommended instead (Gerlt & Starr, 2013).

Menstrual Migraine

A *menstrual migraine headache* refers to a sharp, disabling headache, often accompanied by nausea or vomiting or vision changes, which occurs at the same time as a menstrual flow (Karlı, Baykan, Ertaş, et al., 2012). This is probably caused by the drop in estrogen, which occurs immediately prior to a menstrual flow. Therapy is NSAIDs, which decrease inflammation, or sumatriptan (triptan), which reduces swollen blood vessels. Menstrual migraines seem to be more intense in adolescents taking birth control pills so those who tend to have these should be counseled to use another form of reproductive planning (Hershey, 2012). Any form of migraine headache is frightening because of its sharp intensity; assure girls this is not an uncommon symptom to accompany menstrual flows. Although this doesn't relieve the pain, it can help adolescents not read more into the symptom than it warrants.

Endometriosis

Endometriosis is the abnormal growth of extrauterine endometrial cells, often in the cul-de-sac of the peritoneal cavity or on the uterine ligaments or ovaries, and is one of the main causes of dysmenorrhea in adolescents (Facchin et al., 2015; Kennedy & Koninckx, 2012). This abnormal tissue results from excessive endometrial production and a reflux of blood and tissue through the fallopian tubes during a menstrual flow. The condition tends to occur most often in White nulliparous women, but there is also a familial tendency in which daughters of women with endometriosis develop symptoms of dysmenorrhea early in life.

The excessive production of endometrial tissue can be related to a deficient immunologic response. In many women, it appears to be related to excess estrogen production or a failed luteal menstrual phase caused by not ovulating or ovulating irregularly. The resulting proliferation of tissue forces the menstrual flow into the fallopian tubes.

Dysmenorrhea occurs as the abnormal tissue begins to slough in the same manner as the uterine lining in response to estrogen and progesterone stimulation and withdrawal. This causes inflammation of surrounding tissue in the abdominal cavity and a release of prostaglandins. Abnormal tissue in the pelvic cul-de-sac can cause *dyspareunia* (painful coitus) because it puts pressure on the posterior vagina. Subfertility may result if the fallopian tubes become immobilized and blocked by tissue implants or adhesions, preventing peristaltic motion and transport of ova (see Chapter 9). Adolescents with endometritis may want to consider having children early in life before overgrowth of the endometrium becomes so extensive that it begins to interfere with conception.

Assessment

Pelvic examination may show the uterus is displaced by tender, fixed, palpable nodules. Nodules in the cul-de-sac or on an ovary may be palpable and painful.

Therapeutic Management

Treatment for endometriosis can be medical or surgical, depending on the extent of the condition. Estrogen/progesterone-based oral contraceptives may reduce the amount of extrusion into the peritoneal cavity because the tissue sloughs under the influence of the progesterone. Danazol (Danocrine), a synthetic androgen, can be prescribed to help shrink the abnormal tissue. Administration of a GnRH agonist, such as leuprolide acetate (Lupron), can reduce hormone stimulation and cause the same effect (see Box 47.5). Aromatase inhibitors, which reduce estrogen levels, are still another solution (Agarwal & Foster, 2015). A laparotomy with excision by laser surgery is the most effective measure, but, because this is a highly invasive procedure, a course of conservative medical treatment may be tried first.

Amenorrhea

Amenorrhea, or absence of a menstrual flow, strongly suggests pregnancy but is by no means definitive because it can also result from tension, anxiety, fatigue, chronic illness, extreme dieting, or strenuous exercise. Amenorrhea as a sign of pregnancy is discussed in Chapter 10. Competitive swimmers, long-distance runners (50 to 75 miles weekly), and ballet dancers may notice their intensive training causes menstrual periods to become scant and irregular, a phenomenon related to their low ratio of body fat to body muscle; this leads to excessive secretion of prolactin. An elevation in prolactin then causes a decrease in GnRH from the hypothalamus, followed by declines in follicle-stimulating hormone (FSH), follicular development, and estrogen secretion. Menstrual cycles usually return to normal within a few months after discontinuation of strenuous training and conditioning and an increase in caloric intake (Weiss Kelly & Hecht, 2016).

Adolescents who wish to maintain a normal cycle while training for a sports event may take bromocriptine (Parlodel), which reduces high prolactin levels by its action on the hypothalamus. Many adolescents, however, view the absence of menstrual periods as a benefit of sports training. If a menstrual flow is delayed and pregnancy is suspected, bromocriptine should be discontinued because it is potentially teratogenic.

Amenorrhea also occurs among females who diet excessively, partially as a natural defense mechanism to limit ovulation and also probably as a means of conserving body fluid. Adolescents with *anorexia nervosa* or *bulimia* (eating disorders described in Chapter 54) often develop amenorrhea after approximately 3 months of excessive dieting or binging and dieting; as in athletes, this is caused by an increase in prolactin (Dominé, Dadoumont, & Bourguignon, 2012).

What If . . . 47.2

Navi returns to the clinic in 6 months and tells the nurse she hasn't had a menstrual flow for 3 months. What would the nurse first suspect as Navi's condition? What questions should the nurse ask Navi?

Premenstrual Dysphoric Disorder

Premenstrual dysphoric disorder (PDD) is a condition that occurs in the luteal phase of the menstrual cycle and is relieved by the onset of menses. Because of the variety of possible symptoms, as many as 3% to 8% of women experience some degree of PDD, such as anxiety, fatigue, abdominal bloating, headache, irritability, or depression, and these may begin as early as adolescence. For a small subset of these women, these symptoms become so extreme that they are incapacitating (Hofmeister & Bodden, 2016).

The cause of PDD is unproven, but, contrary to previous beliefs, it must be due to more than a drop in progesterone just before menses. A syndrome similar to PDD can occur in women after tubal ligation; with this, apparently a decrease in the blood supply to the ovary results in decreased luteal function. In some women, a vitamin B–complex deficiency may lead to estrogen excess, causing an abnormal ratio of estrogen to progesterone. Other related causes may be poor renal clearance leading to water retention, or hypoglycemia leading to a surge of epinephrine and low calcium levels and interference with serotonin synthesis.

Because symptoms of PDD vary from cycle to cycle and throughout life, therapy is aimed at correcting specific symptoms (Steinberg, Cardoso, Martinez, et al., 2012). Adolescents who think they have PDD should keep a diary of when symptoms occur. They should be certain their diet is high in vitamins and calcium and low in salt. Agents that suppress ovarian function, such as oral contraceptives or the GnRH agonist leuprolide, may be prescribed. If depression is a major symptom, an antidepressant may be prescribed, although antidepressants (especially serotonin-reuptake inhibitors) are prescribed with caution in adolescents because they may be responsible for an increase in suicidal behavior (Adegbite-Adeniyi, Gron, Rowles, et al., 2012).

ADDITIONAL REPRODUCTIVE DISORDERS IN FEMALES

Female Circumcision

Female circumcision is the incision and removal of the clitoris (Gele, Johansen, & Sundby, 2012). There is no medical reason or advantage of the procedure, but, performed just prior to puberty, it is regarded as a coming of age ritual or religious practice in some cultures. Both a painful and mutilating procedure, it is not legal in the United States. You may, however, see adolescents or women in gynecology and pregnancy care settings who have had this done in another country. A major complication of the procedure is that women may have difficulty with conception or childbirth because of vulvar scarring and perineal contraction.

Imperforate Hymen

The *hymen* is the membranous ring of tissue that partly obstructs the vaginal opening. An *imperforate hymen* totally occludes the vagina, preventing the escape of vaginal secretions and menstrual blood (Cetin, Soysal, Khatib, et al., 2016).

Before menarche, a girl with an imperforate hymen usually has no symptoms. With the onset of menstruation, however, the menstrual flow builds up in the vagina, causing increased pressure in the vagina and uterus and, eventually, abdominal pain. Palpation of the abdomen reveals a lower abdominal mass. On vaginal examination, an intact, bulging hymen is evident. The treatment is surgical incision or removal of the hymenal tissue. The girl may have local pain after the incision, which can be relieved by a mild analgesic and warm baths.

Because most girls of early menstrual age have scant knowledge of anatomy, pictures of the reproductive tract can help to explain that this is a local and minor problem. Once relieved, it will not interfere with sexual relations or future childbearing.

Polycystic Ovary Syndrome

Polycystic ovary syndrome (PCOS) is the most frequent cause of ovulation failure seen today. It is found in about 10% of women of childbearing age (Connor, 2012). Adolescents with the syndrome begin to develop an increased androgen (male hormone) level, which then prevents follicular ovarian cysts from maturing, a situation that leads to typical symptoms of irregular or missed menstrual cycles, acne, excessive hair growth (hirsutism), being overweight, male pattern baldness, type 2 diabetes, and, most important, an absence of ovulation. The androgen increase is usually directly related to obesity and further exacerbates insulin resistance (Spritzer & Motta, 2015).

Assessment for the disorder includes a thorough history and physical exam, a pelvic exam to determine the consistency and size of ovaries, and perhaps an ovarian ultrasound for the same purpose. Serum androgen and glucose levels will also be assessed.

Because the exact cause of polycystic ovaries is not known, treatment is aimed at relieving the symptoms. Many adolescents with the syndrome are obese, therefore, weight loss by increasing lean meat, fruits, and vegetables and decreasing the amount of concentrated carbohydrates in their diet is encouraged. This eating pattern also lowers blood glucose levels, improves the body's use of insulin, and helps to normalize testosterone secretion. If a woman is morbidly obese, bariatric surgery may be recommended because this will achieve the same result.

A COC may be prescribed because this changes the ratio of estrogen and testosterone produced, leading to better regulated menstrual cycles. To prevent type 2 diabetes from developing, metformin (Glucophage) may be prescribed, which is yet another method to reduce blood glucose levels. If the adolescent or woman wants to become pregnant, fertility medications such as a course of clomiphene (Clomid) to stimulate ovulation may be suggested. Two final therapies to help achieve pregnancy are in vitro fertilization (IVF) (see Chapter 7) and ovarian drilling, a surgery technique done by laparoscopy that reduces the size of the ovaries and limits the amount of testosterone the ovaries are able to produce. To decrease hair growth and reduce acne symptoms, antiandrogens

such as spironolactone (Aldactone) or finasteride (Propecia) can be tried. Caution women that finasteride is teratogenic and so should not be used if they intend to become pregnant, and it should be discontinued during pregnancy (Mysore & Shashikumar, 2016).

PCOS is a perplexing disorder because it produces such a wide range of symptoms, and responses to therapy may not be immediate. Support from healthcare providers is important, especially if the woman wants to become pregnant and realizes her condition is not going to readily allow this to happen.

QSEN Checkpoint Question 47.3

QUALITY IMPROVEMENT

The symptoms of PCOS can begin with adolescence. If Navi had this, which of the following facts would a nurse want her to describe after an educational session?
  a. PCOS can be easily treated with an antibiotic.
  b. This condition can cause both obesity and interfere with future fertility.
  c. The condition usually fades with full maturity at the end of adolescence.
  d. Polycystic ovaries are easy to identify because they are so painful.

Look in Appendix A for the best answer and rationale.

Toxic Shock Syndrome

Toxic shock syndrome (TSS) is an infection that is usually caused by toxin-producing strains of *Staphylococcus aureus*. Although organisms can enter the body by other means, they typically enter through vaginal walls that have been damaged by the insertion of tampons at the time of a menstrual period (Edmonds, 2012). Once occurring at epidemic proportions because of superabsorbent tampons, it now can be prevented by simple steps (Box 47.6).

Assessment

The symptoms of TSS are a high temperature (over 102°F [38.9°C]), vomiting and diarrhea, hypotension, severe muscle pain, decreased platelet count, and a macular (sunburn-like) rash that desquamates on palms and soles. As the infection progresses, septic shock develops; renal, liver, and central nervous system functions fail, leading to disorientation and confusion.

Some adolescents have mild diarrhea as a normal accompaniment to dysmenorrhea, but any female who develops fever with diarrhea and vomiting during a menstrual period should suspect TSS and telephone her primary care provider.

Therapeutic Management

Women or adolescents with suspected TSS need a careful vaginal examination and removal of any tampon particles as well as cervical and vaginal cultures for *S. aureus*. Iodine douches may reduce the number of organisms present vaginally. A penicillinase-resistant antibiotic such as the cephalosporins, oxacillins, or clindamycins is prescribed. Intravenous fluid therapy to restore circulating fluid volume or a vasopressor such as dopamine (Intropin) may be necessary to increase blood pressure. Osmotic therapy to shift fluid back

BOX 47.6

Nursing Care Planning to Empower a Family

MEASURES TO PREVENT TOXIC SHOCK SYNDROME

Q. Navi says to you, "I use tampons. How can I make sure I don't get toxic shock syndrome?"

A. The following measures can help prevent the syndrome:

- Use the lowest absorbency tampon possible that is still adequate for your individual flow.
- Alternate use of tampons with use of sanitary pads. Change tampons at least every 4 hours.
- Avoid handling the portion of the tampon that will be inserted vaginally.
- Do not use tampons near the end of a menstrual flow, when excessive vaginal dryness can result from scant flow.
- Do not insert more than one tampon at a time to avoid abrasions and to keep the vaginal walls from becoming too dry.
- Avoid deodorant tampons, deodorant sanitary pads, and feminine hygiene sprays; these products can irritate the vulvar–vaginal lining.
- If fever, vomiting, or diarrhea occurs during a menstrual period, discontinue tampon use and immediately consult your healthcare provider because these are symptoms of TSS.
- Anyone who has had one episode of TSS is well advised not to use tampons again until two vaginal cultures for *Staphylococcus aureus*, the bacteria usually responsible for TSS, are negative.

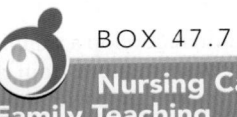

BOX 47.7

Nursing Care Planning Based on Family Teaching

TIPS FOR RELIEVING THE PAIN OF VULVOVAGINITIS

Q. Navi says to you, "My bottom is irritated from my vaginal discharge. What can I do to relieve that?"

A. Here are some tips that might help:

- Wash the area twice a day with mild, nonperfumed soap and water, and pat dry to remove secretions and decrease irritation. Always wash and dry from front to back to prevent spreading rectal contamination forward.
- Take a tub bath or apply warm, moist compresses three times a day to soothe the area and to keep it free of irritating drainage.
- After drying the cleansed area, apply cornstarch for comfort and to absorb residual moisture.
- Avoid bubble baths and feminine hygiene sprays because the ingredients in these may cause additional local irritation as well as may contribute to urinary tract infections.
- Take acetaminophen (Tylenol) or a nonsteroidal anti-inflammatory drug (NSAID) such as ibuprofen every 4 hours. These are both analgesics and so relieve pain and reduce itching, a mild pain sensation.
- Avoid scratching, which may increase abrasions and introduce a secondary infection. Instead, apply a cold compress to relieve the itching sensation.
- Wear cotton underwear, which allows air to circulate and moisture to evaporate rather than nylon or silk, which prevents air circulation and retains moisture.
- Sleep without underwear.
- Use an anesthetic spray or hydrocortisone cream if prescribed.
- If an antibiotic has been prescribed for a vaginal infection, take it conscientiously because only after the infection subsides will the vaginal discharge and itching clear.

into the intravascular circulation is important to prevent renal and cardiac failure. Recovery occurs in 7 to 10 days with adequate therapy; however, fatigue and weakness may last for months.

TSS recurrence can occur probably because the organism was not completely eliminated from the body. That makes it important for girls to complete their entire antibiotic prescription and in the future to use the lowest absorbency tampon appropriate for their individual flow.

Vulvovaginitis

In **vulvovaginitis**, inflammation of the vulva or vagina is accompanied by pain, odor, pruritus, and a vaginal discharge (Rome, 2012). Vaginal bleeding may also be present. The condition may occur in a girl of any age, but it tends to be more frequent as girls reach puberty probably because the change to adult pH and the presence of vaginal secretions make the vagina more receptive to infections. Box 47.7 discusses common measures to relieve vulvovaginal discomfort.

Preschool- and School-Age Children

Vaginal discharge may occur before menarche, but bleeding is rarely seen at this age. If vaginal bleeding does occur, it is usually caused by irritation caused by an inserted foreign object into the vagina, infestation of pinworms, or daily bubble baths (which can lead to urinary tract infections [UTIs] as well as vulvar irritation). It could also be due to urethral bleeding from cystitis (bladder infection) or rectal pruritus, which has led to scratching and rectal bleeding. Precocious puberty is yet another disorder that must be ruled out. Finally, whether sexual maltreatment has occurred must be investigated because it could be a cause of any bleeding, tenderness, or infection (see Chapter 55).

Treatment for pinworm is discussed in Chapter 43. If there is a foreign body in the vagina, it obviously should be removed by a vaginal examination. This may be difficult for young girls to accept because, unless a small speculum is used, vaginal manipulation and stretching can be painful. Application of a local antibiotic ointment or warm baths afterward may be prescribed to prevent infection and inflammation after removal of the object.

A few preschool- or school-age children develop a vaginitis due to *Streptococcus* or to *Escherichia coli* introduced from the anus by improper perineal care after voiding or bowel movements. A tight hymen then traps the microorganisms in the vagina and leads to infection. The girl may need an antibiotic prescribed for this and needs to be reminded to wipe from front to back after voiding or bowel movements to help prevent this from occurring again.

Adolescents

As a girl enters puberty, she may notice a slight vaginal discharge caused by increased vaginal secretions. As long as she has no other symptoms, you can reassure her this is normal. To keep from developing vulvar irritation, caution girls to wear cotton underpants rather than nylon (so that moisture is absorbed better) and to dry the vulva thoroughly after bathing or swimming. Daily washing of the perineum and frequent changing of tampons or sanitary pads during menstruation helps prevent chafing or stasis of menstrual blood and so helps prevent irritation and odor.

Pelvic Inflammatory Disease

Pelvic inflammatory disease (PID) refers to various inflammatory conditions of the genital tract in females: the uterus, fallopian tubes, ovaries, and their supporting structures (Black, 2014). The infection can extend so far it causes pelvic peritonitis. Although sexual transmission accounts for approximately 75% of all instances of PID (gonorrheal and chlamydial organisms are frequently responsible), infections from other causes such as *E. coli* or *Streptococcus* can occur and may be as severe. Adolescents, those with multiple sexual partners, and those who don't use condoms have a higher incidence of PID than other groups (Ross, 2012).

PID usually begins with a cervical infection that then spreads by surface invasion along the uterine endometrium and then out to the fallopian tubes and ovaries. It is most likely to occur at the end of a menstrual period because menstrual blood provides an excellent growth medium for bacteria and there is loss of the normal barrier of cervical mucus during this time.

Assessment

With acute PID, a woman or adolescent notices severe pain in the lower abdomen. She may have an accompanying heavy, purulent discharge. As the infection progresses, she develops a fever, and leukocytosis and an elevated erythrocyte sedimentation rate will be present. During a pelvic examination, any manipulation of the cervix causes severe pain, making it difficult to palpate the ovaries because of tenderness and abdominal guarding. As peritoneal tissue becomes inflamed and edematous, a purulent exudate forms in the tubes. If the process is untreated, it enters a chronic phase and fibrotic scarring with stricture of the fallopian tubes results. With this chronic phase, the abdominal pain lessens but dyspareunia and dysmenorrhea may be extreme. If the ovaries are affected, intermenstrual spotting may occur. A diagnosis can be aided by ultrasound or laparoscopy.

Therapeutic Management

Therapy involves administration of analgesia for comfort plus a broad-spectrum antibiotic such as doxycycline (Vibramycin) or clindamycin (Cleocin). In some women, a pelvic abscess forms and must be drained through the cul-de-sac before healing can occur. Women who have IUDs in place do not need to have them removed because these do not interfere with therapy (Tepper, Steenland, Gaffield, et al., 2013).

Women who have had one episode of PID have an increased chance of a second occurrence because the immune protection of the tubes and ovaries may have been damaged. They should avoid coitus during menstruation, when their protective mechanisms are lowest, and be certain their sexual partner is also not infected with the organism that caused the original infection. Early childbearing or IVF may be necessary for some women because extensive tubal scarring impaired their fertility. It is important for adolescents to recognize the symptoms of PID and to seek early help to avoid these worst case outcomes.

Breast Disorders

Although males have few breast disorders, they can occur in either males or females.

Gynecomastia (enlarged breast tissue) may occur temporarily in preadolescent boys in response to a rising estrogen level. Particularly noticeable in obese males, this enlargement fades with a normal increase in testosterone production with puberty (Dickson, 2012). It may also occur in teens who participate in body-building sports as a result of steroid use. If this is the cause, counseling regarding the danger of performance-enhancing drug use is crucial.

ACCESSORY (SUPERNUMERARY) NIPPLES

As the name implies, *accessory nipples* are additional breast nipples (Marcdante & Kliegman, 2015a). They tend to occur along the mammary lines and can be present in either male or female (Fig. 47.2). They are present from birth but usually are not as protuberant as true nipples; they also lack areolar pigmentation. Parents should be told what they are so they can inform their child later about this because some growth in accessory nipples may occur at puberty or during pregnancy in response to estrogen stimulation. If girls are unaware they have an accessory nipple and think it is a large mole, they may be worried they have skin cancer when these changes occur.

In a few instances, actual breast tissue is present beneath the accessory nipple. If so, it is subject to the same diseases as other breast tissue such as fibrocystic disease or breast cancer (Valeur, Rahbar, & Chapman, 2015). If the accessory nipple or accessory breast tissue is cosmetically distressing to an adolescent, it can be removed by simple surgical excision.

BREAST HYPERTROPHY

Breast hypertrophy (macromastia) is abnormal enlargement of breast tissue. In the average girl, progesterone levels are low until menstruation cycles are fully established. Breast development halts after puberty, as soon as progesterone levels rise to mature strength. If the time span between puberty and maturation is a lengthy one, breast growth lasts for longer than usual, resulting in larger than usual breasts.

Breast hypertrophy can lead to both physical and emotional stress because a girl may feel pain and fatigue in her back or shoulders from the weight of heavy breast tissue.

Figure 47.2 Nipple lines, along which accessory nipples occur.

In addition, she may feel self-conscious and try to minimize her breast size by slouching, resulting in poor posture or rounded shoulders. Pregnancy and lactation may be particularly difficult times because breasts that are already large become even heavier with milk formation. Hearing comments such as "I wish I had your problem" rather than receiving support and understanding from parents, peers, and healthcare providers does not relieve her concerns.

Be certain adolescents with large breasts conscientiously schedule a yearly breast examination with their healthcare provider because it is easier for a cancerous lesion to escape detection in large amounts of breast tissue than in smaller breasts.

If breast hypertrophy is so extreme that it interferes with a girl's physical and emotional well-being, surgical breast reduction is a possibility (Srinivasaiah, Iwuchukwu, Stanley, et al., 2014). Adolescents need to seriously consider the consequences of this procedure, however, before undertaking it at this early age. If a large amount of glandular tissue is removed, breastfeeding might no longer be an option. The adolescent also needs to be told realistically that changing her physical appearance will reduce physical discomfort, but changing her self-concept must come from within.

BREAST HYPOPLASIA

Breast hypoplasia is less-than-average breast size. In most instances, this does not represent a decreased amount of glandular or functional breast tissue but a reduced amount of fatty tissue. If having small breasts interferes with self-esteem, a girl can have surgical augmentation by a silicon or a saline implant inserted under the breast tissue to increase breast size, but, again, this needs careful consideration regarding whether it is necessary at this young age. Be certain the girl understands that her breast tissue is not replaced by the implant,

and that she still needs breast examinations because she could still develop breast cancer in later years.

Breasts with implants in place may feel firmer than usual on palpation due to the formation of a fibrotic band or capsule around the implant. Decreased nipple sensation may be present for approximately 1 year after the procedure.

Breast implants do not interfere with breastfeeding because they are placed behind the milk glands. A traumatic blow to the breast, such as one that could occur from an automobile accident, requires examination by the augmentation surgeon to be certain the implant did not rupture, causing its contents to leak into the bloodstream or breast tissue.

FAT NECROSIS

If breast tissue is struck during a fall or other traumatic injury such as injury from a seatbelt, it can become tender, painful, inflamed, or reddened (Alvarez & Jacobs, 2011). A few days after the injury, necrosis or disintegration occurs in the fatty layer. As the area heals, fibrotic scar tissue forms leaving a firm, palpable lump in the breast. It is not freely movable; it can, however, cause skin or nipple retraction or dimpling on the skin surface. Unlike malignant breast growths that also show this "orange peel" sign, posttraumatic breast lumps tend to be well delineated because of the scar tissue.

It is generally recommended that such fibrotic areas be biopsied and then excised. The procedure is a minor one, usually leaves little scarring, and the adolescent no longer needs to worry about the lump in her breast afterward.

FIBROCYSTIC BREAST DISEASE

Fibrocystic breast disease is the most common benign breast condition in women of all ages (De Silva, 2012). It can occur as early as puberty, when estrogen rises to adult levels. More commonly, however, it is found in older adolescents. Round, fluid-filled, and freely movable cysts form in the connective breast tissue (Fig. 47.3). The consistency of these lesions varies with the menstrual cycle, changing from firm to soft, depending on the amount of serous fluid present. The lesions tend to shrink or disappear during pregnancy and lactation, and they tend to fade with menopause.

Decreased sodium intake or short-term use of a mild diuretic just before menses can reduce fluid retention and the

Figure 47.3 Round, fluid-filled cysts form in breast tissue in fibrocystic breast disease.

size of the cysts. Discontinuing smoking can help as well. Because fibrocystic breasts feel tender and "stretched," this can interfere with active sports and other strenuous activity. This discomfort can usually be relieved with a simple analgesic, such as acetaminophen (Tylenol), an NSAID, or warm compresses, avoidance of trauma, and firm bra support. The formation of fibrocystic lesions may be increased in some women with the use of methylxanthines found in caffeine, theophylline, and theobromine, so avoiding foods such as coffee, cola drinks, tea, chocolate, some toffee candy, and medications that contain caffeine helps reduce pain.

If these measures do not decrease fibrocystic symptoms, cysts may be aspirated under a local anesthetic by injection of a thin sterile needle attached to a small syringe. This procedure not only reduces the size of the cyst but also provides fluid for biopsy (Alvarez & Jacobs, 2011).

In addition to being physically distressed, women with fibrocystic breasts may worry that each lump could be malignant. Breast carcinoma does occur in women with fibrocystic breast disease, but fibrocystic lesions do not directly lead to this. Breast cancer, however, may not be discovered before a woman seeks a health consultation because a woman assumes all her breast lesions are benign. Therefore, in addition to a yearly breast examination, women with fibrocystic breast disease need an annual breast ultrasound or magnetic resonance imaging (MRI) to efficiently locate and identify that the cysts are benign.

FIBROADENOMA

Fibroadenomas are tumors that consist of both fibrotic and glandular components that occur in response to estrogen stimulation (Valeur et al., 2015). They may increase in size during adolescence, during pregnancy and lactation, or when a woman takes an estrogen source such as an oral contraceptive.

Unlike fibrocystic lesions, fibroadenomas feel round and well delineated, are painless and freely movable, and do not tend to cause skin retraction. Occasionally, they calcify and feel extremely hard. Like fibrocystic lesions, the presence of them can be distressing, but they do not appear to become malignant.

Such tumors can be surgically excised so a woman no longer has to worry about them. Because the incision is small, it leaves little scarring at the site.

QSEN Checkpoint Question 47.4

SAFETY

Navi, 15 years of age, asks whether it would be safe for her to have breast augmentation. What advice should the nurse give her?

 a. She would not likely be able to breastfeed after undergoing augmentation.
 b. Breast implants increase her risk of developing fibrocystic disease.
 c. It is safe for girls her age to have this surgery, but careful consideration is needed.
 d. Implants increase her risk of breast cancer in later life.

Look in Appendix A for the best answer and rationale.

MASTITIS

Mastitis is inflammation or infection of the breast. Because this usually occurs as a complication of breastfeeding, it is discussed in Chapter 19.

Sexually Transmitted Infections

Sexually transmitted infections (STIs) are diseases that are spread through sexual contact with an infected partner. They range in severity from easily treated infections, such as trichomoniasis, to HIV infection, which, despite advances in therapy, is life threatening. If these diseases are discovered in young children, the possibility of sexual maltreatment has to be considered (Hornor, 2017). Adolescents account for almost half of the new cases of STIs each year, which includes heterosexual and same-sex transmission (Goyal, Shea, Hayes, et al., 2016).

Abstinence or condom use provides the best protection against STIs. Additional measures include voiding immediately and washing genitals well with soap and water after coitus as well as choosing sexual partners who are at low risk for infection (i.e., avoiding persons who are intravenous drug users or those with multiple sexual partners). Educating adolescents about safer sex practices, including the need for condom use (see Chapter 5) and the importance of health screening for these disorders, is an important nursing responsibility. Pay particular attention to adolescents who do not have a strong family support system because it may be particularly difficult for these youth to receive correct information about preventing STIs (Hudson, 2012).

STIs are becoming more difficult to treat because the causative organisms are becoming increasingly resistant to antibiotics. Always reinforce the fact that little immunity develops from STIs, so such diseases can be contracted repeatedly. In most instances, an infected partner should also be treated or the disease can recur from cross infection.

Several STIs, such as syphilis, are known to be teratogenic. All of them are suspected of being a causative factor of preterm birth. Chapter 12 discusses care for the newborn affected by such diseases.

CANDIDIASIS

Candidiasis is a vaginal infection spread by the fungus *Candida*, an organism that thrives on glycogen (Rome, 2012). Candidiasis is so common that as many as 90% of women will have it sometime in their life. Because oral contraceptives produce a pseudopregnancy state, adolescents using oral contraceptives tend to have frequent vaginal candidal infections. If being treated with an antibiotic for another infection (which destroys normal vaginal flora and lets fungal organisms grow more readily), they are also particularly susceptible to this infection. Incidence is also strongly associated with immune suppression and diabetes mellitus because hyperglycemia provides the perfect glucose-rich environment for candidal growth.

Assessment

Because of the scant mucus production in the period before menses, symptoms may be most acute at this time. The adolescent will notice vulvar and vaginal reddening, burning and itching, and even bleeding from hairline fissures. A thick, cream cheese–like discharge can usually be observed at the vaginal outlet. Internally, the vagina shows white "patches" that cannot be scraped away without bleeding on the walls. There may be accompanying pain on coitus or on tampon insertion. Candidal infections can also be present at other body sites, such as the oral cavity or a moist area such as the umbilicus. In immunosuppressed individuals, candidal infections can become systemic (Edmonds, 2012).

Candidal infections are diagnosed by removing a sample of the discharge from the vaginal wall and placing it on a glass slide. Three or four drops of a 20% potassium hydroxide (KOH) solution are then added, and the mixture is protected by a coverslip. Under a microscope, typical fungal hyphae indicate the presence of *Candida* organisms (Table 47.1). An at-home test kit (Vagisil Screening Kit) is available, which gives results instantly. A woman inserts a pH wand into her vagina and in a few seconds compares the color of the swab to a pH color chart. If the reading is above 5.0, it suggests she may have a bacterial infection and should see her healthcare provider. A pH level of 4.5 plus itching and/or burning, unusual discharge, or a yeasty odor suggests a yeast infection, and it would be all right for her to use an over-the-counter treatment.

Therapeutic Management

Therapy for candidal infections includes vaginal tablets or cream applications of antifungal preparations such as over-the-counter miconazole (Monistat) or clotrimazole (Lotrimin) once a day for 3 to 7 days. Oral fluconazole (Diflucan) can be administered as a one-time dose. Teach women to insert antifungal tablets or creams at bedtime, so the drug does not drain from the vagina immediately afterward. Treatment should not be interrupted until it is complete, even during a menstrual period.

If a girl has frequent candidal infections, her urine should be tested for glucose to rule out diabetes mellitus. If she is using an oral contraceptive, she might be counseled to use another reproductive planning method. If an adolescent is sexually active, treatment of the male partner may be necessary to break a reinfection cycle (McGreal & Wood, 2013).

Pregnancy and Candidiasis

Candidiasis occurs more frequently during pregnancy than usual because the increased estrogen level present during pregnancy causes the vaginal pH to be less acidic and even more favorable for yeast growth. Women with repeated infections should have their urine tested for glucose to determine whether gestational diabetes is present.

Both miconazole (Monistat) for 7 days or a single dose of oral fluconazole (Diflucan) are approved for use during pregnancy. Treating the infection during pregnancy is important not only because the profuse vaginal discharge and pruritus is uncomfortable but also because if the infection is present in the vagina at the time of childbirth, it may cause a candidal infection, or *thrush*, in the newborn (see Chapter 43). Caution pregnant women to call their primary healthcare providers before using an over-the-counter product to double-check that the product is safe to use during pregnancy and also so the primary care provider can know a vaginal infection is occurring (Mashburn, 2012).

What If . . . 47.3

Navi tells the nurse she feels protected from contracting an STI because she knows she is up to date with her immunizations. What patient education would the nurse best provide?

TABLE 47.1 COMMON VULVOVAGINAL INFECTIONS

Causative Agent	Symptoms	Common Therapy
Candida albicans	Vulvar reddening and pruritus; thick, white, cheese-like vaginal discharge	Clotrimazole (Lotrimin) or miconazole (Monistat) vaginal suppositories or fluconazole (Diflucan) orally; bathing with dilute sodium bicarbonate solution may relieve pruritus
Trichomonas	Thin, irritating, frothy, gray-green discharge; strong, putrid odor; itching	Metronidazole (Flagyl) or tinidazole (Tindamax) orally; douching with weak vinegar solution to reduce pruritus
Herpesvirus type 2	Painful pinpoint vesicles on an erythematous base with a watery vaginal discharge possible; voiding may be irritating and painful	Bathing with dilute sodium bicarbonate solution, applying lubricating jelly to lesions, or an oral analgesic such as ibuprofen may be necessary for pain relief; topically applied acyclovir (Zovirax) helps heal lesions
Gardnerella	Edema and reddening of vulva; milky gray discharge; fishlike odor	Metronidazole (Flagyl) or clindamycin
Chlamydia trachomatis	Watery, gray-white vaginal discharge; vulvar itching	Tetracycline or doxycycline; erythromycin during pregnancy
Neisseria gonorrhoeae	Possibly symptomless; may have profuse yellow-green vaginal discharge	Ceftriaxone and doxycycline
Enterobius vermicularis (pinworm)	Rectal pruritus, especially on rising in the morning	Oral administration of an anthelmintic, such as mebendazole (Vermox)
Treponema pallidum (syphilis)	Painless ulcer on vulva or vagina	Benzathine penicillin, administered intramuscularly
Streptococcus	Vaginitis, vulvar itching; edema and reddening of vulva	Antibiotic such as amoxicillin
Foreign body	Vaginal discharge; odor	Removal of foreign body during pelvic examination

TRICHOMONIASIS

Trichomonas vaginalis is a curable STI and has the highest prevalence among adolescents (Swartzendruber, Sales, Brown, et al., 2014). The incubation period is 4 to 20 days. A serious consequence of trichomoniasis is that infection can cause such genital inflammation that it makes it easier for the person to be infected with the HIV virus or to pass the HIV virus on to a sex partner (Centers for Disease Control and Prevention [CDC], 2017).

Assessment

With a trichomonal infection, females may notice only a slight vaginal discharge or else notice extreme vaginal itching and a frothy white or grayish-green vaginal discharge. The upper vagina looks reddened and may have pinpoint petechiae. In some women, these changes can be so extreme, a Pap test taken during this time may be misinterpreted as showing abnormal tissue. Males with the same infection tend not to report any symptoms.

The infection is diagnosed by microscopic examination of a sample of the vaginal discharge; trichomonads typically appear as rounded, mobile structures.

Therapeutic Management

Oral metronidazole (Flagyl) or tinidazole (Tindamax) eradicates trichomonal infections. Use of condoms by sexual partners help prevent recurrence of *Trichomonas* in both parties. Because metronidazole interacts with alcohol (to cause acute nausea and vomiting), caution older adolescents and women to not drink alcoholic beverages during the course of treatment with this drug.

Pregnancy and Trichomoniasis

Trichomoniasis infections are associated with preterm labor, premature rupture of membranes, and postcesarean infection. The drug of choice during pregnancy is single-dose oral metronidazole. Although classified as a Class B pregnancy drug, it may not be prescribed during the first semester of pregnancy to avoid detrimental fetal effects (Karch, 2013).

BACTERIAL VAGINOSIS

Bacterial vaginosis is defined as the absence or deficiency of lactobacilli in the vaginal flora and it occurs frequently among woman of childbearing age (Parma, Vanni, Bertini, et al., 2014). An intensely pruritic vaginal discharge appears milky-white to gray and has a fishlike odor. Microscopic examination of the discharge shows gram-negative rods adhering to vaginal epithelial cells (termed *clue cells*). Like trichomoniasis, bacterial vaginosis can increase a woman's susceptibility to other STIs, such as herpes simplex virus (HSV), chlamydia, and gonorrhea, as well as HIV (Bautista, Wurapa, Sateren, et al., 2016).

The treatment is oral or vaginal metronidazole for 7 days. The woman's sexual partner should also be treated to prevent recurrence of the infection. Therapy with probiotic lactobacilli to change vaginal organisms is a future possibility for prevention (Parma et al., 2014).

Pregnancy and Bacterial Vaginosis

The treatment during pregnancy is oral metronidazole or clindamycin for 7 days in order to prevent preterm labor as well as premature rupture of the membranes (Bennett, 2012).

CHLAMYDIA TRACHOMATIS INFECTION

Chlamydia trachomatis infections have become the most commonly reported bacterial cause of STIs in the United States (Pearson, Gift, Leichliter, et al., 2015). The incubation period is 1 to 5 weeks; symptoms include a heavy, grayish-white discharge and vulvar itching. Diagnosis is made by identification of the organism, which can be done at the point of care with a urethra or cervix swab. A urine specimen can be used as an alternative screening method. Therapy is oral doxycycline for 7 days or azithromycin as a single dose. Because the infection has become so common, most public health departments require that the infection be reported to the health department the same as other STIs such as gonorrhea. Because there is a strong association between gonorrhea and *Chlamydia*, if a chlamydial infection is documented, women are usually tested for gonorrhea as well. Long-term effects of chlamydial infections are PID, possibly leading to subfertility.

Pregnancy and *Chlamydia*

Screening for *Chlamydia* via a vaginal culture is usually done during a woman's first prenatal visit. If a woman has multiple sexual partners, screening may be repeated again in the third trimester. Doxycycline (Vibramycin), the therapy for nonpregnant women, is contraindicated during pregnancy because of possible fetal long-bone deformities; azithromycin (Zithromax) or amoxicillin (Amoxil) are used instead. A woman's partner also should be treated to prevent her from becoming reinfected.

It's important that chlamydial infections be treated during pregnancy because they are associated with premature rupture of the membranes, preterm labor, and endometritis in the postpartum period. An infant who is born while a chlamydial infection is present can develop conjunctivitis or pneumonia after birth (see Chapters 40 and 50).

HUMAN PAPILLOMAVIRUS

The human papillomavirus (HPV) causes fibrous tissue overgrowth (sometimes called genital warts) on the external vulva, vagina, or cervix (condyloma acuminatum). At first, lesions appear as discrete papillary structures; they then spread, enlarge, and coalesce to form large, cauliflower-like lesions. The infection may be present in as many as 10% to 30% of women and is most common in women who have multiple sexual partners. Children (both male and female) who develop an HPV infection should be further investigated for sexual maltreatment (Francis & Katz, 2013). Therapy for such lesions is aimed at dissolving the lesions and also ending any secondary infection present. Small growths often fade by themselves, although they can be removed by applying podophyllin (Podofin), a wart removal medication. Large lesions are removed by laser therapy, cryocautery, laser, or knife excision. With cryocautery, edema at the site is evident immediately; lesions become gangrenous, and sloughing occurs in 7 days, with healing complete in 4 to 6 weeks with only slight depigmentation at the site. Warm baths and a lidocaine cream may be soothing during the healing period.

HPV infections are serious because they are associated with the development of penile and cervical cancer later in life (D'Hauwers, Depuydt, Bogers, et al., 2012). Related to this, women who have had one episode of infection should be conscientious about having yearly Pap tests for the rest of their lives, and men should conscientiously inspect their penis for any abnormal growths or ulcers. The vaccines, Gardasil or Cervarix, are recommended as part of routine administration to both early teenage girls and boys to prevent such infections. Approach the subject of immunization with parents and teenagers with sensitivity because some parents and children are not ready to admit they might be or will soon become sexually active and need this protection (Katz, Oldach, Goodwin, et al., 2014). Immunizing teenagers against an HPV infection should reduce not only the incidence of HPV infections in the future but also the rate of cervical and penile cancer as well (Markman, 2013).

Pregnancy and Human Papillomavirus Infection

HPV lesions tend to increase in size during pregnancy because of the high vascular flow in the pelvic area. They may become secondarily ulcerated and infected; when this occurs, a foul vulvar odor may develop.

Podophyllum is contraindicated during pregnancy because of possible toxic effects on the fetus. Trichloroacetic acid (TCA) or bichloroacetic acid (BCA) applied to the lesions weekly may be effective and can be used during pregnancy. Women who do not find the lesions bothersome may choose to leave them in place until the postpartum period and have them removed then. Remind them, in the meantime, that the lesions are infectious and can spread to a sexual partner.

The presence of vulvar lesions appears to have no effect on the fetus during pregnancy, but if they are so large they obstruct the birth canal for birth, a cesarean birth may be scheduled.

HERPES GENITALIS (HERPES SIMPLEX TYPE 2)

Genital herpes is caused by *herpesvirus hominis* type 2 (also called herpes simplex virus type 2 or HSV-2). This is one of four similar herpesviruses: cytomegalovirus, Epstein–Barr, varicella zoster, and herpes type 1 (HSV-1) and type 2 (HSV-2). Genital herpes occurs in epidemic proportions in the United States, and HSV-1 is becoming more commonly the cause of primary genital infections (Groves, 2016). Although the virus can be contained, unlike most other STIs, there is no known cure. The disease involves a lifelong process, therefore, and, although it may not be

a direct precursor to cervical cancer, women with cervical cancer tend to have more antibodies against herpes genitalis than others or probably have been exposed to the virus more than others. The virus is spread by skin-to-skin contact, entering through a break in the skin or mucous membrane. In the newborn, acquired at birth, the virus can be systemic or even fatal (see Chapter 26).

Assessment

Herpes is diagnosed by culture of the lesion secretion from its location on the vulva, vagina, cervix, or penis or by isolation of HSV antibodies in blood serum. The incubation period is 3 to 14 days. On first contact, extensive primary lesions originate as a group of pinpoint vesicles on an erythematous base. Within a few days, the vesicles ulcerate and become moist, painful, draining, and open lesions. An adolescent may have accompanying flu-like symptoms with increased temperature; vaginal lesions may cause a profuse discharge. Pain is intense on contact with clothing or acidic urine. Diagnosis of the disorder is made by the appearance of the lesions and on the results of a Pap smear and an enzyme-linked immunosorbent assay (ELISA).

After this primary stage, which lasts approximately 1 week, lesions heal but the virus lingers in a latent form in the sensory nerve ganglia. The condition can flare up and become an active infection again during illness, just prior to menstruation, fever, overexposure to sunlight, or stress. This secondary response usually produces only local lesions rather than systemic symptoms.

Therapeutic Management

Both acyclovir (Zovirax) and valacyclovir (Valtrex) are examples of antivirals that can control the virus by interfering with DNA reproduction and decreasing symptoms (Groves, 2016). Topical imiquimod (Aldara) or foscarnet (Foscavir) may be prescribed for resistant lesions. If applying a topical ointment or vaginal gel to a patient, be certain to protect yourself with a finger cot or glove so you do not contract the virus or absorb the drug. Warm baths three times a day may be helpful to reduce discomfort for the patient. An emollient (A&D Ointment) can also reduce discomfort, although its moisture tends to prolong the active period of the lesions. Infected people need to inform their partners when they have any active lesions and either avoid sexual contact or use a condom to decrease the danger of spreading the virus.

Because of the possible association with cervical cancer, any female with genital herpes should have yearly Pap tests for the rest of her life, and men need to self-inspect for recurrent lesions.

Pregnancy and Herpes Simplex Virus Type 2 Infection

If a woman contracts an HSV-2 infection during pregnancy, herpes can be transmitted across the placenta to cause congenital infection in the newborn. If primary or secondary active lesions in the vagina or on the vulva are present at the time of birth, herpes infection can be transmitted to the newborn at birth. When this occurs, a severe systemic infection that is often fatal can result (see Chapter 26). To help avoid transmission, women with active lesions are usually scheduled for cesarean birth (Groves, 2016).

The drug of choice for the treatment of herpes infection during pregnancy is the same as for nonpregnant women (acyclovir [Zovirax] or valacyclovir [Valtrex]) (Karch, 2013). Women can reduce the pain of the lesions by taking baths or applying warm, moist tea bags to the area.

HEPATITIS B AND HEPATITIS C

Both hepatitis B and hepatitis C can be spread by semen as well as blood and therefore are considered STIs. These are discussed in Chapter 45, with other forms of hepatitis. Because hepatitis B can be spread by sexual intercourse, adolescents who did not receive immunization against this as an infant and who are sexually active need immunization.

GONORRHEA

Gonorrhea is transmitted by *Neisseria gonorrhoeae*, a gram-positive diplococcus, which thrives on the mucous membrane of the vagina or penis (O'Connor & Shubkin, 2012). In males, symptoms include *urethritis* (pain on urination and frequency of urination) and a urethral discharge, which appear after a 2- to 7-day incubation period. Untreated, the infection spreads easily among sexual partners and may spread to the testes, scarring the tubules and causing permanent sterility. It often occurs concurrently with a chlamydial infection.

Although symptoms of gonorrhea in females are not as visible, there may be a slight yellowish vaginal discharge. The Bartholin glands may become inflamed and painful. If left untreated, the infection can spread to pelvic organs, most notably the fallopian tubes, can cause PID, and, as in males, tubal scarring with permanent sterility. In both males and females, if systemic involvement occurs, arthritis or heart disease can develop.

Assessment

A urine culture for the gonococcal bacillus, in addition to vaginal, urethral, and perhaps anal and oral cultures, should be obtained on all children with vulvovaginitis or a urethral discharge to rule out gonorrhea because, if gonorrhea is detected, child maltreatment needs to be ruled out.

Therapeutic Management

One intramuscular injection of ceftriaxone (Rocephin) plus 7 days of oral doxycycline (Vibramycin) or azithromycin (Zithromax) is the current recommended therapy because this treatment regimen is effective for gonorrhea, chlamydia, and syphilis (Kransdorf, Kling, & Mayer, 2014). Sexual partners should receive the same treatment (Box 47.8, an interprofessional care map for an adolescent with an STI).

Approximately 24 hours after beginning treatment, gonorrhea is no longer infectious. Approximately 7 days after treatment, however, a patient should return for a follow-up culture to verify the disease has been completely eradicated (few adolescents take this precaution without urging). Most states require gonorrhea be reported to the health department; adolescents are asked to name sexual contacts to help prevent the disease spread. Without being told who put them at risk, these people can then be notified by a health department investigator that they have been exposed to a particular STI and need treatment.

Pregnancy and Gonorrhea

Gonorrhea is associated with spontaneous miscarriage, preterm birth, and endometritis in the postpartum period. Pregnant women cannot be administered doxycycline because it has the potential to be teratogenic. Instead, they are prescribed azithromycin. It is important that gonorrhea is identified and treated during pregnancy because, if the infection is present at the time of birth, it can cause a severe eye infection, which can lead to blindness in the newborn (ophthalmia neonatorum; see Chapter 26).

QSEN Checkpoint Question 47.6

PATIENT-CENTERED CARE

Navi does not seem concerned about the possibility she could contract gonorrhea again. What additional health teaching does she need to better understand how this disease is spread?

   a. The microorganism of gonorrhea can be spread via anal, oral, and vaginal intercourse.

   b. It is possible for the gonorrhea organism to be spread by anal/penile contact.

   c. The low pH of saliva prevents this from being spread by oral/penile contact.

   d. Gonorrhea is a virus that can be treated effectively if diagnosed early.

Look in Appendix A for the best answer and rationale.

SYPHILIS

Syphilis is a systemic disease transmitted by the spirochete *Treponema pallidum* (O'Connor & Shubkin, 2012). Like gonorrhea and chlamydia, its occurrence must be reported to public health departments.

After an incubation period of 10 to 90 days, a deep ulcer (termed a *chancre*), which is usually painless despite its size, appears usually on the genitalia (penis or labia) or in the vagina, on the mouth, lips, or rectal area from oral–genital or genital–anal contact. Swollen lymph nodes may also be present, but these are likely to be less noticed by the affected person. Without treatment, a chancre lasts approximately 6 weeks and then fades.

About 2 to 4 weeks after the chancre disappears, a generalized, macular, copper-colored rash appears. Rare among rashes, it covers the soles and the palms as well as extremities and the body. There may be secondary symptoms of generalized illness, such as a low-grade fever. A serologic test for syphilis taken at this time yields a positive result. With or without treatment, this stage of syphilis also fades.

The next stage is a latency period that may last from only a few years to several decades. The only indication of the disease at this point is a serologic test, which continues to yield a positive result.

The final stage of syphilis is a destructive neurologic disease that involves major body organs, such as the heart and the nervous system, with symptoms such as blindness, paralysis, mental confusion, slurred speech, and lack of coordination. If this third stage is not identified and treated, it can become fatal.

BOX 47.8

Nursing Care Planning

Navi is a 15-year-old female high school student you meet at a pediatric clinic. She describes intense vulvar irritation from a yellowish-green vaginal discharge.

Family Assessment: Navi lives with mother in a studio apartment in inner city. Mother works at home as a freelance journalist. Mother describes finances as "good."

Patient Assessment: Well-proportioned female; sexual maturity Tanner stage 3. Menarche at 12 years; periods every 30 days; duration 6 days. Sexually active for approximately 1 year with same partner. "He doesn't use a condom anymore because I'm the only one he's dating."

Vulva reddened and excoriated. Yellow-green discharge noted at vaginal introitus. Reddened areas noted on vaginal walls. One dose of intramuscular (IM) ceftriaxone (Rocephin), plus oral doxycycline (Vibramycin) prescribed for 7 days. She says, "I think I got this from a towel I borrowed in gym class. Does my boyfriend need treated too?"

Nursing Diagnosis: Deficient knowledge related to cause and treatment of sexually transmitted infection (STI)

Outcome Evaluation: Adolescent states she understands cause of STI; reports boyfriend has an appointment within 48 hours for evaluation.

Team Member Responsible	Assessment	Intervention	Rationale	Expected Outcome
Activities of Daily Living, Including Safety				
Nurse	Assess whether adolescent understands importance of washing hands after using bathroom and avoiding sexual intercourse during treatment.	Discuss how disease can be spread to boyfriend or to other body parts by unclean hands.	Gonorrhea is particularly hazardous because it can cause eye infections with corneal scarring.	Adolescent states she will take precautions to wash hands well; will avoid sexual intercourse until repeat culture.
Teamwork and Collaboration				
Nurse/STI counselor	Confer with STI counselor as to whether disease is a reportable one.	Meet with STI counselor regarding procedure for STI contacts.	Gonorrhea is a reportable disease.	STI counselor assumes responsibility for securing STI contacts.
Procedures/Medications for Quality Improvement				
Nurse	Assess whether adolescent has experience with taking medicine. Assess if a reminder sheet would be helpful.	Administer ceftriaxone (Rocephin) IM; give instructions for oral doxycycline (Vibramycin) for 7 days as prescribed.	The antibiotics chosen for gonorrhea treatment are also effective against chlamydia, which is frequently associated with gonorrhea.	Adolescent accepts IM injection; states she understands importance of taking oral antibiotic for full 7 days.
Nurse	Assess whether adolescent has access to a bathtub at home.	Recommend the use of warm bath before and after school.	Warm baths are soothing and help keep the vulva free of irritation.	Adolescent states she will use home bathtub for sitz baths twice daily and will wash tub well after use.
Nutrition				
Not applicable (N/A)	N/A	N/A	N/A	N/A
Patient-Centered Care				
Nurse	Assess whether adolescent is aware STIs are spread through sexual intercourse not a towel exchange.	Teach adolescent about the cause, means of spread, and treatment for gonorrhea.	Adolescent must be aware of the spread of STIs to prevent them in the future.	Adolescent states she understands STIs are spread by sexual relations.

Continued on following page

BOX 47.8

Nursing Care Planning (continued)

Team Member Responsible	Assessment	Intervention	Rationale	Expected Outcome
Psychosocial/Spiritual/Emotional Needs				
Nurse	Assess intensity of adolescent's pruritus or pain from vulvitis on a scale of 1 to 10.	Discuss the use of acetaminophen or ibuprofen for pain and pruritus as needed.	Acetaminophen and ibuprofen are effective analgesics for mild pain and itching.	Adolescent describes correct dosage of analgesics and states intention to use them.
Nurse/STI counselor	Assess whether adolescent has had sexual contacts other than current boyfriend.	Ask adolescent to name any additional sexual contacts.	Sexual contacts need to be notified so they can also receive treatment.	Adolescent names any other sexual contacts; possibility of rape or sexual maltreatment is ruled out.
Informatics for Seamless Healthcare Planning				
Nurse	Assess whether adolescent understands, in the light of contracting this disease, that she must ask boyfriend to use a condom for sexual relations.	Discuss the possibility that because he contracted an STI, his relationship with her may not be monogamous.	STI was spread to her by a sexual contact.	Adolescent states she will be more conscientious about insisting boyfriend use a condom.
Nurse	Assess whether adolescent or parent has any questions about disease or therapy.	Schedule adolescent for a return appointment in 1 week for repeat culture.	A repeat culture will reveal whether antibiotic therapy has been effective.	Child and parent state they understand the importance of a repeat culture and return appointment.

Assessment

Syphilis is diagnosed by recognition of the various symptoms of the three stages and by serologic serum tests, such as the Venereal Disease Research Laboratory (VDRL) test, the automated reagin test (ART), the rapid plasma reagin (RPR) test, or the fluorescent treponemal antibody–absorption test (FTA-ABS).

Therapeutic Management

Benzathine penicillin G, given intramuscularly in two sites, is effective therapy. For the adolescent who is sensitive to penicillin, either oral erythromycin or tetracycline can be given for 10 to 15 days. Sexual partners are treated in the same way as the person with an active infection. Therapy effectively arrests the disease at whatever stage it has reached. After therapy, adolescents may experience a sudden episode of hypotension, fever, tachycardia, and muscle aches (a Jarisch-Herxheimer reaction caused by the sudden destruction of spirochetes). The reaction lasts about 24 hours and then fades. Because syphilis can be treated so easily, one would think it would be easy to eradicate. In reality, however, because the primary chancre is painless, many people are either unaware of it or choose to ignore it, thereby transmitting the disease to unsuspecting sexual partners. Be certain adolescent are screened for all STIs with both a history and a physical examination, and that sexuality is discussed at healthcare visits (Hsu & Burstein, 2016). They also need to be assured they can report the disease to healthcare personnel and name sexual contacts without fear of being criticized.

Pregnancy and Syphilis

Early in pregnancy (before week 18), the placenta appears to provide some protection against syphilis. After this time, however, the spirochete crosses the placenta freely and may be responsible for spontaneous miscarriage, preterm labor, stillbirth, or congenital anomalies in the newborn (see Chapter 12). All pregnant women are screened for syphilis at a first prenatal visit with a VDRL, ART, or FTA-ABS antibody reaction test. Those who have multiple sexual partners are typically tested again at about week 36 of pregnancy. In some institutions, women are screened again at the beginning of labor, and their newborns are screened for congenital syphilis by a cord blood sample. One injection of benzathine penicillin G is the drug of choice for the treatment of syphilis during pregnancy the same as for those who are not pregnant. If the woman has syphilis, her infant needs penicillin therapy at birth as well (Patel, Klinger, O'Toole, et al., 2012).

If a woman contracted syphilis during pregnancy but it was unrecognized and untreated, and so the newborn is untreated, a congenital form of the disease can occur in the newborn. Severely infected infants will be stillborn; others, less infected, are born with congenital anomalies. Wear gloves to handle such infants because moist lesions (the cord and nasal secretions) may be infectious.

Unlike adults, the infant does not develop a chancre but, about a week after birth, will develop a typical copper-colored rash most prominent over the face, soles of feet, and palms of hands. The infant's nose may show a severe rhinitis (stuffiness). An X-ray of the long bones reveals changes of epiphyseal lines at about 1 to 3 months of age. By 5 to 6 months, these bone changes may no longer be visible and so may be missed.

When the child's permanent teeth erupt at 5 or 6 years of age, the tops may be pegged or notched (Hutchinson's teeth), tend to be of poor quality, and decay easily. If the disease remains untreated even with these symptoms, interstitial keratitis, an inflammatory reaction of the cornea that can result in scarring and blindness, may develop by school age. As the disease progresses further, it may become tertiary or lead to severe neurologic symptoms.

GROUP B STREPTOCOCCAL INFECTION

Although streptococcus B infection is a less publicized disease than STIs such as HSV-2 or gonorrhea, it may actually occur at a higher incidence than those diseases (Page-Ramsey, Johnstone, Kim, et al., 2013). If contracted during pregnancy, consequences can include UTIs, intra-amniotic infections, perhaps preterm birth, and postpartum endometritis.

Pregnant women are generally screened for streptococcus B at 35 to 38 weeks of pregnancy to prevent their newborn from becoming infected from placental transfer or from direct contact with vaginal secretions at birth. If they become infected, neonates can develop severe pneumonia, sepsis, respiratory distress syndrome, or meningitis (see Chapter 26).

A broad-spectrum penicillin such as ampicillin is the treatment of choice. Women who experience rupture of membranes at less than 37 weeks of pregnancy and so have not yet been screened may be treated with intravenous ampicillin during labor to reduce the risk of spreading the infection to the newborn.

HIV

HIV is carried by semen as well as other body fluids, so, although not officially listed as such, is an STI. Invasion of the virus is discussed with other immune system disorders in Chapter 42.

What If . . . 47.4
A nurse is particularly interested in exploring one of the 2020 National Health Goals with respect to reproductive disorders in children (see Box 47.1). What would be a possible research topic pertinent to this goal that would be applicable to Navi's family and would also advance evidence-based practice?

KEY POINTS FOR REVIEW

- Children who are born with a reproductive tract disorder frequently adjust well when young. They may need counseling at puberty or when they become aware of the impact of their disorder on sexual functioning or their ability to reproduce.
- The cause of ambiguous genitalia is unknown but may be related to the level of testosterone produced in utero. The true gender of children is established by a karyotype of chromosomes.
- The development of breast or pubic hair before age 8 years is considered precocious sexual development. Children may be treated with a synthetic analog of GnRH to reduce development. Without effective support, such children are at high risk for disturbed body image.

- Delayed puberty is the failure to develop secondary sex characteristics by the age of 17 years. Girls may be administered estrogen to promote development; boys may be administered testosterone.
- Balanoposthitis (inflammation of the glans and prepuce of the penis) and phimosis (constricted foreskin) occur in boys. Phimosis can be treated with circumcision.
- Cryptorchidism is failure of one or both testes to descend during intrauterine life. The condition is surgically corrected to prevent subfertility and to make it possible to detect testicular cancer later in life.
- Testicular cancer is rare but tends to occur in young men. Boys need to be taught testicular self-examination for early detection.
- Dysmenorrhea, or painful menstruation, occurs frequently in adolescent girls. Therapy is the use of a prostaglandin inhibitor such as ibuprofen.
- Untreated endometriosis (the abnormal growth of extra-uterine endometrial tissue) can lead to subfertility later in life. Therapy is the administration of a synthetic androgen or GnRH receptor inhibitor or surgery to reduce the size of the abnormal tissue.
- Vulvovaginitis (inflammation of the vulva and vagina) and PID are infections that can occur in adolescents. Therapy to prevent fallopian tube scarring and subfertility later in life is essential. In addition, girls need to be taught ways to avoid TSS from the use of menstrual tampons. Vulvovaginitis in young girls needs to be investigated for the possibility of sexual maltreatment.
- Conditions such as fibrocystic breast disease can occur in adolescents. Teaching to reduce the intake of caffeine and sodium can minimize symptoms and also help in planning nursing care that not only meets QSEN competencies but also best meets an adolescent's total needs.
- STIs such as candidiasis, trichomoniasis, *C. trachomatis* infection, genital warts, herpes genitalis, gonorrhea, and syphilis are increasing in incidence in the adolescent population. An important health-teaching area for adolescents is the need to follow safer sex practices.
- When teaching about STIs, it is important to stress that they do not confer immunity and therefore can be contracted more than once. If an STI occurs in a young child, the potential for child maltreatment should be investigated.

CRITICAL THINKING CARE STUDY

Melinda is a 16-year-old teenager you meet at an adolescent clinic. Her parents are divorced and she lives with her father.

1. Melinda is concerned because she has little breast development as of yet and only began having menstrual periods last week. She asks you if she is going to be underdeveloped.
2. Melinda's boyfriend wants to have sex with her. Because he has an unrepaired hypospadias, he has assured her she can't get pregnant. Should she believe him?
3. Melinda tells you she learned everything she knows about sexual relations and contraception from the Internet because her father has difficulty discussing such things with her. Is this a good source of information for her?

RELATED RESOURCES

Explore these additional resources to enhance learning for this chapter:

- Student resources on thePoint, including answers to the What If . . . and Critical Thinking Care Study questions, http://thepoint.lww.com/Flagg8e
- Adaptive learning powered by PrepU, http://thepoint.lww.com /prepu

REFERENCES

Adegbite-Adeniyi, C., Gron, B., Rowles, B. M., et al. (2012). An update on antidepressant use and suicidality in pediatric depression. *Expert Opinion on Pharmacotherapy, 13*(15), 2119–2130.

Agarwal, S. K., & Foster, W. G. (2015). Reduction in endometrioma size with three months of aromatase inhibition and progestin add-back. *BioMed Research International, 2015*, 878517.

Aktaş, D. (2015). Prevalence and factors affecting dysmenorrhea in female university students: Effect on general comfort level. *Pain Management Nursing, 16*(4), 534–543.

Bakke, A. (2016). Empowering our youth: Initiating sexual health education on the inpatient unit for the chronically ill pediatric patient. *Urologic Nursing, 36*(6), 267–288.

Bautista, C. T., Wurapa, E., Sateren, W. B., et al. (2016). Bacterial vaginosis: A synthesis of the literature on etiology, prevalence, risk factors, and relationship with chlamydia and gonorrhea infections. *Military Medical Research, 3*, 4.

Bennett, P. (2012). Preterm labour. In D. K. Edmonds (Ed.), *Dewhurst's textbook of obstetrics & gynaecology* (8th ed., pp. 338–355). Oxford, United Kingdom: Wiley-Blackwell.

Black, A. (2014). Management of pelvic inflammatory disease. *Nurse Prescribing, 12*(9), 443–450.

Braga, L. H., & Lorenzo, A. J. (2017). Cryptorchidism: A practical review for all community healthcare providers. *Canadian Urological Association Journal, 11*(1–2 Suppl. 1), S26–S32.

Centers for Disease Control and Prevention. (2017). *Trichomoniasis fact sheet*. Washington, DC: Author.

Cetin, C., Soysal, C., Khatib, G., et al. (2016). Annular hymenotomy for imperforate hymen. *The Journal of Obstetrics and Gynaecology Research, 42*(8), 1013–1015.

Chien, L. W., Chang, H. C., & Liu, C. F. (2013). Effect of yoga on serum homocysteine and nitric oxide levels in adolescent women with and without dysmenorrhea. *Journal of Alternative and Complementary Medicine, 19*(1), 20–23.

Colaco, M., Heavner, M., Sunaryo, P., et al. (2015). Malpractice litigation and testicular torsion: A legal database review. *The Journal of Emergency Medicine, 49*(6), 849–854.

Connor, E. L. (2012). Adolescent polycystic ovary syndrome. *Adolescent Medicine, 23*(1), 164–177.

De Silva, N. K. (2012). Breast disorders in the female adolescent. *Adolescent Medicine, 23*(1), 34–52.

D'Hauwers, K. W., Depuydt, C. E., Bogers, J. J., et al. (2012). Human papillomavirus, lichen sclerosus and penile cancer: A study in Belgium. *Vaccine, 30*(46), 6573–6577.

Dickson, G. (2012). Gynecomastia. *American Family Physician, 85*(7), 716–722.

Dominé, F., Dadoumont, C., & Bourguignon, J. P. (2012). Eating disorders throughout female adolescence. *Endocrine Development, 22*, 271–286.

Dubowitz, H. (2013). Neglect in children. *Pediatric Annals, 42*(4), 73–77.

Edmonds, D. K. (2012). Benign diseases of the vagina, cervix & ovary. In D. K. Edmonds (Ed.), *Dewhurst's textbook of obstetrics & gynaecology* (8th ed., pp. 706–714). Oxford, United Kingdom: Wiley-Blackwell.

Facchin, F., Barbara, G., Saita, E., et al. (2015). Impact of endometriosis on quality of life and mental health: Pelvic pain makes the difference. *Journal of Psychosomatic Obstetrics & Gynaecology, 36*(4), 135–141.

Fantasia, J., Aidlen, J., Lathrop, W., et al. (2015). Undescended testes: A clinical and surgical review. *Urologic Nursing, 35*(3), 117–126.

Fine, R. G., & Poppas, D. P. (2012). Varicocele: Standard and alternative indications for repair. *Current Opinion in Urology, 22*(6), 513–516.

Francis, S. A., & Katz, M. L. (2013). The HPV vaccine: A comparison of focus groups conducted in South Africa and Ohio Appalachia. *Maternal and Child Health Journal, 17*(7), 1222–1229.

Gaylord, N. M., & Petersen-Smith, A. M. (2013). Genitourinary disorders. In C. E. Burns, A. M. Dunn, M. A. Brady, et al. (Eds.), *Pediatric primary care* (5th ed., pp. 809–843). Philadelphia, PA: Elsevier/Saunders.

Gele, A. A., Johansen, E. B., & Sundby, J. (2012). When female circumcision comes to the West: Attitudes toward the practice among Somali immigrants in Oslo. *BMC Public Health, 12*, 697.

Gerlt, T., & Starr, N. B. (2013). Gynecologic disorders. In E. E. Burns, A. M. Dunn, M. A. Brady, et al. (Eds.), *Pediatric primary care* (5th ed., pp. 844–876). Philadelphia, PA: Elsevier/Saunders.

Gharloghi, S., Torkzahrani, S., Akbarzadeh, A. R., et al. (2012). The effects of acupressure on severity of primary dysmenorrhea. *Patient Preference and Adherence, 6*, 137–142.

Goyal, M. K., Shea, J. A., Hayes, K. L., et al. (2016). Development of a sexual health screening tool for adolescent emergency department patients. *Academic Emergency Medicine, 23*(7), 809–815.

Groves, M. J. (2016). Genital herpes: A review. *American Family Physician, 93*(11), 928–934.

Haugnes, H. S., Bosl, G. J., Boer, H., et al. (2012). Long-term and late effects of germ cell testicular cancer treatment and implications for follow-up. *Journal of Clinical Oncology, 30*(30), 3752–3763.

Hershey, A. D. (2012). Perimenstrual headache in adolescence. *Current Pain and Headache Reports, 16*(5), 474–476.

Hofmeister, S., & Bodden, S. (2016). Premenstrual syndrome and premenstrual dysphoric disorder. *American Family Physician, 94*(3), 236–240.

Hornor, G. (2017). Sexually transmitted infections and children: What the PNP should know. *Journal of Pediatric Health Care, 31*(2), 222–229.

Hsu, K. K., & Burstein, G. R. (2016). Syphilis screening recommendation in nonpregnant adults and adolescents: Still waters run deep. *JAMA Pediatrics, 170*(8), 733–735.

Hudson, A. L. (2012). Where do youth in foster care receive information about preventing unplanned pregnancy and sexually transmitted infections? *Journal of Pediatric Nursing, 27*(5), 443–450.

Alvarez, A., & Jacobs, L. K. (2011). Breast diseases. In K. J. Hurt, M. W. Guile, J. L. Bienstock, et al. (Eds.), *The Johns Hopkins manual of gynecology and obstetrics* (4th ed., pp. 15–32). Philadelphia, PA: Lippincott Williams & Wilkins.

Karch, A. M. (2013). *2013 Lippincott's nursing drug guide*. Philadelphia, PA: Lippincott Williams & Wilkins.

Karlı, N., Baykan, B., Erta , M., et al. (2012). Impact of sex hormonal changes on tension-type headache and migraine: A cross-sectional population-based survey in 2,600 women. *The Journal of Headache and Pain, 13*(7), 557–565.

Katz, M. L., Oldach, B. R., Goodwin, J., et al. (2014). Development and initial feedback about a human papillomavirus (HPV) vaccine comic book for adolescents. *Journal of Cancer Education, 29*(2), 318–324.

Kelvin, J. F. (2015). Sperm banking: Fertility preservation for male patients with cancer. *Clinical Journal of Oncology Nursing, 19*(1), 108–110.

Kennedy, S., & Koninckx, P. (2012). Endometriosis. In D. K. Edmonds (Ed.), *Dewhurst's textbook of obstetrics & gynaecology* (8th ed., pp. 615–616). Oxford, United Kingdom: Wiley-Blackwell.

Kransdorf, L. N., Kling, J. M., & Mayer, A. P. (2014). Treatment of gonococcal infection: When one drug is not enough. *Journal of Women's Health, 23*(7), 627–628.

Lathrop, B. L., Cheney, T. B., & Hayman, A. B. (2014). Ethical decision-making in the dilemma of the intersex infant. *Issues in Comprehensive Pediatric Nursing, 37*(1), 25–38.

Marcdante, K. J., & Kliegman, R. M. (2015a). Assessment of the mother, fetus, and newborn. In K. J. Marcdante & R. M. Kliegman (Eds.), *Nelson essentials of pediatrics* (7th ed., pp. 186–203). Philadelphia, PA: Saunders/Elsevier.

Marcdante, K. J., & Kliegman, R. M. (2015b). Disorders of puberty. In K. J. Marcdante & R. M. Kliegman (Eds.), *Nelson essentials of pediatrics* (7th ed., pp. 589–596). Philadelphia, PA: Saunders/Elsevier.

Marcdante, K. J., & Kliegman, R. M. (2015c). Disorders of sexual development. In K. J. Marcdante & R. M. Kliegman (Eds.), *Nelson essentials of pediatrics* (7th ed., pp. 604–607). Philadelphia, PA: Saunders/Elsevier.

Markman, M. (2013). Risk of cervical cancer after HPV vaccination. *Current Pharmaceutical Design, 19*(8), 1488–1489.

Mashburn, J. (2012). Vaginal infections update. *Journal of Midwifery & Women's Health, 57*(6), 629–634.

Matteson, K. A., Raker, C. A., Clark, M. A., et al. (2013). Abnormal uterine bleeding, health status, and usual source of medical care: Analyses using the medical expenditures panel survey. *Journal of Women's Health, 22*(11), 959–965.

McGreal, S., & Wood, P. (2013). Recurrent vaginal discharge in children. *Journal of Pediatric & Adolescent Gynecology, 26*, 205–208.

McIntosh, L. A., Scrimgeour, D., Youngson, G. G., et al. (2013). The risk of failure after primary orchidopexy: An 18 year review. *Journal of Pediatric Urology, 9*, 759–762.

Menon, P. S., & Vijayakumar, M. (2014). Precocious puberty—perspectives on diagnosis and management. *Indian Journal of Pediatrics, 81*(1), 76–83.

Morris, B. J., Waskett, J. H., Banerjee, J., et al. (2012). A "snip" in time: What is the best age to circumcise? *BMC Pediatrics, 12*, 20.

Munro, M. G. (2012). Classification of menstrual bleeding disorders. *Reviews in Endocrine & Metabolic Disorders, 13*(4), 225–234.

Mysore, V., & Shashikumar, B. M. (2016). Guidelines on the use of finasteride in androgenetic alopecia. *Indian Journal of Dermatology, Venereology, and Leprology, 82*, 128–134.

Navvabi Rigi, S. D., Kermansaravi, F., Navidian, A., et al. (2012). Comparing the analgesic effect of heat patch containing iron chip and ibuprofen for primary dysmenorrhea: A randomized controlled trial. *BMC Women's Health, 12*, 25.

O'Connor, C. A., & Shubkin, C. D. (2012). Adolescent STIs for primary care providers. *Current Opinion in Pediatrics, 24*(5), 647–655.

Page-Ramsey, S. M., Johnstone, S. K., Kim, D., et al. (2013). Prevalence of group B Streptococcus colonization in subsequent pregnancies of group B Streptococcus-colonized versus noncolonized women. *American Journal of Perinatology, 30*, 383–388.

Panabokke, G., Clifford, I. D., Craig, S. S., et al. (2016). Reduction of paediatric inguinal hernias. *Emergency Medicine Australasia,28*(2), 224–227.

Parma, M., Vanni, V. S., Bertini, M., et al. (2014). Probiotics in the prevention of recurrences of bacterial vaginosis. *Alternative Therapies in Health and Medicine, 20*(Suppl. 1), 52–57.

Patel, S. J., Klinger, E. J., O'Toole, D., et al. (2012). Missed opportunities for preventing congenital syphilis infection in New York City. *Obstetrics and Gynecology, 120*(4), 882–888.

Pearson, W. S., Gift, T. L., Leichliter, J. S., et al. (2015). Differences in treatment of *Chlamydia trachomatis* by ambulatory care setting. *Journal of Community Health, 40*(6), 1115–1121.

Rome, E. S. (2012). Vulvovaginitis and other common vulvar disorders in children. *Endocrine Development, 22*, 72–83.

Ross, J. D. C. (2012). Pelvic infection. In D. K. Edmonds (Ed.), *Dewhurst's textbook of obstetrics & gynaecology* (8th ed., pp. 597–606). Oxford, United Kingdom: Wiley-Blackwell.

Russell, S. S. (2014). Testicular cancer: Overview and implications for health care providers. *Urologic Nursing, 34*(4), 172–176.

Rydz, N., & Jamieson, M. A. (2013). Managing heavy menstrual bleeding in adolescents. *Contemporary OB/GYN, 58*(7), 49–52.

Shahid, S. K. (2012). Phimosis in children. *ISRN Urology, 2012*, 707329.

Smith, M. K., & Stepanov, N. (2014). School-based youth health nurses and adolescent decision-making concerning reproductive and sexual health advice: How can the law guide healthcare practitioners in this context? *Contemporary Nurse, 47*(1–2), 42–50.

Spritzer, P. M., & Motta, A. B. (2015). Adolescence and polycystic ovary syndrome: Current concepts on diagnosis and treatment. *International Journal of Clinical Practice, 69*(11), 1236–1246.

Srinivasaiah, N., Iwuchukwu, O. C., Stanley, P. R., et al. (2014). Risk factors for complications following breast reduction: Results from a randomized control trial. *The Breast Journal, 20*(3), 274–278.

Steinberg, E. M., Cardoso, G. M., Martinez, P. E., et al. (2012). Rapid response to fluoxetine in women with premenstrual dysphoric disorder. *Depression and Anxiety, 29*(6), 531–540.

Sung, E. K., Setty, B. N., & Castro-Aragon, I. (2012). Sonography of the pediatric scrotum: Emphasis on the Ts—torsion, trauma, and tumors. *American Journal of Roentgenology, 198*(5), 996–1003.

Swartzendruber, A., Sales, J. M., Brown, J. L., et al. (2014). Correlates of incident *Trichomonas vaginalis* infections among African American female adolescents. *Sexually Transmitted Diseases, 41*(4), 240–245.

Tepper, N. K., Steenland, M. W., Gaffield, M. E., et al. (2013). Retention of intrauterine devices in women who acquire pelvic inflammatory disease: A systematic review. *Contraception, 87*, 655–660.

Twiss, J. (2013). A new look at abnormal uterine bleeding. *The Nurse Practitioner, 38*(12), 22–30.

U.S. Department of Health and Human Services. (2010). *Healthy people 2020*. Washington, DC: Author.

Valeur, N. S., Rahbar, H., & Chapman, T. (2015). Ultrasound of pediatric breast masses: What to do with lumps and bumps. *Pediatric Radiology, 45*(11), 1584–1599.

Weiss Kelly, A. K., & Hecht, S. (2016). The female athlete triad. *Pediatrics, 138*(2), e20160922.

Yang, N. Y., & Kim, S. D. (2016). Effects of a yoga program on menstrual cramps and menstrual distress in undergraduate students with primary dysmenorrhea: A single-blind, randomized controlled trial. *Journal of Alternative and Complementary Medicine, 22*(9), 732–738.

48

Nursing Care of a Family When a Child Has an Endocrine or a Metabolic Disorder

Rob Tebecco is a 16-year-old boy with type 1 diabetes whom you meet in the emergency department, where he was taken after he became comatose while ice skating. His diabetes was diagnosed when he was 7 years old. His records indicate that his disease has generally been under good control over the past years, but in the last 6 months, he has "forgotten" to take his insulin at least once a week. During your assessment, he tells you that ice skating practice every morning and a new girlfriend have occupied his time and interrupted what used to be a strict schedule of home-cooked meals and a rigid routine.

Previous chapters described the growth and development of well children. This chapter adds information about the dramatic changes, both physical and psychosocial, that occur when children develop an endocrine or metabolic disorder. This is important information because it builds a base for care and health teaching.

Is Rob's history unusual for an adolescent? What health teaching do you think will most help him reestablish control?

KEY TERMS

carpopedal spasm

exophthalmos

glycosuria

hormones

hyperglycemia

hypoglycemia

hypothalamus

ketoacidosis

latent tetany

manifest tetany

pedal spasm

polydipsia

polyuria

sella turcica

Somogyi phenomenon

OBJECTIVES

After mastering the contents of this chapter, you should be able to:

1. Describe the structure and function of the endocrine glands and why metabolic illnesses occur.

2. Identify 2020 National Health Goals that nurses can help the nation achieve related to childhood endocrine or metabolic disorders.

3. Assess a child with a disorder of endocrine or metabolic dysfunction.

4. Formulate nursing diagnoses for a child with altered endocrine or metabolic dysfunction.

5. Establish expected outcomes for a child with endocrine or metabolic dysfunction.

6. Help parents to manage seamless transitions across healthcare settings.

7. Using the nursing process, plan nursing care that includes the six competencies of Quality & Safety Education for Nurses (QSEN): Patient-Centered Care, Teamwork & Collaboration, Evidence-Based Practice (EBP), Quality Improvement (QI), Safety, and Informatics.

8. Implement nursing care such as teaching long-term medicine administration to a child with an endocrine or metabolic disorder.

9. Evaluate expected outcomes for achievement and effectiveness of care.

10. Integrate knowledge of endocrine and metabolic disorders with the interplay of nursing process, the six competencies of QSEN, and Family Nursing to ensure quality maternal and child health nursing care.

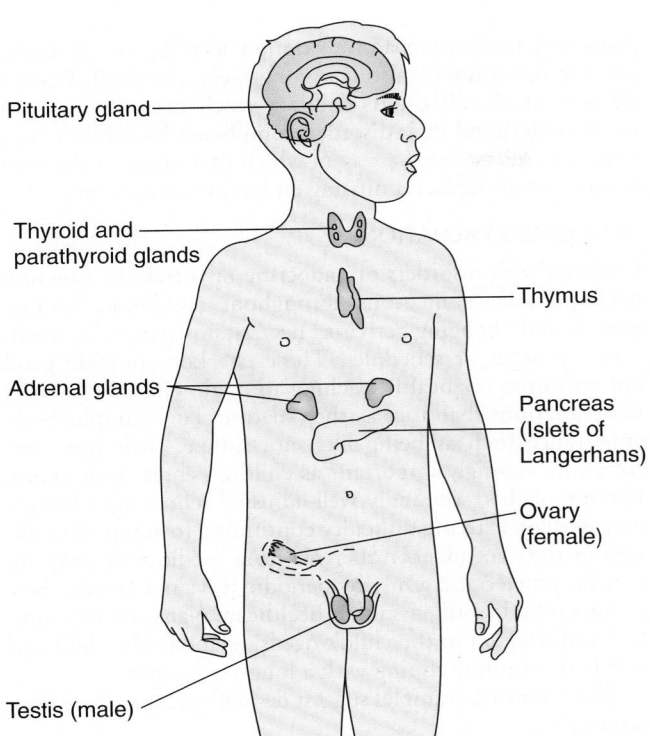

Pituitary gland

Thyroid and
parathyroid glands

Thymus

Adrenal glands

Pancreas
(Islets of
Langerhans)

Ovary
(female)

Testis (male)

Figure 48.1   The location of the endocrine glands.

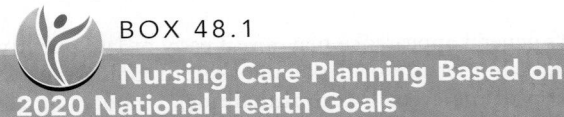

BOX 48.1

Nursing Care Planning Based on 2020 National Health Goals

Endocrine disorders tend to be long term and so cause lifetime consequences. Reducing the incidence of these or improving care has long-term implications. A sample of 2020 National Health Goals related to these include:

- Reduce the diabetes-related death rate from a baseline of 77 per 100,000 to no more than 46 per 100,000 people.
- Increase the proportion of persons with diabetes who receive formal diabetes education from a baseline of 56.8% to a target of 62.5%.
- Reduce the proportion of children aged 3 to 10 years diagnosed with a disorder through newborn blood spot screening who experience developmental delay requiring special education services from 15.1% to a target level of 13.5%.
- Increase the proportion of children with long-term illnesses who have access to a medical home from 57.5% of children under 18 years to 63.3% (U.S. Department of Health and Human Services, 2010; see www.healthypeople.gov).

Nurses can help the nation achieve these goals by educating children with diabetes about their care and being certain newborns receive blood spot testing so children with these disorders not only can be identified as early in life as possible but also can receive continuing care in a "medical home." As the number of home births increases, it's important to evaluate at well-child healthcare visits if a child did receive routine blood spot testing at birth or whether this should be obtained at a later date.

The endocrine system is composed of a small group of ductless glands that work together with the neurologic system to regulate and coordinate all body systems (Fig. 48.1). The glands produce **hormones**, which are secreted into surrounding tissue and picked up by the bloodstream, where their action is to turn on or turn off various organ functions. (The word *hormone* is from the Greek *hormaein*, which means "to set in motion.") Each gland of the endocrine system acts on a specific target (or designated) organ or has specific duties that are necessary for regulating body processes (van Karnebeek & Stockler, 2012).

The inadequate secretion of hormones or dysfunction of the glands results in a variety of disorders, most of which have long-term implications. Parents and children, as soon as they are old enough, need to understand the causes and symptoms of these diseases so they can participate in their long-term plan of care. Box 48.1 shows 2020 National Health Goals related to endocrine and metabolic disorders in children.

Nursing Process Overview

FOR CARE OF A CHILD WITH AN ENDOCRINE OR METABOLIC DISORDER

ASSESSMENT

Endocrine and metabolic disorders, as a group, commonly cause changes in growth and a child's social and physical development and may impair their cognitive development. These disorders are often manifested in growth and development delays, especially during puberty or adolescence. If not identified at birth, the disorder is usually detected when a child's height and weight are measured at a healthcare visit and found to be above or below a typical measurement for that age. An acute loss in weight is often the first symptom of type 1 diabetes mellitus in children. Thyroid deficiencies or type 2 diabetes mellitus (T2D) may be revealed by being overweight. Pituitary difficulties may be revealed by unusually short or tall stature.

To obtain information on activity in the child, take a day history by asking a parent or child to describe all of the child's actions on a typical day because this type of information yields clues that are helpful in distinguishing between a child with a more introverted nature (a "quiet" child) and one who is experiencing inactivity and chronic fatigue as a result of decreased endocrine function. For example, the quiet child lies down after school and reads, whereas the ill child lies down and sleeps. The healthy child appears to "go constantly" but can sit through a favorite television program or a meal. The child with increased thyroid hormone production may be unable to sit quietly at all.

Also assess dietary and elimination habits. Extreme thirst or appetite may occur with an endocrine disorder such as diabetes insipidus or type 1 diabetes mellitus. Frequent voiding in children most often reflects a urinary tract infection, but it may be evidence of excessive urine excretion (**polyuria**), possibly from pituitary dysfunction or diabetes mellitus.

A child's general appearance may reveal early or late puberty changes, scaling or dry or darkening skin, drooping eyelids, protrusion of the eyeballs (**exophthalmos**), or poor muscle tone, all indications of endocrine disorders.

NURSING DIAGNOSIS

Because endocrine glands control vital body functions, nursing diagnoses relevant to children with endocrine or metabolic disorders include both physiologic functions and the child's response to those changes. Some examples of such nursing diagnoses include:

- Deficient fluid volume related to constant excessive loss of fluid through urination
- Risk for imbalanced nutrition, less than body requirements, related to an inability to use glucose because of diabetes mellitus
- Disturbed body image related to abnormal height
- Health-seeking behaviors related to the self-administration of insulin
- Deficient knowledge related to long-term treatment needs
- Fear related to the potential and unknown illness outcome
- Anticipatory grieving related to presumed losses associated with diagnosis of long-term illness
- Interrupted family processes related to the child's chronic illness
- Anxiety related to financial resources required to maintain optimum family health

OUTCOME IDENTIFICATION AND PLANNING

Although most endocrine and metabolic disorders have long-term implications, parents and children may find it easier to work with outcomes that are initially short term—particularly if they are having difficulty accepting the diagnosis and the long-term nature of the disorder. Because symptoms usually are not acute, children may easily forget to take (or parents may forget to give) necessary medications. Helping parents create reminder charts or set alerts on their smartphones are effective measures to increase compliance.

Evaluate both the school and home situation for any child with a chronic illness. You may need to help teachers better understand the child's health problem (with the parents' permission) so that they do not make excessive or inappropriate demands such as insisting that a child with hyperthyroidism submit neat handwriting assignments when the child cannot do so.

Selected organizations that are helpful for referral to parents include the American Diabetes Association (www.diabetes.org), the Congenital Adrenal Hyperplasia Support Group (www.cah.org.uk), Little People of America (www.lpaonline.org), and the National Tay-Sachs and Allied Diseases (www.ntsad.org).

IMPLEMENTATION

Interventions for children with endocrine or metabolic disorders must always be carried out with long-term aspects of care in mind. Bribing children to take medicine, for example, is never good practice with any child. It has no place with children who must continue to take a medication for the rest of their lives (bribery quickly becomes ineffective). Instead, offer the family referrals to age-appropriate support groups within their communities that will serve to build life-long bonding and relationships. Sharing effective treatment plans and medication administration techniques can facilitate successful interventions in long-term care (Bell, Bayliss, Glauert, et al., 2016). As children reach maturity and can better understand their disorder, compliance increases as they begin to understand the way in which their daily medication is necessary to replace a missing endocrine component.

OUTCOME EVALUATION

Children with disorders of endocrine or metabolic function need periodic evaluations throughout childhood because growth and changing activities necessitate changes in medication dosages or schedules. These checkups provide good opportunities for health teaching to equip children to meet new situations that arise as they mature. For example, body appearance such as being like, not unlike, their peers becomes increasingly important as children enter adolescence. Because of this, seemingly well-adjusted school-age children may develop extreme difficulty continuing to accept their illness as they get older. Adherence to a medication program may become erratic. Only by periodic reevaluation can these problems be identified so that healthcare plans can be modified and adapted to the child's needs, enabling the child and family to continue coping with a long-term illness.

The following examples suggest desired outcomes have been achieved:

- The child brings to clinic a written record showing that she took her medication as recommended.
- Parents list developmentally appropriate, not size-appropriate, activities for their child with a short stature.
- The child's blood pressure and pulse remain within normal limits for age, specific gravity of urine is between 1.003 and 1.030, skin turgor is good, and the child states thirst is not excessive.
- Parents demonstrate correct insulin injection technique and state they are comfortable administering an injection to their child.

Health Promotion and Risk Management

Many endocrine and metabolic disorders are inherited; therefore, education and genetic counseling are important preventive measures (Box 48.2).

T2D is strongly associated with obesity so is at an epidemic incidence because obesity in school-age children is also at epidemic proportions (Sherr & Weinzimer, 2012). School nurses can be instrumental not only in counseling and helping students manage this disorder during school hours but also in helping prevent T2D by serving as an advisor to what foods and snacks ought to be available in school settings.

The Pituitary Gland

The work of the pituitary gland is directed by the **hypothalamus**, an organ located in the center of the brain and which serves as the regulator of the autonomic nervous system. About 1 cm long, 1.0 to 1.5 cm wide, and 0.5 cm thick, the pituitary gland rests in the **sella turcica**, a depression of the sphenoid bone.

ASSESSING A CHILD WITH AN ENDOCRINE DISORDER

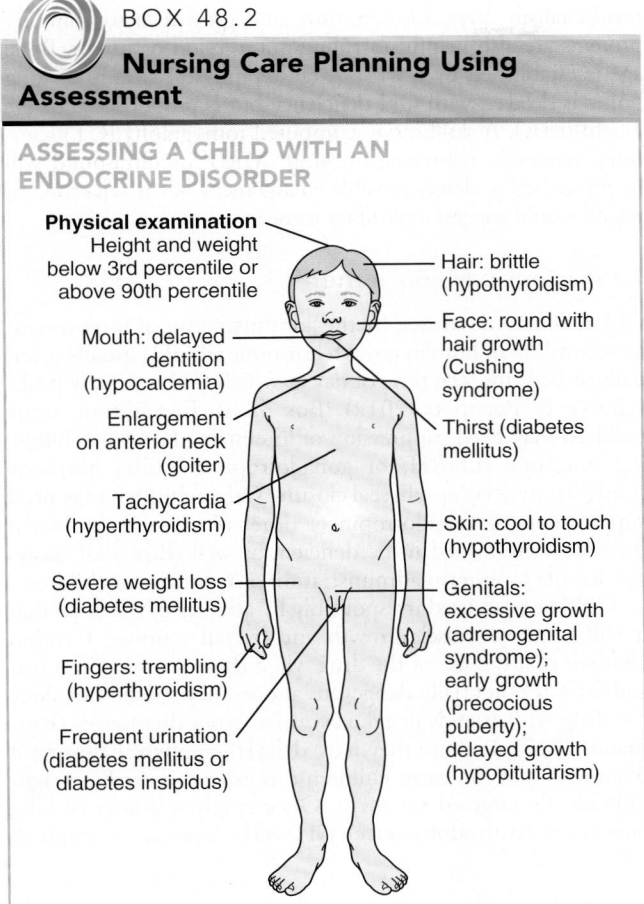

Physical examination
Height and weight below 3rd percentile or above 90th percentile

Mouth: delayed dentition (hypocalcemia)

Enlargement on anterior neck (goiter)

Tachycardia (hyperthyroidism)

Severe weight loss (diabetes mellitus)

Fingers: trembling (hyperthyroidism)

Frequent urination (diabetes mellitus or diabetes insipidus)

Hair: brittle (hypothyroidism)

Face: round with hair growth (Cushing syndrome)

Thirst (diabetes mellitus)

Skin: cool to touch (hypothyroidism)

Genitals: excessive growth (adrenogenital syndrome); early growth (precocious puberty); delayed growth (hypopituitarism)

The gland is divided into several distinct regions: the anterior lobe, or *adenohypophysis*; the posterior lobe, or *neurohypophysis*; and the intermediate lobe, or *pars intermedia*, which lies between the anterior and posterior lobes. Altogether, these divisions store and release eight different hormones. Four of these—the antidiuretic hormone (ADH), thyrotropin, corticotropin, and somatotropin—are prominently involved in childhood illnesses (Table 48.1).

Pituitary Gland Disorders

Illnesses caused by pituitary dysfunction can result from a tumor growing in either the pituitary gland or the hypothalamus, interference with circulation to the gland, trauma, inflammation, structural abnormalities, erratic or nonfunctional feedback mechanisms, and, possibly, autoimmune responses. Interference due to these reasons can result in hypopituitarism (lack of growth hormone), hyperpituitarism (excess secretion of growth hormone), or diabetes insipidus (undersecretion of ADH).

GROWTH HORMONE DEFICIENCY

If production of human growth hormone (GH, or somatotropin) is deficient, children are not able to grow to full size (Dörr, Boguszewski, Dahlgren, et al., 2015). As a result, children may appear well proportioned but measure well below the average on a standard growth chart. Deficient production of GH may result from a nonmalignant cystic tumor of embryonic origin that places pressure on the pituitary gland or from increased intracranial pressure as a result of trauma. In most children with hypopituitarism, however, the cause of the defect is unknown; it may have a genetic origin.

If hypopituitarism is not treated, predicting exactly what height a child will reach is difficult because height varies with each individual. Without treatment, however, most children will not reach more than 3 or 4 ft in height.

Assessment

The child with deficient production of GH is usually normal in size and weight at birth. Within the first few years of life, however, the child begins to fall below the third percentile of height and weight on growth charts. The face appears infantile because the mandible is recessed and immature, and the nose is usually small. The child's teeth may be crowded in a small jaw (and may erupt late). The child's voice may be high pitched, and the onset of pubic, facial, and axillary hair and genital growth will be delayed. The history, physical findings, and a decreased level of circulating GH contribute to the diagnosis.

TABLE 48.1 COMMON PITUITARY HORMONES AND THEIR PURPOSES

Pituitary Hormone	Source and Target Organs	Actions and Effects
Antidiuretic hormone (ADH)	Secreted by the neurohypophysis *Target organ:* kidney	ADH helps regulate fluid volume by regulating urine output. By decreasing urine output, it increases the volume of extracellular fluid volume; when secretion of ADH is low, urinary output increases. Factors such as trauma, pain, anxiety, and exposure to high temperatures all increase ADH release.
Corticotropin (ACTH)	Secreted by the adenohypophysis *Target organ:* adrenal glands	ACTH stimulates the adrenal gland to produce glucocorticoid and mineralocorticoid hormones. Increased production of adrenal gland secretions decreases ACTH production and vice versa.
Somatotropin (growth hormone [GH])	Secreted by the adenohypophysis *Target organ:* none; acts on all body cells	GH increases bone and cartilage growth by increasing the gastrointestinal absorption of calcium. If GH production is inhibited, undergrowth will occur; if GH production is excessive, overgrowth will occur.
Thyrotropin (TSH)	Secreted by the adenohypophysis *Target organ:* thyroid gland	TSH stimulates the thyroid gland to produce thyroid hormones (thyroxine and triiodothyronine). Too little TSH leads to atrophy and inactivity of the thyroid gland; too much TSH causes hypertrophy (increase in size) and hyperplasia (increase in the number of cells) of the gland.

ACTH, adrenocorticotropic hormone; TSH, thyroid-stimulating hormone.

A pituitary tumor must be ruled out as the cause of decreased GH production. Sudden halted growth suggests a tumor; gradual failure suggests an idiopathic involvement. A history of vision loss, headache, an increase in head circumference, nausea, and vomiting (signs of increased intracranial pressure) also suggest a pituitary tumor. Growth failure may be so marked in some children that the parents may be suspected of child neglect.

As part of the history taking, evaluate the family history for traits of short stature or constitutional delay (familial late development). If at all possible, obtain estimates of the parents' height and siblings' height and weight during their periods of growth. Assess the child's prenatal and birth history for any suggestion of intrauterine growth restriction. Assess also for any severe head trauma that could have injured the pituitary gland or chronic illness, such as a heart, kidney, or intestinal disorder that could have contributed to the decreased level of growth. Take a 24-hour nutrition history to see if "picky eating habits" are extensive enough to halt growth. Be certain to assess not only the child's actual height but also his or her feelings about being short.

A physical assessment, including a funduscopic examination, neurologic testing, and blood analysis for hypothyroidism, hy-

poadrenalism, hypoaldosteronism, and growth factor–binding proteins are also helpful in ruling out a lesion or tumor. Bone age is established by a wrist X-ray (epiphyseal closure of long bones is delayed with GH deficiency but is proportional to the height delay). A skull series, computed tomography (CT) scanning, magnetic resonance imaging (MRI), or ultrasound will be prescribed to detect possible enlargement of the sella turcica, which would suggest a pituitary tumor.

Therapeutic Management

GH deficiency is treated by the administration of intramuscular recombinant human growth hormone (rhGH) usually given daily at bedtime, the time of day at which GH normally peaks (Graber & Rapaport, 2012) (Box 48.3). In addition, some children may need suppression of luteinizing hormone–releasing hormone (LHRH, or gonadotropin-releasing hormone [GnRH]) to delay epiphyseal closure. Other children may need supplements of gonadotropin or other pituitary hormones if these are determined to be deficient as well (Box 48.4 shows tips for the long-term administration of medicine to children).

GH has been used irresponsibly by athletes in the hope that it will improve muscle growth and overall stamina. Caution children that the use of the drug when there is no medical reason for it is potentially dangerous and so they should not share the drug with friends or take excessive doses themselves (Baumann, 2012). Because they have delayed epiphyseal closure, if treatment is begun early, children can expect to reach a height individually targeted for them. Once epiphyseal lines of long bones close (with adolescence), GH will be tapered and stopped.

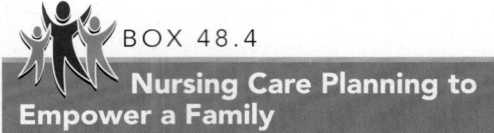

BOX 48.3

Nursing Care Planning Based on Responsibility for Pharmacology

SOMATROPIN (NUTROPIN, HUMATROPE)

Classification: Somatropin is an example of a recombinant human growth hormone (rhGH).

Action: used for the long-term treatment of children who have growth failure from inadequate production of pituitary hormone, renal failure, or Turner syndrome (Baronio, Mazzanti, Girtler, et al., 2017)

Pregnancy Risk Category: C

Dosage: Somatropin dosage is individualized. The drug is administered by injection either SC or intramuscularly.

Possible Adverse Effects: injection site pain, glucose intolerance, hypothyroidism, bone problems (particularly the hip), blood abnormalities, rare intracranial hypertension in first 8 weeks of therapy

Nursing Implications

- Advise parents that X-rays of the wrist or hip will be performed before therapy begins. Thereafter, parents should be alert for limping or knee or hip pain, which should be reported to their primary healthcare provider because slipped capital epiphysis is associated with rhGH supplementation.
- Reinforce the need for periodic thyroid function tests and funduscopic examination to detect rare intracranial hypertension.
- Alert parents that rhGH may interact with glucocorticoid therapy such as prednisone, causing a decrease in the effectiveness of the rhGH. Urge parents to inform all healthcare providers that the child is receiving rhGH to avoid this type of interaction.

BOX 48.4

Nursing Care Planning to Empower a Family

GUIDELINES FOR SUCCESSFUL LONG-TERM MEDICINE ADMINISTRATION

Q. Rob's father asks you, "What are good rules for long-term medicine administration?"

A. To be successful giving medicine over a long period of time, build the administration of it into your family's general routine through such measures as:

- Begin involving your child as early as possible in medicine administration by explaining what it is and why the child needs to take it.
- Plan times for medication administration that allow for a normal lifestyle, such as not having to wake up at 2 AM or having to interrupt a meal for an injection.
- Be aware of the life span of the medicine so that medication does not expire.
- Be certain to anticipate the need to obtain prescriptions before vacations, summer camp, or holidays so medicine is always available.
- If an intramuscular, subcutaneous, or intravenous medication is prescribed, not only the child but also at least one parent should learn the injection technique to ensure adherence.

Nursing Diagnoses and Related Interventions

Nursing Diagnosis: Situational low self-esteem related to short stature

Outcome Evaluation: Child speaks positively about self; identifies friends and activities enjoyed with peers.

If a child has been consistently behind in growth since early life, parents may simply assume in early childhood that the child is going to be short as an adult. The parents then may become concerned that something is wrong only after the child reaches puberty and fails to develop secondary sex characteristics. If an investigation at that time reveals the child's true problem is a lack of GH, parents may feel guilty that they did not become alarmed earlier. They may feel resentment toward healthcare personnel who did not alert them to the problem earlier. Encourage parents to discuss these feelings and provide support to help them

accept their child in this new light as well as participate in making the new plan of care a success (Box 48.5). Children with short stature tend to report feelings of lower quality of life largely related to discrimination (Geisler, Lass, Reinsch, et al., 2012). You may need to remind parents to assign duties and responsibilities to children that match their chronologic age, not their physical size, in order to promote children's feelings of maturity and self-esteem. Because children different in any way from their peers may be the victims of bullying, alert parents to this possibility and assess for this at well-child visits to help protect the child's quality of life (Box 48.6).

GROWTH HORMONE EXCESS

An overproduction of GH usually is caused by a benign tumor of the anterior pituitary (an adenoma). If the overproduction occurs before the epiphyseal lines of the long bones have closed, excessive or overgrowth will result. Weight will become excessive also, but it is proportional to height. The skull circumference typically exceeds usual, and the fontanels may close late or not at all. After epiphyseal lines close, *acromegaly* (enlargement of the bones of the head and soft parts

---

BOX 48.5

Nursing Care Planning Tips for Effective Communication

Rob, a 16-year-old with diabetes, is short in stature. While observing him and his mother, you notice Rob is wearing clothes more suitable for a preteen than an adolescent.

Tip: Explore feelings around stature with both children and their parents. Help parents to understand all children grow older chronologically and need age-appropriate activities and interests even if they still appear young. Because many children with endocrine or metabolic disorders are short in stature, they are viewed as cute and petite by parents, and some parents express that they enjoy their child's short stature; it makes it seem as if the child will remain a child longer and not grow up and become independent. In the following scenario, the nurse gives Rob's mother the opportunity to discuss her feelings further.

Nurse: Mrs. Tebecco, do you have any questions about Rob's care?

Mrs. Tebecco: No. I'm worried, though, that he'll be wanting a driver's license soon. I'm lucky he's so short he can't really drive yet.

Nurse: Is he happy being so short?

Mrs. Tebecco: It made him better at gymnastics than the taller boys. Probably because he looks so much younger than he is.

Nurse: But how does he feel about his size? How do you think he'll feel in the future?

Mrs. Tebecco: I don't even think about that. I don't want to lose my baby.

Nurse: Let's talk a bit about how his growing up makes both of you feel before we review his insulin injection technique.

 BOX 48.6

Nursing Care Planning to Respect Cultural Diversity

The prevalence of endocrine disorders, such as type 2 diabetes, is correlated to nutrition and physical activity factors. The effects of nutrition impact a child's health from conception through adolescence. Nutrition and physical activity vary in families and are often a learned behavior.

Healthcare providers who seek to prevent diabetes and improve diabetes outcomes face challenges related to the disproportionate incidence and prevalence of both diabetes and diabetes-related complications among diverse populations, and each population has its own cultural influences. Culture can be defined by the way people look at the world, how they interact with others, and how they expect others to behave (Hagan, Shaw, & Duncan, 2017). Issues related to nutrition reflect the feeding environment, which includes foods selected, the environment within which food is offered, and the relationship between the caregiver and the child (Hagan et al., 2017). To provide effective patient education on nutrition, the nurse must understand attitudes about body weight and food insecurity. It is important for healthcare providers to respect and appreciate the variety of cultural traditions related to food and the variation in food practices among families, while promoting healthy nutrition and physical activity. Healthcare providers must also examine their own cultural influences and attitudes toward nutrition and physical activity when providing counseling (Hagan et al., 2017).

of the hands and feet) begins to be evident. The tongue can become so enlarged and thickened that it protrudes from the mouth, giving the child a dull, apathetic appearance and making it difficult to articulate words. If the condition remains untreated, a child may reach a height of more than 8 ft.

If X-rays or ultrasounds of the skull reveal that the sella turcica is enlarged or that a tumor is present, laser surgery to remove the tumor or cryosurgery (freezing of tissue) is the primary treatment. If no tumor is present, a GH antagonist such as bromocriptine (Parlodel) taken orally or octreotide (Sandostatin) taken by injection can slow the production of GH. When GH secretion is halted in this way, other hormones may also be affected; therefore, the child may need to receive supplemental thyroid extract, cortisol, and gonadotropin hormones in later life. A more permanent therapy is irradiation or radioactive implants of the pituitary gland, again to halt GH production. It is difficult for a child always to be bigger and taller than playmates, and problems such as buying clothes or fitting into airline seats continue to be very real and distressing in adulthood. Counseling them about maintaining self-esteem and making the adjustments necessary to accommodate their larger-than-usual size is a nursing responsibility.

QSEN Checkpoint Question 48.1

QUALITY IMPROVEMENT

Sandy, Rob's 14-year-old girlfriend, often comes to the pediatric clinic with him. Sandy has hypopituitarism, and she and Rob first met at the endocrine clinic. Which of Sandy's statements would make the nurse believe she needs more education about her disorder? Select all that apply.

a. "Taking growth hormone subcutaneously is a bother; I hope I'll be changed to pills soon."
b. "I know I have to take growth hormone for life but it's okay; I'll be all right."
c. "Growth hormone makes me pee a lot; I asked for a locker near the bathroom."
d. "Growth hormone turned my cheeks red, but I cover it with makeup so it's okay."
e. "I'm determined not to let this take away my quality of life."

Look in Appendix A for the best answer and rationale.

DIABETES INSIPIDUS

Diabetes insipidus is a disease in which there is decreased release of ADH by the pituitary gland (Chamarthi, Morris, Kaiser, et al., 2013). This causes less reabsorption of fluid in the kidney tubules. Urine becomes extremely dilute, and a great deal of fluid is lost from the body. Diabetes insipidus may reflect an X-linked dominant trait, or it may be transmitted by an autosomal recessive gene. It may also result from a lesion, tumor, or injury to the posterior pituitary, or it may have an unknown cause. In a rare type of diabetes insipidus, pituitary function is adequate, but the kidneys' nephrons are not sensitive to ADH (a kidney-related etiology).

Assessment

The child with diabetes insipidus experiences excessive thirst (**polydipsia**) that is relieved only by drinking large amounts of water; there is accompanying polyuria. The specific gravity of the urine will be as low as 1.001 to 1.005 (normal values are more often 1.010 to 1.030). Urine output may reach 4 to 10 L in a 24-hour period (normal range, 1 to 2 L), depending on age.

Because so much fluid is lost, sodium becomes concentrated or hypernatremia occurs with symptoms of irritability, weakness, lethargy, fever, headache, and seizures. The signs and symptoms usually appear gradually. Parents may notice the polyuria first as bed-wetting in a toilet-trained child or weight loss because of the large loss of fluid. If the condition remains untreated, the child is in danger of losing such a large quantity of water that dehydration and death can result.

MRI, CT scanning, or an ultrasound study of the skull reveals whether a lesion or tumor is present. A further test is the administration of vasopressin (Pitressin) to rule out kidney disease. For this, after the child's urine output has been measured to establish a baseline, vasopressin is administered. The drug decreases the blood pressure, alerting the kidney to retain more fluid in order to maintain vascular pressure. If the fault that is causing the dilute urine is with the pituitary gland, not the kidneys, the child's urine output will decrease; if the fault is with the kidneys, urine will remain dilute and excessive in amount because the diseased kidneys cannot concentrate fluid.

Therapeutic Management

Surgery is the treatment of choice if a tumor is present. If the cause is idiopathic, the condition can be controlled by the administration of desmopressin (DDAVP), an arginine vasopressin. In an emergency, this drug can be given intravenously (IV). For long-term use, it is given intranasally or orally (Burke, Vendrame, Pileggi, et al., 2016). If desmopressin is given as an intranasal spray, this may cause nasal irritation; the route will not be effective if the child develops an upper respiratory tract infection with swollen mucous membranes. Caution children that they will notice an increasing urine output just before the next dose is due so they can arrange their day according to where bathrooms are located.

 Nursing Diagnoses and Related Interventions

Nursing Diagnosis: Risk for deficient fluid volume related to constant, excessive loss of fluid through urination

Outcome Evaluation: Child's blood pressure and pulse are within normal limits for age; specific gravity of urine is between 1.003 and 1.030; skin turgor is good; child states thirst is not excessive.

Teach About Long-Term Therapy. Be certain to explain the difference between diabetes insipidus and diabetes mellitus so the family is not confused about the differences in therapy. Help the family establish a routine to ensure the child receives adequate fluid to discourage a feeling of thirst and has access to bathroom facilities possibly more frequently than others. Review suggestions for long-term medicine administration with them (see Box 48.4).

Encourage Communication. Caution parents that when seeking any type of health care, they should always notify healthcare providers that the child has diabetes insipidus. For example, surgery poses particular dangers because of the fluid restrictions that accompany most procedures. Encourage children to wear a medical alert tag identifying them as having diabetes insipidus. Urge parents to inform school personnel that the child may need to use the bathroom frequently and to plan on frequent bathroom stops and adequate fluid intake on long trips or activity-filled days.

Concept Mastery Alert

Hyposecretion of antidiuretic hormone, as seen in diabetes insipidus, results in fluid loss. The symptoms—excessive thirst, frequent voiding, weakness, lethargy, and headache—are related to the loss of fluid.

SYNDROME OF INAPPROPRIATE ANTIDIURETIC HORMONE

The syndrome of inappropriate antidiuretic hormone (SIADH) is a rare condition in which there is overproduction of ADH by the posterior pituitary gland. This results in a decrease in urine production, which leads to water intoxication. As sodium levels fall in proportion to water, the child develops hyponatremia or a lowered sodium plasma level. SIADH can be caused by central nervous system infections such as bacterial meningitis (see Chapter 49), long-term positive pressure ventilation, or pituitary compression such as could occur from edema or a tumor.

Mild symptoms of hyponatremia are weight gain, concentrated urine (increased specific gravity), nausea, and vomiting. As the hyponatremia grows more severe, coma or seizures occur from brain edema.

Therapy consists of restriction of fluid and supplementation of sodium by IV fluid if needed. Demeclocycline (Declomycin), a tetracycline antibiotic that has the side effect of blocking the action of ADH in renal tubules and reducing resorption of water, may be prescribed (Miell, Dhanjal, & Jamookeeah, 2015).

The Thyroid Gland

The thyroid gland, located at the front of the neck, is responsible for controlling the rate of metabolism in the body through the hormones thyroxine (T_4) and triiodothyronine (T_3), which are produced by its follicular cells.

ASSESSMENT OF THYROID FUNCTION

Radioimmunoassay of T_4 and T_3 is a specific blood study to determine how much protein-bound iodine (PBI) is present in serum. Ask if a child has recently taken large amounts of cough medicine containing iodide or underwent a study using an iodine-based contrast medium (e.g., urography, bronchography) recently before the study or PBI levels may be abnormally elevated. The small amount of iodine ingested from iodized salt does not affect PBI levels.

Children who have low circulating albumin levels can have abnormally low PBI levels because iodine is carried bound to protein. Phenytoin (Dilantin), a common anticonvulsant medication prescribed for children with recurrent seizures, may displace T_4 from binding globulin and further contribute to low PBI levels.

Another test of thyroid function is a radioactive iodine uptake test. The child is given an oral dose of a solution containing radioactive iodine (^{123}I). The thyroid gland "traps" this iodine, and, 24 hours later, after the maximum amount has been trapped, the amount of radioactive iodine present can be determined. It is important in this type of test that the child swallows all the solution. In infants, the solution usually is given as a gavage feeding, so that accuracy of the dose can be ensured.

An uptake of less than 10% of the test dose suggests hypothyroidism. If the child vomits after ingesting the substance, this event should be recorded and called to the attention of the laboratory; it will obviously result in a lower uptake value because only a part of the actual dose will be available for uptake. Be certain that the child does not receive iodine or thyroid extract in any other form during the 24-hour test time because this would compete with uptake of the radioactive iodine and, again, produce a falsely low value.

Thyroid Gland Disorders

CONGENITAL HYPOTHYROIDISM

Thyroid hypofunction causes reduced production of both T_4 and T_3. Congenital hypofunction (reduced or absent function) occurs as a result of an absent or nonfunctioning thyroid gland in a newborn. There has been a large increase in the incidence of congenital hypothyroidism in the United States in the last two decades (Kollati, Ambati, Reddy, et al., 2017). Researchers are attempting to determine if this increase reflects a true increase in the disorder possibly due to environmental factors, due to better screening methods, or results from an increase in transient hypothyroidism (lessened thyroid function caused by a low iodine level in the mother or autoimmune antibodies that crossed the placenta). The increased incidence is associated with Whites, is evident more in infant girls than boys, and in newborns of either low birth weight or a birth weight over 4,500 g (LaFranchi, 2014).

Congenital hypothyroidism or an indication that the infant's thyroid is not functioning well may not be noticeable at birth because the mother's thyroid hormones (unless she ingested less than usual amounts of iodine) maintain adequate levels in the fetus during pregnancy. The symptoms of the disorder become apparent during the first 3 months of life in a formula-fed infant and at about 6 months in a breastfed infant. Because congenital hypothyroidism leads to both severe, progressive physical and cognitive challenges, early diagnosis is crucial.

Assessment

A screening test for hypothyroidism is mandatory at birth in the United States in all 50 states (using the same few drops of blood obtained for a phenylketonuria [PKU] blood spot test) (Kollati et al., 2017). If an infant should miss this screening procedure, an early sign that parents report is that their child sleeps excessively, but because the tongue is enlarged, they notice respiratory difficulty, noisy respirations, or obstruction. The child may also suck poorly because of sluggishness or choking from the enlarged tongue. The skin of the extremities usually feels cold, dry, and perhaps scaly, and the child does not perspire. Pulse, respiratory rate, and body temperature all

Figure 48.2 An infant with congenital hypothyroidism. Notice the short, thick neck and enlarged abdomen. (© David/NMSB/Custom Medical Stock Photograph.)

become subnormal. Prolonged jaundice may be present due to the immature liver's inability to conjugate bilirubin. Anemia may increase the child's lethargy and fatigue.

On a physical exam, the hair is brittle and dry, and the child's neck appears short and thick. The facial expression is dull and open mouthed because of the infant's attempts to breathe around the enlarged tongue. The extremities appear short and fat; as muscles become hypotonic, deep tendon reflexes decrease and the infant develops a floppy, rag-doll appearance. Generalized obesity usually occurs. Dentition will be delayed, or teeth may be defective when they do erupt.

The hypotonia affects the intestinal tract as well, so the infant develops chronic constipation; the abdomen enlarges because of intestinal distention and poor muscle tone (Fig. 48.2). Many infants have an umbilical hernia. Infants have low radioactive iodine uptake levels, low serum T_4 and T_3 levels, and elevated thyroid-stimulating factor. Blood lipids are increased. An X-ray may reveal delayed bone growth. An ultrasound reveals a small or absent thyroid gland. Untreated, the condition will result in severe irreversible cognitive deterioration or delay (Kollati et al., 2017).

Therapeutic Management

Transient hypothyroidism usually fades by 3 months' time. The treatment for true hypothyroidism is the oral administration of synthetic thyroid hormone (sodium levothyroxine). A small dose is given at first, and then the dose is gradually increased to therapeutic levels. The child needs to continue taking the synthetic thyroid hormone indefinitely to supplement that which the thyroid does not make. Supplemental vitamin D may also be given to prevent the development of rickets when, with the administration of thyroid hormone, rapid bone growth begins (Kim, 2016).

Further cognitive challenges can be prevented as soon as therapy is started, but any degree of impairment that was already present cannot be reversed, making the disorder one of the most preventable causes of mental development delay known (LaFranchi, 2014).

Be certain the parents know the rules for long-term medication administration with children, particularly the rule about not putting medicine in a large amount of food (T_4 tablets must be crushed and added to food or a small amount of formula or breast milk) and being certain they have medicine

during holidays or vacations. Periodic monitoring of T_4 and T_3 helps to ensure an appropriate medication dosage. If the dose of thyroid hormone is not adequate, the T_4 level will remain low and there will be few signs of clinical improvement. If the dose is too high, the T_4 level will rise and the child will show signs of hyperthyroidism: irritability; fever; rapid pulse; and perhaps vomiting, diarrhea, and weight loss.

ACQUIRED HYPOTHYROIDISM (HASHIMOTO THYROIDITIS)

Hashimoto disease is the most common form of acquired hypothyroidism in childhood; the age at onset is most often 10 to 11 years. There may be a family history of thyroid disease and it occurs more often in girls than in boys. The decrease in thyroid secretion is caused by the development of an autoimmune phenomenon that interferes with thyroid production.

Assessment

The excretion of thyroid-stimulating hormone (TSH) from the pituitary increases when thyroid hormone production decreases in an attempt by the pituitary gland to increase thyroid function. In response to the increased level of TSH, hypertrophy of the thyroid gland (goiter) can occur, and body growth is impaired by a lack of T_4, with prominent symptoms of obesity, lethargy, and delayed sexual development.

Antithyroid antibodies will be present in serum if the illness was caused by an autoimmune process. If the thyroid enlarges, it may become nodular as well. Although in childhood, a nodular thyroid is usually benign, an investigation into the possibility this could be a thyroid malignancy must be considered. For diagnosis, children are administered radioactive iodine. If the nodes are benign, there is generally a rapid uptake of radioactive iodine ("hot nodes"). If there is no uptake ("cold nodes"), carcinoma is a much more likely diagnosis (which is rare at this age).

Therapeutic Management

Treatment for acquired hypothyroidism is the administration of synthetic thyroid hormone (sodium levothyroxine), the same as for congenital hypothyroidism. With adequate dosage, the obesity diminishes and growth begins again. It is important that the disease be recognized as early as possible so there is time to stimulate growth before the epiphyseal lines close at puberty.

If acquired hypothyroidism exists in a woman during pregnancy, her infant can be born cognitively challenged because there was not enough iodine present for fetal growth. It is important, therefore, that girls with this syndrome be identified before they reach childbearing age.

What If . . . 48.1
Rob's mother tells a nurse that her sister (Rob's aunt) is 3 months pregnant and was prescribed levothyroxine (Synthroid) (synthetic thyroid hormone) but "forgets to take it most days and really cannot afford it." What should the nurse do?

HYPERTHYROIDISM (GRAVES DISEASE)

Hyperthyroidism is oversecretion of thyroid hormones by the thyroid gland. Neonatal Graves disease develops in the newborns of 1% to 2% of pregnant women who have the disease.

Like transient hypothyroidism, this usually resolves between 3 to 12 weeks of age with no long-term results as the maternal antibodies are cleared (Rivkees, 2014).

In older children, overactivity of the thyroid gland can occur from the glands being overstimulated by TSH from the pituitary gland due to a pituitary tumor. More frequently, however, hyperthyroidism in children is caused by an autoimmune reaction that results in overproduction of immunoglobulin G (IgG), which stimulates the thyroid gland to overproduce T_4. An exophthalmos-producing pituitary substance causes the prominent-appearing eyes that accompany hyperthyroidism in some children.

Assessment

Some children may have a genetic predisposition to development of the disorder, although Graves disease often follows a viral illness or a period of stress. With overproduction of T_3 and T_4, children gradually experience nervousness, tremors, loss of muscle strength, and easy fatigue. Their basal metabolic rate, blood pressure, and pulse all increase. Their skin feels moist, and they perspire freely. They always feel hungry and, although they eat constantly, do not gain weight and may even lose weight because of the increased basal metabolic rate. On X-ray, bone age will appear advanced beyond the chronologic age of the child. Unless the condition is treated, the child is not likely to reach usual adult height because epiphyseal lines of long bones will close before full height can be attained.

The thyroid gland, which usually is not prominent in children, appears as a swelling on the anterior neck as goiter develops. In a few children, the eye globes become prominent (exophthalmia), giving the child a wide-eyed, staring appearance. Laboratory tests show elevated T_4 and T_3 levels and increased radioactive iodine uptake. TSH is low or absent because the thyroid is being stimulated by antibodies, not by the pituitary gland. Ultrasound will reveal the enlarged thyroid.

Therapeutic Management

Therapy consists first of a course of a β-adrenergic blocking agent, such as propranolol, to decrease the antibody response. After this, the child is placed on an antithyroid drug, such as propylthiouracil (PTU) or methimazole (Tapazole), to suppress the formation of T_4. While the child is taking these drugs, the blood is monitored for leukopenia (decreased white blood cell count) and thrombocytopenia (decreased platelet count)—side effects of these drugs. If either of these results, the drug is discontinued until the white blood cell or platelet count returns to normal, so the child does not develop an infection or experience spontaneous bleeding.

Because the thyroid stores considerable thyroid hormone that must be used up first before T_4 levels decline, it takes about 2 weeks for these drugs to have an effect. The child needs to continue to take the drug for 2 to 3 years before the condition "burns itself out." The exophthalmos may not recede, but it will not become worse once therapy is instituted.

If the child has a toxic reaction to medical management (severely lowered white blood cell count or platelet count) or is noncompliant about taking the medicine, radioiodine ablative therapy with ^{131}I or thyroid surgery to reduce the size of the thyroid gland can be accomplished. This has long-term effects, however, because after both radioiodine ablative therapy and thyroidectomy, supplemental thyroid hormone

therapy may need to be taken indefinitely because the gland is no longer able to produce an adequate amount (Léger & Carel, 2013). It is important that adolescent girls be carefully regulated before they consider childbearing because hyperthyroidism during pregnancy can lead to neonatal hyperthyroidism in a fetus.

 Nursing Diagnoses and Related Interventions

Nursing Diagnosis: Situational low self-esteem related to lack of coordination and presence of prominent goiter or exophthalmia

Outcome Evaluation: Child states positive traits about self and identifies friends and activities enjoyed; is not the victim of bullying because of unusual appearance.

Hyperthyroidism begins gradually and so may become fairly involved before it is detected. Suspect children at puberty of having hyperthyroidism if they are losing weight or have behavior problems in school, which occur because of the hand or tongue tremors that make it hard for them to write or speak and the nervousness that makes them unable to sit still during class.

Offer parents support to supervise medication administration so they can be certain the child takes the prescribed medicine every day. Caution children not to stop taking the medicine abruptly, or a thyroxine crisis (sudden onset of extreme symptoms of hyperthyroidism) can occur. Parents may ask if their child can have surgery as a cure so that long-term administration of medicine will not be required. Help them understand that surgery may not dispel the need for medication; if a large portion of the thyroid gland is removed, it may be necessary for their child to take medicine indefinitely to make up for the missing gland. In any event, it is preferable to try a course of medical management before resorting to surgery.

QSEN Checkpoint Question 48.2

PATIENT-CENTERED CARE

Rob has a cousin who has developed hyperthyroidism with puberty. Which of the effects of this health problem might a school nurse need to support Rob's cousin in dealing with?
a. Slow, lethargic movements
b. Swollen, protuberant abdomen
c. Jittery, nervous mannerisms
d. Reduced intellectual processing

Look in Appendix A for the best answer and rationale.

The Adrenal Gland

The two adrenal glands are located retroperitoneally, just above the kidneys. They are made up of two distinct divisions; together, these divisions protect the body against acute and chronic forms of stress. Three hormones—cortisol (a glucocorticoid responsible for glucose and protein metabolism and preventing inflammation), androgen (a steroid hormone responsible for muscle development), and aldosterone (a mineralocorticoid hormone necessary for sodium and fluid balance) are important in childhood illnesses.

Adrenal Gland Disorders

Disorders of the adrenal glands cause either hypofunction, which can lead to acute or chronic production of necessary hormones, or hyperfunction (overactivity), which most often leads to overproduction of androgen or cortisol.

ACUTE ADRENOCORTICAL INSUFFICIENCY

Insufficiency (hypofunction) of the adrenal gland can occur in either an acute or chronic form. In either type, the function of the entire gland suddenly becomes nonproductive. Usually, this occurs following a severe overwhelming body infection such as meningococcemia. It also can occur when corticosteroid therapy such as prednisone, which has been maintained at high levels for a long period, is abruptly stopped and the gland does not return to usual function.

Assessment

With acute adrenocortical insufficiency, the child's blood pressure drops to extremely low levels, the child appears ashen gray, and the pulse will be weak. Temperature gradually becomes elevated; dehydration and **hypoglycemia** (an abnormally low concentration of blood glucose) become marked because cortisol is no longer present to regulate this. As sodium and chloride blood levels fall from a lack of aldosterone production, the potassium level becomes elevated due to the usual inverse relationship between sodium and potassium values. The child appears prostrate and seizures may occur. Without treatment, death can occur abruptly (Agarwal, Singh, Chowdhury, et al., 2017; Korzeniewski, Grigorescu, Kleyn, et al., 2012).

Therapeutic Management

Acute adrenocortical insufficiency is a medical emergency. Treatment involves the immediate replacement of cortisol (with IV hydrocortisone sodium succinate [Solu-Cortef]); the administration of deoxycorticosterone acetate (DOCA), the synthetic equivalent of aldosterone; and IV 5% glucose in normal saline solution to restore blood pressure, sodium, and blood glucose levels. A vasoconstrictor may be necessary to elevate the blood pressure.

Although acute adrenal insufficiency is seen less often now than in the past because of the availability of antibiotics that quickly halt the course of infectious disease because more conditions are being treated with corticosteroids than ever before, the chance the syndrome will occur from sudden withdrawal of high-dose steroids is actually increasing.

CONGENITAL ADRENAL HYPERPLASIA

Congenital adrenal hyperplasia is a syndrome that is inherited as an autosomal recessive trait and which causes the adrenal glands to not be able to synthesize cortisol. Because the adrenal gland is unable to produce cortisol, the level

of adrenocorticotropic hormone (ACTH) secreted by the pituitary increases in an attempt to stimulate the gland to increase function. Although the adrenals enlarge (hyperplasia) under the effect of ACTH, they still cannot produce cortisol; instead, they overproduce androgen.

Assessment

The excessive androgen production during intrauterine life causes the genital organs in a male fetus to "overgrow," or increase in size; it masculinizes a female fetus (i.e., the clitoris is so enlarged that it appears to be a penis; if the labia are fused, she appears to be a boy with undescended testes and hypospadias (Fig. 48.3) (Graber & Rapaport, 2012). Other female organs appear normal, although a sinus between the urethra and vagina may be present (see the discussion of ambiguous genitalia in Chapter 47). If the condition is not recognized at birth and the child remains untreated, bone age will advance so the epiphyseal lines of the long bones close early, preventing the child from reaching a usual adult height; pubic and axillary hair, acne, and a deep masculine voice will appear precociously. At puberty, there will be no breast development or menstruation.

By 3 or 4 years of age, untreated boys develop acne and a deep, mature voice; pubic hair and still greater enlargement of the penis, scrotum, and prostate occur. In contrast, the testes do not enlarge and so appear small in relation to the size of the penis. Spermatogenesis does not occur with puberty, leaving the child infertile.

It is possible to identify the fetus with congenital adrenogenital hyperplasia as early as 6 to 8 weeks of pregnancy by means of maternal serum analysis and at 15 weeks by amniocentesis (see Chapter 9). Although controversial, treatment of a mother with dexamethasone (a corticosteroid), which crosses the placenta to the fetus, can prevent masculinization in the fetus for the remainder of the pregnancy. The newborn will then need hydrocortisone administration after birth for continuing therapy.

The condition is usually diagnosed not during pregnancy, however, but in infancy by serum analysis, which shows the increased level of androgen. By determining the levels of other adrenal hormones, the exact degree of the metabolic defect in production of cortisol can be measured.

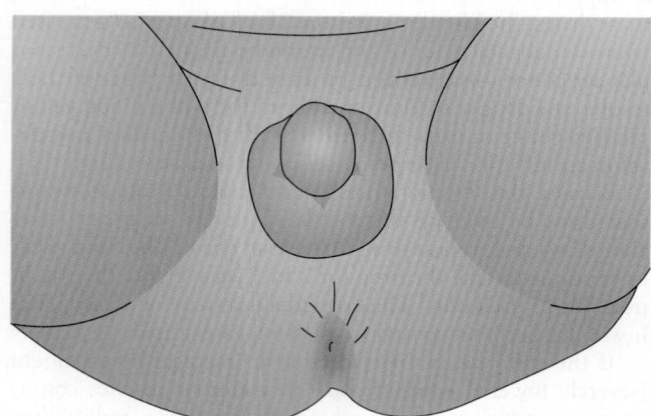

Figure 48.3 A female infant with congenital adrenogenital hyperplasia. Note the fused labia and abnormally enlarged clitoris.

Therapeutic Management

The ultimate goal of therapy is to replace the cortisol that is missing, thereby suppressing ACTH concentrations and normalizing adrenal size and androgen production, a goal that seems quite simple but is actually very difficult to achieve (Léger & Carel, 2013). For therapy, both male and female infants are given a corticosteroid agent, such as oral hydrocortisone, to replace what they cannot produce naturally. When a corticosteroid is given to the child in this way, stimulation by ACTH decreases, the production of androgen returns to normal limits, and no further masculinization occurs. Because corticosteroid therapy needs to continue indefinitely, the child needs periodic analysis of serum cortisol levels and growth measurements to estimate the effectiveness of the therapy. Children may need to have a routine dose increased when they are undergoing periods of stress, such as during surgery or infection. They may need support throughout life if their body image is distorted because of body changes at birth.

Nursing Diagnoses and Related Interventions

Nursing Diagnosis: Situational low self-esteem related to genital formation at variance with true gender

Outcome Evaluation: Child identifies positive traits about self and describes activities enjoyed with peers; expresses satisfaction with gender identity; does not report bullying from peers.

All newborns need an extensive physical examination at birth so chromosomal girls with this syndrome are not wrongly identified as male. It is sometimes recommended to parents that a girl's enlarged clitoris be reduced by plastic surgery in infancy. This treatment is controversial, however, because even with finer surgical techniques, clitoral reduction can also result in reduced clitoral sensation. A girl should have the right to make this decision for herself, however, so, as a rule, surgery is delayed until the girl is old enough to understand what will be the implication of not having clitoral sensation on her sexual enjoyment (Michala, Liao, Wood, et al., 2014).

Parents of females with congenital adrenogenital hyperplasia may need a great deal of support during the first few days of their child's life because they may voice that their child is imperfect in an embarrassing, hard-to-explain way. When they are the results of the chromosome analysis, parents may react with grief for the loss of the son they first thought had been born to them. Parents need support from healthcare personnel who recognize that the child is simply lacking the ability to produce cortisol but is complete in every other way.

SALT-LOSING FORM OF CONGENITAL ADRENOGENITAL HYPERPLASIA

If there is a complete blockage of cortisol formation, aldosterone production will also be deficient. Without adequate aldosterone, salt is not retained by the body, so fluid is not retained. Almost immediately after birth, affected infants begin to have vomiting, diarrhea, anorexia, loss of weight,

and extreme dehydration (Mak, Lee, Chan, et al., 2013). If these symptoms remain untreated, the extreme loss of salt and fluid can lead to collapse and death as early as 48 to 72 hours after birth.

About one third of children with congenital adrenogenital hyperplasia are affected by this complete deficiency. Because boys with this syndrome appear normal at birth, the symptoms may be incorrectly diagnosed as infection or as failure to thrive. In girls, because of the ambiguous genitalia, the correct diagnosis can be made more easily.

Assessment

The salt-losing form must be detected before an infant reaches an irreversible point of salt depletion. (The reason newborns are weighed at birth and again at 24 hours is to detect this condition.) Weighing infants at each well-child health checkup is also important because, in boys, the inability to gain back their birth weight may be the first sign of the syndrome.

Therapeutic Management

Children with this form of congenital adrenogenital hyperplasia need to be supplemented with hydrocortisone, an increased salt intake, and DOCA, a synthetic aldosterone, in order to maintain a balance of fluid and electrolytes. A long-acting form of DOCA can be given once a month intramuscularly. Capsules of DOCA can also be implanted subcutaneously (SC) as another form of long-acting therapy. As the child grows older, fludrocortisone (Florinef), a mineralocorticoid, may be given orally to aid salt retention.

Nursing Diagnoses and Related Interventions

Nursing Diagnosis: Risk for deficient fluid volume related to loss of body fluid

Outcome Evaluation: Child's skin turgor remains good; specific gravity of urine is between 1.003 and 1.030.

Teach parents about the body's critical need to balance aldosterone, salt, and water, so they understand the drastic consequences if their child skips a dose of medication. Otherwise, they may underestimate that salt, although an "extra" in their own diet, is as vital to their child's intake as digitalis is in heart disease or insulin is in diabetes. Help them to set up a schedule as necessary for measuring their child's weight, giving medication, or measuring urine output.

CUSHING SYNDROME

Cushing syndrome is caused by overproduction of the adrenal hormone cortisol; this usually results from increased ACTH production due to either a pituitary or adrenal cortex tumor. The peak age of occurrence is 6 or 7 years, but the syndrome can occur as early as infancy. The inappropriate use of high-potency steroid creams for diaper dermatitis may be a possible cause (Smy, Shaw, Smith, et al., 2015). The overproduction of cortisol results in increased glucose production; this causes fat to accumulate on the cheeks, chin, and trunk, causing a moon-faced, stocky appearance. Cortisol is catabolic, so protein wasting also occurs. This leads to muscle wasting, making the extremities appear thin in contrast to the trunk, and loss of calcium in bones (osteoporosis). Cortisol also suppresses the immune system, so humoral immunity is decreased, leaving children susceptible to infections. Additionally, it causes vasoconstriction, so extreme hypertension may occur.

Yet, other effects are hyperpigmentation (the child's face appears unusually red, especially the cheeks), which occurs from the melanin-stimulating properties of ACTH; abnormal masculinization or feminization, which occurs from overproduction of androgen or estrogen; and poor wound healing, which results from reduced protein regulation. Purple striae resulting from collagen deficit appear on the child's hips, abdomen, and thighs, similar to those seen in pregnancy (Fig. 48.4).

Polyuria begins to develop as the body tries to excrete increased glucose levels. Growth ceases, and, if the condition is not reversed before the epiphyseal lines close, short stature will result.

Children who receive high doses of synthetic corticosteroids, such as prednisone, over a long period may develop the same symptoms as those observed in Cushing syndrome (termed a *cushingoid appearance*). Children who are obese may have elevated levels of plasma corticosteroids and so be wrongly diagnosed as having Cushing syndrome. However, with this, the child's growth is not impaired, so these elevated levels of corticosteroids are secondary to the obesity, not the cause.

Assessment

The serum of children with Cushing syndrome reveals an elevated plasma cortisol and increased urinary free-cortisol levels. A dexamethasone suppression test may be administered for diagnosis. For this test, a child is administered a dose of dexamethasone (a glucocorticoid); if the child has the syndrome, the plasma level of adrenal cortisol will fall. It will not fall in children with adrenocortical tumors because the tumor continues to stimulate the adrenal glands to oversecretion. If cosyntropin (Cortrosyn), a synthetic corticotropin, or ACTH is administered, plasma cortisol levels will normally rise. In children with an adrenal tumor, the gland is already functioning at full capacity, so no cortisol elevation occurs. A CT scan or ultrasound reveals the enlarged adrenal or pituitary gland, confirming the diagnosis.

Therapeutic Management

Treatment of Cushing syndrome is the surgical removal of the causative tumor. The prognosis depends on whether the tumor is benign or malignant because a carcinoma of this type tends to metastasize rapidly. If a major part of the adrenal glands are surgically removed, the child will need replacement cortisol therapy indefinitely.

If a major portion of the pituitary gland is removed because the problem was overproduction of ACTH, the replacement of all pituitary hormones may be necessary. After adrenal surgery, observe the child carefully for signs of shock: Without epinephrine also produced by the gland, the body's ability to maintain blood pressure is severely compromised, and severe hypotension can result.

QSEN Checkpoint Question 48.3

INFORMATICS

Rob has his adrenal gland function assessed through diagnostic testing. What is the effect on a child when sufficient aldosterone cannot be produced?
   a. Substantially fewer red blood cells are produced.
   b. There is an overall decreased urine output.
   c. An excessive amount of sodium is lost in urine.
   d. The child's growth rate increases abnormally.

Look in Appendix A for the best answer and rationale.

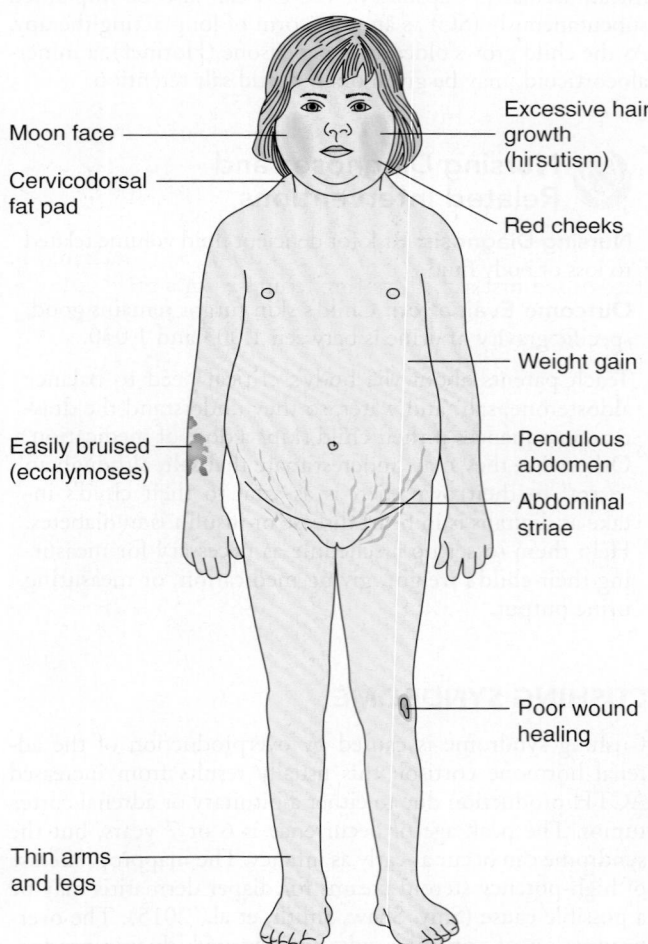

Figure 48.4 Signs and symptoms of Cushing syndrome.

Moon face
Cervicodorsal fat pad
Easily bruised (ecchymoses)
Thin arms and legs
Excessive hair growth (hirsutism)
Red cheeks
Weight gain
Pendulous abdomen
Abdominal striae
Poor wound healing

The Pancreas

The pancreas is a unique organ in that it has both endocrine (ductless) and exocrine (with duct) types of tissue. The *islets of Langerhans* form the endocrine portion, alpha islet cells have the responsibility to secrete glucagon, and beta islet cells secrete insulin.

Insulin is essential for carbohydrate metabolism and is also important in the metabolism of both fats and protein. It is formed from amino acids at a rate between 35 and 50 units per day in adults and proportionately less in children. When serum glucose that passes through the pancreas exceeds 100 mg/dl, beta cells immediately begin insulin production. When serum glucose levels are low, production decreases.

Insulin production is also stimulated by gastrin, a gastrointestinal hormone that rises when the stomach is full as well as the levels of glucagon, cortisol, GH, progesterone, and estrogen. Increasing levels of epinephrine or norepinephrine inhibit the secretion of insulin in order to preserve glucose for "flight or fight."

The principal childhood disorders associated with pancreatic dysfunction are type 1 and type 2 diabetes mellitus and cystic fibrosis. Because the nursing care for children with cystic fibrosis includes many respiratory care procedures, it is discussed in Chapter 40.

TYPE 1 DIABETES MELLITUS

Type 1 diabetes mellitus is a disorder that involves an absolute or relative deficiency of insulin, which is in contrast to type 2, where insulin production is only reduced (Table 48.2). Type 1 diabetes is equal in incidence in boys and girls and affects approximately 1 of every 500 children and adolescents in the United States (Sherr & Weinzimer, 2012).

Etiology

The disease apparently results from immunologic damage to islet cells in susceptible individuals. Why autoimmune destruction of islet cells occurs is unknown, but children with the disorder have a high frequency of certain human leukocyte antigens (HLAs), particularly HLA-DR3 and HLA-DR4, located on chromosome 6, that may lead to susceptibility. If one child in a family has diabetes, the chance that a sibling will also develop the illness is higher than in other families because siblings also tend to have one of the specific HLA that are associated with the disease.

Disease Process

Insulin can be thought of as a compound that opens the doors to body cells, allowing them to admit glucose, which is needed for functioning. It does not play a major role in glucose transport into the brain, erythrocytes, leukocytes, intestinal mucosa, or kidney epithelium. These cells, therefore, can survive insulin deficiency but not glucose deficiency.

If glucose is unable to enter body cells because of a lack of insulin, it builds up in the bloodstream (**hyperglycemia**). As soon as the kidneys detect hyperglycemia (greater than the renal threshold of about 160 mg/dl), the kidneys attempt to lower it to normal levels by excreting excess glucose into the urine, causing **glycosuria**, accompanied by a large loss of body fluid (polyuria). Excess fluid loss, in turn, triggers the thirst response (polydipsia), producing the three cardinal symptoms of diabetes: polyuria, polydipsia, and hyperglycemia.

Because body cells are unable to use glucose but still need a source of energy, the body begins to break down protein and fat. If large amounts of fat are metabolized this way, weight loss occurs and ketone bodies, the acid end product of fat breakdown, begin to accumulate in the bloodstream (creating high serum cholesterol levels and ketoacidosis) and spill into the urine as ketones. Potassium and phosphate, attempting to serve as buffers, pass from body cells into the bloodstream. From there, they are evacuated, causing a loss of these important electrolytes.

Untreated diabetic children, therefore, lose weight, are acidotic due to the buildup of ketone bodies in their blood, are dehydrated because of the loss of water, and experience an electrolyte imbalance because of the loss of potassium and phosphate in urine. Because large amounts of protein and fat are being used for energy instead of glucose, children lack the necessary components for growth; they therefore remain short in stature and underweight.

Assessment

Although children may be prediabetic for some time, the onset of symptoms in childhood is usually abrupt. Parents notice increased thirst and increased urination (which may be recognized first as bed-wetting [enuresis] in a previously toilet-trained child). The dehydration may cause constipation.

TABLE 48.2 COMPARISON OF TYPE 1 AND TYPE 2 DIABETES

Assessment	Type 1	Type 2
Age at onset	5–7 years or at puberty	40–65 years (may occur in adolescents as maturity-onset diabetes of youth [MODY])
Type of onset	Abrupt	Gradual
Weight changes	Marked weight loss often initial sign	Associated with obesity
Other symptoms	Polydipsia and polyphagia	Polydipsia
	Polyuria (often begins as bed-wetting)	Polyuria
	Fatigue (marks fall in school)	Fatigue
	Blurred vision (marks fall in school)	Blurred vision
	Mood changes (may cause behavior problems in school)	Mood changes
Therapy	Hypoglycemia agents never effective; insulin required	Diet, oral hypoglycemic agents, or insulin
	No dietary foods used; should count carbohydrates plus evaluate blood glucose levels to help determine insulin dosage.	Nutrition concentrates on no excess weight gain and balanced intake of carbohydrates, protein, and fat
	Commonsense foot care for growing children	Meticulous skin and foot care necessary
Period of remission	Period of remission for 1–12 months ("honeymoon period") generally after initial diagnosis	Not demonstrable

TABLE 48.3 ACCEPTABLE BLOOD GLUCOSE RANGES FOR CHILDREN WITH TYPE 1 DIABETES

Timing	Value (mg/dl)
Before a meal	70–110
1 hr after a meal	90–180
2 hr after a meal	80–150
Between 2 AM and 4 AM	70–120

Laboratory Studies

In some children, diabetes is detected at a routine health screening. For others, although the disease has been progressing internally for some time, outward symptoms have such an abrupt onset that the child is in a coma from acidosis and hyperglycemia by the time it is detected. Laboratory studies usually show a random plasma glucose level greater than 200 mg/dl (normal range, 70 to 110 mg/dl fasting; 90 to 180 mg/dl not fasting) and significant glycosuria (Table 48.3).

Two diagnostic tests, the fasting blood glucose test and the random blood glucose test, are used to confirm diabetes. A diagnosis of diabetes is established if one of the following three criteria is present on two separate occasions:

- Symptoms of diabetes plus a random blood glucose level greater than 200 mg/dl
- A fasting blood glucose level greater than 126 mg/dl
- A 2-hour plasma glucose level greater than 200 mg/dl during a 75-g oral glucose tolerance test (GTT)

Typically, a GTT involves the oral ingestion of a concentrated glucose solution followed by blood glucose levels drawn at fasting (baseline), after 1 hour, and after 2 hours. The test is difficult for children to undergo because it requires them to fast for 8 hours, drink an overly sweet solution, and submit to painful, intrusive procedures (routine application of lidocaine/prilocaine [EMLA] cream to finger stick or venipuncture sites and use of intermittent infusion devices greatly reduces this problem). Do not take blood for glucose analysis from functioning IV tubing to try to help with pain because the glucose in the IV solution will cause the serum reading to be abnormally high.

Other Diagnostic Tests

If diabetes is detected, the diagnostic workup also usually includes an analysis of blood samples for pH, partial pressure of carbon dioxide (PCO_2), sodium, and potassium levels; a white blood cell count; and a glycosylated hemoglobin (HbA1c) evaluation. Normally, the hemoglobin in red blood cells carry only a trace of glucose. If serum glucose is excessive, however, excess glucose attaches itself to hemoglobin molecules, creating HbA1c. In nondiabetic children, the usual HbA1c value is 1.8 to 4.0. A value greater than 6.0 reflects an excessive level of serum glucose. Measuring HbA1c has advantages because it not only provides information on what is the child's present serum glucose level but what the serum glucose levels have been during the preceding 3 to 4 months (red blood cells have a life span of 120 days).

If the potassium level of the blood is low, a child may need an electrocardiogram to observe for T-wave abnormalities, the mark of potassium deficiency. The white blood cell count of a child with diabetes may be elevated even though no infection is present, apparently as a response to the ketoacidosis.

The presence of infection must always be suspected, however, because it is often a precipitant to a diabetic crisis. For this reason, nose and throat cultures may be obtained as well.

Therapeutic Management

Therapy for children with type 1 diabetes involves five measures: insulin administration, regulation of nutrition and exercise, stress management, and blood glucose and urine ketone monitoring. The standard of care in the United States regarding a child with newly diagnosed diabetes involves a hospital admission of approximately 3 days, which includes extensive education involving caretakers and the child (Schmidt, Bernaix, Chiappetta, et al., 2012).

The Initial Regulation of Insulin

When children are first diagnosed with diabetes, they are usually hyperglycemic and perhaps ketoacidotic. To correct the metabolic imbalance, they are given insulin administered IV at a dose of 0.1 to 0.2 units per kilogram of body weight per hour. This initial IV infusion of insulin is then gradually reduced once the blood glucose level is lower than 200 mg/dl. Ideally, within 12 hours, the acidosis is considerably less than when a child was admitted to the hospital, and the serum glucose level is near the normal range. The insulin given for emergency replacement this way is regular (short-acting) insulin such as Humulin-R because this is the form that takes effect most quickly.

It may seem that in a child with diabetes in a state of acidosis, the administration of glucose would not be warranted. Because the child is being given insulin, however, body cells soon become ready to use glucose, so they require, incorporate, and use available glucose quickly. If more glucose is not provided, cells are forced to continue to break down fats and protein, and the acidosis can increase, not decrease. Glucose, therefore, may be added to the infusion.

After 24 hours, as the child's serum glucose returns to normal, oral feedings may replace the IV route. Further management in the days after this first crucial 24-hour period is based on serum glucose determinations. A child may remain on regular insulin given SC alone (given three or four times a day) for the first 1 or 2 days. Typically, intermediate-acting insulin is then added as soon as oral fluids are taken, usually on the second day of therapy.

Insulin Administration

Types of insulin vary as to their time of onset, peak action, and duration of action (Table 48.4). Children can be regulated on a variety of insulin programs, but typically receive a combined insulin dose of 0.4 to 0.7 units per kilogram of body weight daily in two divided doses (one before breakfast and one before dinner); adolescents may need as much as 1.2 units per kilogram daily divided into the two doses. The most common mixture of insulin used with children is a combination of an intermediate-acting insulin and a regular insulin, usually in a 2:1 ratio or 0.75 units of the intermediate-acting insulin to 0.33 units regular insulin, and given in the same syringe, although this prescription varies for individual children. The morning dose is two thirds of the total daily dose; the evening dose is the remaining one third.

The advantage of using two different types of insulin is that the peak effects occur at different times. Because the peak time of short-acting insulins is 3 to 4 hours, the child

TABLE 48.4 COMMON TYPES OF HUMAN INSULIN

Preparation	Onset	Peak Effect	Duration of Effect (hr)
Lispro (Humalog)	Immediate	30 min–1 hr	3–4
Aspart	15 min	30–40 min	3–5
Regular (Humulin-R)	0.5–1.0 hr	2–4 hr	5–7
Lantus	1 hr	5 hr	24
Humulin-N	1–2 hr	4–12 hr	24+
Humulin-L	1–3 hr	6–14 hr	24+
Humulin-U	6 hr	16–18 hr	36+

From Karch, A. M. (2013). *2013 Lippincott's nursing drug guide.* Philadelphia, PA: Lippincott Williams & Wilkins.

who takes insulin before breakfast will notice a maximum effect between 10 AM and 12 noon. The peak effect period of the intermediate-acting insulin is 8 to 14 hours, or late afternoon, just before dinner. These are important times to remember because these are the times when a child is most apt to experience symptoms of hypoglycemia.

Some children require a program of insulin therapy that includes three or even four injections daily in order to prevent hyperglycemia. Although these regimens are not popular with children, multiple injections allow for greater variation in activity and calorie consumption.

Part of the education of parents is to allow them to vary their child's insulin doses based on an insulin algorithm or protocol influenced by the child's level of activity and the size of meals consumed for that day (referred to as "thinking scales"). The time between the insulin injection and a meal is known as "lag time." If a child's premeal blood glucose level is above a target range, parents learn that increasing the lag time or delaying the meal will help prevent hyperglycemia. If the blood glucose is low at a premeal test, decreasing the lag time could help prevent hypoglycemia. If it is anticipated that the child will eat an unusually large meal such as at a special birthday dinner, parents can increase the size of the premeal regular insulin injection. If the child is to participate in a strenuous sport in the afternoon that will use glucose, the regular insulin injection can be decreased. Insulin glargine injection (Lantus) is a new long-acting insulin that is supplied in an injectable pen and lasts 24 hours. A disadvantage of this insulin is its pH, which is so low it cannot be mixed in a syringe with other insulins. In some children, glucose levels can be regulated on insulin glargine injection (Lantus) plus three doses of regular insulin before meals.

Injection Technique

Teach parents that when insulins are mixed in one syringe, the regular or short-acting insulin should be drawn into the syringe first. Then, if mixing accidentally occurs in the bottle, the time of effectiveness of the short-acting insulin (which needs to be kept short-acting for emergency treatment) will not be lengthened by the addition of the intermediate-acting insulin.

Insulin is always injected SC except in emergencies, when half the required dose may be given IV. Subcutaneous tissue injection sites used most frequently in children include those of the upper outer arms and the outer aspects of the

thighs (Fig. 48.5). The abdominal subcutaneous tissue injection sites commonly used in adults can be adequate sites, but most children dislike this site because abdominal skin is tender. Encourage children or parents to rotate sites in a pattern based on their planned activity. Absorption, for example, is increased if the muscles under the injection site are exercised, so it is best to choose sites that will not be exercised soon after the injection. If a child will be jogging after an injection, for example, the thigh probably should not be used. Similarly, if the child will be playing tennis, the injection probably should not be given in the dominant arm.

Work out a plan of rotation with children so that everyone who will be giving injections knows what injection site should be used next. In the hospital, record the injection site in the child's record or nursing plan, so each nurse can check it before an injection and not repeat an injection site. This is less of a problem now that synthetic human insulin is used, but if the same injection site is used repeatedly, a great deal of subcutaneous atrophy (lipodystrophy) can occur, causing deep pockmarks.

Children quickly learn that if they continuously give injections in the same site, scar tissue (lipohypertrophy) forms there, and no pain will be felt on injection (a situation sometimes called subcutaneous insulin resistance syndrome [SIRS]). This is a dangerous practice, however, because as lipohypertrophy occurs, insulin no longer absorbs well from the site. To be effective, the dose has to be increased beyond what the child actually needs for glucose metabolism because a portion of each dose is "locked" in the tissue. Should the child then inject this larger dose of insulin into a new site, there is a potential for overdose (which would cause hypoglycemia).

Figure 48.5 According to the American Diabetes Association, insulin injection sites in children and adults are the upper outer portions of the arms; the thighs, 4 in. below the hip and 4 in. above the knee (adjusted proportionally for children); and the abdominal area just above and just below the waist. The navel and a circular area just around it are excluded as injection sites. In some children, the abdominal area may not be an appropriate injection site.

Although parents should keep additional bottles of insulin in the refrigerator to increase the insulin's shelf life, insulin should be administered at room temperature because this diminishes subcutaneous atrophy and ensures peak effectiveness.

Because a short needle (less than 0.4 in.) is used, insulin can be injected at a 90-degree angle (Fig. 48.6). Although this is not a usual subcutaneous injection technique, because the needle is so short, the insulin will be deposited into the subcutaneous tissue. This technique is easier for children to learn because it takes less coordination to administer an injection at a 90-degree angle than at a 45-degree subcutaneous angle. Automatic injection devices are available, such as pens and jet injectors, which are easy for children to use, come with prepared doses, promote early independence, and can be given with the 90-degree technique (Fig. 48.7).

Insulin Pumps

An insulin pump is an automatic device approximately the size of an iPhone. It delivers insulin at a constant rate, so it regulates serum glucose levels better than periodic injections (Buchko, Artz, Dayhoff, et al., 2012). To use a pump, a syringe of regular insulin is placed in the pump chamber; a length of thin polyethylene tubing leads to the child's abdomen, where it is implanted into the subcutaneous tissue of the abdomen by a small-gauge needle. Women who develop gestational diabetes also use insulin pumps; therefore, these are illustrated and the care is described in Chapter 20. Most children adjust well to pump therapy and prefer it to daily injections.

Inhalation Insulin

Inhalation insulin is not available as yet but may be in the future; production of it is in experimental trials. Difficulties with development are constructing an accurate delivery system and determining how the development of a cold or allergies that cause edema of the nasal membrane will affect drug absorption (Boss, Petrucci, & Lorber, 2012).

Nutrition

In order to know how much insulin to give before a meal, parents need to learn to count the total carbohydrate amount in food by carefully reading food labels. An insulin-to-carbohydrate ratio is then calculated individually for each child depending on age and activity to guide insulin administration. For example, if a child is prescribed an insulin-to-carbohydrate ratio of 1 unit of insulin to each 10 g of carbohydrates and the meal the child will be served contains 50 g carbohydrates, the parent would administer 5 units of regular insulin before the meal.

An overall meal pattern should include three spaced meals that are high in fiber plus a snack in the midmorning, midafternoon, and evening to keep carbohydrate amounts as level as possible during the day. Most parents need to meet with a nutritionist to discuss what a "meal high in fiber" means, how to become adept at carbohydrate counting, and what meals are best to serve to their age child. General rules are shown in Box 48.7.

Self-Monitoring of Blood Glucose

Children as young as early school age can learn the techniques of finger puncture and reading a computerized monitor. Using a spring-loaded injection pen helps minimize pain; an automatic readout monitor simplifies the procedure (Fig. 48.8). Children are adolescents, however, before they can be counted on to independently monitor their serum glucose levels on a daily basis.

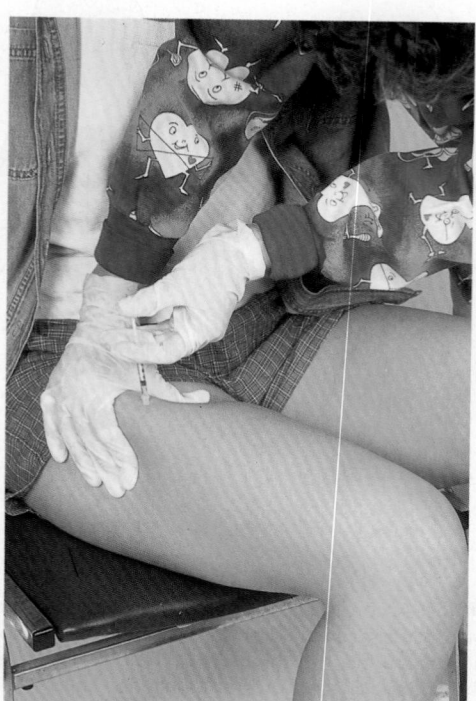

Figure 48.6 Insulin is usually injected at a 90-degree angle with a short needle. This angle places the insulin in the subcutaneous space. (© Lesha Photography.)

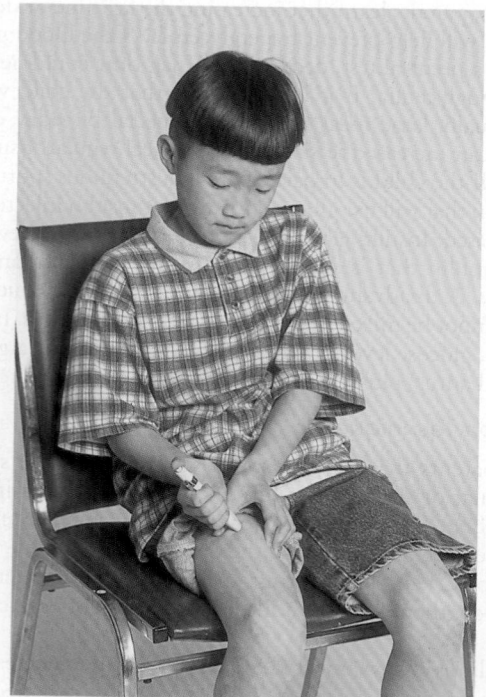

Figure 48.7 The injection of insulin by an automatic device. (© Lesha Photography.)

BOX 48.7

Nursing Care Planning Based on Family Teaching

NUTRITIONAL GUIDELINES FOR CHILDREN WITH TYPE 1 DIABETES

Q. Rob's mother is concerned that Rob, as an adolescent, doesn't eat well. She asks you, "How can we make sure our child, who has diabetes, gets adequate nutrition?"

A. Here are some nutritional guidelines to help you:

- Be certain you understand your child's insulin-to-carbohydrate ratio and how to use this to plan meals. As a rule, foods high in carbohydrates are fruit and vegetables, "starchy foods" such as bread or pasta, milk and yogurt, and "sugary" foods such as candy bars or cake.
- Be aware of food portions. The total carbohydrate on a package of pasta refers to what one serving of pasta will contain, not the whole box of pasta.
- Provide three meals throughout the day, plus three snacks. A total daily caloric intake divided to provide 20% as breakfast, 20% as lunch, 30% as dinner, and 10% as morning, afternoon, and evening snacks help distribute carbohydrates throughout the day.
- Do not use dietetic food. This food is expensive and not necessary.
- Urge your child not to omit meals. Getting him to eat at every meal calls for creative planning so he likes the foods served and eats readily.
- Maintain a positive outlook by stressing the foods your child is allowed to eat, not those he should avoid.
- Steer clear of concentrated carbohydrate sources, such as candy bars, and be sure to include foods with adequate fiber, such as broccoli, because fiber helps prevent hyperglycemia.
- Keep complex carbohydrates available to be eaten before exercise, such as swimming or a softball game, to provide a sustained carbohydrate energy source to prevent hypoglycemia.
- Teach children about carbohydrate counting as early as possible so they can wisely select what to eat at school or at a friend's home and can begin independent self-care.

Urine Testing

Urine testing is not used routinely but is used to test for ketonuria if the child develops a gastrointestinal "flu" and is not able to eat. Acetone revealed by a test strip is a sign fat is being used for energy or that the child is becoming acidotic.

The "Honeymoon" Period

After a child's diagnosis has been confirmed and the blood glucose level has been initially regulated by insulin, a honeymoon period may follow, during which only a minimal amount of insulin, or none at all, is needed for glucose regulation. This apparently occurs because the exogenous insulin stimulates the islet cells to produce a small amount of natural

Figure 48.8 A child uses an automatic lancet for blood sampling *(left)*. Blood glucose level will be determined by the glucometer *(right)*. (© Lesha Photography.)

insulin, as if they are being reminded of their function. After a month or even up to a year, however, the islet cells will begin to fail once again, and diabetic symptoms will recur. This can be upsetting to parents if they began to believe their child was wrongly diagnosed or that a cure had taken place. Caution both the parents and the child that symptoms will inevitably recur.

Stress Adjustment

Whenever children with diabetes undergo a stressful situation, either emotionally or physically, they may need increased insulin to maintain glucose homeostasis. When children are seen at healthcare facilities for periodic checkups, ask them whether they are having any difficulty with blood testing or insulin injection and how things are at home and at school to detect their stress level.

Try to interview children separately from their parents, so they can feel free to talk about anything that may be happening or going wrong. If a child is experiencing stress because of school, parents may have to meet with school officials to help them view the child as well, not ill, so that they will allow participation in all activities, including sports. Sometimes, children are embarrassed to have to do blood glucose testing in school, especially in a public lavatory. It may be easier for them if they can go to the nurse's office for privacy when testing.

Complications

If an infection occurs and the child's temperature rises, insulin resistance increases, causing a need for additional insulin. Teach parents to notify their primary healthcare provider if their child appears to be ill (particularly if the child is nauseated or vomiting) for careful observation and a change in insulin dosage if necessary. If a child with diabetes is scheduled for surgery, careful regulation on the day of surgery and in the immediate postoperative period is essential, especially if oral fluids will be restricted.

Many long-term body changes such as arteriosclerosis (hardening of artery walls), which can lead to general poor circulation and kidney disease, and thickening of retinal capillaries and cataract formation, which ultimately can result in blindness, occurring because of chronic hyperglycemia, are not a major part of disease management in childhood because their onset does not begin until adulthood. It is not too early, however, when discussing hyperglycemia to mention that it does have long-term effects if not regulated beginning in childhood.

Pancreas Transplantation

For children who develop severe kidney disease or arteriosclerosis, pancreas transplantation may be considered to prevent further damage. In contrast to other organ transplantation procedures, the child's pancreas is not removed entirely prior to transplant. This is because the portion that supplies digestive enzymes is still functioning and so is left in place. The digestive enzymes of the new pancreas are diverted into the intestine or bladder, or the pancreatic ducts can be sclerosed, so the digestive enzymes do not leave the transplanted organ. Grafts may be taken from cadavers or from live donors, who can donate up to 45% of their pancreas and still maintain a functioning organ for themselves.

To reduce the child's immune response and protect against graft rejection, drugs such as antilymphocyte globulin, cyclosporine, prednisone, or azathioprine (Imuran) are administered after surgery. If rejection does start to occur, the patient is given monoclonal T-cell antibodies (OKT3) to try to reverse this process.

Pancreatic transplantation is a last resort solution for children because it involves major surgery, the outcome is guarded (about 50% of transplanted organs are rejected), and the result—continuous immunosuppressive medication for life—may not be regarded as a major improvement over the original illness, which requires continuous daily insulin for life. In addition, some pancreatic transplant recipients have a recurrence of diabetes (Burke, Vendrame, Virdi, et al., 2015).

 ## Nursing Diagnoses and Related Interventions

Nursing Diagnosis: Health-seeking behaviors related to self-administration of insulin, balanced exercise, and nutrition

Outcome Evaluation: Child demonstrates insulin injection technique to nurse, describes steps correctly, and discusses plans for an exercise and nutrition program.

Self-Administration of Insulin. From about 8 years of age, children can be taught to administer their own insulin (Fig. 48.9). Many children younger than this do not have the dexterity to handle a syringe or an understanding of the importance of sterile technique and proper dosage. They may skip injections if they are tired or busy.

Figure 48.9 A school-age child practices insulin administration using a teaching doll for practice.

Do not underestimate how difficult it is for children to learn to give injections to themselves. Although it may seem like a two-step process (draw up the medication and then inject it), in actuality, more than 25 steps are involved.

If the child has to mix insulins, the number of steps increases. Besides lacking dexterity and adult-level fine motor skills, children have to face injecting themselves. There is no such thing as getting used to injections. Children grow used to the *idea* of self-injection, not to the injections themselves.

Even if children are taught to give their own insulin from the beginning, at least one adult in the family should be taught to give it as well. There will be days when the child refuses to administer his or her own insulin or is not feeling well and needs to have or appreciates having someone administer it. Parents may have a hard time giving their child a painful injection; teaching them to view it as a helping action helps to alleviate their distress.

Exercise. Exercise is an important component of care because it uses up carbohydrates and helps reduce hyperglycemia. No type of exercise is restricted for children with diabetes. A problem that arises with vigorous exercise, however, is the development of hypoglycemia due to increased absorption of insulin from the injection site and use of glucose by active body cells. One way to minimize this effect is to choose the injection site that is least likely to be exercised. Another method is to eat additional carbohydrates or decrease the regular insulin injection according to an established protocol before exercise.

Teach children to design a consistent daily exercise program such as briskly walking the dog or 10 minutes of aerobics every day before school. Once a daily program is established, the child needs to continue this type of exercise every day (including weekends) to avoid becoming hyperglycemic on days of no exercise. If this process is not explained, parents may attempt to keep the child relatively quiet, unaware that exercise is actually healthful.

Hygiene. Skin care, particularly foot care, is extremely important for adults with diabetes because arterisclerosis causes loss of circulation to the feet, and decreased circulation leads to poor healing ability. This is not as important a concern with children, but they (and all children) should be taught to cut their toenails straight across, to prevent ingrown toenails, and to tend to cuts and scrapes promptly so that healing can begin right away. Properly fitted shoes are essential. Girls may need to be reminded of good perineal care to prevent vaginal infections.

Nursing Diagnosis: Parental anxiety related to newly diagnosed diabetes mellitus in their child

Outcome Evaluation: Parents accurately describe their child's illness and treatment and ways in which the disease will affect their lifestyle. They state a specific plan for daily routine child care and identify potential problems in the schedule and ways they can be managed.

Parents whose child is newly diagnosed with diabetes mellitus have a great deal of new responsibility. Be certain they have the telephone number of the healthcare facility, liaison, or home care person to call during the first days of home management so they have someone to consult before they give insulin the first several times.

Encourage the Expression of Feelings. Although parents may be aware that other family members have the disease, they may be surprised that diabetes has occurred in their child. Both the parents and the child need time to describe their perception of diabetes. If there are other family members with the illness, children may have heard many false stories about the disorder and may have been told how difficult it was in the past to achieve insulin control. These misconceptions need to be corrected so children can begin to accept their diagnosis and view themselves as basically well except for faulty insulin release.

What If . . . 48.2
Rob wants to try out for the soccer team at his school, but the soccer coach thinks children with diabetes should be excluded from sports. Because Rob doesn't always take his insulin reliably, would you agree with the coach?

Establish a Mode of Supervision and Support. Children with diabetes need frequent health supervision visits, approximately every 3 months. Those who appear to accept their diagnosis initially may have difficulty later, when their true feelings about their disorder surface. When they reach adolescence and are rebelling against a multitude of things, they may choose to rebel against blood glucose testing and insulin administration. Assess that children with diabetes have supportive friends to help them through "bad days." Make sure the parents can identify support people and others to contact if they have problems or questions. Sometimes what is needed most from healthcare personnel is understanding and appreciation of the difficulties encountered by children living with diabetes.

Teach Hypoglycemic Management. An episode of hypoglycemia is an extremely serious condition and must be prevented, if possible, because if it is not recognized and treated, it can lead to coma and seizures. Severe glucose depletion can lead to permanent brain damage with mental and motor impairment because brain cells need glucose for metabolism.

Symptoms of hypoglycemia occur when the blood glucose level falls to about 60 mg/dl. At this point, there is no glycosuria. It results from the administration of too much insulin, excessive exercise (because exercise uses up glucose), or failure to eat enough food. Typically, beginning symptoms include nervousness, weakness, dizziness, sweating, or tremors. In many children, the first signs of hypoglycemia are behavior problems: temper tantrums, stubbornness, silliness, irritability, or simply "not acting like usual self." A few children become insensitive to the symptoms of hypoglycemia (termed *hypoglycemia unawareness*) and are then unable to recognize that it is occurring. Such children need more blood glucose determinations built into their routine.

When the signs of hypoglycemia are recognized, a child needs an immediate source of carbohydrates. Fifteen grams of a fast-acting carbohydrate such as that contained in a half glass of orange juice or regular soda is recommended. It is easy for children always to carry glucose tablets or hard candy such as Life Savers with them to have them available for these times. If there is no improvement in symptoms and the blood glucose level has not risen by 15 mg/dl after 15 minutes, more carbohydrates (perhaps juice) should be given.

If the child is comatose when first discovered or is too upset or uncooperative to take oral sugar, parents can inject a specified dose of glucagon hydrochloride intramuscularly. This converts the glycogen that is stored in the liver into glucose. Usually, enough glycogen is converted after the drug injection to bring the child out of the coma, after which an oral form of glucose can be given. The drug will not be effective, however, if the child's supply of glycogen is depleted.

If parents cannot give their child an injection and oral sugar cannot be given, honey, corn syrup, cake icing gel, or glucose can be rubbed onto the gums or inside the cheek (of course, parents should be taught how to prevent aspiration) or corn syrup can be given as an enema. As soon as children are out of the coma or are cooperative, they should take a source of complex carbohydrates, such as crackers or whole wheat toast, to prevent further hypoglycemia. The primary healthcare provider needs to be notified of the incident so that its cause can be determined and steps can be taken to prevent hypoglycemia from occurring again.

Urge parents to anticipate occasions when hypoglycemia is likely to occur and to take preventive measures if possible. Hypoglycemia is most likely to occur, for example, at the peak effective time of the insulins being given, such as just before lunch or just before dinner. This means that many children who are attending school need to be scheduled for the first lunch period, not the second, or need a snack before lunch. Encourage the child and parents to discuss lunch times with the school nurse so appropriate meal planning is coordinated with the child's insulin schedule. Follow-ups at 6-month intervals are important so adjustments to account for changes in growth and school schedules can be made.

If children are going to engage in an active sport, such as swimming, tennis, or basketball, they should ingest a source of sugar before participation. This precaution is extremely important before swimming because a child who suddenly becomes weak in the middle of a pool may be unable to reach the side safely. Although eating before swimming is something that children typically are taught not to do, the child with diabetes must be taught to break this rule. This should be done sensibly, of course—before swimming, the child should eat a complex carbohydrate, such as crackers, not a full meal. Day and residential camps are available to help children learn more about diabetes and common measures other athletic children use to prevent hypoglycemia.

Occasionally, insulin overuse and persistent hypoglycemia cause a rebound hyperglycemic response; this is referred to as the **Somogyi phenomenon**. This phenomenon is suspected when children have nighttime (2 AM or 3 AM) hypoglycemia followed by high early-morning hyperglycemia. These children need to be referred to their healthcare provider because they actually need less insulin rather than more to correct the problem.

Teach Signs of Ketoacidosis. Because hyperglycemia leads to diabetic **ketoacidosis** (DKA), it is a metabolic emergency (Donahey & Folse, 2012). DKA is a serious complication of diabetes that occurs when the body produces high levels of blood acids called ketones. The condition develops when the body can't produce enough insulin and begins to break down fat as fuel. It may be difficult for parents to distinguish between hypoglycemia (occurring from too much insulin) and hyperglycemia (occurring from too little insulin for the level of glucose present

in the bloodstream) because hyperglycemia presents with almost the same symptoms as hypoglycemia: irritability, vomiting and abdominal pain, and behavior changes such as temper tantrums.

If a parent does not know whether the problem is hypoglycemia or hyperglycemia, the child should be offered a carbohydrate, as if the problem were hypoglycemia. This is because the added carbohydrate will do no harm if the problem is already hyperglycemia, whereas giving insulin is harmful if the cause is hypoglycemia. An inability to void is a good clue that the problem is hypoglycemia because with hyperglycemia, urine output is copious—one of the primary signs of diabetes. The real key to differentiating ketoacidosis from hypoglycemia, however, is the blood glucose level. Assessing the blood glucose concentration by finger stick solves the problem of whether symptoms relate to hypoglycemia or hyperglycemia. For quick reference, a comparison of hypoglycemia and hyperglycemia is shown in Table 48.5.

If ketoacidosis is not relieved when it first begins, it becomes severe with deep and rapid respirations (Kussmaul breathing) as the body attempts to "blow off" carbon dioxide and lessen the acidotic state. The child's breath smells sweet because of the presence of ketone bodies, and the pulse rate may be rapid. Signs of dehydration, including dry mucous membranes and skin, sunken eyeballs, and no tears, may be present. This is typically the picture when children are first diagnosed as having diabetes. It is also seen in children with diabetes who develop gastroenteritis and so eat poorly for several meals. Because the child is not eating well, parents may omit giving insulin. In actuality, because of an increased metabolic rate due to fever, parents need to consult with their primary care provider because the child may need more insulin and glucose than usual during these times. Box 48.8 shows an interprofessional care map for a child with diabetes type 1 to show how aspects of care need coordination.

TABLE 48.5 COMPARISON OF HYPOGLYCEMIA AND HYPERGLYCEMIA

Comparison Factor	Hypoglycemia	Hyperglycemia
Cause	Excessive insulin injection	Inadequate insulin injection
	Limited food intake	Excessive food intake
	Excessive exercise	Stress from infection, surgery, etc.
Symptoms	Hunger	Glycosuria and ketonuria
	Lethargy and sensorial changes	Polyuria, polydipsia; vomiting
	Sweating	Kussmaul respirations
	Pallor	Flushing and dehydration
	Seizures	Sweet (acetone) breath
	Coma	Lowered sodium, potassium, bicarbonate, chloride, and phosphate levels; decreased CO_2 combining power
		Coma
Danger	Brain cells need glucose for function and survival	Fatty acids used and ketoacidosis develops
Major nursing interventions	Administration of source of glucose by oral or intravenous route	Reestablishment of electrolyte balance and hydration
	Education to prevent recurrences	Education to prevent recurrences

BOX 48.8

Nursing Care Planning

AN INTERPROFESSIONAL CARE MAP FOR AN ADOLESCENT WITH TYPE 1 DIABETES MELLITUS

Rob Tebecco is a 16-year-old boy with type 1 diabetes whom you meet in the emergency department, where he was taken after he became comatose while ice skating. He has had diabetes since he was 7 years of age; he was managing his insulin administration well up until 6 months ago when he began to "forget" to take his insulin at least once a week. When you ask him about this, he tells you ice skating practice every morning and a new girlfriend have occupied his time and interrupted what used to be a strict schedule of home-cooked meals and a rigid routine.

Family Assessment: Adolescent lives with one younger sister and parents. Father works as Zamboni operator at a professional hockey arena. Mother works part-time at the local post office. Family rates finances as "We have everything we need."

Patient Assessment: Child was skating at local ice rink when he suddenly collapsed. Was brought to the emergency department by the emergency medical technician service, unconscious and breathing deeply. Breath smelled sweet. Blood glucose was 700 mg/dl. Received regular insulin intravenously (IV). As soon as blood glucose returned to normal, he regained consciousness. Arterial blood gases: pH, 7.20; Pco_2, 10 mmHg; HCO_3, 10 mEq/ml. Right heel has red and inflamed ulcer.

Currently takes short-acting and intermediate-acting insulin every morning before breakfast and again before dinner with self-injection device. Child performs finger-stick blood glucose levels four times a day. Blood glucose levels normally range between 105 and 115 mg/dl. Dietary history reveals three meals per day with midmorning, afternoon, and bedtime snack. Rob states, "Okay. I'm ready to do better. That was scary to black out."

Nursing Diagnosis: Health-seeking behaviors related to need to follow a more conscientious diabetes regimen.

Outcome Evaluation: Child and parents voice intention to be more conscientious about insulin administration and serum glucose testing. Child voices willingness to try insulin pump therapy.

Team Member Responsible	Assessment	Intervention	Rationale	Expected Outcome
Activities of Daily Living, Including Safety				
Nurse	Explore with child and parents their understanding of the interrelationship of nutrition, exercise, and diabetes.	Review and reinforce the importance of insulin administration, blood glucose monitoring, and exercise.	Explore and provide baseline information for identifying teaching needs and developing possible strategies.	Adolescent and parent state they understand new regimen; glucose levels do not fluctuate higher than 126 mg/dl.
Teamwork and Collaboration				
Nurse/primary care provider	Assess whether adolescent would be a good candidate for insulin pump therapy to increase adherence.	Consult with diabetic service team to present the new method of insulin administration.	Use of an insulin pump offers a continuous supply of insulin; can be advantageous for busy adolescent.	Diabetic service team meets with adolescent and parent to present possibility of using insulin pump.
Procedures/Medications for Quality Improvement				
Nurse	Assess adolescent's level of understanding about the action of insulin with pump therapy.	Demonstrate and observe the adolescent draw up and refill the insulin syringe and begin insulin pump infusion.	Adolescent's return demonstration best reveals whether he understands how to maintain the insulin pump.	Adolescent demonstrates proper preparation and administration of the insulin pump.
Nutrition				
Nurse/nutritionist	Assess adolescent's usual meal pattern; determine who prepares food and whether adolescent counts carbohydrates.	Review importance of regular meals plus a bedtime snack to keep glucose within consistent levels with the insulin pump.	Irregular meal patterns can cause hypoglycemia with pump therapy.	Parents and adolescent state they will try to estimate carbohydrate count better; adolescent will test blood glucose according to set schedule.

Continued on following page

BOX 48.8

Nursing Care Planning (continued)

Team Member Responsible	Assessment	Intervention	Rationale	Expected Outcome
Patient-Centered Care				
Nurse/diabetic service team member	Assess whether adolescent and parents are aware of actions to take if hypoglycemic symptoms should occur with pump therapy.	Review signs and symptoms of hypoglycemia; review need to always carry a source of carbohydrate.	Having a readily available source of carbohydrate helps raise blood glucose levels quickly should hypoglycemia occur.	Adolescent and parents describe signs of hypoglycemia and action of carbohydrates to prevent this.
Nurse/diabetic service team member	Assess whether adolescent and parents are aware of necessity to safeguard feet against trauma.	Review necessity to wear properly fitting shoes and skates and to clean any cuts or scrapes promptly.	Diabetes can result in decreased circulation to the feet and slowed healing, increasing the possibility for infection, which can ultimately affect glucose control.	Adolescent states he will be more conscientious about foot care; acknowledges foot infection may have contributed to his ketoacidosis episode.
Psychosocial/Spiritual/Emotional Needs				
Nurse/nurse practitioner	Assess whether child's busy schedule allows for adequate diabetic control.	Encourage parents to discuss adolescent's needs with him and ways he could modify his schedule to better accommodate his diabetic routine.	Poor medicine adherence may be a way adolescents express their identity.	Parents and child plot out a weekly schedule that allows both freedom for new activities and for conscientious diabetic care.
Informatics for Seamless Healthcare Planning				
Nurse	Assess whether child has experience with keeping a diabetic care journal.	Suggest the adolescent keeps a written diary of blood glucose levels, dietary intake (including snacks), and any symptoms of hypo- or hyperglycemia.	A written diary provides objective evidence for evaluating the new regimen and can indicate the need for possible changes or adjustments.	Adolescent agrees to keep a detailed journal until returning to clinic for a follow-up visit.
Nurse	Assess whether the adolescent or parents have any additional questions.	Arrange for a follow-up appointment in 1 week; encourage adolescent and parents to call with any questions or concerns.	Follow-up visit provides a means for evaluating the effectiveness of the new regimen and child's adaptation.	Adolescent and parents state they understand importance of follow-up visit for regulation of insulin pump therapy.

QSEN Checkpoint Question 48.4

TEAMWORK & COLLABORATION

Rob tells the nurse that he experienced a "honeymoon" period when he was first diagnosed with diabetes mellitus. The nurse recognizes that this would be demonstrated by which of the following signs?

   a. He developed an unnatural craving for sweets.
   b. His metabolism increased because of glucose stimulation.
   c. He became light-headed or "giddy" every afternoon.
   d. His need for injected insulin was drastically reduced.

Look in Appendix A for the best answer and rationale.

TYPE 2 DIABETES MELLITUS

T2D, characterized by diminished insulin secretion, is a separate disease from type 1 diabetes because it is not caused by autoimmune factors (Sherr & Weinzimer, 2012). Usually, children with T2D do not need daily insulin because their disease can be managed with diet alone or with diet and an oral hypoglycemic agent. Once thought to occur only in older adults, T2D is now seen as early as in overweight school-aged children (Caprio, 2012). Other influencing factors are a strong family history of diabetes; children from African, Hispanic, Asian, or Native Indian descent; those who eat a diet high in fats and carbohydrates; and those who do not exercise regularly. Development of polycystic ovary syndrome (PCOS) (see Chapter 8) is also strongly associated with the disorder. At the time of diagnosis, it may not be possible for the classification to be correctly determined because symptoms and findings are so similar.

Symptoms often become apparent for the first time at puberty because increasing sex hormones naturally increase insulin resistance, creating a need for more insulin production. Children's urine will show glucose but few ketones. Children experience lessened amounts of thirst or increased urination. About 90% of children with T2D have dark shiny patches on the skin (*acanthosis nigricans*), which are most often found between the fingers and between the toes, on the back of the neck ("dirty neck"), and in axillary creases (Stephen, Gungor, & Douty, 2012). Children whose family has a history of T2D, are from susceptible genetic groups, or have symptoms such as acanthosis nigricans or high blood pressure should be screened by a fasting blood sugar test at puberty and again every 2 years.

With this type of diabetes, because the pancreatic islet cells are still able to minimally function, the pancreas continues to secrete at least small amounts of insulin. Therapy, therefore, consists of nutrition and exercise, the same as for type 1 diabetes, combined with an oral antiglycemic agent such as a biguanide (metformin), which decreases the amount of glucose produced by the liver and increases insulin sensitivity in both the liver and muscle cells.

T2D is a chronic condition that will extend into adulthood and be present for life. Eventfully, it leads to atherosclerosis with thickening of arteries and capillaries, kidney disease, poor healing ability, and blindness because of poor circulation to body organs. In order to prevent these complications, children who develop T2D need good instruction in how to manage their illness so, whether they are home with their parents supervising their care or away from home at camp or college, they can prevent hyperglycemia and the irritation to blood vessels which that causes.

QSEN Checkpoint Question 48.5

SAFETY

Rob needs to adjust his regular insulin dose to the amount of carbohydrates he eats in order to prevent dangerous complications of his disease. If his insulin-to-carbohydrate ratio is 1:10, how many units of insulin should he inject if his lunch will consist of a hotdog on a bun (24 g), 1 cup chicken noodle soup (7 g), an apple (19 g), and a glass of milk (25 g)?

a. 3 units
b. 7.5 units
c. 9 units
d. 12 units

Look in Appendix A for the best answer and rationale.

The Parathyroid Glands

The four parathyroid glands, located posterior and adjacent to the thyroid gland, regulate serum levels of calcium in the body by controlling the rate of bone metabolism through the secretion of parathyroid hormone. This hormone is unique in that it is not under the control of the pituitary gland but rather is controlled by a negative feedback from the circulating serum levels of calcium and how much vitamin D is present to allow absorption of calcium from the gastrointestinal tract into the bloodstream.

HYPOCALCEMIA

Hypocalcemia is a lowered blood calcium level that occurs to some extent in all newborns before they begin sucking well. It occurs because phosphorus and calcium levels are always maintained in an inverse proportion to each other in the bloodstream (if phosphorus levels rise, calcium levels decrease, and vice versa). Hypocalcemia may be caused, therefore, by a change in either calcium or phosphorus metabolism (Thomas, Smith, White, et al., 2012).

Assessment

Hypocalcemia tends to occur in infants who experienced birth anoxia (phosphorus is released with anoxia), in immature infants (the parathyroid glands are immature), and in infants of women with diabetes (it tends to accompany the hypoglycemia that occurs in these infants shortly after birth).

The chief sign of hypocalcemia is neuromuscular irritability, referred to as **latent tetany**. This occurs if the blood calcium level falls below 7.5 mg/dl. The newborn will demonstrate jitteriness when handled or if the infant has been crying for an extended period.

Four methods are used to produce the clinical manifestations of tetany for diagnosis, as shown in Table 48.6. Any of these tests are helpful in determining whether a newborn's jitteriness is a result of hypocalcemia or a central nervous system concern.

If the blood calcium level falls well below 7 mg/dl, **manifest tetany** may result, which is commonly observed as muscular twitching and a **carpopedal spasm** (abduction of the hand and flexion of the wrist with the thumb positioned across the palm). In **pedal spasm** (foot spasm), the foot is extended, the toes flex, and the sole of the foot cups. Without therapy at this point, generalized seizures or spasm of the larynx, with the infant emitting a high-pitched, crowing sound on inspiration, can occur. If the spasm is prolonged, respirations may cease.

Therapeutic Management

Treatment is aimed at increasing the calcium level in the blood above the point of latent tetany. This can be administered orally as 10% calcium chloride if the infant can and will suck. Otherwise, it will be given IV as a 10%

TABLE 48.6 TESTS FOR DETECTION OF HYPOCALCEMIA

Sign	Description
Chvostek	When skin anterior to external ear (just over sixth cranial nerve) is tapped, facial muscles surrounding eye, nose, and mouth contract unilaterally.
Trousseau	When upper arm is constricted by tourniquet for 2–3 min and area becomes blanched, carpal spasm is elicited (hand abducts, wrist flexes, thumb is positioned across cupped palm).
Peroneal	When fibular side of leg over peroneal nerve is tapped, foot abducts and dorsiflexes.

solution of calcium gluconate. Newborns who are having generalized seizures may require anticonvulsant therapy in addition to the calcium gluconate to halt the seizures. Emergency equipment for intubation to relieve laryngospasm should be available.

After immediate therapy to increase the low blood calcium levels, infants are given oral calcium therapy until their calcium level stabilizes at greater than 7.5 mg/dl. Because vitamin D is necessary for the absorption of calcium from the gastrointestinal tract, the infant also may be given a vitamin D supplement such as calcitriol.

Metabolic Disorders (Inborn Errors of Metabolism)

Many causes of hormonal deficiency or excess in children are not related to the endocrine glands and the highly complex system of feedback and communication between these glands and the pituitary but rather are due to inherited biochemical disorders that disrupt the metabolism of amino acids, proteins, carbohydrates, or lipids. Many of these disorders are evident at or soon after birth and can cause irreversible cognitive challenge and early death, making early detection and treatment crucial. Gene therapy is expected to be available in the future to reverse symptoms of these disorders (van Karnebeek & Stockler, 2012).

PHENYLKETONURIA

PKU is a disease of metabolism, which is inherited as an autosomal recessive trait. The infant lacks the liver enzyme phenylalanine hydroxylase, which is necessary to convert phenylalanine, an essential amino acid, into tyrosine (a precursor of epinephrine, T_4, and melanin). As a result, excessive phenylalanine levels build up in the bloodstream and tissues, causing permanent damage to brain tissue and leaving children severely cognitively challenged.

The metabolite phenylpyruvic acid (a breakdown product of phenylalanine) spills into the urine to give the disorder its name. It causes urine to have a typical musty or "mousy" odor that is so strong that it often pervades not only the urine but the entire child.

As the disease progresses, because tyrosine is necessary for building body pigment and T_4, the child becomes blue-eyed with very fair skin and light blonde hair. Without adequate T_4, the child fails to meet average growth standards. Many children develop an accompanying seizure disorder. The skin is prone to eczema (atopic dermatitis). There is such a strong association between these two disorders that all infants with atopic dermatitis need to be rescreened for PKU at a well-child visit (Cunningham, Bausell, Brown, et al., 2012).

PKU is found in 1 of every 10,000 births in the United States; it occurs rarely in people of African or Jewish ancestry. If the condition remains untreated, the child will be left with an IQ below 20, muscular hypertonicity and spasticity, and possible recurrent seizures. PKU cannot be detected by amniocentesis as a routine screening measure because the phenylalanine level does not rise in utero while the infant is still under the control of the mother's enzyme system. Recombinant DNA techniques can be used for carrier detection and prenatal diagnosis from maternal serum.

Assessment

Early identification of the disorder is essential to prevent the child from becoming severely cognitively challenged. Because of this, all infants in the United States are screened at birth by blood spot analysis after receiving 2 full days of breast or formula feedings. If an infant is born at home or is discharged from a hospital or birthing center before the second day of life, remind the parents to have the test performed on the second or third day after birth. If a newborn did not suck well, so there is a question as to whether the baby received adequate milk for the test to be effective, the test can be repeated at the second week of life during a healthcare visit.

Therapeutic Management

Dietary restriction has been the main treatment of PKU for over 50 years and still remains the main therapy. In addition to this, large neutral amino acids have been suggested as an alternative treatment to improve outcomes (Miell et al., 2015). The drug sapropterin (Kuvan), which works by increasing tolerance to phenylalanine, has been approved by the U.S. Food and Drug Administration (FDA) for treatment (Cunningham et al., 2012).

To begin dietary regulation, infants in whom this disease is detected during the first few days of life are placed on a formula that is extremely low in phenylalanine, such as Lofenalac. A dietitian may recommend a mother who wants to breastfeed do so on a limited basis so the child does receive some phenylalanine (this essential amino acid is necessary for growth and repair of body cells). Unfortunately, a low amino acid formula can cause stools to be loose and has a rather disagreeable taste; therefore, some infants may resist drinking the formula after tasting breast milk.

Providing nutrition for a child with PKU becomes a difficult task as the child grows older because there is no natural protein with both a low phenylalanine concentration and normal levels of other essential amino acids. This means dietary management of PKU must consist of a balancing act between the child consuming enough nutrition to support growth and development and not consuming enough protein to increase the blood phenylalanine level (MacDonald, Rocha, van Rijn, et al., 2011).

Foods highest in phenylalanine are those that are rich in protein, such as meats, eggs, and milk. Foods low in phenylalanine include orange juice, bananas, potatoes, lettuce, spinach, and peas. A formula such as Lofenalac can be used to prepare treat foods, such as ice cream, milk shakes, birthday cakes, and puddings (foods that would otherwise be forbidden because they are made with milk). Children need their blood and urine monitored frequently for phenylalanine levels (which should be below 8 mg/dl). Hemoglobin levels should also be closely monitored to ensure the child is not becoming anemic because iron is found primarily in protein-rich foods, which the child must avoid. Because the diet tends to be high in carbohydrates to replace protein, children need to be screened for obesity at healthcare visits as well.

Be certain to offer parents the opportunity to express their feelings about the difficulty of maintaining a young child on such a restricted diet. Also assess the child's ability to cope with the illness because by the time they reach adolescence, they tend to grow very tired of the constant testing and restrictive diet.

What If . . . 48.3

A nurse is helping at a preschool and notices a teacher's assistant urging Rob's cousin Mike, who has PKU, to drink his milk. When the nurse suggests that milk might not be good for him, the assistant says, "Of course it is. Milk is nature's perfect food." How should the nurse respond?

At one time, it was thought children could discontinue the diet when they reached adolescence to solve the problem of compliance. The current advice is for children to follow the diet indefinitely, therefore, because discontinuing the diet may lead to some detrimental consequences, such as a lack of muscle strength. A woman who has PKU must anticipate when she wants to have children as an adult; if she has not been following her diet conscientiously, she needs to return to a strict low-phenylalanine diet for about 3 months before conception and must remain on the diet for the duration of pregnancy (see Chapter 13). Otherwise, her fetus will be exposed to high levels of phenylalanine during pregnancy and will be born cognitively challenged.

MAPLE SYRUP URINE DISEASE

Maple syrup urine disease is a rare disorder, inherited as an autosomal recessive trait, in which there is a defect in metabolism of the amino acids leucine, isoleucine, and valine, which leads to cerebral degeneration similar to that observed in children with PKU.

Infants who have the disorder appear well at birth but quickly begin to show signs of feeding difficulty, loss of the Moro reflex, and irregular respirations. The symptoms progress rapidly to *opisthotonos*, generalized muscular rigidity, and seizures. If the condition remains untreated, an infant may die of the disease as early as 2 to 4 weeks of age. Fortunately, prenatal detection is possible by analyzing cells obtained by amniocentesis or from maternal serum (Cunningham et al., 2012). Also, like PKU, all infants in the United States are screened at birth for the disorder (Chen, Mei, Kalman, et al., 2012).

Although the disorder is rare, it is mentioned here because nurses are the healthcare personnel who are often the first ones to detect the disorder because on the first or second day of life, the urine of the child develops the characteristic odor of maple syrup (hence the name of the disease) due to the presence of ketoacids. Being aware of the disorder prevents discounting the pleasant urine odor not as an innocent finding but as the mark of a severe metabolic disorder.

Therapeutic Management

If maple syrup urine disease is diagnosed during the first day or two of life and the child is placed on a well-controlled diet that is high in thiamine and low in the amino acids leucine, isoleucine, and valine, cerebral degeneration can be prevented, just as it can be prevented in PKU. Such a diet is extremely difficult to maintain, however, because of its low protein content. Parents need intensive nutritional counseling. Hemodialysis or peritoneal dialysis may be necessary to temporarily reduce abnormal serum levels at birth or during a childhood infection, when catabolism of cells releases increased amino acids into the bloodstream.

GALACTOSEMIA

Galactosemia is a disorder of carbohydrate metabolism that is characterized by abnormal amounts of galactose in the blood (*galactosemia*) and in the urine (*galactosuria*). It occurs in about 1 in every 60,000 births, most often as an inborn error of metabolism, which is transmitted as an autosomal recessive trait. The child is deficient in the liver enzyme galactose-1-phosphate uridyltransferase (Chen et al., 2012).

Lactose (the sugar found in milk) normally is broken down into galactose and glucose; galactose is then further broken down into additional glucose. Without the galactose 1-phosphate uridyltransferase enzyme, this second step, the conversion of galactose into glucose, cannot take place, and galactose builds up in the bloodstream and spills out into the urine. When it reaches toxic levels in the bloodstream, it destroys body cells.

Assessment

Symptoms appear as soon as the child begins formula or breastfeeding and include lethargy, hypotonia, and perhaps diarrhea and vomiting. The liver enlarges as cirrhosis develops. Jaundice is often present and persistent, and bilateral cataracts develop. If the condition remains untreated, symptoms can worsen so rapidly, a child may die by 3 days of age. Untreated children who survive beyond this time may be cognitively challenged and have bilateral cataracts.

Diagnosis is made by measuring the level of the affected enzyme in the red blood cells. A screening test (the Beutler test) can be used to analyze cord blood if a child is known to be at risk for the disorder.

Therapeutic Management

The treatment of galactosemia consists of placing the infant on a diet free of galactose or giving the child formula made with milk substitutes such as casein hydrolysates (Nutramigen). Once the child's condition is regulated on this diet, symptoms of the disease do not progress; however, any neurologic or cataract damage that is already present will persist. The duration of the restricted diet is controversial but probably should be followed for life.

QSEN Checkpoint Question 48.6

EVIDENCE-BASED PRACTICE

Because parents have so much influence on how children adjust to having a long-term illness, researchers administered a questionnaire to a total of 185 parents with children 1 to 19 years of age divided into three groups: one where the children had either PKU or galactosemia; one where the children were healthy; and a third group where the children had a chronic illness, which was likely to interfere with longevity. Results of the study revealed that the parents of children with PKU or galactosemia rated their quality of life equal with that of parents of healthy children and far above that of parents whose child could have a short life span. Factors that influenced the children's quality of life most were the presence of support people (a positive effect) and loss of friends (a negative effect) (Fidika, Salewski, & Goldbeck, et al., 2013).

Based on this study, which comment by LaRoya, a 12-year-old girl who comes to the clinic because she has galactosemia, would make the nurse believe LaRoya's family's quality life is not ideal?

a. "My mother still loves to cook, although no one comes over anymore."

b. "We go to church every Sunday; my dad helps teach church school."

c. "We've lived in the same house for 10 years; the carpet is getting old."

d. "My grandmother is hard of hearing, so we have to shout so she hears us."

Look in Appendix A for the best answer and rationale.

GLYCOGEN STORAGE DISEASE

Glycogen storage disease refers to a group of genetically transmitted disorders that involve altered production and use of glycogen in the body. Twelve of the 13 described types are inherited as autosomal recessive traits; the other is a sex-linked disorder.

Glycogen is normally stored in the liver to provide a reserve supply of glucose. When the body needs glucose for energy, this glycogen is transformed back to glucose. In children with glycogen storage disease, glycogen is deposited normally, but an enzyme deficiency prevents retransformation of the glycogen back to glucose.

In one form of this disorder (type II, or Pompe disease), children deposit large stores of glycogen not only in the liver but also in the muscle and heart (Rajan & Abdel-Hamid, 2012). The muscles begin to feel hard on palpation due to the deposits of glycogen. The heart becomes enlarged, and often, an arrhythmia will be present. Without therapy, children with this form usually die of heart failure before they reach adulthood.

Assessment

Because the liver must store such a large supply of glycogen, it increases so much in size that the abdomen protrudes. Over a long period, the child's growth will be stunted because there is only glucose available for energy, not for growth. If hypoglycemic episodes have been severe, brain damage may result. Many children have a tendency toward epistaxis or hemorrhage and are at risk when having surgery performed because of an impaired clotting ability due to decreased platelet adhesiveness. They are susceptible to periods of hypoglycemia because their only source of ready glucose is their oral intake. The development of gout from deposition of uric acid crystals in joints may also occur (Kuwahara, Yoshitaka, Tomonori, et al., 2017).

Therapeutic Management

Children with glycogen storage disease need to eat a high-carbohydrate diet with snacks between meals to prevent hypoglycemia. In addition, a continuous glucose nasogastric or gastrostomy feeding during the night may be necessary to prevent hypoglycemia while sleeping. Therapy with diazoxide (Proglycem), an antihypoglycemic drug that inhibits insulin release, may help regulate the glucose level to provide additional growth. Liver transplantation may be a possibility, but it will not cure the basic enzyme deficiency.

TAY-SACHS DISEASE (INFANTILE GM2 GANGLIOSIDOSIS)

Tay-Sachs disease is an autosomal recessively inherited disease in which the infant lacks hexosaminidase A, an enzyme necessary for lipid metabolism. Without this enzyme, lipid deposits accumulate on nerve cells, leading to severe cognitive challenge, due to deposits on brain cells, and blindness, due to deposits on optic nerve cells (Chen et al., 2012).

Tay-Sachs disease is found primarily in the Ashkenazi Jewish population (Eastern European Jewish ancestry). Children generally appear well in the first few months of life except for an extreme Moro reflex and mild hypotonia. If left untreated, at about 6 months of age, they begin to lose head control and are unable to sit up or roll over without support. On an ophthalmoscopic examination, a characteristic cherry-red macula is noticeable (caused by lipid deposits). By 1 year of age, children will have developed symptoms of spasticity and are unable to perform even simple motor tasks. By 2 years of age, generalized seizures and blindness will have occurred. Most children die of cachexia (malnutrition) and pneumonia by 3 to 5 years of age. There is no cure for Tay-Sachs disease. The disorder may be detected in utero by amniocentesis. Carriers for the disease trait may be identified by hexosaminidase. For more information about Tay-Sachs disease and updates on health and family stories, please visit http://curetay-sachs.org/.

What If . . . 48.4

A nurse is particularly interested in exploring one of the 2020 National Health Goals with respect to endocrine or metabolic disorders in children (see Box 48.1). A total of 16.9% of children and adolescents aged 2 to 19 years were considered obese in 2009 to 2012 (www.healthypeople.gov). According to the Healthy People 2020 Leading Indicators, a 14.2% decrease in obesity in children and adolescents is needed by the year 2020. What would be a research topic pertinent to this goal that would be applicable to Rob's family and would also advance evidence-based practice?

KEY POINTS FOR REVIEW

- Endocrine disorders are almost all long-term disorders. Helping parents and children remember to take medicine on a long-term basis is an important nursing responsibility that not only meets QSEN competencies but that also best meets the family's total needs.

- Children with endocrine or metabolic disorders often develop height or weight discrepancies. Help children continue to maintain high self-esteem by concentrating on the things they are able to do despite a growth lag.

- GH deficiency, a pituitary disorder, results in extremely short stature if left untreated. Therapy for children consists of the injection of synthetic GH. Children can experience situational low self-esteem if they do not receive adequate emotional support from significant others.

- Other pituitary disorders include GH excess and diabetes insipidus. With GH excess, there is an overgrowth of body tissues. With diabetes insipidus, there is a decreased release of ADH, which leads to polyuria. Therapy is the administration of desmopressin, an arginine vasopressin.

- Congenital hypothyroidism occurs as a result of an absent or nonfunctioning thyroid gland. The condition is discovered by a blood spot test at birth. Therapy is the oral administration of synthetic thyroid hormone.

- Acquired hypothyroidism (Hashimoto disease) is an autoimmune phenomenon that interferes with thyroid gland function. Therapy is the administration of synthetic thyroid hormone.

- Hyperthyroidism is caused by overproduction of thyroid hormones. It leads to jitteriness and tachycardia. It is treated by medication to suppress thyroxine release.

- Acute adrenocortical insufficiency is an emergency situation in which there is abrupt nonfunction of the adrenal glands. Congenital adrenogenital hyperplasia is an inherited disorder in which girls are born masculinized. Both girls and boys may be unable to retain sodium, resulting in rapid fluid loss. Therapy is the administration of hydrocortisone and also aldosterone if sodium loss is present.

- Cushing syndrome is caused by the overproduction of cortisol by the adrenal gland, which is usually caused by a tumor in the gland. Children appear abnormally obese. Therapy is the surgical removal of the tumor.

- The most frequently occurring pancreatic disorder is type 1 diabetes mellitus, an autoimmune process that destroys insulin-producing islet cells. Therapy is a combination of insulin, diet, and exercise. Type 2 diabetes is now occurring in children, especially those who are obese. Therapy is diet, exercise, and an oral antiglycemic agent.

- Hypocalcemia, a parathyroid gland disorder, results in a lowered blood calcium level, causing tetany to develop. Therapy is the administration of calcium.

- Various disorders of metabolism that interfere with carbohydrate, amino acid, or fat metabolism occur in children. Representative of these are PKU, galactosemia, and Tay-Sachs disease.

CRITICAL THINKING CARE STUDY

Cassie is a 4-year-old child who has hypocalcemia because of inadequate parathyroid function caused by being struck in the neck by a baseball when she was 2 years of age. She takes a daily supplement of both vitamin D and calcium, and she is urged to eat a diet high in calcium. She has begun to be increasingly uncooperative about taking her medication. Her mother worries that, as Cassie grows older, she will refuse her medication completely.

1. Cassie's mother is worried her daughter will gain weight drinking whole milk and so serves her nonfat milk. She adds chocolate syrup to it to change the taste. This morning, she realized Cassie gave her 10-year-old brother her glass of milk to drink. Does serving nonfat milk or adding chocolate to it change the calcium content of milk? What actions could you take to help Cassie's mother increase Cassie's cooperation with drinking more milk?

2. Cassie's mother tells you she is at "the end of her rope" with trying to get Cassie to take her medicine. She's so frustrated that she's stopped trying to give her vitamin D because "it's only a vitamin." What suggestions could you make to help the mother increase Cassie's medicine compliance?

3. The teacher at the preschool Cassie attends has told her mother that Cassie refuses to hold a pencil when it's time to practice alphabet letters. She "acts out" by holding her hands together, "pretending they hurt" instead. She's asked the mother to reinforce with Cassie the importance of learning letters to be ready for kindergarten. How would you suggest the mother handle this?

RELATED RESOURCES

Explore these additional resources to enhance learning for this chapter:

- Student resources on thePoint, including answers to the What If . . . and Critical Thinking Care Study questions, http://thepoint.lww.com/Flagg8e
- Adaptive learning powered by PrepU, http://thepoint.lww.com/prepu

REFERENCES

Agarwal, P. K., Singh, P., Chowdhury, S., et al. (2017). A study to evaluate the prevalence of hypogonadism in Indian males with type-2 diabetes mellitus. *Indian Journal of Endocrinology and Metabolism, 21*(1), 64–70.

Baronio, F., Mazzanti, L., Girtler, Y., et al. (2017). The influence of growth hormone treatment glucose homeostasis in girls with Turner syndrome: A 7 year study. *Journal of Clinical Endocrinology and Metabolism, 102*(3), 878–883.

Baumann, G. P. (2012). Growth hormone doping in sports: A critical review of use and detection strategies. *Endocrine Reviews, 33*(2), 155–186.

Bell, M. F., Bayliss, D. M., Glauert, R., et al. (2016). Chronic illness and developmental vulnerability at school entry. *Pediatrics, 137*(5), e20152475.

Boss, A. H., Petrucci, R., & Lorber, D. (2012). Coverage of prandial insulin requirements by means of an ultra-rapid-acting inhaled insulin. *Journal of Diabetes Science & Technology, 6*(4), 773–779.

Buchko, B., Artz, B., Dayhoff, S., et al. (2012). Improving care of patients with insulin pumps during hospitalization: Translating the evidence. *Journal of Nursing Care Quality, 27*(4), 333–340.

Burke, G. W., III, Vendrame, F., Pileggi, A., et al. (2016). Pancreas transplantation. *American Journal of Transplantation, 16*, 235–245.

Burke, G. W., III, Vendrame, F., Virdi, S. K., et al. (2015). Lessons from pancreas transplantation in type 1 diabetes: Recurrence of islet autoimmunity. *Current Diabetes Reports, 15*(12), 121.

Caprio, S. (2012). Development of type 2 diabetes mellitus in the obese adolescent: A growing challenge. *Endocrine Practice, 18*(5), 791–795.

Chamarthi, B., Morris, C. A., Kaiser, U. B., et al. (2013). Clinical problem-solving. *The New England Journal of Medicine, 369*, 1344–1355.

Chen, B., Mei, J., Kalman, L., et al. (2012). Good laboratory practices for biochemical genetic testing and newborn screening for inherited metabolic diseases. *Morbidity and Mortality Weekly Report, 61*(2), 1–44.

Cunningham, A., Bausell, H., Brown, M., et al. (2012). Recommendations for the use of sapropterin in phenylketonuria. *Molecular Genetics & Metabolism, 106*(3), 269–276.

Dörr, H. G., Boguszewski, M., Dahlgren, J., et al. (2015). Short children with CHARGE syndrome: Do they benefit from growth hormone therapy? *Hormone Research in Paediatrics, 84*(1), 49–53.

Donahey, E., & Folse, S. (2012). Management of diabetic ketoacidosis. *Advanced Emergency Nursing Journal, 34*(3), 209–215.

Fidika, A., Salewski, C., & Goldbeck, L. (2013). Quality of life among parents of children with phenylketonuria (PKU). *Health and Quality of Life Outcomes, 11*, 54.

Geisler, A., Lass, N., Reinsch, N., et al. (2012). Quality of life in children and adolescents with growth hormone deficiency: Association with growth hormone treatment. *Hormone Research in Paediatrics, 78*(2), 94–99.

Graber, E., & Rapaport, R. (2012). Growth and growth disorders in children and adolescents. *Pediatric Annals, 41*(4), e1–e9.

Hagan, J. F., Shaw, J. S., & Duncan, P. M. (2017). *Bright futures: Guidelines for health supervision of infants, children and adolescents* (4th ed.). Elk Grove Village, IL: American Academy of Pediatrics.

Kim, D. (2016) Low vitamin D status is associated with hypothyroid Hashimoto's thyroiditis. *Hormones (Athens)*, *15*(3), 385–393. http://dx.doi.org/10.14310/horm.2002.1681

Kollati, Y., Ambati, R. R., Reddy, P. N., et al. (2017). Congenital hypothyroidism: Facts, facets and therapy. *Current Pharmaceutical Design*. Advance online publication. doi:10.2174/1381612823666170206124255

Korzeniewski, S., Grigorescu, V., Kleyn, M., et al. (2012). Performance metrics after changes in screening protocol for congenital hypothyroidism. *Pediatrics*, *130*(5), 1252–1261.

Kuwahara, E., Yoshitaka, M., Tomonori, O., et al. (2017). Increased childhood BMI is associated with young adult serum uric acid levels: A linkage study from Japan. *Pediatric Research*, *81*, 293–298.

LaFranchi, S. H. (2014). How should we be treating children with congenital hypothyroidism? *Pediatric Journal Clinical Endocrinology & Metabolism*, *4*, 99–363.

Léger, J., & Carel, J. C. (2013). Hyperthyroidism in childhood: Causes, when and how to treat. *Journal of Clinical Research in Pediatric Endocrinology*, *5*(Suppl. 1), 50–56.

MacDonald, A., Rocha, J. C., van Rijn, M., et al. (2011). Nutrition in phenylketonuria. *Molecular Genetics & Metabolism*, *104*(Suppl. 1), S10–S18.

Mak, C. M., Lee, H. C., Chan, A. Y., et al. (2013). Inborn errors of metabolism. *Critical Reviews Clinical Laboratory Sciences*, *50*(6), 142–146.

Michala, L., Liao, L. M., Wood, D., et al. (2014). Practice changes in childhood surgery for ambiguous genitalia. *Journal of Pediatric Urology*, *10*(5), 934–939.

Miell, J., Dhanjal, P., & Jamookeeah, C. (2015). Evidence for the use of Demeclocycline in the treatment of hyponatremia secondary to SIADH: A systematic review. *International Journal of Clinical Practice*, *69*(12), 1396–1417. http://dx.doi.org/10.1111/ijcp.12713

Rajan, D. S., & Abdel-Hamid, H. (2012). Child neurology: Pompe disease: New horizons. *Neurology*, *79*(23), 197–200.

Rivkees, S. A. (2014). Pediatric Graves' disease: Management in the post-propylthiouracil Era. *International Journal of Pediatric Endocrinology*, *2014*(1), 10.

Schmidt, C. A., Bernaix, L. W., Chiappetta, M., et al. (2012). In-hospital survival skills training for type 1 diabetes: Perceptions of children and parents. *Maternal Child Nursing*, *37*(2), 88–94.

Sherr, J., & Weinzimer, S. (2012). Diabetes types 1 and 2 in the pediatric population. *Pediatric Annals*, *41*(2), 1–7.

Smy, L., Shaw, K., Smith, A., et al. (2015). Hair cortisol as a novel biomarker of HPA suppression by inhaled corticosteroids in children. *Pediatric Research*, *78*, 44–47.

Stephen, M. D., Gungor, N., & Douty, D. R. (2012). Type 2 diabetes mellitus in a young girl: Ominous presentation and atypical course. *Journal of Pediatric & Endocrinology Metabolism*, *25*(5–6), 577–580.

Thomas, T. C., Smith, J. M., White, P. C., et al. (2012). Transient neonatal hypocalcemia: Presentation and outcomes. *Pediatrics*, *129*(6), e1461–e1467.

U.S. Department of Health and Human Services. (2010). *Healthy people 2020*. Washington, DC: Author.

van Karnebeek, C. D., & Stockler, S. (2012). Treatable inborn errors of metabolism causing intellectual disability: A systematic literature review. *Molecular Genetics and Metabolism*, *105*(3), 368–381.

49

Nursing Care of a Family When a Child Has a Neurologic Disorder

*T*asha is a 3-year-old girl you meet in an emergency department because she's had a seizure. Her mother grabs your arm, visibly upset. "Her sister has cerebral palsy and seizures. Does this mean Tasha has cerebral palsy too?" she asks you.

Previous chapters described normal growth and development in children and nursing care of children with disorders of other systems. This chapter adds information about the dramatic changes, both physical and psychosocial, that occur when a child is born with or develops a neurologic disorder. Such information builds a base for care and health teaching for children with these disorders.

What education does this parent need about cerebral palsy or recurrent seizures?

KEY TERMS

asterognosis

automatism

autonomic dysreflexia

choreoathetosis

choreoid

decerebrate posturing

decorticate posturing

diplegia

dyskinetic

graphesthesia

hemiplegia

infantile spasms

kinesthesia

paraplegia

pulse pressure

quadriplegia

status epilepticus

stereognosis

OBJECTIVES

After mastering the contents of this chapter, you should be able to:

1. Describe common neurologic disorders in children.
2. Identify 2020 National Health Goals related to neurologic disorders in children that nurses can help the nation achieve.
3. Assess a child with a neurologic disorder.
4. Formulate nursing diagnoses for a child with a neurologic disorder.
5. Establish expected outcomes for a child with a neurologic disorder to help the family manage seamless transitions across differing healthcare settings.
6. Using the nursing process, plan nursing care that includes the six competencies of Quality & Safety Education for Nurses (QSEN): Patient-Centered Care, Teamwork & Collaboration, Evidence-Based Practice (EBP), Quality Improvement (QI), Safety, and Informatics.
7. Implement nursing care, such as monitoring medicine effectiveness, for a child with a neurologic disorder.
8. Evaluate expected outcomes for achievement and effectiveness of care.
9. Integrate knowledge of neurologic disorders and the interplay of nursing process, the six competencies of QSEN, and Family Nursing to promote quality maternal and child health nursing care.

BOX 49.1

Nursing Care Planning Based on 2020 National Health Goals

Neurologic disorders are major causes of long-term disability in children. The 2020 National Health Goals that address these disorders are:

- Increase the proportion of children or youth with disabilities who spend at least 80% of their time in regular education programs from a baseline of 56.8% to a target level of 73.8%.
- Reduce the number of people 21 years of age and younger with disabilities who are in congregate care facilities from a baseline of 28,890 to 26,001.
- Increase the proportion of people with epilepsy or uncontrolled seizures who receive appropriate medical care.
- Reduce emergency department visits for nonfatal traumatic brain injuries from 407.2/100,000 population to 366.3/100,000 (U.S. Department of Health and Human Services, 2010; see www.healthypeople.gov).

Nurses can help the nation achieve these goals through helping to prevent neurologic injury by educating children and parents about the use of helmets for bicycle and motorcycle safety, by administering and teaching paramedical personnel to administer safe care at accident scenes so children's heads and necks are protected, and by decreasing the possible spread of bacterial meningitis through good hand washing and infection control precautions in hospitals.

Neurologic disorders encompass a wide array of problems resulting from congenital disorders, infection, or trauma. Many of these disorders severely alter the child's life; some result in life-threatening complications. Whenever possible, prevention must be the highest priority for keeping the nervous system healthy because, in the future, stem cell research may offer a cure for neurologic disorders, but for now, because neural tissue does not regenerate like other body tissue, any nervous system degeneration is likely to be permanent. Therefore, nursing care focuses on prevention or measures to help the child and family develop strategies for dealing with the associated loss in mental or physical functioning, making the child comfortable, and providing an environment conducive to the child's development and self-esteem (Parachuri & Inglese, 2013). The 2020 National Health Goals related to neurologic disorders in children are shown in Box 49.1.

Nursing Process Overview

FOR CARE OF A CHILD WITH A NEUROLOGIC SYSTEM DISORDER

ASSESSMENT

Neurologic disorders often begin with vague symptoms. Parents may report that their child seems to be "walking strangely" or is "just not herself," making a thorough history and neurologic examination imperative for isolating the cause of the concern.

The neurologic examination covers six areas of neurologic functioning as well as motor and sensory functioning. If more information is needed following an exam, additional diagnostic tests will be prescribed. The parents and child need considerable support throughout the assessment process because, although the neurologic examination can be made "fun" for a child, other procedures such as a computed tomography (CT) scan or lumbar puncture can be frightening. Additionally, the anxiety of not knowing what is wrong and fearing the worst can make the waiting period for test results especially difficult for the child's parents.

NURSING DIAGNOSIS

Nursing diagnoses for children with neurologic disorders vary according to the child's needs and level of functioning. Initially, a child may need emergency care and constant observation; later on, maintenance care to retain function is the priority. If the child has surgery, nursing diagnoses need to address not only immediate preoperative and postoperative care but also long-term care such as rehabilitation and home care. Three common nursing diagnoses that apply to almost all neurologic disorders are:

- Risk for disuse syndrome related to neurologic deficit affecting one area of functioning
- Interrupted family processes related to stress associated with the long-term effects of neurologic involvement
- Health-seeking behaviors related to care of a child with neurologic involvement

Other nursing diagnoses are specific for disorders and thus are described along with specific disorders.

OUTCOME IDENTIFICATION AND PLANNING

Be realistic when establishing expected outcomes because children who have permanent limitations will not be able to achieve progress in all areas. When neurologic disorders are first diagnosed, parents may be so stressed that they may be able to focus only on short-term aspects of care, such as whether the child will survive meningitis or whether the child has stopped convulsing. Later, they'll be able to concentrate on the long-term picture: What type of education setting will be best for their child? What type of exercise program will be required?

Before a diagnosis is confirmed, parents may attribute their child's functional deficits to immaturity (she is not walking yet because she is simply too young). This can make them unable to make plans because they have not fully acknowledged their child's neurologic deficits. Only when parents begin to adjust to the new reality are they ready to participate in planning and problem solving.

Numerous organizations are available for assistance and support, such as the Epilepsy Foundation of America (www.epilepsyfoundation.org), the National Dissemination Center for Children With Disabilities (www.parentcenterhub.org), the Children's Tumor Foundation (www.ctf.org), the United Spinal Association (www.spinalcord.org), and the United Cerebral Palsy Association (www.ucp.org).

IMPLEMENTATION

Nursing interventions for a child with a neurologic problem must address both short- and long-term needs. A lot of nursing care involves modeling care, such as how to gently handle

Figure 49.1 Meninges of the **(A)** brain and **(B)** spinal cord.

an infant with increased intracranial pressure (ICP) and how to turn an infant on the side during a seizure to prevent choking, and reviewing needed medications with parents—actions that give parents confidence to be able to care for their child at home.

OUTCOME EVALUATION

Evaluation of a child with a neurologic disorder should address not only the child's progress in regaining physical function but also the child's level of self-esteem. Some examples indicating achievement of possible outcomes are:

- The child states he or she is aware of potential for injury related to recurrent seizures.
- The parent/caregiver states understanding of potential for injury related to recurrent seizures.
- Family members state they are able to maintain family cohesiveness yet sustain contact with hospitalized child.
- The child practices exercises daily to reduce possibility of contracture from disuse syndrome.

Anatomy and Physiology of the Nervous System

Nerve cells (*neurons*) are unique among body cells in that, instead of being compact, they consist of a cell nucleus and extensions: one axon and several dendrites. The *dendrite* transmits impulses to the cell nucleus; the *axon* transmits impulses away from the cell nucleus to body organs. These cells vary in size, ranging from a few inches to several feet long, reaching from distant body sites such as the feet, through the spinal cord, and to the brain. Although their great length is vital to motor and sensory function, it also makes nerve cells more susceptible than other body cells to injury.

The nervous system is not fully functioning at birth; it continues to mature through the first 12 years of life. Two separate systems are involved: the *peripheral nervous system* (PNS) and the *central nervous system* (CNS). The PNS consists of the cranial

nerves, the spinal nerves, and the somatic and visceral divisions. The CNS includes the brain and the spinal cord (Fig. 49.1) surrounded by the cerebrospinal fluid (CSF), the skull, and three membranes or meninges (the *dura mater*, a fibrous, connective tissue containing many blood vessels; the *arachnoid membrane*, a delicate serous membrane; and the *pia mater*, a vascular membrane) that protect the brain and spinal cord from trauma.

The properties of CSF are shown in Table 49.1. Basically, it is a colorless, alkaline fluid with a specific gravity of approximately 1.004 to 1.008, containing traces of protein, glucose, lymphocytes, and body salts.

Assessing the Child With a Neurologic Disorder

Because neurologic symptoms, such as headache, unsteady gait, or lethargy, are often insidious, both a thorough history and a neurologic examination are needed to reveal the cause and extent of such symptoms (Box 49.2).

HEALTH HISTORY

A child's history may first reveal symptoms of a neurologic disorder. Because many neurologic problems that are evidenced in infants and young children result from injury that occurred in utero, it is important to obtain the mother's pregnancy history as well.

At primary care visits, always ask parents about their child's developmental milestones and ability to perform age-appropriate tasks successfully. A screening test can be used to indicate whether a parent's concern about a preschool child is well founded. The ability to perform well in school is important documentation for an older child.

NEUROLOGIC EXAMINATION

A complete neurologic examination takes at least 20 minutes and requires both patience and skill to keep a child's attention while observing for possible indications of neurologic disease.

TABLE 49.1 NORMAL PROPERTIES OF CEREBROSPINAL FLUID

Parameter	Normal Finding	Abnormal Finding: Possible Significance
Opening pressure	Newborns: 8–10 cm H_2O; children: 10–18 cm H_2O	Lowered pressure usually indicates there is subarachnoid obstruction in the spinal column above the puncture site.
		Elevated pressure suggests intracranial compression, hemorrhage, or infection.
		Pressure increases if a child coughs or pressure is applied to the external jugular vein (Valsalva maneuver).
Appearance	Clear and colorless	If cloudy, indicates possible infection with an increased number of white blood cells (WBCs).
		If reddened, color is probably because of red blood cells (RBCs).
Cell count	0–8/mm³	Granulocytes suggest cerebrospinal fluid (CSF) infection.
		Lymphocytes suggest meningeal irritation and inflammation.
		A few RBCs and WBCs are normally present in the newborn CSF due to the trauma of birth.
Protein	15–45 mg/100 ml	Elevated count (>45/100 ml) occurs if RBCs are present.
		If both protein content and RBC count are elevated, meningitis or subarachnoid hemorrhage is suggested.
		If protein content alone is elevated, it more likely suggests a degenerative process such as multiple sclerosis.
Glucose	60%–80% of serum glucose level	Bacterial meningitis causes a marked decrease in CSF glucose; invasion of fungi, yeast, tuberculosis, or protozoans into the CSF results in some decrease in glucose level.
		Viral infections do not cause a decrease in CSF glucose and may occasionally cause a slight increase.
Albumin/globulin (A/G) ratio	8:1	Increased level suggests infection or an A/G ratio neurologic disorder.

For a full examination, six areas are assessed: cerebral, cranial nerve, cerebellar, motor, sensory, and reflex function.

Cerebral Function

Both general and specific cerebral functions need to be evaluated by assessing level of consciousness, orientation, intelligence, performance, mood, and general behavior (Rust, 2011). Children do best when these types of tests are presented as a game. Be certain to convey that there are no right or wrong answers because children who believe that they have failed these tests may not respond well to further testing.

The best way to evaluate a child's level of *consciousness* is through conversation. Note any drowsiness or lethargy. Allow the child to answer questions without prompting and listen carefully to be certain the answer is appropriate to the question.

Orientation refers to whether children are aware of who they are, where they are, and what day it is (person, place, and time). Be certain to take into account a child's age, making questions age-appropriate to the child's developmental abilities. Children younger than 4 years of age, for example, may not know both their first and last names. Children may be of school age before they know their address. Children younger than 7 or 8 years of age may have difficulty with the days of the week, confusing "yesterday" with "today" or "tomorrow." Intellectual performance (IQ) can be determined by the child's score on a standard intelligence test. Estimates of intellectual function can be made by asking the child questions on common topics.

Immediate recall is the ability to retain a concept for a short time, such as being able to remember a series of numbers and repeat them (a child of 4 years can usually repeat three digits; a child older than 6 years can repeat five digits). *Recent memory* covers a slightly longer period of time. To measure this, show the preschool child an object such as a key and ask the child to remember it because later you will ask him or her to tell you what it was. After about 5 minutes, ask whether the child remembers what object you showed him or her. Ask older children what they ate for breakfast to test recent memory.

Remote memory is long-term recall. Ask preschoolers what they ate for breakfast that morning or for dinner the night before because, for them, that was a long time ago; ask older children what was the name of their first-grade teacher because most people remember this information their whole life.

Specific cerebral function can be measured by assessing language, sensory interpretation, and motor integration. When assessing language, listen to the child's ability to articulate. Remember, when listening to speech, many preschoolers substitute "w" for "r," saying "west time" instead of "rest time"; be aware that pronunciation is altered if English is not the child's primary language.

Stereognosis refers to the ability of a child to recognize an object by touch; it is a test of sensory interpretation. For this, ask a child to close his or her eyes and then place a familiar object, such as a key, a penny, or a bottle cap, in her hand and ask her to identify it. This is a skill even preschoolers are able to do successfully.

Graphesthesia is the ability to recognize a shape that has been traced on the skin. Ask a child to close his or her eyes; trace first a circle and then a square on the back of his or her hand and then ask him or her whether the shapes are the same or different. Be sure the child understands the concept

BOX 49.2

Nursing Care Planning Using Assessment

ASSESSING A CHILD FOR SIGNS AND SYMPTOMS OF A NEUROLOGIC DISORDER

History
Chief concern: Seizure, loss of consciousness, delay in developmental tasks, headache, clumsiness at motor tasks.
Past medical history: Infection during pregnancy; difficult birth; difficulty with initiating respirations at birth; head injury from fall or unintentional injury.
Family medical history: History of seizures or headaches in other family members.

Physical examination

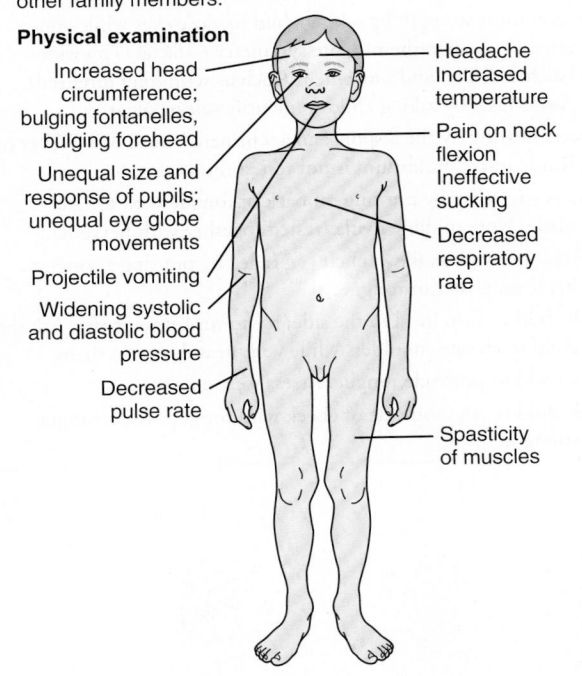

Increased head circumference; bulging fontanelles, bulging forehead

Unequal size and response of pupils; unequal eye globe movements

Projectile vomiting

Widening systolic and diastolic blood pressure

Decreased pulse rate

Headache Increased temperature

Pain on neck flexion Ineffective sucking

Decreased respiratory rate

Spasticity of muscles

of "different" by first showing him or her objects such as two keys and a bottle cap and documenting that he or she is able to identify the keys as being the same and the bottle cap as being different. For older children, trace numbers (8, 3, 0, and 1 work well) and ask the child to identify each one.

Kinesthesia is the ability to distinguish movement. Have a child close her eyes and extend her hands in front of her. Raise one of her fingers and ask her whether it is up or down. Hold the finger by its sides so that your other fingers do not brush against the child's palm or the back of her hand and reveal the finger position. Repeat the same movement with a toe on each foot. For preschoolers, be certain to first determine whether the child understands the concept of up and down.

To measure motor integration, ask a child to perform a complex motor skill, such as folding a piece of paper and putting it into an envelope. A child of 4 years or older should be able to do this neatly.

Remember, children do best when these tests are presented as a game. Be certain to convey that there are no right or wrong answers. A child who believes that he or she has failed these tests may not respond well to further testing.

Cranial Nerve Function

Testing for cranial nerve function consists of assessing each pair of cranial nerves separately. Cranial nerves and methods of cranial nerve testing are described in Table 49.2. Methods to test pupil constriction and ability to follow into fields of gaze are described in Chapter 34.

Cerebellar Function

Tests for cerebellar function are tests for balance and coordination. To test these, observe the child walk to assess whether the walk is natural (most children walk at least a little self-consciously when they know they are being observed, so watch them also as they enter the exam room and move around for other activities). Ask the child to stand on one foot; a child as young as 4 years should be able to do this for as long as 5 seconds. Ask the child to attempt a tandem walk (walk a straight line, one foot directly in front of the other, heel touching toe) (Fig. 49.2A). A child older than 4 years of age should be able to do this for about four consecutive steps. Ask the child to touch his or her nose with his or her finger and then to reach and touch your finger with the same hand (held about 1½ feet in front of the child) (see Fig. 49.2B). Tell the child to repeat this action and move your finger to a new position each time. The average child rarely reaches past your finger or stops before touching it.

Ask the child to pat one knee with the palm of the hand and then quickly turn the hand over and pat the knee with the back of the hand; repeat over and over, one hand at a time. The majority of children are able to do this rapid, coordinated motion without much difficulty. Preschoolers will "mirror" the movement of the actively moving hand by moving the inactive hand as well. Older children should not demonstrate this (or should show only a small amount of movement).

Other tests are to ask the child to touch each finger on one hand with the thumb of that hand in rapid succession or ask the child to run the heel of one foot down the front of his or her other leg while he or she is lying supine (children should be able to do this without "running off" the leg). With the child lying on the examining table, ask the child to close his or her eyes and draw a circle or figure 8 in the air with his or her foot (children should also be able to do this without difficulty).

Tests of cerebellar function such as these are fun for children to do as long as they know that there are no passes or failures. Show approval for effort even if they are having difficulty with a task so that they have confidence to try another one.

Motor Function

Motor function is measured by evaluating muscle size, strength, and tone. Begin by comparing the size and symmetry of extremities. If in doubt about either of these, measure the circumference of the calves and thighs or upper and lower arms with a tape measure. Palpate muscles for tone. Move the extremities through passive range of motion to evaluate symmetry, spasticity, and flaccidity bilaterally. To test for strength, ask the child to extend her arms in front of her and then resist your action as you push down or up on her hands or push them out to the side. Do the same with the lower extremities.

Sensory Function

If children's sensory systems are intact, they should be able to distinguish light touch, pain, vibration, hot, and cold. Have a

TABLE 49.2 CRANIAL NERVE FUNCTION

Cranial Nerve	Function	Assessment
I (olfactory)	Sense of smell	Assess child's ability to recognize common odors such as peanut butter or an orange while eyes are closed.
II (optic)	Vision	Assess vision fields and visual acuity; examine retinas.
III (oculomotor)	Motor control and sensation for eye muscles and upper eyelid	Assess pupillary size, equality, reaction to light, and ability to follow an object in all directions. Note any nystagmus (an abnormal jerking motion).
IV (trochlear)	Movement of major eye globe muscles	As for nerve III
V (trigeminal)	Mastication muscles and some facial sensations	Assess ability to discern light touch to test sensory component; assess symmetry and strength of bite to test motor component.
VI (abducens)	Movement and muscle sense of eye globe	As for nerves III and IV
VII (facial)	Impulses for facial muscles, salivation, and taste	Assess motor strength by asking child to close eyes while you attempt to open them. Note symmetry of facial expression (such as smile) and movement (such as wrinkling forehead). Assess taste by asking child to identify salt or sugar.
VIII (acoustic)	Equilibrium and hearing	Assess hearing by the response to a whispered word or a Weber or Rinne test. Equilibrium is not tested routinely.
IX (glossopharyngeal)	Motor impulses to heart; sensation from pharynx, thorax, and abdominal organs	Assess gag reflex by pressing on back of tongue with tongue blade. Note midline uvula (tested together with nerve X).
X (vagus)	Swallowing and gag reflexes	Assess ability to swallow; elicit gag reflex by pressing a tongue blade on posterior tongue.
XI (accessory)	Impulses to striated muscles of pharynx and shoulders	Ask child to turn head to the side; try to turn it to center. Ask the child to elevate shoulders while you press down on them.
XII (hypoglossal)	Motor impulses to tongue and skeletal muscles; sensation from skin and viscera	Ask child to protrude tongue. Assess for tremors. Ask child to press on side of cheek with tongue; assess tongue strength.

Figure 49.2 Cerebellar function tests. **(A)** A child attempting a tandem walk. **(B)** Nose-to-finger test. (© Lesha Photography.)

child close his or her eyes and then ask the child to point to the spot where you touch him or her with an object. Light touch is tested by using a wisp of cotton, deep pressure by pressure of your finger, pain by a safety pin, and temperature by water bottles filled with hot or cold water. Vibration is tested by touching the child's bony prominences (iliac crest, elbows, knees) with a vibrating tuning fork. Warn the child that on pin testing, he or she will feel a momentary prick. Otherwise, the child may be unwilling to close his or her eyes again for further testing.

Reflex Testing

Deep tendon reflex testing, which is part of a primary physical assessment (see Chapter 34), is also a basic part of a neurologic assessment. In newborns, reflex testing is especially important because the infant cannot perform tasks on command to demonstrate the full range of neurologic function (see Chapter 18).

QSEN Checkpoint Question 49.1

PATIENT-CENTERED CARE

Tasha, 3 years old, is scheduled for a full neurologic examination. What explanation would best prepare her for this?
   a. "You'll need to answer questions carefully so you can pass this test."
   b. "I'll be asking you to move in different ways, almost like a game."
   c. "I need to find out how healthy or unhealthy your brain seems to be."
   d. "Seizures can be caused by a brain tumor, so that needs to be ruled out."

Look in Appendix A for the best answer and rationale.

DIAGNOSTIC TESTING

A variety of diagnostic tests may be prescribed to provide additional information should any abnormalities be detected in the health history, physical examination, or neurologic examination. Many of these tests are invasive, so if you are scheduling these, be certain both the child and family are well prepared for these procedures; try to schedule the least invasive procedures first to better elicit the child's cooperation. So explanations will be well understood, take into account not

only the child's chronologic age but also the child's level of cognitive functioning. Provide an explanation that includes not only physically what will happen but also a description of any sensory experiences the child might undergo such as anything he or she might feel, hear, smell, or taste.

Lumbar Puncture

Lumbar puncture, the introduction of a needle into the subarachnoid space (under the arachnoid membrane) at the level of L4 or L5 to withdraw CSF for analysis, is used most frequently with children to diagnose hemorrhage or infection in the CNS or to diagnose an obstruction of CSF flow. The procedure is contraindicated if the skin over the needle insertion site is infected (to avoid introducing pathogens into the CSF) or if there is a suspected elevation of CSF pressure (if intracranial pressure [ICP] is elevated, the higher pressure in the intracranial space could cause the brainstem to be drawn down into the spinal cord space, compressing the medulla and compromising the action of the cardiac and respiratory centers). To limit pain, EMLA or lidocaine cream should be applied to the puncture site 1 hour before the procedure. Alternatively, the child may be administered conscious sedation for the procedure (see Chapter 39).

For a lumbar puncture, a newborn is seated upright with the head bent forward (Fig. 49.3A). The older infant or child is placed on one side on the examining table. Help the child flex the head forward, flex the knees against the abdomen, and arch the back as much as possible; this position opens the space between the lumbar vertebrae, facilitating needle insertion (see Fig. 49.3B). You might describe the position as "rolling into a ball" or "folding up like an astronaut in a small spaceship" to associate it with something the child knows about. Children younger than school age need to be held in this position because they may be so frightened by someone working on their back unseen that they are unable to hold this arched position (they try to turn over or turn their head to see what is happening). It helps a school-age child or adolescent if you stand by the table facing him or her and gently rest your hand on the back of the head, as a reminder to keep it bent forward. Talking quietly with the child not only assists in calming the child but also helps assess the child's respiratory status as the child is "curled up." Closely observe an infant for any respiratory distress.

Children need good preparation for a lumbar puncture because they cannot see what is happening. Be certain they know the healthcare provider performing the procedure will

Figure 49.3   (A) Positioning an infant for a lumbar puncture. (© Barbara Proud.) **(B)** Positioning an older child for a lumbar puncture.

wash their back with a solution that feels cold and then inject a local anesthetic that might sting for a moment (if an analgesic cream was not applied before the procedure). Caution children they will feel pressure but not pain as the lumbar puncture needle is inserted. Occasionally, the needle will press against a dorsal nerve root and the child will experience a shooting pain down one leg. If this happens, reassure the child this feeling passes quickly and does not indicate an injury.

When the insertion stylette is removed and CSF drips from the end of the needle, the procedure has been successful. An initial pressure reading is made. To confirm the subarachnoid space in the cord is patent with that in the skull, the examiner may ask a child who is older than 3 years of age to cough; for an infant, the examiner may ask you to press on the child's external jugular vein. If either of these measures causes an increase of CSF pressure, it indicates that fluid is flowing freely through the subarachnoid space. Typically, three tubes of CSF, containing 2 to 3 ml each, are collected; a closing pressure reading is taken; and the needle is withdrawn. Samples are usually sent for culture, sensitivity, glucose level, and presence of red blood cells. The first sample obtained may contain blood or skin pathogens from the puncture, so it should not be the sample sent for determination of red blood cell content or culture. Additional evaluations requested might be albumin/globulin ratio or gamma-globulin level (an increased level of gamma-globulin is suggestive of multiple sclerosis or meningitis).

Lumbar puncture involves at least momentary pain, so children need to be comforted afterward. A few children may develop a headache after a lumbar puncture as a result of the reduction in CSF volume or invasion of a small air pocket during the puncture, although this is rare because of the small-sized needle used. Encourage the child to lie flat for at least 30 minutes and to drink a glass of fluid afterward to help prevent cerebral irritation caused by air rising in the subarachnoid space and to help increase the amount of CSF quickly. Encourage parents to hold an infant in a flat position across their knees. If the child develops a headache despite the precautions taken, an analgesic can be given for pain relief.

If a child had minimally increased CSF pressure at the time of the puncture, closely observe the child after the procedure to detect respiratory and cardiac difficulty from medulla pressure. An increase in blood pressure or a decrease in pulse and respiration rates, a change in consciousness, pupillary changes, or a decrease in motor ability are all important signs of increased intracranial compression.

QSEN Checkpoint Question 49.2

TEAMWORK & COLLABORATION

Tasha's diagnostic workup will include a lumbar puncture. When collaborating with the physician to perform this procedure, what nursing action should the nurse prioritize?

a. Explain to Tasha that her back will be washed with a cold liquid.
b. Apply EMLA cream to Tasha's lumbar region 5 to 10 minutes before the procedure.
c. Reassure Tasha that the procedure will not hurt.
d. Help Tasha into a prone position on the procedure table.

Look in Appendix A for the best answer and rationale.

Ventricular Tap

In infants, CSF may be obtained by a subdural tap into a ventricle through the anterior fontanelle. A small space on the scalp over the insertion site is shaved or clipped, and the area is prepared with an antiseptic. The infant's head must be held firmly in a supine position to prevent movement during the procedure so the needle does not strike and lacerate meningeal tissue.

Fluid must always be removed from this site slowly, rather than suddenly, to prevent a sudden shift in pressure that could cause intracranial hemorrhage. After the procedure, a pressure dressing is applied to the site, and the infant is placed in a semi-Fowler's position to prevent additional drainage from the puncture site. After the procedure, comfort the infant or allow the parents to do so to both reduce the stress of a painful procedure and prevent the infant from crying excessively, an action that could increase ICP and loss of additional CSF.

X-Ray Techniques

A flat-plate skull X-ray film may be used to obtain information about increased ICP or skull defects such as fracture or craniosynostosis (premature knitting of cranial sutures). Increased ICP is suggested if skull sutures appear separated on the X-ray. If the ICP is chronic, other subtle changes, such as a flattening of the sella turcica or an increase in the convolutions of the inner table of the skull, may be present.

Cerebral Angiography

Cerebral angiography is an X-ray study of cerebral blood vessels that involves the injection of a contrast material into the femoral or carotid artery. Serial X-rays are then taken as the dye flows through the blood vessels of the cerebrum, and any vessel defects or space-occupying lesions occluding cranial blood vessels are revealed.

Myelography

Myelography is the X-ray study of the spinal cord following the introduction of a contrast material into the CSF by lumbar puncture to reveal the presence of space-occupying lesions of the spinal cord. After the procedure, keep the head of the child's bed elevated to prevent contrast medium from reaching the meninges surrounding the brain and causing irritation.

Computed Tomography and Magnetic Resonance Imaging

Computed tomography (CT) involves the use of X-rays to reveal densities at multiple levels or layers of brain tissue and is helpful to confirm the presence of a brain tumor or other encroaching lesions. Single-photon emission computed tomography (SPECT) is a similar procedure used mainly for blood flow evaluation. Magnetic resonance imaging (MRI) uses magnetic fields to show differences in tissue composition, revealing normal versus abnormal brain tissue. Both CT and MRI are discussed in greater detail in Chapter 37.

Nuclear Medicine Studies (Brain Scan and Positron Emission Tomography)

Brain Scan

For a brain scan, a radioactive material is injected intravenously, and after a fixed time during which the injected material is deposited in cerebral tissue, radioactivity levels over the skull are measured. If the blood–brain barrier is not functioning, the radioactive material will accumulate in specific areas, suggesting possible tumor, subdural hematoma, abscess, or encephalitis.

Positron Emission Tomography

The diagnostic technique of positron emission tomography (PET) involves imaging after injection of positron-emitting radiopharmaceuticals into a vein. These radioactive substances accumulate at diseased areas of the brain or spinal cord. PET is extremely accurate in identifying seizure foci.

Echoencephalography (Ultrasound of Head or Spinal Cord)

Echoencephalography involves the projection of ultrasound (high-frequency sound waves above the audible range) toward the child's head or spinal cord (a type of ultrasound). The technique may be used to outline the ventricles of the brain. Because this technique of scanning is noninvasive, produces no discomfort, and has no known complications, it may be repeated frequently to monitor changes in the size of ventricles or an invading lesion and is particularly effective in infants with open fontanelles. This noninvasive technique is often used in neonatal intensive care units to monitor intraventricular hemorrhages and other problems frequently encountered by preterm infants.

Electroencephalography

The electroencephalogram (EEG) reflects the electrical patterns of the brain summarizing the physical and chemical interactions within the brain at the time of the test (Rapin, 2011). An EEG tracing typically indicates four types of waves: delta (1 to 3 waves per second), theta (4 to 7 waves per second), alpha (8 to 12 waves per second), and beta (13 to 20 waves per second).

To reduce extraneous movements of the eyes, head, or muscles that would affect the tracing, the child must be cooperative and quiet during the procedure. Traditionally, therefore, parents are asked to keep their child up later than usual the night before the exam so the child will fall asleep during the test. Educate children and their families that the room will be darkened to help them rest. Use terminology to describe the procedure in terms that the child can understand depending on age and development. Reassure them that attaching the small suction cups or leads is not painful. Use of terminology that is age appropriate will help to keep the patient and family at ease during the procedure.

Sedation or conscious sedation may be necessary for children who are unable to lie still during the procedure. The goals of sedation are to (a) assure the patient's safety and welfare, (b) assure minimal pain and discomfort during the procedure, (c) control the patient's anxiety with minimal psychological trauma, and (d) modify behavior and movements during the procedure (Coté & Wilson, 2016). For example, chloral hydrate, a frequently used sedative for this procedure, may increase the fast activity of brain waves; chlorpromazine (Thorazine) is known to increase slow activity. Because some seizure medications also cause changes in brain waves, be certain to note on the child's electronic record what medications the child is currently receiving. Parents should receive specific instructions whether antiseizure medication should be given on the morning of testing.

Although EEGs can show important information about brain activity, they are not helpful in all circumstances because about 15% of children who have no cranial trauma or seizure activity demonstrate some abnormality on an EEG. They may not reveal a brain tumor because most brain tumors in children are in the posterior fossa, which is not revealed on an EEG. On inspection of the symmetry of brain waves in different hemispheres, local lesions such as a hematoma may be suggested. An EEG is most beneficial in diagnosing absence seizures. The typical pattern with this disorder is discussed later in this chapter.

Visual stimulation, such as having a child look at a whirling disk, may be used in connection with an EEG because various types of electrical discharges increase with rapid eye movements. In a child who is sensitive to this type of stimulation, the testing may produce a seizure; therefore, it is up to the prescriber to decide if the benefits outweigh the possible effects. Following an EEG, children will be sleepy if they have been sedated or had an EEG while sleep-deprived. Allow them to sleep as long as needed.

Health Promotion and Risk Management

Health promotion for the nervous system begins prenatally with measures to ensure optimal fetal growth and development and prevention of problems associated with anoxia. It continues throughout childhood with routine health maintenance visits, screening for possible neurologic or developmental problems, and timely immunizations to prevent sequelae of childhood infections such as measles or chickenpox. Nurses play a key role in providing education to parents about the importance of prenatal care, obtaining immunizations, and completing medication therapy to ensure complete resolution of an infection.

Nurses are able to provide parents with anticipatory guidance about safety measures to prevent injury, specifically, head and spinal cord injury by the use of seat belts or child restraints while riding in automobiles and protective gear when playing contact sports. Remind parents and children to wear helmets when riding or using anything that can move faster than the child can run such as scooters, roller skates/rollerblades, ice skates, horses, skis, skateboards or snowboards, bicycles, or motorcycles (Riesch, Kedrowski, Brown, et al., 2012). For a child with a long-term neurologic disorder, rehabilitation and early intervention play a major role in reducing the risk of complications and in promoting the child's and family's optimal level of functioning.

Increased Intracranial Pressure

Increased ICP is not a single disorder but a group of signs and symptoms that occur with many neurologic disorders (Table 49.3). It is important to assess for signs and symptoms when caring for a child with a potential neurologic disorder (Sigurtà, Zanaboni, Canavesi, et al., 2013). Increased ICP occurs because of an increase in the CSF volume, blood entering the CSF, cerebral edema, head trauma or infection,

TABLE 49.3 SIGNS AND SYMPTOMS OF INCREASED INTRACRANIAL PRESSURE

Sign or Symptom	Indication of Increased Intracranial Pressure
Increased head circumference	An increase >2 cm per month in first 3 months of life, >1 cm per month in the second 3 months, and >0.5 cm per month for the next 6 months
Fontanelle changes	Anterior fontanelle tense and bulging; closing late
Vomiting	Occurring in the absence of nausea, on awakening in morning or after nap; possibly projectile
Eye changes	Diplopia (double vision) from pressure on abducens nerves; white of sclera evident over pupil (setting sun sign); limited visual fields, papilledema
Vital sign changes	Elevated temperature and blood pressure; decreased pulse and respiration rates
Pain	Headache, often present on awakening and standing; increasing with straining at stool (Valsalva maneuver) or holding breath
Mentation	Irritability, altered consciousness such as sleepiness

space-occupying lesions such as brain tumors, or the development of hydrocephalus or Guillain-Barré syndrome.

The rate at which symptoms develop depends on the cause and the ability of the child's skull to expand to accommodate the increased pressure. Children with open fontanelles, for example, can withstand more pressure without brain damage than older children, whose suture lines and fontanelles have closed.

ASSESSMENT

Assessment of ICP may involve only a few quick procedures, such as obtaining vital signs, evaluating pupil response, and determining levels of consciousness, motor, and sensory function, or it may include more elaborate electronic monitoring.

Because symptoms are subtle at first, the initial signs children may show are headache, irritability, or restlessness. Growing pressure on the brainstem, which controls respiration and cardiac activity, soon causes pulse and respiration rates to slow. Compression of cranial vessels leads to a compensatory increase in blood pressure (or **pulse pressure**, the gap between the systolic and diastolic blood pressures). Pressure on the hypothalamus, the temperature-regulating center of the body, causes an increase in body temperature. An older child may be able to report symptoms such as diplopia (double vision). On funduscopic examination, papilledema may be detected. Compare a new assessment against all recordings taken in the last 24 hours so a progressive change can be detected.

If ocular changes such as a dilated pupil occur, this indicates pressure is increasing posterior to the eye globe, causing compression of the second cranial nerve. Record any tendency toward strabismus, nystagmus (constant eye movement), or "sunset eyes" (white sclera showing over the top of the cornea) or inability to follow the light into any quadrant. Be sure to be specific about what you document. "Inability to follow light," for example, is not as informative as "Inability to follow light into left superior field; vertical nystagmus noted as child follows light into other fields."

An additional test for ICP is a "doll's eye" reflex. If a child lies supine and you turn his or her head gently but rapidly to the right, the eyes will normally turn toward the left, and vice versa. If a child has increased ICP, this phenomenon will be absent (a test useful in assessing a comatose child who is unable to cooperate by following a light).

Assess the child's level of consciousness because if the child is alert but unable to comprehend surroundings, time, or place, this may be the first indication of increased ICP. As pressure continues to increase, a pseudo-awake state will occur, in which the child is awake but unable to follow light or locate a noise. Finally, the child becomes fully comatose, unable to be roused by any stimuli. Levels of coma are rated by the Glasgow Coma Scale, discussed in Chapter 52 in connection with assessment for head trauma.

Children, like adults, generally become disoriented about time first, then place, and then self. Explain to the parent and child that you will be periodically asking seemingly simple questions, such as asking the child for his or her name or to identify the day of the week. Let them know that it is important for the child to answer the questions if the child is able in order to understand the child's level of consciousness.

Be aware that many children, even when healthy, are groggy when they first awaken, especially if they have been dreaming. Make sure children are fully awake, therefore, before attempting to determine level of consciousness. Ask questions appropriate to the child's age. Preschoolers, for example, do not usually know their whole name or the day of the week and may not know concepts such as *morning* or *night*. To assess consciousness in children this age, it is often more productive, every hour, to show them a colored block, a piece of fruit, or a cartoon character known to the child and ask them to name it.

A good way to test an infant's level of consciousness is to determine whether the child responds to sounds, such as a familiar music box or voices, or reaches for an attractive object you offer. Motor ability can be assessed by asking a child to perform some simple motor tasks, such as squeezing your hands, pushing against your hands with both feet, or performing rapid, alternating hand movements, such as turning a hand over and back several times. Evaluate cranial nerves grossly by having the child make a face, close the eyes tightly, or smile. Evaluate whether the facial responses are equal and symmetric bilaterally. Test deep tendon reflexes because these decrease in intensity with decreased level of consciousness.

As a final assessment, carefully observe the child's resting posture because when motor control grows weaker because of loss of cell function, characteristic posturing (primitive reflexes) occurs. Cerebral loss is shown mainly by **decorticate posturing**: the child's arms are adducted and flexed on the chest with wrists flexed, hands fisted; the lower extremities are extended and internally rotated; the feet are plantar flexed (Fig. 49.4A). **Decerebrate posturing**, which occurs when the midbrain is not functional, is characterized by rigid extension

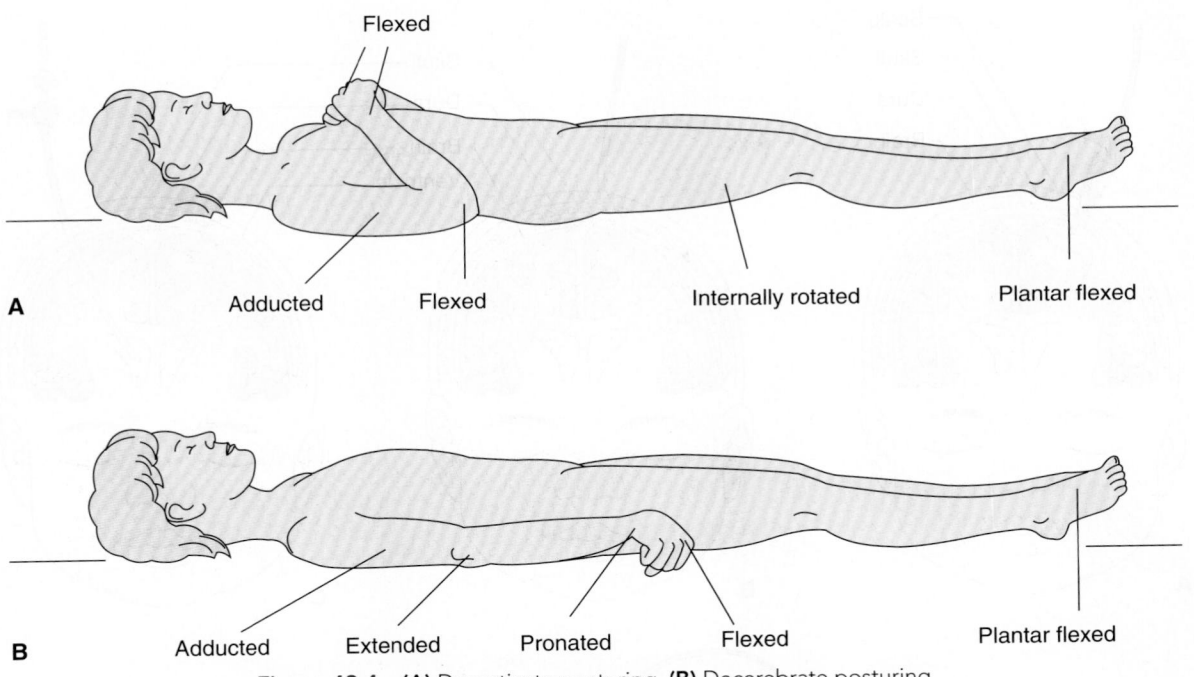

Flexed

A   Adducted   Flexed   Internally rotated   Plantar flexed

B   Adducted   Extended   Pronated   Flexed   Plantar flexed

Figure 49.4   (A) Decorticate posturing. **(B)** Decerebrate posturing.

and adduction of the arms and pronation of the wrists with the fingers flexed; the legs are held extended with the feet plantar flexed (see Fig. 49.4B).

Seizures are a sign of increased ICP, so if these occur, the child's ICP is becoming greatly compromised.

INTRACRANIAL PRESSURE MONITORING

ICP can be measured by several additional methods:
- An intraventricular catheter inserted through the anterior fontanelle
- A subdural screw or bolt inserted through a burr hole in the skull
- A fiberoptic sensor implanted into the epidural space (or the anterior fontanelle in an infant) (Fig. 49.5)

Intraventricular catheters (see Fig. 49.5C) are threaded into the lateral ventricle, filled with normal saline, and then connected to an external pressure monitor (Bailey, Liesemer, Statler, et al., 2012). As pressure in the ventricle fluctuates, it registers through the filled catheter onto an oscilloscope screen plus a written printout. This method is advantageous over simple scanning because it also enables CSF drainage and administration of medication through the catheter.

ICP in children normally ranges from 1 to 10 mmHg; a level greater than 15 mmHg needs further assessment. As blood pressure rises and falls with the influx of blood through vessels, so does ICP. On a monitor, this appears as A waves (plateau waves), B waves (short-duration waves), or C waves (small, rhythmic bursts). If brain ischemia is present, wave patterns change even before there is a deviation in blood pressure or pulse rate (Fig. 49.6). Because A waves appear to reflect brain ischemia, they can be used to signal when a child needs more oxygen.

ICP monitoring also supplies information on cerebral perfusion pressure (CPP) or the amount of cerebral blood flow available to the brain (Box 49.3) because, if ICP ever exceeds arterial blood pressure (arises above about 50 mmHg),

cerebral vessels can become obstructed (Budohoski, Zweifel, Kasprowicz, et al., 2012).

Parents can have difficulty accepting procedures such as the insertion of intraventricular catheters or screws. Explaining the brain's anatomy can help them understand that the catheter or screw is inserted into a hollow space and thus does not puncture or tear brain tissue. Be sure to explain that this type of monitoring is advantageous not only because it enables early detection should problems arise but also because it helps to reduce the risk of further injury or complications.

THERAPEUTIC MANAGEMENT

The cause of ICP must be identified and remedied as quickly as possible to prevent brain injury or compression to the brainstem, which can lead to both cardiac and respiratory failure. Actions such as coughing, vomiting, and sneezing and rapid administration of intravenous (IV) fluid increase ICP. When a parent is burping an infant after a feeding, caution them to be careful not to put pressure on the jugular veins because this is another action that increases ICP. Placing a child in a semi-Fowler's position (use an infant seat for babies) or administering a corticosteroid such as dexamethasone (Decadron) can effectively reduce cerebral edema and its accompanying pressure. An osmotic diuretic, such as mannitol, given IV, causes a shift of fluid from extravascular compartments into the vascular stream (from brain tissue into blood vessels), so it also reduces pressure. Children usually have an indwelling urinary catheter inserted before beginning an osmotic diuretic to ensure that the child's kidneys are able to successfully excrete the intravessel fluid and prevent back pressure on the heart. If the ICP is caused by excessive fluid accumulating in the brain's ventricles, a ventricular tap may be necessary for immediate reduction of pressure.

Because increased ICP is a sign of an underlying disorder, after the pressure is reduced, the underlying cause must then be identified and rectified or the pressure will rise again from the original disorder.

Figure 49.5 Devices used to monitor intracranial pressure. **(A)** Subarachnoid screw. **(B)** Epidural sensor. **(C)** Intraventricular catheter. **(D)** Intraparenchymal monitoring.

Neural Tube Disorders

The neural tube is the embryonic structure that matures to form the CNS. Because this structure first forms in utero as a flat plate and then molds to form the brain and cord, it is susceptible to malformation. The disorders that occur as a result, such as spina bifida, are present at birth and are discussed in Chapter 27.

Neurocutaneous Syndromes

Neurocutaneous syndromes are characterized by the presence of skin or pigment disorders with CNS dysfunction.

STURGE-WEBER SYNDROME

A child with Sturge-Weber syndrome (encephalofacial angiomatosis) has a congenital port-wine birthmark on the skin of the upper part of the face that follows the distribution of the first division of the fifth cranial nerve (trigeminal nerve). Because the lesion is usually unilateral, the port-wine stain ends abruptly at the midline, although it may extend inward at that point to the meninges and choroid plexus. If the disorder is limited to the ophthalmic branch of the fifth nerve, the lesion is usually confined to the upper aspect of the face.

Because of involvement of the meningeal blood vessels, blood flow can be sluggish, and anoxia may develop in some portions of the cerebral cortex. The child will develop symptoms of hemiparesis (numbness) on the side opposite the lesion from destruction of motor neurons. Intractable seizures, a cognitive challenge, or blindness caused by glaucoma may also be present. A CT scan or an MRI of the skull usually demonstrates calcification of the involved cerebral cortex, which appears as a "railroad track" or double-groove pattern on the CT or MRI screen. An EEG usually shows decreased voltage in the affected areas.

When this syndrome is first diagnosed, parents may ask to have the skin lesion surgically removed in the belief that this will correct their child's condition. Unfortunately, because the lesion is not just a surface phenomenon, it's important that parents understand the need for long-term follow-up, particularly if the child has accompanying seizures that require long-term antiseizure therapy (Lo, Marchuk, Ball, et al., 2012).

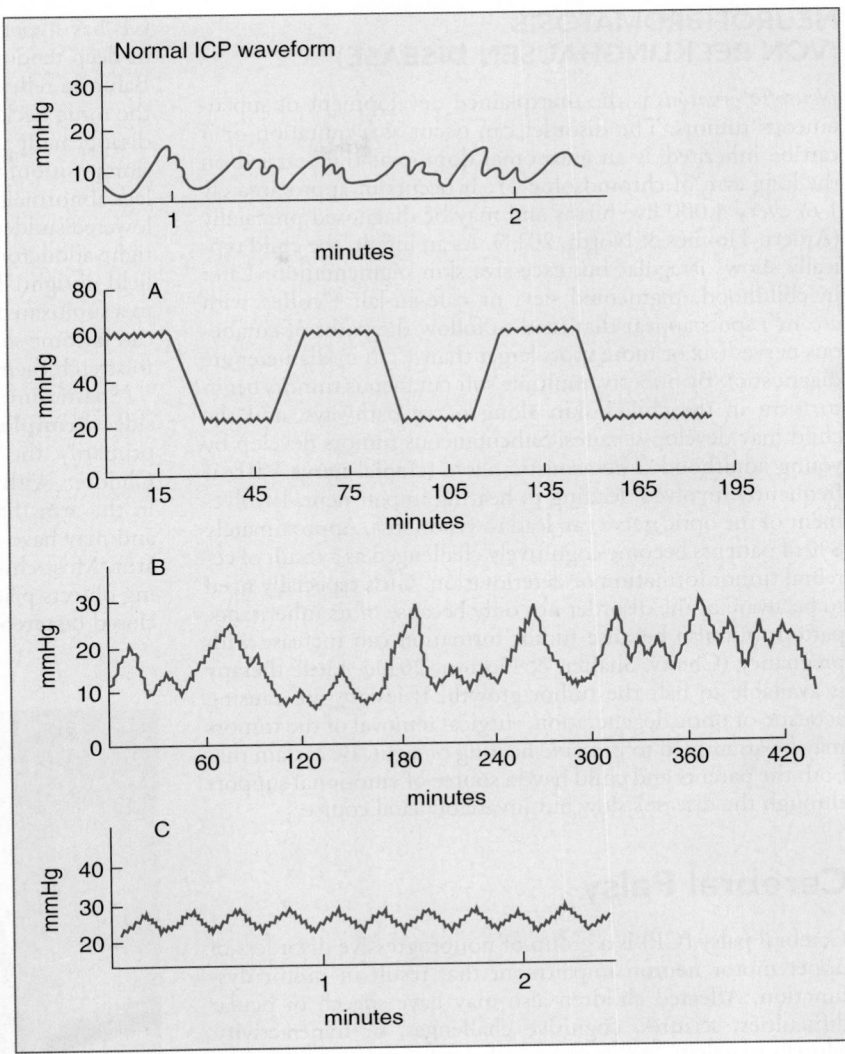

Figure 49.6 Normal intracranial pressure (ICP) waveform and generalized shapes of the three types of ICP waves: A waves or plateau waves, B waves, and C waves.

BOX 49.3

Calculating Cerebral Perfusion Pressure

Cerebral perfusion pressure (CPP) ranges from about 60 to 150 mmHg. If it is too low, it suggests blood is having difficulty circulating to brain cells; if it rises too high, it can also result in brain ischemia from the increased intracranial pressure (ICP). CPP is calculated by subtracting the mean ICP from the mean arterial pressure (MAP) or:

$$MAP - ICP = CPP$$

MAP is determined by subtracting the diastolic blood pressure (DBP) level from the systolic blood pressure (SBP) level, then dividing the result by 3, and adding that sum to 80 or:

$$MAP = \frac{(SBP - DBP)}{3} + 80$$

To calculate CPP in a child with a blood pressure of 100/70 mmHg and an ICP of 10 mmHg, for example, first calculate the MAP:

$$\frac{(100 - 70)}{3} + 80 = 90 \text{ mmHg}$$

Next, calculate the CPP:

$$90 - 10 = 80 \text{ mmHg (the child's CPP or a normal value)}$$

NEUROFIBROMATOSIS (VON RECKLINGHAUSEN DISEASE)

Neurofibromatosis is the unexplained development of subcutaneous tumors. The disorder can occur as a mutation or it can be inherited as an autosomal dominant trait carried on the long arm of chromosome 17. It occurs in approximately 1 of every 4,000 live births and may be diagnosed prenatally (Ardern-Holmes & North, 2011). As an infant, the child typically shows irregular but excessive skin pigmentation. Later in childhood, pigmented nevi or café-au-lait ("coffee with cream") spots appear that tend to follow the paths of cutaneous nerves (six or more spots larger than 1 cm in diameter are diagnostic). By puberty, multiple soft cutaneous tumors begin to form in the child's skin along nerve pathways, and the child may develop seizures. Subcutaneous tumors develop by young adulthood. The acoustic nerve (cranial nerve VIII) is frequently involved, leading to hearing impairment. Involvement of the optic nerve can lead to vision loss. Approximately 8% of patients become cognitively challenged as a result of cerebral tumor formation or deterioration. Girls especially need to be aware of the disorder not only because of its inheritance pattern but also because tumor formation can increase with pregnancy (Chetty, Shaffer, & Norton, 2011). Little therapy is available to halt the tumor growth. If lesions are causing acoustic or optic degeneration, surgical removal of the tumors may be attempted to preserve hearing or sight. Be certain that both the parents and child have a source of emotional support through the disease's slow but invariably fatal course.

Cerebral Palsy

Cerebral palsy (CP) is a group of nonprogressive disorders of upper motor neuron impairment that result in motor dysfunction. Affected children also may have speech or ocular difficulties, seizures, cognitive challenges, or hyperactivity. Muscle spasticity can lead to orthopedic or gait difficulties (Crosbie, Alhusaini, Dean, et al., 2012).

CP is caused by abnormal brain development or damage to the developing brain, leading to cell destruction of the motor tracts. Nutritional deficiencies, drug use, and maternal infections such as cytomegalovirus or toxoplasmosis, as well as direct birth injury, may also contribute to the cause.

CP occurs in approximately 2 of every 1,000 births, most frequently in very-low-birth-weight infants and those who are small for gestational age; it is increasing in incidence because of the number of very-low-birth-weight infants who survive today. Head injury such as from child maltreatment or automobile accidents also may lead to CP symptoms. Infections such as meningitis or encephalitis can result in CP symptoms as well.

TYPES OF CEREBRAL PALSY

There are four main types of CP: a pyramidal or spastic type (approximately 40% of affected children), an extrapyramidal (dyskinetic) type, ataxic, and mixed (Centers for Disease Control and Prevention, 2017).

Spastic Type

Spasticity is excessive tone in the voluntary muscles that results from loss of upper motor neurons. A child with spastic

CP has hypertonic muscles, abnormal clonus, exaggeration of deep tendon reflexes, abnormal reflexes such as a positive Babinski reflex, and continuation of neonatal reflexes, such as the tonic neck reflex, well past the age at which these usually disappear. If infants with CP are held in a ventral suspension position, they arch their backs and extend their arms and legs abnormally. They fail to demonstrate a parachute reflex if lowered suddenly and tend to assume a "scissors gait" because tight adductor thigh muscles cause their legs to cross when held upright. This involvement may be so severe that it leads to a subluxated hip. By school age, tightening of the heel cord can become so severe that children walk on their toes, unable to stretch their heel to touch the ground (Fig. 49.7).

Spastic involvement may affect both extremities on one side (**hemiplegia**), all four extremities (**quadriplegia**), or primarily the lower extremities (**diplegia** or **paraplegia**). Children with hemiplegia usually have greater involvement in the arm than the leg. The involved arm may be shorter and may have a smaller muscle circumference than the other arm. Most children with hemiplegia have difficulty identifying objects placed in their involved hand when their eyes are closed (**astereognosis**).

Figure 49.7 Physical therapy can help a child with cerebral palsy to lengthen the heel cords. (© Tina Manley/Alamy.)

In older children, leg involvement may be detected most easily by examining the child's shoes as, because the child does not put the heel all the way down on the involved side, one shoe heel will be much more worn than the other. On physical examination, it may be difficult to abduct the involved hip fully, extend the knee, or dorsiflex the foot.

A child with quadriplegia invariably has impaired speech (pseudobulbar palsy) but may or may not be cognitively challenged. Swallowing saliva may be so difficult that the child drools and has difficulty swallowing food (Lewis, 2011).

Dyskinetic or Athetoid Type

The athetoid type of CP involves abnormal involuntary movement (*athetoid* means "wormlike"). Early in life, the child appears limp and flaccid. Later, in place of voluntary movement, children make slow, writhing motions. This can involve all four extremities plus the face, neck, and tongue. Because of the poor tongue and swallowing movements, the child drools and speech is difficult to understand. Under emotional stress, the involuntary movements may become irregular and jerking (**choreoid**) with disordered muscle tone (**dyskinetic**).

Ataxic Type

Children with ataxic involvement have an awkward, wide-based gait. On neurologic examination, they are unable to perform fine coordinated motions, the finger-to-nose test, or rapid, repetitive movements (tests of cerebellar function).

Mixed Type

Some children show symptoms of both spasticity and athetoid or ataxic and athetoid movements. This combination obviously results in a severe degree of physical impairment.

ASSESSMENT

The diagnosis of CP is based on history and physical assessment. Any episode of possible anoxia during prenatal life or at birth should be documented. Determining the extent of involvement in an infant is difficult, so the full extent of the disorder may not be recognized until the child attempts complex motor skills, such as walking or coloring.

Children with all forms of CP may have sensory alterations such as strabismus, refractive disorders, visual perception problems, visual field defects, and speech disorders such as abnormal rhythm or articulation. They may show an attention deficit disorder or autism spectrum syndrome. Cognitive challenge and recurrent seizures also frequently accompany all types of the disorder. A skull X-ray or ultrasound may show cerebral asymmetry. An EEG may be abnormal, although the pattern is highly variable.

Nursing Diagnoses and Related Interventions

Parents who are reacting to the news that their child has multiple physical disabilities often find it difficult to make long-range plans. Therefore, try to focus expected outcomes on short-term concerns to assist with family functioning.

Nursing Diagnosis: Deficient knowledge related to understanding of complex disease condition

Outcome Evaluation: Parents state that they understand the cause of the disease is unknown but it is not progressive.

It's important for parents to understand that CP is nonprogressive and that the brain damage that occurred during pregnancy or at birth will not extend. The child's condition may seem to grow more apparent with age, however, as the child is expected to complete fine motor tasks. Without follow-up care, contractures from spasticity can result, further reducing existing motor function.

Caution parents also that CP is a single name for a wide variety of disorders of varying consequence. Although another child they know may have such severe CP that he has no useful function in his extremities, this does not mean their own child will be affected to the same extent. Conversely, although they know someone with CP who is able to hold a full-time job, their child may not be able to do so as well. Each child needs individual assessment so the child's maximum potential can be evaluated.

Nursing Diagnosis: Risk for disuse syndrome related to spasticity of muscle groups

Outcome Evaluation: Child walks with a minimum of support or equipment; skin and tissue remain intact.

Children with CP need promotion of any function that is not already impaired to prevent further loss of function and allow them to master the highest level of self-care, communication, ambulation, education, nutrition, and establishment of self-esteem they can achieve.

Learning to be ambulatory is an important part of self-care because it plays a large role in determining how independent the child can become. Walking can be difficult for the child to master because of lack of muscle coordination. Following surgery to lengthen heel tendons, assisted ambulation devices such as wheeled walkers may be necessary (Fig. 49.8). There are no drugs that cure CP, but a number can help relieve spasticity. Dopaminergic drugs, such as carbidopa/levodopa (Sinemet), widely used in Parkinson disease, increase the level of dopamine and, therefore, reduce rigidity. Muscle relaxants such as baclofen (Lioresal), given either orally or administered continuously by an infusion pump, and benzodiazepines such as diazepam (Valium) can also help with smoother muscle movement (Gray, Morton, Brimlow, et al., 2012). Administration of botulinum toxin (Botox) has been successful in some children to relieve spasticity and aid in walking (Placzek, Siebold, & Funk, 2010). Cerebellar pacemakers and vagal stimulation are future therapy options.

Preventing contractures is vitally important to maintain motor function. To help avoid these, teach parents that the passive exercises and games their child has been prescribed are an important part of their child's therapy and must be done consistently each day. To further prevent contractures, partial lightweight leg braces may be prescribed to encourage children to bring their heels down and to keep heel cords from tightening. If leg braces are prescribed, parents may need some encouragement and support to insist a child wears them because it is the constant stretching that offers best results.

Figure 49.8 Wheeled walkers give a child added stability for walking and keep heel cords from shortening. (© fotosearch.com.)

Nursing Diagnosis: Risk for self-care deficit related to impaired mobility

Outcome Evaluation: Child feeds and dresses self and manages elimination independently.

Children need to learn self-care measures such as dressing, tooth brushing, bathing, and toileting, so they can not only gain self-esteem by accomplishing these tasks but also achieve optimal independence. Modifications such as straps attached to their toothbrush or feeding utensils may be necessary so they can hold them more securely. Advise parents to always supervise children during bathing because lack of coordination could cause them to slip under water and drown. Toileting is often difficult because the child does not have the muscle group coordination necessary to achieve successful bowel evacuation. A high-fiber diet helps prevent constipation and aids bowel evacuation. Voiding may be equally difficult because the child may lack sufficient voluntary muscle control.

Parents may need considerable support and guidance to allow a child to complete self-care tasks independently because doing so often requires extreme patience. Letting a child perform these activities, however, helps to instill confidence and self-esteem in the child and helps allow the child to reach his or her maximum potential.

Nursing Diagnosis: Risk for delayed growth and development related to activity restriction secondary to CP

Outcome Evaluation: Child receives environmental stimulation; expresses interest in people and activities around him or her; attends school setting that is as free of restrictions as possible.

Children with CP may be unable to pursue stimulating activities and surroundings because they are not fully mobile. Therefore, encourage parents to bring these things to them as well as be certain that toys and activities are appropriate to the child's intellectual, developmental, and motor levels, not the child's chronologic age. Some children need more stimulating activities than others because they have difficulty concentrating on one activity for any length of time.

A preschool program is important to provide exposure to the outside world. If at all possible, school-age children with CP should be mainstreamed so that they can learn alongside other children. You may need to advocate that a child be placed in a school setting that is consistent with intellectual abilities.

Nursing Diagnosis: Risk for imbalanced nutrition, less than body requirements, related to difficulty sucking in infancy or difficulty feeding self in an older child

Outcome Evaluation: Child's weight remains within 5th to 95th percentile on height–weight chart; skin turgor remains good; specific gravity of urine is 1.003 to 1.030.

Providing adequate nutrition to children with CP can be difficult because they often have difficulty sucking because uncoordinated movements of the tongue, lips, and jaw and tongue thrusting make this difficult. They may tend to push food out of their mouth (a retained primitive reflex) rather than swallow smoothly. Older children may have difficulty holding and controlling a spoon to bring food to their mouths. Parents may need guidance in finding a feeding pattern that works for their child. Manually controlling the jaw may help control the head, correct neck and trunk hyperextension, and stabilize the jaw to assist with feeding. If a child cannot chew or swallow well, a liquid or soft diet may be necessary. A hyperactive gag reflex or symptoms of gastroesophageal reflux may cause children to vomit after feeding. Positioning infants upright after feeding helps to prevent aspiration if vomiting occurs.

Nursing Diagnosis: Impaired verbal communication related to neurologic impairment

Outcome Evaluation: Child can verbally make needs known to strangers and family members.

Most children with CP benefit from speech therapy, which helps them learn to speak slowly and to coordinate their lips and tongue to form speech sounds. Be patient when talking to them so they feel comfortable taking their time to form words deliberately. For the child who cannot speak clearly, provide an alternative form of communication, such as flash cards, a picture board, or a touch-screen computer, to aid communication.

LONG-TERM CARE

Because CP is not always diagnosed early in infancy, parents may not learn their child has a chronic disorder until 2 to 4 years later. Listen to parents during healthcare visits and encourage them to discuss the difficulties of daily living, such as feeding problems. Offer them support as needed if they grieve because their child is not able to accomplish all of the major things they had wished for during pregnancy or feel defeated by the day-to-day strain of caring for their child's multiple special needs. Care of a child with a chronic illness is discussed further in Chapter 56.

QSEN Checkpoint Question 49.3

INFORMATICS

Tasha's sister Wanda was diagnosed with CP as an infant. What information would the nurse want her parents to know about her prognosis?

a. Symptoms of CP typically begin to wane just after puberty.
b. The severity of cognitive deficits parallels the severity of physical deficits.
c. CP may occasionally be caused by a childhood vaccine reaction.
d. Symptoms may seem to grow worse as fine motor skill is needed.

Look in Appendix A for the best answer and rationale.

Infection

Infection of the nervous system is always potentially serious. It typically occurs from illnesses such as meningitis, encephalitis, Guillain-Barré syndrome, Reye syndrome, and botulism.

BACTERIAL MENINGITIS

Meningitis is, as the name implies, infection of the cerebral meninges. It tends to occur most frequently in children younger than 24 months of age and most often in winter. The organisms most frequently seen are *Streptococcus pneumoniae* or group B *Streptococcus*. In children younger than 2 months of age, *Escherichia coli* is a common cause. If children with myelomeningocele develop meningitis, *Pseudomonas* infection may be the causative agent. Children who have had a splenectomy are particularly susceptible to pneumococcal meningitis unless they have received a pneumococcal vaccine. *Haemophilus influenzae*, once a major cause of meningitis, is now rarely seen because of routine immunization against this organism (Greenberg-Kushnir, Haskin, Yarden-Bilavsky, et al., 2012).

Pathologic organisms usually spread to the meninges from upper respiratory tract infections by lymphatic drainage possibly through the mastoid or frontal sinuses or by direct introduction through a lumbar puncture or skull fracture. Once organisms enter the meningeal space, they multiply rapidly and then spread throughout the CSF to invade brain tissue through the meningeal folds, which extend down into the brain itself. Brain abscess or invasion of the infection into cranial nerves can result in blindness, hearing impairment, or facial paralysis. If a thick exudate accumulates in the narrow

aqueduct of Sylvius, it can cause obstruction leading to hydrocephalus. Brain tissue edema can put pressure on the pituitary gland, causing increased production of antidiuretic hormone, resulting in the syndrome of inappropriate antidiuretic hormone secretion (SIADH), causing hyponatremia.

Assessment

Children usually have had 2 or 3 days of upper respiratory tract infection prior to the development of meningitis. They then grow increasingly irritable because of an intense headache. They experience sharp pain when they bend their head forward. In the newborn, symptoms such as poor sucking, weak cry, or lethargy develop. As the disease progresses, signs of meningeal irritability then occur, as evidenced by positive Brudzinski and Kernig signs.

Children may hold their back arched and their neck hyperextended (opisthotonos). If third and sixth cranial nerve paralysis occurs, a child will not be able to follow a light through full visual fields. If the fontanelles are open, they bulge upward and feel tense; if they are closed, papilledema may develop. If the meningitis is caused by *H. influenzae*, the child may develop septic arthritis. If it is caused by *Neisseria meningitidis*, a papular or purple petechial skin rash may occur (Pace & Pollard, 2012).

After this beginning of a myriad of general symptoms, sudden cardiovascular shock, seizures, nuchal rigidity, or apnea can occur. Because the infant has open fontanelles, nuchal rigidity appears late and is not as useful a sign for diagnosis as in the older child. As a rule, a child with a high temperature who then has a seizure is assumed to have meningitis until CSF findings prove otherwise.

CSF analysis obtained by lumbar puncture confirms the diagnosis. CSF results indicative of meningitis include increased white blood cell and protein levels, increased ICP, and a glucose level less than 60% of blood glucose (because bacteria have fed on the glucose). In addition to supplying blood for glucose level, blood is cultured and examined for increased WBC count. If the child has had close association with someone with tuberculosis, a tuberculin skin test to rule out tuberculosis meningitis will be done. A CT scan, MRI, or ultrasound study will be prescribed to examine for brain abscess.

Therapeutic Management

Antibiotic therapy as indicated by sensitivity studies is the primary therapy. Intrathecal injections (directly into the CSF) may also be necessary, especially because the blood–brain barrier may prevent the chosen antibiotic from passing freely into the CSF. In some children, it takes a month before the CSF cell count returns to normal. A corticosteroid such as dexamethasone or the osmotic diuretic mannitol may be administered to reduce ICP and help prevent hearing loss.

In addition to standard precautions, children with meningitis are placed on respiratory precautions for 24 hours after the start of antibiotic therapy to prevent transmission of the infection to other family members or healthcare providers. In addition, an antibiotic may be prescribed prophylactically for the child's immediate family members or for playmates who have been in close contact with the child.

Meningitis is always a serious disorder because it can run a rapid, fulminating, and possibly fatal course. If symptoms are recognized early and treatment is effective, however, a child will recover with no sequelae. Neurologic sequelae, such as learning problems, seizures, hearing and cognitive challenges, and inability to concentrate urine from lessened antidiuretic hormone secretion, must be assessed in the weeks to come because these can be long-term consequences.

What If . . . 49.1

The cause of Tasha's seizure is found to be bacterial meningitis. Because she has severe neck pain whenever she is moved, her mother asks the nurse not to be so concerned about measuring intake and output, so her daughter can rest. How should the nurse respond? The nurse calls Tasha's name and she does not answer. Why is this a particular cause of concern in a child with meningitis?

Nursing Diagnoses and Related Interventions

If a child has meningitis, the parents may feel responsible for the illness because they knew the child had an upper respiratory infection. They may ask if they could have prevented meningitis if only they had taken the child to their primary care provider as soon as the respiratory symptoms began. You can assure them the symptoms of meningitis occur so insidiously that no one can appreciate what disease process is at work from the first generalized signs.

Be certain to orient parents to infection control techniques if the child is isolated so they can feel comfortable caring for their child.

Nursing Diagnosis: Pain related to meningeal irritation

Outcome Evaluation: Child states pain is tolerable and shows no facial grimacing or other signs of discomfort.

For a child with meningitis, dealing with the number of invasive procedures, such as lumbar puncture, venipuncture, and IV therapy, necessary can make a hospital stay difficult. Remember that children feel pain when their head is flexed forward, so they usually are more comfortable without a pillow. Be careful not to flex their neck forward when turning or positioning them.

Although children would probably benefit from puppet play or coloring, activities that could help them express how they feel about so many intrusive procedures, frequently, they are too uncomfortable to play and thus are not able to be comforted by these measures. Be certain that children receive a good explanation of everything that is happening and extra attention from healthcare personnel not just when they perform painful procedures but so children can feel secure. Help parents understand that their child's acute irritableness is caused by the disease process and not by anything they did or are doing so they can continue to interact with the child. You can assure them that, as their child recovers, irritability will lessen and the child will begin to show more interest in communicating feelings. Promote rest by keeping stimulation in the room to a minimum.

Nursing Diagnosis: Risk for ineffective tissue perfusion (cerebral), related to increased ICP

Outcome Evaluation: Child's vital signs return to normal; child is alert and oriented; motor, cognitive, and sensory functions are within acceptable parameters for the child's age; specific gravity of urine is 1.003 to 1.030.

Observe the child carefully for signs of increased ICP such as increased blood pressure or slowed pulse rate. Carefully monitor the rate of all IV infusions to prevent overhydration and increased ICP. Measure urine specific gravity to detect oversecretion or undersecretion of antidiuretic hormone because of pituitary pressure. Measure the child's head circumference and weigh the child daily. Monitor hearing acuity (reduced if there is compression of the eighth cranial nerve) by asking an older child a question or observing whether an infant listens to a music box or to your voice.

GROUP B STREPTOCOCCAL INFECTION

A major cause of meningitis in newborns is group B streptococci. The organism is contracted either in utero or from secretions in the birth canal. It can spread to other newborns in a hospital nursery if good hand washing technique is not used.

Colonization can result in either an early-onset or a late-onset illness. With the early-onset form, symptoms of pneumonia become apparent in the first few hours of life. The late-onset type leads to meningitis instead of pneumonia.

With meningitis, at approximately 2 weeks of age, the infant gradually becomes lethargic and develops a fever and upper respiratory tract symptoms. The fontanelles bulge from increased ICP. The disease is extremely serious as mortality from the infection is approximately 25%; surviving infants may develop neurologic consequences such as hydrocephalus or seizures (Libster, Edwards, Levent, et al., 2012). Treatment is with antibiotics that are effective against the group B *Streptococcus*, such as ampicillin and cephalosporins. Because it can be difficult for parents to understand how their infant suddenly became so ill, they may need considerable support in immediately caring for the infant or if the infant is left neurologically challenged.

QSEN Checkpoint Question 49.4

QUALITY IMPROVEMENT

Tasha is diagnosed as having bacterial meningitis, and her plan of care is being amended in light of this diagnostic finding. How long should the care team maintain respiratory precautions for this condition after Tasha begins an antibiotic?

a. 4 hours
b. 24 hours
c. Until her core body temperature returns to normal
d. Until her arterial blood gases return to normal

Look in Appendix A for the best answer and rationale.

ENCEPHALITIS

Encephalitis is an inflammation of brain tissue and, possibly, the meninges as well (Kneen, Michael, Menson, et al., 2012). It can arise from protozoan, bacterial, fungal, or viral invasions. Enteroviruses are the most frequent cause, followed by arboviruses. Several encephalitis viruses, such as those that cause St. Louis encephalitis, West Nile encephalitis, and Eastern equine encephalitis, are borne by mosquitoes and thus are seen most often during the summer months. Encephalitis also can result from direct invasion of the CSF during lumbar puncture. Yet, another cause is as a complication of childhood diseases such as measles, mumps, or chickenpox. In order to prevent the disease, therefore, it is crucial children receive immunization against childhood diseases and use mosquito repellents when in mosquito-infested areas.

Assessment

Symptoms of encephalitis begin either gradually or suddenly and include symptoms such as headache, high temperature, ataxia (loss of usual muscle movements), muscle weakness or paralysis, diplopia, confusion, and irritability; if meninges are also involved, signs of meningeal irritation, such as nuchal rigidity and a positive Brudzinski or Kernig sign, may also be present. A child becomes increasingly lethargic and eventually comatose.

The diagnosis is made by the history and physical assessment. CSF evaluation will reveal an elevated leukocyte count and an elevated protein level. An EEG will demonstrate widespread cerebral involvement. A brain biopsy, usually taken from the temporal lobe or infected CSF, identifies the virus.

Therapeutic Management

Treatment for a child with encephalitis is primarily supportive. An antipyretic is prescribed to control fever. Mechanical ventilation may be required to maintain the child's respirations during the acute phase. A variety of medications, such as acyclovir (Zovirax), an antiviral agent, and carbamazepine (Tegretol), an anticonvulsant, may be prescribed. A steroid such as dexamethasone or an osmotic diuretic such as mannitol may be needed to decrease brain edema and ICP.

Encephalitis is always a serious diagnosis because although a child may recover from the initial attack without further symptoms, there can be residual neurologic damage, such as seizures or learning disabilities. Parents may find it hard to believe their child is so seriously ill at first because in the beginning of the illness, their child only seemed tired and had a slight headache. They can find it even harder to accept that permanent impairment, such as a learning disability, could result. This makes follow-up care after hospitalization important both for the child's rehabilitation and to help parents deal with their grief, shock, and possible anger over this devastating turn of events in their life.

REYE SYNDROME

Reye syndrome is acute encephalopathy with accompanying fatty infiltration of the liver, heart, lungs, pancreas, and skeletal muscle. It occurs in children from 1 to 18 years of age regardless of gender (Ninove, Daniel, Gallou, et al., 2011).

The cause is unknown, but symptoms such as lethargy, vomiting, confusion, and combativeness usually occur after a viral infection such as varicella (chickenpox) or influenza that was treated with acetylsalicylic acid (aspirin). Treatment is supportive. Untreated, the condition leads to coma and death. Anticipatory guidance to parents and children about avoiding the use of aspirin during viral infections has almost prevented the syndrome (Bennett, Starko, Thomsen, et al., 2012).

GUILLAIN-BARRÉ SYNDROME

Guillain-Barré syndrome (inflammatory polyradiculoneuropathy) is a perplexing syndrome that occurs in about 1 in every 100,000 children. Both motor and sensory portions of peripheral nerves are affected. Boys develop it more often than girls (Yuki & Hartung, 2012). With successful widespread polio eradication efforts, Guillain-Barré syndrome is now the most common cause of acute and subacute flaccid paralysis in childhood (Rosen, 2012).

The cause of the condition is unknown, but it is suspected that the reaction is immune mediated, occurring after upper respiratory tract or gastrointestinal illnesses or, rarely, immunizations. Inflammation of the nerve fibers apparently causes temporary demyelization of the nerve sheaths.

Assessment

Children experience peripheral neuritis several days after the primary infection. Tendon reflexes begin to decrease and then become absent. Muscle paralysis and paresthesia (loss of sensation) begin first in the legs and then spread to involve the arms, trunk, and head. The symmetric nature of the disorder helps to differentiate it from other types of paraplegia. Cranial nerve involvement leads to facial weakness and difficulty in swallowing. As the respiratory muscles become involved, spontaneous respirations are no longer possible, leading to respiratory involvement severe enough to warrant mechanical ventilation.

A significant laboratory finding is an elevated CSF protein level. An EEG may show denervation and decreased nerve conduction velocity.

Therapeutic Management

Treatment of Guillain-Barré syndrome is supportive until the paralysis peaks at 3 weeks and then is followed by gradual recovery. A course of prednisone to halt the autoimmune response may be tried, but its use is controversial. Plasmapheresis or transfusion of immune serum globulin may shorten the course of the illness. Cardiac and respiratory function must be closely monitored. All patients should be given subcutaneous fractionated or unfractionated heparin and support stockings until they are able to walk independently to prevent deep vein thrombosis.

Other necessary measures include prevention of the effects of extreme immobility while guarding respiratory function. An indwelling urinary catheter is usually inserted to monitor urine output. Enteral or total parenteral nutrition may be used to support protein and carbohydrate needs. If the child has discomfort from neuritis, adequate analgesia is necessary.

To prevent muscle contractures and effects of immobility, turning and repositioning every 2 hours is important in addition to passive range-of-motion exercises about every 4 hours. Be certain to provide adequate stimulation for the long weeks when the child is unable to perform any care independently.

Fortunately, despite the long period of mandatory ventilation therapy, most children recover completely, without any residual effects of the syndrome, although some may continue to have minor problems such as residual weakness.

BOTULISM

Botulism occurs when spores of *Clostridium botulinum* colonize and produce toxins in the intestine. Infant botulism is not transmitted from person to person and occurs predominantly in infants younger than 6 months of age (American Academy of Pediatrics, 2015). Honey has been identified as a common source for infant botulism and should not be given prior to 12 months of age (American Academy of Pediatrics, 2015).

Symptoms occur within a few hours after ingestion of the contaminated food. Almost immediately, there is generalized weakness, hypotonia, listlessness, a weak cry, and a diminished gag reflex, followed by a flaccid paralysis of the bulbar muscles that leads to diminished respiratory function. The organism can be cultured from stools or serum. Electromyography may be helpful to support the diagnosis. Treatment is supportive care. Human-derived botulinum immune globulin may stop the progress of the disease.

Inflammatory Disorders

Two neurologic inflammatory disorders are found frequently in adolescents.

CARPAL TUNNEL SYNDROME

Carpal tunnel syndrome is nerve compression of the median nerve that passes through the carpal tunnel at the wrist (Luckhaupt, Dalhamer, Ward, et al., 2013). Compression of the nerve causes numbness and sharp pain and burning in the thumb and the second, third, and fourth fingers of the hand. Word processing, texting, and video games have turned this previously adult disorder into a disorder that occurs in children as well. Pain usually occurs at night and is enough to keep a child awake. The usual therapy is application of a splint to the wrist, which holds the wrist in a neutral (not flexed and not extended) position. An oral anti-inflammatory medication and perhaps a corticosteroid injection into the inflamed wrist both help to relieve pain. If these therapies are not successful, the stricture at the carpal canal can be relieved surgically.

FACIAL PALSY (BELL PALSY)

Facial palsy is facial paralysis of the seventh (facial) cranial nerve, the nerve that innervates the muscles of facial expression. The syndrome occurs abruptly and may be associated with herpes or Lyme disease infection or occur as a result of cold air from skiing or from riding in a convertible. Therapy in adults consists of prednisone to reduce inflammation and acyclovir if the syndrome is herpes related. In children, prednisone use is variable. If the child is unable to close the eye on the affected side, eye drops three or four times daily will be needed. Although recovery is slow, usually takes about 4 months, most children recover without any permanent disability (McNamara, Doyle, McKay, et al., 2013).

Paroxysmal Disorders

A paroxysmal disorder is one that occurs suddenly and recurrently. Seizures, headaches, and breath-holding spells are the most frequent types seen in childhood.

EPILEPSY (RECURRENT SEIZURES)

A *seizure* is an involuntary contraction of muscle caused by abnormal electrical brain discharges. Approximately 5% of children will have at least one seizure by the time they reach adulthood (Sidhu, Velayudam, & Barnes, 2013). These episodes are always frightening to parents and other children because of the intensity. Although about 50% of seizures are idiopathic (unknown cause), they also can be attributed to infection, trauma, or tumor growth. Familial or polygenic inheritance may be responsible. Because they are not so much a disease as a symptom of an underlying disorder, all seizures need to be investigated.

The term *epilepsy* comes from a Greek word meaning "to take hold of." Because the word has stigmas of cognitive challenge, behavioral disorders, institutionalization, or unexplainable strangeness attached to it, a preferred term is *recurrent seizures* because this term explains the disease process without the effect of discrimination (Box 49.4).

The types and causes of seizures vary with age and are classified into two major categories: partial and generalized seizures. As the name implies, with partial seizures, only one area of the brain is involved; with generalized seizures, the disturbance appears to involve the entire brain; loss of consciousness usually occurs. It's important that seizures be differentiated by their degree of severity and type so that parents can know any special precautions they need to take for their child and appropriate management and drug therapy can be instituted.

Seizures in the Newborn Period

Seizure activity in the newborn period may be difficult to recognize because it may consist only of twitching of the head, arms, or eyes; smacking of the lips; slight cyanosis; and perhaps respiratory difficulty or apnea. Afterward, the infant

BOX 49.4
Nursing Care Planning to Respect Cultural Diversity

The degree of understanding about the cause of disorders such as recurrent seizures varies in different cultures. The often unknown cause of recurrent (idiopathic) seizures has led to them being attributed to an invasion by evil spirits or the effect of curses. Many people today still fear that recurrent seizures will lead to cognitive impairment. Many parents worry that their child will be refused admission to a school or refused a job as an adult because their child is viewed as so unpredictable. Being aware of these common misconceptions can help you appreciate parents' anxiety about the diagnosis of recurrent seizures, an anxiety that can accentuate the need for parent education and careful planning to maintain self-esteem in their child.

may appear limp and flaccid. Whereas seizures in older children are often of unknown cause, 75% of seizures in neonates have a known cause such as trauma and anoxia from intrauterine life or birth; metabolic disorders, such as hypoglycemia, hypocalcemia, or lack of pyridoxine (vitamin B_6); neonatal infection; or acute bilirubin encephalopathy caused by a blood incompatibility.

Because of the nervous system's immaturity, EEGs in the newborn may be normal despite extensive disease. A noticeably abnormal EEG in the newborn period, therefore, generally means a poor prognosis, indicating that involvement this early in life must be severe. Because almost 20% of all newborns have abnormal CSF values compared with adult standards (protein is increased, and there may be a few red blood cells from rupture of subarachnoid capillaries from the pressure of birth), lumbar puncture also is not conclusive.

High doses of antiseizure medication may be needed to control seizures in newborns because they metabolize drugs more rapidly than older children. In adults, for example, phenobarbital may be administered in the range of 1.5 mg/kg body weight per day. In newborns, the dose might be as high as 3 to 10 mg/kg/day.

Seizures in the Infant and Toddler Periods

Seizures commonly seen in this age group are **infantile spasms**, a form of generalized seizure often called "salaam" or "jackknife" seizures, or infantile myoclonic seizures. These are characterized by very rapid movements of the trunk with sudden strong contractions of most of the body, including flexion and adduction of the limbs, or the infant suddenly slumps forward from a sitting position or falls from a standing position. The episode may occur singly or in clusters as frequently as 100 times a day.

In approximately 50% of affected children, there is an identifiable cause such as trauma, a metabolic disease such as phenylketonuria, or a viral invasion such as herpes or cytomegalovirus. In other children, the spasms apparently result from a failure of normal organized electrical activity in the brain. Approximately 90% of infants with this type of involvement will be developmentally delayed as intellectual development appears to halt and even regress after the pattern of seizures begins. Most children with infantile spasms show high-amplitude slow waves and spikes, a chaotic discharge called *hypsarrhythmia* on an EEG tracing.

These seizures occur slightly more often in males than females, occur in 2 to 3 per 10,000 live births, have a family history in 3% to 6% of cases, and only spontaneously stop in 30% of children (Go, Mackay, Weiss, et al., 2012). Because the response to treatment with antiseizure therapy tends to be poor, parenteral adrenocorticotropic hormone (ACTH) therapy, prednisone, or high-dose vigabatrin, an amino acid, are used in its place. High-dose valproate or a newer antiseizure agent such as topiramate (Topamax) may be used in children who do not respond to usual therapy, as well as pyridoxine (vitamin B_6) or a ketogenic diet (see following discussion), but research shows none to be as effective as ACTH, especially for preserving neurodevelopmental outcomes (Go et al., 2012). In most children, the seizure phenomenon seems to "burn itself out" by 2 years of age. Any associated cognitive or developmental delay remains, however, so children need good follow-up planning and care.

Seizures Caused by Poisoning or Drugs

The possibility of poisoning has to be considered in any child who has a first seizure. Although this is most likely to occur between 6 months and 3 years of age, it must be considered again in adolescence, when drugs may be intentionally self-administered. Seizures also can be a late symptom of encephalopathy caused by lead poisoning (see Chapter 52).

Seizures in Children Older Than 3 Years of Age

Febrile Seizures

Seizures associated with high fever (102° to 104°F [38.9° to 40.0°C]) are the most common type seen in preschool children, although these can occur as late as 7 years of age. They are most serious if they occur under 6 months of age. Such seizures may occur after immunization with live vaccines because these most commonly produce fevers. The seizure is usually a generalized tonic–clonic pattern, which lasts for 15 to 20 seconds. An EEG tracing afterward is usually normal. There also is usually a history of other family members having had similar seizures.

The seizure is due to a sudden spike of temperature, not a gradual incline. The seizure only lasts 1 to 2 minutes or less. Further evaluation is necessary after a febrile seizure to exclude underlying conditions or infections (Sidhu et al., 2013).

Prevention of Febrile Seizures

Because these seizures arise with high fever, they are largely preventable. If ibuprofen or acetaminophen is given to keep a developing fever below 101°F (38.4°C), the seizures rarely occur. They happen most often when a child develops a fever at night, when a parent is not aware of it, or when a parent is reluctant to give ibuprofen or acetaminophen in large enough doses to be therapeutic. Because the recommended doses of these medicines vary with the type (liquid or pills), caution parents to read the bottle label carefully before administration to be certain they are administering the correct dosage. Family history and younger age at onset of first seizure are risk factors for reoccurrence of a febrile seizure.

Teach parents that every child who has a febrile seizure must be seen by a healthcare provider to rule out meningitis and to be aware that it will be assumed by emergency room personnel that the child has meningitis until it is ruled out by a complete neurologic workup.

Therapeutic Management

After a febrile seizure subsides, parents should sponge the child with tepid water to reduce the fever quickly. Advise them not to put the child in a bathtub of water to do this because it would be easy for the child to slip under water should a second seizure occur. Caution parents not to apply alcohol or cold water because extreme cooling causes shock to an immature nervous system; in addition, alcohol can be absorbed by the skin or the fumes can be inhaled in toxic amounts, compounding the child's problems. Parents should not attempt to give oral medications such as acetaminophen because the child will be in a drowsy, or *postictal*, state after the seizure and might aspirate the medicine. Suppositories may be given at the appropriate dose. If attempts to reduce the child's temperature by sponging are unsuccessful, advise parents to put cool washcloths on the child's forehead, axillary, and groin areas and transport the child, lightly clothed, to a healthcare facility for immediate evaluation.

At the healthcare facility, a lumbar puncture will be performed to rule out meningitis. If warranted, antipyretic drugs to reduce the fever below seizure levels will be administered. Appropriate antibiotic therapy will be prescribed if an infection is documented.

Many parents need to be reassured that febrile seizures do not lead to brain damage and that the child is almost always completely well afterward.

What If . . . 49.2

Tasha's mother refuses to allow her to play with other children because she's worried Tasha will contract an upper respiratory infection from one of them and then have a febrile seizure. Is the mother taking a safe precaution or overreacting to the possibility of a seizure?

Complex Partial (Psychomotor or Temporal Lobe) Seizures

More than half of children who develop recurrent seizures during school age have an idiopathic type or the cause of the seizures cannot be discovered. Despite this, medication can effectively control these seizures in almost all affected children. Some seizures in this age group occur because of organic causes such as laceration of brain tissue from an automobile accident or fall, an enlarging brain tumor, hemorrhage due to a blood dyscrasia, infection (meningitis or encephalitis), anoxia, or toxic conditions such as lead poisoning that have left residual damage. The possibility that brain trauma could have been caused by child maltreatment is always another possibility to consider.

Complex partial (psychomotor) seizures vary greatly in extent and symptoms and tend to be a difficult type to control. The child may notice a slight *aura*, or sensation a seizure is about to occur, but this is rarely as definite as that seen with tonic–clonic seizures. Results of a CT or MRI scan and EEG will invariably be normal.

This type of seizure often begins with a sudden change in posture, such as an arm dropping suddenly to the side. Other motor, sensory, and behavioral signs might include **automatisms** (complex purposeless movements, such as lip smacking, fumbling hand movements, intense running, or screaming). A few children may then slump to the ground, unconscious. Circumoral pallor develops due to a halt in respirations. The child begins breathing again almost immediately and usually regains consciousness in less than 5 minutes. He or she may feel slightly drowsy afterward but does not have an actual postictal stage or a period of sustained unconsciousness as seen with tonic–clonic seizures.

Common drugs used to treat this type of seizure include carbamazepine (Tegretol) (Box 49.5) or valproate (Depakene). Carbamazepine can lead to neutropenia, so white blood cell counts need to be monitored during therapy. If these drugs are not effective, surgery to remove the epileptogenic focus or the implantation of a vagus nerve stimulator can be used to significantly reduce seizure frequency. If seizures cannot be controlled fully, parents need to anticipate potentially hazardous situations during their child's day, such as having to cross a busy street on the way to school or riding a bicycle.

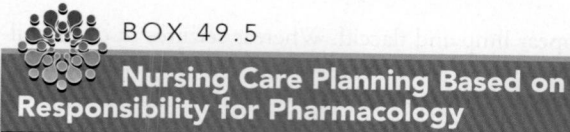

BOX 49.5

Nursing Care Planning Based on Responsibility for Pharmacology

CARBAMAZEPINE (TEGRETOL)

Classification: Carbamazepine is an antiseizure medication.

Action: Exact mechanism of action is unknown, but it is believed to inhibit polysynaptic responses and block post-tetanic potentiation (Karch, 2013).

Pregnancy Risk Category: C

Dosage: Initially in children 6 to 12 years of age, 10 mg/kg/24 hr orally twice a day on the first day (maximum dose 100 mg), increased gradually in 100-mg increments at 1-week intervals until best response is achieved, or 10 to 30 mg/kg/day in divided doses three or four times a day. Not to exceed 1,000 mg/day.

Possible Adverse Effects: Dizziness, drowsiness, behavioral changes, nausea, vomiting, abnormal liver function tests, bone marrow depression, rash, photosensitivity

Nursing Implications

- Advise parents to administer the drug with food to minimize gastrointestinal upset.
- Remind parents to obtain serum drug levels as prescribed to monitor for effectiveness and to prevent possible toxicity; also, obtain liver function studies and blood cell counts to detect marrow depression.
- Suggest that parents obtain a medical alert bracelet and have the child wear it in case of a seizure.
- Instruct parents to not give sleep-inducing or over-the-counter drugs because these can interact with antiseizure medication to cause dangerous synergistic effects. Caution adolescents to avoid alcohol.
- Caution parents not to discontinue the drug abruptly or change the dose unless ordered by the healthcare provider.
- Instruct parents to notify their healthcare provider if the child develops bruising, bleeding, or signs of infection because these could be signs of bone marrow depression.

State regulations vary, but the majority of adolescents are not eligible to secure a permit to drive until they are cleared by their primary care provider (after about a year free of seizures) to protect their own safety and that of others.

Partial (Focal) Seizures

Partial seizures originate from a specific brain area. A typical partial seizure with motor signs begins in the fingers and spreads to the wrist, arm, and face in a clonic contraction. If the movement remains localized, there will be no loss of consciousness. If the spread is extensive, the seizure can cross the midline and become generalized and, at that point, is impossible to differentiate from a full generalized tonic–clonic seizure. This makes it important, therefore, to observe children carefully as a seizure begins to distinguish whether it began with local signs such as numbness, tingling, paresthesia, or pain all associated with one brain area. Documenting the spread can help localize the spot in the brain that first initiated the abnormal electrical discharge or be instrumental in detecting the location of a rapidly growing brain tumor.

Absence Seizures

Absence seizures are one form of generalized seizures, formerly known as petit mal seizures (Sidhu et al., 2013). They occur more often in girls than boys, usually occur in school-age children between 4 and 12 years, and consist of a staring spell that lasts for a few seconds. A child might be reciting in class, for example, when he or she pauses and stares for 1 to 5 seconds and then continues the recitation as if he or she is unaware time has passed. Rhythmic blinking and twitching of the mouth or an extremity may accompany the staring. As many as 100 seizures can occur during a day.

Children with absence episodes usually have normal intelligence but may have failing school marks, be accused of daydreaming in school, or be referred to the school nurse for behavior problems because they miss so many of a teacher's instructions.

On a neurologic exam, the presence of absence seizures can usually be demonstrated by asking a child to hyperventilate while the child counts out loud. If the child is susceptible to such seizures, he or she typically breathes in and out deeply, possibly 10 times, stops and stares for 3 seconds, and then continues to hyperventilate and count, unaware that he or she paused.

No first aid measures are necessary for absence seizures, and downplaying the importance of these episodes helps children maintain a positive self-image. They can be controlled by ethosuximide (Zarontin), valproate, or "off-label" lamotrigine (Robotham, 2011). If seizures are fully controlled by medication, children can participate in normal school activities and ride a bicycle or motorcycle. If seizures cannot be controlled fully, parents need to anticipate potentially hazardous situations during the child's day to prevent risky activities such as swimming alone.

Approximately one third to one half of all children with absence seizures "outgrow" them by adulthood. This does not mean that treatment is not necessary during childhood, however, in order to keep the child safe and maintain self-esteem. Follow-up health supervision is necessary during adolescence because some children's seizure pattern changes from absence involvement to tonic–clonic involvement as they approach adulthood.

Tonic–Clonic Seizures

Typical tonic–clonic seizures (formerly termed grand mal seizures) are generalized seizures usually consisting of three stages: a prodromal period of hours or days or an aura, or warning, immediately before the seizure that a seizure is about to occur; a tonic–clonic stage; and, finally, a postictal stage.

The prodromal period may consist of drowsiness, dizziness, malaise, lack of coordination, or tension. As a child reaches school age, the child may be able to predict from these vague preliminary feelings when a seizure is about to occur.

An aura reflects the portion of the brain in which the seizure originates. Smelling unpleasant odors (often reported as feces) denotes activity in the medial portion of the temporal lobe. Seeing flashing lights suggests the occipital area, repeated hallucinations arise from the temporal lobe, numbness of an extremity relates to the opposite parietal lobe, and

a "Cheshire-cat grin" relates to the frontal lobe. Young children, unable to describe or understand an aura, may scream in fright or run to their parent at its onset. Noting exactly what symptoms the child experiences during this time helps to localize the involved brain portion.

The next phase is the tonic stage. All muscles of the body contract, extremities stiffen, the face distorts, air is pushed through the glottis from contraction of the chest muscles to produce a guttural cry, and the child falls to the ground. Although this phase lasts only about 20 seconds because the respiratory muscles remain contracted during this time, the child may experience hypoxia and begin to appear cyanotic. Contraction of the throat prevents swallowing, so saliva collects in the mouth. A few children bite their tongue when the jaws contract and thus have bleeding from their mouth.

The seizure then enters a clonic stage, in which muscles of the body rapidly contract and relax, producing quick, jerky motions. The child may blow bubbles from foamy or bloody saliva and will be incontinent of stool and urine. This phase usually lasts 20 to 30 seconds.

Following this tonic–clonic period, the child falls into a sound sleep, the *postictal period*. He or she will sleep soundly for 1 to 4 hours rousing only to painful stimuli. When children awake, they often experience a severe headache. They have no memory of the seizure.

In some children, seizures occur only at night. The child wakes in the morning with a sore tongue, blood on the pillow, or a bed wet with urine. In a child with persistent bed-wetting, the possibility this may be occurring from nocturnal seizures should be considered.

Children with this type of seizure may or may not have an abnormal EEG pattern. If an abnormal pattern is found, other family members may be found to have similarly abnormal EEG patterns, although they do not have symptoms.

Therapy includes the daily administration of an antiseizure medication such as valproate (Depakene) and carbamazepine (Tegretol). Phenobarbital may be administered to young children.

Medications are usually continued until the child has been seizure free for 2 to 3 years. No antiseizure medication should be stopped suddenly (it should be tapered) because rapid withdrawal may precipitate a seizure. In addition to medication, some children may be prescribed a ketogenic diet or a diet high in fat and low in protein and carbohydrate. This diet is proven to be highly effective in 40% to 50% of children who are started on it. This diet is difficult for parents to adhere to and to incorporate into the family's lifestyle and may need to be "fine-tuned" to improve seizure control (Selter, Turner, Doerrer, et al., 2014).

Status Epilepticus

Status epilepticus refers to a seizure that lasts continuously for longer than 30 minutes or a series of seizures from which the child does not return to the previous level of consciousness. This is an emergency situation requiring immediate treatment before exhaustion, respiratory failure, permanent brain injury, or death occurs. An IV benzodiazepine drug such as diazepam (Valium) or lorazepam (Ativan) halts seizures dramatically. Diazepam must be administered with extreme caution, however, based on the child's drug history because the drug is incompatible with many other medications, and any accidental infiltration into subcutaneous tissue causes extensive tissue sloughing. Parents can be instructed on how to administer diazepam by enema at home. Lorazepam (Ativan), a long-acting benzodiazepine used for children older than 2 years of age, provides a longer duration of action and also less respiratory depression (Karch, 2013). Both oxygen to relieve cyanosis and administering a medication to halt the seizure may be necessary; obtaining blood to monitor for glucose may reveal that hypoglycemia needs to be corrected.

QSEN Checkpoint Question 49.5

EVIDENCE-BASED PRACTICE

Recurrent seizures can be depressing for children and parents if the seizures are difficult to eliminate with therapy. A 2015 study looked at parents' coping behaviors and stressors, and their ability to care for their child with chronic disease. The parents were given the *Coping Inventory for Parents* (CHIP) survey along with the *Pediatric Inventory for Parents* (PIP). Significant correlations were found in the study showing the need for early identification by nurses of disease-related challenges, stressors, and parental coping methods to improve the outcomes of the children (Senger, Ward, Barbosa-Leiker, et al., 2015).

Based on this study, if Tasha is found to have recurrent seizures, which statement by her mother at a healthcare visit would concern a nurse the most?

 a. "I forgot to give Tasha her medicine twice last week; I have to try harder."
 b. "I feel really sad when children call Tasha names because of her seizures."
 c. "I don't like having to miss work due to Tasha's clinic visits."
 d. "I think Tasha's medicine is giving her headaches; maybe she needs glasses."

Look in Appendix A for the best answer and rationale.

Unfolding Patient Stories: Jackson Webber • Part 2

 Think back to Chapter 31 where you met Jackson Webber. Jackson was diagnosed with generalized seizures 2 years ago at age 3 years. He had another seizure and his mother brought him to the hospital. How would the nurse differentiate tonic–clonic seizures from other types of seizures? Compare and contrast the characteristics of each type of seizure.

Care for Jackson and other patients in a realistic virtual environment: **vSim** *for Nursing* (thepoint.lww .com/vSimMaternityPed). Practice documenting these patients' care in DocuCare (thepoint.lww.com /DocuCareEHR).

Assessment of the Child With Seizures

It's important that a thorough pregnancy history be obtained on any child with seizures. Events that occurred immediately before the seizure and an accurate description of the seizure itself also should be recorded. Investigate the child's overall behavior in the last few weeks such as bed-wetting or failing marks in school because these might be signs of absence or nocturnal seizures that have occurred but gone unnoticed.

A complete physical and neurologic examination and blood studies are necessary to rule out metabolic or infectious processes. Prepare a child for a lumbar puncture to rule out meningitis or bleeding into the CSF. A CT scan, MRI, skull radiograph, or EEG may be obtained as indicated. Caution children during the EEG that they may be stimulated with rhythm patterns or flashing lights or asked to hyperventilate to see whether a seizure can be provoked.

Nursing Diagnoses and Related Interventions

Nursing Diagnosis: Risk for injury related to recurrent seizures

Outcome Evaluation: Child exhibits no signs of aspiration or traumatic injury.

Help a child having a partial seizure to a sitting position to protect against falling. Turn a child who has fallen to the floor onto the side so fluid will drain from the mouth and not be aspirated. Protecting a child from being hurt during a tonic–clonic seizure is crucial, but restraining the child's thrashing extremities is not advisable because it is difficult for an adult to do so and could result in injury to the parent or child because of the amount of force needed to keep the child still (Box 49.6). Do not insert anything between the child's teeth to stop tongue biting because this is rarely necessary and can result in broken and aspirated teeth.

Remaining calm is an important responsibility because it is reassuring for parents to see someone calm and in control of a situation that seems to be very out of control. If the child passes rapidly from one seizure into another (status epilepticus), be prepared to provide supplemental oxygen and administer antiseizure therapy as needed.

Nursing Diagnosis: Interrupted family processes related to diagnosis of long-term illness in child

Outcome Evaluation: Child, parents, and other family members express fears and questions about disease to healthcare team; parents discuss ways to accommodate the illness in their daily life, such as medication schedules, school accommodations, sports activities, plans for vacation, and discipline.

As soon as the diagnosis of a seizure disorder is made, parents and children need to be told that it is likely to signify a long-term disorder because although seizures can be controlled with medication, these do not change or cure the underlying cause of the seizures. Box 49.7 shows an interprofessional care map illustrating both nursing and team planning for a child with recurrent seizures. Most children are given tablets rather than liquid medication because the latter tends to settle at the bottom of the bottle, resulting in over diluted or over concentrated doses that can allow seizures to break

BOX 49.6

Nursing Care Planning Based on Family Teaching

SAFETY DURING SEIZURES

Q. Tasha's mother asks you, "What can we do to be certain she doesn't get hurt during a seizure?"

A. Here are the usual actions to help keep her safe:

- Remain calm.
- Move away furniture or any sharp objects.
- Turn your child gently on her side, or on her abdomen with her head turned to the side, to prevent aspiration of unswallowed mouth secretions.
- Do not restrain her other than to keep her head turned to the side. Restraining a child could result in injury because of the amount of force necessary.
- Do not attempt to place an object between the child's teeth to prevent tongue biting. Trying to force an object into the mouth could break or loosen teeth.
- Be aware that a child having this type of seizure may have some slight cyanosis during the tonic and clonic stages, but these stages are so short that administering oxygen is not needed.
- After any seizure, telephone your primary care provider about the seizure so arrangements for any necessary follow-up care can be initiated.
- If your child should pass rapidly from one seizure into another (status epilepticus), she may need supplemental oxygen or medicine to stop the seizure. If this happens, telephone your emergency medical service number (911).

through at the end of the prescription period. To avoid this happening, caution parents to shake liquid medication thoroughly before every dose. Parents need to establish ways to remember to buy medicine so they always have an adequate supply, especially if they are taking a trip away from home or need to provide enough for holidays.

Be certain the child receives health maintenance care during childhood to be certain that the medication dosage remains adequate with continued growth. To document that serum levels of drugs are adequate, children need periodic blood sampling.

Provide parents with as much information as possible about the cause of their child's seizures because it's almost always easier to deal with a known disease, not an unexplainable and unpredictable one. Although the cause of the seizures is unknown, you can assure them that treatment is known; new antiseizure medications are being introduced yearly into therapy.

General guidelines for safe administration of antiseizure medications to stress with parents include:

- Caution children to be careful around motor vehicles and electrical equipment because many antiseizure medications cause drowsiness.
- Advise the child and parents to observe for easy bruising because some antiseizure medicines may suppress bone marrow function.
- Caution the adolescent to avoid alcohol while taking antiseizure medications because alcohol can potentiate the CNS effects of these medications.
- Use caution when administering antiseizure medications to children with liver disease. Because many of these drugs are metabolized by the liver, they may not be fully effective in such children.

- Caution the child and parents not to discontinue antiseizure therapy abruptly because this may lead to uncontrolled seizures.
- Remind parents about the need for follow-up blood tests to evaluate the drug level. Maintaining a therapeutic blood level enhances the drug's effectiveness and minimizes the risk for toxicity.

Discuss with parents the need to treat children with seizures the same as other family members. Scolding children, asking them to do household chores, or insisting they do their homework will not cause seizures. A few children with absence seizures can initiate them by hyperventilating and may try to manipulate those around them by doing this to gain sympathy. The few children who use this extreme form of manipulation may need to be referred for counseling.

Assure parents also that occasional seizures in children are not harmful. Unless status epilepticus occurs and the child becomes anoxic, the chance their child will be injured during a seizure is remote. Knowing this helps parents not to worry about the child becoming cognitively challenged or about other misconceptions regarding seizures. Although some children who have seizures are cognitively challenged, this impairment and the seizures were caused by the same event; the seizures did not cause the impairment. At every healthcare visit, be certain parents have time to ask questions about their child's care and to express concerns. There are so many "scare stories" about seizures that every parent is likely to believe some of these stories unless counseled otherwise (Box 49.8).

As a rule, children with seizures should attend regular school and participate in physical education classes and active sports (with possible exceptions such as scuba or sky diving or rock climbing). Many teachers are concerned about the responsibility of having a child with seizures assigned to their class. Contact the school nurse (with the parents' permission) to help them learn about the success of modern seizure control.

BOX 49.7

Nursing Care Planning

AN INTERPROFESSIONAL CARE MAP FOR A CHILD WITH RECURRENT SEIZURES

Tasha is a 3-year-old girl who was brought to the emergency department by her mother because she had a seizure. Her mother grabs your arm, visibly upset. "Her sister has cerebral palsy and seizures. Does this mean Tasha has cerebral palsy too?" she asks you.

Family Assessment: Parents are divorced. Child lives in a two-bedroom apartment with mother and a 6-year-old sibling; attends child care daily from 9 AM to 3 PM. Neighbor watches her from 3 to 6 PM, when mother returns from work as a research librarian.

Patient Assessment: Well-proportioned preschooler sleeping soundly on left side since admission. Had first seizure 2 hours ago; a second one 30 minutes ago. Temperature at 103.4°F. Other vital signs within age-appropriate parameters. Reacts to painful stimuli only. Deep tendon reflexes depressed. Mother reports, "I kept her home from child care because she has a cold. Suddenly, she fell to the floor and started shaking. I called 911, and they brought her here." Apparent pain on forward flexion of the neck. Lumbar puncture performed; pressures within normal limits; specimens sent for cell count, glucose, and culture.

Nursing Diagnosis: Risk for injury related to diminished level of consciousness resulting from seizure episode

Outcome Criteria: Child is conscious within the hour. Exhibits no signs of aspiration or traumatic injury.

Team Member Responsible	Assessment	Intervention	Rationale	Expected Outcome
Activities of Daily Living, Including Safety				
Nurse	Assess whether mother was aware child's temperature was elevated. Assess whether child has continued pain on dorsiflexion of neck.	Keep child on side to help ensure an open airway until alert and responsive. Ask if mother has a thermometer to take any future fevers.	Side-lying position reduces risk for aspiration. Pain on dorsiflexion of neck and irritability are symptoms of meningitis.	Mother states she understands importance of taking temperature in the future; difficult to evaluate pain as child is unconscious.
Teamwork and Collaboration				
Nurse/primary care provider	Assess in light of this second seizure and spinal tap results whether neurologic service should be consulted.	Consult with neurologic service, if indicated, about management of child.	A second seizure suggests this may be more than a simple response to elevated fever.	Neurologic service meets with mother and child as appropriate based on findings.
Procedures/Medications for Quality Improvement				
Nurse	Assess whether child has had a lumbar puncture or intravenous (IV) fluid administration before.	Assist with lumbar puncture and specimen collection. Begin IV fluid administration as prescribed.	Lumbar puncture is a frightening procedure for both child and parent. IV line supplies an emergency medicine route if needed for seizure control or infection therapy.	Mother states she understands reason for procedure and gives consent. IV line is established and safeguarded with board for unresponsive child.
Nurse	Assess whether mother understands why respiratory precautions are necessary.	Obtain equipment for respiratory precautions as needed.	Diagnosis could be meningitis, which is contagious by contact with nasal secretions.	Mother states she understands the importance of precautions. Respiratory precautions are readied.

Nutrition

Nurse	Assess child's level of consciousness using a Glasgow Coma Scale.	Do not give anything by mouth until the child is fully awake, alert, and oriented and the gag reflex is intact.	Giving oral fluids too early increases risk for aspiration.	Child receives no oral fluid until she is awake and aware.

Patient-Centered Care

Nurse/nurse practitioner	Assess what mother knows about febrile seizures and meningitis.	Teach that a febrile seizure is more of a symptom of fever than a long-term condition. A meningeal infection could be very serious.	Understanding the basis for febrile seizures and meningitis can help the parent understand the basis for emergency care.	Mother states she understands child's current status and possible future implications.

Psychosocial/Spiritual/Emotional Needs

Nurse	Assess whether mother needs to contact a support person if her child's diagnosis is found to be serious.	Help mother contact a support person if she feels this would be helpful.	A support person can be vital to help a parent withstand an ominous diagnosis.	Mother contacts support person as needed.

Informatics for Seamless Healthcare Planning

Nurse	Assess whether parent has any further questions about child's condition before transfer to pediatric intensive care unit.	Answer any remaining questions to make transfer as comfortable for parent and child as possible.	A parent gains confidence in emergency department staff and may find it difficult to change to new healthcare providers.	Mother states she understands that if meningitis or recurrent seizures are diagnosed, her child needs ongoing care.

BOX 49.8

Nursing Care Planning Tips for Effective Communication

Tasha, 3 years old, had a febrile seizure and was diagnosed as having meningitis. You talk to her mother about the seizure.

Tip: Be sure to identify the parent's concern and attempt to clarify it, providing an opportunity for patient teaching. In the following scenario, the nurse responds with a therapeutic statement ("That must have been frightening.") and identifies a misconception verbalized by the mother.

Nurse: Mrs. Jarman, can you describe what happened?

Mrs. Jarman: She started shaking all over. It was really frightening.

Nurse: Did she voice any symptoms before the seizure?

Mrs. Jarman: No, just started shaking.

Nurse: That must have been frightening.

Mrs. Jarman: Thinking about what it did to her is scarier.

Nurse: Did to her?

Mrs. Jarman: I know seizures cause mental retardation. Our neighbor's son has them, and he's severely retarded.

Nurse: Let's talk about this a little more.

In many children, seizures increase or intensify at puberty, probably as the result of glandular changes or the need for an increased medicine dosage because of preadolescent growth. All antiseizure medications are potentially teratogenic to a fetus, so be certain adolescent girls are aware of this so they can choose to delay childbearing until later in life, when their medication can be reduced or even discontinued.

QSEN Checkpoint Question 49.6

SAFETY

Suppose Tasha has a tonic–clonic seizure while in the hospital. Which of the following items should the nurse keep available at the bedside for a child known to have generalized seizures? (Select all that apply.)
   a. Suction
   b. Tracheostomy tube
   c. Oxygen
   d. Call bell
   e. Padded tongue blade

Look in Appendix A for the best answer and rationale.

BREATH HOLDING

Breath holding is a phenomenon that occurs in young children when they are stressed or angry. The child breathes in and, because of anger or stress, does not breathe out again or else breathes out and then does not inhale again. As brain cells become anoxic, the child appears cyanotic and slumps to the floor, momentarily unconscious. With loss of consciousness, the child begins breathing again, color returns, and the child awakens. Breath holding this way is frightening to parents but results from the immaturity of the child's neurologic control. This differs from a temper tantrum, in which a child deliberately attempts to hold his or her breath and then passes out (see Chapter 30). The child needs no immediate therapy except reassurance the episode is over. Breath holding may be associated with iron-deficiency anemia; if this is discovered, iron supplementation may be prescribed to decrease the breath-holding episodes.

HEADACHE

Headaches in children younger than school age used to be considered rare, but young children can report "hair hurt" or have fussiness from allergies and viral inflammation of the upper respiratory tract that cause headaches. A toddler who has both vomiting and a headache should be evaluated because these are common signs of brain tumor, one of the most common tumors of childhood (Cleves & Rothner, 2011). Headache may also occur with a fever because of increased ICP caused by increased cerebral blood flow. As children reach school age, headaches may occur as a result of conditions as simple as eye-strain and sinusitis or, again, as serious as a brain tumor.

Headache pain results because of meningeal or vascular irritation, not from the brain itself because brain tissue is insensitive to pain. Because of this insensitivity, a cerebral tumor can be present for a lengthy time before meningeal irritation is enough that pain symptoms become apparent. With a brain tumor, pain becomes intense on changing body position, so a young child who reports a headache shortly after getting up in the morning should be carefully evaluated. Pain from a brain tumor is also usually occipital, so asking the child to indicate where it hurts helps determine whether a tumor could be the cause.

Tension or Stress Headache

When children are studying intently or taking a test, contraction of their neck muscles from tension can cause temporary ischemia to the head. This type of headache is usually experienced as a dull, steady pain across the forehead, the temporal area, or the back of the neck. Children with these symptoms should have their vision tested because poor eyesight may be the reason they hunch over their books. Stress headaches are relieved by simple analgesics, such as acetaminophen or ibuprofen, or by sleep or application of a cool compress. Advising children to take frequent "stretches" while studying can help avoid muscle tension and stress and reduce the number of headaches experienced.

Sinus Headache

Sinus headache usually accompanies sinusitis or is associated with inflammation and possible obstruction of the sinuses and is discussed in Chapter 40.

Migraine Headache

Migraine headache refers to a specific type of headache that may or may not begin with an aura or visual disturbance such as diplopia or a zigzag pattern across the visual field. The pain

that follows is usually unilateral and extremely intense, with throbbing that is moderate to severe. The headache is aggravated by routine physical activity or menstrual periods; it may be compounded by nausea and vomiting and intolerance to bright lights and noise (Cleves & Rothner, 2011).

The cause of migraine headache is not well understood but probably results from abnormal constriction of intracranial arteries that temporarily reduces cerebral blood supply. The reduction in blood flow is then followed by compensating over distention of cranial blood vessels. The aura accompanying such headaches results from the temporary ischemia that occurs in between those two processes. Some children who have migraine headaches have an abnormal EEG, but a normal EEG does not rule out the reality of the headaches.

Most children with migraine headache have a positive family history, or someone else in the family also has the same type of headache. A migraine syndrome may be inherited as a dominant trait.

Assessment

To help assess the cause of a headache, obtain a thorough history, including:
- When the headache usually occurs
- The events preceding it (to detect an aura)
- Its usual duration, frequency, intensity, description, and associated symptoms
- Any actions taken to treat the headache

The child needs a thorough physical examination, including funduscopic examination, to rule out papilledema. Blood pressure must be measured to rule out hypertension. If an aura is documented, an EEG will be prescribed to investigate a seizure as the basis of the headache.

Therapeutic Management

At the time of the headache, sleep or lying down may be necessary to relieve the pain and vomiting. Acetaminophen and nonsteroidal anti-inflammatory drugs are the first-line medical treatment for headaches in children, including migraines. Ergotamine tartrate (Cafergot), a vasoconstrictor, may be prescribed in addition for some children. Almotriptan, a member of the triptan family of drugs, is approved by the U.S. Food and Drug Administration for migraine in adolescents and may also be helpful. Frequent headaches interfere with a child's ability to achieve in school. Children may need to be reassured that even though their headaches are intense and even incapacitating, migraine headaches are benign and will not lead to any other condition so they can keep their headaches in perspective. Follow-up visits are necessary to confirm that they are not growing worse so treatment is remaining adequate (El-Chammas, Keyes, Thompson, et al., 2013).

If other family members have migraine headaches, counsel them that their reactions to their headaches influence their child's reaction to a headache. If the mother goes to bed for the day when she has a migraine headache, for example, she cannot expect her child to go to school when the child has a headache.

Spinal Cord Injury

Because of the resilience of their vertebrae, children have fewer spinal cord injuries than adults. However, the incidence among adolescents is increasing, especially among male adolescents, because more teenagers are involved in motor vehicle accidents, particularly motorcycle or off-road vehicle accidents, than previously (Martin-Herz, Zatzick, & McMahon, 2012). Another frequent cause of spinal cord injury is diving into too shallow water at beaches or backyard pools. Spinal cord injury without radiologic abnormality (SCIWORA) syndrome may occur, so any child with a multiple traumatic injury needs to be assessed for spinal cord damage. Stabilizing the neck at the accident scene is the best protection against further injury in these children (Hazinski, 2012).

RECOVERY PHASES

Spinal injuries result when the spinal cord becomes compressed or severed by the vertebrae; further cord damage can result from hemorrhage, edema, or inflammation at the injury site as the blood supply becomes impeded. Table 49.4 summarizes functional ability that will probably be present after spinal cord injury at different vertebral levels. Predictions such as these of useful body function cannot be made accurately at the time of the injury, however. Three phases of recovery must first take place.

First Recovery Phase

Immediately after the injury, the child experiences a *spinal shock syndrome* or loss of autonomic nervous system function (loss of nerve fibers traveling through the anterior horn of the spinal canal), leading to loss of motor function, sensation, reflex activity, and the presence of flaccid paralysis in body areas below the level of the injury. If a cervical or high thoracic injury is present, there will be loss of or decreased respiratory function because of flaccidity of the diaphragm or loss of the accessory muscles of the chest. At all levels, the child has no ability to sweat or shiver to change body temperature below the level of the lesion because of loss of autonomic nerve control; therefore, hypothermia or hyperthermia always becomes

a threat. Blood vessels below the level of the injury are no longer able to constrict, so blood tends to pool in the lower body, leading to yet another concern—upper body hypotension, especially if the upper body is elevated. Loss of bladder control occurs if the bladder is left flaccid (it expands and continually overflows). Loss of control in the bowel allows it to become equally distended; bowel sounds will be absent. This phase of spinal cord injury lasts from 1 to 6 weeks. As a rule, the shorter the phase of spinal shock, the better is the final outcome.

Administration of a corticosteroid can help reduce edema and possibly protect function of the spinal cord during this phase. A vasopressor agent such as dopamine may be prescribed to maintain blood pressure and perfusion to the cord.

Second Recovery Phase

During the second phase of recovery, the flaccid paralysis of the shock phase is replaced by spastic paralysis. Normally, motor impulses begin in the brain cortex and are transmitted to the medulla, where they cross to the opposite side of the cord; they then travel down the descending motor tracts of the spinal cord. They synapse in the anterior horn of the spinal cord and travel by way of the spinal and peripheral nerves to the designated muscle group, which they set in motion. The nerve pathways of the brain and the descending tracts are termed *upper motor neurons*. Those in the anterior horn cells and the spinal and peripheral nerves are termed *lower motor neurons*. Whether a motor neuron has upper or lower function, therefore, does not depend on its height in the spinal tract but rather on its position in relation to an anterior horn: Between the brain and the anterior horn, it is an upper motor neuron; between the anterior horn and the point of innervation, it is a lower motor neuron (Fig. 49.9).

Spasticity in the second phase is caused by the loss of upper level control or transmission of meaningful innervation to the

TABLE 49.4 FUNCTIONAL ABILITY AFTER SPINAL CORD INJURY

Injury Site	Highest Key Functions Still Present	Effects and Possible Interventions
C1–C3	Head and neck muscles intact	Respiratory paralysis from loss of phrenic nerve innervation; will need ventilatory assistance
		No voluntary motion below chin; possibly able to learn to use mouth to control pen for writing and mouth stick to reach objects
C4	Diaphragm intact	Loss of motor function of upper and lower extremities and trunk; able to learn to use abdominal muscles to breathe independently
C5	Shoulder control; biceps, deltoid function	Able to feed self and operate wheelchair if fitted with self-care aids
C6	Forearm pronation; wrist extension	Use of upper extremities for self-care; can transfer to wheelchair and so have increased independence
C7	Triceps function	Able to transfer to wheelchair readily; increasing independence
C8	Thumb and finger function	Able to do fine motor tasks; increases self-care ability
T1–T7	Intercostal muscles (able to breathe with chest, not abdominal, muscles)	Full use of upper extremities but is still dependent on wheelchair
		Possibly able to drive car with hand controls
		Possibly able to have high leg braces fitted for standing
T10–12	Abdominal muscles	Use of long leg braces and four-point crutch to ambulate
L2–L4	Hip flexion	Use of long or short leg braces to ambulate
	Leg extension	
L5–S1	Gluteus maximus muscle function	Able to walk without aids
S4	Bladder and anal sphincter control	Able to control bladder and bowel function
		Penile erection and ejaculation possible

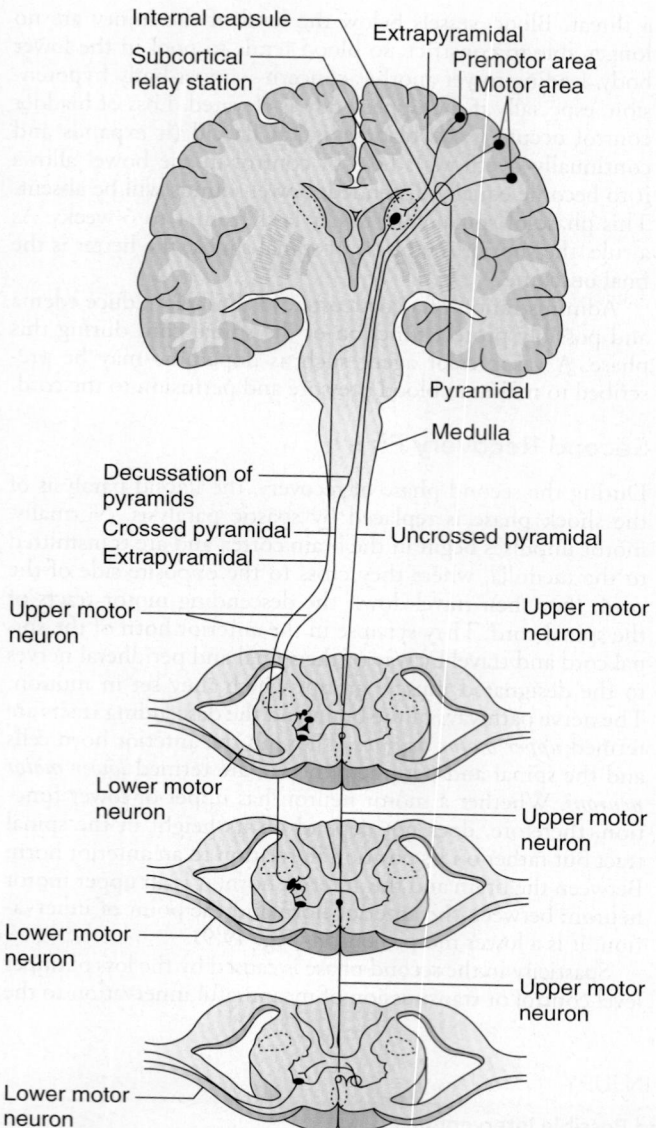

Figure 49.9 Diagram of motor pathways between the cerebral cortex, one of the subcortical relay stations, and lower motor neurons in the spinal cord. Decussation (crossing of fibers) means that each side of the brain controls skeletal muscles on the opposite side of the body.

anterior horn. Lacking upper motor neuron function because of a severed cord, the lower motor neurons or reflex arcs cause the muscles to contract and remain that way. Parents and children are quick to interpret the sudden spastic movement of a lower extremity as meaningful activity. This is particularly easy to believe with infants, who cannot tell you they have no control or cannot stop their legs from contracting. Differences between upper and lower neuron damage are listed in Table 49.5. If the injury is very low in the spinal tract, affecting mostly lower motor neurons, the muscles will remain flaccid because the lower motor neurons cannot send impulses for contraction.

During this phase, if the child's bladder is allowed to fill, the resultant sensory stimulation relayed to the damaged cord can initiate a powerful sympathetic reflex reaction

(**autonomic dysreflexia**). The child will experience extreme hypertension, tachycardia, flushed face, and severe occipital headache. This is an emergency situation because if the severe hypertension is not relieved, cerebrovascular accident can result (Pellatt, 2010). Assess that the child's urinary catheter is not obstructed, so urine can flow freely and reduce the sensory stimulation. Also, frequently assess for signs of urinary tract infection such as elevated temperature or cloudy urine because urinary complications remain the leading cause of morbidity and the most common infection for individuals with spinal cord injury (Eves & Rivera, 2010).

 Concept Mastery Alert

Respiratory function is of great concern in the first stage of recovery. By the second stage, respiratory function should have stabilized and become predicable. Contractures can occur during this stage as the flaccid paralysis of the first stage passes and the spastic paralysis of the second stage begins.

Third Recovery Phase

The third phase of recovery from spinal cord injury is learning to live with the final outcome or permanent limitation of motor and sensory function. If the compression of the spinal cord was only caused by edema that is then relieved, no permanent motor and sensory disability will occur.

ASSESSMENT OF SPINAL CORD INJURY

Cervical and thoracolumbar areas of the spine are the ones most likely to sustain injury, but spinal cord injury should be suspected whenever a child has sustained a forceful trauma of any kind. Do not move a child with suspected spinal cord injury at the scene of the injury until the back and head can be supported in a straight line to prevent further injury to the spinal column from twisting or bending. In the emergency department, as a general rule, do not attempt to move the child from a stretcher to an examining table until spinal X-ray films have been obtained; if helping move the child onto the X-ray table, use a gentle log-rolling technique to avoid additional movement or injury. If resuscitation is necessary, be certain to maintain the child's head in a neutral position, not hyperextended. To keep the neck immobilized, if a child is wearing a football, bicycle, or motorcycle helmet or a neck brace, do not remove these (Nayduch, 2010). Help maintain spinal immobilization during such procedures as obtaining blood samples or a neurologic assessment.

 ## Nursing Diagnoses and Related Interventions

During the first phase of recovery, a child's major problems are those that result from almost complete immobility: pressure ulcers on bony prominences, loss of appetite and subsequent poor nutrition from depression or being kept in a supine position, urinary calculi caused by excessive calcium loss from bones, atrophy of flaccid muscle groups, and urinary retention and bladder infection. These effects of immobility are presented in Figure 49.10.

TABLE 49.5 CHARACTERISTICS OF UPPER AND LOWER MOTOR NERVE INJURY AFTER SPINAL SHOCK PHASE

Finding	Upper Motor Lesion	Lower Motor Lesion
Spasticity	Present	Absent (flaccidity present)
Clonus	Present, increased	Absent
Tendon reflexes	Increased	Absent
Babinski reflex	Present	Absent
Reflexes below level of lesion	Present	Absent
Reflex at level of lesion	Absent	Absent
Atrophy of muscles	Absent or present only to slight degree	Present (muscle fasciculations may be present)

Nursing Diagnosis: Impaired physical mobility related to effects of spinal cord injury

Outcome Evaluation: Child ambulates with a minimum of artificial support and equipment; participates in exercise program within limitations.

To relieve edema at the injury site and prevent further injury, IV corticosteroids will be administered. Children may be placed in cervical traction with Crutchfield tongs and a traction belt (Fig. 49.11) or with halo traction (see Chapter 51). Having tongs inserted into the skull is a very frightening procedure for children because they worry the tongs will burrow into their skull and strike their brain. Encourage parents to stay with children during the procedure both for psychological support and to help them lie still during the procedure.

To promote circulation and prevent loss of calcium that results from inactivity, full range-of-motion exercises must be scheduled approximately three times per day. Assist with these as necessary as they are time-consuming but important to maintain joint function.

During the second phase of recovery, when spasticity of muscle groups occurs, preventing contractures becomes the chief concern. Specialized splints, boots, or even high-top sneakers may be used to prevent foot drop (Fig. 49.12). If children have upper extremity mobility but will be left with lower extremity paralysis, exercises to strengthen the upper extremity muscle groups are needed so children will be strong enough to lift themselves from a bed to a wheelchair or raise themselves with a trapeze over the bed when changing positions. Holding legs and arms at the joints while moving is a good technique to help reduce muscle spasms.

One major problem of ambulation after spinal cord injury is helping a child's body readjust to a vertical position after being maintained in the supine position for so long.

Figure 49.10 Effects of immobilization.

Figure 49.11 Crutchfield tongs used to create spinal traction.

In the new upright position, blood tends to pool in dilated blood vessels below the level of the spinal injury, resulting in a pseudohypovolemia and hypotension. The first time a child sits up or stands may occur to such an extent that the child faints. Gradually increasing the angle of the bed helps the child become acclimated to the upright position without experiencing so much vascular pooling.

Nursing Diagnosis: Self-care deficit related to spinal cord injury

Outcome Evaluation: Child states intention of taking over self-care; practices using equipment for eating, bathing, and toileting; participates in one new aspect of self-care each week.

As soon as possible, children should be introduced to self-help methods for activities of daily living. You may need to encourage parents to allow a child to become as self-sufficient as possible or not to take over complete care.

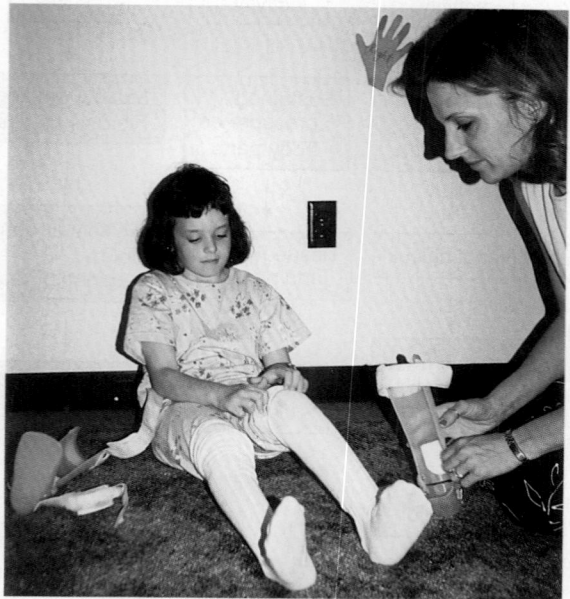

Figure 49.12 Specialized splints are used for a child with a low spinal cord injury to prevent contractures and foot drop. Here, the physical therapist prepares to apply the splint to the child's leg. (Photograph courtesy of Sue Moses.)

The child may well outlive them and will someday need to be able to function as independently as possible without them.

Remember, without autonomic nervous system function, a child is unable to sweat and becomes hyperthermic if covered too warmly; if not covered warmly enough, the capillaries dilate, and the child loses considerable heat into the environment. If the room temperature cools at night, be careful to dress the child appropriately for sleeping.

Specific measures for bowel evacuation may be necessary, depending on the level of the injury. A bowel program incorporating the use of stool softeners, suppositories, and bowel retraining may be required. The child and parents need support and instructions in accomplishing this task and gaining independence as it may take weeks or months to accomplish.

For some children and parents, the first day of using a wheelchair is exciting (proof that the child can be partially ambulatory). For others, it is the day on which they are forced to face the reality that they cannot undo the results of the injury and that their child has a permanent life-long disability. If parents have almost overcome their grief and accepted their child's disability, the introduction of a symbol of disability such as a wheelchair or long leg braces may bring new grieving and a sense of loss.

When the child reaches sexual maturity, limitations in this area may become a child's chief concern. If a male has had an upper motor neuron injury, he will not be able to achieve spontaneous erection or ejaculation. However, with manual stimulation of the penis (stimulation of lower motor neuron function), he may be able to achieve an erection and engage in coitus even though ejaculation and fertility remain limited. With most spinal cord injuries, a female is not able to experience orgasm but is able to conceive and bear children.

The limitations caused by a spinal cord injury become especially evident to the child (and the parents) when choosing a vocation and selecting an appropriate school program (remember children cannot be denied regular schooling by federal law in the United States, even with a severe physical disability). Counseling and rehabilitation are crucial aspects to achieve an optimal level of functioning and independence.

Nursing Diagnosis: Risk for impaired gas exchange related to spinal cord injury

Outcome Evaluation: Respiratory rate is within acceptable parameters; lungs are clear; airway is patent.

If the cervical level of the cord is involved, a child will need ventilatory assistance. The child may be intubated at first, but orotracheal or nasotracheal intubation is only a temporary measure to maintain a patent airway. At a later date, a tracheostomy will be done for long-term airway management and to prevent sloughing of pharyngeal tissue from the constant pressure of the intubation tube. If a tracheotomy tube is required, be certain parents receive thorough instructions on caring for the tracheostomy and, if necessary, working with a mechanical ventilator. A phrenic nerve pacemaker may be used to stimulate the diaphragm to contract and initiate respirations. If the child has a thoracic-level injury (which is rare because the rib cage gives extra strength to thoracic vertebrae), the child will be able to breathe independently but will have reduced vital capacity. Periodic positive-pressure breathing treatments may be necessary to encourage increased lung filling. Be careful when positioning a child not to compromise chest movement with equipment or other restricting objects. Other respiratory care measures, such as suctioning and chest physiotherapy, also help maintain chest function.

Nursing Diagnosis: Risk for impaired skin integrity related to immobility

Outcome Evaluation: Child's skin remains clean, dry, and intact without signs of erythema or ulceration.

To prevent skin breakdown, turn children about every 2 hours (always being certain to logroll or maintain immobilization with a striker frame or a continuously moving, automatically controlled bed). The use of an alternating-pressure mattress may also be helpful. With loss of sensation in body parts, the child is unable to report skin irritation from a wrinkled sheet or wet clothing. If the child is incontinent, change the linen immediately to prevent skin breakdown. Once children are ambulatory by wheelchair, check their legs and buttocks regularly to prevent pressure ulcers caused by sitting or using leg braces (McCaskey, Kirk, & Gerdes, 2011).

Nursing Diagnosis: Risk for impaired urinary elimination related to spinal cord injury

Outcome Evaluation: Child's urine output is adequate for intake; child identifies measures to assist with voiding; child demonstrates procedure for self-catheterization.

To prevent urinary retention during the first phase of recovery, a Foley catheter is usually inserted, or the bladder can be emptied by periodic suprapubic aspiration or intermittent catheterization. Second-stage spasticity causes periodic reflex emptying. The bladder rarely empties completely, however, so problems of stasis and infection continue. To live independently, the child needs to learn self-catheterization to empty the bladder (see Chapter 46).

Nursing Diagnosis: Anticipatory grieving related to loss of function secondary to spinal cord injury

Outcome Evaluation: Child and parents openly discuss their feelings about the injury and its effect on their lives.

The second recovery phase is the time for parents and children to begin thinking about what this degree of disability will mean to them as a family and to face what adjustments they will need to make. Children and parents typically react to the initial diagnosis with grief. They may still be in denial or shock when the second phase begins. With no sudden miracle cure in sight, they may begin to move through stages of anger, bargaining, depression, and then acceptance (the injury happened; we must go on from this point). They need assistance and support to work through all of these feeling, however. Both the parents and the child may need counseling to reach acceptance (Fig. 49.13).

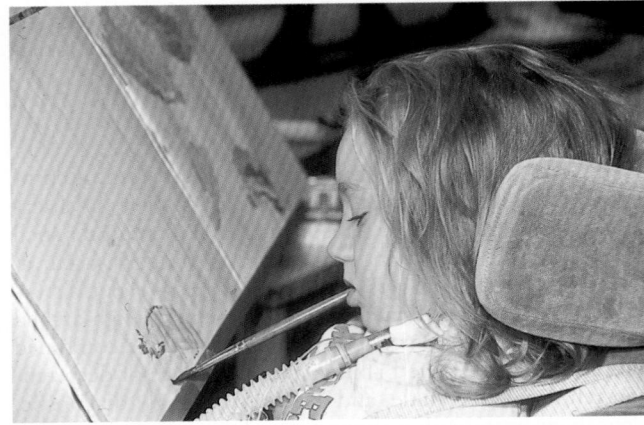

Figure 49.13 A 6-year-old girl with a cervical spine injury adapts to her disability by using her mouth to hold a paintbrush and participate in age-appropriate activities. (© Elisa Peterson/Stock Boston.)

> *What If . . . 49.3*
> **Tasha's father, a high school science teacher, asks the nurse to help him design a program to teach teenagers how to prevent spinal cord injury. What topics would be best to include?**

Ataxic Disorders

Ataxia is failure of muscular coordination or irregularity of muscle action. Ataxic disorders are often manifested by an awkward gait or lack of coordination. Causes of ataxia differ, but degeneration of cerebellar or vestibular function is always involved.

ATAXIA-TELANGIECTASIA

Ataxia-telangiectasia, transmitted as an autosomal recessive trait attributable to a defect of chromosome 11, is a primary immunodeficiency disorder that results in progressive cerebellar degeneration. This is a multisystem disease with neurologic and immunologic aspects. In addition, endocrine abnormalities may occur, and there is an increased risk of cancer, particularly brain tumor. Telangiectasias (red vascular markings) appear on the conjunctiva and skin at the flexor creases (American Academy of Pediatrics, 2012).

Both immunologic and neurologic symptoms of this disorder vary in severity and onset. Serum immunoglobulin A (IgA) and immunoglobulin E (IgE) levels may be low, and there is often evidence of reduced T-cell function. Children develop frequent infections (primarily sinopulmonary) because of the immunologic deficits. Tonsillar tissue in the pharynx appears scant.

Neurologic symptoms caused by the degeneration process can usually be detected in early infancy when developmental milestones are not met. Children develop an awkward gait when they begin to walk. **Choreoathetosis** (rapid, purposeless movements), nystagmus, an intention tremor, or scoliosis may develop. Children may be unable to move their eyes or follow movement through visual fields. Eye changes (conjunctival telangiectasia) develop by 5 years of age. Unfortunately, there is no effective treatment. Children with this disorder often die in late adolescence of infection, respiratory failure, or a malignant brain tumor.

FRIEDREICH ATAXIA

Friedreich ataxia, which is carried on the short arm of chromosome 9 as an autosomal recessive trait, involves a variety of degenerative symptoms (Koeppen, 2011). Symptoms such as progressive cerebellar and spinal cord dysfunction occur in late adolescence. Teenagers develop a progressive gait disturbance, a lack of coordinated arm movements, a high-arched foot (pes cavus), hammer toes, and scoliosis. The combined symptoms of a positive Babinski reflex, absence of deep tendon reflexes in the ankle, and ataxia are strongly diagnostic. Neurologic examination shows difficulty in recognizing foot position (whether the foot is moved up or down). If the ataxia remains untreated, death occurs in young adulthood from myocardial failure. Antioxidant therapy may help to delay this outcome by reducing ventricular hypertrophy (Lynch, Regner, Schadt, et al., 2012).

What If . . . 49.4
A nurse is interested in exploring one of the 2020 National Health Goals related to children with neurologic disorders (see Box 49.1). Most government-sponsored funding for nursing research is allotted based on these goals. What would be a possible research topic pertinent to these goals that would be applicable to Tasha's family and also advance evidence-based practice?

KEY POINTS FOR REVIEW

- Nerve cells are unique in that they do not regenerate if damaged, tending to make neurologic diseases long-term illnesses. Parents and children alike need support from healthcare providers to cope with problems that continue to occur over a long period. Planning nursing care to achieve this not only meets Quality & Safety Education for Nurses (QSEN) competencies but hopefully also meets the family's total needs.
- Increased ICP arises from an increase in the volume of CSF or from blood accumulation, cerebral edema, or space-occupying lesions. Vital sign changes such as increased temperature and blood pressure and decreased pulse and respirations begin as subtle changes. Always compare assessments with previous levels to detect that a consistent, although minor, change is occurring.
- CP is a nonprogressive disorder of upper motor neurons. The exact cause is usually unknown, but the condition is caused by abnormal brain development or damage to the developing brain. Four major types are identified: spastic (excessive tone in the voluntary muscles), dyskinetic or athetoid (abnormal involuntary movement), atonic (decreased muscle tone), and mixed (symptoms of both spasticity and athetoid movements).
- Meningitis is infection of the cerebral meninges, caused most frequently by bacterial invasion. Children need follow-up afterward to monitor for hearing acuity and impaired secretion of antidiuretic hormone.

- Encephalitis is inflammation of brain tissue. This is always a serious diagnosis because the child may be left with residual neurologic damage, such as seizures or learning disabilities.
- Reye syndrome is acute encephalitis with accompanying fatty infiltration of the liver, heart, and lungs; it most frequently occurs if a child with a viral infection is administered acetylsalicylic acid (aspirin) and is the reason children should not be administered aspirin for fever.
- Guillain-Barré syndrome is inflammation of motor and sensory nerves. The reaction may be immune mediated, occurring after an upper respiratory tract illness. Temporary demyelization of the nerve sheaths causes loss of function.
- Botulism occurs when spores of *C. botulinum* produce toxins in the intestine. Because honey can be a source of the organism, it should not be given to infants.
- Recurrent seizures are involuntary contractions of muscles caused by abnormal electrical brain discharges. Common types seen in children include febrile seizures, infantile spasms, partial (focal) seizures, absence seizures, and tonic–clonic seizures. Therapy is administration of antiseizure drugs.
- Spinal cord injury is occurring at increased rates in children involved in sports and motor vehicle accidents. Children pass through a first, second, and third recovery phase after the injury until they reach a final outcome.

CRITICAL THINKING CARE STUDY

Darien Fisher is a 12-year-old boy you see in the emergency room because he was brought to the hospital by ambulance after having a tonic–clonic seizure at basketball practice. His parents are divorced, so Darien lives with his mother and two younger brothers in a trailer park during weekdays. On the weekend, he lives with his father on a houseboat.

1. The emergency room physician asked Mrs. Fisher for permission to do a lumbar puncture on Darien but she refused because she remembered what a terrible headache she had after receiving spinal anesthesia for Darien's birth. Would you agree that lumbar punctures often lead to severe headaches? What are some things you could do to help prevent a headache in Darien?
2. Darien is prescribed carbamazepine (Tegretol) for recurrent seizures. His mother is concerned he won't take it on weekends because his father is "all fun—nothing serious." Would you agree with her that she's right in refusing to allow Darien to visit his father on weekends?
3. Darien is concerned that he won't be allowed to play on his school basketball team if he has another seizure. Are recurrent seizures aggravated by strenuous activity? Would preventing him from playing be good advice?

RELATED RESOURCES

Explore these additional resources to enhance learning for this chapter:
- Student resources on thePoint, including answers to the What If . . . and Critical Thinking Care Study questions, http://thepoint.lww.com/Flagg8e
- Adaptive learning powered by PrepU, http://thepoint.lww.com/prepu

REFERENCES

American Academy of Pediatrics. (2012). *Telangiectasias*. Retrieved from https://pediatriccare.solutions.aap.org/Content.aspx?gbosid=165682

American Academy of Pediatrics. (2015). Botulism and infant botulism. In D. W. Kimberlin, M. T. Brady, M. A. Jackson, et al. (Eds.), *Red book: 2015 Report of the Committee on Infectious Diseases* (30th ed., pp. 294–296). Elk Grove Village, IL: Author.

Ardern-Holmes, S. L., & North, K. N. (2011). Therapeutics for childhood neurofibromatosis type 1 and type 2. *Current Treatment Options in Neurology, 13*(6), 529–543.

Bailey, B. M., Liesemer, K., Statler, K. D., et al. (2012). Monitoring and prediction of intracranial hypertension in pediatric traumatic brain injury: Clinical factors and initial head computed tomography. *Journal of Trauma and Acute Care Surgery, 72*(1), 263–270.

Bennett, C. L., Starko, K. M., Thomsen, H. S., et al. (2012). Linking drugs to obscure illnesses: Lessons from pure red cell aplasia, nephrogenic systemic fibrosis, and Reye's syndrome. A report from the Southern Network on Adverse Reactions (SONAR). *Journal of General Internal Medicine, 27*(12), 1697–1703.

Budohoski, K. P., Zweifel, C., Kasprowicz, M., et al. (2012). What comes first? The dynamics of cerebral oxygenation and blood flow in response to changes in arterial pressure and intracranial pressure after head injury. *British Journal of Anaesthesia, 108*(1), 89–99.

Centers for Disease Control and Prevention. (2017). *Facts about cerebral palsy*. Retrieved from https://www.cdc.gov/ncbddd/cp/facts.html

Chetty, S. P., Shaffer, B. L., & Norton, M. E. (2011). Management of pregnancy in women with genetic disorders: Part 2: Inborn errors of metabolism, cystic fibrosis, neurofibromatosis type 1, and Turner syndrome in pregnancy. *Obstetrics & Gynecology Survey, 66*(12), 765–776.

Cleves, C., & Rothner, A. D. (2011). Headache in children and adolescents: Evaluation and diagnosis, including migraine and its subtypes. In S. J. Tepper & D. E. Tepper (Eds.), *The Cleveland Clinic manual of headache therapy* (pp. 81–92). New York, NY: Springer Publishing.

Coté, C. J., & Wilson, S. (2016). Guidelines for monitoring and management of pediatric patients before, during, and after sedation for diagnostic and therapeutic procedures: Update 2016. *Pediatric Dentistry, 38*(6), 216–245.

Crosbie, J., Alhusaini, A. A., Dean, C. M., et al. (2012). Plantarflexor muscle and spatiotemporal gait characteristics of children with hemiplegic cerebral palsy: An observational study. *Developmental Neurorehabilitation, 15*(2), 114–118.

El-Chammas, K., Keyes, J., Thompson, N., et al. (2013). Pharmacologic treatment of pediatric headaches: A meta-analysis. *JAMA Pediatrics, 167*(3), 250–258.

Eves, F. J., & Rivera, N. (2010). Prevention of urinary tract infections in persons with spinal cord injury in home health care. *Home Healthcare Nurse, 28*(4), 230–241.

Go, C. Y., Mackay, M. T., Weiss, S. K., et al. (2012). Evidence-based guidelines update: Medical treatment of infantile spasms. Report of the Guideline Development Subcommittee of the American Academy of Neurology and the Practice Committee of the Child Neurology Society. *Neurology, 78*(24), 1974–1980.

Gray, N., Morton, R. E., Brimlow, K., et al. (2012). Goals and outcomes for non ambulant children receiving continuous infusion of intrathecal baclofen. *European Journal of Paediatric Neurology, 16*(5), 443–448.

Greenberg-Kushnir, N., Haskin, O., Yarden-Bilavsky, H., et al. (2012). *Haemophilus influenzae* type b meningitis in the short period after vaccination: A reminder of the phenomenon of apparent vaccine failure. *Case Reports in Infectious Diseases, 2012*, 950107.

Hazinski, M. F. (2012). Neurological disorders. In M. F. Hazinski (Ed.), *Nursing care of the critically ill child* (3rd ed., pp. 587–678). St. Louis, MO: Elsevier Health Sciences.

Karch, A. M. (2013). *2013 Lippincott's nursing drug guide*. Philadelphia, PA: Lippincott Williams & Wilkins.

Kneen, R., Michael, D. B., Menson, E., et al. (2012). The management of suspected viral encephalitis in children. Association of British Neurologists and British Paediatric Allergy, Immunology and Infection Group national guidelines. *Journal of Infection, 64*(5), 449–477.

Koeppen, A. H. (2011). Friedreich's ataxia: Pathology, pathogenesis, and molecular genetics. *Journal of the Neurological Sciences, 303*(1–2), 1–12.

Lewis, D. W. (2011). Neurology. In K. J. Marcdante, R. M. Kliegman, H. B. Jenson, et al. (Eds.), *Nelson essentials of pediatrics* (6th ed., pp. 671–700). Philadelphia, PA: Saunders/Elsevier.

Libster, R., Edwards, K. M., Levent, F., et al. (2012). Long-term outcomes of group B streptococcal meningitis. *Pediatrics, 130*(1), e8–e15.

Lo, W., Marchuk, D. A., Ball, K. L., et al. (2012). Updates and future horizons on the understanding, diagnosis, and treatment of Sturge-Weber syndrome brain involvement. *Developmental Medicine & Child Neurology, 54*(3), 214–223.

Luckhaupt, S. E., Dalhamer, J. M., Ward, B. W., et al. (2013). Prevalence and work-relatedness of carpal tunnel syndrome in the working population. *American Journal of Industrial Medicine, 56*(6), 615–624.

Lynch, D. R., Regner, S. R., Schadt, K. A., et al. (2012). Management and therapy for cardiomyopathy in Friedreich's ataxia. *Expert Reviews of Cardiovascular Therapy, 10*(6), 767–777.

Martin-Herz, S. P., Zatzick, D. F., & McMahon, R. J. (2012). Health-related quality of life in children and adolescents following traumatic injury: A review. *Clinical Child and Family Psychology Review, 15*(3), 192–214.

McCaskey, M. S., Kirk, L., & Gerdes, C. (2011). Preventing skin breakdown in the immobile child in the home care setting. *Home Healthcare Nurse, 29*(4), 248–255.

McNamara, R., Doyle, J., McKay, M., et al. (2013). Medium term outcome in Bell's palsy in children. *Emergency Medicine Journal, 30*(6), 444–446.

Nayduch, D. A. (2010). Back to basics: Identifying and managing acute spinal cord injury. *Nursing, 40*(9), 24–31.

Ninove, L., Daniel, L., Gallou, J., et al. (2011). Fatal case of Reye's syndrome associated with H3N2 influenza virus infection and salicylate intake in a 12-year-old patient. *Clinical Microbiology and Infection, 17*(1), 95–97.

Pace, D., & Pollard, A. J. (2012). Meningococcal disease: Clinical presentation and sequelae. *Vaccine, 30*(Suppl. 2), B3–B39.

Parachuri, V., & Inglese, C. (2013). Neurological problems in the adolescent population. *Adolescent Medicine State of the Art Reviews, 24*(1), 1–28.

Pellatt, G. C. (2010). Spinal surgery for acute traumatic spinal cord injury: Implications for nursing. *British Journal of Neuroscience Nursing, 6*(6), 271–275.

Placzek, R., Siebold, D., & Funk, J. F. (2010). Development of treatment concepts for the use of botulinum toxin A in children with cerebral palsy. *Toxins, 2*(9), 2258–2271.

Rapin, I. (2011). Child neurologists as evaluators of developmental disorders. *Seminars in Pediatric Neurology, 18*(2), 104–109.

Riesch, S. K., Kedrowski, K., Brown, R. L., et al. (2012). Health-risk behaviors among a sample of US pre-adolescents: Types, frequency, and predictive factors. *International Journal of Nursing Studies, 50*(8), 1067–1079.

Robotham, D. (2011). Neurology. In K. Arcara & M. Tschudy (Eds.), *The Harriet Lane handbook: A manual for pediatric house officers* (pp. 504–523). St. Louis, MO: Mosby.

Rosen, B. A. (2012). Guillain-Barré syndrome. *Pediatrics in Review, 33*(4), 164–170.

Rust, R. S. (2011). What the child neurologist should know at the conclusion of training: History taking, examination, and formulation (and a few other generalizations). *Seminars in Pediatric Neurology, 18*(2), 59–65.

Selter, J. H., Turner, Z., Doerrer, S. C., et al. (2014). Dietary and medication adjustments to improve seizure control in patients treated with the ketogenic diet. *Journal of Child Neurology, 30*(1), 53–57.

Senger, B. A., Ward, L. D., Barbosa-Leiker, C., et al. (2015). Stress and coping of parents caring for a child with mitochondrial disease. *Applied Nursing Research, 29*, 195–201.

Sidhu, R., Velayudam, K., & Barnes, G. (2013). Pediatric seizures. *Pediatrics in Review, 34*, 333–341.

Sigurtà, A., Zanaboni, C., Canavesi, K., et al. (2013). Intensive care for pediatric traumatic brain injury. *Intensive Care Medicine, 39*(1), 129–136.

U.S. Department of Health and Human Services. (2010). *Healthy people 2020*. Washington, DC: Author.

Yuki, N., & Hartung, H. (2012). Guillain-Barré syndrome. *The New England Journal of Medicine, 366*(24), 2294–2304.

50

Nursing Care of a Family When a Child Has a Vision or Hearing Disorder

Carla Vander, a 6-year-old child, is brought to your pediatric clinic for evaluation. Her mother states, "She was born deaf and with a cataract. Today, she has pain in her ear and her left eye is red. How could a bad eye or an ear without a functioning nerve get infected?"

Previous chapters discussed the growth and development of well children. This chapter adds information about the changes, both physical and psychosocial, that occur when a child develops a disorder of the eyes (vision) or ears (hearing). This is important information because it builds a base for care and health teaching.

How would you answer Ms. Vander? What additional information does she need to know about eye and ear disorders?

KEY TERMS

accommodation	goniotomy	photophobia
amblyopia	hyperopia	ptosis
astigmatism	light refraction	stereopsis
diplopia	myopia	strabismus
enucleation	nystagmus	tympanocentesis
fovea centralis	orthoptics	

OBJECTIVES

After mastering the contents of this chapter, you should be able to:

1. Describe the structure and function of the eyes and ears and disorders of these organs as they affect children.
2. Identify nursing contribution in achieving 2020 National Health Goals related to vision and hearing disorders of children.
3. Assess a child who has a disorder of vision or hearing.
4. Formulate nursing diagnoses related to a child with a disorder of vision or hearing.
5. Establish expected outcomes for a child with a disorder of vision or hearing to help parents manage seamless transitions across differing healthcare settings.
6. Using the nursing process, plan nursing care that includes the six competencies of Quality & Safety Education for Nurses (QSEN): Patient-Centered Care, Teamwork & Collaboration, Evidence-Based Practice (EBP), Quality Improvement (QI), Safety, and Informatics.
7. Implement nursing care to meet the specific needs of a child who has a disorder of the eyes or ears, including patient and parent education.
8. Evaluate effectiveness and achievement of expected outcomes for a child with a vision and/or hearing disorder.
9. Integrate knowledge of childhood disorders of the eyes or ears with the interplay of nursing process, the six competencies of QSEN, and Family Nursing to promote quality maternal and child health nursing care.

Any interference with vision or hearing poses a threat to normal growth and development because so much of what and how a child learns about the world are achieved through these sensory organs. Infants first learn how to interact with others by watching their parents' faces, for example. They learn to speak by listening to words spoken to them. They continue to depend on sensory input for stimulation and to protect their safety throughout life (LaRoche, 2013).

Eye and ear disorders may be transitory. However, they always have the potential for becoming long-term illnesses if they permanently affect vision and hearing. This is an area, therefore, in which health promotion, illness prevention, and health rehabilitation are all vital aspects of nursing care. Because of the importance of vision and hearing, the 2020 National Health Goals have been established in relation to them (Box 50.1).

Nursing Process Overview

FOR CARE OF A CHILD WITH A VISION OR HEARING DISORDER

ASSESSMENT

All newborns should be assessed for their ability to focus on or see an examiner's face and to follow an object from the periphery to the midline. Observe the infant closely to ensure that this response is evoked by sight, not by the sound of your voice. If it's unclear whether a newborn can see, vision can be further tested by optokinetic nystagmus testing.

Assessing newborn infants for hearing loss is an equally important part of newborn care. This can be done by assessing if newborns quiet to the sound of a soothing voice. Most hospitals further routinely test newborns' hearing with otoacoustic emissions and auditory brain stem response (Akinpelu, Peleva, Funnell, et al., 2014).

Throughout childhood, children should be assessed by history for both vision and hearing disorders. In addition, children also should be assessed for their ability to speak clearly and appropriately for their age because language development is influenced by hearing. Because hearing and vision assessment are part of routine physical exams, the techniques of these are discussed in Chapter 34.

NURSING DIAGNOSIS

Teaching health promotion measures to safeguard vision and hearing is one of the most important roles in nursing. Examples of nursing diagnoses in this area include:
- Health-seeking behaviors related to the prevention of trauma to the eyes or ears
- Deficient knowledge related to the importance of early diagnosis and treatment of eye or ear infections
- Self-care deficit related to impaired visual acuity
- Risk for injury related to hearing loss
- Risk for situational low self-esteem related to long-term vision deficit
- Impaired verbal communication related to congenital hearing deficit
- Social isolation related to effects of hearing loss
- Risk for complicated grieving related to child's loss of sight

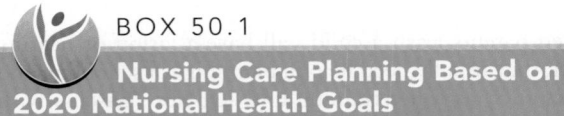

BOX 50.1

Nursing Care Planning Based on 2020 National Health Goals

Adequate vision and hearing ability are necessary for normal growth and development; therefore, several 2020 National Health Goals focus on prevention, early detection, treatment, and rehabilitation of eye and hearing health. These include:

- Increase the proportion of preschool children aged 5 years and younger who receive vision screening from a baseline of 40.1% to 44.1%.
- Reduce blindness and visual impairment in children and adolescents aged 17 years and younger from 28.2 per 1,000 children to 25.4 per 1,000.
- Reduce visual impairment in children aged 12 years and older from 136.1 per 1,000 population to 122.5 per 1,000.
- Increase the use of personal protective eyewear in recreational activities and hazardous situations around the home from 16.5% to 18.2% of children and adolescents aged 6 to 17 years.
- Reduce otitis media in children and adolescents from 246.1 persons per 1,000 persons younger than age 18 years to 221.5 per 1,000.
- Increase the proportion of persons with hearing impairments who have ever used a hearing aid or assistive listening devices or who have cochlear implants (developmental).
- Increase the proportion of persons who have had a hearing examination on schedule from 79.3% to 87.2% of adolescents aged 12 to 19 years (U.S. Department of Health and Human Services, 2010; see www.healthypeople.gov).

Nurses can help the nation achieve these goals by screening for vision and hearing at all well-child assessments, paying particular attention to those children who had low birth weight, were cared for in neonatal intensive care units, or who were excessively exposed to loud noises such as loud music.

- Risk for parental role strain related to responsibilities of caring for a sensory impaired child
- Readiness for enhanced family coping related to child's traumatic injury and subsequent loss of vision in one eye

OUTCOME IDENTIFICATION AND PLANNING

Be certain that expected outcomes established are realistic and address areas in which treatment can have some impact. By listening attentively to the concerns of parents and those of the child and by providing useful anticipatory guidance, you can help to increase a child's ability to function effectively. Because many eye and ear disorders cause pain, helping parents reduce pain in their child is a major nursing responsibility. Be certain that expected outcomes address preventive aspects of care in all areas of daily living.

When parents learn a child will have a vision or hearing disorder, they usually need help in planning for schooling and activities such as toilet training and self-care. Discuss with them the importance of talking to and touching their infant, so the infant learns how to communicate and learn about the world through his or her functioning senses. Most children with sensory disorders benefit from very early preschool education programs because this exposes them to interesting and stimulating tasks while their initiative is strongest.

Many parents whose infant screens positive for hearing loss in the hospital do not follow up with additional hearing screening as recommended probably because of inadequate communication about the concern or a lack of health insurance (Alam, Gaffney, & Eichwald, 2014). Internet resources that can be helpful to parents are the Alexander Graham Bell Association for the Deaf and Hard of Hearing (www.agbell .org), the American Foundation for the Blind (www.afb.org), the American Speech-Language-Hearing Association (www .asha.org), Lighthouse Guild (www.lighthouseguild.org), the National Federation of the Blind (www.nfb.org), Learning Ally (www.learningally.org), and the National Association of the Deaf (www.nad.org).

IMPLEMENTATION

A disorder of the eyes or ears can range from an acute, onetime illness to a chronic and developmentally debilitating condition if steps are not taken to treat the initial problem quickly and completely. However, even the most rigorous preventive care and attention cannot avert the occurrence of some serious disorders affecting vision and hearing. Nursing care must then focus on helping the child and parents adjust to the condition, ensuring that the child receives the stimulation needed to grow and develop on a usual continuum.

Nursing interventions for a child with a disorder of the eyes or ears range from providing anticipatory guidance and teaching children and parents measures to promote eye and ear health to preparing a child for surgery. Nursing interventions also include helping a child and parents adjust to aids that are used to improve hearing, speech, or sight.

OUTCOME EVALUATION

Continuing follow-ups with hearing and vision concerns is essential so self-esteem can be evaluated. Do children think of themselves as well or ill? As people able to do things or as disabled? Some parents may require help with their own feelings of worth (feeling inferior to other parents is common among parents of children with vision and hearing impairment or challenge) before they can help their children. Be certain to evaluate if they're able to "let go" so their child can attend school.

Examples of expected outcomes include:

- Parent states she understands that antibiotics are no longer prescribed for simple otitis media.
- Parents state concrete plans for enrolling child in a hearing-impaired preschool program.
- The child wears corrective lenses for a major portion of each day.
- The child with a hearing disorder communicates effectively with healthcare providers by lip reading or writing out her needs.

Health Promotion and Risk Management

Vision can be assessed shortly after birth by eliciting a blink reflex and the ability to follow a moving object. All babies should be screened by a formal method for hearing loss before leaving the hospital or no later than 1 month of age (Kemper, Crews, Strickland, et al., 2014). Such tests give reassurance to worried parents that their child's vision and hearing is adequate or set the stage for early interventions if their child is visually or hearing challenged. School nurses play a vital role in the continuing assessment and formal screening of vision and hearing as well as being instrumental in laying a foundation for steps that parents and children need to take to maintain vision and hearing health (Box 50.2).

A history and physical examination performed at each health maintenance visit can provide important clues to possible problems or the need for further evaluation. General guidelines for evaluation are listed in Table 50.1. During these visits, be certain to offer parents opportunities to ask questions and voice any concerns they may have regarding their child.

Children with vision or hearing disorders need to attend regular classrooms in school, if possible, so that they can have contact with seeing and hearing children to promote growth and development. If a child has a vision or hearing impairment, assist the parents with measures to adapt the child's

BOX 50.2

Nursing Care Planning Using Assessment

ASSESSING A CHILD FOR VISION OR HEARING DISORDERS

History
Chief concern: Are symptoms of vision or hearing difficulty present—blurriness of vision, squinting, turning head, leaning toward speaker, ignoring instructions?
Past health history: Has child had any exposure to loud noises? Eye trauma? Ear infection?
Family medical history: Do any family members have a hearing disorder? What is the vision level of parents?

Physical assessment
Hair: white forelock (associated with congenital deafness)

Eyes: tearing, crusting of eyelids, uneven size of pupils, improperly formed pupils, squinting, white pupils

Neck: "cocking neck"

Ears: incompletely formed pinna

Speech: unclear

Posture: leaning forward

TABLE 50.1 ASSESSMENT PARAMETERS FOR VISION AND HEARING SCREENING

Age	Vision Assessment Parameters	Hearing Assessment Parameters
Infant	Ability to follow objects	Startle reflex at hearing sound (at birth)
	Corneal (blink) reflex	Ability to track sounds (3–6 months)
	Ability to turn to light stimuli	Ability to recognize sounds (6–8 months)
		Ability to locate sounds (8–12 months)
Toddler	Corneal light reflex	Ability to react to soft sounds (whispers)
	Cover test	Ability to form a noun–verb sentence by 2 years
	Smooth ocular movements	Ability to follow simple directions
	Hand–eye coordination	Awareness of pitch and tone
Preschooler	Corneal light reflex	Pure tone audiometry (starting at age 4 years)
	Cover test	Understandable language with increasing vocabulary
	Snellen E chart, Allen figures (or modification)	
School age	Visual acuity testing every 1–2 years	Pure tone audiometry at ages 6, 8, and 11 years
Adolescent	Visual acuity testing every 1–2 years	Pure tone audiometry at ages 14 and 18 years

environment to meet safety needs while promoting growth, development, and independence as much as possible. Help them to supplement verbal explanations with tactile and visual aids as appropriate as well as allow the child to use drawings, writing, gestures, a talking picture board, text messaging, and/or e-mail to respond and communicate. Assess whether parents are interested in investigating a cochlear implant for a child with hearing impairment. Be certain parents are familiar with measures to prevent eye and ear infections so that these do not lead to long-term problems. Assess that children receive adequate vitamin A because, although not common in the United States, a deficiency of vitamin A may cause diminished night vision or even blindness (Bruins & Kraemer, 2013).

Caution children that exposure to high levels of sound over a period of time can permanently lower the level at which they hear. Music heard through earbuds, for example, is at about 110 dB (compared to 50 to 60 dB, the level of usual conversation). Rock concerts expose listeners to decibels as high as 120 to 140 dB. To lessen the danger of such exposure, urge students to invest in quality earplugs, don't listen through them for long time intervals, and listen to music at the lowest level possible. At music concerts, they should not sit near loud speakers and should wear foam earplugs to decrease the sound level (Box 50.3).

Vision

Vision occurs because light rays reflect from an object through the corneas, aqueous humors, lenses, and vitreous humors to the retinas (Fig. 50.1). If any of these structures have defects, light rays may not be able to reach the retinas or focus correctly there, resulting in a vision disorder. Both retinas are studded with *rods*, which are instrumental for night vision and for detecting movement in the visual field, and *cones*, which register daylight and color vision. The **fovea centralis** (the center of the macula) is an area of closely packed cones on the retinas where color is best perceived.

Each eye globe must not only develop good central and peripheral vision but also learn to work with the other eye to fuse or interpret a dual image as one (*single binocular vision*).

Infants with poor eye alignment cannot establish single binocular vision but have **diplopia**, or double vision, instead.

STEREOPSIS

Stereopsis is depth perception, or the ability to see objects as three-dimensional. Children with vision loss in one eye do not develop stereopsis and, consequently, tend to reach farther or closer than the actual distance of an object when attempting to grasp it. They have difficulty learning to ride a bicycle and have great difficulty driving a car safely. Lack of stereopsis can be detected by a depth perception test such as the *Stereo Fly* dot test, a test where the image of a fly is constructed from a series of colored dots. When asked to touch the fly's wings, a child with good depth perception touches them accurately. A child with poor depth perception touches a spot 2 or 3 in. above the pattern.

ACCOMMODATION

Accommodation is the adjustment the eye makes to focus on a close image. To do this, the eyes converge (look medially) and the pupils constrict. To test for accommodation, ask a child to follow a penlight as you move it in toward the nose, if developmentally appropriate. Children who cannot accommodate are unable to fuse their vision to follow a penlight toward their nose this way; instead, they demonstrate double vision (diplopia). Poor accommodation is important to recognize because it can lead to headaches, poor reading ability, and difficulty achieving in school.

Disorders That Interfere With Vision

Eye disorders in children are always potentially serious because, if permanent vision impairment occurs, a child's functioning at many everyday tasks can be severely compromised.

REFRACTIVE ERRORS

Refractive errors that cause visual impairment are one of the most common visual deficits in school-age children

BOX 50.3

Nursing Care Planning Based on Family Teaching

PROTECTING VISION AND HEARING

Q. Carla's mother says to you, "What can we do to protect our children from having problems with their eyes and ears?"

A. Here are some helpful tips to protect children's vision and hearing:

To protect vision:

- Place infants and small children in a car seat (for older children, use a seat belt). Follow National Highway and Traffic Safety Administration (NHTSA) guidelines when in a car to keep them from hitting the dashboard or front seat in the event of an accident.
- Do not allow infants to hold sharp objects because the object could strike the eye as the infant brings the hand to the mouth to suck his or her thumb.
- Do not allow children to carry sharp objects such as lollipop sticks in their hands while walking. If they fall, the object could puncture their eye.
- Caution older children to use eye-protection measures, such as goggles, when working with projects, such as soldering metal, in school or at home.
- Encourage the use of proper athletic facial protective gear when playing sports.
- Teach children not to place any medication in their eyes that is not prescribed by a healthcare provider; do not use outdated eye medication because it may become contaminated with bacteria or may change in composition with time.
- Wear a hat or ultraviolet (UV) coated lenses when outdoors, especially for children with light-colored eyes.
- Caution children that chemicals can cause burns to the eye; alert them to the emergency shower installations in science rooms that are used to wash away any spilled chemical from their eyes. Chemical burns may be worse in children who have contact lenses in place because chemicals can flow under the lens and remain in contact with the cornea longer.
- Teach children not to wear contact lenses for longer intervals than recommended by the manufacturer to prevent drying and a lack of oxygen supply to the cornea.

To prevent hearing loss:

- Keep children away from high noise levels, such as loud toys or electronic games. While in loud environments, protect ears with earplugs or earmuffs.
- Teach children to avoid chronic exposure to loud noises, such as can occur with radios and earbuds/earphones.
- Secure prompt treatment for pharyngitis (fever and sore throat) because this condition can lead to otitis media (middle ear infection).
- Caution children not to put anything in their ear canals because they could puncture their eardrums.
- Be certain children's immunizations are kept up to date because illnesses such as parotitis (mumps) or bacterial meningitis can lead to hearing loss.

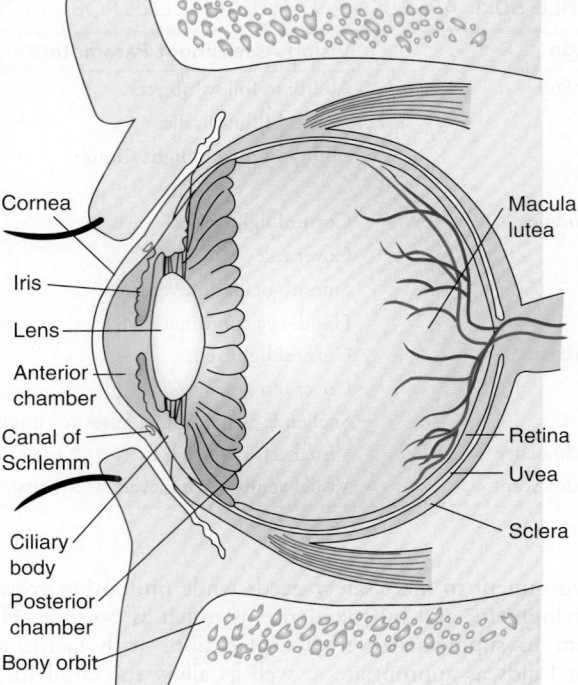

Figure 50.1 The anatomy of the eye.

(Qiu, Wang, Singh, et al., 2014; Wojciechowski, 2011). **Light refraction** refers to the manner in which light is bent as it passes through the lens. Normally, this bending causes a ray of light to fall directly on the retina (Fig. 50.2A). Because the depth of the eye globe in infants and children increases with age, the light rays do not always focus onto the retina accurately as the child grows older, but at a point behind the retina. This results in **hyperopia** (farsightedness), in which vision is blurry at a close range and clear at a far range. It is important to remember that this normal hyperopia of preschoolers needs no correction when performing vision screening with children of this age because at about 5 years of age, as a result of developmental changes, hyperopia will begin to diminish. Some children, however, remain hyperopic. Focusing on close objects requires such strong accommodation that these children often develop headaches or dizziness while doing schoolwork. A finding of hyperopia in a school-age child is cause for referral so that the child can get a prescription for glasses with a convex lens (see Fig. 50.2B).

Myopia (nearsightedness) occurs when light rays focus anterior to the retina, causing objects that are far away to be unfocused. Typically, this develops around age 8 years and then progresses (Belden, DeFriez, & Huether, 2013). These children can read a book or a computer screen immediately in front of them but are unable to read the blackboard clearly from a distance. They have difficulty reading signs across the street or playing baseball. Myopia tends to plateau as the child reaches adolescence. Children with myopia need corrective (concave) lenses to enable them to see at a distance (see Fig. 50.2C).

Myopia has a familial tendency, so if both parents are myopic, their children should be screened yearly during the early school years. Because children with myopia try to focus on objects by squinting or rubbing their eyes, any child who reports difficulty seeing or who shows mannerisms suggestive of

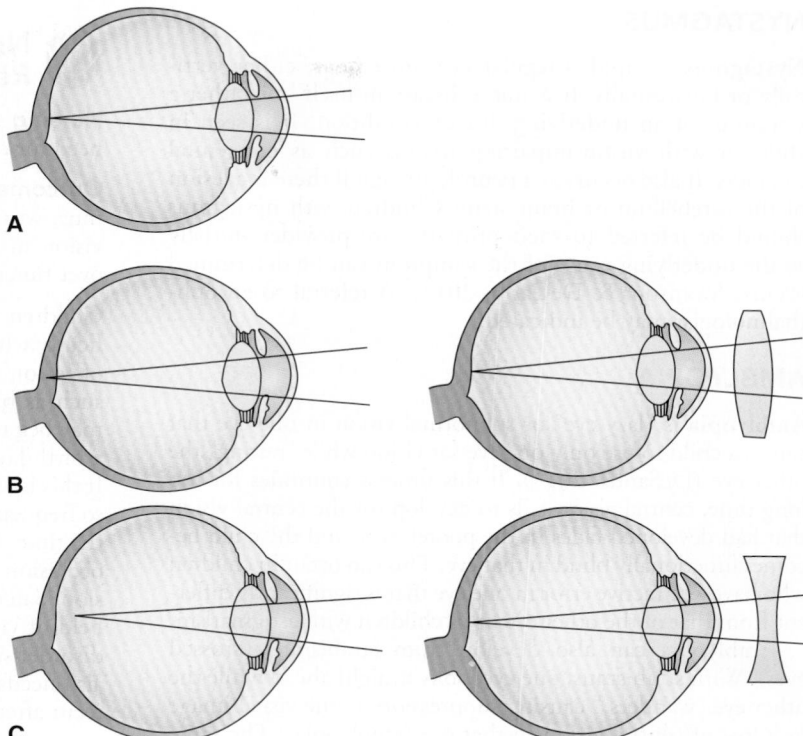

Figure 50.2 Corrective lenses for refractive errors of vision. **(A)** Normal vision. **(B)** Convex lens for hyperopia (farsightedness). **(C)** Concave lens for myopia (nearsightedness).

refraction errors—rubbing the eyes, tearing, blinking, squinting, or pressing on the eyes—should be screened for visual difficulty.

It is possible for contact lenses to be fitted for even young infants. Children as young as 5 years of age are capable of putting them in and taking them out if taught properly. Contact lenses are a big responsibility, however; they require conscientious cleaning or changing to prevent eye irritation or infection. Children are usually about 12 years of age before they can be relied on to take appropriate care of contact lenses independently.

Young children may resist wearing glasses because they're worried they'll be bullied if they wear them. If glasses are needed, however, encourage children to give them a fair try. In most instances, glasses improve vision to such an extent that after trying them, children will appreciate the difference they make and continue to wear them. Some children may need continued encouragement to keep wearing glasses, however, until they are old enough for contact lenses or surgical correction. Advise parents to choose frames fitted with safety glass (shatterproof) lenses so that if the lenses accidentally break, the child's eyes will not be injured.

By late adolescence, children can have laser surgery (known as laser in situ keratomileusis [LASIK] or photorefractive keratectomy [PRK]) to permanently change the contour of the cornea and correct refractive vision errors.

Laser In Situ Keratomileusis and Photorefractive Keratectomy

LASIK and PRK are both laser surgery correction procedures for either myopia or hyperopia (Stahl, 2014). These involve an incision under the cornea to change the contour of the eye globe so that light rays fall more accurately on the retina. Postoperatively, children may have disturbed tear functioning for 1 or more months and so need to instill artificial tears or ointments to prevent surface damage. Because having the procedure carried out before the child's eye globe has reached its adult size would require the surgery to be repeated with maturity, the youngest age at which LASIK therapy is appropriate is controversial; most authorities recommend this not be done before 21 years of age to allow for natural eye contour changes to occur. The exception to this is children who have amblyopia or strabismus (see later in the chapter) (Birch, 2013; Stahl, 2014).

ASTIGMATISM

Astigmatism is an irregular curvature of the cornea, causing light to focus incorrectly on the retina, resulting in an uneven quality of vision. When children with astigmatism look at the letter T, for example, they may see the crossbar but not the letter stem. If they focus on the stem, they cannot see the crossbar. On any given page of print, therefore, they may see only half the letters or can have great difficulty reading or following written instructions. They may report headache and vertigo after doing close work. Even though their vision appears deceptively normal on vision screening tests (they are able to see all of the numbers on a chart by tilting their head), these children need to be referred to an ophthalmologist on the basis of their other problems such as vertigo, headaches, and difficulty with reading. Corrective lenses for close work relieve the symptoms and restore functional vision. Contact lenses may be even more helpful because they actually smooth out the curvature of the cornea. A form of LASIK surgery may be appropriate to correct astigmatism (Ivarsen, Næser, & Hjortdal, 2013).

NYSTAGMUS

Nystagmus is rapid, irregular eye movement, either vertically or horizontally. It is not a disease in itself but rather a symptom of an underlying disease condition. It is seen in children with vision-impairing lesions such as congenital cataracts. It also occurs as a neurologic sign if there is a lesion of the cerebellum or brain stem. Children with nystagmus should be referred to their primary care provider initially so the underlying cause of the symptom can be determined (Penix, Swanson, & DeCarlo, 2015). A referral to an ophthalmologist may be indicated.

AMBLYOPIA

Amblyopia is "lazy eye" or subnormal vision in one eye that causes a child to use only one eye for vision while "resting" the other eye (DeSantis, 2014). If this process continues for too long time, central vision fails to develop (or the central vision that had developed fades in the poorer eye), and the child becomes functionally blind in that eye. This can occur in children who have a refractive error in one eye that is significantly different from that of the other eye or in children with astigmatism.

Amblyopia can also develop from strabismus (crossed eyes). With strabismus, one eye looks straight ahead while the other eye "wanders," causing suppression of one visual image or a loss of central vision in that eye (amblyopia). The same phenomenon can occur if the vision in one eye is obscured by a lid that does not open fully (ptosis).

Assessment

It is recommended that all children between the ages of 3 and 5 years have at least one vision screening to detect amblyopia (Kemper et al., 2014). If a child has amblyopia, a screening exam such as a preschool E chart (see Chapter 34) typically demonstrates 20/50 vision (which is normal for preschool age) in one eye, but the other eye shows lessened vision (perhaps as different as 20/100).

Therapeutic Management

Treatment for amblyopia is most successful among children younger than the age of 7 years, but there is evidence to show a response to treatment for children between 7 and 13 years of age (DeSantis, 2014). Treatment can consist of wearing correcting lenses (glasses), covering the good eye with a patch, or a combination of the two (Holmes, 2014). Wearing a patch over the good eye forces the child to use the poor eye, thus developing vision in that eye. Usually, children have some difficulty initially adjusting to a patch because they are unable to see well from the unpatched eye. They may report headaches or dizziness and notice poor depth perception. Only constant attempts to see with the weaker eye, however, will improve binocular vision, so parents have to enforce patching if prescribed (DeSantis, 2014; Pediatric Eye Disease Investigator Group, 2014).

The patch should be removed for 1 hour each day to prevent amblyopia from developing in the nonamblyopic eye. If patching does not produce the anticipated result, LASIK surgery to improve the refractive error may be indicated. Yet, a further option is the administration of levodopa in addition to occlusion therapy because this almost immediately improves vision in both eyes (Pediatric Eye Disease Investigator Group, 2014).

 Nursing Diagnoses and Related Interventions

Nursing Diagnosis: Deficient knowledge related to the need for consistent wearing of eye patch

Outcome Evaluation: Parents state the reason their child must wear a patch over the functioning eye is to improve vision in the poorly functioning eye. Child wears patch over functioning eye for all but 1 hour per day.

Children with an eye patch in place may have more difficulty with motor coordination due to the decreased field of vision and so need careful supervision with activities such as bicycle riding or crossing a street safely. A child may beg to remove the patch for special occasions, such as a birthday party or a family wedding, or just for an hour. If this is allowed, the "special occasions" may soon become so frequent that the child is wearing the patch for only half the time. Remind parents how important it is to adhere to occlusion therapy so that their child will achieve good vision. Safety may also be a concern due to child's decreased field of vision. If amblyopia occurs secondary to another disorder such as strabismus or ptosis, the primary problem also needs to be corrected. Otherwise, the amblyopia will recur after the patching is completed.

QSEN Checkpoint Question 50.1

PATIENT-CENTERED CARE

Carla, who is 6 years old, has developed amblyopia. Which statement by her mother would assure the nurse that her learning needs are being met?
a. "I place the patch over her weak eye to enhance the vision in her stronger eye."
b. "I place the patch over her good eye to allow the weaker eye to strengthen."
c. "I alternate the patch between eyes every other day so both eyes strengthen."
d. "I can take off the patch while Carla eats to make it easier for her."

Look in Appendix A for the best answer and rationale.

COLOR VISION DEFICIT (COLOR BLINDNESS)

Color deficit is, as the name implies, the inability to perceive color correctly. It occurs in 4% to 8% of boys because one of the sets of cones of the retina that perceive red, green, or blue is absent. It is inherited as a sex-linked disorder, although there is also a high incidence in children with hemophilia (which is also sex linked), congenital nystagmus, or glucose-6-phosphate dehydrogenase deficiency (Rajavi, Sabbaghi, Baghini, et al., 2015).

The vision problem may involve the inability to distinguish red from green or blue from yellow. A small proportion of children are unable to see any colors. It can be detected by the use of color plates or discs for children as young as preschool age. Children with normal vision see numbers or patterns on these plates, whereas children with a color vision deficit see only a jumble of dots or unclear images.

There is currently no therapy for color vision deficit because the condition is caused by a genetic mutation. The deficit is categorized based on severity. It's important that the loss of color perception is detected early so the child is not asked to complete color identification assignments in pre-school and can learn to appreciate color changes in traffic signals or other color-dependent signs necessary for safety.

Some children associate color blindness with total "blindness" and fear they will eventually lose their eyesight. Reassure them that although color blindness means they have a loss of color discrimination, their loss is limited to that one area.

Structural Problems of the Eye

Structural problems of the eye tend to be congenital or already present at birth.

COLOBOMA

A *coloboma* is an example of an incomplete closure of the facial cleft. The incomplete closure may involve only the lower eyelid (there is a notch in the lid). It may involve the iris, giving it the shape of a keyhole rather than a circle (Fig. 50.3). It may involve the ciliary body, the lens, the choroid, the retina, and the optic nerve. Children with any degree of coloboma should be referred to an ophthalmologist for further investigation to determine the extent of the condition. Children with only iris involvement have no decline in vision; those with retina and optic nerve coloboma will have some vision impairment in the affected eye (Braverman, 2012).

HYPERTELORISM

Hypertelorism is congenital, abnormally wide-spaced eyes. Children with wide epicanthal folds by the inner canthus may appear to have wide-spaced eyes, but, when the distance between the pupils is measured and compared with standards for the child's age, the true condition is revealed. Detecting true hypertelorism in children is important because this condition is associated with chromosomal abnormalities, most notably Waardenburg syndrome, which also involves congenital hearing impairment. Children with this syndrome also have a white forelock of hair, different-colored irises,

Figure 50.3 Coloboma involving the iris, showing a "keyhole" appearance. (From Tasman, W., & Jaeger, E. A. [1996]. *The Wills Eye Hospital atlas of clinical ophthalmology.* Philadelphia, PA: Lippincott-Raven Publishers.)

and eyebrows that tend to grow together in the center line, all signs not necessarily noticeable in newborns. Therefore, wide-spaced eyes, because of a broad-bridged nose, are the chief clue in a newborn that the child can hear no sound and will need close follow-up to determine whether cochlear implants or hearing aids can provide their ability to hear.

PTOSIS

Ptosis is the inability to raise the upper eyelid the usual distance, so the eyelid always remains slightly closed. With this, children tend to wrinkle their forehead and raise their eyebrows more than usual in an attempt to lift the eyelid further or cock their heads back to see under the lowered lid. The condition may be congenital (frequently hereditary and bilateral) or acquired (usually unilateral) (Marenco, Macchi, Galassi, et al., 2017). It may be a result of injury to the lid or levator muscle, injury to the third cranial nerve, or from the development of myasthenia gravis (see Chapter 51). If the third cranial nerve has been injured, paralysis of one or more of the other muscles supplied by that nerve will also be affected and a child will exhibit:

- A dilated pupil
- An inability to rotate the eye globe upward, medially, or downward
- Weakness of accommodation (looking at near objects)

After a careful investigation of the cause has been completed, ptosis is corrected surgically. The correction is usually important to the child from a cosmetic standpoint, but if the ptosis is unilateral, and more importantly, if the lid obstructs vision, early surgery is necessary to prevent the development of amblyopia (from a lack of use of the closed eye) (Stein, Kelly, & Weiss, 2014). Be certain that parents understand it's important that ptosis be corrected during the preschool period because although the ptosis can be corrected when the child is older, the amblyopia cannot.

STRABISMUS

Strabismus is unequally aligned eyes (cross-eyes) caused by an imbalance of the extraocular muscles that control the movement of the eye globes, similar to the handling of reins of a horse (Fig. 50.4). Approximately 1% to 2% of children demonstrate some degree of strabismus. The condition does not favor either gender, social status, or geographic area; about 30% of children have a history of a similar strabismus in the family.

With strabismus, the resting position of one eye, instead of facing forward, will be *divergent* (turned out) or *convergent* (turned in). One pupil may appear higher than the other (vertical strabismus). The strabismus may be monocular, in which the same eye deviates constantly, or it may be an alternating strabismus, in which one eye and then the other deviates.

Assessment

Infants' eyes may cross occasionally until 6 weeks of age. If infants demonstrate a constant strabismus, refer them to their primary care provider at any time; if they still demonstrate occasional strabismus past 6 months, refer them at that point.

Definite deviations are obvious at a physical exam (Fig. 50.5). Note if the deviation is *exotropia* (an eye turns out), *esotropia* (an eye turns in), or *hypertropia* (an eye turns up). If the deviation is not so obvious or occurs only when the child is fatigued or ill

Eye muscle	Action	Innervation
Superior rectus	Turns eye up and medially	Oculomotor (third cranial) nerve
Medial rectus	Turns eye inward	Oculomotor (third cranial) nerve
Inferior rectus	Turns eye down and medially	Oculomotor (third cranial) nerve
Lateral rectus	Turns eye out	Abducens (sixth cranial) nerve
Superior oblique	Turns eye down and laterally	Trochlear (fourth cranial) nerve
Inferior oblique	Turns eye up and laterally	Oculomotor (third cranial) nerve

Figure 50.4 The extraocular eye muscles.

and, therefore, less able to maintain fixation, the terms used are *exophoria*, *esophoria*, and *hyperphoria*. If the parents report that the deviation occurs only when the child is tired or sick, attempt to assess the strabismus at such a time because then the deviation will be most striking.

Strabismus may be detected best when children are asked to examine a nearby object because to do this, they must turn both eyes medially, or *converge*, to focus at the short distance. If they are farsighted in one eye, they will have to turn the affected eye in more than the other, causing esotropia. If one eye is nearsighted, they will not need to turn that eye in as far as the other one; this results in divergence or exotropia.

Some children have a latent strabismus or appear to have straight vision. Because they are only able to maintain fusion at the expense of eyestrain; however, they develop symptoms such as headache; tired, irritated eyes; and perhaps even nausea and vomiting.

Children who have flat, broad-bridged noses, a narrow interpupillary distance, an epicanthal fold, or oval-shaped palpebral fissures may appear to have strabismus (pseudostrabismus) because less white sclera is visible in the inner margin of the eye than usual. A cover test reveals the true condition. If pseudostrabismus is present, the covered eye will not move after being uncovered because it only appears to be turned medially due to the obscured sclera at the inner canthus. The Hirschberg test is another method of detecting true strabismus (see Chapter 34).

Once strabismus is detected, it is important to attempt to discern whether it is concomitant (measures the same in all directions of gaze) or nonconcomitant (greater in one direction than in another, often called *paralytic strabismus*). Concomitant (nonparalytic) strabismus is the most usual type found in children. All the muscles of the eye are capable of functioning, but they do not function together. The deviation is equally apparent in all directions of gaze.

Paralytic strabismus is caused by paralysis of a muscle or nerve, perhaps from an injury (such as a birth injury), or an invading lesion. The eyes appear straight except when they are moved in the direction of the paralyzed muscle. Then, double vision occurs, and the crossed eye is evident. Such children often close one eye or tilt their head to decrease the double vision. They may tilt their head so much that they appear to have a torticollis or "wry neck"—an orthopedic rather than an eye problem. They may appear clumsy because of the diplopia. Because they are too young to describe double vision and how nauseated this makes them feel, they may express this by fussiness or whining.

Therapeutic Management

The therapy for strabismus depends on the cause of the problem. If the fusion mechanism is weak, eye exercises (**orthoptics**) can strengthen the weak muscle. If eyes are diverging because of farsightedness or nearsightedness, the child needs glasses or contact lenses to correct the basic visual defect. Surgical treatment can be used to permanently align the extraocular muscles if the cause is due to muscle strength.

A side effect of strabismus can be amblyopia because, to avoid double vision, the child suppresses the vision in one eye. For this reason, eye correction for strabismus must be done early in life, before 7 years of age. Some children, because of an accommodation problem caused by hyperopia in one eye, outgrow the condition as the normal hyperopia of the preschooler lessens. This does not always occur, however. Even if the child's eyes appear to be straighter later, an amblyopia may be present that could have been prevented by earlier treatment.

After strabismus surgery, eye patches are not usually required. Postoperatively, antibiotic ointment is applied to the eye for 2 or 3 days. The child may experience some pain on eye movement for the first day as well as nausea and vomiting. Further nursing care for the child having eye surgery is discussed later in this chapter.

Follow-up visits after surgery are necessary to determine the success of the surgery. Retest children who have had this surgery periodically at health maintenance visits to be certain their vision remains equal and eye alignment remains straight.

Infection or Inflammation of the Eye

Many different types of eye infections or inflammatory conditions can occur in children (Table 50.2). Newborns are at risk for contracting an eye infection from exposure to a variety of organisms while passing through the birth canal (see

Figure 50.5 Strabismus (esotropia) in an infant.

TABLE 50.2 INFECTIOUS AND INFLAMMATORY EYE DISORDERS

Disorder	Description/Cause	Signs and Symptoms	Treatment
Stye	Infection of a ciliary gland (a modified sweat gland) that enters into the hair follicle at the lid margin; most commonly caused by *Staphylococcus*	Pain and redness at a localized point on the lid margin with possible edema of the lid out of proportion to the severity of the disease; preauricular lymph node swelling and tenderness	Hot, moist compresses for 15–20 minutes four times daily; antibiotic ointment application after the compresses (possible); incision and drainage (when the stye points [develops a head]); nose and throat cultures for *Staphylococcus*
			Follow-up evaluation for repeated episodes to rule out other debilitating diseases such as diabetes mellitus or anemia
			Visual acuity assessment (although styes are not associated with refraction error, they occur when children rub their eyes excessively possibly because of problems with visual acuity)
Chalazion	Low-grade granulation tissue tumor of the *meibomian*, or tarsal, gland on the eyelid; cause unknown but may be a result of a low-grade infection produced by retained secretion in the gland	Small, slow-growing, hard, but painless nodule on the lid; skin freely movable over it; absence of inflammation or edema	Nodule may resolve spontaneously, evacuating itself onto the conjunctival surface of the lid; incision and drainage if no spontaneous remission, followed by antibiotic ointment application to prevent secondary gland infection
			If ptosis is present in a child younger than 7–8 years of age, surgical removal is performed to prevent possible subsequent amblyopia.
Blepharitis marginalis	Inflammation of the eyelid margin; usually a local infection caused by *Staphylococcus*; possibly an extension of seborrheic dermatitis (cradle cap)	Eyelid margin reddened, possibly covered by hard, dirty-yellow crusts that stick tenaciously to the lid margin and lashes; styes possibly present secondary to the presence of *Staphylococcus*	Application of an antibiotic ointment six to eight times a day to the lower conjunctival rim; removal of crusts with a moistened cotton applicator after the lid margins have been covered by wet compresses for 10–15 minutes
			If condition persists, systemic antibiotic therapy is used to reduce the presence of *Staphylococcus* on the skin surface.
Conjunctivitis	Inflammation of the conjunctiva; causes are numerous, including ophthalmia neonatorum (exposure to gonococcus bacillus; see Chapter 26) and bacterial, viral, and fungal organisms	Eyes watery with reddened conjunctiva and sensitivity to light; sticking of eyelids with pustular drainage	Application of an antibiotic ointment applied from inner to outer canthus to prevent spread of infection to other eye; follow-up visit is mandatory to be certain infection clears.
Inclusion blennorrhea	*Chlamydia* organism	Acute inflammation usually occurring on the 5th–14th day after birth; conjunctiva reddened with tearing; eye discharge	Systemic antibiotic such as erythromycin
Acute catarrhal conjunctivitis	Commonly called "pinkeye," usually caused by a virus or irritation from a foreign body; most frequently caused by *Haemophilus influenzae* and *Streptococcus pneumoniae*	Conjunctiva fiery red with tearing; mucopurulent or purulent discharge	Antibiotic ointment or drops three to four times daily for 7 days (redness usually disappears within 48 hours); avoid rubbing and transmitting infection to unaffected eye.
			Cool, moist compresses to affected eye
Herpetic conjunctivitis	Herpes simplex viral infection (may occur along with development of facial herpes lesion)	Series of pinpoint vesicles on the conjunctiva; on fluorescein stain, vesicles stain bright green and are readily evident	Referral to ophthalmologist (can spread easily and become a corneal infection with resultant opacity and permanent scarring)
			Antibiotics are ineffective; steroids are avoided.
			Idoxuridine (Herplex), specific for herpesvirus, is possibly effective in limiting corneal involvement.
Allergic conjunctivitis	Hypersensitivity to specific allergen; usually seasonal	Eyelid edema; profuse tearing and severe itching	Treatment of underlying allergy; cool, moist compresses

Continued on following page

TABLE 50.2 INFECTIOUS AND INFLAMMATORY EYE DISORDERS (Continued)

Disorder	Description/Cause	Signs and Symptoms	Treatment
Keratitis	Inflammation and infection of the superficial layers of the cornea; may accompany or be a complication of conjunctivitis; may result when a foreign body strikes the cornea	Acute pain, tearing, photophobia (sensitivity to light), and redness	Referral to ophthalmologist for therapy (infection could lead to corneal scarring, resulting in vision impairment [light rays unable to enter the eye normally])
Periorbital cellulitis	Cellulitis (infection of subcutaneous tissue) most often caused by extension of a superficial infection after an open break in the skin, such as a mosquito bite or scratch near the eye	Swelling around and in the eye with possible damage to eye globe or optic nerve	Intravenous antibiotic therapy
Dacryostenosis	Blockage of the nasolacrimal duct; primarily in newborns because of a membrane obscuring distal end of duct or plugging by epithelial debris	Painless lump in the inner canthus; tearing; usually unilateral	Gentle pressure to inner aspect of each eye at each feeding in attempt to "milk" secretions down into duct; ophthalmologic probing of gland duct if condition not corrected spontaneously after age 6 months
Dacryocystitis	Inflammation of nasolacrimal duct; possibly secondary to dacryostenosis (from fluid stasis) or from nasal mucosal swelling and infected mucus being forced back into duct	Acute pain in inner canthus (from presence of infected sac); complaints of pain in back of eye or possibly in the eye itself	Local and systemic antibiotics; possible probing of duct to free obstruction and allow for free drainage; antihistamines for children with chronic allergies or sinusitis to reduce nasal congestion

Chapter 26). Although it is a controversial practice, in most hospitals, antibiotic ointment is placed in each newborn's eye after birth to prevent serious eye infections (Cotter, Cyert, Miller, et al., 2015). Small children contract infections by rubbing their eyes with unclean hands. School-age children are exposed to many infectious agents from other children in school classrooms or by participating in sports activities. Regardless of how the infection was contracted, be certain parents have specific instructions about instilling eye drops or applying ointment, preventing the transmission of infection, applying compresses, and completing systemic antibiotic therapy. Having eye medication applied can be frightening for children because they worry a healthcare provider's or a parent's hand will slip and cut their eye. If they have pain, they may be especially reluctant to let anyone touch their eye.

QSEN Checkpoint Question 50.2

QUALITY IMPROVEMENT

Carla is diagnosed as having a bacterial conjunctivitis of her right eye, and the unit has a standardized care plan and educational materials that address this common diagnosis. What instruction should the nurse check in these clinical resources?

a. Keep the infected eye tightly closed by covering it with clean gauze.

b. Do not apply the eye drops for more than 3 days in order to prevent a rebound.

c. Clean the eye discharge away from the inner to the outer canthus.

d. Caution Carla not to blow her nose for the next 24 hours.

Look in Appendix A for the best answer and rationale.

Traumatic Injury to the Eye

Children account for 35% of ocular injury in the United States (Li, Zarbin, & Bhagat, 2015). These injuries may be caused by a variety of situations, such as improper use of fireworks, sports injuries, dirt, pieces off toys, fighting with others, and even fingernail scratches (Li et al., 2015).

ASSESSMENT

Children who have eye injuries are usually in acute pain immediately after the injury. Their eyes tear and are sensitive to light, and they blink rapidly. Vision may be blurred or lost in the affected eye. Because of the pain and the fear of not being able to see clearly, most children are very reluctant to let anyone examine or touch their injured eye. A few drops of a topical anesthetic instilled into the eye may be necessary to relieve the pain and allow the eye to be opened for examination. Even after the anesthetic is applied, the child needs a thorough explanation that an examiner is "just looking" (provided this is true). Even after an anesthetic application, a child may not be able to open the eye readily for inspection because the acute pain of the injury can cause either the eyelid to close by reflex spasm or eyelid edema to form so quickly that these interfere with the eye's ability to open. Do not confuse these physical problems with an unwillingness to open the eye.

To visualize the inner surface of the lower lid and the bottom half of the eye globe, press firmly on the lower lid with your fingertip until it turns out. The inner surface of the upper lid and the upper portion of the eye globe can best be visualized if the upper eyelid is everted. Ask the child to look downward. Grasp the eyelashes and gently stretch the upper eyelid downward. Place the stick of a cotton-tipped applicator horizontally against the center of the upper lid. While still grasping the eyelashes, pull the eyelid upward and over

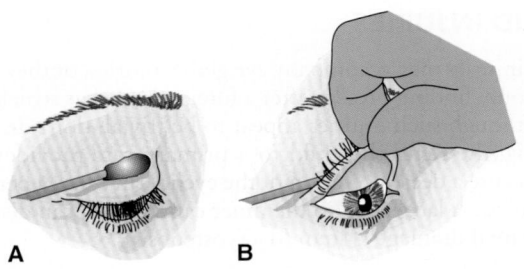

A   **B**

Figure 50.6 The technique for everting the upper eyelid for examination and foreign body removal. **(A)** Place a cotton applicator across the upper eyelid. **(B)** Pull the eyelid outward and upward over the applicator.

the applicator until it is everted (Fig. 50.6). Gently press the everted eyelid against the eyebrow to maintain the everted position. Be careful not to exert pressure on the eye globe during the procedure in case a penetrating injury from a foreign body is present to prevent further embedding the object into the eye globe.

A foreign body, such as a speck of dirt or a fragment of glass, often clings inside of the upper lid and can be readily removed by touching it with a moistened, sterile, cotton-tipped applicator while the lid is everted. Keep an eyelid everted no longer than is necessary while you remove the object because the eye globe begins drying as soon as it is exposed. Magnetic resonance imaging (MRI) and ultrasound are excellent methods for documenting internal eye damage or corneal scarring from an injury (Sung, Nadqir, Fujita, et al., 2014).

 Nursing Diagnoses and Related Interventions

Nursing Diagnosis: Parental role conflict related to feelings of guilt about unintentional injury affecting child's vision

Outcome Evaluation: Parents accurately state child's treatment plan and expected outcome; child and parents talk openly about the injury and ways to prevent future injuries; parents participate actively in child's care and in decision making with healthcare providers regarding follow-up care.

Eye injuries are almost always serious in children because of the pain and the potential threat to vision. Both parents and children are apt to feel guilty that an injury occurred. Parents may have difficulty handling this emergency because they are angry at their child and even angrier at themselves for not supervising the child or teaching the child more about eye safety. Children may need help understanding that although this injury might have been prevented, unintentional injuries do happen. Doing so can help them maintain a sense of self-esteem. Parents also may need counseling to reestablish their feelings of worth as parents (Box 50.4).

After eye trauma, the degree of vision in the child's affected eye as well as the status of the parent–child relationship needs to be evaluated because guilt about the injury, in either the parent or the child, can interfere with this relationship.

Carla's older brother, Jon, a 7-year-old, is brought to the emergency department by his mother after his right eye was hit by a baseball.

Tip: Avoid focusing on assessing the events surrounding the injury so much that you fail to identify the parent's feelings. In the following scenario, the nurse actively listens to the mother and so elicits information not just about the injury but also about her feelings.

Nurse: Hello, Mrs. Vander. How did this injury happen?

Ms. Vander: He was playing catch with his cousin in the backyard.

Nurse: Is he hurt anywhere else?

Ms. Vander: No. I should have been watching him more closely.

Nurse: Watching him more closely?

Ms. Vander: I should have been outside supervising them. What kind of a mother am I?

Nurse: Let's talk a little more about this.

FOREIGN BODIES

Foreign bodies such as sand or dirt that are loose on the conjunctiva can be removed by irrigation with a sterile normal saline solution or by gentle wiping with a well-moistened, sterile, cotton-tipped applicator after the eyelid is everted. After the removal, if the conjunctiva is touched with a strip of filter paper impregnated with fluorescein stain, any corneal ulceration or abrasion from the foreign body will stain green and be readily apparent. If the foreign body is easily removed and no corneal ulceration or injury is present, no further treatment is necessary. The child will blink a few times after the upper lid is returned to its place, but, in a matter of minutes, the child will report feeling "fine" again. If the fluorescein stain shows any corneal ulceration, refer the child to an ophthalmologist for follow-up care.

If a foreign body adheres to the cornea, it needs to be removed by an ophthalmologist because if the foreign body is metallic and has been in contact with the cornea for a period of hours, a rust ring can form around the particle. This rust ring must be removed as well as the object, or it will continue to act as a foreign body. After corneal injury, corneal tissue begins to regenerate. To aid this, the eye is washed with an antibiotic solution and then closed and patched. Assess that the patch is secure enough to keep the eyelid closed yet does not put undue pressure on the eye. Caution the child that the patch must be left in place until it is well healed and secure once more.

This prevents the delicate regenerating corneal epithelium from being rubbed off. If a foreign object is relatively large, such as a BB bullet, lollipop stick, or piece of broken glass, the fact that it has punctured the eye globe is usually apparent on first inspection. In these instances, the child also needs to be examined by an ophthalmologist. Surgery may be necessary to explore the depth of the puncture and to save the child's sight in that eye. Iron or copper fragments must be removed to prevent rust formation and continued irritation.

An extremely serious (although rare) complication called *sympathetic ophthalmia*, or inflammation of the opposite eye, may result if the uveal tract was involved in a penetrating injury. As a result, an autoimmune inflammatory response occurs in the noninjured eye, possibly leading to blindness in that eye. This complication can be prevented by the administration of a corticosteroid and antibiotics to reduce inflammation in the injured eye. If this is unsuccessful, removal (**enucleation**) of the injured eye may be necessary to prevent the other eye from being affected. In either case, the decision is a difficult one for the parents to make because this is a loss for them and their child. Allow the parents to verbalize their feelings and provide support to the parents. Fortunately, immediate treatment with corticosteroids and antibiotics has significantly reduced the incidence of this complication; if these are prescribed, be certain parents understand the importance of giving the full course of these medications (Edelson, 2013).

CONTUSION INJURIES

Many eye injuries happen not from a sharp object striking the eye but from blunt trauma such as being hit in the eye by a baseball, a fist, a soccer ball, or an automobile dashboard. With this type of injury, the eyelid and the surrounding tissue, including the intraorbital tissue, hemorrhage and become edematous (Armstrong, Kim, Linakis, et al., 2013).

The simplest form of contusion injury is a "black eye." When this occurs, the eye globe (including a funduscopic examination) must be assessed. If a vision chart is not available, vision can be assessed by having children tell you how many fingers they can count at a distance of about 6 ft (assuming they are old enough to count accurately) or by having them read a printed page at reading distance (assuming they are old enough to read). Evaluate extraocular eye movements by asking the child to follow a light into all six cardinal positions of gaze (see Chapter 34). Children should be able to look up and down, left and right, upward obliquely, and downward obliquely (LaRoche, 2013).

If there is no apparent eye injury, ocular movement is good, and vision is normal (for that child), the only treatment necessary is an ice pack applied to the eye to minimize swelling (20 minutes on, 20 minutes off, and repeat). The reabsorption of hemorrhage in the tissue surrounding the eye will take place over the next 1 to 3 weeks. Often, tissue hemorrhage extends across the nose and surrounds the other eye the day after the injury. You can assure both the parents and the child that this is not a worsening of the condition but rather mainly evidence of the severity of the initial blow.

Limited eye movement or reports of diplopia (double vision) are strong evidence a "blowout" fracture of the floor of the orbit (the maxillary bone) has occurred, and the fracture line is trapping intraorbital tissue and preventing the eye globe from moving freely. Refer these children to an ophthalmologist because surgery is needed to free the entrapped tissue, prevent interference with vascular flow, and restore normal eye movements.

After a blunt contusion to the eye globe, findings such as a dilated, fixed, or cloudy pupil; a cloudy lens or cornea; a loss of vision in the eye; or visible blood in the anterior chamber (hyphema) indicate that dislocation of the lens or retinal detachment may have occurred. Again, immediate evaluation by an ophthalmologist is necessary.

EYELID INJURIES

Eyelid injuries may accompany eye globe injuries, or they may be the only finding present after a foreign body has struck the eye. Although such injuries appear to be trivial, don't dismiss them lightly. Refer the child to a primary care provider for care because a deep laceration of the eyelid can cause a permanent ptosis. A laceration to the inner canthal area can disrupt the lacrimal drainage system (dacryostenosis).

> *What If . . . 50.1*
> A nurse is asked to teach Carla Vander's first-grade class on ways to prevent eye injuries. What suggestions should the nurse include? How would the nurse's teaching plan be different if the class was for 16-year-old students?

Inner Eye Conditions

Inner eye conditions are those that affect the lens, the retina, or the aqueous humor.

CATARACTS

A *cataract* is marked opacity of the lens. This may be present at birth, or it may become apparent in early childhood. Some children have cataracts as a dominantly inherited condition, whereas in others, it may be as a result of another disease process such as galactosemia or scarring from an injury. A few children develop cataracts as a result of steroid use or radiation exposure. If the opacity occurs on the anterior surface of the lens, the cause is thought to be a birth injury or possibly contact between the lens and the cornea during intrauterine life. If the opacity is located at the edge of the lens, it may be a result of nutritional deficiency during intrauterine life, such as hypocalcemia. A quarter of infants born to women who were exposed to or contracted rubella may develop cataracts (Medsinge & Nischal, 2015).

Assessment

When you inspect the pupil of a child with a cataract, the red reflex elicited by shining a light into the pupil appears white. Older children may report blurred vision because of cataract formation. In the infant, this can be detected by lack of response to a smile or an inability to reach and grasp a nearby object. The infant may also demonstrate nystagmus from being unable to focus the eye on objects. A few other conditions, such as retinoblastoma, retinopathy of prematurity, congenital glaucoma, or an abscess of the posterior chamber, simulate this appearance.

Therapeutic Management

Treatment of childhood cataract is the surgical removal of the cloudy lens, followed by insertion of an internal intraocular lens. If the total lens is involved, this may be done as early as 3 months of age. If this is not done before 6 years of age, amblyopia may result.

With modern surgical techniques, the incision is so small that eye patching is not necessary. Infants may be given a sedative to help them rest for 24 hours to keep them from rubbing their eyes. Introduce fluids cautiously after eye surgery so nausea and vomiting do not occur because vomiting increases intraocular pressure (IOP), which could injure the suture line. Encourage parents to stay with their infant and to help with care so the infant does not cry because crying also increases IOP. Infants can be expected to have some discomfort, but in general, they should not have acute pain after surgery. If they are unusually restless, fussy, or cry as if in pain, report this. Use an appropriate pain assessment scale, such as CRIES or FLACC, to assess pain. Although this could be unrelated to the surgery, it may be a sign of increased IOP from hemorrhage or from occlusion of the canal of Schlemm, causing a developing glaucoma. The child may need to be medicated for pain.

As a rule, children will be given a mydriatic agent to dilate the pupil and steroids to prevent postoperative development of pupillary adhesions. If the eye that had the cataract is now amblyopic, patching the better eye (as with usual amblyopia correction) may be necessary to improve vision. Holding, rocking, and stimulating the child's senses in other ways will help to decrease their fear and anxiety.

Parents of children with congenital cataracts need support to carry out the procedures necessary and to give the long-term medication and corrective measures needed. Outcome evaluations should include children's current vision status and also how they view themselves in light of this early vision problem (Rajavi & Sabbaghi, 2016).

QSEN Checkpoint Question 50.3

SAFETY

If Carla, the 6-year-old who has strabismus, has to have corrective eye surgery, why would the prevention of vomiting from anesthetic be a high priority?
a. Vomitus could be splashed into the eye.
b. Loss of sodium threatens the integrity of the new lens.
c. Vomiting increases IOP.
d. Loss of fluid causes the globe diameter to shrink.

Look in Appendix A for the best answer and rationale.

CONGENITAL GLAUCOMA

Childhood glaucoma is a condition of the eye characterized by increased IOP, potential damage to the optic nerve, and possible vision loss (Giangiacomo & Beck, 2017).

Normally, aqueous humor, produced by the ciliary body, flows from the posterior chamber through the pupil to the anterior chamber; it is excreted through the canal of Schlemm at the lateral angle into the venous circulation (Fig. 50.7). In congenital glaucoma, a developmental anomaly in the angle of the anterior chamber prevents proper drainage into the canal. Later in life, glaucoma can occur when the canal becomes blocked, usually as a result of eye trauma. The increased fluid content that accumulates in the eye causes the globe to increase in size. After it has increased in size to the extent that it can, pressure in the eye globe continues to rise, compressing and ultimately destroying the optic nerve (Yeung & Walton, 2012). Glaucoma (meaning "gray") gets its name from the color of the retina or red reflex (which appears gray to green) in the eye after sight has been lost.

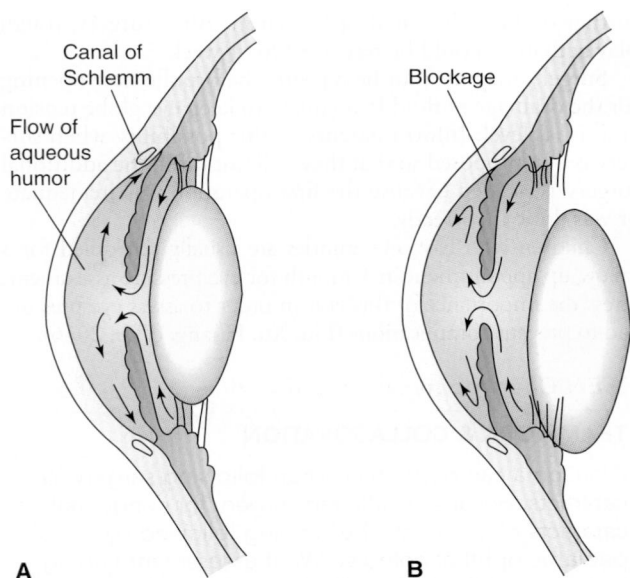

Figure 50.7 **(A)** The circulation of aqueous humor. **(B)** The blockage of the canal of Schlemm in congenital glaucoma.

Assessment

Although congenital glaucoma is a rare disorder, all infants should be assessed for it because the disease accounts for vision disorders in 5% to 13% of children in schools for those with visual impairment. In most infants, the condition is bilateral and is caused by the inheritance of a recessive gene. Symptoms may be noticeable as soon as shortly after birth, and they are readily noticeable at 1 year of age. The condition occurs in about 1 in every 10,000 live births and more often in girls than in boys (Papadopoulos, Brookes, & Khaw, 2013).

The cornea, which appears enlarged, may also be edematous and hazy; it feels tense to finger palpation. There may be accompanying tearing, pain, and **photophobia** (sensitivity to light)—all difficult signs to identify in a newborn.

Eye pressure is measured by means of a *tonometer*, a pressure-sensitive device that is placed against the anterior eye globe and measures eye pressure by a beam of light directed toward the eye. Tension greater than the normal range of 12 to 20 mmHg is suggestive that glaucoma has developed. If local anesthesia is needed for tonometry, caution parents that children should not rub their eyes after the procedure (an infant's arms may need to be gently restrained to prevent eye rubbing for about 4 hours after such an examination). Otherwise, corneal abrasions could occur because of the cornea's temporary lack of sensitivity.

Therapeutic Management

Surgery, such as trabeculotomy and **goniotomy**, laser procedures that create shunts to allow fluid to drain from the eye, as well as medical treatment are used to lower IOP (El Sayed & Gawdat, 2017).

A drug such as acetazolamide (Diamox), a carbonic anhydrase inhibitor that suppresses the formation of aqueous humor, may be used temporarily to reduce eye pressure before surgery can be scheduled.

Before surgery, the infant should not receive any drug, such as atropine sulfate, that dilates the pupil because this will further occlude the canal of Schlemm. After surgery, rough play activities should be restricted for 1 week.

Surgery may need to be repeated before the new opening for the drainage of fluid is adequate to keep eye globe tension at a usual level. Inform parents of this possibility when surgery is first proposed so that they will not think the additional surgery is needed because the first operation was inadequate or was done incorrectly.

Children who have eye injuries are usually scheduled for a follow-up appointment in 1 month for eye pressure assessment. Stress the importance of this visit in order to assess eye pressure and to prevent complications (Lin, Xu, Huang, et al., 2016).

QSEN Checkpoint Question 50.4

TEAMWORK & COLLABORATION

Glaucoma can occur in children following surgery for cataracts. Because Carla had surgery for congenital cataracts as an infant, she is being followed by a pediatric ophthalmologist. What assessment finding from the ophthalmologist's documentation would best reveal that Carla is developing glaucoma?

a. Assessment for migraine headaches
b. Carla's ability to identify colors
c. Results of eye pressure assessment
d. Results of temporal palpation

Look in Appendix A for the best answer and rationale.

The Child Scheduled for Eye Surgery

Inform the parents that surgery for cataracts or glaucoma in childhood is usually performed during the infant period. The preparation for surgery, therefore, primarily consists of helping a baby to adjust to a strange environment and encouraging parents or a primary caregiver to room-in with the infant if possible to decrease anxiety and provide auditory and tactile stimulation. This is particularly important if the eyes will be patched after surgery. Surgery for strabismus is often done during the preschool period. Explaining why the operation is needed can be done by the use of puppets or dolls so that it feels nonthreatening. Manipulation of equipment is also a way children cope with unfamiliar situations. As with all surgical procedures, talk about the child's affected parts (in this case, the eyes) being "fixed" or "made better" but never "cut." Be sure that the language and descriptions are concrete and developmentally appropriate.

Nursing Diagnoses and Related Interventions

Nursing Diagnosis: Anxiety related to lack of knowledge about eye surgery and postoperative experience

Outcome Evaluation: Child asks questions and expresses fears about surgery; child states plans for postoperative period and practices putting on eye patches if these will be used.

Most eye surgery is completed as ambulatory surgery. A major nursing role is preparing the parents to support the child through the procedure.

If the child's eyes are going to be patched after surgery, introduce these preoperatively so the child can become accustomed to the feeling of the patches beforehand. Even when only one eye is going to be operated on, it is not unusual for both eyes to be patched because the eyes move conjugately—that is, when the right eye looks to the right, so does the left. The repaired eye, therefore, will stay immobile under a bandage only if both eyes are patched.

You could show the child a doll with eye patches and let the child practice wearing them. You could play a game such as "pin the tail on the donkey" or "blind man's bluff" to adjust to the sensation of the eyes being covered. Another helpful game is to have the child pull out familiar objects from a paper bag—a key, an orange, a spoon, and a penny—and, with the eyes covered, try to guess what they are.

Postoperatively, check that the young child's favorite toy is within reach if eyes are patched. If a child will require arm restraints to prevent pressing on the eyes or removing patches, introduce these preoperatively as well. Children who awaken from conscious sedation and find their arms tied down can be extremely frightened. Encourage the parents to room-in if possible.

What If . . . 50.2

Carla, a 6-year-old, is scheduled for surgery under conscious sedation to remove a chalazion from her eyelid. Her mother tells the nurse, "She's always good so I'm sure she'll cooperate. If not, we'll just wait until she's older to have it removed." Why might the nurse not be surprised if Carla was not as cooperative as her mother predicts? Is the mother's "plan B" to delay surgery a best plan?

The Hospitalized Child With a Visual Impairment

The National Dissemination Center for Children With Disabilities (NDCCD, 2012) defines *vision impairment* as "vision that, even with correction, adversely affects a child's educational performance." Vision losses of this extent can occur for a multitude of reasons, including congenital cataracts, glaucoma, vitamin A deficiency, inadequately treated eye infections, or corneal scarring (Solebo & Rahi, 2014). Children may be hospitalized because of their primary vision disorder or, like other children, be hospitalized for a disorder such as appendicitis or pneumonia. Severe vision impairment or blindness can make it exceptionally difficult for a child to adjust to a hospital environment.

Nursing Diagnoses and Related Interventions

Nursing Diagnosis: Powerlessness related to difficulty adjusting to strange environment, secondary to vision impairment

Outcome Evaluation: Child identifies specific fears and concerns; child is able to make age-appropriate decisions regarding self-care.

Vision impairments can range from severe disorders to total blindness. Assess children carefully for the degree of their vision impairment to better gauge their abilities so you help them neither too much nor too little. Keep in mind that severe vision impairment can lead to chronic depression as children grow older and begin to realize more and more the many ways their reduction or lack of vision affects their life. To help avoid this, be sure to thoroughly orient them to the hospital experience and their surroundings. Remind them as necessary that their parents are nearby because they may become extremely frightened if they think a parent has left them when the parent has only moved a few feet away or behind a curtain.

Before you approach children who are blind, always speak first to avoid startling them. Children can usually sense another person's presence in the room, so don't attempt to slip into their room quietly to straighten their bed or pick up some equipment without speaking to them.

Common hospital sounds such as beeping infusion pumps, call lights, etc., can be frightening to a child with a visual impairment. Stand by the child's bed and explain the sounds you both hear together because sound is a major way that children with visual impairment experience their environment.

Children who are blind learn self-care the same as other children; they bathe themselves, brush their teeth, and put on clothes the same as other children their age. Toilet training may come later than usual because they cannot see the excretions that parents are asking them to dispose of in a special place.

Children who are blind often want to be told what is on their food tray when it is first presented to them. Name the foods so they can identify tastes with names as well as the location of the foods on the plate. Do not hesitate to use food colors: "Those are green beans; this is an orange; those are red beets" because these words are names as well as colors. Preschoolers with visual impairment enjoy the same finger foods as sighted children. Children with severe vision disorders have difficulty getting food from spoons or forks to their mouths neatly. However, they should not be spoon-fed just because it is neater and faster; eating is an important self-care skill a blind child must learn in order to be independent as an adult.

Be certain to offer frequent descriptions of what is happening or planned for children with visual impairments. They cannot see their surgical dressing, for example, so encourage them to feel it. They cannot see the intravenous infusion, but they can feel the tubing and the arm board that is holding their arm in place.

Parents of a child with severe visual impairment usually plan to room-in with their child during a hospitalization experience. Review with the parents their routine at mealtime and bedtime, their child's favorite toy, what word is used for voiding, and so on, and post it conspicuously or pass this information on to the entire nursing staff. Only when parents have confidence in you and the other staff members will they be able to leave their child in your care to meet their own needs, such as going to a coffee shop for a meal.

Structure and Function of the Ears

Ear anatomy is shown in Figure 50.8. Most diseases of the ear in children involve the external and middle portions.

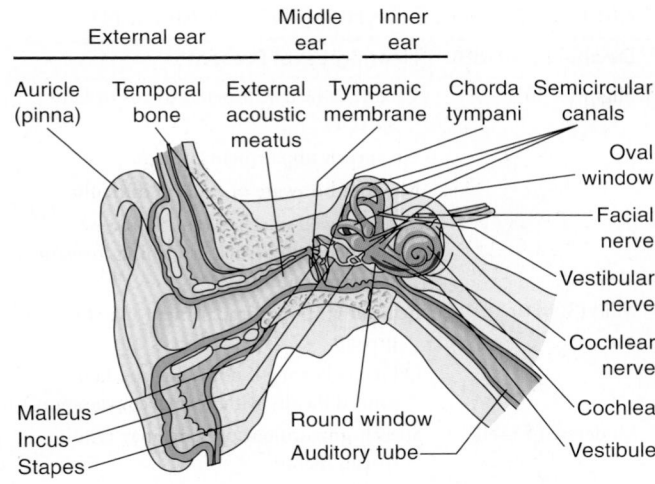

Figure 50.8   The structures of the ear.

THE PHYSIOLOGY OF HEARING LOSS

Hearing loss is termed a *conduction loss* if there is interference with sound reaching the inner ear (difficulty with the external canal, the tympanic membrane, or the ossicles). It is termed *nerve* or *sensorineural loss* if the inner ear or the eighth cranial nerve is affected. Conduction loss occurs in children if the external canal is obstructed with cerumen (wax) or a foreign object, if the tympanic membrane is damaged or immobile, or if the middle ear is filled with fluid, as occurs in *serous otitis media*. Sensorineural loss results from diseases that affect the transmission of sound sensation to the cerebral cortex or because of a pathologic condition of the cochlea. In children, nerve damage is usually congenital, although it can occur after drug therapy, an infection such as meningitis or rubella, or exposure to loud sound (Prosser, Cohen, & Greinwald, 2015).

Because diseases such as Treacher Collins syndrome, otosclerosis, osteogenesis imperfecta, and Waardenburg syndrome that lead to inherited hearing challenges tend to be autosomal dominant, there is a strong chance they will occur in future siblings of the child with hearing impairment. Genetic counseling can aid in increasing parental awareness of this possibility.

HEARING IMPAIRMENT

Approximately 12,000 infants, or 2 to 3 out of 1,000 children born in the United States are hard of hearing or deaf. Without newborn screening, these children may not be diagnosed with hearing loss until 2.5 to 3 years of age when development delays such as a lack of speech are identified (Alford, Arnos, Fox, et al., 2014).

Hearing impairment occurs in many different degrees and is rated by level of severity (Table 50.3). Causes of slight hearing impairment include serous otitis media, trauma from such things as inflating automobile airbags, and untreated acute otitis media with rupture of the tympanic membrane.

The discovery that a child is hearing challenged is almost always a shock to parents because 9 out of 10 children born deaf are born to hearing parents (Poon & Zaidman-Zait,

TABLE 50.3 LEVELS OF HEARING IMPAIRMENT

Decibel Level (dB)	Hearing Level Present
Slight (<30)	Unable to hear whispered words or faint speech
	No speech impairment present
	May not be aware of hearing difficulty
	Achieves well in school and home by compensating (such as leaning forward, speaking loudly)
Mild (30–50)	Beginning speech impairment may be present
	Difficulty hearing if not facing speaker; some difficulty with normal conversation
Moderate (55–70)	Speech impairment present; may require speech therapy
	Difficulty with normal conversation
Severe (70–90)	Difficulty with any sounds but nearby loud voice
	Hears vowels more easily than consonants
	Requires speech therapy for clear speech
	May still hear loud sounds, such as jets or train whistles
Profound (>90)	Hears almost no sound

2014). Children with hearing deficits should be exposed to language programs for children with hearing impairment as soon as possible so they have an optimum chance for language development and effective communication (Fig. 50.9).

For children who have conductive losses, an improvement in hearing usually can be achieved by use of a hearing aid (which intensifies the level of sound waves). Children who have inner ear or nerve deafness, however, cannot expect this kind of improvement. Parents of children with neural deafness need an explanation of the difference so they do not continue to search for a "cure" for their child or spend a great deal of money for hearing aids or alternative therapies, hoping a different brand, model, or technique will help their child.

Figure 50.9 A young girl with hearing impairment learning to use the computer with the aid of a speech therapist. (© Bob Daemmrich/Stock Boston.)

Hearing Aids and Cochlear Implants

Hearing aids pick up sound through a microphone, convert the sound waves into electrical impulses, and amplify them across the tympanic membrane. They are powered by batteries that must be changed periodically.

Hearing aids are designed to be as inconspicuous as possible, so children will not feel self-conscious wearing them. The receiver of the hearing aid may be incorporated into eyeglasses, molded into a plastic form that fits behind or into the ear, or housed in a small box (the size of a cell phone) that children wear on a cord around their neck or carry in a blouse or shirt pocket. Sound amplification systems are available to assist children in the classroom, such as personal frequency modulation systems in which the teacher wears a microphone that transmits directly to the child's hearing device (Kuppler, Lewis, & Evans, 2013). Teach children to remove hearing aids before washing their hair, showering, or swimming and to turn them off when removed to preserve the life of the batteries.

Children with a hearing impairment may grow self-conscious about wearing a hearing aid at school and may be the victims of bullying. Encourage children to report bullying, so it can be stopped. Be certain they value themselves as someone capable of overcoming great odds rather than as someone with a disability to hide.

Cochlear implants are mechanical devices consisting of a microphone, a speech processor, a transmitter/receiver, and an arrangement of electrodes that send impulses from the receiver directly to the auditory nerve. The auditory nerve then transmits the impulses to the brain where they are interpreted as words or common noises. The implant consists of an external portion that sits behind the ear and a second portion that is surgically implanted under the skin (Haynes, Gifford, & Rivas, 2016).

Approximately 38,000 children in the United States have received cochlear implants (National Institute on Deafness and Other Communication Disorders [NIDCD], 2012). These implants do not restore normal hearing but do allow for sounds to be received. Although adequate for communication, many children report hearing with a cochlear implant as sounding "muffled" or "under water." Months of training may be necessary to help a child correctly interpret these distorted impulses. Some adults with hearing impairment are reluctant to consent to a cochlear implant for their child because they believe the change from a child with hearing impairment to a hearing status will remove their child from their deaf culture. Support parents with the choice they make regarding the implant; at the end of adolescence, children who have not received a cochlear implant can independently make the choice whether to have one. Children who spoke with an impediment before cochlear implantation usually need speech therapy afterward to improve their speech pattern because their pronunciation of words is so ingrained at that point.

Speech Therapy

If children who are hearing challenged are to interact as fully as possible with the world around them, they need an intensive program of speech therapy. Whether children should be introduced to sign language early is controversial; some therapists believe learning sign language early is helpful because it allows children to express their needs early, whereas others believe that by learning sign language, children decrease their need to learn to articulate speech sounds or to lip read and, for those reasons, learning sign language should not be encouraged. It is true that for real independence and to perform in regular school classes, children need to communicate by means other than sign language. For children with a profound impairment, however, learning speech sounds may be a long-term process, making sign language necessary for contact with the world around them until they can learn to speak.

What If . . . 50.3

A nurse discovers that Carla, who is hearing challenged, refuses to wear her hearing aid because another child at her school made fun of it. What suggestions could the nurse give her parents to help Carla better accept wearing her hearing aid?

Disorders of the Ear

Ear disorders are always serious in children because hearing is such an important function for the growing child. Methods to assess hearing are discussed in Chapter 34.

EXTERNAL OTITIS

External otitis (otitis externa) is inflammation of the external ear canal. Although external ear inflammation rarely threatens hearing or causes permanent damage, it does cause discomfort in the form of itching and sometimes extreme pain (Marais, 2015).

Assessment

The history of children with external otitis usually reveals that they have recently been swimming, which is why this condition is popularly called *swimmer's ear*. It also can occur if a young child pushes a foreign object into the ear canal. Unlike a middle ear infection (otitis media), there is no history of a recent respiratory infection. Children first notice itching of the canal and then pain. When the external ear is touched, the pain becomes acute. The moisture in the canal left from swimming or from decay of a food substance has caused inflammation, and a secondary infection then can occur in the closed space. *Pseudomonas* and *Candida* are agents frequently involved in these infections. On otoscopic examination, the pain may be found to be due to the sharply localized, tender swelling of a furuncle, or the entire canal may be swollen shut and tender to the touch. Fungal infections tend to turn the canal brown or black; although, if mold forms around a foreign body, such as the tip of a cotton applicator, it may appear white or gray. The skin under the object will be moist, red, and eroded.

If doing a first assessment on a child, be certain to visualize the tympanic membrane if possible to be certain it is intact and that it is not inflamed or to verify if the inflammation is about to extend into the middle ear. Before the tympanic membrane can be visualized clearly, it is often necessary to remove superficial debris from the canal. A Weber test (discussed in Chapter 34) should show that hearing is not decreased in the affected ear. If the sound of a tuning fork vibrates louder in the affected ear, it suggests otitis media is present.

Removing debris by an ear curette from an infected external canal requires both patience and skill. Children must lie still for the procedure to prevent them from suddenly turning their head and causing the curette to puncture the tympanic membrane, and so they may need to be restrained. If the debris in the canal is hard and difficult to remove, it can be softened and loosened by touching it with a hydrogen peroxide–soaked cotton applicator or, alternatively, by dropping 2% acetic acid into the canal and allowing this to stand for a few minutes. Don't irrigate the external canal until it has been shown that the tympanic membrane is intact so that infected material is not washed through a rupture into the middle ear.

Therapeutic Management

The treatment of otitis externa differs according to the organism causing the infection. If the canal is so swollen that ear drops cannot flow back into the canal, a cotton wick moistened with Burow's solution may be threaded into the canal. The cotton extending out into the auricle is kept moistened by rewetting it periodically for the next 24 hours with Burow's solution. This usually reduces the swelling of the canal to a point where further cleaning can be accomplished.

Ear drops containing hydrocortisone, an antibiotic, or an antifungal mixture may be prescribed. Hydrocortisone reduces inflammation, and the antibiotic or antifungal preparation will reduce the infection. If ear pain is present, an analgesic, such as acetaminophen or ibuprofen, may be necessary to control discomfort. It is important that children keep the ear canal dry until the inflammation subsides, so they need to avoid swimming and washing their hair during this time. If they shower, they should first insert ear plugs into the external meatus or wear a shower cap to keep out moisture.

Nursing Diagnoses and Related Interventions

Nursing Diagnosis: Deficient knowledge related to technique for ear drop instillation or other care measures

Outcome Evaluation: Parents demonstrate proper instillation of ear drops; parents state the importance of continuing prescribed treatment to completion.

Administering ear drops can be a challenging task for parents because children invariably are reluctant to have any fluid dripped into their ear. Demonstrate to parents how this is done (see Chapter 38) before they leave the health-care facility. Caution them to give the medication for the full period prescribed. Otherwise, especially if the child is resistant, parents may administer the ear drops only until the pain subsides (24 to 48 hours). As a result, the infection may recur.

Follow-up evaluation after the completion of treatment for external otitis should include assessment of inflammation, pain, and the parents' awareness of prevention strategies. Preventive strategies include avoiding insertion of any object into the ear canal and using ear plugs while swimming. Instillation of a dilute alcohol or acetic acid solution by dropper after swimming is a prophylactic measure that may be recommended for children who swim competitively and spend a great deal of time in water to help keep the ear canal dry.

IMPACTED CERUMEN

Cerumen (earwax) serves the important function of cleansing the external ear canal as it gradually moves outward, bringing with it shed epithelial cells and any foreign object. Parents are often concerned that earwax will lead to a loss of hearing (or they view it as dirty) and so ask healthcare professionals to have it removed. Wax accumulation rarely is extensive enough in children that it interferes with hearing and removing it can diminish its protective function, so it should not be removed routinely. Using cotton-tipped applicators to clean ears as a regular practice can also scratch the ear canal, creating a site for a secondary infection. This practice may also push accumulated cerumen farther into the ear canal, resulting in plugging of wax.

Commercial softeners are available if cerumen accumulates to such an extent that hearing is affected. In some instances, a dilute solution of hydrogen peroxide may be necessary to dissolve cerumen. Again, this should not be done regularly because this will keep the ear canal constantly moist, an environment that leads to external otitis.

QSEN Checkpoint Question 50.5

EVIDENCE-BASED PRACTICE

A concern about the many mobile electronic devices available today is that increased noise exposure will cause neurologic hearing injury. To investigate whether hearing loss was present in teenagers who typically listened to music through earphones, researchers tested the hearing of 381 first-year university students and then asked them to self-report their history of music exposure. The results of the study showed those students with a high level of recreational noise exposure had lower hearing thresholds than those students with less recreational noise exposure (Tung & Chao, 2013).

Based on this study, which action by Carla's teenage brother would cause a nurse the most concern?
a. He listens to music on his computer while he does his homework.
b. He typically listens to sports news on the radio while he eats.
c. He plays varsity basketball in a noisy gymnasium once a week.
d. He listens to music with earbuds when he rides the bus and subway.

Look in Appendix A for the best answer and rationale.

ACUTE OTITIS MEDIA

Inflammation of the middle ear (otitis media) is one of the most prevalent diseases of childhood. It occurs most often in children 6 to 36 months of age and again at 4 to 6 years. Children most susceptible to it are males, Alaskan and Native American children, those with cleft palate, and infants who are formula-fed rather than breastfed. Formula-feeding leads to this because infants are held in a more slanted position while feeding, allowing milk to enter the eustachian tube. The incidence of otitis media is highest in the winter and spring because it frequently follows an upper respiratory infection and is higher in homes in which a parent smokes

cigarettes (Zhang, Xu, Zhang, et al., 2014). Although it occurs frequently, otitis media is a potentially serious disease of childhood because permanent damage can occur to middle ear structures, leading to permanent hearing impairment.

Assessment

Acute otitis media usually occurs following a respiratory tract infection. Children have a "cold," rhinitis, and perhaps a low-grade fever for several days. Suddenly, their fever peaks to about 102°F (38°C), and sharp, constant pain begins in one or both ears. Older children can verbalize they have pain and point to where the pain is felt. Infants, unable to do this, become extremely irritable and frequently pull or tug at the affected ear in an attempt to gain relief from pain. On examination, the external canal is usually free of wax because the warmth of the inflammation and fever melts the wax and moves it more readily out of the canal. In contrast to an external ear canal infection, the discomfort they feel does not increase on manipulation of the auricle. Palpate the mastoid process behind the ear to be certain it doesn't feel tender to your touch. If it does, the infection probably has spread out of the middle ear into the mastoid cells, a very serious complication that may lead to meningitis.

The appearance of a normal eardrum shows the outline of the malleus (see Chapter 34). With an infection, the tympanic membrane appears inflamed or reddened. It may bulge forward into the external canal because of fluid and edema behind it. The landmarks of the tympanic membrane, the malleus and incus, can be visualized only poorly or not at all. The light reflex of the otoscope will not be as definite as usual because of the "pushed out" or convex shape of the eardrum. There is decreased mobility on a pneumatic examination.

Therapeutic Management

Most middle ear infections are caused by *Streptococcus pneumoniae*, *Haemophilus influenzae* (especially in children younger than 5 years of age), or *Streptococcus pyrogenes*. An otitis media infection may resolve spontaneously; however, if it does not, antibiotic therapy may be indicated.

Other pharmacologic agents children may need are an analgesic and antipyretic such as acetaminophen (Tylenol) and decongestant nose drops to open the eustachian tubes and allow air to enter the middle ear. These are given for only 2 to 3 days because if they are given longer, a rebound effect can occur, causing edema and a subsequent increase in mucous membrane inflammation. Providing a smoke-free home environment can help prevent further episodes of otitis media (Zhang et al., 2014).

During the course of otitis media, some children experience a conductive hearing loss; this may last as long as 6 months after the acute infection. Caution parents about this, so they will not think the infection is growing worse if they first notice the impairment. They also need to know about the possibility of hearing loss so that when the child gets hearing screening in school during the 6 months following the infection, they can account for the hearing loss. If a child still has a conductive hearing loss after 6 months (or has other symptoms), the child should be reevaluated to see whether a new infection or serous otitis media has developed. Box 50.5 shows an interprofessional care map illustrating both nursing and team planning for a child with otitis media (Lieberthal, Carroll, Chonmaitree, et al., 2013).

BOX 50.5

Nursing Care Planning

AN INTERPROFESSIONAL CARE MAP FOR A CHILD WITH OTITIS MEDIA

Carla Vander, a 6-year-old, is brought to your pediatric clinic for evaluation. Her mother states, "She was born with a hearing loss and a cataract. Today, her eye is red and she has pain in her ear. Can you see her quickly so I can get an antibiotic for the ear infection before the drugstore closes?"

Family Assessment: Child lives with parents and two brothers, 7 and 14 years old, in three-bedroom suburban cottage. Father works as a travel agent; mother is a grade school librarian. Father describes finances as "middle class."

Patient Assessment: Child has had two previous ear infections in the past 8 months. Child had a clear, watery nasal discharge and slight cough for 2 days. Today has thick, purulent, nasal drainage. Temperature this morning was 102.2°F (39.0°C). Observed tugging vigorously on right ear. On examination, right tympanic membrane is erythematous and bulging, with poor mobility on pneumoscopy. Left ear examination unremarkable. Child is diagnosed with otitis media of the right ear.

Nursing Diagnosis: Pain related to inflammation and erythema secondary to ear infection

Outcome Evaluation: Child no longer tugs at right ear; tympanic membrane no longer reddened or bulging; child rates pain as no higher than 2 on a FACES Pain Rating Scale.

Team Member Responsible	Assessment	Intervention	Rationale	Expected Outcome
Activities of Daily Living, Including Safety				
Nurse	Assess whether child is able to sleep or wakes with pain.	Suggest mother give prescribed antihistamine at bedtime. Urge child to sleep with affected ear up.	Antihistamines can make children sleepy. Sleeping on affected ear can put pressure on eustachian tube, which can increase pain.	Mother reports child is able to sleep through the night.
Teamwork and Collaboration				
Nurse/primary care provider	Assess whether child has susceptibility to ear infections or whether this could be reoccurrence of a former infection.	Meet with ear, nose, and throat service to consult on cause of frequent otitis media.	Otitis media is painful so can affect quality of life.	Consultant meets with mother to discuss cause of frequent ear infections.
Procedures/Medications for Quality Improvement				
Nurse	Assess whether child has experience with taking oral medicine; rate child's level of pain by FACES Pain Rating Scale.	Instruct the mother to administer acetaminophen every 4 hours or ibuprofen every 8 hours and how to instill saline nose drops.	Acetaminophen and ibuprofen are effective analgesics and antipyretics for this degree of pain; nose drops relieve nasal inflammation.	Child is able to take oral medicine cooperatively; rates pain level as not above 2 on FACES Pain Rating Scale.
Nutrition				
Nurse	Assess what soft foods and fluids child likes to eat.	Encourage mother to offer liquids and soft foods.	Movement of the eustachian tube, such as with chewing, may increase pain.	Child names some foods and fluid she is willing to eat; eats less than usual but adequate amount.
Patient-Centered Care				
Nurse	Assess how much mother and child understand about the cause of otitis media and the newer, no-antibiotic approach to treatment.	Educate the mother about the common characteristics of otitis media; reassure mother the infection will resolve without an antibiotic.	Education promotes better understanding of the problem, alleviating some of the stress and anxiety associated with it.	Mother states her prime goal is to get child well again; will follow primary care provider's recommendation for care.

Continued on following page

BOX 50.5

Nursing Care Planning (continued)

Team Member Responsible	Assessment	Intervention	Rationale	Expected Outcome
Psychosocial/Spiritual/Emotional Needs				
Nurse	Assess how much experience mother has with care of an ill child.	Teach mother that otitis media usually resolves without the need for an antibiotic.	Correct information helps mother accept a lack of antibiotic prescription.	Mother states she feels capable of caring for child without antibiotic prescription.
Informatics for Seamless Healthcare Planning				
Nurse	Assess whether child or parents have any questions about care that they still need to be answered.	Instruct the mother to contact the clinic or healthcare provider if there is no improvement within 24 to 48 hours or if the child exhibits increased pain.	Lack of improvement within 24 to 48 hours indicates the need for further evaluation; increased pain may indicate excessive fluid accumulation, which could lead to tympanic rupture.	Mother has clinic telephone number; will telephone if symptoms of complications occur.

OTITIS MEDIA WITH EFFUSION

Otitis media with effusion occurs when otitis media becomes chronic. Normally, the middle ear is an air-filled cavity; air is supplied to it each time the eustachian tube opens with swallowing, yawning, or chewing. If this source of air to the middle ear is closed off due to inflammation or edema of the eustachian tube, the epithelial cells of the middle ear begin to secrete a thin, watery mucus. Over time, the compartment becomes so filled with this and the fluid becomes so thick and tenacious that it appears glue-like. Some children notice a feeling of fullness or the sound of popping or ringing in their ears. There may be a drop in hearing of 20 to 40 dB because of the inability of the ossicles to function effectively. Involvement is usually bilateral. The condition occurs most frequently in children 3 to 10 years of age (Robb & Williamson, 2016).

Assessment

A child experiences muffled hearing and a feeling of pressure in the ear with otitis media with effusion. Otoscopic examination may show a level of fluid behind the tympanic membrane. However, a fluid line will be visible only if there is also a quantity of air in the middle ear to contrast with it. As the collected fluid becomes thick, it tends to retract the eardrum. This makes the malleus more prominent and perhaps displaced to a horizontal angle as the membrane is retracted around it; the light reflex from the otoscope light becomes distorted. If a pneumatic otoscope is used, gentle introduction of air against the eardrum produces no movement of the tympanic membrane (as there would be normally).

Therapeutic Management

Therapy for otitis media with effusion may be long term. If the condition appears to be intensified by inflammation from an allergy, measures to control the allergy must be initiated. These may include avoidance of the allergen, hyposensitization, or pharmacologic alteration of the allergic response (see Chapter 42).

Definitive medical treatment is aimed at supplying air to the middle ear. For mild involvement, the daily administration of an antihistamine or a nasal decongestant to shrink the mucous membrane of the eustachian tube may be enough to achieve an air supply. In a few children, the eustachian tube is blocked by enlarged adenoids, and their removal is indicated. Fluid from the middle ear can be removed by **tympanocentesis** (a needle inserted through the tympanic membrane); however, the fluid usually returns unless some intervention to introduce air into the middle ear (tubal myringotomy) is undertaken.

Tubal Myringotomy

A source of air can be supplied to the middle ear by the insertion of small plastic (Teflon) tubes inserted through the tympanic membrane (tympanostomy). The insertion of such tubes is done by a myringotomy at a point in the tympanic membrane that is not instrumental for hearing, so the tube does not interfere with hearing (Fig. 50.10). Myringotomy tubes can be placed in one or both ears as an ambulatory

Figure 50.10 A myringotomy tube provides air to the middle ear to prevent otitis media with effusion.

procedure after the local injection of lidocaine (Xylocaine). Tubes tend to be extruded after 6 to 12 months. For most children, this period is long enough to halt the secretory process of the middle ear. In others, tubes must be reinserted to continue the aeration.

When myringotomy tubes are in place, the child has to be careful to not allow water to enter the ears. It's better if they bathe rather than shower, but showering is all right if ear plugs are used, especially while washing hair. Similarly, swimming is either contraindicated or allowed only with ear plugs in place.

Because the course of the process is long term, the hearing impairment associated with the condition may also be long term. Urge parents to notify the school nurse that their child has compromised hearing because of the middle ear fluid and has myringotomy tubes in place. Children may need to move to the front of the class to mitigate difficulty hearing and encourage participation in class until the condition improves.

QSEN Checkpoint Question 50.6

INFORMATICS

Carla is diagnosed as having otitis media. When interpreting the documentation in Carla's electronic health record, the nurse should recognize that this diagnosis differs from otitis externa in what way?

   a. Otitis media occurs from swimming; otitis externa typically follows a common cold.

   b. Otitis media involves the middle ear; otitis externa involves the outer canal.

   c. Otitis media involves the eardrum; otitis externa involves the cochlear nerve.

   d. Otitis media does not cause pain; otitis externa produces throbbing pain.

Look in Appendix A for the best answer and rationale.

The Hospitalized Child With a Hearing Impairment

Conversation is usually held between 50 and 60 dB so a hearing loss greater than 49 dB is sufficient enough to interfere with hearing conversation and developing language. Like those who are visually challenged, children with hearing deficits may be hospitalized as a direct consequence of their ear disorder or from other health problems. It can be difficult for parents to prepare children with hearing deficits for hospitalization because they are unfamiliar with words such as "surgery," "tonsils," "hurts," "operating room," and "recovery room." Showing the child illustrated books depicting anatomical landmarks and procedures is helpful. Allowing children time to play with dolls or puppets can help them understand hospital routine. Children who are hearing challenged may have additional challenges during hospitalization.

Always allow children with hearing impairment to see you before you touch them because they will not find this nearly as startling as being touched without warning. If children are sleeping when you approach them, use a light touch to waken them gently. Some children turn off their hearing aid or remove it while they sleep. You may need to turn it on before you call them to wake them, or they may need to replace the hearing aid as soon as they awaken. Children as young as

2 years of age are effective lip readers as long as you are facing them. Position yourself at eye level, so the child can view your face. In a group, help the child follow conversation by directing the child to the person who is speaking. Assign consistent staff members to decrease the number of people with whom the child must attempt to communicate. Have a staff person accompany the child and stay with the child in all departments to help with communication.

Do not underestimate the intelligence level of children with hearing impairment. Because they do not speak clearly, others may assume children with hearing impairment are cognitively challenged. As a result, they may not be given information that the average hearing child receives, such as explanations of how things work. On a hospital unit, children with hearing impairment are unable to express how they feel about procedures especially if providers are not familiar with sign language. They need help from healthcare personnel who understand these challenges and take sufficient time to offer explanations and provide support.

Ask parents of children who are hearing challenged to draw pictures or demonstrate the sign language symbols their children use for important words such as "pain," "drink," and "bathroom." Encourage children to use or draw pictures of what they want if they are still too young to write words and if you cannot understand what they are saying.

Children with hearing impairment have the right to be provided with a sign language interpreter during care. Advocate for this, especially if the parents will not be continually present.

What If . . . 50.4

A nurse is particularly interested in exploring one of the 2020 National Health Goals with respect to vision and hearing disorders in children (see Box 50.1). What would be a possible research topic pertinent to this goal that would be applicable to Carla's family and that would also advance evidence-based practice?

KEY POINTS FOR REVIEW

- Teaching preventive measures to avoid eye and hearing injuries (using proper eye protection during sports or play and wearing goggles or ear protection as appropriate) and screening children for sensory impairments are important nursing roles.

- Refractive errors of vision such as myopia and hyperopia are the most common eye disorders in children. Amblyopia is subnormal vision in one eye. Children with these disorders need correction at the time the disorder is recognized to prevent further vision distortion.

- Coloboma is congenital and involves the incomplete closure of the pupil or lower eyelid. Ptosis is the inability to open the upper eyelid normally. Ptosis needs correction to prevent the development of amblyopia. Strabismus is unequally aligned eyes. Like ptosis, it can lead to amblyopia if not corrected.

- Infections of the lids, such as styes or chalazia, can occur in children. Conjunctivitis (inflammation of the conjunctiva) often manifests with acute symptoms. An antibiotic is necessary for therapy.

- Eye injuries such as penetration by a foreign body need a follow-up after treatment to be certain vision remains adequate.

- Children who are either vision or hearing challenged need special preparation and orientation for a hospital or ambulatory health visit that not only meets QSEN competencies but also best meets a family's total needs.

- Help children who are vision challenged to work through new experiences by letting them feel equipment as much as possible. Guide their hands through the steps of a new procedure you are teaching them.

- Otitis media (a middle ear infection) is a common childhood illness. Some children who have otitis media with effusion have myringotomy tubes inserted to relieve pressure and to supply air access to the middle ear.

- Use photographs, drawings, or demonstrations with children with hearing impairment to help them learn new skills. Contact a sign language interpreter as appropriate to be certain that children understand instructions.

CRITICAL THINKING CARE STUDY

Hannah, 11 years old, wears glasses because of a severe refractive difference in her eyes. She has had a severe hearing impairment since birth and wears a hearing aid. She is admitted to your unit for dehydration secondary to influenza. Her father tells you Hannah is proficient in American Sign Language and can also read lips fairly well.

1. What special precautions do you need to take to ensure Hannah is safe in the hospital environment?

2. Hannah's parents are separated; she spends 1 week a month with her mother and the other 3 weeks with her father. Her father worries she doesn't wear her glasses during the week she's with her mother. Her mother tells you she doesn't wear them when she's with her father. What suggestions could you make to remind her to wear the glasses?

3. You notice Hannah doesn't like the taste of the oral rehydrating solution, which she needs to drink to restore her fluid volume. When you check to see if she drank all of it, even though you know you faced her squarely and spoke loudly, she says she didn't hear you tell her to drink it. What would be a better way to communicate with Hannah?

RELATED RESOURCES

Explore these additional resources to enhance learning for this chapter:

- Student resources on thePoint, including answers to the What If . . . and Critical Thinking Care Study questions, http://thepoint.lww.com/Flagg8e
- Adaptive learning powered by PrepU, http://thepoint.lww.com/prepu

REFERENCES

Akinpelu, O. V., Peleva, E., Funnell, W. R., et al. (2014). Otoacoustic emissions in newborn hearing screening: A systematic review of the effects of different protocols on test outcomes. *International Journal of Pediatric Otorhinolaryngology, 78*(5), 711–717.

Alam, S., Gaffney, M., & Eichwald, J. (2014). Improved newborn hearing screening follow-up results in more infants identified. *Journal of Public Health Management and Practice, 20*(2), 220–223.

Alford, R. L., Arnos, K. S., Fox, M., et al. (2014). American College of Medical Genetics and Genomics guideline for the clinical evaluation and etiologic diagnosis of hearing loss. *Genetics in Medicine, 16*(4), 347–355.

Armstrong, G. W., Kim, J. G., Linakis, J. G., et al. (2013). Pediatric eye injures presenting to United States emergency departments: 2001-2007. *Graefe's Archive for Clinical and Experimental Ophthalmology, 251*(3), 629–636.

Belden, J., DeFriez, C., & Huether, S. E. (2013). The special senses. In S. E. Huether & K. L. McCance (Eds.), *Understanding pathophysiology* (5th ed., pp. 335–339). New York, NY: Elsevier.

Birch, E. E. (2013). Amblyopia and binocular vision. *Progress in Retinal and Eye Research, 33*(2013), 67–84.

Braverman, R. S. (2012). The eye. In W. W. Hay, M. J. Levine, J. M. Sondheimer, et al. (Eds.), *Current pediatric diagnosis & treatment* (20th ed., pp. 401–441). Columbus, OH: McGraw-Hill.

Bruins, M., & Kraemer, K. (2013). Public health programmes for vitamin A deficiency control. *Community Eye Health, 26*(84), 69–70.

Cotter, S. A., Cyert, L. A., Miller, J. M., et al. (2015). Vision screening for children 36 to <72 months: Recommended practices. *Optometry and Vision Science, 92*(1), 6–16.

DeSantis, D. (2014). Amblyopia. *Pediatric Clinics of North America, 61*(3), 505–518.

Edelson, C. (2013). Uveitis. In C. S. Hoyt & D. Taylor (Eds.), *Pediatric ophthalmology & strabismus* (4th ed., pp. 377–392). Philadelphia, PA: Elsevier/Saunders.

El Sayed, Y., & Gawdat, G. (2017). Two-year results of microcatheter-assisted trabeculotomy in paediatric glaucoma: A randomized controlled study. *Acta Ophthalmologica.* Advance online publication. doi:10.1111/aos.13414

Giangiacomo, A., & Beck, A. (2017). Pediatric glaucoma: Review of recent literature. *Current Opinion in Ophthalmology, 28*(2), 199–203.

Haynes, D. S., Gifford, R. H., & Rivas, A. (2016). Introduction to the 14th Symposium on Cochlear Implants in Children, Nashville, TN Papers. *Otology & Neurotology, 37*(2), e12.

Holmes, J. M. (2014). Screening, confirming, and treating amblyopia based on binocularity. *JAMA Ophthalmology, 132*(7), 820–822.

Ivarsen, A., Næser, K., & Hjortdal, J. (2013). Laser in situ keratomileusis for high astigmatism in myopic and hyperopic eyes. *Journal of Cataract & Refractive Surgery, 39*(1), 74–80.

Kemper, A. R., Crews, J. E., Strickland, B., et al. (2014). Vision screening among children aged <6 years—Medical Expenditure Panel Survey, United States, 2009-2010. *MMWR Supplements, 63*(2), 43–46.

Kuppler, L., Lewis, M., & Evans, A. (2013). A review of unilateral hearing loss and academic performance: Is it time to reassess traditional dogmata? *International Journal of Pediatric Otorhinolaryngology, 77*(5), 617–662.

LaRoche, G. R. (2013). Examination, history and special tests in pediatric ophthalmology. In C. S. Hoyt & D. Taylor (Eds.), *Pediatric ophthalmology & strabismus* (4th ed., pp. 45–54). Philadelphia, PA: Elsevier/Saunders.

Li, X., Zarbin, M. A., & Bhagat, N. (2015). Pediatric open globe injury: A review of the literature. *Journal of Emergencies, Trauma, & Shock, 8*(4), 216–223.

Lieberthal, A. S., Carroll, A. E., Chonmaitree, T., et al. (2013). The diagnosis and management of acute otitis media. *Pediatrics, 131*(3), e964–e999.

Lin, Z. J., Xu, S., Huang, S. Y., et al. (2016). Comparison of canaloplasty and trabeculectomy for open angle glaucoma: A meta-analysis. *International Journal of Ophthalmology, 9*(12), 1814–1819.

Marais, A. (2015). Clinical evidence in the management of swimmer's ear. *South African Family Practice, 57*(5), 4–8.

Marenco, M., Macchi, I., Galassi, E., et al. (2017). Clinical presentation and management of congenital ptosis. *Clinical Ophthalmology (Auckland, N.Z.), 11*, 453–463.

Medsinge, A., & Nischal, K. K. (2015). Pediatric cataract: Challenges and future directions. *Clinical Ophthalmology, 9*, 77–90.

National Dissemination Center for Children With Disabilities. (2012). *Categories of disabilities.* Washington, DC: Author.

National Institute on Deafness and Other Communication Disorders. (2012). *Statistics about hearing disorders, ear infections, and deafness.* Hyattsville, MD: National Center for Health Statistics.

Papadopoulos, M., Brookes, J. L., & Khaw, P. T. (2013). Pediatric glaucoma. In C. S. Hoyt & D. Taylor (Eds.), *Pediatric ophthalmology & strabismus* (4th ed., pp. 353–367). Philadelphia, PA: Elsevier/Saunders.

Pediatric Eye Disease Investigator Group. (2014). A randomized trial of atropine versus patching for treatment of moderate amblyopia: Follow-up at 15 years of age. *JAMA Ophthalmology, 132*(7), 799–805.

Penix, K., Swanson, M. W., & DeCarlo, D. K. (2015). Nystagmus in pediatric patients: Interventions and patient-focused perspectives. *Clinical Ophthalmology, 9*, 1527–1536.

Poon, B. T., & Zaidman-Zait, A. (2014). Social support for parents of deaf children: Moving toward contextualized understanding. *Journal of Deaf Studies and Deaf Education, 19*(2), 176–188.

Prosser, J. D., Cohen, A. P., & Greinwald, J. H. (2015). Diagnostic evaluation of children with sensorineural hearing loss. *Otolaryngology Clinics of North America, 48*, 975–982.

Qiu, M., Wang, S. Y., Singh, K., et al. (2014). Racial disparities in uncorrected and undercorrected refractive error in the United States. *Investigative Ophthalmology & Visual Science, 55*(10), 6996–7005.

Rajavi, Z., & Sabbaghi, H. (2016). Congenital cataract screening. *Journal of Ophthalmic & Vision Research, 11*(3), 310–312.

Rajavi, Z., Sabbaghi, H., Baghini, A. S., et al. (2015). Prevalence of color vision deficiency and its correlation with amblyopia and refractive errors among primary school children. *Journal of Ophthalmic & Vision Research, 10*(2), 130–138.

Robb, P. J., & Williamson, I. (2016). Otitis media with effusion in children: Current management. *Pediatrics and Child Health, 26*(1), 9–14.

Solebo, A. L., & Rahi, J. (2014). Epidemiology, aetiology and management of visual impairment in children. *Archives of Disease in Childhood, 99*, 375–379.

Stahl, E. D. (2014). Pediatric refractive surgery. *Pediatric Clinics of North America, 61*(3), 519–527.

Stein, A., Kelly, J. P., & Weiss, A. H. (2014). Congenital eyelid ptosis: Onset and prevalence of amblyopia associations with systemic disorders and treatment outcomes. *The Journal of Pediatrics, 164*(4), 820–824.

Sung, E. K., Nadqir, R. N., Fujita, A., et al. (2014). Injuries of the globe: What can the radiologist offer? *Radiographics, 34*(3), 764–776.

Tung, C. Y., & Chao, K. P. (2013). Effect of recreational noise exposure on hearing impairment among teenage students. *Research in Developmental Disabilities, 34*(1), 126–132.

U.S. Department of Health and Human Services. (2010). *Healthy people 2020.* Washington, DC: Author.

Wojciechowski, R. (2011). Nature and nurture: The complex genetics of myopia and refractive error. *Clinical Genetics, 79*(4), 301–320.

Yeung, H., & Walton, D. (2012). Recognizing childhood glaucoma in the primary pediatric setting. *Contemporary Pediatrics, 29*(5), 32–40.

Zhang, Y., Xu, M., Zhang, J., et al. (2014). Risk factors for chronic and recurrent otitis media-a meta-analysis. *PLoS One, 9*(1), e86397.

51

Nursing Care of a Family When a Child Has a Musculoskeletal Disorder

Jeffrey, a 13-year-old boy, accompanies his mother and 3-year-old sister into the hospital emergency room because his sister has pain in her arm after a fall. As you talk to Jeffrey, you notice his left lower leg is swollen, warm to the touch, and painful. When he takes off his shirt, you notice his spine is not straight. His mother tells you she noticed an infected mosquito bite on his leg 2 weeks ago. After further evaluation, Jeffrey's sister is diagnosed with a fracture of her ulna; Jeffrey is diagnosed with osteomyelitis. His mother asks you, "I know our family is prone to orthopedic problems, but how could a bone infection happen from such a simple thing as an insect bite? Are you sure he's not developing muscular dystrophy like his uncle? Or is he just having growing pains?"

Previous chapters described the growth and development of well children and the nursing care of children with a disorder of other body systems. This chapter adds information about the dramatic changes, both physical and psychosocial, which can occur when a child develops a musculoskeletal disorder.

What other information does Jeffrey's mother need to know about bone infections? How would you explain to her what has happened?

KEY TERMS

apposition

arthroscopy

cartilage

compartment syndrome

diaphysis

distraction

epiphyseal plate

epiphysis

fracture

malleoli

metaphysis

myopathy

periosteum

remodeling

resorption

sequestrum

traction

OBJECTIVES

After mastering the contents of this chapter, you should be able to:

1. Describe common musculoskeletal disorders in children.
2. Identify 2020 National Health Goals related to musculoskeletal disorders in children that nurses can help the nation achieve.
3. Assess a child with a musculoskeletal disorder.
4. Formulate nursing diagnoses related to a child with a musculoskeletal disorder.
5. Establish expected outcomes for a child with a musculoskeletal disorder that help children and parents manage seamless transitions across differing healthcare settings.
6. Using the nursing process, plan nursing care that includes the six competencies of Quality & Safety Education for Nurses (QSEN): Patient-Centered Care, Teamwork & Collaboration, Evidence-Based Practice (EBP), Quality Improvement (QI), Safety, and Informatics.
7. Implement nursing care, such as helping a child with a musculoskeletal disorder meet optimal ambulation capacity.
8. Evaluate expected outcomes for achievement and effectiveness of care.
9. Integrate knowledge of children's musculoskeletal disorders with the interplay of nursing process, the six competencies of QSEN, and Family Nursing to promote quality maternal and child health nursing care.

The skeletal system, composed of more than 200 bones connected by the joints and tendons, provides the structural casing or protective armor for the internal organs of the body and supplies the body with red and white blood cells grown in the central marrow. Skeletal muscles, which are attached to the bones by connective tissue, tendons, and ligaments, allow for voluntary movement, including gross motor activities, such as running, and fine motor activities, such as writing. Together, the skeletal and muscular systems both support the body and make coordinated movement possible.

Because their bones and muscles are still growing, children suffer from disorders of the musculoskeletal system more frequently than do adults. The difference between adults and children is growth. Childhood **fractures** (break in the continuity or structure of bone) heal much more quickly than fractures do in adults and because a child's bone grows from the epiphysis or growth plate, a fracture within this area may cause serious complication, such as a deformity. Nurses play a key role in teaching parents ways to expose children who have muscular or skeletal disorders to the same sorts of stimuli that might be experienced if they were able to move around independently. Because the maintenance of musculoskeletal function and locomotion is so important, these are addressed by 2020 National Health Goals (Box 51.1).

BOX 51.1

Nursing Care Planning Based on 2020 National Health Goals

To maintain a healthy musculoskeletal system, proper exercise is necessary. Several 2020 National Health Goals address this, including:

- Increase the proportion of the nation's public and private schools that require daily physical education for elementary grade students from a baseline of 3.8% to 4.2%.
- Increase the proportion of the nation's public and private schools that require daily physical education for middle or junior high students from a baseline of 7.9% to 8.6% and for senior high students from 2.1% to 2.3%.
- Increase the proportion of adolescents who meet current federal physical activity guidelines for aerobic physical activity and for muscle-strengthening activity (developmental).
- Increase the proportion of children and adolescents aged 2 years through 12th grade who view television, videos, or play video games for no more than 2 hours a day from 78.9% to 86.8%.
- Increase the proportion of trips that children and adolescents make by walking (Developmental) (U.S. Department of Health and Human Services, 2010; see www.healthypeople.gov).

Nurses can help the nation achieve these goals by educating children about the importance of physical activity, serving as consultants for school systems in designing physical education programs, and being certain to ask children about their usual activity level at health maintenance visits.

Nursing Process Overview

FOR CARE OF A CHILD WITH A MUSCULOSKELETAL DISORDER

ASSESSMENT

Unlike many other diseases in children, disorders of the skeletal system usually manifest with specific, localized symptoms; therefore, parents usually bring children to healthcare facilities early in the course of such illnesses. Disorders of the muscles or joints, however, such as juvenile idiopathic arthritis (JIA), may manifest insidiously; when the disorder is diagnosed, parents may feel guilty for not having sought health care earlier.

One condition whose seriousness parents may underestimate is a childhood limp. A limp is never normal, and it may be the first manifestation of a serious hip or knee problem. When weighing or measuring children at healthcare visits, take the opportunity to assess gait (whether a child walks naturally or stiffly, on tiptoes or on the whole foot; whether the feet are in good alignment; and whether the back is held straight). Such assessments may detect that a child brought to a healthcare center because of an upper respiratory condition, for example, has another, perhaps more important, musculoskeletal problem requiring an evaluation. It is also important to note that skeletal injuries can be a sign of child maltreatment; thus, careful history taking is necessary at all health visits (see Chapter 55).

NURSING DIAGNOSIS

The nursing diagnoses most frequently identified for children with musculoskeletal disorders include those that deal with pain, lack of mobility, and, because of immobilization, a need for diversional activities. Children, especially adolescents, who require a walker or other equipment to aid in skeletal support or locomotion may encounter problems with self-esteem. Examples of some typical nursing diagnoses include:

- Pain related to chronic inflammation of joints
- Impaired physical mobility related to a cast on the leg
- Deficient diversional activities related to a need for imposed activity restriction for 4 weeks
- Situational low self-esteem related to the continuous use of a body brace

OUTCOME IDENTIFICATION AND PLANNING

Many musculoskeletal problems in children require long-term care. Despite current therapies, some disorders may leave a child with a permanent disability. Before a child is discharged from an ambulatory or inpatient setting, help parents plan how they will manage any necessary restrictions at home. For example, at first, a cast on an arm seems exciting: It is something for a school-age child to show off and an excuse not to write in school. After a few days, however, the cast may feel more frustrating than enjoyable. Take the time, therefore, to review what wearing the cast will mean to the child in everyday situations. Will the cast fit through required school uniform shirts with tight cuffs? Will a preschooler with a large cast fit into a car seat? If the child must stay home from school, do the parents know how to arrange for tutoring? If both parents work outside their home, will they need to arrange for childcare?

Depending on the child's and family's circumstances, the answers to these problems can differ greatly. Taking the time to sit down with the parents and ask them whether these concerns will pose problems, however, not only initiates problem solving but also allows parents to prepare solutions with a concerned person rather than by themselves at home.

Referral to an appropriate organization can be helpful if a child has a long-term condition. Examples of these are the Arthritis Foundation (www.arthritis.org), The Muscular Dystrophy Association (www.mda.org), the Osteogenesis Imperfecta Foundation (www.oif.org), and the National Scoliosis Foundation (www.scoliosis.org).

IMPLEMENTATION

Many nursing interventions for children with musculoskeletal disorders involve care of a child in a cast or in traction (treatment involving pulling on a body part in one direction against a counter pull exerted in the opposite direction) or teaching about common concerns, such as posture or children's shoes. Parents and children who are kept well-informed in these matters are much more likely to be able to cope with circumstances that occur from growth.

OUTCOME EVALUATION

Children with musculoskeletal disorders invariably need follow-up care after discharge from an ambulatory visit or inpatient care because bone healing is a slow process. Both parents and children may need support at reevaluation visits if they learn that a cast or brace must stay on longer than they thought or if they must continue exercises. Praise for their management so far is an effective intervention for helping parents and the child realize that, because they have coped with the situation so far, they can continue to cope with the situation into the future.

During reevaluation visits, spend time assessing children's body image and self-esteem or the total effect of their condition on growth and development. The success of treatment cannot be achieved if a child's self-concept has been diminished by an injury or disease.

Some examples indicating achievement of outcomes include:

- Child states he feels no pain or numbness in the extremity after the application of a cast.
- Child demonstrates allowable weight-bearing activities with casted lower extremity.
- Parents accurately state the child's care needs both in and out of the hospital.
- Child states positive aspects of self, participates in activities, and establishes friendships with peers.

The Musculoskeletal System

BONES AND BONE GROWTH

Bones are generally classified by their shape as long (those found in extremities), short (those of the wrist or ankle), flat (those of the skull, ribs, scapula, and clavicle), or irregular (the vertebrae, the pelvis, and the facial bones of the skull).

The mark of a long bone is a lengthy central shaft (the **diaphysis**), a rounded end portion (the **epiphysis**), and a thin area between them (the **metaphysis**) (Fig. 51.1). Increases in the length of long bones occur at the **cartilage** (connective tissue) segment (the **epiphyseal plate**), between the epiphysis

Figure 51.1 The structure of a bone.

and the metaphysis. Injury to this area in a growing child is always potentially serious because it may halt growth, stimulate abnormal growth, or cause irregular or erratic growth.

The central shafts of long bones are covered by an outer sensitive layer of **periosteum**. Bone width increases by growth at the inner surface of this. Injury to the periosteum, such as may occur with osteomyelitis, has the potential to also threaten bone growth (Tafin-Kampé & Kamsu-Foguem, 2013). Although it is easy to think of bones as rigid, solid structures, they are, in fact, active living tissue to which nutrients must be supplied for growth. Calcium, one of the main components of bone, is important for both original bone formation, **remodeling** (replacement of old by new bone tissue), and **resorption** (bone breakdown). These processes are strongly influenced by vitamin D and the parathyroid hormone calcitonin. "Bone age" in children can be determined by an X-ray of the wrist that shows the ossification level of the bones.

The inner core of long bones is filled with yellow and red marrow and is responsible for the formation of platelets, red blood cells, white blood cells, and adipose (fat) cells. Red marrow is primarily involved in blood component production, whereas yellow marrow is chiefly involved in adipose cell formation. The blood supply to bones is abundant so that the marrow can actively supply enough blood components for the entire body. As with other tissues, if the blood supply is cut off, bone cells die and blood cell production is hindered.

MUSCLE

The skeletal muscular system is composed of striated muscle (differentiated from the smooth muscle found in body organs, which is responsible for such activities as intestinal peristalsis). Activation of skeletal muscle occurs with innervation from a motor nerve and is under voluntary control. **Myopathy**, or disease of the muscular system, can be inherited (as in muscular dystrophy) or acquired (as in myasthenia gravis).

Assessment of Musculoskeletal Function

In addition to a history and physical examination, diagnostic tests are frequently necessary to detect musculoskeletal dysfunction. These may include X-ray and bone scans, bone and muscle

Nursing Care Planning to Respect Cultural Diversity

Economic globalization has led medical device companies to incorporate cultural diversity into the companies' engineering. Companies are now taking into account how cultural differences will influence effectiveness of medical device use. Depending on the type of medical device and the developmental age of the child, caregivers are likely to be involved. This involvement may seem natural to most, but depending on the relationships between different family members, this is not always straightforward. When educating caregivers on medical devices, always assess the cultural and social context (the relationship between family members). Other cultural needs to be addressed may involve issues that appear simple, such as colors. In certain cultures, colors have significant meaning. For example, in Japan, the color red is associated with prosperity; because of this, the start button on IV pumps is not green but rather red (Liu, Hoelscher, & Yao, 2013).

biopsies, electromyography, and arthroscopy. Ultrasound and magnetic resonance imaging (MRI) studies are used to reveal soft tissue disorders. Furthermore, obtain information on how parents and children are adjusting to a potential disability because poor acceptance of a condition can limit a child's potential as much as the physical involvement (Box 51.2).

RADIOGRAPHY

Because bones are opaque, they outline well on an X-ray or computerized tomography (CT) scan to provide information about a specific bone or a joint. Other tests, however, are indicated to confirm problems with cartilage, tendons, and ligaments. X-rays in children are limited to the least number necessary for diagnosis or prognosis because excessive radiation is associated with the development of malignancies, such as leukemia (Adelstein, 2015). Radiation of epiphyseal plates can lead to uneven growth.

BONE SCAN (SCINTIGRAPHY)

A bone scan is a study of the uptake by bone of intravenously injected radioactive substances (American College of Radiology, 2014). Areas of increased metabolic activity cause the substance to concentrate in that area, often providing information on very early stages of bone disease and healing, possibly before they are visible on an X-ray.

ELECTROMYOGRAPHY

Electromyography studies the electrical activity of skeletal muscle and nerve conduction to determine the location and cause of disorders such as myasthenia gravis, muscular dystrophy, and lower motor neuron and peripheral nerve disorders (Karakis, Liew, Darras, et al., 2014).

For the test, surface electrodes are placed over the muscle or needle electrodes are inserted into the muscle. The electrical activity of the muscle at rest and in motion is then detected

by audio amplification and recorded on an oscilloscope screen. Normally, resting muscle is quiet. If fasciculations are present, abnormal noises or oscilloscope spikes will be observed.

Although the needle electrodes are small, if they are used, the test can be frightening for children because they are pricked by needles. They need support from someone they know during the procedure. Before and after, provide opportunities for therapeutic play so a child can express anxiety and feelings about such an invasive procedure.

MUSCLE OR BONE BIOPSY

Both muscle and bone biopsies involve removal of a tissue sample for examination of its microscopic structure. They can provide evidence about infection, malignant bone growth, inflammation, or atrophy of the area. Either type may be done during surgery or as an ambulatory procedure.

Biopsies of these types are usually done using conscious sedation or a local anesthetic. If local anesthesia is used, caution children they will feel the initial prick of an anesthetizing needle; they will then feel additional momentary pressure as the biopsy needle is inserted. You can assure them the amount of tissue that will be taken from them is no larger than the inner bore of the biopsy needle, comparable to the size of the graphite in a pencil.

ARTHROSCOPY

Arthroscopy involves direct visualization of a joint with a fiber optic instrument. It is usually done under local anesthesia in an ambulatory care setting. Arthroscopy allows a joint, most commonly the knee, but also the hip, shoulder, elbow, or wrist, to be examined without a large incision. It is most often used to diagnose athletic injuries and to differentiate between acute and chronic joint disorders (Jeong, Lee, & Ko, 2012).

Health Promotion and Risk Management

Health promotion for children with musculoskeletal disorders focuses on thorough assessment at all health maintenance visits. A child's ability to achieve developmental milestones, specifically gross and fine motor abilities, provides important information about musculoskeletal function. Screening for musculoskeletal disorders, such as for scoliosis in the prepubescent child and the adolescent, is an extremely important health promotion nursing role.

Safety precautions and anticipatory guidance for parents is essential to minimize the risk of injury, specifically to extremities. As a child grows and becomes active in sports, parental and child education about the importance of using bike helmets for bike riding, or protective gear for organized sports, takes on an even greater role.

Nutrition education is important to ensure adequate calcium and vitamin D intake for bone growth and healing. However, if a child requires bed rest, calcium intake should be moderated to reduce the risk of renal calculi formation resulting from immobilization. The teenage years are an important time for both males and females to build calcium stores to protect against osteoporosis later in life (Matkovic & Visy, 2015).

Therapeutic Management of Musculoskeletal Disorders in Children

Various methods are used as therapy for children with musculoskeletal disorders, including casts, traction, distraction, and open reduction. Amputation, a rare necessity, is discussed in Chapter 53.

CASTING

Casts are used to treat a wide range of musculoskeletal disorders, from simple fractures in the extremities to correction of congenital structural bone disorders.

Cast Application

Casts are created from either plaster of Paris or fiberglass. Fiberglass is an attractive material to use for children's casts because it is light in weight; comes in attractive colors; and, when a special waterproof liner is used, can be immersed in water. Unfortunately, it is more expensive and may not be practical for casts that need frequent changing, such as those used to correct talipes disorders, a common congenital disorder that requires serial casting.

Children need an explanation of what to expect with casting. To maintain alignment of body parts, a healthcare provider may gently exert a pull on the body part being casted during the cast application. If a large body cast is being applied, children may be positioned on a special cast table with a traction apparatus at the chin and pelvis to initiate tension. Allow a support person to accompany children to a cast room to hold their hand or talk to them during the application. Most children (and adults) are unaware that casts are formed from strips or rolls of material impregnated with the casting material. The normal curiosity of children as they watch a cast grow and mold to their body part usually makes casting a pleasant procedure. Some children voice that they regard the cast as a badge of courage, or at least, a conversation piece.

Before a cast is applied, a tube of stockinette is stretched over the area and soft cotton padding is placed over bony prominences. At the end of the application, the stockinette will be pulled up and over the raw edges of the cast to create a smooth, padded surface (Fig. 51.2). If a plaster cast is to be applied, caution children that, at first, the wet strips of plaster of Paris feel cool. Almost immediately, however, the strips begin to generate heat as evaporation begins and body parts start to feel warm. If the cast is a full-body cast, children may become uncomfortably warm, with perspiration possibly running from their forehead. Assure them this feeling of warmth is transient and is never enough to cause a burn.

A plaster cast takes 10 to 72 hours to dry depending on its size. Fiberglass casts usually dry within 5 to 30 minutes. A "window" may be placed in a cast if an infection is suspected, so that the area can be observed. If the child has a body or hip spica cast, windowing can prevent uncomfortable abdominal distention and allow bowel sounds to be assessed.

Compartment syndrome is a phenomenon that can occur when a cast or tight constrictive dressing puts pressure on an enclosed space such as the forearm. This pressure can result in severely decreased blood flow that potentially threatens damage to and necrosis of surrounding soft tissue

Figure 51.2   Cast application. **(A)** A cast is applied to a young boy's leg over a stockinette. **(B)** Casts do not cover the toes so these can be assessed for color and warmth. (© Blend images/Alamy.)

or nerves. The pathophysiology of the condition remains uncertain, although mechanisms involving artery compromise are involved. An injury to a major artery with inadequate collateral circulation can lead to decreased perfusion and ischemia of both capillaries and muscles, resulting in an increase in permeability of the capillary walls and, ultimately, edema (Lee, Lightdale-Miric, Chang, et al., 2014).

Assess fingers or toes carefully for warmth, pain, and function after application of a cast to be certain a compartment syndrome is not developing. If signs of compartment syndrome are present, the cast will need to be released immediately to prevent permanent nerve and tissue damage. A fasciotomy (surgically opening the compartment) may be necessary to further prevent nerve damage.

 ## Nursing Diagnoses and Related Interventions

Nursing Diagnosis: Risk for ineffective peripheral tissue perfusion related to pressure from cast

Outcome Evaluation: Child states she feels no pain or numbness in extremity; distal nail bed blanches and refills in less than 3 seconds; pedal pulses are palpable.

If an extremity has been casted, keep it elevated by a pillow to prevent edema. Check circulation frequently, such as every 15 minutes during the first hour, hourly for the next 4 hours, and then every 4 hours throughout the first day. Assess for color, warmth, presence of pedal or radial pulses, and sensations of numbness or tingling. Signs of impaired neurovascular function include pallor (including blueness or coldness of the distal part), pulselessness, pain in the casted part, paresthesia (numbness or tingling in the part, as if it were "asleep"), and paralysis. Children younger than 6 or 7 years of age have difficulty describing paresthesia; however, they may whine or cry with the discomfort of the sensation. Edema that does not improve with elevation is also an important sign. Any of these symptoms requires immediate attention because neurovascular impairment can lead to nerve ischemia and destruction, possibly causing permanent paralysis of an extremity.

Preventing the flow of urine under the edges of a cast can be a problem with full-body or high-leg casts in non–toilet-trained children. If a cast surrounds the genital area, cover the edges with plastic or waterproof material to help keep it dry. Keeping children in a semi-Fowler position by using pillows or raising the head of the bed helps to direct urine and feces downward and away from the cast. Because a cast is heavy, infants tend to slip down in bed a great deal, so they need frequent repositioning to remain in this raised position.

If young children have a body cast, make certain they have a bib or cover over the top edge of their cast so crumbs or fluids do not spill inside. Choose toys carefully so small parts cannot drop inside. A piece of food inside a cast will mold and macerate the skin; a small part of a toy could cause irritation and a pressure ulcer. If food or fluid is spilled on the outside of the cast, the cast can be cleaned with a damp cloth.

Nursing Diagnosis: Parental health-seeking behaviors related to care of child with cast at home

Outcome Evaluation: Parents state plans for adapting home environment and lifestyle to accommodate child with cast; parents demonstrate measures to check neurovascular status.

If a child has an upper extremity cast, be certain the parents understand how to position the extremity properly, such as with a sling. If the cast is on a lower extremity, be certain parents and the child understand the amount of weight bearing allowed on the affected extremity and how to use crutches safely, if prescribed.

Handling a child in a large cast can seem so overwhelming for parents that they do not see how they will be able to care for their child at home. Assure them the child is quite comfortable in the cast despite its awkward, constricting appearance. Role model moving the child to show them that it is not an impossible task. Be sure to caution them that if an abduction bar is used with a cast, it must never be used as a handle for lifting. Such use can break the bar from the cast or weaken its support.

Parents need to use good body mechanics (lift with the thighs, not the back) when turning or positioning the child in a full-body cast. They may appreciate suggestions on ways to move the child from room to room, such as using a toy wagon with a flat board on top or using a skateboard for children to propel themselves forward.

Point out that all children thrive on being touched. Children in large body casts need their head and arms stroked (or any areas of the body that are not covered by the cast) so they receive this. Demonstrate how even a child in a large hip spica cast can be held, cuddled, and supported for feeding.

Many children report a sensation of itching inside a cast at about the end of the first week. If the area is immediately under the edge of the cast, the itching is probably the result of dry skin caused by the drying effect of the cast. Reaching a hand under the edge of the cast and massaging the area usually relieves the itching. Applying hand lotion may relieve the dryness. If the area is unreachable, blowing cool air through the cast with a fan or a hair dryer set on cool air may relieve the uncomfortable feeling. Caution both the child and parents not to use implements such as a coat hanger or knitting needle to scratch the area. These can injure the skin, causing an infection under the cast (Box 51.3).

BOX 51.3
Nursing Care Planning to Empower a Family

CAST CARE AT HOME

Q. Jeffrey's sister has a fiberglass cast fitted onto her arm. Her mother asks you, "Is there any special things I have to do?"

A. Some helpful tips to care for your child's cast at home include:

- Keep the casted body part elevated on a pillow for the first day to decrease swelling.
- Observe the hands and fingers (the body part distal to the cast) for swelling or blueness and ask your child to move her fingers about every 4 hours for the first 24 hours. If she is unable to move her fingers or if she has swelling, blueness, or pain, telephone your healthcare provider. These signs could mean the cast is pressing on a nerve or constricting a blood vessel.
- Encourage usual activities so your child remains active but monitor strenuous activities, such as roughhousing, while the cast is in place.
- Ask your child to think through how wearing a cast will change her day, such as making it difficult to eat at preschool or to join in play at the playground, and brainstorm how to solve these problems.
- Explain to your child not to put anything inside the cast. If itching occurs, blowing some cool air into it from a hair dryer can be comforting.
- Keep the cast dry (cover it with a plastic bag to shower); no swimming is allowed. Remind her not to use magic markers for autographs because fiberglass is a porous material.
- Keep your return appointment for follow-up care because children can outgrow a cast rapidly. Outgrowing a cast can put pressure on nerves and can lead to permanent disability.

Transporting the child in a car, particularly fitting a bulky cast into an infant car seat, can be a major problem for parents. They may need to purchase a larger car seat than intended for their child to transport the child safely. Before any child with a cast is discharged from a health-care facility, give parents a telephone number to call if they have any questions about cast care or their child's condition because they often do not realize what questions they will have until they return home.

Cast Removal

Most casts remain in place for 4 to 8 weeks and are then removed using an electric cast cutter with a rapidly vibrating, circular disk (Fig. 51.3). Cast cutters are frightening because the disk makes a very loud noise as it cuts through the cast material and also generates heat. To the child, the disk appears capable of cutting through not only the plaster but also an arm or leg as well. The person removing the cast usually demonstrates that the disk does not cut skin by touching a thumb to the edge of it. Not all children are totally convinced by the demonstration, however, and may require additional support while the disk moves from one end of a cast to the other, such as saying, "It's all right to cry; I know this looks scary" or by holding your hands over the child's ears to lessen the noise.

The skin of the child's extremity looks macerated and dirty after a cast is removed; a good bath usually washes away most of this. If an arm has been casted in flexion, the elbow may feel stiff and even sore when the child is asked to extend it for the first time. Children often continue to use extremities with caution after a cast has been removed. Advise parents to allow children to begin using extremities again at their own pace. As children naturally play and reach for objects, they gradually forget to favor the arm or leg, and full function then returns. Once healing has taken place, the extremity is as strong as it was before the fracture. The child does not need to continue to favor the extremity to protect it from a second fracture.

MEDICAL BOOTS (FRACTURE BOOTS) OR SPLINTS

In some instances, a fracture does not require a cast for immobility but can be immobilized by a supportive boot or splint. The child wears the boot or arm splint continuously as if it were a cast; an advantage is that, if a complication should occur, it can be readily removed by its Velcro attachments. Ask at return appointments if children who are prescribed boots or splints are wearing the immobilizer continually. Be certain children who say they take them off "a little" are not actually describing taking them off often and, therefore, are not receiving the support necessary for effective bone healing.

CRUTCHES

Crutches are prescribed for children for one of three reasons: to keep weight off one or both legs, to support weakened legs, or to maintain balance. Usually, a physical therapist measures crutch length and gives beginning instruction in crutch walking. Being familiar with how crutches are measured and having crutch walking supervised not only allows you to offer emotional support to children as they learn to use crutches but also helps you assess progress at follow-up visits.

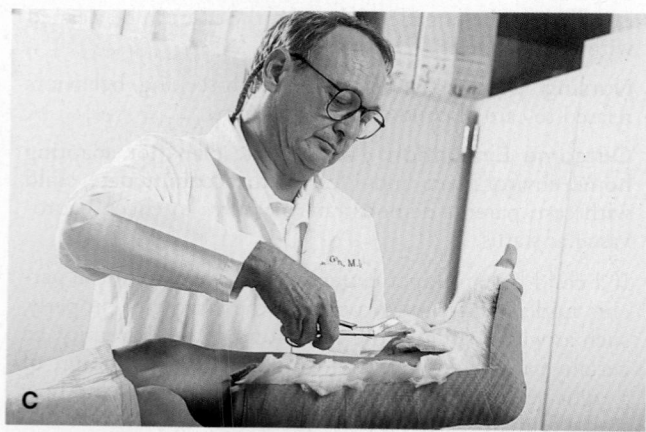

Figure 51.3 Cast removal. **(A)** A cast cutter is used to begin the removal of a fiberglass cast on an adolescent's leg. **(B)** The fiberglass cast is lifted off. **(C)** The underlying stockinette and padding are removed. (© Will and Deni McIntyre/Science Source/Photo Researchers.)

Fit and Adjustment

If crutches are properly fitted, there should be a space of 1 to 1.5 in. between the axilla crutch pad and the child's axilla. When the child stands upright and places his hands on the hand rests of the crutches, the elbows should flex about 20 degrees. This degree of flexion ensures that when the child bears weight on the crutch, the body weight will be borne by the arm, not the axilla. Pressure of a crutch against the axilla could lead to compression and damage of the brachial nerve plexus crossing the axilla, resulting in permanent nerve palsy. Teach children not to rest with the crutch pad pressing on the axilla but to always support their weight at the hand grip.

Always assess the tips of crutches to be certain the rubber tip is intact and not worn through because the tip prevents the crutch from slipping. Be certain the child is walking with the crutches placed about 6 in. to the side of the foot. This distance furnishes a wide, balanced base for support.

Before discharge from a healthcare facility, explore with children any problems crutches may cause with their daily activities. If they carry books to school, for example, they will need to wear a backpack so their hands are free for the hand rests. Caution parents to clear articles such as throw rugs, small footstools, or toys out of paths at home.

Crutch Walking

Two main crutch-walking patterns are used (Fig. 51.4). A two-point gait is used when a child needs support for weakened muscles or balance but may bear weight on both lower extremities. The child places the right crutch and left foot forward, then the left crutch and right foot forward, and so on. Using the crutch opposite a foot provides a wider base of support than using the crutch next to the foot. Caution children to take small steps until they feel confident.

A three-point swing-through gait is used when no weight bearing is allowed on one foot. For this, the crutches are both brought forward. The weight of the body is then shifted forward as both legs are swung through the crutches. The child bears weight on the unaffected (good) leg and moves

the crutches forward again. It takes strong arm support to bear full weight on crutches this way. Be certain the child is bearing weight on the hands and not on the axillae. Some children use a swing-through gait rather recklessly and need to be advised to slow their pace to a safer one.

To walk downstairs using a swing-through gait, children place their crutches on the lower step and then swing the unaffected (good) foot forward and down to that step. To go upstairs, they place their unaffected (good) foot on the elevated step and then raise the crutches onto the step and lift themselves up. To help children remember this pattern, the following saying can be taught: "Angels" (the good foot) go up; "devils" (the bad foot with the crutches) go down.

QSEN Checkpoint Question 51.1

INFORMATICS

Jeffrey is prescribed crutches to take weight off his affected leg. What teaching point should the nurse include in his health education?

a. His crutches should be at least 6 in. longer than he is tall.
b. He should lean forward at a 45-degree angle while walking.
c. He should bear weight on his arms to avoid pressure on his axillae.
d. It is unsafe to walk downstairs with crutches; walking upstairs is acceptable.

Look in Appendix A for the best answer and rationale.

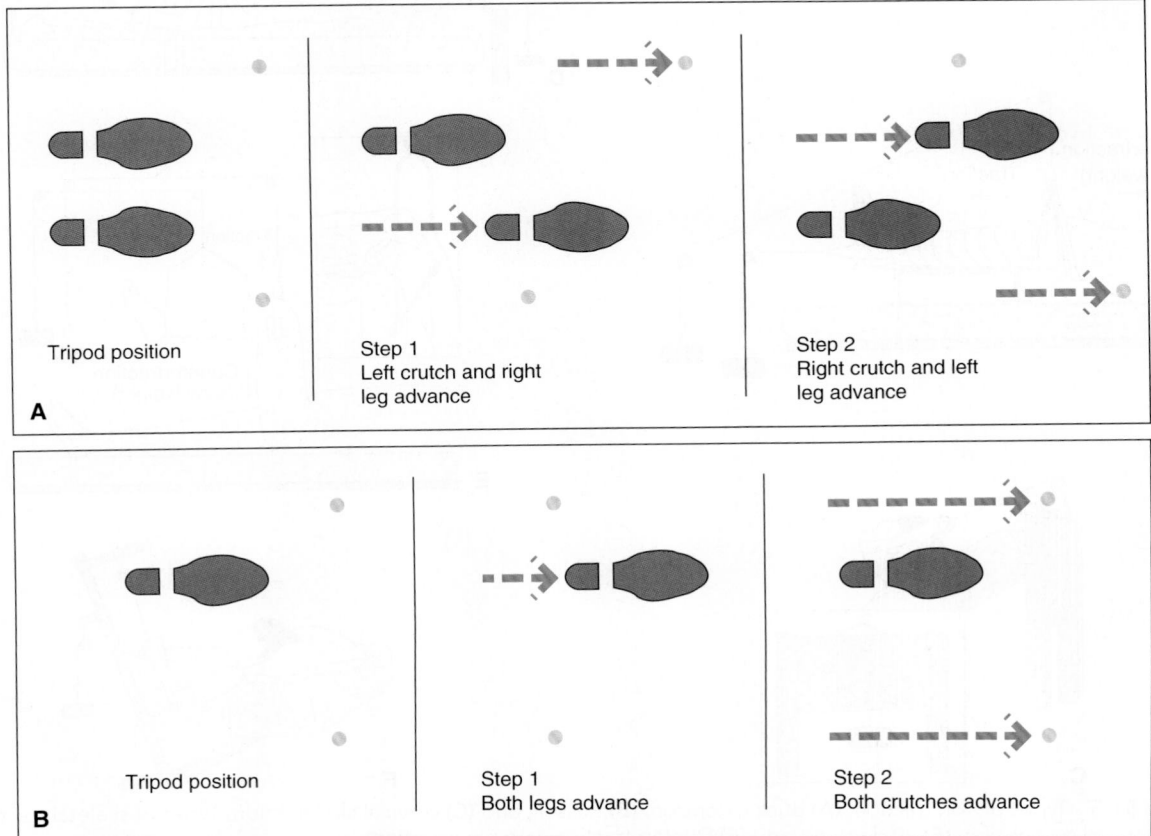

Figure 51.4 Crutch-walking patterns. **(A)** The two-point gait. **(B)** The swing-through gait.

TRACTION

Traction, which is used to reduce dislocations and immobilize fractures, involves pulling on a body part in one direction against a counterpull exerted in the opposite direction. Although still necessary for some conditions, the use of intramedullary rods is making its use unnecessary in many instances. In straight (running) traction, the child's body weight serves as the counterpull. In suspended or balanced traction, the body part is suspended by a sling, and the counterpull and primary pull are accomplished by pulleys and weights. Either skin traction (in which skin provides the counterpull) or skeletal traction (in which bone provides the counterpull) may be used. Skin traction is used if only minimal traction is necessary; the child's skin must be in good condition for this procedure. Skeletal traction is used if a longer period of traction or a greater strength of traction pull is needed. Types of tractions are illustrated in Figure 51.5. Use of traction in the home shortens hospital stays and enables a child to interact with family members, so it should be encouraged when possible.

Skin Traction

Skin traction means a child's extremity is wrapped in a material such as an elastic bandage and then suspended from a nearby pole or frame so the weight of the body part produces traction. Bryant traction, used for fractured femurs in children younger than 2 years of age, is an example of skin traction (Fig. 51.6). It also may be used in preparation for surgical repair of congenital developmental disorders, such as developmental hip dysplasia (see Chapter 27). This type of traction is used less frequently now because the elevation of the extremities causes blood to pool at the hips. This and the possible tourniquet effect of the traction strips, bandages, and traction itself increase the risk for vasospasm and avascular hip necrosis.

Buck extension is an example of skin traction used for immobilizing lower extremity fractures in older children. Dunlop traction is used to immobilize an upper extremity. Cervical skin traction may be used to decrease muscle spasms in the back. This type of traction uses a halter-type device attached to weights. The head of the bed is elevated to provide countertraction.

Figure 51.5 Types of skin traction: **(A)** Buck extension, **(B)** Russell, and **(C)** cervical skin traction. Types of skeletal traction: **(D)** balanced suspension, **(E)** 90 degrees, and **(F)** Dunlop traction with pin insertion.

Figure 51.6   An infant in Bryant traction. It's important that the infant's hips do not rest on the bed due to bulkiness of a diaper. (© BSIP/Custom Medical Stock Photograph.)

Figure 51.7   Children in skeletal traction need engaging activities and therapeutic play so they can remain in this confined position. (© Gary Wagner/Stock Boston.)

Skeletal Traction

Skeletal traction involves the use of a pin, such as a Steinmann pin, or a wire, such as a Kirschner wire, that is passed through the skin into the end of a bone. The pin or wire can be inserted in an emergency department under local anesthesia if the child can hold absolutely still, but usually, it is done under general anesthesia in the operating room. With skeletal traction, ropes strung over pulleys and attached to weights exert a pull on the extremity at the pin site. Cotton gauze squares are usually placed around the ends of the pin on the outside. The sites are cleaned with half-strength hydrogen peroxide using sterile technique to keep them free of drainage. Be certain to observe pin sites daily for drainage because odorous or excessive drainage or local erythema may be a sign of infection.

Traction-Related Care

Children in traction need to be assessed carefully for neurovascular impairment, the same as children in casts. Assess the extremity in traction every 15 minutes during the first hour, hourly for 24 hours, and every 4 hours thereafter for signs of pallor (or blueness), lack of warmth, tingling, absent peripheral pulse, edema, or pain. Traction can lead to hypertension because the head typically is positioned lower than the lower extremities. Assess once a day for this possibility by taking blood pressure readings.

Be extremely careful when changing a child's bed linens or carrying out nursing functions that you do not move the weights or interfere with the traction. Provide good skin care on the child's back, elbows, and heels because they may become irritated from friction against the sheets. A trapeze bar suspended over the bed provides a great deal of mobility and assists children in using a bedpan or positioning themselves in bed.

Being in traction is not as dramatic for children as being placed in a cast. There is an unspoken feeling from other children that "if what you have is really serious, you'd have a cast." Explain to children why this type of treatment is best for them. Keep parents and children informed of X-ray assessments (e.g., "The fracture is being held in just the right position; the bone is beginning to reform"). Although they cannot see progress, this information can help assure them that progress is occurring.

Children in traction usually are not "ill" children. They feel well except for the leg or arm being held in its correct position. Therefore, they have the energy and the need for stimulation of well children. Child life specialists or volunteers can be helpful in keeping them occupied. Being certain they are involved in activities (perhaps using a wireless computer or texting) is an important part of nursing care (Fig. 51.7).

Helping children maintain contact with their school friends through cards, letters, or recorded messages, social media, or texting is also important. If hospitalized, position their bed so they can see unit activities. Whether at home or in the hospital, encourage frequent visitors of their own age to help maintain peer relationships.

DISTRACTION

Distraction is the use of an external device to separate opposing bones, which then encourages new bone growth. It can be used to lengthen a bone if one limb is shorter than the other. It also can be used to immobilize fractures or to correct defects if the bone is rotated or angled.

A device such as the Ilizarov external fixator is used to achieve distraction (Fig. 51.8). It consists of wires that are inserted through the bone then attached to either full or half rings, which are secured to telescoping rods. For bone lengthening, the rods are adjusted approximately 1 mm each day to stimulate bone growth until the desired length is achieved. The device remains in place until consolidation is complete; there is no pain, limp, or edema; and the bone is healed and can bear weight.

Both the child and parents need thorough preparation for the surgery, application of the device, how it will appear, and the usual reaction of others to it (surprise). If it seems important to parents, provide suggestions of ways to minimize the device's appearance, such as wide-legged pants with adjustable closures. If parents will be adjusting the telescoping rods, providing care to the wire insertion sites, or restricting activity, be certain they have full and clear instructions on what to do as well as how to assess for signs and symptoms of infection. Ascertain that they have follow-up appointments because continued care is essential to ensure an optimal outcome for their child.

Figure 51.8 An Ilizarov device in place to treat a comminuted fracture when bone is splintered or crushed.

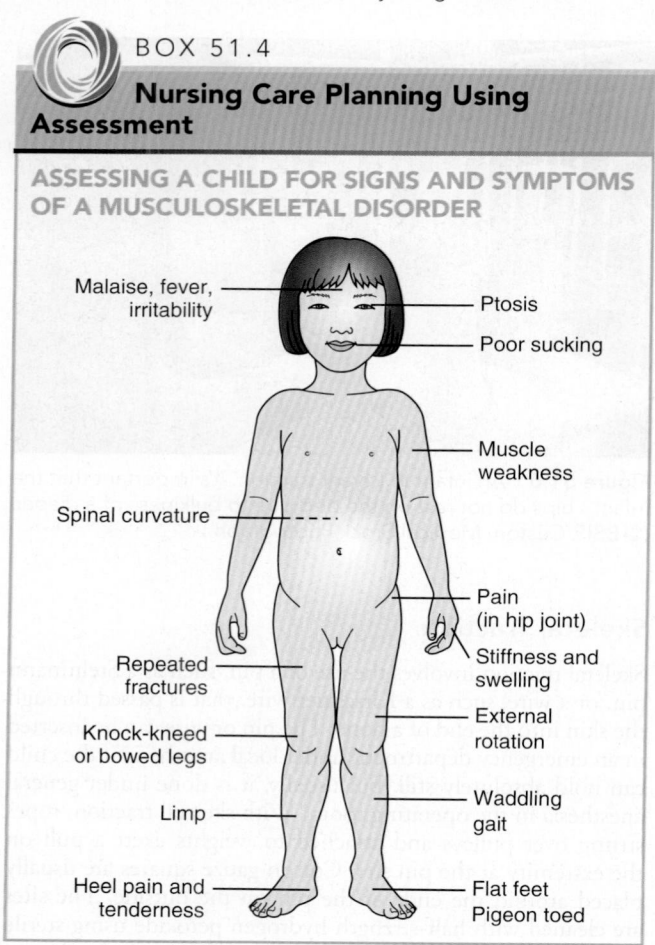

BOX 51.4

Nursing Care Planning Using Assessment

ASSESSING A CHILD FOR SIGNS AND SYMPTOMS OF A MUSCULOSKELETAL DISORDER

OPEN REDUCTION

Open reduction is a surgical technique used to align and repair bone. If there is a spinal fracture or both bones of a forearm or lower leg are fractured, open reduction and insertion of a rod or screw (open reduction) stabilizes the bones.

Once an open reduction is completed, the area usually is casted to provide support. Invariably, at least a small amount of serosanguineous fluid oozes from the open reduction site into the cast. Outline with a ballpoint pen any stain that suggests oozing from a surgical incision, so that an increase in the size of the mark can be detected. Do not use a magic marker for this because the fluid tends to penetrate through the cast (use a pen or crayon). Add the time at which you make the mark so you can tell how rapidly the spot is increasing. Because children with an open reduction are prone to infection, the same as any child with a surgical incision, be aware as well of systemic symptoms (e.g., increased pulse, increased temperature, lethargy) as well as local signs (e.g., edema, pain, tingling, blueness or coolness of the distal extremity) of infection.

Disorders of Bone Development

Many common musculoskeletal disorders in children are first noticed during routine physical exams (Box 51.4).

FLAT FEET (PES PLANUS)

The term *flat feet* refers to relaxation of the longitudinal arch of the foot (American Academy of Orthopaedic Surgeons

[AAOS], 2013). Although it is rare, many parents become concerned because their newborn's foot is flatter and proportionately wider than an adult's foot. In actuality, a transverse arch rarely is visible in newborns, and a longitudinal arch may not be present until the child has been walking for months.

Evaluate children's feet at healthcare visits by having them stand on tiptoe. In this position, a longitudinal arch should be visible. Observing whether children are able to stand on their heels with the soles of the feet off the ground is another good assessment. Lastly, examine the ankle joint to be certain a full range of motion is present and the Achilles tendon is not shortened. Tarsal and metatarsal joints should also show a full range of motion.

Some children experience foot pain at the end of the day because of poor arch development. Their arch can be strengthened and the pain diminished if the child walks on tiptoe for 5 to 10 minutes daily or practices picking up marbles with the toes. For an older child, standing pigeon toed (toes pointed in) and throwing the weight forward onto the lateral aspect of the feet also tends to strengthen arches.

Children do not need a high top or rigid shoe in order for the arch to develop. A sneaker is an example of a shoe that not only offers enough support but that also allows normal arch development.

BOWLEGS (GENU VARUM)

Genu varum is lateral bowing of the tibia. If this is present, the **malleoli** (rounded prominence on either side of the an-

Figure 51.9   **(A)** Genu varum. **(B)** Genu valgum.

kles) will be touching and the medial surfaces of the knees will be more than 2 in. (5 cm) apart (Fig. 51.9A). Children develop this condition as part of normal development; it is seen most commonly in 2-year-olds. It also can occur in athletes who play load-bearing sports such as football (Zbinden, Rutz, Jacobson, et al., 2015).

Record the extent of the bowing at health maintenance visits by approximating the medial malleoli of the ankles and measuring the distance between the patellas (knees) for changes. Genu varum gradually corrects itself in young children by about 3 years of age or, at the latest, by school age. If the problem is unilateral, becomes rapidly worse, or persists beyond this time, the child needs referral to an orthopedist for further evaluation.

KNOCK KNEES (GENU VALGUM)

Genu valgum, or knock knee, is the opposite of genu varum. The medial surfaces of the knees touch, and the medial surfaces of the ankle malleoli are separated by more than 3 in. (7.5 cm) (see Fig. 51.9B).

This is seen most commonly in children 3 to 4 years old and corrects itself by school age as the child grows. Children who continue to have this problem and those in whom the abnormality is unilateral or becomes more pronounced need a referral to an orthopedist for further evaluation because obesity as well as both vitamin D and calcium deficiencies can cause the deformity.

BLOUNT DISEASE (TIBIA VARA)

Blount disease, also known as tibia vara, is a developmental disorder of unknown etiology that primarily affects the posteromedial portion of the proximal tibial growth plate and results in bowed legs. Unlike the normal developmental aspect of genu varum, Blount disease is usually unilateral and is a serious disturbance in bone growth that requires treatment (Sabharwal, 2015).

Because it is not possible to rule out Blount disease by appearance alone, almost all children with bowed legs have an initial X-ray to identify if Blount disease is present. In those with Blount disease, the medial aspect of the proximal tibia will show a sharp, beaklike appearance on X-ray.

Either bracing or osteotomy may be necessary to correct this deformity or prevent it from becoming more severe. Parents may need an explanation of why their child requires treatment or surgery when another child on their block with a similar appearance (developmental genu varum) is predicted to outgrow the problem.

TOEING-IN

Toeing-in may occur as a result of foot, tibial, femoral, or hip displacement. Assess for these conditions if parents describe their child as "always falling over the feet" or "awkward." *Metatarsus adductus* is turning in of the forefoot. The heel is in good alignment; only the forefoot is turned in. This condition may develop or become more pronounced in infants who sleep prone with the feet adducted and in older children who watch television by kneeling and turning their feet in. If you stand the child on a copying machine and make a print, the turning in of the foot can be well demonstrated.

Most instances of metatarsus adductus resolve without therapy. Those that persist beyond 1 year can be corrected by passive stretching exercises; a few infants with extremely rigid, incorrect foot posture may require casts or splints for correction. Early detection of these extreme instances is important because treatment for metatarsus adductus is most effective if it is begun before an infant walks. With early treatment, the prognosis is excellent.

Inward tibial torsion also may be evidenced as toeing-in. This condition is diagnosed when a line drawn from the anterior superior iliac crest through the center of the patella intersects the fourth or fifth toe (or a position even more lateral) (Fig. 51.10) because, ordinarily, such a line should intersect the second toe.

Tibial torsion usually improves as the tibia grows, so this requires no treatment. Parents need a good explanation of why no treatment is necessary, however. Reassure them at periodic health maintenance visits that patience and time will correct tibial torsion (Mudge, Bau, Purcell, et al., 2014). Inward femoral torsion can be detected if you ask a child to lie supine and attempt to rotate the leg internally and then

Figure 51.10   Toeing-in caused by inward tibial torsion. In good alignment, a line drawn from the anterosuperior iliac crest through the patella should intersect the second toe.

externally at the hip. Normally, internal rotation is about 30 degrees, and outward rotation is about 90 degrees. With inward femoral torsion, the internal rotation is closer to 90 degrees. In some children, the femur rotates so far that the patellar bones face each other. As with tibial torsion, no treatment is necessary. Inward femoral rotation will not correct itself, but a compensating tibial torsion will develop and make feet appear straight.

A fourth cause of toeing-in may be improper hip placement or developmental hip dysplasia, a problem that is very serious and needs early therapy for correction (see Chapter 27).

GROWING PAINS

Listen to parents carefully when they state their child has "growing pains" because what they are reporting may be symptoms indicative of rheumatic fever or JIA rather than a simple, transient phenomenon. Growing pains occur most frequently in the muscle of the calf, never in a joint. They are reported most often in preschool- and school-age children, who wake at night because of the pain. Such cramping usually follows a day of vigorous activity or wearing new shoes with a heel of a different height than before. Some children, especially adolescents, who report they have growing pains may actually be reporting restless leg syndrome. This syndrome (involuntary leg movements that cause insomnia) is thought to be associated with genetics and brain iron deficiency that causes decreased dopamine production (Hoogwout, Paananen, Smith, et al., 2015; Stehlik, Ulfberg, Hedner, et al., 2014).

OSTEOGENESIS IMPERFECTA

Osteogenesis imperfecta is a connective tissue (collagen) disorder in which fragile bone formation leads to recurring (pathologic) fractures (Morello & Esposito, 2012). Although as many as eight types have been identified, the disease occurs most frequently as a severe autosomal dominant form that is recognized at birth (osteogenesis imperfecta type I) or an autosomal recessive form where symptoms, including hearing and cardiovascular anomalies, develop later in life (osteogenesis imperfecta type III).

Children with type I disease may be born with countless fractures already present from the force of birth. They develop many more fractures from the everyday activities of childhood. X-rays reveal a particular ribbonlike or mosaic pattern in their bones, which aids in diagnosis. The sclera of the eye is unusually blue because of poor connective tissue formation.

Children with the type III form may have associated deafness and dental deformities (Morello & Esposito, 2012). In both instances, the major clinical manifestation is a tendency for bones to fracture easily because of the poor collagen formation. In some children, the bones are so fragile that fractures can result not only from trauma, such as a fall, but also from simple walking. Because the child has such frequent injuries, parents may be accused of child maltreatment before the child's condition is firmly diagnosed and documented (Morello & Esposito, 2012).

As the child grows older, the multiple breaks tend to cause limb and spinal column deformities, interfering with alignment or growth. Lessened rib motility leads to interference with respirations. Bisphosphonates are widely used in the palliative treatment of osteogenesis imperfecta with the intention of reducing fracture risk. Bisphosphonates increase bone mineral density (BMD) but do not prevent fractures (Hald, Evangelou, Langdahl, et al., 2015). Lightweight leg braces or intramedullary rod insertion techniques may also be prescribed (Morello & Esposito, 2012).

Parents need to protect children from trauma, fractures need to be aligned and casted, and children need to be educated about a lifestyle that is productive yet minimizes the risk of trauma. Always be careful when caring for a child with this disorder not to cause any trauma to bones. Be certain to raise side rails on cribs or beds. Keep floors dry, and remove objects that could cause falls. Always lift children gently and avoid lifting them by a single arm or leg to avoid placing strain on a bone.

What If . . . 51.1

Jeffrey's parents report that he has been waking up at night because of "growing pains." Is there such a thing? What might "growing pains" actually suggest?

LEGG-CALVÉ-PERTHES DISEASE (COXA PLANA)

Legg-Calvé-Perthes disease is avascular necrosis (a lack of blood flow resulting in destruction) of the proximal femoral epiphysis (AAOS, 2015b). The disorder occurs more often in boys than in girls and has a peak incidence between 4 and 12 years of age. It usually occurs unilaterally but may occur bilaterally.

A child with Legg-Calvé-Perthes disease looks well and often has no fever. The child is ambulatory and can have a limp, which may be subtle. There is little pain on motion of the hip, but there is guarding of the hip while moving it (Cook, 2014). X-ray studies distinguish the condition from simple synovitis (inflammation of the hip joint), which begins with the same symptoms. X-ray changes may not be apparent when a child is first seen, but they appear after about 3 weeks. For this reason, most children seen for synovitis of the hip joint are asked to return in 3 weeks for a repeat film.

Children with Legg-Calvé-Perthes disease pass through four stages. First is the synovitis stage or a period of painful inflammation. Next is a necrotic stage, during which bone in the femur head shrinks in size and shows increased density on an X-ray. This stage lasts 6 to 12 months. The third stage is a fragmentation stage; resorption of dead bone occurs over a 1- to 2-year period. The fourth stage, a reconstruction stage, marks the final healing, with deposition of new bone.

Treatment for Legg-Calvé-Perthes disease in children younger than 6 years of age usually focuses on pain reduction with nonsteroidal anti-inflammatory drugs (NSAIDs) plus keeping the head of the femur within the acetabulum by a containment device. The acetabulum then acts as a mold to preserve the shape of the femoral head and maintain range of motion. In children older than 6 years of age, reconstructive surgery (an osteotomy to center the femur head in the acetabulum followed by cast application) is most often prescribed. This technique returns the child to normal activity within 3 to 4 months in contrast to many months of restricted activity required by non–weight-bearing devices (AAOS, 2015b).

Parents and children need thorough education about treatment and care because most of this occurs on an ambulatory basis. It can be difficult for young children to accept the extended treatment period involved with this disorder. Be certain that both parents and children understand there are long-term consequences if rest is not followed conscientiously. Without treatment, the femur head tends to remold into a mushroom shape, making the hip unstable thereafter and leading to degenerative changes later in life, which lead to chronic pain, reduced mobility of the hip joint, and possibly permanent disability. Parents may need assistance with devising appropriate activities for the child during the time that activity is limited and weight bearing is not allowed.

OSGOOD–SCHLATTER DISEASE

Osgood–Schlatter disease is the thickening and enlargement of the tibial tuberosity resulting from microtrauma probably caused from overuse (AAOS, 2015a). It occurs more often in boys than girls and at preadolescence or early adolescence probably because of rapid growth at these times. Children notice pain and swelling just below the knee that is aggravated by running or squatting.

Therapy depends on the extent of the bone changes. Administration of NSAIDs, ice, and limiting strenuous physical exercise may be all that is necessary for effective healing (Kabiri, Tapley, & Tapley, 2014). Occasionally, immobilization of the leg in a walking cast or immobilizer for about 6 weeks may be required.

SLIPPED CAPITAL FEMORAL EPIPHYSIS

Slipped capital epiphysis is, as the name implies, a slipping or displacement of the capital femoral epiphysis (femoral head) from the femoral neck (metaphysis) through the epiphyseal plate (Bennison & Horn, 2015). The proximal femoral head displaces posteriorly and inferiorly, allowing an avascular necrosis—similar to that observed in Legg-Calvé-Perthes disease—to begin. If the cartilage covering the femur head is destroyed, permanent loss of motion of the femoral head in the acetabulum can result. Surgical reconstruction of the hip joint will then be necessary to correct the problem (Loder & Dietz, 2012).

This disorder occurs twice as frequently in young Blacks than in children of other races and twice as frequently in boys as in girls. It occurs most frequently in preadolescence and its highest incidence is in obese children. This suggests that it occurs because of the influence of growth hormone and excessive weight bearing on the hip joint.

The onset of symptoms occurs gradually. Children begin to limp as well as hold the leg on the affected side externally rotated to relieve stress and pain in the hip joint. Although the involvement is actually in the hip, they may report pain first in the knee because favoring the hip joint puts abnormal stress on the knee. On physical examination, internal rotation of the hip is difficult and painful. An X-ray reveals the slipped epiphysis at the femoral head.

Early detection of the condition is important because correction is easiest if it is attempted before the necrosis has progressed to epiphyseal destruction. Percutaneous in situ fixation remains the standard of care for stable slipped capital femoral epiphysis. The goal of this treatment is to prevent further slippage and achieve stable closure of the proximal femoral physis while avoiding potentially devastating complications such as osteonecrosis and chondrolysis (Escott, De La Rocha, Jo, et al., 2015). In some children, a total hip replacement is advised to fully restore hip function (Traina, De Fine, Abati, et al., 2012). With either surgery, the child will have activity restrictions for an extended time afterward.

Because the disease is most common in preadolescence, help children to understand the potential seriousness of the condition. Although they may not like being restricted or confined to bed, supportive communication and education can help them accept the treatment as necessary to maintain good healing and function of their hip joint. Encourage frequent visits and telephone calls with friends to provide optimal growth and development.

Although this condition usually is unilateral, some children later develop the same condition in the opposite hip. All children with a slipped capital epiphysis, therefore, need follow-up care, with careful attention to the condition of the opposite hip. If children are obese, they need nutritional counseling to bring weight back to a healthy level and to relieve strain on the lower extremities.

What If . . . 51.2
A nurse notices Jeffrey is overweight. He also rarely eats green vegetables. Although he just participated in a 2-mile school walkathon, he said it wasn't as much fun as he thought it would be. Which of his features make him at highest risk for developing slipped capital epiphysis?

Infectious and Inflammatory Disorders of the Bones and Joints

All bone infections are potentially dangerous because bones have such a rich blood supply that infection can easily spread and become systemic (septicemia).

OSTEOMYELITIS

Osteomyelitis is an infection of the bone (Tafin-Kampé & Kamsu-Foguem, 2013). Acute osteomyelitis is often the result of a hematogenous spread of bacteria such as *Staphylococcus aureus* in older children and by *Streptococcus pyogenes* in younger children. Children with sickle-cell anemia have a special susceptibility to *Salmonella* invasion in long bones. The infection may occur after extensive impetigo, burns, or something as simple as a furuncle (skin abscess) when the infectious organism is then carried through the blood supply to the bone. It also may occur directly by outside invasion from a penetrating wound, open fracture, or contamination during surgery.

The age of the child often determines where the infection will take place. In children younger than 1 year of age, the capillaries near the epiphysis are often the transport for bacteria. In older children, the rich sluggish blood flow makes the metaphysis the most common site based on the location of the vascular sinusoids (Schreiber, Illingworth, & Ward, 2016).

Assessment

Osteomyelitis usually begins with acute symptoms. Children show systemic malaise, fever, and irritability. They experience sharp pain at the bone metaphysis site. By the second day, the area of skin over the infected bone feels warm to the touch, and edema is also usually present. Edema formation is serious because it reduces the blood supply to a large expanse of bone, causing the death of bone tissue. This dead bone tissue, which appears dense on an X-ray, is called **sequestrum** and is an important marker for diagnosis. An MRI can be helpful to reveal if the infection has spread to nearby soft tissue (Kim & Rosenblum, 2014).

Diagnostic labs will reveal an increased white blood cell count, C-reactive protein level, and sedimentation rate; blood culture results usually are positive for the offending organism. CT scans are helpful to demonstrate early-stage bone changes. Simple X-rays, in contrast, may not reveal bone changes (the formation of sequestrum) until 5 to 10 days after the beginning of the infection.

Therapeutic Management

Medical therapy includes a limitation on weight bearing on the affected part, bed rest, immobilization, and a short administration of an intravenous (IV) antibiotic such as oxacillin, as indicated by the blood culture. IV therapy is usually initiated in the hospital and then continued at home for as long as 2 weeks by use of an intermittent infusion device or peripherally inserted central catheter (PICC). After this, the child will be prescribed an oral antibiotic for 3 to 4 more weeks.

If pus forms under the periosteum, it may be aspirated using a technique similar to bone marrow aspiration. After the procedure, a catheter may be inserted into the area for instillation of an antibiotic solution. A drainage tube may be inserted and attached to suction to evacuate the subperiosteum area.

 ### Nursing Diagnoses and Related Interventions

Nursing Diagnosis: Parental health-seeking behaviors related to care of the child with osteomyelitis

Outcome Evaluation: Parents accurately identify child's care needs in the hospital and at home; parents demonstrate procedure for IV antibiotic administration.

When planning care for a child with osteomyelitis, because of the long-term immobilization that may be necessary, parents may need to make major changes in their lifestyle such as taking a temporary leave from work or employing a home care nurse.

Parents usually have many questions when osteomyelitis is diagnosed because the defect may not initially show on a routine X-ray. This can leave them puzzled as they hear their primary healthcare provider advising them about the need for 6 weeks of antibiotic therapy. They need support and education to make an informed decision about treatment because they may be suspicious, anxious, and afraid that hospitalization and administration of IV antibiotics are excessive. Keep in mind that young children are active even if they are on bed rest and need age-appropriate activities so they maintain rest, not activity. If a child had surgery and drainage tubes are in place, institute infection-control precautions because the drain

evacuates infected material. Always handle the extremity gently when giving care because movement can cause pain. Provide instructions to the parents about good food sources of calcium and protein for bone healing.

When the child is discharged from the hospital, review measures to care for the antibiotic IV line with parents if this will be continued at home. Also, review the signs and symptoms of reinfection, measures for wound care and infection control, and possible adverse effects of the prescribed antibiotic (see Box 51.5, an interprofessional care map for a child with osteomyelitis). Ask if parents would like a referral for home care follow-up to ensure continued support and education.

Most children recover without serious consequences; however, if osteomyelitis is not entirely eradicated with the initial treatment, it will return and result in a chronic infectious process with open, draining sinuses and bone deformity in years to come. Growth plates can be destroyed, leading to shortening of the affected extremity.

QSEN Checkpoint Question 51.2

SAFETY

A nurse is planning care for Jeffrey, who has osteomyelitis. Which of the following interventions should the nurse prioritize in the care plan?
a. Maintain Jeffrey's IV antibiotic therapy.
b. Teach his parents about the root causes of his infection.
c. Restrict his fluid intake to increase his hematocrit level.
d. Fully assist Jeffrey with his activities of daily living.

Look in Appendix A for the best answer and rationale.

TRANSIENT SYNOVITIS

Transient synovitis is an acute, nonpurulent inflammation of the synovial membrane of a joint that occurs most commonly in the hip joint in children, with an age of incidence between 2 and 10 years, peaking at age 6 years. The exact etiology is unknown; however, there is usually a prodrome of upper respiratory symptoms (Cook, 2014). Children notice pain in the groin, in the lower portion of the thigh or knee, or in the buttocks. Pain is intense and is most noticeable in the morning when they first awaken. Children may wake at night or in the morning, crying from the pain of turning over. Pain again becomes worse later in the day when the child becomes tired.

Aside from the localized pain, children feel well except they usually hold the joint flexed in a position of comfort. On physical examination, a child with transient synovitis will look well, often playing with toys in the examination room but not moving the hip. There is no or, at most, low-grade fever (<38°C). There can be pain of the hip with passive range of motion. Unlike a child with a septic hip who refuses to walk, the child with transient synovitis may also refuse to walk or will walk with a limp (Cook, 2014). A pelvic X-ray or MRI may reveal capsular swelling at the involved joint.

BOX 51.5

Nursing Care Planning

AN INTERPROFESSIONAL CARE MAP FOR A CHILD WITH OSTEOMYELITIS

Jeffrey, a 13-year-old boy, accompanied his mother and 3-year-old sister into the hospital emergency room because his sister had pain in her arm after a fall. As you talked to Jeffrey, you noticed his left lower leg was swollen, warm to the touch, and painful. When he took off his shirt, you noticed his spine was not straight. His mother said she noticed an infected mosquito bite on his leg 2 weeks ago. Jeffrey is diagnosed with osteomyelitis and admitted to the hospital for intravenous antibiotic therapy. His mother asks you, "How could he get a bone infection from such a simple thing as an insect bite? Are you sure he's not just having growing pains?"

Family Assessment: Child lives with 10 and 3-year-old sisters and two parents. Father works as a family court judge. Mother works part time as a court reporter. Child rates finances as, "Okay. Although I'd like a better bicycle."

Patient Assessment: Left lower extremity pale but warm; pedal pulses present. Capillary refill time in toes is 3 seconds. States he had pain on admission, rated at 4 on a numerical scale of 1 to 10. Relieved with prescribed ibuprofen. During morning assessment, child states, "I'm so bored. If I have to stay in bed for a whole week, I'll go stir crazy." Child normally enjoys playing baseball with friends and video games.

Nursing Diagnosis: Risk for peripheral neurovascular dysfunction related to the effects of bone infection

Outcome Criteria: Child's extremity remains pink and warm with palpable pedal pulses and capillary refill time of 3 seconds or less; pain is no more than 2 on a scale of 1 to 10; states he is complying with bed rest by choosing activities carefully.

Team Member Responsible	Assessment	Intervention	Rationale	Expected Outcome
Activities of Daily Living, Including Safety				
Nurse	Assess whether child understands he should not bear weight on affected leg.	Review with child the importance of not bearing weight on infected leg.	Infected bone is weakened, and so it could fracture more easily than usual.	Child states he understands he should not put pressure on leg.
Teamwork and Collaboration				
Nurse/primary healthcare provider	Assess whether orthopedic service will be needed to consult on antibiotic therapy.	Consult with orthopedic service if needed to assure antibiotic regimen is adequate.	Bone infections are deep seated, so antibiotics must be selected for specific organisms and tissue penetration.	Orthopedic service consults as necessary to help decide best therapy.
Procedures/Medications for Quality Improvement				
Nurse	Assess whether child has past experience with intravenous (IV) therapy.	Orient child to IV therapy and importance of small armboard to guard against infiltration.	Infiltration interferes with antibiotic infusion and can cause tissue necrosis.	Child states he understands importance of continuous IV therapy and will work to guard site.
Nutrition				
Nurse/nutritionist	Meet with child to discuss what are his favorite foods.	Discuss importance of not gaining weight while on bed rest.	Child will be fitted with an orthopedic brace for his back. Gaining weight will interfere with correct fit.	Child states he understands the importance of not gaining weight and will cooperate with nutritionist's recommendations.
Patient-Centered Care				
Nurse	Assess what child understands about the cause of bone infections.	Review association between skin infection and osteomyelitis.	Osteomyelitis is often caused by extension of a skin infection such as impetigo or infected insect bite.	Child and mother state they understand outcome should not result in loss of function.

Continued on following page

BOX 51.5

Nursing Care Planning (continued)

Team Member Responsible	Assessment	Intervention	Rationale	Expected Outcome
Psychosocial/Spiritual/Emotional Needs				
Nurse	Assess what activities child would enjoy during bed rest.	Talk to child about importance of keeping busy because he will not feel systemically ill during this time.	Bed rest is difficult for children when they feel well except for one body part.	Child names at least two activities besides schoolwork he could do to keep busy and help relieve boredom.
Informatics for Seamless Healthcare Planning				
Nurse	Assess whether child has had experience taking oral medication at home.	Explain necessity to continue antibiotics even though symptoms are lessening.	If child does not understand purpose of long-term therapy, he may neglect to take antibiotic once symptoms fade.	Child and mother state they understand importance of continuing antibiotic and will keep the return appointment.

Because this is inflammation, not infection, the treatment of synovitis is the prescription of an NSAID such as ibuprofen (Motrin) and limited activity until muscle spasm from the pain has passed. In most children, a few days of rest reduces the synovitis. Some children, however, may need as many as 10 to 14 days of rest and a short course of oral corticosteroids to completely reduce the symptoms.

Synovitis must be differentiated from septic arthritis or Legg-Calvé-Perthes disease based on child's age, presentation, and diagnostic markers. Septic hip tends to occur in younger children (<2 years), and Legg-Calvé-Perthes typically occurs between the ages of 4 and 9 years. Children with septic hip typically look ill, and the joint will be held in a position that maximally increases the volume of the affected joint (Cook, 2014). Children with Legg-Calvé-Perthes disease look well and often do not have fever. The child is ambulatory and can have a limp, which may be subtle. There is little pain on motion of the hip, but there is guarding of the hip while moving it (Cook, 2014).

Explain to both children and parents that synovitis, although painful, is a simple inflammation process that will heal without sequelae. Rest is important for this recovery, however, so they must be prepared to enforce this (which is not easy to do with active children).

APOPHYSITIS

Calcaneal apophysitis (sever injury/disease) is considered an overuse injury that is self-limiting. It is a common injury in active, often overweight, predominantly male children. Symptoms usually start between the age of 8 and 15 years in boys and 8 and 13 years in girls (Aiyer & Hennrikus, 2014; Wiegerinck, Zwiers, R., Sierevelt, et al., 2016).

Pain usually can be relieved by adding a lift or cup to the heel of shoe on the affected side, thus reducing the tension on the heel cord and bone. Other helpful treatment modalities include ice application before and after athletic events, nonsteroidal anti-inflammatory medications, and possible activity modification. After the pain has subsided, the adolescent needs to practice exercises to stretch the heel cord, such as standing on a slanting board that elevates the foot and toes above the level of the heel for 20 minutes about three times a day.

Although not a serious condition, it can be debilitating for adolescents who want to excel in sports because it may recur.

Disorders of Skeletal Structure

Spinal disorders in children may include kyphosis (an outward curvature of the cervical spine) or lordosis (an inward curving of the lumbar spine), but idiopathic scoliosis (an S-shaped curve) is the most commonly seen type of these disorders.

FUNCTIONAL (POSTURAL) SCOLIOSIS

Scoliosis is a three-dimensional spine deformity characterized by lateral and rotational curvature of the spine (AAOS, 2015c). The spinal deformity is characterized by a lateral (sideways) curve of the spine of 10 degrees or more (Hresko, 2013). Scoliosis affects the spine in all three planes: axial, coronal, and sagittal. It may involve all or only a portion of the spinal column, such as the thoracic vertebrae. It may be functional (a nonrotated spinal curve caused by a secondary problem, such as a leg length discrepancy) or structural (a primary deformity such as an underlying neuromuscular disorder). Scoliosis may also be the initial presenting sign of underlying conditions such as heritable collagen diseases, neurologic conditions, or skeletal dysplasia that may have been undetected until adolescence (AAOS, 2015c).

STRUCTURAL SCOLIOSIS

The most common form of scoliosis occurs in or near adolescence and is termed *idiopathic scoliosis* (Fig. 51.11). The primary curve is often a right thoracic convexity. As the original curve becomes severe, rotation and angulation of vertebrae also occur. The thoracic rib cage rotates to become very protuberant on the convex curve. Vertebral growth may halt because of extreme pressure changes.

A family history of curvature of the spine is found in up to 30% of children with scoliosis, although no specific inheritance pattern has been documented. It is 5 times more common in girls than in boys and has a peak incidence at 8 to 15 years of age. As long as the child is growing, the spinal

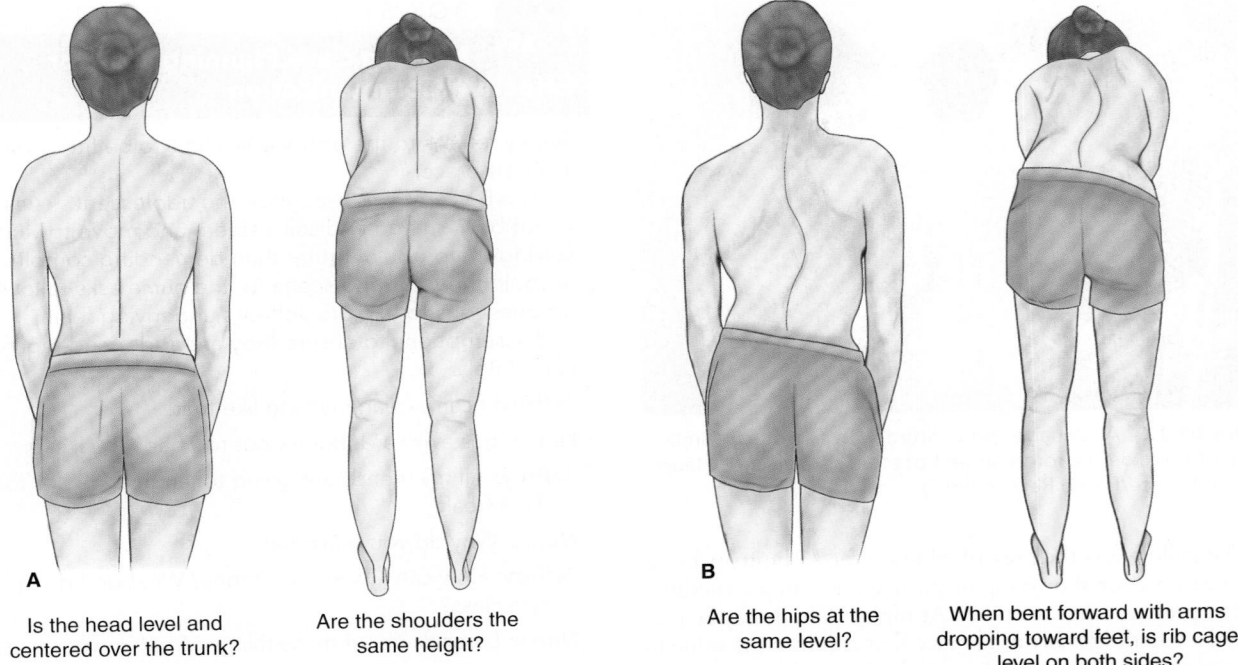

A

Is the head level and
centered over the trunk?

Are the shoulders the
same height?

B

Are the hips at the
same level?

When bent forward with arms
dropping toward feet, is rib cage
level on both sides?

Figure 51.11 Assessing scoliosis. **(A)** Normal position and spinal curves. **(B)** Scoliosis indicators.

curves will become more severe, which is why the symptoms become most marked at prepuberty (a time of rapid growth). If the child bends forward (Adams test), the curve becomes even more noticeable.

Assessment

Screening examinations for spine deformity occur at different locations and remain controversial because prospective, randomized, controlled studies on population screening for scoliosis have not been done. The Scoliosis Research Society (SRS), AAOS, Pediatric Orthopaedic Society of North America (POSNA), and American Academy of Pediatrics (AAP) believe that screening examinations for spine deformity should be part of the medical home preventive services visit for females at age 10 and 12 years and for males at age 13 or 14 years (see Chapter 34). Often, the condition develops insidiously and is prominent before it is noticed because of the preadolescent's and adolescent's need for privacy and the lack of pain that accompanies the condition. A parent might notice when doing laundry that a daughter's bra straps are adjusted to unequal lengths. A girl may find it difficult to buy jeans that fit correctly because of uneven iliac crests or she may notice that a skirt or dress hangs unevenly.

A scoliometer is a commercial device that can be used to document the extent of a spinal curve. With this device (a specialized inclinometer), a reading greater than 7 degrees equals a 20-degree scoliotic curve detected by an X-ray.

MRIs, X-rays, and CT scans all play a role in estimating the extent of the deformity and in providing a baseline description. If the child has a vertebral rotation causing rib imbalance, pulmonary function studies and a chest X-ray may be obtained to document the effect on lung capacity. Children's bone age is established by an X-ray of the left wrist or iliac bones. If bone growth is complete or almost complete and the curve is less than 50 degrees, little more deformity will result, so no correction may be necessary. If the child has

1 to 2 years of bone growth remaining, however, some correction most likely will be recommended.

Therapeutic Management

Usually, if the spinal curve is less than 20 degrees, no therapy is required except for close observation and X-rays about every 6 months until the child reaches growth maturity. If the curve is greater than 20 degrees, treatment can consist of a conservative, nonsurgical approach using a body brace; it could include surgery or a combination of both surgical and nonsurgical measures. Curves greater than 40 degrees may require surgery with spinal fusion. The goal of both surgery and mechanical bracing is to maintain spinal stability and to prevent further progression of the deformity until bone growth is complete. Because of this, regardless of the type of treatment chosen, the child and family must be prepared for long-term treatment.

During prepuberty and adolescence, children tend to be very concerned about body image and so can become very impatient with scoliosis correction. Offering them a great deal of support at healthcare visits to help them cope can be an important nursing contribution.

Bracing

For slight spinal curves in a child who is still skeletally immature, bracing—one of the oldest forms of correction—is still a prime intervention (AAOS, 2015c). The Milwaukee brace was the first type used for this purpose, so, although today's braces look much different, they may still be referred to by this name. Originally, these braces extended to the neck and were almost impossible to conceal under clothing; today, they are underarm thoracolumbar supports (e.g., a Boston brace) that fit under clothing (Fig. 51.12). Braces are now designed by computer-aided techniques to ensure that the brace will be both comfortable and will accomplish maximum correction (Cobetto, Aubin, Parent, et al., 2016).

Figure 51.12 A teenage girl is fitted with a thoracic-lumbar-sacral orthotic device for treatment of scoliosis. (© Aaron Haupt/Science Source/Photo Researchers.)

The child wears the prescribed brace for 23 hours per day, removed only for showering or participation in a structured athletic program such as soccer. At night, a child may be prescribed a Charleston bending brace that confines the spine to an overcorrected position. Assess whether children and parents know how to safely apply these braces. Frequent follow-up healthcare visits are necessary to check that the device still fits snugly without rubbing on bony prominences, such as the iliac crests. Caution children and parents not to loosen straps if rubbing occurs because this causes the brace to fit loosely, thus not allowing for it to exert adequate compression and traction on areas that are curved. Alert parents and children to notify their healthcare provider instead.

Assess that the child is wearing the brace over a T-shirt to prevent the plastic pads from touching skin surfaces and causing skin excoriation. During the first couple of weeks they wear a brace, children may notice slight muscle aches resulting from the new straighter back alignment. A mild analgesic such as acetaminophen (Tylenol) will decrease this discomfort in most children. Rest also provides considerable relief. Caution children not to remove the brace during this time because taking it off compounds the problem of discomfort by prolonging the period of adjustment.

 ## Nursing Diagnoses and Related Interventions

Nursing Diagnosis: Situational low self-esteem related to obviousness of the brace used for scoliosis correction

Outcome Evaluation: Child states positive aspects of self; participates in activities; establishes friendships with peers.

Adjusting to wearing a brace may be a major problem for some children. Help them to concentrate on things they can do with the brace in place, such as having a friend over or going to the movies, rather than those things they cannot do because of the brace (e.g., playing a contact sport) (Box 51.6).

Encourage children to remain as socially active as possible. They may comment at first that they feel awkward or "so much taller" that they are afraid they will fall. However, the only way to get comfortable with a brace is to walk and get used to the new sensation of actually being a

Jeffrey returns to the orthopedic clinic to be fitted with a scoliosis brace.

Tip: Be careful to recognize the adolescent's cues about body image and self-esteem and move toward solving the problem rather than demanding compliance. In the following scenario, the nurse asks follow-up questions to explore Jeffrey's underlying fears and assumptions to ensure they are addressed more completely.

Jeffrey: I can't wear anything like that!

Nurse: It is awkward, but it's not too bad. You'll see.

Jeffrey: All my friends are going to laugh at me! I'll look like a freak!

Nurse: Why do you think that?

Jeffrey: How can I wear my clothes? What do I do in gym class?

Nurse: Let's talk about those things. What do you usually wear to school for a start?

little taller. Braces may be awkward at school if chairs are attached to desks. Advocate for the child with the school nurse for seating arrangements that are comfortable.

Friends typically ask questions about why the child needs the brace. The sooner children expose the brace to friends and family, the sooner these questions cease. A brace may need adjustment about every 3 months to accomplish more alignment, and even more frequent visits may be required so children can express the problems they are having with social and school adjustment. Do not underestimate, however, an adolescent's ability to adjust to new situations. Children can see by looking in a mirror that their spine is curved, and they want this corrected. They will endure necessary discomfort if they have hope they will emerge at the end of the correction period without an obvious physical deformity.

In some instances, parents must be firm about insisting their child continuously wears the brace. Be certain children do not envision spinal surgery (which they will need if bracing is ineffective) as a simple and quick procedure, similar to an appendectomy, because, if they think this, they may deliberately avoid wearing the brace, hoping that surgery will then be prescribed. Do not, however, depict spinal surgery as horrible. In some children, even with conscientious bracing, the scoliosis continues to worsen, and surgery will still be necessary.

Scoliosis braces are typically worn until children's spinal growth stops (about 24 months postmenarche in girls, 16.5 years in boys), as demonstrated by a spinal X-ray. The child is usually weaned from the brace gradually because some demineralization and weakening of vertebrae may have occurred during the long period of bracing. Gradual resumption of activity and wearing the brace for a shorter period of time each day allows both remineralization and continued spinal support.

Halo Traction

Halo traction is the use of opposing forces to straighten and reduce spinal curves that are severe when first diagnosed (over 80 degrees) or that are progressing despite bracing. Halo traction is achieved using a ring of metal (a halo) held in place with about four stainless steel pins inserted into the skull bones (Koller, Zenner, Gajic, et al., 2012). Counter-traction is applied by pins inserted into the distal femurs or the iliac crests (Fig. 51.13). A halo traction apparatus is bulky and looks frightening. Children cannot help but worry that when the pins are inserted into their skull (under general anesthesia), they will slip and penetrate their brain. They may worry the apparatus will be so heavy it will strain or break their neck.

Halo traction is typically used for those children who have such severe scoliosis that they experience respiratory involvement or cervical instability or have a high thoracic deformity or decreased vital capacity from severe spinal curvature and rotation. If at all possible, children need to see photographs of the apparatus or should be able to talk to children who have the apparatus in place before having it applied. This gives them time to express their feelings about being placed in such a cumbersome device. Because it is so cumbersome, some children react to the apparatus physically, with nausea or diarrhea, or emotionally, with chronic sadness, until they realize they can adjust to it. Be certain that orientation is as thorough for the parents as it is for the child. Otherwise, parents may also show symptoms of stress for the first few days after the application of such traction. After application, parents may feel unsure and appreciate practical pointers in how to care for their child. Emphasizing positive aspects, such as what the child can do, and explaining how the traction will help the spinal curvature is helpful to allow both children and parents to accept such extreme traction.

Halo traction is prescribed until optimal spinal correction is achieved. For the first 24 hours after application, most children experience a nagging level of pain at the pin insertion sites and perhaps in their back; offer analgesia as prescribed.

Children in halo traction need frequent care at the pin sites according to practitioner or hospital policy. In the absence of skin sensitivity, pin sites should be cleaned once weekly using an alcoholic chlorhexidine solution and nonshedding gauze

(McClung, 2015). Encourage children to be self-sufficient and do as many things as they are able.

After optimal spinal correction has been achieved with the device, the equipment is easily removed. The pin sites in the skull heal within 1 week without obvious scarring.

Surgical Intervention: Spinal Instrumentation

Surgical correction usually is necessary if the spinal curvature is greater than 40 degrees. Instruments such as rods and screws are placed next to the spinal column to provide firm reduction of the curvature; the spine is then fused in the corrected position (Fig. 51.14A). A disadvantage of fusion is that it prevents further spinal growth and limits motion of the lumbar section if involved—a concern that can be solved by the use of fusionless interventions such as intervertebral stapling or expandable rods (Dede, Demirkiran, & Yazici, 2014). Although this is back surgery, the surgical approach may be either from the back (posterior) of the child or from the front (anterior) through the abdomen.

A

B

Figure 51.14 (A) Cotrel-Dubousset rods to correct scoliosis. A short distraction rod is linked to a longer one to correct the major curve. A convex rod is then applied. **(B)** Preparing to log roll. Two nurses use a draw sheet to roll the child in one coordinated movement to the side-lying position.

Figure 51.13 A 9-year-old girl in halo traction. (© Caroline Brown, RNC, MS, DEd.)

Preoperative Nursing Care

Before spinal instrumentation, extensive X-rays are taken to plan the exact location of instrumentation, such as rods and screws or staples. Ensure children have a good explanation of what they can expect before and after surgery (see Chapter 36). Deep-breathing exercises will be particularly important for children whose scoliosis has caused chronically reduced lung capacity, so introduce these plus incentive spirometry preoperatively. A nasogastric tube usually is inserted before surgery to prevent abdominal distention because major surgery may cause temporary paralytic ileus and a lack of bowel tone. Because this surgery involves major muscle and tendon shifts, the child will have pain afterward. It is a major operation, so they can also expect to feel tired and "not themselves" for several days. Young adolescents appreciate learning about these feelings before surgery as well as appreciate being treated like adults. Be aware, however, that early adolescents are not adults, and, although they seem eager to breathe deeply and cooperate with routines before surgery, these requests can be overwhelming for them postoperatively; their behavior postoperatively may not be nearly as mature as they anticipated it would be. Epidural anesthesia offers a great deal of pain relief. Allowing children to use an IV or epidural patient-controlled analgesia system offers both pain relief and a feeling of control.

Postoperative Care

Following surgery, repositioning is important to prevent pressure areas and to maintain care of instrumentation. Repositioning may be performed by using a log-roll technique (see Fig. 51.14B). Along with postoperative assessment of the incision and/or drainage, assess vital signs and pain per hospital policy. Some children spend the first 24 hours in the pediatric intensive care setting for pain management and frequent assessment. Neurologic complications (e.g., nerve root, cauda equina, spinal cord deficit) are not common, but neurologic assessment is essential following spinal surgery. Careful neurologic assessment of upper and lower extremity function should be continued for at least 48 hours after surgery. Delayed neurologic complications may be caused by progressive spinal cord ischemia secondary to traction or to the development of an epidural hematoma. Blood pressure should be monitored carefully and mean arterial blood pressure should be maintained at greater than 80 mmHg to help maintain spinal cord perfusion (Stepanovich, Mundis, & Yaszay, 2015). Another rare complication following surgery may involve proximal small intestinal obstruction due to increased pressure generated by contraction of the angle between the superior mesenteric artery and the aorta (Keskin, Akgül, Bayraktar, et al., 2014). Circulatory pressure changes resulting from realignment of the chest cage and reduced rotation of the spine may result in circulatory impairment. There is usually extensive blood loss during spinal fusion surgery, which may cause shock and hypotension. A drainage system, such as a Hemovac, may be inserted next to the incision to evacuate any accumulating blood. The amount collected from this needs to be recorded. Other postoperative complications include wound infection, ileus, and atelectasis.

Children are usually prescribed nothing by mouth until bowel sounds return (usually 12 to 24 hours). An indwelling urinary catheter, placed during surgery, is usually left in place for 24 hours because voiding may be difficult. This also allows for an assessment of kidney function.

Although a child's parents have been prepared for the fact that spinal rod insertion is major surgery, they may still be shocked by the child's appearance after surgery. They may be afraid to touch their child at a time when the child would probably enjoy being hugged because of feeling so ill and frightened. Role model touching and talking to the child to help parents overcome their concern as quickly as possible.

As soon as bowel sounds are present, a child can begin to take fluids and then solids. Usually on day 1 postop, physical therapy is initiated to help children learn how to change position and ambulate. They may feel dizzy at first; therefore, allow them to get used to sitting by attempting it for only short periods at a time at first. Activity is then increased to a normal level with few restrictions.

Because removing rods is as extensive a procedure as inserting them, instrumentation rods are left in place permanently unless they cause irritation or infection later. The average child becomes unaware the rods are in place.

Children may be afraid to move freely after rod insertion or stapling because if they have worn a brace beforehand, they have been in some type of restraining device for a long time. They may need to be reassured frequently that, following surgery, their scoliosis is corrected with an "internal" brace or instrumentation.

What If . . . 51.3

Jeffrey, who was diagnosed with having scoliosis, was prescribed a brace to wear 23 hours a day. During the past month, he dropped out of the school band and the one after-school club to which he belonged. He tells the nurse he dropped these activities "to have more time to study." Why might the nurse be concerned?

Disorders of the Joints and Tendons: Collagen Vascular Disease

Collagen is composed of bundles of protein-rich fibers that form the connective tissue of tendons, ligaments, and bones. Because this tissue is found throughout the body, collagen diseases are systemic. They tend to be painful, involve inflammation, and are long term.

JUVENILE IDIOPATHIC ARTHRITIS

JIA, also called simply juvenile arthritis (JA) or juvenile rheumatoid arthritis (JRA), primarily involves the joints of the body, although it also affects blood vessels and other connective tissues. Three groups have developed sets of criteria to classify children with arthritis:

- American College of Rheumatology (ACR)
- European League Against Rheumatism (EULAR)
- International League of Associations for Rheumatology (ILAR)

The ACR-accepted terminology for JIA includes children younger than 16 years of age who have chronic arthritis (swelling or effusion, or presence of two or more of the following signs: limitation of range of motion, tenderness or pain on motion, and increased heat) in one or more joints (lasting more than 6 weeks) and in whom no other specific cause of arthritis can be identified. Onset type is defined by type of disease in the first 6 months. The organization recognizes the following three subtypes:

- *Polyarticular*: five or more inflamed joints, often involving weight-bearing joints. Rheumatoid nodules may be seen in patients with rheumatoid factor (RF)-positive disease and symmetrical involvement of small joints in the hands.
- *Pauciarticular*: less than five inflamed joints. Large, weight-bearing joints, such as the knees and ankles, are typically affected.
- *Systemic*: arthritis in one joint for at least 6 weeks' duration in a child age 16 years with or preceded by fever of at least 2 weeks' duration that is documented to be daily ("quotidian") for at least 3 days and accompanied by one or more of the following: evanescent erythematous rash, generalized lymphadenopathy, hepatomegaly or splenomegaly, and serositis (Ringold, Weiss, Beukelman, et al., 2013)

Three separate subtypes of JA exist (Table 51.1).

The ILAR classification of JIA includes the following six categories:

- *Systemic-onset JIA*: characterized by spiking fevers, typically occurring once or twice each day, at about the same time of day, with temperature returning to normal or below normal
- *Oligoarticular JIA*: oligoarthritis (pauciarticular disease): less than five inflamed joints. Large, weight-bearing joints, such as the knees and ankles, are typically affected.
- *Polyarticular JIA*: polyarthritis: five or more inflamed joints, often involving weight-bearing joints. Rheumatoid nodules may be seen in patients with RF-positive disease and symmetrical involvement of small joints in the hands.
- *Psoriatic arthritis*: usually mild. Onset of arthritis precedes that of psoriasis in approximately half of children.

- *Enthesitis-related arthritis*: frequently presents as evening and postexercise pain. Attention should be given to buttock pain and back pain that improves with activity (inflammatory back pain). These children cannot lie in bed all morning but have to get up due to back pain.
- *Undifferentiated arthritis*: diagnosed if the patient's manifestations either do not fulfill the criteria for any one category or fulfill the criteria for more than one (Sherry, Bhaskar, Poduval, et al., 2016)

The EULAR proposed the term *juvenile chronic arthritis* (JCA) for the heterogeneous group of disorders that manifest as JA. The diagnosis requires that the arthritis begins before age 16 years and lasts for at least 3 months. The EULAR criteria for JCA recognize the following subtypes based on characteristics at onset:

- Pauciarticular (one to four joints)
- Polyarticular (five or more joints)
- Presence of RF (two positive tests at least 3 months apart)
- Systemic onset with characteristic features
- Positivity for RF
- Juvenile ankylosing spondylitis
- Juvenile psoriatic arthritis

The cause of JA is unknown, although it is thought to be an autoimmune process in which a child develops circulating antibodies (immunoglobulins) against body cells. This is revealed by the presence of antinuclear antibodies (ANA), RF, and human leukocyte antigen (HLA)-B27 in blood serum. A genetic predisposition may also be present and increases the risk in some children (Soep, 2012).

Assessment

Children with systemic JA are usually brought to a healthcare facility because of a persistent fever and rash, symptoms that present even before the pain and stiffness of joint involvement begins. Regardless of the type of JA, assess children for

TABLE 51.1 COMPARING DIFFERENT TYPES OF JUVENILE ARTHRITIS

Characteristic	Polyarticular	Pauciarticular	Systemic Onset
Number of joints involved	Five or more	Four or less	Any number
Joints affected	Small joints of fingers and hands, also possibly weight-bearing joints	Usually large joints, such as knees, ankle, or elbow	Any joint
	Often same joint on both sides of body	Usually one joint on one side of body	
Gender affected	More girls than boys	More girls than boys (most common type)	Boys and girls equally
Body temperature	Low-grade fever	Low-grade fever	High spiking fever lasting for weeks or months
Other symptoms	Stiffness and minimal joint swelling, leading to limited motion	Eye inflammation; painless joint swelling with little redness	Macular rash on chest, thighs
	Rheumatoid nodules or bumps on elbow or other body area receiving pressure from chairs, shoes, or other object	(+)ANA titer (possible)	Inflammation of heart and lungs
	(+)Rheumatoid factor (in approximately 20% of children)	(+)HLA antigen (possible in boys)	Anemia
	(+)ANA titer (possible)		Enlarged lymph nodes, liver, and spleen
	Elevated white blood cell count, complement, and sedimentation rate		Rarely + rheumatoid factor and ANA titer
			Elevated white blood cell count

ANA, antinuclear antibody; HLA, human leukocyte antigen.

the effect their disease is having on self-care. Do they need help eating, dressing, ambulating, or toileting? Also, assess the child's and parents' understanding of the illness and the therapy planned because children and parents will typically bear the major responsibility of evaluating further symptoms and for carrying out therapy at home.

Children with pauciarticular arthritis need screening with a slit-lamp examination every 6 months for uveitis (inflammation of the iris, ciliary body, and choroid membrane of the eye) because severe uveitis can lead to blindness (Soep, 2012).

Therapeutic Management

Because JA is a long-term illness, therapy includes a balanced program of exercise, rest, and medication administration to relieve pain, restore function, and maintain joint mobility.

Daily Activities and Exercise

An activity such as sitting on the toilet may be uncomfortable if hip and knee joints are painful. Using an elevated toilet seat can be helpful because it reduces the amount of bending required at the knee. Children may also be unable to dress themselves because they are unable to button or zipper due to painful finger joints. Modifying these activities by using loops or Velcro strips not only helps children feel good about themselves but also increases their overall level of activity despite joint involvement (Fig. 51.15).

Because a set exercise program has the potential to help preserve muscle and joint function, children are prescribed a set program of daily range-of-motion exercises designed to strengthen muscles and put joints through their full range of motion. They can do these independently, although participating in a group is usually appealing to children at this age.

It is best if these exercises can be incorporated into a dance routine or a game, such as Simon Says because this not only makes exercises enjoyable but can also make the exercise a family participation time to be anticipated rather than a dull routine that must be followed daily. Swimming and tricycle or bicycle riding are excellent exercises because they provide smooth joint action. Also, encourage children to do as much self-care as they can because the natural motions of activities such as dressing and brushing teeth exercise joints. In contrast,

to reduce joint destruction, activities that place excessive strain on joints, such as running, jumping, prolonged walking, and kicking, should be avoided. School-age children can cooperate to avoid these activities. Parents of preschool children need to create interesting alternative activities, so the child avoids such motions.

Children should continue to attend school if at all possible because this increases activity that hopefully leads to fewer contractures and less decalcification of bones. Children with JA fatigue easily, however, so they may need a shortened school day; moving their starting time to midmorning can be a way to implement this. This late start can allow a child time for a warm bath in the morning, an activity that not only reduces pain but also increases movement in the involved joints.

Heat Application

Heat reduces pain and inflammation in joints and so increases comfort and motion. Heat can be applied by the use of a heating pad or warm water soaks for 20 to 30 minutes. Paraffin soaks can be useful for wrist and finger inflammation. Caution parents that young children frequently play with the controls on a heating pad, so they should tape the control to its medium temperature to help guard against burns.

Medication

NSAIDs such as ibuprofen (Motrin) or naproxen (Naprosyn) are the analgesics of choice for children with JA because they not only control pain and inflammation, thereby reducing joint swelling, joint discomfort, and morning stiffness, but also may contribute to improvement in malaise and irritability. NSAIDs are taken about four times a day and must be taken for at least 6 to 8 weeks to ensure effectiveness.

Because taking so many NSAIDs can cause gastrointestinal upset and bleeding, be certain parents know to always give the medication with food. Most parents think of NSAIDs as a drug to give children only when they have pain. Teach that they should continue to give the drug even if the child has no noticeable pain at the time of administration because the drug's anti-inflammatory action is just as important as its pain prevention.

Slow-acting antirheumatic drugs (SAARDs), also called *disease-modifying antirheumatic drugs* (DMARDs), can be used if NSAIDs are ineffective. In contrast to the immediate pain relief or anti-inflammatory effect of NSAIDs, these drugs modify the natural progress of the disease over weeks to months (Ringold, Weiss, Colbert, et al., 2014).

Methotrexate, a cytotoxic drug, is the second drug usually prescribed. Steroids, such as prednisone, are only added to the drug therapy if the disease is extremely severe or is an incapacitating systemic disease that has not responded to other anti-inflammatory agents. Steroids are injected directly into the affected joint. The first biologic medication, etanercept (Enbrel), was approved to treat JIA in the United States in 1999. Therapies continue to include the administration of medications called tumor necrosis factor (TNF) inhibitors, such as etanercept (Enbrel) or infliximab (Remicade). These drugs reduce inflammation by blocking the action of TNFs, which cause inflammation. Etanercept is subcutaneously injected every week, so parents need detailed instructions on the technique to do this as well as the importance of guarding against infections because children are more susceptible

Figure 51.15 The knees of a child with juvenile arthritis. Note the degree of joint enlargement and swelling. (Photograph courtesy of A. I. duPont Institute, Children's Hospital, Wilmington, DE.)

to infection than usual while taking these drugs. Infliximab is given IV and so usually requires a short-term healthcare facility stay for safe administration. The newest targets for arthritis treatment are the kinase inhibitors, such as tofacitinib. Tofacitinib is an oral medication that has shown clinical response in as little as 2 weeks with sustained response up to 12 months. Other orally bioavailable therapeutic treatments are also in trials for clinical effectiveness.

Nutrition

Children with JA, like those with other chronic diseases, may eat poorly because of joint pain and fatigue. Some children experience mild gastric irritation from NSAID therapy. Help parents plan mealtimes at the "best times" of the day to overcome these problems.

Nursing Diagnoses and Related Interventions

Nursing Diagnosis: Deficient knowledge related to care necessary to manage disease symptoms

Outcome Evaluation: Parents and child follow instructions regarding exercise and medication.

Help parents and children to understand the necessity for them to take an active role in therapy by planning exercise and medication programs around school or other activities. Children with JA commonly experience irritability and fatigue, which may interfere with plans. Assist them with devising a schedule that allows for a balance of rest periods with exercise to maximize the possibility of success.

Evaluate how well children are managing their symptoms in addition to how they view themselves (hopefully feeling well after a long period of pain and illness). The few children who develop joint contractures may require soft-tissue surgery, such as contracture release, tendon reconstruction, and synovectomy, or orthopedic surgery, such as equalization of leg length or orthoplasty, at a later date. Surgery of these types are usually delayed until growth is complete, so further growth will not influence the outcome.

About half of children with JA recover at the end of adolescence. The others will continue to have the disease into adulthood. Until the disease does reach remission, children need a great deal of support to perform exercises and take daily medication as prescribed.

QSEN Checkpoint Question 51.3

PATIENT-CENTERED CARE

Jeffrey's 10-year-old sister has JA, and her mother is eager to explore alternative methods of pain control in addition to standard approaches of analgesia. The standard approach to analgesia with JA is:

a. Applying ice to painful joints to reduce inflammation
b. Having joints scraped biannually during an arthroscopy
c. Applying topical hydrocortisone to affected joints
d. Taking an NSAID on a daily basis

Look in Appendix A for the best answer and rationale.

Disorders of the Skeletal Muscles

MYASTHENIA GRAVIS

For nerve conduction to cause muscles to contract effectively, a neurotransmitter, acetylcholine (ACh), must be released at synaptic junctions. The release of ACh is governed by the enzyme cholinesterase. With myasthenia gravis, there is interference in ACh processing, which leads to symptoms of progressive muscle weakness or inability to contract. The fault may be impaired synthesis or storage of ACh, insufficient ACh release, inadequate ACh receptors present at motor end plates, opposition of ACh by an anti-ACh factor, or excessive cholinesterase. In adults, the defect is probably most often a motor end plate insufficiency (a decreased number of ACh receptors are present). In children, myasthenia gravis probably occurs most often from an autoimmune process (autoantibodies may block receptor sites for ACh or other receptors such as muscle-specific kinase (MuSK) receptors (VanderPluym, Vajsar, Jacob, et al., 2013).

The disease occurs in three forms in childhood: neonatal transient myasthenia, congenital myasthenia, and juvenile myasthenia.

Assessment

With neonatal transient myasthenia, the mother has myasthenia gravis and the infant demonstrates transient disease symptoms at birth because of the transfer of antibodies from the mother. The newborn appears "floppy," sucks poorly, and has weak respiratory effort. Ptosis (drooping eyelids) may be present. The symptoms disappear within 2 to 4 weeks, but if they are not recognized when present, they could prove fatal because of respiratory muscle dysfunction.

Congenital myasthenia appears to be an inherited disorder that results in faulty ACh transmission or reception. Juvenile myasthenia gravis is an autoimmune process that occurs most typically at 10 to 13 years of age and in girls more frequently than in boys. Most children with this form have thymus hypertrophy; this sign helps document the autoimmune process (VanderPluym et al., 2013).

With all forms, children gradually begin to develop double vision (diplopia) and ptosis because of weakness of the extraocular muscles. Symptoms grow intense as facial, neck, jaw, swallowing, and intercostal muscles become affected. Fatigue is extreme, becoming more noticeable as a day progresses. All symptoms increase with emotional stress, fatigue, menstruation, respiratory infections, and alcohol intake. In the most severe form, all muscles, including those of respiration, become unable to contract.

Obtaining an accurate history, especially documenting whether a child can perform repetitive movements, is important. Ask a child to look upward and hold that position. Children with myasthenia gravis, unlike others, will gradually demonstrate ptosis. Other repetitive motions, such as walking up stairs or clapping, may also be tested, although the time spent doing this should not be prolonged because it is tiring and does not reveal much more information. Most children have myography performed to document their poor muscle function. An MRI or a CT scan demonstrates the enlarged thymus gland.

Edrophonium (Tensilon) is a drug that prolongs the action of ACh and therefore increases muscle strength. If the child's muscle strength improves moments after an injection, the child's diagnosis is positive for myasthenia gravis (Karch, 2016).

Therapeutic Management

The goal of treatment for myasthenia gravis is to improve the strength and endurance of a patient by facilitating neuromuscular transmission (Liew, Powell, Sloan, et al., 2014). Myasthenia gravis is treated by the administration of neostigmine (Prostigmin) or pyridostigmine bromide (Mestinon), acetylcholinesterase inhibitors that prolong the action of ACh (Box 51.7). The dosage of these agents must be individually determined. If toxicity occurs, symptoms similar to those of the original disease occur because excessive ACh leads to

---

BOX 51.7

Nursing Care Planning Based on Responsibility for Pharmacology

NEOSTIGMINE (PROSTIGMIN)

Classification: Neostigmine is a cholinesterase inhibitor that acts as an antimyasthenic agent.

Action: Neostigmine increases the concentration of acetylcholine at nerve endings, prolonging and exaggerating its effects and facilitating neuromuscular transmission (Karch, 2016).

Pregnancy Risk Category: C

Dosage: orally, 2 mg/kg daily in divided doses every 3 to 4 hours; or 0.01 to 0.04 mg/kg per dose intramuscularly, intravenously, or subcutaneously every 2 to 3 hours, as needed

Possible Adverse Effects: salivation, dysphagia, increased peristalsis, cardiac arrhythmias, increased respiratory secretions, urinary frequency, pupil constriction, and diaphoresis

Nursing Implications

- Assess the child for increased muscle weakness, indicating possible cholinergic crisis. Keep atropine sulfate readily available as the antidote.
- If giving neostigmine orally, administer the drug with food or milk to minimize gastrointestinal upset. Instruct parents to administer the drug exactly as prescribed.
- Plan to administer larger portions of the divided doses approximately one-half hour before anticipated times of greater fatigue.
- Advise parents to watch for signs of excessive salivation, emesis, or frequent urination and to notify their healthcare provider if these occur.
- Encourage parents to control the child's environmental temperature as much as possible to prevent diaphoresis from too hot or too humid an environment.
- Inform parents an increase in muscle weakness may be related to either drug overdose or exacerbation of the disease. Urge them to report any signs of increased weakness to their healthcare provider immediately.

---

continued neurotransmitter stimulation and the inability of muscles to repolarize for a new contraction. In some children, prednisone or an immunosuppressant such as azathioprine may be added to their medication regimen to decrease the amount of anticholinesterase medication required. In still others, plasmapheresis to remove immune complexes from the bloodstream or the administration of IV immunoglobulin to provide immune suppression will reduce symptoms (Bird, 2016).

Excision of the thymus gland may also effectively reduce symptoms, although this is a last resort because it may leave the child open to additional autoimmune disorders in the future.

Teach parents and children that symptoms become worse under stress; therefore, parents need to adequately prepare children for new experiences such as menstruation, high school, a parental divorce, or surgery in order to minimize stress. Help children plan their day to include rest periods, possibly advocating for a special school schedule if necessary. If chewing and swallowing are difficult, ensure a rest period before meals. Even so, children may need to take their medication about an hour before mealtime, eat a soft diet, and learn to eat slowly and cautiously to avoid choking and aspiration. If symptoms of muscle weakness suddenly become very severe, parents should call 911 because the loss of function of intercostal muscles may lead to respiratory arrest. Atropine, an anticholinergic agent and the antidote for an overdose of anticholinesterase drugs, should be available to administer as necessary both for parents at home and on a hospital unit that cares for children with this disease.

DERMATOMYOSITIS

Dermatomyositis occurs from the degeneration of skeletal muscle fibers. The cause of the disorder is unknown, although either a viral infection or an autoimmune basis is suspected. It is more common in girls than in boys and occurs between the ages of 5 and 14 years (Soep, 2012). Symptoms usually begin insidiously, with muscle weakness that presents with difficulty in swallowing or that prevents children from performing tasks they could manage previously, such as competing in gym classes, lifting objects, or climbing onto a high stool. Skin symptoms such as swollen and discolored upper eyelids, a confluent rash on the cheeks that increases to become telangiectatic, and scaling begin to develop. Subcutaneous calcifications may appear, making the skin feel unusually firm. Muscle breakdown leads to the appearance of creatine phosphokinase and aldolase in the serum. A muscle biopsy or electromyography reveals a lack of electrical activity in muscle fibers.

High-dose corticosteroids, methotrexate, or specific immunosuppressants are the drugs of choice to improve muscle strength. Children who survive beyond the first year after diagnosis have a good prognosis for prolonged remissions, although they are more susceptible to developing cancer later in life.

THE MUSCULAR DYSTROPHIES

The muscular dystrophies are a group of more than 30 genetic diseases characterized by progressive weakness and degeneration of the skeletal muscles that control movement. Duchenne muscular dystrophy is caused by an absence of dystrophin (a protein in the muscles) that is necessary for muscle contraction due to genetic mutation (The Muscular Dystrophy Association, 2016).

Types

Muscular dystrophies seen in children are classified into three main types: congenital myotonic dystrophy, facioscapulohumeral muscular dystrophy, and pseudohypertrophic muscular dystrophy (Duchenne disease).

Congenital Myotonic Dystrophy

Congenital myotonic dystrophy is inherited as an autosomal dominant trait. Because the disease process begins in utero, the infant may already have severe myotonia (muscle weakness) at birth. Muscle degeneration continues until adequate respiratory muscle movement becomes difficult. Diagnosis is by serum enzyme analysis and muscle biopsy. Most of these infants die before they are 1 year old because they cannot sustain respiratory function.

Facioscapulohumeral Muscular Dystrophy

Facioscapulohumeral muscular dystrophy is inherited as a dominant trait carried on chromosome 4. Symptoms begin after the child is 10 years old. The predominant symptom is facial weakness. The child becomes unable to wrinkle the forehead and cannot whistle. Serum enzyme analysis and muscle biopsy are used in diagnosis. The symptoms usually progress so slowly a normal life span is possible.

Pseudohypertrophic Muscular Dystrophy (Duchenne Disease)

Duchenne disease, the most common form of muscular dystrophy, is inherited as a sex-linked recessive trait. Therefore, it occurs only in boys, although a mother who carries the gene may demonstrate some symptoms. Symptoms are usually apparent by 3 years of age.

Assessment

Children with Duchenne muscular dystrophy usually have a history of meeting motor milestones, such as sitting, walking, and standing, but they reach these milestones later than does the average infant. By about 3 years of age, symptoms become acute and obvious as boys develop a waddling gait and have difficulty climbing stairs. They can rise from the floor only by rolling onto their stomachs and then pushing themselves to their knees. To stand, they press their hands against their ankles, knees, and thighs (they "walk up their front"), called a Gower sign. They may walk on their toes, which leads to the development of a short heel cord. Speech and swallowing become difficult. It may be awkward to lift a young child with this condition by placing your hands under the axillae because the child seems to slip through your hands due to the lax shoulder muscles. In contrast, calf muscles are hypertrophied (measure larger than normal) because the muscles become so degenerated they are replaced by fat and connective tissue.

As the disease progresses, muscle weakness becomes more and more pronounced. Scoliosis of the spine and fractures of long bones may occur from abnormal muscle tension and lack of muscle support. By junior high school age, most boys become wheelchair dependent. Tachycardia can occur as the heart muscle weakens and enlarges. Pneumonia develops easily as the child's cough reflex becomes weak and ineffective. Death from pulmonary dysfunction tends to occur at about 20 years of age.

The diagnosis is based on the history and physical findings, a muscle biopsy showing fibrous degeneration and fatty deposits, electromyography showing a decrease in amplitude and duration of motor unit potentials, an increased concentration of serum creatine phosphokinase, and genetic analysis.

Therapeutic Management

Encourage boys with muscular dystrophy to remain ambulatory for as long as possible by a program of active and passive daily range-of-motion exercises. Splinting and bracing may be necessary to maintain lower extremity stability and to avoid contractures. If children become overweight, remaining ambulatory becomes even more difficult for them. Therefore, encourage a low-calorie, high-protein diet to avoid excessive weight gain. In addition, to prevent constipation because of poor abdominal muscle tone, encourage a high intake of fiber and fluids. Advocate for a stool softener if necessary. In the meantime, corticosteroid therapy is helpful to increase function and strength at least on a short-term basis; help parents understand the importance of this and have a set schedule of administration. Newer therapies include cell repair, gene transfer, and stem cell (Strehle & Straub, 2015).

The average life expectancy of these patients has doubled and now stands at about 25 years (Strehle & Straub, 2015). Because the disease is progressive, assist the child and family with achieving the optimal level of activity within the child's limitations. Provide support for parents to assist them with coping because they can become depressed as disease symptoms progress.

QSEN Checkpoint Question 51.4

QUALITY IMPROVEMENT

Jeffrey's mother said she was worried her son might be developing muscular dystrophy. A clinical care map for children who have this disease should prioritize which action?

a. Urging them to rest most of the day to avoid systemic fatigue
b. Helping them to avoid weight gain so they can be mobile longer
c. Cautioning them not to eat foods that contain purines
d. Encouraging a diet rich in calcium to prevent osteoporosis

Look in Appendix A for the best answer and rationale.

FRACTURES

A fracture is a break in the continuity or structure of bone. Because children experience falls during their growth years, fractures of long bones are common childhood injuries. Various types are described in Table 51.2. Fractures in children tend to be different than in adults because:

- Bone in childhood is fairly porous, allowing bones to bend rather than break.
- The periosteum is thick, so the bone may not break all the way through.
- Epiphyseal lines may cushion a blow so that the bone does not break.
- Healing is rapid as a result of overall increased bone growth.

TABLE 51.2 COMMON FRACTURES IN CHILDREN

Type of Fracture	Description
Plastic deformation (bend)	Bone bends, causing a microscopic fracture line that does not cross the bone; most common in the ulna and fibula
Buckle (torus)	Fracture on the tension side of the bone near softened metaphyseal bone, causing a buckling and raised area on the harder diaphyseal bone (opposite side)
Greenstick	Bone bent with fracture beginning but not crossing through the bone
Complete	Bone divided (either transversely [crosswise at right angle to long axis of bone], obliquely [slanted but straight], or spirally [slanted and circular]); bone remnants possibly attached by a periosteal hinge

Because of the high resilience of immature bone, many fractures in early childhood are the greenstick variety (one side of a bone is broken; the other is only bent). These fractures cause minimal pain, swelling, or deformity, the usual hallmarks of a fracture.

Many fractures in children, however, occur at the epiphyseal line. These types of fractures can be serious because bone growth occurs at this point. Damage to the area can lead to undergrowth, overgrowth, or uneven growth, resulting in angulation. If a fall occurred from a high distance or was caused by a violent force, such as a speeding automobile, breaks may be complex, or the formation may be compounded (the bone pierces the skin) or comminuted (parts of the bone are fragmented). These injuries are always serious because the severed bone may lacerate nerves or blood vessels. The open wound may become infected, and correction will most likely involve surgery with the risks of anesthesia.

The healing of bone is relatively slow compared with other body injuries. Immediately after a fracture, a hematoma forms at the site of the break; over the next several days, granulation tissue is laid down. Over the next several weeks, osteoblasts invade this new tissue, and calcium is deposited (termed *callus*) to form new bone. By the time a callus formation is extensive (enough for movement at the fracture site to be impossible), clinical healing or clinical union has occurred. Complete healing does not occur until all of the temporary callus formation has been replaced by mature bone cells and the bone has once more regained its normal shape and contour.

Several complications may occur during this process. One is fat embolus, which is the release of fat from the marrow of the broken bone into the bloodstream. This embolus then travels to the cerebral vessels and causes symptoms such as confusion or hallucinations as the oxygen supply to brain cells is shut off. It also could become a pulmonary embolus, producing

dyspnea, tachycardia, and cyanosis. A second problem that can occur is *compartment syndrome*, which was discussed previously (Najarian, 2013).

If there is a great deal of edema present in the injured part, a splint or a cast may be applied but split or bivalved on each side to allow for swelling to decrease to avoid compartment syndrome. If the growth plate was severely involved in the injury, some children may need bone-lengthening or bone-shortening procedures later in life to assure equal and adequate bone growth.

Assessment

When children are seen in an emergency department for multiple trauma, observe the extremities closely for the hallmark signs of fracture (deformity, edema, and pain). If you do suspect a fracture, splint the extremity to avoid further trauma. Splinting also reduces pain because it prevents further movement of the bone. Splints should extend from a joint above to a joint below the suspected fracture site to prevent movement and muscle tension, which could cause further dislocation of the fracture. For example, for a fracture of the forearm, the splint should reach from above the elbow to below the wrist. If an extremity is so seriously deformed by the break that it will not conform to the contour of a splint, do not attempt to move it into a splint position. Immobilize the extremity by placing sandbags on the sides of the arm or leg and leave it in that position.

Perform a thorough history of how the fracture occurred. Some fractures in childhood occur from child maltreatment. This must be ruled out for all unintentional injuries.

Therapeutic Management

All children with a suspected fracture need an X-ray to confirm the diagnosis and to determine the alignment and

apposition (the amount of end-to-end contact there is of the bone fragments). Apposition is not as important in children as it is in adults, so bayonet or side-to-side apposition may be established for children up to 10 or 12 years old. With this, as the child grows and remodeling occurs, the bone will develop with normal contour and length. Side-to-side apposition has the advantage of allowing for a rapid, strong union and actually is the preferred position for some fractures.

If skin over the fracture site has been broken, the child may need tetanus prophylaxis and IV antibiotics. A hematocrit determination to estimate blood loss and cross-matching for replacement therapy may be necessary if a long bone such as a femur was fractured in trauma.

All children with fractures are in some pain. Usually, they are frightened not only from the pain, the appearance of the fracture, and their inability to use the extremity but also from the frightening situation that led to the fracture such as a fall from a bunk bed or an automobile accident. Spend time comforting and helping children to realize they are now safe and will not be injured further. Provide analgesia so they can relax enough to not move the fractured extremity, decreasing the pain. Reassure both children and parents that, unless the bone has been crushed, bone fragments can be brought back into line, allowing the break to heal with the same strength the bone had prior to being fractured.

Types of Fractures

Forearm Fractures

Because children often fall on an outstretched arm, fractures of the forearm are a common type. Most forearm fractures in children involve the distal third; a smaller number of such accidents occur in the middle or proximal third. Only the radius, both the radius and ulna, or a displacement of the epiphyseal plate of the radius may be involved. In young children, the injury usually is a greenstick or an incomplete fracture.

If a greenstick fracture is slight so that the degree of angulation is not great, it may not be reduced or brought into a straight line; as callus is formed and the bone remodels itself, it will naturally straighten into good alignment. Sometimes, greenstick fractures are broken completely before casting to prevent the bone's resuming its "bent" position within the cast. Refer to this as "straightening" the bone rather than "breaking" the bone so it sounds less frightening.

If the fracture is complete and overriding is excessive, traction to the fingers may be used as a part of the cast. This "banjo" traction is cumbersome and limits the child's use of that hand. You may need to reassure parents that, although the cast is more cumbersome than they anticipated, their child will be able to manage it well with a little practice.

Elbow Fractures

If a child falls and stops the fall with a hand, the elbow may hyperextend, transmitting the force of the blow to the distal humerus and causing a supracondylar fracture of the humerus. Fractures of this kind are reduced and stabilized with an arm cast, a splint, traction, or open surgery depending on the position of the fracture. Elevating the cast on pillows or suspending the hand by a strip of gauze or traction apparatus reduces edema. Although the fracture may be minor, the child needs to be assessed carefully for signs of blood vessel or nerve compression (Volkmann contracture).

Volkmann Ischemic Contracture

When an arm is flexed and put into a cast, the radial artery and nerve can be compressed at the elbow, causing nerve injury or severe impairment of circulation. If symptoms of compression are present but not detected within 6 hours, Volkmann contracture and possible permanent damage to the arm will result. The arm is left permanently flexed at the elbow. The wrist is hyperextended, and the fingers assume a flexed, clawlike, and useless position. If a child is going to be discharged from a healthcare facility after application of a cast, inform parents about the symptoms of compression so they can continue to assess for its development. If a child is admitted to the hospital after cast application, the radial pulse (if palpable at the edge of the cast) should be taken hourly, along with checks for coldness, blanching, and color of the fingers, during the first 8 hours. In some instances, a cast is applied incompletely for 24 hours, the elbow portion being simply splinted and wrapped with elastic bandages. After 24 hours, when edema has subsided and the chance of compression is less, the rest of the arm is then casted.

Epiphyseal Separations of the Radius

If a child breaks a fall with an outstretched arm, the separation of the epiphysis of the distal radius may result. When this occurs, the wrist must be casted to restabilize the epiphysis. Although epiphyseal injuries are always serious, distal radial injury rarely causes serious sequelae in children. Advise parents, however, that it is important to keep appointments for follow-up visits so that growth disturbances can be detected early. Stapling the epiphysis or stimulation of the epiphyseal line may be done to arrest abnormal growth if it occurs.

Clavicle Fractures

When young children catch themselves during a fall with an outstretched arm, the force of the blow can be transmitted to the clavicle, causing a fracture of the clavicle or dislocation at the sternal joint. Clavicles also may be fractured during birth and are often fractured playing football. These fractures need to be evaluated carefully because they also could be a mark of child maltreatment.

QSEN Checkpoint Question 51.5

TEAMWORK & COLLABORATION

A nurse is collaborating with a licensed practical nurse in the care of a child with an elbow cast. What information about an elbow cast should all care team members to be aware of?

   a. The cast must be constructed from fiberglass, not plaster of Paris.

   b. Edema at the elbow from a too tight cast can cause severe nerve damage.

   c. The child should expect to have low-grade pain following application.

   d. These casts often get dirty and so lead to humeral osteomyelitis.

Look in Appendix A for the best answer and rationale.

Swelling is often present at the site of the break. In the newborn, a Moro reflex can only be demonstrated on the unaffected side. An older child refuses to use the arm, leaving it hanging at the side. Crepitus (crackling) can be felt over the clavicle. After an X-ray diagnosis, if the bone fragments are not displaced, the child is placed in a commercially manufactured or figure-of-eight splint or stockinette placed over the shoulders and under the axilla, which keeps the arm adducted and flexed across the chest. Caution the parents to keep the splint dry—no swimming or showering during this time—and how to observe it every morning to check that it is firmly in place or if it needs tightening. Because the splint is left in place for about 3 weeks, the wrap becomes extremely soiled. Parents are usually apologetic about the appearance of the splint when they return for a repeat X-ray. They may be worried the soiled appearance of the splint reflects the quality of their housekeeping or child care. You can assure them that a soiled appearance is expected and proof they followed instructions well to leave the splint in place.

Some parents may need reassurance that a simple splint is adequate therapy. Acknowledge their concern but also assure them that treatment for nondisplaced broken clavicles are the exception to the usual fracture treatment. Indications for operative treatment include fractures that are open, complicated comminuted fractures, and fractures with neurovascular compromise or greater than 100% displacement (width of the clavicle) where skin is tented (Arora, Fichadia, Hartwig, et al., 2014).

Dislocation of the Radial Head

If a small child is lifted by one hand, as happens when a parent pulls on one arm to lift the child over a curb or up a step, the head of the radius may escape the ligament surrounding it and become dislocated (nursemaid's elbow) (Vitello, Dvorkin, Sattler, et al., 2014). The child holds the arm flexed at the elbow with the forearm pronated. The child winces with pain when the radial head is palpated.

A simple dislocation of the radial head can be reduced in an emergency room by gentle pressure on the radial head while the arm is flexed and supinated. Relief of pain is immediate, and the child begins to use the arm again.

Parents feel guilty because they caused this dislocation. You can reassure them that this is a common injury in small children but that they need to avoid lifting their child in this manner again. Be aware, however, that a dislocation of the radial head can occur from extremely rough handling, as is seen in child maltreatment. Investigate the circumstances of the injury closely (Cicero, 2013).

QSEN Checkpoint Question 51.6

EVIDENCE-BASED PRACTICE

Young children between the ages of 1 and 4 years frequently sustain dislocation of the radial head at the elbow that is often associated with the history of a pull to the arm, such as when a child is lifted by their arm or pulled at the wrist to prevent a fall. This is often referred to as a nursemaid's elbow or a radial head subluxation. The left arm is affected more often than the right in both males and females, likely due to right hand dominance; and for unclear reasons, females are at greater risk for sustaining the injury (Vitello et al., 2014).

Based on this literature, which activity should the nurse advise Jeffrey not to do with his preschool sister?
   a. Swinging her by the arms to make her laugh
   b. Encouraging her to practice hip-hop dancing
   c. Helping her to fly her kite on a windy afternoon
   d. Helping her take off a tight sweater or shirt

Look in Appendix A for the best answer and rationale.

Fracture of the Femur

Children who are involved in automobile accidents or who fall from considerable heights and land on their feet may suffer a fractured femur. Child maltreatment should be considered in an infant who sustains a fractured femur because there are few normal instances when a fracture of this magnitude should occur in an infant. That the break was caused by the presence of a bone malignancy (see Chapter 53) is a third possibility.

Even with closed femoral fractures, blood loss can be extensive because of the size of the bone broken. As the child lies on the examining table in the emergency department, the child tends to hold the leg externally rotated and the thigh may appear abnormally short or deformed. Often, the child is in a great deal of pain, possibly with signs of shock from pain and blood loss. Children are frightened as well by the force of the accident that caused such a severe injury.

In the past, fractured femurs were not casted immediately because strong tendon spasms cause poor alignment and overriding of the femur segments. Only after the muscle spasm had been reduced enough by skeletal or Bryant traction to allow close approximation of the bone edges (7 to 14 days) was the child removed from traction and placed in a hip spica cast. Today, a child may be taken to surgery immediately to have an intramedullary rod placed to align and stabilize the fracture. No cast may be required. Help children and families identify ways for children to continue contact with friends or enjoy usual activities during the time of restricted activity.

What If . . . 51.4

A nurse is particularly interested in exploring one of the 2020 National Health Goals with respect to musculoskeletal disorders in children (see Box 51.1). What would be a possible research topic pertinent to this goal that would be applicable to Jeffrey's family and that would also advance evidence-based practice?

KEY POINTS FOR REVIEW

- Bone and muscle disorders tend to be long-term disorders. Help children and their families to think about how the disorder will affect tasks of daily living to help a child better adjust to interventions such as a cast or brace. Help children plan self-diversional activities as necessary, so they can continue to grow developmentally while confined to a cast or traction.

- As a rule, children with a broken bone need additional calcium in their diet to aid bone healing. If they are on strict bed rest, however, this should only be a moderate addition to their diet to prevent renal calculi from forming.

- Many children have casts applied to allow broken bones to heal. If broken bones cannot be easily aligned, children are placed in traction.

- Developmental disorders that occur in children include flat feet (pronation), genu varum (bowlegs), and genu valgum (knock knees). The majority of these disorders are corrected naturally by normal growth.

- Slipped capital epiphysis is the slipping of the femur head in relation to the neck of the femur at the epiphyseal line. It occurs most frequently in obese or rapidly growing boys. It may require surgery or possibly a total hip replacement for treatment.

- Osteomyelitis is an infection of the bone. Because it can result in extensive destruction of bone, both IV and oral antibiotic therapy is necessary.

- Scoliosis is a lateral curvature of the spine. It is treated by bracing or surgery.

- JIA occurs in several different forms: polyarticular, pauciarticular, and systemic onset. Therapy includes exercise, heat application, and the administration of medications such as NSAIDs or methotrexate. Stressing the importance of these measures helps in planning nursing care that not only meets Quality & Safety Education for Nurses (QSEN) competencies but also best meets a family's total needs.

- Myasthenia gravis can occur in three types: neonatal transient myasthenia, congenital myasthenia, and juvenile myasthenia. Anticholinesterase drugs such as neostigmine, which prolong ACh action, are used.

- Muscular dystrophies are a group of disorders that lead to progressive degeneration of skeletal muscles. Common types that occur in children include congenital myotonic, facioscapulohumeral, and pseudohypertrophic. Children and parents need support throughout this long-term illness.

- A fracture or bruise of soft tissue can result from any trauma, including child maltreatment. Be certain to secure a detailed history of all injuries to be certain the history is consistent with the degree of injury.

- Volkmann ischemic contracture is a complication that occurs when an arm is casted in a bent position, which causes the radial artery and nerve to become compressed at the elbow. Frequent assessments of finger color and warmth are safeguards to detect if this is occurring when an arm cast is in place.

CRITICAL THINKING CARE STUDY

Bonnie Sue is a 12-year-old who is discovered to have scoliosis during a routine school nurse assessment. She lives with her mother and stepfather on her family's dairy farm. Her chores include helping with milking two times a day and keeping her own room clean. Her mother had "slight scoliosis" as a teenager, which didn't require treatment.

1. Bonnie's mother is concerned that her daughter developed scoliosis because she insists on wearing sneakers plus she doesn't get enough exercise because she rides a bus to school. Could these factors have contributed to the development of her scoliosis?

2. Bonnie is fitted with a spinal brace. When you see her at a return appointment, her mother tells you Bonnie has to take the brace off at night to be able to sleep and sometimes during the day because it gets too hot. What further health teaching does this family need?

3. When you ask if Bonnie Sue drinks milk daily, her mother answers, "We live on a dairy farm. What do you think?" When you ask if Bonnie Sue is able to do her usual chores, her stepfather answers, "Well, she doesn't help with milking anymore." Could you be certain from these answers that Bonnie Sue is receiving a good source of calcium necessary for strong bone growth and is adjusting well to wearing her brace?

RELATED RESOURCES

Explore these additional resources to enhance learning for this chapter:
- Student resources on thePoint, including answers to the What If . . . and Critical Thinking Care Study questions, http://thepoint.lww.com/Flagg8e
- Adaptive learning powered by PrepU, http://thepoint.lww.com /prepu

REFERENCES

Adelstein, S. J. (2014). Radiation risk in nuclear medicine. *Seminars in Nuclear Medicine, 44*(3), 187–192.

Aiyer, A., & Hennrikus, W. (2014). Foot pain in the child and adolescent. *Pediatric Clinics of North America, 61*(6), 1185–1205.

American Academy of Orthopaedic Surgeons. (2013). *Flexible flatfoot in children*. Retrieved from http://orthoinfo.aaos.org/topic.cfm?topic =a00046

American Academy of Orthopaedic Surgeons. (2015a). *Osgood-Schlatter disease (knee pain)*. Retrieved from http://orthoinfo.aaos.org/topic .cfm?topic=a00411

American Academy of Orthopaedic Surgeons. (2015b). *Perthes disease*. Retrieved from http://orthoinfo.aaos.org/topic.cfm?topic=A00070

American Academy of Orthopaedic Surgeons. (2015c). *Position statement: Screening for the early detection of idiopathic scoliosis in adolescents*. Retrieved from https://posna.org/POSNA/media/Documents/Position %20Statements/1122-Screening-for-the-Early-Detection-of-Idiopathic -Scoliosis-in-Adoles_12-28.pdf

American College of Radiology. (2014). *Practice parameter for the performance of skeletal scintigraphy (bone scan)*. Retrieved from http://www .acr.org/~/media/839771405B9A43F7AF2D2A9982D81083.pdf

Arora, R., Fichadia, U., Hartwig, E., et al. (2014). Pediatric upper-extremity fractures. *Pediatric Annals, 43*(5), 196–204.

Bennison, J. M., & Horn, P. L. (2015). Pediatric patients with slipped capital femoral epiphysis with knee pain. *The Journal for Nurse Practitioners, 11*(10), 954–959.

Bird, S. J. (2016). *Treatment of myasthenia gravis*. Retrieved from https:// www.uptodate.com/contents/treatment-of-myasthenia-gravis

Cicero, M. X. (2013). Musculoskeletal injuries. In D. Cline & O. J. Ma (Eds.), *Tintinalli's emergency medicine* (7th ed., pp. 287–293). New York, NY: McGraw-Hill.

Cobetto, N., Aubin, C. E., Parent, S., et al. (2016). Effectiveness of braces designed using computer-aided design and manufacturing (CAD/CAM) and finite element simulation compared to CAD/CAM only for the conservative treatment of adolescent idiopathic scoliosis: A prospective randomized controlled trial. *European Spine Journal, 25*(10), 3056–3064.

Cook, P. (2014). Transient synovitis, septic hip, and Legg-Calve-Perthes disease: An approach to the correct diagnosis. *Pediatric Clinics of North America, 61*, 1109–1118.

Dede, O., Demirkiran, G., & Yazici, M. (2014). 2014 Update on the 'growing spine surgery' for young children with scoliosis. *Current Opinion in Pediatrics, 26*(1), 57–63.

Escott, B. G., De La Rocha, A., Jo, C., et al. (2015). Patient-reported health outcomes after in situ percutaneous fixation for slipped capital femoral epiphysis: An average twenty-year follow-up study. *The Journal of Bone and Joint Surgery. American Volume, 97*(23), 1929–1934.

Hald, J., Evangelou, E., Langdahl, B., et al. (2015). Bisphosphonates for the prevention of fractures in osteogenesis imperfecta: Meta-analysis of placebo-controlled trials. *Journal of Bone and Mineral Research, 30*(5), 929–933.

Hoogwout, S., Paananen, M., Smith, A., et al. (2015). Musculoskeletal pain is associated with restless legs syndrome in young adults. *BMC Musculoskeletal Disorders, 16*, 294.

Hresko, M. T. (2013). Idiopathic scoliosis in adolescents. *New England Journal of Medicine, 368*, 834–841.

Jeong, H. J., Lee, S. H., & Ko, C. S. (2012). Meniscectomy. *Knee Surgery & Related Research, 24*(3), 129–136.

Kabiri, L., Tapley, H., & Tapley, S. (2014). Evaluation and conservative treatment for Osgood-Schlatter disease: A critical review of the literature. *International Journal of Therapy & Rehabilitation, 21*(2), 91–96.

Karakis, I., Liew, W., Darras, B. T., et al. (2014). Referral and diagnostic trends in pediatric electromyography in the molecular era. *Muscle & Nerve, 50*, 244–249.

Karch, A. M. (2016). *2016 Lippincott's nursing drug guide.* Philadelphia, PA: Wolters Kluwer.

Keskin, M., Akgül, T., Bayraktar, A., et al. (2014). Superior mesenteric artery syndrome: An infrequent complication of scoliosis surgery. *Case Reports in Surgery, 2014*, 1–5.

Kim, P., & Rosenblum, B. (2014). Diagnosing osteomyelitis. *Podiatry Management, 33*(6), 99–102.

Koller, H., Zenner, J., Gajic, V., et al. (2012). The impact of halo-gravity traction on curve rigidity and pulmonary function in the treatment of severe and rigid scoliosis and kyphoscoliosis. *European Spine Journal, 21*(3), 514–529.

Lee, C., Lightdale-Miric, N., Chang, E., et al. (2014). Silent compartment syndrome in children: A report of five cases. *Journal of Pediatric Orthopaedics, Part B, 23*, 467–471.

Liew, W. M., Powell, C. A., Sloan, S. R., et al. (2014). Comparison of plasmapheresis and intravenous immunoglobulin as maintenance therapies for juvenile myasthenia gravis. *JAMA Neurology, 71*, 575–580.

Liu, L., Hoelscher, U., & Yao, Z. (2013). *Cultural diversity—new challenge to medical device use safety for international markets.* Retrieved from https://www.researchgate.net/profile/Long_Liu6/publication/272029595_Cultural_Diversity_-New_Challenge_to_Medical_Device_Use_Safety_for_International_Markets/links/54d9ab070cf24647581f06e1/Cultural-Diversity-New-Challenge-to-Medical-Device-Use-Safety-for-International-Markets.pdf?origin=publication_detail

Loder, R. T., & Dietz, F. R. (2012). What is the best evidence for the treatment of slipped capital femoral epiphysis? *Journal of Pediatric Orthopedics, 32*(Suppl. 2), S158–S165.

Matkovic, V., & Visy, D. (2015). Nutrition and bone health during skeletal modeling and bone consolidation of childhood and adolescence. In M. F. Holick & J. W. Nieves (Eds.), *Nutrition and bone health* (2nd ed., pp. 199–216). New York, NY: Springer Publishing.

McClung, A. (2015). Preoperative and postoperative care including use of halo-gravity traction. In Y. Wang, O. Boachie-Adjei, & L. Lenke (Eds.), *Spinal osteotomy* (pp. 239–244). Dordrecht, Netherlands: Springer Publishing.

Morello, R., & Esposito, P. W. (2012). *Osteogenesis imperfecta.* Retrieved from http://cdn.intechweb.org/pdfs/28140.pdf

Mudge, A., Bau, K., Purcell, L., et al. (2014). Normative reference values for lower limb joint range, bone torsion, and alignment in children aged 4-16 years. *Journal of Pediatric Orthopaedics, Part B, 23*(1), 15–25.

Najarian, S. L. (2013). Compartment syndrome. In D. Cline & O. J. Ma (Eds.), *Tintinalli's emergency medicine* (7th ed., pp. 615–616). New York, NY: McGraw-Hill.

Ringold, S., Weiss, P. F., Beukelman, T., et al. (2013). 2013 Update of the 2011 American College of Rheumatology recommendations for the treatment of juvenile idiopathic arthritis: Recommendations for the medical therapy of children with systemic juvenile idiopathic arthritis and tuberculosis screening among children receiving biologic medications. *Arthritis and Rheumatism, 65*, 2499–2512.

Ringold, S., Weiss, P. F., Colbert, R. A., et al. (2014). Childhood Arthritis and Rheumatology Research Alliance consensus treatment plans for new-onset polyarticular juvenile idiopathic arthritis. *Arthritis Care & Research, 66*(7), 1063–1072.

Sabharwal, S. (2015). Blount disease. An update. *Orthopedic Clinics of North America, 46*, 37–47.

Schreiber, V., Illingworth, K., & Ward, W. (2016). Treating orthopaedic infections in pediatric patients. *Operative Techniques in Orthopaedics, 26*(1), 12–19.

Sherry, D. D., Bhaskar, A. R., Poduval, M., et al. (2016). *Juvenile idiopathic arthritis.* Retrieved from http://emedicine.medscape.com/article/1007276

Soep, J. B. (2012). Rheumatic diseases. In W. W. Hay Jr., M. J. Levin, R. R. Deterding, et al. (Eds.), *Current diagnosis & treatment: Pediatrics* (21st ed., pp. 889–896). New York, NY: McGraw-Hill/Lange.

Stehlik, R., Ulfberg, J., Hedner, J., et al. (2014). High prevalence of restless legs syndrome among women with multi-site pain: A population-based study in Dalarna, Sweden. *European Journal of Pain, 18*(10), 1402–1409.

Stepanovich, M., Mundis, G., & Yaszay, B. (2015). Complications of the treatment of adolescent idiopathic scoliosis. *Seminars in Spine Surgery, 27*, 58–61.

Strehle, E., & Straub, V. (2015). Recent advances in the management of Duchenne muscular dystrophy. *Archives of Disease in Childhood, 100*(12), 1173–1177.

Tafin-Kampé, K., & Kamsu-Foguem, B. (2013). Acute osteomyelitis due to Staphylococcus aureus in children: What is the status of treatment today? *Pediatric Infectious Disease, 5*(3), 122–126.

The Muscular Dystrophy Association. (2016). *Duchenne muscular dystrophy (DMD).* Retrieved from https://www.mda.org/disease/duchenne-muscular-dystrophy

Traina, F., De Fine, M., Abati, C. N., et al. (2012). Outcomes of total hip replacement in patients with slipped capital femoral epiphysis. *Archives of Orthopedic Trauma Surgery, 132*(8), 1133–1139.

U.S. Department of Health and Human Services. (2010). *Healthy people 2020.* Washington, DC: Author.

VanderPluym, J., Vajsar, J., Jacob, F., et al. (2013). Clinical characteristics of pediatric myasthenia: A surveillance study. *Pediatrics, 132*(4), E939–E944.

Vitello, S., Dvorkin, R., Sattler, S., et al. (2014). Epidemiology of nursemaid's elbow. *Western Journal of Emergency Medicine, 15*, 554–557.

Wiegerinck, J., Zwiers, R., Sierevelt, I., et al. (2016). Treatment of calcaneal apophysitis: Wait and see versus orthotic device versus physical therapy: A pragmatic therapeutic randomized clinical trial. *Journal of Pediatric Orthopaedics, 36*(2), 152–157.

Zbinden, I., Rutz, E., Jacobson, J. A., et al. (2015). Tibial bowing in children—what is normal? A radiographic study. *European Radiology, 25*, 3459–3471.

52

Nursing Care of a Family When a Child Has an Unintentional Injury

Jason Varton is 10 years old; his sister Sage is 4 years old. An electrical fire started while the Varton family was sleeping. Jason jumped out of a window and hit his head on a cement walkway when the carpet caught on fire. Although his only visible sign of trauma is a reddened edematous area on his forehead, his temperature is 99.4°F (37.5°C); respirations are 18 breaths/min; pulse is 62 beats/min; and blood pressure is 110/62 mmHg. His left pupil appears more dilated than his right, and it reacts sluggishly to light. The children's father was able to rescue Sage and exit the house through the door but not before she suffered third-degree burns on her arms, hands, and neck.

Previous chapters described the growth and development of well children and care of children with disorders of specific body systems. This chapter adds information about the characteristic changes, both physical and psychosocial, that occur when children experience an unintentional injury.

Suppose you are a triage nurse. Would you rate Jason and Sage as children who need to be seen immediately, or could they be given second priority?

OBJECTIVES

After mastering the contents of this chapter, you should be able to:

1. Describe the causes and consequences of common unintentional injuries in childhood and measures to prevent them.

2. Identify 2020 National Health Goals related to children who have experienced trauma that nurses can help the nation achieve (Box 52.1).

3. Assess a child with unintentional injuries.

4. Formulate nursing diagnoses related to an unintentionally injured child.

5. Establish expected outcomes for an unintentionally injured child that can help parents manage seamless transitions across differing healthcare settings.

6. Using the nursing process, plan nursing care that includes the six competencies of Quality & Safety Education for Nurses (QSEN): Patient-Centered Care, Teamwork & Collaboration, Evidence-Based Practice (EBP), Quality Improvement (QI), Safety, and Informatics.

7. Implement nursing care for a child with an unintentional injury, such as providing pain relief.

8. Evaluate expected outcomes for achievement and effectiveness of care.

9. Integrate knowledge of unintentional injury in children with the interplay of nursing process, the six competencies of QSEN, and Family Nursing to achieve quality maternal and child health nursing care.

BOX 52.1

Nursing Care Planning Based on 2020 National Health Goals

Because prevention of unintentional injuries could have both immediate and long-term effects on the nation's health, several 2020 National Health Goals are concerned with preventing unintentional injuries in children:

- Reduce the number of drowning deaths each year from a baseline of 1.2 per 100,000 to 1.1 per 100,000.
- Reduce sports and recreational injuries from 46.6 per 100,000 to 41.9 per 100,000.
- Reduce the rate of firearm-related deaths from a baseline of 10.2 per 100,000 to 9.2 per 100,000.
- Prevent an increase of poisonings deaths from a baseline of 13.1 per 100,000 (maintain baseline value).
- Reduce the number of deaths caused by suffocation in infants age 0 to 12 months from a baseline of 22.5 per 100,000 to 20.3 per 100,000 infants.
- Reduce unintentional injury deaths from 40.1 per 100,000 to 36.0 per 100,000 (U.S. Department of Health and Human Services, 2010; see www.healthypeople.gov).

Nurses can help the nation achieve these goals by providing counseling on safety precautions to parents and children. Always help assess whether injuries were unintentional or possibly a result of child maltreatment or self-injury.

According to the Centers for Disease Control and Prevention (CDC, 2017) Childhood Injury Report updated in 2015, the leading cause of morbidity and mortality among children in the United States is unintentional injuries caused by burns, drowning, falls, poisoning, and motor vehicle accidents. More than 12,000 children die and 9.2 million are treated in emergency departments due to unintentional injuries yearly in the United States. For this reason, all healthcare providers must be aware of how to prevent, care for, and treat childhood injuries.

The National Action Plan for Child Injury Prevention was developed by the CDC to help raise awareness about child injuries and how they affect our nation, highlighting prevention goals and strategies, and to mobilize coordinated efforts to reduce childhood injuries (see the CDC website for additional information at www.cdc.gov/safechild/publications.html) (CDC, 2016b).

Nursing Process Overview

FOR CARE OF A CHILD WITH AN UNINTENTIONAL INJURY

ASSESSMENT

When children are seen at healthcare facilities because of unintentional injuries, neither they nor their parents may be functioning at their optimal level because of the stress of the situation. Both may be apprehensive and frightened not only about what *has* happened but also about what could have happened. Children often feel guilty and worry they will be scolded or punished. Their parents can feel equally guilty because they realize they could have been watching more

closely, causing them to act defensively. Remember people under stress do not process information well, so parents may not perceive the information you give them correctly. All information you supply in an emergency department, therefore, may need to be repeated after the immediate care is completed.

Children are likely to be in pain and may be confused because they count on their parents to keep them safe, but yet they have been hurt. Trust is momentarily broken. How can they be safe in the hospital if their parents are no longer protecting them?

NURSING DIAGNOSIS

Nursing diagnoses need to address not only the physical injury a child sustained but also the psychological or emotional trauma both the child and the parents are experiencing. Examples of possible nursing diagnoses are:

- Pain related to fractured tibia from sports injury
- Ineffective airway clearance related to effect of burned esophageal tissue
- Impaired physical mobility related to severe burn injury
- Disturbed body image related to change in physical appearance from thermal injury
- Parental fear related to outcome after head injury in child
- Interrupted family processes related to child's unintentional injury
- Anxiety related to apprehension and lack of knowledge regarding medical treatment of child

OUTCOME IDENTIFICATION AND PLANNING

Parents in an emergency department are rarely ready for long-term planning; they often have great difficulty in just answering the most straightforward, immediate questions. As a result, long-term planning may have to be delayed until the shock of the injury has passed.

On discharge from the emergency department, be certain parents have printed as well as oral instructions about the child's care, the name and number of the person to contact if they have questions about care or progress, and an appointment (or the number to call for a return appointment) for follow-up care. If a child is admitted to the hospital from the emergency department, it's helpful if the nurse who cared for the child in the emergency department can accompany the child to the hospital unit because the first person who cares for a child after an injury assumes a very important role to the child and parents because that person was the first one to recognize their distress. A transition period, or "passing on of care," helps a parent accept the child's new caregivers as being as dependable and trustworthy as the emergency department staff.

A key component of nursing intervention in an emergency department is to help parents understand why an injury happened and plan ways to make their immediate or community environment safe for children. Organizations that might be appropriate for referral are the American Association of Poison Control Centers (www.aapcc.org), the American Burn Association (www.ameriburn.org), the American Academy of Pediatrics (www.aap.org), and, for advice on cardiac resuscitation, the American Heart Association (www.heart.org).

IMPLEMENTATION

The extent of a child's injury depends on the injuring agent, the part of the body that was injured, and often the immediate care, including both physical and psychological management that a child receives.

Be certain to maintain standard infection precautions in emergency situations the same as at any other time. Remember parental consent must be obtained for treatment procedures even in an emergency, except for lifesaving actions, such as cardiopulmonary resuscitation (CPR) (it is assumed parents would consent to lifesaving procedures, and delaying procedures until they can be located could result in permanent disability or death).

OUTCOME EVALUATION

After an injury, children need follow-up care to be certain the immediate interventions were adequate and successful healing is taking place. Evaluation visits are also a time to determine whether the child's environment has been changed so the child is safer now than at the time of the injury (if applicable).

If an injury could not have been anticipated, parents appreciate hearing one more time that such an injury could not have been avoided and that they are good parents because this helps them maintain adequate self-esteem to continue to function well as parents.

Examples of expected outcomes suggesting achievement of goals are:

- The child swallows fluids without distress after esophageal burns.
- The child states pain is at tolerable level within 20 minutes after administration of pain medication.
- The child demonstrates full range of motion in hand after thermal injury.
- The child states he understands that wearing a seat belt is an important safety measure.
- The child states she will wear a helmet when riding a bicycle in the future.

Health Promotion and Risk Management

In every care setting, nurses have the important opportunity among healthcare professionals to provide child and family teaching concerning the prevention of unintentional injuries. After an injury has occurred, nurses can provide valuable instruction to families about safeguarding their children against future injuries. This chapter will discuss safety tips after each section that can help prevent injuries during childhood.

QSEN Checkpoint Question 52.1

EVIDENCE-BASED PRACTICE

As children develop new skills and attempt new activities, they are at increased risk for unintentional injuries. Damashek and Corlis (2017) interviewed mothers to obtain a history of their child's injuries to identify whether the behavior of the mother had a predictive relationship on the frequency of the child's injuries. Injury severity scales and measures of supervision were obtained. Supervision was defined with the following three categories: proximity, visual, and auditory. The results found that visual and proximity in combination are predictive in preventing injuries. More specifically, if the mother was near the child and in view of the child, injuries were less frequent than

any single or different combination of supervision. As the number of children in the household increased, the frequency of unintentional injuries increased.

Sage is 4 years old and sustained a burn that required hospitalization when her 10-year-old brother attempted to cook a meal while their mother was in the living room watching television. The nurse is preparing Sage for discharge from the hospital. Based on the evidence presented, the most effective advice the nurse could give to the mother to prevent future unintentional injuries is to:

a. Discuss that it is difficult to supervise children's activities when they are out of sight.
b. Inform her that a 10-year-old is not old enough to cook.
c. Suggest in the future that she keep the volume on the television low, so that she can hear what the children are doing.
d. Ask her if she has working smoke detectors and a fire extinguisher in the home.

Look in Appendix A for the best answer and rationale.

The Injured Child

Because the emergency department nurse is often the first person who sees a child after an injury, nurses need to be prepared to make a preliminary assessment of the extent of a child's injuries. Remember that children may be seriously hurt but not crying because they are in shock. They may be hemorrhaging, but if they are bleeding internally, no blood may be visibly evident. Unintentional injuries become fatal when lung, heart, or brain function becomes inadequate. These three body systems, therefore, must be evaluated first (airway, breathing, circulation, and disability, or an ABCD evaluation). Table 52.1 lists signs and symptoms to assess when determining the respiratory, cardiovascular, and neurologic status of an injured child.

TABLE 52.1 IMPORTANT ASSESSMENTS ON INITIAL EXAMINATION OF AN INJURED CHILD

Body System	Assessment
Respiratory system	Rate and quality of respirations
	Any sound of obstruction (wheezing, stridor, retractions, coughing?)
	Color (cyanotic?)
	Oxygen hunger (restlessness, inability to lie flat?)
Cardiovascular system	Color (pallor from hemorrhage or cardiovascular collapse?)
	Evident bleeding
	Pulse rate (increases with hemorrhage)
	Blood pressure (decreases with hemorrhage)
	Feeling of apprehension from altered vascular pressure
Nervous system	Level of consciousness (child answers questions coherently, infant attunes to parent's voice?)
	Pupils (equal and reacting to light?)
	Bumps or bruises on head or spinal column
	Loss of motion or sensory function in a body part

While conducting a preliminary assessment of a child's major body systems, take a brief history of the injury. What happened? How long ago did it happen? Was the child using protective equipment such as a helmet or a secured seat belt? What have the parents done? If the child fell, how far was the fall? On what body part did the child land? What do the parents think is the child's major injury (children may report one body part hurts at first but then a small cut elsewhere begins to bleed, and they focus on the minor bleeding as their major injury). If parents say, "At first, he acted as if his stomach hurt," this may be the first suggestion that he has a serious abdominal injury such as splenic rupture.

Evaluating children in an emergency department is difficult because they may be unconscious, too young to communicate, or so frightened that they cannot stop crying to report which body parts are painful or to indicate which parts should be assessed first. Spend a few minutes attempting to calm children and get them past this initial fright, unless symptoms of major body system disturbances require you to direct your immediate efforts elsewhere. Parents need frequent explanations while their child is being evaluated because as long as parents are worried and tense, children cannot be calmed easily.

A proportion of unintentional injuries in children result from child maltreatment. Conflicting histories (a parent and child recounting different stories) are a hallmark of maltreatment. Nurses are mandated reporters of child maltreatment. If you suspect an injury is intentional, a report must be made to the abuse registry so that child protection specialists can further explore the incident (see Chapter 55).

Head Trauma

Head injuries occur commonly in childhood, and most head trauma in children is minor and not associated with brain injury or long-term consequences.

Children often receive head injuries when they are involved in multiple-trauma injuries, such as motor vehicle accidents, or when they fall from swing sets, windows, or bunk beds. Other children receive head injures by being struck on the head by an object such as a baseball, rock, or hockey puck or by falling off a bicycle, especially if they're not wearing a protective helmet. Falls are the leading cause of traumatic brain injuries followed by unintentional blunt trauma and thirdly motor vehicle accidents (CDC, n.d.-b).

When providing patient education, head injury prevention tips to share with parents and children include:

1. Children should always wear a helmet when riding a bicycle, skating, or skiing.
2. Watch children closely while biking.
3. Bicycling on the street requires good bike control and ability to follow traffic rules. Young children should never be allowed to ride on the street.
4. Install car seats correctly and use the seat every time the child rides in a car.
5. Children under 4 ft 9 in. tall must sit on a car/booster seat when riding in a car.
6. Use window gates and guards to protect children from falling out.
7. Teach children how to cross the street safely by looking both ways for cars (CDC, 2017).

Head injuries are always potentially serious not only because the immediate injury can be life-threatening to the child but also because the injury can lead to complications that can be equally severe. Following a depressed skull fracture, for example, recurrent seizures and abnormalities on an electroencephalogram (EEG) as a result of scar tissue may occur.

Some children experience minor personality changes, memory deficits, or symptoms such as headache, irritability, and blurry vision (CDC, n.d.-a).

Behavioral manifestations may also include aggressiveness or poor school performance, although it may be difficult to determine whether these symptoms are organic or the result of being treated differently than before the injury by anxious parents.

IMMEDIATE ASSESSMENT

All children with head trauma need to have their neck stabilized with a brace until cervical trauma has been ruled out. They also require a neurologic assessment as soon as they are seen and again at frequent intervals to detect signs and symptoms of increased intracranial pressure (ICP) because increasing pressure puts stress on the respiratory, cardiac, and temperature centers, causing dysfunction in these areas. The mark of increased pressure is a decrease in pulse and respiratory rate and an increase in temperature and pulse pressure (the distance between the diastolic and systolic pressure). The child's pupils also become slow or unable to react immediately. Level of consciousness and motor ability also decrease.

Important assessments include vital signs, observation of the child's pupils to be certain they are equal and react to light, level of consciousness, and motor function.

IMMEDIATE MANAGEMENT

After a head injury, brain edema is likely to occur because fluid rushes into the inflamed and bruised area. ICP monitoring should be initiated (see Chapter 49). A computed tomography (CT) scan or magnetic resonance imaging (MRI) will determine areas of edema or bleeding. A central venous or central arterial line may be inserted, so pressure can be reduced with the administration of a hypertonic intravenous (IV) solution such as mannitol. As this is infused, it increases intravascular pressure and causes the edema fluid to shift back into the blood vessels. Administration of a steroid such as dexamethasone and keeping the child's head elevated are other ways to decrease inflammation and edema and lower ICP.

 Nursing Diagnoses and Related Interventions

Nursing diagnoses for children with head injuries address both the physical abnormalities that need to be corrected and the psychosocial stress that such a serious injury generates.

Nursing Diagnosis: Risk for excess fluid volume related to administration of hypertonic solution

Outcome Evaluation: Child's respiratory rate remains between 16 and 24 breaths/min; specific gravity of urine is between 1.003 and 1.030; pulse remains between 60 and 100 beats/min; blood pressure remains consistent for height and age; lungs are clear to auscultation.

When hypertonic solutions are infused intravenously to reduce cerebral edema, fluid shifts from interstitial spaces into the bloodstream, possibly resulting in blood volume overload. To detect this, assess vital signs frequently. The body evacuates this fluid by the kidneys, so it is important to keep an accurate intake and output record to ensure the kidneys are functioning; test the specific gravity of urine to detect whether pituitary compression is leading to over- or underproduction of antidiuretic hormone.

Nursing Diagnosis: Risk for delayed growth and development related to late sequelae of head injury

Outcome Evaluation: Child shows no evidence of any alteration in thought processes, seizure activity, or memory at follow-up visits. Cognitive and physical development proceed appropriately.

Caring for a child after a head injury can be difficult for parents because they are so worried about the child's condition. To help them feel a sense of control, offer information on the child's progress as it becomes available. Help parents become partners in the care of their child during the hospitalization.

SKULL FRACTURE

A skull fracture is a crack in one of the bones of the skull. Detecting skull fractures in children is important because associated cerebral injury often occurs under the fracture. Many fractures are simple linear types; most involve the parietal bones. In some children, instead of a bone fracturing, the suture lines separate. This occurs more commonly in the lambdoid suture line; a coronal suture separation is rare and, if present, indicates severe trauma (Fig. 52.1).

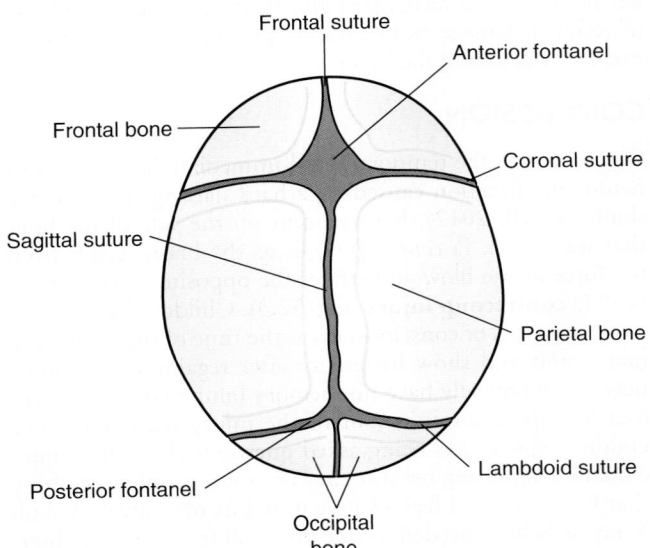

Figure 52.1 Location of suture lines of the skull.

Assessment

Skull fractures are confirmed by a skull X-ray. Make sure you have a thorough history of the injury so the mechanism of injury can be determined. If the base of the skull is fractured, a child usually exhibits ecchymosis around the eyes or behind an ear. **Rhinorrhea** or **otorrhea** (clear fluid draining from the nose or ear, respectively) may be noticeable. The fluid is cerebrospinal fluid (CSF) and is a serious finding because it means that the child's central nervous system is open to infection. If it is not clear whether the fluid is CSF or rhinitis from an allergy, test the fluid with a glucose reagent strip. CSF will test positive for glucose, whereas the clear, watery drainage from an upper respiratory tract infection or allergy will not.

If a skull fracture is linear with no underlying pathology, no treatment except observation and prescription of an analgesic is necessary. In about 3 weeks, a repeat X-ray will confirm that healing has taken place. You can assure parents that a second X-ray this soon is not harmful but necessary.

If a fracture is depressed (a bone fragment is pressing inward) or compounded (bone is broken into pieces), surgery will be necessary to remove or repair broken fragments and halt any bleeding that is occurring from a blood vessel being cut by a bone fragment. Cranial surgery of this type is discussed in Chapter 49.

Therapeutic Management

If CSF is draining from the nose or ear, a child will be admitted to the hospital for observation because this implies the force of the blow was severe. Keep the child in a semi-Fowler's position so fluid drains out, not inward, to reduce the possibility of introducing infection. Make certain children do not hold their nose or pack their nostrils with something to halt the drainage so the amount escaping can be judged. If the drainage is excoriating to the upper lip, coat the space with an ointment such as petrolatum. Children may be prescribed a prophylactic antibiotic to reduce the risk of meningitis. If the drainage does not stop within a few days, surgery will be necessary to repair the fracture and reduce the danger of meningitis. Air that entered intracranial spaces at the time of the injury usually is absorbed rapidly. If X-rays at 72 hours still show air in the cerebral spaces, this implies a skull defect remains, and surgery may be indicated to close the defect.

Potential Complications

A long-term complication of even a linear fracture of the skull may be a *leptomeningeal cyst*. This results from projection of the arachnoid membrane into the fracture site. With the interfering tissue, bone cannot heal and actually erodes, so the fracture site becomes progressively larger, not smaller. The follow-up X-ray will help determine if a leptomeningeal cyst is occurring. If a child develops focal seizures or symptoms of increased ICP after a skull fracture, a leptomeningeal cyst should be suspected. The defect may be palpated on the skull as an underlying indentation. Surgical resection is necessary to remove the cyst.

SUBDURAL HEMATOMA

Subdural hematoma is venous bleeding into the space between the dura and the arachnoid membrane (Fig. 52.2A). Subdural hematomas tend to occur in infants more often

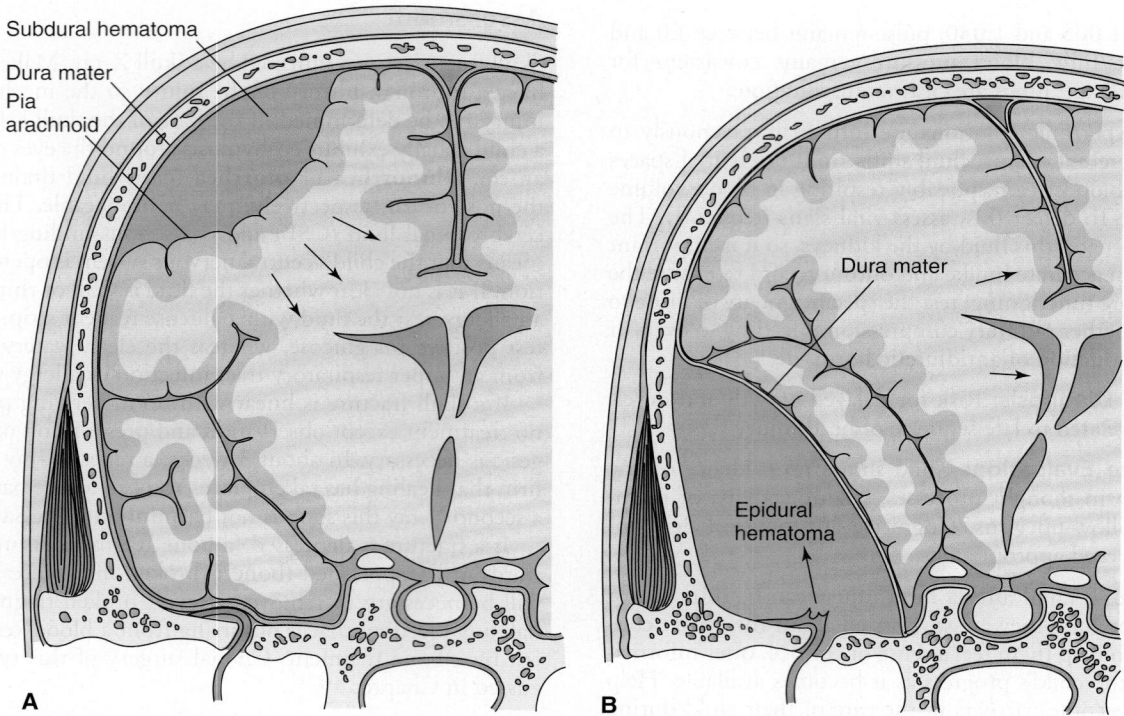

Figure 52.2 **(A)** Subdural hematoma. The red area in the upper left area of the drawing is the hematoma. Note the shift of structures. **(B)** Epidural hematoma. The red area in the lower left area of the drawing is the hematoma. Note the broken blood vessel and the shift of midline structures.

than in older children. Symptoms can occur within 3 days or as late as 20 days after trauma. Infants usually have symptoms of increased ICP, such as seizures, vomiting, hyperirritability, and enlargement of the diameter of the head. Anemia caused by the substantial blood loss may occur. Angiography, MRI, or ultrasound will reveal the extent of the hematoma.

In infants, accumulated subdural blood is removed by a subdural puncture through the anterior fontanelle, if it is still patent, by a procedure similar to a lumbar puncture. Infants receive conscious sedation for the procedure and must be held extremely still so that they do not move and cause the aspiration needle to be inserted incorrectly.

Subdural punctures may need to be repeated daily to empty the subdural space. If bleeding is still present after 2 weeks, surgery usually is necessary to reduce the space and halt bleeding. In older children, surgery usually is necessary from the beginning because the anterior fontanelle is closed and the space cannot be reached by puncture.

EPIDURAL HEMATOMA

Epidural hematoma is bleeding into the space between the dura and the skull and occurs when head trauma is severe (see Fig. 52.2B). Whereas subdural hemorrhage is usually venous bleeding, epidural hemorrhage is usually a result of rupture of the middle meningeal artery and thus is arterial bleeding. The bleeding can be severe and cause rapid brain compression.

At the time of the injury, children are apt to become momentarily unconscious. They then regain consciousness and, to the untrained eye, appear to be well for minutes or hours. Then, signs of cortical compression, such as vomiting, loss of

consciousness, headache, seizures, or hemiparesis (paralysis on one side), begin to develop. On physical examination, unequal dilation or constriction of the pupils may be present. Decorticate posturing (see Chapter 49) may be seen, indicating extreme pressure on upper cortical centers. If the pressure is allowed to continue unchecked, it may grow so great that brain stem, respiratory, or cardiovascular function become impaired.

The treatment is surgical removal of the accumulated blood and cauterization or ligation of the torn artery. The earlier the process is recognized and treated, the less likelihood of residual damage from extreme pressure or anoxia to the involved portion of the brain.

CONCUSSION

Concussion is the temporary and immediate impairment of neurologic function caused by a hard, jarring shock to the skull (Purcell, 2012). It may occur on the side of the head that was struck (a *coup injury*) or as the brain recoils from the force of the blow and strikes the opposite surface of the skull (a **contrecoup injury**; Fig. 52.3). Children have at least a transient loss of consciousness at the time of the injury and may vomit and show irritability after regaining consciousness. They typically have no memory (amnesia) of the event that led up to the injury or of the injury itself. For some children, this makes being asked questions about the injury extremely upsetting because they do not remember anything that happened and feel a frightening loss of control. A skull X-ray or MRI is needed to rule out skull fracture, and observation for 24 hours is needed to rule out severe brain trauma, edema, or laceration. A child can be observed at home by

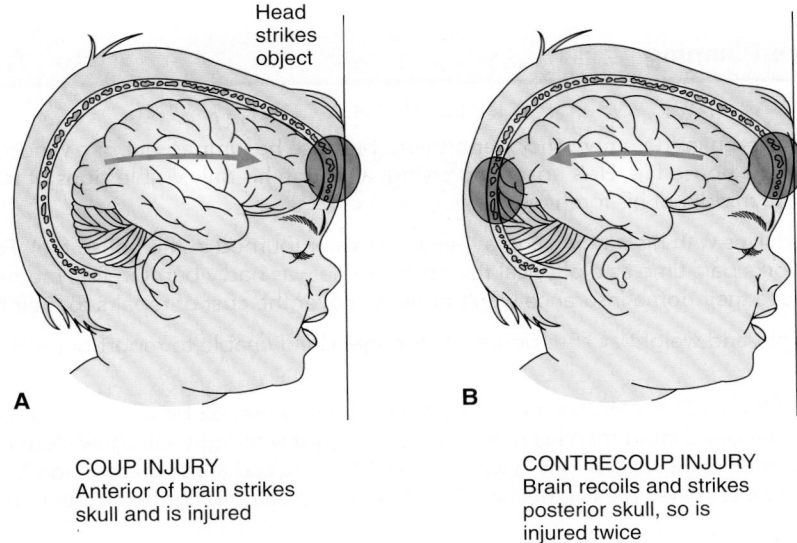

Figure 52.3 Etiology of (A) coup and (B) contrecoup injuries.

the parents if they are able to assess the child's level of consciousness every 1 to 2 hours while the child is awake. Parents usually are instructed not to keep waking children during the night because multiple wakings are disorienting and can make it difficult to tell if the child is confused or not. Parents should wake the child at least once during the night, however, and to be certain they are conscious, ask them to name a familiar object, such as a favorite toy, or to name the color of some object shown to them. Being able to tell parents their name or where they live is equally revealing.

There is an old belief that if children fall asleep after a head injury, they will die in their sleep; this belief can cause parents to keep shaking their child awake or to make the child walk continually. Be certain they understand that it is okay for children to sleep, but they must wake them at least once to assess their status (see Box 52.2 for an interprofessional care map for a child with a concussion). As a final instruction, be certain parents have a telephone number to call if they have any questions or worries about their child's care.

CONTUSION

A brain *contusion* occurs when there is tearing or laceration of brain tissue (Fig. 52.4). It is also known as bruising on the brain. The symptoms are the same as for a concussion but more severe. In addition, symptoms related to the specific brain area that is lacerated such as a focal seizure, eye deviation, or loss of speech will occur. Surgery may be necessary to halt bleeding. The child's prognosis depends on the extent of the injury.

What If . . . 52.1

In the emergency department, after Jason's head injury, his parents tell the nurse they both had a gastrointestinal "flu" last week. They assure the nurse that the reason Jason is vomiting now is probably because "he's caught their flu." How could the nurse evaluate whether the vomiting is from the head injury or a gastrointestinal infection?

COMA

Coma (unconsciousness from which a child cannot be roused) or **stupor** (grogginess from which a child *can* be roused) may occur in children after severe head trauma. Because these are both symptoms of underlying disorders, it's important to obtain a thorough history of the injury so treatment can be directed specifically toward the cause.

Assessment

For assessment, obtain a history from a parent or an observer of the event that caused the injury to determine what happened immediately before the time the child became comatose (e.g., the child fell, was choking, or took a recreational drug).

Undress the child completely so you can inspect all body parts. Although head injury is most likely to be the underlying cause of coma or seizure, metabolic disturbances such as diabetes mellitus, dehydration, severe hemorrhage from another body part, or drug ingestion also must be considered as possible causes. Count respirations and pulse and measure blood pressure to establish baseline values because changes in these values often provide good clues as to the cause of coma. A child with increased ICP, for example, will show decreased pulse and respiratory rates and increased blood pressure. The child with diabetes, in contrast, will develop increased respirations. Internal hemorrhage will lead to an increased pulse rate and decreased blood pressure. Drug ingestion may lead to either increased or decreased measurements, depending on the drug ingested.

Always turn an unconscious child on the side because if brain stem compression is present, the child cannot swallow effectively; lying on the side allows saliva to drain from the mouth to prevent aspiration. Observe the child's eyes for signs of dilated pupils, which could indicate increased ICP. If both pupils are dilated, irreversible brain stem damage is suggested, although such a finding may also be present with poisoning with an atropine-like drug. Pinpoint pupils suggest barbiturate or opiate intoxication. One pupil dilated or one eye deviated downward or laterally more than the other

BOX 52.2

Nursing Care Planning

AN INTERPROFESSIONAL CARE MAP FOR A CHILD WITH A CONCUSSION

Jason, a 10-year-old boy, is seen in the emergency department because he jumped out of a window and hit his head on a cement walkway escaping a house fire. He's upset and crying, although his only visible signs of trauma are a reddened and edematous area on the middle of his forehead.

Family Assessment: Child lives with his parents and a 4-year-old sister (burned in the house fire). Father is an insurance salesman; mother works part-time as a physical therapist. Home was badly burnt in fire; mother describes present finances as "shaky" because their home insurance won't begin to cover the cost of repairs to their home.

Patient Assessment: Height and weight at 75th percentile for age. Child unable to report or recall anything about the incident.

Vital signs: Temperature, 99.4°F (37.5°C); respirations, 18 breaths/min; pulse, 62 beats/min; and blood pressure, 110/62 mmHg. Left pupil is more dilated than his right; it reacts sluggishly to light. Glasgow Coma Scale score is 10. Alert enough to name baseball cards he brought in with him. A 1.5-cm raised area noted on forehead. Skin intact without evidence of bleeding. Child cries when area is touched. Negative otorrhea or rhinorrhea. Able to move all extremities through range of motion.

Nursing Diagnosis: Risk for injury related to effects of concussion

Outcome Criteria: Child remains alert and oriented; easily arousable. Pupils equal, round, react to light and accommodation; vital signs within age-acceptable parameters; exhibits no signs or symptoms of neurologic dysfunction.

Team Member Responsible	Assessment	Intervention	Rationale	Expected Outcome
Activities of Daily Living, Including Safety				
Nurse	Take history of injury; document distance child fell.	Assess child's vital signs, level of consciousness, and neurologic function initially and then every 30 minutes until discharge.	Changes in vital signs, level of consciousness, or neurologic function could indicate increasing intracranial pressure.	Parent describes injury and reactions of child since injury.
Teamwork and Collaboration				
Nurse/primary care provider/ trauma care team	Assess who is available from trauma team for consult; assess if child has ever had magnetic resonance imaging (MRI) before.	Help trauma care team assess child because child has been told not to talk to strangers. Accompany child to MRI service.	Symptoms of concussion can develop slowly over the next few hours after injury. MRI can help detect bleeding and edema.	Trauma care team examines child; prescribes follow-up care. Child cooperates with MRI.
Procedures/Medications for Quality Improvement				
Nurse/primary care provider	Assess whether child's demeanor (crying) is from fright or pain.	Institute measures to calm the child. Encourage the parents to hold and reassure him.	Crying increases intracranial pressure. Involving the parents provides them with a concrete activity, helping to provide some sense of control over the situation.	Parents are able to calm child to allow for better evaluation of condition.
Nutrition				
Nurse	Assess whether child has vomited since head injury.	If not nothing by mouth (NPO), offer clear fluid to be certain child does not have vomiting.	Vomiting is a symptom of increased intracranial pressure.	Child drinks some fluid without vomiting.

Patient-Centered Care

Nurse	Assess what parents understand about concussion in children.	Teach parents how contrecoup injuries occur and what symptoms they cause.	A contrecoup injury causes injury or edema to the posterior brain.	Parents state they understand why their child has posterior (eye control) symptoms and the assessment they will need to continue after discharge.
Nurse	Children often have no memory of events with concussion. Orientation and explanation help to minimize a child's fear of the unknown and of his situation.	Parents and child state they understand procedures being carried out. Voice confidence in care.		

Informatics for Seamless Healthcare Planning

Nurse/primary care provider	Assess whether parents understand why child will be admitted to observation unit overnight.	Child needs continuing care such as being roused every 2 hours during night to ensure he is conscious.	Assessing consciousness is important to assess whether complications are occurring.	Parents state one of them will remain with child in hospital to help reduce child's fear of strangers and better accept needed procedures.

suggests third cranial nerve compression or a tentorial tear (laceration of the membrane between the cerebellum and cerebrum) with herniation of the temporal lobe into the torn membrane. This situation requires immediate surgery to correct temporal compression.

Lack of a doll's eye reflex (see Chapter 49) suggests compression of the oculomotor nerves (third, fourth, or sixth)

Intracerebral hemorrhage

Figure 52.4 Intracerebral hemorrhage. The central large dark area represents the hemorrhage. Note the midline shift.

or brain stem involvement. Observe for posturing, such as decerebrate posturing, which suggests cerebral compression and dysfunction. If the retina of the eye reveals papilledema (swelling), it suggests that increased ICP has been long-standing (more than 24 to 48 hours).

Metabolic or renal disorders that cause unconsciousness are revealed by blood analysis; therefore, studies such as blood glucose, electrolytes, blood urea nitrogen (BUN), liver function tests, blood gas studies, and toxicology tests may be prescribed to rule out possible causes. A lumbar puncture and a CT or MRI will be done if a head injury is the most likely cause (Sigurtà, Zanaboni, Canavesi, et al., 2013).

Lumbar puncture may have little value at first in predicting the severity of a head injury. The procedure is contraindicated if increased ICP is present because release of fluid with the puncture could cause brain stem compression into the cord, a serious complication.

Coma is graded according to a standard scale so that changes in the level of consciousness can be evaluated and deterioration or improvement can be documented. Figure 52.5 shows the Glasgow Coma Scale, the most commonly used evaluation system for coma (Rhine, Wade, Makoroff, et al., 2012). Because this system was devised as an adult assessment scale, it must be modified for use with children or infants. Such a modification is shown in Box 52.3.

On the scale, a score of 3 to 8 suggests severe trauma (a number less than 5 suggests a very severe prognosis); a score of 9 to 12, moderate trauma; and 13 to 15, slight trauma.

Therapeutic Management

If children are unconscious for longer than a transient period, they usually are admitted to an observation unit for further assessment. An IV route is established so that, when specific

Glasgow Coma Scale			AM			PM				AM					
Assessment	Reaction	Score	8	10	12	2	4	6	8	10	12	2	4	6	8
Eye opening Response	Spontaneously	4	X						X	X	X	X	X		
	To speech	3		X				X							
	To pain	2			X	X	X								
	No response	1													
Motor response	Obeys verbal command	6	X						X	X	X	X	X		
	Localizes pain	5		X	X										
	Flexion withdrawal	4				X	X								
	Flexion	3						X							
	Extension	2													
	No response	1													
Verbal response	Oriented ×3	5	X						X	X	X	X	X		
	Conversation confused	4		X				X							
	Inappropriate speech	3			X										
	Incomprehensible sounds	2				X	X								
	No response	1													

Figure 52.5 Glasgow Coma Scale scoring for a child. A score of 3 to 8 denotes severe trauma; 9 to 12, moderate trauma; 13 to 15, slight trauma. Notice the gradual improvement from coma in this example.

measures such as blood replacement, electrolyte replacement, or fluid replacement are needed, a route for immediate administration is available. Oral suctioning to remove mucus from the mouth and pharynx may be necessary. Measure oxygen saturation by pulse oximetry. If a child has acute signs of respiratory difficulty or oxygen saturation is low, endotracheal intubation may be necessary to ensure respiratory function.

Obtain the child's vital signs and assess neurologic status, such as state of consciousness and the ability of pupils to react to light, every 15 to 20 minutes or as prescribed, so a picture of gradual change can be detected.

A child's prognosis after coma depends on the initial cause of the coma and the immediate care the child receives. If the increased ICP can be relieved before any permanent brain damage results, the effects of the coma will be transient. Prognosis is always guarded, however, because coma is a serious, possibly life-threatening, response until ruled otherwise.

Nursing Diagnoses and Related Interventions

Care of the child in coma is directed toward maintaining body function in an optimal state until the child reawakens.

Nursing Diagnosis: Risk for ineffective airway clearance related to brain stem pressure

Outcome Evaluation: Child's respiratory rate remains between 16 and 20 breaths/min; no retractions or signs of obstruction are present.

Some children who are comatose require endotracheal intubation or tracheotomy with mechanical ventilation to ensure an open airway and adequate oxygenation. An endotracheal tube may be replaced with a tracheotomy after 3 to 7 days to prevent necrosis of the pharynx from pressure of the endotracheal tube.

Nursing Diagnosis: Risk for impaired skin integrity related to lack of mobility

Outcome Evaluation: Child exhibits no areas of broken or irritated skin.

Bathe children who are comatose daily to stimulate skin circulation; include the hair as part of the bath about every 3 days. Change the child's position at least every 2 hours to prevent pressure ulcer formation or development of hydrostatic pneumonia from pooled secretions in the lungs. Keep the linen on the bed dry and free from wrinkles. Use of a sheepskin, an egg-carton foam, or an alternating-pressure or water mattress can help to decrease skin pressure. Perform thorough passive range-of-motion exercises to maintain muscle tone and prevent contractures.

Nursing Diagnosis: Risk for imbalanced nutrition, less than body requirements, related to inability to take in oral food or fluid

Outcome Evaluation: Child has good skin turgor; weight is not falling percentiles on the growth curve; hourly urine output remains greater than 1 ml/kg.

Children who are unconscious cannot be fed orally due to the risk of aspiration into the lungs. Therefore, nutrition is maintained by nasogastric (NG) or gastrostomy tube feedings, IV fluid administration, or total parenteral nutrition (TPN). IV fluid is only a short-term option,

BOX 52.3

Scoring for Glasgow Coma Scale

EYE OPENING

4. Child opens eyes spontaneously when you approach.
3. Child opens eyes in response to speech (spoken or shouted).
2. Child opens eyes only in response to painful stimuli, such as pressure on a nail bed.
1. Child does not open eyes in response to painful stimuli.

MOTOR RESPONSE

6. Child can obey a simple command such as "hand me a toy" (infant smiles or attunes).
5. Child moves an extremity to locate a painful stimulus applied to the head or trunk and attempts to remove the source.
4. Child attempts to withdraw from the source of pain.
3. Child flexes arms at the elbows and wrists in response to painful stimuli to the nail beds (decorticate rigidity).
2. Child extends arms (straightens the elbows) in response to painful stimuli (cerebrate rigidity).
1. Child has no motor response to pain on any extremity.

VERBAL RESPONSE

5. Child is oriented to time, place, and person (child >4 years old knows name, date, and where he or she is; infant appears to recognize parent).
4. Child is able to converse, although not oriented to time, place, or person (does not know who or where he or she is; infant says words but does not appear to differentiate parents from others).
3. Child speaks only in words or phrases that make little or no sense ("I want frazzle no"; infant's vocabulary is less than it is normally).
2. Child responds with incomprehensible sounds, such as groans.
1. Child does not respond verbally at all.

Modified from Teasdale, G., & Bennett, B. (1974). Assessment of coma and impaired consciousness: A practical scale. *Lancet*, *2*(7872), 81–84.

because adequate protein and fat cannot be supplied solely by this route. Always aspirate NG or gastrostomy tubes for stomach contents before giving a feeding to check tube placement and assess gastric residual amounts. As a rule, return any amount of stomach residue aspirated because if this is discarded each time, a child will lose a large amount of stomach acid, possibly leading to alkalosis. Because children's stomach size is small, check whether the amount of the feeding should be reduced by the amount of fluid remaining in the stomach before feeding the full amount of prescribed formula.

Give mouth care at least twice daily with clear water and a padded tongue blade. Coat lips with petrolatum or a commercial ointment to prevent drying and cracking. If a child's eyes tend to be dry, close them to prevent corneal ulceration. Artificial tears (methylcellulose) may be prescribed to keep eyes from drying until the child regains consciousness.

QSEN Checkpoint Question 52.2

PATIENT-CENTERED CARE

Jason's parents are in distress because they fear that his ICP is increasing. The nurse wants to reassure his parents that Jason is being monitored closely. Which event would be most indicative that his ICP is increasing?

a. Jason refuses to let the nurse assess his tympanic temperature.
b. Jason asks the nurse to read the same story to him over and over.
c. Jason can't remember a thing about how his injury happened.
d. Jason's temperature and blood pressure are both slowly increasing.

Look in Appendix A for the best answer and rationale.

Abdominal Trauma

Abdominal trauma can result from an object such as a baseball bat, a high-speed motor vehicle accident without restraint or with a seat belt without a shoulder strap, child maltreatment, or a fall from a height greater than 20 ft (Klimek, Lutz, Stranzinger, et al., 2013). Children are more apt to experience injury to their spleen and liver than adults because these organs are more exposed in children than they are in adults. The injury may be difficult to detect, however, because, unlike obvious signs of head or respiratory injuries, abdominal trauma usually presents with much more subtle signs.

ASSESSMENT

To detect abdominal trauma, assess vital signs for a baseline and then continue measurements to reveal whether abdominal hemorrhage could be occurring; rapid respirations, hypotension (less than 80 mmHg systolic pressure in an older child; less than 60 mmHg in an infant), and increasing pallor usually suggest that hidden internal bleeding is present. An additional suggestion that internal bleeding is present is that a low blood pressure shows little improvement when IV fluid is administered.

If abdominal trauma is suspected, an NG tube may be passed. Stomach contents are then aspirated to be assessed visually for fresh and occult blood, and the tube is then attached to low intermittent suction to allow for continued stomach observation. An indwelling urinary (Foley) catheter may be inserted into the bladder to evaluate urine for blood and urine output; evidence of blood in the urine suggests bladder damage, and a decreased output suggests accompanying kidney trauma. A paracentesis (introduction of a catheter into the abdomen to aspirate for the presence of blood) is another way to detect internal bleeding. Keep in mind that procedures such as NG tube or catheter placement are extremely frightening for young children (unsure of their anatomy, they have no clear idea where the tubes are going). Developmentally appropriate education prior to the procedure will help remove some of the fear (Box 52.4).

Nursing Care Planning Tips for Effective Communication

Jason, 10 years old, has no memory of how he sustained a head injury and thus needs additional assessments to rule out other trauma.

Tip: Be sure to help establish a sense of support and trust in addition to obtaining consent for procedures. Nurses sometimes focus on getting needed care done while failing to recognize the fear, apprehension, and loss of self-esteem the parent is feeling. In the following scenario, the nurse listens and thus recognizes and attends to the parent's fears.

Mr. Varton: Why are you looking at his belly? He didn't hurt that.

Nurse: He needs a thorough assessment to be sure there aren't any other problems. Next, I'll be putting in an IV line and urinary catheter and then taking him for an MRI.

Mr. Varton: How much will all that cost?

Nurse: I can see you have a lot of worries and concerns on your mind, your son's health, your home, being able to pay for health care, and having a place to live. This must be an extremely stressful time for you.

Mr. Varton: My daughter is burned. My house is ruined. I should have been able to get the children out before they got injured.

Nurse: Would you like to speak to a trauma counselor? It may help to organize your thoughts about all of the events that have occurred in such a tragic situation.

An abdominal X-ray, MRI, or ultrasound may help rule out a ruptured liver or spleen or a fractured pelvis, all conditions that could be contributing to blood loss. Air under the diaphragm on an X-ray suggests gastric or intestinal rupture with escape of air from these organs into the peritoneal cavity. Free fluid in the abdomen suggests leakage of bowel fluid, liver or splenic rupture, and pooling of blood.

Parents may not seek immediate medical attention after abdominal trauma because they are unaware a serious injury has resulted. Because often, there are no obvious signs of injury with abdominal trauma, it is vital to educate parents and patients on the degree of concern with abdominal bleeding and the need to perform diagnostic procedures to help determine the severity of the injury.

⬡ Nursing Diagnoses and Related Interventions

Major features of abdominal injury are pain and a feeling of "fullness," both from edema and possibly internal bleeding. If parents did not recognize their child was injured, guilt and fear on their part may compound the child's care. Goal setting is usually concerned with the immediate diagnostic procedures or anticipated surgery. Interventions differ according to the specific injury present.

Nursing Diagnosis: Pain related to abdominal injury

Outcome Evaluation: Child states that level of pain is tolerable or rates it as low on a pain rating scale; does not grimace or guard when abdomen is palpated.

Routinely, analgesics are not administered to children after abdominal trauma, unless their pain is severe, to avoid masking increasing pain and, also, because the location of the pain can help identify which organ may be injured. Offer support until analgesia can be given. Being held by a parent or lying absolutely still on an exam table helps prevent abdominal organs from shifting and thus may help reduce the degree of pain.

SPLENIC RUPTURE

In children, the spleen is the most frequently injured organ when there is abdominal trauma because of its location under the lower left ribs (McCance & Grey, 2012). Frequent causes of injury involving the spleen are inappropriately applied seat belts in automobiles, handlebar injuries in bicycle accidents, or skateboard or snowboard accidents. The child will have tenderness in the left upper quadrant of the abdomen, especially on deep inspiration, when the diaphragm moves down and touches the spleen. The child may hold the left shoulder elevated so that the diaphragm is raised on the left side to keep this from happening or report radiated left shoulder pain while lying in a supine position (Kehr sign).

An X-ray will show little about the spleen itself but may reveal a broken rib over the spleen, suggesting the extent of the trauma to that area. An MRI will rule out damage not only to the spleen but also to the left kidney just behind the spleen, which may also have suffered trauma. A complete blood count is done to detect blood loss and determine kidney involvement. An IV line is begun immediately and blood is typed and cross-matched, so that blood can be readied for replacement if necessary. Children with suspected splenic injury are usually admitted to an observation unit if the blood loss from rupture appears to be mild. If bleeding is severe, immediate surgery, such as a partial or total splenectomy, may be necessary to halt the bleeding and save the child's life.

After a splenectomy, children are very susceptible to infection. Vaccines such as *Haemophilus influenzae* type b, pneumococcal, and meningococcal are recommended to protect these children against bacterial infections.

LIVER RUPTURE

The liver is also more prone to rupture in children than in adults because the liver, like the spleen, is not completely sheltered by the rib cage in children (Shao, Zou, Li, et al., 2013).

Children with liver rupture or laceration usually have severe abdominal pain that is most marked on inspiration, when the diaphragm descends and touches the liver. They also show symptoms of blood loss, such as tachycardia, hypotension, anxiety, and pallor. Their hematocrit level will be low or falling. Such children need to be prepared for immediate surgery because the liver is a highly vascular organ, and blood loss can be life-threatening.

Occasionally, a communication between an artery and the bile duct occurs at the time of liver trauma. In this situation, symptoms are not immediate, but gastrointestinal (GI) bleeding, such as hematemesis (vomiting blood) or melena (blood in stool), may be seen a few days after the injury. The child may report colicky upper abdominal pain relieved by emesis. An MRI plus a liver study, such as a liver arteriogram, is necessary to reveal the extent of the injured artery.

After either liver or spleen surgery, children need careful observation for return of bowel function, assessment for the possibility of peritonitis, and slow reintroduction of oral nutrition.

When providing patient education, abdominal trauma prevention tips for parents and children include:

1. Using guards on windows, stair gates, and guard rails to prevent children from dangerous tumbles
2. Checking that playground equipment is well maintained and supervising young children at all times when they are out at play
3. Knowing how to install and use car seats, booster seats, and seat belts appropriately
4. Using car seats on every trip no matter how short
5. Setting a good example by always using a seat belt yourself (CDC, 2016a)

Dental Trauma

Injuries to teeth occur most often from falls in which a child strikes the upper front incisors or from blows to the face by objects such as baseball bats or hockey sticks. Such injuries are always potentially serious because they can lead to aspiration of the injured teeth or malalignment of future teeth. If a tooth is knocked out of the mouth, parents should rinse the tooth in water, drop it in a salt solution or milk, and bring it to the emergency department with them. Deciduous teeth may not be replaced, but if a permanent tooth can be saved, washed with saline or an antiseptic in the emergency department and then replaced and wired into place, there is a good chance it will reimplant successfully (McTigue, 2013).

The child will usually be prescribed a course of oral antibiotic, such as penicillin, to prevent infection. Stress to the parents the importance of giving the full course of the antibiotic and allowing only soft food until the tooth has firmly adhered (approximately 2 weeks).

If a blow to a child's teeth was extensive, an X-ray may be necessary to rule out an accompanying mandibular or maxillary fracture. If a portion of a tooth cannot be located, the possibility of aspiration must be considered and confirmed or ruled out by a chest X-ray. In young children, often a tooth is not knocked free but is pushed back up into the gum. These teeth gradually regrow, and although they may darken in color, they usually are healthy. If the affected tooth is a deciduous tooth, the permanent tooth is rarely injured even though it is already formed underneath in the gum. At the appropriate time, the permanent tooth will erupt without difficulty.

When providing patient education, dental trauma prevention tips for parents and children should focus on using mouth guards and face protection when playing contact sports.

Drowning

Drowning is death caused by suffocation from submersion in liquid when the inhaled water fills the lungs and therefore blocks the exchange of oxygen in the alveoli. More than 3,500 children die from drowning annually, making it one of the most frequent causes of death by unintentional injury among children in the United States (CDC, 2016d).

When providing patient education, drowning prevention tips for parents and children should include:

1. Use secure fencing and gating around swimming pools.
2. Ensure adequate adult supervision at all times with all children during all water activities.
3. Use flotation devices while swimming or boating.
4. Toddlers can drown in shallow areas, including toilets and buckets and therefore should always be adequately supervised (CDC, 2016d).

Most infant drownings occur in bathtubs; 1- to 4-year-old children most frequently drown in artificial pools; older children most frequently drown in bodies of fresh water. The majority of drowning injuries that take place outside the home occur in the summer months, when more children are swimming and boating. These may occur in young children because parents overestimate the child's swimming ability (Morrongiello, Sandomierski, Schwebel, et al., 2013). In older children, male adolescents are particularly at risk, although both sexes may take dares to swim farther than they are capable of or may swim under the influence of alcohol, which impairs their decision-making ability and their physical coordination.

PATHOPHYSIOLOGY OF DROWNING

When a child's head is submerged and water inhalation occurs, the natural response is to cough to remove the irritation in the nose and throat caused by the water. If the child cannot get the head out of the water at this point, water enters the larynx, causing the larynx to spasm and prevent any further water from entering. This mechanism unfortunately also prevents air from entering the trachea, resulting in asphyxia. If ventilation occurs at this point, the likelihood of effective treatment is good because there is little water in the lungs.

If ventilation is not given at this point, the larynx relaxes from the asphyxia and water enters the lungs. Oxygen can no longer be exchanged as the alveoli fill with water. Hypoxia deepens, and cardiac arrest occurs.

Additional changes that occur when water enters the lungs depend on whether the water is fresh or salt. Salt water is hypertonic, so fluid osmoses from the bloodstream into the alveoli in an attempt to dilute the aspirated water, increasing the amount of fluid in lung tissue and increasing hypoxia. Blood viscosity increases as shown by an increased hematocrit level; both tachycardia and decreased blood pressure from hypovolemia result.

Fresh water is hypotonic, causing the aspirated water to shift from the lungs into the bloodstream, again, because of osmotic pressure. This can lead to hemolysis of the red blood cells, a dilution of plasma, and possibly hypervolemia with tachycardia and increased blood pressure. If the release of potassium from destroyed red blood cells is large enough with fresh-water drowning, cardiac arrhythmias may occur. In both instances, loss of surfactant from lung alveoli, caused by introduction of the water (adult respiratory distress syndrome), can lead to alveolar collapse on expiration (CDC, 2016d).

When very young children dive into very cold water, a mammalian diving reflex occurs that helps them survive drowning (immediately after plunging into cold water, a lifesaving bradycardia and shunting of blood away from the periphery of the body to the brain and heart occur). This reflex is triggered when water is 70°F (21°C) or less and the face is submerged first. The phenomenon explains why very young children survive more often than older children after being submerged in icy wintertime water.

EMERGENCY MANAGEMENT

When a child is pulled from the water after drowning, mouth-to-mouth resuscitation and CPR should be started at once (discussed in Chapter 41). This is an exception to the advice to use hands-only resuscitation as the child's lungs are filled with water, which must be displaced (CDC, 2016d). Assuming CPR is effective, the child then needs follow-up care at a healthcare facility because the child is certain to be acidotic from accumulated carbon dioxide and hypoxic from lack of oxygen caused by water retained in the alveoli. There also is a high risk for respiratory infection from contaminants in the water.

Follow-up care aims to increase the child's oxygen and carbon dioxide exchange capacity by using the lung areas that are not filled with water. Attach a pulse oximeter to monitor oxygen saturation. If respiratory efforts remain severely compromised, a child is intubated with a cuffed intratracheal tube; mechanical ventilation with positive end-expiratory pressure may be necessary to force air into the alveoli. A cuffed tube is used because water that has been swallowed will be vomited as the child revives and the cuff will prevent vomitus from being aspirated. The child is usually given 100% oxygen so that as much space as possible in the available lung alveoli can be used. In addition, an NG tube is inserted to decompress the stomach, prevent vomiting, and free up breathing space. A bronchodilator such as albuterol may be administered by aerosol to prevent bronchospasm and, again, to allow the child to make maximum use of the oxygen administered. If the child aspirated salt water, plasma may be administered to replace protein being lost into the lungs and prevent hypovolemia.

If the child's body temperature is very low, it is generally better to allow gradual warming (not using a warming blanket) so the child's metabolic requirement does not rise sharply before alveolar space is ready to accommodate this increased oxygen need. Extracorporeal membrane oxygenation (ECMO) may be necessary when most of the lung has water aspiration.

Unfortunately, a danger of drowning is that neurologic damage can occur due to the amount of oxygen deprivation to the brain. If the child is awake or only lethargic at the scene of the injury and immediately afterward in the hospital, the prognosis is greatly improved over that of the child who is comatose.

 Nursing Diagnoses and Related Interventions

Drowning has both physical (lack of oxygen) and emotional (extreme fright) components, so both areas need to be addressed in planning care.

Nursing Diagnosis: Risk for infection related to foreign substance in respiratory tract

Outcome Evaluation: Child's tympanic temperature remains within normal parameters; rales are absent on lung auscultation; respiratory rate is within age-acceptable parameters.

After drowning, a child is usually prescribed prophylactic antibiotic therapy to prevent pneumonia or additional airway interference. Assess vital signs and auscultate lung sounds frequently for adventitious sounds, such as rales or fine rhonchi. Turning the child every 2 hours if on bed rest and encouraging deep breathing and incentive spirometry every hour to help aerate the lungs fully and prevent the accumulation of fluid, which promotes infection.

Nursing Diagnosis: Fear related to drowning experience

Outcome Evaluation: Child discusses fear; states she understands that although frightening, the experience is over, and she is now safe.

Children may be admitted to an observation unit for monitoring of oxygenation until water from the alveoli is absorbed and they once again can ventilate effectively on their own. Nightmares that revisit the drowning episode may occur and interfere with the child's sleep. Encourage children to verbalize the fright they feel about the experience. Assure them they are now safe and definitely out of the water. Because drowning is such a frightening experience, a child may need support from parents before they are willing to try swimming again. The goal is to get the child to an emotionally comfortable state where he or she can regain confidence with swimming. Encourage solid swimming skills to help prevent future drowning experiences.

Poisoning

According to the American Association of Poison Control Centers, there are more than 1 million reported poison exposures among children younger than 6 years of age yearly. For children 6 years and older, the estimated yearly reported exposures drops to about 300,000. Because many poisoning exposures are not reported, these numbers are most likely an underestimate. Poisoning occurs in all socioeconomic groups, and 90% of the time it occurs in the child's home. The substances most frequently ingested in children 5 years and younger include cosmetics/personal care products, household cleaning products, analgesics, foreign bodies such as toys, and topical preparations. Children younger than 6 years of age are at high risk for ingesting pharmaceutical agents. Nearly 9,500 children will be hospitalized yearly for unsupervised ingestion of prescription medications. The most commonly ingested medications include opioids and benzodiazepines, acetaminophen, cough and cold remedies, ibuprofen, and diphenhydramine.

Reference from: AAPCC.org (American Association of Poison Control Centers)

When providing patient education, poison prevention tips for parents should include (www.aapcc.org):

1. Keep medicines and toxic products locked and away from children.
2. Add the poison control number (1-800-222-1222) in your cell phone and make sure all caretakers do the same.
3. Call the poison control center if you think your child has ingested anything that may be poisonous. Keep in mind that the child may be awake and alert and acting normally.

4. If your child has ingested a poisonous product and collapses or stops breathing, call 911.
5. When administering medications, be sure to read labels carefully and to administer the appropriate amount.
6. Safely dispose unused, unneeded, or expired medications and vitamins (CDC, 2015).

 ## Nursing Diagnoses and Related Interventions

Poisoning tends to occur when parents are preoccupied or highly stressed; nursing planning needs to address not only immediate care measures but also education to prevent poisoning from occurring again.

Nursing Diagnosis: Risk for injury related to young maturational age of child and presence of unsecured poisons in the home

Outcome Evaluation: Parents identify poisonous and toxic items in the home and describe how they are stored safely; parents state local poison control center number; parents describe measures to take if poisoning occurs.

EMERGENCY MANAGEMENT OF POISONING AT HOME

If poisoning occurs, parents should telephone the National Poison Control Center (1-800-222-1222) to ask for advice regarding what to do. Instructions are specific to what the child ingested. The parent should be prepared to provide the following information to the poison control center:

- What was swallowed; if the name of a medicine is not known, what it was prescribed for and a description of it (color, size, shape of pills)
- The child's weight and age and how long ago the poisoning occurred
- The route of poisoning (oral, inhaled, sprayed on skin)
- An estimation of how much of the poison the child took (a bottle of cleaner or medicine should say how many pills or how much liquid it originally contained)
- The child's present condition (sleepy, hyperactive, comatose)

If the poison was in pill form, parents should check whether there are pills scattered under a chair before they assume they were swallowed. If one child in a family has swallowed a poison, parents should investigate whether other children have also poisoned themselves because a preschooler often shares "candy" with a younger sibling. If the poison control center advises parents to make the child vomit, the best way to do this is to place a finger at the back of the child's throat. Old remedies such as giving mustard or salty water are not that effective and waste time that could be spent telephoning an emergency service (911) for help or transporting the child to the hospital.

🌿 *What If . . . 52.2*
A nurse has learned that Jason's younger sister, Sage, 4 years old, suffered a mouth burn a year ago when she sprayed her mouth with oven cleaner. What preventive tips and patient education could the nurse provide to Sage and her mother?

EMERGENCY MANAGEMENT OF POISONING AT THE HEALTHCARE FACILITY

In the emergency department, the best method to deactivate a swallowed poison is the administration of activated charcoal either orally or by way of an NG tube to halt the action of the poison.

Activated charcoal is supplied as a fine black powder that is mixed with water for administration. Adding a sweet syrup to the mixture can make it more palatable. Caution parents that, as the charcoal is excreted through the bowel over the next 3 days, stools will appear black so they do not mistake the color for blood (Box 52.5).

ACETAMINOPHEN POISONING

Acetaminophen (Tylenol) is an over-the-counter medication that is frequently involved in childhood poisoning today because parents use acetaminophen to treat childhood fevers and have it readily available in the home. They may delay bringing the child for emergency care, thinking it is a harmless drug. Acetaminophen in large doses, however, is not innocent; it can cause extreme permanent liver destruction (Ogilvie, Rieder, & Lim, 2012).

Immediately after ingestion, the child develops symptoms of anorexia, nausea, and usually vomiting. Serum aspartate transaminase (AST [SGOT]) and serum alanine transaminase (ALT [SGPT]), liver enzymes, rise. The liver may feel tender on palpation as liver toxicity occurs.

 ### BOX 52.5

Nursing Care Planning Based on Responsibility for Pharmacology

ACTIVATED CHARCOAL

Classification: Activated charcoal is an antidote for poisoning.

Action: absorbs toxic substances that have been swallowed to prevent them from being absorbed by the stomach (Karch, 2013)

Pregnancy Risk Category: C

Dosage: provided as a powder that must be mixed with water and administered orally or by way of nasogastric (NG) tube

Possible Adverse Effects: vomiting, diarrhea, black stools

Nursing Implications
- Administer orally to conscious victims only.
- Give the drug as soon as possible after poisoning.
- Store the drug in a closed container because if it absorbs gases from the air, it is inactivated.
- Recognize that the solution feels gritty and tastes disagreeable so young children often have difficulty swallowing it, which is why it may have to be administered by NG tube.
- Caution child and parents that stools will be black for several days after administration.

In the emergency department, activated charcoal or acetylcysteine, a mucolytic agent and also the specific antidote for acetaminophen poisoning, will be administered. Acetylcysteine prevents hepatotoxicity by binding with the breakdown product of acetaminophen so that it will not bind to liver cells. Unfortunately, acetylcysteine has an offensive odor and taste. Administering it in a small amount of a carbonated beverage can help the child to swallow it. For small children, it may be administered directly into an NG tube to avoid this difficulty. If the child is admitted to an observation unit, continue to observe for jaundice and tenderness over the liver and assess ALT and AST levels.

 ## Nursing Diagnoses and Related Interventions

Parents feel guilty after acetaminophen poisoning because they realize they should have been more careful with storing all medicine out of their child's reach. Be aware that, because it is a drug commonly available in the average home, acetaminophen poisoning may be the cause of unidentified coma or self-injury.

Nursing Diagnosis: Situational low self-esteem of parents related to child's poisoning

Outcome Evaluation: Parents state guidelines for continued assessment of child at home; state ways they can improve "childproofing."

After the child is stabilized following the poisoning episode, take some time to talk with the parents about the event. Remember, poisoning tends to happen in homes where there is stress. If stress was already present, how has this poisoning event added to it?

Before the child is discharged from a healthcare facility, be certain the parents are comfortable with any further assessment measures they will need to continue at home, such as temperature taking and pushing high fluid intake. Be certain they understand the importance of liver function tests for follow-up care to detect any long-term liver injury.

QSEN Checkpoint Question 52.3

QUALITY IMPROVEMENT

The nurse notices that Sage was seen in the emergency department last year for acetaminophen poisoning. The hospital's algorithm for dealing with acetaminophen overdose should specify what action?

a. Advise the parents their child must never take acetaminophen again.
b. Be prepared to administer either acetylcysteine or activated charcoal.
c. Palpate the child's abdomen to assess whether the bladder feels tender.
d. Administer potassium chloride elixir immediately.

Look in Appendix A for the best answer and rationale.

CAUSTIC POISONING

Ingestion of a strong alkali, such as lye, which is contained in certain toilet bowl cleaners or hair care products, causes burns and tissue necrosis in the mouth, esophagus, and stomach. It's very important that parents do not try to make a child vomit after ingestion of these substances because they can cause additional burning as they are vomited (Rumack & Dart, 2012).

Assessment

After a caustic ingestion, the child has immediate pain in the mouth and throat and drools saliva because of oral edema and an inability to swallow. The mouth turns white immediately from the burn and the child may vomit blood, mucus, and necrotic tissue. The loss of blood from the denuded, burned surface may lead to systemic signs of tachycardia, tachypnea, pallor, and hypotension. Tissue in the mouth turns brown as edema and ulceration develop. At times, there may be such marked edema of the tongue that it is difficult to examine past the lips. Activated charcoal should not be administered because it is ineffective and obstructs an endoscopic view.

Therapeutic Management

When parents whose child has ingested a caustic substance call a poison control center to ask for advice on how to proceed, they will be advised to immediately take the child to a healthcare facility for treatment because there is a high possibility that pharyngeal edema will become severe enough to obstruct the child's airway. This can occur as quickly as 20 minutes after a burn and is why ingestion of caustic substances can be life-threatening.

In the emergency department, relieving the child's pain is a first step. Advocate for a strong analgesic, such as IV morphine, to achieve pain relief for this level of injury. A chest X-ray may then be prescribed to determine whether the aspirated poison has caused an esophageal perforation that will allow swallowed fluid to seep from the injured esophagus into the mediastinum. A laryngoscopy and esophagoscopy under conscious sedation or general anesthesia may be done to assess the lungs and esophagus, although these must be done cautiously because of the possibility that an examining scope could perforate the burned esophagus or trachea.

Assess vital signs, especially the respiratory rate, and attach a pulse oximeter to establish a baseline and for continued monitoring to help detect if edema of the pharynx is obscuring the child's airway. In infants, increasing restlessness is an important accompanying sign of oxygen deprivation. For some children, intubation or a tracheotomy may be necessary to provide a patent airway, although, again, any intubation must be done cautiously because the throat is edematous and could be injured easily. To protect against stomach reflux to the burned esophageal area, a proton pump inhibitor may be prescribed intravenously. Even though the child has denuded mouth or throat areas, prophylactic antibiotic therapy is not usually necessary. Once a mainstay of therapy to reduce esophageal stricture, the use of a corticosteroid such as dexamethasone (Decadron) is now controversial and may or may not be prescribed.

Nursing Diagnoses and Related Interventions

Poisoning with a caustic substance is a true emergency because care must be initiated to preserve the child's airway. Providing adequate nutrition is a second concern because the child is unable to swallow through an edematous throat or esophagus.

Nursing Diagnosis: Risk for imbalanced nutrition, less than body requirements, related to esophageal stricture from burn scarring

Outcome Evaluation: Child's diet meets recommended daily allowance requirements for age.

Oral intake commonly will be a problem for the first week, following a caustic injury because of soreness in the child's mouth; an NG tube is contraindicated, so the child may be fed by TPN or gastrostomy feedings during this time. After about a week, liquids are introduced because liquid passing through the burned and scarred esophagus can help maintain esophageal patency or be therapeutic for the burn as well as nutritious for the child. Observe children carefully the first time they attempt to drink something for coughing, choking, or cyanosis, which are signs that suggest the liquid is not able to pass through the esophagus and is being aspirated into the lungs. Be certain parents have clear explanations of how to offer soft food for as long as the child's mouth or throat is sore and the need for follow-up care to be certain the child's esophagus has not stenosed. After 2 weeks, a barium swallow or esophagoscopy will be performed to reveal the final extent of the esophageal burns and determine any further therapy needed. Some children require periodic dilation of the esophagus by endoscopy during the first year after the injury. To correct complete obstruction, repeated surgical procedures such as transplantation of intestinal tissue or a synthetic graft will be required to replace the obstructed esophagus. Because there is a correlation with the development of esophageal carcinoma later in life in individuals who swallowed a caustic substance, both the parents and the child need to be alerted to this possibility and to the signs of esophageal cancer (e.g., weight loss, difficulty swallowing) (Mas, Breton, & Lachaux, 2012).

IRON POISONING

Iron is frequently swallowed by small children because it is an ingredient in vitamin preparations, particularly in prenatal vitamins. When ingested, a large amount of iron is corrosive to the gastric mucosa and leads to signs and symptoms of severe gastric irritation in the child (Chang & Rangan, 2011).

The immediate effects include nausea and vomiting, diarrhea, and abdominal pain. After 6 hours, however, these symptoms seem to fade, and the child's condition appears to improve. Internally, however, hemorrhagic necrosis of the lining of the GI tract continues to occur. By 12 hours, melena (blood in stool) and hematemesis (blood in emesis) are revealed. Lethargy and coma, cyanosis, vasomotor collapse, coagulation defects, and hepatic injury may also occur. Hypovolemic shock may result from blood loss and decreased cardiac output. Long-term effects include gastric scarring from fibrotic tissue formation.

Assessment

It is difficult to estimate the amount of iron a child has swallowed because the amount of elemental iron in compounds varies and parents can only guess at the number of pills that were in the bottle before the ingestion. Obtaining blood for a serum iron level analysis should be performed to establish a baseline.

Therapeutic Management

In the emergency department, activated charcoal is not given because it is not effective at neutralizing iron. Stomach lavage is done instead to remove any pills not yet absorbed. A cathartic may be given to help the child pass enteric-coated iron pills before they can be activated. A soothing compound such as Maalox or Mylanta (aluminum hydroxide and magnesium hydroxide) or a proton pump inhibitor can help decrease gastric irritation and pain.

If a child has ingested a potentially toxic dose of iron, an exchange transfusion can be used to remove excess iron from the body. Administration of a chelating agent such as IV or intramuscular (IM) deferoxamine can also be effective because this combines with the iron and allows it to be excreted harmlessly from the body in the urine. To avoid concern, caution parents that deferoxamine causes urine to turn orange. Parents may be asked to test the stool for 3 days for occult blood to assess for stomach irritation and subsequent GI bleeding. Be certain that parents understand how to do this accurately.

For follow-up, an upper GI X-ray series and liver studies may be performed 1 week after the ingestion to screen for long-term effects. The goal is that the iron load is removed from the stomach in time so that not all of it gets absorbed and long-term effects are prevented.

 Nursing Diagnoses and Related Interventions

Many parents are unaware that iron can be toxic because they have been told so often that iron is necessary for good blood cell formation.

Nursing Diagnosis: Deficient parental knowledge related to the danger of iron as a poison

Outcome Evaluation: Parents state they understand the danger of iron ingestion for children; state ways they have safeguarded their child from future iron exposure.

Pregnant women may not realize prenatal vitamins contain high levels of iron (25 to 60 mg compared to 18 mg in children's vitamins) and thus may not be as conscientious about storing these in a safe place, an action that can lead to iron poisoning in a child. Because many children's vitamins are manufactured in the shapes of familiar television or cartoon characters, children can think of these as candy and overdose on them if not supervised.

Whenever you instruct parents on taking an iron supplement for themselves or their children, stress that overdoses can be fatal to small children. Help them think of iron as they would any other medicine and keep it out of the reach of small hands.

LEAD POISONING

When lead enters the body, it interferes with red blood cell function by blocking the incorporation of iron into the protoporphyrin compound that makes up the heme portion of hemoglobin in red blood cells and leads to a hypochromic, microcytic anemia (Lee & Marcdante, 2011). In addition, kidney destruction may occur, causing excess excretion of amino acids, glucose, and phosphates in the urine. The most serious effect, however, is lead encephalitis or inflammation of brain cells because of the toxic lead content. Lead poisoning (**plumbism**), like all forms of poisoning in children, tends to occur most often in children younger than 6 years of age. Children living in poverty and in older housing are at greater risk.

When providing patient education, lead prevention tips for parents should include:

1. Keep children away from peeling paint or chewable surfaces painted with lead-based paint.
2. Children should not be present in homes built before 1978 that are undergoing renovation.
3. Use contact paper or duct tape to cover holes in the walls or to block children's access.
4. Regularly wash children's hands and toys with water.
5. Regularly wet-mop floors and wet-wipe windows/windowsills to avoid lead dust from surfacing on the objects and floors in the home.
6. Take off shoes when entering the house to prevent bringing in lead from the outdoors.
7. Keep children from playing in bare soil and away from the sides of the house.
8. Test all children for lead at 1 and 2 years of age and anytime there is reason to suspect lead poisoning (CDC, 2016c).

Assessment

There is no safe level of lead accumulation in a child's body. Lead poisoning is said to be present when the child has two successive blood serum lead levels greater than 5 μ/dl (CDC, 2012). Ingestion of lead and chronically elevated lead levels can be identified through radiology of the intestinal tract and long bones (Fig. 52.6). The usual sources of ingested lead are lead-based paint and lead-contaminated dust. Lead was banned from paint in 1978. More than 4 million homes in the United States have lead-contaminated paint and dust and have one or more young children living in them (CDC, 2014, 2016c).

Paint tastes sweet, so a child will repeatedly pick up paint chips off the floor or off the walls to taste them. If a crib rail or a windowsill is painted with lead paint, a child can ingest it by teething the rail or sill. In fishing communities, swallowing lead sinkers can be a common source. Restoring an older home saturates the air with lead dust. In such homes, lead plumbing also may contaminate the drinking water.

Studies have shown that even low lead levels in children can affect the child's IQ and cause learning disability and behavioral attention problems. The effects of the lead exposure cannot be corrected; therefore, preventing lead exposure before it causes any harm is the goal.

Therapeutic Management

A child with a blood lead level over 5 μg/dl needs to be rescreened to confirm the level and then active interventions are required to prevent further lead exposure such as removal of the child from the environment containing the lead source

Figure 52.6 **(A)** Ingested paint chips (white crescents) in the intestinal tract. **(B)** A radiograph of the long bones of a child with chronic lead ingestion showing the characteristic "lead line" or white marking at the epiphyseal line. (Radiographs courtesy of Dr. Jerald P. Kuhn, Children's Hospital, Buffalo, NY.)

or removal of the source of lead from the child's environment. Removal of the lead source is not an easy task in homes because simple repainting or wallpapering does not necessarily remove the source of peeling paint adequately. After some months, the new paint will begin to peel because of the defective paint underneath. The walls must therefore be covered by paneling or drywall or other solid protective material in order to completely remove the lead exposure in the home.

Some children with lead levels greater than 10 to 20 μg/100 ml will be prescribed an oral chelating agent such as dimercaptosuccinic acid (DMSA) or succimer. Children with blood lead levels of greater than 45 μg/100 ml are treated with stronger chelation therapy such as dimercaprol (British anti-Lewisite [BAL]) or edetate calcium disodium (CaEDTA) (Karch, 2013).

Chelating agents (except BAL) remove the lead from soft tissue and bone (although not from red blood cells), allowing it to be eliminated in the urine. CaEDTA can be given intravenously or by IM injection into a large muscle mass. IM injection of CaEDTA is painful and should be combined with 0.5 ml of procaine for administration. BUN, serum creatinine, and protein in urine are assessed to ensure kidney function is adequate because CaEDTA can lead to nephrotoxicity or kidney damage if it cannot be excreted. Be certain to measure intake and output to assess that kidney function is adequate to excrete the lead.

CaEDTA is so effective as a chelating agent that it unfortunately has the side effect of also removing calcium from the body; children who receive CaEDTA, therefore, must have serum calcium measured periodically to determine whether their calcium level is adequate.

BAL has the advantage over CaEDTA of being able to remove lead from red blood cells as well as other tissues, but because of the danger of severe toxicity, it is prescribed only for children who have severe forms of lead intoxication.

 ## Nursing Diagnoses and Related Interventions

Care planning can be difficult when a child is diagnosed with lead poisoning because parents are immediately upset at learning their child has been exposed to a source of lead. They may experience a loss of self-esteem and a sense of powerlessness as they realize their housing situation has hurt their child.

Nursing Diagnosis: Deficient knowledge related to the dangers of lead ingestion

Outcome Evaluation: Parents state they understand the importance of preventing further lead exposure; identify measures to take to reduce lead in the environment.

Parental education about the risk of lead poisoning is crucial. Parents may have to move to a new home or locale or extensively renovate their home. As temporary measures, placing the television or an overstuffed chair against a lead-based windowsill or placing the child's crib about 3 ft away from the walls can be helpful to prevent the child from picking at loose wallpaper or exposed lead-based plaster. Be certain parents understand that all children with elevated lead levels need careful follow-up to determine the seriousness of their condition and to ensure they are being kept away from the lead source. Because children who recover from symptomatic lead poisoning have a high incidence of permanent neurologic damage, all children with elevated blood lead levels need appropriate follow-up care to evaluate development and intelligence (CDC, 2016c).

QSEN Checkpoint Question 52.4

INFORMATICS

Sage is found to have an elevated serum lead level. What is the most common source of lead poisoning in young children that would contribute to this assessment finding?

- a. Smelling lead fumes from cooking utensils
- b. Swallowing batteries that fall out of toys
- c. Drinking lead-contaminated drinking water
- d. Chewing on chips of flaking lead-based paint

Look in Appendix A for the best answer and rationale.

Foreign Body Obstruction

Foreign bodies can become lodged in a child's esophagus, ear canals, nostrils, or lungs, causing direct obstruction of the airway or long-term stasis of secretions and infection. Whether a foreign substance is inhaled or embedded elsewhere, nursing interventions should focus first on comforting the child and aiding in removal of the object and later on teaching the child and parents ways to avoid such occurrences in the future.

FOREIGN BODIES IN THE EAR

Any child with a history of draining exudate from the ear canal needs an otoscopic examination to determine the cause. With toddlers and preschoolers, the drainage often is the result of a foreign body such as a small toy, a piece of paper, a small battery, or food, such as a peanut that gets pushed into the ear canal (Sharpe, Rochette, & Smith, 2012).

Removal of a foreign body from the ear can be difficult. Fear of the instruments being used and pain make it difficult for children to keep still during the procedure. Often, it is better to wait for an otolaryngologist to care for the child because trauma to the ear canal during an attempt to remove a foreign body can cause edema and make removal even more difficult.

In many instances, if the object is in the outer canal, it can be grasped by forceps and easily removed. If the tympanic membrane is intact, irrigating the object from the ear canal with a syringe and normal saline may be possible, although this should not be done if the object is a substance that will swell when wet, such as a peanut. If there is a possibility that the tympanic membrane is ruptured, the ear canal should not be irrigated or fluid will be forced into the middle ear, possibly introducing infection (otitis media).

FOREIGN BODIES IN THE NOSE

Foreign objects stuffed into the nose eventually cause inflammation and purulent discharge from the nose. The odor accompanying such impaction is often the first sign noticed by the parent. Objects pushed into the nose usually can be removed with forceps. A local antibiotic might be necessary after removal if ulceration resulted from the local irritation.

FOREIGN BODIES IN THE ESOPHAGUS OR STOMACH

Children tend to not chew food well or to swallow portions that are too big to pass safely through the esophagus when they are in a hurry. Pieces of candy, such as Life Savers, are common objects caught in the esophagus in young children; coins may be swallowed by adolescents playing drinking games. Wires of orthodontic appliances that dislodged are also frequently swallowed. The mark of an object lodged in the esophagus is intense pain at the site where the object is located. If the object is one that will dissolve, such as a Life Saver or a piece of digestible meat, offer the child fluid to drink to help flush the object into the stomach. Even after the object dissolves or passes into the stomach, the child will feel transient pain at the original site of the obstruction.

Magnets, particularly those in watches or hearing aids, are also frequently swallowed by young children. These need to be removed by endoscopy as soon as possible because they can lead to bowel perforation or volvulus from their acid content. Objects, such as a part of a toy, a chicken bone, or a large coin that will not dissolve or be passed, are also removed by endoscopy (Avey, Euathrongchit, & Stern, 2012).

Small coins, such as pennies and dimes, usually pass by themselves without difficulty. Parents and older children need to observe stools over several days to determine that the coin does pass through the GI tract (about 48 hours after ingestion). Without frightening them, caution parents to observe for signs of bowel perforation or obstruction, such as vomiting or abdominal pain, until the coin has passed. If there is any doubt, an X-ray taken 3 to 7 days after ingestion will establish whether the coin has been evacuated from the body.

SUBCUTANEOUS OBJECTS

Children get many wood splinters in the hands and feet. These items can be removed easily with a probing needle and tweezers after cleaning with an antiseptic solution. If the penetrating object is metal, such as a sewing needle or nail, its presence can be detected by X-ray. If the object is one that would have been in contact with soil, such as a rusty nail, the child will need tetanus prophylaxis after extraction of the object if the child's tetanus immunization is not current.

What If . . . 52.3
Sage's mother tells the nurse she thinks the reason Sage has an elevated lead level is because she swallowed a penny a month ago and it must still be inside her. What additional information would the nurse request from the mother? What patient education would the nurse provide?

Bites

Children are bitten by snakes and animals such as dogs or raccoons; they occasionally are bitten by other children. In an emergency room, the source of a bite needs to be documented because human bites can also result from child maltreatment.

MAMMALIAN BITES

Dog bites account for approximately 90% of all bites inflicted on humans, and children and adolescents are involved in one third to one half of reported incidents. The dog is usually one owned by the child's family. Cat bites, wild animal bites, and human bites also constitute a threat, although these are less common in children. All of these bites can cause abrasions, puncture wounds, lacerations, and crushing injuries related to the size of the animal and the location of the bite (Dyring-Andersen, Menne, & Skov, 2012).

The biggest concerns associated with animal bites are the scarring and disfigurement and the possibility of infection, especially rabies, from the presence of microorganisms in the animal's mouth. Rabies and the vaccine for rabies are discussed in Chapter 43.

SNAKEBITE

Snakebites tend to occur during the warm months of the year, from April to October. A few fatal bites in the United States occur from cottonmouth moccasins or coral snakes

(both found in southeastern states), but the majority of fatal snakebites (envenomations) are from copperheads or rattlesnakes. Copperheads are found in eastern and southern states; rattlesnakes are found in almost every state. The effect of the bite of a rattlesnake, copperhead, or cottonmouth moccasin (all pit vipers) is the almost immediate failure of the blood coagulation system (Warrell, 2012).

Coral snakes are known for the small coral, yellow, and black rings encircling their body. Fortunately, they are shy and seldom bite. However, the venom injected through the bite of these snakes leads to neuromuscular paralysis.

Assessment

Immediately after a pit viper bite, a white wheal surrounding the puncture marks begins to appear, accompanied by excruciating pain at the site. Purplish erythema and edema extend rapidly from the site.

By the time a child is seen at a healthcare facility, sanguineous fluid may be oozing from the bite. Systemic symptoms, such as dizziness, vomiting, perspiration, and weakness, may be present. Because snake venom interferes with blood coagulation, the child may have hematemesis or bleeding from the nose, intestines, or bladder because of subcutaneous or internal hemorrhage. The pupils may be dilated, showing the potent effect on cerebral centers. If the envenomation is not treated, seizures, coma, and death may result.

Emergency Management at the Scene

At the scene of a snakebite, parents should apply a cold compress to the bite because this can decrease the spread of the venom and reduce edema formation. Urging the child to lie quietly, with the bitten extremity dependent also helps to slow circulation. Commercial snakebite kits have rubber suction cups in them that can be used to suction out the venom, so if available, they should be used. Excising the bite with a knife and sucking out the venom orally (often shown in old western movies) is of questionable value and if the person administering the treatment has open mouth lesions, such as carious teeth, the procedure could be dangerous to that person (venom is not dangerous when swallowed, only when absorbed through open lesions). Excising the bite also may lead to secondary infection and, if done too vigorously, may injure tendon or muscle. It is vital to transport the child to a healthcare facility as quickly as possible.

Emergency Management at the Health Facility

In the emergency department, ask the child or the caretaker to describe the snake. In areas where snakebites are frequent, keep available photographs of the venomous snakes commonly found because even a preschooler may be able to identify the snake by pointing to a photograph. Specific antivenin depending on the type of snake is then administered. Because rattlesnakes, copperheads, and cottonmouth moccasins are all one type of snake (pit vipers), one form of antivenin acts against all of these bites. Specific antivenin is prepared for coral snake or cobra bites (not typically kept in emergency departments but obtained from most zoos). If a child receives antivenin promptly after a bite, the prognosis for full recovery is good.

Antivenin may contain a horse-serum base. Therefore, before the serum is injected intramuscularly or intravenously, a skin test may need to be performed to prevent a possible anaphylactic reaction to the horse serum. If giving the serum IM, do not inject it into an edematous body part because medication will be poorly absorbed from edematous tissue; you may need to assure the parents that giving antivenin into the limb opposite the bitten limb is just as effective as administering it into the bitten limb. If the child's immunization status is unknown or it has been more than 10 years since a tetanus immunization was given, ask if tetanus prophylaxis should be administered.

 ### Nursing Diagnoses and Related Interventions

Snakebites are frightening; therefore, nursing diagnoses need to address both calming the child and parents as well as administering immediate interventions.

Nursing Diagnosis: Fear related to seriousness of child's condition

Outcome Evaluation: Parents and child state they are able to cope with the degree of fear present.

Following a venomous snakebite, children need a great deal of support from healthcare personnel because their parents may be too frightened to offer adequate support. As a final care measure, teach children the following common safety rules for avoiding snakebites:

- Look for snakes before stepping into underbrush.
- Be aware that snakes sun on warm rocks.
- Do not lift up rocks without looking at what could be under them.
- Listen for the telltale sound of a rattlesnake.
- Know the markings of poisonous snakes to help avoid them.

Athletic Injuries

Although participating in athletics promotes growth and development and teaches concepts of teamwork and perseverance, this can unfortunately also lead to injury. More than 2.6 million children each year are treated in emergency departments for sports and recreational related injuries (CDC, 2016c).

Playing on backyard trampolines, in particular, is a dangerous activity for children because neck and spine injuries can result (American Academy of Pediatrics Council on Sports Medicine and Fitness, 2012). Strategies to prevent sports injuries include preparticipation health examinations, proper coaching, attention to safety, adequate hydration, proper officiating, availability of first aid and medical coverage at all sporting events, and proper equipment and field or surface playing conditions.

KNEE INJURIES

Participation in sports such as football, skateboarding or snowboarding, skiing, soccer, and track running is a frequent cause of knee injuries in children that usually involve the ligaments surrounding the knee—the medial, lateral, posterior, and cruciate ligaments. Immediately after the injury, the child reports severe pain in the knee, and localized edema becomes evident. An X-ray or MRI will be done to rule out fracture and the extent of the ligament damage. If the injury is mild (only a few torn fibers), bed rest with an ice pack applied to the knee is often the only therapy needed. After 24 hours, heat is applied to the knee to hasten healing.

If the injury is more severe, the knee joint may fill with fluid. In addition to bed rest and an ice pack applied to the joint, the abnormal synovial fluid may be aspirated and a compression dressing applied to discourage accumulation of further fluid. After 24 hours, heat treatments hasten healing.

If the injury is severe, arthroscopy is necessary to visualize and surgically repair the knee ligaments. Arthroscopic surgery makes repair of ligaments or cartilage a minor procedure and limits the necessity for immobilization and a cast. Children who have one anterior cruciate ligament injury need to be aware that they may suffer another in their other knee and may be more prone to osteoarthritis in the affected knee later in life (Smith, Vacek, Johnson, et al., 2012).

If a child experiences a severe twisting motion to the knee, a dislocation of the patella (kneecap) can result (the kneecap moves to the posterior surface of the knee). The knee appears immediately deformed, and the child feels acute pain. An ultrasound or MRI will reveal if there is accompanying ligament damage. Immediate treatment for a dislocated kneecap is to slide the patella back to the front of the knee. After this realignment, the pain subsides, but the child may have to be fitted with a leg immobilizer for about 1 week to keep the kneecap in good alignment. Quadriceps exercises (straight-leg raising) are important to prevent the dislocation from reoccurring. These exercises strengthen the leg muscles and tendons. If the problem becomes chronic or occurs frequently, surgery to strengthen the knee ligaments may be necessary (Felus & Kowalczyk, 2012).

THROWING INJURIES

Throwing an object such as a baseball places repeated stress on an upper extremity, particularly the elbow joint. The injury that occurs is caused either by the forward motion of the arm or during the follow-through. After the injury, a child is unable to extend the elbow completely because of minute tears and fibrous contractures in the muscle that can occur for 24 to 48 hours postinjury. Pain and tenderness are marked. Resting the arm and applying ice packs for 15 to 20 minutes three times a day relieve the pain. An anti-inflammatory agent (nonsteroidal anti-inflammatory drug) will also relieve the pain. A limited number of cortisone injections into the elbow musculature may be necessary for complete healing. Exercises to strengthen flexor muscles help to prevent this type of injury.

"Little leaguer's elbow" is epiphysitis (inflammation) of the medial epicondylar epiphysis caused by repeated throwing motion. An X-ray of the elbow will reveal increased growth, separation, and fragmentation of the medial epicondylar epiphysis. Children need extra protection against this type of injury by limiting the amount of time spent in practice or games until the epiphyseal growth centers at the elbow have fused. This typically occurs between 14 to 17 years of age (Hoang, Coel, Vidal, et al., 2012).

Treatment for little leaguer's elbow is rest and immobilization until pain, tenderness, and limitation of movement has resolved. This is important because if the injury is not treated adequately, permanent damage to the epiphyseal line and elbow deformity can occur (Fleisig & Andrews, 2012).

Injuries of the Extremities

FINGER INJURIES

It is common for a child to sustain a finger injury from a slammed car door. This injury, which causes a crushing blow to the tip of the finger, is excruciatingly painful. The fingernail may be lacerated and detached. As blood accumulates under the fingernail, pain continues to increase unless an incision under the distal end of the nail or a stab wound through the nail helps to relieve the pain. Fingernails often are lost after these injuries, but they grow back readily with little scarring. You can assure parents that although the fingernail may be lost, the cosmetic effect will invariably not be a problem.

Parents may feel embarrassed and guilty when they bring a child to a healthcare facility for this type of injury. The injury usually occurred because they closed a door without looking out for the child's finger. They appreciate how much this hurts and are angry for being so careless. Reassure parents that this is a common childhood injury and unintentional injuries do happen.

An X-ray of the fingertip may be obtained to be certain the tip of the distal phalanx is not broken. The rule, "If the child can bend it, it's not broken," does not apply to this injury because the fracture may be distal to the last phalangeal joint. The open wound needs to be cleaned well. If the distal phalanx is fractured, the finger needs a splint applied to stabilize the bone. A follow-up visit will be necessary to ensure healing has occurred.

STRAINS AND SPRAINS

A **strain** is a muscle–tendon injury. A **sprain** is a ligament injury. Strained or sprained ankles are common and slow-to-heal childhood injuries (Tiemstra, 2012). Immediately after an injury, the affected joint feels painful and gets swollen. Such injuries typically occur from inline skating or snowboarding or skateboarding. When X-ray reveals no fracture, a child may feel as though someone has said the injury is not serious but "just a sprain." This makes the extent of the swelling and pain baffling.

Help the child and parents to understand that strains and sprains are truly painful. Because a cast is not used and the ankle is not immobilized but just wrapped in an elastic bandage, strains and sprains can be more painful than fractures.

If the injury is recent, apply an ice pack for approximately 20 minutes to reduce edema at the site; repeat this for 4 to 7 days at home. The child may be fitted for crutches to limit weight bearing for the next 3 or 4 days or fitted with a supportive medical boot. Make certain the parents understand how the elastic bandage is applied so that it can be rewrapped if it loosens and be certain the child is using the crutches or boot properly before being discharged from the emergency department.

When providing patient education, sports injury prevention tips for parents should include:

1. Make sure children wear protective equipment that fits appropriately and correctly at all times during sports and recreational activities.
2. Make sure children are well hydrated with water (avoid sugary drinks) and appropriately dressed to avoid heat-related injuries or illness.
3. Parents should be good role models and wear helmets and protective equipment when participating in sports and recreational activities (CDC, 2016c).

Thermal Injuries

Thermal injuries include those caused by either cold (frostbite) or excessive heat (burns).

FROSTBITE

Frostbite is tissue injury caused by freezing cold; the extreme cold causes peripheral vasoconstriction, cutting off the oxygen supply to surrounding cells (Castellani & Young, 2012). In children, the body parts involved usually are the nose, fingers, or toes.

Assessment

The severity of frostbite is classified by degree:

- First degree: mild freezing of epidermis; appears erythematous with edema
- Second degree: partial- or full-thickness injury; appears erythematous; blisters and pain occur after re-warming
- Third degree: full-thickness injury (epidermis, dermis, and subcutaneous tissue); appears white
- Fourth degree: complete necrosis with gangrene and possible ultimate loss of body part

Frostbite occurs most frequently in children who have been skiing, snowmobiling, or snowboarding for long periods. Frostbite of the lips or tongue can occur from sucking on a popsicle and from inhalant abuse. Always explore the cause and circumstances of frostbite with careful history taking because it can also result from neglect or child maltreatment.

Therapeutic Management

Always warm frostbitten areas gradually because sudden warming increases the metabolic rate of cells which can cause additional damage. Administration of a vasodilator and use of hyperbaric oxygen may help reduce the effect on body cells.

 Nursing Diagnoses and Related Interventions

Frostbite may not be recognized immediately. Children generally have pain and blistering by the time they are seen for emergency care.

Nursing Diagnosis: Pain related to damage of cells because of freezing temperature

Outcome Evaluation: Child states that pain is controlled at a tolerable level.

As soon as warming of the frostbitten body part begins, the part becomes extremely painful because the cells that are injured register their anoxic state. Pain management is essential at this time.

During the next few days after severe frostbite, necrosis of destroyed tissue occurs; the affected tissue then sloughs away. Apply or change dressings as necessary to avoid secondary bacterial contamination of the necrotic injury site. Assess body temperature frequently to detect early symptoms of infection. Be certain that children understand the cause of the injury so they take more precautions against cold injury in the future.

BURNS

Burns are injuries to body tissue caused by excessive heat (heat greater than 104°F [40°C]). Burns are the second most common unintentional injuries seen in children 1 to 4 years of age and the third most common cause in children 5 to 14 years of age. Every day, there are more than 300 children treated in emergency rooms for burn-related injuries. Younger children are most at risk for scald burns that are caused by hot liquids or steam. Older children are more apt to be burned from flames after they move too close to a campfire, heater, or fireplace; touch a hot curling iron; or play with matches or lighted candles (CDC, 2016c). Eye burns occur from splashed chemicals doing home projects or in science classes. Always keep in mind when evaluating burns that some (particularly scalding) can also be caused by child maltreatment (Blackburn, Levitan, MacLennan, et al., 2012).

Burn injuries tend to be more serious in children than in adults because the same size burn covers a larger surface of a child's body. Many burns can be prevented with improved parent and child education. When providing patient education, burn prevention tips for parents include:

1. Install smoke alarms in the home, on every floor, and near all rooms in which family members sleep.
2. Maintain smoke alarms by testing them monthly to make sure they are working properly and by using long-life batteries.
3. Create a family fire escape plan, involve the children in the planning, and practice frequently.
4. Never leave food unattended on the stove and always supervise or restrict the use of stoves, ovens, and microwaves with children.
5. Check the water heater temperature and make sure that the thermostat is set to 120°F or lower. Always test the water before children enter the bathtub or shower (CDC, 2016c).

Assessment

Because burns are classified as to degree, when children with a burn injury are brought to a healthcare facility, the first questions asked must be "Where is the burn?" and "What are its extent and depth?" (Nicole & Huether, 2012). Along with the size and depth, be certain to assess and document the location of the burn. Face and throat burns, for example, are particularly hazardous because there may be accompanying but unseen burns in the respiratory tract that could lead to respiratory tract obstruction. Hand burns are also hazardous because if the fingers and thumb are not positioned properly during healing, adhesions will inhibit full range of motion in the future. Burns of the feet carry a high risk for secondary infection. Genital burns are also hazardous because edema of the urinary meatus may prevent a child from voiding.

With adults, the "rule of nines" is a quick method of estimating the extent of a burn. For example, each upper extremity represents 9% of the total body surface; each lower extremity represents two 9s, or 18%, and the head and neck represent 9%. Because the body proportions of children are different from those of adults, this rule does not always apply and is misleading in the very young child. Data for determining the extent of burns in children are shown in Figure 52.7. Computer analysis is now available to rapidly assess the extent of burns.

Depth of Burn

When estimating the depth of a burn, use the appearance of the burn and the sensitivity of the area to pain as criteria. Descriptions of tissue at various burn depths are shown in Table 52.2 and illustrated in Figures 52.8 through 52.11.

Many burns are compound, involving first-, second-, and third-degree burns, or there may be a central white area insensitive to pain (third degree), surrounded by an area of erythematous blisters (second degree), and surrounded by another area that is erythematous only (first degree).

Be certain to undress children with burns completely in order to inspect the entire body. Because a first-degree burn is painful and a third-degree burn is not, a child may be crying from a superficial burn that is obvious on the arm, although the condition needing the most immediate attention is a third-degree burn on the chest covered by a jacket.

Be certain to ask what caused the burn because different materials cause different degrees of burn. Hot water, for example, causes scalding, a generally lesser degree of burn than one caused by flaming clothing. Ask where the fire happened because fires in closed spaces are apt to cause more respiratory involvement than those in open areas.

Lastly, determine whether other family members were burnt as well. Parents, for example, may have burned hands from putting out the fire on the child's clothes and need equal care, but in their anxiety about the child's condition, they do not mention this. If they picked up and brought the burned child to the hospital quickly, they may have left other children unprotected at home. They also may be so concerned about the burn that they neglect to mention the child has a secondary health concern such as diabetes or allergy to a common drug unless specifically asked.

Emergency Management for Minor Burns

All burns, including minor burns, need immediate care because of the potential pain involved (Mandt & Grubenhoff, 2012). Although minor burns (typically first-degree partial-thickness burns) are the simplest type of burn, they involve pain and death of skin cells and therefore must be treated seriously. Immediately apply cool water to cool the skin and prevent further burning. Application of an analgesic–antibiotic ointment and a gauze bandage to prevent infection is usually the only additional treatment required. Be certain that parents have a follow-up appointment in about 2 days to have the dressing changed and the area inspected for a secondary infection. Caution parents to keep the dressing dry (no swimming or getting the area wet while bathing until the burn is healed—about 1 week).

Emergency Management for Moderate Burns

Moderate or second-degree burns typically are blistered. Do not rupture these blisters because doing so denudes the site and invites infection. The burn should be covered with a topical antibiotic such as silver sulfadiazine and a bulky dressing to prevent damage to the burned site and promote healing. The child usually is asked to return in 24 hours to assess that pain control is adequate and there are no signs and symptoms of infection. Broken blisters may be debrided (cut away) to remove possible necrotic tissue as the burn heals.

AREA	BIRTH	AGE 1 YEAR	AGE 5 YEARS
A = 1/2 of head	9 1/2	8 1/2	6 1/2
B = 1/2 of one thigh	2 3/4	3 1/4	4
C = 1/2 of one leg	2 1/2	2 1/2	2 3/4

AREA	AGE 10 YEARS	AGE 15 YEARS	ADULT
A = 1/2 of head	5 1/2	4 1/2	3 1/2
B = 1/2 of one thigh	4 1/2	4 1/2	4 3/4
C = 1/2 of one leg	3	3 1/4	3 1/2

Figure 52.7 Determination of extent of burns in children.

TABLE 52.2 COMMON CLASSIFICATIONS AND DESCRIPTIONS OF BURNS

Degree	Description	Common Cause
First degree	Involves the epidermis or outer layer of skin. Appears reddened, dry, and feels mildly painful. Heals by simple regeneration so takes 1–10 days to heal.	Sunburn (Fig. 52.9A)
Second degree	Involves the epidermis and part of the dermis layer of skin. Appears red, blistered, and may be swollen. Very painful. Heals by regeneration of tissue over 2–6 weeks.	Scalding (Fig. 52.9B)
Third degree	Involves the epidermis and full extent of the dermis. Appears white or charred and lacks sensation as the nerve endings are destroyed. Skin grafting is usually necessary, and healing takes months. Scar tissue will cover the final healed site.	Flames (Figs. 52.10 and 52.11)
Fourth degree	Full-thickness burn extending into muscle or bone. Skin grafting is necessary; muscle and bone may be permanently damaged; scarring will cover the healed site.	High-voltage electric or severe fire

Depths of burns

Skin grafts

Superficial
(1st degree)

Partial
thickness
(2nd degree)

Full
thickness
(3rd degree)

Epidermis

Split
thickness

Full
thickness

Dermis

Subcutaneous
tissue

Figure 52.8   Depths of burns.

Figure 52.9   Partial-thickness burns. **(A)** An infant with a first-degree burn on the arm and chest caused by scalding with hot water. **(B)** A toddler with a second-degree burn caused by scalding. The area appears severely reddened and moist with some blistering. (**A**, © Dr. P. Marazzi/SPL/Science Source/Photo Researchers. **B**, © NMSB/Custom Medical Stock Photograph.)

Figure 52.10   Full-thickness (third-degree) burn of the foot. Both layers of skin are involved with this type of burn. (© Dr. Michael English/Custom Medical Stock Photograph.)

Figure 52.11 **(A)** An adolescent's hand scarred from third-degree burns. Note the proper extension and alignment of the hand and fingers, which were maintained by the use of splints during healing **(B)**. (© Dr. P. Marazzi/SPL/Science Source/ Photo Researchers.)

QSEN Checkpoint Question 52.5

SAFETY

A nurse is with Jason when he spills scalding hot water onto his hand. Which of the following would be the best emergency action?
  a. Apply a layer of vegetable oil over his hand.
  b. Cover his hand with a gauze dressing.
  c. Pour cool water from a faucet over his hand.
  d. Apply soothing hand lotion to keep the area moist.

Look in Appendix A for the best answer and rationale.

Emergency Management for Severe Burns

The child with a third-degree or fourth-degree burn is critically injured and requires immediate care. Sure care, including fluid therapy, systemic antibiotic therapy, pain management, and physical therapy. The goal is to prevent disability caused by scarring, infection, or contracture.

Emergency Management for Electrical Burns of the Mouth

If a child puts the prongs of a plugged-in extension cord into the mouth or chews on an electric cord, the mouth can be burned severely. When electrical current from a plug is conducted for a distance through the skin and underlying tissue it can cause an ulcer (Yeroshalmi, Sidoti, Adamo, et al., 2011). If blood vessels were burned, active bleeding from the lesion will be present.

The immediate treatment for electrical burns of the mouth is to unplug the electric cord and control bleeding if present. This can be done by pressing a towel against the burn site. In the emergency room, pain management and wound care are essential. Clean the wound with an antiseptic solution, such as half-strength hydrogen peroxide, or as otherwise prescribed to reduce the possibility of infection (a real danger in this area due to the amount of bacteria present in the mouth).

Most children with electric burns are admitted to an observation unit for at least 24 hours because edema in the mouth could lead to airway obstruction. Eating will be a challenge for the next week because the child's mouth is so sore. Soft foods and fluids may be easiest to swallow.

Electrical burns of the mouth turn black as local tissue necrosis begins. They heal with white, fibrous scar tissue, possibly leaving a deformity of the lips or cheeks and difficulty speaking clearly afterward. This can be minimized by using a mouth appliance, which helps maintain lip contour. Many children need follow-up care by a plastic surgeon to restore the lip contour.

🔥 Nursing Diagnoses and Related Interventions

Because pain and anxiety often accompany burn care, relieving them is always an important concern in burn care.

Nursing Diagnosis: Pain and anxiety related to thermal damage to body cells

Outcome Evaluation: Child states that pain and anxiety are at a tolerable level; rates pain at 2 or below on a pain rating scale.

Morphine sulfate IV or via epidural injection is commonly the agent of choice for pain relief. Performing burn care such as debridement (the removal of necrotic tissue from a burned area) may be done with the use of patient-controlled analgesia or conscious sedation.

In addition to having pain from a burn, children may be required to remain in awkward positions to keep joints overextended so the skin over them does not heal with a contracture. If the anterior throat is burned, for example, the child's head needs to be hyperextended to keep the scar tissue that forms on the anterior neck from pulling the chin down against the chest in a permanent position. If children have burns over extremity joints, they may have splints applied over their burn dressings to maintain the joints in extension. This will help decrease contractures from developing. Be certain parents understand the importance of keeping the splint in place at all times.

Encourage children to talk about their injury and how it occurred (a form of debriefing) so they can integrate this unexpected event into their life.

Although most children are awake and very aware of the pain and treatments involved, children who experience smoke inhalation from the fire that caused their injury may become unconscious from brain anoxia. After the first week following a major burn, some children develop symptoms of delirium, seizures, and coma that result from toxic breakdown of damaged cells, sensory deprivation, isolation, and lack of sleep. Nursing care aimed at reducing unnecessary stimuli and providing adequate pain relief helps to prevent these late symptoms from occurring.

Nursing Diagnosis: Deficient fluid volume related to fluid shifts from severe burn

Outcome Evaluation: Skin turgor remains good; hourly urine output is greater than 1 ml/kg, with specific gravity between 1.003 and 1.030; vital signs are within acceptable parameters for child's age.

Immediately after a severe burn, there is an increased permeability of capillaries (or direct damage to capillaries). This leads to a loss of plasma, which oozes from blood vessels into the burn site and then sequesters in edematous tissue surrounding the site resulting in hypovolemia. The phenomenon is most marked during the first 6 hours after a burn. It continues to some extent for the first 24 hours.

In addition to hypovolemia, because so much of the child's skin surface may be exposed for examination, a child is prone to hypothermia (keep body parts not burned well covered). Children may also develop a severe anemia following a burn because of injury to red blood cells caused by the heat and loss of blood at the wound site. The large amount of sodium lost from the bloodstream into the edematous burn fluid and the release of potassium from damaged cells can lead to both immediate hyponatremia and hyperkalemia (Table 52.3).

To detect whether extreme hypovolemia is occurring, monitor vital signs closely even with relatively minor

burns; lactated Ringer's solution is the commercially available solution most compatible with extracellular fluid, so that or normal saline will be administered for fluid replacement. A child may also need plasma replacement and a source of glucose such as 5% dextrose in water. Do not administer a potassium additive immediately after a burn until kidney function is evaluated to be certain extra potassium can be eliminated. IV fluid is usually administered by the most convenient venous access, so that an analgesic for pain can be administered. A more stable fluid line may then be inserted.

The amount of fluid necessary is calculated carefully based on predicted insensible fluid loss and loss that can be predicted because of the burn (2,000 ml/m² of body surface per 24 hours plus 5,000 ml/m² of body surface burned over 24 hours). Fluid is administered rapidly for the first 8 hours (half of the 24-hour load) and then more slowly for the next 16 hours (the second half). It is important that fluid administration is continued beyond the time of increased capillary permeability (at least the first 24 hours), so be certain to protect the administration site to prevent infiltration. A central venous pressure or pulmonary artery catheter may be inserted to determine hemodynamic and fluid volume status and evaluate that the child is receiving adequate fluid. If many red blood cells were destroyed at the burn site, the child may need packed red blood cells to maintain an adequate hemoglobin level.

About 48 hours after the burn, as inflammation decreases, the extracellular fluid at the burn site begins to be reabsorbed into the bloodstream. Edema at the burn site begins to subside; the child begins diuresis and loses weight. The heart rate increases because of temporary hypervolemia. The hematocrit level will be low because red blood cells are diluted. The child needs frequent evaluation of electrolyte levels to determine if the hypervolemia is not overwhelming. Potassium supplements may be necessary to maintain normal heart function because although potassium is released into the serum from destroyed cells, it is rapidly excreted by the kidneys.

Nursing Diagnosis: Risk for ineffective tissue perfusion related to cardiovascular adjustments after burn injury

Outcome Evaluation: Child's vital signs stay within normal limits for age; hourly urine output remains greater than 1 ml/kg of body weight per hour.

A complete blood cell count, blood typing and crossmatching, electrolyte and BUN determinations, and blood gas studies to ascertain blood levels of oxygen and carbon dioxide are important to obtain to monitor the shifts in fluid and electrolytes that occur.

Take height, weight, and vital signs on admission of a child with a burn and continue to take vital signs every 15 minutes until they are stable. Once these are stabilized, record pulse, blood pressure, and central venous pressure closely until the child passes the immediate danger of shock (at least 24 hours). Another important monitoring period occurs at 48 hours after the injury when fluid is returning to the bloodstream. Remember that gradual but persistent changes in blood pressure may be as informative as sudden changes.

TABLE 52.3 FLUID SHIFTS AFTER BURN INJURY

Fluid Shifts in First 24 Hours	Remobilization of Fluid After 48 Hours
Burn	Edematous tissue surrounding burn area
↓	↓
Increased capillary permeability	Intravascular compartment
↓	↓
Hypoproteinemia	Hypervolemia
Hyponatremia	Hypernatremia
Hyperkalemia	Hypokalemia
Hypovolemia	

Nursing Diagnosis: Risk for ineffective breathing patterns related to respiratory edema from burn injury

Outcome Evaluation: Child's respiratory rate remains within normal range for age; lung auscultation remains bilaterally clear without adventitious sounds.

If a child inhaled smoke from a fire, the injury from the smoke inhalation can be more serious than the skin surface burns received because smoke coming from a fire is at the temperature of the fire or is the same as exposing the upper respiratory tract to open flame. In addition, toxic substances and soot given off by the fire may cause local irritation to the respiratory tract. If carbon monoxide is inhaled with the smoke, it enters red blood cells in place of oxygen, shutting off the oxygen supply to body cells. If this is extensive, it can lead to loss of consciousness because of cerebral anoxia. If the trachea is burned, edema fluid will pass into the injured bronchioles and trachea, causing pulmonary edema or obstruction and limiting air inflow, leading to dyspnea and stridor. About 1 week after the smoke inhalation, the child is at risk for the development of pneumonia because of infection of the denuded tracheal and bronchial tract areas. Because parents are usually relieved that their child has suffered only smoke inhalation from a fire, they may need an explanation of the physiologic consequences that can result from pulmonary injury and why hospitalization is necessary.

To help rule out smoke inhalation, obtain a history to assess whether the fire occurred in a closed space, such as a garage. Assess for burns of the face, neck, or chest, which would indicate the fire was near the nose and respiratory tract. Assess the quality of the child's voice (it will be hoarse if the throat is irritated from smoke). Carefully monitor the respiratory rate of all burned children because respiratory rate increases with respiratory obstruction. A child also may become restless and thrash about because of lack of oxygen. Measurement of oxygen saturation will demonstrate the degree of hypoxia present from carbon monoxide intoxication. The best therapy for displacing carbon monoxide and providing adequate oxygenation to body cells is the administration of 100% oxygen. The child may need endotracheal intubation or a tracheostomy with assisted ventilation to ensure adequate oxygen is reaching the lungs. Intubation is best because tracheostomies can lead to infection, and this child is at a much higher risk for pneumonia than the average child.

Bronchodilators and antibiotics may be prescribed as a prophylactic measure because symptoms of smoke inhalation may not occur immediately but only 8 to 24 hours after the burn when the child's temperature increases or a chest X-ray reveals collecting edematous fluid and decreased aeration. High-frequency ventilation may be helpful to keep alveoli functioning. Some children need ECMO support because smoke inhalation has compromised their lung function to such a great extent.

Nursing Diagnosis: Risk for impaired urinary elimination related to burn injury

Outcome Evaluation: Child's urine output is greater than 1 ml/kg of body weight per hour.

Because the child's blood volume can decrease immediately after a burn, renal function can be threatened just when it is needed in order to rid the body of breakdown products from burned cells. Monitor blood volume conscientiously to detect whether hypovolemia is occurring and maintain IV fluid administration so urinary output can be maintained at about 1 ml/kg of body weight per hour. Monitor the specific gravity of urine as well to determine whether the kidneys are able to concentrate urine to conserve body fluid (failing kidneys lose this ability rapidly). In the days after the burn, because products of necrotic tissue and toxic substances must be evacuated by the kidneys and antidiuretic hormone and aldosterone levels may increase in response to low blood pressure, kidney function may fail again. If free hemoglobin from destroyed red blood cells plugs kidney tubules (acute tubular necrosis), urine color will turn red or black because of the hemoglobin present.

Because maintaining kidney function is so important, throughout the child's hospital stay, observing urinary output is a major nursing responsibility. An indwelling urinary (Foley) catheter should be inserted in the emergency department for a child with a large burn to obtain a baseline urine for analysis and allow for continued specimens to be obtained. If hemoglobin in tubules becomes a threat, a diuretic may be administered to flush this from the kidneys (urine will turn to its usual straw color if this is effective).

Nursing Diagnosis: Risk for imbalanced nutrition, less than body requirements, related to burn injury

Outcome Evaluation: Child's weight remains within 1 standard deviation from prior age-appropriate growth percentiles; skin turgor remains good; urine specific gravity remains between 1.003 and 1.030.

After burns, the metabolic rate increases in children as the body begins to pool its resources to adjust to the insult. If children do not receive enough calories in IV fluid to accommodate this increased metabolic need, their body will begin to break down protein for use, a particularly dangerous problem because the child needs protein to be available for burn healing. Additionally, if the breakdown of protein is extreme, it can lead to severe acidosis.

After a severe burn, some children feel nauseated because bowel peristalsis halts (paralytic ileus) from the systemic shock. Symptoms of intestinal obstruction, such as vomiting, abdominal distention, and colicky pain, follow within hours of the burn. To prevent aspiration of vomitus, an NG tube will be inserted and attached to low, intermittent suction. It then remains in place until bowel sounds are detected to make certain that the GI tract is again functioning (as long as 24 to 72 hours in severely burned children). Fluid suctioned from an NG tube may appear blood tinged (coffee-ground fluid) because of bleeding caused by stomach vessel congestion. Closely observe this drainage for a change to fresh bleeding, which can be caused by the development of a stress ulcer (Curling ulcer) from the overall trauma of the burn. This type of ulcer can be prevented by administering a histamine-2 receptor antagonist, such as cimetidine (Tagamet) or a proton pump inhibitor such as omeprazole (Prilosec), which reduce gastric acidity (Pilkington, Wagstaff, & Greenwood, 2012). If a bleeding ulcer does occur, gastric lavage with iced saline may be necessary. Blood for transfusion should be readily available because the blood loss from a GI ulcer can be rapid and severe.

Because of these potential GI concerns, children with severe burns usually are placed on nothing by mouth (NPO) for 24 hours. After this time, most children are able to eat, and oral feedings are begun as soon as possible. To supply adequate calories for increased metabolic needs and spare protein for repair of cells, the diet is high in calories and protein (Medlin, 2012). Children may also need supplemental vitamins (particularly B and C), iron supplements, and high-protein drinks between meals to ensure an adequate protein intake (Latenser, 2013).

In addition to this oral intake, it may be necessary to supplement the child's diet with IV or parenteral nutrition solutions or gastrostomy tube feedings. As methods of stimulating interest in eating, encourage school-age children to help add intake and output columns, help the dietitian add a calorie-count list, or keep track of their own daily weight (taken at the same time each day in the same clothing). It may be helpful to make contracts with older children to agree to eat at least some of each food offered on their plate.

Nursing Diagnosis: Risk for injury related to effects of burn, denuded skin surfaces, and lowered resistance to infection with burn injury

Outcome Evaluation: Child's temperature remains at 98.6°F (37°C); skin areas surrounding burned areas show no signs of infection such as erythema or warmth.

There appears to be some defect in the ability of neutrophils to phagocytize bacteria after burn injury, and the formation of immunoglobulin G antibodies also apparently fails. For these reasons, a child has reduced protection against infection for some time after a severe burn. *Staphylococcus aureus* and group A β-hemolytic streptococci are the gram-positive organisms and *Pseudomonas aeruginosa* is the gram-negative organism most likely to invade burn tissue. In addition to bacteria, fungi such *Candida* also may invade burns (White, Swales, & Butcher, 2012). Children are usually prescribed an antibiotic to prevent these infections and tetanus toxoid to prevent tetanus.

Bacteria and fungi can penetrate the burn eschar readily, so this tissue offers little protection from infection, necessitating nose, throat, and wound cultures to be done immediately and then daily to detect whether offending organisms are present. Fortunately, granulation tissue, which forms under the eschar 3 to 4 weeks after the burn, is resistant to microbial invasion.

Systemic antibiotics are not totally effective in controlling burn-wound infection, probably because the burned and constricted capillaries around the burn site cannot carry the antibiotic to the area. For this reason, any equipment used at the burn site must be sterile to avoid introducing infection. Children are placed on a sterile sheet on the examining table, and personnel caring for the severely burned child should wear caps, masks, gowns, and gloves, including during emergency care.

Even if their burns are covered by gauze dressings, children usually are cared for in private rooms to help reduce the possibility of infection. Helping children maintain their self-esteem and keeping them from withdrawing from social contacts when such strict infection control precautions are a challenge and must be addressed creatively within nursing care.

QSEN Checkpoint Question 52.6

TEAMWORK & COLLABORATION

A nurse is helping a fellow nurse care for Sage, Jason's younger sister who has a third-degree burn on her arms and neck. Which statement by the fellow nurse on the second day of Sage's care would alert the nurse that the care team needs more instruction on burn management?

a. "I'm guarding her IV site so she has an open route for pain management."
b. "I'm measuring her oral and IV fluid intake to help prevent hypervolemia."
c. "I'm monitoring urine output so I can be certain her kidneys are functioning."
d. "I'm urging her not to talk so she doesn't relive the house fire over and over."

Look in Appendix A for the best answer and rationale.

Therapy for Burns

Second- and third-degree burns may receive open treatment, leaving the burned area exposed to the air, or closed treatment, in which the burned area is covered with an antibacterial cream and many layers of gauze. These two methods are compared in Table 52.4. As a rule, burn dressings are applied loosely for the first 24 hours to prevent interference with circulation as edema forms. Be certain not to allow two burned body surfaces, such as the sides of fingers or the back of the ears and the scalp, to touch, because, as healing takes place, webbing will form between these surfaces. Do not use adhesive tape to anchor dressings to the skin; it is painful to remove and can leave excoriated areas, which provide additional entry sites for infection. Netting is useful to hold dressings in place because it expands easily and needs no additional tape.

TABLE 52.4 COMPARING OPEN AND CLOSED BURN THERAPY

Method	Description	Advantages	Disadvantages
Open	Burn is exposed to air; used for superficial burns or body parts that are prone to infection, such as perineum	Allows frequent inspection of site; allows child to follow healing process	Requires strict isolation to prevent infection; area may scrape and bleed easily and impede healing
Closed	Burn is covered with antibiotic cream and nonadherent gauze; used for moderate and severe burns	Provides better protection from injury; is easier to turn and position child; allows child more freedom to play	Requires dressing changes that can be painful; possibility of infection is still present because of dark, moist environment

Topical Therapy

Silver sulfadiazine (Silvadene) is the drug of choice for burn therapy to limit infection at the burn site in children. It is applied as a paste to the burn, and the area is then covered with a few layers of mesh gauze. Because silver sulfadiazine has a sulfa base, it is an effective agent against both gram-negative and gram-positive organisms and even against secondary infectious agents, such as *Candida*. It is soothing when applied and tends to keep the burn eschar soft, making debridement easier. It does not penetrate the eschar (the tough, leathery scab that forms over moderately or severely burned areas) well, however, which is its one drawback.

If *Pseudomonas* is detected in cultures, nitrofurazone (Furacin) cream may be applied. If a topical cream is not effective against invading organisms in the deeper tissue under the eschar, daily injections of specific antibiotics into the deeper layers of the burned area may be necessary.

If a burned area, such as the female genitalia, cannot be readily dressed, the area can be left exposed. The danger of this method is the potential invasion of pathogens.

Escharotomy

As natural protection for a burned area, a rigid scab (an eschar) forms over moderately or severely burned areas. Fluid accumulates rapidly under an eschar, putting pressure on underlying blood vessels and nerves. If an extremity or the trunk has been burned so that both anterior and posterior surfaces both have eschar formation, a tight band may form around the extremity or trunk, cutting off circulation to distal body portions. If distal parts feel cool to the touch and appear pale, any tingling or numbness is present, pulses are difficult to palpate, and capillary refill is slow (longer than 5 seconds), an **escharotomy** (cut into the eschar) may be performed (Kupas & Miller, 2010). Some bleeding will occur after escharotomy. Packing the wound and applying pressure usually relieves this.

Debridement

Debridement is the removal of necrotic tissue on which microorganisms could thrive from a burned area to reduce the possibility of infection. This may be done using collagenase (Santyl), an enzyme that dissolves devitalized tissue, or manually. For manual debridement, children may have 20 minutes of hydrotherapy beforehand to soften and loosen eschar, which then can be gently removed with forceps and scissors. Debridement is painful, and some bleeding occurs with it. Premedicate the child with a prescribed analgesic and help the child use a distraction technique during the procedure to reduce the level of pain. Transcutaneous electrical nerve stimulation (TENS) therapy or patient-controlled analgesia also can be helpful pain management measures. Extensive debridement is done using conscious sedation. Praise any degree of cooperation. Plan an enjoyable activity afterward to aid in pain relief and also to help reestablish some sense of control over the situation (Fig. 52.12).

If burned areas are debrided in this manner day after day, granulation tissue forms underneath. When a full bed of granulation tissue is present (about 2 weeks after the injury), the area is ready for skin grafting. In some burn centers, this waiting period is avoided by immediate surgical excision of eschar and placement of skin grafts.

Figure 52.12 A nurse provides comfort and support to a child before debridement. (© Kathy Sloane/Science Source/Photo Researchers.)

Grafting

Allografting is the placement of skin (sterilized and frozen) from cadavers or a donor on the cleaned burn site. These grafts do not grow but provide a temporary protective covering for the area. In small children, *xenografts*, or skin from other sources, such as porcine (pig) skin, may be used. **Autografting** is a process in which a layer of skin of both epidermis and a part of the dermis (called a *split-thickness graft*) is removed from a distal, unburned portion of the child's body and placed over the prepared burn site, where it will grow and replace the burned skin (Coruh & Yontar, 2012). The advantage of both types of grafting is that they reduce fluid and electrolyte loss, pain, and the chance of infection.

Skin for a split-thickness graft is removed from the buttocks or inner thigh under general anesthesia. Large burn areas may require mesh grafts (a strip of partial-thickness skin is slit at intervals so that it can be stretched to cover a larger area; Fig. 52.13).

After the grafting procedure, the burned area is covered by a bulky dressing. The donor site on the child's body is also covered by a gauze dressing. So that the growth of the newly adhering cells underneath will not be disrupted, don't remove or change the dressings. To detect infection at the sites, observe both the donor and graft dressings for fluid drainage and odor, and assess for pain and body temperature, all of which might indicate infection. Autograft sites heal so quickly that they can be reused every 7 to 10 days, so any one site can provide a great deal of skin for grafting.

Full-thickness grafts involve both layers of the skin and are used for deep or very severe burned areas. Skin for these is usually removed from the back or abdomen; because the amount of skin removed is so extensive, the donor site may require a split-thickness graft for healing. An alternative to skin grafting in a child who doesn't have enough unburned skin surface for autografting is the technique of using artificial skin to cover the burn. Artificial skin consists of synthetic fibers that, when placed over the denuded burn area, are filled in by

Figure 52.13 Mesh grafting is necessary to cover large areas of the body such as in this young child with third-degree burns. (© CC Studio/SPL/Photo Researchers Inc.)

fibroblasts and blood vessels and nerve fibers from surrounding healthy tissue to create a new dermal layer. Artificial skin is not rejected as is an allograft or a xenograft but is dissolved as the new skin replaces it. Another option is removing a small number of the child's skin cells and allowing them to grow in a culture laboratory until they can be used as a graft. Because skin cells grow fairly rapidly, this supplies an unlimited supply of available skin for large burn areas.

 ## Nursing Diagnoses and Related Interventions

For children who survive the immediate insult of a large burn, infection becomes their chief threat.

Nursing Diagnosis: Social isolation related to infection control precautions necessary to control spread of microorganisms

Outcome Evaluation: Child states he understands the reason for infection control precautions; accepts it as a necessary part of therapy.

Infection control measures involved in the care of children with major burns consist of more than just placing the child in a private room. Aseptic technique and appropriate barriers are necessary to reduce the risk of exposing the child to infection by the use of gowns, masks, caps, and sterile gloves by healthcare providers, creating a situation where the child is doubly isolated—by distance and by never being touched directly.

It is easy for children with burns (who were told measures such as not to play with matches or go too close to the fireplace) to interpret confinement in a room as punishment. Make every effort to make the child's environment as

warm and comforting as possible despite infection control procedures. Place children's beds so they can see as much unit activity as possible. Decorate walls in front of them with cards they receive or with a changing gallery of pictures drawn by staff members of things in which the child appears interested.

Provide time for children to discuss their feelings about being kept in a room by themselves. A question such as "It's hard to understand a lot of things about a hospital; do you understand why your bed is in this special room?" gives children a chance to express their feelings.

Show parents how to put on gowns, gloves, and masks if required so they can feel comfortable participating in the child's care. Parents may not offer to help with care when their child is severely burned because they are still in a state of shock or grief. They may perceive the bulky dressings as making it impossible for them to hold the child. You can assure them the closed bulky dressings on the burned area are what make it *possible* for them to hold the child. If it is not possible for them to do this, help them see how stroking their child's face or touching a hand (even with gloves in place) gives the child a feeling of still being loved and not totally removed from warm contact.

Remember that, even if children's chests, abdomens, and hands are burned, they do not stop thinking and thus need stimulation in their restricted environment. A television set is good for passing time, but for longer than 1 day, it is not adequate as the child's main communication with the outside world. Listening to favorite music with them, reading stories to them, talking about what is going on at home or what they normally do at school, and doing schoolwork are also important.

Make certain to visit a child in isolation to talk or play a game at times other than procedure or treatment times so the child can view the nursing staff as friends and caregivers, not as busy people who can't be interrupted. Frequent visits also convey that the child is not alone and others are aware of important needs.

Nursing Diagnosis: Interrupted family processes related to the effects of severe burns in a family member

Outcome Evaluation: Family members state that they are able to cope effectively with the degree of stress to which they are subjected; family demonstrates positive coping mechanisms.

Children with severe burns always have a difficult hospitalization because of the pain, restrictions, and (at some point) awareness of the disfigurement that accompanies major burns. Some parents have exceptional difficulty adjusting to what has happened because they are grieving so deeply over the child's condition or are so concerned with other upsetting factors in their lives (many burns happen because of situational crises in the family; the family may have lost their home and possessions to the fire that burnt the child) that their interaction with the child seems to falter or be very difficult for them. Because they may not be able to stay with the child constantly because they also have to meet with financial advisors, insurance inspectors, or home construction people to begin to get their home back in repair, assure them their child is in good hands during the time they must be away to help relieve stress at least in this one area.

Nursing Diagnosis: Disturbed body image related to changes in physical appearance with burn injury

Outcome Evaluation: Child expresses fears about physical appearance; demonstrates desire to resume age-appropriate activities.

Children with burns are often forced to become extremely dependent on the nursing staff because of the position in which they must lie and because the bulky dressings that cover their arms or hands prevent them from feeding themselves. They respond to this forced dependence at first with gratitude. They are hurt, and someone is taking care of them. After a period, however, their response may become less healthy; young school-age children or preschoolers may revert to bed-wetting or baby talk. Older children may respond by open aggressiveness such as refusing to eat or to lie in a position that is best for them in order to reestablish independence and counteract their feelings of helplessness. To help avoid these reactions, make certain to allow independent decision making whenever possible. Be careful to avoid questions such as "Can I change your dressing now?" or "Will you swallow this pill?" because these imply choices when there really are none as these measures are important for healing.

Allow secondary choices instead. Children, for example, must take the 10 o'clock medicine, but they can choose the fluid they want to swallow after it. They must be fed meals because of the bulky dressings over their hands, but they can decide which food they will eat first. They must have their dressings changed, but they can choose the story you will read them afterward.

Immediately after a severe burn, children (if they are old enough to understand) and their parents are most concerned with whether the child will live. After body systems have stabilized and the parents have been assured the child will live, thoughts turn to the child's cosmetic appearance. At first, it is easy for children and parents to ignore this problem because the burned areas are covered by dressings. Even when the dressings are removed for debridement or whirlpool therapy, it's easy for children to assume the appearance of the burned area is only temporary and that the area will eventually heal and have a good appearance. They have probably never seen anyone with a scar from a second- or third-degree burn and have no reason to worry about it.

When children begin to see others on the hospital unit with burn scars, however, they do begin to realize that healing may result in permanent scarring (Fig. 52.14). Parents and children need time to talk about their feelings about this because they may feel a great deal of guilt about the incident and ways they could have prevented the burn from happening (Bakker, Van Loey, Van Son, et al., 2010).

Both boys and girls are concerned about whether their face will be scarred. A girl may be extremely concerned if her chest is burned because she is worried breast tissue will not develop (a very real concern, depending on the extent of the burn).

Figure 52.14 Extensive scarring on the chest of a 9-year-old boy following a third-degree burn. (© Dr. P. Marazzi/SPL/Science Source/Photo Researchers.)

Children watch you as you care for them to see if you find them unattractive. As dressings are removed, children may expose parts of their body seemingly inappropriately to see if you are shocked or revolted by them. It is easy to think that you will not react this way, but for everyone, the first sight of a severe burn is a shock and it is difficult not to react accordingly. Imagining how children feel and realizing that this mutilated skin is their skin can help healthcare providers maintain a professional attitude. As a rule, the appearance of scar formation can be improved by the application of pressure dressings that the child wears 24 hours a day.

Returning to school can be difficult for all children who have been hospitalized or have been receiving home care for a long time. Their old friends have new friends, so they may feel cut out of school activities. It may be particularly difficult if the child is left with burn scars. Ask how the child is adjusting at follow-up visits. Some children need referral for formal counseling to help rebuild their self-image. Some parents need formal counseling also to help them accept their child's changed appearance and work through lingering guilt.

What If . . . 52.4

A nurse is particularly interested in exploring one of the 2020 National Health Goals related to unintentional injury in children (see Box 52.1). What would be a possible research topic pertinent to this goal that would be applicable to Jason's family and also advance evidence-based practice?

KEY POINTS FOR REVIEW

- Children need total body assessment after an unintentional injury because they may be unable to describe other injuries besides the primary one they have suffered.

- Be aware that some trauma in children occurs as a result of child maltreatment. Screen for this by history and physical examination. Make sure to assess the entire body for physical findings.

- Head injuries are always potentially serious in children. Many different types such as skull fractures, subdural hematomas, epidural hematomas, concussions, and contusions can occur. Coma (unconsciousness from which a child cannot be roused) may be present after severe head trauma.

- Abdominal trauma can result in rupture of the spleen or liver and may occur in connection with multiple trauma.

- Drowning can occur in either salt or fresh water. The physiologic basis for complications after drowning differs depending on the type of water in which the child was submerged.

- Children place anything in their mouth. Common substances children swallow that result in poisoning include prescription medications, over-the-counter medications, and caustic substances. Teach parents to keep the number of the National Poison Control Center next to their telephone or as a contact number in their cell phone (1-800-222-1222) and always call first for advice before administering an antidote for poisoning.

- Lead poisoning most frequently occurs from the ingestion of paint chips in older housing units. Educating parents on how they can prevent this is a major nursing responsibility.

- Burns are classified as first, second, third, and fourth degree—depending on the depth of the burn. Use sterile technique when caring for a child who has been burned to prevent infection. Be aware that burns produce systemic body reactions and require long-term nursing care.

CRITICAL THINKING CARE STUDY

Meredith is a 2-year-old girl you see in an emergency room. Meredith lives with her mother, Antoinette, and her mother's boyfriend in a three-bedroom suburban home. Meredith swallowed three of her mother's birth control pills earlier this evening. On the way to the hospital, Antoinette ran her car into a pick-up truck. Meredith was thrown out of the car and trapped against the exhaust pipe of the truck. The dress she was wearing is partially burned away; her chest is reddened and blistered and weeping fluid. She's obviously in pain. "Can anything else go wrong?" Antoinette asks you. "I received my divorce papers today. My college loan wasn't approved. And now my car is ruined."

1. Antoinette doesn't understand why Meredith swallowed the pills. She says, "I've told her over and over medicine is for grown-ups." What factors in this family's background made this a day when poisoning was apt to occur? Did Antoinette take the best first-aid step for an unintentional poisoning?

2. Meredith has a second-degree burn on her chest, so insertion of an IV line with an infusion of normal saline is

prescribed. You're concerned that, because the burned area is losing fluid, Meredith needs electrolytes replaced as well as fluid. What do you need to know to safely add a potassium supplement following a severe burn?

3. While hospitalized for her burn, Meredith had her serum lead level assessed, and it was found to be 15 μg/dl. What is the safe level of lead in children? If Meredith is prescribed CaEDTA to be infused IV, what do you need to know before administration? What is the purpose of this drug?

RELATED RESOURCES

Explore these additional resources to enhance learning for this chapter:

- Student resources on thePoint, including answers to the What If . . . and Critical Thinking Care Study questions, http://thepoint.lww.com/Flagg8e
- Adaptive learning powered by PrepU, http://thepoint.lww.com/prepu

REFERENCES

American Academy of Pediatrics Council on Sports Medicine and Fitness. (2012). Trampoline safety in childhood and adolescence. *Pediatrics, 130*(4), 774–779.
Avey, G., Euathrongchit, J., & Stern, E. J. (2012). Simultaneous cases of traumatic coin aspiration. *Current Problems in Diagnostic Radiology, 41*(4), 118–119.
Bakker, A., Van Loey, N. E., Van Son, M. J., et al. (2010). Brief report: Mothers' long-term posttraumatic stress symptoms following a burn event of their child. *Journal of Pediatric Psychology, 35*(6), 656–661.
Blackburn, J., Levitan, E. B., MacLennan, P. A., et al. (2012). The epidemiology of chemical eye injuries. *Current Eye Research, 37*(9), 787–793.
Castellani, J. W., & Young, A. J. (2012). Health and performance challenges during sports training and competition in cold weather. *British Journal of Sports Medicine, 46*(11), 788–791.
Centers for Disease Control and Prevention. (2012). *Childhood lead poisoning data, statistics, and surveillance.* Atlanta, GA: Author.
Centers for Disease Control and Prevention. (2014). *Prevention tips.* Retrieved from https://www.cdc.gov/nceh/lead/tips.htm
Centers for Disease Control and Prevention. (2015). *Tips to prevent poisonings.* Retrieved from https://www.cdc.gov/homeandrecreationalsafety/poisoning/preventiontips.htm
Centers for Disease Control and Prevention. (2016a). *Fall prevention.* Retrieved from https://www.cdc.gov/safechild/falls/index.html
Centers for Disease Control and Prevention. (2016b). *National action plan for child injury prevention.* Retrieved from https://www.cdc.gov/safechild/nap/index.html
Centers for Disease Control and Prevention. (2016c). *Prescription drug take-back day.* Retrieved from https://www.cdc.gov/healthywater/observances/pill_disposal.html
Centers for Disease Control and Prevention. (2016d). *Unintentional drowning: Get the facts.* Retrieved from https://www.cdc.gov/homeandrecreationalsafety/water-safety/waterinjuries-factsheet.html
Centers for Disease Control and Prevention. (2017). *Injury prevention & control.* Retrieved from https://www.cdc.gov/injury/index.html
Centers for Disease Control and Prevention. (n.d.-a). *Signs and symptoms.* Retrieved from https://www.cdc.gov/traumaticbraininjury/symptoms.html
Centers for Disease Control and Prevention. (n.d.-b). *TBI: Get the facts.* Retrieved from https://www.cdc.gov/traumaticbraininjury/get_the_facts.html
Chang, T. P., & Rangan, C. (2011). Iron poisoning: A literature-based review of epidemiology, diagnosis, and management. *Pediatric Emergency Care, 27*(10), 978–985.
Coruh, A., & Yontar, Y. (2012). Application of split-thickness dermal grafts in deep partial- and full-thickness burns: A new source of auto-skin grafting. *Journal of Burn Care & Research, 33*(3), e94–e100.
Damashek, A., & Corlis, M. (2017). The role of proximal maternal supervision in children's risk for injury in a low-income sample. *Journal of Pediatric Psychology.* Advance online publication. doi:10.1093/jpepsy/jsx044

Dyring-Andersen, B., Menne, T., & Skov, L. (2012). Sharply demarcated incisions caused by rat bites. *Archives of Dermatology, 148*(10), 1209–1210.

Felus, J., & Kowalczyk, B. (2012). Age-related differences in medial patellofemoral ligament injury patterns in traumatic patellar dislocation: Case series of 50 surgically treated children and adolescents. *American Journal of Sports Medicine, 40*(10), 2357–2364.

Fleisig, G. S., & Andrews, J. R. (2012). Prevention of elbow injuries in youth baseball pitchers. *Sports Health, 4*(5), 419–424.

Hoang, Q. B., Coel, R. A., Vidal, A., et al. (2012). Sports medicine. In W. Hay, M. Levin, R. Deterding, et al. (Eds.), *Current diagnosis & treatment pediatrics* (21st ed., pp. 849–880). New York, NY: McGraw-Hill/Lange.

Karch, A. (2013). *2013 Lippincott's nursing drug guide.* Philadelphia, PA: Lippincott Williams & Wilkins.

Klimek, P. M., Lutz, T., Stranzinger, E., et al. (2013). Handlebar injuries in children. *Pediatric Surgery International, 29*(3), 269–273.

Kupas, D. F., & Miller, D. D. (2010). Out-of-hospital chest escharotomy: A case series and procedure review. *Prehospital Emergency Care, 14*(3), 349–354.

Latenser, B. A. (2013). Burn treatment guidelines. In E. T. Bope & R. D. Kellerman (Eds.), *Conn's current therapy* (pp. 1111–1115). Philadelphia, PA: Elsevier/Saunders.

Lee, K. J., & Marcdante, K. J. (2011). The acutely ill or injured child. In K. J. Marcdante, R. M. Kliegman, H. B. Jenson, et al. (Eds.), *Nelson essentials of pediatrics* (6th ed., pp. 141–166). Philadelphia, PA: Saunders/Elsevier.

Mandt, M. J., & Grubenhoff, J. A. (2012). Emergencies & injuries. In W. Hay, M. Levin, R. Deterding, et al. (Eds.), *Current diagnosis & treatment pediatrics* (21st ed., pp. 316–338). New York, NY: McGraw-Hill/Lange.

Mas, E., Breton, A., & Lachaux, A. (2012). Management of caustic esophagitis in children. *Archives of Pediatrics, 19*(12), 1362–1368.

McCance, K. L., & Grey, T. C. (2012). Altered tissue & cellular biology. In S. E. Huether & K. L. McCance (Eds.), *Understanding pathophysiology* (5th ed., pp. 59–97). New York, NY: Elsevier.

McTigue, D. J. (2013). Overview of trauma management for primary and young permanent teeth. *Dental Clinics of North America, 57*(1), 39–57.

Medlin, S. (2012). Nutrition for wound healing. *British Journal of Nursing, 21*(12), S11–S15.

Morrongiello, B. A., Sandomierski, M., Schwebel, D. C., et al. (2013). Are parents just treading water? The impact of participation in swim lessons on parents' judgments of children's drowning risk, swimming ability, and supervision needs. *Accident Analysis and Prevention, 50*(1), 1169–1175.

Nicole, N. H., & Huether, S. E. (2012). Structure, function & disorders of the integument. In S. E. Huether & K. L. McCance (Eds.), *Understanding pathophysiology* (5th ed., pp. 1038–1069). New York, NY: Elsevier.

Ogilvie, J. D., Rieder, M. J., & Lim, R. (2012). Acetaminophen overdose in children. *CMAJ: Canadian Medical Association Journal, 184*(13), 1492–1496.

Pilkington, K. B., Wagstaff, M. J., & Greenwood, J. E. (2012). Prevention of gastrointestinal bleeding due to stress ulceration: A review of current literature. *Anaesthesia and Intensive Care, 40*(2), 253–259.

Purcell, L. K. (2012). Evaluation and management of children and adolescents with sports-related concussion. *Paediatrics & Child Health, 17*(1), 31–34.

Rhine, T., Wade, S. L., Makoroff, K. L., et al. (2012). Clinical predictors of outcome following inflicted traumatic brain injury in children. *Journal of Trauma & Acute Care Surgery, 73*(4, Suppl. 3), S248–S253.

Rumack, B. H., & Dart, R. C. (2012). Poisoning. In W. Hay, M. Levin, R. Deterding, et al. (Eds.), *Current diagnosis & treatment pediatrics* (21st ed., pp. 339–366). New York, NY: McGraw-Hill/Lange.

Shao, Y., Zou, D., Li, Z., et al. (2013). Blunt liver injury with intact ribs under impacts on the abdomen: A biomechanical investigation. *PLoS One, 8*(1), e52366.

Sharpe, S. J., Rochette, L. M., & Smith, G. A. (2012). Pediatric battery-related emergency department visits in the United States, 1990–2009. *Pediatrics, 129*(6), 1111–1117.

Sigurtà, A., Zanaboni, C., Canavesi, K., et al. (2013). Intensive care for pediatric traumatic brain injury. *Intensive Care Medicine, 39*(1), 129–136.

Smith, H. C., Vacek, P., Johnson, R. J., et al. (2012). Risk factors for anterior cruciate ligament injury: A review of the literature—part 2: Hormonal, genetic, cognitive function, previous injury, and extrinsic risk factors. *Sports Health, 4*(2), 155–161.

Tiemstra, J. D. (2012). Update on acute ankle sprains. *American Family Physician, 85*(12), 1170–1176.

U.S. Department of Health and Human Services. (2010). *Healthy people 2020.* Washington, DC: Author.

Warrell, D. A. (2012). Venomous bites, stings, and poisoning. *Infectious Disease Clinics of North America, 26*(2), 207–223.

White, R., Swales, B., & Butcher, M. (2012). Principles of infection management in community-based burns care. *Nursing Standard, 27*(2), 64–68.

Yeroshalmi, F., Sidoti, E. J., Jr., Adamo, A. K., et al. (2011). Oral electrical burns in children: A model of multidisciplinary care. *Journal of Burn Care & Research, 32*(2), e25–e30.

53

Nursing Care of a Family When a Child Has a Malignancy

KEY TERMS

biopsy

chemotherapeutic agent

Ewing sarcoma

leukemia

lymphoma

metastasis

neoplasm

nephroblastoma

neuroblastomas

oncogenic virus

osteogenic sarcoma

rhabdomyosarcoma

sarcomas

tumor staging

OBJECTIVES

After mastering the contents of this chapter, you should be able to:

1. Describe usual cellular growth and theories that explain why cells alter to become malignant in children.

2. Identify 2020 National Health Goals related to the care of the child with a malignancy that nurses can help the nation achieve.

3. Assess a child with a common malignant process, such as a rhabdomyosarcoma, neuroblastoma, nephroblastoma, or leukemia.

4. Formulate nursing diagnoses related to a child with a malignancy.

5. Establish expected outcomes for a child with a malignancy to help parents manage seamless transitions across differing healthcare settings.

6. Using the nursing process, plan nursing care that includes the six competencies of Quality & Safety Education for Nurses (QSEN): Patient-Centered Care, Teamwork & Collaboration, Evidence-Based Practice (EBP), Quality Improvement (QI), Safety, and Informatics.

7. Implement nursing care for a child with a malignancy, such as explaining why chemotherapy is important.

8. Evaluate expected outcomes for achievement and effectiveness of care.

9. Integrate knowledge of malignancy in children with the interplay of nursing process, the six competencies of QSEN, and Family Nursing to achieve quality maternal and child health nursing care.

Gerri is a 6-year-old boy you meet at a health maintenance organization clinic when he arrives for a well-child checkup. His mother tells you that Gerri wakes up every morning with a headache and vomits soon after waking; he is then able to have a normal breakfast and seems fine. The problem began just after he started a new school in the fall, so the mother is certain the vomiting is related to this. His teacher has suggested that Gerri needs an eye examination because he cocks his head to see the chalkboard. When you weigh him, you notice he has lost weight. "What do I do for school phobia?" his mother asks you.

Previous chapters described the growth and development of well children and disorders associated with specific body systems. This chapter adds information about the dramatic changes, both physical and psychosocial, that occur when children develop a malignancy, a phenomenon that can happen in any body system. Such information forms a base for care and health teaching.

Is Gerri's mother describing school phobia, or is this something more serious? What additional questions would you want to ask to help discover whether you need to alert her primary care provider of your concern?

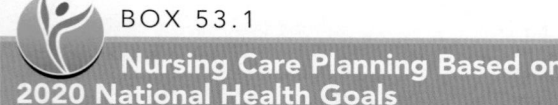

Nursing Care Planning Based on 2020 National Health Goals

Several 2020 National Health Goals concern cancer prevention and children:

- Reduce the overall cancer death rate from a baseline of 178.4 per 100,000 to 160.6 per 100,000 of the population.
- Increase the proportion of adolescents in grades 9 through 12 who follow protective measures that may reduce the risk of skin cancer from 9.3% to 11.2%.
- Reduce the rate of melanoma cancer deaths from a baseline of 2.7 per 100,000 to a target level of 2.4 per 100,000 of the population (U.S. Department of Health and Human Services, 2010; see www.healthypeople.gov).

The health goals don't speak to leukemia because there is no screening test available as yet for hematologic types. Nurses can help the nation achieve these goals by careful history taking at health assessments to reveal the symptoms of leukemia, which are often subtle in children, and by active teaching of available self-screening measures, such as testicular examination, and preventive measures, such as avoiding excessive sun exposure.

The terms *malignant* and *cancerous* describe cells that are growing and proliferating in a disorderly, chaotic fashion. In adults, cancer usually occurs in the form of a solid tumor. In children, the most frequent type of cancer is that of immature white blood cell (WBC) overgrowth, or **leukemia** (Brown & Hunger, 2013).

Many parents assume that a diagnosis of cancer means their child's life will be very limited. Because of the tremendous advances in cancer research and treatment over the past 20 years, however, the prognosis for children and the chances for a cure improve daily. Up to 95% of children with the most common form of leukemia, for example, can expect to be cured. To help both parents and children adjust to this serious illness, however, nursing support is necessary from the time of diagnosis throughout the long-term therapy required. Because decreasing the incidence of cancer is important to the nation, 2020 National Health Goals related to malignancies and children address this concern and are shown in Box 53.1.

Nursing Process Overview

FOR CARE OF A CHILD WITH A MALIGNANCY

ASSESSMENT

The symptoms of malignancy in children are often insidious and difficult to identify because headaches or pain at a particular body site can often be explained away by other factors, such as a sports injury or fatigue. Weight loss, however, is a symptom of some forms of childhood cancer, and unintentional weight loss is never normal in healthy children. Therefore, at every healthcare visit, plot and analyze a child's height and weight carefully to document evidence of this important finding.

NURSING DIAGNOSIS

Nursing diagnoses established for the child with a malignancy address specific symptoms caused by the malignancy itself, side effects of therapy, or coping abilities of the child and family. Examples include:

- Pain related to neoplastic process in bone
- Imbalanced nutrition, less than body requirements, related to mucositis from radiation therapy
- Risk for infection related to immunosuppressive effects of chemotherapy
- Disturbed body image related to loss of hair after radiation treatment or chemotherapy
- Compromised family coping, related to long-term chemotherapy regimen

OUTCOME IDENTIFICATION AND PLANNING

When a neoplasm (abnormal growth that does not respond to normal growth-control mechanisms) is first diagnosed in their child, parents may be able to deal only with short-term outcomes and plans. They may concentrate on learning about the effect or toxic properties of a particular chemotherapeutic drug prescribed for their child, or they may ask how long the child's surgical incision will be. Dealing with such specifics helps them to control their anxiety because it prevents them from dealing with the overall picture or prognosis—that their child has a potentially life-threatening illness.

Be certain the family has an overall picture of the treatment protocol. Explain measures they will need to take to make their child more comfortable during therapy such as not forcing food if their child is nauseated and playing games or reading stories while an intravenous (IV) chemotherapy agent is administered.

Parents are usually eager for results of diagnostic tests. They may need support while waiting until all the findings have been assembled for an accurate assessment of staging and prognosis. Establishing a primary relationship with both the child and the parents is important so that, no matter how many hospitalizations are necessary, they know a support person is waiting to help them through this long-term illness. Be certain the child's siblings are considered in planning care, because the treatment will be long term, putting stress on the entire family.

Parents can be expected to experience grief if they learn their child's prognosis is poor and move through stages of denial, anger, bargaining, depression, and, hopefully, acceptance. During planning, be certain to take into account their current stage of grief so planning can be successful (see Chapter 56).

Organizations that may be helpful for referral are the American Cancer Society (ACS) (www.cancer.org), the National Cancer Institute (www.cancer.gov), the Children's Oncology Group (www.childrensoncologygroup.org), CureSearch (www.curesearch.org), Candlelighters for Children with Cancer (www.4kidswithcancer.org), and the Leukemia & Lymphoma Society (www.lls.org).

IMPLEMENTATION

Nursing interventions for a child with cancer include supporting the child and parents from the time of diagnosis through procedures such as surgery, radiation therapy, chemotherapy, and continued health supervision. Increasingly, cancer treatment is offered on an ambulatory basis to keep hospitalization to a minimum, so many nursing interventions include teaching the parents how to give care or monitor for side effects while at home. Nurses play a critical role in ensuring that the parents are aware of signs and symptoms, and of steps to take, should the child develop emergent issues such as bleeding or fever while at home.

Keep in mind that the stress of long-term treatment can put the child and family at risk for developmental or family coping problems. You can be a positive force in encouraging healthy adaptation to the demands of the child's illness and in reassessing the situation periodically during therapy to be certain the child is receiving appropriate stimulation for developmental growth. Providing comfort and alleviating pain are often primary concerns in oncology nursing. Measures for pain relief are discussed in Chapter 39.

OUTCOME EVALUATION

Because cancer therapy includes long-term care, children need to be evaluated periodically to be certain projected outcomes are being met and are still current. Some examples indicating outcome achievement are:

- Child keeps all appointments for chemotherapy treatments.
- Child maintains passing grades in school despite interruptions for therapy.
- Parents state they are able to keep anxiety at an acceptable level between clinic appointments.

Children with cancer need much of the same well-child maintenance care that all children do, with one exception. While they are undergoing chemotherapy, which causes a decreased immune response, they should not receive routine vaccines. The siblings in the home can receive all non-live vaccines and the entire family (including the child undergoing treatment) are encouraged to receive a yearly flu vaccine.

Follow-up visits are usually anxiety filled for both the parents and the child. The child seems well, but parents may be apprehensive while a healthcare provider palpates the child's abdomen or blood specimens are obtained. Some parents may find the strain of returning for follow-up visits too great and miss appointments (not knowing seems better than to be told bad news). Such parents need help in understanding that initial remissions can be maintained and second remissions can be achieved, so maintenance therapy must be continued. Because a child who is treated for cancer is at risk for developing long-term complications from therapy, they should have appropriate follow-up and screening according to the Children's Oncology Group Guidelines (www.survivorship.org). If a child dies, parents may feel a need to return to the healthcare agency for support. This provides an opportunity to evaluate their adjustment and refer to a social work professional if concerns are identified. Siblings should also be assessed by a provider to assure they are coping in a developmentally appropriately way with the death of a brother or sister.

Health Promotion and Risk Management

Because childhood cancers do not seem to arise from environmental contaminants as some adult cancers do, methods to reduce the risk are not as well defined. Urging parents to reduce children's exposure to secondary cigarette smoke and urging adolescents not to begin smoking, including the use of tobacco alternatives, can help reduce the incidence of lung cancer when they reach adulthood. Although it is not yet known how much sunscreen actually reduces the risk of melanoma, applying sunscreen, reducing the overall time of sun exposure, and avoiding tanning salons are measures to help reduce the development of skin cancer in later life (Quatrano & Dinulos, 2013). Children who receive chemotherapy or radiation for one cancer have a higher incidence of developing another cancer later in life. Therefore, urging these children to continue health appointments so that any additional tumor development can be discovered as soon as it occurs is another important preventive measure. Reminding parents that both boys and girls should receive the vaccine against human papillomavirus (HPV) is an important preventive measure to reduce the incidence of cervical cancer (Petrosky, Bocchini, Hariri, et al., 2015).

Parents of a child with cancer may seek health maintenance care or evaluation for their other children more often than other parents would because they are worried that what seems like just a minor symptom is actually a sign of cancer in that child. They may need greater amounts of reassurance that their other children are well, reflecting the overall stress they feel (Cernvall, Carlbring, Ljungman, et al., 2013).

Neoplasia

All body tissue undergoes continuing growth to develop into and maintain that specific type of tissue. Normally, the body is able to balance the proliferation necessary to replace old cells that die plus produce new cells for physical growth needs. Cancerous, or malignant, tissue, however, is unable to maintain this balance and begins to proliferate in disorderly, chaotic ways.

The word **neoplasm** means "new growth," although it is typically used to refer to a new *abnormal* growth that does not respond to normal growth-control mechanisms. Whether this process is one that produces a solid tumor or one that involves blood-forming elements, growth begins insidiously and usually has been happening for some time before the parents or child realize it is present. Even after they are aware a change exists, some time may pass before they realize the few symptoms they feel are serious enough to require health care (Box 53.2).

Although cancer in children is rare compared to unintentional injury or infection, it is a leading cause of death among children younger than 15 years of age. Fortunately, the overall survival rate for children with cancer today has improved. The overall 5-year survival rate is 83%, and for acute lymphoblastic leukemia (the most common form of childhood cancer), the 5-year survival is 90% (Ward, DeSantis, Robbins, et al., 2014).

CELL GROWTH

The normal cell cycle consists of two main divisions: an interphase (resting) phase and a mitosis (dividing) phase. The interphase has four separate stages: G0, G1, S, and G2. Activity during these periods is summarized in Table 53.1. The time span of a cell's life cycle varies based on the type of tissue involved. The rate of the cycle is slowed or increased by outside stimuli, such as hypoxia, genetic and immunologic

BOX 53.2

Nursing Care Planning to Respect Cultural Diversity

Nurses frequently care for patients from differing cultural backgrounds and practices. An understanding of how these cultural variations impact the delivery of care is important to determine early on and should be communicated to the healthcare team at large. Some aspects of care may be easily identified, for example, food preferences or specific holiday observances. Other cultural differences may be more difficult to ascertain and may require ongoing discussions to fully appreciate, for example, beliefs about the cause of disease and talking to the child about his or her disease. Many institutions have an international department which may be accessed to help promote communications and cultural sensitivity.

People in various cultures have differing beliefs regarding what causes cancer, ranging from evil spirits or evil past lives to totally environmental, genetic, or psychological causes. Talking with the parents and the child, if old enough, about what they think is the cause of cancer can help practitioners to understand their reactions to procedures or medicine and to provide explanations that are more meaningful because they are geared to fit within the patient's and parents' beliefs.

factors, and physical and chemical agents. Normally, an organ has some cells in both resting and active cells.

Cells have the ability to recognize their own type, possibly by recognizing surface enzymes or glucose particles on cell membranes. As a result, cells of like type do not migrate away from each other but instead recognize and adhere to each other to form a solid mass. In contrast, neoplastic cells seem to lose this ability to adhere to one another (they are autonomous cells). The reason for this is not well documented but may be related to decreased calcium in the cell

TABLE 53.1 PHASES OF THE CELL CYCLE

Phase	Activity
G	Gap, or the phase between mitosis and synthesis
G0	Cell at rest. Cells remain in this state until some stimulant, such as death of surrounding cells, triggers the cell to enter an active phase; it is difficult to destroy cells in this resting state.
G1	Period until DNA stabilization is complete; it remains difficult to destroy cells in this phase.
S (synthesis)	Period (6–8 hr) during which DNA and chromosomes are duplicated or a cell readies itself for division into two daughter cells
G2	Cell doubling in size as preparation for dividing into two daughter cells; if protein synthesis can be stopped at this point so that the cell cannot reach a "critical mass," mitosis (cell division) cannot take place.
M (mitosis)	Period of cell division into two like daughter cells

membrane or to an increased negative charge that repels other cells rather than bonds them together (Cooper & Hausman, 2016).

Another feature of healthy cells is that they appear to be able to recognize when they are being crowded for the space they must occupy and, at that point, are able to halt growth to reduce overcrowding. Neoplastic cells do not respond to this communication or cannot receive it, so, despite how crowded they become, they continue to grow. By the time a tumor mass is detected by palpation, it is probably about 30 times the size of its original aberrant cell (Harrington, Bristow, Hill, et al., 2013).

NEOPLASTIC GROWTH

Neoplasms are either *benign* (growth is limited) or *malignant* (cancerous or with unlimited growth). Even when a tumor is benign, however, it doesn't mean it is completely harmless because it can cause damage by pressing on adjacent tissue. For example, brain tumors in children are often benign, but they may cause life-threatening neurologic complications by compressing other areas of the brain.

Causes of Neoplastic Growth

The exact origin of neoplastic growth is unknown, and any growth may actually involve more than one cause. As more and more evidence is compiled on the nature of genes, specific markers in tumors that apparently fail to suppress, or stimulate, cancer-causing genes are being identified; almost all childhood cancers have such markers or a genetic trigger or predisposition to cancer.

In adults, tumors may grow because normal cell growth has been altered by environmental exposures, such as chronic exposure to chemical irritants or cigarette smoke. In adults, the skin, bladder, lungs, and intestines involve organs exposed to such outside influences and irritation and thus become common sites for abnormal growths. In children, in contrast, tumors most frequently occur in organs unexposed to the environment such as leukemia of the bone marrow, nephroblastoma of the kidney (Wilm tumor), tumors of the brain, or neuroblastoma in the abdomen, and because many tumors occur in children younger than 5 years of age who haven't had long-term exposure to environmental carcinogens, this cause of tumors is probably not a great influence in childhood cancer (Pizzo & Poplack, 2015).

Somatic mutation theory postulates that an accumulation of mutations in the cell is what ultimately results in the transformation to a neoplastic state. This theory explains why the growth of neoplastic cells is not reversible (the cells cannot return to a normal state because they are intrinsically changed at the genomic level) and why neoplasms occur in some people but not in others (both an intrinsic and an extrinsic factor, or an inherited tendency and an environmental insult, must be present). It is difficult to document this process, however, because if there is a lengthy time span between these steps, the cause-and-effect relationship is difficult to trace and in general is more pertinent to adult cancers in which decades of time contribute the amount of potential mutations (Kennedy, Loeb, & Herr, 2012).

In other cancers, **oncogenic viruses** (cancer-causing virus) such as HPV may be directly responsible for tumor growth (Gao & Smith, 2016). According to this viral theory, oncogenic viruses have the ability to change the structure of DNA or RNA in cells. C-type RNA viruses, for example, have been implicated in leukemia. The Epstein–Barr virus (EBV) is associated with Burkitt lymphoma. This theory is supported by the fact that an immunodeficient state appears to increase the risk for development of a neoplastic growth. In some children, because of their genetics, tumor suppressor cells may not be present, allowing abnormal growth stimulated by viruses to continue.

Assessing Children With Cancer

The incidence of various types of childhood cancers is shown in Figure 53.1. Because these cancers involve different body systems, signs and symptoms can vary greatly (Box 53.3).

HISTORY

Many of the early symptoms of childhood cancer mimic other common childhood illnesses, and cancer is rarely the immediate differential diagnosis for a routine sick visit to the pediatrician. Thorough history taking at healthcare visits is necessary to reveal the symptoms that may point to a malignancy; an abnormal intensity or duration rule may help identify the most concerning symptoms. Abnormal intensity of symptoms refers to symptoms that seem more extreme than would be expected, for example, a simple lower extremity injury that is associated with more pain than typical. Abnormal duration refers to symptoms that have lingered or increased over an unusually long period, for example, a fever that has not responded to antibiotics and has lasted longer than expected for recovery from an acute illness. Also important is discovering and appreciating systemic effects such as cachexia (loss of weight and anorexia) because these can occur if the tumor is growing so rapidly it is taking nutrients away from normal cells. Other systemic symptoms occur because of excessive hormone production (e.g., overproduction of antidiuretic, thyroid, or adrenocorticotropic hormone), which results from tumor growth in a specific body area (Box 53.4).

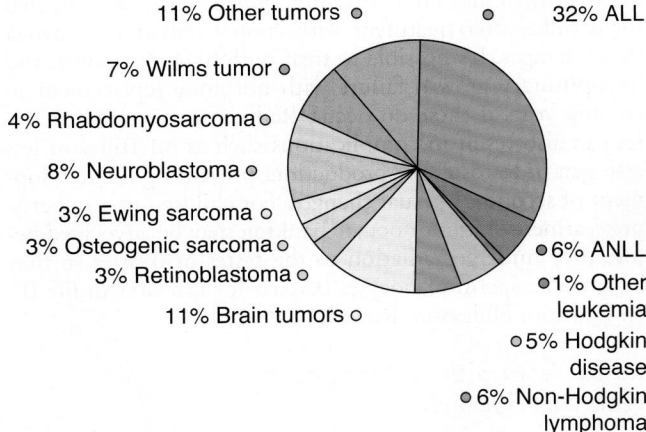

Figure 53.1 Approximate incidence of common childhood cancers. ALL, acute lymphocytic leukemia; ANLL, acute nonlymphocytic leukemia.

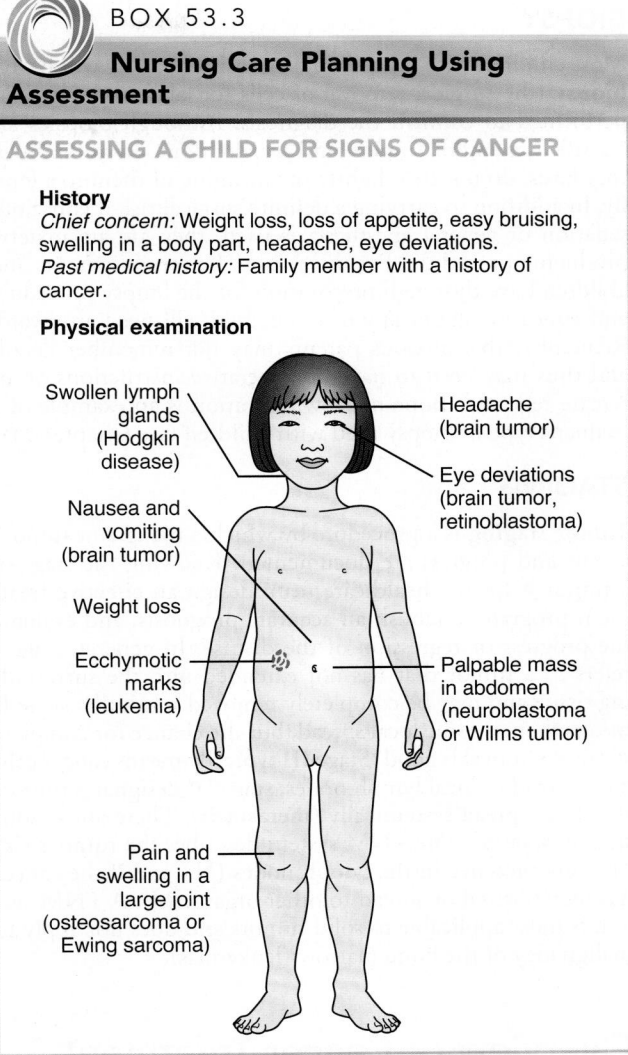

PHYSICAL AND LABORATORY EXAMINATION

Assessing height and weight followed by a thorough physical examination of children are instrumental measures in discovering malignancy. To confirm a diagnosis, a number of further diagnostic procedures may be used, including X-ray, ultrasound, magnetic resonance imaging (MRI), blood analysis, and biopsy.

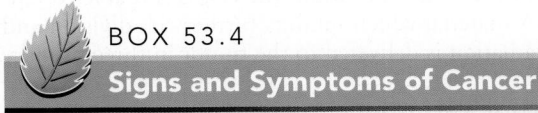

BOX 53.4
Signs and Symptoms of Cancer

GENERAL SIGNS AND SYMPTOMS OF CANCER
- Unexplained fever
- Bleeding/bruising
- Morning headaches and neurologic changes
- Palpable abdominal mass
- Swollen lymph nodes
- Bone and joint pain
- Fatigue

BIOPSY

Most children with a possible diagnosis of cancer will have a **biopsy** (the surgical removal of cells for laboratory analysis) performed to confirm the diagnosis. Although biopsies are classified as minor surgery and usually done on an ambulatory basis, do not treat lightly the meaning of them to a family. In addition to carrying a definite surgical risk if conscious sedation or general anesthesia is used, they are an anxiety-producing procedure. For this reason, be certain parents and children have thorough preparation for the biopsy procedure and education about any care the child will need afterward. Remember that anxious parents may not remember details and thus may need to have postoperative instructions or aftercare repeated. Bone marrow aspiration is an example of a frequent type of biopsy used with children (see Chapter 44).

STAGING

Tumor staging is a procedure by which a malignant tumor's extent and progress are documented. Knowing the stage of a tumor helps the healthcare team design an effective treatment program, establish an accurate prognosis, and evaluate the progress or regression of the disease. In general, stage I refers to a tumor that has not extended into the surrounding tissue and may be completely removed surgically; stage II means there is some local spread, but the chance for complete surgical removal is good. Stage III typically means cancer cells have spread to local lymph nodes; stage IV designates tumors that have spread systemically (**metastasis**). There are various staging systems. The TNM system describes the tumor's size (T), any presence in the lymph nodes (N), and if the cancer has metastasized or spread to other organs (M). A TNM system is most applicable to solid tumors and does not apply to malignancy of the bone marrow (leukemias).

Overview of Cancer Treatment Measures Used With Children

Therapy for a child with cancer focuses on devising ways to kill the growth of the abnormal cells while protecting the normal surrounding cells. Treatment may include any one or a combination of surgery, radiation, chemotherapy, stem cell transplantation, and immunotherapy (biologic response modifiers).

RADIATION THERAPY

Radiation therapy changes the DNA component of a cell's nucleus and prevents replication; the cell is not able to replicate DNA material which inhibits further cell division and growth. Radiation is delivered to the tumor in three primary ways:
1. External beam radiation
2. Brachytherapy
3. Stereotactic radiosurgery

External beam radiation delivers high-energy particles (photons, electrons, protons) from outside the body to the tumor. External beam radiation is administered in one to two treatments per day over several days to a week. Brachytherapy delivers radiation via implants directly to the tumor site (interstitial, intracavitary, or on the surface). Radioactive material is then loaded into the implant, typically over a 4- to 6-day period. Stereotactic radiosurgery delivers a single high dose of radiation to the tumor using three-dimensional (3-D) imaging to target the exact tumor space (Ermoian, Fogh, Braunstein, et al., 2016).

Side Effects

Radiation has both systemic and localized immediate effects. Radiation sickness (fatigue, anorexia, nausea, vomiting) is the most frequently encountered systemic effect. This occurs most frequently if the gastrointestinal (GI) tract is irradiated. It also occurs to a lesser degree as a result of the release of toxic substances from destroyed tumor cells, so children may have these symptoms even when the GI tract is not in the radiation field. To counteract this, a child is often prescribed an antiemetic before each radiation treatment. Skin reactions, such as erythema and tenderness, are typical local effects. Maintaining good skin hygiene and use of mild soaps or moisturizers (non-fragrant) may help preserve skin integrity.

The long-term side effects of radiation are becoming more apparent as increasing numbers of children who have undergone intense radiation therapy survive years beyond the radiation. Because radiation damages all cells in its path toward the tumor to some extent, any body tissue in the radiation field has the possibility of long-term complications or malignant transformation.

Long-Term Side Effects on Bone

Asymmetric growth of bones, easy fracturing, scoliosis, kyphosis, and hypoplasia (not reaching full growth potential) are effects that can occur in bones. Bone tissue is most vulnerable during times of rapid growth, such as during the first years of life or during a prepubertal growth spurt. Scoliosis and kyphosis can be avoided if the entire vertebra tis irradiated rather than only one side or the other; this means a larger area of bone may be irradiated than was done formerly, so that both sides of the vertebra are in the radiation path.

Long-Term Side Effects on Hormones

Radiation to the head and neck can result in long-term thyroid, hypothalamic, and pituitary gland dysfunction, resulting in growth hormone deficiency, hyperprolactinemia, central adrenal insufficiency, or gonadotropin deficiency (Rose, Horne, Howell, et al., 2016). For this reason, children's growth and endocrine function need to be evaluated for decades after treatment with cranial radiation to detect these changes. It's possible to treat both hypothyroidism and hypopituitary growth failure with hormone replacement in coming years if these do occur. Radiation to ovaries or testes can also result in complications such as infertility or less estrogen or testosterone production, preventing the development of secondary sexual changes. For children past puberty, pretreatment sperm or oocyte banking may be advocated before they undergo radiation to the testes or ovaries so they have viable sperm or oocytes banked for use later in life (E. K. Johnson, Finlayson, Rowell, et al., 2017).

Long-Term Side Effects on the Nervous System

Long-term effects of radiation to the nervous system are demyelination and necrosis of the white matter of the brain, which results in symptoms of lethargy, sleepiness, and possibly seizures, and effects on the gray matter, which can result in learning disabilities. Careful history related to school and learning issues is critical; neuropsychological testing is recommended to identify any weakness and assist in the development of individual education plans. In addition, children may experience headaches, cataracts, salivary gland damage, and a chronic change in or loss of taste.

Long-Term Side Effects on the Organs of the Chest and Abdomen

Extensive radiation to the lungs can result in a chronic pneumonitis and pulmonary fibrosis, resulting in obstructive or restrictive chronic lung disease. Heart effects may include left ventricular dysfunction, valve abnormalities, early coronary artery disease, or conduction abnormalities. Radiation to the GI system can result in chronic malabsorption from changes in intestinal villi; hepatic fibrosis can result in reduced liver function. Radiation to the kidney and bladder can result in nephritis and chronic cystitis.

If the child's head area is involved in therapy, permanent alopecia (hair loss), impaired growth of teeth, or reduced salivary gland function (leading to a constantly dry mouth) may result. Radiation to bone marrow may depress the production of both WBCs and platelets. The possibility of these long-term effects of radiation should be explained to parents when radiation is initially discussed, as a part of obtaining informed consent. At the early stage of diagnosis, however, parents rarely are concerned with these long-term effects. Their thoughts are understandably filled with such short-term outcomes as the achievement of a remission or destruction of the tumor.

🔥 Nursing Diagnoses and Related Interventions

Nursing diagnoses related to radiation therapy should include not only the physical preparation or aftercare necessary but also the stress such a procedure places on families.

Nursing Diagnosis: Parental and child anxiety related to radiation therapy

Outcome Evaluation: Parents state they understand the necessity of the therapy and will help support the child during therapy.

Before Treatment. The points where radiation therapy will be directed are usually marked on the child's skin in indelible ink or tattoo. As a rule, parents shouldn't apply any cream or lotion to the marked areas until the treatment series is complete because if a cream contains a metal base, it could distort or interfere with the entrance of radiation. If the head will be irradiated, a dental consultation may be necessary because radiation therapy can slow healing if a tooth extraction is necessary.

During Treatment. Most children have previously had X-ray films taken by the time that radiation therapy is begun, so they're already familiar with thinking of the radiation machine as a giant nonthreatening camera. Because the procedure requires them to lie still for a period

of time, possibly on an uncomfortable table in a room isolated from personnel or their parents, they may experience extreme fear. Reassure the parents and the child that during the treatment, just as there is no sensation from X-ray exposure, the child will experience no sensation from radiation. Infants and young children are usually sedated or have general anesthesia before therapy to ensure they are able to lie still during the needed time interval. To make this approach effective, if only a sedative will be given, keep the child fairly active early in the day and introduce calming activities after the sedative is administered so the child will be sleepy and fall asleep during irradiation. An older child may want to plan an activity to think about during irradiation, such as selecting 10 people to take on a camping trip (and why), or choosing 10 places to visit next year—mental activities that require no movement but are still stimulating.

After Treatment. Children undergoing radiation therapy need their white blood cell and platelet counts monitored periodically for changes; careful assessment of skin in the radiation field is also crucial. Teaching points for parents to help their children during therapy are summarized in Box 53.5.

🌿 *What If . . . 53.1*
The nurse finds Gerri's mother scrubbing her son's head to remove the purple marks inked there by the radiation department. How should the nurse best respond?

CHEMOTHERAPY

A **chemotherapeutic agent** is a drug that is capable of destroying malignant cells. In most instances, several chemotherapeutic agents of differing mechanisms are used to ensure maximal tumor cell death. Like radiation, chemotherapy is scheduled at intervals that increase the ability to destroy malignant cells throughout the cell cycle.

Types of Chemotherapeutic Agents

Chemotherapeutic agents (Table 53.2) fall into a number of different categories and may be administered intravenously, orally, or intramuscularly/subcutaneously. Typically, any agent that needs mixing for hospital use is prepared under a specialized hood in the pharmacy to prevent unintentional exposure. When administering such agents, wear gloves and wash your hands well afterward to prevent skin exposure and absorption of the drug. Chemotherapy drugs should be considered hazardous substances and have special handling procedures (hospital specific protocols should be followed). Caution parents, when administering such drugs at home, to use similar precautions.

Chemotherapy Protocols

Chemotherapy is scheduled for children at set times and days and by various predetermined routes. At first, children may remain in the hospital for a few days of treatment; later, they may report on a specific day for therapy, or parents may

BOX 53.5

Nursing Care Planning Based on Family Teaching

CARING FOR THE CHILD RECEIVING RADIATION THERAPY

Q. Gerri's mother asks you, "What sorts of things do we need to do when Gerri begins receiving radiation therapy?"

A. In addition to preventing infection, you need to take some special actions to meet your child's needs. Here are some tips designed to promote radiation's therapeutic benefits and minimize its adverse effects.

Skin Care

- If the area to be radiated is marked on the child's skin, do not erase the marks.
- Expose irradiated area to air but not to direct heat or sunlight.
- Avoid lengthy soaks in bath water or swimming pools.
- If the head is irradiated, use mild shampoo on hair and rinse gently with water. Air dry or pat excess moisture gently. Avoid rough towels and hair dryers.
- Supply a soft toothbrush to protect gums and oral mucous membranes. Keep the mouth moist by offering frequent sips of water—particularly if radiation decreases salivary gland secretions.
- Encourage clothing that fits loosely over irradiated areas.
- Because some skin preparations are drying and some interfere with radiation, do not apply creams or lotions to the irradiated area unless prescribed.

Nutrition

- To promote retention of nutrients, administer antiemetics as prescribed.
- Encourage high-calorie meals when child is least likely to be nauseated. Praise the child's efforts to eat. Strive for peaceful and pleasant meal and snack times.
- Provide foods identified by child as special favorites. Serve easy-to-swallow foods at best liked temperatures.

Hydration

- Reduce amounts of fresh fruit and vegetables rich in cellulose and eliminate apple juice from the child's diet because these may contribute to diarrhea and subsequent fluid loss if the gastrointestinal tract is in the radiation field.
- If diarrhea occurs, administer antidiarrheal medication as prescribed.

Activity

- Provide adequate rest periods. Schedule activities to avoid waking the child frequently at night.
- Structure the child's activities to be stimulating but not physically tiring.
- Recommend mild activity that does not stress bones that may be weakened by radiation and, therefore, easily fractured (if applicable).

Instruction and Distraction

- Prepare the child for the effects of radiation therapy, particularly hair loss (if cranial radiation), in case they occur. Some comfort measures may include wearing a wig or special cap; introducing play things, such as dolls without hair; and most important, stressing that people like people for themselves, not for their appearance.
- Schedule a tour of the radiation department. If possible, let the child play–act and become familiar with the equipment. Provide ample time to answer questions.
- Help the child devise "mind games" to play during the procedure such as listing 10 friends to take camping, 10 activities to do, or 10 favorite games to play so the procedure is not boring but a learning experience.

TABLE 53.2 TYPES OF CHEMOTHERAPEUTIC AGENTS

Chemotherapeutic Agents	Mechanism of Action	Exemplar Drug
Alkylating agents	Cell-cycle specific; effective against cells in the G1 and S phases of growth	Cyclophosphamide (Cytoxan)
Antimetabolites	Interrupts the cells metabolic processes; effective in S phase	Methotrexate
Plant alkaloids	Interferes with cell mitosis; effective in M phase	Vincristine
Antitumor antibiotics	Impairs DNA synthesis; not cell cycle–specific, effect in resting and dividing cycles	Doxorubicin (Adriamycin)
Nitrosoureas	Disrupts protein production/DNA synthesis; crosses the blood brain barrier	Lomustine (CCNU)
Corticosteroids	Binds to DNA to inhibit mitosis and probably RNA synthesis	Prednisone
Immunotherapy	Stimulates body's immune system to destroy foreign (malignant) cells	Chimeric antigen receptor T cells (CAR-T)

administer the designated therapy at home. Parents must learn about the child's treatment protocol so that they know which drug the child will be receiving each day and on which day each drug must be administered. Knowing the protocol and the specific drug therapy not only helps with accurate dosing but also helps parents begin to prepare the child for administration of a particular drug, such as increasing fiber in the child's diet for a few days before the beginning of a constipation-causing drug like vincristine.

Caution parents, while children are receiving chemotherapy, not to give them nonsteroidal anti-inflammatory drugs as they may interfere with blood coagulation, a problem that may already be present because of lowered thrombocyte levels. Instead, suggest they use acetaminophen (Tylenol) to relieve a headache or to reduce fever and ensure they inform their oncology team of fever because infection in a child receiving cancer treatment may be life-threatening and is considered an emergency while immunocompromised. A parent who wants to give a child vitamins should check with their child's primary healthcare provider to be certain the vitamin preparation will not interfere with a chemotherapeutic agent. Administration of a vitamin that contains folic acid, for example, could interfere with the effectiveness of methotrexate, a folic acid antagonist.

A child receiving chemotherapy is particularly susceptible to contracting an infection and thus should be kept away from people with known infections. Zoster immune globulin may be administered if the child has not been immunized against varicella and is exposed to chickenpox during chemotherapy. Caution parents that live-virus vaccines should not be given during chemotherapy because, if the child's immune mechanism is deficient, these vaccines could cause widespread viral disease. Non-live vaccines are also not given while receiving chemotherapy since the immune system cannot mount the response necessary to create immunity.

Side Effects and Toxic Reactions to Chemotherapy

All chemotherapeutic agents have both side effects and toxic effects. Table 53.3 lists commonly used chemotherapeutic agents, their specific side effects, and their potential toxic effects. Malnutrition, nausea and vomiting, hair loss, mucositis (mouth irritation), constipation, diarrhea, cushingoid effects, and susceptibility to infection are side effects common to most of these agents. Some chemotherapy agents are referred to as vesicants and may cause extensive tissue sloughing and damage if infiltrated into the subcutaneous tissue. Therefore, monitor IV infusions of chemotherapeutic vesicants carefully, especially if not administered through a central line, to prevent tissue infiltration. All hospitals should have an extravasation policy that should be reviewed before administration of a vesicant chemotherapy drug.

QSEN Checkpoint Question 53.1

EVIDENCE-BASED PRACTICE

Following discharge from the hospital, parents assume the responsibility of administering chemotherapy at home. To determine whether parents followed adequate protection for themselves while handling chemotherapy drugs, researchers asked 50 parents of children with acute lymphoblastic leukemia to fill in a questionnaire asking about their experience with chemotherapy drugs. Seventy-two percent of parents reported receiving instruction on safe handling of oral chemotherapy. Ninety percent of parents, however, reported they did not use protective gear such as gloves during preparation of oral chemotherapy. Although tablet crushers were designated for use with oral chemotherapy by 61% of parents, 22% used the same device to crush other nonchemotherapy medications. Over 50% of parents disposed of medication waste with regular garbage or poured the remainder down the sink (Held, Ryan, Champion, et al., 2013).

Based on this study, which statement by Gerri's mother would cause the nurse to believe she needs additional education about safe administration of Gerri's oral chemotherapy?

a. "I'll call for advice if Gerri vomits a pill or refuses to take one."
b. "I know his pills' side effects and will observe for them carefully."
c. "I know I have to give the medicine according to a schedule."
d. "I know to wash my hands before handling his pills."

Look in Appendix A for the best answer and rationale.

Nursing Diagnoses and Related Interventions

As with radiation therapy, nursing diagnoses related to chemotherapy need to address both physical and psychosocial aspects of care.

Nursing Diagnosis: Imbalanced nutrition, less than body requirements, related to nausea, vomiting, or anorexia resulting from chemotherapy

Outcome Evaluation: Child is able to eat frequent, small meals; calorie intake is adequate for age and size; child maintains percentile place on growth curve.

It is easy for a child with cancer to become malnourished as the fast-growing malignant cells take more than their share of nutrients from normal cells. Nausea and vomiting resulting from chemotherapy add to the difficulty of maintaining an adequate oral intake. If stomatitis (intestinal mucosal irritation) or mucositis (mouth irritation) occurs as a result of chemotherapy, eating becomes exceedingly difficult because of mouth pain (Hartnett, 2015).

If the effect of the chemotherapy is extreme, stomach and intestinal ulcers can develop and interfere with absorption. Changes in fatty acid metabolism may alter the responsiveness of body cells to insulin metabolism. Unable to use glucose effectively, cells cannot function at an optimum level, and a chronic feeling of fatigue results. Anorexia may occur from a factor produced by the tumor that acts directly on the center for hunger in the hypothalamus or from nausea produced by chemotherapy. Cyclophosphamide, a commonly used chemotherapeutic agent to treat leukemias or lymphomas, is associated with taste changes. Many children taking this drug report that foods

TABLE 53.3 COMMONLY USED CHEMOTHERAPEUTIC AGENTS

Drug	Classification	Side Effects and Toxic Effects	Special Considerations
L-Asparaginase (Elspar)	Enzyme; deprives cancer cells of asparagine, leading to cell death	Anorexia, weight loss, nausea, vomiting, hepatotoxicity, central nervous system toxicity, anaphylactic reaction	Staying with child for first hour of infusion is important; take vital signs every 15 min for first hour to detect anaphylactic reaction.
Cisplatin (Platinol)	Alkylating agent; reacts with and injures cell nucleus	Bone marrow depression, nephrotoxicity (renal dysfunction), nausea, vomiting, loss of taste, tinnitus, high-frequency hearing loss	Infusion bag must be covered with aluminum foil or commercial cover to keep out light, or decomposition can result.
Cyclophosphamide (Cytoxan)	Alkylating agent (nitrogen mustard derivative)	Bone marrow depression, anorexia, nausea, vomiting, mucositis, alopecia, cystitis, (hemorrhagic) hepatotoxicity	Encourage high fluid intake; maintain IV line to limit bladder irritation; test urine for blood and specific gravity.
Cytarabine (Ara-C)	Antimetabolite (pyrimidine analog)	Nausea, vomiting, bone marrow depression, mucositis, alopecia, photosensitivity	Child may need to wear sunglasses in bright light.
Dactinomycin (Cosmegen)	Antibiotic; inhibits DNA synthesis	Nausea, vomiting, bone marrow depression, mucositis	Extreme tissue inflammation occurs if it extravasates into tissue.
Daunorubicin (DaunoXome)	Antibiotic; vesicant	Alopecia, bone marrow depression	Extravasation causes severe tissue damage.
Etoposide (Toposar)	Mitotic inhibitor; inhibits DNA synthesis	Fatigue, alopecia, nausea and vomiting	Slow IV administration is necessary to avoid irritation.
Doxorubicin (Adriamycin)	Antibiotic; inhibits DNA synthesis; vesicant	Nausea, vomiting, bone marrow depression, alopecia, mucositis, possible heart toxicity	Urine may turn red; take pulse for full minute to detect arrhythmia; tissue necrosis occurs if extravasated.
Ifosfamide (Ifex)	Alkylating agent; interferes with DNA synthesis	Leukopenia, alopecia, hemorrhagic cystitis	Maintaining hydration is important to prevent cystitis.
Lomustine (CCNU; CeeNu)	Alkylating agent (nitrosourea compound)	Nausea, vomiting, bone marrow depression (after 3–4 wk)	Administration on an empty stomach enhances absorption.
Mercaptopurine (Purinethol)	Antimetabolite (purine analog)	Bone marrow depression, nausea, vomiting, mucositis, hepatotoxicity	Allopurinol delays the degradation of mercaptopurine and thus increases toxicity; question prescription if both are to be administered.
Methotrexate (MTX)	Antimetabolite	Mucositis, bone marrow depression, nausea, vomiting, alopecia, hepatotoxicity, nephrotoxicity at high dosage	Decreased effect occurs if administered with salicylates; often followed by leucovorin to decrease toxicity to normal cells
Prednisone	Corticosteroid; suppresses lymphocyte production	Weight gain, cushingoid facies, depressed systemic response to infection	Child may need support to accept changed appearance.
Procarbazine (Matulane)	Antineoplastic; interferes with DNA and RNA synthesis	Nausea, vomiting, bone marrow depression	Drug may cause blurriness of vision; avoid foods with high tyramine content.
Thioguanine	Antimetabolite	Bone marrow suppression	Monitoring of hepatic function tests is necessary.
Vincristine (Oncovin)	Plant alkaloid; vesicant	Constipation, alopecia, joint and muscle pain, muscle weakness	Paresthesia of fingers and toes; foot drop may occur; may need stool softener; tissue necrosis occurs if infiltrated.

Additional Agents

Drug	Classification	Side Effects and Toxic Effects	Special Considerations
Allopurinol (Lopurin, Zyloprim)	Antigout agent	Nausea, vomiting	Prevents uric acid formation from destroyed cells
Leucovorin (Wellcovorin)	Folic acid derivative		Neutralizes the toxicity of methotrexate.
Interferon	Antiviral agent	Fever	Blocks virus replication
Filgrastim (Neupogen)	Granulocyte colony-stimulating factor	Nausea, vomiting	Leukocyte count increases.
Epoetin alfa (Procrit)	Recombinant human erythropoietin	Hypertension; headache	Red blood cell count increases.

taste bitter or do not describe foods as sweet until they are very sweet. Because of these taste changes, foods the child used to enjoy may no longer be enjoyable. Unwilling to try new foods, the child decreases oral intake.

To counteract these taste changes, you may need to suggest different foods or methods of food preparation or include a dietitian as a health team member. Chicken, for example, may taste less bitter than beef or pork. Sprinkling brown sugar on cereal may offer a sweeter taste than plain sugar. However, do not recommend honey as a sweetener. Botulism organisms can grow in honey, placing the immunosuppressed child at risk for infection. Be certain they continue careful cleaning of their teeth after eating to prevent tooth decay.

Urge parents to be careful that mealtime remains a pleasant time, even if the child isn't eating well. Encourage them to allow the child to make choices whenever possible. Offer small portions because a small meal fully finished is usually more satisfying than a large meal half finished. Being certain snack foods are nutritious (perhaps a malted milkshake rather than a cola beverage) is another way to increase nutrient intake. Suggest eating larger meals early in the day before chemotherapy begins, when the child is less likely to be nauseated (Fig. 53.2).

Nursing Diagnosis: Risk for deficient fluid volume related to nausea and vomiting resulting from chemotherapy

Outcome Evaluation: Skin turgor remains good; mucous membranes are moist; vomiting does not occur more than once a day.

Nausea and vomiting are common side effects of almost all chemotherapy agents. Nausea and vomiting may be prevented by administering an antiemetic, such as hydroxyzine (Atarax) or ondansetron (Zofran), before chemotherapy and at 4- to 8-hour intervals during the course of therapy (Box 53.6). These drugs work best in children to prevent nausea; they do not necessarily relieve it once it is present. Thus, begin these medications prophylactically or before chemotherapy begins for best results.

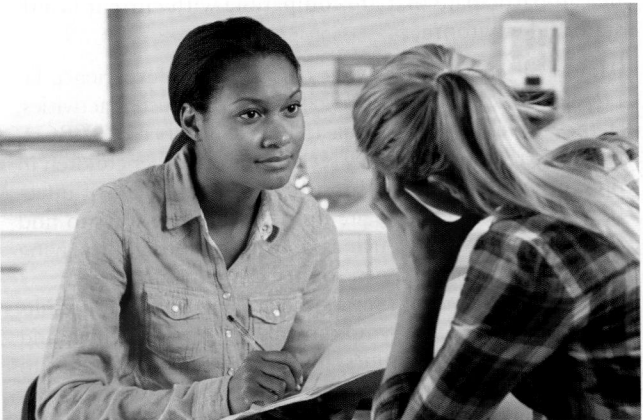

Figure 53.2 Children receiving radiation or chemotherapy often have reduced appetites. Here, a healthcare professional discusses nutrition and food choices with a 15-year-old with leukemia. (Monkey Business Images/shutterstock.com)

Intravenous fluids are often necessary to maintain optimal hydration during chemotherapy. Careful I & O's or urine specific gravity monitoring during treatment helps to determine if the child is appropriately hydrated.

Nursing Diagnosis: Risk for disturbed body image related to changes in physical appearance caused by chemotherapy

Outcome Evaluation: Child discusses feelings about appearance changes with nurse and parents; child states that, although she does not like them, she understands any changes are temporary.

Because chemotherapy causes changes in body appearance, both children and their parents can benefit from a frank discussion of symptoms and their feelings about these changes both before chemotherapy begins and during the therapy.

Alopecia. Alopecia, or hair loss, is a side effect that occurs with almost all chemotherapeutic drugs because hair cells are fast-growing and easily killed as they incorporate the drug. Even when forewarned that such a consequence is likely, most children and parents are surprised at the suddenness of the hair loss (clumps of hair may fall out at one time, and a child can become totally bald in 1 to 3 days). If a child feels self-conscious, suggest a wig, scarf, or baseball cap. Introducing a doll without hair and reminding the child that those who love the child love the whole person, not just the packaging, are also helpful (Fig. 53.3).

BOX 53.6

Nursing Care Planning Based on Responsibility for Pharmacology

ONDANSETRON HYDROCHLORIDE (ZOFRAN)

Classification: Ondansetron is an antiemetic agent.

Action: Blocks central and peripheral serotonin receptor sites to prevent chemotherapy-induced nausea and vomiting in adults and children older than 3 years of age (Karch, 2013).

Dosage: Dependent on weight of child. Typically, 4 mg orally three times daily, first dose administered 30 minutes before beginning chemotherapy, with subsequent doses at 4 and 8 hours after chemotherapy continued every 8 hours for 1 to 2 days after chemotherapy treatment; or three doses of 0.15 mg/kg IV, first dose started 20 minutes before chemotherapy and given over 15 minutes, with subsequent doses at 4 and 8 hours.

Possible Adverse Effects: Dizziness, headache, pruritus, myalgia, pain at injection site

Nursing Implications
- Be aware of timing of chemotherapeutic treatment to ensure that first dose is given 20 to 30 minutes before beginning chemotherapy.
- Instruct parents to continue oral form for 1 to 2 days after completion of chemotherapy to maximize effect.
- Advise parents to administer the oral drug every 8 hours around the clock for maximum results.

Figure 53.3 A nurse uses a doll to help prepare a child for the hair loss that accompanies chemotherapy.

Cushingoid Appearance. Children receiving long-term corticosteroid (prednisone) therapy develop a typical "moon face," red cheeks, and a stocky build. Like the loss of hair, a cushingoid appearance can be devastating to children or parents, the final insult in light of all the other things happening to them. Provide support and reassurance that this appearance is only temporary and will fade after they are no longer on therapy.

Nursing Diagnosis: Impaired oral mucous membrane related to effects of chemotherapy

Outcome Evaluation: Child states mouth discomfort is at a tolerable level, no signs of ulceration are present, and the child is able to eat and drink normally.

Mucositis (ulcers of the gum line and mucous membranes of the mouth) is another frequent effect of chemotherapy (Bennett, 2016). Because chewing is painful, the child needs soft foods with low acidity prescribed. Brushing, flossing, and fluoride supplements should continue when possible. Brushing teeth with a soft swab rather than a toothbrush may feel more comfortable for some children. If the child has ulcers present, an antibacterial mouthwash may be prescribed (be certain that the child understand the wash should be spit out afterward, not swallowed; demonstrate this to very young children if necessary so you're certain they understand what "don't swallow" means).

Another caution is to be aware that mucous membrane ulcers can occur throughout the GI tract. Rectal temperatures should be avoided in children being treated for cancer to avoid further trauma to the tissue and to reduce the risk of infection or bleeding. General measures to reduce mucositis are summarized in Box 53.7.

Nursing Diagnosis: Risk for constipation or diarrhea related to effects of chemotherapeutic agents

Outcome Evaluation: Child maintains usual pattern of bowel elimination; child reports (and parent confirms) no existence of hard or loose stools. Some chemotherapeutic agents, particularly vincristine, cause constipation. Record the frequency of bowel movements so that constipation is recognized early in its course. Anticipate the need for increasing the intake of fluids and dietary roughage and prescribing of a

BOX 53.7

Nursing Care Planning to Empower a Family

TIPS FOR RELIEVING THE DISCOMFORT OF MUCOSITIS

Q. Gerri's father tells you, "Our son has developed ulcers in his mouth from the chemotherapy. What can we do to help him feel more comfortable?"

A. Continuing oral care despite discomfort is important to minimize the number of germs in the mouth and ideally prevent infection. Here are some tips for relieving the discomfort:

- Use a soft toothbrush.
- Try to make oral hygiene fun. Make up a game about mouth care such as "Simon Says" (and he says "brush") that the whole family can play.
- Encourage your child to rinse his mouth with lukewarm water about three times a day for comfort and to encourage healing.
- Serve soft foods such as mashed potatoes and pudding rather than hard ones, such as toast crusts or crunchy cereal, to avoid further abrasions to tender gum lines.
- Provide nonacidic foods, such as gelatin instead of orange juice, which can sting if sores are present.
- Encourage your child to drink as much fluid as possible because proper hydration helps to keep lips from cracking.
- Keep lips well lubricated with petroleum jelly or a commercial product. This care also prevents cracking.

stool softener, such as docusate sodium (Colace), to prevent hard stools from exacerbating rectal ulcers. Diarrhea needs to be identified early to prevent dehydration. Care of a child with diarrhea is discussed in Chapter 45.

Nursing Diagnosis: Risk for deficient diversional activity related to hospitalization or side effects of treatment

Outcome Evaluation: Child identifies activities in which he can participate that are compatible with current health state and environment.

Almost all children receiving chemotherapy experience fatigue and are unable to participate in their usual activities. If they develop neutropenia (reduced number of WBCs), they may require temporary seclusion from other children to prevent exposure to and subsequent development of infection. Help children who are restricted in these ways to find an activity they enjoy, such as drawing, coloring, or playing handheld electronic games, so they can remain active.

Vincristine, a drug used as therapy for leukemias, results in specific neurologic symptoms of weakness, tingling, and numbing of the extremities and sometimes the inability to walk because of a condition called foot drop. In some children, physical therapy may be needed along with special braces or boots to prevent this. While taking the drug, children may be unable to hold a pen or pencil or maneuver small parts of toys because their fingers are so affected. These symptoms typically subside after the medication is discontinued, but in the meantime, help the child think of games that can be accomplished without fine motor control.

Nursing Diagnosis: Risk for infection related to therapy-induced depression of immune system

Outcome Evaluation: Child's temperature is no higher than 98.6°F (37.0°C); no areas of erythema or other signs or symptoms of infection are present.

Children with cancer are susceptible to infection, not only because their immune system is depressed by chemotherapy but also because they may develop a degree of malnutrition that decreases the effectiveness of macrophage and phagocytosis functions and possibly lowers the production of interferon, which is important for destroying viral invaders. A malignant process in the body also decreases the body's overall ability to recognize foreign invaders and respond with the usual efficient rejection process. IV insertion sites, disrupted mucous membranes, and ulcer formation throughout the GI tract provide ready sites for invasion of microorganisms.

Administration of a colony-stimulating factor such as filgrastim (Neupogen) can help the body quickly begin replacing damaged WBCs (Mhaskar, Clark, Lyman, et al., 2014). Even with the use of this agent, however, gram-negative bacteria such as *Escherichia coli*, *Pseudomonas aeruginosa*, and *Klebsiella pneumoniae* and gram-positive bacteria such as *Staphylococcus aureus* and streptococci commonly cause infections. Viral infections such as varicella (chickenpox), varicella zoster (shingles), herpes simplex, viral hepatitis, and cytomegalovirus also are common invaders.

Pneumocystis carinii pneumonia (PCP, normally a very rare pneumonia) may occur from protozoal invasion. Antibiotic prophylaxis, typically sulfamethoxazole/trimethoprim, is prescribed to prevent PCP during immunosuppression. Treating bacterial infections with antibiotics can cause overgrowth of fungal infections such as candidiasis or aspergillosis.

If infection is discovered in a child with cancer, the causative agent is identified by culture. Specific antibiotics are then prescribed. Box 53.8 identifies interventions to reduce the possibility of infection occurring in a child with a low WBC count (neutropenia).

What If . . . 53.2

Gerri's mother tells the nurse that she does not want her child to have an antiemetic drug before chemotherapy because the nausea and vomiting are proof the chemotherapy is working. What action would the nurse take in response to Gerri's mother's perception?

BOX 53.8
Nursing Care Planning Based on Family Teaching

PREVENTING INFECTION IN THE CHILD WITH NEUTROPENIA

Q. Gerri's mother asks you, "What special things should I do to help prevent my child from developing an infection until his white blood cell count returns to normal?"

A. Here are some suggestions to help prevent infection:

- Arrange for your child to sleep in a single bed and room, if possible, to avoid close contact with other family members who might have infections.
- Limit the child's exposure to large crowds, such as those at movie theaters.
- Screen and prohibit visitors who have signs of infection such as runny nose, oral herpes, or rashes; who have been exposed to a communicable disease, such as chickenpox; or who have recently been vaccinated.
- Wash your hands frequently before child care and after handling potentially contaminated items such as tissues or diapers.
- Urge the child to wash hands well after using a bathroom and before eating.
- Keep child's immediate surroundings free of plants, flowers, and goldfish, all of which could harbor mold spores.
- Be sure the child has a daily bath or shower. Clean mouth with soft toothbrush to reduce opportunity for bacteria, which are always present in the mouth, to invade.
- Inspect mouth daily for breaks in the tissue, bleeding, or white patches that suggest oral thrush (*Candida*) infection. Apply a moisturizing and protective barrier, such as petroleum jelly, to the lips to help prevent them from cracking.
- Take temperature daily or if the child feels warm. Avoid taking rectal temperatures to protect against injuring rectal tissue.
- Inspect all skin surfaces daily for scratches that could become entrances for infection. Include intravenous or intramuscular injection sites, venous access device insertion sites, and the diaper area.
- Administer stool softeners, if prescribed, to promote soft stools and bowel movements and avoid rectal tears.
- Provide high-calorie, high-protein foods and food supplements to promote healing. Avoid raw fruits and vegetables because they have the potential to harbor infectious organisms.
- Assess for respiratory tract infection by listening for cough; inspect throat for redness and nasal passage for discharge.
- Assess for possible genitourinary tract infections. Note the color, clarity, frequency, and concentration of urine. If necessary, obtain a urine specimen using a clean-catch method for testing. Promote increased fluid intake to keep urine flowing. Advise girls to wipe from front to back after voiding or defecating to avoid bringing organisms forward to the urethra. If a girl is menstruating, urge her to change pads or tampons frequently (every 4 hours).
- Avoid the administration of any vaccine until the child's immune system has recovered (exception: flu vaccine).

STEM CELL TRANSPLANTATION

Transplantation of stem cells from the bone marrow of a well person to a child with cancer has become a frequently used treatment. The procedure allows higher doses of chemotherapy and radiation to be used because, in the event of severe bone marrow depression, the child can have healthy marrow restored. Immune cells in the transplanted marrow may actually help to kill remaining cancer cells in the child's circulation.

If stem cells are donated by someone who is histocompatible (immune compatible) with the child, this is an *allogeneic* transplant. If the child's own cord blood was preserved and frozen since birth or removed prior to chemotherapy, this is an *autologous* transplant. A *syngeneic* transplant is one between twins.

Before transplantation, the child receives a chemotherapy agent, such as cyclophosphamide, or total-body irradiation to kill as many T cells as possible, suppress the child's immune response to the transplanted tissue, and create space in the bone marrow to allow the newly transplanted cells to implant.

Stem cells are removed from the circulating blood of the designated donor or from cord blood. They are then processed and transfused into the child intravenously. The new stem cells enter the bone marrow and begin to function after about 3 weeks. Until this time, a child is at extreme risk for infection. Everyone coming in contact with the child must wash their hands well, and specific infection control precautions must be maintained. Transfusion of blood products may be necessary to maintain functional blood components until the transplanted marrow begins to function (Carson, Stanworth, Roubinian, et al., 2016).

Not all medical centers perform stem cell transplantation, so a family may have to travel a distance for the therapy. Complications of stem cell transplantation are discussed in Chapter 44 because this technique also is used for children with blood dyscrasias.

PAIN ASSESSMENT

Because growing tumors impinge on normal tissue, pain is a common symptom experienced by children with cancer. Methods to assess pain and interventions to help children deal with pain are discussed in Chapter 39.

The Leukemias

Leukemia is the distorted and uncontrolled proliferation of WBCs (leukocytes) and is the most frequently occurring type of cancer in children.

ACUTE LYMPHOCYTIC (LYMPHOBLASTIC) LEUKEMIA

Acute lymphocytic leukemia (ALL) accounts for 75% of leukemias (Brown & Hunger, 2013) and involves lymphoblasts (immature lymphocytes). Because of the rapid proliferation of so many immature lymphocytes, the production of red blood cells (RBCs) and platelets declines. The abnormally proliferating cells are so immature that they may be identifiable as an immature "blast cell."

The highest incidence of ALL is in children between 2 and 6 years of age. The prognosis in children younger than 1 year or older than 10 years at the time of first occurrence is not as good as in those between 2 and 10 years of age. The prognosis in children who have a WBC count higher than 50,000/mm^3 or who have more than 10% L2 cells (see classification of cells described later) in bone marrow at the time of diagnosis is not as good as in those with a lower WBC count and fewer L2 cells at first diagnosis. The incidence of ALL is slightly higher in boys than in girls, and the disease is seen more often in Hispanic and White children than in children of other races (Vrooman & Silverman, 2016).

Although it can be shown that leukemia in mice and cats is of viral origin, the cause of leukemia in children is unknown. Radiation, exposure to chemicals, or genetic factors may have some influence on the occurrence as children with Down syndrome are more likely to develop leukemia than other children.

Assessment

With ALL, because the bone marrow overproduces lymphocytes and therefore is unable to continue normal production of other blood components, the first symptoms of ALL in children usually are those associated with decreased RBC production (anemia) such as pallor, low-grade fever, and lethargy. A low thrombocyte (platelet) count will lead to petechiae and bleeding from oral mucous membranes and cause easy bruising on arms and legs. As the spleen and liver begin to enlarge from infiltration of abnormal cells, abdominal pain, vomiting, and anorexia occur. As abnormal lymphocytes invade the bone periosteum, the child experiences bone and joint pain. Central nervous system (CNS) invasion leads to symptoms such as headache or unsteady gait.

On physical assessment, painless, generalized swelling of lymph nodes is revealed. Laboratory studies reveal an elevated leukocyte count with cells almost stopped at the blast cell stage. The platelet count and hematocrit value will be low; RBCs that are present are normocytic and normochromic (of normal size and color) but few in number. A lumbar puncture may show evidence of blast cells in the cerebrospinal fluid (CSF).

A bone marrow aspiration (performed at the iliac crest) will be prescribed to identify the type of WBC involved, which documents the type of leukemia.

QSEN Checkpoint Question 53.2

INFORMATICS

The child in the room next to Gerri's is a boy with ALL. Although his parents knew he wasn't well, they had no idea his diagnosis would be leukemia. A review of this boy's electronic health record would most likely note what early signs commonly seen in a child with ALL?

 a. Nodules and an abdominal rash
 b. Headaches and sleepiness
 c. Fatigue and leg bruises
 d. Joint pain and coughing

Look in Appendix A for the best answer and rationale.

Therapeutic Management

Up to 95% of children with ALL will achieve a first remission. If a child experiences a relapse, the chances of long-term survival are reduced and bone marrow transplantation may be required to achieve long-term survival.

Disease Classification and Prognosis

Leukemia is classified to define subgroups of cells and to predict the response to treatment. Blasts with B-lymphocyte cell characteristics can be recognized by the presence of immunoglobulin and antigen–antibody receptors on their surfaces. B-lymphocyte cell types account for about 85% of instances of ALL; the other 15% of children have T-lymphocyte cell involvement (Hunger & Mullighan, 2015).

Cure as Goal

The goal of therapy for leukemia is complete cure, typically achieved with chemotherapeutic agents and without radiation. Prognostic factors of the disease and presentation will be discussed with the family at diagnosis. Adherence to therapy increases the chance of cure and should be stressed when discussing home-administered chemotherapy.

A chemotherapy program is aimed at, first, achieving a complete remission or absence of leukemia cells (induction phase); second, preventing leukemia cells from invading or growing in the CNS (sanctuary or consolidation phase); third, administering delayed intensive therapy; and fourth, maintaining the original remission (maintenance phase).

Chemotherapy in children is often administered by means of a central venous catheter or port because administration of drugs into a major vessel helps prevent irritation to the vessel walls. Central catheters are usually in place for the duration of treatment and parents may have maintenance responsibilities while the child as at home; for example, flushing with heparin or changing dressings for external lines. Portacaths are inserted below the skin and accessed with a needle when needed. They do not require home maintenance and allow for the greatest freedom between treatments.

The drug regimen frequently used to initiate a remission includes vincristine, prednisone or dexamethasone, L-asparaginase, and doxorubicin given over a period of 4 weeks. Because so many cells are destroyed by chemotherapy. During rapid cell destruction, a high level of uric acid must be excreted by the kidneys during treatment. To prevent kidney damage the child will be kept well hydrated or a drug such as allopurinol will be initiated to help reduce the formation of uric acid.

Although a chemotherapy protocol will achieve disease remission in 95% of children, because many chemotherapy drugs do not cross the blood–brain barrier in effective concentrations, leukemic cells in the CNS can continue to flourish. Intrathecal administration (injection of methotrexate into the CSF by lumbar puncture) is instituted to eradicate this source of leukemic cells. Cranial radiation, once used extensively for this purpose, is rarely used today due to the learning disorders that may result.

The third phase of therapy (intensification phase) strengthens the assault against leukemic cells again using chemotherapeutic agents such as vincristine, prednisone, L-asparaginase, doxorubicin, and methotrexate. A drug such as leucovorin (often called leucovorin rescue) may be administered after systemic methotrexate to neutralize its action and protect normal cells from the effect of the drug (Box 53.9).

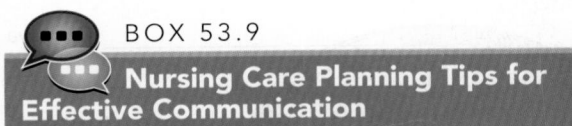

BOX 53.9
Nursing Care Planning Tips for Effective Communication

Gerri, 6 years old, was diagnosed with a brain tumor 3 months ago. His mother brings him into the emergency room because of a severe nosebleed. While you are putting pressure on his nose, you notice his eyes seem to have poor alignment.

Tip: When talking with parents, determine whether they are using any alternative therapies. Patients and families may seek out alternative therapies during cancer treatment. Some of them do no harm, so parents can continue to give them along with proven therapies. Others actually interfere with the action of a chemotherapy drug and are contraindicated.

In the scenario below, the parent has chosen an unproven regimen that closely resembles L-asparaginase. The nurse prioritizes current patient care but acknowledges the information given with a plan to follow up with patient education. Ignoring the possibility that this choice may be an unhelpful one (L-asparaginase does not come from asparagus) and denying the potential discovery of the recurrence of cancer would not be therapeutic and could be detrimental in the long term.

Nurse: Is Gerri still receiving chemotherapy, Mrs. Miller?

Mrs. Miller: No. He's in remission.

Nurse: Is he taking anything that would lower his platelet count or clotting factors?

Mrs. Miller: He takes asparagus powder we get from Mexico.

Nurse: Asparagus powder?

Mrs. Miller: It's the same as L-asparaginase. And so much cheaper.

Nurse: Let's get this nosebleed stopped. Then, we can take a minute to talk about what chemotherapy means.

Maintenance and Monitoring

Maintenance chemotherapy aims to eliminate completely any remaining leukemic cells. Standard maintenance therapy includes a combination of daily mercaptopurine, weekly methotrexate, sporadic vincristine and prednisone, and intrathecal methotrexate and may be continued for 2 to 3 years. During the maintenance phase, the child's blood values must be monitored and are usually in a safe range, allowing the child to return to most of their pretreatment activities, including school and social activities. If there is serious bone marrow depression, medication levels may be reduced.

Complications

Throughout therapy, the healthcare team and family need to be alert for complications of leukemia or of the therapy. Among the problems seen long term are CNS, renal, and reproductive system disorders.

Central Nervous System Involvement

If CNS involvement occurs, it can cause significant complications. Blindness, hydrocephalus, and recurrent seizures are

Figure 53.4 An Ommaya reservoir. Medication injected into the reservoir flows down to the ventricle and enters the cerebrospinal fluid.

possible, although the meninges and the sixth and seventh cranial nerves are the structures most often affected. With meningeal involvement, the child develops nuchal rigidity, headache, irritability, and perhaps vomiting and papilledema. A lumbar puncture will reveal the presence of blast cells in the CSF. If these are discovered, the child will be treated with radiation in conjunction with intrathecal injections of chemotherapy. Always check that a child is not prescribed oral and IV methotrexate at the same time because some of the dose of intrathecal methotrexate will be absorbed systemically and could lead to a toxic reaction. Insertion of silicon tubing into a cerebral ventricle and threading it under the scalp (an Ommaya reservoir) is sometimes employed and provides easy access to the CSF for sampling or injection without the need for repeated lumbar punctures (Fig. 53.4).

Renal Involvement

Kidney involvement, resulting from invasion of leukemia cells or obstruction of renal tubules with uric acid crystals, is another serious complication. The kidneys enlarge, and their function will be impaired. The development of renal involvement or impairment may limit the use of chemotherapeutic agents because the metabolites of these can no longer be excreted effectively.

Testicular Invasion

Males are at risk for testicular invasion with leukemic cells which may not be destroyed with chemotherapy. Careful physical exam of the testes is necessary throughout and after treatment to identify signs of testicular involvement. If the testes are found to have leukemic invasion, local radiation is necessary for effective treatment. If a boy is past puberty and is producing sperm, sperm banking may be suggested before chemotherapy and radiation to preserve sperm for reproduction later in life (Babayev, Arslan, Kogan, et al., 2013).

 Nursing Diagnoses and Related Interventions

Nursing care for a child with leukemia centers on administering chemotherapy, providing supportive care for prevention and treatment of side effects, and helping the young child and parents adjust to the illness.

Nursing Diagnosis: Risk for infection related to immunosuppressive effects of therapy

Outcome Evaluation: Child's temperature remains lower than 98.6°F (37.0°C); no areas of erythema or drainage are present.

Because the number of functioning WBCs is reduced and the drugs used for treatment are immunosuppressive, children with leukemia are at high risk for infection during chemotherapy. Infection in immunosuppressed children may be life-threatening and is a significant cause of mortality in this population.

While children are receiving care at home, teach parents to observe them carefully and to promptly report any indication of infection such as low-grade fever or behavior that does not seem typical of the child because the sooner the symptoms are reported, the sooner anti-infective therapy can begin.

Some children may be prescribed prophylactic antibiotics to reduce the possibility of infection. Parents may be advised to limit visitors, especially anyone with an infection, until the child's functioning WBC count improves.

Nursing Diagnosis: Risk for bleeding due to diminished platelet production

Outcome Evaluation: No evidence of hemorrhage is present (no epistaxis, hematuria, or hematemesis); pulse rate and blood pressure remain within parameters for age group.

Because platelet production is limited, children with leukemia are also prone to hemorrhage. Epistaxis (nosebleed) is the most common kind of bleeding; GI, renal, or CNS bleeding also may occur.

Digital pressure against the nose is usually effective to stop epistaxis, although the application of Gelfoam soaked in topical thrombin may be necessary. In some children, postnasal packing will be necessary, and the child will be transfused with packed RBCs to replace the lost blood volume. Platelet transfusion may be prescribed to improve the platelet count. Because the life span of transfused platelets is short (1 to 3 days), platelets may be infused frequently.

After an intramuscular (IM) injection or the removal of an IV needle, always apply firm pressure to the injection site to prevent bleeding from these sites. Because children with leukemia have blood samples drawn frequently, receive transfusions, and have IV chemotherapeutic drugs administered, provide opportunities for them for therapeutic play with empty, clean syringes or IV tubing so they can work through some feelings about these intrusive procedures (Jibb, Nathan, Stevens, et al., 2015). Advocate for intermittent infusion devices such as heparin locks or multilumen central venous catheters to minimize the need for repeated venipunctures.

Nursing Diagnosis: Pain related to invasion of leukocytes and replacement of marrow with leukemic cells

Outcome Evaluation: Child rates pain as not above 2 on a pain rating scale (if infant, child is not crying).

Children with acute leukemia experience pain because of the vast number of WBCs that invade the periosteum of the bones. Always assess pain using a validated scale for accuracy. Handle legs and arms gently to minimize pain on movement. Use an alternating mattress or sheepskin underneath body joints to help reduce skin irritation caused by resting in a constant position. Administer analgesia as needed.

Nursing Diagnosis: Ineffective health maintenance related to long-term therapy for leukemia

Outcome Evaluation: Parents and child state importance of regular health maintenance visits; child continues chemotherapy regimen at home and keeps all ambulatory appointments.

During the maintenance phase of therapy, children can participate in usual activities and should attend regular school. Because chickenpox is serious to a child who is immunosuppressed, parents should ask the child's school to notify them if any other child in the school develops this disease so appropriate intervention can be administered. If the child has not received immunization against varicella (chickenpox) before this, varicella immune globulin will need to be administered if exposure does occur.

Evaluation of children at follow-up visits includes not only the state of their blood counts but also whether they are making forward-thinking plans or beginning to think of themselves as well children again. Parents may continue to need a great deal of support during the maintenance phase of therapy as they live from day to day, hoping the remission period will not end (Davies, Young, & Salmon, 2016).

ACUTE MYELOID LEUKEMIA

Acute myeloid leukemia (AML) involves the overproliferation of granulocytes (neutrophils, basophils, and eosinophils). It is most often seen in adults and accounts for only about 20% of all childhood leukemias. The frequency of the disorder increases in late adolescence (Madhusoodhan, Carroll, & Bhatla, 2016).

With AML, granulocytes grow so rapidly that they are forced out into the bloodstream while still in the blast stage; these immature cells are not able to carry out normal immune functions and put the child at risk for infection. As with ALL, the overproliferation of granulocytes limits the production of RBCs and platelets.

Assessment

Children with AML have the same symptoms as those with ALL. Comprehensive history and physical examination focused on local or systemic infections is warranted.

Therapeutic Management

The diagnosis is established by bone marrow aspiration and biopsy. After diagnosis, chemotherapy to effect remission begins. Cytarabine (Ara-C), etoposide (VePesid), and daunorubicin (DaunoXome) make up the drug regimen commonly used for therapy. It may take 1 to 2 months to reach a full remission. Bone marrow transplantation may be attempted after the initial remission to ensure a sustained remission (Taga, Tomizawa, Takahashi, et al., 2016).

The Lymphomas

Lymphomas are malignancies of the lymph or reticuloendothelial system; they account for about 11% of all malignancies and are categorized broadly as Hodgkin or non-Hodgkin lymphomas. Non-Hodgkin lymphomas are more common worldwide in children (about 60% vs 40% Hodgkin). Both types occur more frequently in males than in females (Armitage, Gascoyne, Lunning, et al., 2017).

HODGKIN DISEASE

With Hodgkin disease, lymphocytes proliferate in the lymph glands, and special *Reed-Sternberg cells* (large, multinucleated cells that are probably nonfunctioning monocyte-macrophage cells) develop. Although these lymphocytes are capable of DNA synthesis and mitotic division, they are abnormal because they lack both B- and T-lymphocyte surface markers and cannot produce immunoglobulins as do usual B-lymphocytes (Diefenbach, Connors, Friedberg, et al., 2017).

As with all neoplastic diseases, the etiology of Hodgkin disease is unknown, but both genetic and environmental factors probably play a part. It is rarely seen in children younger than 7 years of age, with the incidence increasing greatly during adolescence and young adulthood. Metastasis is through lymphatic channels. Untreated, late in the disease process, it spreads to lung, liver, and bone marrow.

Assessment

Symptoms of Hodgkin disease usually begin with the enlargement of only one painless, enlarged, rubbery lymph node. Other nodes then become involved and potentially spread to the liver, spleen, and bone marrow. The child may report accompanying symptoms of anorexia, malaise, night sweats, and loss of weight. Fever may be present. The sedimentation rate is elevated as well as other markers of inflammation.

Hodgkin disease is confirmed by biopsy of the lymph nodes. Further studies (bone marrow analysis, liver function tests, chest and abdominal computed tomography [CT] or MRI scans, lymphangiography, and abdominal biopsy) are done to classify the clinical stage of the disorder. The chest CT scan may reveal enlarged mediastinal nodes; the abdominal CT may reveal enlarged lymph nodes of the abdomen.

Positron emission tomography–computed tomography (PET-CT) is typically used to stage and monitor response to Hodgkin disease treatment. The PET-CT is a nuclear medicine scan that uses a radionuclide injected into the body which is taken up by metabolically active tissue. Because cancer cells are very metabolically active, the uptake of the trace is an accurate way to identify sites and size of disease. Children diagnosed with Hodgkin disease will have intermittent PET-CTs to gauge the response to treatment and determine the amount of therapy needed (P. Johnson, Federico, Kirkwood, et al., 2016). Preparation for the scan will include a period of fasting (usually 6 to 8 hours).

Therapeutic Management

Although the main subcategories of Hodgkin disease are lymphocyte predominant and nodular sclerosing, mixed cellularity and lymphocyte depletion also occur. The disease is staged according to regional involvement revealed by a PET-CT scan or MRI, followed by lymph node and bone marrow biopsies.

Treatment depends on the clinical stage of the disease at the time of diagnosis. Although Hodgkin disease once was treated mainly with radiation therapy, today the standard of care is combination chemotherapy using the agents cyclophosphamide, vincristine, procarbazine, and prednisone; with radiation reserved for those who have a limited response to chemotherapy or those with recurrent/progressive disease. Current therapy results in a 98% 5-year survival rate for children, and up to 50% for those with relapsed or refractory disease. If a relapse occurs, additional chemotherapy, radiation, or bone marrow transplantation will be scheduled (Kelly, 2015).

Nursing Diagnoses and Related Interventions

The nursing diagnoses often used with Hodgkin disease address the child's impaired immune defenses and risk for infection, fear and feelings about the diagnosis, or changed body image (particularly in an adolescent). Both the parents and the child need opportunities to express their feelings about the seriousness of this disease and how this has changed their life.

Nursing Diagnosis: Risk for powerlessness related to fear of disease recurrence

Outcome Evaluation: Child states he feels healthy during remission; participates in school and extracurricular activities; voices confidence in healthcare team to treat symptoms if they recur.

For adolescents (in whom the disease is most prevalent), some live from day to day wondering whether symptoms will recur. Encourage adolescents to attend regular school after remission, so that they can lead a normal life. Both adolescents and their parents need continued support from healthcare personnel during the long course of therapy because they worry symptoms could return (Morgan & Soanes, 2016).

QSEN Checkpoint Question 53.3

PATIENT-CENTERED CARE

Gerri's father is a Hodgkin lymphoma survivor, having experienced the active disease as an adolescent. Because of his disturbing memories of having this disease, he is highly anxious that the care team assess Gerri for Hodgkin lymphoma. What is the most likely first sign that Hodgkin lymphoma is beginning to develop in Gerri?

  a. A single, enlarged submaxillary lymph node
  b. Sharp pain in joints from blocked lymph drainage
  c. Easy bruising from a shortage of platelets and RBCs
  d. Discolored fingernails from clotting in distal extremities

Look in Appendix A for the best answer and rationale.

NON-HODGKIN LYMPHOMA

Non-Hodgkin lymphomas are malignant disorders of the lymphocytes (either B or T cells) and occur in a number of forms. Unlike Hodgkin disease, spread from the original site is through the bloodstream rather than directly by lymph flow, making the course of the disease unpredictable. Metastatic spread to CNS may occur early in the disease, with the common age of occurrence at 5 to 15 years.

The cause of non-Hodgkin lymphomas is undocumented, but viruses such as EBV, which causes mononucleosis; *Helicobacter pylori*, which causes stomach ulcers; and HIV have all been linked to the occurrence of lymphomas. That is not to say that the viruses cause the lymphoma, only that the viruses were recently present or are present at the same time the lymphoma develops (Rochford & Moorman, 2015). Lymphomas also occur with increased frequency in children who are receiving long-term immunosuppressive therapy, such as those who received organ transplantation (Morscio & Tousseyn, 2016).

Assessment

Non-Hodgkin lymphomas tend to involve the lymph glands of the neck and chest most commonly, although axillary, abdominal, or inguinal nodes may be the first involved. If mediastinal lymph glands are swollen, the child may notice a cough or chest "tightness." Because mediastinal nodes press on the veins returning blood from the head, edema of the face may result. Diffuse, undifferentiated types manifest most commonly with an abdominal mass. Children notice abdominal pain; they may have diarrhea or constipation, and a mass may be palpable on examination.

To establish the diagnosis, biopsy of the affected lymph nodes and bone marrow is performed. Both are needed because it is often difficult to distinguish between undifferentiated lymphoma cells and ALL; if a bone marrow biopsy shows more than 25% blasts, the diagnosis is acute leukemia; fewer than this is suggestive of lymphoma. Areas of metastases are identified by X-ray, PET-CT, or CT scan.

Therapeutic Management

Non-Hodgkin lymphomas are treated with systemic chemotherapy, similar to that used for ALL. The initial phase of therapy is an induction phase (a time during which the child is put into remission or no tumor can be detected by clinical examination); this is followed by a maintenance phase of up to 2 years. The common drug regimen used is cyclophosphamide, doxorubicin (Adriamycin), vincristine (Oncovin), and prednisone (CHOP therapy). Intrathecal chemotherapy may be included because of the tendency for non-Hodgkin lymphoma to invade the CNS. Because the breakdown of cells is so rapid with chemotherapy, frequent blood analysis for electrolyte imbalances will be necessary. Anticipate that allopurinol may be added to the therapy to prevent uric acid accumulation and blocking of kidney tubules.

Burkitt Lymphoma

Burkitt lymphoma (a non-Hodgkin lymphoma involving B-lymphocyte cells) is a rarer form of lymphoma in the United States; it is seen much more commonly worldwide. Children 2 to 14 years of age have the highest incidence, with a peak at 7 years. The same associations as in non-Hodgkin lymphoma exist regarding infection with *H. pylori*, HIV, or EBV.

The first indicators of disease are enlarged lymph nodes of the neck or abdomen. They are typically painless unless they have grown to a large size and are impinging on surrounding tissues. The abnormal cells may grow so rapidly that the cell mass may double in size in as few as 24 hours, so early diagnosis and treatment are important. Surgery may be used to remove the primary tumor or for diagnostic evaluation only. This is followed by administration of the same chemotherapy regimen used with other non-Hodgkin lymphomas. To prevent CNS involvement, intrathecal methotrexate may be given (Cortelazzo, Ferreri, Hoelzer, et al., 2017).

Because Burkitt lymphoma can be such a rapidly growing tumor, the condition responds dramatically to chemotherapy (the cells are almost always in a susceptible state). As with other lymphomas, tissue breakdown may be so voluminous that the uric acid level may cause renal tubule obstruction unless the child is kept well hydrated and a drug such as allopurinol is administered concurrently.

Neoplasms of the Brain

Brain tumors are the second most common form of cancer and the most common solid tumor in children. Tumors tend to occur between 1 and 10 years of age, with 5 years being the peak age of incidence. In children, brain tumors tend to occur at the midline in the brainstem or cerebellum and be located beneath the tentorial membrane, a contrast to the usual site in adults, which is lateral and above the tentorial membrane. This feature is what makes brain tumors particularly difficult to remove in children without damage to normal brain tissue (Segal & Karajannis, 2016).

TYPES OF BRAIN TUMORS

Common sites for brain tumors in children are shown in Figure 53.5. The most common brain tumors are cerebellar astrocytomas, medulloblastomas, and brainstem gliomas.

Astrocytomas are slow-growing, cystic tumors that arise from the glial or support tissue surrounding neural cells. They account for about one fourth of all brain tumors in children. The peak age of incidence is 5 to 8 years.

Medulloblastomas are fast-growing tumors found most commonly in the cerebellum. The peak age of incidence

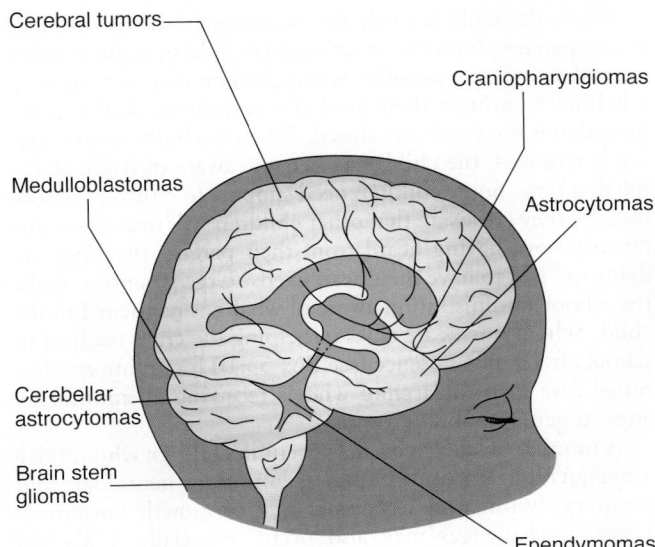

Figure 53.5 Common sites for brain tumors in children.

is 5 to 10 years. Usually found at the midline, they cause fourth-ventricle compression and disturbances in the flow of CSF. Brainstem gliomas often cause paralysis of the 5th, 6th, 7th, 9th, and 10th cranial nerves. They may produce symptoms of ataxia, nystagmus, and changes in respiratory and pulse findings because of pressure on these centers.

ASSESSMENT

Children with any form of brain tumor develop symptoms of increased intracranial pressure: headache, vision changes, vomiting, an enlarging head circumference, or papilledema. Lethargy, projectile vomiting, and coma are late signs.

The headache associated with brain tumor usually occurs on arising in the morning. It may be intermittent throughout the day because of pressure changes related to position and the ability of the cranium to expand to some degree and temporarily relieve the associated pressure. It becomes intense on straining, such as occurs with coughing or bowel movements. A parent may report these symptoms as an increasingly irritable young child who is constipated because of reluctance to strain to pass stool. With some tumors, the pain is occipital. This is an important finding because this is an unusual location for a headache from any other cause.

Vomiting, like headache, most commonly occurs on arising. Unlike the child who vomits because of GI distress, the child with a brain tumor is not usually nauseated and will eat immediately afterward. Vomiting may eventually become projectile; projectile vomiting, however, is not an initial symptom. Vomiting early in the morning is easily discounted by parents as school phobia (reluctance to attend school) because the child is able to eat again immediately and seems to recover about half an hour after getting out of bed (at the same time the school bus leaves).

Diplopia or ptosis because of cranial nerve involvement or strabismus because of suppression of vision in one eye may begin to be noticeable as the tumor continues to grow. Children may tilt their head to the side or develop a torticollis (wry neck) to compensate for the suppression and strabismus. Papilledema (swelling of the optic nerve) may be evident on funduscopic examination.

Apart from these generalized symptoms of increased intracranial pressure, a growing tumor produces specific localized signs, such as nystagmus (constant horizontal movement of the eye) or visual field defects. As tumor growth continues, symptoms of ataxia, personality change (e.g., emotional lability, irritability), and seizures may occur.

Weeks to months may pass from the time of initial symptoms until symptoms become localized enough to arouse suspicion of a brain tumor. When this suspicion arises, a child needs a thorough neurologic examination; a bone scan, ultrasound or MRI, cerebral angiography, or a CT scan will be performed as needed. Myelography may be done to identify tumors that could have spread into the spinal column. Lumbar puncture must be done cautiously because the release of CSF can cause the brainstem (under pressure from the tumor) to herniate into the spinal cord, interfering with respiratory and cardiac function.

THERAPEUTIC MANAGEMENT

Therapy for brain tumors includes a combination of surgery, radiation, and chemotherapy, depending on the location and extent of the tumor (Segal & Karajannis, 2016). Because they are located so deeply, many tumors cannot be completely surgically removed, making radiation and chemotherapy increasingly important. Radiation therapy is carefully staged because, if tumor tissue is not rapidly proliferating, cells are not easily destroyed. Chemotherapy is also limited because many chemotherapeutic agents do not readily cross the blood–brain barrier. Typical drugs used are carboplatin or a combination of thioguanine, procarbazine, lomustine, and vincristine. Administration of drugs directly into the ventricular system via a reservoir (Ommaya) may increase drug effectiveness.

The diagnosis of brain tumor at any age is always serious and stressful for parents. Closely observe a child who is admitted to the hospital for a possible diagnosis of brain tumor to detect signs of increased intracranial pressure or new localizing signs as they occur. Record pulse rate, blood pressure, and respiratory rate with extreme accuracy, so that subtle changes are apparent. Note and document episodes of irritability, drowsiness, speech difficulty, and eye involvement. Statements such as "Child says he sees two forks when I show him one" or "Child is unable to see objects held out on her left side" are much more meaningful to a neurologic exam than "Child has difficulty seeing." Completely describe any seizure activity observed as well, particularly the beginning movements of the seizure, because these can help localize the point of maximum brain pressure. Be certain side rails are in place for protection in case a seizure should occur while the child is in bed.

Preoperative Care

Before brain surgery, a child will usually receive a stool softener to prevent straining with bowel movements. Dexamethasone (Decadron) may be prescribed to reduce cranial edema. An anticonvulsant will be prescribed if the child is experiencing seizures or if surgery is apt to induce seizures. Before surgery, a portion of the child's head is shaved. Prepare the child for this by emphasizing that this is necessary and hair grows back very rapidly. If the child will be cared for in an intensive care unit (ICU) for the first few days after surgery, include a preoperative visit to meet the ICU staff if at all possible.

Postoperative Care

Following cranial surgery, position the child as prescribed by the surgical team, as the best position for the child depends on the location of the tumor and the extent of surgery. In general, a child is positioned on the side opposite the surgical incision. Keep the bed flat or only slightly elevated, again, as prescribed, because this helps to reduce intracranial pressure from accumulation of fluid in the surgical area. Note carefully how much movement of the child's neck is allowed. If surgery was in the low occipital area, the surgeon may want the child to be moved as though the head and neck were a single body part. A neck brace or cast may be applied to stabilize the head and neck and prevent movement.

You can expect the child to be heavily sedated or extremely lethargic for several days after surgery because of brain irritation and edema. In addition, a child may require mechanical ventilation because of pressure on the respiratory center. Many children have such extreme facial edema that they cannot close their eyelids completely or their nasal breathing space is impaired. Cool compresses over the eyes may help

to reduce edema. Saline eye drops or eye dressings (with the eyes carefully closed under the dressings) may be prescribed to keep the cornea from drying and ulcerating.

Carefully assess the pulse and respiratory rates, pupillary size and ability to react to light, muscle strength (ask children to squeeze your hands), and level of consciousness (ask their name or give a simple instruction to follow) about every 15 minutes until vital signs are stable and there is no apparent increase in intracranial pressure. A child's temperature may be either elevated or decreased immediately postoperatively because of the effect of the edema on the hypothalamus. Measures to reduce hyperthermia (sponging, antipyretics given by gavage or rectal administration because of lethargy or coma, or a hypothermia blanket) may be necessary to reduce the temperature to less than 101°F (38.4°C).

Be certain to regulate the rate of IV fluid infusions carefully because an increase in the infusion rate has the potential to increase intracranial pressure. Children with increased pressure may have infusions of mannitol or hypertonic dextrose prescribed to aid in evacuating the cerebral hemispheres of edematous fluid. As the child regains consciousness, small amounts of oral fluid can be introduced. Make certain, when introducing fluid, the child is free of nausea from the anesthetic, to help prevent vomiting because this increases intracranial pressure.

Observe head dressings carefully for any drainage. A wet dressing is no longer a sterile dressing because pathologic organisms can filter through its folds to reach the meninges and cause meningitis. Place a sterile towel, therefore, under a wet dressing or reinforce the dressing with sterile compresses. Report signs of drainage and estimate the extent of the seepage so that you can tell later whether seepage has increased or stopped.

Children regaining consciousness after brain surgery usually are confused regarding time and place; they may have difficulty performing simple tasks they could do easily before. As the cerebral edema subsides and they begin to regain consciousness, they may need a parent to stay with them or to be restrained to stop them from touching their head dressing or IV line. Use as few restraints as possible, however, because fighting restraints is yet another way to cause intracranial pressure to increase. Help the child gradually regain independence in self-care.

When the child is ready for discharge from the hospital, talk to parents about encouraging their child to begin as near-normal activities as possible. Some children may need to wear a helmet to protect their head if a section of skull was removed or is not yet firmly closed. When the bulky head dressing is removed, the child may become aware of baldness for the first time. Some children need support to return to school because they are aware that other children will treat them differently now, having heard from their parents that they are dying or "had to have their head fixed." Urge parents to make the school administration aware of what has happened to the child. School nurses are allies in helping the child readjust to school after a long absence (see Box 53.10 for an interprofessional care map for a child who is receiving chemotherapy after surgery for a brain tumor).

A number of late effects may occur in children who survive a malignant brain tumor, such as long-term neurologic and pituitary dysfunction (especially lack of growth hormone). Learning challenges may also occur, especially if a child received high doses of cranial radiation at a very young age.

BOX 53.10

Nursing Care Planning

AN INTERPROFESSIONAL CARE MAP FOR A CHILD RECEIVING CHEMOTHERAPY

Gerri, 6 years old, has had surgery to remove a brain tumor. He is now on ambulatory care receiving additional chemotherapy postoperatively. His father states, "He refuses to take his antinausea medicine, so he's vomiting all the time. He says he's never going back to school because he looks so funny. This cure is worse than the disease."

Family Assessment: Child lives with parents and two sisters (ages 2 and 12 years) in four-bedroom first-floor home. Father is manager of a local computer store. Mother used to work as a manicurist but is stay-at-home mom since Gerri was diagnosed with cancer. Father rates finances as, "Okay. If nothing unexpected happens."

Client Assessment: Sad and pale-appearing school-age child with bald head and recent surgical scar. Weight decreased 5 lb in last 2 weeks. Skin turgor sluggish. Oral mucous membranes red and irritated. Two ulcers noted on inner aspect of left cheek at gum line. Child states, "I look like an old man."

Nursing Diagnosis: Disturbed body image related to hair loss and nausea secondary to the effects of chemotherapy

Outcome Criteria: Child states effect of hair loss on appearance and feelings; verbalizes measures to cope with hair loss; child discusses reasons for not taking anti-emetic and develops strategy for coping with nausea; reports continued participation in age-appropriate activities.

Team Member Responsible	Assessment	Intervention	Rationale	Expected Outcome
Activities of Daily Living, Including Safety				
Nurse	Assess whether child is capable of self-care in light of changes that have occurred with chemotherapy.	Encourage child to perform as many self-care activities as he did before becoming ill.	Maintaining self-care activities is a way of maintaining self-esteem and competence.	Child states that although he doesn't feel well, he will try to do self-care.
Teamwork and Collaboration				
Nurse/oncology nurse specialist	Assess whether oncology nurse specialist is available for consult with parents and child.	Contact oncology nurse, if desired, to review problems with nutrition, self-image, and mouth care during chemotherapy.	An expert can help parents to determine more effective strategies to combat and accept the nausea and appearance caused by chemotherapy.	Oncology nurse specialist arranges a home visit to review child's situation and suggest improvements in quality of life.
Procedures/Medications for Quality Improvement				
Nurse	Assess oral mucous membrane to document oral lesions.	Review importance of oral care with parents. Advise using a soft toothbrush or swabs to cleanse teeth.	Good oral care is essential to prevent further ulceration.	Child is able to maintain nutrition despite oral lesions; cooperates with toothbrushing three times daily.
Nutrition				
Nurse/primary care provider	Assess whether child is taking prescribed antiemetic and has had any relief at all.	Review with parents importance of giving antiemetic 30 minutes before chemotherapy and every 8 hours.	Antiemetics administered before chemotherapy help to prevent nausea and vomiting.	Child states he will take antiemetic as prescribed to give it a "fair chance" to work.
Nurse/nutritionist	Assess child's intake by a 24-hour recall history.	Encourage parent to offer food early in the day before chemotherapy. Suggest frequent, high-calorie snacks, such as high-energy snack bars.	Eating before chemotherapy enhances nutrition because the child is less likely to be nauseated at this time.	Parent states she will try to have child eat highly nutritious snacks during times he is not nauseated to optimize nutrition intake.

Continued on following page

BOX 53.10

Nursing Care Planning (continued)

Team Member Responsible	Assessment	Intervention	Rationale	Expected Outcome
Patient-Centered Care				
Nurse	Assess parents' and child's understanding of the action of chemotherapy.	Teach parents about the type of medications child is receiving and their usual actions and side effects.	Understanding that side effects are expected, not unique, can help parents and child accept the appearance changes that occur.	Parents/child state they understand what changes to expect and they understand these are temporary.
Psychosocial/Spiritual/Emotional Needs				
Nurse	Assess whether child can devise any measures that would make him feel better about his changed appearance.	Brainstorm with child and parents about measures such as wearing a scarf or cap or modeling an action figure.	Fostering a positive outlook can help child accept changed appearance as a mark he is managing a stressful time of life very well.	Child states he will try to view hair loss as a positive feature, not a detrimental one.
Informatics for Seamless Healthcare Planning				
Nurse	Assess whether parents or child have any further questions before leaving clinic and have appointment for return visit.	Urge parent to contact clinic if child develops further ulcerations or experiences continued weight loss or an increase in nausea and vomiting.	Continued nausea and vomiting, weight loss, or development of more ulcers requires further evaluation and follow-up to minimize the risk of additional concerns for the child.	Parents and child state they feel confident in managing nutrition adequately during remainder of chemotherapy and will keep return appointment.

Nursing Diagnoses and Related Interventions

Because a diagnosis of brain tumor is so frightening to parents and the child, nursing diagnoses need to include both physical and psychosocial aspects.

Nursing Diagnosis: Fear related to diagnosis of brain tumor

Outcome Evaluation: Parents and child continue to maintain function as a family, visit in hospital, and plan appropriately for discharge and continued care.

Because parents bring their child to a healthcare facility in response to insidious symptoms such as vomiting, headache, or strabismus, they may not be prepared for the severity of their child's diagnosis. This can cause such distress at the time of the initial diagnosis that they cannot think of questions to ask. In the hours or days after the diagnosis, however, they often have a great need to talk to healthcare professionals who are familiar with the care of children with brain tumors to ask questions about surgery or their child's prognosis.

Most parents want to hear a definite statement about prognosis—for example, "All of the tumor can be removed;

your child will be as good as new" or "Your child's chances are 1 in 4 of surviving surgery (or of having permanent effects)." Because the type of tumor, its exact location, and its extent are not fully known until surgery, these predictions are difficult to make with more than an uninformed guess. You can assure parents it is normal in these instances for a surgeon not to give more definitive information; this vagueness does not reflect an unwillingness to offer a definite prognosis or lack of interest. They also may need assurance that if they had realized their child's symptoms were serious earlier, it would not have made a difference in the final outcome. Such assurance is what makes it possible for them to live with themselves afterward and not be overwhelmed by guilt, thinking they could have prevented a bad outcome. Symptoms of brain tumor are insidious, and parents cannot be expected to recognize them for what they represent.

Help parents also to understand that because of the importance of brain tissue, brain surgery is never minor. Be certain they understand their child will have a large, bulky head dressing; may be drowsy or unresponsive; and possibly have extensive facial edema afterward. The child may be intubated and ventilated. Even parents who are well prepared are likely to be shocked at the actual sight of their child. Before you take them to the child's room after surgery, review with them once more how the child will look to be certain they are prepared for the changed appearance of their child.

Some parents may not "hear" the full extent of their child's diagnosis before surgery. After surgery, when they are told some of the tumor had to be left to preserve the brain tissue nearby, a very genuine grief reaction can occur. As a result, it may be difficult for them to sit and hold the child's hand or read to the child because their minds have already jumped ahead to the time when the child might die. The child may have difficulty relating to them because they are no longer acting like the parents the child knew before surgery. Offering parents support from the time a child is first seen, through the days of surgery, chemotherapy, and any remission, is an important nursing responsibility.

Children as young as 5 years old are aware their brain is important for functioning. They become very aware of the tone they detect in the words of parents and health-care personnel when they talk about a brain tumor. Because they undergo several diagnostic studies, followed by surgery and prolonged therapy, provide children with opportunities to express their feelings about intrusive procedures through play with puppets or hospital equipment. Remember that, when a person becomes unconscious, hearing is often the last sense lost. Although children do not appear to respond after surgery, they may be able to hear what is said in the room.

Figure 53.6 **(A)** The diaphysis (midshaft) is one of the most frequent sites of Ewing sarcoma. **(B)** The epiphysis of a bone is a common site of osteogenic sarcoma.

QSEN Checkpoint Question 53.4

QUALITY IMPROVEMENT

Gerri had surgery for a brain tumor 2 weeks ago. The care unit protocol specifies that the administration of stool softeners be given before and after surgery when not contraindicated. What is the rationale for this protocol?

   a. Constipation stimulates the release of pituitary hormones.

   b. Straining with bowel movements increases intracranial pressure.

   c. Constipation can lead to anal fissures, which can be a source of infection.

   d. Children in Trendelenburg positions cannot effectively move their bowels.

Look in Appendix A for the best answer and rationale.

Bone Tumors

Tumors derived from connective tissue, such as bone and cartilage, muscle, blood vessels, or lymphoid tissue, are termed **sarcomas**. They are the second most frequently occurring neoplasms in adolescents (only lymphomas occur more frequently). Bone tumors may arise during adolescence because rapid bone growth is occurring at this time. Because girls have a puberty growth spurt a year or two earlier than boys, bone tumors tend to occur slightly earlier in girls than in boys (13 compared with 14 or 15 years of age). The two most frequently occurring types are osteogenic sarcoma and Ewing sarcoma (Fig. 53.6).

OSTEOGENIC SARCOMA

An **osteogenic sarcoma** is a malignant tumor of long bone involving rapidly growing bone tissue (mesenchymal-matrix forming cells). It occurs more commonly in boys than in girls and in children who have had radiation for other malignancies as a later life effect. The most common sites of occurrence are the distal femur, the proximal tibia, and the proximal humerus, and the tumor is often associated with locoregional pain and swelling (HaDuong, Martin, Skapek, et al., 2015). Children with a specific genetic syndrome have a higher incidence than usual of developing an osteosarcoma, so a hereditary predisposition may be present.

Metastasis occurs early with bone tumors because of the extensive vascular system in bones. Metastasis to the lungs is very common; as many as 25% of adolescents will have lung metastasis already by the time of initial diagnosis. Other common sites of metastasis are brain and other bone tissue.

Assessment

The area may be painful and swollen; it may be inflamed and feel warm because tumors are highly vascular and therefore call increased blood into the area. Children may report a history of recent trauma to the site such as a fall playing basketball or a bump to their knee during soccer practice and attribute pain in the knee to this injury for some time. To prevent the adolescent from thinking he caused the tumor, be certain he and his parents understand trauma did not cause the process; it merely called attention to the leg or arm where a malignant process was at work.

Features of osteosarcoma are visible on radiologic studies such as MRI, but a biopsy will be done of the suspicious site to confirm the diagnosis. To determine metastasis, a complete blood cell count, urinalysis, chest X-ray, chest CT scan, and bone scans will be done. Caution children not to bear weight on an affected leg while waiting for tests or surgery because if the bone has become weakened by the growing tumor, weight bearing could result in a fracture at the tumor site.

Therapeutic Management

Chemotherapy is prescribed to shrink the tumor before surgery. If parents are concerned with this delay, explain that, with a bone tumor, this is a helpful intervention because it will make removal of the tumor more successful. A common chemotherapy drug regimen used for treatment includes methotrexate, cisplatin, doxorubicin, and ifosfamide.

When at all possible, surgical procedures will attempt to remove the tumor without amputation. These surgeries are referred to as limb salvage. The bone that is removed is typically replaced by cadaver or man-made prosthesis (Jackson, Bittman, & Granowetter, 2016). Rarely, if the tumor is extensive at the time of diagnosis, the extremity may be amputated at the joint above the tumor.

Only a few years ago, a diagnosis of osteogenic sarcoma was ominous; few children survived into adulthood. Today, 70% of adolescents in whom the diagnosis is made early and who are treated rigorously can be cured (Brown & Hunger, 2013).

Nursing Diagnoses and Related Interventions

Diagnosis of malignant bone tumor is a shock to both parents and children because the symptoms began so insidiously the diagnosis doesn't seem real. You can assure parents that any delay in seeking treatment would not have had a marked effect on the chances for a cure. Neither the adolescent nor the parents could have been expected to seek medical attention any earlier than they did. This is important assurance because it can help parents function more effectively to help their child through the illness.

It may be particularly difficult for the patient and family to accept certain aspects of the disease and its impact on the future. For example, depending on the tumor site, there may be limitations to participating in specific sports or physical activities. Supporting the child and family while they incorporate their new reality is an important aspect of nursing care.

Nursing Diagnosis: Risk for injury related to surgery and bone prosthesis

Outcome Evaluation: Extremity distal to surgical incision remains warm to touch; capillary filling is less than 5 seconds.

The major danger associated with surgery for excising osteosarcoma and placement of a bone prosthesis (limb salvage surgery) is that the swelling that occurs during surgery or immediately afterward can disrupt neurologic or circulatory function to the lower leg. Always position and handle the leg carefully to prevent further disruption. Assess frequently for signs the neurologic and circulatory systems are intact distal to the surgery (toes are warm and pink; capillary filling is less than 5 seconds; adolescent reports no numbness or tingling).

QSEN Checkpoint Question 53.5

TEAMWORK & COLLABORATION

Gerri's school nurse informs another nurse that his mother forbids him to play basketball because she heard a friend's son developed osteosarcoma when he was injured playing the sport. The nurses collaborate to plan a unified response to her concerns. What would be the best advice to give Gerri's mother regarding her understanding of osteosarcoma?

a. Evidence has shown that bone cancer is associated with active, organized sports.

b. Osteosarcoma more often occurs in girls, so the boy's diagnosis is unusual.

c. The sports injury more likely led to diagnosis of the tumor but was not the cause of it.

d. The boy's inadequate calcium intake was a more likely cause of his health problem.

Look in Appendix A for the best answer and rationale.

EWING SARCOMA

Ewing sarcoma is a malignant bone tumor; it occurs most frequently in the bone marrow of the diaphyseal area (midshaft) of long bones and spreads longitudinally through the bone (see Fig. 53.6). Ewing sarcoma may also present as a primary site outside the skeletal system where it is referred to as a primitive neuroectodermal tumor (PNET). Ewing sarcoma of the bone occurs primarily in young adolescents and older school-age children; it is slightly more common in boys than in girls. Metastasis is usually present at the time of diagnosis, with the lungs, other bones, the CNS, and lymph nodes being the most common sites (Jackson et al., 2016).

Assessment

Most children have had pain at the site of the tumor for some time before seeing a primary healthcare provider. At first, the pain is intermittent, and the child attributes it to an injury (perhaps a friend punched his leg or the child bumped it against a footstool). Finally, the pain becomes constant and so severe the child cannot sleep at night. X-rays will reveal an unusual "onion-skin" reaction (overlapping fine lines disclosed on the X-ray film) surrounding the invading tumor cells. A bone scan, bone marrow aspiration and biopsy, CT scan of the lungs, and MRI will be done to determine the extent of the tumor and whether metastasis has occurred. A biopsy of the tumor site will be done for a definite diagnosis. During tests, urge the child to avoid bearing weight on the affected extremity because this could cause a pathologic fracture at the site.

Therapeutic Management

With Ewing sarcoma, therapy consists of a combination of surgery to remove the primary tumor, radiation, and chemotherapy. The drug regimen often used includes vincristine, dactinomycin, cyclophosphamide, doxorubicin, etoposide, and ifosfamide. Radiation is typically used only when surgical resection is not possible or incomplete (Jackson et al., 2016).

About 50% of children survive for at least 5 years; older children have a better survival rate than younger children. Caution adolescents to continue to be careful about activities that cause stress on an extremity that has received radiation (e.g., football or weight lifting) because it may not be as strong as usual afterward.

Other Childhood Neoplasms

NEUROBLASTOMA

Neuroblastomas are tumors that arise from the cells of the sympathetic nervous system; cells are highly undifferentiated and invasive, occur most frequently in the abdomen near the adrenal glands or spinal ganglia, and are the most common abdominal tumor in childhood (Matthay, Maris, Schleiermacher, et al., 2016). Neuroblastoma occurs primarily in infants and preschool children; it is slightly more common in boys than in girls. These tumors may occur so early in life, in fact, that they may be detected by fetal ultrasound or shortly after birth. Common sites of metastasis include the bone marrow, liver, and subcutaneous tissue.

Assessment

The growing tumor is most often discovered on abdominal palpation as an abdominal mass after general symptoms of weight loss and anorexia are noticed. Pressure on the adrenal glands from the tumor may cause excessive sweating, flushed face, and hypertension. Abdominal pain and constipation may also be present. Compression on the spinal nerves or invasion into the intervertebral foramina may cause loss of motor function in lower extremities.

If the primary lesion is in the upper chest, children will report dyspnea; swallowing may be difficult, and neck and facial edema may occur from compression on the vena cava. If liver metastasis is present, children may have jaundice. If metastasis to the skin has occurred, blue or purplish nodules (prominent raised areas) on arms or legs may be seen.

The extent of the tumor and any metastases present are identified by MRI or ultrasound (a mass growing on an adrenal gland just above the kidney will demonstrate kidney compression); an arteriogram (neuroblastomas are vascular tumors and incorporate veins and arteries into their structure as they grow); ultrasound, CT, or MRI scan of the chest, abdomen, and pelvis; a gallium bone scan; or bone marrow aspiration and biopsy. If an adrenal tumor is present, it will stimulate production of adrenal gland hormones or catecholamines. To detect these substances, a urine sample will be tested for the presence of vanillylmandelic acid and homovanillic acid (the breakdown products of catecholamines). A biopsy of the tumor site will be planned so the tumor can be definitely identified.

Therapeutic Management

Infants in the initial stages of disease may require observation only as some of these tumors will regress without intervention. If the tumor is localized (stage I or II), therapy will consist of surgical removal of the primary tumor. If the tumor is stage III (lymph nodes are involved) or stage IV (metastasis has occurred), surgery will be followed by chemotherapy combinations using agents such as doxorubicin, cyclophosphamide, etoposide, and carboplatin (Pinto, Applebaum, Volchenboum, et al., 2015).

A "second look" surgical procedure may be scheduled within several months to determine the effectiveness of therapy and to attempt the possible removal of further tumor. Immunotherapy is another possibility to eliminate residual disease after chemotherapy (Park, Bagatell, London, et al., 2013).

Stage IV disease is a unique form because it has a high rate of spontaneous regression. This occurs because the tumor either spontaneously degenerates or undergoes differentiation to normal tissue (Matthay et al., 2016).

Overall, children with neuroblastoma have a 5-year survival rate of 70% to 90%. Although most children have a positive initial response to therapy, recurrence is common within the first year. The prognosis is better in children diagnosed before 1 year of age.

RHABDOMYOSARCOMA

A **rhabdomyosarcoma** is a tumor of striated muscle (Williams, Fernandez-Pineda, & Gosain, 2016). It arises from the embryonic mesenchyme tissue that forms muscle, connective, and vascular tissue. The peak age of incidence of these tumors is 2 to 6 years, with a second peak occurring during puberty. Common sites of occurrence include the eye orbit, paranasal sinuses, uterus, prostate, bladder, retroperitoneum, arms, and legs. CNS invasion occurs from direct tumor extension, resulting in cranial nerve palsy, nuchal rigidity, bradycardia, or bradypnea (because of brainstem compromise). Distant metastasis most commonly occurs in lungs, bone, or bone marrow.

Assessment

The symptoms relate to the site of the tumor (Table 53.4). A biopsy specimen of the tumor is taken and examined for tissue identification. Metastasis is ruled out by bone scan, chest X-ray, CT scan, MRI, and bone marrow aspiration.

TABLE 53.4 COMMON SITES AND ASSOCIATED SYMPTOMS OF RHABDOMYOSARCOMA

Site of Tumor	Symptoms
Orbit	Proptosis (extruding eye); visible and palpable conjunctival or eyelid mass
Neck	Hoarseness, dysphagia; visible and palpable mass in neck
Nasopharynx	Airway obstruction, epistaxis, dysphagia, visible mass in nasal or nasopharyngeal passages
Paranasal sinuses	Swelling, pain, nasal discharge, epistaxis
Middle ear	Pain, chronic otitis media, hearing loss, facial nerve palsy, mass protruding into external ear canal
Bladder and prostate	Dysuria, urinary retention, hematuria, constipation, palpable lower abdominal mass
Vagina	Mass protruding from uterus or cervix into vagina, abnormal vaginal bleeding
Trunk, extremities	Visible and palpable soft-tissue mass
Testicles	Visible and palpable soft-tissue mass

Therapeutic Management

The primary treatment is surgical removal of the tumor, followed by chemotherapy combinations with agents such as vincristine, dactinomycin, cyclophosphamide, doxorubicin, etoposide, topotecan, and ifosfamide. The child receives chemotherapy every 3 to 4 weeks for 18 to 24 months. If CNS extension has occurred, intrathecal chemotherapy may be included in the regimen. Radiation is frequently used for local control of disease with intensity-modulated radiotherapy (IMRT) employed to reduce the long-term complications to surrounding tissue (Hiniker & Donaldson, 2015).

A child's prognosis depends on the size of the tumor and whether metastasis was present at the time of initial diagnosis. If the entire tumor was removed and no lymph node metastasis has occurred, the chances are as high as 80% that the tumor will not recur. If some of the tumor had to be left because of its size or location, the chance of recurrence rises to about 50%. If metastasis to the lungs or bone was present at the time of the initial diagnosis, the prognosis drops still further; about 20% of children in this situation have long-term survival. Among children who do survive, long-term complications such as cardiomyopathy and infertility may occur from the side effects of chemotherapy.

NEPHROBLASTOMA (WILMS TUMOR)

Nephroblastoma (Wilms tumor) is a malignant tumor that rises from the metanephric mesoderm cells of the upper pole of the kidney (Malkan, Loh, Bahrami, et al., 2015). It accounts for 20% of solid tumors in childhood, and overall survival rates are greater than 90%. It may occur in association with congenital anomalies such as aniridia (lack of color in the iris), cryptorchidism, hypospadias, pseudohermaphroditism, cystic kidneys, hemangioma, and talipes disorders. A number of gene mutation has been identified as associated with the disease. Without therapy, metastatic spread by the bloodstream is most often to the lungs, regional lymph nodes, liver, bone, and, eventually, brain.

Assessment

A nephroblastoma is usually discovered early in life (6 months to 5 years; peak at 3 to 4 years), although it apparently arises from an embryonic structure present in the child before birth. Nephroblastomas distort the kidney anteriorly so that the tumor is felt as a firm, nontender abdominal mass. Parents are aware their infant has a mass in the abdomen but bring the infant to their healthcare provider thinking that it is hard stool from chronic constipation. Parents often report that the mass seemed to appear overnight. This actually can happen, because tumors can hemorrhage into themselves, doubling their size in a matter of hours. If this happens, accompanying signs may be hematuria and a low-grade fever. The child may be anemic from blood loss and lack of erythropoietin formation by the diseased kidney. Although hypertension may also occur because of excessive renin production, blood pressure is not taken routinely in children of this age, so the tumor is rarely discovered by this method.

A CT scan or ultrasound reveals the primary tumor and any points of metastasis. Kidney function studies, such as glomerular filtration rate or blood urea nitrogen, will be done to assess function of the kidneys before surgery. Little time, however, can be allotted for preoperative testing, because

these tumors metastasize rapidly as a result of the large blood supply to the kidneys and adrenal glands.

Therapeutic Management

Nephroblastomas are staged to predict therapy and prognosis. The tumor will be removed by nephrectomy (excision of the affected kidney). This is usually followed immediately by chemotherapy with dactinomycin, doxorubicin, or vincristine, cyclophosphamide, and etoposide. Chemotherapy may be given at varying intervals for as long as 15 months. Radiation is usually limited to high-risk disease (anaplastic histology) or advanced disease (Dome, Graf, Geller, et al., 2015).

If tumor involvement is bilateral, the operative decisions obviously become more complex. If the tumors are small, both tumors may be removed, leaving functioning kidney on both sides intact. In other children, the kidney with the larger tumor is removed and the tumor site in the remaining kidney is then treated with both radiation and chemotherapy.

Complications such as nephritis, small bowel obstruction, and hepatic damage caused by fibrotic scarring from radiation or scar tissue from surgery can occur. In girls, radiation-related damage to the ovaries may result in sterility. Radiation to the lungs may result in interstitial pneumonia.

QSEN Checkpoint Question 53.6

SAFETY

A child on the hospital unit is undergoing chemotherapy for newly diagnosed leukemia and is neutropenic. A visit arrives on the unit with a plant and flowers to put in the child's room. What should the nurse do to ensure the immunocompromised patient remains safe?

  a. Let the child have the plant in the room but place it far away from the bed.

  b. Let the child have the plant to help cheer the child up.

  c. Tell the visitor that the plant/flower may harbor fungus or other infectious materials and unfortunately can't be allowed in the room.

  d. Allow the visitor to place the plant/flower at the nurse's station so that it can be enjoyed by the patient without being placed in the room.

Look in Appendix A for the best answer and rationale.

RETINOBLASTOMA

Retinoblastoma is a malignant tumor of the retina of the eye. A rare tumor, it accounts for only 1% to 3% of childhood malignancies. In about 10% of children, these tumors develop because of an inherited autosomal dominant pattern that causes an alteration of chromosome 13. Parents who have one child with retinoblastoma have about a 4% chance of having a second child with a similar tumor. If two or more children have the tumor, the parents are probably carriers, and it can be predicted that up to 50% of their children will be affected. Because of the dominant pattern of inheritance, a person who survives retinoblastoma has an elevated chance of having a child with a similar tumor. Parents who may be carriers and children who survive the disease need genetic counseling so that they are aware of the risk to their children.

Because the 5-year survival rate for children with retinoblastoma is good (at least 90%), this is an important counseling role (Rowland & Metcalfe, 2013).

Retinoblastoma occurs most often, however, as spontaneous development, not the inherited type. Children with the inherited type tend to develop bilateral disease; those with the spontaneous type may or may not have the tumor in both eyes.

Assessment

Retinoblastoma occurs early in life, from about 6 weeks of age through the preschool period. It occurs equally in boys and girls, and there is no preference for either the right or the left eye. One tumor or many individual tumors may be present. Tumors are located on the retina or in the vitreous fluid or may extend backward into the choroid, the optic nerve, and the subarachnoid space.

On examination, the child's pupil appears white (the red reflex is absent) or is described as a typical "cat's eye." The child develops strabismus as the eye becomes nonfunctional. This tumor metastasizes readily along the course of the optic nerve to the subarachnoid space and brain; it can quickly involve the second eye. Metastasis to distant body sites, such as bone marrow and liver, is possible.

Children with a family history should have an ophthalmic exam usually under general anesthesia or conscious sedation at least three times yearly until they reach 5 years of age. CT scanning, MRI, and ultrasound may all be prescribed to detect intraocular calcification or the presence of tumor. The possibility of distant metastasis is evaluated by lumbar puncture, liver and skeletal survey, MRI, or bone marrow biopsy.

Therapeutic Management

Retinoblastomas, if allowed to grow, will cause blindness. An important goal for children with retinoblastoma is to preserve as much vision as possible for as long as possible. If the tumor is very small at the time of diagnosis, it may be treated with cryosurgery (freezing the tumor to destroy local cells), hopefully preserving partial vision in the eye. Photocoagulation using laser surgery to destroy the blood vessels supplying the tumor or localized radioactive applicators or plaques sutured to the sclera over the tumor may also be used. If the tumor has metastasized, the child may also receive radiation treatment and chemotherapy (vincristine, cyclophosphamide, doxorubicin, carboplatin, and etoposide are components of commonly used regimens).

If the tumor is large when first discovered, enucleation of the eye may be necessary. After enucleation, the child has a large pressure dressing applied to the empty socket. Observe for bleeding on the dressing and assess vital signs frequently. To keep young children from tugging at the dressing and removing it, they may need to be restrained if a parent cannot be with them constantly. After about 48 hours, the pressure dressing is removed and a small eye patch is applied. Irrigation of the empty socket with normal saline solution or application of an antibiotic ointment may be prescribed with dressing changes.

An eye prosthesis is fitted about 3 weeks after surgery. Prostheses in children do not need to be removed and cleaned daily, and in children this young, leaving the prosthesis in place prevents the child from removing and playing with it (an interesting, colorful, round ball).

Evaluation of the child after retinoblastoma must include not only whether metastasis can be detected but also whether the child is adjusting to any loss of vision. Children who do not have binocular vision this early in life usually do not have difficulty adjusting. They notice it most at school age when they may have difficulty participating in sports that require 3-D sight, such as baseball. If radiation was used for therapy, cataracts may develop several years later. The increased incidence of osteogenic and soft-tissue sarcomas that occur following retinoblastoma may result from the therapy or an underlying genetic predisposition.

 ## Nursing Diagnoses and Related Interventions

A diagnosis of retinoblastoma is a devastating one for parents because, at best, it threatens their child's vision. At worst, it can be fatal.

Nursing Diagnosis: Decisional conflict related to approval of enucleation to save child's life

Outcome Evaluation: Parents and child state they can accept enucleation to save child's life.

With the diagnosis of retinoblastoma, parents may be asked to make a most difficult decision. To save their child's life, they must agree to the removal of an eye. Even after this procedure, the second eye may become involved or distant metastasis may be detected. Offer parents support in the decision they make because, if there is metastasis at a later date, they may feel guilty they agreed to enucleation, believing they have put the child through surgery without achieving a benefit. They may need help managing the degree of guilt they feel because they noticed their child's eye was abnormal but delayed seeking health care. Be certain parents understand fully what the word enucleation means (loss of the eye) before surgery. Provide time for discussion to help them work through this very emotional time in their life.

What If . . . 53.3

Gerri's mother shows the nurse a photo she took of their family, and the nurse notices that only the pupil of the left eye of Gerri's 2-year-old sister shows a typical red reflex; the other pupil appears white. Why might the nurse be concerned?

SKIN CANCER

One in five people in the United States develop skin cancer in their lifetime (Apalla, Nashan, Weller, et al., 2017). Three common types are involved: basal cell carcinoma (a surface epithelial growth that appears as a small ulcer that does not heal), squamous cell carcinoma (a tumor of the epidermis that appears as a white scaly lesion), and malignant melanoma (a tumor originating in melanocytes or nevi) that appears as a mole changing in appearance. All three types of skin cancer are increasing in incidence, and although the symptoms usually do not appear until late adolescence, the chief cause (excessive sun exposure) begins in childhood (Nahar, 2013). In addition, skin cancer is a leading second malignancy seen after treatment of childhood cancer.

MALIGNANT MELANOMA

Melanomas can be differentiated from benign moles by an A-B-C-D assessment: **a**symmetry, **b**order irregularity, **c**olor (variable or dark pigmentation), and **d**iameter (over 6 mm). Melanomas are treated with surgery, radiation, and immunotherapy to improve overall survival. Nurses can play a major role in helping to reduce the incidence of skin cancer by teaching parents and adolescents ways to identify these malignancies and better protect against excessive sun exposure using measures such as:

- Apply a sunscreen or wear protective clothing if a child will be out in the sun for longer than 20 minutes.
- Avoid indoor tanning beds or ultraviolet light. If used, maintain the same precautions as with sunlight.
- Avoid sunburn because there is a direct association between two or more episodes of sunburn in adolescence and the development of malignant melanoma in young adulthood (ACS, 2015).

What If . . . 53.4

A nurse is particularly interested in exploring one of the 2020 National Health Goals that address malignancies in children (see Box 53.1). What would be a possible research topic pertinent to this goal that would be applicable to Gerri's family and also advance evidence-based practice?

KEY POINTS FOR REVIEW

- After a diagnosis of malignancy, parents and children should be informed that current treatment strategies provide long-term survival for the majority of patients.
- Therapy for childhood cancer may be very disruptive to family life and requires support of the entire family.
- Radiation is an important treatment modality in cancer therapy. Immediate side effects include anorexia, nausea, vomiting, and hair loss if radiation is to the head. Long-term effects may include growth restriction or learning disabilities.
- A chemotherapeutic agent is one that is capable of destroying malignant cells. Common acute side effects are similar to those of radiation therapy. Help children to use time during chemotherapy treatments in constructive ways, such as playing a game, to keep them mentally stimulated and distracted from negative associations.
- Be aware of the need to use protective equipment when preparing to administer a chemotherapy drug to protect yourself from adverse effects of the medication.
- Leukemia is the distorted and uncontrolled proliferation of WBCs and is the most frequently occurring type of cancer in children. About 90% to 95% of children will achieve remission and have a good prognosis for long-term survival.
- Hodgkin disease and non-Hodgkin lymphomas are malignancies of the lymphatic system. Hodgkin disease occurs most often in adolescents; the initial symptom is a painless, enlarged lymph node. Therapy including chemotherapy and radiation is used for advanced or slow responding disease.
- Brain tumors are the most common solid tumors occurring in childhood. Beginning symptoms are usually those of increased intracranial pressure. Therapy may include a combination of surgery followed by radiation and chemotherapy.
- Bone tumors occur in two main forms: osteogenic sarcoma and Ewing sarcoma. They can occur in any bone but often occur in extremities. Therapy consists of surgery followed by radiation and chemotherapy.
- Neuroblastomas are tumors that arise from the cells of the sympathetic nervous system. They are the most common abdominal tumor in childhood. Therapy is surgery and chemotherapy.
- Rhabdomyosarcomas are tumors of striated muscle. The peak age of incidence is 2 to 6 years. Therapy is surgery and chemotherapy.
- Nephroblastoma (Wilms tumor) is a malignancy that arises from the metanephric mesoderm cells of the kidney. It is usually discovered early in life. Therapy is surgery followed by chemotherapy and radiation for high-risk or advanced stage disease.
- Retinoblastoma is a malignant tumor of the retina of the eye. It may be inherited as an autosomal dominant pattern. Therapy is aimed at local control and preservation of vision; enucleation may be necessary if the tumor is large.
- Skin cancer is a type of malignancy that can be prevented beginning in childhood. Cautioning children about sensible sun exposure can be an important health promotion role for nurses.

CRITICAL THINKING CARE STUDY

Jack is a previously active 4-year-old who has been running a fever on and off for the last 2 weeks. In addition, Jack's mother has noticed that he is much more tired than usual and has developed bruising and petechiae on his extremities and trunk. Jack and his parents have just been told by the oncologist that he likely has leukemia and that further workup will be necessary before he can be treated.

1. Jack's parents are very worried. What could have caused Jack to develop leukemia? Is there a risk that his brothers and sisters could catch the disease?
2. What additional tests will likely be done to further diagnose Jack's leukemia?
3. What kind of treatments will Jack likely need and for how long?

RELATED RESOURCES

Explore these additional resources to enhance learning for this chapter:
- Student resources on thePoint, including answers to the What If . . . and Critical Thinking Care Study questions, http://thepoint.lww.com/Flagg8e
- Adaptive learning powered by PrepU, http://thepoint.lww.com/prepu

REFERENCES

American Cancer Society. (2015). *Does UV radiation cause cancer?* Retrieved from https://www.cancer.org/cancer/cancer-causes/radiation-exposure/uv-radiation/uv-radiation-does-uv-cause-cancer.html
Apalla, Z., Nashan, D., Weller, R. B., et al. (2017). Skin cancer: Epidemiology, disease burden pathophysiology, diagnosis and therapeutic approaches. *Dermatology and Therapy, 7*(Suppl. 1), 5–19.

Armitage, J. O., Gascoyne, R. D., Lunning, M. A., et al. (2017). Non-Hodgkin lymphoma. *The Lancet*. Advance online publication. doi:10.1016/S0140-6736(16)32407-2

Babayev, S. N., Arslan, E., Kogan, S., et al. (2013). Evaluation of ovarian and testicular tissue cryopreservation in children undergoing gonadotoxic therapies. *Journal of Assisted Reproduction & Genetics, 30*(1), 3–9.

Bennett, M. (2016). Pain management for chemotherapy-induced oral mucositis. *Nursing Children & Young People, 28*(10), 25–29.

Brown, P., & Hunger, S. P. (2013). Acute leukemia in children. In E. T. Bope & R. D. Kellerman (Eds.), *Conn's current therapy* (pp. 769–775). Philadelphia, PA: Elsevier/Saunders.

Carson, J. L., Stanworth, S. J., Roubinian, N., et al. (2016). Transfusion thresholds and other strategies for guiding allogeneic red blood cell transfusion. *Cochrane Database of Systematic Reviews*, (10), CD002042.

Cernvall, M., Carlbring, P., Ljungman, G., et al. (2013). Guided self-help as intervention for traumatic stress in parents of children with cancer: Conceptualization, intervention strategies, and a case study. *Journal of Psychosocial Oncology, 31*(1), 13–29.

Cooper, G. M., & Hausman, R. (2016). *The cell: A molecular approach* (7th ed.). Sunderland, MA: Sinauer Associates.

Cortelazzo, S., Ferreri, A., Hoelzer, D., et al. (2017). Lymphoblastic lymphoma. *Critical Reviews in Oncology/Hematology, 113*, 304–317.

Davies, S., Young, B., & Salmon, P. (2016). Towards understanding problems in the parent-practitioner relationship when a child has cancer: Meta-synthesis of qualitative literature. *Psycho-oncology, 25*(11), 1252–1260.

Diefenbach, C. S., Connors, J. M., Friedberg, J. W., et al. (2017). Hodgkin lymphoma: Current status and clinical trial recommendations. *Journal of the National Cancer Institute, 109*(4), 1–12.

Dome, J. S., Graf, N., Geller, J. I., et al. (2015). Advances in Wilms tumor treatment and biology: Progress through international collaboration. *Journal of Clinical Oncology, 33*(27), 2999–3007.

Ermoian, R. P., Fogh, S. E., Braunstein, S., et al. (2016). General principles of radiation oncology. In P. A. Pizzo & D. G. Poplack (Eds.), *Principles and practice of pediatric oncology* (7th ed.). Philadelphia, PA: Lippincott Williams & Wilkins.

Gao, G., & Smith, D. I. (2016). Human papillomavirus and the development of different cancers. *Cytogenetic Genome Research, 150*(3–4), 185–193.

HaDuong, J. H., Martin, A. A., Skapek, S. X., et al. (2015). Sarcomas. *Pediatric Clinics of North America, 62*(1), 179–200.

Harrington, L., Bristow, R. G., Hill, R. P., et al. (2013). Introduction to cancer biology, In I. Tannock, R. Hill, R. Bristow, et al. (Eds.), *The basic science of oncology* (5th ed., pp. 1–5). New York, NY: McGraw-Hill.

Hartnett, E. (2015). Integrating oral health throughout cancer care. *Clinical Journal of Oncology Nursing, 19*(5), 615–619.

Held, K., Ryan, R., Champion, J. M., et al. (2013). Caregiver survey results related to handling of oral chemotherapy for pediatric patients with acute lymphoblastic leukemia. *Journal of Pediatric Hematology & Oncology, 35*(6), e249–e253.

Hiniker, S. M., & Donaldson, S. S. (2015). Recent advances in understanding and managing rhabdomyosarcoma. *F1000Prime Reports, 7*, 59.

Hunger, S. P., & Mullighan, C. G. (2015). Acute lymphoblastic leukemia in children. *The New England Journal of Medicine, 373*(16), 1541–1552.

Jackson, T. M., Bittman, M., & Granowetter, L. (2016). Pediatric malignant bone tumors: A review and update on current challenges, and emerging drug targets. *Current Problems in Pediatric and Adolescent Health Care, 46*(7), 213–228.

Jibb, L. A., Nathan, P. C., Stevens, B. J., et al. (2015). Psychological and physical interventions for the management of cancer-related pain in pediatric and young adult patients: An integrative review. *Oncology Nursing Forum, 42*(6), 339–357.

Johnson, E. K., Finlayson, C., Rowell, E. E., et al. (2017). Fertility preservation for pediatric patients: Current state and future possibilities. *Journal of Urology*. Advance online publication. doi:10.1016/j.juro.2016.09.159

Johnson, P., Federico, M., Kirkwood, A., et al. (2016). Adapted treatment guided by interim PET-CT scan in advanced Hodgkin's lymphoma. *The New England Journal of Medicine, 374*(25), 2419–2429.

Karch, A. (2013). *2013 Lippincott's nursing drug guide*. Philadelphia, PA: Lippincott Williams & Wilkins.

Kelly, K. M. (2015). Hodgkin lymphoma in children and adolescents: Improving the therapeutic index. *Hematology American Society Hematology Education Program, 2015*, 514–521.

Kennedy, S. R., Loeb, L. A., & Herr, A. J. (2012). Somatic mutations in aging, cancer and neurodegeneration. *Mechanisms of Ageing and Development, 133*(4), 118–126.

Madhusoodhan, P. P., Carroll, W. L., & Bhatla, T. (2016). Progress and prospects in pediatric leukemia. *Current Problems in Pediatric and Adolescent Health Care, 46*(7), 229–241.

Malkan, A. D., Loh, A., Bahrami, A., et al. (2015). An approach to renal masses in pediatrics. *Pediatrics, 135*(1), 142–158.

Matthay, K. K., Maris, J. M., Schleiermacher, G., et al. (2016). Neuroblastoma. *Nature Reviews Disease Primers, 10*(2), 16078.

Mhaskar, R., Clark, O. A., Lyman, G., et al. (2014). Colony-stimulating factors for chemotherapy-induced febrile neutropenia. *Cochrane Database of Systematic Reviews*, (10), CD003039.

Morgan, S., & Soanes, L. (2016). Nursing young people with cancer: What is "different" about it? *Bulletin du Cancer, 103*(12), 999–1010.

Morscio, J., & Tousseyn, T. (2016). Recent insights in the pathogenesis of post-transplantation lymphoproliferative disorders. *World Journal of Transplantation, 6*(3), 505–516.

Nahar, V. K. (2013). Skin cancer prevention among school children: A brief review. *Central European Journal of Public Health, 21*(4), 227–232.

Park, J. R., Bagatell, R., London, W. B., et al. (2013). Children's oncology group's 2013 blueprint for research: Neuroblastoma. *Pediatric Blood & Cancer, 60*(6), 985–993.

Petrosky, E., Bocchini, J. A., Jr., Hariri, S., et al. (2015). Use of 9-valent human papillomavirus (HPV) vaccine: Updated HPV vaccination recommendations of the advisory committee on immunization practices. *Morbidity and Mortality Weekly Report, 64*(11), 300–304.

Pinto, N. R., Applebaum, M. A., Volchenboum, S. L., et al. (2015). Advances in risk classification and treatment strategies for neuroblastoma. *Journal of Clinical Oncology, 33*(27), 3008–3017.

Pizzo, P. A., & Poplack, D. G. (2015). *Principles and practice of pediatric oncology* (7th ed.). Philadelphia, PA: Wolters Kluwer Health.

Quatrano, N. A., & Dinulos, J. G. (2013). Current principles of sunscreen use in children. *Current Opinion in Pediatrics, 25*(1), 122–129.

Rochford, R., & Moorman, A. M. (2015). Burkitt's lymphoma. *Current Topics in Microbiology and Immunology, 390*(Pt. 1), 267–285.

Rose, S. R., Horne, V. E., Howell, J., et al. (2016). Late endocrine effects of childhood cancer. *Nature Reviews Endocrinology, 12*(6), 319–36.

Rowland, E., & Metcalfe, A. (2013). Communicating inherited genetic risk between parent and child: A meta-thematic synthesis. *International Journal of Nursing Studies, 50*(6), 870–880.

Segal, D., & Karajannis, M. A. (2016). Pediatric brain tumors: An update. *Current Problems in Pediatric and Adolescent Health Care, 46*(7), 242–250.

Taga, T., Tomizawa, D., Takahashi, H., et al. (2016). Acute myeloid leukemia in children: Current status and future directions. *Pediatric International, 58*(2), 71–80.

U.S. Department of Health and Human Services. (2010). *Healthy people 2020*. Washington, DC: Author.

Vrooman, L. M., & Silverman, L. B. (2016). Treatment of childhood acute lymphoblastic leukemia: Prognostic factors and clinical advances. *Current Hematologic Malignancy Reports, 11*(5), 385–394.

Ward, E., DeSantis, C., Robbins, A., et al. (2014). Childhood and adolescent cancer statistics, 2014. *CA: A Cancer Journal for Clinicians, 64*(2), 83–103.

Williams, R. F., Fernandez-Pineda, I., & Gosain, A. (2016). Pediatric sarcomas. *Surgical Clinics of North America, 96*(5), 1107–1125.

UNIT 8

The Nursing Role in Restoring and Maintaining the Mental Health of Children and Families

UNIT 8

The Nursing Role in Restoring and Maintaining the Mental Health of Children and Families

Nursing Care of a Family When a Child Has an Intellectual or Mental Health Disorder

*Y*ou meet Todd, a kindergartner who was diagnosed last year with autism spectrum disorder, who is admitted to your ambulatory care unit to have plaque removed from his teeth under conscious sedation. You observe Todd coloring, repetitively drumming on the table, opening and closing the door, and lacking interest in the other children in the room. His sister Cheyenne, 15 years old, who seems very underweight, tells you she is "at her wits' end" trying to babysit Todd in the evenings because of his short attention span and disruptive behavior. Todd's father tells you he's proud that his son is "all boy."

Previous chapters described the normal growth and development of well children and the care of children with physiologic disorders. This chapter provides additional information about the dramatic changes that can occur when children exhibit symptoms of an intellectual or mental health disorder. Such information builds a base for care and health teaching.

What additional education does Todd's family need to understand him better? Does his older sister need counseling as well?

KEY TERMS

anhedonia
binge eating
catatonia
choreiform movements
complex motor tics
complex vocal tics
coprolalia
Diagnostic and Statistical Manual of Mental Disorders (5th ed.; *DSM-5*)

echolalia
flat affect
hyperactivity
labile mood
palilalia
purging
simple motor tics
simple vocal tics

OBJECTIVES

After mastering the contents of this chapter, you should be able to:

1. Describe common intellectual and mental health disorders that occur in children.
2. Identify 2020 National Health Goals related to intellectual or mental health disorders that nurses can be instrumental in helping the nation achieve.
3. Assess a child for an intellectual or mental health disorder.
4. Formulate nursing diagnoses related to the intellectual or mental health disorders in childhood.
5. Establish expected outcomes for a child with an intellectual or mental health disorder that help parents manage seamless transitions across differing healthcare settings.
6. Using the nursing process, plan nursing care that includes the six competencies of Quality & Safety Education for Nurses (QSEN): Patient-Centered Care, Teamwork & Collaboration, Evidence-Based Practice (EBP), Quality Improvement (QI), Safety, and Informatics.
7. Implement nursing care for a child with an intellectual or mental health disorder, such as explaining ways to remember to take medicine long term.
8. Evaluate expected outcomes for achievement and effectiveness of care.
9. Integrate knowledge of children with an intellectual challenge or mental illness with the interplay of nursing process, the six competencies of QSEN, and Family Nursing to achieve quality maternal and child health nursing care.

Children who are mentally healthy typically master the tasks of each developmental phase of childhood, achieving new adaptive and appropriate self-regulatory skills, and grow up to possess a positive self-concept and sense of contentment within their own limits. In addition, children who display adequate mental health often benefit from a positive emotional relationship between the parents and the child and have a sense of safety and security in their home environment. Therefore, promoting suggestions for healthy individual self-regulation and family functioning during healthcare visits, providing anticipatory guidance about normal achievement of developmental milestones and needs, and listening carefully to both children and parents are important nursing actions to foster both the physical and mental health of children and families.

Sound mental health implies that a child is able to be flexible and adaptive and use coping skills that promote self-regulation appropriately in order to meet the normal, or even extreme, stressors of life. When stressors—whether increasing school work, social pressure, or more significant trauma such as acute illness, hospitalization, abuse, natural disasters, or chronic illness—exceed a child's ability to effectively self-regulate or extend beyond a family's resources, many children and parents are unable to cope adequately, which can result in emotional dysregulation, family dysfunction, and/or maladaptive coping, such as self-harm, addiction, or eating disorders, and ultimately lead to a mental health diagnosis. It is important for nurses to be able to recognize how environmental stressors can overwhelm a child's self-regulatory skills and affect children and their families and to be prepared to provide interventions, improve coping skills, and provide necessary community referrals for support (Brosbe, Faust, & Gold, 2013).

Children can develop the same mental health disorders that affect the adult population, such as depression, anxiety, and psychotic- and stress-related disorders; however, children's symptoms present differently than symptoms in adults. In addition, several disorders such as autism spectrum disorder or separation anxiety are typically best assessed during early childhood. Current research attributes the development of some disorders that occur in children to genetic vulnerability and others to disruption in family life, child temperament, inadequate parent–child bonding and attachment, or a combination of any of the above. For best results, children with mental illness, whatever the cause, should be evaluated and treated by specialists in the child mental health field as early in their symptomology as possible. A child health nurse is often the first healthcare provider to become aware of such symptoms, and he or she can be instrumental, through brief psycho-education and appropriate community referrals, in helping a child and family to access appropriate mental health resources.

Because mental health is important to the nation, Box 54.1 shows intellectual and mental health disorders addressed by the 2020 National Health Goals.

BOX 54.1

Nursing Care Planning Based on 2020 National Health Goals

Intellectual and mental health disorders in children produce major costs to the nation, as well as to individual families, because these disorders have the potential to reduce the earning power and contributions of the nation's future citizens. Examples of 2020 National Health Goals that speak to this are:

- Decrease the proportion of adolescents 12 to 17 years of age who experience major depressive episodes from a baseline of 8.3% to a target level of 7.4%.
- Increase the proportion of children with mental health problems who receive effective treatment from a baseline of 68.9% to 75.8%.
- Prevent inappropriate weight gain (excessive or inadequate) in adolescents 12 to 18 years of age.
- Increase the incidence of primary care physicians who screen youth age 12 to 18 years for depression during office visits from 2.1% to 2.3% (U.S. Department of Health and Human Services, 2010; see www.healthypeople.gov) (Weersing, Brent, Rozenman, et al., 2017).

Nurses can help the nation achieve these goals by educating parents about nutrition and inadequate weight gain; educating families about ways to reduce stress; and helping to identify children in school and healthcare settings who demonstrate a high level of stress, depression, or other symptoms of mental illness.

Nursing Process Overview

FOR CARE OF A CHILD WITH AN INTELLECTUAL CHALLENGE OR MENTAL ILLNESS

ASSESSMENT

Both personality and mental growth potential in a child are influenced by several factors, including genetic makeup, cultural background, family environment, socioeconomic status, and access to community resources and support. It is essential that all of these are taken into account when assessing a child's intellectual or mental health. As a child health nurse, be certain to assess children for emotional as well as physical problems at regular health maintenance visits. If a mental health or intellectual problem is suspected, obtain a detailed history of the presenting concern, including onset of symptoms, current stressors, the child's developmental history including school and social aspects, family dynamics, family history of mental illness, and finally current barriers or access to community resources and supports.

NURSING DIAGNOSIS

Nursing diagnoses established for children who are ill often also address mental health or the response of children and their families due to their medical condition or treatment. Examples of mental health diagnoses due to a medical condition that can affect children and their families include:

- Ineffective coping related to a medical diagnosis, surgery, or prognosis
- Caregiver role strain related to potential loss of independence secondary to traumatic injury

- Significant low self-esteem related to disfiguring scars after accident
- Dysfunctional or interrupted family processes related to accident or sudden change of independence and control in hospital environment

Examples of additional nursing diagnoses, which need to be added if a concern of intellectual or mental health is present, include:

- Knowledge deficit related to intellectual testing and subsequent diagnosis, communication disorders, autism spectrum, attention deficit hyperactivity, and motor disorders
- Impaired personal identity related to depression, anxiety, or underlying mental health condition
- Risk for caregiver role strain related to stress- and trauma-related disorders
- Impaired or dysfunctional impulse-control

OUTCOME IDENTIFICATION AND PLANNING

Although the diagnosis of a mental health disorder or referral to a child mental health or psychiatric clinic does not carry the stigma it once did, many parents still worry such a referral is a mark of inadequacy or a sign of failure for themselves as a child's guardian. Help them to see that this type of referral is in their child's best interest and is no different from a referral to any specialist, such as a cardiologist or orthopedist for a purely physical reason. In fact, current research indicates that approximately 13% of children ages 8 to 15 years had a mental health diagnosis within the previous year, and a 46% lifetime prevalence for children ages 13 to 18 years (Centers for Disease Control and Prevention, 2013).

Parents can be hesitant to pursue mental health services for a child for various reasons. Nurses can reassure parents that today's world puts many pressures and stresses on children and families that they cannot control or prevent completely. Ensure parents that contact with a child mental health clinic, psychologist, or psychiatrist will be kept confidential and offer support that healthcare personnel making the referral will continue to offer episodic or health maintenance care—they are not being "transferred out" but asked to seek additional help only in this one area. Furthermore, providing additional access to psycho-educational resources can help the families understand their child's current experiences and mental health needs at the community, state, and national level.

IMPLEMENTATION

Often, what parents and children need most when an intellectual or mental health disorder is identified is an empathic, nonjudgmental person to listen to their story objectively and to provide emotional support for them as they try to resolve and manage the situation to a conclusion satisfactory for the family. Serving in this capacity, the nurse can be a comfort to families and also personally satisfying.

OUTCOME EVALUATION

Children who have an intellectual or mental health disorder need ongoing evaluation by healthcare personnel at routine visits because symptoms can be long term and the presentation can change through different developmental stages. In addition, it's important to determine whether any circumstance that might have led to a temporary problem has truly been corrected or only superficially changed because, if the circumstance remains the same, the child's problem may return or be manifested later in another way.

Examples suggesting achievement of expected outcomes are:

- Parents report reduction in overall anxiety symptoms to improve daily functioning due to compliance with treatment.
- Child reduces the number of self-harm behaviors during the coming month.
- Parents report decrease in child's disruptive behavior since child started therapy and/or prescription medication.
- Child with eating disorder increases daily caloric intake with no binge eating more days than not.
- Parents verbalize confidence in the care of child with an intellectual disorder and follow through with referrals and resources given, understanding child's full capabilities and limitations.

Health Promotion and Risk Management

Nurses play a key role in assessing and promoting the mental and intellectual health of children and their families at health maintenance visits, establishing environments for children and families that can foster mental health. Although it is impossible to keep children, like adults, completely shielded from stress, preventive education and actions can be taken to increase the capacity of children and families to better cope with life's stressors and the difficulties that follow. Table 54.1 lists some helpful observational and interview data for assessing these areas.

Various factors have been associated with an increased risk for mental health disorders in children, including trauma, poverty or neglect, difficult temperament or attachment problems, medical illness, or major losses to the family such as divorce or death. A thorough assessment of the child and family can provide clues to the existence of such possible risk factors and suggest strategies to reduce their impact through counseling or early intervention programs, helping to minimize the overall effects of the disorder on the child and family.

Classification of Mental Health Disorders

Psychopathology in children is classified according to the American Psychiatric Association (APA) and described in the ***Diagnostic and Statistical Manual of Mental Disorders*** **(5th ed.; *DSM-5*)** (APA, 2013). The *DSM-5* is the fifth and newest revision of the manual that is used to facilitate a classification system for more reliable diagnoses. The manual was created in harmony with the World Health Organization's *International Classification of Diseases*, or ICD-10 (APA, 2013). The *DSM-5* is not only an important manual in the standardization of language and understanding of important health diagnoses; it is essential for billing and insurance purposes and therefore treatment of children

TABLE 54.1 GUIDELINES FOR THE MENTAL HEALTH INTERVIEW OF A CHILD

Observational Data	Examples of Possible Findings
General appearance	Height, weight, grooming and hygiene, nutrition, physical health, rhythmic movement or tics
Motor behaviors	Fine and gross balance, unusual motor activity
Speech and language	Receptive, expressive; content, tone, and articulation
Affect	Predominant emotion (depressed, angry, anxious, happy, labile), emotional reactions to content of interview (appropriate, inappropriate, congruent)
Thought process	Estimated intellectual level via language and knowledge base (organization and thought content); orientation (to person, place, time); perceptual distortions (hallucinations, illusions, obsessions, delusions); attention span, learning disabilities
Ability to relate to evaluator	Eye contact; attitude toward interviewer (negative, positive, shy, suspicious, withdrawn, friendly, self-centered)
Behaviors displayed during interview	Impulsivity, aggression, inhibition, distractibility, low frustration tolerance, ability to have fun, sense of humor, creativity
Interview Data	
Interpersonal relationships	Attitudes toward and perceptions of family, siblings, peers, transitional objects (inanimate objects used to allay anxiety); social skills and relationships with peers, parents, and siblings; conflicts; behavior problems; adjustment to changes in routine or new situations
Self-concept and image	Self-appraisal (does child like self?), comparison of self with others (siblings, peers). What would the child like to change about self? Sense of pride in accomplishments, sex role, and gender identity
Conscience or moral reasoning	Understands right and wrong; is able to express common judgments or values.

and families with these disorders. The *DSM-5* is organized into groups of conditions based on common features including period of onset and intellectual, behavioral, and psychological symptoms.

Neurodevelopmental Disorders

Neurodevelopmental disorders, although not related by etiology, typically share a common feature in that there is a delay in one or more areas of development such as attention span, cognition, language, affect, and social or moral behavior. Because these behaviors are interrelated, a delay in one area co-occurs with development in another area in approximately 50% of cases (The Arc, 2016). This category includes intellectual disability, communication, autism spectrum, attention deficit hyperactivity, specific learning, and motor disorders.

INTELLECTUAL DISABILITY

Intellectual disability is commonly defined based on two criteria: intellectual functioning significantly below average—an IQ of 70 to 75 or lower with onset during the developmental period—and concurrent deficits in adaptive functioning in conceptual, social, and practical domains (APA, 2013). The IQ level of 70 to 75 was chosen as the upper limit of intellectual disorder because most children who score below this level are so limited in functioning that they require special services, protection, and schooling. For infants, because available intelligence tests do not yield numerical values, a clinical judgment of significant sub-average mental status function is necessary.

Approximately 1% to 3% of children in the United States are diagnosed with intellectual disability (APA, 2013; The Arc, 2016). This does not occur as the result of a single cause but

from genetic abnormalities such as fragile X syndrome and trisomy 21 (Down syndrome) or metabolic disorders such as untreated congenital hypothyroidism. In addition, brain malformations; maternal disease such as measles and meningitis; environmental influences such as alcohol, drugs, or other toxins while in utero; or the interplay of several genes with environmental factors (multifactorial causes) are possible sources in some children (APA, 2013) (Box 54.2).

Children with intellectual and adaptive functioning deficits are seen in healthcare settings for their specific diagnosis. They continue to come to healthcare settings throughout their lives for the same reasons as all children—for well-child

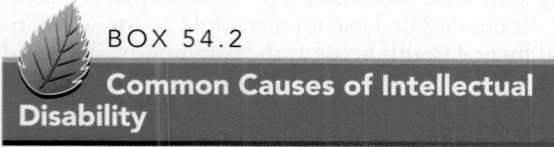

BOX 54.2

Common Causes of Intellectual Disability

- Chromosomal abnormalities such as Down syndrome and fragile X syndrome
- Infection in utero, such as rubella or cytomegalic inclusion disease
- Anoxia at birth from such causes as umbilical cord compression
- Fetal alcohol spectrum disorder
- Inherited metabolic disorders such as phenylketonuria or Tay-Sachs disease
- Head trauma, lead poisoning, or hypothyroidism
- Brain malformations such as anencephaly
- Very low birth weight
- Infections such as measles encephalitis
- Autism spectrum disorder

or ambulatory health maintenance visits, for treatment of lacerations or urgent care needs in emergency departments, or for treatment of ongoing medical or surgical needs in-patient care units. For these reasons, nurses need to be skilled in meeting the needs of children with intellectual disability.

Classification

It is unfair to categorize children only according to the results of intelligence tests; therefore, intellectual disability is determined by both IQ testing that assesses intellectual functioning and careful clinical evaluation that assesses adaptive functioning. Diagnosis is specified as mild, moderate, severe, or profound, defined on the basis of adaptive functioning, as this determines the number of supports required such as communications, social ability, and independent living (APA, 2013). As a child health nurse, assessing for physical illness in children with intellectual disability is challenging because they may not appreciate the seriousness of symptoms or be able to report them as well as other children.

Mild Intellectual Disability

About 85% of children who are diagnosed with mild intellectual disability have an IQ range between 50 and 70. During preschool age, these children exhibit difficulties in acquisition of academic skills, such as reading, writing, math, time, or money, and are typically more concrete in their problem solving (APA, 2013). Socially, they are observed as less mature, have a limited understanding of risk, and demonstrate poorer affect regulation than their similarly aged peers. As adults, they can usually achieve adequate social and vocational skills for minimum self-support and independent living but need guidance and assistance with complex daily living tasks, such as grocery shopping, banking, health decisions, or childcare.

Moderate Intellectual Disability

Children in this category have an IQ ranging between 35 and 49 and represent about 10% of children with moderate intellectual disability. For these children, language and preacademic skills develop slowly during preschool age, and continue to advance slowly through school, typically peaking with academic skills at the elementary level (APA, 2013). Socially, communication is much less complex with poor interpretation of social cues when compared to peers of a similar age (APA, 2013). Through adolescence and into adulthood, simple activities of daily living such as dressing, eating, hygiene, and household chores can be learned through extended periods of teaching and caregiver support (APA, 2013). As adults, they may be able to contribute to their own support by performing unskilled or semiskilled work under close supervision.

Severe Intellectual Disability

Children in this group have an IQ range between 20 and 34 and represent only about 4% of children with severe intellectual disability. These children develop a limited understanding of language and academic skills, with minimal acquisition of communicative speech, such as with single words and phrases, or augmented means (APA, 2013). They require parental support in all activities of daily living, such as eating, bathing, and hygiene, and constant supervision is mandatory to ensure safety.

Profound Intellectual Disability

The IQ of children in this group is less than 20. Less than 1% of children with intellectual disability fall into this group. Children demonstrate only minimal capacity for sensorimotor functioning and are nonverbal and nonsymbolic in communication (APA, 2013). Some are able to respond to training in minimal self-care, such as tooth brushing, but only very limited self-care is possible. They need a highly structured environment and are dependent on others for activities of daily living, help, and supervision for safety.

Assessment

Assessment for children with suspected intellectual disability is completed through individualized IQ testing, culturally sensitive standardized measures, and careful clinical evaluation and judgment. Early assessment is key and should be done as soon as healthcare providers or parents become aware of a delay in motor, language, or social milestones. Early assessment and diagnosis allow parents to appreciate and understand the needs of their child, adopt realistic expectations of their child, and identify and implement appropriate resources and supports.

Intelligence is routinely measured with individualized, standardized tests and must be interpreted with sound clinical judgment by professionals in the mental health field. Adaptive behavioral functioning, which may vary in different environments, is judged according to several methods, including standardized instruments for assessing mental status, social maturity, and adaptive skills with respect to cultural differences. A composite picture of life functioning is drawn from these multiple sources including family members, teachers, or childcare providers.

Parents may initially react to the diagnosis of intellectual disability in the same way as those who have been told that their child has a chronic or fatal illness—with a grief reaction. This may manifest as denial, anger, bargaining, or depression. This grief reaction may resurface among parents, particularly at times when the child would have reached milestones in life, such as the first day of school or at the age the child would have obtained a driver's license. Be certain when working with such families to help them develop plans that are realistic for their individual child that maximize the child's capabilities and opportunities for success (Yildirim, Hacihasanoğlu Aşilar, & Karakurt, 2013).

Therapeutic Management

To aid in planning, parents need a realistic prognosis for their child. This may be difficult to offer in early life because infant intelligence tests are not accurate and more sophisticated tests are difficult to administer until the preschool years. Because prediction based on these early tests involves some subjective input, a child's potential may be overrated or underrated when using these. Once parents have a realistic expectation based on the best judgment possible, however, they are ready, with guidance, to help their child achieve his or her full potential. Encourage parents to seek early intervention, education, and support in their community through involvement in support groups, parent education, agencies like The Arc (http://www.thearc.org), and their local chapters. Furthermore, validate parents' and caregivers' own needs, such as encouraging respite care through trusted family members, friends, or their local department of social services.

Nursing Diagnoses and Related Interventions

Parents of children with intellectual disability have several important decisions to make concerning care of their child.

Nursing Diagnosis: Parental knowledge deficit related to healthcare needs for a child with an intellectual disability

Outcome Evaluation: The parents will be able to verbalize and identify the child's healthcare needs and demonstrate strategies to meet those needs.

Home and Family Environment. Children with intellectual disabilities are ideally cared for best in a consistent, nurturing, family environments with emphasis on developing their social skills, receiving adequate stimulation, appropriate supervision to monitor at-risk behaviors, and achieving mastery in their activities and skills.

This type of home environment requires parents to allocate a great deal of time, effort, and responsibility, which increases as both the child and the parents age. Parents find that their freedom to go on vacation or to have an adult life apart from the child may be restricted, and disproportionate time spent with the child may leave other children in the family feeling left out, unloved, or burdensome.

The nurse can provide parents the opportunity to discuss the challenges they have in meeting their child's needs in a nonjudgmental manner and discuss options available to the family if they are unable to care for a child at home. An in-home health aid, suitable foster home placement, or group home (6 to 12 children living in a home with assigned counselors) may be necessary to best provide a care setting congruent with the child's needs. Finally, connect families with children with intellectual disabilities to community supports and resources.

Health Maintenance Needs. Children with intellectual disability need the same health maintenance supervision as all other children. At healthcare visits, reinforce and review precautions against unintentional injuries. Remind parents to treat their child according to the child's intellectual age, not the chronologic age. For instance, all 2-year-old children might turn on the burners of the stove to see the flame if they could reach them. Most 2-year-olds are unable to do this, however, because they cannot reach that high. In contrast, a child who is 6 years old but operates at a 2-year-old level can reach the burners, so parents have to maintain constant vigilance to prevent that from happening.

Illness. Children with intellectual disabilities are at increased risk to develop a degree of depression by school age as they attempt to fit into a school system geared for higher functioning children (McGillivray & Kershaw, 2013). It may be more difficult to detect this or other illness in children than usual because they may not communicate the severity of symptoms or be able to describe symptoms clearly. For example, children experiencing pain may respond to it by generalized crying, the same as infants, because they do not know the terms sharp, nagging, or aching. For older children, a pain scale with faces can be a helpful indicator of pain (Wong & Baker, 1988). Encourage parents to carefully observe their child for symptoms such as tugging at an ear, refusing to swallow food, rapid breathing, or limping because these symptoms will help to localize the affected area of discomfort. When they call healthcare personnel, parents may be apologetic about their lack of ability to judge their child. Let them know you understand that detecting illness in their child can be challenging. Reassure them they have done the correct thing by calling and reporting their concern.

When children with an intellectual disability are seen in an emergency department or an ambulatory setting for care, they may need more explanations of what is expected of them than other children. The average 6-year-old child, for example, sees you with a thermometer in your hand and thinks, "I'm going to have my temperature taken." When you explain what you are going to do, it is not really news, only a confirmation of what the child had already guessed. A child who is intellectually disabled may not be able to make this association between the thermometer and what you are going to do; your explanation, therefore, is the first introduction to the event, so it is necessary for it to be thorough and appealing.

When children are admitted to the hospital for continued care, be certain your nursing plan of care, again, considers the child's intellectual age, not the chronologic age, because this can help you decide the appropriate and necessary safety precautions, such as side rails or restraints or the way you explain preparations for procedures.

When children with intellectual disabilities are discharged from the healthcare facility, review with parents the signs and symptoms to look for to help ensure continued good health. Remember that such signs may be more difficult for parents to elicit, depending on the degree of the child's intellectual disability. Be sure parents have a telephone number they can call to seek further information or advice if they are unsure of their own observations in the period immediately after discharge.

Education. Most children who are intellectually disabled do well in preschool programs, possibly giving them a head start in learning to socialize with peers and to develop fine and gross motor coordination.

The school chosen for the child depends both on the degree of intellectual delay and on the school settings available in the community. Whenever possible, it is mandatory that children with intellectual disabilities be included in regular classes (termed inclusion or main streaming) to provide access to important educational and social experiences (Fig. 54.1) because this arrangement offers children maximum stimulation for learning. The arrangement also helps them learn to work and socialize with peers, something they will need to do for the rest of their lives. It may be necessary to advocate for a child to be reevaluated or included in a usual school classroom. By federal law, children have the right to be educated in the least restrictive environment possible. They need an individualized education plan (IEP)

Figure 54.1 A young man with Down syndrome at work. With appropriate training and support, individuals with Down syndrome can grow up to find meaningful employment and make valuable contributions to their communities. (Courtesy of Getty Images.)

based on their individual learning style and projected capabilities. In addition, they need safety instructions such as how to locate the correct bus for the trip home from school and education to report bullying if this should occur.

Nursing Diagnosis:

- Impaired growth and development related to intellectual disability
- Impaired verbal communication related to intellectual disability
- Risk for injury related to aggressive behavior imbalance or physical impairments

- Impaired social interaction related to difficulty speaking and adapting socially
- Interrupted family processes related to having a child with intellectual disability
- Self-care deficit related to changes in physical mobility and/or lack of developmental maturity

Outcome Evaluation:

- Child performs self-care within limits of disorder; expresses feelings of mastery with accomplishments.
- Families and children are able to identify coping strategies for successful communication and a safe environment for the child with an intellectual disability.
- Families are able to identify the resources in the community to care for the child with intellectual disability.

The overall goal of self-care may not be to help the child become completely independent but to help the child function at the maximum capability able to be achieved and develop sense of self-efficacy.

Self-Care Activities. Learning the maximum amount of self-care possible provides children with intellectual disability with a sense of control and accomplishment, essential in child development. Carefully assess at healthcare visits whether children may benefit from adaptive equipment to achieve activities of daily living, such as brushing teeth, combing hair, taking a bath, and eating, in order to develop mastery of these important skills. Even after children learn how to perform these skills, remind parents they may need to provide continued reminders or review of the skill. Additionally, if children are hospitalized, allow them to continue these skills as much as possible, in order to reinforce already mastered self-care activities (Box 54.3).

Play. Children with intellectual disabilities enjoy play like any child. Play is an important activity to help children develop mastery, self-esteem, and problem-solving skills. Caution parents to provide toys that are appropriate both for the child's developmental age and chronologic age. In addition, be certain children are guided toward active as well as sedentary play experiences so they do not become

BOX 54.3

Nursing Care Planning Based on Family Teaching

TEACHING GUIDELINES FOR THE CHILD WHO IS INTELLECTUALLY DISABLED

Q. Todd's mother says to you, "How can we make sure our son learns as much as he's able?"

A. Here are some guidelines for teaching and learning:

- Break a task down into separate small steps because short-term memory is often possible when long-term memory is not. Feeling success at learning a small step can provide motivation to continue to the next step.
- Demonstrate the skill to be learned. Seeing a skill performed is generally better than just hearing it explained.
- Reduce the number of extra stimuli present. Faced with too many stimuli, a child cannot focus attention on the task to learn (or realize the task is more important than surrounding stimuli).
- Introduce motivators for learning, such as generous praise. Remember that accomplishing even the most simple skill may be very difficult for your child. Learning to tie shoes may take the same effort as another child spends learning mathematics.
- Keep things simple. Children with intellectually disability may have difficulty with learning principles or abstractions. They may be able to learn to wash their hands, for example, but not why they should wash them (other than that it pleases you).
- Remember to be patient and flexible with the child and the task at hand. If possible, work in collaboration with the child to problem solve and improve success.

obese from inactivity, a concern for children with intellectual disabilities (Casey & Rasmussen, 2013).

Social Relationships. Children with intellectual disabilities may become aggressive in social situations because they are unable to communicate or compete readily with peers due to delayed language development (Davies & Oliver, 2013). For some children, speech therapy may be necessary to help them articulate sounds correctly to improve these skills. Talking picture boards (boards with pictures on them, available commercially or made by parents), to which children can point if they want something, is a way for parents to help vocabulary building and effective communication.

Encourage parents to enroll children in preschool programs to help them learn to be comfortable with other children at the earliest time possible, if appropriate. For a school-age child, participating in organized groups such as Girl Scouts or Special Olympics is an excellent way to give them the opportunity to interact with others and feel successful, important tasks for any child. Teach parents to be sensitive to their child's risk of becoming victims of bullying. Review with all parents the importance of telling their child to report bullying to them so action against this can be taken and making relationships with teachers and advocates for the child at the school as well. Children with intellectual disabilities may not be able to advocate for themselves; children need to be aware of their responsibility to report bullying to protect these special children (Starke, 2011).

Preparation for Adulthood. As children reach adolescence, they need orientation to sexual responsibility, the same as all children. Girls are able to understand a simple explanation of menstruation and necessary menstrual hygiene. Both boys and girls need explanations of how pregnancy occurs and the measures they need to take to prevent this as well as socially acceptable sexual activities and safer sex practices.

Adolescents can be prescribed contraceptives if needed. Be mindful the level of supervision and assistance required and available. If she lives with a responsible adult, an oral contraceptive to be given to her daily by that adult. Longer acting contraceptives, such as subdermal progestin implants, which do not require daily administration, also are available. Sterilization is not recommended because adolescents with intellectually disability may not appreciate the full implications of the procedure, and therefore, consent is not fully informed. If pregnancy should occur, an adolescent with an intellectual disability can be counseled regarding the pregnancy. Should the adolescent decide to continue the pregnancy, assisting her through the pregnancy and planning safe care for her child is an important nursing responsibility.

 What If . . . 54.1

Todd, who has intellectual limitations and autism spectrum disorder, is admitted to the hospital because he is critically ill with pneumonia. The nurse recognizes there might be other underlying reasons for the delay in care. What reasons might explain the parents' actions?

QSEN Checkpoint Question 54.1

PATIENT-CENTERED CARE

Parents of children like Todd, who has a moderate intellectual disability, often develop chronic sorrow or complicated grieving. Which of the following events would most likely increase sorrow for Todd's parents?

   a. After an extended time alone as a family, such as a vacation
   b. When Todd receives his scheduled immunizations
   c. When children Todd's age reach a milestone that Todd does not achieve
   d. After spending time with Todd's extended family

Look in Appendix A for the best answer and rationale.

AUTISM SPECTRUM DISORDER

Autism spectrum disorder (ASD) is marked by difficulties in three main areas: social deficits, communications issues, and restricted behaviors, with onset in the early developmental stages, that impair everyday functioning (The Arc, 2016). Within the first 36 months of life, children with ASD often lack responsiveness to people around them, display gross impairment in communication skills, and produce bizarre responses to various aspects of the environment. It occurs in 1% of U.S. children or occurs as frequently as 1 in 68 children and more commonly in males (The Arc, 2016). As many as 50% of children with the disorder are also diagnosed with intellectual disability; many have coexisting mental health diagnoses (Stafford, Talmi, & Burstein, 2012; The Arc, 2016). Any concern that immunization may precede or cause the disorder has now been ruled out (Kirkland, 2012). Nurses should counsel parents about these misconceptions and educate them about evidence-based immunization data.

Assessment

Common symptoms of ASD are summarized in Box 54.4. ASDs often are typically recognizable in children between 12 and 24 months but may be noticed earlier if the condition is more severe (APA, 2013). The first symptoms of ASD noticed by parents are delay in language development, odd communication, lack of social interest, or unusual interactions, such as avoiding eye contact, and unusual play, with

BOX 54.4

Common Symptoms in the Child With Autism Spectrum Disorder

- Failure to develop social relations
- Stereotyped behaviors such as hand gestures
- Extreme resistance to change in routine
- Abnormal responses to sensory stimuli
- Decreased sensitivity to pain
- Inappropriate or decreased emotional expressions
- Specific, limited intellectual problem-solving abilities
- Stereotyped or repetitive use of language
- Impaired ability to initiate or sustain a conversation

repetitive play and preference becoming more apparent as the child ages (APA, 2013). Parents may bring a child to a healthcare facility for the first time due to difficulties establishing relationships, delay in communication, or odd play; however, these may be caused by other disorders such as hearing impairment, language, communication, or movement disorders; attention deficit hyperactivity disorder; or prodromal schizophrenia and therefore should be ruled out (APA, 2013).

The impairment in communication includes both verbal and nonverbal skills, and communication may be totally absent. For children with ASD who do speak, deficiencies in grammatical structure, an inability to name objects (nominal aphasia), and abnormal speech melody, such as question-like rises at the end of statements, may exist. **Echolalia** (repetition of words or phrases spoken by others) and concrete interpretation are also common findings. Nonverbal deficiencies include abnormal eye contact, poor use and understanding of body movements and gestures, and lack of facial expressions (APA, 2013).

Bizarre responses to the environment may include intense reactions to minor changes in the environment (perhaps screaming if a toy box is moved across the room), attachment to odd objects such as always carrying a string or a shoe, and a rigid demand for routine. For children with ASD, a minor disruption in their day, such as having a substitute teacher, may cause a physical or emotional breakdown. Signs in children prior to school age include repetitive hand movements (clapping or flapping) and constant body rocking; in these cases, early assessment is advised. It may be difficult to gain the child's attention as the child becomes intensely preoccupied by music or objects that revolve, such as a fan, the swirling water in the toilet bowl, or a spinning top. Aggressive actions, such as hitting, head banging, and biting, or the inability to feel pain, may also be present.

Children are said to have a **labile mood** (crying occurs suddenly and is followed immediately by giggling or laughing or vice versa). They may overrespond to sensory stimuli, such as light or sound, but then be unaware of a major event in the room, such as the sound of a fire alarm.

In contrast to these mannerisms, long-term memory and "savant" skills (exceptional skills such as virtuoso piano playing) may be excellent (Bölte, Duketis, Poustka, et al., 2011). For example, children with ASD may be able to recall dates and spoken words from conversations that took place years before. This excellent memory previously led to the belief that most of these children have usual intelligence, but around 50% of children with ASDs have an intellectual disability as well (APA, 2013).

Therapeutic Management

ASD is a perplexing condition because of the extreme variability a child may exhibit. Primary treatment for children with ASD includes educational, compensatory, and behavior modalities, such as the evidence-based applied behavior analysis (ABA) treatment based on the associations between behavior and learning (The Arc, 2016). Treatment such as ABA is typically very intensive and can involve the entire family, taking place in the home, at agencies, at school, or in the community; although treatment is unique to each child, parental involvement is essential to facilitate development of self-care skills and process with therapy (Carter, Lane, Cooney, et al., 2013). No specific medications are approved

for the treatment of ASD; however, medications may be used to modify troublesome symptoms, such as high energy, inability to focus, depression, or seizures (Autism Speaks, n.d.).

Atypical antipsychotic medications, such as risperidone (Risperdal) and aripiprazole (Abilify), are approved by the U.S. Food and Drug Administration (FDA) for children and teens with ASD. Advantages of these agents include improving sociability while decreasing tantrums, aggressive outbursts, and self-injurious behavior (Volkmar, Siegal, Woodbury-Smith, et al., 2014). "Off-label" medications may be selected to relieve significant suffering in persons with ASD in the absence of significantly large and targeted studies. These medications include selective serotonin reuptake inhibitors (SSRIs), α2 agonists, antipsychotics, mood stabilizers, and selective norepinephrine reuptake inhibitors (SNRIs) (Volkmar et al., 2014). Melatonin is an over-the-counter medication that may be recommended to reduce sleep difficulties (Scheffer, 2011).

It is important for nurses to ask at healthcare visits whether parents are finding time for both care of their child and themselves because there is a danger that excessive parental stress can lead to child maltreatment (Hall & Graff, 2012). Encourage parents of children with ASD to seek support through organizations in the community to help support their own mental well-being and that of their families.

As children mature, they develop greater awareness of and attachment to parents and other familiar adults. A day care program can help promote social awareness. Some children may eventually reach a point where they can become passively involved in loosely structured play groups. A small number of children, typically with higher levels of functioning, may be able to lead independent lives, although social ineptness and awkwardness may continue, especially if accompanied by intellectual disability. Box 54.5 shows an interprofessional care map for a child with ASD.

QSEN Checkpoint Question 54.2

INFORMATICS

Todd has symptoms of autism spectrum disorder. When reviewing Todd's electronic health record, which of these symptoms does the nurse recognize as being most consistent with this disorder?

a. Lack of short-term memory
b. Audio hallucinations
c. Constant whirling around in a circle
d. Severe depression or emotional lability

Look in Appendix A for the best answer and rationale.

SPECIFIC DEVELOPMENTAL DISORDERS

Developmental disorders in children can include all or any of the following: learning disorders, communication disorders, and motor skills disorders. They can be diagnosed at varying times during childhood.

Learning disorders occur in approximately 5% to 15% of children in the United States. Although the degree may vary, the disorders involve a discrepancy between actual achievement and what is expected based on the child's chronologic age and intelligence (APA, 2013). Learning disorders affect

BOX 54.5

Nursing Care Planning

AN INTERPROFESSIONAL CARE MAP FOR A SCHOOL-AGE CHILD WITH AUTISM SPECTRUM DISORDER

Todd, a kindergartner, is admitted to the 1-day surgery unit to have plaque removed from his teeth under conscious sedation. You observe Todd drumming on the table, running to the door, opening and closing the door, and then throwing pamphlets out of an information rack. His sister, who seems very underweight, tells you she is "at her wits' end" trying to babysit Todd in the evenings while their mother works because his behavior is so disruptive. Todd's father tells you he's proud that his son is "all boy."

Family Assessment: Child lives with two parents and sister in three-bedroom condominium. Father works as a sail maker; mother works part-time in local fish market. Father rates finances as "Not good. My wife wants to work more, but we can't find anyone to watch Todd; he's such a handful."

Patient Assessment: A 5-year-old, slightly overweight male grasping toy dog tightly in his arms. Mother states, "He talks to the dog when he's upset." Tends not to interact with other children. Often repeats himself, asking "What's your name?" and "How old are you" over and over. Mother feeds him mainly fast-food meals because he throws food if he doesn't like the taste. Toilet trained but sometimes has accidents as he "forgets" to go. Needs supervision dressing because he loses track of task at hand. Refuses to let mother brush teeth. Mother says, "He gets upset and cries easily if his routine changes." Attends special class in public school, as he was too disruptive in regular classroom.

Nursing Diagnosis: Impaired social interaction related to easy distractibility

Outcome Criteria: Child cooperates to extent possible with intravenous (IV) therapy and bed rest after conscious sedation.

Team Member Responsible	Assessment	Intervention	Rationale	Expected Outcome
Activities of Daily Living, Including Safety				
Nurse	Assess what self-care activities child completes for himself.	Allow child to wear own clothes until under conscious sedation to avoid confrontation.	Self-care can offer a sense of control unless it becomes frustrating.	Child cooperates to help with self-care to the extent he is capable.
Teamwork and Collaboration				
Nurse/childcare specialist	Assess whether childcare specialist is available for consultation.	Consult with childcare specialist about what activities would be best for child who is easily distracted.	Games can become frustrating if they can't be completed in a short time period.	Childcare specialist visits with child and suggests at least two activities for period before surgery.
Procedures/Medications for Quality Improvement				
Nurse	Assess whether child has past experience with IV therapy and whether he took prescribed medication today.	Begin IV line in nondominant hand. Document medication given at home.	Use of nondominant hand allows child to complete small, frequent tasks. Documentation will help avoid medication toxicity.	Mother remains with child to ensure child does not remove IV line.
Nutrition				
Nurse/nutritionist	Assess what mother means by "fast-food" meals.	Discuss a diet with mother that doesn't involve so many fatty foods because child is overweight.	Child is overweight, a finding that can be caused by eating fat-heavy, fast-food meals.	Mother states she will try to find healthier foods that child will eat.

Patient-Centered Care

Nurse	Assess what parent understands about good tooth care.	Talk to mother about techniques to make brushing teeth a game, not a chore.	Plaque will form again on teeth if they are not brushed after this procedure.	Mother suggests two different ways, such as playing "Simon Says," that she could use to interest child in brushing teeth.
Nurse/primary healthcare provider	Assess what parents understand about autism spectrum disorder and if they have enough support to care for child with a potentially disruptive disorder.	Educate parents that autism is a disorder, not normal boyish behavior. Explore whether the family is aware of "respite" services in community.	As long as one parent continues to think of the child's behavior as within usual limits, it will be difficult for them to be consistent in care.	Mother and father state they understand their son's condition is one that needs therapy.

Psychosocial/Spiritual/Emotional Needs

Nurse	Assess whether child can take favorite toy to operating room.	Respect that toy dog is favorite toy and important to child.	Children can find comfort and security in a favorite toy.	Toy is respected by hospital and surgery personnel.

Informatics for Seamless Healthcare Planning

Nurse	Assess whether parents have any questions about care at home after dental procedure.	Discuss that child will be sleepy for remainder of day after conscious sedation.	Conscious sedation is necessary because of child's resistance to new procedures.	Mother repeats care needed for next 24 hours to safeguard a still sleepy child.

keystone academic skills in reading, mathematics, or writing (Batorowicz, Missiuna, & Pollock, 2012). Children need IEPs to help them achieve at the highest level possible and prevent low self-esteem or deficits in social skills (DuPaul, Gormley, & Laracy, 2013).

Communication disorders involve problems of speech (expressive production); language (form, function, and use) including expressive disorders, phonologic disorders, and stuttering; and communication, both verbal and nonverbal (APA, 2013). Like learning disorders, these conditions can lead to a lack of self-esteem unless a child receives support and encouragement from parents, teachers, and healthcare providers. Speech therapy is usually effective to improve these disorders and allow children to achieve sufficiently to become successful adults, and early prevention is best.

Attention Deficit and Disruptive Behavior Disorders

All children can be disruptive and oppositional sometimes, particularly when tired, hungry, stressed, or upset; this type of behavior is not diagnostic of psychopathology (Melnyk & Jensen, 2013). Disruptive behaviors need to be evaluated thoroughly, and other causes ruled out. They are a diagnosis of exclusion. Attention deficit hyperactivity disorder and the disruptive behavior disorders may begin with behavior problems that are more frequent and more severe than typically observed in individuals at a comparable level of development (APA, 2013). As a result, parents may be initially unaware of the need for interventions. By the time they do seek help, they may be extremely distressed about the seeming unmanageability of their child.

Like ASD, these disorders need to be diagnosed as early as possible, before the child's behavior leads to a deteriorating level of self-esteem, compromised social skills, and complications in family functioning. The severity of behaviors associated with disruptive disorders, including attention deficit hyperactivity disorder, oppositional defiant disorder, and conduct disorder, can be specified as mild, moderate, and severe (APA, 2013). Additionally, a large percentage of individuals diagnosed with a disruptive behavior disorder may also have comorbid conditions or may be at risk for learning disorders, depression, anxiety, substance use or abuse, or ASDs (APA, 2013). As a nurse, it is important to recognize the unique characteristics of every child and adolescent and plan accordingly. It may be helpful to consider the process of eliminating other explanations for disruptive behavior when evaluating these children and adolescents (Fig. 54.2).

ATTENTION DEFICIT HYPERACTIVITY DISORDER

Attention deficit hyperactivity disorder (ADHD) is one of the most common neurobiologic conditions in childhood that can also persist into adulthood. It is a persistent pattern of inattentive or impulsive symptoms, or both, present before the age of 12 years, that causes impairment in at least two settings (APA, 2013). Conservative estimates suggest 4% to 12% of school-age children are diagnosed with ADHD, with boys affected more frequently than girls. Although the cause is unknown, environmental (such as very low birth weight [<1,500 g]), genetic, and physiologic factors can contribute to ADHD; in fact, ADHD is higher in families with a biologic history of the disorder (APA, 2013). Therefore, environmental and behavior modification as well as pharmacologic therapy can be used with success, a fact that may support the theory of varying causes.

Figure 54.2 Severity continuum of symptoms in evaluating disruptive disorders. (Adapted from Lusk, P. [2013]. Disruptive disorders in children and adolescents. In B. M. Melnyk & P. Jensen (Eds.), *A practical guide to child and adolescent mental health screening, early intervention, and health promotion* [p. 179]. New York, NY: National Association of Pediatric Nurse Practitioners.)

The disorder is characterized by three major behaviors—inattention, impulsiveness, and hyperactivity—and can present differently, depending on the age at presentation. Inattention can include symptoms such as difficulty organizing tasks and a reluctance to do tasks that require mental effort over time. Impulsiveness includes a child acting before thinking and therefore having difficulty with such tasks as waiting his or her turn, blurting answers before a question is completed, and interrupting or intruding on others' conversations. With **hyperactivity**, children may shift excessively from one activity to another and can be described as "on the go" or "acts as if driven by a motor."

Assessment

Many parents recognize excessive motor activity when the child is a toddler, although symptoms are difficult to distinguish from normative behavior until the age of 4 years. Although the preschool-age child often presents with hyperactivity and impulsivity, as the child ages and moves through older grades, inattention may become the predominant manifestation. During adolescence, symptoms of hyperactivity are usually limited to fidgeting or an inner feeling of restlessness or impatience (APA, 2013). According to population studies, ADHD is more common in males than females, with a ratio of 2:1 in children and 1.6:1 in adults. In women, inattentive features are more common during presentation and may escape diagnosis because of less disruptive behavior (APA, 2013).

The criteria for diagnosis of ADHD includes a thorough initial history, physical examination, and completion of evidence-based rating scales by an individual who is familiar with the child, such as parents, teachers, primary care providers, and other caretakers (Melnyk & Jensen, 2013). A good initial history should include a complete birth history and environmental history and consider developmental milestones, dietary history, social history (including child abuse, neglect, and foster care), and past infections such as encephalitis. Additionally, a family history is important to review, as

ADHD is more common in first-degree relatives. The physician or nurse will perform the physical examination, which is designed to rule out other causes of behavior problems. For example, a child with visual impairment who is unable to see the board may not have ADHD but gets "off-task" because he or she cannot see assignments clearly. Other medical causes will need to be examined, and testing will vary depending on the information gained from the history. Evaluations include height, weight, body mass index (BMI), vision, hearing, complete blood count (CBC) with differential (to rule out anemia), a thyroid-stimulating hormone (TSH) and free thyroxine (T_4) test (to rule out thyroid disorders), a lead screen, a genetic screen, and a toxicology screen. The physical exam is also important to assess for comorbid conditions that are common with ADHD, including specific learning disabilities (10% to 40%), oppositional-defiant disorder (30% to 60%), depression/anxiety disorders, bipolar disorders, fetal alcohol affect, Tourette syndrome, and psychosocial morbidities.

As a rule, children with ADHD do not have a deficit in intelligence, although they may seem to because of their impulsive behavior and an unawareness that their behavior is upsetting to family, friends, and teachers. On physical assessment, they often show many "soft" neurologic signs, such as difficulty performing tests such as a finger-to-nose test or rapid hand movements (touching one finger after another with the thumb). Children with ADHD also tend to show "mirroring" with these movements (their second hand imitates what the first hand is doing). Cerebellar difficulty may be evidenced by the inability to perform a tandem walk or a heel-to-shin test. Children may not show the normal responses of graphesthesia (ability to recognize a shape that has been traced on the skin) or stereognosis (ability to recognize an object by touch). When asked to stand with arms outstretched, **choreiform movements** (aimless movements), such as rising of the fingers, are often present. More definite neurologic signs, such as a unilateral Babinski reflex, may also be present. Testing children through the use of games may be necessary so that their attention is maintained long enough to complete the assessment.

IQ testing is used to document intelligence. The Wechsler Intelligence Scale for Children (WISC), the test most often chosen, consists of two portions: a verbal scale and a performance scale. A child is given three final scores: verbal IQ, performance IQ, and a combination or full-scale IQ. The child with perceptual and motor deficits tends to do poorly on the performance scale but average or better on the verbal scale. Children with language difficulty typically do poorly on the verbal scale but average or greater on the performance scale. Children with ADHD show a "scatter" pattern on both performance and verbal portions, doing well on some portions and poorly on others. Because they have difficulty filtering out stimuli, they tend to do poorly on group-administered intelligence tests. For this reason, test results are more accurate if they take IQ tests individually. Be certain that neurologic examinations are performed in rooms free of distractions such as attractive toys for this same reason. Children's behavioral and emotional functioning skills are also assessed across a variety of settings with checklists (completed by children, parents, and teachers) and/or direct observation in classroom and home settings. Completion of evidence-based rating scales is important during the diagnostic phase as well to monitor progress with the treatment plan.

Children with ADHD are often referred to a healthcare facility by school personnel due to difficulty achieving in school. Parents may notice their child's difficulty settling down to tasks and use excuses such as "he's adventurous" or "every child is different." Parents may need time to accept the child's diagnosis as one that interferes with learning. Because caring for the child can be exhausting, parents may be unaware themselves of the strain the child's symptoms have produced in their family system.

Therapeutic Management

A variety of treatment methods are used, often in combination, in the management of children with ADHD.

Environmental Modification

Construction of a stable learning environment is crucial for children with ADHD so instruction can be free from the distractions of an entire class. Some parents may have difficulty accepting special schooling for their child (the intelligence test, after all, said their child was normal or even above average). In the school environment, ADHD may negatively affect academic performance. Children and teens with ADHD may miss important educational concepts, exhibit inconsistent development of skills, and lack organizational skills. Many children and teens with ADHD may benefit from educational accommodations provided under the federally mandated 504 Plan. These might include preferential seating, extended time for test taking, a written list of assignments and due dates, and note-taking support. Healthcare personnel can be instrumental in helping parents understand that their child's condition interferes with school functioning and that a special program will offer their child the best chance to succeed. Parents and teachers can help the child manage the specific challenges of ADHD. The main goal of behavior management is to increase appropriate behavior and decrease negative behavior. Children and teens with ADHD respond best in an environment, both at home and at school, that is structured and predictable, with clear and consistent rules and expectations. Encourage parents to be fair but firm and to set consistent limits to reduce arguments. Teach parents to give instructions slowly and to make certain they have their child's attention before beginning instructions, such as kneeling down to eye level. Breaking down a chore into several steps may help (get the toy box is one step; pick up the toys is a second). Consequences need to be established and discussed ahead of time and delivered immediately. If a child has difficulty making decisions because of easy distractibility, a question such as "Do you want to wear your red or your blue shirt today?" is less effective than a statement such as "Here is your blue shirt to wear today." Also encourage parents to understand, when they correct behavior, that anger is normal but should be directed at the child's disruptive behavior and not at some incident that happened because of the child's inability to sequence, filter, or integrate concepts. Urge parents to make sure their child recognizes their anger is at the behavior, not the child. It is easy for children with ADHD to develop poor self-esteem because, although they are intelligent, they face extra challenges in order to succeed. Helping parents build, not hinder, their child's self-esteem at every developmental stage possible is an important nursing action.

Family Support

Parents of a child with ADHD may have more frequent healthcare encounters because of unintentional injuries, such as lacerations or simple burns. Ask parents at these visits if they are having difficulty managing the challenge of raising a child who exhibits so much activity. Help them to understand that because of a very complex and as yet ill-understood syndrome, the behavior is the best their child can achieve. Organizations such as Children and Adults with Attention-Deficit/Hyperactivity Disorder (CHADD), Attention Deficit Disorder Association (ADDA), and the Attention Deficit Information Network (AD-IN) may have local, community chapters and may also be available online.

Although hyperactivity fades with late adolescence, some children and teens with ADHD continue to experience problems with impulsivity and inattention into adulthood. They may need counseling to find a career that fits with these behaviors and allows them to succeed as adults.

Medication

Medication management is a proven treatment for many individuals with ADHD, but not all children and teens with ADHD need to take medication. Those with milder forms may be successful with a structured environment and firm, but fair types of discipline and reward. The decision to use medication is the parent's personal decision, and the nurse can support the parents by providing accurate information about the medications, expected response, and side effects. Several medications are helpful in reducing the excessive activity of children with ADHD as well as lengthening attention span and decreasing distractibility so they can function in school (Box 54.6). Stimulant medications, methylphenidate, and amphetamines are the most frequently prescribed for individuals with ADHD. There are short-, intermediate-, and long-acting formulations as well as methylphenidate transdermal (Daytrana) in a patch form. Stimulants work by stimulating dopamine receptors so there is more regular nerve transmission, which results in increased attention span. Unfortunately, the drug has side effects of insomnia and anorexia. Administering the drug early in the day may relieve the insomnia and decreased appetite can be addressed by administering the medication before breakfast and offering nutritionally sound snacks between meals. The nurse should be aware of the type of dosage, whether it is a prompt-release, intermediate-release, or extended-release preparation. Most prescribers will start with a prompt-release preparation and switch to an extended release product once the maintenance dose is determined. One advantage of extended-release preparation is single, daily dosing, which may eliminate the lunchtime dose and the need for a visit to the school nurse. There is a "black box warning" from the FDA regarding the risk of stimulants in those with a structural heart defect and should not be used in those with a history of alcohol or substance abuse. A thorough history should be completed and documented. Be certain at healthcare visits to measure height and weight to assess if long-term appetite suppression is causing weight loss. Caution parents that this drug offers a "high" to children who do *not* have ADHD, so their child must be conscientious that the medication is not stolen by other children to use for an euphoria effect (Viana, Trent, Tull, et al., 2012).

BOX 54.6

Nursing Care Planning Based on Responsibility for Pharmacology

STIMULANT MEDICATION

1. Methylphenidate hydrochloride (Ritalin, Concerta, Daytrana), dexmethylphenidate (Focalin)
2. Dextroamphetamine (Dexedrine), dextroamphetamine mixed salts (Adderall), lisdexamfetamine (Vyvanse)

Classification: Central nervous system stimulants

Action: Acts paradoxically in children with attention deficit hyperactivity disorder, possibly by stimulating dopamine receptors to calm rather than stimulate activity (Martinez-Raga, Ferreros, Knecht, et al., 2017)

Pregnancy Risk Category: C; Schedule II

Dosage:

1. Methylphenidate: Start with a prompt release formulation; once the maintenance dose is determined, an extended-release may be indicated. The starting dose is approximately 0.3 mg/kg before breakfast and lunch. Dosage can be increased by 0.1 mg/kg weekly and should not exceed 60 mg/kg/day. The transdermal system methylphenidate hydrochloride (Daytrana) is approved for children aged 6 to 17 years; initially apply one 10-mg patch for 9 hours; this may be titrated based on response and tolerability. Dosage can be increased by 5 mg weekly. Patches are available in 15-, 20-, and 30-mg doses. The patch should be applied 2 hours before the desired effect and removed 9 hours after application.
2. Dextroamphetamine, dextroamphetamine mixed salts: 0.3 to 1.5 mg/kg/day given one to three times daily. The starting dose for lisdexamfetamine is 30 mg/day in children ages 6 years and older; the dosage can be adjusted in increments of 10 to 20 mg weekly to a maximum of 70 mg/day.

Possible Adverse Effects: Nervousness, insomnia, anorexia, pulse rate changes, hypertension or hypotension, tachycardia, leukopenia, anemia, and growth suppression. Excessive use with caffeine-containing products (coffee, cola, tea) may cause increased central nervous system (CNS) stimulation.

Nursing Implications

- Administer the drug exactly as prescribed and instruct parents to do the same. Reinforce proper administration of once-daily extended-release form.
- Instruct parents to have child swallow extended-release tablets whole and to refrain from chewing or crushing them; however, dextroamphetamine (Dexedrine Spansules), dextroamphetamine mixed salts (Adderall XR), and lisdexamfetamine (Vyvanse) capsules can be opened and sprinkled on applesauce or yogurt for children who are unable to swallow pills or capsules.
- Instruct the parents to administer oral doses of the drug before 6 PM to prevent interference with sleep.
- Advise the parents and child to avoid over-the-counter drugs, such as cold remedies and cough syrups that contain alcohol.
- Obtain baseline vital signs, including height and weight, and monitor changes at follow-up visits.
- Arrange for follow-up laboratory tests, including complete blood count, differential, and platelet count for children on long-term therapy.
- Stress the need for adequate nutrition by offering snacks between meals in light of possible anorexia.
- The safety of using methylphenidate for children younger than 6 years of age has not been established.
- The U.S. Food and Drug Administration (FDA) has approved short- and intermediate-acting dextroamphetamines for children as young as 3 years of age.

NONSTIMULANT MEDICATION

1. **Atomoxetine (Strattera)**

Classification: Selective norepinephrine reuptake inhibitor (SNRI)

Action: Selectively inhibits the presynaptic transporter of norepinephrine to increase attention span

Pregnancy Risk Category: C

Dosage: In individuals weighing <70 kg, 0.5 mg/kg/day initially; may increase the dose every 3 days to a daily target dose of 1.2 mg/kg, given once or twice daily; for individuals >70 kg, initially 40 mg daily and may increase the dose every 3 days to a target daily dose of 80 mg/day given once or twice daily.

Possible Adverse Effects: Dizziness, fatigue, insomnia, nausea and vomiting, constipation, decreased appetite, and suicidal thoughts

Nursing Implications

- Monitor blood pressure, pulse, and growth (body weight and height).
- There is an FDA "black box warning" for suicidal ideation; monitor for notable changes in behavior that could indicate the emergence of suicidal thoughts.

2. Guanfacine (Tenex [immediate-release], Intuniv [extended-release])

Classification: α_2-Adrenergic agonists

Action: Facilitates neurotransmitter release to the prefrontal cortex, which is responsible for activities related to executive function, such as increasing attention and decreasing impulsivity

Pregnancy Risk Category: B

Dosage: Starting dose is 1 mg to maximum of 4 mg

Possible Adverse Effects: Hypotension, bradycardia, drowsiness, trouble sleeping, stomach pain, constipation, and dizziness

Nursing Implications

- Immediate-release and extended-release preparations should not be interchanged.
- Monitor blood pressure and pulse, particularly during any dose adjustment.
- Monitor attention span, impulse control, and interactions with others.

3. Clonidine hydrochloride (Kapvay)

Classification: α_2-Adrenergic agonists

Action: Facilitates neurotransmitter release to the prefrontal cortex, which is responsible for activities related to executive function, such as increasing attention and decreasing impulsivity

Pregnancy Risk Category: C

Dosage: 0.1 mg daily at bedtime; can increase the dose by 0.1 mg and increase the frequency to twice daily; maximum dose is 0.4 mg/day

Possible Adverse Effects: Drowsiness, dry mouth, and constipation

Nursing Implications

- Swallow extended-release tablets whole; do not crush, break, or chew.
- Advise patients to avoid driving or other activities requiring mental alertness until response to the medication is known.
- The medication should not be stopped abruptly because of the risk of withdrawal; the dose should be tapered slowly.

Other medications that may be used for ADHD include nonstimulant medications, atomoxetine (Strattera), SNRIs, and centrally acting adrenergic agents, guanfacine (Intuniv, Tenex) and clonidine. Atomoxetine may be a first-line medication for children with ADHD who cannot tolerate stimulants. Atomoxetine must be used cautiously with children because of a "black box" warning about the increased risk of suicidal ideation. Additionally, it takes approximately 6 weeks for the full effect to be realized; if there is an adverse effect (AE), it could take longer to resolve than an AE with a stimulant (Klykylo, Bowers, Weston, et al., 2014). Centrally acting adrenergic agents work by strengthening actions in the prefrontal cortex, which includes regulation of attention, planning, impulse control, and processing (Strange, 2008). Guanfacine is available in both immediate- and extended-release formulations. Kapvay, an extended-release clonidine, has been approved by the FDA for monotherapy or adjunctive to stimulants (Hejazi, 2012).

OPPOSITIONAL DEFIANT DISORDERS

Oppositional defiant disorders (ODDs) consist of a pattern of irritability, defiant behaviors, and vindictiveness that result in disturbed functioning in academic and social domains. Children and adolescents with ODD typically have difficulty controlling their temper; such anger is often directed at an authority figure. It is important to distinguish behavior that is within normal limits from behavior that is symptomatic. The frequency and intensity of the disruptive outbursts should be considered as well as the distress associated with those in an individual's social context (family, peer group, work colleagues), although distress can be isolated toward family interactions only (non-sibling). The disorder develops most frequently in late preschool or early school age and rarely later than early adolescence. The cause may be a combination of temperament, inheritance, and adverse social factors. Evidence-based tools, including the Vanderbilt and the Connor Rating Scale for ADD, include items that screen for ODD and include specific rating scales for parents and teachers (Lusk, 2013). Behavioral therapy and cognitive behavioral therapy (CBT) are individually designed to meet the needs of the child and includes such techniques as family therapy and anger management (Fraire & Ollendick, 2012). The treatment of ODD and other disruptive disorders may be "particularly problematic" and often requires a multidisciplinary and multimodal approach, including psychosocial interventions and occasionally medication (American Academy of Child and Adolescent Psychiatry [AACAP], 2007b). Collaborative Problem Solving and Creating Opportunities for Personal Empowerment (COPE) are two evidence-based treatment programs for teens with ODD (Melnyk, 2003). These programs help the teen learn new tools and skills to positively influence their thoughts, emotions, and behaviors. Parent management training focuses on effective disciplining and age-appropriate supervision to increase support for positive social behavior. Recommended parent management training programs include Triple P (http://www.triplep.net/), The Incredible Years (http://www.incredibleyears.com/), and The REACH Institute (http://thereachinstitute.org/help-for-families).

Medication may be an additional component to psychosocial treatment for the symptoms of aggressive behavior and to treat comorbid conditions; it should *not*, however, be the only treatment intervention. Treatment with medications must include the teen's assent in order to have a positive outcome. Some of the medications used include stimulants and atomoxetine to treat comorbid ADHD; mood stabilizers and atypical antipsychotics are commonly prescribed to address maladaptive aggression (AACAP, 2007b). The nurse should explain the importance of compliance with the medication regimen, as abruptly stopping them increases the risk of a rebound reaction. Nurses should educate the patient and the family about side effects and can monitor metabolic assessments and laboratory evaluations that are clinically relevant, comprehensive, and based on established guidelines (Center for Education and Research on Mental Health Therapeutics, 2010)

Conduct Disorders

ODD has milder symptoms and is sometimes a precursor to conduct disorder (CD) (APA, 2013). The symptoms of CD differ from ODD in that the child/adolescent with CD demonstrates a lack of empathy and guilt and violates age-appropriate social norms and rights (APA, 2013). Symptoms of CD that begin at a younger age are associated with a poor long-term outcome. CDs are persistent antisocial acts that involve violations of personal rights or societal rules, such as disobedience, stealing, fighting, destruction of property, fire setting, and early sexual behavior (Buitelaar, Smeets, Herpers, et al., 2013). Symptoms can be clustered as involving aggression toward people and animals, destruction of property, deceitfulness and theft, and serious violations of family and community rules.

CDs are seen in about 2% to 10% of children and occur more frequently in males than in females, particularly if property or violent crimes are involved (APA, 2013). The prevalence of CDs among girls is increasing, however, so the male predominance may reduce over time (APA, 2013). Children with the disorder seem to develop an increasing loss of self-regulation or an inability to know when to stop a disruptive action.

A number of etiologic factors are suggested as the cause of the disorder, including genetic predisposition, neurologic deficit correlates, and sociologic factors related to poverty and cultural disadvantage. The home environment may be characterized by rejection, frustration, and harsh and inconsistent discipline. Parents may have marital conflicts or substance abuse problems or children may have had a series of inconsistent caretaking by stepparents or foster parents or a history of institutional living (AACAP, 2013).

Therapy for children with CDs needs to be individualized and focus on modifying the home environment and educating the child and parent in social skills, anger management, and problem-solving skills so children can appreciate how their behavior affects others. Learning problem-solving skills can also help children learn to generate alternative solutions to situations, sharpen thinking about the consequences of choices, and evaluate responses. In most instances, parental education is essential, but this can be difficult to achieve until the parents realize this is a family concern, not an isolated child concern. If the home environment cannot be changed, removing the child from the home to a structured, consistent, and caring day care environment may produce better results.

As with ODD, treatment with medication is used to decrease explosive outbursts and decrease aggressive behaviors. Medications such as carbamazepine (Tegretol), propranolol (Inderal), and lithium carbonate may be prescribed to reduce the aggressive behavior. Long-term therapy with an agent such as buspirone (BuSpar) may be effective in helping children control temper or explosive outbursts. Nurses need to be cognizant of providing a safe environment for the affected youth and the community at large as well as themselves. Those with CD have a lower threshold for disruptive (and perhaps violent) behavior and lack the capacity to feel guilt or remorse for their actions. Healthcare providers, including nurses, have a "duty to warn" an identified target. If a patient with CD shares a desire to hurt/harm another person, that patient's right to confidentiality is not as great as the protection of a potential target. When working with families, make sure to put a safety plan in place, such as leaving the house and going to a neighbor's house to call emergency medical service (EMS). Homicidal behavior requires emergency psychiatric intervention.

Anxiety Disorders

A certain degree of fear and anxiety can be a normal part of child development and should not interfere with functioning or persist beyond developmentally appropriate times. Fear is defined as "the emotional response to a real or perceived impending threat," whereas anxiety is the "anticipation of a future threat" (Melnyk & Jensen, 2013). Children and teens with anxiety disorders experience severe and persistent distress that interferes with their daily lives. Anxiety disorders are associated with other major classes of disorders, including bipolar and related disorders, depressive disorders, disruptive disorders, eating disorders, and substance use disorders. It is important for children and teens with anxiety disorders to receive treatment, as emerging evidence shows that anxiety disorders may be part of a developmental progression in which anxiety is expressed early in life, followed by depression in adulthood (Merikangas, Nakamura, & Kessler, 2009). The spectrum of anxiety disorders can include separation anxiety, specific phobias, and social anxiety (middle childhood); panic attack or disorder and agoraphobia (late adolescence); and general anxiety disorder (GAD) into late adolescence.

Because childhood anxieties such as stranger anxiety in the 6- to 12-month-old child (discussed in Chapter 29), separation anxiety in the toddler (discussed in Chapter 30), fear of mutilation and fear of the dark in the preschooler (discussed in Chapter 31), and performance anxiety or school avoidance in the school-age child (discussed in Chapter 32) are considered part of usual development, other anxiety disorders in children may be overlooked. If these disorders are left untreated, however, children may cope with their fear by becoming overly dependent on others for support or by turning away from the problem and withdrawing into themselves, leaving them socially immature and unable to achieve in school. The development of anxieties involves a complex interaction of the environment and genetic traits, possibly related to an overactive amygdala, the part of the brain that controls the fear response (Beesdo, Knappe, & Pine, 2009).

Childhood and the teen years compose the core phase with the highest risk to develop anxiety symptoms and syndromes, ranging from transient mild symptoms to full-blown anxiety disorders (Beesdo et al., 2009). Anxiety disorders among children and adolescents include separation anxiety disorder, specific phobia, social anxiety disorder, agoraphobia, panic disorder, and GAD.

Separation anxiety is considered a disorder when an older child shows excessive anxiety about separation or the possibility of separation from parents. This causes them to be so worried they have difficulty falling asleep at night or insist on sleeping with their parents or just outside their parents' bedroom door. They experience acute distress and perhaps frequent nightmares about separation and, when separated, show somatic symptoms of nausea, vomiting, or crying to such a degree that it prevents them from visiting at friends' houses, enjoying a camp experience, or actively participating in school (Santucci & Ehrenreich-May, 2013). A child with a specific phobia is characterized by a marked fear or anxiety about a specific object or situation, such as a fear of heights or animals, which usually starts before the age of 12 years. Social phobias, including selective mutism, occur in late childhood and early adolescence. Panic disorder, agoraphobia, and GAD have their roots in later adolescence, but a discussion of those conditions is beyond the scope of this chapter. It is important to recognize and treat children with anxiety disorder, as convincing evidence shows that anxiety disorders are associated with an increased risk of depression (APA, 2013). Risk factors for anxiety disorders include family history, negative experiences, temperament, new social or work demands, and health conditions that may draw attention, such as a physical disability. These disorders occur slightly more frequently in girls than in boys.

Treatment for anxiety disorders begins with individual therapy, such as CBT or behavioral skill building, such as COPE (Melnyk, 2003). Family interventions are focused on educating parents about anxiety management and helping them to gain greater insight into the dynamics of the problem and aid the child to gain more confidence in the ability to function independently. Nurses can educate parents and children about common signs and symptoms of anxiety and can promote environmental changes. Promoting good sleep habits, adequate nutrition (especially limiting caffeine intake), regular exercise, and the establishment of predictable routines are important for successful outcomes (Melnyk & Jensen, 2013). For some children, medication can be helpful. SSRIs and antianxiety medications such as

buspirone (BuSpar) are generally the first pharmacologic agents used. Remind parents that when children take antidepressant medication, they need to be observed closely because the use of antidepressants is associated with increased thoughts of suicide (Adegbite-Adeniyi, Gron, Rowles, et al., 2012). The increasing use of antidepressant medications, including SSRIs, calls for an increased level of vigilance in monitoring the effects of these medications (Mojtabai & Olfson, 2014). Children and teens started on SSRIs should have weekly follow-ups with the prescriber, and nurses monitor for signs and symptoms of suicidality. Other medications may include SNRIs venlafaxine (Effexor), benzodiazepines, and clonazepam (Klonopin) (Melnyk & Jensen, 2013).

POSTTRAUMATIC STRESS DISORDER

Posttraumatic stress disorder (PTSD) occurs in children who have experienced or witnessed a traumatic event, such as child abuse, neglect, domestic violence, a natural disaster such as a hurricane, a harrowing accident such as a house fire, a home robbery, or a near-fatal illness. A diagnostic criterion for PTSD includes symptoms that occur 1 month following the initial event. Acute stress disorder describes similar symptoms experienced several days to 1 month following the experience or witness of a traumatic event. Children continue to have recurring recollections or dreams of the event or demonstrate intense psychological symptoms, if a reminder of the initiating event occurs. They may feel guilt they survived the event if a close family member or friend did not.

Absence of effective support can contribute to, and even exacerbate, symptoms. Therapy for children and adolescents consists of trauma-focused CBT, integrated play therapy, eye movement desensitization and reprocessing (EMDR), and family therapy. Psychological debriefing immediately following a traumatic event can help a child better understand the event and reduce the feeling of threat (Gillies, Taylor, Gray, et al., 2012).

Eating Disorders

The *DSM-5* states that "feeding and eating disorders are characterized by persistent disturbance of eating or eating-related behavior that results in altered consumption or absorption and significantly impairs physical health or psychosocial functioning" (APA, 2013). These include pica, rumination, and food aversion in young children and anorexia nervosa and bulimia nervosa in older children.

PICA

Pica is the Latin word for magpie (a bird that is an indiscriminate eater). Pica in children is the persistent eating of non-food substances such as dirt, clay, paint chips, crayons, yarn, or paper (Bryant-Waugh, Markham, Kreipe, et al., 2010). It is a potential dangerous disorder because of the possibility of unintentional poisoning. Other complications include constipation, gastrointestinal malabsorption, fecal impaction, and intestinal obstruction. The disorder is seen predominantly between the ages of 2 and 6 years, although it may be present in adolescence, particularly with pregnancy. Often, it is not diagnosed until a child presents with a pica-induced complication, such as lead poisoning (see Chapter 52).

The prevalence of pica is high in children who have an intellectual disability, and it increases with severity of the disability, possibly because of their inability to distinguish edible from inedible substances. Environmental factors, including neglect or lack of supervision, are other prognostic factors. It is highly associated with and may be caused by iron-deficiency anemia (which is why it occurs with a high incidence in pregnant teenage girls, who also may be iron deficient) (Young, 2010). In most instances, correcting the anemia also corrects the pica. In the meantime, individualized therapy, parental education, and a safety plan can help to keep the child from ingesting inedible substances until the phenomenon fades.

RUMINATION DISORDER OF INFANCY

The term *rumination* comes from the Latin word for "chewing the cud" (as cattle do). It is the act of repeated regurgitation and then reswallowing of previously ingested food. A rare disorder that usually affects infants between the ages of 3 and 12 months, it is seen most often in children with intellectual disability and appears to be a pleasurable act (Bredenoord, 2011). Both organic and environmental theories have been investigated to explain the disorder. In some children, an accompanying gastroesophageal reflux disorder may be implicated and is one medical condition that needs to be excluded. It has also been postulated that rumination is a form of self-stimulation by the infant, similar to actions such as head banging and body rocking. It also may be related to a lack of stimulation in the environment, although attempts to implicate the role of the primary caregiver in contributing to the disorder are not apparent. Attachment between the child and the parents, however, may be at risk because of the anxiety experienced by parents from their infant's constant regurgitation of food and consequent lack of growth.

A parent may report a child is constantly "spitting up" or vomiting or that the child's breath smells sour. Children can lose so much fluid and electrolytes through this process that they show signs of failure to thrive (a distinct problem of under nutrition discussed in Chapter 55). Distracting infants by holding, rocking, and talking to them tends to decrease rumination. Offering cereal thickened with formula or expressed breast milk may be effective in reducing rumination because this is more difficult to regurgitate than simple milk. Parents may need support, reassurance, and education to help them maintain or reestablish a bond with the child.

AVOIDANT OR RESTRICTIVE FOOD INTAKE DISORDERS

Food avoidance or restrictive intake is, as the name implies, failure to eat adequately because of lack of interest in food, sensory characteristics of the food, or related to aversive consequences (APA, 2013). The persistent failure to eat eventually results in significant failure to gain weight or actual weight loss, although no medical reason or lack of food appears to be present. The disorder begins in infancy and is usually seen in children younger than 6 years of age. Infants and young children may present as too sleepy, upset, or stressed to feed. In older children and teens, food avoidance or restriction may be associated with emotional difficulties that do not meet criteria for anxiety, depression, or bipolar and related disorders. Because the child does not eat, mealtime becomes a battlefield as parents insist on the child's eating and the child persistently refuses food or exhibits extremely faddish or bizarre food preferences.

Therapy is a combination of counseling for the parents, to help them appreciate that food refusal used this way can be a potent controlling measure, and CBT for the child, to learn to recognize hunger as a stimulant to eating rather than using food refusal as a controlling or attention-getting mechanism. By late school age, food aversion seems to fade and, along with it, the parent–child conflict.

ANOREXIA NERVOSA

Anorexia nervosa is characterized by refusal to maintain a minimally usual body weight because of a disturbance in perception of the size or appearance of the body (Clarkin, 2012). It may be genetically based and includes three separate features: self-induced starvation to a significant degree, a relentless drive for thinness, and medical signs and symptoms resulting from starvation. In an era when healthcare providers concentrate on reducing obesity, it is easy to miss that underweight can be just as unhealthy as overweight (Bonsergent, Agrinier, Thilly, et al., 2013).

Specific characteristics of a child or teen with anorexia nervosa that are usually present include:
- Severely distorted body image
- BMI less than 17.5 kg/m^2 or less than 85% of expected weight
- Intense fear of gaining weight or becoming fat even though underweight
- Refusal to acknowledge seriousness of weight loss

Anorexia nervosa occurs most often in girls (90%), usually at puberty or during adolescence. It is also more common in lesbian, gay, bisexual, transgender, or questioning/queer (LGBTQ) youth (Austin, Nelson, Birkett, et al., 2013) and among sisters and daughters of mothers who also had the disorder (Box 54.7). Children or teens with the disorder think of themselves as overweight even though their weight is adequate and thus severely limit their intake, begin excessive exercise, or use emetics, laxatives, enemas, or diuretics (**purging**) to better reduce their weight to what they envision their weight should be (Sigel, 2012).

Multifactorial risk factors exist for anorexia nervosa, including temperament, environment, genetics, and physiology. Children who develop an eating disorder this way may have a genetic susceptibility to the illness. Stressors in their environment such as parental divorce, social pressure to lose weight, and personal psychological trauma such as sexual assault or abuse can then set into motion a chain reaction that, coupled with the genetic tendency, leads to the development of the eating disorder. Adolescents who are "overachievers" or strive to be the best academically or at sports may develop the disorder as a way of helping them improve a poor self-image or feelings of inadequacy (they cannot live up to their own or their parents' expectations) because excessive dieting can offer them a sense of control they otherwise don't feel. Lack of nutrition can become so extreme in these children that it causes delayed pubertal development. They develop a starved appearance and significant symptoms of dehydration and acidosis. They may develop severe osteoporosis from loss of calcium from bones (Swenne & Stridsberg, 2012).

BOX 54.7

Understanding Gender Identify and Sexual Orientation

Although society has embraced technological and healthcare delivery advances, it has been more resistant to accepting individuals who do not adhere to convention such as those who identify as lesbian, gay, bisexual, transgender, or questioning/queer (LGBTQ) (see Chapter 2) (Mead, Dana, & Carson, 2017). Approximately 4% to 10% of the U.S. population comprises the LGBTQ population (Moe, Finnerty, Sparkman, et al., 2015); however, they are at high risk for poor mental health across developmental stages. Data from studies of adults indicate elevated rates of depression and mood disorders (Bostwick, Boyd, Hughes, et al., 2010), alcohol use and abuse (Burgard, Cochran, & Mays, 2005), and suicidal thoughts or attempts (Mustanski, Garofalo, & Emerson, 2010). When comparing these findings with mental health diagnosis rates within the general population, the contrast is drastic: Almost 18% of LGBT youth met the criteria for major depression and 11.3% for post-traumatic stress disorder (PTSD), and 31% reported suicidal behavior at some point in their life. Contrast this to national rates for these diagnoses and behaviors among youth at 8.2%, 3.9%, and 4.1%, respectively (Kessler, Avenevoli, Costello, et al., 2012; Nock, Green, Hwang, et al., 2013).

Additionally, contemporary youth are disclosing their sexual or gender identities ("coming out") at a younger age. In the 1970s, the average age of coming out was 20 years (Troiden, 1979), whereas data from samples collected since 2000 show an average age of coming out at 14 years old (Floyd & Bakeman, 2006). This has implications, as adolescents are not financially independent and still maturing socially and developmentally. Previous studies have demonstrated disproportionate rates of distress, symptomology, and behaviors related to mental health disorders among LGBTQ youth prior to adulthood (Fish & Pasley, 2015; Needham, 2012).

It is important for nurses to identify their own biases as well as acknowledge the health care and mental healthcare needs of persons who identify as LGBTQ in order to provide quality care. As advocates, nurses can screen for alcohol and substance abuse, depression, and other mental health issues brought on by social stigma (Mead et al., 2017) and can encourage healthcare systems to include:

- Brochures and educational material for LGBTQ patients
- Assessment forms with neutral terms
- Adding transgender to the gender box on intake forms
- Asking about relationship status rather than marital status
- Displaying visible safe-space and nondiscrimination policies
- Making community resources available to patients (Matza, Sloan, & Kauth, 2015)

Assessment

Because of their intense fear of becoming obese, children with anorexia come to perceive food as revolting and nauseating; they refuse to eat or else vomit food immediately after eating. Always ask whether, in addition to not eating, the child is using a laxative, diuretic, or enemas or is extensively exercising to further lose weight. Physical examination findings and laboratory abnormalities may be present. The most remarkable finding on the physical exam is emaciation, although accompanied by a distorted body image that he or she is "fat." The nurse may also observe significant hypotension, hypothermia, and bradycardia. If the process is allowed to continue without therapy, it can lead to starvation, serious health problems, and even death. Some individuals may develop lanugo, fine downy body hair, as well as a yellowing of the skin associated with hypercarotenemia. Laboratory analysis may reveal anemia and leukopenia, elevated blood urea nitrogen (BUN) and creatinine levels, hypercholesterolemia, and elevated liver enzymes; endocrine studies may reveal a low triiodothyronine (T_3) and T_4, whereas reverse T_3 levels may be elevated. An electrocardiogram commonly demonstrates bradycardia and may include arrhythmias or a prolonged QTc interval. A dual-energy X-ray absorptiometry (DEXA) scan, which measures bone mineral density, may reveal osteopenia or osteoporosis, which increases the risk of fracture in affected individuals (APA, 2013).

By the time most children/teens are seen at healthcare facilities, they are already extremely underweight, pale, and lethargic, and amenorrhea may be present in girls. Often, the child's parents have tried various methods of getting the child to eat, such as threatening, coaxing, and punishing; as a result, parent–child relationships may be strained. Parents may feel guilty for insisting their child lose weight if the girl was once overweight.

Therapeutic Management

The treatment for anorexia nervosa requires the reestablishment of dietary intake to restore physical health followed by mental health treatments. Planning and outcome identification for a child with anorexia nervosa requires a multidisciplinary team. Although the condition began as a psychosocial problem, by the time a child is seen for care, physical starvation and its effects have become a second important component. A person who has become accustomed to fasting will not be able to eat typically "normal" amounts of food. Smaller meals offered more frequently are often necessary. For some patients, hospitalization may be needed due to extreme weight loss and electrolyte imbalance, and total parenteral nutrition or enteral feeding via nasogastric tube may be necessary to provide necessary fat, protein, and calories. Teens usually accept total parenteral nutrition well because they view it as "medicine," not as food. In addition, identification of emotional triggers and education about normal nutritional needs is an important aspect of therapy. Nurses are an integral part of the multidisciplinary team in establishing trust and effective communication, which are crucial measures to help the child resolve interpersonal issues that are present (Box 54.8).

The goal of therapy is gradual weight gain (1 to 3 lb/week) because a rapid gain of weight can cause a child to begin dieting to reduce this weight gain. Weighing once a week is better than every day to reduce the focus on weight. There are no medications specifically prescribed for the treatment of anorexia

BOX 54.8

Nursing Care Planning Tips for Effective Communication

Cheyenne, 15 years old, is 5 ft 8 in. tall and weighs 95 lb. She is diagnosed with anorexia nervosa.

Tip: Attempt to obtain more information about the patient, her image of herself, and her diet in the hope that when the nurse knows more about the patient, she can help her eat more.

Nurse: Let's talk about your weight, Cheyenne.

Cheyenne: I know I'm fat. Look at this belly of mine.

Nurse: You feel fat?

Cheyenne: I am fat. I pig out constantly.

Nurse: What did you pig out on for breakfast this morning?

Cheyenne: Well, nothing this morning, but I was in a hurry.

nervosa. Medications, such as antidepressants or antianxiety medications may be used to treat accompanying depression, anxiety, and/or obsessive-compulsive disorder. SSRIs such as fluoxetine (Prozac), citalopram (Celexa), sertraline (Zoloft), paroxetine (Paxil), fluvoxamine (Luvox), and escitalopram (Lexapro) may be used to address comorbid anxiety or depression. Atypical antipsychotics such as risperidone (Risperdal) and quetiapine (Seroquel) may be helpful in persons with bipolar and related disorders. Children and teens who have had anorexia nervosa need continued follow-up after weight is regained to be certain they do not revert to their former dieting pattern (Fig. 54.3). Counseling may need to be continued for 2 to 3 years to be certain self-image is maintained. With adequate counseling, most teens learn more appropriate responses to stress and achieve full recovery with adulthood.

What If . . . 54.2

Every time the nurse sees Todd's family at the clinic, his teenage sister, Cheyenne, appears more and more underweight. Her mother tells the nurse that Cheyenne has lost 20 lb in the past 6 months. "She's the perfect daughter, always getting straight A's in school," the mother adds. Should the nurse be worried about Cheyenne?

BULIMIA NERVOSA

Bulimia refers to recurrent and episodic binge eating and purging by vomiting, accompanied by awareness that the eating pattern is abnormal yet the individual is not able to stop the pattern (Lock, 2013). Eating is considered "**binge eating**" when large amounts of food are consumed in a relatively short period of time, followed by inappropriate compensatory measures to prevent weight gain, typically within 2 hours. These actions can include self-induced vomiting; misuse of laxatives, diuretics, or other medications; fasting; or excessive exercise (APA, 2013). A period of depression or guilt usually follows the period of bingeing. Like anorexia nervosa, bulimia typically is seen in adolescence or early adult life and predominantly in girls. Individuals with bulimia are often a normal weight or slightly overweight, and therefore, the problem may escape notice from friends and family. The teen may frequently worry

or complain about being fat, may not want to eat in public or in front of others, and may go to the bathroom during a meal or immediately afterward. The disorder may last for months or years with periods of normal eating interspersed between bulimic ones, and the risk of death is significant. Some teenagers with the disorder rely on laxatives and diuretics and excessive exercise in place of vomiting to maintain their weight (a non-purging type) (Sigel, 2012). With either type, the combination of frequent vomiting and use of laxative or diuretics can result in such serious physical complications, notably electrolyte abnormalities, which can ultimately lead to effects as severe as cardiac arrest. Adolescents with purging may develop severe erosion of their teeth because of the constant exposure to acidic gastrointestinal juices from vomiting. Russell's sign, scars or calluses on the dorsal side of the hand from repeated contact of the teeth while inducing vomiting, might be present in those who engage in purging behavior. Esophageal tears may also result from forceful vomiting.

Factors associated with the development of bulimia include being female, age (late teen to early adulthood), and having a first-degree relative with a history of an eating disorder.

Psychological and emotional problems such as anxiety, depression, and low self-esteem may increase the risk of bulimia. There are also societal pressures, including the media and activities that stress physical appearance, such as modeling.

Treatment focused on restoring nutritional balance and keeping a structured nutritional intake is key for successful mental health counseling. CBT concentrates on improving the person's distorted self-image, uncontrollable and excessive eating, and guilt and embarrassment associated with bingeing and purging.

Family counseling can address concerns about how the bulimia is affecting the teen's development and family functioning. The use of medications usually includes antidepressants or other medications to address the obsessive thinking and compulsive behaviors. The antidepressant, anti–obsessive-compulsive, and antiemetic actions of fluoxetine are linked to the inhibition of neuronal reuptake of serotonin in the central nervous system (CNS). Fluoxetine (Prozac) is the only SSRI that has the FDA indication for treatment of bulimia, and the failure of a patient to respond to treatment is evident in approximately 3 weeks (Sysko, Sha, Wang, et al., 2010).

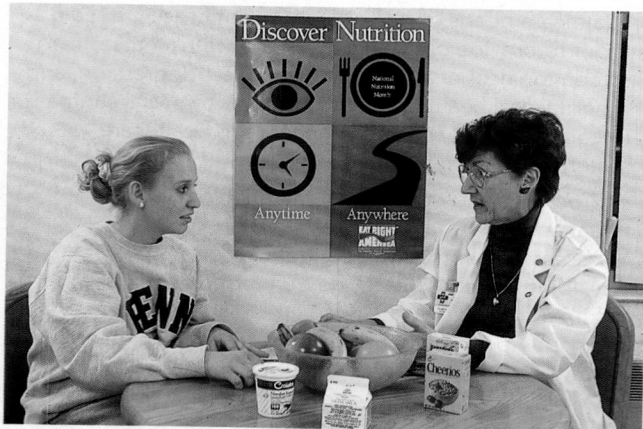

Figure 54.3 This anorexic teen, who is in the later stages of treatment, continues to meet with a counselor to discuss her food choices, exercise program, and overall well-being. (© Barbara Proud.)

EVIDENCE-BASED PRACTICE

Eating disorders have a high incidence in adolescents. To see if this also exists in teenage athletes, researchers asked 966 first-year high school students to complete a questionnaire and then sit for an interview as to whether they have or ever had an eating disorder. Results of the study showed that the prevalence of eating disorders was higher in athletes compared to nonathletes (6.9% versus 2.3%). It was also higher in female than male athletes (13.5% versus 3.2%) (Martinsen & Sundgot-Borgen, 2013).

Based on the previous study, which statement by Cheyenne, Todd's adolescent sister, would make her at highest risk for developing an eating disorder?

a. "I hate sports. Nothing more athletic than poker interests me."
b. "I've played basketball for 2 years; I like the way I look in uniform."
c. "I don't play a whole lot of sports, but I love watching football games."
d. "I don't know why girls play sports like tennis; they all look so skinny."

Look in Appendix A for the best answer and rationale.

Tic Disorders

A tic is a sudden, rapid, recurrent, nonrhythmic motor movement or vocalization (APA, 2013). Four diagnostic categories are used, based on the presence of motor and/or vocal tics, duration of symptoms, and age at onset when other medical causes have been excluded. The hierarchical ranking of tic disorders is described as provisional tic disorder, persistent (chronic) motor or vocal tic disorder, and Tourette disorder. The pathophysiology of tic disorder involves a complex pathway involving the basal ganglia and neurotransmitters and interaction with motor, sensory, limbic, and executive networks (Yael, Vinner, & Bar-Gad, 2015). The neurotransmitters may be misfiring or not communicating correctly causing tics. They may be motor (such as rapid eye blinking or facial twitching) or vocal (throat clearing or twitching) and can be described as transient/provisional or chronic.

Provisional tic disorder describes single or multiple motor and/or vocal tics, onset before age 18 years, and duration of symptoms less than 1 year. Chronic tics are diagnosed when certain criteria are met, including an occurrence of symptoms almost every day for more than a year, no "tic-free" period longer than 3 months, and a diagnosis before the age of 18 years (APA, 2013). They usually become more pronounced during periods of stress and diminish during sleep. Tics can further be described as "**simple motor tics**," which have a short duration (milliseconds). **Simple vocal tics** include coughing, throat clearing, snorting, and barking. **Complex motor tics** have a longer duration and often include a combination of simple tics, such as head turning and shoulder shrugging. They may appear purposeful and include facial gestures, grooming behaviors, jumping, touching, and smelling objects. Children are most prone to these disorders before the onset of puberty, with peak severity between 10 and 12 years of age. They occur more frequently in boys than in girls and more frequently in children who demonstrate obsessive-compulsive behavior or ADHD. Some instances tend to be familial, possibly because of dopamine receptor inhibition. They occur so frequently that as many as 15% of children experience some form of transient tic disorder (Plessen, 2013).

Because transient tics are associated with high stress, treatment usually focuses on reducing areas of stress in the child's life. Pointing out the mannerism to the child is not usually helpful and may intensify the frequency of the manifestation if it increases stress. Behavior modification may be successful in eliminating a particular tic. If the stress is not removed, however, the child may substitute another compulsive mechanism for the original tic. Treatment of persistent/chronic tic disorder depends on the severity of symptoms as the degree of socially disruptive behavior and is similar to the treatment of Tourette syndrome.

TOURETTE SYNDROME

Although persistent/chronic tic disorder is either vocal or motor tics, Tourette syndrome is an inherited syndrome of motor and one or more phonic vocal tics (Wu & Gilbert, 2013). It occurs three times more frequently in boys than in girls, and because it is inherited, often, there is some other form of movement disorder in another family member. Typically, the age at onset is between 4 and 6 years, peaking in severity around the ages of 10 to 12 years, with motor tics usually occurring before vocal tics. **Complex vocal tics** include the repeated use of words or phrases out of context—specifically, **coprolalia** (use of socially unacceptable words, usually obscenities), **palilalia** (repeating one's own words), and echolalia (repeating others' words). Some children with this syndrome have nonspecific electroencephalographic abnormalities and soft neurologic signs that aid in diagnosis. Although most children can suppress their tics for short periods, giving into a tic brings a sense of relief. Children with Tourette syndrome can develop low self-esteem because of their uncontrollable actions before the syndrome is fully diagnosed. Treatment for Tourette syndrome, including comprehensive behavioral intervention for tics (CBIT), is associated with an improvement in symptoms. In CBIT, children and teens are taught to recognize the urge to tic and to use a replacement response instead of the tic (Piacentini, Woods, Scahill, et al., 2010). This syndrome responds to medications that alter the effects of dopamine, such as haloperidol (Haldol), pimozide (Orap), or risperidone (Risperdal).

QUALITY IMPROVEMENT

Cheyenne tells the nurse she had a transient tic disorder when she was in grade school. The nurse would rate Cheyenne's subsequent care as most adequate if it included assessment for which of the following?

a. Signs she has developed a convulsive disorder
b. Lack of sensitivity to pain from autistic disorder
c. Gastrointestinal symptoms because she likely has pica
d. Depression because she has a loss of self-esteem

Look in Appendix A for the best answer and rationale.

Depression, Psychiatric, and Bipolar and Related Disorders Affecting Children

Three mental health illnesses typically thought of as occurring in adults—depression, bipolar disorder, and schizophrenia—have their roots in childhood.

CHILDHOOD DEPRESSIVE EPISODES

Children and adolescents can experience depressive episodes similar to those experienced by adults (Hagerty, 2012). A significant way depression can be differentiated from "usual" sadness is when children report they cannot remember the last time they felt happy or had a good time (**anhedonia**) (Fig. 54.4). The incidence ranges from 1% to 3% before puberty and 3% to 6% among adolescents, as likelihood of onset increases with puberty. A child is considered to have a major depressive disorder when symptoms such as loss of interest or pleasure, significant weight loss or gain, depressed mood, insomnia, psychomotor agitation, feelings of worthlessness or excessive or inappropriate guilt, diminished concentration, recurrent thoughts of death, and suicidal ideation exist for 2 weeks or longer. A family history of depression is the number 1 risk factor for a major depressive disorder. Persistent depression disorder has a reported prevalence of 1.6% to 8%. Persistent depression disorder differs from a major depressive disorder in the length of time; the child/teen must have symptoms for 1 year. Underlying factors that lead to extended depression in children are marital discord or violence, paternal anxiety, and lack of family or social support (Fatori, Bordin, Curto, et al., 2013). Because these symptoms are easily missed, a history should be taken from the child as well as from the parents at well-child healthcare visits. The AACAP has issued practice parameters for the assessment and treatment of depressive disorders in children and adolescents

Figure 54.4 Symptoms of depression are easily missed in school-age children unless history taking is thorough. (© Caroline Brown, RNC, MS, DEd.)

because early identification and treatment of depression has a significant impact on the child/teen and family functioning (AACAP, 2007a). Several evidence-based screening tools can easily be administered to youth and adult guardians and take only a few minutes to complete, such as the Children's Depression Inventory, or CDI-2. Children diagnosed with depression need CBT or psychotherapy, such as individual or family counseling, to help children regain self-esteem and to help the family to understand the level of depression that has occurred. Those with mild symptoms of depression can benefit from psychoeducation, active support, and exercise therapy. In addition to counseling, some children require antidepressant therapy with an SSRI to relieve the symptoms. Observe carefully any child who is prescribed an antidepressant to detect deepening depression or emerging suicidal behavior because this is associated with antidepressant use in children. Adolescent self-injury as a result of depression is discussed in Chapter 33 with concerns of the adolescent.

What If . . . 54.3

The parents of Cheyenne, Todd's sister, tell the nurse that Cheyenne seems increasingly tired, so much so that she sleeps almost all day every weekend. Is this usual teenage behavior, or does Cheyenne need a referral to detect whether she is depressed?

BIPOLAR AND RELATED DISORDERS

Bipolar and related disorders serve as the bridge between depression and schizophrenia in terms of symptomology, history, and genetics and include bipolar I, bipolar II, and cyclothymia (APA, 2013). Although children and adolescents are unlikely to be diagnosed with bipolar disorder, they may experience bipolar-like symptoms. Bipolar I disorder requires at least one manic episode, which is an elevated, expansive, or irritable mood, such as grandiose behavior, little need for sleep, increased goal-directed activity, distractibility, or a flight of ideas (APA, 2013). Although the mean age at onset is typically 18 years, children who experience a manic episode may present with repeated episodes of extreme silliness or happiness in an inappropriate setting, beyond what is developmentally expected of the child; children can also present with an overestimation of skills or ability, such as being the very best, or unstoppable (APA, 2013). The same is true for bipolar II disorder, although there is no presence of mania, but rather hypomania, a less severe, shorter period of increased energy, mood, and activity. Cyclothymic disorder is the presence of hypomanic and depressive periods that do not meet full criteria for bipolar I or II and persist for at least 1 year in children or adolescents (APA, 2013). Nurses should consider family history of bipolar disorder, as genetic predisposition is the most consistent and strongest risk factor for the diagnosis, and monitor for suicidal ideation in children with family history and/or suspected bipolar disorder due to the increased risk of suicide in individuals with bipolar.

CHILDHOOD SCHIZOPHRENIA

Schizophrenia is actually a group of disorders of thought processes characterized by the gradual disintegration of mental functioning; it occurs in about 2 of every 10,000 children (Miller & Buckley, 2013). It is a devastating mental illness that most commonly strikes in adolescence or young adulthood, and onset prior to adolescence is rare (APA, 2013). Symptoms until that time may be undifferentiated or ill defined. Despite years of investigation, the cause of schizophrenia is unknown. Current evidence suggests there may be both genetic and environmental foundations for the disorder. Magnetic resonance imaging (MRI) has shown that cerebral involvement, such as enlarged ventricles, decreased blood to the frontal lobe, or cortical cell loss, may begin the disorder. Neurochemical mediators may influence or prolong the disorder. The use of functional brain imaging, including positron emission tomography (PET) and single-photon emission computerized tomography (SPECT), may lead scientists to be able to classify and diagnose various psychiatric disorders and possibly predict therapeutic effect. (Drug Addiction & Alcoholism Treatment Centers, 2013). Children with schizophrenia experience hallucinations (hear or see people or objects that other people cannot) and may display rambling or illogical speech patterns. They may not be responsive (have a **flat affect**), may withdraw into themselves so completely they are stuporous (**catatonia**), or be so extremely suspicious that others want to harm them (paranoia) that it is difficult for them to function. Although schizophrenic manifestations may occur suddenly after a major stress in a child's life (such as rejection by a boyfriend or girlfriend), subtle signs of mental illness have usually been present for some time.

The diagnosis of a psychotic disorder of this extent is often a shock to parents. Fortunately, therapy with modern antipsychotic drugs such as clozapine is effective in reducing children's hallucinations and bizarre thought processes. Many children who are diagnosed as having schizophrenia in childhood continue to have mental illness as adults, making continuing support and long-term follow-up essential (Malone-Cole, 2012).

QSEN Checkpoint Question 54.6

TEAMWORK & COLLABORATION

Symptoms of schizophrenia often begin in adolescence, so the nurse reviews Cheyenne's history with a psychiatric–mental health nurse. Which statement by Cheyenne would signal to the nurses she is developing symptoms of schizophrenia?

   a. "I absolutely hate babysitting for my younger brother on week nights."
   b. "Both my English and math teachers gave me bad marks last quarter. I got so mad."
   c. "My father seems more worried about his health than he does about mine."
   d. "At night, I can hear my friends plotting against me through the water pipes."

Look in Appendix A for the best answer and rationale.

Elimination Disorders

Elimination disorders include functional enuresis (involuntary loss of urine) and encopresis (involuntary loss of feces). Developmental enuresis is discussed in Chapter 31 with the development of the preschooler.

ENCOPRESIS

In children ages 4 years and older, loss of feces is *encopresis* if there is repeated passage of feces at least once a month for at least 3 months in places not culturally appropriate for that purpose. It is more common in boys than in girls and considered primary if the child was never fully toilet trained and secondary if the problem began after effective training (Coehlo, 2011). It is diagnosed only after medical causes such as lactase deficiency, thyroid disease, hypercalcemia, Hirschsprung disease, and infectious diarrhea have been ruled out. Between 1.5% and 7.5% of children ages 6 to 12 years old have encopresis, and it is 6 times as common in boys as in girls (Ortiz & Stratis, 2013).

Isolated occurrences of encopresis may happen when a sibling is born (as part of an overall regression reaction) or when a child is visiting at a strange house and is too shy to ask for the bathroom. It can occur in a new school because a child is unable to locate the bathroom in time or cannot use a bathroom because it is "owned" by a school gang.

In a few instances, encopresis occurs because hard bowel movements cause anal fissures. Because it then hurts to move the bowels, children avoid bowel movements, leading to chronically distended rectums. They are then no longer able to sense when they need to defecate, so involuntary or overflow defecation occurs.

Assessment

To document encopresis, take a careful history of usual bowel evacuation habits, the number of bowel accidents, and the times at which they occur. Additionally, a dietary history including fiber and fluid intake is important. Investigate any recent changes or stress factors in the child's environment. A physical examination that includes a rectal examination should be done to establish whether there is proper anal sphincter control. If anal fissures are present, the possibility of child maltreatment needs to be investigated, although encopresis alone does not substantiate sexual abuse.

Therapeutic Management

Once diagnosed, the treatment of encopresis begins with a therapeutic regimen to empty the bowels of impacted stool, most often with laxatives, enemas, or a combination of both (Mosca & Schatz, 2013). Behavior interventions are centered on habit relearning. Reserving time in a busy household for children to evacuate their bowels about two times daily (in the morning and after dinner) may create new "habit" periods for them. It is especially advantageous if they are able to evacuate their bowels before they leave for school in the morning because then they are less likely to experience encopresis and embarrassment in school. The administration of a stool softener such as lactulose, a high-fiber diet, or 1 to 6 tablespoons of mineral oil daily for 2 or 3 months often softens stools so bowel movements are not painful. Remind parents that children receiving long-term mineral oil therapy also need to take water-soluble forms of vitamins A, D, and K because these vitamins tend to be removed from the gastrointestinal tract with the mineral oil. Emphasize to parents that children should not be punished for encopresis. Encourage them to pay as little attention as possible to bowel accidents and to give praise for days when encopresis does not occur.

ENURESIS

Enuresis is defined as repeated involuntary or intentional urination during the day or at night after an age at which a child has attained or should have attained control over bladder function, when no organic cause for the problem can be found (Deshpande, Caldwell, & Sureshkumar, 2012). Chronologic age (or developmental level) is at least 5 years (APA, 2013), and there is a positive family history in many instances. Although stress may be a factor in occurrences of enuresis, its primary cause is unknown. Most children outgrow the problem by adolescence. It is important to treat enuresis to minimize embarrassment and anxiety of the child and frustration experienced by parents and/or caregivers. The most serious result of enuresis is related to the child's feelings of failure with each occurrence and associated rejection by peers. All this contributes to a lowered sense of self-esteem. The problem and associated nursing diagnoses are described in more detail in Chapter 46. Treatment focuses on behavioral management and positive reinforcement (Walle, Rittig, Tekgül, et al., 2017). Enuresis alarms can be beneficial in the short and long term; however, their use can be labor intensive and time-consuming. Success is more likely with strong family support and a positive attitude. A medication such as desmopressin (DDAVP), a synthetic analogue of antidiuretic hormone (ADH), is a first-line pharmacologic agent used in children over the age of 5 years. It can be used for short-term treatment for children hesitant to be away from home overnight, for example, at a slumber party or overnight camp.

What If . . . 54.4
The nurse is particularly interested in exploring one of the 2020 National Health Goals related to mental illness in children (see Box 54.1). What would be a possible research topic pertinent to this goal that would be applicable to Todd and Cheyenne's family and also advance evidence-based practice?

KEY POINTS FOR REVIEW

- Both intellectual and mental health disorders pose long-term care concerns for children and their families.
- For children with intellectual disability, a stigma still may be present in many communities, although less so than previously. Help parents to gain the insight that intellectual disabilities occur in a proportion of infants in every population and that having a child with this problem merely reflects a chance occurrence not a reflection of their family's capabilities.
- Mental health disorders often begin subtly in children and are often first manifested as behavior problems in school or with personal relationships. Assess thoroughly any child who is referred for disruptive behavior or interpersonal distress in a school class for the possibility the child has a serious mental health problem in order to not only meet QSEN competencies but also best meet the family's total needs.
- Autism spectrum disorder is a pervasive developmental disorder that has a range of behaviors, including fascination with movement, impairment of communication skills, and insensitivity to pain.

- Attention deficit and disruptive behavior disorders, such as oppositional defiant and conduct disorders, may occur in childhood. Children with ADHD may be treated with stimulant or nonstimulant medication to reduce the hyperactivity and allow them to achieve better in school and interact successfully at home.
- Eating disorders seen in childhood include pica, rumination, anorexia nervosa, and bulimia. All of these disorders can lead to loss of weight and electrolyte imbalances if left unrecognized and untreated.
- Tic disorders such as Tourette syndrome are abnormalities of semi-involuntary movement that are thought to result from dysfunction of the basal ganglia or distorted dopamine reception.
- Children with depressed mood are at high risk for self-injury. They need thorough assessment and close observation to be certain that this does not happen. Monitor children carefully who are prescribed antidepressants to relieve depression because these may actually increase self-injury attempts.
- Schizophrenia often begins in adolescence. It usually presents as disorganized behavior. Long-term therapy with antipsychotic drugs is necessary.
- Encopresis is the repeated passage of feces in places not culturally appropriate for that purpose. Therapy is both physiologic and psychological.

CRITICAL THINKING CARE STUDY

Leonette is an 8-year-old child you see at an ambulatory clinic. She began loud lip smacking and shouting, "Hey! Hey! Hey!" almost constantly when she was 4 years old. The timing coincided with her parents' divorce, so her mother thought for a long time that her behavior was a reaction to the divorce. A childcare teacher suggested that it might be something more significant, and Leonette was diagnosed with Tourette syndrome. Today, she takes haloperidol and still has those mannerisms, but they only occur when she is in a new or stressful situation. Leonette lives with her mother; a new stepfather; two stepbrothers, ages 12 and 14 years; and a new baby sister, age 2 months. Because the house is small, Leonette and her two brothers share a bedroom and bathroom. "Not a good arrangement," Mrs. Firestone tells you, "but workable." Mrs. Firestone works as a teller at a local bank; she has just returned to work after a 10-week maternity leave; her husband sells real estate.

1. "Take Your Daughter to Work Day" is next week, so you ask Leonette's mother if she is going to take Leonette to the bank with her. Mrs. Leonette looks uncomfortable at your question and replies quickly, "No. It's not allowed, because we handle money and everything." Leonette looks disappointed. Would you suggest that Mrs. Firestone take Leonette, or would the visit be too upsetting to suggest?

2. Leonette's mother brought her to the clinic today because she's had two episodes in the past month where the school called her to take Leonette home because of encopresis. When you ask the mother when was the last time Leonette moved her bowels at home, her mother

answers, "No idea. I don't have time to keep track of who's going to the bathroom or not." How could you help this family?

3. You notice that Leonette is afraid to leave her mother's side to come into an examining room so you can take her blood pressure. Her mother tells you she has had to stay home from work for the past 3 days because Leonette refused to go to school and even refuses to leave her side, following her from room to room in the house and sleeping on the floor at the foot of her bed. "Her teacher said it's separation anxiety from the new marriage and will pass," the mother tells you. Would you be concerned that this is not as simple a problem as the mother suggests?

RELATED RESOURCES

Explore these additional resources to enhance learning for this chapter:

- Student resources on thePoint, including answers to the What If . . . and Critical Thinking Care Study questions, http://thepoint.lww.com/Flagg8e
- Adaptive learning powered by PrepU, http://thepoint.lww.com /prepu

REFERENCES

Adegbite-Adeniyi, C., Gron, B., Rowles, B. M., et al. (2012). An update on antidepressant use and suicidality in pediatric depression. *Expert Opinion in Pharmacotherapy, 13*(15), 2119–2130.

American Academy of Child and Adolescent Psychiatry. (2007a). Practice parameters for the assessment and treatment of children and adolescents with depressive disorders. *Journal of the American Academy of Child and Adolescent Psychiatry, 46*(11), 1503–1526.

American Academy of Child and Adolescent Psychiatry. (2007b). Practice parameters for the assessment and treatment of children and adolescents with oppositional defiant disorder. *Journal of the American Academy of Child and Adolescent Psychiatry, 46*(1), 126–141.

American Academy of Child and Adolescent Psychiatry. (2013). *Conduct disorder.* Retrieved from http://www.aacap.org/AACAP/Families_and _Youth/Facts_for_Families/FFF-Guide/Conduct-Disorder-033.aspx

American Psychiatric Association. (2013). *Diagnostic and statistical manual of mental disorders* (5th ed.). Arlington, VA: Author.

Austin, S. B., Nelson, L. A., Birkett, M. A., et al. (2013). Eating disorder symptoms and obesity at the intersections of gender, ethnicity, and sexual orientation in US high school students. *American Journal of Public Health, 103*(2), e16–e22.

Autism Speaks. (n.d.). *Medicines for treating autism's core symptoms.* Retrieved from https://www.autismspeaks.org/what-autism/treatment/medicines -treating-core-symptoms

Batorowicz, B., Missiuna, C. A., & Pollock, N. A. (2012). Technology supporting written productivity in children with learning disabilities: A critical review. *Canadian Journal of Occupational Therapy, 79*(4), 211–224.

Beesdo, K., Knappe, S., & Pine, D. S. (2009). Anxiety and anxiety disorders in children and adolescents: Developmental issues and implications for DSM-5. *The Psychiatric Clinics of North America, 32*(3), 483–524.

Bölte, S., Duketis, E., Poustka, F., et al. (2011). Sex differences in cognitive domains and their clinical correlates in higher-functioning autism spectrum disorders. *Autism, 15*(4), 497–511.

Bonsergent, E., Agrinier, N., Thilly, N., et al. (2013). Overweight and obesity prevention for adolescents: A cluster randomized controlled trial in a school setting. *American Journal of Preventive Medicine, 44*(1), 30–39.

Bostwick, W. B., Boyd, C. J., Hughes, T. L., et al. (2010). Dimensions of sexual orientation and the prevalence of mood and anxiety disorders in the United States. *American Journal of Public Health, 100*(3), 468–475.

Bredenoord, A. J. (2011). Belching, aerophagia, and rumination. *Journal of Pediatric Gastroenterology Nutrition, 53*(Suppl. 2), S19–S21.

Brosbe, M. S., Faust, J., & Gold, S. N. (2013). Complex traumatic stress in the pediatric medical setting. *Journal of Trauma Dissociation, 14*(1), 97–112.

Bryant-Waugh, R., Markham, L., Kreipe, R. E., et al. (2010). Feeding and eating disorders in childhood. *International Journal of Eating Disorders, 43*(2), 98–111.

Buitelaar, J. K., Smeets, K. C., Herpers, P., et al. (2013). Conduct disorders. *European Child & Adolescence Psychiatry, 22*(Suppl. 1), S49–S54.

Burgard, S. A., Cochran, S. D., & Mays, V. M. (2005). Alcohol and tobacco use patterns among heterosexually and homosexually experienced California women. *Drug Alcohol Dependency, 77*(1), 61–70.

Carter, E. W., Lane, K. L., Cooney, M., et al. (2013). Parent assessments of self-determination importance and performance for students with autism or intellectual disability. *American Journal of Intellectual Developmental Disabilities, 118*(1), 16–31.

Casey, A. F., & Rasmussen, R. (2013). Reduction measures and percent body fat in individuals with intellectual disabilities: A scoping review. *Disability & Health Journal, 6*(1), 2–7.

Center for Education and Research on Mental Health Therapeutics. (2010). *Treatment of Maladaptive Aggression in Youth (T-May): Rutgers CERTs pocket reference guide for primary care clinicians and mental health specialists.* New Brunswick, NJ: Rutgers University.

Centers for Disease Control and Prevention. (2013). Mental health surveillance among children — United States 2005–2011. *Morbidity and Mortality Weekly Report, 62*(2), 1–35.

Clarkin, A. (2012). Eating disorders: Anorexia nervosa and bulimia nervosa. In K. M. Fortinash & P. A. Holoday Worret (Eds.), *Psychiatric mental health nursing* (5th ed., pp. 416–436). St. Louis, MO: Elsevier/Mosby.

Coehlo, D. P. (2011). Encopresis: A medical and family approach. *Pediatric Nursing, 37*(3), 107–112.

Davies, L., & Oliver, C. (2013). The age related prevalence of aggression and self-injury in persons with an intellectual disability: A review. *Research in Developmental Disabilities, 34*(2), 764–775.

Deshpande, A. V., Caldwell, P. H., & Sureshkumar, P. (2012). Drugs for nocturnal enuresis in children (other than desmopressin and tricyclics). *Cochrane Database of Systematic Reviews,* (12), CD002238.

Drug Addiction & Alcoholism Treatment Centers. (2013). *fMRI brain scans may diagnose mental illness.* Retrieved from https://www.promises.com /articles/mental-health/fmri-brain-scans-may-diagnose-mental-ill

DuPaul, G. J., Gormley, M. J., & Laracy, S. D. (2013). Comorbidity of LD and ADHD: Implications of DSM-5 for assessment and treatment. *Journal of Learning Disabilities, 46*(1), 43–51.

Fatori, D., Bordin, I. A., Curto, B. M., et al. (2013). Influence of psychosocial risk factors on the trajectory of mental health problems from childhood to adolescence: A longitudinal study. *BMC Psychiatry, 13*(1), 31.

Fish, J. N., & Pasley, K. (2015). Sexual (minority) trajectories, mental health, and alcohol use: A longitudinal study of youth as they transition to adulthood. *Journal of Youth and Adolescence, 44*, 1508–1527.

Floyd, F. J., & Bakeman, R. (2006). Coming-out across the life course: Implications of age and historical context. *Archives of Sexual Behavior, 35*, 287–296.

Fraire, M. G., & Ollendick, T. H. (2012). Anxiety and oppositional defiant disorder: A transdiagnostic conceptualization. *Clinical Psychology Reviews, 33*(2), 229–240.

Gillies, D., Taylor, F., Gray, C., et al. (2012). Psychological therapies for the treatment of post-traumatic stress disorder in children and adolescents. *Cochrane Database of Systematic Reviews,* (12), CD006726.

Hagerty, B. M. (2012). Mood disorders, depression, bipolar, and adjustment disorders. In K. M. Fortinash & P. A. Holoday Worret (Eds.), *Psychiatric mental health nursing* (5th ed., pp. 218–258). St. Louis, MO: Elsevier/ Mosby.

Hall, H. R., & Graff, J. C. (2012). Maladaptive behaviors of children with autism: Parent support, stress, and coping. *Issues in Comprehensive Pediatric Nursing, 35*(3–4), 194–214.

Hejazi, N. (2012, September). *Pediatric focused safety review Kapvay™ (clonidine hydrochloride).* Paper presented at the Pediatric Advisory Committee Meeting of the U.S. Food and Drug Administration, Silver Spring, MD.

Kessler, R. C., Avenevoli, S., Costello, J., et al. (2012). Prevalence, persistence, and sociodemographic correlates of DSM-IV disorders in the National Comorbidity Survey Replication adolescent supplement. *Archives of General Psychiatry, 69*(4), 372–80.

Kirkland, A. (2012). Credibility battles in the autism litigation. *Social Studies of Science, 42*(2), 237–261.

Klykylo, W. M., Bowers, R., Weston, C., et al. (2014). *Green's child and adolescent clinical pharmacology* (5th ed.). Philadelphia, PA: Lippincott Williams & Wilkins.

Lock, J. (2013). Bulimia nervosa. In E. T. Bope & R. D. Kellerman (Eds.), *Conn's current therapy* (pp. 930–932). Philadelphia, PA: Elsevier/Saunders.

Lusk, P. (2013). Disruptive behaviors in children and adolescents. In B. M. Melnyk & P. Jensen (Eds.), *A practical guide to child and adolescent mental health screening, early intervention and health promotion* (pp. 177–199). New York, NY: National Association of Pediatric Nurse Practitioners.

Malone-Cole, J. A. (2012). Schizophrenia and other psychotic disorders. In K. M. Fortinash & P. A. Holoday Worret (Eds.), *Psychiatric mental health nursing* (5th ed., pp. 259–297). St. Louis, MO: Elsevier/Mosby.

Martinez-Raga, J., Ferreros, A., Knecht, C., et al. (2017). Attention-deficit hyperactivity disorder medication use: Factors involved in prescribing safety aspects and outcomes. *Therapeutic Advances in Drug Safety, 8*(3), 87–99.

Martinsen, M., & Sundgot-Borgen, J. (2013). Higher prevalence of eating disorders among adolescent elite athletes than controls. *Medicine and Science in Sports and Exercise, 45*(6), 1188–1197.

Matza, A. R., Sloan, C. A., & Kauth, M. R. (2015). Quality LGBT health education: A review of key report and webinars. *Clinical Psychological Science Practices, 22*(2), 127–144.

McGillivray, J. A., & Kershaw, M. M. (2013). The impact of staff initiated referral and intervention protocols on symptoms of depression in people with mild intellectual disability. *Research in Developmental Disabilities, 34*(2), 730–738.

Mead, D. R., Dana, R. C., & Carson, C. A. (2017). *The primary care approach to lesbian, gay, bisexual, transgender and queer/questioning populations.* Retrieved from http://www.consultant360.com/articles/primary-care-approach-lesbian-gay-bisexual-transgender-and-queerquestioning-populations

Melnyk, B. M. (2003). *Creating Opportunities for Personal Empowerment for children, adolescents, and young adults.* Powell, OH: COPE2Thrive.

Melnyk, B. M., & Jensen, P. (Eds.). (2013). *A practical guide to child and adolescent mental health screening, early intervention, and health promotion* (2nd ed.) New York, NY: National Association of Pediatric Nurse Practitioners.

Merikangas, K. R., Nakamura, E. F., & Kessler, R. C. (2009). Epidemiology of mental disorders in children and adolescents. *Dialogues in Clinical Neuroscience, 11*(1), 7–20.

Miller, B., & Buckley, P. (2013). Schizophrenia. In E. T. Bope & R. D. Kellerman (Eds.), *Conn's current therapy* (pp. 952–956). Philadelphia, PA: Elsevier/Saunders.

Moe, J. L., Finnerty, P., Sparkman, N., et al. (2015). Initial assessment and screening with LGBTQ clients: A critical perspective. *Journal of LGBT Issues in Counseling, 9*(1), 36–56.

Mojtabai, R., & Olfson, M. (2014). National trends in the long-term use of antidepressant medications: Results from the US national health and nutrition examination survey. *Journal of Clinical Psychiatry, 75*(2), 169–177.

Mosca, N. W., & Schatz, M. L. (2015). Encopresis: Not just an accident. *NASN School Nurse, 28*(5), 218–221.

Mustanski, B. S., Garofalo, R., & Emerson, E. M. (2010). Mental health disorders, psychological distress, and suicidality in a diverse sample of lesbian, gay, bisexual, and transgender youths. *American Journal of Public Health, 100,* 2426–2432.

Needham, B. L. (2012). Sexual attraction and trajectories of mental health and substance use during the transition from adolescence to adulthood. *Journal of Youth and Adolescence, 41,* 179–190.

Nock, M. K., Green, J. G., Hwang, I., et al. (2013). Prevalence, correlates, and treatment of lifetime suicidal behavior among adolescents: Results from the National Comorbidity Survey Replication Adolescent Supplement. *JAMA Psychiatry, 70,* 300–310.

Ortiz, C., & Stratis, A. (2015). Pediatric elimination disorders. In R. Flanagan, K. Allen, & E. Levine (Eds.), *Cognitive and behavioral interventions in the schools* (pp. 199–218). New York, NY: Springer Publishing.

Piacentini, J., Woods, D. W., Scahill, L., et al.(2010). Behavior therapy for children with Tourette disorder: A randomized controlled clinical trial. *JAMA, 303*(19), 1929–1937.

Plessen, K. J. (2013). Tic disorders and Tourette's syndrome. *European Child & Adolescent Psychiatry, 22*(Suppl. 1), S55–S60.

Santucci, L. C., & Ehrenreich-May, J. (2013). A randomized controlled trial of the child anxiety multi-day program (CAMP) for separation anxiety disorder. *Child Psychiatry and Human Development, 44*(3), 439–451.

Scheffer, R. (2011). Psychiatric disorders. In K. J. Marcdante, R. M. Kliegman, H. B. Jenson, et al. (Eds.), *Nelson essentials of pediatrics* (6th ed., pp. 63–80). Philadelphia, PA: Saunders/Elsevier.

Sigel, E. J. (2012). Eating disorders. In W. Hay, M. Levin, R. Deterding, et al. (Eds.), *Current diagnosis & treatment pediatrics* (21st ed., pp. 167–178). New York, NY: McGraw-Hill/Lange.

Stafford, B., Talmi, A., & Burstein, A. (2012). Child & adolescent psychiatric disorders & psychosocial aspects of pediatrics. In W. Hay, M. Levin, R. Deterding, et al. (Eds.), *Current diagnosis & treatment pediatrics* (21st ed., pp. 179–222). New York, NY: McGraw-Hill/Lange.

Starke, M. (2011). Young adults with intellectual disability recall their childhood. *Journal of Intellectual Disabilities, 15*(4), 229–240.

Strange, B. C. (2008). Once-daily treatment of ADHD with guanfacine: Patient implications. *Neuropsychiatric Disease and Treatment, 4*(3), 499–506.

Swenne, I., & Stridsberg, M. (2012). Bone metabolism markers in adolescent girls with eating disorders and weight loss: Effects of growth, weight trend, developmental and menstrual status. *Archives of Osteoporosis, 7,* 125–133.

Sysko, R., Sha, N., Wang, Y., et al. (2010). Early response to antidepressant treatment in bulimia nervosa. *Psychological Medicine, 40*(6), 999–1005.

The Arc. (2016). Retrieved from http://www.thearc.org

Troiden, R. R. (1979). Becoming homosexual: A model of gay identity acquisition. *Psychiatry, 42*(4), 362–373.

U.S. Department of Health and Human Services. (2010). *Healthy people 2020.* Washington, DC: Author.

Viana, A. G., Trent, L., Tull, M. T., et al. (2012). Non-medical use of prescription drugs among Mississippi youth: Constitutional, psychological, and family factors. *Addictive Behavior, 37*(12), 1382–1388.

Volkmar, F., Siegal, M., Woodbury-Smith, M., et al. (2014). Practice parameters for the assessment and treatment of children and adolescents with autism spectrum disorders. *Journal of the American Academy of Child and Adolescent Psychiatry, 53*(2), 237–257.

Walle, J. V., Rittig, S., Tekgül, S., et al. (2017). Enuresis: Practical guidelines for primary care. *British Journal of General Practice.* Advance online publication. doi:10.3399/bjgp17X691337

Weersing, V. R., Brent, D. A., Rozenman, M. S., et al. (2017). Brief behavioral therapy for pediatric anxiety and depression in primary care: A randomized clinical trial. *JAMA Psychiatry.* Advance online publication. doi:10.1001/jamapsychiatry.2017.0429

Wong, D., & Baker, C. (1988). Pain in children: Comparison of assessment scales. *Pediatric Nursing, 14*(1), 9–17.

Wu, S. W., & Gilbert, D. L. (2013). Gilles de la Tourette syndrome. In E. T. Bope & R. D. Kellerman (Eds.), *Conn's current therapy* (pp. 605–607). Philadelphia, PA: Elsevier/Saunders.

Yael, D., Vinner, E., & Bar-Gad, I. (2015). Pathophysiology of tic disorders. *Movement Disorders, 30*(9), 1171–1178.

Yildirim, A., Hacihasanoğlu Aşilar, R., & Karakurt, P. (2013). Effects of a nursing intervention program on the depression and perception of family functioning of mothers with intellectually disabled children. *Journal of Clinical Nursing, 22*(1–2), 251–261.

Young, S. L. (2010). Pica in pregnancy: New ideas about an old condition. *Annual Review of Nutrition, 30*(8), 403–422.

55

Nursing Care of a Family in Crisis: Maltreatment and Violence in the Family

KEY TERMS

KEY TERMS

abusive head trauma

factitious disorder

failure to thrive

hebephile

incest

intimate partner violence

learned helplessness

maltreatment

mandatory reporters

molestation

pedophile

permissive reporters

rape trauma syndrome

sexual maltreatment

*H*illary Landstrum is a 3-year-old you see in an emergency department. Her mother, who is the city mayor, tells you Hillary fell off a swing in the backyard. Hillary has a broken forearm, a broken rib, and multiple bruises on her chest and back. You notice in her electronic record that Hillary was seen in the same emergency room a month ago for a burn on her hand. When you mention to her mother that Hillary's injuries seem extreme for a simple fall, her mother says, "She isn't very pretty. I guess she's also clumsy."

Previous chapters described the normal growth and development of children and care of children with disorders of specific body systems. This chapter adds information about the effect on children when child maltreatment or intimate partner violence occurs in a family. Such information can build a base for care and for putting into place ways to prevent further maltreatment or violence.

You suspect Hillary is a victim of child maltreatment. What additional questions would you want to ask her mother to help determine whether this is so? What should you do if you feel certain Hillary has been maltreated?

OBJECTIVES

After mastering the contents of this chapter, you should be able to:

1. Discuss the types of child maltreatment or intimate partner violence seen in families and the theories explaining their occurrence.

2. Identify 2020 National Health Goals related to child maltreatment or intimate partner violence that nurses can help the nation achieve.

3. Assess a family that has experienced physical or emotional child maltreatment or intimate partner violence.

4. Formulate nursing diagnoses related to a family in which child maltreatment or intimate partner violence is present.

5. Develop expected outcomes for a family that has experienced child maltreatment or intimate partner violence to help them manage seamless transitions across differing healthcare settings.

6. Using the nursing process, plan nursing care that includes the six competencies of Quality & Safety Education for Nurses (QSEN): Patient-Centered Care, Teamwork & Collaboration, Evidence-Based Practice (EBP), Quality Improvement (QI), Safety, and Informatics.

7. Implement nursing care for a family in which child maltreatment or intimate partner violence has occurred, such as ways to role model developmentally age appropriate parenting.

8. Evaluate expected outcomes for effectiveness and achievement of care.

9. Integrate knowledge of family child maltreatment or intimate partner violence with the interplay of nursing process, the six competencies of QSEN, and Family Nursing to promote quality maternal and child health nursing care.

Child protective services in the United States receive 3.4 million reports of children being maltreated or neglected per year, with about 683,000 of those children determined to have been maltreated (U.S. Department of Health and Human Services, Administration for Children and Families, Administration on Children, Youth and Families, Children's Bureau, 2017). A nationally representative sample determined that 10.2% of U.S. children are maltreated in some way, and the lifetime cost in medical bills and lost productivity is over $210,000 per child, making the total economic cost of maltreatment as much as $585 billion a year nationally (Fang, Brown, Florence, et al., 2012).

Child maltreatment is associated with stress and has been linked with the inability of a family to handle external and internal stressors. Accordingly, maltreatment or violence in a family is rarely an isolated event but rather an indication of many other factors that require intervention (McCloskey, 2013).

Maltreatment, formerly termed *abuse*, is defined as the "willful injury by one person of another" (Helfer & Kempe, 1987) and takes many forms: physical or emotional maltreatment, neglect or sexual maltreatment, intimate partner violence, and maltreatment or violence of the elderly. Maternity, child health, and family care nurses need to be especially observant for signs of possible maltreatment or violence in a family because these increase during pregnancy and possibly during the care of an ill child. In all instances, the victim's safety is paramount, but ensuring this safety must be done with sensitivity to the importance of maintaining and improving overall family functioning.

Child maltreatment has long-term consequences; as many as 30% of children from families where there is child maltreatment become maltreating parents themselves (A. J. Lang, Gartstein, Rodgers, et al., 2010; Valentino, Nuttall, Comas, et al., 2012). It also predisposes victims to numerous psychological problems and induces a persistent sensitization of the stress-response system (Heim, Shugart, Craighead, et al., 2010). Box 55.1 shows 2020 National Health Goals related to child maltreatment and intimate partner violence.

Nursing Process Overview

FOR CARE OF A FAMILY THAT HAS EXPERIENCED CHILD MALTREATMENT OR INTIMATE PARTNER VIOLENCE

ASSESSMENT

Nurses are often the first individuals to identify symptoms of possible child maltreatment or intimate partner violence in a family because they are often the first to take a health history or see a child or woman undressed at a healthcare visit and recognize significant bruising; they are also often the person to whom a pregnant woman or child confides the problem. If maltreatment or violence in any form is suspected, it is essential to get as full a picture as possible. If child maltreatment is suspected, talk with the parents first, without the child, and then interview the child separately to help uncover any inconsistencies in the parents' explanations. Remember, however, you are *not* investigating the concern—you are doing an initial screening to assess the need for referral and reporting. Your agency's patient protective services department will do the actual investigation.

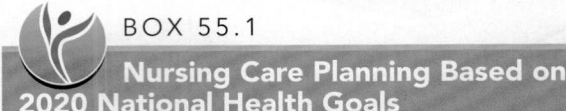

BOX 55.1

Nursing Care Planning Based on 2020 National Health Goals

The mark of a developed nation is the ability to protect the health of its most vulnerable members. This makes both child maltreatment and intimate partner violence national health concerns. Examples of 2020 National Health Goals that specifically address these issues are:

- Reduce the rate of maltreatment of children younger than 18 years of age from a baseline of 9.4 per 1,000 to a target level of 8.5 per 1,000.
- Reduce the rate of child maltreatment fatalities from a baseline of 2.4 per 100,000 to a target level of 2.2 per 100,000.
- Reduce the rate of physical, sexual, and psychological violence by current or former intimate partners.
- Reduce stalking by former or present intimate partners.
- Reduce abusive sexual conduct and rape (U.S. Department of Health and Human Services, 2010; see www.healthypeople.gov).

Nurses can help the nation achieve these goals by educating parents about how to parent more effectively and by identifying children or adults in school or healthcare agency settings who have been maltreated, neglected, or victim of violence.

NURSING DIAGNOSIS

Nursing diagnoses associated with child maltreatment or family violence should address both the physical and the emotional results of the concern. Some examples are:

- Pain related to burn on hand from documented child maltreatment
- Risk for injury related to previous intimate partner violence
- Risk for other-directed violence related to admitted poor self-control
- Impaired parenting related to high level of stress
- Compromised family coping as manifested by child maltreatment related to alcohol use by father
- Disturbed self-esteem related to stalking and sexual maltreatment

OUTCOME IDENTIFICATION AND PLANNING

Planning must center first on ensuring the safety of the maltreated family member and minimizing the effects of trauma. Second comes reporting the discovery to authorities as nurses are mandated by law to report child maltreatment. Long-term planning includes helping a maltreated family member find safe refuge and re-establishing self-esteem through a self-help or advocacy program. Teaching empowerment, or the ability to take charge of one's life, is particularly important for older children and women in families where there is maltreatment or violence. In addition, the person who maltreated a child or woman needs a program of therapy to help prevent future offenses.

The following organizations can be helpful for referral: Parents Anonymous (www.parentsanonymous.org), the Child

Abuse Prevention Network (www.child-abuse.com), the National Coalition Against Domestic Violence (www.ncadv.org), and Women Organized Against Rape (www.WOAR.org).

IMPLEMENTATION

The most important intervention related to family child maltreatment or intimate partner violence is prevention. Nurses can do much in all settings to be particularly observant for families who seem to be at risk for maltreatment or violence and role model optimal ways to handle family stress. Further education is an intervention that can help parents who may not recognize their children's needs or normal child behavior to learn healthy patterns of childrearing.

OUTCOME EVALUATION

Expected outcomes should focus on specific examples of improved family interaction, such as:

- The parent holds baby in a caring manner and maintains good eye contact.
- The parent attends full series of counseling sessions on learning better parenting.
- The parent states she has the Crisis Center telephone number on her cell phone and will call for help if she feels under threat by her partner.
- The adolescent states she can still think of herself with high self-esteem despite rape by stepbrother.
- The parent attends monthly meetings of Parents Anonymous.

Health Promotion and Risk Management

Prevention must be the goal of healthcare providers to reduce the incidence of child maltreatment (Box 55.2). Because many adults who maltreat children were maltreated themselves, stopping the cycle of abuse will help prevent maltreatment in generations to come.

Identifying parents who may be at risk for maltreating their child is a necessary step in prevention. Listen carefully to the way pregnant women or their partners talk about the child they are expecting. A parent who is overly concerned about the physical appearance or sex of the child ("This had better be a girl" or "He'd better not have his father's nose" or "She better have good hair") may have difficulty accepting a child who does not meet these expectations. Listen for a parent who is concerned about "not letting children get the upper hand" or who says a child "had better be good." Such parents may be conveying worry about how they will act when a child is "bad."

During the postpartum period, be aware of parents who do not touch their infant within 24 hours and those who make disparaging remarks about the child's appearance, as this lack of contact could signal risk. Remember, though, not all parents immediately bond or react warmly to their newborns. Many may only tentatively touch or pick up their infant immediately.

Parents may also be identified as being able to maltreat children during health maintenance visits. By the time a baby is brought to a healthcare agency for the initial health maintenance visit, you should be able to see that positive parent–child

interaction has begun. Listen for parents who say the baby is "nothing but trouble," "cries all the time," or "is bad." Ask new parents how it feels to be a new parent. "I'm exhausted but enjoying it" is a different answer from "It takes too much time" or "It's not much fun." Specific observations to make during postpartum and pediatric healthcare checkups are summarized in Box 55.3.

Helping parents to seek assistance from support people is another necessary step in prevention. Home visits, family counseling and therapy, and referral to organizations for parents who maltreat children, such as Parents Anonymous, can be highly effective in encouraging parents to reach out for help in times of crisis.

Another nursing responsibility aimed at preventing child maltreatment is helping young parents learn about normal growth and development of children and how to better respond to the child's behavior (Fig. 55.1). Courses in high school or college that describe sound parenting and review normal growth and development and the responsibilities involved in parenting are additional measures in preventing child maltreatment. Parenting classes conducted in high-risk prenatal settings might also have an impact.

BOX 55.2

Measures to Prevent Child Maltreatment or Intimate Partner Violence

1. Advocate for high school or college courses on parenting and growth and development of children so young parents are familiar with typical growth and development of children.
2. Help children learn problem-solving techniques so they are not overwhelmed by mounting problems when they become adults.
3. Foster high self-esteem in children and women so they are not dependent on others but are assertive (to prevent them from becoming passive observers to maltreatment or violence).
4. Help parents with responsible reproductive planning, so children are intended and desired.
5. Help parents locate support people in their community, such as crisis centers or Parents Anonymous or religious or social contacts, so they have ready support people to help them manage stress.
6. Role model caring behaviors with children for parents.
7. Identify children who may be viewed as special in some way by parents, such as those who were separated from the family at birth, were premature, or are physically or cognitively challenged, because these children are at high risk to be victims of maltreatment.
8. Identify parents who were maltreated as children and offer specific help to them to break the chain of child maltreatment.
9. Advocate and support laws that implement the "No Hit Zone" in public places such as hospitals and school settings.

Questions to Ask to Detect the Potential for Child Maltreatment in New Parents

1. Is the parent enjoying this new role?
2. Does the parent establish eye contact with the baby?
3. How does the parent talk to the baby? Is everything expressed as a demand?
4. Are most of the parent's verbalizations about the child negative?
5. Does the parent remain disappointed about the child's sex or appearance?
6. Are the parent's expectations for the child's development far beyond the child's capabilities?
7. Is the parent very bothered by the baby's crying? Does he or she ignore the baby's demands to be fed? When the baby cries, is the parent able to comfort the child?
8. What is the parent's reaction to the task of changing diapers? Is the parent repulsed by the messiness?
9. Can the parents name a support person they can turn to for advice or assurance?
10. Is sibling rivalry a problem? Is the husband jealous of the baby's claim on the mother's time and affection?
11. When a parent brings the child for health care, does the parent become involved with the baby's needs during the examination and while in the waiting room? Or does the parent relinquish control to the healthcare provider or nurse such as undressing the child, holding the child, or allowing the child to express fears?
12. Can attention be focused on the child in the parent's presence? Can the parent see something positive in that focus?
13. Does the parent report nonexistent symptoms in the baby? Describe the child in terms that you do not recognize at all? Call with strange stories, such as the child has stopped breathing, changed color, or is doing something "on purpose" to aggravate the parent?

Figure 55.1 Teaching that all children have unique characteristics helps to prevent child maltreatment. Here, new parents explore the already noticeable unique aspects of their newborn.

Child Maltreatment

Because parenting is not an easy task and good parenting is not an automatic or truly instinctive ability, children in every community are injured because of maltreatment. This may be physical (the child is beaten or burned), it may be neglect (the child is not fed, clothed, supervised properly, or offered medical care or educational opportunities), or it also could be psychological or emotional (a child is made to feel unintelligent or inadequate). In some instances, women who threatened the health of their fetus by abusing drugs during pregnancy have been viewed by some courts as being guilty of child maltreatment (Goodwin, 2011).

Maltreatment not only places a child at immediate risk for harm but can also lead to long-term effects. For example, physically maltreated children are found to be more angry, noncompliant, and hyperactive than others; they may demonstrate poor self-control and low self-esteem. Children whose parents do not interact with them (emotional maltreatment) are apt to be more withdrawn and to have a flatter affect than others. Because a family where maltreatment occurs is a disrupted one, children often have undiagnosed medical problems, such as anemia, otitis media, or lead poisoning. Children who suffer sexual maltreatment can develop sexually transmitted infections or have long-term effects of depression, guilt, and difficulty enjoying sexual relations (Hornor, 2010).

In addition, when children reach adulthood and begin parenting, they tend to rear their children in basically the same way as they were reared. Parents who themselves received little love or were maltreated as children may never form a basic sense of trust and so may not be able to form a sense of intimacy or the ability to care for others as late adolescents.

THEORIES OF CHILD MALTREATMENT

The most commonly accepted theory regarding why child maltreatment occurs is that a special triad of circumstances develops (Helfer & Kempe, 1987):

- A parent has the potential to maltreat a child (special parent).
- A child is viewed as "different" in some way by the parent (special child).
- An event or circumstance brings about the maltreatment (special circumstance).

Some health practices or illnesses can be confused with child maltreatment and thus are important to remember in assessment. For example, coin-rolling, a type of massage to draw illness out of the body used by some Asian cultures (a coin is heated and then vigorously rubbed over the body), leaves red welts on the back similar to those that would appear on a child who has been struck repeatedly.

Some infants may bump their head while learning to walk; most toddlers have some ecchymotic spots on their legs from bumping into tables or chairs during normal toddler activities, and preschoolers who actively play may have bruises on multiple bony spots (shin, elbows, knees, etc.). Some childhood diseases, such as leukemia or purpura, begin with easy bruising, which can mimic marks from maltreatment. Children with osteogenesis imperfecta have frequent broken bones as a natural consequence of their disease. Because of inadequate fact finding in these instances, false reports do occur. When this happens, it can lead to severe stress on the family that has been falsely accused and can interfere with the relationship between the parents of an ill child and the healthcare personnel who will then give care to the child. Being aware of a practice such as coin-rolling and usual symptoms of illnesses aids understanding of the meaning of illness to parents and helps prevent false reports of child maltreatment.

There are, however, classic "red flags" of nonaccidental trauma that are important to keep in mind, such as spiral fractures of bones (from a twisting force—envision an adult twisting a child's arm, hard) and skull fractures. There are times when these injuries are unintentional injuries, such as a spiral fracture of the leg because the child slipped when climbing down the bunk-bed ladder and the leg was caught while the body twisted and fell, but these injuries always need to be reviewed carefully with an increased index of suspicion. Any fracture in a nonmobile infant is suspicious, especially long bone fractures (Sullivan, 2011). Always assess for injuries that do not match a child's developmental level or abilities or injuries that do not match the explanation of how the injury occurred.

Special Parent: Parents Who Maltreat

Risk factors for parents who maltreat children include substance abuse, mental health issues, young age, low education and income, single parent status, and having multiple dependent children (Fortson, Klevens, Merrick, et al., 2016). Many of these parents were maltreated as children. They may be unfamiliar with the normal growth and development of children and so have unrealistic expectations of a child. They also may be socially isolated, with no support readily available, and can become overwhelmed by childrearing. The isolation may be by distance (a parent separated from other people in a farmhouse miles from neighbors) or it may be the type that exists in communities or apartment houses where neighbors do not routinely speak to one another. Maltreatment is strongly associated with excessive parental use of drugs such as alcohol, substances that remove inhibitions and self-control. Studies have found that areas with an increased amount of bars per square mile have increased amounts of child neglect, whereas areas with more off-premises alcohol outlets/liquor stores have increased amounts of child maltreatment, possibly because some parents who drink in bars leave children home alone, whereas some parents who drink at home are more likely to maltreat when the child "misbehaves" (Freisthler, 2011).

Special Child: Children Who Are Maltreated

Maltreated children tend to be viewed by parents as somehow "different." They may be more or less intelligent than other children in the family; they may have been unplanned, or they just may not live up to their parents' expectations in some way. Studies suggest that lesbian, gay, and bisexual (LGB) children and adolescents are also at greater risk of child maltreatment compared to non-LGB kids. These children and adolescents are 3.8 times more likely to experience sexual abuse and 1.2 times more likely to be physically abused compared to their heterosexual peers (Friedman, Marshal, Guadamuz, et al., 2011). Additionally, children with gender nonconformity are at increased risk of child maltreatment during childhood (Roberts, Rosario, Corliss, et al., 2012).

Children younger than 4 years of age are at greater risk for child abuse then older children as are those who require an increased caregiver burden such as children with disabilities, mental retardation, mental health issues, and chronic illness (Fortson et al., 2016). Without an effective relationship, when a child is injured, parents who are unable to deal with stress may not show the usual degree of compassion for their child's pain or offer comfort. They may appear more concerned with how the injury affects them than how it affects the child, saying, "Don't cry. You'll make me look like a bad parent," rather than, "It's okay to cry. I know that hurts." They may not seek treatment for an injury in an expected amount of time.

To prevent maltreatment, a child may assume a role reversal with the parent or become the comforting, solacing person. They recognize very early in life that when a parent is upset, they will be hurt. They learn to comfort the parent and reduce the parent's stress and anxiety, thereby avoiding the hurt. For this reason, it is important to assess who is comforting whom when a childhood injury occurs.

Special Circumstance: Stress

The third factor in child maltreatment is stress, which may be a response to an event that would not necessarily be stressful for an average parent. It might be something as common as a blocked toilet, an illness in the family, a lost job, a landlord asking for the rent, or a rainstorm that cancels a picnic. Child maltreatment crosses all socioeconomic levels because stress of this nature occurs at all levels. Stress generally has a greater impact on individuals who do not have strong support people around them. Families whose internal support system is faulty or who have not formed outside support systems are apt to have a higher incidence of maltreatment.

REPORTING SUSPECTED CHILD MALTREATMENT

State laws typically identify two levels of responsibility for reporting child maltreatment: mandatory reporters and permissive reporters. **Permissive reporters** are encouraged to report suspected child abuse but are not required by law. **Mandatory reporters** are professionals who are mandated by law to report child maltreatment. Nurses are included in the mandatory category in most states; this means they *must* report suspected child maltreatment when they identify it. Failure to do so can result in a fine, jail time, or loss of nursing licensure. The fact that the information was given in a confidential interview does not free a nurse from this responsibility (it is an exception under the confidentiality rules of the Health Insurance Portability and Accountability Act [HIPAA]) (Fraser, Mathews, Walsh, et al., 2010).

All healthcare institutions and agencies have protocols on how the reporting of child maltreatment should be managed. It is important to learn the protocol required by your particular agency, community, and state. After an official report of child maltreatment has been made to a child protection agency, a hospital has the right, in most instances, to hold the child for 72 hours for protection to give an appointed caseworker time to investigate whether maltreatment has occurred. After the 72 hours, a court proceeding will determine whether the child should be returned to the parents' care or kept in a safer location. Because child maltreatment is a crime, the healthcare record of the child can be subpoenaed and displayed in court. Be certain, therefore, when charting information related to child maltreatment that you make specific and factual notes (observations, not interpretations), such as "Parent spoke loudly and slurred his words," rather than "Parent was intoxicated," or "Mother stated, 'This child is nothing but trouble,'" not "I think this mother dislikes this child." Photographs of physical maltreatment enhance the strength of the testimony of maltreatment, so these are usually taken.

A second provision in state laws is protection from having a lawsuit brought against a healthcare provider for reporting suspected maltreatment "in good faith" that is then proved false. In other words, the laws are written to make it better to err on the side of reporting suspected maltreatment rather than not reporting it, from both a child safety standpoint and a legal perspective. When maltreatment is officially reported, parents need to be told child maltreatment is suspected because open lines of communication with parents are important to both protect the child and to arrange counseling for the parent who has maltreated the child. Remember when taking history that maltreatment is not always done by parents, so a parent could really not know how an injury occurred. Alternate caregivers such as daycare workers, a babysitter, or a nonbiologic parental figure (the new spouse) could be the person at fault.

PHYSICAL MALTREATMENT

Physical maltreatment is the action of a caregiver that causes physical injury to a child. It is commonly revealed by burns or by injuries to the head or hands (Box 55.4).

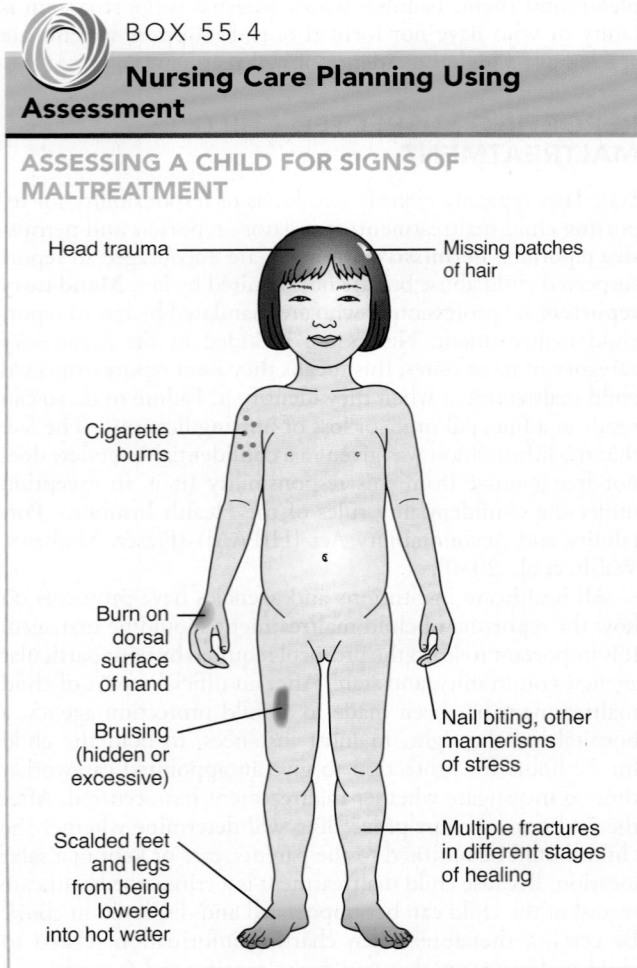

BOX 55.4

Nursing Care Planning Using Assessment

ASSESSING A CHILD FOR SIGNS OF MALTREATMENT

- Head trauma
- Missing patches of hair
- Cigarette burns
- Burn on dorsal surface of hand
- Bruising (hidden or excessive)
- Nail biting, other mannerisms of stress
- Scalded feet and legs from being lowered into hot water
- Multiple fractures in different stages of healing

Assessment

When taking history, always ask caregivers to account for any injury to a child's body. Remember, however, that most childhood injuries are the result of unintentional injuries caused by the child's inability to distinguish safe situations from dangerous ones or by parents' overestimating their child's ability to do such things as lighting a fire to burn trash or using a saw for a wood project.

An important mark of maltreatment in contrast to an unintentional injury is that the injury is out of proportion to the history given by the parent or caregiver (Fig. 55.2). The parent or caregiver, for example, may report that the child was playing underneath the coffee table when he reared up quickly and hit his head to explain the large hematoma and temporary loss of consciousness the child is experiencing or that the infant "rolled off the couch" but now has two broken arms. In other instances, the parents may give conflicting stories (the mother says the child fell, but the father says the child broke his arm while throwing a baseball) or they may give no reason for the injury ("He woke up from his nap and couldn't move his arm; I have no idea what could have happened.").

Ask children about the injury as well as the parents because if they did not hear the parent's explanation of the injury, they may say something that is inconsistent with the parent's explanation. They also may cry little in response to a painful procedure, such as an injection, because they are not used to receiving comfort for pain. They may draw back from an examiner more than the average child because they are afraid of adults. These are very subjective observations, however, because children react in different ways to the fear produced by a recent injury or a health examination.

It is often difficult to remain objective when talking to the parents of a child who has been maltreated when you believe the parent is the one who is guilty of the maltreatment. Emotional involvement is not constructive, however; it rarely helps the parents to change, and it may cause them to avoid seeking health care in the future, leaving the child totally unprotected, especially if they were not the one who hurt the child.

To remain objective, always assume the parents have done the best they could under the circumstances in which they found themselves. The fact they have brought the child for care means they are seeking help; it may be their way of saying, "Help me; I don't want this to happen again." In many instances, child maltreatment is not an isolated phenomenon or a parent is also a victim and needs as much help and protection as the child.

Physical Examination

When children are examined at a well-child visit or because of illness, be certain they are fully undressed (including removing all bandages and adhesive bandage) so their entire body can be observed. Plot height and weight on a standard growth chart. Delays in growth may suggest neglect.

Several injuries in children clearly signal probable child maltreatment. Most parents protect their children's hands carefully; in contrast, children who are maltreated have a higher incidence of hand injury. Children who are beaten with electrical cords, belts, or clotheslines have peculiar circular and linear lesions (see Fig. 55.2). Children who are beaten with a belt buckle may have additional curved lacerations from the imprint of the buckle; few other objects produce

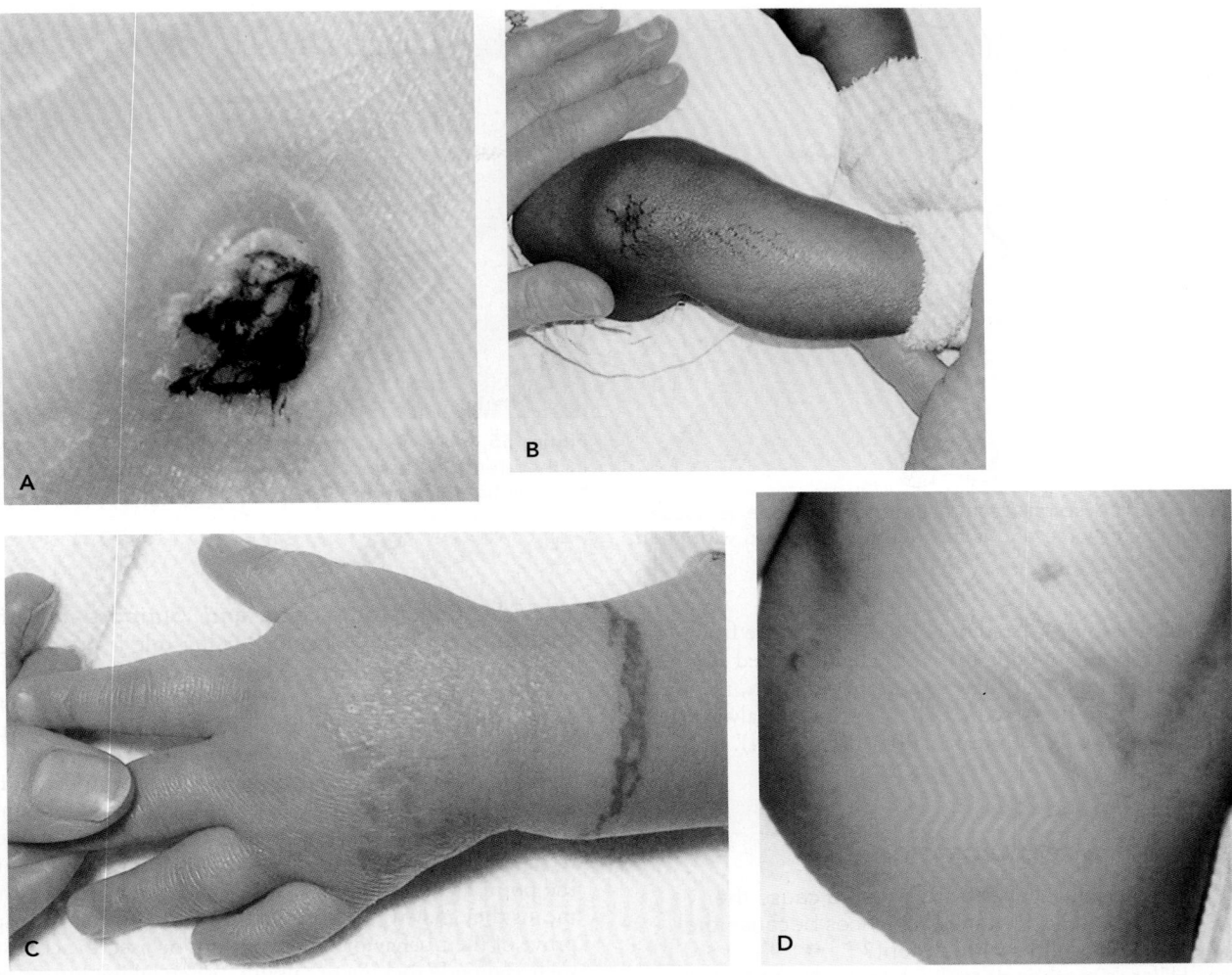

Figure 55.2 (A) Cigarette burn on child's foot. **(B)** Branding injury showing imprint of radiator cover. **(C)** Rope burn with edema and skin breakdown from being tied to crib rails. **(D)** Imprint marks from beating with a looped electrical cord. (From Zitelli, B. J., & Davis, H. W. [1997]. *Atlas of pediatric physical diagnosis* [3rd ed.]. St. Louis, MO: Mosby–Year Book, Inc.)

such contusions. Abrasions or ecchymotic areas on the wrists or ankles may be present if the child was tied to a bed or against a wall.

Burns or scalds are frequent injuries in maltreated children. The peak age at which children unintentionally burn themselves is 2 years; the peak age of burns related to maltreatment is closer to 3 years. When children burn their hand by accident, they usually burn the palm; burns from maltreatment are often on the dorsal surface. Scalding with hot water can occur from a child pulling a hot cup of coffee or a coffee maker off a table. This can, however, be child maltreatment (an adult deliberately scalded the child). Young children do unintentionally step into bathtubs containing water that is hot enough to burn. When this happens, however, the child usually falls forward and so also has burns on the hands and splash marks on the chest or face. If a child is lowered into scalding water as punishment, only the feet and the skin up to the knees are scalded. A child who is placed in a tub of hot water buttocks first by an angry parent usually has no burn in the center of the buttocks because the buttocks touched the bottom of the tub creating a ring of burns or a "doughnut-hole" effect.

Cigarette burns are another common finding on the bodies of physically maltreated children. A fresh cigarette burn causes a blister that resembles the scab of impetigo; differentiation at this stage is often difficult. Impetigo lesions, however, heal without scarring. Cigarette burns heal with a definite circular scar.

Human bites or chunks of hair pulled off the scalp are other signs of maltreatment. Head injuries and broken bones are also frequent findings. Children who are preschool age and younger usually do not fall far enough under normal circumstances to break bones; a broken bone at this age, therefore, suggests the child was thrown or struck so hard the bone broke. Other common findings include multiple fractures in different stages of healing, rib or occipital fractures, and metaphyseal–epiphyseal injuries. Bones are not always broken if a child is shaken roughly, but the periosteum may be torn so that an X-ray reveals a strange haziness along both sides of the bone shaft. Tibial torsion (twisting) is also often seen (Fig. 55.3).

Deliberate poisoning is yet another form of child maltreatment; this usually occurs in a child younger than 2.5 years of age. Bruises on a child who is too young to walk also are

Figure 55.3 A spiral fracture around the bone is caused by a wrenching force and is frequently associated with child maltreatment.

Figure 55.4 Large bruises on a child's body. With this type of injury, carefully assessing the history of the traumatic event would be essential. (© Biophoto Associates/Photograph Researchers.)

highly suspicious because those bruises only come from outside sources. Remembering the 3 *B*s, a light-hearted although meaningful phase for such an important situation, may help with assessment: **B**ruises on **B**abies are nearly always **B**ad (Lazoritz, Rossiter, & Whiteaker, 2010) (Fig. 55.4).

QSEN Checkpoint Question 55.1

TEAMWORK & COLLABORATION

Which finding in Hillary's history would cause the nurse to alert Child Protective Services because the nurse suspects child maltreatment?

a. Hillary's mother described her as "not pretty."
b. Hillary has a previous health visit for "multiple bruises."
c. Hillary's mother is under severe stress because of her job.
d. Hillary's mother described her as "clumsy."

Look in Appendix A for the best answer and rationale.

 ### Nursing Diagnoses and Related Interventions

Nursing Diagnosis: Risk for injury related to documented maltreatment by parent

Outcome Evaluation: Child has no further physical injuries identifiable as being inflicted by parent.

Prevent Further Maltreatment. When child maltreatment is discovered, it would be ideal if the person responsible for the maltreatment could change behavior, and thus, the relationship could be kept intact. In most cases, however, once child maltreatment has been discovered, either the child or the abuser usually must be removed from the home to keep the child safe from being maltreated again. Even so, it may be impossible to reverse the damage that has been done to the child's sense of trust and self-esteem.

Provide Consistent Care and Support for the Maltreated Child. A major nursing role is providing a consistent, caring adult presence for a maltreated child where the child can feel safe. Box 55.5 shows an interprofessional care map illustrating both nursing and team planning for a child who has been maltreated.

Use a primary or case management type of nursing care assignment to offer consistency and the security of a one-to-one relationship. Many maltreated children are used to playing by themselves, not with an adult, and only to the point at which a parent wants them to continue; this means they may watch you carefully for signs that you approve of their behavior. They may not be used to activities such as quietly rocking or talking. When taking history, be careful not to imply that any one answer to your question will be the correct one. Otherwise, maltreated children may supply what they think you want to hear rather than the truth. (A question such as "That feels better, doesn't it?" may be followed by an instant "yes" even though the child feels no improvement in symptoms.)

Evaluate and Promote Family Health. An important factor to help evaluate is whether a child will be safe remaining in the parents' care. When parents who are suspected child abusers visit the healthcare facility, be certain they are given the same welcome and orientation to the facility and procedures as other parents. When caring for a child, point out positive characteristics about the child, as well as growth and development markers and realistic expectations of the child's age, because lack of knowledge of normal growth and development may have contributed to the maltreatment. Take some time as well to talk to the parents away from the child so that your total attention is focused on them. Praise them for the things they have done well to lay a foundation for them to accept counseling and hopefully change.

For many parents, the response to a charge of child maltreatment is anger. For others, it is relief; now, an unwanted child will be taken away from them. In some instances, the diagnosis of maltreatment will force a passive partner to make some important decisions about whether to continue a marriage or relationship with the abusive

BOX 55.5

Nursing Care Planning

AN INTERPROFESSIONAL CARE MAP FOR A CHILD WHO HAS BEEN MALTREATED

Hillary is a 3-year-old you see in the emergency department. She has a broken forearm, a broken rib, and multiple bruises on her chest and back. She was seen in the same emergency room a month ago for a burn on the palm of her hand. When you mention to her mother that Hillary's injuries seem extreme for a simple fall, her mother says, "Hillary isn't very pretty. I guess she's also clumsy." You suspect Hillary may be a victim of child maltreatment.

Family Assessment: Hillary is an only child. Mother works long hours as city mayor; father (computer consultant) provides child care most evenings. Finances rated as "good." When primary healthcare provider suggested the child may have been beaten and maltreated, she stated, "Neither of us would ever do that. Not with me running for reelection."

Patient Assessment: A 3-year-old girl dressed in wool coat and cap even though outside temperature is 80°F. Father protested removal of the child's clothing for examination. Child's right forearm is misaligned and swollen; 3 × 4-in. bruise on right side of anterior ribs, four ½-in. diameter circular lesions on right arm; large 4-cm ecchymotic area on both buttocks and anterior left thigh. Sharp, pointed, triangular blistering and inflamed area noted on back of left hand mother states are "mosquito bites"; mark on hand is a "birthmark." Child remained passive while being examined but drew back when mother approached.

Nursing Diagnosis: Fear related to repeated episodes of maltreatment

Outcome Criteria: Child expresses fears verbally and through play; interacts with caregivers appropriately; demonstrates positive age-appropriate coping behaviors.

Team Member Responsible	Assessment	Intervention	Rationale	Expected Outcome
Activities of Daily Living, Including Safety				
Nurse	Assess what self-care activities child is able to complete after right arm is casted.	Assist child as necessary with self-care.	Maltreated children may lack self-esteem; allowing them to do as much self-care as able can help improve self-esteem.	Child names tasks she thinks she can do herself; asks for appropriate help for others.
Teamwork and Collaboration				
Nurse/primary healthcare provider	Assess physical and history findings to establish suspicion of maltreatment.	Contact hospital child maltreatment team and alert them to suspicious findings.	Child healthcare providers have an obligation to report maltreatment to proper authorities.	Child maltreatment team meets with parents; documents or rules out maltreatment.
Procedures/Medications for Quality Improvement				
Nurse/nurse practitioner	Assess whether child has ever had a full physical examination and full-body photographs before.	Perform or assist with a complete physical exam and photographs to document child's injuries.	Physical examinations can refresh memories of maltreatment; photographs document extent and type of injuries.	Child cooperates with physical exam and photographer. Photographs are obtained.
Nutrition				
Nurse	Assess whether child is able to manage fork and spoon with cast in place.	Offer help with eating as necessary.	Eating is a self-care activity that can increase self-esteem.	Child demonstrates ability to eat satisfactorily with cast in place.
Patient-Centered Care				
Nurse/primary healthcare provider	Assess whether parent understands the seriousness of the diagnosis of child maltreatment and need for hospitalization.	Explain the reporting procedures and actions that accompany a child maltreatment report.	The parent's cooperation is essential for a successful outcome.	Mother states she will cooperate with procedures. Child understands she will remain in hospital overnight.

Continued on following page

BOX 55.5

Nursing Care Planning (continued)

Team Member Responsible	Assessment	Intervention	Rationale	Expected Outcome
Psychosocial/Spiritual/Emotional Needs				
Nurse	Assess which nurse would be the best primary nurse provider for the child.	Arrange for a primary nurse provider; assure child she is now in safe hands.	Removing the child from the threatening environment and providing a consistent caretaker can help reduce fear.	Child states she feels safe in the hospital; participates in therapeutic play.
Informatics for Seamless Healthcare Planning				
Nurse/child maltreatment team	Assess whether parent would like a referral to Parents Anonymous.	Make a referral as appropriate for support group for family. Explain why a restraining order may be issued to prevent one or both parents from visiting child.	Family needs continued follow-up and support because investigation of child maltreatment can be lengthy. Passive parent needs counseling as well as potential maltreating parent.	Parents are cooperative with maltreatment investigation; will attend at least one parents' group meeting.

partner. These are not easy decisions to make; if decision making of any kind were easy for this parent, the circumstances probably would never have reached the point at which child maltreatment occurred.

In some instances, a maltreated child will be removed temporarily from a home and only returned to the home after the person responsible for the maltreatment has been removed or after the stress that led to the maltreatment has been resolved. Such children need careful follow-up because an offending parent may return to the home while waiting trial and, if stress occurs again, revert to a maltreatment pattern.

If a child was injured seriously enough to be hospitalized and has had to be removed permanently from the parents' care, urge the foster family to visit before discharge to make the transition less frightening for the child. Children who are being removed from their parents in this way can feel an acute sense of loss and may grieve for the non-abusing parent or siblings very much. You may also find maltreated children grieving for an abusing parent, especially if they are convinced that they were the one responsible for the maltreatment or that the parent was not to blame.

Outcome evaluation for maltreated children must include not only whether they are physically safe but also whether they are developing emotional well-being. Children who are maltreated oftentimes suffer from post-traumatic stress disorder that can affect them throughout adulthood if not addressed earlier.

What If . . . 55.1

A nurse overhears Hillary keep repeating to her mother that she knows the fall was her own fault and her mother shouldn't be mad because everything will be all right. Is this a typical sign of maltreatment?

ABUSIVE HEAD TRAUMA

Abusive head trauma, previously known as shaken baby syndrome, is the repetitive, violent shaking of a small infant by the arms or shoulders, causing a whiplash injury to the neck, edema to the brainstem, possibly subdural hemorrhage, and distinctive hemorrhages to the retinas (Hitchcock, 2012). A controversial diagnosis, and one difficult to prove, it is a particularly insidious form of child maltreatment because the damage inflicted on the infant is not readily apparent. Increased use of computed tomography (CT) scans and magnetic resonance imaging is helping to detect children with these internal symptoms. Parents may bring a child for care because they have used a covert camcorder ("a Nanny cam") to reveal that a caregiver shook their baby this way.

RITUAL MALTREATMENT

Ritual maltreatment is cult-based or religiously, spiritually, or satanically motivated and typically involves physical, sexual, or psychological maltreatment with bizarre or ceremonial activities. With this type of maltreatment, multiple perpetrators may maltreat multiple victims over an extended period (Schwecke, 2011).

PHYSICAL NEGLECT

Physical neglect is a more subtle form of maltreatment than physical maltreatment, but it can be just as damaging to a child's welfare. A neglected child may appear unwashed, thin, and malnourished or be dressed inappropriately, such as without mittens, a coat, or shoes in cold weather. In some families, no one has a warm coat to wear or receives enough food because there is no money for these things; that is, different from the family in which parents do have these things, but the children or one particular child does not.

Failing to bring a child for medical attention or failing to seek early medical care for an infection are other signs of neglect. Not requiring a child to attend school, deliberately keeping a child out of school without setting up a home school program, or allowing a child to go unsupervised after school may also be interpreted as neglect. Such actions may be willful or they may occur if parents simply do not realize the developmental needs of a child. Use of electronic records allowing a child's total healthcare history to be examined has made identifying neglected children easier (Tonmyr, Jack, Brooks, et al., 2012). Many parents need anticipatory guidance from healthcare personnel to better understand their child's needs and developmentally appropriate parenting skills.

PSYCHOLOGICAL MALTREATMENT

Psychological maltreatment includes constant belittling or threatening, rejecting, isolating, or exploiting a child or is the absence of positive parenting. Children who are psychologically maltreated this way are likely to have difficulty becoming emotionally confident adults. This type of maltreatment is the most difficult form of maltreatment to detect because it may occur only in the home, and its effects, although severe, may be subtle. It can result, however, in the same type of inability to achieve that occurs in children who are physically maltreated.

Be sure to include enough growth and development questions during a health assessment to assess for it; observe the parent–child interaction to determine whether it is positive and healthy or negative and potentially unhealthy. Some indicators of emotional abuse include:

- Developmental delays
- Bed-wetting without medical cause
- Frequent psychosomatic complaints
- Severe depression
- Anxiety or aggression
- Self-destructive behaviors such as self-harming
- Overly compliant child

Children who are emotionally abused may model negative behaviors and language from their parent, which can be witnessed when they are playing with other children.

FACTITIOUS DISORDER

Factitious disorder, formally known as Munchausen syndrome by proxy, refers to a parent who repeatedly brings a child to a healthcare facility and reports symptoms of illness when, in fact, the child is well (Kucuker, Demir, & Oral, 2010). For example, a parent might report symptoms such as seizures, excessive sleepiness, or abdominal pain in a child. Because of these symptoms, the child is submitted to needless diagnostic procedures or therapeutic regimens. Another parent might go so far as to deliberately inflict injury on a child, such as giving a laxative to induce diarrhea or slowly poisoning the child with a prescription drug. Two classic findings of the syndrome are usually present: First, the symptoms are not easily detected by physical examination, only by history; and second, the symptoms are present only when the person initiating the symptoms is providing care (they disappear when care is provided by another person). The parent usually has some degree of medical or childcare knowledge obtained through formal education, reading, or Internet browsing. In the hospital, the parent tends to stay with the child constantly, offering to give the majority of care. This makes a difficult to detect form of maltreatment because wanting to stay and give care is also the hallmark of a very conscientious and caring parent.

To diagnose this disorder, covert video surveillance may be necessary. Because this syndrome reveals distorted perceptions on the part of the parent, it is almost always necessary to remove the child from the home to protect the child, even if the parent receives counseling.

QSEN Checkpoint Question 55.2

SAFETY

If Hillary had been maltreated as an infant, she might have experienced abusive head trauma (shaken baby syndrome). Which finding is common with this syndrome and would indicate a baby should be evaluated for medical and safety reasons?

   a. A baby is fearful of strangers.
   b. Retinal hemorrhages develop.
   c. A baby develops Crohn disease.
   d. A major bone has been broken.

Look in Appendix A for the best answer and rationale.

FAILURE TO THRIVE (REACTIVE ATTACHMENT DISORDER)

Failure to thrive is a unique syndrome in which an infant falls below the 5th percentile for weight and height on a standard growth chart or is falling in percentiles on a growth chart. The condition is usually divided into two categories: One where severe loss of weight can be explained because of organic causes, such as cardiac disease, and a second that occurs because of a disturbance in the parent–child relationship, resulting in maternal role insufficiency (a nonorganic cause). Sometimes, both forms combine to play a role in failure to thrive (Jaffe, 2011).

The nonorganic type is considered a form of child neglect, although this represents a very complex interplay between parent and child. In many instances, the parent feels little emotional attachment to the child and often has a history of frequent moves and little family support. The parent may not be offering enough food because of the lack of attachment, he or she is not aware of the hunger cues the infant is offering, or the parent does not have enough concern for the child to offer food regularly. A child may contribute to the poor parenting interaction by being an irritable, fussy, colicky, or "difficult" child. Some infants are offered sufficient food, but the emotional deprivation they sense makes them so lethargic they do not eat enough. In other instances, the child has a minimal neurologic dysfunction and thus does not respond in a way that is developmentally appropriate for the child's age. The mother may interpret this lethargic behavior as lack of response to her and thus does not interact or nurture the infant adequately.

Failure to thrive begins with subtle signs that need to be identified and taken seriously because the syndrome can lead to cognitive impairment in the child and even death if allowed to continue.

Assessment

Take a detailed pregnancy history of children at routine health assessments because in many instances, a breakdown in the development of parenting began in the prenatal period because of such factors as a pregnancy that was unintended or not accepted, a partner who left during the pregnancy, an economic catastrophe such as loss of a job, or a long-distance move that left support people behind.

Always weigh children at routine assessments and plot and compare their weight with standard growth curves so children who are failing to thrive can be identified at the earliest point possible. On physical examination, these infants usually demonstrate typical characteristics such as:

- Lethargy with poor muscle tone, a loss of subcutaneous fat, or skin breakdown (Fig. 55.5)
- Lack of resistance to the examiner's manipulation, unlike the response of the average infant
- Rocking on all fours excessively, as if seeking stimulation
- Possibly a greater reluctance to reach for toys or initiate human contact than is demonstrated by the average infant; diminished or nonexistent crying
- Staring hungrily at people who approach them as if they are starved for human contact
- Little cuddling or conforming to being held
- Delays in sitting, pulling to a standing position, crawling, and walking because the child spends so much time alone
- Markedly delayed or absent speech because of the lack of interaction

With advanced failure to thrive, the child's nutritional status may be so extremely poor that the infant is near acidosis from starvation. If an upper respiratory tract infection should develop, the child's resistance to infection may be so low that it could result in death from secondary infections such as pneumonia.

Figure 55.5 The child with failure to thrive experiences a loss of subcutaneous fat, muscle wasting, and skin breakdown. (From Zitelli, B. J., & Davis, H. W. [1997]. *Atlas of pediatric physical diagnosis* [3rd ed.]. St. Louis, MO: Mosby–Year Book, Inc.)

Therapeutic Management

With rare exceptions, children with failure to thrive need to be removed from the parents' care and hospitalized for evaluation and therapy. Otherwise, the syndrome may lead to permanent neurologic damage or leave a child cognitively challenged because of protein deficits and interference with brain metabolism. If an infant is admitted to a hospital, studies other than routine admission blood work and urinalysis are usually delayed to avoid submitting such an understimulated child to pain or unnecessary manipulation.

Infants are immediately placed on a diet appropriate for their ideal weight (the weight they would have been normally for their age). Rapid weight gain on this diet is diagnostic that their presenting illness was nonorganic failure to thrive.

Nursing Diagnoses and Related Interventions

Nursing Diagnosis: Imbalanced nutrition, less than body requirements, related to inadequate intake secondary to emotional deprivation

Outcome Evaluation: Child shows interest in bottle feedings; child is able to establish a regular eating pattern; child begins to gain weight.

Be certain the plan of care designed for the family of a child who is failing to thrive is realistic because parents cannot be made to form a bond with a child instantly, particularly if lack of bonding has gone on for some time. Don't give up hope, however, that this will happen. With the proper support and guidance over time, and when obstacles to bonding are removed, a healthy child–parent relationship could still develop.

Ensure Adequate Nutrition. Keep a careful record of intake and output so the number of calories being consumed every day can be effectively calculated. Assess stools for pH and reducing substances (glucose) to be certain the infant is absorbing nutrients. If a stool tests positive for glucose or has an acid pH (less than 7.0), it suggests that carbohydrates, the easiest food to absorb, are being processed.

Evaluate how well the infant sucks or is able to take food from a spoon and swallow to be certain these reflexes are intact. Record any symptoms, such as pulling up the legs or crying after eating, that suggest gastrointestinal discomfort.

Nurture the Child. Because infants with failure to thrive are suffering from emotional deprivation, they need effective nurturing from the nurses who care for them. This does not mean everyone who passes the crib should stop and play with the child for a few minutes; it means one member of the nursing team should be chosen to care for the child during the hospital stay (a primary nursing or case management pattern of assignment). It is important this nurse reserves time for providing active interactions with the child such as rocking and talking, giving a leisurely bath, offering toys, and "parenting" as passive rocking without talking to the child may be no different than the parents' care.

Support and Encourage the Parents. Encourage the parents of children with failure to thrive to visit as much as possible while the child is hospitalized or in foster care because without encouragement, these parents may visit little or not at all. When they do visit, encourage them to feed and interact with the infant. Parents cannot change their feelings about a child overnight, however, so telling them they ought to pick up the baby more or hold the infant while feeding may only increase the parents' feelings of inadequacy. Giving some suggestions about how the baby tries to communicate with them may be more effective; for example. "Do you know what I think he's trying to say when he stops sucking like that? I think he's saying he's ready to be burped." and "Look how he turns his head at the sound of your voice. He recognizes you."

Occasionally, parents are so distraught by such factors as the illness or death of an older child or relative they simply have become unaware of how much energy is being drained from them by these events. These parents quickly can become good parents to a deprived child as soon as they realize what has been happening. More often, however, the disturbance in a parent–child interaction began long before or is so great that a parenting bond cannot be established. If the infant is discharged from the hospital to the parents' care, the parents will need effective follow-up in the months to come to see that they maintain parenting skills that will keep the infant thriving and safe. There is a very thin line between the child who fails to thrive and one who is maltreated causing some of these children to be placed in foster homes for their own safety and to ensure that they receive adequate care.

Help Prevent Poor Parenting. Parents who may be at risk for lacking adequate parenting skills and support systems need to be identified during pregnancy, so they can receive counseling and close follow-up in the postnatal period. Some parents who are overwhelmed by the task of parenting may need respite care for their children and extended counseling to prevent future parenting breakdown.

What If . . . 55.2
A nurse weighs Hillary's baby cousin at a well-child visit and discovers that the infant's weight has fallen below the 2nd percentile on a standardized growth chart. What questions should the nurse ask the mother? What particular areas would the nurse assess on a physical examination?

Sexual Maltreatment

Sexual maltreatment is broadly defined as any sexual contact between a child and an adult (Neutze, Grundmann, Scherner, et al., 2012). Child sexual abuse is evident when the activity is intended to gratify or satisfy the needs of the other person. Such a scenario can include an adult or another child who is in a relationship of trust or power due to age. This type of relationships includes but is not limited to the coercion of a child to engage in any unlawful sexual activity or the exploitation of a child in prostitution or pornographic performances and materials (Legano, McHugh, & Palusci, 2009). It involves the coercion of dependent, developmentally immature children or adolescents in sexual activities that they do not fully comprehend, to which they are unable to give informed consent, or that violate the social taboos of society.

Sexual abuse is a problem of epidemic proportions with 25% of girls and 16% of boys in the United States sexually abused before the age of 18 years (Hornor, 2011). Adolescents have a higher rate of rape or sexual maltreatment than any other age group (8% to 10%) (Delacroix, Brown, Kadenhe-Chiweshe, et al., 2011). It's important to remember that boys, as well as girls, can be sexually maltreated. Although their abusers may be seemingly trustworthy coaches or teachers, they also may be people inside the family such as an older sibling, a parent, or a stepparent (Carlson, 2011). Abusers may contact children online through chat rooms, making the monitoring of websites an important preventive measure for parents (Briggs, Simon, & Simonsen, 2011). Health professionals who care for children with cognitive disabilities must be especially watchful to protect these vulnerable children from sexual maltreatment (Koetting, Fitzpatrick, Lewin, et al., 2012).

Sexual maltreatment is physically and emotionally destructive because it leaves children unable to trust others and may result in a sense of ambivalence toward intimacy and an overall sense of worthlessness. Remind parents to teach children by preschool age that their bodies are their own and to report anyone who tries to touch them in their private parts (Fig. 55.6). Children who have been sexually maltreated may be identified because they have a sexual vocabulary beyond that expected of a child their age. On physical exam, girls will have tears or inflammation of the vagina or perineum; both sexes may have rectal tears or symptoms of a sexually transmitted disease. Nurses need to keep in mind that less than 5% of children who are sexually abused will have a physical finding upon examination. This is due to the noninvasive forms of abuse, the elasticity of the hymen and other ano-genital structures, and the rapid healing of ano-genital injuries without residual injury (Hornor, 2011).

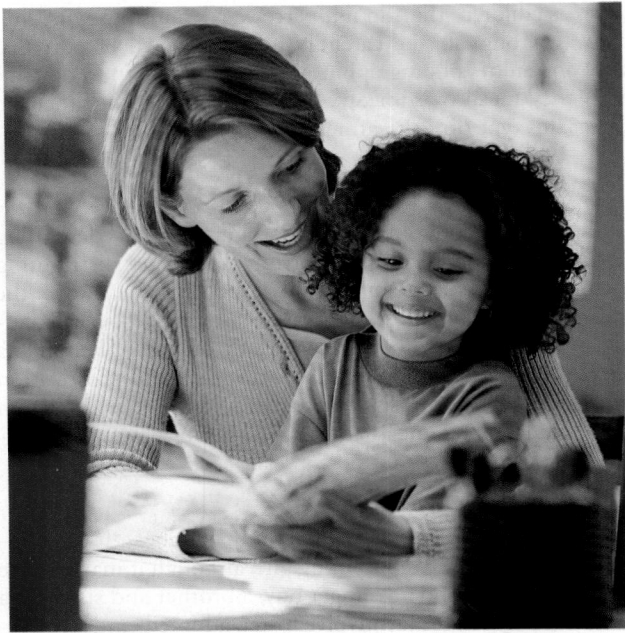

Figure 55.6 Teach children their bodies are their own and they have to give permission before anyone can touch them.

Megan's Law is a federal law that requires law enforcement authorities to report to neighbors when a sexual abuser moves into a neighborhood. Parents need to be aware of this law and insist that it should be enforced so they can take appropriate precautions to protect their children's safety (Neutze et al., 2012). Sexual predators are also listed on websites and thus can be tracked by parents. Additional laws parents need to be aware of to keep their children safe are child pornography laws. In some states, for example, "sexting" (texting sexually explicit photos) to friends may violate such laws—even though a minor is doing the texting. Their child could forever be classified as a sexual abuser and listed under Megan's Law (Wastler, 2010).

TYPES OF SEXUAL MALTREATMENT

Sexual maltreatment involves a wide range of diagnoses from molestation to vaginal penetration.

Molestation

Molestation is a vague term that includes "indecent liberties" such as oral–genital contact, genital fondling and viewing, or masturbation. A **pedophile** is an adult who seeks out prepubescent children (Tanner stage 0 to 1, usually younger than 12 years of age) for sexual gratification, whereas a **hebephile** seeks out pubescent children (Tanner stage 1 to 4, usually age 11 to 15 years) (Neutze et al., 2012). In contrast to a rapist, whose crime is violent, both pedophiles and hebephiles may be very gentle and limit the involvement to molestation. Such persons are usually male, but sometimes female; they may have suffered sexual maltreatment as a child and thus repeatedly select children or young adolescents who are of the same age at which the maltreatment occurred. The relationship may involve people with either homosexual or heterosexual orientations. Many pedophiles or hebephiles take photos or videos of their activities with children to use for sexual gratification at a later date.

Rehabilitation of pedophiles/hebephiles is difficult because they are fixated emotionally at a childhood level (seeing themselves as children, they do not perceive relationships with children as wrong). Listen carefully to children who report that someone enjoys photographing them; ask children to describe what they mean by someone "touching" or "feeling" them to detect this type of maltreatment.

Pornography and Prostitution

Child pornography involves photographing or describing sexual acts by any medium involving children or distributing such material in person or by mail, fax, cell phone, or over the Internet. Child prostitution involves arranging or participating in sexual acts with children. Both of these phenomena are demeaning to children and are illegal. Child prostitution carries the additional risks of sexually transmitted infection and violence, the same as adult prostitution.

Incest

Incest is sexual activity between family members. It often involves an older man and a young girl, although it may involve an older woman and a younger boy, a brother and sister, or a same-sex partner. It may involve foster, adopted, and stepchildren. Incest is a deviation from the norm and is so strongly viewed as such by most people that incest taboos are common

to most cultures (Carlson, 2011). Incest results in a destructive relationship because it causes a great deal of guilt and loss of self-esteem in both the abusing and the maltreated person. The abuser is aware that this act is not culturally approved but still is unable to end the relationship; the victim recognizes this act as wrong but is unable to resist the advances. Other members of the family are likely to suspect the maltreatment is occurring but are helpless to do anything about it; this leads to guilt and feelings of worthlessness on their part for not being able to protect the victim.

Children do not typically report incest because they have been told by the abuser to keep the activity a secret. In some cases, it is first revealed on a routine health examination by either history or physical findings of vaginal or rectal lesions.

QSEN Checkpoint Question 55.3

EVIDENCE-BASED PRACTICE

It is difficult to know the true incidence of sexual maltreatment in adolescents because it is suspected that many adolescents never report the abusive incident. To investigate whether adolescents who are sexually maltreated confide in their parents, researchers interviewed 800 male and female adolescents ages 13 to 16 years to identify if they had been the victim of sexual maltreatment. One hundred and seventy-seven adolescents in the study revealed they had been sexually maltreated. Of that number, 81% of the participants disclosed the maltreatment to a friend and 70% disclosed to a friend within a month of the incident. Sixty-three percent disclosed to more than one person (Lam, 2014).

Mrs. Landstrum's adolescent sister, Andrea, is examined in the emergency room because she has pain and a vaginal discharge. Based on the previous study, the nurse determines which person (aside from Andrea herself) as most likely to be the most reliable reporter as to whether Andrea has been sexually maltreated?

  a. Andrea's mother, because Andrea says she respects her
  b. Megan, a soccer teammate and close friend of Andrea
  c. Andrea's father, because he is the patriarch of the family
  d. Andrea's soccer coach, because she sees Andrea daily

Look in Appendix A for the best answer and rationale.

ASSESSMENT

Signs of sexual maltreatment are shown in Box 55.6. In addition to physical signs, a suspicion of sexual maltreatment may first be revealed by a young girl worrying she is pregnant or a child's abnormal anxiety about a parent returning home from a hospital stay or being left with or cared for by a particular individual in the family (Box 55.7). Young children who are the victims of this type of relationship typically have extremely low self-esteem and may believe they are so inadequate they deserve to be treated this way.

Allowing young children to play with anatomically correct dolls is a common method for determining whether sexual

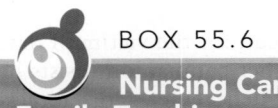

BOX 55.6

Nursing Care Planning Based on Family Teaching

IDENTIFYING SIGNS OF SEXUAL MALTREATMENT

Q. Hillary's mother asks you, "What signs should I look for if I suspect my daughter is being sexually maltreated?"

A. Here are some general indications that a child is being sexually maltreated:

- The child reports she has had sexual activity with an adult.
- The child demonstrates an awareness of sex or a sexual vocabulary beyond her age expectations.
- The child participates in sexual expression with dolls.
- A girl younger than 15 years of age is pregnant.
- A perineal, vaginal, or anal exam reveals inflammation or vaginal tears or anal fissures.
- A child younger than 15 years of age has a sexually transmitted infection.
- A child has a history of symptoms of increased anxiety such as a sleep disturbance, development of nervous tics, nail biting, or stuttering.
- There is a change in school performance, school phobia, or truancy.
- The child voices a fear of being left alone with a certain adult.
- A child reports vague abdominal pain or demonstrates acting-out behavior.

BOX 55.7

Nursing Care Planning Tips for Effective Communication

You notice during history taking that Hillary uses several swear words to describe where she hurts.

Tip: Help parents identify signs of potential child maltreatment. Remain nonjudgmental and encourage parents to ask questions or to discuss any concerns they may have.

Nurse: Mrs. Lindstrum, your daughter seems to know some words that are unusual for a 3-year-old.

Mrs. Lindstrum: She gets that from watching cartoons on TV.

Nurse: Cartoon characters don't usually say the words she uses.

Mrs. Lindstrum: We're proud she's advanced for her age.

Nurse: Using words with sexual connotations doesn't necessarily mean her vocabulary is advanced. It means she most likely keeps company with an adult who speaks that way.

Mrs. Lindstrum: That's probably her uncle. He babysits once a week.

Nurse: Does she mind staying with him?

Mrs. Lindstrum: Does it matter? A free babysitter doesn't happen every day.

Nurse: Let's talk some more about her vocabulary, especially in light of her infection.

maltreatment is occurring (Hlavka, Olinger, & Lashley, 2010). The average reaction of a preschooler or young school-age child who has not been maltreated, for example, is to undress the dolls, giggle for a moment or two about how they look, and then redress or put them aside. The child who is involved in an incestuous relationship may make the dolls perform a sexual act, such as placing the male doll's penis into the female doll's mouth. The use of such dolls is controversial because there is a concern that without a common protocol for their use, the child's actions could be misinterpreted. Asking the child to draw a picture of what happened may also be an effective way of revealing sexual maltreatment.

THERAPEUTIC MANAGEMENT

Sexual maltreatment, like physical maltreatment, must be reported because this is a criminal offense. It's important, as with all child maltreatment, that information about the maltreatment is collected objectively so the adult's rights are respected and the testimony is therefore admissible in court.

Both the adult and the child involved in a sexual maltreatment relationship need psychological counseling—the child to improve self-esteem and the adult to channel sexual expression to less destructive outlets. To improve the child's self-esteem, the adult in the relationship needs to admit the fault was the adult's, not the child's. Follow-up care is best done by one of the providers who sees the child initially, so that the child does not have to recount the incident to strangers again and again. Treatment for sexually transmitted infections or protection against pregnancy should be provided as needed.

Parents may need as much counseling as the child when their child has been sexually maltreated, so they can help the child work through feelings about the situation. In many instances, because the offender is a family member or a trusted outsider and the relationship has been occurring for some time before it is reported, parents may feel guilty they allowed the family member to have access to the child or did not listen to a child's protestations that being alone with this family member was uncomfortable for the child. If incest involves a parent or marriage or relationship partner, it may be extremely difficult for parents or partners to continue to relate to each other effectively enough to help the child. Review with parents and encourage parents to teach children simple rules to help children avoid sexual maltreatment (see Chapter 32, Box 32.4).

QSEN Checkpoint Question 55.4

QUALITY IMPROVEMENT

A member of the child maltreatment team offers Hillary anatomically correct male and female dolls for her to play with. When Hillary begins playing, she places the male doll's penis in the female doll's mouth. How should the nurse best respond?

    a. "Do you think it's wrong that the dolls do that?"
    b. "I bet you're playing a game you've seen on TV."
    c. "Are the dolls playing a game? Tell me about it."
    d. "Okay, can you please put the dolls down now?"

Look in Appendix A for the best answer and rationale.

Rape

Rape is sexual activity such as intercourse or penetration of a body orifice by a penis or other object under actual or threatened force. *Statutory rape* is sexual activity with a person under the age of consent (in most states, younger than 18 years of age) and is considered to have occurred regardless of the apparent willingness of the underage person. *Sexual assault* is typically used to refer to other forced sexual acts, such as oral–genital or anal–genital acts (Hornor, 2011).

Rape is a crime of violence, not of passion, and includes "date rape," a situation in which an individual forces a date or casual friend into having coitus despite a voiced unwillingness or inability to consent (D. L. Lang, Sales, Salazer, et al., 2011). The increasing misuse of flunitrazepam (Rohypnol), a drug easily dissolved in a drink, has led to an increase in the incidence of date rape because it leaves a victim with little or no memory of the event (see Chapter 33). It may be very difficult for the victim of date rape to find a sympathetic ear if her companion insists he meant no harm; he simply didn't believe her. Urge adolescents to be aware of the danger of the drug and to say "no" convincingly (Makin-Byrd & Bierman, 2013).

Both rape and sexual assault represent deviant behavior. They lack privacy and mutual consent, which are the elements of "normal" or usual sexual behavior, and include violence, causing them to be degrading and dehumanizing and leaving the victim feeling helpless and victimized. Review with teenagers of both sexes ways to prevent rape at routine health visits (Box 55.8).

Determining the actual incidence of rape is difficult; it seems to be more prevalent than formerly but that may be because more people report it. Many adolescents want to avoid the secondary, but no less severe, trauma associated with reporting rape and therefore do not report it. This leaves them, unfortunately, without the immediate

---

BOX 55.8

Nursing Care Planning to Empower a Family

GUIDELINES FOR THE PREVENTION OF RAPE IN ADOLESCENTS

Q. Hillary's mother is concerned about the incidence of rape in her community. She asks you, "What should I teach my adolescent sister to help her avoid rape?"

A. A number of suggestions are:

Home

1. Do not advertise that you stay home alone while a parent works or is on vacation.
2. Do not allow anyone to your house when you are home alone, even meter readers or repairmen who produce identification.
3. Insist on adequate lighting for hallways in an apartment building or streetlights around your home.
4. Have your house key in your hand when you approach your door; do not stand fumbling for it by the doorway.
5. Keep your doors and windows locked when you are alone at home.

Car

1. Avoid isolated parking places; park near a building or in a lot with a parking attendant.
2. Lock your car when waiting in it and after parking it.
3. Look in the backseat before unlocking and entering your car to be sure no one is there.
4. Have your car key ready when you approach your car; do not stand fumbling for it.

Work or School

1. Do not enter an elevator with a stranger.
2. Lock the outside door and do not admit people you do not know when working alone in an office or classroom at night.
3. Ask for security protection to walk out to your car after hours.
4. When going to and from school or work after dark, walk in the street rather than next to shrubs or dark buildings.

Social Settings

1. Be clear with your date that when you say no, you mean no.
2. Limit alcohol use because it can lead to risk-taking behavior.
3. Make it clear you consider date rape the same as any rape and you will press charges.
4. Flunitrazepam (Rohypnol) is a sedative, known as a "date rape" drug. Do not date any individual who brags that he knows how to obtain it or use it.

Personal Actions

1. Do not wear chains around your neck that could be used to strangle you.
2. Learn self-defense; scratch the attacker to obtain skin and blood specimens under fingernails.
3. Be aware that an attacker could take any weapon you hold away and use it on you; use caution carrying a weapon or mace.
4. If an attack occurs, observe the attacker's appearance as carefully as possible. Note identifying characteristics, such as a birthmark, scar, tattoo, words, or manner of speech, to be able to identify the individual later.
5. Press charges in court to make rape a crime of extreme magnitude and as an opportunity to fight back.
6. Work to provide rape prevention information and a united front against rape in your community.

treatment and follow-up care that are so important to a complete recovery.

Although victims can be of any age and either male or female, the average rape victim is an adolescent girl. The rapist may be a relative or family friend, and rapists frequently commit the act in the neighborhood where they live. Up to 75% of girls know their attacker. Based on arrest data, the average rapist is a late adolescent man with a background of aggressive behavior. His motivation usually relates to expressions of power or anger; sexual satisfaction does not appear to be a dominant motive. An excessive amount of alcohol intake often precedes rape (Thompson, McGee, & Mays, 2012). Rape tends to be a repetitive, planned activity on the part of the attacker rather than an isolated event.

ASSESSMENT

Many rape victims demonstrate immediate physical and emotional symptoms that can last for weeks. These symptoms constitute what has been termed **rape trauma syndrome**, a form of posttraumatic stress syndrome, and they usually occur in two stages: disorganization and reorganization. In the immediate *disorganization phase*, victims feel a combination of humiliation, shame and guilt, embarrassment, anger, and vengefulness. They feel that their lives have been completely disrupted by the crisis because they were unable to protect themselves from the assault. They may tremble from fear or be in great pain from perineal lacerations and are apt to startle visibly at the sound of anyone approaching or touching them. They need gentle, sympathetic support in the days after the event to allow them to feel safe. They may have nightmares of the attack occurring again. This immediate stage of disruption and disorganization usually lasts about 3 days.

The second stage of rape trauma syndrome, termed the *reorganization phase*, may last for months or years. Many rape victims report recurring nightmares, perhaps sexual dysfunction, and continuing inability to relate to the opposite sex or to face new and surprising situations. They may continue to have a great deal of difficulty discussing the rape. Many rape victims, trying to escape, change their residence at great sacrifice to finances and lifestyle. If not offered constructive counseling, victims may still feel guilt or shame when thinking about the rape as long as 20 to 30 years later.

EMERGENCY CARE

Although most large-city police forces have special officers assigned to investigate rape charges, victims can be confused and further traumatized by police officers who imply they provoked the attack because of their manner of dress or could have done more to resist or prevent the event. This increases a victim's feelings of shame and degradation. It may be especially harmful to adolescents because people they have been taught to respect have no concept of the degree of fright they have experienced or the strength of their attacker. Healthcare providers usually are the second group of people victims see after an attack. It is vital that healthcare providers are extremely cautious to not show this same type of callous behavior.

Most healthcare agencies where many rape victims are seen have a rape trauma team, including specially educated counselors to talk to victims immediately after a rape and to offer long-term counseling as needed. Nurses serve as important members of such teams and may provide primary care after a rape. Any nurse should be able to offer emergency support because it might be a long time before a specifically designated staff member arrives, and such services are not available in every community.

Because rape is a crime, the electronic record of a rape victim is often displayed as part of a court procedure. For the victim to bring charges against the attacker, information concerning the victim's appearance and history needs to be detailed in the record. For that reason, a sexual assault nurse examiner (SANE nurse) should be called if available. Pediatric nurses trained as sexual assault examiners are called P-SANE nurses and are a crucial part of properly examining a child assault victim. Make sure to involve child advocacy centers (CACs) if available in your area to consult with and examine child maltreatment and child sexual assault victims. If available, *stop* after the initial basic exam and call the CAC team so they can properly interview and examine the victim, observing local laws and evidence requirements.

Table 55.1 summarizes common tests and procedures for emergency care of rape victims. If no CAC team is available, be certain statements you make in a record are accurate and unbiased. Quote the victim's exact words whenever possible. Describe the victim's physical appearance in unbiased detail, including the presence and location of injuries, such as bruises, lacerations, teeth marks, or abrasions, and the condition of clothing. Be certain to ask whether the victim bathed or washed before coming for care because this can obscure evidence and obliterate the presence of sperm or DNA material. Ask whether the woman was menstruating or using a tampon as the force of penis penetration with rape can cause a tampon to tear through the posterior vaginal wall into the abdominal cavity, causing an extreme loss of blood internally.

After preliminary observations, a gynecologic or anal examination will be done to evaluate the physical condition of the victim and to document that rape occurred by the presence of any vaginal or perineal lacerations or sperm or DNA left behind by the assailant on the perineum or in the vagina or rectum. Acid phosphate, a component of prostatic fluid, is a substance that is not normally present in vaginal or rectal secretions but is present in semen. Determining the presence of acid phosphate can be extremely important, therefore, if the attacker is infertile or sterile, making DNA analysis difficult. Its presence may be the best evidence that rape occurred. Vaginal and anal cultures are taken for gonorrhea, and a Pap test is also performed. Blood is drawn for a pregnancy test and a Venereal Disease Research Laboratory (VDRL) test for syphilis if appropriate. Prophylactic administration of antibiotics against gonorrhea and syphilis may be necessary. If the woman is not menstruating, she may be given "morning after" therapy to avoid pregnancy. The victim may have a baseline blood sample drawn to diagnose HIV and hepatitis B status.

Be certain during emergency care to provide privacy. Many people may want to ask the victim questions, including police officers or detectives, the victim's family, a rape trauma team, and an examining primary healthcare provider. Describing the experience is good, but lack of privacy during a perineal examination demonstrates little concern for the victim's self-esteem. Many female victims are uncomfortable with a male

TABLE 55.1 COMMON SPECIMEN PROCEDURES AFTER RAPE

Procedure	Purpose
Oral washing	Help patient rinse mouth with 5 ml sterile water, which is then collected in test tube, analyzed for blood group antigens, or sperm or DNA of attacker.
Fingernail scraping	Scrape under all of patient's fingernails so scrapings can be analyzed for blood, skin, DNA, and clothing fibers of attacker.
Blood Venereal Disease Research Laboratory (VDRL), HIV, and hepatitis B surface antigen (HBsAg)	Draw blood for antibody titer for syphilis, HIV, and hepatitis B and typing to differentiate it from attacker's type.
Pregnancy test	Obtain blood for analysis; complete vaginal examination before woman voids.
Hair samples	Remove both scalp and pubic hairs of patient (about 10) to be compared with attacker's.
Vaginal smear for sperm and DNA	Swab vagina with a dry applicator and smear onto slide so sperm and DNA analysis can be performed.
Gonococcus smear	Culture the patient's cervix, vagina, and rectum (also throat if oral coitus was attempted).
Vaginal washing	Place 5 ml of sterile saline into patient's vagina and aspirate again to detect sperm, DNA, and acid phosphate.
Skin washings	Touch any dried stains of blood or semen on the patient's skin or clothing with a moistened cotton swab to be analyzed for attacker's blood, semen, or DNA.
Clothing	Save any clothing stained or torn as evidence of violent attack.

Label all specimens carefully, indicating where they were obtained, to aid medical therapy and provide legal evidence.

examiner after rape because they are temporarily fearful of men. Having a female nurse remain with the victim during this time may be helpful. A male nurse can be equally supportive, however, because it is not the male–female contrast that a victim is seeking so much as a contrast between aggression and caring.

What If . . . 55.3

Hillary's physical examination reveals she has purulent vulvovaginitis, and a culture reveals this is caused by gonorrhea. What questions should the nurse ask Hillary to determine how she contracted the infection? Would the fact that Hillary's mother is influential in the city influence what questions the nurse asks?

LEGAL CONSIDERATIONS

Nurses working in emergency departments may be asked to testify in court about a rape victim's appearance after the assault, although the documentation in the record is usually all that is necessary. Many victims, especially adolescents, do not press charges against their assailants because they were too frightened or unable at the time to observe the assailant's appearance and therefore cannot identify him later. They may fear that if they name him in court, he will return and kill them. Whether victims follow through with a legal action or not is their choice, but the incidence of rape might be reduced if rapists were aware they are not apt to escape without a penalty for their crime. For that reason, some states have prosecutors press charges even if the victim declines, as with domestic violence charges. Taking the rapist to court may be an opportunity and appropriate time for victims to "fight back" and therefore not be as helpless as they were forced to be during the attack.

QSEN Checkpoint Question 55.5

INFORMATICS

Hillary's mother reveals that she was raped when she was a teenager. What is the most important question to ask before beginning a physical assessment for an adolescent who has been raped?

a. "Have you bathed or showered since the attack?"
b. "Did the rape feel more sexual or more violent?"
c. "Was anything stolen from you during the attack?"
d. "Can you think of a way you could have prevented this?"

Look in Appendix A for the best answer and rationale.

Nursing Diagnoses and Related Interventions

Nursing Diagnosis: Anxiety related to recent rape

Outcome Evaluation: Victim is able to discuss what happened and voice intense feelings about the crime; victim states ability to move forward with life.

One of the major needs of any victim after a violent act is to talk about what happened because a person who can describe an incident can also begin to "put a fence around" the event or bring the event down from "something terrible has happened," a situation that leaves the person with a continuing high anxiety level, to "this specific thing has happened," a situation that allows the traumatic event to be examined and managed (something that is concrete and describable is rarely as frightening as "something out there").

Ask the victim to describe the incident to you with an introduction such as "Most people find it helps to talk about what happened to them." Be certain victims have a support person to accompany them home. Be sure they know that, if their distress becomes acute, they can return as needed to the healthcare facility for additional care or counseling. Be certain as well that they have the telephone number of a counseling service.

Because genital bruising may not be apparent until 24 hours after the rape, victims may be asked to return for a re-examination the next day so this can be documented. Syphilis will not be apparent for up to 6 weeks in serum, so they should return for a repeat VDRL at that time. They may be advised to return in 6 weeks and again in 6 months for HIV testing.

Nursing Diagnosis: Disabled family coping related to recent rape of family member

Outcome Evaluation: Partner or other family members express feelings about the rape to healthcare provider; family members state confidence in ability to support rape victim.

In many instances, the victim's usual sexual partner has difficulty being a support person after a rape because this person has as much difficulty dealing with the rape as the victim. Not infrequently, a relationship that was meaningful before the rape deteriorates because the partner mistakenly believes the victim was somehow responsible for the trauma or actually enjoyed the experience. In other instances, the partner may become so overprotective (not allowing the victim to go out alone; checking on her constantly) that she is not free to maintain her identity. Parents of a young adolescent may feel the same way. Counseling for the victim's partner or family may be necessary to help them to be truly supportive (Box 55.9).

Intimate Partner Violence

Intimate partner violence is maltreatment by a family member against another adult living in the household, such as a spouse or significant other. Spouse or partner maltreatment and child maltreatment may both exist in a family. It is vital for nurses to provide family-centered care to help identify and intervene with these situations. As many as 20% to 30% of women seen in emergency departments are there because they have been maltreated by their intimate partner. Common injuries suffered include burns, lacerations, bruises, and head injuries. Asking all women at physical examinations to account for any bruise they have helps detect physical maltreatment. Asking them whether they are ever concerned about their safety or well-being during well visits helps detect and prevent this type of maltreatment.

Like child maltreatment, intimate partner violence affects all ethnic and social groups. If it appears to be more prevalent in lower socioeconomic neighborhoods, it is because these families are more visible to service organizations and law enforcement officials. When it occurs in middle or upper class houses, wives are often too embarrassed to let people know and tend to keep the violence hidden longer.

> **BOX 55.9**
> ### Goals of Crisis Intervention for Families of Rape Victims
>
> - Help the family be supportive of and reassuring to the victim to help initiate problem-solving techniques.
> - Explain the possibility of future psychological and somatic symptoms that characterize a rape trauma syndrome and what the family can do to minimize these symptoms.
> - Eliminate the family's sense of guilt for not protecting the victim by assuring them they could not have anticipated or prevented the rape.
> - Educate the family about rape as a *violent crime*, not a sexually motivated act, to eliminate a focus on the victim's guilt or responsibility.
> - Discourage violent, destructive, or irrational retribution toward the rapist (under the guise of being on the victim's behalf) by encouraging sharing of feelings of helplessness, sadness, hurt, and anger.
> - Encourage discussion of the sexual relationship between partners; suggest that the victim's partner let her know (a) that his or her feelings have not changed (if this is true) and that she is still sexually desirable, (b) that the partner will wait for her to approach, and (c) that sex therapy is available if they have persistent difficulties and want assistance in reestablishing usual sexual relations.
> - Explain the possibility of sexually transmitted disease and pregnancy that may result from a rape, the preventive care necessary for the victim and spouse or sexual partner, and the follow-up care indicated.
> - Refer the family for counseling if members' shared responses to the crisis interfere with their ability to cope adaptively.
> - Identify how the family has handled crises in the past and encourage members to use adaptive coping mechanisms for this crisis. Encourage contact with persons identified as supportive to the family and offer to contact such persons.

It occurs at a higher rate during pregnancy than other times, so including questions about this in pregnancy health histories is especially important (Hellmuth, Gordon, Stuart, et al., 2013). The rate of intimate partner violence is so high during pregnancy that homicide from intimate partner violence is the number one cause of death in pregnant women, a finding that probably occurs because stress (from pregnancy) can be a trigger to violence.

Maltreated women may have an unintended and unwanted pregnancy because they were unable to fight off sexual advances from their abusive partner. Other women may desire the pregnancy because they believe having a child will change the partner and make him a better person or having an infant will offer her someone who loves her.

The reason why intimate partner violence occurs is perplexing, but violent family situations can be divided into two groups: those in which violence preceded the relationship or children and those in which the violence developed after the relationship was established or children were born.

In the first situation, which is more common, violence is usually brought into the family by a man with a history of violence (although women may also be offenders). His violence-prone characteristics usually erupt early in the courtship and grow progressively worse as he uses violence to handle even small conflicts, which instills a pervasive feeling of powerlessness in the people around him. Such men usually have a history of early and prolonged exposure to family violence as children; alcohol is frequently associated with the expression of violence (Gómez, 2011).

A cycle of violence often follows three phases: tension-building, acute violence, and a "honeymoon" or tranquil, loving phase. During the first phase, the offender displays actions such as anger, arguing, and blaming the victim for external problems or for provoking the violence. The acute violence phase can be triggered by a response from the intimate partner or by an external crisis and can result in extreme physical harm to the victim. The tranquil, loving phase, characterized by kind and contrite behavior, follows the violence, lulling the victim into forgiveness and a wish to continue the relationship. Without intervention, however, this phase ends at some point, and the cycle of violence repeats (Kuijpers, van der Knaap, & Winkel, 2012).

Partners react to the situation in three phases (Table 55.2). During the impact phase (stage I), or the light level of violence, the victim uses denial as a defense mechanism. By not stopping or facing what is happening, however, she is indirectly giving the offender permission to continue. During the second stage, the victim can no longer deny the violence is occurring. At the same time, she cannot stop it because she does not provoke the violence; she is only a convenient recipient of poorly controlled extreme behavior. She is forced to use coping mechanisms such as becoming very obedient and cooperative and doing everything her partner asks in a desperate effort to reduce the violence. The woman is forced to become isolated; she sinks into hopelessness and depression. This phase is often referred to as psychological infantilism or **learned helplessness**. To stop the cycle from repeating after a period of calm, she needs healthcare personnel to recognize her circumstances and offer her help.

Although it is impossible to predict how any individual woman will respond, pregnant maltreated women may demonstrate typical behaviors that reveal violence. A woman may come for care late in pregnancy or not at all, for example, because her partner controls her transportation or money; she may have been pretending the pregnancy did not exist to reduce stress in her home. She may be noticeable in a prenatal setting because she has purchased no maternity clothing (she has no funds for herself and asking for money may incite violence). For the same reason, she may decline laboratory tests if they involve additional transportation or money.

A maltreated woman may have difficulty following recommended pregnancy nutrition (she must cook what her partner wants or she will be beaten). She may grow anxious if her appointment is running late (she must be home to cook dinner or risk a beating). She may call and cancel appointments frequently (or simply not keep appointments) because she has an obvious black eye or a bleeding facial laceration she does not want to reveal. She may dress inappropriately for warm weather, wearing long-sleeved, tight-necked blouses to cover up bruises on her neck or arms. When undressed for a physical examination, there may be bruises or lacerations on her breasts, abdomen, or back she cannot explain. Her neck may reveal linear bruises from strangulation. Give thoughtful consideration as to whether the explanation the woman gives for a bruise or laceration correlates with the extent and placement of the injury.

A woman who has experienced recent violence may be anxious to listen to the baby's heartbeat or have fundal height measured at prenatal visits because she is worried the fetus may have been hurt. If abdominal trauma is present, an ultrasound may be prescribed to further assess fetal health. If an ultrasound reveals minimal placental infarcts from blunt abdominal trauma, this can lead to poor placental perfusion, low birth weight, or pregnancy loss.

QSEN Checkpoint Question 55.6

PATIENT-CENTERED CARE

Through history taking, the nurse discovers that Hillary's mother is a victim of intimate partner violence. When addressing this issue, what typical characteristic of an intimate partner who is violent toward a female partner should the nurse be aware of?

   a. A man has been raised in a family where the father was violent.
   b. A man wants to earn more money but has no education.
   c. A man is under severe psychological stress.
   d. A man has more than three children younger than 10 years old.

Look in Appendix A for the best answer and rationale.

Nursing Diagnoses and Related Interventions

Nursing diagnoses for a woman who has experienced intimate partner violence may pertain to physical injuries sustained, but they should also address the emotional manifestations of violence. Some examples include:

- Powerlessness related to perception that it is impossible to break away from abusing partner
- Fear related to constant threat of violence
- Social isolation related to patient's need to hide evidence of intimate partner violence
- Ineffective denial related to inability to face the fact that partner is sexually violent
- Compromised family coping related to dysfunctional relationship between patient and abusive partner

TABLE 55.2 TYPICAL LEVELS OF INTIMATE PARTNER VIOLENCE

Level	Description
I	Maltreatment is occasional; consists of slapping, punching, kicking, verbal maltreatment. Contusions occur.
II	Maltreatment is becoming more frequent; beatings are sustained and cause fractures, such as a broken jaw or rib fracture.
III	Maltreatment is even more frequent, perhaps daily. A weapon, such as a gun, baseball bat, or broom handle, may be used. Permanent disability or death from injuries, such as intracranial hemorrhage or concussion, may occur.

Expected outcomes should address specific tasks a woman could accomplish to keep herself safe from further intimate partner violence, such as:

- Patient carries with her telephone numbers of emergency services and a shelter for women who have experienced intimate partner violence.
- Patient and abusive partner continue to attend counseling sessions.
- Patient states she has filed a restraining order against abusive partner.
- Patient states she feels secure living at a safe house.

It may be difficult to understand why a woman elects to stay in a violent intimate partner relationship. A common finding is that a woman is unable to leave because the guilt and low self-esteem she feels have led her to believe she deserves to be treated this way or because of fear the abusive person will find her and kill her. To free herself from this emotional paralysis, she needs outside help. Unfortunately, she doesn't seek this because her low self-esteem and depression lead her to believe that no one would be interested in helping her.

Until she can develop better self-esteem, a woman may need support to make even simple decisions. Any ability she has to make constructive decisions should be supported and reinforced. Be familiar with shelters for women who have experienced intimate partner violence in your community; discuss with her how she can call the police at any time and they will take her to the shelter. Help her to file charges or obtain a restraining order to keep the abusive person from coming near her again if this is necessary.

Be careful not to blame the victim or leave a woman who has found the courage to leave her abuser without a support system because without effective support, she may decide that self-injury or returning to the intimate partner is her best recourse. If a woman does return to live with an abusive partner, both she and the infant need frequent healthcare visits scheduled so their health and welfare can be monitored. A child raised in a home where a member is violent will learn that this is acceptable conduct, and the violence may extend to yet another generation.

Children who have a parent who is violent may be identified because of behavior problems, noncompliance, and aggression in school. They may develop low levels of empathy or they may display distress behaviors such as clinging, crying, abdominal pain, or sleeping disorders. Effects may be long term if the violence causes teenage girls to shy away from relationships with boys, afraid they will be exposed to the same level of violence as their mother.

What If . . . 55.4

A nurse is interested in exploring one of the 2020 National Health Goals regarding violence toward or maltreatment of children and families (see Box 55.1). Most government-sponsored funding for nursing research is allotted based on these goals. What would be a possible research topic pertinent to these goals that would be applicable to Hillary's family and also advance evidence-based practice?

Recall Charlie Snow, a 6-year-old boy with a known hypersensitivity to dyes, perfumes, and peanuts, whom you first met in Chapter 42. Since living with his aunt and uncle while his parents are in the military, he has been treated for a skin reaction and is now hospitalized with an anaphylactic reaction from peanut ingestion. How would the nurse determine if Charlie is at risk for maltreatment or neglect? What measures can the nurse take to assure his safety at home?

Care for Charlie and other patients in a realistic virtual environment: *vSim for Nursing* (thepoint.lww.com /vSimMaternityPed). Practice documenting these patients' care in DocuCare (thepoint.lww.com /DocuCareEHR).

KEY POINTS FOR REVIEW

- Child maltreatment can exist in many forms. It may be physical, emotional, or sexual and may encompass neglect.
- A high suspicion for child maltreatment should be present if burns, head injury, or rib fractures are present or if the history of the accident seems out of proportion to the injury.
- Abusive head trauma, previously known as shaken baby syndrome, involves repetitive, violent shaking of a small infant by the arms or shoulders, causing a whiplash injury to the neck, edema to the brainstem, and distinct retinal hemorrhages.
- A triad of "special parent, special child, special circumstance" is characteristic of the family in which child maltreatment occurs.
- Failure to thrive is a syndrome in which an infant falls below the 5th percentile for weight and height on a standard growth chart. It may be associated with a disturbance in the parent–child relationship.
- Children who comfort parents in emergency settings may just be sensitive children or they may be demonstrating role reversal, a behavior characteristic of maltreated children.
- In families in which a child is maltreated, a parent may also be a victim of maltreatment. Ask about safety in the home at healthcare visits to be certain that this problem does not exist as well as help plan nursing care that not only meets Quality & Safety Education for Nurses (QSEN) competencies but also best meets the family's total needs.
- Child maltreatment is reportable by law. Nurses can initiate reporting as an independent action or through their health agency's referral network.
- Methods to prevent maltreatment in which nurses can actively participate include teaching about the expected growth and development of children, educating parents for parenting roles, and teaching empowerment or a sense that children and adults have control of their own lives.
- Sexual maltreatment of children can be prevented by teaching children to recognize abnormal advances and to empower the child to speak out if touched in private parts or forced to perform any inappropriate acts.

- Maltreatment is a family problem, not an individual problem. Therapy must include all family members to be effective.
- Rape is a crime of violence, not of sexual intent. Rape victims need both short- and long-term counseling.
- Pregnant women with traumatic injuries need to be carefully assessed to determine whether intimate partner violence was the cause of the trauma.

CRITICAL THINKING CARE STUDY

Nick is 6 years old; his brother Sam is 13 months old. Emergency medical technicians (EMTs) brought them into your emergency room by ambulance after a minor automobile accident involving their family car. They are alert, were in child booster seats with seat belts, and appear uninjured. However, when examined at the accident scene, the EMTs found bruises in various stages of healing on the children. Some were in expected areas, but others indicated potential child maltreatment.

1. Sites of "expected bruising" change with developmental level. How would they differ between Nick, a 6-year-old, and his 13-month-old brother?

2. When the boys' father arrives, you hear him tell the boys, "Don't say a word about the accident." Is this a clue the boys have been maltreated? If these two boys are being maltreated, would they have been so carefully protected by seat belts in the car?

3. Should you alert your agency's child protection team based on the stated findings that you suspect child abuse or wait until you talk to the mother to see if there is another side of this story?

RELATED RESOURCES

Explore these additional resources to enhance learning for this chapter:
- Student resources on thePoint, including answers to the What If . . . and Critical Thinking Care Study questions, http://thepoint.lww.com/Flagg8e
- Adaptive learning powered by PrepU, http://thepoint.lww.com/prepu

REFERENCES

Briggs, P., Simon, W. T., & Simonsen, S. (2011). An exploratory study of Internet-initiated sexual offenses and the chat room sex offender: Has the Internet enabled a new typology of sex offender? *Sexual Abuse, 23*(1), 72–91.

Carlson, B. E. (2011). Sibling incest: Adjustment in adult women survivors. *Families in Society, 92*(1), 77–83.

Delacroix, J., Brown, J., Kadenhe-Chiweshe, A., et al. (2011). Rectal perforation secondary to rape and fisting in a female adolescent. *Pediatric Emergency Care, 27*(2), 116–119.

Fang, X., Brown, D. S., Florence, C. S., et al. (2012). The economic burden of child maltreatment in the United States and implications for prevention. *Child Abuse & Neglect, 36*(2), 156–165.

Fortson, B. L., Klevens, J., Merrick, M. T., et al. (2016). *Preventing child abuse and neglect: A technical package for policy, norm, and programmatic activities.* Retrieved from https://www.cdc.gov/violenceprevention/pdf/CAN-Prevention-Technical-Package.pdf

Fraser, J., Mathews, B., Walsh, K. M., et al. (2010). Factors influencing child abuse and neglect recognition and reporting by nurses: A multivariate analysis. *International Journal of Nursing Studies, 47*(2), 146–153.

Freisthler, B. (2011). Alcohol use, drinking venue utilization, and child physical abuse: Results from a pilot study. *Journal of Family Violence, 26*(3), 185–193.

Friedman, M. S., Marshal, M. P., Guadamuz, T. E., et al. (2011). A meta-analysis of disparities in childhood sexual abuse, parental physical abuse, and peer victimization among sexual minority and sexual nonminority individuals. *American Journal of Public Health, 101*(8), 1481–1494.

Gómez, A. M. (2011). Testing the cycle of violence hypothesis: Child abuse and adolescent dating violence as predictors of intimate partner violence in young adulthood. *Youth & Society, 43*(1), 171–192.

Goodwin, M. B. (2011). Precarious moorings: Tying fetal drug law policy to social profiling. *Rutgers Law Journal, 42*(3), 659–694.

Heim, C., Shugart, M., Craighead, W. E., et al. (2010). Neurobiological and psychiatric consequences of child abuse and neglect. *Developmental Psychobiology, 52*(7), 671–690.

Helfer, R. E., & Kempe, R. S. (Eds.). (1987). *The battered child* (4th ed.). Chicago, IL: University of Chicago Press.

Hellmuth, J. C., Gordon, K. C., Stuart, G. L., et al. (2013). Risk factors for intimate partner violence during pregnancy and postpartum. *Archives of Women's Mental Health, 16*(1), 19–27.

Hitchcock, J. (2012). The debate over shaken baby syndrome. *Journal of Neonatal Nursing, 18*(1), 20–21.

Hlavka, H. R., Olinger, S. D., & Lashley, J. L. (2010). The use of anatomical dolls as a demonstration aid in child sexual abuse interviews: A study of forensic interviewers' perceptions. *Journal of Child Sexual Abuse, 19*(5), 519–553.

Hornor, G. (2010). Child sexual abuse: Consequences and implications. *Journal of Pediatric Health Care, 24*(6), 358–364.

Hornor, G. (2011). Medical evaluation for child sexual abuse: What the PNP needs to know. *Journal of Pediatric Health Care, 25*(4), 250–256.

Jaffe, A. C. (2011). Failure to thrive: Current clinical concepts. *Pediatrics in Review, 32*(3), 100–107.

Koetting, C., Fitzpatrick, J. J., Lewin, L., et al. (2012). Nurse practitioner knowledge of child sexual abuse in children with cognitive disabilities. *Journal of Forensic Nursing, 8*(2), 72–80.

Kucuker, H., Demir, T., & Oral, R. (2010). Pediatric condition falsification (Munchausen syndrome by proxy) as a continuum of maternal factitious disorder (Munchausen syndrome). *Pediatric Diabetes, 11*(8), 572–578.

Kuijpers, K. F., van der Knaap, L. M., & Winkel, F. W. (2012). Risk of revictimization of intimate partner violence: The role of attachment, anger and violent behavior of the victim. *Journal of Family Violence, 27*(1), 33–44.

Lam, K. Y. (2014). Factors associate with adolescents' disclosure of sexual abuse in Hong Kong. *Journal of Sexual Abuse, 23*(7) 768–791.

Lang, A. J., Gartstein, M. A., Rodgers, C. S., et al. (2010). The impact of maternal childhood abuse on parenting and infant temperament. *Journal of Child and Adolescent Psychiatric Nursing, 23*(2), 100–110.

Lang, D. L., Sales, J. M., Salazer, L. F., et al. (2011). Rape victimization and high risk sexual behaviors: Longitudinal study of African-American adolescent females. *Western Journal of Emergency Medicine, 12*(3), 333–342.

Lazoritz, S., Rossiter, K., & Whiteaker, D. (2010). What every nurse needs to know about the clinical aspects of child abuse. *American Nurse Today, 5*(7), 1–3.

Legano, L., McHugh, M. T., & Palusci, V. (2009). Child abuse and neglect. *Current Problems in Pediatric and Adolescent Health Care, 39*(2), 31.e1–31.e26.

Makin-Byrd, K., & Bierman, K. L. (2013). Individual and family predictors of the perpetration of dating violence and victimization in late adolescence. *Journal of Youth and Adolescence, 42*(4), 536–550.

McCloskey, L. A. (2013). The intergenerational transfer of mother-daughter risk for gender-based abuse. *Psychodynamic Psychiatry, 41*(2), 303–328.

Neutze, J., Grundmann, D., Scherner, G., et al. (2012). Undetected and detected child sexual abuse and child pornography offenders. *International Journal of Law and Psychiatry, 35*(3), 168–175.

Roberts, A. L., Rosario, M., Corliss, H. L., et al. (2012). Childhood gender nonconformity: A risk indicator for childhood abuse and posttraumatic stress in youth. *Pediatrics, 129*(3), 410–417.

Schwecke, L. H. (2011). Beyond childhood sexual abuse: Ritual abuse-torture and human trafficking. *Journal of Psychosocial Nursing and Mental Health Services, 49*(1), 8–10.

Sullivan, C. M. (2011). Child abuse and the legal system: The orthopaedic surgeon's role in diagnosis. *Clinical Orthopaedics and Related Research*, *469*(3), 768–775.

Thompson, N. J., McGee, R. E., & Mays, D. (2012). Race, ethnicity, substance abuse, and unwanted sexual intercourse among adolescent females in the United States. *The Western Journal of Emergency Medicine, 13*(3), 283–288.

Tonmyr, L., Jack, S. M., Brooks, S., et al. (2012). Utilization of the Canadian Incidence Study of Reported Child Abuse and Neglect by child welfare agencies in Ontario. *Chronic Disease & Injury in Canada, 33*(1), 29–37.

U.S. Department of Health and Human Services. (2010). *Healthy people 2020*. Washington, DC: Author.

U.S. Department of Health and Human Services, Administration for Children and Families, Administration on Children, Youth and Families, Children's Bureau. (2017). *Child maltreatment 2015*. Retrieve from https://www.acf.hhs.gov/sites/default/files/cb/cm2015.pdf

Valentino, K., Nuttall, A. K., Comas, M., et al. (2012). Intergenerational continuity of child abuse among adolescent mothers: Authoritarian parenting, community violence, and race. *Child Maltreatment, 17*(2), 172–181.

Wastler, S. (2010). The harm in "sexting": Analyzing the constitutionality of child pornography statutes that prohibit the voluntary production, possession, and dissemination of sexually explicit images by teenagers. *Harvard Journal of Law & Gender, 33*(2), 687–702.

56

Nursing Care of a Family When a Child Has a Long-Term or Terminal Illness

Charlie is a 3-year-old who has had a relapse after 18 months of chemotherapy for leukemia. You meet him in the emergency department because he has developed a severe cough and high fever. He is diagnosed as having pneumonia. "We're all so tired," her mother tells you. "And he's been sick for so long. How could he develop something else?"

Previous chapters described the growth and development of well children and the care of children with specific disorders. This chapter adds information about the care of chronically and terminally ill children. This is important information because it builds a base for care and health teaching and support for the parents and child.

How could you best help this parent? What would be important topics to talk to her about?

KEY TERMS

anticipatory grief

complicated grief

death

grief process

vulnerable children

OBJECTIVES

After mastering the contents of this chapter, you should be able to:

1. Describe common concerns of parents of children with a long-term or terminal illness.
2. Identify nursing contributions in achieving 2020 National Health Goals related to children with long-term or terminal illnesses.
3. Assess the adjustment of a child or family to a long-term or terminal illness.
4. Formulate nursing diagnoses for a child with a long-term or terminal illness to help him or her manage seamless transitions across differing healthcare settings.
5. Identify expected outcomes for a child with a long-term or terminal illness.
6. Using the nursing process, plan nursing care that includes the six competencies of Quality & Safety Education for Nurses (QSEN): Patient-Centered Care, Teamwork & Collaboration, Evidence-Based Practice (EBP), Quality Improvement (QI), Safety, and Informatics.
7. Implement nursing care for a child with a long-term or terminal illness, such as helping parents with time management and identification of resources.
8. Evaluate effectiveness and achievement of expected outcomes for a child with a long-term or terminal illness and their families.
9. Integrate knowledge of long-term or terminal illness with the interplay of nursing process, the six competencies of QSEN, and Family Nursing to promote quality maternal and child health nursing care.

When children have an acute illness, both they and their parents become frightened by the sudden onset and severity of symptoms. Because human beings have a great capacity for coping with stress, however, as long as they are given adequate support, they can usually adjust to the strain of disrupted daily routines, hospital visits, and home care.

When a child's illness becomes long term or is one that is projected to have a terminal outcome, a family's capacity to cope can become stretched beyond its limits. Support is essential for such a family if it is to survive under this level of pressure and stress (Nikkola, Kaunonen, & Aho, 2013).

People cope with situations depending on their perception of the event, the type and kind of support they receive from people around them, and the ways they have found to be successful in coping with stressful situations in the past. When working with parents of a child with a long-term or terminal illness, discovering how the parents perceive the problem, what resources they have available, and how they plan to use these resources are crucial in planning effective nursing care.

Whether the medical diagnosis involves a permanent disability or impending death, parents' first response may be grief. The parents have either lost the "perfect" child imagined during pregnancy or the well child they had up to the time of diagnosis. Depending on their age and maturity, children may also experience a grief response. Quality of life in children with long-term or terminal conditions is important to the overall health of children; therefore, the related 2020 National Health Goals are shown in Box 56.1.

Nursing Process Overview

FOR CARE OF A FAMILY WITH A CHILD WHO HAS A LONG-TERM OR TERMINAL ILLNESS

ASSESSMENT

Because a family's coping abilities are best assessed gradually and over a period of many contacts, nurses' assessments of the degree of a family's coping are often the most thorough and meaningful of all healthcare providers.

Observing children at home, where they are most comfortable, or at school in a familiar atmosphere often reveals a great deal more about a child's present disease status or coping potential than does a formal test situation. Children with a long-term illness, on the whole, have been through multiple tests and procedures in the process of diagnosis; they may have come to think of healthcare providers as people who hurt them, not people from whom they wish to receive care. Changing their perception may require maintaining a reassuring, gentle manner during assessment and subsequent care procedures.

NURSING DIAGNOSIS

A long-term illness can take many forms. A condition that requires daily attention, such as diabetes mellitus (e.g., managing an insulin pump), but is relatively stable may not be as stressful to parents as an illness, such as muscular dystrophy, that may require many adjustments in care due to its slow progression. In the former, although the child and family must adjust their lifestyle to incorporate the child's

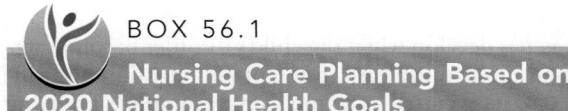

BOX 56.1

Nursing Care Planning Based on 2020 National Health Goals

Long-term illness or early death in children is a major cost to the nation and individual families because it has the potential to reduce the earning power and contribution of future citizens. Examples of 2020 National Health Goals that address this include:

- Increase the proportion of youth with special healthcare needs whose healthcare provider has discussed transition planning from pediatric to adult health care from a baseline of 41.2% to a target level of 45.3%.
- Increase the proportion of children with disabilities from birth through age 2 years who receive early intervention services in home or in community-based settings from 91% to 95%.
- Reduce the rate of infant deaths from a baseline of 6.7 per 1,000 live births to a target rate of 6.0 per 1,000.
- Reduce the death rate for children 1 to 4 years of age from a baseline of 28.6 per 100,000 to no more than 25.7 per 100,000 children and for children aged 5 to 9 years from a baseline of 13.7 per 100,000 to 12.3 per 100,000.
- Reduce the death rate for children 10 to 14 years of age from a baseline of 16.9 per 100,000 to no more than 15.2 per 100,000 and the death rate for adolescents 15 to 19 years of age from a baseline of 61.9 per 100,000 to 55.7 per 100,000 (U.S. Department of Health and Human Services, 2010; see www.healthypeople.gov).

Nurses can help the nation achieve these goals by educating women to seek care during pregnancy so that congenital anomalies, a common cause of infant morbidity and mortality, are less frequent and to teach unintentional injury prevention and the importance of immunizations so unintentional injuries and infectious diseases that can lead to long-term illness, such as rubeola and meningitis, can be reduced.

daily needs, they feel more in control of the illness and the child's overall health. In the latter, the child and family feel powerless because they lack the ability to alter the course of the disease; they must simply be prepared for the next acute crisis to develop. Nursing diagnoses for children with long-term or terminal illnesses need to address both the child and the family and the stage of illness. Some examples of nursing diagnoses when a long-term illness is present include:

- Interrupted family processes related to recent diagnosis of chronic illness in the child
- Compromised family coping related to the child's disability
- Disabling family coping related to the parents' inability to accept the child's long-term illness
- Anticipatory grieving related to chronicity of the child's illness
- Risk for delayed growth and development due to decreased mobility because of disability

New issues develop when the child's disorder becomes terminal. The family must learn to accept not only the child's illness but also its eventual outcome. Some examples of nursing diagnoses when a terminal illness is present include:

- Hopelessness related to steady progression of the child's disease
- Anticipatory grieving related to the child's terminal illness
- Powerlessness related to inability to change the course of the child's illness
- Decisional conflict related to treatment options and choice of setting for the child's final care

OUTCOME IDENTIFICATION AND PLANNING

Be certain when planning care for children with a chronic or fatal illness that the outcomes established are realistic. You probably cannot alter the course of a child's illness, but you can help parents cope with signs and symptoms of the illness or the impending death.

Parents who have not yet accepted the seriousness of their child's illness—who hold on to the hope that their child will eventually be cured or restored to full health—may make plans that the child cannot accomplish. Sometimes, this level of denial is necessary for the development of coping strategies to deal with the child's daily needs and the needs of the rest of the family. If parents believe they must shield the child or other family members from the truth, it can be hard for them to plan effective outcomes. Focusing on hopeful but realistic outcomes, such as the desire the child will not experience pain or the child will learn how to move about independently in a wheelchair, can help a family move forward toward acceptance of the seriousness of the child's illness.

Referrals can be made to helpful organizations such as the Candlelighters for Children With Cancer (www.4kidswithcancer.org), The Compassionate Friends (www.compassionatefriends.org), and the National Association of School Psychologists (www.nasponline.org).

IMPLEMENTATION

Parents can become overprotective of children who have a long-term or terminal illness, which may discourage their development. Helping parents recognize their child's capabilities and arrange appropriate activities for the child are ways in which nurses can facilitate parents' acceptance of the diagnosis and the road ahead. Suggestions for helping children achieve developmental milestones are discussed for each age group in Chapters 29 through 33.

Helping parents develop coping strategies and establish effective ways to manage the complex medical needs of the child, maintain quality care despite the burdens of care, and maintain a balanced life that includes self-care are other important measures.

OUTCOME EVALUATION

Children with a long-term or terminal illness need periodic follow-up care because children's needs across the life span changes. Plans made in the early school years may need to be modified by the time the child is 12 years of age, and they must change again with adolescence. You may need to remind parents that in addition to health care by a specialty clinic, children also need routine health maintenance care.

Otherwise, children will be well protected from the complications of their special illness but unprotected from common childhood illnesses.

An evaluation of whether expected outcomes for the family and child are achieved will identify discrepancies between what families hope for and what is realistic given the child's condition. When discordance is identified, and outcomes are not achieved, healthcare providers have an opportunity to strengthen their understanding of the effect of chronic illness or the death of a child on families.

Some examples suggesting achievement of outcomes include:

- Parents state realistic plans for their child regarding school placement.
- Parents state they have been able to deal with their grief over their child's diagnosis to maintain near-normal family functioning.
- Parents state they are able to cope with present stressors and can specify coping strategies they utilize.
- The child states he is aware his illness is chronic (long term) but thinks of himself as a person who will be able to accomplish many things in life.

The Child With a Long-Term Illness

Families have different resources, and everyone reacts to situations differently. Each child with a long-term illness and the family need to be assessed individually for their potential to cope with the illness and to provide necessary care. Through such an assessment, appropriate interventions to help the family adapt can be started early in the course of the illness (Longden, 2011).

THE PARENTS' ADJUSTMENT

Children need support in adjusting to stressful events and parents can serve as role models while providing the emotional and instrumental support the child needs. Therefore, an assessment begins with an examination of the parents' response to the stress of a long-term illness. Responses from caregivers can vary based on the relationship and dynamics between the caregiver and the child. This relationship can be based on family structure and emotional stability of the family and on differences in the typical behavior of mothers, fathers, sons, and daughters. Questions by the nurse should seek to elicit responses by each family member and identify the different relationships that exist in the family.

Chronic health conditions affect the entire family. The nurse should support each family member as their reactions and needs may vary because each person's response is individualized. The nurse should seek to:

- Answer the family's questions or seek assistance from the medical team in answering their questions.
- Identify and address the needs of the family and child.
- Assist the family in meeting the physical needs of the child, including pain relief and symptom management.
- Assist the family with advanced care planning, including the inevitable effect on the physical and mental health of parents, siblings, and extended family.
- Identify and assist with psychological and spiritual support.
- Assist with care coordination.

TABLE 56.1 THE STAGES OF GRIEF

Stage	Parents' Reaction	Description
1	Denial	Parents have difficulty realizing what has occurred. They ask, "How could this have happened?"
2	Anger	Parents react to the injustice of being singled out this way. They say, "It isn't fair this is happening."
3	Bargaining	Parents attempt to work out a "deal" to buy their way out of the situation. They say, "If my child gets well, I'll devote the rest of my life to doing good."
4	Depression	Parents begin to face what is happening. They feel sad and unprotected.
5	Acceptance	Acceptance is being able to say, "Yes, this is happening, and it is all right it is happening." With a child who has a long-term illness, parents may never reach this stage but will always remain in the chronic sorrow of the depression stage.

Based on Kübler-Ross, E. (1969). *On death and dying.* New York, NY: Macmillan.

The Grief Response

Parents can be expected to experience a **grief process**, or the regulated steps in grieving, after diagnosis of a terminal illness and physical or cognitive challenges their child will experience. The most commonly accepted steps or stages of grief are those outlined by Kübler-Ross (1969). Table 56.1 summarizes these stages. Many parents with a child who is physically or cognitively challenged never arrive at the final stage of acceptance or they spend years with chronic sorrow (also called **complicated grief**) (Whittingham, Wee, Sanders, et al., 2013). Reaching a final stage may be particularly difficult when parents grieve in different ways or at different paces (Wender, 2012).

During the first stage of grief (shock or denial), parents are usually unable to plan past immediate or short-term actions (e.g., learning to change a dressing, what pills to give each day). Trying to establish long-term outcomes at this point (e.g., what type of school the child will attend, future surgery that will be needed) is rarely productive because this must all be done again when parents are truly ready to look this far ahead. During the second stage (anger), parents may be unwilling to concentrate on goals (e.g., the whole thing is so unfair; planning is asking too much of them; besides, if you were really helpful, you would cure their child and not talk about ways they have to adjust). Therefore, this may also be a time of waiting. During the bargaining stage of grief, parents are still not ready to plan. They believe that if their bargain is fulfilled (e.g., if their child is able to walk, and they promise to spend the rest of their life doing good), they do not have to make plans such as purchasing a wheelchair because these will be unnecessary after their wish is granted and the child's condition improves.

During the next stage of grief (depression), parents are ready to make plans but need a great deal of support because they feel sad and fatigued. During this phase, it is critical to make plans *with* them not *for* them. Many parents of children who are physically or cognitively challenged develop low self-esteem as well as depression. Their low confidence in their parenting abilities may make them believe your suggestions are superior to their own. Upon their return home, they are the ones who must implement these plans and mitigate challenges they will experience so they need to participate in the planning process.

Even after parents reach the final stage of grief (acceptance), some parents need guidance in making plans to avoid ignoring the needs and wishes of other family members. For example, parents may spend every waking moment with their ill child. Talking to them about the importance of self-care and the burdens of caregiving are helpful. Help them approach their child's care with moderation and allow time for all family members as well. Helping them to plan a respite from the care of a sick child, such as an evening out while a babysitter cares for the child, could be part of this approach (Thomas & Price, 2012).

If parents had a chronically ill child late in life, by the time the child is school age, parents need to face one more step in their development as parents of a chronically ill child: to begin to make some concrete plans as to who will care for the child in the event of their death. Like the steps that came before it, this is very difficult for parents; it asks them to contemplate not only their child's vulnerability but also their own. They might consult with family members about guardianship and with a lawyer to help them write a will that will provide future caretaking and economic support for the chronically ill child when they are no longer able to do so.

Factors Influencing Parental Adjustment

Certain circumstances, such as the degree and timing of their child's illness, the experience of the parents, the availability of support, and the ability to make long-term plans, appear to increase parents' ease or difficulty in adjusting to their child's disabling or long-term illness.

The Degree of Illness

The seriousness of an illness affects the ability of parents to adjust (Whittingham et al., 2013). A child who needs total care, for example, requires a much more radical readjustment of the parents' lives than a child who only needs additional speech therapy for an hour a day. In most instances, the parents' perception of the child's illness is as important as the child's condition itself (Fig. 56.1). For example, a parent who envisioned a son as someday becoming an Olympic runner may perceive a son with developmental hip dysplasia as having a serious physical challenge; a parent whose mental image of the child was that of a lawyer mainly doing desk work may not view the hip problem as a serious illness.

Many parents have hopes and dreams for their child, once women realize they are pregnant. Hidden desires are often revealed if you ask parents, "If things could have been different, what kind of person would you have liked your child to be?" A parent who answers "A kind person" can still have that wish fulfilled no matter what the degree of illness. A parent who says "I always assumed my child would take over the family business someday" may have some major mental readjustments to make.

Figure 56.1 A parent's perception of a child's disability is important to how well the family adjusts. Often, it is easier to accept a disability that allows for greater functioning in everyday activities. (© Bill Bachman/Science Source/Photo Researchers.)

Whether an illness is noticeable (cerebral palsy) or not noticeable (controlled seizures) also can make a difference in how parents adjust to the illness. A mother who takes her child with cerebral palsy shopping, during which the child walks unsteadily and knocks over a display, may hear other shoppers say, "Wouldn't you think a mother would watch her child more carefully?" On days that her child uses a wheelchair, however, shoppers' comments are more apt to be, "Poor little thing. Isn't it wonderful his mother brings him shopping with her?" She is happy to have a signal (the wheelchair) that announces that her child is different and cannot be held to the same standards as other children. Other parents might be more grateful that a child's illness is not a visible one: It makes the illness seem lesser in extent and therefore easier for them to accept.

The Relationship With Own Parents

When adults are able to relate well to their parents, it suggests they were raised in an atmosphere of love or were able to develop a sense of trust (Erikson, 1993). People with a sense of trust are able to form a firm sense of intimacy as adults and so be better able to give love to children even when the children have challenges in some way.

The Onset of the Illness

Whether a condition is apparent at birth (such as a myelomeningocele) or occurs at a later time (a child is struck by a car at school age or who develops autism spectrum disorder) is another factor that may make a difference in parents' ability to adjust. In either situation, the long-term care of a child will totally change the parents' lifestyle. As an example, when a child has a physical handicap, parents may have to change their living arrangements to accommodate for the needs of the child. These changes may impact housing, transportation, and work schedules and cause financial constraints due to the cost of care of a chronically ill child.

The Effect of Parental Experience

First-time parents may have more difficulty caring for a child with a long-term illness than older, more experienced parents

because all phases of parenting are new and unique for them. On the other hand, first-time parents may have no preconceived opinions and so may be more flexible than other parents or able to adjust more readily to a change in routine. A young parent who has just this one child may have more time to spend in a daily exercise program than does a parent with four other children.

The Availability of Support People

Adjusting to illness in a child for a family with few close friends and relatives at a distance may be more difficult than a family that has close support system. People who can locate secondary support systems in their community, such as an organization for parents of children who are physically or cognitively challenged or a local church or synagogue, or who can depend on healthcare resources usually do better than parents who are without these resources. Whether a family can depend on healthcare resources is related to:

- The availability of transportation (e.g., it is difficult to take a child in a 50-lb cast on a bus)
- A language barrier (e.g., it is frustrating to go for care and be unable to make your needs known)
- Finances and insurance coverage (e.g., it is disturbing for parents to be told their child needs to see a specialist when they have no money or health coverage to pay for one)
- Past experience with healthcare providers can set the stage for a distrustful relationship between the provider and parent.

Life Events

A child's illness usually appears to be more acute at times when the child would normally reach developmental milestones than when the child reaches traditional milestones such as obtaining their driver's license or participating in a bar mitzvah. When the child does not reach these traditional milestones, it reminds parents about their child's illness in a particularly painful way. Factors that indicate a family will probably be able to adjust to caring for a child with a long-term illness are summarized in Table 56.2.

QSEN Checkpoint Question 56.1

INFORMATICS

A nurse is reviewing the electronic notes of the social worker who has been involved with the family's care of Charlie, 3 years of age. What noted factor is most apt to help Charlie's parents cope with the stress of his long-term illness?

a. The parents believe in alternative therapies and consequently have many options.
b. Both parents have a good relationship with their own parents.
c. The parents are wealthy, so are not distressed by the cost of his care.
d. The family is private, so they cannot compare Charlie's condition to other ill children.

Look in Appendix A for the best answer and rationale.

TABLE 56.2 FACTORS THAT EASE PARENTAL ADJUSTMENT TO A CHILD'S LONG-TERM ILLNESS

Factor	Rationale
Support people are available.	Caring for a child is a series of crises during which support people become very important.
A strong marital bond exists between the parents.	A marriage partner can serve as the strongest support person.
A good relationship exists between the child's parents and their parents.	The parents have a firm sense of trust and the ability to give care to another and child has the support of the extended family.
The child is other than the first born.	The parents have had practice parenting.
The family lives close to shopping, schools, and transportation.	The family is not isolated.
The family has a strong spiritual faith or community contacts.	Secondary support systems are important in times of stress.
The parents are told of the child's disability as soon as possible.	A handicap may be easier to accept if the parents never thought of the child as totally well.

THE CHILD'S ADJUSTMENT

A child's reaction to being physically or cognitively challenged or to having a long-term illness is strongly influenced by the family's reaction to the illness. This may range from overprotectiveness to rejection and from denial to acceptance. The child's adjustment may also be influenced by peers and other support people, such as school personnel or healthcare providers. Social exclusion, discrimination, and physical barriers at school or in the community make it difficult for a child to adjust to a physical challenge or a long-term illness. Inclusion in school and social activities, acceptance by peers and support people, and the ability to function as normally as possible help the child adjust (Crosland & Dunlap, 2012).

A child's ability to cope is further influenced by personal attitude and temperament, self-concept, age and development, understanding of the condition, and degree of the disorder. As the child grows and life situations change, the ability to cope may improve or worsen. For example, an adolescent who is physically challenged may have a more positive outlook on life with a chronic illness because she is successfully working at her first job; another adolescent may become angered by his deteriorating condition because he is suddenly confined to a wheelchair.

The degree of fatigue that a child experiences is also instrumental in how well they adjust to a chronic illness because chronic fatigue can play a large role in making even simple tasks seem monumental (Fisher & Crawley, 2013).

Nursing interventions to help a child better adjust to a chronic condition include encouraging optimal growth and development (see Chapters 29 to 33), promoting self-care activities, enhancing self-esteem, preventing social isolation, providing health education, preventing fatigue, and supporting the child and family to identify strategies to adapt to living with the child's condition.

SIBLINGS' ADJUSTMENT

Siblings' reactions to a child with a long-term or terminal illness are influenced by individual circumstances; however, their chief reaction is most profoundly affected by the reactions and perceptions of the parents. Without counseling, siblings may react with jealousy, anger, hostility, resentment, competition, guilt, or withdrawal. They may feel they take second place to the sibling who needs more care. These reactions are common when parents focus most of their attention on the ill child, allow the health problem and its treatment to disrupt family life significantly, or grant the ill child special privileges and minimal discipline.

With counseling and support, however, siblings can develop acceptance, care, concern, and cooperation (Vermaes, van Susante, & van Bakel, 2012). Such reactions are common when parents make it a point to set aside time each day for special activities with the well siblings such as playing a table game, walking in the park, teaching a child to swim, carefully explaining the condition and the necessity for their sibling's special care, including them in the care of the ill child, providing them with respite from care if needed, and establishing realistic rules for all family members.

At any one time, the siblings may experience a mixture of feelings. For example, if a boy's parents must take his sister for chemotherapy during his swim meet, the boy may feel both resentment that his parents missed the meet and sadness that his sister could not compete in that meet or in any others.

THE NURSE AND THE ILL CHILD

Caring for children with long-term illnesses can be a stressful role for nurses (St. Ledger, Begley, Reid, et al., 2012). Nurses help the parents and child with a long-term illness review specific aspects of the child's condition and the possible complications that could occur. Over a period of years, parents become experts in the care of a child with a particular condition (Box 56.2). This can make them grow impatient with healthcare providers who appear to be unaware of things they know well. When young children are seen at an ambulatory care setting or are admitted to a hospital for care, review with the parents their routines and techniques so that you can continue to care for their child in the same way. As the child grows older and more independent in managing their care, include the child in these discussions. Be available, however, to show a parent or a child an easier way to do something if it seems appropriate. Frankly admitting to parents "You're more familiar with Jennifer's care than I am; you'll have to teach me some things" is a refreshing approach; it not only allows parents to feel confidence in you, but your honesty also increases their self-esteem.

Familiarize yourself as well with the community resources that are available for children with long-term illnesses. Advising parents to see a dentist who specializes in caring for children with autism spectrum disorder when there is no one

Charlie is admitted to the hospital, and intravenous therapy is begun. You notice his skin is unusually reddened where the adhesive tape was removed. He cries when you touch the irritated site.

Tip: It is easy to believe that a fellow nurse who has spent a great deal of time caring for a child has become an expert in that child's care. It is often more difficult to remember that a parent can become this type of expert also. Remember to ask parents of children with a long-term illness for their input. This can not only simplify care but also add to the parents' feeling of self-esteem, thus improving their parenting.

Nurse: Look at Charlie's skin. It looks so red and sore.

Mrs. Circuso: That's from the adhesive tape.

Nurse: Has Charlie had this type of reaction before?

Mrs. Circuso: It has happened before.

Nurse: I should have been more specific when I asked about allergies. I'll make a note in his patient record.

Figure 56.2 Therapy dogs can be helpful to keep children with a long-term illness active and in touch with usual events. (© Marmaduke St. John/Alamy.)

of that description less than 200 miles away, for example, is not only helpful but it can also be destructive because it raises expectations in parents that cannot be met, thus accentuating a problem.

Most parents of a chronically ill child adhere well to instructions and keep healthcare appointments consistently. Sometimes, however, you will find parents who do not follow this pattern. This inability to adhere usually is related to their stage of adjustment to the illness. As long as denial, anger, bargaining, or depression is present, coming in for health care or an evaluation is viewed as a major demand. Each visit is more of a reminder of the child's illness than a time of reassuring health assessment.

Developmental Tasks

Children with long-term illnesses often do not meet developmental milestones on schedule because achieving developmental tasks takes practice. When you are helping parents teach a child who is physically or cognitively challenged a new skill, such as toilet training or using a spoon, help them break the task down into its component parts (e.g., reach for the spoon, grasp it, push it under the chosen food, lift it toward the mouth). Breaking a task down into steps in this way allows parents to appreciate that they are asking their child to learn a task that, although it looks easy, actually encompasses 20 or more coordinated motions. Helping them learn this technique enables them to be patient in teaching additional tasks in future years.

The unique concerns of children who are physically or cognitively challenged and ways to help them achieve developmental tasks are discussed in Chapters 29 to 33. For healthcare providers, exposing them to usual events during a hospital stay or an ambulatory healthcare visit can help expand their world (Fig. 56.2).

Education

Children with a long-term illness often need special education programs or at least separate hours of individualized instruction to succeed in school. Most children benefit from preschool programs because these programs offer them a head start. Children with a long-term illness tend to miss school more often than do their healthier classmates because of healthcare visits and exacerbations of their illness. This can cause them to fall behind in school unless individualized plans to keep them with their school group are made. By federal law (Public Law No. 99-457, Education of the Handicapped Amendment), a school system must provide educational opportunities in the least structured setting possible for physically and cognitively challenged children, beginning with preschool. You may have to be a strong child advocate to see that the best educational program available is being provided for an individual child (Kirk, Beatty, Callery, et al., 2012).

Home Care

Most children with a long-term illness may be hospitalized for a short term but then receive the bulk of their care at home (Newton & Lamarche, 2012).

Planning for home care is discussed in Chapter 4. Important aspects to consider include the best school setting (home or traditional school), ways to involve the family in community activities, ways to include the child in a play group if possible, how much self-care the child can achieve, and future plans, such as preparing a child for puberty or enrolling in college. Home care or community health nurses can be instrumental in identifying goals for self-care and planning school or community activities (Peacock & Stanik-Hutt, 2013).

Many parents today seek complementary or alternative therapies for children with long-term illnesses in home care. Always ask what therapies and medications they are using to document the full extent of treatment that a child is receiving (Braga & Almgren, 2013).

What If . . . 56.1

A nurse arranges for Charlie's mother to spend an afternoon shopping so she can have some respite time away from her ill child, but she spends the time cleaning her kitchen cupboards instead. How might the nurse advise Charlie's mother?

Unfolding Patient Stories: Brittany Long • Part 2

Think back to Brittany Long, whom you met in Chapter 38. Brittany is a 5-year-old Black girl diagnosed with sickle cell anemia who lives with her mother, 7-year-old sister, and grandmother. Her pain crises are mostly managed at home, and she has been hospitalized three times. How can the nurse help Brittany and her family cope with a long-term illness and the management of acute crises? How can the reactions of family members influence Brittany's adjustment to sickle cell disease? What effect can a long-term illness have on the sister and what actions can support her understanding and cooperation?

Care for Brittany and other patients in a realistic virtual environment: *vSim for Nursing* (thepoint.lww.com/vSimMaternityPed). Practice documenting these patients' care in DocuCare (thepoint.lww.com/DocuCareEHR).

The Child Who Is Terminally Ill

Death can come suddenly to some families, such as when adolescents choose to harm themselves or take their own life or when a child is killed in an automobile accident or random shooting, providing no time for parents to prepare for the death (Bogle & Go, 2015). Parents of terminally ill children need to make end-of-life preparations for their child. Nurses can be an integral part of this planning. This can be one of the hardest tasks in nursing because most people are raised to accept the fact that elderly people die, but such people have also lived a long life. Most people can accept the death of middle-aged people with the same philosophy—they experienced at least a portion of their life. It is often more difficult to accept the death of children because they have had so

little opportunity to live. It is imperative for nurses to work through their own feelings about a child's dying so they can find the strength to care for the child and support the parents.

PARENTAL GRIEF RESPONSES

Although the reaction to learning that a child has a terminal illness can be culturally influenced, each family reacts in a unique way. Being aware of the usual grief response that occurs in anticipation of a child's death helps in recognizing such a response as grief and supporting a family through this very difficult period (Box 56.3).

Stage 1: Denial

A parent's usual response to the diagnosis of a terminal illness in a child is denial, the same as with long-term illness (see Table 56.1). Although people are aware that children die, most proceed through life thinking and hoping for a cure or minimal challenges. When they realize they might lose their child, they respond with disbelief. The likelihood of this response is enhanced by the fact that many terminal illnesses, such as a brain tumor or leukemia, begin insidiously allowing little opportunity for parents to be mentally prepared (e.g., "How can a few black-and-blue marks be the symptoms of a potentially terminal disease?").

How the parents handle this initial disbelief has a great deal to do with their relationship with healthcare personnel. If they have a trusting relationship with healthcare providers from past experiences, they are more likely to seek information and support from the providers. If they lack trust in the providers, they may not believe the diagnosis and feel the need to obtain a second opinion. Although this often involves considerable expense, for many parents, it is a necessary step in moving past this first reaction. Parents who feel a need for a third, fourth, or fifth opinion may be having an unusually difficult time resolving a "surely not me" response. Be certain they have received factual explanations and evidence of the diagnosis such as through a copy of the blood or the pathologist's biopsy report.

BOX 56.3

Nursing Care Planning to Respect Cultural Diversity

The way death is viewed and the manner in which people express grief differ greatly across cultures. Some people express grief very loudly and openly, whereas others are very restrained. The way a child's body is handled after death also differs. Some religions, for example, forbid organ donations or transplants. Autopsies are not approved because it is important that a child be buried quickly. Cremation may or may not be permitted. Being aware that people have different expectations for final care and that grief is expressed differently by different cultures enables better understanding of parents' concerns and reactions during a child's terminal illness and when death occurs. Don't depend on stereotypical descriptions of how parents should react; ask them if they need help resolving a cultural conflict or if there is a care measure based on their cultural beliefs that they would like you to include in care.

Urge them to talk about how they feel and ask questions. Facts regarding the illness, the challenges it may present and also the terminal nature of it will assist parents to accept the diagnosis and identify strategies to adapt.

During this stage of denial, you may find the parents' downplaying their child's illness. It is easy to view such denial as a step that should be hurried because parents cannot begin to deal with the problem as long as they deny there is a problem. Denial is a temporary pain-relief measure and a necessary step on the way to acceptance, and individuals will move through this stage at different speeds.

Stage 2: Anger

Parents can be expected to enter a stage of anger soon—a change from "Surely not me" to "It's not right this is happening to me." When parents are angry about a diagnosis, they may be unable to direct their anger appropriately. One parent may be angry with the other (e.g., criticizing the other for reckless driving or for eating a fattening food for lunch). They may be angry with you (e.g., for not answering the child's call light immediately). They may be angry with the medical, X-ray, laboratory, and dietary staff or with the entire healthcare system. It can be difficult to react to this kind of anger because it seems unjustified. Be certain your first reaction is not to be angry in response.

A more therapeutic reaction is to accept the parents' explicit emotions and anger and respond with empathy and acceptance.

Some parents may seek out another healthcare provider during this stage, although their reaction will depend to a great extent on their experience with death in the past.

When you ask grieving parents to talk, therefore, they may talk not about the child but about how they felt when a parent died, how hard their job is for them, or how they worry that their marriage is failing. This is part of grief: gathering resources, reworking stress from the past, and arming themselves to face present stress and what to except in the future. Parents often receive support from other parents in the hospital whose children are also terminally ill. Interacting with parents of other children and learning about ways they have adjusted to the effects of a terminal illness will be helpful.

What If . . . 56.2

Charlie's parents, who are both 50 years old and live on a ranch, tell the nurse their two grown children have expressed resentment at the amount of time and money they have spent trying to find a cure for Charlie. Charlie's parents have no health insurance, so finances are always tight. How should the nurse respond to Charlie's parents?

Stage 3: Bargaining

Although not everyone progresses through a grief response in a linear fashion, and instead vacillates between stages, bargaining often follows anger. This is a time when parents try to correct or change the course of illness by bargaining. They vow to be better people or to function in a different way in exchange for their child's life. When parents realize that bargaining is ineffective, it brings them to a very low point because they are let down not only by healthcare providers but also by the superior power with whom they tried to bargain. They may need more support after bargaining fails than at any other point.

Stage 4: Depression

When parents have passed through the stages of denial, anger, and bargaining, developing awareness of the reality of this diagnosis will usher them into the stage of depression. This is a change from "I can keep it from happening" to "It is happening." Frequent crying or projecting an overall sad countenance is the most common sign that this stage has been reached. Parents may ask more questions about care, procedures, or medications than they did before. Be careful you do not interpret this questioning as criticism. Parents' questions stem from the full awareness of the serious implication of the chronic illness.

At this stage, parents may work through the expected challenges that lie ahead by talking about their plans for the child. They may suddenly shower the child with expensive gifts or trips and have difficulty leaving a hospitalized child to go home to care for other children or to report for work. On the surface, all the questions and demands may imply they are taking a step backward. Actually, this reflects their appreciation of the diagnosis and its magnitude and should be seen as a step forward.

At about this stage, parents need to think about preparing other children in the family for the challenges the ill child will face. If the ill child is hospitalized and siblings have not been allowed to visit, siblings may misinterpret the hospital experiences of the ill child and also the reasons why visitation may be restricted. You may need to advocate for sibling visitation to overcome this misinterpretation and to allow the sibling to observe the hospital setting first hand.

Some siblings feel responsible for the death of the ill child. All children wish at one time or another that a sibling were dead (or would simply disappear) so they could have a bedroom all to themselves or so they could have the other child's bicycle. Maybe they were told not to wrestle with the ill sibling, but they did anyway. These children need reassurance that the sibling's death is not a result of their musings but an expected result of the child's illness. Assure them that they need not feel guilty.

Stage 5: Acceptance

The acceptance stage of the grief process is resolution that the child has an illness that may be fatal. Some parents do not reach this stage until the time of the child's death; working through grief will need to continue for years after the child has died.

QSEN Checkpoint Question 56.2

PATIENT-CENTERED CARE

Charlie's parents are grieving because they fear he will not survive this recurrence of his illness. The nurse is planning Charlie's care with the knowledge that the family is experiencing intense sadness. During which stage of grief do parents usually feel the most intense depression?

a. The first stage, because everything is such a shock
b. The last stage, because they fully accept the death
c. The fourth stage, as they realize death is happening
d. The stage at which the child begins to talk about death

Look in Appendix A for the best answer and rationale.

PARENTAL COPING RESPONSES

Throughout the stages of grieving, parents develop important coping mechanisms to help them through this crisis in their life. Even if they have already learned to cope positively with their child's illness and treatment measures, the determination that the illness is now terminal requires yet another step. Promoting the development of positive coping strategies while being sensitive to the unique needs of each family member is an important nursing responsibility. It may be difficult to determine when a coping strategy is truly helpful and when it has become maladaptive. For instance, seeking information, such as surfing the Internet and asking to have medical library access, is generally a very useful strategy for parents with ill children. Knowing what to expect reduces anxiety. Some parents, however, continue these seeking procedures past the point at which information is helpful to them, believing if they only look hard enough or long enough, they will discover a way to cure their child (prolonged denial), or they may "overintellectualize" their child's illness and impending death to block out their feelings of sadness.

Problem solving is always an effective coping strategy as long as the parents are realistic about which problems they can solve. Seeking the support of others, including healthcare providers and families with similar needs, is encouraged. Providing the names of support groups or individual families (with their permission) who have gone through similar experiences can also be helpful. You may also need to help parents who are not comfortable accepting the help of others to learn how to do so or to simply learn how to feel comfortable expressing their feelings to others.

Many parents are able to cope by searching for the meaning of life or death in philosophical, spiritual, or religious terms. For these parents, body organ donation may be a meaningful way to give themselves some solace that their child will in some way continue to live and contribute to others. Assuring parents that their child will be kept comfortable and will not suffer at the end of life can be extremely comforting.

Anticipatory Grief

Parents who have been warned that their child's death should be expected from the time the child's illness is diagnosed may begin a preparatory or **anticipatory grief** phase in which they gradually incorporate the reality of their child's fate into their thoughts (Yang, Mu, & Wang, 2016). Anticipatory mourning in this way can prepare parents for their child's death and spare them the abrupt, devastating, and intolerable grief reaction that comes to parents whose child dies suddenly from trauma, such as in a car accident or sudden infant death syndrome (see Box 56.4, an interprofessional care map on nursing and team responsibility for care of children when illness has become terminal).

Although anticipatory grief does not shield parents from experiencing renewed grief at the time of their child's death, it can be a useful process for them. A danger of anticipatory grief is that a parent may reach the acceptance stage of the grief process too far in advance of the child's death. If this happens, parents may begin to treat the child as if the child has already died. They stop visiting, or when they do visit, they spend most of their time visiting other children on the unit or sitting in the waiting room talking to other parents. Once they spent time comforting their child; now, they may fail to rock or touch the child as much. They may clean out the child's room and throw out or give away toys. They are gradually drawing back from emotional attachment to shield themselves from the abrupt, stabbing pain that death will bring.

Children need a great deal of support if anticipatory grieving blocks out communication this way, just as they did during the initial denial stage. Parents cannot help that the grief process did not coincide with the child's death. Extend understanding and do not provide criticism for this reaction.

For some parents, because of anticipatory grief, the event seems anticlimactic when the child actually dies. They have anticipated death so long that when it does occur, they cannot believe it has actually happened. They may be so used to thinking constantly about their child's needs and having their child dependent on them that they feel lost or feel as if there is a hole in their thoughts and life. Some parents are reluctant to leave the hospital this final time because leaving with the child's possessions is the step that will make the death real.

Vulnerable or Fragile Child Syndrome

When anticipatory grief proceeds so effectively that parents begin to think of a youngster as already dead but then the child does not die, parents may find their grief reaction was so complete that they are unable to reverse it and they cannot view the child in the same way as they did before. Instead, they begin to treat the child in a cold and unfeeling way, as if the child were not really there but had actually died. Such children are termed **vulnerable children**, or fragile children (Green & Solnit, 1964). They may develop behavior problems as they grow older (e.g., acting out behavior, such as temper tantrums; stealing in school; shoplifting as adolescents) as if to say, "Notice me! I'm not dead!" They may require skilled counseling so they can feel secure that they are still loved and can learn to react effectively with others.

CHILDREN'S REACTIONS TO IMPENDING DEATH

Children's reactions to death are strongly influenced by the previous experiences and the family's attitude toward death. For instance, death can be a new or frightening phenomenon if a child has never had a pet die, was forbidden from visiting a dying relative, or was discouraged from discussing the death of a loved one. Children's reactions to death are also influenced by their stage of development and cognitive ability.

Infants and Toddlers

Infants and toddlers are certainly too young to appreciate that their death is imminent. If the person who cared for them dies, they experience a deep loss and a void in their life. If such a loss interferes with the development of a sense of trust, its implications for the child's ability to achieve warm, close relationships could last a lifetime.

Preschoolers

Preschoolers cannot always differentiate what is real from what is make-believe play. This is a normal part of development and extends to abstract concepts such as illness and death. They envision death as temporary and therefore may not have the same fears adults may have about death.

BOX 56.4

Nursing Care Planning

AN INTERPROFESSIONAL CARE MAP FOR THE FAMILY OF A CHILD WITH A POTENTIALLY FATAL ILLNESS

Charlie is a 3-year-old who has had a relapse after 18 months of chemotherapy for leukemia. His parents have arranged for hospice care for him at home. They state, "He's been through so much already. It's very hard on us but we want him to die at home, close to us."

Family Assessment: Child lives with parents on their llama ranch. Two older siblings (brother, age 20 years, and sister, age 26 years) have left home. Parents report finances as "tight." Family has no health insurance because they are self-employed.

Patient Assessment: Child is cachexic. Skin cool, damp, and mottled. Pulse rate, 62 beats/min and weak; respirations, 8 breaths/min. Rattling sounds noted from chest. Responsive only to deep pain stimuli. Parents at bedside; older siblings absent.

Nursing Diagnosis: Anticipatory grieving related to impending death of child

Outcome Criteria: Parents express feelings about anticipated death; demonstrate positive coping mechanisms.

Team Member Responsible	Assessment	Intervention	Rationale	Expected Outcome
Activities of Daily Living, Including Safety				
Nurse	Assess whether the parents have any concerns or special wishes about child's final days of care.	Stay with the family and sit with them quietly if they prefer not to talk and allow them to cry.	Your presence demonstrates caring and concern for their well-being and wishes and offers support.	Parents discuss any concerns or wishes they have with care.
Teamwork and Collaboration				
Nurse/hospice care staff	Assess whether the parents would like a final visit from their clergy or other support person.	Arrange for visit by the support person if desired.	A visit by the family's support people can provide the family with final needed support.	Parents state whether a support person's visit would be helpful to them. Help plan arrangements.
Procedures/Medications for Quality Improvement				
Nurse	Assess whether the child appears comfortable.	Provide for the child's comfort, including positioning, turning, changing linen, applying lotion, and alleviating pain.	Providing comfort to the child is comforting to the family as well as the child.	Parents state they feel the child is comfortable.
Nurse	Ask whether the parents would like to provide final care.	Allow family members to provide care as desired without forcing them.	Allowing family participation in care provides them with some sense of control over the situation, decreasing their feelings of powerlessness.	Parents state they feel they have had a voice in and are satisfied with child's care.
Nutrition				
Nurse	Assess the child's appetite and whether he could be hungry.	The child's mental state is not appropriate for oral feeding; intravenous (IV) fluid prescribed only as maintenance.	Hunger is an uncomfortable sensation, and feeding is a basic need per Maslow's hierarchy of needs.	Parents agree they feel the child is comfortable and no food is needed.

Patient-Centered Care

Nurse	Assess whether parents have any questions about what actions they should take at the time of death.	Inform the family about what to expect and explore their expectations and clarify any misconceptions.	Providing information helps to ease the family's fears and anxiety about the unknown.	Parents state they feel comfortable caring for child in final minutes and immediately afterward.

Psychosocial/Spiritual/Emotional Needs

Nurse	Assess whether parents need any type of additional emotional support and if appropriate question why older siblings are not present.	Explore as far as parents are willing whether support from their other children would be helpful.	Close family members can supply the most meaningful type of emotional support.	Parents state that although they are disappointed in older siblings' reactions, they understand everyone grieves differently and are managing well.
Nurse	Ask whether parents have begun "grief work" such as reviewing and preserving memories of the child.	Provide the family with opportunities to review special memories or experiences with the child.	Reviewing memories and special experiences provides a positive method for coping with grief.	Parents report they have begun a scrapbook of favorite photos they anticipate will give them solace in years to come.

Informatics for Seamless Healthcare Planning

Nurse	Assess whether parents have made final arrangements for the child's burial and responsibility for reporting death to hospice group.	Assist the family with making arrangements for what to do when the child dies.	Assistance with planning provides support and aids in grieving, allowing time to be spent with the child rather than on arrangements.	Parents state that they understand obligations for reporting death and have good relationship with the hospice group to answer questions.
Nurse	Assess whether parents have contacted a community support group other than hospice group.	If parents feel they need this, initiate referral to a community organization for additional support.	Community organizations can supply long-term support after the child dies.	Parents state they have the name of a community support group and will contact group if they feel a need in the future.

This view of death is sometimes interpreted as unfeeling. For example, the first response of a child who is told his brother has just been killed in an automobile accident might be to ask if he can have his brother's cell phone. This happens because he thinks of his brother as being gone for only a short time, making this a chance to take advantage of his property. The understanding of death as temporary may be strengthened by fictional depictions of death in children's animation or stories in which sometimes characters that are killed come back to life.

The separation anxiety preschoolers experience can complicate their response to death. When confronted with their own death, their main concern may be separation from their parents. Constant reassurances and having a caregiver present with the child helps mitigate these fears.

School-Age Children

School-age children begin to have additional experiences with death, so their knowledge of its finality increases. They may think of it, however, as something that happens only to adults. Children's books tend to deal only superficially with the subject, although many books that deal specifically with death are available for children (Box 56.5). As children near

BOX 56.5

Books About Death for Children

Brown, L. K., & Brown, M. (1996). *When dinosaurs die: A guide to understanding death*. Boston, MA: Little, Brown.
Davis, C. (1997). *For every dog an angel*. Portland, OR: Lighthearted Press.
Farrant, N. (2013). *After Iris*. New York, NY: Dial Press.
Isherwood, S., & Isherwood, K. (2000). *Remembering Granddad*. London, United Kingdom: Oxford Press.
Koppens, J., & van Lindenhuizen, E. (2013). *Goodbye, fish*. New York, NY: Clavis.
Millis, J. C. (2003). *Gentle Willow: A story for children about dying*. Warminster, PA: Marco.
Spergel, H., & Stylou, G. (2013). *Cloud City: A child's journey through bereavement*. Upper Montclair, NJ: Turn the Page.
Tott-Rizzuti, K. (1992). *Mommy, what does dying mean?* Pittsburgh, PA: Dorrance.
Weitzman, E. (1996). *Let's talk about when a parent dies*. New York, NY: Rosen Group.

8 or 9 years of age, they begin to appreciate that death is permanent. They may experience the same feeling of loneliness experienced when they went away to camp or just for a weekend, but this time, the separation will be permanent.

Most school-age children are aware of what is happening to them when their disorder has a fatal prognosis. Unfortunately, they may learn of this prognosis from other children on the unit or at school, from their parents' unusual responses to questions, or from overhearing conversations about reports or physical findings. Children are accustomed to adapting to new situations (e.g., starting school, visiting a museum for the first time, boarding an airplane for the first time), and they are able to effectively cope with these experiences as long as they know someone they care about will be there to support them. Dying can be viewed as another new experience, which they are able to cope with as long as they know they will have someone with them. If the parents are unable to relate to a child because of their grief, a nurse may need to step in and fill the gap (Fig. 56.3).

Many children associate death with sleep, so they may be afraid to fall asleep without someone near them and will need to have you sit with them while they fall asleep. They may need the light left on at night because they associate death with darkness. Considering how busy a unit nurses' station can be, a child who is dying may be moved to the end of the hallway, away from the nurses' station. However, this further isolates both a child who needs support and the child's parents, who also need your support and your presence nearby. Advocate as necessary for both the child and the parents so they can have continued interaction not just with each other but also with outside sources.

Adolescents

During adolescence, the capacity to think in abstract terms grows and an adolescent has a realistic perspective on death. However, adolescents have an unrealistic view of their own mortality and see themselves as invincible. Risky activities such as driving at high speeds reflect this judgment. They may deny symptoms that reveal their condition is worsening for longer than you'd expect because they believe it is impossible that anything serious could be happening to them. They appreciate time provided for discussion of how they have contributed to their family or community while their own death is imminent. Continuing to participate in favorite activities helps them maintain a sense of control.

Figure 56.3 A one-to-one nursing relationship helps children with terminal illnesses to not feel deserted.

QSEN Checkpoint Question 56.3

QUALITY IMPROVEMENT

Charlie, 3 years old, asks the nurse what it feels like to die. Keeping in mind the goal to improve the way sensitive topics are discussed with children, which response by the nurse is best?
a. "I think it's like going into a long white tunnel."
b. "It doesn't hurt if you're worrying about that."
c. "Everything probably goes black like it does at night."
d. "Why are you asking a question about dying?"

Look in Appendix A for the best answer and rationale.

ENVIRONMENT FOR DEATH

The environment in which children die can influence their and their family's acceptance of death.

The Hospital

A number of children die each year in emergency departments from unintentional injuries such as automobile accidents or from severe infections (Allareddy, Anderson, Lee, et al., 2015). Children with a terminal illness have many medical needs (e.g., a new tracheotomy, lung ventilation), and their complex medical care may necessitate they remain in an acute care setting. Their family may not have the skills or resources to manage the complex medical needs at home. In a hospital setting, be certain that visiting hours are adequately extended for parents and other family members so that children are not left alone when they need people around the most. Be certain also that children have opportunities to maintain contact with peers.

The Home

Today, most children with terminal illnesses are not kept in the hospital when it is determined that therapy is no longer effective. Many families prefer that their child die at home, surrounded by family and familiar possessions rather than in a hospital. Time spent discussing arrangements—such as who the parents should contact if the child suddenly decompensates, how they will manage periodic checkups, or how they will purchase medicine or supplies—is important preparation for home care. Assess how the family will schedule leisure time so they can balance the care of the ill child and their self-care.

Including safeguards in the home plan of care will involve interventions for caregivers' emotional and physical health (discussed further in Chapter 4).

The Hospice

In 1967, St. Christopher's Hospice in London opened as a facility for people who wanted to die in a homelike setting while still receiving skilled professional health care. Most large communities today have hospice settings, although places specifically for children, and especially infants, are still not available in many communities (Price, Dornan, & Quail, 2012).

In a hospice, friends, family, and even younger children and pets are allowed unlimited visiting. Children are invited to bring possessions with them that are important to them. They are given choices regarding the degree of pain relief they want. Strong analgesia is often used to make a child pain free.

The philosophy of hospice care is that death is an extension or part of life, not a separate entity; therefore, it can be accepted not with separate or awkward rituals but with the same warm concern as other situations in everyday life. For many children, hospice care is furnished as part of home care so that they are not separated from their families (Robert, Zhukovsky, Mauricio, et al., 2012).

QSEN Checkpoint Question 56.4

TEAMWORK & COLLABORATION

Charlie's parents were told by his medical care team that he was going to die, but he doesn't. What is an unexpected consequence of anticipatory grieving a nurse would want their nursing colleagues to know when planning subsequent care for the family?

    a. It will have minimal effect because he did not die.
    b. It could disrupt the parents' relationship with Charlie.
    c. It teaches the child that heathcare providers can be wrong.
    d. It breaks the parents' confidence in healthcare procedures.

Look in Appendix A for the best answer and rationale.

PREPARATION FOR A NURSING ROLE WITH DYING CHILDREN AND THEIR FAMILIES

End-of-life care for children can be an emotionally distressing experience for healthcare providers as well as family members (Forster & Hafiz, 2015). Although it is best that nursing assignments be consistent so a child has meaningful support, there is a point at which a healthcare provider may need a respite from caring for the child or providing support for the parents.

Self-Awareness

Before you can offer support to children in any circumstance, be aware of your own reactions and feelings. To offer support to a child who is dying, one must recognize their own feelings, values, and beliefs about death of children.

Fear

Fear is a natural response to death, and to overcome this fear, it should be put into perspective. In nursing, you care for many people who have illnesses and experiences you will never have, so caring for people with experiences beyond your own is not really strange but almost routine.

People who have never seen someone die may fear the moment of death and how they will respond to it. People who were declared dead and then resuscitated by heroic measures report that death was not at all frightening but actually involved a feeling of exceptional calm and comfort; people have reported afterward they wished they had been allowed to die rather than being called back to their body because death seemed so appealing (Facco & Agrillo, 2012).

Failure

Some healthcare professionals find themselves drawing back from caring for dying children because death symbolizes failure to them. Remind yourself that death is the ultimate outcome for everyone. At the point that death becomes unpreventable, the only failure that can exist is the failure of healthcare professionals to help a child die with dignity and consideration and free of pain.

Grief

Nursing care is so intense that the relationship formed between a nurse and a child may be closer than you realize until a child is diagnosed as having a terminal illness or dies and only then do you experience the depth of the relationship. Because nurses develop such close bonds with terminally ill children, they may experience profound grief when a child dies or no longer requires their care. The grief that accompanies caring for dying children can be broken down into the same stages of grief experienced by the children themselves when they learn they are dying.

Denial

There is a danger that a nurse who is in a stage of denial may care for children without mentioning they have more than a simple illness. This includes omitting the use of such common expressions as "How are you this morning?" to avoid having to hear the answer. Denial may be so extensive that you avoid going into a child's room unless an important procedure must be done. This is unfortunate because it can be confusing and lonely for children because they miss the normal exchange of conversation and contact. The moral distress felt by nurses after the death of a child to whom they felt close may result in them reevaluating the profession and whether they want to continue this career.

Anger

Anger may be intense when a young child dies because the death seems so unfair. Feelings of anger cause difficulty in offering effective care. Anger also clouds nursing judgment, such as to which analgesic would be best to administer or whether a change in vital signs is important. It is disappointing from a child's perspective because dying children may not fully grasp the anger in caregivers and identify its origin. They may feel lonely and perhaps feel guilty that they caused this anger.

Bargaining

Caregivers begin to bargain for life, just as children do. A statement such as "If Tommy just makes it through the weekend while I'm off, I'll spend all my extra time with him next week" is a bargaining statement. Bargains of this kind are easy to overlook in your coworkers or yourself. Listening for them helps you to evaluate when a fellow worker is having difficulty caring for a particular child and perhaps needs a change in assignments. Hearing yourself express these sentiments should alert you that you may be more involved with a child than you perhaps have realized. It's a warning that you need to talk to someone about your feelings or ask for help. Remember that when bargaining fails, people reach their lowest point in grief. Recognizing bargaining statements in yourself, therefore, helps you prepare for the sadness that may follow.

Depression

Nurses who enter this phase may be ineffective caregivers because depression may cloud judgment and result in inadequate problem-solving skills. It's easy for nurses to make unwise decisions in their personal lives as a result of the ineffective problem solving.

Depression is twice as destructive because when you are depressed, your reasoning processes are so distorted that you lose the ability to recognize that depression is the problem. When caring for a child who is expected to die, monitor your behavior to see if you are following your usual pattern. If irregularities occur (e.g., changes in sleeping pattern or loss of appetite), assess whether depression may be the underlying cause. If you feel you are depressed, try to make no major decisions for at least a week or you may find later you have made an unwise, irreversible decision.

Acceptance

The average person can reach a stage of acceptance in grief because people are subjected to few true losses in a lifetime. A nurse on a unit, where many terminally ill children come for care, may find him or herself facing loss or death repeatedly. Therefore, a stage of acceptance may not be reached fully. A caregiver who cannot reach a stage of acceptance is left in a stage of distress and may have difficulty functioning.

To achieve a stage of acceptance, you may need to modify your perspective. You may not be able to accept the unfairness of death in children, but you can accept your ability to offer care that facilitates death with dignity and compassion and maintains quality of life. It is important for parents to take care of their own emotional health, and they will improve their ability to care for others as they nurture themselves and their child.

What If . . . 56.3

A nurse has been caring for Charlie for an extended period. Would the nurse feel grief over Charlie's condition? How might this grief be expressed?

Caring for the Dying Child

A child may live for days, weeks, or even months at the end-of-life stage. Attentive physical and emotional care is essential for a child to maintain a sense of security and positive self-esteem during this time. It is also essential to assess if parents are coping well if this period is prolonged. Frequent and substantive communication is a major part of providing this care. Children, like their parents, need the opportunity to talk about their fears and feelings about death. Practicing good communication skills when providing any care such as when administering pain medication, starting intravenous lines, or providing basic comfort measures such as a bath help to establish a trusting relationship with the child, hopefully making the child feel more comfortable about openly sharing their feelings with you (Fig. 56.4). Box 56.6 provides some specific guidelines about communicating with a child who is dying.

The Child's Family

For many children, terminal illness involves a series of hospital admissions interspersed with ambulatory care or home

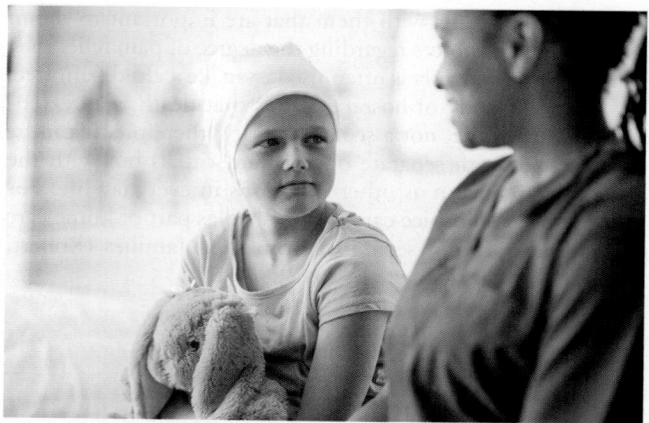

Figure 56.4 Good communication skills help build a trusting relationship, allowing a child to share feelings about being terminally ill. (iStock.com/FatCamera)

visits. Parents need time during these visits to talk about the problems they are having, not only with physical care (e.g., Should the child attend regular school? Could he come on vacation? How many times a day are we supposed to give the immunosuppressant?) but also about how it feels to live with a child who is dying (e.g., How should they answer the child's

---

BOX 56.6

Nursing Care Planning to Establish Therapeutic Relationships

MEASURES TO HELP COMMUNICATION WITH CHILDREN WHO ARE TERMINALLY ILL

1. *Continue active conversation.* Children who are dying need to be stimulated and kept engaged.
2. *Use moments of silence therapeutically.* Such moments occur normally. Do not feel obligated to chatter to fill quiet intervals. Silence allows for processing and reflection.
3. *Use the words "death" and "dying" as appropriate in conversation.* Trying to avoid a word makes interchanges awkward. The word "death" or "dying" can be mentioned without hesitation in sentences as appropriate.
4. *Preserve dying children's defenses.* If they are using denial or bargaining, do not try to push them to the next step of grieving by confrontation. Children will move on to the next step when they are psychologically ready.
5. *Terminally ill children may feel more vulnerable at night.* They may be comforted by having someone sit beside them until they fall asleep.
6. *Be supportive, not trite.* A statement such as "All of us are dying" is true but not helpful. A supportive statement such as "This must be hard for you" is more appropriate.
7. *Be aware that not all people's beliefs are the same as yours.* Statement such as "God works in mysterious ways," which may explain death for the person saying it, may evoke an angry response from you. People grieve and react to grief in many different ways.

or siblings' questions about death?). Although many parents are reluctant to tell a child that he is dying, this is probably the soundest course once the child can see that his or her condition is deteriorating because there is often less anxiety in knowing what is happening than in hearing people whispering or spelling out words.

If a child with a chronic illness experiences an exacerbation of the disease, parents may again begin an anticipatory grief reaction: anger, bargaining, depression, and acceptance. The process will be cut short by improvement, only to begin again at the next exacerbation. For this reason, the parents of a child who is being admitted to the hospital for the 12th time for a fatal illness may be in the same stage of grief as the parents of a child with a newly diagnosed fatal illness.

During health supervision visits, ask parents how other children in the family are managing. The parents may need to be reminded that, although the dying child does need a lot of their time, other children find this illness in a sibling just as baffling as the parents. When the ill child dies, siblings need the same active support to help them grieve (Siegel, Alpert, & Goldstein, 2011).

QSEN Checkpoint Question 56.5

EVIDENCE-BASED PRACTICE

Helping parents survive the death of a child can be a challenging experience in nursing. Two hundred parents were studied to investigate what parents believe their role is when caring for seriously ill children. The study concluded that parents saw their role as ensuring their child felt loved, followed by focusing on the child's health, making informed medical care decisions, and advocating for their child with medical staff (Feudtner, Walter, Faerber, et al., 2015).

Based on this study, which action would probably give Charlie's mother the most satisfaction with his end-of-life care?

a. Participating in keeping him clean and comfortable
b. Being allowed to inspect his health record on a regular basis
c. Interacting with the nursing staff on a personal or friendly level
d. Providing counseling to other parents on the unit

Look in Appendix A for the best answer and rationale.

The Onset of Death

As death nears in children, physiologic changes, such as slowed metabolism, decreased cell oxygenation, and cell dysfunction, begin to occur, thus changing children's appearance.

Stroke volume of the heart decreases, so the power to circulate blood is reduced. The child's skin feels cool and may appear mottled or cyanotic because blood can no longer be pushed to distal sites. Just before death, blood begins to pool in dependent body parts, making them appear purple. As circulation fails, absorption of a drug from a muscle becomes virtually impossible; if emergency drugs need to be administered, they need to be injected intravenously or often don't have an effect.

As peripheral circulation fails, less heat is lost from the body and the internal temperature rises. The child's body compensates for this by increased perspiration to increase heat loss through evaporation. This makes the child's skin feel cool and damp. You may need to change linens frequently because of the increased moisture on the skin. Because perfusion of distal body parts is impaired, turn the child slowly to allow the circulatory system to accommodate to the change in position.

Slowed respirations lead to increased secretions in the lungs and the appearance of rales, the sound of air being pulled through fluid in the alveoli. To compensate for a few minutes of very slow respirations, a child may take several quick or extremely deep inhalations periodically. Be certain the child's chest is not compressed so that the child has optimal lung expansion to do this.

A decrease in muscular function leads to severe weakness and fatigue. More and more, children maintain the exact position into which they were placed. As the throat muscles become lax, the possibility of aspiration increases. Offer only a small amount of oral fluid until you're certain the child's swallowing reflex is intact before offering a full glass. If the gag or swallowing reflex is impaired, position the child on the side to allow saliva to drain from the mouth to prevent aspiration.

A loss of consciousness occurs as children grow closer and closer to death, although they may remain perfectly alert until seconds before death. Vision apparently blurs because children tend to turn their head toward a light. Touch seems to remain intact as they often quiet to a gentle stroking of the arm or shoulder, and they will grasp your hand meaningfully, as if touch is appreciated and felt. Because hearing is one of the last senses lost, you may need to remind family members and, on occasion, other healthcare personnel, that the child may not be able to respond but may be able to hear. Continue to explain procedures to unconscious children as if they were conscious because they undoubtedly do hear you. Never make any comment in their presence that you would not make if they were alert. Continue to use the same gentle touch and nonverbal communication motions, such as holding a hand or brushing hair from the forehead as if children were fully conscious because they may be fully aware of your actions even though they can give no indication of it.

Another body function that slows is digestion as total body metabolism slows. Constipation because of poor bowel tone and decreased peristaltic action will occur. The abdomen may become distended from intestinal flatus. Dehydration with dry mucous membranes and conjunctivae will occur unless intravenous fluid replacement is initiated. Mouth dryness will lead to cracking, secondary infection, and pain; prevent this by frequently cleaning the mucous membrane with clear water and with the application of an ointment to the lips. If the conjunctivae appear dry, ask for a prescription of moistening eye drops, and keep any crusting at the eyelids washed away so that optimal vision is possible.

Be certain to keep skin surfaces from rubbing against one another by using supportive pillows and good positioning. Keep the skin free of urine or feces from incontinence to prevent painful ulcers. These are concerns in that are due to the decreased peripheral blood perfusion. Assess for indications of pain (e.g., thrashing, moaning) and provide relief with appropriate comfort measures.

QSEN Checkpoint Question 56.6

SAFETY

Children's body functions grow increasingly weaker as death approaches. What safety precaution would the nurse want to remember when caring for Charlie?

a. Children may aspirate easily as their gag reflex begins to fade.
b. Children who are unconscious cannot hear and so like the room quiet.
c. Turning and repositioning children can cause more harm than good.
d. To help them cope, you should avoid asking parents to give any final care.

Look in Appendix A for the best answer and rationale.

Documentation of Death

Defining when death occurs is controversial and involves both legal and ethical issues. As a child nears death, ethical committees may be used to assist families in decision making. Signs of death in a child not receiving ventilatory or mechanical assistance are the same as in adults:

- Absence of respirations
- No audible heart sounds by stethoscope
- No pulse by palpation
- No apparent blood pressure
- Absence of body movement or reflexes
- Dilated, fixed pupils

Death is officially determined by a lack of receptivity and responsivity, no spontaneous muscular movement or breath, no reflex response, and a flat electroencephalogram—again, the same as in adults.

Organ Donation

Parents may be asked by their primary healthcare provider or by a specifically designated transplantation team before a child's death to grant permission for body organs to be transplanted into other children after death occurs (Weiss, Hornby, Witteman, et al., 2016).

This is particularly important for liver and kidney transplants because it is difficult to transplant adult-size organs into children. If parents decide to allow organ donation, document this information on the child's electronic record and alert the primary care provider about the decision. When death does occur, the child's body will be maintained on life support to ensure that the organ remains perfused until it can be removed. The donation of body organs is not something that all parents can agree to, but it can help parents who choose the option to accept their child's death more easily because it allows them to feel that their child has helped another person live. Donating their child's organs is not a practice for everyone (Siebelink, Albers, Roodbol, et al., 2012).

Aftercare

Before beginning any aftercare for a child who has died in a healthcare facility or at home, check with family members to see if they want to spend a few minutes with the child or if there are any religious rites they want to complete before the body is transported to the morgue or funeral parlor. Some parents need

this time for closure. Some people have special prayers or traditions and rituals they need to follow; others want to say a final, private goodbye. Check that the child's bed and room is orderly before you ask a family whether they would like to spend some time in the room, particularly if the death was following an unsuccessful resuscitation attempt.

Remain in the room with the family in case they need your support, but be unobtrusive. Some parents fear touching a child's body after death, but touch is a strong and intimate gesture that a family member may need to be encouraged to make. Some parents may seem unable to leave the room or to let go of the child's hand. It may be necessary for you to gradually separate their hands while showing empathy for what they are experiencing. This helps parents begin to accept the fact that, in more than a physical sense, it is time to let go.

Crying is helpful for parents. You may need to reassure them that crying is not a sign of weakness but a normal response to a loved one's death. Do not, however, interpret a lack of tears as a lack of feeling because crying is not everyone's response to death. It is not unprofessional for nurses to cry when a child dies. A parent's warmest memory of a hospital experience may be that a nurse cried as she said goodbye to their child—the implication being the child made an important impact on people other than the family.

Autopsy Permission

State laws vary, but generally, if a child's death is a result of homicide, suicide, death within 24 hours after a hospital admission, suspected harmful death, or death in an institution or home where the child was not under the care of a primary healthcare provider, an autopsy is required by law and parents have no input regarding whether this is done or not. In other instances, it would be helpful to medical progress or to research if an autopsy could be done. In these instances, parents must give permission for this. Parents may refuse to allow an autopsy for a child, believing that doing so will protect the child from any more hurt or because of spiritual convictions. Autopsies advance medical science, so they should be done if at all possible; however, parents have every right to refuse permission without being made to feel guilty for their actions, so you may need to advocate for them.

What If . . . 56.4

A nurse is particularly interested in exploring one of the 2020 National Health Goals related to chronic or terminal illness in children (see Box 56.1). What would be a possible research topic pertinent to this goal that would be applicable to Charlie's family and that would also advance evidence-based practice?

KEY POINTS FOR REVIEW

- Children with long-term illnesses need continual reassessment because, like all children, their needs change as they grow older. Larger doses of medicine may become necessary or additional muscle-strengthening exercises may be necessary.
- Factors that make it easier for parents to accept a long-term illness in a child include having support people present and being told about the child's condition as early as possible.
- Long-term illness in a child is often most difficult for parents to accept at times when the child would have been achieving specific milestones of development such as a time that would

have been the first day of school for the child. Extra support for both the parents and the child may be necessary during these challenging times not only because it meets QSEN competencies but also because it meets a family's needs.

- Help children with a long-term disorder to do as much care for themselves as possible within the limits of their illness. Self-care empowers them to be as independent as possible.

- Children are about 9 years old before they are able to understand the meaning of death and that it is permanent. A child and parents can be expected to move through the stages of grief (denial, anger, bargaining, depression, and acceptance) on learning about a potentially fatal diagnosis.

- Children and parents are apt to need help to face a terminal diagnosis in a child. Urge the parents and the child to ask for help to see them through this very difficult time in their lives.

CRITICAL THINKING CARE STUDY

"Skater" is a 16-year-old gang member you meet in the emergency room. He is unconscious from a gunshot wound to his head, which was suffered while he was robbing a convenience store. The police officer who accompanied the ambulance tells you Skater was shot by the store owner. A fellow gang member tells you Skater shot himself to keep from being arrested.

1. Skater was diagnosed with autism spectrum disorder when he was 4 years old. He dropped out of school last year because "he didn't like being told what to do." If you were assigned to accompany him to the X-ray department for a cranial magnetic resonance imaging (MRI), would you need to explain to him what is happening (he doesn't like instructions and he's unconscious)?

2. Skater's mother rushes into the emergency room and describes her son as "a precious child" whom she wants to live. His older brother describes him as "nothing but trouble his whole life" and adds that the family would be better off if Skater died. Would these conflicting opinions affect your care? Would the dispute over whether he was shot or shot himself influence care?

3. Skater's mother and sibling seem to have totally different opinions about the effect Skater has had on his family, probably based on actions related to him being autistic. Why do you suppose these two people have formed such different opinions of Skater?

RELATED RESOURCES

Explore these additional resources to enhance learning for this chapter:
- Student resources on thePoint, including answers to the What If . . . and Critical Thinking Care Study questions, http://thepoint.lww.com/Flagg8e
- Adaptive learning powered by PrepU, http://thepoint.lww.com/prepu

REFERENCES

Allareddy, V., Anderson, I. M., Lee, M. K., et al. (2015). Hospital-based emergency department visits in children with motor vehicle traffic accidents: Estimates from the nationwide emergency department sample. *World Journal of Pediatrics, 11*(3), 261–266.

Bogle, A. M., & Go, S. (2015). Breaking bad (news) death-telling in the emergency department. *Missouri Medicine, 112*(1), 12–16.

Braga, S. F., & Almgren, M. M. (2013). Complementary therapies in cystic fibrosis: Nutritional supplements and herbal products. *Journal of Pharmacy Practice, 26*(1), 14–17.

Crosland, K., & Dunlap, G. (2012). Effective strategies for the inclusion of children with autism in general education classrooms. *Behavior Modification, 36*(3), 251–269.

Erikson, E. (1993). *Childhood and society* (3rd ed.). New York, NY: W.W. Norton.

Facco, E., & Agrillo, C. (2012). Near-death experiences between science and prejudice. *Frontiers in Human Neuroscience, 6*, 209.

Feudtner, C., Walter, J., Faerber, J., et al. (2015). Good-parent beliefs of parents of seriously ill children. *JAMA Pediatrics, 169*(1), 39–47.

Fisher, H., & Crawley, E. (2013). Why do young people with CFS/ME feel anxious? A qualitative study. *Clinical Child Psychology & Psychiatry, 18*(4), 556–573.

Forster, E., & Hafiz, A. (2015). Paediatric death and dying: Exploring coping strategies of health professional and perceptions of support provisions. *International Journal of Palliative Nursing, 21*(6), 294–301.

Green, M., & Solnit, A. (1964). Reactions to the threatened loss of a child: A vulnerable child syndrome. Pediatric management of the dying child, part III. *Pediatrics, 34*, 58–66.

Kirk, S., Beatty, S., Callery, P., et al. (2012). Perceptions of effective self-care support for children and young people with long-term conditions. *Journal of Clinical Nursing, 21*(13–14), 1974–1987.

Kübler-Ross, E. (1969). *On death and dying*. New York, NY: Macmillan.

Longden, J. V. (2011). Parental perceptions of end-of-life care on paediatric intensive care units: A literature review. *Nursing Critical Care, 16*(3), 131–139.

Newton, K., & Lamarche, K. (2012). Take the challenge: Strategies to improve support for parents of chronically ill children. *Home Healthcare Nurse, 30*(5), E1–E8.

Nikkola, I., Kaunonen, M., & Aho, A. L. (2013). Mother's experience of the support from a bereavement follow-up intervention after the death of a child. *Journal of Clinical Nursing, 22*(7–8), 1151–1162.

Peacock, J., & Stanik-Hutt, J. (2013). Translating best care practices to improve nursing documentation regarding pediatric patients dependent on home mechanical ventilation and tracheostomy tube support: A quality improvement initiative. *Home Healthcare Nurse, 31*(1), 10–17.

Price, J., Dornan, J., & Quail, L. (2012). Seeing is believing—reducing misconceptions about children's hospice care through effective teaching with undergraduate nursing students. *Nurse Education in Practice, 13*(5), 361–365.

Robert, R., Zhukovsky, D. S., Mauricio, R., et al. (2012). Bereaved parents' perspectives on pediatric palliative care. *Journal of Social Work in End-of-Life & Palliative Care, 8*(4), 316–338.

Siebelink, M. J., Albers, M. J., Roodbol, P. F., et al. (2012). Children as donors: A national study to assess procurement of organs and tissues in pediatric intensive care units. *Transplant International, 25*(12), 1268–1274.

Siegel, B. S., Alpert, J. J., & Goldstein, R. (2011). Palliative care & end-of-life issues. In K. J. Marcdante, R. M. Kliegman, H. B. Jenson, et al. (Eds.), *Nelson essentials of pediatrics* (6th ed., pp. 8–12). Philadelphia, PA: Elsevier/Saunders.

St. Ledger, U., Begley, A., Reid, J., et al. (2012). Moral distress in end-of-life care in the intensive care unit. *Journal of Advanced Nursing, 69*(8), 1869–1880.

Thomas, S., & Price, M. (2012). Respite care in seven families with children with complex care needs. *Nursing Children and Young People, 24*(8), 24–27.

U.S. Department of Health and Human Services. (2010). *Healthy people 2020*. Washington, DC: Author.

Vermaes, I. P., van Susante, A. M., & van Bakel, H. J. (2012). Psychological functioning of siblings in families of children with chronic health conditions: A meta-analysis. *Journal of Pediatric Psychology, 37*(2), 166–184.

Weiss, M. J., Hornby, L., Witteman, W., et al. (2016). Pediatric donation after circulatory determination of death: A scoping review. *Pediatric Critical Care Medicine, 17*(3), e87–e108.

Wender, E. (2012). Supporting the family after the death of a child. *Pediatrics, 130*(6), 1164–1169.

Whittingham, K., Wee, D., Sanders, M. R., et al. (2013). Predictors of psychological adjustment, experienced parenting burden and chronic sorrow symptoms in parents of children with cerebral palsy. *Child: Care, Health & Development, 39*(2), 366–373.

Yang, B. H., Mu, P. F., & Wang, W. S. (2016). The experiences of families living with the anticipatory loss of a school-age child with spinal muscular atrophy—the parents perspectives. *Journal of Clinical Nursing, 25*(17–18), 2648–2657.

Answers to QSEN Checkpoint Questions

CHAPTER 1
A Framework for Maternal and Child Health Nursing

1.1 **C.** The nurse should inform the team members that a Magnet hospital is one that stresses exemplary nursing care. It does not necessarily denote care for acute patients. This designation is not conferred by the American Medical Association.

1.2 **C.** The nurse explains that the perinatal period is the time between 20 weeks of pregnancy and 4 to 6 weeks following birth.

1.3 **C.** The trend toward quality improvement through technology can become overwhelming for families if nursing support is not included in care. Premature infants require extensive care, and there are no immunizations for all childhood diseases. Nursing is predicted to maintain an important role in health care.

1.4 **A.** The nurse should assess if Mr. Chung is open to trying skin-to-skin contact with his newborn. Skin-to-skin contact is important for newborns and may help fathers bond with their infants. It would be incorrect to withhold this until after discharge.

1.5 **B.** The nurse should acknowledge the patient's concerns while affirming her efforts rather than downplaying her concerns or providing false assurance.

1.6 **D.** The nurse should explain that consent is required for all patients regardless of age and the amount of pain involved in the procedure and can be given by telephone or e-mail for long distance consultation.

CHAPTER 2
Diversity and Maternal Child Nursing

2.1 **B.** The nurse assessing a family's structure and decision-making norms is a component of culturally competent care. These patterns of behavior differ significantly between cultures. Nurses should avoid assumptions that may border on being stereotypes, such as equating a preference for tacos with a patient who is Hispanic.

2.2 **A.** The nurse should encourage the care provider to communicate as naturally and clearly as possible; imitating Maria's accent is inappropriate. There is no particular need to avoid pop culture references if these are contextually appropriate.

2.3 **D.** It is important for the nurse to avoid interactions between home remedies and prescribed medicine. For the nurse to use the words "you people" is a term of disrespect.

2.4 **B.** It would be discriminatory for the nurse to presume that Maria will not "fit in" by virtue of her ethnicity.

2.5 **D.** The nurse respecting food choices is a way of respecting cultural diversity. The nurse addressing the taste of the food does not focus on Maria's concerns.

2.6 **B.** The nurse should reinforce the results of the study and state that "Children raised in same-sex parent houses do just as well as children raised with different sex parents." Questioning whether Sofia will be a good parent based on sexual orientation, defining the situation as a challenge to raising a child, or assuming the child needs a male figure is disrespectful to the family structure.

CHAPTER 3
The Childbearing and Childrearing Family in the Community

3.1 **B.** The nurse should address that fact that because women earn less than men and single-parent families are usually headed by women, finances are a common concern. Communication, emotional engagement, and education are not necessarily lacking as often.

3.2 **B.** The nurse should be aware that the person who allows information in or out of a family is the gatekeeper.

3.3 **D.** The nurse knows that the oldest child marks a family stage; because the Hanovans' oldest child is 17 years of age, they are at a family with an adolescent stage.

3.4 **D.** The nurse should teach parents that automobile accidents are a major cause of death in adolescents. Rates of such accidents exceed those among younger children.

3.5 **B.** The nurse should ensure the parents are aware that teenagers need responsible adult supervision in both custodial settings. It would be inappropriate for the nurse to suggest shared custody, to suggest quitting work, or to assume that the situation will be independently resolved.

3.6 **C.** The nurse should teach parents that the AAP recommends television viewing be restricted until a child is 2 years of age to reduce exposure to violence and stimulate language development.

CHAPTER 4
Home Care and the Childbearing and Childrearing Family

4.1 **C.** The nurse could suggest that Lisa needs a sedentary activity to interact with friends. Shouting for basketball teams or joining in with cheerleading would contradict bed rest. She is unable to safely go on outings due to her activity restriction. Journaling does not meet her socialization needs.

4.2 **A.** The nurse's first visit will involve gathering a health history, so having a parent present would be helpful. The nurse should not dictate a time because this is not an effective way to empower or involve a patient in planning care.

4.3 **D.** The nurse should always call for help if he or she feels in danger. Leaving the home would leave the patient still in danger. Changing the locks would not solve the immediate problem. It is difficult and often unsafe to reason with angry people.

4.4 **A.** The nurse should assure Lisa that privacy rules apply to home care as well as hospital care; health records are not copyrighted.

4.5 **C.** The nurse should suggest drinking more fluid as an adequate fluid intake helps prevent constipation. Walking is contraindicated as Lisa is on bed rest. The size of meals or calcium intake shouldn't make a difference.

4.6 **A.** Lisa's community is probably safe enough for her to stay alone. The nurse should worry about the mother "trying to quit smoking" because it is not enough to prevent exposure to secondary smoke and toxic tobacco contaminants because smoke particles cling to clothing. If the mother "usually" smokes outside, then this implies that she is sometimes smoking in the home.

CHAPTER 5
The Nursing Role in Reproductive and Sexual Health

5.1 **C.** The nurse should teach the client that thelarche refers to breast development. Adrenarche is development of other secondary sex characteristics; menarche is the first menstrual period.

5.2 **C.** The nurse should state that because the vas deferens is easy to locate, it is the organ blocked/ligated for a vasectomy.

5.3 **D.** The nurse should explain that cystocele is herniation of the bladder into the vagina and can lead to urinary tract infection.

5.4 **D.** The nurse could help the patient calculate the ovulation date by teaching that ovulation usually occurs on the 14th day from the end of the menstrual cycle, or in this instance, 14 from 34 or on the 20th day.

CHAPTER 6
Nursing Care for the Family in Need of Reproductive Life Planning

6.1 **B.** The nurse should teach Dana that cervical mucus is thin and watery at ovulation. Subjective sensations of warmth, breast tenderness, and emotional lability are not safe and reliable indicators.

6.2 **B.** The nursing care plan for Dana should include teaching her that female condoms should be inserted before any sexual contact, they should not be reused, and they already contain a spermicide.

6.3 **D.** The nurse should have Dana report severe migraine headaches because they are a contraindication to COCs.

6.4 **B.** Intramuscular injections (DMPA) are associated with osteoporosis, so recommending a high calcium intake is important.

6.5 **A.** The nurse should teach Dana that tubal ligation is a minor surgical procedure in which the fallopian tubes are occluded by cautery, crushed, clamped, or blocked, thereby preventing passage of both sperm and ova.

6.6 **C.** Having access to multiple methods, reliable methods, and highly effective methods of birth control caused a 36% decrease in the pregnancy rate among adolescents from 2007 to 2012. Teens were not likely to decrease sexual activity or more likely to use abortion. Although community influence may play a role in the rates of adolescent pregnancy, that was not measured in this study.

CHAPTER 7
Nursing Care of the Family Having Difficulty Conceiving a Child

7.1 **C.** The nurse should state that a year is the typical time to wait as, after trying to conceive unsuccessfully for 1 year, a couple is said to be subfertile. Acknowledging the reality of regretting a decision does not directly address her concerns.

7.2 **C.** The nurse should remind couples with reduced fertility that just because they are no longer using a contraceptive method, they still need to follow safer sex precautions.

7.3 **A.** Patient teaching should include the fact that mild cramping may occur during the procedure. X-ray is not used; no bleeding should result.

7.4 **D.** The nurse should document endometriosis on the health record because this condition can affect fertility by blocking fallopian tubes and interfering with sperm or ovum transport.

7.5 **C.** The nurse should state that patients who are to undergo intrauterine insemination receive an injection of clomiphene (Clomid) or FSH 1 month prior to the procedure. Estrogen, bedrest, and genetic testing are not indicated.

7.6 **C.** The nurse should tell Cheryl that women begin breastfeeding effectively but may need additional support to continue it long term. Telling someone to not worry is not effective counseling. IVF does not preclude normal breastfeeding.

CHAPTER 8
The Nursing Role in Genetic Assessment and Counseling

8.1 **D.** The nurse providing health information in a relevant and appropriate manner is an important component of high-quality care. False hope must be avoided. Journals and websites are not substitutes for health education provided by nurses and may not meet Amy's learning needs.

8.2 **D.** The nurse should recommend that in order for Mrs. Alvarez to make an informed choice about her future, talking to other parents might be helpful. False hope should be avoided, and the nurse's own personal views are not relevant.

8.3 **B.** The nurse should inform team members that infants with Down syndrome have one palm crease instead of the usual three. Babies tend to be hypotonic, not hypertonic. Sole creases are an indication of any mature fetus.

CHAPTER 9
Nursing Care During Normal Pregnancy and Care of the Developing Fetus

9.1 **D.** The nurse should state to team members that the baby is an embryo during the period between implantation and 5 to 8 weeks. After that, it is a fetus.

9.2 **B.** The nurse's assessment findings of a normal umbilical cord would be one vein and two arteries. Other patterns are associated with cardiac or chromosomal disorders.

9.3 **A.** The nurse should explain that surfactant, a phospholipid substance, is formed and excreted by the alveolar cells of the lungs beginning at approximately the 24th week of pregnancy. This decreases alveolar surface tension on expiration, preventing alveolar collapse and improving the infant's ability to maintain respirations in the outside environment at birth.

9.4 **A.** The study reveals alcohol consumption, low socioeconomic status, and depression contribute to smoking. The nurse should counsel the client regarding the effects of smoking and alcohol on the fetus.

9.5 **C.** The nurse should teach that a full bladder improves the accuracy of the scan. There is no pain involved.

9.6 **A.** If the client is having the amniocentesis after week 20 of pregnancy, the nurse should ensure the client voids prior to the amniocentesis to prevent puncturing the bladder.

CHAPTER 10
Nursing Care Related to Psychological and Physiologic Changes of Pregnancy

10.1 **A.** The nurse is aware that women in the study reacted both positively and negatively at the thought of a second pregnancy. Lauren's paradoxical response represents this.

10.2 **B.** The nurse counsels Lauren that ensuring safe passage for the fetus consists of accepting the pregnancy (first trimester), accepting the coming baby (second trimester), and preparing for parenthood (third trimester).

10.3 **C.** The nurse would tell the unlicensed care provider that narcissism refers to interest in yourself in contrast to interest in others.

10.4 **D.** The nurse should teach that the three positive signs of pregnancy are fetal heartbeat heard by examiner or seen on sonogram and fetal movement felt by examiner.

10.5 **D.** The nurse should explain that Chadwick's sign is a color change in the vagina from pink to purple because of increased formation of blood vessels and blood flow.

10.6 **A.** The nurse should state that with insulin becoming ineffective, glucose levels rise, serving to safeguard the fetus from hypoglycemia. Maternal insulin does not cross the placenta.

CHAPTER 11
Nursing Care Related to Assessment of a Pregnant Family

11.1 **C.** The nurse should explain that the odds of experiencing a medication-free birth are far higher when a nurse-midwife leads care. It is inaccurate to characterize nurse-midwives as always being more "patient-friendly," and it is not appropriate to wholly defer teaching or advice when the patient initiates.

11.2 **C.** The nurse should state that prenatal care is a prime time for health education; during this time, nurses play an important role in effective prenatal care. Ultimately, this promotes safe pregnancy, labor, and delivery. This is more important than collecting statistical data or promoting social interaction. Allergies are not correlated with preterm labor. Despite the patient's wishes, regular prenatal care should be strongly encouraged.

11.3 **B.** The nurse should ask Sandra about past surgery because surgery such as for appendicitis can leave adhesions, which then might interfere with uterine growth. Risks of uterine rupture and preterm labor are not higher in women with a surgical history.

11.4 **D.** The nurse should teach that palmar erythema commonly occurs from increasing estrogen levels. It is not a result of Rh incompatibility, edema, or anxiety.

11.5 **D.** The nurse should know that relaxation is important to reduce pain with a pelvic examination and teach her to breathe slowly and evenly when being examined. Holding the breath or pushing down on the diaphragm does not relax abdominal muscles.

11.6 **C.** The nurse should have Sandra report a weight gain more than 3 lb a week during the second trimester as this would be a potential sign of gestational hypertension. The other listed changes do not constitute safety risks.

CHAPTER 12
Nursing Care to Promote Fetal and Maternal Health

12.1 **C.** The nurse should teach Julberry that she can still contact a sexually transmitted infection, so she still needs to use precautions. However, a condom would not tear the membranes. Julberry's other responses reflect a sound understanding or self-care during pregnancy.

12.2 **A.** The nurse should recognize that jogging is not recommended during pregnancy because the extra weight of the pregnancy can cause knee injuries. The other health promotion statements are accurate.

12.3 **C.** The nurse assesses that all of the things Julberry describes are concerns, but it is the accumulation of symptoms that apparently leads to depression.

12.4 **D.** The nurse should counsel Julberry to use witch hazel as it feels cool and may shrink hemorrhoids. Mineral oil is contraindicated because it prevents absorption of vitamin A; eating fiber should not be omitted because it is helpful in preventing constipation; she can't lie on her stomach because she is pregnant.

12.5 **C.** The nurse would recognize that Julberry has read the correct information on ankle edema. Ankle edema is a common occurrence in pregnancy and occurs from increased pressure on lower extremity veins. It can be relieved by resting with feet elevated.

12.6 **C.** The nurse should teach that pregnant women should check with their healthcare provider before taking medicine during pregnancy. All over-the-counter medicine is not safe; measles vaccine contains a live virus so is contraindicated during pregnancy.

CHAPTER 13
The Nursing Role in Promoting Nutritional Health During Pregnancy

13.1 **B.** The team should recommend that Tori gain 15 to 25 lb during her pregnancy because she is slightly overweight.

13.2 **D.** The nurse should confirm that iron is absorbed best from an acid medium. Crushing the pills or taking them with milk or carbonated beverages is not advised.

13.3 **C.** The nurse should recommend leafy green vegetables to eat during pregnancy. Leafy green vegetables are rich in many of the dietary components that are lacking women's diets. Protein, fiber, and iron are all important during pregnancy so should be encouraged. Dieting should normally be discouraged.

13.4 **C.** The assessment document should specify a 24-hour recall history to secure the most accurate nutrition pattern.

13.5 **A.** The nurse identifies eating erasers as a sign of pica. Some women report a craving for foods such as oranges or chocolate. Women with pica, however, crave a non-food substance, in this case, an eraser. Typically, these cravings include clay, dirt, cornstarch, or ice cubes.

13.6 **D.** The nurse would note that vitamin B_{12} is found only in animal sources and would be omitted in a vegetarian diet.

CHAPTER 14
Preparing a Family for Childbirth and Parenting

14.1 **D.** The nurse recognizes that the statement that best assures a workable birth plan is keeping the plan "flexible." Rigid expectations can lead to disappointment and anxiety. The partner's wishes are indeed secondary, but they should not be wholly rejected. Interventions such as opioids should not be included solely on the recommendation of a parent.

14.2 **B.** The nurse should suggest squatting or tailor sitting to tighten perineal muscles. Tightening and relaxing them (Kegel exercises) would also strengthen them. The nurse should not recommend vigorous exercise and bearing down forcefully as these actions carry safety risks.

14.3 **C.** The nurse should make Elena aware that women who give birth in upright positions have fewer obstetric and anal sphincter injuries. Voicing the fact that she is willing to try different positions should achieve this. Media presentations of labor are not always realistic.

14.4 **A.** The Lamaze philosophy is based on the gate control theory of pain perception, which states that pain sensations can be interrupted. This philosophy does not deny the reality of pain or the inevitability of pain during labor.

14.5 **D.** The nurse should teach that slow breathing is adequate for early contractions; a cleansing breath is always important. Hypoventilation is relieved by breathing into a paper bag. Rapid breathing is contraindicated.

14.6 **C.** The nurse should emphasize that emergency care is more readily available in a hospital setting than in other birth settings. Childbirth is not pain-free, and the cost of present-day hospital stays is typically high. Hospitals, like all birth settings, are not sterile environments.

CHAPTER 15
Nursing Care of a Family During Labor and Birth

15.1 **A.** The nurse is aware that an occipitoanterior position means the lie is cephalic—the back of the baby's head is facing the right anterior quadrant of the mother's pelvis. Full flexion means the smallest diameter of the fetal head is presenting to the cervix. This position is considered to be ideal and is most conducive to a healthy delivery that requires fewer interventions.

15.2 **D.** An important teaching point for Celeste would have been that cervical dilation is a mark of true labor. For the mucus plug to be loosened, cervical dilatation must be occurring.

15.3 **A.** The nurse should be most concerned that Celeste is "losing a grasp on things." In the study, a feeling of loss of control severely affected women's impressions of whether labor was traumatic or not.

15.4 **D.** The nurse should assure her that a placenta loosens quickly so waiting time will not be long. Pulling on the cord, pushing on the uterine fundus, or hard pushing could all cause additional bleeding. The placenta must normally be delivered spontaneously.

15.5 **B.** The nurse should report a contraction 70 seconds long as it is long enough to compromise fetal oxygenation. In the context of labor, pain is not necessarily indicative of pathophysiology.

15.6 **B.** The nurse would document FHR decreasing in rate 30 seconds after the start of a contraction as a late deceleration. A late deceleration means the FHR decreases as a contraction ends, rather than at the beginning of a contraction, as is usual.

CHAPTER 16
The Nursing Role in Providing Comfort During Labor and Birth

16.1   **C.** The nurse's best answer would be that a doula is a second support person in labor. She doesn't replace a woman's partner and does much more than time contractions. The use of a doula is an individual choice.

16.2   **D.** Based on the study, the nurse could confirm that music is best used in early labor to help a woman relax.

16.3   **C.** The nurse should recommend slow breathing. Slow breathing calls for concentration. Consequently, it can be used as a distraction technique. Women should not lie on their back during labor in order to prevent hypotension. Women should not hold their breath as long as possible, and rapid breathing should not be encouraged.

16.4   **B.** The nurse should state that warm water is comforting during labor; it may be contraindicated if membranes are ruptured because of the increased risk of infection.

16.5   **A.** The nurse should inform Jonny that peripheral relaxation can lead to systemic hypotension with epidural anesthesia. A slowed second stage of labor also may occur.

16.6   **C.** The nurse should have a drug to speed gastric emptying on hand in case of general anesthesia use. A drug to increase gastric emptying helps to avoid vomiting. The other listed drugs do not have this therapeutic effect.

CHAPTER 17
Nursing Care of a Postpartal Family

17.1   **C.** The taking-hold phase means a woman is interested in actively caring for her baby. The nurse should encourage her to participate in the care of her baby by bathing the baby. Telling her she did well or encouraging the naming of the baby does not help to usher in the taking-hold phase.

17.2   **A.** The nurse assesses that an "en face" position suggests she is interested in becoming acquainted with the newborn.

17.3   **A.** The nurse should teach Leana that tampons should not be used postpartum to help prevent infection.

17.4   **B.** If the uterine fundus does not grow firm with massage, extreme atony, possibly retained placenta fragments, or an excess amount of blood loss may be occurring; the nurse should notify the woman's primary care provider. A uterine fundus decreases in size at a rate of one fingerbreadth a day. The fundus should be located midline. Firm massage will result in pain, but this is not acceptable nursing practice.

17.5   **D.** The nurse worries about Leana's comment that the baby will sleep fine. This statement may suggest that Leana is unprepared for the fact that her infant may spend more time crying than sleeping. Her expectations for her own levels of rest may be unrealistic.

17.6   **B.** The nurse records that Leana's uterine fundus sinks below the symphysis pubis at about 10 days after birth. This is a normal finding.

CHAPTER 18
Nursing Care of a Family With a Newborn

18.1   **D.** The nurse is aware that conduction is the transfer of body heat to a cold object that touches the infant. Each of the other factors can result in heat loss, but none involves heat loss by conduction.

18.2   **C.** The nurse should lift the baby's head and allow it to fall back 1 in. to elicit a Moro reflex. This action best initiates a Moro reflex. Making a noise or shaking a crib is less effective way to test the reflex.

18.3   **A.** Using the apgar test, the nurse assesses heart rate, respiratory effort, muscle tone, reflex irritability, and color.

18.4   **A.** The nurse should advice Beth that milia spots will disappear on their own, so she doesn't need to take any action.

18.5   **C.** The nurse would confirm that a week is an average time for a dried cord to detach.

18.6   **C.** Shaking infants is potentially dangerous because it can cause head injury; the nurse educating about newborn abilities helps parents better understand a newborn reacts the way he or she does. This approach is likely more effective than the nurse immediately addressing shaken baby syndrome, which may be a premature and "heavy-handed" approach. A sedative is contraindicated with breastfeeding.

CHAPTER 19
Nutritional Needs of a Newborn

19.1   **A.** Nursing assessment of infant nutrition begins during pregnancy with assessment of the mother's and her partner's attitudes and choices about infant feeding. This is an important aspect of patient-centered care and should normally precede other assessments.

19.2   **A.** The nurse sees having prenatal care as an indication that Linda will successfully breastfeed. Prenatal care is associated with success at exclusive breastfeeding. Smoking, young age, and low income are negatively associated.

19.3   **B.** The nurse should teach Linda that breast milk provides not only nutrition but also aspects of immunity. Breastfeeding may reduce the risk of obesity but does not ensure the infant will never become obese. It does not necessarily prevent cancer.

19.4   **C.** The nurse determines that Linda stating that she should drink 12 glasses of fluid a day warrants further teaching. Drinking 12 glasses of fluid a day is extreme; 6 to 8 is a better recommendation.

19.5   **A, B, D.** The nurse should teach that breastfeeding exclusively for 6 months can reduce the risk of obesity later in life and decrease the risk of breast and ovarian cancer for the mother, and a pacifier can be used to decrease the risk of sudden infant death syndrome once breastfeeding is established. Formula feeding does not increase calcium density of the spine.

19.6   **D.** Educational literature should include the fact that discarding leftover milk discourages the growth of pathogens. The presence of yellowish stools is consistent with breast milk. A microwave should not be used to warm breast milk, and propping a bottle risks for aspiration.

CHAPTER 20
Nursing Care of a Family Experiencing a Pregnancy Complication From a Preexisting or Newly Acquired Illness

20.1 **C.** An appropriate nursing action for Angelina is allowing her to choose a subcutaneous site for the injection. Heparin is administered subcutaneously. Hemoglobin levels and WBC do not need to be monitored during therapy.

20.2 **C.** The nurse is alerted to the fact that the woman is taking an iron pill every day. Women with sickle-cell anemia are not prescribed iron pills during pregnancy because sickle cells are unable to incorporate as much iron in their structure as normal red cells. The woman's other statements reflect a sound understanding of sickle cell disease.

20.3 **C.** Nurses should emphasize that good perineal care, a generous fluid intake, wearing cotton underwear, and avoiding bath salts are common ways to avoid urinary tract infections so should be followed during pregnancy.

20.4 **A.** The nurse should alert care team members that because the fetus requires calcium to build bones, calcium-surrounded tuberculosis lesions can be activated if a woman doesn't ingest adequate calcium.

20.5 **B.** The nurse should explain that continuous insulin administration with no food intake can lead to hypoglycemia. Women should typically eat a high-protein/complex carbohydrate snack such as peanut butter and celery before bedtime to prevent fetal hypoglycemia from ingesting little food during the night.

20.6 **A.** The nurse should be concerned about Angelina wanting to "shed some pounds." Concerns about gaining weight and having to have a cesarean birth were the two factors most associated with depression following pregnancy with gestational diabetes. Wanting to "shed some pounds" is suggestive of earlier weight gain that is perceived as being excessive.

CHAPTER 21
Nursing Care of a Family Experiencing a Sudden Pregnancy Complication

21.1 **C.** The nurse should advise saving any clots or material passed to help the healthcare provider assess the amount of bleeding and whether the miscarriage process is incomplete or complete and allows them to be assessed for the possibility of gestational trophoblastic disease. A woman should not use a tampon, so the amount of bleeding she is having can be evaluated. Vaginal bleeding always needs to be investigated during pregnancy.

21.2 **B.** The nurse should check if Beverly received Rh immune globulin (RhIG or RhoGAM) because it is the medication used to minimize the risk of isoimmunization.

21.3 **C.** It is important for the nurse to assess for vaginal bleeding and clear fluid leakage every shift. Vaginal examinations are contraindicated as this procedure may cause bleeding. If the previa is not total, a cesarean birth may not be necessary.

21.4 **B.** The nurse identifies assessing FHR and whether she is having contractions as the best first actions. Walking stimulates contractions. Hydration, not dehydration, may reduce contractions.

21.5 **D.** The nurse recognizes that edema is often a first symptom of gestational hypertension a woman notes. The edema associated with gestational hypertension can be separated from the typical ankle edema of pregnancy because it begins to accumulate in the upper part of the body as well. Beverly's other statements are not necessarily indicative of gestational hypertension.

21.6 **B.** The nurse is aware that activities at work were not associated with development of hypertension of pregnancy. Not taking time to eat regularly could lead to fetal hypoglycemia and would be a significant concern that the nurse should address.

CHAPTER 22
Nursing Care of a Pregnant Family With Special Needs

22.1 **C.** The nurse should support Mindy in her attempts to take responsibility for her own care. Pregnant adolescents are emancipated minors so are capable of and appreciate support for making healthcare decisions. It would be unwise for the nurse to create a climate that would alienate the mother as, although an emancipated minor, Mindy will still need the support and help of her mother.

22.2 **C.** The nurse should check Mindy's lab results. Reticulocytes are immature red blood cells that will start to grow rapidly if sufficient iron is available. Mindy's oral report may or may not be reliable. Urine testing and assessment of her nail beds are not reliable indicators.

22.3 **D.** Nurses should be aware that gestational hypertension is caused by marked vasospasm and monitor women over the age of 40 years. Hypertension becomes even more acute if blood vessels have limited elasticity, as in older individuals.

22.4 **C.** It is imperative for the nurse to provide information that is appropriate to the patient's cognitive level. The patient herself must not be excluded from education. Written material is unlikely to be ideal.

22.5 **D.** The nurse should refer Mindy to addictions support services. Substance dependence is such an all-encompassing phenomenon, and such women need support from an interprofessional team because pregnancy is a long time to remain drug free. Toxicology testing will confirm the type of substance being abused but will not give Mindy support to quit. The nurse telling her to quit without providing support would be futile.

22.6 **B.** The nurse should halt bleeding by putting pressure on the edges of the laceration as the priority nursing action. This may be difficult to achieve in the lower extremities because venous pressure is so greatly increased in the legs during pregnancy. After cleansing and applying lidocaine, the area can be sutured through each layer of tissue involved to approximate the edges.

CHAPTER 23
Nursing Care of a Family Experiencing a Complication of Labor or Birth

23.1   **D.** It would be important for the nurse to document the characteristics of Rosann's contractions to see if they are irregular; even though ineffective, they are still painful so she needs pain relief.

23.2   **C.** The nurse would question her labor augmentation with oxytocin because with a large fetus cephalopelvic disproportion may be present. Amniocentesis, elevated blood pressure, and ruptured membranes do not contraindicate the use of oxytocin.

23.3   **C.** Discontinuing the oxytocin infusion would be the nurse's first step in the management of Rosann's change in labor progress. Turning to the left side and increasing fluid are second and third steps.

23.4   **D.** Although not evidence based, the nurse would want team members to know a hands-and-knees position appears to aid fetal occipital rotation more than the other listed positions.

23.5   **C.** The research results revealed an increase in shoulder dystocia, which can result in diaphragmatic paralysis. Because this affects breathing, it is the nurse's primary assessment taken after the birth.

CHAPTER 24
Nursing Care of a Family During a Surgical Intervention for Birth

24.1   **C.** A danger of amniotomy is that the fetal cord can prolapse which will interfere with fetal circulation. This makes the nurse's immediate assessment of the fetal heart rate important.

24.2   **A.** The urinary catheter inserted by the nurse will keep the bladder empty. Oxytocin contracts the uterus, not the bladder. Restricting fluid and administering a diuretic could lead to fluid volume deficit.

24.3   **C.** Moja will want her dominant hand free to hold her baby after birth, so the nurse needs to identify this. The nurse giving Moja this choice exemplifies patient-centered care.

24.4   **A.** The nurse's priority in this situation is to protect confidential health information. Leaving or minimizing the record until the nurse who left it open returns may expose Moja's health information. Reporting this error to the nurse-manager is not the immediate priority.

24.5   **C.** Women rated spontaneous vaginal birth as the most satisfying type. Nurses should be knowledgeable about best evidence and use this knowledge to guide their practice. A coworker's personal experience might not be a reliable opinion. Instrumental vaginal births were rated lower than cesarean sections, so it would be inaccurate to describe all vaginal births as being more satisfying than all cesarean births.

24.6   **D.** Moja needs reassurance from the nurse that incisional pain only lasts about 7 days following surgery. Although women need to be comfortable while breastfeeding, many medications are contraindicated. Referral to a lactation consultant may or may not be necessary, and the nurse should not insist on this action.

CHAPTER 25
Nursing Care of a Family Experiencing a Postpartum Complication

25.1   **D.** The nurse should assess uterine tone and height for the potential to prevent uterine hemorrhage. Collection of this assessment datum is a priority over assessing the patient's perineal care, oxygen saturation, or skin integrity.

25.2   **C.** The nurse would expect a human chorionic gonadotropin test to reveal a retained fragment is present. Human chorionic gonadotropin hormone is produced by the placenta. As a result, it will be present as long as any placenta is present. Estrogen, progesterone, and oxytocin levels are not assessed for this purpose.

25.3   **A.** The nurse should advise that an upright position prevents pooling of infected lochia. Supine, prone, and Trendelenburg positions should be avoided.

25.4   **D.** The nurse should promote early ambulation as a safeguard against the development of blood stasis, which could lead to a blood clot. None of the other listed measures is a prevention against venous thromboembolism.

25.5   **B.** The nurse is aware that according to the study, a depressed person would be more likely to be withdrawn in behavior with the infant. In this case, the father is not talking to the baby yet. Misunderstanding an explanation does not necessarily suggest a lapse in memory. The other statements are not suggestive of depressed mood.

25.6   **C.** The nurse is aware that postpartum psychosis means a woman has separated from reality, such as stating "I'm happy not to have any children." Each of the other statements can be linked to Bailey's current reality.

CHAPTER 26
Nursing Care of a Family With a High-Risk Newborn

26.1   **C.** It is critical to guard against hypothermia in low–birth-weight infants because they are unable to increase their metabolic rate to warm themselves. The study revealed that stockinette caps alone are not adequate to do this. The nurse should provide teaching to Mrs. Atkins regarding precautions to prevent hypothermia.

26.2   **C.** Developmental care is aimed at instilling a sense of safety and security into the child by reducing stimuli such as loud noise or bright lights. The nurse recommending a homemade blanket could give him a feeling of being sheltered. None of the other listed actions would have this beneficial effect.

26.3   **B.** The nurse should teach Mrs. Atkins that surfactant is not a relaxant, and it does not influence respiratory rate. It acts on the surface of the alveoli to help them not to stick together upon expiration. Without surfactant, the sticky alveoli collapse, the sides stick together, and are very difficult to inflate.

26.4   **B.** The nurse should flick the foot gently to stimulate the infant to remember to breathe. Theophylline would not be an initial intervention. Both rectal temperature assessment and vigorous suctioning can produce a vagal stimulation causing bradycardia. In addition, the infant should only be suctioned as needed, not every 2 hours.

26.5 **B.** Nurses should urge all mothers to breastfeed early. Early feeding enhances bilirubin clearance. Infants should be in a well-lit environment to enhance binding of bilirubin. Phototherapy is not initiated until the infant's total serum bilirubin level rises to a specific age- and gestational age–dependent level. An older therapy, phenobarbital is rarely used today to combat neonatal jaundice.

26.6 **A.** The nurse should explain that if a woman with diabetes has hyperglycemia during pregnancy; her baby is apt to be born large and lethargic—facts that are a potential source of stress. The infant will not necessarily have diabetes, impaired respiratory function, or cognitive deficits.

CHAPTER 27
Nursing Care of the Child Born With a Physical or Developmental Challenge

27.1 **A.** The nurse should teach Maia to perform baby neck stretching exercises. Simple neck stretching should relieve torticollis in infants. Giving aspirin with each feeding would result in an overdose and would not alleviate the problem. Application of a warm towel is insufficient.

27.2 **C.** Pavlik harnesses seem simple, but because they hold the hip in adduction, they are very effective. The nurse should state that they should be worn constantly except for bathing. Looking at blog sites for specific care advice could supply misinformation.

27.3 **B.** The nurse should role-model better interaction with the infant to demonstrate warmer parent–child interactions. Although the mother may not realize she is not reacting warmly to her child, people do not usually change behavior simply by being told to change it.

27.4 **D.** The nurse should keep the herniated intestines moist to keep them from drying. Warmth is important but not by a radiant heater because this would dry the bowel. Resting on the abdomen could cause intestine to twist.

27.5 **C.** The nurse sitting the infant in an infant chair encourages the herniated bowel to sink against the diaphragm, freeing up lung space. Lying on the left side allows getter respirations in the unaffected lung.

27.6 **C.** The nurse should report changes in vital signs. Changes in vital signs with increased cranial pressure are easy to remember because they move in opposite directions: Temperature and blood pressure increase, and pulse and respiratory rate decrease.

CHAPTER 28
Principles of Growth and Development

28.1 **B.** The nurse should explain that the lymphatic system reaches such a peak in early school-age children; their throats appear to be "all tonsils."

28.2 **B.** Young children in the study recognized what overweight was but were unable to apply the concept

to themselves. The nurse recognizes John's inability to connect his own appearance with the pictures is consistent with this tendency.

28.3 **C.** The interprofessional team should recognize that Freud stressed that school age is a latent stage and that it is not a stage of great advancement.

28.4 **D.** The nurse should choose health promotions activities for John based on Erikson's theory that the developmental task of the school-age child is to learn industry or to do things well.

28.5 **A.** The nurse recognizes that ascribing human properties to inanimate objects is indicative of magical thinking.

28.6 **C.** The nurse understands that conservation is learning that two different shapes can actually be equal in mass or volume, and John has not yet learned this concept.

CHAPTER 29
Nursing Care of a Family With an Infant

29.1 **C.** Infants sit steadily at 8 months of age.

29.2 **A.** Children at 12 months usually say two words beside "ma-ma" and "da-da." They are not incapable of understanding, but they cannot express their needs verbally.

29.3 **A.** Infants understand permanence when they look for someone or something out of sight.

29.4 **D.** A mother who "always has a hot cup of coffee in her hand" could easily spill that on the infant while giving care or holding the infant.

29.5 **D.** Aspiration and falls are the most frequent unintentional injuries in infants.

29.6 **D.** Focusing on abilities rather than inabilities promotes efficacy and well-being among the family members of a child with unique needs. This practice exemplifies patient-centered care. Lowering the family's expectations is normally inappropriate and unnecessary.

CHAPTER 30
Nursing Care of a Family With a Toddler

30.1 **B.** The nurse should reaffirm with Jason's father that toddlers typically walk with a wide-based gait. Strong arch support would not make a difference.

30.2 **B.** The nurse would expect 2-year-olds to speak with two-word, noun–verb sentences.

30.3 **D.** The nurse should teach that television viewing for toddlers should be carefully limited; they need supervision to prevent pulling a television onto themselves.

30.4 **D.** The nurse should teach that locking medicine or placing it out of reach is the best safeguard. Young children can occasionally open childproof caps.

30.5 **A.** The nurse enforces the rule that a child should sit still in time-out for as many minutes as his age. This seems like a short time, but for a 2-year-old, sitting still for 2 minutes is a long time.

30.6 **C.** The nurse should advise that reducing the number of questions asked reduces the number of times a toddler can say no. Reasoning with toddlers or mimicking behavior is rarely effective.

CHAPTER 31
Nursing Care of a Family With a Preschool Child

31.1 **C.** Although this is variable, the nurse should point out that preschoolers typically ask 300 to 400 questions a day.

31.2 **B.** The nurse should suggest that watching chosen DVDs could improve the quality of video material to which Cathy is exposed. Cartoons are often violent. TV should be carefully limited but does not necessarily need to be withheld until age 5 years.

31.3 **C.** Allowing a child to use a night-light, inspecting the child's room for objects that look particularly scary after dark, and limiting the child's television viewing to programs not as frightening are recommendations that the nurse can make to help decrease a child's fears.

31.4 **D.** The nurse should advise the parents to instruct their child not to leave daycare with anyone but them or a designated person. If the parents wish, it is acceptable to have a child's fingerprints taken and recorded. It is not likely necessary to limit Cathy to her own home. Describing kidnapping is likely to elicit fear.

31.5 **A.** It is important for the nurse to encourage women to maintain contact with their preschooler during the short time they are hospitalized for the new birth. This fosters family cohesion. Each of the other teaching points may be necessary, but none so clearly promotes family bonding.

31.6 **C.** The nurse should state that sexual education should be approached in a clear but age-appropriate manner. At this age, it is not normally necessary to address sexual intercourse and its consensual nature.

CHAPTER 32
Nursing Care of a Family With a School-Age Child

32.1 **D.** The nurse can establish a sense of industry in Shelly by encouraging her to complete small projects or tasks that offer a reward when completed.

32.2 **C.** The school nurse could state that clubs can potentially foster social interaction between children whose interests are similar. Clubs are frequently single-gender, and they do not always have formal rules and regulations.

32.3 **A.** The nurse should advise that heavy backpacks can put unnecessary strain on the back of school-age children. School-age children still need assistance with evaluating illness. Eating healthy to avoid being overweight should start before 18 years of age. Booster seats are usually unnecessary at this age.

32.4 **D.** The study documents the fact that injuries occur in cheerleading activities. However, the nurse should state that taking part is likely of benefit, provided Shelly is cognizant of some of the risks. No mention is made of weight or calcium intake.

32.5 **B.** The nurse should teach that candy that dissolves rapidly remains in contact with teeth for the shortest time. This may be associated with a reduced risk of dental caries.

32.6 **C.** The nurse should acknowledge that smoking is viewed as an adult activity; therefore, adopting the habit can be considered a giant step on the road to adulthood. Antismoking interventions must acknowledge this reality. The media are not known to have exaggerated the risks of smoking.

CHAPTER 33
Nursing Care of a Family With an Adolescent

33.1 **B.** The nurse should teach that apocrine glands, found predominantly in the axilla and groin, are responsible for body odor. This problem does not result from sebaceous activity or ethnicity, and hygiene is not the major contributing factor.

33.2 **A, B, C, D.** The nurse recognizes that all the options represent tasks adolescents must complete to achieve a sense of identity: emancipation, body image, values, and career choice.

33.3 **B.** The nurse should counsel that medications should not be shared with other people. The nurse should also teach the warnings and precautions involved with the administration of this drug, including the fact that it is a teratogen.

33.4 **C.** The nurse would note that whether stalking is done in person or by the Internet, continuous, unwelcome actions are stalking.

33.5 **C.** The nurse is aware that alcohol is identified as the gateway drug or is the one which is most apt to lead to further substance use disorders, especially if parents condone early use.

33.6 **D.** The nurse is aware that sniffing cocaine can cause loss of nasal hair. Upon assessment, the absence of nasal hair would suggest more extensive cocaine use.

CHAPTER 34
Child Health Assessment

34.1 **C.** The nurse should teach the father that household products were swallowed most commonly by young children. These are often stored below sinks in bathrooms or kitchens. The nurse should question if these cabinets are locked if they contain household products.

34.2 **B.** Parents may be unwilling to discuss a chief concern until they feel comfortable with an interviewer. The nurse should provide an open-ended invitation to address any outstanding issues that can sometimes reveal important data.

34.3 **B.** Blood pressure is routinely assessed beginning at 3 years of age; therefore, the nurse can exclude this assessment in this case.

34.4 **B.** The nurse should be aware that gagging a child who has a swollen epiglottis can cause the epiglottis to obstruct breathing.

34.5 **D.** The nurse identifies the fourth or fifth left intercostal space at the nipple line as the best place to assess mitral heart valve closing, although this is not its anatomical position.

34.6 **D.** The nurse teaches the father that human papillomavirus virus (HPV) vaccine is typically administered at 11 to 12 years of age.

CHAPTER 35
Communication and Teaching With Children and Families

35.1 **D.** The nurse should perform teaching in personal space, which is a distance of about 18 in. to 4 ft, or conversational space. It is most appropriate for face-to-face teaching.

35.2 **C.** The nurse should be guided by the principle that technology has the potential to enhance learning and communication, but it cannot wholly substitute for the nurse's sophisticated and thoughtful interpersonal communication skills.

35.3 **B.** The nurse is teaching using cognitive learning, which is learning facts or increasing knowledge. A and D are affective learning; C is psychomotor or skill learning.

35.4 **A.** Video resources must be vetted by the nurse to ensure that the material presented is evidence-based, safe, and age-appropriate.

35.5 **C.** Neither the Web-based/DVD program nor the face-to-face instruction was demonstrably superior; therefore, the nurse could allow the child to choose which delivery method he or she preferred.

35.6 **C.** When teaching a 3-year-old, the nurse would probably do best by playing a game. Lecture, group discussion, and reading a pamphlet are all more advanced than this child's age level.

CHAPTER 36
Nursing Care of a Family With an Ill Child

36.1 **A.** The nurse confirms that Becky's symptoms of anxiety may indicate separation anxiety. Protest, the first stage of separation anxiety, is marked by loud, intense crying.

36.2 **D.** The most significant outcome of teaching patients and their families about the perioperative process was a reduction in their anxiety. As an outcome of education, this is more important than being able to adhere to instructions, describe asepsis, or explain the rationale for surgery. While providing teaching, the nurse should also focus on reducing anxiety for the child and caregivers.

36.3 **B.** School children do best with small tasks and a feeling of reward. The nurse should use a collaborative approach with the caregivers to encourage Becky to drink more water in small glasses, which is also more likely to prevent nausea and vomiting. Warning her of negative consequences is less likely to result in positive outcomes.

36.4 **D.** A children's hospital playroom is designated as a "pain-free" zone to help the child cope with the stressors of hospitalization. Reducing the ill effects of separation and hospitalization to the extent possible should be a high priority for the nurse. The nurse should encourage parents to stay whenever possible and tell the child if they need to be separated from them for a time. The nurse should ensure all procedures are performed in the treatment room, not at bedside, so the child feels comfortable in the hospital room.

36.5 **D.** The nurse is aware that blocks that are 1-in. square are the smallest items that can fit in a toddler's mouth easily. The nurse should teach the parents that any item smaller than the internal roll on toilet paper is a dangerous size to be aspirated. The other listed toys do not pose a serious risk of aspiration.

36.6 **B.** The nurse could have Becky handle a bandage to address specifically what is happening to Becky. She can apply it to the foot and become more comfortable with the concept of a bandage. Therapeutic play materials are best if they are most relevant to a child's condition or procedures.

CHAPTER 37
Nursing Care of a Family When a Child Needs Diagnostic or Therapeutic Modalities

37.1 **C.** The nurse should provide support during procedures using the least amount of restraint possible. In this case, the help of another nurse to hold the hand steady is the best choice. The mother may not be capable of restraining the child during the procedure in a safe manner.

37.2 **D.** Most parents are anxious to have diagnostic tests done so their child's illness can be identified. The nurse should ask her why she feels the way she does, which might reveal that she needs a better understanding of what an MRI involves.

37.3 **C.** The commercial device reduced pain by serving as a distraction. The nurse should collaborate with the mother to select a distraction technique that would be effective with Felipe because his mother may know what will work most best. Pre- and postprocedure assessment will not necessarily reduce his anxiety and pain. The nurse telling him that he or she will try to distract him may be counterproductive.

37.4 **B.** The nurse giving Felipe a choice of fingers to use can interest him in the procedure. Comparing him to other children his age or threatening the withholding of privileges or treats is inappropriate nursing responses.

37.5 **A.** The nurse should start the 24-hour urine collections from the discard of the first urine to ensure it is truly a 24-hour specimen.

37.6 **A.** Measuring the amount a child vomits (emesis) can be challenging if it spills onto clothing or bed linen. When this happens, the nurse should estimate the amount in relation to the amount of food or fluid the child recently ate and include the number of episodes and a description of the vomitus. The nurse should not delegate estimating the quantity of the vomitus to Felipe's mother.

CHAPTER 38
Nursing Care of a Family When a Child Needs Medication Administration or Intravenous Therapy

38.1 **C.** Any drugs are transported attached to plasma proteins; a deficit of these can interfere with medication distribution. ABGs, gallbladder function, and renal function are important assessments, but none directly gauges drug distribution.

38.2 **C.** In the absence of an ID band, the nurse should ask a parent to identify her. Children may lie about their name or give a false name out of fear or being playful.

38.3 **C.** The nurse should recommend that using something that dissolves easily, like ice, can allow children to practice swallowing in a safe and effective way. Drawing a picture or tipping the child's head forward is not effective. The nurse should never refer to medicine as candy.

38.4 **D.** The nurse should keep the child's head turned to the side to allow the medication to stay in the ear longer and increase absorption. Self-administration is unsafe and impractical. For a child older than age 2 years, the nurse should pull the ear pinna up and back.

38.5 **D.** The nurse is aware that the point of watching television is to create a distraction. If Terry is absorbed in her watching her present program, changing the channel could exacerbate her pain by removing the distraction.

38.6 **A.** Reading a story to Terry is an appropriate distraction. To help guard the stability of the intravenous site while still meeting her psychosocial needs, Terry needs the nurse to initiate an activity which is quiet and which does not include use of her hands.

CHAPTER 39
Pain Management in Children

39.1 **B.** The nurse would document somatic pain. Bone pain is somatic pain. Cutaneous pain is skin pain; visceral is pain from body organs.

39.2 **B.** The nurse ensuring that the doses are correct is a priority; drug doses are based on weight, not age. Site compatibility is irrelevant because the two drugs have two different routes.

39.3 **A.** The nurse knows that the advantage of a patient-controlled pump is that it offers the child a sense of control and rapid analgesia. Nursing care is not reduced, and there is still a chance of adverse effects.

39.4 **D.** The nurse should instruct colleagues to tell the child she will be sleepy but able to talk. This is a comforting and accurate explanation. It is inappropriate to tell a child that he or she will be "knocked out." A description of analgesia and anesthetic is too technical for a 3-year-old.

39.5 **C.** Distraction techniques need to be individualized; therefore, that nurse should ask the mother what technique is apt to be most successful. Reassuring the parents before the procedure so they do not radiate extensive fear would be a better action than asking them to leave or not talk.

39.6 **C.** Imagery requires a child to be able to replace a painful image with a nonpainful one. This requires a working imagination, which is a characteristic of childhood.

CHAPTER 40
Nursing Care of a Family When a Child Has a Respiratory Disorder

40.1 **A.** The nurse should advise the parent to pinch the lower part of the nose (alae nasi) for 10 minutes without releasing pressure. The nurse should also advise the parent to keep the child in an upright position with his head tilted slightly forward to minimize the amount of blood pressure in nasal vessels and to keep blood moving forward, not back into the nasopharynx.

40.2 **B.** Choanal atresia is blockage of the posterior nares in newborns. The nurse may assess this health problem by holding the newborn's mouth closed, then gently compressing first one nostril, and then the other. If atresia is present, infants will struggle as they experience air hunger when their mouth is closed.

40.3 **C.** The nurse should teach the parents a full course of prescribed antibiotics is necessary to prevent glomerulonephritis or rheumatic fever.

40.4 **D.** Cold decreases edema and promotes healing. Foods that are salty, have sharp edges, or tarts are difficult to swallow and should be avoided.

40.5 **D.** Because initiating gagging may cause further airway closure, the nurse should never elicit a gag reflex on children with a high fever, barky cough, and sore throat. Instead, the nurse should assess his throat with simple inspection.

40.6 **C.** The nurse should instruct the child who is undergoing peak flow testing to place the meter in his or her mouth and blow out as hard and fast as possible.

CHAPTER 41
Nursing Care of a Family When a Child Has a Cardiovascular Disorder

41.1 **D.** The nurse would be alerted to the mother's comment that nausea and vomiting are expected side effects for the first few weeks of treatment. Although nausea and vomiting are side effects of digoxin (and many medications), the child would not automatically experience these symptoms after initiation of the medication. If the child does experience these symptoms, the provider should be contacted immediately and the family should not wait several weeks. All of the other statements are true.

41.2 **B.** Henry's surgery to repair his VSD is open-heart surgery, performed through the breastbone, and he does require cardiopulmonary bypass. But overall, children who have a VSD repaired do very well. There was a recent study in 2017 where the researchers noted that VSD surgeries overall go very well and infrequently have significant complications. They did note that children with genetic syndromes and low weight for age at the time of surgery do tend to have prolonged ICU stays with longer mechanical ventilation times, but they ultimately did well. Therefore, Henry may need his breathing tube in the ICU for a few days, but he should recover without major complications.

41.3 **D.** The nurse should emphasize that after heart surgery requiring a median sternotomy approach, infants and children will require 6 weeks for the sternum to heal. Limiting participation in physical activities and heavy lifting (including heavy backpacks for school) will ensure strong healing of the bone and minimal pain for the child. During this time, children should not be lifted under their arms or pulled by the arms as this will cause significant pain for the child. Infants should be scooped behind the neck and under their bottoms. Children should be assisted by supporting behind the back. Surgeries that required a lateral thoracotomy approach are also very painful, and maintaining these same guidelines is appropriate.

Regardless of the surgical approach, all children should use car seat belts, booster seats, or car seats as recommended. Appropriate placement and fit of these safety restraints will not harm the child after surgery.

41.4 **B.** The nurse notes that this heart rate is exceptionally high for a child of this age. This rate and rhythm meet all of the criteria for SVT: The rate is greater than 160 bpm, it is a narrow complex that does not change with activity level, and the P waves are not visible. Sinus tachycardia would most likely not have a rate this high, and the P waves would be visible. Torsades de pointes is a chaotic and pulseless rhythm so the child would not have other vital signs that were life sustaining. Ventricular tachycardia in children is typically a very wide complex rhythm; it may or may not have associated vital signs that are near normal. This child has presented with classic symptoms, ECG, and onset pattern of SVT.

41.5 **D.** The nurse knows that regardless of the child's underlying medical disorder or etiology of a pediatric arrest, ensuring a patent airway and providing appropriate respirations is paramount. Children more frequently experience a pure respiratory decompensation or arrest prior to any cardiac involvement, even in children with underlying cardiac disorders. Positioning the child in a sniffing position to ensure an optimal airway and providing respiratory support through bag/mask ventilation will likely reverse the bradycardia. Regardless, the nurse should begin with respiratory support and provide cardiac support with compressions once the nurse is able or when help arrives. The nurse should never leave a child who is decompensating to retrieve equipment or personnel. As more personnel arrive, they will fill the other necessary roles of CPR provider, documentation, medications, and medical support.

41.6 **C.** It is important for the nurse to include the child when discussing management strategies. Adolescents (and many school-age children) are quite capable of participating in conversations about their health and wellness, and any treatment plan will be better followed if the child was included in its development or has an understanding of the importance of such a plan. Charlene needs to address not only her diet but also her weight and most likely her activity level. By working with both Charlene and her mother, the nurse's treatment strategies are more likely to be effective.

CHAPTER 42
Nursing Care of a Family When a Child Has an Immune Disorder

42.1 **D.** The nurse is aware that repeated exposures to latex can create allergies in sensitive children. Distraction does not help protect his safety, and the use of a new blood pressure cuff does not prevent allergic reactions.

42.2 **A, C.** A complete blood count with differential is always the best starting point to evaluate a child like Dexter. Allergic children generally have a higher number or proportion of eosinophils in the blood. Children with immunodeficiencies may have elevated neutrophil counts if they have an active bacterial in-

fection. At baseline, a reduced lymphocyte count or percentage may be a "red flag" for an immunodeficiency. Allergic children generally have elevated IgE levels, both the overall serum IgE as well as allergen-specific IgE.

42.3 **C.** The nurse should teach that hyposensitization increases the number of IgG immunoglobulins, which then block the action of IgE immunoglobulins that are involved in an allergic response. Immunotherapy does not improve the broader function of the immune system or protect against infection.

42.4 **C.** Epinephrine is the drug of choice for an anaphylactic reaction because it quickly causes bronchodilation, immediately enlarging a constricted airway. The nurse would administer 0.3 mg of the drug.

42.5 **A.** The nurse would deem treatment successful if the child is able to maintain age-appropriate activities despite having allergies. "Curing" allergies is not always a possibility.

42.6 **B.** The nurse knows that many accidental ingestions occur because food was offered by another person. A willingness to share may include sharing food and a consequent allergic reaction that would best be treated by an EpiPen.

CHAPTER 43
Nursing Care of a Family When a Child Has an Infectious Disorder

43.1 **B.** The nurse should stress handwashing and the role parents have in setting a good example with this practice. Parents' hand-washing practices were noted to influence handwashing in their children. Frequent reminders, teaching children about bacteria, and characterizing hand hygiene as "grown up" were not specifically noted to be effective interventions.

43.2 **C.** The nurse knows that coughing and sneezing requires droplet precautions (gloves, mask, and gown). If Jack wears a mask, there may be contaminated surfaces in the room so the nurse needs to guard against these surfaces.

43.3 **B.** Although rating his pain would be informative, to stop the itching, administration of an antihistamine by the nurse would be most effective. Children need their hands free to facilitate self-care.

43.4 **B.** The nurse would assess for mono by evaluating the spleen by nontouching maneuvers using the scratch test. The spleen enlarges to destroy the affected cells, so the spleen could rupture easily on pressure. Petechiae should not be massaged; percussion and the use of a Doppler are unnecessary during assessment.

43.5 **C.** Mumps cause a parotid gland enlargement without skin erythema in the majority of patients. This enlargement will obscure the angle of jaw and therefore is helpful from differentiating it from submaxillary adenitis (inflammation of lymph nodes). The best method of differentiation is to place a hand along the jaw line. If the major amount of swelling is above the hand, it is probably mumps.

43.6 **D.** The nurse would inform the school nurse that scarlet fever is contagious for 1 to 7 days after the appearance of disease symptoms, so Jack will no longer be infectious after a week. A faster return to school may result in the infection of other children.

CHAPTER 44
Nursing Care of a Family When a Child Has a Hematologic Disorder

44.1   **B.** The nurse reassuring Lana's mother that the consequent risks of infection will be addressed acknowledges potential risks while still providing reassurance. It would be inappropriate for the nurse to have the child's mother restrain her during a painful procedure. It would also be inaccurate to reassure her that this is a one-time event.

44.2   **A.** The nurse knows the mother understands iron chelation therapy when she states that the drug acts to remove excess iron from her child. Iron chelation therapy removes excess iron from the body to prevent hemosiderosis. The mother needs to assess voiding, not pulse, before administration.

44.3   **B.** The nurse could suggest that swimming would be a healthy and low-risk activity. To protect the father, playing football would be inadvisable. Sedentary activities are not an advantage for either father or son.

44.4   **B.** Pain control is paramount during sickle-cell crises. As a result, evidence of adequate pain control is a nursing priority over positive expressions about his time in hospital, even though these are certainly desirable. The nurse should perform health education also, but pain control is the priority.

44.5   **D.** The nurse should inform the team members that autoimmune acquired hemolytic anemia affects red blood cell counts and a CBC should be performed promptly.

44.6   **A.** Idiopathic thrombocytopenia purpura (ITP) is a deficiency of platelets so the nurse should caution Lana and her mother that Lana will bruise easily. Assessments related to blood glucose levels, headache, and proteinuria are not priorities.

CHAPTER 45
Nursing Care of a Family When a Child Has a Gastrointestinal Disorder

45.1   **C.** The nurse would expect metabolic alkalosis, which occurs because of the loss of gastric acid that occurs with emesis.

45.2   **C.** The nurse should teach that raw chicken is a potential source of *Salmonella*. None of the other listed actions prevents this foodborne illness.

45.3   **A.** The nurse should assess the baby for vomiting immediately after feeding because that is a symptom of pyloric stenosis. The vomiting occurs due to the thickened pylorus muscle causing a delay in gastric emptying.

45.4   **B.** The nurse recognizes that hepatitis A can be transmitted via fecally contaminated shellfish. The nurse should advise parents to carefully consider the origin of sushi or shellfish served to their family.

45.5   **A.** The nurse should keep the parents informed by encouraging daily interaction with the medical team.

45.6   **C.** Kwashiorkor results from a deficiency of protein in the diet; therefore, the nurse would anticipate the dietitian to prioritize quality protein in the diet.

CHAPTER 46
Nursing Care of a Family When a Child Has a Renal or Urinary Tract Disorder

46.1   **C.** The nurse should keep in mind that because preschoolers have recently been taught that voiding is a private activity, voiding while an X-ray is taken may feel uncomfortable. Dye capsules are not used, and the test does not occur in a metal tube.

46.2   **C.** The nurse realizes that the grandmother received adequate education on the prevention of UTIs when she says she will be certain to administer all the antibiotic pills prescribed. Taking the full antibiotic prescription helps prevent recurrence of infection. Avoidance of dairy and exercise is unnecessary. The use of bath salts is not recommended.

46.3   **B.** The nurse recognizes that the first symptom of post-streptococcal glomerulonephritis is often bright red hematuria. Abdominal pain and joint pain are atypical.

46.4   **C.** The nurse teaches the grandmother that testing for urine protein is important with nephrotic syndrome because a large amount of protein is lost in urine. The other listed actions do not directly address this health problem.

46.5   **A, B, C, E.** The following findings suggest to the nurse that Carey's kidneys are failing: Anemia develops from a lack of erythropoietin and vitamin D cannot be synthesized, phosphorus cannot be excreted, and fluid overload causes hypertension. Creatinine levels increase, not decrease, in cases of renal failure.

46.6   **A.** Parents thought support from healthcare professionals was important; therefore, it was an appropriate action for the nurse to assure the grandmother that she can call the clinic any time with questions. Asking the grandmother to keep a journal or ignore family members could make her time management even more stressful.

CHAPTER 47
Nursing Care of a Family When a Child Has a Reproductive Disorder

47.1   **C.** The nurse would teach the parents that although children with precocious puberty appear older, they function at their chronologic age. Both sexes can be fertile even at such a young age. Dietary and activity restrictions are unnecessary.

47.2   **C.** The nurse would recommend that Navi participate in an exercise program. Yoga may be an effective measure to reduce symptoms of dysmenorrhea. Increased exercise intensity is not a guarantee of a proportionate reduction in pain. The benefits of yoga were not limited to improved coping.

47.3   **B.** The nurse should teach Navi that polycystic ovary syndrome leads to obesity, hirsutism, irregular menstrual cycles, and subfertility. It is not easy to reverse the syndrome.

47.4   **C.** The nurse should counsel Navi that if having small breasts interferes with self-esteem, a girl can have surgical augmentation, but this needs careful consideration regarding whether it is necessary at this young age. There is no increase in disease risk, and breastfeeding is unaffected.

47.5 **C.** The nurse would refer the adolescent for further treatment if she had a white, cheese-like vaginal discharge. Candidal vaginal infections usually cause a thick, pruritic, white vaginal discharge. All of the listed complaints warrant follow-up, but they are not indicative of candidiasis.

47.6 **A.** The nurse needs to teach Navi that gonorrhea may be spread by singular sexual contact. The disease has a bacterial etiology. All forms of sexual contact carry risks, and saliva is not bactericidal.

CHAPTER 48
Nursing Care of a Family When a Child Has an Endocrine or a Metabolic Disorder

48.1 **A, B.** The nurse should teach that growth hormone is an injectable and can be discontinued in adolescence when full growth is achieved. It is not recommended to take in the oral form.

48.2 **C.** The school nurse should be aware that hyperthyroidism increases metabolism, so it leads to rapid, jittery movements.

48.3 **C.** A function of aldosterone is to retain sodium in the body.

48.4 **D.** The nurse understands that when children with diabetes first begin injections of insulin, it "reminds" their pancreas to produce insulin, so for a short period, the child may not need exogenous insulin administered or may need minimal amounts.

48.5 **B.** The total amount of carbohydrates included in this lunch is 75 g. At a ratio of 1:10, he would inject 7.5 units of regular insulin.

48.6 **A.** Based on the study, the nurse would believe LaRoya's family situation is not ideal because she has lost friends. The study found that loss of friends had a negative effect on quality of life. The other statements do not reflect an influence on quality of life.

CHAPTER 49
Nursing Care of a Family When a Child Has a Neurologic Disorder

49.1 **B.** Neurologic examinations are lengthy so it's difficult to keep children's attention unless the nurse presents the examination as being interesting. There is no "pass" or "fail." Alluding to the possibility of tumors or an "unhealthy brain" will likely cause undue anxiety.

49.2 **A.** The nurse should inform Tasha that before a lumbar puncture is performed, the lumbar region is cleansed with a solution that creates a temporary sensation of cold. The procedure is not necessarily painless, and EMLA should be applied approximately 1 hour beforehand. A side-lying position is used to perform a lumbar puncture.

49.3 **D.** The nurse should teach the parents that as the child needs fine motor control to achieve at writing or ambulating, the loss of function may seem more acute. Cognitive and physical effects of the disease do not necessarily exist in the same degree. Vaccinations do not cause cerebral palsy.

49.4 **B.** The nursing team should maintain respiratory precautions for at least 24 hours following the beginning of antibiotic therapy.

49.5 **B.** The nurse should suspect depression when Tasha's mother expresses sadness. None of the other listed statements is as clearly suggestive of depression.

49.6 **A, C, D.** It is not likely a child would require a tracheostomy. The nurse should have the call bell, suction, and supplementary oxygen available to maintain safety and the integrity of the child's airway.

CHAPTER 50
Nursing Care of a Family When a Child Has a Vision or Hearing Disorder

50.1 **B.** The nurse notes that the mother covering the stronger eye will encourage central vision to develop in the weaker eye. Each of the other actions is counterproductive.

50.2 **C.** The nurse teaches that wiping infectious discharge away from the other eye prevents infection from spreading to the second eye. The other listed actions are not indicated.

50.3 **C.** The nurse should prevent vomiting because increased intraocular pressure from vomiting could disrupt a suture line.

50.4 **C.** The nurse is aware that the hallmark of glaucoma is increased intraocular pressure.

50.5 **D.** The nurse would be concerned that he listens to music with earbuds. The study showed that long exposure to loud noise may be responsible for lowering hearing level in teenagers. An individual is more likely to listen at high volume when using earphones (as when on a bus or in a subway car). Listening to computer speakers may not be as loud.

50.6 **B.** The nurse recognizes that otitis media is an infection of the middle ear; otitis externa is infection of the ear canal. Both diagnoses can be painful.

CHAPTER 51
Nursing Care of a Family When a Child Has a Musculoskeletal Disorder

51.1 **C.** The nurse should teach Jeffrey that it's important to bear weight on his arms, not his axillae, so nerves and blood vessels that cross at the axilla are not injured. If crutches are properly fitted, there should be a space of 1 to 1½ in. between the axilla crutch pad and the child's axilla. The nurse should ensure that when Jeffrey stands upright and places his hands on the hand rests of the crutches, the elbows flex about 20 degrees. Stairs present a fall risk.

51.2 **A.** Osteomyelitis is a severe bone infection that needs IV antibiotic therapy to ensure that microorganisms do not cause chronic infection and deformity. The nurse's vigilant administration of antibiotics is thus a priority over health education, even though this should be performed. ADLs should be encouraged within his current limitations. Fluid restriction is not indicated.

51.3 **D.** Application of heat and administration of a nonsteroidal anti-inflammatory agent are first-line therapies for children with juvenile arthritis.

51.4 **B.** The nurse should prioritize preventing weight gain and encouraging the child to be as mobile as possible to prolong function in muscular dystrophy as muscles weaken. Purines and calcium are not focuses of dietary modifications.

51.5 **B.** The team members should be aware that an elbow cast that is too tight can lead to compartment syndrome and result in permanent nerve damage. Frequent neurovascular assessment is necessary, and this could be safely performed by the LPN. Sepsis is not likely, and cleanliness of cast is not a priority over neurovascular assessment.

51.6 **A.** The nurse should advise Jeffrey not to swing his sister by the arms. Holding preschoolers by the arm and swinging them is the most common cause of a traction injury. The other listed activities are not considered to be high risk.

CHAPTER 52
Nursing Care of a Family When a Child Has an Unintentional Injury

52.1 **A.** Based on Damashek and Corlis (2017) study, visual and proximity in combination are predictive in preventing injuries

52.2 **D.** The nurse is aware that increasing temperature and blood pressure are marks of increasing intracranial pressure. Amnesia is frequently seen with a head concussion.

52.3 **B.** The appropriate nursing action is to administer acetylcysteine or activated charcoal. Acetylcysteine is the specific antidote for acetaminophen poisoning; activated charcoal may be given if no acetylcysteine is immediately available. Educating the parents is important but is not the immediate priority.

52.4 **D.** The nurse would assess for paint chips in the home. Paint chips taste sweet so children enjoy their taste; they are the most common source of lead poisoning in children.

52.5 **C.** The nurse would recommend applying cool water to reduce the water temperature and stop the burning as well as reduce the pain.

52.6 **D.** The nurse would instruct the care team to allow Sage to speak of the incident. Being burned is such a frightening event, children need "debriefing" afterward, so they are assured they are now safe and healing. The other listed actions are appropriate.

CHAPTER 53
Nursing Care of a Family When a Child Has a Malignancy

53.1 **D.** The nurse confirms that hand hygiene prevents the mother from spreading microorganisms to her son, but it does not protect her from the possible effect of handling toxic drugs. The nurse needs to tell her to wear gloves to handle oral chemotherapy agents. The other listed actions are appropriate.

53.2 **C.** The nurse would confirm the early signs of ALL are fatigue and leg bruises. Because so many white blood cells are produced in cases of ALL, red blood cell and platelet production falls leading to fatigue and bleeding disorders.

53.3 **A.** The nurse would confirm Hodgkin disease usually presents with a single isolated lymph node and suspect its development. The other listed signs and symptoms are not closely associated with this disease.

53.4 **B.** The nurse explains that straining to pass stool causes increased ICP. A Trendelenburg position would rarely be used because this would increase ICP.

53.5 **C.** The nurse should inform Gerri's mother that osteosarcoma is often discovered when a sports injury causes an athlete to report pain or a swelling at the injury site for some time, but sports injury is not the cause of osteosarcoma. Calcium intake is unrelated.

53.6 **C.** The nurse should keep the child's immediate surroundings free of plants, flowers, and goldfish, all of which could harbor mold spores. If the child comes in contact with the flowers at the nurse's desk, it could still be an infection risk.

CHAPTER 54
Nursing Care of a Family When a Child Has an Intellectual or Mental Health Disorder

54.1 **C.** The nurse understands that chronic sorrow is apt to be most acute at the time of developmental milestones such as beginning first grade or high school graduation.

54.2 **C.** The nurse recognizes that repetitive movements such as whirling, rocking, or watching a spinning top are common symptoms of autistic spectrum disorder. The other listed symptoms are not consistent with this health problem.

54.3 **C.** The nurses know that the most common side effects of methylphenidate hydrochloride (Ritalin) are insomnia and lack of appetite. Weight gain and iron-deficiency anemia are atypical.

54.4 **B.** Eating disorders in the study occurred more often in female athletes than in nonathletes.

54.5 **D.** The nurse would check if Cheyenne received an assessment for depression. Because tics are poorly understood, children who have them can be the victim of bullying or teasing and develop low self-esteem.

54.6 **D.** The nurse would suspect schizophrenia after Cheyenne says she hears her friends plotting against her at night. Hearing voices, or hallucinations, is a prominent symptom of schizophrenia. The other listed statements are not consistent with this disorder.

CHAPTER 55
Nursing Care of a Family in Crisis: Maltreatment and Violence in the Family

55.1 **A.** The average parent describes their child in a positive manner. Stating that a child is "not pretty" would alert the nurse to assess for child maltreatment because it is considered to be more negative than describing her as "clumsy."

55.2 **B.** The nurse would be alerted to shaken baby syndrome if retinal hemorrhages develop. Shaking a baby causes small hemorrhages in the retina of the eye as well as possibly more serious injuries such as subdural hematoma. Broken bones are associated with maltreatment but not specifically with shaking.

55.3 **B.** According to this study, most adolescents reveal sexual maltreatment to a trusted peer.

55.4 **C.** Children who have been physically maltreated may reveal the maltreatment through having dolls simulate a sex act. The nurse should want to learn more about their reaction, not stop the play.

55.5 **A.** The nurse should counsel that it is important to preserve any DNA evidence that could reveal the identity of the rapist so a woman should not bath or shower until after an internal examination. Property loss is comparatively insignificant, and it would be highly inappropriate to address prevention at this time.

55.6 **A.** The nurse should be aware of the fact that intimate partner violent offenders are often men who were raised in a household with violence.

CHAPTER 56
Nursing Care of a Family When a Child Has a Long-Term or Terminal Illness

56.1 **B.** The nurse is aware that as with any crisis, support people can offer help and guidance. Privacy and a belief in alternative therapies may not necessarily enhance their coping skills. Wealth can be an asset

during treatment but does not necessarily help the family cope with the child's illness.

56.2 **C.** The nurse assesses that the parents are in the fourth stage of grief or depression. This is the stage when parents start to realize death will happen.

56.3 **D.** The nurse notes that this is a mature question for a 3-year-old. Before answering, it would be important to know why the child is asking the question. Has he heard he is dying or just interested in what happened to a favorite cartoon character he just saw "die" on television?

56.4 **B.** The nurse should inform nursing colleagues that anticipatory grieving can make it hard for parents to relate to their child because they have already grieved as if the child were dead.

56.5 **A.** The study revealed parents wanted most to just continue to be effective parents. The nurse should promote enhancing his comfort by keeping him neat and clean as the sort of activity that might meet that need. None of the other listed actions would be normally appropriate.

56.6 **A.** The nurse should be aware that if a gag reflex is not intact, children can aspirate easily. Hearing may not be lost; parents usually appreciate giving final care.

Index

NOTE: Page numbers followed by *f* indicate figures, page numbers followed by *t* indicate tables, and page numbers followed by *b* indicate boxes.

A

Abandonment
  children's fear of, 47–48, 845–846
  maternal feelings of, 401–402
Abdomen
  child, examination of, 940, 940*f*
  discomfort, in pregnancy, 268–269
  exercises for, 313
  infant, 940
  in labor
    assessment of, 348
    contour of, 346, 346*f*
  newborn, 440*t*, 448–449, 940
  preschooler and school-age child, 940
  radiation therapy and, 1505
  support, after cesarean birth, 640, 640*f*
  toddler, 812, 813*f*
  trauma to
    in children, 1475–1477
    in pregnancy, 587–588, 588*f*, 591
Abdominal circumference, 929
Abdominal massage (effleurage), 317, 318*f*, 379
Abdominal muscle contractions, 313
Abdominal pain
  chronic recurrent, 1287
  in colic, 804, 805*b*–806*b*
  in pregnancy, 252–253, 587
Abdominal pregnancy, 535
Abdominal reflexes, 942
Abdominal thrusts, for aspiration, 1112, 1112*f*
Abdominal wall defects, 449, 731–738
Abduction, 451, 452*b*, 838, 846
ABE. See Acute bilirubin encephalopathy
Abilify (aripiprazole), 1539
Abnormal uterine bleeding (AUB), 1330
ABO incompatibility, 704
Abortion, 529
  induced, 126–129, 155
  septic, 533
  spontaneous, 529–533 (*See also* Miscarriage)
Abruptio placentae, 527*t*, 540–541, 540*f*, 541*t*
Abscess
  brain, 1391
  breast, 662
  osteomyelitis and, 1447
  pelvic, 661, 1334
  perineal, 657, 658
  retropharyngeal, 1108
  staphylococcal, 1220
Absence seizures, 1397
Absorption, drug, 1053
Abstinence, 104, 105*t*, 106*b*
Abstract thought, 773
Abuse. *See* Maltreatment, child
Abusive head trauma, 459, 1566
Acanthosis nigricans, 1369
Accelerations, in fetal heart rate, 357–358

Acceptance, in grief, 1583, 1583*t*, 1588, 1594
Acceptance, in pregnancy, 204*t*, 205–206, 224, 579
Accessory nipples, 448, 1334, 1335*f*
Accommodation, cognitive, 773, 864
Accommodation, visual, 1413
Acculturation, 27*b*
Acesulfame-K (Ace K), 292
Acetaminophen
  in children
    for ear infections, 1428
    for fever, 1030–1031, 1395
    for headache, 1402
    for hemophilia, 1253
    for idiopathic thrombocytopenic purpura, 1251
    for infectious mononucleosis, 1215
    for Kawasaki disease, 1161
    for postoperative pain, 1302–1303
    for sickle-cell anemia, 1246
    for streptococcal infections, 1216
    for viral exanthems, 1205, 1206, 1208
  in fibrocystic breast disease, 1336
  poisoning, 1479–1480
  in pregnancy, 270
Acetazolamide, 739, 1423
Acetylcholine, 1457–1458
Acetylcholinesterase, 197
Acetylcysteine, 1480
Achilles reflex, 942, 945*f*
Achondroplasia, 450, 718–719
Acid–base imbalance, 1261
Acidosis
  fetal, 346, 346*f*
  metabolic, 1261, 1264
  respiratory, in high-risk newborn, 673, 687
Acinetobacter, multidrug-resistant, 1202
AcipHex (rabeprazole), 1267
Acme, in uterine contraction, 339, 339*f*
Acne, 887, 898–899, 898*f*, 900*b*
Acoustic impedance testing, 951
Acoustic stimulation, of fetus, 192–194
Acquired aplastic anemia, 1239
Acquired heart disease, in children, 1126–1127, 1159–1165
Acquired immune deficiency syndrome. *See* HIV/AIDS
Acrocyanosis, 431, 437, 441, 497, 681, 693, 1131
Acromegaly, 1352
Acromion process (A), fetal position and, 332–334
ACTH. *See* Adrenocorticotropic hormone
Activated charcoal, 1479, 1479*b*, 1480
Active immunity, 956, 956*b*
Active phase, of labor, 341
  protracted, 600*t*, 601
Activity level, 760
Acupressure, 380, 1087
Acupuncture, 17, 380, 1087

Acute adrenocortical insufficiency, 1356
Acute bilirubin encephalopathy (ABE), 441, 677, 686
Acute blood-loss anemia, 1238
Acute herpetic gingivostomatitis, 1211
Acute herpetic vulvovaginitis, 1211
Acute infection, anemia of, 1238
Acute lymphocytic (lymphoblastic) leukemia (ALL), 1512–1515
Acute myeloid leukemia (AML), 1515
Acute nasopharyngitis, 504, 1107
Acute otitis media, 1428
Acute pain, 1074
Acute poststreptococcal glomerulonephritis, 1308–1309
Acute renal failure, 1315
Acyanotic heart disease, 1140
Acyclovir, 272, 708, 1178, 1208, 1209, 1339, 1340, 1393
Adaptability, 761
Adaptive immunity, 1201–1202
Adenoidectomy, 1108
Adenosine (Adenocard), 1159
ADHD. *See* Attention deficit hyperactivity disorder
Adolescence, definition of, 567, 886
Adolescent Pediatric Pain Tool (APPT), 1079, 1080*f*
Adolescents, 885–913
  abstinence education for, 104, 106*b*
  acne in, 887, 898–899, 898*f*, 900*b*
  alcohol intake of, 765
  assessment of, 886
  body image of, 890–891
  breasts of, 887–888, 889*f*, 936–937
  bullying or sexually aggressive, 973
  career decisions of, 891
  cognitively challenged, 1538
  contraception for, 109, 119, 120, 123, 125*b*–126*b*, 568, 572
  culture and, 890*b*
  death of
    causes of, 14, 14*b*, 894, 906
    reaction to impending, 1592, 1592*f*
  depression and self-injury in, 906–909
  development of, 887–893
    cognitive, 772*t*, 773, 893
    emotional, 888–892
    moral, 891, 893
    promoting in daily activities, 895–896
    psychosexual, 769*t*
    psychosocial, 769*t*, 771, 771*f*, 888–892
    spiritual, 893
  diagnostic and therapeutic procedures for, 1025
  dress of, 895
  emancipation from parents, 891–892
  exercise for, 896
  eyes of, 932, 946
  family functioning and, 896

inguinal, 941, 1282–1283, 1328
umbilical, 449, 732, 940
Heroin, 274, 586, 710, 905, 906*t*
Herpes labialis, 1211
Herpes simplex virus, 1211
conjunctivitis, 1419*t*
genital (HSV-2), 14, 243, 272, 433, 708, 1211, 1337*t*, 1339–1340
oral (HSV-1), 272, 1211
Herpes zoster, 1208–1209, 1209*f*
Herpetic gingivostomatitis, 1211
Heterosexual, 34, 35*b*
Heterozygous, 158
Hiatal hernia, in pregnancy, 508–509
Hib. *See Haemophilus influenza* type B vaccine
Highly active antiretroviral therapy (HAART), 1176–1177
High-risk newborns, 671–713
airway of, 674–675, 674*f*, 675*f*
developmental care for, 691–693, 692*b*
developmental needs of, anticipating, 679–680
discharge of, 692
drug therapy for, 676
extrauterine circulation in, establishing, 676
fluid and electrolyte balance in, 676–677, 687–689
follow-up at home, 680, 692
infection prevention for, 679, 689
lung expansion in, 675–676, 675*f*
maltreatment of, 680
maternal illness and, 708–710
maternal infection and, 707–708
nursing diagnoses for, 672–673
nursing process for, 672–673
nutrition for, 678–679, 679*f*, 687–689, 688*f*
parent–infant bonding for, 679, 689–690, 690*b*, 690*f*
postpartum care for mother, 422–423
priorities in first days of life, 673–680
regionalization of care, 17, 17*f*
respiration in, 673–676, 686–687
respiratory difficulties in, predisposing factors for, 674*b*
resuscitation of, 673–676, 687
skin-to-skin contact for, 677–678, 689
substance dependence and, 709–710, 709*b*
temperature regulation for, 677–678, 677*f*, 689
ventilation maintenance in, 676
waste elimination in, establishing, 679
High-risk pregnancy, 251, 252*t*, 492. *See also* Pregnancy, complications in
adolescent, 568, 569*f*
nursing diagnoses in, 490–491
procedures during birth, 625–627
Hind milk, 469
Hip
child, examination of, 942
developmental dysplasia of, 720–723, 720*f*, 721*f*, 722*b*, 723*f*
newborn, 450, 450*f*
Hip subluxation, 450
HIPAA. *See* Health Insurance Portability and Accountability Act
Hirschberg test, 931, 931*f*
Hirschsprung disease, 1283–1284, 1283*f*
Histamine, 1180
Histamine 2 receptor antagonist, 298, 631
Histocompatibility antigens, 1318
HIV/AIDS, 14, 1343
in adolescents, 901
CD4 cells (T cells) in, 1172, 1178–1179
in childbirth, management of, 1178–1179
in children, 1175–1178
circumcision and, 457
immunization in, 1177, 1178
lymphoma in, 1516

neonatal infection, 708, 1176, 1178
newborn bathing and, 456
opportunistic infections in, 1178–1179
in pregnancy, 1177–1179
prenatal screening for, 250, 271, 1178
substance abuse and, 584, 586
Hives (urticaria), 1186
HLAs. *See* Human leukocyte antigens
Hobbies, prenatal question on, 231*t*
Hodgkin disease, 1515–1516
Holter/event monitor, 1133
Homans sign, 412
Home births, 15, 318, 321
Home care, 58–73
advantages of, 60
assessment for, 59, 61–62
by age of child, 62, 63*t*
environmental, 62, 62*t*, 64–65
health history and physical exam in, 62
interview in, 61–62
bed rest in, ensuring, 66, 68*f*, 69*b*
beginning, 63–72
care map for pregnant adolescent on, 67*b*–68*b*
for child with long-term or terminal illness, 1586–1587
child's caregiver in, identifying primary, 65–66
communication in, 64*b*, 71
cultural considerations in, 61*b*
definition of, 59
depression in adolescents on, 61–62, 69
direct care in, 61
disadvantages of, 60
family's health literacy in, 66
features of, 61
frequency of, 61
health intervention in, 69–71
health maintenance in, 66–68
health promotion in, 65–66
health rehabilitation in, 71
health teaching in, 66–71
healthy family functioning in, 66
incorporation into family routine, 65*f*
increasing reliance on, 18
indirect care in, 61
legal and ethical considerations in, 63
long-term, 71–72, 71*f*
National Health Goals and, 59*b*
nursing diagnoses for, 59
nursing process for, 59–60
nutrition in, 67*b*, 70–71
online resources for, 59
pain management in, 71, 1088
resources in, 62, 66
safe medicine administration in, 70, 70*b*
safety in, 62*t*, 63, 63*t*
Home care assistants, 65
Home pregnancy tests, 205, 210–212
Home visit, 63–65
Homeless youth, 909–910
Homeschooling, 877
Homicide, child and adolescent, 14
Homosexual, 34, 35*b*. *See also* LGBT issues
Homozygous, 158
Honeymoon behavior, of adopted child, 47
"Honeymoon" cystitis, 1304
"Honeymoon" period, in diabetes mellitus, 1368
Hookworms, 1225
Hordeolum, 931, 1419*t*
Horizontal lie, 331
Hormonal contraception, 106*t*, 113–119
Hormone(s), 1347
adrenal, 1355–1356
disorders of, 1347 (*See also specific disorders*)
pituitary, 138, 1349, 1349*t*
placental, 177, 178–179
postpartum changes in, 405

radiation therapy and, 1504
thyroid, 1353
Hormone replacement therapy, 36*b*
Hospice care, 59, 1592–1593
Hospitalized children. *See* Ill children
Hostile work environment, 97
Hot tubs, 261
hPL. *See* Human placental lactogen
HPV. *See* Human papillomavirus
"Huffing," 274, 586, 879–880
Human bites, 1563
Human chorionic gonadotropin (hCG)
in advanced maternal age, 577
in ectopic pregnancy, 534–535
in gestational trophoblastic disease, 536–537
in ovulation induction, 141
postpartum change in, 405
in pregnancy, 177, 178–179, 196, 210–212
in retained placenta, 654
in threatened miscarriage, 531
Human Genome Project, 155
Human immunodeficiency virus. *See* HIV/AIDS
Human leukocyte antigens (HLAs), 1273, 1317–1318, 1359
Human papillomavirus (HPV), 457, 1211–1212, 1338–1339, 1502
Human papillomavirus (HPV) vaccine, 233, 958, 1212, 1339
Human placental lactogen (hPL), 177, 179, 405
Humatrope (somatropin), 1350, 1350*b*
Humidifiers, 1100
Humility, cultural, 27*b*
Humor, 967
Humoral immunity, 1171, 1172–1173, 1173*f*, 1174*f*, 1175
Hutchinson teeth, 273, 1343
Hyaline membrane disease. *See* Respiratory distress syndrome
Hyaluronidase, 176
Hydatiform mole. *See* Gestational trophoblastic disease
Hydralazine, 552–553, 553*t*, 1310
Hydramnios, 179. *See also* Polyhydramnios
Hydrocele, 941, 1328
Hydrocephalus, 617, 738–744, 739*b*, 739*f*, 741*b*–742*b*
Hydrocodone-acetaminophen, abuse of, 393
Hydrocortisone sodium succinate, 1356
Hydrocortisone-pramoxine, 267
Hydrolaparoscopy, transvaginal, 142–143
Hydromorphone (Dilaudid), 1083–1085
Hydronephrosis, 1304, 1305–1306
Hydrops fetalis, 704
Hydrotherapy, in childbirth, 323, 378–379, 379*f*
Hydroxyurea, 1247
Hydroxyzine, 382, 1509
Hygiene. *See also* Bathing
adolescent, 887, 895
in cesarean birth, 631
in child health assessment, 919
in diabetes mellitus, 1364–1365
hand, 1200
perineal, during pregnancy, 260
postpartum, 414
in preschoolers, 840–842
in school-age children, 868
Hymen, 85
Hymen, imperforate, 85, 1329, 1332
Hyperactive bladder, in pregnancy, 502
Hyperactivity, 1542. *See also* Attention deficit hyperactivity disorder
Hyperactivity, fetal, 346, 346*f*
Hyperalgesia, 1074
Hyperbilirubinemia, 184, 441, 687, 695, 703–706
Hypercholesterolemia, 289. *See also* Dyslipidemia
Hyperemesis gravidarum, 70, 251, 297, 304–305

Self-feeding, 800, 800f, 819
Self-injury, 906–909
Sella turcica, 1348
Selsun shampoo, 1226
Semen analysis, 138, 138b
Seminal vesicles, 82f, 84
Semi-vegetarians, 302
Senses, 435–436, 789–790. *See also specific senses*
Sensorimotor phase, 771–773, 772t, 816
Sensorineural hearing loss, 1425
Sensory deprivation, 1011
Sensory function assessment, 942, 1380–1382
Sensory overload, 1012
Separation anxiety, 825–826, 845–846, 994–995, 1002–1003, 1547
Sepsis, 1202
Septal defects, 1141–1143, 1141f, 1142f, 1154
Septic abortion, 533
Septic shock, 1202
Septicemia, 656, 1222
Septra. *See* Trimethoprim-sulfamethoxazole
Septum-dividing uterus, 90, 90f
Sequestration crisis, 1246
Sequestrum, 1448
Seroquel (quetiapine), 1550
Serous cystadenoma, 236t
Serous otitis media, 1425
Sertraline, 1550
Serum studies, in pregnancy, 155, 165t, 191b, 196, 250, 577
Severe combined immunodeficiencies (SCID), 1175
Sex assigned at birth, 36, 81
Sex chromosomes, 86, 157, 157f, 176, 185, 1324–1326
Sex determination, 176, 185
Sex education
  for adolescents, 901, 901b
  for LGBT youth, 877
  for preschoolers, 848–849, 849f, 1569, 1569f
  for school-age children, 877
Sexual activity
  adolescent, 892, 901, 901b
  cognitive challenge and, 1538
  postpartum, 417–418
  pregnancy and, 260, 260b
Sexual assault, 901, 1572–1575
Sexual counseling, 98b–99b
Sexual desire, 99, 209–210
Sexual harassment, 97
Sexual health. *See* Reproductive and sexual health
Sexual history, 79, 80b, 146b, 234–236
Sexual maltreatment, 849, 865, 867b, 941, 1561, 1569–1571, 1571b
Sexual maturation, 857–859, 887–888. *See also* Puberty
Sexual orientation, 34–36, 35b, 1549b. *See also* LGBT issues
Sexual partner notification, 1340
Sexual response, 96–97
Sexual violence, 97, 901, 1572–1575, 1572b, 1574t, 1575b
Sexually aggressive adolescent, 973
Sexually transmitted infections (STIs), 79–80, 901, 1322b, 1336–1343, 1341b–1342b. *See also specific infections*
SGA. *See* Small for gestational age
Shaken baby syndrome, 459, 1566
Shared feelings, 966
Shared personal ideas, 966
Sharing, difficulty with, 846
Shigellosis, 1266
Shingles (herpes zoster), 1208–1209, 1209f
Shirodkar procedure, 537

Shock
  anaphylactic, 1184–1186, 1184b, 1185f, 1186b
  hypovolemic, 526–529, 528f, 528t, 1481
  septic, 1202
  spinal, 1403
Shoplifting, 879, 895
Short-bowel/short-gut syndrome, 1277
Shoulder dystocia, 616–617, 694
Shoulder presentation, 332, 334f, 335t
"Show," 278t, 279
Shy child, 972
SIADH. *See* Syndrome of inappropriate antidiuretic hormone
Sibling rivalry, 847, 848b
Siblings
  adjustment to long-term or terminal illness, 1585
  ill children and, 1003
  infant safety with, 795
  postpartum visitation of, 401, 401f
  preparing preschooler for, 847, 847f
Sickle-cell anemia
  in children, 1243–1248
    communication about, 1244b
    National Health Goals for, 1231b
    pain management in, 1246–1247
    school safety precautions for, 1248b, 1254
  ethnicity and, 156b, 1231, 1243–1244
  exercise and, 1244
  genetic screen for, 250
  in pregnancy, 499–500
Sickle-cell crisis, 1243, 1244–1246, 1244b, 1245b–1246b, 1247–1248
Sickle-cell trait, 250, 499, 1243–1244
Side effects, of drugs, 1192
SIDS. *See* Sudden infant death syndrome
Sign language, 582, 583, 1426–1427, 1431
Sildenafil, 139
Silence, 970
Silicon, 767t
Silver sulfadiazine (Silvadene), 1494
Silverman-Andersen index, 437, 438f
Simian crease, 450, 942
Simple motor tics, 1551
Simple vocal tics, 1551
Sims position, 261, 262f, 267, 366
Sinciput, 331, 331f
Sinemet (carbidopa/levodopa), 1389
Single-mother family, 45
Single-parent family, 41, 45
Single-parent fathers, 45
Single-photon emission computed tomography (SPECT), 1032, 1382
Single-ventricle heart defects, 1147–1150
Sinus arrhythmia, 938, 1158
Sinus bradycardia, 1158
Sinus headache, 1402
Sinus tachycardia, 1158
Sinuses, prenatal assessment of, 241t
Sinusitis, 1110
Sinusoidal pattern, in fetal heart rate, 359
SIRS. *See* Subcutaneous insulin resistance syndrome
Sitting position, 784–785, 784f, 785f
Six-week examination, postpartum, 421–422, 422t
Skeletal disorders, congenital, 716–723
Skeletal muscle, 1436
Skeletal muscle disorders, 1457–1459
Skeletal traction, 1443
Skene glands, 85, 85f, 235t, 243
Skin
  adolescent, 930
  child, examination of, 929–930, 930t
  development of, 185

fetal, labor and, 345
infant, 930
integrity, maintaining in home care, 66
newborn, 440–444, 930
postpartum changes in, 406
pregnancy and changes in, 211t, 212f, 213t, 217–218, 217f
prenatal assessment of, 238, 241t
preterm infant, 681
spinal cord injury and, 1407
toddler, preschooler, and school-age child, 930
viral infections of, 1211–1212
Skin cancer, 1525–1526
Skin lesions, 1203, 1205f
Skin rashes (exanthems), 1199, 1203–1210, 1206f
Skin testing, in allergies, 1181, 1181f
Skin traction, 1442, 1442f
Skin turgor, 444, 693, 929
Skin-to-skin contact, 18, 471, 677–678, 689, 790
Skull
  fetal, 329–330, 329f, 330f
  newborn, 445, 930
  sutures of, 329, 329f, 445, 718, 930
Skull fracture, 1469, 1469f
Skyla IUD, 119–120
Sleep
  for adolescent, 895–896
  in child health assessment, 919
  for ill children, 1009–1011, 1009t, 1010f
  for infants, 801
  for newborns, 458–459
  non–rapid eye movement (NREM), 1009, 1009t, 1010f
  postpartum, 413–414
  during pregnancy, 261–262, 262f
  for preschoolers, 840
  rapid eye movement (REM), 1009, 1009t, 1010f
  for school-age children, 868
  for toddlers, 821–822
Sleep apnea, 1010–1011
Sleep deprivation, 1009–1010
Sleep talking, 1010
Sleeping position
  for newborns/infants, 254, 456–457, 701, 803, 930
  for pregnant women, 261, 262f
Sleepwalking, 1010
Slipped capital femoral epiphysis, 1447
SLIT. *See* Sublingual immunotherapy
Slow-acting antirheumatic drugs (SAARDs), 1456
Slow-reacting substance of anaphylaxis (SRS-A), 1180
Slow-to-warm-up child, 762b
Small for gestational age (SGA), 555, 680, 681t, 693–694, 709
Smallpox, 958, 1209
Smart infusion pumps (SIPs), 1065
Smell, sense of, 436, 790
Smile, social, 790, 790f
Smoking
  adolescents and, 903
  and labor/childbirth, 393
  in pregnancy, 188–190, 231t, 274–275, 276b–277b, 303
    decreasing, 276b–277b
    nutritional effects of, 303
    prenatal questions on, 231t
    teratogenicity of, 274–275, 303
  school-age children and, 880
Snakebite, 591, 1484–1485
SNAP (Supplemental Nutrition Assistance Program), 294